Elaine S. Jaffe, MD
Pathologist
Bethesda, Maryland

Daniel A. Arber, MD
Donald West and Mary Elizabeth King Professor and
Chair
Department of Pathology
University of Chicago
Chicago, Illinois

Elias Campo, MD, PhD
Senior Consultant and Professor
Department of Anatomic Pathology
Hospital Clinic of Barcelona
Institute for Biomedical Research August Pi i Sunyer
(IDIBAPS)
University of Barcelona
Barcelona, Spain

Attilio Orazi, MD, FRCPath
Professor and Chair
Department of Pathology
Texas Tech University Health Sciences Center
El Paso, Texas

Leticia Quintanilla-Martinez, MD
Professor of Pathology
Institute of Pathology
University Hospital Tübingen
Eberhard-Karls-University Tübingen
Tübingen, Germany

Lisa M. Rimsza, MD
Professor and Consultant
Department of Laboratory Medicine and Pathology
Mayo Clinic
Scottsdale, Arizona

Steven H. Swerdlow, MD
Emeritus Professor of Pathology
University of Pittsburgh School of Medicine
Pittsburgh, Pennsylvania

HEMATOPATHOLOGY

THIRD EDITION

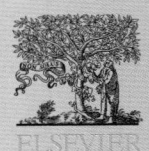

ELSEVIER

Elsevier
1600 John F. Kennedy Blvd.
Ste 1800
Philadelphia, PA 19103-2899

HEMATOPATHOLOGY, THIRD EDITION

ISBN: 978-0-323-83165-9

Notice

Previous editions copyrighted 2017 and 2011.

Executive Content Strategist: Belinda Kuhn
Senior Content Development Manager: Kathryn DeFrancesco
Publishing Services Manager: Catherine Jackson
Senior Project Manager: Daniel Fitzgerald
Designer: Ryan Cook

Printed in India.

Last digit is the print number: 9   8   7   6   5   4   3   2   1

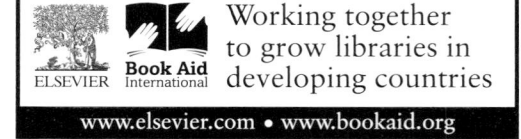

Contributors

Daniel A. Arber, MD
Donald West and Mary Elizabeth King Professor and Chair
Department of Pathology
University of Chicago
Chicago, Illinois

Adam Bagg, MD
Professor
Department of Pathology and Laboratory Medicine
University of Pennsylvania
Philadelphia, Pennsylvania

Govind Bhagat, MD
Professor of Pathology and Cell Biology at CUIMC
Division of Hematopathology
Department of Pathology and Cell Biology
Columbia University Irving Medical Center
New York, New York

Michael J. Borowitz, MD, PhD
Professor
Department of Pathology and Oncology
Johns Hopkins Medical Institutions
Baltimore, Maryland

Laura E. Brown, MD
Assistant Clinical Professor
Laboratory Medicine
University of California, San Francisco
San Francisco, California

Russell K. Brynes, MD
Professor of Clinical Pathology
Department of Pathology
Keck School of Medicine of the University of Southern California
Los Angeles, California

Katherine R. Calvo, MD, PhD
Acting Chief
Hematology Section
Department of Laboratory Medicine
National Institutes of Health Clinical Center
Bethesda, Maryland

Elias Campo, MD, PhD
Senior Consultant and Professor
Department of Anatomic Pathology
Hospital Clinic of Barcelona
Institute for Biomedical Research August Pi i Sunyer (IDIBAPS)
University of Barcelona
Barcelona, Spain

Gabriel C. Caponetti, MD
Associate Professor
Department of Pathology and Laboratory Medicine
Hospital of the University of Pennsylvania
Philadelphia, Pennsylvania

Devon Chabot-Richards, MD
Associate Professor of Pathology
University of New Mexico
Director
Molecular Diagnostics and Oncology
Tricore Laboratories
Albuquerque, New Mexico

John K.C. Chan, MBBS, FRCPath, FRCPA
Consultant Pathologist
Department of Pathology
Queen Elizabeth Hospital
Kowloon, Hong Kong

Yi-Hua Chen, MD
Professor
Department of Pathology
Northwestern University Feinberg School of Medicine
Chicago, Illinois

Sindhu Cherian, MD
Professor
Department of Laboratory Medicine and Pathology
University of Washington
Seattle, Washington

James R. Cook, MD, PhD
Hematopathology Section Head
Department of Laboratory Medicine
Cleveland Clinic
Professor of Pathology
Cleveland Clinic Lerner College of Medicine
Cleveland, Ohio

Magdalena Czader, MD, PhD
Virgil Moon Professor of Pathology
Department of Pathology and Laboratory Medicine
Indiana University
Indianapolis, Indiana

Laurence de Leval, MD, PhD
Director of the Institute of Pathology
Department of Laboratory Medicine and Pathology
University Hospital of Lausanne
Full Professor of Pathology
University of Lausanne
Lausanne, Switzerland

Amy S. Duffield, MD, PhD
Professor of Pathology, Molecular and Cell-Based
Medicine
Director of Hematopathology
Mount Sinai Hospital
New York, New York

Eric Duncavage, MD
Professor, Director of Molecular Oncology
Department of Pathology and Immunology
Washington University School of Medicine
St. Louis, Missouri

Caoimhe Egan, MB BCh BAO
Consultant Haematopathologist
Haematopathology and Oncology Diagnostic Service
Cambridge University Hospitals NHS Foundation Trust
Cambridge, United Kingdom

Fabio Facchetti, MD, PhD
Full Professor
Department of Molecular and Translational Medicine—
Pathology Section
University of Brescia School of Medicine
Chief
Department of Pathology
Spedali Civili Brescia
Brescia, Italy

Andrew L. Feldman, MD
Professor of Laboratory Medicine and Pathology
Department of Laboratory Medicine and Pathology
College of Medicine
Mayo Clinic
Rochester, Minnesota

Falko Fend, MD
Full Professor and Chair
Institute of Pathology and Neuropathology
University Hospital Tübingen
Tübingen, Germany

Sebastian Fernandez-Pol, MD, PhD
Clinical Assistant Professor
Department of Pathology
Stanford University
Stanford, California

Judith A. Ferry, MD
Director of Hematopathology and Nancy Lee Harris,
MD, Endowed Chair in Pathology
Department of Pathology
Massachusetts General Hospital
Professor of Pathology
Department of Pathology
Harvard Medical School
Boston, Massachusetts

Armando C. Filie, MD
Senior Research Physician
Laboratory of Pathology
National Cancer Institute
Bethesda, Maryland

Kathryn Foucar, MD
Distinguished Professor of Pathology
University of New Mexico
Albuquerque, New Mexico

Philippe Gaulard, MD
Professor
Department of Pathology
Hôpital Henri Mondor
Créteil, France

Tracy I. George, MD
Professor
Department of Pathology
University of Utah School of Medicine
Chief Scientific Officer and President, Innovation
Business Unit
ARUP Laboratories
Salt Lake City, Utah

Sarah E. Gibson, MD
Associate Professor of Pathology
Department of Laboratory Medicine and
Pathology
Mayo Clinic in Arizona
Phoenix, Arizona

Blanca Gonzalez-Farré, MD, PhD
Department Consultant of Laboratory of Anatomic
Pathology
Hospital Clinic of Barcelona
Barcelona, Spain

Dita Gratzinger, MD, PhD
Professor
Department of Pathology
Stanford University
Stanford, California

Ashley S. Hagiya, MD
Assistant Professor of Clinical Pathology
Department of Pathology
Keck School of Medicine of University of Southern
California
Los Angeles, California

Sylvia Hartmann, MD
Department of Pathology
Goethe University
Frankfurt, Germany

Robert P. Hasserjian, MD
Director, Hematopathology Fellowship
Department of Pathology
Massachusetts General Hospital
Professor of Pathology
Harvard Medical School
Boston, Massachusetts

Hans-Peter Horny, MD
Professor
Institute of Pathology
Ludwig Maximilians University
Munich, Germany
Institute of Pathology
University Hospital Salzburg
Paracelsus Medical University
Salzburg, Austria

Eric D. Hsi, MD
Professor and Chair
Department of Laboratory Medicine and
Pathology
Mayo Clinic
Rochester, Minnesota

Giovanni Insuasti-Beltran, MD
Associate Professor of Pathology
Wake Forest University School of Medicine
Winston-Salem, North Carolina

Elaine S. Jaffe, MD
Pathologist
Bethesda, Maryland

Patty M. Jansen, MD, PhD
Department of Pathology
Leiden University Medical Center
Leiden, The Netherlands

Pedro Jares, PhD
Department of Anatomic Pathology
Hospital Clinic de Barcelona
University of Barcelona
Barcelona, Spain

Dragan Jevremovic, MD, PhD
Professor
Laboratory Medicine and Pathology
Mayo Clinic
Rochester, Minnesota

Marshall E. Kadin, MD
Professor
Department of Pathology
University of Virginia
Charlottesville, Virginia
Department of Dermatology
Boston University
Boston, Massachusetts

Werner Kempf, MD
Co-Director
Kempf und Pfaltz
Histologische Diagnostik
Professor and Consultant Physician
Department of Dermatology
University Hospital
Zurich, Switzerland

Rebecca L. King, MD
Professor
Division of Hematopathology
Mayo Clinic
Rochester, Minnesota

Wolfram Klapper, MD
Professor
Department of Pathology, Hematopathology Section
University Hospital Schleswig-Holstein (UKSH),
Christian-Albrechts University of Kiel
Kiel, Germany

Young Hyeh Ko, MD, PhD
Department of Pathology
Cheju Halla General Hospital
Jeju, South Korea
Emeritus Professor
Department of Pathology
Sungkyunkwan University
Seoul, South Korea

Ralf Küppers, PhD
Institute of Cell Biology (Cancer Research)
University of Duisburg-Essen, Medical School
Essen, Germany

Hans Michael Kvasnicka, MD, PhD
Professor of Pathology
Chair
Institute of Pathology and Molecular Pathology
University Clinic Wuppertal
Wuppertal, Germany

Laurence Lamant-Rochaix, MD, PhD
Senior Pathologist
Department of Pathology
Institut Universitaire du Cancer Toulouse Oncopole
Toulouse, France

Camille Laurent, MD, PhD
Senior Pathologist
Department of Pathology
Institut Universitaire du Cancer Toulouse Oncopole,
CHU
Toulouse, France

Philip E. LeBoit, MD
Professor of Pathology and Dermatology
Department of Pathology and Dermatology
University of California, San Francisco
San Francisco, California

Michael A. Linden, MD, PhD
Professor and Director of Hematopathology
Department of Laboratory Medicine and Pathology
University of Minnesota
Minneapolis, Minnesota

Laura Llao-Cid
Institut d'Investigacions Biomèdiques August Pi i
Sunyer (IDIBAPS)
Barcelona, Spain

Robert B. Lorsbach, MD, PhD
Director of Hematopathology
Division of Pathology & Laboratory Medicine
Cincinnati Children's Hospital Medical Center
Clinical Professor
Department of Pathology
University of Cincinnati
Cincinnati, Ohio

Abner Louissant, Jr., MD, PhD
Aziz and Nur Hamzaogullari Endowed Scholar in
Hematologic Malignancies
Associate Pathologist
Department of Pathology
Massachusetts General Hospital
Associate Professor of Pathology
Department of Pathology
Harvard Medical School
Boston, Massachusetts

Manuela Mollejo, PhD
Complejo Hospitalario Toledo
Department of Pathology
SESCAM
Toledo, Spain

William G. Morice, II, MD, PhD
Professor
Laboratory Medicine and Pathology
Mayo Clinic
Rochester, Minnesota

Krzysztof Mrózek, MD, PhD
Research Scientist
Comprehensive Cancer Center
Clara D. Bloomfield Center for Leukemia Outcomes
Research
The Ohio State University
Columbus, Ohio

Megan Nakashima, MD
Assistant Professor
Department of Laboratory Medicine
Cleveland Clinic Foundation
Cleveland, Ohio

Alina Nicolae, MD, PhD
Associate Professor
Department of Pathology
Hautepierre Hospital, CHU Strasbourg
University of Strasbourg
Strasbourg, France

Attilio Orazi, MD, FRCPath
Professor and Chair
Department of Pathology
Texas Tech University Health Sciences Center
El Paso, Texas

Ilske Oschlies, MD
Professor
Department of Pathology, Hematopathology Section
University Hospital Schleswig-Holstein (UKSH),
Christian-Albrechts University of Kiel
Kiel, Germany

German Ott, MD
Professor of Pathology
Department of Clinical Pathology
Robert-Bosch-Krankenhaus
Stuttgart, Germany

Tony Petrella, MD
Pathology
Hospital Maisonneuve-Rosemont
Montreal, Quebec, Canada

Laura B. Pincus, MD
Professor of Dermatology and Pathology
Department of Dermatology and Pathology
University of California, San Francisco
San Francisco, California

Miguel A. Piris, MD
Emeritus Researcher
Department of Pathology
Fundacion Jimenez Diaz
Madrid, Spain

Stefania Pittaluga, MD, PhD
Senior Research Physician
Laboratory of Pathology
National Cancer Center
Bethesda, Maryland

Anna Porwit, MD, PhD
Professor Emerita
Department of Clinical Sciences
Division of Oncology and Pathology
Lund University
Faculty of Medicine
Lund, Sweden

Sonam Prakash, MBBS
Health Sciences Clinical Professor
Laboratory Medicine
University of California, San Francisco
San Francisco, California

Leticia Quintanilla-Martinez, MD
Professor of Pathology
Institute of Pathology
University Hospital Tübingen
Eberhard-Karls-University Tübingen
Tübingen, Germany

Frederick Racke, MD, PhD, FACP
Medical Director
Advanced Diagnostics, Hematopathology and Coagulation
Quest Diagnostics
San Juan Capistrano, California

Mark Raffeld, MD
Senior Research Physician
Laboratory of Pathology
National Cancer Institute, NIH
Bethesda, Maryland

Karen L. Rech, MD
Laboratory Medicine and Pathology
Mayo Clinic
Rochester, Minnesota

Kaaren K. Reichard, MD
Professor
Department of Laboratory Medicine and Pathology
Mayo Clinic
Rochester, Minnesota

Lisa M. Rimsza, MD
Professor and Consultant
Department of Laboratory Medicine and Pathology
Mayo Clinic
Scottsdale, Arizona

Heesun J. Rogers, MD, PhD
Staff Hematopathologist
Department of Laboratory Medicine
Cleveland Clinic
Associate Professor
Department of Pathology
Cleveland Clinic Lerner College of Medicine
Cleveland, Ohio

Nancy S. Rosenthal, MD
Professor of Pathology
Wake Forest University School of Medicine
Winston-Salem, North Carolina

Jonathan W. Said, MD
Professor of Pathology
Vice Chair Research
Chief of Hematopathology
Department of Pathology
David Geffen School of Medicine and UCLA Medical Center
Los Angeles, California

Itziar Salaverria, PhD
Molecular Genetics of Pediatric Lymphomas
Institute for Biomedical Research August Pi i Sunyer (IDIBAPS)
Barcelona, Spain

Kristian T. Schafernak, MD, MPH
Staff Pathologist
Department of Pathology and Laboratory Medicine
Phoenix Children's Hospital
Associate Professor of Child Health and Pathology
University of Arizona College of Medicine—Phoenix
Associate Clinical Professor of Pathology
Creighton University College of Medicine
Assistant Professor of Laboratory Medicine and Pathology
Mayo Clinic College of Medicine
Phoenix, Arizona

Anne M.R. Schrader, MD, PhD
Department of Pathology
Leiden University Medical Center
Leiden, The Netherlands

David W. Scott, MBChB, PhD
Clinician Scientist
Centre for Lymphoid Cancer
BC Cancer
Associate Professor
Department of Medicine
University of British Columbia
Vancouver, British Columbia, Canada

Min Shi, MD, PhD
Professor
Laboratory Medicine and Pathology
Mayo Clinic
Rochester, Minnesota

Reiner Siebert, MD
Professor
Institute of Human Genetics
Ulm University & Ulm University
Medical Center
Ulm, Germany

Oscar Silva, MD, PhD
Clinical Assistant Professor
Department of Pathology
Stanford University
Stanford, California

Aliyah R. Sohani, MD
Hematopathologist
Department of Pathology
Massachusetts General Hospital
Professor of Pathology
Harvard Medical School
Boston, Massachusetts

Karl Sotlar, MD
Professor
Head of the Department
Institute of Pathology
University Hospital Salzburg
Paracelsus Medical University
Salzburg, Austria

Steven H. Swerdlow, MD
Emeritus Professor of Pathology
University of Pittsburgh School of
Medicine
Pittsburgh, Pennsylvania

Wayne Tam, MD, PhD
Senior Director
Division of Hematopathology
Department of Pathology and Laboratory Medicine
Northwell Health
Greenvale, New York
Professor
Department of Pathology and Laboratory Medicine
Donald and Barbara Zucker School of Medicine at
Hofstra/Northwell
Hempstead, New York

Alexandar Tzankov, MD
Professor
Head Histopathology and Autopsy
Institute of Medical Genetics and Pathology
University Hospital Basel
Basel, Switzerland

Peter Valent, MD
Professor
Department of Internal Medicine I
Division of Hematology and Hemostaseology and
Ludwig Boltzmann Institute for Hematology and
Oncology
Medical University of Vienna
Vienna, Austria

Girish Venkataraman, MD, MBBS
Professor of Pathology
Section of Hematopathology
University of Chicago Medical Center
Chicago, Illinois

Maria (Ria) E. Vergara-Lluri, MD
Associate Professor of Clinical Pathology
Department of Pathology
Keck School of Medicine of University of Southern
California
Los Angeles, California

Anjanaa Vijayanarayanan, MD
Hematopathology Fellow
Laboratory Medicine
University of California
San Fransisco, California

Hao-Wei Wang, MD, PhD
Associated Research Physician
Laboratory of Pathology
Center for Cancer Research
National Cancer Institute
National Institutes of Health
Bethesda, Maryland

Sa A. Wang, MD
Professor
Hematopathology
MD Anderson Cancer Center
Houston, Texas

Olga K. Weinberg, MD
Hematopathologist
Associate Professor
Department of Pathology
UT Southwestern
Dallas, Texas

Rein Willemze, MD, PhD
Department of Dermatology
Leiden University Medical Center
Leiden, The Netherlands

Tadashi Yoshino, MD, PhD
Specially Appointed Professor
Department of Pathology
Okayama University Medical School
Okayama, Japan

Constance M. Yuan, MD, PhD
Associate Research Physician
Laboratory of Pathology
Center for Cancer Research
National Cancer Institute
National Institutes of Health
Bethesda, Maryland

Qian-Yun Zhang, MD, PhD
Professor of Pathology
University of New Mexico
Albuquerque, New Mexico

Lawrence R. Zukerberg, MD[†]
Hematopathologist and Gastrointestinal Pathologist
Department of Pathology
Massachusetts General Hospital
Associate Professor of Pathology
Harvard Medical School
Boston, Massachusetts

---

† Deceased.

The first edition of *Hematopathology* was published in 2011, shortly after the introduction of the fourth edition of the *WHO Classification of Tumours of Haematopoietic and Lymphoid Tissues*. The second edition was coordinated with the release of the revised fourth edition *Bluebook* in 2017. The third edition is being released at a critical time in the evolution of the classification of hematolymphoid neoplasms, as for the first time in nearly 30 years the field has seen the publication of two major classifications in 2022. Most of the principal editors of the 3rd and 4th edition WHO Classifications collaborated to produce the International Consensus Classification (ICC) in 2022, under the auspices of the Society for Hematopathology and the European Association for Haematopathology. The classification was developed following a Clinical Advisory Committee meeting, with the participation of more than 200 pathologists, clinicians, and scientists from 24 countries in September 2021, and published in a series of articles in *Blood* in 2022.[1-4] Concurrent with these events, the International Agency for Research on Cancer (IARC) invited a panel of editors and authors to develop the 5th edition of the WHO Classification, published in draft form in *Leukemia* in 2022.[5,6] The third edition of *Hematopathology* has adopted the ICC system to present the basic framework for the discussion of neoplastic disorders of lymphoid, myeloid, and histiocytic neoplasms. However, each chapter will present key synonyms, where appropriate, for the WHO 5th edition, and importantly discuss the rationale for the preferred terminology adopted in the book.

The reader will find not only the most current terminology, but also a discussion of key changes in the classification of lymphomas and leukemias and of histiocytic disorders. Thus this book will be a valuable resource for the pathologist trying to keep up with this rapidly changing field.

Hematopathology is a discipline in which traditional methods of clinical and morphologic analysis are interwoven with newer, biologically based studies to achieve an accurate diagnosis. Scientific advances are proceeding at a rapid pace, with a greater emphasis today on the integration of newer genomic studies as a basis for diagnosis, and, in many cases, treatment. Studies of hematologic malignancies have been at the forefront in applying the principles of basic research to the understanding of human disease. All cancers are increasingly recognized as genetic diseases, with precise genetic alterations often defining entities. Advances in immunologic and molecular genetic technology have rapidly migrated to the clinical laboratory, where they play a role in routine diagnosis, and the introduction of next-generation sequencing is changing the face of molecular diagnostics. The reader will find valuable guidance in how to integrate these new advances in daily practice.

The discussion of each disease includes a description of morphologic, immunophenotypic, and clinical features, along with relevant genetic findings. These data inform our understanding of disease pathogenesis and provide valuable and often critical adjuncts to diagnosis and treatment. The goal is to provide concise, up-to-date, and practical information that is easily accessed by the reader. Equally relevant to the diagnostic pathologist is an appreciation of the spectrum of reactive and inflammatory lesions of hematolymphoid tissues occurring in immunocompetent patients and in those with altered immune states. Thus the reader will find a discussion of reactive lymphadenopathies and primary and iatrogenic immunodeficiency disorders. Additional chapters deal with the bone marrow response to inflammatory, infectious, and metabolic diseases; germline changes impacting hematopoiesis myeloid neoplasia; and the impact of therapy on bone marrow morphology. The book offers a comprehensive guide to benign and malignant hematopathology that will be a valued resource for the practicing pathologist, hematologist, and oncologist.

It is increasingly important that clinicians be aware of basic principles of hematopathology diagnosis; hematologists and hematopathologists must work as a team to achieve the correct diagnosis. Just as the pathologist must use clinical data to make an accurate diagnosis, the clinician should have sufficient knowledge of diagnostic principles to appreciate when the pathologic diagnosis just does not quite fit.

The Editors appreciate that the reader needs to have access to key source material and that a richly referenced book provides important information for those who wish to delve further into the topic. The scientific literature is voluminous, and we thought it was important to include older historical references, as well as the most recent scientific data. All the references are accessible on the Elsevier eBooks+ website, with the benefit of electronic access to the PubMed links instantaneously. However, the authors provide key references in print in each chapter to provide the reader with the most useful sources to examine the topic in greater depth.

We were delighted to add several new experts to the editorial team for the third edition. Two international experts in lymphoid diseases, Lisa Rimsza and Steven Swerdlow, have joined as editors. Dr. Rimsza is a leader in the integration of new biological approaches to diagnosis, while Dr. Swerdlow was a key figure in the development of the modern lymphoma classification. Attilio Orazi, an international expert in myeloproliferative and myelodysplastic diseases, joins Dan Arber to complete the bone marrow and myeloid squadron.

We acknowledge the valuable contributions of Nancy Lee Harris and James Vardiman, who were editors for earlier editions and were critical in establishing this book as the classic reference in its field. We hope this book will prove to be a constant and valued resource for pathologists and clinicians dealing with hematologic diseases and will ultimately benefit patients and their families.

Elaine S. Jaffe, MD

Daniel A. Arber, MD

Elias Campo, MD, PhD

Attilio Orazi, MD, FRCPath

Leticia Quintanilla-Martinez, MD

Lisa M. Rimsza, MD

Steven H. Swerdlow, MD

REFERENCES

1. Campo E, Jaffe ES, Cook JR, et al. The International Consensus Classification of Mature Lymphoid Neoplasms: a report from the Clinical Advisory Committee. *Blood.* 2022;140:1229–1253.
2. Arber DA, Orazi A, Hasserjian RP, et al. International Consensus Classification of Myeloid Neoplasms and Acute Leukemias: integrating morphologic, clinical, and genomic data. *Blood.* 2022;140:1200–1228.
3. de Leval L, Alizadeh AA, Bergsagel PL, et al. Genomic profiling for clinical decision making in lymphoid neoplasms. *Blood.* 2022;140:2193–2227.
4. Duncavage EJ, Bagg A, Hasserjian RP, et al. Genomic profiling for clinical decision making in myeloid neoplasms and acute leukemia. *Blood.* 2022;140:2228–2247.
5. Alaggio R, Amador C, Anagnostopoulos I, et al. The 5th edition of the World Health Organization Classification of Haematolymphoid Tumours: Lymphoid Neoplasms. *Leukemia.* 2022;36:1720–1748.
6. Khoury JD, Solary E, Abla O, et al. The 5th edition of the World Health Organization Classification of Haematolymphoid Tumours: Myeloid and Histiocytic/Dendritic Neoplasms. *Leukemia.* 2022;36:1703–1719.

Contents

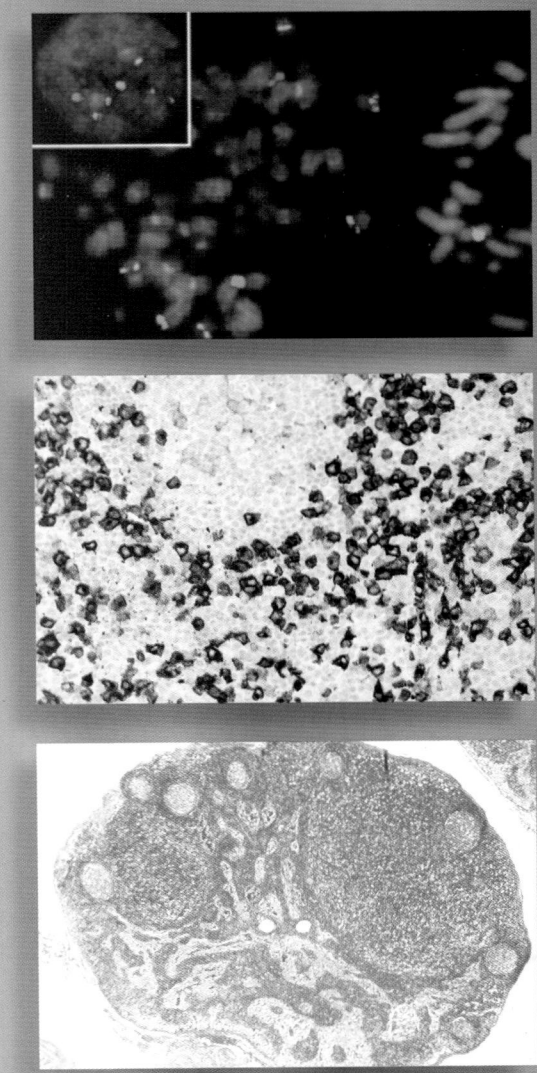

PART I

Technical Aspects

Chapter 1

Processing of the Lymph Node Biopsy Specimen

Sebastian Fernandez-Pol, Dita Gratzinger, and Oscar Silva

A multiparameter approach that integrates clinical, histologic, immunophenotypic, cytogenetic, and molecular data for precise diagnostic classification is central to the World Health Organization (WHO) and International Consensus Classification (ICC) schemes of hematolymphoid tumors.[1,2] Other than clinical information, all of the information necessary for the correct diagnosis depends on the availability of an adequate quantity of appropriately processed tissue.[3] If the initial processing of a lymph node biopsy specimen is not performed correctly, all subsequent morphologic, immunophenotypic, cytogenetic, and molecular studies are compromised, potentially leading to a nondiagnostic result that may necessitate a follow-up procedure, a delay in diagnosis, increased patient anxiety, and increased costs. With the current mandate to provide cost-effective health care and with mounting pressure to diagnose based on needle aspirations and cytologic preparations, repeating an open lymph node biopsy procedure is not trivial. Thus it is imperative that the pathologist play an active role in optimal handling, triaging, and processing of lymph node specimens. In particular, when small pieces of tissues are available, pathologists may play a pivotal role in deciding which ancillary studies should be prioritized to maximize the likelihood of achieving a definitive diagnostic, prognostic, or theranostic result.

The lymph node presents certain unique challenges for pathologists and histotechnologists because of its innate organizational structure.[4] It is composed of millions of small cells held together by fine strands of connective tissue surrounded by a fibrous capsule that is relatively impervious to fixation and to processing chemicals. Histologic sections of excellent quality can be obtained only if each step in the processing of a lymph node is handled with care and knowledge of the underlying factors that result in optimal preparations. This chapter reviews the essential steps for triage, handling, and stewardship of lymph node tissue for a variety of morphologic, immunophenotypic, molecular, and other ancillary techniques that are crucial to optimal patient care.

ASSESSING AND PRIORITIZING FRESH TISSUE

Knowledge of the patient's clinical history and the suspected or differential diagnosis facilitates the targeting of a lymph node that best represents the underlying pathologic process. Despite the obvious appeal of convenient access, minimal discomfort, and the procedural simplicity of excising a superficial lymph node, these are not always of diagnostic value. Given that most lymphomas are fluorodeoxyglucose (FDG) avid, combined imaging modalities such as 18F-fluorodeoxyglucose positron-emission tomography/computed tomography (^{18}F-FDG PET/CT) have revolutionized the targeting, staging, and monitoring of lymphomas.[5,6] By assessing the standardized uptake value (SUV), a surgeon may target highly FDG-avid lymph nodes, which are accessible and safe for sampling (Fig. 1-1). Radiologic assistance to guide optimal acquisition of lymph nodes is particularly relevant in cases of suspected large cell transformation and is recommended by the International Conference on Malignant Lymphomas Imaging Working Group.[7] This approach should lead to a precise, targeted lymph node excision and avoids the erroneous sampling of nondiagnostic tissue.

Excisional biopsy of an entire lymph node has the significant benefit of providing a complete view of the lymph node architecture, which can reveal patterns of malignant cell involvement that serve as diagnostic and histologic features to

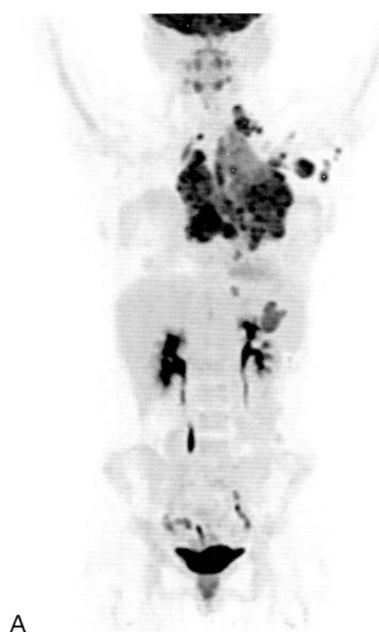
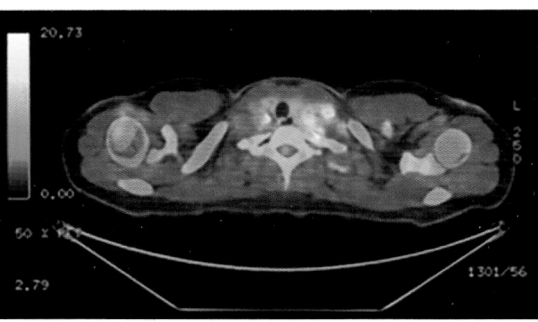
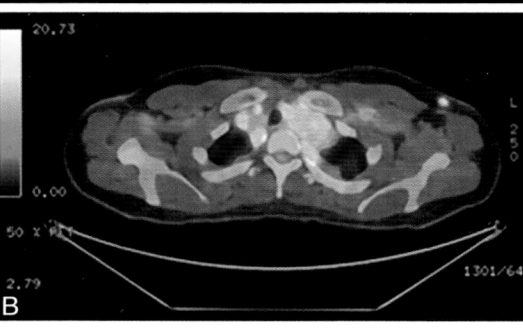

A

B

Figure 1-1. Using PET-CT to aid in the selection of a lymph node for biopsy. A, Coronal positron-emission tomography (PET) scan showing increased fluorodeoxy-glucose (FDG) avidity *(black)* in the left cervical, left axillary, medias-tinum, and hilar lymph nodes. **B,** Axial PET-computed tomography (CT) scan showing increased FGD avidity *(yellow)* in the left cervi-cal lymph nodes *(upper)* and me-diastinum *(lower).* By selecting a PET-avid lymph node with a high standardized uptake value (SUV), the likelihood of obtaining a diag-nostic specimen may be higher, es-pecially when evaluating for large cell transformation.

lead to the correct diagnosis. The benefit of excisional lymph node biopsy is especially relevant at initial diagnosis, whereas smaller-volume biopsies may be sufficient in patients with some forms of recurrent lymphoma.[8,9] Excisional biopsies are particularly preferred when diagnostic cells are admixed in a reactive background, as, for example, in nodular lymphocyte predominant B-cell (Hodgkin) lymphoma (NLPBL)[10]; when intact architecture contributes substantially to diagnosis because of substantial overlap with other malignant or benign entities, such as follicular helper T-cell lymphoma (TFH) of the angioimmunoblastic-type (AITL)[11]; or when there is partial involvement of lymphoma. When an infectious cause is suspected, the surgeon should submit a portion from one pole of the lymph node for appropriate microbiological studies directly from the sterile environment of the operating room. It should be noted, however, that such specimens are prone to contamination.[12]

In all other circumstances, the intact specimen should be submitted fresh to the pathologist in a specimen container and immersed in saline or a culture medium such as RPMI (Roswell Park Memorial Institute) medium to ensure the specimen does not dry out during transit. Wrapping the specimen or laying it on gauze, sponges, or towels should be avoided, because this leads to desiccation of the lymph node cortex, especially when the specimen is exposed to air. Request for a "lymph node workup" should be clearly indicated on the requisition slip, specimen tag, or both. Ideally, the pathologist should be notified at the time of the biopsy to avoid a delay in the handling of the specimen. When a delay in delivery to the pathologist is anticipated, the specimen should be refrigerated to minimize autolysis. Storage at 4° C for up to 24 hours can yield satisfactory but not optimal morphologic, immunohistochemical, and genetic preservation.[13] When long delays are expected before the pathologist receives the specimen, the surgeon may be instructed to bisect the lymph node and make air-dried imprints, after which the fresh specimen can be sliced thinly, a portion placed in a culture

medium such as RPMI for flow cytometry, and the remaining portion placed in buffered formalin for fixation. Certain specific clinical situations call for very specific handling and apportionment of fresh tissue, as when breast implant-associated anaplastic large cell lymphoma is suspected.[14]

A general workflow for lymph node tissue appropriation and processing is depicted in Figure 1-2 and discussed in detail herein.

Once a well-targeted lymph node is excised within the operative room, a sterile intraoperative specimen can be submitted for cultures if infection is a clinical consideration. The specimen should be transported in saline or RPMI medium to the pathologist for gross processing, cytologic preparation, and possible intraoperative consultation (frozen section). A fresh portion should be provided in RPMI medium for flow cytometry, fluorescence in situ hybridization (FISH), or molecular assays. The remaining tissue should be fixed in formalin for generation of formalin-fixed paraffin embedded (FFPE) tissue blocks for histology (hematoxylin and eosin [H&E]), immunohistochemistry (IHC), FISH, and select molecular assays.

GROSS PROCESSING OF THE LYMPH NODE BIOPSY

Gross Examination

The gross appearance of lymph nodes, including their color, consistency, and changes in contour, may provide useful information about the diagnosis and should be recorded during gross inspection of the fresh specimen (Fig. 1-3). Preservation of the hilus and the presence or absence of nodularity and fibrosis can offer important diagnostic clues. Preservation of the hilus is rare in lymphomas, and its presence suggests a reactive process (Fig. 1-3A and B). Necrosis within the node indicates the possibility of an infectious process and may prompt microbiological studies. Adherence of the node

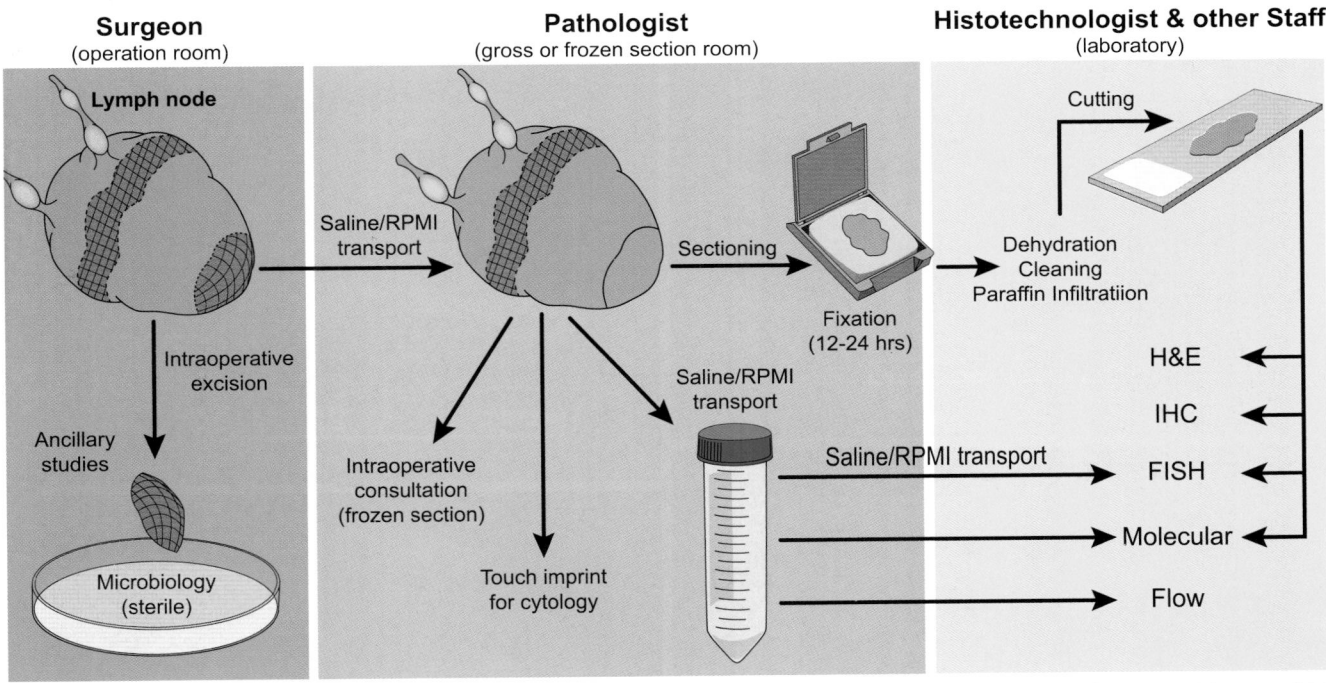

Figure 1-2. Appropriation of lymph node tissue. *FISH,* Fluorescence in situ hybridization; *H&E,* hematoxylin and eosin; *IHC,* immunohisto-chemistry; *RPMI,* Roswell Park Memorial Institute medium.

to the surrounding fat may denote extracapsular extension of disease and should also be noted in the gross description. Most lymphomas completely efface the nodal architecture, and a nodular appearance or fibrosis can be seen on gross examination (Fig. 1-3C to E).

Although gross findings can be helpful in narrowing the differential diagnosis, an accurate pathologic diagnosis is virtually never possible based on gross findings alone. Thus, these findings must be interpreted in conjunction with microscopic features and immunophenotypic and genetic studies to establish a definitive diagnosis.

Intraoperative Consultation

The diagnosis of lymphoid malignancies can be challenging even on permanent sections. Because of the numerous artifacts generated during the preparation of a frozen section, a diagnosis of lymphoma based on frozen tissue is perilous and best avoided; moreover, even after fixation, previously frozen tissue contains artifacts that can influence diagnostically relevant features, including cell size and chromatin characteristics. In addition, frozen tissue cannot be used for flow cytometry immunophenotyping. Although certain lymphomas can be distinguished on frozen sections, clinical colleagues should be advised of the unreliability of frozen sections for the accurate diagnosis and classification of lymphoma. In the rare event that a rapid interpretation is necessary for patient care, cytologic preparations (touch imprints or scrape preparations, as appropriate) should be examined in conjunction with frozen sections. Imprints require a negligible amount of material, thus preserving tissue for ancillary studies and yielding cytologic details that may not be appreciated on frozen tissue sections.[15]

The appropriate use of cytologic preparations, including touch or scrape imprints, and/or frozen sections of lymph node biopsy specimens is to estimate the adequacy of the tissue for diagnosis and to assess for morphologically evident non-hematolymphoid processes such as metastatic carcinoma. Touch imprints and/or frozen sections also offer pathologists the opportunity to allocate tissue for ancillary studies based on the preliminary differential diagnosis. This allows for rapid initiation of microbiological, cytogenetic, or flow cytometry studies with optimal preservation of cell viability. If the changes seen on touch imprint and/or frozen sections suggest a reactive process in a patient in whom there is a strong clinical suspicion of lymphoma, the surgeon or interventional radiologist can be advised to sample further to obtain diagnostic tissue.

Cytologic Preparations

The utility of cytologic preparations in the evaluation of lymphoid lesions should not be underestimated. Cytologic touch imprint or scrape preparations complement tissue diagnosis and are useful both at the time of frozen section and when examining permanent tissue sections. Touch and scrape imprints are encouraged for all intraoperative consultations for lymphoid lesions and should be examined in conjunction with the frozen tissue sections. Imprints can also facilitate the intraoperative assessment of hematolymphoid lesions of bone when frozen sections cannot be obtained.

When cytologic imprints are prepared from lymph node specimens, it is best to prepare and label six to eight slides ahead of time. For touch imprints, the cut surface of the lymph node should be positioned on a flat surface, such as a towel (Fig. 1-4A). While the slide is held firmly at one end, it is gently lowered and brought into contact with the cut surface

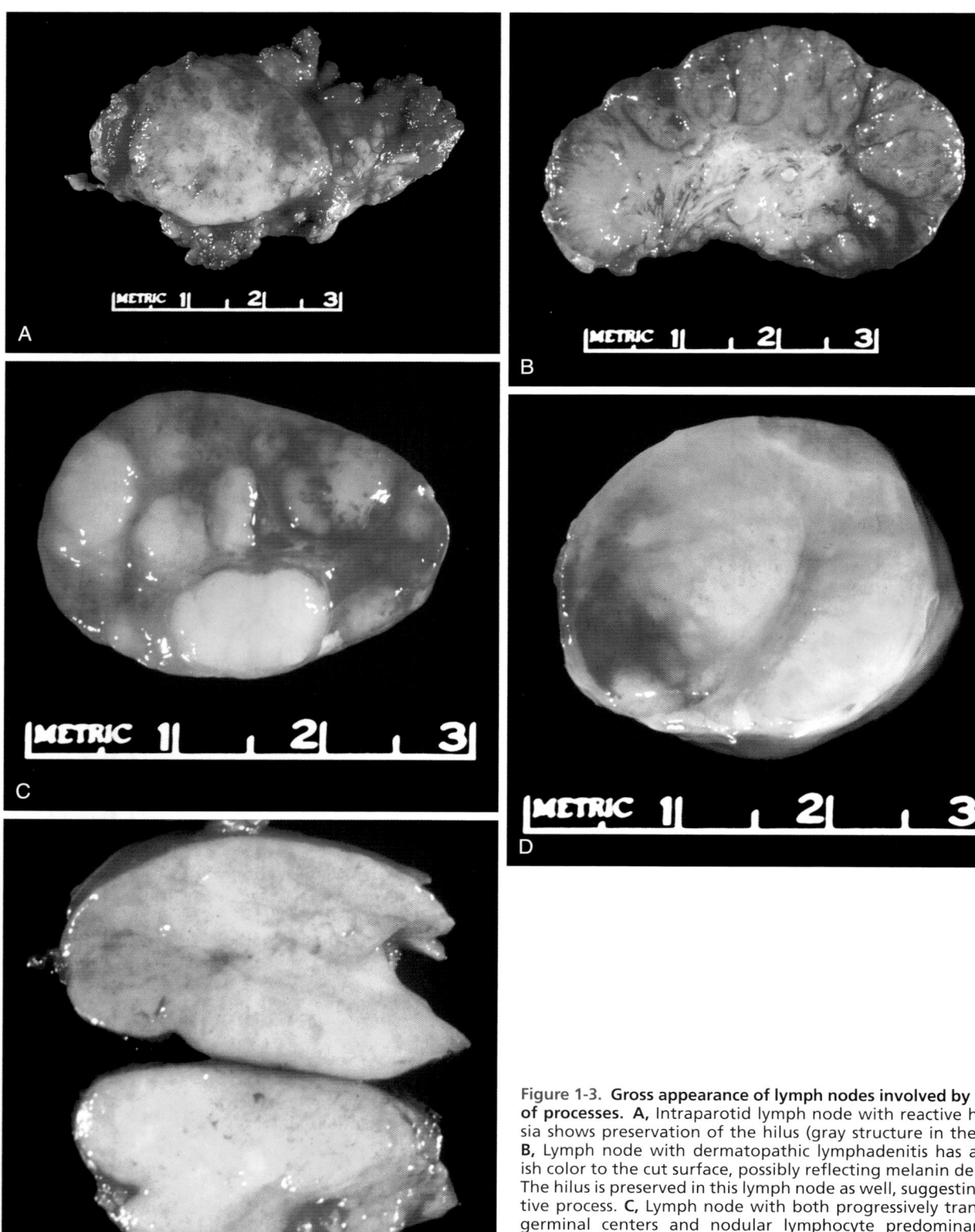

Figure 1-3. Gross appearance of lymph nodes involved by a variety of processes. A, Intraparotid lymph node with reactive hyperplasia shows preservation of the hilus (gray structure in the center). **B,** Lymph node with dermatopathic lymphadenitis has a brownish color to the cut surface, possibly reflecting melanin deposition. The hilus is preserved in this lymph node as well, suggesting a reactive process. **C,** Lymph node with both progressively transformed germinal centers and nodular lymphocyte predominant B-cell lymphoma has an obviously nodular architecture on cut section. **D,** Lymph node containing nodular sclerosis classic Hodgkin lymphoma has fibrous bands traversing the cut surface. **E,** Lymph node involved by follicular lymphoma has a homogeneous, fleshy cut surface with obliteration of the hilus, which is typical of lymphomatous involvement.

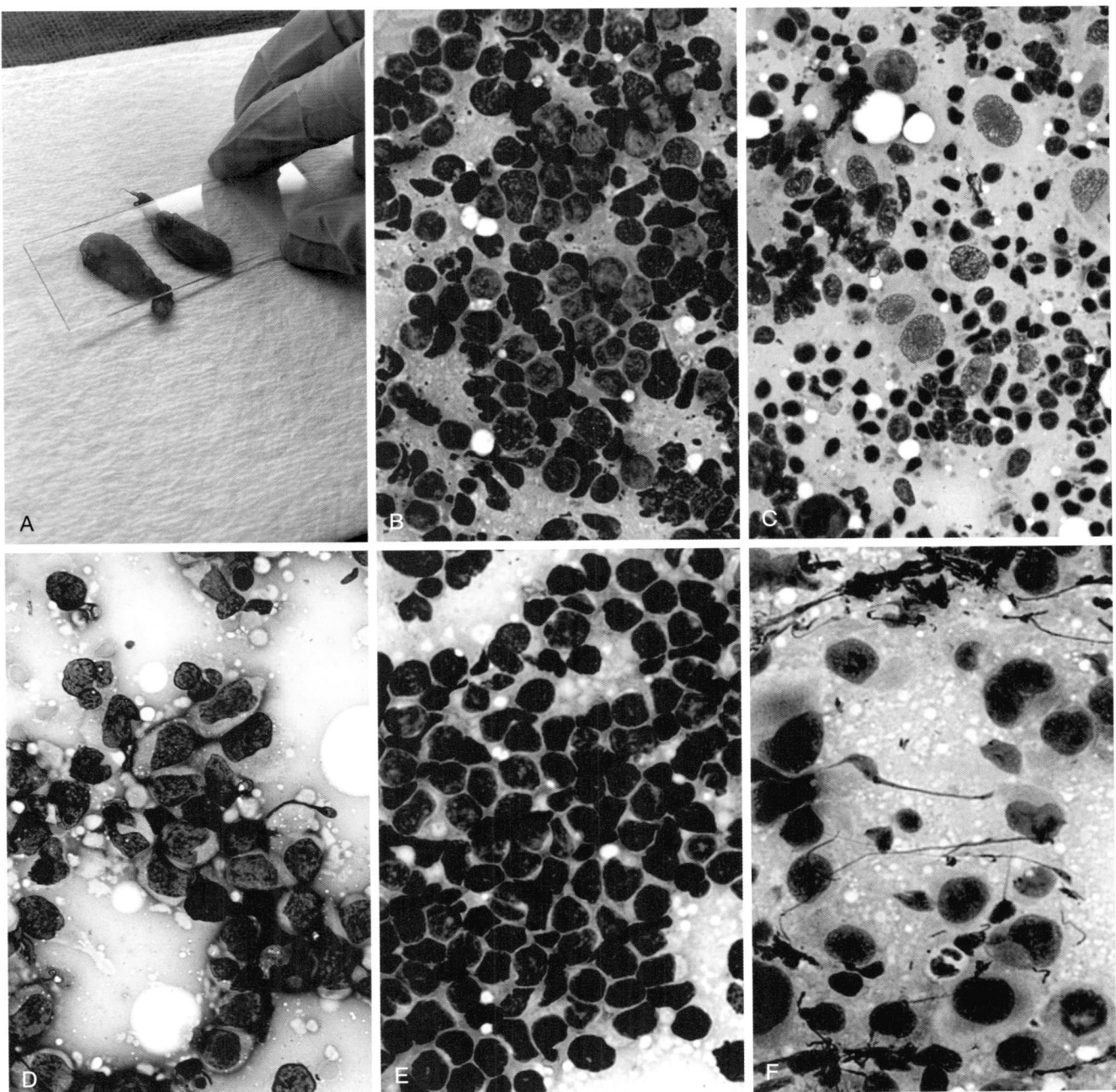

Figure 1-4. **A,** Example of touch imprint technique. **B,** Microscopic images of B-lymphoblastic lymphoma. **C,** Classic Hodgkin lymphoma. **D,** Diffuse large B-cell lymphoma. **E,** Follicular lymphoma. **F,** Metastatic poorly differentiated carcinoma of unknown primary site.

of the node, avoiding smearing or sideways movement. This process can be repeated three to five times, creating a series of touch imprint slides. The imprint slide should immediately be placed in a Coplin jar with 95% alcohol. Buffered formalin or formaldehyde can also be used as a fixative. A few imprint slides may be air dried. Although there is almost always enough material available to make touch imprints without compromising specimen integrity, scrape preparations may not be necessary if touch preparations are informative and are best avoided when dealing with very small samples to prevent inadvertent crushing or distortion of the tissue. For scrape preparations, the fresh-cut surface of the lymph node is gently scraped with the edge of a slide or the blunt edge of a scalpel and immediately smeared onto a previously labeled slide. Alcohol-dried and air-dried slides can be generated as for touch imprints.

A Wright-Giemsa or Diff-Quik stain is best for identifying and characterizing cells of the hematopoietic system and tumors derived from them, but the Papanicolaou stain is useful for assessing nuclear details such as membrane irregularity, chromatin configuration, and nucleoli. When necrosis and inflammatory cells are present, a Gram stain can be helpful to highlight bacterial organisms. In general, aspirations of lymph nodes are highly cellular and are characterized by a dispersed cell pattern and lymphoglandular bodies (detached cytoplasmic fragments of lymphoid cells). In aggressive lymphomas, the presence of monotonous sheets of medium-sized to large-sized cells, especially when associated with karyorrhexis and apoptosis, suggests the differential diagnosis of lymphoblastic, Burkitt, or large cell lymphoma (Fig. 1-4A). Similarly, imprints can be helpful in highlighting Reed-Sternberg cells (Fig. 1-4C) or high-grade cytologic features in diffuse large B-cell lymphoma (Fig. 1-4D). Indolent lymphomas composed of predominantly small cells or a mixed cellular milieu are much more difficult to diagnose on cytologic preparations than are aggressive lymphomas. Reactive follicular hyperplasia can be nearly impossible to distinguish from follicular lymphoma (Fig. 1-3E) on cytologic imprints, although the presence of a limited range of maturation together with the absence of tingible body macrophages favors a malignant diagnosis. Cytologic preparations can also be useful in the diagnosis of metastatic melanoma and carcinoma (Fig. 1-4F) and of non-neoplastic lesions in the lymph node, such as granulomatous and Kikuchi lymphadenitis. Lesions associated with significant sclerosis seldom yield sufficient material for cytologic preparations.

Sectioning

The two most important initial steps in the processing of a lymph node specimen are sectioning (blocking) and fixation. Blocking should be performed promptly and should precede fixation, because an intact lymph node capsule is impervious to fixation. In addition, touch and scrape imprints are best obtained fresh. The objective of good lymph node sectioning is to provide an undisrupted section that maintains the overall architecture of the tissue and is thin enough to yield significant cytologic detail. Sections should also preserve the relationship between the capsule and the remainder of the lymphoid compartments (Fig. 1-5). The best cross-section of a lymph node results from sectioning perpendicular to the long axis of the node with a sharp knife in one continuous sweep. This technique facilitates excellent preservation of the nodal architecture. For lymph nodes less than 1 cm in diameter, a single cut along the long axis is recommended; such small specimens may be crushed when attempting to perform cross-sections perpendicular to the long axis. The entire specimen should be sectioned in 2- to 3-mm slices and then placed promptly in fixative. Portions of lymph nodes should never be left unfixed or fixed without slicing. Because the fibrous tissue in the capsule may contract when exposed to fixatives, scoring of the capsule by introducing small cuts with a sharp scalpel blade may prevent distortion during processing (Fig. 1-5A). When lymph node specimens are fixed whole or when the central portion of the section is too thick, uneven fixation results (Fig. 1-6). This may lead to autolysis of the central areas or retraction of the tissue, causing erosion or cracking of the sections upon cutting with a microtome blade.

Thin slices of 2 to 3 mm should be placed in shallow plastic cassettes (used in most modern surgical pathology laboratories) to allow adequate penetration by fixation and processing reagents. Thorough—if not complete—sampling of the lymph node specimen is essential. This practice prevents sampling errors in disorders that may only partially

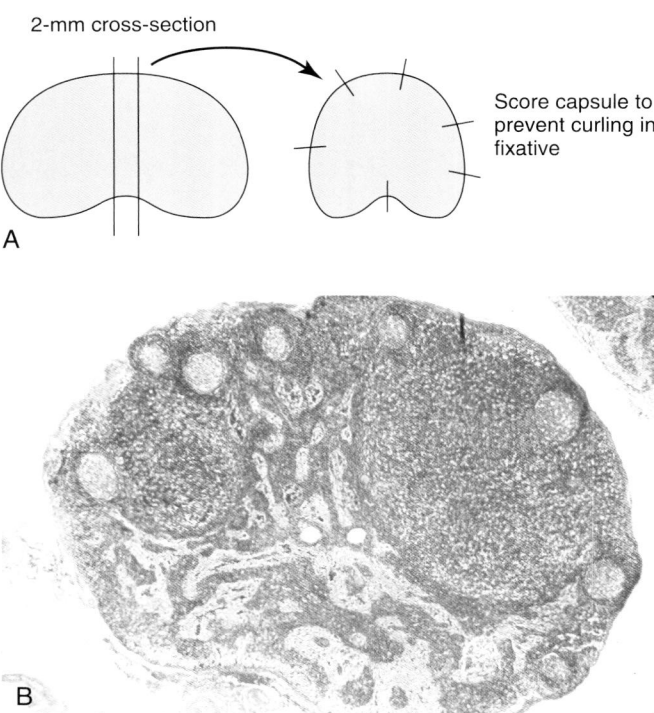

Figure 1-5. Lymph node sectioning. Lymph nodes should be sectioned to provide a complete cross-section that allows an appreciation of architecture. **A,** Schematic diagram shows that the lymph node is cut perpendicular to the long axis of the node (best for specimens >1 cm in diameter). The lymph node capsule can be scored with several small cuts before placing the section in fixative; this prevents curling as the capsule retracts on exposure to fixative. **B,** Low-power photomicrograph of a properly oriented lymph node section shows the capsule, cortex, paracortex, and medulla.

involve the lymph node, such as NLPBL in patients with progressive transformation of germinal centers and in cases of grade variations or focal progression of a low-grade lymphoma (e.g., follicular lymphoma). Under most circumstances, once portions of the lymph node specimen have been removed for ancillary studies, the specimen is small enough to be submitted entirely in a few cassettes. When multiple lymph nodes are submitted or when a lymph node is so large that 10 or more cassettes are required to submit the entire specimen, knowledge of the clinical differential diagnosis and good gross examination skills are helpful. Multiple sections at 2- to 3-mm intervals should be made throughout the specimen, and sections from various portions should be submitted. It is always preferable to err on the side of submitting too much adequately fixed tissue rather than not having enough to establish a definitive diagnosis or perform ancillary studies. In any lymph node biopsy in which microscopic examination of the initially submitted sections does not yield a definitive diagnosis, all the remaining tissue should be promptly submitted for microscopic examination.

Fixation

Fixation is the point of no return in the processing of a lymph node specimen. Although subsequent steps, including infiltration, clearing, and dehydration, can be repeated, if necessary, inadequate fixation cannot be reversed. Inadequate

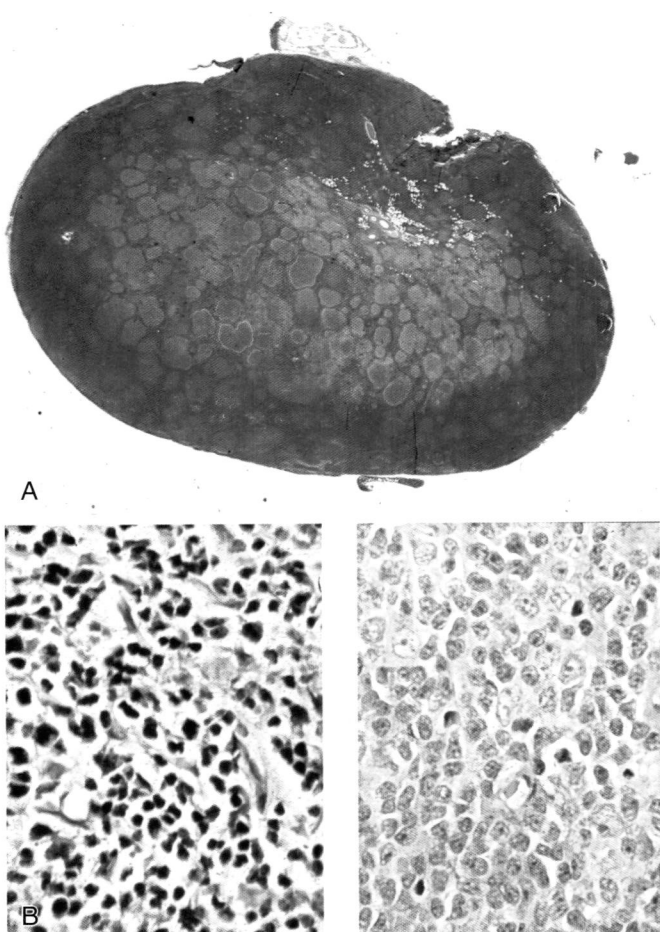

A

B

Figure 1-6. Lymph node fixation. This lymph node was placed in fixative without first cutting thin sections. **A,** Only the outer 1.0 mm of this paraffin section stained with hematoxylin and eosin is well fixed and stained; the center shows fainter staining and evidence of cell retraction. **B,** At high magnification, the center of the node *(left)* is autolyzed, with suboptimal cellular detail; the periphery *(right)* shows good cellular detail.

fixation may lead to a significant delay in patient care if attempts are made to reprocess a poorly fixed specimen, ancillary studies fail, or the poorly processed specimen is sent for expert consultation to avoid a repeat biopsy.

Excellent-quality slides can be prepared from lymph node specimens using a number of different fixatives as long as the proper volume and strength of fixative are used and, most importantly, adequate time is allowed for fixation.[16] The advantages and disadvantages of the most commonly used fixatives for lymph node specimens are outlined in Table 1-1. Neutral buffered formalin has the advantage of both excellent morphologic detail and adequate preservation of antigens for IHC and nucleic acids for in situ hybridization and next-generation sequencing assays. In most laboratories, assays to assess expression of proteins and ribonucleic acid (RNA) and the presence of genetic abnormalities are validated for use in FFPE specimens; therefore fixation in neutral buffered formalin is preferred. Some laboratories may use a combination of neutral buffered formalin and a metal-based fixative; one or two slices are fixed in a metal-based fixative for speed of fixation and optimal morphology, and the remainder are fixed in formalin for preservation of DNA and long-term storage. Although pathologists' preferences for metal fixatives vary, B5, neutral Zenker's solution, and zinc sulfate formalin are the most commonly used. Although B5 fixative renders excellent nuclear detail (Fig. 1-7), several factors make its routine use problematic. These include the relatively high cost, the time-sensitive nature of fixation (2–4 hours), and the need to remove mercuric chloride crystals from the sections and dispose of the mercury, an environmental hazard. Zinc formalin is an alternative to B5 fixative; it offers good nuclear detail, is less costly, and requires no special procedures for handling and disposal as it contains no mercuric chloride. Fixatives that are highly acidic, such as Zenker's, B5, Bouin's, and Carnoy's, are unsuitable for molecular diagnostic studies because they compromise the efficiency of polymerase chain reaction (PCR) amplification by decreasing the ability of the DNA within tissue to function as a template for the amplification of DNA fragments of desirable length.

Table 1-1 Advantages and Disadvantages of Commonly Used Fixatives[13,17]

Fixative	Optimal Length of Fixation (hrs)*	Morphologic Preservation	Immunopreservation	Molecular Preservation	Stability	Cost	Hazard
Neutral buffered formalin	12+	Excellent	Excellent	Excellent	Long	Low	Low
B5	2-4	Excellent Nuclear detail	Variable	Undesirable	Short (hours)	High	Moderate-high
Alcohols	<24	Moderate-excellent	Variable	Excellent	Long	Moderate	Low
Bouin's solution	<24	Excellent	Moderate	Undesirable	Short (days)	Low	Low
Neutral Zenker's solution	<24	Excellent Nuclear detail	Variable	Undesirable	Short (days)	Low	Moderate-high
Zinc formalin	6-8	Excellent Nuclear detail	Excellent	Undesirable	Short (days)	Low	Low
Carnoy's solution	<4	Moderate	Variable	Undesirable	Long	Moderate	Low

*Time is dependent on the size and thickness of the tissue and other factors.

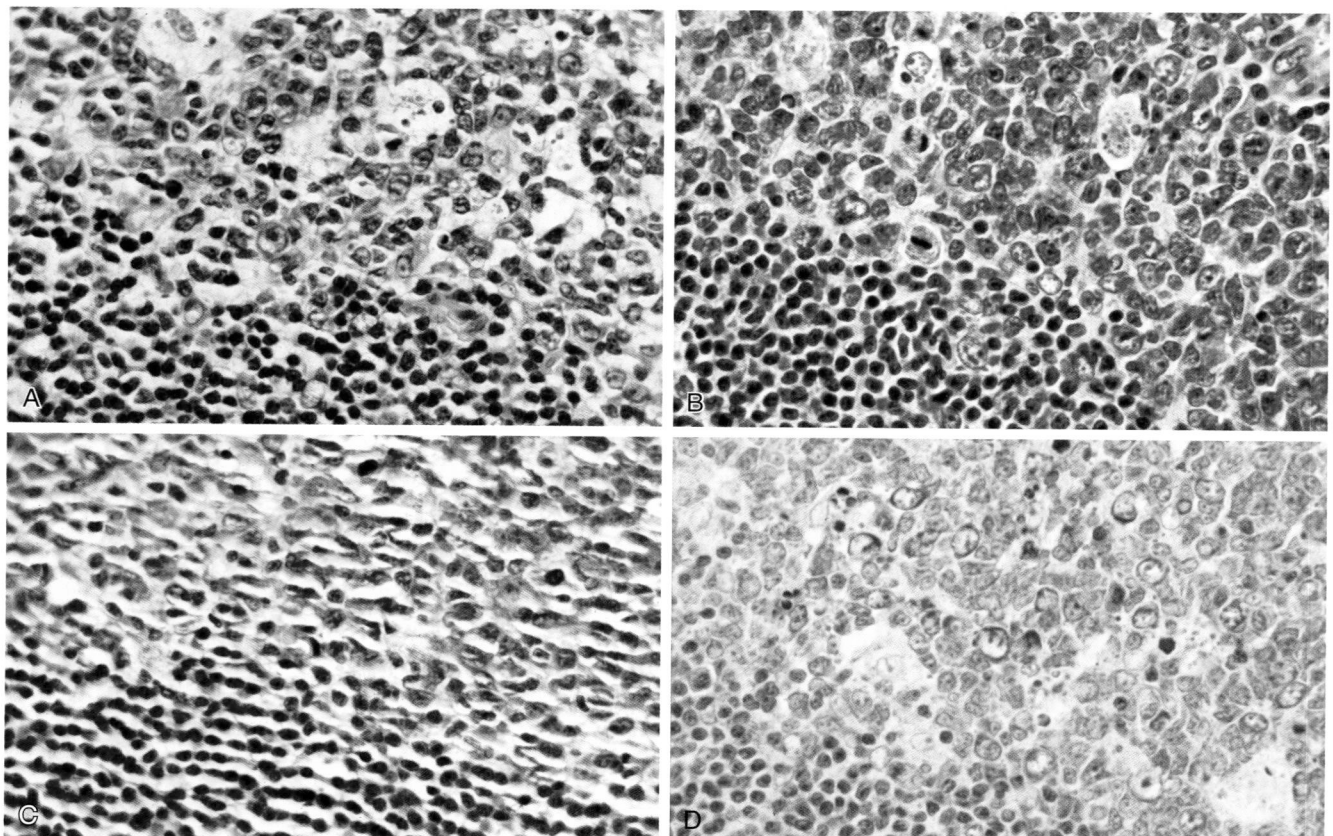

Figure 1-7. Lymph node germinal center showing the effects of different fixatives, cutting techniques, and staining. A, Specimen fixed in formalin for 24 hours and stained with hematoxylin and eosin (H&E) shows adequate fixation but some cytoplasmic retraction. **B,** Specimen fixed in B5 and stained with H&E shows crisp nuclear detail and better preservation of the cytoplasm. **C,** The same field and paraffin block as in **A** was cut by an inexperienced technician. Marked chatter artifact makes the recognition of cellular detail impossible. The section in **A** was cut by the same technician the next day after reviewing the initial slide with the pathologist. **D,** The same germinal center shown in **B** stained with Giemsa stain. The clear chromatin structure, peripheral nucleoli, and cytoplasmic basophilia of centroblasts are now more clearly delineated and contrast with the dispersed chromatin and pale cytoplasm of centrocytes.

We find that 10% neutral buffered formalin offers the best overall results by furnishing excellent morphologic preparations with good preservation of immunoreactivity and suitability for molecular diagnostic studies (Table 1-2). The standard use of FFPE tissue has the benefit of being in line with tissue handling and processing and ancillary study validation across the anatomic pathology laboratory. In addition, neutral buffered formalin provides the best method for long-term storage of fixed tissue, a particularly important consideration in storing archival material for research purposes. For good morphology, though, fixation in formalin requires at least 12 hours, with a maximum of about 48 hours for optimal morphology and tissue preservation for IHC.[17]

Contribution of the Histotechnologist

Once thinly sliced tissue sections are well fixed, the subsequent steps, including dehydration, clearing and infiltration by paraffin, and sectioning, depend on the expertise of the histotechnologist. The histotechnologist is responsible for ensuring the quality and combination of solutions used in tissue processors and for changing those solutions frequently enough to avoid dilution or contamination. It is particularly important to dehydrate the specimen without a trace of moisture before clearing with xylene and infiltration by paraffin. Blocks can be difficult to section if these steps are inadequately performed, resulting in cracking of the blocks, disintegration, or wrinkling of sections in the water bath.

Well-fixed and well-processed paraffin-embedded lymph node tissue should be cut at no more than 3- to 4-μm sections for microscopic slides. The best cytologic details are obtained when lymph node sections are uniformly one cell layer thick. Such sections provide remarkable details regarding the texture of the chromatin, the irregularities of the nuclear membrane, the presence or absence of nucleoli, and other features that enhance diagnostic capability. A sharp microtome blade, maintenance of the water bath at the optimal temperature, addition of appropriate detergents, and good mounting techniques are some of the key elements in obtaining a perfect microscopic section[23] (Fig. 1-7A and C). The College of American Pathologists (CAP) and the National Society for Histotechnology (NSH) Committee publish practical and up-to-date guides to specimen handling in surgical pathology that can serve as a histology laboratory resource.[24]

Table 1-2 Specimen Types Suitable for Ancillary Diagnostic Studies[18-22]

Study	Fresh Tissue	Frozen Tissue	Formalin-Fixed Paraffin Embedded Tissue	Imprints/Cytospin Preparations
Microbiological cultures	+*	−	−	−
Immunophenotypic studies				
Flow cytometry	+	−	−	−
Immunohistochemistry	+	+	+	+
Genetic studies				
In situ hybridization	+	+	+	+
Cytogenetic studies				
Karyotyping	+	−	−	−
FISH	+	+	±	+
Chromosomal microarray	+	+	+	−
Molecular diagnostic studies				
PCR	+	+	+	−
Next-generation sequencing	+	+	+	−
RNAseq	+	+	+	−
Mass spectrometry (amyloid subtyping)			+	

*Submit under sterile conditions.
+Suitable; −, unsuitable; ±, suboptimal but acceptable for study because of altered or destroyed antigens, with limited success using selected probes or antibodies. *FISH*, fluorescence in situ hybridization; *PCR*, polymerase chain reaction.

Whole Slide Imaging

Whole slide imaging (WSI) is at the core of the move to digital pathology and, in many ways, improves downstream workflows by increasing access to microscopic images and facilitating review of current and historic cases for second opinions and clinical and educational conferences.[25,26] WSI has good performance characteristics for primary lymphoma diagnosis, but it has limitations related to resolution (e.g., not optimal for detection of microorganisms), a fixed z-plane (inability to focus up and down), and differences in the ease and speed of slide manipulation, all of which can cause occasional diagnostic discrepancies compared with glass slide review.[27] Processing of the lymph node biopsy, including section thickness and staining characteristics, should be optimized as part of the WSI validation process, as it can have significant downstream effects on the quality of the scanned image.[28] The CAP recommendations for validation of WSI stress the importance of validating the entire process in a manner as similar as possible to real-world clinical use, including using at least 60 sample cases per general application (such as H&E-stained fixed tissue) and an additional 20 cases for additional applications (such as IHC and special stains).[29]

ROUTINE HISTOLOGIC, HISTOCHEMICAL, AND SPECIAL STAINS

H&E-stained sections are sufficient for the assessment of many lymphoid lesions. The Giemsa stain highlights nuclear features such as chromatin texture, nucleoli, and cytoplasmic granules, especially in myeloid and mast cells, and demonstrates cytoplasmic basophilia in cells such as centroblasts, immunoblasts, and plasma cells (Fig. 1-7D). Periodic acid–Schiff (PAS) stain is helpful in highlighting mucin, glycogen, and the basement membrane of blood vessels, and it is particularly useful in assessing the architecture of the spleen, where it highlights the fenestrated basement membrane of the sinuses. Cytoplasmic and nuclear immunoglobulin (Ig) inclusions, particularly IgM and IgA, which are rich in carbohydrate moieties, also stain with PAS.

Enzyme histochemical stains have been largely replaced by more specific and reliable immunohistologic and flow cytometric immunophenotyping methods in the diagnosis of lymph node specimens.

Microbiological Evaluation of Fixed Lymph Node Tissue

On H&E-stained sections, if necrosis or granulomas are identified, special stains for pathogenic organisms are routinely undertaken and correlated with microbiological cultures. Even dispersed histiocytic infiltrates may be a subtle sign of an infectious process in the setting of a blunted immune response, as in the setting of adult-onset immunodeficiency associated with neutralizing anti-interferon-gamma autoantibodies, which can mimic AITL, classic Hodgkin lymphoma, and other malignant and nonmalignant hematolymphoid processes.[30,31] PCR-based methods are highly sensitive and specific for detection and speciation of various microorganisms, even on FFPE tissue, and should be considered depending on the clinical setting and histologic findings. For necrotizing granulomatous processes, we routinely use Grocott-Gomori methenamine silver (GMS) and acid-fast bacillus (or Fite) stains to rule out fungal organisms and acid-fast bacilli; we also use PAS stain, which is helpful in the diagnosis of Whipple disease and for the identification of fungi. Of note, when fungal elements are identified and concomitant fungal cultures are not available, PCR-based methods should be used to identify the genus and species of the fungus. Similarly, sensitive PCR-based techniques can allow identification and speciation of mycobacterial organisms in FFPE tissue.[32,33]

In necrotizing lymphadenitis, a modified Gram stain (Brown and Hopps) can be used to detect gram-positive organisms. When an infectious gram-negative organism, such as *Bartonella henselae* (cat scratch disease), or a spirochete is suspected, a silver stain such as Steiner or Warthin-Starry stain can highlight the organisms; however, interpretation is difficult as a result of scant organisms and common confounding precipitate, which may lead to false positives. An

Table 1-3 Role of Immunohistochemistry, In Situ Hybridization, and Flow Cytometry Immunophenotyping in the Lymph Node Workup

Ancillary Study	Target	Roles
Immunohistochemistry	Proteins in fixed tissue	Therapeutic targets (e.g., CD30[37])
		Expression of normal and aberrant antigens (B, T, NK, myeloid)
		Prognostication (e.g., Ki67 in mantle cell lymphoma[38])
In situ hybridization	mRNA in fixed tissue	Diagnosis (e.g., EBER for PTLD[39])
		Highly sensitive detection of low-level mRNA for diagnosis (e.g., HTLV-1 integration in ATLL[40])
Flow cytometry immunophenotyping	Proteins in fresh tissue	Expression of normal and aberrant antigen expression (B, T, NK, myeloid)
		Minimal residual disease studies (usually in BM or PB specimens)
		Quantitation of antigen expression to predict response to therapy (e.g., CD19 for CAR-T[41] therapy)

ATLL, Adult T-cell leukemia/lymphoma; *BM,* bone marrow; *CAR-T,* chimeric antigen receptor T-cell; *EBER,* Epstein-Barr virus–encoded small RNA; *HTLV-1,* human T-cell leukemia virus type I; *mRNA,* messenger ribonucleic acid; *PB,* peripheral blood; *PTLD,* posttransplant lymphoproliferative disorder.

immunohistochemical stain is also available for *B. henselae,* but it is likely less sensitive than PCR on FFPE tissue.[34] Gram-negative organisms of the *Brucella* genus may be visualized using McCullum-Goodpasture or Giemsa stain and can be identified and speciated in FFPE tissue with PCR.[35]

Immunohistochemistry, In Situ Hybridization, and Flow Cytometry Immunophenotyping

Lymph node diagnoses benefit from multiple complementary approaches (Table 1-3) allowing for characterization of protein or mRNA expression patterns either on the slide (IHC and in situ hybridization) or in disaggregated fresh cells (flow cytometry immunophenotyping). Though the number of immunohistochemical stains used in clinical laboratories can number from 1 to 200, in situ hybridization markers are more limited. Commonly used examples of in situ hybridization stains include markers for Epstein-Barr virus (EBV) and kappa and lambda light chains. IHC and in situ hybridization performed on unstained slides cut from FFPE tissue allow interpretation of protein or mRNA expression in the context of a counterstain highlighting the nuclei of tissue cells. A large number of immunohistochemical stains for membrane, cytoplasmic, and nuclear antigens are in routine clinical use and, in combination with histologic features, can support the diagnosis and correct classification of many common lymphomas and lymphadenopathies.

Flow cytometry is recommended when sufficient fresh tissue is available and is particularly helpful in demonstrating light chain restriction in B-cell lymphomas and in identifying immunophenotypic aberrancies in potentially neoplastic T-cell populations.[36] When there is a need to quantitate the number

of cells stained or the antigen density within a population, for example, in measuring the level of expression or the percent of lymphoma cells expressing a potential therapeutic target, flow cytometry is the technique of choice. In addition, flow cytometry provides a means of analyzing multiple antigens simultaneously and of assessing small samples, which is particularly helpful for the measurement of minimal residual disease and for fine-needle aspirates. Because flow cytometry studies can be completed within a few hours from the time of tissue procurement, this method is preferred when rapid diagnosis of a suspected hematolymphoid lesion is needed. For sections to be generated for immunohistologic staining on FFPE tissue, an overnight step in the tissue processor is often necessary, although more rapid processors are coming into use at some institutions.

Occasionally, the diagnosis may necessitate a particular type of study that is best achieved with either flow cytometry or the use of FFPE tissue. For example, for the definitive diagnosis of mantle cell lymphoma, immunoreactivity for cyclin D1 is best assessed by paraffin-section IHC, because flow cytometry for cyclin D1 and other nuclear antigens is less than optimal. In suspected posttransplant or other immunodeficiency-related disorders or extranodal NK/T cell lymphoma, nasal type, demonstration of EBV by EBV-encoded small RNA (EBER) in situ hybridization is helpful for diagnosis. In the case of some small B-cell lymphomas that do not aberrantly co-express CD5 or CD10, diagnosis on FFPE tissue alone may be challenging because of the suboptimal ability to distinguish light chain restriction by IHC.

Cytogenetic and Molecular Studies

The roles of cytogenetic and molecular studies in diagnosis, prognosis, and treatment planning are summarized in Table 1-4. Cytogenetic studies—including routine karyotyping of cultured cells, FISH, and chromosomal microarrays—assess for changes in the location, arrangement, and copy number of segments of chromosomes. Molecular genetic studies assess for qualitative and/or quantitative changes in DNA. Examples include allele-specific PCR, T-cell receptor or Ig gene rearrangement testing by multiplex PCR or next-generation sequencing (NGS), somatic mutation panel testing by NGS, and RNA sequencing to detect mutations and gene fusions. Many of these assays are discussed in detail in Chapter 6. If lymphoblastic lymphoma or myeloid neoplasia is suspected, retention of a portion of fresh tissue for cytogenetic studies is highly desirable, as karyotyping of cultured cells is still the gold standard. Furthermore, FISH panels are often validated for metaphase cultures and not for interphase FISH on FFPE tissue. Likewise, molecular assays applicable to acute leukemias may not be validated for FFPE tissue. Most FISH tests and other molecular tests applicable to mature lymphoma can, by contrast, be performed on either fresh or fixed tissue.

The choice of assays is large and the pace of change in the sensitivity, speed, and scope of the various technologies is rapid. Nevertheless, more is not necessarily better; not only may low-yield testing deplete precious material that may be needed at a later point for other targeted testing as new treatment options or clinical trials become available, but also unexpected or false-positive results may lead to delays in diagnosis, additional unnecessary testing, and even misdiagnosis. The choice of cytogenetic and molecular studies should focus

Table 1-4 Role of Cytogenetic and Molecular Studies in Diagnosis, Prognosis, and Treatment Planning

Ancillary Study	Role
Karyotype	Lymphoblastic lymphoma or myeloid neoplasia classification and risk stratification
FISH	Specific rearrangements, fusions, or deletions (e.g., *CCND1* rearrangement in mantle cell lymphoma)
Chromosomal microarray	Variable, nonreciprocal cytogenetic abnormalities (e.g., large cell lymphoma with 11q aberration)
Allele-specific PCR	Specific somatic mutations (e.g., $BRAF^{V600E}$ mutation in hairy cell leukemia)
T-cell receptor[42] or immunoglobulin gene[43] rearrangement	Distinguishes lymphoma from reactive proliferations; favors T versus B lineage; assessment for recurrent disease
NGS somatic mutation panels	Aid in diagnosis (e.g., $RHOA^{G17V}$ in AITL[44]) and subclassification (e.g., $MYD88^{L265P}$ in LPL)[45] and identify targetable mutations
RNA sequencing	Combined detection of mutations and gene fusions[46]; does not replace FISH[47]

AITL, Angioimmunoblastic T-cell lymphoma; *FISH,* fluorescence in situ hybridization; *LPL,* lymphoplasmacytic lymphoma; *NGS,* next-generation sequencing; *PCR,* polymerase chain reaction; *RNA,* ribonucleic acid; *RT-PCR,* reverse transcription PCR.

on rendering a definitive diagnosis and on providing the additional prognostic and therapeutically relevant information appropriate to the patient based on the clinical setting and evidence-based guidelines. Communication with the treating oncologist is key in prioritizing the choice of ancillary studies to ensure efficient and appropriate patient management.

REPORTING THE LYMPH NODE BIOPSY

The diagnosis of lymphoid malignancies uses a multiparameter approach that includes many ancillary studies that contribute to a comprehensive definitive diagnosis. Although the histopathologic findings, together with the immunophenotypic results, may be available within 1 or 2 days after a biopsy procedure, FISH, cytogenetic, and molecular genetic studies may not be available for 1 to 2 weeks. In these cases, a preliminary diagnosis based on the information at hand should be rendered, with ancillary studies reported in the form of an addendum to the original report. However, when the ancillary studies are necessary for even a preliminary diagnosis, the clinician treating the patient should be informed of the situation, and the report may be delayed until the results of ancillary studies are available.

The final lymph node biopsy report should include all relevant information for a comprehensive and complete diagnosis, including the results of all pertinent ancillary studies, such as IHC, cytogenetic, and molecular studies. There are several advantages to this practice. First, such a report facilitates continuity of care when patients are seen in follow-up or when relapses of disease occur. Second, it permits easy comparison of prior and subsequent immunophenotypic and molecular data in the detection of posttreatment minimal residual disease. When ancillary studies are performed in multiple specialized laboratories or sent off site, the issuing of multiple addenda when these results become available may be cumbersome. An accurate and efficient data-management system that allows easy access to ancillary test results may be a reasonable alternative to an integrated pathology report. It is imperative that the pathologist ensure that a system is in place to link the results of ancillary studies to the original specimen and to provide an interpretation that relates to the original diagnosis.

Increasingly, core needle biopsies with or without fine-needle aspiration are being used both for initial assessment of adenopathy and in the setting of known lymphoma with adenopathy concerning for residual or transformed disease.

Such biopsies are often convenient, fast, cost-efficient, and minimally invasive, making them ideal for fast-moving patient-centered care. Nevertheless, the limited sample volume can cause false-negative results from a lack of diagnostic material and can also raise the risk of misclassification of entities for which architecture plays a role in diagnosis and/or for which diagnostic features are rare, such as in NLPBL.[10] Though these small samples are frequently diagnostic, care must be taken to communicate the need for repeat biopsy if there is a discrepancy between the clinical suspicion and pathologic diagnosis. In addition, a low threshold for recommending a larger biopsy is warranted for cases in which there is concern that the small biopsy will not be representative or sufficient for diagnosis.

Pearls and Pitfalls

Before the biopsy
- Communicate need for fresh tissue for flow immunophenotyping.

During the intraoperative consultation
- Attempt touch preparation first to preserve tissue for morphology and flow cytometry immunophenotyping.

In the gross room
- If received fresh, make touch preparation.
- Fresh material should be set aside in RPMI medium for possible flow cytometry.
- Formalin fixation is preferred to preserve nucleic acids.

In the histology lab
- Consider cutting unstained slides up front for small/core needle biopsies.

At the microscope
- Triage studies in view of all ancillary studies are required for clinical decision-making.
- Steward tissue so that material is left in block for future needs (e.g., clinical trial eligibility).

KEY REFERENCES

1. Alaggio R, Amador C, Anagnostopoulos I, et al. The 5th edition of the World Health Organization Classification of Haematolymphoid Tumours: lymphoid neoplasms. *Leukemia.* 2022;36(7):1720–1748.
2. Campo E, Jaffe ES, Cook JR, et al. The International Consensus Classification of mature lymphoid neoplasms: a report from the Clinical Advisory Committee. *Blood.* 2022;140(11):1229–1253.
3. Kroft SH, Sever CE, Bagg A, et al. Laboratory workup of lymphoma in adults: guideline from the American Society

for Clinical Pathology and the College of American Pathologists. *Arch Pathol Lab Med.* 2021;145(3):269–290.

4. Loo E, Siddiqi IN. Processing the lymph node biopsy. In: Day CE, ed. *Histopathology.* Vol. 1180. New York: Springer; 2014:271–282.

13. Bass BP, Engel KB, Greytak SR, Moore HM. A review of preanalytical factors affecting molecular, protein, and morphological analysis of formalin-fixed, paraffin-embedded (FFPE) tissue: how well do you know your FFPE specimen? *Arch Pathol Lab Med.* 2014;138(11):1520–1530.

17. Compton CC, Robb JA, Anderson MW, et al. Preanalytics and precision pathology: pathology practices to ensure molecular integrity of cancer patient biospecimens for precision medicine. *Arch Pathol Lab Med.* 2019;143(11):1346–1363.

24. Lott R, Tunnicliffe J, Sheppard E, et al. *Practical Guide to Specimen Handling in Surgical Pathology.* College of American Pathologists. https://documents.cap.org/documents/practical-guide-specimen-handling.pdf.

29. Pantanowitz L, Sinard JH, Henricks WH, et al. Validating whole slide imaging for diagnostic purposes in pathology: guideline from the College of American Pathologists Pathology and Laboratory Quality Center. *Arch Pathol Lab Med.* 2013;137(12):1710–1722.

46. Crotty R, Hu K, Stevenson K, et al. Simultaneous identification of cell of origin, translocations, and hotspot mutations in diffuse large B-cell lymphoma using a single RNA-sequencing assay. *Am J Clin Pathol.* 2021;155(5):748–754.

Visit Elsevier eBooks+ for the complete set of references.

Chapter 2

Fine-Needle Aspiration of Lymph Nodes

Magdalena Czader and Armando C. Filie

Fine-needle aspiration (FNA) of superficial and deep-seated lymph nodes is a well-established and safe method for assessing lymphadenopathy in adult and pediatric patients.[1-14] Patients with primary or recurrent lymphoma frequently undergo FNA, and this diagnostic modality is even more common in suspected reactive or metastatic lymphadenopathy. Using FNA as a first-line procedure has obvious benefits, such as rapid turnaround time, low cost, and low morbidity. The cytomorphologic diagnosis is relatively straightforward in the majority of cases of reactive lymphadenopathy and non-hematopoietic metastatic disease. The diagnostic accuracy of FNA in lymphoma cases is variable and dependent on lymphoma type and concurrent use of ancillary studies.[4,8-11,13,15-26] The latter significantly enhances diagnostic sensitivity and specificity beyond that obtained with cytomorphologic evaluation alone.[22,26] Nevertheless, the inability to assess architectural features and limited immunohistochemistry (IHC) can be challenging. Therefore, the application of FNA to establish a primary diagnosis of lymphoma is controversial.[15,17,18,27] With few exceptions, FNA has been used predominantly as a screening tool with a final diagnosis and lymphoma classification often requiring lymph node excision or biopsy.[17,27] The Sydney system for cytopathologic evaluation of lymphadenopathy has shown high sensitivity, specificity, and positive predictive value and slightly lower negative predictive value.[28,29] This proposed system combines clinical information, imaging findings, cytopathological features, and ancillary techniques with the goal of standardizing the cytopathologic diagnosis and reporting of lymph nodes and provides an algorithm for patient management. Nevertheless, in clinical practice, a final diagnosis of lymphoma is rarely solely based on FNA, with the exception of cases in which excision or incisional biopsy is medically contraindicated. FNA without a follow-up biopsy is more commonly used for diagnosis of progression, transformation, or recurrent disease in patients with a previously documented history of lymphoma and to procure fresh material for specialized studies such as genetic testing for targeted therapy.

The effectiveness of FNA as a diagnostic procedure in hematopoietic neoplasms is dependent on a dedicated multidisciplinary team of highly specialized experts in cytopathology and hematopathology, and experienced aspirators. This integrated approach will ensure the procurement of an adequate FNA specimen and analysis by appropriate cytomorphologic, immunophenotypic, and molecular techniques. When core needle biopsy (CNB) is procured concurrently with FNA, correlating results obtained from both samples is strongly recommended. A detailed clinical history should be reviewed at the time of FNA. An on-site evaluation provides information regarding the cellularity of a sample, guides selection of additional testing, and in cases with scant cellularity, allows one to prioritize ancillary studies. If an adequate sample is available and there is suspicion of a lymphoproliferative process, material should be reserved for flow cytometry (FCM) and cell block for IHC or molecular studies. When a definitive diagnostic immunophenotype is not provided by FCM or other ancillary studies, such as immunocytochemistry (ICC)/IHC, a lymph node excision is recommended.

This chapter focuses on the cytomorphologic diagnoses of the most common reactive and neoplastic lymphoid proliferations as seen on FNA smears. Cell block preparations are referenced primarily when IHC is discussed as a diagnostic aid; however, for a complete discussion of immunophenotypic and genetic features, the reader is referred to the chapters discussing individual lymphoma entities. We provide a brief guide for the optimal processing and evaluation of cytologic

Table 2-1 Approach to Lymphoma Diagnosis Using Fine-Needle Aspiration: Recommendations and Limitations

Process	Recommendations/Limitations
Sample collection	On-site evaluation of specimen adequacy by a pathologist or cytotechnologist is highly recommended. If on-site evaluation is not available, perform additional passes until solution is cloudy. Perform multiple passes (>3) from different parts of lymph node. Prepare cell block for immunocytochemistry (critical in cases with rare neoplastic cells that may be difficult to immunophenotype by FCM, such as cHL).
Case sign-out	Correlate cytomorphology with ancillary studies. Consider possibility of false-positive and false-negative results of ancillary studies. In challenging cases or in cases with discrepant results, discuss cytomorphology with flow cytometrist, who may prompt additional gating. If cytologic findings do not correlate with clinical presentation, recommend lymph node excision or biopsy.
Evaluation of high-grade B-cell lymphoma and high-grade transformation*	Large lymphocyte count >20% is highly predictive of large cell lymphoma (in practice, >25%). If large cell count is >25% but <50%, correlate cytomorphology with clinical and immunophenotypic findings. Biopsy/excision may be required in discrepant cases.

*High-grade B-cell lymphomas include entities with blastoid morphology.
cHL, Classic Hodgkin lymphoma; FCM, flow cytometry.

samples obtained by FNA of lymph nodes (Table 2-1). A role of CNBs in lymphoma diagnosis is also discussed, as these biopsies are frequently procured at the time of FNA to provide a more robust assessment of architectural and cytomorphologic features. Nevertheless, CNBs did not provide as complete an evaluation as lymph node excisions,[30] and an excision remains the gold standard in lymphoma diagnosis.

SPECIMEN COLLECTION AND PROCESSING

The proper handling and processing of a lymph node aspirate is imperative for an accurate diagnosis. In general, at least three separate passes should be executed.[31] Nonaspiration technique, performed using only a needle or a needle attached to a syringe without a plunger (to minimize bleeding and sample mixing with peripheral blood), can be applied for cytologic evaluation of lymph nodes. On-site Coulter counters can be used to ensure collection of a minimum of 10 million cells for adequate FCM.[15] An on-site assessment for specimen adequacy should be performed by a pathologist or a cytotechnologist. This is most easily accomplished with a Wright's-Giemsa–type stain (usually a Diff-Quik [DQ]) carried out on an air-dried smear, which allows a detailed visual evaluation of the cytoplasm and nuclei of the lymphoid cells; this is imperative for classification. Although DQ stain, comparable to the Romanowsky and Giemsa stains used in clinical hematology laboratories, is generally preferred for cytologic evaluation, some authors believe alcohol-fixed slides stained with Papanicolaou (Pap) stain should also be prepared to provide enhanced nuclear detail. Techniques that use alcohol fixation with Pap staining, including monolayer technologies, are insufficient for demonstration of cytoplasmic features and should not be used as the only stain when hematopoietic processes are evaluated. If desired, these approaches can be used in addition to air-dried Giemsa-stained material. Air-dried Giemsa-stained cytospins may be particularly helpful because the cell morphology on the cytospin may be superior to that on the smear owing to the flattening and enlarging effect of cytocentrifugation (Fig. 2-1). Sample collection for monolayer preparations is easy and may be a viable alternative,[32] especially when on-site assessment is not available. Liquid-based cytology has been shown to perform well while using the Sydney system.[33] However, such preparations are known to increase the risk of false-negatives and should not be used without accompanying FNA smears.[34]

Once a differential diagnosis is formulated based on cytomorphology and clinical history, a portion of a sample should be placed in cell culture media such as RPMI (Roswell Park Memorial Institute) medium to assure preservation of cell viability. From this aliquot, cells can be submitted directly for FCM and molecular diagnostics. A cell block prepared from tissue fragments embedded in paraffin[35] or a cytospin can be used for ICC/IHC, fluorescence in situ hybridization (FISH), or in situ hybridization for Epstein-Barr virus (EBV) with the EBV-encoded small RNA (EBER) probe.

ANCILLARY STUDIES

Immunocytochemistry

ICC can be performed on air-dried cytospins or smears on charged slides that have been stored desiccated and refrigerated, and are postfixed in acetone before staining. The staining protocols used for air-dried cytospins are similar to those used for frozen section material (see Chapter 4). Cell block sections can also be used for immunohistochemical studies with a staining protocol similar to that used for tissue sections.[19,34,36] If cellular material is limited, it may be preferable to prepare cytospins rather than attempting a cell block with potentially insufficient material. Of note, alcohol fixation may affect the performance of some lymphoid markers.

ICC on cytospins may be as effective as FCM for the immunophenotyping of cytologic specimens and may be particularly suited for samples with an insufficient number of cells for FCM analysis.[37,38] One distinct benefit of ICC on cytospins is the detailed visualization of cell size in conjunction with immunophenotypic staining patterns, particularly with mixed cell populations.

Flow Cytometry

FCM is an indispensable ancillary technique that significantly enhances the sensitivity and specificity of lymphoma diagnosis in cytologic material.[26,27,39-41] The combination of FCM and cytomorphology can lead to a specific lymphoma classification with a rapid turnaround time of less than 24 hours. Commonly available multiparameter FCM instruments

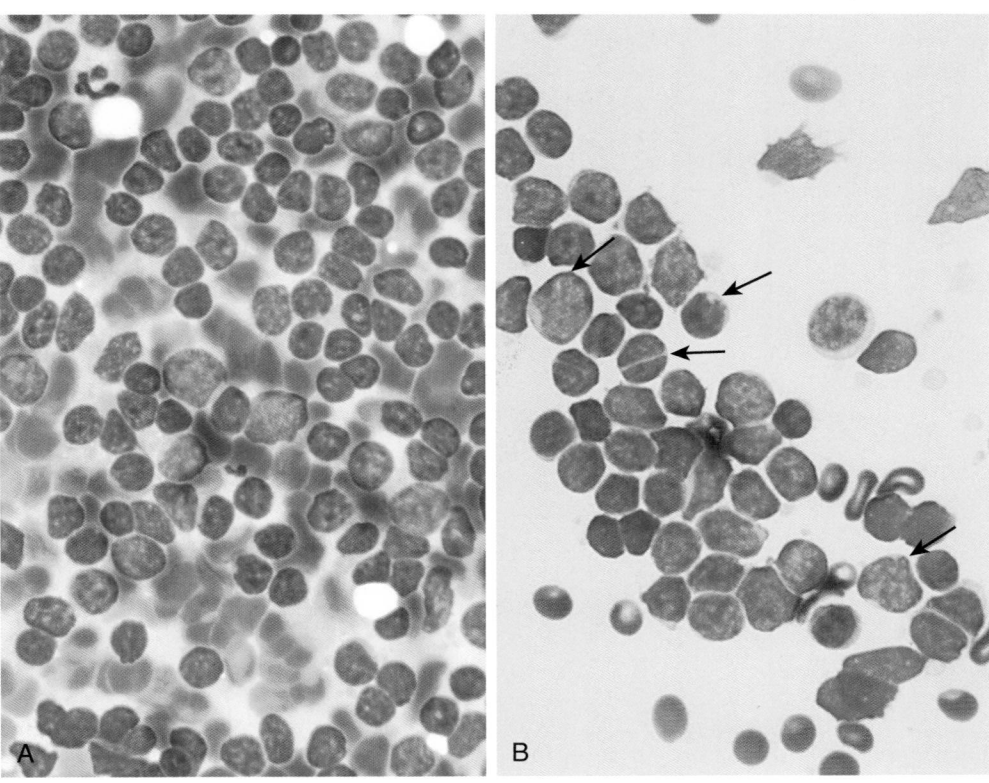

Figure 2-1. A, Smear of chronic lymphocytic leukemia/small lymphocytic lymphoma showing mostly small, atypical lymphoid cells with scant cytoplasm and round, slightly irregular nuclei with occasional nuclear clefts. **B,** Cytospin preparation for the same case showing the flattening and enlarging effect of atypical lymphoid cells, accentuating the nuclear irregularity and clefts *(arrows)* (Diff-Quik).

analyze numerous markers simultaneously and allow comprehensive immunophenotyping of a wide variety of samples, including paucicellular specimens. This obviates the need to prioritize markers on the basis of a cytomorphologic triage. Optimally, several million cells are needed to analyze an expression of 10 to 20 antigens. In scant samples, immunophenotyping can be performed on as few as 50,000 cells, provided the cell viability is not compromised. In these cases and in those with a suspicion of rare types of lymphoma, close communication between the cytopathologist and the hematopathologist performing the FCM may help design a more specific antibody panel and facilitate incorporation of FCM results in the cytomorphologic diagnosis.

Sample type and processing can significantly influence cellular yield and viability. In our experience, FNA yields a superior material for FCM in comparison with CNBs, which are often procured at the same time.[42] Some advocate obtaining cell suspensions using a rinse technique and have reported it provides FCM material comparable to an FNA or disintegrated CNB.[43] The FCM sample should be placed in RPMI medium with 10% fetal bovine serum immediately after procurement and stored at 4° C. Samples of select, highly proliferative lymphomas will deteriorate rapidly, even if stored in a protective media; thus, a specimen should be stained promptly whenever possible to avoid cell loss. If rapid analysis is not feasible, a stained sample can be fixed and analyzed the next day.

Results of FCM must be interpreted within the context of cytomorphology and clinical information because of the possibility of false-negative or false-positive results.[40] A false-negative immunophenotype occurs most commonly in limited paucicellular samples because of necrosis and fibrosis or cell loss during processing. It may also be challenging to identify a malignant clone in cases in which neoplastic cells are accompanied by a rich reactive background or aggregating with reactive lymphocytes, as seen in classic Hodgkin lymphoma (cHL). False-positive results may be encountered in reactive lymphoid processes with a skewed kappa-lambda light chain ratio, which is primarily seen in follicle center lymphocytes or in cases with an abnormal T-cell immunophenotype. An interpretation of atypical T-cell immunophenotype has become easier as a result of FCM evaluation of T-cell receptor constant beta chain-1 (TRBC1), which allows confirmation of the clonality of T-cell proliferation.[44] Of note, minor immunophenotypic abnormalities should not be interpreted as evidence of a neoplastic process unless supported by cytomorphologic findings and clinical presentation. Additional studies may be warranted when a false-negative or false-positive result is suspected.

When a definitive diagnostic immunophenotype is not provided by FCM and other ancillary studies (such as ICC or IHC) are not conclusive, a lymph node excision is recommended as the gold standard for lymphoma diagnosis. The latter may also be required in cases in which there are discrepancies among clinical presentation, cytomorphology, and FCM immunophenotype. When a lesion is not easily accessible, such as in deep-seated lymph nodes, CNBs may be attempted.

Molecular Studies

In the past, molecular studies were most commonly performed in FNA cases in which a conclusive diagnosis could not be reached with a combination of cytomorphology and immunophenotyping. As the number of lymphomas defined by molecular genetic abnormalities increases, molecular genetic studies are routinely used for lymphoma classification.[45,46]

The majority of molecular studies can be performed on fresh or archival FNA samples.[47,48] Alcohol-fixed, air-dried, and stained FNA slides can be used to scrape off material to extract DNA and RNA using the method of choice.[49] Similar to FCM, the results of the molecular studies should be interpreted in the context of morphologic findings and clinical data because of potential false-positive and false-negative assays.

Interphase FISH has added tremendously to the diagnostic specificity of FNA. Numerous commercially available probes allow for interrogation of lymphoma-associated rearrangements, and a few are specific for certain lymphoma subtypes.[16,22,50-56] Cytospins or smears prepared from FNA material are ideally suited for FISH because scoring of fluorescent signals is easier in a cell population dispersed as a monolayer.[54] Both fresh, ethanol-fixed, and archival (Pap-stained and DQ-stained) slides can be used. The adequacy of hybridization varies in published reports, with the highest success rates at approximately 95%. FISH with lymphoma type-specific probes is predominantly used for the classification of lymphoid neoplasms.[55,56] Of note, only select translocations (e.g., *IG::CCND1* for mantle cell lymphoma and *NPM1::ALK* for anaplastic large cell lymphoma [ALCL]) are specific for a particular entity and allow for a definitive classification in the context of appropriate cytomorphology and immunophenotype. Many other genetic alterations can occur in several histologically and immunophenotypically defined entities and thus are not diagnostic of a specific lymphoma type. A demonstration of these genetic abnormalities by FISH can still be used as a proof of clonality and can support a diagnosis of lymphoma in cases with equivocal cytomorphology and/or immunophenotyping.

The importance of saving additional unstained smears for molecular assays has been emphasized by some cytopathologists, and the triage of FNA material based on on-site evaluation has been proposed.[14,55,56] It remains to be seen whether FNA with stepwise application of ancillary techniques, including molecular studies, is the most accurate and cost-effective approach to diagnose and classify lymphomas at the time of initial diagnosis, particularly in cases involving peripheral lymph nodes that are amenable to excision.

NON-NEOPLASTIC ASPIRATES

Lymph node enlargement can be secondary to lymphadenitis, an inflammatory or infectious process or reactive lymphoid hyperplasia secondary to a variety of immune stimuli. Lymphadenitis is broadly divided into acute and chronic (granulomatous and nongranulomatous).[57] The inflammatory or infectious processes can be readily identified in aspirated samples based on the composition of the cellular population. In such instances, FNA can also be procured for additional studies, including microbiology studies. The presence of atypical lymphoid cells in an otherwise inflammatory background, however, raises the possibility of lymphoma.

Aspirates of reactive hyperplasia are diverse and diagnostically challenging (Fig. 2-2). The pattern and distribution of the lymphoid population vary according to the stage of the reactive process and the primary lymph node compartment affected by it—lymphoid follicles or paracortex. Paracortical hyperplasia is characterized by

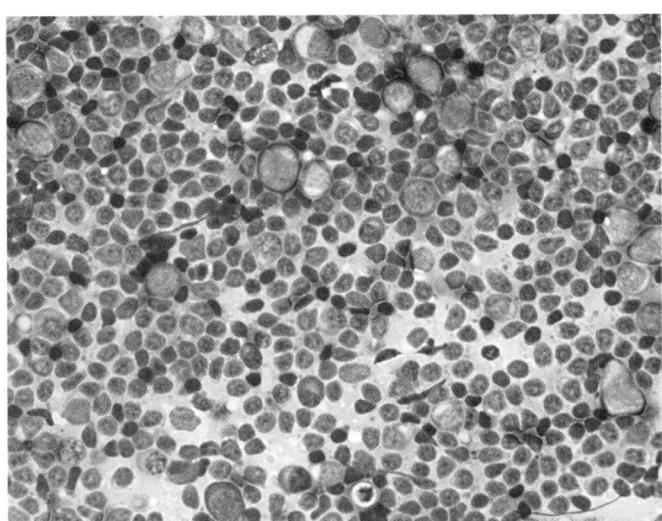

Figure 2-2. Reactive lymphoid hyperplasia. Polymorphous population of lymphocytes composed of numerous small mature lymphocytes, centrocytes, and centroblasts. Background shows rare plasma cells, lymphoglandular bodies, and scattered red blood cells (Diff-Quik, smear).

a polymorphous population of lymphoid cells, ranging from small lymphocytes to immunoblasts, and other inflammatory cells including plasma cells, histiocytes, and eosinophils. Follicular center cells associated with tingible body macrophages and follicular dendritic cells (FDCs) predominate in follicular hyperplasia. The lymphoid cells are frequently seen in aggregates, embedded in a meshwork formed by the FDCs and their processes.[58] The FDC aggregates are composed of large cells with ovoid to coffee-bean shaped nuclei with small central nucleoli, fine nuclear membranes, and clear cytoplasm. Some lymphomas are associated with a polymorphous background and may mimic an inflammatory process. High proliferative activity favors lymphoma but can also be seen in some reactive conditions, such as infectious mononucleosis.[59]

ASPIRATES OF LYMPHOID NEOPLASMS

The World Health Organization (WHO) classification and International Consensus Classification include a wide variety of B-cell, T-cell, and histiocytic-dendritic–cell neoplasms.[45,46,60] Reviewing the cytologic features of all tumor types is beyond the scope of this chapter. Our goal is to focus on the cytomorphologic features of the most common types of B-cell and T-cell lymphomas encountered in clinical practice (Table 2-2).

Mature B-Cell Neoplasms

The most common cell types seen in B-cell lymphomas include centrocytes, centroblasts, and immunoblasts (Fig. 2-3). The range of cytologic appearances is exceedingly broad and reflects the spectrum of B-cell differentiation. Immunophenotypic and molecular features useful in differential diagnosis are listed in the chapters reviewing individual disease entities, and this information will not be duplicated here unless unique to cytologic preparations.

Table 2-2 Cytomorphologic Features of Common Types of Lymphoma

Lymphoma Diagnosis	Cytomorphologic Features
Chronic lymphocytic leukemia/small lymphocytic lymphoma	The majority of neoplastic lymphocytes are small with round to oval nuclei, coarsely clumped chromatin, occasional nucleoli, and scant cytoplasm. Admixed prolymphocytes are larger with round nuclei with a vesicular chromatin, prominent nucleoli, and a moderate to abundant amount of cytoplasm. A monomorphic population of large transformed lymphoid cells is consistent with Richter transformation.
Marginal zone lymphoma	Intermediate-sized lymphoid cells with mild atypia including slightly irregular nuclei, condensed chromatin, indistinct nucleoli, and moderate to abundant cytoplasm. Plasmacytoid features and typical plasma cells may be present.
Follicular lymphoma	Heterogeneous population of centrocytes and centroblasts in varying proportions, dependent on histologic grade. Centrocytes are medium sized with irregular nuclear outlines, condensed chromatin, and scant cytoplasm. Centroblasts are large with oval to round nuclei, dispersed chromatin, several nucleoli, and moderate cytoplasm. Follicular dendritic cell meshworks are apparent with adherent lymphocytes.
Mantle cell lymphoma	Classic variant: a monotonous population of small to medium-sized lymphoid cells with delicate nuclear clefts, finely stippled chromatin, inconspicuous nucleoli, and distinct pale or basophilic cytoplasm. Blastoid variant: intermediate-sized to large lymphoid cells with slightly irregular nuclei, evenly distributed chromatin, small nucleoli, and scant pale blue cytoplasm (Diff-Quik). Pleomorphic variant: Large lymphoid cells with pleomorphic nuclei with hyperchromasia and moderate cytoplasm.
Diffuse large B-cell lymphoma	Abundant large lymphoid cells, frequently with centroblast or immunoblast features, and prominent lymphoglandular bodies; pleomorphic nuclei may be seen.
Primary mediastinal large B-cell lymphoma	Scattered medium-sized to large lymphoid cells with round to oval or multilobated nuclei, smooth to irregular nuclear contours, one or more visible nucleoli, and scant to abundant pale blue or basophilic cytoplasm. Vacuoles may be identified. Background may include connective tissue fragments admixed with single lymphocytes or groups of lymphocytes.
Burkitt lymphoma	Medium-size lymphoid cells with round nuclei, finely granular to coarse chromatin, several nucleoli, and abundant, deeply basophilic cytoplasm with small cytoplasmic vacuoles. The background includes tingible body macrophages, apoptotic bodies, lymphoglandular bodies, and a watery, basophilic proteinaceous matrix.
Classic Hodgkin lymphoma	Large, pleomorphic, and often binucleated or multinucleated cells (Hodgkin and Reed-Sternberg cells) with prominent nucleoli and abundant cytoplasm in a polymorphous reactive background including small lymphocytes, histiocytes, eosinophils, and plasma cells.
Nodular lymphocyte predominant large B-cell lymphoma	Large pleomorphic lymphoid cells with multilobated nuclei, vesicular chromatin, delicate nuclear membrane, and abundant cytoplasm ("popcorn" cells) in a background rich in small lymphocytes and epithelioid histiocytes.
Peripheral T-cell lymphoma, not otherwise specified	Variable cell size and cytomorphology, from small to large with nuclear pleomorphism. Hodgkin-like cells can be seen. Background can include epithelioid histiocytes, eosinophils, plasma cells, and fragments of vessels.
Follicular helper T-cell lymphoma, angioimmunoblastic-type	Small and medium-sized atypical lymphoid cells with abundant clear cytoplasm on a background of small lymphocytes, histiocytes, plasma cells, B immunoblasts, follicular dendritic cells, and fragments of vessels. Aggregates of lymphocytes associated with follicular dendritic cells can be frequent and are termed *dendritic cell–lymphocyte complexes.*
Anaplastic large cell lymphoma	Cytomorphology dependent on morphologic variant. Most frequently, atypical large pleomorphic lymphoid cells with abundant, variably staining cytoplasm with vacuoles, azurophilic granules, or cytoplasmic blebbing. The nuclei can be horseshoe shaped or wreath-like ("hallmark cells"). Lymphoid cells with multiple nuclei are also seen. Admixed small and medium-sized plasmacytoid cells are abundant in the small cell variant. The background contains lymphoglandular bodies, small lymphocytes, histiocytes, and neutrophils.
Lymphoblastic lymphoma	Monotonous population of medium-sized lymphoid cells with round to irregular nuclei with speckled chromatin and scant agranular cytoplasm, which may contain small vacuoles. The background includes variable lymphoglandular bodies, tingible body macrophages, necrosis, and mitotic figures.

Chronic Lymphocytic Leukemia/Small Lymphocytic Lymphoma

Cytomorphology

Aspirates of chronic lymphocytic leukemia/small lymphocytic lymphoma (CLL/SLL) are composed of two cell populations (Fig. 2-4). Most cells are small with round to oval nuclei, coarsely clumped chromatin, occasional nucleoli, and scant cytoplasm (Fig. 2-1). Prolymphocytes are fewer in number and are larger with round nuclei, a vesicular chromatin pattern, prominent nucleoli, and a moderate to abundant amount of cytoplasm.[4,61] A uniform population of large transformed cells suggests Richter transformation.[62-64] Other cytologic features suggestive of progression are an increased number of intermediate-sized or plasmacytoid cells, mitotic figures, the presence of apoptotic bodies and necrosis, and a myxoid and dirty

background.[62] The latter features are also more frequently observed in the accelerated phase; however, a definitive cytomorphologic definition of accelerated CLL/SLL remains to be determined. In rare cases of Hodgkin lymphoma (HL) (Richter) transformation, isolated large bilobated or multilobated cells on a background of histiocytes and poorly formed granulomata are identified.[65] The cytologic appearance should be correlated with clinical features indicative of transformation.

Ancillary Studies

The cytomorphologic diagnosis requires confirmation by immunophenotyping, most commonly by FCM. FISH studies can be performed on FNA material; however, they are of limited diagnostic value and are typically used for a prediction of prognosis in individual patients.[22] There is accumulating evidence that Richter transformation includes clonally related

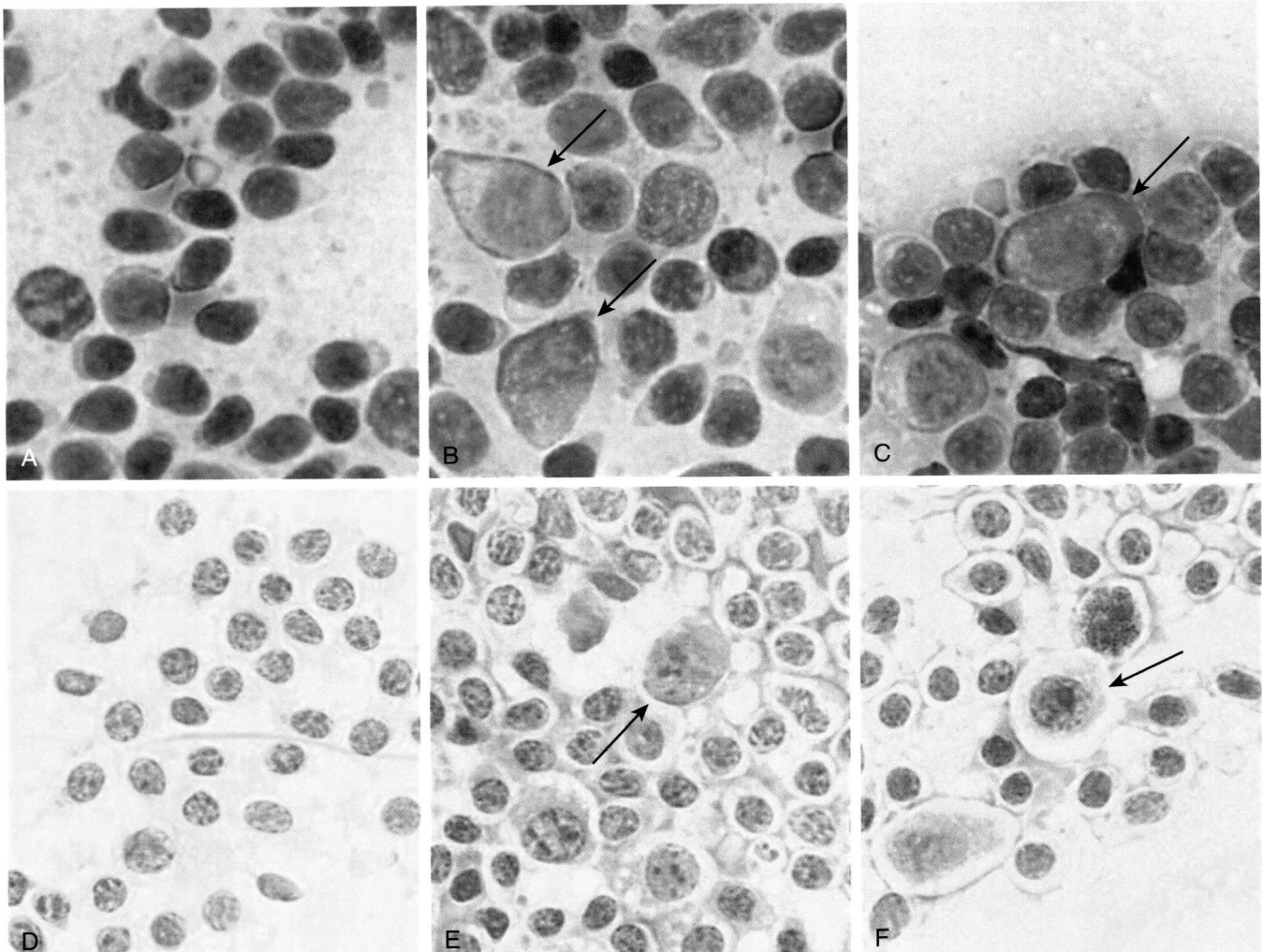

Figure 2-3. Common cellular components of B-cell lymphomas. A, Centrocytes with clumped chromatin and scant cytoplasm (Diff-Quik, smear). **B,** Centroblasts *(arrows)* with enlarged round nuclei, visible nucleoli, and moderate amounts of basophilic cytoplasm (Diff-Quik, smear). **C,** Immunoblast *(arrow)* shows an enlarged round nucleus, a single prominent nucleolus, and a deep blue cytoplasm (Diff-Quik, smear). **D,** Centrocytes with round nuclei, coarsely clumped chromatin, and scant cytoplasm (Pap smear). **E,** Large centroblast *(arrow)* in a background of small centrocytes. The centroblast shows an enlarged nucleus, dusty chromatin, and a moderate amount of cytoplasm (Pap smear). **F,** Immunoblast *(arrow)* with an enlarged round nucleus, a prominent eosinophilic nucleolus, and dense cytoplasm (Pap smear).

and unrelated (de novo) lymphoid neoplasms, a distinction that has prognostic significance.[66] FNA is an excellent tool to obtain diagnostic material to study clonal relationships at the time of progression.

Differential Diagnosis

The differential diagnosis includes reactive lymphoid hyperplasia, follicular lymphoma, mantle cell lymphoma, marginal zone lymphoma, and lymphoplasmacytic lymphoma. Differentiation of these entities is relatively straightforward based on immunophenotype. On the contrary, a tissue-based monoclonal B-cell lymphocytosis with CLL/SLL immunophenotype is challenging to diagnose without lymph node excision.[67,68] Similarly, an accelerated phase of CLL/SLL has been primarily defined on lymph node histology, and careful attention to detail is required to avoid diagnosis of large

cell transformation when evaluating histologic progression in CLL/SLL.

Marginal Zone Lymphoma

Cytomorphology

Aspirates of nodal marginal zone lymphoma and extranodal marginal zone lymphoma of mucosa-associated lymphoid tissue (MALT lymphoma) usually display a population of numerous intermediate-sized lymphoid cells with mild atypia (round to slightly irregular nuclei, condensed chromatin, and indistinct nucleoli) (Fig. 2-5).[61,69,70] The cytoplasm is moderate to abundant. Neoplastic cells may have a plasmacytoid appearance.[71-73] The background contains small lymphocytes, plasmacytoid lymphocytes, plasma cells, and occasional immunoblasts.[71,74] These heterogeneous features

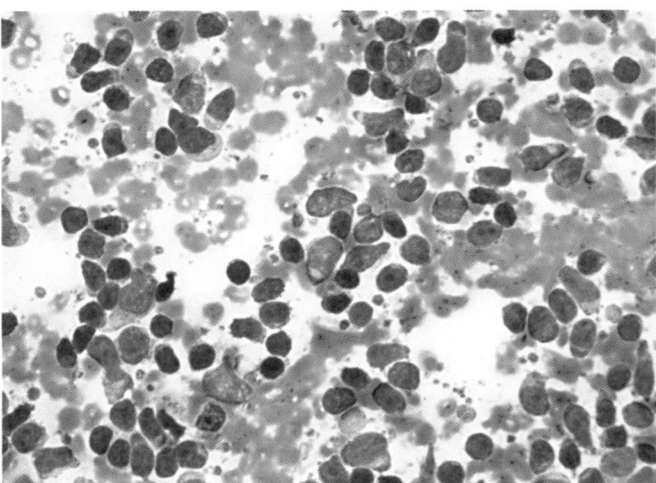

Figure 2-4. **Small lymphocytic lymphoma.** Numerous small, atypical lymphoid cells with mostly round nuclei, coarsely clumped chromatin, and scant amounts of cytoplasm. Scattered larger prolymphocytes with open chromatin, nucleoli, and basophilic cytoplasm are also shown (Diff-Quik, smear).

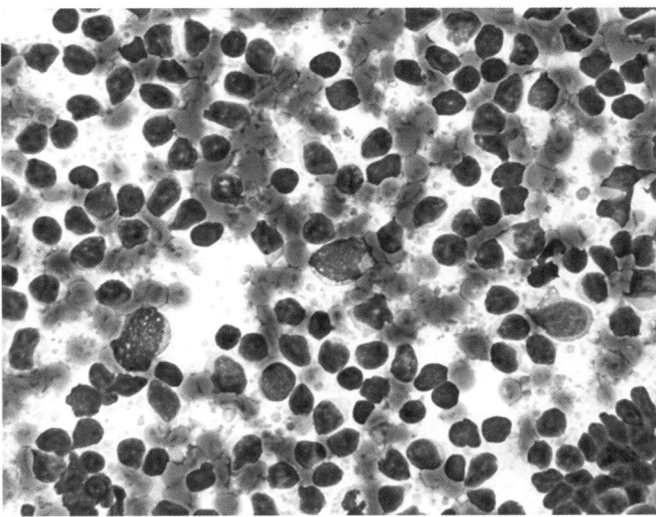

Figure 2-6. **Follicular lymphoma.** Follicular lymphoma (grade 1 to 2) composed predominantly of small to intermediate-sized atypical centrocytes and a few atypical centroblasts simulating a polymorphous lymphoid population seen in a reactive process (Diff-Quik, smear).

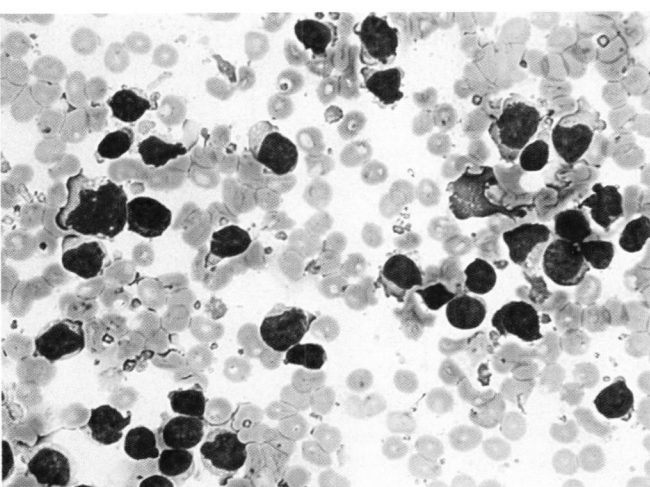

Figure 2-5. **Marginal zone lymphoma.** Atypical small to intermediate-sized lymphoid cells with slightly enlarged irregular nuclei and variable amounts of basophilic cytoplasm. Isolated benign centrocytes and a plasma cell are also shown (Diff-Quik, smear).

can make marginal zone lymphoma difficult to distinguish from a reactive process.[70]

Ancillary Studies

Nodal marginal zone lymphoma is often a diagnosis of exclusion because of a lack of specific immunophenotypic or cytogenetic features. An addition of CD43, NMDA and IRTA1 antigens may be helpful along with negative markers, which are typically specific in other B-cell lymphomas, such as cyclin D1, SOX11, follicular center cell markers, CD5, and LEF1.[75] The nodal marginal zone lymphoma shows no recurrent gene rearrangements, however, t(11;18)(q12;q21) is frequently detected in pulmonary and gastric MALT lymphomas, and rearrangement of *MALT1* can be detected by interphase FISH with break-apart probe on cytospin preparations.[22,71] Specific translocations are not detected in nodal marginal

zone lymphoma.[22] The reported mutations also differ among nodal variants and individual sites of extranodal marginal zone lymphoma.[76]

Differential Diagnosis

The differential diagnosis includes reactive hyperplasia, follicular lymphoma, mantle cell lymphoma, lymphoplasmacytic lymphoma, and small lymphocytic lymphoma. In cases with extreme plasma cell differentiation, a distinction from plasmacytoma may be difficult on cytologic material.

Follicular Lymphoma

Cytomorphology

Follicular lymphoma aspirates contain a mixed population of centrocytes and centroblasts in varying proportions (Fig. 2-6).[61,77] It is important not to confuse centroblasts with FDCs, which are normal occupants of lymphoid follicles. FDCs have oval to coffee-bean shaped nuclei, with smooth nuclear membranes and indistinct cytoplasm (Fig. 2-7).[77] The atypical lymphoid cells may be seen in tight clusters, in fragments of follicles, or adherent to the FDCs. Follicular structures may also be seen in reactive hyperplasia. Occasionally, tingible body macrophages are seen, but they are less frequent than in reactive lymph nodes.[78]

Grading

Although architectural assessment cannot be achieved on aspirates, grading of FNA samples using the counting method of Mann and Berard on entire smears or solely on follicular structures has been the subject of investigation using Pap-stained or Pap/DQ-stained cytologic material.[77,79-82] The investigators agree that the discrimination of large centrocytes from centroblasts is facilitated by use of the Pap stain. Discrimination of centroblasts from FDCs is particularly important, as it can lead to erroneous grade assignment.[83] Although Sun and coworkers[84] were able to discriminate intact follicular structures in smears and

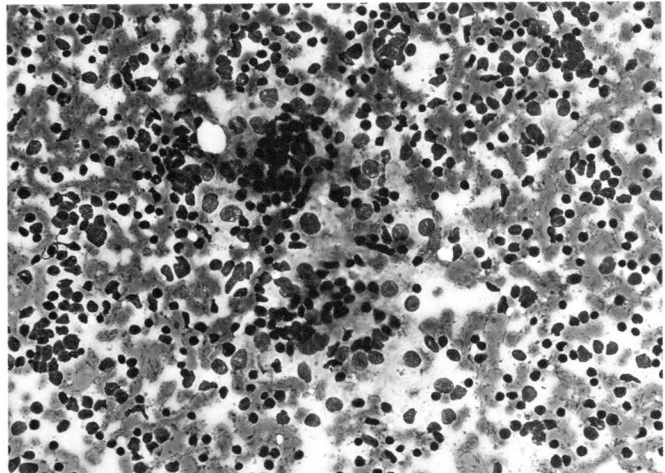

Figure 2-7. Follicular lymphoma. Lymphoid fragments with numerous follicular dendritic cells and aggregates of lymphocytes. Follicular dendritic cells have abundant syncytial cytoplasm and histiocyte-like nuclei. Note the paucity of tingible body macrophages (Diff-Quik, smear).

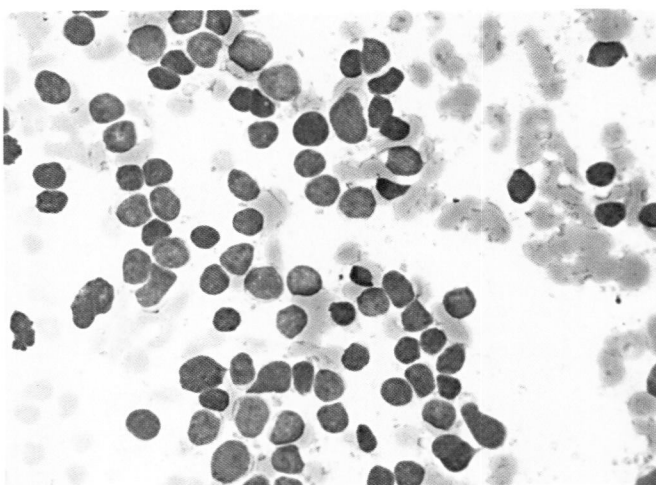

Figure 2-8. Mantle cell lymphoma. Monotonous population of atypical small to intermediate-sized lymphocytes with slightly enlarged nuclei, dispersed chromatin pattern, scattered nuclear clefts, and scant pale cytoplasm (Diff-Quik, smear).

use them for a centroblast count, Young and colleagues were unable to make this discrimination reliably on any material other than cell blocks and used the entire smear for centroblast counting.[80]

The 2016 WHO classification did not require the distinction of grades 1 and 2, which historically was challenging in both tissue sections and cytologic preparations.[82] In the 2004 study by Sun and coworkers,[84] a minimum of 200 cells was counted in 6 to 10 intact lymphoid follicular structures at 40× magnification. The number of large cells or centroblasts was expressed as a percentage of the total number of cells counted within the follicles and graded accordingly. In grade 3, they identified 48.4 ± 7.5% centroblasts, which is readily distinguished from significantly fewer centroblasts in grades 1 and 2 (9.7 ± 2.9% and 24.7 ± 5.6%, respectively). Brandao and coworkers were able to grade follicular lymphoma on Pap-stained monolayer preparations by counting the number of centroblasts in 300 lymphoid cells or 10 high-power fields.[85] The most recent edition of the WHO classification abandoned morphologic grading on histologic material as a result of the debatable clinical differences between grade 1 to 2 and grade 3A.[45] The histologic grading has remained in use in the International Consensus Classification, with emphasis on distinction of the grade 3B, which seems to be the most clinically relevant.[46] The distinction between grades 3A and 3B has not been studied by cytomorphology and may be challenging considering a lack of architecture assessment. Similarly, discrimination between grade 3B and diffuse large B-cell lymphoma (DLBCL) is not feasible without the context of nodal architecture seen on histology.

Ancillary Studies

Both FCM and interphase FISH for *IG::BCL2* rearrangement can be used to support a diagnosis of follicular lymphoma in cytologic preparations. The sensitivity and specificity of FCM in detecting a neoplastic population varies depending on the assay and can approach 94% to 100%.[26] Similarly, Richmond et al. showed 81% sensitivity and 100% specificity for detection of the *IG::BCL2* rearrangement on archival Pap-stained cytologic smears.[53] Of note, t(14;18)(q32;q21) can also be detected on Giemsa-stained smears by PCR-based techniques; however, it is generally less sensitive than the FISH-based approach.[22] Of note, a small proportion of follicular lymphomas, including those involving both nodal and cutaneous sites, and pediatric follicular lymphomas are negative for *BCL2* rearrangement, as are some grade 3 cases. Therefore, lack of t(14;18)(q32;q21) does not exclude a follicular lymphoma diagnosis. Some translocation-negative cases may contain rearrangements of *BCL6*, which can also be assessed. In addition, FISH for *IRF4/MUM1* rearrangement may be indicated to exclude large B-cell lymphoma with *IRF4* rearrangement.

Differential Diagnosis

Included in the differential diagnosis are variants of follicular lymphoma such as diffuse and pediatric follicular lymphoma, large B-cell lymphoma with *IRF4* rearrangement, reactive hyperplasia, mantle cell lymphoma, marginal zone lymphoma, small lymphocytic lymphoma, and DLBCL, not otherwise specified. A diagnosis of in situ follicular neoplasia requires correlation with histology.

Mantle Cell Lymphoma

Cytomorphology

Mantle cell lymphoma aspirates often show a monotonous population of small to intermediate-sized lymphoid cells with delicate nuclear clefts, dispersed or finely stippled chromatin, inconspicuous nucleoli, and distinct pale or basophilic cytoplasm (Fig. 2-8).[61,86-88] Two variants of mantle cell lymphoma—blastoid and pleomorphic—have potential clinical significance. The blastoid variant exhibits intermediate-sized to large lymphoid cells with enlarged, slightly irregular nuclei, evenly distributed chromatin, and small nucleoli (Fig. 2-9). The cytoplasm on DQ-stained material is scant and pale blue. Apoptotic and lymphoglandular bodies may be present in the background.[87] In the pleomorphic or anaplastic variant, the atypical lymphoid cells are larger, with more nuclear irregularity and hyperchromasia.[61]

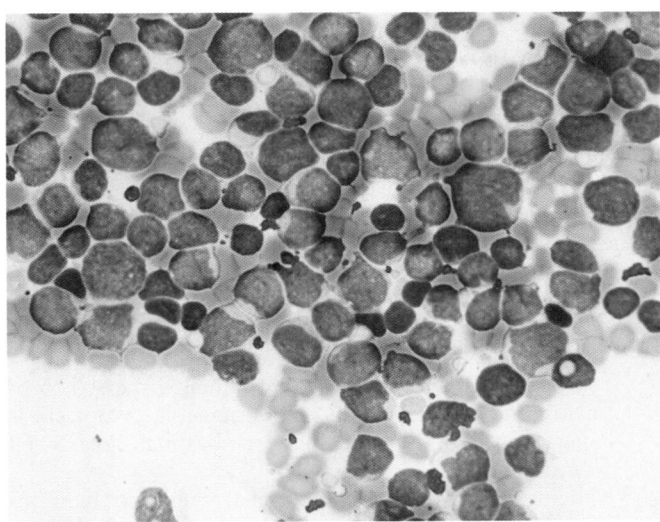

Figure 2-9. Blastoid variant of mantle cell lymphoma. Atypical intermediate-sized to large lymphocytes with enlarged irregular nuclei and small amounts of pale blue cytoplasm (Diff-Quik, smear).

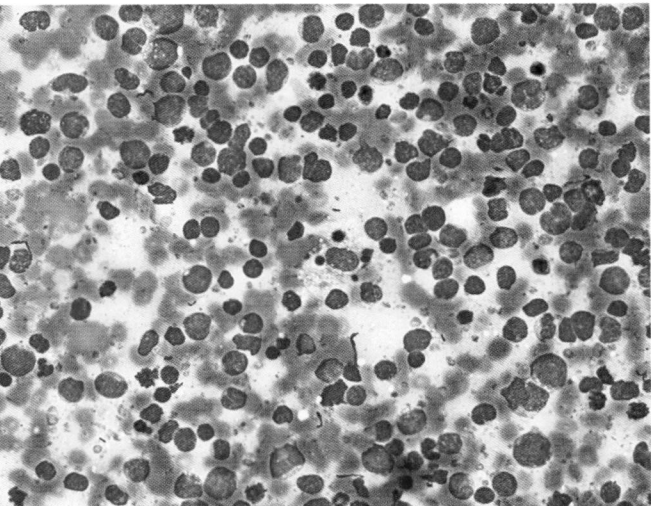

Figure 2-10. Diffuse large B-cell lymphoma, not otherwise specified. Predominant population of large atypical centroblasts with basophilic cytoplasm admixed with benign centrocytes and centroblasts, lymphoglandular bodies, and a single tingible body macrophage. Apoptotic cells are noted (Diff-Quik, smear).

Ancillary Studies

The t(11;14)(q13;q32) is present in the vast majority of cases and can be detected by FISH on cytospins of FNA material.[22,50] ICC/IHC for SOX11 may be informative in cases negative for *IG::CCND1* rearrangement.[22] A confirmation of *CCND2* and *CCND3* rearrangements by FISH or sequencing is recommended in these cases, as they should be classified as mantle cell lymphoma.[89]

In addition, the National Comprehensive Cancer Network (NCCN) recommends assessing the proliferative activity by Ki67 immunostain and evaluating the *TP53* status, preferably by sequencing, both of which are used for prognostication and therapy assignment.[90]

Differential Diagnosis

The differential diagnosis includes reactive hyperplasia, follicular lymphoma, marginal zone lymphoma, small lymphocytic lymphoma, and lymphoblastic lymphoma. A diagnosis of in situ mantle cell neoplasia requires correlation with histology.

Diffuse Large B-Cell Lymphoma, Not Otherwise Specified

Cytomorphology

DLBCL is characterized by the presence of a significant number of discohesive large lymphoid cells (Figs. 2-10 and 2-11). Smear preparations showing cohesive clusters of large lymphoid cells mimicking carcinoma cells may also be seen.[91] Cytoplasmic fragments, so-called *lymphoglandular bodies,* are usually abundant (Figs. 2-10 and 2-11). The majority of cells on FNA smear preparations are centroblasts. These cells have a vesicular chromatin pattern, distinct nuclear membranes, prominent nucleoli, and basophilic cytoplasm. The immunoblastic variant of DLBCL shows a predominance of lymphoid cells (immunoblasts) with large round nuclei, single prominent nucleoli, and abundant plasmacytoid or clear to pale cytoplasm.[4,61,74] Atypical large cells may display pleomorphic multilobated nuclei, similar to ALCL. In cell block preparations, the presence of "sheets" of large lymphoid

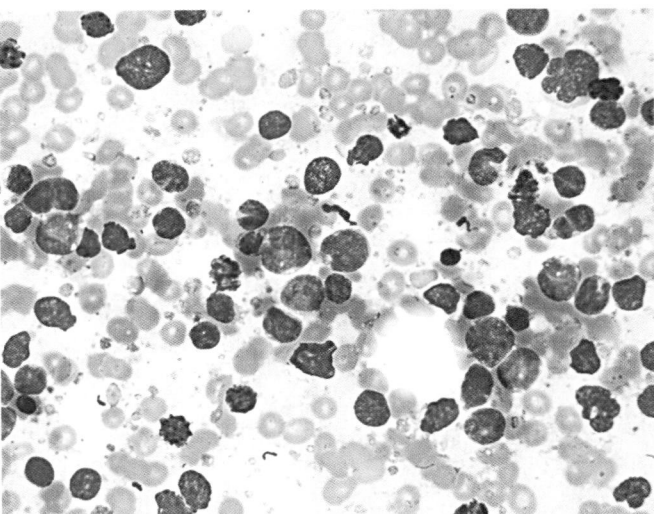

Figure 2-11. Diffuse large B-cell lymphoma, not otherwise specified. Large atypical centroblasts with enlarged nuclei, prominent nucleoli, and basophilic cytoplasm. Some atypical centroblasts display irregular nuclear membranes. The background contains a few benign centrocytes and centroblasts and lymphoglandular bodies (Diff-Quik, smear).

cells may be an indication of a primary diagnosis of large cell lymphoma or transformation of a small cell lymphoma.[61]

Differential Diagnosis

The differential diagnosis includes, but is not limited to, grade 3 follicular lymphoma, large B-cell lymphoma with *IRF4* rearrangement, HL, Burkitt lymphoma, histiocytic sarcoma, myeloid sarcoma, malignant melanoma, seminoma, and metastatic carcinoma. Distinctive cytologic features of nonlymphoid malignancies include:

- Metastatic carcinoma—presence of atypical cells in clusters and absence (usually) of lymphoglandular bodies in the background

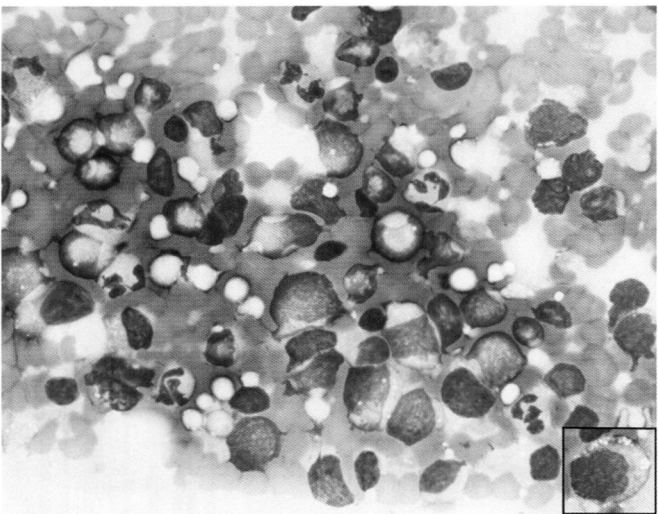

Figure 2-12. Primary mediastinal (thymic) large B-cell lymphoma. Large atypical lymphoid cells with enlarged round to irregular nuclei and variable amounts of cytoplasm in a background of mostly red blood cells. Inset shows a large, atypical lymphocyte with moderate amounts of basophilic cytoplasm and small vacuoles (Diff-Quik, smear).

- Metastatic melanoma—presence of pigment and intranuclear cytoplasmic inclusions
- Seminoma—presence of a "tigroid" background on DQ with scattered small, mature lymphocytes; there may be multinucleated giant cells
- Myeloid sarcoma—lack of lymphoglandular bodies; cytoplasmic granules may be present, including Auer rods (rarely); nuclear chromatin is finely distributed, with prominent and usually central nucleoli in blasts; myeloid maturation may be present.

Primary Mediastinal (Thymic) Large B-Cell Lymphoma

Cytomorphology

Aspirates of primary mediastinal large B-cell lymphoma show predominantly single, medium-sized to large lymphoid cells with round to oval nuclei, smooth to irregular nuclear contours, one or more visible nucleoli, and scant to abundant cytoplasm (Fig. 2-12). In some cases, the atypical lymphoid cells show markedly lobulated nuclei.[92-94] The cytoplasm is pale blue or deeply basophilic (DQ-stained slides), and vacuoles may be identified.[94] The background may contain connective tissue fragments admixed with single or groups of lymphocytes. These lymphocytes may have a distorted or elongated morphology as a result of fibrosis.[93] Some aspirates may show scant cellularity with a few atypical lymphoid cells.[88]

Ancillary Studies

The confirmation of B-cell origin and presence of associated markers such as CD23, MAL (myelin and lymphocyte), CD200, cREL, TRAF1, TNFAIP2 and pSTAT6 by FCM or ICC are helpful in a differential diagnosis.[95] The majority of primary mediastinal large B-cell lymphomas do not express surface immunoglobulins, which, by definition, are atypical and indicative of a lymphoma diagnosis.[92]

Cytomorphologic diagnosis can also be supported by rearrangements of *CIITA* (*C2TA*) and abnormalities of the *JAK2/PDCD1LG2/CD274* locus at 9p24.1.[95]

Differential Diagnosis

The differential diagnosis of tumors in this anatomic location includes cHL, lymphoblastic lymphoma, thymoma, and poorly differentiated carcinoma. Distinctive cytologic features of these most common differential diagnoses include:
- cHL—presence of classic Reed-Sternberg cells in a background of lymphocytes, plasma cells, and eosinophils
- Lymphoblastic lymphoma—presence of intermediate-sized atypical lymphoid cells with finely dispersed chromatin and inconspicuous, small nucleoli; cytoplasm is sparse (in contrast to primary mediastinal large B-cell lymphoma)
- Thymoma—presence of epithelial cells and lymphocytes; keratinaceous debris may be present if there is cystic degeneration
- Poorly differentiated carcinoma—atypical cells are cohesive, and lymphoglandular bodies are often absent.

Burkitt Lymphoma

Cytomorphology

The lymphoid cells in Burkitt lymphoma are intermediate in size with round nuclei, a finely granular to coarse chromatin pattern, several nucleoli, and abundant, deeply basophilic cytoplasm with small cytoplasmic vacuoles (Fig. 2-13).[96,97] The background shows tingible body macrophages, apoptotic bodies, lymphoglandular bodies, and a watery, basophilic proteinaceous matrix.[61,96,97] Usually, there are only a few reactive lymphocytes in the background. Similar cytomorphology with slightly more pleomorphic neoplastic lymphoid cells can be encountered in large B-cell lymphoma with 11q aberration (synonym: high-grade B-cell lymphoma with 11q aberrations). The tingible body macrophages seen in the latter entity show numerous coarse apoptotic bodies (Fig. 2-12).[98]

Ancillary Studies

ICC and FCM can be helpful in distinguishing Burkitt lymphoma from CD10-positive DLBCL; however, the definitive confirmation of the diagnosis requires a demonstration of *MYC* translocation in the absence of other common genetic abnormalities, such as rearrangements of *BCL2* and *BCL6*.[22] The t(8;14)(q24;q32) and variant translocations of the *MYC* gene can be detected by FISH on cytospins and cell block sections of FNA material.[97]

Differential Diagnosis

The differential diagnosis includes DLBCL, myeloid sarcoma, lymphoblastic leukemia/lymphoma, and other subtypes of high-grade B-cell lymphomas.

Hodgkin Lymphoma

Diagnosis of both cHL and nodular lymphocyte predominant B-cell lymphoma (synonym: nodular lymphocyte predominant Hodgkin lymphoma) can be challenging on cytologic material alone. The paucity of neoplastic cells,

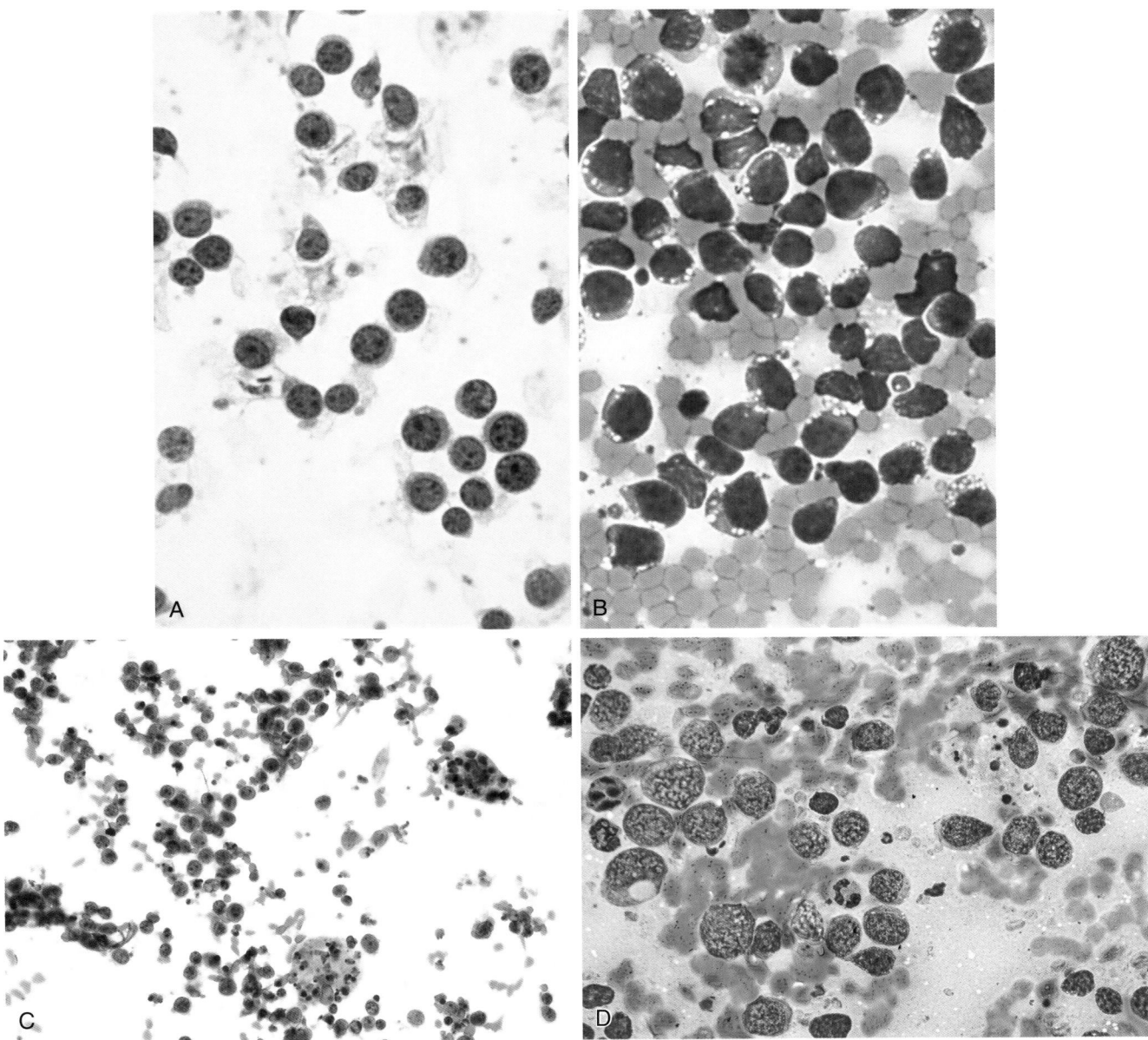

Figure 2-13. Burkitt lymphoma and large B-cell lymphoma with 11q aberration. Burkitt lymphoma shows uniform population of atypical lymphoid cells of intermediate size with enlarged round nuclei, coarse chromatin, prominent nucleoli, and homogeneous, well-defined cytoplasm. Some atypical cells display small vacuoles in the cytoplasm. **A,** Pap smear. **B,** Diff-Quik smear. **C, D,** Large B-cell lymphoma with 11q aberration shows more pleomorphic lymphoid cells and tingible body macrophages with prominent coarse apoptotic debris (**C,** Pap smear. **D,** Diff-Quik smear).

rich polymorphous background, cytomorphologic features overlapping with other lymphomas, and difficulties in immunophenotyping by FCM limit the utility of FNA for the initial diagnosis of HL. In the majority of cases, a follow-up biopsy or lymph node excision are recommended. In patients with a prior history of HL, FNA may be helpful in confirmation of a recurrent disease.

Classic Hodgkin Lymphoma

Cytomorphology

FNA smears of cHL show large pleomorphic and Hodgkin and Reed-Sternberg (HRS) cells in a polymorphous reactive background including small lymphocytes, histiocytes, eosinophils, and plasma cells (Fig. 2-14).[99-101] The HRS cells, pathognomonic for cHL, are binucleated with prominent nucleoli and abundant cytoplasm. Hodgkin cells and their variants can be mononuclear or multinucleated, with abundant cytoplasm and nucleoli ranging from small, single, and inconspicuous to large, multiple, and prominent. It has been suggested that a number of neoplastic cells encountered in FNA smears and a type of non-neoplastic component correspond to specific types of cHL. For example, nodular sclerosis cHL frequently shows paucicellular smears with HRS cells, fibroblasts, eosinophils, and fibrous strands.

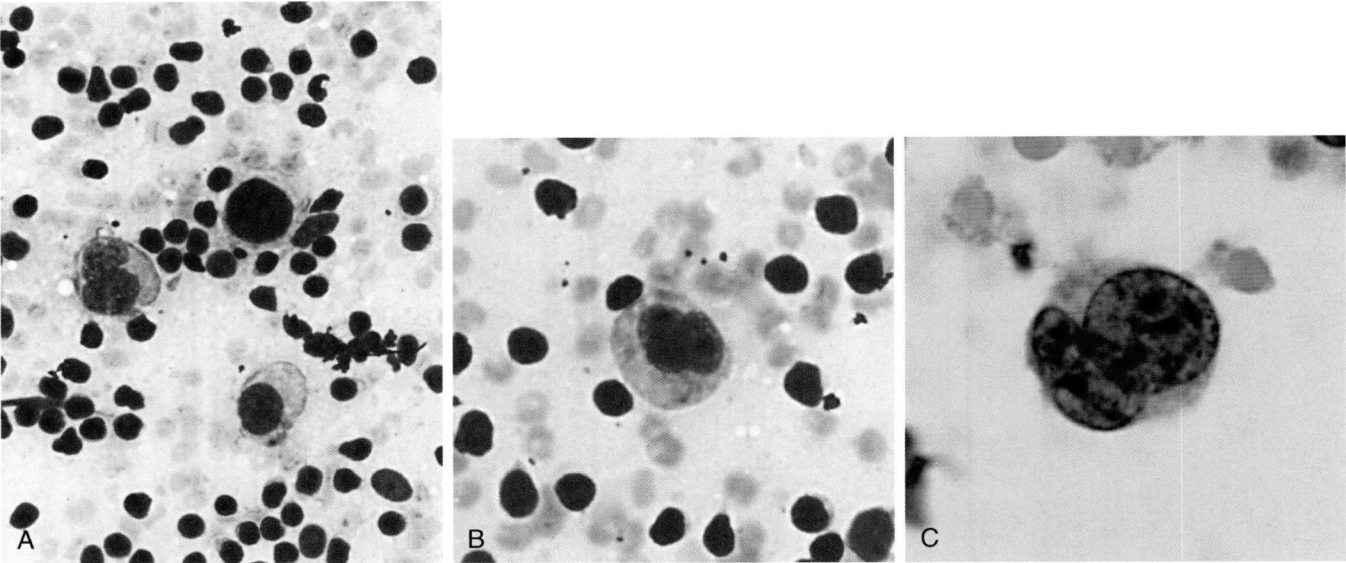

Figure 2-14. Classic Hodgkin lymphoma. A, Reed-Sternberg cell, mononuclear Hodgkin cells, and numerous small lymphocytes in the background (Diff-Quik, smear). **B,** Classic binucleated Reed-Sternberg cell with prominent nucleoli and abundant pale cytoplasm (Diff-Quik, smear). **C,** Reed-Sternberg cell seen in Pap smear.

Ancillary Studies

Immunophenotyping can be performed on smears/cytospins or cell blocks; however, in clinical practice, the definitive diagnosis of cHL relies on tissue histology supported by IHC whenever possible.

Differential Diagnosis

Because of the overlapping cytomorphology of neoplastic cells and polymorphous inflammatory background, the differential diagnosis of cHL is broad and includes a number of reactive conditions such as infectious mononucleosis, granulomatous lymphadenitis, and suppurative lymphadenitis. Infectious mononucleosis, ALCL, and T-cell/histiocyte-rich large B-cell lymphoma can be distinguished from cHL only with the help of ICC/IHC. Differential diagnosis also includes metastatic poorly differentiated carcinoma, melanoma, and germ cell tumors.

Nodular Lymphocyte Predominant B-Cell Lymphoma (Synonym: Nodular Lymphocyte Predominant Hodgkin Lymphoma)

Cytomorphology

Neoplastic cells of nodular lymphocyte predominant B-cell lymphoma have a multilobated nucleus with complex folds ("popcorn" cells). The "popcorn" morphology is best appreciated in histologic sections. The chromatin is vesicular with a delicate nuclear membrane, multiple small nucleoli, and scant cytoplasm.[102] The cytology of neoplastic cells may vary, however, and may include cells more closely mimicking HRS cells and their variants. The background is rich in small lymphocytes and epithelioid histiocytes.[102]

Ancillary Studies

Ancillary studies are marginally helpful, as this lymphoma displays a B-cell immunophenotype similar to other large B-cell lymphomas. Definitive diagnosis requires lymph node excision because it is predominantly based on architectural features.

Differential Diagnosis

Given the rarity of neoplastic cells in the reactive background, the cytologic diagnosis is challenging, and the differential diagnosis is similar to that of cHL.

Mature T-Cell Neoplasms

Diagnosis and classification of T-cell lymphomas can be challenging because of polymorphous cytomorphology, commonly a non-specific immunophenotype, and a low index of suspicion resulting from the low frequency of these disorders. A significant admixture of cells typically seen in reactive lesions such as macrophages, epithelioid histiocytes, plasma cells, eosinophils, and a few small background lymphocytes may suggest reactive lymphadenopathy. We discuss here the cytomorphologic and ancillary features of the most common T-cell lymphomas.

Peripheral T-Cell Lymphoma, Not Otherwise Specified

Cytomorphology

Aspirates of lymph nodes involved by peripheral T-cell lymphoma, not otherwise specified (PTCL, NOS) are typically highly cellular and show a spectrum of cytomorphology (Fig. 2-15).[103,104] The atypical lymphoid cells range from small to large. The small lymphoid cells are larger than a mature small lymphocyte and show more abundant cytoplasm. There is variable nuclear irregularity with indentations and protrusions and coarse chromatin, which are better visualized on Pap stain. The nucleoli can be inconspicuous or prominent. Large lymphoid cells have round to irregular nuclei, finely granular chromatin, and prominent nucleoli.

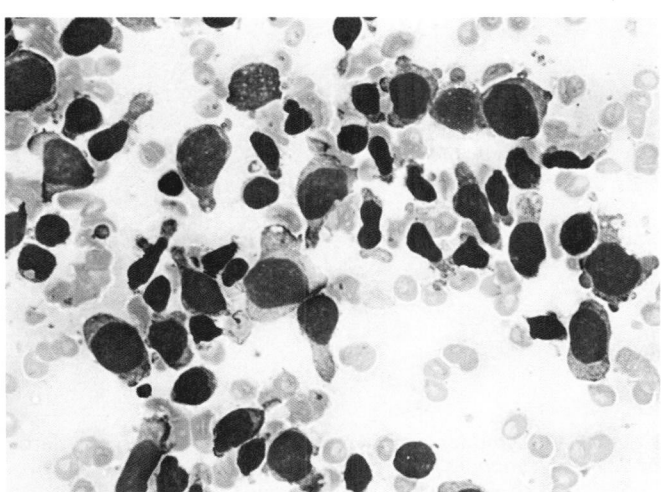

Figure 2-15. Peripheral T-cell lymphoma, not otherwise specified. Medium-sized to large atypical lymphocytes with irregular nuclear outlines and scant cytoplasm (Diff-Quik, smear).

Large pleomorphic cells resembling Hodgkin cells can be seen; however, binucleated or multinucleated forms are uncommon. Cases with a polymorphous cytomorphology, including medium-sized to large lymphoid cells, are not infrequent. Epithelioid histiocytes, eosinophils, plasma cells, and fragments of vessels can be seen in a background of neoplastic cells. These heterogeneous cytologic features coupled with a low frequency of PTCL, NOS make a conclusive diagnosis and classification challenging, even when supported by ancillary studies.

Ancillary Studies

The atypical immunophenotype includes a loss of various T-cell markers, most commonly CD7, and is best seen by FCM. A simplified method to detect T-cell clonality by FCM based on the T-cell receptor (TR) constant beta chain-1 can also be applied.[44] TR gene rearrangement studies by PCR or sequencing can also be performed on cytologic preparations; however, the definitive confirmation of the PTCL, NOS diagnosis is best performed on a lymph node excision.[48,55]

Differential Diagnosis

A differential diagnosis based on cytomorphology alone is broad and includes reactive lymphoid hyperplasia, follicular lymphoma, marginal zone lymphoma, and DLBCL. In select cases with large pleomorphic cells, HL, poorly differentiated carcinoma, and melanoma should be excluded based on the results of flow cytometric immunophenotyping, ICC, or IHC, if a cell block is available.

Follicular Helper T-Cell Lymphoma, Angioimmunoblastic-Type (Synonyms: Nodal T-Follicular Helper Cell Lymphoma, Angioimmunoblastic-Type; Angioimmunoblastic T-Cell Lymphoma)

Cytomorphology

Similar to PTCL, NOS, the cytomorphology of angioimmunoblastic T-cell lymphoma (AITL) is heterogeneous because of a significant component of non-neoplastic small

lymphocytes, histiocytes, plasma cells, B immunoblasts, FDCs, and fragments of vessels.[105,106] Small and medium-sized atypical lymphoid cells are found in all reported cases. Lymphoid cells with abundant clear cytoplasm, similar to those seen in histologic sections, have been reported. The lymphocytes are often found associated with aggregates of FDCs, an arrangement termed *dendritic cell-lymphocyte complexes*. FDCs have an amphophilic cytoplasm with ragged outlines, an oval nucleus, a thin nuclear membrane, and a small nucleolus. Vessels can be seen in tissue fragments on FNA smears or on cell block sections. The heterogeneous population described earlier and the absence of tingible body macrophages, follicle center cells, and Reed-Sternberg cells can suggest a diagnosis of AITL in patients with typical clinical presentation.

Ancillary Studies

Multiparameter FCM confirms the presence of a neoplastic T-cell population in both lymph node and peripheral blood.[107,108] Utilization of markers associated with follicular helper T cells, such as PD1 (CD279), ICOS, CXCL13, CD10, and BCL6, is required. Clonal TR gene rearrangements can be accompanied by clonal IG gene rearrangements, and therefore are best interpreted in the context of histologic evaluation of a lymph node excision.[109,110]

Differential Diagnosis

Differential diagnosis includes reactive lymphoid hyperplasia, especially mixed lymphoid hyperplasia, paracortical hyperplasia, or dermatopathic lymphadenopathy, which are characterized by paracortical expansion and vascular proliferation. Cytomorphology in conjunction with clinical information serves as a screening tool to exclude cases of reactive lymphadenopathy and, if suspicious, to recommend lymph node excision. HL and T-cell/histiocyte-rich large B-cell lymphoma are also included in the differential diagnosis because of the presence of a polymorphous background cell population.

Anaplastic Large Cell Lymphoma

Cytomorphology

FNA smears of ALCL are variably cellular and show a discohesive population of cells. Cytomorphology is dependent on the histologic variant, and in the most common variant, it includes numerous atypical large pleomorphic lymphoid cells with abundant, variably staining cytoplasm (Fig. 2-16).[111-113] Vacuoles, azurophilic granules, or cytoplasmic blebbing can be seen. The nuclei are often horseshoe shaped or wreath-like and correspond to nuclei of "hallmark cells." Lymphoid cells with multiple nuclei are also seen. Nuclei show finely condensed chromatin, well-defined, irregular membranes, and centrally or eccentrically placed prominent nucleoli. Small and medium-sized plasmacytoid cells are admixed.[111,112] The latter are particularly abundant in the small-cell variant. The background may contain lymphoglandular bodies, small lymphocytes, histiocytes, and neutrophils.

Ancillary Studies

The cytologic diagnosis requires confirmation by immunophenotyping. The most useful is demonstration of the classical strong membranous and paranuclear dot

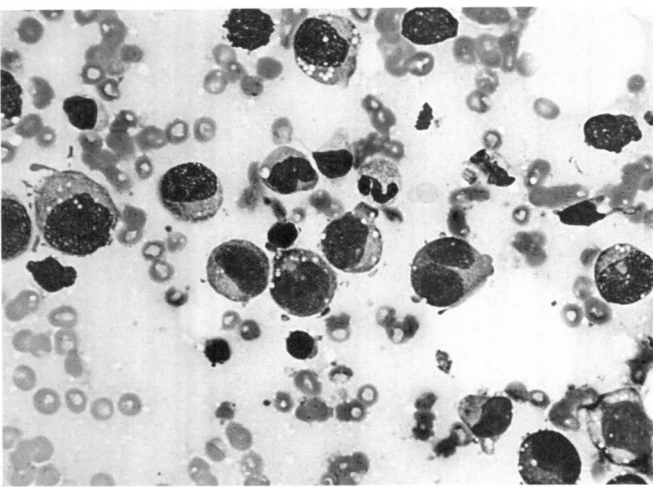

Figure 2-16. Anaplastic large cell lymphoma. Large atypical lymphoid cells with pleomorphic nuclei, occasional binucleation, and pale basophilic cytoplasm. Background shows rare small lymphocytes, red blood cells, and debris (Diff-Quik, smear).

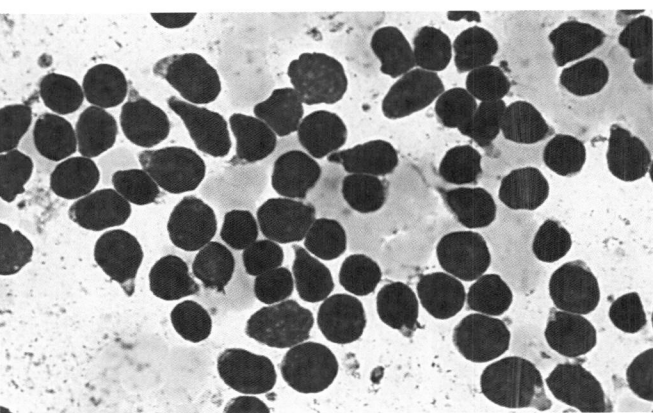

Figure 2-17. Lymphoblastic lymphoma. Monotonous population of atypical lymphoid cells (twice the size of small benign lymphocytes) with enlarged, round to oval nuclei, high nuclear-to-cytoplasmic ratio, and scant amount of pale basophilic cytoplasm (Diff-Quik, smear).

pattern of CD30 by IHC, coupled with the absent B-cell and non-hematopoietic antigens. ALK positivity and/or FISH demonstrating rearrangement of the *ALK* gene are useful in ALK-positive ALCL.

Differential Diagnosis

The differential diagnosis includes HL, histiocytic sarcoma, DLBCL, poorly differentiated carcinoma, malignant melanoma, and sarcoma. The erroneous diagnosis of HL has been reported as one of the common major discrepancies between cytology-based and histology-based diagnoses.[114] Certain cytomorphologic features, such as abundant eosinophils and neutrophils seen in cHL or melanin pigment in melanoma, can help in differentiating ALCL from other entities; however, the definitive diagnosis is based on adequate IHC/ICC. In the absence of a convincing immunophenotype, lymph node excision is recommended.

Lymphoblastic Leukemia/Lymphoma

Cytomorphology

FNA samples of lymphoblastic leukemia/lymphoma (LBL) of either B-cell or T-cell origin show similar features (Fig. 2-17). The aspirates contain a monotonous population of immature lymphoid cells that are frequently larger than a small mature lymphocyte and have a high nuclear-to-cytoplasmic ratio.[115] The cytoplasm is scant, agranular, and may contain small vacuoles. Nuclei can be round or irregular, with nuclear clefts and convolutions. The chromatin is finely dispersed, similar to other immature cells, and may be more condensed than that of myeloid blasts. The background shows variable amounts of lymphoglandular bodies, tingible body macrophages, and necrosis.[116] Mitoses may be frequent.

Ancillary Studies

A definitive diagnosis requires immunophenotyping, preferably by FCM, to confirm a homogeneous population of immature T cells or B cells and to exclude rare cases of mixed-phenotype acute leukemia, which can also involve lymph nodes and is challenging to diagnose using IHC.

Thymocytes in thymic hyperplasia or thymoma show an immunophenotype consistent with a spectrum of maturation.

Differential Diagnosis

The differential diagnosis includes lymphomas composed of small and medium-sized lymphocytes, including mantle cell lymphoma (blastoid variant). Other neoplasms presenting as mediastinal mass, such as thymoma and small cell carcinoma, should be considered. Myeloid sarcoma occasionally involves lymph nodes and can have a cytomorphology similar to that of LBL.

LIMITATIONS OF FINE-NEEDLE ASPIRATION

Limitations of lymph node FNA are related to technical issues associated with the procedure itself or are intrinsic to entities that are difficult to diagnose based on cytomorphology without the context of architectural features. Poor sampling resulting in a paucicellular specimen that is insufficient for ancillary studies and sampling error are procedure-related problems that are also encountered in FNA of other organs. Missing a lymph node or FNA of a highly fibrotic lesion can result in low or no cellularity. Similarly, inadequate sampling with only a few passes may yield a sample that is not representative of a disease process when a lymph node is partially involved by lymphoma or shows focal transformation. Entities characterized by a rich reactive background with only a few neoplastic cells, such as HL and T-cell/histiocyte-rich large B-cell lymphoma, are also a potential diagnostic challenge.[114,117] These two entities and other lymphomas with a polymorphous population of cells, such as select T-cell lymphomas, are most confidently diagnosed within the context of nodal architecture. Similarly, a follicular or diffuse growth pattern cannot be evaluated in cytology preparations other than a cell block section in some cases. The ability to determine follicular architecture is clinically significant in grade 3 follicular lymphoma versus DLBCL of follicle center cell origin. CNBs (see discussion in next section) accompanying aspiration may partially mitigate some of these limitations; however, in difficult cases, the threshold to recommend lymph node excision should be low.

It is generally agreed that FNA can be used with confidence to distinguish between benign/reactive and malignant

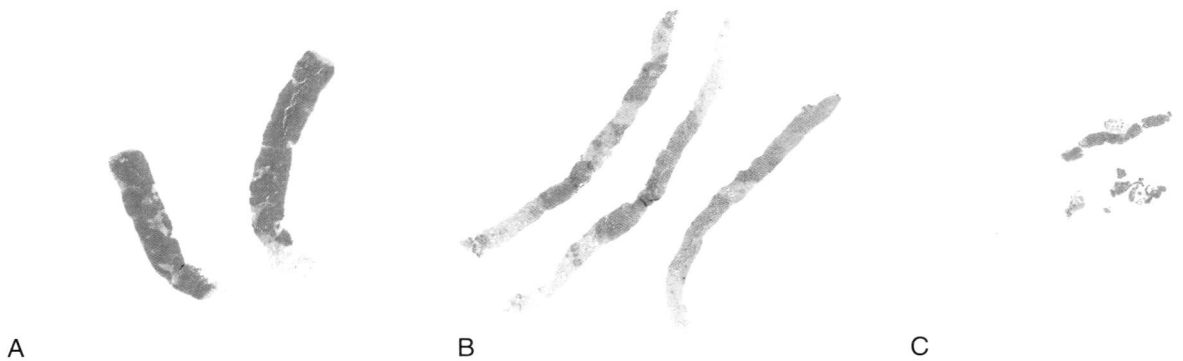

Figure 2-18. Examples of core needle biopsies performed with different gauge needles. A, 14-gauge core needle biopsy (CNB) of axillary lymph node. **B,** Optimal CNB sample including several tissue fragments procured with 18-gauge needle. **C,** CNB inadequate for evaluation because of small, fragmented sample (20-gauge needle).

lymphoid processes and for the diagnosis of recurrent disease or staging.[27,118,119] However, there is no consensus regarding use of FNA for primary lymphoma diagnosis.[27] Reported diagnostic sensitivity varies greatly, and precise classification can be achieved in less than 80% of cases.[17,27,120] This is partially related to the FNA limitations discussed in the previous paragraph and is also dependent on a variable level of expertise in the diagnosis and current classification of hematologic neoplasms among the cytopathology community. Cytopathologists must be familiar not only with the cytomorphologic evaluation of lymphoid neoplasms; they must also integrate the results of a variety of highly specialized ancillary studies, such as FCM and molecular assays. These studies are typically performed by hematopathologists and molecular pathologists; therefore, effective communication among the team testing individual FNA samples is critical. Close communication with an attending clinician is also important because the knowledge of the clinical context is essential both for an on-site evaluation and at the time of sign-out. The more challenging cases, at least, should be thoroughly discussed within the team before a final cytology diagnosis is issued. Whenever the cytomorphologic diagnosis is inconsistent with the clinical presentation or results of ancillary studies, a lymph node excision or multiple CNBs for inaccessible sites are advised.

ROLE OF CORE NEEDLE BIOPSY IN LYMPHOMA DIAGNOSIS

CNBs are increasingly procured at the time of FNA in an attempt to improve diagnostic sensitivity and provide additional material for ancillary studies. Because of the ease of procurement and low morbidity associated with the procedure, there have been suggestions that CNB can supplement or replace FNA or even lymph node excision in the evaluation of lymphadenopathy. The reported accuracy of CNB in the diagnosis of lymphoma appears superior to FNA alone.[121,122] A modest improvement in accuracy has been reported when CNB is added to FNA.[123,124] The advantage of adding CNB was most pronounced in cases involving DLBCL and cases in which FNA material was not sufficient for diagnosis. Small B-cell lymphomas showed similar diagnostic accuracy when evaluation was based on FNA alone and FNA accompanied by CNB.

It is challenging to determine whether CNB can replace lymph node excision and become a diagnostic standard. The NCCN and European Society of Medical Oncology guidelines recommend excision or incisional biopsy for lymphoma diagnosis.[90,125-127] Nevertheless, the number of CNBs increases each year owing to the low morbidity of the procedure, ease of performance, and decreased expense.[121,122,128-130] In large multi-institutional series or in the referral lymphoma network setting, CNB can provide a definitive diagnosis in 70% to 90% of cases.[30,42,131] The diagnostic accuracy may differ depending on the regional versus referral setting, use of ancillary studies, and a primary versus recurrent diagnosis.[131,132] Nevertheless, the number of cases with nondefinitive diagnoses is higher for CNB than for lymph node excisions. A comparison of CNB and paired excision samples showed a major diagnostic discrepancy in approximately 10% of cases. This number may be higher when excisions are specifically requested after diagnostic difficulties encountered on preceding CNBs. Specifically, diagnostic challenges related to CNB are common in PTCL and especially angioimmunoblastic T-cell lymphoma, for which the evaluation of architectural features is paramount. In addition, HL, nodular lymphocyte predominant large B-cell lymphoma, T-cell/histiocyte-rich large B-cell lymphoma, and nodal marginal zone lymphoma can be challenging to diagnose based on CNB. Studies have shown that approximately 20% of CNBs yield material insufficient for diagnosis. One multi-institutional study reported significant differences in aggregate core length among institutions.[42] Not surprisingly, longer cores and larger needle gauges were associated with a definitive diagnosis on CNB and fewer diagnostic discrepancies.[42] The standardization of CNB and quality control may improve diagnostic yield. Obtaining several cores with needles that are 18-gauge or larger may provide reasonable material for an initial diagnosis, at least in select subtypes of lymphoma (Fig. 2-18). It is questionable whether CNB samples will be sufficient for potential future ancillary studies such as molecular genetic testing, evaluation of tumor microenvironment, and other tests required for clinical trial qualification and novel therapies. Therefore, lymph node excision or incisional biopsy remains the standard for lymphoma diagnosis.

Pearls and Pitfalls

- Diagnostic accuracy of FNA in lymphoma cases is variable and is significantly increased by the use of ancillary studies such as FCM, ICC, and molecular testing.
- Standardized protocol for the collection and processing of FNA samples is recommended to procure sufficient material and eliminate delays in ancillary studies.
- On-site evaluation, including a detailed review of clinical history, guides the selection of additional testing and, in cases with scant cellularity, allows one to prioritize ancillary studies.
- Addition of air-dried Giemsa-stained cytospins may be helpful, as the cell cytology is superior on cytospins because of the flattening and enlarging effect of cytocentrifugation.
- Alcohol fixation with Pap staining, including monolayer technologies, is insufficient for demonstration of cytoplasmic features, may increase the risk of false-negative diagnoses, and should not be used as the only stain when evaluating hematopoietic processes.
- In our experience, FNA yields superior material for FCM when compared with CNBs, which are often procured at the same time.
- Results of FCM must be interpreted within the context of cytomorphology and clinical information because of the possibility of false-negative or false-positive results.
- When a definitive diagnostic immunophenotype is not available in cases with cytomorphologic features of lymphoma, a lymph node excision is recommended.
- Cytomorphologic diagnosis of lymphoma is challenging in cases with polymorphous populations of cells, including cells typically seen in reactive lesions such as macrophages, epithelioid histiocytes, plasma cells, and eosinophils. Such cases are most confidently diagnosed within the context of nodal architecture.
- Evaluation of growth pattern (follicular vs. diffuse) and distinction between grade 3A and grade 3B follicular lymphomas are not feasible in cytologic material. In these cases, the threshold to recommend lymph node excision or biopsy should be low.
- Differential diagnosis of cHL, nodular lymphocyte predominant large B-cell lymphoma, T-cell/histiocyte-rich large B-cell lymphoma, and ALCL may be challenging because of a polymorphous cell population and frequently noncontributory FCM.
- Close communication with attending clinicians, hematopathologists, and molecular pathologists is critical in cytomorphologic evaluation of cases of suspected lymphoma.
- For a definitive lymphoma classification and whenever the cytomorphologic diagnosis is inconsistent with the clinical presentation or results of ancillary studies, a lymph node excision or incisional biopsy is advised.

KEY REFERENCES

17. Hehn SG T, Miller T. Utility of fine-needle aspiration as a diagnostic technique in lymphoma. *J Clin Oncol.* 2004;22(15):3046–3052.
18. Austin RM, Birdsong GG, Sidawy MK, Kaminsky DB. Fine needle aspiration is a feasible and accurate technique in the diagnosis of lymphoma. *J Clin Oncol.* 2005;23(35):9029–9030: author reply 9030-1.
26. Barrena S, Almeida J, Del Carmen Garcia-Macias M, et al. Flow cytometry immunophenotyping of fine-needle aspiration specimens: utility in the diagnosis and classification of non-Hodgkin lymphomas. *Histopathology.* 2011;58(6):906–918.
27. Wakely P. The diagnosis of non-Hodgkin lymphoma using fine-needle aspiration cytopathology. *Cancer Cytopathol.* 2010:238–243.
42. Czader M, Chiu A, Perkins S, Hasserjia R. Core needle biopsy in lymphoma diagnosis: a multiinstitutional study. 27:344A.
60. Swerdlow SHCE, Harris NL, et al. *WHO Classification of Tumors of Haematopoietic and Lymphoid Tissues;* 2016.
74. Meda BBDW RD, et al. Diagnosis and subclassification of primary and recurrent lymphoma. *Am J Clin Pathol.* 2000;113:688–699.
114. Landgren O, Porwit MacDonald A, Tani E, et al. A prospective comparison of fine-needle aspiration cytology and histopathology in the diagnosis and classification of lymphomas. *Hematol J.* 2004;5(1):69–76.
102. DeMay RM. *The Art & Science of Cytopathology.* 2nd ed. 2011.
118. Young NM,A, Haja J, et al. Fine-needle aspiration biopsy of lymphoproliferative disorders—interpretations based on morphologic criteria alone. *Arch Pathol Lab Med.* 2006;130:1766–1771.

Visit Elsevier eBooks+ for the complete set of references.

Chapter 3

Immunohistochemistry for the Hematopathology Laboratory

Girish Venkataraman and Karen L. Rech

INTRODUCTION

Perhaps in no other subspecialty of pathology does immunohistochemistry (IHC) play as important a role in the accurate diagnosis and definition of disease subtypes as it does in hematopathology. Before the development of this technology, the diagnosis of lymphoproliferative diseases depended on classification systems based solely on morphologic differences. The subjective use of morphologically based classification schemes led to difficulty in defining biologically different entities, and the morphologic categories were often difficult to reproduce, even among expert hematopathologists. The advent of IHC allowed the objective identification of specific phenotypic characteristics associated with different lymphoid proliferations. Such phenotypic markers provide information about the cell lineage and origin of the hematopoietic neoplasm, the production of characteristic oncogenic proteins, and the proliferative characteristics of the tumor. IHC is increasingly being used to identify underlying molecular alterations to aid in diagnosis and guide therapy decisions. By integrating IHC studies with morphologic characteristics, more reproducible and biologically relevant classification schemes were developed, reaching their current level of sophistication with the most recent iteration of the World Health Organization Classification and International Consensus Classification of myeloid/lymphoproliferative diseases.[1,2] The goal of this chapter is to introduce the reader to the practice of IHC and to the wide range of antigenic targets that have proved useful in hematopathology.

BASIC IMMUNOHISTOCHEMISTRY

In theory, IHC is a simple technology that requires only three basic elements: a cellular antigen of interest, a primary antibody targeting the antigen, and a detection system to visualize the location of the antibody-antigen complex. In actual practice, the production of an optimally immunostained slide is much more problematic and depends on the condition of the tissue antigen; the type, specificity, and affinity of the primary antibody; and the detection system used. The interpretation of IHC stains requires knowledge of and control over these elements and an experienced pathologist.

Antigens

At the heart of IHC is the antigen-antibody reaction; therefore, it is crucial that the antigenic epitopes recognized by the cognate diagnostic antibody maintain their reactive conformation. The specific antigenic epitopes present on any given protein or carbohydrate moiety are subject to enzymatic degradation that begins immediately after biopsy or resection and to further conformational changes resulting from fixation. To ensure preservation of the antigen of interest, rapid tissue fixation is important. Some antigenic epitopes, such as those on keratin proteins and other structural proteins of the cell, are relatively resistant to degradation; other antigens, such as phosphoepitopes on signaling proteins, undergo rapid degradation within minutes to hours.[3,4]

Although prompt tissue fixation is essential to preserve antigenicity, the specific fixative and the fixation process itself can interfere with antigenicity by causing conformational changes in antigenic molecules or by chemically modifying the antigenic epitopes. Traditionally, tissues have been fixed in neutral buffered formalin (pH 7.0) because it is inexpensive, has sterilizing properties, and preserves morphologic features well. The exact chemical reactions that occur in tissues are not well understood, but it is generally assumed that formalin's ability to cross-link aldehyde groups in proteins is responsible for its fixative properties. This mode of action is potentially deleterious to antigenic structure, and although some antigenic epitopes may not be affected significantly by formaldehyde cross-linking, these chemical modifications clearly have an adverse effect on many antigens. As formalin penetrates tissues slowly and the chemical reactions are complex, the number of modifications that take place is time dependent. In practice, this means that antigens fall into three basic categories: formalin-resistant epitopes, highly formalin-sensitive epitopes, and epitopes with a time-dependent sensitivity to formalin fixation. Although there have been attempts to generate antibodies specific to formalin-resistant epitopes,[5] most of the antibodies found to react with formalin-resistant epitopes have been identified through large-scale screenings of available antibody preparations.

Over the years, there has been great interest in identifying methods to overcome or reverse the deleterious effects of formalin fixation. The earliest attempts to retrieve antigenicity used proteolytic enzymes,[6] which presumably act by breaking formaldehyde-induced methylene cross-links in the antigenic molecules, thereby relaxing some of the conformational constraints on the protein epitopes. Such proteolytic methods continue to be used in many IHC laboratories and are particularly useful for recovering the reactivity of the cytokeratins. Nonetheless, proteolytic methods are difficult to control, and careful attention is needed to optimize their retrieval effect and avoid tissue destruction.

Despite some successes with proteolytic methods, the major breakthrough that brought IHC into widespread use was the development of heat-induced epitope retrieval (HIER) procedures.[7] This technique involves heating fixed tissue sections in buffered solutions at or above 100° C for several minutes to more than 30 minutes. HIER methods vary in terms of the recommended buffer solutions and the mode of heating, but the basic formula of applying wet heat over a period of time is universal.[8,9] The exact mechanism by which HIER reverses the loss of antigenicity in formalin-fixed tissue is unknown. However, hydrolytic cleavage of formaldehyde-related chemical groups and cross-links, the unfolding of inner epitopes, and the extraction of calcium ions from coordination complexes with proteins are among the hypothesized mechanisms.[10,11]

The advent of HIER methods revolutionized IHC and greatly expanded the number of antibodies that react in formalin-fixed, paraffin-embedded tissue sections.[7,11,12] HIER has also improved the sensitivity of antibodies directed to formalin-resistant epitopes and has enabled the routine assessment of a wide spectrum of antigens in epoxy resin–embedded bone marrow sections.[13] Appropriate antigen retrieval can minimize many of the problems related to preanalytic factors, reducing differences in immunostaining that result from the variations in fixation time in the clinical laboratory.[14]

The major disadvantage of HIER is that the high heat can cause considerable tissue damage, particularly when the tissue is underfixed or has a high collagen content, the antigen-retrieval time is prolonged, and the buffers contain ethylenediaminetetraacetic acid (EDTA) or have a high pH. Tissue damage can be minimized by ensuring tissues are optimally fixed, reducing the antigen-retrieval time, or changing the retrieval buffer. Despite this potential problem, the ability to detect otherwise nondetectable antigens far outweighs the potential for occasional damage of tissue sections.

Primary Antibodies

There are two major categories of primary antibodies used in diagnostic pathology: monoclonal antibodies and polyclonal antibodies. Polyclonal antibodies are generated by injecting an animal (most commonly a rabbit or goat) with the antigenic preparation of interest and harvesting the animal's serum once an immune response is detected. The serum is subjected to antibody purification and sometimes to differential adsorptions to eliminate unwanted reactivity, but it always contains a spectrum of antibody molecules originating from multiple unrelated antibody-producing cells (hence the term *polyclonal*). The specificity of a polyclonal antibody preparation is highly dependent on the purity of the initial antigenic preparation and how extensively adsorbed it is. Obtaining highly specific preparations is difficult, and background problems can be troublesome, especially when applied to IHC. Further, because the antibody response is variable over time and from one individual animal to another, complete standardization of antibody composition is not possible. Although developments in recombinant DNA and protein synthesis technology have greatly improved the specificity of polyclonal antibodies by providing tools to generate highly purified protein immunogens or even specific immunogenic peptides, polyclonal antibodies may still contain unwanted specificities.

Monoclonal antibodies, in contrast, are the product of a single immortalized antibody-producing cell, thus avoiding most problems related to antibody heterogeneity and specificity inherent in polyclonal antibody preparations. The hybridoma technology pioneered by Kohler and Milstein[15] in the 1970s allows the immortalization of a single antibody-producing mouse plasma cell by fusing it with a mouse plasmacytoma cell line. Individual hybrid mouse cells can be clonally expanded in tissue culture or in mice as tumors, providing a continuous source of antibody of known composition and reactivity. Because of their high quality and specificity, monoclonal antibodies were rapidly developed as diagnostic reagents in hematopathology and for other clinical applications that require standardized reagents. The specificity advantage of the monoclonal antibody, however, can also be a disadvantage when applied to denatured proteins in tissue sections. Because a polyclonal antibody preparation generally contains a mixture of antibodies reacting to multiple epitopes, it does not matter if some of the epitopes are rendered inactive by the fixation process, as long as one epitope remains in its reactive conformation. However, if the single epitope recognized by a monoclonal antibody is affected by the fixation process, the antibody cannot be used for IHC. A second disadvantage of mouse monoclonal antibodies is that they generally have weaker affinity constants than do comparable polyclonal rabbit antibody preparations. This led to the development of rabbit plasmacytoma cell lines that could be used as fusion partners to generate high-affinity rabbit monoclonal antibodies. These high-affinity rabbit monoclonal antibodies have improved the detection of some antigens, such as cyclin D1, and permitted detection of others that were heretofore unavailable with murine antibodies, such as CD103.

Regardless of which type of antibody is chosen for an IHC procedure, careful control over the development and use of the antibody must be maintained. Although antibody specificity is best demonstrated by immunoblotting or immunoprecipitation, this type of biochemical analysis is required only during the initial development of the antibody by the commercial vendor. However, before placing any antibody into clinical use, extensive validation of its efficacy and staining characteristics on tissue sections in the individual laboratory is necessary. This should include extensive testing of normal and tumor tissues to assess the specificity and sensitivity of tissue staining. The use of tissue microarrays can be helpful during this stage. Once the antibody has been validated and placed in service, the continued use of positive controls is mandatory with each test sample. The use of on-slide quality control tissue is an optimal practice that uses tissues known to contain the antigen of interest. As an alternative to on-slide quality control tissues, many hematopathology antigens are expressed on internal control cells within most tissues (e.g., cyclin D1 stains endothelial and stromal cells, and CD15 stains granulocytes).

Detection Systems

Detection systems contain an enzyme, a chromogenic substrate, and a link or bridge reagent that brings the enzyme into proximity with the primary labeling antibody. The choice of detection system is of great importance, and each method has its own advantages and disadvantages. Factors influencing the selection of a detection method are related to the type of tissue, the cellular target, its abundance and localization, and laboratory-specific issues (e.g., complexity, time requirements, reagent costs). Detection systems based on avidin-biotin immunoperoxidase complexes (ABC) have been largely replaced by polymer-based detection systems that avoid the possibility of high backgrounds in tissues rich in endogenous biotin.[16,17] As in biotin-based systems, an unlabeled primary antibody is used first, followed by a modified polymer (e.g., dextran) that is linked to a large number of secondary link antibodies and enzyme (peroxidase) molecules. Thus, one reagent contains both a species-specific secondary anti-immunoglobulin linking antibody and the chromogen developing enzyme. Newer detection systems have also been developed to increase the sensitivity for detecting antigens expressed at very low levels or to improve the detection of low-affinity primary antibodies. These systems involve a tyramide-based signal amplification method known as the *catalyzed reporter deposition (CARD)* or *catalyzed system amplification (CSA)* method.[18,19] All present-day clinical IHC is performed on automated instruments; hence, knowledge of the design of the amplification systems and postprimary options is critical for optimizing immunostains on a day-to-day basis.

Interpretive Problems

It is necessary to distinguish specific and non-specific signals when interpreting IHC. There are many sources of false-positive results, including endogenous biotin or peroxidase, inappropriately high antibody concentrations, poor technique (e.g., excessive antigen retrieval, drying artifacts, prolonged detection), or interpretive errors such as mistaking endogenous pigment for the chromogenic reaction product. Endogenous biotin reactivity can be a serious problem because of its variable occurrence in tumors. This biotin positivity is often amplified by retrieval techniques and presents as a granular pattern that can be difficult to distinguish from other granular cytoplasmic staining.[20] Failure to block biotin can lead to problems with interpretation and the reporting of false-positive results.[21,22] Use of one of the newer polymer-based detection systems that avoids the use of a biotin-avidin link can eliminate this problem. There are also myriad reasons for false-negative results, the most frequent of which are inadequate antigen retrieval, suboptimally fixed tissue, inappropriate primary antibody, or other technical staining issues.

It cannot be overemphasized that the accurate interpretation of IHC stains requires knowledge of the laboratory's methods, the antibodies used, and the expected staining pattern for each antibody. Different antibody preparations to the same antigen may show various patterns and intensities of non-specific or even specific staining. For instance, monoclonal antibodies targeting different epitopes of the Treg-associated marker FOXP3 have been shown to stain different subpopulations of cells in comparative studies in paraffin sections.[23] As another example, the anti–Ki-67 monoclonal antibody MIB-1 has been reported to stain the cell membrane of some tumor types, whereas other monoclonal antibodies to the same antigen do not show this type of aberrant staining.[24] Knowledge of the subcellular staining location of the targeted antigen is crucial, including nuclear, cytoplasmic, membranous, Golgi, and extracellular compartments and combinations of these stereotypical patterns (Fig. 3-1). An unexpected staining localization should immediately raise a red flag and should not be considered positive in any situation. For example, nucleolar staining for CD20 is seen when secondary antibody cross-reacts with nuclear histones, but non-specific staining in neutrophils may be seen for TIA1 in decalcified marrows.

Special Considerations for Immunostaining Bone Marrow Biopsies

Examination of bone marrow trephine biopsies is an integral component of the assessment of hematologic disorders and other diseases affecting hematopoiesis. It is particularly useful for the evaluation of marrow cellularity, cell distribution, and the relationship between different cell types. Its role is critical when evaluating patients with a "dry tap"—that is, when examination of the aspirate is unsuccessful owing to fibrosis or other infiltrative processes.

For tissue morphology to be preserved, the length and type of fixation, tissue processing, sectioning, and quality of staining are crucial. Decalcification procedures represent an additional variable that may influence the staining pattern and affect the preservation of antigenicity in IHC.[25] A variety of fixatives are available, including buffered formalin, mercury-containing solutions such as Zenker's or B5, or a combination based on acetic acid–zinc–formalin (AZF) as proposed by the Hammersmith protocol[26,27]; the last provides a morphologic quality comparable to B5, but with superior antigen and

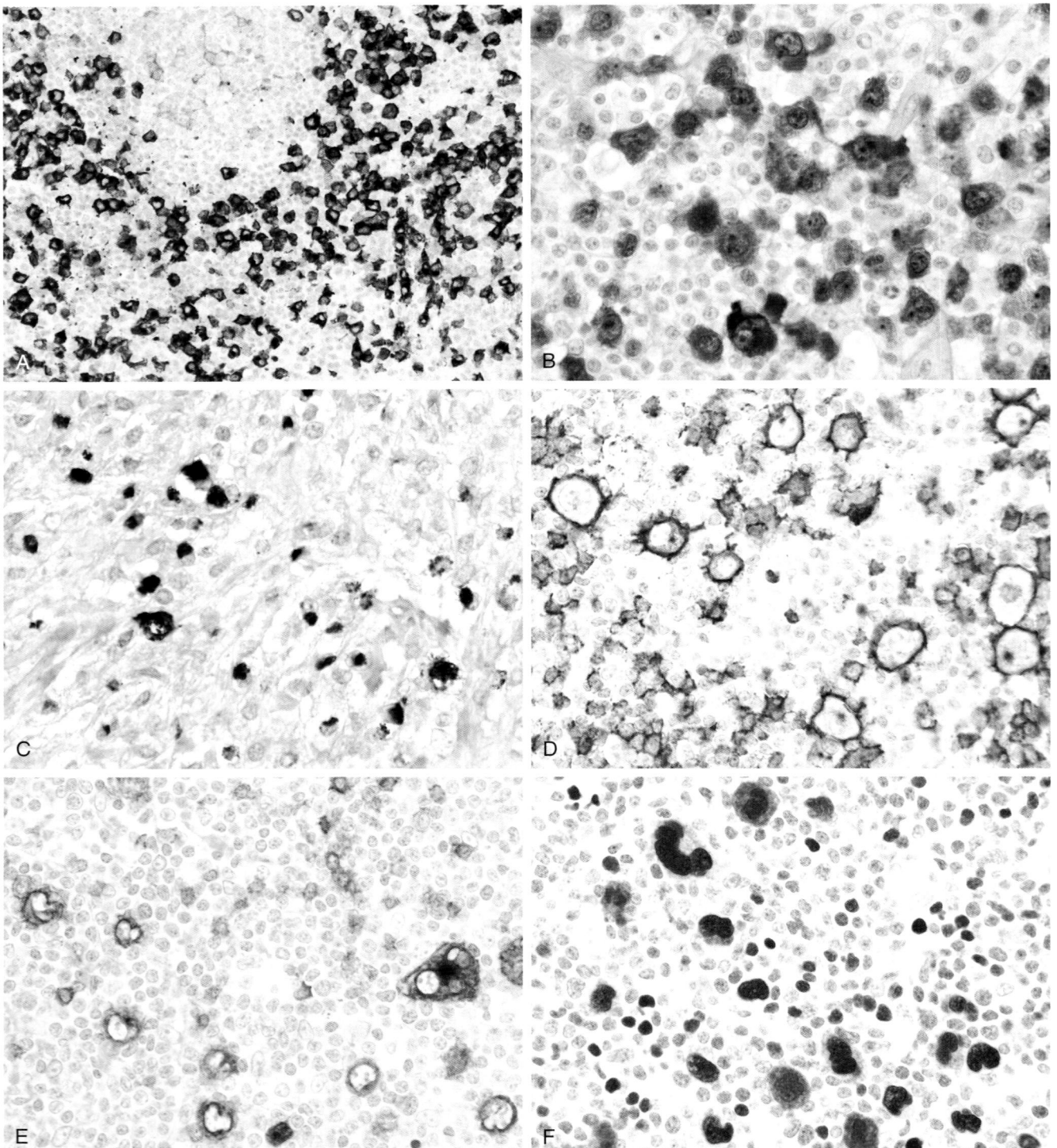

Figure 3-1 Representative patterns of cell-associated immunohistochemical staining in different cellular compartments (U-view/DAB detection, Ventana, Tucson, AZ; plus hematoxylin counterstain). **A-C,** Examples of immunohistochemical targeting of antigen expression in a case of anaplastic lymphoma kinase (ALK)-positive anaplastic large cell lymphoma. **A,** Membranous and Golgi staining pattern with a monoclonal antibody against CD30. **B,** Nuclear and cytoplasmic staining pattern characteristic of a monoclonal antibody against ALK. **C,** Cytoplasmic granular staining pattern characteristic of a monoclonal antibody against TIA-1. **D,** Membranous staining pattern with a monoclonal antibody against CD20 in nodular lymphocyte-predominant Hodgkin lymphoma. **E** and **F,** Examples of immunohistochemical targeting of antigen expression in a case of nodular lymphocyte-predominant Hodgkin lymphoma (termed more recently as nodular lymphocyte predominant B-cell lymphoma). **E,** Cytoplasmic staining pattern with membranous and perinuclear accentuation with a polyclonal antibody against immunoglobulin D. **F,** Nuclear and cytoplasmic staining with a monoclonal antibody against OCT-2.

Table 3-1 Recommended Immunohistochemistry Panels for Lymph Nodes and Lymphoma Diagnosis

Diagnostic Panel	Antibodies
Small B-cell lymphomas	CD20, CD79a, CD3, CD5, CD10, CD23, CD21, BCL2, BCL6, cyclin D1, IgD, kappa and lambda light chains, Ki-67, LEF1, MUM1, SOX11
Aggressive B-cell lymphomas	CD20, CD3, CD5, BCL2, BCL6, CD10, IRF4/MUM1, MYC, EBER ISH
Plasma cell neoplasms, plasmablastic neoplasms	CD20, CD79a, CD3, kappa and lambda light chains, Ig heavy chains, CD56, CD138, MUM1, ALK, EMA, EBER ISH, HHV8
Classic Hodgkin lymphoma	CD20, CD3, CD30, CD45, CD15, PAX5, OCT2, BOB.1, EBER ISH, LMP1
Nodular lymphocyte-predominant B-cell lymphoma	CD20, CD3, IgD, OCT-2, BCL6, CD21, PD-1
Peripheral T-cell lymphoma (nodal)	CD20, CD3, CD5, CD4, CD8, CD2, CD7, CD10, CD21, CD25, CD30, TIA-1, PD-1, BCL6, CXCL13, ICOS, ALK, EBER ISH
Peripheral T-cell lymphoma (extranodal)	CD20, CD3, CD5, CD4, CD8, CD2, CD7, CD25, CD30, CD56, TIA-1, granzyme B, β-F1, ALK, TCR delta, EBER ISH

nucleic acid preservation (if followed by formic acid decalcification).[26] Subsequent to fixation, the bone marrow trephine needs to undergo decalcification with either calcium-chelating agents such as EDTA or acid-based agents. EDTA decalcification usually lasts 48 to 72 hours; with acid-based solutions, the decalcifying time is shorter (1 to 2 hours or up to 6 hours when 10% formic acid and 5% formaldehyde are used). Usually, each laboratory has a standardized procedure whereby bone marrow biopsies are monitored during fixation and decalcification to ensure morphologic preservation and the best conditions for IHC and molecular techniques.

Since the introduction of antigen retrieval and improvements in decalcification, the number of antibodies that can be used on bone marrow trephine biopsies has grown dramatically from a few in the early 1990s to more than 100 today. The staining procedures and detection systems are similar to those already described for other formalin-fixed, paraffin-embedded tissue sections. The vast majority of antibodies used on lymph node biopsies can also be applied to bone marrow biopsies. Each IHC test that will be used on bone marrows should be specifically validated for that specimen type, with changes to optimize the protocol if necessary, prior to using it for clinical testing.

ANTIGENS OF HEMATOPATHOLOGIC INTEREST

The complexity of hematopathologic neoplasms parallels the complexity of the hematopoietic and immune cells from which they derive, and accurate diagnosis frequently requires the assessment of multiple diverse phenotypic markers. Commonly targeted markers include those related to cell lineage, degree of cellular differentiation, cell function, altered gene products associated with lymphomagenesis, and proliferative activity. The sum of this information allows the hematopathologist to categorize diseases in phenotypic groups that correspond to clinically relevant diagnostic entities. In addition to the characterization of lesional tumor cells, analysis of the microenvironment, which plays an important role during the development and differentiation of hematopoietic and immune cells, can provide diagnostic or prognostic information.

Immunohistochemical Characterization of Lymphoid Malignancies

The use of cell lineage and differentiation markers to assist in making a diagnosis is best illustrated with lymphomas; it has been predicated in large numbers of studies that have validated the concept that the various lymphoma subtypes arise from or at least appear to reflect different stages of normal lymphocyte development. Coordinated and unique programs of gene expression occur during both B-cell and T-cell differentiation, producing unique combinations of stage-specific protein expression that can be exploited by immunologic techniques, including IHC, to characterize these cell populations; these combinations can also be used to assist in the diagnosis of corresponding lymphomas.

In any given case, the panel of targets assessed by IHC should be based on the differential diagnosis formulated after a review of the section stained with hematoxylin and eosin. Successive panels should be ordered in a stepwise fashion to further refine the diagnosis based on initial results. Although this approach may delay the final diagnosis by 1 or 2 days, the process is cost-effective and efficient while still retaining adequate tissue for possible genetic studies (such as clonality studies and next-generation sequencing [NGS] [*MYD88*, *TP53* mutations] for lymphoplasmacytic lymphoma or mantle cell lymphoma [MCL], in which this is mandatory in the frontline setting). One should never order an IHC stain without an understanding of how the result will be used or how it will affect the diagnostic decision process. Table 3-1 outlines some recommended panels for lymph node diagnosis based on common diagnostic questions. The immunophenotypic characteristics of each of the entities are discussed in subsequent chapters; therefore, extensive discussion of the immunoprofiles of individual diseases is deferred.

For many hematopoietic tumors, tumor-associated oncogene products provide unique and sometimes specific targets for IHC interrogation, although their expression may not have diagnostic value; one such gene is *TP53*. *TP53* mutations or deletions have been described in numerous subtypes of mature B-cell and T-cell lymphomas, and they are usually considered a secondary event associated with a more aggressive clinical course. Especially in low-grade lymphomas such as chronic lymphocytic leukemia (CLL) and MCL, there is a critical need to assess *TP53* alterations either via fluorescence in situ hybridization (FISH) or NGS prior to therapy with Bruton's tyrosine kinase (BTK) inhibitors. Deletion of one allele of *TP53* is often associated with mutation in the other allele, resulting in strong P53 detectable by immuhistochemistry.[28,29] The exact thresholds of p53 immunopositivity that correlate with any underlying mutations (often missense mutations) vary across each lymphoma, and one must be aware of this before using binary cutoffs for p53 IHC.

Historically, one of the first examples of a tumor-associated oncogene product that proved useful in hematopathologic diagnosis was BCL2. BCL2 was discovered as a result of its involvement in the follicular lymphoma–associated t(14;18)(q32;q21) translocation, which juxtaposes the *BCL2* gene to the immunoglobulin heavy-chain locus, resulting in its overexpression.[30] BCL2 resides primarily on the mitochondrial membrane and is the prototypic member of a large family of apoptosis-related proteins.[31] Reactive germinal-center B cells do not express BCL2; therefore, detection of this protein is useful for distinguishing reactive from neoplastic follicles. Certain B-cell lymphomas may harbor mutations in the *BCL2* gene in regions encoding the portions of the protein recognized by the common clone 124. Such cases should be tested using an alternative BCL2 clone such as E17 or SP66 before determining BCL2 IHC to be negative.[32]

Overexpression of cyclin D1 as a result of the t(11;14)(q13;q34) translocation is the hallmark of MCL, involving the immunoglobulin heavy-chain locus and the *CCND1* locus located on 11q13.[33] Most MCL expresses strong cyclin D1 consequent to the translocation, allowing distinction from CLL and marginal zone lymphoma.[34] Cyclin D1 expression can also be detected in multiple myeloma carrying the t(11;14) translocation. Expression is also seen in hairy cell leukemia and Langerhans cell histiocytosis,[35] unrelated to a specific *IGH* translocation but rather consequent to upregulated mitogen-activated protein (MAP) kinase signaling. In addition to cyclin D1, antibodies to LEF1 and SOX11 have been developed and help support diagnoses of CLL and MCL, respectively, in the setting of atypical CD5-positive small to medium B-cell lymphoproliferations.[36]

B-cell lymphomas that have *MYC* gene rearrangements will almost invariably show strong MYC protein expression by IHC.[37] However, the identification of high-level MYC protein expression does not necessarily reflect an *MYC* rearrangement in all B-cell lymphomas, and it typically does not correlate with an *MYC* translocation in T-cell lymphomas.[38] Programmed death receptor-ligand 1 (PD-L1) amplifications are frequent in classic Hodgkin lymphoma and primary mediastinal large B-cell lymphoma, resulting in overexpression of PD-L1, although immunostaining for PD-L1 is not critical for diagnosis or prognosis in these settings.[39,40]

In contrast to the majority of translocations in B-cell lymphomas, the anaplastic large cell lymphoma (ALCL)–associated translocation involving the anaplastic lymphoma kinase *(ALK)* gene located on 2p23 results in a fusion protein with a variety of partner genes on different chromosomes.[41] The ALK protein is normally expressed only in the brain, so it is a highly specific target for diagnostic application. The most frequent translocation involves the *ALK* gene and the nucleophosmin *(NPM1)* gene encoding for a nucleolar phosphoprotein with a chaperone function. This leads to a fusion protein that contains the amino-terminal portion of *NPM1* fused to the intracytoplasmic portion, including the catalytic domain of the ALK protein. As a result of the t(2;5)(p23;q35) translocation, the ALK protein is expressed in the nucleus and cytoplasm of the malignant ALCL T cells and can be detected by monoclonal antibodies.[42] In cases with variant translocations, the staining pattern of ALK can be cytoplasmic or membranous; the latter staining pattern is usually associated with the t(2;X)(p23;q11-12) translocation involving the moesin *(MSN)* gene. The expression of ALK can also be detected in rare cases of diffuse large B-cell lymphoma with immunoblastic or plasmablastic features, but these cases usually show a granular cytoplasmic staining, lack CD30, express B-cell markers, and may be IgA positive. In addition, some non-hematopoietic neoplasms such as rhabdomyosarcomas, inflammatory myofibroblastic tumors, and a small subset of lung adenocarcinomas express ALK, but they are easily distinguished morphologically and immunophenotypically from ALCL. Expression of ALK is also prognostically relevant, as ALK-positive ALCLs have vastly superior outcomes with front cyclophosphamide, hydroxydaunorubicin, vincristine, and prednisone (CHOP)-based regimens compared with ALK-negative ALCLs.[43]

Evaluation of the proliferative rate of the lymphoid populations is also diagnostically useful in many settings. Among the proliferation markers, Ki-67 is by far the most widely targeted antigen in pathology. Although the original Ki-67 antibodies were not immunoreactive in formalin-fixed, paraffin-embedded tissue sections, other investigators were successful in generating the now widely used Ki-67 MIB-1 antibody clone. MIB-1 staining can assist in the distinction between follicular hyperplasia and follicular lymphoma; in the former, the reactive germinal centers have a higher proliferative rate with orderly polarization compared with low-grade follicular lymphomas.

Within a particular subtype of lymphoma, an increased number of actively proliferating tumor cells is usually associated with a more aggressive clinical course, although the prognostic significance of Ki-67 staining is not always consistent among studies. There are numerous possible explanations for the lack of concordance among studies, including technical variations and differences in scoring criteria and cutoff values.[44-46] MIB-1 staining is particularly sensitive to preanalytic factors related to fixation, decalcification (especially in bone marrow biopsies) and the type of antigen-retrieval procedure used. The poor reproducibility in diffuse large B-cell lymphoma is particularly evident in multicenter studies, where interlaboratory variations play a greater role, whereas the Ki-67 index tends to maintain its significance in defining high-risk groups in series published from single institutions.[45] Furthermore, when Ki-67 immunostaining was assessed in the context of the "proliferation signatures" generated by gene-expression studies in MCL, transformed follicular lymphoma, and nodal peripheral T-cell lymphoma, it has generally shown excellent correlation.[47-49] Along these lines, Ki-67 proliferation used in the MCL International Prognostic Index indicates three risk groups based on cut-off points of <10%, 10% to 30%, and >30%.[50]

Immunohistochemical Characterization of Myeloid Leukemias, Myelodysplastic Disorders, and Other Myeloproliferative Diseases

In the diagnosis of acute leukemias, immunophenotyping of bone marrow trephine biopsies is usually complementary to flow cytometry, which uses large panels to characterize the

Table 3-2 Recommended Panels for Bone Marrow Immunohistochemistry

Panel	Antibodies
Acute leukemias	CD34, CD117, TdT, CD3, CD19, CD20, CD10, MPO, CD33, CD61 (or CD42b), hemoglobin A, glycophorin A or C, PAX5; also CD123, NPM1, CD68, lysozyme, P53
MDS/MPN	CD34, CD117, CD61, MPO, CD33, mast cell tryptase, hemoglobin A
Plasma cell disorders	CD138, kappa, lambda, CD56, CD20, cyclin D1
Histiocytic (macrophage or dendritic) neoplasms	CD4, CD11c, CD14, CD68, CD163, S100, OCT2, CD1a, CD207 (langerin), lysozyme, BRAF V600E, cyclin D1
Mastocytosis	Mast cell tryptase, CD117, CD25, CD2; also CD34, CD3, CD20

MDS/MPN, Myelodysplastic syndrome/myeloproliferative neoplasms.

neoplastic populations, identify their lineages, and detect aberrant antigenic expression patterns that can be used in diagnosis and to monitor residual or recurrent disease (see Table 3-2 for a list of useful panels). The role of IHC in most immature myeloid and lymphoid neoplasms is valuable in two scenarios: (1) testing antigens not widely examined by flow cytometry (such as mutant NPM1, p53 IHC) or (2) to quantitate disease burden in hemodilute marrow aspirate samples consequent to fibrosis (such as CD34 in fibrotic myeloid neoplasms, CD138 kappa/lambda in myeloma). Another situation arises in patients treated with targeted agents such as anti-CD19 (blinatumomab), anti-CD22 (inotuzumab), and anti-CD38 (daratumumab), when flow antibodies targeting these antigens are unable to detect surface expression of these antigens, thereby necessitating alternate immunostains (CD138, CD79a, kappa, lambda) for detection of minimal disease.

The identification of blasts is critical in the characterization of all potential leukemias and myelodysplastic/myeloproliferative disorders, and this is easily achieved with antibodies against CD34 and CD117. However, it should be noted that, in about 25% of cases of acute myeloid leukemia (AML), the blasts do not express CD34. The addition of myeloperoxidase (MPO), glycophorin A or C, hemoglobin, and CD61 is helpful for assessing the distribution and number of different cell types and to identify morphologically abnormal forms such as micromegakaryocytes.

A panel including CD34, TdT, MPO, CD33, CD68 (KP-1 and PGM-1), glycophorin A, CD61, CD20, CD79a, PAX5, CD3, and CD1a is useful to distinguish AML from lymphoblastic leukemia. In cases with monocytic differentiation, additional markers include CD11c, CD14, CD64, CD4, CD163, and lysozyme. In AML, immunophenotyping can be used to identify specific subgroups. Typically, AML with the t(8;21) (q22;q22) translocation is characterized by expression of CD34, CD13, CD33, MPO, and human leukocyte antigen (HLA)-DR and often aberrantly co-expresses CD56 and the B-cell markers PAX5, CD79a, and CD19, whereas AML with the t(15;17)(q22;q12) translocation typically expresses myeloid antigens, MPO, CD13, and CD33; lacks expression of HLA-DR; shows negative to weak CD34; and may aberrantly coexpress CD2, particularly in the microgranular variant.[51] Aberrant co-expression of CD2 can also frequently be seen in AML with the inv(16) or t(16;16) translocation and thus is not specific to a particular AML subtype. Immunostains for p53 and mutated NPM1 are becoming relevant as reliable surrogates of entities with underlying mutations in the respective genes, *TP53* and *NPM1.*[52,53]

Immunohistochemical Characterization of Histiocytic, Dendritic, Mast Cell, and Other Tumor Cell Types

The neoplastic cells of histiocytic sarcoma may express macrophage or dendritic cell antigens such as CD68, CD163, CD11c, CD14, lysozyme, CD4 and PU.1.[54,55] As many of these markers are not lineage specific, expression of at least two markers is recommended to confirm a histiocytic phenotype. Several markers are useful in the differential diagnosis of Langerhans cell proliferations (CD1a, CD207 [langerin], BRAF-V600E, and cyclin D1)[35] and follicular dendritic cell sarcoma (CD21, CD35, CXCL13, clusterin).[56]

All mast cell proliferations can be identified by IHC with an antibody against mast cell tryptase (also effective on bone marrow specimens), irrespective of their degree of maturation.[57] However, CD117 on bone marrow biopsies is particularly useful to identify early erythroid precursors, promyelocytes, and mast cells (which stain rather strongly). Most cases of systemic mastocytosis can be picked up using an initial CD117, but additional CD25 helps confirm neoplastic phenotype in mast cells.

The tumor cells of the blastic plasmacytoid dendritic cell neoplasm express CD4, CD43, and CD56 in addition to CD123 and TCL-1/TCF4.[58]

BEYOND DIAGNOSTICS: THE EVOLVING ROLE OF IMMUNOHISTOCHEMISTRY

Until recently, IHC had primarily been a tool for pathologists to assist in the differential diagnosis of specific disease entities. However, the role of IHC has been evolving and its application is becoming much broader. The information the IHC laboratory provides now extends well beyond diagnostics, contributing prognostic and predictive information and informing therapeutic decision-making. These newer roles of IHC have been created by rapid advances in three areas: (1) progress in our understanding of molecular mechanisms that underlie tumor cell biology, including host tumor interactions, (2) identification of cancer-associated mutations in critical genes involved in cell growth, and (3) rapid development of targeted cancer therapies. We now know many of the genes implicated in the majority of human cancers and the precise molecular aberrations affecting those genes. We have a much better understanding of the intricate molecular mechanisms used by tumors to evade the immune response. This increase in our understanding of cancer biology has provided a foundation for the rapid development of targeted cancer therapies. Precise identification of the specific cellular lesions is required in each instance for selection of the correct drug. IHC has a major role in meeting this requirement, whether it is identifying a mutated oncogene, a cell surface molecular target for a therapeutic antibody or cytotoxic T cell, or a critical molecule involved in suppression of immune responses.

Rituximab (anti-CD20) was the first widely applied antibody-directed targeted therapy used for lymphoma. Although hematopathologists initially used anti-CD20 antibodies as a diagnostic tool to identify B-cell lymphomas, verification of CD20 expression soon became a requirement for treatment with the therapeutic antibody. Today, multiple cell surface antigens have been targeted by antibodies in B-cell and T-cell neoplasias, with varying degrees of success, including CD20, CD22, CD19, CD138, CD2, CD3, CD4, CD52, CD25, CD30, and CD194 (CCR4).[59-61] In some cases, the therapeutic antibodies are "naked" or unconjugated (e.g., rituximab), but in other cases, the antibodies may be structurally modified to activate effector functions (e.g., anti-CCR4) or conjugated to a radiochemical or toxin (e.g., antibodies to CD22, CD25, and CD30) to elicit target-cell killing. In addition to the cell-lineage–specific or B-cell/T-cell–restricted antigens, antibodies to markers such as CD123[62] and CD30 have been developed and are currently in clinical trials. Trials with toxin-conjugated antibodies to CD30 (brentuximab vedotin) in both Hodgkin lymphoma and T-cell neoplasms such as ALCL and ATL have shown promising results.[63,64]

Similarly, genetically engineered T-cell transfer immunotherapy using chimeric antigen receptor (CAR) is becoming more common, and protocols targeting CD19 and CD22 have been developed for the treatment of B-cell neoplasms expressing these antigens.[65] In particular, data from CD19 CAR T-cell trials in B-cell acute lymphoblastic leukemia (B-ALL) and CLL have been encouraging.[66] Similar trials targeting the plasma cell antigen B-cell maturation antigen (BCMA) have shown promising results thus far in multiple myeloma and other plasma cell neoplasms.[67] As serum BCMA is easily measured prior to trial enrollment, immunostaining for BCMA has not gained traction.

New research into the immune checkpoints (ICs) that control the reactivity of cytotoxic T cells against self-antigens coupled with the concurrent development of therapeutic antibodies that interfere with these IC proteins has provided pathologists with a completely different set of antigenic targets to evaluate. Programmed death receptor-1 (PD-1) and its ligand (PD-L1) are two checkpoint proteins that have gained attention.[68] Especially for PD-L1, several antibody clones have been developed and received U.S. Food and Drug Administration approval as companion diagnostic tests. Testing for PD-L1 via IHC and quantitation of tumor and immune cell expression of PD-L1 has been critical for solid tumors, including lung and bladder cancer, where there is a significant linear correlation between expression and response to IC inhibitors. In the realm of hematopathology, many B-cell lymphomas have been shown to harbor PD-L1 alterations, including classic Hodgkin lymphoma and primary mediastinal large B-cell lymphoma. Pembrolizumab and nivolumab are two widely used IC inhibitors that have shown promising results for relapse and even as front-line treatment.[69] Testing for PD-L1 via IHC is not critical to determine eligibility for IC inhibitor therapy in most lymphomas. However, data indicates that PD-L1 addicted non-germinal center diffuse large B-cell lymphoma (DLBCL) (detected via IHC) may benefit from adding IC inhibitors to an R-CHOP backbone.[70]

Knowledge of the molecular pathways and genetic lesions responsible for tumor cell growth provides investigators and oncologists with yet a different set of signaling pathways and proteins to inhibit, and for pathologists, another set of targets to evaluate. There are clinically useful antibodies that are commercially available and capable of identifying mutations in several genes (BRAF V600E is a notable one). BRAF V600E mutations occur in nearly all cases of hairy cell leukemia and in over 50% of cases of Langerhans cell histiocytosis and Erdheim-Chester disease. The IHC laboratory can play a critical role in identifying the presence of this mutation. The BRAF inhibitor, vemurafenib, has shown durable response in Langerhans cell histiocytosis, Erdheim-Chester disease, and hairy cell leukemia.[71,72] Antibodies to IDH1 R132H are also available and can be used to identify cases of AML known to carry this mutation.[73] Newer antibodies to less common IDH1 variants and to IDH2 R172 mutations, common in both AML and in angioimmunoblastic T-cell lymphoma (AITL), have already been reported in the literature (Fig. 3-2).[74] Other common mutations that are potentially amenable to IHC targeting include the JAK2 V617F mutation, which is common in a variety of myeloproliferative diseases, and the MYD88 L265P mutation, which is characteristic of lymphoplasmacytic lymphoma (LPL) and a fraction of marginal zone lymphomas and the activated B-cell subtype of DLBCL.

IN SITU HYBRIDIZATION

Although this chapter's focus is IHC, a few words regarding the role of in situ hybridization (ISH) in hematopathology are warranted. These technologies have similarities in that they both interrogate targets in situ—that is, on frozen or paraffin-embedded tissue sections—and they have similar detection systems. The type of target and the chemistry of its identification are the major differences. ISH is a simple and sensitive technique that permits direct assessment of DNA or RNA targets within tissue sections (both frozen and formalin-fixed), single-cell suspensions, and cytogenetic preparations, whereas IHC targets proteins.

The application of ISH in hematopathology is particularly useful when antibodies are not available, have limited sensitivity, or are associated with high background staining (e.g., kappa and lambda light chain immunostains).[75] It may also be indicated when proteins are rapidly secreted and are not stored within cells or when nucleic acids are more abundant than proteins. The major technical limitations are related to the abundance and preservation of target sequences within cells; thus, preanalytic factors such as fixation and tissue processing can have a significant effect on target-sequence detection by ISH.

Similar to IHC, a primary incubation is performed, substituting DNA or RNA probes instead of a primary antibody. Reactivity (hybridization) is based on complementarity between the sequence of interest and the designed probe, rather than on antigen-antibody recognition. Detection of the annealed products was originally based on the use of

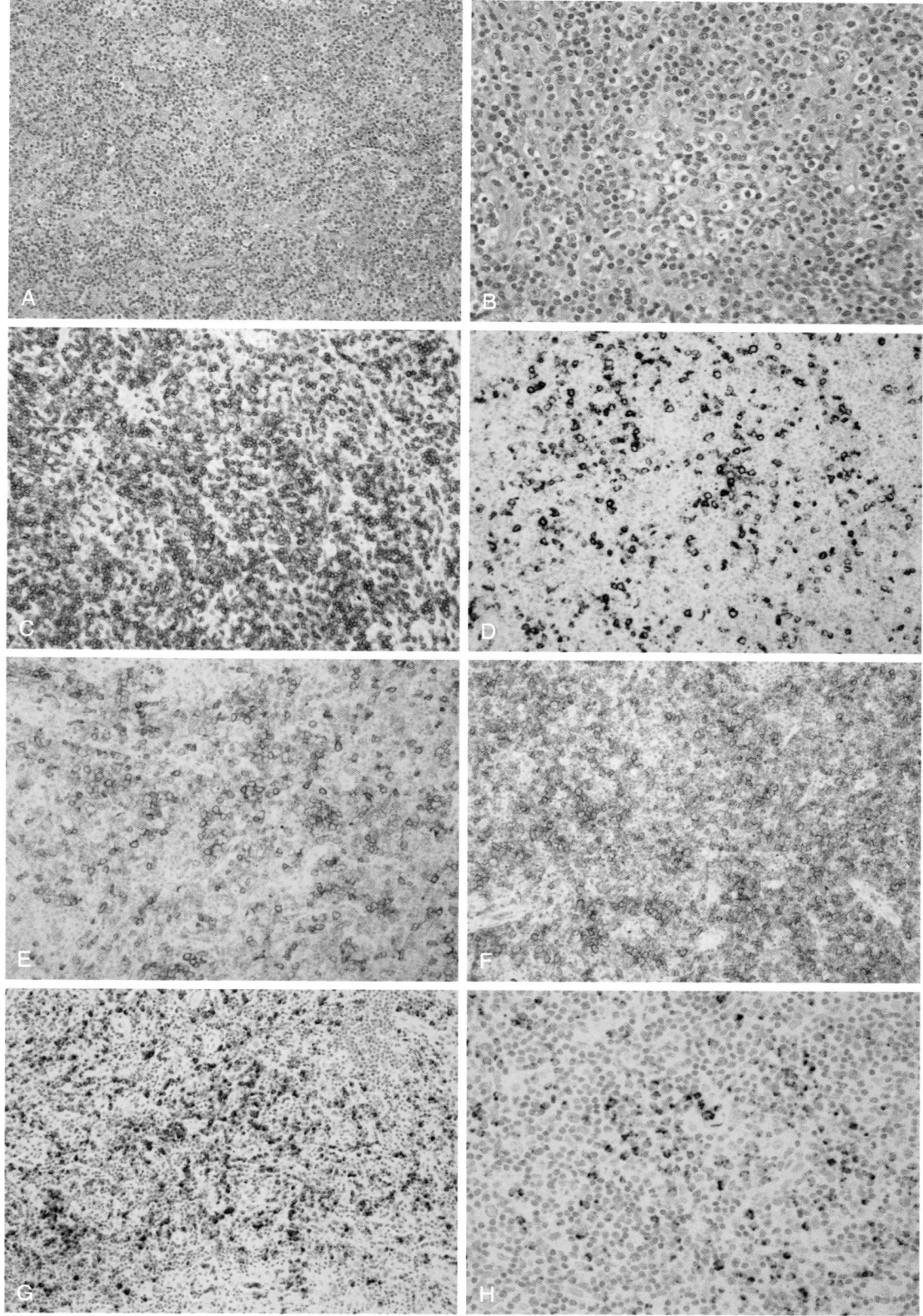

Figure 3-2 **Immunostains in T-follicular helper (TFH)-cell neoplasm.** **A and B,** Low-power and medium-power images depicting angioim-munoblastic T-cell lymphoma with a polymorphic population of small-sized to medium-sized lymphoid cells. **C,** These lymphoma cells are positive for CD3 and express TFH markers, including **D,** CD10 (abnormal and bright); **E,** programmed death receptor-1 (PD-1); **F,** ICOS; and **G,** CXCL13. Although not shown, there is focal expression of BCL6, which also supports TFH designation. Most nodal TFH lymphomas harbor mutations related to the DNA methylation pathway *(DNMT3A, TET2)* in addition to *RHOA* and, frequently, *IDH2*. **H,** The cells are immunopositive for antibody specific to mutant *IDH2* R172K.

radiolabeled probes, which were visualized by slide emulsion autoradiography. Currently, especially in the clinical setting, radioisotopes have been replaced by nonisotopic detection methods. In chromogen-based ISH (CISH), a biotin-labeled or digoxigenin-labeled probe is detected with a secondary antibody and a chromogenic detection system similar to that in IHC. In FISH techniques, signals are detected with a fluorophore-labeled probe in a darkfield setting. These methods offer significant advantages over radioisotope-based ISH, including improved probe stability without waste-disposal issues (other than DAB), shortened assay time, excellent sensitivity, superior tissue preservation, and more accurate subcellular localization.

The primary CISH assay used by hematopathologists is for the detection of kappa and lambda immunoglobulin light chains as an assessment of B-cell clonality. Indications for its use are limited to situations in which IHC is not feasible, such as when there is high background in the IHC stain owing to the presence of high levels of interstitial immunoglobulins from serum or when there is high expression of immunoglobulin light chain proteins, such as in some plasma cell dyscrasias or B-cell neoplasms showing plasmacytic differentiation. The applicability of CISH for kappa and lambda detection extends to bone marrow sections. ISH in some settings is preferable to kappa or lambda IHC because the problem of background staining from serum immunoglobulins is eliminated. However, sensitivity with current probes is not necessarily increased. Use of optimized antigen-retrieval techniques can reduce the high background staining seen in light chain IHC and can permit identification of light chain restriction in up to 80% of B-cell lymphomas.[76]

CISH is also widely used for the detection of infectious agents, particularly viruses, within cells or tissues. One of the most common clinical CISH tests is the detection of Epstein-Barr virus (EBV) in infected cells. In this test, the targets are EBV-encoded RNAs (EBERs), which are short nuclear transcripts that are present early in latent infection and in high copy number (approximately 10 copies/cell). Because of these characteristics and their minimal homology to cellular RNA, EBERs are an excellent target for the detection of EBV-infected cells by ISH on formalin-fixed, paraffin-embedded tissue sections and are preferable to the commonly used IHC target, latent membrane protein (LMP). From an interpretive perspective, pathologists must always make sure that intact RNA is detectable in the tissue of interest using the polyuridine probe against the poly A tail of mRNA ("RNA control").

APPROACH TO USING IMMUNOHISTOCHEMISTRY

There is wide variation in the use of IHC in the context of hematopoietic neoplasms. In general, for leukemic processes

where the majority of phenotyping is performed via flow cytometry, additional immunostains performed on the core biopsy should only reflect markers not performed by flow cytometric analysis (NPM1, P53, etc.). In the context of lymphomas, beyond flow cytometry, c-Myc, Bcl-2, Ki-67, cyclin D1, and CD30 are useful in the context of B-cell lymphomas. However, additional immunostains may be required in the case of nodal T-cell lymphomas, especially with small cell cytomorphology, as flow cytometry may not pick abnormal T-cell populations that could easily be missed. Multiple iterative rounds of immunostains based on diagnostic possibilities in sync with the clinical picture is the most ideal approach toward using immunostains. Familiarity with patterns of staining with specific markers (Fig. 3-3) and awareness of the pitfalls (Fig. 3-4) are both critical for effective use of IHC in diagnostic hematopathology. Table 3-3 lists top-level, high-yield immunostain panels (of up to eight markers per scenario) targeting differential diagnostic possibilities in three different scenarios (elderly pancytopenia, blastic processes, and recurrent reactive adenopathy) commonly encountered by most practicing hematopathologists.

Pearls and Pitfalls

- Always use coated or charged slides and bake the slides for 1 or preferably 2 hours at 60° C to enhance tissue adhesion.
- Cut paraffin tissue sections may lose their antigenicity over time. Unstained slides expire after 3 months.
- Once the primary antibody is applied, do not allow the section to dry, or non-specific staining will occur.
- Inconsistent results are most frequently caused by poor control over preanalytic parameters, especially the antigen-retrieval step.
- Antigen-retrieval conditions vary depending on the target antigen. Nuclear antigens often benefit from high pH retrieval, though membrane antigens are better with low pH (pH 6) protocols.
- Overdigestion or excess HIER may result in non-specific staining or unacceptable morphology.
- Positive and negative controls should be run with all test cases, but, for some lymphoid specimens, the tissue itself may serve as an internal control owing to the presence of normal hematolymphoid elements.
- Positive control tissues should express low levels of the target antigen so that immunoreactivity can be appropriately assessed to ensure optimal sensitivity.
- Controls should be handled in the same preanalytic manner as patient samples in terms of fixation and processing.
- Avoid interpreting interstitial staining as membranous. This frequently happens with IgG, kappa, and lambda immunostains (see Table 3-4 for additional technical and interpretive points on some antibodies).
- The absence of staining may be real, whereas diffuse staining of all tissue elements is likely to be an artifact.

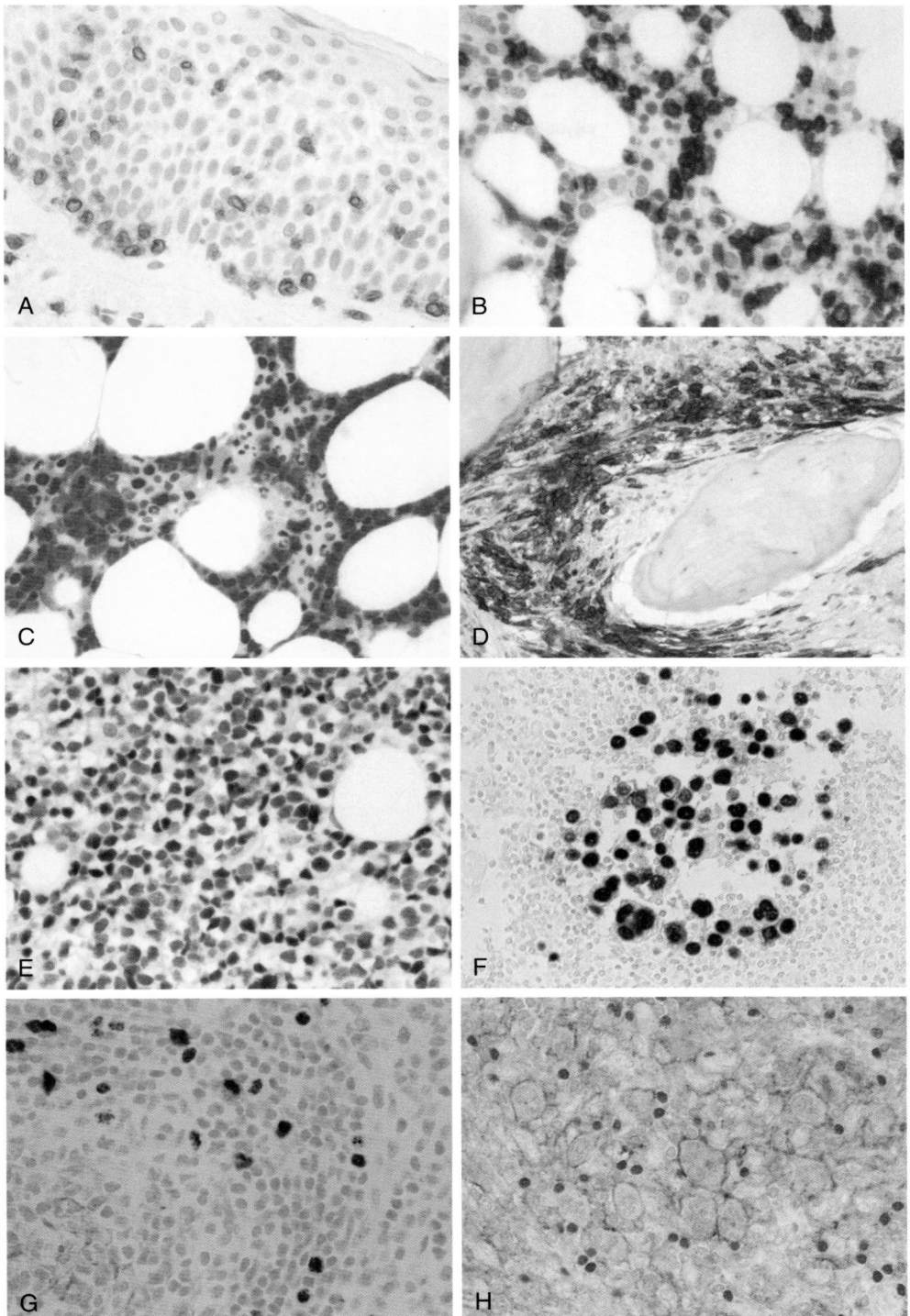

Figure 3-3 Staining patterns useful in immunochemistry diagnosis. A, CD3 immunohistochemistry decorating abnormal CD3-positive T cells in a "string of pearls" pattern in a skin biopsy with mycosis fungoides. Oftentimes, these abnormal cells are scarce and visible only on immunohistochemistry; hence, a high degree of clinical suspicion is necessary. **B,** Sinusoidal CD8-positive T-cell infiltrate in a patient with T-cell large granular lymphocytic leukemia. These infiltrates are often not visible on the hematoxylin and eosin slide, so CD3 and CD8 immunostains are useful in patients with pancytopenia. **C,** Mutant NPM1-specific immunohistochemistry in a patient with *NPM1* exon 12 mutation showing abnormal cytoplasmic staining of blastic cells. Scattered cells with wild-type isolated nuclear staining are seen in the center of the biopsy. **D,** CD117-positive paratrabecular clusters of spindly mast cells in systemic mastocytosis. CD25 is additionally useful to corroborate neoplastic phenotype in mast cells. **E,** Strong p53 expression in a patient with hypodiploid precursor B-cell acute lymphoblastic leukemia with Li-Fraumeni syndrome. Strong expression usually correlates with underlying missense mutations. **F,** Epstein-Barr virus in situ hybridization (EBER) expression in neoplastic germinal center B cells in a patient with germinotropic lymphoproliferative disorder. **G,** Scattered single HHV8-positive plasmablasts within the mantle zones of a secondary lymphoid follicle with regression in a patient with HIV-related HHV8-positive multicentric Castleman disease. The cells additionally expressed IgM with monotypic lambda light chain. **H,** Double immunostain for programmed death receptor-ligand 1 (PD-L1) *(brown)*/PAX5 *(red)* in a patient with classic Hodgkin lymphoma. The Hodgkin cells express weak PAX5 with membranous expression of PD-L1 while the surrounding normal small B cells express strong PAX5 without membranous staining for PD-L1.

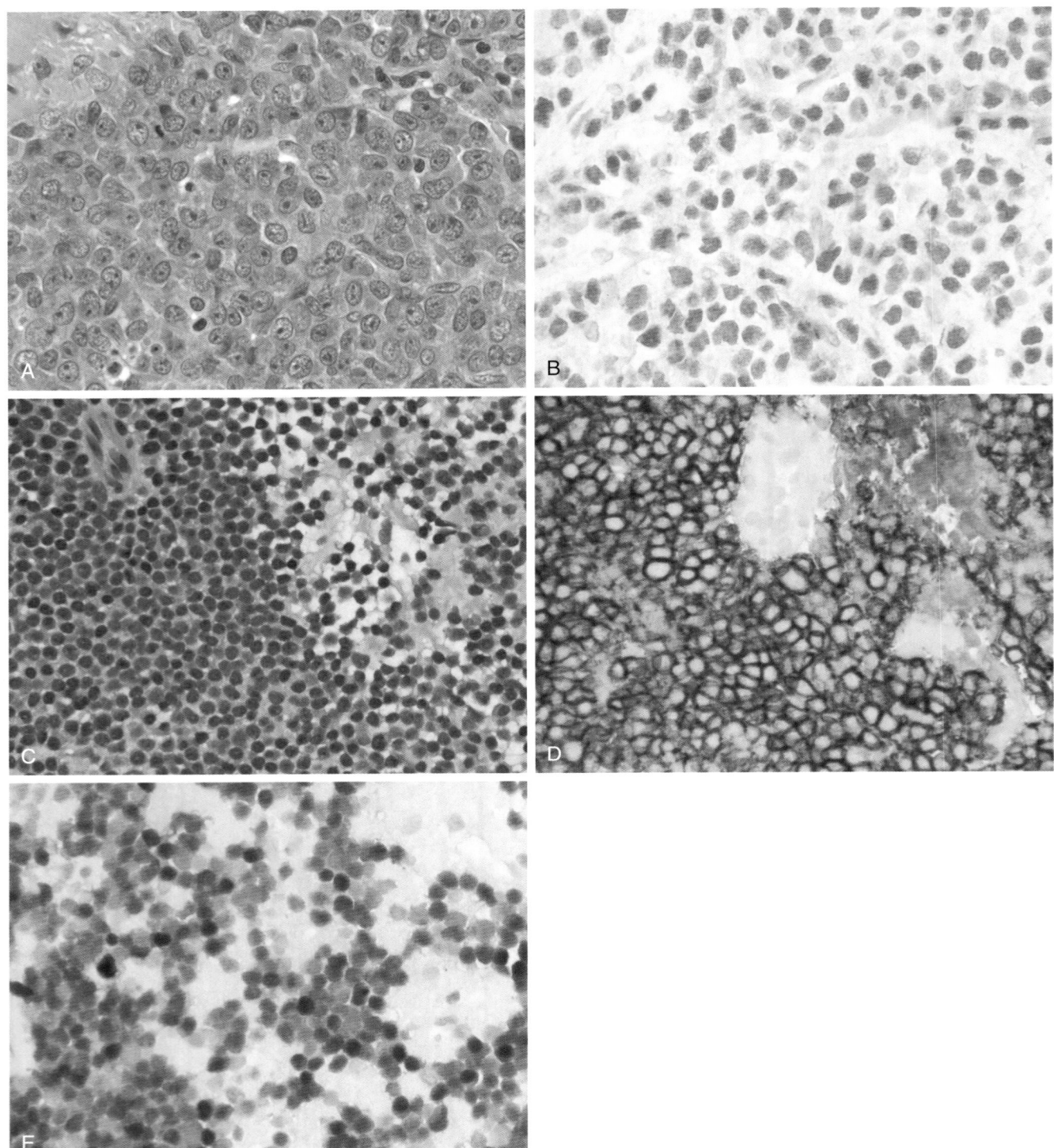

Figure 3-4 Pitfalls in immunohistochemistry. A, Medium-sized to large-sized monomorphic infiltrate of blastic cells in extramedullary soft tissue mass. **B,** The cells in this case express uniform PAX5, giving the impression of B lymphoblastic leukemia. However, there was underlying *RUNX1-RUNX1T1* fusion with expression of myeloid markers, confirming the diagnosis of acute myeloid leukemia (AML) with t(8;21). Rarely, these tumors may also express weak CD19; one must be careful not to make a diagnosis of mixed phenotype acute leukemia, B/ myeloid. **C-E,** Second case with extramedullary involvement by sheets of medium-sized lymphoid cells **(C).** The cells are strongly positive for CD20 (not shown) based on strong staining for cyclin D1 **(E).** This was initially thought to be mantle cell lymphoma, but additional CD138 expression **(D)** was strongly positive with expression of CD56, warranting reclassification as myeloma expressing cyclin D1. Often, myeloma expressing cyclin D1 is known to express CD20 in addition to PAX5 with frequent lymphocyte-like cytomorphology, posing diagnostic confusion.

Table 3-3 Common Clinical and Morphologic Scenarios, Respective Top Differentials, and Pertinent First Round of Immunostains

Presenting Features	Differential	Key Top-Level Stains
Elderly pancytopenia (BM)	MDS	CD34, P53
	HCL/SMZL/THRBCL	CD20
	T-negative LGL leukemia	CD3
	HLH	CD30 (ALCL), EBER
Adenopathy (reactive)	EBV reactivation	EBER
	CMV infection	CMV
	IgG4-related adenopathy	IgG4
Blastoid infiltrate	AML	CD33, CD34, NPM1
	ALL (B-cell and T-cell)	CD3, PAX5, TdT
	BPDCN	CD123
	Plasmablastic lymphoma	MUM1, CD138
	Blastoid lymphoma (MCL, Burkitt)	CD20, Cyclin D1, MYC (>80%)

ALCL, Anaplastic large cell lymphoma; *ALL,* acute lymphoblastic leukemia/lymphoma; *BPDCN,* blastic plasmacytoid dendritic cell neoplasm; *EBV,* Epstein-Barr virus; *HCL,* hairy cell leukemia; *HLH,* hemophagocytic lymphohistiocytosis; *LGL,* large granular lymphocytic; *MCL,* mantle cell lymphoma; *MDS,* myelodysplastic syndrome; *SMZL,* splenic marginal zone lymphoma; *THRBCL,* T-cell/histiocyte-rich large B-cell lymphoma.

Table 3-4 Specific Technical and Interpretive Pearls With Respect to Common Antibodies and Antibody Combinations in Hematopathology

Antibody	Pearls/Pitfalls to Remember
CD20	About the only B-cell marker that works well, even on necrotic tissues.
OCT2	Useful for nodular lymphocyte predominant B-cell lymphoma and plasmablastic processes that lose B-cell antigens
CD3	Often aberrantly positive in HHV8-positive B-cell lymphomas
CD45	Not a great marker for hematopoietic neoplasms such as plasmablastic lymphoma and ALCL; often can be negative in these
Cyclin D1	Useful for MCL, cyclin D1-positive myeloma, HCL, and LCH
CD34	Separate protocols may be needed for bone marrow to stain blasts
CD5	Look for biphasic dim staining in CLL and bright staining in T cells
MUM1	Great stain to identify rare classic Hodgkin cells after therapy/relapse
IgG4/EBER/CMV	Useful trio for seemingly reactive large nodes in the right setting
EBER ISH	Do not order on very necrotic tissues, as RNA is degraded. IHC for EBV-LMP1 or EBNA2 is useful in this setting.
HHV8	Always check HIV history and order before dismissing as a reactive node

ALCL, Anaplastic large cell lymphoma; *CLL,* chronic lymphocytic leukemia; *EBNA2,* Epstein-Barr virus nuclear antigen 2; *EBV-LMP1,* Epstein-Barr virus latent membrane protein 1; *HCL,* hairy cell leukemia; *IHC,* immunohistochemistry; *LCH,* Langerhans cell histiocytosis; *MCL,* mantle cell lymphoma.

KEY REFERENCES

1. Alaggio R, Amador C, Anagnostopoulos I, et al. The 5th edition of the World Health Organization classification of haematolymphoid tumours: lymphoid neoplasms. *Leukemia.* 2022;36(7):1720–1748.

2. Arber DA, Orazi A, Hasserjian RP, et al. International Consensus Classification of myeloid neoplasms and acute leukemias: integrating morphologic, clinical, and genomic data. *Blood.* 2022;140(11):1200–1228.

11. Taylor CR, Shi SR, Chaiwun B, et al. Strategies for improving the immunohistochemical staining of various intranuclear prognostic markers in formalin-paraffin sections: androgen receptor, estrogen receptor, progesterone receptor, p53 protein, proliferating cell nuclear antigen, and Ki-67 antigen revealed by antigen retrieval techniques. *Hum Pathol.* 1994;25(3):263–270.

15. Kohler G, Milstein C. Continuous cultures of fused cells secreting antibody of predefined specificity. *Nature.* 1975;256(5517):495–497.

27. Naresh KN, Lampert I, Hasserjian R, et al. Optimal processing of bone marrow trephine biopsy: the Hammersmith Protocol. *J Clin Pathol.* 2006;59(9):903–911.

32. Adam P, Baumann R, Schmidt J, et al. The BCL2 E17 and SP66 antibodies discriminate 2 immunophenotypically and genetically distinct subgroups of conventionally BCL2-"negative" grade 1/2 follicular lymphomas. *Hum Pathol.* 2013;44(9):1817–1826.

45. de Jong D, Xie W, Rosenwald A, et al. Immunohistochemical prognostic markers in diffuse large B-cell lymphoma: validation of tissue microarray as a prerequisite for broad clinical applications (a study from the Lunenburg Lymphoma Biomarker Consortium). *J Clin Pathol.* 2009;62(2):128–138.

51. Ossenkoppele GJ, van de Loosdrecht AA, Schuurhuis GJ. Review of the relevance of aberrant antigen expression by flow cytometry in myeloid neoplasms. *Br J Haematol.* 2011;153(4):421–436.

72. Evseev D, Kalinina I, Raykina E, et al. Vemurafenib provides a rapid and robust clinical response in pediatric Langerhans cell histiocytosis with the BRAF V600E mutation but does not eliminate low-level minimal residual disease per ddPCR using cell-free circulating DNA. *Int J Hematol.* 2021;114(6):725–734.

76. Marshall-Taylor CE, Cartun RW, Mandich D, et al. Immunohistochemical detection of immunoglobulin light chain expression in B-cell non-Hodgkin lymphomas using formalin-fixed, paraffin-embedded tissues and a heat-induced epitope retrieval technique. *Appl Immunohistochem Mol Morphol.* 2002;10(3):258–262.

Visit Elsevier eBooks+ for the complete set of references.

Chapter 4

Flow Cytometry

Constance M. Yuan, Sindhu Cherian, and Hao-Wei Wang

Multiparametric flow cytometry (FCM) is invaluable in the diagnosis and classification of hematolymphoid neoplasms, determining prognosis, and monitoring response to therapy. FCM is especially suited for immunophenotypic analysis of blood, fluids (e.g., cerebrospinal fluid [CSF], pleural fluid), and aspirations of bone marrow and lymphoid tissue. FCM is also ideal in small samples; its multiparametric nature allows the concurrent staining of cells with multiple antibodies complexed to different fluorochromes, thus maximizing data obtained from few cells. FCM can characterize surface, cytoplasmic, or nuclear antigen expression. Furthermore, FCM can provide highly accurate quantitation of cellular antigens/molecules. With increasing use of antigen-directed targeted therapies such as rituximab, ofatumumab (anti-CD20), epratuzumab, inotuzumab (anti-CD22), gemtuzumab (anti-CD33), and blinatumomab (CD19-directed CD3 T-cell engager) and cellular therapies, including T cells genetically engineered to express chimeric antigen receptors (CAR T cells), the use of FCM is likely to increase. FCM identifies therapeutic targets on the surface of malignant cells, thus informing the potential utility of antibody-targeted therapy in a given patient. Once a diagnosis is established, FCM provides high sensitivity in the detection of minimal/measurable disease (MRD). FCM can detect MRD with a sensitivity of 1 in 10^4 to 10^6, allowing for a precise assessment of disease progression and/or the effect of prior therapy and providing valuable prognostic information.

GENERAL PRINCIPLES

In a flow cytometer, cells rapidly pass single file through a series of finely focused lasers. The cell momentarily breaks the laser beam as it passes, scattering light at a low angle (also called *forward scatter*). This forward scatter/low-angle scatter (FSC) is proportional to the cell volume/size. Laser light is simultaneously scattered at a high/wide-angle (*side scatter* [SSC]) by intracellular and nuclear components. This SSC is proportional to the complexity of a cell, which is determined by the type and amount of cytoplasmic granularity, cytoplasmic membrane irregularities (e.g., villous or "hairy-appearing" projections), and nuclear characteristics. Light scatter characteristics are also useful in restricting analysis to single cells (e.g., excluding doublets [two adherent cells]). These physical scatter properties accurately identify cell types and are the basis for many commercial hematology analyzers that provide automated differential cell counts.[1]

In addition to FSC and SSC properties, cells are further characterized by staining with multiple fluorescent markers, such as antibodies conjugated to fluorochromes or DNA-binding dyes. An antigen on the cell surface binds to a fluorochrome-conjugated antibody, which emits light at a particular wavelength that is measured by detectors. When used in combination with DNA-binding dyes, the DNA content can also be determined, yielding cell cycle data. Multiple fluorochromes (sometimes referred to as *colors*), each with uniquely identifiable spectral emissions, are simultaneously measured with multiple detectors. Most clinical laboratories use six-color to eight-color FCM, with some using 10 or more colors.[2] Four is generally considered the minimally acceptable number of colors to ensure reliable discrimination of neoplastic cell populations in a broad range of sample types.[3,4]

Traditionally, FCM was used to determine the presence or absence of lineage-specific or lineage-associated antigens; however, immunophenotypic interpretation has evolved from a simplistic "positive" or "negative" approach for a given antigen to an assessment of the degree and pattern of antigen expression. This approach is highly reliable in discriminating cell types and identifies characteristic immunophenotypic features and patterns unique to certain hematolymphoid neoplasms. The antigen expression of many hematolymphoid neoplasms overlap with their normal counterparts, making diagnosis a challenge. The ability of multiparametric FCM to highlight subtle differences in the patterns of antigen expression (aberrant antigen expression or changes in intensity, for instance) makes it extremely powerful in the diagnosis of neoplasia.

TECHNICAL CONSIDERATIONS

General

Appropriate samples for FCM include blood, bone marrow, lymph node samples, extranodal tissue biopsies, fine-needle aspirates (FNA), and body fluids (e.g., pleural, peritoneal, CSF). International consensus guidelines on medical indications for FCM are available and based on patient history and presenting symptoms.[5]

Timely processing of samples is necessary to maximize cell yield, maintain cell viability and integrity, and prevent loss of abnormal cells of interest (see Stetler-Stevenson et al.[4] for recommendations). Blood and bone marrow specimens must be collected in a tube containing an appropriate anticoagulant, such as sodium heparin or ethylenediaminetetraacetic acid (EDTA). Lysis is the preferred approach for removing excess erythrocytes (see Stetler-Stevenson et al.[4] for recommendations). In patients with an inaspirable marrow or "dry tap" (i.e., a fibrotic marrow or a marrow packed with neoplastic cells), submission of core biopsy material for FCM is appropriate. These cores are disaggregated to release cells into fluid suspension for FCM.[4]

If possible, portions of tissue for FCM should represent an area that is also being submitted for histology to minimize discordance as a result of sampling. Intact portions of solid tissue (such as biopsies of bone marrow, lymph nodes, or other tissue masses) must be made into cell suspensions for FCM. Mechanical tissue disaggregation is a fairly simple and rapid procedure that leaves cells relatively unaltered. It is achieved by slicing, mincing, and teasing apart the tissue with commercial devices or manual tools.[4] Enzymatic dissociation methods are also described for processing fibrotic tissue; however, they can alter antigen expression and decrease viability.

Antibody-staining protocols differ according to application and specimen type. Successful panel design requires an in-depth understanding of antigen-expression patterns in both normal and neoplastic cells. Antibody panels assess lineage and maturation patterns of normal cellular components

and characterization and classification of neoplastic cells. The emission spectra of fluorochromes vary, and antibody-fluorochrome conjugates should be used to maximize detection. For example, antibodies conjugated to bright fluorochromes may improve detection and visualization of dimly expressed antigens, and strongly expressed antigens, such as CD3 on T cells, may be adequately visualized on-scale with fluorochromes of only moderate brightness. Multiple antibodies are required for lineage assignment; many are not cell lineage–specific, and neoplastic cells may lack one or more antigens of a particular lineage. Overall, the number of reagents in a panel should be sufficient to allow the recognition of all abnormal and normal cells in the sample; conversely, limiting the number of antibodies may compromise diagnostic accuracy.[3] In general, higher sensitivity and specificity of detection and characterization is achieved with a larger antibody panel. By international consensus, the number of reagents needed to adequately evaluate a specimen for potential hematologic neoplasms is dependent on the presenting symptoms.[3,6] In addition, markers of potential prognostic utility should be included.

Viability

Regarding viability, no set cutoff exists that dictates automatic specimen rejection for FCM testing. General guidelines suggest rejecting replaceable specimens (such as peripheral blood, which may be redrawn from the patient) if the viability is less than 75%. A variety of viability dyes and instrumentation are commercially available to determine viability.

An important consideration, though, is that many samples submitted for FCM testing are considered irreplaceable specimens. These are specimens either obtained by an invasive procedure with significant trauma to the patient or obtained from a site that is difficult, if not impossible, from which to recollect. In addition, some peripheral blood specimens obtained at certain timepoints in treatment are unique in that the timing is critical for information regarding clinical management and are irreplaceable. In such cases, every effort should be made to obtain diagnostic information, and the results from FCM testing, even on specimens of decreased viability, may still prove valuable.

To maximize the information obtained from low-viability specimens by FCM, all cells are acquired from the sample and exported into the list mode data file. Any removal of non-specific debris events is performed post-acquisition only to avoid missing potentially useful data. Gating for single cells (doublet discrimination) may be performed by examining the forward scatter-height (FSC-H) (and/or forward scatter-width [FSC-W]) versus the forward scatter-area (FSC-A) parameters, as doublets exhibit disproportionately large FSC-W and FSC-A relative to FSC-H compared with single cells.

Viability gating based on scatter properties is helpful, as nonviable cells show decreased FSC resulting from loss of integrity of the cell membrane. Examination of CD45 versus FSC and CD45 versus SSC may help account for (and potentially remove by gating) small red blood cells, platelets, and debris from relevant cell populations. It is important to be aware that the nonviable cells may bind antibodies non-specifically, causing artifacts that may interfere with accurate immunophenotyping. Decreased sample viability is also commonly observed in solid-tissue samples and aggressive lymphomas (such as Burkitt lymphoma), where the metabolic rate and cell kinetics are quite high. Nevertheless, a low-viability sample composed of many neoplastic cells can still yield meaningful results. In irreplaceable specimens with decreased viability, any abnormal populations should still be reported, though care should be taken to avoid misinterpretation of non-specific antibody staining of nonviable tissue. In poorly viable specimens in which no abnormal population is identified, it is prudent to include a comment noting suboptimal specimen viability. The results from such a sample should not be viewed as a true negative,[4] as subsequent testing may be informative.

Small Specimens

Diagnosis of hematolymphoid malignancies, and in particular lymphoma, is frequently based on evaluation of small biopsies, FNA, and body fluids (e.g., CSF, vitreous humor, effusions). Small samples can provide sufficient cells for FCM, even when cell numbers are too low to count using conventional methods. FCM can be more sensitive than morphology, especially when neoplastic cells are admixed with normal counterparts or associated with a brisk inflammatory response, as in extranodal marginal zone lymphoma of mucosa-associated lymphoid tissue (MALT)[7] or gastric lymphoma in endoscopic biopsies.[8]

FCM increases the sensitivity of detection of hematolymphoid neoplasia in specimens of limited cellularity such as bronchoalveolar lavage specimens[9] and FNA.[10-12] The immunophenotypic information obtained from FCM assists in both detection and diagnostic subclassification of lymphoma.[10,11,13-15]

Involvement of the CSF by hematopoietic malignancies may be difficult to document by morphology alone. FCM improves the detection sensitivity of non-Hodgkin lymphoma in CSF[16-19] and is vital in the diagnostic evaluation of high-grade lymphomas. In a study assessing FCM in evaluating CSF in patients at risk for central nervous system (CNS) involvement in aggressive B-cell lymphoma, FCM was significantly more sensitive than cytology alone in disease detection and prognostication. Large cell lymphoma is susceptible to increased selective cell loss with red blood cell lysis procedures; therefore, processing CSF without red blood lysis will improve sensitivity of detection in such instances. FCM is also useful in identifying CNS leukemia and increases the detection rate over cytology alone.[19,20] Thus, FCM is crucial in the evaluation of CSF for hematolymphoid malignancies.[18] Studies report a rapid decline in CSF cell numbers within the first 30 minutes of sampling, and immediate stabilization with serum-containing media or commercially available stabilizers is vital to preserve the specimen until it reaches the FCM laboratory.[19,21]

MATURE B-CELL NEOPLASMS

FCM detection of malignant B-cell populations requires extensive knowledge of normal B-cell antigen expression and light scatter characteristics. Markers of B-cell neoplasia include light chain restriction, abnormally large B cells (as demonstrated by an increase in forward light scatter properties), abnormal levels of antigen expression, absence of normal antigens, and presence of antigens not normally present on mature B cells.

Evaluation of Light Chain Expression

B-cell neoplasms are typically characterized by monotypic light chain expression. It should be noted, however, that monotypic B-cell populations may be seen in patients with no evidence of lymphoma.[22-24] In some cases, this finding may represent early, preclinical detection of a B-cell malignancy[25] or, in rare instances, may be seen in reactive settings.[22]

A monotypic B-cell population is characterized by the expression of a single immunoglobulin (Ig) light chain by a B-cell population,[26] resulting in positive staining with only one light chain reagent (e.g., kappa-positive/lambda-negative population, or vice versa) (Fig. 4-1, middle row, kappa-vs.-lambda dot plot showing an example of lambda light chain restriction). In normal/benign lymphoid tissue, individual B cells express a single light chain Ig, and the ratio of kappa-expressing to lambda-expressing B cells is approximately 60% to 40%.[27] Lack of surface Ig among mature B cells or a deviation from this normal ratio (for example, a predominance of lambda-expressing B cells) should prompt a diligent search for an underlying monotypic B-cell population that may be discriminated by CD19, CD20, CD22, or other antigens.

FCM is advantageous because it can identify monotypic B cells, even in B-cell lymphopenia, by facilitating rapid analysis of large numbers of acquired B cells; it can also detect neoplastic B cells in a background of polyclonal B cells[26,27] by detecting aberrant antigens on the neoplastic cells. Antibody panels can be designed to exploit the expression of disease-characterizing antigens, such as CD5 in mantle cell lymphoma or CD10 in follicular lymphoma.[28] By examining B-cell subsets with differential CD19, CD20, or CD22 expression and/or aberrant antigen expression, a monotypic B-cell population may be discovered.[26,29] Figure 4-1 shows an example peripheral blood sample involved by chronic lymphocytic leukemia (CLL). Normal B cells with appropriate intensity of CD19, CD20, and CD22 are present (*blue*) and demonstrate a polyclonal pattern of surface light chain Ig. CLL (*orange*) is identified by the aberrant expression of CD5 on the CD19-positive B cells, along with the expression of dim CD20 and dim CD22, dim compared with the intensity of CD20 and CD22 on normal B cells. These features allow the CLL cells to be captured by gating; subsequently, they are shown to be monotypic B cells expressing lambda surface light chain, which is also slightly dimmer in intensity compared with the level of lambda expression of polyclonal B cells within the sample.

Absence of surface Ig may also be a feature of both indolent and aggressive mature B-cell neoplasms,[30,31] but caution is imperative when interpreting the significance of such a population. In bone marrow aspirates, normal plasma cells and most normal immature B cells (hematogones; benign precursor B cells) also lack surface Ig. In lymph node and lymphoid tissues, reactive germinal-center B cells (GCBs) with dim surface Ig may be mistaken for neoplasm. For this reason, it is important to understand the normal patterns associated with lymph node and lymphoid tissue.

The FCM patterns demonstrated in normal lymph node and lymphoid tissue are consistent and reproducible and reflect the cellular compartments of normal lymph

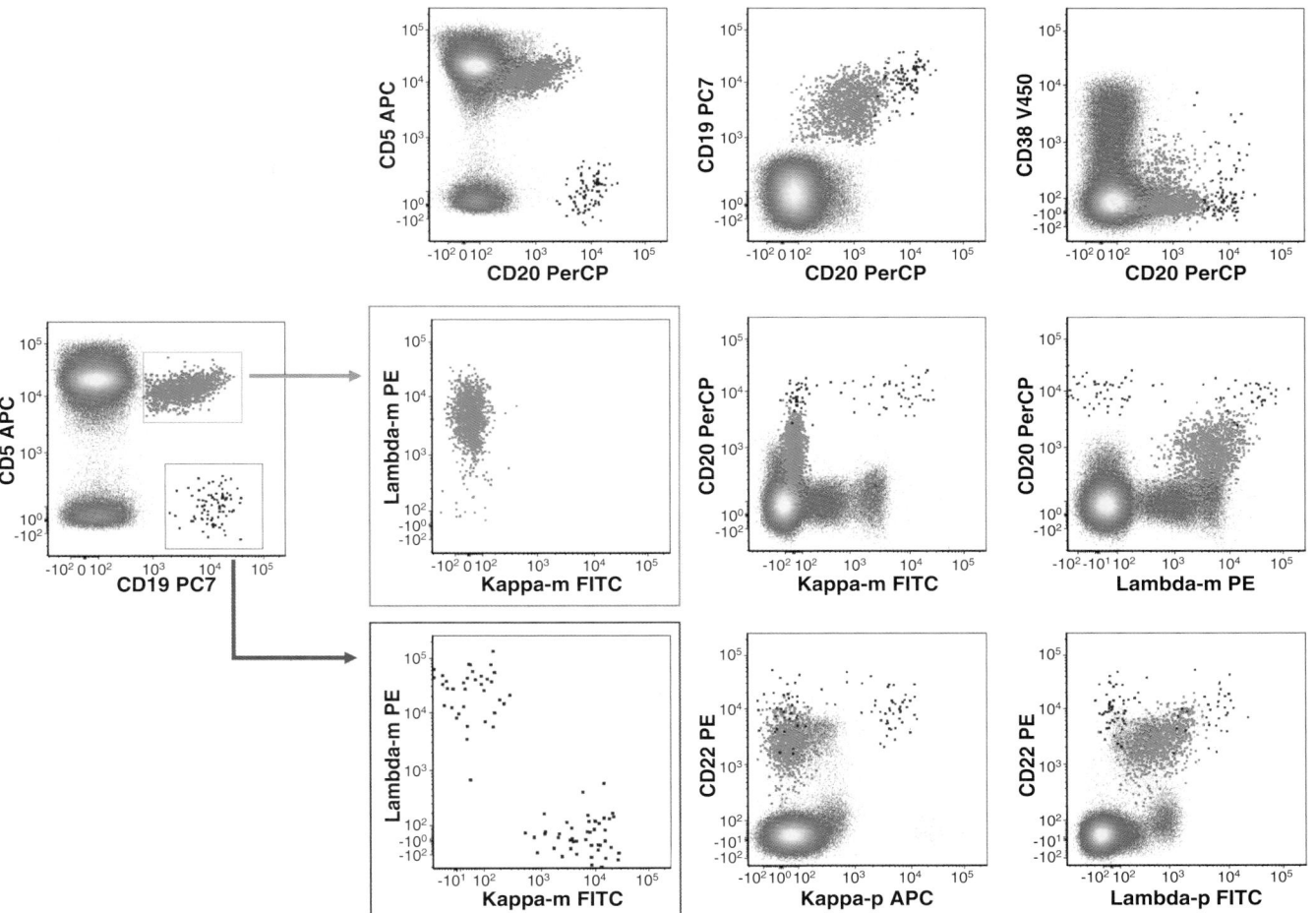

Figure 4-1. Flow cytometry detection of chronic lymphocytic leukemia (CLL) in peripheral blood. A significant population of B cells with aberrant CD5 expression *(orange)* corresponding to CLL are detected, along with fewer normal (CD5-negative) B cells *(blue)*; CD5-positive CD19-negative T cells are also present *(gray, far left dot plot)*. The CLL cells *(orange)* demonstrate dim CD20 *(top row, middle row)* and dim CD22 *(bottom row)* compared with normal B cells *(blue)*. The CLL cells are monotypic and demonstrate lambda light chain restriction *(orange, middle row, kappa-vs.-lambda dot plot)*; the normal B cells demonstrate an appropriate polyclonal pattern of both kappa and lambda light chain expression *(blue, bottom row, kappa-vs.-lambda dot plot)*. The differing intensities of CD20, CD22, kappa surface Ig, and lambda surface Ig can be simultaneously appreciated in both the CLL cells *(orange)* and normal B cells *(blue)* *(middle row, bottom row)*.

node architecture. CD19 is an excellent marker of B cells; however, the use of CD20 for B-cell characterization in FCM evaluation of lymph node and lymphoid tissues (Fig. 4-2) adds the advantage of clearly distinguishing the different morphologically recognized cellular components of the lymph node. Using CD20 expression, lymphocyte populations can be divided into T cells from the paracortical region (T: CD20 negative), mantle zone B cells (MB: moderately CD20 positive) and GCBs (bright CD20 positive) (Fig. 4-2, photomicrographs and upper row of dot plots). GCBs are distinguished by higher levels of CD20, higher levels of CD38, CD10 expression, and a slight increase in FSC (larger cell size/volume) compared to MB (Fig. 4-2, top and middle rows of dot plots). GCBs also express IgG heavy chain, in contrast to MB, which predominantly express IgD heavy chain, IgM heavy chain, and to a much lesser extent, IgA heavy chain (Fig. 4-2, bottom row of dot plots). In GCBs, kappa and lambda surface Ig expression is typically dim,

especially compared with the polyclonal pattern of kappa and lambda surface Ig in MB; this dim light chain expression is better appreciated compared with Ig-negative T cells within the sample (Fig. 4-2, middle row of dot plots).[32] In follicular hyperplasia, increased GCBs with dim surface Ig may be so prominent as to be mistaken for a B-cell neoplasm, such as follicular lymphoma or CD10-expressing large cell lymphoma; however, knowledge of the normal patterns and intensity of antigen expression of GCBs, including absence of intracellular BCL-2, can prevent misdiagnosis.[33-35]

Technical Considerations in Demonstration of Light Chain Restriction

Technical factors, such as antibody choice and cytophilic antibody artifact, can affect a laboratory's ability to assess surface light chain.[26] Cytophilic antibodies may be passively absorbed by Fc receptors present on natural killer

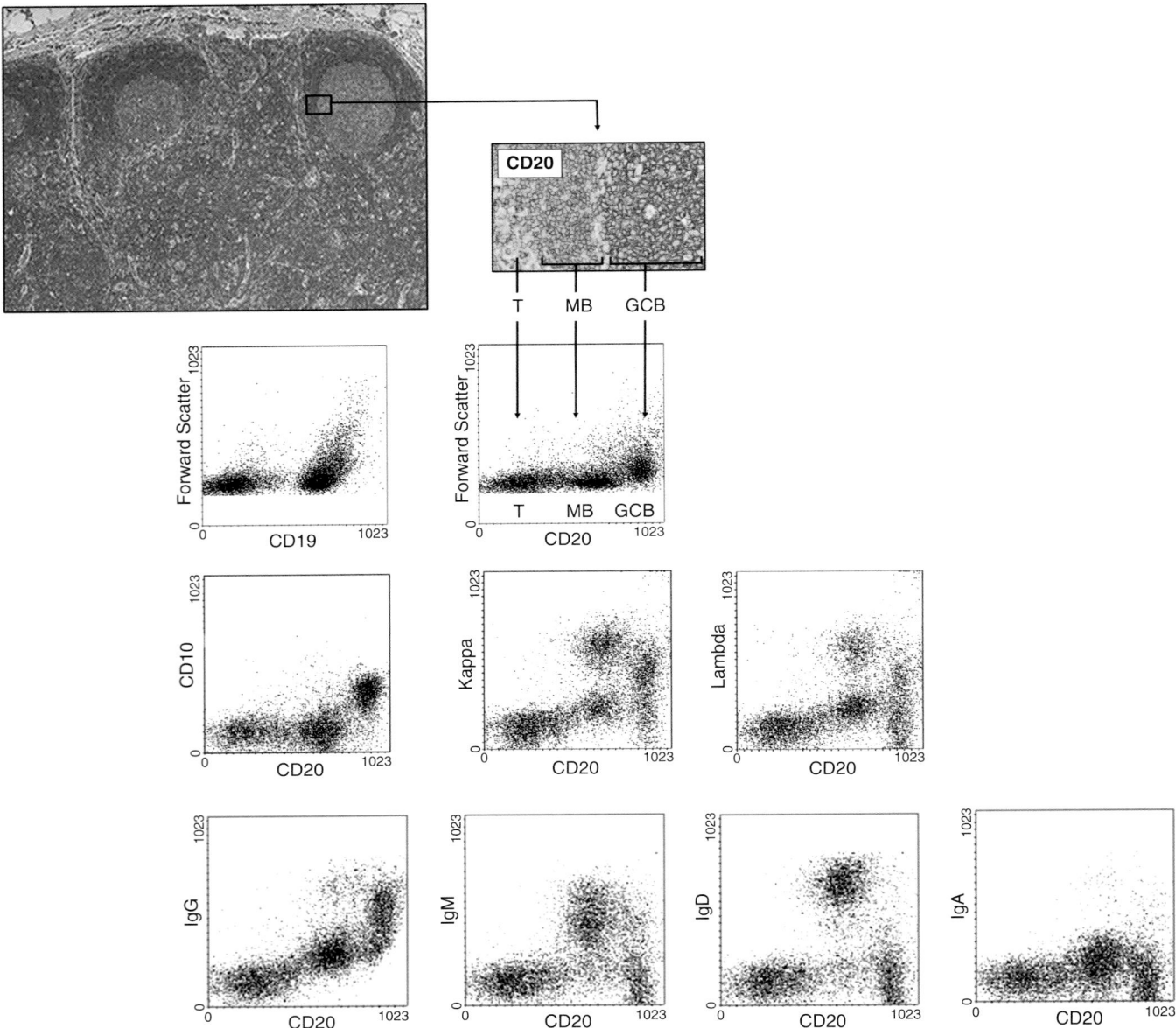

Figure 4-2. Flow cytometry evaluation of normal lymph node. H&E (hematoxylin and eosin) stained section of normal lymph node architecture with focus on portion of lymph node follicle *(top row, left photomicrograph, low power)*; CD20 immunohistochemistry shows CD20-negative T cells (T), CD20-positive B cells of the mantle zone (MB) and bright CD20-positive germinal-center B cells (GCBs) *(top row, right photomicrograph, high power)*. These normal cellular compartments are also clearly identified by flow cytometry (FCM) evaluation of CD20 and forward light scatter *(upper middle row, right dot plot)*, with GCBs showing brighter CD20 expression than MB and increased forward light scatter properties, which reflect the larger size of GCBs. CD20 is superior to CD19 *(upper middle row, left dot plot)* for discrimination of T, MB and GCB lymphoid compartments. GCBs are also distinguished by expression of CD10 *(middle row, left dot plot)* and dim surface light chain immunoglobulin (Ig) compared with the intensity of kappa and lambda staining of polyclonal MB *(middle row, center, and right dot plots)*. GCBs also express IgG heavy chain *(bottom row, left dot plot)* in contrast to MB, which predominantly express IgD and IgM heavy chain and, to a much lesser extent, IgA heavy chain *(bottom row, center, right, and far right dot plots)*. *(Data courtesy of Dr. Raul C. Braylan.)*

(NK) cells, activated T cells, monocytes, granulocytes, and some B cells, resulting in apparent surface light chain expression. Washing a specimen with phosphate-buffered saline (PBS) before staining, either at room temperature or 37° C, is sufficient to eliminate this artifact in most cases.[26]

Neoplastic B cells may express light chain epitopes not readily detected by some antibodies. Incorporation of two sets of light chain reagents, including both monoclonal and polyclonal antibodies, may improve the sensitivity of monotypic B-cell detection.[26,36]

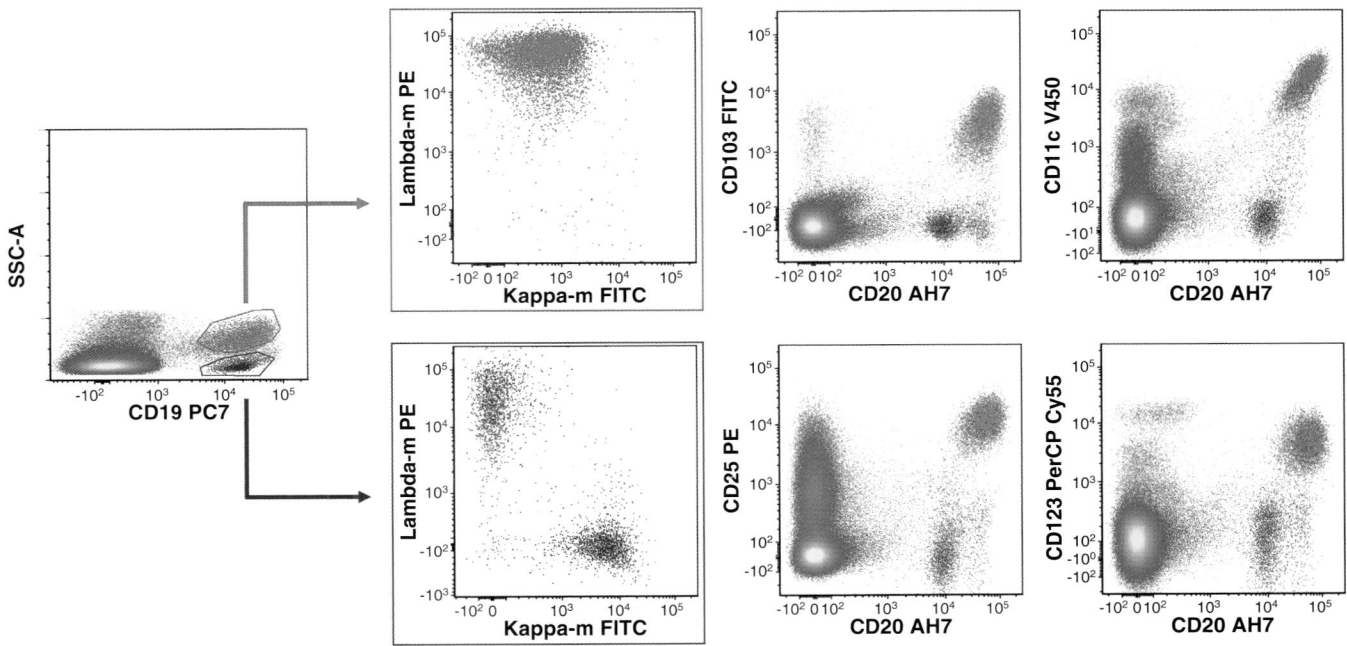

Figure 4-3. Flow cytometry evaluation of hairy cell leukemia (HCL). Detection of HCL is usually performed by gating on bright CD20-positive B cells with CD103, bright CD11c, bright CD25, and bright CD123 expression, with subsequent demonstration of monotypic light chain expression. However, this unique case illustrates an example of HCL *(red)* with distinctively increased side scatter-area (SSC-A) that is fully distinguished from normal B cells of low SSC-A *(blue)* within the sample *(far left dot plot)*. The HCL cells *(red)* show restricted expression of bright lambda surface light chain *(top row, kappa-vs.-lambda dot plot)*, in contrast to the polyclonal pattern of surface light chain expression of normal B cells *(blue, bottom row, kappa-vs.-lambda dot plot)*. In addition to the expression of CD103, bright CD11c *(top row, center, and right dot plots)*, bright CD25, and bright CD123 *(bottom row, center, and right dot plots)*, the HCL cells *(red)* also show brighter expression of CD20 compared with the intensity of CD20 on normal B cells *(blue)*.

Additional Immunophenotypic Characteristics of Mature B-Cell Neoplasms

Abnormalities in B-cell antigen expression can be used to identify malignant B cells.[37] Mature normal B cells express CD19, CD20, and CD22, and except for plasma cells, failure to express one of these antigens is abnormal. An important caveat is a history of monoclonal antibody therapy (e.g., rituximab, ofatumumab), as the therapeutic antibody may mask detection of the targeted antigen. For example, CD20 expression cannot be detected on B cells (normal and malignant) post-treatment with rituximab, and this may persist for 6 months or longer after cessation of rituximab therapy.[38]

The detection of aberrant antigens (not normally expressed on B cells) is a notable feature of malignant B cells. Aberrant expression of T-cell markers (such as CD2, CD4, CD7, and CD8) may be observed in B-cell non-Hodgkin lymphoma.[39-41] Abnormal intensity of antigen expression (e.g., abnormally dim or bright expression) is also diagnostically important and aids in subclassification. CLL is characterized by dim CD20 expression, dim CD22 expression, and CD5 expression (Fig. 4-1). Hairy cell leukemia is characterized by expression of CD103, bright CD20, bright CD22, bright CD11c (Fig. 4-3, top row), bright CD25, and bright CD123 (Fig. 4-3, bottom row).[42] Follicular lymphoma frequently exhibits dim expression of CD19, along with expression of CD10.[43]

In addition, light scatter characteristics may aid in detecting neoplastic B-cell populations. Abnormally high FSC is observed in large cell lymphoma (Fig. 4-4, top row, upper left dot plot showing CD19 vs. FSC), reflecting an increase in the neoplastic cell's size/volume. Abnormally increased SSC is a notable feature of hairy cell leukemia (Fig. 4-3, left dot plot showing CD19 vs. SSC); it is comparable to the SSC exhibited by monocytes and reflects the membrane irregularities that are characteristic of this disease. Increased FSC is also a helpful feature of primary effusion lymphoma (PEL), which lacks expression of CD19, CD20, CD22, cytoplasmic CD79a, and other B-cell antigens. Morphologically, the size of a PEL cell may be tremendously larger than that of a small lymphocyte (Fig. 4-3, upper and lower right micrographs). PEL may only express CD45 (often dim), along with only a few of the following antigens: CD38, CD138, VS38c, HLA-DR, and CD30.[13,44] The increased FSC is a helpful identifying feature; PEL cells may be so large as to compress near the visible edge or "hit the ceiling" of the dot plot, depending on how the data is visually scaled (Fig. 4-5, top row, FSC vs. CD45 dot plot).

Another area where the FSC parameter is helpful is in the FCM evaluation of B-cell lymphoma, especially lymphoplasmacytic lymphoma, in the bone marrow. Bone marrow contains many precursor B cells with normal, variable expression patterns of CD10, CD20, and CD45. In addition, plasma cells in bone marrow express a normal and heterogeneous pattern of CD19 and CD45. Both precursor B

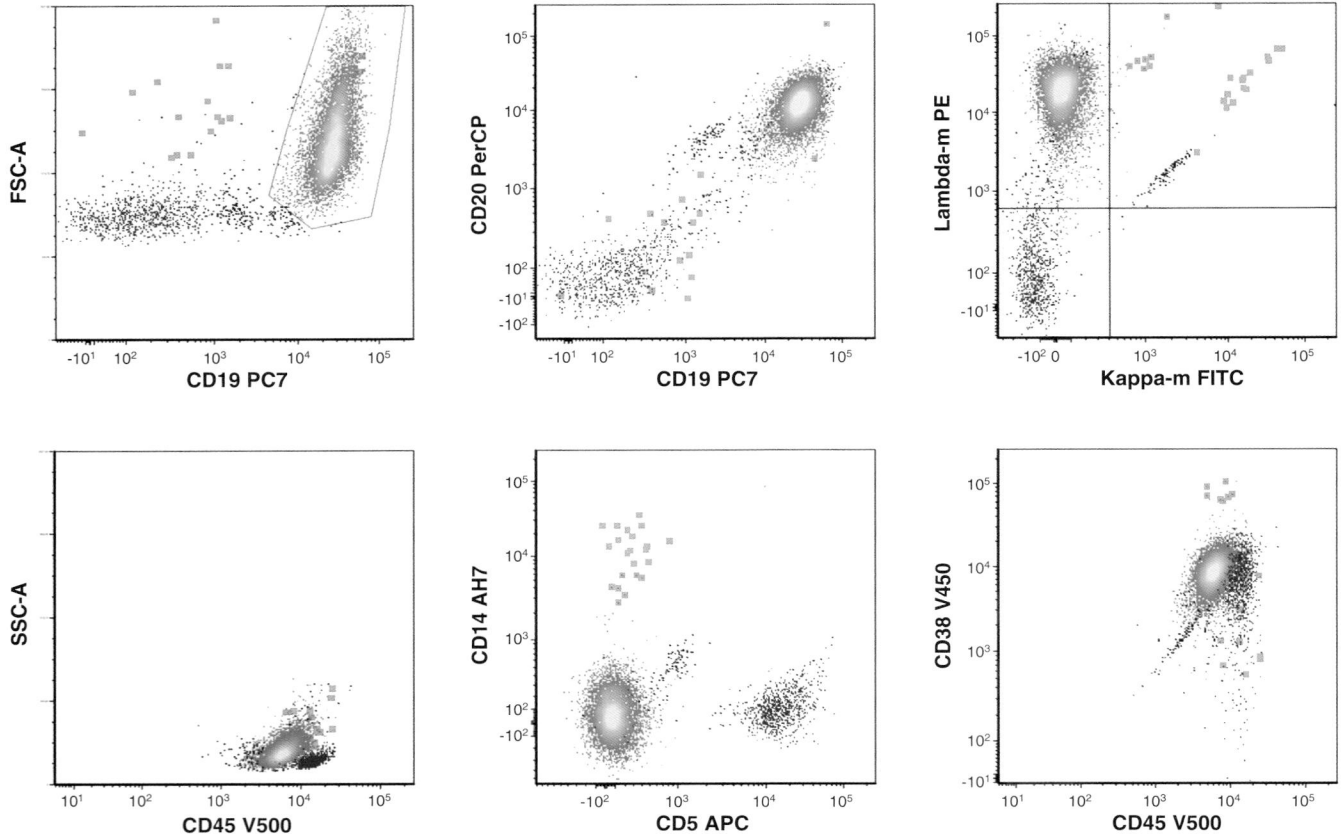

Figure 4-4. Flow cytometry evaluation of cerebrospinal fluid involved by diffuse large B-cell lymphoma. The specimen was processed without red blood cell lysis, and CD45-negative small red blood cells were initially gated out of the analysis post-acquisition. Next, a population of CD19-positive B cells is identified *(red)* with abnormally increased forward scatter-area (FSC-A), consistent with B cells of increased size/volume *(top row, left dot plot)*. The FSC-A of the B cells is much larger than that of CD5-positive T cells *(blue)* and equivalent to the FSC-A of CD14-positive monocytes *(aqua)* that are also present in the sample *(bottom row, center dot plot)*. The abnormal B-cell population expresses CD20 *(top row, center dot plot)*, CD45 at a slightly dimmer intensity than T cells *(blue)* and monocytes *(aqua, bottom row, left and right dot plots)*, and demonstrates monotypic expression of lambda surface light chain *(top row, right dot plot)*.

cells with appropriately progressive maturation and normal plasma cells can obscure identification of B-cell lymphoma and especially of lymphoplasmacytic lymphoma, which contains both monotypic mature B-cell and plasmacytic-cell components.[45,46] Analysis strategies that examine the FSC of B cells along with CD19, CD20, CD45, and CD38 can often help delineate the normal from abnormal B cells more clearly. Precursor B cells are small cells with distinctly low FSC, whereas plasma cells have slightly higher FSC and distinctly bright CD38. Accounting first for the normal B-cell and plasma-cell compartments subsequently facilitates the identification of B-cell lymphoma in the marrow.[47]

In FCM, an increase in FSC reflects an increase in cellular volume. Thus, cells with increased amounts of cytoplasm, such as normal plasma cells of bone marrow, may exhibit slightly higher FSC and appear "large" as a result of the increased volume of cytoplasm; however, plasma cells are not considered "large" cells in the traditional histopathologic context, which is based on evaluation of nuclear size on hematoxylin and eosin (H&E)-stained slides. When interpreting FCM data, this distinction is important to bear in mind.

Emerging Role of Flow Cytometry in the Diagnosis of Hodgkin Lymphoma

So far, we have discussed the utility of FCM exclusively in non-Hodgkin B-cell lymphoma and lymphoproliferative disorders. Historically, FCM evaluation was considered suboptimal for evaluation of classic Hodgkin lymphoma (cHL) because of the apparent lack of sensitivity of FCM to detect Hodgkin and Reed-Sternberg (HRS) cells within a heavily infiltrated background of inflammatory cells. This may have been caused by the rarity of HRS cells, the difficulty in aspirating HRS cells from within the fibrotic bands of the nodular sclerosis-subtype of this disease, and/or their fragility/susceptibility to being lost during FCM cell processing.

FCM evaluation for assessment of Hodgkin lymphoma has become increasingly sophisticated. The ability to use a greater numbers of markers, modern instrumentation (6 to 9 colors or more), specific methods for tissue processing and disaggregation, increased number of acquired cells for analysis, and a specifically tailored gating strategy have improved detection of HRS cells.[48,49] Modern methods of cHL detection boast a diagnostic sensitivity of 89% and specificity

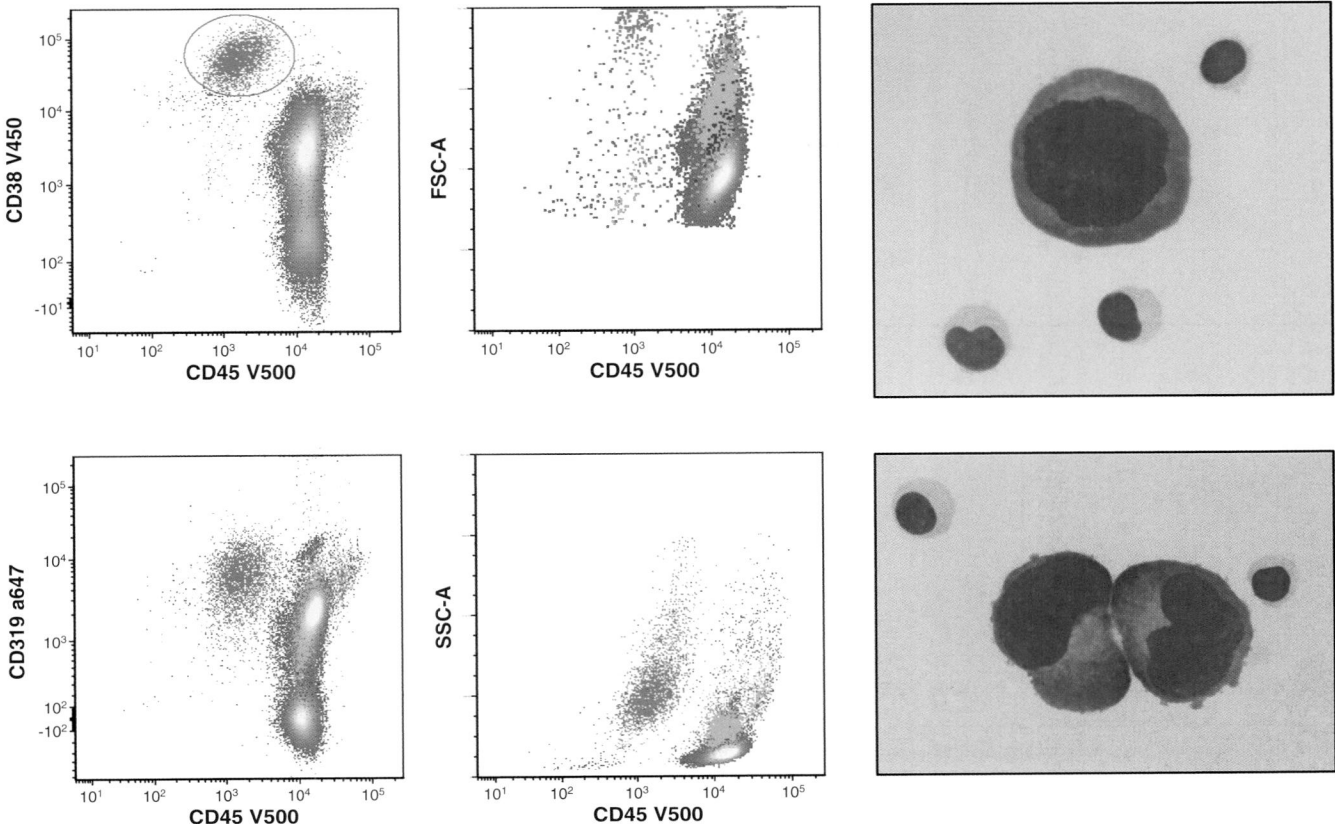

Figure 4-5. Flow cytometry evaluation of primary effusion lymphoma (PEL). A population of PEL cells is identified by expression of CD38, dim CD45 *(top row, left dot plot)* and CD319 *(bottom row, left dot plot)*, with atypical side scatter-area (SSC-A; *bottom row, center dot plot)* and markedly increased forward scatter-area (FSC-A; *top row, center dot plot)*. Cytologic evaluation identifies malignant PEL cells that are significantly larger than small lymphocytes *(top row, right photomicrograph; bottom row, right photomicrograph).*

approaching 100%, even though HRS cells typically contain less than 1% of the total specimen cellularity.[50]

In cHL, HRS cells show distinctively increased side scatter (compared with small lymphocytes within the sample) and expression of CD15, CD30, bright CD40, CD71, and CD95, along with dim/negative expression of CD20.[50,51] Furthermore, FCM reveals T-cell rosettes (T cells forming a ring around HRS cells), a common histopathologic feature of this disease.[52,53] HRS cells express CD54 and CD58, mediating T-cell binding to the HRS cell surface; FCM identifies HRS T-cell rosettes by their co-expression of both bright CD45 and bright CD5 in a reproducible, slightly diagonal-appearing pattern.[48,51] Certain features of the reactive background cellular infiltrate are also associated with cHL. The CD4-positive T cells in cHL are associated with characteristically bright CD7 and bright CD45 expression[54,55] and contain increased immunosuppressive T-regulatory cells.[56,57] Pioneering work continues to explore the role of FCM, not only in diagnosis of cHL, but in nodular lymphocyte predominant B-cell lymphoma (NLPBL) (synonym and related term: nodular lymphocyte predominant Hodgkin lymphoma [NLPHL], World Health Organization [WHO] Classification)[58] and other related entities.[59,60]

PLASMA CELL NEOPLASMS

Plasma cell neoplasms (PCNs) are a group of disorders with a spectrum of clinical presentations from the asymptomatic

monoclonal gammopathy of uncertain significance (MGUS) and smoldering multiple myeloma (SMM) to the symptomatic multiple myeloma (MM) (synonym and related term: plasma cell myeloma [PCM], WHO classification). Although diagnosis is based on serum M (monoclonal) spike, extent of plasma cell involvement of the bone marrow, and presence of end organ damage, FCM characterization and quantification of neoplastic plasma cells have been used in the diagnosis, prognostication, and monitoring of PCN.[46,61-63] In patients with reactive bone marrow plasmacytosis, FCM can distinguish normal from neoplastic plasma cells. FCM is vital in the diagnosis of unusual cases of myeloma, such as IgM myeloma (differentiating these cases from other IgM secretory diseases) and rare cases of nonsecretory myeloma.[64] FCM is also useful in differentiating myeloma from lymphoplasmacytic lymphoma (LPL) and other non-Hodgkin lymphomas, as the monotypic CD38-positive cells in lymphoma typically are CD19-positive and CD45-positive and lack expression of CD56, an immunophenotypic profile that is uncommon in myeloma.[46,61] Plasma cells are fragile and may deteriorate rapidly and/or be susceptible to loss during processing for FCM.[65] In addition, plasma cell infiltrates in MM may be focal and/or show a patchy distribution in the bone marrow; as such, immunohistochemistry is better suited to visualize and quantitate plasma cells on the bone marrow core biopsy. Nevertheless, FCM detection of plasma cells demonstrates increased sensitivity over immunohistochemistry in MGUS and SMM and is consistent

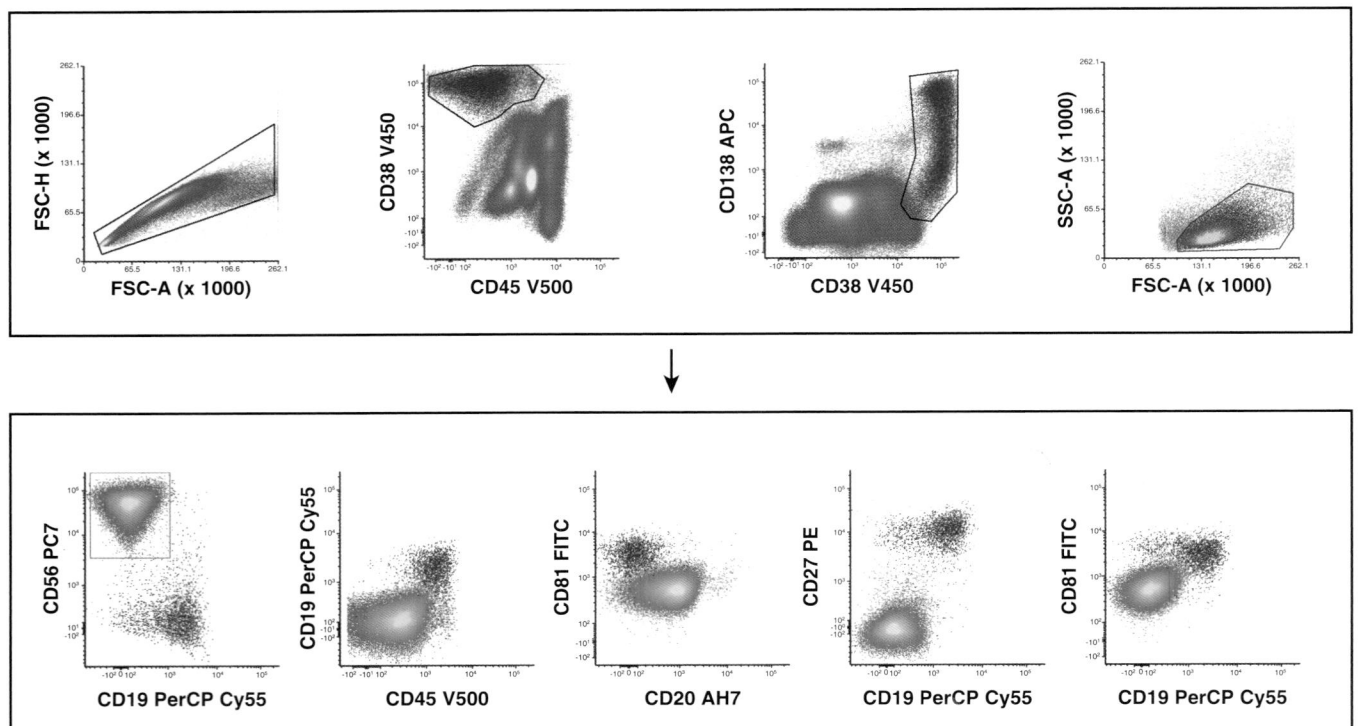

Figure 4-6. Flow cytometry evaluation of plasma cells. Both normal and neoplastic plasma cells *(purple)* are captured for analysis using a combination of gates to include single cells *(top row, far left dot plot)* that demonstrate bright CD38 expression, moderate-to-low CD45 expression, and variable CD138 expression *(top row, center left and center right dot plots)* that fall within a generous forward and side scatter gate appropriate for plasma cells *(top row, right dot plot)*. The neoplastic plasma cells are distinguished from normal plasma cells by differential surface expression of CD19, CD45, CD56, CD20, CD27, and CD81. The neoplastic plasma cells *(red)* that aberrantly express CD56 *(bottom row, far left dot plot)* show aberrant CD20 expression, abnormally dim CD81 expression, and lack of CD19, CD45, and CD27. The remaining plasma cells are normal plasma cells *(purple, bottom row)* with appropriate expression of CD19, CD45, CD81, and CD27 and are appropriately negative for CD20 and CD56.

and reproducible, regardless of the choice of anticoagulant, biopsy site, or pull sequence in unilateral and bilateral bone marrow sampling.[66] FCM determination of the proportion of plasma cells that are phenotypically aberrant allows risk stratification of progression of MGUS and SMM to overt MM and is prognostically valuable.[67-73] FCM studies also help predict response to autologous stem cell transplantation.[73-75] In addition, FCM can detect circulating abnormal plasma cells in the peripheral blood, which affects progression-free survival (PFS) and overall survival (OS).[72,76-78] FCM MRD detection post-therapy in MM has been demonstrated to be a robust independent predictor of PFS and OS in prospective studies.[79-84] An FCM-negative MRD study in MM is one of the most relevant prognostic factors for patients undergoing autologous stem cell transplantation and for patients treated with novel agents.[81-84] This led the FDA to adopt the viewpoint that FCM detection of myeloma MRD is a mature technology with proven prognostic value in predicting PFS and OS and is therefore an acceptable surrogate endpoint in clinical trials.[85,86]

When designing panels, antibody cocktails must contain CD19, CD38, CD45, and CD138 to adequately identify plasma cells and CD27, CD56, CD81, and CD117 to accurately distinguish between normal and neoplastic plasma cells in the sample.[62,87-90] Intracellular light chain evaluation is appropriate at diagnosis but may be optional post-therapy,

as abnormal plasma cells can be identified by surface antigen expression alone; examination of surface CD19, CD38, CD45, CD56, CD138, CD27, CD81, and CD117 is important for identification of subpopulations of clonal plasma cells.[62,67,89,91-94]

Consensus guidelines for PCM MRD detection by FCM highlight special considerations for specimen processing (red cell lysis and cell concentration prior to staining), demonstration of specimen quality (viability and presence of normal marrow elements), the number of cells acquired (2 million minimum, up to 5 million optimal), gating strategies (based on CD38, CD45, CD138, and light scatter), and the definition of malignant plasma cells based primarily on abnormal surface antigen expression.[65,95,96] Plasma cell analysis and gating must be performed with caution to ensure inclusion of plasma cells with aberrant antigen expression (Fig. 4-6). Light scatter characteristics are used to select single cells (also referred to as doublet discrimination) and exclude debris while taking care not to exclude hyperdiploid or tetraploid plasma cells, which have abnormally high FSC and SSC.[96] Gating subsequently captures cells with positive expression of CD138 and bright CD38 (Fig. 4-6, top row). Special attention should be focused on examination of plasma cells that may express dimmer-than-normal CD38 and CD45. Once an analysis gating strategy is delineated, neoplastic plasma cells are defined based on their variation from normal plasma cells (Fig. 4-6, bottom row). Neoplastic plasma cells are characterized by expression of CD38 (frequently dimmer than in normal plasma cells), CD138, monotypic cytoplasmic Ig, diminished CD27 and/or CD81 expression, absence of CD19 and CD45, and aberrant expression of antigens, including (but not limited to) CD56, CD20, CD28, and CD117.

Normal plasma cells exhibit a highly conserved surface antigen immunophenotype.[87-90,97] Minor subsets of normal plasma cells can immunophenotypically overlap with aberrant plasma cells in expression of single markers; however, this issue is overcome when a larger number of markers are considered for analysis. Normal plasma cells show heterogeneous, moderate-intensity expression of CD45 and CD19 and bright expression of CD27 and CD81 (although rare normal plasma cells with dim-to-negative CD27 and CD81 expression maybe observed with very high acquisition numbers). They are negative for CD20 and CD117. CD56 and CD28 expression can be observed in a small subset (between 5% and 20%) of normal plasma cells with higher frequency in post-treatment bone marrow samples, but they will demonstrate a polyclonal pattern of intracellular light chain Ig.

Daratumumab, a therapeutic anti-CD38 monoclonal antibody used for treatment of PCM, obscures detection of plasma cells by causing them to appear dim or negative for CD38 expression when FCM is performed. This hinders traditional methods of plasma cell detection, especially if CD138 expression (which can be labile) is decreased in plasma cells. Strategies to improve FCM detection of plasma cells in this particular context have explored the use of alternative markers. These include detection of CD319,[98,99] intracellular IRF4, intracellular CD38,[100] multi-epitope CD38,[101] and intracellular VS38c, which detects cytoskeleton-associated protein 4 (CKAP4).[102,103] These approaches have been met with success and are promising alternatives to the use of traditional anti-CD38 antibody.

The increasingly widespread availability of clinical flow cytometers with 8-color and 10-color capabilities (or more) has allowed for validated panels for PCM MRD testing to include all appropriate antibodies in as little as one or two antibody cocktails. In addition, acquisition of up to 10 million events has improved MRD detection sensitivity.[101,104-107] This type of high sensitivity FCM for myeloma MRD detection shows performance comparable to that of next-generation sequencing (NGS) for the detection of IgH gene rearrangements; although FCM requires the use of a fresh sample (whereas NGS can be performed on DNA from archived, formalin-fixed samples), it offers quick test turn-around, and clonal plasma cells are detectable without the need for comparison to a diagnostic and/or previously characterized disease clone.[108] Efforts continue to further explore and standardize FCM detection of PCM MRD, which will ultimately improve the quality of the testing and its utility in patient care.

MATURE T-CELL NEOPLASMS

FCM immunophenotyping is useful in the evaluation of mature T-cell neoplasms, including initial diagnosis, subclassification, staging, prognostication, monitoring, and identification of therapeutic targets (e.g., for immunotherapy). In general, detection of T-cell neoplasia by FCM is often more challenging than detection of B-cell neoplasia. Typically, T cells are examined for abnormal cell clusters compared with normal T cells by light scatter and/or antigen expression. A variety of phenotypic abnormalities, including a restricted or abnormal CD4/CD8 pattern, abnormal (absent, diminished or increased) expression of pan–T-cell antigens, the presence of aberrant antigens, and expansion of normally rare T-cell populations, may be indicators of T-cell neoplasia.[109,110]

Initial examination of CD4 and CD8 can be informative. Normal reactive lymphoid populations contain a mixture of CD4-positive and CD8-positive cells, with a predominance of CD4-positive cells. The average CD4-to-CD8 ratio is around 1.5 in normal blood, slightly above 1 in the bone marrow, and approximately 3.5 in lymph nodes.[111-113] Mature clonal T-cell populations are restricted to either CD4 or CD8 expression (Fig. 4-7, top row, center right and far right dot plots), co-expression of both CD4 and CD8, or lack of CD4 and CD8 (less frequently observed). Caveats include viral infections, which are often characterized by a dramatic increase in CD8-positive T cells, usually in association with other indications of T-cell activation such as increased CD2 expression, decreased CD7 expression, and expression of activation markers.[114] Also, a history of HIV infection may diminish or obliterate the number of CD4-positive T cells.[111]

A significant population of T cells lacking both CD4 and CD8 is abnormal and may be compatible with T-cell lymphoma; however, other non-neoplastic conditions should be excluded first. The majority (70%) of TCRγδ T cells are CD4-negative CD8-negative, and 30% are CD4-negative CD8-positive; rarely (1%), they are CD4-positive CD8-negative.[115] TCRγδ T cells normally constitute only a minor subset (<10%) in peripheral blood but are more abundant in certain tissue (e.g., 25% to 60% in the gut) and may be expanded in various reactive conditions. A reactive increase in CD4-negative CD8-negative TCRγδ T cells should not be interpreted as a T-cell lymphoproliferative disorder.[116] CD4-negative CD8-negative T cells are also present in some immunodeficiency states and are a hallmark of autoimmune lymphoproliferative syndrome (ALPS).[117]

Co-expression of CD4 and CD8 is less common in mature T-cell neoplasms. Although it can occur, often in T-prolymphocytic leukemia, occasionally in proliferations of T-cell large granular lymphocytes, and rarely in adult T-cell leukemia/lymphoma, this finding necessitates excluding T lymphoblastic leukemia/lymphoma (T-ALL) or normal cortical thymocytes, especially if the specimen is from the mediastinum. FCM can distinguish a neoplastic T-cell process from normal cortical thymocytes in thymoma or thymic hyperplasia if normal T-cell maturation subsets are examined, as evidenced by pattern and intensity of CD2, CD3, CD4, CD5, CD7, CD8, CD10, CD34, and CD45.[118,119] In addition, increased CD4-positive CD8-positive T cells (>10% of T cells) are commonly found in lymph node specimens involved by NLPBL and progressive transformation of germinal centers.[120,121] The presence of this CD4-positive CD8-positive population should not be misinterpreted as a T-cell or composite neoplasm. Finally, apparent double positives can be a technical artifact in staining of unwashed blood and should be interpreted with care.[122]

Because mature T-cell neoplasms frequently exhibit abnormal (absent, diminished, or increased) expression of at least one T-cell antigen (i.e., CD2, CD3, CD5, or CD7), analysis of pan–T-cell antigens is an essential component of the analysis.[109,123] It is important to include multiple T-cell

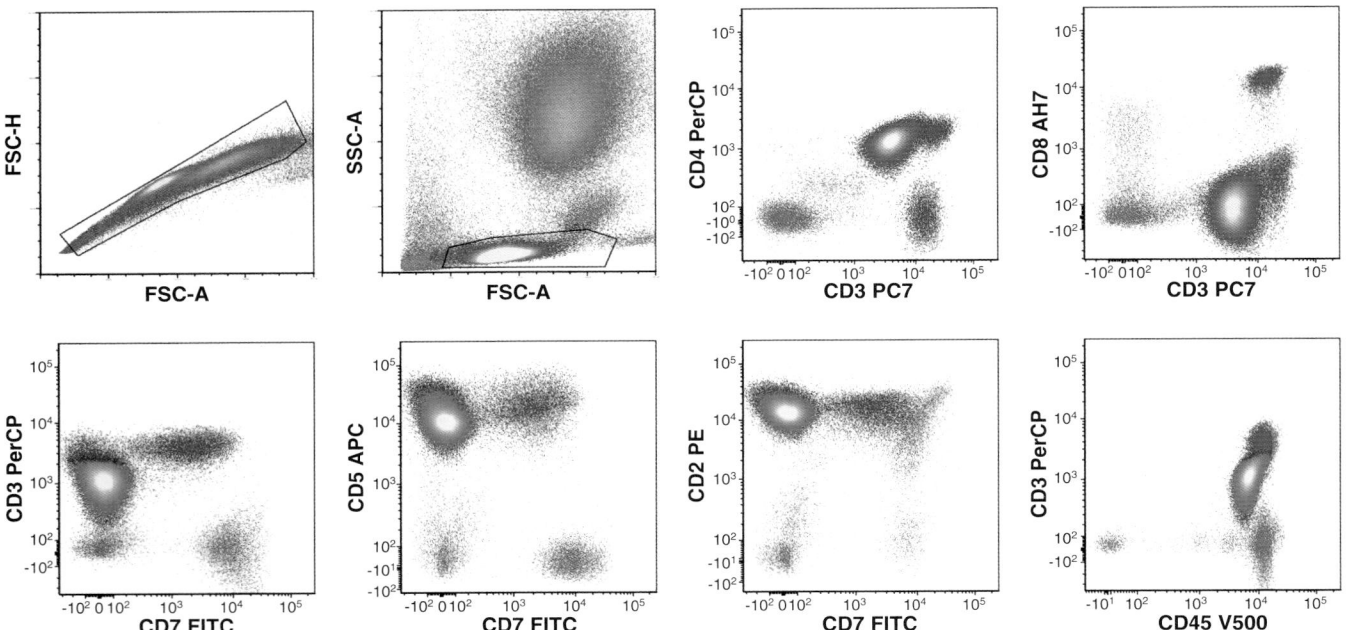

Figure 4-7. Flow-cytometric detection of abnormal T-cell populations. Lymphoid cells are identified by gating for single cells and subsequently on cells with appropriate forward scatter (FSC) and side scatter (SSC) characteristics *(top row, middle left and far left dot plots)*. The majority of the abnormal cells are CD4-positive and CD8-negative T cells *(violet)*, and a small population of normal CD4-positive and CD8-positive T cells are present *(green, top row, middle right and far right dot plots)*. The CD4-restricted T cells *(violet)* demonstrate abnormally dim CD3 expression *(top row, middle right and far right dot plots; bottom row, far right and far left dot plots)* compared with the residual normal T cells within the sample *(green)*; the abnormal T cells are CD5-positive, CD2-positive, and CD7-negative *(bottom row, middle right and middle left dot plots)*.

antigens (CD2, CD3, CD5, and CD7) in a diagnostic panel to ensure sensitivity in detection. When interpreting data, one must first recognize the intrinsic heterogeneous patterns in normal T cells. Normally, a small percent of peripheral blood CD3-positive T cells are CD7-negative, and a subset of TCRγδ cells does not express CD5. However, large numbers of CD7-negative CD4-positive CD5-negative T cells (e.g., non–gamma delta T cells) are abnormal. CD2-negative T cells are rare, and absence of surface CD3 is distinctly abnormal. The intensity of the T-cell markers is not uniform among subsets. Notably, TCRγδ T cells express a brighter CD3 than TCRαβ T cells. Among the TCRαβ T cells, CD4-positive T cells express a higher level of CD3 and CD5 than do CD8-positive T cells. The normal CD7-negative T cells typically express slightly higher levels of CD2 and CD5.[124] CD2 expression is often upregulated in reactive T cells.[125]

As opposed to the expected normal heterogenous patterns, neoplastic T cells may be detected as a homogeneous population with an abnormal level of antigen expression (e.g., abnormal CD2, CD3, CD5, CD7, or CD45).[109,123] For example, CD3 may be expressed at a higher or lower level than normal as measured by staining with anti-CD3. Dim CD3 expression is characteristic of Sézary cells and adult T-cell leukemia/lymphoma.[126,127] Diminished or absent CD3 is also a typical feature of follicular helper T-cell lymphoma, angioimmunoblastic type (also known as angioimmunoblastic T-cell lymphoma, WHO classification 4th edition, and nodal T-follicular helper cell lymphoma, angioimmunoblastic type, WHO classification 5th edition).[128,129] T-cell large granular lymphocytic leukemias typically have abnormally dim levels of

CD5 expression. Abnormal levels of CD2 and CD7 expression may also be observed in T-cell lymphoproliferative processes.

A subgroup of clonal T-cell processes is characterized by increased numbers of T-cell subpopulations normally present in low numbers. In T-cell large granular lymphocytic leukemia, CD8-positive T cells co-expressing CD57, CD56, or CD16 are increased. Dim CD5 expression and absence of normal T-cell antigens, such as CD7 and CD2, assist in the diagnosis. CD20, considered a B-cell antigen, is expressed by a small subgroup of normal T cells. However, detection of a significant population of CD20-positive T cells is highly abnormal.

In addition, T-cell lymphoma may occasionally show aberrant expression of non–T-cell lineage antigens. Aberrant expression of myeloid markers such as CD13 and/or CD33 may be seen in ALK-positive anaplastic large cell lymphoma.[130] Rare peripheral T-cell lymphomas may show aberrant B-cell markers, including CD19.[131] Those cases are generally rare, but the aberrant phenotype may become a diagnostic pitfall.

In all T-cell neoplasms, correlation with patient history and morphology is essential. When the vast majority of cells are neoplastic by morphology, a corresponding aberrant immunophenotype can be easily interpreted. Caution should be exercised when interpreting single immunophenotypic abnormalities, as these can be found in benign T-cell populations that are highly activated or when subsets are present in numbers increased above normal (e.g., increased gamma delta T cells, loss of CD7 on T cells in Epstein-Barr virus [EBV] infection). Neoplastic T cells usually have multiple abnormalities in antigen expression and light scatter

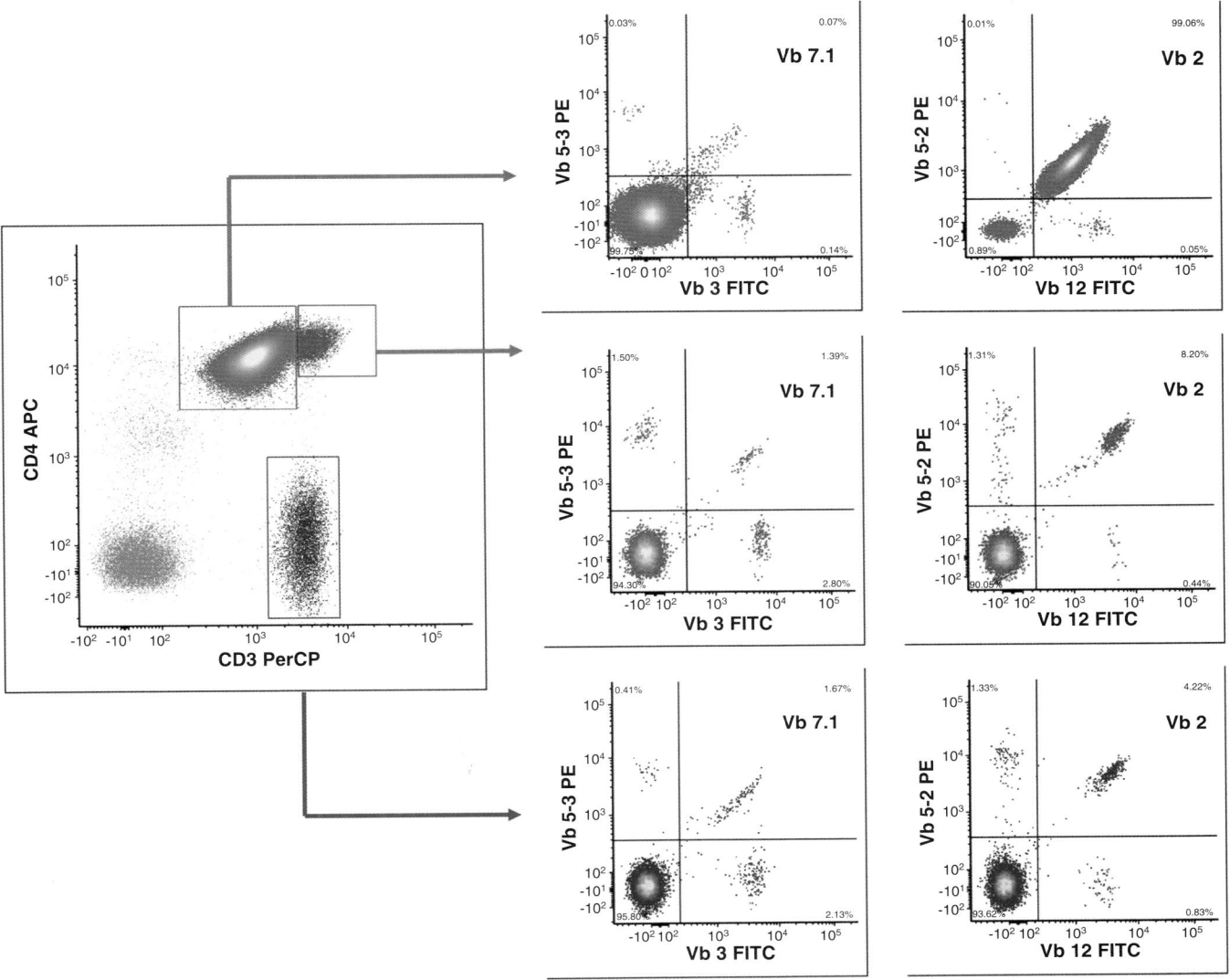

Figure 4-8. T-cell receptor Vβ repertoire flow cytometry analysis to identify a clonal T-cell population. Three populations of T cells are discriminated by expression patterns of CD3 and CD4 *(far left dot plot)*. The majority of the T cells are abnormal and express dim CD3 and CD4 *(violet)*. Normal T cells with appropriate intensity of CD3 that are either CD4-positive *(green)* or CD4-negative *(blue)* are also present. The abnormal T cells *(violet)* demonstrate uniform expression of a single Vβ family, consistent with a clonal T-cell population *(top row)*. Normal T cells expressing CD4 *(green)* demonstrate nonrestricted/non-clonal Vβ family usage *(middle row)*. Similarly, normal T cells that are CD4-negative, likely corresponding to normal CD8-positive T cells *(blue)*, also demonstrate nonrestricted/non-clonal Vβ family usage *(bottom row)* and serve as an internal control.

properties, which, because of the multiparametric nature of FCM, can be detected in the same cell, differentiating these cells from normal cells.

In addition, as in clonality analysis in B-cell neoplasms, T-cell clonality can be directly assessed by FCM analysis of the β-chain variants of the T-cell receptor (TCR Vβ).[132,133] Commercial antibodies are available against approximately 70% of the human class-specific sequences among the TCR Vβ segments. Normal T cells have a relatively stable distribution of the Vβ repertoire, which is well defined,[134] but a clonal T cell population has the same variable, diversity, and joining segments and hence a restricted Vβ expression pattern. An abnormal expansion of a Vβ-expressing population is consistent with a clonal T-cell population. A panel of

antibodies can be combined with anti-Vβ antibodies to detect abnormal T-cell populations and determine the clonality of the immunophenotypically defined abnormal T cells (Fig. 4-8). This TCR Vβ repertoire analysis can be used to establish an initial diagnosis of T-cell neoplasia and to monitor MRD.[132,133,135-137]

Alternatively, T-cell clonality can be examined by analyzing the expression pattern of the TCR β-chain constant region 1 (TRBC1),[138-140] which is less laborious and costly than Vβ repertoire analysis. The TCR β-chain constant region is encoded by two mutually exclusive T-cell receptor β-chain constant region genes: TRBC1 and TRBC2. The utilization of TRBC1 or TRBC2 during TCR gene rearrangement is a random process, and thus normal T cells express a mixture of TRBC1 and TRBC2, whereas a clonal T-cell population

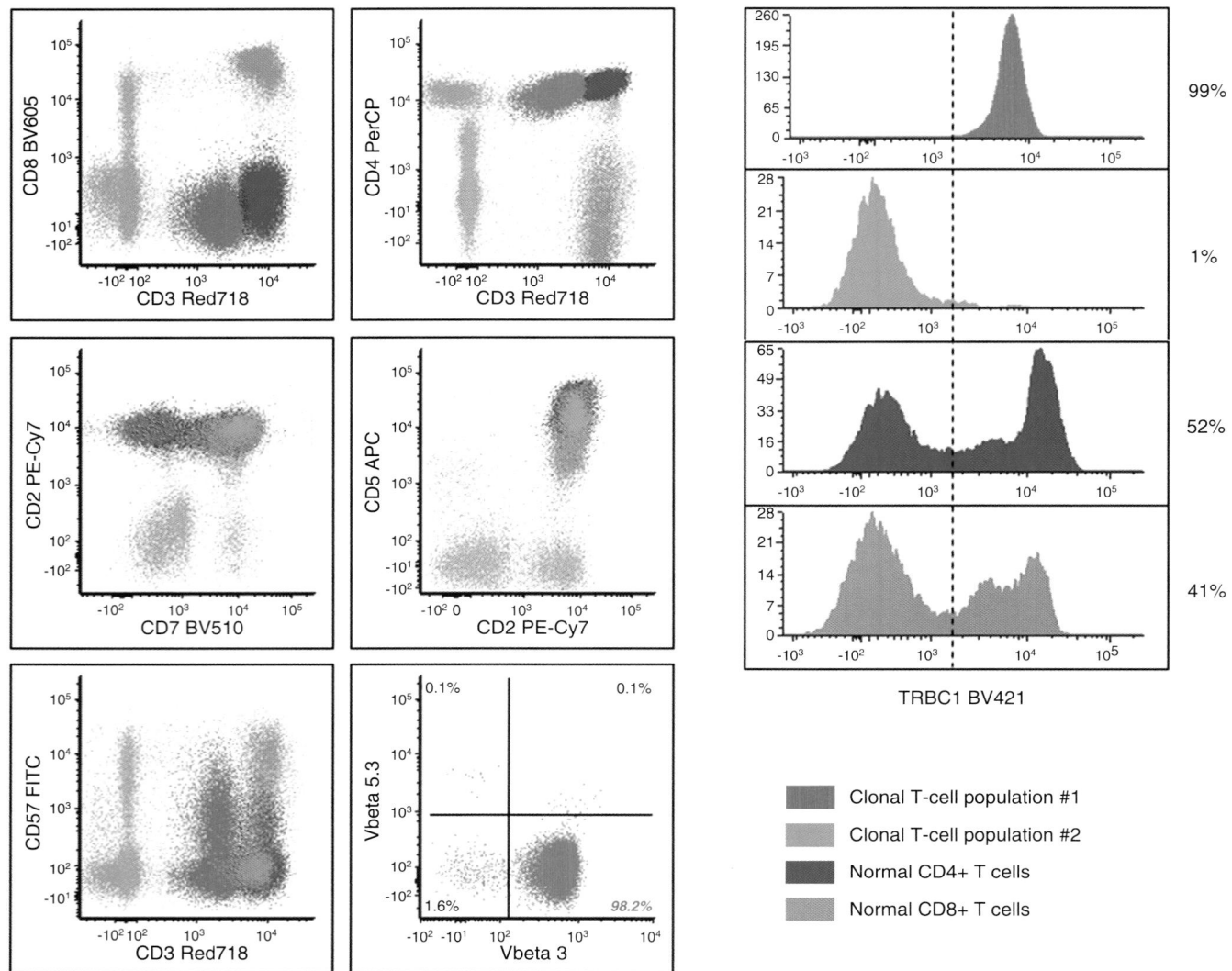

Figure 4-9. Flow cytometric evaluation of T-cell receptor β-chain constant region 1 (TRBC1) expression for assessment of T-cell clonality. Two abnormal T-cell populations with an aberrant phenotype are identified in this peripheral blood specimen. One population *(red)* demonstrates abnormally dim CD3 and partial CD57, lacks CD7, and expresses CD2, CD4, CD5, and a monotypic TRBC1 pattern (99% positive). Concurrent Vβ repertoire shows restricted expression of Vβ-3, supporting a clonal T-cell population. An additional abnormal T-cell population *(green)* lacks surface CD3, expresses CD2, CD4, CD5 and CD7, and is negative for TRBC1 expression. The normal CD4-positive *(blue)* and CD8-positive *(purple)* T cells show a polytypic TRBC1 expression pattern.

exhibits restricted expression of either TRBC1 or TRBC2. Monoclonal antibody is currently available to detect TRBC1 by FCM. In combination with a panel of antibodies, analysis of the TRBC1 expression pattern allows clonality assessment on immunophenotypically defined abnormal T cells. Figure 4-9 shows an example of peripheral blood that contains two clonal T-cell populations with a monotypic TRBC1 expression pattern (the red population is TRBC1 positive; the green is TRBC1 negative); the normal T cells in the background demonstrate a polytypic pattern.

NATURAL KILLER CELL NEOPLASMS

Normal NK cells are characterized by the expression of CD16 and/or CD56, and they also express a subset of T-cell antigens, including CD2 and CD7. Unlike T cells, NK cells only express subunits of the CD3 complex, including the epsilon and zeta chains (CD3ε and CD3ζ); they lack the gamma and delta chains (CD3γ and CD3δ) and are unable to form CD3 heterodimers.[141,142] Thus, NK cells are usually CD3 negative by FCM immunophenotyping assays using anti-CD3 antibodies that recognize assembled CD3 heterodimers and are often CD3-positive by immunohistochemical assays that typically use anti-CD3ε antibodies. This difference in the pattern of CD3 expression is useful in distinguishing NK-cell neoplasms from T-cell neoplasms.[143]

NK cells express neither TCRαβ nor TCRγδ and have the TCR genes in the germline configurations. They are usually negative for CD4 and CD5 and often show partial and dim expression of CD8. Normal NK cells usually exhibit a heterogeneous pattern of CD16, CD56, and CD57. The bright CD56-positive and dim CD16-negative NK cells are found primarily in the second lymphoid tissue and are abundant cytokine producers with limited cytotoxic activity. Dim CD56-positive and bright CD16-positive NK cells are the major circulating subset and act primarily as cytotoxic effector cells.[144,145]

Although no specific immunophenotypic markers exist that accurately distinguish reactive from neoplastic NK cells, changes in the pattern of surface antigen expression may be helpful to identify abnormal NK cells.[146] CD16 may appear unusually homogeneous, and CD56 may be abnormally bright or uniformly dim, as has been observed in chronic lymphoproliferative disorders of NK (CLPD-NK) cells (synonym and related term: NK-large granular lymphocytic leukemia, WHO classification).[147] Diminished expression of CD2 or CD7, aberrant expression of CD5, and a homogeneous pattern of CD8 expression may also be helpful features. In addition, the number and proportion of NK cells and the NK-cell FSC properties (presence of large cells) also help the diagnosis, especially in extranodal NK/T-cell lymphoma, which has a marked inflammatory background.

Both extranodal NK/T-cell lymphoma and aggressive NK-cell leukemia often exhibit a bright CD56-positive, dim to negative CD16 phenotype, reflecting the possible origin from this NK-cell subtype.[148] CLPD-NK cells have been shown to consist of two major entities: one subtype is characterized by signal transducer and activator of transcription (STAT) pathway activation, including STAT3/5B variants, and exhibit a bright CD16-positive immunophenotype; the other subtype demonstrates loss of function, *TET2* mutation, and a dim CD16 phenotype.

Confirming clonality in NK cells in the clinical laboratory setting is often challenging. Unlike T-cell neoplasms, a true NK-cell neoplasm will exhibit germline configuration of the T-cell receptor gene. Human NK cells express multiple receptors that recognize specific ligands on target cells, such as the major histocompatibility complex (MHC) class I molecules, and deliver inhibitory or activating signals to finetune the cells' cytotoxic activity. FCM analysis of NK-cell receptors, including the killer-cell Ig-like receptors (KIRs) and the C-type lectin receptors, such as CD94/NKG2 heterodimers and CD161, have been applied to evaluate NK-cell neoplasms.[149,150] Individual NK cells express different sets of KIR molecules, and the combinational diversity of KIRs leads to a broad range of NK-cell specificity.[151] Thus, analysis of the repertoire of KIRs (e.g., CD158a, CD158b, and CD158e) in a normal NK-cell population yields an unrestricted distribution of KIR expression, but a clonally expanded NK-cell population may demonstrate a restricted or skewed pattern.[152] It should be noted that the KIR expression patterns are mainly determined epigenetically through DNA methylation and can be stably maintained over multiple cell generations,[153] allowing the use of KIR repertoire analysis to investigate NK-cell clonality.

In contrast to KIRs, the C-type lectin receptors CD94/NKG2 and CD161 are not clonally expressed. Nonetheless, these NK-cell receptors may still be useful in evaluating NK-cell neoplasms. Bright expression of CD94 and NKG2A has been shown to distinguish CLPD-NK from a reactive NK-cell population.[154] Diminished CD161 expression is also frequent in CLPD-NK.[146,152,154] However, these findings are not specific and have also been described in viral processes and EBV-driven lymphoproliferations,[155-157] so clinicopathologic correlation should be used and care should be exercised in their interpretation. Currently, these modalities are limited in availability and are not routinely used in clinical FCM laboratories.

FLOW CYTOMETRY IN DIAGNOSIS AND CLASSIFICATION OF ACUTE LEUKEMIA

The approach to diagnosis of acute leukemia by FCM often begins with evaluation of a CD45-versus-SSC plot. Most abnormal progenitor or blast populations have decreased CD45 and intermediate SSC and can be recognized as an expanded population in a CD45-versus-SSC–defined "blast gate"[158] (Fig. 4-10A and B). As the CD45-versus-SSC–defined blast gate also contains cells that are not blasts (these include basophils, plasmacytoid dendritic cells, plasma cells, hypogranular neutrophils, and immature monocytes), any suspected blast population should be evaluated by a panel that will (1) allow definition of a population as a blast with specific markers and (2) allow lineage assignment. Some populations of blast equivalents fall outside the typical CD45-versus-SSC–defined blast gate (Fig. 4-10C and D); therefore, the evaluation for leukemic blasts should not be limited to this region. As true myeloid leukemias can aberrantly express lymphoid markers, and vice versa, the use of a comprehensive panel is vital for accurate lineage assignment.[3,13,159-161] The WHO and International Consensus Classification (ICC) diagnostic classification systems incorporate specific genetic alterations and characteristic translocations that carry prognostic and sometimes therapeutic implications into the classification of leukemia.[13,162,163] Associations between specific genetic and immunophenotypic features in acute leukemia have been described, and FCM may provide the first clue to the presence of a specific underlying genetic alteration. In addition, FCM MRD detection carries important prognostic implications and may guide further therapeutic options.

Acute Myeloid Leukemia

FCM immunophenotyping plays an important role in the WHO classification of acute myeloid leukemias. FCM is highly sensitive and specific in differentiating acute myeloid leukemia (AML) from acute lymphoblastic leukemia (ALL) and in identifying granulocytic, monocytic, erythroid, and megakaryocytic differentiation. In general, blasts in AML express a combination of antigens associated with an immature phenotype (which may include CD34 and/or CD117)[13,159,161] in conjunction with myeloid antigens (which may include CD13, CD33, CD15, and myeloperoxidase). Aberrant expression of lymphoid markers (such as CD2, CD5, CD7, CD19, or CD56) may be seen in some cases as well.[13,159,161] A typical example of AML is illustrated in Figure 4-10E to H. The patterns of antigen expression that characterize neoplastic blasts generally differ from that seen on normal regenerating myeloid blasts; for this reason, an understanding of normal antigen expression patterns is critical in differentiating leukemic blast populations from marrow regeneration. This is particularly important in the setting of MRD detection post-therapy.

In addition to the standard myeloid blast seen in most subtypes of AML, blast equivalents may include abnormal promyelocytes (seen in acute promyelocytic leukemia) or

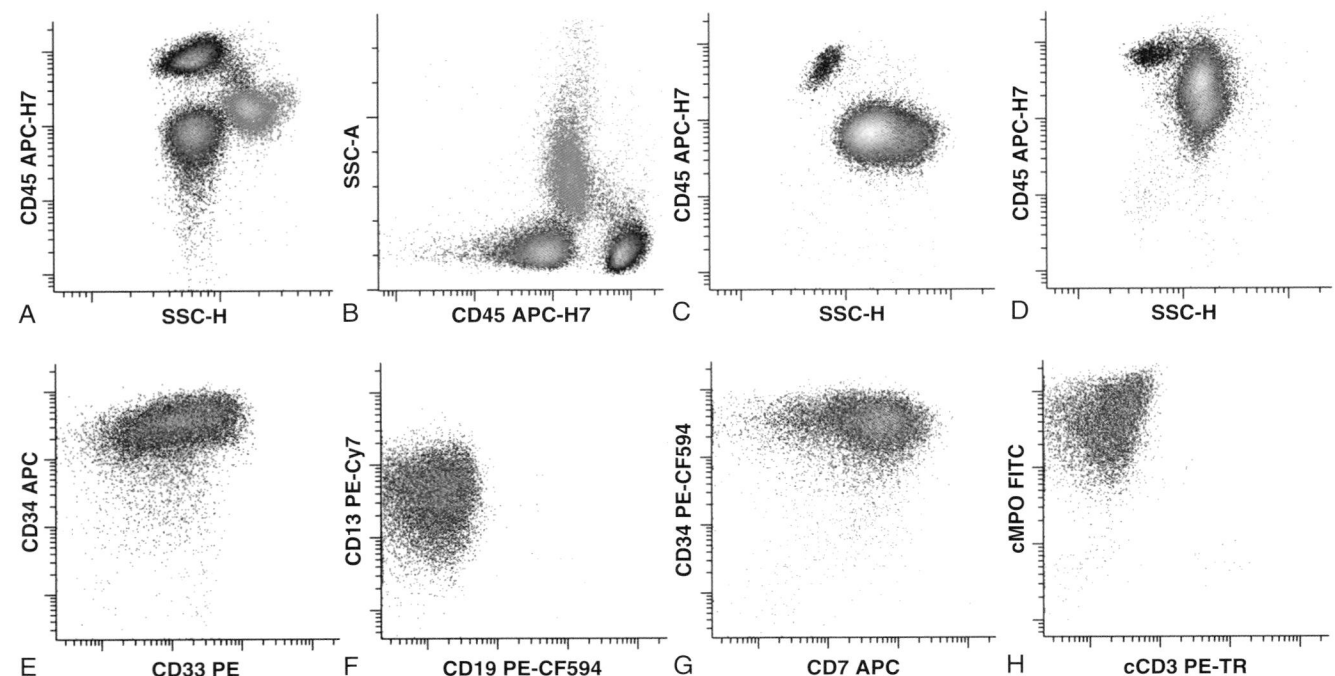

Figure 4-10. Acute leukemia. A CD45-versus-SSC plot from a bone marrow specimen involved by acute myeloid leukemia (AML) is shown in panels **A** and **B**. All viable cells are displayed. **A** shows CD45 on the *y*-axis and side scatter (SSC) height (log scale) on the *x*-axis. Panel **B** shows SSC area on the *y*-axis (linear scale) and CD45 on the *x*-axis. Blasts in both histograms *(red)* are identified as a population with decreased CD45 and intermediate SSC. Mature lymphoid cells *(blue)*, monocytes *(pink)*, and granulocytes *(green)* are shown. **C** and **D**, All viable cells are displayed. Blast equivalents are shown *(red)*. **C**, As the blast equivalent in acute promyelocytic leukemia has higher SSC than a typical myeloid blast, the neoplastic promyelocytes may overlay the area of normal granulocytic cells on a CD45-versus-SSC plot. **D**, The blast equivalent in monocytic leukemias may express increased CD45 compared with a typical myeloid blast and may overlap with the typical position of monocytes on a CD45-versus-SSC plot. Panels **E-H** show blasts from the case depicted in panels **A** and **B**. These are myeloid blasts expressing CD34 and with CD13, variable CD33, and cytoplasmic MPO. The blasts are negative for CD19 and cytoplasmic CD3 but aberrantly express CD7, an antigen typically expressed on T-cell and NK-cell populations. Aberrant expression of a marker of a different lineage is an abnormality that may be seen in leukemic blasts.

immature monocytic cells (monoblasts or promonocytes that are seen in AML with monocytic differentiation). These blast equivalents are more differentiated than typical myeloid blasts and may not fall in the standard CD45-versus-SSC–defined blast gate (Fig. 4-10C and D). For instance, compared with typical myeloid blasts, abnormal promyelocytes generally have increased SSC, and immature monocytic cells may have higher CD45.

In the current WHO and ICC classifications, a few notable subtypes of AML are described with "recurrent genetic abnormalities," or characteristic genetic features. These include several AML subtypes with balanced translocations that respond well to therapy, have a high rate of complete remission, and carry a favorable prognosis. Because some of these AML subtypes exhibit a characteristic immunophenotype as well, FCM often provides the first clue that a case of AML may fall into a favorable subgroup and can prompt appropriate molecular and cytogenetic studies/correlation.

The immunophenotype of AML with t(8;21)(q22;q22.1) (AML with *RUNX1::RUNX1T1* fusion in the WHO 5th edition) translocation is usually CD34-positive, with expression of CD13 and CD33. Frequently, the B-lymphoid marker CD19

is co-expressed on a subset of the blasts.[164,165] CD56 may also be co-expressed, though less frequently than CD19, and may portend a poor prognosis, perhaps due in part to an association with *KIT* mutations.[166-168]

Among the acute myeloid leukemias with characteristic genetic abnormalities, the diagnosis of acute promyelocytic leukemia (APL, AML with *PML::RARA* fusion in the WHO 5th edition) carries with it specific clinical, prognostic, and therapeutic implications, setting it apart from other AML subtypes. APL carries an increased risk of disseminated intravascular coagulation, and the microgranular variant is known to present with a high white blood cell count and rapid doubling time. Despite this, APL is sensitive to treatment with agents including all-trans retinoic acid and arsenic trioxide and, if identified and treated in a timely fashion, carries a favorable prognosis. The leukemic promyelocytes exhibit a characteristic immunophenotype: (1) CD33 expression is usually bright and homogeneous; (2) CD13 is expressed in a heterogeneous fashion; (3) HLA-DR and CD34 are usually absent or may be dimly expressed on a minor subset; and (4) in contrast to normal promyelocytes, which show strong CD15 expression, CD15 is negative or only dimly expressed on abnormal promyelocytes. In the microgranular variant of

APL, the leukemic promyelocytes frequently co-express CD2 and may express CD34 at some level.[169,170]

Blast equivalents in AML with monocytic differentiation may exhibit brighter CD45 expression and may overlap with the location of normal monocytes on the CD45-versus-SSC plot. In monocytic differentiation, cells initially express HLA-DR, CD33, and CD64, and with maturation to mature monocytic cells, acquire high levels of CD14 and CD300e. Acute monoblastic and monocytic leukemia can express such monocytic antigens to varying degrees. Other characteristic antigens may be expressed, such as CD4, CD11b, CD11c, CD35, CD36, and lysozyme. Monocytic and myeloid cells share expression of many common antigens (e.g., CD13 and CD33); however, the normal maturation patterns are distinct and exhibit subtle differences in the timing and intensity of expression.[171,172] Expression of antigens typically associated with a different lineage may be seen in monocytic leukemia. For instance, aberrant expression of CD56 may be seen in AML with monocytic differentiation.[168] It is important to note, however, that CD56 may also be expressed in reactive monocytic populations and is not sufficient in isolation to denote neoplasia.[173] CD2 co-expression may be observed in AML with inv(16)(p13.1q22) (AML with *CBFB::MYH11* fusion in the WHO 5th edition), a subtype of AML with an expanded abnormal eosinophil component that often shows myelomonocytic maturation and carries a favorable prognosis.[159,174]

In addition to cytogenetic abnormalities, AML can be associated with gene mutations that carry prognostic significance. For instance, *FLT3* internal tandem duplications confer a poor prognosis, whereas *NPM1* mutations in the absence of *FLT3* mutations are associated with a favorable prognosis.[13] Detection of such abnormalities can be particularly helpful for prognostication in normal-karyotype AML. FCM may provide a clue to gene mutations in some cases. For example, in AML, blasts with cuplike nuclear indentations by morphology in conjunction with myeloperoxidase expression and decreased or absent CD34 and HLA-DR expression have been associated with *FLT3* and *NPM1* mutations.[175-177]

True pure erythroid leukemia is a rare entity. Immunophenotypically, it can be highlighted by bright expression of CD71 and glycophorin A. Erythroid blasts in pure erythroid leukemia with less evidence of maturation may lack glycophorin A. CD36 is also expressed in erythroid progenitors and may be observed in erythroid leukemia.[13,159] Interpretation, however, should be made with care, as both CD36 and CD71 are not lineage-specific. In addition, as glycophorin A is positive on mature red blood cells, lysis of red blood cells before staining is critical to avoid a false-negative result.

Blasts of acute megakaryoblastic leukemia characteristically express CD36 and can exhibit high FSC as a result of the larger size and volume of the cell relative to typical myeloblasts. Expression of CD36, the platelet glycoproteins, CD41, CD61, and CD42 (to a lesser extent) are also noted. Myeloid antigens CD13 and CD33 may be expressed. Because this entity is uncommon among AML cases (<5%), it is important to fully exclude the consideration of an undifferentiated acute leukemia, another subtype of AML, a plasmacytoid dendritic-cell neoplasm, or lymphoblastic leukemia in the immunophenotypic workup.[13] Careful examination of lymphoid markers, terminal deoxynucleotidyl transferase (TdT), and myeloperoxidase may be helpful. Also, care should be taken in the interpretation of CD41, CD42, and CD61, as platelets adhering to the surface of blasts or monocytes may lead to a false-positive result with these reagents.[13,159]

A recognized group of AML in children that may occasionally be associated with megakaryocytic differentiation is AML with an RAM immunophenotype (RAM are the initials of the first patient in whom this immunophenotype was described).[168,178] This subset of AML is characterized by expression of bright CD56 with dim-to-absent CD45 and CD38 without HLA-DR. AML with an RAM immunophenotype is sometimes associated with a *CBFA2T3–GLIS2* fusion, and studies suggest this subtype has a poorer overall prognosis.

Finally, when considering an AML diagnosis, one entity that may be included in the differential diagnosis is a blastic plasmacytoid dendritic-cell neoplasm (BPDCN). These are neoplasms of plasmacytoid dendritic cells (PDCs) that typically involve the skin, blood, and marrow. Both normal and neoplastic PDCs usually occupy the standard CD45-versus-SSC–defined "blast region" and express high levels of CD123 with HLA-DR and CD4. Unlike normal mature PDCs, neoplastic PDCs associated with BPDCN usually express strong CD56. A thorough immunophenotypic profile is needed to identify and definitively distinguish this entity from other CD56-positive hematopoietic neoplasms, including some AMLs and neoplasms of NK/T-cell origin.

B Lymphoblastic Leukemia/Lymphoma

The blasts of B lymphoblastic leukemia/lymphoma (B-ALL) typically express B-cell markers (CD19, CD22, cCD79a), with markers denoting immaturity (CD10, TdT, CD34, dim CD45). Surface Ig is almost always negative (though rare exceptions are described), and CD20 is often negative but may be expressed, often at a low level. Normal bone marrow contains B-cell precursors (hematogones) that can be increased in children and in the setting of bone marrow regeneration.[179] Hematogones demonstrate coordinated expression of many of the same markers listed earlier in very conserved patterns associated with normal B-cell maturation,[179,180] whereas B-ALL typically expresses patterns of antigen expression that deviate from that seen on normal hematogones (Fig. 4-11).[181] An understanding of normal hematogone antigen expression is critical for distinguishing a leukemic blast from a regenerating hematogone and is particularly important in the setting of MRD detection.

Similar to AML, there are some immunophenotypic correlates with genotype. For instance, in B-ALL with a t(1;19)(q23;p13.3) translocation fusing the *TCF3* and *PBX* genes, there is often a relatively mature immunophenotype (increased CD45, decreased CD34, and expression of cytoplasmic mu chain) and co-expression of CD9.[13] An association also exists between B-ALL lacking expression of CD10 and CD24 and aberrant expression of CD15 and 11q23 translocations involving the *KMT2A* gene, a poor prognostic feature.[13] Conversely, intense co-expression of CD10 with dim-to-absent expression of both CD9 and CD20 is characteristic of the prognostically favorable t(12;21)(p21;q22) *ETV6::RUNX* translocation.[13,182,183] Identification of these immunophenotypic features provides the first clue that cytogenetic studies may yield prognostically important information and prompt appropriate clinicopathologic correlation.

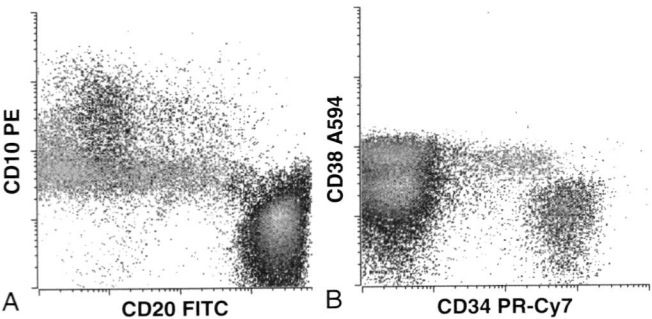

Figure 4-11. Residual disease in acute leukemia. The histograms depicted in panels **A** and **B** show all CD19-positive B cells from a bone marrow specimen of a patient with a history of B lympho-blastic leukemia/lymphoma. Normal mature B cells *(dark blue)*, normal hematogones *(aqua)*, and abnormal blasts *(red)* are shown. Normal hematogones have a predictable and conserved pattern of expression of antigens including CD10, CD20, CD34, and CD38; ab-normal blasts are easily identified, as they express abnormally high CD10 and CD34 and lack CD38. This pattern is not seen with normal hematogone maturation and allows separation of the abnormal blasts from the normal mature and maturing B cells. Additional examples of minimal residual disease (MRD) in acute leukemia are seen in Chapter 56 (Evaluation of Bone Marrow After Therapy).

T Lymphoblastic Leukemia/Lymphoma

In T-ALL, blasts typically express T-cell markers in conjunction with markers of immaturity.[13,159,160] The most commonly expressed T-lineage markers are cytoplasmic CD3 and CD7, though variable expression of CD2, CD5, and occasionally surface CD3 may be seen. CD4 and CD8 may be double positive, double negative, or singly expressed. TdT is typically expressed and indicates immaturity. Occasionally, CD34 expression can be seen as well. CD1a and CD10 may be expressed in some cases, and aberrant myeloid antigen expression, most commonly CD13 and/or CD33, has been observed.

Normal T-cell precursors are not present in significant numbers in the bone marrow; however, T-cell precursors are abundant in thymic tissue. Thymic T cells (as may be seen in a normal thymus, thymic hyperplasia, or thymoma) show a spectrum of maturation with highly conserved patterns of antigen expression. In contrast to normal thymic tissue, in which a spectrum of maturation is seen, T-ALL shows both aberrant antigen expression and relatively homogeneous antigen expression, allowing distinction of T-ALL and thymic tissue in most cases.[118,119]

One subtype of T-ALL that can be distinguished by FCM is the early T-cell precursor (ETP) subtype. ETP T-ALL has been associated with poorer response to induction therapy and poor prognosis in some, though not all, studies and has a distinctive immunophenotype with lack of CD8, lack of CD1a, and expression of myeloid and/or stem-cell antigens (CD13, CD33, CD34, CD117, and/or HLA-DR).[184,185] Although initial studies describing this entity indicated CD5 is characteristically dim or absent, more recent studies suggest a lesser significance to the pattern of CD5 expression.[186,187]

Acute Leukemia of Ambiguous Lineage

Occasionally, an acute leukemia may defy classification as AML or ALL. One may consider such cases as undifferentiated acute leukemia or mixed phenotype acute leukemia (MPAL). Before a diagnosis of undifferentiated acute leukemia or MPAL is rendered, an extensive FCM panel is required and should include the lineage-specific markers cytoplasmic CD3 and MPO, monocytic markers, and several B-cell markers.[13,162,163] A designation of MPAL may be considered when two distinct blast populations of different lineages are present or if a single blast population is present expressing antigens of more than one lineage (often myeloid or monocytic and lymphoid). In the later situation in which a single blast population is present, criteria for assigning lineage are well defined in the WHO 5th edition. To assign B-cell lineage, strong expression of CD19 with one additional strongly expressed B-cell antigen (CD10, CD22, or CD79a) or weak expression of CD19 with two additional strongly expressed B-cell antigens is required. Assignment of myeloid lineage requires expression of myeloperoxidase (with intensity of expression in part exceeding 50% of that expressed by a mature neutrophil) or expression of two or more monocytic antigens (non-specific esterase, CD11c, CD14, CD64, or lysozyme). Finally, T-lineage assignment requires strong expression of CD3 (surface or cytoplasmic). For lymphoid antigens, strong expression is defined as expression exceeding in part at least 50% of that of mature B or T lymphoid cells. Though the WHO 5th edition provides guidelines for intensity of antigen expression, a percentage threshold for positivity has not been specified. When undifferentiated acute leukemia is a consideration, evaluation of antigens to definitively exclude megakaryocytic, erythroid, and PDC differentiation is recommended as well.

Measurable Residual Disease Testing in Acute Leukemia After Therapy

MRD testing is emerging as a powerful prognostic factor in ALL and AML in both pediatric and adult populations.[188-192] In general, MRD detection by FCM relies on the principle that normal populations have very conserved and predictable patterns of antigen expression that accompany normal maturation. In neoplastic cells, these normal patterns are altered secondary to underlying mutations, leading to immunophenotypes not seen in normal healthy tissue. FCM allows for recognition of abnormal cells in the setting of normal background tissue, such as resting or regenerating marrow, on the basis of these immunophenotypic abnormalities. The two primary approaches to identifying MRD are the difference from normal (DfN) approach and the leukemia associated immunophenotype (LAIP) approach. In the DfN approach, normal maturation patterns are established using a standardized antibody panel, and leukemic cells are defined by their differences from normal patterns. In the LAIP approach, immunophenotypic abnormalities associated with leukemic cells are established at the time of diagnosis, and subsequent time points are evaluated for these abnormal populations. Most effective strategies incorporate elements of both approaches, and a combined approach is recommended by the European LeukemiaNet (ELN).[193] MRD testing allows for identification of abnormal blast populations at very low levels (often less than 1 cell in 10,000 can be detected).[194-196] This topic will also be discussed in Chapter 57: Evaluation of the Bone Marrow After Therapy.

Modern therapeutic regimens for acute leukemia often incorporate antigen-directed targeted therapies. Overlap may exist between targeted antigens and antigens used for gating or assessing populations by FCM in the post-therapy setting. Awareness of therapies used and the potential effect they may have on the immunophenotypic characteristics of normal and leukemic cells is critical for accurate interpretation of FCM data in the post-therapy setting.[197]

CHRONIC MYELOID NEOPLASMS

The use of FCM in evaluating chronic myeloid stem neoplasms (MSNs), such as myelodysplastic syndromes/neoplasms and myeloproliferative neoplasms, has grown significantly. Advances in this area have paralleled the increase in our understanding of normal patterns of antigen expression on myeloid progenitors and maturing myeloid forms and the routine use of multiparametric FCM in clinical laboratories. As has been noted, very conserved and synchronized patterns of antigen expression accompany normal maturation, and such patterns are disrupted in MSNs. Identifying aberrant antigen expression by FCM can aid in the diagnosis of MSN and, in some cases, FCM may provide additional prognostic data. Similar to MRD testing, it is worth emphasizing that experience and knowledge of how normal antigenic patterns can shift in various reactive states (for instance, growth factor administration or with bone marrow regeneration after a toxic marrow insult) is critical for accurate interpretation of FCM data.[171]

Myelodysplastic Syndromes/Neoplasms

Although bone marrow morphology with concurrent cytogenetic study remains the gold standard for the diagnosis of myelodysplastic syndromes/neoplasms (MDS), a significant number of patients have blood and bone marrow findings that make diagnosis and classification difficult.

Studies have demonstrated that FCM is useful in distinguishing MDS and non-MDS cytopenias,[198] with some studies suggesting the presence of abnormalities by FCM in patients with cytopenias correlates with morphologic dysplasia, genetic data, and risk of progression. For this reason, FCM is increasingly being used in diagnostic evaluation of potential MDS cases in an attempt to increase sensitivity and specificity of diagnosis.[199-201] This is reflected in the inclusion of FCM in the minimal diagnostic criteria for MDS developed at a 2006 international working conference.[202] Moreover, the 2016 *WHO Classification of Tumours of Haematopoietic and Lymphoid Tissues* recognized the utility of FCM in the evaluation of MDS.[13] Specific recommendations have not yet been provided in the WHO 5th edition or ICC classification systems. The ELN provides suggested standardized strategies for incorporation of FCM data into the diagnostic workup of MDS.[203,204]

Normal hematopoiesis is characterized by conserved changes in the appearance of cells that are predictable and orderly and accompany different stages of maturation. In MDS, normal hematopoiesis is rendered ineffective, leading to dysplastic changes that alter normal morphology. Similarly, this ineffective hematopoiesis leads to alterations in the normally highly conserved patterns of antigen expression accompanying normal maturation. Such changes in antigen expression can be detected by FCM and may be seen in a variety of lineages ranging from myeloid blasts to maturing granulocytic, monocytic, and erythroid cells.

No single MDS-specific immunophenotype exists; rather, it is a difference from normal that characterizes MDS. In addition, identifying MDS by FCM is best approached by considering several populations (e.g., myeloid progenitors, maturing myeloid forms, monocytic forms, erythroid forms). The types of abnormality seen on myeloid blast typically fall into one of four categories: (1) abnormal intensity of antigen expression; (2) dyssynchronous expression of mature and immature antigens; (3) homogeneous expression of an antigen normally expressed at varying levels during maturation; and (4) expression of an antigen of a different lineage (e.g., expression of CD5, CD7, or CD56 on myeloid blasts). Maturing granulocytic forms may show decreased SSC (Fig. 4-12A and

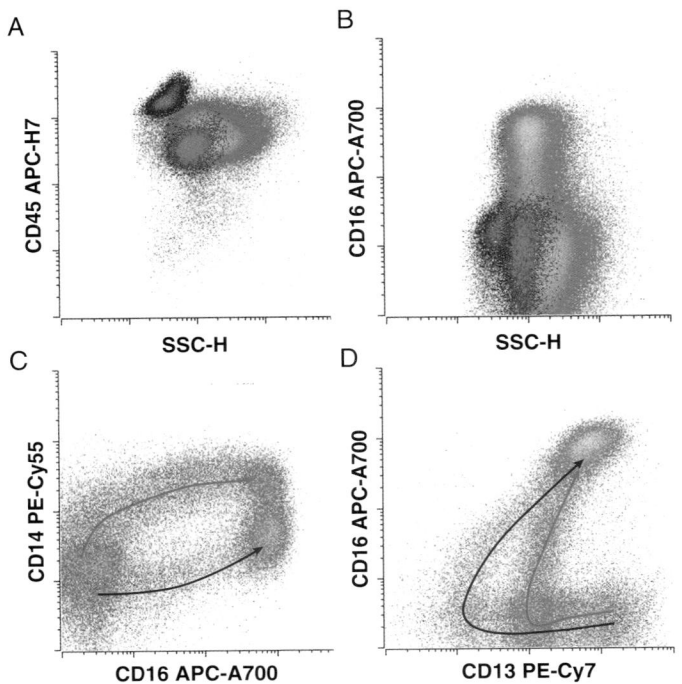

Figure 4-12. Flow cytometry in myelodysplastic syndrome (MDS). A and **B,** Decreased side scatter (SSC) on neutrophils. Dot plots show all viable cells from a bone marrow specimen involved by MDS. Lymphoid cells *(blue)* and maturing granulocytic cells *(green)* are shown. Myeloid blasts *(red)* are highlighted for emphasis. The maturing granulocytic population has variable SSC in this case, with the SSC of a major subset of granulocytic cells overlapping with the position of blasts and monocytic cells on the CD45-versus-SSC plot. The mature neutrophils (myeloid forms with the highest levels of CD16) have very low SSC (similar to that of the myeloid blasts). This finding is analogous to the neutrophil cytoplasmic hypogranulation seen in some cases of MDS. **C** and **D,** Abnormal patterns of antigen expression on maturing granulocytic forms. Dot plots show all maturing granulocytic cells from a bone marrow specimen involved by MDS. Normal granulocytic cells show conserved and variable expression of CD13, CD14, and CD16 markers, with maturation from the promyelocyte stage to the mature neutrophil. In this specimen, two separate lines of maturation can be appreciated. The *blue arrows* follow normal patterns of antigen expression with maturation, but in this case, a second, aberrant clone is present with increased expression of CD13 and CD14 *(red arrows)*.

B), paralleling the decreased cytoplasmic granularity seen in dysplastic neutrophils by morphology. In addition, maturing myeloid or monocytic forms may show aberrant patterns of antigen expression (e.g., an aberrant pattern of CD11b or CD13 vs. CD16 (Fig. 4-12C and D) or an increase or decrease in the intensity of a normally expressed antigen. Detection of the multiple characteristic immunophenotypic abnormalities that have been described in MDS depends on incorporation of large numbers of antibodies in a multiparameter panel. Antigens that are useful in detecting MDS on myeloid progenitors, maturing myeloid populations, and monocytic populations include, but are not limited to, CD5, CD7, CD10, CD11b, CD13, CD14, CD16, CD33, CD34, CD38, CD56, CD117, and HLA-DR.[171,198-201,205-209] Occasional associations between genotype and immunophenotype have also been described in MDS.[210]

Evaluation of erythroid precursors can be challenging, in part because specimen preparation often involves red cell lysis; however, several abnormalities have been described by FCM in association with erythroid maturation and include aberrancies in expression of CD36, CD71, and CD117.[206,211,212]

Myeloproliferative Neoplasms

Many patients with chronic-phase chronic myeloid leukemia (CML) are easily monitored for residual disease by molecular methods, typically fluorescence in situ hybridization (FISH), to detect the t(9;22) translocation. Virtually little-to-no role exists for FCM in a patient with chronic-phase CML with stable white blood cell counts. However, FCM can provide accurate blast characterization and an approximate enumeration of blasts and basophils for patients with increasing white blood cell counts who may be undergoing disease progression or entering blast phase.

The role of FCM is limited in uncomplicated polycythemia vera or essential thrombocythemia. In fact, neither isolated thrombocytosis nor polycythemia is considered an indication for FCM per the 2006 Bethesda International Consensus Recommendations for FCM or the American Society of Clinical Pathology Choosing Wisely recommendations for peripheral blood FCM.[5,213]

In cases of myelofibrosis, either primary or secondary to a preceding myeloproliferative neoplasm, abnormalities are often seen by FCM and are typically similar to those described regarding MDS.[172,200] There appears to be some relationship between the presence of cytogenetic abnormalities and FCM abnormalities in non-CML myeloproliferative neoplasms[172]; however, further study is needed to clarify the role of FCM in these diseases.

Acknowledgements

The authors wish to acknowledge Dr. Raul C. Braylan, Dr. Jonni Moore, Dr. Maryalice Stetler-Stevenson, and Dr. Brent Wood for their mentoring of colleagues and influential work in applying FCM to the diagnosis of hematolymphoid disorders.

Pearls and Pitfalls

Pearls	Pitfalls
Mature B-Cell Neoplasia	
• Blood and bone marrow may contain excess serum Ig that binds anti-kappa and anti-lambda antibodies, preventing binding to cells. Serum Ig bound to Fc receptors on cells also stains positive with anti-kappa and anti-lambda, interfering with detection of a possible B-cell clone. Washing blood or bone marrow specimens with room temperature or 37° C PBS eliminates free serum Ig and removes Ig bound to the cell surface.	• With small samples (e.g., CSF), cell loss during washing with PBS may be considerable. In the absence of significant serum contamination (e.g., no blood), consider reducing or eliminating washing.
• When polyclonal B cells are abundant, they obscure detection of abnormal B cells. Gating on large cells (with increased FSC), cells with abnormal antigen intensity, or cells expressing specific antigens (e.g., CD10) allows detection of monotypic B cells.	• Normal germinal-center B cells (often increased in follicular hyperplasia) are larger cells (with increased FSC) expressing bright CD20, CD10, CD38, and dim but present surface Ig. Recognition of this characteristic pattern will prevent misdiagnosis of B-cell lymphoma.
• Malignant B cells are frequently missing a normal antigen (e.g., CD19, CD20, CD22).	• Normal plasma cells are usually CD20-negative and CD22-negative. B cells are CD20-negative after rituximab therapy.
• Monotypic light chain expression (positive expression of only kappa or lambda surface Ig) is a characteristic feature of B-cell neoplasms.	• Normal plasma cells are surface-Ig negative but have intracellular light chain Ig expression. Germinal-center B cells have dim surface light chain Ig.
Plasma Cell Neoplasms	
• Plasma cells are detected based on expression of bright CD38 and CD138.	• CD38 expression can be dim in myeloma, and CD138 is labile. As myeloma characteristically has dim-to-negative CD45, by examining CD45 versus CD38, the abnormally dim CD38 myeloma cells can be detected.
• Plasma cell myeloma is detected based on an abnormal pattern of surface antigen expression. Frequently observed abnormalities include CD19-negative, dim or negative CD27, CD45-negative, CD56-positive, dim or negative CD81, CD117-positive.	• Plasma cells are present in lower numbers in FCM specimens. A large number of events must be acquired (minimum of 2 million, 3-5 million recommended); otherwise, an abnormal plasma cell population may be missed.
• Plasma cells will appear dim or negative CD38 after treatment with daratumumab, a monoclonal antibody therapy targeting CD38.	• To avoid missing dim or negative CD38 plasma cells in this scenario, consider alternative reagents to detect plasma cells (CD319, intracellular VS38c, intracellular IRF4, intracellular CD38, multiepitope CD38).

Continued

Pearls and Pitfalls—cont'd

Pearls	Pitfalls
Mature T-Cell Neoplasms	
• Failure to express a T-cell antigen (CD2, CD3, CD5, CD7) is a feature of 75% of T-cell malignancies. • Malignant T cells frequently demonstrate abnormal levels of antigen expression (too bright or too dim). • T-cell clonality is detectable by Vβ repertoire or TRBC1 analysis.	• CD7-negative T cells are a normal subset and can increase with infection. A subset of normal γδ T cells is frequently CD5-negative. • Levels of expression of some antigens, such as CD2, are affected by inflammation. • A background of normal T cells may obscure a clonal T-cell population. In such cases, gating on abnormal T cells with subsequent Vβ repertoire or TRBC1 analysis reveals the T-cell clone.
Acute Leukemia	
• A "blast cell" can be defined based on dim expression of CD45 with low/intermediate SSC. • Abnormal antigen expression characterizes and distinguishes abnormal blasts from normal blasts. • Lineage infidelity can be observed in acute leukemias (e.g., CD13-positive or CD33-positive ALL or CD7-positive AML). • Immunophenotype can predict genotype and may correlate with prognosis in some cases of acute leukemia.	• Some populations of blast equivalents (abnormal promyelocytes, promonocytes, monoblasts) may not fall in the CD45-versus-SSC–defined blast gate. Furthermore, some cells that fall within the blast gate are not blasts (plasmacytoid dendritic cells, basophils, plasma cells). • Knowledge of normal antigen expression patterns—on myeloid blasts and hematogones in the bone marrow and thymocytes in thymic tissue—is important to accurately identify abnormal blasts. • A complete immunophenotypic panel, including lineage-specific markers, is required to distinguish aberrant antigen expression of a different lineage from true mixed-phenotype acute leukemia. • The immunophenotypic changes seen generally reflect underlying genetic alterations. FCM should not be interpreted in isolation but should be used in conjunction with complete clinical, morphologic, and genetic data in the workup of acute leukemia.

FSC, Forward light scatter; *Ig,* immunoglobulin; *PBS,* phosphate-buffered saline; *sIg,* surface immunoglobulin; *SSC,* side or orthogonal light scatter.

KEY REFERENCES

4. Stetler-Stevenson M, Ahmad E, Barnett D, et al. In: Stetler-Stevenson M, Ahmad E, Barnett D, et al., eds. *Clinical Flow Cytometric Analysis of Neoplastic Hematolymphoid Cells; Approved Guideline-Second Edition. CLSI Document H43-A2.* Wayne, Pennsylvania, 19087-1898 USA: Clinical and Laboratory Standards Institute; 2005.

5. Davis BH HJ, Bene MC, Borowitz MJ, et al. *2006 Bethesda International Consensus Recommendations on the Flow Cytometric Immunophenotypic Analysis of Hematolymphoid Neoplasia: Medical Indications Cytometry Part (Clinical Cytometry).* ;72B. ; 2007:S5–S13.

6. Wood BL, A.M, Barnett D, et al. 2006 Bethesda international consensus recommendations on the immunophenotypic analysis of hematolymphoid neoplasia by flow cytometry: optimal reagents and reporting for the flow cytometric diagnosis of hematopoietic neoplasia. *Cytometry B Clin Cytometry.* 2007;72B:S14–S22.

36. Horna P, et al. Flow cytometric analysis of surface light chain expression patterns in B-cell lymphomas using monoclonal and polyclonal antibodies. *Am J Clin Pathol.* 2011;136(6):954–959.

41. Shao H, et al. Distinguishing hairy cell leukemia variant from hairy cell leukemia: development and validation of diagnostic criteria. *Leuk Res.* 2013;37(4):401–409.

46. Seegmiller AC, et al. Immunophenotypic differentiation between neoplastic plasma cells in mature B-cell lymphoma vs plasma cell myeloma. *Am J Clin Pathol.* 2007;127(2):176–181.

50. Fromm JR, Thomas A, Wood BL. Flow cytometry can diagnose classical Hodgkin lymphoma in lymph nodes with high sensitivity and specificity. *Am J Clin Pathol.* 2009;131(3):322–332.

101. Flores-Montero J, et al. Next Generation Flow for highly sensitive and standardized detection of minimal residual disease in multiple myeloma. *Leukemia.* 2017;31(10):2094–2103.

104. Roshal M, et al. MRD detection in multiple myeloma: comparison between MSKCC 10-color single-tube and EuroFlow 8-color 2-tube methods. *Blood Adv.* 2017;1(12):728–732.

119. Li S, et al. Flow cytometry in the differential diagnosis of lymphocyte-rich thymoma from precursor T-cell acute lymphoblastic leukemia/lymphoblastic lymphoma. *Am J Clin Pathol.* 2004;121(2):268–274.

123. Jamal S, et al. Immunophenotypic analysis of peripheral T-cell neoplasms. A multiparameter flow cytometric approach. *Am J Clin Pathol.* 2001;116(4):512–526.

128. Chen W, et al. Flow cytometric features of angioimmunoblastic T-cell lymphoma. *Cytometry B Clin Cytom.* 2006;70(3):142–148.

133. Tembhare P, et al. Flow cytometric immunophenotypic assessment of T-cell clonality by Vbeta repertoire analysis: detection of T-cell clonality at diagnosis and monitoring of minimal residual disease following therapy. *Am J Clin Pathol.* 2011;135(6):890–900.

143. Shi M, et al. Cytoplasmic expression of CD3epsilon heterodimers by flow cytometry rapidly distinguishes between mature T-cell and natural killer-cell neoplasms. *Am J Clin Pathol.* 2020;154(5):683–691.

146. Morice WG. The immunophenotypic attributes of NK cells and NK-cell lineage lymphoproliferative disorders. *Am J Clin Pathol.* 2007;127(6):881–886.

171. Kussick SJ, Wood BL. Using 4-color flow cytometry to identify abnormal myeloid populations. *Arch Pathol Lab Med.* 2003;127(9):1140–1147.

192. Short NJ, et al. Association of measurable residual disease with survival outcomes in patients with acute myeloid leukemia: a systematic review and meta-analysis. *JAMA Oncol.* 2020;6(12):1890–1899.

195. DiGiuseppe JA, Wood BL. Applications of flow cytometric immunophenotyping in the diagnosis and posttreatment monitoring of B and T lymphoblastic leukemia/lymphoma. *Cytometry B Clin Cytom.* 2019;96(4):256–265.

196. Chen X, Wood BL. Monitoring minimal residual disease in acute leukemia: technical challenges and interpretive complexities. *Blood Rev.* 2017;31(2):63–75.

203. Porwit A, et al. Revisiting guidelines for integration of flow cytometry results in the WHO classification of myelodysplastic syndromes-proposal from the International/European LeukemiaNet Working Group for Flow Cytometry in MDS. *Leukemia.* 2014;28(9):1793–1798.

Visit Elsevier eBooks+ for the complete set of references.

Chapter 5

Molecular Pathology of Hematologic Neoplasms

Eric Duncavage, Gabriel C. Caponetti, and Adam Bagg

INTRODUCTION

The understanding of the biological basis of hematopoietic diseases in general and neoplasia in particular has been significantly enhanced by the application of genetic and especially molecular techniques to the study of these diseases. The use of Southern blotting hybridization analysis, although now obsolete, initiated the integration of molecular biological techniques into hematopathology and substantially contributed to understanding the clonality status of lymphoproliferative disorders. The availability of molecular probes to the antigen receptor loci facilitated identification and molecular cloning of partner genes involved in chromosomal translocations underlying the pathogenesis of several lymphoid neoplasms. The advent of the polymerase chain reaction (PCR) had a dramatic effect on the ability to interrogate primary tissue samples for molecular aberrations, including refinement of the understanding of clonality in lymphoproliferative disorders and detection of translocations. The versatility of PCR resulted in adaptations including rapid amplification of cDNA from both 5′ and 3′ ends for the identification of genes involved in chimeric fusions driving hematopoietic neoplasia. The implementation of PCR-cycle sequencing profoundly enhanced the ability to identify somatic point mutations in a variety of neoplasms and tracking of clonal genetic aberrations after therapy and in tumor progression. The advent of next-generation (also referred to as massively parallel or high throughput) sequencing (NGS) has offered the most detailed view of genetic aberrations in hematologic neoplasms, with an acute myeloid leukemia (AML) genome being the first cancer genome to be sequenced.[1] This development led to the refinement of our understanding of the genetic basis of most hematologic neoplasms and facilitated diagnoses and recognition of prognostically relevant subgroups. Today the identification of recurrent genomic findings is required for the accurate classification of many myeloid neoplasms and has an increasing role in the assessment of a number of lymphoid neoplasms.[2-5] Sequencing-based diagnostics have been rapidly adopted by most laboratories, with applications extending into risk-stratification, therapy selection, and tracking disease after therapy. A summary of the major genomic methods and their features is presented in Table 5-1.

BIOLOGICAL AND TECHNOLOGIC ISSUES

Nucleic Acid Isolation and Tumor Enrichment

The successful implementation of molecular techniques depends on the reliable and robust extraction of nucleic acids. The protocols implemented depend on the specimen type and quantity and on the quality and amount of nucleic acid required for the assay. PCR now permits the analysis of a wide variety of specimens, including fresh whole blood, bone marrow aspirates, plasma, serum, fine-needle aspirates, tissue biopsies, cultured cells, cerebrospinal fluid, dried aspirates, and fixed paraffin-embedded tissues. Microdissected cells or ethanol-fixed cells scraped from cytologic slide preparations may have DNA or RNA extracted that is readily interrogated by molecular techniques. For most clinical applications, filtration column-based DNA/RNA extraction methods are preferred over simpler ethanol precipitation methods which tend to result in lower DNA/RNA purity. In general, DNA or RNA extracted from fresh (nonfixed) samples is preferable to

Table 5-1 General Features, Advantages, and Limitations of Comprehensive Genomic Methods

	CG	FISH	CMA	PCR	RT-PCR	WGS	WTS	Targeted NGS Panels	
Analyte	Chromosomes in dividing cells	DNA in interphase nuclei and metaphases	DNA	DNA	RNA	DNA	RNA	DNA	RNA
Coverage	Unbiased	Targeted	Unbiased	Targeted	Targeted	Unbiased	Unbiased	Targeted	Targeted
Need for viable cells	Yes	No	No	No	No	No	No	No	No
Resolution	~5 Mb	100–200 kb	20–100 kb	1b p	1 bp	1 bp	1 bp	1 bp	1 bp
Distinction of individual cell clones	Yes	Yes	No	No	No	No	No	No	No
TAT (days)	2–21	<1–2	3–7	<1–3	<1–5	3–14	14–21	7–14	7–14
Unmapped region detection	Yes	No	No	No	No	No	No	No	No
Ability to multiplex	Low	Low	High	High	High	High	High	High	High
Analytical sensitivity (%)	5	1–10	10–20	~0.01	~0.01	5–20	1–10	<1–10	5–10
SVs	Yes	Yes	No	Yes	Yes	Yes	Yes	No	Yes
CNAs	Yes	Yes	Yes	No	Limited	Yes	Limited	Limited	Limited
SNVs	No	No	No	Yes	No	Yes	Yes	Yes	Yes
ARGRs	No	No	No	Yes	Yes	Yes	No	Yes	Yes
Application	D, R, M	D, R, M	D, R	D, R, M, MRD	D, R, M, MRD	D, R	D, R	D, R, M, MRD	D, R, M, MRD
Availability	High	High	Moderate	High	High	Low	Low	High	High
Cost	$$	$$	$$$	$$	$$	$$$$	$$$$	$$$	$$$

ARGR, Antigen receptor gene rearrangements; *b,* base; *CG,* cytogenetics; *CMA,* chromosomal microarray; *CNA,* copy number alterations; *D,* diagnosis; *FISH,* fluorescence in situ hybridization; *kb,* kilobase; *M,* monitoring; *Mb,* megabase; *MRD,* measurable residual disease; *NGS,* next-generation sequencing; *PCR,* polymerase chain reaction; *R,* relapse; *RT-PCR,* reverse transcription PCR; *SNV,* single nucleotide variants; *SV,* structural variants; *TAT,* turnaround time (actual TAT availability and cost may vary significantly by region and laboratory); *WGS,* whole genome sequencing; *WTS,* whole transcriptome sequencing.
Data from references 5 and 402.

formalin-fixed samples; fixation results in extensive nucleic acid cross-linking and lower (often <200 base pairs [bp]) fragment sizes.[6]

Antigen Receptor Gene Rearrangements

B cells and T cells exhibit the unique characteristic of undergoing somatic DNA rearrangements of their antigen receptor gene loci to produce functional immunoglobulin (IG) and T-cell receptor (TR) molecules, respectively. The rearrangements provide a critical mechanism for generation of a significant component of the diversity of the IG and TR genes involved in the specificity of the immune response.[7]

Immunoglobulin Gene Rearrangement

The IG genes encode IGs that are produced exclusively by B cells. IG molecules are heterodimeric proteins consisting of two identical heavy chains linked with two identical light chains, kappa (κ) and lambda (λ). The IG genes are located on different chromosomal loci: the IG heavy (IGH) chain gene is located on 14q32, the IG kappa on 2p12, and the IG lambda on 22q11.

In the germline configuration, the antigen receptor loci are composed of noncontiguous segments of DNA grouped into variable (V), diversity (D), joining (J), and constant (C) regions. All three IG genes contain V, J, and C regions, but only IGH genes contain D regions (Fig. 5-1A). The IGH region contains approximately 45 functional V region segments and approximately 23 DH and 6 JH segments. The human IG constant region contains 11 C region segments that define nine functional IG classes and subclasses (IgM, IgD, IgG1, IgG2, IgG3, IgG4, IgA1, IgA2, and IgE). Early in B-cell development in the bone marrow, genetic recombination events occurring at the DNA level result in the initial joining of a single D segment with a J segment, followed by rearrangement of the partially rearranged D-J region to a V segment (Fig. 5-1B). These events are mediated by the recombination activating gene (RAG1/RAG2) complex. The fused V-D-J region is transcribed and joined to the Cμ (IgM) constant region segment at the RNA level. Successful rearrangement of one of the IGH loci is followed by light chain gene rearrangement, which entails direct joining of the V to J region segments because the light chain genes lack D segments. IGK rearrangement typically precedes IGL rearrangement. Further combinatorial diversity is generated by addition of nongermline palindromic (P) nucleotides through nonhomologous end joining and incorporation of nontemplated (N) nucleotides by the enzymatic activity of DNA terminal deoxynucleotidyl transferase (TdT).

The IGH genes are subjected to somatic hypermutation (SHM), which occurs when naïve B cells migrate to germinal centers of peripheral lymphoid tissues such as lymph nodes and is generally followed by class-switch recombination (CSR), where the IGH V-D-J segment is fused to a G, A, or E constant

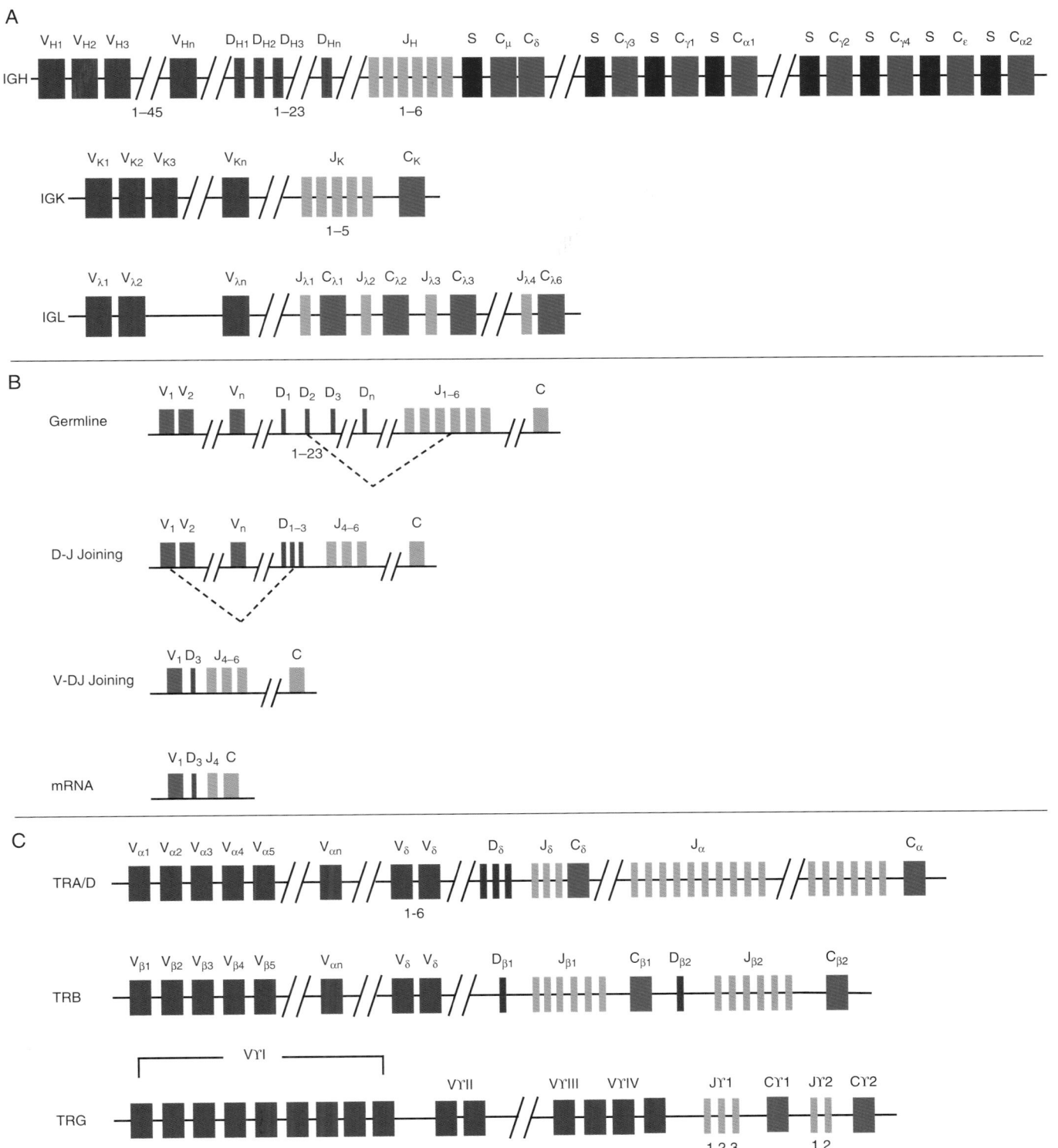

Figure 5-1. Structure of antigen receptor gene rearrangements and detection of clonal populations by polymerase chain reaction and next-generation sequencing (NGS). A, Schematic representation of germline configurations of immunoglobulin heavy chain and kappa (κ) and lambda (λ) light chain loci. *Top panel,* Immunoglobulin heavy (IGH) chain locus contains variable (V) region genes, diversity (D) region, joining (J) region, and constant (C) region segments. *Middle panel,* IG light chain kappa locus contains V, J, and C regions but no D regions. *Bottom panel,* IG lambda light chain locus contains V, J, and multiple C loci and no D regions. **B,** Genetic recombination events occur at the DNA level, resulting in rearrangement of the D segment with a J segment, followed by rearrangement of the partially rearranged D-J region to a V segment. In loci containing V, D, J, and C regions, the process begins with a D-J (partial) rearrangement, followed by a V-D-J or V-J (complete) recombination. This process is mediated by the RAG1/2 recombinases and results in deletion of all intervening segments and juxtaposition of V-D-J or V-J segments that are otherwise distantly (several kilobases) located from one another in the genome. **C,** Schematic representation of germline configurations of the T-cell receptor (TR) TRA/D, TRG, and TRD genes. Note the absence of D region segments in the TRG genes.

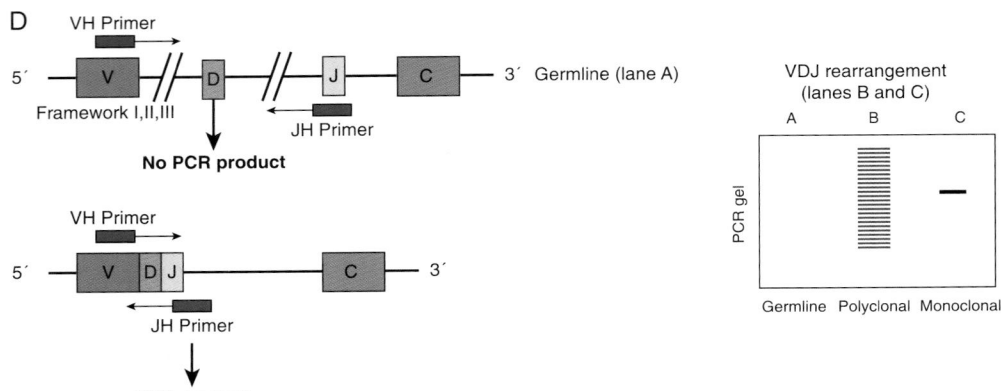

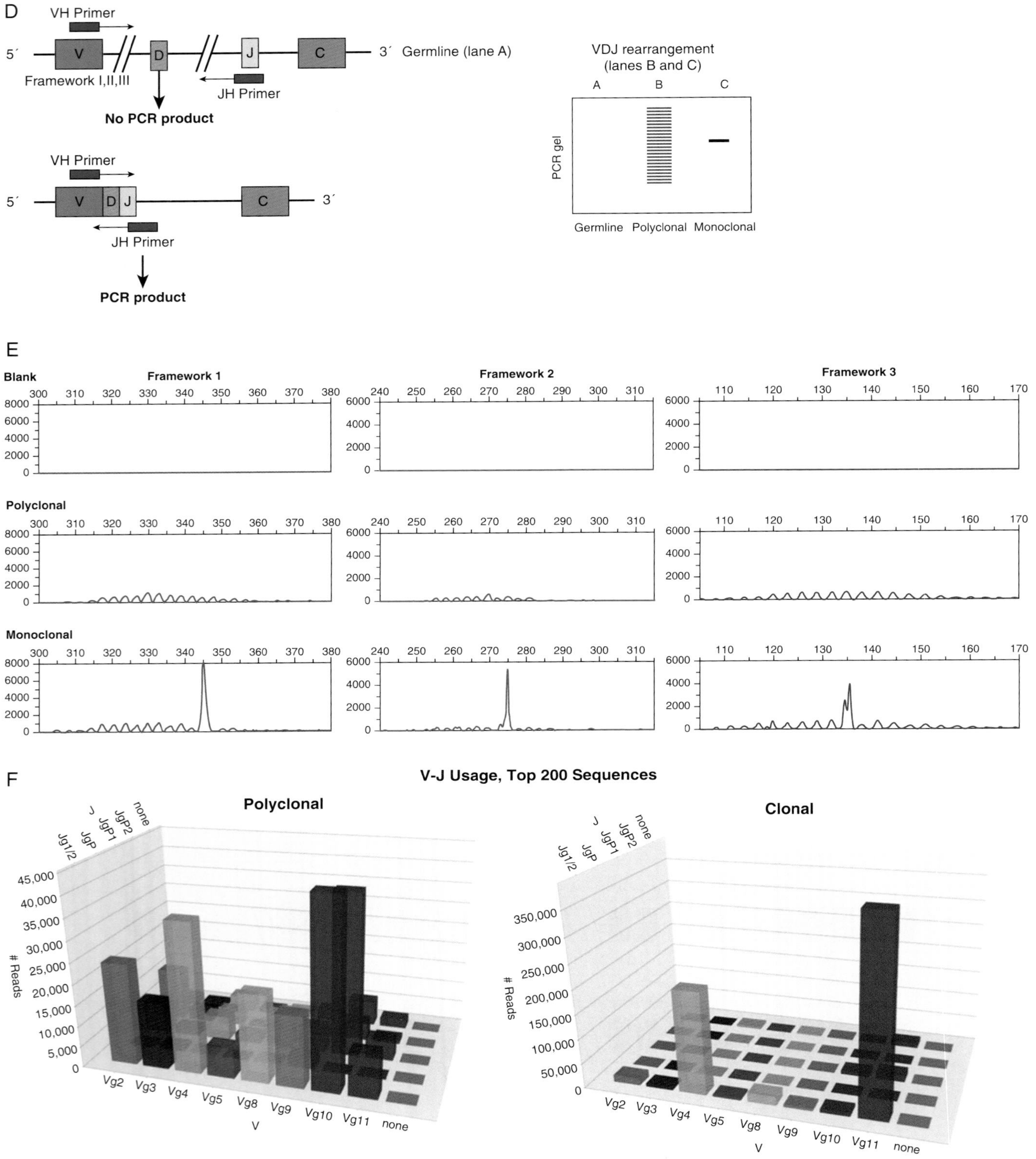

Figure 5-1, cont'd. D, Schematic representation of antigen receptor gene rearrangement detection by the polymerase chain reaction (PCR) and gel electrophoresis. Illustrated example is representative of PCR for clonality analysis of IGH gene showing V, D, J, and C regions separated by several kilobases. Consensus primers complementary to the V segment framework regions are used to recognize the majority of V regions. Similarly, primers recognizing the J region genes are used in the PCR amplification. No amplification occurs in the germline configuration from nonlymphoid cells because the V and J region genes are located several kilobases apart (lane A). A similar pattern would be observed in a no-template (H$_2$O only) control. In reactive conditions, each B cell has a unique (V-D-J or V-J) rearrangement and thus when resolved by gel electrophoresis yields a polyclonal ladder pattern reflective of the different recombination event (lane B). By contrast, clonal B-cell populations yield a single or two prominent bands on gel electrophoresis (lane C). **E,** Capillary electropherogram depicting IGH PCR clonality assay. *Top panel,* Template-free control. *Middle panel,* Polyclonal control showing multiple peaks distributed over a broad size range. *Bottom panel,* Single dominant peak in all three framework panels. **F,** TR clonality testing by NGS. This is similar to PCR-based testing, except that detection of PCR products is performed by sequencing instead of amplicon sizing by gel or capillary electrophoresis (CE). In this example, the plot on the left shows results from a reactive lymph node. Similar to electrophoretic detection, a number of peaks are seen representing various combinations of V (x-axis) and J (z-axis) regions. The height of the plot (y-axis) represents the number of reads (abundance). The plot on the right shows a T-cell lymphoma. Note that essentially all observed sequences are accounted for by two bars indicating a clonal cell population with two rearranged TRG loci. *(Image F courtesy of Bijal Parikh, MD PhD.)*

region segment, leading to expression of the gamma (γ), alpha (α), or epsilon (ε) heavy chains, respectively, in the B cells, although there is also evidence that CSR can occur prior to SHM.[8] Both of these processes are mediated by activation-induced cytidine deaminase.[7] SHM refines the specificity of the antibodies, with the highest level occurring in the third complementarity-determining region (CDR3). Thus primers for IGH gene rearrangements by PCR are designed to anneal to the framework regions where the hypermutation rate is lowest.

T-Cell Receptor Gene Rearrangement

The TCR is a heterodimeric protein comprising either an alpha (α) and beta (β) chain or a gamma (γ) and delta (δ) chain. A mature T cell expresses only either an $\alpha\beta$ or a $\gamma\delta$ TCR heterodimer. The TCR alpha (TRA) and delta (TRD) genes are located on chromosome 14q11.2. Indeed, the entire TRD gene is located within the TRA locus. The TRB encodes the TCRβ protein and is located at chromosome 7p34, and the TRG gene encodes TCRγ and is located at 7p14.

Precursor T cells migrate from the bone marrow to the thymus to undergo maturation into competent peripheral (postthymic) T cells. The hierarchy of the TCR gene rearrangements occurring during T-cell development is such that the TRD genes are the first to undergo rearrangement, followed by the TRG genes. As a result of these rearrangements, a small proportion of T cells express $\gamma\delta$ TCRs. The TRB genes are the next to undergo rearrangement.[9] This is detectable in the CD4-positive CD8-positive cortical thymocyte stage. The TRA genes are the next to rearrange, and this leads to deletion of the TRD locus that is located within the α locus. Successful TRB and TRA rearrangements lead to expression of TCR$\alpha\beta$ protein expression. T-cell maturation occurs with further thymic selection and egress of the mature T cells out of the thymus to the periphery.[10] This sequence of rearrangements has practical implications for T-cell clonality assays because although most T-cell lymphomas express TCR$\alpha\beta$, most of these will have undergone rearrangements of the TRG genes. The TCR gene rearrangement process is similar to that which occurs at the IG loci (Fig. 5-1C). Notably, however, SHM does not occur in the TCR genes and thus does not contribute to diversity of the T-cell repertoire, and CSR does not occur either.

Determination of Clonality in Lymphoid Proliferations

The expression of IG light chain molecules in mature B cells provides an avenue for convenient immunophenotypic assessment of clonality status in mature B-cell populations. Thus whereas clonality may be readily determined in mature B cells by immunophenotypic methods, determination of clonality by immunophenotyping of T cells has been technically challenging,[11] although more user-friendly flow cytometric assays have become available.[12] Clonality assays are frequently used in clinical contexts to establish the monoclonal status of suspicious lymphoid proliferations. Notwithstanding their utility in this setting, it is important to recognize that monoclonality is not equivalent to malignancy, and all laboratory results should be interpreted within relevant clinicopathologic contexts. Conversely, the inability to detect clonality does not exclude the presence of (lymphoid) malignancy, since these assays have a well-documented low rate of false negativity.

PCR (which will be discussed in detail) is the main approach for the detection of clonal lymphoid proliferations. The assay design uses consensus V region and J region primers in PCR amplification followed by electrophoresis. Because each lymphocyte harbors a unique IG or TR gene rearrangement, clonality analysis of polyclonal populations yields multiple products distributed over a size range within the amplicon detection limit of the PCR assay. This was historically visualized as a smear in agarose gels, a ladder pattern on polyacrylamide gels (Fig. 5-1D), or a multipeak pattern in capillary gels that are capable of single-base resolution. Protocols for the assessment of clonality evaluating the IGH, IGK, and IGL loci have matured to routine use and standardization in clinical laboratories.[13] Similarly, standardized T-cell clonality assays assessing the TRG, TRB, and TRD have also been successfully implemented.[14]

Capillary electrophoresis (CE), which separates products based on nucleotide number (amplicon size), has emerged as a reliable platform for the analysis of products from clonality PCR assays. Other options have included denaturing gradient gel electrophoresis and heteroduplex analysis on polyacrylamide gels that discriminate PCR products based on denaturation parameters, such as melting temperature, reflecting their nucleotide composition. Polyclonal B- or T-cell populations yield a pseudo-gaussian distribution of peaks when analyzed by CE (Fig. 5-1E). Each of the discrete peaks represents many antigen receptors that yield amplicons of identical size.[13,15,16]

Digital sequencing methods (i.e., NGS) have begun to replace CE for detection of clonal PCR products. Rather than relying on fragment size, sequencing-based detection determines the actual clonal sequence of the rearranged IG or TR locus and can be useful in resolving oligoclonal patterns caused by similarly sized PCR products that may represent different rearranged sequences (Fig. 5-1F).[17,18]

Interpretation

Monoclonal populations are identified with CE when one or two dominant peaks substantially above that of the next highest background peak are observed. The sensitivity of clonality assays by PCR and CE reliably permits detection of neoplastic populations at a 5% level in the background of polyclonal lymphocytes. Detection of clonal populations by sequencing generally involves counting the number of unique clonal sequences generated to determine whether any one (or two) sequences represents a larger than expected fraction (generally >3%–5%) of total observed sequences. A major advantage of sequencing-based detection is that the exact clonal sequence can be compared with previous cases, allowing for distinction between new primary lymphomas versus recurrences.[18] Sequencing-based detection can also be used for measurable residual disease (MRD) detection by simply querying all reads to determine whether a previously identified clonal sequence is present. These methods can be used from blood, marrow, or cell-free DNA to detect MRD in mature and precursor lymphoid neoplasms.[19,20]

Major Molecular Methodologies

Polymerase Chain Reaction

The PCR is primer-directed amplification of nucleic acid using a thermostable polymerase and thermal cycling to generate exponential copies from a DNA template.[21] In most protocols, the PCR requires template DNA, thermostable DNA polymerase, oligonucleotide primers that are designed to be complementary to target sequence, deoxynucleoside triphosphates (dNTPs) from each base (dATP, dTTP, dGTP, dCTP), and Mg^{2+}. For amplification of RNA, a cDNA synthesis step precedes the PCR amplification. The amplification reaction entails multiple cycles of denaturation, primer annealing, and extension. For conventional PCR, postamplification analysis involves electrophoresis of the products generated from the amplification reaction. Authentication of the product generated is based on visualization of bands or peaks of expected size for the amplicon. An alternative and popular quantitative format is real-time PCR, wherein homogeneous assays are performed with amplification product synthesis and analysis simultaneously occurring in a closed-tube format. A perfectly efficient PCR assay (i.e., doubling of DNA copy number every cycle) in one 30-cycle reaction yields approximately 10^9 (or more accurately $1,073,741,824 = 2^{30}$) copies of product. This amplification capacity renders PCR extremely sensitive and well suited for the molecular diagnosis and monitoring of hematopoietic neoplasms that carry characteristic genetic aberrations, such as translocations. Accordingly, PCR is more sensitive than conventional cytogenetics or fluorescence in situ hybridization (FISH) analysis and can detect 1 neoplastic cell in a background of 1000 normal cells when interrogating antigen receptor gene rearrangements or 1 copy of mutant DNA in a background of approximately 10^5 wild-type DNA sequences.

Real-Time Polymerase Chain Reaction

Real-time PCR is used to describe a technique wherein nucleic acid synthesis is monitored during amplification rather than at the end point. The technique incorporates fluorescent reporters into the amplification reaction and is monitored by use of thermal cyclers integrated with devices configured to monitor fluorescence. Fluorescence monitoring during the amplification reaction permits identification and quantification of the PCR product.[22] Because amplification and detection occur simultaneously in the same tube, real-time PCR is advantageous in that the process is rapid and less subject to the risk of contamination arising from liberation of amplicons from opening tubes before electrophoresis. Further, the ability to perform accurate relative and absolute quantification has favored the use of this approach in many applications in the clinical laboratory.

The fluorescent reporters used in real-time PCR assays are broadly classified into two major categories: non-specific nucleic acid binding dye-based and specific probe-based methods. The profile of real-time PCR resembles a logistic regression curve wherein there is an initial lag phase followed by a log-linear or exponential phase and finally a plateau phase. Efficient PCR is associated with doubling of the number of copies of the target, and this is reflected in a flat linear phase. At a critical fractional cycle number known as the cycle threshold (C_T), there is an exponential increase in product abundance reflected as geometric increases in the fluorescence levels above background. Accordingly, the C_T is defined as the number of cycles required for the fluorescent signal to exceed the background signal. C_T levels vary in inverse proportion to the starting quantity of the target nucleic acid in the sample, that is, the C_T value is lower when the initial quantity of the

template DNA is most abundant. Conversely, lower levels of input template will yield higher C_T values.

Three basic fluorescence chemistries are used in real-time monitoring of amplification reactions: double-stranded DNA binding dyes (generally no longer used in the clinical laboratory), fluorescently labeled primers, and target-specific probe-based detection.

Fluorescently Labeled Primers

Oligonucleotide primers labeled with fluorophores at the 5′ end may be used in real-time PCR assays.[23] In the simplest configuration, a primer can be labeled with one fluorophore at the 5′ end, and amplification results in increased synthesis of labeled template accompanied by changes in fluorescence that occur with hybridization. In another design, a primer can be labeled both with a fluorophore on the 5′ of a hairpin and a fluorescence quencher toward the 3′ end. During PCR, the primer undergoes conformational changes that result in separation of the fluorophore from the quencher, leading to an increase in fluorescence during each round of extension in the amplification reaction. Use of different-colored fluorescently labeled primers offers the ability to perform multiplex assays because the different products may be monitored in different fluorescence channels.

Target-Specific Probe Detection

Target-specific probes that are complementary to a sequence within the amplicon may be incorporated into PCR. The use of target-specific probes provides an additional level of specificity for detection of the authentic product. In general, three specific probe chemistries may be used in target-specific probe-based amplification reactions: hybridization probes, hydrolysis probes, and dual-mechanism probes. The target-specific probe-based mechanisms depend on fluorescence resonance energy transfer (FRET) occurring between donor and acceptor fluorophores, and fluorescence emissions from the reporter probe may be monitored as an index of amplicon synthesis during PCR.

Hybridization Probes. In this design, two oligonucleotide probes are included in the amplification reaction. Both probes are complementary to an internal sequence within the target and hybridize to the template. The 5′ probe has a donor fluorophore on its 3′ end, and the second probe carries the acceptor (reporter) fluorophore on its 5′ end (the interfluorophore distance is optimally ≤1 nucleotide). Excitation of the donor fluorophore with light leads to emission with FRET transfer to the acceptor fluorophore. The transferred energy results in the release of light at a longer wavelength that is then detected. This approach provides high specificity of identification of the target amplicon because fluorescence is a FRET–based event requiring hybridization of the probes to the template. Hence, low background levels are observed, ensuring high signal discrimination from background noise. The hybridization probe-based formats also offer the opportunity for further verification of the identity of the product by probe melting curve analysis. Despite this advantage and the exquisite specificity associated with this design, the requirement for a total of four oligonucleotides in the amplification reaction results in a higher level of complexity in hybridization probe-based assays.

Hydrolysis Probes. Target-specific probe-based systems may also be designed with fluorescently labeled probes configured with a donor fluorophore conjugated to the 5′ end of the probe and a quencher at the 3′ end. Because of the 5′ → 3′ exonuclease function of Taq polymerase, the probe is hydrolyzed and the donor fluorophore is separated from the influence of the quencher, leading to fluorescence. Because the target-specific probes are hydrolyzed, probe-melting analysis for verification of the identity of the amplicon is not reliably performed with this probe design. However, minor-groove binders functioning as hybrid stabilizing agents can be incorporated with the probe to improve the robustness of this system. Overall, the simplicity (only three oligonucleotides in the reaction for detection of one target) and specificity provided by this design favor its use in routine clinical settings.

Dual-Mechanism Probes. Several probe designs incorporate both hybridization and hydrolysis mechanisms. These include the hairpin probe-based system that incorporates a design wherein the loop portion of the hairpin is complementary to a specific target sequence and the stem sequences are a shorter segment on either end of the probe with base complementarity to one another. The 5′ end of the hairpin is labeled with a donor fluorophore and the 3′ end with a quencher. Hybridization separates the donor from the quencher and results in fluorescence. This approach is highly specific because fluorescence is based on a hybridization event to the authentic target.

Product Detection and Quantification

Real-time PCR provides an analytically precise and technically robust approach for quantification of nucleic acid species in a sample. The quantitative applications of real-time PCR take advantage of the large dynamic range of more than five orders of magnitude. Quantification by real-time PCR is most often achieved by determination of the C_T. The C_T represents a fractional cycle number obtained by interpolation of the amplification profile of the PCR. The C_T may be calculated by a variety of approaches, including the threshold analysis method, in which a baseline level of fluorescence is selected (typically from the early amplification cycles) and adjusted by arithmetic or proportional adjustment methods to represent a normalized baseline. This approach suffers the drawback of yielding less reliable results if sample fluorescence levels are low, as might occur in samples with low copy numbers of the intended target. An alternative and suitable approach not requiring such normalization is the *second derivative* maximum method. In the second derivative maximum method, calculation of the fractional cycle number takes the shape of the amplification curve into consideration. This is advantageous in that there is no requirement for baseline corrections or normalization of fluorescence values. Regardless of method used, well-optimized amplification reactions double template copy numbers with each cycle, and the C_T is inversely related to the logarithm of the initial template concentration (Fig. 5-2). Thus a log-fold increase in copy numbers between samples is reflected in a 3.3 cycle number decrease in CT ($2^{3.3} = 10 = 1$ log). Quantitative real-time PCR assays are continually used for the quantification of fusion transcripts such as *BCR::ABL1* in routine clinical diagnostics.

A more recent modification of real-time PCR is droplet digital PCR (ddPCR).[24] Using this approach, single DNA or cDNA molecules along with primers, fluorescently labeled probes, and PCR reagents are added and emulsified in individual nanoliter-sized droplets through the use of microfluidics. PCR

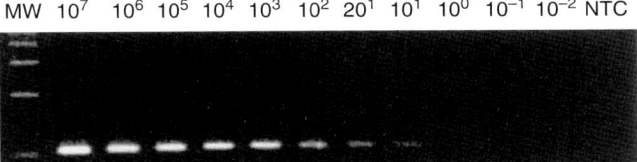
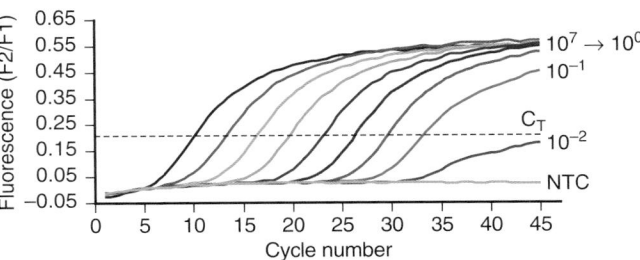

Figure 5-2. Quantitative polymerase chain reaction (PCR). *Upper panel,* Conventional quantitative PCR. Serial dilutions of template DNA are amplified over a range of initial template abundance from 10^7 to 10^{-2} copies. Amplification product is visible at 10^1 copies. Such "end-point"–based assays are more susceptible to quantification error because quantification may be performed at the nonlinear points of PCR amplification. *Lower panel,* Quantitative real-time PCR. Serial dilutions as in the upper panel. Crossing thresholds (C_T) increase in magnitude inversely to initial template quantity; although the specimens with 10^7 to 10^0 copies yield similar end-point amounts after 45-plus cycles, those with greater initial template amounts cross the C_T earlier. For example, the C_T value for the *dark blue line* (reflecting 10^7 copies) is approximately 10, whereas that for the *brown line* (reflecting 10^2 copies) is approximately 25.

is carried out on a standard thermocycler and the droplets are then read by a fluorescent reader to determine whether they are positive (amplified DNA present) or negative (no amplified DNA present). Each ddPCR reaction typically contains more than 10,000 droplets that are read individually. Unlike qPCR, the amount of template DNA with a mutation is not measured based on the number of PCR cycles (C_T value), but is instead calculated based on the abundance of droplets containing the amplified product with the mutation relative to those without the targeted mutation after a fixed number of PCR cycles. The large number of "digital" observations allows for more accurate quantification of targeted regions in the original template DNA, which can be calculated using a Poisson distribution. ddPCR can also be used to detect low abundance mutations such in *JAK2* p.V617F or *KIT* p.D816V in myeloproliferative or mast cell neoplasms, respectively, with sensitivities of 0.1% or better.[25]

Sequencing

Sanger Sequencing

Sanger sequencing is a method of DNA sequencing that uses nonextendable dideoxynucleotide incorporation by a DNA polymerase.[26] The classical dideoxy chain termination method includes a DNA fragment of interest, a DNA primer, a DNA polymerase, and deoxynucleoside triphosphates (dATP, dGTP, dCTP, and dTTP). One of four of the dideoxynucleoside triphosphates (ddATP, ddGTP, ddCTP, or ddTTP) is added to each reaction; the other three nucleotides are the standard unmodified deoxynucleoside triphosphates. PCR cycle sequencing entailing repeated denaturation, annealing, chain

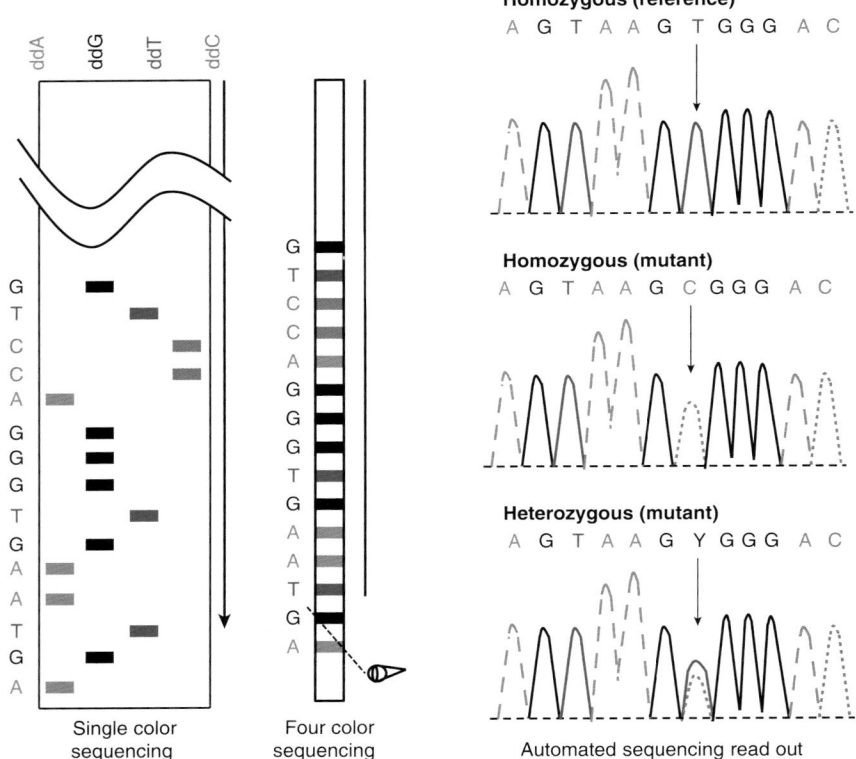

Figure 5-3. Sanger sequencing and next-generation sequencing (NGS) workflow. Schematic representation of Sanger sequencing using single-color and four-color sequencing. *Left panel,* Sanger sequencing with all dideoxynucleoside triphosphates labeled with the same single-color fluorophore (single color) and run on four parallel lanes on a sequencing (slab) gel. Chain termination at different lengths results in each lane's yielding polynucleotides of different lengths ending with the dideoxynucleotide containing the same base. The DNA sequence of the target is read by progressive identification of sequences with increasing lengths until the last base is reached. *Right panel,* Sanger sequencing with all dideoxynucleoside triphosphates labeled with distinct fluorescence tags: dideoxyadenosine (ddA), dideoxyguanosine (ddG), dideoxythymidine (ddT), and dideoxycytidine (ddC) and products run on one lane. Each base is discriminated by color, and sequencing is by progressive length based on migration time through a capillary that is read by a fluorescence detector positioned to detect changes in fluorescence. These changes are reflected as colored peaks identifying each base. *Right panel,* Sequencing electrophe-rogram showing base-specific color peaks representing bases in their respective positions. *Upper right panel,* Reference sequence. *Middle right panel,* Homozygous T-C transition (single-base substitution). *Bottom right panel,* Heterozygous T-C transition showing superimposed peaks representative of both bases.

extension, and termination steps is used to generate amplicon fragments of different lengths by incorporation of one of the four dideoxynucleotide base analogs (Fig. 5-3). The pentose ring in the dideoxynucleotide analogs lacks the 3′ hydroxyl and the 2′ hydroxyl groups. Given that DNA chain extension requires the 3′ hydroxyl group, incorporation of such a base terminates further chain elongation. The fragments generated are fluorescently labeled either by fluorescently labeled primers or by fluorescently labeled dideoxynucleotide terminators. In modern sequencers, the products of cycle sequencing are resolved with denaturing polyacrylamide gels or, more frequently, CE. Detection is achieved by interrogation of fluorescence signals as the DNA fragments traverse the gel past a detector. When fluorescently labeled primers are used to label the amplified fragments, four tubes are required for separate termination reactions. In assay configurations wherein one color is used, each dideoxy termination reaction mixture is subjected to electrophoresis in a separate lane or capillary. Alternatively, if four fluorophores are used, the termination reactions may be combined in one tube during electrophoresis and resolved with only one capillary. Conventional Sanger sequencing permits routine analysis of DNA fragments of up

to 800 to 1000 bases in multiwell plate assays containing 96 or 384 samples in a 2-hour analytical run. Sanger sequencing is capable of reliable detection of mutant alleles constituting 20% of the allele burden in somatic conditions (neoplasms) with heterozygous mutations (Fig. 5-3).

Next-Generation Sequencing

Next-generation sequencing (NGS) is arguably the most disruptive of technologic advances in molecular biology since the development of PCR and has dramatically transformed the landscape of molecular diagnostics testing. NGS has also been referred to as massively parallel sequencing or high throughput sequencing. Typical workflow for the role of NGS for the clinical diagnostics laboratory is represented in Figure 5-4. In the research setting, NGS is used for de novo genome assembly, DNA resequencing, transcriptome and exome sequencing, and epigenomics studies that continue to reveal novel insights in constitutional genetics and the genetic basis of disease.[27] NGS is not a single technology, but represents multiple sequencing approaches that rely on massive parallelization of the sequencing process to generate massive amounts of sequencing data for comparatively little

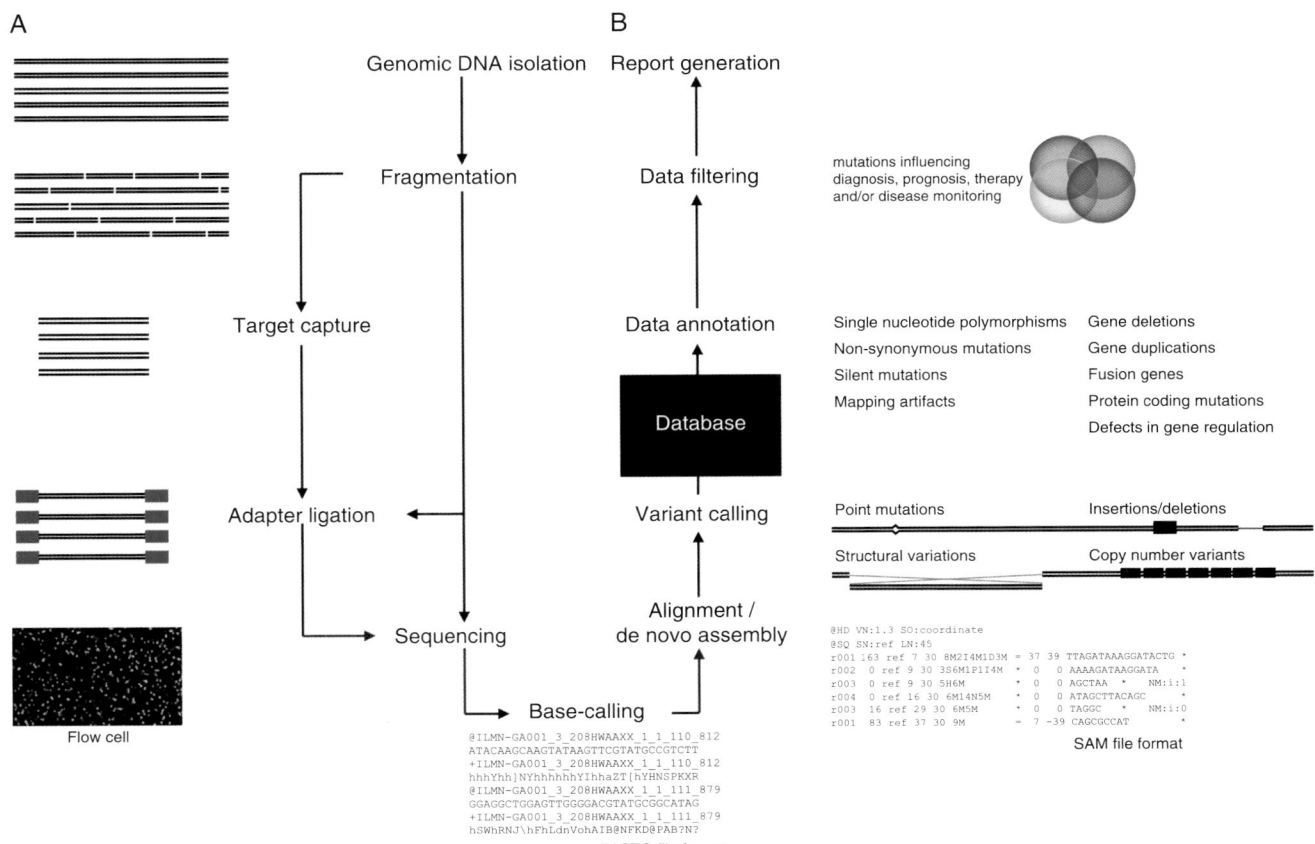

Figure 5-4. Next-generation sequencing (NGS) workflow. A, Extracted nucleic acid is fragmented by one of several methods (e.g., shearing or ultrasonic fragmentation). This is followed by ligation of adapter sequences (oligonucleotide sequences that permit universal amplification) onto the ends of the DNA fragments. Nucleic acid (DNA or cDNA) templates are generated from the libraries, which are then clonally amplified for subsequent sequencing. When sequencing is complete, the analysis pipeline for NGS data includes a preprocessing step to remove adapter sequences, end trimming and removal of low-quality reads, mapping to the reference genome, or de novo alignment and alignment of compiled sequences. **B,** Sequence analysis includes base-calling, detection of single nucleotide variants and insertion/deletion variants, chimeric fusion sequences (RNA sequencing), and juxtaposed genomic sequences from noncontiguous loci resulting from large structural variations such as deletions, insertions, and translocations. Sequence variants are annotated in a first step, and secondary annotation is achieved by conversion of the nucleic acid variants to amino acid sequences. Further annotation may be performed, including prediction of the functional consequences of DNA or encoded amino acid variations (e.g., deleterious). Interrogation of databases to catalog variants and to assess association with specific clinical end points, such as diagnostic, prognostic, and therapeutic implications, may be performed and indicated in an integrated report.

cost.[27] Historically, most NGS technologies have relied on short-read sequencing approaches, where read lengths are generally shorter (75–400 bp) than those generated by Sanger sequencing. However, newer approaches now facilitate read lengths of >10 kb, allowing for sequencing of low complexity parts of the genome and providing the ability to phase genomes by reconstructing haplotypes.[28] Clinical diagnostic sequencing is currently dominated by two platforms, one made by Illumina Inc. (San Diego, CA) and the other by Thermo Fisher Scientific (Waltham, MA). However, with expiration of key patents in the field, it is expected that new companies and technologies will enter the space, further driving down the cost of sequencing.

The Illumina series of instruments use a sequencing-by-synthesis approach coupled with reversable fluorescent dye terminators. With this chemistry, DNA libraries are flowed over a glass substrate called a *flow cell* where they bind fixed oligonucleotides complementary to either the 3′ or 5′ end of the library.[29] The affixed DNA is then amplified in situ in a process known as *bridge amplification* to produce clusters of replicated DNA molecules attached to the flow cells. Fluorescently labeled dNTPs (four colors to one color per base in older chemistries, or two colors in newer sequencing by synthesis chemistries) are added to the flow cell along with DNA polymerases; these dNTPs are modified with a reversible terminator so that only a single fluorescently labeled dNTP can be added to the newly synthesized strand. Once the dNTP is added to the synthesized DNA molecule attached to the flow cell, the flow cell is scanned with a laser to determine the color (identity) of the incorporated base. The reversable block on the incorporated nucleotide is then removed, completing the sequencing cycle, and the process repeated, allowing for reads as long as 300 bp. Illumina sequencing is also capable of paired-end sequencing where the library is sequenced from both the 3′ and 5′ directions, which allows for better read-mapping during analysis.

The Thermo Fisher Ion Torrent sequencing approach is similar in that it also uses a sequencing-by-synthesis approach but uses a unique semiconductor pH-based detection method instead of fluorescently labeled bases. In this approach,

DNA template molecules are confined to nano wells on the sequencing chip and deoxyribonucleotide triphosphate bases are added one at a time (as opposed to Illumina chemistry, where all four bases are added during each sequencing cycle). If the added base is incorporated into the synthesized DNA molecule, a proton (H+) and pyrophosphate molecule are released. Release of the proton is measured by detecting a change in pH in the nano well using a complementary metal oxide semiconductor (CMOS) sensor embedded below. The order that bases are added to the flow cells is called the *flow space* and is recorded in the sequencing data file along with the identity of the incorporated base called the *base space*. Advantages of this approach over fluorescently labeled nucleotide include more rapid data acquisition and less reagent consumption. Disadvantages include difficulty resolving long homopolymer runs (>7 bp) and lower overall throughput compared with dye-labeled methods.

In addition to commonly used Illumina and Thermo Fisher sequencing approaches, several other technologies have entered the clinical market. PacBio HiFi sequencing (Menlo Park, CA) allows for accurate single molecule read lengths of >15 kb and has found utility in phasing genomes and sequencing in difficult-to-resolve, low-complexity areas of the genome.[30] Oxford Nanopore Technologies sequencing (Oxford, UK) uses a α-hemolysin-like protein nanopore to generate real-time sequencing data by passing single DNA molecules through the pore and measuring changes in charge across the pore. Charge profiles are specific for each base and allow for rapid real-time sequencing without the need for chemical detection systems, which allows for much smaller instrument sizes. Nanopore sequencing can generate long reads and directly detect methylated cytosine bases, similar to PacBio. Disadvantages of the Nanopore approach include higher error rates than other methods and lower overall throughput than competing methods.

Multiple other sequencing platforms are beginning to enter the market, including MGI Tech (Shenzhen, China), Ultima Genomics (Newark, CA), Roswell Biotechnologies (San Diego, CA), and Element Biosciences (San Diego, CA). Regardless of platform, all sequencing methods first require library preparation, which can include targeting of specific regions of the genome.

Sequencing Concepts

One of the most important sequencing concepts is coverage or sequencing depth, which refers to the number of reads that span a given position in the genome. To a large extent the sensitivity or limit of detection of an NGS assay is based on the amount of coverage obtained. Sequencing coverage is ultimately determined by the user and is a function of both the sequencing instrument and the number of samples in each run. Coverage can be further divided into total coverage and unique coverage, which reflects the number of nonduplicate reads. Unique coverage is related to the number of DNA molecules present in the library and determines the limit of detection for a particular sample.

Another important sequencing concept is the variant allele frequency (VAF). The VAF is simply a measure of abundance for a particular mutation or variant and is calculated by dividing the number of reads with a particular mutation by the total number of reads that span the position. For inherited or germline variants, VAF are either 50% (heterozygous) or 100% (homozygous); however, for somatic (acquired) variants, mutation VAFs can range from <1% to 100%, the latter when there is a concurrent copy number alteration.

DNA Library Preparation

An important first step in library preparation involves DNA fragmentation by acoustic sonication or enzymatic methods, followed by DNA repair and end polishing. Synthetic DNA adapters are then covalently ligated to each 3′ and 5′ end of the genomic DNA, termed an *insert*, by a DNA ligase enzyme to create a library. These adapters are platform-specific universal sequences that are used for amplification of the library fragments and are required to anneal the libraries to the flow cell. DNA libraries prepared from genomic DNA can be used directly for whole genome sequencing (WGS) or enriched for exome or targeted sequencing. During the library preparation step, sample-specific indexes (usually 8–10 bp DNA oligonucleotides) can be added to one or both ends of the library. Sample indexes allow for multiple libraries to be sequenced in a single run, optimizing throughput and reducing overall costs. Once sequencing data is generated, reads can be demultiplexed based on the sample index. The use of multiplex sequencing is common in clinical applications. Libraries may also be modified to include unique molecular identifiers (UMIs, also called *molecular barcodes*). UMIs are generally synthesized as random (degenerate) oligonucleotides ranging from 8 to 16 bp, but they may also represent fixed sequences in some implementations. UMIs allow for tracking of individual DNA molecules throughout the amplification and sequencing process and are typically used for high sensitivity sequencing applications where low background error rates are required.

Whole Genome Sequencing

WGS provides a comprehensive annotation of the genome of an individual or sample. WGS provides a detailed map of the structural variations occurring in a genome, including complex and large structural aberrations such as translocations and rearrangements, copy number variations including whole chromosomal additions and losses, loss of heterozygosity, small insertions and deletions, and single nucleotide variations (e.g., point mutations), all within a single assay.[31] While WGS is the simplest NGS method to implement in the clinical laboratory because of the lack of enrichment steps, until recently WGS was limited to research studies because of the high cost of sequencing and complexity of data analysis. Continued reductions in sequencing costs, coupled with cloud-based and hardware-accelerated informatics platforms, have now made it possible to perform clinical WGS from blood or marrow in as little as 3 days at a cost comparable with conventional multiplatform genomic evaluation.[32] As sequencing costs continue to drop, it is expected that WGS will ultimately replace current cytogenetic testing for hematologic neoplasms.

Transcriptome Sequencing

Transcriptome (RNA) sequencing (RNA-Seq) is a large-scale and comprehensive analytical interrogation of the transcriptome.[32] RNA-Seq entails isolation of RNA, from which a library of cDNA fragments is generated. Adapters are ligated to one or both ends of the cDNA fragments, and each molecule is then sequenced in a massively parallel fashion. Short polynucleotide sequences varying in length from 30 to 400 base pairs are obtained from one end in single-end sequencing or from both ends in paired-end sequencing. RNA-Seq entails conversion of isolated RNA (total or subspecies such as poly[A]+) into a cDNA library to which adapters are attached. The reads obtained from sequencing may be aligned to a reference genome or transcripts or assembled de novo to generate a genome-level transcription map that includes the transcriptional architecture and expression levels of each gene. The flexibility of NGS platforms permits powerful applications, such as massively parallel cDNA sequencing or RNA-Seq, which has led to significant advances in the characterization and quantification of transcriptomes. Unlike gene expression arrays, RNA-Seq is not limited to detection of known transcripts and thus, RNA-Seq can offer information on small RNAs, such as microRNAs, PIWI-interacting RNAs, and short interfering RNAs with greater dynamic range.[33-35] RNA-Seq also permits characterization of alternative splicing events and gene-fusion identification.[35] RNA-Seq–based gene-fusion identification has been pivotal in the identification of novel gene fusions that are oncogenic drivers in many forms of human cancer, including many hematologic neoplasms.[36-38]

Accordingly, several algorithms have been developed to facilitate the identification of chimeric fusions from RNA-Seq data. These include TopHat-Fusion,[39] ChimeraScan,[40] and deFuse,[41] among others. Although WGS and some targeted sequencing panels can also detect translocations from DNA, this requires sequencing of large intronic regions to identify DNA-level breakpoints, making RNA-Seq more efficient in terms of sequencing usage. Potential disadvantages of RNA-based fusion detection include preanalytic variability in RNA preservation leading to false negative results and the inability to detect translocations that do not result in fusion gene products (e.g. *IGH::MYC*).[42] RNA-Seq has also been applied for detection of mutations,[43] but this is subject to variations in the abundance of transcripts. Targeted multiplex panels focusing on multiple recurrently translocated genes that participate as fusion partners in several neoplastic conditions can be configured for diagnosis.

Whole Exome Sequencing

Whole exome sequencing (WES) involves the massively parallel sequencing of protein-coding regions of the genome. This method has dramatically facilitated the investigation of genomic alterations that lead to mutations in coding sequences that are associated with diseases. The human exome contains ~30 million base pairs, thus constituting approximately 1% of the human genome (~3 billion base pairs) and representing approximately 180,000 exons. Both mendelian and somatic genetic abnormalities underlying human diseases are readily identifiable by exome sequencing. WES requires use DNA capture to enrich for protein-coding sequences in genomic DNA. An important consideration is that there is no formal definition of the exome, and exome reagents vary by manufacturer in terms of exactly what regions are included.

The sensitivity of exome sequencing varies depending on the depth of coverage but typically ranges from 2% to 5% VAF given mean coverages of 100× to 500×. Although WES covers all coding regions and is therefore useful for the discovery of coding region mutations, exome sequencing cannot detect structural variants such as translocations,

because breakpoints generally occur in intronic regions. Depending on the analysis methods used, exome sequencing may be able to detect copy number alterations (CNAs); however, there may be difficulty in detecting smaller CNAs in regions of the genome in which there are few or widely spaced gene exons.[44]

Targeted Sequencing

Targeted sequencing panels make up the vast majority of clinical NGS tests performed for hematologic neoplasms. Targeted sequencing methods are similar to exome methods in that they require enrichment of sequencing libraries for specific target genes or regions. The number of targeted genes varies greatly depending on the application but typically ranges from 5 to 1000 genes. Enrichment technologies can be divided in to two main categories: PCR enrichment (amplicon-based), which is generally faster and suited to small (<50 gene) panels; and capture-based enrichment, which is well suited to larger panels (Fig. 5-5). The genes or regions targeted by the panel can be chosen by the laboratory or may be part of a vendor-supplied kit. The major advantages of targeted panels over broader sequencing approaches such as WES or WGS is lower cost and higher sensitivity. By focusing sequencing on clinically significant genes, it is possible to obtain high coverages (500×–1000×) for minimal cost.

Sequencing for Measurable Residual Disease

Advances in sequencing methods, especially error-corrected sequencing using UMIs, have allowed for ultrasensitive sequencing to evaluate for measurable (previously termed *minimal*) residual disease in follow-up blood, marrow, or cell-free DNA (cfDNA) specimens. The limit of detection for these methods typically ranges from 0.1% VAF for detection of somatic mutations in AML to <10^{-6} for detection of clonal IG or TCR sequences in B-lymphoblastic leukemia/lymphoma (B-ALL) or T-ALL. In general, mutations are first identified in a diagnostic sample and subsequent posttreatment samples are evaluated to determine the extent to which these mutations have been cleared. Mutation clearance has become an important biomarker for many hematologic neoplasms and can be used to assess patient relapse risk or response to a specific therapy.[45-47]

Optical Genome Mapping

Optical genome mapping (OGM) is a technique that allows for detection of structural variants in DNA including translocations and CNAs. In this approach DNA is not directly sequenced and is instead digested by multiple restriction enzymes and stained with a fluorescent dye, creating a fragment map of the genome from which structural variants can be inferred. Modern OGM methods use microfluidics to create restriction maps from numerous single DNA molecules, which are then analyzed to create a high-resolution consensus map. Similar to WGS, OGM has been shown to be more sensitive than conventional G-banded cytogenetics to detect structural variants in myeloid neoplasms.[48,49] OGM is currently less expensive than WGS, making it a potentially appealing technology for clinical laboratories. Limitations of OGM include the requirement for ultrahigh molecular weight DNA and the inability to detect gene-level mutations, including single nucleotide variants and insertions/deletions, the latter of which necessitates running

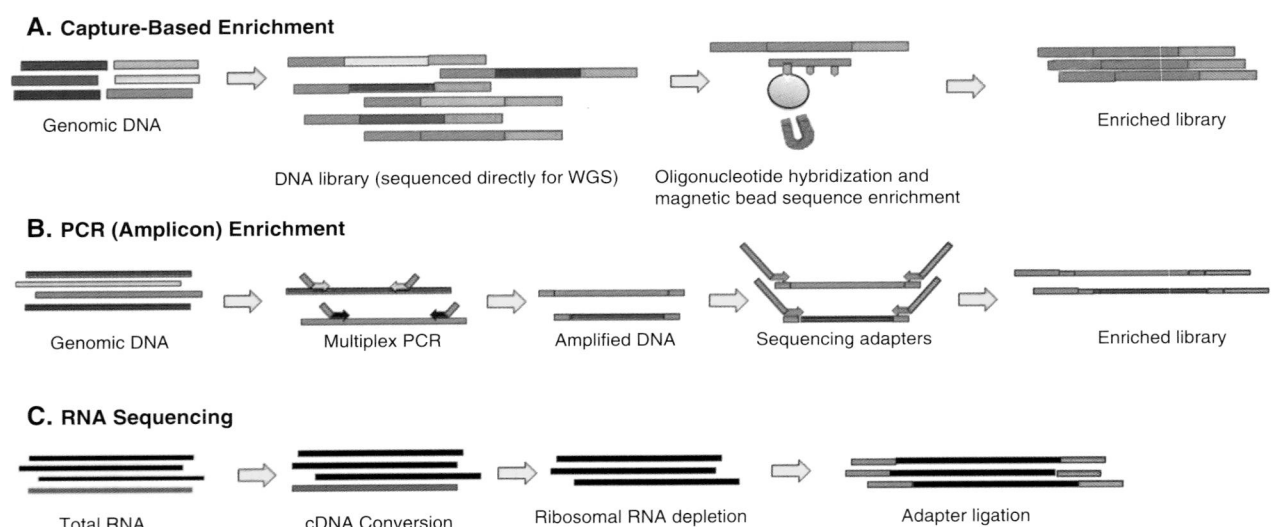

A. Capture-Based Enrichment

Genomic DNA

DNA library (sequenced directly for WGS)

Oligonucleotide hybridization and magnetic bead sequence enrichment

Enriched library

B. PCR (Amplicon) Enrichment

Genomic DNA

Multiplex PCR

Amplified DNA

Sequencing adapters

Enriched library

C. RNA Sequencing

Total RNA

cDNA Conversion

Ribosomal RNA depletion

Adapter ligation

Figure 5-5. Capture-based versus amplicon-based enrichment for next-generation sequencing (NGS). A, Capture-based enrichment is the most common approach for most clinical sequencing applications. Genomic DNA is generally first fragmented by either mechanical or enzymatic methods. Adapter sequences (specific to the sequencing platform) are then ligated on to the 3′ and 5′ ends of DNA inserts to make a library. This library can be sequenced directly for whole genome sequencing (WGS). The library can also be enriched using oligonucleotide probes to target genes or regions of interest. The probes then bind DNA inserts by sequence-complementary hybridization. Probes are synthesized to contain biotin molecules, allowing for magnetic bead enrichment when coming after the addition of streptavidin-coated magnetic beads. DNA not bound to probes is washed away, leaving a library enriched for specific sequences of interest. **B,** Amplicon-based sequencing can be implemented in a variety of ways. In the simplest approach, genomic DNA is amplified using primers that target genes or regions of interest, often using multiplex PCR reactions. PCR primers are typically tailed with a short motif that can be recognized by a second set of longer primers with sequencer specific adapters. **C,** RNA sequencing libraries can be prepared multiple ways. In general, total RNA is extracted and converted to cDNA using random hexamer primers. The resulting cDNA is then depleted of ribosomal RNA, and sequencing adapters are added. Similar to DNA, cDNA libraries can be enriched by hybrid capture to focus sequencing to specific regions, permitting for targeted translocation detection or detection of specific transcripts.

OGM in parallel with panel-based NGS testing for complete genomic evaluation.

Epigenomics

The role of epigenetic changes is increasingly being recognized in the pathogenesis of cancers.[50] The implementation of NGS–based methods may be used for assessing DNA methylations status, mapping of transcription factor occupancy, and evaluation of histone modification. Genome-wide interrogation of DNA methylation can be performed by sequencing libraries before and after treatment with sodium bisulfide. Methylated cytosines will be converted to uracil (thymidine). Post-bisulfide-treated DNA can then be compared with pretreatment data to determine how many cytosine bases have been replaced by thymidine, indicating the presence of methylation at that position. Less expensive but informative alternative strategies, such as reduced representation bisulfite sequencing and targeted enrichment followed by bisulfite treatment, can also be used.[51,52] Affinity enrichment-based methods with methylcytosine-specific antibodies (MeDIP-Seq) and recombinant methyl binding domains of proteins[53] enable identification of genome regions that are modified by methylation. It is important to note that newer sequencing technologies such as PacBio and Oxford Nanopore instruments can detect methylated cytosines directly and do not require bisulfite sequencing.

Single-Cell Sequencing

Sequencing-based evaluation can now be performed on the single-cell level, allowing for more granular evaluation of genomic events, including dissection of clonal hierarchies. Although not currently used in the clinical setting, single-cell sequencing can identify RNA expression patterns or DNA mutations within individual cells.[54,55] This can be used to define how specific mutations drive changes in gene expression. Single-cell methods have also been adapted to measure protein expression (CITE-Seq) by coupling antibodies to oligonucleotide tags that can be detected by the sequencer in conjunction with DNA or RNA sequencing data.[56]

Bioinformatics and Computational Methods for Next-Generation Sequencing

Bioinformatic analysis remains a challenge and bottleneck in the interpretation of NGS data. Many of the analytical programs still require command line computer languages and can be difficult for bioinformatics nonexperts to use. Nevertheless, several programs now exist to simplify NGS data analysis by provision of easy-to-use graphical interfaces.

In general, the primary data outputs from each platform typically consist of text files containing sequence reads and the quality scores for each base (typically a FASTQ file). Reads are then aligned to a reference genome in a computationally intensive step using algorithms such as BWA (Burrows-Wheeler Alignment), MAQ (Mapping and Assembly with Quality), Bowtie, and Novoalign to produce a binary BAM or CRAM file.[57-59] The data can be visualized in genome browsers such as IGV (Integrative Genomics Viewer).[60] The next step is to identify sequence variations from reference with specialized algorithms. These algorithms generally use Bayesian rules that compute the probability of a variant's occurring at a specific position while taking into account the known polymorphism rate and sequencing errors. Typically, multiple different variant callers will be used to identify the full spectrum of mutations, including single nucleotide variants, indels, CNAs, and translocations. Variant detection is followed by annotation with gene and transcript identifiers and prediction of the functional consequences of the variants (i.e., nonsynonymous; missense, stop, or frameshift mutations). Once functional annotation is complete, genotypic-phenotypic associations of the individual variants can be determined by querying the published literature or websites that contain information about mutations and disease association (e.g., OMIM for mendelian diseases and COSMIC for cancer). An important consideration in cancer sequencing is separating inherited (germline) variants from somatically acquired variants. This can be accomplished by comparing cancer data to paired normal tissue or more frequently comparing variant data to population databases such as gnomAD to remove polymorphisms,[61] with testing of uninvolved and blood-uncontaminated tissue (such as cultured skin fibroblasts or hair follicles) being the recommended gold standard.

LYMPHOID NEOPLASMS

Mature Lymphoid Neoplasms

Molecular technologies have a variety of roles in the evaluation of mature and immature lymphoid neoplasms of B-cell, T-cell, and NK-cell lineage, ranging from documenting clonality in morphologically or immunophenotypically equivocal cases to facilitating the diagnosis of specific entities and determining prognosis to defining targets of and responses to therapy.

Mature B-Cell Lymphomas/Leukemias

Chronic Lymphocytic Leukemia/Small Lymphocytic Lymphoma

Cytogenetic abnormalities in chronic lymphocytic leukemia/small lymphocytic lymphoma (CLL/SLL) mostly encompass numerical abnormalities that are better detected by FISH than by metaphase cytogenetics and are relevant for risk stratification. Del(13q), del(11q), trisomy 12, del(17p), and del(6q) are the most common.[62-64] When seen in isolation and in <60% of nuclei, del(13q14) portends a favorable prognosis, whereas trisomy 12 predicts an intermediate prognosis; del(11q22-q23) and del(17p13) correlate with aggressive behavior.[63,64] FISH for del(17p13)(TP53) is recommended prior to therapy initiation.[64] A complex karyotype (≥3 chromosomal abnormalities) may be a stronger predictor of poor outcomes than del(17p) or TP53 mutation in patients treated with ibrutinib-based regimens, while a highly complex karyotype (≥5 chromosomal abnormalities) is an even more robust adverse prognostic factor.[62,63] Patients with unmutated IGHV (≥98% germline sequence homology) have a poorer outcome than those with SHM.[62-64] VH3-21 usage (of stereotype subset 2) correlates with unfavorable prognosis independent of the IGHV mutational status.[63] Cases carrying the R110-mutated lambda V3-21 light chain gene defines a subgroup with specific biological features and an unfavorable prognosis independent of IGHV mutational status.[65]

The most commonly mutated genes in CLL/SLL include NOTCH1, ATM, SF3B1, TP53, BIRC3, POT1, and MYD88 (Table 5-2) and, with the exception of MYD88, they portend unfavorable prognosis.[63,64,66,67] TP53 mutations are also associated with resistance to cytotoxic chemotherapy independent of 17p chromosome status, and patients with this mutation (or del17p) are instead treated with BTK or BCL2 inhibitors or immunotherapy.[62-64] BTK, PLCG2, and CARD11 mutations confer resistance to BTK inhibitors,[68] while BCL2 mutations and other mechanisms may underlie resistance to venetoclax.[69] Risk-stratifying prognostic scores incorporate several of the earlier mentioned genomic prognostic markers.[62,63] Genetic testing in CLL/SLL is also of value in determining whether diffuse large cell lymphomas arising in this setting are clonally related (true Richter transformation) or de novo, which is of prognostic relevance, noting that even the latter may show mutational profiles reminiscent of those seen in CLL/SLL.[70]

Follicular Lymphoma

Follicular lymphoma (FL) is characterized by the presence of t(14;18)(q32;q21) in ~85% of cases, which juxtaposes BCL2 next to IGH, leading to BCL2 overexpression and apoptosis inhibition.[71-73] FISH/karyotypic evaluation for BCL2 translocation is not necessary for diagnosis of FL as long as BCL2 immunohistochemical positivity is demonstrated in germinal center B cells. FL grade and the presence of a BCL2 translocation are inversely related.[4,74] BCL2 rearrangements are not specific for FL.[72,75-77] Some subtypes of FLs either lack the BCL2 translocation (testicular FL, pediatric-type FL), or display it in only in minor subsets (primary cutaneous follicle center lymphoma, PCFCL).[78,79]

Certain deletions and gains, biallelic B2M mutations/deletions, TP53 or PIM1 mutations, and other genomic abnormalities may associate with a higher risk of transformation to diffuse large B-cell lymphoma (DLBCL).[80] The rare acquisition of MYC rearrangement in FL is currently not sufficient for the diagnosis of high-grade B-cell lymphoma,[81] although these cases might have more adverse outcomes[4] or develop the so-called "lymphoblastic transformation" of FL.[82] BCL6 translocations (seen in 10%–15% of cases) appear to predict an aggressive course[71,72]; association with high histologic grade FL is controversial.[74]

Genes involved in epigenetic regulation (KMT2D, EZH2, CREBBP, and EP300) are frequently mutated in FL (Table 5-2).[71,72,78,83] Other frequently mutated genes in FL include BCL2, TNFRSF14, ARID1A, CARD11, STAT6, MEF2B, and IRF8.[71,72,78] Although uncommon, TP53 mutations/deletions and CREBBP deletions are associated with decreased overall survival (OS).[78,83,84] Mutational status of EZH2, ARID1A, MEF2B, EP300, FOXO1, CREBBP, and CARD11 helps predict treatment outcome of front-line immunochemotherapy.[71,72,83] The mutational profile of FL may also help tailor treatment with targeted therapies. Mutations of histone modifiers render the disease amenable for treatment with histone deacetylase inhibitors, and EZH2-activating mutations (Y641) predict response to EZH2 inhibition.[71]

Genomic features may help distinguish less-common types of FL that tend to lack BCL2 rearrangements from systemic (nodal) FL. PCFCL shows no BCL6 translocations, and displays del(1p36) in 10%.[72,78] The presence of two or more mutations in CREBBP, KMT2D, EP300, and EZH2 and the presence of a BCL2 translocation can help distinguish secondary cutaneous involvement by systemic (nodal) FL from PCFCL.[79] In pediatric-type FL, the most common genomic abnormalities include del(1p36) and TNFRSF14, MAP2K1,

Table 5-2 Recurrent Somatic Mutations and Associated Pathways in Small B-Cell Neoplasms

Genes	Frequency	Pathway and Cellular Processes	Genes	Frequency	Pathway and Cellular Processes
Chronic Lymphocytic Leukemia/Small Lymphocytic Lymphoma			TET2	17%	Epigenetic regulation
ATM	5%–36%	DNA repair/cell cycle control	SPEN	17%	Epigenetic regulation
NOTCH1	5%–22%	Notch signaling	KMT2D	34%	Epigenetic regulation
SF3B1	4%–15%	RNA splicing and processing	LRP1B	15%	Receptor-mediated endocytosis, cellular signaling
TP53	4%–8%	DNA damage response/cell cycle control	PRDM1	15%	Loss of tumor suppressor
MYD88	2%–4%	Toll-like receptor signaling	EP300	13%	Epigenetic regulation
BIRC3	3%–6%	Apoptosis inhibition	TNFRSF14	11%*	NF-κB signaling
POT1	3%–5%	Telomeric processing/genomic stability	NOTCH1	11%	Notch signaling
			NOTCH2	<5%–11%	Notch signaling
Follicular Lymphoma			B2M	10%*	Association with MHC class I heavy chain
CREBBP	45%–83%	Epigenetic regulation	MYD88	6%–7%†	Toll-like receptor signaling
KMT2D	36%–82%	Epigenetic regulation	KLF2	6%	NF-κB signaling
BCL2	10%–76%	Transcriptional regulation	**Nodal Marginal Zone Lymphoma**		
TNFRSF14	20%–47%	NF-κB signaling	KMT2D	34%	Epigenetic regulation
EZH2	9%–30%	Epigenetic regulation	NOTCH2	20%–25%	Notch signaling
SOCS1	2%–22%	JAK/STAT pathway	KLF2	17%–20%	NF-κB signaling
IRF8	6%–21%	B cell development	PTPRD	14%–20%	Loss of tumor suppressor
MEF2B	0%–21%	Epigenetic regulation	TNFAIP3	9%	NF-κB signaling
STAT6	5%–19%	JAK/STAT pathway	MYD88	~5%	Toll-like receptor signaling
TP53	0%–18%	DNA damage response/cell cycle control	**Splenic Marginal Zone Lymphoma**		
EP300	0%–18%	Epigenetic regulation	KLF2	20%–40%	NF-κB signaling
CARD11	10%–15%	BCR signaling, NF-κB signaling	NOTCH2	10%–25%	Notch signaling
ARID1A	0%–15%	Transcriptional regulation	MYD88	15%	Toll-like receptor signaling
TNFAIP3	3%–15%	NF-κB signaling	TP53	15%	DNA damage response/cell cycle control
MAP2K1	0%–12%	RAS/MAPK pathway	NOTCH1	5%	Notch signaling
CCND3	0%–10%	Cell cycle regulation	**Lymphoplasmacytic Lymphoma**		
HIST1H1B	0%–7%	Epigenetic regulation	MYD88	>90%	Toll-like receptor signaling
Mantle Cell Lymphoma			CXCR4	23%–30%	Chemokine signaling
ATM	44%–56%	DNA repair/cell cycle control	KMT2D	24%	Epigenetic regulation
CCND1	12%–44%	Cell cycle regulation	ARID1A	5%–17%	Epigenetic regulation
TP53	27%–35%	DNA damage response/cell cycle control	TP53	7%–10%	DNA damage response/cell cycle control
NSD2 (WHSC1)	7%–31%	DNA repair, epigenetic regulation	**Hairy Cell Leukemia**		
CDKN2A	21%–24%	Cell cycle regulation	BRAF	~100%	RAS/MAPK pathway
KMT2D	12%–23%	Epigenetic regulation	TP53	2%–28%	DNA damage response/cell cycle control
BIRC3	5%–22%	RNA splicing and processing	KLF2	13%–16%	NF-κB signaling
NOTCH1	5%–14%	Notch signaling	CDKN1B	10%–16%	Cell cycle
Extranodal Marginal Zone Lymphoma of Mucosa-Associated Lymphoid Tissue			MAP2K1	0%–22%‡	RAS/MAPK pathway
TNFAIP3	29%	NF-κB signaling	KMT2C	15%	Epigenetic regulation
CREBBP	22%	Epigenetic regulation	NOTCH1	4%–13%	Notch signaling
KMT2C	19%	Epigenetic regulation			

*Includes deletions.
†Mainly in ocular MALT lymphoma.
‡Mainly in IGHV4-34-positive hairy cell leukemia and hairy cell leukemia variant.
BCR, B-cell antigen receptor; *JAK/STAT*, Janus kinase/signal transducer and activator of transcription; *NF-κB*, nuclear factor kappa B; *RAS/MAPK*, rat sarcoma virus/mitogen-activated protein kinase.

and *IRF8* mutations.[72] *BCL2*-rearrangement-negative, *CD23*-positive follicle center lymphoma, a provisional new entity in the 2022 ICC, presents with localized inguinal involvement, often a predominantly diffuse growth pattern, and harbors frequent *STAT6* mutations.[4,85]

In situ follicular neoplasia (ISFN) is an incidental early germinal-center lymphoid neoplasia that shares many genomic aberrancies with FL, including the presence of t(14;18)(q32;q21)/IGH::BCL2, del(1p36), and *EZH2, TNFRSF14*, and *KMT2D* mutations.[72]

Although FL is among the lymphomas with the lowest levels of circulating tumor DNA (ctDNA), evaluation of ctDNA in FL appears to be promising in predicting prognosis, evaluating MRD, and assessing tumor volume.[86]

Mantle Cell Lymphoma

Mantle cell lymphoma (MCL) is characterized by the presence of t(11;14)(q13;q32)/IGH::CCND1 in >90%.[73,87,88] FISH is far superior to PCR for the detection of *CCND1* translocations.[89] FISH/karyotypic evaluation for *CCND1* translocation is not necessary for diagnosis of MCL as long as CCND1 immunohistochemical positivity is demonstrated. In cases in which cyclin D1 overexpression is observed (typically by immunohistochemistry), but no *IGH::CCND1* fusion is detected by FISH, the possibility of *IGK::CCND1* or *IGL::CCND1* rearrangements should be suspected[90,91]; a subset of these rearrangements is cryptic, even to FISH.[92] *CCND2* or *CCND3* is translocated predominantly with IG light chain genes or their enhancers in the majority of the rare cases of MCLs without *CCND1* rearrangements.[91,93]

Nodal and leukemic nonnodal MCL are two subtypes of the disease that differ clinically, immunophenotypically, and in their development.[88] Conventional nodal MCL typically shows unmutated IGHV; mutations in *ATM, CDKN2A, TP53, RB1, KMT2D, CCND1,* and *BIRC3* (Table 5-2); and a variety of copy number abnormalities (CNAs), while the more indolent leukemic nonnodal variant of MCL exhibits mutated IGHV, a comparatively stable genome, fewer epigenetic modifications, more frequent del(8p21.3), and +8q.[94]

Disease progression in MCL is associated with acquisition of mutations in *ATM, TP53, CDKN2A,* and *CCND1.*[87] *TP53* abnormalities, *MYC* translocations, complex karyotypes [≥3 chromosomal abnormalities in addition to t(11;14)(q13;q32)], a higher number of CNAs, and the degree of DNA methylation is associated with poor outcomes.[87,88,94-96] The prognosis of leukemic nonnodal MCL can be negatively affected because of a high number of DNA methylation changes, mutations in *TP53* and *ATM,* or del(13q14).[88,97] *TP53* mutations confer resistance to both chemotherapy and ibrutinib in MCL.[87,88] Mutations in *CCND1* and in genes involved in chromatin modification, oxidative phosphorylation, or the noncanonical NK-κB pathway have also been implicated in resistance to ibrutinib or disease progression.[87,88]

Currently, real-time quantitative PCR amplification of clonal IGH or *IGH::CCND1* rearrangements is the gold standard for MRD monitoring in MCL; however, ddPCR may be a technically advantageous methodology with better quantification.[98,99] The detection of ctDNA appears to be a promising methodology for the assessment of prognosis and MRD.[87,88,99]

Marginal Zone Lymphoma

Marginal zone lymphoma (MZL) subtypes include extranodal MZL of mucosa-associated lymphoid tissue (MALT lymphoma), nodal MZL (NMZL), splenic MZL (SMZL), primary cutaneous marginal zone lymphoproliferative disorder (PCMZLPD) (which has been reclassified as no longer being termed a lymphoma), and pediatric MZL (PMZL).[73]

The majority of MZLs show SHM of IGVH indicative of transit through the germinal center.[100,101] The presence of the ongoing mutations and the biased usage of certain IGHV segments, seen in all MZL subtypes, suggest that lymphomagenesis in MZL may be antigen-driven.[100,101] MZLs display a variety of recurrent chromosomal translocations, mostly seen in MALT lymphomas (but not in other MZL subtypes),[101] and numerical abnormalities.[101-103]

Extranodal Marginal Zone Lymphoma of Mucosa-Associated Lymphoid Tissue. The translocations associated with MALT lymphomas mainly include t(11;18) (q21;q21), t(1;14)(p22;q32), t(14;18)(q32;q21), and t(3;14) (p14.1;q32); the frequencies with which these occur vary

markedly with the primary site of disease and the putative etiology (Fig. 5-6).[73]

t(11;18)(q21;q21)/*BIRC3::MALT1* is specific for MALT lymphoma[100] and is detected in 40% to 50% of gastric, intestinal, and pulmonary cases, and less commonly in other organs.[101] Testing for *BIRC3::MALT1* at diagnosis may help guide treatment as it is associated with lack of tumor response to alkylating agents and eradication of *H. pylori.*[101] t(14;18)/*IGH::MALT1* is detectable in 3% to 20% of MALT lymphomas, typically in the ocular adnexa, lung, liver, salivary glands, and skin.[101,103] t(1;14)(p22;q32)/*IGH::BCL10* is observed in <5% of MALT lymphomas from various anatomic sites.[101,103,104] t(3;14)(p14.1;q32)/*IGH::FOXP1* is found in ~10% of MALT lymphomas, mainly from the thyroid, ocular adnexa, and skin.[101] Numerical chromosomal abnormalities in MALT lymphoma more frequently include +3 (<85% of cases), +18 (~20%), and various gains and losses.[101]

Mutations in MALT lymphoma mainly affect *TNFAIP3, CREBBP, KMT2C, TET2, SPEN, KMT2D, LRP1B,* and *PRDM1* (Table 5-2)[101,105,106] and these vary according to the anatomic locations involved (Fig. 5-6).[73,101] *TP53* abnormalities and t(3;14)(p14.1;q32)/*IGH::FOXP1* portend high-grade transformation of MALT lymphomas.[101,107] TNFAIP3 inactivation is associated with reduced lymphoma-free survival in ocular adnexal MALT lymphoma.[101]

Nodal Marginal Zone Lymphoma. Trisomy of 3 and 18, gains of 2p15, 3p25, and 3p14, and losses of 1p36, 1p21, 6q23, and 12q21 are the most frequent cytogenetic abnormalities in NMZL.[102] The most common mutations involve *PTPRD, NOTCH2,* and *KLF2* (Table 5-2).[100,105] *PTPRD* mutations are almost exclusively seen in NMZL.[100,108]

Splenic Marginal Zone Lymphoma. SMZL commonly displays a variety of cytogenetic abnormalities including a complex karyotype, del(7q31), +18, and gains of 3q.[102,109] The most frequent mutations affect *KLF2, NOTCH2, TP53,* and *TNFAIP3* (Table 5-2), the latter three of which predict transformation.[105,108]

Lymphoplasmacytic Lymphoma

The detection of an *MYD88* L265P mutation that is present in >90% of lymphoplasmacytic lymphomas (LPLs) is a useful diagnostic tool in the appropriate context[110,111]; however, it is not completely specific for LPL as it can be identified in other B-cell neoplasms[108] and in non-neoplastic mature and immature B cells.[112] The lack of a *MYD88* L265P is an adverse prognostic factor in LPL.[113,114] *CXCR4* mutations, seen in a subset of cases of LPL (Table 5-2), predict more aggressive disease and resistance to ibrutinib.[110,115] The combination of *MYD88* L265P and *CXCR4, KNMT2D, or ARID1A* mutations appears to be diagnostic of LPL.[108]

Hairy Cell Leukemia

Hairy cell leukemia (HCL) harbors the *BRAF* V600E mutation (exon 15) in >95% of cases and lacks recurrent cytogenetic abnormalities.[116] The identification of *BRAF* V600E mutation may predict response to *BRAF* inhibitors. *BRAF* mutations in exon 11 have been identified in some cases without the V600E mutation.[116] A search for *TP53* mutations and/or del(17p) is recommended in cases resistant to therapy with purine analogs.[116] Additional mutations can also be observed in HCL (Table 5-2).[116] A high prevalence of *MAP2K1* mutations is observed in IGHV4-34-positive HCL and HCL-variant,

Sites   Genetics

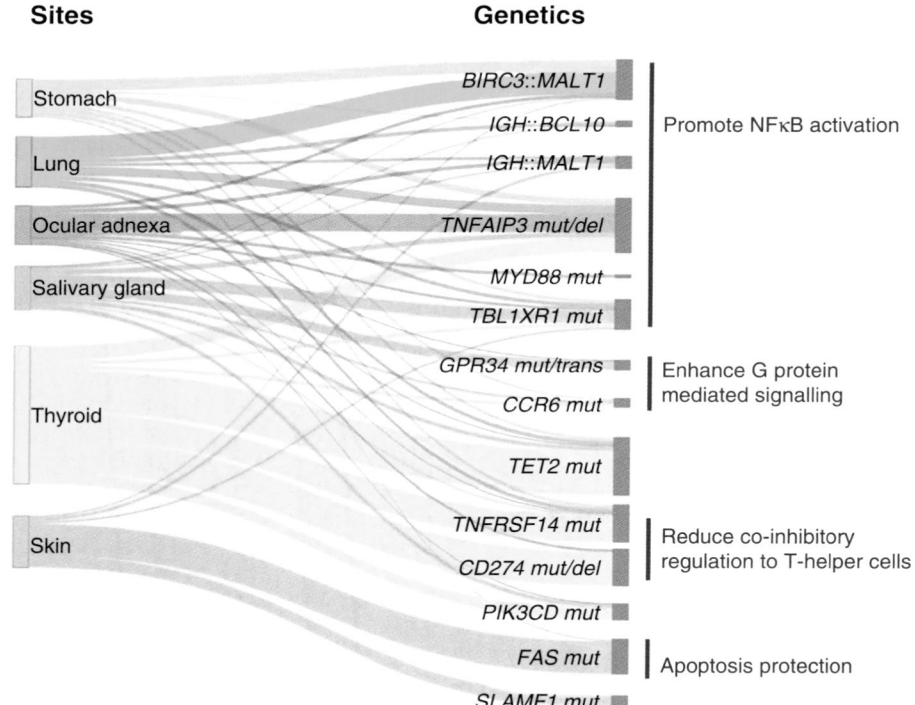

Figure 5-6. Recurrent genetic abnormalities in extranodal marginal zone lymphoma (EMZL). Note the association of certain abnormalities with various anatomic sites. Because many of the genes involved in EMZL have not been uniformly investigated in these different anatomic locations, only those genetic abnormalities that are recurrent and fundamental to the understanding of the pathogenesis of these lymphomas are depicted. The height of the boxes under sites does not reflect the frequencies of these lymphomas. *del*, Deletion; *mut*, mutation; *trans*, translocation. *(Reproduced and modified with permission from Alaggio R, Amador C, Anagnostopoulos I, et al. The 5th edition of the World Health Organization Classification of Haematolymphoid Tumours: Lymphoid Neoplasms. Leukemia. 2022;36[7]:1720-1748. https://doi.org/10.1038/s41375-022-01620-2.)*

whereas they are rare in IGHV4-34-negative cases.[116] IGHV4-34-positive HCL and HCL-variant lack *BRAF* V600E mutation and are associated with more aggressive disease.[116]

Diffuse Large B-Cell Lymphoma

There are numerous subtypes of DLBCL, with the most common category, DLBCL, not otherwise specified (NOS), classified according to its cell of origin (COO) by gene expression profiling (GEP) into the germinal center B-cell (GCB) and activated B-cell (ABC) subtypes, though 10% to 20% of cases are unclassifiable.[117] Because GEP is not widely available for clinical use, surrogate immunohistochemical algorithms have been developed for its classification. This COO–based classification is relevant for prognosis and was thought to be of value in prediction of response to therapy: the 5-year OS of patients treated with R-CHOP is longer in patients with the GCB subtype of DLBCL,[118] while DLBCLs of the ABC subtype show frequent response to BTK inhibitors.[117,119] Molecular approaches have helped define novel DLBCL genomic subgroups.[119-123] Among these, GEP studies performed on the GCB subtype of DLBCL identified an association of the double-hit signature (DHIT) in GCB cases with an outcome similar to that of cases of the ABC subtype.[124,125]

The most frequently translocated genes in DLBCL are *BCL6* (20%–30%), *BCL2* (13%–20%), and *MYC* (8%–15%) (Table 5-3),[125-127] with the IG loci (IGH, IGK, and IGL) their predominant partners.[127,128] Partners of *MYC* other than the IG loci include *PAX5, BCL6, BCL11A, IKZF1,* and *BTG1.*[127]

BCL2 and *MYC* translocations associate with the GCB subtype, while *BCL2* amplifications, *BCL6* translocations, and *CDKN2A* deletions are more frequent in the ABC subtype (Table 5-3).[125,127,129,130]

The mutational profile in the ABC subtype of DLBCL includes frequent mutations in *CD79B/A, CARD11, MYD88, BCOR, ETV6, PRDM1/BLIMP1, PIM1, CDKN2B,* and *CDKN2A,* while in the GCB subtype the most frequent mutations include *EZH2, KMT2D, CREBBP, BCL2, TNFRSF14, B2M, FOXO1, ACTB, SOCS1, GNA13,* and *GNA12* (Table 5-3).[129,130] DLBCLs of immune privileged sites (including those of the CNS and testes), a group of lymphomas that shares immunophenotypic and genomic features with the ABC subtype of DLBCL, are characterized by concomitant *MYD88* and *CD79B* mutations.[73,131]

DLBCL can also be further stratified into distinct genomic subgroups with the GenClass and LymphGen algorithms (MCD, N1, BN2, EZB, A53, and ST2)[117,124] or in genetic clusters (1 through 5),[128] within which cases share genetic features, GEP signatures, and clinical outcomes. Certain subgroups identified with the GenClass algorithm have cluster equivalents (MCD/C5, EZB/C3, BN2/C1).[126,127,132] An additional molecular classification based on massively parallel sequencing results identified five molecular subtypes (*MYD88, BCL2, SOCS1/SGK1, TET2/SGK1,* and *NOTCH2*), along with an unclassified group (Fig. 5-7). MCD, N1, and A53 subgroups, and EZB and ST2 subgroups, tend to predominantly contain ABC and GCB cases, respectively, whereas BN2 associates with all three GEP-defined

Table 5-3 Key Features Distinguishing Different Subtypes of Diffuse Large B-Cell Lymphoma

	GCB	ABC	PMBL
Cell of Origin	Germinal center B cell	Late/post–germinal center B cell	Thymic B cell
Prognosis	Favorable	Adverse	Favorable
Key Genetic Events	BCL2 and MYC rearrangements, PTEN deletion	BCL2 amplification, BCL6 rearrangement, and CDKN2A deletion	+9p24 (JAK2, PDL1, PDL2); gain of REL; CIITA rearrangement
Most Frequent Mutations	EZH2, GNA13, BCL6, TNFSR14, FOXO1, ACTB, SOCS1, BCL2, SGK1, KMT2D, CREBBP, EP300, TP53, HST1H1E/C, B2M	MYD88, CD79A/B, CARD11, TNFAIP3, PIM1, NOTCH1, SPIB, PRDM1, HLA1, TP53, MEF2B, NOTCH2, BTG1/2, SOCS1, DTX, SPEN, TNFAIP3, TMSB4X	TNFAIP3, NFKBIE, PTPN1, SOCS, STAT6, IL4R, CIITA, B2M, IRF1, IRF4, IRF8, IRF2BP2A, GNA13, ITPKB

ABC, Activated B cell; *GCB,* germinal center B cell; *PMBL,* primary mediastinal large B-cell lymphoma.

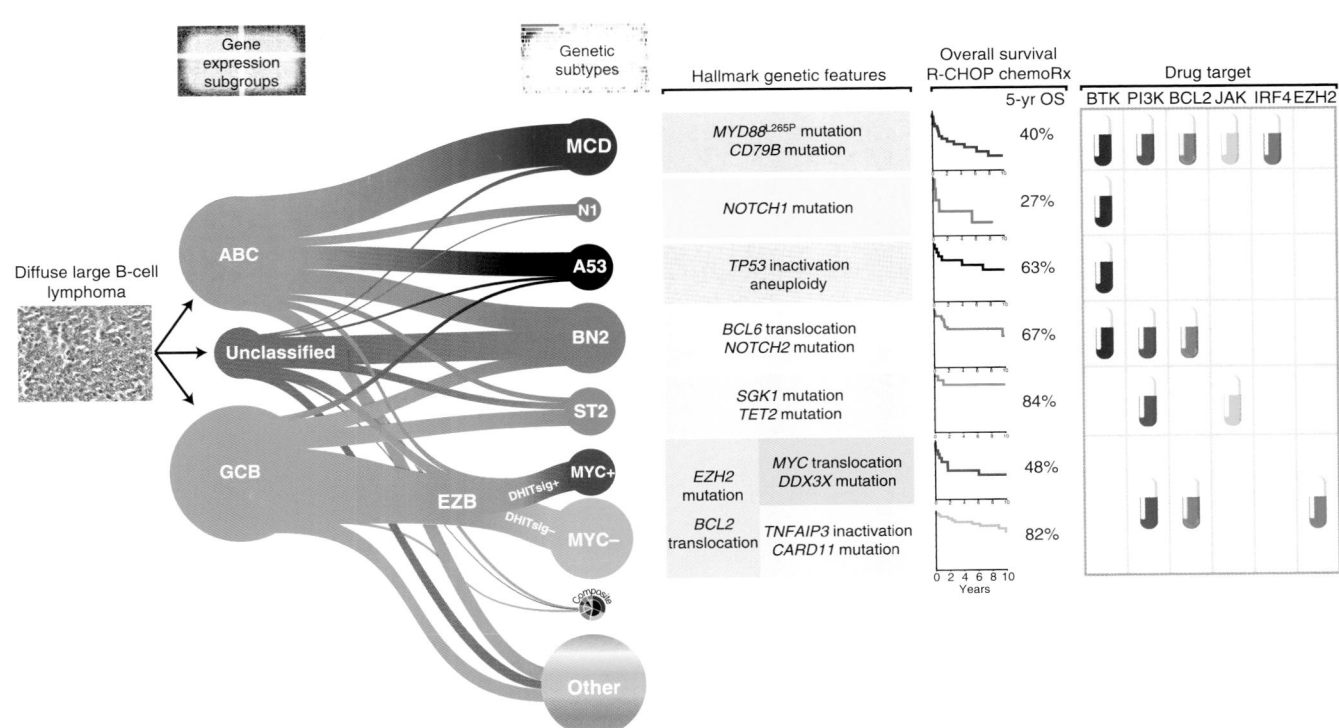

Figure 5-7. Genetic subgroups of diffuse large B-cell lymphoma (DLBCL) illustrated using the LymphGen algorithm. This shows the relationships between cell of origin (COO) and the probabilistic assignments to genetics-based subgroups. The size of the subgroup circles approximates the proportions of patients in each group,[117] adjusted for a population-based distribution of COO subgroups. Tumors assigned with high confidence to two or more subgroups are assigned to the composite group, while ~37% of tumors are not assigned to any subgroup with sufficient confidence (Other). The hallmark genetic features are those that are frequent within that subgroup but they are not required for that assignment. Overall survival after R-CHOP chemoimmunotherapy along with inferred drug targets are shown. *(Reproduced with permission from de Leval L, Alizadeh AA, Bergsagel PL, et al. Genomic profiling for clinical decision making in lymphoid neoplasms.* Blood. *2022;140[21]:2193-2227. https://doi.org/10.1182/blood.2022015854.)*

subgroups.[117,124] The majority of DLBCLs with a DHIT signature are either EZB or genetically composite cases of EZB and A53, and frequently bear *MYC* translocations, amplifications or mutations, *TP53* mutations or deletions, and mutations in *GNA13, DDX3X,* and *FOXO1.*[124]

The genetic classification of DLBCL also helps further refine the prognosis within the GEP-defined subgroups. Within the ABC DLBCLs, the BN2 subgroup has a significantly better survival than in the rest, while in GCB DLBCLs the survival of EZB cases tends to be shorter than in other subgroups.[117,124] In addition, only within the EZB subset of GCB, the survival of cases with a DHIT signature is significantly worse than in those without it.[124] This genetic classification of DLBCL may also help predict therapeutic response (Fig. 5-7).[124] Among

ABC DLBCLs, impressive outcomes have been observed in young patients with the MCD or N1 subtypes treated with R-CHOP and ibrutinib.[119,132]

DLBCLs with expression of ALK kinase are rare aggressive lymphomas with translocations of *ALK.*[133] The most common partner of *ALK* in these cases is *CLTC* (~70% of cases) because of the t(2;17)(p23;q23).[134] The identification of *ALK* rearrangements in DLBCL is prognostically and therapeutically relevant.[134,135]

Large B-cell lymphoma with 11q aberration (LBL-11q, formerly known as Burkitt-like lymphoma with 11q aberration) typically presents in the young with localized lymphadenopathy, shares morphologic, immunophenotypic, and gene expression features with BL but lacks *MYC* translocations and, instead, carries proximal gains and telomeric losses in 11q.[4,73] Frequent additional CNAs are also identified.[136,137] The most common mutations in LBL-11q involve *BTG2, DDX3X, EP300, ETS1, GNA13, TTN,* and *FAT4,* while the *ID3, TCF3,* and *SMARCA4* mutations commonly found in BL are not observed.[73] In order to identify LBL-11q cases, FISH studies with the 11q probe or copy number arrays are recommended in cases arising in young patients that are morphologically compatible with BL, DLBCL, or HGBL with a GCB immunophenotype, display a very high Ki67 (>90%), and lack a *MYC* translocation.[4,73,133,134]

High-Grade B-Cell Lymphoma, NOS or With MYC and BCL2 or BCL6 Rearrangements

High-grade B-cell lymphomas (HGBL) encompass tumors with morphology of DLBCL, blastoid cytology, and features intermediate between DLBCL and Burkitt lymphoma (BL).[129] Other B-cell lymphomas (e.g., follicular lymphoma or MCL) with *MYC* translocations are excluded from this category.

Among HGBLs with *MYC* and *BCL2* or *BCL6* rearrangements, the majority of cases harbor *BCL2* rearrangements, less commonly *BCL6* rearrangements, and rarely concurrent *BCL2* and *BCL6* rearrangements.[138,139] *MYC* partners include both IG and non-IG genes (*PAX5, IKAROS, BCL6,* and *BCL11A*).[138,139] Although *BCL2* is typically translocated with the IGH enhancer, *BCL6* can involve a variety of partners, including all three IG loci.[138] Because no morphologic or immunophenotypic features reliably predict *MYC, BCL2,* or *BCL6* translocations, all aggressive B-cell lymphomas with a diffuse pattern should be evaluated by FISH for these abnormalities. A cost-effective approach to the diagnosis of this entity involves initial evaluation for *MYC* rearrangements, with subsequent evaluation for *BCL2* and *BCL6* only in *MYC*-translocated cases. Though break-apart FISH probes are considered the most sensitive for detection of these translocations, false negatives can occur depending on the breakpoint. For this reason, the addition of dual-fusion probes for IGH/*MYC*, IGK/*MYC*, and IGL/*MYC* can improve the sensitivity of the study and identify *MYC* translocations that are missed with the *MYC* break-apart probe. Of note, ~30% of HGBLs with *MYC* and *BCL2* or *BCL6* translocations are not diagnosed as such because of the presence of translocations that are cryptic to FISH studies, or because of focal *MYC* and *MIR17H* copy number gains, or focal deletion of the *PVT1* promoter.[140] HGBLs with *MYC* and *BCL2* or *BCL6* rearrangements recurrently harbor complex karyotypes.[139]

HGBLs with *MYC* and *BCL2* translocations are enriched in mutations affecting *CREBBP, KMT2D, EZH2, TP53,* and *TNFRSF14,* while *CCND3* and *UBE2A* are the most common mutations in HGBLs with *MYC* and *BCL6* translocations.[139,140] In HGBLs with *MYC, BCL2,* and *BCL6* translocations, the most frequent mutations affect *KMT2D, CCND3,* and *IRF8.*[139]

HGBLs with *MYC* and *BCL2* or *BCL6* rearrangements have a worse prognosis with standard therapy than DLBCL, while cases of HGBLs with *MYC* and *BCL6* rearrangements appear to have outcomes intermediate between HGBLs with *MYC* and *BCL2* rearrangements and DLBCL without *MYC* rearrangement and data suggest that they may not, in fact, reflect a distinct entity.[129]

HGBL, NOS, currently largely a diagnosis of exclusion based upon morphologic features, harbors isolated *MYC, BCL2,* and *BCL6* rearrangements in ~40%, <10%, and <10%

Table 5-4 Genetic Features of Burkitt Lymphoma (BL), High-Grade B-Cell Lymphoma (HGBL), and Diffuse Large B-Cell Lymphoma (DLBCL)

	BL	HGBL	DLBCL
MYC rearrangement	Yes (~90%)	Common (~40%)	Rare (~10%)
IG-*MYC**	Yes	Sometimes	Rare
Non–IG-*MYC*	No	Sometimes	Rare
BCL2 but no *MYC* rearrangement	No	Rare	Occasional
BCL6 but no *MYC* rearrangement	No	Rare	Occasional
MYC with *BCL2* or *BCL6* rearrangement	No	Common	No
MYC simple karyotype[†]	Yes	Rare	Rare
MYC complex karyotype[†]	Rare	Common	Common
CCND3, TCF3, ID3 mutations	Common	Common	Rare
MYC mutations	Common	Common	Rare
EZH2, BCL2, CREBBP mutations	Rare	Common	Common
KMT2D, EP300, MEF2B, SGK1 mutations	Rare	Rare	Common

*IG-*MYC*, juxtaposition of *MYC* to one of the immunoglobulin loci: IGH at 14q32, IGK at 2p12, or IGL at 22q11. Non-IG-*MYC* tumors contain a *MYC* rearrangement with juxtaposition to genes other than one of the immunoglobulin loci.
†Simple karyotype: No or only few cytogenetic or chromosomal microarray abnormalities other than the *MYC* rearrangement. Complex karyotype: Six or more abnormalities.

of cases, respectively. As in the case of HGBLs with *MYC* and *BCL2* or *BCL6* rearrangements, HGBL, NOS often shows a complex karyotype, a feature that that may help distinguish those with an isolated *MYC* rearrangement from BL (Table 5-4). In HGBL, NOS, an isolated *MYC* rearrangement or lack of *MYC, BCL2,* or *BCL6* rearrangements confers a trend toward inferior survival.[141]

Burkitt Lymphoma

BL is an aggressive germinal center-derived mature B-cell lymphoma characterized by translocations involving *MYC* and IG loci.[142-144] The translocation t(8;14)(q24;q32) is found in 70% to 80% of cases, while t(2;8)(p12;q24) and t(8;22)(q24;q11) are found in 10% to 15%.[145] Although BL usually presents with a simple karyotype, there is a high prevalence of non-random additional CNAs.[145] Tetrasomy 1q resulting from supernumerary idic(1)(p12) or i(1)(q10) in BL can make it difficult to distinguish immunophenotypically from B-lymphoblastic leukemia/leukemia.[146,147]

MYC is also the most commonly mutated gene in BL.[137,143,144] Other commonly mutated genes are *BACH2, DDX3, DNMT1, HIST1H1E, BCL7, ID3, CCND3, TP53, FBX011, SMARCA4,* and *TCF3.*[137,143,144] Certain mutations associate with BL subtype and EBV status.[143,144]

FISH studies for the identification of *MYC* translocations are necessary for the diagnosis of the majority of cases of BL. Although *MYC* translocations can be identified on metaphase analyses, FISH studies are preferred given their faster turnaround time and higher sensitivity, and also because not all t(8;14)(q24;q32) translocations involve *MYC* and IGH.[148] *MYC* break-apart probes are recommended for the detection of *MYC* rearrangements; however, 4% of

Table 5-5 Genetic Abnormalities in Classic Hodgkin Lymphoma

Gene	Chromosome Location	Frequency	Genetic Alteration	Effect of Genetic Lesion
B2M	15q21	21%–70%	Mutation	Modulation of tumor microenvironment
CD58	1p13.1	~23%	Deletion	
JAK2	9p24	5%–56%	Copy gain/amplification/polysomy	Activation of JAK/STAT pathway
PD-L1/PD-L2	9p24	38%–92%	Copy gain/amplification/polysomy	Induction of PD-1 signaling with inhibition of T-cell activation/proliferation
SOCS1	16p13	~52%	Mutation	Impaired JAK2 degradation, and hence activation of JAK/STAT pathway
REL	2p13	28%–70%	Amplification	Activation of NF-κB pathway
TNFAIP3	6q23-q25	40%–45% and 21%–60%, respectively	Mutation and deletion, respectively	Activation of NF-κB pathway
NFKBIA	14q13	15%–40%	Mutation	Activation of NF-κB pathway
NFKBIE	6p21	17%–27%	Deletion	Activation of NF-κB pathway
TNFRSF14	1p36.32	13%–42%	Deletion	Activation of NF-κB pathway
STAT6	12q13	~32%	Mutation	Activation of JAK/STAT pathway
GNA13	17q24	~24%	Mutation	Loss of Gα13 signaling
PTPN1	20q13	~20%	Mutation	Activation of JAK-STAT pathway
XPO1	2p15	~18%	Mutation	Inhibition of tumor suppressors
ITPKB	1q42	~16%	Mutation	Activation of PI3K-AKT pathway
FAS	10q24	~10%	Mutation	Evasion of apoptosis
MDM2	12q13-q14	~60%	Gain	p53 inactivation
MAP3K14	17q21-q22	~25%	Gain	Activation of NF-κB pathway
ETS1	11q23	~65%	Deletion	Decreased transcription factor function
TRAF3	14q32	~15%	Deletion	Loss of inhibition of CD40 signaling
CIITA	16p13	~15%	Translocation	Downregulation of surface HLA class II expression and overexpression of CD273 and CD274, modulating immunogenicity
IGH SHM	14q32	~25%	"Crippling" SHM	Indicates that the neoplastic cells are B-cells and of germinal center or post–germinal center origin

IGH, Immunoglobulin heavy chain; SHM, somatic hypermutation.

MYC-positive cases are not detected with this method and a subset of these can be detected with MYC/IGH fusion probes instead.[149] Cryptic insertions of MYC into IGH and vice versa, functionally equivalent to the IGH::MYC translocation, have been described.[150,151] In general, the identification of MYC translocations by PCR is hampered by the scattering of the breakpoints on both of the affected chromosomes and is hence not used in the clinical setting.[150]

Hodgkin Lymphoma

Hodgkin lymphoma (HL) includes classic Hodgkin lymphoma (cHL) and nodular lymphocyte predominant Hodgkin lymphoma (NLPHL), with the latter renamed nodular lymphocyte predominant B-cell lymphoma (NLPBL) by the ICC but not the 5th edition of the WHO classification.[4,73]

In cHL, Hodgkin/Reed-Sternberg (HRS) cells carry clonally rearranged, somatically hypermutated, and class-switched IG, which indicates their B-cell lineage and their passage through the germinal center reaction.[152] Several genomic alterations are responsible for the loss of the B-cell phenotype of the HRS cells, including crippling IG mutations and lack of BCR expression caused by aberrant AID-mediated SHM, and epigenetic silencing through promoter hypermethylation with dysregulation of the expression of genes involved in B-cell differentiation.[152,153]

Multiple genomic abnormalities promote survival and immune escape of HRS cells (Table 5-5). Constitutive

activation of the NF-κB pathway can be mediated by gain/amplification of REL, MAP3K14, and BCL3, and deletions and loss-of-function mutations in negative regulators (TNFAIP3, NFKBIA, and NFKBIE).[152,154] Genomic abnormalities that constitutively activate the JAK-STAT pathway in cHL include SOCS1 loss-of-function mutations, STAT6 gain-of-function mutation, PTPN1 gain-of-function and loss-of-function mutations, and JAK2 amplification/gain.[154-156] HRS cells evade the immunosurveillance through mutations in PTPN1 and B2M, translocations of CIITA, +9p24/9p24 amplification (PDL1 and PDL2), and loss of TNFRSF14.[152,154,156] PDL1 and PDL2 amplification in HRS cells and the consequent overexpression of PDL1 and PDL2 has been effectively exploited therapeutically with the use of PD1 blockers.[157] Several other mutations in cHL affect other pathways (Table 5-5).[153,156,158]

Metaphase analysis of cHL has demonstrated occasional aneuploidy and hypertetraploidy, but no recurrent or specific chromosomal abnormalities,[159] while comparative genomic hybridization techniques have identified frequent CNAs.[153] Metaphase analyses and CGH studies in NLPHL/NLPBL show frequent complex karyotypes and non-specific CNAs.[160-162] BCL6 rearrangements are identified in 17% to 50% of cases.[160,163,164] The mutational landscape of the LP cells includes frequent PAX5, PIM1, MYC, RHOH, SGK1, DUSP2, JUNB, and SOCS1 mutations[164] and uncommon TNFAIP3 and NFKBIA mutations.[165]

Although biologically intriguing, none of the genomic abnormalities in HL are currently used for routine diagnostic use. Detection and quantitation of cHL–associated ctDNA with techniques such as ddPCR has the potential to complement the prognostic utility of FDG-PET scanning in the evaluation of residual cHL after therapy.[152,153] The detection of specific mutations (e.g., XPO1 E571K) in plasma cell-free DNA by digital PCR has been proposed as a biomarker for the detection of MRD.[166]

Plasma Cell Neoplasms

Plasma cell neoplasms (PCNs) harbor complex heterogeneous genomic changes occurring during disease progression from monoclonal gammopathy of uncertain significance (MGUS) and smoldering multiple myeloma to multiple myeloma (MM) and plasma cell leukemia.

Genomic abnormalities in PCNs are classified into primary and secondary.[167-169] Primary genomic abnormalities initiate the process of plasma cell immortalization and development of MGUS (which contains these abnormalities in ~50% of cases), while the secondary genomic abnormalities occur later in the disease and determine whether the plasma cell clone progresses to MM or remains at an earlier evolutionary step.[167,169]

Primary genomic abnormalities in PCNs broadly classify cases into the hyperdiploid and non-hyperdiploid groups. The hyperdiploid group (~50% of PCNs) is characterized by trisomy of one or more odd-numbered chromosomes, and more favorable outcomes.[167-169] The non-hyperdiploid group typically harbors the juxtaposition of IGH next to an oncogene such as CCND1 (11q13) (~20% of MM cases), CCND3 (6p21) (~2%), FGFR3 and NSD2 (4p16) (~15%), MAF (16q23) (5%–10%), or MAFB (20q12) (~1%).[167-169] While t(4;14)(p16.3;q32.3), t(14;16)(q32.3;q23), and t(14;20)(q32;q12) have poor prognosis, the effect of t(11;14)(q13;q32) and t(6;14)(p21;q32) on prognosis is neutral.[168] Despite the association of t(4;14) with poor prognosis, treatment with bortezomib results in improved survival.[168,169] t(11;14)(q13;q32) in MM correlates with small plasma cell morphology, cyclin D1 and CD20 expression, and response to venetoclax.[170]

Secondary genomic abnormalities in PCNs mainly include translocations of MYC, CNAs, somatic mutations, and DNA hypomethylation.[167-169] MYC translocations (~15% of MM cases) most frequently partner with the IG loci, FAM46C, FOXO3, and BMP6, and constitute an adverse prognostic factor.[167,168] Among CNAs, deletion of TP53, +1q, and del(1p) are the most frequent.[167] TP53 deletion is associated with increased risk of mutation of the remaining TP53 allele, rapid disease progression, and poor prognosis, particularly if the fraction of myeloma cells with del(17p) is >55%.[167,168] del(1p) and +1q are collectively seen in almost a quarter of MM, and are also associated with adverse prognosis.[168,171] del(13q) (45%–50% of cases) may lack prognostic significance.[168]

FISH studies have greater sensitivity than metaphase analysis for the detection of cytogenetic abnormalities in PCNs because plasma cells are typically averse to division ex vivo, and their detection rate is enhanced with plasma cell enrichment (CD138 cell selection).[167,169] The results of FISH studies are one of the components of the Revised International Staging System (R-ISS) used for risk stratification. Chromosome 1

abnormalities will likely be incorporated into future MM risk stratification models as high-risk abnormalities.[171,172]

RAS mutations (up to 40% of MM) are frequently subclonal, and predict adverse outcomes.[167,168] KRAS mutations associate with TP53 mutations and t(11;14), while NRAS mutations correlate with decreased response to bortezomib.[167] Less-common mutations affect FAM46C and DIS3 (~11% each), TP53 (8%), and BRAF (6%).[167] Constitutively, activation of the NF-κB pathway (caused by TRAF2, TRAF3, CYLD, and BIRC2/BIRC3 loss-of-function mutations, and NFKB1, NFKB2, CD40, LTBR, TACI, and NIK gain-of-function mutations) occurs in at least 50% of MM, although it does not appear to influence survival.[167,168,173]

Mature T-Cell and NK-Cell Lymphomas/Leukemias

T-Cell Prolymphocytic Leukemia

Metaphase analysis and FISH can help establish the diagnosis of T-cell prolymphocytic leukemia (T-PLL). T-PLL commonly demonstrates complex karyotypes (in up to 80%) and the genomic hallmark inv(14)(q11q32.1) or t(14;14)(q11;q32.1)] (~80% of cases), which involves TRA on 14q11 and the TCL1A/TCL1B loci on 14q32.1, and leads to TCL1 overexpression.[174] This TCL1 overexpression can be identified by immunohistochemistry, and in the context of a T-cell neoplasm, these cytogenetic/FISH or immunohistochemistry findings are considered diagnostic of T-PLL. Approximately 20% of cases harbor a t(X;14)(q28;q11) involving MTCP1 on Xq28 and TRA on 14q11, while rare cases harbor the t(X;7)(q28;q35) with resultant juxtaposition of MTCP1 next to TRB on 7q35, each resulting in MTCP1 overexpression.[174,175] Recurrent mutations and deletions frequently affect a variety of pathways in T-PLL (Table 5-6) such as DNA repair, DNA damage response, proteasomal degradation, JAK-STAT pathway, and epigenetic regulation.[176,177]

Adult T-Cell Leukemia/Lymphoma

Adult T-cell leukemia/lymphoma (ATLL) is driven by human T-lymphotropic virus type-1 (HTLV-1) infection, which integrates into the T-cell genome and disrupts gene regulation. The infrequent neoplastic transformation of HTLV-1 infected T-cells requires accumulation of additional genomic abnormalities, which occur progressively.[178,179]

Genomic analyses in ATLL have demonstrated a high frequency of mutations in genes involved in the TR and NF-κB signaling pathways, T-cell trafficking, and immunosurveillance (Table 5-6).[178-180] Gain-of-function PRKCB mutations appear to be relatively specific to ATLL.[180] Mutational differences have been described between North American and Japanese cases.[180] Deletions at the NRXN3 locus are thought to be pathognomonic for ATLL.[181] Frequent CTLA4::CD28 and ICOS::CD28 fusions have been described in Japanese cases.[180,181]

The total number of genomic abnormalities is higher in aggressive (acute and lymphomatous) subtypes, with higher frequency of TP53 and IRF4 mutations and CNAs (including PD-L1 amplifications and CDKN2A deletions), than in the indolent (chronic and smoldering) variants, whereas STAT3 mutations are more characteristic of the latter.[179,182] CNAs of cell cycle-related genes (CDKN2A, TP53) and CD58 predict transformation of chronic into acute forms of ATLL.[180] Genomic studies have classified ATLL into two groups with

Table 5-6 Recurrent Somatic Mutations and Associated Pathways in Mature T-Cell and NK-Cell Neoplasms

T-Cell Neoplasm Subtype	Most Commonly Mutated Genes	Frequency	Pathway and Cellular Processes	Other Mutated Genes
T-Cell Prolymphocytic Leukemia	ATM	73%–90%	DNA repair/cell cycle control	SAMHD1, CHEK2, MSH6, MSH3, KMT2D, KMT2C, KDM6A, KDM6B
	JAK3	21%–36%	JAK/STAT pathway	
	TP53	14%–31%	DNA damage response/cell cycle control	
	STAT5B	7%–19%	JAK/STAT pathway	
	TET2	17%	Epigenetic regulation	
	EZH2	13%	Epigenetic regulation	
	BCOR	9%	Epigenetic regulation	
	FBXW10	8%	Proteasomal degradation	
	JAK1	6%	JAK/STAT pathway	
Adult T-Cell Leukemia/ Lymphoma	PLCG1	36%–38%	T-cell signaling pathway	
	CCR4	29%–35%	PI3K/AKT activation	
	PRKCB	31%–33%	Apoptosis	
	TET2	8%–32%	Epigenetic regulation	
	CIC	31%	Transcriptional repression	
	CARD11	24%–27%	BCR signaling, NF-κB signaling	
	STAT3	22%–27%	JAK/STAT pathway	
	TP53	8%–22%	DNA damage response/cell cycle control	
	GATA3	15%–20%	Th2 cytokine gene expression	
	VAV1	15%–18%	T-cell signaling, other	
	NOTCH1	15%–18%	NOTCH signaling	
	TBL1XR1	~17%	Epigenetic regulation	
	IRF4	~14%	Toll-like receptor signaling	
	CCR7	11%–13%	T-cell chemotactic response and migration	
T-Cell Large Granular Lymphocytic Leukemia	STAT3	27%–72%	JAK/STAT pathway	TNFAIP3, PTPRT, BCL11B, PTPN14, PTPN23, FLT3, KRAS, ADCY3, ANGPT2, PTK2, ANGPT2, KDR/ VEGFR2, and CD40LG
	STAT5B	0%–55%*	JAK/STAT pathway	
Anaplastic Large Cell Lymphoma, ALK-Positive	PRF1	25%	Lymphocyte-mediated cytolysis	KMT2C, KMT2D, TET2
	LRP1B	19%	Diverse, receptor-mediated endocytosis, cellular signaling	
	NOTCH1	15%	NOTCH signaling	
	STAT3	13%	JAK-STAT pathway	
	TP53	11%	DNA damage response/cell cycle control	
	EP300	11%	Epigenetic regulation	
Anaplastic Large Cell Lymphoma, ALK-Negative	STAT3	Up to 38%	JAK/STAT pathway	
	JAK1	Up to 26%	JAK/STAT pathway	
	TP53	23%	DNA damage response/cell cycle control	
	KMT2D	20%	Epigenetic regulation	
	MSC	15%	Transcriptional repression	
Breast Implant-Associated Anaplastic Large-Cell Lymphoma	STAT3	20%–64%	JAK/STAT pathway	SOCS1, SOCS3, PTPN1, DNMT3A, STAT5B
	KMT2C	26%	Epigenetic regulation	
	JAK1	7%–18%	JAK/STAT pathway	
	CREBBP	15%	Epigenetic regulation	
	CHD2	15%	Epigenetic regulation	
	TP53	12%	DNA damage response/cell cycle control	
	EOMES	12%	Transcriptional regulation	
	KMT2D	9%	Epigenetic regulation	
Extranodal NK/T-Cell Lymphoma, Nasal Type	TP53	8%–43%	DNA damage response/cell cycle control	NOTCH2
	BCOR	0%–32%	Epigenetic regulation	
	STAT3	3%–23%	JAK/STAT pathway	
	DDX3X	4%–20%	RNA helicase family	
	ECSIT	19%	Toll pathway	
	KMT2C	15%	Epigenetic regulation	
	MSN	8%–14%	Cell-cell signaling	

Continued

Table 5-6 Recurrent Somatic Mutations and Associated Pathways in Mature T-Cell and NK-Cell Neoplasms—cont'd

T-Cell Neoplasm Subtype	Most Commonly Mutated Genes	Frequency	Pathway and Cellular Processes	Other Mutated Genes
	EPHA1	13%	RAS/MAPK pathway	
	KMT2D	13%	Epigenetic regulation	
	JAK3	3%–13%	JAK/STAT pathway	
	JAK2	11%	JAK/STAT pathway	
	PTPRK	10%	JAK/STAT pathway	
	MAP3K5	10%	RAS/MAP kinase pathway	
	CIITA	10%	MHC class II gene expression regulation	
	NOTCH1	10%	NOTCH signaling	
	TET2	9%	Epigenetic regulation	
	MGA	8%	MYC repression, transcriptional regulation, and cellular proliferation	
	EP300	8%	Epigenetic regulation	
	BRAF	8%	RAS/MAPK pathway	
	ARID1A	7%	Epigenetic regulation	
Follicular Helper T-Cell Lymphoma: Angioimmunoblastic-Type/Follicular Type, and NOS Type	TET2	47%–82%	Epigenetic regulation	FYN, VAV1, KMT2D, STAT3
	IDH2 R172K	20%–45%	Epigenetic regulation	
	RHOA	50%–72%	Epigenetic regulation	
	DNMT3A R882H	14%–40%	Epigenetic regulation	
	PLCG1	11%–14%	T-cell signaling pathway	
	CD28 T195/D124	4%–14%	T-cell signaling pathway	
Peripheral T-Cell Lymphoma, Not Otherwise Specified	TP53	7%–45%	DNA damage response/cell cycle control	
	FAT1	40%	Cell migration, cell-cell adhesion	
	KMT2C	32%	Epigenetic regulation	
	TET2	12%–22%	Epigenetic regulation	
	CREBBP	16%	Epigenetic regulation	
	ATM	15%	DNA damage response/cell cycle control	
	TP63	13%	DNA damage response/cell cycle control	
	KMT2A	11%	Epigenetic regulation	
	SETD2	10%	Epigenetic regulation	
	ASXL3	8%	Transcriptional regulation	
	DNMT3A	6%–8%	Epigenetic regulation	
	CHD1	7%	Epigenetic regulation	
	MBD4	7%	Epigenetic regulation	
	RHOA (mainly non-G17V type)	7%	Inhibits GTP binding	
Hepatosplenic T-Cell Lymphoma	SETD2	25%	Epigenetic regulation	
	INO80	21%	Epigenetic regulation	
	STAT5B	29%–31%	JAK/STAT pathway	
	ARID1B	19%	Epigenetic regulation	
	TET3	16%	Epigenetic regulation	
	SMARCA2	12%	Epigenetic regulation	
	STAT3	10%	JAK/STAT pathway	
	PIK3CD	10%	PI3K–AKT–mTOR pathway	
	TP53	10%	DNA damage response/cell cycle control	
	UBR5	10%	Cell signaling and proteostasis	
	IDH2	6%	Epigenetic regulation	
Enteropathy-Associated T-Cell Lymphoma	JAK1	15%–75%	JAK/STAT pathway	
	STAT5B	0%–29%	JAK/STAT pathway	
	JAK3	0%–27%	JAK/STAT pathway	
	STAT3	12%–25%	JAK/STAT pathway	
	KRAS	20%	RAS/MAPK pathway	
	SETD2	0%–15%	Epigenetic regulation	
	SOCS1	12%	JAK/STAT pathway	
Monomorphic Epitheliotropic Intestinal T-Cell Lymphoma	STAT5B	35%–60%	JAK/STAT pathway	
	JAK3	33%–46%	JAK/STAT pathway	
	SH2B3	20%	Negative regulation of several signaling pathways	
	JAK1	10%–30%	JAK/STAT pathway	
	STAT3	10%–15%	JAK/STAT pathway	
	TP53	33%	DNA damage response/cell cycle control	
	BRAF	10%–26%	RAS/MAPK pathway	

Table 5-6 Recurrent Somatic Mutations and Associated Pathways in Mature T-Cell and NK-Cell Neoplasms—cont'd

T-Cell Neoplasm Subtype	Most Commonly Mutated Genes	Frequency	Pathway and Cellular Processes	Other Mutated Genes
Indolent Clonal T-Cell Lymphoproliferative Disorder of the Gastrointestinal Tract	KRAS	10%–20%	RAS/MAPK pathway	
	NRAS	10%	RAS/MAPK pathway	
	GNAI2	0%–24%	G-protein-coupled receptor signaling	
	SETD2	70%–93%	Epigenetic regulation	
	CREBBP	26%–30%	Epigenetic regulation	
	STAT3	30%	JAK/STAT pathway	
	TNFAIP3	10%	NF-κB signaling	
	TET2	20%	Epigenetic regulation	
	KMT2D	20%	Epigenetic regulation	
	DNMT3A	10%	Epigenetic regulation	
	DIS3	10%	RNA processing	
	MAPK1	10%	RAS/MAPK pathway	
	TP53	10%	DNA damage response/cell cycle control	
	POLE	10%	DNA repair	
	SMAD4	10%	TGFB and BMP signaling	
	SF3B1	10%	RNA processing	
	CDKN2A	10%	Cell cycle regulation	
	MCM5	10%	Cell cycle regulation	
Indolent NK-cell Lymphoproliferative Disorder of the Gastrointestinal Tract	JAK3 K563_C565del	30%	JAK/STAT pathway	PTPRS, AURKB, AXL, ERBB4, IGF1R, PIK3CB, CUL3, CIC, CHEK2, RUNX1T1, SMARCB1, SETD5
Primary Cutaneous Anaplastic Large Cell Lymphoma	STAT3	14%	JAK/STAT pathway	
	JAK1	14%	JAK/STAT pathway	
	MSC	6%	Transcriptional repression	
Mycosis Fungoides	MAKP1	25%	RAS/MAPK pathway	
	KMT2C	13%	Epigenetic regulation	
	KMT2D	13%	Epigenetic regulation	
	STAT3	13%	JAK/STAT pathway	
	PREX2	13%	PI3K pathway, G protein-coupled receptor regulation	
Sézary Syndrome	TP53	16%	DNA damage response/cell cycle control	SETD1A, SMARCA, MLL3
	PLCG1	up to 12%	T-cell signaling pathway	
	KDM6B	16%	Epigenetic regulation	
	TET2	12%	Epigenetic regulation	
	CREBBP	8%	Epigenetic regulation	
	CHD3	8%	Epigenetic regulation	
	BRD9	8%	Epigenetic regulation	
	PRKG1	8%	Nitric oxide/cGMP signaling pathway	
	CARD11	Up to 8%	BCR signaling, NF-κB signaling	

*Varies depending on immunophenotype; see text for details.

distinct clinical and prognostic features.[179] Almost all genomic abnormalities recurrently identified in ATLL are subclonal, a finding that suggests that targeted therapies for specific genomic alterations may exert only partial effect.[180] However, the presence of gain-of-function *CCR4* mutations/CCR4 overexpression may predict response to mogamulizumab with improved OS.[180] While the occasional PD-L1 overexpression may serve as the rationale for therapeutic purposes, rapid progression after PD-1 blockade may occur.[180] Analysis of tumor cfDNA is a promising methodology for monitoring the disease, particularly the lymphomatous type of ATLL.[178]

T-Cell Large Granular Lymphocytic Leukemia

Demonstration of T-cell monoclonality, although not specific, is necessary for the diagnosis of T-cell large granular

lymphocytic leukemia (T-LGL). This can be achieved through the evaluation of one of the TR genes by PCR or NGS, or by flow cytometry with monoclonal antibodies against the variable regions of the TCR beta chain.[183]

STAT3 mutations are frequent in T-LGL (Table 5-6); >70% involve hotspots Y640 and D661 in the SH2 domain[175,184] and they are linked to symptomatic disease and reduced OS.[184] While *STAT3* Y640F mutations are thought to predict complete response to treatment with methotrexate, cases with other *STAT3* mutations or without *STAT3* mutations display variable therapeutic response.[175] Both the presence and number of *STAT3* mutations correlate with concomitant rheumatoid arthritis.[175] *STAT5B* mutations are rare in CD8+ CD4− T-LGL,[184] but more common in CD4+ CD8+ and CD4+ CD8− T-LGLs and TCR gamma-delta T-LGLs,[184,185] and may associate with an aggressive clinical course in CD8+ T-LGL[184,186] but not in CD4+ T-LGL.[185] Mutations other than *STAT3* and *STAT5* are less common (Table 5-6).[184,187]

Anaplastic Large Cell Lymphoma

Anaplastic large cell lymphoma (ALCL) includes four entities: (1) ALCL, ALK-positive, (2) ALCL, ALK-negative, (3) primary cutaneous ALCL (PCALCL), and (4) breast implant–associated ALCL (BIA-ALCL).

Anaplastic Large Cell Lymphoma, ALK-Positive

By definition, ALCL ALK-positive has a rearrangement of the *ALK* gene with one of various partner genes, most commonly *NPM1* [t(2;5)(p23;q35)] (>80%)] or *TPM3* [t(1;2)(q25;p23)] (13%).[175,188,189] Other partners are rare (≤1%).[188,189] FISH/karyotypic evaluation for *ALK* translocation is not necessary for diagnosis of ALCL ALK-positive as long as ALK immunohistochemical positivity is demonstrated in a mature T-cell lymphoma. The ALK immunohistochemical patterns vary with the fusion partner.[188] RT-PCR assays for the detection of *ALK* rearrangements are of limited diagnostic value but they may play a role in the identification of measurable disseminated/residual disease.[190] A variety of genes are mutated in ALCL ALK-positive (Table 5-6).[188,191] While the prognosis of ALCL ALK-positive is favorable, cases with *TP53* mutations or measurable disseminated/residual disease are associated with inferior outcomes.[190,191]

Anaplastic Large Cell Lymphoma, ALK-Negative

By definition, ALCL ALK-negative lacks *ALK* rearrangements and ALK expression. Instead, *IRF4-DUSP22* and *TP63* translocations have been described in 18% to 30% and 8% of cases, respectively.[188,189] Rarely, these translocations coexist.[192,193] *IRF4-DUSP22* most commonly translocates with *FRA7H* [t(6;7)(p25.3;q32.3)], while the most common partner of *TP63* is *TBL1RXR1* [inv(3)(q26q28)].[194] Rare cases of ALCL ALK-negative harbor other fusion genes such as *NFKB2::ROS1*, *NCOR2::ROS1*, *NFKB2::TYK2*, and *PABPC4::TYK2*.[175,188,194] *IRF4-DUSP22* and *TP63* translocations are not specific for ALCL ALK-negative.[188,195] Because of the genomic proximity of the *TP63* and *TBL1RXR1* loci, FISH with dual-fusion probes for *TBL1RXR1* and *TP63* is recommended in those cases in which the results of the FISH studies with a break-apart *TP63* probe cases are positive or equivocal.[196] Of note, immunohistochemistry for p63 is not specific, and therefore cannot replace FISH studies.[194]

STAT3, *JAK1*, and *MSC* mutations are common in ALCL ALK-negative (Table 5-6),[188,191,194] while they lack *STAT5B*, *JAK3*, or *RHOA* mutations.[197] *MSC* E116K mutations are nearly exclusively seen in *IRF4-DUSP22*-translocated cases.[194,198] ALCL ALK-negative with *IRF4-DUSP22* translocations correlates with a favorable prognosis, similar to that of ALCL ALK-positive, whereas translocations of *TP63* predict an adverse outcome.[194] Those without either translocation have an intermediate prognosis. *STAT3* and *TP53* mutations and loss of *TP53* and *PRDM1/BLIMP1* predict inferior outcomes in ALCL ALK-negative.[175,191]

Extranodal NK/T-Cell Lymphoma, Nasal Type

Gene mutations in extranodal NK/T-cell lymphoma, nasal type (ENKTL) mainly affect the JAK/STAT pathway, NF-κB pathway, epigenetic modifiers, the RNA helicase family, the RAS/MAP kinase pathway, tumor suppressors, immune evasion, NOTCH signaling, and cell-cell signaling, among others (Table 5-6).[199,200] Although most studies have not found or evaluated differences in the genomic landscapes of ENKTL of T-cell lineage versus NK-cell lineage, some have demonstrated distinct profiles, with ENKTL of NK-cell lineage harboring mutations/CNVs of *STAT3*, *DDX3X*, *KMT2C*, *JAK2*, *KMT2D*, *EP300*, *STAT5B*, and *STAT5A*, and amplification of 9p24.1/*PD-L1/2*, with ENKTL of T-cell lineage displaying mutations/CNVs of *EPHA1*, *TP53*, *ARID1A*, *PTPRQ*, *NCOR2*, *PPFIA2*, *BCOR*, *PTPRK*, and *HDAC9*, without amplification of 9p24.1/*PD-L1/2*.[201,202] TR gene rearrangement studies show evidence of monoclonality in up to 40% of cases of ENKTLs, even if cases do not express TCR proteins,[199] and can be used to differentiate NK from T-cell lineage.[201] Rare intravascular NK/T-cell lymphomas carry *HIST1H2AM*, *HIST1H2BE*, *HIST1H2BN*, and a variety of other mutations.[203]

Follicular Helper T-Cell Lymphomas

Three types of follicular helper T-cell lymphomas (FHTL) are recognized: (1) FHTL, angioimmunoblastic type, also referred to as angioimmunoblastic T-cell lymphoma (AITL); (2) FHTL, follicular type; and (3) FHTL, NOS.[4] AITL is characterized by high-frequency mutations in epigenetic modifiers (*TET2*, *IDH2* R172K, and *DNMT3A* R882H), in *RHOA*, and in members of the T-cell signaling pathway (*CD28* T195/D124 and *PLCG1*) (Table 5-6).[204,205] *RHOA* G17V mutations account for >90% of all *RHOA* mutations and most co-occur with *TET2*, *DNMT3A*, or *IDH2* mutations.[175,206] Among T-cell lymphomas, *RHOA* G17V and *IDH2* R172K mutations are exclusively found in FHTL.[205,206] AITL with *TET2* or *DNMT3A* mutations may develop from a background of clonal hematopoiesis.[207,208] The non-specific *CTLA4::CD28* gene fusion has been identified in >50% of AITL in an Asian cohort.[205,209] While the *ITK::SYK* fusion is extremely rare in AITL, and more prevalent in other FHTLs, gains of *ITK* and *SYK* have been identified in 38% and 14% of AITL, respectively.[204]

Peripheral T-Cell Lymphoma, Not Otherwise Specified

GEP studies have identified three peripheral T-cell lymphoma, NOS (PTCL-NOS) subgroups (GATA3, TBX21, and unclassified) with distinct signatures and prognoses.[210-212] An immunohistochemistry algorithm can also be used to classify PTCL-NOS into these subgroups.[211,212] Although the GATA3 subgroup has an inferior clinical outcome than the TBX21 subgroup, a subset within the TBX21 subgroup with a cytotoxic gene signature also has poor clinical outcomes.[210,211] The distinction between these subgroups is relevant for prognostication and possibly therapy selection.[212]

The most frequently mutated genes in PTCL-NOS include tumor suppressor genes, epigenetics modifiers, *VAV1*, and genes of the NOTCH and JAK/STAT pathways (Table 5-6).[206,213,214] *RHOA*, *DNMT3A* or *TET2* mutations are less frequent in PTCL-NOS than in T-cell lymphomas with TFH phenotype, while *IDH2* mutations are absent.[206,213] The vast majority of the *RHOA* mutations found in PTCL-NOS are of non-G17V type. Deletions of *PTEN* and *CDKN2A* are frequent in PTCL-NOS and, if concurrent, they appear to be highly specific for PTCL-NOS.[206,215] Alterations of *TP53* and *CDKN2A*, and mutations in *FAT1*, *IKZF2*, genes associated with immune evasion, epigenetics modifiers, and genes of the TCR signaling/NF-κB pathways correlate with an adverse prognosis.[206,213,215]

Hepatosplenic T-Cell Lymphoma

Mutations in chromatin-modifying genes are seen in >60% of hepatosplenic T-cell lymphoma (HSTL), while other less-frequent mutations affect genes of the JAK/STAT and PI3K-AKT-mTOR pathways, *TP53*, *UBR5*, and *IDH2* (Table 5-6).[216] The most common chromosomal abnormalities in HSTL involve chromosome 7 (47%–100%), mainly isochromosome 7q [i(7)(q10)], typically with –7p and +7q, followed by +8 or 8q amplifications (31%–87%), with these CNAs being associated with worse outcomes.[217,218]

Primary Intestinal T-Cell Lymphomas

Enteropathy-Associated T-Cell Lymphoma. Enteropathy-associated T-cell lymphoma (EATL) is closely, but not exclusively, linked to celiac disease (CD)[219,220] and often preceded by type 2 refractory CD (RCD) and, infrequently, type 1 RCD.[220,221] While in RCD, type 1 TR gene rearrangement studies by PCR most commonly yield polyclonal results, and genetic or gene sequencing analyses reveal no abnormalities, in RCD type 2 monoclonal TR gene rearrangements, CNAs, and *JAK1* and *STAT3* mutations are frequent,[219,221] noting that clonal TR gene rearrangements in small intestinal biopsies are not specific for RCD type 2.[222] No CNAs appear to be specific for EATL, as they can also be found in MEITL.[220,223] However, losses of 3p21.31 (SETD2) have not been described in EATL, a fact which may aid in the distinction from MEITL.[224,225] Mutations in EATL mainly involve the JAK/STAT and RAS pathways, while a small proportion of cases exhibit *SETD2* loss-of-function mutations (Table 5-6).[220,223,226] The mutational profile of EATL substantially overlaps with that of MEITL.

Monomorphic Epitheliotropic Intestinal T-Cell Lymphoma. Monomorphic epitheliotropic intestinal T-cell lymphoma (MEITL), unlike EATL, shows no association with CD.[219] Mutations in MEITL mainly involve the JAK/STAT, RAS/RAF/MAPK, and G-protein-coupled receptor pathways, *TP53*, and chromatin modifier/potential tumor suppressor genes (Table 5-6).[220,223] The mutational profile of MEITL significantly overlaps with that of EATL.[223,224,227] The most common CNAs in MEITL include loss of 3p21 (*SETD2*), a feature that distinguishes it from EATL, and 9p21.3 (*CDK2A/B*).[223,224,227]

Cutaneous T-Cell Lymphoma

Primary Cutaneous Anaplastic Large Cell Lymphoma. *IRF4-DUSP22* and *TP63* translocations can be found in 20% to 30% and 5% of cases, respectively.[188,189] Although PCALCL has traditionally been considered to lack *ALK* translocations,[194] rare primary cutaneous tumors associated with insect bites that resemble PCALCL may harbor these translocations.[188] *JUNB* amplification has been noted in the majority of PCALCL,[228] while *STAT3*, *JAK1*, and *MSC* mutations are found in minor subsets (Table 5-6).[198] Although the presence of a *IRF4-DUSP22* translocations does not appear to effect prognosis,[188] *TP63* translocations may correlate with aggressive behavior.[189]

Mycosis Fungoides. TR gene rearrangement studies are frequently positive for monoclonality in mycosis fungoides (MF), although the specificity and sensitivity of these studies are relatively low in early MF, particularly when reviewed in the absence of immunophenotypic results.[229] The dominant clone may be accompanied by additional reactive clones.[230]

The specificity of the TR gene rearrangement studies in blood in early-stage disease can be improved by comparing the results to those from diagnostic skin biopsies.[231] Concurrent monoclonal TR gene rearrangements in skin and lymph nodes predict inferior outcomes.[231] Mutations in MF involve epigenetic modifier genes, and genes of various signaling pathways, including *MAKP1*, *STAT3*, and *PREX2*, among others (Table 5-6).[232] MF displays a complex and heterogeneous cytogenetic profile, with deletion of negative regulators of the JAK/STAT pathway (*SOCS1*), and recurrent translocations of *ARHGAP26*, *ATXN1*, *CLEC16A*, *ELF1*, *EYS*, *RBPJ*, *RPS6KA3*, *SLC24A2*, and *SSH2*, many of which lead to deletion of genes involved in cell cycle control, chromatin regulation, and the PI3K pathway.[175]

Sézary Syndrome. Sézary syndrome (SS) is a rare aggressive leukemic form of cutaneous T-cell lymphoma. Inferior OS can be predicted if TR gene rearrangement studies document monoclonality in both skin and lymph nodes.[231] The most frequently mutated genes are *TP53*, *PLCG1*, epigenetic modifier genes, and genes of several signaling pathways (Table 5-6).[232] A variety of fusions have been identified: *TPR::MET*, *MYBL1::TOX*, *DNAJC15::ZMYM2*.[233]

Precursor Lymphoid Neoplasms

B-Lymphoblastic Leukemia/Lymphoma

Nascent genomic interrogation has led to the discovery of increasing numbers of distinct categories of B-lymphoblastic leukemia/lymphoma (B-ALL/LBL) that are occasionally differently designated by the ICC and WHO classification schemes (Tables 5-7 and 5-8). Metaphase analysis and FISH are routinely used to identify some of these recurrent genetic abnormalities, which aid in the diagnosis, risk stratification, and therapy selection. In addition, gene sequencing, including whole transcriptome sequencing, RT-PCR, or commercially available FISH probes can help refine the detection of B-ALL/LBL subtypes.[4,73] Fundamental strides have been made in deepening our understanding of the role of the genomic landscape affecting outcomes in B-ALL/LBL and they may continue to further inform future classification schemes.[234]

Although almost all cases of B-ALL/LBL demonstrate monoclonal IGH rearrangements by PCR, concurrent illegitimate monoclonal TR gene rearrangements are also frequently observed.[235] Therefore such analyses are unreliable for the assignment of the lineage of lymphoblasts, although they may provide additional targets for MRD assessment.

T-Lymphoblastic Leukemia/Lymphoma

T-ALL/LBL harbor translocations in ~50%, most commonly involving 14q11 (TRA and TRD) 7p14.1(TRG), and 7q34 (TRB) regions, juxtaposing the TR genes to pivotal transcription factor genes, such as *TAL1*, *TAL2*, *LYL1*, *OLIG2*, *LMO1*, *LMO2*, *TLX1* (*HOX11*), *TLX3* (*HOX11L2*), *NKX2-1*, *NKX2-2*, *NKX2-5*, *HOXA*, *MYC*, and *MYB* (Table 5-9).[232,236,237] Also, *ABL1* may be cryptically rearranged with *NUP214*, *EML1*, and *ETV6*, and the resultant gene fusions may be amenable to TKI therapy.[236] Most frequent mutations and CNAs in T-ALL/LBL involve *NOTCH1*, *FBXW7*, and *MYB*, genes involved in cell cycle regulation (*CDKN2A* and *CDKN2B*), genes involved in the JAK-STAT, RAS/PI3K/AKT, and NF-κB pathways; epigenetic modifier genes; transcription regulator genes; and genes involved in mRNA maturation and ribosomal activity (Table 5-9).[175,232,236] Among

Table 5-7 Cytogenetic Abnormalities Defining Categories of B-ALL/LBL With Recurrent Genetic Abnormalities

B-ALL/LBL Category	Frequency (Age Group)	Comments	Most Common Co-Occurring Genomic Abnormalities	Prognosis
B-ALL/LBL with hyperdiploidy	Up to 30% (pediatric) <10% (adult)	Gain of ≥5 chromosomes, total of >50 chromosomes, characteristically displays trisomies; distinction from low hypodiploid or near-haploid B-ALL/LBL with masked hypodiploidy is critical	Histone modifiers (*CREBBP*, *WHSC1*, *SUV420H1*, *SETD2*, and *EZH2*), RTK-RAS pathway (*FLT3*, *NRAS*, *KRAS*, and *PTPN11*)	Excellent prognosis, particularly in cases with +17 or +18, although +5 and +20 may predict poorer outcomes
B-ALL/LBL with low-hyperdiploidy	Up to 11% (pediatric) Up to 15% (adult)	47–50 chromosomes		Data regarding prognosis is controversial
B-ALL/LBL with hypodiploidy	High-hypodiploid: <7% (pediatric and adult) Low-hypodiploid: 0.5% (pediatric) 4% (adult) Near-haploid: 0.5% (pediatric)	<46 chromosomes, 80% are near-diploid (45 chromosomes); the rest are strictly hypodiploid (≤44 chromosomes), which includes high-hypodiploid (40–44 chromosomes), low-hypodiploid (30–39 chromosomes), and near-haploid (24–29 chromosomes) subgroups. Low-hypodiploid: testing for germline *TP53* mutations is recommended; low hypodiploid and near-haploid may be misdiagnosed as high-hyperdiploid or triploid karyotype ("masked hypodiploidy")	High-hypodiploid: complex karyotypes Low-hypodiploid: *CREBBP*, *RB1*, *IKZF2*, *CDKN2A/2B*, *TP53* Near-haploid: *NRAS*, *FLT3*, *KRAS*, *PTPN11*, *NF1*, *PAG1*, *IKZF3*, *CDKN2A/B*, *RB1*, *CREBBP*, and histone cluster at chromosome 6p22	Near-diploid: prognosis is less adverse than strict hypodiploidy Strict hypodiploidy: adverse prognosis Concurrent gene fusions (*BCR::ABL1*, *TCF3::PBX1*, and *ETV6::RUNX1*) may alter the prognosis of hypodiploid cases
B-ALL/LBL with *BCR::ABL1* fusion	≤4% (pediatric) ~25% (adult)	*BCR::ABL1* fusion results in the production of p190 or p210 proteins. p190 protein is more frequent, especially in children; this must be distinguished from the lymphoid blast phase of chronic myeloid leukemia, particularly in children, as management of these entities differs in this age group	Deletions of the *IKZF1*, *PAX5*, *EBF1* and *CDKN2A/2B*	Adverse outcome, although the prognosis has improved with the use of TKIs
B-ALL/LBL, *BCR::ABL1*-like	15%–21% (pediatric) ~24% (adult)	Gene-expression profile similar to that of B-ALL/LBL with *BCR::ABL1* fusion but lack this fusion	Three different subtypes: (1) ABL-1 class rearranged, (2) JAK-STAT activated, and (3) NOS. B-lymphoid transcription factor genes (*IKZF1*, *PAX5*), genes deregulating cytokine receptor and tyrosine kinase signaling, *CRLF2* translocations (*IGH::CRLF2*, *2RY8::CRLF2*)	*CRLF2* translocations are associated with poor prognosis, especially if there is a concurrent *IKZF1* deletion; the three subtypes dictate different management strategies
B-ALL/LBL with *KMT2A* translocations	~50% (infant) 5% (pediatric other than infant) 10% (adult)	*KMT2A* fuses with >90 partner genes, most commonly *AFF1*, *MLLT3*, and *MLLT1*	Mutations in *KRAS*, *NRAS*, *FLT3*, *NF1*, *PTPN11*, and *PIK3R1*	Poor prognosis, particularly in translocations with *AFF1* as a result of t(4;11)(q21;q23)
B-ALL/LBL with *ETV6::RUNX1* fusion	~25% (pediatric) <1% (adult)	The fusion arises from t(12;21)(p13;q22), which is cytogenetically cryptic and requires FISH or RT-PCR studies for its detection	*ETV6*, *PAX5*, *ATF7IP*	Excellent prognosis
B-ALL/LBL with iAMP21	<2% (pediatric)	Defined as ≥3 extra copies of RUNX1 on a single chromosome 21 (≥5 RUNX1 signals/cell) typically detected with *RUNX1* FISH probes	Gains of X, 10, or 14; deletions of 7/7q, 11q, *ETV6*, and *RB1*; mutations in genes of the RAS signaling pathway; *P2RY8::CRLF2* fusion	Poor prognosis; can be improved with intensive chemotherapy
B-ALL/LBL with *TCF3::PBX1* fusion	<6% (pediatric)	t(1;19)(q23;p13) results in this fusion	Unknown	Historically associated with adverse prognosis, but modern intensive chemotherapy has reverted this
B-ALL/LBL with *TCF3::HLF* fusion	<1% (pediatric)	Translocations of *HLF* with *TCF3* (or *TCF4*) can be detected with a break-apart *HLF* FISH probe, and/or WTS	Deletions of *PAX5* and *VPREB1*, and aberrations in genes of the RAS pathway	Very poor prognosis
B-ALL/LBL with *IGH::IL3* fusion	<1% (adolescents and young adults)	The t(5;14)(q31.1;q32.1) juxtaposes the IGH enhancer to *IL3*, or *IL3* is cryptically inserted into IGH, resulting in increased IL3 production and eosinophilia	*IKZF1* deletions	Intermediate prognosis

FISH, Fluorescence in situ hybridization.

Table 5-8 Comparison of Selected Entities Listed Under "New Entities in B-ALL/LL Defined by Structural Alterations" and "Classification of Acute Lymphoblastic Leukemia" by the 2022 ICC and as "B-ALL/LBL With Other Defined Genetic Abnormalities" by the 2022 WHO Classification

ICC Nomenclature and Disease Classification	WHO Nomenclature and Disease Classification
B-ALL with *MYC* rearrangement*	B-ALL/LBL with *IG::MYC* fusion*
B-ALL with *DUX4* rearrangement*	B-ALL/LBL with *DUX4* rearrangement*
B-ALL with *MEF2D* rearrangement*	B-ALL/LBL with *MEF2D* rearrangement*
B-ALL with *ZNF384(362)* rearrangement*	B-ALL/LBL with *ZNF384* rearrangement*
B-ALL with *NUTM1* rearrangement*	B-ALL/LBL with *NUTM1* rearrangement*
B-ALL with *HLF* rearrangement*	B-ALL/LBL with *TCF3::HLF* fusion*
B-ALL with mutated *PAX5* P80R*	B-ALL/LBL with *PAX5* p.P80R (NP_057953.1) abnormalities*
B-ALL, *ETV6::RUNX1*-like[†]	B-ALL/LBL with *ETV6::RUNX1*-like features*
B-ALL, with *PAX5* alteration[†]	B-ALL/LBL with PAX5alt*
B-ALL, with mutated *ZEB2* (p.H1038R)/*IGH::CEBPE*)[†‡]	
B-ALL, *ZNF384* rearranged-like[†‡]	
B-ALL, *KMT2A* rearranged-like[†‡]	
B-ALL with mutated *IKZF1* N159Y*[‡]	
B-ALL with *UBTF::ATXN7L3/PAN3,CDX2* ("CDX2/UBTF")*[‡]	

*Definite entity.
[†]Provisional entity.
[‡]Not classified in the 2022 WHO Nomenclature and Disease Classification.

these, activating *NOTCH1* mutations and loss-of-function mutations of FBXW7 are the most frequent,[232,238] followed by del(9p21) and altered methylation of *CDKN2A* and *CDKN2B*.[175] No specific mutations appear to correlate with patient outcome in T-ALL/LBL.[232] Early T-cell precursor ALL (ETP-ALL) is a distinct form of T-ALL/LBL with an immunophenotype and a GEP similar to those of hematopoietic stem cells.[175,236] ETP-ALL harbors mutations in genes of multiple pathways, including early hematopoietic and lymphoid development; RAS, cytokine receptor and kinase signaling and epigenetic regulators.[4,175,236] *DNMT3A* and *RUNX1* mutations in ETP-ALL may predict poor OS.[232] Although almost all cases of T-ALL/LBL demonstrate monoclonal TR gene rearrangements by PCR, concurrent illegitimate monoclonal IGH gene rearrangements may also be identified in ~20% of cases.[238,239]

MYELOID NEOPLASMS

The full spectrum of technologies available in the clinical laboratory is routinely applied to the characterization of myeloid neoplasms. Although these have evolved through classical cytogenetics, FISH, PCR-based approaches, and NGS, they all still largely remain complementary, with each having different roles in different contexts, albeit with some appropriate built-in redundancy that is useful for confirmation of diagnostic aberrations. Broadly considered, the myeloid neoplasms comprise three major groups: AMLs, myeloproliferative neoplasms (MPNs), and myelodysplastic syndromes (MDSs). Others include overlap syndromes, those associated with eosinophilia and specific genetic aberrations, mast cell neoplasms, dendritic cell neoplasms, and those with a germline predisposition.

Acute Myeloid Leukemias

Karyotypic Abnormalities

AML is an extremely heterogeneous disease at the genetic level, with at least 300 different but recurrent structural cytogenetic abnormalities observed.[240] Of all of the

parameters that are integrated to yield a final diagnosis and appropriate classification of AML, the most relevant are the genetic abnormalities.[241] Large multicenter cooperative studies and organizations have identified broad prognostic groups based on cytogenetics, although molecular abnormalities have also been appropriately incorporated. In addition to their prognostic relevance, many of the recurrent translocations in AML are used to define specific entities in the ICC and WHO classification (Table 5-10). Accordingly, the identification of these is germane to the contemporary diagnosis of AML. In addition to these recurrent cytogenetic abnormalities, mutational analysis plays a key role in AML classification such that both are now central to contemporary classification in which they are hierarchically stratified (Fig. 5-8).[2,242]

t(15;17)(q24.1;q21.2)

Among all acute leukemias, acute promyelocytic leukemia (APL) is the one with the most compelling genotype–morphologic phenotype correlation in that the genetics can frequently be "predicted" on the basis of the characteristic morphology, be it in the classic hypergranular form with abundant Auer rods or in the hypogranular variant with "cottage loaf" or "kagami mochi" nuclei. It also remains paradigmatic with regard to the use of targeted therapy.[243] Accounting for ~5% to 10% of translocations in AML as a whole, the t(15;17)(q24.1;q21.2) is seen in ~99% of APLs. In this prototypic translocation, *RARA* (on 17q21.2) is fused to *PML* (on 15q24.1). Although the involvement of RARA is central to neoplastic transformation, the disruption of PML also plays a role in leukemic transformation. In the approximate 1% of remaining cases, interesting variant translocations are present, with approximately 10 different fusion partners other than *PML*. For all of these, the common denominator is the disruption of the *RARA* gene at 17q21.2, converting a transcriptional activator into a repressor.[244] However, these variants are no longer considered definitional of APL because not all are as exquisitely responsive to all-*trans* retinoic acid (ATRA) and arsenic [i.e., t(11;17)(q23;q21.2), *RARA-ZBTB16*]. Thus from a molecular diagnostic perspective, it is

Table 5-9 Common (≥5%) Recurrent Genetic Abnormalities in T-ALL/LBL

Gene	Chromosome Location	Frequency	Genetic Alteration	Biological Function of Protein	Effect of Genetic Lesion	Clinical Effect
CDKN2A/2B	9p21	~70%	Deletion/ hypermethylation	Negative cell cycle regulator	Loss of inhibition of cyclin-dependent kinases, leading to increased cell-cycle progression	Unfavorable
NOTCH1	9q34	~55%	Mutation	Membrane receptor needed for normal lymphocyte function	Activation of NOTCH1 pathway, resulting in impaired intercellular signaling and development	Favorable (in children); co-occurrence with FBXW7 mutations especially favorable
TLX3::BCL11B	t(5;14)(q35;q32)	~20%	Translocation	Transcription factor	Deregulation of TLX3 with downregulation of target genes	Unfavorable
TAL1	del(1)(p32)	~25%	Deletion resulting in fusion to STIL	Transcription factor for hematopoietic differentiation	Overexpression of TAL1, causing epigenetic dysregulation	Unclear
FBXW7	4q31	~20%	Mutation	Component of ubiquitin protein ligase that degrades activated NOTCH1	Activation of NOTCH1 pathway	Favorable (in children); co-occurrence with NOTCH1 mutations especially favorable
PHF6	Xq26	~20%	Mutation	Potential role in transcriptional regulation or chromatin remodeling	Unclear, putative tumor suppressor	Unfavorable
RUNX1	21q22	~20%	Mutation	Transcription factor	Dominant negative effect leading to decreased transcription	Unfavorable
LEF1	4q23	~20%	Mutation and microdeletion	Component of Wnt signaling pathway	Impaired Wnt signaling	Unclear
JAK1	1p21	~15%	Mutation	Tyrosine kinase	Increased JAK-STAT signaling	Unfavorable
PTEN	10q23	~15%	Mutation	Protein and lipid phosphatase; tumor suppressor	Loss of function, leading to increased cell-cycle progression	Unfavorable
TCRAD::TAL1	t(1;14)(p32;q11)	~15%	Translocation	Transcription factor for hematopoietic differentiation	Overexpression of TAL1, causing epigenetic dysregulation	Favorable
SET-NUP214	del(9) (q34.11q34.13)	~10%	Translocation	Fusion protein may activate members of the HOXA cluster	Elevated expression of HOXA genes	Unclear
IL7R*	5p13	~10% (45%)	Mutation	Receptor for IL-7	Gain of function important for lymphoid differentiation	Unfavorable
BCL11B	14q32	~10%	Mutation	May be involved in TP53 signaling pathway	Impaired differentiation and cell-cycle arrest	Unclear
ETV6	12p13	~10%	Mutation	ETS family transcription factor	Loss of function; exact effect unclear	Unclear
MYB	6q22-q23	~10%	Duplication	Transcriptional activator	Increased proliferation	Unclear
ABL1	9q34	~5%	Most often fusion with NUP214 and episomal amplification	Tyrosine kinase	Kinase activation, leading to increased proliferation	Unclear; sensitive to tyrosine kinase inhibition
PTPN2	18p11	~5%	Deletion	Tyrosine phosphatase	Increased proliferation and cytokine sensitivity	Unclear
FLT3*	13q12	~5% (~40%)	Point mutations and internal tandem duplications	Class III receptor tyrosine kinase that regulates hematopoiesis	Constitutive activation of signal transduction, increased proliferation, and decreased apoptosis	Unfavorable in ETP

*IL7R and FLT3 mutations are enriched in early T-cell precursor ALL (ETP-ALL) with the higher frequencies in parentheses reflecting this. They are uncommon in other forms of T-ALL/LBL; conversely, NOTCH1 and FBXW7 mutations are rare in ETP-ALL compared with the other forms.

Table 5-10 Acute Myeloid Leukemia Entities Defined by Recurrent Cytogenetic Abnormalities*

Cytogenetic Abnormality	Genes Involved
t(15;17)(q24.1;q21.2)[†]	*PML::RARA*
t(8;21)(q22;q22.1)	*RUNX1::RUNX1T1*
inv(16)(p13.1q22) or t(16;16) (p13.1;q22)	*CBFB::MYH11*
t(9;11)(p21.3;q23.3)	*MLLT3::KMT2A*
Other 11q23.3 rearrangements	*KMT2A* and another gene
t(6;9)(p22.3;q34.1)	*DEK::NUP214*
inv(3)(q21.3q26.2) or t(3;3) (q21.3;q26.2)	*GATA2; MECOM*
Other 3q26.2 rearrangements	*MECOM* and another gene
t(9;22)(q34.1;q11.2)	*BCR::ABL1*
Myelodysplasia-related cytogenetic abnormalities[‡]	Variable
Other rare recurring translocations[§]	Variable

*With the exception of t(9;22)(q34.1;q11.2)/*BCR::ABL1* and myelodysplasia-related cytogenetic abnormalities, both of which require ≥20% blasts to diagnose AML, ≥10% blasts are sufficient to render a diagnosis of AML with these abnormalities.

[†]This is specifically associated with acute promyelocytic leukemia (APL). A number of other *RARA* translocations are also described, including those involving 1q42.3/*IRF2BP2*; 5q35.1/*NPM1*; 11q23.2/*ZBTB16*; cryptic inv(17q) or del(17) (q21.2q21.2)/*STAT3* or *STAT5B*; 3q26.3/*TBL1XR1*, 4q12/*FIP1L1*; Xp11/*BCOR*.

[‡]Defined by detecting a complex karyotype (≥3 unrelated clonal chromosomal abnormalities in the absence of other class-defining recurring genetic abnormalities), del(5q)/t(5q)/add(5q), −7/del(7q), +8, del(12p)/t(12p)/add(12p), i(17q), −17/add(17p) or del(17p), del(20q), or idic(X)(q13) clonal abnormalities.

[§]The other rare recurring translocations and genes involved are t(1;3) (p36.3;q21.3)/*PRDM16::RPN1*, t(3;5)(q25.3;q35.1)/*NPM1::MLF*, t(8;16)(p1 1.2;p13.3)/*KAT6A::CREBBP*, t(1;22)(p13.3;q13.1)/*RBM15::MRTF1*, t(5;11) (q35.2;p15.4)/*NUP98::NSD1*, t(11;12)(p15.4;p13.3)/*NUP98::KMD5A*, t(11p15.4)/*NUP98* and other partners, t(7;12)(q36.3;p13.2)/*ETV6::MNX1*, t(10;11)(p12.3;q14.2)/*PICALM::MLLT10*, t(16;21)(p11.2;q22.2)/*FUS::ERG*, t(16;21)(q24.3;q22.1)/*RUNX1::CBFA2T3*, inv(16)(p13.3q24.3)/*CBFA2T3::GLIS2*.

important to identify these rare variants because not all such patients will benefit from ATRA therapy. t(11;17)-positive leukemic cells tend to have regular nuclei, with an increased number of Pelger-Huët–like cells.

Although typically identifiable by metaphase analysis, the relatively slow turnaround time of this approach and need for prompt initiation of therapy have led to the routine use of more rapid FISH or RT-PCR. Rarely, the translocation may be cryptic, being detected by FISH or RT-PCR but missed on metaphase analysis.[245] The use of dual-color break-apart FISH probes not only allows the identification of the t(15;17) but also can recognize variant translocations, albeit without identifying the *RARA* partner. With regard to RT-PCR for the common t(15;17), the breakpoints in *RARA* are well conserved in intron 2, whereas there are two major intronic and one intronic breakpoints in the *PML* gene. Thus a single downstream *RARA* primer and two upstream *PML* primers will detect most (>95%) of *PML::RARA* fusion transcripts.

FLT3 internal tandem duplication (ITD) mutations are enriched in t(15;17) AML, occurring in 30% to 40% of cases; whereas these mutations are typically associated with a poor prognosis in other settings, their prognostic effect in this context is unclear.[246] By contrast, *FLT3* tyrosine kinase domain (TKD) mutations that occur in 10% are associated with an adverse outcome. Up to 50% of patients with APL may harbor mutations in genes encoding epigenetic modifiers that portend a poor prognosis.[247] Rarely, *RARA* or *PML* mutations occur and can be associated with the development

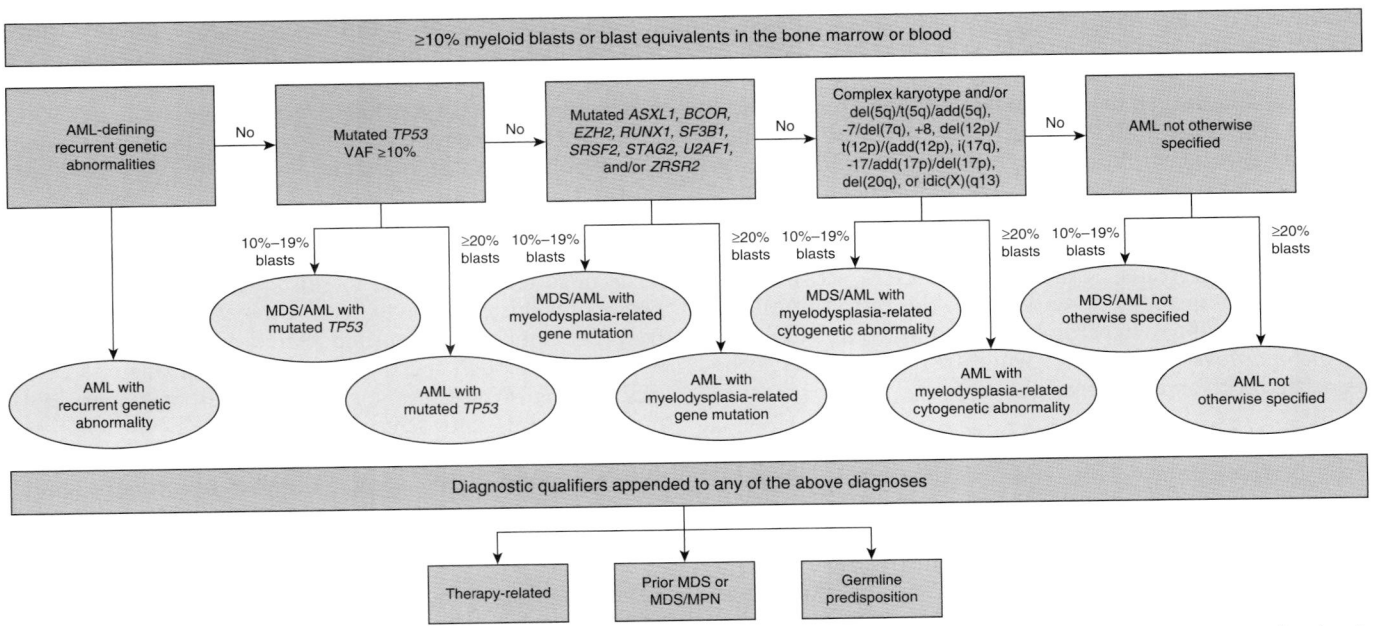

Figure 5-8. Hierarchical classification of the International Consensus Classification of acute myeloid leukemia (AML). The classification is hierarchical (i.e., AML with recurrent genetic abnormalities takes precedence over all other categories; among the remaining categories, AML with mutated *TP53* supersedes AML with myelodysplasia-related gene mutations, and the latter supersedes AML with myelodysplasia-related cytogenetic abnormalities. *AML,* Acute myeloid leukemia; *MDS,* myelodysplastic syndrome. (*Reproduced with permission from Döhner H, Wei AH, Appelbaum FR, et al. Diagnosis and management of AML in adults: 2022 recommendations from an international expert panel on behalf of the ELN. Blood. 2022;140[12]:1345-1377. https://doi.org/10.1182/blood.2022016867.)*

of resistance, and it may become important to test for their presence in relapsing patients.[248,249]

t(8;21)(q22;q22.1)

This translocation is seen in ~5% to 10% of AMLs. The translocation fuses part of the *RUNX1* gene (formerly *AML1* or *CBPA2*) on 21q22.1 with part of the *RUNX1T1* (formerly *ETO*) gene on 8q22.[250] *RUNX1* is half of the heterodimer core binding factor (CBF) that is a crucial transcription factor in hematopoiesis. This half directly contacts DNA, whereas the β-subunit facilitates DNA binding. The two genes that encode the two components of this CBF transcriptional factor are common targets of translocations in AML and pediatric ALL and are collectively disrupted in ~20% to 25% of each of these major types of acute leukemia. When *RUNX1* is translocated, the subsequently generated fusion protein acts in a dominant negative fashion, inhibiting the transcription of a number of important hematopoietic target genes, including *MPO, GM-CSF, IL-3,* and *TRB.* By contrast, AMLs with *RUNX1::RUNX1T1* fusions upregulate expression of B-cell genes, and hence these AMLs typically co-express one or more of CD19, CD79a, PAX5, and TdT.

The breakpoints cluster within a single intron of both genes, so that similar chimeric transcripts are usually generated in every case. Thus a simple RT-PCR assay, with a *RUNX1* primer and a *RUNX1T1* primer, is able to detect this translocation at a molecular level and can be used diagnostically. FISH can also easily detect the translocation. Leukemias harboring a t(8;21) translocation evince particular sensitivity to and substantial benefit from therapeutic regimens containing high-dose cytosine arabinoside. In addition, so-called CBF leukemias [that include those with this translocation and those with inv(16)(p13.2q22)/t(16;16)(p13.3;q22)] show increased sensitivity to monoclonal antibody therapy directed at CD33. Whereas this good prognostic association appears to be well established in adult AML, this is less clear in pediatric AML. Cooperative mutations commonly seen in *RUNX1::RUNXT1* AMLs are those that affect the *KIT* gene, which result in constitutive activation of the encoded receptor tyrosine kinase and are associated with a relatively poor outcome, although this may depend on the site of the mutation, with those in exon 17 adverse while those in exon 8 are not.[251] *ASXL2* mutations are also recurrent in this form of AML (second only to *KIT* mutations); whereas they have no effect on OS, there may be a greater incidence of relapse.[252] *CCND1* and *CCND2* mutations are also enriched in this form of AML.[253] Coexisting del(9q), hyperdiploidy, and hypodiploidy may predict improved survival,[254] while trisomy 8 tends to be associated with an inferior prognosis.[255]

inv(16)(p13.1q22)/(16;16)(p13.1q22)

This pericentric inversion, and the molecularly identical t(16;16), is seen in ~5% to 10% of AMLs. It is characteristically associated with acute myelomonoblastic leukemia with abnormal eosinophils and their precursors that contain abnormally large basophilic granules. The inversion fuses parts of the *CBFB* gene (formerly *PEBP2B*) on 16q22 with parts of one of the myosin heavy chain genes, *MYH11* (previously *SMMHC*) located at 16q11. The inv(16) can sometimes be quite subtle at the karyotypic level and may on occasion be missed, particularly if the metaphase preparations are suboptimal. Of note, +22 is the most common associated

abnormality in patients with inv(16) but is uncommon in other situations.[256] Thus the presence of an apparently isolated +22 should alert one to the presence of a possible cryptic *CBFB::MYH11* fusion. Accordingly, molecular studies have a particularly relevant role in the detection of this abnormality. Interestingly, the presence of +22 in an inv(16)-positive AML predicts for a better outcome compared with those lacking +22, according to most but not all studies.[254] Though the presence of a *FLT3*-ITD mutation in core binding factor (CBF) AMLs is associated with inferior outcomes, this is abrogated by the coexistent trisomy 22 in *CBFB::MYH11* AML.[257] As noted, AMLs with the *CBFB::MYH11* fusion show increased sensitivity to immunotherapy directed at CD33,[258] and hence it is important to detect for this reason.

The inversion/translocation is detectable by both FISH and RT-PCR. Whereas 99% of breakpoints in *CBFB* occur in intron 5 of that gene, the breakpoint heterogeneity is quite marked in the *MYH11* gene, with seven different exons (7 through 13) variably included in the fusion transcripts. This complexity notwithstanding, the most common form, designated type A, accounts for ~90% of cases with this genetic fusion; two other transcripts (types D and E) account for an additional 5%. Whereas +22 might predict a better outcome, the presence of *FLT3*-TKD and *KIT* mutations predicts a worse outcome, while the effect of +8 is unclear.[254] *RAS* mutations are common in this form of AML (~50% of cases) and do not have well established prognostic significance, although some studies suggest a favorable association.[255]

11q23.3 Translocations

KMT2A (formerly *MLL*) at chromosome 11q23.3 is one of the most promiscuous genes in the human leukemic genome and is involved in at least 160 different translocations, and these are seen in both AML and ALL.[259] One specific translocation, which fuses *KMT2A* with *MLLT3* as a consequence of the t(9;11)(p22;q23.3), is now recognized as a distinct entity with an intermediate prognosis to distinguish it from other *KMT2A* translocations that typically portend an adverse prognosis.[260] In general, *KMT2A* translocations in AML are associated with monoblastic differentiation and prior therapy with topoisomerase II inhibitors.

The breakpoints in *KMT2A* tend to cluster in a relatively small (8.3-kb) area spanning exons 5 to 11, referred to as a breakpoint cluster region. *KMT2A* translocations seen in de novo leukemias tend to cluster in the 5′ region of the breakpoint cluster region, whereas those seen in both infantile B-ALL/LBL and therapy-related AML occur more often in the 3′ region. Although specific fusions are amenable to specific FISH and RT-PCR assays, a single *KMT2A* break-apart FISH probe can be used for screening purposes.

The intermediate prognosis association of the t(9;11) translocation has not been confirmed in pediatric AML; however, other interesting prognostic associations have been observed with other *KMT2A* translocations in this age group.[261] Thus the t(6;11)(q27;q23.3) is associated with a particularly dismal prognosis, whereas the t(1;11)(9q21;q23.3) portends an especially good outcome, with a more than 90% event-free survival.[261]

t(6;9)(p23;q34.1)

This translocation is quite rare, occurring in ~1% of AMLs. Frequently associated with basophilia and multilineage dysplasia, this disease entity has an adverse prognosis. The translocation disrupts the *DEK* gene on chromosome 6p23 and the *NUP214* (formerly *CAN*) gene on chromosome 9q34.1.[262] The breakpoints cluster within a single intron of both *DEK* and *NUP214*, allowing convenient analysis by RT-PCR. Metaphase analysis and FISH are also used in the diagnosis of this entity. *FLT3*-ITD mutations are highly enriched in AMLs with this translocation, occurring in up to 90% of cases.[263]

inv(3)(q21.3q26.2)

The inv(3) and the related t(3;3) are found in ~1% to 2% of AML cases that may display megakaryocytic differentiation, dysplastic changes (binucleated megakaryocytes), and an elevated platelet count.[264] They are typically associated with a poor clinical outcome. These chromosome 3 abnormalities are centered on the dysregulation of *EVI1* on 3q26, which has a variety of alternative splice forms including one variant that results in the endogenous (nonpathogenic) fusion of *EVI1* with an adjacent gene called *MDS1*, resulting in the gene's name being modified to *MECOM* (*MDS1* and *EVI1* complex locus). In contrast to all the other recurrent translocations in AML, inv(3)/t(3;3) does not generate a fusion protein; rather, it results in the inappropriate overexpression of *MECOM*. The involved gene at 3q21.3 had historically been thought to be *RPN1*; however, subsequent studies incriminated *GATA2* as being more pertinent, with its transcriptional machinery driving unregulated *MECOM* expression. Given the absence of a bona fide fusion gene and transcript, RT-PCR–based assays have been difficult to develop. However, a FISH assay for *MECOM* is available and appears more accurate than conventional chromosomal analysis. The gene encoding the core RNA splicing factor *SF3B1* is mutated in >30% of AMLs with inv(3)/t(3;3), which leads to aberrant *EVI1* splicing and contributes to its pathogenesis.[265]

t(9;22)(q34.1;q11.2)

This translocation, fusing *BCR* on 22q11.2 and *ABL1* on 9q34.1, more characteristically associated with CML and ALL, may also reflect a distinct subtype of AML.[266,267] These cases tend to have a poor outcome. Deletion of the IGH gene may be a characteristic finding that might help distinguish de novo cases from those that reflect AMLs developing from CML. Metaphase analysis, FISH, and RT-PCR can be used to detect this translocation. FISH on nonblast cells in this form of AML (and ALL) may be valuable in distinguishing de novo AML from CML in blast phase, with the *BCR::ABL1* fusion more likely to be seen in differentiating granulocytic cells in the latter, but not in de novo AML.

Rationale for Performing Molecular Genetic Studies for Translocations in AML

Whereas all of the recurrent translocations may be readily discernible with metaphase/karyotypic studies, these cytogenetic analyses have a variable false negativity rate. Some of these are truly cryptic in nature in that they are submicroscopic; however, other false-negative results may have a technical basis. For example, there are well-documented reports of false-negative cytogenetics for the three most frequent translocations in AML, t(15;17)/*PML::RARA*, t(8;21)/*RUNX1::RUNX1T1*, and inv(16)/*CBFB::MYH11*. Given the importance of the detection of each in appropriate AML classification and therapy, it might be prudent to screen

all newly diagnosed AMLs for the presence of these lesions, at the molecular genetic level.[268,269] RT-PCR assays are available, and they may be multiplexed. Novel ligase-dependent PCR assays might allow the simultaneous detection of more than 50 translocations.[270] An additional reason for performing FISH or RT-PCR is the superior turnaround time these assays provide compared with metaphase analysis, so that appropriate therapy can be instituted without substantial delay.[271] Even in those scenarios in which cytogenetics easily detect these translocations at diagnosis, it is reasonable to perform the appropriate molecular genetic studies ab initio. The rationale for this is that a disease-specific molecular lesion needs to be identified so that it can be subsequently exploited as a sensitive target for the detection of MRD after therapy.[272]

Mutations

In addition to gross chromosomal abnormalities including the cytogenetically detectable translocations discussed earlier, some of which require molecular genetic analysis for accurate detection, a variety of subchromosomal lesions (in particular mutations) are frequently encountered in AML.[273-275] They are (unsurprisingly but conveniently) enriched in cytogenetically normal AMLs. Thus these molecular abnormalities can be identified in more than 95% of cytogenetically normal AMLs, which account for ~45% of all AMLs. NGS has led to an explosion in the discovery of mutations that play a role in the pathogenesis of AML and that have diagnostic, prognostic, and therapeutic relevance.[276,277]

Nearly all AMLs have mutation in one of eight categories of genes that are almost certainly relevant for pathogenesis, including *NPM1* (~30%), tumor-suppressor genes (~15%), DNA methylation–related genes (~45%), signaling genes (~60%), chromatin-modifying genes (~30%), myeloid transcription factor genes (~20%), cohesin complex genes (~15%), and spliceosome complex genes (~15%) (Fig. 5-9).[261] Another study, which has identified 16 genetic classes of AML, relies on data from both cytogenetics and mutations in 32 genes.[278] Some of the more frequently detected mutations are summarized in Table 5-11, with a subset of these described in more detail here. Patterns of cooperation and mutual exclusivity suggest strong biological relationships among several of the genes and categories. For example, *FLT3*, *NPM1*, and *DNMT3A* tend to occur together, whereas the transcription factor fusions arising as a consequence of some of the aforementioned translocations and mutations of *NPM1*, *RUNX1*, *TP53*, and *CEBPA* are mutually exclusive. *IDH1/IDH2* and *TET2* mutations also tend to be mutually exclusive, although this is not always the case. One study identified 11 classes of AML based upon their genetics, with some overlap with the above, with three new categories emerging[279]: AML with mutations in genes encoding chromatin regulators (such as *ASXL1*), RNA-splicing regulators (such as *SRSF2*), or both (in 18% of patients); AML with *TP53* mutations, chromosomal aneuploidies, or both (in 13%); and, provisionally, AML with *IDH2* (R172) mutations (in 1%). There are currently four AML categories that are defined by the presence of mutations, namely those affecting *NPM1*, *CEBPA*, and *TP53*, as well as those that have one of nine myelodysplasia-related gene mutations. They will be discussed here, followed by a discussion of a number of other relevant, but not disease-defining, mutations.

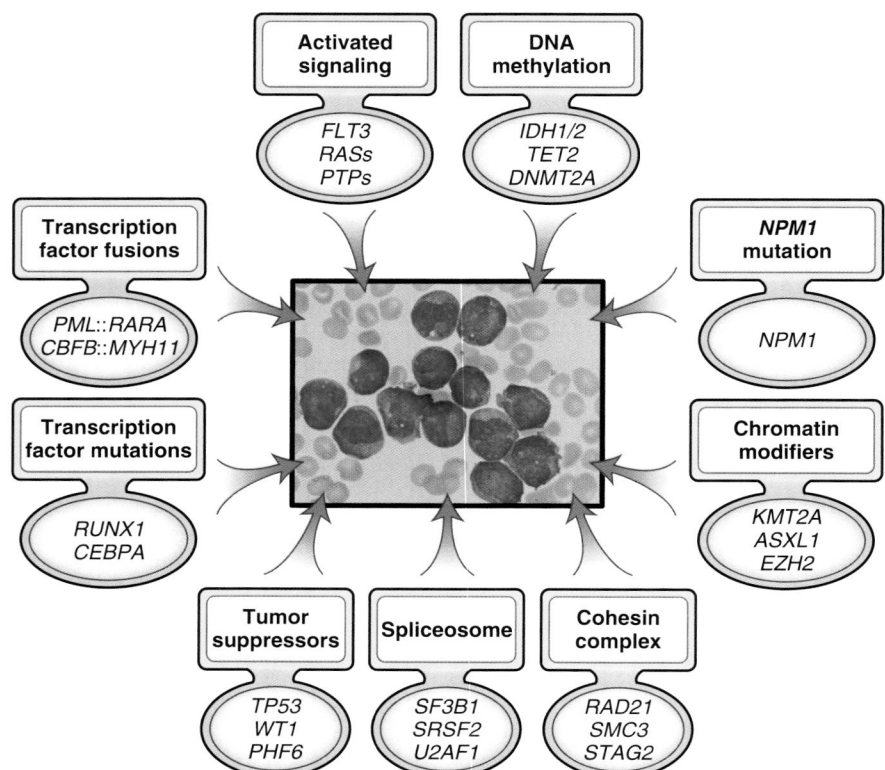

Figure 5-9. Molecular basis of acute myeloid leukemia (AML). Virtually all AMLs harbor a mutation in one of eight genetic categories or transcription factor translocations that are central to their pathogenesis. Seven of the eight mutational categories contain a number of genes, and typically no more than one member of each group is mutated in AML. One group contains only a single gene: *NPM1*. The noted recurrent translocations (the ninth category in the figure) lead to the disruption of cellular differentiation by abrogating the function of transcription factors.

Table 5-11 Examples of Recurrent Mutations in Acute Myeloid Leukemia (AML)

Gene	Approximate Frequency*	Prognostic Significance	Putative Consequence/Altered Biological Mechanism	Associations
NPM1	30%	Good	Cytoplasmic mislocalization; dysregulated P53	Cuplike nuclear invaginations, CD34−, FLT3-ITD
FLT3	20%	Poor (ITD only)	↑ Signal transduction	Cuplike nuclear invaginations, *NPM1* mutations
DNMT3A	20%	Poor	Epigenetic (DNA methylation)	Poor prognosis diminished with increased dose of doxorubicin
RAS	15%	None	↑ Signal transduction	CBF AML
WT1	10%–15%	Poor	↓Transcription	—
TET2	10%–15%	Poor	Epigenetic (DNA methylation)	—
CEBPA	10%	Good	↓Transcription	Co-expression of T-cell antigens
ASXL1	10%	Poor	Chromatin modification	—
RUNX1	10%	Poor	↓ Transcription	Minimal differentiation
IDH1	5%–10%	Unclear/poor	Oncometabolite; epigenetic (DNA methylation)	Cuplike nuclear invaginations
IDH2	5%–10%	Unclear/good	Oncometabolite; epigenetic (DNA methylation)	Cuplike nuclear invaginations
TP53	5%–10%	Poor	Tumor suppressor	More common (70%) in AMLs with a complex karyotype
KIT	5%	Poor	↑ Signal transduction	CBF AML
KMT2A partial tandem duplication	5%	Poor	Chromatin modification	Trisomy 11

*Frequency of some mutations may be up to twofold higher in cytogenetically normal AML. See text for details.
CBF, Core binding factor; *ITD,* internal tandem duplication.

NPM1

The gene encoding nucleophosmin (*NPM1*) is, according to most but not all studies, the most frequently mutated gene in AML.[280,281] *NPM1* mutations (typically small insertions of 4 bp, sometimes up to 11 bp) in the coding region of the terminal exon (exon 12 in DNA, designated as exon 11 in RNA), occur in ~ 60% of cytogenetically normal AMLs, equivalent to ~30% of all AMLs. It appears that *NPM1* mutations are orchestrated by the ability of TdT to add N-nucleotides.[282] A normal karyotype is seen in ~82% of *NPM1*-mutated AMLs. The protein functions as a chaperone, actively shuttling between the nucleolus, nucleoplasm, and cytoplasm; however, it is predominantly found in the nucleolus. It is involved in promoting cell growth, in part through its mediation of ribosomal biogenesis and by its functional interactions with the tumor suppressors CDKN2A/p14^ARF, *TP53*, and NF-κB. Mutations alter tryptophan residues required for proper nucleolar localization and create a putative nuclear export signal at the C terminus of the protein. Consequently, the mutant nucleophosmin protein is predominantly localized to the cytoplasm and through dimerization causes the mislocalization of the wild-type protein as well. This leads to the mislocalization and destabilization of p14^ARF and to the inhibition of *TP53* activity. In addition to this interesting pathobiology, the mislocalization may be exploited diagnostically because cytoplasmic nucleophosmin can be detected immunohistochemically, ideally with a mutation-specific antibody.[283,284] Some novel (nonexon 12) mutations and gene fusions are missed with standard PCR assays, yet can still be detected immunohistochemically.[285]

NPM1 mutations increase disease-free and OS in patients with AML. This benefit, however, is affected by the *FLT3* status. *FLT3* ITDs are enriched in AMLs with *NPM1* mutations in that they are seen twice as often in this group compared with AMLs with wild-type *NPM1*. Indeed, ~40% of *NPM1*-mutated AMLs also harbor an *FLT3* ITD, and their presence abrogates the good prognostic connotations of *NPM1* mutations. The OS of patients with an AML that is *NPM1* mutation-positive and *FLT3* mutation-negative approaches that of patients with AMLs that harbor karyotypes correlated with a favorable prognosis, such as t(8;21), t(15;17), or inv(16), and for whom bone marrow transplantation may not have survival benefit. It has also been suggested that *NPM1* mutations are only good when accompanied by *IDH2* mutations. Combining the status of these two "dueling" mutations (of *NPM1* and *FLT3*) allows stratification into three prognostic groups. Accordingly, patients may be assigned into good (*FLT3*-ITD–/*NPM1*+), intermediate (*FLT3*-ITD–/*NPM1*– or *FLT3*-ITD+/*NPM1*+), and poor (*FLT3*-ITD +/*NPM1*–) categories. Although typically associated with a good prognosis, one study has suggested that high VAFs (>44%) of mutated *NPM1* predict an unfavorable outcome.[286] A variety of different but simple molecular assays to detect *NPM1* mutations (either DNA or RNA based) are routinely available in most clinical laboratories. NPM1-positive AMLs tend to lack CD34 expression but express CD33 rather brightly; they are also associated with cuplike nuclear morphology.

CEBPA

CEBPA (CCAAT enhancer binding protein alpha) encodes a key transcription factor that regulates myeloid cell differentiation and proliferation. Mutations of the gene are heterogeneous but are concentrated at the amino and carboxyl terminals of the gene. Mutations are seen in ~10% of all AMLs, typically with relatively well-preserved platelet counts, and are associated with a favorable prognosis. While it was previously noted that this favorable association only occurred when the mutations are biallelic (compound heterozygous, with an N-terminal mutation affecting 1 allele and a C-terminal mutation affecting the other),[287] it has subsequently been demonstrated that only

in-frame mutations affecting the bZIP domain (C-terminus) are required to predict a positive outcome and define this entity, without the need for biallelic mutations.[288-290] In the pediatric setting, co-occurring *CSF3R* mutations appear to nullify this favorable prognostic effect.[288] Germline mutations of *CEBPA* predispose to the development of AML. These mutations are associated with a 100% risk for development of AML with a median age at presentation of 24 years; although recurrences (that are clonally distinct) are common, the outcomes are good.[291]

TP53

The gene encoding this prototypic tumor suppressor is mutated in ~5% to 10% of de novo AMLs, but it is mutated much more frequently in the setting of complex cytogenetics (in particular when associated with a monosomal karyotype), prior cytotoxic chemotherapy, increasing age, and in erythroleukemia. AML with mutated *TP53* was recognized as a separate entity within a larger umbrella category of myeloid neoplasms with *TP53* mutations that include MDS and MDS/AML with such mutations.[2] It has been suggested that *TP53* mutations are not directly induced by cytotoxic chemotherapy.[292] Rather, they are likely to reflect rare age-related (or CHIP, see later) mutations that are resistant to chemotherapy and that expand preferentially after treatment. AML with mutated *TP53* is associated with an especially poor outcome. Immunohistochemistry for *TP53* may provide a reasonable surrogate screen for underlying mutations, both missense mutations that lead to overexpression, and truncating mutations that result in lack of expression.[293]

Myelodysplasia-Related Gene Mutations

In addition to the presence of cytogenetic abnormalities that allow for the recognition of a category of AMLs that are myelodysplasia-related, a panel of mutated genes had been identified to be strongly associated with evolution from an underlying MDS, with these two categories (AML with myelodysplasia-related cytogenetic abnormalities and AML with myelodysplasia-related gene mutations) replacing the previous entity of AML-MRC. The genes, mutations of any one of which will allow entry into this category, are *ASXL1*, *BCOR*, *EZH2*, *RUNX1*, *SF3B1*, *SRSF2*, *STAG2*, *U2AF1*, and *ZRSR2*.[279,294,295] Of note, this group now encompasses (and removes as a sole consideration) the previously designated provisional entity of AML with mutated *RUNX1*.

FLT3

FLT3 is a class III receptor tyrosine kinase and IG receptor superfamily member that is expressed by hematopoietic progenitor cells and downregulated during differentiation. Once physiologically activated through *FLT3* ligand binding, phosphorylation of regions in the juxtamembranous domain leads to growth induction and apoptosis inhibition through STAT5 and MAPK signaling. Two major types of genetic abnormalities of *FLT3* have been described: ITD of the juxtamembranous domain and a missense mutation resulting in the amino acid change at D835 that together occur in ~30% of cytogenetically normal AMLs and ~20% of all AMLs.[296] The ITD is more common, occurring in ~23%, with the point mutation seen in ~7% of cytogenetically normal AMLs. As in *NPM1* mutations, TdT appears to be mechanistically involved in *FLT3*-ITD mutations by priming replication slippage.[297]

Functionally, these lesions result in the constitutive activation of the TKDs through autophosphorylation, leading to a persistent "on" signal in the transformed leukemic cell; clinically, however, only the ITDs consistently appear to have prognostic relevance.

Importantly, from a clinical perspective, FLT3 dysregulation has been shown to be one of the single most pertinent prognosticators for OS in AML patients. Additionally important, from a molecular diagnostic perspective, these abnormalities are easily discerned by PCR and other mutational detection systems. A number of variables appear to affect the prognostic associations of FLT3 ITDs. Thus only when the mutant allele burden is greater than the wild-type allele, that is, >50% (typically a consequence of acquired uniparental disomy), does its prognostic pertinence appear to emerge; however, this cut-off is not universally agreed upon and even very small FLT3 ITD mutations (clone size of 0.2% to 2%) are important to detect because they may survive chemotherapy and expand over time.[298] Indeed, in the 2022 ELN recommendations allelic ratio (AR) is no longer considered in risk classification.[242] Also, insertion of the ITD into the beta1 sheet of the TKD 1 and, controversially, the length of the mutation are associated with a particularly adverse prognosis,[299,300] although the latter may be overcome with targeted therapy.[301-303] Further, the presence of >1 ITD is an adverse prognosticator and the class of ITD also predicts outcomes with regard to response to FLT3 inhibitors. Thus typical ITDs (in which the mutated sequence matches the wild-type sequence) do better than those that are atypical (where exogenous nucleotides are incorporated).[304] A described third class of FLT3 mutations reflects deletional mutations.[305] Although the current gold standard for detecting FLT3 mutations involves PCR with fragment analysis by CE, from which ARs are derived, other technologies are also used, including MPS, in which VAFs are measured, noting that these two metrics (AR and VAF) are not equivalent; in addition, these two approaches have advantages and disadvantages and hence might be best considered complementary rather than equivalent alternative assays.[306] Similar to the association with NPM1 mutations, blasts of AMLs with FLT3 mutations tend to show cuplike nuclear invaginations.[307]

FLT3 inhibitors have been used in the therapy of patients with (and sometimes without) such mutations. Interestingly but perhaps unsurprisingly, resistance develops because of the expansion of mutant clones, in particular those occurring in and around D835 and those with gatekeeper mutations affecting F691.[308,309] Resistance to FLT3 inhibition may also occur because of the emergence of RAS pathway mutations, as well as with the acquisition of BCR::ABL1.[310] Importantly, while FLT3 mutations are clearly central to the pathogenesis of (and targeted therapy for) AML, they do not define an AML entity because they are not deemed to be primary drivers of the disease, but it is nevertheless essential to test for them for both prognostic and therapeutic reasons.

IDH1/IDH2

IDH1 and IDH2 are NADP-dependent enzymes that convert isocitrate to alpha-ketoglutarate in the Krebs cycle (in the cytoplasm and mitochondria, respectively). The consequence of mutations is the creation of a neomorphic enzyme that generates 2-hydroxyglutarate instead, and this oncometabolite ultimately inhibits the function of TET2, accounting for the usual but not invariable mutual exclusivity

of mutations of their respective genes.[311] This may also be the case with WT1 and the other two mutations so that all three tend to be mutually exclusive.[312] In some studies, IDH2 mutations, particularly those affecting p.R172, associate with improved OS. Inhibitors to both mutant IDH1 and IDH2 are now available for clinical use. As with FLT3 mutations, while IDH mutations do not define AML entities, they are important to detect to direct targeted therapy. Also as with FLT3 inhibitors, resistance to these therapies may emerge.[313] Immunohistochemical detection of mutant proteins may provide a useful surrogate for the presence of mutations.[284]

Other Genetic Abnormalities in AML

Whereas a variety of other genetic abnormalities that have biological relevance have been described in AML and contribute to leukemogenesis, none of these is currently routinely evaluated in the clinical setting. These include increased expression of intact genes, copy number variations detected by array comparative genomic hybridization and single nucleotide polymorphism arrays, epigenetic perturbations, and microRNAs.

Myeloproliferative Neoplasms

Genetic studies have a central and ever-expanding role in the diagnosis and classification of the MPNs, not only in the four classical MPNs (CML, polycythemia vera [PV], primary myelofibrosis [PMF], and essential thrombocythemia [ET]) but also in the more recent entries into this umbrella category (chronic neutrophilic leukemia, chronic eosinophilic leukemia, and MPN, unclassifiable) as well as other separately classified chronic myeloid neoplasms (Fig. 5-10).[314]

Chronic Myeloid Leukemia

The identification of the Philadelphia chromosome (Ph) in 1960 heralded the era of cancer cytogenetics that has come full circle with the use and unprecedented success of rational, targeted therapy (initially imatinib, as well as other tyrosine kinase inhibitors) directed against the molecular consequence (chimeric BCR::ABL1 oncoprotein) of the pathognomonic t(9;22)(q34.1;q11.2). This oncoprotein dysregulates multiple pathways that lead to a variety of biological effects, such as increased proliferation, resistance to apoptosis, adhesion defects, and genomic instability, with a latter central to the inexorable disease progression that occurs in untreated patients.[315]

Molecular testing in CML is indicated in three scenarios: at diagnosis, to monitor responses to therapy, and to detect mutations that may induce resistance to therapy. Depending on the denominator, ~95% of patients with a substantial clinical and hematologic diagnostic consideration of CML, in particular based on the complete blood count and peripheral blood smear findings, will be cytogenetically positive for the presence of the defining t(9;22)(q34.1;q11.2); of the ~5% remaining, half (i.e., ~2.5% overall) are positive only at the submicroscopic (molecular genetic) level by either FISH or RT-PCR for the BCR::ABL1 fusion. Whereas the other 2.5% had historically been designated Ph-negative CML, these cases are now classified as atypical CML (aCML) or chronic myelomonocytic leukemia (CMML), both of which are myelodysplastic/MPNs. Accordingly, CML is essentially defined by the presence of a BCR::ABL1 fusion that is usually

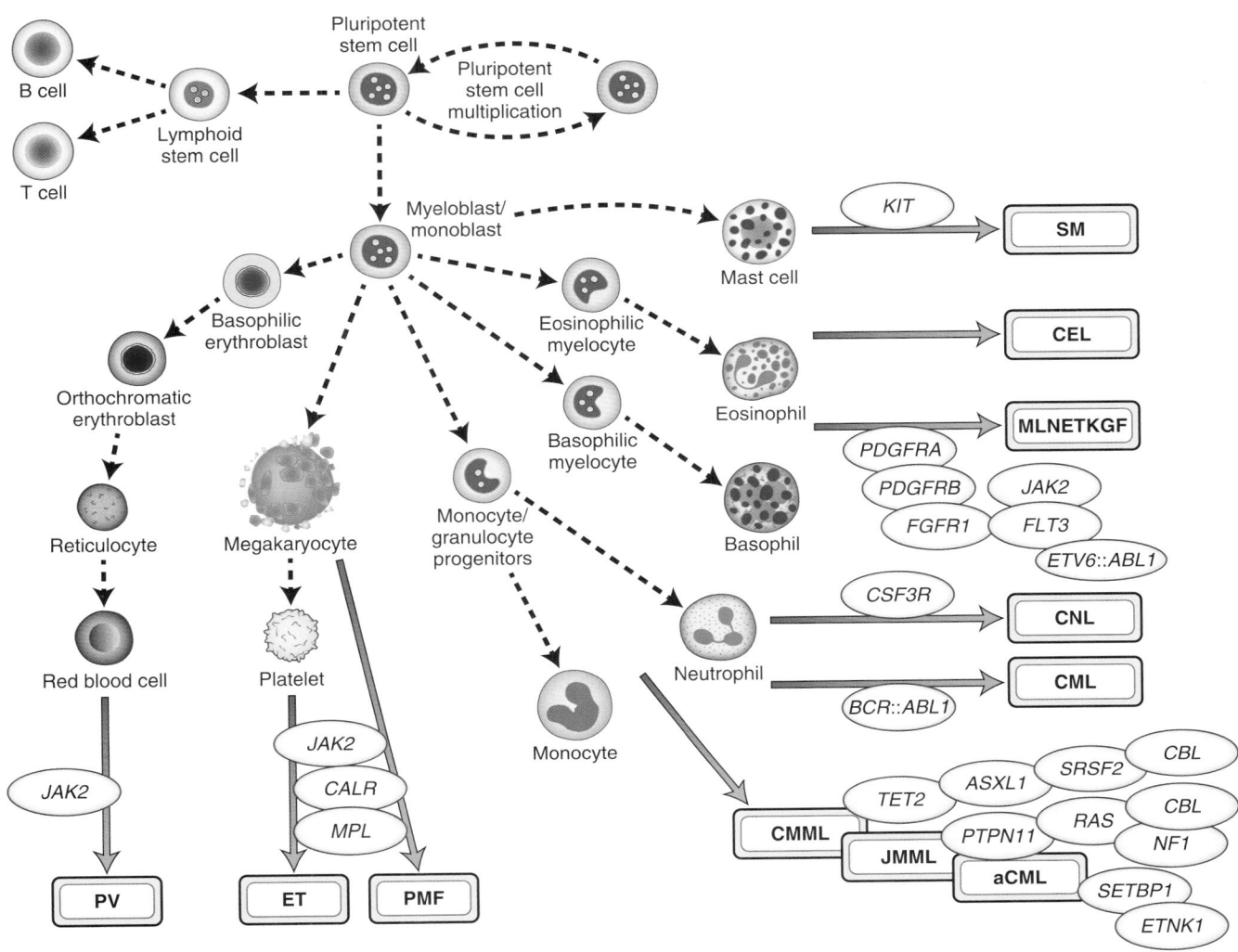

Figure 5-10. Molecular basis of the myeloproliferative neoplasms (MPNs) and related disorders. Different recurrent mutations and translocations, mostly occurring in pluripotent hematopoietic stem cells and hence in all neoplastic progeny, are associated, to variable degrees, with the development of myeloproliferative (and related) neoplasms that tend to be associated with the somewhat limited expansion of a specific hematopoietic lineage (*clockwise, from top right:* SM, systemic mastocytosis; CEL, chronic eosinophilic leukemia, the only category currently without a well-defined specific associated molecular abnormality; MLNETKGF, myeloid and lymphoid neoplasms with eosinophilia and tyrosine kinase gene fusions; CNL, chronic neutrophilic leukemia; CML, chronic myeloid leukemia; CMML, chronic myelomonocytic leukemia; JMML, juvenile myelomonocytic leukemia; aCML, atypical chronic myeloid leukemia; PMF, primary myelofibrosis; ET, essential thrombocythemia; PV, polycythemia vera). The detection of these molecular abnormalities is essential for the diagnosis of some of these neoplasms, whereas in others, they can be used as major diagnostic criteria.

but not always accompanied by the classical karyotypically determined translocation, in the appropriate clinical and hematologic context.

Even if the cytogenetic data are unequivocal, it is necessary to document the presence of the fusion by FISH and RT-PCR. This is important not only to indicate that the target of planned tyrosine kinase inhibitor therapy is indeed present but also to discern the specific molecular fingerprint (based on the location of the breakpoints on qualitative RT-PCR analysis) that may be important for the subsequent tracking of MRD. As a corollary, even if there is molecular genetic validation of the diagnosis, it is necessary to perform conventional cytogenetics, both at diagnosis and during the course of the disease, to evaluate for additional chromosomal abnormalities (ACAs) that have prognostic and diagnostic significance (disease metamorphosis to accelerated or blast phase, which is almost invariably heralded by cytogenetically discernible clonal evolution), or for

the emergence of Ph-negative clones, which have been reported in ~5% to 10% of patients treated with imatinib.[316,317] There are six ACAs that may be used as criteria for accelerated phase: an additional Ph chromosome, +8, iso(17q), +19, complex cytogenetics, and abnormalities of 3q26.2. Different ACAs are associated with different frequencies of transformation to blast phase.[318] The emergence of ACAs in Ph-negative clones is of uncertain significance because very few are associated with the development of another overt hematologic neoplasm; however, while –Y may be inconsequential, –7 or del(7q) may be associated with the development of AML or MDS.[319,320]

Broadly, the major indications for *BCR::ABL1* testing are in the specific differential diagnostic contexts of CML versus a leukemoid reaction (noting that morphologic clues ought to be most useful) and in CML versus other MPNs and some other chronic myeloid neoplasms. The translocation is not specific for CML; it is also seen in a number of other leukemias, particularly adult B-ALL/LBL, in which it is the most common cytogenetic abnormality. It can also be seen, albeit rarely, in AML. The breakpoints in the *ABL1* gene are usually consistent in both CML and ALL (typically 5′ of *ABL1* exon 2, but occasionally 5′ of exon 3), but they vary in the *BCR* gene. The breakpoints in the *BCR* gene in CML are usually homogeneous, mostly occurring after exon 13 or exon 14, in the M-bcr region of the gene. Thus a simple qualitative RT-PCR assay with a single upstream *BCR* exon 13 primer and a single downstream *ABL1* exon 2 (a2) primer suffices for the molecular detection of this event in virtually all cases of CML. Although there are abundant studies assessing the effect of the site of the M-bcr breakpoint with variable findings, there appears to be no definitive clinical or biological significance, with some of the differences reflecting technical factors[321]; however, because of alternative splicing, an intron 14 break may yield transcripts containing both e13 and e14 (equivalent to b2 and b3). Indeed, ALL-type transcripts (e1a2) may also be identified in the context of bona fide CML, unrelated to an e1 breakpoint; rather, this too is a manifestation of alternative splicing. However, rare cases (~1%–2%) of CML do harbor e1 *BCR* breakpoints. Such cases are more likely to be associated with a monocytosis, and they are important to recognize because they may not respond well to tyrosine kinase inhibitors and might have an adverse prognosis, and have the potential to be misdiagnosed as CMML.[322] Another noteworthy additional breakpoint, the μ(micro)-bcr, is that occurring after e19, associated with CML with neutrophilia, which must be distinguished from chronic neutrophilic leukemia. Breakpoints other than those occurring in the regions noted here can lead to alternative product sizes or false-negative molecular results; while these are rare, it is important to be aware of them (that ought to be positive by FISH or karyotyping), since they are not trackable by standard quantitative assays.

Whereas the *BCR::ABL1* oncogene has historically been interpreted to be the sole driver of seemingly genetically homogeneous CML, NGS has shown that numerous mutations accompany this in chronic phase. These include those affecting *ASXL1* (which appears to be the most frequently mutated gene in CML), *TET2, RUNX1, DNMT2A, EZH2,* and *TP53*, with *TET2* and *DNMT3A* sometimes detected in *BCR::ABL1*-negative ancestral clones, possibly reflecting clonal hematopoieis.[323] Some of these and other mutations are seen in advanced phase, with *RUNX1* (33%) often mutated in myeloid and *IKZF1* (70%) and *CDKN2A* (50%) deleted in lymphoid blast transformation.

In addition to the value of RT-PCR testing at the time of diagnosis of CML (when a *qualitative* assay is essential to determine the site of the *BCR* breakpoint), such testing is mandated to monitor MRD after therapy in patients treated with tyrosine kinase inhibitors and after stem cell transplantation (SCT). For this monitoring, *quantitative* assays are essential.[324-326] Because there is high concordance between peripheral blood and bone marrow testing, the less invasive former procedure suffices for monitoring MRD. Most patients are RT-PCR-positive in the first 6 months after SCT, and this is not of consequence because graft-versus-leukemia can be slow to develop; by contrast, RT-PCR positivity beyond 6 months after SCT is associated with a high risk of relapse.[327] However, some patients may show persistent low levels of disease up to 10 years after transplantation without relapse. With regard

to responses to tyrosine kinase inhibitors, the primary goal for some time has been the attainment of a major molecular response (MMR), defined as a greater than 3-log reduction (equivalent to ≤0.1%) in the amount of transcript compared with a standardized control by 12 or 18 months, although it has also been asserted that this has no added value over and above achieving a complete cytogenetic remission by 12 months in predicting prolonged survival. Earlier goals that have clinical relevance include a greater than 1-log reduction (≤10%) at 3 months, also referred to as early molecular remission (EMR) and a greater than 2-log (≤1%) reduction by 6 months. Some studies suggest that reducing *BCR::ABL1* levels by more than 50% by as early as day 10 is a robust predictor of sustained treatment free remission.[328] Although occasionally still used in the literature, the term *complete molecular remission* should be avoided, with the preferred term being *deep molecular remission (DMR)*, qualified by the sensitivity of the assay; if a greater than 4-log reduction (≤0.01%) is attained this is designated as DMR[4] and if a greater than 4.5-log reduction (≤0.0032%) is attained this is designated as DMR[4.5]. Attainment of sustained DMR is a criterion for consideration of cessation of TKI therapy. In addition to monitoring response to therapy, quantitative monitoring (be it by RT-PCR or ddPCR, with the latter showing greater analytic sensitivity and predictive value[329]) can also be used to predict relapse; this is usually defined as a 10-fold (1 log) or greater increase in *BCR::ABL1* levels determined by a minimum of two consecutive analyses, with this being more pertinent when it is associated with loss of MMR. FISH does not play a well-established role in monitoring MRD, but may be of some value in patients with variant breakpoints that may not be amenable to quantitative RT-PCR.

A critical issue with regard to quantitative *BCR::ABL1* testing had been tremendous variability in how the assay is performed and limited availability of an international standard to allow expression of levels on the International Scale (IS). This has been overcome by the generation and availability of secondary standards and commercial kits or systems that have been calibrated to WHO-generated reference material.[330] Alternatively, clinical laboratories could use the secondary reference materials to align their laboratory-developed *BCR::ABL1* test to the IS, through a conversion factor, which is analogous to the international normalized ratio used in coagulation testing.[331] Other emerging technologies in addition to ddPCR include DNA (rather than RNA/cDNA) patient-specific PCR that might be able to detect 7-log reductions.[332]

A large number (>50) of mutations in the *ABL1* component of the fusion gene have been described, which may lead to resistance to imatinib and other tyrosine kinase inhibitors.[333] However, only a handful (approximately six) of these mutations are common and together account for approximately two-thirds of cases. Nevertheless, different mutations result in variable degrees of resistance to specific TKIs. Many laboratories are now able to test for these mutations, the presence of which may then mandate a change in therapy. This change may not necessarily be the need to switch to an alternative tyrosine kinase inhibitor, such as second-generation agents like dasatinib or nilotinib; some mutations will respond to increasing the dose of imatinib, whereas others might be best dealt with by SCT or the use of a third-generation drug like ponatinib or novel agents such as asciminib for the T315I mutation. Compound mutations are emerging as a therapeutic challenge, with some of these conferring ponatinib resistance.[334] There are a number of defined triggers for mutation testing, including the loss of hematologic, cytogenetic, or molecular responses. Despite its relative insensitivity (~10%–20%), Sanger sequencing had been the preferred technology for mutational analysis; however, this is now being superseded by NGS to afford the early detection of minor clones that are poised to expand.[335] Testing is indicated in response to the noted triggers and seems not yet to be of value at initial diagnosis in patients in the chronic phase, although it is in the accelerated and blast phase.

Classic Myeloproliferative Neoplasms Other Than Chronic Myeloid Leukemia

Three of the other classical MPNs, namely PV, ET, and PMF, are variably associated with three hallmark driver mutations: JAK2, CALR, and MPL.[314,336,337]

JAK2 encodes an intracellular kinase that mediates signal transduction from cytokine receptors, including the erythropoietin receptor in red cell precursors and the thrombopoietin receptor in megakaryocyte precursors. JAK2 V617F mutations occur in the vast majority (over 90%) of patients with PV and ~60% of patients with ET and PMF. JAK2 V617F mutations lead to ligand-independent proliferation of cells that harbor them and are central to the genesis of these MPNs. Putative explanations as to how the same mutation leads to three distinctive neoplasms include the amount of the mutant allele with acquired uniparental disomy more commonly observed in PV than in ET and PMF, the cellular target of the initiating mutation, the presence of additional mutations, and the order in which additional mutations (in particular those affecting TET2 or DNMT3A) develop.[338]

JAK2 V617F mutations occur in exon 14 of the gene; different mutations, occurring in exon 12, are also seen in PV but not in ET and PMF. Thus almost 100% of patients with PV harbor a JAK2 mutation, either in exon 14 or exon 12 (~4%). Although qualitative assays suffice, there might be a role for quantitative testing for JAK2 mutations because measurement of VAF at diagnosis may become relevant and, more important, to gauge response to therapy; while JAK2 inhibitors typically fail to elicit a substantial reduction in mutational levels, testing for molecular responses and MRD is of value in the SCT setting and with the use of interferon.

Mutations in CALR (encoding calreticulin, a calcium-binding protein that interacts with the endoplasmic reticulum) occur in ~20% to 25% of cases of PMF and ET but not in PV. There are two major mutations, type 1 (a 52-bp deletion, ~65% of cases) and type 2 (a 5-bp insertion, ~32% of cases), that might have different clinicopathologic associations, with PMF more likely with type 1 and ET more likely with type 2 mutations.[339] A minor subset of cases of ET (1%–4%) and PMF (5%–8%) harbor mutations in the MPL gene, which encodes the thrombopoietin receptor.

Patients with CALR mutations appear to have a less-aggressive form of PMF with a median survival of approximately 18 years compared with those with mutations of JAK2 or MPL; by contrast, those PMFs that are triple-negative, namely, lacking mutations in all three of these genes (now accounting for only ~5% to 10% of patients), tend to have a more aggressive clinical course with a median survival

of only approximately 3 years.[340] In PMF, type 1 (or type 1-like) CALR mutations are associated with better outcomes than those with type 2 (or type 2-like) CALR mutations.[341]

The mutations in these three genes tend to be focused in particular regions of the genes. Thus JAK2 mutations are primarily located in exons 12 and 14, CALR mutations in exon 9, and MPL mutations in exon 10. Accordingly, most mutational assays target these specific regions. However, such an approach may lead to occasional activating (so-called "noncanonical") mutations being missed.

A variety of other mutations have been described in MPNs, with virtually all harboring one or more of these mutations in addition to one of the three hallmark mutations. Many of these are not restricted to MPNs in that they are also seen to variable degrees in other myeloid neoplasms, such as AML and MDS. Certain additional mutations in PMF are considered "high molecular risk" and predict poor outcomes; they include those affecting ASXL1, EZH2, SRSF2, TF53, IDH1, and IDH2.[342] Other mutations that negatively affect prognosis include those of RAS, TET2, and U2AF1 (in particular Q157 mutations).[343] Either single gene assays or multitarget NGS panels may be used to detect these mutations and facilitate the diagnosis of these MPNs. It is important for these assays to be highly sensitive, with the ability to detect VAFs as low as 1%. While single gene assays can be used, panels may be of added value because they can establish clonality in triple-negative MPNs and identify additional mutations that are prognostically pertinent. It may also be of value to perform BCR::ABL1 testing to exclude CML. It has provocatively been suggested that these non-CML MPNs could be classified (with an associated individualized prognosis) in the absence of morphology and bone marrow studies, with eight genomic subgroups: (1) TP53 disruption or aneuploidy; (2) chromatin or spliceosome mutation; (3) CALR mutation; (4) MPL mutation; (5) homozygous JAK2 or NFE2 mutation; (6) heterozygous JAK2 mutation; (7) other driver mutation such as TET2 or DNMT3A; and (8) no known driver mutation.[344]

Despite the major advances derived from these molecular abnormalities, there is still a role for metaphase analysis. Thus certain karyotypic abnormalities in PMF are reported to have prognostic implications. For example, +9, −13q, and −20q tend to portend a favorable outcome, whereas abnormalities of chromosomes 5, 7, inv(3), 11q23, and 17 (among others) predict an adverse prognosis.

Chronic Neutrophilic Leukemia

This MPN that may display toxically granulated neutrophils is associated with CSF3R mutations in the majority of cases.[345] The gene encodes the granulocyte colony-stimulating factor receptor. As is becoming thematic, a number of other mutations are present, including SETBP1, SRSF2, and ASXL1, some of which might be prognostically detrimental. There are two major classes of acquired CSF3R mutations; most in chronic neutrophilic leukemia are membrane proximal (typically T618I), whereas those that are intracytoplasmic are rare. These have therapeutic (and prognostic, with T618I being adverse) relevance because the former are sensitive to JAK2 inhibitors (such as ruxolitinib), whereas the C-terminal truncating mutations (that are activating because of the loss of negatively regulating elements) respond to dasatinib (that is also effective in CML).[346] CSF3R mutations are not present in all cases (80%–90% have these mutations), so their absence does not exclude the diagnosis; nevertheless, this should prompt careful review of the diagnosis. C-terminal truncating mutations also develop in patients with severe congenital neutropenia that typically occurs as a consequence of germline *ELANE* mutations. When acquired *CSF3R* mutations arise in the setting of severe congenital neutropenia, they are associated with the development of acute leukemia.

Chronic Eosinophilic Leukemia, Not Otherwise Specified

This is an MPN with eosinophilia that does not meet criteria for other MPNs and in particular must be distinguished from myeloid and lymphoid neoplasms associated with eosinophilia and tyrosine kinase gene fusions. Though they do not have any of these specific disease-defining genetic abnormalities, they do have another clonal genetic aberration detected by targeted MPS analysis[347] and are often accompanied by morphologic abnormalities.[348] By contrast, idiopathic hypereosinophilic syndrome is likely a constellation of non-neoplastic and nonfamilial disorders with eosinophilia and end organ damage but without an identified genetic lesion. There is also a lymphoid variant of hypereosinophilic syndrome associated with an indolent expansion of sometimes monoclonal CD3-negative CD4-positive T cells.[349]

Myeloid and Lymphoid Neoplasms Associated With Eosinophilia and Tyrosine Kinase Gene Fusions

This group of neoplasms was previously referred to as myeloid and lymphoid neoplasms associated with eosinophilia and gene rearrangements. The initially recognized group comprised three members with translocations involving one of *PDGFRA*, *PDGFRB*, or *FGFR1*.[350] The first two are especially important to recognize as they are sensitive, sometimes exquisitely so, to imatinib. All three can be detected with appropriate FISH probes, which are particularly valuable in detecting *PDGFRA* rearrangements that are often cytogenetically cryptic. Subsequent additions to this category include those with t(8;9) that fuses *JAK2* with *PCM1* (other *JAK2*-rearranged neoplasms, including those involving *ETV6* or *BCR*, show less distinctive features but are considered to be genetic variants[351]), t(9;12) that fuses *ETV6* with *ABL1,* and those with *FLT3* translocations,[352] the most common being t(12;13), which involves *ETV6*.

Mast Cell Neoplasms

These include a spectrum of numerous different disease subtypes, with variable frequencies of sometimes different *KIT* mutations.[353] Whereas the hallmark D816V mutation affecting the second intracellular TKD (exon 17) is particularly common (~90% of adult cases) in the various forms of systemic mastocytosis (SM), this mutation is seen in only ~30% of cases with pediatric/primary cutaneous mastocytosis that, by contrast, are more likely to have *KIT* mutations affecting the extracellular domain, encoded by exons 8 and 9. D816V mutations are resistant to imatinib but respond to other kinase inhibitors, such as midostaurin. Rare SM patients with a different *KIT* mutation (in the juxtamembranous or extracellular domain) or with no *KIT* mutation may respond to imatinib. Highly sensitive allele-specific oligonucleotide or ddPCR assays can detect the hallmark mutation in the peripheral blood of most patients with SM, and quantitative assays measuring allelic burden can be used to monitor the natural course of the

disease or during therapy. Quantification is also prognostic at the time of diagnosis as the allelic burden is a surrogate for the degree of multilineage involvement, which is a key criterion for disease progression. Standard NGS panels are considered to have insufficient sensitivity to detect mutations in many patients with SM. Additional mutations seen in SM include those affecting *SRSF2, ASXL1, RUNX1, NRAS, DNMT3A,* and *EZH2* that are associated with more aggressive disease.

Myelodysplastic Syndromes/ Myeloproliferative Neoplasms

These reflect a group of neoplasms that display features of both MDS (see later) and MPN, and include CMML, aCML, and MDS/MPN with thrombocytosis and *SF3B1* mutation. Juvenile myelomonocytic leukemia (JMML) is included in this category by the WHO[354] but not the ICC.[2] CMML is associated with a variety of mutations; the most common are those affecting *SRSF2, CBL, TET2, RUNX1, SETBP1,* and *ASXL1*, with the big three of *TET2, ASXL1,* and *SRSF2* each being mutated in around 50% of cases.[355] Mutations of *ASXL1* predict a poor prognosis. *NPM1* mutations are rarely seen in CMML (3%–5%) and they predict an aggressive clinical course; their presence in this setting of known CMML cannot be used to define de novo AML with an *NPM1* mutation. The myeloproliferative subtype of CMML is often associated with other mutations, such as those affecting the RAS pathway (*NRAS, KRAS,* and *CBL*) and *JAK2* or *SETBP1*. aCML is associated with mutations in *SETBP1*, albeit in only a minority of cases (~25%).[356] *ETNK1* that encodes an ethanolamine kinase is mutated in ~10% of aCMLs and rarely in CMML (3%). JMML is characterized by mutations in the RAS signaling pathway, affecting *PTPN11, NF1, NRAS,* and *KRAS*. The presence of *SETBP1, RUNX1,* and *EZH2* mutations in cases of MDS/MPN may be predictive of failure to respond to hypomethylating agents.[357] MDS/MPN with isolated isochromosome 17q may represent a distinct clinico-biological subset.[358]

Histiocytic and Dendritic Cell Neoplasms

Syndromic diseases such as Langerhans cell histiocytosis (LCH), Erdheim-Chester disease, Rosai-Dorfman-Destombes disease, and juvenile xanthogranuloma were once thought to be reactive inflammatory disorders. However, they are now known to represent neoplasms with, for example, ~50% of cases of LCH and Erdheim-Chester disease harboring *BRAF* V600E mutations, or other mutations in the RAS-MAPK pathway, including those affecting *MAP2K1*.[359] *MAP2K1* encodes MEK1 that is just downstream of RAF in this signaling pathway. Less commonly encountered are mutations in the PI3K pathway. Rosai-Dorfman-Destombes disease is also enriched in similar mutations.[360] In addition to mutations, fusions affecting *BRAF, ALK,* and *NTRK1* may also be seen in LCH.[361] ALK-positive histiocytosis, with *ALK* fusions, in particular *KIF5B::ALK* fusions, is a distinct entity that is frequently characterized by neurologic involvement.[362]

Myelodysplastic Syndromes

The MDSs are clonal hematopoietic stem cell disorders that are mechanistically distinct from most other hematologic malignant neoplasms, with ineffective hematopoiesis accounting for the apparently paradoxical coexistence of peripheral cytopenias despite a typically hypercellular bone marrow.[363] Akin to AML, MDS can arise de novo (primary) or as a result of inciting toxic agents, including some chemotherapeutic drugs, as well as chemical or radiation exposure (secondary). There are characteristic dysplastic morphologic features, present in variable degrees, in both the bone marrow and peripheral blood, associated with a variably expanded blast population.

Recurrent cytogenetic abnormalities are associated with MDS and are an integral component of the diagnosis.[364] Although present in the majority of cases of secondary MDS (>80% of cases), these cytogenetic abnormalities are seen in only ~50% of cases of primary MDS, thereby limiting their diagnostic utility. In contrast to many of the cytogenetic alterations described in other hematologic malignant neoplasms that are typically balanced translocations without a net gain or loss of genetic material, unbalanced numeric chromosomal abnormalities predominate in MDS, hinting at alternative genetic mechanisms. More commonly identified aberrations include –5/del(5q), –7/del(7q), +8, del(20q), and complex karyotypes. However, neither +8 nor del(20q) can be used to facilitate a diagnosis of MDS. Independent of complex karyotypes, a monosomal karyotype also predicts inferior outcomes as in AML. These cytogenetic features are an integral facet of the International Prognostic Scoring System and have assumed an even greater role in the Revised International Prognostic Scoring System (IPSS-R), in which the number of different cytogenetic aberrations has tripled (Table 5-12).

It is generally (but not universally) thought that FISH analysis provides no significant added value over and above a good-quality conventional cytogenetic analysis.[365,366] FISH is of utility, however, only in the context of karyotypic failure. FISH on CD34-enriched peripheral blood cells seems to have added value but is labor-intensive.[367]

Isolated del(5q), which defines a specific subtype of MDS (and currently the only one that is defined by its cytogenetic abnormality), is typically associated with a good prognosis and response to lenalidomide. However, TP53 mutations are not uncommon in this subtype (seen in ~20% of cases) and predict a poor prognosis, and hence it may be important to test for such mutations even in this form of MDS.[368] Specific genetic targets in MDS with isolated del(5q) have been sought, and they include RPS14,[369] SPARC, CSNK1A1,[370] CTNNA1, and LMNB1, with the latter loss accounting for the characteristic nuclear hypolobation of neutrophils.[371] Of note, not all MDS cases with 5q-negative have MDS with del(5q). In general, MDS with del(5q) targets more distal regions (5q33), where both RPS14 and SPARC reside. In addition, in this entity there can be no more than one additional cytogenetic abnormality [except –7/del(7q)] or multihit TP53 mutations.[2]

With the advent of high-throughput MPS technologies, it is now possible to evaluate MDS specimens for a number of key mutations that may have relevance diagnostically, prognostically, and therapeutically.[372-374] Point mutations have been identified in more than 90% of patients with MDS. Some of the more frequently mutated genes are detailed in Table 5-13 and illustrated in Figure 5-11. The IPSS-R has been updated to incorporate mutational analysis, is designated the IPSS-M, with M for molecular,[375] and includes an analysis of up to 31 genes (16 of which are considered main effect genes), allowing for six risk categories with an open access online calculator that accounts for missing values (https://mds-risk-model.com). The six most frequently mutated genes (seen in >10% of patients) in MDS are TET2, ASXL1, SF3B1, DNMT3A, SRSF2, and RUNX1. Whereas other studies have identified mutations in ASXL1, TP53, EZH2, ETV6, and RUNX1 as predictors of poor OS, according to the IPPSS-M, TP53 (multihit), FLT3, and KMT2A (partial tandem duplication) are the top genetic predictors of adverse outcomes. The frequency of mutations of IDH1, IDH2, FLT3, and those in the RAS pathway increases at the time of transformation to AML, with mutations affecting signaling pathways leading to convergent clonal evolution, a hallmark of progression.[376] Unlike in AML, where a single TP53 mutation is prognostically adverse, in MDS TP53 defects need to be multihit to be prognostic and indeed definitional of TP53 mutated MDS. Multihit TP53 requires the presence of two or more distinct TP53 mutations (VAF ≥10%), or a single TP53 mutation associated with either: (1) a cytogenetic deletion involving the TP53 locus at 17p13.1; (2) a VAF of >50%; or (3) copy-neutral loss of heterozygosity (LOH) at the 17p TP53 locus.[377,378] In the absence of LOH information, the presence of a single TP53 mutation in the context of any complex karyotype is considered equivalent to a multihit TP53.

A third category of MDS that is now recognized by virtue of its genetic features [in addition to those with del(5q) and multihit TP53 mutations] is that associated with SF3B1 mutations, which defines a more homogeneous group than that originally defined by the presence of ring sideroblasts.[379] Mutations of this spliceosome gene leads to the mis-splicing of several genes, with effects on MAP3K7 leading to anemia[380] and those on ABCB7 and TMEM14C associated with the characteristic ring sideroblasts.[381] While this form of MDS and SF3B1 mutations are characteristically associated with a good prognosis, other factors can overcome this association and may indeed lead to poor outcomes; these include scenarios

Table 5-12 Cytogenetic Abnormalities That Affect Prognosis in Myelodysplastic Syndromes (Revised International Prognostic Scoring System)

Prognostic Group	Cytogenetic Abnormality	Median Survival (Years)	AML Evolution (25%, Years)	Hazard Ratio (Overall Survival)
Very good (~4%)	–Y, del(11q)	5.4	NR	0.7
Good (~69%)	Normal, del(5q), del(12p), del(20q), double abnormalities including del(5q)	4.8	9.4	1
Intermediate (~16%)	del(7q), +8, +19, i(17q), any other single or double independent abnormalities	2.7	2.5	1.5
Poor (~4%)	–7, inv(3), double including –7/del(7q), three abnormalities	1.5	1.7	2.3
Very poor (~7%)	>Three abnormalities	0.7	0.7	3.8

AML, Acute myeloid leukemia; *NR*, not reached.

Table 5-13 Examples of Recurrent Mutations in Myelodysplastic Syndromes

Gene Target	Approximate Frequency in MDSs	Prognostic Significance	Putative Consequence/Altered Biological Mechanism	Associations
SF3B1	~20%–25%	Good	RNA splicing	Ring sideroblasts (~80%)
TET2	~20%–25%	Possibly good	Epigenetic (DNA methylation)	Predicts response to hypomethylating agents, more frequent in CMML (~50%)
RUNX1	~15%	Poor	↓ Transcription	—
ASXL1	~15%	Poor	Chromatin modification	More frequent in CMML (~50%)
SRSF2	~10%	Poor	RNA splicing	More frequent in CMML (~50%)
DNMT3A	~10%	Poor	Epigenetic (DNA methylation)	Predicts response to hypomethylating agents
TP53	~5%–10%	Poor	Loss of DNA damage repair, apoptosis	More frequent in secondary MDS (~20%)
NRAS	~5%–10%	None	↑ Signal transduction	—
U2AF35	~5%–10%	None	RNA splicing	—
EZH2	~5%	Poor	↓ Histone methylation	—
SETBP1	~5%	Poor	Unclear	More frequent in aCML (~25%)

aCML, Atypical chronic myeloid leukemia; *CMML,* chronic myelomonocytic leukemia; *MDS,* myelodysplastic syndromes.

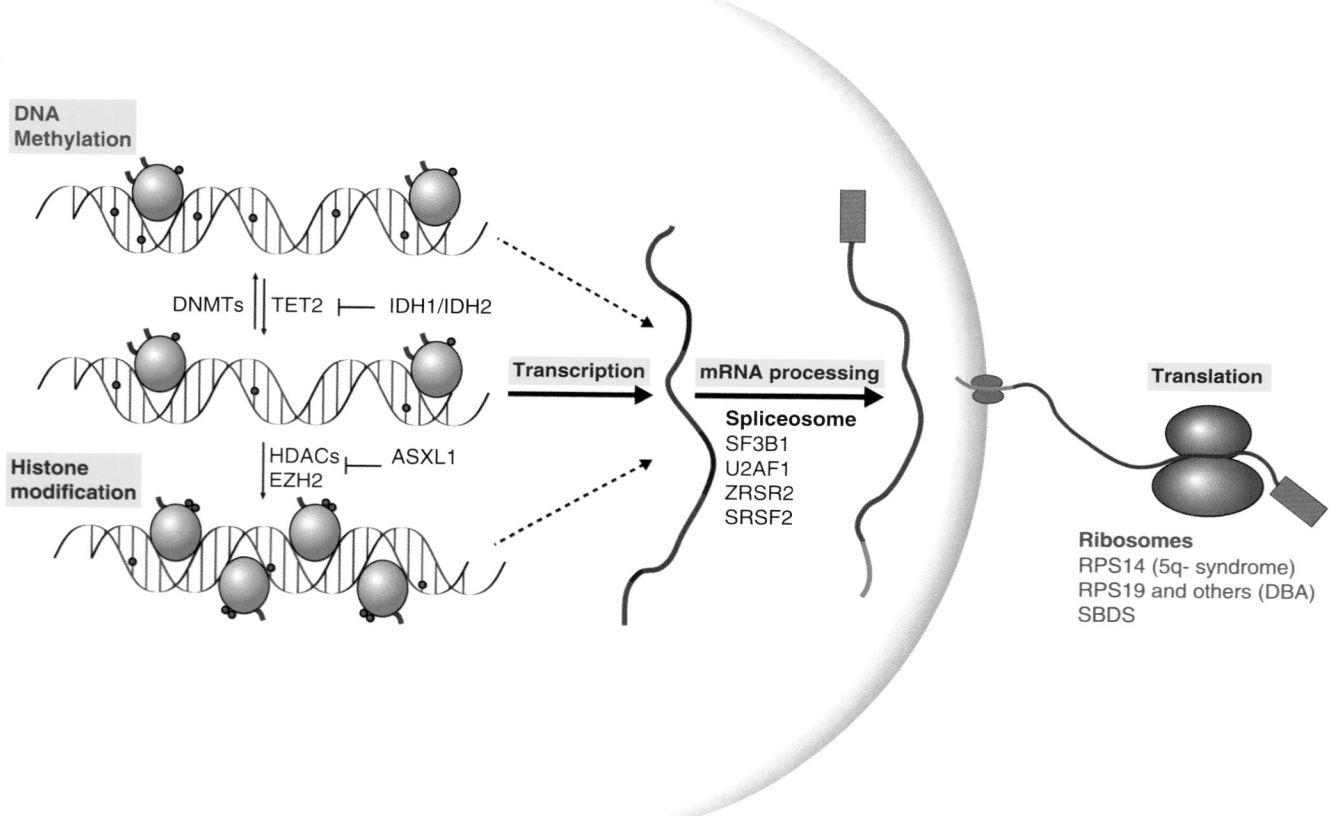

Figure 5-11. Molecular basis of the myelodysplastic syndromes (MDSs). Many of the mutations affect the fundamental pathway of transcription, RNA splicing, and ribosomal biogenesis. DNA in a steady state of transcriptional regulation *(middle)* is subject to methylation *(top)* and histone modification *(bottom)*. DNA methyltransferases (DNMTs) methylate DNA, reducing transcription; mutation of *DNMT3A* (one of the genes encoding a DNMT) affects this process. *TET2* mediates a step in the opposite process, removing DNA methylations; mutations of the *TET2* gene lead to a loss of this demethylation function. *IDH1/2* mutations result in altered enzymatic function and production of 2-hydroxyglutarate, which inhibits *TET2*. Histones *(green balls)* reduce transcription through increased binding. Histone deacetylases (HDACs) and *EZH2* modify histone acetylation *(red lines)* and methylation *(magenta circles)*, resulting in increased histone avidity for DNA and reduced transcription. Mutations of *EZH2* and *ASXL1* lead to dysregulation of histone modification. The spliceosome processes mRNA, removing introns *(blue lines)*; genes encoding proteins that constitute the splicing machinery (*SF3B1, U2AF1, ZRSR2,* and *SRSF2*) are mutated in MDS and may result in aberrant splicing. mRNA processing adds the 5′ methyl guanine cap *(tan box)* and the polyalanine tail *(green line)*. Ribosomal proteins, including RPS14 [MDS with del(5q)], RPS19 (Diamond-Blackfan anemia), and SBDS, play roles in ribosomes *(blue ovals)*, translating mRNA into protein; these ribosomal genes are targeted in MDS with del(5q) and in hereditary bone marrow failure syndromes (e.g., Diamond-Blackfan anemia and Shwachman-Diamond syndrome [Shwachman–Bodian–Diamond syndrome]). *(Modified with permission Nybakken GE, Bagg A. The genetic basis and expanding role of molecular analysis in the diagnosis, prognosis, and therapeutic design for myelodysplastic syndromes.* J Mol Diagn JMD. *2014;16[2]:145-158. https://doi.org/10.1016/j.jmoldx.2013.11.005.)*

in which the mutation is seen in the context of excess blasts, commutated with *ASXL1, RUNX1,* or *EZH2,* or when the *SF3B1* mutation affects K666 (rare, seen in 1%–2% of cases) rather than the canonical K600 mutation (seen in 97% of cases).[382]

Unsurprisingly, sequencing in morphologically nondiagnostic marrows can identify patients who are at heightened risk for development of MDS; in contrast to the CHIP mutations seen in aging individuals (see "Potential Pitfalls of Molecular Testing" section), these have a higher allelic frequency (~40% versus ~10%) and likelihood of more than one mutation (~65% versus ~10%). Mutational testing on peripheral blood appears to be as informative as that on bone marrow, perhaps precluding the need to perform this invasive procedure for these analyses.[383] *ATRX* mutations in MDS lead to the development of acquired alpha-thalassemia and should be considered when an MDS is associated with microcytosis (in contrast to the usual macrocytosis).

Hematologic Neoplasms With Germline Predisposition

Once considered to be quite rare and restricted to younger individuals, particularly pediatric patients with AML or MDS, such conditions are increasingly recognized in all age groups and to extend beyond myeloid neoplasms, in that it is posited that ~8% of adults with cancer have a pathogenic germline variant.[384] Although not designed to specifically detect *germline* mutations, the widespread adoption of panels used to detect *somatic* mutations has led to an increased awareness and recognition of these entities. Their identification has numerous ramifications, and is crucial for not only correct diagnosis and initial management of the afflicted patient, including the selection of therapeutic conditioning, should SCT be considered, but also for screening of related donors for SCT, and genetic counseling for both the patient and affected family members.[385] While there may be clues (family history, syndromic stigmata, and findings from somatic panels, such as VAFs of mutated genes >30%, "biallelic" mutations, two mutations in the same gene, and persistence of the mutation at high VAF in remission, among others), many of these disorders may lack some of these features, and hence it has been suggested that germline predisposition risk should be considered for all patients diagnosed with a hematologic neoplasm regardless of age, since some germline predisposition alleles, like those in *DDX41,* can drive hematopoietic malignancies in older age.[386] Indeed, reliance upon the interpretation of VAFs from somatic panels is fraught, because a variety of potentially confounding phenomena including somatic genetic rescue in which correction of the germline mutation may occur.[387] Of course testing for these mutations should be performed on uninvolved specimens uncontaminated by blood, ideally from cultured skin fibroblasts or hair bulbs, since somatic testing panels cannot be relied upon to exclude their consideration.

The ICC category of hematologic neoplasms with germline predisposition includes four major subgroupings,[2] namely those: (1) without a constitutional disorder (e.g., *CEBPA, DDX41*); (2) with a constitutional platelet disorder (e.g., *RUNX1, ANKRD26, ETV6*); (3) with a constitutional disorder affecting multiple organ systems (e.g., *GATA2, SAMD9, SAMD9L*), classical bone marrow failure syndromes (e.g., Fanconi anemia, Shwachman-Diamond syndrome, dyskeratosis congenita), neurofibromatosis, Noonan and Noonan-like syndrome, and Down syndrome; and (4) associated with, in particular, acute lymphoblastic leukemia (e.g., *IKZF, PAX5*). The recognition of these disorders is an evolving field without clearly established guidelines, but it is anticipated that future studies will lead to the development of a comprehensive list of all predisposition genes.[388,389]

POTENTIAL PITFALLS OF MOLECULAR TESTING

Having detailed the virtues and advantages of molecular analysis in hematologic neoplasms, it is essential to be cognizant of a number of limitations of such testing.

Antigen Receptor Gene Rearrangements

False-positive results may occur for antigen receptor gene rearrangement studies in small samples or samples with very few lymphocytes (pseudoclonality).[390] Routine duplicate testing of these specimen types can identify these spurious positive, and nonreproducible, results. Monoclonal antigen receptor gene rearrangements may also be seen in a variety of reactive and inflammatory conditions that include *H. pylori*–induced gastritis, hepatitis C and other viral infections, Sjögren syndrome, and rheumatoid arthritis. These are typically a reflection of bona fide oligoclones that, unlike pseudoclonality, may remain constant with duplicate testing. Many of these scenarios, of course, are associated to a variable degree with the subsequent development of bona fide (typically B-cell) lymphomas. Other examples in which apparent clonal antigen receptor gene rearrangements are identified, in the absence of neoplasia, include canonical TR gamma chain rearrangements involving the Vγ9 segment that is associated with aging, immune reconstitution after bone marrow transplantation, and immune response to tumors. An additional caveat is that antigen receptor gene rearrangements may not be specific for definition of lineage of neoplastic populations because in immature lymphoid malignant neoplasms, cross-lineage rearrangements may occur with those of IGH occurring in T-lymphoblastic leukemia and those of TR occurring in B-lymphoblastic leukemia.[391]

False-negative molecular genetic studies of antigen receptor gene rearrangements can be caused by technical or biological factors. Technical factors include oversimplified approaches, for example, the use of single V region consensus primers and the use of CDR3-only upstream primers to detect IGH gene rearrangements that ought not to be in contemporary clinical assays. Whereas PCR is highly sensitive, the consensus primers used amplify rearranged IG genes from normal B cells and TR genes from normal T cells in the sample as well as from the clonal population, and a small clonal population may not be identifiable because of the polyclonal background. Thus the sensitivity of the assay is highly dependent on the proportion of background normal lymphocytes present in the sample. The biological phenomena that may elicit false-negative IGH PCR results are somewhat different, depending on the specific neoplasms. In the context of precursor B cells, a variety of factors may confound the ability to detect IGH gene rearrangements. These include the presence of partial D-J (rather than complete V-D-J) rearrangements, which would be missed with upstream V primers; oligoclonal rearrangements, which are seen in up to one-third of precursor B-cell ALLs; and ongoing rearrangements at the time of relapse. With regard to more mature B-cell neoplasms, passage through the germinal center, with the induction of SHM, is associated with a greater degree of IGH PCR false negativity, a problem particularly prevalent in FLs. Many of the shortcomings of antigen receptor PCR assays have been overcome with the introduction of the standardized BIOMED-2 reagents, in particular the use of IGH D-J and IGK primers. NGS-based approaches that extend beyond the limited assessment of the size (base pair length) of rearrangements by also determining sequences (base constituents) appear to offer a superior approach for the assessment of these gene rearrangements, and are poised to replace capillary or gel electrophoresis-based assays.[392]

Translocations and Mutations in Normal Individuals

There is an ever-expanding list of leukemia- or lymphoma-associated translocations being detected by ultrasensitive PCR or RT-PCR techniques in "normal" individuals with neither concurrent nor subsequent development of malignant disease (Table 5-14).[393] The biological significance of these is uncertain, although they do suggest that many of these translocations are indeed "necessary, but not sufficient" for the full neoplastic phenotype. The t(14;18) fusion, which is evident in the peripheral blood of up to 60% of normal individuals, is positively correlated with age, heavy smoking, hepatitis C virus infection, and pesticide exposure. It has been suggested that once circulating *IGH::BCL2* levels exceed 1:10,000, there is indeed a heightened risk (23-fold) for the development of lymphoma. The t(11;14) fusions are less frequent, occurring in ~5% of normal individuals, and they can persist for long periods.

From a clinical laboratory perspective, the presence of such translocations in the normal population should elicit some caution but certainly not undue concern. The reasons for this include the fact that many of these have been detected only with hypersensitive assays detecting these fusions at levels so low ($\sim 10^{-6}$ to 10^{-8}, equivalent to 0.0001% to 0.000001%) that they are irrelevant diagnostically and unlikely to be relevant even in the context of contemporary MRD testing, in which approximately 10^{-4} to 10^{-5} appears to be the usual degree of sensitivity required.

Although biologically fascinating, more potentially troublesome from a diagnostic point of view is the detection of mutations seen in a spectrum of myeloid neoplasms occurring in normal individuals and increasing with age at levels much higher (and thus detectable in many standard assays) compared with the low-level translocations described. Such mutations by definition have VAFs of >2% and occur in the absence of a myeloid neoplasm and cytopenias, and are termed clonal hematopoiesis of indeterminate potential (CHIP).[394] These studies show that approximately ~2% of the general population harbor these mutations in the peripheral blood, with frequencies of less than 1% for age younger than 50 years (although they occur in individuals as young as 25 years), ~10% in those older than 65 years, and ~20% in those older than 90 years. With more sensitive assays with lower VAFs, CHIP is virtually universal by middle age. The most frequently mutated genes are *DNMT3A* > *TET2* > *ASXL1* (the top three), *JAK2*, *TP53*, *GNAS*, *PPM1D*, *BCORL1*, and *SF3B1*, with those affecting *TP53* and *PPM1D* expanding in the setting of cytotoxic therapy (especially platinum-based therapies) with the potential to elicit therapy-related myeloid neoplasms.[395-397] There are a total of approximately

Table 5-14 **Examples of Translocations Detected in Normal Individuals**

Translocation	Genes Fused	Tumor Association
t(14;18)	*BCL2::IGH*	Follicular lymphoma
t(11;14)	*CCND1::IGH*	Mantle cell lymphoma
t(8;14)	*MYC::IGH*	Burkitt lymphoma
t(9;22)	*BCR::ABL1*	Chronic myeloid leukemia, B-lymphoblastic leukemia/lymphoma
t(2;5)	*NPM1::ALK*	Anaplastic large cell lymphoma, ALK-positive
inv(2)	*ATIC::ALK*	Anaplastic large cell lymphoma, ALK-positive
t(12;21)	*ETV6::RUNX1*	B lymphoblastic leukemia/lymphoma

20 genes that are recurrently mutated in CHIP, as currently defined. Individuals with CHIP mutations have a 10- to 15-fold increased risk for development of a hematologic neoplasm, increased all-cause mortality, and increased risk of inflammation-associated diseases such as cardiovascular disease, gout, and chronic obstructive pulmonary disease (COPD).[398,399] These observations underscore the fact that the detection of these mutations cannot be used to diagnose MDS, although the opposite may be true, namely, that the absence of a mutation may render a diagnosis of MDS unlikely but not impossible. There are three genomic features, particularly in the setting of clonal cytopenias of undetermined significance (CCUS), that are likely to predict an increased likelihood of progression to a neoplasm: (1) the gene affected, such as *U2AF1*, *SF3B1*, *SRSF2*, *IDH1*, *IDH2*, and *TP53*, more risky; (2) the number of genes mutated, with two or more worse than one; and (3) the VAF, when greater than 10%. Whereas CHIP is by definition unaccompanied by cytopenias, CCUS[400] is, and this expands the risk for developing bona fide neoplasms. Because *DNMT3A*, *ASXL1*, and *TET2* mutations are so frequent in CHIP and MDS, a mutation in one of these genes cannot always be considered diagnostically useful nor indeed of value in tracking MRD in AML. In contrast, genes that are less frequently mutated in CHIP (such as *U2AF1*, *TP53*, and *RUNX1*) might retain some specificity in the appropriate clinical context. CHIP and CCUS are essentially analogous to MGUS, MBL, and FL-like B cells of undetermined significance in the setting of myeloma, CLL, and FL, respectively, reflecting precursor lesions, albeit with an apparently relatively low risk (~1%/year) of progressing to an overt neoplasm.

Similar mutations have also been described in up to almost 50% of cases of aplastic anemia, perhaps limiting their use in distinguishing this group of bone marrow failure syndromes from hypocellular MDS. Mutations include those affecting *ASXL1*, *TET2*, *DNMT3A*, *BCORL1*, and *BCOR*. *ASXL1* and *DNMT3A* mutant clones expand over time and *ASXL1* mutations are (as is characteristic) associated with a poor prognosis and increased risk for development of MDS.[401] *TET2* mutations portend a better prognosis and are associated with longer survival in aplastic anemia.

There is tremendous overlap in diseases in which many of these mutations occur. There is a growing list of mutations that are seen not only in AML, MPN, and MDS but also in lymphoid neoplasms[402] and indeed a number of non-hematologic neoplasms, highlighting the fact that most of the mutations encountered are not disease specific, although clear associations have emerged. In addition, an increasing number of mutations is encountered in what are currently considered to be "benign" diseases, blurring the diagnostic lines between the traditional separation of neoplastic versus reactive.[403] The presence of CHIP can also cause confusion in the interpretation of ctDNA studies and solid tumor sequencing panels, with the latter potentially confounded by blood contamination. This highlights the important fact that most if not all molecular abnormalities should never be interpreted in isolation, and the need to correlate all molecular data with available morphologic and immunophenotypic data cannot be overemphasized.

SUMMARY AND CONCLUSIONS

Insights into the vast spectrum of genetic abnormalities that are required to initiate and to sustain hematologic neoplasms continue to evolve from fragmented accounts based on restricted lines of investigation into a much more comprehensive view of how the multitude of facets (gene fusions and dysregulation through gross chromosomal abnormalities, mutations, epigenetic transcription control through DNA and chromatin modifications, and alterations in the noncoding genome, among others) interact. Disruptive technologies such as NGS have dramatically altered our understanding by facilitating an assessment of the panoply of genetic aberrations that drive hematologic neoplasms, opening the door to a more refined manner in which we can diagnose, prognosticate, monitor, and treat these neoplasms with tumor-specific and precision therapies.

Acknowledgments

The authors express their profound appreciation to Insuk Choe, JD for excellent editorial assistance.

Pearls and Pitfalls

- The incremental adoption of disruptive technologies in the evaluation of hematologic neoplasms has facilitated our understanding of the genetic basis of many of these neoplasms. Not only is the judicious use of these tools central to the diagnosis of a subset of lymphomas, leukemias, and other hematologic neoplasms, but they also inform prognosis and targeted therapeutic approaches.
- Despite the high throughput, precision, and sensitivity of nascent technologies such as NGS, time-honored tools, such as conventional metaphase cytogenetic analysis, still retain diagnostic and prognostic relevance in contemporary practice.
- Some hematologic neoplasms are essentially defined, in the appropriate clinicopathologic context, by specific generic aberrations, such as the *BCR::ABL1* fusion in chronic myeloid leukemia. In contrast, others, although highly associated with a hallmark genetic abnormality, such as the t(14;18)/*IGH::BCL2* in follicular lymphoma, can be diagnosed in the absence of this abnormality, which is also not diagnostically specific for follicular lymphoma.
- Certain mutations, initially described in the setting of a specific neoplasm, for example, acute myeloid leukemia (AML), have subsequently been detected not only in a spectrum of other myeloid neoplasms (such as the myelodysplastic syndromes [MDSs] and myeloproliferative neoplasms [MPNs]) but also in lymphoid and in non-hematologic neoplasms, thus highlighting the notion that these mutations cannot be exclusively used to render specific diagnoses and should be interpreted in combination with other pathologic data in appropriate clinical contexts.
- The increasing detection of a plethora of disease-associated genetic aberrations in normal (but occasionally restricted, e.g., the aging) populations reinforces the need for the rational use and contextual interpretation of the ever-expanding menu of molecular tests.

KEY REFERENCES

3. de Leval L, Alizadeh AA, Bergsagel PL, et al. Genomic profiling for clinical decision making in lymphoid neoplasms. *Blood.* 2022;140(21):2193–2227.
5. Duncavage EJ, Bagg A, Hasserjian RP, et al. Genomic profiling for clinical decision making in myeloid neoplasms and acute leukemia. *Blood.* 2022;140(21):2228–2247.
27. McCombie WR, McPherson JD, Mardis ER. Next-generation sequencing technologies. *Cold Spring Harb Perspect Med.* 2019;9(11):a036798.
124. Wright GW, Huang DW, Phelan JD, et al. A probabilistic classification tool for genetic subtypes of diffuse large B cell lymphoma with therapeutic implications. *Cancer Cell.* 2020;37(4):551–568.e14.
232. Bigas A, Rodriguez-Sevilla JJ, Espinosa L, Gallardo F. Recent advances in T-cell lymphoid neoplasms. *Exp Hematol.* 2022;106:3–18.
236. Iacobucci I, Mullighan CG. Genetic basis of acute lymphoblastic leukemia. *J Clin Oncol Off J Am Soc Clin Oncol.* 2017;35(9):975–983.
242. Döhner H, Wei AH, Appelbaum FR, et al. Diagnosis and management of AML in adults: 2022 recommendations from an international expert panel on behalf of the ELN. *Blood.* 2022;140(12):1345–1377.
277. El Achi H, Kanagal-Shamanna R. Biomarkers in acute myeloid leukemia: leveraging next generation sequencing data for optimal therapeutic strategies. *Front Oncol.* 2021;11:748250.
393. Miller PG, Steensma DP. Implications of clonal hematopoiesis for precision oncology. *JCO Precis Oncol.* 2020;4:639–646.
403. Akkari YMN, Baughn LB, Dubuc AM, et al. Guiding the global evolution of cytogenetic testing for hematologic malignancies. *Blood.* 2022;139(15):2273–2284.

Visit Elsevier eBooks+ for the complete set of references.

Chapter 6

Important Chromosomal Aberrations in Hematologic Neoplasms and Key Techniques to Diagnose Them

Itziar Salaverria, Reiner Siebert, and Krzysztof Mrózek

TYPES OF CHROMOSOMAL ABERRATIONS IN HEMATOLOGIC MALIGNANCIES

Introduction to Human Chromosomes

In 1888, Waldeyer was first to introduce the term *chromosome* (meaning "stainable body," from the Greek *chroma,* meaning "color," and *soma,* meaning "body"). Waldeyer referred to Walther Flemming, who coined the terms *chromatin* and *mitosis* in 1879 at Kiel University. Flemming was also first to describe germinal centers. Since the pioneering studies by Flemming and Waldeyer, a wealth of knowledge on the composition and function of chromosomes has emerged. Each chromosome consists of a DNA double helix bearing a linear sequence of genes, coiled and recoiled around aggregated proteins called *histones.* Two sister chromatids (each constituting half of a chromosome) are joined together at a junction called a *centromere* (primary constriction). The full chromosome containing both joined sister chromatids becomes visible only during mitosis, in a phase known as *metaphase.* Regular human cells have 23 pairs of chromosomes (22 pairs of autosomes, numbered consecutively from 1 to 22, and 1 pair of sex chromosomes, i.e., XX in females and XY in males). Thus a normal human somatic cell has two complements of 23 chromosomes (2n) for a total of 46 chromosomes, in contrast to a germ cell, which only has one chromosomal complement (1n) of 23 chromosomes. By convention, chromosomes are numbered in descending order according to their size and the position of the centromere (arm ratio) and are arranged into seven groups (from A to G) (Denver classification). On the basis of the centromere location, there are three main types of chromosomes: *metacentric,* with their arms roughly equal in length; *submetacentric,* with one arm clearly shorter than the other; and *acrocentric,* with a centromere located near one end of the chromosome. A *band* is defined as part of the chromosome that is clearly distinguishable from its adjacent parts by appearing darker or lighter with one or more banding techniques. This banding pattern, to some extent, reflects the base pair and histone composition of the different chromosome parts. Bands are grouped in regions delimited by specific landmarks and numbered consecutively from the centromere outward along each chromosome arm, with the first number specifying region and the second band within this region; if sub-bands are discernible, they are numbered with the third number (and fourth in some instances) placed behind a period. Letters *p* (from French, *petite*) and *q* are used to designate, respectively, the short and long arm of each chromosome. For designation of a particular band, four items are required: (1) chromosome number, (2) arm designation (*p* or *q*), (3) region number, and (4) band number within that region. For details on banding patterns, naming of chromosomes, and their parts, please refer to the International System of Cytogenetic Nomenclature (ISCN).[1]

Chromosomal aberrations (or abnormalities) are changes in the number of chromosomes (numerical abnormalities; also named *aneuploidy* when one or a few chromosomes are gained or lost) or in their structure (structural abnormalities). In cancer cytogenetics, somatic (i.e., acquired, tumor-associated) aberrations have to be clearly differentiated from constitutional (i.e., germline) abnormalities. In principle, a chromosomal alteration—particularly if detected in all cells of an investigated individual—could represent a constitutional aberration, as long as its constitutional appearance is compatible with life.[2] Some common examples of constitutional alterations recurrently detected during tumor genetic workup are numeric changes in the sex chromosomes (e.g., XXY in patients with Klinefelter's syndrome), Robertsonian translocations [e.g., t(13;14)(q10;q10)], balanced translocations in phenotypically normal carriers [e.g., t(11;22)(q23;q11)], trisomy 21 in individuals with Down syndrome, or germline uniparental disomy (i.e., two different chromosomes from the same parent). The constitutional nature of a suspected abnormality should be confirmed or refuted with cytogenetic analysis of phytohemagglutinin (PHA)-stimulated culture of blood and/or cultured fibroblasts, or another alternative cell system (e.g., buccal swap, sedimented cells from urine). Moreover, occasionally somatically acquired alterations may also occur independently from tumorigenesis. Examples include loss of the Y chromosome in marrow or blood of older male patients or T-cell receptor (TR) gene loci rearrangements.

Clones and Clonal Evolution

A *clone* is a cell population derived from a single progenitor cell. At the cytogenetic level, a clone is defined as two metaphase cells with the same structural abnormality or gain of the same chromosome, or three cells with loss of the same chromosome. The presence of a cytogenetically aberrant clone (or clones) at diagnosis usually indicates a neoplastic process. However, a clone does not necessarily prove the presence of a neoplastic disease, as occasionally, a clonal abnormality may be present in non-neoplastic cells, such as in the case of the aforementioned clonal loss of chromosome Y during aging. Moreover, a tumor population is not always homogeneous, and in addition to the most basic clone of a tumor cell population, termed *stemline,* one or more subclones (termed *sidelines*), containing new abnormalities in addition to the ones present in the stemline, can appear during tumor development (clonal evolution). Non-clonal aberrations (i.e., those occurring in single cells) are usually not listed in the karyotype description, but if they are indicated, it is done separately from the clonal abnormalities. A single-cell abnormality can sometimes be judged to be of a clonal origin if it represents a typical, cancer-associated aberration and/or its clonality is corroborated by alternative techniques (e.g., fluorescence in situ hybridization [FISH]), or it is found at other time points (e.g., at relapse).

Chromosomal instability is a transient or persistent state that causes a series of mutational events leading to gross genetic alterations. Multiple whole chromosome gains and losses and structural abnormalities present in more than one clone and in non-clonal cells are common manifestations of genomic instability. Determination of chromosomal instability requires approaches capable of monitoring cell-to-cell variability and/or the rate of both numerical and structural chromosomal changes. The most commonly used methods to determine chromosomal instability are conventional cytogenetics, FISH, or copy number (CN) array-based procedures.[3] Nevertheless, new more molecular-oriented technologies like optical mapping or genome sequencing approaches (particularly using long reads) might increasingly supplement the conventional (molecular) cytogenetics technologies in the future.

Alterations of Cell Ploidy

Cell ploidy alterations are changes in the number of chromosome complements. As outlined earlier, the basic set of human chromosomes is called *haploid* and contains 23 chromosomes: one copy of each of the 22 autosomes and one sex chromosome. A haploid chromosome set is characteristic for germ cells. A normal somatic human cell has two haploid sets and is called *diploid* (2n = 46 chromosomes). Cells with an increased number of chromosome sets are called *triploid* (3n = 69 chromosomes), *tetraploid* (4n = 92 chromosomes), and so on (Table 6-1).

Systematic cytogenetic analysis of solid tumors and hematologic malignancies has revealed that the chromosome

Table 6-1 Relationship Between Modal Number and Ploidy Level

Ploidy Level	Modal Number	Number of Chromosomes
Near-haploid	**23±**	**≤34**
Hypohaploidy		<23
Hyperhaploidy		24–34
Near-diploid	**46±**	**35–57**
Hypodiploidy		35–45
Hypertriploidy		45–57
Near-triploid	**69±**	**58–80**
Hypotriploidy		58–68
Hypertriploidy		70–80
Near-tetraploidy	**92±**	**81–103**
Hypotetraploidy		81–91
Hypertetraploidy		93–103
Near-pentaploidy	**115±**	**104–126**
Hypopentaploidy		104–114
Hyperpentaploidy		116–126
Near-hexaploidy	**138±**	**127–149**
Hypohexaploidy		127–137
Hyperhexaploidy		139–149
Near-heptaploidy	**161±**	**150–172**
Hypoheptaploidy		150–160
Hyperheptaploidy		162–172
Near-octaploidy	**184±**	**173–195**
Hypooctaploidy		173–183
Hyperoctaploidy		185–195

Data from McGowan-Jordan J, Hastings RJ, Moore S, eds. *ISCN (2020): An International System for Human Cytogenomic Nomenclature (2020).* Basel: Karger; 2020.

number in cancer cells can be highly variable, ranging from hypodiploidy (<46 chromosomes) to tetraploidy (4n = 92) or even pentaploidy (5n = 115), hexaploidy (6n = 138), or octaploidy (8n = 184). The modal number is the most common chromosome number in a tumor cell population. All changes in chromosome number should be expressed in relation to the appropriate ploidy level. A hyperdiploid karyotype characterizing a subset of acute lymphoblastic leukemia (ALL) patients is thought to arise from a single-step mechanism. Unscheduled tetraploidy can arise by one of three main mechanisms: cell fusion, mitotic slippage, or a failure to undergo cytokinesis. Maintenance of heterozygosity has been demonstrated, suggesting that the hyperdiploidy does not arise from a near-haploid precursor.

Aneuploidy: Monosomy and Trisomy

Monosomy is a term to describe the absence of one member of a chromosome pair, resulting in a clone with 45 chromosomes in the case of a single monosomy. Conversely, the term *trisomy* describes the presence of an extra chromosome (three copies instead of one pair); a single trisomy results in cells with 47 chromosomes. In the karyotype, a monosomy is usually denoted with a minus sign (e.g., –7 meaning *monosomy* 7) and a trisomy with a plus sign (e.g., +8 meaning *trisomy* 8).

Balanced Chromosomal Alterations (Reciprocal Translocations, Insertions, and Inversions)

Balanced chromosomal changes include reciprocal translocations, insertions, and inversions. Reciprocal translocations are interchromosomal abnormalities resulting from the exchange of chromosomal material between two chromosomes without apparent gain or loss of chromosome material. Insertions are created when a segment of one chromosome is excised and inserted into one of the arms of another chromosome, whereas inversions constitute intrachromosomal aberrations derived from a 180-degree rotation of a segment within a single chromosome. The majority of recurring reciprocal translocations and inversions in hematologic neoplasms are considered to be primary events. They can lead to generation of gene fusions encoding chimeric transcripts, which contain sequences from both fused genes, or to deregulation of wild-type genes located next to a breakpoint by either promoter substitution or novel regulatory context. Several of these translocations and inversions are highly conserved and can be present in a majority of tumors of a given subtype. This makes various primary genetic alterations valuable diagnostic markers. Few cases carry three-way translocations that similarly involve three chromosomes with one breakpoint in each.

Unbalanced Chromosomal Aberrations (Deletions, Duplications, and Unbalanced Translocations)

In addition to a whole chromosome gain (trisomy), chromosomal segments can be gained through unbalanced translocations or intrachromosomal duplications. Massive gain of a large number of copies of a small chromosomal region is called *amplification*, which cytogenetically is manifested as a homogeneous staining region (HSR) if the amplicon sticks together at one chromosomal site or as small acentric structures called *double minutes (dmin)*. Amplifications are known to activate oncogenes and constitute a genetic mechanism leading to the overexpression of the amplification target gene(s). In this sense, several loci of recurrent amplification have been identified in different leukemia and lymphoma types as amplifications of *REL/BCL11A* at 2p16, *BCL2* at 18q21, or *MYC* at 8q24. The border between chromosome material gain and amplification is sometimes difficult to establish. Complex rearrangements containing amplification of two loci juxtaposed by a chromosomal translocation have been named *complicons*.[4,5]

Structural abnormalities resulting in loss of a chromosomal segment are intrachromosomal deletions and unbalanced translocations. The major consequences of deletions in cancer cells are the loss and/or inactivation of tumor suppressor genes, although occasionally deletions can lead to gene fusions and oncogene activation. The most prominent example of deletions in both lymphoid and myeloid neoplasms with a complex karyotype is loss of the short arm of chromosome 17 (17p), which contains the locus of the tumor suppressor gene *TP53*. Losses of 6q are present in many types of aggressive lymphoma, such as diffuse large B-cell lymphoma (DLBCL), follicular lymphoma (FL), or mantle cell lymphoma (MCL). In patients with these deletions, the other allele of the target gene is frequently inactivated by a mutation. In some other cases, a homozygous deletion (i.e., deletion of both alleles) can occur. This is recurrently the case in chromosomal region 9p21, in which homozygous deletions involving the *CDKN2A* gene can be detected in several types of lymphoma and ALL.[6,7] However, for many recurring deletions, genes presumed to be targets of deletions have not been hitherto identified. It has been suggested that such deletions can play a role in leukemogenesis through haploinsufficiency, that is, decreased expression of genes mapped to the lost segments because of the presence of only one functional allele following a deletion of the second.[8]

In myeloid and lymphoid neoplasms with reciprocal translocations or inversions as primary abnormalities, unbalanced aberrations associated with gain and loss of chromosome material usually represent secondary genetic events and might be present only in a subset of cells of a given tumor. In contrast, in patients diagnosed with acute myeloid leukemia (AML) or myelodysplastic syndrome (MDS) with a complex karyotype, unbalanced aberrations predominate and have presumed primary significance.[8-10]

Copy-Neutral Loss of Heterozygosity

Loss of heterozygosity (LOH) means that a constitutionally heterozygous locus loses one allele. The reason for such loss can be a deletion (which is a copy-associated LOH) or LOH without chromosomal loss because of gain of the other allele in the form of a (partial) isodisomy. For this second kind of event, the term *copy-neutral-LOH* (CN-LOH) has been introduced. In this sense, consequences of loss of one allele and duplication of the mutated allele can be functionally similar to a homozygous mutation. CN-LOH is a recurrent oncogenic event in lymphomas and AML. The regions affected by CN-LOH in lymphomas usually include such tumor suppressor genes as *TP53*[11] or *TNFRSF14*,[12] whereas in AML, CN-LOH often results in homozygous mutations at loci frequently mutated in this disease, such as *CEBPA, FLT3, RUNX1,* and *WT1.*[13-14] Its identification has been useful for characterizing tumor stages and progression in different cancer types.[13-16] As the gene dosage is not altered, CN-LOH cannot be detected by conventional cytogenetics, FISH, or comparative genomic hybridization (CGH) array analysis.

Chromothripsis

Chromothripsis is a phenomenon identified in cancer cells by whole-genome sequencing that produces catastrophic chromosome reorganization of one or a small number of chromosomes at a single point in time.[17] Some distinctive features of chromothripsis are: (1) alternating regions of CN aberration with a minimal number of CN states (one and two copies in its simplest form); (2) LOH of the lower CN state; (3) derivation of each "new derivative" chromosome from one or a small number of chromosomes. Features 1 and 2 can be assessed by CN array, but this approach does not reveal the full complexity of the interchromosomal rearrangements. Chromothripsis escapes conventional cytogenetic detection but can be suspected in complex karyotypes with one to three chromosomes participating in complex rearrangements. Multicolor FISH (M-FISH) or spectral karyotyping (SKY) can also identify the involvement of a minimal number of chromosomes (feature 3), but at low resolution. Nevertheless, a combination of both CN array and multicolor karyotyping techniques or analysis by Optical Genome Mapping (OGM) or (long-read) sequencing are currently the possible strategies for detection of chromothripsis in routine diagnosis.[18,19]

Moreover, Baca et al.[20] also introduced the term *chromoplexy* to describe another type of coordinated structural genome rearrangement that, differently from chromothripsis, can occur in different steps in the evolution of the tumor, not in one single catastrophic event, and the breakpoints are unclustered and include multiple chromosomes. These changes have been identified in chronic lymphocytic leukemia (CLL).[21,22]

CONVENTIONAL CYTOGENETIC METHODS

Conventional cytogenetics analysis is based on the study of metaphase chromosomes obtained from viable, dividing cells from bone marrow, peripheral blood, lymphoid tissue, or other tumor-containing tissue with staining techniques. This method has become a routine test in the management of hematologic malignancies. The main banding techniques are those that produce the so-called *quinacrine (Q), Giemsa (G), centromeric (C),* and *reverse (R)* banding. In Q-banding, the chromosomes are stained with quinacrine hydrochloride, which reveals a consistent and reproducible banding pattern of brighter fluorescence in A-T–rich regions and dull fluorescence in G-C–rich regions.[23] Q-banding is especially suitable to identify the Y chromosome in both metaphase and interphase nuclei. In G-banding, the chromosome preparation is subjected to treatment with sodium salt citrate at a warm temperature or to a mild treatment with an enzyme such as trypsin, followed by staining with a weak solution of Giemsa or Wright stain. This procedure also reveals transverse dark and light bands that correspond, respectively, to the brightly fluorescent and dully fluorescent bands produced by Q-banding.[23,24] Currently, most laboratories routinely use G-banding for the diagnosis of hematologic neoplasms (Fig. 6-1A).

There are different techniques to obtain R-banded chromosomes like fluorescent R-banding or incubation of the chromosome preparation in very hot phosphate buffer, followed by Giemsa staining.[25] R-banding yields a banding pattern that is the reverse of G-banding, that is, dark bands in G-banded chromosomes stain light with R-banding, and vice versa. R-banding is useful for identifying deletions or translocations that involve the telomeric regions of chromosomes and the late-replicating, inactive X chromosome.

C-banding involves short treatment of the chromosomes with a weak solution of alkali, such as barium hydroxide, followed by Giemsa staining.[26] C-banding suppresses staining all along the chromosome except at the centromeric heterochromatin regions.

Given the importance of cytogenetic analysis, it is important to obtain chromosome preparations of good quality. Every specimen can have specific culture requirements. For example,

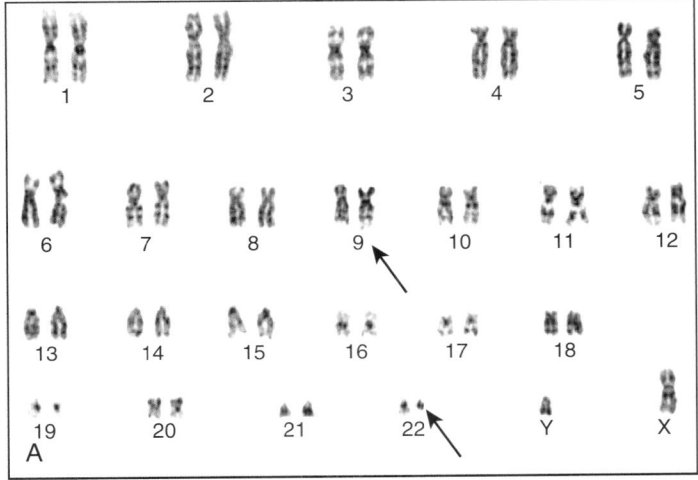
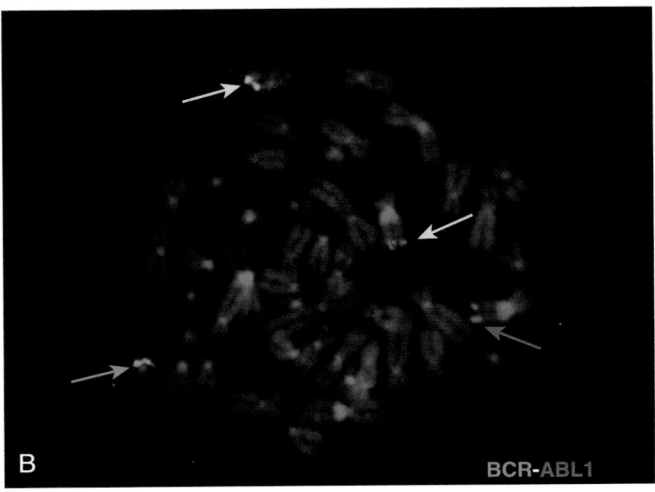

Figure 6-1. A, G-banded karyotype showing 46,XY,t(9;22)(q34;q11.2). **B,** Fluorescence in situ hybridization (FISH) with dual-color dual-fusion *BCR::ABL1* Vysis probe. Fusion is indicated with yellow arrowheads. *(Kindly provided by Dr. Dolors Costa, Hospital Clínic Barcelona.)*

precursor B lymphoblastic leukemia/lymphoma (B-ALL) or T lymphoblastic leukemia/lymphoma (T-ALL) specimens that have a high mitotic index can be grown in direct culture for 1 to 6 hours, whereas most neoplasms require a short-term, unstimulated culture (24–48 hours). Stimulation with mitogens (e.g., 3 days) is necessary in such chronic lymphoproliferative disorders as CLL (e.g., with DSP30 or CpG-oligonucleotide/ interleukin 2) or T-cell leukemias (with PHA). Technical details can be obtained from *The AGT Cytogenetics Laboratory Manual,* which is the standard reference.[27]

To describe chromosomes and their aberrations, the ISCN is applied. It is based on the results of several international conferences, the first of which took place in 1960 in Denver, Colorado. ISCN is periodically updated on the basis of new information and constitutes the widely accepted standard for chromosome and chromosome abnormalities description.[1] In the karyotype description, the first item is the total number of chromosomes followed by sex chromosomes and a description of chromosome abnormalities with ISCN-approved abbreviations. The symbol identifying the type of rearrangement (e.g., t = translocation, inv = inversion, or del = deletion) is followed by the chromosome number(s) involved in this rearrangement placed in parentheses, and then designation of breakpoints within the rearranged chromosome(s) in a second set of parentheses, for example, inv(16)(p13.1q22). If two or more chromosomes are altered, a semicolon is used to separate their designation. The number of cells constituting each clone is given in square brackets at the end. For example, two clones from a male patient carrying a t(8;21) translocation as a sole abnormality in a stemline and together with a loss of the Y chromosome in a sideline, identified in 13 and 10 metaphase cells, respectively, is reported as follows: 46,XY,t(8;21)(q22;q22)[13]/45,X,–Y,t(8;21)(q22;q22)[10].[1]

Conventional cytogenetic analysis is a powerful tool for characterizing tumor karyotypes. However, it is time-consuming, technically demanding, and requires dividing cells to obtain metaphases. In many hematologic malignancies, particularly lymphomas, the mitotic index is often low and the quality of metaphases poor. In addition, the karyotypes of many advanced lymphoid tumors are highly complex and cannot be completely resolved by conventional cytogenetic analysis. Another limitation of conventional cytogenetic analysis is its inability to distinguish molecularly distinct rearrangements that appear to be cytogenetically identical. For example, the t(14;18)(q32;q21) translocation is observed in FL and extranodal marginal zone lymphoma of mucosa-associated lymphoid tissue (MALT), but the genes at 18q21 deregulated by the translocation are different. The fusion product in FL is *IGH::BCL2,* whereas in MALT it is *IGH::MALT1.* It is important to distinguish between these translocations because each is associated with a distinct histologic subtype. Another limitation of conventional cytogenetic analysis is its inability to detect cryptic translocations involving telomeric parts of the chromosome, such as the t(6;14)(p25;q32)/*IGH::IRF4* translocation typically present in plasma cell myeloma (PCM), also named multiple myeloma (MM),[28] and in a subset of germinal-center–derived B-cell (GCB) lymphomas.[29]

MOLECULAR CYTOGENETIC METHODS

Because of the aforementioned limitations, investigators searched for alternative molecular methods that would enable the analysis of non-dividing cells and offer better resolution. FISH was the first such molecular method developed, and several others, namely SKY or M-FISH, and CN analysis, including CGH array, single-nucleotide polymorphism (SNP) array, and molecular inversion probe (MIP) assays, followed rapidly.[30,31] The applications, advantages, and disadvantages of these methods in comparison to conventional G-banding are summarized in Table 6-2.

Fluorescence in Situ Hybridization

In FISH, fluorescently labeled DNA probes are hybridized to interphase nuclei or metaphase spreads prepared for standard cytogenetic analysis. FISH can also be applied to a wide range of cellular preparations such as banded slides, air-dried bone marrow or blood smears, fresh tumor touch prints, frozen or paraffin-embedded tissue sections, or nuclear isolates from fresh or fixed tissues.

A variety of FISH probes, each targeting a specific region or the entire chromosome, are available. Probes routinely used in the analysis of hematologic malignancies include chromosome-specific enumerator (i.e., mostly centromeric) probes, gene- or locus-specific probes, whole chromosome painting (WCP) probes, arm-specific sequence probes, and telomeric probes.

Chromosome-specific centromeric probes are derived from the highly repetitive, mostly alpha-satellite DNA sequences located within the centromeres. Because the target size is several hundred kilobases (kb) in length, the probes exhibit bright, discrete signals and are easy to evaluate in both metaphase and interphase nuclei. Centromeric probes are useful in identifying numerical abnormalities (aneuploidy), dicentric chromosomes, and the origin of marker chromosomes. Clinically important aberrations such as trisomy 12 in CLL, monosomy 7 in AML, and (high) hyperploidy in ALL—all of which are detected at a lower incidence by conventional cytogenetics owing to low mitotic index or poor morphology—are routinely evaluated by FISH in many clinical laboratories. Another example is the use of differentially labeled probes specific for chromosomes X and Y in monitoring engraftment in sex-mismatched allogeneic stem cell transplantation.

WCP or arm-specific sequence probes use mixtures of fluorescently labeled DNA sequences derived from the entire length of the specific chromosome or one of its arms.[30,31] They are helpful in characterizing complex rearrangements and marker chromosomes. However, cryptic rearrangements affecting terminal regions may remain undetected because of suppression of the repetitive DNA sequences within these regions. The application of chromosome painting probes is limited to metaphase analysis because the signals are often large and diffuse in interphase. Chromosome-specific telomeric or subtelomeric probes are derived from DNA sequences located at or adjacent to the telomeres and are effective in detecting terminal, interstitial, and cryptic translocations that are below the resolution of conventional cytogenetics and/or are undetectable by WCP.

Gene-specific or locus-specific probes are derived from unique DNA sequences or loci within the chromosome. With banding techniques on highly extended chromosomes, the smallest detectable chromosome abnormality is 2000 to 3000 kb, whereas gene- or locus-specific probes can routinely

Table 6-2 Comparison of Conventional and Molecular Cytogenetic Techniques

Feature	G-Banding	SKY/M-FISH	FISH	CGH	CGH Array	SNP Array	MIP Assay Array	OGM
Resolution	>5 Mb	>2 Mb	50 kb	3–10 Mb	3 kb Agilent 1M array	10–20 kb SNP6	50–100 kb	
Identification								
Balanced translocations	Yes	Yes	Yes*	No	No	No	No	Yes
Unbalanced translocations	Yes	Yes	Yes*	?	?	?	?	Yes
Structural rearrangements within a single chromosome	Yes	Sometimes	Yes*	No	No	No	No	Yes
Origin of marker chromosome	No	Yes	No	?	?	?	No	?
Copy number changes	Yes	Yes	Yes	Yes	Yes	Yes	Yes	Yes
Deletions <10 Mb	Sometimes	Sometimes	Yes	No	Yes	Yes	Yes	Yes
Allelic loss	No	No	Yes	No	No	Yes	Yes	Yes
Copy number neutral loss of heterozygosity	No	No	No	No	No	Yes	Yes	No
High-level amplification	Sometimes‡	Sometimes‡	Yes*	Yes	Yes	Yes	Yes	Yes
Subtelomeric rearrangements	No	No	Yes*	No	No	No	No	Yes
Resolves complex and cryptic chromosomal alterations	No	Yes	Yes*	No	No	No	No	Yes
Pros and Cons								
Requires specifically labeled probes	No	Yes	Yes	Yes	No	No	No	No
Requires prior knowledge of DNA sequences of the aberration	No	No	Yes	No	No	No	No	No
Scans the entire genome	Yes	Yes	No	Yes	Yes	Yes	Yes	Yes
Identifies tumor heterogeneity	Yes	Yes	No	No	Yes	Yes	No	Yes
Requires viable cells	Yes	Yes	No	No	No	No	No	Optimally yes
Requires tumor metaphase spreads	Yes	Yes	No	No	No	No	No	No
Applicable to interphase nuclei and nondividing cells	No	No	Yes	No	No	No	No	No
Applicable to DNA extracted from archived tissue (FFPE)	No	No	No	Yes	Yes	No	Yes	No
Labor-intensive	Yes	Yes	No	No	No	No	No	No
Interpretation highly dependent on experience and knowledge	Yes	Yes	Yes	Yes	No	No	No	No
Expensive for small diagnostic laboratories	No	Yes	No	Yes	Yes	Yes	Yes	Yes
Applicable and cost-effective as a routine screening method	Yes	No	Yes	No	No	No	No	Limited
Turnaround time (days)	3–10	2–7	2–7	2–3	3–4	3–4	3–4	4–6

*Only with appropriately designed probes.
‡When present in the form of a homogeneous staining region or double minutes.
CGH, Comparative genomic hybridization; FFPE, formalin-fixed paraffin embedded; FISH, fluorescence in situ hybridization; kb, kilobase; Mb, megabase; M-FISH, multicolor FISH; MIP, molecular inversion probe; OGM, Optical Genome Mapping; SKY, spectral karyotyping; SNP, single nucleotide polymorphism.

detect regions as small as 0.1 kb.[31] As such, these probes have wide application in both basic and clinical research. Gene-specific or locus-specific probes have been extremely useful in gene mapping and in defining structural rearrangements, amplifications, and origin of marker chromosomes in both metaphase chromosomes and interphase nuclei.

In lymphoid malignancies, locus- or gene-specific probes have also been effective in delineating minimal regions of deletion (e.g., on chromosomes 6q,[32] 11q,[33] and 13q[34]) and in demonstrating monoallelic losses of such genes as RB1 and TP53.

Although the FISH probes can be easily applied to and analyzed on cytogenetic preparations, paraffin-embedded or frozen tissue sections can be difficult to work with and require additional standardization techniques. Loss of signal because of low hybridization efficiency and high non-specific background autofluorescence can lead to atypical signal patterns, making signal interpretation difficult. Nevertheless, adapted FISH protocols have been successfully implemented in the routine diagnosis (Fig. 6-2).[35] The major limitation of detecting losses by FISH in paraffin-embedded tissues is that part of the cell can be lost during the sectioning process, leading to false-positive results. Therefore for detection of deletions, the cutoff value (i.e., a minimal percentage of cells with deletion detected for calling the case positive) has to be established at a higher level and appropriate negative controls

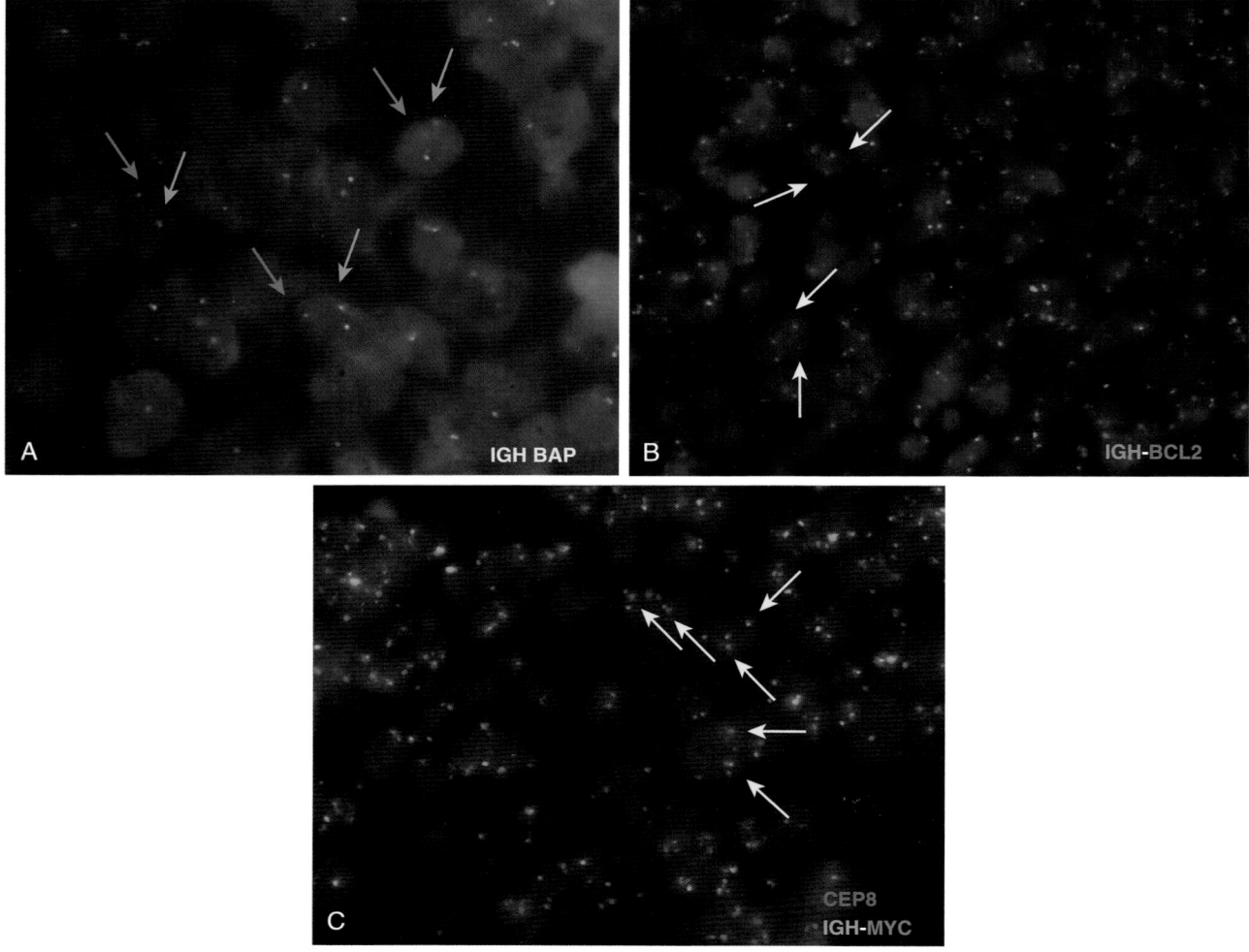

Figure 6-2. Fluorescence in situ hybridization (FISH) analysis of 14q32 (IGH)-associated translocations in B-cell lymphomas on formalin-fixed paraffin embedded (FFPE) and frozen material. A, Analysis of IGH breaks with break-apart IGH probe (Vysis) on FFPE sections from a mantle cell lymphoma case. Breaks are indicated with green and red arrows. **B and C,** FISH analysis with dual-color dual-fusion *IGH::BCL2* (Vysis) and *IGH::MYC* (three-color DCDF, Vysis) on frozen tissue sections from follicular lymphoma and Burkitt lymphoma cases. Fusions are indicated with yellow arrows. *(Kindly provided by Dr. Cristina Lopez, Institute of Human Genetics, Kiel.)*

have to be evaluated.[35] Consequently, commercial FISH probes designed for evaluation of losses usually include an internal FISH hybridization control labeled with a different fluorochrome that usually hybridizes to the centromere of the chromosome with the locus of interest, or to a distal region of the same chromosome expected to be preserved if the deletion occurs. In the analysis of deletions by FISH, the evaluation by two different observers is highly recommended, as it is for the evaluation of translocations.

For the detection of translocations, two types of FISH probes are widely used, break-apart probes (BAPs) and dual-color dual-fusion (DCDF) probes. The BAPs detect gene rearrangements with differently labeled DNA probes that are complementary to sequences distal and proximal to the breakpoint within the target gene. The DCDF are designed for proving the juxtaposition of two loci and are used for the identification of reciprocal translocations. For this purpose, two DNA probes labeled with different colors located at the respective breakpoints of both translocation partners are used.

The juxtaposition of both genes is translated into a third color under the microscope (fusion signal) (Fig. 6-1B; Fig. 6-2B and C). BAP probes are less informative than DCDF probes because although they can reveal breakage within a specific locus, they do not define the other gene involved. In addition, because they flank the locus of interest, small insertions could remain unidentified. Nevertheless, their advantage lies in their ability to detect translocations involving different partners of such promiscuous genes as *MYC, KMT2A* (formerly known as *MLL*), or *BCL6*, and they are easier to evaluate because the separation of two signals is easily recognizable. However, because some normal signals can be vaguely separated when BAP probes are used, the normal signal pattern has to be carefully defined according to probe design, locus interrogated, the material investigated, and so on. On the other hand, a positive result with DCDF probes consists of two fusion signals, an event that is very unlikely to occur by chance. For both kinds of probes, variant signal constellations caused by complex or unbalanced changes need to be considered.

Among the critical factors affecting an accurate interpretation of FISH is the establishment of proper cutoff values for the different probes used. For DCDF, the cutoff is usually clearly below 5%, but it might be significantly higher for some variant signal patterns, for example, when it is caused by the loss of one derivative chromosome involved in the translocation. On the other hand, because BAPs are variable based on the location of the breakpoints and the probe design, the FISH evaluator needs to visually estimate the relative distance between the different color probes in normal controls. A break is usually recognized if the distance between the two signals is at least twice the estimated signal diameter. Ideally, the BAP cutoff should be between 1% and 5%, although it might be higher, again depending on the probe design and locus investigated.

ISCN standard nomenclature is also established for description of chromosomal changes detected by FISH. In interphase FISH, the abbreviation *nuc ish* is followed by the locus designation in parentheses, a multiplication sign (×), and the number of signals seen: for example, nuc ish(D13S319×2). The presence of an extra signal is reported as nuc ish(D13S319×3), whereas loss of one copy is reported as nuc ish(D13S319×1). If loci of two separate chromosomes are tested and they are juxtaposed (translocation), the results are expressed as follows: nuc ish(ABL1×2),(BCR×2),(ABL1 con BCR×1); or, alternatively, nuc ish(ABL1,BCR)×2(ABL1 con BCR×1).[1]

Probe sets for the detection of most rearrangements associated with specific subtypes of leukemia or lymphoma are now available commercially and routinely used in cytogenetic laboratories to establish a diagnosis, select therapy, and monitor the effects of therapy. However, it is important to underline that in contrast to conventional cytogenetic analysis, which allows the simultaneous recognition of all microscopically detectable abnormalities in tumor cells regardless of whether they are numerical, structural, balanced, or unbalanced, FISH can be currently used only to detect the presence or confirm the absence of specific abnormalities that the probes used are designed to identify.

Similar to FISH, the chromogenic in situ hybridization (CISH) technique relies on the ability of DNA probes to hybridize specifically to complementary target DNA, but for signal identification CISH uses chromogens instead of the fluorochromes used by FISH. An advantage of CISH is that evaluation can be performed with a conventional bright-field light microscope instead of fluorescence microscopy with multiband pass filters. This allows comparison of CISH results with the tumor area routinely stained. The limitations of CISH include a relatively low number of commercially available probes and, in contrast to FISH, difficulty in evaluating more than two different probes simultaneously.[36]

FISH can also be combined with immunophenotyping, which is particularly useful in identifying the cell lineage of a cytogenetically aberrant neoplastic clone. Simultaneous fluorescence immunophenotyping (FICTION technique) allows visualization of antigen expression of cells with chromosomal aberrations directly correlating phenotypic and genotypic cell features.[37] Different studies have demonstrated the application of combining FISH and cell-sorting techniques, such as magnetic-activated cell sorting (MACS), in the diagnosis of plasma cell myeloma.[38]

Multicolor Fluorescence in Situ Hybridization Techniques

SKY and M-FISH enable the simultaneous visualization of each of 22 pairs of autosomal chromosomes and both sex chromosomes in different colors. To prepare probes used for multicolor hybridizations, flow-sorted chromosomes are labeled with one to five fluorochromes to create a unique color for each chromosome pair. In SKY, image acquisition is based on a combination of epifluorescence microscopy, charge-coupled device imaging, and Fourier spectroscopy.[39] In M-FISH, separate images are captured for each of five fluorochromes with narrow band-pass microscope filters; these images are then combined by dedicated software. Both methods have the ability to characterize complex rearrangements, define marker chromosomes, and identify cryptic translocations (Fig. 6-3).[39-41]

Multicolor images of metaphase cells hybridized with the SKY/M-FISH probe mixture are analyzed together with electronically inverted and contrast-enhanced DAPI (4′,6-diamidino-2-phenylindole) images producing G-banding–like patterns that enable specific breakpoint assignments both in interchromosomal and intrachromosomal rearrangements. The final identification of chromosome aberrations and assignment of breakpoints in structural rearrangements is based on a combination of spectral classification and G-banding (Fig. 6-4). Additional FISH experiments are often required to clarify ambiguous results, and to confirm or refute the suspected involvement of specific genes located near breakpoints in structural abnormalities. The resolution of SKY/M-FISH for the detection of interchromosomal rearrangements is between 500 and 2000 kb and depends significantly on the quality of the metaphases and the resolution of the chromosomes involved in the rearrangement. As with banding techniques, subtle, subtelomeric translocations cannot be detected by SKY or M-FISH.

Comparative Genomic Hybridization

CGH is designed to scan the entire genome for gains, losses, and amplifications.[42] In this method, test (tumor) and reference (normal) DNAs are differentially labeled and cohybridized to normal metaphase spreads (chromosomal CGH) or to microarrays (array CGH).

CGH has the advantage of requiring only tumor DNA extracted from either fresh or archived material. The reference DNA does not need to be from the same patient. The tumor DNA is usually labeled with a green fluorochrome (FITC/spectrum-green), and the reference DNA is labeled with a red fluorochrome (TRITC/spectrum-red). The differences in CN between the tumor and normal DNA are reflected by differences in green and red fluorescence along the length of the chromosome. A number of hematologic malignancies have been analyzed by chromosomal CGH to identify genomic imbalances. One valuable finding has been the identification of high-level amplification of genes such as *REL*, *MYC*, and *BCL2* in B-cell lymphomas.[43-46] The importance of gene amplification as a genetic mechanism in the biology of lymphomas remained unrecognized by studies with banding-analysis alone. A caveat related to this assay is its inability to detect balanced genomic aberrations. Moreover, to be reliably detected, a gain or loss must usually be present in at least 35%

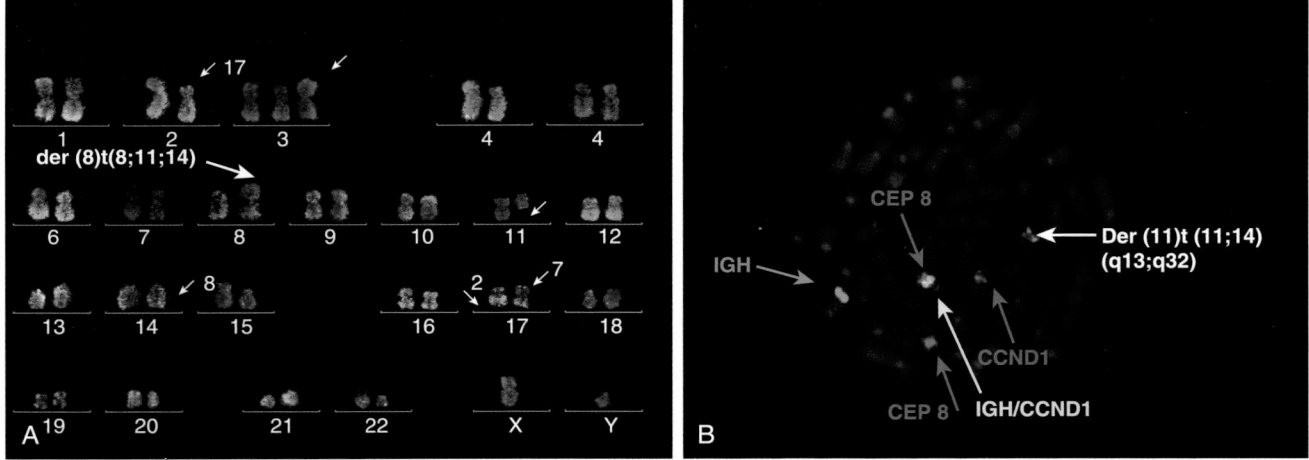

Figure 6-3. A, Multicolor fluorescence in situ hybridization (M-FISH) of a primary case of mantle cell lymphoma carrying a cryptic t(11;14)(q13;q32) translocation involving chromosome 8. The karyotype was 47,XY,t(2;17)(p11;q13)[6],+3[6],t(8;11;14)(11qter→11q13::14q32::8p11→8qter;11pte r→11q13::14q32→14qter;14pter→14q32::8p11→8pter)[6], der(17)t(7;17)(p15;p13)[6],-21[3]/46,XY[2] [cp8]. **B,** FISH demonstrating the presence of *IGH::CCND1* fusion in derivative chromosome 8. Aberrations are indicated by arrows. *(From Salaverria I, Espinet B, Carrió A, et al. Multiple recurrent chromosomal breakpoints in mantle cell lymphoma revealed by a combination of molecular cytogenetic techniques.* Genes Chromosomes Cancer. *2008;47:1086–1097.)*

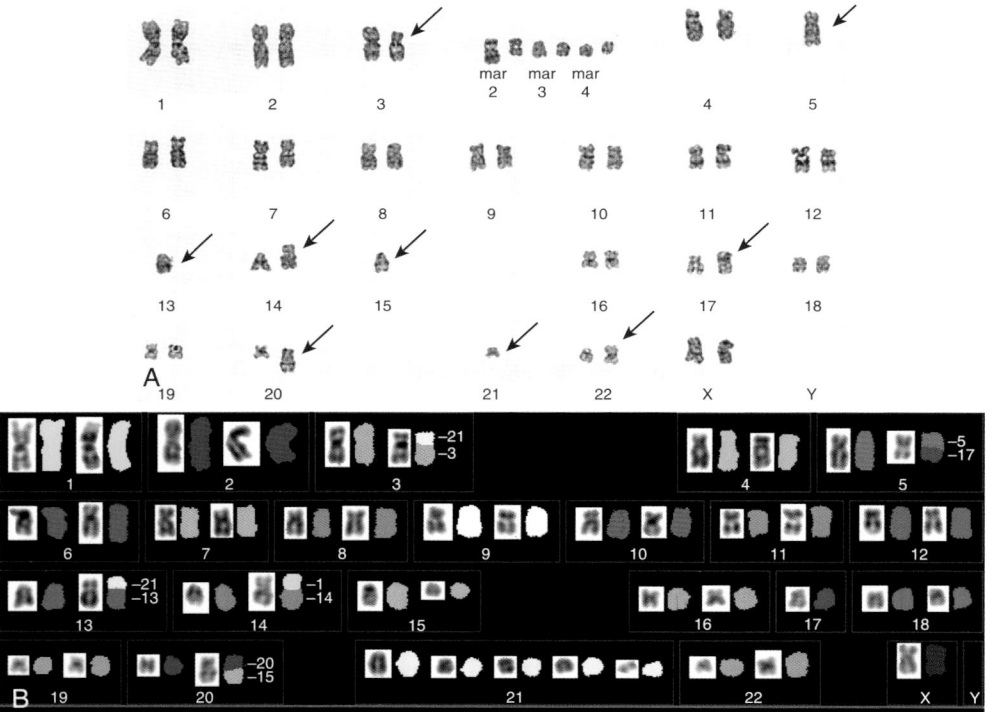

Figure 6-4. Standard cytogenetic and spectral karyotyping (SKY) analysis of a complex karyotype detected in a patient with de novo acute myeloid leukemia (AML). A, G-banded karyotype interpreted as 48,XX,del(3)(p1?1p2?1), −5, −13,add(14)(p13), −15,add(17)(p11.2),add(20) (q13.?3), −21,i(22)(q10),+mar1,+mar2,+mar3,+mar4. Arrows indicate chromosome abnormalities. **B,** Spectral karyotype from the same patient. Each chromosome is represented twice, by G-banding–like inverted and contrast-enhanced 4′,6-diamidino-2-phenylindole (DAPI)–stained image *(left)* and SKY image shown in spectra-based classification colors *(right)*. SKY enabled determination of the origin of marker chromosomes and unidentified material in unbalanced translocations. Notably, SKY revealed high-level amplification of 21q material present in der(3)t(3;21), der(13) and four marker chromosomes. The final karyotype interpretation was 48,XX,der(3)t(3;21)(p1?1;q?),der(5)t(5;17)(q11;q1?1),der(13)(21q11→21q22::13p1?1→13qter),der(1 4)t(1;14)(p32;p11),del(15)(q1?5),−17,der(20)t(15;20)(q15;q13.3),der(21)t(21;21;21), +der(21)t(21;21) x2,+ider(21)t(21;21),idic(22)(p11). Loss of one chromosome X in the depicted cell is random.

of the tumor cells, and the altered regions must be at least 10 Mb. For detection of high-level amplifications, the size of a given amplicon must amount to at least 2 Mb.[47]

Array-Based Copy Number Determination

Genetic complexity of cancer cells requires use of sensitive techniques that facilitate detection of small genomic changes in a mixed cell population and segmental regions of homozygosity. Akin to conventional CGH, CGH arrays rely on the difference in the CN between differentially labeled test and reference DNAs. The spots on the array are either DNA isolated from clones, such as bacterial artificial chromosomes (BACs) containing human genomic DNA or oligonucleotides synthesized directly on the glass slide. For the CGH array, the DNAs are directly labeled with Cy3 and Cy5 fluorescent dyes, for example, with display tumor DNA pseudocolored red and reference DNA green. Again, through competition between test and control, a scanner detects the ratios of the fluorescence intensities of both dyes at each spot.

High-density oligonucleotide arrays have improved the ability to detect gains and losses of fewer than 5 kb, thus permitting the identification of smaller amplicons and microdeletions that were previously undetectable (Fig. 6-5A).[48] Moreover, application of paired germline DNA from the same individual can exclude germline variants, and differences will reflect only somatic lesions acquired by the tumor cells. Nevertheless, one of the limitations of the CGH arrays is that they do not allow detection of regions of homozygosity. The genome-wide SNP arrays rely on oligonucleotide probes corresponding to the allelic variants of selected SNPs covering the whole genome. Hybridization of test DNA to both probe variants indicates heterozygosity, whereas the signal for only one allele is consistent with homozygosity. The fluorescence

emitted from individual probes allows the analysis of gene CN (Fig. 6-5B, *upper panel*). The major advantage of SNP arrays over other CN platforms is the ability to detect diploid stretches of homozygosity (Fig. 6-5B, *lower panel*). The detection of LOH and other chromosomal changes with large numbers of SNP markers has enabled identification of patterns of allelic imbalances with potential prognostic and diagnostic utility.

MIP technology offers a potential solution to the challenges of CN and genotype assessment in formalin-fixed paraffin embedded (FFPE)-derived DNA samples. The small intact target DNA sequence footprint required by MIP probes (~40 base pairs [bp]) makes the MIP platform well suited to work with degraded FFPE DNA.[49] The OncoScan assay uses MIP technology, which has been optimized for highly degraded FFPE samples (probe interrogation site of just 40 bp). Assay performance has been extensively validated with archived FFPE samples (10 years or older) and has been shown to be compatible with all major solid-tumor tissue types.

Application of these CN technologies, which use only single indirectly labeled tumor DNA for hybridization, has revealed that many normal CN variations occur throughout the genome within the general population.[50] Information on these regional variations must be taken into account when normal DNA from the patient whose tumor sample is tested is not available.

Although many molecular cytogenetic techniques are available, conventional cytogenetics and FISH are the most widely used techniques in the clinic (see Table 6-2). Nevertheless, CN arrays initially introduced in prenatal and postnatal diagnosis are increasingly used in the diagnosis of hematologic and oncologic disorders, especially in hematologic malignancies with a low mitotic index that does not allow conventional cytogenetics analysis. Moreover, CN arrays allow the detection of segmental regions of homozygosity and small

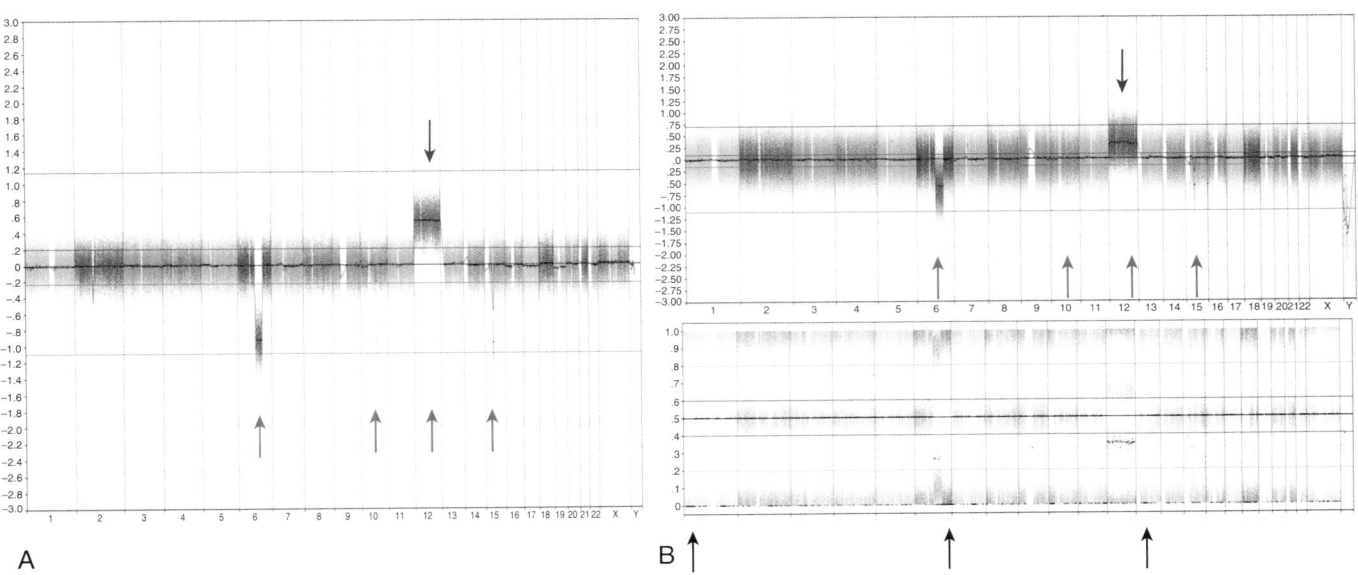

Figure 6-5. Copy number profiles for a chronic lymphocytic leukemia case analyzed by both Agilent 1M array CGH **(A)** and SNP–Array, Affymetrix 6.0 **(B)**. Data are displayed as whole-genome "rainbow" plots in which each chromosome is denoted by a different color. **B,** Copy number information *(upper panel)* and allelic ratio information *(lower panel)* are shown. Red arrows indicate losses, blue arrows indicate gains, and black arrows indicate copy-neutral loss-of-heterozygosity regions. Several types of software are available for generation of copy number profiles. In this example, Nexus BioDiscovery (El Segundo, CA) software was used to analyze both types of arrays.

genomic changes in a mixed cell population, and their use has identified novel genomic abnormalities that escaped detection with other methods. Moreover, CN arrays are a comprehensive tool for identification of chromothripsis, which requires the detection of at least seven switches between two or more CN states detected on an individual chromosome.[51,52]

Thus these array-based technologies have become a complementary tool in cases with existing cytogenetic information and are used as the diagnostic tool (together with FISH) in cases without dividing cells. CN arrays specifically designed for analyzing CN and LOH alterations on DNA from FFPE (MIP-assay) have been introduced.

Optical Genome Mapping

OGM has emerged as a robust technology to diagnose, in a single step numerical and structural, both balanced and unbalanced, chromosome aberrations.[53] This technique relies on high-throughput imaging of high molecular weight DNA (>250 Kb) fluorescently labeled at a specific 6 bp sequence motif that occurs 15 times per 100 Kb in the human genome. The unique labeling pattern allows identification of the genomic location of every molecule, generating a consensus map that can be compared with a reference genome. This approach detects both balanced and unbalanced structural variants from single molecules, from 500 bp resolution and down to 1% allele fraction. In addition, genome coverage depth information is also used for the detection of CN alterations and whole-chromosome aneuploidies. OGM does not require any cell culture before sample processing and results may be available in 4 to 6 days (the time required for the isolation and labeling of the DNA and its subsequent analysis). Several studies used OGM to analyze samples from patients with ALL,[54,55] AML,[56-59] MDS,[58-60] and CLL.[19,61] Thus, it has been suggested that OGM could replace other cytogenetic assays we described (e.g., conventional cytogenetics, FISH, and CN arrays) in the evaluation of hematologic disorders.[19,54,59] However, OGM seems to have some technical and diagnostic limitations. Because OGM uses the CN variation (CNV)-pipeline, which uses quantification of uniquely attributable genetic material to detect variants, the detection of numerical chromosomal aberrations, triploidy, and higher-order polyploidy is difficult.[53] The other important limitation is the need for a significant amount of fresh and frozen blood cells for its performance because the analysis of previously extracted DNA is not suitable.

Whole Genome Sequencing and Karyotyping

In principle, different types of whole genome sequencing (WGS) analyses ranging from shallow to full, deep genomic sequencing and short-read to long-read analyses are able to also provide a gross karyotype-like overview, with current limitations in repetitive sequence areas like centromeres.[62] Akkari et al.[63] exhaustively reviewed advantages and limitations of several novel technologies, including OGM and WGS.[62] After consideration of clinical, logistic, technical, and financial implications, the authors concluded that despite undisputable clinical usefulness of WGS, the immediate implementation of this technology by clinical laboratories worldwide is rather

unlikely. At least in the near future, standard chromosome banding analysis, FISH, and SNP arrays will remain the gold standard of cytogenetic testing in hematologic neoplasms.[63]

CLINICAL RELEVANCE OF CHROMOSOMAL ABNORMALITIES IN HEMATOLOGIC MALIGNANCIES

Detection of chromosomal abnormalities helps to identify distinct disease entities and is useful in establishing diagnosis, classification, prognostication, therapy selection, monitoring of disease progression, and evaluation of response to therapy. Several aberrations and their molecular counterparts have been included in the previous editions and the 5th edition of the WHO Classification of Hematologic Neoplasms/ Haematolymphoid Tumors and the International Consensus Classification of Leukemias and Lymphomas.[64-68] Together with morphology, immunophenotype and clinical features are used to define distinct clinical entities with unique patterns of responses to treatment (Table 6-3).[65-68] The most important aberrations will be discussed in the respective chapters. Importantly, cytogenetic investigations are a mandatory part of the diagnostic workup for patients with MDS, AML, ALL, and chronic myeloid leukemia (CML), and are strongly recommended for patients with primary myelofibrosis (PMF) according to recommendations of the National Comprehensive Cancer Network (NCCN) Clinical Practice Guidelines in Oncology[69-72] and the European LeukemiaNet (ELN).[73-76] Pretreatment karyotypic findings are among the most important independent prognostic factors in MDS,[77,78] AML,[79-83] and ALL[79,84-87] and, together with molecular genetic findings, are used to determine choice of therapy in patients with these diseases.[88-90] In CML, cytogenetic testing is also recommended for assessment of response to treatment with tyrosine kinase inhibitors along with molecular determination of BCR::ABL1 transcript levels by standardized quantitative reverse-transcription polymerase chain reaction.[72,75]

Myeloproliferative Neoplasms

Among several entities included in the *myeloproliferative neoplasms* category in the current myeloid neoplasms classifications,[66,68] only CML is strongly associated with a specific chromosome abnormality, t(9;22)(q34;q11.2), which creates the BCR::ABL1 fusion gene whose chimeric protein product is a target of therapy with tyrosine kinase inhibitors. The derivative chromosome 22 generated by the t(9;22) translocation is, for historical reasons, named the *Philadelphia chromosome* and designated as *Ph*. A vast majority of CML patients, approximately 90% to 95%, carry a standard t(9;22) translocation at diagnosis,[91] whereas in the remaining patients, BCR-ABL1 arises as a result of either three-way or even four-way variant translocations involving, respectively, one additional chromosome, for example, t(1;9;22)(p36;q34;q11.2), or two extra chromosomes, for example, t(3;17;9;22) (q26;q21;q34;q11.2); or through cryptic insertions such as ins(9;22)(q34;q11.2q11.2) or ins(22;9)(q11.2;q34q34).[92] These cryptic insertions can be detected with FISH or PCR.[75] At diagnosis, secondary abnormalities accompanying the t(9;22) translocation or variants, such as −Y, +8, i(17)(q10), +19, and +der(22)t(9;22)(q34;q11.2), are rare and are only detected

Table 6-3 Entities Within International Consensus Classification of Myeloid Neoplasms and Acute Leukemias That Are Delineated Based on the Presence of Specific Chromosome Abnormality (Part A) and Those Within the 5th Edition of the World Health Organization Classification of Haematolymphoid Tumours (Part B)

A. International Consensus Classification of Myeloid Neoplasms and Acute Leukemias

Myeloproliferative Neoplasms (MPN)

Chronic myeloid leukemia, BCR::ABL1–positive*

Myelodysplastic Syndrome (MDS)

MDS with del(5q)[†]

MDS, unclassifiable without dysplasia, −7/del(7q) or complex karyotype

Myelodysplastic/Myeloproliferative Neoplasm (MDS/MPN)

New provisional subentity: MDS/MPN with isochromosome (17q)[‡]

Acute Myeloid Leukemia (AML)[§]

Acute promyelocytic leukemia (APL) with t(15;17)(q24.1;q21.2)/PML::RARA

APL with other RARA rearrangements, including:
t(1;17)(q42.3;q21.2)/IRF2BP2::RARA; t(5;17)(q35.1;q21.2)/NPM1::RARA; t(11;17)(q23.2;q21.2)/ZBTB16::RARA; cryptic inv(17q) or del(17)(q21.2q21.2)/STAT5B::RARA, STAT3::RARA; other genes rarely rearranged with RARA::TBL1XR1 (3q26.3), FIP1L1 (4q12), BCOR (Xp11.4)

AML with t(8;21)(q22;q22)/RUNX1::RUNX1T1

AML with inv(16)(p13.1q22) or t(16;16)(p13.1;q22)/CBFB::MYH11

AML with t(9;11)(p21.3;q23.3)/MLLT3::KMT2A

AML with other KMT2A rearrangements, including:
t(4;11)(q21.3;q23.3)/AFF1::KMT2A[ǁ]; t(6;11)(q27;q23.3)/AFDN::KMT2A; t(10;11)(p12.3;q23.3)/MLLT10::KMT2A; t(10;11)(q21.3;q23.3)/TET1::KMT2A; t(11;19)(q23.3;p13.1)/KMT2A::ELL; t(11;19)(q23.3;p13.3)/KMT2A::MLLT1

AML with t(6;9)(p23.3;q34.1)/DEK::NUP214

AML with inv(3)(q21.3q26.2) or t(3;3)(q21.3;q26.2)/GATA2; MECOM(EVI)

AML with other MECOM rearrangements, including:
t(2;3)(p11~23;q26.2)/MECOM::?; t(3;8)(q26.2;q24.2)/MYC, MECOM; t(3;12)(q26.2;p13.2)/ETV6::MECOM; t(3;21)(q26.2;q22.1)/MECOM::RUNX1

AML with other rare recurring translocations, including:
t(1;3)(p36.3;q21.3)/PRDM16::RPN1; t(3;5)(q25.3;q35.1)/NPM1::MLF1; t(8;16)(p11.2;p13.3)/KAT6A::CREBBP; t(1;22)(p13.3;q13.1)/RBM15::MRTF1[ǁ]; t(5;11)(q35.2;p15.4/NUP98::NSD1[ǁ]; t(11;12)(p15.4;p13.3)/NUP98::KMD5A[ǁ]; abnormalities creating fusions involving NUP98 and other partners[ǁ]; t(7;12)(q36.3;p13.2)/ETV6::MNX1[ǁ]; t(10;11)(p12.3;q14.2)/PICALM::MLLT10; t(16;21)(p11.2;q22.2)/FUS::ERG; t(16;21)(q24.3;q22.1)/RUNX1::CBFA2T3; inv(16)(p13.3q24.3)/CBFA2T3::GLIS2[ǁ]

AML with t(9;22)(q34.1;q11.2)/BCR::ABL1[¶]

AML with myelodysplasia-related cytogenetic abnormalities[#]
Defined by the presence of a complex karyotype (≥3 unrelated clonal chromosome abnormalities in the absence of other class-defining recurring genetic abnormalities), del(5q)/t(5q)/add(5q), −7/del(7q), +8, del(12p)/t(12p)/add(12p), i(17q), −17/add(17p) or del(17p), del(20q), and/or idic(X)(q13)

B. The 5th Edition of the World Health Organization Classification of Haematolymphoid Tumors

Myeloproliferative Neoplasms

Chronic myeloid leukemia, defined by the BCR::ABL1 fusion resulting from t(9;22)(q34;q11)

Myelodysplastic Neoplasms (MDS)

MDS with low blasts and isolated 5q deletion (MDS-5q)[†]

MDS with low blasts and SF3B1 mutation (MDS-SF3B1), absence of 5q deletion; −7, or complex karyotype

AML With Defining Genetic Abnormalities

Acute promyelocytic leukemia with PML::RARA fusion

AML with RUNX1::RUNX1T1 fusion

AML with CBFB::MYH11 fusion

AML with DEK::NUP214 fusion

AML with RBM15::MRTFA fusion

AML with BCR::ABL1 fusion**

AML with KMT2A rearrangement

AML with MECOM rearrangement

AML with NUP98 rearrangement

AML with NPM1 mutation

AML with CEBPA mutation**

AML with other defined genetic alterations[††]

Table 6-3 Entities Within International Consensus Classification of Myeloid Neoplasms and Acute Leukemias That Are Delineated Based on the Presence of Specific Chromosome Abnormality (Part A) and Those Within the 5th Edition of the World Health Organization Classification of Haematolymphoid Tumours (Part B)—cont'd

AML, myelodysplasia-related[‡‡]
Defined by the presence of the following cytogenetic abnormalities: a complex karyotype (≥3 abnormalities), 5q deletion or loss of 5q because of unbalanced translocation, monosomy 7, 7q deletion, or loss of 7q caused by unbalanced translocation, 11q deletion, 12p deletion or loss of 12p because of unbalanced translocation, Monosomy 13 or 13q deletion, 17p deletion or loss of 17p caused by unbalanced translocation, Isochromosome 17q, idic(X)(q13).
Also, defined by the presence of somatic mutations in the following genes: *ASXL1, BCOR, EZH2, SF3B1, SRSF2, TAG2, U2AF1* and/or *ZRSR2*.

*In approximately 90% to 95% of patients, *BCR::ABL1* fusion is created by t(9;22)(q34;q11.2), whereas the remaining cases harbor three- or four-way balanced translocations invariably involving chromosomes 9 and 22 and one or two other chromosomes, or carry cryptic insertions or translocations between chromosomes 9 and 22.
†del(5q) can be accompanied by one additional abnormality, with the exception of –7/del(7q).
‡i(17q) can occur with one other additional abnormality other than –7/del(7q).
§≥10% of blasts are required for diagnosis of most listed categories, unless indicated otherwise.
¶≥20% of blasts are required for diagnosis. The category of "MDS/AML" will not be used for AML with *BCR::ABL1* because of its overlap with progression of *BCR::ABL1*-positive CML.
‖Occurs predominantly in infants and children.
#Patients with ≥20% of blasts are diagnosed with AML and those with 10% to 19% of blasts with MDS/AML.
**At least 20% blasts are required for diagnosis.
††At present, subtypes under this heading include AML with rare genetic fusions.
‡‡To diagnose AML, myelodysplasia-related in patients with 20% of blasts in their bone marrow or blood, the presence of at least one of the listed cytogenetic or molecular abnormalities and/or history of myelodysplastic or myeloproliferative neoplasm are required.
Data from Arber et al.[66] and Khoury et al.[68]

Table 6-4 Most Common Recurrent Balanced Chromosome Aberrations in Myelodysplastic Syndromes

Chromosome Abnormality	% of Patients With the Abnormality as the Sole Chromosome Aberration (No. With Sole Aberration/ Total No. of Patients)	Chromosome Abnormality	% of Patients With the Abnormality as the Sole Chromosome Aberration (No. With Sole Aberration/ Total No. of Patients)
Balanced Structural Abnormalities			
t(1;3)(p36.3;q21.1)	67% (14/21)	t(6;9)(p23;q34)	100% (8/8)
t(3;21)(q26.2;q22.1)	36% (10/28)	t(2;11)(p21;q23)	28% (5/18)
inv(3)(q21q26.2)	47% (23/49)	t(9;11)(p22;q23)	83% (5/6)
t(3;3)(q21;q26.2)	30% (7/23)	t(11;16)(q23;p13.3)	75% (3/4)
t(3;12)(q26;p13)	33% (2/6)		
t(3;8)(q26;q24)	29% (4/14)		

Data from the Mitelman Database,[92] which consisted of 4846 patients with myelodysplastic syndromes and abnormal karyotype as of October 17, 2022.

in approximately 5% to 10% of patients.[93-95] However, their presence has been reported to represent a poor prognostic factor in patients treated with imatinib because patients who harbored any secondary abnormality had lower overall cytogenetic and molecular response rates and longer time to response to therapy.[95] Patients who had the so-called *major route abnormalities*, that is, +8, i(17)(q10), +19 and +der(22)t(9;22), also had significantly shorter progression-free and overall survival (OS).[94] Acquisition of chromosomal abnormalities, especially the major route ones, in a clone with a t(9;22) translocation during therapy with tyrosine kinase inhibitors (i.e., clonal cytogenetic evolution) indicates disease acceleration[75] and has been associated with shorter OS in patients receiving imatinib.[96] On the other hand, clonal chromosome aberrations, most often –Y and +8, occurring in cells without the t(9;22) translocation in 5% to 10% of CML patients during treatment with a tyrosine kinase inhibitor, appear not to affect patient outcomes. However, acquisition of –7 has been linked to increased risk for developing MDS or AML,[97] thus indicating the need for more-frequent cytogenetic monitoring of such patients.

Myelodysplastic Syndromes

General Cytogenetic Features

Clonal chromosome abnormalities are found in approximately 52% of patients diagnosed with de novo MDS,[98] but their frequency is higher, 76% to 97%, in treatment-related MDS and AML.[99] The frequencies of abnormal karyotypes in larger series of MDS patients have varied between 38% and 73%,[98] likely because the proportions of patients with particular subtypes of MDS included in these studies differed, as does the incidence of abnormal karyotypes among specific MDS entities.[98]

Cytogenetically, MDS is very heterogeneous, with over 100 chromosome aberrations hitherto recognized as recurrent,[92] but the involvement of specific chromosomes in structural and numerical abnormalities is highly non-random. Tables 6-4 and 6-5 contain lists of the most frequent of these recurrent abnormalities. Balanced rearrangements, such as t(1;3) (p36.3;q21.1), inv(3)(q21q26.2)/t(3;3)(q21;q26.2), t(3;21) (q26.2;q22.1), t(6;9)(p23;q34), and translocations involving the *KMT2A* gene—t(2;11)(p21;q23), t(9;11)(p22;q23), and (11;16)(q23;p13.3)—are relatively rare, and each of them have also been reported in AML (Table 6-4). A vast majority of cytogenetically abnormal MDS patients carry unbalanced abnormalities: deletions, most commonly of 5q, 20q, 7q, 11q, 13q, and 12p; unbalanced translocations, such as der(1;7)(q10;p10) that result in simultaneous 7q loss and 1q gain; isochromosomes, such as i(17)(q10), idic(X)(q13) or i(14)(q10); and whole-chromosome gains (e.g., +8, +21, and +11) and/or losses (e.g., –7, –5, –Y, and –X) (Table 6-5).[92]

Table 6-5 Most Common Recurrent Unbalanced Chromosome Aberrations in Myelodysplastic Syndromes

Unbalanced Structural Abnormality	Unbalanced Structural Abnormality
der(1;7)(q10;p10)	del(9)(q13-22)
dup(q12-32q24-44)	del(11)(q11-24q22-25)
del(3)(p21)	del(12)(p11-13p11-p13)
del(3)(q21)	del(13)(q11-22q14-34)
del(4)(q21-31)	i(14)(q10)
del(5)(q11-31q31-q35)	del(17)(p11-13p13)
dic(5;17)(q11;p11)	i(17)(q10)*
der(5)t(5;17)(q11-21;q11-21)†	del(20)(q11-13q12-13)
del(6)(q13-21q23-24)	idic(X)(q13)
del(7)(q11-34q22-36)	

Numerical Abnormality: Trisomy	Numerical Abnormality: Trisomy
+2	+14
+6	+15
+8	+19
+9	+21
+11	

Numerical Abnormality: Chromosome Loss	Numerical Abnormality: Chromosome Loss
−5	−X
−7	−Y

*Also described as der(17)t(5;17)(p11-12;p11-13) or der(5;17)(p10;q10).
†Includes a very similar idic(17)(p11).
Data from the Mitelman Database,[92] which consisted of 4846 patients with MDS and abnormal karyotype as of October 17, 2022.

Associations Between Cytogenetic Findings and Clinical Outcome of Myelodysplastic Syndrome Patients

Pretreatment karyotypic findings in MDS patients have been repeatedly associated with both survival and risk for evolution to AML.[77,78,98,100-103] Several recurring abnormalities and a normal karyotype have been incorporated into scoring systems for evaluation of prognosis for MDS patients, which also include hematologic and clinical features in addition to karyotype.[102,103] Introduced in 2012, the Revised International Prognostic Scoring System (IPSS-R)[78] categorizes cytogenetics into five prognostic subgroups: "very good" indicates an isolated −Y and del(11q) (score value 0); "good" indicates a normal karyotype, isolated del(5q), del(12p), del(20q), and two cytogenetic abnormalities that include del(5q) (score 1); "intermediate" indicates isolated del(7q), +8, +19, i(17)(q10) or any other single- or double-chromosome abnormalities (score 2); "poor" indicates isolated −7, inv(3)(q21q26.2)/t(3;3) (q21;q26.2), del(3q), two chromosome abnormalities that include −7/del(7q), and a complex karyotype with three abnormalities (score 3); and "very poor" indicates a complex karyotype with four or more abnormalities (score 4).[103] The other prognostic variables included in the IPSS-R are percent of bone marrow blasts (scores from 0 to 3), hemoglobin level (scores 0 to 1.5), platelets (scores 0 to 1), and absolute neutrophil counts (scores 0 to 0.5). By combining the risk scores for cytogenetic subgroup, bone marrow blast percentage, and cytopenias, MDS patients can be stratified into five risk groups as follows: "very low," overall score ≤1.5; "low," score >1.5 to 3; "intermediate," score >3 to 4.5; "high," score >4.5 to 6; and "very high," score >6. The respective median survival

times of patients classified into these risk groups in the study by Greenberg and colleagues[103] were as follows: "very low," 8.8 years; "low," 5.3 years; "intermediate," 3 years; "high," 1.6 years; and "very high," 0.8 years. The times for 25% of the patients to undergo evolution to AML were: "very low," >14.5 (median not reached) years; "low," 10.8 years; "intermediate," 3.2 years; "high," 1.4 years; and "very high," 0.7 years.[103]

The usefulness of the IPSS-R in predicting clinical outcome in MDS patients has been tested and confirmed by several studies,[104-106] including a study of MDS patients who received allogeneic stem cell transplantation.[106] Two of these studies[104,105] found IPSS-R to have better predictive power than the earlier IPSS system.[101] This, in part, has been attributed to refinements in cytogenetic categorization of MDS and increasing the effect of cytogenetics within IPSS-R.[103]

Acute Myeloid Leukemia

General Cytogenetic Characteristics

Pretreatment cytogenetic analysis of bone marrow or blood detects clonal chromosome abnormalities in 55% to 60% of adults[79-82] and 76% to 78% of children[107,108] with AML, with the remaining patients having an entirely normal karyotype, that is, cytogenetically normal AML (CN-AML). Moreover, the frequencies of specific chromosome abnormalities differ between adult and childhood AML. For example, balanced rearrangements involving 11q23/KMT2A are four times less common in adults than in children,[79] and their incidence decreases with age from approximately 50% in infants younger than 1 year[109] to approximately 40% in children age 1 to 2 years,[110] approximately 9% in older children,[110] approximately 4% of adults in general,[79,82] to less than or equal to 3% of patients older than 60 years.[111,112] Similarly, a cryptic t(5;11)(q35;p15)/NUP98::NSD1 is seven times less frequent in adults than in children,[113] and a rare t(1;22) (p13;q13)/RBM15::MRTFA translocation does not occur in adults at all, being found mostly in children younger than 2 years.[114] On the other hand, inv(3)(q21q26.2) and t(3;3) (q21;q26.2) are almost never found in childhood AML,[107,108] and del(5q) and other abnormalities resulting in loss of 5q, and complex karyotype with greater than or equal to five aberrations, are more frequent in adults than in children.[79]

Cytogenetically, AML is a remarkably heterogeneous disease, with greater than 300 recurrent abnormalities identified to date.[92] Aberrations that are sometimes found as sole chromosome alterations and are infrequently (or never) detected in other hematologic neoplasms or solid tumors are considered to be primary abnormalities that play an important role in leukemogenesis and often heavily influence clinical characteristics of patients carrying them.[79] The more common presumed primary structural aberrations are listed in Tables 6-6 and 6-7. They include balanced abnormalities (i.e., reciprocal translocations, inversions, and insertions) (see Table 6-6) and those unbalanced ones (deletions, isochromosomes, and unbalanced translocations) that have been recurrently observed as the only chromosome aberrations (see Table 6-7). Numerical aberrations can also be considered to be of primary importance when they are found as the sole alteration. The most frequent sole trisomy is +8, detected in approximately 4% of AML patients, followed by +11, +13, +21, and +4, whereas the most common sole monosomy is −7, followed by −Y.

Table 6-6 More Frequent Balanced Chromosome Abnormalities With Presumed Primary Significance in AML and the Associated Non-random Secondary Aberrations

Chromosome Abnormality	Gene(s) Rearranged	% of Patients With the Abnormality as the Sole Chromosome Aberration (No. With Sole Abnormality/ Total No. of Patients)	Recurring Secondary Abnormalities*
t(1;3)(p36.3;q21.1)	RPN1::PRDM16	61% (34/56)	del(5q)
t(1;22)(p13;q13)	RBM15::MRTFA	63% (40/64)	+19
t(2;3)(p15-21;q26-27)	MECOM	38% (8/21)	−7
inv(3)(q21q26.2)	GATA2::MECOM RPN1::MECOM	35% (137/391)	−7
t(3;3)(q21;q26.2)†	GATA2::MECOM RPN1::MECOM	41% (70/170)	−7
t(3;12)(q26;p13)	ETV6::MECOM	62% (28/45)	−7
t(3;21)(q26.2;q22)	RUNX1::MECOM or RUNX1::RPL22P1	44% (31/70)	−7
t(3;5)(q25;q34)‡	MLF1::NPM1	80% (62/78)	+8
t(6;9)(p23;q34)	DEK::NUP214	72% (84/116)	None
t(5;11)(q35;p15)	NUP98::NSD1 or STIM1::NSD1	69% (29/42)	del(9q) and +8
t(7;11)(p15;p15)	HOXA9::NUP98 or HOXA11::NUP98 or HOA13::NUP98	78% (62/79)	None
t(8;16)(p11;p13)	KAT6A::CREBBP	58% (86/148)	None
t(9;22)(q34;q11.2)	BCR::ABL1	44% (133/302)	−7, +8 and +der(22)t(9;22)
t(8;21)(q22;q22)	RUNX1::RUNX1T1	42% (743/1768)	−Y§, −X‖ and del(9q)
t(10;11)(p11-15;q13-23)	MLLT10::PICALM	49% (44/89)	+4
t(1;11)(q21;q23)	MLLT11::KMT2A	71% (22/31)	+19
t(2;11)(p21;q23)	KMT2A	50% (13/26)	del(5q)
t(4;11)(q21;q23)	KMT2A::AFF1	49% (10/39)	+8
t(6;11)(q27;q23)	KMT2A::AFDN	81% (96/118)	None
t(9;11)(p22;q23)	KMT2A::MLLT3	67% (310/462)	+8
ins(10;11)(p11-13; q23q13-25)	KMT2A::MLLT10	45% (15/33)	+8
t(10;11)(p11-13;q23)	KMT2A::MLLT10	48% (29/60)	+8
t(11;17)(q23;q12-21)	KMT2A::MLLT6	81% (54/67)	+8
t(11;17)(q23;q25)	KMT2A::SEPT9	67% (30/45)	+8
t(11;19)(q23;p13.1)	KMT2A::ELL	85% (58/69)	None
t(11;19)(q23;p13.3)	KMT2A::MLLT1	40% (19/47)	+8
t(4;12)(q11-12;p13)	CHIC2::ETV6	71% (22/31)	−7
t(7;12)(q36;p13)	MNX1::ETV6	7% (2/29)	+19 and +8
t(12;22)(p12-13;q11-13)	ETV6::MN1	21% (6/29)	+8 and −7
t(15;17)(q22;q12-21)¶	PML::RARA	70% (966/1380)	+8
inv(16)(p13.1q22)	MYH11::CBFB	68% (682/1003)	+22 and +8
t(16;16)(p13.1;q22)	MYH11::CBFB	83% (43/52)	+22
inv(16)(p13q24)#	CBFA2T3::GLIS2	69% (22/32)	None
t(16;21)(q24;q22)	CBFA2T3::RUNX1	29% (9/31)	+8
t(16;21)(p11;q22)	FUS::ERG	67% (42/63)	+10

*Only those secondary abnormalities that occur in ≥10% of patients with a given primary abnormality are listed.
†This abnormality was also interpreted as ins(3;3)(q21;q21q26).
‡This translocation was also reported as t(3;5)(q21;q31).
§−Y is detected in approximately 60% of male patients with t(8;21).
¶The breakpoints in t(15;17) have been variously assigned to 15q22 or 15q24, and to 17q11, 17q12, 17q21, or 17q22.
‖−X is detected in approximately 33% of female patients with t(8;21).
#This abnormality is cryptic, and the Mitelman Database[92] does not list individual patients with this inversion. The numbers provided are from Masetti et al.[148] and Gruber et al.[147]
AML, Acute myeloid leukemia.
Data from the Mitelman Database,[92] which consisted of 21,062 patients with AML and abnormal karyotype as of October 17, 2022.

Primary abnormalities can be accompanied by secondary chromosome changes, which are generally less specific, are usually unbalanced, and can occur together with several distinct primary aberrations in AML or even with primary aberrations in other leukemia types or non-hematologic malignant disorders.[79] The most widespread secondary change is +8, which can be recurrently found in AML patients with t(3;5)(q25;q34), t(5;11)(q35;p15), t(9;22)(q34;q11.2), t(12;22)(p12-13;q11-13), t(15;17)(q22;q12-21), inv(16)(p13.1q22), t(16;21)(q24;q22), and these rearrangements involving 11q23/*KMT2A*: t(4;11) (q21;q23), t(9;11)(p22;q23), ins(10;11)(p11-13;q23q13-25), t(10;11)(p11-13;q23), t(11;17)(q23;q12-21), t(11;17) (q23;q25), and t(11;19)(q23;p13.3) (Table 6-6), as well as in patients diagnosed with MDS, ALL, lymphoma, and solid tumors.[92] As shown in Table 6-6, secondary abnormalities accompany some primary changes more often than others. For example, at least one secondary alteration is detected in 60% to 70% of patients with inv(3)(q21q26.2)/t(3;3)(q21;q26.2), t(8;21)(q22;q22), or t(9;22)(q34;q11.2), whereas this is the case in only approximately one-third of patients with t(15;17)

Table 6-7 Unbalanced Chromosome Abnormalities With Presumed Primary Significance in Acute Myeloid Leukemia

Chromosome Abnormality	Chromosome Abnormality
Resulting in Loss of a Chromosomal Segment	
del(1)(p12-34p34-36)	del(9)(q11-34q12-34)
del(1)(q12-32q25-44)	del(11)(p11-14p13-15)
del(2)(p11-23p13-25)	del(11)(q13-23q22-25)
del(2)(q11-34q13-37)	del(12)(p11-13p12-13)
del(3)(p11-25p14-26)	del(13)(q11-22q14-34)
del(3)(q11-27q21-29)	del(15)(q11-22q14-34)
del(5)(q12-31q31-35)	del(16)(q12-22q21-24)
del(6)(p12-p22p23-25)	del(17)(p11-13p12-13)
del(6)(q13-24-q21-27)	del(17)(q11-23q21-25)
del(7)(p11-21p14-22)	del(20)(q11-13q12-13)
del(7)(q11-34q22-36)	del(21)(q11-22q21-q22)
del(8)(q11-24q22-24)	del(22)(q11-13q13)
del(9)(p11-22p13-24)	del(X)(q13-24q24-28)
Resulting in Gain of a Chromosomal Segment	
dup(q11-32q24-44)	+i(4)(p10)
+i(q10)	+i(12)(p10)
Resulting in Both Loss and Gain of a Chromosomal Segment	
der(1;7)(q10;p10)	der(16)t(1;16)(q21-32;p13)
i(7)(p10)	der(16)t(1;16)(q11-25;q11-24)
i(7)(q10)	i(17)(q10)
der(13)t(1;13)(q11-24;p11-13)	i(21)(q10)
i(13)(q10)	idic(X)(q13)
i(14)(q10)	

Only aberrations reported as the only chromosome alterations in at least three patients with AML are included.
Data from the Mitelman Database,[92] which comprised 21,062 patients with AML and abnormal karyotype as of October 17, 2022.

(q22;q12-21), t(16;21)(p11;q22), or inv(16)(p13.1q22), and in approximately 15% of patients with t(3;5)(q25;q34), t(6;9) (p23;q34), t(6;11)(q27;q23), t(7;11)(p15;p15), or t(11;19) (q23;p13.1).

Correlations Between Cytogenetic Findings and Clinical Outcome of Patients With Acute Myeloid Leukemia

Large collaborative studies conclusively showed that pretreatment cytogenetic findings constitute one of the most important independent determinants for attainment of complete remission (CR), and duration of disease-free survival (DFS) and OS in AML patients,[80-82,107,108,111,112] and proposed prognostic classifications assigning AML patients into favorable, intermediate, or unfavorable risk groups based on the pretreatment karyotype (Table 6-8). Although there are some differences among these classifications, several chromosome abnormalities are almost uniformly assigned to these categories: favorable-risk, for example, t(15;17), t(8;21) and inv(16)/t(16;16); intermediate-risk, for example, –Y, +8; and adverse-risk, for example, inv(3) or t(3;3), –7, and a complex karyotype.

Acute Promyelocytic Leukemia With *PML::RARA* Fusion/t(15;17)(q22-24.1;q21.2) or With Variant *RARA* Rearrangements

Currently, the most prognostically favorable subset of AML is acute promyelocytic leukemia (APL) with the *PML::RARA* fusion/t(15;17) because the use of targeted treatment regimens containing all-*trans*-retinoic acid

(ATRA) and/or arsenic trioxide (ATO) result in CR rates of 85% to 100% and a cure rate of up to 97% in studies.[115] It is important to determine whether the newly diagnosed APL patient carries the most common t(15;17)/*PML::RARA* or any of the rare variant *RARA* rearrangements, in which chromosomes other than chromosome 15 are involved, for example, t(1;17)(q42;q21)/*IRF2BP2::RARA*, t(3;17) (q26;q21)/*TBL1XR1::RARA* or *FNDC3B::RARA*, t(4;17) (q12;q21)/*FIP1L1-RARA*; t(5;17)(q35;q21)/*NPM1::RARA*, t(11;17)(q23;q21)/*ZBTB16::RARA*, t(11;17)(q13;q12-21)/ *NUMA1::RARA*, t(X;17)(p11.4;q21)/*BCOR::RARA*, or a submicroscopic rearrangement of chromosome 17 resulting in the *STAT5B::RARA* fusion.[89,92] ATRA has been effective in patients with the classic t(15;17)/*PML::RARA* and in patients with variant fusions between *RARA* and the *BCOR*, *FIP1L1*, *FNDC3B*, *IRF2BP2*, *NPM1*, *NUMA1*, and *PRKAR1A* genes.[116] In contrast, patients with t(11;17)(q23;q21)/*ZBTB16::RARA*, t(3;17)(q26;q21)/*TBL1XR1::RARA* and *STAT5B::RARA* are resistant to ATRA and have a poorer prognosis. Moreover, thus far only APL with the *PML::RARA*, *TBL1XR1::RARA*, *IRF2BP2::RARA*, *PRKAR1A::RARA*, and *FNDC3B::RARA* fusions have been responsive to treatment with ATO.[116] The presence of abnormalities secondary to t(15;17) does not seem to affect patient prognosis,[82] although in two studies,[117,118] a complex karyotype with ≥3 aberrations was associated with a lower CR rate[117] and shorter event-free survival (EFS)[118] and OS[117] in patients with APL treated with regimens containing ATO.

"Core Binding Factor" Acute Myeloid Leukemia With *RUNX1::RUNX1T1* Fusion/t(8;21)(q22;q22.1) or *CBFB::MYH11* Fusion/inv(16)(p13.1q22)/t(16;16) (p13.1;q22)

Two abnormalities consistently associated with a relatively favorable prognosis,[80-82,119-122] especially when repetitive cycles of high-dose cytarabine are administered as postremission therapy,[123,124] are t(8;21)(q22;q22.1) and inv(16)(p13.1q22)/t(16;16)(p13.1;q22). They are related at the molecular level because the former disrupts the *RUNX1* gene and the latter the *CBFB* gene encoding the α and β subunits, respectively, of the core binding factor (CBF) complex, a heterodimeric transcription factor regulating transcription of genes encoding proteins involved in hematopoietic differentiation. Patients with either cytogenetic rearrangement have similar, high CR rates of 85% to 89% and cure rates of 55% to 60%,[121,122] and their prognosis can be further improved by the addition of dasatinib, a multikinase inhibitor, to intensive chemotherapy.[125,126] The clinical outcome of t(8;21)-positive patients does not seem to be affected by secondary aberrations, whereas in inv(16)/t(16;16)-positive patients, +22 has been associated with a lower relapse risk, longer OS, and, in patients with internal tandem duplication of the *FLT3* gene (*FLT3*-ITD), lengthened relapse-free survival (RFS) and +8 with a shorter OS.[121,122,127] In both cytogenetic types of CBF-AML, *KIT* mutations have been demonstrated to constitute a poor prognostic factor.[128,129]

Acute Myeloid Leukemia With *DEK::NUP214* Fusion/t(6;9)(p23.3;q34.1) or With *MECOM* Rearrangement/inv(3)(q21.3q26.2)/t(3;3) (q21.3;q26.2)

Two other rearrangements that denote specific entities within the category of "Acute myeloid leukemia with defining

Table 6-8 Prognostic Categorizations of Cytogenetic Findings by Main Collaborative Studies of Adult Acute Myeloid Leukemia and by the 2022 European LeukemiaNet Classification

Cytogenetic Risk Group	Younger Adult Patients*		Older Adult Patients†			Adults, No Age Limit Specified‡			
	SWOG/ECOG‡,80	MRC82	MRC119	AMLSG112	Eleven Italian Centers120	CALGB§,81 — CR Rate	CALGB§,81 — CIR	CALGB§,81 — OS	ELN#,73
Favorable	t(15;17), t(8;21) [if del(9q) or complex karyotype not present], inv(16)/t(16;16)/ del(16q)	t(15;17), t(8;21), inv(16)/t(16;16)	t(15;17), t(8;21), inv(16)/t(16;16)	t(15;17), inv(16)/t(16;16)	t(8;21), inv(16)/t(16;16)	t(8;21), inv(16)/t(16;16)		t(8;21), inv(16)/t(16;16), del(9q)¶	t(8;21), inv(16)/t(16;16)
Intermediate	Normal karyotype, +6, +8, −Y, del(12p)	Normal karyotype, Abnormalities other than favorable or adverse	Normal karyotype, +8 sole, abnl(11q23), abnls other than favorable or adverse	Normal karyotype, t(8;21), t(11q23),+8 within a non-complex karyotype, and +11 within a non-complex karyotype	Normal karyotype, abnl(11q23), +8, del(7q), "other numerical," "other structural"	Normal karyotype, −Y, del(5q), t(6;9), t(6;11), −7, loss of 7q, +8 sole, +8 with 1 other abnl, del(9q), t(9;11), del(11q), +11, t(11;19) (q23;p13.1), +13, del(20q), +21		Normal karyotype, −Y, del(5q), t(9;11), del(9q), +8 sole, +8 with 1 other abnl, +11, +13	t(9;11) (p22;q23), abnls other than favorable or adverse
Adverse	−5/del(5q), −7/ del(7q), abnl(3q), abnl(9q), abnl(11q), abnl(20q), abnl(21q), abnl(17p), t(6;9), t(9;22), complex karyotype (≥3 abnl)	abnl(3q) [excluding t(3;5)], inv(3)/t(3;3), add(5q)/del(5q)/−5, add(7q)/del(7q)/−7 (excluding patients with favorable karyotype), t(6;11), t(10;11), t(11q23) [excluding t(9;11) and t(11;19)], t(9;22), −17/ abnl(17p), complex karyotype (≥4 abnl, excluding patients with favorable or adverse changes)	−7,del(5q)/−5, abnormal (3q) alone and in combination with up to 3 other cytogenetic abnormalities; complex karyotype (≥5 abnl)	+4, +14, +21, +22, del(5q)/−5, abnl(12p), del(13q), −17/ del(17p), −18, −20/del(20q), complex karyotype [≥3 abnl, in the absence of t(8;21), t(11q23), t(15;17), or inv(16)/t(16;16)]	del(5q), −7, abnl(3) (q21q26), t(6;9) complex karyotype (>3 unrelated cytogenetic abnormalities)	−7, +21, complex karyotype [≥3 abnl, excluding patients with t(8;21), inv(16)/t(16;16) or t(9;11)]		inv(3) or t(3;3), t(6;9), t(6;11), −7, +8 sole, +8 with 1 other with t(11;19) (q23;p13.1), complex karyotype [≥3 abnl, excluding patients with t(8;21), inv(16)/t(16;16) or t(9;11)]	inv(3)/t(3;3), t(6;9), t(v;11) (v; q23) [excluding t(9;11)], t(9;22), t(8;16), t(3;v) (q26.2;v), −5 or del(5q), −7, −17 or abnl(17p), complex karyotype,** monosomal karyotype††

*The SWOG/ECOG study[80] included patients between 15 and 55 years of age, and the MRC study[82] included patients between 16 and 59 years.

†The MRC study[119] included patients aged between 44 and 91 years (median age, 66 years), and the AMLSG study[112] included patients older than 60 years.

‡All abnormalities that are not listed were considered to have unknown risk.

§Abnormalities not specified as conferring favorable, intermediate, or adverse risk were not included in the risk-assessment model.

¶Favorable for a group of 13 patients with del(9q) that included 6 who underwent transplantation off-protocol; intermediate for nontransplanted patients treated with chemotherapy only.

#In addition to cytogenetic findings, 2022 ELN classification uses these molecular genetic alterations (irrespective of cytogenetic findings) to categorize patients as follows: mutated NPM1 without FLT3-ITD or bZIP in-frame mutated CEBPA into a favorable group; wild-type NPM1 with FLT3-ITD or mutated NPM1 with FLT3-ITD into an intermediate group; and mutated ASXL1, BCOR, EZH2, RUNX1, SF3B1, SRSF2, STAG2, U2AF1, or ZRSR2 (unless they coexist with favorable-risk AML subtype) and mutated TP53 at a variant allele fraction of ≥10%.

**Defined as ≥3 unrelated chromosome abnormalities in the absence of other class-defining recurring genetic abnormalities, [73] excludes hyperdiploid karyotypes with ≥3 trisomies (or polysomies) in the absence of structural abnormalities.

††Defined as a karyotype with ≥2 autosomal monosomies or one autosomal monosomy and ≥1 structural chromosome abnormality other than inv(16)/t(16;16) or t(8;21).

abnl, Abnormality; AMLSG, German-Austrian Acute Myeloid Leukemia Study Group; CALGB, Cancer and Leukemia Group B; CIR, cumulative incidence of relapse; CR, complete remission; ECOG, Eastern Cooperative Oncology Group; ELN, European LeukemiaNet; FLT3-ITD, internal tandem duplication of the FLT3 gene; MRC, Medical Research Council; OS, overall survival; SWOG, Southwest Oncology Group.

genetic abnormalities" are t(6;9)(p23.3;q34.1)/*DEK::NUP214* and MECOM rearrangements by inv(3)(q21.3q26.2)/ t(3;3)(q21.3;q26.2), which portend a very poor prognosis.[80-82,120,130,131] In approximately 85% of patients with t(6;9), the translocation is an isolated cytogenetic aberration, but in two-thirds of the patients it is accompanied by a molecular alteration—the *FLT3*-ITD, a known adverse prognostic factor in AML.[130,131] Nevertheless, the presence or absence of *FLT3*-ITD does not appear to influence a very poor outcome of both adults and children treated with chemotherapy.[130,131] However, patient prognosis can be improved by allogeneic stem cell transplantation,[132,133] which also seems to be the only treatment option for patients with inv(3)/t(3;3),[134] whose clinical outcome has been dismal regardless of the presence of –7, a secondary abnormality present in approximately 50% of patients (Table 6-6). However, in one study, patients with –7 fared even poorer than those without.[135]

Acute Myeloid Leukemia With *BCR::ABL1* Fusion/t(9;22)(q34.1;q11.2)

A poor clinical outcome has also been associated with AML with t(9;22)(q34.1;q11.2)/*BCR::ABL1*.[80,82] To date, a diagnosis of AML in patients carrying the t(9;22) translocation has been somewhat controversial because such patients often are considered to suffer not from AML but CML in myeloid blast phase, occurring after an unrecognized chronic phase. Careful comparisons of clinical, cytogenetic, and molecular genetic characteristics of patients with t(9;22)-positive AML and those with CML in myeloid blast crisis revealed several features that help distinguish both entities.[136-138] In contrast to patients with CML, AML patients had a higher percentage of blood blasts[137]; had less likely splenomegaly or peripheral basophilia; rarely[136] or never[137,138] had major route secondary abnormalities characteristic for CML blast phase, but sometimes had abnormalities of chromosome 7 [–7/del(7q)][136]; and occasionally had *NPM1* mutations (~20%),[137] a cryptic gain of chromosomal material from 19p,[138] frequent loss of the *IKZF1* and/or *CDKN2A* genes, cryptic deletions within the immunoglobulin (IG) and TR genes, and a specific genome signature.[138] Recognition of AML with t(9;22)/*BCR::ABL1* is important because of the availability of targeted therapy with tyrosine kinase inhibitors.

Acute Myeloid Leukemia With a Complex Karyotype

Another cytogenetic subset consistently associated with a very poor prognosis is a complex karyotype, found in 10% to 12% of all AML patients (if complex karyotype is defined as ≥3 aberrations), or in 8% to 9% (if defined as ≥5 aberrations).[9] Patients with a complex karyotype had CR rates between 10% and 40% and 5-year OS rates of less than 10%.[9] Notably, *complex karyotype* was defined differently among studies, as ≥5 unrelated chromosome abnormalities,[119] >3 abnormalities,[120] ≥4 abnormalities after exclusion of specific aberrations that confer favorable or adverse prognosis[82] or ≥3 abnormalities, usually excluding t(8;21), inv(16)/t(16;16), and t(15;17).[80,81,112] Complex karyotypes can comprise various numbers of chromosome aberrations in individual patients that occasionally may reach approximately 30, but the occurrence of particular structural and numerical abnormalities is not random.[9] Balanced rearrangements are rare, and most aberrations are unbalanced, leading to loss of

chromosome material, most often from chromosome arms (in decreasing order) 5q, 17p, 7q, 18q, 16q, 17q, 12p, 20q, 18p, and 3p. Less frequent recurrent gains, often hidden in marker chromosomes or partially identified abnormalities, mainly involve 8q, 11q, 21q, 22q, 1p, 9p, and 13q.[9] Approximately 5% of complex karyotype patients have only numerical abnormalities (e.g., +8, +13, +21, +14, +10, and +19), and such patients were reported to have had better OS than patients with a hyperdiploid complex karyotype with one or more structural abnormalities.[139] Moreover, a study designated complex karyotypes with loss of 5q, 7q, and/or 17p as typical, and complex karyotypes with ≥3 abnormalities that do not include loss of 5q, 7q, and/or 17p as atypical, and demonstrated that both pretreatment characteristics and outcomes differ between patients with these two complex karyotype subtypes.[10] Patients with the atypical complex karyotype were younger, had higher white blood cell (WBC) counts and percentages of bone marrow and blood blasts, carried *TP53* mutations less often (10% versus 67%), and more often had tyrosine kinase domain mutations in the *FLT3* gene (*FLT3*-TKD) and mutations in the *MED12*, *NPM1* and *PHF6* genes than those with the atypical complex karyotype. Relevantly, the former had higher CR rates and longer OS.[10]

Although the molecular consequences of most chromosome alterations found in AML patients with complex karyotypes are still not well-characterized, the association between 17p abnormalities and loss of and/or mutations in the *TP53* gene is well-documented.[140] The presence of *TP53* alterations makes the dismal clinical outcome of patients with a complex karyotype even worse, and it was associated with significantly lower CR rates and shorter RFS and OS compared with patients without *TP53* alterations.[140] In up to 50% of patients with *TP53* mutations, a complex karyotype can be created by chromothripsis.[51] *TP53*-mutated patients with chromothripsis have a poorer prognosis than those without evidence of chromothripsis.[51]

Acute Myeloid Leukemia *KMT2A* Rearrangement

Patients with the t(9;11)/*KMT2A::MLLT3* translocation, which is the most common of more than 120 cytogenetic aberrations disrupting band 11q23 and the *KMT2A* gene,[141] have usually been classified in the intermediate cytogenetic-risk category[73,81,82] because their outcome is better than the outcome of patients with other rearrangements involving 11q23/*KMT2A*,[142,143] who are typically included in the adverse-risk group.[80,82] However, the more favorable prognosis of patients with t(9;11) seems to be characteristic of adults younger than 60 years, whereas t(9;11)-positive patients age 60 years or older have a very poor outcome that is comparable to the outcome of patients with other 11q23/*KMT2A* rearrangements.[83,144,145] In two-thirds of the patients, t(9;11) is the only chromosome change, whereas approximately 20% of patients have a secondary +8 and 4% to 5% of patients harbor secondary +19 or +21.[92] A large pediatric study found that 11q23/*KMT2A* patients with a secondary +8 had a lower relapse incidence, whereas +19 was an independent adverse prognostic factor for not only incidence of relapse but also EFS and OS.[146]

Cytogenetically Normal Acute Myeloid Leukemia

The largest cytogenetic subset of AML is CN-AML. It is detected in 40% to 45% of adults and 22% to 24%

of children[79,10,108] and consists of patients without any clonal chromosome abnormality. In childhood AML, a fraction of patients with a normal karyotype on standard cytogenetic analysis may harbor cryptic rearrangements like a prognostically adverse *NUP98* rearrangement, for example from t(5;11)(q35;p15)/*NUP98::NSD1* fusion,[113] or inv(16)(p13.3q24.3)/*CBFA2T3::GLIS2*,[147,148] but these rearrangements are very rare (the former) or do not occur (the latter) in adults with AML. As a group, patients with CN-AML have intermediate prognosis in all major cytogenetic-risk classifications because their CR, DFS, and OS rates are worse than those of adequately treated patients with t(8;21), inv(16), or t(15;17), but better than outcomes of patients with unfavorable aberrations.[79,82] However, CN-AML is very heterogeneous molecularly, with several molecular alterations having prognostic significance.[149,150] A favorable outcome was associated with mutations in *NPM1*, *CEBPA* bZIP in-frame mutations, and high expression of *miR-181a*, whereas adverse prognosis was associated with *FLT3*-ITD, a partial tandem duplication of *KMT2A* [*KMT2A*-PTD]; mutations in *DNMT3A* (both R882 and non-R882 mutations), *IDH1*, *IDH2* (R172 mutations), *TET2*, *ASXL1*, *RUNX1*, *WT1*, and *BCOR*; expression of *GAS6*; and high expression of *BAALC*, *ERG*, *MN1*, *SPARC*, *DNMT3B*, *miR-3151*, and *miR-155*.[149-151] Mutations in *NPM1* and in-frame bZIP *CEBPA* mutations denote separate entities in both the current 5th edition of the WHO Classification of Haematolymphoid Neoplasms[68] and the International Consensus Classification of Myeloid Neoplasms and Acute Leukemias.[66] *RUNX1* mutations occur not only in 6% to 25% of mostly older patients with CN-AML, who usually do not harbor concurrent *NPM1* or *CEBPA* mutations,[152-154] but they also can be detected in up to one-third of AML patients with non-complex karyotypes and such recurrent abnormalities as –7/del(7q), +8, +11, or +21,[152,155] and are especially frequent in patients with sole +13 (~90% of patients).[152] In CN-AML, more than one prognostic mutation and gene-expression change can often be found in the same patient, thus making it necessary to investigate how multiple molecular genetic alterations affect patient prognosis.

The European LeukemiaNet Prognostic Classifications of Acute Myeloid Leukemia

The first ELN genetic-risk classification in 2010 divided AML patients into four genetic groups: favorable, intermediate I, intermediate II, and adverse, based on a combination of pretreatment cytogenetic findings and such molecular genetic markers as *FLT3*-ITD, and *CEBPA* and *NPM1* mutations, which were assessed only in patients with CN-AML.[156] Thereafter, the ability of the four ELN genetic groups to predict treatment outcome has been confirmed[144,157] and shown to be independent from other established prognostic factors.[144] Because percentages of patients younger than 60 years and those age 60 years and older differed in the favorable, intermediate II, and adverse genetic groups, and older patients had poorer outcomes than younger patients for each ELN group, older and younger patients were recommended to be analyzed separately.[144] The ELN classification was first modified in 2017,[158] and again in 2022.[73] The 2022 ELN classification includes only one intermediate group and increased the number of gene mutations, whose testing is no longer limited to patients with CN-AML, in the prognostic stratification of AML.[73] Details of 2022 ELN classification are provided in Table 6-8. Whether these changes have improved the ability of outcome prediction of the 2022 ELN genetic-risk classification remains to be determined, although a study found no advantage of the 2022 ELN classification over the previous one published in 2017.[159]

Precursor Lymphoid Neoplasms

Chromosome abnormalities are one of the most important prognostic factors in ALL. The majority of patients exhibit an abnormal karyotype, and the changes are either numerical (aneuploidy) or structural; the latter consist mainly of translocations and deletions. The recurring abnormalities are associated with morphology and immunophenotype and define subsets of patients with different responses to therapy and prognosis. There are two groups of precursor cell neoplasms presenting as lymphoblastic leukemia/lymphoma (ALL) based on cell lineage: B-cell ALL (B-ALL) and T-cell ALL (T-ALL), respectively. Substantial differences are seen in the incidence of recurring abnormalities between pediatric and adult ALL.[160]

Among the various recurring abnormalities associated with prognosis, ploidy, t(9;22)(q34;q11.2), t(4;11)(q21;q23), t(12;21)(p13;q22), and t(1;19)(q23;p13) are the most important, and, together with clinical features (e.g., age, WBC count), are used in risk assessment and therapeutic decision-making.[79,84-87,161-163]

Some of the other recurring abnormalities associated with poor or intermediate risk are low hyperdiploidy (47 to 50 chromosomes), –5/del(5q), +8, +21, del(1p), del(6q), del/t(9p), and del(12p). Because these abnormalities often occur in addition to other recurring translocations or abnormalities, their true influence on outcome has been difficult to determine. Abnormalities of the TR locus have been described in 4% to 6% of adult T-ALL, and t(10;14)(q24;q11) is the most common among them. Patients with this translocation have an excellent prognosis when treated with conventional multiagent regimens.[84,162]

B Lymphoblastic Leukemia/Lymphoma

t(9;22)(q34.1;q11.2)/BCR::ABL1

The presence of t(9;22)(q34;q11.2)/*BCR::ABL1* in ALL patients is relatively more common in adults than in children (25% versus 9%). In both age groups, the presence of the t(9;22)/*BCR::ABL1* translocation has been historically associated with poorer prognosis, though nowadays it offers the option of targeted therapy with tyrosine kinase inhibitors associated with improved outcome. In children, percentage and WBC count and response to therapy can be indicators of more favorable prognosis.

t(v;11)(v;q23)/KMT2A Rearranged

KMT2A rearrangements are the most common findings in leukemia in infants younger than 1 year and are mostly associated with the t(4;11) translocation in this age group. Similar to AML, these rearrangements are less frequent in older children, and their frequency in ALL increases with age in adults. These patients present with high WBC and frequent CNS involvement. Several *KMT2A* translocations have been observed in ALL. The most recurrent partner is *AFF1* (*AF4* at 4q21). Other common partner genes are *MLLT1*

(*ENL* at 19p13.3) and *MLLT3* (*AF9* at 9p22). *KMT2A::MLLT1* fusions are more frequent in T-ALL. Patients with t(4;11) (q21;q23)/*KMT2A::AFF1* have a poor prognosis.[164]

t(12;21)(p13;q22)/ETV6::RUNX1 (TEL::AML1)

The t(12;21)(p13;q22) translocation is common in pediatric patients (age 1 to 10 years) with B-ALL, and it is not seen in T-ALL. Many patients with B-ALL fall into a high-risk group using standard risk factors and are therefore treated aggressively. The presence of t(12;21)(p13;q22) distinguishes a subset of children with a favorable prognosis who thus might benefit from less-toxic and less-intensive therapy. This translocation is not detectable with standard cytogenetic analysis because of the similar morphology of the juxtaposed segments from 12p and 21q, and molecular cytogenetic methods are required to detect this rearrangement.[79,162,163]

t(5;14)(q31;q32)/IGH::IL3

The t(5;14)(q31;q32) translocation juxtaposes the IGH gene to the interleukin-3 gene (*IL3*). The presence of this translocation is rare, accounting for less than 1% of ALL and is associated with an increase in circulating eosinophils. It is present in both children and adults. Clinical characteristics are similar to other ALLs.[6]

t(1;19)(q23;p13.3)/TCF3(E2A)::PBX1

The t(1;19)(q23;p13.3) translocation identifies a subgroup of patients who are at high risk and typically fail treatment early and thus require intensive multiagent therapy.[165] This translocation is more common in pediatric B-ALL. In one large study, the adverse outcome of B-ALL with t(1;19)(q23;p13.3) remained significant, even after adjustment for recognized adverse clinical features, indicating that it is an independent risk factor.[79,166]

High Hyperdiploidy

High hyperdiploidy denotes karyotypes with multiple chromosome gains and a chromosome number of 50 to 66, usually without structural abnormalities. The distribution of specific extra chromosomes is non-random, with chromosomes X, 4, 14, and 21 being the ones most commonly gained.[167] High hyperdiploidy is common in children and is associated with the most favorable prognosis and cure rates exceeding 90%. Adults, however, do not show the excellent outcome observed in children.

T Lymphoblastic Leukemia/Lymphoma

Translocations Involving T-Cell Receptor Gene Loci

The t(10;14)(q24;q11)/*TR::TXL1* translocation occurs in 7% and 30% of childhood and adult T-ALL patients, respectively, whereas the t(5;14)(q11;q35)/*TR::TXL3* translocation is present in 30% of childhood patients and 10% to 15% of adult patients. Both translocations have prognostic significance, with t(10;14)/*TR::TLX1* being associated with a favorable outcome[168] and t(5;14)/*TR::TLX3* with a poorer outcome.[169]

Copy Number Alterations With Prognostic Significance in Acute Lymphoblastic Leukemia

CGH-array analyses of both pediatric and adult B-ALL and T-ALL have shown that the frequencies of genomic gains and losses vary among the cytogenetically defined subgroups.[170,171]

Pediatric B-ALL with (high) hyperploidy frequently exhibited genomic amplification, but this was rarely observed in other subgroups. Genomic loss was detected in all subgroups, with the highest frequency noted in the t(12;21)(p13;q22) and hypodiploid subgroups and the lowest frequency in the 11q23/*KMT2A*-rearranged subgroup. For both adult and pediatric B-ALL, intrachromosomal genomic loss occurred at a higher frequency than gain, and the majority of deletions had an average size of less than 1 Mb, thus being cytogenetically cryptic. Importantly, a high frequency of genomic alterations involving key genes that regulate B-cell differentiation was evident in B-ALL, suggesting that these genomic imbalances play a role in disease pathogenesis. This is evidenced by the microdeletion including the *IKZF1* locus at 7p12, which has now been identified as deleted in more than 80% of the t(9;22)(q34;q11.2) subgroup of ALL patients and is also associated with transformation of CML to ALL (lymphoid blast crisis).[172,173]

Mature Lymphoid Neoplasms

Mature lymphoid neoplasms are an extremely heterogeneous group of diseases. Lymphomas derived from the B-cell lineage constitute 85% of these tumors, and much of the currently available information on cytogenetics comes from these B-cell non-Hodgkin lymphomas (NHLs). The remaining 15% are derived from T-cell or natural killer (NK)-cell lineage and, owing to their rarity and the difficulty of obtaining appropriate tumor samples, remain cytogenetically ill defined. The majority of lymphomas are characterized by complex karyotypes with multiple abnormalities, and a number of recurring translocations, gains, losses, and amplifications have been identified. Although not unique, the recurring translocations are associated with specific diseases (Table 6-9). Here we describe in detail the most common recurrent cytogenetic markers associated with the diagnosis of B-cell mature lymphoid neoplasms, mainly IG translocations that lead to activation of oncogenes.

Mature B-Cell Neoplasms

Absence of Primary Aberrations in Chronic Lymphocytic Leukemia

The majority of mature lymphoid neoplasms are associated with specific IG chromosomal translocations, whereas comparable rearrangements in CLL are rare. Early studies suggesting that t(11;14)(q13.3;q32.3) involving the IGH and *CCND1* locus was common in CLL mainly included cases of leukemic MCL or splenic lymphoma, and the translocation has not been found in *bona fide* CLL. Nevertheless, IG translocations do occur in CLL, albeit at low frequency; approximately less than 2% of all cases have been reported to involve *BCL2*, *BCL3*, and *BCL11A*, among others. The pathologic consequences of these translocations are deregulated expression of the oncogene caused by the physical juxtaposition of the IG enhancers.[174] Instead, CLL is characterized by a recurrent pattern of chromosomal imbalances, namely deletion in 13q14, gain of 12q13 (mostly as trisomy 12), deletion in 11q22.3, and deletion in 17p13.[175] Several of these changes, particularly the 13q14 deletions, can derive from non-recurrent translocations with breakpoints in the respective regions.[21,176] By conventional cytogenetic analysis, only a subset of cases shows aberrant

Table 6-9 Recurring Clonal Chromosomal Abnormalities With Diagnostic and Prognostic Significance in Mature B-Cell Neoplasms (Non-Hodgkin Lymphoma)

Histologic Subset	Diagnostic	Progression/ Transformation	Intermediate or Adverse Outcome	Favorable Outcome
Chronic lymphocytic leukemia, small lymphocytic lymphoma		+12, del(11q), del(6q), del(17p), t/der(14)(q32)	+12, del(11q), del(17p)	del(13q)
Plasma cell myeloma (multiple myeloma)	t(11;14)(q13;q32) t(4;14)(p16;q32) t(14;16)(q32;q23) t(6;14)(p21;q32) t(6;14)(p25;q32) t(14;20)(q32;q11)	Dup(1q), t(8;14)(q24;q32)	−13/del(13q), t(4;14)(p16;q32)	t(11;14)(q13;q32)
Extranodal marginal zone lymphoma of MALT	t(11;18)(q21;q21) t(1;14)(p22;q32) t(14;18)(q32;q21)		t(11;18)(q21;q21) t(1;14)(p22;q32)	
Follicular lymphoma	t(14;18)(q32;q21)*	t/der(1q), +7, del(6q), del(17p), t(8;14) (q24;q32)	del(17p), t(8;14)(q24;q32)	
Mantle cell lymphoma	t(11;14)(q13;q32) CCND2, CCND3 translocations†		dup(3q26), dup(12q14), del(8p21), del(9p21), del(9q22), del(13q14), del(17p13),t(8;14)(q24;q32)	
ABC, diffuse large B-cell lymphoma		der(q21), del(6q), del(9p21), del(17p)	der(q21), del(6q), t(8;14) (q24;q32)	
GCB, diffuse large B-cell lymphoma	t(14;18)(q32;q21)* IRF4 translocations	der(q21), +7, del(6q), del(17p)	der(1q)(21), del(6q), del(9p21), t(8;14)(q24;q32)	
Large B-cell lymphoma with IRF4	IRF4 translocations			
Burkitt lymphoma	t(8;14)(q24;q32)‡	dup(1q), del(17p), +21	dup(1q), dup(7q) del(13q)	
High-grade B-cell lymphoma/ large B-cell lymphoma with 11q aberration	dup/inv(11q)			
Anaplastic large-cell lymphoma	t(2;5)(p23;q25)§ t(6;7)(p25.3;q32.3)		TP63 rearrangements	t(2;5)(p23;q25)§

*Includes variants t(2;18)(p12;q21) and t(18;22)(q21;q11).
†Mainly translocations of CCND2 and CCND3 with immunoglobulin light chains.
‡Includes variants t(2;8)(p12;q24) and t(8;22)(q24;q11).
§Includes variants of t(2;5): t(1;2)(q25;p23), inv(2)(p23;q35), t(2;2)(p23;p23), t(2;3)(p23;q21), t(2;19)(p23;p13), and t(X;2)(q11-12;p23).
ABC, Activated B-cell like; ALK, anaplastic lymphoma kinase; GCB, germinal-center B-cell like; MALT, mucosa-associated lymphoid tissue.

karyotypes, though this can be enhanced by stimulation (e.g., with CpG oligonucleotides). Nevertheless, particularly the 13q14 losses, which are present in around half of CLL cases, frequently are cytogenetically cryptic. The detection of a complex karyotype in CLL is an indicator of poor prognosis, mostly linked to deletion of 17p affecting the TP53 gene.[177,178] Loss or mutation of TP53 is the most informative unfavorable prognostic marker. Overall, because of its biologic and genetic peculiarities, CLL is more suitable to FISH diagnostics with a panel of probes directed to the recurrent aberrations than it is the domain of conventional cytogenetics. Alternatively, some proposals of array-based diagnostic tools for CLL aberrations have been described.[179-181]

Plasma Cell Myeloma/Multiple Myeloma Primary Aberrations

PCM, also named MM, is a heterogeneous genetic disease. Cytogenetic studies have shown that many of the specific translocations affect the IGH locus (55% to 70% of tumors), with some being cryptic and detectable only by FISH analysis. The most frequent abnormalities involve these oncogenes: CCND1 (15% to 18%), MAF (5%), FGFR3/MMSET (NSD2) (15%), CCND3 (3%), and MAFB (2%).[64] Translocations in the IRF4 gene have also been described in MM.[28] The remaining

cases are mostly hyperdiploid and associated most frequently with gains of chromosomes 5, 9, 15, and 19 and are classified as "MM with recurrent cytogenetic abnormalities." Both IGH rearrangements and hyperdiploidy seem to be early genetic events.[6] Deletion of 13q is the most common change in MM and, if detected by cytogenetics, is associated with poor prognosis. Like CLL, MM is more suitable to FISH diagnostics on immunologically defined plasma cells (e.g., MACS or FICTION) than conventional cytogenetics. FISH panels usually include the detection of the prognostic IGH translocation, hyperploidy, 13q deletions, 17p deletions, and progression markers like MYC breaks and 1q gains. In terms of association with prognosis, myeloma cases can be separated in two big groups according to genetic features, a non-hyperdiploid subtype (mainly cases harboring IGH translocations and associated with more aggressive behavior), and a hyperdiploid subtype, a more indolent form of disease.[182]

MYC Translocations: The t(8;14)(q24;q32) Translocation and Variants

The t(8;14)(q24;q32) translocation or its variants, which juxtapose the locus of the MYC gene and one of the three IG loci, are present in almost all Burkitt lymphoma (BL) cases. In endemic BL, most IG::MYC translocations affect the VDJ region because of aberrant somatic hypermutation, whereas in sporadic cases, the translocations are mediated by IG class-switch recombination of the IGH locus at 14q32.[183] The *MYC* breakpoints can be located up to 1 Mb centromeric of *MYC* in t(8;14) and telomeric of *MYC* in t(8;22)(q24;q11) and t(2;8) (p12;q24).[184]

The common functional effect of these translocations is that the *MYC* gene undergoes constitutive expression in tumor cells. The *MYC* translocation is not a genetic lesion exclusive of BL. An *MYC* break has been observed in up to 15% of patients with classical DLBCL, usually associated with complex karyotypes and very poor outcome. Some of these cases can be classified as molecular BL based on gene-expression profiles.[185,186] Other cases frequently carry a t(14;18)(q32;q21) translocation associated with the t(8;14) or variant *MYC* translocation and are clinically aggressive with poor response to current therapies. These cases are called DLBCL/high-grade B-cell lymphoma (HGBL) with *MYC* and *BCL2* rearrangements (or *double-hit lymphomas*) in the WHO 5th edition and just HGBL with *MYC* and *BCL2* rearrangements in the International Consensus Classification

(ICC) independently of the cytological variant. Similarly, double hits involving the *MYC* and *BCL6* genes are recurrently observed, which form a group of lymphomas clinically and pathologically distinct from the *MYC* and *BCL2* double hits. Acquisition of an *MYC* translocation has been observed as a secondary event in MCL with blastoid or pleomorphic features, and FL is frequently associated with transformation to DLBCL.[187,188]

Gain and Loss 11q Pattern in High-Grade/Large B-Cell Lymphoma With 11q Aberration(s)

The high-grade/large B-cell lymphoma with 11q aberrations entity, according to the WHO 5th edition and ICC terminology, respectively, defines a subset of tumors with a spectrum of morphology from intermediate/blastoid or Burkitt-like morphology to large B-cell morphology, germinal center phenotype and very high proliferation (>90%), and negative for *MYC* rearrangements.[65,67,189] Those cases are characterized by a prototypical alteration of chromosome 11 including 11q23.2-q23.3 gain and 11q24-qter loss (Fig. 6-6A). Of note, cytogenetic studies have shown that the gained region

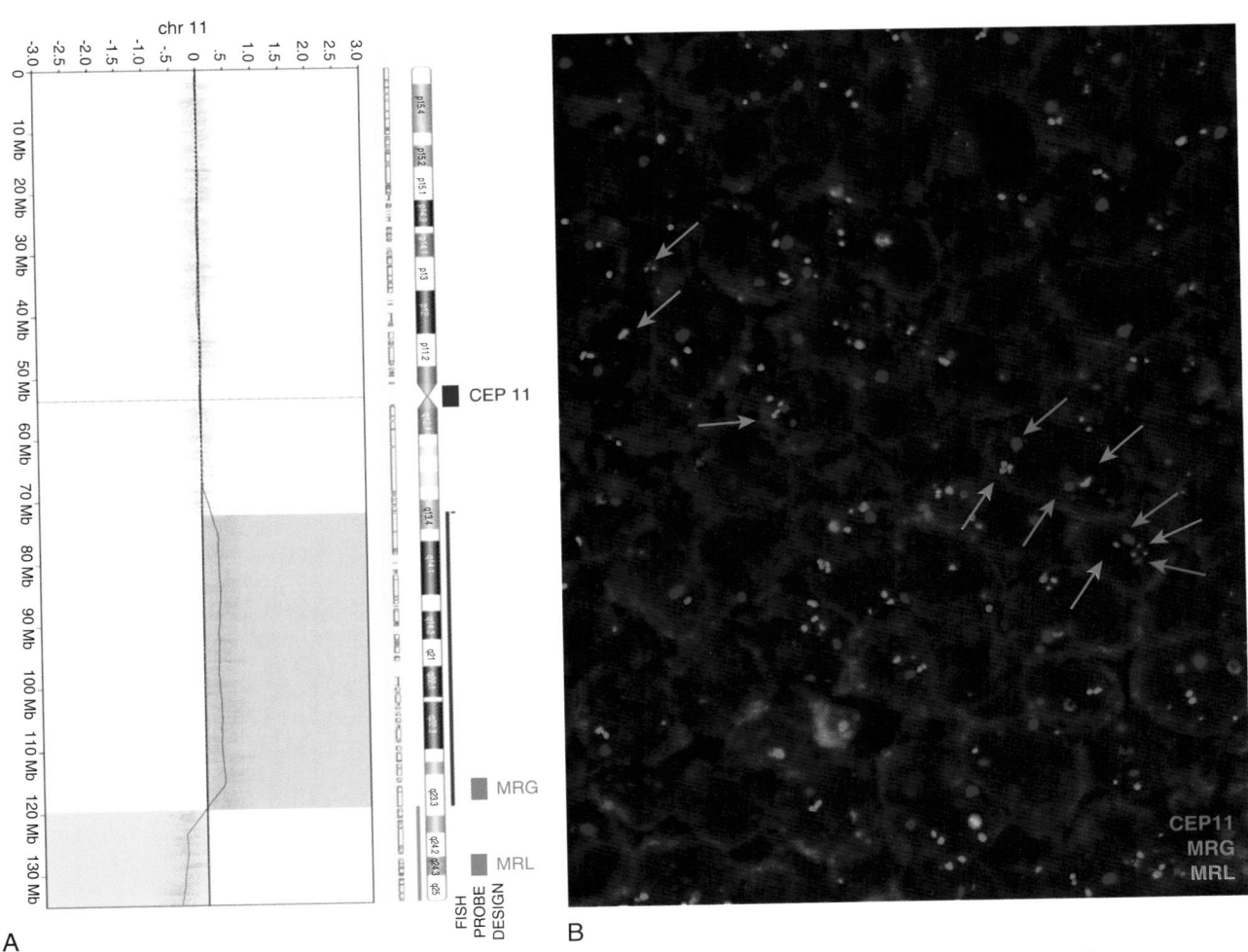

Figure 6-6. High-grade/large B-cell lymphoma with 11q aberration(s). A, Chromosomal view of chromosome 11 copy number profile analyzed by CytoScan array, depicting gains of 11q13.4-q23.3 in blue and terminal losses of 11q23.3-q25 in red. **B,** FISH constellation of 11q aberration using a custom probe combining CEP11 (spectrum aqua), RP11-414G21 (spectrum green, MRG), and RP11-629A20 (spectrum red, MRL) bac clones. Two blue signals are observed per cell corresponding to the two chr11 centromeres (blue arrows); the presence of three green signals per cell indicates 11q gain (bold green arrows) and the presence of only one red is indicative of the 11q terminal loss (red arrows). *CEP 11,* Centromeric probe chr11; *MRG,* minimal region of gain; *MRL,* minimal region of loss.

is frequently inverted.[190,191] This alteration can be detected by specific FISH probes for the commonly gained and lost regions (Fig. 6-6B) and an appropriate control. Because isolated cases have been shown to depict single terminal losses or, alternatively, proximal gains together with terminal CN-LOH, the use of CN arrays is recommended.[191-193]

The t(14;18)(q32;q21)IGH::BCL2 Translocation

Around 80% to 90% of FLs carry a t(14;18)(q32;q21) translocation or one of its variants, t(2;18)(p12;q21) or t(18;22)(q21;q11), that juxtaposes the BCL2 oncogene, an inhibitor of apoptosis, next to the IGH or the IG light chain loci, respectively. This translocation has to be distinguished from the t(14;18)(q32;q21) translocation involving MALT1 at the same chromosome 18q band (IGH::MALT1) that occurs in extranodal marginal zone lymphomas. The different involved genes at 18q21 can be recognized by FISH with specific probes. In nodal FL, the translocation is more frequent in grade 1 to 2 than in grade 3, particularly grade 3B, and it is extremely rare or virtually absent in patients with FL younger than 14 years.[194-196] Breakpoints of BCL2 in translocations with light chain genes are located in the 5′ end of the BCL2, similar to MYC translocations. Because of their rarity, the clinical implications of the variant translocations are not well defined. About 20% to 30% of DLBCLs show the presence of the t(14;18) translocation. These cases are predominantly centroblastic and belong almost exclusively to the GCB DLBCL subtype.

BCL6 Translocations

Translocations of the 3q27 locus where BCL6 is localized are found in around 30% of DLBCLs. Translocations of BCL6 have also been detected in FL, mainly in grade 3B/follicular large B-cell lymphoma cases, which resemble DLBCL in many features.[197] The breakpoint in 3q27 occurs within the major translocation cluster of BCL6. As a result, either one of the three IG genes or a variable non-IG gene is juxtaposed to the coding region of BCL6. The variability of the partner chromosomes juxtaposed to BCL6 suggests that this gene belongs to a group of promiscuous genes. The substitution of BCL6 promoter by heterologous regulatory sequences causes deregulation of BCL6 expression in DLBCL carrying these rearrangements. One feature shared by all these promoters linked to rearranged BCL6 alleles is that they are physiologically active in normal B cells. These translocations could prevent BCL6 downregulation blocking differentiation from GCB to plasma cell.

IRF4 Translocations

The t(6;14)(p25;q32) translocation juxtaposes the IGH gene to the IRF4 (formerly MUM1) gene, leading to activation of the transcription factor IRF4. This translocation, first described in PCM/MM,[28] has also been observed in a subtype of mature B-cell lymphomas.[29] Specifically, IGH::IRF4 and its variant fusions are associated with a subgroup of GCB lymphomas characterized by FL grade 3 or centroblastic DLBCL morphology, co-expression of IRF4 and BCL6 in the absence of PRDM1/BLIMP1, a specific gene-expression profile, and a disease onset predominantly in the head and neck region of children or young adults (mean age, 12 years).[198] Although the number of cases reported is still limited, IG::IRF4-positive lymphomas are associated with a significantly better prognosis

after treatment.[29,199,200] Deletions of 17p locus, frequently found in the context of isochromosome 17, and 11q12-qter gains are characteristic of this entity.[201,202] The category of large B-cell lymphoma with IRF4 rearrangement is included in the current classifications of lymphoid neoplasms to recognize these cases.[65,67]

TBL1XR1::TP63 Gene Fusion

The TBL1XR1::TP63 gene fusion, initially observed on RNA-sequencing data, has been detected in 5% of de novo GCB DLBCLs. The fusion appears exclusive to GCB and was not seen in non-GCB cases examined.[203] The TBL1XR1::TP63 gene fusion is predicted to give rise to a unique chimeric protein, in contrast to the deregulated expression of wild-type BCL6, BCL2, and MYC that result from other DLBCL translocations. Although the function of this fusion protein is not yet elucidated, the recurrence, subtype enrichment, and conservation of the TP63 portion of the fusion suggest an important functional role in lymphomas carrying this fusion and may be a novel target for therapeutic intervention.

The t(11;14)(q13;q32)/IGH::CCND1, CCND2 and CCND3 Translocations

Virtually all cases of MCL carry the t(11;14)(q13;q32) translocation, leading to the juxtaposition of the CCND1 gene at 11q13 to the IGH joining region at 14q32, which results in the constitutive overexpression of cyclin D1. The t(11;14) translocation is detected in approximately 65% of MCLs by conventional cytogenetics, but it can be identified in virtually all cases by FISH with probes involving the IGH and CCND1 regions. Very few cases with variant CCND1 translocations with IG light chains have been reported. Similar to other B-cell lymphomas with variant translocations involving oncogenes, there is also a variation in breakpoints affecting CCND1 and in the IG light chain translocations in MCL, with breakpoints occurring in the 3′ region of the CCND1 gene.[188] Chromosomal rearrangements of the CCND2 locus have been detected in 55% of cyclin D1–negative MCLs. These translocations are mainly with IG light chains (IGK and IGL).[204] In addition, whole-genome/exome sequencing has allowed the identification of cryptic insertions of light chains near CCND3 that have been associated with cyclin D3 overexpression. By specific FISH probes, including the IGK enhancer region, additional cryptic IGK juxtapositions to CCND3 and CCND2 in MCL that overexpressed these cyclins, respectively, have been described.[205] This similar approach has also allowed the identification of cryptic insertions of IG light chains in the CCND1 locus in MCL expression cyclin D1.[206] From a clinical point of view, detection of these translocations is important to differentiate MCL from other low-grade B-cell lymphomas, in particular when the immunophenotype is inconclusive.

MALT Lymphoma Translocations

There are three translocations associated with MALT lymphoma: t(11;18)(q21;q21)/API2::MALT1, t(14;18)(q32;q21)/IGH::MALT1, and t(1;14)(p22;q32)/IGH::BCL10. All these alterations are associated with activation of the NF-κB pathway, suggesting that this deregulation is essential for MALT lymphoma development. An additional translocation, t(3;14)(p14.1;q32), has also been observed in MALT lymphomas.

This translocation brings the *FOXP1* gene under the control of an IGH enhancer, resulting in its overexpression.[207] It has also been observed in other B-cell neoplasms, mainly DLBCL.[208] In gastric MALT lymphoma, t(11;18)(q21;q21) and t(1;14) (p22;q32) are typically seen in patients with advanced disease who do not respond to antibiotic therapy. In an analysis of 111 patients with *Helicobacter pylori*–positive gastric MALT lymphomas, only 4% of the patients who responded exhibited t(11;18)(q21;q21), as opposed to 67% who failed to respond.[209] Although the t(11;18)(q21;q21) translocation is associated with adverse clinical features, it is seldom found in transformed MALT lymphoma.[210]

Mature T-Cell Neoplasms

Anaplastic large-cell lymphoma (ALCL) anaplastic lymphoma kinase (ALK)-positive is genetically characterized by the t(2;5) (p23;q25) translocation and its variants t(1;2)(q25;p23), inv(2)(p23q35), t(2;2)(p23;p23), t(2;3)(p23;q21), t(2;19) (p23;p13), and t(X;2)(q11-12;p23), which result in expression of the ALK protein. Patients with these tumors are significantly younger (mean age, 22 years) and have a low International Prognostic Index (IPI) score and a more favorable prognosis compared with ALCL ALK-negative.[65,67] Multivariate analysis has shown that the favorable prognosis in patients with ALK-positive systemic ALCL is not merely because of their younger age or low-risk IPI group.[211] A subset of large B-cell lymphomas expressing the ALK kinase with t(2;17)(p23;q23)/*CLTC::ALK* or other ALK translocations has also been described.[212,213]

In the subgroup of ALK-negative ALCL, t(6;7)(p25.3;q32.3) disrupting the *IRF4/DUSP22* locus on 6p25.3 and adjoining the *FRA7H* fragile site on 7q32.3 has been identified in 30% of the cases. This translocation has been associated with downregulation of *DUSP22* and upregulation of microRNA miR-29a on 7q32.3.[214] Also, translocations involving *TP63* have been identified in 8% of ALK-negative ALCLs.[215] *DUSP22*-rearranged cases have favorable outcomes similar to ALK-positive ALCLs, whereas *TP63* rearrangements have been associated with poorer outcomes.[216]

Hepatosplenic T-cell lymphomas typically carry gains of chromosomes 7 and 8, mostly presenting as isochromosome 7q and trisomy 8.[217] T-cell prolymphocytic leukemia is characterized in around 80% of cases by an inv(14)(q11q32) or t(14;14)(q11;q32) juxtaposing the *TCL1* oncogene next to the TRA/TRD locus, or by its variant, t(X;14)(q28;q11) involving the *MTCP1* gene in Xq28.[218,219]

Hodgkin Lymphoma

Conventional cytogenetic and FISH studies have shown the presence of aneuploidy and hypertetraploidy in Hodgkin lymphoma (HL) cells. This finding is consistent with the presence of multinucleation in neoplastic cells. Nevertheless, these techniques failed to identify recurrent or specific chromosomal translocations in Hodgkin and Reed-Sternberg (HRS) cells, but IGH breakpoints were observed in 17% of these cases.[220] Moreover, structural chromosomal changes involving the *PDL2* locus in 9p23 or the *C2TA* locus in 16p are common in classic HL.[221] Breaks affecting the *BCL6* locus have also been recurrently described in nodular lymphocyte predominant HL, nowadays also called nodular lymphocyte predominant B-cell lymphoma.[222]

Copy Number Alterations With Prognostic Significance in Lymphoid Neoplasms

Most of the described chromosome translocations in lymphomas are insufficient to induce malignancy by themselves. One evidence is that *BCL2*-translocated and *CCND1*-translocated B cells are circulating at very low levels in the peripheral blood of healthy individuals.[223,224] Studies of genetic alterations other than translocations with conventional cytogenetics, FISH, CGH, CGH array, or SNP array have revealed that patients with the same disease entity may show different secondary genomic alterations. The profile of these alterations is relatively characteristic of each disease, and some of them may have prognostic significance (Table 6-9). These regions may contain genes that confer growth advantages, or the possibility of escaping apoptosis or cell-cycle arrest triggered by the genomic instability. In some of these regions, several target tumor-suppressor genes or oncogenes have been identified, such as *TP53* at 17p13, *CDKN2A/B* at 9p21, and *RB1* at 13q14.[225] The genetic profiles of lymphoma entities are constantly being refined based on new technologies becoming available. Moreover, the application of genome-wide analysis to FFPE materials has revealed the genetic profiles of rare subgroups of these diseases. Unfortunately, comparisons of genetic complexity among lymphoma types based on CN array studies are difficult because of different resolution and analysis algorithms.

In CLL, several studies that used FISH to estimate the incidence of del(13q), del(11q), +12, and del(17p) have shown that del(11q) and del(17p) identify subgroups of patients with rapid disease progression and short survival, respectively. Patients with del(13q) as a single defect have the longest survival.[226-228] In FL, cytogenetic studies have repeatedly correlated deletions of 1p and 17p with poor prognosis.[229,230] Molecular cytogenetics studies including CGH and CGH arrays have shown 6q25-q27 deletions,[231] 9p losses, and gains of 11q as unfavorable prognostic markers.[232] One SNP array study determined that the abnormalities more frequent in transformed FL samples are gains of 3q27.3-q28 and chromosome 11, and losses of 9p21 and 15q, whereas gains of X or Xp and losses of 6q predicted OS.[233] Comparison based on CGH data has shown that MCLs have a higher number of genomic aberrations per tumor than other B-cell malignancies.[225] Gains of 3q, 7p, and 12q, and losses of 17p are significantly more frequent in blastoid and pleomorphic versus classical variants. Alterations in several chromosomal regions were related to poor survival, as gains of 3q26 and 12q14, losses of 8p21, 9p21, 9q22, 13q14, and 17p13, and an increased number of chromosomal imbalances (≥3) have been associated with shorter OS.[234] In addition, the CN profiles of cyclin D1–negative MCL resemble those of cyclin D1–positive cases.[204]

In DLBCL, specific CN alterations were associated with the different molecular subtypes.[235,236] Common findings in activated B-cell (ABC) DLBCLs are frequent gains of 3q, 18q, and 19, and losses of 9p and 6q. GCB-DLBCLs shows gains of the mir-17-92-supercluster on chromosome 13, gains of *REL* on chromosome 2, and losses of 10q including *PTEN*.[237,238] As in other lymphomas, there is evidence that deletions of 17p and 9p21 are associated with poor prognosis.[239] CN studies in BL have described gains of 1q, 8q24, and 12q, and losses of 13q31-q32 and 17p13 as the most frequent alterations.[240-242] Abnormalities in 1q and 7q have been associated with poor outcome.[240] Secondary alterations in MM include −13 or del(13q) found in 50% of the cases. Other secondary aberrations, such as *TP53* deletions or gain and loss of 1q and 1p have also been observed.[65,67]

Finally, the CN studies in HL are limited because of the low content of the neoplastic HRS cells in the affected tissues. Therefore the information on CN alterations of HL has been historically based on the study of cell lines.[243,244] Nevertheless, improvements in laser-capture microdissection and linear nucleic acid amplification techniques have unraveled a complex pattern of recurrent changes and defined regions of chromosomal gain or loss harboring potential oncogenes and tumor-suppressor genes such as *IKBKB, CD40, MAP3K14, CDKN2B,* and *TNFRSF14.*[245,246] Moreover, gains of 16p11.2-13.3 have been significantly more frequently found in pretreatment and relapse biopsies of unresponsive patients and associated with shortened disease-specific survival.[246]

CONCLUSION

Cytogenetic analysis of leukemias and lymphomas has been instrumental in identifying recurring translocations and inversions, and establishing the principle that these balanced rearrangements cause deregulation of genes at the breakpoints, leading to aberrant cell function and initiation of neoplastic proliferation. By pointing to the genes involved, recurrent chromosome rearrangements have provided critical insights into the biology of neoplastic transformation and normal hematopoiesis.

The introduction of molecular cytogenetic methods has significantly expanded the application of chromosome analysis in both clinical and basic research. In addition to conventional cytogenetics, molecular cytogenetics including FISH and CN arrays are methods for the routine detection of chromosomal changes in lymphomas. The application of both standard karyotyping and these molecular techniques has also shown that specific chromosome changes are associated with treatment outcomes, thereby enabling therapeutic decisions based on the results of chromosome analysis. This has led to a better understanding of the disease and better patient management.

Pearls and Pitfalls

- Conventional and molecular cytogenetic techniques are key elements in elucidating the pathogenesis of a large number of hematologic neoplasms and providing information relevant to their diagnosis and prognosis.
- The ICC and the 5th edition of the WHO Classification of Haematolymphoid Tumours include a number of entities defined in part by specific genetic abnormalities, particularly chromosome translocations, deletions, and gene mutations. As a result, genetic studies must be a routine part of the diagnostic workup of these neoplasms to adhere to up-to-date classifications.
- Different genetic techniques are available for clinical practice. The most applicable and cost-effective routine screening methods are conventional G-banding and FISH. Other molecular techniques are powerful research tools and can resolve the complexity of genetic alterations in hematologic neoplasms.
- The clinical relevance of many recurring abnormalities observed in complex karyotypes remains contentious. The new array-based molecular genetics technologies now applicable to archived materials are continuously providing new information that will help determine the biologic and clinical significance of these alterations.

Acknowledgments

The authors gratefully acknowledge Dr. Gouri Nanjangud, Dr. Nallasivam Palanisamy, Dr. Jane Houldsworth, and Dr. R.S.K. Chaganti for their many helpful suggestions. IS was supported by a Miguel Servet II contract (MS18/00015) from the Carlos III Health Institute and the European Regional Development Fund "A Way of Making Europe." KM gratefully acknowledges Dr. Clara D. Bloomfield, who died on March 1, 2020, for her constant help and encouragement over the years. The support of the cytogenetic and molecular cytogenetic groups of the authors is gratefully acknowledged as is the continuous support from various granting agencies.

KEY REFERENCES

1. McGowan-Jordan J, Hastings RJ, Moore S, eds. *ISCN (2020): An International System for Human Cytogenomic Nomenclature (2020)*. Basel: Karger; 2020.
27. Ashram MS, Barch MJ, Lawce HJ, eds. *The AGT Cytogenetics Laboratory Manual*. 4th ed. Hoboken, NJ: Wiley-Blackwell; 2017.
42. Kallioniemi A, Kallioniemi OP, Sudar D, et al. Comparative genomic hybridization for molecular cytogenetic analysis of solid tumors. *Science*. 1992;258:818–821.
63. Akkari YMN, Baughn LB, Dubuc AM, et al. Guiding the global evolution of cytogenetic testing for hematologic malignancies. *Blood*. 2022;139:2273–2284.
73. Döhner H, Wei AH, Appelbaum FR, et al. Diagnosis and management of AML in adults: 2022 ELN recommendations from an international expert panel. *Blood*. 2022;140(12):1345–1377.
82. Grimwade D, Hills RK, Moorman AV, et al. Refinement of cytogenetic classification in acute myeloid leukemia: determination of prognostic significance of rare recurring chromosomal abnormalities among 5876 younger adult patients treated in the United Kingdom Medical Research Council trials. *Blood*. 2010;116:354–365.
103. Greenberg PL, Tuechler H, Schanz J, et al. Revised international prognostic scoring system for myelodysplastic syndromes. *Blood*. 2012;120:2454–2465.
144. Mrózek K, Marcucci G, Nicolet D, et al. Prognostic significance of the European LeukemiaNet standardized system for reporting cytogenetic and molecular alterations in adults with acute myeloid leukemia. *J Clin Oncol*. 2012;30:4515–4523.
226. Döhner H, Stilgenbauer S, Benner A, et al. Genomic aberrations and survival in chronic lymphocytic leukemia. *N Engl J Med*. 2000;343:1910–1916.
236. Lenz G, Wright GW, Emre NC, et al. Molecular subtypes of diffuse large B-cell lymphoma arise by distinct genetic pathways. *Proc Natl Acad Sci USA*. 2008;105:13520–13525.

Visit Elsevier eBooks+ for the complete set of references.

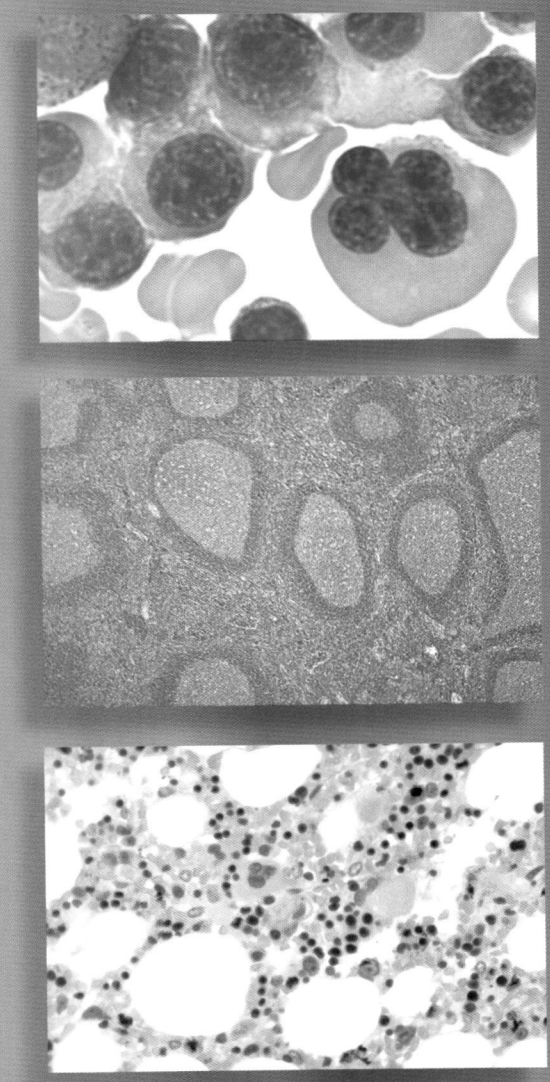

PART II

Normal and Reactive Conditions of Hematopoietic Tissues

Chapter 7

Normal Lymphoid Organs and Tissues

Laura Llao-Cid, Ralf Küppers, and Elias Campo

Lymphoid tissues are the sites where precursor cells mature into immunocompetent lymphoid cells and where immune reactions to antigens occur. The lymphoid tissues and the stages of lymphocyte differentiation and maturation have an anatomy—they occur at specific sites in the body. They have an architecture—each lymphoid tissue is organized in a specific way, and cellular differentiation and reactions occur in specific sites within this organized tissue. They have a specific cellular morphology—the cells change size, shape, and other features as they mature and react to antigen and other stimuli. They undergo specific genetic and biological changes—lymphoid cells alter their genes, their gene expression, and the proteins they produce and respond to at the various stages of differentiation and maturation. Understanding these normal structures and their alterations during lymphoid cell development and activation and during immune responses is important for pathologists who must diagnose reactive and neoplastic conditions of lymphoid tissues and cells.

Superimposed on this lymphoid tissue anatomy is the biology of the immune system. The function of the immune system is to defend the body against infection. Its cellular components include myeloid cells (granulocytes such as neutrophils, eosinophils, and basophils; monocytes; and histiocytes or macrophages), lymphocytes (T, B, plasma, and natural killer [NK] cells), and professional antigen-presenting cells (histiocytes, dendritic cells, and B cells). There are two distinct types of immune reactions: innate or natural immune responses and acquired or adaptive immune responses (Box 7-1).[1]

NORMAL LYMPHOID TISSUES

Lymphoid tissues are divided into two major compartments according to lymphoid cell differentiation stages and functional interactions: central or primary lymphoid tissues and peripheral or secondary lymphoid tissues. The terms *tertiary lymphoid organs* and *ectopic lymphoid structures* refer to organized lymphoid tissue formed at sites of chronic inflammation. The central lymphoid tissues are the bone marrow and thymus. These organs contain the precursor

lymphoid cells and sustain the cells' initial antigen-independent differentiation process from the immature stage to the mature stage, at which they can perform their function in response to antigens. The peripheral or secondary lymphoid organs are the lymph nodes, spleen, and mucosa-associated lymphoid tissue (MALT), where the mature lymphoid cells encounter antigens and develop different types of immune responses. These compartments are highly organized microenvironments of different cell populations, vascular structures, and stromal components that maximize the selective interactions between lymphocytes and antigens for the initiation and expansion of the immune responses.[2,3]

Primary (Central) Lymphoid Tissues

Bone Marrow

Bone marrow is the source of self-renewing populations of hematopoietic stem and precursor cells and early common lymphoid B-cell and T-cell precursors. The early B-cell differentiation program continues in the bone marrow, whereas the precursor elements committed to T-cell differentiation migrate to the thymus to complete the T-cell maturation process. Bone marrow is also a repository for plasma cells (and some memory B cells [MBCs]) that migrate back to the bone marrow after being generated in peripheral lymphoid organs and tissues. B-cell development in the bone marrow is dependent on the interactions of precursor lymphoid cells with stromal cells in different topographic niches, which provide specific contacts and signals to maturing lymphoid cells. The most immature hematopoietic cells are in the endosteal niche close to the interior surface of the bone, where osteogenic cells seem to provide signals for the development of B cells; subsequently, they move to central regions of the bone marrow close to periarteriolar and sinusoidal cells. Cytokines and chemokines influence B-cell differentiation and trafficking in the bone marrow (Table 7-1). Two of the major players are CXCL12, also known as stromal cell–derived factor-1 (SDF-1), and its receptor, CXCR4. CXCL12 is expressed by osteoblasts, bone marrow stromal cells, and

Box 7-1 *Innate and Adaptive Immune Response Systems*

Innate
- Defensive system developed very early in evolution.
- Mediated by phagocytes, dendritic cells, NK cells, and some T cells, including γ-δ T cells.
- These cells always respond to antigens in the same way, regardless of prior exposure to the antigen.
- The receptors that recognize antigens in these cells are encoded by the germline DNA without subsequent modifications.
- Antigens recognized by this system contain highly conserved structures that are present on common pathogens but not in host cells.
- Innate immune cells perform their effector functions immediately upon receptor engagement.
- Cells of the innate immune system initiate and regulate adaptive immune responses by presenting antigens and activating signals to T and B cells.

Adaptive
- Immune system developed in vertebrates.
- Mediated by B and T lymphocytes.
- The cell surface antigen receptors (B and T cell receptors) are highly specific and encoded by somatically rearranged immunoglobulin and T-cell receptor loci. B cells typically undergo further affinity selection of their B-cell receptor upon exposure to antigens.
- Cells expressing receptors against self-antigens must be selected against.
- Cells recognizing foreign antigens first proliferate to expand the few antigen-specific B or T cells (clonal selection).
- The adaptive system generates memory cells and improves in efficiency and specificity during the life of the individual owing to repeated exposure to antigens.

Table 7-1 Chemokines and Chemokine Receptors Implicated in Lymphoid Tissue Organization

Cell Source	Chemokine	Chemokine Receptor	Cell Expressing Receptor
Bone marrow Osteoblasts	CXCL12 (SDF-1)	CXCR4	CD34+ cells Precursor lymphoid cells
Endothelium Stromal cells Splenic red pulp Stromal cells Dark-zone stromal cells	IL-7	IL-7R	Plasma cells Centroblasts
Follicular dendritic cells Follicular stromal cells Follicular T-helper cells	CXCL13	CXCR5	B and T lymphocytes Follicular helper T cells
Interdigitating dendritic cells High endothelial venules Stromal cells in T areas Thymic medullary epithelium	CCL19 CCL21	CCR7	CD4 and CD8 thymic cells Mature T cells Mature dendritic cells
Enterocytes	CCL25	CCR9	IgA-secreting cells Mucosal T lymphocytes

endothelial cells. CXCR4 is present in hematopoietic stem cells and in early stages of B-cell differentiation, whereas it is downregulated in pre-B cells and mature B cells in peripheral lymphoid organs. CXCR4 is upregulated again in mature cells after antigen stimulation and plasma cell differentiation, which may explain the homing back of these cells to the bone marrow. Late progenitor B (pro-B) and precursor B (pre-B) cells require interleukin (IL)-7 generated by different stromal cells in the endosteal and central niches. Later stages of differentiation in the marrow are less dependent on contact with stromal cells, allowing them to leave these niches and continue their maturation in secondary lymphoid organs.[4]

Precursor B lymphocytes or lymphoblasts are not easily detected morphologically in normal bone marrow. These cells have round nuclei with dispersed chromatin and small nucleoli. They may be seen more commonly in regenerating bone marrow, where they are called *hematogones*.[5] These cells express immature lymphoid markers, may be numerous—particularly in autoimmune disorders, human immunodeficiency virus, and other viral infections—and are associated with neoplasia. Caution is needed to avoid misinterpreting these cells as neoplastic lymphoid cells.[5]

Thymus

The thymus, located in the anterior mediastinum, is where precursor cells that migrate from the bone marrow undergo maturation and selection to become mature, naïve T cells that can respond to foreign antigens (Fig. 7-1). The thymus

is critical to the development of a normal T-cell repertoire in early life, and there is evidence that it continues to function in T-cell development throughout life.[1,6]

The thymus has a central lymphoid compartment—the thymic epithelial space—and a peripheral compartment—the perivascular space.[6] The thymic epithelial space is divided into a cortex and a medulla; each is characterized by specialized epithelium and accessory cells, which provide the milieu for T-cell maturation. The cortex contains cortical epithelial cells, which are large cells with vesicular chromatin, prominent nucleoli, and pale cytoplasm that form a reticular 3-dimensional supporting meshwork and express high levels of major histocompatibility complex (MHC) class II. Phagocytic histiocytes (macrophages) are also present in the cortex, where they both present antigen and phagocytize apoptotic thymocytes. The medullary epithelial cells are coarser and express MHC classes I and II. In central areas, these cells form spherical whorls with central keratinization known as Hassall corpuscles. The medulla contains dendritic cells that are similar to cutaneous Langerhans cells and lymph node interdigitating dendritic cells. Perivascular spaces are present in both the cortex and medulla.

The lymphocytes of the cortex (cortical thymocytes) range in morphology from medium-sized blastic cells with dispersed chromatin and nucleoli in the outer cortex to somewhat smaller, more mature-appearing round lymphocytes in the inner cortex. The immunophenotype of most cortical thymocytes is that of precursor T cells (TdT positive, CD1a positive, CD4 positive, CD8 positive). Medullary thymocytes

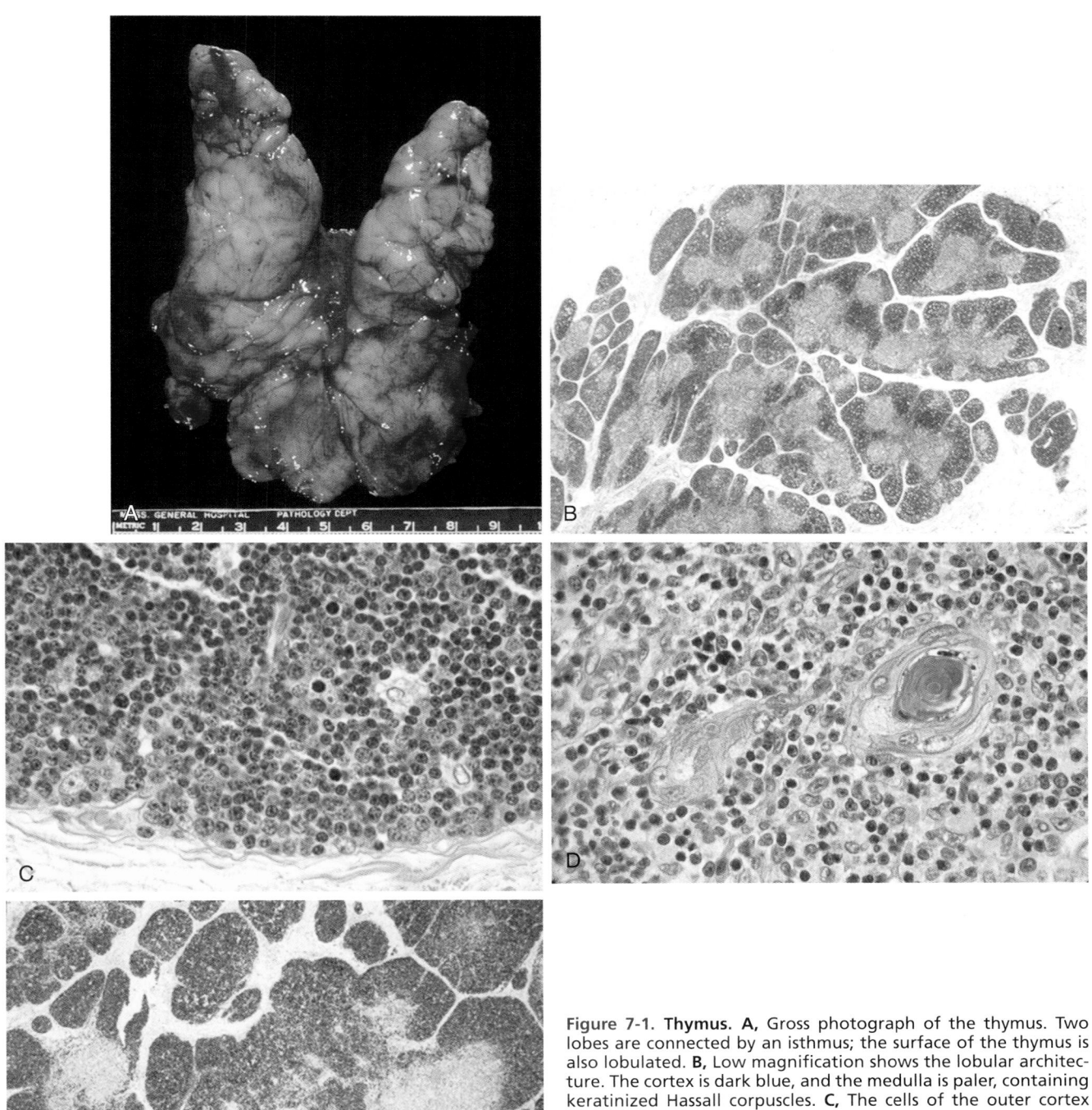

Figure 7-1. Thymus. A, Gross photograph of the thymus. Two lobes are connected by an isthmus; the surface of the thymus is also lobulated. **B,** Low magnification shows the lobular architecture. The cortex is dark blue, and the medulla is paler, containing keratinized Hassall corpuscles. **C,** The cells of the outer cortex are medium-sized blastic cells with rather dispersed chromatin. Large oval cortical epithelial cells are visible, with distinct nucleoli and indistinct cytoplasm. **D,** The cells of the medulla are mature-appearing lymphocytes, associated with more spindle-shaped epithelial cells. **E,** With immunostaining for terminal deoxynucleotidyl transferase, the cortical thymocytes are stained, and the medullary thymocytes are negative.

are small, mature-appearing lymphocytes with round or slightly irregular nuclei and inconspicuous nucleoli. Lymphocytes in the perivascular spaces resemble those in the medulla.[6] Both have the immunophenotype of mature T cells (TdT⁻, CD1a⁻, CD3⁺, CD4⁺, or CD8⁺).

The thymic medulla also contains a particular population of B cells with dendritic morphology that expresses mature B-cell markers CD23, CD37, CD72, CD76, immunoglobulin (Ig)M, and IgD. These cells form rosettes with non-B cells and have been called asteroid cells. The close relationship with T cells and epithelial thymic cells suggests that they may play a functional role in the T-cell differentiation process.[7,8] These asteroid cells may be the cell of origin for primary mediastinal large B-cell lymphoma.

The thymic epithelial space begins to atrophy at 1 year; it shrinks by about 3% per year through middle age and then by 1% per year thereafter[6]; concomitantly, the perivascular space increases. The "fatty infiltration" noted in the adult thymus occurs in the perivascular space.[6]

Secondary (Peripheral) Lymphoid Tissues

Lymph Nodes

Lymph nodes are strategically located at branches of the lymphatic system throughout the body to maximize the capture of antigens and chemokines present in lymph drained from most organs via the afferent lymphatics (Fig. 7-2). The lymph nodes are protected by an external fibrotic capsule with internal prolongations that form trabeculae, providing the basic framework for the organization of the different cellular, vascular, and specialized stromal components.

The cellular compartments are distributed among three discrete but not rigid regions: the cortex, paracortex, and medullary cords. The cortex or cortical area is the B-cell zone and contains the lymphoid follicles; the paracortex contains mainly T cells and T-cell antigen-presenting cells. The medullary cords in the inner area of the lymph node contain B cells, T cells, plasma cells, macrophages, and dendritic cells.

Cortical Area

The initial cortical structure is the primary lymphoid follicle, composed of aggregates of naïve B cells with a small network of follicular dendritic cells (FDCs) (Fig. 7-2B).[9-11] The lymphoid cells are small and have round nuclei with dense chromatin and scant cytoplasm. These cells express mature B-cell markers, IgM, IgD, CD21, and CD23. Antigen stimulation of B cells generates the expanded and highly organized secondary lymphoid follicle with a mantle cell corona, a germinal center, and a dense meshwork of FDCs (Figs. 7-2C–F and 7-3).

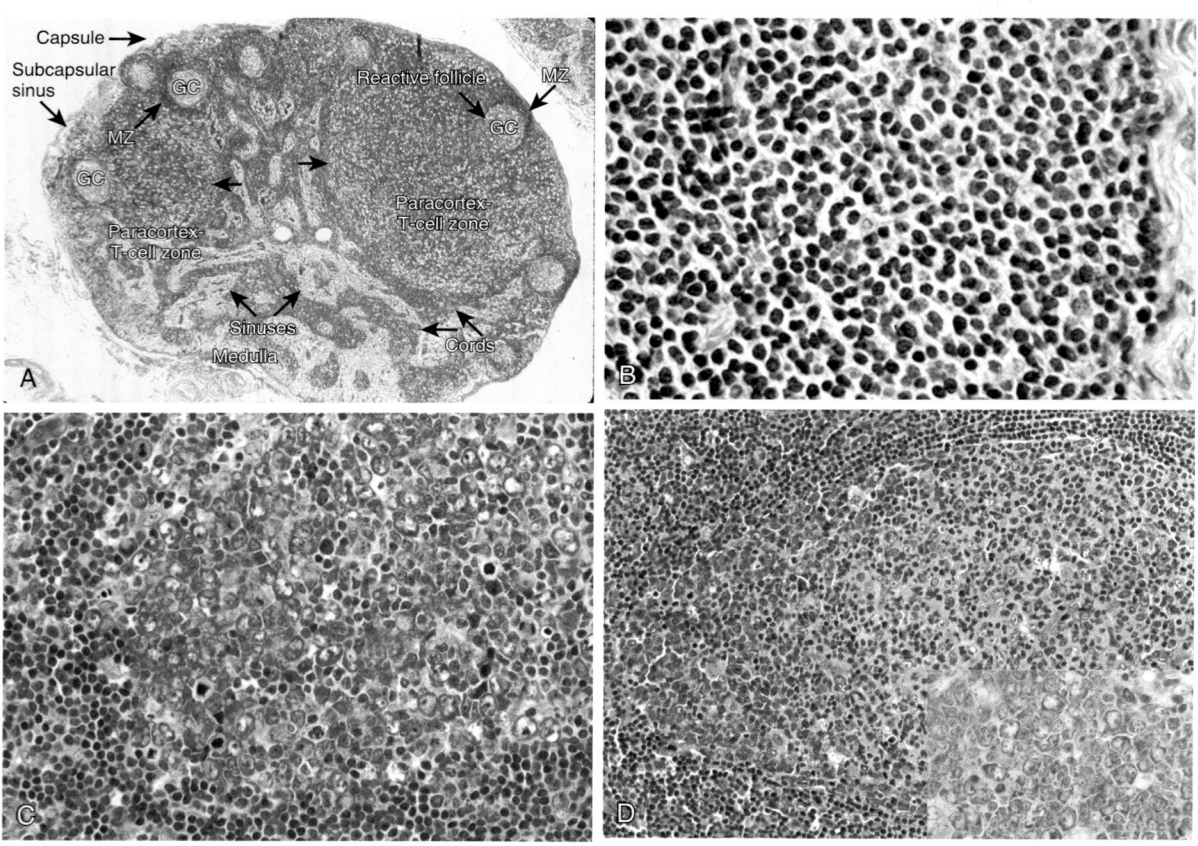

Figure 7-2. Lymph node. A, Low magnification illustrates the architecture of a reactive lymph node. Lymph nodes have a capsule, a cortex, a medulla, and sinuses (subcapsular, cortical, and medullary). The sinuses contain histiocytes (macrophages), which take up and process antigens, which are then presented to lymphocytes. The cortex is divided into follicular *(long, thin arrows)* and paracortical *(short, thick arrows)* regions, and the medulla is divided into medullary cords and sinuses. Both T-cell and early B-cell reactions to antigens occur in the paracortex, and the germinal-center reaction occurs in the follicular cortex. Plasma cells and effector T cells generated by immune reactions accumulate in the medullary cords and exit via the medullary sinuses. **B,** Primary follicle composed of small, predominantly round lymphocytes arranged in a cluster that appears somewhat 3-dimensional. These cells express IgM, IgD, and CD23. **C,** Secondary follicle with an early germinal center predominantly contains centroblasts—large blast cells with vesicular chromatin, one to three peripherally located nucleoli, and basophilic cytoplasm. Occasional centrocytes are present—medium-sized cells with dispersed chromatin, inconspicuous nucleoli, and scant cytoplasm that is not basophilic (Giemsa stain). **D,** The germinal center has polarized into a light zone and a dark zone, surrounded by a mantle zone of small lymphocytes. The dark zone contains mostly centroblasts, with admixed and closely packed centrocytes *(inset)* (Giemsa stain).

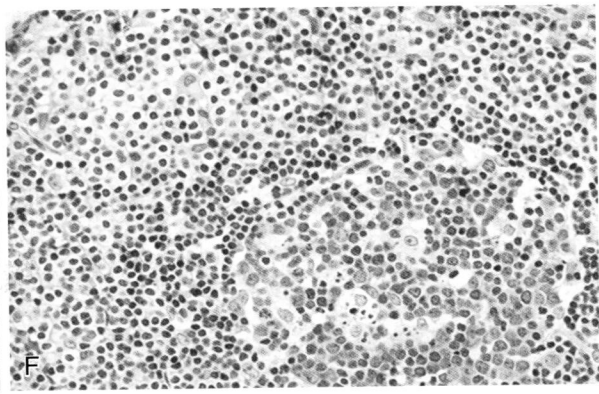

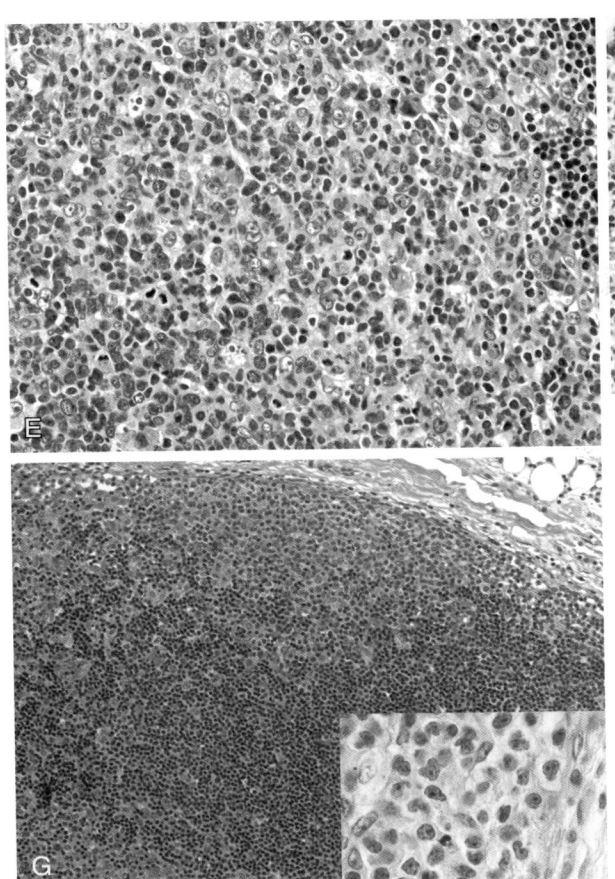

Figure 7-2, cont'd. E, The light zone contains centrocytes, numerous T cells, and many follicular dendritic cells with oval, vesicular nuclei that are often bilobed or binucleate. **F,** Follicle from a mesenteric lymph node has an expanded marginal zone composed of cells with centrocyte-like nuclei and pale cytoplasm. **G,** Lymph node with a monocytoid B-cell aggregate forming a pale band beneath the subcapsular sinus. Inset shows the cells at higher magnification; they have folded, monocyte-like nuclei and abundant pale-to-eosinophilic cytoplasm. *GC,* Germinal center; *MZ,* mantle zone.

The mantle zone is composed mainly of the small B cells of the primary lymphoid follicle that are pushed aside by expansion of the germinal center. Like primary follicle B cells, mantle zone B cells express IgM, IgD, CD21, and CD23. Occasional B cells co-expressing CD5 are also located in this area but are difficult to identify in routine histologic sections. The mantle corona also contains MBCs when the outer marginal zone is not developed.

The germinal center is a specialized lymphoid compartment in which the humoral T-cell–dependent immune response occurs.[9-11] This structure sustains the proliferative expansion of antigen-activated B-cell clones and the generation of high-affinity antibodies by the induction of antigen-driven somatic hypermutation of the Ig heavy and light chain variable region genes. Ig heavy chain constant region genes also undergo the class or isotype switch recombination from IgM and IgD (which can be co-expressed as a result of differential splicing) to IgG, IgA, or IgE. This process is not exclusive to the germinal centers; it may occur in other sites, to a lesser degree, in the T-cell–independent response. The germinal center also provides a microenvironment that selects the antigen-stimulated clones that produce high-affinity antibody, whereas B cells that do not produce high-affinity antibody to the specific antigen undergo apoptosis. Antigen-selected cells then exit the germinal center, becoming MBCs or long-lived plasma cells.

Morphologically, the early germinal center contains predominantly small and large centroblasts. These cells are medium-sized to large-sized B cells with an oval-to-round vesicular nucleus containing one to three small nucleoli close to the nuclear membrane and a narrow rim of basophilic cytoplasm; these features are best seen on Giemsa staining (Fig. 7-2C). After several hours or days, the germinal center becomes polarized into two distinctive areas: the dark zone and the light zone (Fig. 7-2D). The dark zone is composed predominantly of centroblasts. Mitotic figures are common in this area. Closely packed centrocytes are also present in the dark zone (Fig. 7-2D, *inset*). Centrocytes are small-to-large B cells with irregular, sometimes deeply cleaved nuclei, dense chromatin, inconspicuous nucleoli, and scant cytoplasm that is not basophilic on Giemsa staining. Macrophages phagocytizing apoptotic nuclear debris are also present (tingible body macrophages). The light zone contains predominantly quiescent centrocytes.

The light zone also contains a high concentration of FDCs, and their vesicular and often double nuclei with small nucleoli are easily seen in this area (Fig. 7-2E). Contrary to other dendritic cells, FDCs are derived from mesenchymal cells and are important organizers of the germinal centers and the T-cell–dependent immune response. These cells express a profile of molecules that attract B and T cells and facilitate the antigen-presenting process. Thus, FDCs secrete CXCL13, a chemokine that recruits B and T cells expressing CXCR5 (Table 7-1). They also express CD23, the adhesion molecules ICAM-1 and VCAM-1, and complement receptors (CD21, CD35) that fix immunocomplexes (Fig. 7-3). It is important to note that, whereas conventional dendritic cells present antigenic peptides bound to MHC class II molecules

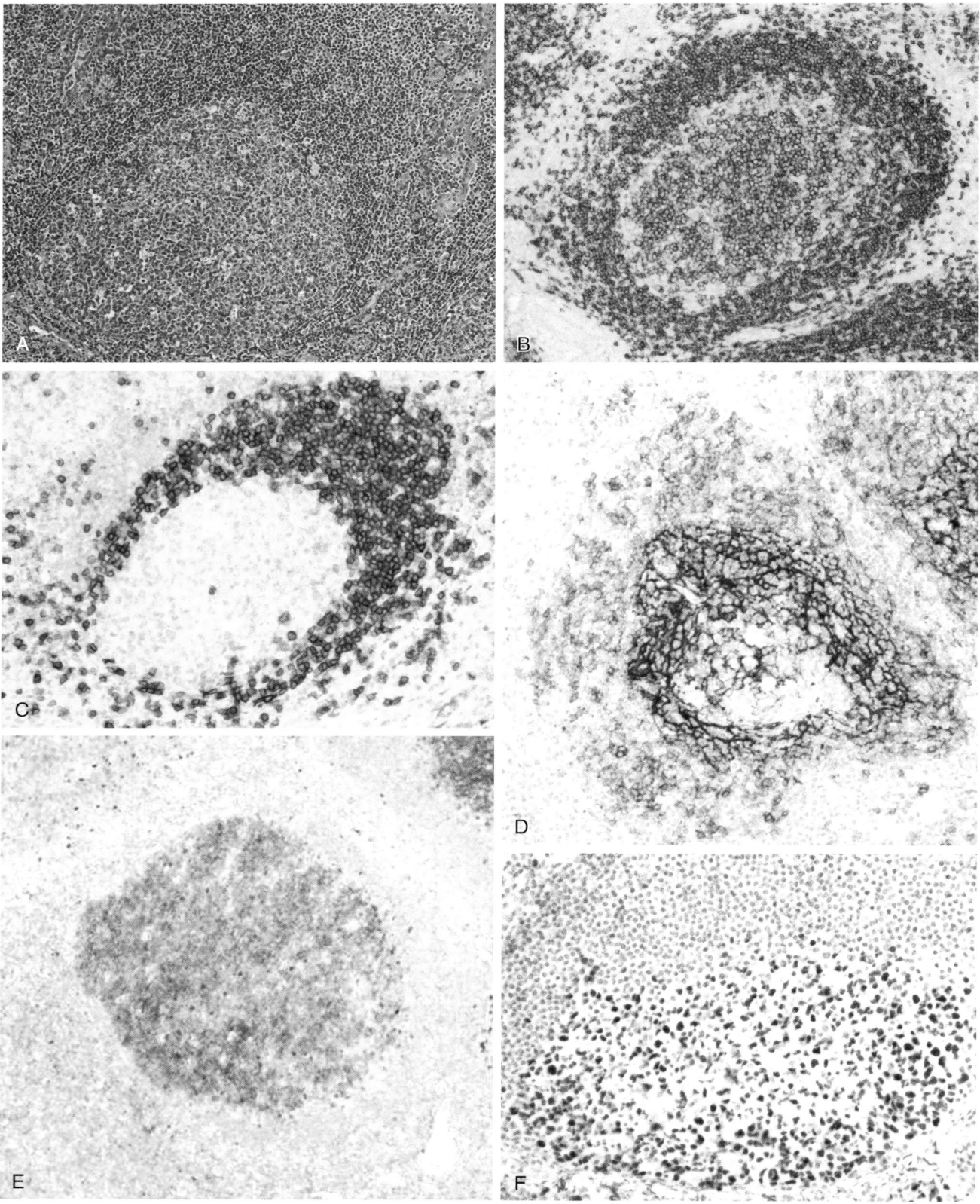

Figure 7-3. Secondary follicle. A, Reactive follicle with a polarized germinal center *(dark zone to the left and light zone to the right)* and a mantle zone area more developed near the light zone of the germinal center. **B,** Immunostain for CD20 shows staining of both the mantle zone and the germinal center. **C,** Immunostain for IgD shows staining of the mantle zone lymphocytes. **D,** CD23 stains follicular dendritic cells (FDCs) predominantly in the light zone in addition to mantle zone B cells. **E,** CD10 highlights the germinal center. **F,** BCL6 shows nuclear staining of most germinal-center cells.

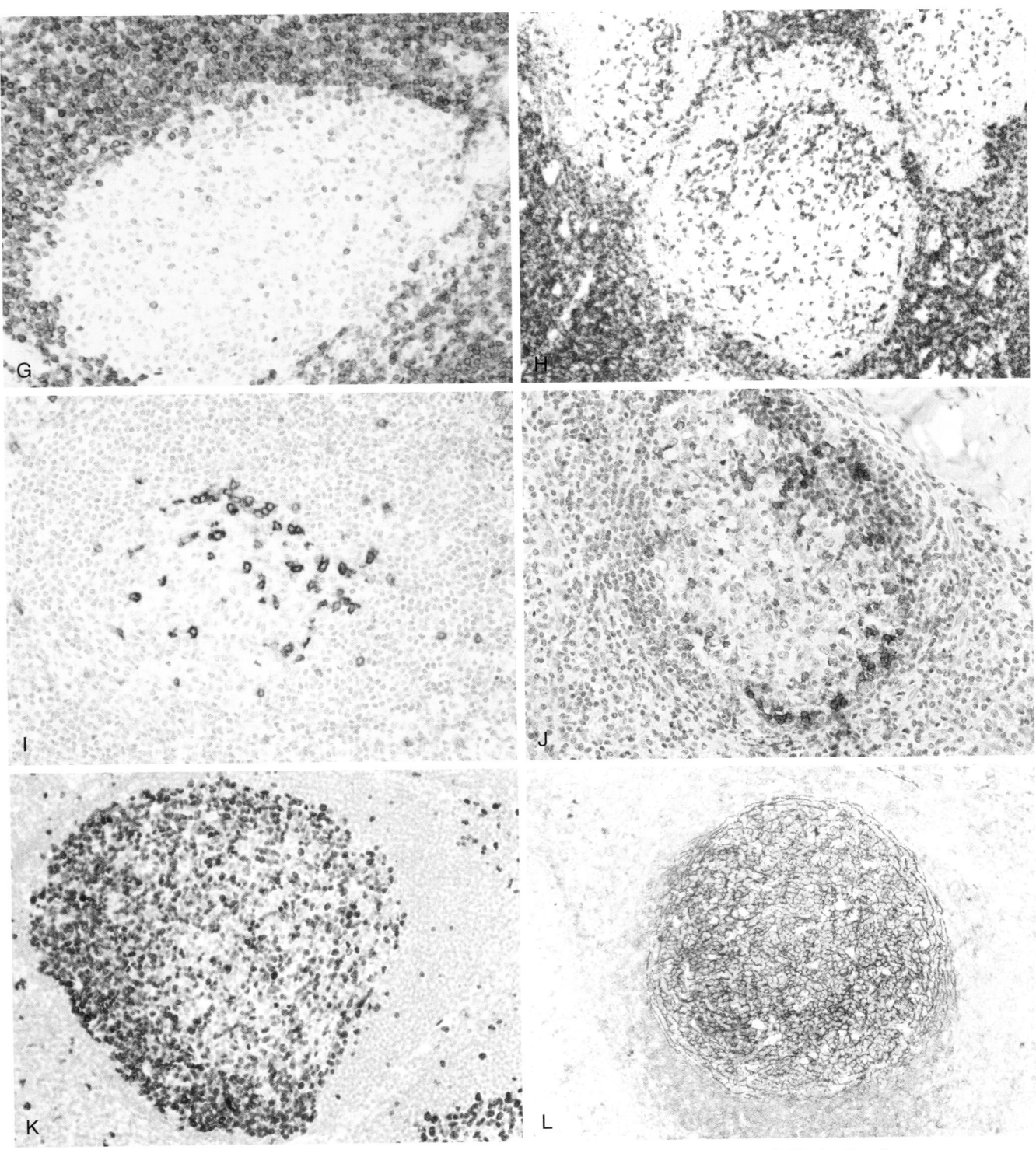

Figure 7-3, cont'd. G, BCL2 is expressed by mantle zone B cells and some intrafollicular T cells, but germinal-center B cells are negative. **H,** CD3 stains the T cells in the paracortex and numerous T cells within the germinal center. They are more numerous in the light zone than in the dark zone and form a crescent at the junction of the germinal center and the mantle zone. **I,** CD57 is expressed by a subset of germinal-center T cells. **J,** CD279 (PD1) is expressed by germinal-center T cells of the follicular helper subset. **K,** The majority of cells in the dark zone are in cycle, staining for Ki-67, whereas fewer cells in the light zone are proliferating. **L,** CD21 stains FDCs predominantly in the light zone and mantle zone B cells.

to CD4-positive T cells, FDCs do not express MHC class II. Therefore FDCs present unprocessed antigen-antibody immune complexes to the B cells either bound to complement or to membranous Fc receptors.

Phenotypically, both centroblasts and centrocytes express mature B-cell antigens (CD19, CD20, CD22, CD79) and germinal-center markers such as BCL6, CD10, LMO2, MEF2B, and HGAL (Fig. 7-3). Centroblasts express Ig at low levels, which may aid in the replacement of the former Ig by modified Ig upon somatic hypermutation. They express high CXCR4 and are negative or low for CD83 and CD86. Surface Ig is re-expressed by centrocytes so that these cells can be selected for having Ig with higher affinity for the driving antigen. Centrocytes are positive for CD83 and CD86 but negative or low for CXCR4. BCL6 is an essential nuclear zinc-finger transcription factor required for germinal-center formation and the T-cell–dependent immune response. It is expressed in germinal-center B and T follicular helper (T_{FH}) cells but not in naïve B cells, mantle zone B cells, MBCs, plasma cells, or other T cells.[10,12] CD10 is a membrane-associated molecule (also known as common acute lymphoblastic leukemia antigen [CALLA]) that is normally expressed in early pro-B cells in the bone marrow but is lost in naïve cells and re-expressed in germinal-center cells. Its function is not well known, but it seems to be indispensable for germinal-center formation. CD10-positive mature lymphoid cells are restricted to germinal centers, and their identification outside this compartment should suggest the presence of a follicular lymphoid cell-derived neoplasm. LIM-only transcription factor 2 (LMO2) and human germinal-center–associated lymphoma (HGAL) are more recently identified genes expressed in germinal-center B cells. LMO2 is a transcription factor that plays an important role in hematopoiesis, and in the bone marrow it is normally expressed in myeloid, erythroid, and lymphoid cells, but in peripheral tissues it is only expressed in germinal-center B cells. HGAL is a highly evolutionary conserved gene that is highly expressed in the cytoplasm of normal and neoplastic germinal-center B cells, whose function is not well understood.[13,14] Myocyte Enhancer Factor 2B (MEF2B) is a transcription factor that interacts with BCL6 and regulates a gene program involved in germinal center formation, particularly the dark zone.[15] It is expressed exclusively in the nucleus of germinal-center B cells but, contrary to BCL6, it is not detected in germinal-center T cells.[16] An important functional phenotypic change in germinal-center B cells is the downregulation of the antiapoptotic molecule BCL2, constitutively expressed in naïve and memory lymphoid cells.[9,10] Thus, these cells are susceptible to death through apoptosis, and only the clones binding the specific antigens will be rescued and survive in this microenvironment. Germinal-center B cells also express surface molecules involved in interactions with FDCs and T cells. In particular, CD40, CD86, and CD71 facilitate the association with T cells, whereas CD11a/18 and CD29/49d recognize the FDC ligands CD44, ICAM-1, and VCAM-1.[10-12]

Germinal centers contain specialized subpopulations of T cells that play an important role in the regulation of the B-cell differentiation process and T-cell–mediated immune response (Fig. 7-3). T_{FH} cells are mainly localized in the light zone and in the mantle zone area and express CD4, CD57, ICOS, CXCL13, PD-1 (programmed death-1, or CD279), and CXCR5, the receptor for the CXCL13 chemokine also secreted by FDCs.[17] T_{FH} cells promote B-cell differentiation through induction of activation-induced cytidine deaminase (AID) expression by B cells, which is needed for Ig class switch. Germinal centers also contain a subset of T regulatory (Treg) cells that express CD4, CD25, and FOXP3 and play a role in preventing autoimmunity and limiting T-cell–dependent B-cell stimulation. These cells also seem to directly suppress B-cell Ig production and class switch.[18] Treg cells are also found in interfollicular areas.

Marginal zones are sometimes seen around follicles in lymph nodes, although these are usually not as prominent as those in the spleen; they are often more conspicuous in mesenteric lymph nodes (Fig. 7-2F). Marginal zone B cells have nuclei that resemble those of centrocytes but with more abundant pale cytoplasm; they appear to be a mixture of naïve B cells and MBCs. In some reactive conditions, slightly larger B cells with even more abundant pale-to-eosinophilic cytoplasm appear in aggregates between the mantle zone and cortical sinuses; these are known as monocytoid B cells (Fig. 7-2G). Neutrophils are frequently intermingled with expanded marginal zone cells. A subset of neutrophils is able to stimulate the antibody production by marginal zone cells, suggesting a possible bridge between innate and adaptive immune response.[19]

Paracortex

The paracortex is the interfollicular T-cell zone (Fig. 7-2A). This compartment contains mainly mature T cells and dendritic cells of the interdigitating cell subtype that specialize in presenting antigens to T cells (Fig. 7-4A). This area is organized by the production of the chemokines CCL19 and CCL21 by stromal cells of the paracortex, particularly fibroblastic reticulum cells and endothelial cells of the high endothelial venules (HEVs) present in this area. These chemokines recruit the T cells and dendritic cells expressing their receptor, CCR7. The T cells in these areas are heterogeneous, with a predominance of CD4-positive cells; some CD8-positive and Treg cells are also found. The interdigitating cells are positive for S100, MHC class II, CD80, CD86, and CD40 but negative for CD1a, CD21, and CD35; they have complex interdigitating cellular junctions. In some reactive conditions, particularly those associated with rashes, the paracortical areas contain Langerhans cells that have migrated from the skin.

Interfollicular areas also contain isolated large B or T cells with immunoblastic morphology; these cells may be numerous in some reactive conditions. B-immunoblasts are large cells similar in size to centroblasts but with prominent single nucleoli and more abundant basophilic cytoplasm (Fig. 7-4B). These cells express mature B-cell markers and abundant cytoplasmic Igs and are considered intermediate steps toward plasma cells. In some reactive situations, these cells may be abundant, express CD30, and downregulate mature B-cell transcription factors such as PAX5, mimicking Hodgkin cells. However, CD15 is negative and polytypic light chain expression is common.[20] A less-frequent subset of large B cells with a dendritic morphology has been identified in nodal T-cell areas.[21] These cells carry Ig somatic mutations and express mature B-cell markers and CD40 but are negative for germinal-center markers (BCL6 and CD10), CD30, and CD27. The functional role of these cells is not known, but they resemble the thymic asteroid cell.

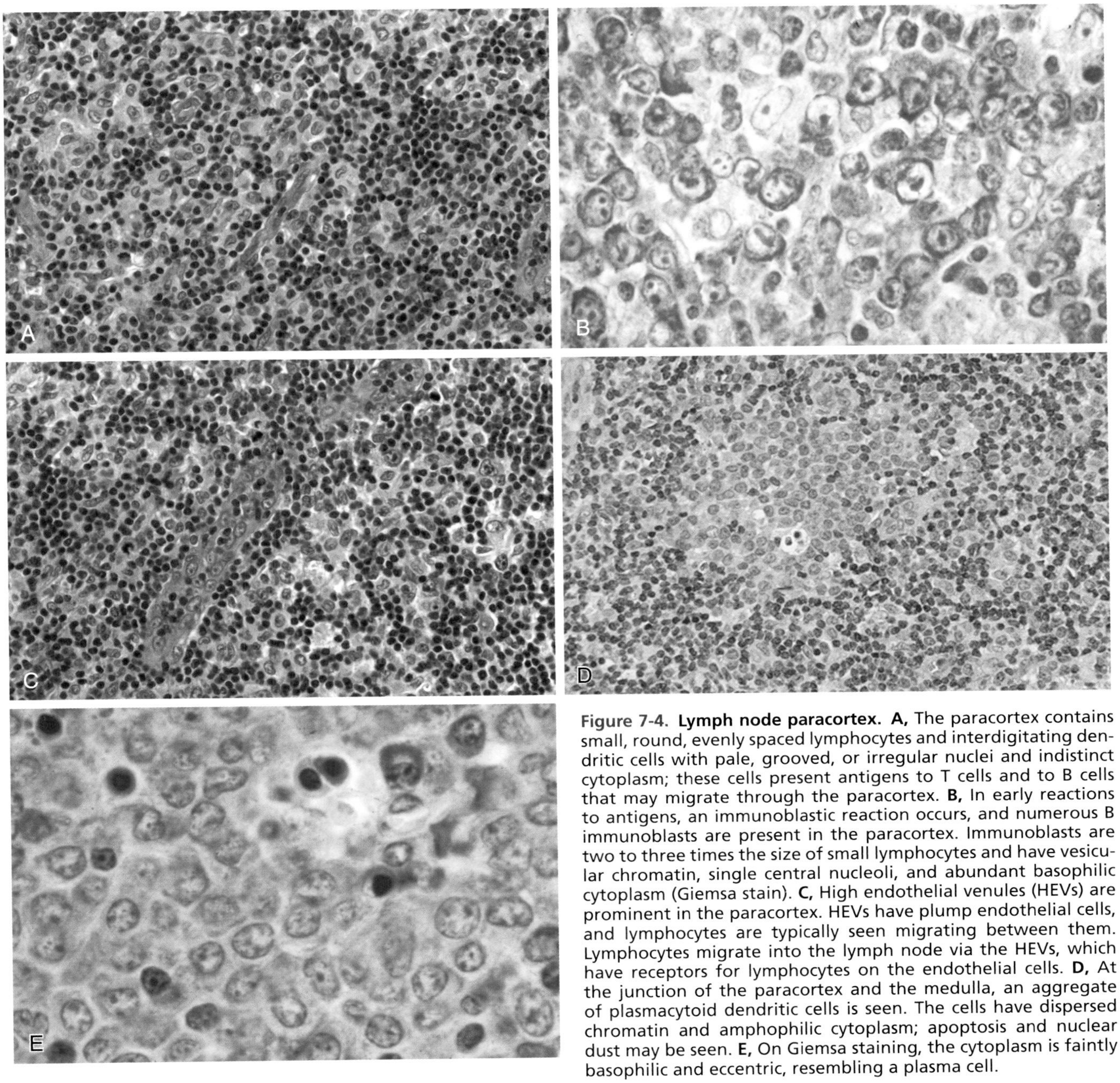

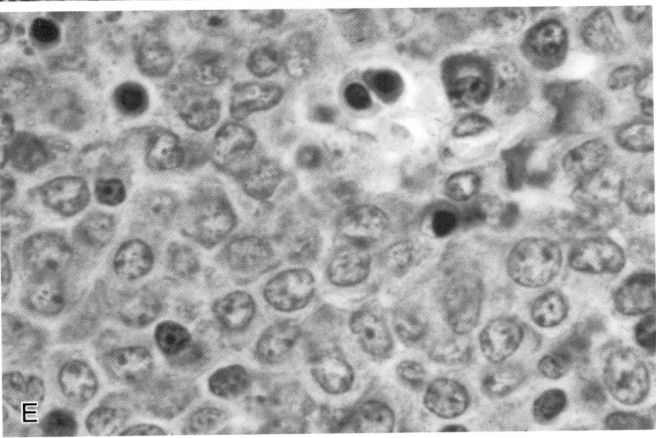

Figure 7-4. Lymph node paracortex. A, The paracortex contains small, round, evenly spaced lymphocytes and interdigitating dendritic cells with pale, grooved, or irregular nuclei and indistinct cytoplasm; these cells present antigens to T cells and to B cells that may migrate through the paracortex. **B,** In early reactions to antigens, an immunoblastic reaction occurs, and numerous B immunoblasts are present in the paracortex. Immunoblasts are two to three times the size of small lymphocytes and have vesicular chromatin, single central nucleoli, and abundant basophilic cytoplasm (Giemsa stain). **C,** High endothelial venules (HEVs) are prominent in the paracortex. HEVs have plump endothelial cells, and lymphocytes are typically seen migrating between them. Lymphocytes migrate into the lymph node via the HEVs, which have receptors for lymphocytes on the endothelial cells. **D,** At the junction of the paracortex and the medulla, an aggregate of plasmacytoid dendritic cells is seen. The cells have dispersed chromatin and amphophilic cytoplasm; apoptosis and nuclear dust may be seen. **E,** On Giemsa staining, the cytoplasm is faintly basophilic and eccentric, resembling a plasma cell.

The paracortex contains HEVs, postcapillary venules through which both T and B lymphocytes enter the lymph node from the blood (Fig. 7-4C).[22] HEVs have large, plump endothelial cells whose nuclei often appear to virtually occlude the lumen. HEVs are also found in other secondary lymphoid tissues except spleen tissue and in tertiary lymphoid structures. These endothelial cells express adhesion molecules that anchor circulating lymphocytes and also act as tissue-specific recognition molecules (called *addressins*) that bind to specific molecules on the lymphocytes (called *homing receptors*). These include E-selectin, P-selectin, VCAM-1, ICAM-1, ICAM-2, peripheral node addressin (peripheral lymph nodes), and mucosal addressin (mesenteric lymph nodes) cell adhesion molecules (MAdCAMs). The addressins bind to L-selectin (CD62L) and $\alpha_4\beta_7$-integrins on the lymphocytes. Postcapillary

venules in other tissues do not express lymphocyte adhesion molecules unless they are stimulated by inflammatory mediators; however, those in the lymph nodes express them constitutively and thus recruit lymphocytes continuously.[23] The HEVs usually contain lymphocytes both within the lumen and infiltrating between the endothelial cells and the basement membrane.

Under some circumstances, collections of plasmacytoid dendritic cells may be found in the paracortex, usually at its junction with the medullary cords. These are medium-sized cells with dispersed chromatin, small nucleoli, and eccentric, amphophilic cytoplasm; they typically occur in small clusters, sometimes with apoptotic debris and histiocytes, mimicking a small germinal center. These cells produce high amounts of interferon-α and function in the regulation of T-cell responses.

They express CD4, CD68, granzyme B, CD123, TCL1, and CLEC4C (BDCA2) and lack specific markers of T-cell, B-cell, or myeloid differentiation.[24-26]

Lymph Node Vasculature and Conduit System

The interaction among lymph, blood, and the different cell components of the lymph node is facilitated by a highly organized vascular system. Blood arrives via arteries at the hilus and branches to reach the subcapsular area and paracortex, where the capillaries form loops and specialize into postcapillary HEVs. Lymph arrives through the afferent lymphatic vessels at the opposite pole of the node, which open to the subcapsular sinus, and flows through the trabecular and medullary sinuses toward the efferent lymph vessels at the hilus. Macrophages in the subcapsular sinuses capture large antigens, immune complexes, and viruses and may present them to nearby B and T cells in the primary follicles in the cortical areas. Small soluble antigens may diffuse through the sinus wall and reach the cortical areas.[27]

The nodal conduit system is a specialized structure that connects the lymphatic sinuses with the walls of the blood vessels, particularly the HEVs in the paracortex, allowing the rapid movement of small antigenic particles (around 5.5 nm and 70 kDa) and cytokines from the afferent lymph deep into the portal of entry of lymphocytes to the nodal parenchyma.[2,28] This structure consists of small conduits composed of a core of type I and III collagen fibers associated with cross-linked microfibrils of fibromodulin and decorin, all of them surrounded by a basal membrane of laminin and type IV collagen. This entire conduit system is generated and wrapped by fibroblastic reticular cells. These cells are positive for vimentin, smooth muscle actin, desmin, and keratins 8 and 18. They also express CCL19/CCL21, serving as a homing mechanism for B cells and T cells expressing the receptor CCR7.[3] Some studies suggest that these cells may acquire FDC markers under certain T-cell stimuli and may be the origin of the expanded meshwork of FDCs that surrounds the HEV in angioimmunoblastic T-cell lymphoma.[3]

Spleen

The spleen has two major compartments—red pulp and white pulp—related to its two major functions as a blood filter for damaged elements of the blood and a defense against blood-borne pathogens, respectively. The white pulp organization is similar to that of the lymphoid tissue of lymph nodes (Fig. 7-5A–F). Follicles and germinal centers are found in the Malpighian corpuscles, and T cells and interdigitating cells are found in the adjacent periarteriolar lymphoid sheath (PALS). The red pulp also contains antigen-presenting cells; lymphocytes, particularly a subset of γ-δ T lymphocytes; and plasma cells. A distinctive feature of the spleen is the presence of a prominent marginal zone that surrounds both the B-cell and T-cell zones (Fig. 7-5D).[29,30]

White Pulp

The B-cell and T-cell areas in the spleen are organized around the branching arterial vessels (Fig. 7-5A–F). Similar to the lymph nodes, the T-cell and B-cell compartments are recruited and maintained by specific chemokines. CCL19 and CCL21 are produced mainly by stromal cells in the T-cell areas, and the FDCs secrete CXCL13; these chemokines recruit cells expressing the receptors CCR7 and CXCR5, respectively

(Table 7-1). T cells surround the arterioles in a discontinuous manner, whereas B-cell follicles may be found adjacent to the T-cell sheaths or directly attached to the arteriole without a T-cell layer (Fig. 7-5F). A distinctive area of the splenic white pulp is the marginal zone, which is more evident in follicles with an expanded germinal center and plays a role in T-cell independent immune response with rapid production of plasmablasts. B cells in this area have slightly irregular nuclei, resembling those of centrocytes but with more abundant pale cytoplasm, and express CD21 and IgM, but contrary to mantle cells, IgD expression is negative or weak (Fig. 7-5D). The marginal zone has two subpopulations of macrophages that constitute an innate immune barrier: the marginal zone and metallophilic macrophages. The marginal zone macrophages in the outer area express CD68, C-type lectins (DC-SIGN/SIGNR1), and the scavenger receptor MARCO that can bind bacterial polysaccharide antigens. Metallophilic macrophages are located in the inner area of the marginal zone, express CD169, and can bind sialic acid-containing molecules on immune cells and some pathogens. They also express Toll-like receptors. The human marginal zone is surrounded by a perifollicular area with more widely separated fibers and capillaries sheathed by abundant macrophages that are positive for sialoadhesin. A large amount of the splenic blood passes through this area, where the flow seems to be retarded. This anatomic relationship between an open blood area and the marginal zone seems to facilitate direct contact between blood-borne antigens and B cells.[29,30]

Red Pulp

The red pulp is composed of sinuses and cords (Billroth cords). The sinuses form an interconnected meshwork covered by a layer of specialized sinusoidal endothelial cells (littoral cells) and surrounded by annular fibers of extracellular matrix; these annular fibers may be seen on periodic acid–Schiff staining (Fig. 7-5G). The cells have cytoplasmic stress fibers that regulate the passage of blood cells. The capillaries open into the cords, and the blood cells that cannot pass through the sinusoidal cells are destroyed by the abundant macrophages resident in the cords. Sinusoidal blood flows into the venous system. The sinusoidal littoral cells have a specific phenotype with expression of CD8 and factor VIII but negative for CD34 (Fig. 7-5H). The red pulp cords also contain plasmablasts and plasma cells. Upregulation of CXCR4 in these cells may play a role in this movement because it binds to the CXCL12 expressed in the red pulp; on the contrary, CXCR5 and CCR7, which bind to the white pulp chemokines CXCL13, CCL19, and CCL21, are downregulated in these cells (Table 7-1).[29,30]

Figure 7-5. Spleen. A, At low magnification, the white pulp contains a reactive follicle with a germinal center *(left)* and a T-cell zone *(right);* both are surrounded by a pale-staining marginal zone. **B,** CD20 staining highlights the B-cell nodules. **C,** Splenic follicle contains a germinal center, a mantle zone, and a pale-staining marginal zone composed of medium-sized cells with abundant pale cytoplasm. **D,** Marginal zone area of the B-cell follicle. The cells have pale cytoplasm. **E,** T-cell zone has an appearance similar to that of the nodal paracortex, with interdigitating dendritic cells present in a background of small lymphocytes. **F,** CD3 stains the periarteriolar T cells. **G,** Periodic acid–Schiff stain highlights the basement membrane of the sinuses, which are fenestrated, allowing nucleated red blood cells to be trapped in the cords. **H,** CD8 strongly stains the red pulp sinusoidal cells.

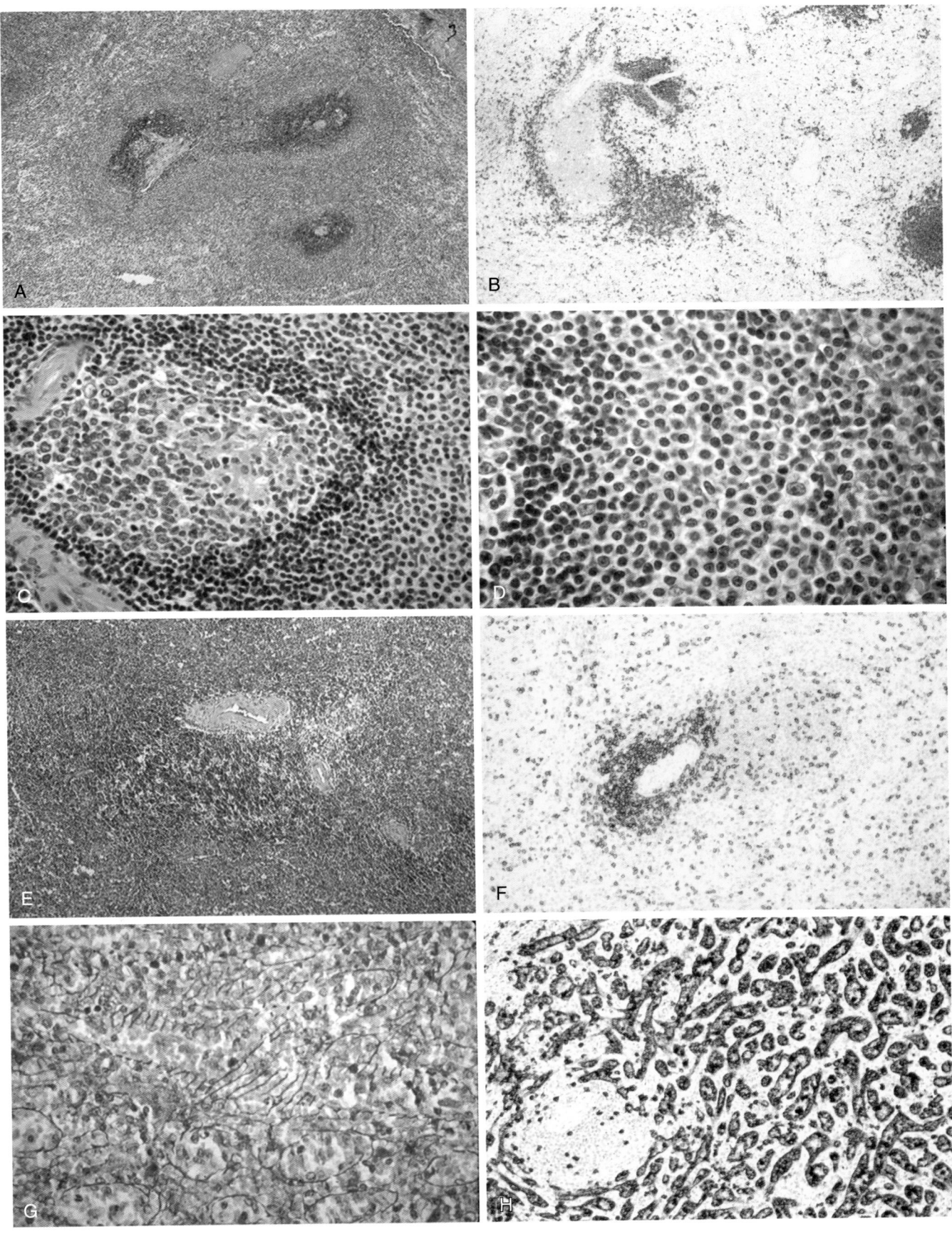

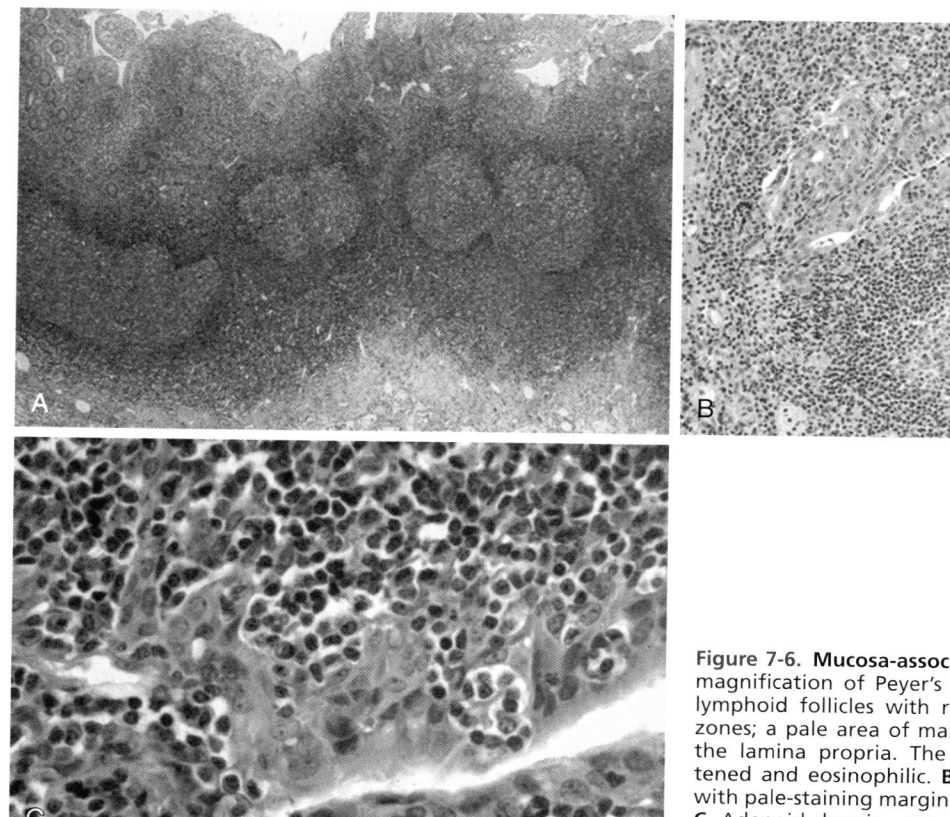

Figure 7-6. Mucosa-associated lymphoid tissue (MALT). A, Low magnification of Peyer's patches of the terminal ileum shows lymphoid follicles with reactive germinal centers and mantle zones; a pale area of marginal zone cells extends upward into the lamina propria. The overlying mucosa is somewhat flattened and eosinophilic. **B,** Adenoid showing a reactive follicle with pale-staining marginal zone cells extending toward a crypt. **C,** Adenoid showing marginal zone cells within the epithelium (lymphoepithelium).

Mucosa-Associated Lymphoid Tissue and Tertiary Lymphoid Organs

Specialized lymphoid tissue is found in association with certain epithelia, in particular the gastrointestinal tract (gut-associated lymphoid tissue—Peyer's patches of the distal ileum, mucosal lymphoid aggregates in the colon and rectum), the nasopharynx and oropharynx (Waldeyer's ring—adenoids, tonsils), and in some species, the lung (bronchus-associated lymphoid tissue). Collectively, this is known as MALT. In each territory, MALT contains four lymphoid compartments: organized mucosal lymphoid tissue, lamina propria, intraepithelial lymphocytes, and regional (mesenteric) lymph nodes (Fig. 7-6).[31] The organized lymphoid tissue is exemplified by Peyer's patches of the terminal ileum and is also found in Waldeyer's ring. The lymphoid follicles are structurally and immunophenotypically similar to those found in lymph nodes. The only difference here is the expanded marginal zone, which tends to reach the superficial epithelium. MALT marginal zone cells are morphologically like those found in the spleen. The interfollicular areas are occupied by T cells and interdigitating dendritic cells. The lamina propria contains mature plasma cells and macrophages and occasional B and T lymphocytes. These plasma cells secrete mainly dimeric IgA, but small populations producing IgM, IgG, and IgE are also present. The dimeric IgA and pentameric IgM are secreted into the intestinal lumen bound to the secretory component, a glycoprotein produced by the enterocytes. The T lymphocytes in the lamina propria are a mixed population of CD4-positive and CD8-positive cells, with a slight predominance (2:1 to 3:1) of the former. Intraepithelial lymphocytes are observed between the epithelial cells and are composed of a heterogeneous population of T cells. The predominant cells are CD3 positive, CD5 positive, and CD8 positive, whereas 10% to 15% are CD3 positive and double negative for CD4 and CD8. CD3-positive CD4-positive cells are a minority, and only rare cells are CD56 positive.[32] Most of the T cells express the α-β form of the T-cell receptor (TCR), and around 10% of the cells are TCR γ-δ. The epithelium above the Peyer's patches contains clusters of B cells and specialized epithelial cells called membranous or microfold cells (M cells). These cells are also found more dispersed in other parts of the gastrointestinal tract and other mucosal sites, particularly in the epithelium over lymphoid follicles.[33] M cells play a sentinel role for the mucosal immune system by capturing luminal antigens and delivering them to the underlying immune cells. The basic structure of mesenteric lymph nodes is similar to that of other lymph nodes, but the marginal zone surrounding the follicles is usually expanded and visible.

The organization of the immune system in mucosal sites is orchestrated by the coordinated action of several adhesion molecules, chemokines, and their respective receptors. Lymphoid cells that respond to antigens in the MALT acquire homing properties that enable them to return to these tissues.[34,35] This homing is mediated in part by expression of high levels of $\alpha_4\beta_7$-integrin, which binds to MAdCAM-1 on HEVs in gut-associated lymphoid tissue.[23] In addition, the MALT immune cells express $\alpha_E\beta_7$-integrin (CD103), whose

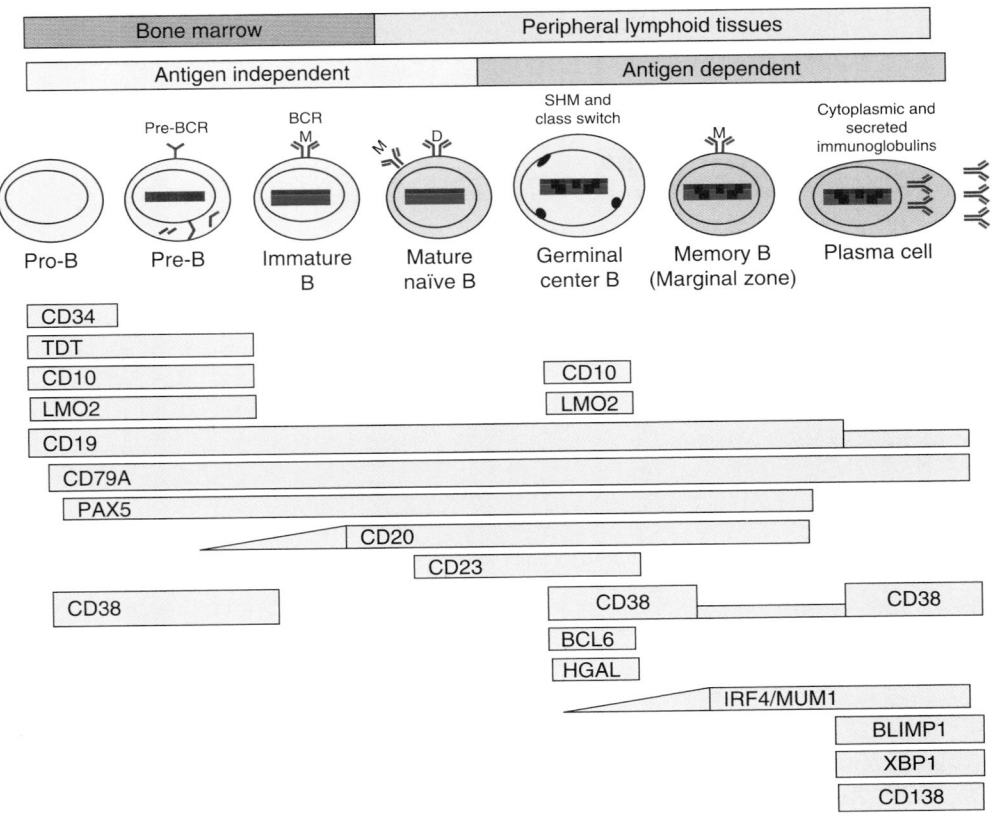

Figure 7-7. Schematic diagram of B-cell differentiation. Early B-cell precursors express CD34, terminal deoxynucleotidyl transferase (TDT), LMO2, and CD10. CD19 is an early B-cell differentiation antigen that is maintained during the entire B-cell differentiation program, and its expression is attenuated in plasma cells. CD79A and PAX5 appear at nearly the same time as heavy-chain gene rearrangement. CD20 is not expressed until the stage of light-chain rearrangement. Germinal-center cells are positive for BCL6 and HGAL and re-express CD10, LMO2, and CD38. The plasma cell differentiation program is characterized by the downregulation of PAX5 and the expression of CD138, BLIMP1, and XBP1. *BCR,* B-cell receptor of mature B cells; *pre-BCR,* pre–B-cell receptor consisting of a heavy chain and the surrogate light chain (which is composed of two linked small peptides, Vpre-B and λ5, represented in *green*); *SHM,* somatic hypermutation; *red bar, IgH* gene rearrangement; *blue bar, IGL* gene rearrangement; *red bar and blue bar with black insertions,* rearranged *IgH* and *IgL* genes with somatic mutations.

ligand E-cadherin is expressed on the basolateral surface of the epithelial cells. Epithelial cells also secrete CCL25, which recruits T cells expressing its receptor CCR9 (Table 7-1).[36]

Tertiary Lymphoid Organs

Tertiary lymphoid organs are organized lymphoid tissue formed at sites of chronic inflammation to develop an adaptive immune response in front of different causes such as infectious, autoimmune, or neoplastic disorders.[37] They have follicular structures and T-cell compartments with HEV and antigen-presenting cells. Contrary to lymph nodes, these areas are not encapsulated and may resolve once the initial stimuli disappear. The initial steps in the genesis of these structures are the priming of resident fibroblastic cells by inflammatory stimuli such as IL-12, IL-17, and IL-22 with production of CXCL13, CCL19, and CCL21, which will attract lymphoid cells, and progressive formation of follicular structures with FDCs and development of HEV.

B-CELL AND T-CELL DIFFERENTIATION

In both the T-cell and B-cell systems, there are two major phases of differentiation: foreign antigen-independent and

foreign-antigen dependent (Figs. 7-7 and 7-8). Foreign antigen-independent differentiation occurs in the primary lymphoid organs—the bone marrow and thymus—without exposure to foreign antigens. This produces a pool of lymphocytes that are capable of responding to foreign antigens (naïve T and B cells) and in general do not respond to self-antigens or autoantigens. The early stages of foreign antigen-independent differentiation involve hematopoietic stem cells and lymphoblasts (blast or progenitor cells of the entire lymphoid line), which are self-renewing; the latter stages involve resting cells with a finite life span ranging from weeks to years. Naïve B and T cells carry surface molecules that are receptors for antigens (surface Ig and the T-cell receptor, respectively). On exposure to antigens, naïve lymphocytes transform into large, proliferating blast cells (immunoblasts for progenitor cells of immune effector cells or centroblasts for blast cells of the germinal center). These blasts give rise to progeny that are capable of direct activity against the inciting antigen: antigen-specific effector cells. The early stages of both antigen-independent and antigen-dependent differentiation involve proliferating cells; the fully differentiated effector cells do not divide unless they are stimulated by an antigen.

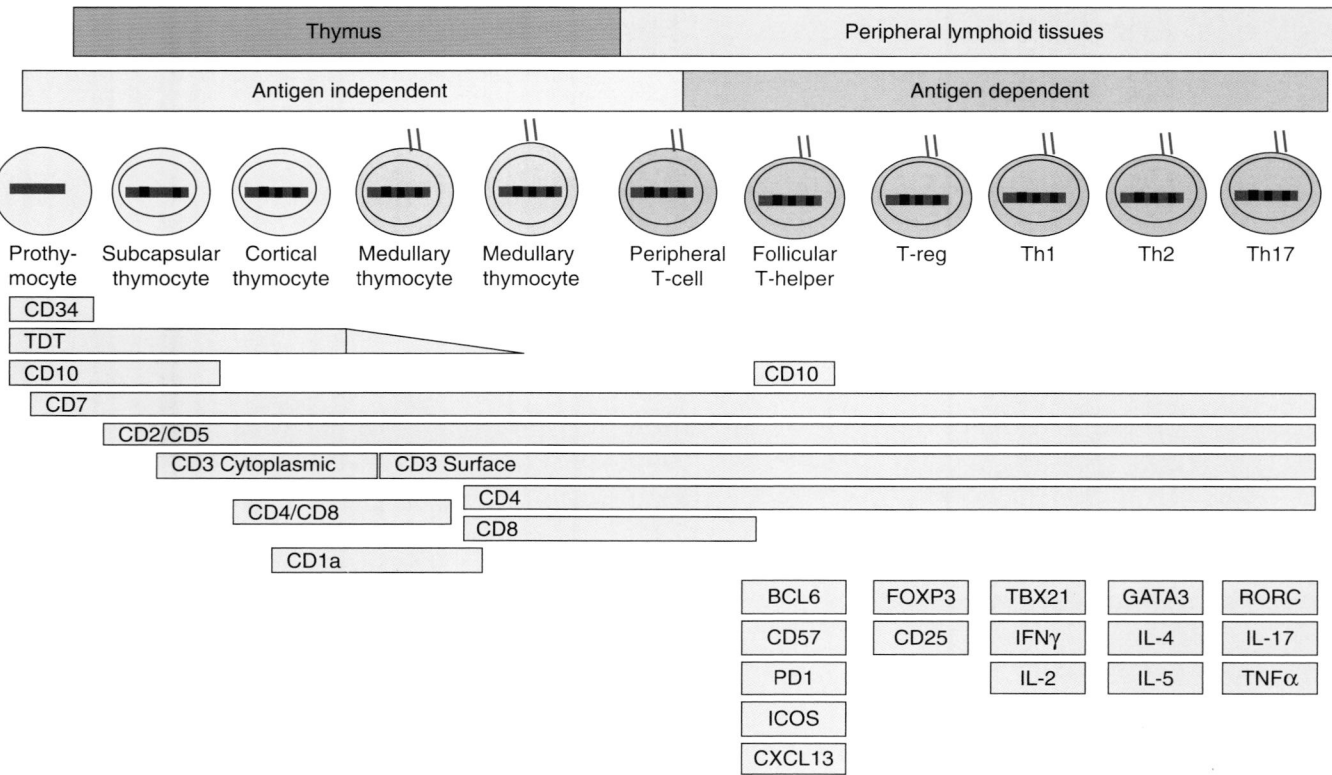

Figure 7-8. Schematic diagram of T-cell differentiation. Early T-cell precursors express CD34, terminal deoxynucleotidyl transferase (TDT), and CD10. CD7 is the first T-cell–specific antigen expressed, followed by CD2/CD5 and cytoplasmic CD3. Cortical thymocytes are double positive for CD4 and CD8 and express CD1a. Medullary thymocytes are already positive for either CD4 or CD8 and express surface CD3. Different subpopulations of mature T cells have been recognized. This simplified diagram illustrates follicular T-helper (Th) cells that express CD10, BCL6, CD57, PD1, and ICOS. T-regulatory cells and Th1, Th2, and Th17 CD4-positive cells are characterized by expression of the transcription factors FOXP3, TBX21, GATA3, and RORC, respectively. Germline T-cell receptor (TCR) genes are represented schematically with a *solid red bar*. Additional *blue* segments represent gene rearrangements. The TRG gene is the first one rearranged, followed by TRB and TRD. The α-β T cells delete the TRD gene during the TRA rearrangement, as delta segments are included in the TRA locus. The γ-δ T cells may have TRB gene rearrangements without assembly of a complete α-β TCR. These gene rearrangements generate two main populations of T cells—α-β and γ-δ—with expression of the TCR complex in the cell membrane (represented here as *double solid bars*).

B-Cell Differentiation

Antigen-Independent B-Cell Development

Precursor B Cells

Precursor B cells develop from hematopoietic stem cells and differentiate in the bone marrow before they migrate to the peripheral lymphoid tissues as naïve mature B lymphocytes. Fetal early B-cell development occurs in the liver, bone marrow, and spleen, whereas in adults it is restricted to the bone marrow. B-cell differentiation produces a broad repertoire of B-cell antigen receptors by the recombination of the variable (V), diversity (D), and join (J) segments of the Ig genes. In this process, the gene segments V, D, and J are joined to encode the heavy-chain (H) variable region that is then joined to the constant region upon RNA splicing.

Cells in the earliest stages are called pro-B cells; they retain some self-renewal capacity and start the rearrangement of the Ig heavy chain.[1] These cells first carry out DH-JH rearrangements, followed by a VH rearrangement to the DH-JH element. The key enzymes for the V(D)J recombination process are the recombination activating genes (RAG) 1 and 2. Some of the common chromosomal translocations in B-cell lymphomas occur at this stage of differentiation when the cell is initiating the Ig rearrangement. As the ends of the rearranging V, D, and J genes are trimmed and additional nongermline encoded nucleotides may be added in the recombination process, there is about a 66% chance that a rearrangement is out-of-frame and thus nonproductive. In such an instance, a second attempt can be made on the second Ig heavy chain allele. If the rearranged V-region gene is in-frame and can be expressed as a μ heavy chain, the cells enter the next pre–B-cell stage in which they synthesize the μ heavy chain protein. At this stage, the cells also synthesize a surrogate light chain composed of two linked small peptides consisting of a variable region (V_{pre-B}) and a constant region (λ5) (pre–B-cell receptor). If this initial receptor is functional, it delivers signals to the cells to proliferate and reactivate the recombination machinery for the kappa light chain gene rearrangements. If no functional kappa light chain rearrangements are generated, the cells perform lambda light chain gene rearrangements. The light chain V-region genes are composed of only two segments, a V and a J segment; D elements are missing. When light-chain rearrangement is complete, a complete surface B-cell receptor (BCR) is expressed as an IgM molecule, and the cell becomes an immature B cell. This population of immature B cells has a vast repertoire of receptors with different antigen specificities, including recognition of antigens in normal cells of the human body (self-reactive cells). The BCRs that recognize these self-antigens generate negative signals to the cells that are induced to die, to became inactivated (anergic), or to perform novel light chain gene rearrangements to replace the original light chain with a new one (light chain editing). In the latter case, further development is possible if the new BCR is no longer autoreactive. Finally, the mature cells that do not react, or that react with very low affinity, with self-antigens leave the bone marrow, now expressing both IgM and IgD.

The pro-B cell expresses CD19 and the precursor markers CD34, CD10, CD127, and HLA-DR. The transcription factors E2A and EBF are also induced at this stage and regulate the machinery for the BCR rearrangements, particularly RAG1, RAG2, and PAX5, a master transcription factor that maintains the B-cell differentiation program through all the B-cell stages up to the plasma cell differentiation stage.[38] These cells also express the terminal deoxynucleotide transferase (TdT) that mediates the addition of nongermline encoded nucleotides (N nucleotides) during the heavy and light chain rearrangements. Pre-B cells lose CD34 and CD127 expression and upregulate CD79a and CD79b, molecules associated with surface Ig and involved in signal transduction after engagement with antigen,[39,40] analogous to CD3 and the TCR molecule. Expression of MHC class II antigens persists throughout the life of the B cell and is important in interactions with T cells; in contrast, TdT is lost before the cells leave the bone marrow. The mature B-cell antigen CD20 is expressed weakly in pre-B cells and increases in immature B cells.

Naïve B Cells

The newly formed B cells that leave the bone marrow are called *transitional B cells*. These cells already co-express IgM and IgD, are CD5 positive, and show high level expression of CD10, CD24, and CD38. In mice, some of these cells are still autoreactive, express AID, and tend to migrate to the spleen where they may undergo negative selection. The differentiation processes of human transitional B cells into mature B cells are less well understood. The newly formed mature B cells that have not yet encountered foreign antigens are called *naïve B cells*. They have rearranged but unmutated Ig and express IgM/IgD, but they are negative for CD27.[41] Several subpopulations of naïve B cells have been recognized.[42,43] *Mature naïve B cells* express pan–B-cell antigens (CD19, CD20, CD22, CD40, CD79a), HLA class II molecules, complement receptors (CD21, CD35), CD23, CD44, and L-selectin and downregulate CD10 and CD38. Many of the surface antigens expressed by mature B cells are involved in "homing" or adhesion to vascular endothelium, interaction with antigen-presenting cells, and signal transduction. Surface Ig, CD79a, CD19, and CD22 are involved in the BCR signaling; CD40 is involved in interaction with T cells, providing a required costimulatory signal for B-cell activation.[44,45] Resting B cells also express the BCL2 protein, which promotes survival in the resting state.[46] A subset of human naïve B cells expresses CD5 and resembles murine *B1 cells* in several aspects. Whether

the human mature CD5-positive B cells are a separate B-cell lineage, as the murine B1 cells, with particular roles in T-cell independent immune responses is unclear.

Morphologically, naïve B cells are small resting lymphocytes. In fetal tissues, they are the predominant lymphoid cell in the spleen; in children and adults, they circulate in the blood, where they typically encompass 50% to 60% of the B cells and constitute a majority of the B cells in primary lymphoid follicles and follicle mantle zones.[47] Studies of single cells picked from the mantle zones of reactive follicles show that they are clonally diverse and contain unmutated Ig genes, consistent with naïve B cells.[48]

Chronic lymphocytic leukemia (CLL) and mantle cell lymphoma (MCL) were traditionally considered neoplasms of naïve B cells but are now interpreted as derived from CD5-positive B cells that have experienced antigens, possibly having passed through the germinal center or matured through an extrafollicular pathway (Table 7-2).[49-51]

Antigen-Dependent B-Cell Differentiation

T-Cell–Independent B-Cell Reaction

Some antigens can trigger a B-cell immune reaction without T-cell cooperation. Large nonprotein antigens interact with the BCRs and toll-like receptors (TLRs), a group of pattern recognition receptors, providing two activating signals to naïve cells. Large antigens with repeat structures may also activate naïve B cells by strong crosslinking of BCR molecules. These activated cells transform into proliferating blast and short-lived plasma cells, producing the IgM antibody of the primary immune response.[52] In general, such immune responses do not give rise to long-lived MBCs. Class-switching can occur in some of the activated B cells in T-cell–independent immune responses. This response is rapid, but the antibodies have a lower affinity for antigens than the antibodies generated in T-cell–dependent immune reactions, as Ig somatic hypermutation is not induced or occurs at a low level. Cells activated by these T-cell–independent mechanisms may receive accessory signals from myeloid cells, particularly neutrophils and macrophages, mediated by BAFF and APRIL (a proliferation-inducing ligand), which stimulate the nuclear factor-κB (NF-κB) pathway in the activated B cells.[53] These signals likely have an effect similar to CD40L-CD40 interactions in the germinal center.

T-Cell–Dependent Germinal-Center Reaction

Later in the primary response (within 3 to 7 days of antigen challenge in experimental animals) and in secondary responses, the T-cell–dependent germinal-center reaction occurs. The mechanisms triggering this response may depend on the type of antigen and requires simultaneous stimulation of the BCR and cognate activation of the B cells by T_{FH} cells mediated by CD40L, IL-4, IL-21, and further coactivating factors.[54] Each germinal center is formed by a few to dozens of naïve B cells and ultimately contains approximately 10,000 to 15,000 B cells; thus, more than 10 generations are required to form a fully developed germinal center.[48] Proliferating IgM-positive B blasts formed from naïve B cells that have encountered antigens in the T-cell zone (paracortex) migrate into the center of the primary follicle and fill the FDC meshwork about 3 days after antigen stimulation, forming a germinal center.

Table 7-2 Immunohistologic and Genetic Features and Postulated Normal Counterparts of Common B-Cell Neoplasms

Neoplasm	Postulated Normal Counterpart	sIg; cIg	CD20	CD5	CD10	CD23	CD43	CD103	Cyclin D1	SOX11	LEF1	CD38/CD138	Genetic Abnormality	Mutated Genes
Chronic lymphocytic leukemia	Antigen-experienced B cell	+; -/+	+ (weak)	+	-	+	+	-	-	-	+	-	Trisomy 21; del(13q); del(11q); del(17p)	NOTCH1 ATM SF3B1 BIRC3 TP53 MYD88
Lymphoplasmacytic lymphoma	Postfollicular B cell that differentiates to plasma cell?	+; +	+	-	-	-	+/-	-	-	-	-	+	del 6(q23)	MYD88 CXCR4
Hairy cell leukemia	Memory B cell?	+; -	+	-	-	-	+	++	+/-	-/+	-	-	None known	BRAF CDKN1B
Follicular lymphoma	Germinal-center B cell	+; -	+	-	+/-	-/+	-	-	+/-	-	-	-	t(14;18); BCL2	KMT2D CREBBP EZH2 FOXO1 MEF2B TNRSF14 RRAGC
Mantle cell lymphoma	Mantle zone B cell, Antigen-experienced cell	+; -	+	+	-	-	+	-	+	+*	-	-	t(11;14); CCND1	ATM TP53 NSD2 HNRNPH1 NOTCH1/2
Splenic marginal zone lymphoma	Marginal zone B cells	+; -/+	+	-	-	-	-	+	-	-	-	-	del 7(q31-32)	KLF2 NOTCH2 TP53 BIRC3 TNFAIP3
Nodal marginal zone lymphoma	Marginal zone B cell	+; +/-	+	-	-	-/+	-/+	-	-	-	-	-		KLF2 NOTCH2 TP53 TNFAIP3 BIRC3 BRAF PTPRD
MALT lymphoma	Marginal zone B cell	+; +/-	+	-	-	-/+	-/+	-	-	-	-	-	Trisomy 3 t(11;18); t(14;18) MALT1; t(1;14) BCL10; t(3;14) FOXP1	TNFAIP3 FAS (skin)
Diffuse large B-cell lymphoma GCB subtype	Germinal-center B cell	+/-	+	-	+/-	NA	-	NA	-	-	-	-	t(14;18), t(8;14), t(3q27); BCL2, MYC, BCL6,	KMT2D EZH2 CREBBP SGK1 TET2

Entity	Cell of origin										Genetics	Genes
Diffuse large B-cell lymphoma ABC subtype	Activated B cell	+/–; –/+	+	–	NA	–	NA	–	–/+	–	t(3q27) BCL6; +3q; +18q; –9p. –6q21	MYD88, CD79B, BLIMP1, TNFAIP3, CARD11, BCL6, NOTCH1
Burkitt lymphoma	Germinal-center B cell	+; –	+	–	–	+	NA	–	–	–	t(8;14), t(2;8), t(8;22), MYC, EBV –/+	TCF3, ID3, CCND3
Plasmablastic lymphoma	Plasmablast	+	–	–/+	–	–	–	+	–	+	t(8;14), MYC; EBV+	STAT3, NRAS, KRAS, TP53, CARD11, SOCS1, TET2
Plasma cell myeloma	Bone marrow plasma cell	–/+	+/–	–/+	+/–	–/+	–	–/+	–	+	Hyperdiploidy, CCND translocations, MAF translocations, NSD2 translocations, t(8;14), MYC	TP53, NRAS, KRAS, FAM46C
Nodular lymphocyte predominant B-cell (Hodgkin) lymphoma#	Germinal center cell	–	+	–	–	+	–	–	–	–	BCL6 translocation, REL gains	DUSP2, SGK1, JUNB
Classic Hodgkin lymphoma +	Germinal center cell	–	–	–	–	–	–	–	–	–	Aneuploidy, REL, MAP3K14, JAK, PDL1/2 amplification	SOCS1, STAT6, B2M, NFAIP3, NFKBIA, NFKBIE

*Leukemic non-nodal MCL is SOX11 negative.

#NLPBL Phenotype: PAX5+, CD30+, CD15–, EMA +.

+Classic Hodgkin phenotype: PAX5 + weak, CD30+, CD15–; IRF4+, EBV +/–.

+, >90% positive; +/–, >50% positive; –/+, <50% positive; –, <10% positive.

cIg, Cytoplasmic immunoglobulin; EBV, Epstein-Barr virus; MALT, mucosa-associated lymphoid tissue; NA, not available; sIg, surface immunoglobulin.

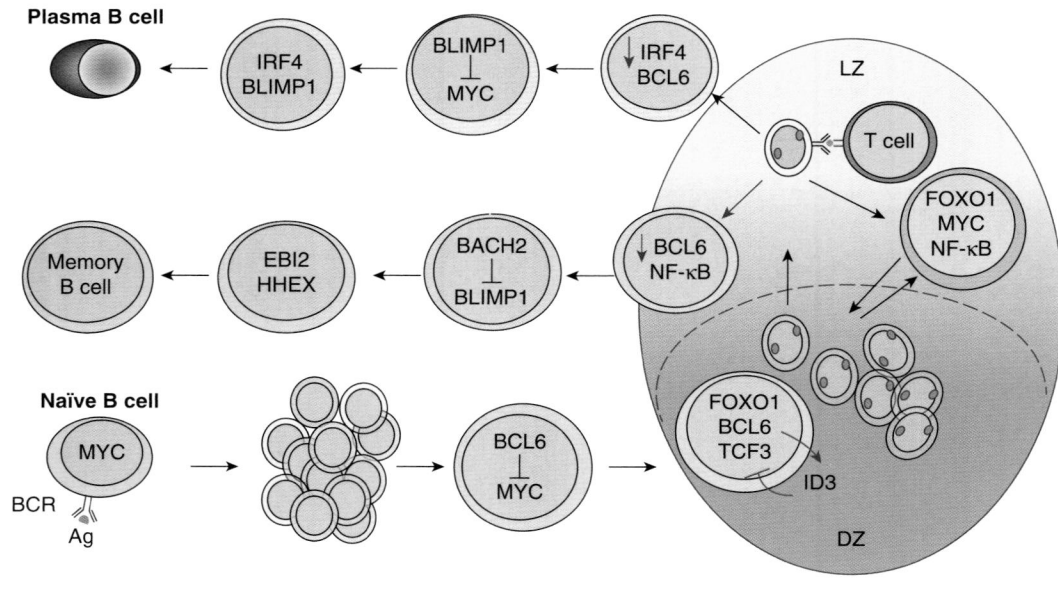

Figure 7-9. Interactions between different transcription factors in germinal-center formation and B-cell differentiation. MYC is initially expressed in naïve B cells that have interacted with antigens and T cells.[56] The subsequent BCL6 expression represses MYC and turns on the germinal-center formation. The proliferation program in the dark zone is maintained by activation of the TCF3 program. The inhibitory loop between ID3 and TCF3 attenuates the proliferation and allows the cells to move toward the light zone of the germinal center. Here, depending on the intensity of the T_{FH} activation, the cells will follow different pathways.[53] A weak T-cell signal resulting from low affinity of the B-cell receptor (BCR) will trigger low NF-κB activation, downregulation of BCL6, and expression of BACH2, leading to memory B-cell differentiation. A moderate T signal will lead to expression of FOXO1 and MYC and re-entry of the centrocytes to the dark zone to follow subsequent rounds of proliferation and somatic mutations of the immunoglobulin genes. If the T signal is very strong because of high affinity of the BCR, the cell will express IRF4 and BLIMP1 and exit the germinal center to differentiate toward a memory or plasma cell.

Movement from the T cell to the follicular area is determined by the upregulation of CXCR5 in the primed B and T cells. This receptor binds to the CXCL13 ligand produced by the FDCs and adjacent stromal cells (Table 7-1). The germinal-center reaction is an efficient mechanism to generate expanded B-cell clones with a highly selected antigen receptor and two types of effector cells—MBCs and long-lived plasma cells. This process includes four major steps: proliferation, induction of Ig somatic hypermutation and class switch, selection, and differentiation.[55]

An important event in the early phase of germinal-center formation is the expression of MYC in the naïve B cell, induced by interaction with the antigen and T cells (Fig. 7-9).[56] This expression is transient but essential for the germinal-center formation. MYC regulates proliferation through activation of cyclin D2 and D3 and E2F1 that in turn induces the expression of EZH2, further promoting proliferation by suppressing the expression of CDK inhibitors and phosphorylation of RB, among others.[53] In a subsequent step, BCL6 is expressed and represses MYC by binding to its promoter. BCL6 is expressed by centroblasts, centrocytes, and germinal-center T cells, but not by naïve B cells, MBCs, mantle zone B cells, or plasma cells.[10,11,55] BCL6 upregulation is necessary for germinal-center formation and maintenance, and its transcription program targets a series of genes directly involved in the germinal-center reaction.[55] BCL6 downregulates genes involved in negative cell cycle regulation and the genotoxic

response. One of the major targets is *TP53*. Its inhibition in the germinal center leads to the downregulation of the cell cycle inhibitor *CDKN1A* (p21) and consequently facilitates proliferation. In addition, the downregulation of *TP53*, *ATM*, and *ATR*, genes involved in the cell response to DNA damage, facilitates the germinal-center cells' tolerance to the DNA breaks and rearrangements that occur during the somatic hypermutation and class-switch processes. Finally, BCL6 represses the differentiation of centrocytes to plasma cells and MBCs, particularly by inhibiting the plasma cell differentiation transcription factor BLIMP1, among others. Other transcription factors required for germinal-center formation are FOXO1 and MEF2B.[10,11,55] FOXO1 regulates a program overlapping in part with BCL6. It is essential for the development of the dark zone, promoting proliferation and reducing affinity maturation, and it is downregulated when the cells move to the light zone.[53] MEF2B collaborates with BCL6 in germinal-center formation.[55]

T_{FH} cells are important modulators of germinal-center B-cell responses, mainly mediated by IL-4, IL-21, and CD40L, cooperating with BCR signaling.[57] They participate in the initial steps of B-cell stimulation, class-switch recombination, and selection in light zones. Their function is negatively modulated by TNFRS14 (HVEM), which is expressed in B cells and binds to BTLA in T_{FH} cells. These interactions prevent uncontrolled expansion of B cells in the germinal center.[58] Frequent inactivation of *TNFRS14* in follicular lymphoma

B cells seem to favor lymphomagenesis by disrupting this negative control of T_{FH} cells on B cells.[59]

Proliferation. The antigen-stimulated B blasts differentiate into centroblasts, which appear at about 4 days and accumulate in the dark zone.[10,11,55] These cells are highly proliferative, with inactivation of cell-cycle inhibitors and expression of cell-cycle activators. The proliferation program of these cells seems orchestrated by the transcription factor TCF3 (E2A), which is highly expressed in the cells of the dark zone. TCF3 induces genes required for the proliferation, such as *CCND3* and *E2F2*. It also induces its own inhibitor, ID3, which creates an autoregulatory loop that attenuates the TCF3 proliferative program, allowing the cell to move toward the light zone of the germinal center. The proliferation program of germinal-center cells differs from that of proliferative cells in other tissues. Thus, centroblasts activate telomerase to prevent the shortening of telomeres in each cell cycle, downregulate antiapoptotic genes such as *BCL2* and other members of the family, and upregulate proapoptotic molecules such as CD95 (FAS). The effect of this proapoptotic default program is to facilitate the survival of only those cells that will be rescued by the generation of highly selected receptors to the specific antigen present in the germinal center.[10,11,55]

Somatic Hypermutation and Class Switch. Centroblasts undergo somatic hypermutation of the Ig heavy and light chain V-region genes, which alters the antigen affinity of the antibody produced by the cell.[10,11,55] This process requires the activity of AID, which is induced in these cells by IL-4 and CD40L. Somatic hypermutation results in marked intraclonal diversity of antibody-combining sites in a population of cells derived from only a few precursors. Studies of single centroblasts picked from the dark zone of germinal centers suggest that, in the early stages, a germinal center may contain about 5 to 10 clones of centroblasts, which show only a moderate amount of Ig V-region gene mutation; later, the number of clones diminishes to as few as three, and the degree of somatic mutation increases.[48] This process introduces somatic mutations in other genes expressed in the germinal center, such as *BCL6*, although at a much lower frequency than is seen in the Ig genes.[60-62] In some types of germinal-center–associated B-cell lymphomas, the targeting of non-Ig genes is further deregulated, causing targeting of more genes, including several protooncogenes. This lymphoma-associated extensive targeting of non-Ig genes has been termed *aberrant somatic hypermutation*.

Class-switch recombination is a further AID-mediated process that allows replacement of the heavy chain isotype. This process had been considered to occur in light zone centrocytes. However, evidence from murine studies suggests that this phenomenon mainly occurs very early after the initial antigen activation of B cells, before entering the germinal center and starting somatic hypermutation.[63] This sequence of events may explain the observations, in some lymphomas, of translocations between Ig genes and different oncogenes mediated by AID and aberrant class-switched mechanisms in cells with unmutated Ig (occurring prior to the germinal-center reaction).[64]

Selection. Centroblasts mature to nonproliferating centrocytes, which accumulate in the opposite pole of the germinal center—the light zone. Centrocytes express the somatically mutated Ig genes and now need to be selected for expression of a BCR with improved affinity.[48] Centrocytes whose Ig-gene mutations have resulted in *decreased* affinity for antigens

rapidly die by apoptosis; the prominent "starry sky" pattern of phagocytic macrophages seen in germinal centers at this stage is a result of the apoptosis of centrocytes. In contrast, centrocytes whose Ig-gene mutations have resulted in *increased* affinity are able to bind to native, unprocessed antigens trapped in antigen-antibody complexes by the complement and Fc receptors on the processes of FDCs. The centrocytes are able to process the antigen and present processed peptides on MHC class II molecules to T cells in the light zone of the germinal center. The activated T cells express CD40L, which can engage CD40 on the B cell, "rescuing" them from apoptosis.[10,11,55]

Selected cells in the light zone typically undergo several cycles of recirculating backward to the dark zone, allowing additional rounds of proliferation and Ig somatic mutations to create antibodies of higher affinity and further expand clonally. This re-entry to the dark zone requires downregulation of BCL6 that allows the transient re-expression of MYC in a subset of the light-zone cells (Fig. 7-9). An important step preparing the cell to re-enter the dark zone is the activation of the mTORC1 pathway in positively selected B cells, increasing the anabolic metabolism necessary for cell growth and subsequent proliferation.[53,65] Once the cell enters the dark zone, it again upregulates BCL6 and TCF3 and downmodulates MYC and mTORC1.[56]

Differentiation. Termination of the germinal-center program and post–germinal-center differentiation of selected centrocytes into plasma cells or MBCs require inactivation of the master regulator BCL6. The increasing signaling activity from the selected high-affinity BCR induces the ubiquitination of BCL6 and subsequent degradation. Similarly, the CD40-CD40L activation of B cells induces NF-κB activation and expression of the transcription factor IRF4, which in turn represses BCL6.[55] Centrocytes of the light zone may be directed to exit the germinal center and become MBCs or plasma cells. IRF4 and BLIMP1 seem to cooperate as potent inductors of plasma cell differentiation, whereas PAX5, which has maintained the B-cell program from the early stages of B-cell differentiation, needs to be shut off to allow plasma cells to develop. The transcription of BLIMP1 is negatively regulated by BCL6, and this inhibition is released by the downregulation of BCL6 at the end of the germinal-center program. BLIMP1, in turn, represses PAX5, opening the pathway to plasma cell differentiation and MYC, preventing centrocytes from re-entering the dark zone of the germinal center. BLIMP1 also stimulates the transcription of XBP1, which is required to maintain and tolerate the endoplasmic reticulum stress signals that appear during the secretory phenotype of the plasma cells.[53,55,66]

Most B-cell lymphomas originate in cells derived from the germinal center and carry mutations in key genes involved in the normal development of the cells in this structure (Table 7-2).[55,67-70]

Memory B Cells. MBCs have the capacity to survive long term and to rapidly differentiate into antibody-secreting cells upon antigen re-encounter, therefore conferring life-long immunity. T-cell dependent memory cells are generated in the light zone of the germinal center, preferentially in the early phases of the immune response, and typically carry lower levels of somatic mutation and show less affinity maturation relative to plasma cells.[53,54] Cells in the light zone seem to differentiate to memory cells when they receive moderate levels of T-cell activation that prevents the activation of MYC and re-entry to the dark zone. The low levels of IL-4 and IL-21 also reduce the expression of *BCL6* required to exit the germinal center. Downregulation of BCL6 allows the expression of EBI2 and HHEX, two transcription factors that promote MBC differentiation and exit of the germinal center. Expression of the BACH2 transcription factor is also crucial to direct the cell to the memory differentiation, as it downregulates cell cycle elements and prevents the BLIMP1 expression required for plasma cells differentiation (Fig. 7-9). MBCs leave the follicle and are detectable in the peripheral blood and different tissue compartments, including the marginal zones. Studies in mice showed that some antigen-activated B cells, after first interaction with T cells in the primary reaction in the T-cell area of lymph nodes, had already differentiated into MBCs without even entering the germinal center and undergoing somatic hypermutation there. The small subset of human MBCs with unmutated IgV genes may mostly derive from this differentiation pathway, assuming it also exists in humans.

Human MBCs are a heterogeneous population, usually expressing CD27 with variable expression of other markers. Two major subsets have been recognized that express either IgM or IgG/IgA. Upon antigen rechallenge, IgG or IgA memory cells mostly differentiate rapidly into plasmablasts, whereas IgM memory cells preferentially proliferate and generate a new germinal-center reaction.[71] IgM memory cells represent 10% to 20% of all B cells in the peripheral blood of adults, whereas the class-switched cells account for 15% to 25% and the naïve cells for about 50% to 70%. Similar IgM memory cells are present in tissues, particularly in splenic and MALT marginal zones, tonsils, and lymph nodes.

Most of the IgM-positive CD27-positive B cells with mutated IgV genes co-express IgD. These cells are present in the peripheral blood and are the dominant B-cell subset populating the splenic marginal zone. There is still some controversy about the origin and identity of these cells. Some minimally mutated IgM-positive IgD-positive CD27-positive B cells are detectable in patients with hyper-IgM syndrome owing to a CD40-CD40L genetic deficiency in whom classical germinal-center reactions are absent. Because of their resemblance to murine marginal zone B cells, which are typically involved in T-cell–independent immune responses, it is postulated that these are MBCs generated in a similar T-independent pathway, with somatic hypermutation outside of germinal centers. However, other features of these cells argue that they are bona fide germinal-center–derived MBCs.[72-74] They frequently carry mutations in the *BCL6* gene, which should only occur in germinal-center B cells where BCL6 is transcribed. They often form common clones together with classical class-switched MBCs. Genealogic trees of such clones show an intermingling of IgM-positive IgD-positive and class-switched B cells, strongly indicating an origin from a common mutating germinal-center B-cell clone. They also show a transcriptome more similar to IgG/IgA MBCs than to naïve B cells. Perhaps, early in life, a first subset of IgM-positive IgD-positive CD27-positive B cells with no or very few Ig mutations is generated in a germinal-center–independent pathway, but with increasing age, these cells are replaced by post–germinal-center IgM-positive IgD-positive CD27-positive MBCs.

Nodal, extranodal, and splenic lymphomas carrying IgV mutations consistent with germinal-center exposure and antigen selection resembling normal marginal zone and monocytoid B cells have been described (Table 7-2).[75,76] In addition, about 50% of CLLs and 10% of MCLs have mutated Ig V-region genes and appear to derive from a CD5-positive memory-like B-cell subset.[77]

Plasma Cells. Plasma cells are heterogeneous. The precursor of a mature, antibody-secreting plasma cell is a cell that retains proliferating activity, known as a plasmablast. Mature plasma cells are divided into short-lived and long-lived subsets.[66] Plasmablasts express MHC class II but lose mature B-cell markers such as CD20 and PAX5 and the CXCR5 and CCR7 receptors that maintain the lymphoid cells in the B-cell and T-cell compartments in response to CXCL13, CCL19, and CCL21. Plasmablasts acquire CXCR4, which attracts the cells to the CXCL12-secreting tissues in the bone marrow and other plasma cell niches such as the lymph node medullary cords and splenic red pulp cords.[66]

Short-lived IgM-secreting plasma cells are generated in the T-cell–independent immune response and reside in secondary lymphoid organs, whereas long-lived IgM-positive and class-switched plasma cells are effector cells of the T-cell–dependent immune response. IgG-producing plasma cells accumulate in the lymph node medulla and splenic cords. From there, it appears the predecessors of the bone marrow plasma cell leave the nodes and spleen and migrate to the bone marrow.

Plasma cells lose surface Ig (although IgM and IgA plasma cells retain some surface BCR expression),[78] pan–B-cell antigens, HLA-DR, CD40, and CD45 and accumulate cytoplasmic IgM, IgG, or IgA. Plasma cells also express CD138 (syndecan) and higher levels of CD38 than germinal-center B cells. PAX5 is lost at the plasma cell stage, whereas BLIMP1, XBP1, and IRF4/MUM1 are expressed.

Tumors of bone marrow–homing plasma cells correspond to osseous plasmacytoma and multiple myeloma (Table 7-2). Some aggressive lymphomas have the morphology and cell-proliferation activity of centroblasts or immunoblasts but the immunophenotype of plasma cells and may correspond to the malignant counterpart of plasmablasts (Table 7-2). These lymphomas include plasmablastic lymphoma, primary effusion lymphoma, and large B-cell lymphomas associated with multicentric Castleman disease.[79]

Mucosa-Associated Lymphoid Tissue. A subset of B cells is programmed for gut-associated rather than nodal lymphoid tissue. In these tissues (Waldeyer's ring, Peyer's patches, mesenteric nodes), similar responses to antigens occur, but both the intermediate and end-stage B cells that originate in the gut or mesenteric lymph nodes preferentially return there rather than to the peripheral lymph nodes or bone marrow. Thus, the plasma cells generated in gut-associated lymphoid tissue home preferentially to the lamina propria rather than to the bone marrow.[34,35] The mechanisms facilitating this tissue-specific traffic of effector cells include chemokines and their receptors and different adhesion molecules. Many extranodal low-grade B-cell lymphomas are thought to arise from MALT and have somatically mutated V-region genes, consistent with an antigen-selected post–germinal-center B-cell stage (Table 7-2).[80-82]

T-Cell Differentiation

Antigen-Independent T-Cell Differentiation

Cortical Thymocytes

The earliest antigen-independent stages of T-cell differentiation occur in the bone marrow; later stages occur in the thymic cortex. The cells entering the thymus are common lymphoid progenitors with potential to differentiate to several lymphoid lineages. They express CD34, CD45RA, CD7, CD44, and CD25.[1,83] The expression of NOTCH1 by the precursor cell and the ligand by thymic cortical epithelial cells determine the commitment to the T-cell lineage.[84] The initial T cells are negative for CD4 and CD8 (double negative). These cells express RAG1, RAG2, and TdT and rearrange the β chain of the TCR expressed in the cytoplasm but not on the surface. CD3 is also expressed in the cytoplasm. Subsequently, they acquire CD1a, CD2, and CD5 and lose CD25 and CD44 expression. At this stage, the cells express first the CD4 and then the CD8 antigen together (double positive). The α chain of the receptor is rearranged and expressed with the β chain and CD3 on the surface. Cortical thymocytes express CD45RO instead of CD45RA. At this stage, T cells undergo a positive selection if they recognize the HLA molecules. T cells recognizing MHC class I become CD8-positive T cells (single positive), whereas T cells recognizing MHC class II differentiate into CD4-positive T cells (single positive). Subsequently, a negative selection occurs if they recognize self-antigens. The final selected cells express increased levels of surface CD3, acquire CD27, switch their CD45 isotype from RO back to RA, lose CD1a, express BCL2, and become mature naïve T cells.[1,83]

Naïve T Cells

Mature, naïve T cells are small lymphocytes with low proliferation fraction that lack TdT and CD1 and express either CD4 or CD8 in addition to surface CD3, CD5, CD7, CD2, and CD45RA and the costimulatory receptors CD27 and CD28 (Fig. 7-10).[1,83] These cells leave the thymus and can be found in the circulation, in the paracortex of lymph nodes, and in the thymic medulla. These are migratory cells with a surveillance function. They arrive at the secondary lymphoid tissues via the bloodstream and exit the circulation through HEVs in the nodes and MALT and through the sinusoids in the spleen. Naïve T cells express CCR7 and CD62L (L-selectin), which are instrumental at these sites by recognizing the CCL21 and vascular addressins, respectively, expressed by the HEVs. Some cases of T-cell prolymphocytic leukemia may correspond to naïve T cells (Table 7-3).

Antigen-Dependent T-Cell Activation

A complex interaction of T-cell surface molecules with molecules on the surface of antigen-presenting cells is required for T-cell activation in response to antigens. The complex of CD3, the coreceptor molecules CD8 or CD4, and the T-cell receptor (which may be either γ-δ or α-β and has a combining site that "fits" the specific peptide antigen) binds to the antigen-MHC complex on the antigen-presenting cell. CD4 and CD8 T cells bind to MHC class II or I molecules, respectively. The adhesion molecule LFA-1 on the T cell binds to ICAM-1 on the antigen-presenting cell; the activation-associated molecule CD40L on CD4-positive T cells binds to CD40; CD28 and CTLA-4 on the T cell bind to B7-1 (CD80) and B7-2 (CD86) on the antigen-presenting cell.[1] The interaction of CD40-CD40L provides an activation stimulus for both the T cell and the antigen-presenting cell, and binding of CD28 to CD80/CD86 provides a crucial second stimulus for the T cell.[85] CTLA-4 also binds to CD80/CD86 but provides an inhibitory signal to the T lymphocyte that limits its activation. CD4-positive T cells primarily interact only with professional antigen presenting cells that express MHC class II (dendritic cells, macrophages, B cells). CD8-positive T cells can principally interact with all nucleated cells, as all cells express MHC class I, an important means to scan the cells in the body, for example, for a viral infection.

T Immunoblasts

On encountering antigens, mature T cells transform into immunoblasts, which are large cells with prominent nucleoli and basophilic cytoplasm that may be morphologically indistinguishable from B immunoblasts. T immunoblasts, in contrast to T lymphoblasts (thymocytes), are TdT negative and CD1 negative, strongly express pan–T-cell antigens, and continue to express either CD4 or CD8. Activated or proliferating T cells express HLA-DR in addition to CD25 (IL-2 receptor) and both CD71 and CD38. Antigen-dependent T-cell reactions occur in the paracortex of lymph nodes, the periarteriolar lymphoid sheath of the spleen, and at extranodal sites of immunologic reactions.

Effector T Cells

Activated CD4 and CD8 T cells become effector cells with different functions and phenotypes, and a small proportion of them will become memory cells. After clearance of the pathogens, most T cells undergo apoptosis. However, a small subset of memory T cells persists for a long time, often for the life of the host.

Antigen-stimulated T cells switch CD45RA to CD45RO. CD4 effector T cells typically act as helper cells, and CD8 effector T cells are cytotoxic and kill other cells. Activated CD8-positive cells produce interferon-γ and have cytoplasmic cytotoxic granules containing several types of granzymes, perforin, and TIA-1.

Different subsets of specialized CD4-positive effector cells are now recognized.[86] The major subsets are T-helper 1 (Th1), Th2, and Th17 cells and are induced by distinct interleukins and involved in the production of different cytokines. These states display a high degree of plasticity, changing form one to another under specific stimuli. Th1 cells are generated by IL-12 and secrete interferon-γ. They are important activators of macrophages, NK cells, and CD8-positive T cells. Th2 cells are generated by IL-4 and secrete IL-4, IL-5, IL-6, IL-13, and IL-25. These cells are involved in allergic reactions and mobilize B cells, eosinophils, basophils, mast cells, and alternatively, activated macrophages. Th17 cells produce IL-17 and tumor necrosis factor-α (TNF-α) and regulate acute inflammation. The differentiation of these Th1, Th2, and Th17 cells is mediated by the transcription factors TBX21(T-bet), GATA3, and RORC, respectively. Other subsets have been recognized with the expression of specific cytokines such as Th22 producing IL-22 and Th9 producing IL-9.

CD4 cells involved in the germinal-center B-cell response are a specific subset of T$_{FH}$ cells. BCL6 is the crucial transcription factor required for T$_{FH}$ differentiation. These cells express CXCR5 and are recruited into B-cell follicles by CXCL13 produced in the germinal centers by FDCs. T$_{FH}$ cells also express the costimulatory molecule ICOS, CXCL13, and the receptor PD1, and a subset is CD57 positive. They produce IL-21 and IL-4 and express CD40L, which stimulates B cells.

Table 7-3 Immunohistologic and Genetic Features and Postulated Normal Counterparts of Common T-Cell Neoplasms

Neoplasm	Postulated Normal Counterpart	CD3 (S;C)	CD5	CD7	CD4	CD8	CD30	CXCL13	CD56	TCR	NK (16, 56)	Cytotoxic Granule*	EBV	Genetic Abnormality	Mutated Genes
T-PLL	Naïve T lymphocyte	+	−	+, +	+/−	−/+	−	−	−	αβ	−	−	−	inv14 t(14;14) Trisomy 8q	JAK1, JAK3; STAT5B
T-LGLL	Naïve T lymphocyte	+	−	+, +	−	+	−	−	−	αβ	+, −	+	−	None known	STAT3, STAT5B
NK-LGLL	NK cell	−	−	+, −	−	+/−	−	−	+	−	−, +	+	+	None known	STAT3 TET2 CCL22
Extranodal NK/T-cell lymphoma	NK cell	−; +	−	−/+	−	−	−	−	+	−	NA, +	+	++	None known	STAT3, JAK3 TP53 DDX3X, KMT2D
Hepatosplenic T-cell lymphoma	γ-δ T cell	+	−	+	−	−	−	−	+/−	γδ > αβ	+, −/+	+	−	Iso 7q Trisomy 8	STAT5B STAT3
Enteropathy-type T-cell lymphoma	Intraepithelial T lymphocyte	+	+	+	−	+/−	+/−	−	−	αβ >> γδ	−	+	−	+ 9q + 1q32.2-q41 + 5q34-q35.2	STAT3 JAK1 KMT2D TET2
Monomorphic epitheliotropic intestinal T-cell lymphoma	Intraepithelial T lymphocyte	+	+	+	−	+	+	−	+	γδ > αβ	+	+	−	+ 9q	STAT5B JAK3 SETD2
Mycosis fungoides	Mature skin-homing CD4+ T cell	+	+	−/+	+	−	−	−	−	αβ	−	−	−	None known	PLCG, JAK1/3 STAT3/5
Subcutaneous panniculitis-like T-cell lymphoma	Mature cytotoxic α-β T cell	+	+/−	+/−	+/−	−	++	−	−	αβ	−	−/+	−	None known	
Primary cutaneous γ-δ T-cell lymphoma	γ-δ T cell	+	+	+	−	+	−/+	−	+	γδ	−, +/−	+	−	None known	
PTCL, NOS	Mature T cell	+/−	+/−	+/−	+/−	−/+	−/+	−	−	αβ > γδ	−/+	−/+	−/+	inv 14, complex	TP53, CDKN2A/B RB1
T follicular helper lymphoma (angioimmunoblastic T-cell lymphoma)	Follicular T-helper cell	+	+	+	+/−	−/+	−	+	−	αβ	−	NA	+/−	None known	TET2, DNMT3A IDH2, RHOA
ALK+ ALCL	?	+/−	+/−	NA	−/+	−/+	++	−	−	αβ	−	+	−	t(2;5); NPM/ALK	JAK1 STAT3
ALK− ALCL	?	+/−	+/−	NA	−/+	−/+	++	−	−	αβ	−	−(DUSP22) +	−	DUSP22-R TP63-R	MSC JAK1 STAT3

*Cytotoxic granule = TIA-1, perforin, and/or granzyme.
+, >90% positive; +/−, >50% positive; −/+, <50% positive; −, <10% positive.
ALCL, Anaplastic large cell lymphoma; ALK, anaplastic lymphoid kinase; C, cytoplasmic; EBV, Epstein-Barr virus; Ig, immunoglobulin; NK, natural killer; NK-LGLL, NK-cell large granular lymphocytic leukemia; NOS, not otherwise specified; PTCL, peripheral T-cell lymphoma; R, rearranged; S, surface; TCR, T-cell receptor gene; T-LGLL, T-cell large granular lymphocytic leukemia; T-PLL, T-cell prolymphocytic leukemia.

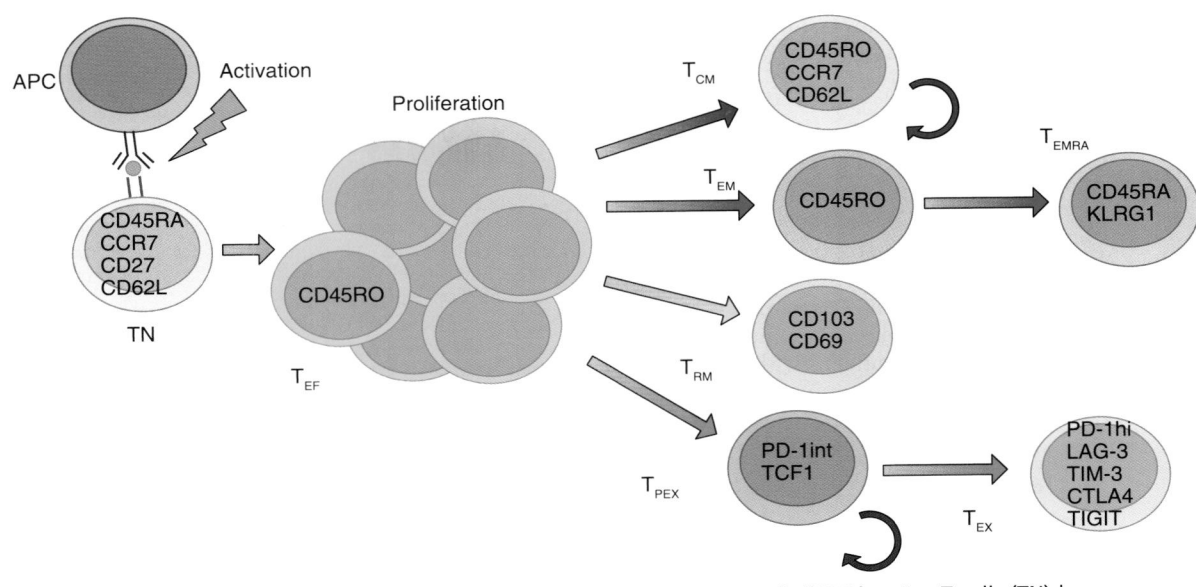

Figure 7-10. Upon antigen recognition in antigen presenting cells (APCs), naïve T cells (TN) become activated, proliferate, and differentiate into effector T cells (T_{EF}) to kill target cells.[83] Once the pathogenic agent is cleared, effector T cells undergo apoptosis, and only a small population of cells persists as memory T cells. Central memory T cells (T_{CM}) maintain self-renewal capacities and reside in the secondary lymphoid organs. Effector memory T cells (T_{EM}) provide rapid protection against secondary exposure to the same pathogen and differentiate into terminally differentiated effector memory cells re-expressing CD45RA (T_{EMRA}). Tissue-resident memory T cells (T_{RM}) reside in nonlymphoid tissues. The signals that regulate fate decision, i.e., the acquisition of a given memory phenotype, are largely unknown. Chronic antigen exposure drives an alternative differentiation program in which precursor exhausted T cells (T_{PEX}) produce an expanded pool of terminally exhausted (T_{EX}) progeny that is unable to clear the established infection or tumor.

CD4-positive Treg cells are an important element in limiting the expansion of immune responses. Treg cells express CD25 and the inhibitory receptor CTLA4, secrete IL-10, and are generated by the activity of the transcription factor FOXP3.

Most cases of peripheral T-cell lymphoma (PTCL) correspond to stages of antigen-dependent T-cell differentiation (Table 7-3).[87] Nodal T_{FH} cell lymphoma is the malignant counterpart of T_{FH} cells.[87] However, the relationship between neoplastic and normal T cells is not nearly as well understood as that in the B-cell system.

Memory T Cells, Exhaustion, and Senescence. A subpopulation of T cells differentiates to memory T cells after antigen recognition and activation (see Fig. 7-10). These cells are long-lived and can quickly expand after re-exposure to their antigens, again becoming effector T cells. Memory T cells may be either CD4 positive or CD8 positive and maintain CD45RO expression, and most of them lack CD45RA. Depending on the cell surface expression of certain receptors and ligands, these cells may migrate to different tissues. Expression of CD62L (L-selectin) and CCR7 facilitates homing to lymph nodes, whereas selectin P ligand (CLA) guides lymphocytes to the skin and α4β7 integrin and CCR9 lead to the small intestine.[88] Several subpopulations of T memory cells have been recognized with similar phenotypes within the different subsets of CD4-positive and CD8-positive cells.[86,89] *Central memory T cells* (T_{CM}) express CD62L (L-selectin) and CCR7 and have high proliferative potential, resistance to apoptosis, and self-renewal properties (see Fig. 7-10). These cells maintain and supply new generations of memory T cells, although they have a limited immediate effector function. Upon antigen stimulation, they may differentiate to T effector cells (see Fig. 7-10).

Effector memory T cells (T_{EM}) lack expression of CCR7 and CD62L and are found mainly in the peripheral circulation and nonlymphoid tissues. Upon antigen stimulation, they have a rapid effector response with production of cytokines and cytotoxic granules. *Terminally differentiated effector memory cells re-expressing CD45RA* (T_{EMRA}) are a subpopulation of T_{EM} cells that have a potent effector function but decreased proliferative capacity with a tendency toward apoptosis or senescence. Contrary to naïve T cells, this subpopulation lacks CCR7 and CD62L and the costimulatory molecules CD27 and CD28. They tend to be excluded from lymphoid organs but are present in peripheral blood and nonlymphoid tissues. *Tissue-resident memory T cells* (T_{RM}) can be either CD4-positive or CD8-positive lymphocytes, are present in nonlymphoid tissues, and can promptly respond when re-exposed to their antigens, providing protective immunity independently of T cells newly recruited from peripheral blood. This subpopulation seems to have a relevant role in antitumor functions.

After chronic antigen stimulation, memory T cells may become dysfunctional, acquiring an exhausted or senescence state in which the cells lose their proliferative and functional properties.[86] *Exhausted T cells* (T_{EX}) may be recognized by the expression of a constellation of inhibitory receptors that include high PD-1, TIM-3, CTLA-4, LAG-3, or TIGIT. Exhausted cells express more than one of these markers. Precursor T_{EX} cells still maintain proliferative capacity and may reverse the exhausted state when treated with immunotherapy strategies with monoclonal antibodies targeting some of these receptors (e.g., anti-PD-1, anti-PD-L1, or anti-CTLA-4).[90] Senescent cells are more resistant to apoptosis, and it is a nonreversible state. These cells express KLRG1 and CD57, lose costimulatory receptors such as CD27 and CD28, and lack the migratory signals CD62L and CCR7.

Differentiation of Cells of the Innate Immune Response

The innate immune system is conserved through evolution and constitutes a first line of defense that is based on relatively non-specific germline-encoded receptors.[1] The cells involved in the innate immune response are localized mainly in barriers such as the mucosa and skin and do not require antigen-presenting cells or the association of antigens with MHC. The main lymphoid cells involved in innate immune responses are γ-δ T cells and NK cells. Phagocytes, mast cells, eosinophils, and basophils are also involved in innate responses.

γ-δ T Cells

Mature γ-δ T cells express these two chains of the TCR. The γ-δ TCR binds directly to the antigens and does not require specialized antigen processing and presentation by the HLA system, as α-β T cells do. The γ-δ T cells are mainly present in mucosa, skin, and splenic red pulp but are rare in lymphoid organs. These cells are generated in the thymus, most of them already with effector capacity and little plasticity in the periphery. They are positive for CD3, CD2, and CD7 but negative for CD4 and CD8, and they express cytotoxic granules in the cytoplasm. These cells participate in rapid innate immune responses and also in tissue repair by expressing epithelial growth factors.[91,92] Hepatosplenic γ-δ T-cell lymphoma and primary cutaneous γ-δ T-cell lymphoma are considered neoplasms derived from these cells (Table 7-3).[87]

Natural Killer Cells

NK cells appear to derive from a progenitor common with T cells. They can kill certain targets such as virus-infected self–class I MHC molecules on the surfaces of cells through killer cell Ig-like receptors (KIRs), and they kill cells that lack these antigens.[93] A main function of NK cells is to detect and eliminate virus-infected cells that have been instructed by viral factors to downregulate MHC class I as a viral strategy to evade recognition by cytotoxic CD8-positive T cells. Activated NK cells express the epsilon and zeta chains of CD3 in the cytoplasm, but these cells do not rearrange their TCR genes or express TCRs or surface CD3. They are characterized by certain NK-cell–associated antigens (CD16, CD56, CD57), which can also be expressed on some T cells; they also express some T-cell–associated antigens (CD2, CD5, CD28, CD8). Similar to γ-δ T cells, NK cells have cytotoxic granules that specifically contain granzyme-M. NK cells appear in the peripheral blood as a small proportion of circulating lymphocytes; they are usually slightly larger than most normal T and B cells, with abundant pale cytoplasm containing azurophilic granules—so-called "large granular lymphocytes". Nasal NK/T-cell lymphoma, aggressive NK-cell leukemia, and possibly NK-cell large granular lymphocytic leukemia are thought to be neoplasms of NK cells[87] (Table 7-3).

Acknowledgements

We thank Drs. Elaine S. Jaffe and Nancy L. Harris, previous authors of this chapter, for the information provided.

Pearls and Pitfalls

- The immune system has two differentiated arms: the innate and the adaptive systems. The innate system is a first line of defense mediated by cells that express germline-coded receptors, recognize a wide but relatively non-specific number of antigens, and do not generate immunologic memory. The adaptive system reacts specifically against antigens presented to lymphocytes, in most instances associated with MHC. The immune cells of the adaptive immune system express specific receptors encoded by somatically rearranged genes that may recognize a virtually universal spectrum of antigens and generate cells with immunologic memory.
- Lymphoid tissues are highly organized microenvironments in which different cell populations, vascular structures, and stromal components facilitate the selective interactions between lymphocytes and antigens for the initiation and expansion of immune responses.
- The follicular lymphoid germinal center is a complex structure in which cells of the adaptive immune system expand clonally and the IgV genes are somatically mutated to select high-affinity antigen receptors. The Ig heavy chain gene also undergoes idiotype switch, and the cell commits to an MBC or plasma cell.
- The high proliferation and DNA breaks that occur in germinal-center B cells are mechanisms that facilitate the development of lymphoid neoplasms. Most B-cell lymphomas carry somatically mutated IgV genes, indicating they derive from cells with germinal-center experience.
- Most lymphoid neoplasms are related to a normal cell counterpart of the immune system. Some lymphomas, however, do not correspond to a known normal stage of differentiation, and others display aberrant phenotypes, lineage heterogeneity, or changes in cell lineage that may represent the malignant counterpart or the physiologic plasticity of the immune cells.

KEY REFERENCES

10. Victora GD, Nussenzweig MC. Germinal centers. *Annu Rev Immunol*. 2022;26(40):413–442.
17. Vinuesa CG, Tangye SG, Moser B, Mackay CR. Follicular B helper T cells in antibody responses and autoimmunity. *Nat Rev Immunol*. 2005;5:853–865.
27. Batista FD, Harwood NE. The who, how and where of antigen presentation to B cells. *Nat Rev Immunol*. 2009;9:15–27.
44. Seda V, Mraz M. B-cell receptor signalling and its crosstalk with other pathways in normal and malignant cells. *Eur J Haematol*. 2015;94:193–205.
49. Sutton LA, Agathangelidis A, Belessi C, et al. Antigen selection in B-cell lymphomas—tracing the evidence. *Semin Cancer Biol*. 2013;23:399–409.
53. Laidlaw BJ, Cyster JG. Transcriptional regulation of memory B cell differentiation. *Nat Rev Immunol*. 2021;21:209–220.
54. Vinuesa CV, Chang PP. Innate B cell helpers reveal novel types of antibody responses. *Nat Immunol*. 2013;14:119–126.
56. Dominguez-Sola D, Victora GD, Ying CY, et al. The proto-oncogene MYC is required for selection in the germinal center and cyclic reentry. *Nat Immunol*. 2012;13:1083–1091.
66. Ise W, Kurosaki T. Plasma cell differentiation during the germinal center reaction. *Immunol Rev*. 2019;288:64–74.
71. Kurosaki T, Kometani K, Ise W. Memory B cells. *Nat Rev Immunol*. 2015;15(3):149–159.
86. Brummelman J, Pilipow K, Lugli E. The single-cell phenotypic identity of human CD8+ and CD4+ T cells. *Int Rev Cell Mol Biol*. 2018;341:63–123.
93. Cheent K, Khakoo SI. Natural killer cells: integrating diversity with function. *Immunology*. 2009;126:449–457.

Visit Elsevier eBooks+ for the complete set of references.

Chapter 8

Reactive Lymphadenopathies

Rebecca L. King and Eric D. Hsi

The major question that confronts the surgical pathologist when examining a lymph node biopsy is whether the process is benign or malignant.[1] The pathologist must be familiar with the histologic changes of a diverse group of non-neoplastic disorders in order to differentiate them from lymphoma and to render a specific diagnosis or a differential diagnosis on morphologic grounds. A specific diagnosis often requires correlation with the clinical history and the results of additional studies such as immunohistochemistry, stains for microorganisms, cultures, serologic studies, and molecular analysis for microbial genetic material.

We group the reactive lymphadenopathies into four major categories according to their predominant architectural histologic pattern: follicular/nodular, sinus, interfollicular or mixed, and diffuse. Although this approach is convenient, multiple nodal compartments may be involved in a single process, and variation exists from case to case. Furthermore, reactive conditions of the lymph node are dynamic processes, and the predominant pattern may differ, depending on the time during the course of the disease at which the biopsy is performed.

Box 8-1 lists the major reactive conditions that cause lymph node enlargement and that may result in lymph node biopsy. Several benign disorders and borderline lesions such as immune deficiency-related lymphadenopathy, sinus histiocytosis (SH) with massive lymphadenopathy, and the plasma cell and plasmablastic variants of Castleman disease are covered in other chapters.

FOLLICULAR AND NODULAR PATTERNS

Follicular Hyperplasia

Follicular hyperplasia (FH) is defined as an increase in the number and usually in the size and shape of secondary lymphoid follicles (Fig. 8-1). It is among the most common reactive patterns encountered by the surgical pathologist. The antigens responsible are usually not known. Hyperplastic follicles contain germinal centers (GCs) with a mixture of centroblasts (noncleaved cells) and centrocytes (cleaved cells), which vary in proportion depending on the duration of immune response. Tingible body macrophages containing apoptotic cellular debris are common and impart a starry-sky pattern to the GC (Fig. 8-1A and B). The prominence of the starry-sky pattern correlates with the proliferative index in the GC. Typically,

I. Follicular and Nodular Patterns

Follicular hyperplasia
Autoimmune disorders (rheumatoid arthritis)
   Luetic lymphadenitis
   Castleman disease, hyaline vascular type
   Progressive transformation of germinal centers
   Mantle zone hyperplasia
   Mycobacterial spindle cell pseudotumor

II. Predominantly Sinus Patterns

Sinus histiocytosis
   Non-specific
   Specific etiology—lymphangiogram, storage disease,
     prosthesis, Whipple disease
Vascular transformation of sinuses
Hemophagocytic lymphohistiocytosis

III. Interfollicular or Mixed Pattern

Paracortical hyperplasia and dermatopathic reaction
Granulomatous lymphadenitis
   Nonnecrotizing granulomas
   Necrotizing granulomas
     Tuberculosis
     Fungal infection
     Cat scratch disease
IgG4-related lymphadenopathy
Kimura disease
Toxoplasmic lymphadenitis
Systemic lupus erythematosus
Kikuchi lymphadenitis
Kawasaki disease
Inflammatory pseudotumor
Bacillary angiomatosis

IV. Diffuse Pattern

Infectious mononucleosis
Cytomegalovirus infection
Herpes simplex lymphadenitis
Dilantin lymphadenopathy

some follicles show polarization of the GC with the proliferative dark zone, composed mostly of centroblasts, located toward the medullary side of the GC and an apical light zone, containing a predominance of centrocytes, located on the capsular side of the follicle (Figs. 8-1C and 8-2A). Proliferation and somatic hypermutation of GC B cells occurs in the dark zone while affinity maturation occurs in the light zone.[2] Early in a hyperplastic reaction, GCs may consist almost exclusively of centroblasts (Fig. 8-3). The high proliferative index is highlighted by staining with MIB-1 (Ki-67) (Fig. 8-1D and Fig. 8-3B). Centrocytes, plasma cells, varying numbers of follicular helper T cells (TFH) (CD4-positive, CD57-positive, PD1-positive, ICOS-positive), and follicular dendritic cells (FDC) are present in the light zone.[3] FDC have intermediate-sized, pale nuclei, which contain a small central nucleolus; many are binucleated, with apposing nuclear membranes appearing flattened (Fig. 8-2B). A variably prominent mantle zone composed of small lymphocytes surrounds the GC. In a polarized GC, the mantle zone is expanded around the light zone (Fig. 8-1C). Other features of FH include large, irregular GCs with oddly shaped geographic outlines (Fig. 8-1B) and, occasionally, follicular lysis (Fig. 8-4). The latter is characterized by disrupted GCs because of infiltration by mantle zone lymphocytes. The interfollicular area may show variable expansion with scattered transformed cells, small lymphocytes, plasma cells, and high endothelial venules.

GCs are composed predominantly of CD20+ B cells, with varying numbers of CD4+/CD57+/PD1+/ICOS+ TFH. These PD1-positive T cells tend to be present at the periphery of the GC.[4] BCL2 is not expressed by reactive GC B cells, whereas BCL6 and CD10 are expressed in both benign and neoplastic GC B cells. Other GC B-cell markers such as GCET1, HGAL, and LMO2 are also expressed in reactive and neoplastic GC B cells.[5,6]

Differential Diagnosis

The main differential diagnosis in FH is follicular lymphoma. Features that favor a benign process include polarization, tingible body macrophages with a starry-sky pattern, the presence of plasma cells within follicles, and a well-defined mantle zone. Immunostains show a lack of BCL2 protein in B cells.[7,8] Because T cells express BCL2, this stain should always be interpreted in conjunction with B-cell and T-cell markers so that relative percentages of each type of cell can be determined, allowing appropriate interpretation of the BCL2 stain. Although the t(14;18)(q32;q21) translocation, characteristic of follicular lymphoma, may be detected in hyperplastic lymph nodes by polymerase chain reaction (PCR),[9] this finding does not appear to be a significant problem with assays that have sensitivity of one in 10^4 or less.[10] An uncommon incidental finding in the setting of FH is strong CD10-positive/BCL2-positive co-expression of follicular B cells that represents in situ follicular neoplasia. This finding is characterized by lack of architectural distortion with involvement (often partial) in only a minority of follicles.[11] This occurs in approximately 2% of reactive lymph nodes and is likely associated with a low risk for development of overt follicular lymphoma.[12]

Pediatric-type follicular lymphoma (PTFL), a variant of follicular lymphoma, may also rarely enter the differential diagnosis. PTFL occurs predominantly in young males with localized disease and histologically demonstrates effacement of the lymph node by large ill-defined follicles with a starry-sky pattern. They are composed of sheets of large centroblasts. Although monoclonal, BCL2 protein is not expressed and *BCL2* translocation is absent. Prognosis is excellent even with conservative management.[13,14]

Lack of surface immunoglobulin light chain on a B-cell population by flow cytometry is considered an abnormal finding and seen in more than 5% of cases of small lymphocytic leukemia/chronic lymphocytic leukemia, follicular lymphoma, and diffuse large B-cell lymphoma. However, it can rarely be seen in reactive lymph nodes, particularly in the setting of HIV.[15,16] By immunostaining, kappa- or lambda-restricted plasmacytic cells can be seen in scattered reactive GCs and likely reflects local clonal dominance as a result of affinity maturation and selection, rather than emerging lymphoma. The cells represent plasma cells and centrocytes/centroblasts with plasmacytic differentiation. There is always a mixture of polytypic and monotypic GCs with the latter in the minority or isolated.[17] Clinical correlation is important; when in doubt, observation and repeat biopsy of persistently enlarge lymph nodes may be a

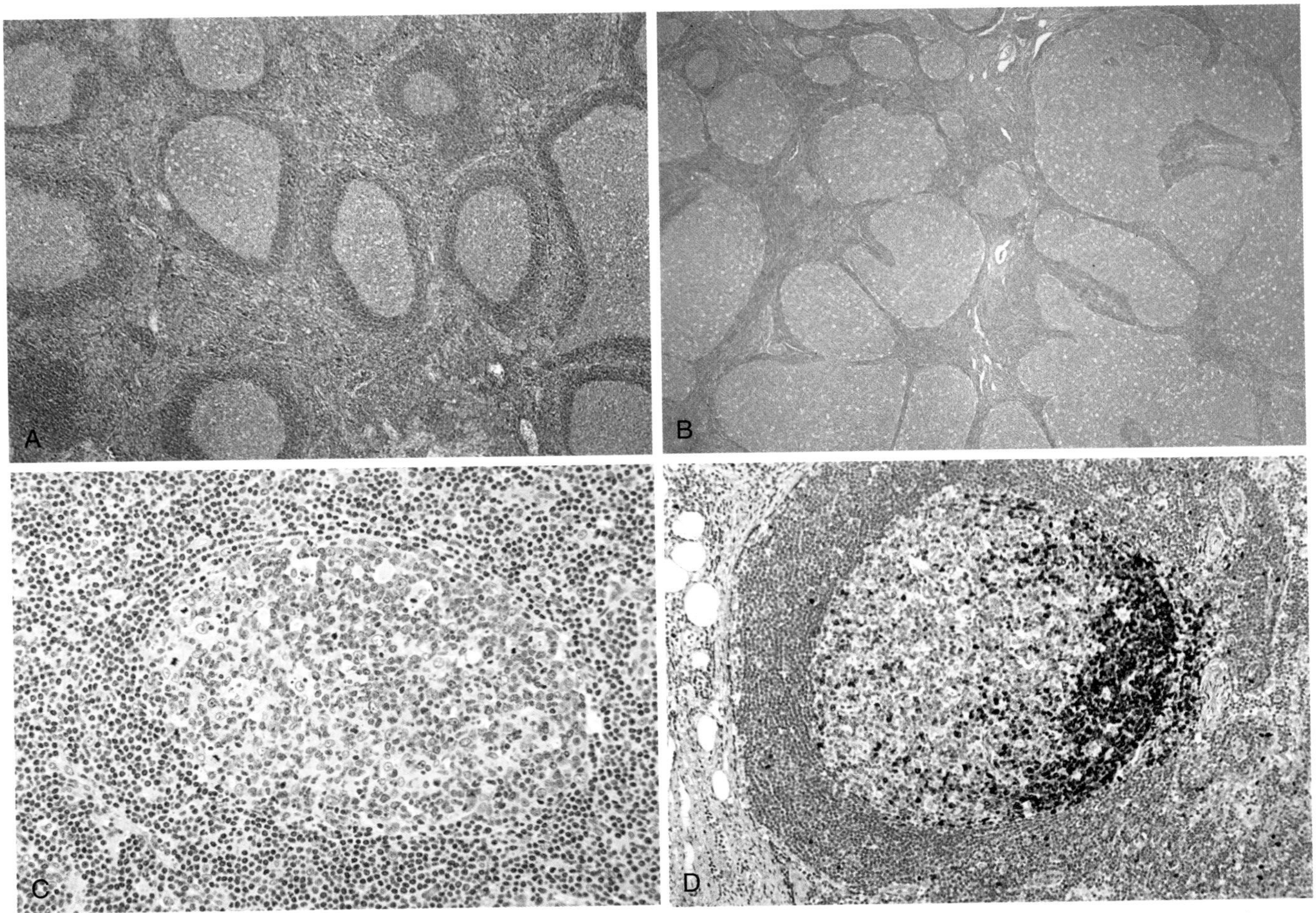

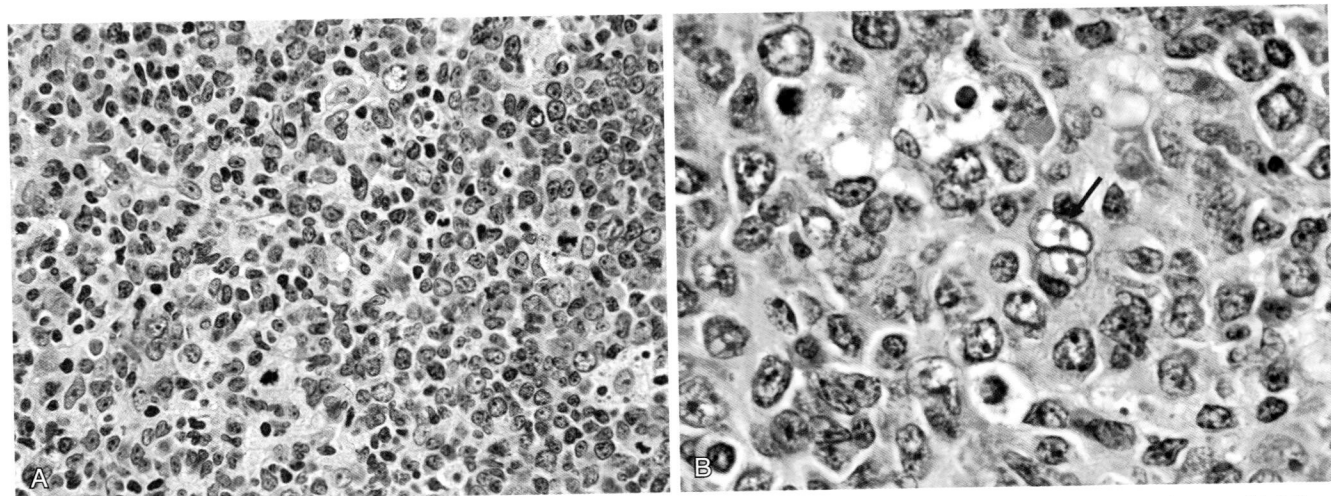

Figure 8-1. Follicular hyperplasia. A, Increased numbers of follicles with large irregular germinal centers (GCs), preserved mantle zones, and ample interfollicular areas (hematoxylin and eosin [H&E], ×35). **B,** GCs may be large and form irregular large, bizarre structures (H&E, ×90). **C,** Polarization of GC with a dark zone composed of centroblasts and tingible body macrophages and a light zone with a predominance of centrocytes (H&E, ×330). **D,** MIB-1 stain showing that almost all cells in the dark zone are positive. The mantle zone is expanded adjacent to the light zone (MIB-1, ×70).

Figure 8-2. A, Higher magnification of a GC. The light zone *(left)* shows a predominance of centrocytes, while the dark zone *(right)* contains mostly centroblasts interspersed by tingible body macrophages (H&E, ×500). **B,** A follicular dendritic cell is shown *(arrow)*. These cells have clear chromatin with a small central nucleolus and often appear bilobed with flattening of opposing nuclear membranes (H&E, ×500).

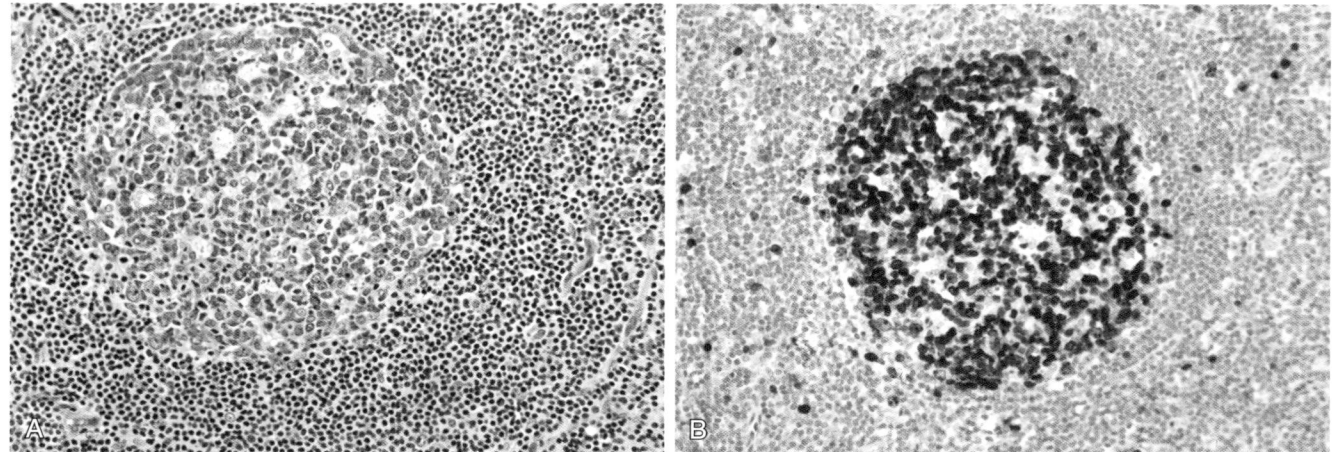

Figure 8-3. A, GC consisting almost exclusively of centroblasts. Tingible body macrophages are scattered throughout (H&E, ×330). **B,** MIB-1 staining of the GC in **A** showing positivity in all centroblasts, indicating that these cells are proliferating (MIB-1, ×400).

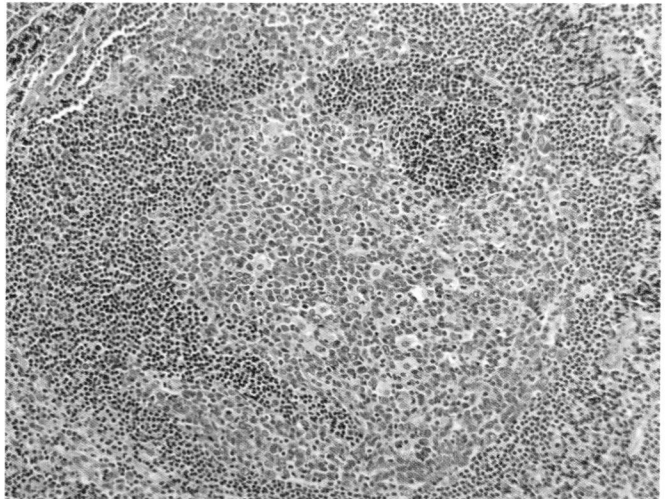

Figure 8-4. Follicular lysis of a germinal center. Mantle cell lymphocytes infiltrating into and disrupting the GC (H&E, ×100).

reasonable approach (particularly in the context of a needle biopsy).

Monocytoid B-Cell Proliferation

FH may be associated with proliferation of monocytoid B cells in and around cortical sinuses, around venules, or in a parafollicular location.[18-20] Although this proliferation may be associated with non-specific FH (Fig. 8-5), it is characteristic of toxoplasmic lymphadenitis, HIV-associated lymphadenopathy, cytomegalovirus (CMV) lymphadenitis, and disorders associated with suppurative granulomas, especially cat scratch disease (CSD).[21] Monocytoid B cells are medium-sized cells with abundant pale to clear cytoplasm and round to slightly indented nuclei with moderately dispersed chromatin. Neutrophils and immunoblasts are usually scattered among the monocytoid cells (Fig. 8-5). The differential diagnosis when the monocytoid B-cell proliferation is prominent includes marginal zone lymphoma. Although this differentiation may be difficult in some cases, evidence of clonality supports a diagnosis of lymphoma and can be

established by demonstrating light chain restriction in paraffin sections or by immunoglobulin gene rearrangement molecular studies. Morphologic features favoring lymphoma include partial effacement of the architecture by the monocytoid B-cell proliferation and increased numbers of large cells with an increased mitotic index. BCL2 expression has been suggested to be useful in distinguishing marginal zone lymphoma (positive) from marginal zone hyperplasia (negative), but hyperplastic processes in the spleen, abdominal lymph nodes, and ileum have been shown to express BCL2. Thus it is considered a soft criterion.[22,23] Molecular genetic analysis for immunoglobulin gene rearrangement by PCR may be helpful if other features are not diagnostic. Follicular lymphoma with marginal zone differentiation may also be considered. In this situation, there are increased numbers of follicles composed of monotonous centrocytes surrounded by a rim of monocytoid B cells several layers thick. Demonstration of BCL2-expressing GC B cells, monoclonality, or presence of a *BCL2::IGH* translocation support this diagnosis.

Autoimmune Disorders (Rheumatoid Arthritis)

Patients with autoimmune disorders such as rheumatoid arthritis (RA), juvenile RA, and Sjögren syndrome often develop lymphadenopathy, which is characterized by FH.[24-27] Although biopsies are not ordinarily performed in these patients, they may be done if there is a clinical suspicion of lymphoma. The features of RA-associated lymphadenopathy are well characterized. We will focus primarily on RA.

The lymph node histologic changes seen in RA are FH, interfollicular and intrafollicular plasmacytosis, and neutrophils within sinuses (Fig. 8-6).[24,27] The lymph node capsule may be thickened but is not infiltrated by plasma cells. Expansion of the lymphoid reaction into perinodal tissue may occur and does not necessarily connote malignancy. Compared with non-specific FH, the reactive GCs of RA were found to be smaller and more regularly spaced, with a predominance of centrocytes exhibiting less mitotic activity.[27] Sarcoidal granulomas and focal deposition of PAS-positive hyaline material in the interfollicular areas, which may become calcified, can be seen.[28] Immunohistochemical

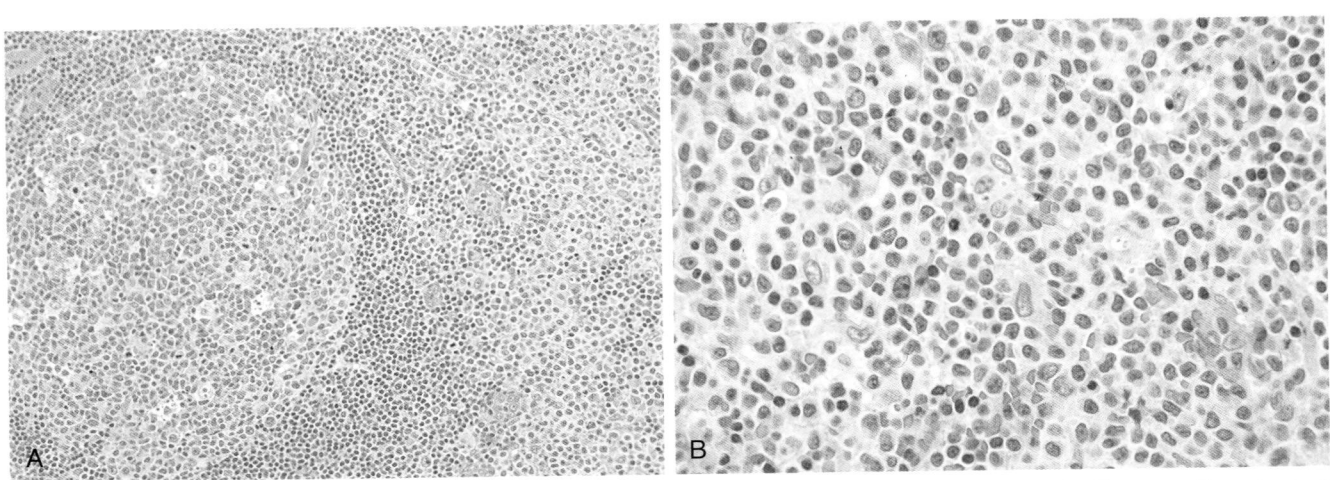

Figure 8-5. **A,** Reactive follicle with adjacent monocytoid B-cell proliferation (H&E, ×100). **B,** The monocytoid cells are medium sized with slightly indented nuclei and ample cytoplasm. Neutrophils are scattered among the monocytoid cells (H&E, ×400).

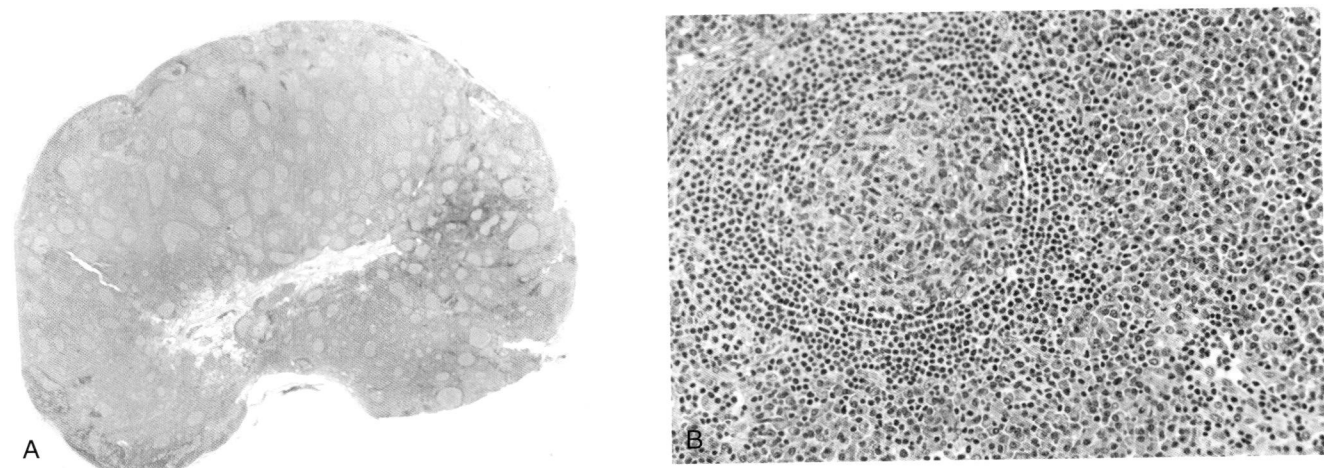

Figure 8-6. Follicular hyperplasia in a lymph node from a patient with rheumatoid arthritis. A, Follicles with enlarged GCs varying in size and shape are present throughout cortex and medulla (H&E, ×5). **B,** Follicle surrounded by sheets of plasma cells (H&E, ×250). *(From Schnitzer, B, Pathology of lymphoid tissue in rheumatoid arthritis and allied diseases. In Glynn LE, and Schlumberger HD, eds: Bayer Symposium VI, Experimental Models of Chronic Inflammatory Diseases. New York, Springer-Verlag, 1977, pp. 331-348; and from Schnitzer, B: Reactive lymphoid hyperplasia. In Jaffe ES, ed: Surgical Pathology of the Lymph Nodes and Related Organs. Philadelphia, W.B. Saunders Company, 1985, pp. 22-56.)*

studies have shown CD4-positive T cells to predominate in the interfollicular areas with CD8-positive T cells within GCs.[24,27] Increased numbers of polytypic CD5-positive B cells, which can be expanded in autoimmune disorders, may also be seen.[24] These features may also be seen in other disorders such as Sjögren syndrome; however, monocytoid B-cell hyperplasia is more frequent in the latter.

In some RA patients, an atypical proliferation that is unlike the typical FH with plasmacytosis can occur. It has been divided into three types. The first resembles multicentric Castleman disease with hyaline vascular lymphoid follicles, interfollicular polytypic plasmacytosis, and vascular proliferation. The second is a paracortical hyperplasia and has well-formed lymphoid follicles with GCs. The paracortex is expanded by polyclonal CD4-positive T cells with varying degrees of atypia, plasma cells, immunoblasts, and histocytes. Epstein-Barr virus (EBV) is absent in the few cases reported. The third type is an atypical lymphoplasmacytic, immunoblastic proliferation, and occasional Hodgkin-like cells.[29] This latter type may be akin to the atypical, usually EBV-driven, proliferations seen in the setting of methotrexate or other immune modulatory drugs.

Still disease is an acute febrile form of juvenile RA characterized by high-spiking fever, skin rash, arthralgia, arthritis, polyserositis, hepatosplenomegaly, lymphadenopathy, leukocytosis, elevated erythrocyte sedimentation rate (ESR), polyclonal hypergammaglobulinemia, and absence of autoantibodies. Adult-onset Still disease (AOSD) occurs and represents 5% of fevers of unknown origin. Lymph node findings overlap with that describe for RA. Small series describe four features, the most common of which is paracortical hyperplasia with vascular proliferation, admixed B and T immunoblasts, and infiltration by reactive lymphocytes and inflammatory cells. Paracortical hyperplasia, lack of follicles, SH, and S100-positive histocyte aggregates are uncommonly seen. A third pattern consisting of an exuberant but patchy paracortical T-immunoblastic reaction (polyclonal) should be differentiated from lymphoma (monoclonal).

CD30 may be expressed in a subset of immunoblasts. The fourth pattern consists of FH. Few scattered EBV-positive small lymphocytes may be seen, and are not associated with a specific pattern. Cases with dermatopathic features or resembling histiocytic necrotizing lymphadenitis have been reported, and increased expression of chemokines CXCL10 and CXCR3 by immunohistochemistry has been suggested to be helpful in distinguishing AOSD from mimics such as PTCL and histiocytic necrotizing lymphadenitis.[30]

The differential diagnosis of FH associated with RA also includes FH due to other causes. Appropriate clinical history and laboratory findings should help confirm the diagnosis of RA-associated lymphadenopathy.

Syphilis may show histologic features similar to those in RA. However, in contrast to RA, the capsule is often thickened and infiltrated by plasma cells and lymphocytes, especially around small vessels. In addition, epithelioid granulomas may be present in interfollicular areas. Also, endarteritis and venulitis are typically found. Special stains for spirochetes may be diagnostic. HIV infection, particularly early in its course, may show histologic changes similar to those in RA. Follicular lymphoma might also be considered in the differential diagnosis. Demonstration of BCL2 protein positive GC B cells or the presence of the t(14;18)(q32;q21) translocation would confirm the diagnosis of follicular lymphoma, although its absence does not negate such a diagnosis.[31]

In FH associated with Sjögren syndrome, marginal zone lymphoma should be excluded. Features suggesting lymphoma include large confluent areas of monocytoid B cells. Demonstration of monoclonality may be necessary to confirm the diagnosis in cases of FH with extensive monocytoid B-cell proliferation.[32]

Luetic (Syphilitic) Lymphadenitis

Although lymph node biopsy does not play a significant role in the diagnosis of syphilis, the localized or generalized lymphadenopathy of primary and secondary syphilis may be clinically suspicious for lymphoma, and, therefore, biopsies may be performed.[33] The typical histologic picture is FH with interfollicular plasmacytosis, similar to that seen in RA-associated lymphadenopathy.[33,34] Features that point to luetic lymphadenitis include capsular and trabecular fibrosis with infiltration by plasma cells and lymphocytes, especially around capillaries (Fig. 8-7). Sarcoidal-type or, rarely, suppurative granulomas in the paracortex, clusters of epithelioid histiocytes, and endarteritis or venulitis with clusters of neutrophils around small vessels may be present.[35] Rarely,

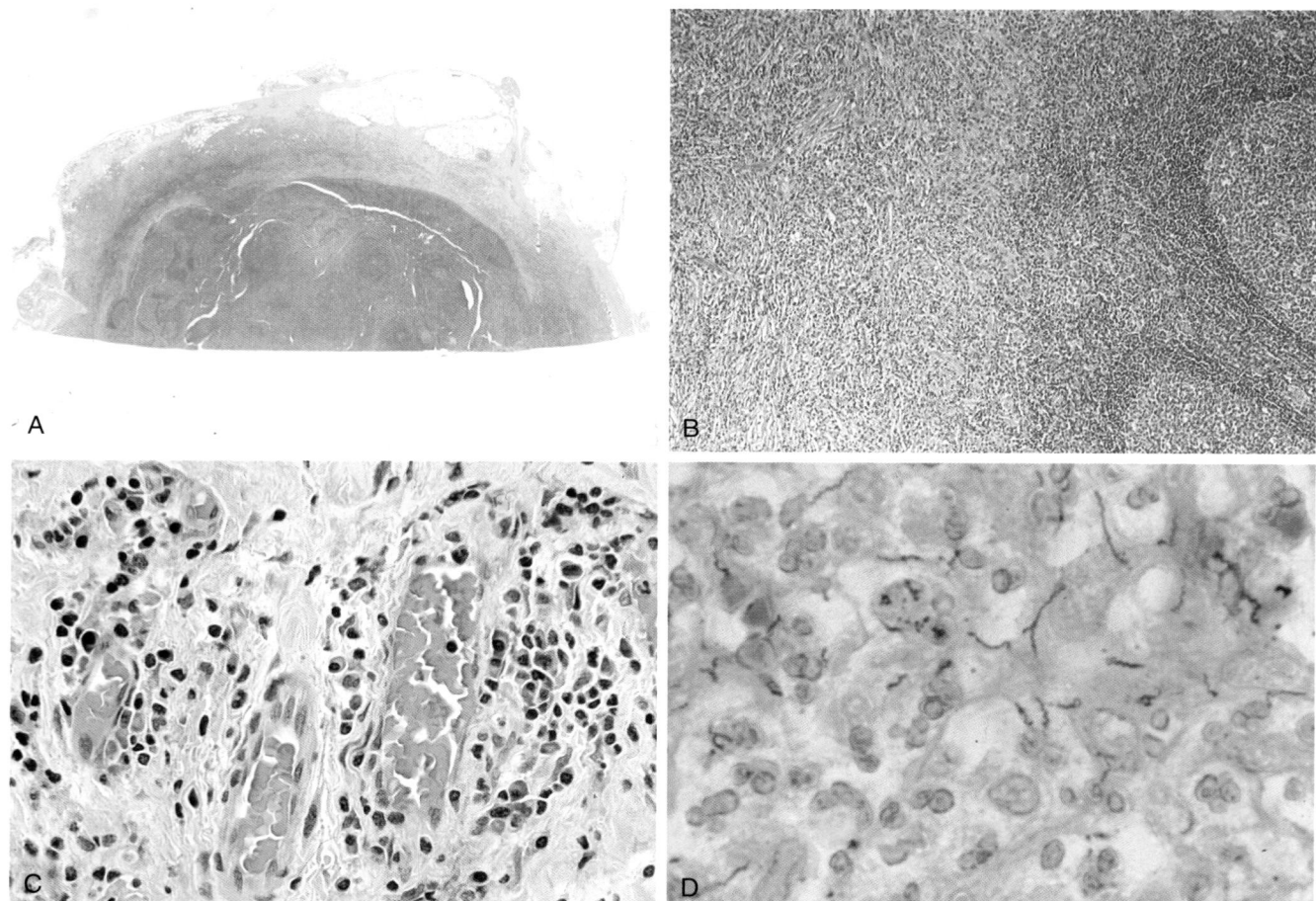

Figure 8-7. Syphilitic lymphadenitis. A, The thickened, fibrotic capsule is infiltrated by chronic inflammatory cells. Follicular hyperplasia (FH) and interfollicular plasmacytosis are present (H&E, ×5). **B,** Higher magnification of heavily inflamed fibrotic capsule and two large reactive follicles (H&E, ×45). **C,** The vessels in the capsule are surrounded by plasma cells along with lymphocytes (H&E, ×500). **D,** Steiner stain shows numerous spirochetes in a case of necrotizing syphilitic lymphadenitis. *(D, Courtesy Dr. Judith A. Ferry, Pathology, Massachusetts General Hospital.)*

a suppurative form of syphilitic lymphadenitis produces a necrotizing lymphadenitis. Stains such as Warthin-Starry or Steiner stains may demonstrate spirochetes anywhere in the lymph node but most consistently within the walls of blood vessels and epithelioid histiocytes.[33] Spirochetes may be difficult to identify, but serologic studies should be positive.[36] Immunohistochemistry is extremely helpful in detection of the organisms.[37]

Another described manifestation of syphilitic disease in lymph nodes is luetic inflammatory pseudotumor (IP) of lymph node,[38] described later in this chapter.

The differential diagnosis includes other causes of FH, and because of the increased number of plasma cells, autoimmune disorders such as RA.

Castleman Disease, Hyaline Vascular Type (Angiofollicular Lymphoid Hyperplasia)

Castleman disease may be either localized (unicentric) or one of the multicentric types. Unicentric Castleman disease is typically the hyaline vascular Castleman disease (HVCD), but the plasma cell variant may also be localized. HVCD is typically a disease of young adults, although it can affect patients of any age. Clinically it presents as a localized mass, with the mediastinal and cervical lymph nodes being the most common sites involved. Patients with HVCD are usually asymptomatic, unlike those who have the plasma cell type, and are not infected with HIV.[39] In general, localized CD can be successfully treated with surgical resection, whereas multicentric forms require systemic therapy.[40]

Often considered a hyperplastic or reactive process, reports of stromal tumors arising in patients with HVCD as well as karyotypic abnormalities have led to the hypothesis that HVCD is a monoclonal proliferation. A study examining cases of HVCD in female patients using human androgen receptor assays have detected monoclonality in a high proportion of cases and correlation with size of the tumor. While no immune receptor gene rearrangements were seen, cytogenetic abnormalities in stromal cells were seen, suggesting that HVCD may be a neoplasm of lymph node stromal cells.[41] This is supported by a whole exome sequencing study that identified a recurrent activating *PDGFRB* mutation in 17% of cases of UCD cases, localizing the mutation to CD45-negative stromal cells.[42]

Histology

The histologic features of HVCD include numerous small, regressively transformed GCs surrounded by expanded mantle zones, and a hypervascular interfollicular region (Fig. 8-8A and B).[43] The cells within the regressively transformed GCs are predominantly FDC and endothelial cells. Relatively few follicle center B cells remain. The mantle cells tend to form concentric rings lined up along FDC processes, imparting an onion-skin pattern. Blood vessels from the interfollicular area may penetrate at right angles into the GC to form a lollipop follicle (Fig. 8-8C). The interfollicular area contains increased numbers of high endothelial venules and varying numbers of small lymphocytes. A useful diagnostic feature is the presence of more than one GC within a single mantle (twinning) (Fig. 8-8D). Occasional clusters of plasmacytoid dendritic cells are

found. The relative numbers of follicular and interfollicular components may vary from case to case. Sclerosis in the form of perinodal fibrosis and fibrous bands, often perivascular, within the lesion is common.

A stroma-rich variant of HVCD has been described, with stromal cells consisting of an angiomyoid component expressing actins. This variant is also clinically benign.[44,45] In some cases, there may be atypical FDCs with enlarged, irregular nuclei, which some investigators regard as dysplastic.[46] Clonal karyotypic abnormalities in these dendritic cell proliferations have also been seen.[47] Although the exact relationship is not known, these cells may be precursors to FDC tumors and sarcomas that have been reported in patients with HVCD.[44,48,49] Plasma cell Castleman disease (PC-CD) may be localized (approximately 10% of localized Castleman disease). It may be associated with constitutional symptoms that may resolve with resection. The predominant features of PC-CD are FH with dense interfollicular plasmacytosis. The plasma cells are not cytologically atypical. A mixed or transitional type of Castleman disease may be diagnosed when occasional hyaline vascular-type follicles are present.

Immunophenotype

The immunophenotype of the follicles in HVCD is like that of reactive follicles. Expanded, concentric meshworks of FDCs stain with antibodies to CD21 or CD23; multiple GCs may be found within a single expanded FDC meshwork.[50] The expanded mantle zone B cells express CD20 and may express CD5 in approximately one-third of cases when sensitive staining protocols are used.[51] Terminal deoxynucleotidyl transferase (TdT)-positive T-lymphoblastic populations of cells can be seen in most cases (75%) of HVCD as rare individual cells or, less commonly, in patchy clusters in interfollicular areas.[52] Flow cytometric studies show these cells may be double positive or double negative for CD4 and CD8 and rarely may be CD4-negative/CD8-positive.[53] Patches of plasmacytoid dendritic cells are highlighted by stains for CD123, CD68, and CD43.[54] Staining for human herpesvirus 8 (HHV-8) is typically negative in HVCD. Plasma cells in localized PC-CD are generally polytypic plasma cells; however, as with multicentric PC-CD, monotypic plasma cells may be present.

Differential Diagnosis

The morphologic features of HVCD are not entirely specific, and the differential diagnosis includes late-stage HIV-associated lymphadenopathy, early stages of follicular T-cell lymphoma (TFH) of angioimmunoblastic type (AITL), follicular or mantle cell lymphomas, and non-specific reactive lymphadenopathy. Clinical history and serologic testing can exclude HIV infection. AITL is typically a diffuse process containing expanded meshworks of FDCs outside of B-cell follicles, highlighted by CD21 or CD23 staining. However, atrophic GCs may occasionally be present. In early stages, the atypical infiltrate of AITL may be interfollicular, and the proliferation of high endothelial venules may resemble the hypervascular interfollicular region of HVCD. Atypia of the lymphoid cells, including characteristic clear cells, is usually seen, and CD10+/PD1+/BCL6+/ICOS+/CXCL13+ T cells outside of GCs are characteristic of the follicular T-helper cell origin of AITL.[55,56] In-situ hybridization for EBV-EBV encoded RNA

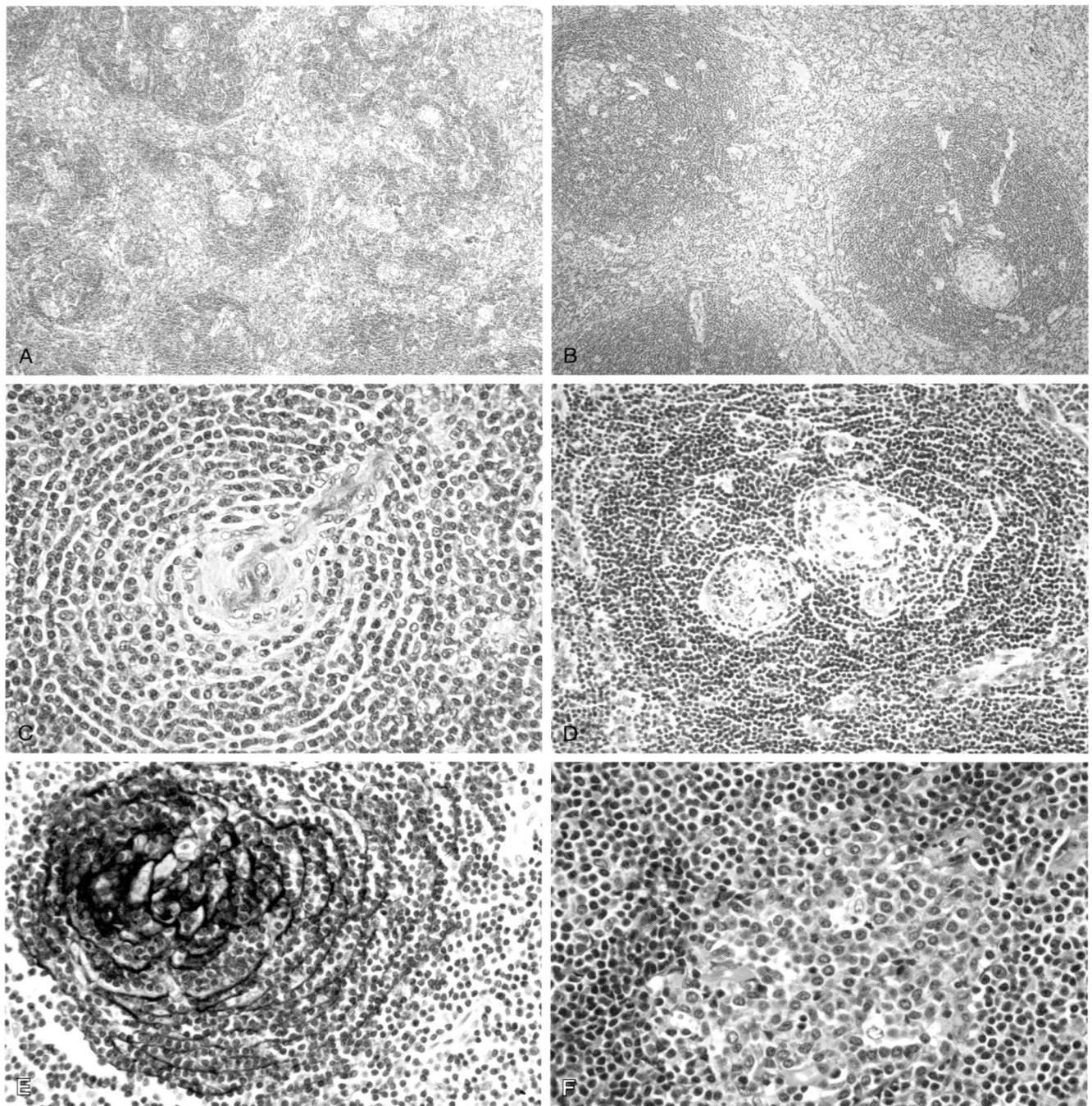

Figure 8-8. Hyaline vascular Castleman disease. A, Follicles with expanded mantle zones containing regressively transformed GCs. Interfollicular vascular proliferation is prominent (H&E, ×25). **B,** Higher magnification of expanded mantle zones penetrated by vessels from the interfollicular areas and atrophic GCs (H&E, ×90). **C,** Residual GC penetrated at right angle by hyalinized vessel rendering a lollipop appearance to the follicle. Small lymphocytes palisade around the GCs (onion-skin appearance) (H&E, ×330). **D,** Two atrophic GCs within a single mantle zone (H&E, ×180). **E,** CD21 staining shows the tight follicular dendritic meshwork within the atrophic GC extending in a loosely arranged pattern into the mantle zone. (CD21 immunostain, ×20). **F,** A cluster of plasmacytoid dendritic cells that is characteristically seen in hyaline vascular Castleman disease (HVCD) (H&E ×180).

(EBER) may reveal EBV-positive B immunoblasts in the interfollicular region in early AITL; however, these cells should not be present in HVCD.

The mantle zone pattern of MCL may mimic HVCD. However, the lymphoid component in MCL is atypical, monotypic, and expresses cyclin D1. The characteristic interfollicular vascularity of HVCD is absent. Small follicles of FL can be mistaken for the regressively transformed GCs of HVCD. However, immunostains demonstrate the typical phenotype of FL (CD20-positive, CD10-positive, BCL2-positive). Exclusion of autoimmune processes such as RA or HIV infection is important when considering a diagnosis of PC-CD.

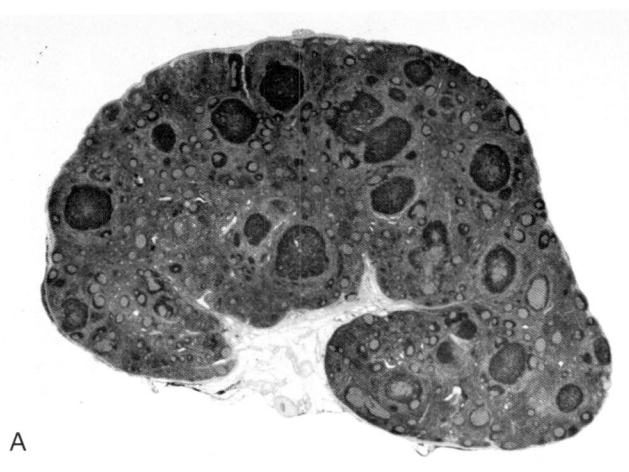
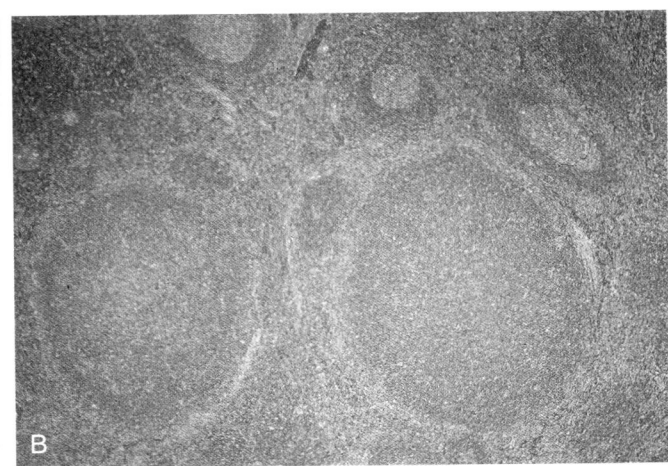

Figure 8-9. Progressive transformation of germinal centers. A, FH characterized by increased numbers of reactive follicles among progressively transformed GCs that are recognized by their large size (CD20, ×5). **B,** Reactive follicles and two large progressively transformed GCs that are composed predominantly of small lymphocytes (H&E, ×10).

Progressive Transformation of Germinal Centers

Progressive transformation of GCs (PTGC) is a pattern of reactive lymphadenopathy that often presents as a single enlarged lymph node in asymptomatic young adults (peak incidence in the second decade and predominantly in males), although it is also seen in children. Cervical and axillary lymph nodes are most commonly involved.[57-59] The few cases studied by FDG-PET have shown increased uptake. PTGC has been shown to be associated with autoimmune phenomena in a pediatric population.[60]

PTGC occurs as macronodules scattered in the background of typical FH (Fig. 8-9). The nodules are usually at least twice as large as, and often much larger than, the hyperplastic follicles and are composed predominantly of small lymphocytes with scattered follicle center cells present singly or in small clusters. Five patterns of PTGC have been described that range from nodules resembling FH, to those that resemble large primary follicles. Pattern 1 shows scalloped mantle zones with budding of the GCs into mantle zones. Pattern 2 shows incomplete septum-like protrusion of mantle zone cells into the residual GCs, while pattern 3 is completely dissected by variably thick septae of expanding mantle zone cells. Patterns 4 and 5 show few or no remnants of residual GC cells. In practice, these patterns are not generally reported, but help in understanding the spectrum of PTGC.[61] In most cases, a single or a few PTGCs are present in a lymph node. However, florid PTGC, in which numerous progressively transformed GCs are present, may occur, especially in young males.[62] Even in these cases, typical reactive follicles are always present between PTGC. Epithelioid histiocytes may occasionally be seen surrounding the follicles. Immunophenotypically, the small cells are predominantly IgM-positive, IgD-positive, mantle zone B cells.[63] Concentric, smooth meshworks of CD21-positive, CD23-positive FDCs outline the follicles. PD1-expressing T cells are increased both within the nodules and in extrafollicular areas.[3,4]

Differential Diagnosis

The main differential diagnostic consideration is nodular lymphocyte predominant B-cell (Hodgkin) lymphoma (NLPBL). NLPBL and PTGC resemble one another, and both may occur in the same lymph node. NLPBL may be present focally in cases of florid PTGC; in such cases, it is imperative that the entire lymph node be submitted for histologic examination. Like PTGC, NLPBL contains macronodules, but in contrast to those in PTGC, they efface the nodal architecture and lack interspersed reactive follicles. As in PTGC, the nodules also consist predominantly of small B cells with scattered large cells. However, the large cells in NLPBL are Reed-Sternberg cell variants also known as popcorn cells or LP cells. The LP cells, unlike the centroblasts in nodules of PTGC, have large, lobulated nuclei and variably sized nucleoli. T cells and CD57-positive/PD1-positive (CD279) TFH are often present in small clusters in NLPBL, whereas they are more uniformly scattered in PTGC. A feature useful in the differential diagnosis is the rosetting of CD3 and PD1-positive TFH around the neoplastic CD20-positive LP cells in NLPBL,[64] a finding typically absent in PTGC. Popcorn cells are EMA-positive in some cases of NLPBL, whereas residual centroblasts in PTGC are negative. In addition, the nodules in PTGC usually have sharply defined borders, while in NLPBL the nodules have ragged, "moth-eaten" edges.[65] These features are accentuated in sections stained with CD20 or CD79a. Epithelioid histiocytes are also commonly seen, not only around but also within the nodules in NLPBL. The presence of epithelioid histiocytes within nodules should raise suspicion for NLPBL rather than PTGC. To rule out NLPBL, morphologic and immunophenotypic features should be carefully evaluated in areas in which the nodules are closely packed.

A PTGC-like pattern of immunoglobulin G4 (IgG4)–related lymphadenopathy has been described.[66] Thus, in patients with known extranodal IgG4-related disease or with the clinical signs/symptoms of IgG4-related disease (particularly in elderly males), such as generalized lymphadenopathy and the common laboratory abnormalities associated with IgG4-related disease (elevated ESR, hypergammaglobulinemia, increased serum IgG4, IgG, and IgE, but not IgA or IgM), and circulating autoantibodies, immunostaining for IgG and IgG4 may be indicated.

Although surgical excision is often curative, PTGC may recur in the same site. Indeed, repeat biopsies after a diagnosis of PTGC were done in 11/29 patients in one report. It showed many recurring instances of PTGC.[60] Some investigators suggest a histogenetic relationship between PTGC and NLPBL, since PTGC can be seen preceding, simultaneously present with, or after a diagnosis of NLPBL.[58,60,67] Most studies show that the risk of development of NLPBL in a patient with PTGC is low, but the magnitude of risk is not known.[62] Thus, patients with florid or recurrent PTGC, particularly in the context of prior NLPBL, should be followed closely and suspicious lymph nodes should be biopsied to rule out development of NLPBL.[57,68]

Mantle Zone Hyperplasia

Mantle zone hyperplasia (MZH) rarely causes lymph node enlargement.[69] Mantle zones may be expanded around either hyperplastic or atrophic GCs. MZH may arouse suspicion for HVCD, mantle cell, or marginal zone lymphomas. The interfollicular vascularity seen in Castleman disease is lacking. Mantle cell lymphoma (mantle zone pattern) usually involves a majority of the lymph node, whereas MZH is most often limited to the cortex or involves only selected follicles (Fig. 8-10). Fusion of adjacent mantle zones may be present in MCL. Stains for CD5, CD43, cyclin D1, and immunoglobulin light chains may be useful in excluding mantle cell or marginal zone lymphoma; rarely, gene rearrangement analysis may be required to exclude lymphoma.[69] Mantle cell lymphoma in situ is recognized by cyclin D1-positive mantle zone B cells limited to mantles and is generally not part of the differential diagnosis of MZH, since the architecture of the lymph node is not altered and the mantle zone is generally not expanded.

Mycobacterial Spindle Cell Pseudotumor

Mycobacterial spindle cell pseudotumor (MP) is a spindle cell lesion sometimes occurring in HIV-positive patients.[70] These rare tumors usually involve lymph nodes but can be seen in other sites such as skin. Histologically, they appear as nodules within the lymph node, which may replace the normal architecture. The nodules are composed of bland spindle cells that form fascicles or take on a storiform pattern. These cells are histiocytes expressing CD68 and contain mycobacterial organisms that can be demonstrated with acid-fast stains.[70,71]

The differential diagnosis, particularly in the clinical setting of HIV infection, is Kaposi sarcoma (KS). KS cells may also form spindle cell tumors but can be distinguished from MP by their immunohistochemical profile (CD34-positive/CD31-positive). KS cells also contain HHV-8.

PREDOMINANTLY SINUS PATTERN

Sinus Histiocytosis

SH is a common, non-specific reaction that is characterized by expansion of sinuses by histiocytes. It is often seen in lymph nodes draining a tumor. Its prognostic significance (a marker of immune response) in this setting has been debated in older literature, with some studies suggesting a better survival when SH was present. SH may also be a reaction to recent surgery for a malignancy such as breast cancer.[72]

SH is a non-specific and benign finding in a clinically enlarged lymph node.[73-77] The degree of histiocytic reaction is variable. Cytologically, the histiocytes are bland (Fig. 8-11), without mitoses, which is a key distinguishing feature between this entity and sinusoidal involvement by malignancies such as melanoma, mesothelioma, and anaplastic large cell lymphoma. These malignancies may preferentially involve the sinuses with an infiltrate of noncohesive cells. In contrast to SH, they are composed of cytologically atypical cells. Uncommonly, SH may take on a signet ring appearance and mimic metastatic adenocarcinoma.[77] Immunohistochemistry for markers specific for these tumors and for histiocytes (CD68) can be used to sort out rare problematic cases.

Histiocytic Expansion Caused by a Specific Cause (Storage Disease, Lymphangiogram, Prosthesis, Whipple Disease)

Histiocytic reactions involving lymph nodes, although they may not primarily manifest as sinusoidal histiocytosis, may sometimes be attributed to specific causes, which are briefly described here.

Lymphangiogram, performed in the past for staging of lymphomas, produced large vacuoles formed by lipid-rich contrast material, resulting in the formation of lipogranulomas

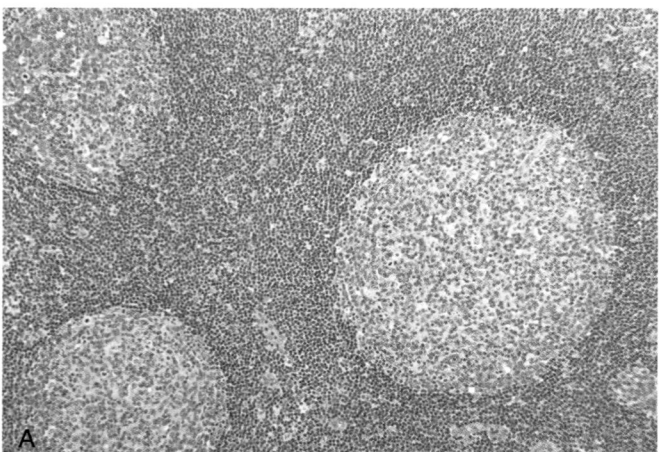
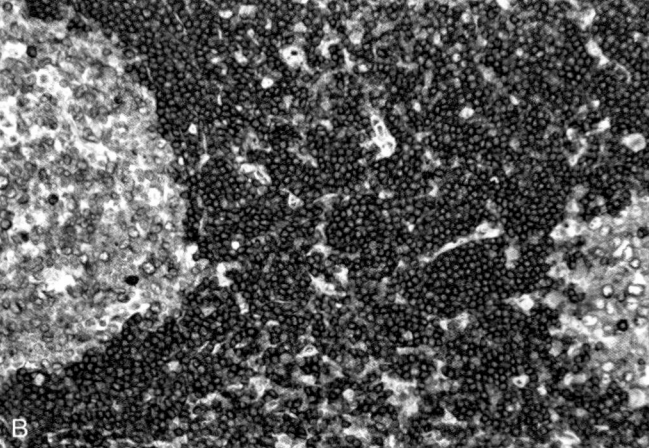

Figure 8-10. Mantle zone hyperplasia. A, Three follicles with expanded mantle zones that have virtually replaced the interfollicular area (H&E, ×70). **B,** CD79a stain shows positive mantle zone B cells with absence of interfollicular areas and parts of two GCs (CD79a, ×90).

and foamy histiocytes in sinuses and foreign body giant cells (Fig. 8-12).[78]

Histiocytic reactions may result from release of foreign material from deteriorating joint or silicone prostheses and also can cause regional lymphadenopathy.[79-83] Foreign material may be present in the regional lymph node in sinuses with extension into the paracortex and granuloma formation. Metal fragments and refractile prosthetic material can be demonstrated in the histiocytes. Silastic prostheses have been reported to produce granulomas with multinucleated giant cells containing yellow refractile, nonbirefringent silicone.[84] Breast implants may also result in lymphadenopathy with diffuse infiltrates of vacuolated and foamy histiocytes along with large cystic spaces containing silicone.[83] Polarized light examination may be helpful in demonstrating certain types of material such as polyethylene.[85]

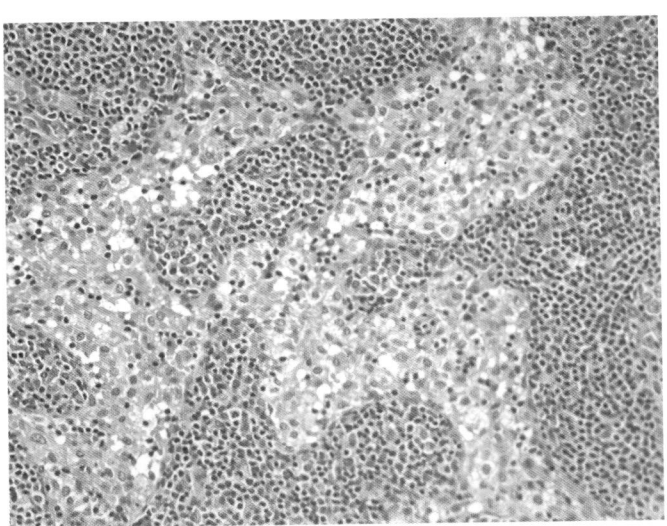

Figure 8-11. Sinus histiocytosis. The sinus is distended with histiocytes that have ample cytoplasm and bland-appearing nuclei without nucleoli (H&E, ×200).

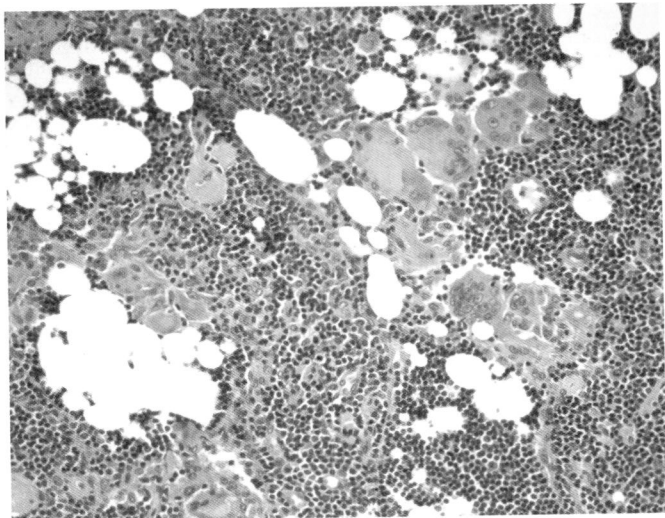

Figure 8-12. Abdominal lymph node from a patient who had a lymphangiogram. The sinuses are distended by large vacuoles surrounded by sinus histiocytes and foreign body-type giant cells (H&E, ×350).

Hereditary storage diseases such as Gaucher and Niemann-Pick diseases may also be associated with nodal infiltrates of storage-product-laden macrophages. The histiocytes retain the characteristics of the particular disease seen in other sites (e.g., tissue-paper appearance in Gaucher disease).[59,86]

Whipple Disease

Whipple disease, first described by George Whipple in 1907,[87] is an infection caused by the bacterium *Tropheryma whipplei* (formerly *T. whippelii*).[88,89] It occurs most commonly in middle-aged males with symptoms of weight loss, diarrhea, abdominal pain, and often arthralgia. Abdominal lymphadenopathy is usually present, with peripheral or mediastinal lymphadenopathy in about 50% of cases. Although Whipple disease is often diagnosed by small bowel biopsy, a lymph node may be the first tissue biopsied, especially in patients without abdominal complaints.

Lymph node sinuses contain large, pale-staining, finely vacuolated histiocytes that harbor diastase-resistant, PAS-positive sickle-form structures and large cystic vacuoles (Fig. 8-13). Electron microscopy confirms the presence of bacteria.[87,90,91] Not all cases have the characteristic findings; some cases have nonnecrotizing granulomas resembling sarcoidosis.[92,93] The PAS stain may be only focally positive when few organisms are present.[88] A high degree of suspicion is required in order not to miss this diagnosis.

The differential diagnosis of Whipple disease includes lymphangiogram effect, mycobacterial infection such as *Mycobacterium avium-intracellulare* (MAI), sarcoidosis, and leprosy.[94] The latter can show diffuse infiltrates of histiocytes with abundant vacuolated cytoplasm. Cystic spaces, however, are absent. In MAI, the organisms are both PAS and acid-fast positive, whereas in leprosy the organisms are acid-fast positive but PAS negative.[95] The presence of *T. whipplei* in fixed tissues can be confirmed by PCR.[87] Immunostaining has also been used to detect the organism in tissue section.[96]

Vascular Transformation of Sinuses

Vascular transformation of sinuses (VTS) (stasis lymphadenopathy, nodal angiomatosis, or hemangiomatoid plexiform vascularization) is an uncommon vasoproliferative lesion that occurs in patients of all ages; it is usually an incidental finding in a lymph node removed for other reasons. Histologically, subcapsular sinuses and, less frequently, other sinuses are expanded by thin-walled blood vessels lined by flat endothelial cells. The vascular spaces are more cellular in the intermediate sinuses and become ectatic and less cellular in the subcapsular sinuses (Fig. 8-14).[97] Arborizing slitlike spaces may also be formed. The histologic appearance varies, some cases having a more solid appearance because of plump endothelial cells and smaller vascular spaces. A plexiform variant consists of dilated and anastomosing spaces with flat lining cells. Extensive VTS may form spindle cell nodules.[97-100] Immunophenotypic analysis shows some loss of the lymphatic marker D2-40 in cells lining these spaces.[101]

The pathogenesis of VTS is thought to be lymphatic or vascular obstruction.[98-100,102] The differential diagnosis includes KS, hemangioma, and bacillary angiomatosis (BA). KS involves subcapsular sinuses in its early stages and is composed of slitlike vascular spaces. The nodal capsule, which is often involved in KS, is never infiltrated in VTS.

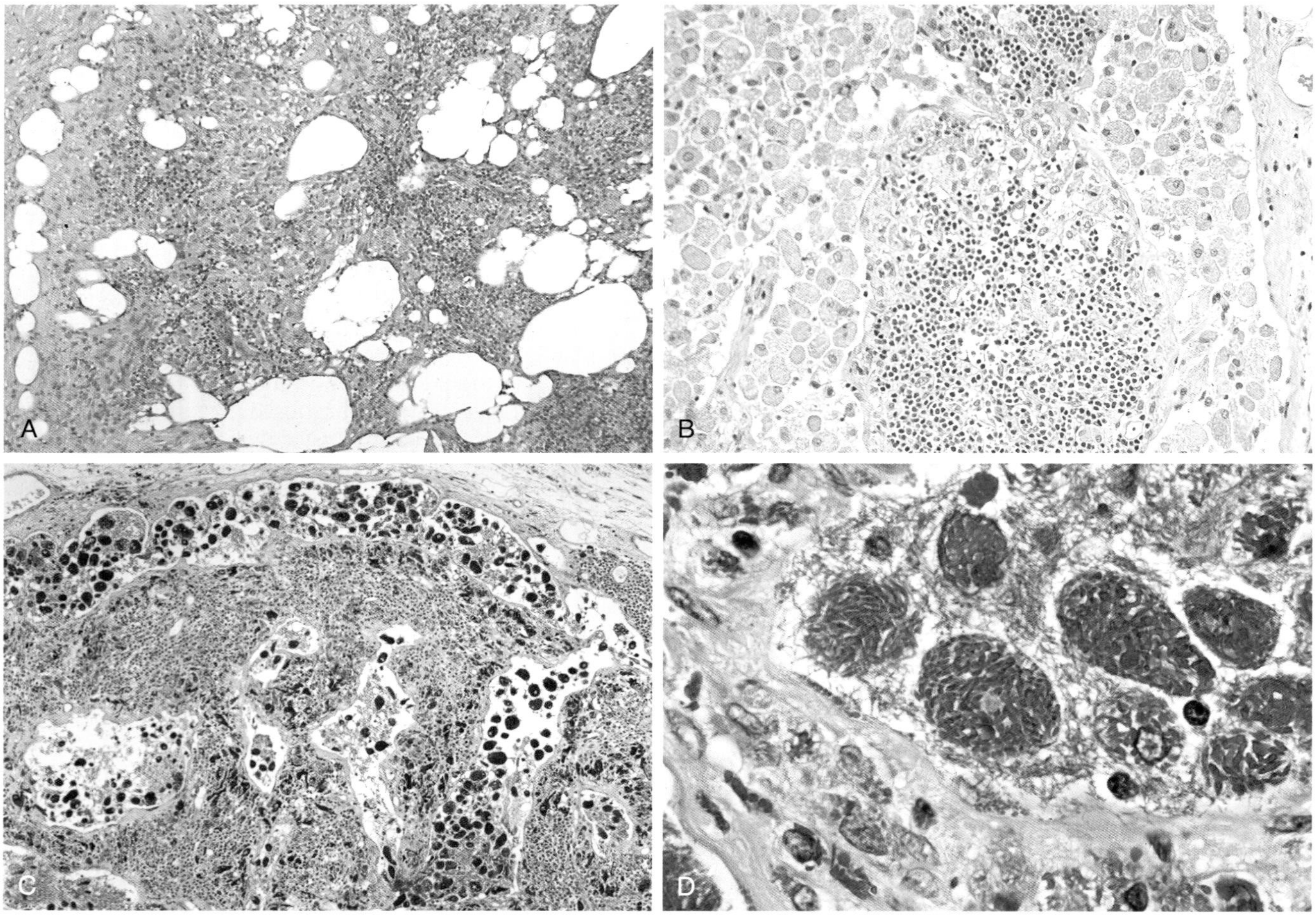

Figure 8-13. Whipple disease involving a lymph node. A, Sinuses contain varying-sized vacuoles and few histiocytes (H&E, ×25). **B,** Sinuses filled with large, pale-staining histiocytes (H&E, ×140). **C,** PAS-positive histiocytes fill sinuses (PAS, ×25). **D,** High magnification of histiocytes filled with PAS-positive sickle-form particles (PAS, ×700).

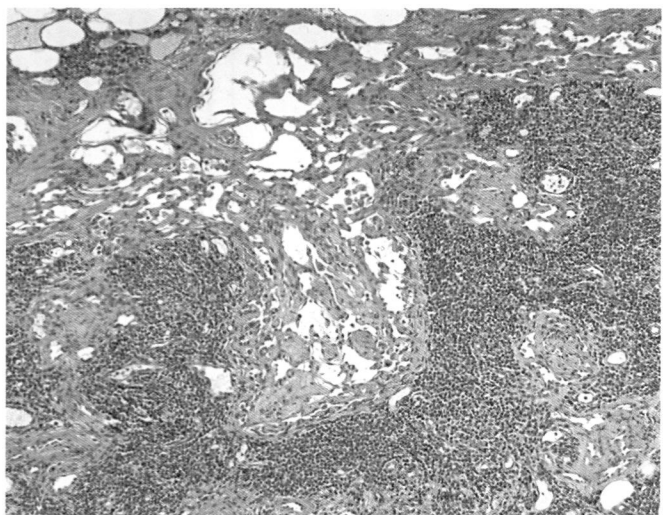

Figure 8-14. Vascular transformation of sinuses. The subcapsular and intermediate sinuses are replaced by vascular structures ranging from slitlike spaces, especially in the intermediate sinus, to ectatic vessels in the subcapsular sinus and associated fibrosis (H&E, ×25).

Sclerosis is minimal in KS, and there are long spindle cell fascicles, whereas BA, as discussed, forms nodules, and contains granular eosinophilic material and neutrophilic

debris not seen in VTS. Hemangiomas have well-developed vascular spaces and form nodules.[103,104]

Hemophagocytic Lymphohistiocytosis

Hemophagocytic lymphohistiocytosis (HLH) is a potentially fatal disorder of immune regulation characterized by abnormal activation of macrophages and lymphocytes, production of proinflammatory cytokines, and tissue infiltration of histiocytes that demonstrates hemophagocytosis. It can be classified into primary and secondary forms. Primary (genetic) forms of HLH are often associated with familial HLH (*PRF1, UNC13D, STS11,* and *STXP2* mutations), albinism syndromes (*RAB27A, LYST,* and *AP3B1*), or immune deficiencies (*SH2DIA, XIAP, ITK, MAGT1,* and *CD27* defects). Secondary causes include infections (often viral), autoimmune disorders (often termed *macrophage activation syndrome* in this setting), immunosuppression, malignancy, and rare metabolic disorders.[105] Lymphomas, especially T- and NK-cell lymphomas, may be complicated by HLH, a combination associated with a very poor prognosis. Primary cutaneous gamma/delta T-cell lymphoma is particularly associated with HLH.[105-108] Patients are constitutionally ill, usually with organomegaly, fever, and skin rash. Common laboratory findings include hyperlipidemia, cytopenias, and elevated ferritin. More detailed information on the classification, pathogenesis, and clinicopathologic characteristics of HLH are covered in Chapter 28 and 52.

Bone marrow aspiration and biopsy are the most performed procedures to document the presence of hemophagocytosis and to exclude leukemia as a cause for the HLH. Lymph node or tissue biopsy is usually avoided, except to exclude other malignancies. Of note, by revised diagnostic criteria for HLH diagnosis, demonstration of hemophagocytosis by bone marrow, spleen, or lymph node biopsy is not absolutely required if other criteria are met.[109]

Regarding lymph node pathology, there is a proliferation of benign histiocytes present in sinuses. There may be an immunoblastic proliferation or, alternatively, the lymph node may be depleted of lymphocytes. The histiocytes may be stuffed with erythrocytes, but other hematopoietic cells may also be phagocytized (Fig. 8-15). This latter feature may be seen especially clearly in smears of bone marrow aspirates.[110,111] In lymphoma-associated HLH, there may or may not be involvement of the lymph node by neoplasia.

Lack of evidence of malignancy in the lymph node does not exclude the possibility of a lymphoma-associated HLH.[112,113]

The differential diagnosis includes SH with massive lymphadenopathy (Rosai-Dorfman disease). This disorder is characterized by a sinusoidal infiltrate of large histiocytic cells with prominent nucleoli demonstrating emperipolesis of lymphocytes and occasionally plasma cells, rather than true cytophagocytosis.[114] The histiocytes are strongly S100 positive, while the histiocytes in HPS or SH are S100 negative or variably and weakly positive (see Chapter 52 for more detailed information).

Cells of Langerhans cell histiocytosis (LCH) also involve sinuses, but are CD1a and langerin positive, in addition to being S100 positive. Furthermore, the nuclei of the LCH cells have a characteristic nuclear groove/crease and are accompanied by an inflammatory infiltrate that often includes eosinophils (see Chapter 52 for more detailed information).

INTERFOLLICULAR OR MIXED PATTERNS

Paracortical Hyperplasia and Dermatopathic Reaction

Paracortical hyperplasia, or expansion of the paracortical (T-zone) region of the lymph node, may be a cause of lymphadenopathy. Causes include response to viral infection, reaction to a nearby malignancy, and autoimmune disease, although frequently the pathologist is not able to identify a specific etiology.[115-117] Histologically, there is a mixed population of small lymphocytes with variable numbers of immunoblasts and plasma cells. There may be admixed histiocytes, prominent vascularity (high endothelial venules), and interdigitating dendritic cells.[118-120]

Dermatopathic lymphadenitis is a specific type of paracortical hyperplasia that typically manifests in lymph nodes draining areas of chronic skin irritation. Histologically, there are vague paracortical lymphoid nodules that are composed of small lymphocytes admixed with increased numbers of interdigitating dendritic cells, Langerhans cells, and histiocytes containing melanin, or, less commonly, iron (Fig. 8-16). The various populations of histiocytes and dendritic cells have a mottled appearance at low magnification.

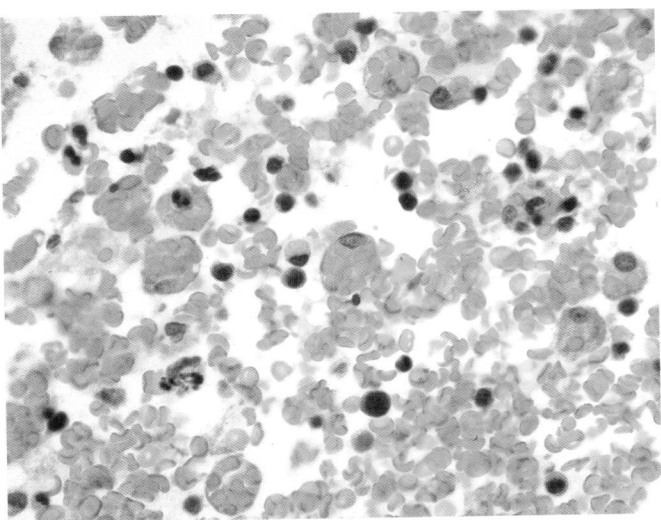

Figure 8-15. Lymph node from a patient with hemophagocytic lymphohistiocytosis. The distended sinus contains histiocytes engorged with phagocytized red blood cells (H&E, ×625).

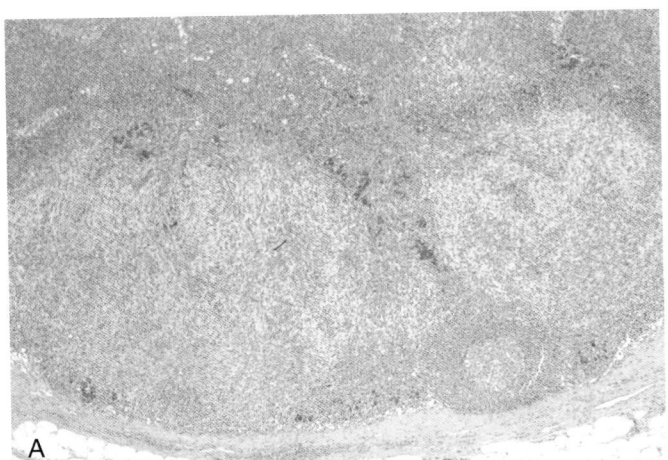
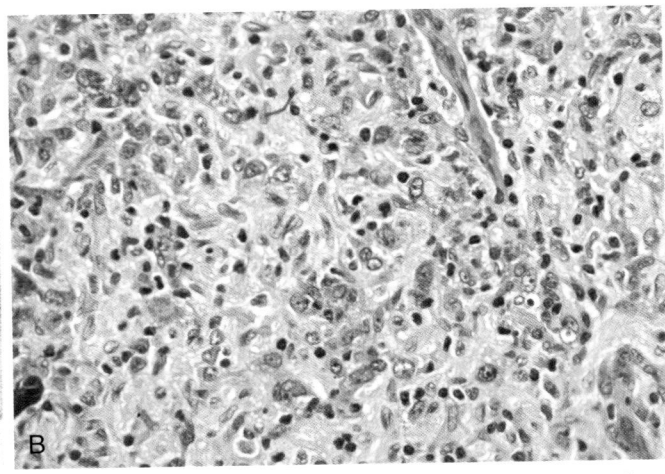

Figure 8-16. Dermatopathic lymphadenitis. A, Two pale-staining nodules in the expanded paracortex composed of Langerhans cells and histiocytes, some containing melanin. A follicle is compressed adjacent to the capsule (H&E, ×25). **B,** Higher magnification showing mixtures of pigment containing macrophages and Langerhans cells (H&E, ×400).

Both interdigitating dendritic cells and Langerhans cells are positive for S100 protein, and Langerhans cells also express CD1a and langerin. The histiocytes are positive for CD68. Studies have shown that dermatopathic changes can often occur in the absence of dermatitis.[121] The lymphocytes present within the nodules are predominantly T cells, which lack significant cytologic atypia. In most instances, there is no need for extensive immunophenotypic evaluation of lymph nodes with dermatopathic change. One pitfall is that these nodules should not be confused for involvement by LCH. The paracortical pattern (rather than sinusoidal as in LCH) and lack of eosinophilic infiltration can provide clues to the dermatopathic nature of the infiltrate.

The major differential diagnosis is with lymph node involvement by mycosis fungoides (MF), in which dermatopathic change is common. Lymph node involvement by MF may take several forms, ranging from the presence of atypical cells in clusters without obvious effacement of the lymph node architecture to diffuse involvement by lymphoma that may even resemble classic Hodgkin lymphoma (CHL).[122] Scoring systems to grade this involvement and predict behavior have been suggested,[123] but multivariate survival analysis calls into question their utility.[124] If there is a clinical history of MF, more extensive phenotyping of the T cells and careful morphologic evaluation should be performed. Gene rearrangement studies may be helpful in evaluating histologically equivocal cases and predicting outcome.[125,126]

Granulomatous Lymphadenitis

Granulomatous lymphadenitis can be divided into nonnecrotizing, necrotizing, and suppurative forms. Although a specific cause often cannot be determined, specific causes of granuloma formation in lymph nodes are presented here.

Nonnecrotizing Granulomas

Nonnecrotizing epithelioid granulomas are often seen as non-specific reactions to malignancy such as lymphoma or carcinoma. The lymph node may or may not be involved with the malignancy.[86,127,128] Types of lymphoma particularly associated with granulomas include CHL, nodular lymphocyte predominant B-cell lymphoma, lymphoplasmacytic lymphoma, and some peripheral T-cell lymphomas (Lennert lymphoma), although clusters of histiocytes smaller than granulomas are more characteristic of the latter. Metastatic nasopharyngeal carcinoma may be associated with a florid granulomatous reaction that obscures the tumor.

Sarcoidosis involving the lymph node results in discrete, well-formed epithelioid granulomas with or without multinucleated giant cells and scattered lymphocytes. The granulomas first involve the paracortical regions but often become confluent and can eventually replace the entire lymph node (Fig. 8-17). Schaumann, asteroid, and Hamazaki-Wesenberg bodies may be seen but are not specific for sarcoidosis.[129-132] PAS-positive and acid-fast Hamazaki-Wesenberg bodies (1–15 μm ovoid to spindle-shaped intracellular and extracellular structures) should not be mistaken for microorganisms.[132] The granulomas may be surrounded and replaced by fibrous tissue. Immunophenotyping shows a predominance of CD4-positive T cells.[133] Although almost any tissue can be involved, lung and mediastinal lymph nodes are most commonly affected. Cultures and special stains for microorganism should be done

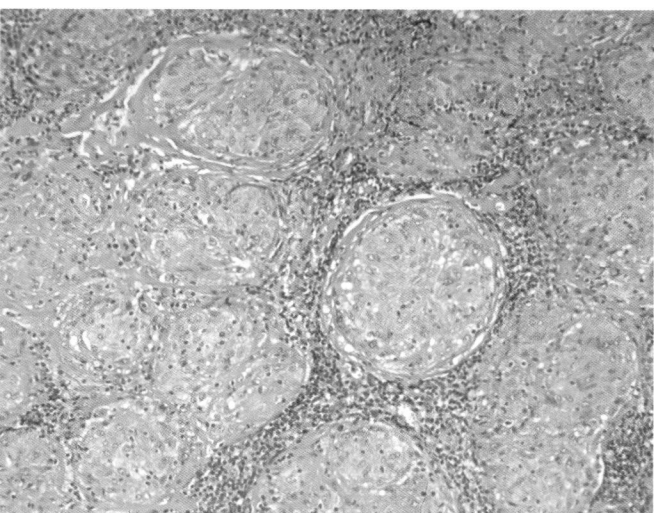

Figure 8-17. Sarcoidosis in a lymph node characterized by epithelioid granulomas, some surrounded by delicate fibrous bands (H&E, ×140).

to exclude infectious etiologies, particularly looking for fungi and acid-fast organisms.[134]

Necrotizing Granulomas (Tuberculosis, Fungal Infections, Cat Scratch Disease)

Necrotizing granulomas are caused by a variety of infectious organisms including mycobacteria, fungi, and bacteria. Some show characteristic histologic features.

Tuberculosis

Mycobacterial infections, particularly *Mycobacterium tuberculosis*, are common throughout the world.[135] After increasing incidence in the 1980s and 1990s, the numbers in the United States have stabilized at 6.8/100,000 per year.[135,136] In tuberculosis patients who present with peripheral lymphadenopathy, cervical lymph nodes are most commonly involved.[137] Cervical lymphadenopathy may also be the presenting feature in atypical mycobacterial infection with organisms such as *Mycobacterium scrofulaceum*, particularly in children.[138,139] Epitrochlear, axillary lymph, or inguinal nodes may be infected with *Mycobacterium marinum* from cutaneous lesions (swimming pool granulomas).

Histologically, lymph nodes infected by mycobacteria of any kind contain multiple well-formed granulomas consisting of epithelioid histiocytes and multinucleated giant cells. Caseating necrosis is often seen. In immunocompromised patients, the granulomas may not be well formed and may contain neutrophils. Mycobacterial organisms may be demonstrated in the granulomas with acid-fast stains. Culture is usually required to definitively identify species, although PCR has also been used.[140,141] Brucellosis (infection by the *Brucella* species bacteria) may cause a granulomatous lymphadenitis similar to that seen in tuberculosis; organisms are difficult to demonstrate in tissue sections.

Fungal Infection

Fungal infections of lymph nodes typically cause granulomatous lymphadenitis that may be necrotizing and indistinguishable from mycobacterial infection. Fibrosis and calcification may occur in older lesions. In

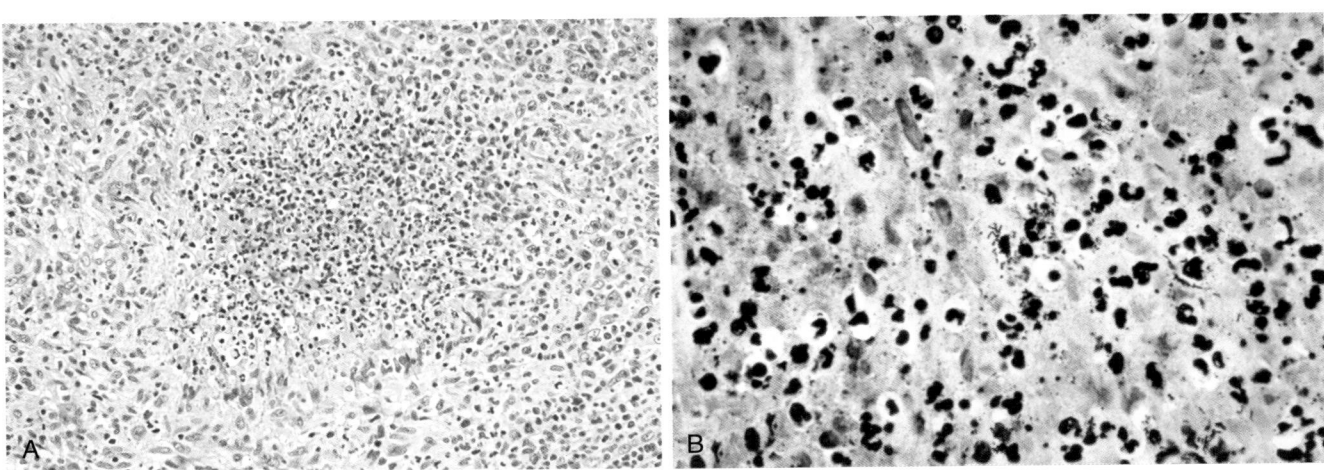

Figure 8-18. Lymph node from a patient with cat scratch disease. A, Suppurative granuloma with central area composed predominantly of neutrophils surrounded by palisading histiocytes and fibroblasts (H&E, ×250). **B,** Warthin-Starry stain showing the causative *Bartonella henselae* organisms (Warthin-Starry, ×700).

general, the lymphadenitis occurs as part of pulmonary-based disease or a disseminated infection. Disseminated infections usually occur in immunocompromised patients, either in the setting of HIV infection, malignancy, or in iatrogenically immunosuppressed patients.[135,142,143] In immunocompromised patients, the granulomas may not be well formed. In a large series of cases, *Histoplasma capsulatum* was the most common fungal infection in immunocompetent patients.[134] Gomori methenamine silver (GMS) or PAS stains will aid in identification of the organisms, although organisms are often absent in older lesions. The differential diagnosis includes necrotizing granulomas caused by an infectious cause such as mycobacteria.

Cat Scratch Disease

CSD, caused by *Bartonella henselae,* is histologically characterized by suppurative granulomas.[144,145] It is likely underrecognized and may be one of the more common causes of chronic lymph node enlargement in children.[146] Patients usually present with axillary or cervical lymphadenopathy and mild fever of 1 to 2 weeks' duration.[146,147] As cats are the reservoir of the causative organism, there is often, but not always, a history of exposure to cats, particularly kittens, which have higher levels of bacteremia and are more likely to scratch than adult cats.[146] The disease usually resolves spontaneously in several months.

The histologic features of CSD are characteristic but not entirely specific. Well-developed lesions are characterized by FH, monocytoid B-cell reaction, and suppurative granulomas (Fig. 8-18). Suppurative granulomas consist of a central necrotic focus containing abundant neutrophils and neutrophilic debris surrounded by palisaded macrophages forming the classic stellate microabscess.[144] Various stages in the development of the characteristic suppurative lesion are often seen in the same node. Early lesions show small foci of necrosis within clusters of monocytoid B cells, containing small clusters of neutrophils. Later lesions are surrounded by histiocytes. Very old lesions may contain central areas of caseation, similar to that seen in mycobacterial infection. Although the stellate microabscess (suppurative granuloma) is characteristic, over 40% of cases may not have these characteristic features, and instead may show features

mimicking other reactive patterns including those of fungal/mycobacterial disease, Kikuchi disease, and toxoplasma.[148]

The bacilli in CSD can be identified within the granulomas or walls of vessels with a Warthin-Starry stain, although these stains are challenging to interpret.[145] They are most readily seen in early lesions, where they tend to cluster in the walls of blood vessels (Fig. 8-18). Cultures are rarely definitive, but PCR tests in fixed tissue have been successful in detecting the organism.[148,149] Confirmation of the diagnosis by acute and convalescent serologic testing is recommended.

The differential diagnosis of suppurative granulomas includes other infectious agents such as *Chlamydia trachomatis* (lymphogranuloma venereum), *Francisella tularensis* (tularemia), *Yersinia pseudotuberculosis* (mesenteric lymphadenitis), *Listeria monocytogenes* (listeriosis), *Burkholderia mallei* (glanders), and *Burkholderia pseudomallei* (melioidosis). Many of these disorders are rare but have a specific clinical picture or a history of exposure to animals to aid in the clinical diagnosis, when combined with appropriate microbiological studies.[150-154] Potential uses of some of these agents in bioterrorism have raised awareness of their virulence and manifestations.[155,156]

Immunoglobulin G4–Related Disease

IgG4-related disease is a fibro-inflammatory disorder consisting of tumefactive lesions in multiple sites and a dense[157] plasmacytic infiltrate containing numerous IgG4-positive plasma cells, eosinophils, obliterative phlebitis, and storiform fibrosis (Fig. 8-19).[158,159] Serum IgG4 levels are often, but not always, increased. IgG4-related disease can involve virtually any organ, but is frequently seen in the pancreas and salivary and lacrimal glands. In addition, lymph nodes are frequently involved, although the features are less specific than those seen in extranodal sites with storiform fibrosis and obliterative phlebitis being rarely seen.[157] Axillary, mediastinal, and intraabdominal nodes are most commonly affected. There are five different, but sometimes overlapping, histologic patterns in lymph nodes: type I, multicentric Castleman-like disease; type II, FH; type III, interfollicular expansion; type IV, PTGC; and type V, IP-like. Only type

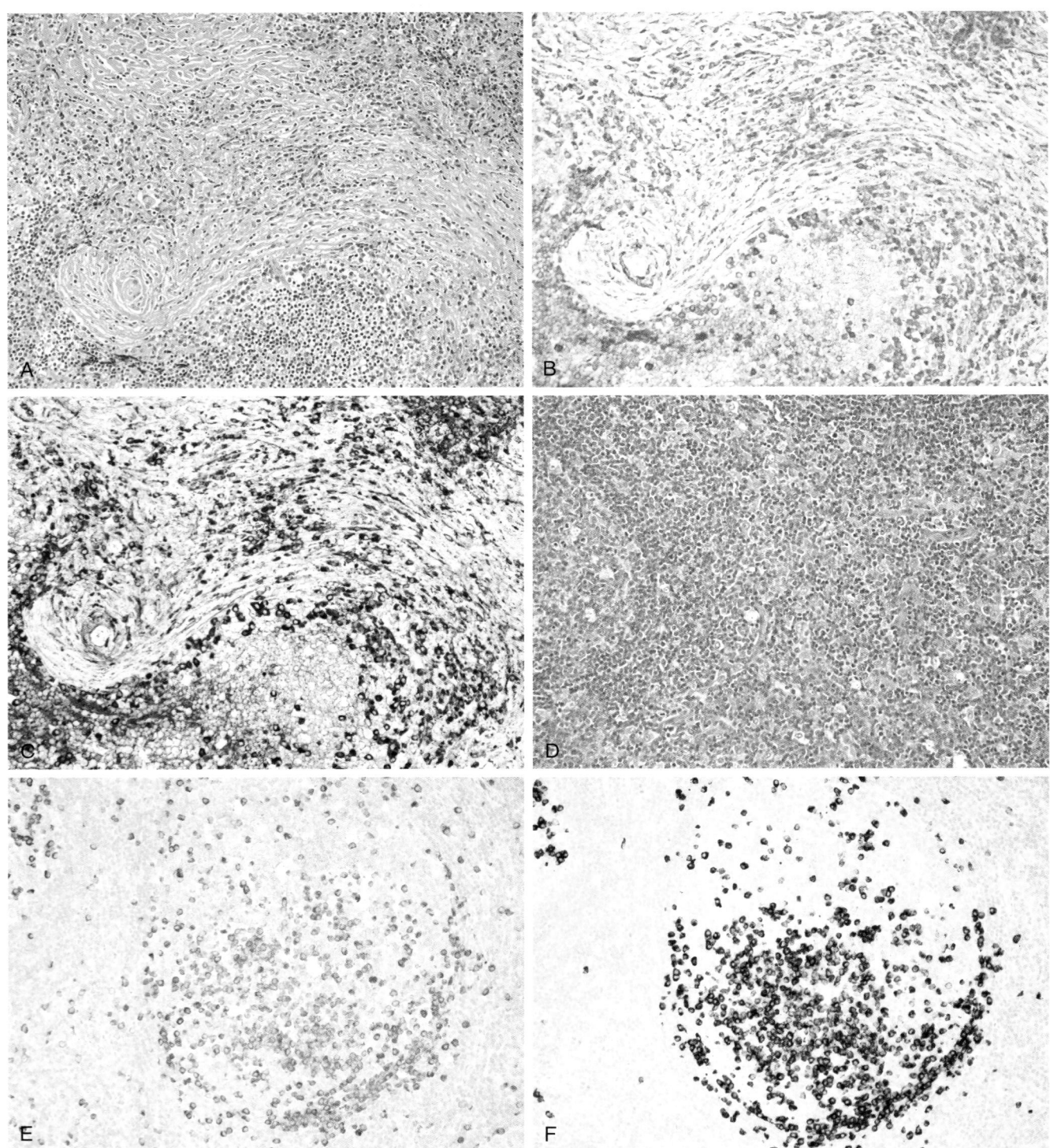

Figure 8-19. Features of immunoglobulin G4–related disease involving lymph nodes. A, Storiform fibrosis with increased plasma cells (H&E, ×200). **B,** Immunoglobulin G (IgG) stain highlighting plasma cells within fibrosis (×200). **C,** IgG4 stain showing IgG4/IgG ratio of close to 100% (×200). **D,** Follicular and paracortical hyperplasia with increased paracortical eosinophils and plasma cells is a common finding in lymph nodes from patients with IgG4-related disease but is non-specific (H&E, ×100). **E,** IgG stain showing increased intrafollicular plasma cells (×200). **F,** IgG4 stain showing elevated IgG4/IgG ratio (×200).

V is specific for IgG4-related disease, and is the least common pattern.[66,160] Overlapping patterns may be seen in types I and II, I and III, and between II and IV. All five of these types show an increase in IgG4 plasma cells (often >100 per high power field) and IgG4/IgG ratio (>40%).[66,158,161-163] However, these features are not specific for IgG4-related lymphadenopathy. Guidelines from the American College of Rheumatology recommend against the use of a lymph node to fulfill the histologic criteria for a diagnosis of IgG4-related disease.[157]

Type I pattern resembles multicentric Castleman disease or autoimmune-associated lymphadenopathy. The lymph node architecture is retained, and hyperplastic follicles and regressed follicles are present. Some of the follicles are radially penetrated by high endothelial venules (lollipop appearance) that are abundant in the interfollicular regions, together with numerous mature plasma cells and scattered eosinophils.

Type II pattern shows FH, interfollicular plasmacytosis, and plasma cells in GCs, with occasional eosinophils. Similar findings are seen in rheumatoid lymphadenopathy and other autoimmune disorders.

Type III pattern shows a prominent expansion of the interfollicular zones. Some follicles may be penetrated by high endothelial venules from the interfollicular areas (lollipop appearance), which, in addition, contain mature plasma cells, plasmablasts, immunoblasts, and eosinophils. The latter pattern may resemble TFH AITL. However, in contrast to AITL, there is no cellular atypia, no foci of clear cells, no aberrant immunophenotype, and no increased CD21-positive follicular dendritic meshworks around blood vessels. Increased numbers of EBV-infected cells that are seen in AITL have also been reported in IgG4-related lymphadenopathy, mostly in the PTGC type.[164] In addition, there are increased IgG4-positive cells and an increased IgG4/IgG ratio, both of which are absent in AITL.

Type IV pattern shows a preservation of architecture with reactive-appearing follicles and large PTGCs (3 to 4 times the size of reactive GCs) in various stages of transformation characterized by infiltration of mantle cells from a thickened mantle zone into the GCs, disrupting and eventually replacing them. Some of the reactive follicles and the PTGCs may be infiltrated by plasma cells and eosinophils.

Type V pattern is the rarest.[157] It is characterized by a storiform pattern of collagen fibers that are infiltrated by plasma cells and lymphocytes. It is similar to the process found in extranodal sites.

Although the numbers of IgG4-positive plasma cells and the IgG4/IgG ratio are increased, they are insufficient for a definitive diagnosis because other conditions, such as RA, Kimura disease, multicentric Castleman disease, Rosai-Dorfman disease, and other conditions may show the same findings. Therefore it is of utmost importance that both clinical correlations be applied when evaluating a lymph node specimen for IgG4-related disease.[157]

Kimura Disease

Kimura disease is a chronic inflammatory condition of unknown cause that affects young to middle-aged patients, most often males of Asian descent.[165] Patients usually present with a mass in the head and neck region with involvement of subcutaneous tissue, soft tissue, salivary glands, and single or multiple regional lymph nodes. Peripheral blood examination shows an eosinophilia and increased serum IgE levels. The disease is self-limited, although recurrences can occur over a period of years.[165]

Key histologic features include florid FH that may contain a proteinaceous precipitate (IgE in a follicular dendritic network pattern) and vascularization of the GCs (Fig. 8-20). The interfollicular areas show prominent high endothelial venules with a mixture of lymphocytes, plasma cells, eosinophils,

and mast cells. Follicle lysis is often present, and eosinophilic abscesses are characteristic within GCs and in the paracortex. Polykaryocytes are usually seen in GCs and paracortex. A varying degree of fibrosis is seen.

Immunohistochemistry is of minimal utility in this disease, but may help in excluding other disorders. Because of similar Th2 T-cell responses that promote eosinophil proliferation and class switching of plasma cells to IgE and IgG4, lymph nodes in Kimura disease may have increased IgG4-positive plasma cells and patients may have increased serum IgG4.[166,167] Staining for IgE to identify proteinaceous deposits in GCs has been proposed as a useful diagnostic tool for Kimura disease, but is not specific for this entity.[168]

In lymph nodes, the differential diagnosis includes other entities associated with eosinophilia including allergic/hypersensitivity reactions and parasitic infestation, as well as IgG4-related disease. These disorders less frequently will show eosinophilic abscesses of follicles and paracortex.

The entity most likely to be confused with Kimura disease is angiolymphoid hyperplasia with eosinophilia (ALHE), which also involves the head and neck region. Long thought to be synonymous with Kimura disease, ALHE is a vascular neoplasm characterized by the proliferation of blood vessels lined by plump endothelial cells with abundant eosinophilic cytoplasm, imparting a hobnail appearance. This lesion is part of the spectrum of what have been called *histiocytoid* or *epithelioid hemangiomas*, and is a low-grade vascular tumor. There is a dense, mixed inflammatory cell infiltrate consisting of lymphocytes, plasma cells, and eosinophils. The prominent histiocytoid endothelial cells seen in ALHE are not seen in Kimura disease, and the presence of this feature is the most reliable distinction between these two entities.[165,169-171]

Toxoplasma Lymphadenitis

Infection by *Toxoplasma gondii* in the immunocompetent patient results most commonly in solitary cervical lymphadenopathy. The organism has a worldwide distribution, with 30% to 40% of adults in the United States having been exposed to it.[172] Patients with an acute infection may be asymptomatic, or, less frequently, they may have non-specific symptoms such as malaise, sore throat, and fever, a constellation of symptoms similar to those found in infectious mononucleosis (IM). In addition, reactive lymphocytes may be found in peripheral blood smears, thus clinically resembling the features of IM.[172-174] The disease is self-limited, but immunodeficient patients may develop severe complications such as encephalitis. Infection during pregnancy may result in birth defect or fetal loss.

Histologically, lymph nodes show prominent FH with expansion of monocytoid B cells in a sinusoidal and perisinusoidal pattern. Small clusters of epithelioid histiocytes in the paracortex encroach upon and are present within GCs (Fig. 8-21). The GCs have ragged, "moth-eaten" margins, and contain numerous tingible body macrophages. Granulomas and multinucleated giant cells are absent. Parasitic cysts are seen only rarely, and earlier attempts to detect the organisms by PCR were mostly unsuccessful.[175,176] Serology is the primary means for confirmation of the diagnosis.[174] However, a study showed a PCR detection rate of 83% in cases with the histologic triad of florid reactive FH, clusters of epithelioid histiocytes, and focal sinusoidal distention by monocytoid B cells.[177]

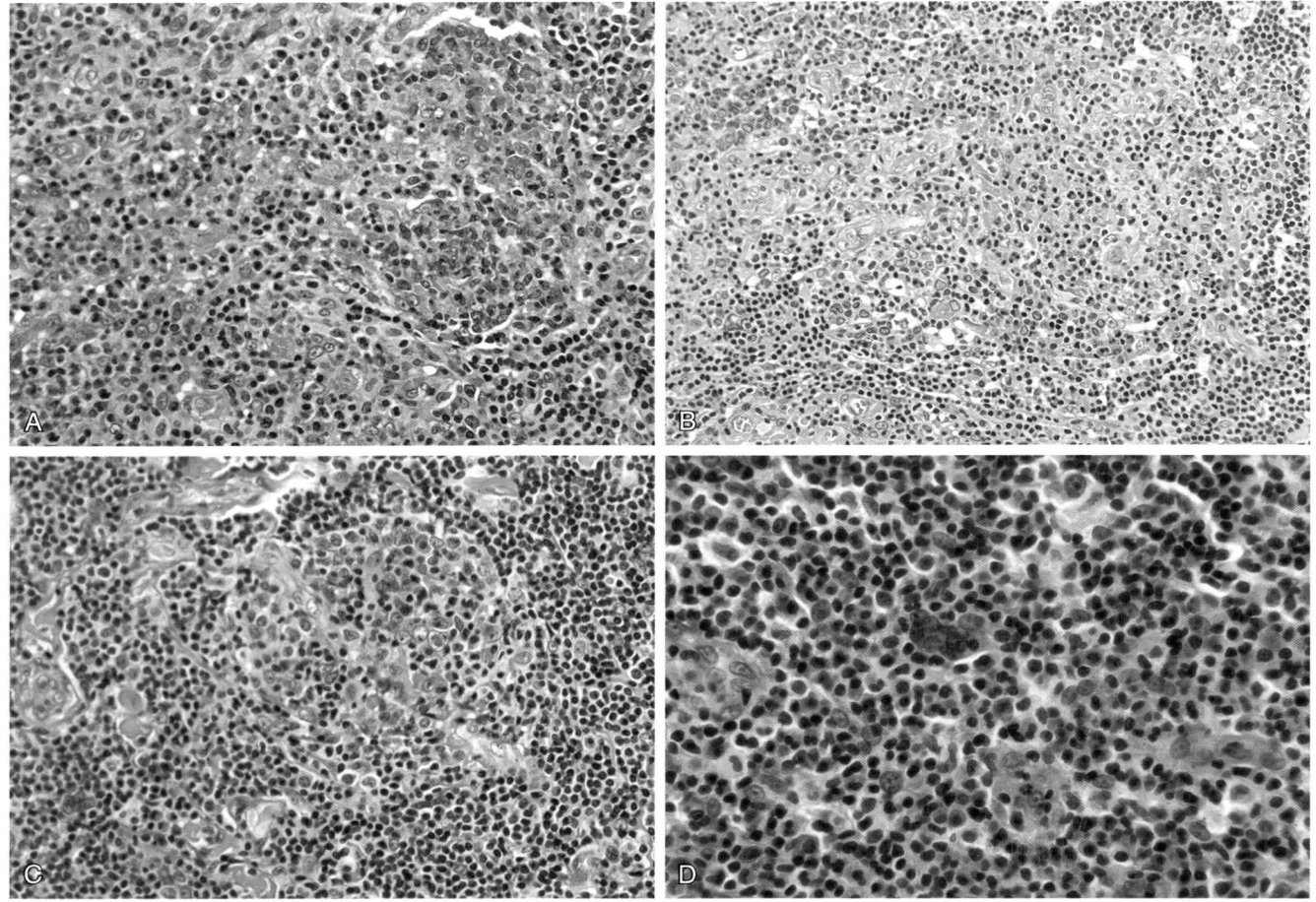

Figure 8-20. Kimura disease in a lymph node biopsy from a young man with a mass in the parotid gland region. A, Follicular lysis with eosinophils in a hyperplastic GC (H&E, ×330). **B,** Eosinophilic abscess in a GC. Residual clusters of large GC cells are present (H&E, ×330). **C,** Vascularization of a GC and high endothelial venules in the paracortex (H&E, ×330). **D,** Numerous eosinophils in the paracortex along with a polykaryocyte (H&E, ×500).

Although the histologic features are characteristic of toxoplasma lymphadenitis, the differential diagnosis includes leishmanial lymphadenitis, which can result in a histologic picture similar to toxoplasmosis. In leishmaniasis, organisms may be seen in the granulomas. Ultrastructurally, leishmaniasis can be distinguished from toxoplasma by the presence of kinetoplasts and basal bodies in the former.[178] Early stages of CSD, IM, and CMV lymphadenitis may also have morphologic features similar to that of toxoplasma lymphadenitis.

Systemic Lupus Erythematosus

Patients who have systemic lupus erythematosus (SLE) are at increased risk for development of lymphoma, and lymphadenopathy is present in up to 60% of the patients, most commonly involving cervical and mesenteric nodes.[179,180] The histologic features of lymph nodes in SLE include nonspecific FH, with or without an interfollicular expansion of lymphocytes and immunoblasts, often with numerous plasma cells both within GCs and in the medullary cords. A characteristic feature of lupus lymphadenitis is coagulative necrosis, often involving large areas of the lymph node (Fig. 8-22).[179,181-183] The necrotic areas contain ghosts of lymphoid cells, often abundant karyorrhectic debris, and histiocytes; segmented neutrophils are scant, but may be

present, in contrast to Kikuchi lymphadenitis. The presence of hematoxylin bodies, extracellular amorphous hematoxyphilic structures probably composed of degenerated nuclei that have reacted with antinuclear antibodies, is specific for SLE. The hematoxylin bodies are found in areas of necrosis and in sinuses. Hematoxylin bodies are absent in Kikuchi disease.

Kikuchi Lymphadenitis (Kikuchi-Fujimoto Lymphadenitis, Histiocytic Necrotizing Lymphadenitis)

Histiocytic necrotizing lymphadenitis, also known as Kikuchi or Kikuchi-Fujimoto lymphadenitis, was described in Japan in 1972.[184,185] It has a worldwide distribution and predominantly affects young adults, especially young women of Asian descent. The disease in most instances resolves spontaneously within several months. Patients most often present with cervical lymphadenopathy, sometimes associated with fever and leukopenia. Three histologic subtypes, probably representing various stages in the evolution of the disease, have been described: proliferative stage, necrotizing stage, and xanthomatous stage.[186]

The earliest proliferative stage is characterized by the presence of numerous immunoblasts with prominent

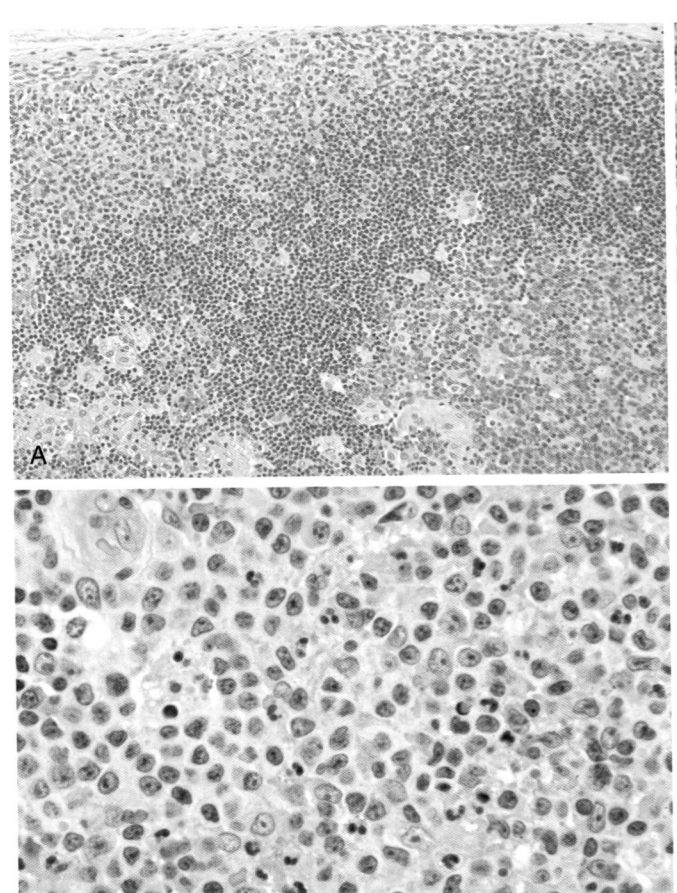

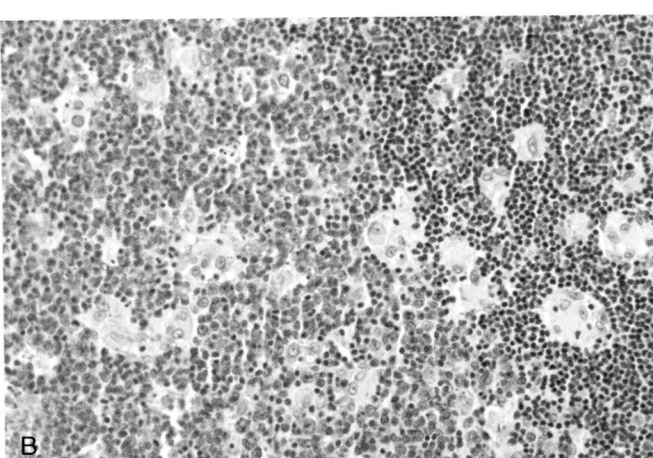

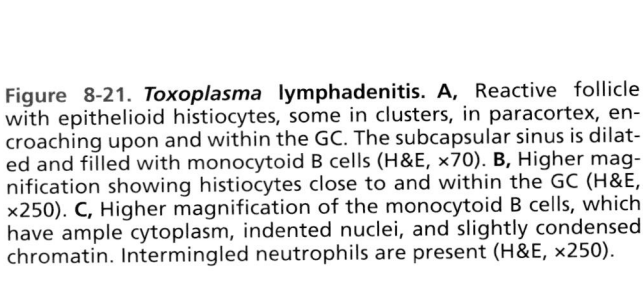

Figure 8-21. *Toxoplasma* **lymphadenitis. A,** Reactive follicle with epithelioid histiocytes, some in clusters, in paracortex, encroaching upon and within the GC. The subcapsular sinus is dilated and filled with monocytoid B cells (H&E, ×70). **B,** Higher magnification showing histiocytes close to and within the GC (H&E, ×250). **C,** Higher magnification of the monocytoid B cells, which have ample cytoplasm, indented nuclei, and slightly condensed chromatin. Intermingled neutrophils are present (H&E, ×250).

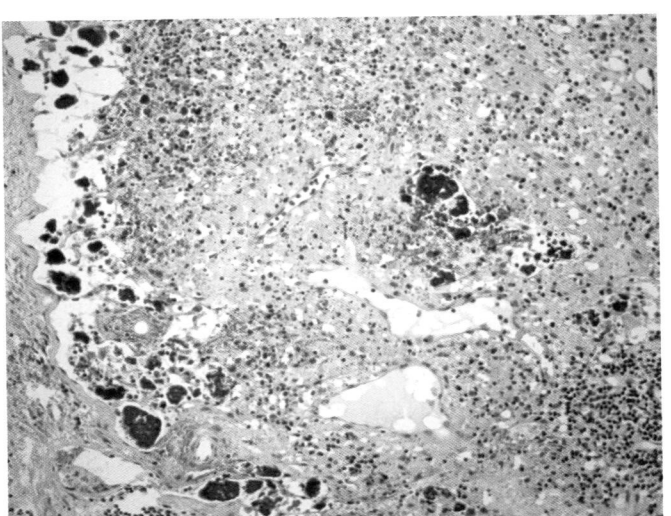

Figure 8-22. Lymph node from a patient with systemic lupus erythematosus. Extensive necrosis with apoptotic debris and hematoxylin bodies found predominantly within sinuses. Neutrophils are absent (H&E, ×100).

nucleoli and basophilic cytoplasm in the paracortex, raising the differential diagnosis of large-cell lymphoma. The immunoblasts are admixed with large mononuclear cells including histiocytes, some with curved nuclei (crescentic histiocytes) and some with twisted nuclei, and aggregates of

plasmacytoid dendritic cells may be prominent. The latter cells are intermediate-sized with round-to-oval nuclei and granular chromatin, placed eccentrically within an amphophilic cytoplasm. They are often difficult to identify within the mixture of cells. Karyorrhectic bodies are often interspersed among the plasmacytoid dendritic cells, and the necrosis seen in Kikuchi disease often appears to begin in nests of these cells.

The necrotizing stage, which is seen in most cases, is characterized by patchy areas of necrosis within the paracortex (Fig. 8-23). The necrosis contains no neutrophils, has abundant karyorrhectic nuclear debris, and is surrounded by a mixture of mononuclear cells identical to those found in the proliferative type. The karyorrhectic debris is both extracellular and phagocytized by histiocytes.

The xanthomatous stage is the least common and most likely represents the healing phase of this entity. It contains many foamy histiocytes and fewer immunoblasts than the other stages. Necrosis may or may not be present in the xanthomatous type.

Minimum criteria for the diagnosis of Kikuchi lymphadenitis include paracortical clusters of plasmacytoid dendritic cells admixed with karyorrhectic bodies and crescentic histiocytes.[187] The noninvolved parts of the node show a mottled appearance caused by the presence of immunoblasts scattered among small lymphocytes. Reactive lymphoid follicles may be seen. There is also a proliferation of

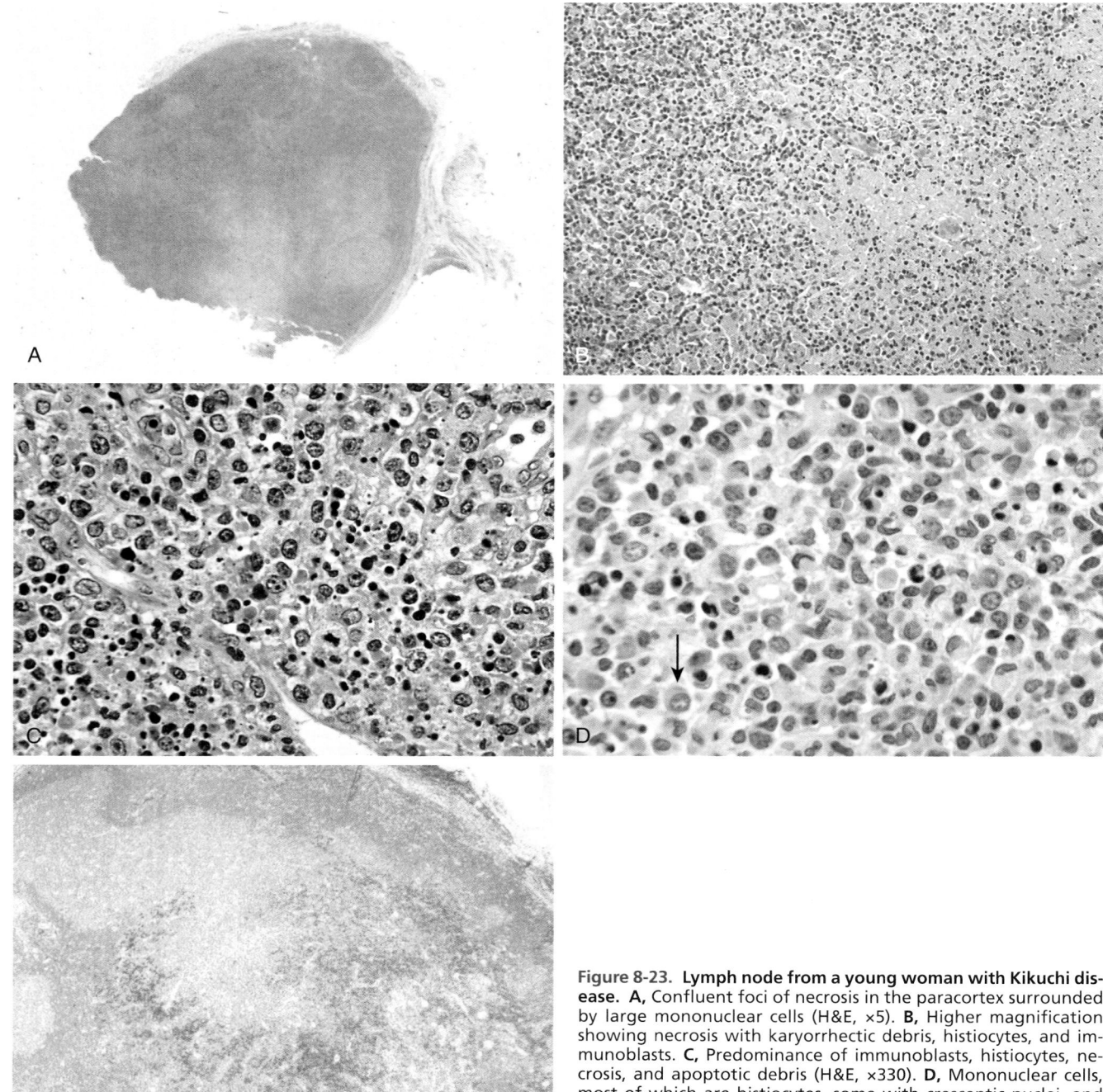

Figure 8-23. Lymph node from a young woman with Kikuchi disease. A, Confluent foci of necrosis in the paracortex surrounded by large mononuclear cells (H&E, ×5). **B,** Higher magnification showing necrosis with karyorrhectic debris, histiocytes, and immunoblasts. **C,** Predominance of immunoblasts, histiocytes, necrosis, and apoptotic debris (H&E, ×330). **D,** Mononuclear cells, most of which are histiocytes, some with crescentic nuclei, and plasmacytoid dendritic cells *(arrow)* and immunoblasts (H&E, ×330). **E,** CD123 staining shows plasmacytoid dendritic cells surrounding an area of necrosis (×40).

high endothelial venules.[187] This histologic picture resembles that seen in viral-associated lymphadenopathy.

The immunoblasts are typically CD8-positive T cells but may be a mixture of T and B cells. This is a pitfall that can lead to misdiagnosis as an aggressive lymphoma if the characteristic constellation of findings for Kikuchi is not recognized. Plasmacytoid dendritic cells can be best recognized by staining for CD123, but also express CD68, CD4, and CD43 (Fig. 8-23E). CD68 and CD163 stain histiocytes. Myeloperoxidase-positive histiocytes are frequently present

but lack specificity.[188] Typically, there is not a prominent B-cell infiltrate.

The differential diagnosis includes lupus lymphadenitis and non-Hodgkin lymphoma. The findings in Kikuchi lymphadenitis may be indistinguishable from those of lupus, and some investigators have raised the possibility of a relationship between the two; however, cases reported as Kikuchi lymphadenitis in association with SLE are almost certainly lupus lymphadenitis misdiagnosed as Kikuchi lymphadenitis.[181,189] Extensive necrosis, the presence of hematoxylin bodies, and plasma cells or occasional neutrophils favor SLE.[181] Most patients with Kikuchi lymphadenitis lack antinuclear antibodies.[187] Because of the difficulty in distinguishing histologically between the two, whenever a diagnosis of Kikuchi lymphadenitis is made, serologic testing for SLE is advisable; if tests are positive, the diagnosis is lupus lymphadenitis.

Cases with abundant immunoblasts may be mistaken for lymphoma. Patchy involvement of the lymph node, abundant karyorrhectic debris, a mixed cell population including the crescentic histiocytes, the absence of B-cell markers on the immunoblasts, and lack of a B- or T-cell receptor gene rearrangement favor Kikuchi lymphadenitis.[181]

Kawasaki Disease (Mucocutaneous Lymph Node Syndrome)

Kawasaki disease is an acute exanthematous childhood disease of unknown etiology,[190] a male-to-female ratio of 1.5:1 and a peak age of 3 to 4 years.[191,192] Diagnosis rests on the presence of five of the six following features not attributable to other causes: fever unresponsive to antibiotics, bilateral conjunctivitis, oral mucositis, distal extremity cutaneous lesions, polymorphous skin exanthems, and cervical lymphadenopathy.[193] The disease appears to be a systemic vasculitis, and the term *juvenile polyarteritis nodosa* has been proposed. Although most children recover, patients are at high risk for coronary artery aneurysm. Sudden death occurs in approximately 1% of patients.[194,195] Histologically, the lymph nodes show nongranulomatous foci of necrosis, with or without neutrophils, associated with vasculitis and thrombosis of small vessels. Scattered lymphocytes, plasma cells, and immunoblasts are seen in the background. The overall nodal architecture is often effaced. The differential diagnosis is extensive and includes other entities with necrosis such as SLE and Kikuchi lymphadenitis.[181,196] Observation of fibrin thrombi in nodal vessels with the appropriate clinical history would strongly favor Kawasaki lymphadenitis.

Inflammatory Pseudotumor

IP is an idiopathic reactive condition of lymph nodes affecting young adults (median age 33) without gender predilection.[197] Patients have constitutional symptoms and often laboratory abnormalities such as hypergammaglobulinemia, elevated ESR, and anemia. Single peripheral or central, or multiple lymph node groups, and the spleen may be involved.[198,199] IP can spontaneously resolve; surgical excision or antiinflammatory agents can relieve symptoms.[199]

The key histologic feature is a fibro-inflammatory reaction of the connective tissue framework of the lymph node with extension into the perinodal soft tissue. The capsule, trabeculae, and hilum are involved by a proliferation of small vessels, histiocytes, and myofibroblastic cells with admixed lymphocytes, plasma cells, eosinophils, and neutrophils. The myofibroblastic cells are spindly to polygonal with bland nuclei and abundant cytoplasm. They can form ill-defined fascicles or appear in a storiform pattern. Fibrinoid vascular necrosis, karyorrhexis, and focal parenchymal infarction may be seen. Invasion and destruction of medium-sized vessels may be present. Lymphoid follicles are uncommon.[197,198,200,201] Immunophenotyping shows that the lymphoid cells are predominantly T cells. CD68-positive histiocytes and vimentin-positive/actin-positive

spindle cells are present, supporting the fibrohistiocytic nature of the proliferation.[198,200,201] As the lesions age, the node becomes replaced by fibrotic tissue with a scant inflammatory infiltrate.[198]

The differential diagnosis includes KS, FDC tumors, hypocellular anaplastic large-cell lymphoma, and syphilis infection. Early involvement by KS shows capsular, subcapsular, and trabecular spindle cell areas that may suggest the connective tissue framework pattern of IP. Vascular structures are poorly formed in KS, in contrast to their appearance in IP. The PAS-positive hyaline globules of KS are not present. The bland cytologic features of IP, the lack of a mass-forming nodule, and the absence of FDC markers such as CD21 and CD35 aid in making the distinction from FDC tumors.[202,203] Hypocellular anaplastic large-cell lymphoma has an edematous fibromyxoid background with scattered myofibroblastic cells that may form fascicles, mimicking IP. CD30 and ALK expression in atypical cells that tend to cluster around vessels confirm lymphoma and exclude IP.[204] Syphilis infection can also result in an IP-like lesion. Thus all IPs should be investigated for spirochetes using *Treponema* immunohistochemistry. Features that might suggest syphilis include pronounced FH and capsular fibrosis with plasma cell infiltrate and neutrophilic infiltrates around small vessels.[38]

Bacillary Angiomatosis

BA caused by infection with *B. henselae* or, less commonly, *Bartonella quintana*[205-207] may cause lymphadenopathy in immunocompromised patients, particularly those infected with HIV. Patients present with skin lesions, lymphadenopathy, and occasionally hepatosplenomegaly.

The lymph nodes demonstrate single or confluent nodules composed of small blood vessels lined by plump endothelial cells, interstitial granular eosinophilic material, and varying numbers of neutrophils with leukocytoclasis. Warthin-Starry staining demonstrates tangles of bacilli in the eosinophilic material,[208,209] and organisms may be detected by *Treponema* immunohistochemistry and PCR (Fig. 8-24).[210,211]

The differential diagnosis includes other vasoproliferative disorders.[103] In immunocompromised patients, KS must be considered. In KS, the vascular structures are less well formed, and the fascicular pattern and hyaline globules of KS are not seen in BA. The endothelial cells of BA are positive for *Ulex europaeus* and factor VIIIRA, whereas they are negative in KS. Detection of bacteria in BA and HHV-8 in KS is helpful.

DIFFUSE PATTERN

Diffuse paracortical proliferations are the most difficult benign lymphadenopathies to differentiate from lymphomas because there is often subtotal effacement of the nodal architecture. There are prominent immunoblasts with atypical cytologic features, occasionally mimicking large cell or Hodgkin lymphomas. Clinical history, results of laboratory studies, immunophenotyping, and molecular analysis are crucial in distinguishing benign from malignant proliferations.

Infectious Mononucleosis

IM caused by EBV infection commonly produces lymphadenopathy and enlargement of tonsils in adolescents

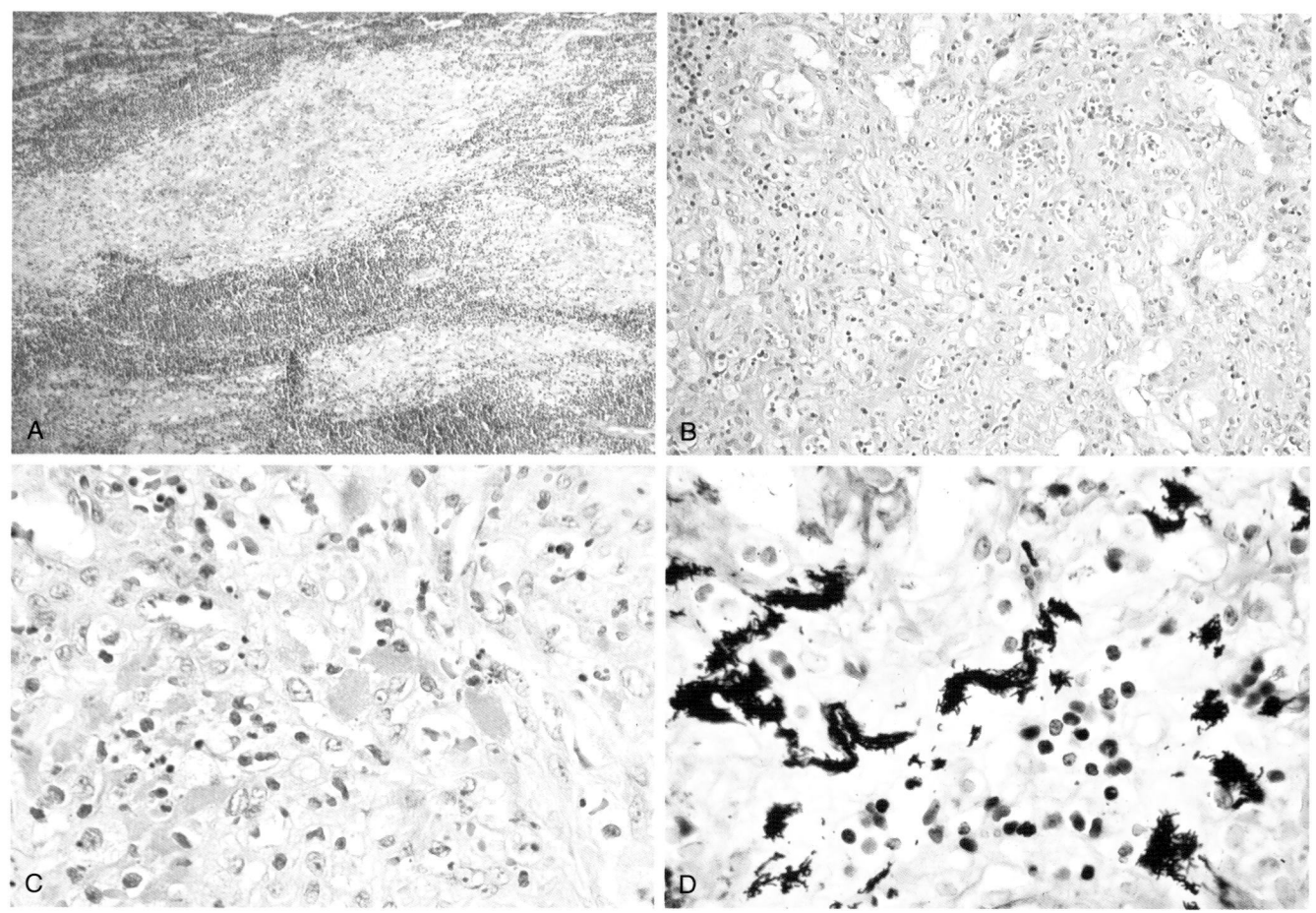

Figure 8-24. Bacillary angiomatosis involving a lymph node. A, Multiple coalescent nodules of proliferated blood vessels (H&E, ×5). **B,** Blood vessels, some barely canalized, lined by plump endothelial cells with pale cytoplasm (H&E, ×140). **C,** Amphophilic material representing tangles of bacteria among endothelial cells (H&E, ×250). **D,** Tangles of *Bartonella henselae* (Warthin-Starry, ×250).

and young adults, although older adults may also be affected. Clinical features including pharyngitis, fever, cervical lymphadenopathy of short duration, splenomegaly, and laboratory features such as reactive peripheral blood lymphocytes and the presence of heterophile antibody usually lead to a diagnosis without a lymph node biopsy. However, lymph nodes may be biopsied to exclude the diagnosis of lymphoma, and tonsils may be removed for relief of airway obstruction.

The histologic features vary during the course of the disease.[19,120,212-214] Early in the disorder, there is FH often with monocytoid B-cell aggregates and epithelioid histiocytes, resembling toxoplasmic lymphadenitis. Later, expansion of the paracortex predominates. Although the architecture of the lymph node or tonsil may be distorted, it is not totally effaced. There is a polymorphous paracortical infiltrate with a mottled pattern caused by the presence of large immunoblasts in a background of medium-sized and small lymphocytes and plasma cells (Fig. 8-25). There may be atypical immunoblastic cells that are occasionally binucleate and resemble classic Reed-Sternberg cells. In areas, there may be a diffuse proliferation of immunoblasts resembling a large cell lymphoma. However, in contrast to large cell lymphoma, intermediate-sized lymphocytes,

plasma cells, and plasmacytoid cells are present among the immunoblasts, high endothelial venules are often prominent, and single-cell necrosis is common. The sinuses are often distended and filled with monocytoid B cells, small lymphocytes, and immunoblasts.

Immunophenotyping shows both T- and B-cell immunoblasts, with B-cell immunoblasts usually predominating.[215] The immunoblasts, including Reed-Sternberg–like cells, often express CD30, but they are usually CD15 negative (Fig. 8-25).[216] CD8-positive T cells typically outnumber CD4-positive T cells. In situ hybridization for EBER shows numerous positive immunoblasts, plasma cells, and B cells in the paracortex. Monocytoid B cells may also contain EBER.[217,218] LMP-1 protein is also expressed and may be related to p53 accumulation within the cells, because the two proteins appear to colocalize.[219,220] In addition, in acute IM EBNA2 is positive and shows the typical EBV latency III of the acute episode. CD21 staining may reveal an underlying distorted but retained FDC network not readily apparent on hematoxylin and eosin staining.

The most important differential diagnoses are diffuse large B-cell lymphoma, peripheral T-cell lymphoma, and CHL. Morphologic features favoring a benign process include incomplete architectural effacement,

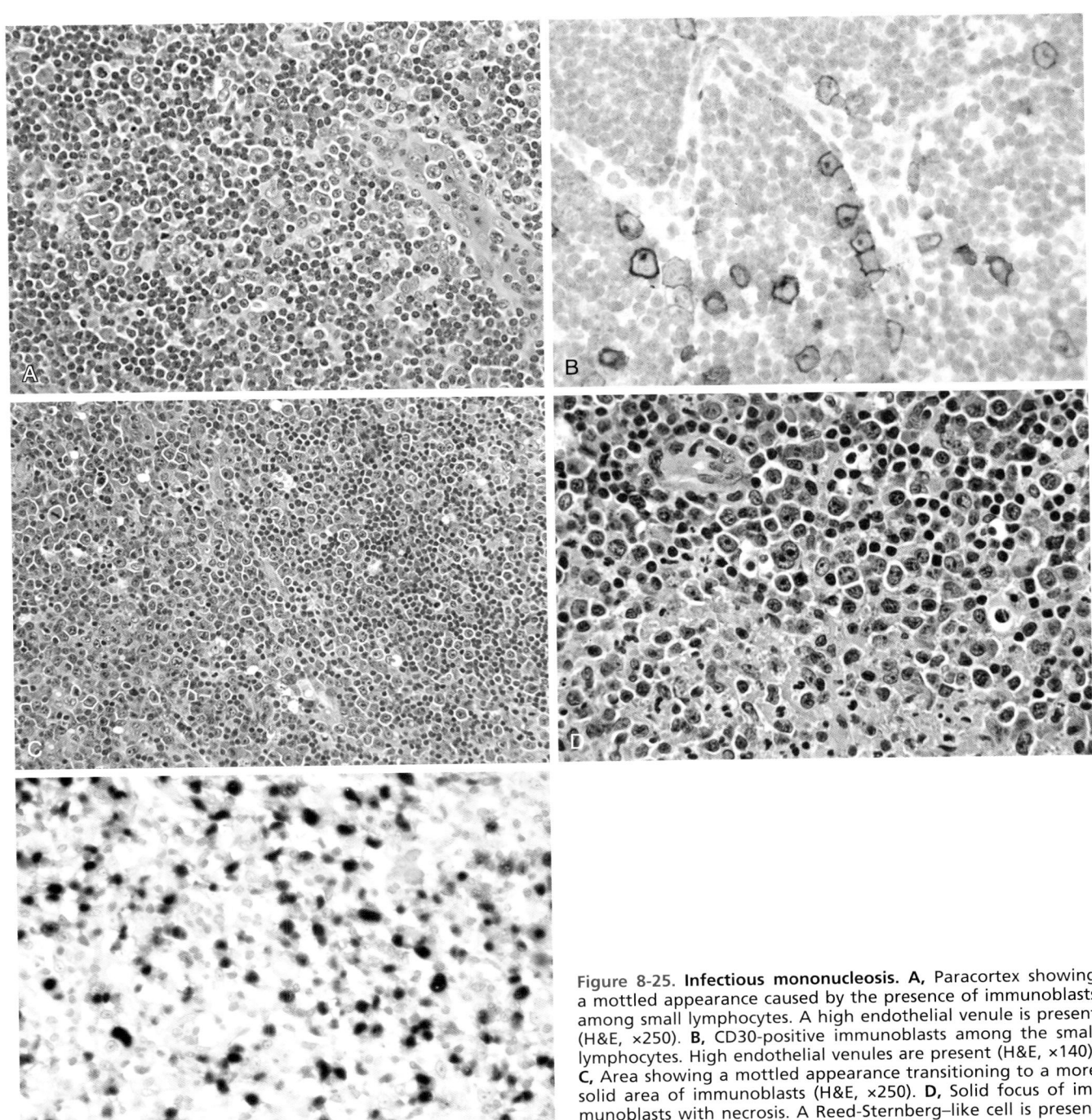

Figure 8-25. **Infectious mononucleosis. A,** Paracortex showing a mottled appearance caused by the presence of immunoblasts among small lymphocytes. A high endothelial venule is present (H&E, ×250). **B,** CD30-positive immunoblasts among the small lymphocytes. High endothelial venules are present (H&E, ×140). **C,** Area showing a mottled appearance transitioning to a more solid area of immunoblasts (H&E, ×250). **D,** Solid focus of immunoblasts with necrosis. A Reed-Sternberg–like cell is present (H&E, ×300). **E,** Epstein-Barr encoded RNA in situ hybridization showing numerous Epstein-Barr virus–infected cells.

a mixed cellular infiltrate, patent lymph node sinuses, and the presence of high endothelial venules among the large cells. The presence of geographic necrosis in the polymorphous infiltrate is another clue to the diagnosis of IM. Immunohistochemical features include the presence of both B- and T-cell immunoblasts, and a predominance of CD8-positive T cells. The presence of classic Reed-Sternberg–like cells may suggest CHL, but these cells lack expression of CD15, mark with either B- or T-cell antibodies, and are usually CD45 positive. In addition,

they are not in the cellular environment of one of the subtypes of CHL. Another difference between CHL and IM is that EBV-positive cells are almost exclusively limited to the RS cells in CHL, whereas they are found in numerous large, activated immunoblasts and in small lymphocytes and plasma cells in IM. Tonsillar location and young patient age should prompt a conservative approach and testing for EBV.

Other viral infections such as CMV and herpes simplex may resemble IM. The presence of characteristic viral inclusions or

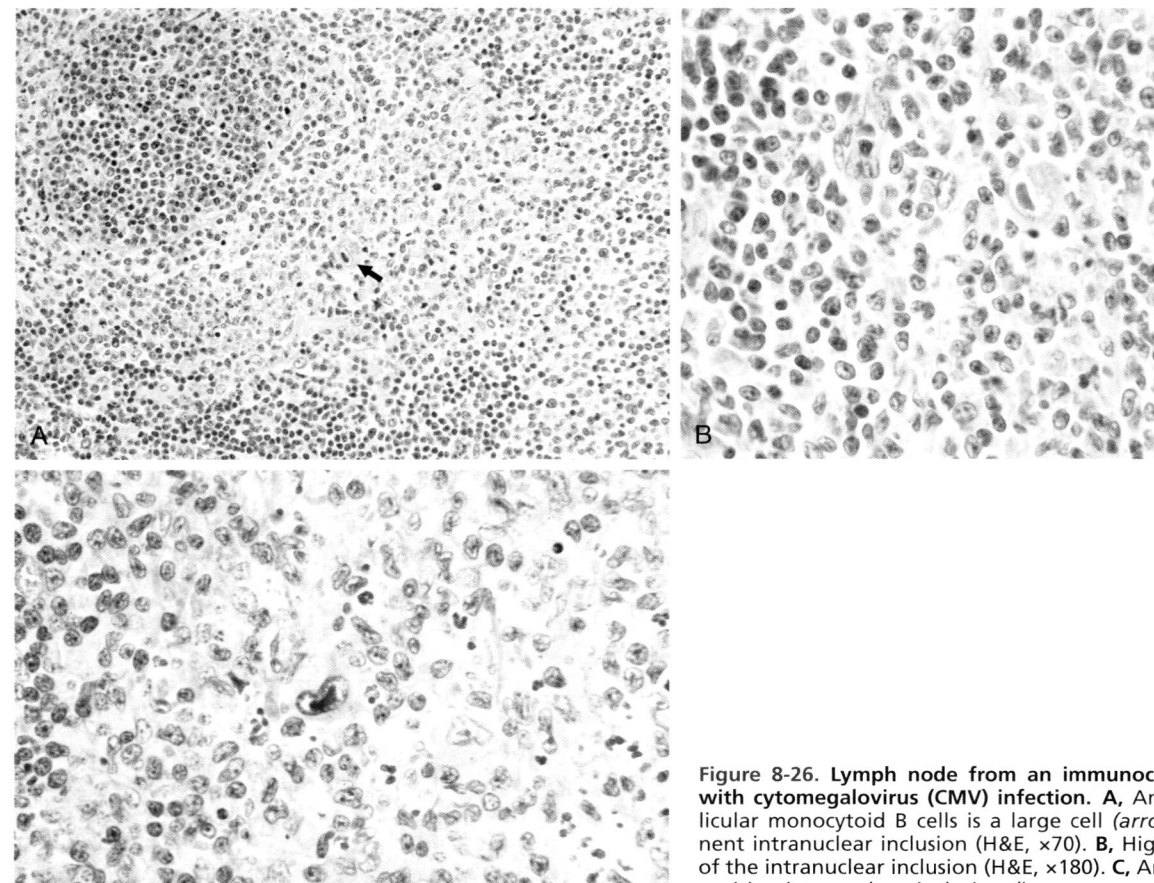

Figure 8-26. **Lymph node from an immunocompetent patient with cytomegalovirus (CMV) infection. A,** Among the parafollicular monocytoid B cells is a large cell *(arrow)* with a prominent intranuclear inclusion (H&E, ×70). **B,** Higher magnification of the intranuclear inclusion (H&E, ×180). **C,** Anti-CMV antibody-positive intranuclear inclusion (immunoperoxidase [anti-CMV], ×500).

the demonstration of viral proteins by immunohistochemistry aids in distinction from IM.

Cytomegalovirus Infection

CMV infection may resemble the clinical picture of IM, but the heterophile antibody test is negative.[221] The infection affects both immunosuppressed and immunocompetent individuals. Lymph nodes show follicular or paracortical hyperplasia with scattered immunoblasts, which may resemble RS cells.[222] A hallmark feature is monocytoid B-cell hyperplasia along sinuses (Fig. 8-26). CMV-infected cells are usually found among the monocytoid B cells. The infected cells contain large acidophilic and intranuclear viral inclusions and multiple small cytoplasmic inclusions. Less frequently, viral inclusions are seen in endothelial cells. In immunocompetent individuals, the inclusions may be sparse, but if present are in T cells (both CD4- and CD8-positive) but not in B cells.[223] They should be diligently searched for in a lymph node biopsy with an unexplained prominent monocytoid B-cell proliferation.

CMV-infected cells may express CD15 in their cytoplasm, but not on their membranes. This phenotype and the presence of large inclusion-bearing cells may cause confusion with CHL.[224] In contrast to CMV-infected cells, classical RS cells express membrane CD15 and cytoplasmic positivity. In addition, the absence of the typical background of CHL

favors CMV lymphadenitis. CMV antigens may be confirmed by immunohistochemistry or by in situ hybridization, both of which are useful, especially in cases without well-developed inclusions.[225]

Herpes Simplex Lymphadenitis

Herpes simplex (Type I or II) produces a lymphadenitis that is most often localized to inguinal lymph nodes but may also be disseminated, and seen predominantly, but not exclusively, in immunocompromised hosts, including patients with chronic lymphocytic leukemia (CLL).[226] When an area of necrosis is found in a lymph node involved by CLL, herpes simplex infection should be ruled out.

The histologic picture varies. There may be FH with expansion of the paracortex by a proliferation of immunoblasts, resembling other viral infections. Monocytoid B cells may be prominent and mimic marginal zone lymphoma.[227] Usually, foci of necrosis are present containing neutrophils and varying numbers of large cells with margination of nuclear chromatin and prominent nuclear inclusions resulting in a ground-glass appearance (Fig. 8-27). Intranuclear eosinophilic inclusions with clear halos have also been reported. Histiocytes often surround necrotic foci, but granulomas are absent.[227] The diagnosis can be confirmed by immunostaining, serology, or in situ hybridization.[228,229]

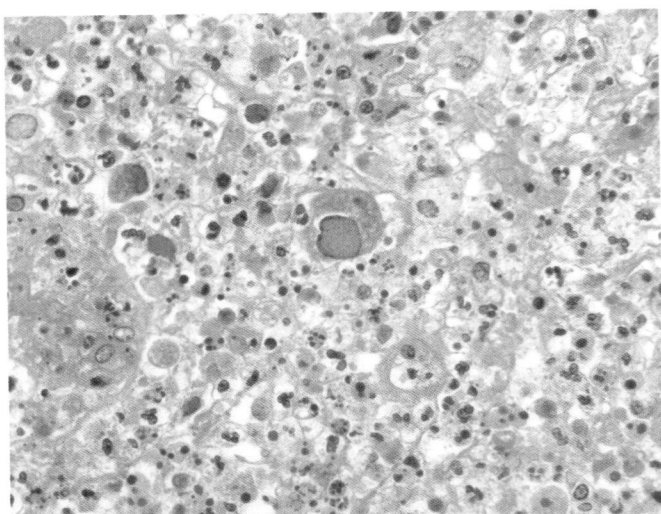

Figure 8-27. Lymph node from a patient with chronic lymphocytic leukemia shows a focus of necrosis containing large cells with margination of nuclear chromatin and a ground-glass nucleus characteristic of herpes simplex infection (H&E, ×625).

Drug-Associated Lymphadenopathy

Lymphadenopathy associated with anticonvulsant therapy (diphenylhydantoin most commonly, less often carbamazepine)[230,231] has been the subject of numerous individual case reports and a few larger series. Since its description a similar pattern has been seen in association with other drugs, including various antibiotics. Rarely, cases of lymphoma have developed in patients using diphenylhydantoin,[232] but a causal role of diphenylhydantoin in the development of lymphoma has not been demonstrated.[233] The syndrome associated with this reaction has been termed drug-induced hypersensitivity syndrome (DIHS) and drug reaction with eosinophilia and systemic symptoms (DRESS). Most patients with suspected DRESS have been on therapy for a prolonged period (median of 2 years), although some

have been treated for less than 6 months. Common symptoms include fever, rash, weight loss, fatigue, organomegaly, and eosinophilia. Lymphadenopathy may be localized or generalized.[233]

The histologic appearance is variable. The most common feature is paracortical expansion by a polymorphous population of immunoblasts, plasma cells, histiocytes, and eosinophils, together with high endothelial venules; Reed-Sternberg–like cells may be found (Fig. 8-28).[35,59] There is variable FH, and some cases show regressed GCs.[233] Immunophenotyping usually shows an intact immunoarchitecture, and many of the immunoblasts are B cells.

The differential diagnosis includes both CHL and non-Hodgkin lymphomas, and viral and autoimmune lymphadenitis. Although the immunoblasts, including Reed-Sternberg–like cells, may express CD30, they are CD15 negative and CD45 positive, which helps exclude a diagnosis of CHL. When immunoblasts predominate, gene rearrangement studies can be useful to assess clonality[234,235]; however, rare cases of anticonvulsant-related lymphadenopathy can be monoclonal. The bone marrow may also be involved, making the diagnosis of a benign condition even more problematic. Viral-induced lymphadenopathy usually lacks eosinophils in the nodal infiltrate and there is no peripheral blood eosinophilia. The clinical history is essential to making this diagnosis. Cessation of the drug should result in resolution of the lymphadenopathy within several weeks.[62,236]

Pearls and Pitfalls

- Knowledge of the spectrum of reactive changes that occur in lymph nodes is essential for accurate diagnosis of both benign and malignant entities.
- A pattern-based approach to reactive lymphadenopathy provides a framework for establishing a differential diagnosis, ancillary study selection, and guiding clinical management.
- Clonality studies and immunohistochemical stains should be used with caution and interpreted in the context of morphologic findings to avoid overdiagnosis of malignancy.

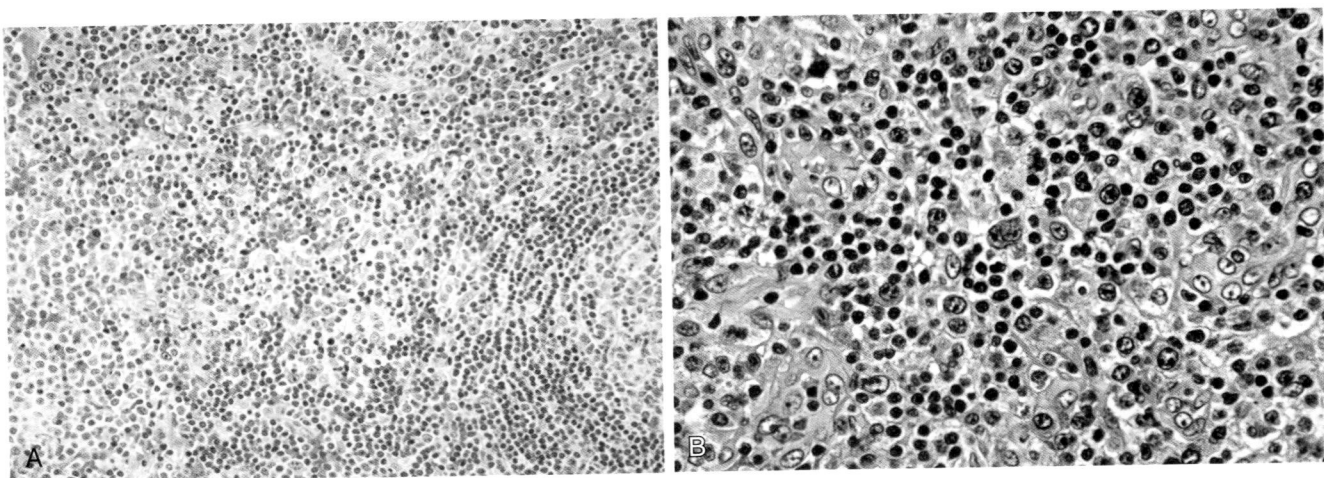

Figure 8-28. Lymph node from a patient taking Dilantin for epilepsy. A, The interfollicular area is expanded by a polymorphous infiltrate. A portion of a follicle is present on the right (H&E, ×40). **B,** Interfollicular area containing lymphocytes, immunoblasts, histiocytes, eosinophils, and high endothelial venules. A Reed-Sternberg–like cell is present (H&E, ×330).

KEY REFERENCES

2. Mesin L, Ersching J, Victora GD. Germinal center B cell dynamics. *Immunity*. 2016;45(3):471–482.
3. Gars E, Butzmann A, Ohgami R, Balakrishna JP, O'Malley DP. The life and death of the germinal center. *Ann Diagn Pathol*. 2020;44:151421.
15. Horna P, Olteanu H, Kroft SH, Harrington AM. Flow cytometric analysis of surface light chain expression patterns in B-cell lymphomas using monoclonal and polyclonal antibodies. *Am J Clin Pathol*. 2011;136(6):954–959.
16. Zhao XF, Cherian S, Sargent R, et al. Expanded populations of surface membrane immunoglobulin light chain-negative B cells in lymph nodes are not always indicative of B-cell lymphoma. *Am J Clin Pathol*. 2005;124(1):143–150.
32. McCurley TL, Collins RD, Ball E, Collins RD. Nodal and extranodal lymphoproliferative disorders in Sjogren's syndrome: a clinical and immunopathologic study. *Hum Pathol*. 1990;21(5):482–492.
47. Cronin DM, Warnke RA. Castleman disease: an update on classification and the spectrum of associated lesions. *Adv Anat Pathol*. 2009;16(4):236–246.
61. Hartmann S, Winkelmann R, Metcalf RA, et al. Immunoarchitectural patterns of progressive transformation of germinal centers with and without nodular lymphocyte-predominant Hodgkin lymphoma. *Hum Pathol*. 2015;46(11):1655–1661.
89. Arnold CA, Moreira RK, Lam-Himlin D, De Petris G, Montgomery E. Whipple disease a century after the initial description: increased recognition of unusual presentations, autoimmune comorbidities, and therapy effects. *Am J Surg Pathol*. 2012;36(7):1066–1073.
160. Deshpande V, Zen Y, Chan JK, et al. Consensus statement on the pathology of IgG4-related disease. *Mod Pathol*. 2012;25(9):1181–1192.
186. Kuo TT. Kikuchi's disease (histiocytic necrotizing lymphadenitis). A clinicopathologic study of 79 cases with an analysis of histologic subtypes, immunohistology, and DNA ploidy. *Am J Surg Pathol*. 1995;19(7):798–809.

Visit Elsevier eBooks+ for the complete set of references.

Chapter 9

The Normal Bone Marrow

Sonam Prakash, Anjanaa Vijayanarayanan, and Laura E. Brown

INTRODUCTION

Meaningful examination and interpretation of a bone marrow specimen requires an adequate and well-prepared sample and knowledge of normal hematopoiesis as well as normal bone marrow composition and architecture. The definition of "adequacy" depends on the clinical indication for the examination. For example, for staging metastatic disease or lymphoma, a bilateral bone marrow core biopsy is superior to a unilateral biopsy[1-3]; thus for this purpose, a bilateral biopsy defines adequacy. In contrast, for the diagnosis of acute leukemia, a unilateral bone marrow aspiration and core biopsy are usually sufficient, in conjunction with appropriate immunophenotyping and genetic studies. This chapter outlines how to collect and process an adequate bone marrow specimen and describes the features of normal bone marrow and hematopoiesis.

MEDICAL INDICATIONS FOR BONE MARROW EXAMINATION

In general, a bone marrow examination is called for when there are hematologic abnormalities that cannot be explained by available clinical and laboratory data. A peripheral blood smear should always be evaluated before deciding whether a bone marrow examination is necessary. Aside from the diagnostic purposes outlined in Table 9-1, staging for metastatic disease and monitoring therapy for antineoplastic effects and/or hematologic toxicity constitute the other two broad indications for bone marrow evaluation.

If the peripheral blood has a sufficient quantity of blasts to meet the diagnostic criteria for acute leukemia and allow other ancillary studies, it has been suggested that a bone marrow examination is superfluous. This approach may save time and money and it is attractive to spare the patient from the discomfort of an invasive procedure. However, subsequent evaluation of postchemotherapy marrow requires knowledge of the preinduction bone marrow landscape and blast proportion.

Comorbid conditions such as coagulopathy, infection close to the proposed biopsy site, or prior radiation to the biopsy site should be carefully assessed before performing a bone marrow biopsy. However, such factors are not necessarily contraindications to biopsy, and the procedure can often be modified to accommodate these circumstances. For example,

Table 9-1 Indications for Bone Marrow Examination

Diagnostic Purposes	Staging for Malignant Disease	Monitoring
• Unexplained cytopenia or cytosis • Diagnosis of hematopoietic and lymphoid neoplasms • Workup of unexplained blasts or other abnormal cells in the blood suggestive of bone marrow pathology • Evaluation of mastocytosis, amyloidosis, and metabolic storage disorders • Workup of monoclonal gammopathy • Workup of fever of unknown origin • Workup of unexplained splenomegaly or other organomegaly	• Staging of lymphoma • Detection of metastatic tumor, in particular small cell tumors of childhood	• Follow-up after induction of chemotherapy for acute leukemia and, less often, before and during consolidation or maintenance chemotherapy • Restaging after treatment for lymphoma • Follow-up after hematopoietic stem cell transplantation • Follow-up in patients with aplastic anemia, Fanconi anemia, paroxysmal nocturnal hemoglobinuria, and other bone marrow failure syndromes to monitor for the possible development of myelodysplastic syndromes

factor replacement or reversal of anticoagulant therapy may be implemented in the case of severe coagulopathy. The sternum may be selected as the marrow aspiration site if infection or radiation to the pelvis is a concern. Of note, thrombocytopenia is a common indication for bone marrow examination and is not usually in itself a contraindication to bone marrow aspiration as long as pressure is meticulously applied for hemostasis afterward. Thus, when bone marrow examination is truly justified, the aspiration and biopsy can usually be accomplished safely.

COMPONENTS OF A BONE MARROW EVALUATION

A thorough bone marrow examination includes both marrow aspiration and trephine biopsy. A bone marrow aspirate is required for accurate blast enumeration, differential count, and evaluation of dysplasia, as well as for ancillary studies including flow cytometric immunophenotyping and cytogenetic/molecular genetic studies. A trephine biopsy is required for the assessment of cellularity, architecture of the marrow, fibrosis, and stromal changes, as well as for immunohistochemical studies. For focal processes involving the marrow, such as metastatic tumors, both aspirate smears and trephine biopsies should be evaluated. In a study of more than 4000 diagnostic bone marrow specimens over a 10-year period, approximately 30% of carcinomas would have been missed if only the aspirate had been examined. Conversely, in 9% of bone marrow specimens positive for metastatic carcinoma, the diagnosis was made on the aspirate alone.[1] The benefit of examining both the marrow aspirate and core biopsy also applies to the diagnosis of less focal processes, particularly during follow-up. For example, Barekman and colleagues[1] reported positive findings in the biopsy but not in the aspirate in 20 of 576 marrow specimens obtained as follow-up for acute leukemia. Occasionally, despite a marrow "packed" with leukemic blasts at diagnosis, the aspirate may be sparsely cellular and diagnosis and phenotypic characterization rest on the trephine biopsy. Taken together, these data justify the collection of both marrow aspiration and core biopsy. In general, a bilateral biopsy is recommended to detect marrow involvement by lymphoma, metastatic tumor, or other focal infiltrative processes. Bilateral aspiration may also be considered, especially for staging small cell tumors of childhood.

In addition to obtaining aspirate and trephine biopsy samples for morphologic examination, consideration should be given to procuring sufficient samples for ancillary studies necessary for accurate diagnosis or prognosis. Diagnosing hematopoietic disorders requires a multiparametric approach that includes morphology, immunophenotype, genetic features, and clinical features.[4,5] In general, if the differential diagnosis includes a malignancy, aspirate samples should be obtained for flow cytometric immunophenotyping, cytogenetic, and molecular genetic analyses. Samples for bacterial, mycobacterial, fungal, or viral cultures should be collected if an infectious process is suspected. Consideration should be given to selecting the anticoagulant that is best suited to performance of these various studies.

COLLECTION OF BONE MARROW ASPIRATE AND CORE BIOPSY

Anatomic Sites

In both adults and children, the posterior superior iliac crest is preferred because of its relative distance from other vital structures and its relatively large surface area, which allows the maneuvering of biopsy and aspiration needles. An alternative site in adults is the sternum, but only marrow aspiration can be performed at this location; core biopsies cannot be performed at the sternum. Sites within previous fields of radiation should be avoided as radiation-induced hypocellularity may persist for years.

Collection Procedures

Whether trephine biopsy or aspirate should be performed first is a matter of debate; however, each sample should be obtained through a separate bone puncture 0.5 to 1 cm away from each other and with a separate and appropriate needle to minimize morphologic distortion from hemorrhage.[6,7] Detailed instructions on how to perform the bone marrow core biopsy and aspiration are beyond the scope of this chapter. Importantly, informed patient consent must be obtained after a careful discussion of the risks and benefits. The following discussion focuses on aspects of the procedure that are relevant to the handling of specimens.

General Approach

Because sterile techniques minimize infectious complications, it is helpful to work with a trained medical technician or technologist who can assist with the handling. Once the

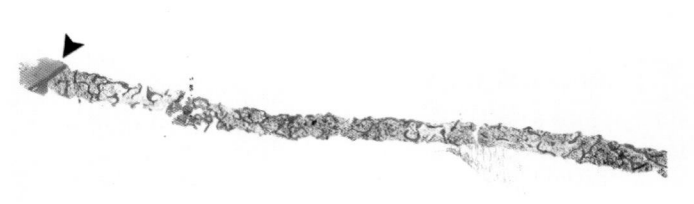

Figure 9-1. An example of an excellent core biopsy (>1 cm long) consisting of mostly marrow, with very little cortical bone or periosteal soft tissue *(arrowhead)*, and with minimal crush artifact or hemorrhage.

procedure begins, it is important to proceed quickly and efficiently to minimize patient discomfort and the clotting of specimens. It is important to plan for the number of core biopsies needed, aspirate volumes, and types of anticoagulants necessary for all required laboratory testing, and, because each successive aspirate becomes more hemodiluted, the sequence in which the various aspirate samples are to be obtained. It is generally recommended that the first aspirate be reserved for morphology.[8] Samples obtained for morphology should ideally be collected without anticoagulant, but if smears for examination cannot be prepared immediately, the aspirated marrow can be placed in ethylenediaminetetraacetic acid (EDTA), with the caution that prolonged exposure to EDTA beyond 2 hours can cause morphologic distortion.[7] Heparin should be avoided, as it may also induce morphologic abnormalities. Specimens for flow cytometric immunophenotyping may be collected in EDTA, or alternatively in sodium heparin or acid citrate dextrose. DNA- and RNA-based molecular assays typically require collection in EDTA, while preservative-free heparin is preferred for cytogenetic studies (karyotype and fluorescence in situ hybridization [FISH]). It is important that the individual performing the aspiration and core biopsy procedure be familiar with the specimen requirements of each specialty laboratory so that the correct anticoagulants are used.

Bone Marrow Trephine Biopsy Procedure and Touch Imprints

Several versions of the Jamshidi biopsy needle are available for procuring the core biopsy. Most adult patients require a 4-inch, 11-gauge needle. When patients are osteopenic, a larger bore needle (8-gauge) allows the collection of an intact core biopsy while minimizing crush artifact. For pediatric patients, a 2- or 4-inch 13-gauge biopsy needle is sufficient. Sola and associates[9] described a bone marrow biopsy technique for neonates in which a 1/2-inch, 19-gauge Osgood needle is used, but in practice, neonatal bone marrow collection is limited to aspiration in some centers. Various powered devices for accessing the bone marrow and procuring core biopsies have become increasingly popular because of a reduction in patient-perceived pain, longer core biopsies, and decreased procedure time.[10]

With the exception of young pediatric patients, an adequate core biopsy prior to fixation should be at least 1.6 cm to 2.0 cm long exclusive of cortical bone, periosteum, and cartilage, and should be free of crush artifact or fragmentation (Fig. 9-1).[5] Some studies have suggested that the number of intertrabecular 40× areas of evaluable marrow might be a better predictor of adequacy than core biopsy length.[11] In a study of 470 core biopsies, O'Neill et al. demonstrated that cores with ≥5.5 intertrabecular areas were contributory to diagnosis.[11] Grossly, cores of marrow have a finely mottled, deep red color and a gritty texture. When the marrow is severely hypoplastic the core may appear pale yellow but should still have a gritty surface. Marrow completely replaced by leukemia, lymphoma, or other neoplasms may appear white. Cortical bone, in contrast, often has an ivory color with a hard, smooth surface, and cartilage is gray-white and glistening, characteristics that should prompt the operator to make another attempt. If an adequate aspirate cannot be obtained, collection of multiple core biopsies may be considered to increase the amount of material available for ancillary studies, particularly in cases of suspected hematopoietic neoplasm that do not significantly involve the peripheral blood.

Touch preparations are a valuable adjunct to morphologic examination of the bone marrow aspirate and are particularly valuable if an adequate bone marrow aspirate cannot be obtained. There are several ways to prepare touch imprints. First, the core can be gently blotted to remove adherent blood. Several clean glass slides are then touched gently to the marrow core. One can also touch the cores to the glass slides. Alternatively, the core is gently rolled between two glass slides, which may yield more cells but carries a higher risk of fragmentation of the core and crush artifact. Once touch imprints have been prepared, the core biopsy should be immediately placed in fixative.

Bone Marrow Aspiration Procedure

For collection of the bone marrow aspirate, although the needle is advanced through the same skin incision used for the biopsy, the site of bone puncture should be separate from the site of the trephine biopsy, preferably 0.5 to 1.0 cm away. This minimizes the risk of obtaining an aspirate composed only of clotted blood, as well as the risk of core biopsy distortion by hemorrhage. Because each successive aspiration becomes more hemodiluted, a rapid and forceful aspiration of 0.5 to 1.0 mL should be obtained first for morphologic examination. Additional aspirations can be obtained, in sequence, for flow cytometry followed by cytogenetics, molecular diagnostic evaluation, and culture, as applicable. The needle used to collect the samples for morphologic examination should be free of anticoagulant, whereas the syringes used for other studies should be coated in the appropriate anticoagulant. Undiluted bone marrow aspirate is deep red in color and slightly thicker than blood, and flecks of marrow spicules may be visible.

PROCESSING OF MARROW TREPHINE BIOPSY AND ASPIRATE

Trephine Biopsy

The following discussion applies to paraffin embedding only.

Fixation

Accurate microscopic evaluation of the bone marrow core biopsy can direct the appropriate selection of ancillary immunohistochemistry and other special studies or may even obviate their need (Fig. 9-2). It is important to recognize the essential role of the core biopsy for immunophenotypic characterization of myeloid and lymphoid neoplasms when the aspiration yields a dry tap, or the aspirate is hemodiluted. Optimal fixation of the core biopsy for preservation of morphologic detail and preservation of tissue for subsequent immunohistochemical studies is essential.

Mercury-based fixatives such as Zenker's and B5 solutions were previously used as they provided excellent cytologic detail. However, they are now unavailable in many countries because of their mercuric chloride content.[12] In laboratories where bone marrow trephine biopsies are processed along with other surgical specimens, neutral buffered formalin is often used. Excellent morphologic detail can be achieved with this fixative,[13] but care should be taken to ensure adequate fixation time relative to the diameter of the biopsy. Zinc acid

formalin also provides excellent morphologic detail and has a somewhat shorter fixation time. Core biopsies should be placed in 10 to 20 mL of fixative. The recommended fixation time for neutral buffered formalin is 8 to 72 hours[12] and for zinc formalin, at least 2 hours but ideally overnight to 72 hours.[12]

Decalcification

After fixation, the core biopsy is removed from the fixative, rinsed with several changes of water, and then decalcified. Several types of decalcification solutions exist, which vary in their decalcification times and degree of preservation of antigenic epitopes and nucleic acids. While hydrochloric-acid based decalcification solutions offer the most rapid decalcification, they are also the least likely to preserve nucleic acids, although antigenic epitopes for immunohistochemistry are generally retrievable. EDTA-based formulas offer the best preservation of nucleic acids for molecular studies and FISH, but the long decalcification time required may result in longer turnaround times for core biopsies. Formic acid–based solutions occupy a middle ground, offering both a moderate degree of nucleic acid preservation as well as a reasonably short decalcification time.[12,14] Some laboratories may prefer to use rapid decalcification for most routine cases in which sufficient fresh aspirate is available for ancillary testing, reserving the use of solutions with longer turnaround time for those specimens with limited alternative material for special studies (e.g., dry tap). Following decalcification, the biopsy should again be washed in several changes of water before being placed in neutral buffered formalin for processing in an automated tissue processor.

Sectioning

Ideally, the paraffin-embedded core biopsies should be sectioned in thicknesses of 3 μm and preferably no more than 4 μm. The importance of adequate sampling cannot be overemphasized, especially if marrow involvement by a focal process such as metastatic disease is a consideration. Statistical modeling has shown that false-negative rates for

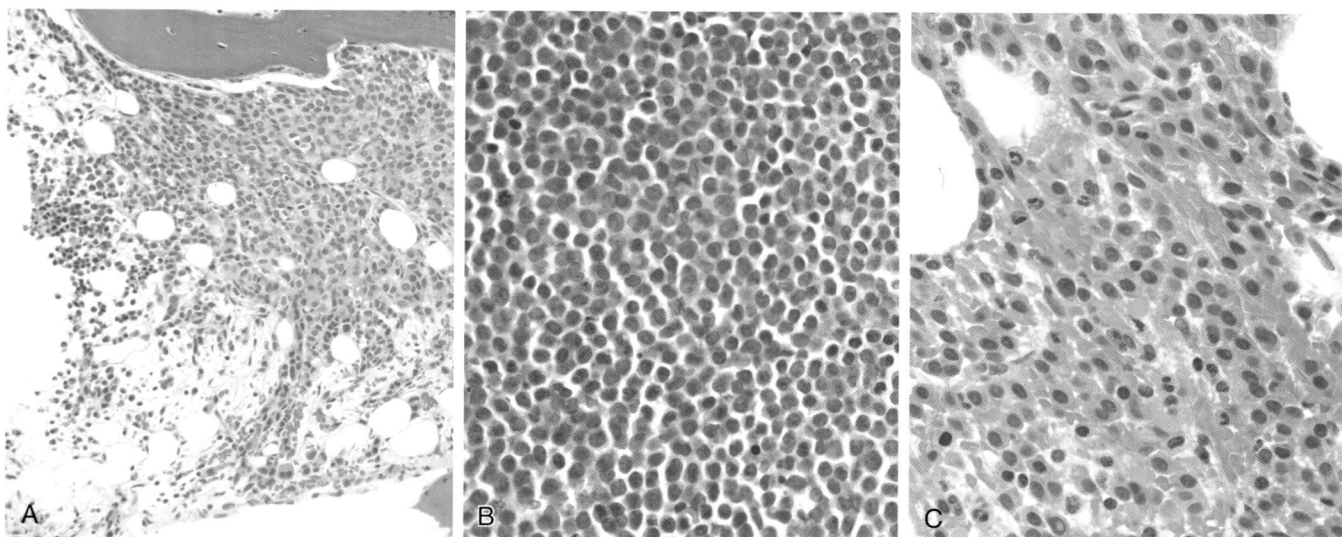

Figure 9-2. Hematoxylin-eosin–stained trephine sections of bone marrow specimens. A, Metastatic carcinoma involving bone marrow. **B,** Acute myeloid leukemia. **C,** Marrow infiltration by plasma cells in a patient with a plasma cell neoplasm.

the detection of metastatic tumor in bone marrow biopsies is inversely proportional to the number of sections examined.[15] While the appropriate number of sections to be prepared also depends on several factors, including laboratory resources and the types of diseases likely to be encountered, at a minimum, several step sections should be mounted for microscopic examination.

Staining

If the core biopsy has been well-fixed, decalcified, processed, and sectioned, routine hematoxylin-eosin staining provides excellent histologic detail. Depending on the individual laboratory and patient population, other stains may be routinely performed. Periodic acid–Schiff (PAS) stains provide a means of evaluating morphology and simultaneously visualizing fungal organisms and may be helpful in institutions with large populations of immunocompromised patients. In cases of myeloproliferative neoplasms, assessment of marrow fibrosis is best done with a silver impregnation stain for reticulin; the normal presence of reticulin fibers around arterioles serves as an internal positive control (Fig. 9-3). Collagenous fibrosis is uncommon in the bone marrow and should be looked for on a case-by-case basis. Giemsa stain can be helpful in highlighting mast cells and plasma cells and in distinguishing myeloblasts from proerythroblasts. There is a high false-negative rate with iron stains of decalcified core biopsy sections, caused by chelation of iron during decalcification[16]; therefore routine iron staining of the core biopsy is not recommended.

Bone Marrow Aspirate

From the 0.5 to 1.0 mL of fluid marrow aspirate obtained for morphologic examination, several preparations can be made that allow the maximal use of all components of the sample: direct smears, particle crush preparations, and particle clot sections. Buffy coat smears are labor intensive and may not

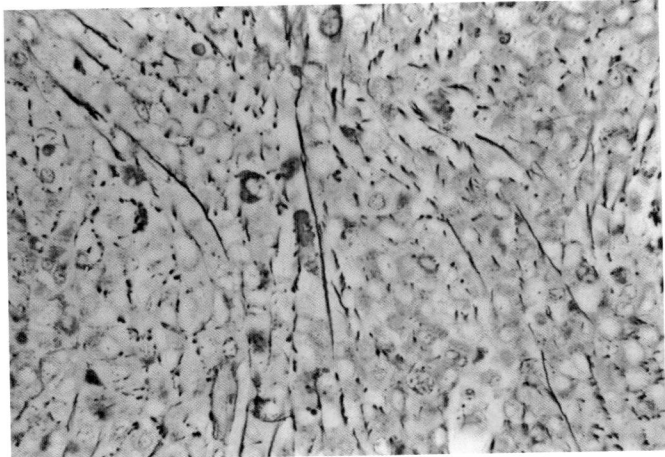

Figure 9-3. Reticulin stain of the bone marrow core section of a patient with chronic myeloid leukemia showing increased reticulin fibers *(brown-black lines)* within the marrow interstitium, away from the expected normal perivascular location *(Wilder reticulin stain).*

add much to the morphologic evaluation; therefore they are not commonly performed.[17]

Direct Smears

As soon as possible, after the 0.5 to 1.0 mL of the first non-anticoagulated fluid marrow is aspirated, most of it is transferred to an EDTA-containing tube. The tube should be inverted several times to ensure adequate mixing. This anticoagulated tube can be used for preparation of additional aspirate smears for morphology and other studies such as iron stains and cytochemistry; if applicable it can also be used to prepare buffy coat smears.

From the remaining non-anticoagulated fluid, individual drops of marrow are quickly placed directly on 6 to 10 glass slides, and a spreader device is used to create aspirate smears. These smears are dried quickly for the preservation of cytologic detail.

Particle Crush Preparation

For particle crush preparation, contents of the EDTA-anticoagulated tubes are placed in a clean Petri dish. Marrow spicules should be picked up, placed on three to four clean glass slides, and gently squashed by placing another glass slide on top and pulling the two slides apart in opposite but parallel directions.

Particle Clot Sections

Any marrow spicules that remain in the Petri dish are rinsed with 0.015 M calcium chloride and pushed close together to form a clot. These particle clots are processed similarly to the core biopsy, but without decalcification. Alternatively, all remaining marrow spicules and fluid can be mixed and dispersed in formalin, filtered, and embedded as a cytoblock. Since marrow clots or cytoblocks are not decalcified, in addition to providing morphologic information, they are also suitable for FISH or molecular studies and can serve as archival material for such studies.

Relative Utility of Different Marrow Aspirate Preparations

Not all these aspirate preparations are necessary for every case, and their contribution to the bone marrow examination sometimes overlaps. On one hand, the direct smears provide excellent cytologic detail with minimal distortion by anticoagulation or centrifugation. On the other hand, examination of a hypocellular specimen can be tedious, and the cell distribution may be uneven. The particle crush preparation bears the closest resemblance to marrow tissue in vivo and allows an approximation of cells' spatial relationship, but also results in more damaged nuclei.

Table 9-2 summarizes the different components of a bone marrow examination and the various types of stains and studies applicable to the specific preparations.

Finally, when staining marrow touch imprints and aspirate preparations for routine morphologic examination, the laboratory should save several unstained preparations for potential additional but unforeseen studies that may arise during the course of the diagnostic evaluation, such as esterase or myeloperoxidase cytochemistry. Molecular testing can also often be successfully carried out using DNA extracted from scrapings of unstained aspirate smears.

Dry Tap

Approximately 2% to 7% of attempts at marrow aspiration yield no fluid, resulting in the so-called "dry tap."[18] In a review of over 1000 bone marrow aspirations and biopsies, Humphries found that faulty technique accounted for just 6.9% of dry taps.[18] Common reasons for dry tap include underlying bone marrow damage or diseases such as aplastic anemia, hairy cell leukemia, advanced-stage myeloproliferative neoplasms, acute megakaryoblastic leukemia, mastocytosis, or acute leukemia, among others. In these circumstances, one should ensure that sufficient touch imprints are made for cytologic examination, and if feasible, additional core biopsies should be obtained for special studies such as cytogenetics, flow cytometry immunophenotyping, and molecular genetics.

Table 9-2 Components of a Bone Marrow Examination and Applicable Stains and Studies

Examination Component	Stain and Method of Analysis
Bone marrow trephine biopsy	H&E Reticulin PAS Immunohistochemistry When freshly collected and prior to fixation, can also be used for cytogenetics, flow cytometry immunophenotyping analysis, molecular diagnostics, and cultures in case of a "dry tap"
Marrow touch imprint	Wright-Giemsa Cytochemistry If unfixed and unstained, can be scraped for DNA extraction for molecular diagnostics
Bone marrow aspirate fluid	Flow cytometry immunophenotyping analysis Cytogenetics Molecular diagnostics Cultures
Bone marrow aspirate smear	Wright-Giemsa Cytochemistry Prussian blue If unfixed and unstained, can be scraped for DNA extraction for molecular diagnostics
Particle clot section	H&E PAS Immunohistochemistry In situ hybridization (FISH or CISH) Prussian blue Molecular diagnostic studies

H&E, Hematoxylin and eosin; *PAS,* periodic acid–Schiff.

Staining of Bone Marrow Aspirate Smears

Wright-Giemsa Stain

The importance of a well-stained marrow aspirate smear cannot be overemphasized (Figs. 9-4 and 9-5). A poorly stained aspirate smear can mislead and frustrate. For air-dried marrow touch imprints and aspirate preparations, a Romanowski-type stain such as Wright-Giemsa or May-Grünwald-Giemsa is often used for morphologic evaluation. With either staining method, for optimal results, slides should be stained within 24 hours of preparation. Slides previously poorly stained with Wright-Giemsa can sometimes be salvaged by restaining within 1 to 2 months from the time of collection.

Iron Stains

For the assessment of storage iron, a Prussian blue stain can be performed on any marrow aspirate preparations with identifiable macrophages (see Fig. 9-6A). It is essential that adequate marrow particles be examined to avoid a false-negative interpretation. Although stainable iron may be found in a single particle, it is recommended that a minimum of seven particles be examined to accurately establish the absence of storage iron.[19] A grading system for iron assessed on bone marrow aspirate smears was proposed by Gale et al. (Table 9-3).[20] If necessary, an iron stain can be performed on the particle clot sections (Fig. 9-6B). The interpretation of iron stores on decalcified core biopsy sections should be undertaken with caution because the absence of storage iron

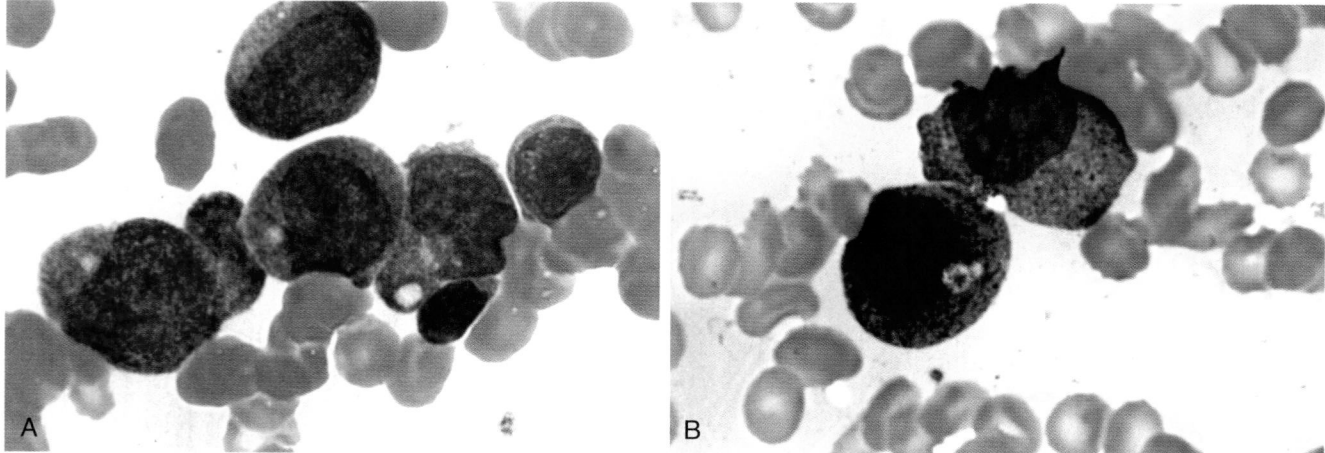

Figure 9-4. Wright-Giemsa–stained bone marrow aspirate smears of agranulocytosis in a patient who presented with profound neutropenia. A, The original stained smear shows a hypocellular specimen with a relative preponderance of early myeloid precursors, raising the differential diagnosis of blasts versus neutrophilic promyelocytes. **B,** Restaining of the smear with Wright-Giemsa shows the presence of azurophilic granules within the precursors, indicative of neutrophilic promyelocytes. Cytogenetic analysis subsequently revealed a normal karyotype. The neutrophil count recovered within 1 week.

in these specimens may be artifactual rather than true iron depletion.[16] Smears previously stained with Wright stain can be superimposed with Prussian blue reagent to assess storage iron and sideroblastic iron.

BONE MARROW EVALUATION

Hematopoiesis

Adequate evaluation of the bone marrow requires a basic understanding of normal hematopoiesis and normal bone marrow composition and architecture.

Although hematopoietic stem cells circulate in small numbers, hematopoiesis, in steady-state conditions in adult life, is largely confined to the bone marrow. All hematopoietic cells are ultimately derived from pluripotent hematopoietic stem cells, which give rise to common lymphoid stem cells and multipotent myeloid stem cells.[21] The multipotent myeloid stem cells in turn give rise to lineage-committed progenitors. None of the stem cells or progenitor cells are morphologically distinguishable from one another, but some can be putatively identified clinically on the basis of immunophenotyping by flow cytometry or other methods. Stem cells in the marrow are located in stem cell "niches" adjacent to either bone or blood vessels, where they maintain a close relationship with stromal cells. With the exception of a subset of platelets derived from megakaryocytes lodged in the lungs, all mature blood cells in healthy adults are produced in the bone marrow (Fig. 9-7).

Bone marrow hematopoiesis occurs in a specific microenvironment: in the intertrabecular spaces occupied by stroma and hematopoietic cells and surrounded by bony trabeculae. The stroma is composed of stromal cells and a

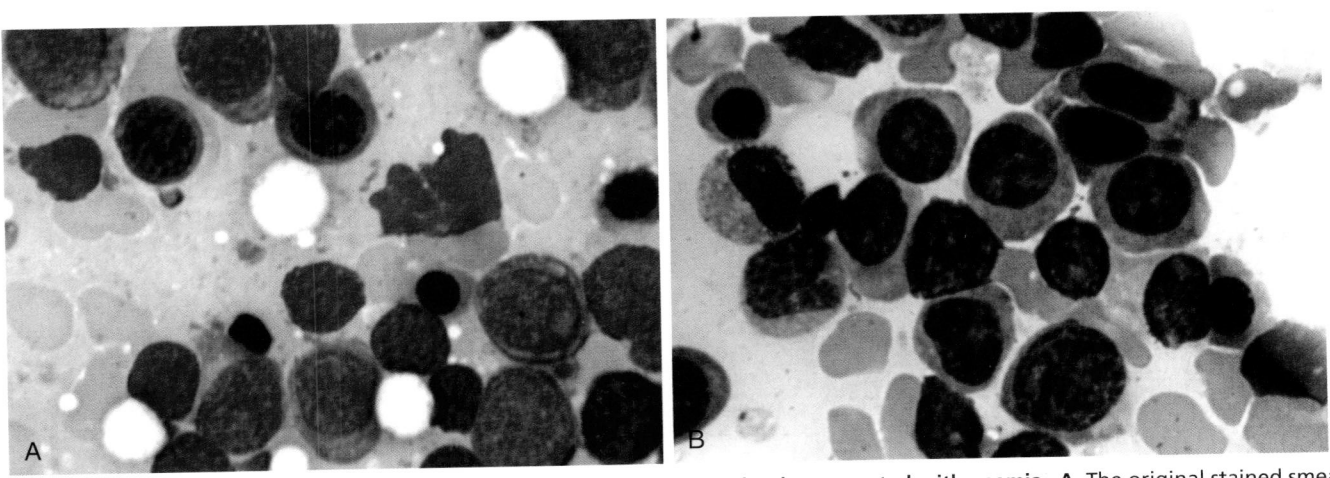

Figure 9-5. Wright-Giemsa–stained bone marrow aspirate smears of an adult who presented with anemia. A, The original stained smear shows an increased proportion of abnormal cells with overlapping features between plasma cells and basophilic normoblasts. Several polychromatophilic erythroblasts are also present. **B,** Restaining of the smear with Wright-Giemsa confirms the presence of abnormal plasma cells. Subsequent immunohistochemical studies of the core biopsy showed kappa-restricted plasma cell myeloma.

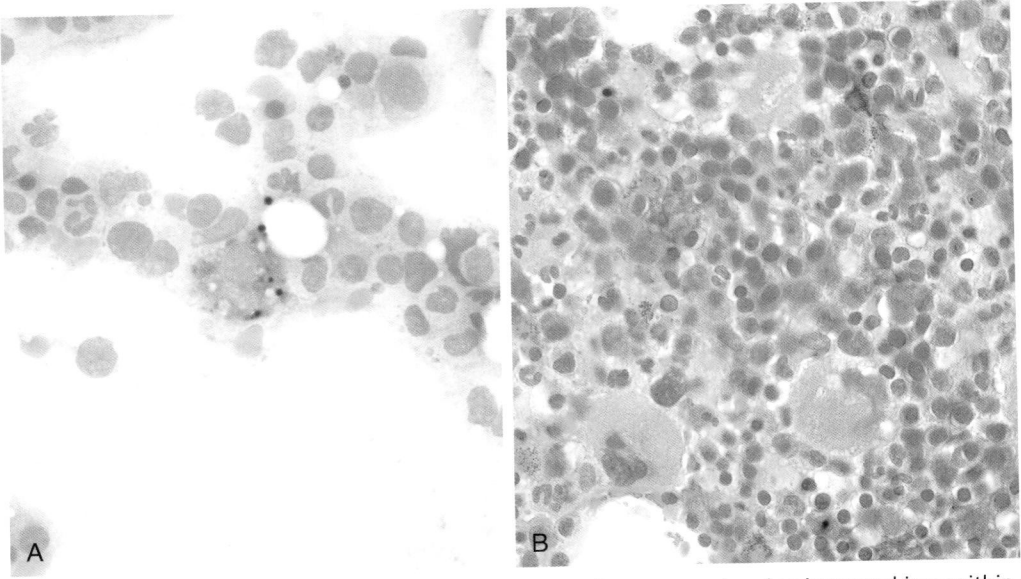

Figure 9-6. Iron stains of bone marrow. A, Perls stain of a bone marrow aspirate smear showing increased iron within a macrophage. **B,** Prussian blue reaction of a clot section.

Table 9-3 Grading of Iron in Bone Marrow Aspirate Smears

Grade	Description
0	No visible iron under oil immersion
1 +	Small iron particles just visible in macrophages under oil immersion
2 +	Small, sparsely distributed iron particles usually visible under low power magnification
3 +	Numerous small particles present in macrophages throughout the marrow particles
4 +	Larger particles throughout the marrow, with tendency to aggregate into clumps
5 +	Dense large clumps of iron throughout the marrow
6 +	Very large deposits of iron, both intracellular and extracellular, which obscure cellular detail in the marrow particles

Modified from Gale E, Torrance J, Bothwell T. The quantitative estimation of total iron stores in human bone marrow. *J Clin Invest*. 1963;42(7):1076-1082.

matrix of proteins such as laminin, thrombospondin, and fibronectin. Recognizable stromal elements and cells include blood vessels, nerves, adipocytes, other mesenchymal cells (e.g. reticular cells, macrophages, fibroblasts), and a delicate fiber network. The earliest recognizable granulocyte precursors—myeloblasts and promyelocytes—are located abutting the endosteum and surrounding arterioles. Myelocytes, metamyelocytes, and neutrophils are each found progressively farther from the endosteum. In contrast, the distribution of eosinophilic cells is random, and that of basophils is unknown. Maturing erythroid cells are found centrally in the intertrabecular space, forming erythroid islands in which erythroid cells of varying maturity surround a central macrophage. Megakaryocytes are also found centrally in the intertrabecular space, preferentially adjacent to sinusoids. Other cellular components of the marrow include mast cells, lymphocytes, plasma cells, monocytes, and macrophages. The normal bone marrow architecture is shown diagrammatically in Figure 9-8.

The regulation of hematopoiesis is highly complex, involving the interaction of adhesion molecules on hematopoietic cells with their ligands on stromal cells, and the action of hematopoietic growth factors such as stem cell factor, interleukin (IL)-3, IL-4, IL-5, IL-6, granulocyte-macrophage colony-stimulating factor, granulocyte colony stimulating factor, monocyte colony-stimulating factor, erythropoietin, and thrombopoietin.[22] Growth factors may be secreted locally by bone marrow cells (e.g., granulocyte-macrophage colony-stimulating factor) or they may be secreted at distant sites (e.g., erythropoietin) (Fig. 9-7). The ultimate effects of growth factors on hematopoiesis are mediated by transcription factors, which coordinate the proliferation and differentiation signals that reach the cell and establish the ultimate characteristics and phenotype of the mature cell. Although diagrams of hematopoiesis often suggest a unidirectional differentiation along one lineage, evidence suggests that it may be possible to reprogram cells of one lineage to differentiate into another by altering the expression of various transcription factors.[21] It is unclear, however, whether this takes place in normal hematopoiesis, only under experimental conditions or in pathologic situations.

Bone marrow cellularity in healthy people is dependent on age. The proportion of the marrow cavity occupied by hematopoietic and lymphoid cells rather than adipose cells varies from essentially 100% at birth to between 30% and 65%

after age 80 years. Between ages 30 and 70 years, cellularity is of the order of 40% to 70%. Except at the extremes of age, a rough estimation of expected cellularity can be derived by subtracting a patient's age from 100. An adequate core biopsy is required for the assessment of marrow cellularity. Subcortical bone marrow is normally hypocellular, and therefore, the first three subcortical spaces are usually not considered in the estimation of cellularity. Figure 9-9 shows a bone marrow biopsy section with normal cellularity in comparison with hypocellular and hypercellular bone marrow specimens.

After assessment of bone marrow cellularity, the three main cell lineages—granulocytic, erythroid, and megakaryocytic—should be evaluated and quantified. The normal bone marrow shows a granulocytic:erythroid ratio of 2 to 3:1. Enumeration of cell types and evaluation of cellular details is best performed on the aspirate smears. Evaluation of tissue architecture and cellular distribution is performed on the bone marrow core biopsy.

Erythropoiesis

The morphologic features of erythroid precursors in bone marrow smears and sections are summarized in Table 9-4 and illustrated in Figures 9-10 to 9-14. It must be remembered that cellular maturation is a continuum rather than a discrete, sudden change from one stage to the next. In normal bone marrow, cells of each successive stage of maturation are more numerous than those of the preceding. Erythroid islands may be noted in bone marrow aspirates (Fig. 9-15), but are more readily apparent in trephine biopsy sections, where they are localized to the intertrabecular space, away from the surface of the bone (Fig. 9-16). In trephine biopsy sections, an artifactual halo around round erythroid nuclei can aid in their identification.

Complete assessment of erythropoiesis in aspirate films requires not only a Romanowsky stain (e.g., Wright-Giemsa or May-Grünwald-Giemsa), but also a Perls Prussian blue stain to assess storage iron and determine the presence, number, and distribution of erythroblast siderotic granules. Perls stain identifies hemosiderin, but not ferritin. Normal late erythroblasts and occasional intermediate erythroblasts have a small number of scattered fine hemosiderin granules (Fig. 9-17). A Perls stain on trephine biopsy sections may be informative on plastic-embedded sections to detect abnormal sideroblasts; however, it is less reliable on paraffin-embedded decalcified biopsies as siderotic granules cannot be assessed and storage iron may have been removed by the process of decalcification.

Granulopoiesis

The morphologic features of granulocytic (specifically neutrophil) precursors in bone marrow smears and sections are summarized in Table 9-5 and illustrated in Figures 9-18 to 9-21. Maturing cells of eosinophil and basophil lineage can be recognized morphologically from the myelocyte stage onward in aspirate smears. In trephine biopsy sections, eosinophils, neutrophils, and their precursors can be identified, but cells of basophil lineage cannot be easily recognized because their granules are lost during processing.

Megakaryopoiesis

Three stages of megakaryocyte maturation can be recognized in normal bone marrow. All recognizable normal

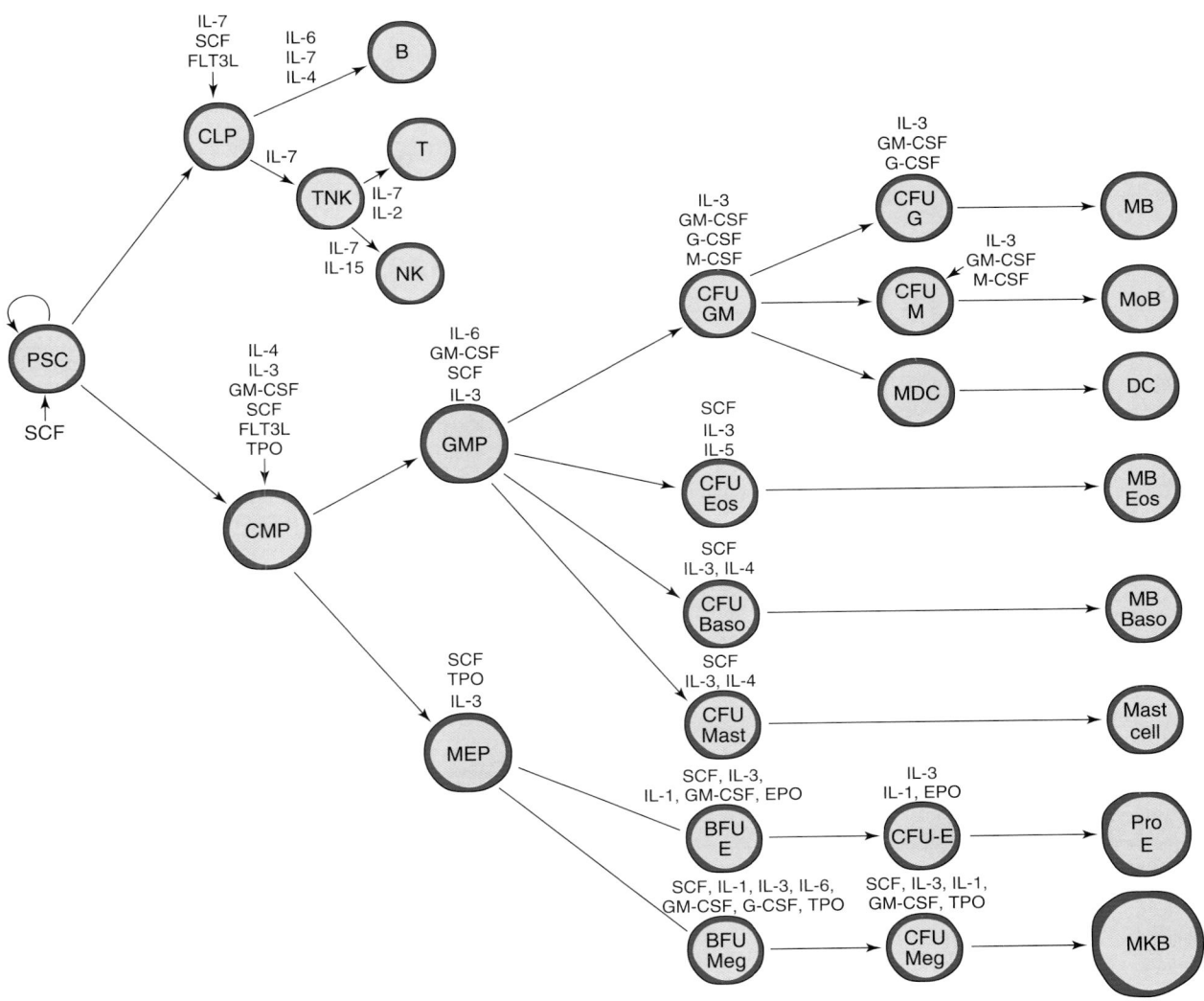

Figure 9-7. Diagrammatic representation of one proposed scheme of the stem cell hierarchy[1] showing the growth factors thought to operate at each stage. Alternative models of hematopoiesis have been proposed,[20,21] including one in which the common erythroid and megakaryocytic progenitor arises directly from the pluripotent lymphoid-myeloid stem cell (PSC; also known as the common lymphoid-myeloid progenitor) rather than from the common myeloid progenitor (CMP; also known as *multipotent myeloid stem cells*). *B*, B lymphocyte; *Baso*, basophil; *BFU*, burst-forming unit; *CFU*, colony-forming unit; *CLP*, common lymphoid progenitor; *CMP*, common myeloid progenitor; *DC*, dendritic cell; *E*, erythroid; *Eos*, eosinophil; *EPO*, erythropoietin; *FLT3L*, ligand of FLT3; *G*, granulocyte (neutrophil); *G-CSF*, granulocyte colony-stimulating factor; *GM*, granulocyte-macrophage; *GM-CSF*, granulocyte-macrophage colony-stimulating factor; *GMP*, granulocyte-monocyte progenitor; *IL*, interleukin; *M*, macrophage; *Mast*, mast cell; *MB*, myeloblast; *M-CSF*, monocyte colony-stimulating factor; *MDC*, myeloid dendritic cell; *Meg*, megakaryocyte; *MEP*, myeloid-erythroid progenitor; *MKB*, megakaryoblast; *MoB*, monoblast; *NK*, natural killer; *ProE*, proerythroblast; *PSC*, pluripotent lymphoid-myeloid stem cell; *SCF*, stem cell factor; *T*, T lymphocyte; *TNK*, T/NK cell progenitor; *TPO*, thrombopoietin.

megakaryocytes are large polyploid cells. The smallest immature megakaryocytes measure 30 μm or more in diameter and have a high nuclear-to-cytoplasmic ratio and basophilic cytoplasm, often with cytoplasmic "blebbing." Mature megakaryocytes are large, up to 160 μm in diameter, with a lobulated nucleus and pink or lilac granular cytoplasm (Fig. 9-22); sometimes platelets are apparent, budding from the surface. A late megakaryocyte (Fig. 9-23) is similar in size to an immature megakaryocyte because virtually all the cytoplasm has been shed as platelets, leaving a somewhat pyknotic nucleus with a thin rim of cytoplasm. Caution should be exercised in interpreting cytologic features of megakaryocytes because they are prone to crushing during preparation, which may cause the nucleus to fragment or

be extruded. The cytoplasm of megakaryocytes occasionally may appear to contain intact cells of other lineages; these are actually within the surface-connected canalicular system. This phenomenon is known as *emperipolesis* (Fig. 9-24) and is physiologic but may be exaggerated in various pathologic states. In histologic sections, mature megakaryocytes are readily recognized by their large size, abundant cytoplasm, and lobulated nuclei (Fig. 9-25). They can be highlighted by a Giemsa stain or a PAS stain. Late megakaryocytes are recognized as apparently bare megakaryocytic nuclei, which are larger than the nuclei of bone marrow cells of other lineages. Early megakaryocytes can be more difficult to recognize because they are not much larger than other bone marrow cells and their features are not very distinctive. They

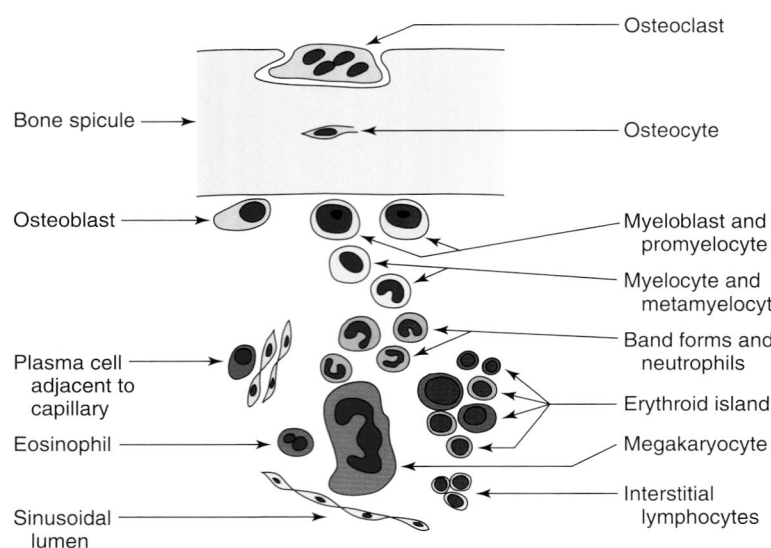

Figure 9-8. Diagrammatic representation of the topography of normal bone marrow. Osteoclasts, osteoblasts, myeloblasts, and promyelocytes are adjacent to the spicule of bone. Deeper in the intertrabecular space are maturing cells of neutrophil lineage, erythroid islands with a central macrophage, and interstitial lymphocytes. Eosinophils and their precursors are apparently randomly scattered, plasma cells are interstitial or form a sheath around capillaries, and megakaryocytes abut a sinusoid at one extremity of the cell.

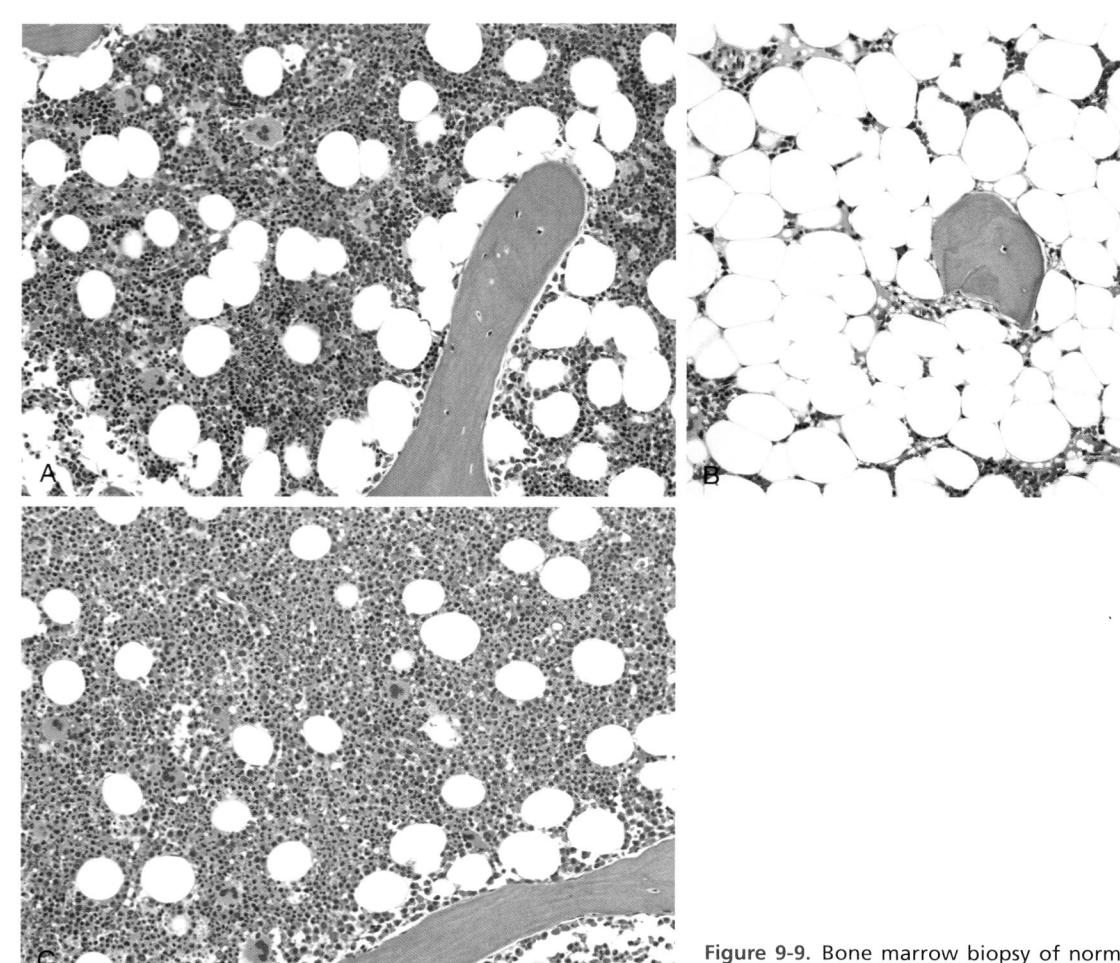

Figure 9-9. Bone marrow biopsy of normal cellularity **(A)** compared with hypocellular **(B)** and hypercellular **(C)** biopsies.

are more readily identified by immunohistochemistry directed to platelet antigens such as CD61 for platelet glycoprotein IIIa (Fig. 9-26) or CD42b for platelet glycoprotein Iba. Care should be taken in interpreting apparent abnormalities of nuclear lobation (e.g., monolobation) in examination of core biopsies, as tissue sectioning often results in an inability to visualize the entirety of a given megakaryocyte.

In the normal marrow, the megakaryocytes are adjacent to sinusoids and are not found in a paratrabecular localization. Determining whether the number of megakaryocytes present

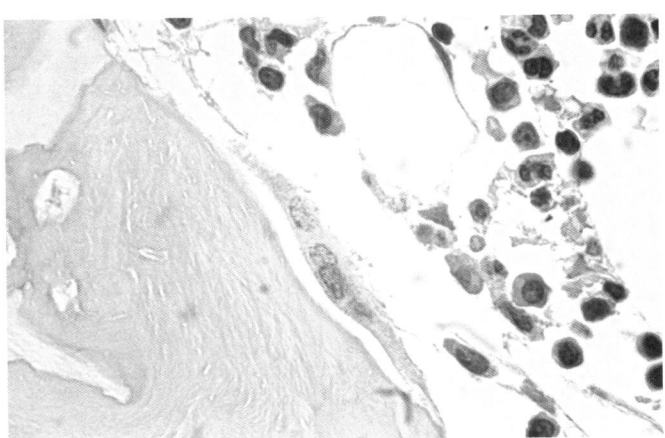

Figure 9-30. Osteoclast adjacent to a bony spicule in a section of a trephine biopsy specimen from a child.

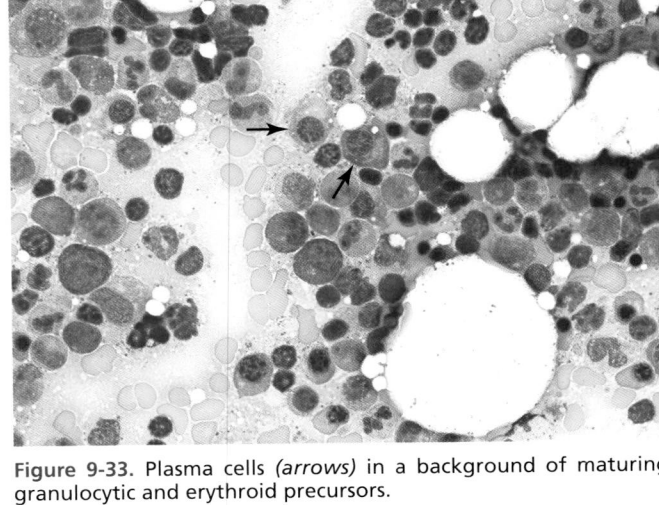

Figure 9-33. Plasma cells *(arrows)* in a background of maturing granulocytic and erythroid precursors.

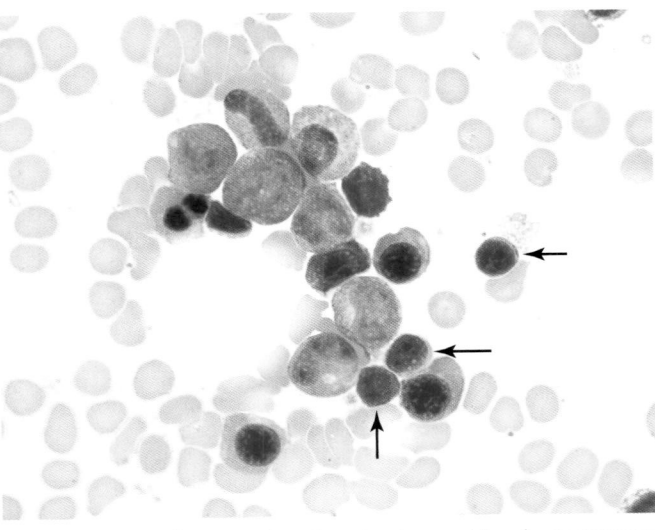

Figure 9-31. Small mature lymphocytes *(arrows)* in a bone marrow aspirate smear.

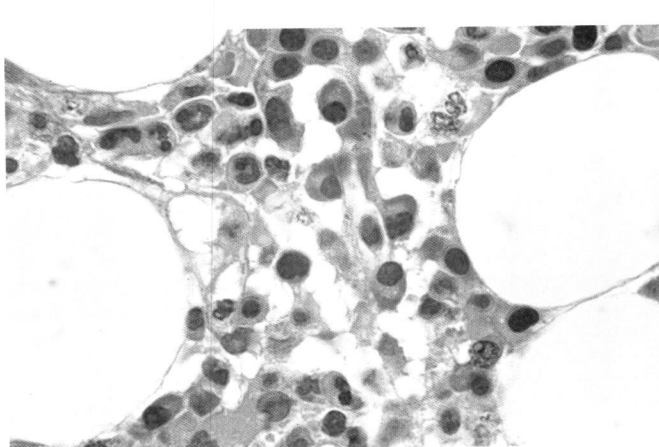

Figure 9-34. Pericapillary plasma cells in a section of a trephine biopsy specimen.

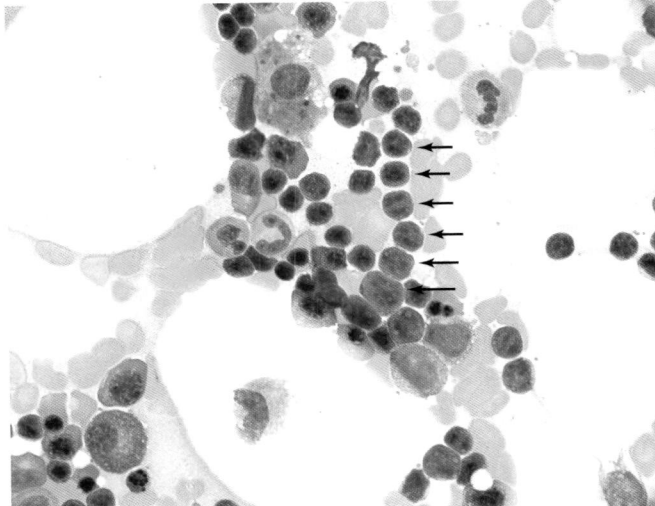

Figure 9-32. **Hematogones *(arrows)* in a bone marrow aspirate smear.** Note the spectrum of size and nuclear maturation.

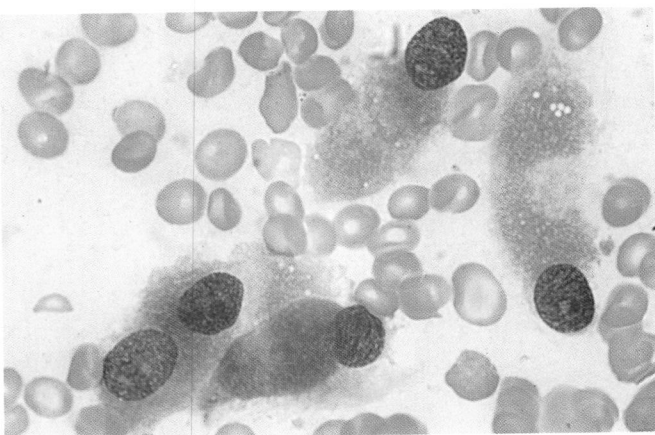

Figure 9-35. A cluster of osteoblasts in a bone marrow aspirate from a child.

Although not specifically discussed in this chapter, examination of a peripheral blood smear is an integral component in the evaluation of any hematologic abnormality, and indeed it is often an abnormality in the blood that triggers a bone marrow examination. Occasionally, the blood may show a greater proportion of blasts, more readily apparent dysgranulopoietic features, or a greater degree of differentiation of leukemic cells than the marrow. It is most efficient to obtain blood smears at the time of bone marrow aspiration and biopsy. If a blood smear is not available to the pathologist, at a minimum, hemogram data should be reviewed.

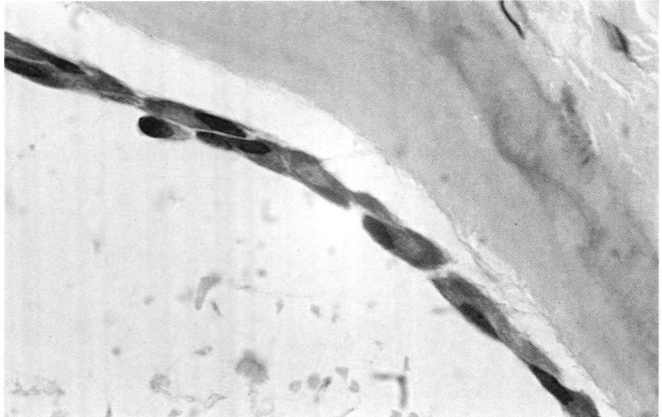

Figure 9-36. Osteoblasts lining bone in a section of a trephine biopsy specimen.

A detailed differential count of the marrow aspirate or blood is not always required to be included in the report, as in the case of examination for metastatic disease, when the hemogram is otherwise normal, when cellularity is markedly low, or there is severe pancytopenia. When a differential count may provide useful information but is not integral to diagnosis or subclassification, the International Council for Standardization in Hematology (ICSH) has indicated that a 300-cell count of the nucleated bone marrow cells is sufficient.[8] However, when the diagnosis or classification of a disease process, such as acute leukemia or myelodysplastic syndrome, relies on knowledge of the proportions of blasts and other abnormal cells, more detailed differential counts are justified. Differential counts of 200 leukocytes in the blood and 500 cells in the marrow are recommended for determining the percentage of blasts,[4] with additional cells counted or additional smears examined if the proportion is at a "critical threshold" or if there is an uneven distribution of such cells.[8] The ICSH recommends that the bone marrow differential counts include blasts, promyelocytes, myelocytes, metamyelocytes, band forms, segmented neutrophils, eosinophils, basophils, mast cells, promonocytes, monocytes, lymphocytes, plasma cells, and erythroblasts. The nucleated cell count should not include megakaryocytes, macrophages, osteoblasts, osteoclasts, stromal cells, smudged cells, or non-hematopoietic cells such as metastatic tumor cells. If lymphoid aggregates are present, they should not be included in the count, but their presence should be commented upon.[8]

The suggested components that should be included in the bone marrow report are listed in Box 9-1. The clinical

Table 9-6 Cytochemical Stains in Bone Marrow Aspirate

Stain	Reactivity in Normal Bone Marrow	Comments
Perls Prussian blue	Hemosiderin in macrophages and developing erythroid cells	Diagnostically important for evaluation of normoblastic and storage iron
Myeloperoxidase	Primary granules of promyelocytes and all later cells of neutrophil lineage (myeloblasts may have scattered fine granules); primary and secondary granules of cells of eosinophil lineage, from promyelocyte stage onward; granules of basophil myelocytes but not normal mature basophils; granules of monocytes, finer and less numerous than granules of neutrophils	Immunophenotyping with antimyeloperoxidase antibodies is more sensitive than a cytochemical reaction dependent on enzyme activity; uncommonly, there is a congenital peroxidase deficiency in hematologically normal subjects
Sudan black B	Stains lipids present in the primary and secondary granules of granulocytes and monocyte lysosomes	Immunophenotyping is more sensitive for detecting granulocytic differentiation; Sudan black B staining is negative in individuals with a congenital peroxidase deficiency
Naphthol AS-D chloroacetate esterase (specific [neutrophil] esterase)	Granules of neutrophils and their precursors from promyelocyte stage onward (normal eosinophils are negative); mast cell granules	Less sensitive than myeloperoxidase or Sudan black B for detecting granulocytic differentiation; immunophenotyping is also more sensitive
Alpha naphthyl acetate esterase (non-specific esterase)	Granules of monocyte precursors, monocytes, and macrophages; granules of megakaryocytes and platelets; many T lymphocytes are positive; normal neutrophils and erythroblasts are negative	Immunophenotyping is an alternative means of demonstrating monocytic differentiation (e.g., with CD14 monoclonal antibodies) and megakaryocytic differentiation (e.g., with CD42 and CD61 monoclonal antibodies)
Alpha naphthyl butyrate esterase (non-specific esterase)	Granules of monocyte precursors, monocytes, and macrophages; some T lymphocytes show focal paranuclear positivity	More specific for monocyte lineage than alpha naphthyl acetate esterase
Toluidine blue	Granules of mast cells and basophils	
Periodic acid–Schiff (PAS)	Neutrophil lineage, strongest in mature cells; eosinophil cytoplasm is positive, but granules of normal eosinophils are negative; basophil cytoplasm may show large, irregular positive blocks, but granules are negative; monocytes show variable diffuse plus granular positivity; megakaryocytes and platelets usually show strong diffuse plus granular or block positivity; plasma cells have strong diffuse positivity; some lymphocytes show granular positivity	Normal erythroblasts are PAS negative

Table 9-7 Histochemical Stains in Bone Marrow Trephine Biopsy Sections

Stain	Reactivity in Normal Marrow	Comments
Perls Prussian blue stain	Hemosiderin in macrophages	More useful in aspirate, as long as it contains bone marrow particles; decalcification procedure may remove iron from bone marrow trephine biopsy specimens
Gomori or Gordon-Sweet stain for reticulin	Scattered linear reticulin with no intersections; normal presence of reticulin fibers around arterioles	Important for highlighting abnormal areas of collagen type III in bone marrow and in the diagnosis of myeloproliferative neoplasms
Masson trichrome	Perivascular collagen	Important for highlighting collagen type I in the diagnosis of myeloproliferative neoplasms
Periodic acid–Schiff (with or without diastase)	Highlights plasma cells, megakaryocytes, and granulocytic cells	Can highlight organisms in immunosuppressed patients
Congo red	None	Amyloid shows positive staining with apple-green birefringence under polarized light

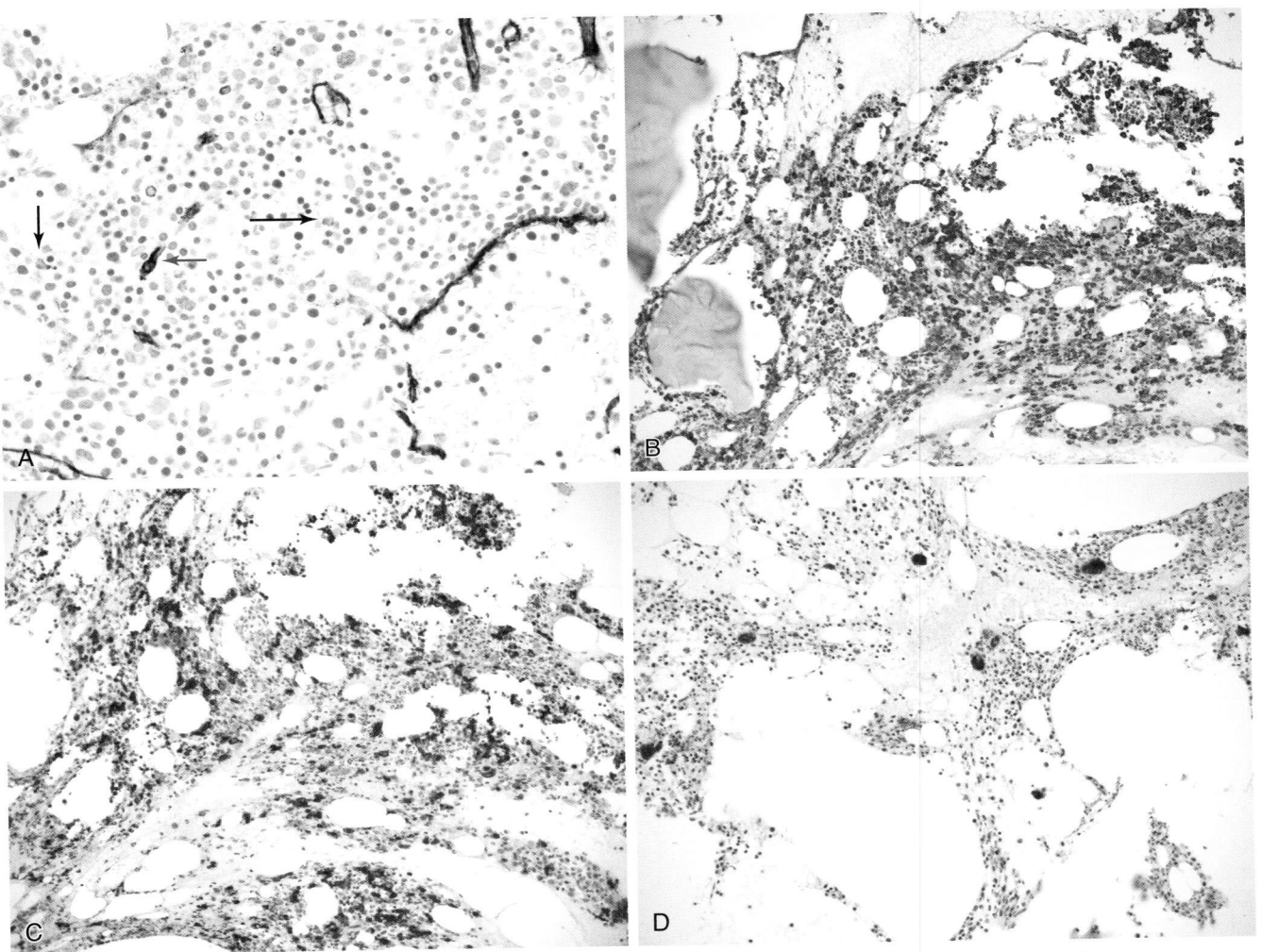

Figure 9-37. Immunohistochemistry of normal bone marrow. A, CD34 immunohistochemical stain highlighting endothelial cells *(blue arrow)* and rare weakly positive blasts *(black arrows).* **B,** Myeloperoxidase immunohistochemical stain highlighting granulocytic precursors. **C,** CD71 immunohistochemical stain highlighting erythroid precursors. **D,** CD61 immunohistochemical stain highlighting scattered megakaryocytes.

Box 9-1 *Components of a Bone Marrow Report*

A brief clinical history including indication for bone marrow examination

Peripheral blood smear review including concurrent complete blood count (CBC) data

Bone marrow aspirate smear

Adequacy and relative cellularity

Granulocytic to erythroid ratio

Granulocyte precursors

Relative percentage, maturation, presence/absence of dysplasia

Percentage of blasts, morphologic description if increased

Erythroid precursors

Relative percentage, maturation, presence/absence of dysplasia

Megakaryocytes

Relative number and morphology

Other cell types: lymphocytes, plasma cells, monocytes, mast cells, eosinophils, and basophils

Differential cell count, if indicated

Bone marrow trephine biopsy or clot

Adequacy and marrow cellularity, including percentage and comparison to age expected cellularity: normocellular/hypocellular/hypercellular for age

Proportion of granulocytic (myeloid) and erythroid cells and relative number of megakaryocytes

Features of bone trabeculae

Stromal elements

Abnormal cellular infiltrates: granulomas, lymphocytic infiltrate, increased plasma cells, and metastatic tumor

Results of cytochemical, histochemical, or immunohistochemical stains, if performed

Results of flow cytometric immunophenotyping, if performed

Results of cytogenetic/molecular genetic studies, if performed

Can be reported as an addendum; however, the list of tests performed should be included in the initial report

Final diagnosis

Tissue examined and site of biopsy

Diagnostic interpretation including all available results of ancillary studies

Classification system used to render diagnosis, if applicable

Pearls and Pitfalls

- Before performing the marrow, determine what samples to collect. How many cores? Bilateral or unilateral? How many aspirate samples, for what studies, in what types of anticoagulant, and in what sequence?
- Obtain additional cores for special studies if the aspiration is hemodiluted or if it yields a dry tap.
- Smear should be made within 2 hours of aspirate collection in EDTA to avoid morphologic distortion.
- Dry all smears rapidly. A small tabletop fan can help when the humidity is high.
- The trephine biopsy should be adequately fixed. Sections must be sufficiently thin (≤4 μm) to permit the recognition of individual cells.
- Differential counts should be performed on well-stained marrow aspirate smears.
- Hemodiluted aspirate smears, thick smears, or poorly stained smears can lead to incorrect interpretation.
- Examine and report on both the aspirate and the core biopsy. Indicate the status of samples that have been sent to specialty laboratories.
- The pathologist must be totally familiar with the appearance of all normal cells that can be found in the bone marrow.
- The morphologic findings in the marrow must be interpreted in conjunction with the peripheral smear and in light of the clinical history.

indication for the bone marrow examination, a complete hemogram, morphologic findings on the peripheral blood smear, bone marrow aspirate smear, and core biopsy, as well as results of all ancillary studies, should be included.

CONCLUSION

Meaningful evaluation of the bone marrow requires a bone marrow specimen that is adequate for the clinical scenario, and which is well prepared. Correct and complete interpretation then relies on the integration of the morphologic findings of the bone marrow aspirate, trephine core biopsy, and peripheral blood with review of relevant ancillary studies and clinical data. Rigorous monitoring of the collection, processing, and staining processes ensures specimen adequacy and accurate morphologic evaluation. In interpreting the marrow, the pathologist should be aware of the range of normality and have a thorough knowledge of the cytologic and histologic features of bone marrow in a healthy subject.

Acknowledgments

The authors graciously appreciate and acknowledge the work from the prior authors, Dr. Phuong Nguyen and Dr. Barbara Bain, which has inspired and contributed significantly to this updated chapter.

KEY REFERENCES

1. Barekman CL, Fair KP, Cotelingam JD. Comparative utility of diagnostic bone-marrow components: a 10-year study. *Am J Hematol.* 1997;56(1):37–41.
4. Arber DA, Orazi A, Hasserjian RP, et al. International consensus classification of myeloid neoplasms and acute leukemias: integrating morphologic, clinical, and genomic data. *Blood.* 2022;140(11):1200–1228.
8. Lee SH, Erber WN, Porwit A, Tomonaga M, Peterson LC, International Council for Standardization in Hematology. ICSH guidelines for the standardization of bone marrow specimens and reports. *Int J Lab Hematol.* 2008;30(5):349–364.
11. O'Neill SS, Wong TC, Parris J, et al. Revisiting bone marrow core biopsy adequacy criteria in the era of extensive ancillary testing. *Clin Lab.* 2019;65(9).
12. Torlakovic EE, Brynes RK, Hyjek E, et al. ICSH guidelines for the standardization of bone marrow immunohistochemistry. *Int J Lab Hematol.* 2015;37(4):431–449.
14. Naresh KN, Lampert I, Hasserjian R, et al. Optimal processing of bone marrow trephine biopsy: the Hammersmith Protocol. *J Clin Pathol.* 2006;59(9):903–911.
19. Hughes DA, Stuart-Smith SE, Bain BJ. How should stainable iron in bone marrow films be assessed? *J Clin Pathol.* 2004;57(10):1038–1040.
21. Orkin SH, Zon LI. Hematopoiesis: an evolving paradigm for stem cell biology. *Cell.* 2008;132(4):631–644.
26. Peterson LC, Agosti SJ, Hoyer JD. Hematology clinical microscopy resource committee, members of the cancer committee, college of American pathologists. Protocol for the examination of specimens from patients with hematopoietic neoplasms of the bone marrow: a basis for checklists. *Arch Pathol Lab Med.* 2002;126(9):1050–1056.
27. Sever C, Abbott CL, de Baca ME, et al. Bone marrow synoptic reporting for hematologic neoplasms. *Arch Pathol Lab Med.* 2016;140(9):932–949.

Visit Elsevier eBooks+ for the complete set of references.

Chapter 10

Evaluation of Anemia, Leukopenia, and Thrombocytopenia

Maria (Ria) E. Vergara-Lluri, Ashley S. Hagiya, and Russell K. Brynes

Quantitative and qualitative abnormalities of the peripheral blood are routinely detected with an automated complete blood count (CBC) and examination of a peripheral blood smear. The peripheral blood evaluation serves as a screening test for potential bone marrow abnormalities and diseases that affect bone marrow function. When peripheral blood abnormalities are identified, the decision to perform an invasive bone marrow procedure is influenced by a moderate number of quantitative findings from the CBC and a greater number of qualitative abnormalities upon inspection of the peripheral blood smear. The decision also relies on a carefully obtained history, thorough physical examination, evaluation of current and historical laboratory values, and imaging studies. The utility of a thorough history in the evaluation of bone marrow specimens cannot be overemphasized. The history should include information about present and past illnesses, including how and when the cytopenia or cytosis presented and how it was discovered. Occupational history and a history of exposure to therapeutic or recreational drugs, alcohol, and toxins should be sought. Physical examination often provides a critical clue to the responsible mechanism or disease process. Other laboratory studies pertinent to the case (e.g., inflammatory markers, autoantibodies, immunoglobulin levels, microbiologic studies) must be reviewed. Finally, in certain cases, review of radiologic data may yield additional useful information. Without integration of these various essential elements, interpretation of the bone marrow findings is often incomplete or misleading. This chapter focuses on nonmalignant anemia, leukopenia, and thrombocytopenia. The differential diagnosis of increased and decreased numbers of clonal red blood cells (RBCs), leukocytes, and platelets is discussed elsewhere in this book.

EVALUATION OF ANEMIA

The World Health Organization (WHO) defines anemia as a hemoglobin concentration of less than 12 g/dL in women, less than 13 g/dL in men, less than 11 g/dL in children aged 6 months to 6 years, and less than 12 g/dL in children aged 6 to 14 years.[1] Age-adjusted charts are available for the pediatric population. It is important to note that racial differences exist. Compared with individuals of European descent of similar age and sex, hemoglobin concentrations of individuals of African descent are almost 1 g/dL lower.[2] The effects of altitude should also be considered, as those residing at higher altitudes exhibit higher hemoglobin levels. The initial evaluation of anemia begins with the CBC data and comprehensive examination of a well-prepared peripheral blood smear. The blood smear should initially be evaluated at scanning power to detect abnormalities such as rouleaux formation and RBC agglutination, followed by observation of individual RBCs with a high-powered lens. Review of pertinent history and physical findings can help determine what additional laboratory tests are needed and whether a bone marrow examination is required to further define the process.

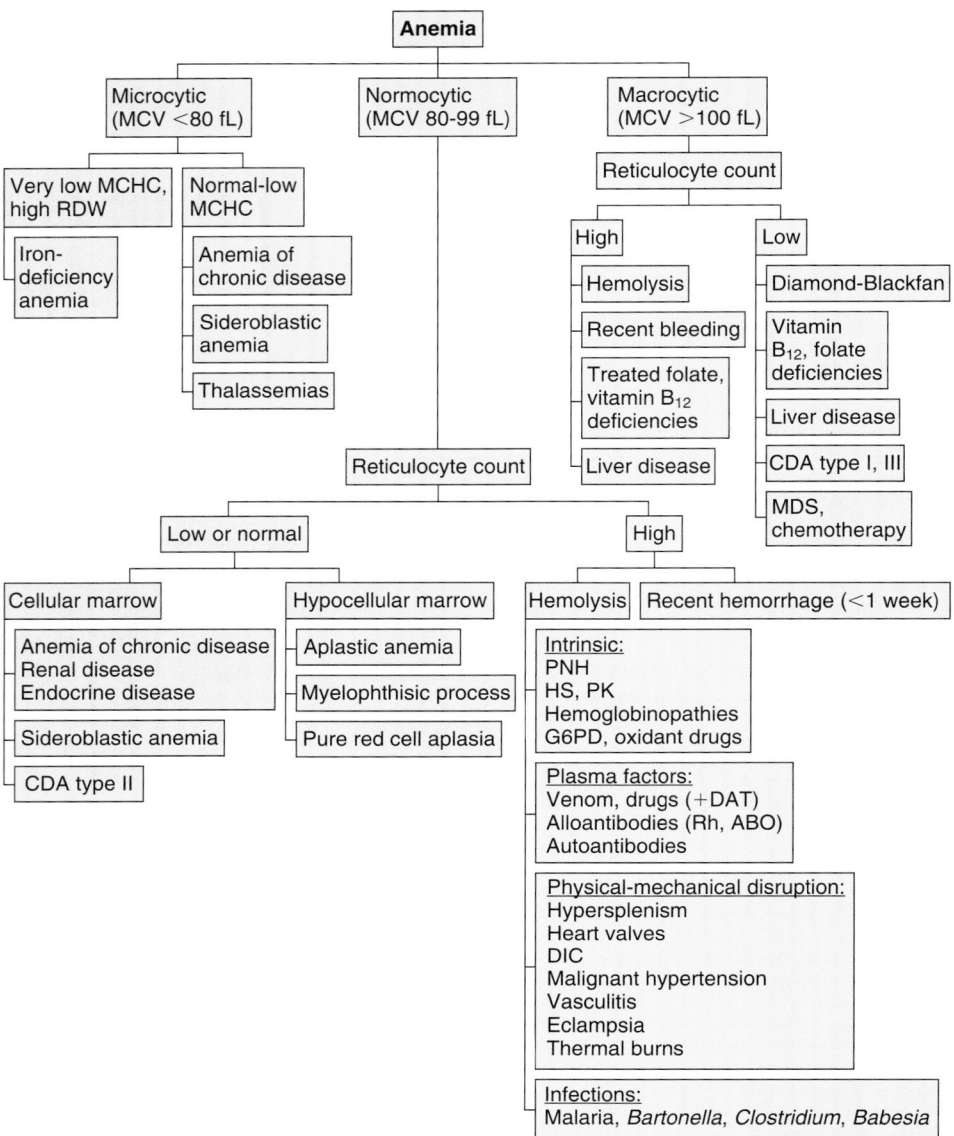

Figure 10-1. Anemia algorithm. Mean corpuscular volume (MCV) is based on adult values; reference ranges must be considered for pediatric patients. *CDA,* Congenital dyserythropoietic anemia; *DAT,* direct antiglobulin test; *DIC,* disseminated intravascular coagulation; *G6PD,* glucose-6-phosphate dehydrogenase; *HS,* hereditary spherocytosis; *MCHC,* mean corpuscular hemoglobin concentration; *MDS,* myelodysplastic syndrome; *PK,* pyruvate kinase deficiency; *PNH,* paroxysmal nocturnal hemoglobinuria; *RDW,* red cell distribution width.

Anemias can be divided into those caused by production problems with insufficient or ineffective erythropoiesis and those caused by either blood loss or decreased RBC survival. The reticulocyte count is the best test to differentiate between abnormalities of production and survival, and it is often the first test considered in algorithms for the evaluation of anemia. Because the reticulocyte count may not be high during the initial stages of hemolysis and blood loss, anemia may be better stratified first by the CBC data, with size (mean corpuscular volume [MCV]), hemoglobinization (mean corpuscular hemoglobin concentration [MCHC] and mean corpuscular hemoglobin [MCH]), RBC count, and degree of anisocytosis (red cell distribution width [RDW]) (Fig. 10-1). This approach can then be extended with an algorithm that adds reticulocyte count, serum iron studies, and vitamin B$_{12}$ and folate values, as needed. With this algorithm, bone marrow examination is required most frequently for normocytic or

macrocytic anemias with low reticulocyte counts that cannot be explained by vitamin B$_{12}$ or folate deficiency, liver disease, drug or alcohol effects, or other clearly defined causes. Bone marrow examination is essential in the diagnosis of aplastic anemia (AA), myelodysplastic syndromes (MDS), and myelophthisic anemia. Of course, anemia is quite common in patients undergoing bone marrow examination for other indications, such as tumor staging.

Microcytic Anemia

In microcytic anemia, the MCV is less than the normal laboratory reference range, generally less than 80 fL for adults and dependent on age for children. The small RBCs result from defective or ineffective production of hemoglobin. Heme, the iron-containing porphyrin ring component of hemoglobin, is synthesized from succinyl coenzyme A (CoA) and glycine

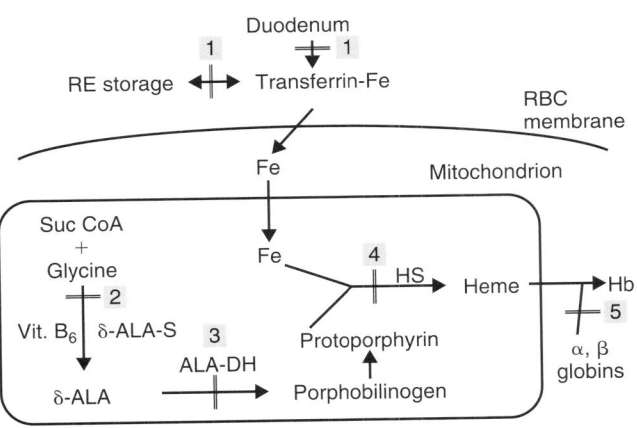

Figure 10-2. Defects causing microcytic anemias. Ferric iron is absorbed by the duodenum and transported via ferroportin receptors to serum transferrin (measured as total iron-binding capacity). Hepcidin, produced by the liver, regulates iron (Fe) uptake and transport through ferroportin in response to iron stores, inflammation, erythropoiesis, and hypoxia. The strongest extrahepatic hepcidin suppressor—erythroferrone (ERFE)—is secreted by more mature erythroid precursors stimulated by erythropoietin (EPO) production, thereby playing a key role in maintaining iron homeostasis. Most serum iron is delivered to the bone marrow for red blood cell (RBC) production. Erythroid precursors have classic transferrin receptors that selectively bind and internalize diferric transferrin. When transferrin saturation exceeds 60%, iron is shunted into histiocyte storage in the bone marrow, spleen, and liver. **1,** Hepcidin excess leads to blockade of this pathway and inability to mobilize iron back into the serum through ferroportin receptors on histiocyte surfaces and on duodenal enterocytes. It is characteristic of anemias of chronic disease. Deficiency or blockade of key steps in heme synthesis by heavy metals and various drugs (e.g., isoniazid) causes iron to accumulate within mitochondria, producing sideroblastic anemias. **2,** Congenital deficiency and heavy metal (lead) inhibition of aminolevulinic acid dehydratase (ALA-DH) **(3)** or heme synthetase (HS) **(4)** produce a similar effect. **5,** Decreased synthesis of globin chains contributes to the microcytosis of thalassemia syndromes. Blood loss or dietary deficiency of iron ultimately produces iron-deficiency anemia. *Hb,* Hemoglobin; *RE,* reticuloendothelial.

through a series of enzymatic steps that occur in the mitochondria (Fig. 10-2). Disorders affecting heme synthesis, the globin genes, iron acquisition by erythroid precursors, or iron availability prevent adequate hemoglobinization and maturation of RBC cytoplasm, resulting in hypochromic microcytic cells.[3,4] Table 10-1 lists additional findings for hypochromic microcytic anemias.

Iron Deficiency

Iron homeostasis, including iron uptake from the intestine and release from stores, is regulated by the liver-secreted protein hepcidin.[5] Iron deficiency occurs when iron utilization or loss exceeds iron absorption and results in depletion of body stores. Early in iron deficiency, iron stores are decreased, but the red cells are morphologically unaffected. Serum ferritin (normally 12 ng/mL to 300 ng/mL) is in equilibrium with tissue stores and serves as an indirect measure of the body's iron stores in uncomplicated cases; indeed, in the absence of inflammation, serum ferritin levels below the reference range are indicative of iron deficiency. However, ferritin is an acute-phase protein, and patients with chronic inflammation

or liver disease may have elevated values even in the presence of iron deficiency. After iron stores are depleted, serum iron drops and the iron transport protein, transferrin, increases so that the total iron-binding capacity is increased. The red cells become microcytic and normochromic, then finally microcytic and hypochromic (Fig. 10-3).[6] Serum iron concentration has diurnal variation and should be measured in the morning, when it is at its highest level. Transferrin saturation (serum iron/total iron binding capacity) of less than 15% is virtually diagnostic of iron deficiency. The sensitivity and specificity of the CBC, transferrin saturation, and ferritin values are usually sufficient to make the diagnosis of iron deficiency without the need to perform a bone marrow study. Serum-soluble transferrin receptor (sTfR) levels, which are elevated in iron deficiency but usually unaffected by inflammation, and the sTfR-ferritin index (sTfR/log ferritin) may be helpful in interpreting iron status in patients with inflammatory disease; however, these tests are not widely available or standardized and are often not needed in routine practice.[7] Although many advances have been made in our understanding of iron metabolism and hepcidin, measurement of serum hepcidin levels continues to be mostly limited to research settings as a result of analytic challenges and difficulties in interpretation; however, it may be useful in assessing iron status and erythropoietin resistance in states of inflammation and in determining the optimal route of iron supplement administration.[8-11] In ambiguous cases, such as patients with elevated acute-phase proteins or hepatic disorders, a bone marrow evaluation for iron assessment is indicated. Bone marrow iron stores and sideroblast iron should be evaluated on an aspirate smear (Fig. 10-4A and B) because iron is chelated by acidic decalcifying agents and is generally underestimated in clot or trephine biopsy sections. In normal bone marrow, one or two small siderotic granules are normally identifiable in at least 10% of the normoblasts (Fig. 10-4A and B). In iron deficiency, the Perls Prussian blue stain demonstrates loss of reticuloendothelial marrow stores and iron incorporation into normoblasts (Fig. 10-4C and D; Table 10-1). The absence of iron stores differentiates iron deficiency from advanced anemia of chronic disease, which may mimic an iron deficiency state. However, some authors suggest the evaluation of multiple marrow spicules before declaring the marrow as iron deficient, as the iron may be irregularly distributed.[12] If recent parenteral iron or RBC transfusion has been given to an iron-deficient individual, these findings may be misleading, because the bone marrow iron stores may appear adequate. Parenteral iron shows a characteristic staining pattern with numerous uniform fine particles that tend to form curvilinear arrays within reticuloendothelial/stromal cells in essentially all marrow spicules.[13] Bone marrow morphology is otherwise non-specific in iron deficiency. In severe anemia, the erythroid precursors may appear smaller, with only a narrow rim of cytoplasm. Rarely, individuals have iron-refractory iron-deficiency anemia that is congenital and caused by defects in the *TMPRSS6* gene that lead to uninhibited hepcidin production.[14] Some cases result from gene mutations involving the transferrin gene or iron transport genes (*TF, DMT1*).[15] Celiac disease, *Helicobacter pylori* gastritis, and autoimmune gastritis can also cause iron deficiency anemia that is refractory to oral iron treatment.[16] As iron is not normally excreted by the body, except in menstrual periods, the etiology for blood loss should be

Table 10-1 **Classification of Hypochromic Microcytic Anemia**

Disorder	Features	Comments
Iron deficiency	CBC: ↓ RBCs, ↓↓ MCHC, ↓↓ MCH, ↓ MCV, ↑ RDW, normal-↓ platelets, ↓ reticulocytes PBS: anisopoikilocytosis, especially elliptocytes ("cigar" or "pencil" cells), prekeratocytes, occasional target cells Iron studies: ↑ TIBC, ↓ TSAT, ↓ serum iron, ↓ ferritin Iron stain patterns on BM aspirate smear: 0 storage iron, 0 incorporated (sideroblast) iron	Iron required for rate-limiting step in heme synthesis Deficiency caused by chronic blood loss (especially menstrual), GI dietary deficiency (breastfed children aged 6 months to 2 years at risk), postgastrectomy (gastric acid required for iron absorption), upper GI malabsorption, *Helicobacter pylori* infection
Iron refractory iron deficiency anemia	CBC: ↓ RBCs, ↓↓ MCHC, ↓↓ MCH, ↓ MCV Iron studies: ↓ serum iron, ↓ TSAT, ↓-normal ferritin Iron stain patterns on BM aspirate smear: ↓-absent storage iron, 0 incorporated (sideroblast) iron	*TMPRSS6* mutation leads to uninhibited hepcidin production Unresponsive to oral iron
β-Thalassemia	CBC: normal-↑ RBCs, ↓↓ MCV, ↓-normal MCHC, normal-↑ RDW PBS: target cells, coarse basophilic stippling	Absent or ↓ synthesis of β globin chains caused by gene mutations Frequent in Mediterranean populations ↑ HbF has heterogeneous distribution in RBCs
α-Thalassemia	Similar to β-thalassemia	Absent or ↓ synthesis of α globin chains caused by gene deletions Frequent in Southeast Asian and African populations
Anemia of inflammation (also known as anemia of chronic disease)	CBC: ↓ RBCs, normal-↓ MCV, normal-↓ MCHC, ↓-normal MCH, normal-↑ RDW PBS: possible hypochromic cells even if normocytic Iron studies: ↓ serum iron, ↓-normal TSAT, ↑ serum ferritin Iron stain patterns on BM aspirate smear: normal-↑ storage iron, ↓ incorporated (sideroblast) iron	More often presents as a normochromic normocytic anemia, caused by excess hepcidin secondary to cytokines (IL-6) Normal-↓ serum iron, normal transferrin saturation
Sideroblastic anemia	PBS: Dimorphic RBCs, moderate poikilocytosis, hypochromic teardrop forms, coarse basophilic stippling, Pappenheimer bodies Iron stain patterns on BM aspirate smear: ring sideroblasts	See Box 10-1 ↓ Reticulocyte count Variable anisocytosis, but may be marked

↑, Increased; *↓,* decreased or low; *↓↓,* very decreased or low; *BM,* bone marrow; *CBC,* complete blood count; *GI,* gastrointestinal; *Hb,* hemoglobin; *IL,* interleukin; *MCHC,* mean corpuscular hemoglobin concentration; *MCH,* mean corpuscular hemoglobin; *MCV,* mean cell volume; *PBS,* peripheral blood smear; *RBC,* red blood cell; *RDW,* red cell distribution width; *TIBC,* total iron binding capacity; *TSAT,* % transferrin saturation.

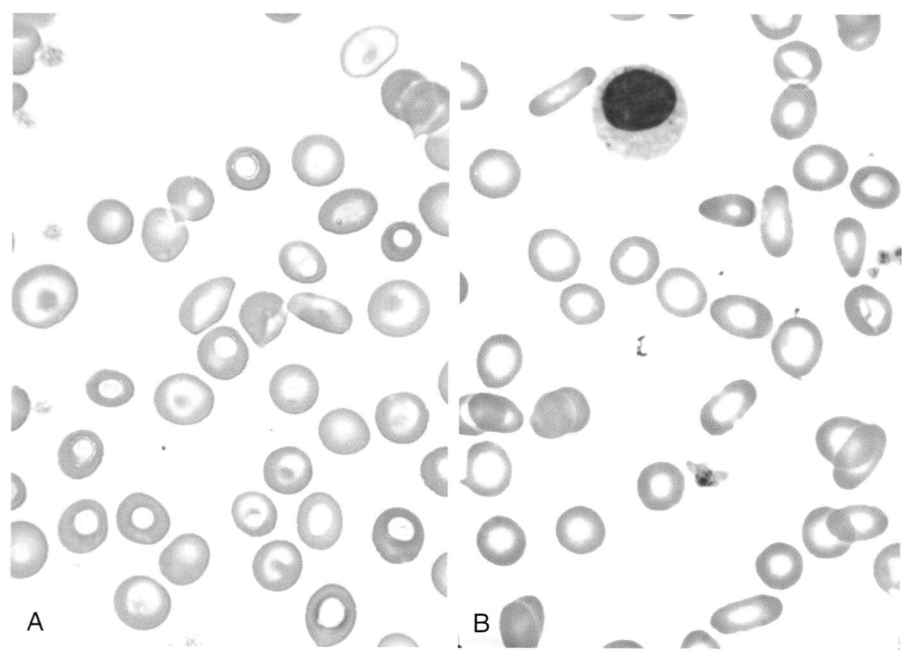

Figure 10-3. A, Iron-deficiency anemia in a child. The red blood cells are hypochromic and microcytic. Note the many target cells, a feature reported in long-standing iron deficiency. **B,** Severe iron-deficiency anemia. The red blood cells are hypochromic and microcytic. Their small size is apparent compared with the nucleus of the lymphocyte. Hypochromic elliptocytes are common in iron-deficiency anemia.

carefully sought. The leading cause of iron-deficiency anemia in adults is occult bleeding from the gastrointestinal tract. Exclusion of *H. pylori* infection as a cause of unexplained iron-deficiency anemia is also important because eradication of the organisms leads to amelioration of the anemia.[17]

Thalassemias

Thalassemias are a common cause of hypochromic microcytic anemia in which adult hemoglobin (HbA [$\alpha_2\beta_2$]) synthesis is quantitatively affected by decreased α or β globin chain

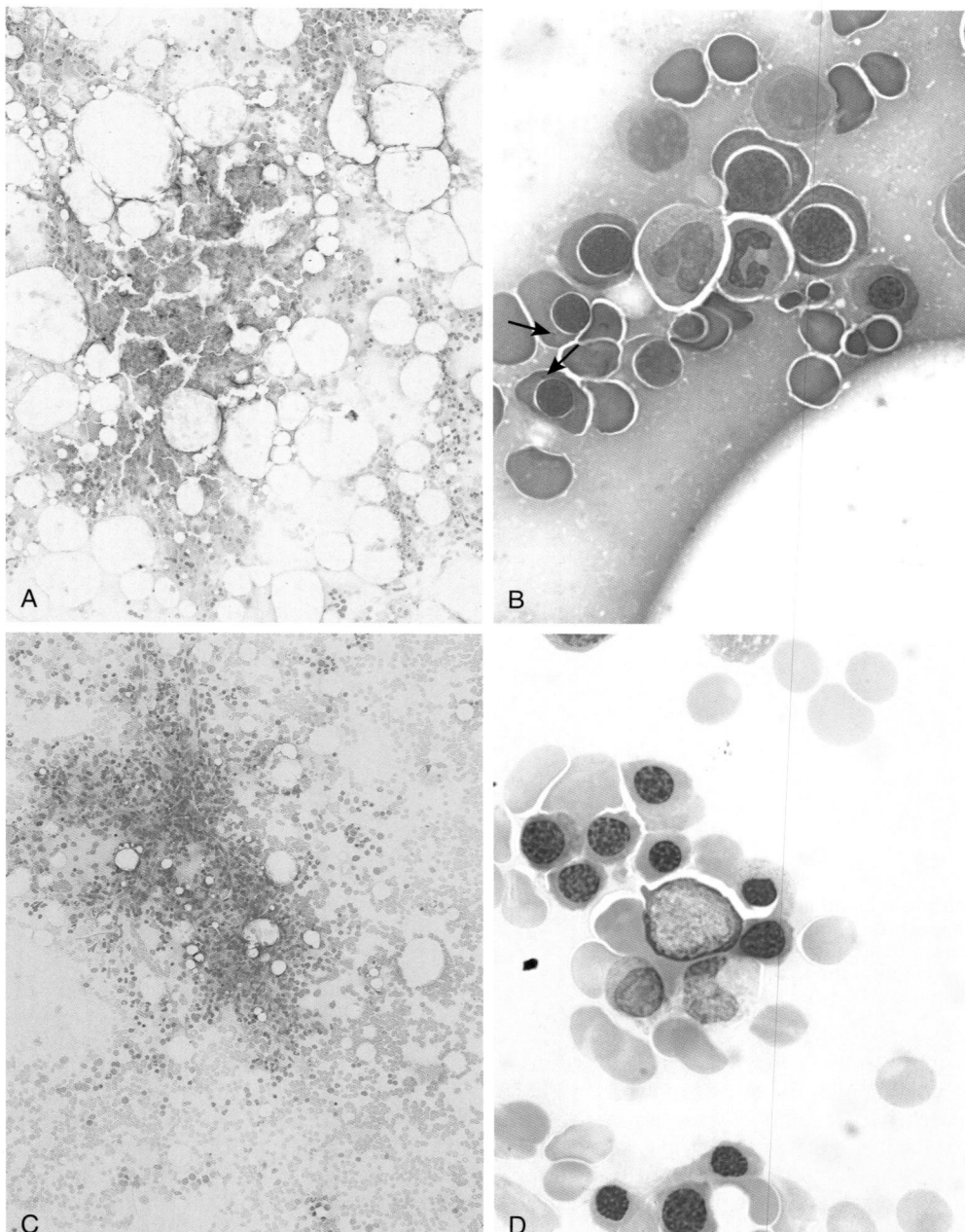

Figure 10-4. Bone marrow particle smear with normal iron stores and incorporation. A, Storage iron in stromal histiocytes stains blue with the Perls Prussian blue stain. **B,** Sideroblast (incorporated) iron granules *(arrows)* are seen in 10% to 20% of normoblasts. In a bone marrow particle smear in iron-deficiency anemia, both storage **(C)** and sideroblast **(D)** iron are absent.

synthesis (Table 10-2; Fig. 10-2).[18,19] Thalassemia is common in Mediterranean regions, tropical Africa, and Asia; β-thalassemia is also seen in the Middle East and India. The diagnosis of β-thalassemia and severe forms of α-thalassemia is best made by high-performance liquid chromatography (HPLC) or electrophoretic techniques such as isoelectric focusing or capillary zone electrophoresis.[20,21] HPLC has been widely adopted worldwide.[22] However, these methods are not as useful in detecting milder forms of α-thalassemia; in these cases, molecular testing may be the only means for definitive diagnosis and may be indicated for genetic counseling.[22]

β-thalassemia is caused by more than 350 different mutations that affect one or both of the β globin chain genes on chromosome 11.[23] These are primarily point mutations affecting transcription, splicing, or translocation of β globin messenger RNA. In its most benign form (β-thalassemia minor; Fig. 10-5A and B), only one of the two genes is mutated, causing either decreased (β^+) or absent (β^0) β globin protein synthesis by the affected allele.[18] The normally produced α chains have insufficient β chains with which to pair, and the excess combine with δ chains to produce HbA$_2$ ($\alpha_2\delta_2$). A mild elevation in fetal hemoglobin (HbF; $\alpha_2\gamma_2$) is also found in about one-third of patients. If both β chain genes are mutated, scant ($\beta^+\beta^+$ or $\beta^0\beta^+$) or no β chains ($\beta^0\beta^0$) are made, causing a serious childhood anemia, β-thalassemia major (Cooley's anemia). This is usually diagnosed in the first year of life

Table 10-2 Hemoglobin Types and Concentrations in Thalassemia

	HbA ($\alpha_2\beta_2$)	HbA$_2$ ($\alpha_2\delta_2$)	HbF ($\alpha_2\gamma_2$)	HbH (β_4)	Hb Barts (γ_4)
Normal adult	97%	2%	1%		
β-Thalassemia minor (high HbA$_2$)	Decreased	>2.5% (4%-8%)	<5% Nl or Sl ↑		
β-Thalassemia minor (high HbF)	Decreased	2%	8%-30%		
β^0-Thalassemia major	0	Variable	>95%		
β$^+$-Thalassemia major	Remainder	≥2%	30%-90%		
α-Thalassemia minor	Normal	Normal	Normal		
HbH disease	70%-90%	≤2%	Normal	5%-30%	
α-Thalassemia major	0	0	0	0	100%

Hb, Hemoglobin.

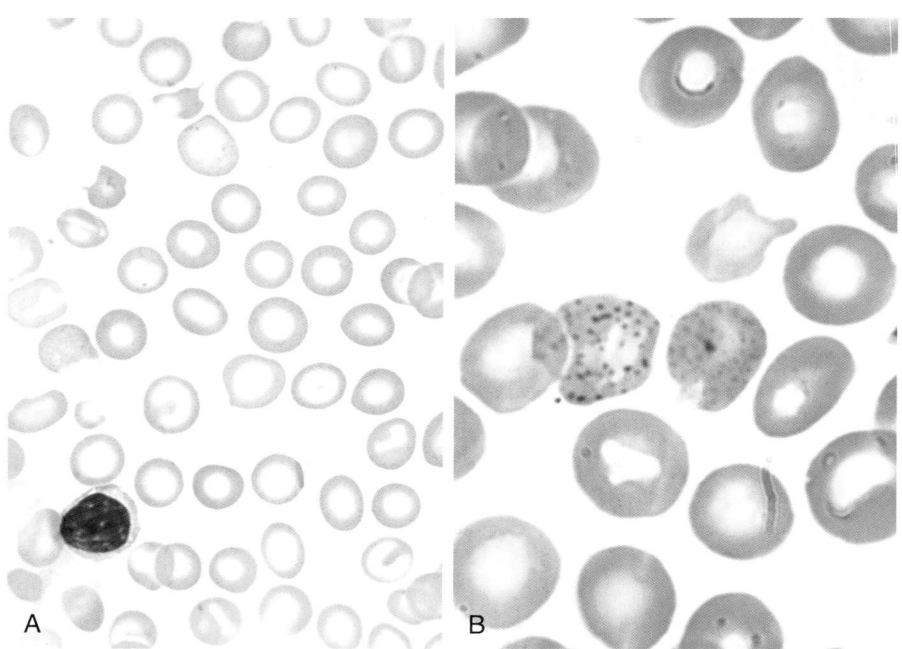

Figure 10-5. A, Blood smear in β-thalassemia minor illustrates hypochromic, microcytic red blood cells. Target cells are increased. **B,** Coarse basophilic stippling is a characteristic feature of β-thalassemias.

as hemoglobin switches from HbF to HbA. It is associated with severe microcytic anemia, marked hemolysis, marked erythroid hyperplasia, hepatosplenomegaly, and failure to thrive. Leukopenia and thrombocytopenia may occur with progressive splenomegaly. Patients who are not transfusion dependent or who are diagnosed later in life are classified clinically as having β-thalassemia intermedia. Methyl violet highlights insoluble α chain inclusion bodies in the red cells, resembling Heinz bodies. They also occur in hemoglobinized erythroid precursors in the marrow and result in ineffective erythropoiesis. Erythropoiesis is also affected by red cell membrane abnormalities in the developing cells (abnormal ratios of spectrin to band 3 and abnormal band 4.1) that promote increased intramedullary death of the red cell precursors. In addition to erythroid hyperplasia, the bone marrow may demonstrate erythrophagocytosis and increased hemosiderin as a result of excessive absorption of dietary iron, secondary to decreased hepcidin levels.[24]

The α-thalassemias are primarily caused by deletions of one, two, or three of the four α chain ($\alpha\alpha/\alpha\alpha$) genes located on chromosome 16.[18] The number of deleted loci determines disease severity. A silent carrier has only one deleted gene ($-\alpha/\alpha\alpha$), and the blood picture is normal. When two genes are involved ($-\alpha/-\alpha$ in African populations or $--/\alpha\alpha$ in

Asian populations), a mild hypochromic microcytic anemia is generally present (α-thalassemia trait) (Fig. 10-6A). Only one functioning α chain ($--/-\alpha$) results in HbH (β_4) disease (Fig. 10-6B). Neonates with this disorder have excess unpaired γ globin chains that form tetramers, called *hemoglobin Barts* (γ_4). They also produce small amounts of HbF until β chain synthesis develops and replaces γ chain synthesis. Adults and older children form β chain tetramers (HbH) with normal amounts of HbF. HbH disease is most common in Asian populations because of deletions of α chain genes in the cis configuration ($--/\alpha\alpha$).[19] They present with variable symptoms and usually moderate hypochromic microcytic anemia with reticulocytosis, although severe anemia similar to β-thalassemia major may be seen. RBCs have HbH inclusions that can be seen best with brilliant cresyl blue or new methylene blue stains. Unlike the globin precipitates of β-thalassemia major, these β globin inclusions are not seen in bone marrow erythroid precursors. The remaining bone marrow findings are similar. Deletion of all four α chain genes (hydrops fetalis) is incompatible with life (Fig. 10-6C). With the absence of α chain production, only hemoglobin Barts is formed. This abnormal hemoglobin has very high oxygen affinity and deprives fetal tissues of needed oxygen. An acquired form of α-thalassemia may develop in elderly patients with myelodysplastic syndrome (MDS) and an

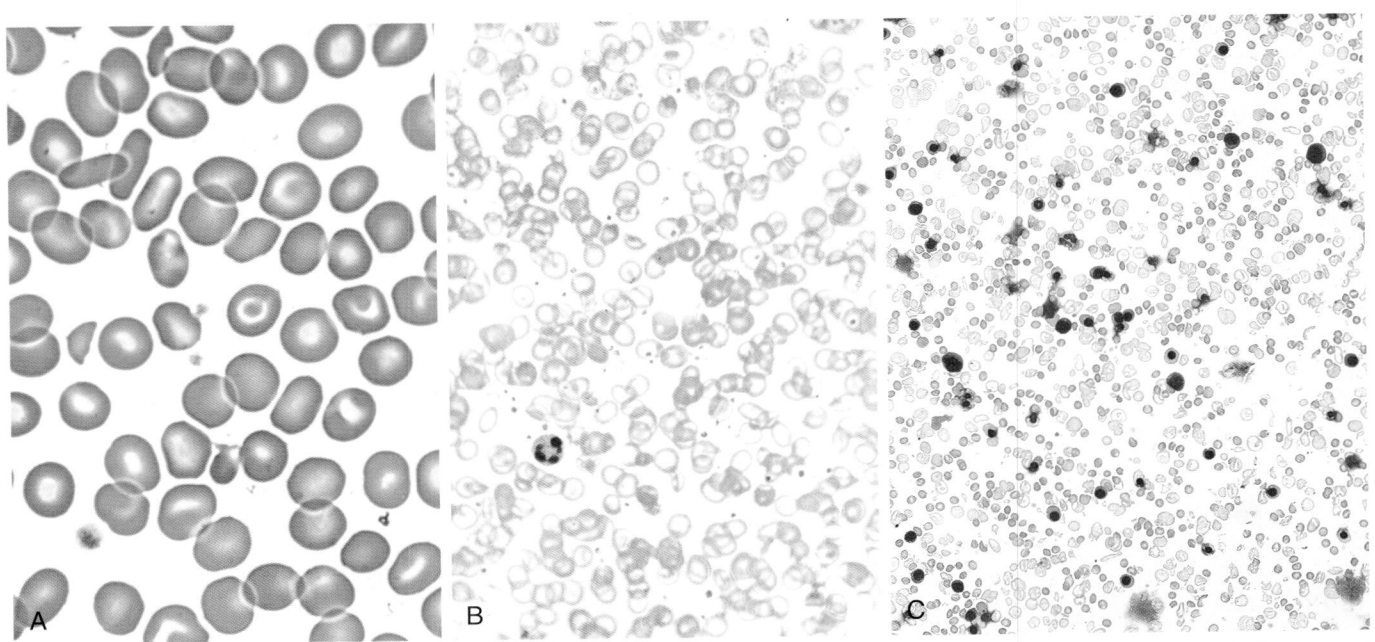

Figure 10-6. A, Blood smear in α-thalassemia minor (– –/αα or –α/–α) is slightly hypochromic or normochromic and microcytic. Rare target cells and spherocytes may be found in some cases. **B,** α-Thalassemia major or HbH disease (– –/–α) produces moderate anemia characterized by hypochromic microcytic red blood cells. Precipitated β globin chains can be detected with brilliant cresyl blue supravital staining. **C,** Hydrops fetalis results from the functional absence of all α chain genes (– –/– –) and the production of hemoglobin Barts (γ4). It is associated with severe hypochromic microcytic anemia. Target cells and normoblasts may be numerous. Spherocytes are also present in this case. Precipitated hemoglobin Barts is easily detected in the red blood cells with brilliant cresyl blue supravital staining.

associated *ATRX* gene mutation that downregulates α chains.[25] In addition, microcytosis associated with abnormal α chain synthesis has been described in cases of classic Hodgkin lymphoma.[26]

A third form of thalassemia, termed *δβ-thalassemia,* is caused by deletions of large segments of DNA on chromosome 11, including both δ and β genes. Heterozygotes present as thalassemia minor with microcytosis and no anemia. Their HbF ($\alpha_2\gamma_2$) levels are typically elevated (5% to 20%), and HbA2 ($\alpha_2\delta_2$) is normal or low.[27] Patients homozygous for the δ-β mutation have 100% HbF and clinical findings similar to those of thalassemia intermedia. Rarely, patients have a thalassemic picture as a result of structurally abnormal hemoglobins, such as hemoglobins Constant Spring, Lepore, and HbE.[28]

Normochromic Normocytic Anemia or Hypochromic Microcytic Anemia

The following anemias are most often normochromic and normocytic but may occasionally be hypochromic and microcytic.

Anemia of Inflammation

Anemia of inflammation (AoI), also known as *anemia of chronic disease (ACD),* is second only to iron-deficiency anemia in frequency. It is observed in patients with infectious, inflammatory, traumatic, or neoplastic disorders and is thus common among hospitalized patients. AoI is characterized by a low serum iron concentration in the face of normal or increased iron stores. It results from cytokine-induced hepcidin production that suppresses erythropoiesis and causes a mild shortening of RBC life

span, impaired mobilization of iron from reticuloendothelial stores to erythroid precursors, lower than expected erythropoietin production, decreased erythrocyte survival, and an inadequate response of erythroid precursors to erythropoietin.[29] The relative contribution of each of these findings may vary according to the underlying disease. For instance, in chronic renal failure, the anemia often has a multifactorial cause, including the effect of certain still ill-defined plasma factors. However, a primary cause is underproduction of erythropoietin by the damaged kidneys.

The liver peptide hormone hepcidin is a major regulator of iron homeostasis and plays a central role in the pathogenesis of AoI.[10] Hepcidin blocks the activity of ferroportin, a transport protein that facilitates basolateral movement of iron from the intestinal apical cells and from histiocytes. Thus, an increase in hepcidin in inflammation leads to hypoferremia, impaired delivery of iron to erythroid precursors, and hyperferritinemia (Fig. 10-2).[29] The expression of hepcidin is upregulated by interleukin (IL)-6 (which can be increased by IL-1) and inhibited by tumor necrosis factor-α and by erythroferrone, the erythroblast-produced modulator of iron homeostasis.[5]

Suppression of erythropoiesis in AoI may be reversible by exogenous erythropoietin (or derivatives), but responses depend on the type of cytokines involved in stimulating hepcidin production.[30] For example, erythropoietin treatment is less effective for correcting the anemia of malignancy than for treating the anemia of chronic renal failure.[31] The beneficial or detrimental effects of providing supplemental iron also appear to depend on the underlying condition.[32] Hepcidin antagonists are being explored as promising therapies for AoI.[29,33,34] Erythroferrone, the strongest extrahepatic negative regulator of hepcidin, may also be a candidate therapeutic target.[5,35]

The normochromic normocytic form of AoI is generally mild to moderate and is far more prevalent than the hypochromic microcytic type, which is usually seen with progression and exacerbation of the underlying disease (Fig. 10-7A). Iron studies are helpful to exclude iron deficiency. However, ferritin can be difficult to interpret, because it is an acute phase protein; a ferritin level greater than 60 μg/L should be considered indicative of adequate iron stores. The bone marrow is usually normocellular, with normal or slightly decreased numbers of erythroid precursors (Fig. 10-7B). Bone marrow examination is helpful primarily in assessing the iron status when iron studies are indeterminate. A Prussian blue stain of the aspirate shows increased accumulation of reticuloendothelial iron stores in histiocytes and decreased sideroblast iron (Fig. 10-8; Table 10-1). This staining pattern excludes iron deficiency; chronic blood loss also becomes a less likely cause.

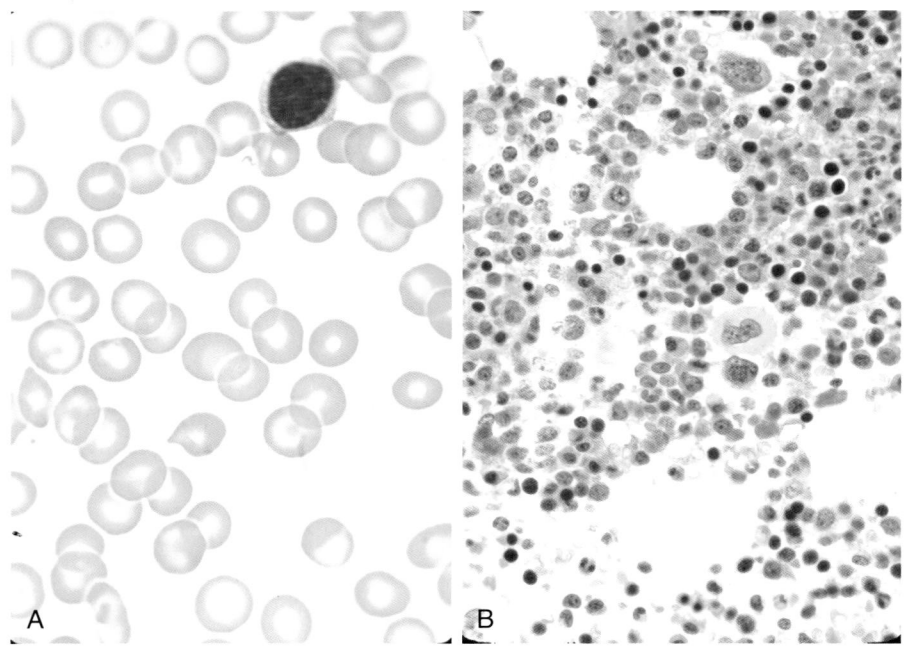

Figure 10-7. A, Slightly hypochromic normocytic red blood cells in anemia of inflammation associated with rheumatoid arthritis. **B,** Bone marrow erythroid precursors are present in normal numbers.

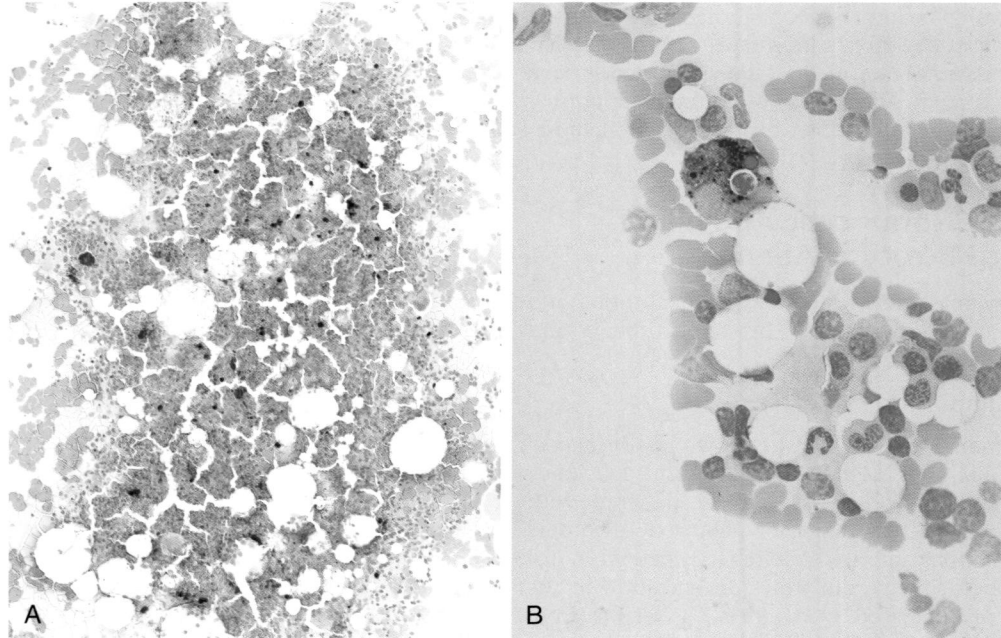

Figure 10-8. A, Anemia of inflammation, iron stores are increased in stromal histiocytes. **B,** Erythroid iron incorporation is decreased or undetectable.

Sideroblastic Anemias

Sideroblastic anemias are a heterogeneous group of disorders that are unified pathologically by abnormal accumulation of mitochondrial iron and impaired heme synthesis. The blood film often shows a striking dimorphic RBC picture with varying numbers of hypochromic and normochromic RBCs (Figs. 10-9 and 10-10). The constellation of blood findings (Table 10-1)

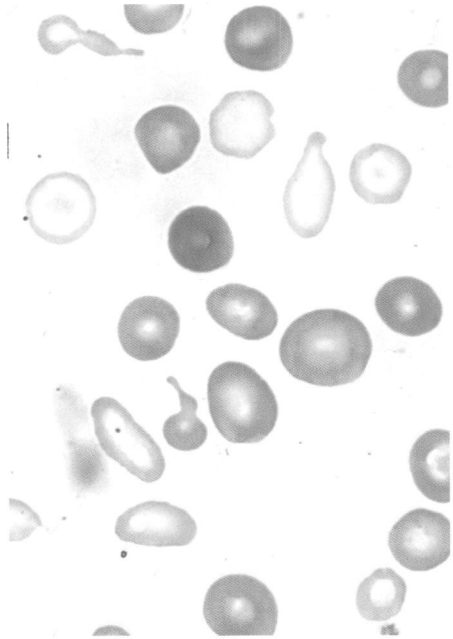

Figure 10-9. Pyridoxine-responsive sideroblastic anemia showing a dimorphic population of normochromic normocytic red blood cells and hypochromic microcytes. Hypochromic teardrop forms are common in sideroblastic anemia.

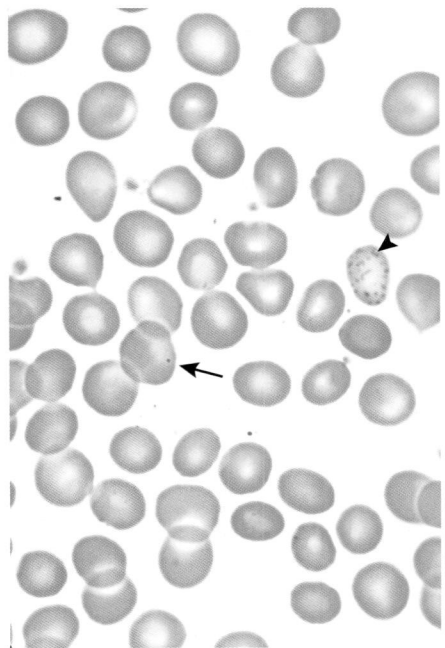

Figure 10-10. Coarse basophilic stippling *(arrowhead)* and Pappenheimer granules *(arrow)* are seen in this case of sideroblastic anemia associated with lead poisoning.

merits a bone marrow examination for definitive diagnosis. The bone marrow exhibits erythroid hyperplasia with normoblastic to megaloblastic maturation (Figs. 10-11 and 10-12). Occasional dysplastic changes are seen, especially in the acquired clonal disorders. In some congenital disorders, such as Pearson marrow-pancreas syndrome, large coalescent vacuoles may be found in the cytoplasm of bone marrow precursors (Fig. 10-13). The diagnostic feature is the presence of increased iron stores and ring sideroblasts, in which five or more large, siderotic granules are found in a perinuclear ring around one-third or

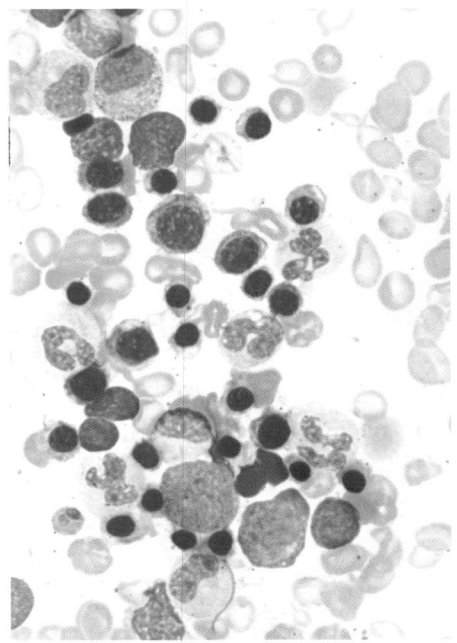

Figure 10-11. Ineffective erythropoiesis produces erythroid hyperplasia in most cases of sideroblastic anemia.

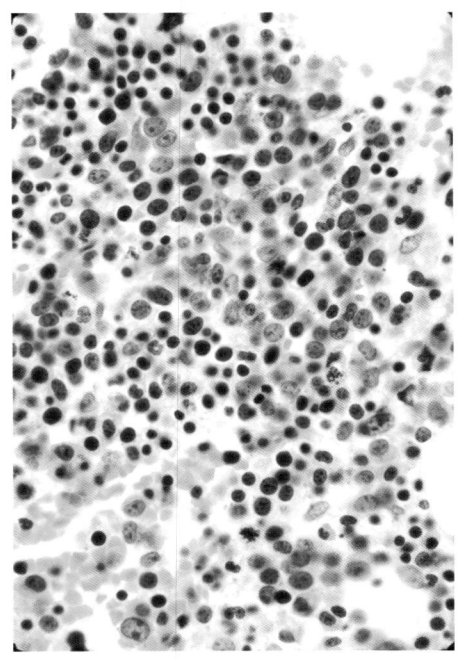

Figure 10-12. Markedly hypercellular bone marrow with erythroid hyperplasia in pyridoxine-responsive sideroblastic anemia.

more of the nucleus (Fig. 10-14). Sideroblastic iron granules are often more numerous and larger than normal. When examined by electron microscopy, large electron-dense deposits are found within mitochondria. Ineffective hematopoiesis is the primary cause of the anemia. Although the mechanisms responsible for sideroblastic anemia are not fully understood, the adverse effects of excess iron on mitochondrial heme synthesis and pyridoxine metabolism play a large role.[36]

Sideroblastic anemias can be classified as congenital or acquired (Box 10-1). The congenital sideroblastic anemias

(CSAs) are most common in children, presenting soon after birth to later in childhood. They most often affect males and show an X-linked pattern of inheritance. The most common form of X-linked sideroblastic anemia is caused by a mutation in the gene that encodes δ-aminolevulinic acid (ALA) synthetase, an enzyme important in the early steps of heme synthesis (Fig. 10-2).[37] The mutation affects the enzyme's affinity for its cofactor, pyridoxal-5′-phosphate. Some patients with this abnormality may respond to pyridoxine; in others, the mutation decreases the stability of the enzyme, and they are resistant

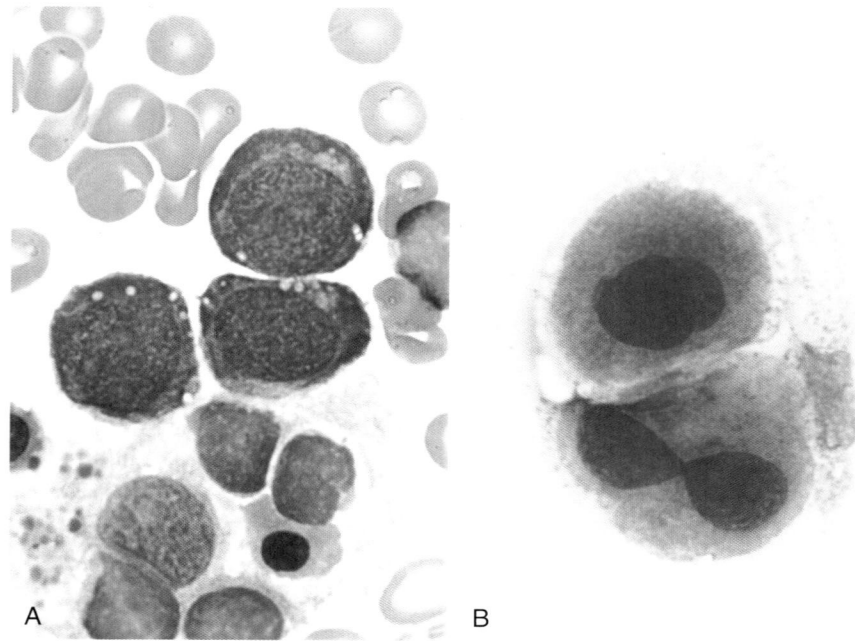

Figure 10-13. Cytoplasmic vacuoles in pronormoblasts **(A)** and megakaryocytes **(B)** are often found in Pearson marrow-pancreas syndrome. This rare form of sideroblastic anemia is associated with exocrine pancreas failure and is caused by deletions or duplications of mitochondrial DNA.

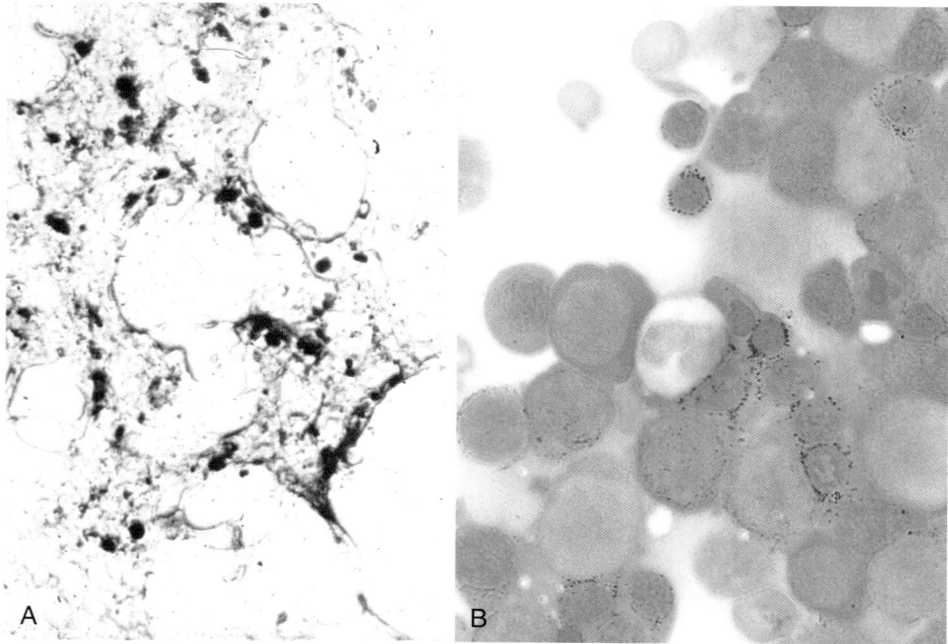

Figure 10-14. Increased iron stores **(A)** and numerous ring sideroblasts **(B)** are the diagnostic hallmarks of all forms of sideroblastic anemia.

to pyridoxine therapy. Another form, X-linked sideroblastic anemia with ataxia, is caused by a mutation in the gene that encodes the transporter protein ABCB7.[37] Autosomal recessive forms include sideroblastic anemias caused by defects in heme synthesis or iron-sulfur biogenesis. CSAs caused by abnormal mitochondrial protein synthesis have been identified.[37] Perhaps the best example is Pearson marrow-pancreas syndrome (Fig. 10-13), which occurs sporadically and is characterized by lactic acidosis, exocrine pancreatic insufficiency, sideroblastic anemia, and large deletions or duplications in mitochondrial DNA (mtDNA).[38] Another CSA, mitochondrial myopathy with

lactic acidosis and ring sideroblasts, is caused by defective mitochondrial protein expression.[39] Point mutations in mtDNA have also been rarely reported.[37] Sideroblastic anemia, immunodeficiency, fevers, and developmental delay is a recently recognized entity caused by defects in cytosolic and mitochondrial protein translation.[37]

The primary or idiopathic acquired forms of sideroblastic anemia include clonal disorders that fall in the spectrum of MDS and MDS/myeloproliferative neoplasms (MPN), which are often associated with somatic mutations in *SF3B1*.[40] They are discussed in Chapter 44 and Chapter 48, respectively.

The secondary and less common forms of acquired sideroblastic anemia are the result of drugs and exposure to toxins, many of which have been characterized. For example, the drug isoniazid inhibits pyridoxine metabolism, lead inhibits δ-ALA dehydratase and heme synthetase, and alcohol produces a direct toxic effect on erythroid precursors (found in 30% of hospitalized alcoholics). The anemia can be reversed by administration of pyridoxal phosphate and discontinuation of the offending drug. Copper deficiency anemia, often secondary to zinc overload, displays red cells that may be microcytic, normocytic, or macrocytic.

Normochromic Normocytic Anemia, Underproduction

The normochromic normocytic anemias are characterized by red cells of normal size and hemoglobin content. They are most easily divided by reticulocyte count into disorders of underproduction (low or normal reticulocyte count) and increased production (high reticulocyte count) (Fig. 10-1).

Pure Red Cell Aplasia

Pure red cell aplasia is an isolated failure of erythropoiesis that results in anemia with reticulocytopenia in the setting of normal neutrophil and platelet counts. The marrow shows absent or diminished erythroid precursors, often with a

---

> **Box 10-1** *Classification of Sideroblastic Anemias*
>
> **Congenital**
> - X-linked sideroblastic anemia (XLSA)
>   - XLSA caused by ALAS2 deficiency
>   - XLSA with ataxia caused by ABCB7 deficiency
> - Autosomal recessive sideroblastic anemia (ARSA)
>   - ARSA caused by mutations in *SLC25A38, GLRX5*
>   - Thiamine responsive megaloblastic anemia caused by mutations in *SLC19A2*
> - Mitochondrial DNA mutations or deletions
>   - Pearson marrow-pancreas syndrome
>   - Mitochondrial myopathy with lactic acidosis and ring sideroblasts (MLASA) caused by mutations in *PUS1* or *YARS2*
>
> **Acquired**
> - Clonal (Often associated with *SF3B1* mutations)
>   - Myelodysplastic syndromes
>   - Myelodysplastic/myeloproliferative neoplasms
> - Non-clonal
>   - Drugs* (isoniazid, chloramphenicol, cycloserine, penicillamine, azathioprine)
>   - Alcohol
>   - Lead poisoning, arsenic
>   - Copper deficiency

* Drug list is not all-inclusive.

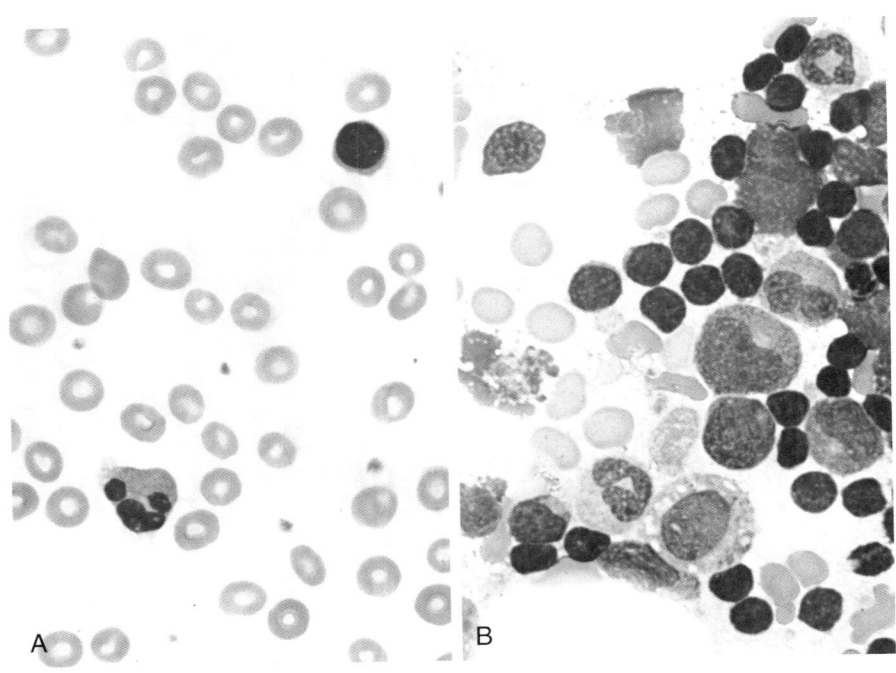

Figure 10-15. A, Severe anemia with reticulocytopenia was the presenting feature in this child with pure red cell aplasia. **B,** The bone marrow aspirate shows an absence of erythroid precursors. Granulocytic maturation is normal. Increased numbers of hematogones are present.

left shift in erythroid maturation (Fig. 10-15). Pure red cell aplasia can be classified as congenital or acquired (Box 10-2). The congenital form, Diamond-Blackfan anemia (DBA), is classified as a macrocytic anemia. The acquired forms of pure red cell aplasia more frequently present with normochromic normocytic anemia and have been associated with autoimmune/collagen vascular disorders, lymphoproliferative disorders, infections, pregnancy, myeloid malignancies, non-hematologic neoplasms, drugs, and toxic agents.[41] The anemia may be acute and transient or chronic, depending on the cause.

Parvovirus B19 is the most common identifiable cause of red cell aplasia in children and immunocompromised adults.[42] The virus selectively invades and replicates in erythroid progenitor cells, causing direct cytotoxic effects with interruption of erythrocyte production. In children, it is associated with erythema infectiosum (fifth disease),

a transient, asymptomatic drop in hemoglobin of about 1 g/dL, with recovery in 10 to 19 days. Children with a hemolytic disorder that shortens the RBC life span, such as red cell enzyme deficiencies, membrane abnormalities, hemoglobinopathies, or malaria infection, often have a more profound anemia and "aplastic crisis" (Fig. 10-16). Parvovirus B19 may persist in immunocompromised individuals who fail to produce neutralizing antibodies to eradicate the virus. Infection manifests as a chronic instead of acute pure red cell aplasia unless patients are treated with intravenous immunoglobulin therapy.[42] Bone marrow findings depend on the timing of the evaluation. Initial RBC depletion may be followed by a wave of early progenitors without maturation. Giant pronormoblasts with intranuclear viral inclusions are transient but may be occasionally identified, particularly in immunocompromised individuals. Viral-associated suppression of myelopoiesis and megakaryopoiesis occurs with rare cases of marrow necrosis. Serum polymerase chain reaction studies for parvovirus B19 DNA, elevated IgM antibody titers, and immunostaining for parvovirus on marrow biopsy sections are diagnostic.

The sudden onset of pure red cell aplasia is often associated with a history of recent respiratory or gastrointestinal viral infection or the use of drugs administered for infectious or inflammatory conditions. Box 10-2 provides a partial list of drugs that may be responsible, with resolution of the aplasia typically occurring with drug cessation. The rare formation of anti-erythropoietin antibodies secondary to erythropoietin treatment in patients with renal failure has been described. This phenomenon was eventually linked to the use of leachates in uncoated rubber stoppers of prefilled syringes; upon recognition, it is now even more rare.[41,43] Transient erythroblastopenia of childhood is an uncommon, acute, and transient anemia characterized by reduced or absent mature erythroid precursors in normocellular bone marrow.[44,45] The cause remains elusive.[41]

Most chronic, acquired pure red cell aplasia cases are idiopathic and believed to be caused by a cytotoxic T-cell mediated process resulting from unknown triggers, with destruction of early erythroid precursors.[43] Classic associations

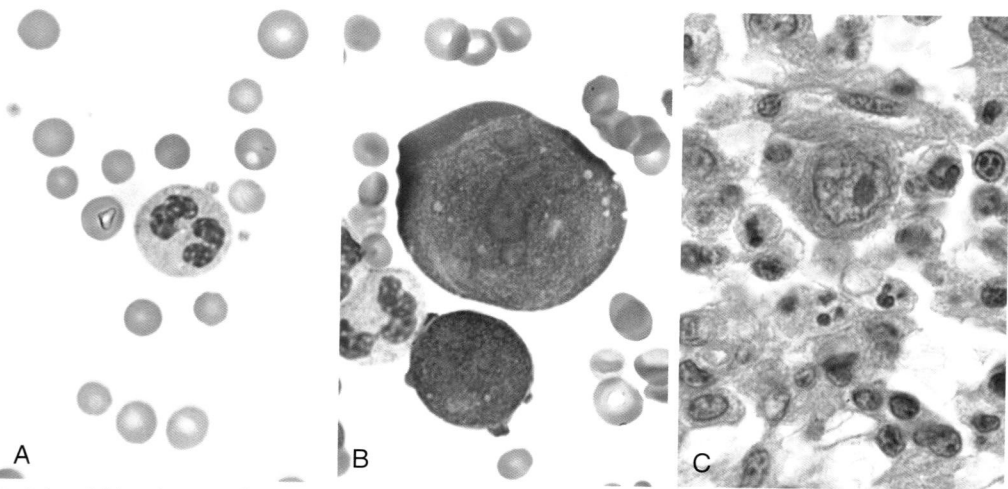

Figure 10-16. A, Peripheral blood smear from a patient with hereditary spherocytosis who developed severe anemia from a parvovirus B19–associated "aplastic crisis." The bone marrow aspirate **(B)** and trephine biopsy **(C)** contained giant pronormoblasts with large, nucleoli-like parvovirus inclusions.

include thymoma, hematologic malignancies, and systemic autoimmune disorders. Despite the clearly established association between red cell aplasia and thymoma, less than 10% of individuals with aplasia are found to have thymomas upon radiographic evaluation. A significant proportion of idiopathic cases is likely secondary to the frequently underdiagnosed T-cell large granular lymphocyte leukemia (Chapter 30), a clonal proliferation of cytotoxic T-cells.[46] In refractory patients without a clear underlying cause and normal cytogenetic studies, pure red cell aplasia may be the initial presentation for MDS.[47,48]

Aplastic Anemia

Aplastic anemia usually presents with pancytopenia and is discussed in this chapter's section on bone marrow failure syndromes.

Myelophthisic Anemias

Myelophthisic anemias are caused by replacement of normal marrow cells by metastatic tumor cells or other types of malignancy, granulomas, histiocytes in storage disease, or fibrosis and usually exhibit bicytopenia or pancytopenia. Although the anemia is typically normochromic and normocytic, red cell fragmentation, spherocytes, and teardrop forms are frequently encountered. Normoblasts and left-shifted granulocyte precursors produce a "leukoerythroblastic" blood picture in most cases associated with a metastatic tumor or fibrosis (Fig. 10-17). Bone marrow evaluation is essential to identify the underlying disorder.

Normochromic Normocytic Anemia, High Output

The remaining normochromic normocytic anemias, which include acute posthemorrhagic anemia and hemolytic anemias, show increased erythropoiesis with elevated reticulocyte counts.

Posthemorrhagic Anemia

Posthemorrhagic anemia caused by recent blood loss is normochromic and normocytic and is accompanied by a reticulocytosis that first manifests 3 to 5 days after blood loss. By 7 to 10 days, the reticulocytes may be so numerous that they increase the MCV up to 100 to 110 fL. Shortly after the hemorrhage, the first notable change in the blood is thrombocytosis, followed by demargination of neutrophils from the release of adrenergic hormones. Finally, the hemoglobin falls as extravascular fluids enter the vascular space.

Hemolytic Anemias

Hemolytic anemias are usually normochromic normocytic anemias in which an elevated reticulocyte count reflects compensation for increased RBC destruction. The process may be episodic or persistent. Hemolysis is caused by four basic abnormalities: intrinsic red cell defects, plasma factors, disruption of the cells by mechanical or thermal damage, and infectious agents (Table 10-3; Fig. 10-1). Patients with hemolytic anemia often have similar clinical and laboratory findings: normochromic normocytic anemia, reticulocytosis, shortened red cell life span, elevated erythropoietin level, increased indirect bilirubin, increased lactate dehydrogenase, markedly decreased haptoglobin, and jaundice. Those with chronic extravascular hemolysis also develop splenomegaly and gallstones. Bone marrow evaluation invariably shows erythroid hyperplasia, even in patients with only mild compensated hemolysis. Circulating red cells with characteristic shape changes (e.g., sickle cells, spherocytes, or schistocytes) are helpful in the diagnosis, whereas the erythroid precursors in the marrow usually have an unremarkable appearance. Identifying or confirming the cause of a hemolytic anemia relies on the patient's history (including the family history) and on definitive laboratory studies, as summarized in Table 10-3.

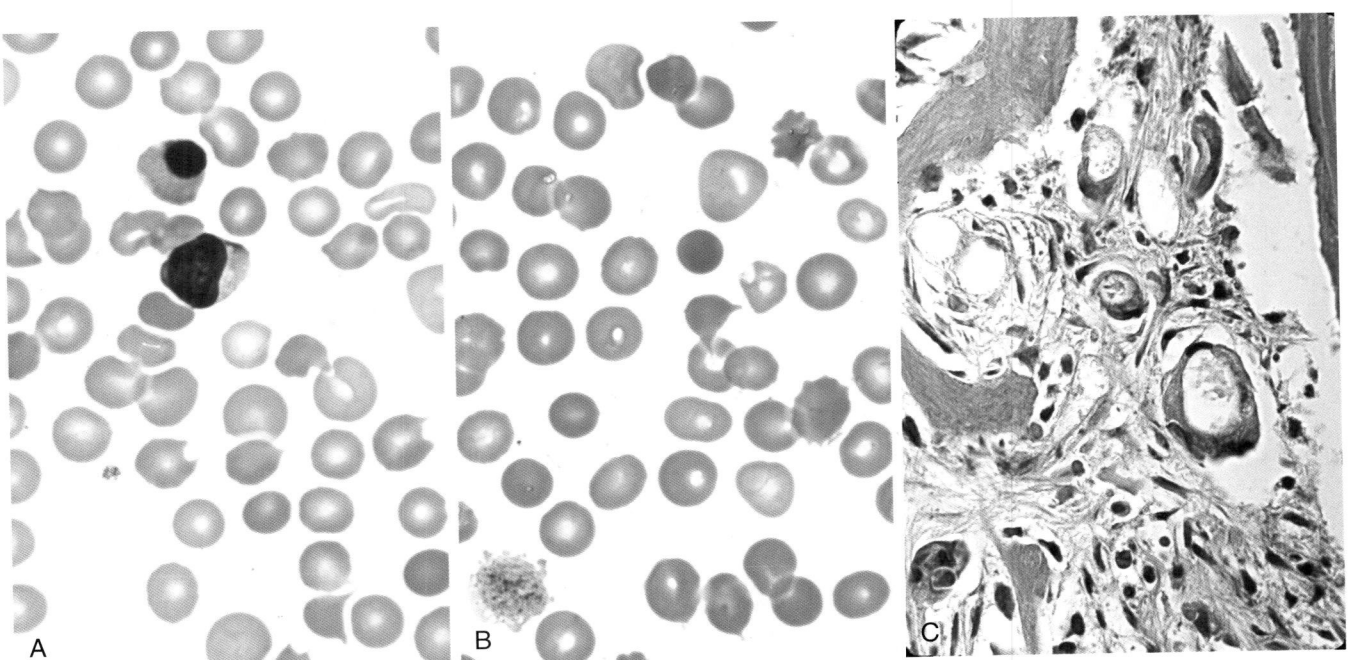

Figure 10-17. A, Myelophthisic anemia typically shows circulating normoblasts and red blood cell fragmentation. A left shift in all cell lines is common. **B,** Note the giant platelet. **C,** Metastatic adenocarcinoma produced the myelophthisic picture.

Table 10-3 Hemolytic Anemias

Cause	Disorder	Diagnostic Test
I. Intrinsic Red Blood Cell Defects		
1. RBC Membrane Defects		
Structural defects	Hereditary spherocytosis	Flow cytometric analysis of eosin-5′-
	Hereditary elliptocytosis	maleimide–labeled RBCs
	Hereditary pyropoikilocytosis	Incubated osmotic fragility
Transport defects	Hereditary stomatocytosis	Glycerol lysis test
		Cryohemolysis test
		Osmotic gradient ektacytometry
		Negative direct antiglobulin test
		Normal glucose-6-phosphate dehydrogenase
		Membrane protein analysis or quantification
		Genomic DNA analysis
2. RBC Enzyme Defects		
HMPS	Glucose-6-phosphate dehydrogenase	Quantitative enzyme assays
	Rare: GSH synthetase, γ-glutamylcysteine synthetase, glutathione reductase	Fluorescent screening tests
		Genomic DNA analysis
Glycolytic pathway*	Pyruvate kinase	
	Rare: hexokinase, aldolase, glucose phosphate isomerase, phosphofructokinase, triose phosphate isomerase, phosphoglycerate kinase	
3. Abnormal Hemoglobin		
Altered solubility	Hemoglobin SS, SC, S/D, S/O-Arab, DD, EE, S/β-thalassemia	High-performance liquid chromatography
		Hemoglobin electrophoresis
Oxidative susceptibility	Unstable hemoglobins (100 variants)	Isopropanol stability test
Abnormal structure	Thalassemias	Genomic DNA analysis
II. Plasma Factors		
1. Immune-mediated		
AIHA	Idiopathic, infection, autoimmune disorders, malignancy	Direct antiglobulin test
Alloimmune	Hemolytic disease of the newborn	ABO and Rh testing
2. Drug-induced		
3. Direct toxic effect		
Spider bites		Coagulation tests
Bee, snake (cobra) venom		
III. Mechanical or Thermal Damage		
Burns, heart valves, vasculitis, eclampsia, malignant hypertension, TTP, DIC, HUS		PT, PTT, D-dimer, fibrinogen, BUN, creatinine
IV. Infection		
Malaria, *Babesia*, *Bartonella*, *Clostridium perfringens*		Peripheral blood smears, cultures
V. Splenic Sequestration		
Hypersplenism—usually distribution abnormality		Physical examination, radiographic studies

*Embden-Meyerhof.
AIHA, Autoimmune hemolytic anemia; *BUN,* blood urea nitrogen; *DIC,* disseminated intravascular coagulation; *GSH,* reduced glutathione; *HMPS,* hexose monophosphate shunt; *HUS,* hemolytic uremic syndrome; *PT,* prothrombin time; *PTT,* partial thromboplastin time; *RBC,* red blood cell; *TTP,* thrombotic thrombocytopenic purpura.

Hemolysis Caused by Intrinsic Red Cell Disorders

As these anemias are inherited, a history of lifelong anemia or a family history of anemia, cholelithiasis, jaundice, or mild splenomegaly is helpful in the diagnosis. A notable exception is paroxysmal nocturnal hemoglobinuria (PNH), an acquired defect described later in this chapter's section on bone marrow failure syndromes.

Red Blood Cell Membrane Disorders

Many advances have been made in understanding the molecular basis of a number of RBC membrane disorders (Table 10-4).[49-51] The red cell membrane is composed of a lipid bilayer, a network of "horizontally" positioned skeletal proteins on the inner surface, and transmembrane proteins that "vertically" traverse the lipid bilayer. The skeletal proteins maintain shape and deformability, and the transmembrane proteins provide membrane cohesiveness. Among the more than 50 transmembrane proteins are transport proteins, receptors, and antigens. Mutations in genes encoding key membrane proteins, particularly spectrin, ankyrin, protein 4.1R, protein 4.2, and band 3, lead to inherited red cell membrane disorders. Membrane disorders can be caused by structural defects or defects in membrane transport.

Hereditary Spherocytosis

Hereditary spherocytosis (HS) is a common cause of nonimmune hemolytic anemia caused by abnormalities in the RBC transmembrane proteins.[49] The defect leads to

Table 10-4 Red Blood Cell Membrane Disorders

Disorder	Defect (Inheritance)	RBC Morphology	Comments
Hereditary spherocytosis	Ankyrin (AD, AR): *ANK-1* mutation Band 3 (AD): *SLC4A1* β spectrin (AD): *SPTB* α spectrin (AR): *SPTA1* Protein 4.2 (AR): *EPB42*	Spherocytes + acanthocytes (5%-10%) Spherocytes, microspherocytes, poikilocytes Spherocytes Few spherocytes, ovalocytes, stomatocytes Spherocytes + "pincered" cells (<5%) "Mushroom" shape in cases of band 3 defect	All ethnic groups, ↑ in those of northern European ancestry (1/2000 incidence), North American, Japanese 75% AD; 25% AR or sporadic 50% ankyrin or combined ankyrin-spectrin protein deficiency
Hereditary elliptocytosis	α spectrin (AD) β spectrin (AD) Protein 4.1 (AD) Glycoprotein C (AD)	Elliptocytes—usually >25% of RBCs If moderate-to-severe anemia: schistocytes, budding RBCs	Heterogeneous clinical, genetic disorder ↑ in those of African and Mediterranean ancestry Majority—partial α and β spectrin deficiencies 10% isolated spectrin deficiency
Southeast Asian ovalocytosis	Band 3 (AD)	Ovalocytes (20%-50%) with 1-2 transverse bars or single longitudinal slit	Very rigid red cell membrane but mechanically stable Little hemolysis
Hereditary pyropoikilocytosis	α spectrin (AR)	Fragile cells fragment into bizarre shapes in circulation, including budding, fragments, spherocytes, triangulocytes	Subset of hereditary elliptocytosis ↑ in those of African ancestry Infants and children present with severe hemolytic anemia and develop associated complications (e.g., growth retardation, bone abnormalities) Cells have ↑ thermal sensitivity
Hereditary stomatocytosis Four subtypes: Dehydrated hereditary stomatocytosis (DHSt) Overhydrated hereditary stomatocytosis (OHS) Cryohydrocytosis (CHC) Familial pseudohyperkalemia (FP)	PIEZO (AD); *PIEZO* in DHSt1 Gardos Channel (AD); *KCNN4* in DHSt2 Rh-associated glycoprotein (AD); *RHAG* in OHS Band 3 (AD); *SLC4A1* in CHC ABCB6 (AD); *ABCB6* in FP	Stomatocytes, target cells, schistocytes, spiculated cells DHSt: MCHC increased, slightly increased MCV OHS: MCHC decreased, high MCV (>110 fL) CHC: MCV normal, MCHC normal FP: MCV normal-high, MCHC normal	DHSt has a mild-to-moderate phenotype, whereas OHS causes the most severe hemolytic anemia

AD, Autosomal dominant; *AR,* autosomal recessive; *RBC,* red blood cell; *MCV,* mean corpuscular volume; *MCHC,* mean corpuscular hemoglobin concentration.

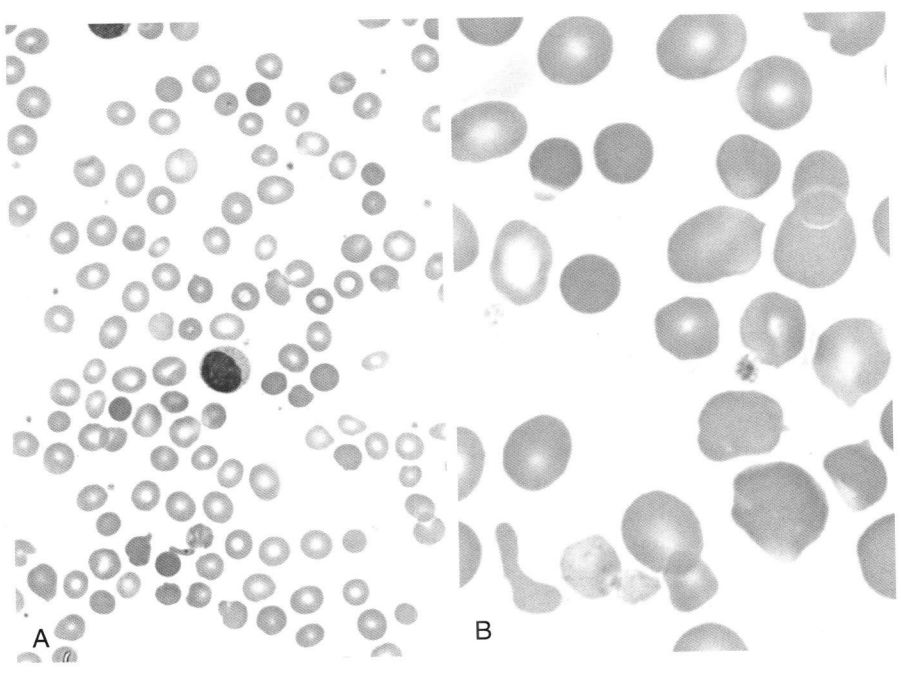

Figure 10-18. A, In this case of hereditary spherocytosis, the number of red blood cells is moderately decreased, and spherocytes are readily apparent. **B,** Spherocytes are smaller and stain more darkly than the surrounding normocytes and large polychromatophilic red blood cells.

local discohesion of the membrane skeleton from the lipid bilayer, which creates a microvesicle with subsequent loss of membrane and formation of a spherocyte. Spherocytosis is the hallmark of HS and should be suspected if the red cell indices include a normal or low MCV and the MCHC after warming remains 36 g/dL or greater (Fig. 10-18). The less deformable spherocytes are selectively trapped in the spleen and are vulnerable to further surface membrane loss and destruction. Genetic defects vary among different racial groups, and heterogeneous molecular abnormalities are often family specific. Gene mutations typically shift the normal reading frames or introduce premature stop codons that result in mutant alleles that fail to produce protein. The specific gene involved (i.e., the molecular phenotype) may not strictly relate to the biochemical phenotype (i.e., the abnormal protein produced).[52] For example, an ankyrin gene defect may manifest as a spectrin protein deficiency. It is usually the spectrin content of the red cell that best correlates with the degree of anemia, percentage of circulating spherocytes, reticulocyte count, and increased osmotic fragility.

Clinically, anemia is the presenting feature in nearly half of patients with HS, although disease severity varies widely among individuals. Mild compensated hemolysis is observed in about 20% of individuals, with most affected people (60%) having moderate hemolysis with a hemoglobin level of 8 to 11 g/dL and reticulocyte percentage generally higher than 8%. At birth, patients with HS usually have a normal hemoglobin value that may sharply and transiently decrease during the first 20 days of life to a level that requires blood transfusions.[53] The more asymptomatic forms of HS may not be identified until a hemolytic crisis develops during childhood, often triggered by a viral infection. Less commonly, an aplastic crisis develops secondary to parvovirus B19 infection (Fig. 10-16). Although a family history of HS is often elicited in individuals suspected of having HS, the most severe forms of the disease are recessive and associated with α-spectrin and some ankyrin defects.[54] Sporadic mutations are particularly common in the autosomal recessive forms of HS. Several diagnostic methods for HS are available, including osmotic fragility studies, flow cytometric analysis of eosin-5'-maleimide (EMA)-labeled RBCs, and osmotic gradient ektacytometry; yet, each test may have considerable false positives and false negatives. Osmotic gradient ektacytometry has the advantage of producing distinct deformability profiles for several types of red cell disorders, but it is not widely available.[55] EMA analysis exhibits the greatest disease specificity for HS at 98%; however, a subset of cases of HS may still be unrecognized with this test alone.[56] Although EMA binds specifically with band 3 protein, membrane protein abnormalities in HS other than band 3 deficiency affect binding and therefore the fluorescent intensity of the dye measured by flow cytometry. Coupled with peripheral blood smear review and depending on availability of testing, the recommended laboratory tests include flow cytometry for EMA binding and the cryohemolysis test.[57] A recently proposed diagnostic algorithm suggests using a combination of EMA testing, osmotic fragility testing, and/or acidified glycerol lysis tests in combination with genetic testing for difficult cases; however, not all of these tests are widely available.[58] Splenectomy has been the primary mode of therapy, but it is not without complications.[59]

Hereditary Elliptocytosis and Hereditary Pyropoikilocytosis

Hereditary elliptocytosis (HE) and hereditary pyropoikilocytosis (HPP) were originally described as distinct entities, but molecular studies have established that HPP is a subset of HE (Tables 10-3 and 10-4).[60] They are caused by defects in the horizontal protein interactions that hold the membrane skeleton together. The abnormality that best correlates with disease severity is a failure of spectrin homodimers to self-associate into heterodimers, the basic building blocks of the

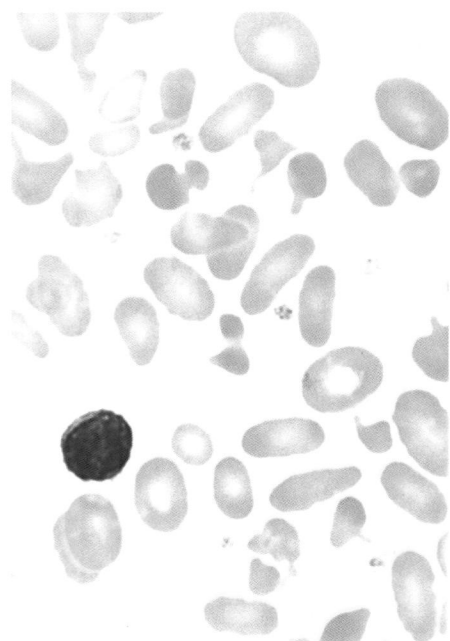

Figure 10-19. Hereditary pyropoikilocytosis. Numerous elliptocytes, fragmented red blood cells, and teardrop forms were found in this child's blood. The mother's blood looked similar. The father's blood was normal.

membrane skeleton. Differences in the clinical severity of HE cannot always be explained by a specific genetic defect. The most prevalent form of the disease is a single gene defect (heterozygous) that causes the red cells to elongate and form elliptocytes in circulation, without anemia or significant splenomegaly. The more severe form of the disease, HPP, is caused by a combination of two defective membrane protein genes that result in marked spectrin deficiency in addition to functionally abnormal proteins. The MCV may be very low because of marked RBC fragmentation, rendering the clinical presentation atypical for a hemolytic anemia, with possible microcytic rather than normocytic RBC indices (Fig. 10-19). A disorder related to HE called *Southeast Asian ovalocytosis* is found in people from Malaysia, Indonesia, the Philippines, and Papua New Guinea.[61] Only a subset of affected individuals has hemolytic anemia, with distinctive oval stomatocytes and theta cells, which have two central pallors.[62] This variant red cell may protect individuals against cerebral malaria.

Hereditary Stomatocytosis Syndromes. Hereditary stomatocytosis syndromes are a group of disorders of the RBC membrane characterized by a mouth-shaped central area of pallor and abnormal permeability to sodium and potassium (Fig. 10-20).[63] This rare red cell disorder is subdivided into four entities: xerocytosis or dehydrated hereditary stomatocytosis (DHSt), overhydrated hereditary stomatocytosis (OHS), cryohydrocytosis (CHC), and familial pseudohyperkalemia (FP).[49,55] Loss of potassium leads to RBC dehydration and mild-to-moderate anemia in the more frequent form, DHSt. Automated counts show an increased MCHC and normal MCV (falsely elevated on some automated counters). A misdiagnosis of atypical HSt is often made. Mutations in *PIEZO1* and *KCNN4* have been identified in DHSt.[49] The PIEZO protein may play a critical role in red cell cation and volume homeostasis. The second subtype, OHS, caused by mutations

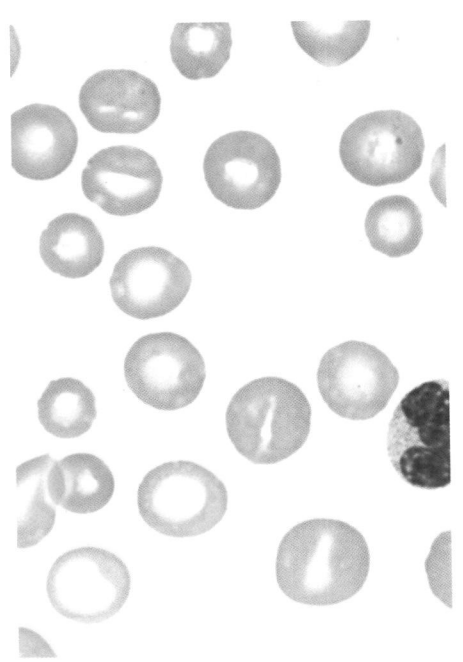

Figure 10-20. Hereditary stomatocytosis. Stomatocytes are often darker than surrounding red blood cells and have a slitlike central pallor from the loss of intracellular fluid.

Table 10-5 Common Glucose-6-Phosphate Dehydrogenase (G6PD) Variants

Isoform	Ethnic Group	Comments
G6PD B	All	Most common, normal variant
G6PD A	African descent (20%)	Normal variant, no hemolysis
G6PD A−	African descent (11%)	Group of variants with same mutation as G6PD A, but with one additional mutation Moderate hemolysis Unstable enzyme, ↑ decay
G6PD^MED	Greek, Arabian, Sicilian, Sephardic Jewish descent	Severe hemolysis Protects against *Plasmodium falciparum*
G6PD^CANTON	Asian descent	Moderate hemolysis

in *RHAG*, is rare and leads to a severe hemolytic phenotype. It is characterized by a 20-fold to 40-fold increase in cation leak, leading to hydrated red cells, a large increase in MCV, and decreased MCHC. Patients with DHSt and OHS have severe thrombotic complications after splenectomy; thus, avoidance of this procedure is important.[55] CHC is characterized by increased permeability to sodium and potassium at low temperatures. Gain-of-function mutations in *SLC4A1* are associated with CHC.[64] FP is an asymptomatic trait caused by mutations in the *ABCB6* gene, which presents with artifactually high potassium levels resulting from red cell leak at low temperatures.[49,55] Of note, stomatocytes can also be seen as an artifact of slowly dried peripheral blood smears.

Red Blood Cell Enzyme Defects. RBC energy requirements are met primarily through the metabolism of glucose by the Embden-Meyerhof glycolytic pathway. Alternatively, approximately 10% of glucose is metabolized by the hexose monophosphate shunt. Erythrocyte disorders caused by enzyme deficiencies of the glycolytic pathway are extremely rare, and approximately 90% of these are deficiencies of pyruvate kinase caused primarily by *PK-LR* gene mutations on chromosome 1q21 (Table 10-3).[65] The majority are inherited as autosomal recessive traits and first detected in infancy or childhood with the clinical presentation of chronic hemolysis. Pyruvate kinase deficiency can be diagnosed by enzyme analysis and DNA studies. The direct antiglobulin test (Coombs test), hemoglobin electrophoresis, and osmotic fragility are normal. The peripheral blood film shows normochromic normocytic RBCs without spherocytes. The remaining morphologic findings are non-specific but include reticulocytosis and erythroid hyperplasia.

Hereditary disorders of the hexose monophosphate shunt enzymes are also rare, except glucose-6-phosphate dehydrogenase (G6PD) deficiency. G6PD deficiency is one of the most prevalent inborn errors of metabolism.[66] There

are at least 230 variants of G6PD with known mutations; all but two of them are either missense mutations or small in-frame deletions (Table 10-5). It is particularly prevalent in populations from geographic areas with endemic malaria, suggesting evolutionary polymorphisms developed to counteract the effects of this parasite. The *G6PD* gene is carried on the X chromosome, and full expression of G6PD deficiency is found only in males; female carriers may have partial deficiency. Clinical manifestations of G6PD deficiency include neonatal jaundice and hereditary nonspherocytic hemolytic anemia. The most serious consequence of G6PD deficiency is neonatal jaundice leading to kernicterus, which is worsened by associated Gilbert's disease.[67] Although a few patients have chronic hemolytic anemia, the majority have episodic anemia induced by increased oxidative stress in erythrocytes from certain foods (fava beans), a number of drugs (sulfonamides, nitrofurans, quinine derivatives, aspirin, rasburicase), and chemicals (naphthalene, toluidine blue).[68,69] Erythrocytes deficient in G6PD are unable to maintain sufficient reduced glutathione for the generation of nicotinamide adenine dinucleotide + hydrogen (NADH), a cofactor that maintains hemoglobin integrity. The WHO has classified G6PD variants based on their degree of enzyme deficiency and severity of hemolysis: class I, less than 10% enzyme activity with severe chronic (nonspherocytic) hemolytic anemia, to class V, increased enzyme level with no hemolysis or clinical sequelae. Oxidant damage is reflected by marked anisopoikilocytosis with "bite" cells and increased polychromatophilia on the peripheral blood film (Fig. 10-21). Supravital staining demonstrates denatured hemoglobin precipitates (Heinz bodies) (Fig. 10-22). The bone marrow most commonly demonstrates erythroid hyperplasia.

Hereditary pyrimidine 5′-nucleotidase deficiency is the third most common cause of chronic nonspherocytic hemolytic anemia related to red cell enzyme defects, after deficiency of PK and G6PD. The peripheral blood smear is characterized by red cells with prominent coarse basophilic stippling secondary to accumulation of precipitated pyrimidine nucleotides.[70,71]

Hemoglobinopathies. Hemoglobinopathies are abnormalities of hemoglobin structure caused by abnormal amino acid sequences in either the α or β globin chains. The most prevalent abnormal hemoglobin is HbS, produced by the substitution of glutamate for valine at the sixth position of the β globin chain. The gene for HbS has autosomal dominant inheritance and is found in areas of the world where malaria

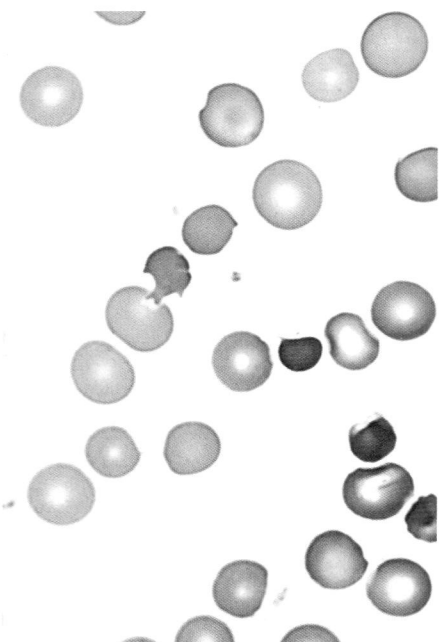

Figure 10-21. Oxidant hemolysis causes hemoglobin to precipitate at the cell membrane. The spleen removes the aggregates of hemoglobin and associated membrane, producing "bite" cells and spherocytes.

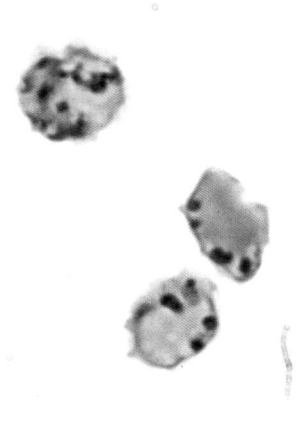

Figure 10-22. This wet mount stained with methylene blue illustrates membrane-associated Heinz bodies seen in oxidant hemolysis.

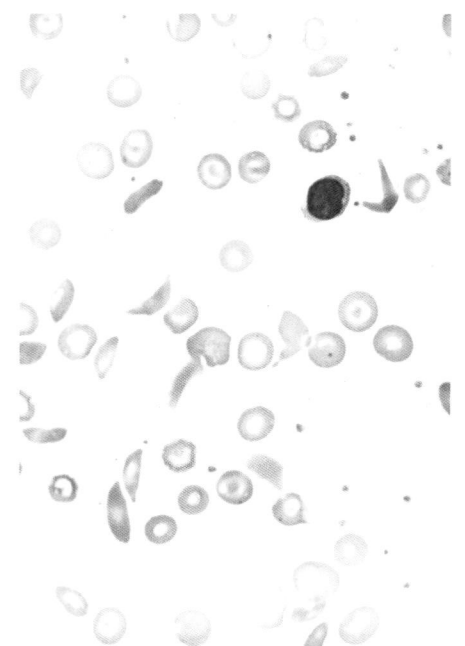

Figure 10-23. Numerous sickled red blood cells and target cells are seen in this patient with sickle cell anemia.

is common.[72] Approximately 8% to 10% of the African American population carries at least one HbS gene.[73] Sickle cell disease occurs in individuals with homozygous sickle mutations (termed *HbSS* or *sickle cell anemia*) or compound heterozygous mutations, most commonly sickle cell β-thalassemia or hemoglobin S-C (HbSC) disease. RBC sickling is induced under conditions of deoxygenation, vasoconstriction, acidosis, increased HbS concentration, and infection. The clinical symptoms of the sickle cell disorders vary greatly in severity among individuals,[74] but they are often a result of the increased tendency of sickle cells to adhere to vascular endothelium and to the ensuing vaso-occlusive complications.[75] Cells become irreversibly sickled and are removed by the reticuloendothelial system. The hallmark of these disorders is morphologically altered red cells (Fig. 10-23). In addition to the sickle cells, irregularly shaped cells, targets, spherocytes, and polychromatophilic cells may be found on the blood film. Howell-Jolly bodies are usually identified in older individuals as a result of autosplenectomy. A left-shifted neutrophilia with toxic features and thrombocytosis are common during an acute crisis. Heterozygous disorders may additionally show microcytosis (Sβ-thalassemia) or intracellular crystals (HbSC disease) (Fig. 10-24). Patients with sickle cell anemia may also develop acute splenic sequestration, parvovirus-related red cell aplasia, and bone marrow necrosis. In addition to erythroid hyperplasia, bone marrow biopsies frequently show increased arterial fibrosis.[76] Patients with sickle cell disease with a genotype other than HbSS (e.g., Sβ-thalassemia) appear to be at risk for bone marrow necrosis and fat embolism syndrome.[77]

Among the numerous other known hemoglobinopathies, HbC and HbE are the next most common causes of chronic hemolysis. The *HbC* gene mutation is most prevalent in people of West African ancestry; the *HbE* gene is found primarily in people of Southeast Asian ancestry. Homozygous HbE is unusual in its presentation as a mild-to-moderate hypochromic microcytic anemia (MCV 50 to 65 fL). HbC is recognized morphologically by the unique intracellular crystalline structures in erythrocytes on the blood film (Fig. 10-25).

Immune-Mediated Hemolytic Anemia

Autoimmune Hemolytic Anemias. Autoimmune hemolytic anemias (AIHAs) are categorized by the temperature at which

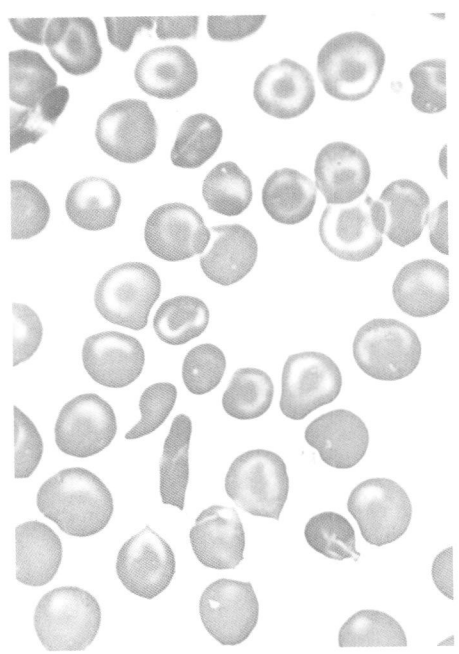

Figure 10-24. In hemoglobin S-C (HbSC) disease, target cells predominate, and plump, darkly stained cells contain precipitated HbS and HbC.

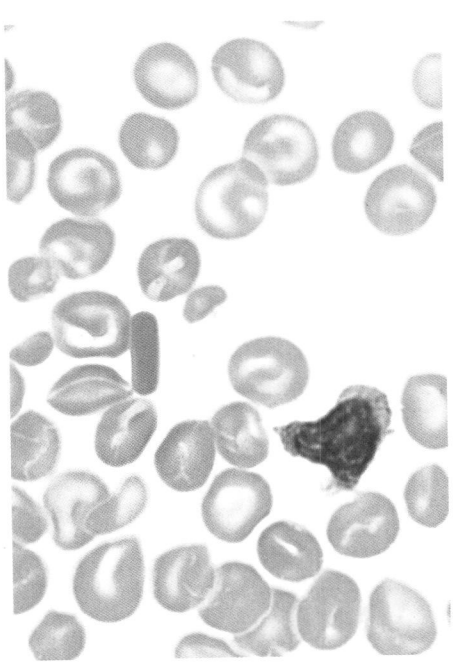

Figure 10-25. In hemoglobin C disease, target cells are numerous. Note the rod-shaped crystal in the "boxcar" cell.

the autoantibody has the greatest avidity for the target red cell antigen, and they are detected by a positive direct antiglobulin test.[78] Warm AIHA is most common (70% of AIHAs) and is clinically significant because it occurs at body temperature. IgG antibody (or occasionally IgA antibody) coated RBCs act to bind Fc receptors on splenic macrophages and, with or without subsequent complement fixation, are removed from circulation. Partial phagocytosis of the RBC membrane produces spherocytes (Fig. 10-26). Cold AIHA is caused by

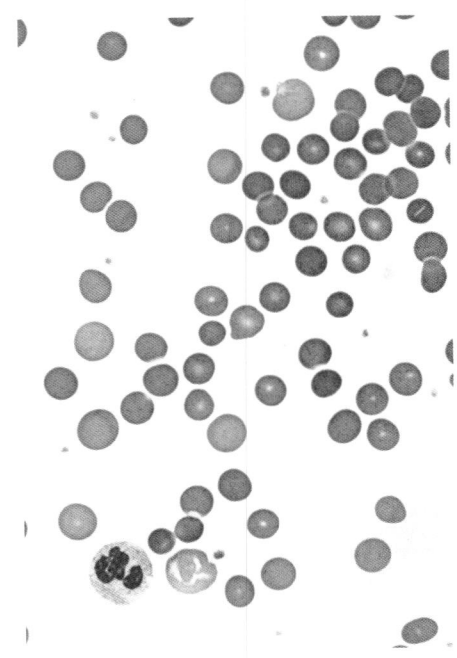

Figure 10-26. In warm antibody hemolytic anemia, numerous spherocytes are seen.

IgM coating of red cells at low temperatures, leading to RBC agglutination and complement fixation.[79] The antibody is most often directed at the I antigen on the red cell membrane. Some hemolysis occurs secondary to intravascular destruction of the agglutinated cells. However, if the antibody is active at temperatures approaching 37° C, complement becomes activated, and clinically significant intravascular and sometimes extravascular complement-mediated hemolysis occur in the liver (80% of the time).[80] Smears typically show agglutinated cells unless the blood tube was previously warmed; spherocytes are less frequent (Fig. 10-27). Autoantibody formation in both warm-type and cold-type AIHA most likely represents a derangement of normal immune function. Approximately 50% of AIHA is idiopathic (primary) and observed in older patients.[81] In contrast, secondary AIHA develops in patients with underlying disease, predominantly lymphoproliferative disorders but also autoimmune disorders, infections, and carcinoma. Young patients, in particular, develop a self-limited cold-type AIHA after *Mycoplasma pneumoniae* infection or infectious mononucleosis.

Drug-Induced Immune Hemolysis. Drug-induced immune hemolysis occurs through three main mechanisms: autoantibody formation (warm-type AIHA), often directed at the Rh locus of the red cell; hapten formation with IgG antibody to the drug that is adsorbed on the red cell surface; and drug–antibody complex that attaches to the RBC surface and activates complement.[82] Examples of drugs that typify these mechanisms are α-methyldopa; penicillin and cephalosporins; and quinine, isoniazid, and insulin, respectively. Certain drugs, such as the cephalosporins and methyldopa (Aldomet), can alter RBC membranes, causing non-specific binding of IgG or IgM. RBCs are lost through splenic sequestration and destruction. The direct antiglobulin test is positive, and bone marrow evaluation is not required.

Hemolysis Caused by Physicomechanical Disruption. Hemolysis caused by physicomechanical disruption

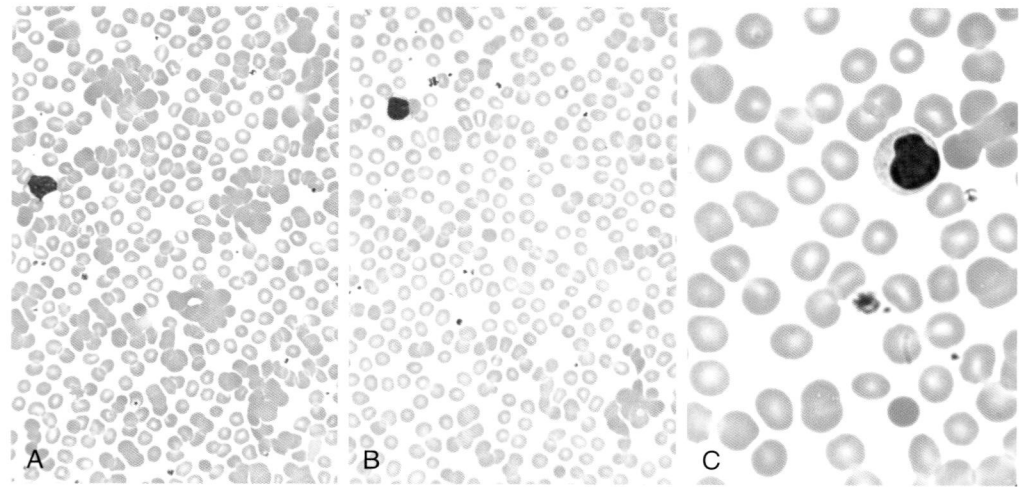

Figure 10-27. A, In cold agglutinin disease, numerous aggregates are seen in blood smears made from blood at room temperature. **B,** When the blood is warmed to 37° C, the agglutination phenomenon is reversed. Red cell morphology is essentially normal in cold agglutinin disease. **C,** Only a rare spherocyte is seen.

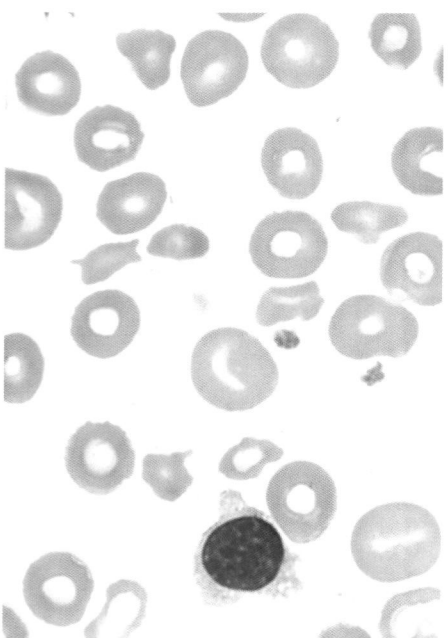

Figure 10-28. Fragmentation syndrome produced by a defective prosthetic aortic valve.

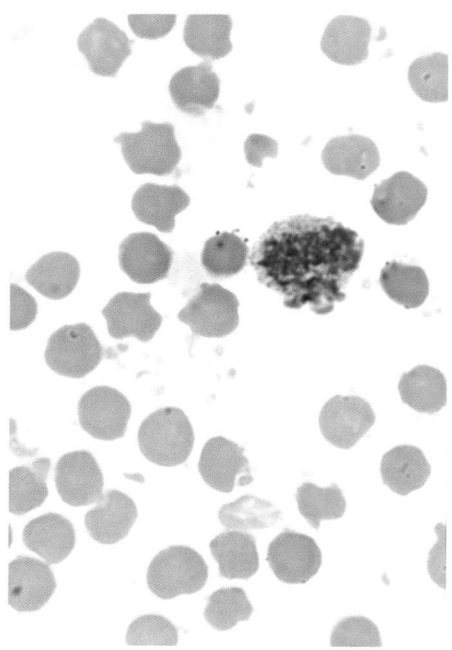

Figure 10-29. This blood smear was made from a specimen inadvertently exposed to high temperatures in a defective pneumatic tube system adjacent to a steam line. Numerous spherocytes, cytoplasmic red blood cell fragments, and a degenerating white blood cell are present.

develops when red cells are exposed to mechanical trauma or to heat above body temperature. Mechanical trauma occurs through a variety of mechanisms, including disruption by fibrin strands in disseminated intravascular coagulation, vasculitis, possibly thrombotic thrombocytopenic purpura, and the effects of vortexing in aortic insufficiency, malignant hypertension, and eclampsia. The blood smear typically contains numerous schistocytes and small numbers of spherocytes (Fig. 10-28). These anemias are commonly referred to as *microangiopathic hemolytic anemia,* even though red cell destruction may occur in the left ventricle, aorta, or other large vessels. When blood is heated to greater than 50° C, red cells fragment into microspherocytes (Fig. 10-29). This phenomenon is typical of patients suffering severe thermal burns of the skin.

Infection-Associated Hemolytic Anemia. Infection-associated hemolytic anemia is caused by organisms that parasitize or otherwise disrupt the RBCs, such as malaria (Fig. 10-30), babesiosis, and bartonellosis.

Macrocytic Anemia

Macrocytic anemia is defined as an MCV greater than 99 fL in adults and is dependent on age for infants and children. Because reticulocytes are larger than normal red cells, a mild degree of macrocytosis (MCV rarely >110 fL) may be seen after recent hemorrhage (>1 week), hemolytic anemia, or

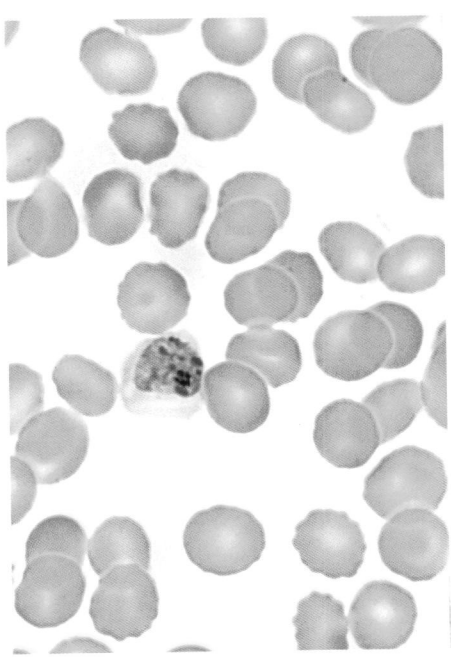

Figure 10-30. Mature schizont of *Plasmodium vivax.*

treated anemia with a brisk reticulocyte response. Secondary reticulocytosis is observed in a subset of patients with liver disease; the RBCs have increased membrane cholesterol and lecithin incorporation, producing thin macrocytes and target cells that have a shortened life span.[83] The increase in reticulocytes in all these processes is reflected by a high RDW. The remaining macrocytic anemias (Table 10-6) exhibit decreased or ineffective hematopoiesis, with low reticulocyte numbers and a frequently normal RDW.

Megaloblastic Anemias

Megaloblastic anemias are the most common macrocytic anemias, particularly those caused by vitamin B_{12} (cobalamin) or folate deficiency (Table 10-6). Megaloblastic anemias are the consequence of ineffective erythropoiesis resulting from defects in DNA synthesis.[84,85] The coenzyme form of folate is an important cofactor in the rate-limiting step and many additional steps of DNA (pyrimidine) synthesis; cobalamin plays an interdependent role involving methionine synthesis and the conversion of methylmalonyl CoA to succinyl CoA. Enlargement or "gigantism" of hematopoietic precursors is seen because cytoplasmic maturation proceeds while cell division is delayed by the lack of sufficient DNA to undergo mitosis. Increased intramedullary cell death ensues, with compensatory erythroid hyperplasia and the development of anemia characterized by oval macrocytes. Anemia is often a late event in folate or vitamin B_{12} deficiency; hypersegmentation of neutrophils usually appears earlier (Figs. 10-31 to 10-34). The hematologic findings in patients with megaloblastic anemia are readily identified (Table 10-6). Bone marrow examination is usually not required but may be performed for the evaluation of pancytopenia (which rarely can also occur in the presence of vitamin B_{12} deficiency) or when the typical peripheral blood findings are masked by concurrent iron-deficiency anemia or a constitutional microcytic anemia. It is extremely important to recognize that severe megaloblastic anemia may have sufficiently bizarre cells and increased pronormoblasts to be

mistaken for MDS or acute erythroid leukemia. The absence of trilineage dysplasia or an increase in myeloblasts helps make this distinction. Abnormally low serum and red cell folate and serum vitamin B_{12} levels further support megaloblastic anemia.

Folate deficiency is most commonly nutritional in origin and is most prevalent in alcoholics, indigents, and the elderly. Mood disorders, particularly in elderly patients, may be attributed to undiagnosed folate deficiency. A normal diet contains a sufficient amount of vitamin B_{12}; thus total body stores of cobalamin are abundant. The most common cause of cobalamin deficiency in the Western world is pernicious anemia. Under normal conditions, cobalamin complexes with intrinsic factor, a product of gastric parietal cells, binds to intrinsic factor receptors in the terminal ileum.[86] In pernicious anemia, parietal cells are destroyed through autoimmune mechanisms, and little or no cobalamin is absorbed. In contrast to folate deficiency, cobalamin deficiency also causes a demyelinating disorder with numerous neurologic manifestations. Controversy exists regarding the best diagnostic approach to identifying these vitamin deficiencies. The most commonly used indicators of deficiency are the red cell folate level and serum cobalamin; however, these tests are not entirely specific or sensitive. Serum cobalamin levels may be normal or only slightly reduced in some patients with vitamin B_{12} deficiency. Additional tests currently used include serum or plasma methylmalonic acid and plasma homocysteine levels, which better detect low tissue cobalamin stores among individuals with early deficiencies.[85,86] However, hyperhomocysteinemia may also be seen in folate deficiency. The measurement of serum holotranscobalamin II, the active form of cobalamin, is also a good marker of early vitamin B_{12} deficiency in patients with normal renal function.[84] Pernicious anemia is associated with several autoantibodies: measurement of parietal cell and intrinsic factor antibodies is diagnostically helpful in the absence of B_{12} absorption assays.[86] RBC folate levels correlate with long-term folate intake, whereas serum folate reflects recent folate intake. The U.S. Food and Drug Administration required the addition of folic acid to all breads, cereals, flours, corn meal, pasta products, rice, and other cereal grain products in the United States. National Health and Nutrition Examination Survey (NHANES) results showed marked improvements in folate status, correlating with success of folate fortification. However, the prevalence of low RBC folate (<140 ng/mL) differed by sex, race, and ethnicity; low levels were most pronounced among non-Hispanic women of African descent compared with non-Hispanic White women and women of Mexican descent.[87] A retrospective review of Mayo Medical Laboratories' folate testing in a 10-year period (1999–2009) indicated that true folate deficiency is exceedingly rare in the current postfortification era[88]; furthermore, they concluded that routine ordering of RBC folate and serum folate together is unnecessary, because they provide equal diagnostic information in almost all situations.[89] On the other hand, testing must be undertaken judiciously based on the patient demographic served by each institution.[90]

Drugs that cause megaloblastic anemia are those that act primarily on DNA synthesis and include antifolates (e.g., methotrexate), purine analogues, pyrimidine analogues (e.g., zidovudine), and ribonucleotide reductase inhibitors (e.g., hydroxyurea). In addition, the metabolism of a number of anticonvulsant and antidepressant drugs is dependent on adequate folic acid for appropriate drug response.[85,91]

Table 10-6 Causes of Macrocytic Anemia

Disorder	Bone Marrow Morphology	Comments
Congenital Disorders		
Diamond-Blackfan anemia	Isolated profound ↓ in erythroid elements, defective erythroid maturation, ↑ hematogones	Familial: AD (40%-45%) Sporadic or familial with different inheritance types Familial cases associated with anomalies (e.g., short stature, abnormalities of head and upper limbs)
CDA I	Megaloblastic maturation, 1%-10% erythroid precursors have internuclear bridging, binucleation with different size and shape, or nuclear budding	*CDAN1* (15q15.1-q15.3), *C15ORF41* (15q14); AR Moderate-to-severe anemia
CDA II (HEMPAS)	Normoblastic or megaloblastic, 10%-40% erythroid precursors have binucleation or multinucleation with equal nuclear size, karyorrhexis	*SEC23B* (20q11.2), AR Mild to severe anemia
CDA III	Megaloblastic maturation, 10%-40% erythroid precursors are multinucleated, including giant erythroblasts (up to 12 nuclei); karyorrhexis	*KIF23* (15q21-25), AD (familial form) Variable inheritance (sporadic form), unknown mutations Absent-to-moderate anemia
CDA IV	Erythroid precursors are binucleated or multinucleated, internuclear bridging	*KLF1* (19p13.2), AD Unlike the other CDAs, reticulocyte count normal or slightly increased Generally severe anemia
X-linked thrombocytopenia with or without dyserythropoietic anemia	Dyserythropoiesis Decreased MKs MKs with cytoplasmic vacuoles and an absence of platelet membrane demarcation	*GATA1* (Xp11.23), XLR Clinically heterogeneous Mild-to-severe anemia
CDA variants		Isolated or syndromic CDA-like conditions X-linked dominant macrocytic dyserythropoietic anemia with iron overload, *ALAS2* (Xp11.21) Majeed syndrome; AR, *LPIN2* (18p11.31) Early infantile epileptic encephalopathy-50, *CAD* (2p23.3) Dyserythropoiesis associated with exocrine pancreatic insufficiency and calvarial hyperostosis, *COX412* (20q11.21) CDA and mevalonate kinase deficiency, *MVK* (12q24.11)
Megaloblastic Disorders		
Cobalamin (vitamin B$_{12}$) deficiency	Dyssynchronous nuclear-cytoplasmic maturation Erythroid and often myeloid hyperplasia—↓ myeloid-erythroid ratio	Caused by inadequate intake (strict vegan diet) or impaired absorption (pernicious anemia, gastrectomy, fish tapeworm [*Diphyllobothrium latum*], ileal resection or disease, pancreatic insufficiency, blind loop syndrome)
Folate deficiency	Erythroid lineage—larger cells with immature nucleus (open chromatin) compared with cytoplasmic maturation, possible multinucleation, abnormal nuclear configurations, Howell-Jolly bodies, basophilic stippling, Cabot rings	Caused by inadequate intake (poor diet, premature infant, hemodialysis), impaired absorption in small intestine (celiac sprue, enteritis, resection), increased utilization (chronic hemolysis, pregnancy, chronic infections)
Drugs	Myeloid lineage—giant serpentine bands and metamyelocytes, hypersegmented neutrophils (6 lobes)	Inhibitors of DNA metabolism (deoxynucleotide synthesis inhibitors, antimetabolites, dihydrofolate reductase inhibitors), anticonvulsants, oral contraceptives
Inborn errors	MKs large with multiple lobes, large platelets	Congenital deficiencies (intrinsic factor, transcobalamin II), errors of metabolism, hereditary orotic aciduria, Lesch-Nyhan syndrome
Other		Liver disease, thyroid disease, toxins, alcohol, aplastic anemia

AD, Autosomal dominant; *AR*, autosomal recessive; *CDA*, congenital dyserythropoietic anemia; *HEMPAS*, hereditary erythroblastic multinuclearity with positive acidified serum; *MK*, megakaryocyte; *XLR*, X-linked recessive.

Constitutional Causes

Constitutional causes of macrocytic anemia are much less common. DBA is a heterogeneous genetic disorder that usually presents within the first few months of life and by 1 year of age in 90% of cases (Table 10-6).[92] It is the first human disease found to be caused by mutations in a ribosomal structural protein (*RPS19* gene on chromosome 19q13.2).[93] Mutations of this gene are found in 25% of sporadic and familial cases. Additional genes that encode ribosomal proteins have been implicated (e.g., *RPS24*). Mutations in nonribosomal protein genes (i.e., *GATA1*, *TSR2*, *EPO*, *ARA2*), in association with a DBA-like phenotype, have also been described. To date, no mutation could be identified in 20% of patients with DBA.[93] The failure of erythroid production is hypothesized to be caused by faulty ribosome production, leading to apoptosis of erythroid precursors. Not surprisingly, the clinical manifestations of the disorder are heterogeneous. Affected family members may have dramatically different degrees of anemia, responses to therapy, and presence of congenital anomalies. Most commonly, the disease presents as a nonresolving severe macrocytic anemia with reticulocytopenia. Bone marrow specimens demonstrate few or no erythroid precursors (erythroblastopenia).[94] Some cases exhibit increased numbers of hematogones. Circulating red cells contain increased HbF (heterogeneous distribution) and have a fetal distribution of intracellular enzymes. In addition to the blood and marrow findings, increased erythropoietin, elevated red cell adenosine deaminase levels, and i antigen expression help support the diagnosis.[93]

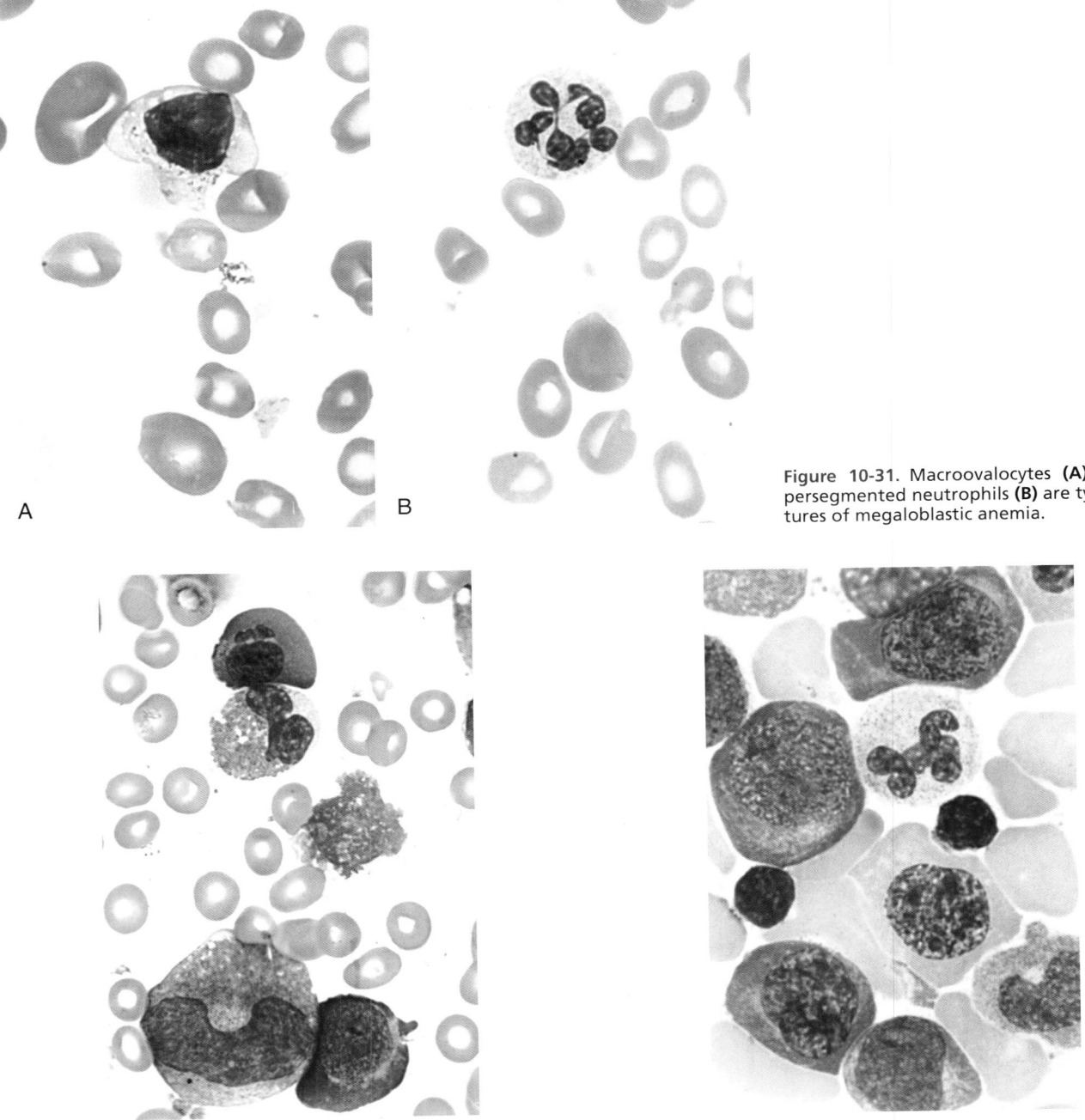

Figure 10-31. Macroovalocytes **(A)** and hypersegmented neutrophils **(B)** are typical features of megaloblastic anemia.

Figure 10-32. Bone marrow aspirate from a patient with cobalamin deficiency illustrates a giant C-shaped neutrophil band and megaloblastic normoblasts.

Figure 10-33. Bone marrow aspirate from a patient with pernicious anemia shows dyssynchrony of nuclear and cytoplasmic maturation in megaloblasts. Band neutrophils often have serpentine nuclear contours.

Congenital Dyserythropoietic Anemias

Congenital dyserythropoietic anemias (CDAs) are rare hereditary disorders characterized by abnormalities of erythropoiesis.[95] The three classically described forms, CDA I, II, and III, are defined by distinctive morphologic abnormalities of erythroblasts (Table 10-6). Additional rare, unique types and variant forms are also recognized, some of which are present as a part of a syndrome. The morphologic hallmark of CDA is prominent erythroid hyperplasia and striking dyserythropoiesis, with normal myeloid and megakaryocytic lineages (Figs. 10-35 to 10-37). Erythropoiesis is ineffective, as manifested by reticulocytopenia, with variable degrees of anemia. Unlike CDA I, II, and III, CDA IV is characterized by a normal or slightly increased reticulocyte count with respect to the degree of anemia, along with generally severe hemolytic anemia and markedly elevated HbF.[95,96] Anisopoikilocytosis is common to all types. Circulating RBCs occasionally have basophilic stippling, cytoplasmic vacuolization, or Cabot rings. Patients with CDA II have strong expression of protein antigens i and I on their RBCs. In general, the clinical findings are those associated with a chronic hemolytic anemia, including increased lactate dehydrogenase and bilirubin levels, jaundice,

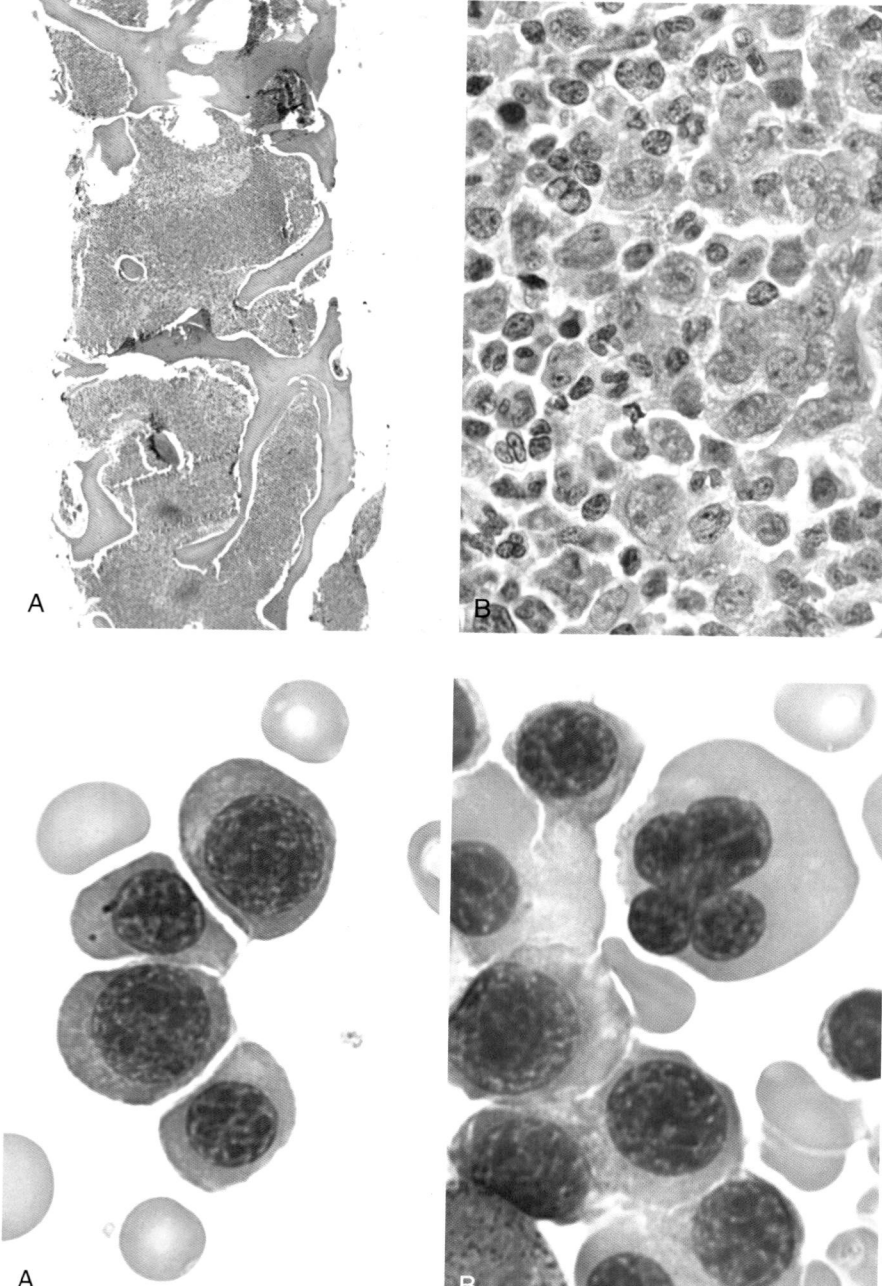

Figure 10-34. The trephine biopsy section of pernicious anemia is often markedly hypercellular **(A)** and contains clusters of large pronormoblasts **(B)**. It is important to distinguish this picture from myelodysplastic syndromes and acute erythroid leukemia.

Figure 10-35. Bone marrow aspirate of congenital dyserythropoietic anemia type I shows megaloblastic maturation, intranuclear bridging by chromatin filaments **(A)**, and multinucleation **(B)**.

splenomegaly, tendency to form gallstones, and iron overload. CDA II is the most common CDA and may be the most frequently misdiagnosed; the correct diagnosis is often not made until patients are teenagers, or even adults, despite the identification of a chronic hemolytic anemia earlier in life.[95] Unlike the other CDAs, CDA II may have associated microspherocytes and a positive osmotic fragility test, suggesting a diagnosis of HS.[95] This can be resolved by genetic testing, which has become a frontline method for evaluation. In the past, CDA II was also misdiagnosed as PNH as a result of a positive Ham acidified serum lysis test (*CDA II* has been called *HEMPAS,* or hereditary erythroblastic multinuclearity with positive acidified serum), but this is no longer an issue, as PNH is now diagnosed by flow cytometry.[97] The presence of hypoglycosylated band 3 is a pathognomonic biochemical feature of the membrane

proteins isolated from CDA II.[95] Treatment with interferon-α has been effective in a few patients with CDA I with *CDAN1* mutations.[95] Activin receptor ligand traps (e.g., luspatercept, sotatercept), which target ineffective erythropoiesis, are being studied as potential therapies for CDA II. Hematopoietic stem cell transplant is another option in severe cases.

EVALUATION OF LEUKOPENIA

Neutropenia

Neutrophils are the most prevalent leukocyte in circulation before 1 week and after approximately 5 years of age. Neutropenia is therefore the most common cause for a decreased white blood cell count. Yet, it is notable that only 3% to 5% of all neutrophils

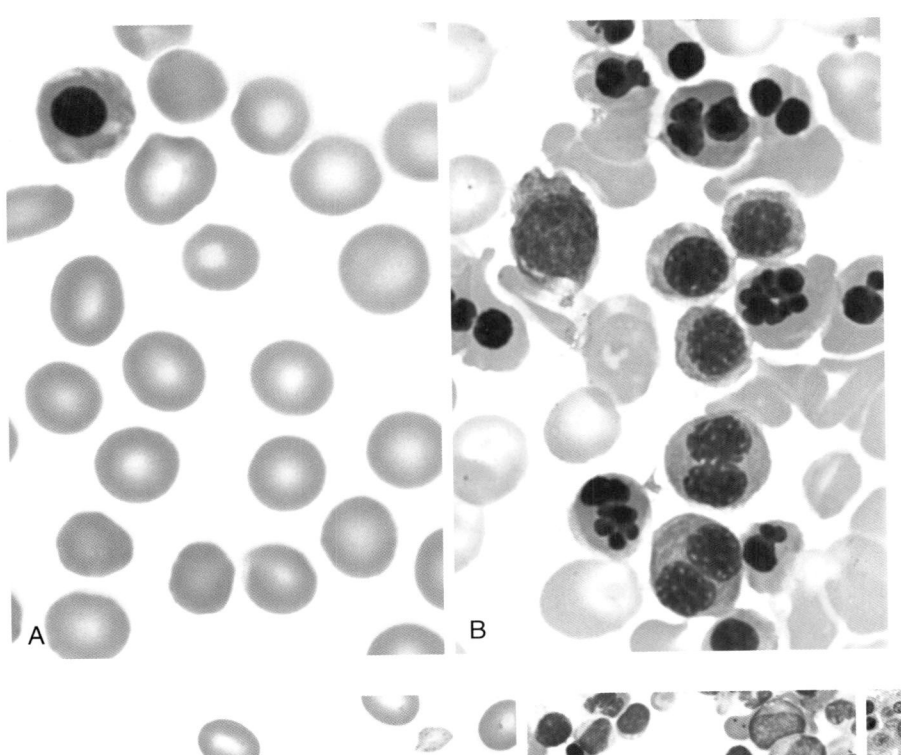

Figure 10-36. A, Peripheral blood smear from a 16-year-old girl with congenital dyserythropoietic anemia type II (hereditary erythroblastic multinuclearity with positive acidified serum [HEMPAS]) shows mild normochromic normocytic anemia and a normoblast. The patient underwent a bone marrow study for unrelated tumor staging. **B,** Numerous binucleated and multinucleated normoblasts were found. Her younger brother had similar changes. Both had a positive acidified serum test.

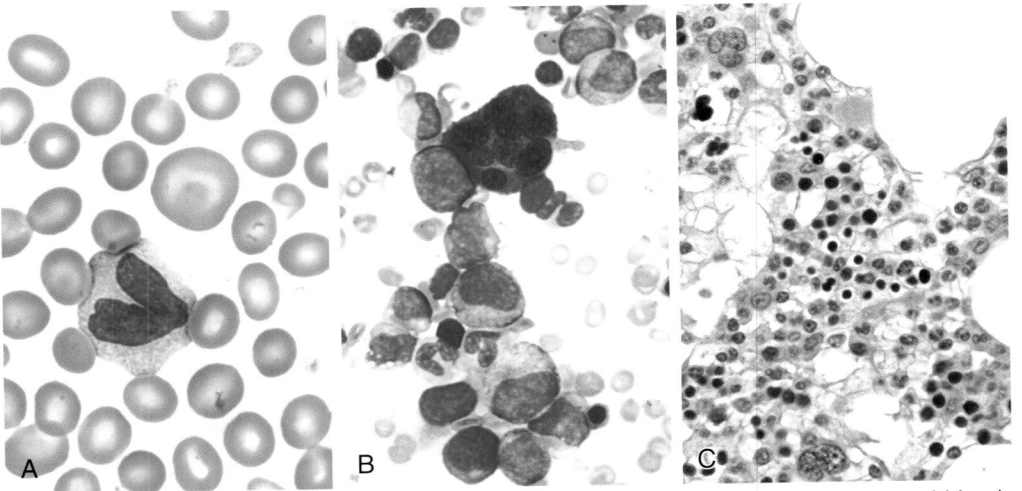

Figure 10-37. A, Peripheral blood smear of congenital dyserythropoietic anemia type III shows macrocytic red blood cells and a megaloblastic neutrophil band. **B,** The bone marrow smear contains a gigantoblast with eight nuclei. **C,** Occasional multinucleated erythroid precursors are seen in the trephine biopsy section.

are present in the peripheral blood, while the majority are in the bone marrow storage pool, ready to be mobilized when the need arises.[98,99] Thus, the adequacy of bone marrow reserve plays a large role in whether the neutropenic patient is at risk for adverse events, such as severe infection.

Age, sex, and ethnic background affect neutrophil counts, and appropriate reference ranges must be considered. Without taking into account sex and ethnic differences, neutropenia is usually present if absolute neutrophil counts (ANCs) are less than 0.7 $\times$ 10^9/L in newborns, less than 2.5 $\times$ 10^9/L in infants, and less than 1.5 $\times$ 10^9/L in children and adults. Compared with Whites, Latinos have slightly higher neutrophil counts, and persons of African descent and some Middle Eastern ethnic groups have slightly lower neutrophil counts, owing to differences in myeloid production or regulation of neutrophil storage.[100] Among healthy individuals of African ancestry, 25% to 50% have ANCs of 1.0 to 1.5 $\times$ 10^9/L that are linked to Duffy antigen receptor chemokine (*DARC*) gene polymorphisms. The *DARC*-null genotype plays a

role in *Plasmodium vivax* malaria resistance and possibly other endemic infections.[101] This normal variant has been designated as "Duffy-null associated neutrophil count" (DANC) or "typical neutrophil count with Fy(a-b-) status." Thus, as an isolated laboratory finding in certain ethnic populations (including African Americans, Africans, Bedouin Arabs, Ethiopian and Yemenite Jews), ANCs at this level are clinically inconsequential and do not lead to increased risk of infection; instead, they are considered a **normal variant with ANC <1.5 $\times$ 10^9/L**—the terminology preferred to the previous designation of "benign ethnic neutropenia" or "benign familial neutropenia."[102,103] Any individual with severe neutropenia (<0.5 $\times$ 10^9/L) that persists for more than a few days has a significant risk for developing a life-threatening infection, particularly from endogenous bacteria. Neonates are particularly vulnerable, because they have qualitative neutrophil defects, a limited bone marrow neutrophil storage pool, and an inability to rapidly increase neutrophil production. Up to 38% of septic neonates become neutropenic.[104]

Several classifications for neutropenia exist. One relies on ANC levels to predict infection risk (i.e. mild, moderate, severe). Others classify based on congenital/constitutional versus acquired or primary versus secondary causes for neutropenia.[105] Another schema is based on normal/increased versus decreased bone marrow reserve, particularly helpful to the laboratorian who reviews bone marrow biopsies.[99] If the bone marrow biopsy displays normal/increased bone marrow reserve, then the neutropenia is likely caused by extrinsic factors from immune-mediated destruction with decreased neutrophil survival, increased neutrophil utilization or neutrophil redistribution, or ineffective trafficking. Neutropenia with decreased bone marrow reserve could be caused by an intrinsic maturation or proliferation defect in myelopoiesis (i.e., through germline or somatic gene variants), increased apoptosis or secondary to conditions that suppress granulopoiesis by direct toxic effects by free radicals or metabolites, or immune-mediated destruction.

Yet another classification is an age-related schema, as some conditions are seen more commonly in infancy, childhood, or adulthood.[99,106] An age-related problem-solving approach combines more clinically based algorithms: exploring worrisome signs and symptoms of low bone marrow reserve, observing the pattern of historical and/or prospectively collected CBC data (i.e., Is the onset of neutropenia acute or chronic? Is neutropenia steady or cyclical?), and examining the blood smear for possible clues to the diagnosis (Fig. 10-38).[98,99,105-107] Laboratory testing would be geared toward suspicion of various etiologies: infection (i.e., microbiologic cultures, serologic studies, polymerase chain reaction [PCR], etc); autoimmune disease (e.g., antineutrophil antibodies, rheumatoid factor, C-reactive protein [CRP], erythrocyte sedimentation rate [ESR], etc.); neoplasms/malignancy (e.g., bone marrow biopsy, flow cytometry, etc.), nutritional deficiencies (e.g., B_{12}, folate, homocysteine, methylmalonic acid, copper, zinc); immunodeficiencies (e.g., immunoglobulins, immune evaluation for detection of cellular or humoral immunity); and congenital/constitutional disorders (e.g., molecular/genetic testing for bone marrow failure syndromes, etc.). Although specialized neutrophil antibody testing (e.g., granulocyte agglutination test, granulocyte indirect immunofluorescence test) have been referenced in the past, these tests are available in very few clinical laboratories, and results are generally considered not helpful in the diagnosis and management of patients.[108-110]

In general, patients with ANC >1.0×10^9/L can be managed as outpatients, while febrile patients with severe neutropenia (ANC <0.5×10^9/L) are admitted for intravenous antibiotics. The latter are assumed to be at high risk for marrow hypoplasia and severe infection; presumptive management with parenteral antibiotics in these instances is prudent.

Neutropenia in the Neonatal Period, Infancy, and Childhood

Causes of neutropenia in neonates depend on maternal factors, genetics, immunologic factors, and postnatal infections, the latter being the most common cause of neutropenia in this age group. In infancy and childhood, neutropenia is often transient or chronic and self-resolving; causes are typically infectious or immunologic in nature (Box 10-3).

Neonatal Alloimmune Neutropenia

Neonatal alloimmune neutropenia is caused by transplacental passage of maternal IgG antibodies that are sensitized to paternally inherited human neutrophil antigens (HNAs) on fetal granulocytes.[111,112] The number of postpartum women with HNAs is significantly higher than the incidence of neutropenia, suggesting that many of the antibodies are clinically irrelevant. Neutropenia varies from relatively mild to severe; thus, an affected infant may be either asymptomatic or septic in extremely severe cases. The neutropenia resolves spontaneously in 6 to 11 weeks after decay of maternal antibodies but may last as long as 6 months.[109] Severe neutropenia is ameliorated by administration of granulocyte colony-stimulating factor (G-CSF). A bone marrow examination, although not normally required, shows normal-to-increased cellularity with a decrease in mature neutrophils.

Primary Autoimmune Neutropenia

Primary autoimmune neutropenia (AIN), or AIN of childhood, is the most common cause of chronic neutropenia in infants and children when not associated with other pathology. This condition affects children younger than 38 months, with spontaneous resolution in 90% of cases by 2 to 3 years of age, with the remainder recovering by age 11.[113] Infectious complications are usually less severe than expected for the degree of neutropenia.[114] A bone marrow examination is usually not required, but if performed, the bone marrow is often normocellular or hypercellular with left-shifted myeloid hyperplasia. Neonates can also develop AIN secondary to placental transfer of autoantibodies when the mother has AIN.

A transient neutropenia of unknown mechanism can be seen in small-for-gestational-age newborns or neonates of hypertensive women.[112]

If older children develop chronic AIN, evaluation for a congenital immunologic disorder such as common variable immunodeficiency should be considered.

Infection-Related Neutropenia in Infancy/Childhood

Three days after birth, neutropenia is more commonly associated with necrotizing enterocolitis or nosocomial infection. Vertical transmission of human immunodeficiency virus (HIV) infection should also be considered in newborns with unexplained neutropenia. Acute isolated neutropenia in children is most often the consequence of a recent viral infection. Neutropenia develops within 48 hours of infection and may persist for up to 6 days. In a cohort of immunocompetent hospitalized children with neutropenia (range, 0 to 16 years), more than 80% were age 3 years or younger. In addition, infectious etiologies were uncovered in 29% of cases, including brucellosis, rickettsiosis, respiratory syncytial viral infection, and others.[115] In addition to primary loss by extensive neutrophil infiltration into infected tissue, splenic sequestration or antineutrophil antibody formation (with Epstein-Barr virus [EBV] infection) may accelerate neutrophil destruction. Monitoring blood counts for evidence of recovery is usually all that is required.

Neutropenia in Adults

Neutropenia in adults has a large number of causes (Box 10-3), most of which are secondary to an associated condition (see Secondary Autoimmune Neutropenia section for further discussion). In contrast to the pediatric population, a bone marrow examination is often required in adults when the clinical history and physical examination do not elicit a likely neutropenic etiology, and particularly when other cell lineages are affected. The cause of neutropenia is often multifactorial.

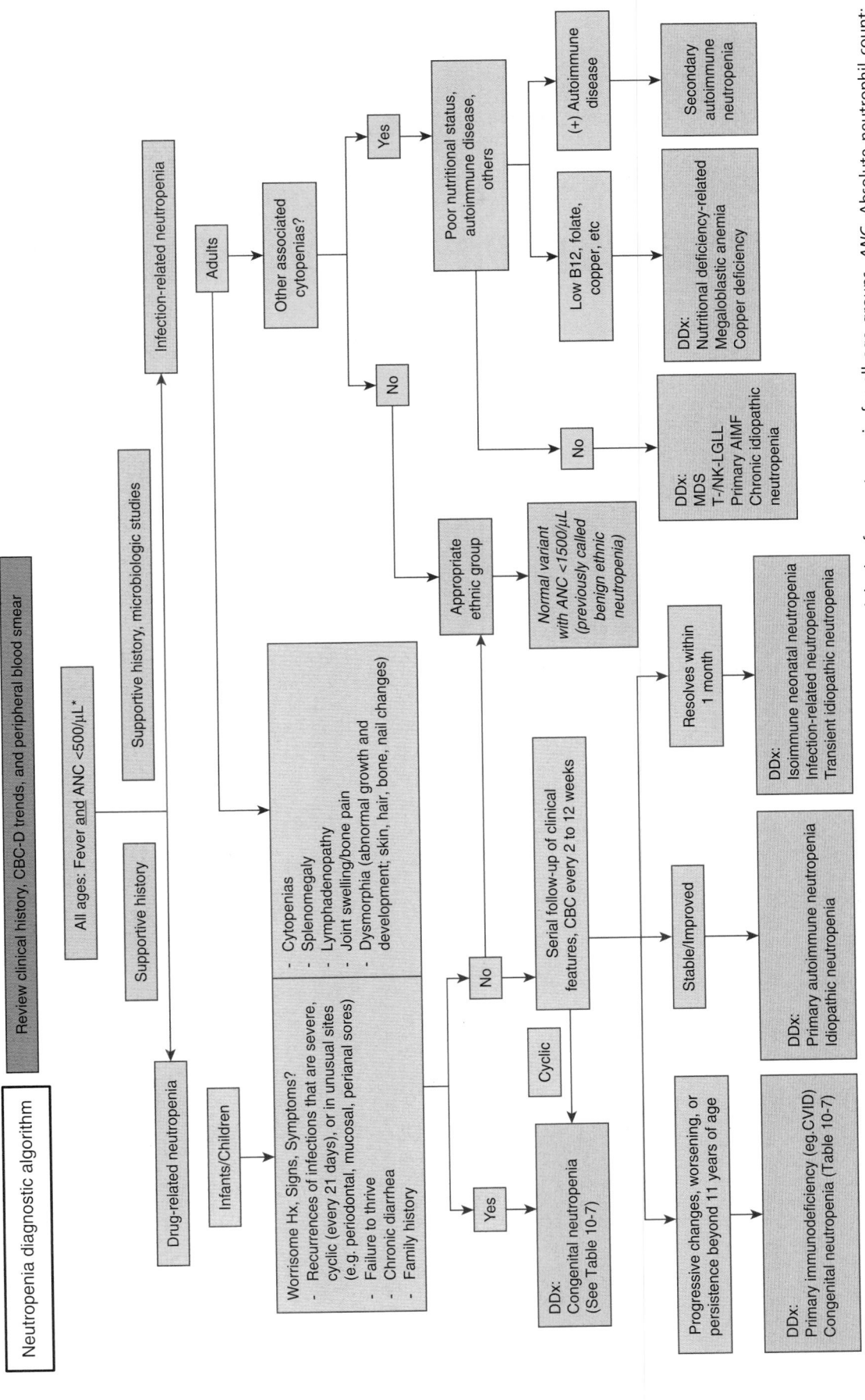

Figure 10-38. Neutropenia algorithm. Drug-induced and infection-related are the most common etiologies for neutropenia for all age groups. *ANC,* Absolute neutrophil count; *BMBx,* bone marrow aspirate and biopsy; *CBC-D,* complete blood cell count with differential.

Drug-Induced Neutropenia

Drug-induced neutropenia is the most common cause of neutropenia in adults. Neutropenia secondary to chemotherapy or radiotherapy shows a dose-dependent relationship. An idiosyncratic drug reaction is the most common cause for an unexpected isolated neutropenia in an outpatient setting. Idiosyncratic drug-induced agranulocytosis (ANC <0.5 × 10⁹/L) is defined as an adverse reaction in an abnormally

susceptible individual with previously normal neutrophil counts.[116] Individuals with mild-to-moderate neutropenia (ANC 0.5 to 1.5 × 10⁹/L) are alternatively referred to as having *drug-induced neutropenia*. The onset of neutropenia is unpredictable in these processes but usually occurs 1 to 2 weeks after initial drug exposure or immediately after drug reexposure. Almost any drug can be involved.[116] Common offending drugs causing severe neutropenia are clozapine, methimazole, sulfasalazine, trimethoprim-sulfamethoxazole, and cocaine (levamisole-tainted).[117] Some of these medications, in addition to posttransplant immunosuppressive agents, also induce pseudo–Pelger-Huët changes, mimicking neutrophilic dysplasia[118] (Fig. 10-39).

Late-onset neutropenia is seen with the monoclonal antibody (mAb) anti-CD20 (rituximab)[119] and with the chimeric antigen receptor T-cell therapy (CAR-T), which may have other cytopenias.[120] Causative mechanisms differ depending on the drug involved and are often incompletely understood. Roles for immune-mediated (immune complex, hapten, or autoimmune) or nonimmune-mediated mechanisms, such as active drug metabolite toxicity to neutrophils or marrow stroma, have been described. The incidence of drug-induced neutropenia increases with age, likely reflecting the higher use of multiple medications in the elderly. Greater susceptibility of some individuals to idiosyncratic reactions is hypothesized to relate to increased myeloid precursor sensitivity to a normal drug concentration or to gene polymorphisms that alter drug metabolism or drug pharmacokinetics. If a severe, drug-related neutropenia is suspected, all nonessential drugs and over-the-counter medications should be discontinued, with substitution of essential medications. Drug-induced agranulocytosis may be fatal with continued exposure to the drug.

Box 10-3 *Causes of Acquired Neutropenia**

Drug Induced Causes That Overlap With Secondary Immune-Mediated Mechanisms
- Antibiotics (sulfasalazine), antifungals, antimalarials
- Anticonvulsants
- Anti-inflammatories
- Antipsychotics (clozapine)
- Antithyroid agents (thionamides)
- Antidepressants
- Sedatives
- Cardiovascular drugs
- Diuretics
- Other: levamisole, rituximab

Primary Immune Mediated
- Neonatal alloimmune neutropenia
- Autoimmune neutropenia of childhood
- Transfusion reaction

Secondary Immune Mediated
- Autoimmune disorders: rheumatoid arthritis, systemic lupus erythematosus, primary biliary cirrhosis, polyarteritis nodosa, scleroderma, Castleman disease, Sjögren syndrome
- Infection: *Helicobacter pylori*, HIV, parvovirus B19
- Neurologic diseases: multiple sclerosis
- Malignancy: Hodgkin lymphoma, T-cell large granular lymphocytic leukemia, Wilms' tumor
- Drug induced: rituximab, fludarabine, propylthiouracil
- Transplantation: stem cell, bone marrow, kidney
- Bone marrow injury: aplastic anemia, paroxysmal nocturnal hemoglobinuria

Other
- Chronic idiopathic neutropenia (likely immune mediated)
- Infection (most common cause)
  - Viral: human immunodeficiency virus; respiratory syncytial virus; cytomegalovirus; Epstein-Barr virus; hepatitis A, B, or C; influenza; measles; mumps; rubella; yellow fever; varicella; herpes simplex virus
  - Bacterial: rickettsia, typhoid, miliary tuberculosis, tularemia, brucellosis, streptococcus, staphylococcus, *Escherichia coli*, *Klebsiella* spp.
  - Protozoan: malaria, kala-azar, trypanosomiasis
  - Fungal: histoplasmosis, *Candida* spp.
- Nutritional deficiencies: vitamin B₁₂ (cobalamin), folic acid, copper, severe caloric deprivation
- Bone marrow infiltration: carcinoma, leukemia, lymphoma, myeloma, granulomatous diseases, fibrotic processes
- Endocrine or metabolic disorders: Addison disease, hyperthyroidism, hypopituitarism, hyperglycemia, acidemia, tyrosinemia, glycogen storage disease type 1B
- Hypersplenism
- Radiation
- Toxins, alcohol
- Hemodialysis
- Maternal hypertension

* List is not all-inclusive and instead represents major causes.

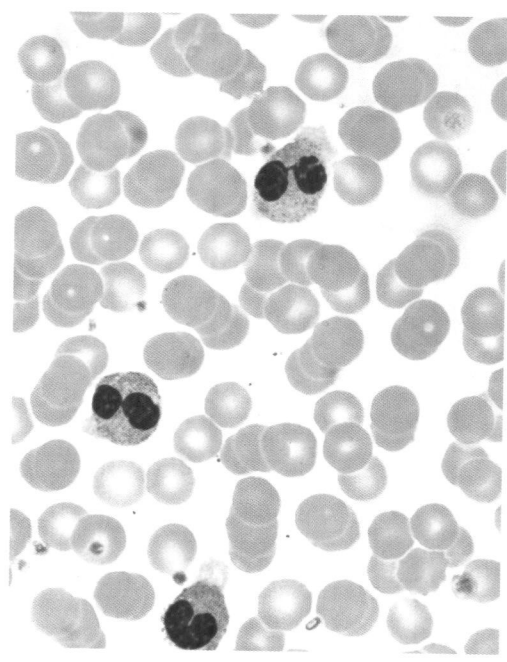

Figure 10-39. Peripheral blood smear of acquired pseudo–Pelger-Huët anomaly in a lung transplant recipient treated with mycophenolate mofetil. Two of the neutrophils feature symmetric bilobed nuclei with so-called "pince nez" morphology.

Secondary Autoimmune Neutropenia

Autoimmune neutropenia (AIN) is more often secondary rather than primary in adults. Secondary AIN is associated with systemic autoimmune disorders, infectious diseases, neoplasms, neurologic disorders, organ transplants, and certain medications.[105] Concurrent thrombocytopenia or hemolytic anemia may be seen, and the neutropenia is often multifactorial in etiology. A bone marrow evaluation may be required to exclude a neoplastic process or aplasia. Physical findings and specific immunologic tests supporting an autoimmune disorder usually suffice to make the diagnosis.[103] Neutropenia associated with systemic autoimmune disorders (e.g., lupus, primary biliary cirrhosis, Sjögren syndrome) may track with disease activity and is rarely severe, except in association with Felty syndrome (i.e., triad of rheumatoid arthritis, neutropenia, and splenomegaly). Both Felty syndrome and T/natural killer (NK)-cell large granular lymphocytic (LGL) leukemia with rheumatoid arthritis have an inherited DR4 haplotype in a majority of cases and are part of the same disease process.[121] Neutropenia occurs in 70% to 80% of patients with LGL leukemia and is of multifactorial origin, with a role for antineutrophil autoantibodies, myelopoiesis inhibition by cytokines, soluble Fas ligand-mediated apoptosis (shed from LGLs), and splenic sequestration. In addition to morphologic evaluation, immunophenotyping for LGLs and identification of a TCR gene rearrangement confirms the diagnosis.

Chronic Idiopathic Neutropenia

Chronic idiopathic neutropenia is defined as a persistent (>3 months), non-oscillating, and unexplained reduction in neutrophils.[122] This is essentially a diagnosis of exclusion after extensive evaluation for other causes. Middle-aged females are primarily affected, particularly those with an HLA-DRB1*1302 genetic predisposition who may have concurrent mild anemia, thrombocytopenia, osteopenia, or osteoporosis. Spontaneous remissions occur rarely among adults. The bone marrow is typically normocellular with a slightly decreased myeloid-to-erythroid ratio caused by mild T-cell and cytokine-mediated suppression of granulopoiesis.

Infection-Related Neutropenia

Infection-related neutropenia may be caused by a large number of infectious agents, including almost any type of viral infection (Box 10-3). Postinfectious neutropenia, although more common in children, is usually self-limited unless the patient is septic or has persistent neutropenia associated with EBV or HIV infections. A number of different mechanisms are involved in the pathogenesis, including infection of progenitor or endothelial cells, immunologically mediated bone marrow suppression (particularly viral infections), excessive cellular destruction (especially bacteremia with endotoxemia), increased neutrophil adherence to the endothelium, development of antineutrophil antibodies, and enhanced neutrophil utilization at the site of infection.[103,105]

Nutritional Deficiency–Related Neutropenia

The myeloid cells in the bone marrow generally show normal morphology in the majority of acquired neutropenias. Notable exceptions include megaloblastic anemia (Table 10-6) and copper deficiency. Neutropenia associated with vitamin B_{12} or folate deficiency rarely occurs without anemia and macrocytosis. Copper deficiency should be considered when cytoplasmic vacuoles are present in myeloid (particularly promyelocytes and myelocytes) and erythroid precursors.[123] The bone marrow may be variably cellular with myeloid and erythroid dyspoiesis, ring sideroblasts, and increased hematogones. Patients have concurrent normocytic, macrocytic, or microcytic anemia, neurologic disorders, and rarely, thrombocytopenia. Copper deficiency occurs secondary to excess zinc intake (through supplements, medications, or denture fixatives), total parenteral nutrition, and gastrointestinal disorders (e.g., partial gastric resection). Mild neutropenia is also observed with severe caloric deprivation, as in anorexia nervosa.

Congenital Neutropenia

Congenital neutropenia refers to neutropenias with genetic mutations and not simply those that are present at birth. Many of these disorders have intrinsic defects that cause premature apoptosis of cells, ineffective neutrophil production, and recurrent infections. The Severe Chronic Neutropenia International Registry (SCNIR) and other national registries recommend identification of mutations in the more than 25 genes that affect the neutrophil differentiation program.[124] A subset of these is discussed here and summarized in Table 10-7.

Severe Congenital Neutropenia

Severe congenital neutropenia (SCN) represents a heterogeneous group of disorders characterized by inherited mutations that result in severe neutropenia and a maturation arrest in neutrophilic myeloid production. Patients present with acute and life-threatening bacterial and fungal infections often involving the skin, oropharynx, and lung. Advancements in next-generation sequencing (NGS) technology have uncovered mutations associated with SCN, yet the genetic cause is still unknown in more than 20% of cases.[124] Molecular classification in the remaining cases is important for risk stratification, treatment, and prognosis. The most frequent pathogenic alterations in patients with SCN are autosomal dominant, heterozygous *ELANE* mutations that present with severe pyogenic infections in early infancy; unless treated with G-CSF or hematopoietic stem cell transplantation, they are fatal by 3 years of age. More than 100 distinct *ELANE* mutations have been described in congenital neutropenias.[124] *ELANE* mutations produce a misfolded neutrophil elastase protein that activates the unfolded protein response mechanism, leading to neutrophil apoptosis. Mutations of *GFI-1* cause a rare autosomal dominant form of disease also associated with lymphopenia. Kostmann originally described an autosomal recessive form of SCN in 1956, classically known as Kostmann neutropenia. It is associated with *HAX1* mutations and is seen in Swedish, Turkish, and Middle Eastern populations, accounting for 15% of SCNs, second in frequency only to *ELANE* mutations.[124] Infants present in the first weeks of life with severe bacterial infections, and a subset develops neurologic symptoms (epilepsy, cognitive defects, mental retardation) caused by an additional *HAX1* isoform expressed in neurons. Autosomal recessive disease caused by mutations of *G6PC3* and *VPS45* are rare, as is X-linked disease.

SCN is considered a preleukemic condition, with one review describing a 21% cumulative incidence of transformation to MDS or acute myeloid leukemia (AML) after 15 years.[124] Clones with acquired *CSF3R* and subsequent *RUNX1* mutations have been identified in patients who progressed to MDS or AML[125,126] (Fig. 10-40). G-CSF is the treatment of choice in SCN and ameliorates neutropenia, reduces infection risk, and improves quality of life in more than 90% of patients with SCN through increased neutrophil survival.[124] However, progression to MDS or AML is more frequent in patients requiring high doses of G-CSF; the current hypothesis is that poor response to G-CSF therapy likely identifies an "at risk" group of SCN individuals that are likely to have adverse clinical outcomes with G-CSF.

Cyclic Neutropenia

Cyclic neutropenia is an autosomal dominant disorder caused by *ELANE* mutations associated with low propensity for leukemic progression and milder disease than SCN such that some patients are not diagnosed until adulthood.[124,127] Patients have neutrophil counts that oscillate at 21-day intervals (intervals vary from 14 to 36 days) between normal and almost absent levels. The marrow exhibits a myeloid maturation arrest before the period of severe peripheral neutropenia. Accelerated apoptosis of bone marrow progenitor cells is found in all stages of the cycle, with insufficient myeloid output.[124] The diagnosis is established by monitoring serial neutrophil counts over a 6-week to 8-week period. G-CSF provides effective therapy without a significant risk for MDS or leukemic transformation.[107,125] Symptoms often improve as an individual grows older.

Shwachman-Diamond Syndrome

Shwachman-Diamond syndrome (SDS) is a rare, autosomal recessive, multisystem disorder that usually presents in the first few years of life.[128,129] Affected infants invariably have malabsorption, steatorrhea, and failure to thrive, with ultimate growth retardation. Increased infections are caused by neutropenia with impaired neutrophil chemotaxis and, commonly, T-cell and B-cell defects. The diagnosis is made based on identification of exocrine pancreatic dysfunction and intermittent or persistent neutropenia. Biallelic mutations of the Shwachman-Bodian-Diamond syndrome gene (*SBDS*) located on 7q11 are found in 90% of individuals, although some patients with clinical disease do not have these mutations. An additional three genes have been associated with an

Table 10-7   Causes of Constitutional Neutropenia With Associated Peripheral Blood and Bone Marrow Findings

Disorder (Inheritance/ Frequency)	Peripheral Blood Findings	Bone Marrow Findings	Additional Features and Most Common Molecular Abnormalities
Severe congenital neutropenia (AR, AD, XL, S; 1-2/million)	Chronic, marked neutropenia (<0.2 × 10⁹/L) Often monocytosis, eosinophilia	Normocellular with maturation arrest at promyelocyte stage Increased monocytes, eosinophils, macrophages, plasma cells	Severe neonatal neutropenia AD: *ELANE* or *GFI1* mutations AR: *HAX1*, *G6PC3*, or *VPS45* mutations XL: *WAS* mutations Acquired *CSF3R* and *RUNX1* mutations found in cases that progressed to MDS or AML
Cyclic neutropenia (AD, S; 1-2/million)	Cyclic, marked neutropenia at nadir of cycle (<0.2 × 10⁹/L) Oscillations in neutrophil, monocyte, reticulocyte, and platelet counts	Myeloid aplasia or hypoplasia with marked left-shift prior to periods of marked neutropenia	Febrile episodes every 21 days; skin and otolaryngeal infections *ELANE* mutations 10% fatal infections Leukemic transformation is rare G-CSF shortens cycle length and increases neutrophil counts
Shwachman-Diamond syndrome (SDS; AR, S; estimated 1:76,000)	Neutropenia (88%-100% of patients), ⅓ chronic, ⅔ intermittent Anemia with reticulocytopenia (up to 80%) Thrombocytopenia (24%–88%)	Variable cellularity Myeloid hypoplasia with possible left shift Possible mild dyspoiesis in all lineages May develop aplasia Prominent multilineage dysplasia may signify MDS or AML	Exocrine pancreatic dysfunction, short stature, skeletal abnormalities, bone marrow stromal defects Increased hemoglobin F (subset of patients) Biallelic *SBDS* mutations in >90% of patients Mutations in *DNAJC21*, *EFL1*, *SRP54* produce SDS-like phenotype
Chédiak-Higashi syndrome (AR; <500 cases reported)	Chronic neutropenia, large cytoplasmic inclusion bodies in granulocytes and precursors, large granular lymphocytes	Cytoplasmic azurophilic granules or inclusion bodies are myeloperoxidase and CD63 positive Found in neutrophils, other myeloid cells, and lymphocytes	*LYST* mutations; missense mutations— milder disease, truncated mutations—severe early disease; protein regulates lysosome-related organelle size and trafficking
WHIM syndrome (myelokathexis) (AD; very rare, estimated at 0.2 per million live births)	Chronic, severe neutropenia Abnormal neutrophil segmentation with thin filamentous strands connecting pyknotic nuclear lobes; hypersegmentation with cytoplasmic vacuoles; lymphopenia	Hypercellular, increased abnormal and hypersegmented neutrophils with apoptotic features, fine interlobar bridging, and cytoplasmic vacuolation	Heterozygous mutations in *CXCR4* lead to abnormal ↑ CXCR4 function Retention, senescence, and apoptosis of mature neutrophils in marrow Improved neutrophil release with G-CSF or GM-CSF therapy; CXCR4 antagonist therapy (e.g., plerixafor in clinical trials)

AD, Autosomal dominant; *AML*, acute myeloid leukemia; *AR*, autosomal recessive; *G-CSF*, granulocyte colony-stimulating factor; *GM-CSF*, granulocyte-macrophage colony-stimulating factor; *MDS*, myelodysplastic syndrome; *S*, somatic; *WHIM*, warts, hypogammaglobulinemia, infections, and myelokathexis; *XL*, X-linked.

SDS-like phenotype: DnaJ heat shock protein family member C21 (*DNAJC21*),[130,131] elongation factor-like 1 (*EFL1*),[131,132] and signal recognition particle 54 (*SRP54*).[133] All genes associated with SDS are involved in ribosome biogenesis, further advancing the concept that SDS is a ribosomopathy.[134] Disease phenotype and bone marrow findings vary with time in individuals and among patients, making the diagnosis challenging in some cases.[135] Symptoms include intermittent anemia and thrombocytopenia, neurocognitive deficits, skeletal abnormalities such as metaphyseal dysostosis, and hepatomegaly.

About 15% to 20% of individuals are diagnosed with MDS or AML at SDS presentation.[136] However, cytogenetic changes are common and not necessarily harbingers of malignancy, including isochromosome 7q and 20q11 deletion.[128,129] Thus, chromosomal abnormalities in isolation (in the absence of prominent or progressive morphologic features of dysplasia

or persistently increased numbers of blasts) should not automatically lead to a diagnosis of MDS or AML. Children with SDS do advance to bone marrow failure with progressive cytopenias and aplastic anemia,[128,129] with malignant transformation reported in 5% to 36% of patients.[136] Lifelong periodic bone marrow assessment is essential to monitor for these changes.

Chédiak-Higashi Syndrome

Though the exact prevalence is unknown, Chédiak-Higashi syndrome (CHS) is a rare disorder, with fewer than 500 cases reported in the literature. It exhibits diverse clinical manifestations related to abnormally enlarged lysosomes or lysosome-related organelles in cells (Fig. 10-41).[137] More than 60 different *LYST* mutations on chromosome 1q42.1-q42.2 are described. The type of mutation commonly affects the phenotype.[138] Improper cellular regulation and

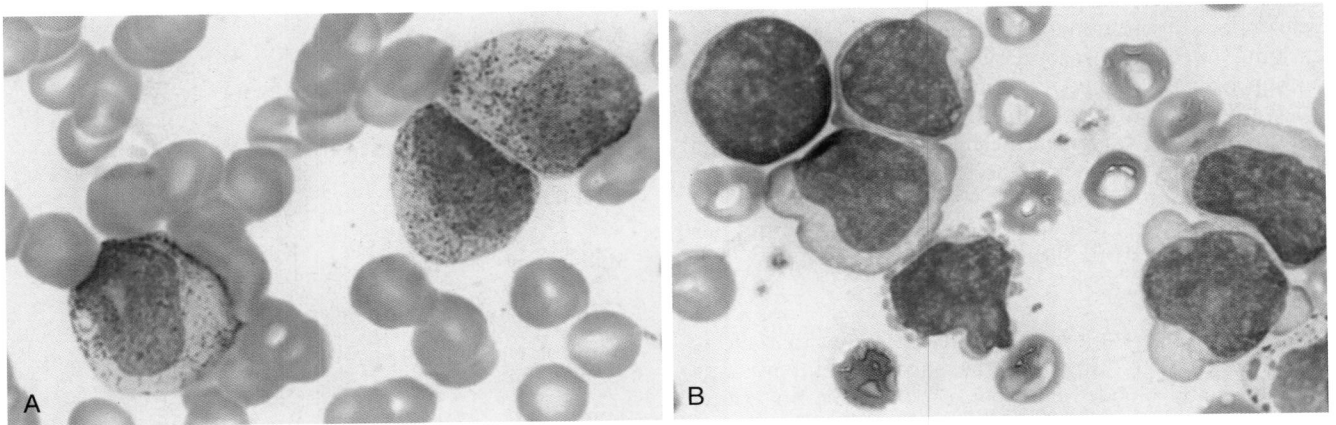

Figure 10-40. A, Bone marrow smear of severe congenital neutropenia in a 3-year-old boy illustrates a maturation arrest at the promyelocyte stage of development. **B,** Ten years later, after repeated poor response to therapy with high-dose granulocyte colony-stimulating factor (G-CSF), he developed acute myeloid leukemia. Point mutations in the G-CSF receptor gene were detected.

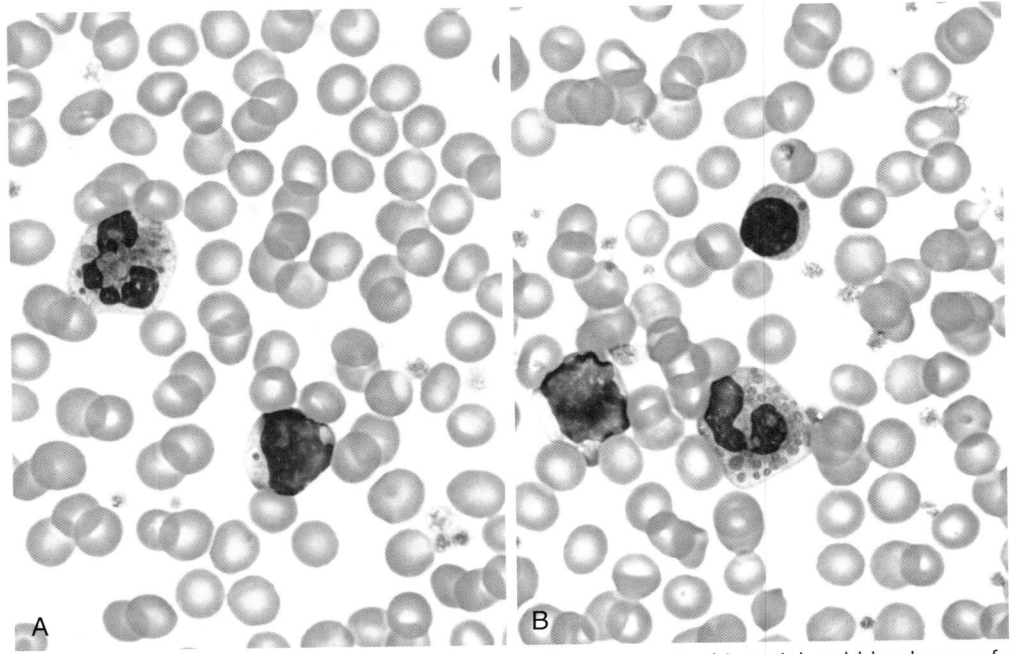

Figure 10-41. Giant neutrophil **(A)** and eosinophil **(B)**; secondary granules are seen in this peripheral blood smear from a patient with Chédiak-Higashi syndrome. Note the abnormal large primary granules in the lymphocytes.

function of lysozymes and related organelles lead to severe immunodeficiency, mild coagulation defects, variable oculocutaneous albinism, progressive neurologic dysfunction, periodontal disease, and defective plasma membrane repair. Faulty neutrophil chemotaxis and function lead to frequent and severe pyogenic infections that characterize this disorder, whereas a deficiency in platelet-dense bodies contributes to the tendency for easy bleeding. The classic (i.e., childhood-onset) form of CHS develops into the so-called "accelerated phase," which is fulminant hemophagocytic lymphohistiocytosis/hemophagocytic syndrome (HLH).[137] Without bone marrow transplantation for classic CHS, the disease is often fatal in the first decade of life.[139]

Myelokathexis

Myelokathexis is a histologic pattern of increased myeloid cells with excessive neutrophil apoptosis in the bone marrow. It is associated with the immunodeficiency disorder WHIM (warts, hypogammaglobulinemia, infections, and myelokathexis) syndrome.[140] Patients with WHIM have recurrent infections secondary to neutropenia, B-cell lymphopenia, and hypogammaglobulinemia. They are particularly susceptible to human papilloma virus infection and require careful surveillance. This is the first example of a disease mediated by a chemokine receptor (CXCR4). *CXCR4* mutations on chromosome 2q21 are believed to increase intracellular signaling that allows for retention of neutrophils in bone marrow or tissue sites.[141]

Additional Disorders

Dyskeratosis congenita is a multisystem disorder that affects tissues with a high turnover rate, such as skin, mucous membranes, and blood. Neutropenia is often the presenting hematologic manifestation. As 80% to 90% of patients develop bone marrow failure, this disorder is more fully described later in this chapter in the section Evaluation of Specific Bone Marrow Failure Syndromes.

Neutropenia may also be a presenting feature of other congenital disorders including Fanconi anemia, reticular dysgenesis, cartilage-hair hypoplasia, Hermansky-Pudlak syndrome type 2, Griscelli syndrome type 2, *LAMTOR2* deficiency, Barth syndrome, AK2 deficiency, poikiloderma, CD40LG deficiency, Cohen syndrome, *GATA2* deficiency, Pearson marrow-pancreas syndrome, *STK4* deficiency, and glycogen storage disease type IB.[124]

Lymphopenia

Lymphopenia or lymphocytopenia is defined as an absolute lymphocyte count of less than 1.5×10^9/L in adults and less than 2.0×10^9/L in young children. It may occur in isolation or as part of pancytopenia. Lymphopenia can be further categorized as decreased B cells, T cells, NK cells, or their subsets. The causes of lymphopenia are extensive and include a variety of infectious, drug-related, autoimmune, and congenital processes (Box 10-4).

Infection-Related Lymphopenia

Lymphopenia is seen in a number of viral, fungal, bacterial, mycobacterial, and parasitic infections.[142] Reactive lymphocyte morphology in these disorders provides a clue to underlying infection. A decreased lymphocyte count is the hematologic

---

Box 10-4 *Causes of Lymphopenia*

Infections
- HIV
- SARS coronavirus, including coronavirus disease 2019 (COVID-19) caused by the novel SARS-coronavirus-2 (SARS-CoV-2)
- Influenza
- Respiratory syncytial virus
- Ebola
- Anaplasmosis (ehrlichiosis)
- *Legionella pneumophila*
- Tuberculosis
- Sepsis-induced immunosuppression

Therapy
- Steroids
- Rituximab
- Chemotherapy, especially purine analogues and alkylating agents
- Antibiotics
- Antithymocyte globulin
- Immunosuppressive therapy
- Radiation therapy

Autoimmune
- Systemic lupus erythematosus
- Rheumatoid arthritis
- Crohn disease
- Vasculitis

Malignancy
- Carcinoma
- Hodgkin and non-Hodgkin lymphoma

Hematologic Disorders
- Aplastic anemia

Congenital
- Severe combined immunodeficiency
- DiGeorge syndrome (thymic aplasia)
- Wiskott-Aldrich syndrome
- Primary immunodeficiency syndromes

Other
- Physiologic stress
- Idiopathic CD4 lymphocytopenia

HIV, Human immunodeficiency virus; SARS, severe acute respiratory syndrome.
* List is not all-inclusive and instead represents major causes.

---

hallmark of HIV infection. The destruction of CD4+ memory T cells, followed by increased memory T-cell turnover and damage to the thymus and other lymphoid tissues, results in profound lymphopenia.[143]

The emergence of the highly transmissible novel coronavirus, severe acute respiratory syndrome coronavirus 2 (SARS-CoV-2), in December 2019 led to a global pandemic with devastating morbidity and mortality, termed coronavirus disease 19 (COVID-19). As of August 2022, over 500 million cases had been reported worldwide, with the vast majority experiencing mild-to-moderate disease. Yet over the same period, severe infections have led to more than 6 million deaths caused by COVID-19.[144,145] In severe disease, not only is the respiratory system affected; there is marked inflammatory response, multiorgan dysfunction with renal, neurologic, and cardiovascular effects, and derangements in the coagulation and fibrinolytic pathways, leading to thromboembolic events.[146] The most notable CBC abnormalities are lymphopenia and neutrophilia at hospital admission, both of which are associated with increased odds of progression to severe disease and death.[147] Striking peripheral CD4 and CD8 T-lymphopenia in patients with severe COVID-19 is hypothesized to occur via diversion of T-cells into infected organs and activation-induced exhaustion, apoptosis, or pyroptosis.[148] A broad spectrum of peripheral blood smear findings has been described in patients with COVID-19, including abnormalities in neutrophils, lymphocytes, monocytes, and platelets.[146,149] Several reports discuss the finding of circulating reactive "atypical" lymphocytes and/or lymphoplasmacytoid cells[150-152] (so-called "covidocytes"); some investigators report their association with better clinical outcomes (Fig. 10-42).[150]

Drug-Related Lymphopenia

Some therapeutic agents are associated with decreased lymphocyte counts. Within hours of administration, corticosteroids initiate lymphopenia, primarily of T cells, through a glucocorticoid receptor–associated apoptotic mechanism.[153] Chemotherapeutic agents, particularly alkylating agents and purine analogues, also induce lymphocyte depletion through several different apoptotic mechanisms. The CD4 T cells are especially sensitive, and lymphopenia a therapy may be prolonged.[154] The anti-CD20 mAb rituximab binds to B cells and produces cell death by complement-mediated lysis and apoptosis.[155]

Congenital Immunodeficiency Disorders

Lymphocytopenia in congenital immunodeficiency diseases and frequent viral, fungal, or protozoal infections suggest a T-cell disorder; on the other hand, abnormal serum immunoglobulin levels and recurrent infections with encapsulated bacteria point toward a B-cell disorder or antibody deficiency.[156,157] Severe combined immunodeficiencies (SCID) are rare disorders of humoral and cellular immunity, classified by the affected lymphocyte subsets (T-cell, B-cell, NK-cell).[157,158] They present as recurrent severe infections with unusual pathogens in young infants. Nearly half of SCID cases are X-linked. Molecular defects in the following genes have been described in patients with SCID: *IL-2RG* (most prevalent), *JAK3, RAG1, RAG2, DCLRE1C, PRKDC, IL7R, CD3D, CD3E, CD247, PTPRC, CORO1A, ADA,* and *AK2.*[158] The most common chromosomal microdeletion disorder, 22q11.2 deletion syndrome (22q11.2DS), is a T-cell deficiency disorder. Initially dubbed "DiGeorge syndrome" in the 1960s for patients presenting with a clinical triad (immunodeficiency, congenital heart defects, and hypoparathyroidism), 22q11.2DS is much more heterogeneous than originally described. Its presentation may also include variable degrees of thymic hypoplasia, other congenital abnormalities (such as palatal, gastrointestinal, and renal), variable cognitive and developmental delays, neuropsychiatric illnesses, and predisposition to infections and autoimmune diseases.[159]

Reactive Lymphopenia

Stress lymphopenia is seen in the setting of myocardial infarction, major surgery, trauma, sickle cell crisis, acute stroke, and intense exercise.[160-162] Release of cortisol with subsequent apoptosis results in decreased lymphocyte numbers.[163] Idiopathic CD4 lymphopenia is a rare disease associated with

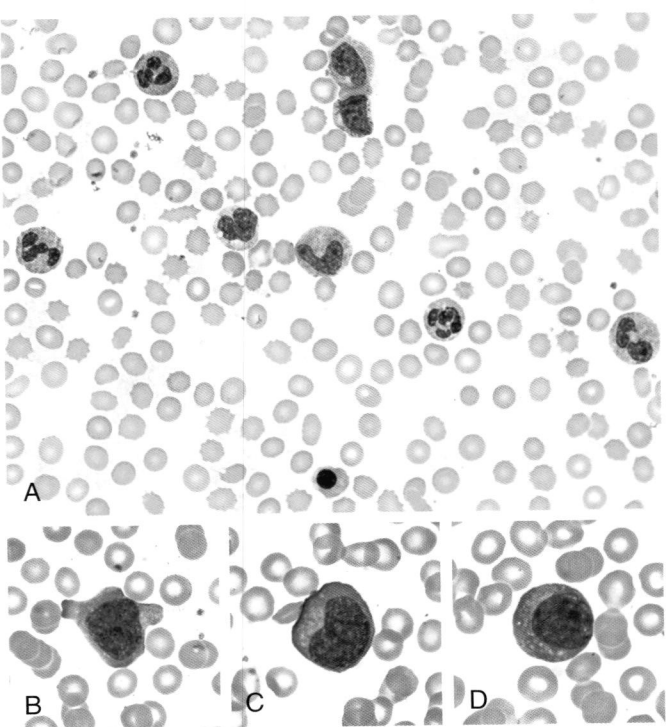

Figure 10-42. Peripheral blood smears from two patients with COVID-19. A, Left-shifted neutrophilia and marked lymphopenia are observed in the blood of an intubated 58-year-old man with severe pneumonitis who had not been vaccinated against SARS-CoV-2. **B-D,** Lymphoplasmacytoid cells (covidocytes) were seen in the blood smear of a 25-year-old woman recovering from severe infection.

persistent lymphopenia (CD4-positive cells $<0.3 \times 10^9$/L) in the absence of HIV infection or other recognized causes of low CD4 cell counts. The pathogenesis is unclear, but it is postulated to occur through redistribution into tissues (such as lymph nodes and spleen) or decreased CD4 T-cell production from disturbed thymic maturation, increased apoptosis via the Fas pathway, or defective interferon-γ production.[164]

Lymphopenia Secondary to Autoimmune Disorders

Decreased lymphocyte count is a criterion for the diagnosis of systemic lupus erythematosus (SLE) (Fig. 10-43) and is encountered in other autoimmune diseases as well, particularly rheumatoid arthritis, Crohn's disease, and vasculitis.[165] Although the exact links between lymphopenia and autoimmune diseases have yet to be elucidated, key mechanisms for immune dysregulation have been proposed with a "double hit hypothesis."[166] The first hit is an autoimmune genetic propensity that, in lymphopenic states, leads to expansion of auto-reactive T cells via lymphopenia-induced proliferation (LIP). This is achieved with increased IL-7 availability signaling through the IL-7 receptor, Akt and JAK-STAT5 activation pathway, and BCL2 antiapoptotic pathway. The second hit is thought to occur when TGF-β signaling, which normally inhibits self-reactive T-cell proliferation, is suppressed in lymphopenic conditions.[167]

EVALUATION OF THROMBOCYTOPENIA

Thrombocytopenia is a decrease in the circulating platelet count to less than 150×10^9/L. It is encountered frequently

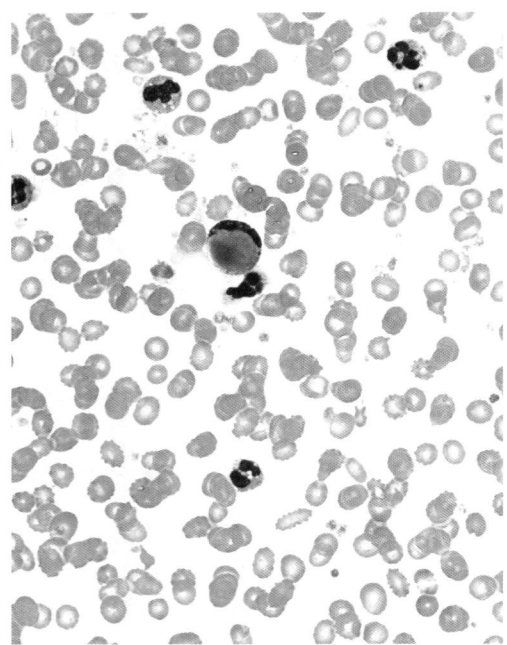

Figure 10-43. Peripheral smear from a patient with systemic lupus erythematosus (SLE). The lupus erythematosus (LE) cell contains phagocytized homogeneous purple nuclear material, which compresses the neutrophil nucleus.

in clinical practice, and when severe, is a common cause of hemorrhage. Thrombocytopenia is the result of decreased production, increased destruction or utilization, or abnormal distribution of platelets. Evaluation of megakaryocytes in patients with unexplained thrombocytopenia is one of the most common indications for a bone marrow examination in clinical practice.[168] An important caveat before bone marrow evaluation is to confirm that the platelet count is not spuriously low as a result of in vitro platelet clumping. This phenomenon is most commonly caused by naturally occurring antibodies directed against a normally hidden platelet epitope (glycoprotein IIb/IIIa complex) that becomes exposed in the presence of ethylenediaminetetraacetic acid (EDTA). Blood collection in sodium citrate or an alternative anticoagulant may alleviate the problem.[169] Additional causes for platelet clumping include inadequate anticoagulant or improper mixing, cold agglutinin, and excessive trauma during venipuncture with release of thrombin. Review of the blood film before bone marrow evaluation is essential to look for platelet clumps and to evaluate for platelet rosetting around white blood cells (satellitism) and platelet–white blood cell aggregates.

Evaluation of bone marrow megakaryocytes is an important initial step in the workup for unexplained thrombocytopenia. Decreased megakaryocytes are indicative of decreased platelet production, whereas normal or increased megakaryocytes point toward ineffective megakaryopoiesis (intramedullary cell death or excessive apoptosis) or loss of platelets from the circulation.

Table 10-8 lists the differential diagnoses for thrombocytopenia when megakaryocytes are absent or decreased. Age is an important consideration; an isolated loss of megakaryocytes (amegakaryopoiesis) suggests a congenital or, rarely, an autoimmune process with anti-megakaryocyte

or anti-thrombopoietin antibodies. Identifying the cause of an underlying bone marrow failure disorder or other process (e.g., Fanconi anemia, acute leukemia) may be a challenge when isolated thrombocytopenia is the presenting finding. Evaluation for subtle dysplasia, viral effects, or abnormal cellular infiltrates is required. Cytogenetic evaluation, chromosome breakage studies (Fanconi anemia), and expanded molecular analysis with NGS for genes associated with bone marrow failure syndromes are warranted, as clinically indicated. Chemotherapy, toxin exposure, or prolonged use of certain drugs can selectively affect the megakaryocytes in some patients. Chronic platelet destruction or consumption may rarely induce amegakaryopoiesis.

Causes of acquired and congenital thrombocytopenia when the bone marrow megakaryocytes are normal or increased in number are listed in Tables 10-9 and 10-10, respectively. A compensatory increase with greater numbers of immature and/or earlier forms of megakaryocytes ("left shift") is often present during times of increased platelet destruction or utilization (Fig. 10-44). Younger megakaryocytes are often smaller and exhibit less nuclear lobation than mature forms. Platelets produced from these younger megakaryocytes are larger than the typical platelet diameter of 4 μm to 7 μm. In this setting, platelet accumulation in bone marrow sinuses also suggests increased platelet consumption when bone marrow artifacts or a myeloproliferative neoplasm are excluded.

Acquired Thrombocytopenia

Immune-Mediated Thrombocytopenia

Immune thrombocytopenia (also called *immune thrombocytopenic purpura* or *ITP*) is the most frequent cause for platelet destruction. The 2011 American Society of Hematology guidelines for ITP (which largely adopted the International Working Group's recommendations for standardizing terminology and definitions)[170] were updated in 2019[171] with a focus on various management approaches, though most of the 2011 nomenclature was retained. The disease may be primary or secondary and is classified by phase: newly diagnosed (0 to 3 months), persistent (3 to 12 months), chronic (>12 months), or refractory (failure to respond to splenectomy or relapse after).[170] Disease severity is based on bleeding symptoms, not platelet count. Platelet antibody testing is not recommended because of poor sensitivity and specificity. Glucocorticoids are used as first-line therapy; however, if disease relapses soon after glucocorticoid therapy, then thrombopoietin receptor agonists (TPO-RA) (eltrombopag or romiplostim), rituximab, and/or splenectomy may be considered.[172] A small number of patients has been reported to develop moderate-to-severe marrow reticulin and/or collagen fibrosis with TPO-RA therapy, with reversal after drug discontinuation.[173-176] On the other hand, a Danish national patient registry reported moderate-to-severe fibrosis in a similar small number of chronic patients with ITP who had not undergone treatment with TPO-RA,[177] suggesting development of fibrosis in chronic ITP may be part of the spectrum of autoimmune myelofibrosis (Chapter 11).

Primary Immune Thrombocytopenia

Primary ITP is defined as an acquired isolated thrombocytopenia with no identifiable associated medical condition. The pathogenesis is primarily IgG autoantibody–mediated platelet

Table 10-8 Thrombocytopenias With Decreased or Absent Bone Marrow Megakaryocytes

Disorder	Comments
Constitutional	
Thrombocytopenia with absent radii (TAR)	*RBM8A* mutation/del(1q21.1), AR Normal-to-small PLTs Reduced MKs in BM; small immature MKs, if present. Bilateral radial aplasia with absence of upper limbs in some Other skeletal, renal, and cardiac anomalies Platelet counts improve by 1 year, possible mild intermittent thrombocytopenia later
Congenital amegakaryocytic thrombocytopenia (CAMT)	*MPL* mutation, AR No physical abnormalities Isolated marked thrombocytopenia at birth, normal-to-small PLTs Absent-to-reduced MKs in BM with development of trilineage BM aplasia in childhood or adolescence Reduced MPL on platelets affects thrombopoietin degradation
Congenital autosomal recessive small-platelet thrombocytopenia (CARST) or *FYB*-related thrombocytopenia	*FYB* mutation, AR Small PLTs, mild iron deficiency Significant bleeding tendency Reduced numbers of mature MKs in BM
BM failure syndromes* (dyskeratosis congenita, Fanconi anemia, Shwachman-Diamond syndrome†)	May present initially with isolated thrombocytopenia
Acquired	
Infection	Viral (rubella, rubeola, varicella, EBV, CMV, hantavirus, HIV, parvovirus B19, dengue, hepatitis, adenovirus, mumps) *Mycoplasma,* mycobacteria, ehrlichiosis, malaria
Immune-mediated destruction	Autoimmune disease, T-cell large granular lymphocyte disorders, some cases of chronic ITP
Toxins/drugs	Alcohol; chemotherapy; drugs, especially after prolonged use (thiazide diuretics, chloramphenicol, estrogen, prednisone, progesterone); ionizing radiation
Nutritional deficiency	Vitamin B$_{12}$ or folate deficiency
Bone marrow replacement	Leukemia, metastatic carcinoma, myeloma, granuloma, fibrosis
MDS	May initially present with isolated thrombocytopenia, dysplastic MKs
Aplastic anemia*	
Paroxysmal nocturnal hemoglobinuria*	

*See Table 10-11 for additional information.
†See Table 10-7 for additional information.
AML, Acute myeloid leukemia; *AR,* autosomal recessive; *BM,* bone marrow; *CMV,* cytomegalovirus; *EBV,* Epstein-Barr virus; *HIV,* human immunodeficiency virus; *ITP,* immune thrombocytopenic purpura; *MDS,* myelodysplastic syndrome or myelodysplastic neoplasm; *MK,* megakaryocyte; *PLT,* platelet.

destruction, with complement-mediated opsonization or cell lysis, defects in T-cell regulation, and plasma effects on megakaryocyte production contributing to the decrease in platelets.[178] Increased T- and NK-large granular lymphocytes (T/NK-LGLs) are seen in patients with chronic ITP. Approximately 30% of children have a chronic form more similar to adult ITP.[179] These children usually present without a viral prodrome, and constitutional platelet disorders need to be excluded. Testing for *Helicobacter pylori* infection, antiphospholipid antibodies, and antinuclear antibodies (ANA) is advocated.[171]

Secondary Immune Thrombocytopenia

Secondary ITP is associated with a wide range of primary diseases, and terminology to describe the disease association is recommended in the diagnosis (e.g., secondary ITP [specific disease or drug-associated]). Some conditions linked to secondary ITP include rheumatologic disorders (e.g., antiphospholipid syndrome, SLE), medications, immunodeficiencies (e.g., common variable immunodeficiency, autoimmune lymphoproliferative syndrome), and infections (*H. pylori*, *Rickettsia*, viral).[180,181] Despite the extensive list of drugs known to be implicated, the diagnosis is frequently difficult and often becomes one of exclusion. The immune

mechanisms involved are also varied and drug dependent, but they act primarily to increase peripheral platelet clearance, with some drugs also causing marrow suppression.[181]

Heparin-Induced Thrombocytopenia

Heparin-induced thrombocytopenia may be immune or nonimmune mediated. The latter is caused by platelet activation developing within days of heparin exposure that often resolves during continued therapy. Immune-mediated heparin-induced thrombocytopenia (HIT) occurs in 0.5% to 5% of individuals after receiving unfractionated or, less frequently, low–molecular-weight heparin for at least 4 days (Table 10-9).[182] Surgical patients are at greater risk than patients receiving heparin for medical interventions; HIT is rare in pediatric and obstetric patients. Antibodies against heparin/platelet factor 4 (heparin-PF4) immune complexes engage with platelet and monocyte Fc receptors, causing cellular activation, procoagulant microparticle release, and thrombin generation.[183] Venous or arterial thrombosis occurs in 17% to 53% of patients with isolated HIT. Clinical scoring systems have been developed to determine the likelihood of HIT given the significant mortality that is associated with misdiagnosis and overdiagnosis in patients receiving heparin.[184] The 4Ts score for evaluating the pretest risk of HIT

Table 10-9 **Acquired Thrombocytopenia With Normal-to-Increased Megakaryocytes**

Mechanism	Disease/Cause	Comments
Increased Destruction or Utilization		
Immunologic	Primary immune thrombocytopenia	Children: acute onset, 60% occurs 2-4 weeks after viral infection or immunization (especially MMR); 50% have PLTs <10 × 10³/L; 80% resolve within 6-12 months; slight PLT enlargement Adults: insidious onset; often PLT 30-50 × 10³/L at presentation; chronic course common; young females present during first trimester of pregnancy; treatment tailored to individual patient
	Secondary immune thrombocytopenia	Immune-mediated thrombocytopenia with associated medical condition
	Rheumatologic, hematologic, or immunologic diseases	Autoimmune collagen vascular disorders (e.g., SLE), rheumatoid disorders, lymphoproliferative disorders (e.g., CLL, lymphoma, T-LGL leukemia), antiphospholipid syndrome, thyroid disease, solid tumors, common variable immunodeficiency disorder, ALPS, autoimmune hemolysis/Evans syndrome
	Drugs, including heparin (HIT)	A number of drugs involved; variety of mechanisms, including hapten-dependent antibody formation, drug–glycoprotein complex antibody formation, autoantibody formation, ligand-induced binding site creation, drug-specific antibody formation, and immune complex–mediated antibody formation; circulating antibodies to PF4-heparin complexes Thrombocytopenia and/or thrombosis at 5-14 days after heparin initiation in heparin-naïve patient; acute thrombocytopenia after heparin reexposure; >30% drop in PLT count from baseline; possible necrotic skin lesions at injection site or anaphylactoid reactions after IV heparin bolus
	Infection	HIV, *Helicobacter pylori*, HCV, VZV; generates antibodies that cross-react with platelet antigens or immune complexes that bind PLT Fc receptors
	Neonatal alloimmune thrombocytopenia	IgG alloantibodies transferred from maternal circulation to baby, formed against incompatible paternal PLT antigens on fetal PLTs; 80% of Caucasians have antibodies to HPA-1a; can present with severe bleeding and marked thrombocytopenia hours to days after birth
	Platelet transfusion	Alloantibodies mounted against a common HPA antigen in the transfused donor PLTs are thought to lead to destruction of host PLTs; develops 5-14 days after transfusion
Thrombotic microangiopathies	Thrombotic thrombocytopenic purpura (TTP)	Increased in women in third to fourth decades of life; rare in children Pentad of findings: thrombocytopenia, microangiopathic hemolytic anemia, fever (25%), neurologic abnormalities (70%-80%), and renal dysfunction (40%); complete pentad is rarely seen in patients. Antibody to ADAMTS13 is causative (often IgG) in immune-mediated TTP (iTTP) Idiopathic (80%); secondary to infection, drugs, pregnancy, other (10%-15%); congenital (<5%) Congenital disorder (Upshaw-Schulman syndrome): *ADAMTS13* gene mutations resulting in severely deficient ADAMTS13 activity; chronic relapsing disease, presents at any age; can be treated by repleting deficient ADAMTS13 by plasma infusion, plasma exchange, recombinant ADAMTS13 in clinical trials.
	Hemolytic uremic syndrome (HUS)	Similar clinical symptoms to TTP but less extensive and predominantly involves the kidneys; common cause of acute renal failure in children Normal ADAMTS13 levels; often treated with supportive care Triggered by infection with Shiga toxin–producing bacteria Atypical HUS (10% of cases) associated with gene mutations that regulate the complement and coagulation pathways in adults and children
	Disseminated intravascular coagulation (DIC)	Syndrome seen in a variety of diseases or with marked tissue damage; thrombohemorrhagic disorder secondary to intravascular activation of coagulation (with fibrin thrombi deposition) and simultaneous consumption of coagulation factors, fibrinolytic agents, and PLTs
Other	HELLP syndrome	Hemolysis, elevated liver enzymes, low PLT counts Develops in pregnant, often White, multiparous women older than 25 years of age
	Mechanical injury	Prosthetic heart valves, burns, malignant hypertension, vasculitis, transplantation-associated microangiopathy
	Kasabach-Merritt syndrome	Vascular lesion causes PLT trapping and activation, with severe thrombotic coagulopathy that occurs in the presence of enlarging vascular tumors; may result in multiorgan hemorrhage in infants; lesions may regress with age
Ineffective Megakaryopoiesis	Infection	HIV, CMV, other
Abnormal Distribution	Splenomegaly	Increased splenic sequestration of up to 80%-90% of circulating PLTs (normal, 30%-35%); chronic liver disease, pediatric sickle cell disease, hemoglobinopathies, chronic infection, myeloproliferative neoplasms, lymphomas, storage diseases
	Hypothermia	Pooling of PLTs in splenic sinusoids, especially at body temperature <25° C
	Massive transfusion	Hemodilution
	Gestational thrombocytopenia	PLT count >70,000/μL in healthy pregnant woman; accounts for 75% of thrombocytopenia in pregnant women; pathogenesis is unclear but probably related to hemodilution and increased PLT clearance

ALPS, Autoimmune lymphoproliferative syndrome; *CLL,* chronic lymphocytic leukemia; *CMV,* cytomegalovirus; *HCV,* hepatitis C virus; *HELLP,* hemolysis, elevated liver enzymes, low platelet count; *HIT,* heparin-induced thrombocytopenia; *HIV,* human immunodeficiency virus; *HPA,* human platelet antigen; *MMR,* measles-mumps-rubella; *PF,* platelet factor; *PLT,* platelet; *SLE,* systemic lupus erythematosus; *T-LGL,* T-cell large granular lymphocytic; *VZV,* varicella-zoster virus.

Table 10-10 Representative List of Constitutional/Inherited Thrombocytopenias With Normal-to-Increased Megakaryocytes

Disease/Syndrome	Gene Mutation, Inheritance	Morphology	Comments
Platelet Adhesion Defect			
Bernard-Soulier syndromes (BSS), including bBSS mBSS GFI1B-related thrombocytopenia	GP9, AR: BSS GP1BB, AR/AD: bBSS, mBSS	BSS: Giant PLTs bBSS/mBSS: Giant/large PLTs Large MKs with increased ploidy, mild to marked thrombocytopenia	Rare; reduced GP Ib-IX-V (CD42a-d) on PLTs Abnormal MK membrane maturation Early childhood mucocutaneous bleeding Severe bleeding during surgery or trauma Defective ristocetin-induced PLT aggregation (bBSS)
Platelet-type von Willebrand disease (PTvWD)	GP1BA, AR/AD: bBSS/mBSS/PTvWD	bBSS/mBSS/PTvWD: Giant/large/normal PLTs	Spontaneous binding of mutated vWF to PLT GP Ibα enhances ADAMTS13 cleavage of large vWF multimers
vWD type 2B (and variant: Montreal platelet syndrome)	VWF, AD	Large PLTs, sometimes circulating PLT aggregates, variable thrombocytopenia	Defective vWF-dependent PLT function Defective ristocetin-induced PLT aggregation
Secretion Defects			
Gray platelet syndrome	NBEAL2, AR	Large "gray" agranular PLTs Progressive thrombocytopenia BM reticulin fibrosis Extensive emperipolesis	Absence of PLT α-granules EM: empty α-granules Bleeding disorder with several PLT aggregation defects Defect in MK maturation
Wiskott-Aldrich syndrome	WAS, XLR Decreased WAS protein	Smaller-than-normal PLTs Mild thrombocytopenia at birth, with progression Premature proplatelet formation of MKs and ectopic PLT shedding in the BM	Severe immunodeficiency, recurrent infections, eczema Autoimmune hemolytic anemia Propensity to develop lymphomas Circulating autoantibodies with splenic engulfment of PLTs
GATA1-associated thrombocytopenia (also XL thrombocytopenia, XL thrombocytopenia with thalassemia)	GATA1, XL	Small PLTs Hypercellular BM with increased or decreased large MKs with nuclear abnormalities	Imbalanced globin chain synthesis Splenomegaly May present with congenital erythropoietic porphyria (see Table 10-6)
Cytoskeletal Defects			
MYH9-related disorders (previously thought to be distinct entities May-Hegglin anomaly, Sebastian, Epstein, and Fechtner syndromes)	MYH9, AD	Giant PLTs, leukocytes with Döhle-like bodies, variable thrombocytopenia	Spectrum of disease, from mild manifestations of peripheral smear findings to more significant presentations of sensorineural hearing loss, chronic kidney disease, cataracts, and/or elevations of liver enzymes
ACTN1-related thrombocytopenia	ACTN1, AD	Large PLTs Isolated mild thrombocytopenia	Absent or mild bleeding diathesis Defect in PLT production and clearance
TUBB1-related thrombocytopenia	TUBB1, AD	Large PLTs Isolated mild thrombocytopenia	Absent or mild bleeding diathesis
Familial Platelet Disorder With Propensity for Malignancy (FPD-PM)			
RUNX1-related thrombocytopenia	RUNX1, AD	Small, normal, or slightly enlarged PLTs Hypo- or normocellular BMs Dysmorphic MKs: small, hypolobated; microMKs BM eosinophilia	Highly variable clinical presentation, from normal and asymptomatic to mild to moderate thrombocytopenia with bleeding tendency FPD-PM with some patients presenting with MDS/AML at initial presentation Mutational defect in megakaryopoiesis
ETV6-related thrombocytopenia	ETV6, AD	Normal-sized PLTs Mild to moderate thrombocytopenia Small, hypolobated MKs Mild myeloid nuclear hypolobation and hypogranulation Mild dyserythropoiesis	Mild to moderate bleeding symptoms; may be initially misdiagnosed as ITP FPD-PM, most commonly B-ALL, although other myeloid malignancies (MDS, AML, CMML, PV) can occur as well
ANKRD26-related thrombocytopenia	ANKRD26, AD	Normal-sized PLTs Usually isolated mild to moderate thrombocytopenia Hypercellular BM with dysmorphic MKs: small, hypolobated; micro MKs	Mild bleeding phenotype FPD-PM
Other			
CYCS-related thrombocytopenia	CYCS, AD	Normal-sized PLTs Isolated mild thrombocytopenia	Absent or mild bleeding diathesis

AD, Autosomal dominant; AML, acute myeloid leukemia; AR, autosomal recessive; B-ALL, B-lymphoblastic leukemia/lymphoma; bBSS, biallelic Bernard Soulier syndrome; BM, bone marrow; BMF/AA, bone marrow failure/aplasia; CMML, chronic myelomonocytic leukemia; EM, electron microscopy; FPD-PM, familial platelet disorder with propensity for malignancy; GP, glycoprotein; mBSS, monoallelic Bernard Soulier syndrome; MDS, myelodysplastic syndrome/myelodysplastic neoplasm; MK, megakaryocyte; PLT, platelet; PV, polycythemia vera; RBC, red blood cell; vWD, von Willebrand disease; vWF, von Willebrand factor; XL, X-linked; XLR, X-linked recessive.

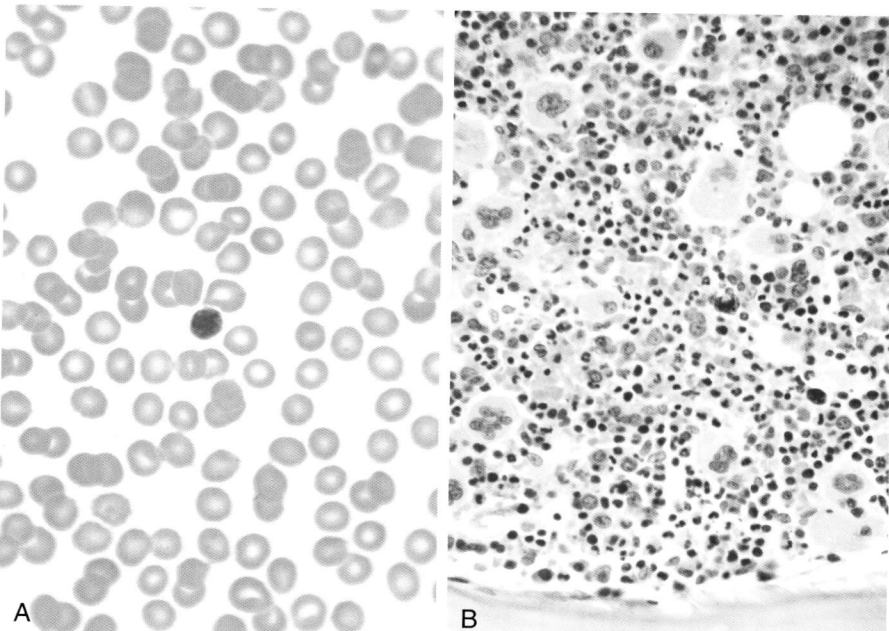

Figure 10-44. A, Peripheral blood smear of immune thrombocytopenic purpura. A single large platelet is seen at the center. Large platelets reflect early release from the bone marrow. **B,** The bone marrow trephine biopsy section contains increased numbers of megakaryocytes.

assigns points in four parameters (i.e., thrombocytopenia, timing of platelet count fall, thrombosis or other sequelae, and other causes of thrombocytopenia) and has been shown to have a very high negative predictive value for HIT when the 4Ts score is less than 4. However, positive predictive values for high or intermediate 4Ts scores are unsatisfactory; thus, this system performs best to exclude HIT. Testing with immunoassay for heparin-PF4 complex antibodies has high sensitivity (>90%) and low specificity, necessitating functional assay testing in some individuals with intermediate clinical findings. Bone marrow examination is required only when platelet counts do not normalize after discontinuation of heparin. Thrombocytopenia in HIT is typically less severe than that seen in classic drug-induced immune thrombocytopenia (DITP). The median nadir platelet counts are less than 20×10^9/L, translating into a high risk of hemorrhagic events in DITP.[185]

Infection-Associated Thrombocytopenia

Infection, especially viral infection, is a frequent cause of thrombocytopenia through direct infection of megakaryocytes, the toxic effects of organism proteins or cytokines, secondary hemophagocytosis, or immune-mediated destruction from antiplatelet antibodies. HIV-associated thrombocytopenia was reported in 5% to 30% of infected individuals before the advent of highly active antiretroviral therapy (HAART), though this has significantly decreased in the post-HAART era.[186] HIV-associated thrombocytopenia involves multiple mechanisms. Immune-mediated platelet destruction occurs after specific or non-specific binding of anti-HIV antibodies or immune complexes to platelets (e.g., glycoprotein IIb/III). The virus directly infects megakaryocytes through CD4 and CXCR4 receptors, which causes ineffective platelet production. Megakaryocytes also undergo increased intramedullary apoptosis[187] and appear pyknotic, with near-naked hyperchromatic nuclei that have scant associated cytoplasm (Fig. 10-45).[188,189]

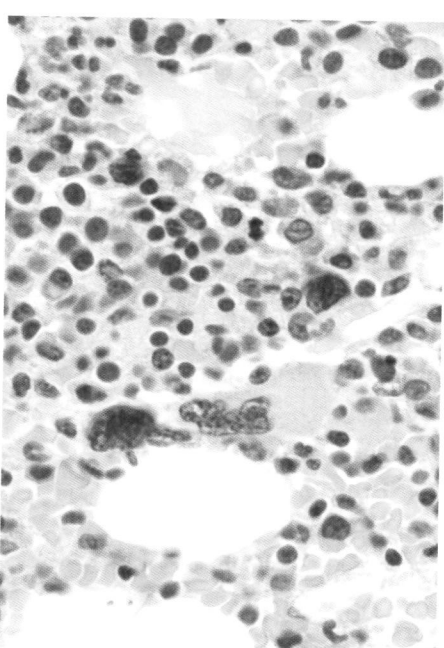

Figure 10-45. Several apoptotic megakaryocytes with high nuclear-to-cytoplasmic ratios are seen in this bone marrow biopsy section from a patient with HIV-associated thrombocytopenia.

H. pylori infection is associated with ITP. Some patients have secondary ITP (*H. pylori* associated), whereas others have primary ITP with a coincidental *H. pylori* infection.[190] The prior explains improvement in platelet counts among thrombocytopenic adults after *H. pylori* eradication programs in some regions of the world, such as Italy and Japan, but not the United States. One trigger initiating the antiplatelet autoantibody response is modulation of the Fcγ receptor balance of monocytes/macrophages through inhibition of the immunosuppressive FcγRIIB signal.

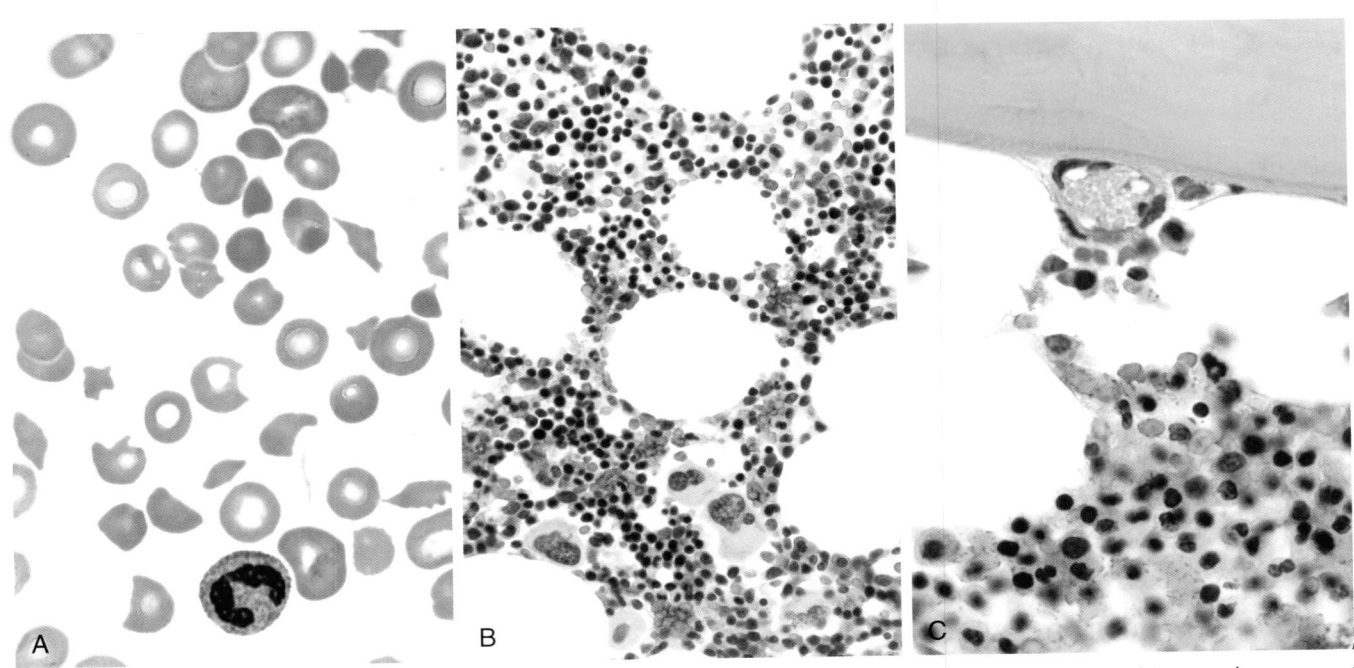

Figure 10-46. **A,** Peripheral blood smear of thrombotic thrombocytopenic purpura. Numerous red cell fragments (schistocytes) are present. No platelets are seen in this field. **B,** The bone marrow trephine biopsy section shows increased numbers of megakaryocytes. **C,** A platelet thrombus is seen in a small vein of the trephine biopsy section.

Neonatal Thrombocytopenia

In newborns, thrombocytopenia caused by perinatal complications such as infection or asphyxia rarely requires bone marrow evaluation before platelet counts resolve. Severe platelet reductions in the first month of life are usually caused by alloimmunization with platelet-specific antigens that are incompatible between mother and child. This diagnosis of neonatal alloimmune thrombocytopenia (NAIT) is best made by examination for platelet antibodies in conjunction with parental and fetal platelet genotyping demonstrating incompatibility.[191]

Thrombocytopenia Secondary to Microangiopathic Processes

Microangiopathic processes are associated with thrombocytopenia, but the anemia and red cell fragmentation (i.e., schistocytes) may not be evident until a few days after the initial clinical presentation (Fig. 10-46). Mechanical fragmentation of erythrocytes occurs during flow through partially occluded high-shear microvessels. The partial arteriolar and capillary occlusion results from excessive platelet deposition or the formation of thrombi in disorders such as thrombotic thrombocytopenic purpura (TTP) and hemolytic uremic syndrome (HUS, including atypical HUS).[192,193] Although disseminated intravascular coagulation (DIC) is typically discussed alongside thrombotic microangiopathies (TMAs)—because of their similarities in causing microvascular thrombosis in association with thrombocytopenia, hemorrhagic risk, and organ failure—only DIC exhibits activation of multiple systems (i.e., coagulation cascade, fibrinolytic pathway, and platelets); only marked platelet activation is seen in TMAs.[194]

Circulating autoantibodies that inhibit ADAMTS13 or increase its clearance cause immune-mediated TTP (iTTP). The metalloproteinase ADAMTS13 regulates von Willebrand factor (vWF) multimers by cleaving ultralarge forms released by the endothelium that induce vessel wall platelet aggregation. Severe ADAMTS13 deficiency (<10%) is characteristic of hereditary TTP, but evaluation of levels is often insensitive for treatment purposes. Any patient with microangiopathic hemolytic anemia and thrombocytopenia without apparent alternative etiology is usually treated with plasma exchange and immunosuppression, because iTTP has a 90% fatality rate without appropriate therapy.[195] Immunosuppression with corticosteroids and rituximab are initiated early in the acute stage of disease. A humanized, bivalent variable-domain-only immunoglobulin fragment of vWF (caplacizumab) has transformed acute therapy for iTTP with its ability to rapidly normalize platelet counts, lower TTP-associated mortality, and decrease the rate of recurrent TTP.[196] Caplacizumab's mechanism of action is inhibition of the interaction between the vWF multimers and platelet GPIb, thereby reducing platelet consumption and thrombus formation.

Children with HUS present with a history of bloody diarrhea secondary to Shiga toxin-producing organisms, most commonly enterotoxigenic *Escherichia coli* (O157:H7 or O104:H4) or *Shigella*. Atypical HUS is usually not associated with diarrhea, and a majority of patients have alternative complement pathway or coagulation pathway mutations.[192,193] Secondary HUS may be seen in a number of disorders (malignant hypertension, autoimmune disorders, chemotherapy, pregnancy) and should be considered part of the primary disease.

Bone marrow examination for a microangiopathic process is usually reserved for questionable diagnoses or for evaluations of an underlying immune disorder such as SLE.

Splenic Sequestration

Splenic pooling of platelets causes their displacement from peripheral circulation; the platelets are not destroyed and remain exchangeable with the peripheral pool. Therefore, megakaryocytes may not increase in number. This condition is most often seen in patients with chronic liver disease with portal hypertension and splenomegaly,[197] and it may explain in part the loss of circulating platelets in some patients with Wiskott-Aldrich syndrome.[198]

Constitutional Thrombocytopenia

Mild forms of inherited thrombocytopenia (IT) may be inconspicuous, and adults are at risk for a misdiagnosis of ITP unless blood films or previous records that show subnormal platelet counts are reviewed. An appropriate diagnosis of IT avoids unnecessary procedures and treatments, and in more severe forms of IT, can provide access to appropriate therapeutic options. With the aid of NGS studies (including whole exome sequencing and RNA profiling), investigations have identified at least 40 novel disorders affecting platelet production and/or function.[199,200] These include varying clinical presentations of disease that involve one gene (e.g., *MYH9, GP1BB, WAS*); gene mutations that increase the risk for aplastic anemia/bone marrow failure syndromes (e.g., *MPL, THPO, HOXA11*) and/or predispose to myeloid or lymphoid malignancies (*RUNX1, ANKRD26, ETV6*)[201] (see Chapter 45 for further discussion; mutations associated with additional clinically relevant congenital defects (e.g., *GATA1, FLI1, RBM8a*); and others that present solely with thrombocytopenia (e.g., *NBEAL2, GP9, ACTN1, TUBB1, CYCS*).[200] The discovery of new mutations has debunked long-held beliefs and led to paradigm shifts about ITs: they are more frequent; most have mild-to-moderate thrombocytopenia; and most patients will have little-to-no bleeding tendency. In an Italian cohort, the six most common ITs (namely, Bernard Soulier syndrome [BSS], *MYH9*-related disease [*MYH9*-RD], *ANKDR26*-related thrombocytopenia [*ANKDR26*-RT], *ACTN1*-RT, *TUBB1*-RT, *CYCS*-RT) account for 75% of ITs and are not associated with severe bleeding diatheses.[200]

Review of the blood film for platelet size, compared with RBCs, helps in the diagnosis.[202] Giant platelets are seen in *MYH9*-RD (Fig. 10-47) and BSS (biallelic forms) (Fig. 10-48). Large platelets are found in *NBEAL2*-mutated gray platelet syndrome (Fig. 10-49), BSS (monoallelic forms), Paris-Trousseau syndrome, and multiple rare ITs with varying mutations (i.e., *TUBB1, FLNA, GFI1b, ITBA2B/B3, ACTN1, GATA1*).[203,204] Normal-sized platelets are present in congenital amegakaryocytic thrombocytopenia (CAMT), thrombocytopenia with absent radii (TAR), and radioulnar synostosis with amegakaryocytic thrombocytopenia. Smaller-than-normal platelets are associated with Wiskott-Aldrich syndrome and congenital autosomal recessive small platelet-thrombocytopenia (CARST) (Table 10-8).[199,203,204] Only a minor subset of the ever-growing list of ITs with normal-to-increased megakaryocytes is included in Table 10-10. Four disorders previously thought to be distinct (May-Hegglin anomaly, Sebastian, Fechtner, and Epstein syndromes) are now collectively termed *MYH9*-RD, as it became apparent that these different clinical manifestations represent the same disease.[205] Neutrophil inclusions with clumps of MYH9

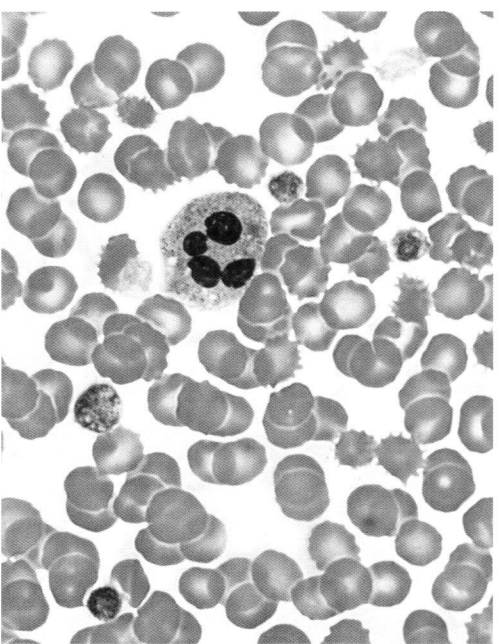

Figure 10-47. *MYH9*-related disease is characterized by large platelets and blue, round or crescent-shaped cytoplasmic deposits of MYH9 protein (May-Hegglin anomaly). Superficially, they resemble Dohle bodies seen in infection.

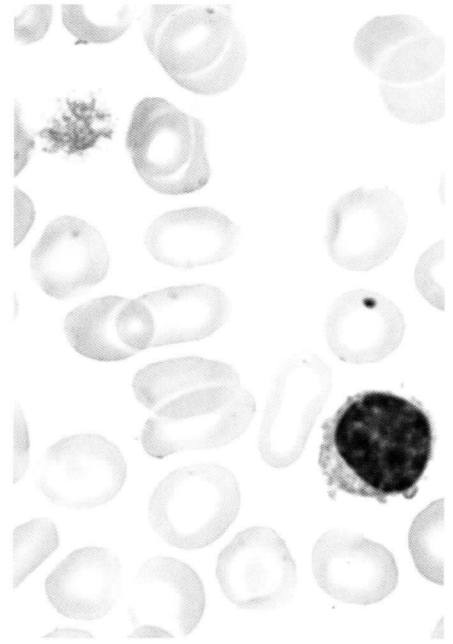

Figure 10-48. Peripheral blood smear of Bernard-Soulier syndrome. The large platelets in this disorder have absent or dysfunctional glycoprotein Ib-IX-V receptors. The patient also has β-thalassemia minor.

protein (round or spindle shaped) help identify this disorder (Fig. 10-47). Additional abnormalities seen on blood films include pale, agranular platelets in gray platelet syndrome; vacuolated platelets and red cell anisocytosis in *GATA1*-related diseases; and stomatocytosis in sitosterolemia (i.e., hypercholesterolemia caused by aberrant accumulation of plant

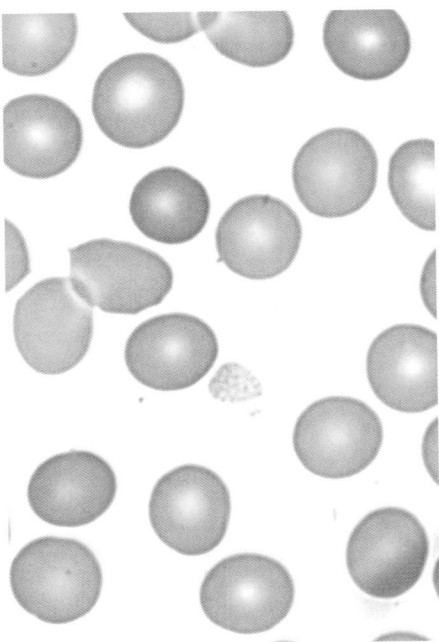

Figure 10-49. Peripheral blood smear of gray platelet syndrome. The large platelet is agranular as a result of the absence of α granules.

sterols, leading to premature atherosclerosis) with *ABCG5* or *ABCG8* mutations. A number of congenital platelet disorders (e.g., Glanzmann thrombasthenia) are caused by qualitative defects in platelets in the absence of thrombocytopenia.[204]

EVALUATION OF SPECIFIC BONE MARROW FAILURE SYNDROMES

Bone marrow hypoplasia involving more than one lineage, also termed *bone marrow failure,* is discussed in this section and includes congenital disorders, acquired aplastic anemia (AA) and PNH (Table 10-11). Acquired multilineage cytopenias may also be caused by nutritional deficiencies (copper, vitamin B_{12}, folate), drug reactions, toxic effects (alcohol), and infections (especially viral); these are discussed in other sections of this chapter.

Select Acquired and Constitutional Bone Marrow Failure Syndromes

Paroxysmal Nocturnal Hemoglobinuria

PNH is a disease of hematopoietic stem cells that have acquired a somatic mutation in the phosphatidylinositol glycan class A (*PIG-A*) gene.[206] These cells have a growth or survival advantage over normal hematopoietic stem cells during immune-mediated bone marrow injury, with further genetic or epigenetic events enhancing their clonal proliferation. The progeny of PNH stem cells have reduced or absent glycosylphosphatidylinositol-anchored proteins (GPI-AP). More than 20 GPI-APs are expressed by hematopoietic cells and include important complement regulatory proteins such as CD55 and CD59 on erythrocytes. Flow cytometric analysis to detect the loss of these GPI-APs or a fluorescein-labeled proaerolysin variant (FLAER) that binds to the GPI anchor

is diagnostic (Fig. 10-50).[207] The International PNH Interest Group subcategorized the disorder based on the size of the mutant clone and clinical findings into: (1) classical PNH (hemolysis and/or thrombosis), (2) PNH associated with AA or MDS, and (3) subclinical PNH with no clinical or laboratory evidence of hemolysis or thrombosis (PNH clone usually <1%).[208] The anticomplement 5 (C5) mAbs eculizumab and ravulizumab are approved to treat classical PNH.[209]

Aplastic Anemia

AA is an acquired immune-mediated disorder of variable severity with predisposing genetic and environmental factors that trigger disease.[210] Acquired AA is multifactorial in etiology but is most commonly idiopathic. Patients present with symptoms of anemia or with bleeding and are found to be pancytopenic with hypocellular bone marrows. Severe AA is characterized by a markedly hypocellular bone marrow (<25% of normal for age or 25% to 50% of normal with <30% hematopoietic cells) accompanied by two of the following: neutrophils <0.5 × 10^9/L; platelets <20 × 10^9/L; or reticulocyte count <20 × 10^9/L (Fig. 10-51).[211] Very serious disease is particularly ominous and further defined by neutrophils <0.2 × 10^9/L with low bone marrow myeloid reserves; consequently, infection is the major cause of death in these patients.[212] AA is thought to be caused by diminished self-renewal and repopulation capacity of hematopoietic stem cells.[213] T-cell–targeted apoptosis of CD34-positive stem cells and aberrant T-cell activation likely play a role through cytokine-mediated suppression and triggering of immune response pathways. Telomere length may be decreased as a result of increased mitotic demand on a limited pool of stem cells.[213]

AA is considered a non-neoplastic hematologic disorder, yet somatic mutations are common, with clonal hematopoiesis observed in more than 70% of patients.[210] Mutations typically are seen within 6 months of immunosuppressive therapy but can also be present at diagnosis. The most common somatic mutations are found in *PIG-A* and *HLA*. Other mutations are frequently seen in *BCOR*, *BCORL*, *DNMT3A*, and *ASXL1*. These findings may create diagnostic uncertainty and raise the possibility of refractory cytopenia of childhood (RCC) and hypoplastic MDS (hMDS) in all ages.[214,215] Although morphologic criteria have been proposed to distinguish AA from myeloid neoplasia (or to predict risk of malignant transformation in AA) in adults[216] and pediatric patients,[215,217] subsequent studies demonstrate interobserver variability and the challenge in distinguishing these entities[218,219] (Chapter 44 and Chapter 45). Megakaryocytic or granulocytic dysplasia, an increase in blasts, and MDS-defining cytogenetic abnormalities (such as monosomy 7) are not characteristic of AA and may be helpful in differentiating between AA and hMDS.[210,214,215] Given that 15% to 20% of patients with AA develop MDS/AML by 10 years of follow-up, periodic bone marrow surveillance (for dysplasia, increased CD34-positive cells, or progressive karyotypic abnormalities) is essential. Increased disease duration, older age, relapsed/refractory disease, accelerated telomere attrition, and certain genetic alterations have been associated with increased risk of progression to MDS or AML.[210]

Severe AA requires immunosuppressive therapy or hematopoietic cell transplantation to stop the immune-mediated destruction. Small PNH clones in 50% to 60%

Table 10-11 Acquired and Constitutional Bone Marrow Failure Syndromes

Disorder	Inheritance/Defect	Morphology	Clinical Features	Comments
Paroxysmal nocturnal hemoglobinuria (PNH)	Acquired: somatic X chromosome *PIGA* gene mutation; loss of GPI-APs on RBCs, neutrophils, monocytes, platelets	Classical PNH: Normochromic, normocytic anemia with increased polychromasia. Normocellular or hypercellular bone marrow. Erythroid hyperplasia, normal morphology	Florid intravascular hemolysis (hemoglobinuria), thrombosis (40%), smooth muscle dystonias, abdominal pain	All ages and ethnic groups, less common in children; thrombosis main cause of morbidity and mortality. Complement-mediated lysis of GPI-AP–deficient cells. Flow cytometry: often >50% of PMNs and monocytes are GPI-AP deficient. Neutrophils may have short telomeres
	In setting of other bone marrow failure syndrome	Evidence of concomitant syndrome (often aplastic anemia or low-grade MDS)	Intermittent hemolysis or no hemolysis (subclinical)	Usually <30% of PMNs are GPI-AP deficient, or <1% of PMNs are GPI-AP deficient
Aplastic anemia (AA)	Acquired: cytotoxic T-cell–induced apoptosis of CD34+ stem cells. Mutations in *PIG, HLA, BCOR, BCORL, DNMT3A,* and *ASXL1*	Cytopenias—slowly progressive (idiopathic) or abrupt (secondary). Bone marrow hypoplasia (often <10%), lymphocytes, plasma cells, hematogones (children), ± mast cells. Possible dyserythropoiesis, but no significant dysplasia in myeloid or megakaryocytic lineages; no increase in CD34+ cells	Development of infections, bleeding, cardiac output failure. Possible evolution to PNH, MDS, or AML. Higher risk if >45 years old	Majority (60%) idiopathic; may be triggered by drugs, chemotherapy, radiation, idiosyncratic drug or chemical reactions, infections (especially seronegative hepatitis), immune disorders. Increased frequency in Southeast Asia and Far East; patients with HLA-DR2 or genetic polymorphisms for drug/toxin clearance
Fanconi anemia	AR, except *FANCB* (XL recessive) and *FANCF/RAD51* (AD). 22 known genes are involved in the Fanconi anemia pathway including breast cancer genes; *FANCA* most common (60%)	Neutropenia and thrombocytopenia may precede anemia; possible macrocytosis; gradual development of pancytopenia and aplasia (90% by 40 years); MDS or AML may develop. AA or, rarely, AML may be the presenting feature	25% lack anomalies. Skin discoloration (40%), skeletal anomalies (51%), abnormal thumbs (35%), abnormal reproductive organs (50%), facial dysmorphic features (26%), short stature, gastrointestinal anomalies, renal malformations	Median age at diagnosis is 7 years (range, 0-49 years); 33% cumulative probability of leukemia and 28% cumulative probability of non-hematologic malignancy by age 40-50 years, especially squamous cell carcinoma of head, neck, esophagus; increased MDS or AML. Increased chromosome breakage with mitomycin C or diepoxybutane and demonstration of FA gene mutations diagnostic
Dyskeratosis congenita	XL: *DKC1* (30%). AR: *NOP10, NHP2, TERT, WRAP53*. AD: *TERC* (10%), *TERT, TINF2*. Mutated genes are involved in telomere maintenance. No mutation identified (40%-50%)	Progressive neutropenia and/or thrombocytopenia followed by pancytopenia; initial compensatory hypercellularity, megaloblastic changes, with progressive loss of cellularity. Aplastic anemia in 33% of X-linked, may be the presenting feature	Reticular pigmentation, nail dystrophy, oral leukoplakia, pulmonary fibrosis, liver disease, neuropsychiatric disorders, premature hair graying. Significant mortality with bone marrow transplantation	Median age at diagnosis is 15 years (range, 0-74 years); 50% are older than 15 years. Diagnosis: gene mutation tests; screening for short telomeres in all leukocyte subsets; diagnostic if <1% length for age. Cumulative incidence of MDS (30%), AML (10%), carcinoma (20%-30%), especially squamous cell

AA, Aplastic anemia; *AD,* autosomal dominant; *AML,* acute myeloid leukemia; *AR,* autosomal recessive; *FA,* Fanconi anemia; *GPI-AP,* glycosylphosphatidylinositol-anchored protein; *MDS,* myelodysplastic syndrome/neoplasm; *PMN,* polymorphonuclear neutrophil; *PNH,* paroxysmal nocturnal hemoglobinuria; *RBC,* red blood cell; *XL,* X-linked.

of patients with AA have been associated with better responsiveness to immunosuppressive therapy in some studies. An erythrocyte PNH clone size of 3% to 5% and a granulocyte PNH clone size of 20% to 25% best predict development of clinical PNH in these patients.[220]

Approximately 25% of children and up to 10% of adults with AA have inherited bone marrow failure syndromes. Pancytopenia is the usual presentation for patients with Fanconi anemia or dyskeratosis congenita. The other congenital syndromes more commonly present with anemia (DBA), neutropenia (SCN, Kostmann syndrome, SDS), or thrombocytopenia (thrombocytopenia with absent radii, congenital amegakaryocytic thrombocytopenia), and they tend to remain single-lineage disorders (Tables 10-6 to 10-8 and 10-10).

In addition to Fanconi anemia and dyskeratosis congenita, patients with SDS and CAMT develop secondary AA; these patients have an increased risk for progression to MDS or AML.

Fanconi Anemia

Fanconi anemia is the most prevalent of the constitutional syndromes and presents as AA in the first decade of life in 90% of cases.[221] Up to 25% of young patients diagnosed with Fanconi anemia have no discernible physical abnormalities.[222] Chromosome fragility testing of blood lymphocytes remains

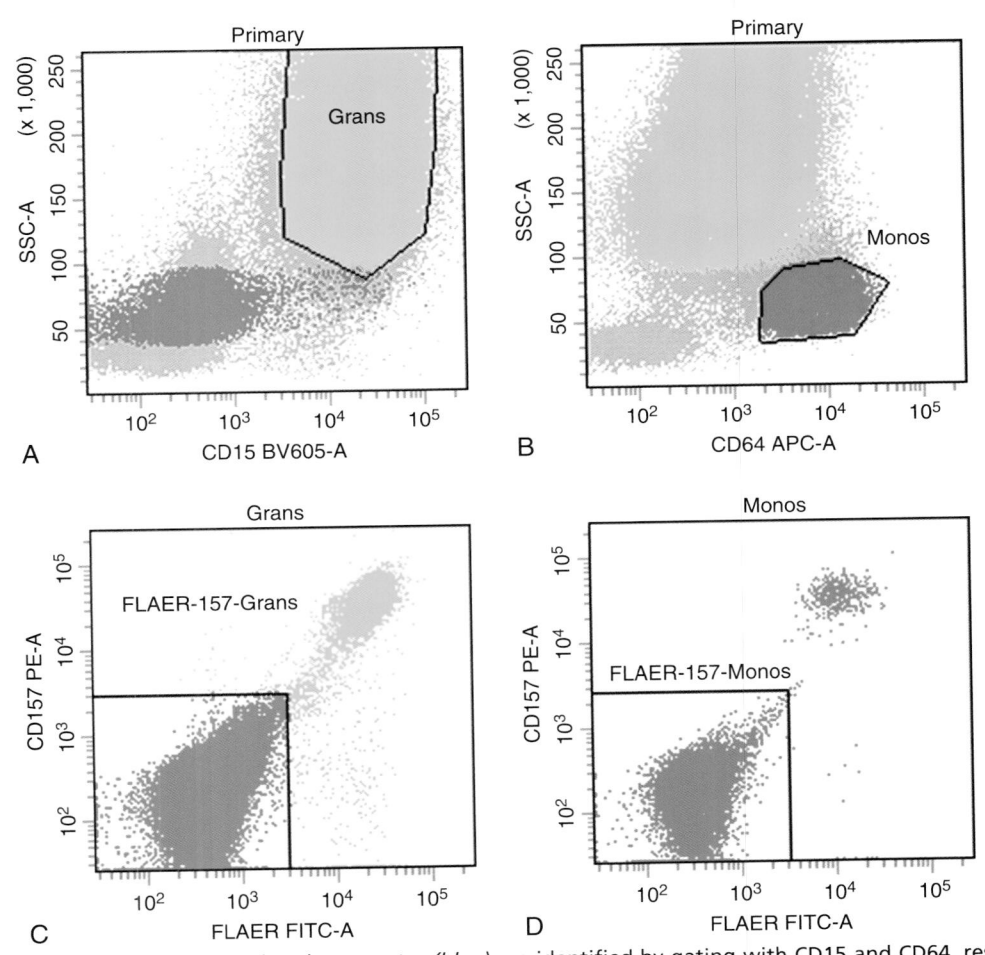

Figure 10-50. A and **B,** Granulocytes *(yellow)* and monocytes *(blue)* are identified by gating with CD15 and CD64, respectively. **C** and **D,** In paroxysmal nocturnal hemoglobinuria, they fail to stain with fluorescein-labeled proaerolysin variant (FLAER) and glycosylphosphatidylinositol-anchored CD157 *(red populations).* Significant numbers of normally expressing granulocytes and monocytes *(yellow and blue populations, respectively)* are also present.

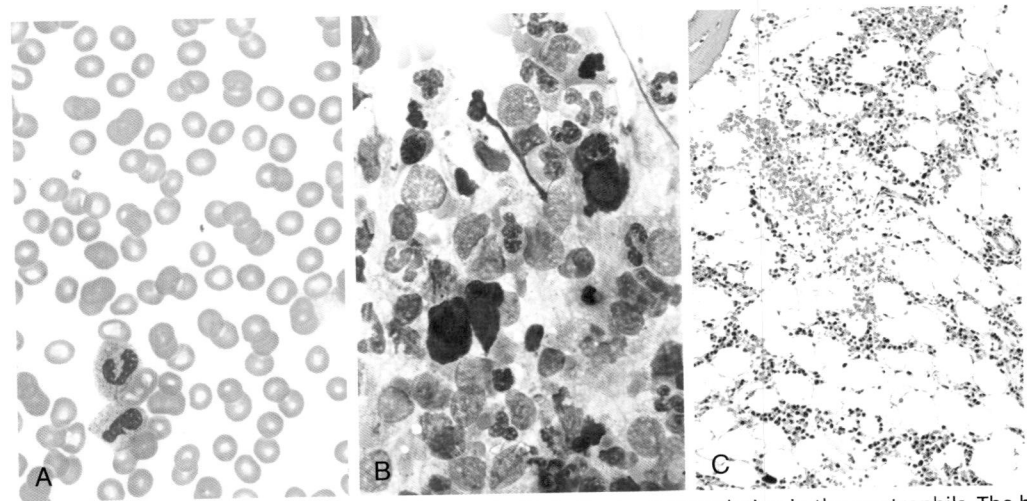

Figure 10-51. A, Pancytopenia in measles-associated aplastic anemia. Note the toxic granulation in the neutrophils. The hypocellular bone marrow smear contains numerous mast cells **(B),** and the trephine biopsy reflects subtotal aplasia **(C).**

a useful diagnostic test, alongside sequencing for Fanconi anemia genes. Chromosomal fragility testing quantifies chromosomal breakage in Fanconi anemia cells with increased hypersensitivity to DNA cross-linking agents (e.g., diepoxybutane, mitomycin). The hypersensitivity results in frequent chromosomal abnormalities, which may wax and wane, and difficulty tolerating therapeutic alkylating agents.[223] Excessive cellular apoptosis and consequent malfunction

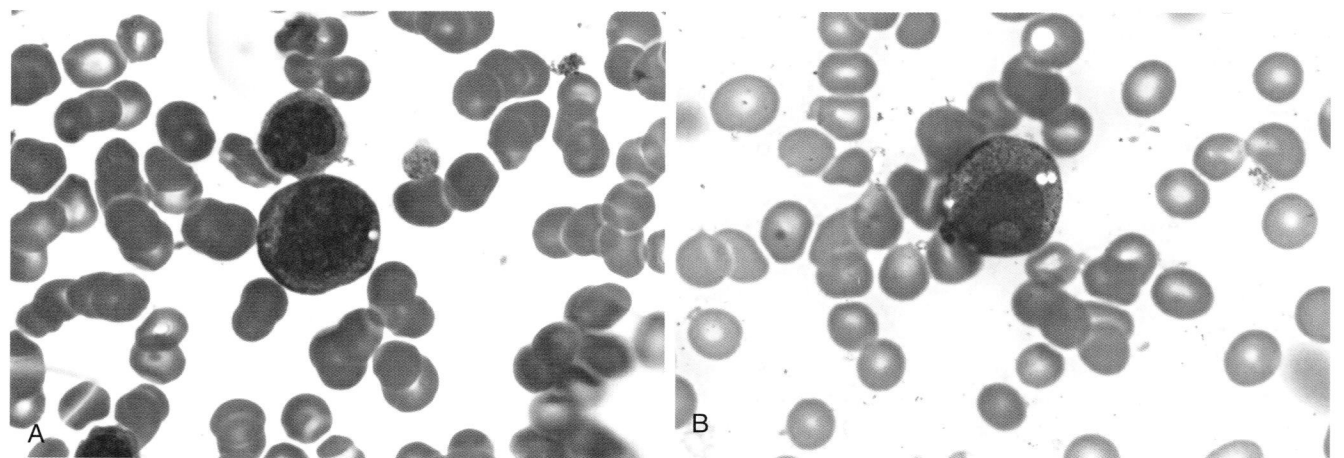

Figure 10-52. Bone marrow aspirate smear in VEXAS syndrome. Sharply punched-out cytoplasmic vacuoles are seen in an erythroblast **(A)** and promyelocyte **(B)**.

of stem cells lead to progressive bone marrow failure.[224] It has been speculated that *MYC* overexpression impairs stem cell function and contributes to bone marrow exhaustion.[225] Mutations in 22 different genes of the Fanconi anemia pathway have been identified.[226] This pathway functions as a DNA damage sensor and repair initiator and regulates oxidative stress. Stem cell transplantation has raised the life expectancy for patients with Fanconi anemia; however, the timing of transplantation is critical, as the development of solid tumors remains a significant problem.[227]

Dyskeratosis Congenita

Dyskeratosis congenita is a genetically heterogeneous telomere maintenance disorder.[228] Low telomerase activity leads to accelerated telomere shortening, decreased proliferative capacity among affected hematopoietic progenitors, and features of a premature aging syndrome. The age of onset, severity, and clinical manifestations vary.[228] Individuals with the classic X-linked form of disease (*DKC1* mutation) present with lacy reticular pigmentation, dysplastic nails, and oral leukoplakia. Severe childhood variants, such as Hoyeraal-Hreidarsson and Revesz syndromes, have associated cerebellar hypoplasia and developmental dysfunction. Some patients with minimal physical findings reach adulthood before diagnosis. The initial clinical presentation may be bone marrow failure, especially in patients with *TERC, TERT,* or *TIN2* mutations, and screening for short telomeres is indicated in these patients. Most boys with X-linked disease develop bone marrow failure by 20 years of age. The estimated cumulative incidence of marrow failure is 80% by 30 years of age.

VEXAS Syndrome

VEXAS (vacuoles, E1 enzyme, X-linked autoinflammatory, somatic) syndrome is a newly recognized adult-onset, treatment-refractory, rheumatologic/bone marrow failure disorder caused by mutations of the X-linked *UBA1* gene. Patients present with a variety of progressive autoinflammatory and hematologic manifestations, including chondritis, fevers, cytopenias (especially macrocytic anemia, lymphopenia, and monocytopenia), neutrophilic dermatoses, lung involvement, thrombosis, vasculitis, and dysplastic marrow containing hallmark cytoplasmic vacuoles in myeloid and erythroid precursors.[229] A significant proportion of patients present with or develop MDS (30-50%), multiple myeloma/monoclonal gammopathy of undetermined significance (MGUS) (25%), or monoclonal B-cell lymphocytosis[230] (see Chapter 45).

Mutations in the ubiquitin activating enzyme-1 (*UBA1*) gene, which encodes a key ubiquitylation pathway enzyme, are found in hematopoietic myeloid and lymphoid progenitors but not in mature lymphocytes or fibroblasts.[231] Many of the autoinflammatory symptoms likely result from dysregulation of inflammation pathways disrupted by mutated myeloid cells. The disorder is rare, and its incidence has been estimated at 1/4200 men aged 50 years or older.[232]

Macrocytosis is seen in nearly all patients, and left-shifted neutrophils are found in half of all cases. The immature neutrophils often contain sharply punched-out vacuoles, and segmented neutrophils show hypogranular and/or hypolobated (pseudo–Pelger-Huët) changes. Lymphopenia, monocytopenia, and mild-to-moderate thrombocytopenia are often present.[230]

Bone marrow aspirate smears show vacuolation in myeloid and erythroid precursors, including myeloblasts (Fig. 10-52). Vacuoles are not seen in lymphocytes. Megakaryocytes generally lack vacuoles, but along with myeloid and erythroid precursors show dysplastic changes. Biopsies are hypercellular with granulocytic hyperplasia and erythroid hypoplasia. Dysplastic changes in more than 10% of any cell line are only found in cases meeting the WHO MDS criteria.[230] Half of patients with MDS exhibit abnormal cytogenetics and/or molecular genetic abnormalities, including mutations in *DNM3A, GNA11, CSF1R,* and *EZH2*.[230] Cases with plasma cell dyscrasias show morphology typical for multiple myeloma or MGUS.

A limited number of disorders demonstrate prominent cytoplasmic vacuoles. These include copper, folate, and vitamin B_{12} deficiencies, acute alcohol toxicity, antibiotic therapy, MDS, and smears prepared from old EDTA-anticoagulated specimens. The constellation of autoinflammatory manifestations, macrocytic anemia, and/or myelodysplasia with associated vacuolated myeloid and erythroid precursors should prompt *UBA1* mutation analysis.

Pearls and Pitfalls

- Most isolated acquired anemias can be diagnosed based on peripheral blood smears, clinical history, physical examination, and laboratory findings.
- RBC size is extremely helpful in narrowing the differential diagnosis for hypoproliferative anemias (i.e., inadequate reticulocyte response).
- Schistocytes associated with microangiopathic processes may not be evident until a few days after the initial clinical presentation. In particular, the absence of increased schistocytes does not exclude the possibility of disseminated intravascular coagulation.
- Patients with acquired red cell aplasia need to be evaluated for parvovirus infection, recent or remote thymoma, underlying neoplasm, or lymphoproliferative disorders (particularly T-cell large granular lymphocytic leukemia).
- Iron stores may appear adequate in iron-deficient individuals who have recently received parenteral iron therapy or red cell transfusions.
- Children who develop profound pure red cell aplasia from parvovirus B19 infection should be evaluated for an underlying congenital hemolytic disorder, such as hereditary spherocytosis.
- Patients with intravascular hemolysis or cytopenias and bone marrow hypocellularity should be screened for paroxysmal nocturnal hemoglobinuria.
- Evaluation for T-cell large granular lymphocytic leukemia is recommended in cases of idiopathic red cell aplasia or in patients with autoimmune disorders who have unexplained chronic cytopenias.
- Nutritional deficiencies (cobalamin, folate, copper) may mimic myeloid neoplasms.
- Congenital disorders causing ineffective or reduced hematopoiesis are more likely to present in infancy or childhood but may not be identified until adulthood in some patients.
- Congenital dyserythropoietic anemia type II may be misdiagnosed as chronic hemolytic anemia with microspherocytes and a positive osmotic fragility test. Bone marrow evaluation is required to make the correct diagnosis.
- Only 3% to 5% of all neutrophils are present in the peripheral blood. The majority are in the bone marrow storage pool, ready to be mobilized when the need arises; thus, the adequacy and functionality of the bone marrow myeloid reserve determines the risk of infection in a neutropenic patient.
- Absolute neutrophil counts below $1500/\mu L$ ($1.5 \times 10^9/L$) are a normal variation in persons of African descent and other specific ethnic groups.
- The most common form of neutropenia in adults is drug induced.
- Neonates often become neutropenic when septic; infection-related neutropenia is a common etiology of neutropenia in childhood.
- Peripheral smear evaluation for platelet clumps or satellitism is required to exclude pseudothrombocytopenia.
- Mild thrombocytopenia may be seen during pregnancy and usually resolves after delivery.
- Congenital platelet disorders should be considered in thrombocytopenic patients with increased large platelets on smear review and no hematologic findings suggestive of an associated myeloid neoplasm.
- Large platelets may be inaccurately gated and undercounted by automated hematology analyzers using an impedance method.
- Leukemic cytoplasmic tags, cryoglobulin deposits, and microspherocytic and/or red cell fragments can spuriously elevate platelet counts in automated hematology analyzers using an impedance method. Laboratory protocols (such as manual peripheral blood smear review, manual hemocytometer platelet counts, fluorescence platelet counts) should be in place to confirm automated platelet counts.
- Megakaryocytes may not be increased in individuals with thrombocytopenia secondary to splenic pooling of platelets.
- Iron should be evaluated in aspirate smears or touch preparations instead of biopsies, as acid decalcifying agents cause iron chelation.
- Clonal hematopoiesis is common in aplastic anemia and, in isolation, should not be considered evidence of myeloid neoplasia. Bone marrow features of aplastic anemia overlap those of hypocellular myelodysplastic syndrome (in all ages) and refractory cytopenia of childhood.
- Children and young adults with idiopathic aplastic anemia should be evaluated for an inherited bone marrow failure syndrome, particularly Fanconi anemia and dyskeratosis congenita.
- Fanconi anemia may not be associated with identifiable physical abnormalities in 25% of cases.

KEY REFERENCES

29. Weiss G, Ganz T, Goodnough LT. Anemia of inflammation. *Blood.* 2019;133:40–50.
38. Ducamp S, Fleming MD. The molecular genetics of sideroblastic anemia. *Blood.* 2019;133:59–69.
43. Gurnari C, Maciejewski JP. How I manage pure red cell aplasia in adults. *Blood.* 2021;137:2001–2009.
49. Ialascon A, Andolfo I, Russo R. Advances in understanding the pathogenesis of red cell membrane disorders. *Br J Haematol.* 2019;187:13–24.
82. Fattizzo B, Barcellini W. Autoimmune hemolytic anemia: causes and consequences. *Expert Rev Clin Immunol.* 2022:1–15.
95. Iolascon A, Andolfo I, Russo R. Congenital dyserythropoietic anemias. *Blood.* 2020;136:1274–1283.
105. Connelly JA, Walkovich K. Diagnosis and therapeutic decision-making for the neutropenic patient. *Hematology Am Soc Hematol Educ Program.* 2021;1:492–503.
118. Wang E, Boswell E, Siddiqi IN, et al. Pseudo-Pelger-Huet anomalies from medications. *Am J Clin Pathol.* 2011;135:291–303.
124. Skokowa J, Dale DC, Touw IP, et al. Severe congenital neutropenias. *Nat Rev Dis Primers.* 2017;3:17032.
192. Kottke-Marchant K. Diagnostic approach to microangiopathic hemolytic disorders. *Int J Lab Hematol.* 2017;39(suppl 1):69–75.
199. Warren JT, Di Paola J. Genetics of inherited thrombocytopenias. *Blood.* 2022;139:3264–3277.
200. Balduini CL, Melazzini F, Pecci A. Inherited thrombocytopenias—recent advances in clinical and molecular aspects. *Platelets.* 2017;28:3–13.
204. Nurden AT, Nurden P. Inherited thrombocytopenias: history, advances and perspectives. *Haematologica.* 2020;105:2004–2019.
210. Sun L, Babushok DV. Secondary myelodysplastic syndrome and leukemia in acquired aplastic anemia and paroxysmal nocturnal hemoglobinuria. *Blood.* 2020;136:36–49.
221. Dokal I, Tummala H, Vulliamy T. The inherited bone marrow failure syndromes. *Blood.* 2022;140:556–570.

Visit Elsevier eBooks+ for the complete set of references.

Chapter 11

Bone Marrow Findings in Inflammatory, Infectious, and Metabolic Disorders

Giovanni Insuasti-Beltran and Nancy S. Rosenthal

This chapter addresses the peripheral blood and bone marrow response to a variety of non-malignant conditions. In inflammatory or metabolic disorders, the bone marrow findings may be consistent with the underlying disease, suggestive of a complication of the disease, or related to treatment. Although performed less commonly now because of more advanced imaging studies, a bone marrow examination may be performed to evaluate a fever of unknown origin, looking for a specific infectious cause.[1]

Reactive proliferations of leukocytes (i.e., leukocytosis) and their associated differential diagnoses are discussed first, followed by specific findings in infectious, inflammatory, and metabolic disorders.

REACTIVE NEUTROPHILIA

Neutrophilic hyperplasia is usually caused by the endogenous secretion of granulocyte-macrophage colony-stimulating factor or granulocyte colony-stimulating factor in response to inflammation. Common causes are infection, systemic rheumatic disease, and malignancy (Box 11-1).[2] Demargination of neutrophils into the circulating pool, and subsequent doubling of the neutrophil count, can be seen after acute stress or epinephrine administration. Corticosteroid therapy increases neutrophils in the peripheral blood because of their early release from marrow stores. Exogenous growth factor therapy may also cause a rise in the neutrophil count. It may be difficult in some cases to distinguish between reactive neutrophilic hyperplasia and a myeloproliferative process (typically chronic myeloid leukemia).[3] Morphologic findings such as a basophilia, abnormal megakaryocytes, and marrow fibrosis may be helpful, but genetic analysis may be needed to determine the diagnosis.[4]

In reactive neutrophilia, examination of the peripheral blood smear shows an increase in the absolute neutrophil count. The white blood count rarely exceeds 50×10^9/L. Circulating immature neutrophils, termed a *left shift*, are often present,[5] and morphologic abnormalities such as toxic granulation, cytoplasmic vacuolization, and Döhle bodies are seen (Fig. 11-1). Marrow aspirate smears show an increased myeloid-to-erythroid ratio and, in some cases, a relative increase in myelocytes and promyelocytes. Increased cytoplasmic granularity may be noted. Marrow tissue sections may show increased cellularity, with an increased myeloid-to-erythroid ratio. Early granulocytic precursors are typically seen in paratrabecular areas. In some cases, this proliferation is so exuberant that it can be mistaken for a neoplastic process and can even mimic metastatic carcinoma (Fig. 11-2).

REACTIVE LYMPHOCYTOSIS

An increase in lymphoid cells in the peripheral blood is associated with a variety of underlying conditions, most commonly related to viral infections (Epstein-Barr virus [EBV], cytomegalovirus [CMV], hepatitis, human herpesvirus 6, human immunodeficiency virus [HIV]) or drug reactions,[6]

Box 11-1 *Causes of Reactive Neutrophilia*

- Infection
- Autoimmune disorders
- Systemic rheumatic disease
- Malignancy
- Exogenous growth factor therapy (granulocyte colony-stimulating factor)
- Acute stress
- Obesity
- Drugs
- Epinephrine administration
- Corticosteroid therapy
- Lithium
- Smoking

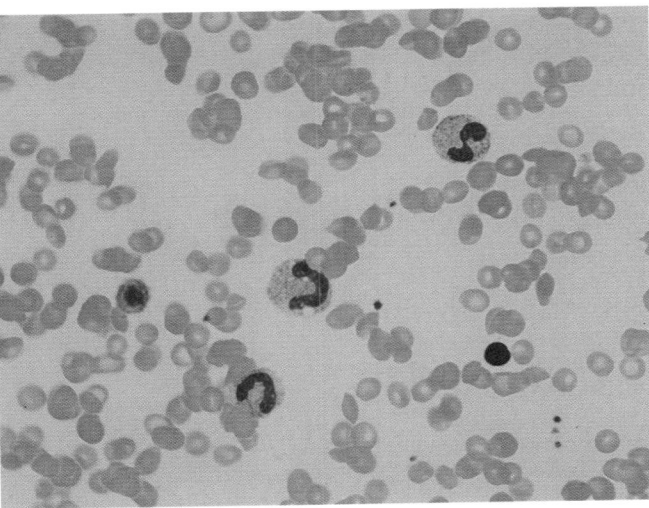

Figure 11-1. Toxic granulation and vacuolization in peripheral blood neutrophils caused by infection.

but it may also be seen in stress conditions.[7,8] The latter conditions may be related to endogenous epinephrine release.[9] Rare cases of polyclonal T-cell lymphocytosis have been described in patients with thymomas.[10] The peripheral lymphocytosis secondary to infection is predominantly a T-cell reaction.[11] An increase in large granular lymphocytes may be seen after bone marrow transplantation.[12]

Reactive marrow lymphocytosis is characterized by an increase in benign-appearing lymphocytes. The increase may or may not be associated with a peripheral lymphocytosis and may be caused by either an interstitial increase in lymphoid cells or an increase in lymphoid aggregates. Increased precursor B-lymphoid cells (hematogones) may be seen in a variety of conditions, especially in children, but they are common after chemotherapy in both adults and children (Fig. 11-3). These cells may be morphologically similar to lymphoblasts in B-lymphoblastic leukemia (see Chapter 42). Flow cytometric or immunohistochemical evaluation is helpful in distinguishing the two. The patient's age is important in determining whether lymphoid cells are increased because children normally have more lymphocytes (up to 35%) in the bone marrow.[13] In adults, the normal value for lymphocytes on the aspirate smear is approximately 6% to 25%.[14]

Persistent polyclonal B-cell lymphocytosis is a rare disorder seen primarily in young women who are often cigarette smokers (Box 11-2).[15,16] Patients are typically asymptomatic and rarely have lymphadenopathy or splenomegaly.[17] There is an association with human leukocyte antigen-DR7 (HLA-DR7).[18] EBV has been found in the peripheral blood cells of rare patients, and the cells appear to have a defective CD40 activation pathway.[19,20] Increased polyclonal immunoglobulin M (IgM) is found in the serum.

The peripheral blood shows increased lymphocytes with moderate amounts of cytoplasm and bilobed nuclei (Fig. 11-4). These cells may be seen in the bone marrow aspirate smear and biopsy, typically in an intrasinusoidal or intravascular pattern.[21] Immunophenotypic evaluation shows a polyclonal proliferation of B cells that are often CD19-positive, CD20-positive, FMC7, IgD-positive, and CD27-positive; multiple *IGH::BCL2* rearrangements have been detected.[15,22] Isochromosome i(3q) with a *MECOM* gene amplification is present in some cases.[23-25] The lymphoid proliferation may persist for many years without any clinical evidence of the development of malignancy.

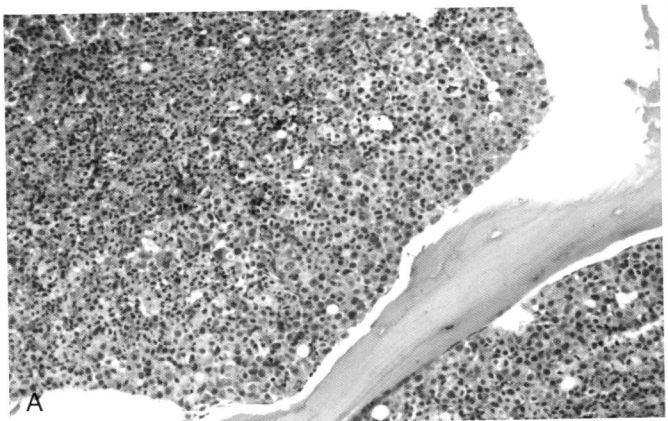
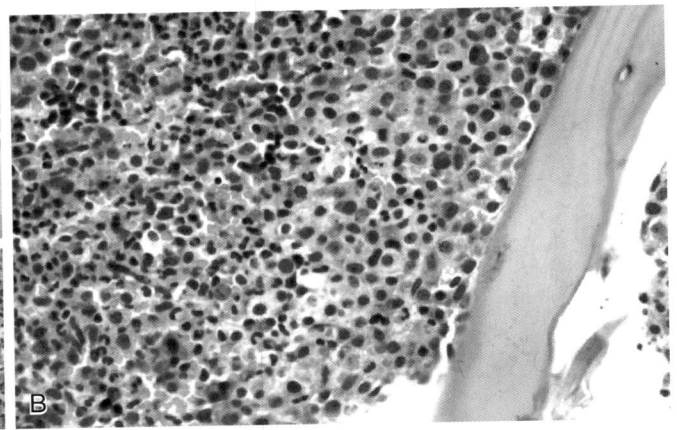

Figure 11-2. Paratrabecular myeloid precursors in bone marrow biopsy at low power **(A)** and high power **(B)**, resembling metastatic carcinoma.

REACTIVE EOSINOPHILIA

Reactive eosinophilia is caused by a wide variety of underlying conditions (Box 11-3).[26-47] Mild elevations in the eosinophil count are usually because of allergic conditions; moderate eosinophilia is more common in lymphomas, rheumatoid

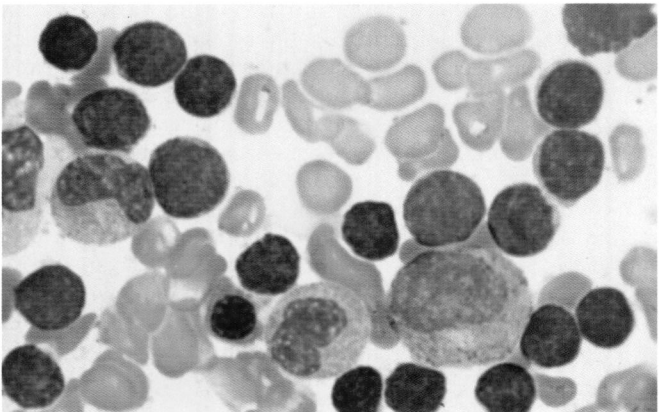

Figure 11-3. Precursor B cells (hematogones) in the bone marrow aspirate from a child with neutropenia. The cells have a high nuclear-to-cytoplasmic ratio, with condensed chromatin and no nucleoli.

Box 11-2 *Characteristics of Persistent Polyclonal B-Cell Lymphocytosis*

Clinical Findings
- Female predominance
- Age 20–40 years
- Asymptomatic
- Cigarette smoker

Laboratory Findings
- Peripheral lymphocytosis
- Bilobed lymphocytes
- Increase in polyclonal serum immunoglobulin M
- Multiple *IGH::BCL2* gene rearrangements
- Polyclonal immunophenotype—memory B cells
- Increased frequency of human leukocyte antigen-DR7
- Isochromosome i(3q)

---

arthritis (RA), and non-hematologic malignancies; and severe elevations are seen in parasitic infections, pulmonary eosinophilia, and clonal eosinophilic disorders.[48,49] Rarely, reactive eosinophilia has been reported as a constitutional abnormality; two of the reported patients had a chromosomal abnormality—a pericentric inversion of chromosome 10.[47]

In cases of reactive eosinophilia, the marrow aspirate smears show increased eosinophils and precursors, usually greater than 5% of the bone marrow nucleated cells.[50] Eosinophilic myelocytes frequently show small basophilic granules. Such myelocytes represent a normal stage of eosinophil development, and the basophilic granules likely represent eosinophil primary granules.[51] In tissue sections of the bone marrow, there is often a diffuse increase in eosinophils and precursors, but focal eosinophilia may be seen surrounding the lesions of marrow involvement by Hodgkin lymphoma, malignant lymphoma, benign lymphoid aggregates, systemic mast cell disease, and Langerhans cell histiocytosis (Fig. 11-5).[52,53] In these cases, increased eosinophils may not be seen in the peripheral blood or in the aspirate smear.

A more detailed discussion of the evaluation of patients with non-neoplastic and neoplastic eosinophilia can be found in Chapter 50.

Box 11-3 *Causes of Reactive Eosinophilia*

- Atopic disorders: allergy, asthma, eczema[26-28]
- Parasitic infections: *Toxocara canis* most common in the United States[29]
- Autoimmune disease[30]
- Drug reactions[31,32]
- Hematopoietic growth factor therapy[34]
- Inflammatory skin disorders[35]
- Carcinoma[36]
- T-cell malignancies
  - Acute lymphoblastic leukemia with t(5;14)(q31;q32)[37]
  - Mycosis fungoides[38]
  - Peripheral T-cell lymphoma[39,40]
- B-cell lymphomas[41]
- Hodgkin lymphoma[42]
- Pulmonary eosinophilic syndromes[43]
- Transplant rejection[44]
- Vasculitis[45,46]
- Constitutional abnormality[47]

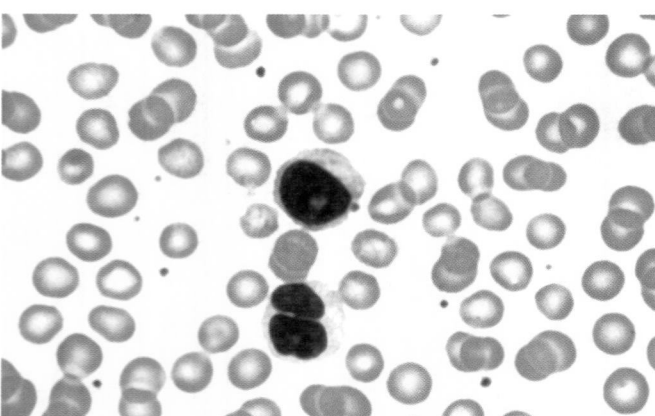

Figure 11-4. Polyclonal B-cell lymphocytosis in a peripheral blood smear. Atypical bilobed lymphocytes are seen. *(Courtesy Linda Sandhaus, MD.)*

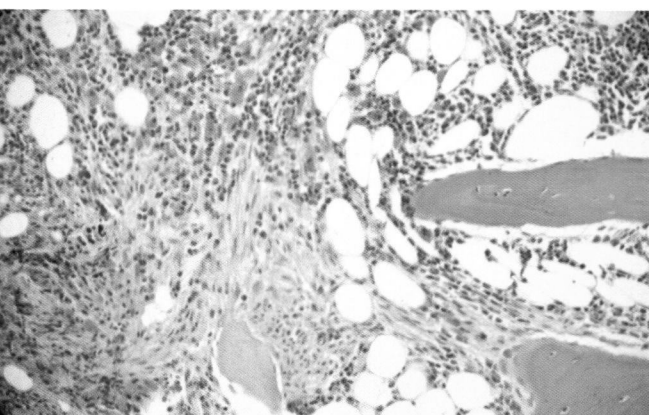

Figure 11-5. Increased eosinophils are seen surrounding a bone marrow lesion of systemic mastocytosis.

- Acute and chronic inflammation
- Acute myocardial infarction
- Autoimmune disorders
- Carcinoma
- Hodgkin lymphoma
- Hypothyroidism
- Neutropenia
- Splenectomy

REACTIVE BASOPHILIA

Reactive basophilia is not a common finding. In some cases, it may be seen with a reactive eosinophil proliferation. Peripheral blood findings show an absolute basophil count greater than 0.2×10^9/L. Bone marrow aspirate smears show an increase in basophils and precursors, accounting for more than 2% of cells.

Commonly associated conditions are allergies, carcinoma, chronic inflammation, malignant lymphoma, plasma cell myeloma, radiation, and renal failure.[54,55]

REACTIVE MONOCYTOSIS

A peripheral blood monocytosis is defined as a monocyte count greater than 1×10^9/L; an increased monocyte level in a bone marrow aspirate smear is often defined as greater than 3% of the differential count.[14] Associated conditions include acute and chronic inflammation, autoimmune disorders, acute myocardial infarction,[56] carcinoma,[57] hypothyroidism,[58] and splenectomy[59] (Box 11-4). Monocytes are also commonly increased in the presence of neutropenia after chemotherapy or because of a congenital deficiency.[60]

BONE MARROW IN INFECTIOUS DISORDERS

Bacterial Infection

Bacterial infections often cause an increase in neutrophils in the peripheral blood, with an increase in immature myeloid cells, or a left shift. Exceptions are seen in neonates and in older adult or debilitated patients who cannot mount a neutrophilic response. Morphologic changes associated with bacterial infection include toxic granulation, Döhle bodies, and cytoplasmic vacuolization. In rare cases, bacteria may be seen within neutrophils and monocytes. An increase in circulating neutrophils results in a subsequent increase in myeloid precursors in the bone marrow.

Rare bacterial infections such as pertussis may cause a lymphocytosis in the peripheral blood, which consists of predominantly CD4-positive cells (Fig. 11-6).[61] In children, these lymphocytes often have irregularly shaped, often clefted (i.e., cleaved) nuclei, similar to the cells seen in peripheralization of follicular lymphoma. Neutropenia may be seen with *Salmonella* or *Brucella* infections. Uncomplicated tuberculosis infection does not typically cause a change in the neutrophil count.

Red cell abnormalities are rarely seen in bacterial infections. *Mycoplasma* pneumonia can lead to the development of a cold agglutinin. Severe hemolysis can be seen in *Clostridium* infection owing to the presence of a hemolysin, phospholipase C.[62]

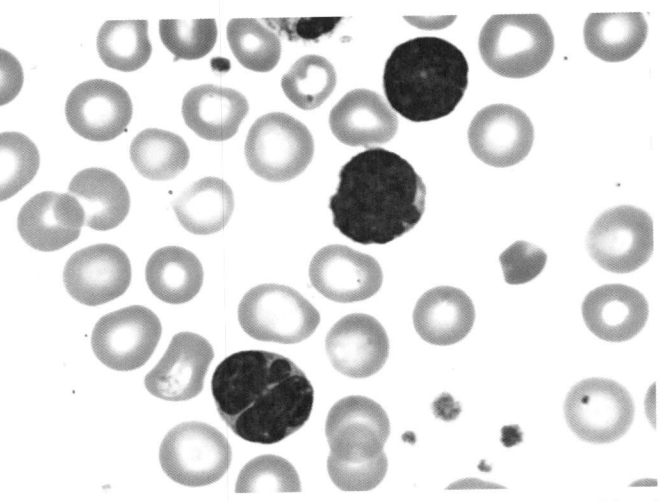

Figure 11-6. Small-clefted lymphocytes in the peripheral blood smear from a child with pertussis infection.

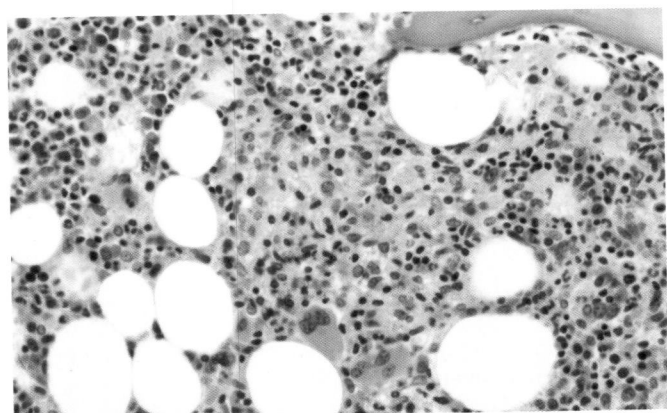

Figure 11-7. Non-caseating granuloma in a bone marrow core biopsy from a patient with brucellosis.

The only bacterial infections diagnosed with any frequency within the bone marrow are those caused by mycobacteria. Rare cases of infection with *Tropheryma whipplei*, the causative agent of Whipple disease, have been described.[63] Periodic acid–Schiff–positive, diastase-resistant organisms are seen within marrow macrophages. Confirmation can be accomplished by polymerase chain reaction (PCR). *Salmonella typhi* infection has been associated with pancytopenia caused by hemophagocytosis,[64,65] granulomas, ring granulomas, or bone marrow necrosis.[66] *Salmonella* organisms may be seen within neutrophils and monocytes. Bone marrow involvement by lepromatous leprosy is characterized by a proliferation of foamy histiocytes that contain the bacilli or by the presence of bacilli lying free in the marrow interstitium.[67] Brucellosis can cause marrow granulomas, hemophagocytosis, and peripheral pancytopenia (Fig. 11-7).[68]

Mycobacterial infection of the bone marrow is most commonly caused by *Mycobacterium tuberculosis* or *Mycobacterium avium* complex. The incidence of the latter infection, mostly seen in severely immunosuppressed individuals, is significantly decreased with effective antiretroviral therapy for HIV infection. Rare cases of infection with other mycobacteria have been described.[69] Patients with pulmonary tuberculosis may have thrombocytosis, leukocytosis, or monocytosis.[70,71] Peripheral

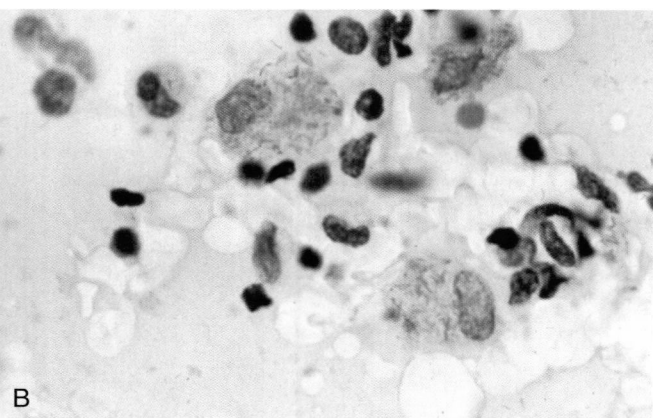

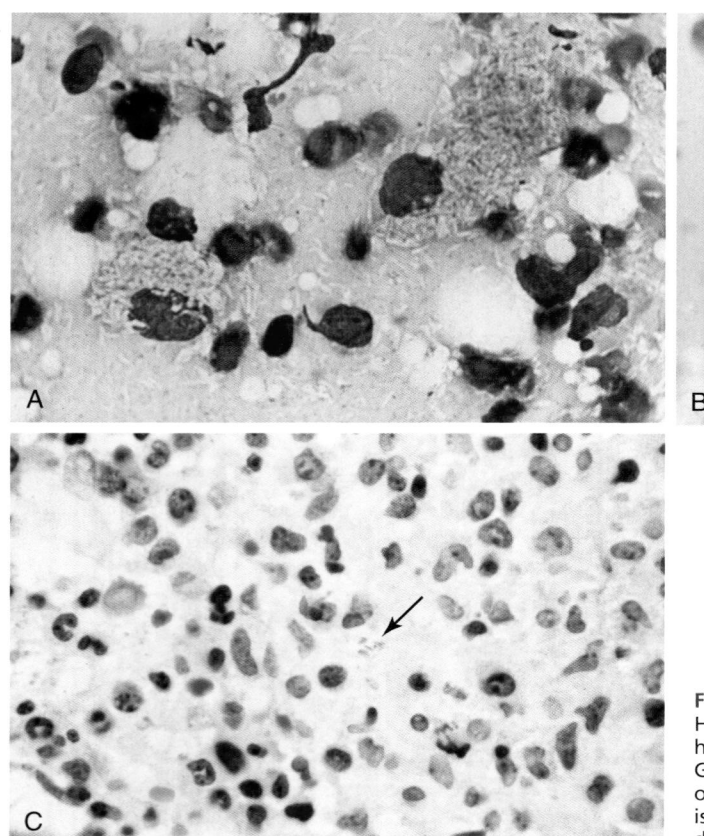

Figure 11-8. **A,** Touch preparation of bone marrow from an HIV patient with *Mycobacterium avium* complex infection. The histiocytes show linear, negatively stained inclusions on Wright-Giemsa stain. **B,** The inclusions in **A** are seen to be mycobacteria on the acid-fast stain. **C,** Rare *Mycobacterium tuberculosis* organisms are identified on this acid-fast stain in a granuloma from a different patient *(arrow).*

blood abnormalities in miliary tuberculosis include the anemia of chronic inflammation, leukopenia, thrombocytopenia, and pancytopenia. Peripheral lymphopenia or thrombocytopenia suggests marrow involvement by granulomas in *M. tuberculosis.*[72] Patients with *M. avium* complex infection may have peripheral blood abnormalities associated with an underlying HIV infection. Negatively stained linear inclusions may be seen within histiocytes on Wright-stained preparations in *M. avium* complex infection (Fig. 11-8A–B).[73] Granulomas can rarely be found on an aspirate smear but are typically detected on the clot section or core biopsy. Caseation within marrow granulomas is rare, but when present it is highly suggestive of infection with *M. tuberculosis.* In *M. avium* complex infection, the granulomas may not be well formed, or there may be diffuse infiltration by histiocytes. Special stains for acid-fast bacilli show rare organisms in *M. tuberculosis* (Fig. 11-8C); the bacilli are more easily found in cases of *M. avium* complex infection and may be numerous. Blood cultures are a more sensitive technique for detecting mycobacteria, especially in the setting of HIV infection,[74] and it has been argued that bone marrow examination has limited value in this setting.[75] Detecting the organism with an acid-fast bacilli stain can significantly shorten the time it takes to make a diagnosis, which may have a positive clinical effect.[76] Rarely, granulomas and organisms can be found in culture-negative patients.[77]

Rickettsial Infection

Rickettsial infections, including Q fever, ehrlichiosis, and anaplasmosis are diseases caused by bacteria spread by ticks

and mites. They have been diagnosed in the bone marrow and blood. Infection with *Coxiella burnetii* causes Q fever, which leads to a characteristic donut or ring granuloma in bone marrow clot sections or core biopsies. The granuloma consists of a ring of epithelioid histiocytes and neutrophils surrounding a central vacuole with an outer fibrin ring (Fig. 11-9).[78,79] These granulomas are not specific for Q fever and have been seen in CMV infection, Hodgkin lymphoma, EBV infection, and typhoid fever.[80]

Human ehrlichiosis and anaplasmosis are caused by infection with *Ehrlichia chaffeensis, Anaplasma phagocytophilum,* or, less commonly, *Ehrlichia ewingii.*[81] The first organism infects monocytes, and the other two infect granulocytes. Any of these infections can cause leukopenia, with a left shift, and thrombocytopenia.[82] A white blood count greater than 11×10^9/L and a platelet count greater than 300×10^9/L are associated with an extremely low yield for anaplasmosis based on PCR testing.[83] Fever and elevated hepatic transaminases may also be seen. The organisms can be identified in the peripheral blood smear, in which small clusters of darkly stained bacteria may be found rarely in monocytes or more commonly in neutrophils.[84] Bone marrow pathology has been better studied in monocytic ehrlichiosis. Granulocytic hyperplasia is common; organisms may be seen within histiocytes in the aspirate, and 67% of patients have granulomas on biopsy sections (Fig. 11-10).[85] The bone marrow in patients infected with *Anaplasma* is either normocellular or hypercellular, with rare infected cells present.[86] Lymphoid aggregates, plasmacytosis, and erythrophagocytosis may be seen.[87] PCR testing of peripheral blood will confirm the diagnosis.[88]

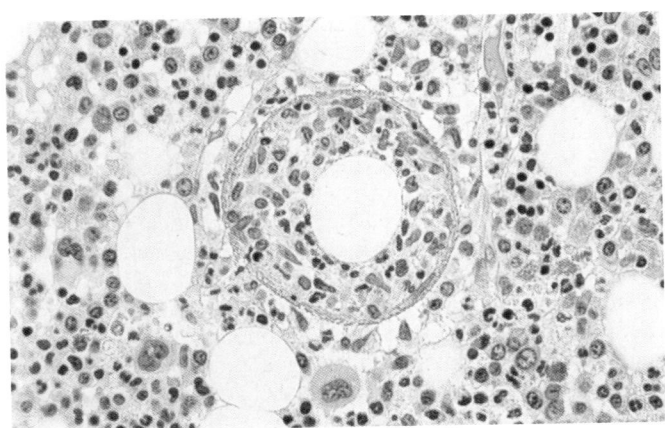

Figure 11-9. Fibrin ring granuloma on a bone marrow core biopsy from a patient with Q fever.

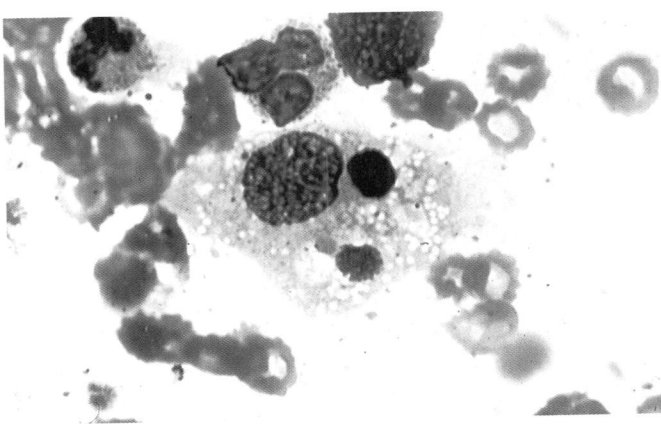

Figure 11-10. Bone marrow aspirate smear showing ehrlichiosis. The organisms are contained within histiocytes.

Parasitic Infection

Infections with tissue-invasive parasites result in an increased eosinophil count in the peripheral blood and bone marrow. *Toxoplasma gondii* pseudocysts have been seen in association with bone marrow necrosis in patients with HIV infection.[89]

Leishmaniasis is a severe disease caused by *Leishmania* species found in endemic areas, but it is also an opportunistic infection in immunocompromised individuals, including those with HIV infection or organ transplantation.[90,91] Clinical findings include fever, hepatosplenomegaly, and pancytopenia. A reactive increase in plasma cells is seen on the aspirate smear. Leishman-Donovan bodies can be seen within macrophages in patients with leishmaniasis. Granulomas may be seen on the core biopsy or clot section. The amastigotes are typically visible within histiocytes. The cytoplasm of the amastigote stains blue, with a red nucleus and a rod-shaped kinetoplast.[92]

Viral Infection

Cytomegalovirus

CMV is a DNA virus that is a member of the herpes family. Acute CMV infection may be associated with a proliferation of reactive lymphocytes in the peripheral blood, similar to those seen with infectious mononucleosis caused by EBV infection (Fig. 11-11).[93] In rare cases, CMV-infected cells with abundant cytoplasm and nuclear inclusions may be seen in the peripheral blood.[94] These cells are most easily seen in the feathered edge of the blood smear. Other peripheral blood findings include hemolysis, neutropenia, and thrombocytopenia.[95-97]

Bone marrow biopsy abnormalities include granulomas or ring granulomas.[98] Rarely, large intranuclear inclusions can be seen in endothelial cells (Fig. 11-12). A myeloid maturation arrest leading to neutropenia can also be seen on the aspirate smear. CMV is one of the causes of hemophagocytic syndrome.

In infants, either congenital or acquired CMV infection can mimic some or most of the clinical features of juvenile myelomonocytic leukemia (JMML).[99] Genetic evaluation for RAS pathway, NF1 or PTPN11 mutations, or monosomy 7 may be required for a definitive final diagnosis of JMML.[100] CMV infection has also been reported to mimic myelodysplasia in adults who present with thrombocytopenia.[101] CMV infections can be seen in patients infected with HIV. Rare intranuclear inclusions may be present, but no other specific findings can be attributed to CMV infection. CMV infection after stem cell transplantation can lead to delayed engraftment, especially with respect to recovery of platelet counts.[102] Similar bone marrow suppression can be seen with human herpesvirus 6 infection.[103]

Epstein-Barr Virus

EBV infection causes peripheral blood and bone marrow abnormalities. The most characteristic finding in the peripheral blood in patients with infectious mononucleosis is an absolute lymphocytosis with many reactive appearing lymphocytes. These are usually larger than normal and a proportion of them may display one or more prominent nucleoli and abundant deeply basophilic cytoplasm. Older patients often have fewer reactive lymphocytes in the peripheral blood.[104] Immunophenotypically, the circulating lymphoid cells are predominantly CD8-positive T cells.[105] Apoptosis of lymphoid cells is also a frequent finding (Fig. 11-13A–C).[106] In addition to exhibiting lymphocytosis, patients may be anemic or thrombocytopenic. In rare patients with EBV infection, hemolytic anemia develops because of a cold agglutinin. If the patient develops hemophagocytic syndrome or bone marrow suppression secondary to EBV, pancytopenia may be present. Rare cases of atypical myelomonocytic proliferations have been seen secondary to EBV infection; this in young children may be clinically confused with JMML.[107] Aplastic anemia has also been described as a sequela of EBV infection.[108,109]

EBV is associated with malignant lymphoid proliferations, including Burkitt lymphoma, lymphomatoid granulomatosis, and immunodeficiency lymphoproliferative disorders, which are discussed in other chapters.

Studies to determine whether a patient has EBV infection should be performed on the peripheral blood. A monospot test for the detection of heterophil antibodies that become positive during the second week of illness, may be used to confirm the diagnosis. This test is more likely to be negative in young children and older adults, owing to the limited production of heterophil antibodies in these age ranges. If the monospot test is negative and the clinical picture is consistent with mononucleosis, additional tests for specific

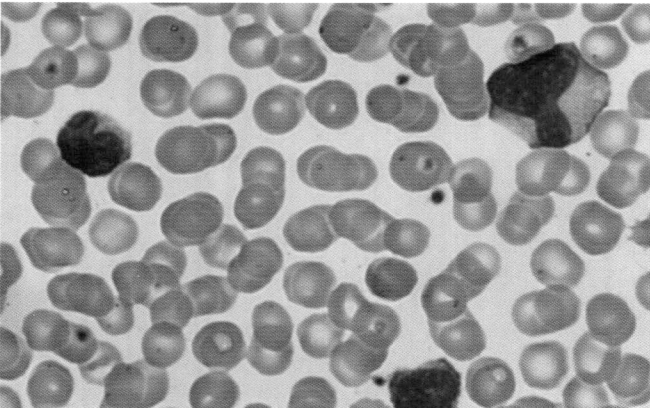

Figure 11-11. Peripheral blood smear showing reactive lymphocytes from a patient with cytomegalovirus infection.

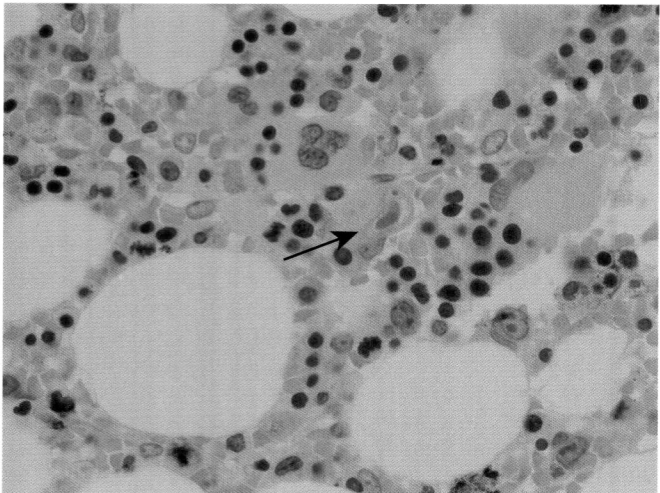

Figure 11-12. Bone marrow core biopsy showing a large eosinophilic cytomegalovirus inclusion (arrow).

viral antibodies directed against viral capsid antigen, early antigen, and Epstein-Barr nuclear antigen should be performed.

Bone marrow examinations are generally not done in patients with infectious mononucleosis; however, when bone marrow biopsies have been performed, benign lymphoid aggregates and non-caseating granulomas without giant cells have been described.[110] In situ hybridization studies for EBV-encoded RNA (EBER) may be performed on biopsy tissue to substantiate the diagnosis (see Fig. 11-13D–E). Marrow aplasia and hemophagocytic histiocytes are seen if aplastic anemia or hemophagocytic syndrome complicates acute EBV infection.

Human Immunodeficiency Virus

Numerous hematologic abnormalities have been described in patients with HIV infection including anemia, granulocytopenia, lymphopenia, and thrombocytopenia.[111] These abnormalities have been lessened with the advent of highly active retroviral therapy (HAART).[112] The anemia is typically caused by chronic disease but may also be caused by infection, nutritional deficiency, medication, or malignancy.[113]

Thrombocytopenia can be because of medications, thrombotic microangiopathy, or immune causes. The degree of neutropenia is related to the severity of the disease. Circulating reactive lymphocytes may be seen at any time during the course of the disease.

Bone marrow features include hypercellularity, serous fat atrophy, lymphoid aggregates, reactive plasmacytosis, eosinophilia, megakaryocytic abnormalities including increased megakaryocyte apoptosis (manifested as naked nuclei), and increased iron stores (Fig. 11-14). Giant pronormoblasts may be seen in parvovirus B19 infection. Granulomas and involvement by lymphoma may also be seen. Stains for acid-fast bacilli and fungi should be performed in all patients regardless of the presence of granulomas; however, the presence of infection has decreased substantially.[114]

Hepatitis

Acute viral hepatitis may be associated with reactive lymphocytosis in the peripheral blood. Hepatitis A, B, C, D, E, and G have been associated with the development of aplastic anemia.[115] Patients with hepatitis C develop a variety of hematologic complications, including monoclonal gammopathies and cryoglobulinemia; they also have an increased risk for low-grade lymphoproliferative disorders.[116] Type II mixed cryoglobulinemia has been associated with atypical lymphoid aggregates in the bone marrow. These aggregates often consist of monomorphic small lymphocytes and may be paratrabecular in location (Fig. 11-15).[117] Immunophenotyping reveals the cells to be B cells that express BCL2, and they may show light chain restriction. Molecular analysis shows an oligoclonal expansion of B cells in many cases. Care should be taken in diagnosing lymphomatous involvement in the bone marrow in the absence of other clinical or molecular evidence of lymphoma.[118]

Hantavirus

Hantavirus pulmonary syndrome was first described in 1993 in the southwestern United States. The infection is caused by Sin Nombre virus.[119] In the prodromal phase, thrombocytopenia is the only finding.[120] The peripheral blood findings that accompany the pulmonary leak syndrome are thrombocytopenia, hemoconcentration, leukocytosis with a left shift, and lymphopenia with more than 10% immunoblasts. Immunoblasts may also be seen in the bone marrow.[121]

Parvovirus B19

The bone marrow findings associated with parvovirus B19 are found in Chapter 11.

COVID-19

Severe acute respiratory syndrome coronavirus 2 (SARS-CoV-2) is the causative organism of the coronavirus disease 2019 (COVID-19) pandemic, a disease with a broad spectrum of clinical presentations and severity.[122] Aside from the well-known pulmonary manifestations, a variety of hematologic findings have been described in patients affected by COVID-19, including increased risk for thrombotic events (at both major and micro vascular levels) and changes in CBC parameters.[123] The latter include thrombocytopenia, apoptosis-mediated lymphopenia, and neutrophilia.[124] These quantitative alterations are more commonly seen in severely

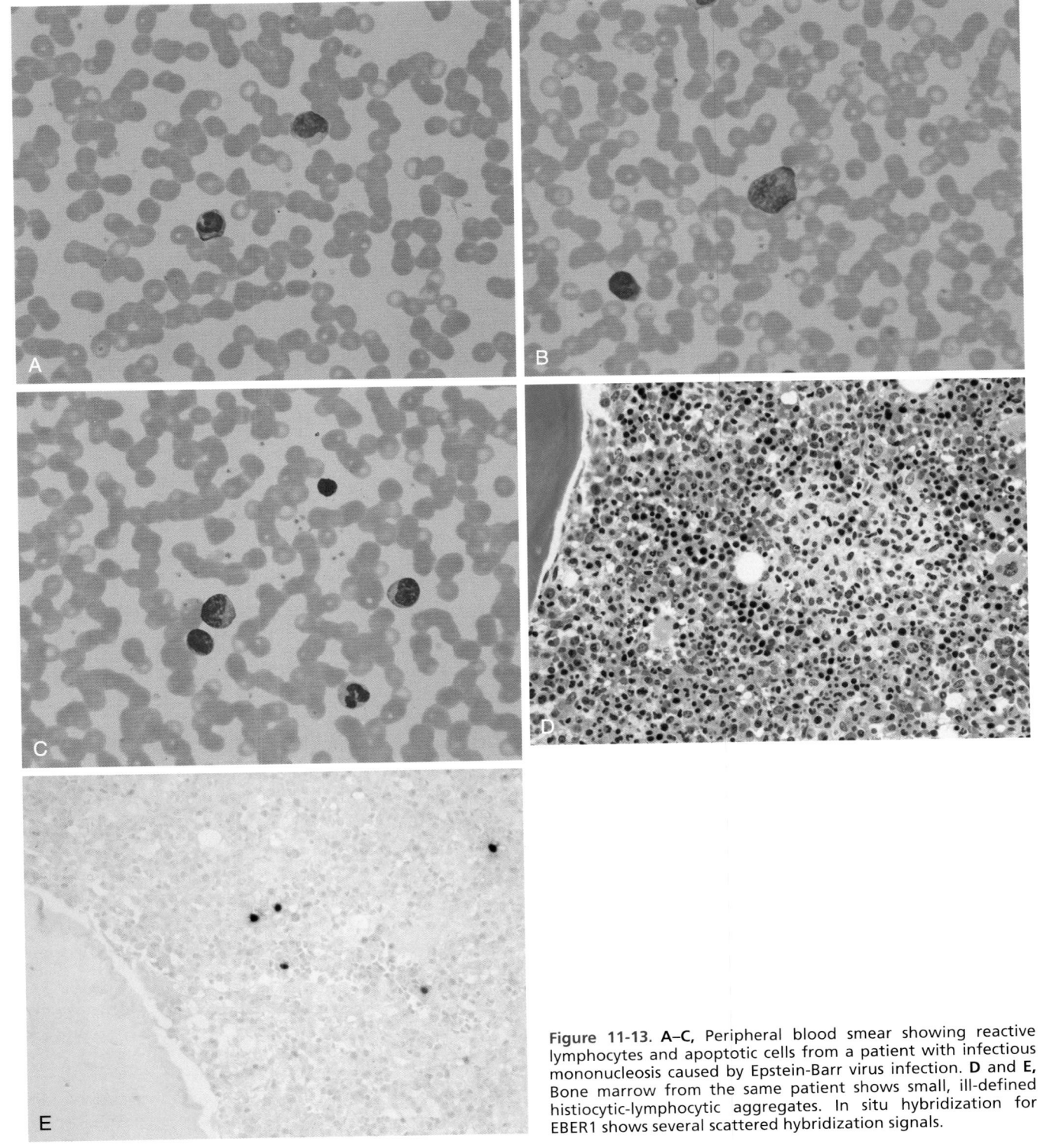

Figure 11-13. A–C, Peripheral blood smear showing reactive lymphocytes and apoptotic cells from a patient with infectious mononucleosis caused by Epstein-Barr virus infection. **D** and **E,** Bone marrow from the same patient shows small, ill-defined histiocytic-lymphocytic aggregates. In situ hybridization for EBER1 shows several scattered hybridization signals.

affected patients. Important morphologic changes described range from increased monocyte vacuolization and expansion of atypical lymphocytes in initial stages or mild disease; more severe or advanced disease has been associated with loss of these changes in the setting of increased neutrophilia and left-shifted maturation.[125]

Fungal Infection

Fungal infections of the bone marrow are most often caused by *Histoplasma* or *Cryptococcus*[126] and are most common in patients with underlying immunodeficiencies.[127] Other fungal infections such as coccidioidomycosis, blastomycosis, and aspergillus have rarely been described. In patients with

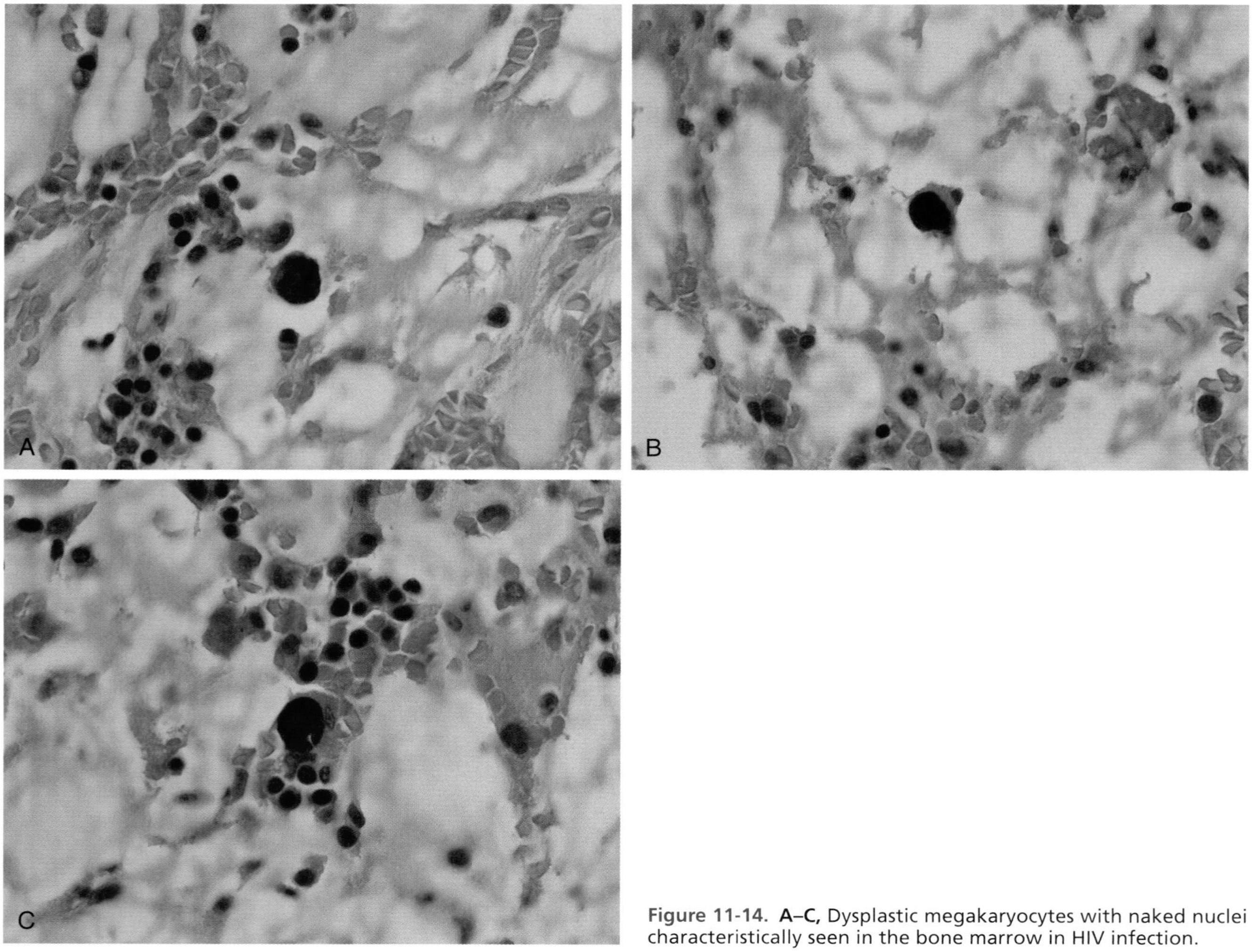

Figure 11-14. A–C, Dysplastic megakaryocytes with naked nuclei characteristically seen in the bone marrow in HIV infection.

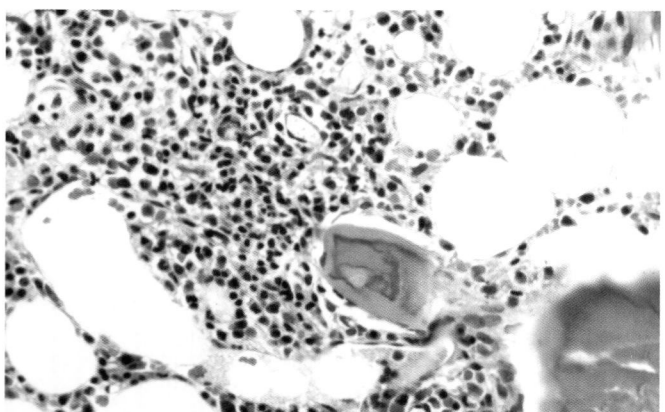

Figure 11-15. Bone marrow core biopsy showing atypical lymphoid aggregates from a patient with hepatitis C infection.

histoplasmosis, peripheral blood findings may include anemia, thrombocytopenia, and leukopenia. In disseminated infection, fungemia may be present, and *Histoplasma* organisms can be seen in circulating monocytes or neutrophils (Fig. 11-16A). Hemophagocytic syndrome has been described

in HIV patients with disseminated histoplasmosis[128] and in rare patients with cryptococcal meningitis.[129]

Bone marrow examination is often useful for the evaluation of disseminated histoplasmosis, particularly in the setting of HIV infection, in which case the marrow is involved in up to 80% of patients.[123] Wright stain can identify organisms in the aspirate smear in many cases (see Fig. 11-16B).[130] Rarely the organisms are confined to the megakaryocytes owing to emperipolesis.[131] Granulomas may be seen on the clot section or core biopsy. *Histoplasma* organisms are positive for both periodic acid–Schiff and Gomori methenamine silver. Cryptococcal organisms can also be recognized on Wright-stained aspirate smear material as variably sized budding yeasts (Fig. 11-17). Granulomas can be seen on histologic sections, and a Gomori methenamine silver or mucin stain can be used to stain the organism. Confirmation by antigen testing can be done on a urine specimen for histoplasmosis or on serum for *Cryptococcus*. Coccidioidomycosis is also a rare cause of granulomas within the bone marrow.

Bone Marrow Necrosis

Bone marrow necrosis is defined as necrosis of hematopoietic tissue and marrow stroma without necrosis of the adjacent

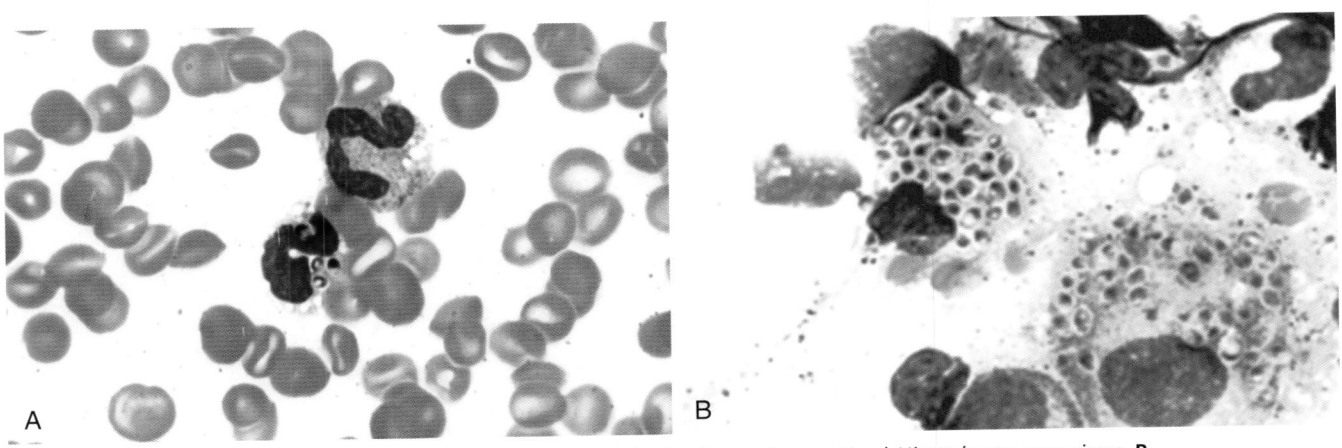

Figure 11-16. A, Peripheral blood neutrophils that have phagocytized *Histoplasma* organisms. **B,** Histiocytes in the bone marrow stuffed with the same organism.

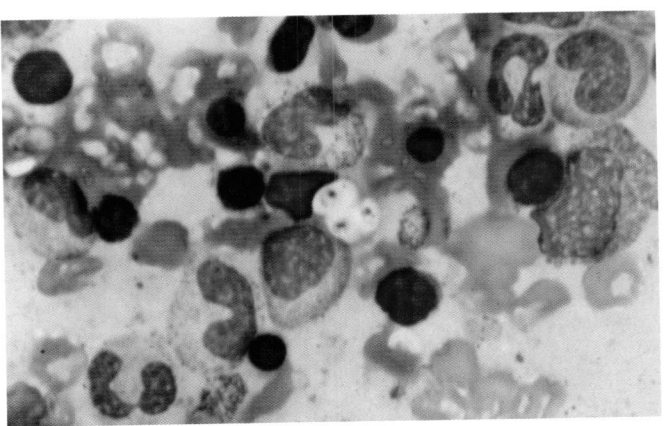

Figure 11-17. Bone marrow touch preparation from a patient with underlying chronic lymphocytic leukemia and *Cryptococcus* infection. Several encapsulated yeasts are seen.

bone. An increase in interleukins with increased apoptosis is postulated as the mechanism. It can be seen in severe infections, hemoglobinopathies, and in disseminated intravascular coagulation, although it is more commonly documented with malignancies.[132,133] The most common malignancies are hematologic, including B-lymphoblastic leukemia, acute myeloid leukemia, and lymphoma. Necrosis because of carcinoma is less common but has been described with lung, stomach, breast, and prostate carcinomas. In many cases, the site of the primary tumor is not identified.[134] Severe bone pain is the most common symptom. Other findings associated with the patient's underlying disease, such as fever, weight loss, malaise, and night sweats, are also common. Bone tenderness may be evident on physical examination. The prognosis depends on the underlying disorder.

The most common peripheral blood findings are anemia, thrombocytopenia, and a leukoerythroblastic reaction.[132] However, the findings depend on the underlying disease and the extent of the necrosis. Elevated lactate dehydrogenase levels and ferritin are often present.

On gross examination, the bone marrow aspirate may appear brown with poorly defined particles. The Wright-stained aspirate shows eosinophilic, necrotic cells in a granular background (Fig. 11-18A). The clot section and core biopsy

show necrotic smudgy cells with nuclear pyknosis (see Fig. 11-18B). The necrosis may be extensive or focal, with viable normal marrow present in the remainder of the biopsy.

The underlying abnormality in bone marrow necrosis is thought to be occlusion of small blood vessels, leading to disruption of blood supply to the marrow.

Fever of Unknown Origin

Determination of a hematologic malignancy is much more likely than an infectious etiology if a bone marrow is performed for a fever of unknown origin.[135] Some studies have shown no increased yield compared with blood culture, whereas others show a higher yield with bone marrow culture.[136]

BONE MARROW IN NON-INFECTIOUS SYSTEMIC AND INFLAMMATORY DISORDERS

Non-infectious Granuloma

Granulomas in the bone marrow have a variety of non-infectious causes, including Hodgkin lymphoma, non-Hodgkin lymphoma, non-hematopoietic malignancies, sarcoidosis, drug reactions, and a variety of autoimmune diseases.[137] Five percent of patients with Hodgkin lymphoma have granulomas,[138] as do 2% to 3% of those with non-Hodgkin lymphoma,[139,140] regardless of whether the marrow is involved by lymphoma. Granulomas have been described with numerous other malignancies, including B-lymphoblastic leukemia, acute myeloid leukemia, plasma cell myeloma, and lung, colon, ovarian, and breast carcinoma[141-143]; as in lymphomas, granulomas may be seen regardless of whether the marrow is involved by disease. Drugs most often implicated are procainamide and amiodarone; many others, including penicillamine, chlorpropamide, and tolmetin have been associated with granuloma formation.[144-147] A wide variety of autoimmune diseases have been associated with granulomas, although most reports are of isolated cases. Patients with granulomatous hepatitis may also have non-caseating granulomas within the bone marrow.[148] Small non-caseating granulomas, which are likely non-specific in nature, are often seen in the marrow after stem cell transplantation.[149]

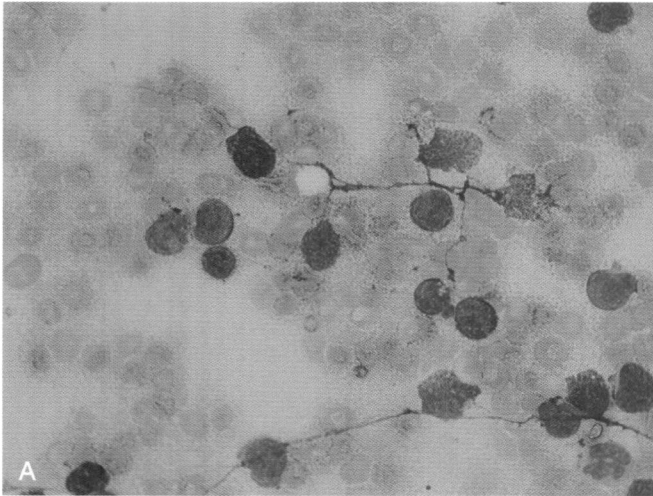
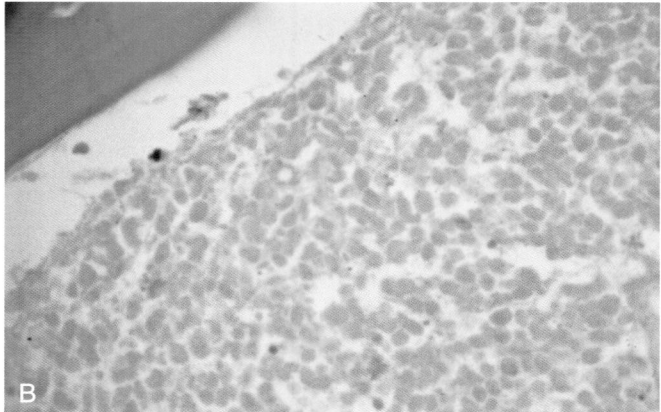

Figure 11-18. Bone marrow aspirate smear **(A)** and core biopsy **(B)** showing severe marrow necrosis. Only degenerated cellular material is seen.

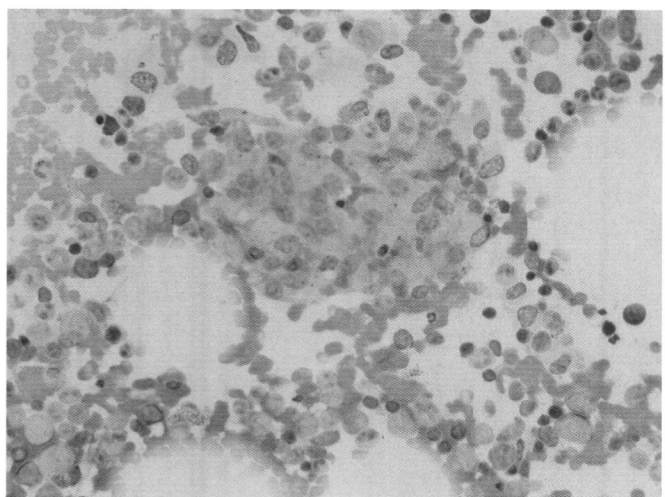

Figure 11-19. Bone marrow aspirate smear with a small granuloma.

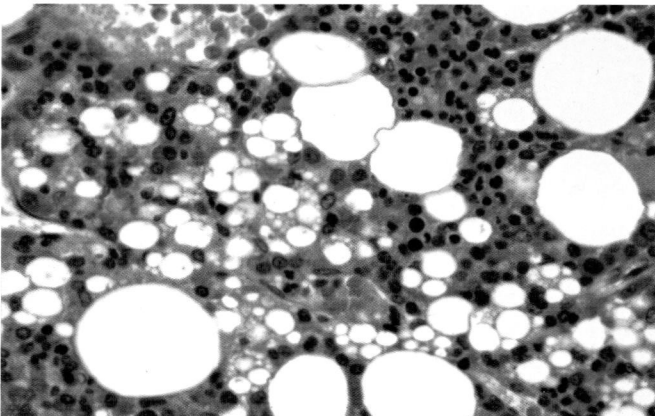

Figure 11-20. Bone marrow core biopsy showing a typical lipogranuloma consisting of histiocytes, lymphocytes, and small fat cells.

In up to 13% of patients with granulomas, no apparent cause is identified.[147]

Non-caseating granulomas are seen primarily on clot and core biopsy sections, although in rare cases aspirate smears contain granulomas (Fig. 11-19). No characteristic morphologic findings have been associated with any of the aforementioned underlying causes. Special stains for acid-fast bacilli and fungi should be performed on these specimens to eliminate the possibility of an underlying infectious disease. Repeat biopsy with culture may be needed if an infectious cause is suspected.

Lipogranulomas may be seen in up to 4% of marrow biopsies.[150] These collections of microvesicular fat, lymphocytes, and histiocytes are often associated with benign lymphoid aggregates (Fig. 11-20). These granulomas have no clinical significance, and no further evaluation is required.

The differential diagnosis of granulomatous lesions within the bone marrow includes the lesions of systemic mastocytosis, marrow involvement by Hodgkin lymphoma, non-Hodgkin lymphoma (particularly T-cell and T-cell–rich B-cell lymphomas), and focal involvement by hairy cell leukemia.

Systemic Rheumatic Disease

Peripheral blood and bone marrow abnormalities have been associated with a variety of systemic rheumatic diseases, including systemic lupus erythematosus (SLE), RA, mixed connective tissue disease, systemic sclerosis, Sjögren syndrome, and polymyositis.[151] These patients have a variety of abnormalities in the peripheral blood and bone marrow that may be related to their underlying disease or its treatment (Box 11-5).

Cytopenias are common in patients with systemic rheumatic diseases. In SLE, there may be a variety of underlying causes (Box 11-6).[152] Anemia may be caused by chronic inflammation, renal insufficiency, immune hemolysis, and, in rare cases, pure red cell aplasia.[153] Neutropenia and thrombocytopenia may also be seen.[154] A microangiopathic hemolytic anemia and thrombocytopenia may be seen in thrombotic thrombocytopenic purpura, which has been reported in association with SLE.[155] Thrombocytopenia may also be a complication of vasculitis with peripheral consumption of platelets.[156] Rare cases of amegakaryocytic thrombocytopenia have also been described in SLE, systemic

Systemic Rheumatic Disease and the Bone Marrow

Laboratory Findings
- Anemia
  - Anemia of chronic inflammation
  - Hemolytic anemia
  - Red cell aplasia
- Immune-mediated neutropenia
- Steroid-induced neutrophilia
- Eosinophilia
- Thrombocytopenia
  - Immune mediated
  - Amegakaryocytic thrombocytopenia
- Thrombocytosis

Morphologic Findings
- Variable cellularity
- Megaloblastic change
- Lymphoid aggregates
- Plasmacytosis
- Increased iron stores
- Granulomas
- Bone marrow fibrosis

Box 11-6 *Hematologic Findings in Systemic Lupus Erythematosus*

- Anemia
  - Anemia of chronic inflammation
  - Autoimmune hemolytic anemia
  - Renal-insufficiency anemia
  - Pure red cell aplasia
  - Microangiopathic hemolytic anemia
- Neutropenia
- Thrombocytopenia
- Myelofibrosis
- Hemophagocytic syndrome
- Necrosis

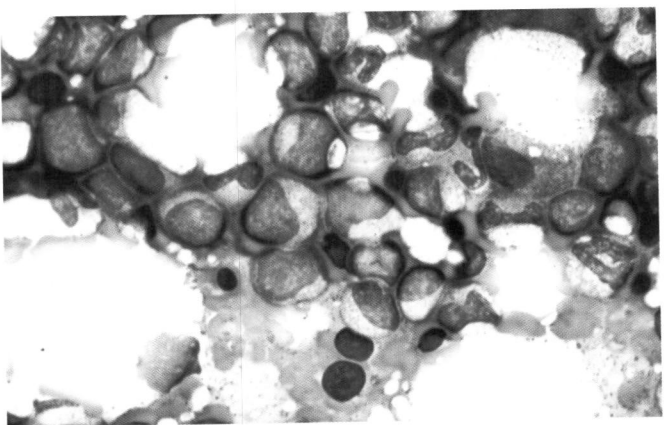

Figure 11-21. Bone marrow touch preparation showing a maturation arrest of the myeloid cell line in a patient with Felty's syndrome.

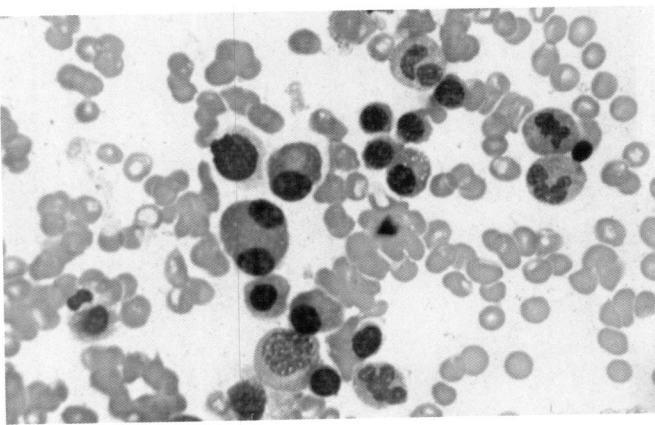

Figure 11-22. Increased reactive plasma cells are seen in the aspirate smear from a patient with rheumatoid arthritis.

sclerosis, and adult onset Still disease caused by immune-mediated suppression of megakaryocyte-colony formation.[157] Small platelets are typically seen on the peripheral blood smear owing to decreased production within the bone marrow.

In RA, the most common cause of anemia is anemia of chronic inflammation, and the severity parallels the disease activity. Neutropenia is seen in Felty's syndrome, which consists of neutropenia, splenomegaly, and RA. Neutrophil counts range from 0.5 to 2.5 × 10⁹/L. The bone marrow is typically hypercellular, with a maturation arrest at the myelocyte stage of development (Fig. 11-21). A proliferation of large granular lymphocytes with a T-cell phenotype may be found in patients with Felty's syndrome, and Felty's syndrome and large granular lymphocytic leukemia and have very similar presentations; however, T-cell clonality and *STAT3* gene mutations are much more common in the latter.[158]

Thrombocytosis may be seen in patients with chronic inflammatory conditions. Typically, platelet counts are less than 1 million, and thrombocytosis is not associated with an increased risk for either thrombosis or hemorrhage.

Leukocytosis is frequently present in patients with polymyalgia rheumatica, Still disease, and Behçet disease, which may be because of increased cytokine (granulocyte colony-stimulating factor) activity.[159]

Bone marrow specimens from patients with any of the systemic rheumatic diseases may contain benign lymphoid aggregates and increased reactive plasma cells (Fig. 11-22). Granulomas are rarely seen and are typically non-infectious; however, care must be taken to exclude an infectious cause, because these patients are often immunosuppressed. Rheumatoid nodules can rarely be seen within the marrow space. Increased polyclonal plasma cells have been rarely described in IgG4-related disease.[160]

Other bone marrow findings include dyserythropoiesis, megaloblastic change, serous fat atrophy, necrosis, and hemophagocytosis.[161,162] Macrophage activation syndrome, which is similar to hemophagocytic lymphohistiocytosis, is associated most commonly with juvenile arthritis.[163] Necrosis has been documented as a complication of antiphospholipid antibody syndrome.[164]

Patients have been described with autoimmune myelofibrosis (AIMF).[165] These patients may have SLE or progressive systemic sclerosis, but they may also have non-specific immune symptoms such as hemolytic anemia or synovitis. The bone marrow is variably cellular. In some cases,

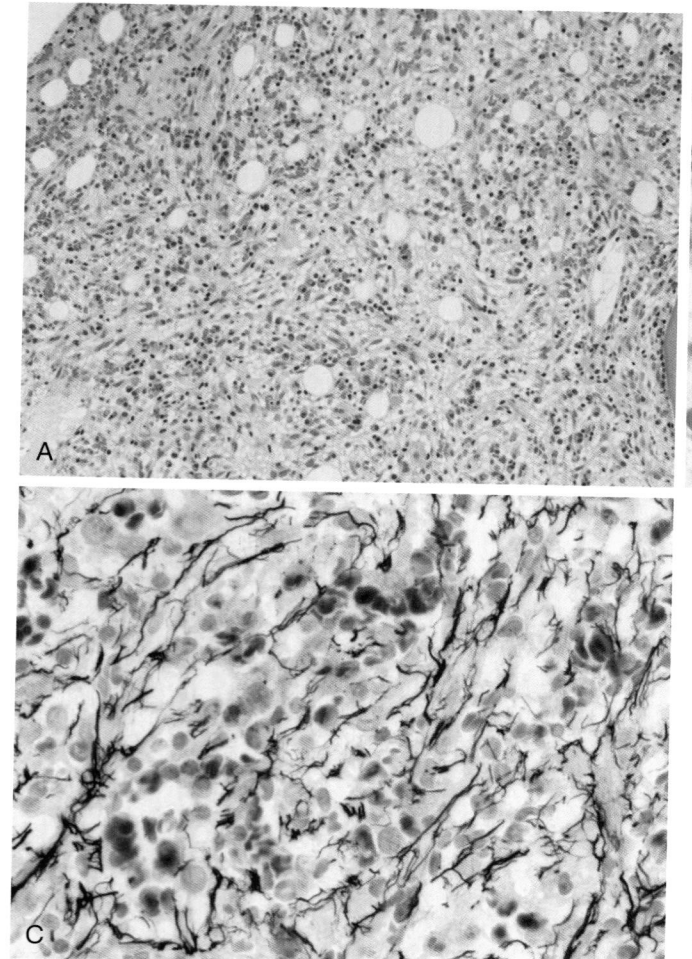

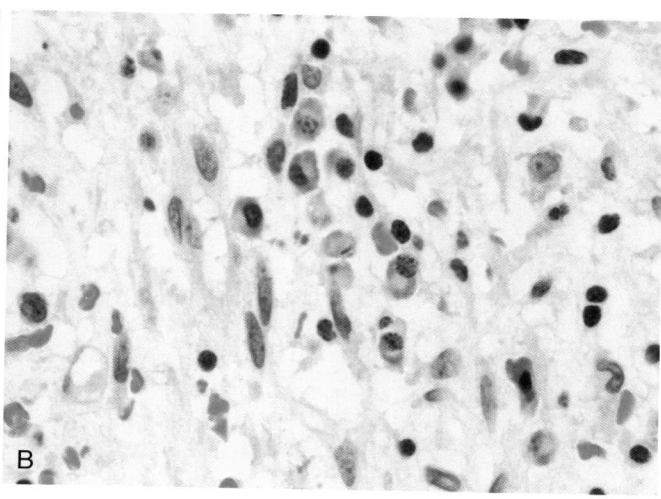

Figure 11-23. A–C, Hypocellular bone marrow from a patient with systemic lupus erythematosus who developed pancytopenia. The marrow is depleted but shows numerous plasma cells, sometimes associated with vessels, and reticulin fibrosis.

the bone marrow may be depleted (Fig. 11-23), whereas in others the marrow is cellular and even has prominent megakaryocytic hyperplasia, which raises the possibility of a myeloproliferative neoplasm. In the latter case, however, the megakaryocytes are not clustered or atypical, as is commonly observed in myeloproliferative neoplasms, and basophilia is not seen. Marrow reticulin but not collagen fibrosis is present; cytopenia(s) in AIMF patients responds to corticosteroid therapy.[166] Benign lymphoid aggregates and plasmacytosis, particularly in perivascular locations, may accompany the fibrosis. Prior to making this diagnosis, testing for JAK2, calreticulin, and MPL mutations should be performed.

Systemic therapy for rheumatic disease may also cause peripheral blood and bone marrow abnormalities. Corticosteroid therapy is associated with a peripheral neutrophilia caused by increased release from bone marrow stores. Lymphopenia is caused by apoptosis of lymphocytes. Eosinophils may also be decreased. Gastrointestinal blood loss caused by non-steroidal anti-inflammatory medications may cause iron-deficiency anemia. Azathioprine can cause leukopenia, thrombocytopenia, or pancytopenia and can give the bone marrow a dysplastic appearance.[167] Methotrexate causes an increase in mean corpuscular volume in 50% of patients treated with this drug. Leukopenia and thrombocytopenia may also occur. Pancytopenia can also

rarely be seen.[168] Alkylating agent chemotherapy is associated with myelodysplastic syndrome and acute myeloid leukemia caused by DNA damage by these drugs.[169,170]

Sarcoidosis

Patients with sarcoidosis may have anemia and leukopenia.[171] Increased eosinophils are common but rarely constitute more than 10% of the peripheral white blood cell count.[172] Peripheral blood eosinophilia does not correlate with tissue eosinophilia in sarcoidosis.

Bone marrow biopsies may contain granulomas and the incidence varies depending on the study, age, gender, and ethnicity.[173] Granulomas can be singular, multiple, or confluent within the marrow biopsy (Fig. 11-24). The granulomas are typically non-caseating and composed of epithelioid histiocytes. Asteroid bodies, Schaumann bodies, and calcium oxalate crystals may be seen. Stains for acid-fast bacilli and fungi are negative. Hemophagocytosis has been described in rare patients.[174]

Alcohol Abuse

Ethanol abuse causes numerous hematologic effects that often overlap with the findings in liver disease. Laboratory studies show anemia with macrocytosis caused by the direct toxic effect

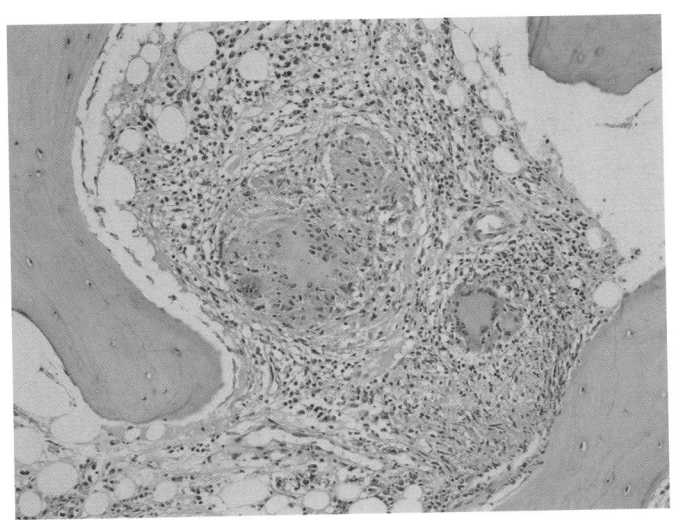

Figure 11-24. Bone marrow core biopsy showing a non-caseating granuloma with a multinucleated giant cell from a patient with sarcoidosis.

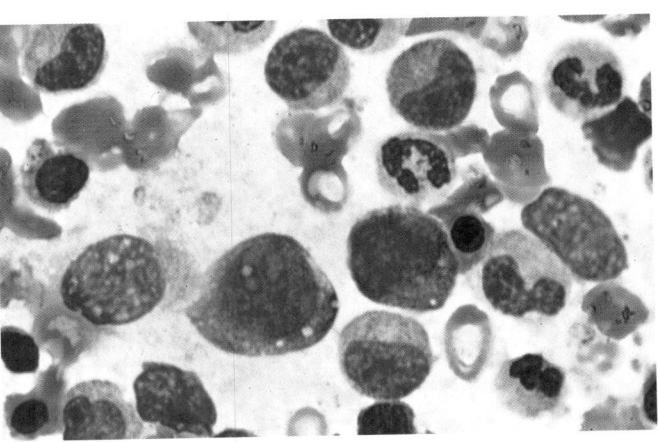

Figure 11-25. Bone marrow aspirate smear showing vacuolated erythroid precursors caused by alcohol abuse.

of ethanol, liver disease, or concomitant folate deficiency[175]; stomatocytes may also be seen. Granulocytopenia and impaired function of granulocytes may be seen leading to an increased risk of infection.[176] Thrombocytopenia is caused by the direct toxic effect of ethanol on megakaryocytes or increased splenic sequestration. Leukopenia can be a result of splenic sequestration or a maturation arrest at the promyelocyte stage. Leukoerythroblastosis may be found if alcoholic hepatitis is present.[177]

Bone marrow aspirate smears show a decreased myeloid-to-erythroid ratio, vacuolated erythroid and myeloid precursors,[178,179] megaloblastic change, and multinucleated erythroid precursors (Fig. 11-25).[180] Megakaryocytes may be decreased or absent. Ring sideroblasts are often seen.[181,182] Plasma cells are often increased and stain for cytoplasmic iron, a finding almost exclusively found in chronic alcoholism. Iron stores are often increased. If bleeding leads to iron deficiency, storage iron is absent.

Bone marrow sections may show decreased cellularity, a rare finding.[183] Precursor vacuolization, ring sideroblasts, and hypoplasia may resolve with abstinence from alcohol.[184,185]

Hepatic Disease

Numerous peripheral blood and bone marrow findings have been described in patients with liver disease (Box 11-7). Some of these findings overlap with the hematologic effects of alcohol. Anemia because of bleeding is common in these patients because of coagulation abnormalities and esophageal or gastric varices.[186] Macrocytic anemia is often present, with target cells seen. Severe liver disease may lead to hemolytic anemia, in which numerous acanthocytes or spur cells may be seen on the peripheral blood smear (Fig. 11-26). The development of hemolysis is associated with a poor prognosis.[187] Hypersplenism caused by portal hypertension can cause pancytopenia.

Hypersplenism is often associated with hypercellular bone marrow in which all three hematopoietic cell lines are increased. Aplastic anemia has been described in

---

Box 11-7 *Hepatic Disease and the Bone Marrow*

- Macrocytic anemia
- Thrombocytopenia
- Pancytopenia
- Aplastic anemia
- Hypersplenism
- Hemolytic anemia

---

patients with viral hepatitis and after orthotopic liver transplantation.[188,189]

Renal Disease

Peripheral blood and bone marrow abnormalities in patients with both acute and chronic renal insufficiency have been described. Patients with chronic renal failure are anemic primarily because of erythropoietin deficiency. Other causes include iron and folate deficiency, aluminum overload, hemolysis, and secondary hyperparathyroidism with osteitis fibrosa.[190] Patients also may have a bleeding diathesis caused by abnormalities of platelet function. Neutropenia may be seen after kidney transplant, related to drug therapy or an immune mechanism.[191] Treatment with recombinant erythropoietin therapy has lessened transfusion dependency in these patients.

Acute renal failure can also lead to impaired erythropoietin production, but anemia is typically related to the disorder causing the renal impairment. For example, hemolytic uremic syndrome, thrombotic thrombocytopenic purpura, and systemic vasculitis cause hemolysis, and red blood cell fragmentation can be seen on the peripheral blood smear.

The anemia of chronic renal insufficiency is normochromic and normocytic, with burr cells or echinocytes seen on the peripheral blood smear. The white blood cells and platelets are normal in number and morphologically unremarkable.

The erythroid precursors may be slightly decreased on the aspirate smear but are morphologically normal. Biopsy sections may reveal bony abnormalities caused by secondary hyperparathyroidism. Bone changes that have been described include paratrabecular fibrosis, widened osteoid seams, and increased bony remodeling (Fig. 11-27). The amount of fibrosis can be extensive and lead to pancytopenia in some

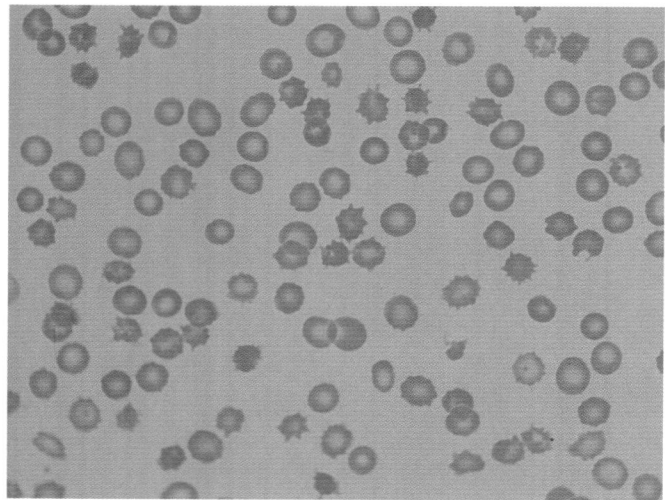

Figure 11-26. Peripheral blood smear with numerous acanthocytes caused by severe liver disease.

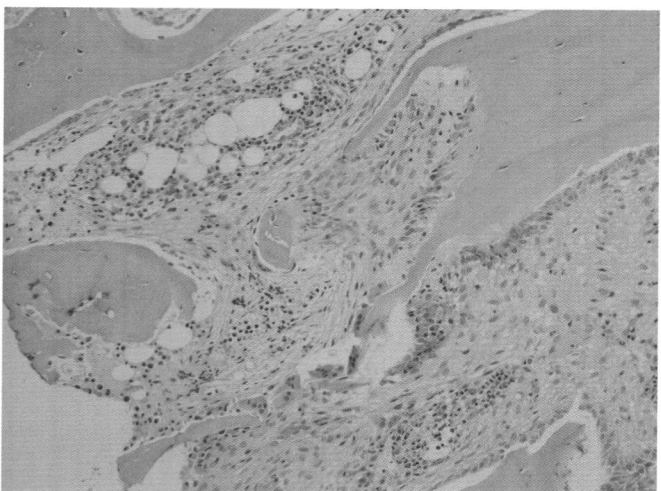

Figure 11-27. Bone marrow core biopsy showing widened osteoid seams and paratrabecular fibrosis in a patient with chronic renal failure.

cases. The myeloid-to-erythroid ratio is often slightly high, and there is an increase in storage iron. Exogenous erythropoietin decreases the myeloid-to-erythroid ratio owing to an increase in erythroid precursors and an increase in overall marrow cellularity.[192,193] Patients with extensive marrow fibrosis because of hyperparathyroidism may be resistant to treatment with erythropoietin.[194] Storage iron in the bone marrow may be completely or relatively depleted after treatment with recombinant erythropoietin, and iron replacement therapy may be needed.[195]

Hypothyroidism

Hematologic findings in hypothyroidism mainly include macrocytosis with or without anemia, decreased reticulocytes, and decreased plasma levels of erythropoietin.[196] Rarely, in severe hypothyroidism, all hematopoietic cell lines can be affected, resulting in pancytopenia. Bone marrow biopsy

may reveal hypoplasia.[197] In myxedema, findings similar to gelatinous transformation of the bone marrow may be seen.[198]

Hyperthyroidism

The hyperthyroid state causes anemia and neutropenia that reverses with treatment. Microcytosis is common, with or without anemia. Graves' disease may lead to autoimmune hemolytic anemia. Treatment with propylthiouracil and methimazole can cause agranulocytosis. Exposure to radioactive iodine (^{131}I) has not been shown to increase the risk for leukemia or myelodysplastic syndromes.[199]

CONCLUSION

In this chapter, a wide variety of findings in inflammatory, infectious, and metabolic conditions have been discussed. In many cases, the findings are non-specific, but often the bone marrow findings are indicative of a specific cause. Clinicopathologic correlation is essential to an accurate diagnosis of these disorders.

Pearls and Pitfalls

- Atypical lymphoid aggregates morphologically suggestive of lymphoma are seen in patients with viral infections such as Epstein-Barr virus or hepatitis C virus.
- Marrow dyspoiesis suggestive of a myelodysplastic syndrome can be seen with cytomegalovirus infection or treatment with immunosuppressive agents.
- Small-clefted (cleaved) lymphocytes, suggestive of follicular lymphoma, may be seen in peripheral blood in *Bordetella pertussis* infection.
- Reactive lymphocytosis is almost always composed predominantly of T cells.
- Persistent polyclonal B-cell lymphocytosis is often characterized by lymphocytes with moderate amounts of cytoplasm and bilobed nuclei; in the bone marrow they may occur in an intrasinusoidal or intravascular pattern.

KEY REFERENCES

5. Chabot-Richards DS, George TI. Leukocytosis. *Int J Lab Hematol.* 2014;36:279–288.
12. Wolniak KL, Goolsby C, Chen YH, et al. Expansion of a clonal CD8+, CD57+ large granular lymphocyte population after autologous stem cell transplant in multiple myeloma. *Am J Clin Pathol.* 2013;139:231–241.
17. DelGuidice I, Pileri S, Rossi M, et al. Histopathological and molecular features of persistent polyclonal B-cell lymphocytosis (PPBL) with progressive splenomegaly. *Br J Haematol.* 2009;144:726–731.
48. Shomali W, Gotlib J. World Health Organization-defined eosinophilic disorders: 2022 update on diagnosis, risk stratification and management. *Am J Hematol.* 2022;96:129–148.
81. Dumler JS, Madigan JE, Pusterla N, et al. Ehrlichioses in humans: epidemiology, clinical presentation, diagnosis and treatment. *Clin Infect Dis.* 2007;45(suppl 1):S45–S51.
123. Rahi MS, Jindal V, Reyes S-P, et al. Hematologic disorders associated with COVID-19: a review. *Ann Hematol.* 2021;100:309–320.

132. Deucher A, Wool GD. How I investigate bone marrow necrosis. *In J Lab Hematol.* 2019;41:585–592.

135. Ben-Baruch S, Canaani J, Braunstein R, et al. Predictive parameters for a diagnostic bone marrow biopsy specimen in the work-up of fever of unknown origin. *Mayo Clin Proc.* 2012;87:136–142.

137. Brackers de Hugo L, French M, Broussolle C, et al. Granulomatous lesions in bone marrow: clinicopathologic findings and significance in a study of 48 cases. *Eur J Intern Med.* 2013;24:468–473.

154. Hunt KE, Salama ME, Sever CD, et al. Bone marrow examination for unexplained cytopenias reveals nonspecific findings in patients with collagen vascular disease. *Arch Path Lab Med.* 2013;137:948–954.

Visit Elsevier eBooks+ for the complete set of references.

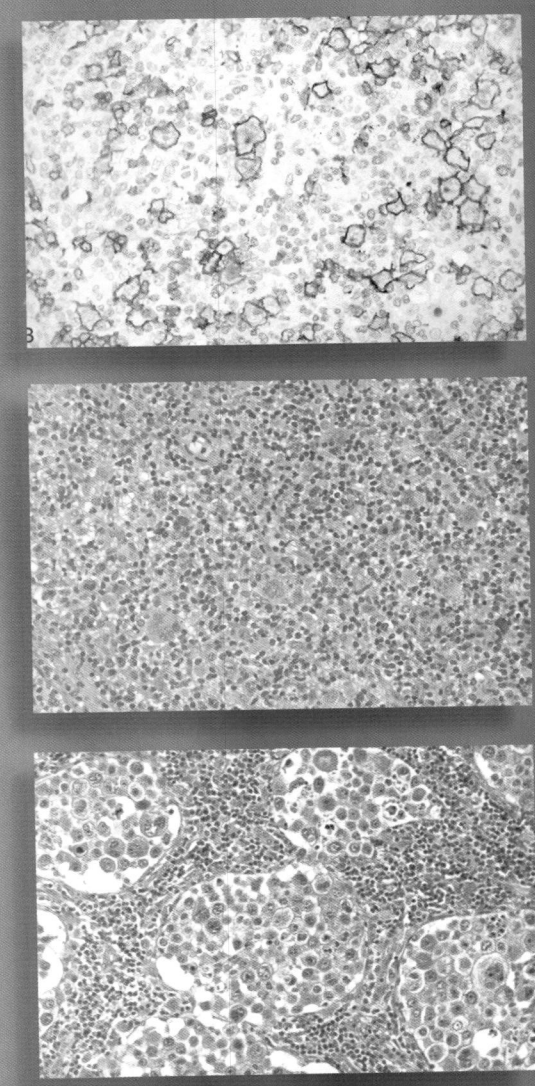

PART III

Lymphoid Neoplasms

Chapter 12

Principles of Classification of Lymphoid Neoplasms

Steven H. Swerdlow, Elias Campo, Leticia Quintanilla-Martinez, and Elaine S. Jaffe

INTRODUCTION

This chapter will set the stage for the subsequent chapters that examine mature lymphoid neoplasms. It will discuss the historical background of the classification of lymphomas, and the biological principles used today to define lymphoid neoplasms. This book uses the *2022 International Consensus Classification* as the primary basis for the discussion of neoplastic disorders of lymphoid, myeloid, and histiocytic neoplasms.[1] However, the text will provide synonyms, where appropriate, for the World Health Organization (WHO) 5th edition classification based on the published overview,[2] and briefly explain where there are significant differences. The actual 5th edition WHO *Blue Book* is not yet published in final form (as this chapter goes to press). Therefore there could be changes from what is included here, which is based solely on the overview of the 2022 WHO classification as published by Alaggio et al.[2]

The *2022 International Consensus Classification* was coordinated by the European Association for Haematopathology (EA4HP) and Society for Hematopathology (SH). It represents a revision of the 2016 WHO classification and relies heavily on decisions made at a September 2021 Clinical Advisory Committee (CAC) meeting, following the basic process established in the mid-1990s for the modern WHO classifications.[1] Each of those proposals were published as review articles, following the respective CAC meetings, and in the 3rd, 4th, and revised 4th editions of the *WHO Classification of Tumours of Haematopoietic and Lymphoid Tissues*.[3-8]

HISTORICAL BACKGROUND

As lymphoma classification has evolved from the functional lymphoma classifications that related lymphomas, where possible, to the normal cells they most closely resembled, with recognition of new entities and new solutions for problematic categories, the basic principles underlying the modern WHO classifications and now the ICC are essentially unchanged from those of the Revised European American Lymphoma (REAL) classification of lymphoid neoplasms published by the International Lymphoma Study Group (ILSG) in 1994.[9] The REAL classification represented a new paradigm in the classification of lymphoid neoplasms (Fig. 12-1), focusing on the identification of "real" diseases rather than a global theoretical framework such as survival, as had been used in the working formulation,[10] or cellular differentiation, as had been applied in the Kiel[11,12] and Lukes-Collins[13] classification systems. Key events in the evolution of the classification of lymphoid malignancies are summarized in Table 12-1.[14-50]

The REAL classification defined distinct entities with a constellation of features: morphology, immunophenotype, genetic features, and clinical presentation and course. Each of these elements plays a part, and no one feature takes precedence over the others consistently. For some diseases, morphology is highly characteristic, although at least phenotypic studies are required prior to making a definitive diagnosis. Most cases of chronic lymphocytic leukemia (CLL) or follicular lymphoma (FL) presenting in lymph nodes fall into this category. For other diseases, knowledge of the underlying genetics may be essential, such as in the diagnosis of anaplastic lymphoma kinase (ALK)–positive anaplastic large-cell lymphoma (ALCL) (Fig. 12-2). The relative importance of each of these features varies among diseases, depending on the state of current knowledge, and there is no one gold standard by which all diseases are defined. Still, lineage is a defining feature and forms the basis for the classification system's structure, recognizing B-cell, T-cell, and natural killer (NK)-cell neoplasms. In addition, a basic premise is the distinction between precursor lymphoid neoplasms and those derived from mature lymphoid cells.

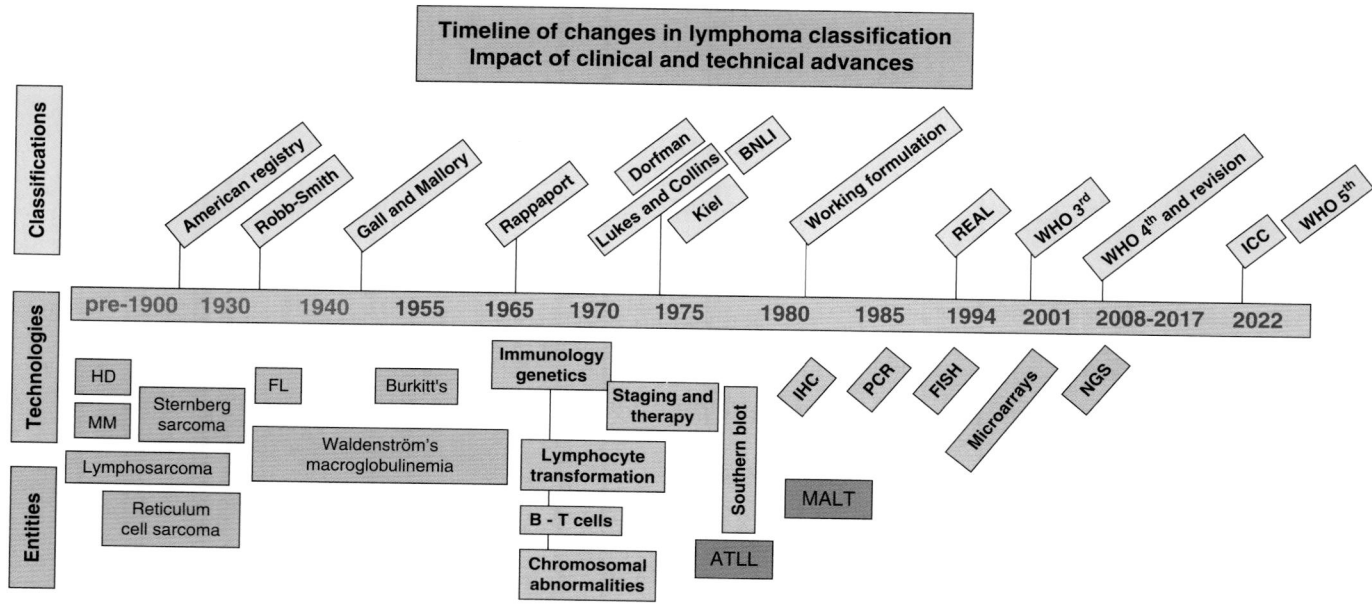

Figure 12-1. Diagram illustrating advances in the classification of lymphoid malignancies *(above the time line)* and corresponding events *(below the time line)* related to insights into the biology of lymphoid cells, the recognition of significant clinicopathologic entities, and advances in treatment and clinical evaluation. Technologic advances identifying the heterogeneity of lymphoid cells in the 1960s and 1970s precipitated a flurry of new classification systems that related lymphoid malignancies to the normal cells of the immune system. Improvements in the treatment and clinical evaluation of patients with lymphoid malignancies facilitated the recognition of clinical correlations and made accurate classification essential for patient management. The Revised European American Lymphoma (REAL) and World Health Organization (WHO) classifications represented a new perspective, emphasizing the recognition of disease entities and integrating morphologic, immunophenotypic, molecular, and clinical data. The introduction of NGS methodology in the last decade has facilitated increasingly rapid discovery of genetic aberrations on clinical samples. This multiparameter approach provides objective criteria for diagnosis, facilitating reproducibility and consensus. *ATLL,* Adult T-cell leukemia/lymphoma; *BNLI,* British National Lymphoma Investigation; *FISH,* fluorescence in situ hybridization; *FL,* follicular lymphoma; *HD,* Hodgkin disease; *ICC,* International Consensus Classification; *IHC,* immunohistochemistry in frozen and, later, paraffin-embedded sections; *MALT,* marginal zone lymphoma of mucosa-associated lymphoid tissue; *MM,* multiple myeloma; *NGS,* next-generation sequencing; *PCR,* polymerase chain reaction studies (for rearrangements of immunoglobulin and T-cell receptor genes).

In the twentieth century, the field of immunology shed light on the functional and immunophenotypic complexity of the immune system.[51] Traditional morphologic approaches were recognized as insufficient to decipher the many benign and malignant cellular components of lymphoid malignancies. Monoclonal antibody technology provided a seemingly endless array of immunophenotypic markers that could delineate the various cell types,[52] and technologic advances soon permitted the immunohistochemical detection of most relevant antigens in routinely processed formalin-fixed, paraffin-embedded sections.[53] Many lymphoid malignancies have characteristic immunophenotypic profiles, but even among some very homogeneous entities, immunophenotypic variation may be seen. For instance, not all cases of CLL are CD5 positive and CD23 positive; not all FLs are BCL2 positive or CD10 positive. CD5 may be expressed in otherwise classical FL. Expression of ALK is essential for the diagnosis of ALK-positive ALCL, but it is also expressed in ALK-positive large B-cell lymphoma and some histiocytic and mesenchymal tumors, mainly in children. Thus knowledge of the immunophenotype is a highly effective tool, but one that must be used in context.

There has been equally dramatic progress in understanding the genetics of lymphoid malignancies. Recurrent cytogenetic

abnormalities have been identified for many lymphoma subtypes. The first to be recognized were the t(14;18)(q32;q21) translocation of FL and the t(8;14)(q24;q32) translocation of Burkitt lymphoma (BL).[34,35,44] Subsequent studies led to the cloning of the genes involved in these translocations. The laboratories of Leder and Croce in 1982 both identified *MYC* as the gene that was translocated into the immunoglobulin genes in human BL[42,43]; other similar discoveries soon followed, such as *IGH::BCL2* in FL[54] and *IGH::CCND1* in mantle cell lymphoma.[55,56] The most common paradigm for translocations involving the immunoglobulin heavy-chain gene, IGH at 14q24, is that a cellular proto-oncogene comes under the influence of the IGH promoter. The list of important chromosomal aberrations in B-cell neoplasms has continued to rapidly expand and become integrated into clinical practice, such as the *IRF4* translocations in large B-cell lymphoma with *IRF4* rearrangement—a distinct clinicopathologic entity.[57,58] There are also less frequent but parallel alterations involving the T-cell receptor genes in T-cell malignancies, as well as other chromosomal aberrations.

The REAL classification recognized the importance of genetic abnormalities in defining disease entities. However, it has become clear that a purely genetic approach to defining diseases is not feasible. Although the *MYC* translocation is

Table 12-1 Milestones in the Evolution of the Classification of Lymphoid Neoplasms

Year	Reference	Principal Contributors	Event
1806	14	Alibert	Clinical description of mycosis fungoides
1828	15	Carswell	"Cancer cerebriformis of the lymphatic glands and spleen"—first case of what was later recognized as Hodgkin disease
1832	15	Hodgkin	"On some morbid appearances of the absorbent glands and spleen"—clinical report of what would later be known as Hodgkin disease
1845 1863	16	Virchow	Description of both leukemia and lymphosarcoma
1865	15	Wilks	Proposal of eponym *Hodgkin disease*
1898 1902	15	Sternberg Reed	Definition of microscopic features of neoplastic cell of Hodgkin disease, establishing an accurate microscopic description of the disease—the first lymphoma to be defined histologically
1914 1928 1930	16	Ewing Oberling Roulet	Description of *reticulosarcomas* (reticular cell sarcomas) of bone and lymphoid organs
1916	16	Sternberg	Description of *leukosarkomatose*, a process with characteristic features of precursor T-lymphoblastic lymphoma
1925 1927	17-19	Brill Symmers	Description of *giant follicle hyperplasia* and *follicular lymphadenopathy*—processes with features of follicular lymphoma and florid follicular hyperplasia
1934	16	Callender	American Registry of Pathology (AFIP) classification
1938	16	Robb-Smith	Robb-Smith classification of reticulosis and reticulosarcoma
1941 1942	20,21	Gall Mallory	Accurate description of follicular lymphoma and proposal of first modern lymphoma classification system
1947	16	Jackson Parker	Proposal of classification of Hodgkin disease
1956	26,27	Rappaport	Proposal of alternative classification for "non-Hodgkin" lymphoma
1958	22	Burkitt	Description of clinical syndrome of Burkitt lymphoma in African children
1960	23	Nowell	Phytohemagglutinin used to "transform" lymphocytes in vitro
1961	24	O'Conor	Histopathologic description of Burkitt lymphoma
1964	25	Epstein	Description of viral particles (Epstein-Barr virus) in cultured cells from Burkitt lymphoma
1966	28	Lukes, Butler	Proposal of modern classification of Hodgkin lymphoma
1972	29	Stein	Identification of high levels of IgM in "histiocytic" lymphomas
1973	16	Lennert	Lennert and colleagues meet to form European Lymphoma Club, predecessor of European Association for Haematopathology
1974	30	Lennert	Proposal of Kiel classification of lymphoma
1974	13	Lukes, Collins	Proposal of Lukes-Collins classification of lymphoma
1974	31	Taylor, Mason	Immunohistochemical detection of immunoglobulin in cells in formalin-fixed, paraffin-embedded sections
1974	32	Jaffe	Identification of complement receptors on cells of "nodular lymphoma," linking them to lymphoid follicle
1975	10	NCI	Failed consensus meeting of proponents of lymphoma classification systems, leading to working formulation study by NCI
1975	33	Southern	Development of Southern blot technique to separate and analyze DNA fragments
1976	34	Klein	Identification of t(8;14)(q24;q32) as recurrent translocation in Burkitt lymphoma
1979	35	Fukuhara, Rowley	Identification of t(14;18)(q32;q21) as recurrent translocation in "lymphocytic lymphoma" (follicular lymphoma)
1979	36	McMichael	Discovery of first monoclonal antibody to human leukocyte differentiation antigen, later defined as CD1a
1980–1982	37-40	Stein, Poppema, Warnke, Mason	Characterization of lymphoid cells by immunohistochemistry on frozen and paraffin sections
1982	41	Bernard, Boumsell	First international workshop on human leukocyte differentiation antigens
1982	42,43	Leder, Dalla-Favera, Croce	Cloning of *MYC* gene; identification of *MYC* and IGH as reciprocal partners in t(8;14)
1982	44	Yunis	Identification of recurrent translocations in follicular lymphoma, Burkitt lymphoma, and chronic lymphocytic leukemia
1982	10	Berard, Dorfman, DeVita, Rosenberg	Publication of NCI-sponsored working formulation for clinical classification of non-Hodgkin lymphomas
1985	45	Mullis	Development of polymerase chain reaction technique for amplification of specific DNA sequences

Continued

Table 12-1 Milestones in the Evolution of the Classification of Lymphoid Neoplasms—cont'd

Year	Reference	Principal Contributors	Event
1986	46	Cremer	Development of in situ hybridization techniques for analysis of chromosome aberrations in interphase nuclei
1991–1992	47	Isaacson, Stein	Founding of ILSG and publication of consensus report on mantle cell lymphoma
1994	48	Kuppers, Rajewsky	Identification of IGH gene rearrangements in Reed-Sternberg cells picked from tissue sections of classic Hodgkin lymphoma
1994	9	Harris, ILSG	Publication of REAL classification of lymphoid neoplasms
1997	49	Armitage	Validation of REAL classification by International Lymphoma Classification Project study
2000	50	Staudt	Application of gene expression profiling to human lymphomas
2001	6	EA4HP and SH	Publication of WHO monograph: *Pathology and Genetics: Tumours of Hematopoietic and Lymphoid Tissues* (3rd ed.)
2008	7	EA4HP and SH	Publication of *WHO Classification of Tumours of Haematopoietic and Lymphoid Tissues* (4th ed.)
2016	5,8	EA4HP and SH	Publication of the revised 4th ed *WHO Classification of Tumours of Haematopoietic and Lymphoid Tissues*
2022	1	EA4HP and SH	Publication of the 2022 International Consensus Classification
2022	2	IARC	Publication of overview of upcoming 5th edition of the WHO Classification of Haematolymphoid Tumours

Adapted from Jaffe ES, Harris NL, Stein H, Isaacson PG. Classification of lymphoid neoplasms: the microscope as a tool for disease discovery. *Blood.* 2008;112:4384-4399 (and subsequent updates).

EA4HP, European Association for Haematopathology; *ILSG,* International Lymphoma Study Group; *NCI,* National Cancer Institute; *REAL,* Revised European American Lymphoma; *SH,* Society for Hematopathology; *WHO,* World Health Organization.

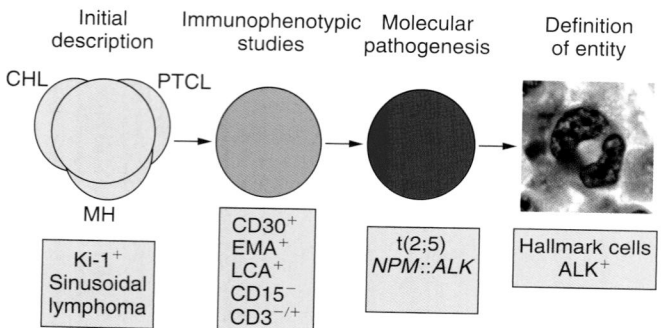

Figure 12-2. The recognition of anaplastic lymphoma kinase (ALK)-positive anaplastic large-cell lymphoma (ALCL) is emblematic of the stepwise advances in the identification of new disease entities. ALCL was first recognized by distinctive morphologic features. The identification of a characteristic immunophenotype, with strong expression of CD30, led to better recognition of the entity and facilitated studies to determine its molecular pathogenesis. Identification of the nucleophosmin *NPM::ALK* translocation, with high levels of ALK expression, led to the development of polyclonal and, later, monoclonal antibodies to identify ALK in formalin-fixed, paraffin-embedded sections. These tools, when incorporated into daily practice, both broadened and narrowed the original concept of ALCL as a morphologic entity. Small-cell variants were included, whereas highly anaplastic and Hodgkin-like forms were largely excluded from the disease spectrum. *CHL,* Classic Hodgkin lymphoma; *MH,* malignant histiocytosis; *PTCL,* peripheral T-cell lymphoma.

nearly universally present in BLs, *MYC* translocations involving the immunoglobulin genes are found as either secondary or, less commonly, primary genetic abnormalities in other lymphoid malignancies, including some diffuse large B-cell lymphomas (DLBCLs), plasmablastic malignancies, and some cases of B-lymphoblastic leukemia/lymphoma. Similarly, *IGH::BCL2* is found in 85% to 90% of FLs and is present in up to 25% to 30% of de novo DLBCLs with no prior clinical evidence of FL.

Even more recently, there is an ever-growing contribution of molecular genetic studies in understanding lymphomas, in helping to better define both older and newer distinct entities and of increasing utility as prognostic/predictive markers important for the practice of precision medicine. They are being integrated more and more into clinical practice, although much remains to be learned. Though not common, some entities are strongly associated with specific mutations such as *BRAF* V600E mutations in hairy cell leukemia and *MYD88* L265P mutations in lymphoplasmacytic lymphoma (LPL). However, similar to what we have learned from other phenotypic and cytogenetic findings, none of these can be interpreted in isolation. *BRAF* V600E mutations are seen in a variety of lymphoid and non-lymphoid malignancies, and *MYD88* L265P mutations are seen in a variety of DLBCL that are not related to LPL. Although not quite ready for incorporation into our classification at this time, there is great interest in the use of molecular/cytogenetic categorization of DLBCLs via high throughput sequencing as reported by several different groups of investigators[59-63] that do not all directly correlate with the distinction of GCB and ABC DLBCL and which have both prognostic and predictive implications. It has been said that "It seems inevitable, on the basis of the results of the [molecular genomic] classification studies, that a more detailed genetic subclassification is poised to supersede the COO [cell of origin] framework."[64] Consistent with this, the ICC report indicates that "cell-of-origin is retained for the present time with the expectation that transition to a molecular genetic classification will be feasible in the near future." Use of such a molecular genomic classification for the DLBCL also may lead to reorganization of some entities that we currently recognize as distinct, but which share an important molecular landscape. Newer molecular studies also are greatly affecting the area of T- and NK-cell neoplasms. For instance, the concept of follicular helper T-cell lymphomas is strongly supported by their overlapping characteristic mutational findings (e.g., with *TET2, DNMT3A,* and *RHOA* mutations).[65] Interestingly, some mutations, such as IDH2[R172], may be associated with distinctive morphologic features within the angioimmunoblastic subtype.[66,67] Nevertheless, individual mutations by themselves cannot be used to define an entity. Finally, the inclusion of clinical criteria was one of the novel aspects of the ILSG approach.[68] The REAL classification recognized that the site of presentation is often a signpost for underlying biological distinctions, such as in extranodal lymphomas of mucosa-associated lymphoid tissue (MALT),[69] primary mediastinal large B-cell lymphoma, and many types of T/NK-cell lymphomas. Even very recently, the importance of a mediastinal location in what is now known as mediastinal gray-zone lymphomas (MGZL) provided evidence that this entity should be segregated from other aggressive B-cell neoplasms with Hodgkin-like cells that had also been considered to have "gray zone" features, with mediastinal and non-mediastinal cases manifesting different genetic profiles.[70-72] The ILSG appreciated that accurate diagnosis cannot take place in a vacuum and requires knowledge of the clinical history, because biologically distinct entities may appear cytologically similar. Integration of clinical features is an essential aspect in the definition of disease entities and in accurate diagnosis in daily practice. The pathologist must be provided with relevant clinical details to arrive at a correct diagnosis, and it is the pathologist's responsibility to insist on sufficient clinical data if it is not provided. Each of the chapters covering the lymphoid neoplasms emphasizes the pertinent clinical features, knowledge of which contributes to an accurate diagnosis. It is also evident that clinical features are important prognostic indicators, and in many instances, the treatment approach chosen is based on the clinical setting in conjunction with the pathologic diagnosis. For instance, some patients with FL can be followed with a "watch and wait" approach, whereas in others a heavy tumor burden at diagnosis mandates immediate therapy. Response to therapy is influenced not only by underlying clinical features but also by biological and prognostic factors. Cytologic grade varies in many disease entities and is discussed in the chapters that follow. Other prognostic factors are based on tumor cell biology[73,74] or host factors, such as the tumor microenvironment.[75] For this reason, it is not possible to stratify lymphoma subtypes in a linear fashion according to their clinical aggressiveness. The pathologist and clinician are part of a management team that determines the therapeutic approach in each case.

The REAL classification was based on the building of consensus, and it recognized that a comprehensive classification system was beyond the experience of any one individual or a small group of individuals. The 19 members of the ILSG contributed their diverse perspectives to achieve a unified point of view. In addition, the ILSG made the decision to base its classification exclusively on published data; thus for an entity to be included in the REAL classification, it had to be validated in more than one publication.

Recognition that the development of classification systems should be a cooperative effort was expanded with the 3rd edition of the WHO classification.[6] Contacted by Dr. L. Sobin and subsequently Dr. P. Kleihues, Dr. E. S. Jaffe, President-Elect of the SH, was invited in 1994 to develop the WHO classification for the 3rd edition of the WHO *Blue Book* tumor series, which, for the first time, would integrate molecular and cytogenetic features, together with clinical, morphologic, and phenotypic features in defining disease entities. The leadership of the SH recognized achieving a broad international perspective was important and invited the EA4HP to join in the effort. This unified EA4HP and SH effort represented the

first true worldwide consensus classification of hematologic malignancies and ultimately was the culmination of the efforts of a 7-member steering committee, 11 pathology committee chairs, 75 author contributors, and 44 clinician participants in a critical clinical advisory committee meeting. In 2008, the 4th edition of the WHO classification involved the efforts of 138 authors and 2 clinical advisory committees comprising 62 clinical specialists with expertise in lymphoid and myeloid disorders. The clinical advisory committee meetings were organized around a series of issues, including disease definitions, nomenclature, grading, and clinical relevance. As with the 3rd edition, the effort was coordinated by the EA4HP and the SH, led by the eight editors who served as a steering committee. This model was maintained for the revision of the 4th edition, with a clinical advisory committee meeting held in 2014 to address newly emerging issues related to the definition of specific entities and with the revised WHO classification published in manuscript form in 2016 and the subsequent WHO *Blue Book* in 2017.[5,8]

Since those publications, there have been many advances in hematopathology, in part because of an explosion in molecular/cytogenetic data and newer therapeutic strategies, so the classification needed to be revised once again. Discussions about the next revision began with IARC in 2019; however, there were some major differences of opinion about how to proceed. Consistent with former revisions, the process led by the SH and EA4HP started with planning for a session that was held at the 2021 EA4HP meeting to begin to get broad-based input from the international hematopathology community. Realizing the continued critical nature of consensus also from clinical hemato-oncologists, the EA4HP and SH once again organized a hybrid CAC with 149 international participants that was held in September 2021 (delayed from 2020 because of the COVID pandemic). This led to the revised classification being published as the *International Consensus Classification*,[1] with additional details provided in a special issue of *Virchows Archiv*.[76] The ICC lymphoma classification was authored by 73 pathologists, clinicians, and biologists representing 20 countries from Europe, North and South America, Asia, and Australia. Unfortunately, in spite of ongoing efforts for a reconciliation, IARC rejected this process. They used an 18-person standing editorial board (which includes 1 hematopathologist) chaired by Dr. I. Cree, IARC Branch Head for Evidence Synthesis and Classification Section, together with a 24-person expert editorial board appointed based on "bibliometrics" and the recommendation of the standing editorial board members, to develop a proposal for the 5th edition of the WHO classification.[2] This proposal presumably will form the basis for the upcoming 5th edition of the WHO *Blue Book*. Although the two separate revisions have many similarities to each other and to the 2016 WHO classification, as highlighted in Table 12-2, there are some major differences between all three classifications, not only in terminology but also in some important concepts.

THE ICC AND WHO 5TH ED. PROPOSALS: SIMILARITIES AND DIFFERENCES

There are important changes in the 2022 ICC[1] and differences from the proposed 2022 WHO[2] that will be discussed in greater detail in the chapters that follow, not all of which are included here. Key changes in terminology are highlighted

Table 12-2 Comparison of Classification Systems for Lymphoid Neoplasms

International Consensus Classification	WHO Classification, Revised 4th Edition	WHO Classification, 5th Edition
Mature B-Cell Neoplasms		
Chronic lymphocytic leukemia/small lymphocytic lymphoma	Chronic lymphocytic leukemia/small lymphocytic lymphoma	Chronic lymphocytic leukemia/small lymphocytic lymphoma
Monoclonal B-cell lymphocytosis	Monoclonal B-cell lymphocytosis	Monoclonal B-cell lymphocytosis
B-cell prolymphocytic leukemia	B-cell prolymphocytic leukemia	**Entity deleted**
Splenic marginal zone lymphoma	Splenic marginal zone lymphoma	Splenic marginal zone lymphoma
Hairy cell leukemia	Hairy cell leukemia	Hairy cell leukemia
Splenic B-cell lymphoma/leukemia, unclassifiable	*Splenic B-cell lymphoma/leukemia, unclassifiable*	Splenic diffuse red pulp small B-cell lymphoma
• *Splenic diffuse red pulp small B-cell lymphoma*	• *Splenic diffuse red pulp small B-cell lymphoma*	**Splenic B-cell lymphoma/leukemia with prominent nucleoli**
• *Hairy cell leukemia-variant*	• *Hairy cell leukemia-variant*	(encompasses hairy cell leukemia-variant and some cases of B-cell prolymphocytic leukemia)
Lymphoplasmacytic lymphoma	Lymphoplasmacytic lymphoma	Lymphoplasmacytic lymphoma
IgM MGUS	IgM MGUS	IgM MGUS
• **IgM MGUS, plasma cell type**		
• **IgM MGUS, NOS**		
Primary cold agglutinin disease		**Cold agglutinin disease**
Heavy Chain Diseases		
Mu heavy chain disease	Mu heavy chain disease	Mu heavy chain disease
Gamma heavy chain disease	Gamma heavy chain disease	Gamma heavy chain disease
Alpha heavy chain disease	Alpha heavy chain disease	Alpha heavy chain disease
Plasma Cell Neoplasms		
Non-IgM MGUS	Non-IgM MGUS	Non-IgM MGUS
		Monoclonal gammopathy of renal significance
MM (Plasma cell myeloma)	Plasma cell myeloma	Plasma cell myeloma
• **MM, NOS**		
• **MM with recurrent genetic abnormality***		
• **MM with CCND family translocation**		
• **MM with MAF family translocation**		
• **MM with *NSD2* translocation**		
• **MM with hyperdiploidy**		
	Plasma cell neoplasms with associated paraneoplastic syndrome	Plasma cell neoplasms with associated paraneoplastic syndrome
	• POEMS syndrome	• POEMS syndrome
	• TEMPI syndrome	• TEMPI syndrome
		• **AESOP syndrome**
Solitary plasmacytoma of bone	Solitary plasmacytoma of bone	Solitary plasmacytoma of bone
Extraosseous plasmacytoma	Extraosseous plasmacytoma	Extraosseous plasmacytoma
Monoclonal immunoglobulin deposition diseases	Monoclonal immunoglobulin deposition diseases	Monoclonal immunoglobulin deposition diseases
• **Immunoglobulin light chain amyloidosis (AL)**	• Primary amyloidosis	• **Immunoglobulin-related (AL) amyloidosis**
• **Localized AL amyloidosis***	• Light chain and heavy chain deposition disease	• **Monoclonal immunoglobulin deposition disease**
• Light chain and heavy chain deposition disease		
Mature B-Cell Lymphomas		
Extranodal marginal zone lymphoma of mucosa-associated lymphoid tissue	Extranodal marginal zone lymphoma of mucosa-associated lymphoid tissue	Extranodal marginal zone lymphoma of mucosa-associated lymphoid tissue
Primary cutaneous marginal zone LPD	Not previously included (originally included under "extranodal marginal zone lymphoma of mucosa-associated lymphoid tissue")	**Primary cutaneous marginal zone lymphoma**
Nodal marginal zone lymphoma	Nodal marginal zone lymphoma	Nodal marginal zone lymphoma
• *Pediatric-type nodal marginal zone lymphoma†*	• *Pediatric nodal marginal zone lymphoma*	• Pediatric nodal marginal zone lymphoma
Follicular lymphoma	Follicular lymphoma	Follicular lymphoma
• In situ follicular neoplasia	• Testicular follicular lymphoma	• In situ follicular B-cell neoplasm
• Duodenal-type follicular lymphoma	• In situ follicular neoplasia	• Duodenal-type follicular lymphoma
	• Duodenal-type follicular lymphoma	• **Follicular large B-cell lymphoma**
		• **Follicular lymphoma with uncommon features**

Table 12-2 Comparison of Classification Systems for Lymphoid Neoplasms—cont'd

International Consensus Classification	WHO Classification, Revised 4th Edition	WHO Classification, 5th Edition
BCL2-R-negative, CD23-positive follicle center lymphoma * (Overlapping features with the diffuse variant of follicular lymphoma in the WHO classification)		
Primary cutaneous follicle center lymphoma	Primary cutaneous follicle center lymphoma	Primary cutaneous follicle center lymphoma
Pediatric-type follicular lymphoma	Pediatric-type follicular lymphoma	Pediatric-type follicular lymphoma
Testicular follicular lymphoma	Considered a subtype of follicular lymphoma	Not separately designated
Large B-cell lymphoma with *IRF4* rearrangement	*Large B-cell lymphoma with* IRF4 *rearrangement*	Large B-cell lymphoma with *IRF4* rearrangement‡
Mantle cell lymphoma	Mantle cell lymphoma	Mantle cell lymphoma
• In situ mantle cell neoplasia	• In situ mantle cell neoplasia	• In situ mantle cell neoplasm
• Leukemic non-nodal mantle cell lymphoma	• Leukemic non-nodal mantle cell lymphoma	• Leukemic non-nodal mantle cell lymphoma
Large B-Cell Lymphomas		
DLBCL, NOS	DLBCL, NOS	DLBCL, NOS
• Germinal center B-cell subtype		• Germinal center B-cell subtype
• Activated B-cell subtype		• Activated B-cell subtype
Large B-cell lymphoma with 11q aberration	*Burkitt-like lymphoma with 11q aberration*	**High-grade B-cell lymphoma with 11q aberrations**
Nodular lymphocyte predominant B-cell lymphoma	Considered a Hodgkin lymphoma subtype	Considered a Hodgkin lymphoma subtype
T-cell/histiocyte-rich large B-cell lymphoma	T-cell/histiocyte-rich large B-cell lymphoma	T-cell/histiocyte-rich large B-cell lymphoma
Primary DLBCL of the central nervous system	Primary DLBCL of the central nervous system	**Primary large B-cell lymphoma of immune-privileged sites (includes central nervous system, testis, and vitreoretina)**
Primary DLBCL of the testis		
Primary cutaneous DLBCL, leg type	Primary cutaneous DLBCL, leg type	Primary cutaneous DLBCL, leg type
Intravascular large B-cell lymphoma	Intravascular large B-cell lymphoma	Intravascular large B-cell lymphoma
HHV-8 and EBV-negative primary effusion-based lymphoma		**Fluid overload-associated large B-cell lymphoma**
EBV-positive mucocutaneous ulcer	EBV-positive mucocutaneous ulcer	EBV-positive mucocutaneous ulcer
EBV-positive DLBCL, NOS	EBV-positive DLBCL, NOS	**EBV-positive DLBCL**
DLBCL associated with chronic inflammation	DLBCL associated with chronic inflammation	DLBCL associated with chronic inflammation
• Fibrin-associated DLBCL	• Fibrin-associated DLBCL	
		Fibrin-associated large B-cell lymphoma
Lymphomatoid granulomatosis	Lymphomatoid granulomatosis	Lymphomatoid granulomatosis
EBV-positive polymorphic B-cell LPD, NOS *		
ALK-positive large B-cell lymphoma	ALK-positive large B-cell lymphoma	ALK-positive large B-cell lymphoma
Burkitt lymphoma	Burkitt lymphoma	Burkitt lymphoma
High-grade B-cell lymphoma, with *MYC* and *BCL2* rearrangements	High-grade B-cell lymphoma with *MYC* and *BCL2* and/or *BCL6* rearrangements	**Diffuse large B-cell lymphoma/high grade B-cell lymphoma with *MYC* and *BCL2* rearrangements**
High-grade B-cell lymphoma with MYC ***and BCL6 rearrangements***		Cases with *MYC* and *BCL6* rearrangements are classified either as a subtype of DLBCL, NOS or HGBL, NOS according to their cytomorphological features
HGBL, NOS	HGBL, NOS	HGBL, NOS
Primary mediastinal large B-cell lymphoma	Primary mediastinal large B-cell lymphoma	Primary mediastinal large B-cell lymphoma
Mediastinal gray-zone lymphoma	B-cell lymphoma, unclassifiable, with features intermediate between DLBCL and classic Hodgkin lymphoma	**Mediastinal gray-zone lymphoma**
Plasmablastic lymphoma	Plasmablastic lymphoma	Plasmablastic lymphoma
HHV-8-associated lymphoproliferative disorders	HHV-8-associated lymphoproliferative disorders	KSHV/HHV-8-associated B-cell lymphoid proliferations and lymphomas
• Multicentric Castleman disease	• HHV-8-positive germinotropic LPD	• KSHV/HHV-8-associated multicentric Castleman disease
• HHV-8-positive germinotropic LPD	• HHV-8-positive DLBCL, NOS	• KSHV/HHV-8-positive germinotropic LPD
• HHV-8-positive DLBCL, NOS	• Primary effusion lymphoma	• KSHV/HHV-8-positive DLBCL
• Primary effusion lymphoma		• Primary effusion lymphoma
Mature T-Cell and NK-Cell Lymphomas		
T-prolymphocytic leukemia	T-prolymphocytic leukemia	T-prolymphocytic leukemia
T-cell large granular lymphocytic leukemia	T-cell large granular lymphocytic leukemia	T-large granular lymphocytic leukemia
Chronic LPD of NK cells	Chronic LPD of NK cells	**NK-large granular lymphocytic leukemia**
Adult T-cell leukemia/lymphoma	Adult T-cell leukemia/lymphoma	Adult T-cell leukemia/lymphoma

Continued

Table 12-2 Comparison of Classification Systems for Lymphoid Neoplasms—cont'd

International Consensus Classification	WHO Classification, Revised 4th Edition	WHO Classification, 5th Edition
Sézary syndrome	Sézary syndrome	Sézary syndrome
EBV-Positive T-Cell and NK-Cell Neoplasms		
Hydroavacciniforme–like LPD • **Classic*** • **Systemic***	Hydroavacciniforme–like LPD	Hydroavacciniforme LPD
Severe mosquito bite allergy	Severe mosquito bite allergy	Severe mosquito bite allergy
Chronic active EBV disease, systemic (T- and NK-cell phenotype)	Chronic active EBV infection of T- and NK-cell type, systemic form	**Systemic chronic active EBV disease**
Systemic EBV-positive T-cell lymphoma of childhood	Systemic EBV-positive T-cell lymphoma of childhood	Systemic EBV-positive T-cell lymphoma of childhood
Extranodal NK/T-cell lymphoma, nasal type	Extranodal NK/T-cell lymphoma, nasal type	**Extranodal NK/T-cell lymphoma**
Aggressive NK-cell leukemia	Aggressive NK-cell leukemia	Aggressive NK-cell leukemia
Primary nodal EBV-positive T/NK-cell lymphoma	(Formerly included in PTCL NOS)	EBV-positive nodal T- and NK-cell lymphoma
Primary Cutaneous T-Cell Lymphomas		
Primary cutaneous CD4-positive small/medium T-cell LPD	*Primary cutaneous CD4-positive small/medium T-cell LPD*	Primary cutaneous CD4-positive small or medium T-cell LPD
Primary cutaneous acral CD8-positive T-cell LPD	*Primary cutaneous acral CD8-positive T-cell lymphoma*	**Primary cutaneous acral CD8-positive LPD**
Mycosis fungoides	Mycosis fungoides	Mycosis fungoides
Primary cutaneous CD30-positive T-cell LPD: • Lymphomatoid papulosis • Primary cutaneous anaplastic large cell lymphoma	Primary cutaneous CD30-positive T-cell LPD: • Lymphomatoid papulosis • Primary cutaneous anaplastic large cell lymphoma	Primary cutaneous CD30-positive T-cell LPD: • Lymphomatoid papulosis • Primary cutaneous anaplastic large cell lymphoma
Subcutaneous panniculitis-like T-cell lymphoma	Subcutaneous panniculitis-like T-cell lymphoma	Subcutaneous panniculitis-like T-cell lymphoma
Primary cutaneous gamma/delta T-cell lymphoma	Primary cutaneous gamma/delta T-cell lymphoma	Primary cutaneous gamma/delta T-cell lymphoma
Primary cutaneous CD8-positive aggressive epidermotropic cytotoxic T-cell lymphoma	*Primary cutaneous CD8-positive aggressive epidermotropic cytotoxic T-cell lymphoma*	Primary cutaneous CD8-positive aggressive epidermotropic cytotoxic T-cell lymphoma
		Primary cutaneous peripheral T-cell lymphoma, NOS
Intestinal T-Cell and NK-Cell Lymphoid Proliferations and Lymphomas		
Indolent clonal T-cell LPD of the gastrointestinal tract	Indolent T-cell lymphoproliferative disorder of the gastrointestinal tract	**Indolent T-cell lymphoma of the gastrointestinal tract**
Indolent NK-cell LPD of the gastrointestinal tract	Entity not previously described	**Indolent NK-cell LPD of the gastrointestinal tract**
Type II refractory celiac disease*		
Enteropathy-associated T-cell lymphoma	Enteropathy-associated T-cell lymphoma	Enteropathy-associated T-cell lymphoma
Monomorphic epitheliotropic intestinal T-cell lymphoma	Monomorphic epitheliotropic intestinal T-cell lymphoma	Monomorphic epitheliotropic intestinal T-cell lymphoma
Intestinal T-cell lymphoma, NOS	Intestinal T-cell lymphoma, NOS	Intestinal T-cell lymphoma, NOS
Other Nodal and Extranodal T-Cell Lymphomas		
Hepatosplenic T-cell lymphoma	Hepatosplenic T-cell lymphoma	Hepatosplenic T-cell lymphoma
Peripheral T-cell lymphoma, NOS	Peripheral T-cell lymphoma, NOS	Peripheral T-cell lymphoma, NOS
Follicular helper T-cell lymphoma		**Nodal TFH cell lymphoma**
• **Follicular helper T-cell lymphoma, angioimmunoblastic type**	Angioimmunoblastic T-cell lymphoma	• **Nodal TFH cell lymphoma, angioimmunoblastic-type**
• **Follicular helper T-cell lymphoma, follicular type**	Follicular T-cell lymphoma	• **Nodal TFH cell lymphoma, follicular-type**
• **Follicular helper T-cell lymphoma, NOS**	Nodal peripheral T-cell lymphoma with TFH phenotype	• **Nodal TFH cell lymphoma, NOS**
Anaplastic large cell lymphoma, ALK-positive	Anaplastic large cell lymphoma, ALK-positive	ALK-positive anaplastic large cell lymphoma
Anaplastic large cell lymphoma, ALK-negative	Anaplastic large cell lymphoma, ALK-negative	ALK-negative anaplastic large cell lymphoma
Breast implant-associated anaplastic large cell lymphoma	Breast implant-associated anaplastic large cell lymphoma	Breast implant-associated anaplastic large cell lymphoma
Hodgkin Lymphoma		
Nodular sclerosis classic Hodgkin lymphoma	Nodular sclerosis classic Hodgkin lymphoma	Nodular sclerosis classic Hodgkin lymphoma
Lymphocyte-rich classic Hodgkin lymphoma	Lymphocyte-rich classic Hodgkin lymphoma	Lymphocyte-rich classic Hodgkin lymphoma
Mixed cellularity classic Hodgkin lymphoma	Mixed cellularity classic Hodgkin lymphoma	Mixed cellularity classic Hodgkin lymphoma
Lymphocyte-depleted classic Hodgkin lymphoma	Lymphocyte-depleted classic Hodgkin lymphoma	Lymphocyte-depleted classic Hodgkin lymphoma

Table 12-2 Comparison of Classification Systems for Lymphoid Neoplasms—cont'd

International Consensus Classification	WHO Classification, Revised 4th Edition	WHO Classification, 5th Edition
	Nodular lymphocyte predominant Hodgkin lymphoma	Nodular lymphocyte predominant Hodgkin lymphoma
Immunodeficiency-Associated Lymphoproliferative Disorders	**Immunodeficiency-Associated Lymphoproliferative Disorders**	**Lymphoid Proliferations and Lymphomas Associated with Immune Deficiency and Dysregulation**§
PTLD • Non-destructive PTLD • Plasmacytic hyperplasia PTLD • Infectious mononucleosis PTLD • Florid follicular hyperplasia PTLD • Polymorphic PTLD • Monomorphic PTLD • Classic Hodgkin lymphoma PTLD Other iatrogenic immunodeficiency-associated LPD Lymphoproliferative diseases associated with primary immune disorders	PTLD • Non-destructive PTLD • Plasmacytic hyperplasia PTLD • Infectious mononucleosis PTLD • Florid follicular hyperplasia PTLD • Polymorphic PTLD • Monomorphic PTLD • Classic Hodgkin lymphoma PTLD Other iatrogenic immunodeficiency-associated lymphoproliferative disorders Lymphoproliferative diseases associated with primary immune disorders	**Hyperplasias arising in immune deficiency/dysregulation**§ **Polymorphic lymphoproliferative disorders arising in immune deficiency/dysregulation**§ **Lymphomas arising in immune deficiency/dysregulation**§ **Inborn error of immunity-associated lymphoid proliferations and lymphomas**

The listing of the WHO Classification, 5th edition, is that published by Alaggio, et al.,[2] as the WHO 5th edition *Blue Book* was not yet published in the final form when this chapter was finalized. The final fifth edition WHO classification is expected to include some changes from the listing here.
Red and blue indicate those entities that differ between the International Consensus Classification (in red) and the World Health Organization (WHO), 5th edition (in blue).
In **bold**, those entities that introduce significant changes with respect to the WHO 4th edition, revised classification are highlighted.
In *italics*, the provisional entities from the International Consensus Classification.
The listing of diseases differs from that in the published ICC,[1] as it was minimally reorganized to allow comparison among the different classifications.
*Entities only present in the *International Consensus Classification*.
†"Pediatric-type follicular lymphoma with marginal zone differentiation" has been proposed as a more accurate name for the provisional entity "Pediatric nodal marginal zone lymphoma" as designated in the ICC classification, and slightly modified here to "Pediatric-type nodal marginal zone lymphoma."
‡This is listed among the large B-cell lymphomas in the WHO classification, 5th edition.
§The 5th edition of the WHO lymphoma classification adopts the nomenclature proposed at the "Workshop on Immunodeficiency and Dysregulation" organized by the Society of Hematopathology and the European Association for Haematopathology in 2015. In this classification, the nomenclature of lymphomas and lymphoid proliferations associated with immunodeficiency and dysregulation is constructed based on a 3-tier structure as follows:
1. Histologic diagnosis according to accepted criteria and terminology
2. Presence or absence of one or more oncogenic virus(es)
3. The clinical setting/immunodeficiency background.
ALK, Anaplastic lymphoma kinase; *DLBCL,* diffuse large B-cell lymphoma; *EBV,* Epstein-Barr virus; *HGBL,* high-grade B-cell lymphomas; *HHV-8,* human herpesvirus 8; *IgM,* immunoglobulin M; *KSHV,* Kaposi sarcoma-associated herpesvirus; *LPD,* lymphoproliferative disorder; *MALT,* mucosa-associated lymphoid tissue; *MGUS,* monoclonal gammopathy of undetermined significance; *MM,* multiple myeloma; *NK,* natural killer; *NOS,* not otherwise specified; *PTLD,* post-transplant lymphoproliferative disorders; *TFH,* T-follicular helper; *WHO,* World Health Organization.

in Table 12-2 and in the ICC publication.[1] To assist in understanding the evolution in terminology, the terms used in the revised 4th edition of the WHO classification are shown (center column) in comparison to the ICC on the left, and the proposed WHO 5th edition on the right. Terms in bold print indicate a change from the WHO 4th edition classification. New ICC entities proposed as provisional are shown in italics. Text shown in red (ICC) as opposed to blue (WHO 5th) indicate differences between the two classification systems. However, as this volume goes to print, the final version of the WHO 5th is uncertain. We have relied on the proposed classification as published by Alaggio et al.,[2] but terminology and definitions may differ in the final *Blue Book* publication.

Some of the key differences will be discussed.

Mature B-Cell Neoplasms

- Clinical participants at the CAC strongly preferred the term *multiple myeloma* (formerly known as plasma cell myeloma). The ICC also requires cytogenetic analysis for subclassification of multiple myeloma for clinical management, although the 2022 WHO proposal from Alaggio et al.[2] does not.
- Consistent with the criteria of the second International Workshop on Waldenström's macroglobulinemia,[77] the ICC now permits the diagnosis of LPL in the bone marrow, even with <10% involvement, as long as the biopsy

demonstrates neoplastic lymphoplasmacytic aggregates with evidence of clonal B cells and plasma cells.
- Two types of IgM MGUS are now recognized in the ICC but not in the 2022 WHO. One subtype of IgM MGUS has the *MYD88* L265 mutation and is considered a precursor to Waldenström macroglobulinemia.
- The 2022 ICC retains the categories of *B-cell prolymphocytic leukemia* and *hairy cell leukemia variant*. The 2022 WHO no longer recognizes the terms, but puts the latter and some of the former cases into a new category of *splenic B-cell lymphoma/leukemia with prominent nucleoli*.
- Both classifications now segregate what has been called *primary cutaneous marginal zone lymphoma* from other extranodal marginal zone lymphomas. In addition, the ICC names this lesion as *primary cutaneous marginal zone lymphoproliferative disorder (LPD)*, rather than *lymphoma* because of its very indolent behavior. As with other entities labeled as *LPD*, there is a desire to avoid labeling patients with a malignant lymphoma diagnosis when not warranted based on clinical outcome data.
- Though the ICC approach to FL remains relatively similar to that of the revised 4th edition, as strongly supported by the clinicians of the CAC, the 2022 WHO recognizes the FL family as including FL, in situ follicular B-cell neoplasm, pediatric-type FL (which is a separate distinct entity in the 2016 WHO and 2022 ICC with a very distinctive molecular

landscape), and duodenal-type FL. The WHO recognizes classic FL, which apparently must have an *IGH::BCL2* fusion and be in part follicular, but rejects the concept of grading within the category of *classic FL*. Alternatively, the WHO segregates follicular large B-cell lymphoma, which appears to correspond to grade 3B FL and includes a new category of *FL with uncommon features*. The latter includes cases that either have blastoid or large centrocyte cytologic features or a predominantly diffuse growth pattern. The ICC, on the other hand, retains the grading of FL as stipulated in the WHO revised 4th edition, but advises that ancillary studies (FISH for *BCL2R* and immunohistochemistry) be implemented to assist in the recognition of grade 3A versus 3B.

- The 2022 ICC includes a new provisional entity of *BCL2-rearrangement negative, CD23-positive follicle center lymphoma*, which has distinctive clinical and genetic findings and should be segregated from other FL. These cases often have a predominantly diffuse growth pattern, but purely follicular cases exist.
- The ICC also considers *testicular FL* a distinct entity rather than just a subtype of typical FL. Large B-cell lymphoma with *IRF4* rearrangement is now considered a definite entity in the ICC and thought to be among the group of pediatric lymphomas with a follicular growth pattern.
- The ICC proposes the term *nodular lymphocyte predominant B-cell lymphoma (NLPBCL)* to replace the prior term *nodular lymphocyte predominant Hodgkin lymphoma*. The conclusion reached at the CAC meeting was that NLPBCL is more properly included among the B-cell lymphomas based on its biological features, clinical behavior, and current therapeutic strategies, which differ from those used for classic Hodgkin lymphoma (CHL). While undoubtably there will be a learning curve for acceptance of the new terminology, clinicians at the CAC meeting opined that this change would help ensure appropriate therapy for this disease.
- The ICC now recognizes *primary DLBCL of the testis* as a distinct entity, which has features overlapping those of *primary DLBCL of the central nervous system* and some other extranodal DLBCL of ABC type with the MCD/C5 molecular/genomic features.[60] The 2022 WHO groups testicular, CNS, and vitreoretinal DLBCL together as *primary large B-cell lymphoma of immune-privileged sites* (a category that does not include other lymphomas that may also share similar molecular/cytogenetic features). This was a topic of extensive discussion at the CAC, but the creation of a new umbrella category—that would be larger than just CNS and testicular DLBCL—was felt to be premature.
- Though both the ICC and WHO revised the name for Burkitt-like lymphoma with 11q aberration because it is not related to Burkitt lymphoma, the ICC considers it a type of large B-cell lymphoma (*large B-cell lymphoma with 11q aberration*) and the WHO, a type of high-grade B-cell lymphoma.
- The ICC uniquely introduced the term *EBV-positive polymorphic B-cell lymphoproliferative disorder, not otherwise specified (NOS)*, described in Chapter 28. The term captures a spectrum of EBV-driven lesions that are distinct from post-transplant lymphoproliferative disorders (PTLD) but fall short of criteria for the diagnosis of EBV-positive DLBCL.
- The ICC segregated *high-grade B-cell lymphoma (HGBL) with MYC and BCL2 rearrangements* (with or without *BCL6* rearrangements) from a new provisional category of *HGBL with MYC and BCL6 rearrangements*. The 2022 WHO does not consider the latter a specific category, believing such cases should be included in DLBCL, NOS. The ICC also now recognizes that some HGBL may express terminal deoxynucleotidyl transferase (TdT) without necessitating the diagnosis of a B-lymphoblastic neoplasm.
- Both new classifications eliminated the unwieldy name of *B-cell lymphoma, unclassifiable with features intermediate between DLBCL and classic Hodgkin lymphoma*, but continue to recognize the category of *MGZL*. In the ICC, non-mediastinal cases with similar morphology are subsumed as variants of DLBCL, based on significant clinical and biological differences from MGZL.

Mature T- and NK-Cell Neoplasms

- Both classifications downgraded *primary cutaneous acral CD8-positive T-cell lymphoma* to a LPD (although the WHO overview dropped "T-cell" from the name).
- Both classifications now recognize *indolent T-cell and NK-cell LPDs of the GI tract* and both acknowledge greater concern for possible progression among the T-cell–derived cases. The ICC preferred the term *indolent clonal T-cell LPD of the gastrointestinal tract* over *indolent T-cell lymphoma of the gastrointestinal tract*, as an indication that these lesions should not be approached clinically as conventional T-cell lymphomas.
- The ICC added *type II refractory celiac disease* to the classification as a precursor lesion for enteropathy-associated T-cell lymphoma.
- Both classifications recognize a largely unified group of *follicular helper T-cell lymphomas*, with three subtypes specified as (1) angioimmunoblastic, (2) follicular, and (3) NOS.

Immunodeficiency Disorders

- The ICC approach to the *immunodeficiency-associated LPDs* is similar to that of the 2016 WHO. The category of *post-transplant LPDs (PTLDs)* is retained, with the suggestion to classify non–post-transplant iatrogenic immunodeficiency-associated LPDs using similar principles. The ICC places major emphasis on the underlying disorder leading to immune deficiency because this has a major effect on clinical management and on the pathobiology of the subsequent B-cell or T-cell proliferation. In contrast, the 2022 WHO has eliminated the category of *PTLD* from its classification, refocusing the cause of the immune deficiency to a secondary factor. The WHO proposal combines all *lymphoid proliferations and lymphomas associated with immune deficiency and dysregulation* under a common heading, which is then further subdivided into (1) hyperplasias, (2) polymorphic LPDs, (3) lymphomas arising in immune deficiency/dysregulation, and (4) those occurring in the setting of inborn errors of immunity.

This approach had been rejected by the 2021 CAC and ICC because of the clinical importance of a PTLD diagnosis, the extensive PTLD literature that does not necessarily pertain to the other immune deficiency–associated LPDs, difficulties sometimes with the subjective assessment of histologic type of PTLD, the major differences between many of the iatrogenic-associated LPDs and HIV-associated lymphomas, and the fact that some PTLDs are of T-cell type. These issues are more fully discussed in Chapters 28, 53, and 54.

CONCLUSION

The ICC classification is a continuation of the successful international collaboration among pathologists, biologists, and clinicians interested in the hematologic malignancies.[1] The 2001 WHO classification was rapidly adopted for clinical trials and successfully served as a common language for scientists comparing genetic and functional data. The explosion of data derived from high-throughput genomic studies conducted over the past few years addressed many ambiguities in the classification, although advances will continue to occur. The chapters that follow embrace these new data and provide guidelines for accurate diagnosis and patient management.

Pearls and Pitfalls

- The accurate diagnosis of lymphoid neoplasms requires integration of morphologic immunophenotypic, genetic, and clinical features.
- Obtaining an adequate clinical history is a key part of the diagnostic process. If you do not get an adequate clinical history, ask for it.
- Properly fixed and sectioned material is essential for accurate histologic interpretation.
- Making the primary diagnosis of lymphoma on a core biopsy specimen may be hazardous. If the biopsy specimen is insufficient, defer your final diagnosis.
- Order sufficient immunohistochemical stains to address the differential diagnosis, but do not order a huge panel of stains irrelevant to the diagnostic question.
- The judicious use of cytogenetic and genetic sequencing studies may be key to the recognition of some disease entities.

KEY REFERENCES

1. Campo E, Jaffe ES, Cook JR, et al. The International Consensus Classification of mature lymphoid neoplasms: a report from the clinical advisory committee. *Blood*. 2022;140(11):1229–1253.
2. Alaggio R, Amador C, Anagnostopoulos I, et al. The 5th edition of the *World Health Organization Classification of Haematolymphoid Tumours:* lymphoid neoplasms. *Leukemia*. 2022;36(7):1720–1748.
3. Harris NL, Jaffe ES, Diebold J, et al. World Health Organization classification of neoplastic diseases of the hematopoietic and lymphoid tissues: report of the Clinical Advisory Committee meeting—Airlie House, Virginia, November 1997. *J Clin Oncol*. 1999;17(12):3835–3849.
6. Jaffe ES, Harris NL, Stein H, Vardiman JW, eds. *Pathology and Genetics of Tumours of Haematopoietic and Lymphoid Tissues*. Lyon: IARC Press; 2001.
8. Swerdlow SH, Campo E, Harris NL, et al., eds. *WHO Classification of Tumours of Haematopoietic and Lymphoid Tissues*. Revised 4th ed. Lyon: IARC; 2017.
9. Harris NL, Jaffe ES, Stein H, et al. A revised European-American classification of lymphoid neoplasms: a proposal from the International Lymphoma Study Group. *Blood*. 1994;84:1361–1392.
11. Stansfeld A, Diebold J, Kapanci Y, et al. Updated Kiel classification for lymphomas. *Lancet*. 1988;1:292–293.
13. Lukes R, Collins R. Immunologic characterization of human malignant lymphomas. *Cancer*. 1974;34:1488–1503.
63. Morin RD, Arthur SE, Hodson DJ. Molecular profiling in diffuse large B-cell lymphoma: why so many types of subtypes? *Br J Haematol*. 2022;196(4):814–829.
76. Arber DA, Campo E, Jaffe ES. Advances in the classification of myeloid and lymphoid neoplasias. *Virchows Arch*. 2023;482(1):1–9.

Visit Elsevier eBooks+ for the complete set of references.

Chapter 13

Chronic Lymphocytic Leukemia/Small Lymphocytic Lymphoma, Monoclonal B-Cell Lymphocytosis, and B-Cell Prolymphocytic Leukemia

Devon Chabot-Richards, Qian-Yun Zhang, and Kathryn Foucar

CHRONIC LYMPHOCYTIC LEUKEMIA/SMALL LYMPHOCYTIC LYMPHOMA

Synonyms

- Chronic lymphocytic leukemia/Small lymphocytic lymphoma (International Consensus Classification [ICC])[1,2]
- Chronic lymphocytic leukemia/Small lymphocytic lymphoma (proposed World Health Organization [WHO] 5th edition)[3,4]

Definition of Disease

B-cell chronic lymphocytic leukemia (B-CLL) is a clonal disorder of mature B lymphocytes with specific immunophenotypic features. Updates to the diagnosis, classification, and workup of lymphoid neoplasms, including chronic lymphocytic leukemia (CLL), have been made.[1,2,3,5] CLL is heterogenous and encompasses a diverse spectrum of morphologic, immunophenotypic, and genetic variants (see Table 13-1).[1,6-9]

The CLL leukemia cells are characterized by small, round nuclei; highly condensed chromatin; inconspicuous nucleoli; scant cytoplasm; and unique immunophenotype (IP). Admixed are occasional large prolymphocytes with prominent nucleoli, which usually account for less than 10% of leukemic cells.[1,2,7]

Peripheral blood and bone marrow are typically involved in CLL. Lymph node is, by definition, the primary site of involvement in small lymphocytic lymphoma (SLL). Liver and spleen are also often involved; involvement of other extranodal sites occurs less frequently.[2,10]

Diagnostic criteria for CLL per ICC and proposed WHO guidelines include that, in the absence of extramedullary tissue involvement, there must be a sustained, persistent monoclonal lymphocytosis of $\geq 5.0 \times 10^9$/L with a CLL IP in the peripheral blood (PB).[1,3] Although bone marrow lymphocytosis is also present, bone marrow examination is often not required for a diagnosis of CLL.[7] Exceptions include patients with unexplained cytopenias in whom bone marrow evaluation is indicated.[11] Many CLL cases can be successfully diagnosed by morphologic review of blood smears with immunophenotypic

Table 13-1 Primary Entities and Variants/Subtypes

Entity	Variants/Subtypes
CLL/SLL[†]	Atypical CLL (morphology) Atypical CLL (immunophenotype) Accelerated CLL CLL with Hodgkin (Reed-Sternberg) cells Transformations of CLL/SLL
Monoclonal B-cell lymphocytosis	Low count and high count
B-prolymphocytic leukemia	*MYC* or *TP53* mutation(s) subtypes Not recognized as such in proposed WHO 5th edition

[†]Borderline with monoclonal B lymphocytosis in blood, bone marrow, and lymph node important to appreciate.
CLL/SLL, Chronic lymphocytic leukemia/small lymphocytic lymphoma.
Data from Sander B, Campo E, Hsi ED. Chronic lymphocytic leukaemia/small lymphocytic lymphoma and mantle cell lymphoma: from early lesions to transformation. *Virchows Arch.* 2023 Jan;482(1):131-145. *Erratum in: Virchows Arch.* 2023 Jan 12; Agbay RL, Jain N, Loghavi S, et al. Histologic transformation of chronic lymphocytic leukemia/small lymphocytic lymphoma. *Am J Hematol.* 2016 Oct;91(10):1036-1043; Giné E, Martinez A, Villamor N, et al. Expanded and highly active proliferation centers identify a histological subtype of chronic lymphocytic leukemia ("accelerated" chronic lymphocytic leukemia) with aggressive clinical behavior. *Haematologica.* 2010 Sep;95(9):1526-1533; Sorigue M, Junca J. Atypical chronic lymphocytic leukemia: Brief historical overview and current usage of an equivocal concept. *Int J Lab Hematol.* 2019 Feb;41(1):e17-e19; Xiao W, Chen WW, Sorbara L, et al. Hodgkin lymphoma variant of Richter transformation: morphology, Epstein-Barr virus status, clonality, and survival analysis—with comparison to Hodgkin-like lesion. *Hum Pathol.* 2016 Sep;55:108-116; Autore F, Strati P, Laurenti L, et al. Morphological, immunophenotypic, and genetic features of chronic lymphocytic leukemia with trisomy 12: a comprehensive review. *Haematologica.* 2018 Jun;103(6):931-938.

confirmation.[7,10] Prognostic workup is also typically done on the PB.

The term *SLL* is used for non-leukemic cases (i.e., below 5.0×10^9/L threshold) with the tissue morphology and IP of CLL.[1,2] The distinction between CLL versus SLL is based primarily on disease distribution and the number of circulating leukemia cells. Disorders with a predominant extramedullary disease distribution and $<5.0 \times 10^9$/L circulating leukemia cells in blood are termed *SLL* (see Box 13-1).[2] Within the lymph node, larger cells (so-called "prolymphocytes/paraimmunoblasts") often form pale foci called *proliferation centers* in a background of monotonous small lymphocytes.

CLL and SLL have been generally regarded as the same disease with different manifestations, although differences in chemokine and integrin expression, as well as genetic differences, may explain why some cases are primarily "leukemia" and others "lymphomatous."[12]

Richter transformation (RT) is defined as transformation of CLL into a more aggressive lymphoma. It occurs in 2% to 10% of CLL/SLL patients. The vast majority of transformations are to diffuse large B-cell lymphoma (RT-DLBCL), although transformation to Hodgkin lymphoma (RT-HL) sometimes occurs.[2,13,14] Rarely, transformation to other types of lymphomas may occur.[14-21]

Epidemiology and Incidence

CLL is the most common leukemia of adults in Western countries. Because of prolonged survival rates, the prevalence of CLL is steadily increasing.[22] CLL is also the most common familial leukemia.[1,22-24] The incidence of CLL rises dramatically with age, and the incidence reaches 50 per 100,000 in men older than 80. CLL is more common in men than in women, with a male-to-female ratio of 1.9:1.[25] It is most commonly

Box 13-1 *Major Diagnostic Criteria of Chronic Lymphocytic Leukemia/Small Lymphocytic Lymphoma*

CLL
- Sustained absolute mature, monoclonal lymphocytosis $\geq 5 \times 10^9$/L
- Monoclonal B cell with mature phenotype, CD5 and CD23 co-expression, weak CD20, weak CD22, weak SIg (IgM/IgD)

SLL
- Extramedullary sites of disease predominate, especially lymph node
- Diffuse infiltrate of small lymphocytes, proliferation centers
- Monoclonal B cells $<5.0 \times 10^9$/L in blood
- Monoclonal B cell with mature phenotype, CD5 and CD23 co-expression, weak CD20, weak CD22, weak SIg (IgM/IgD)

CLL, Chronic lymphocytic leukemia; *IgD,* immunoglobulin D; *IgM,* immunoglobulin M; *SLL,* small lymphocytic lymphoma.
Data from Sander B, Campo E, Hsi ED. Chronic lymphocytic leukaemia/small lymphocytic lymphoma and mantle cell lymphoma: from early lesions to transformation. *Virchows Arch.* 2023 Jan;482(1):131-145. *Erratum in: Virchows Arch.* 2023 Jan 12.

diagnosed in the 70-to-79 years age group, with a median age at diagnosis of 73 years.[7,23,25,26] A study on CLL in patients younger than 55 years reveals slightly different biology and clinical course than CLL in older patients.[27] Younger patients are more likely to have Rai stage I or II disease, with immunoglobulin heavy chain variable region genes (IGHV) unmutated, and ZAP70 expression. The time to treatment is shorter compared with older patients. Although survival of CLL patients younger than 55 years is longer than older CLL patients, their survival is profoundly shortened compared with the age-matched and sex-matched normal population.[27] CLL has also been reported in adolescents and young adults (AYA).[28] In one large series of AYA patients, disease course and outcome generally correlated with similar prognostic markers as seen in older patients. Factors linked to overall survival (OS) included advanced stage, elevated beta2-microglobulin level, unmutated IGHV, del(11q) and del(17p).[28] CLL is very rare in the Asian population, although data have shown an increase in incidence, suggesting an environmental role.[29]

Environmental, medical, and occupational risk factors for CLL have been extensively studied with inconclusive results. Studies linking CLL with radiation exposure have had inconsistent findings as well. Most studies on populations exposed to environmental, medical, or occupational sources of ionizing radiation have not found evidence of a connection.[30-32] Chemical exposures do appear to be associated with increased risk for developing CLL, particularly in farmers and other agricultural workers, rubber workers, and petroleum workers.[33]

Genetic factors play a role in the pathogenesis of CLL. Family history of CLL or other related diseases—such as monoclonal B-lymphocytosis (MBL) and non-Hodgkin lymphoma, especially low-grade B-cell lymphoma—is one of the strongest risk factors for the development of CLL.[7,24] In epidemiologic case-control and cohort studies, the relative risk for CLL in first-degree relatives of CLL patients is increased 6-fold to 12-fold.[34] The risk for developing other lymphoproliferative neoplasms (LPNs) and MBL is also increased.[35,36] Familial CLL patients present about 10 years earlier than those with sporadic CLL and may have a more aggressive clonal expansion.[24]

Clinical Features

CLL typically occurs in older adult patients who usually have an indolent clinical course. Up to 80% of patients are asymptomatic at presentation, and the disease is discovered incidentally by routine complete blood count (CBC) and blood smear review.[1,37] Other patients may present with various signs and symptoms, including peripheral lymphadenopathy, hepatosplenomegaly, autoimmune cytopenia, systemic symptoms (weight loss, fever, night sweats), or cytopenia-related symptoms (weakness, fatigue, or bleeding). Low-level monoclonal paraprotein may present in up to 50% of CLL patients.[38]

Cytopenia is often related to leukemic infiltrate of the bone marrow, leading to compromised hematopoiesis. Cytopenia can also be secondary to autoimmune phenomenon, hypersplenism, treatment, or non–CLL-related etiology. Autoimmune complications are seen in 4% to 25% of CLL/SLL patients and include autoimmune hemolytic anemia (AIHA), immune thrombocytopenic purpura (ITP), pure red cell aplasia, and autoimmune agranulocytosis.[39-41] AIHA is reported in 2% to 25% of CLL patients, whereas ITP is seen in approximately 2% of CLL patients.

CLL is associated with a profoundly impaired immune system resulting in recurrent infections or failure of antitumor immune response. CLL patients have a decreased number and function of B cells, resulting in defective humoral immunity. These patients also have defective cell-mediated immunity with decreased T-cell subsets and natural killer (NK) cells. Abnormalities in complement activity, in monocytes, and in neutrophils are also common. CLL patients may also have an increased number of regulatory T cells and nurselike cells.[42,43] Hypogammaglobulinemia is common in CLL and is a contributing factor to recurrent infections. Its severity increases with duration and stage of the disease.[40] Although there is still limited understanding of the initiating events of immunodeficiency in CLL, reports indicate that progressive loss of plasmacytoid dendritic cell (pDC) function underlies the major immunodeficiency affecting CLL patients.[44] pDCs are highly specialized immune cells that play a major role in promoting innate and adaptive immune responses. Decreased pDC function results in decreased interferon alpha (IFNα) production, and the latter is a cytokine that is critical in immunity and has well-described antitumor activity.[44]

Morphology

Lymph Node

SLL accounts for about 5% to 10% of CLL/SLL overall.[10] Genetic abnormalities [a high incidence of trisomy 12 and lower incidence of del 13(q)] are more common in lymph node in CLL patients than in bone marrow. These differences may underlie the different clinical presentations.[12]

Lymph node involvement in CLL/SLL is generally characterized by diffuse effacement of the architecture with variably preserved sinuses.[1,2,10] The infiltrate consists of small, round lymphocytes with condensed chromatin and scanty amounts of cytoplasm, imparting a dark color on low magnification. Mitotic activity is virtually absent in these areas. Interspersed among these diffuse sheets of small, round lymphocytes are proliferation centers that produce a vague, pale, nodular pattern (Fig. 13-1A).[2,10] On high magnification,

proliferation centers are composed of larger lymphoid cells (so-called "prolymphocytes" and "paraimmunoblasts") with more abundant cytoplasm and more conspicuous nucleoli (Fig. 13-1B–C). By assessment of DNA synthesis such as Ki67 staining, these proliferation centers represent the mitotically active portion of the neoplastic clone. It is important to recognize that proliferation centers may be cyclin D1 positive in ~20% of cases.[45] Although lacking *CCND1* translocations, this cyclin D1 expression may mislead the diagnostician into considering a diagnosis of mantle cell lymphoma (MCL). Enhanced MYC expression protein has also been documented in proliferation centers in CLL/SLL lymph nodes, also not associated with rearrangement or gain of function of the *MYC* gene.[46]

Occasionally, proliferation centers may be very large and confluent, raising concern for transformation to large cell lymphoma (Fig. 13-2).[10,47] In these lymph node sections, proliferation centers are expanded and contain larger lymphoid cells with increased mitotic activity (Fig. 13-2C).[47] Low magnification assessment is essential to detect the vague macronodular appearance of these expanded proliferation centers to avoid an incorrect diagnosis of overt diffuse large cell lymphoma, RT, in these cases. Although expanded accelerated proliferative centers are linked to a more aggressive disease course and a higher rate of overt large cell lymphoma transformation, distinction from overt large cell lymphoma is still important. Studies report that artificial intelligence–assisted mapping of proliferation centers can aid in the distinction of this process from overt diffuse large cell lymphoma.[48]

In a minority of CLL/SLL cases, the pattern of lymph node infiltration is interfollicular or exhibits a perifollicular/marginal zone-type pattern, resulting in potential differential diagnostic confusion with MCL, marginal zone lymphoma (MZL), or other B-cell neoplasms.[49] Likewise, some cases exhibit greater nuclear irregularity of the small lymphocytes, reminiscent of MCL or even follicular lymphoma (FL).[10] However, the presence of proliferation centers, the distinctive immunophenotypic profile including LEF1 expression, and the absence of cyclin D1 and SOX11 expression support a diagnosis of CLL/SLL, as long as cyclin D1 expression in proliferation centers is taken into account (see the section on differential diagnosis).[2,10,45,50,51] In some lymph node biopsy specimens assessed by upfront flow cytometric immunophenotyping (FCI), a small CLL/SLL-type clone will be detected that is not apparent on morphologic review. Inconspicuous, small lymph node infiltrates of CLL/SLL cells that are found in lymph nodes that are not enlarged, do not form proliferation centers, and do not efface architecture, are regarded as nodal monoclonal B lymphocytosis.[1,2] However, in patients with multiple sites of nodal enlargement, there is the possibility that overt CLL is present in other sites.

Spleen

Although the degree of splenomegaly is highly variable in CLL patients, some patients exhibit significant and symptomatic splenic involvement. Splenic involvement by SLL/CLL is characterized by white pulp expansion producing a miliary micronodular appearance grossly (Fig. 13-3).[52] The white pulp infiltrates consist of small, round lymphocytes with scant cytoplasm similar to those seen in lymph node (Fig. 13-4). Although occasional prolymphocytes and paraimmunoblasts

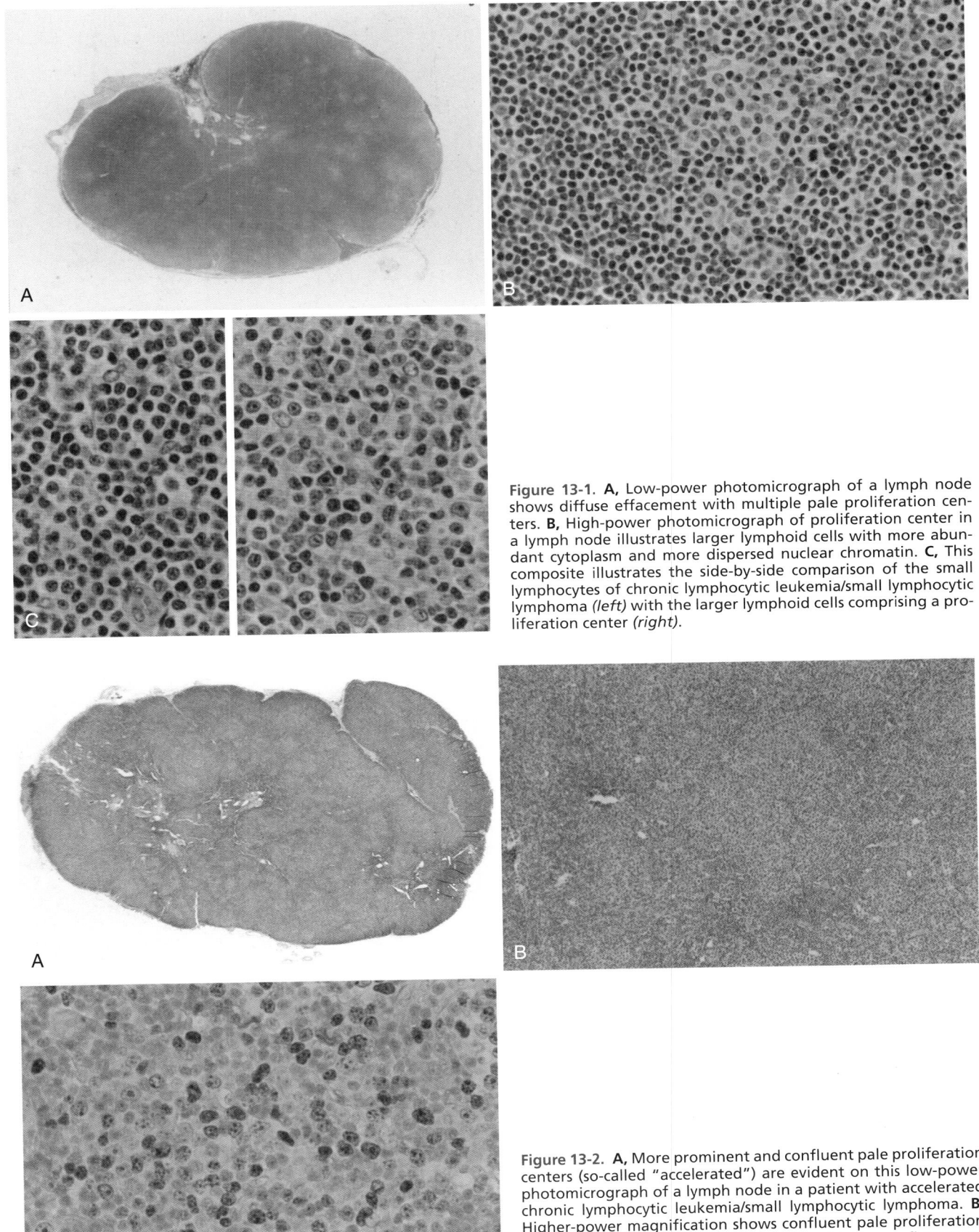

Figure 13-1. A, Low-power photomicrograph of a lymph node shows diffuse effacement with multiple pale proliferation centers. **B,** High-power photomicrograph of proliferation center in a lymph node illustrates larger lymphoid cells with more abundant cytoplasm and more dispersed nuclear chromatin. **C,** This composite illustrates the side-by-side comparison of the small lymphocytes of chronic lymphocytic leukemia/small lymphocytic lymphoma *(left)* with the larger lymphoid cells comprising a proliferation center *(right).*

Figure 13-2. A, More prominent and confluent pale proliferation centers (so-called "accelerated") are evident on this low-power photomicrograph of a lymph node in a patient with accelerated chronic lymphocytic leukemia/small lymphocytic lymphoma. **B,** Higher-power magnification shows confluent pale proliferation centers. **C,** Ki67 positivity is fairly prominent in the confluent proliferation centers in this case (H&E and Ki67 stains by immunoperoxidase).

may be present, typical proliferation centers generally are not readily apparent. Extension of the lymphoid infiltrate into the periarteriolar lymphoid sheath, along the splenic trabeculae, and into both the red pulp cords and sinuses is common.[52]

Blood

A mature lymphocytosis is a diagnostic requirement for CLL, with at least 5.0×10^9/L as a minimum absolute monoclonal lymphocyte count with CLL IP (see Box 13-1).[1,2] These lymphocytes are typically monotonous with relatively homogeneous features, including small, round nuclei with highly condensed nuclear chromatin and inconspicuous nucleoli (Fig. 13-5). The exaggerated chromatin clumping may give a "cracked mud/soccer ball" appearance to these nuclei. These leukemic lymphocytes are easily disrupted during smear preparation, creating smudge cells, which may be numerous (Fig. 13-6). Larger lymphoid cells or lymphocytes with irregular nuclear contours may be evident, but these cells usually comprise less than 2% of the leukemic population (Fig. 13-7). In cases in which these "atypical" forms are conspicuous, a diagnosis of atypical/mixed CLL or CLL/prolymphocytic may be preferred to convey to the clinician these aberrant morphologic features (see the section on morphologic variants).[53] In general, the agranular cytoplasm is scant, but some CLL cases will demonstrate moderate

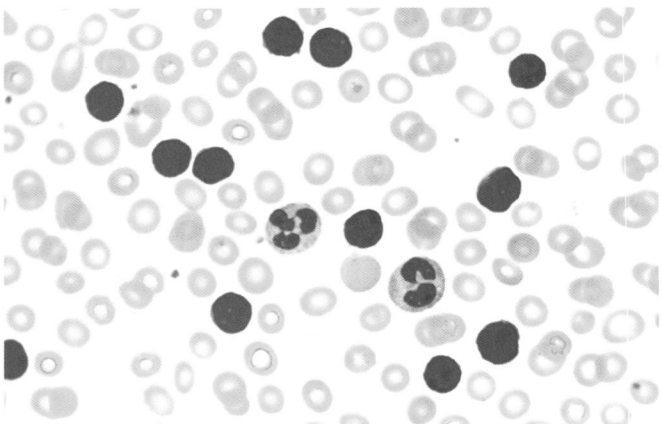

Figure 13-5. A marked mature lymphocytosis characterized by round nuclei with highly condensed chromatin and scant cytoplasm is evident in blood from a patient with chronic lymphocytic leukemia (Wright's stain).

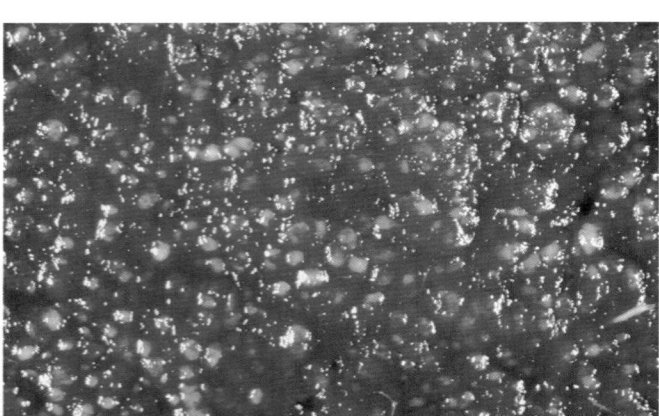

Figure 13-3. Photograph of a spleen in a patient with chronic lymphocytic leukemia/small lymphocytic lymphoma shows a miliary white-pulp pattern of infiltration (Gross).

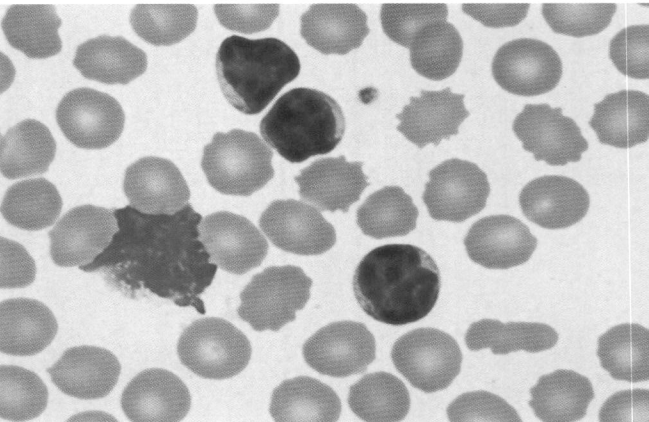

Figure 13-6. Broken chronic lymphocytic leukemia (CLL) cells (so-called "smudge cells") are evident on this peripheral blood smear from a patient with CLL. Smudge cells consist largely of nuclear material (Wright's stain).

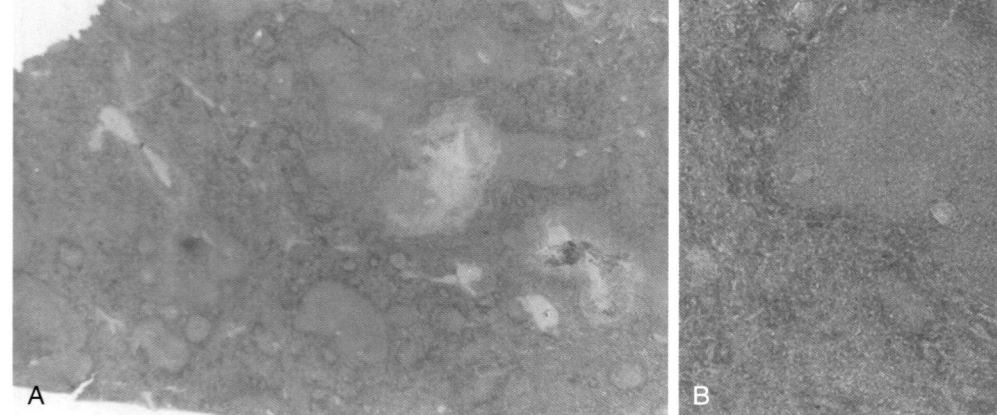
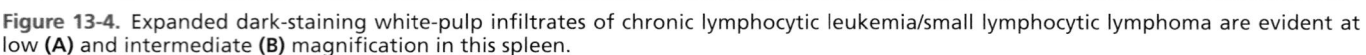

Figure 13-4. Expanded dark-staining white-pulp infiltrates of chronic lymphocytic leukemia/small lymphocytic lymphoma are evident at low **(A)** and intermediate **(B)** magnification in this spleen.

amounts of cytoplasm. Distinctive cytoplasmic vacuoles, crystals, or globules are noted occasionally.[54]

The number of prolymphocytes, clonal cells with a larger nuclear size and a single, distinct nucleolus, should be assessed (see Fig. 13-7). In some patients, an increasing proportion of prolymphocytes may be a harbinger of clonal transformation, whereas other stable CLL cases demonstrate consistently high numbers of prolymphocytes.[55,56] Any significant change in the blood picture should prompt reevaluation of the patient's disease status.

Bone Marrow

Although not usually necessary for diagnosis, bone marrow examination in CLL patients may be useful in assessing residual hematopoiesis and in determining the pattern and extent of bone marrow effacement. On aspirate smears, CLL cells exhibit similar cytologic features to circulating clonal cells (see Box 13-2).[56] These small, mature lymphocytes are generally abundant on aspirate smears, although variability is expected because of the multifocal nature of neoplastic infiltration of the bone marrow. The extent of bone marrow replacement by CLL generally parallels the proportion of lymphocytes on differential cell counts, although the extent of disease is best assessed on core biopsy specimens. In most cases, there is substantial residual preserved hematopoiesis, reflecting the typical blood finding of normal red blood cell, neutrophil, and platelet counts.

On core biopsy sections, the pattern of bone marrow infiltration may be useful for both distinction of CLL from other differential diagnostic considerations and in possibly providing prognostic information.[56-58] In CLL, the bone marrow core biopsy may exhibit a range of infiltration patterns including focal, non-paratrabecular nodules; an interstitial infiltrate in which CLL cells are admixed with hematopoietic elements; and effacing diffuse solid lesions (Figs. 13-8 and 13-9). Multiple patterns may be evident in a single core biopsy specimen. The typical nodular infiltrates of CLL are readily apparent on low magnification because their dark appearance is quite distinct from paler normal hematopoietic cells. This dark appearance is caused by closely packed nuclei with scant cytoplasm that typifies this disorder (see Box 13-2). On high magnification, the densely packed nuclei exhibit round contours and minimal, if any, mitotic activity. The borders of these non-paratrabecular nodules may show infiltrative margins with diffusion of lymphocytes into adjacent hematopoietic tissues. Likewise, diffuse interstitial infiltrates of CLL may be evident throughout the bone marrow widely separated from discrete nodular lesions. In these interstitial areas, adipose cells and hematopoietic elements are at least partially preserved; note that the CLL infiltrates impart a darker appearance on low magnification than uninvolved bone marrow (see Fig. 13-8). The most extensively effaced bone marrow core biopsy sections are characterized by solid areas of complete replacement of both hematopoietic and fat cells by CLL filling the entire hematopoietic cavity between bone trabeculae. The presence of extensive diffuse, solid infiltrates would predict for cytopenia(s) and, consequently, higher clinical stage. Similarly, a diffuse pattern of bone marrow infiltration has also been linked to ZAP70 expression.[58] The extent of bone marrow effacement in CLL is best estimated from technically optimal core biopsy specimens of at least

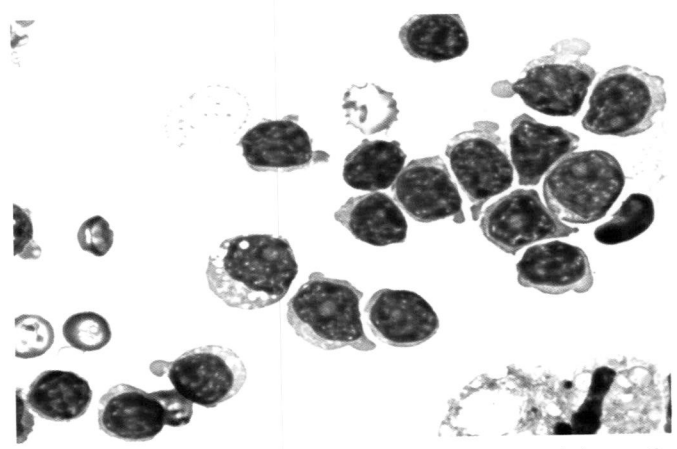

Figure 13-7. Larger lymphoid cells with more dispersed chromatin and distinct nucleoli (so-called "prolymphocytes") are evident on this cytospin in blood from a patient with chronic lymphocytic leukemia (Wright's stain).

Box 13-2 *Bone Marrow in Chronic Lymphocytic Leukemia*

Morphology
- Small lymphoid cells with round nuclear contours, condensed chromatin, and inconspicuous nucleoli analogous to appearance in blood
- Extent of bone marrow involvement variable; ≥30% lymphocytes is considered characteristic

Core Biopsy
- Non-paratrabecular lymphoid nodules with closely packed round nuclei, scant cytoplasm, and minimal mitotic activity
- No predilection for paratrabecular localization
- May also see a diffuse increase in interstitial lymphocytes admixed with hematopoietic elements
- Diffuse solid bone marrow effacement relatively uncommon
- Proliferation centers may be present, but true germinal centers only rarely described

Data from: Sander B, Campo E, Hsi ED. Chronic lymphocytic leukaemia/small lymphocytic lymphoma and mantle cell lymphoma: from early lesions to transformation. *Virchows Arch.* 2023 Jan;482(1):131-145. *Erratum in: Virchows Arch.* 2023 Jan 12; Foucar K. Mature B- and T-cell lymphoproliferative neoplasms. In: Foucar K, Reichard R, Czuchlewski D. *Bone Marrow Pathology,* 4th ed. ASCP Press.

---

10 mm in length that do not consist of significant portions of hypocellular subcortical regions.

Although proliferation centers are a readily apparent, typical feature of nodal infiltrates of CLL/SLL, proliferation centers in bone marrow core biopsy/clot sections in CLL patients are not as distinct of a finding, possibly because of issues of specimen size and quality (Fig. 13-10). In one study, proliferation centers were evident on scanning in 75% of cases; no correlation was found between BM proliferation centers and any CLL parameters including flow cytometric IP and genetic features in this study.[59] Only very rarely are true germinal centers evident in bone marrow specimens from CLL patients; the presence of these germinal centers should prompt systematic exclusion of other B-chronic lymphoproliferative neoplasms (B-CLPNs).[60] In rare CLL patients, foci of large cell lymphoma transformation will be first appreciated in

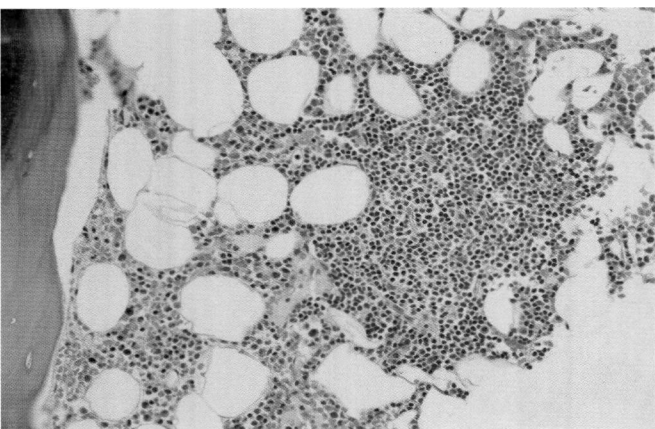

Figure 13-8. Bone marrow core biopsy section from a patient with chronic lymphocytic leukemia (CLL) illustrates a focal, non-paratrabecular infiltrate of leukemia. Note the dark blue color of this infiltrate caused by the back-to-back nuclei that typify CLL infiltrates.

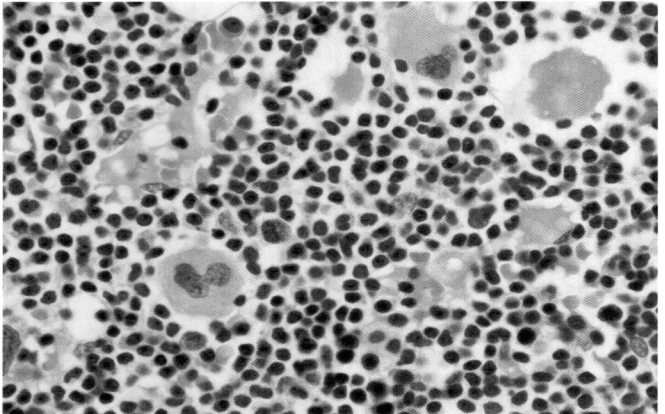

Figure 13-9. Bone marrow biopsy section from a patient with chronic lymphocytic leukemia illustrates the diffuse, interstitial infiltration that can occur in some patients. Note abundant preserved megakaryocytes.

bone marrow specimens. Because of the large overall cell size and the presence of moderate amounts of cytoplasm, these large cell lymphoma infiltrates are quite distinct, even on low magnification in which they are a pale pinkish color (see the section on transformation).

Other Organs

Infiltrates of CLL in a variety of extramedullary/extranodal sites have been well described in autopsy reports and individual site-specific studies (Figs. 13-11 and 13-12).[61] Leukemic infiltrates as a cause of disease manifestations have more recently focused on cases of CLL in the skin and central nervous system (CNS). Unique features of leukemia cutis include prevalence in cartilage-rich sites (ear, nostrils), likely association with prior cutaneous infections, and genetic features including trisomy 12, t(14;18) (*IGH::BCL2*), and *NOTCH1* mutations.[62] Cutaneous CLL usually manifests at disease presentation in otherwise low-stage CLL. Most cases showed dermal infiltrates of small lymphocytes with CLL IP; rare cases of cutaneous large cell lymphoma have also been reported in CLL patients.

Similarly, both CLL and RT (also called transformation) have been reported in the CNS.[63,64] CNS involvement by CLL is rare, about 4% of CLL cases, and is usually diagnosed by flow cytometry of CSF or by imaging studies with biopsy. The outcome of CLL patients with CNS involvement is better for previously untreated CLL patients and generally parallels the molecular genetic characteristics of the CLL (Fig. 13-12).[64]

Morphologic Variants

Atypical/Mixed Chronic Lymphocytic Leukemia

Any discussion of so-called "atypical CLL" (aCLL) must begin by pointing out that the term *aCLL* has been applied to cases based on either morphology or immunophenotyping (see Box 13-3). In addition, the definition of aCLL based on either morphology or immunophenotyping is neither standardized nor applied consistently.[53] Nonetheless, diagnosticians are very familiar with cases of likely CLL in which the morphology shows larger cells, prolymphocytes, or cells with nuclear irregularity, or the flow cytometry shows bright monotypic

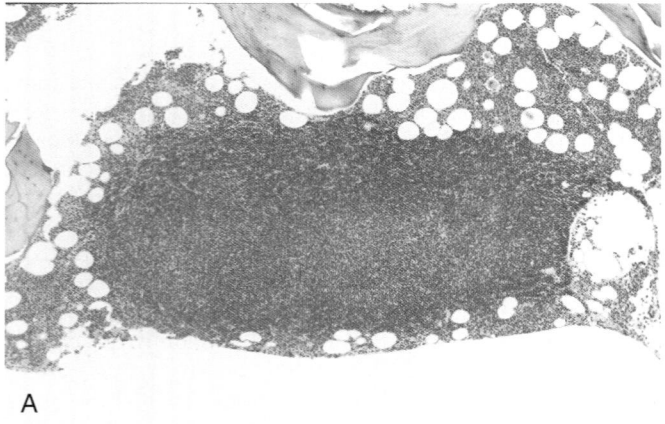
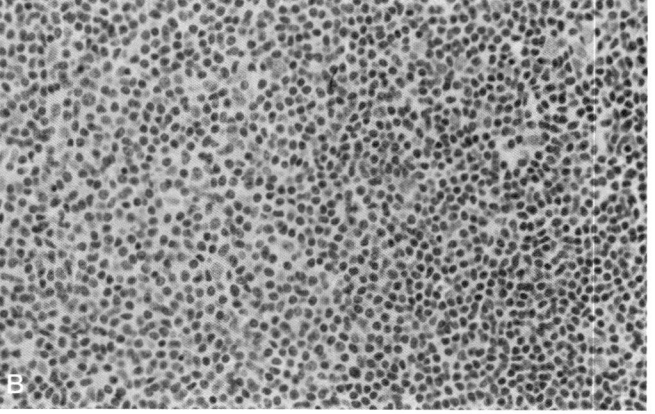

Figure 13-10. A, Low-power photomicrograph of a bone marrow core biopsy from a patient with chronic lymphocytic leukemia (CLL) illustrates a large focal infiltrate with a pale central proliferation center, a less common finding in bone marrow specimens than in lymph nodes. **B,** High-power photomicrograph shows the larger prolymphocyte-like cells *(left)* making up the proliferation center compared with the small, dark typical CLL cells *(right)* with scanty cytoplasm and highly condensed chromatin.

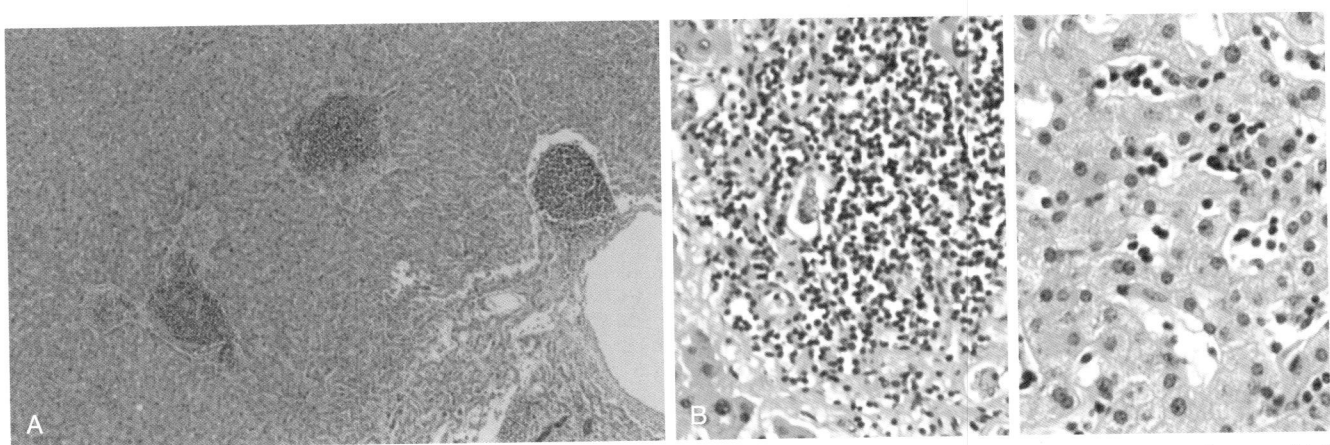

Figure 13-11. A, Low-power photomicrograph of liver from a patient with chronic lymphocytic leukemia (CLL) shows distinctive portal infiltrates. **B,** Composite of liver sections illustrates both portal and sinusoidal infiltrates in a patient with CLL/small lymphocytic lymphoma (SLL).

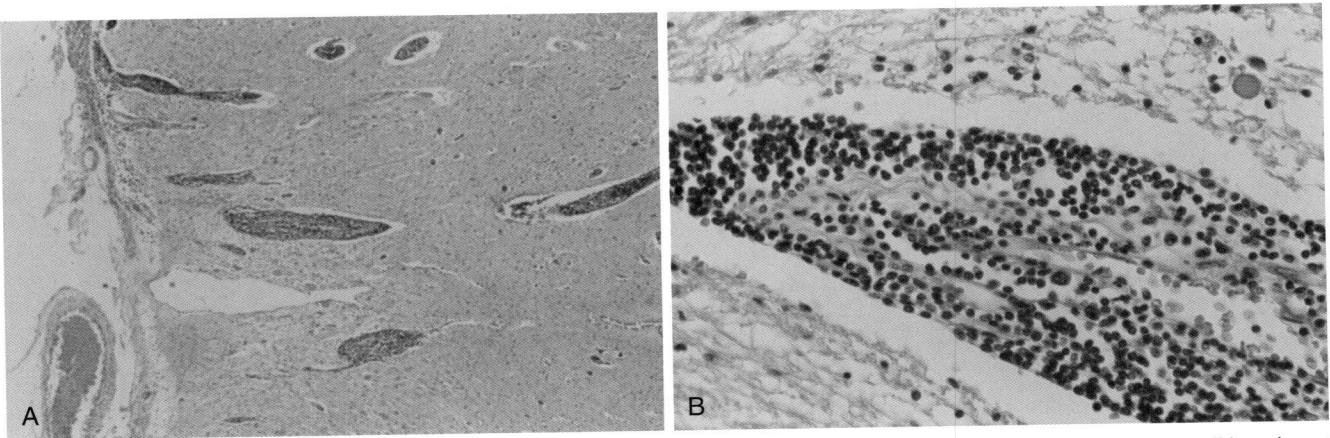

Figure 13-12. A, Low-power photomicrograph of brain from an autopsy on a patient with chronic lymphocytic leukemia/small lymphocytic lymphoma (CLL/SLL) shows prominent infiltration of dark lymphoid cells in Virchow-Robin spaces. **B,** On high power, the lymphoid infiltrate consists of small, round, mature lymphocytes with scanty cytoplasm typical of CLL/SLL.

light chain expression or other aberrancies from the classic CLL flow profile (Figs. 13-13 and 13-14).[53,55] Morphologic or immunophenotypic aberrancies should prompt consideration of other differential diagnoses, as well as prompting a thorough molecular genetic assessment to possibly delineate a genetic finding, such as trisomy 12 and $TP53^m$, that are both linked to aCLL (either morphologic or immunophenotypic).[55,65-67] The diagnostician rendering a diagnosis of "atypical" should explain the justification for this label and indicate additional studies that could identify a genetic cause for the atypical diagnosis.

Accelerated Chronic Lymphocytic Leukemia/Small Lymphocytic Lymphoma

As discussed, some cases of CLL/SLL show confluent and expanded proliferation centers with increased prolymphocytes and paraimmunoblasts or increased mitotic activity >40%[2,4,47] (see Fig. 13-2 and Box 13-3). These cases are designated as accelerated CLL/SLL.[2] Although distinction from overt RT is important, the outcome for cases with this "accelerated" morphology is more adverse than prototypic CLL/SLL.[2,4,47]

CLL/SLL With Hodgkin (Reed-Sternberg) Cells

Hodgkin (Reed-Sternberg)–like cells can be encountered in CLL/SLL in two general patterns. One group manifests the

clinical and hematologic features of straightforward stable CLL/SLL and the Hodgkin (Reed-Sternberg) cells are encountered as an incidental finding admixed with the sheets of small round lymphocytes that typify CLL/SLL (see Box 13-3 and Fig. 13-15).[68] In other patients, the detection of Reed-Sternberg–like cells within CLL/SLL infiltrates is more suggestive of an overt transformation analogous to Hodgkin-type RT.[68] In the former group of cases, Hodgkin (Reed-Sternberg) cells are sparsely dispersed among extensive infiltrates of small, round lymphocytes, whereas more discrete areas of overt Hodgkin-like transformation may be encountered in the second group (see Fig. 13-21). In a single large series, including both patterns, overall outcome was similar in both groups. The Hodgkin (Reed-Sternberg) cells were typically Epstein-Barr virus (EBV) positive in both groups, and the incidence of clonality between the CLL and the Hodgkin cells was similar in both groups.[68]

Immunophenotype

Immunophenotypic assessment in CLL is essential not only in establishing the diagnosis but to assess for prognostic factors and distinguish CLL from other B-CLPN (see Table 13-2). The classic immunophenotypic profile of CLL is best determined

Box 13-3 *Morphologic Variants of Chronic Lymphocytic Leukemia/Small Lymphocytic Lymphoma*

"Atypical"/Mixed CLL

- Term generally applied to CLL cases in which nuclear irregularity is fairly prominent or increased numbers of lymphocytes with distinct nucleoli are present
- Cases exhibit morphologic and immunophenotypic spectrum with some, but not all, features of classic CLL/SLL; overlap with other B-CLPN is common
- Atypical features noted in both blood and lymph node specimens
- May be linked to distinct genotypic subtypes
- Linked to more advanced stage, adverse outcome, and rapid disease progression

Accelerated CLL

- Expanded proliferation centers with increased mitotic activity
- Linked to increased risk of overt Richter transformation

CLL With Reed-Sternberg (Hodgkin) Cells

- Large, pleomorphic cells with morphologic features of Reed-Sternberg cells may be admixed sparsely with otherwise typical CLL/SLL or compose a distinct type of lesion
- Hodgkin-like overt transformation; both groups are linked to adverse outcome
- Clonal link to background CLL/SLL established in some, but not all cases

B-CLPN, B-chronic lymphoproliferative neoplasms; *CLL*, chronic lymphocytic leukemia; *CLPN*, chronic lymphoproliferative neoplasm; *SLL*, small lymphocytic lymphoma.
Data from: Campo E, Jaffe ES, Cook JR, et al. The International Consensus Classification of Mature Lymphoid Neoplasms: a report from the Clinical Advisory Committee. *Blood.* 2022 Sep 15;140(11):1229-1253; Sander B, Campo E, Hsi ED. Chronic lymphocytic leukaemia/small lymphocytic lymphoma and mantle cell lymphoma: from early lesions to transformation. *Virchows Arch.* 2023 Jan;482(1):131-145. *Erratum in: Virchows Arch.* 2023 Jan 12; Cook JR. Nodal and leukemic small B-cell neoplasms. *Mod Pathol.* 2013 Jan;26 Suppl 1:S15-28; Giné E, Martinez A, Villamor N, et al. Expanded and highly active proliferation centers identify a histological subtype of chronic lymphocytic lymphoma ("accelerated" chronic lymphocytic leukemia) with aggressive clinical behavior. *Haematologica.* 2010 Sep;95(9):1526-1533; Sorigue M, Junca J. Atypical chronic lymphocytic leukemia: Brief historical overview and current usage of an equivocal concept. *Int J Lab Hematol.* 2019 Feb;41(1):e17-e19; Oscier D, Else M, Matutes E, et al. The morphology of CLL revisited: the clinical significance of prolymphocytes and correlations with prognostic/molecular markers in the LRF CLL4 trial. *Br J Haematol.* 2016 Sep;174(5):767-775; Soliman DS, Al-Kuwari E, Siveen KS, et al. Downregulation of lymphoid enhancer-binding factor 1 (LEF-1) expression (by immunohistochemistry and/ flow cytometry) in chronic Lymphocytic leukemia with atypical immunophenotypic and cytologic features. *Int J Lab Hematol.* 2021 Jun;43(3):515-525; Fiorcari S, Benatti S, Zucchetto A, et al. Overexpression of CD49d in trisomy 12 chronic lymphocytic leukemia patients is mediated by IRF4 through induction of IKAROS. *Leukemia.* 2019 May;33(5):1278-1302; Xiao W, Chen WW, Sorbara L, et al. Hodgkin lymphoma variant of Richter transformation: morphology, Epstein-Barr virus status, clonality, and survival analysis-with comparison to Hodgkin-like lesion. *Hum Pathol.* 2016 Sep;55:108-116.

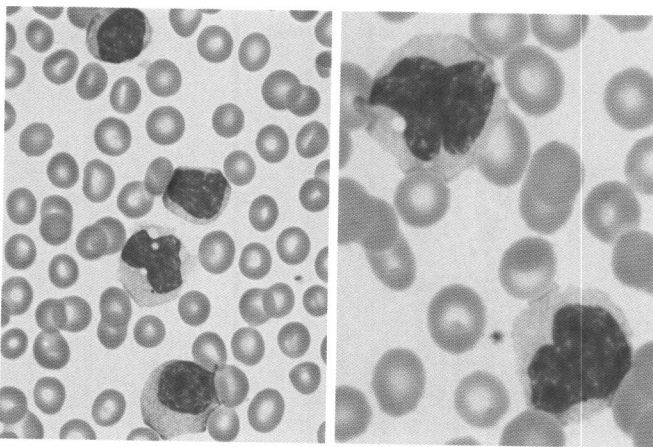

Figure 13-13. A composite of peripheral blood shows the range of atypical cells evident in two atypical/mixed chronic lymphocytic leukemia (CLL) cases. Cases of atypical CLL are linked to specific genetic abnormalities (Wright's stain).

by multicolor flow-cytometric immunophenotyping with evaluation of both intensity of antigen expression as well as patterns of antigen co-expression.[1,2,4,10,56] Prototypic CLL cases are characterized by expression of weak monotypic surface immunoglobulin (SIg), weak CD20, weak CD22, and weak-to-negative CD11c, CD79b, CD25, CD103, CD81, and FMC7, whereas moderate expression of CD19, CD5, CD23, CD200, and ROR-1 is detected (Fig. 13-16).[2] Rare biclonal CLL cases have been described, although some of these cases may represent CLL and MBL.[69]

Diagnostic difficulties occur when cases exhibit some but not all of the immunophenotypic features of classic CLL, and the term *aCLL* may be applied to these cases (see Fig. 13-14).[53,56] In these cases, other differential diagnostic considerations should be systematically excluded; correlation of IP with clinical and morphologic parameters is essential. Some otherwise straightforward CLL cases will exhibit an atypical immunophenotypic profile including either bright surface immunoglobulin, bright CD20, FMC7 expression, and, rarely, absent CD5 co-expression. However, the proportion of seemingly bona fide CLL cases that lack CD5 expression is low.[70] The diagnosis of CD5-negative CLL should be considered only after systematic exclusion of other B-CLPNs. Some bona fide CLL cases can exhibit a flow cytometry IP indistinguishable from MCL, especially when more limited flow studies are performed.[71]

Immunohistochemical (IHC) staining can also be used to assess CLL/SLL infiltrates in bone marrow and other sites (Fig. 13-17). Strong expression of nuclear LEF-1 is highly characteristic of CLL; LEF-1 is not expressed in other mature B-cell leukemia/lymphomas, but T cells are LEF-1 positive.[10,72] SOX11 is typically negative in CLL and positive in MCL, although SOX11 negative MCL has been reported.[72,73] The intensity of CD20 and CD5 expression can be assessed by IHC, although evaluation by flow-cytometric immunophenotyping is more optimal for this type of qualitative assessment. Importantly, cyclin D1 assessment by IHC is essential to detect cases of MCL, although the diagnostician must be aware that proliferation centers in CLL/SLL may show dim cyclin D1 positivity in about 20% of cases.[45] Other potential challenges in the IHC assessment for CLL/SLL are that rare cases of MCL may be CD23 and CD200 positive, and cases of SOX11-negative MCL have also been reported, especially in non-nodal leukemic MCL, which is often the main differential diagnostic consideration in blood and bone marrow specimens.[73,74]

In addition to establishing the diagnosis of CLL/SLL, multiparameter FCI provides substantial prognostic information (see Tables 13-2 and 13-4) (see the section on clinical course and prognosis). The flow-cytometrically detected antigens of greatest prognostic significance are CD38, ZAP70, and CD49d.[75-80] Overexpression (≥30% of leukemia cells) of any of these antigens is linked to adverse outcome (Fig. 13-18). Assessment of CD38 and ZAP70 has been largely replaced by CD49d assessment, since multi-institutional

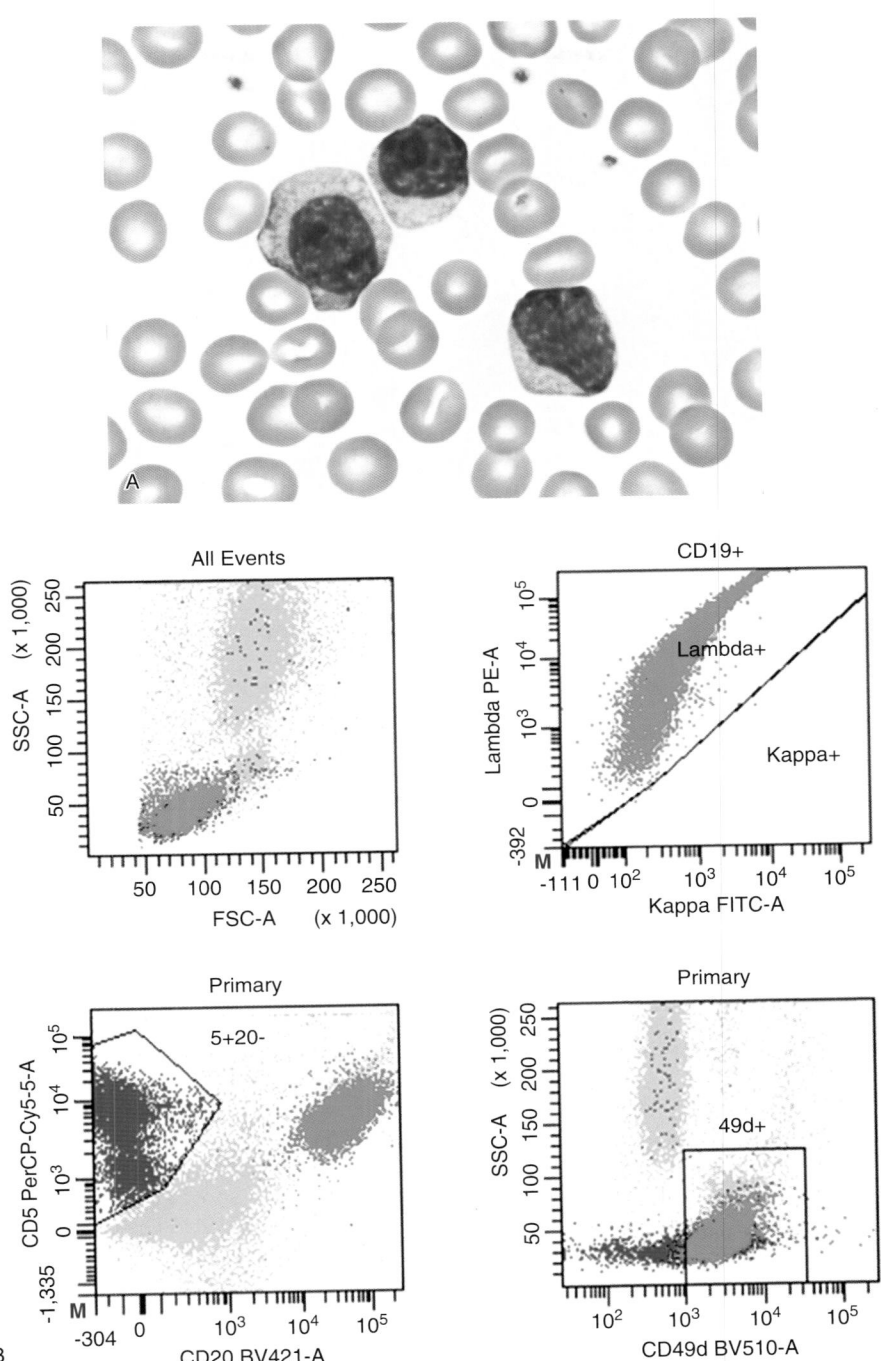

Figure 13-14. A composite of blood smear and associated flow-cytometric immunophenotyping in a patient with atypical chronic lymphocytic leukemia illustrates the atypical morphology and immunophenotypic profile in the case with trisomy 12. Note bright lambda and CD20, along with CD49d positivity (Wright's stain).

studies indicate that CD49d expression is the most significant and robust flow prognosis marker.[75]

Genetic and Molecular Features

Genomic abnormalities in CLL have been demonstrated to have important implications for disease behavior, prognosis, and treatment decisions. At minimum, complete workup of CLL requires assessment of cytogenetic abnormalities, IGHV mutational status, and identification of *TP53* mutations.[1,81,82]

Additional information can be gained from assessment of BCR stereotypes and assessment of additional genomic alterations including mutations in *NOTCH1, BIRC3, SF3B1, BTK, PLCG2,* and *BCL2.*[2,3,83-86] Cytogenetic and fluorescence in situ hybridization (FISH) studies for recurrent abnormalities are well-recognized customary components of the workup for CLL. Commercial FISH panels are available to assess for the most common recurrent abnormalities. More than 80% of CLL cases have acquired chromosomal abnormalities, including deletions of 13q14, 17p13, 11q22-23, and trisomy

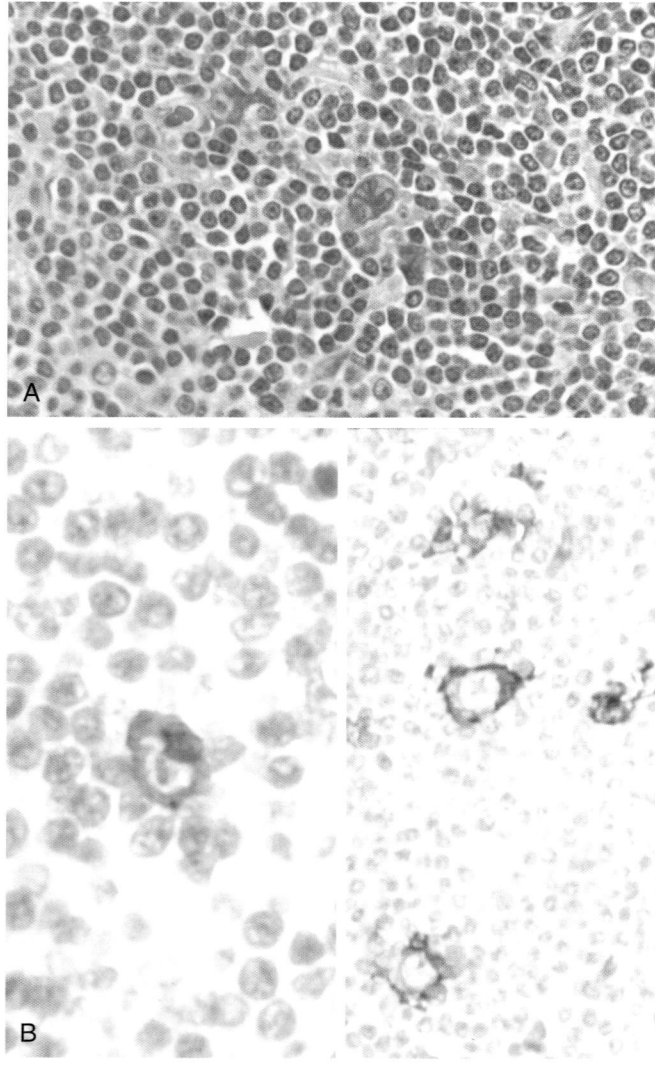

CD30   CD15

Figure 13-15. A, High-power photomicrograph of a lymph node from a patient with long-standing chronic lymphocytic leukemia (CLL) illustrates rare isolated, large Hodgkin (Reed Sternberg)-cells. **B,** Composite highlighting CD30 expression *(left)* and CD15 expression *(right)* in Hodgkin-like cells in a patient with long-standing CLL (H&E and immunoperoxidase stain for CD30 and CD15).

12 (Table 13-3).[87] These alterations are neither sensitive nor specific for a CLL diagnosis, as they are absent in 20% of CLL cases and may be seen in other malignancies, including B-cell lymphomas, and have also been identified in normal patients.[88] Standard karyotype can identify additional abnormalities to those detected by commonly used FISH panels, including deletion of 6q21, gain of 2p, and recurrent translocations such as t(14;19). In addition to assessment of cytogenetic abnormalities, testing for IGHV mutational status is a standard of care in CLL providing key prognostic information. This testing can also identify specific variant chain usage, which plays a role in disease pathogenesis and clinical behavior.[9,89-91] TP53 aberrations, including mutational status, have been established as a key driver of poor prognosis and resistance to treatment.[8,92] Although not formally incorporated into current risk stratification schemes and treatment guidelines,

identification of BCR stereotyped receptors, which use a restricted set of IGH gene segments, can predict response to treatment with BCR inhibitors such as ibrutinib.[8,91] Somatic mutations in a number of genes, including *SF3B1, ATM, NOTCH1,* and *TP53,* have been identified as having diagnostic or prognostic effect and are increasingly being incorporated into the clinical workup of CLL.[9] These mutations are generally associated with unfavorable prognosis and poor treatment response. *TP53* mutations, for example, are associated with poor outcomes and have been formally incorporated into National Comprehensive Cancer Network and European Research Initiative on CLL guidelines.

Cytogenetic Abnormalities

Because the neoplastic cells in CLL are resistant to replication in culture, older studies of CLL underestimated the number of cytogenetically abnormal cases. Introduction of B-cell mitogens has improved the ability of conventional karyotyping to detect clonal abnormalities in CLL.[93] With these methods, abnormalities may be detected at a rate similar to that of interphase FISH.[94] However, the use of FISH panels allows consistent detection of even small deletions, and these panels are standardly used in the workup for CLL. The most common abnormalities are deletion of 13q, trisomy 12, deletion of 11q, and deletion of 17p. Karyotyping and other methods of chromosome evaluation such as microarray and optical genome mapping can demonstrate additional recurrent abnormalities, most commonly deletion of 6q, gain of 2p, and translocations, and can also identify cases with complex karyotypes. These additional abnormalities are associated with adverse outcome. The ability to detect recurrent abnormalities by conventional karyotyping or FISH testing has allowed more refined risk stratification and is recommended at diagnosis or disease progression in CLL.[95]

13q Deletion

Deletion of 13q14 is the most common cytogenetic abnormality in CLL and is seen in 50% to 80% of cases either as the sole abnormality or with other alterations.[96] Deletion of 13q is more common with PB involvement than in tissue disease. The deletion may be monoallelic or biallelic, with a subset of cases showing a mixture of both monoallelic and biallelic deleted cells. This suggests that loss of the second copy may represent a clonal evolution in a subpopulation of cells, although biallelic deletion does not consistently correlate with more advanced or aggressive disease. Deletion of 13q14 occurs in other hematopoietic neoplasms, including MCL and myeloma. Deletion of this region can occur through multiple pathways, including complete loss of the chromosomal arm, interstitial deletion ranging in size from 300 Kb to more than 70 Mb, loss of heterozygosity, and through unbalanced translocations.[97] In addition, epigenetic modifications may silence genes in this region. Cases with high percentage of 13q deletion have shorter time to first treatment and shorter OS; however, the percentage used to define this group has not been consistent between studies.

Genes and microRNA coding regions of interest are located in this region and may play a role in the pathogenesis of CLL. The best studied of these is the *RB1* tumor suppressor gene, although it has been demonstrated that this gene is preserved in the characteristic microdeletion type of 13q14 deletion.[98] It is therefore not believed to be a key player in CLL

Table 13-2 Immunologic Comparison of Chronic Lymphocytic Leukemia/Small Lymphocytic Lymphoma and Mantle Cell Lymphoma

IP	CLL/SLL	MCL	Comments
CD20	Usually weak	+	Weak CD20, CD22, and CD79b reflect BCR defect in CLL
CD22	Usually weak	+	Defect in BCR in CLL
CD79b	Weak		Defect in BCR in CLL
CD23	+	−	Rare cases of CD23+ MCL
CD43	+	+	Positive in other neoplasms and benign T cells, histiocytes, other myeloid cells
CD5	+	+	T cells also positive
LEF1	Nuclear +	−	Negative in most other mature, small B-cell neoplasms; positive in >95% CLL/SLL Positive in T cells
CD200	+	−/+	Expressed in spectrum of immature and mature B-cell and plasma-cell neoplasms; negative in B-PLL and most MCL; may be positive in leukemic, non-nodal MCL
SOX11	−	+ most cases	SOX11–negative MCL linked to a more indolent disease course with blood, BM involvement (leukemic non-nodal MCL)
FMC7	−/weak	+	FMC7 brightly expressed in MCL
Cyclin D1	− (Exception: some proliferation centers are weakly cyclin D1 positive)	+	Cyclin D1–positive proliferation centers in SLL are both t(11;14) and SOX11 negative
CD10	−	−	Germinal center cell antigen
BCL6	−	−	Germinal center cell antigen
BCL2	+	+	Upregulated BCL2 because of microRNA deletion in CLL

B-PLL, B-prolymphocytic leukemia; *BCR,* B-cell receptor; *BM,* bone marrow; *CLL/SLL,* chronic lymphocytic leukemia/small lymphocytic lymphoma; *IHC,* immunohistochemical stain; *IP,* immunophenotype; *MCL,* mantle cell lymphoma.
Data from: Sander B, Campo E, Hsi ED. Chronic lymphocytic leukaemia/small lymphocytic lymphoma and mantle cell lymphoma: from early lesions to transformation. *Virchows Arch.* 2023 Jan;482(1):131-145. *Erratum in: Virchows Arch.* 2023 Jan 12; Lim M, et al., Chronic lymphocytic leukemia, in: *WHO Classification of Tumours Series,* 5th Edition, Volume 11, 2023 (in press), International Agency for Research on Cancer, Lyon (France); Gradowski JF, Sargent RL, Craig FE, et al. Chronic lymphocytic leukemia/small lymphocytic lymphoma with cyclin D1 positive proliferation centers do not have CCND1 translocations or gains and lack SOX11 expression. *Am J Clin Pathol.* 2012 Jul;138(1):132-139; Tandon B, Peterson L, Gao J, et al. Nuclear overexpression of lymphoid-enhancer-binding factor 1 identifies chronic lymphocytic leukemia/small lymphocytic lymphoma in small B-cell lymphomas. *Mod Pathol.* 2011 Nov;24(11):1433-1443; Chen YH, Gao J, Fan G, et al. Nuclear expression of sox11 is highly associated with mantle cell lymphoma but is independent of t(11;14)(q13;q32) in non-mantle cell B-cell neoplasms. *Mod Pathol.* 2010 Jan;23(1):105-112; Foucar K. Mature B- and T-cell lymphoproliferative neoplasms. In: Foucar K, Reichard R, Czuchlewski D. *Bone Marrow Pathology,* 4th Ed. ASCP Press; Kern W, Bacher U, Schnittger S, et al. Flow cytometric identification of 76 patients with biclonal disease among 5523 patients with chronic lymphocytic leukaemia (B-CLL) and its genetic characterization. *Br J Haematol.* 2014 Feb;164(4):565-569; Rangan A, Reinig E, McPhail ED, et al. Immunohistochemistry for LEF1 and SOX11 adds diagnostic specificity in small B-cell lymphomas. *Hum Pathol.* 2022 Mar;121:29-35; Hu Z, Sun Y, Schlette EJ, et al. CD200 expression in mantle cell lymphoma identifies a unique subgroup of patients with frequent IGHV mutations, absence of SOX11 expression, and an indolent clinical course. *Mod Pathol.* 2018 Feb;31(2):327-336; Laurent C, Cook JR, Yoshino T, et al. Follicular lymphoma and marginal zone lymphoma: how many diseases? *Virchows Arch.* 2023 Jan;482(1):149-162.

development. Deletion of *RB1* is detected in 41% of cases.[99] Studies have shown conflicting clinical effects of loss of the *RB1* gene, with some showing deletion correlating with shorter time to first treatment and lower OS[100] and others showing no effect.[99,101,102] Other genes in this region, including *DLEU1* and *DLEU2,* have also been investigated.

DLEU1 and *DLEU2* may function as tumor suppressors.[9] Research has focused on two microRNAs (miRNAs) in the minimal deleted region with tumor suppressor activity, *MIR-15A* and *MIR-16-1,* which are located in this area. Although these sequences are not always deleted in small 13q deletions, they may also be silenced via epigenetic modification, and their expression is decreased in many CLL cases.[103] These miRNAs play a role in modulating the translation mRNA of many genes, including downregulation of BCL2.[9,104] Loss of these miRNAs, therefore, leads to increased BCL2 signaling and inhibition of apoptosis. CLL cases with monoallelic deletion of 13q14 show decreased miRNA expression compared with controls, and cases with biallelic deletion show even lower levels.[105] These miRNAs have also been demonstrated to be deleted in cases without detectable 13q deletion by FISH or cytogenetics, including cases with other recurrent abnormalities such as 11q deletion, 17p deletion, and trisomy 12.[106]

Gene-expression profiling studies demonstrate two distinct groups of 13q14 deletion CLL, correlating with the percentage of cells showing the deletion, with larger clone size correlating with worse outcomes.[107] Patients with deletion in more than 80% of cells show deregulation of genes related to cell proliferation, apoptosis, and cell signaling, and deregulated miRNAs. The gene expression signature in cases with more than 80% deletion is similar to that seen in patients with deletion of 11q and 17p and correlates with poor prognosis. Other studies have suggested a lower threshold, with >60% of cells showing deletion of 13q correlating with shorter treatment free survival.[102]

Deletion of 13q14 is associated with normal CLL morphology, absence of CD38 expression, and hypermutated IGHV. Both monoallelic and biallelic deletions are associated with a favorable prognosis; however, when the deletion is present in a high percentage of cells (>65%), there is shorter time to first treatment.[101]

Trisomy 12

Trisomy 12 is seen in 10% to 20% of CLL cases and appears to represent a heterogeneous clinical entity with regard to clinical behavior and outcome (Fig. 13-19). The effects of trisomy 12 may be caused by gene dosage effect, with increased expression of a number of genes, including *HIP1R, CDK4,* and *MYF6,* located on chromosome 12.[108] The clinical significance of these genes in CLL is unknown; however, CDK4 overexpression may lead to increased transcription factor signaling and proliferation.[109] In addition, these cases show

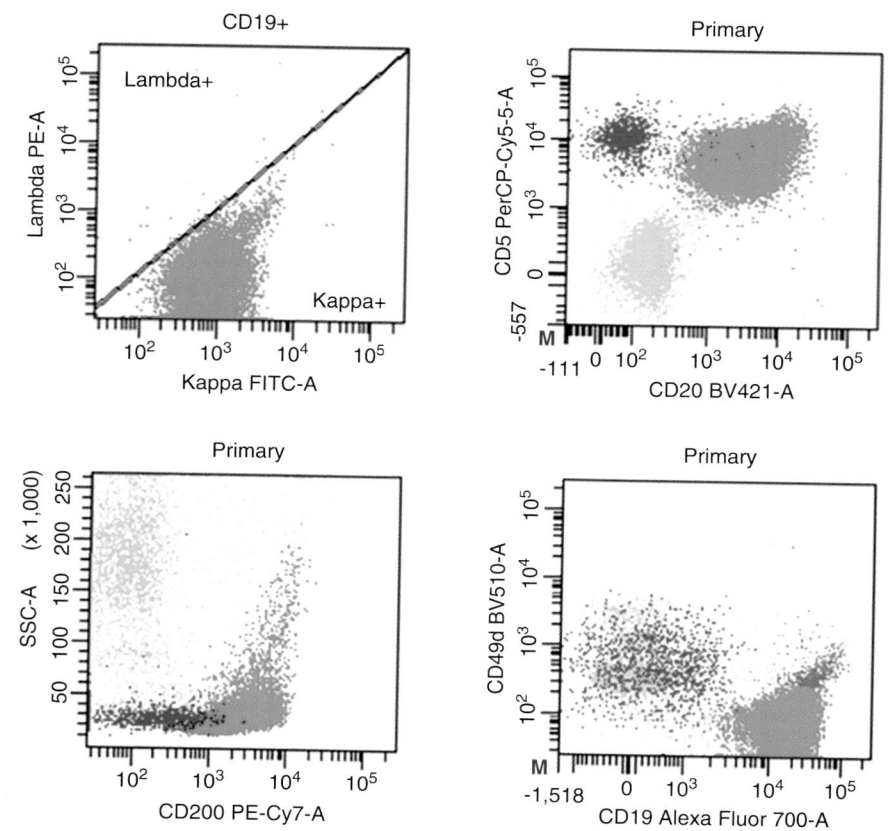

Figure 13-16. **This flow-cytometric histogram illustrates the classic immunophenotypic profile of CLL/SLL, including dim kappa restriction, CD5 co-expression, and CD200 positivity.** Note that CD49d is expressed on <30% of CLL cells.

decreased expression of *P2RY14* and *CD200*, genes located on chromosome 3. A large fraction (25%–30%) of cases with trisomy 12 are associated with deletions of the miR-15a/16-1 cluster located on chromosome 13, leading to overexpression of BCL2.[106] These deletions vary in size and may be too small to be identified by routine FISH techniques.

Trisomy 12 is associated with mutations in the *NOTCH1* gene, located on chromosome 9, although the mechanism underlying this relationship is not clear.[110] Cases with both trisomy 12 and *NOTCH1* mutation show worse outcomes compared with cases without *NOTCH1* mutation.

Trisomy 12 is linked to aCLL morphology and bright CD20 expression.[111] There is also an association with increased CD49d expression.[112] Trisomy 12 is more common in SLL, where it is seen in 30% of cases. It is also associated with RT.[113] Patients with trisomy 12 have an overall intermediate prognosis.

11q22-23 Deletion

Deletions of 11q22.3-23 in CLL are large in size and encompass a number of protein-coding genes, including the tumor suppressor gene *ATM*. This gene functions in DNA damage detection and is known to be involved in lymphomagenesis.[114] CLL cases with deletion of 11q22-23 are associated with chromosomal instability, possibly as a result of decreased *ATM* DNA damage detection.[115] A subset of CLL patients show *ATM* mutation, and these cases are clinically similar to those with 11q22 deletion.[116] Gene expression profiling shows downregulation of genes located in the deleted region, including *ATM* and *DDX10*.[117]

Although *ATM* is the best characterized gene in the region, numerous other genes are included in the deleted region and may play a role in pathogenesis, such as *RDX, RAB39, CUL5, ACAT1, NPAT, KDELC2, MRE11, H2AFX,* and *BIRC3*. Mutation or deletion of the *BIRC3* gene, located near the *ATM* gene at 11q22, is associated with a very high-risk subgroup. *BIRC3* is a negative regulator of the NF-κB signaling pathway, and loss of gene function leads to constitutive NF-κB signaling.[118] Although mutations in *BIRC3* are rare at diagnosis, they are more commonly identified later in the disease course. Mutations in this gene are associated with aggressive disease and resistance to treatment with fludarabine. In addition, *BIRC3* mutation or deletion is mutually exclusive with *TP53* abnormalities.[119]

11q23 deletion is associated with high white blood cell count, splenomegaly, and lymph node involvement. Many studies have demonstrated a shorter survival and adverse prognosis in patients with 11q deletion. These cases are more likely to show unmutated IGHV.[115,120]

17p13 Deletion

17p13 deletion is associated with loss of the *TP53* tumor suppressor gene and is found in 3% to 8% of patients at diagnosis of CLL. This incidence increases to 40% after chemotherapy in treatment-refractory patients and up to 60% in patients with RT.[121] Patients with deletion of 17p13 harbor mutations in the remaining *TP53* gene in 67% of cases.[122] Patients may also harbor mutations in both copies of the gene in the absence of 17p13 deletion. There is evidence that loss of 17p13 follows mutation in the *TP53* gene because

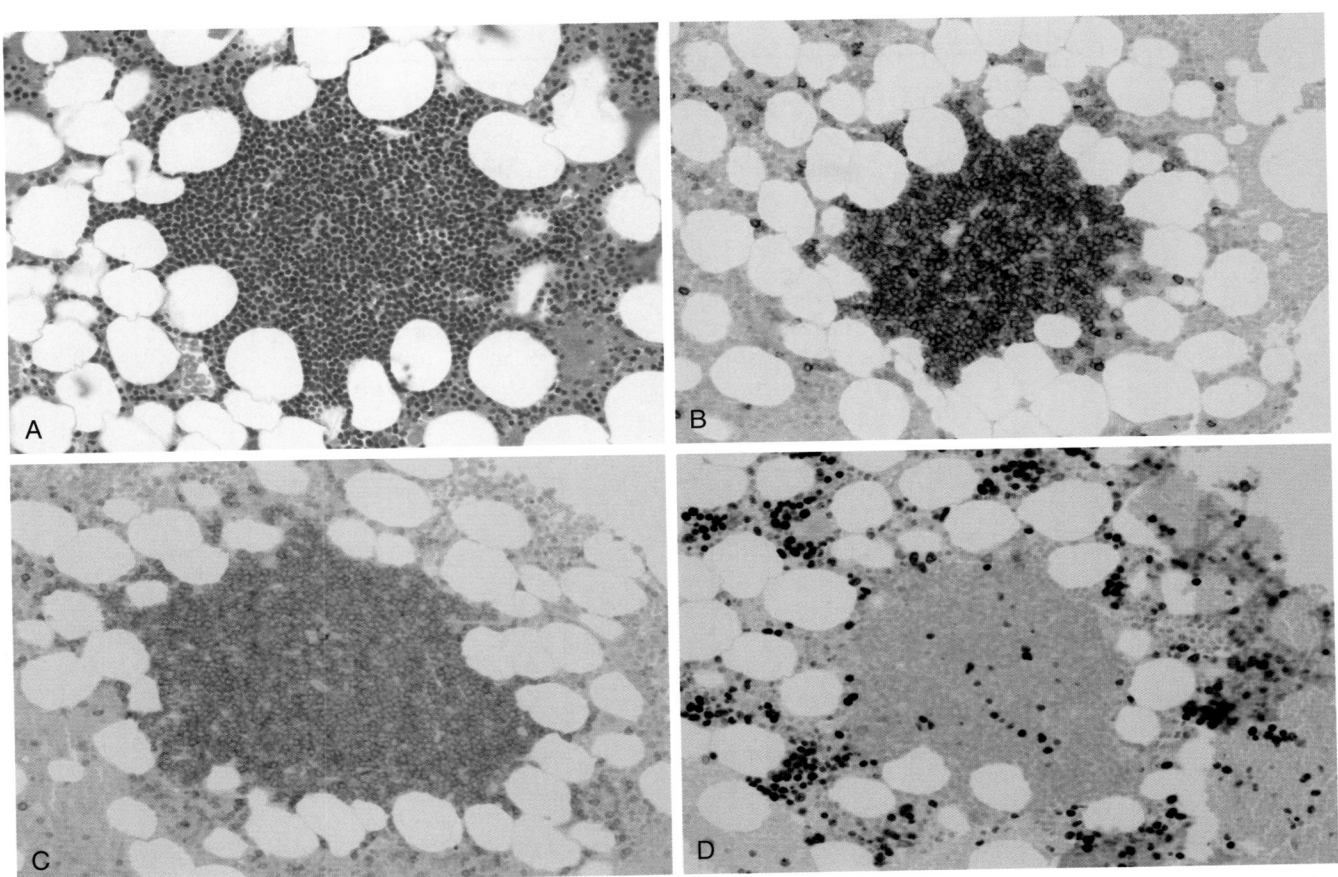

Figure 13-17. A, A composite of chronic lymphocytic leukemia (CLL) in a bone marrow biopsy illustrates morphology; **B,** bright CD20 expression; **C,** dim CD5 expression; and **D,** minimal mitotic activity with comparison to Ki67 positivity in the adjacent normal bone marrow (H&E, CD20, CD5, and Ki67 stains).

of increased genomic instability.[123,124] *TP53* is an important regulator of cell cycle control and functions in DNA damage detection, causing cell arrest and DNA repair or apoptosis. This function may underlie the resistance of 17p13-deleted CLL to alkylating therapies, which cause DNA damage and rely on activation of the apoptosis pathway. *TP53* mutation or deletion is associated with presentation in advanced stage, rapidly progressive disease, treatment refractoriness, and RT.[125,126] There is correlation between the percent of cells with 17p deletion and outcome, with higher percentages associated with worse prognosis.[127,128] One study reports that a cutoff range of 10% to 20% for the number of cells that are *TP53* positive by conventional cytogenetics or FISH as the lower limit linked to adverse outcome, although this is not widely applied in clinical practice.[128]

Gene expression profiling shows numerous changes in 17p13 deleted cases, including downregulation of tumor suppressor genes and genes involved in mRNA and protein processing, such as *DPH1, GABARAP, GPS2, NCOR1, NLRP1,* and *CAMTA2.* Additional genes are overexpressed, including *CCND2,* which is increased in cell cycle progression, and *NME1* and *STT3A,* which have been demonstrated to be overexpressed in other neoplasms.

Cases with 17p13 deletion may show aberrant (i.e., atypical) IP with bright CD20, FMC7, and surface immunoglobulin expression. It is associated with other poor prognostic markers such as CD38 and ZAP70 expression and unmutated

IGHV.[129] Patients with 17p deletion and *TP53* mutation may be considered for stem cell transplant.[130]

Other Cytogenetic Abnormalities

Additional recurrent cytogenetic abnormalities, including translocations, not covered by the typical FISH panel, have been well described in CLL, although the significance of these findings is uncertain in most cases. These findings may represent sole abnormalities or be associated with other more common changes. Around 30% of CLL cases with normal FISH studies harbor abnormalities not identified by the standard panel, including 14q deletions, 7q deletions, 6q deletions, 14q32 translocations, and 3q deletions.[131] 14q deletions are heterogeneous in size and may or may not involve the IGH gene at 14q32. These deletions are associated with typical CLL IP and unmutated IGHV.[132] Patients with 6q deletion may represent a clinically distinct group with higher white blood cell count, splenomegaly, atypical morphology, positive CD38 expression, and intermediate prognosis.[133,134]

Translocations are seen in approximately 8% of CLL cases. Of cases with translocations, 74% are balanced and 26% are unbalanced.[135] Translocations involving IGH at 14q32 have been best studied. The prognostic significance of these translocations is governed by the partner gene. The t(14;19) (q32;q13) creates an *IGH::BCL3* fusion gene with *BCL3* protein overexpression. These cases have atypical morphology and IP, association with trisomy 12 and complex karyotype, and

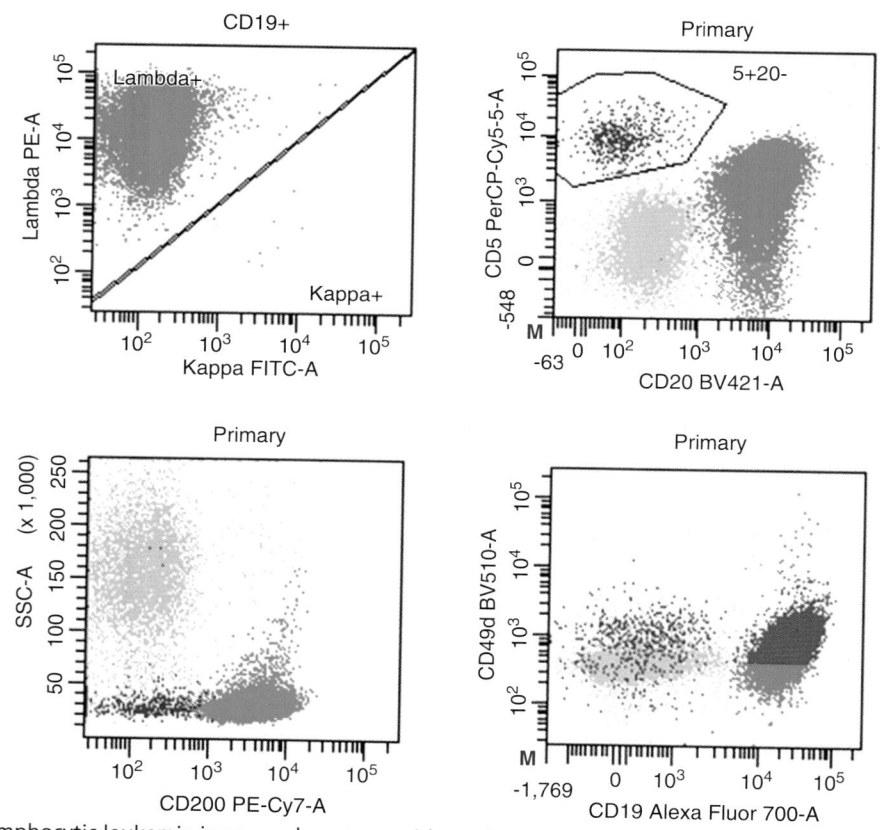

Figure 13-18. Chronic lymphocytic leukemia immunophenotype with moderate SIg, weak CD20, co-expression of CD5, and CD200. CD49d expression is evident, which is associated with adverse prognosis.

unmutated IGHV.[136] *MYC* translocations are also rarely seen in CLL and correlate with poor prognostic features including increased prolymphocytes, 17p deletion, and complex karyotype.[137]

Complex karyotype is defined as three or more structural or numerical abnormalities. It has been associated with aggressive disease and treatment resistance; however, there is evidence that the specific abnormalities and number of changes present may influence the specific prognosis. High complexity karyotypes, with five or more abnormalities, have been identified as an independent marker of poor prognosis. Cases with three or four trisomies in the absence of other changes, however, have a more indolent course.[95] Cases with three or four abnormalities show a stronger correlation with worse prognosis in the presence of *TP53* loss caused by deletion or mutation.

Somatic Mutations and Genomic Profiling

In addition to the well-studied chromosomal abnormalities, increasing numbers of somatic gene mutations have been identified that may be useful in the diagnosis and risk stratification of CLL.[138-141] In general, the frequency of somatic mutations in CLL cases increases with the length of disease, and these mutations are thought to be acquired over the course of disease.

Alterations, including mutations, in the *TP53* tumor suppressor gene have been incorporated into prognostic systems for CLL, including the National Comprehensive Cancer Network and the European Research Initiative on CLL (ERIC) guidelines.[82,97] *TP53* aberrancies are associated

with poor outcomes because of resistance to standard chemotherapeutic regimens, and patients show markedly decreased OS times compared with those without *TP53* aberration.[142]

Though cytogenetic and FISH techniques identify deletion of the *TP53* gene region, use of molecular sequencing techniques identifies mutations causing loss of gene function and use of both methods is recommended for complete assessment prior to starting treatment, and with disease progression necessitating a change in therapy.[92] Mutations are identified in 90% of patients with *TP53* deletion identified by FISH or karyotype; however, approximately 5% of CLL patients have *TP53* mutation without deletion at diagnosis and these patients have similar prognosis to those with 17p deletion. The prevalence of *TP53* mutations is increased in patients with clinically aggressive and treatment refractory disease.[86] Assessment by next generation sequencing methods is generally more sensitive than by Sanger sequencing and may identify smaller clones of clinical importance. At minimum, mutation assessment should include exons 4 to 10, which include the DNA binding domain and oligomerization domain, however, sequencing of all protein coding exons 2 to 11 is preferred for complete assessment.

Single-gene sequencing techniques are often used for targeted sequencing of *TP53*; however, new high-throughput sequencing technologies have identified mutations in a number of other genes with diagnostic and prognostic relevance, and distinct mutation profiles in cases with hypermutated IGHV compared with unmutated cases. *MYD88* and *KLH6* mutations are associated with IGHV hypermutation, whereas *NOTCH1*

Table 13-3 Selected Cytogenetic and Molecular Features of Chronic Lymphocytic Leukemia

Cytogenetics/Molecular	% Incidence	Risk Stratification	Common Associated Features
13q14 deletion (sole cytogenetic abnormality)	55	Favorable	Normal morphology CD38 negative Hypermutated IGHV
11q22-23 deletion	18	Unfavorable	Unmutated IGHV
Trisomy 12	16	Intermediate	Atypical morphology Bright CD20 High WBC count Splenomegaly Lymphadenopathy Unmutated IGHV
17p13 deletion	7	Unfavorable	Rapid disease progression Bright CD20 CD38 positive Unmutated IGHV *TP53* mutation
6q deletion	7	Intermediate	Atypical morphology High WBC count Splenomegaly Lymphadenopathy CD38 positive Unmutated IGHV
t(14;19)(q32;q13)	1	Unfavorable	Atypical morphology Bright CD20, FMC7 positive Unmutated IGHV Trisomy 12 or complex karyotype
MYC translocation	<1	Unfavorable	Increased prolymphocytes RT 17p deletion Complex karyotype
Complex karyotype (≥3 abnormalities)	40	Unfavorable	CD38 positive Unmutated IGHV
TP53 mutation	16.5	Unfavorable	Incidence increases with disease progression
ATM mutation	9.9	Intermediate	More common in advanced disease
NOTCH1 mutation	15	Intermediate	CD38 positive Unmutated IGHV
BIRC3 mutation	3	Unfavorable	
SF3B1 mutation	5–10	Intermediate	Unmutated IGHV

IGHV, Immunoglobulin heavy chain variable region; *RT,* Richter transformation; *WBC,* white blood cell.
Data from: Sander B, Campo E, Hsi ED. Chronic lymphocytic leukaemia/small lymphocytic lymphoma and mantle cell lymphoma: from early lesions to transformation. *Virchows Arch.* 2023 Jan;482(1):131-145. *Erratum in: Virchows Arch.* 2023 Jan 12; Lim M, et al., Chronic lymphocytic leukemia, in: *WHO Classification of Tumours Series,* 5th Edition, Volume 11, 2023 (in press), International Agency for Research on Cancer, Lyon (France); Nadeu F, Delgado J, Royo C, et al. Clinical impact of clonal and subclonal TP53, SF3B1, BIRC3, NOTCH1, and ATM mutations in chronic lymphocytic leukemia. *Blood.* 2016 Apr 28;127(17):2122-30; Blakemore SJ, Clifford R, Parker H, et al. Clinical significance of TP53, BIRC3, ATM and MAPK-ERK genes in chronic lymphocytic leukaemia: data from the randomised UK LRF CLL4 trial. *Leukemia.* 2020 Jul;34(7):1760-1774; Puiggros A, Collado R, Calasanz MJ, et al. Patients with chronic lymphocytic leukaemia and complex karyotype show an adverse outcome even in absence of TP53/ATM FISH deletions. *Oncotarget.* 2017 Apr 21;8(33):54297-54303.

and *XPO1* are seen in unmutated cases.[143] In addition to *TP53*, commonly mutated genes in CLL include *NOTCH1* and *SF3B1*. Other recurrently mutated genes include *ATM, BIRC3, POT1*, and *XPO1*, Notch pathway genes, and several other less commonly mutated genes.

NOTCH1 mutations are found in 10% to 14% of CLL cases at diagnosis, increasing to 20% in advanced disease and 30% in RT. The *NOTCH1* gene encodes a transcription factor that functions in cell differentiation, proliferation, and apoptosis. The most frequently identified mutations in this gene create a more stable protein that is resistant to degradation, leading to increased expression of genes in the signaling pathway and increased cell survival and resistance to apoptosis.[144] Cells with dysregulation of the Notch signaling pathway show increased expression of the *MYC* oncogene. In addition to mutations in the *NOTCH1* gene, mutations in other genes regulating the Notch pathway including *FBXW7* and *MED12*

are found in 2% to 5% of CLL cases and result in similar outcomes and response to therapy.[145] *NOTCH1* mutations are correlated with unmutated IGHV and increased ZAP70 and CD38 expression and decreased CD20 expression. These patients have more aggressive disease, resistance to treatment, particularly with anti-CD20 immunotherapy,[146] a greater risk for RT and poor outcome.[147-149] *NOTCH1* mutations are seen in association with trisomy 12 but are rare in del(13q).[150] *NOTCH1* and other Notch pathway mutations may provide a target for therapy.[151]

SF3B1 encodes a part of the spliceosome, the complex responsible for removing introns from RNA to allow proper protein translation. Mutation in this gene leads to atypical RNA transcripts, typically with premature stop codons. The incidence of mutation in CLL is from 7% to 15% at diagnosis, increasing to 20% in patients with advanced disease. *SF3B1* mutations are associated with aggressive

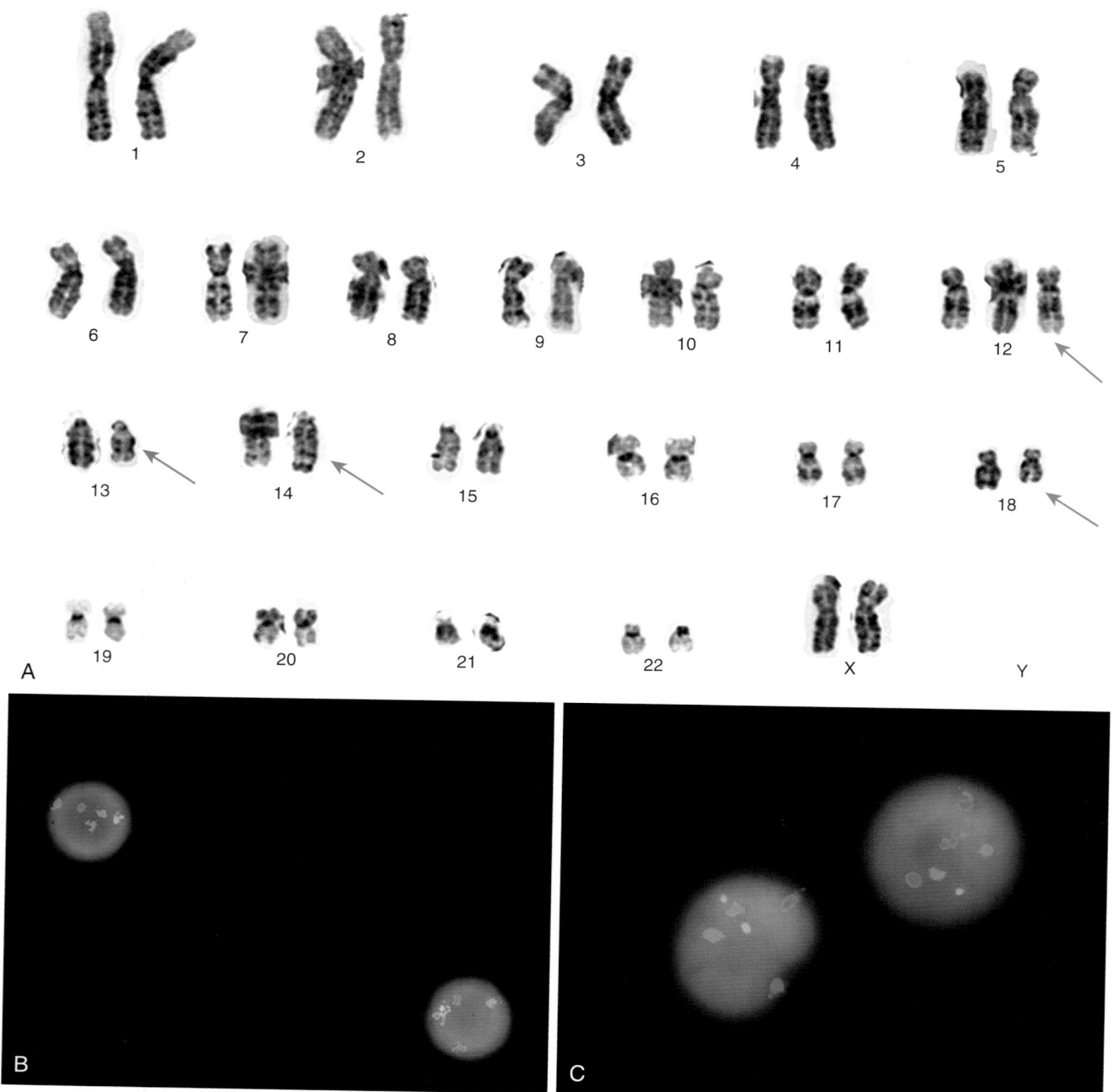

Figure 13-19. A, This karyotype shows trisomy 12 and deletion of 13q, which were seen on a concurrent chronic lymphocytic leukemia (CLL) fluorescence in situ hybridization (FISH) panel. In addition, there is a t(14;18)(q32;q21) that was not tested for and was therefore missed by FISH. **B,** FISH for the 13q14.3 region *(red signal)* shows only one copy of the region, consistent with monoallelic deletion of the region. **C,** FISH for the centromere of chromosome 12 *(green signal)* shows three signals, consistent with trisomy 12.

disease and short survival, a higher white blood cell and leukemic cell count, CD38 positivity, and unmutated IGHV.[152] Interestingly, these mutations are not seen in patients with RT. In addition, these mutations are associated with specific variable chain usage and are more common in IGHV3-21 and possibly IGHV1-69 and are mutually exclusive of IGHV1-2. These mutations are more common in patients with normal karyotype or del(11q) and are not seen in patients with trisomy 12.[150]

The *ATM* gene, located on chromosome 11q, is mutated in 10% to 21% of CLL. The *ATM* gene functions in DNA damage

response. These mutations are more common in cases with del(11q), resulting in loss of both copies of the gene. The prognostic significance of *ATM* mutations has not been fully explored; however, some studies suggest an association with more aggressive disease.[120]

BIRC3 is also located in the commonly deleted area on chromosome 11q and functions in the NF-κB pathway. Mutations have been associated with more aggressive disease, although this may be mitigated with newer treatments such as venetoclax and ibrutinib.[152] Other recurrently mutated genes in CLL include *POT1* and *XPO1*.[153]

Chronic Lymphocytic Leukemia Immunoglobulin Structure and Stereotyped Receptors

B-cell immunoglobulin genes undergo rearrangement in vivo, allowing generation of a large spectrum of unique proteins, each recognizing a different antigen. This rearrangement uses VDJ chains, which are combined in a semirandom fashion and are different in individual cells. Certain chains are associated with increased affinity for certain antigens. After exposure to antigen, somatic hypermutation occurs, leading to further increased antigen affinity. CLL demonstrates both unmutated and hypermutated Ig genes. CLL clones show a preferential usage of certain V regions, with VH4-34 often seen in cases with hypermutation and VH1-69 and VH4-39 seen in unmutated cases.

In addition, 30% of CLL cases show highly similar amino acid sequences in their B-cell receptors, referred to as *stereotyped receptors*.[90,91] Based on these sequences, cases can be divided into subsets that share common clinical and molecular features and associate with different outcomes. For example, subset 2 is associated with poor prognosis and *SF3B1* mutation, while subset 8 is associated with poor prognosis, the highest risk of RT, and *NOTCH1* mutation.[154,155] The findings of recurrent variable chain usage and stereotyped receptors indicate that antigen stimulation by specific structures is likely a key component in CLL pathogenesis. Several possibilities have been explored to identify these antigens. In some cases, autoantigens have been implicated including epitopes that may be exposed during apoptosis.[156] Superantigens including *Staphylococcus aureus* protein A and CMV phosphoprotein pUL32 have also been suggested.[6]

Postulated Cell of Origin and Normal Counterpart Cell

Both IGHV unmutated and hypermutated cases are believed to originate from mature, antigen-experienced B cells. One review detailed B-cell maturation pathways that can give rise to the memory B cell–like cells that could be the cell of origin in CLL.[89] The pathways include classic T-cell dependent germinal center pathway, T-cell dependent extrafollicular pathway, and T-cell independent extrafollicular pathway. The classic germinal center pathway gives rise to IGHV-mutated memory B cells, while the other two pathways often give rise to IGHV-unmutated memory B cells. However, other studies suggested that CLL may originate at the stem cell stage.[13,38,89,157-159] CLL cells show downregulation of surface IgM but not IgD, a feature seen in cells that have been exposed to antigen and are anergic. Gene-expression profiling shows that both types of CLL show similar expression of activation and proliferation markers as memory and marginal zone B cells. CD5-positive B cells are normally found in very low numbers in the PB of adults. CD5-positive B cells are also found in fetal blood and lymphoid tissue.[160]

Clinical Course and Prognosis

CLL is generally an indolent disease. However, the clinical course is highly varied and some patients may have much shorter time to first treatment and a more aggressive clinical course (Table 13-4).[7,8] The International Prognosis Index for CLL (CLL-IPI) was developed as a prognostic model to discriminate different prognostic subgroups.[161] The CLL-IPI

Table 13-4 Prognostic Markers in Chronic Lymphocytic Leukemia

	Clinical	Laboratory	Genetic
Adverse	Male sex Age >65 High clinical stage	CD49d positive CD38 positive ZAP70 positive Elevated β2-microglobulin	IGHV unmutated IGHV3-23 usage 17p13 deletion *TP53* mutation t(14;19)(q32;q13) *MYC* translocation Complex karyotype *NOTCH1* mutation *SF3B1* mutation
Favorable	Female Low clinical stage Age <65	CD49d negative CD38 negative ZAP70 negative	IGHV hypermutated 13q14 deletion (sole abnormality)

CLL, Chronic lymphocytic leukemia; IGHV, immunoglobulin heavy chain variable region.

Data from: Sander B, Campo E, Hsi ED. Chronic lymphocytic leukaemia/small lymphocytic lymphoma and mantle cell lymphoma: from early lesions to transformation. *Virchows Arch.* 2023 Jan;482(1):131-145. *Erratum in: Virchows Arch.* 2023 Jan 12; International CLL-IPI Working Group. An international prognostic index for patients with chronic lymphocytic leukaemia (CLL-IPI): a meta-analysis of individual patient data. *Lancet Oncol.* 2016 Jun;17(6):779-790; Parviz M, Brieghel C, Agius R, et al. Prediction of clinical outcome in CLL based on recurrent gene mutations, CLL-IPI variables, and (para)clinical data. *Blood Adv.* 2022 Jun 28;6(12):3716-3728; Bomben R, Rossi FM, Vit F, et al. TP53 mutations with low variant allele frequency predict short survival in chronic lymphocytic leukemia. *Clin Cancer Res.* 2021 Oct 15;27(20):5566-5575; Nadeu F, Delgado J, Royo C, et al. Clinical impact of clonal and subclonal TP53, SF3B1, BIRC3, NOTCH1, and ATM mutations in chronic lymphocytic leukemia. *Blood.* 2016 Apr 28;127(17):2122-30; Blakemore SJ, Clifford R, Parker H, et al. Clinical significance of TP53, BIRC3, ATM and MAPK-ERK genes in chronic lymphocytic leukaemia: data from the randomised UK LRF CLL4 trial. *Leukemia.* 2020 Jul;34(7):1760-1774; Puiggros A, Collado R, Calasanz MJ, et al. Patients with chronic lymphocytic leukemia and complex karyotype show an adverse outcome even in absence of TP53/ATM FISH deletions. *Oncotarget.* 2017 Apr 21;8(33):54297-54303.

analyzed genetic, biochemical, and clinical parameters and came up with five independent prognostic factors: *TP53* status [no abnormality versus del(17p) or *TP53* mutation or both], IGHV mutational status (mutated versus unmutated), serum β2-microglobulin concentration (≤3.5 mg/L versus >3.5 mg/L), clinical state (Binet A or Rai 0 versus Binet B–C or Rai I–IV), and age (≤65 years versus >65 years). CLL-IPI predicts time to first treatment and OS. Each parameter is weighted and the final scores separate patients into low, intermediate, high, and very-high risk categories with a 5-year survival rate at 93.5%, 79.3%, 63.3%, and 23.3%, respectively.

Other methods to predict clinical outcomes are used in certain regions of the world (Table 13-4). A machine-learning technology using three classes of variables, including recurrent gene mutations, CLL-IPI variables, and (para)clinical data is predictive of individual risk in four clinical outcomes: death, treatment, infection, and the combined outcome of treatment or infection within both a short-term, 2-year outlook and a long-term, 5-year outlook.[162,163] In this model, the predictive performance of CLL-IPI is improved by adding baseline clinical data. In addition, the risk factors predictive of death within a 5-year outlook are mostly similar to risk factors predictive of infection within a 2-year outlook. The IGHV test is only available in a small subset of patients with CLL around the globe. In most parts of the world, especially in resource-limited settings, IGHV is not practical. Alternative systems have been sought for these regions. One such example is lymphocyte doubling time (LDT), which is proposed in place of IGHV mutation status to predict the clinical outcome of CLL patients.[163] Tumor mutation load using next-generation

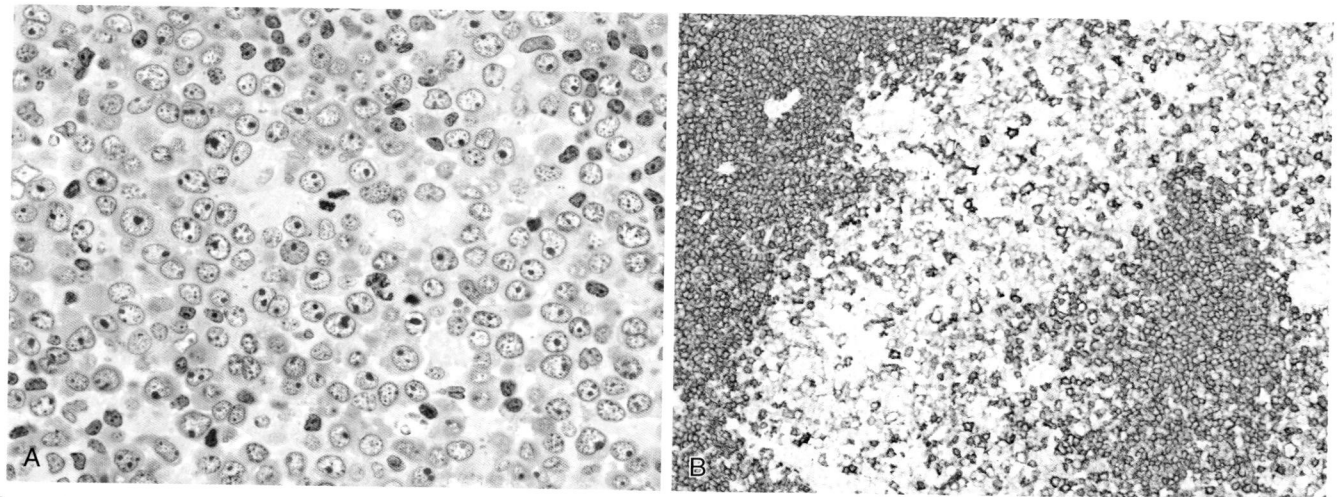

Figure 13-20. **A,** Lymph node biopsy from a patient with chronic lymphocytic leukemia (CLL) transformed to diffuse large B-cell lymphoma (DLBCL) illustrates solid sheets of large lymphoma cells *(center)* with background CLL on both sides. **B,** A CD20 stain of lymph nodes on another case with more focal Richter's involvement reveals weaker CD20 expression in the large transformed cells (H&E and CD20 stains).

sequencing is also a strong predictor of time to first treatment in CLL and monoclonal B-cell lymphocytosis, independent of CLL-IPI.[164] Even low variant allele frequency *TP53* mutations are also predictive of short survival in CLL; one study proposed a 10% to 20% threshold for *TP53* abnormalities detected by standard karyotyping or FISH.[128,165]

Translocations are less common in CLL and are reported in approximately ~3% to 8% (range 1.9%–26.1%) of CLL patients in various studies.[166,167] T(14;18) *IGH::BCL2,* t(14;19) *IGH::BCL3,* t(8;14) *MYC::IGH,* and t(2;14) *BCL11A::IGH* are among the most commonly reported of these generally rare translocations. Reciprocal translocations involving immunoglobin genes, most commonly the immunoglobin heavy chain (IGH) located at 14q32, translocate genes under active regulatory sequences on 14q32, which results in constitutive activation of the translocated genes. Results are mixed; some studies did not find prognostic significance of the translocations, although one study identified *IGH::BCL3* translocation as prognostically important. It is associated with shorter time to first treatment, short 5-year survival rate and OS rate, and is more likely to have high and very high CLL-IPI.[166]

Serum-free light chain and IgM peak have been proposed as prognostic markers.[168-171] Increased serum thymidine kinase and β2-microglobulin levels are associated with poor prognosis.[172-174] Lactate dehydrogenase (LDH) is a useful indicator for tumor turnover. Expression of CD49d or CD38 by flow-cytometric immunophenotyping in ≥30% of clonal B cells is linked to more aggressive clinical course. CD49d is a subunit of cell surface adhesion molecule integrin and is an independent prognostic marker. CD49d expression is associated with shorter time to treatment and decreased OS. Similarly CD38 positivity is also linked to adverse outcome and can also predict unmutated IGHV gene mutation status in most cases. Zeta-chain-associated protein of 70 kiloDalton (kDa) (ZAP70) expression is a surrogate for IGHV mutation status, and ZAP70 positivity is linked to unmutated IGHV status and predicts aggressive clinical course.

The causes of death in CLL patients include disease progression, CLL unrelated causes, second malignancy,

unknown cause, and infection, in descending order.[175,176] Patients in high or very-high risk categories are more likely to have disease progression and die of the disease, while patients in low or intermediate risk categories are more likely to die with the disease.

Transformation

RT is defined as transformation of CLL/SLL into more aggressive lymphomas and is mostly represented by DLBCL (Fig. 13-20), which accounts for 95% to 99% of transformation cases and occurs in 2% to 10% of CLL patients.[2,27,177] Transformation to classic Hodgkin lymphoma is much less frequent, occurring in approximately 0.5% of patients (Fig. 13-21).[68,178] Transformation to lymphoblastic leukemia/lymphoma, histiocytic/dendritic cell sarcoma, high grade T-cell lymphoma, hairy cell leukemia (HCL), plasmablastic transformation, or prolymphocytic leukemia have been reported as case reports (Fig. 13-22).[14-19,179,180]

Risk factors for RT include genetic findings, laboratory parameters, and clinical characteristics. Mutations or deletions of *TP53, CDKN2A,* and *NOTCH1* genes are associated with increased risk of RT. Unmutated IGHV status or stereotyped B-cell receptor subset 8 are also linked to RT. In addition, complex karyotype, 11q deletion, and trisomy 12 are known risk factors for RT. Overexpression of ZAP70 and CD38, elevated LDH, Binet stage B–C or advanced Rai stage at diagnosis, and lymphadenopathy are recognized risk factors as well.[19] Treatment of CLL with purine nucleoside analogs also significantly increases the risk for RT.[177]

Two main genetic pathways are involved in the transformation of CLL to RT-DLBCL.[181] The first pathway involves either acquisition of aberrations in tumor suppressor gene *TP53* or mutations in cyclin-dependent kinase inhibitor 2A (*CDKN2A*). Oncogene *MYC* is activated in a subset of patients with *TP53* aberration. These alterations usually occur at transformation. This pathway appears to be the most common genetic aberration leading to RT-DLBCL; it contributes to the development of RT-DLBCL in 50% of cases. *TP53* is one of the most prominent tumor suppressor genes

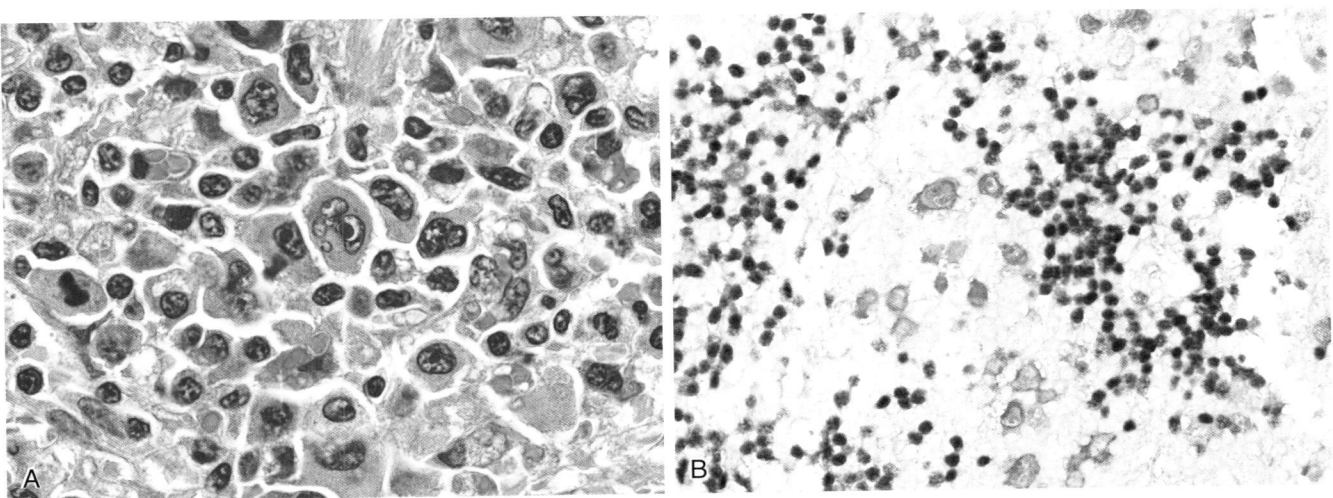

Figure 13-21. A, Spleen from a patient with chronic lymphocytic leukemia (CLL) transformed to Hodgkin lymphoma illustrates scattered Reed-Sternberg cells and Hodgkin cells. A few small lymphocytes and histiocytes are in the background. **B,** PAX5/CD30 stain reveals weak PAX5 nuclear and CD30 cytoplasmic and membrane staining in Reed-Sternberg and Hodgkin cells (H&E and PAX5/CD30 stains).

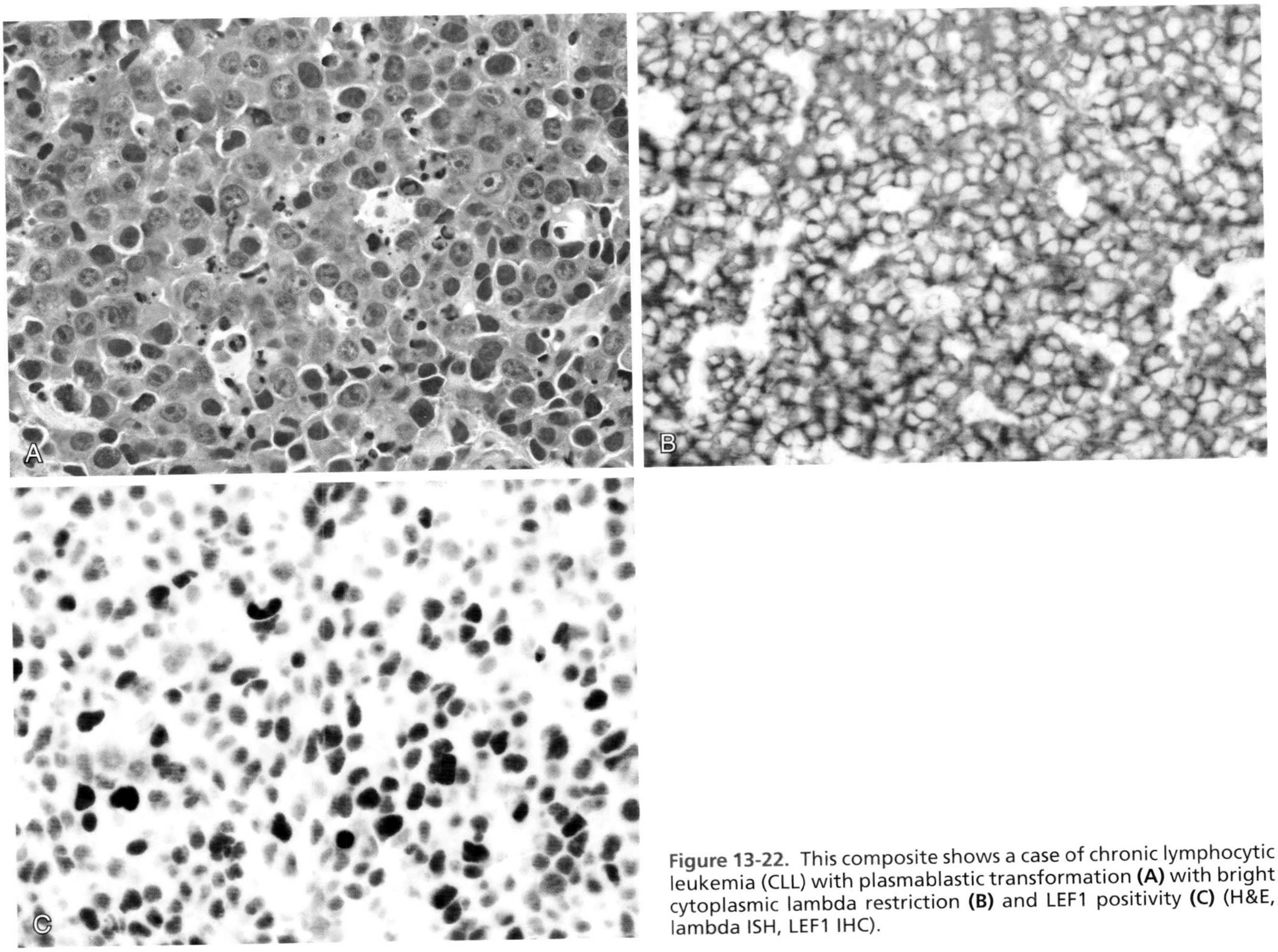

Figure 13-22. This composite shows a case of chronic lymphocytic leukemia (CLL) with plasmablastic transformation **(A)** with bright cytoplasmic lambda restriction **(B)** and LEF1 positivity **(C)** (H&E, lambda ISH, LEF1 IHC).

and p53 protein has a critical role in guarding the integrity of the genome. *CDKN2A* encodes protein p16INK4A, which negatively regulates progression of G1 to the S phase in the cell cycle via inhibition of Cdk4 and Cdk6 kinase. *CDNK2A* also encodes P14ARF, a MDM2 inhibitor. The loss of *CDNK2A*

is often secondary to 9p21 deletion. *MYC* alteration usually occurs via translocation and less commonly because of amplification of 8q24. Activation of *MYC* significantly affects cell proliferation, metabolism, cell adhesion, and cellular function. The second pathway occurs in approximately 30%

of RT cases and involves activation of the *NOTCH1* pathway through somatic mutations. These two pathways appear mutually exclusive. *NOTCH1* mutations occur most frequently in CLL stage in patients with trisomy 12, unmutated IGHV, and ZAP70 positivity. Patients with *NOTCH1* mutations have a 45% chance of developing RT within 15 years. *NOTCH1* encodes a transmembrane receptor that in turn affects cell proliferation and apoptosis through downstream genes, including *CCND1, MYC,* and *BCL2.* The remaining 20% of patients with RT have heterogeneous genomic aberrations.

RT-DLBCL developing while on novel therapeutic agents has become more common.[17,182-190] *TP53, CDKN2A, MYC,* and *NOTCH1* are common aberrations in these cases. Over 70% of patients who developed RT on ibrutinib had associated *TP53* alterations. *BTK* and *PLUG2* mutations are also reported in patients who developed RT on ibrutinib. *TP53* alterations are also observed in over 70% of patients who developed RT on venetoclax. This study also showed that RT genomic profiling is intermediate between CLL and de novo DLBCL and that *CDKN2A* inactivation through DNA loss or mutations is the most frequently acquired lesion at the time of transformation.[181]

It is important for the diagnostician to be aware that RT-like proliferations can develop after cessation of ibrutinib, a phenomenon termed "pseudo-Richter transformation."[1,2] These proliferations regress with reinstitution of BTK inhibitor therapy.

Non-germinal center (non-GCB) phenotype is overrepresented in RT-DLBCL.[13] Biologically RT-DLBCL can be clonally related or unrelated to CLL. Clonally related RT-DLBCL is the most common type (~70% of all RT-DLBCL) and is more commonly seen in IGVH unmutated cases. It carries a very poor prognosis and is often chemotherapy resistant. Clonally unrelated DLBCL is more often seen in IGHV mutated cases and shows a prognosis identical to de novo DLBCL in the setting of immune dysregulation.[181] EBV-associated large B-cell lymphoma occurs in a subset of usually clonally unrelated RT-DLBCL, ranging from 6% to 29%,[21,191,192] particularly in the anti-CD52 antibody alemtuzumab treatment setting, similar to lymphomas arising in the immunodeficiency setting.[193,194]

Clonally related RT-HL is less common and only accounts for ~40% of RT-HL. The majority of RT-HL are clonally unrelated. The risk factors and molecular aberrations of RT-HL are less well understood. The IP of RT-HL is similar to de novo HL and the majority are EBV positive (70%).[17,68]

The median OS for RT-DLBCL is 9 to 12 months, while the median OS for clonally unrelated RT-DLBCL is 62.5 months. The median OS for RT-HL is about 33.5 months.[195,196]

Differential Diagnosis

A spectrum of disorders can manifest PB lymphocytosis. In children and young adults, lymphocytosis is more likely to be benign, whereas in older adults, lymphocytosis is more likely to be neoplastic. Reactive lymphocytosis is typically seen in viral infection, vaccination, autoimmune disorders, or presence of other types of malignancies. The lymphocytes exhibit a heterogeneous morphology ranging from small, mature lymphocytes to large, activated lymphocytes with abundant cytoplasm. A rare phenomenon called benign B-cell polyclonal lymphocytosis reveals stable persistent

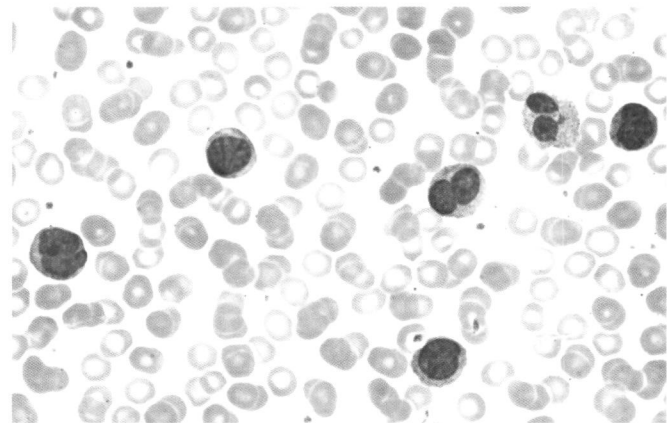

Figure 13-23. Peripheral blood smear from a middle-aged female with polyclonal lymphocytosis illustrates small lymphocytes with scant cytoplasm and condensed chromatin. Occasional bilobed lymphocytes are also present (Wright's stain).

lymphocytosis.[197-199] The lymphocytes in this disorder are small with scant cytoplasm and round nuclei, with occasional binucleated forms (Fig. 13-23). This phenomenon is more commonly seen in young to middle-aged females who often are smokers, and morphologically it is indistinguishable from CLL. Chromosome 3 abnormalities, including isochromosome of the long arm of chromosome 3 and trisomy 3, have been described in a subset of cases.[200,201] An association with the HLA-DR7 haplotype has also been reported.[202-204] In adults with a sustained unexplained lymphocytosis, clinical correlation and workup including flow-cytometric analysis initially, and potential cytogenetic and molecular studies, may be needed to exclude or confirm a neoplastic process, though morphologic and clinical correlation is generally sufficient in children and adults in whom a clinical cause for the lymphocytosis is apparent.

When FCI confirms a B-cell neoplasm, differential diagnostic considerations include other lymphocytic leukemias and lymphomas (Tables 13-5, 13-6, and 13-7). Cell morphology is a helpful feature to predict a CLL diagnosis, which typically shows small and uniform lymphocytes, a scant to moderate amount of cytoplasm, highly condensed chromatin with a characteristic "soccer ball" pattern, and inconspicuous nucleoli.[56] Although morphology is highly characteristic in classic CLL cases, flow-cytometric analysis is required to confirm the diagnosis. MCL usually exhibits a spectrum of morphology ranging from small to intermediate to large lymphoma cells. These cells have irregular nuclear contours, and a subset has prominent nucleoli. However, MCL cells may mimic CLL morphologically, presenting a diagnostic challenge (Fig. 13-24). There is also significant morphologic overlap between CLL cases with prolymphocytoid transformation and de novo B-cell prolymphocytic leukemia (B-PLL), which is a diagnosis of exclusion in ICC.[2] Prior history of CLL is very useful in making this distinction.

Other B-cell neoplasms in the differential diagnosis of CLL include FL with blood involvement. FL cells demonstrate a spectrum of cell size with characteristic deeply cleaved nuclear membranes, and blood involvement typically occurs late in the disease course of these patients. Both morphology and IP distinguish HCL, HCL variant (HCLv), and MZL from CLL because of more abundant cytoplasm of these neoplastic cells

Table 13-5 Comparison of Morphologic Features of B-Chronic Lymphoproliferative Neoplasms in Lymph Node and Spleen

Feature	CLL/SLL	MCL*	FL*	MZL/SMZL*	HCL*
Nuclei	Small round	Small, irregular	Small, clefted	Small, round to reniform	Small reniform
Cytoplasm	Scant	Scant	Scant	Moderate to abundant	Moderate to abundant
Mitotic activity	Minimal	Variable	Minimal	Minimal	Minimal
Pattern of LN infiltration	Diffuse with proliferation centers; some cases with expanded and highly active proliferation centers linked to adverse outcome	Nodular or diffuse; may show spared germinal centers	Follicular	Variable, usually nodular; may show marginal zone pattern with spared germinal centers and mantle zones or sinusoidal pattern; follicle colonization often present	Diffuse, occasionally medullary
Pattern of splenic infiltration	Primarily white pulp with secondary involvement of red pulp	Primarily white pulp with spared germinal centers	Primarily white pulp	Primarily white pulp with variable pattern, often including marginal zone pattern with compartmentalization/zoning of white pulp	Red pulp with erythrocyte lakes and attenuated white pulp

*See relevant chapters in this book.
B-CLPN, B-chronic lymphoproliferative neoplasm; *CLL/SLL*, chronic lymphocytic leukemia/small lymphocytic lymphoma; *FL*, follicular lymphoma; *HCL*, hairy cell leukemia; *LN*, lymph node; *MCL*, mantle cell lymphoma; *MZL/SMZL*, marginal zone lymphoma including splenic MZL.
Data from Sander B, Campo E, Hsi ED. Chronic lymphocytic leukaemia/small lymphocytic lymphoma and mantle cell lymphoma: from early lesions to transformation. *Virchows Arch.* 2023 Jan;482(1):131-145. *Erratum in: Virchows Arch.* 2023 Jan 12; Cook JR. Nodal and leukemic small B-cell neoplasms. *Mod Pathol.* 2013 Jan;26 Suppl 1:S15-28; Foucar K. Mature B- and T-cell lymphoproliferative neoplasms. In: Foucar K, Reichard R, Czuchlewski D. *Bone Marrow Pathology*, 4th ed. ASCP Press; Laurent C, Cook JR, Yoshino T, et al. Follicular lymphoma and marginal zone lymphoma: how many diseases? *Virchows Arch.* 2023 Jan;482(1):149-162; Nadeu F, Martin-Garcia D, Clot G, et al. Genomic and epigenomic insights into the origin, pathogenesis, and clinical behavior of mantle cell lymphoma subtypes. *Blood.* 2020 Sep 17;136(12):1419-1432.

Table 13-6 Pattern and Morphology of Bone Marrow Involvement in B-Chronic Lymphoproliferative Neoplasms

Disorder	Aspirate Morphology	Core Biopsy Features
CLL/SLL	Monotonous small round lymphocytes with scant cytoplasm	Focal non-paratrabecular infiltrates predominate but may see either diffuse interstitial or diffuse solid infiltrates
B-PLL	Intermediate-sized lymphocytes exhibiting round nuclei with relatively condensed nuclear chromatin and prominent central nucleoli	Usually diffuse, interstitial
MCL*	Small to intermediate-sized lymphocytes with variably condensed chromatin and irregular nuclear contours; a variable number of cells may exhibit either prolymphocytic or blastic features	Usually focal non-paratrabecular and paratrabecular infiltrates evident, although interstitial and diffuse lesions also described
FL*	Variable, but small cleaved lymphoid cells typically predominate	Focal paratrabecular lesions predominate
MZL* (including splenic MZL)	Variable with admixture of plasmacytic forms; some cells may exhibit shaggy cytoplasmic contours that tend to be bipolar	Variable, sinusoidal infiltrates common but usually in association with discrete focal lesions; may see "naked" germinal centers
LPL*	Spectrum of lymphoplasmacytic cells and plasma cells; Dutcher bodies; may see abundant mast cells	Focal, interstitial, or diffuse lesions may be noted; may see amyloid deposition
HCL*	Distinctive cell with oblong to reniform nuclei, spongy "checkerboard" nuclear chromatin, and moderate to abundant amounts of slightly basophilic cytoplasm exhibiting shaggy contours	Diffuse interstitial and sinusoidal infiltrates characteristic; can be very subtle and is best appreciated by immunophenotypic assessment

*See relevant chapters in this book.
B-PLL, B-prolymphocytic leukemia; *CLL/SLL*, chronic lymphocytic leukemia/small lymphocytic lymphoma; *FL*, follicular lymphoma; *HCL*, hairy cell leukemia; *LPL*, lymphoplasmacytic lymphoma; *MCL*, mantle cell lymphoma; *MZL*, marginal zone lymphoma.
Data from Sander B, Campo E, Hsi ED. Chronic lymphocytic leukaemia/small lymphocytic lymphoma and mantle cell lymphoma: from early lesions to transformation. *Virchows Arch.* 2023 Jan;482(1):131-145. *Erratum in: Virchows Arch.* 2023 Jan 12; Cook JR. Nodal and leukemic small B-cell neoplasms. *Mod Pathol.* 2013 Jan;26 Suppl 1:S15-28; Foucar K. Mature B- and T-cell lymphoproliferative neoplasms. In: Foucar K, Reichard R, Czuchlewski D. *Bone Marrow Pathology*, 4th ed. ASCP Press; Laurent C, Cook JR, Yoshino T, et al. Follicular lymphoma and marginal zone lymphoma: how many diseases? *Virchows Arch.* 2023 Jan;482(1):149-162.

on PB smear, and FCI features. Rare cases of T-prolymphocytic leukemia (T-PLL) may have a similar presentation and morphologically mimic CLL.

In the bone marrow, CLL may exhibit different patterns including non-paratrabecular lymphoid nodules, interstitial infiltrate, and diffuse effacement of the marrow (Table 13-6). The bone marrow architecture can be preserved in the early phase of the disease with only interstitial infiltrate, and IHC stain with B-cell markers such as CD20 may be required to reveal the infiltrate. The differential diagnosis in the BM includes MCL, HCL, LPL, HCLv, B-PLL, and SMZL. HCL usually exhibits characteristic "chicken wire" or "fried egg" appearance because of abundant cytoplasm. LPL reveals a spectrum of small lymphocytes, plasmacytoid lymphocytes, plasma cells, and increased mast cells. Dutcher bodies may be observed in the plasma cells. HCLv and SMZL may show interstitial or intrasinusoidal infiltrates; discrete lymphoid aggregates may also be seen in SMZL. MCL usually demonstrates paratrabecular and non-paratrabecular lymphoid aggregates. Of particular note, indolent leukemic, non-nodal MCL with interstitial bone marrow involvement may closely mimic CLL and poses a particular differential diagnostic challenge (Fig. 13-25). This type of leukemic, non-nodal MCL is usually associated with a good prognosis.[2,205,206]

Table 13-7 Classic Immunophenotypic Profile of B-Chronic Lymphoproliferative Neoplasms

Disorder	SIg	CD20	CD22	CD23	CD25	CD5	FMC7	CD11c	CD10	CD79b	CD103	CD200	LEF1	Cyclin D1	SOX11
CLL/SLL	w	w	w	+	–	+	–/w	w	–	–/w	–	+ bright	+	–*	–
B-PLL	+	+	+	–	–	v	v	–	–	+	–	–/+	U	–	U
MCL	+	+	+	–, w	–	+	+	–	–	+	–	–/+	–	+	+/–
FL	+	+	+	–	–	–	+	–	+	+	–	+ dim/mod	–	–	–
SMZL	+	+	+	–	–	v	+	v	v	+	–	+ dim/mod	–	–	–
HCL	+	+	+	–	+	–	+	+	s	–	+	+ bright	–	+s	–
LPL	+/CIg+	+	+	–	–	–	–	–	–	+	–	+/– dim	–	–	–

*Proliferation centers in CLL/SLL may be weakly cyclin D1 positive.

+s, Subset of cases positive; *B-PLL*, B-prolymphocytic leukemia; *CIg*, cytoplasmic immunoglobulin; *CLL/SLL*, chronic lymphocytic leukemia/small lymphocytic lymphoma; *FL*, follicular lymphoma; *HCL*, hairy cell leukemia; *LPL*, lymphoplasmacytic; *MCL*, mantle cell lymphoma; *SMZL*, splenic marginal zone lymphoma; *U*, unknown; *v*, variable expression; *w*, weakly expressed.

Data from Sander B, Campo E, Hsi ED. Chronic lymphocytic leukaemia/small lymphocytic lymphoma and mantle cell lymphoma: from early lesions to transformation. *Virchows Arch.* 2023 Jan;482(1):131-145. *Erratum in: Virchows Arch.* 2023 Jan 12; Falini B, Martino G, Lazzi S. A comparison of the International Consensus and 5th World Health Organization classifications of mature B-cell lymphomas. *Leukemia.* 2022 Dec 2; Cook JR. Nodal and leukemic small B-cell neoplasms. *Mod Pathol.* 2013 Jan;26 Suppl 1:S15-28; Gradowski JF, Sargent RL, Craig FE, et al. Chronic lymphocytic leukemia/small lymphocytic lymphoma with cyclin D1 positive proliferation centers do not have CCND1 translocations or gains and lack SOX11 expression. *Am J Clin Pathol.* 2012 Jul;138(1):132-139; Foucar K. Mature B- and T-cell lymphoproliferative neoplasms. In: Foucar K, Reichard R, Czuchlewski D. *Bone Marrow Pathology*, 4th Ed. ASCP Press; Laurent C, Cook JR, Yoshino T, et al. Follicular lymphoma and marginal zone lymphoma: how many diseases? *Virchows Arch.* 2023 Jan;482(1):149-162.

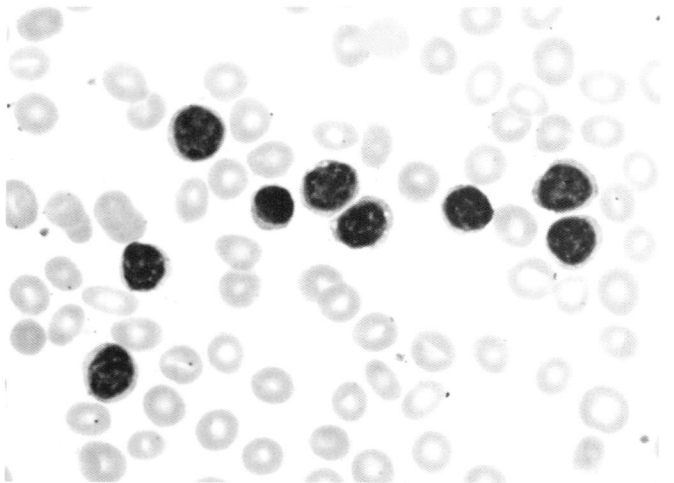

Figure 13-24. Peripheral blood smear from a patient with mantle cell lymphoma reveals uniform lymphoma cells that morphologically mimic chronic lymphocytic leukemia (Wright's stain).

FL reveals a characteristic paratrabecular infiltrate. The morphologic pattern of bone marrow involvement in B-CLPN is summarized in Table 13-6.[2,4,10,56,207]

In the lymph node, CLL exhibits diffuse effacement with scattered proliferation centers, while MCL and FL usually have a nodular pattern. MZL/splenic MZL (MZL/SMZL) demonstrates expansion of the marginal zone. Rarely, HCL may involve lymph nodes with either diffuse replacement or medullary infiltration.

In the spleen, CLL exhibits primarily white pulp disease with secondary red pulp involvement. MCL and FL also typically involve white pulp, while SMZL also involves white pulp with expansion of the marginal zone. Importantly, both HCL and HCLv involve primarily red pulp with distinctive blood lake formation in HCL. The morphologic features of B-CLPN in the lymph node and spleen are summarized in Table 13-5.[1,2,10,47,56,207]

IP is critical to distinguish these entities. CLL and MCL characteristically co-express CD5. Flow-cytometric analysis is helpful in most cases to distinguish CLL from MCL with dim surface immunoglobulin, dim CD20 expression, presence of CD23 and CD200, and absence of FMC7. In a minority of cases, distinction between CLL and non-nodal leukemic MCL is challenging in that these leukemic MCL cells can be CD23 positive, CD200 positive, and SOX11 negative or FMC7 negative, closely mimicking CLL.[74,208,209] The major immunologic differences of CLL and MCL are summarized in Table 13-2. Cytogenetic assessment for t(11;14) is essential in these cases to confirm MCL. Co-expression of CD10 and absence of CD5 by IP is most supportive of a diagnosis of FL. HCL, HCLv, and SMZL are typically CD5 negative and CD10 negative. Flow-cytometric IP reveals expression of T-cell lineage markers in T-PLL. The classic immunophenotypic profile of B-CLPN is summarized in Table 13-7.[1,2,56,207]

Accurate diagnosis of CLL is paramount in guiding clinical management of the patient. Despite the characteristic morphologic and immunophenotypic findings in most cases, a small subset may have atypical morphology or IP and pose a diagnostic challenge.

MONOCLONAL B-CELL LYMPHOCYTOSIS

Definition of Disease

The widespread use of sensitive flow cytometric screening techniques has enabled the detection of small monoclonal B-cell populations in healthy individuals. The term *monoclonal B-cell lymphocytosis (MBL)* is used to describe asymptomatic clonal expansions of B cells where the neoplastic cell count is less than 5×10^9/L.[1,3,210] MBL is the precursor lesion for CLL.[1,3] The majority of MBL cases show an IP that is indistinguishable from CLL, whereas smaller subsets have an aCLL IP or a non-CLL IP. ICC also includes a tissue-based MBL as an incidental nodal finding of an infiltrate of CLL-type cells without proliferation centers in individuals without significant lymphadenopathy.[1,30,31,46] The ICC and proposed WHO 5th ed. separate MBL into low-count MBL of $<0.5 \times 10^9$/L and high-count CLL/SLL-type MBL when the cell count is >0.5 and $<5 \times 10^9$/L.[1,3]

The majority of these clones exhibit an IP similar to that seen in CLL and share many of the same chromosomal and molecular abnormalities.[1] However, cases corresponding to aCLL and other B-cell neoplasms have been identified. Many cases, particularly those with low counts, do not progress to CLL and may represent a normal progression of immunosenescence. The relative risk to progression to overt CLL is approximately 1%/year.[211] Monoclonal B-cell populations can be found in as many as 3.5% of individuals over the age of 40. As the immune system ages, the B-cell population becomes more limited in its immunoglobulin gene repertoire. This leads to an increased incidence of observed clonal populations in chronic infection such as hepatitis C.[212] Monoclonal T-cell populations are also observed in MBL patients, further indicating the presence of immune system dysregulation.[6]

Diagnosis of MBL is more challenging with bone marrow or lymph node involvement. Bone marrow and tissue may show infiltrates of neoplastic B cells with CLL features in the absence of PB involvement or significant lymphadenopathy.[2,31] Patients should not be symptomatic or have lymphadenopathy or other evidence of lymphoma. Specific morphologic features supporting a diagnosis of tissue-based MBL are discussed further. Only a small fraction of patients with MBL progress to CLL; however, retrospective analysis of blood samples obtained prior to diagnosis from CLL patients demonstrates B-cell clones consistent with MBL in the majority of specimens. Patients with low-count MBL are unlikely to progress to overt leukemia/lymphoma, with a risk of 4.3-fold compared with the general population. CLL/SLL-type high count MBL patients have a significantly increased risk of progression of 75-fold, and require clinical monitoring.[210]

Epidemiology and Incidence

Population screening demonstrates that 3% to 4% of healthy adults have monoclonal B-cell populations in the PB. Interestingly, this incidence increases strikingly with age, with MBL being virtually non-existent in individuals younger than 40 years, slowly increasing to nearly 30% of individuals in their 80s, but present in 42% of patients older than 90 years.[210] The true incidence of MBL is difficult to determine, as the greater the sensitivity of the assay used for detection, the greater the number of cases with very low monoclonal B-cell counts identified. For example, a population study using four-color flow cytometry with a minimum of 200,000 events identified a frequency of 3.5% in patients older than 40 years,[213] whereas a study using eight-color flow and analyzing 5×10^6 events report a frequency of 12% in the same age group.[214] The majority of MBL cases have low neoplastic cell counts and no absolute lymphocytosis. A study looking only at cases with borderline or elevated lymphocyte count identified an incidence rate of 3.5 per 100,000.[215] There is an increased risk of MBL in family members of patients with sporadic CLL and in families with inherited CLL predisposition.[211,216]

Clinical Features

MBL occurs by definition in an asymptomatic individual, and is therefore usually an incidental finding. A subset of patients is identified because of detection of lymphocytosis on a routine CBC. The majority of patients, however, do not exhibit an absolute lymphocytosis and are detected by flow cytometry. Clinically, these patients are often monitored for progression to overt CLL; however, the utility of close follow-up in low-count MBL is low.

Morphology

Peripheral Blood

In the PB, MBL is characterized by mature lymphocytes, which are usually similar to those identified in CLL, with homogeneous features; small, round nuclei; condensed nuclear chromatin; and scant cytoplasm. Because of the lower

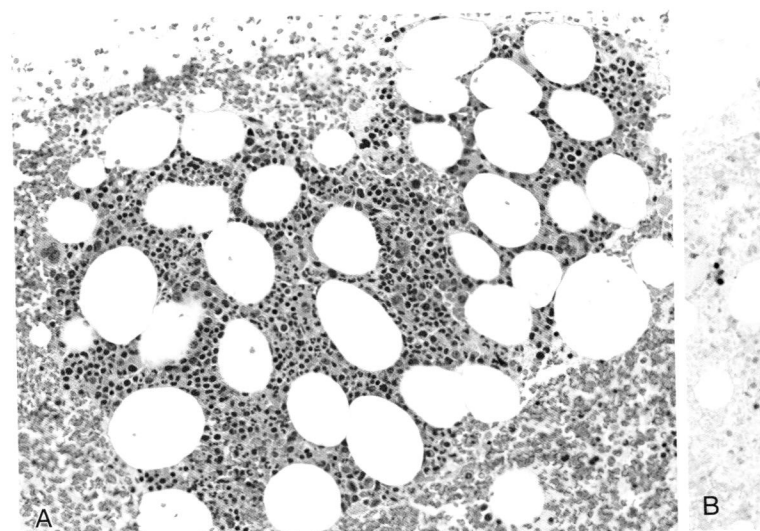
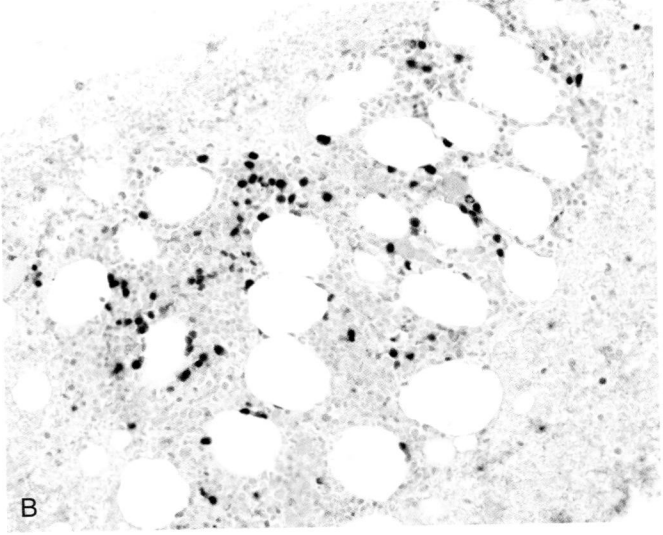

Figure 13-25. A, Clot section from a patient with clinically indolent mantle cell lymphoma (MCL) illustrates bone marrow with trilineage hematopoiesis an obvious lymphoid infiltrate. **B,** Cyclin D1 stain of the clot sections exhibits scattered positive MCL cells (H&E and cyclin D1 stain).

neoplastic cell counts in MBL, however, the neoplastic cells are generally inconspicuous on peripheral smear review.

Bone Marrow

Bone marrow biopsy is not generally performed in patients with MBL; however, MBL in the bone marrow may be identified as an incidental finding in biopsies performed for other indications. Patients with PB MBL almost always exhibit identifiable bone marrow involvement.[31] Neither the ICC nor the proposed WHO 5th ed. define limits of bone marrow involvement by monoclonal B cells that support a diagnosis of CLL versus MBL, and in some cases of MBL with <5 × 10⁹/L PB involvement there is significant disease in the marrow. In the ICC, the finding of cytopenias with bone marrow involvement by monoclonal B cells supports a diagnosis of CLL rather than MBL. Percent of bone marrow involvement in MBL is highly variable, ranging between 4.5% and 81% in one study of 30 cases.[31] Multiple patterns of infiltration in the core biopsy specimen have been identified, with most cases exhibiting either small, interstitial foci of neoplastic cells or scattered neoplastic cells identifiable only by immunohistochemistry (Figs. 13-26 and 13-27). Occasional cases may show a focal interstitial infiltrate. Diffuse involvement has been rarely identified. The pattern of infiltration may differ with the IP of the neoplastic cells, although this association has not been confirmed in all studies. CD5-negative MBLs are more common in the bone marrow than in the PB.[217] The presence of bone marrow involvement by known MBL or identification of small monoclonal populations of B cells in the marrow in the absence of other suspicion for lymphoma should not prompt a diagnosis of lymphoma.

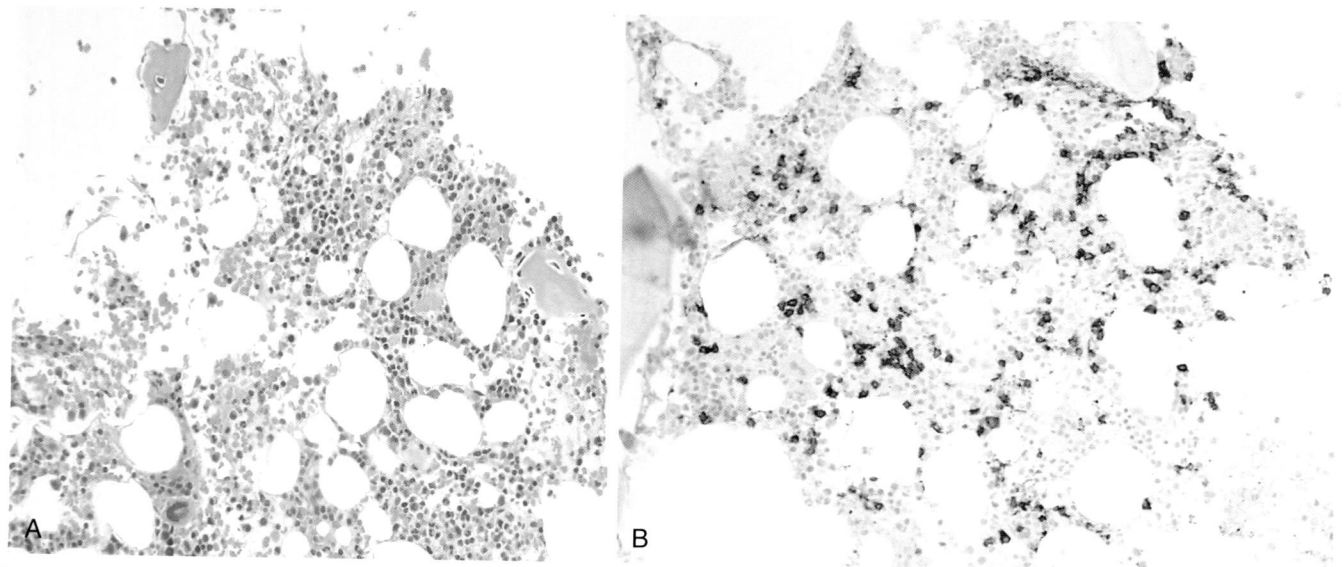

Figure 13-26. A, Bone marrow core biopsy from a patient with monoclonal B-cell lymphocytosis shows no obvious morphologic involvement by neoplastic lymphocytes. **B,** CD20 immunostain highlights increased numbers of scattered B cells, which were monoclonal by flow cytometry (H&E and CD20 stain).

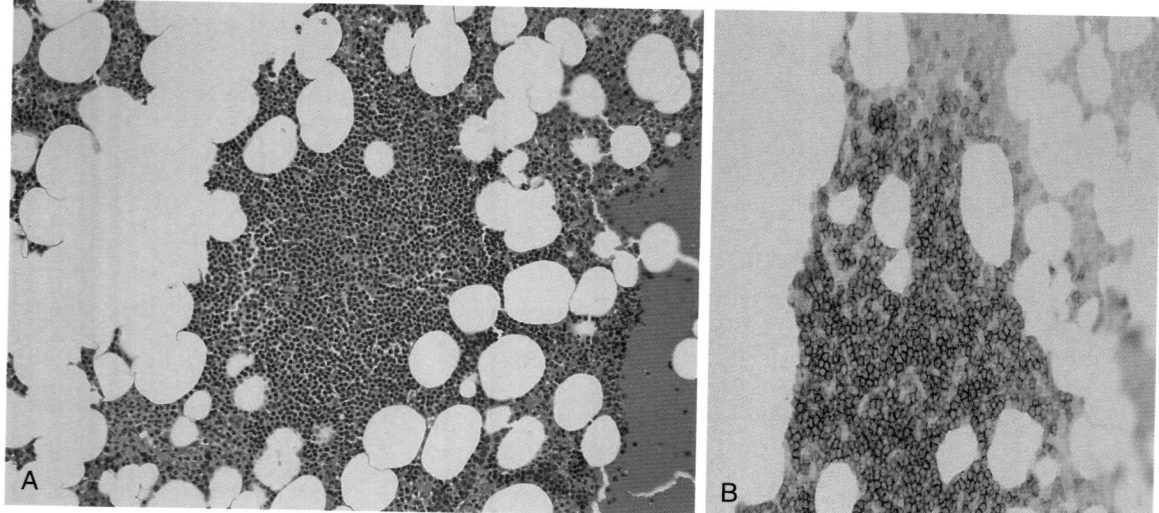

Figure 13-27. A, Bone marrow clot section from a patient with monoclonal B-cell lymphocytosis shows rare small, well-circumscribed nonparatrabecular lymphoid aggregates. Other features of lymphoma were not present. **B,** CD19 immunostain highlights a predominance of B cells in the aggregate, which were monoclonal by flow cytometry (H&E and CD19 stain).

Lymphoid aggregates are seen in approximately half of patients with MBL and are usually small, well circumscribed, and non-paratrabecular; composed of small lymphocytes; and account for less than 5% of marrow cellularity. In most cases, these aggregates appear to be composed of mixed B cells and T cells and are indistinguishable from benign lymphoid aggregates in the absence of supporting flow-cytometric or IHC confirmation of aberrant phenotype. A subset of cases shows B-cell predominance in the aggregates suspicious for lymphoma.[217] Rare cases of MBL may show significant involvement, and firm cutoffs for percent involvement in the bone marrow have not been validated.

Lymph Node

The diagnosis of MBL in lymph node specimens can be problematic because of concern for SLL. In lymph nodes with MBL, the nodes are generally removed for other reasons including staging for carcinoma, as the presence of lymphadenopathy caused by the B-cell population precludes the diagnosis of MBL. Lymph nodes should be less than 1.5 cm in size and usually show infiltration by small, mature lymphocytes with round nuclei and clumped chromatin. These cells are difficult to distinguish by morphology alone and are typically identified by flow cytometry or IHC. There should be no distortion of architecture and an interfollicular and intersinusoidal pattern with preservation of follicles and sinuses is most common.[30,31] Occasional cases show a follicular pattern with infiltration of germinal centers. The presence of proliferation centers with CLL IP supports a diagnosis of overt SLL. Other morphologic features, including percentage of lymph node involvement, do not correlate with disease behavior and should not be used to distinguish between SLL and MBL.[46]

Immunophenotype

The majority of MBL exhibit an IP similar to that seen in CLL, with expression of CD5, CD23, dim CD20, and dim surface immunoglobulin (Fig. 13-28). Additional cases show a pattern similar to that seen in aCLL, with expression of CD5 and bright CD20 and variable CD23, with bright surface immunoglobulin. Finally, cases may show a "non-CLL" phenotype with negative CD5. These cases may represent a similar population to CD5-negative CLL or may correlate with a marginal zone B-cell process. There should not be immunophenotypic markers specific for a lymphoproliferative disorder such as HCL. Expression of ZAP70 and CD38 may correlate with progression to CLL.[31]

Genetic and Molecular Features

In general, MBL cases, including both low-count and high-count cases, show the same cytogenetic abnormalities at similar rates as those seen in CLL in most studies, including 13q deletion, trisomy 12, del11q, and del17p.[218] Although individual studies have identified differences in the incidence of specific cytogenetic abnormalities in low-stage CLL and MBL, these have not been confirmed by other studies.[219-221] In addition, cytogenetic abnormalities do not clearly predict MBL progression to overt CLL, although trisomy 12 may be associated with shorter time to treatment.[31,212]

Studies of somatic gene mutations in MBL have demonstrated mutations in similar genes and frequencies as in CLL, including in *SF3B1*, *NOTCH1*, *DDX3X*, *BIRC3*, and *ATM*.[31,222,223] Mutations in *NOTCH1*, *TP53*, and *XPO1* seem to be present at a lower frequency than in CLL.[224,225] This finding is not unexpected, as the frequency of these mutations is low at diagnosis of CLL and increases over the disease course. These driver mutations are more common in high-count MBL. Identification of clonal expansion can distinguish cases of MBL with increased risk of progression to overt leukemia/lymphoma.[224]

Although the cytogenetic and somatic mutation profiles of MBL and CLL are similar, there are differences in immunoglobulin variant chain usage and IGHV mutational status. MBL cases show hypermutation in 70% of cases and hypermutation is more frequent in low-count MBL. The most frequently used IGHV segment in MBL is IGHV4-59/61, which is rarely seen in overt CLL. The segments commonly seen in CLL, IGHV4-34 and IGHV1-69, are only infrequently seen in MBL.[226] In addition, low-count MBL cases do not show the phenomenon of stereotyped receptors as observed in CLL; however, their usage can be identified in high-count MBL.[227] This may provide opportunity for identifying patients who may benefit from closer monitoring because of usage of CLL-associated IGHV segments or presence of stereotyped receptors.

Clinical Course and Prognosis

The vast majority of MBL cases, particularly those with low lymphocyte counts, remain stable over time and do not progress to CLL. The 5-year risk for needing therapy has been reported to be 7% in low count MBL (~1% per year) compared with 14% (~5% per year) for Rai 0 stage CLL.[228] In earlier studies, high count MBL carried a risk for progressing to CLL requiring treatment of about 1% per year.[159] The presence of cytogenetic or molecular abnormalities does not reliably correlate with the risk for progression; however, the specific IGHV segments used in the clone may provide some indication of likelihood of progression. Clonal expansion does correlate with progression.[224,229] Currently, the most reliable predictive factor is the absolute monoclonal lymphocyte count.

Although overt immune dysregulation and increased infection support a diagnosis of CLL and should not be present in MBL, MBL patients show an increased rate of hospitalization for infection compared with unaffected individuals. This risk is greater than the risk for progression to CLL, and MBL patients may benefit from increased surveillance for infection rather than lymphocyte count.[230] In addition, MBL patients show decreased vaccine response and may require additional doses to achieve seroconversion.[231]

B-CELL PROLYMPHOCYTIC LEUKEMIA

B-PLL is a topic of ongoing debate. The two newly published hematolymphoid classification systems have provided different opinions on this entity. The ICC[1,2] has retained this entity as a diagnosis of exclusion. However, the proposed WHO 5th ed.[3] has deleted this entity and has reassigned most of these cases into three categories: MCL, prolymphocytic progression

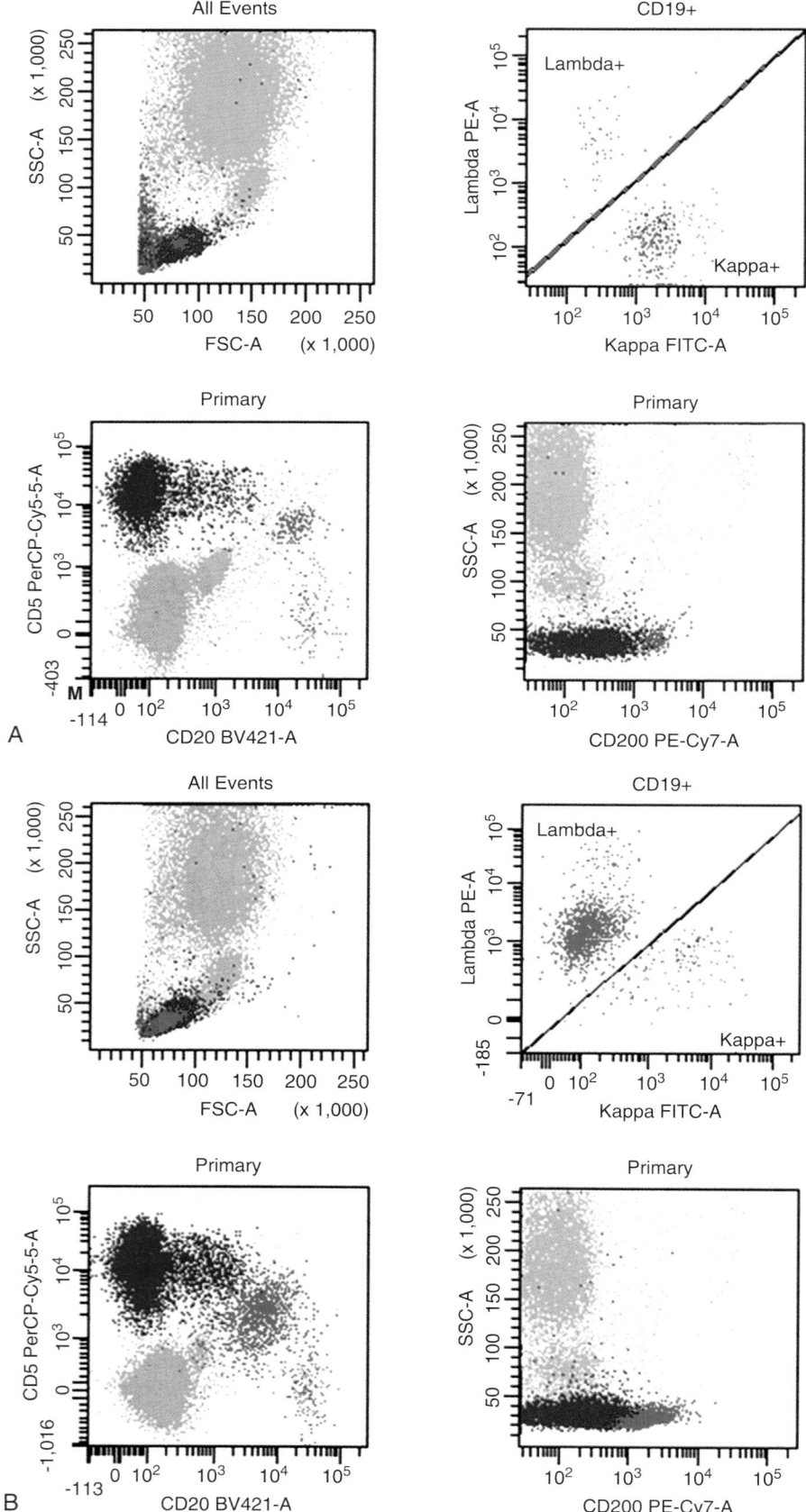

Figure 13-28. Low **(A)** and high **(B)** count monoclonal B lymphocytosis are illustrated. Patients with high count MBL should be monitored for possible progression to CLL.

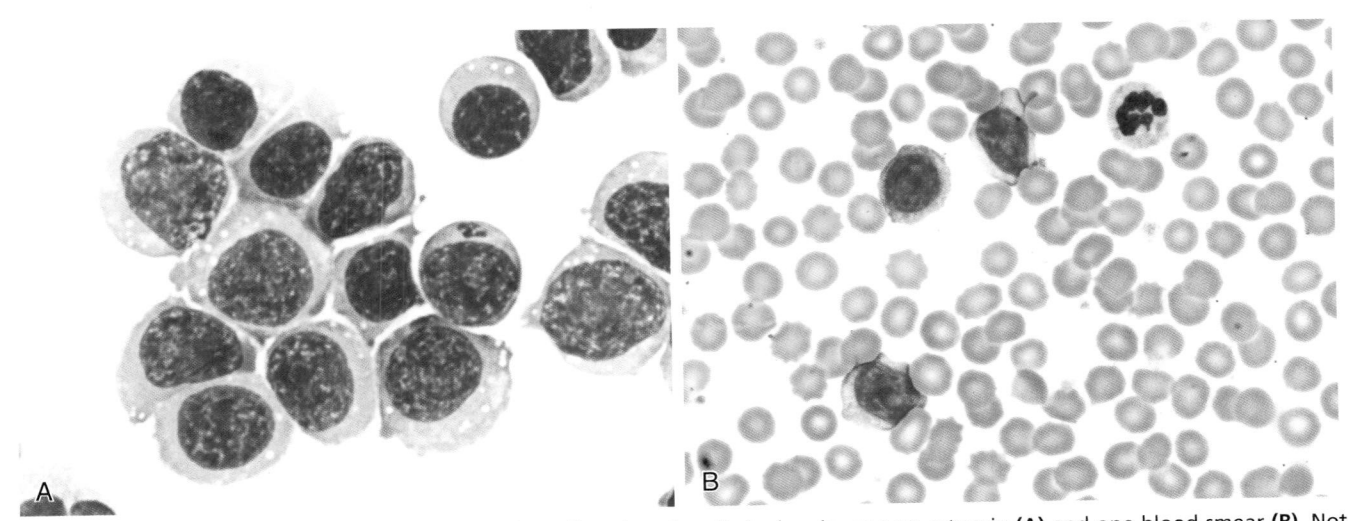

Figure 13-29. This composite illustrates two cases of B-cell prolymphocytic leukemia, one on cytospin **(A)** and one blood smear **(B)**. Note predominance of prolymphocytes (Wright's stain).

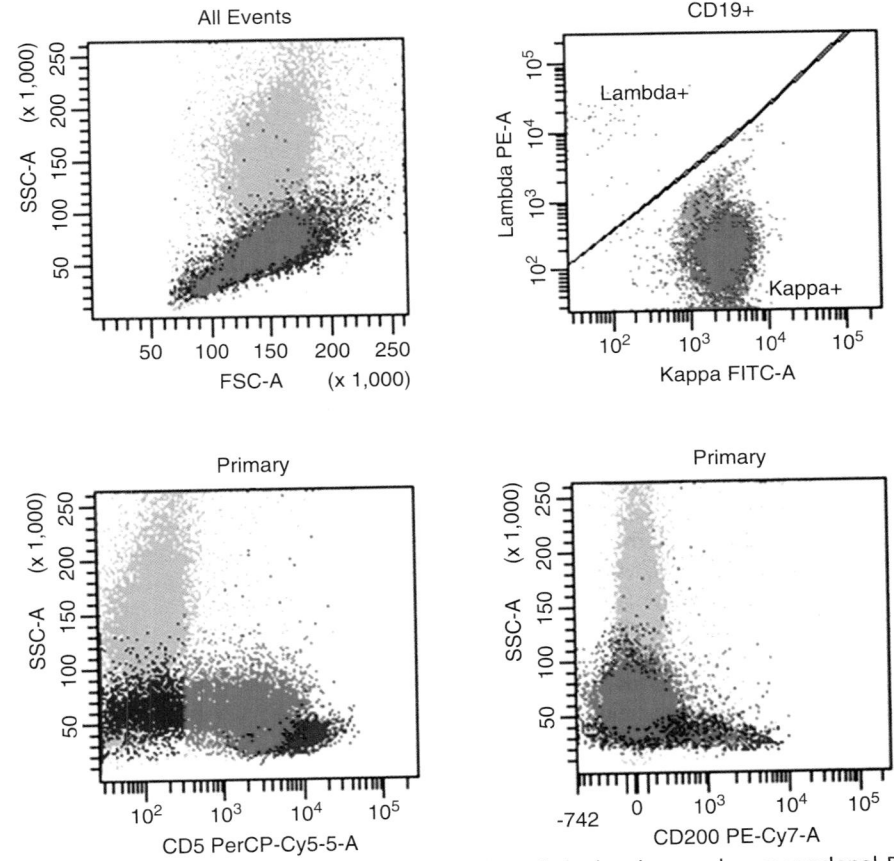

Figure 13-30. Flow cytometric immunophenotyping in B-cell prolymphocytic leukemia reveals a monoclonal B-cell population without distinctive features; this case shows CD5 co-expression, which is seen on about 30% of cases. CD200 is negative.

of CLL (with >15% of prolymphocytes in the blood), and the new entity splenic B-cell lymphoma/leukemia with prominent nucleoli.[3]

Definition: B-PLL is a neoplasm of B prolymphocytes affecting the PB, bone marrow, and spleen. Prolymphocytes must exceed 55% of lymphoid cells in the PB (Fig. 13-29).[2]

Clinical presentation: Patients with B-PLL typically present with rapid onset of B symptoms, marked lymphocytosis (usually >100 × 10^9/L), and massive splenomegaly. Lymphadenopathy is usually not prominent. CNS involvement is rare. A small subset of patients may experience insidious onset of disease and may have a more indolent disease course. The median age at diagnosis is ~72 years old with slight male predominance (60%) and ~82.6% of patients are White.[232,233]

Diagnosis: B-PLL is a diagnosis of exclusion. The diagnosis is made by integrating morphology, IP, and applying genetic assessment. The criteria require >55% prolymphocytes on the PB smear review. Prolymphocytes are intermediate to large cells with moderate light blue cytoplasm, mostly round to occasionally irregular nuclei, slightly open chromatin, and usually prominent central nucleoli. IP of B-PLL shows clonal B-cells with bright CD20 and surface immunoglobulin (SIg). They express surface IgM, CD19, CD22, HLA-DR, CD79b, and FMC7. CD5 is expressed in 20% to 30% and CD23 is expressed in 10% to 20% of cases (Fig. 13-30). The IP is not specific, and it overlaps with CLL and many other B-cell non-Hodgkin lymphomas (B-NHL).

Genetics: Chapiro et al.[233] conducted the largest B-PLL case series with genetic characterization. In this study karyotype, FISH, whole-exome sequencing, targeted deep sequencing, IGHV analysis, RNA sequencing, and in vitro cell viability and programmed cell death assays were performed in 34 patients with B-PLL. Complex karyotype (>3 abnormalities) was present in 73% of patients. High complex karyotype (>5 abnormalities) was seen in 45%. Translocations of *MYC* were the most frequent aberrations (62%), followed by 17p deletion (38%), trisomy 18 (30%), 13q deletion (29%), trisomy 3 (24%), trisomy 12 (24%), and 8p deletion (23%). Twenty-six patients (76%) exhibited *MYC* translocations or gains, which are mutually exclusive.

Molecular studies: Whole exome sequencing identified frequent mutations in *TP53, MYD88, BCOR, MYC, SF3B1, SETD2, CHD2, CXCR4,* and *BCLAF1*. The majority of cases (79%) were IGHV mutated and most cases used IGHV3 or IGHV4 subgroups.

Differential diagnosis: The main differential diagnosis includes CLL with prolymphocytoid transformation, leukemic, non-nodal MCL, lymphoplasmacytic lymphoma, HCL, HCL variant, and SMZL. A comprehensive approach including morphology, IP, cytogenetic studies, and molecular studies is used to exclude these better characterized entities.

Prognosis: The prognosis of B-PLL is largely dependent on the *TP53* mutational status. *TP53* aberration is associated with chemotherapy resistance and worse outcome. The presence of anemia and marked lymphocytosis (>100 × 10⁹/L) are also associated with adverse prognosis. IGHV mutations status and expression of ZAP70 or CD38 have no prognostic significance. In an earlier study, the median OS is about 3 years.[234,235] With the incorporation of small molecule targeted therapy, the OS has improved substantially. In Chapiro's cohort, the median OS for the entire cohort was 125.7 months. Patients with B-PLL with *MYC* aberrations have inferior OS compared with patients whose B-PLL lacked *MYC* aberration. Patients with both *MYC* and 17p deletion had the shortest OS. Patients with *MYC* but not 17p deletion have intermediate OS and patients without either aberration have the best prognosis.[233]

Treatment: The treatment of B-PLL is largely based on *TP53* status. Patients with wild-type *TP53* B-PLL should be considered for chemoimmunotherapy. Patients with *TP53* mutations are typically resistant to chemotherapy and targeted therapy with small molecules should be considered.[235] A combination of ibrutinib, idelalisib, or venetoclax with OTX015 yielded better efficacy than individual agent therapy, particularly in patients with *MYC* translocations. Patients who were treated with ibrutinib alone or in combination with other agents had a variable outcome.[236-238]

Pearls and Pitfalls

Pearls

- Successful diagnosis of chronic lymphocytic leukemia/small lymphocytic lymphoma (CLL/SLL) requires the integration of morphologic and immunophenotypic properties (especially multicolor flow-cytometric immunophenotyping)
- Cyclin D1 expression has a high sensitivity and reasonable high specificity for mantle cell lymphoma (MCL); diffuse cyclin D1 positivity excludes a diagnosis of CLL/SLL and B-cell prolymphocytic leukemia (B-PLL); proliferation centers in CLL/SLL may be weakly cyclin D1-positive
- Proliferation centers in lymph node sections are a reasonably specific feature of CLL/SLL, even if some nuclear irregularity is noted; proliferation centers are less commonly noted in bone marrow core biopsy sections
- Expanded, highly proliferative proliferation centers are an adverse feature in lymph nodes involved by accelerated CLL/SLL
- Prognostic assessment is essential in CLL and requires integration of CD49d/CD38 status by flow cytometry with multiple cytogenetic/molecular features
- Genetic prognostic factors are linked to clonal transformation
- CLL cases can acquire additional genetic mutations during the disease course
- Full genetic risk assessment is optimally performed at the time that the patient requires therapy
- CLL can undergo transformation to large B-cell lymphoma which is usually genetically associated with the underlying CLL—so-called "Richter transformation" (RT)
- Many adverse genetic features of the underlying CLL are linked to RT

Pitfalls

- In blood, bone marrow, and lymph node, it is critical to distinguish CLL/SLL from MCL
- Leukemic, non-nodal MCL can show substantial immunophenotypic overlap with CLL; consequently, FISH testing for t(11;14) should be considered in all cases in conjunction with the CLL FISH panel
- Leukemic MCL cases may be CD23 positive, CD200 positive, and SOX11 negative
- CLL and leukemic non-nodal MCL can also show significant morphologic overlap in blood and bone marrow
- Proliferation centers in CLL/SLL may be cyclin D1 positive
- Rare CLL cases with admixed Hodgkin (Reed-Sternberg) cells in tissue sections should be distinguished from overt Hodgkin lymphoma transformation; both of these CLL morphologic subtypes with Hodgkin (Reed-Sternberg) cells are linked to adverse outcome
- Leukemic, non-nodal MCL and prolymphocytic transformation of CLL must be excluded before a diagnosis of B-PLL is made

KEY REFERENCES

2. Sander B, Campo E, Hsi ED. Chronic lymphocytic leukaemia/small lymphocytic lymphoma and mantle cell lymphoma: from early lesions to transformation. *Virchows Arch.* 2023;482(1):131–145. *Erratum in: Virchows Arch.* 2023.

7. Kay NE, Hampel PJ, Van Dyke DL, et al. CLL update 2022: a continuing evolution in care. *Blood Rev.* 2022;54:100930.

9. Crassini K, Stevenson WS, Mulligan SP, Best OG. Molecular pathogenesis of chronic lymphocytic leukaemia. *Br J Haematol.* 2019;186(5):668–684.

19. Douglas M. Richter transformation: clinical manifestations, evaluation, and management. *J Adv Pract Oncol.* 2022;13(5):525–534.

35. Habermehl GK, Durkin L, Hsi ED. A tissue counterpart to monoclonal B-cell lymphocytosis. *Arch Pathol Lab Med.* 2021;145(12):1544–1551.

36. Ryder CB, Oduro KA, Moore EM. Monoclonal B-cell lymphocytosis in the bone marrow: revisiting the criteria for chronic lymphocytic leukemia/small lymphocytic lymphoma. *Hum Pathol.* 2022;125:108–116.

91. Vlachonikola E, Sofou E, Chatzidimitriou A, et al. The significance of B-cell receptor stereotypy in chronic lymphocytic leukemia: biological and clinical implications. *Hematol Oncol Clin North Am.* 2021;35(4):687–702.

92. Liu YC, Margolskee E, Allan JN, et al. Chronic lymphocytic leukemia with TP53 gene alterations: a detailed clinicopathologic analysis. *Mod Pathol.* 2020;33(3):344–353.

95. Baliakas P, Espinet B, Mellink C, et al. Cytogenetics in chronic lymphocytic leukemia: ERIC perspectives and recommendations. *Hemasphere.* 2022;6(4):e707.

154. Agathangelidis A, Chatzidimitriou A, Chatzikonstantinou T, et al. The European Research Initiative on CLL. Immunoglobulin gene sequence analysis in chronic lymphocytic leukemia: the 2022 update of the recommendations by ERIC, the European Research Initiative on CLL. *Leukemia.* 2022;36(8):1961–1968.

162. Parviz M, Brieghel C, Agius R, et al. Prediction of clinical outcome in CLL based on recurrent gene mutations, CLL-IPI variables, and (para)clinical data. *Blood Adv.* 2022;6(12):3716–3728.

163. Lad DP, Tejaswi V, Jindal N, et al. Modified CLL International Prognostic Index (CLL-LIPI) using lymphocyte doubling time (LDT) in place of IgHV mutation status in resource-limited settings predicts time to first treatment and overall survival. *Leuk Lymphoma.* 2020;61(6):1512–1515.

192. Abrisqueta P, Delgado J, Alcoceba M, et al. Clinical outcome and prognostic factors of patients with Richter syndrome: real-world study of the Spanish Chronic Lymphocytic Leukemia Study Group (GELLC). *Br J Haematol.* 2020;190(6):854–863.

196. King RL, Gupta A, Kurtin PJ, et al. Chronic lymphocytic leukemia (CLL) with Reed-Sternberg-like cells vs classic Hodgkin lymphoma transformation of CLL: does this distinction matter? *Blood Cancer J.* 2022;12(1):18.

223. Tang C, Shen Y, Soosapilla A, et al. Monoclonal B-cell lymphocytosis—a review of diagnostic criteria, biology, natural history, and clinical management. *Leuk Lymphoma.* 2022;63(12):2795–2806.

224. Barrio S, Shanafelt TD, Ojha J, et al. Genomic characterization of high-count MBL cases indicates that early detection of driver mutations and subclonal expansion are predictors of adverse clinical outcome. *Leukemia.* 2017;31(1):170–176.

233. Chapiro E, Pramil E, Diop M, et al. The Groupe Francophone de Cytogénétique Hématologique (GFCH); the French Innovative Leukemia Organization (FILO). Genetic characterization of B-cell prolymphocytic leukemia: a prognostic model involving MYC and TP53. *Blood.* 2019;134(21):1821–1831.

Visit Elsevier eBooks+ for the complete set of references.

Chapter 14

Lymphoplasmacytic Lymphoma and Waldenström Macroglobulinemia

Aliyah R. Sohani

DEFINITION OF THE DISEASE

Lymphoplasmacytic lymphoma (LPL) is defined by the 2022 International Consensus Classification (ICC) as a mature small B-cell neoplasm composed of lymphocytes, plasma cells, and plasmacytic lymphocytes that does not meet criteria for any of the other small B-cell lymphomas that may also exhibit plasmacytic differentiation.[1] It typically involves bone marrow (and any amount of marrow involvement by abnormal lymphoplasmacytic aggregates qualifies for the diagnosis), but peripheral blood, lymph nodes, and spleen may also be involved. Waldenström macroglobulinemia (WM) is defined as LPL involving bone marrow associated with an IgM monoclonal paraprotein of any concentration and is found in the majority of patients with LPL. Many studies of LPL are reported as WM. There are LPL, however, that express IgG or IgA heavy chain, but they are less common. Most LPL cases lack expression of a specific immunophenotype related to antigens commonly assessed in the workup of B-cell malignancies, including CD5, CD10, CD23, and CD103.[1,2] Because of this feature and because plasmacytic differentiation may be seen in a number of small B-cell lymphomas, most commonly one of the subtypes of marginal zone lymphoma, a specific diagnosis of LPL may not always be possible, and some cases are best diagnosed as a small B-cell lymphoma with plasmacytic differentiation with a differential diagnosis provided. However, the diagnosis can be established with greater certainty by molecular analysis through the identification of a *MYD88* L265P somatic mutation, a recurrent finding in greater than 90% of LPL/WM and found in only a small proportion of marginal zone lymphomas.[3-5]

SYNONYMS AND RELATED TERMS

WHO revised 4th edition: Lymphoplasmacytic lymphoma
WHO proposed 5th edition: Lymphoplasmacytic lymphoma/Waldenström macroglobulinemia
Both the 2022 ICC and WHO revised 4th edition include Waldenström macroglobulinemia in the classification indented under LPL.

Related Entities

2022 International Consensus Classification: Immunoglobulin M (IgM) monoclonal gammopathy of undetermined significance (MGUS), plasma cell type and not otherwise specified (NOS)
WHO revised 4th edition: IgM MGUS
WHO proposed 5th edition: IgM MGUS

2022 International Consensus Classification: Primary cold agglutinin disease
WHO revised 4th edition: Associated B-cell lymphoma classified as LPL in subset of cases
WHO proposed 5th edition: Cold agglutinin disease

EPIDEMIOLOGY

LPL/WM is an uncommon lymphoid neoplasm, representing approximately 2% of non-Hodgkin lymphoma cases diagnosed in the United States between 1988 and 2007 according to Surveillance, Epidemiology and End Results (SEER) registry data.[6] The median age at diagnosis is 73 years with a male predominance.[6-8] The overall age-adjusted incidence is 3.8 per 1 million persons per year and incidence increases sharply with age.[6,7,9] A role for genetic factors in the pathogenesis of LPL/WM is suggested based on numerous reports of familial occurrence in case-control and larger cohort studies.[10-13] A study from Asia found lower incidence rates in Japan and Taiwan compared with rates reported in the literature for Asians living in the United States, suggesting that both environmental and genetic factors are involved in LPL/WM development.[9] Among environmental factors, chronic antigenic stimulation secondary to various autoimmune diseases or other inflammatory conditions has been implicated.[14] An etiologic role for hepatitis C virus (HCV) has also been suggested; however, this has not been shown in all studies, and a large study with both serologic and molecular genetic methods for HCV detection found no association with LPL/WM.[15]

CLINICAL FEATURES

The clinical manifestations of LPL/WM can be attributed to two main factors: the effects of the monoclonal IgM paraprotein and tissue infiltration by neoplastic cells. The monoclonal IgM paraprotein causes morbidity via several mechanisms related to its biochemical and immunologic properties, non-specific interactions with other proteins, antibody activity, and propensity to deposit in tissues.[16] The high concentration of monoclonal IgM molecules and their tendency to form pentamers can lead to serum hyperviscosity through binding of water and erythrocyte aggregation. Symptomatic hyperviscosity is seen in 10% to 30% of WM patients, and serum viscosity increases sharply at IgM concentrations of greater than 3 g/dL, with most patients manifesting symptoms at levels greater than 5 g/dL. Symptoms of hyperviscosity include headaches, visual disturbances, mental status changes, and, in severe cases, intracranial hemorrhage.[17-19] Cryoprecipitation of the monoclonal IgM (type I cryoglobulinemia) may be seen in up to 20% of patients, with a minority of such patients exhibiting symptoms of Raynaud phenomenon, acrocyanosis, or, less frequently, renal manifestations.[16,20] In other patients, the monoclonal IgM may behave as a type II cryoglobulin and demonstrate IgG autoantibody activity, leading to symptoms of purpura, arthralgias, renal insufficiency, and peripheral neuropathy.[16,21] Other autoantibody effects of the monoclonal IgM against red blood cell antigens may result in cold agglutinin hemolytic anemia, whereas binding of peripheral nerve constituents may lead to a sensorimotor neuropathy.[22-24] The latter manifestation is relatively common in WM, reported in 25% to nearly 50% of patients in some series.[23-25] Peripheral neuropathy may also be mediated by nonautoimmune effects

of the monoclonal IgM protein, secondary to fibrillar or tubular deposits in the endoneurium, amyloid deposition within nerves, or direct infiltration of nerve structures.[16] The monoclonal protein may also deposit in various other tissues as amorphous aggregates leading to dysfunction of affected organs.[16] Deposition of monoclonal light chain in the form of amyloid (primary amyloid light chain [AL] amyloidosis) is much less common in patients with WM, but may lead to similar types of organ dysfunction.[26]

Direct tissue infiltration by neoplastic cells is most common in the bone marrow, leading to peripheral cytopenias. At the time of presentation, the degree of anemia is typically more profound than other cytopenias, because the anemia in WM/LPL is multifactorial in nature and due in large part to increased plasma viscosity leading to inappropriately low erythropoietin production.[27] Other factors contributing to anemia include hemolysis, plasma volume expansion, and gastrointestinal blood loss in patients with involvement of that site.[16] Nodal and splenic involvement may be present, but bulky lymphadenopathy is uncommon and splenomegaly, if present, is typically mild to moderate in degree. Extramedullary and extranodal sites of disease involvement by LPL that have been reported include lung, soft tissue, skin, gastrointestinal and hepatobiliary tracts, kidney, and central nervous system (CNS).[28-32] Pulmonary involvement, seen in less than 5% of patients, may be in the form of nodules, masses, diffuse infiltrates, or pleural effusions, and results in symptoms of cough (most commonly), dyspnea, and chest pain.[29] Gastrointestinal disease may involve the stomach, duodenum, or small intestine, resulting in malabsorption, bleeding, or obstruction, whereas cutaneous involvement may result in chronic urticaria or in the formation of plaques or nodules.[16] Direct infiltration of the CNS, known as *Bing-Neel syndrome*, is a rare complication of LPL/WM that is characterized clinically by a variety of neurologic signs and symptoms, including mental status changes, headache, motor dysfunction, vertigo, impaired hearing, and, in some cases, coma.[16,29] Unlike in multiple myeloma, lytic bone lesions are not seen, and hypercalcemia is rare.

MORPHOLOGY

Peripheral Blood

Lymphocytosis may be present, but the absolute lymphocyte count is usually lower than in chronic lymphocytic leukemia (CLL) (Box 14-1). Circulating neoplastic cells have plasmacytic features with clumped chromatin, eccentric nuclei, and moderately abundant basophilic cytoplasm, occasionally with a paranuclear hof (Fig. 14-1).[33] Red cell agglutination and rouleaux formation may be present in patients with serum hyperviscosity caused by elevated IgM paraprotein.[34]

Bone Marrow

Bone marrow aspirate smears demonstrate lymphocytosis with a morphologic spectrum that includes small, round lymphocytes with clumped chromatin, plasmacytic lymphocytes, and plasma cells (Fig. 14-2A–B). Varying patterns of bone marrow involvement may be observed in core biopsy specimens, with interstitial and nodular infiltrates most commonly reported.[35-37] Less frequently, pure paratrabecular or diffuse patterns of marrow involvement may

Box 14-1 *Major Diagnostic Features of Lymphoplasmacytic Lymphoma*

Morphology
- Spectrum of small, round lymphocytes with clumped chromatin, lymphoplasmacytic cells, and plasma cells. Russell and Dutcher bodies may be present. Abnormal lymphoplasmacytic aggregates often associated with increased mast cells.
- Bone marrow: Interstitial and nodular infiltrates; paratrabecular or intrasinusoidal growth patterns rare.
- Peripheral blood: Circulating neoplastic cells have plasmacytic features with clumped chromatin, eccentric nuclei, and moderately abundant basophilic cytoplasm with occasional paranuclear hofs; cytoplasmic projections absent.
- Lymph node: Some cases with interfollicular infiltrates with subtotal architectural effacement and retention of primary or secondary follicles and preserved or dilated sinuses; other cases with complete architectural effacement and vaguely nodular growth occasionally with variable follicular colonization and focal monocytoid or marginal zone-like morphology.

Immunophenotype
- Lymphocytic component: Moderate expression of pan–B-cell antigens and monoclonal surface immunoglobulin.
- Plasmacytic/plasma cell component: Positive for cytoplasmic immunoglobulin and CD19, IRF4/MUM1, and CD138 of variable intensity in all or a subset of cells; negative for CD56.
- Moderate expression of CD200 by flow cytometry; CD25 and CD38 frequently expressed; typically negative for phenotypically distinctive markers of other small B-cell neoplasms, including CD5, CD10, CD23, CD103, LEF1, cyclin D1, SOX11, and DBA.44.
- Rare cases may be positive for CD5 or CD10. CD23 may also be expressed.
- Staining of other cell types: CD117-positive/tryptase-positive mast cells, CD21-positive or CD23-positive follicular dendritic cell aggregates.

Genetics
- *MYD88* L265P mutation most common and characteristic, although not specific for LPL: may be seen with relatively high frequency in other B-cell neoplasms, particularly diffuse large B-cell lymphoma (DLBCL) of immune-privileged sites, but infrequent in other small B-cell neoplasms.
- A minority of bona fide LPL lacks *MYD88* mutations, so its absence does not exclude the diagnosis. However, be more cautious in these cases to exclude other B-cell neoplasms with plasmacytic differentiation, particularly marginal zone lymphomas.
- *CXCR4* nonsense and frameshift mutations identified with relatively high frequency, usually in *MYD88*-mutated cases. *CXCR4* nonsense mutations associated with clinically aggressive disease and lower responsiveness to BTK inhibitors.
- Other commonly mutated genes include *ARID1A, TP53, CD79B, KMT2D,* and *BTK. TP53*-mutated cases are associated with clinically aggressive disease and shorter overall survival but remain responsive to ibrutinib. *BTK*-mutated and *MYD88* wild-type cases are less responsive to BTK inhibitors. Wild-type *MYD88* cases contain mutations downstream of BTK and have a higher risk of transformation to DLBCL.
- Other abnormalities associated with more aggressive disease include chromosome 6q deletion spanning a region that encodes for several regulatory genes involved in B-cell receptor signaling and apoptosis; 17p deletion resulting in *TP53* loss of heterozygosity; and karyotypic complexity.

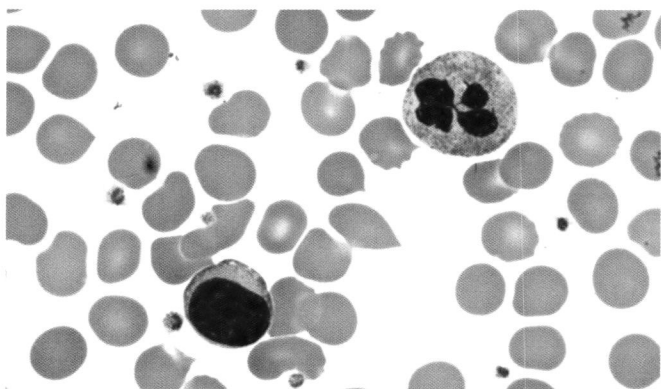

Figure 14-1. Peripheral blood findings in lymphoplasmacytic lymphoma. A circulating neoplastic lymphocyte *(bottom left)* shows features of plasmacytic differentiation with clumped chromatin, nuclear eccentricity, and moderately abundant cytoplasm with a paranuclear hof.

be seen.[35,36] The lymphoid aggregates are composed mainly of small lymphocytes with variable numbers of plasmacytic lymphocytes and plasma cells (Fig. 14-2C–E).[1,2] Plasmacytic differentiation may be reflected by the presence of Russell or Dutcher bodies (Fig. 14-3).[33] Increased mast cells are almost always present in association with the lymphoid aggregates, and their identification may be facilitated by tissue Giemsa stain or CD117 immunohistochemistry; however, this finding is not considered specific for the diagnosis of LPL (see Figs. 14-2F and 14-3B).[1,2,38]

The extent of marrow involvement by abnormal lymphoplasmacytic aggregates typically exceeds 10% of cellularity; however, in keeping with the diagnostic criteria proposed by the 2nd International Workshop on Waldenström Macroglobulinemia, the diagnosis may be made in cases with *any* amount of abnormal lymphoplasmacytic aggregates in the marrow and evidence of B-cell and plasma cell clonality, because even patients with limited marrow involvement may have symptoms of WM related to the monoclonal paraprotein or bone marrow infiltration.[39]

The pattern of bone marrow involvement may raise the differential diagnosis of other small B-cell neoplasms that more commonly involve the bone marrow, including CLL and follicular lymphoma. Distinction from these entities can be made readily on the basis of the immunophenotype of the neoplastic cells as noted (see "Immunophenotype"). In addition, although nodular aggregates may extend to paratrabecular locations and infrequent LPL cases with predominant paratrabecular patterns of involvement have been described, these paratrabecular aggregates are generally not associated with linear growth along bony trabeculae or fibrosis, as seen in bone marrow involvement by follicular lymphoma (see Fig. 14-2C).[35] Bone marrow involvement by marginal zone lymphoma presents a more challenging distinction, given its shared immunophenotype with LPL. Interstitial involvement is more commonly seen in LPL compared with marginal zone lymphoma.[35] In contrast to bone marrow involvement by splenic marginal zone lymphoma (SMZL), intrasinusoidal involvement is rare in LPL.[35,36] Assessment for the presence of the *MYD88* L265P mutation is helpful in difficult cases.[5] Cases with prominent plasmacytic differentiation may raise the differential diagnosis of multiple myeloma, particularly the small cell variant with

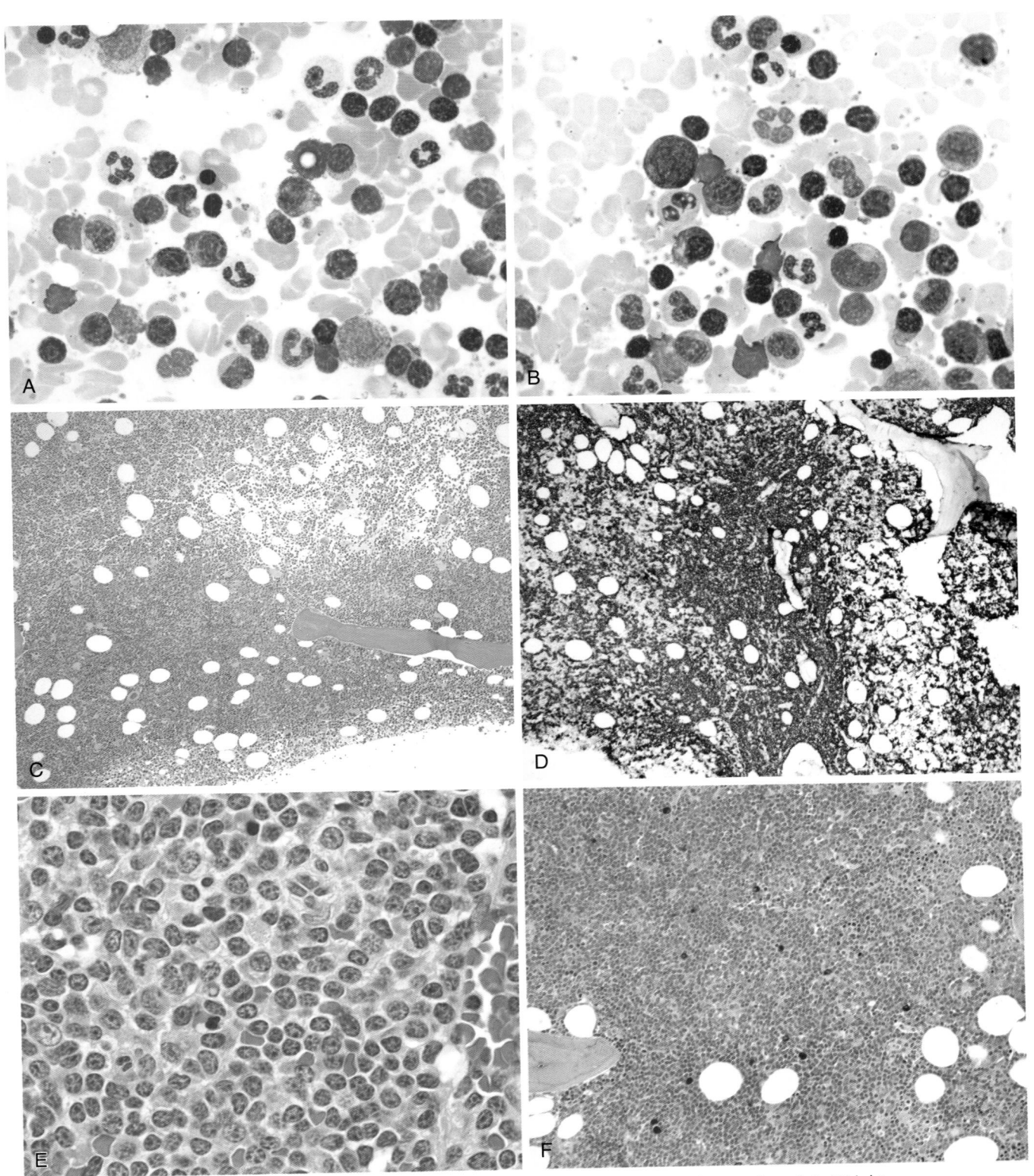

Figure 14-2. Bone marrow involvement by lymphoplasmacytic lymphoma. A and **B,** Wright-Giemsa–stained bone marrow aspirate smears demonstrate a lymphocytosis consisting of small, mature-appearing lymphocytes with clumped chromatin, including many plasmacytic forms. Rare plasma cells are present. **C,** Low magnification evaluation of the corresponding core biopsy specimen shows both interstitial and nodular lymphoid infiltrates, including a loose paratrabecular aggregate. **D,** CD20 immunohistochemical stain highlights the variable patterns of bone marrow involvement, as well as the extent of marrow disease in this case. **E,** Higher magnification demonstrates small lymphocytes with clumped chromatin, occasional plasmacytic lymphocytes, and rare plasma cells. **F,** Increased numbers of mast cells are highlighted by this Giemsa stain.

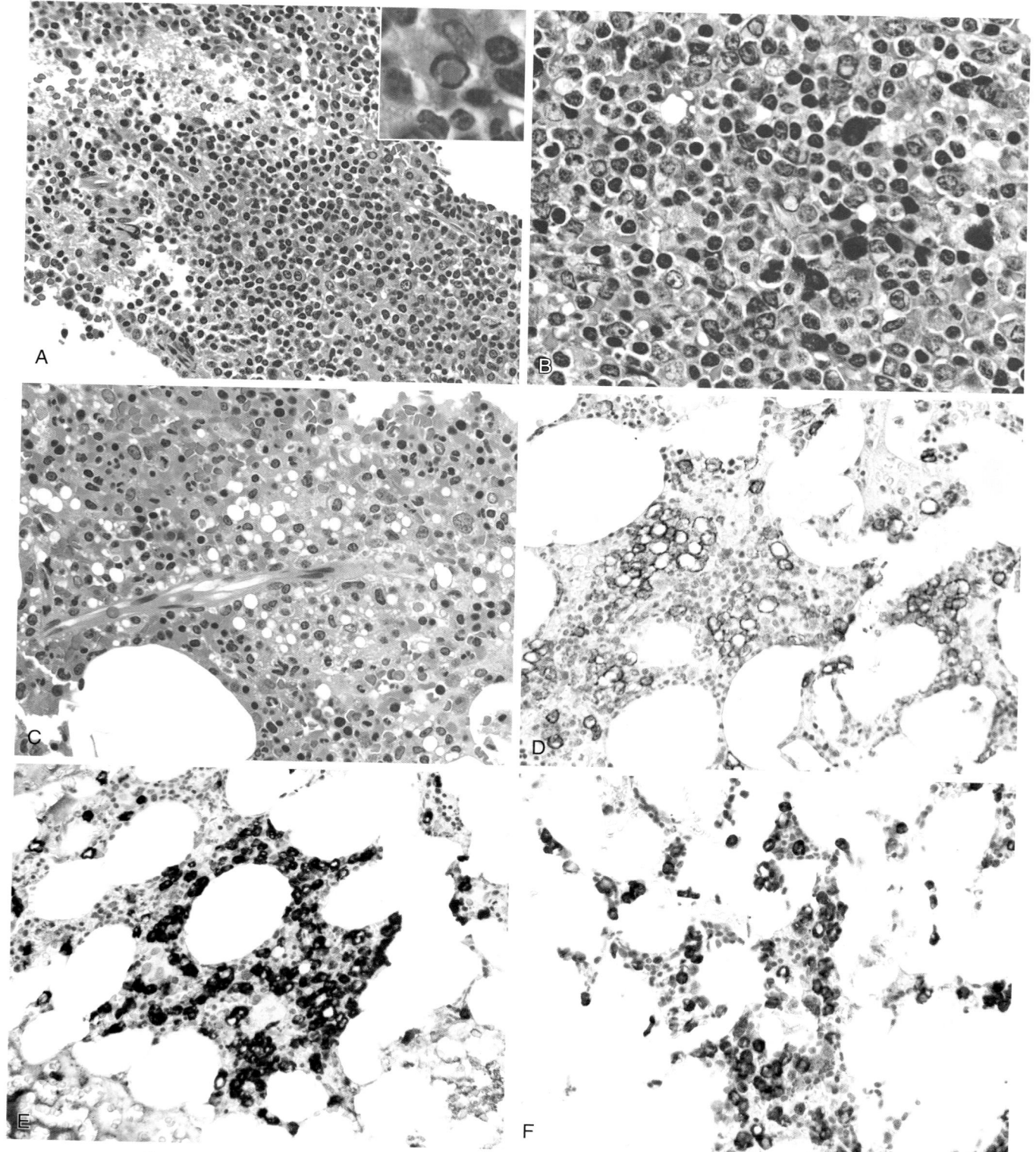

Figure 14-3. Examples of lymphoplasmacytic lymphoma with conspicuous plasmacytic differentiation. A, H&E-stained bone marrow core biopsy specimen of a case of lymphoplasmacytic lymphoma with noticeable immunoglobin pseudoinclusions overlying lymphocyte nuclei; these Dutcher bodies are positive on periodic acid–Schiff (PAS) stain (**A,** *inset*). **B,** Giemsa-stained bone marrow biopsy highlights frequent eccentric nuclei with paranuclear hofs and conspicuous mast cells. **C,** A different case of lymphoplasmacytic lymphoma with prominent clear cytoplasmic immunoglobulin deposits (Russell bodies) imparting a signet-ring appearance to the neoplastic cells. The lymphoplasmacytic cells were positive for CD138 **(D),** IgM **(E),** and kappa light chain **(F),** and were negative for lambda light chain (not shown).

lymphoplasmacytic morphology. The latter is distinguishable from LPL on the basis of its CD45-negative, CD19-negative, CD56-positive immunophenotype and frequent cyclin D1 positivity by immunohistochemistry corresponding to an underlying *CCND1* rearrangement detectable by fluorescence in situ hybridization (FISH).[40-43]

Lymph Nodes

In the classic pattern of nodal involvement, there is subtotal architectural effacement with retention of small primary or enlarged reactive follicles and patent or dilated sinuses (Fig. 14-4A).[2,4,28,33,37,44] The interfollicular areas contain a relatively monomorphic infiltrate of small lymphocytes, plasmacytic lymphocytes, and plasma cells, generally without prominent follicular colonization (Fig. 14-4B).

Following the identification of *MYD88* L265P mutation as being characteristic of LPL, mutational analysis in nodal lymphomas initially diagnosed as LPL, nodal marginal zone lymphoma (NMZL), and small B-cell lymphoma with plasmacytic differentiation have helped to refine the morphologic spectrum of nodal LPL. These studies show that some *MYD88* L265P–mutated cases demonstrate complete nodal architectural effacement, a vaguely nodular growth pattern, variably prominent follicular colonization, or focal areas containing pale monocytoid or marginal zone B cells (see Fig. 14-4C–F).[4,45] Cases harboring the *MYD88* L265P mutation had significantly more common bone marrow involvement, elevated serum IgM levels, and presence of a serum M component, suggesting that they represent true LPL cases despite the presence of morphologic features previously thought to be more characteristic of NMZL.[4,45]

In both the classic and effaced patterns, Dutcher bodies, increased numbers of mast cells, or hemosiderin deposition may be present. Only rare large transformed cells resembling immunoblasts are typically seen; these may be more numerous in some cases, but should not form large aggregates or sheets, in which case a diagnosis of transformation to diffuse large B-cell lymphoma (DLBCL) should be considered.[46] Other possible morphologic findings include the presence of extracellular deposits of immunoglobulin, in the form of amyloid or, more commonly, amorphous Congo red–negative amyloid-like material, or crystal-storing histiocytes. Pseudofollicles or proliferation centers, as seen in CLL/small lymphocytic lymphoma (SLL), are not a typical feature.

Spleen and Other Tissues

Splenic involvement by LPL has not been well described, but older published series and illustrated reviews support the presence of nodular and diffuse infiltrates of lymphoplasmacytic cells involving the red pulp, in a similar distribution to other small B-cell neoplasms with a leukemic pattern of dissemination.[28,47-49] The morphologic spectrum of the lymphoma cells, including small lymphocytes, plasma cells, and intermediate forms, is analogous to that seen in bone marrow and lymph node specimens (Fig. 14-5). This cytologic appearance may give rise to the differential diagnosis of SMZL, which may demonstrate plasmacytic differentiation in some cases. Pathologic features favoring a diagnosis of LPL over SMZL include relative sparing of the white pulp with absence of a marginal zone growth pattern,

absence of monocytoid or marginal zone–type cytology, and conspicuous plasmacytic differentiation that is usually readily apparent by both morphology and on immunohistochemical or in situ hybridization studies of tissue sections (see Fig. 14-5B–E).[48] In addition, LPL patients typically have higher IgM paraproteinemia and more extensive disease involving the bone marrow or lymph nodes, with secondary splenic involvement resulting in a milder degree of splenic enlargement compared with SMZL. Other small B-cell lymphoma entities with diffuse red pulp involvement that may enter into this differential diagnosis include hairy cell leukemia (HCL) and splenic diffuse red pulp small B-cell lymphoma (SDRPSBL). Distinction between LPL and HCL is usually straightforward on clinical, morphologic, and immunophenotypic grounds.[50] Although SDRPSBL cases may show subtle plasmacytic features, they usually lack strong features of plasmacytic differentiation such as cytoplasmic immunoglobulin deposition by immunohistochemistry or in situ hybridization.[51]

Common sites of extramedullary and extranodal disease were described (see "Clinical Features" above). Among the few histologic descriptions in the literature, LPL involving extramedullary sites may show some features that overlap with extranodal marginal zone lymphoma of mucosa-associated lymphoid tissue (EMZL), including the presence of nodular and diffuse infiltrates of lymphoplasmacytic cells, focal clusters of monocytoid B cells, and presence of Dutcher bodies.[28,30] However, in gastrointestinal sites such as the stomach and colon, lymphoepithelial lesions and colonization of preexisting follicles have not been described.[28,30] Skin biopsies have been reported to show interstitial, nodular, or diffuse dermal infiltration by lymphoplasmacytic cells with perinodal and periadnexal accentuation; focal epidermal ulceration may be present in rare cases.[28,52,53] Hepatic involvement, reported most often in cases with splenic disease, shows expansion of portal tracts and sinusoids by small plasmacytic lymphocytes (Fig. 14-6).[28] In cases of CNS involvement (Bing-Neel syndrome), cytologic evaluation of cerebrospinal fluid (CSF) specimens may show a lymphocytic pleocytosis consisting of plasmacytic lymphocytes and plasma cells, similar to the spectrum of cell populations seen in other tissues (Fig. 14-7A–B). Laboratory evaluation of such specimens via flow cytometry, electrophoresis, immunofixation, and *MYD88* L265P mutation analysis may help confirm the diagnosis (see Fig. 14-7C–F).[32,54,55] In some cases, however, the paucity or absence of neoplastic cells in CSF specimens, as in other subtypes of lymphoma involving the CNS, may preclude a definitive diagnosis, requiring brain biopsy.

IMMUNOPHENOTYPE

The lymphocytic component of LPL expresses moderate levels of pan–B-cell antigens, including CD19, CD20, CD22, CD79a, PAX5, and FMC7, as well as monotypic surface light chain (see Figs. 14-2D and 14-6D). The plasmacytic component of the tumor expresses cytoplasmic immunoglobulin and other markers of plasma cell differentiation, including CD138 (variable) and IRF4/MUM1 (see Fig. 14-8C). There is moderate expression of CD200 by flow cytometry.[56] Unlike the neoplastic plasma cells of multiple myeloma, CD19 expression is usually retained on the plasmacytic component and CD56 is negative. CD25 and CD38 are frequently, although not

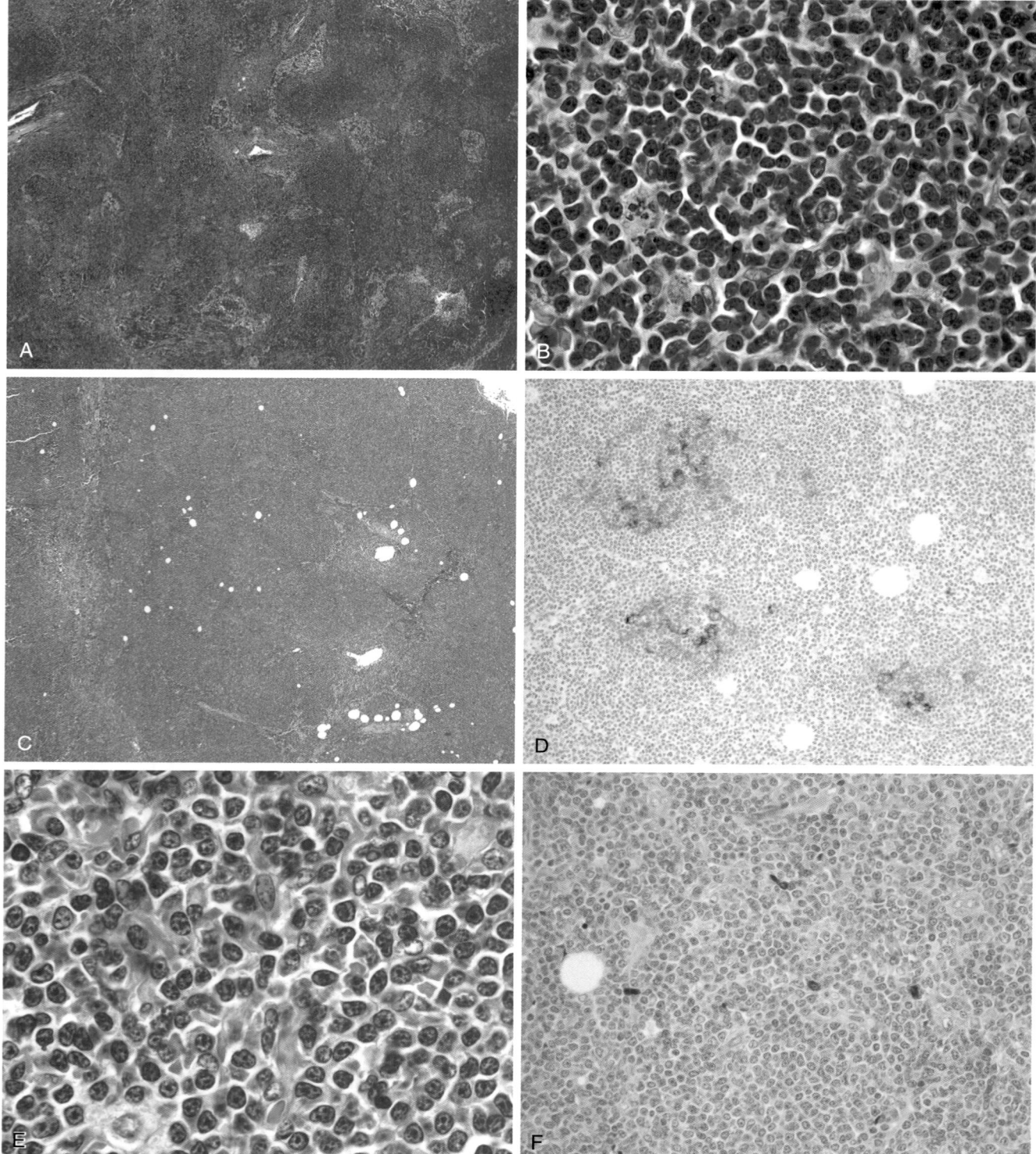

Figure 14-4. Spectrum of nodal involvement by lymphoplasmacytic lymphoma. A and **B,** Case illustrating the "classic" pattern of nodal involvement with subtotal architectural effacement and patent sinuses on low magnification **(A),** and an interfollicular infiltrate of monomorphic small cells with clumped chromatin associated with extracellular hemosiderin deposition on high magnification **(B). C–F,** A case demonstrating more complete nodal architectural effacement **(C)** associated with colonized follicles as shown on CD21 stain **(D).** Plasmacytic differentiation is appreciated on high magnification **(E),** and scattered mast cells are present, as highlighted by Giemsa stain **(F).** Both cases were positive for the *MYD88* L265P mutation on molecular genetic analysis.

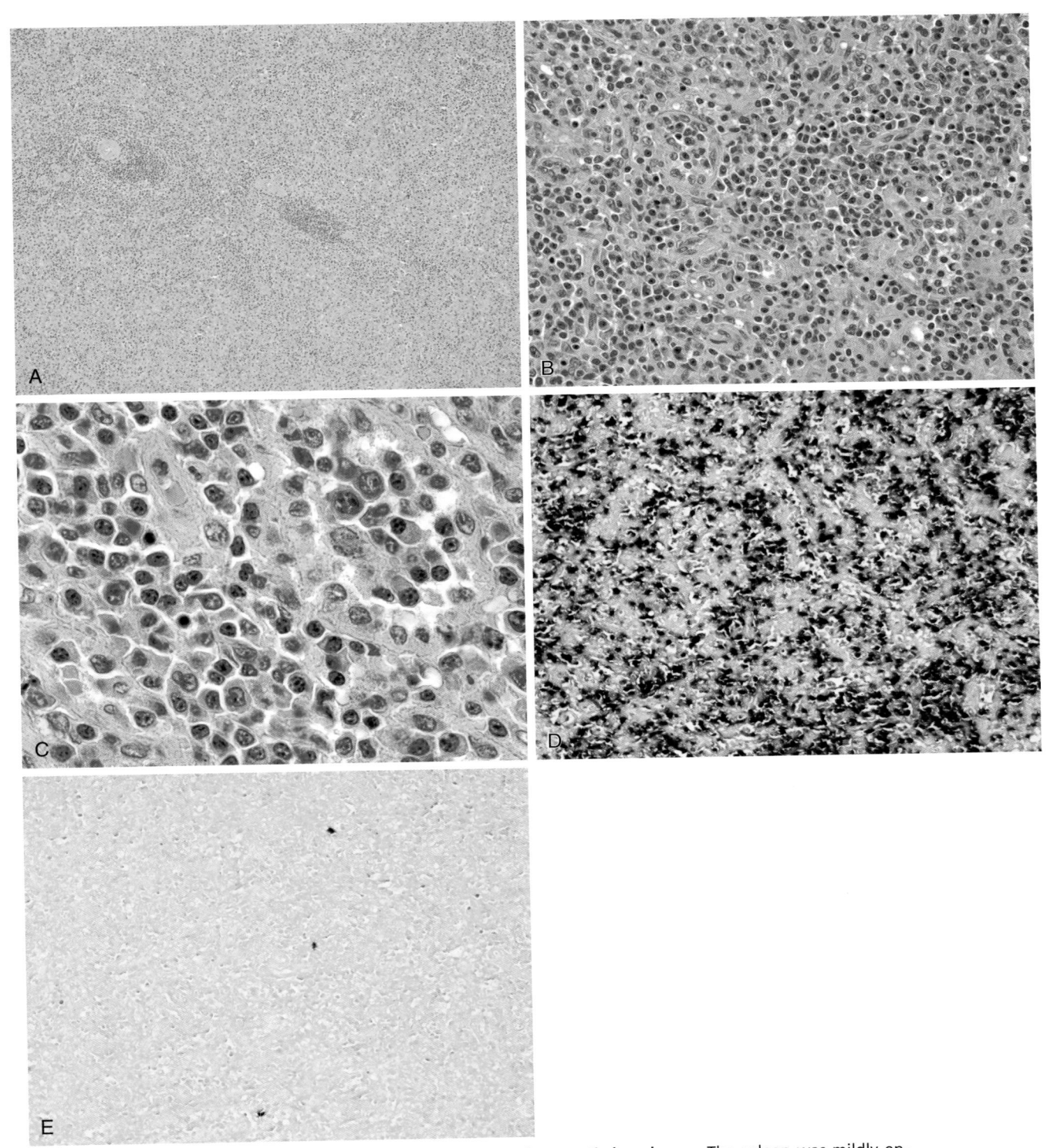

Figure 14-5. Splenic involvement by lymphoplasmacytic lymphoma. The spleen was mildly enlarged, weighing 260 grams. **A,** The lymphoma predominantly involves the red pulp, whereas the white pulp is spared and appears atrophic, as seen at low magnification. **B** and **C,** Red pulp sinuses contain small lymphocytes and conspicuous mature plasma cells, as well as many intermediate forms. **D** and **E,** Plasmacytic differentiation is further evidenced by in situ hybridization demonstrating marked kappa light chain **(D)** predominance over lambda **(E).** *(A–C Used with permission from Sohani AR, Zukerberg LR. Lymphomas of the spleen. In: Ferry JA, ed.* Extranodal Lymphomas. *Philadelphia: Elsevier, 2011. p. 204, Fig. 6.6.)*

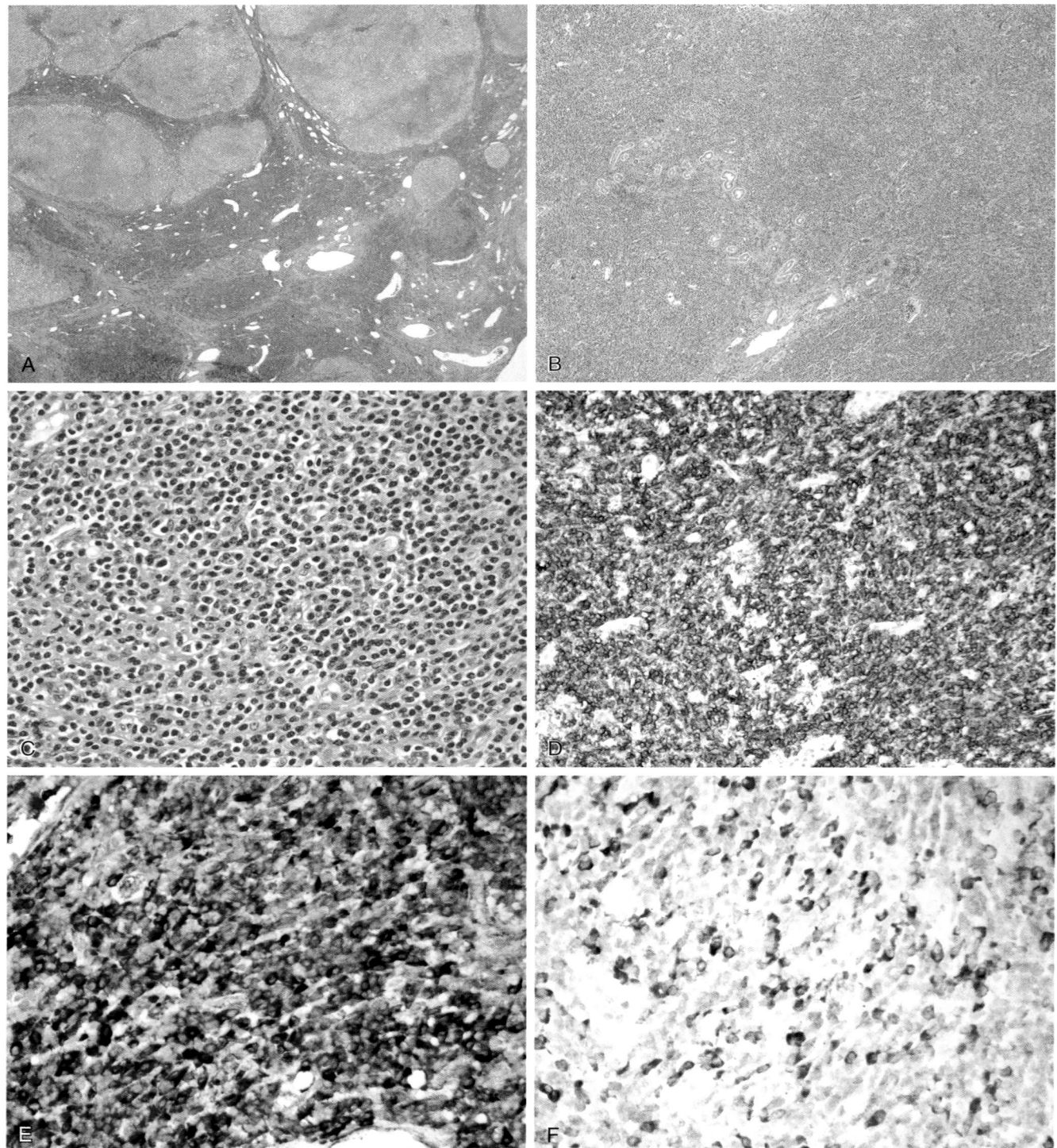

Figure 14-6. Hepatic involvement by lymphoplasmacytic lymphoma. A, Low-magnification view of a cirrhotic explanted liver in a patient with a history of *MYD88*-mutated lymphoplasmacytic lymphoma shows marked expansion of portal tracts by dense collections of lymphocytes surrounding residual bile ducts, but without evident lymphoepithelial lesions **(B). C,** On high magnification, the lymphocytes exhibit characteristic features of lymphoplasmacytic lymphoma with a spectrum of small lymphocytes with clumped chromatin and occasional plasmacytic forms with eccentric nuclei. Note, however, that occasional cells have moderate clear cytoplasm reminiscent of monocytoid B cells. **D,** The lymphoma cells are strongly and diffusely positive for CD20 with restricted expression of IgM heavy chain **(E)** and kappa light chain **(F)**, and negative staining for lambda light chain (not shown).

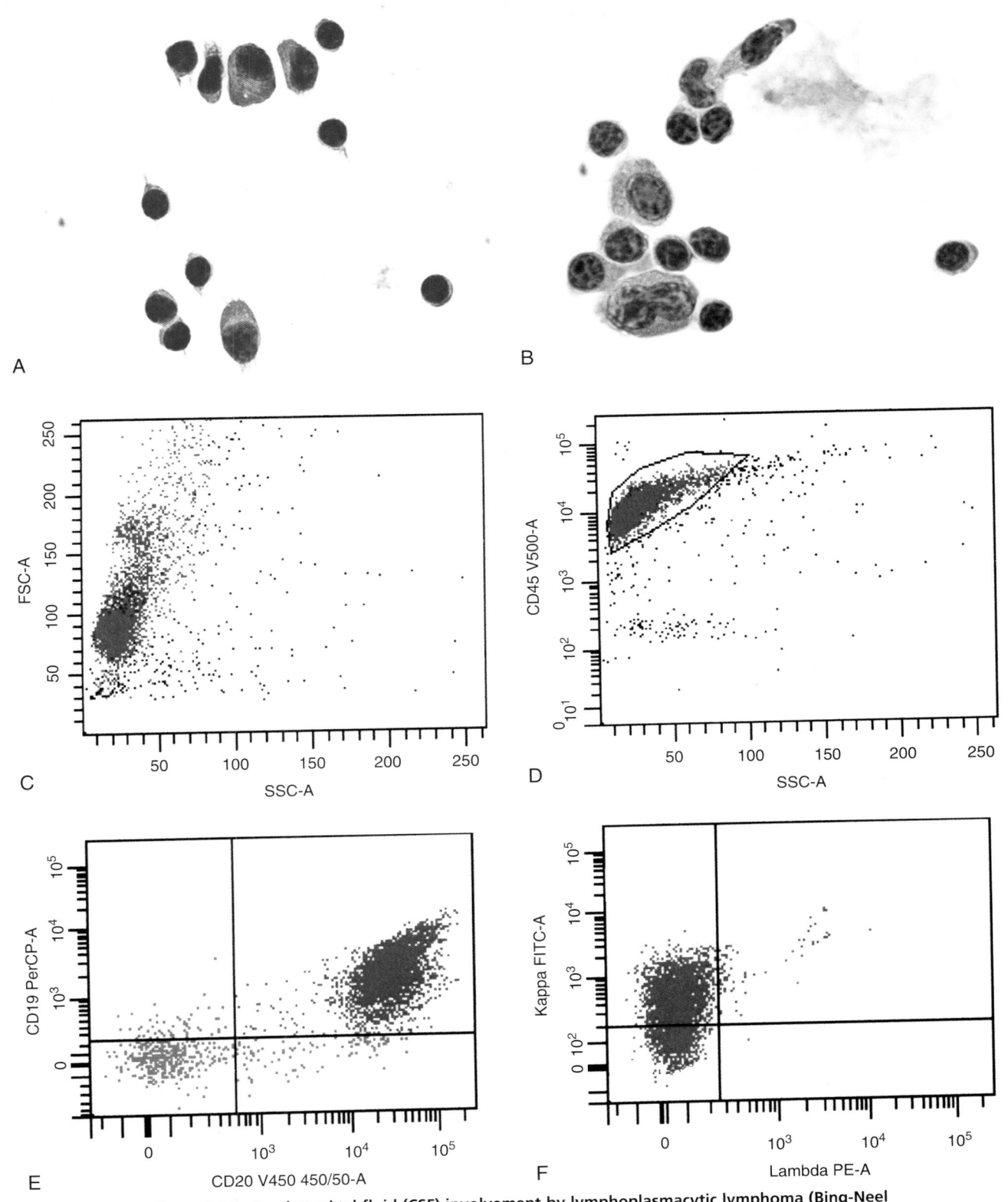

Figure 14-7. Cerebrospinal fluid (CSF) involvement by lymphoplasmacytic lymphoma (Bing-Neel syndrome). Diff-Quik **(A)** and Papanicolaou **(B)** stains show a population of small lymphocytes with condensed or clumped chromatin and larger plasmacytic forms. **C–F,** CSF flow-cytometric analysis confirms the presence of a CD45-positive, CD19-positive, CD20-positive B-cell population with kappa light chain restriction *(blue).* By light-scatter analysis **(C),** a subset of the clonal B cells shows high forward scatter, corresponding to the larger plasmacytic and plasma cells.

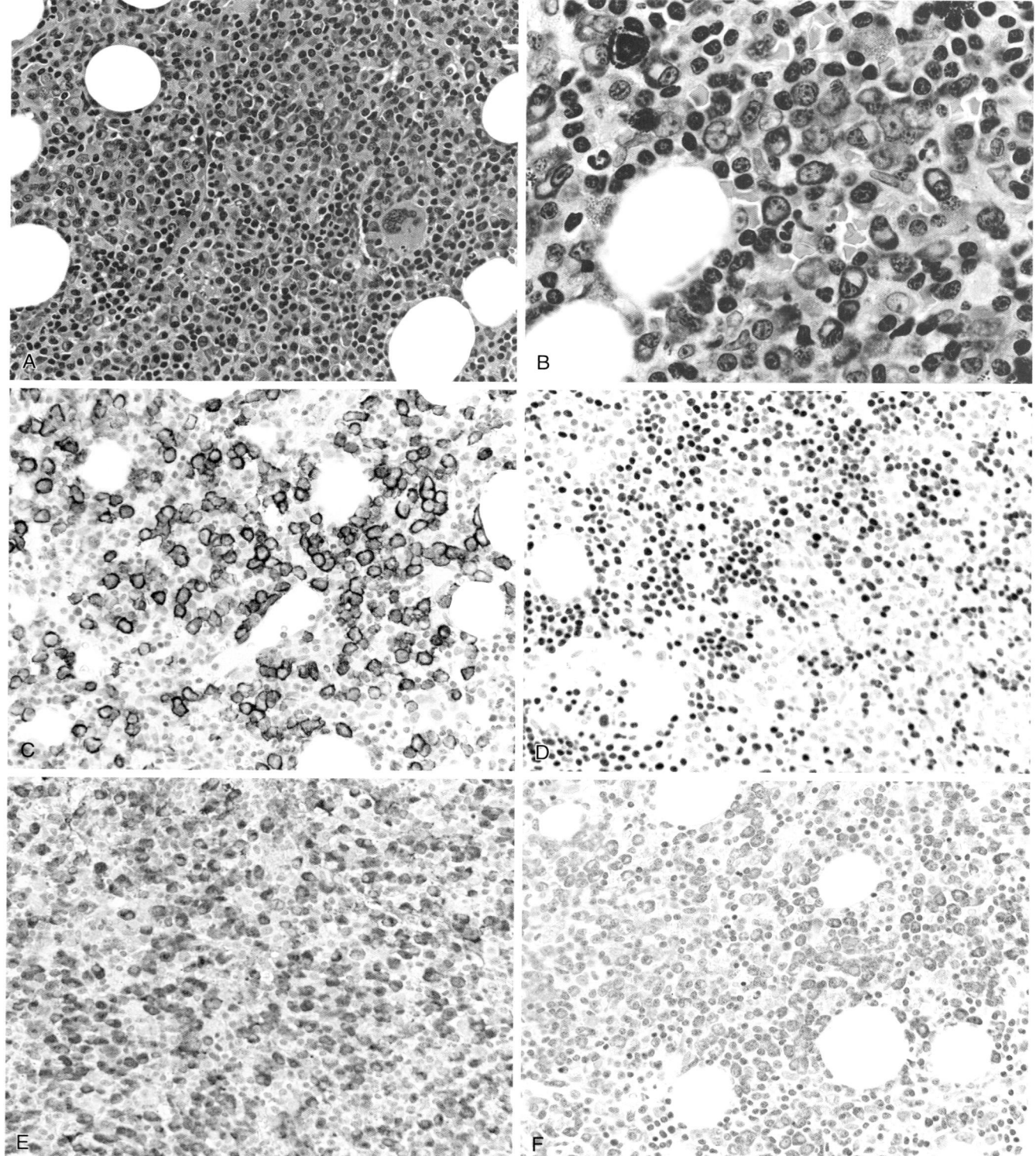

Figure 14-8. IgG-positive lymphoplasmacytic lymphoma with *MYD88* L265P mutation. H&E-stained **(A)** and Giemsa-stained **(B)** bone marrow core biopsy specimen shows a dense lymphoid infiltrate with marked plasmacytic differentiation, as confirmed by CD138 immunohistochemical stain **(C)**. **D,** A stain for PAX5 indicates the presence of many small B cells. The lymphoplasmacytic cells express IgG heavy chain **(E)** and lambda light chain **(F)** and were negative for IgM and kappa light chain (not shown).

always, expressed, and neoplastic cells are typically negative for other phenotypically distinctive markers, including CD5, CD10, CD23, CD103, and DBA.44. Occasional CD5-positive cases have been reported, which can generally be distinguished from CLL/SLL and mantle cell lymphoma by the presence of strong cytoplasmic immunoglobulin expression in a significant subset of cells and the absence of LEF1 or cyclin D1 and SOX11 expression. Similarly, rare CD10-positive cases can be distinguished from follicular lymphoma based on the degree of plasmacytic differentiation, absence of other germinal-center–associated antigens such as BCL6 and LMO2, and pattern of staining with follicular dendritic cell antigens (CD21 or CD23). CD23 may also be positive in some LPL but other features will help exclude CLL/SLL.

MOLECULAR GENETIC FINDINGS

MYD88 L265P Mutation

In 2012, whole-genome sequencing studies of bone marrow lymphoplasmacytic cells in LPL/WM patients identified a somatic T to C point mutation in the myeloid differentiation primary response 88 gene (*MYD88*) on chromosome 3p22.2 that predicted a leucine-to-proline amino acid change at position 265.[3] In the initial study, the *MYD88* L265P point mutation was verified by Sanger sequencing and found to be present in 91% of LPL/WM patients,[3] and in subsequent studies by various groups it was confirmed to be present in up to 95% to 97% of IgM-secreting LPL/WM cases.[5,57-62] Up to 80% of non-IgM LPL cases, including those with extensive plasmacytic differentiation, harbor the *MYD88* L265P mutation (Fig. 14-8).[63,64] Compared with IgM LPL patients, non-IgM LPL patients have lower rates of neuropathy and hyperviscosity, more frequent extramedullary involvement, and a shorter median time to treatment, but similar overall survival.[63,65] The mutation has been identified in 50% to 90% of cases of IgM monoclonal gammopathy of undetermined significance (MGUS), supporting it to be an early genetic event in LPL pathogenesis.[57,58,60,64,66-68] The functional significance of the mutation in the pathogenesis of LPL/WM is discussed in greater detail (see "Postulated Normal Counterpart and Pathogenesis" below).

The high prevalence of *MYD88* L265P in LPL has led to its routine incorporation in the diagnostic workup of small B-cell lymphomas with the development of allele-specific polymerase chain reaction (PCR)-based assays in molecular genetic laboratory settings for use in bone marrow, paraffin-embedded tissue biopsy, and peripheral blood specimens.[4,5,60,69] Assessment of *MYD88* mutational status has been incorporated into multigene high-throughput sequencing panels. However, such targeted next-generation sequencing strategies may fail to detect *MYD88* mutations in up to one-third of patients, particularly those with low bone marrow disease burden.[70] Therefore, testing via allele-specific PCR or, where available, digital droplet PCR is recommended to optimize sensitivity.[64,70,71] It is also important to note that the *MYD88* L265P mutation is not specific to LPL and has been described in other B-cell neoplasms, such as activated B-cell (ABC)-type DLBCL as defined by gene-expression profiling,[72,73] DLBCL of non–germinal-center origin as defined by immunohistochemistry,[74] other subtypes of DLBCL of immune-privileged sites including

primary DLBCL of the CNS,[75-77] primary DLBCL of the testis,[76,78] and primary cutaneous DLBCL, leg type,[79,80] as well as rare cases of CLL and marginal zone lymphomas. Despite a reported prevalence of 40% to 90% in various DLBCL subtypes, the presence of this mutation generally does not pose a diagnostic issue in DLBCL cases, which are readily distinguishable from LPL on histologic grounds. The mutation is found in less than 5% of CLL cases, which are reported to have distinct clinicopathologic features, including younger age at diagnosis, mutated IGHV, and lack of CD38 and ZAP70 expression.[58,81,82] In addition, *MYD88* L265P–positive CLL cases do not typically exhibit plasmacytic differentiation, and only a minority (approximately 10% in one series) are reported to have a small M component.[81] *MYD88* L265P has been identified in a minority of small B-cell lymphomas with plasmacytic differentiation other than LPL that often enter into the differential diagnosis of LPL, including EMZL (7% of cases), SMZL (0% to 10% of cases), and NMZL (0% to 24% of cases).[3,4,45,57,58,83,84] Such cases have been shown to have higher serum IgM levels, and there is additional evidence in some of these reports that they exhibit clinical and laboratory features more akin to LPL, suggesting that they may have been misdiagnosed as marginal zone lymphoma based on standard histopathologic criteria.[3,4,45,83] The mutation has not been identified in multiple myeloma, including cyclin D1–positive cases and rare IgM-positive cases, or in cases of IgG or IgA MGUS.[3,5,58,68,85]

Other Somatic Mutations

Other somatic mutations that have been identified with a relatively high frequency in LPL/WM include C-X-C motif chemokine receptor 4 (*CXCR4*) nonsense and frameshift mutations, found in 30% to 40% of LPL patients.[61,62,86,87] AT-rich interaction domain 1A (*ARID1A*) mutations have been identified in 17% of patients, and additional less common somatically mutated genes include *TP53*, *CD79B*, *KMT2D*, *MYBBP1A*, *BTK*, and *PLCG2*.[3,62,86] Among these, *CXCR4* mutations have been studied in other B-cell lymphomas: they are rare in SMZL and DLBCL, and absent in CLL, HCL, multiple myeloma, and IgG or IgA MGUS.[87] However, given that *CXCR4* mutations occur almost exclusively in tumors that also harbor the *MYD88* L265P mutation, the diagnostic utility of *CXCR4* mutations in discriminating LPL from other entities in the differential diagnosis is limited.[61] The functional, prognostic, and predictive significance of these various mutations in LPL/WM is discussed in greater detail (see "Postulated Normal Counterpart and Pathogenesis" and "Clinical Course, Treatment, and Prognosis").

Cytogenetic Abnormalities

A number of numerical and structural aberrations have been observed. Most common among these are deletions involving the long arm of chromosome 6 in the 6q21-22 region, identified in 40% to 60% of cases,[88-93] although its prevalence appears to be much lower when analysis is restricted to nodal LPL.[44,94] A commonly deleted gene in this region includes *ARID1B*, which is thought to participate in p53 signaling and which, interestingly, is found in patients both with and without visible 6q loss.[86] This region of chromosome 6 also encodes for a number of regulatory genes whose targets are involved B-cell receptor signaling, including Bruton tyrosine kinase (BTK) and nuclear factor (NF)-κB, and apoptosis, including BCL2 and FOXO1.[95] Numerical aberrations that have been identified include gains of chromosomes 3, 4, 5, 12, and 18, and losses of chromosomes 8, 16, 18 to 22, X, and Y.[16,44,90,91,96-101] A study demonstrating a significantly greater frequency of certain copy number abnormalities, including +4, del(6q23.3-6q25.3), +12, and +18q11-18q23, in symptomatic WM versus IgM MGUS, suggests a multistep transformation process that involves specific cytogenetic lesions.[102] Importantly, however, many of these cytogenetic abnormalities are not specific to LPL and have been reported in marginal zone lymphomas of extranodal, nodal, and splenic subtypes.[88] Early reports identified t(9;14)(p13;q32)/IGH::PAX5 as a common recurrent translocation in LPL,[103,104] but this association was not substantiated in subsequent studies showing rearrangements involving the IGH locus to be infrequent in this neoplasm.[44,89,91,105,106]

POSTULATED NORMAL COUNTERPART AND PATHOGENESIS

The lymphocytes of LPL are post–germinal-center B cells capable of spontaneous differentiation to plasma cells in vitro.[107] Molecular genetic analyses of LPL/WM and IgM MGUS have demonstrated the presence of extensive somatic hypermutation within the IGH gene, consistent with derivation from a post–germinal center B cell. There is little evidence of intraclonal variation, and most reports indicate that the tumor cells have failed to undergo heavy chain class switching, with some suggestion that they may be defective in this capacity. These findings suggest that the tumor derives from an IgM-positive memory B cell whose normal counterpart localizes in the bone marrow to mature to an IgM-secreting plasma cell, and that the transformation event occurs after affinity maturation prior to isotype switching.[108-114] Mast cells, which are often increased in tissues involved by LPL, are thought to play a permissive role in LPL development via the elaboration of inflammatory cytokines and CD40 ligand–dependent signaling.[115,116]

Studies unearthing the genetic landscape of LPL/WM have helped to shed further light on its molecular pathogenesis and identify targeted therapeutic approaches. MYD88 encodes a protein involved in toll-like receptor and interleukin-1 receptor signaling that undergoes homodimerization upon receptor activation. It mediates downstream signaling via BTK and a complex of interleukin-1 receptor–associated kinases (IRAKs), ultimately leading to phosphorylation of IκBα and release and activation of NF-κB.[3] L265P is a gain-of-function mutation that promotes cell survival by allowing spontaneous MYD88 homodimerization, BTK activation, and IRAK complex assembly, leading to constitutive NF-κB activation.[72,117,118] Inhibition of MYD88 signaling has been shown to decrease NF-κB nuclear translocation and activity in both MYD88 L265P–mutated ABC-type DLBCL and WM cell lines.[3,72] Blockade of IκBα by proteasome inhibitors is associated with high response rates in WM patients.[119-123] Ibrutinib, a selective BTK inhibitor, showed high activity in MYD88 L265P–mutated cell lines,[117] and has emerged as a preferred first-line treatment option in symptomatic patients

with a MYD88 mutation, the presence of which is predictive for a therapeutic response.[123] The second-most-commonly mutated gene in LPL/WM, CXCR4, is implicated in LPL pathogenesis through AKT activation and mitogen-activated protein (MAP) kinase signaling, which facilitates WM cell migration, adhesion, and homing.[86,124] Loss-of-function CXCR4 mutations result in impaired receptor internalization and have an activating role in WM, as shown by tumor growth, extramedullary dissemination, and decreased survival in transfected mouse models, effects that were abrogated after use of an anti-CXCR4 monoclonal antibody.[87,125] ARID1A, the third-most-common single nucleotide variant in LPL/WM, encodes for a chromatin-remodeling protein, and its family member, ARID1B, resides on chromosome 6q and is frequently lost LPL/WM.[86] Both ARID1A and ARID1B mutations have been described in other malignancies, and are thought to exert their effects via p53 and cyclin-dependent kinase inhibitor 1A (CDKN1A) regulation, important mediators in cell-cycle control and DNA damage response.[126-128] TP53 itself has been found to be mutated in approximately 7% of LPL/WM cases.[86,129] Clonal 6q deletions also result in loss of negative regulators of BTK (IBTK), BCL2 (BCLAF1), and NF-κB (HIVEP2, TNFAIP3).[94] Together, these findings imply that multiple somatic point mutations and deletions exist in LPL/WM that cooperate to promote lymphomagenesis via a variety of mechanisms, including NF-κB–dependent prosurvival signaling, BCL2-dependent antiapoptotic signaling, cell migration and homing, and cell-cycle dysregulation.

CLINICAL COURSE, TREATMENT, AND PROGNOSIS

Like most other low-grade B-cell lymphomas, the clinical course in LPL/WM is generally indolent, with most patients experiencing slowly progressive disease and treatment refractoriness.[16] The median overall survival in large series ranges from 5 to 10 years, with variability in outcome reported based on a number of clinical and laboratory prognostic factors.[130,131] An International Prognostic Scoring System for WM has been developed that takes into account the following five adverse characteristics in determining prognosis and optimizing initial therapy: age greater than 65 years, hemoglobin less than or equal to 11.5 g/dL, platelet count less than or equal to 100×10^9/L, β$_2$-microglobulin greater than 3 mg/L, and serum monoclonal protein concentration greater than 7.0 g/dL.[130] Five-year survival for low-risk patients aged less than or equal to 65 years and with zero or one adverse characteristic is 87% versus 36% for high-risk patients with more than two adverse characteristics.[130] The remaining patients with two adverse characteristics or age greater than 65 years belong to an intermediate-risk group with a 5-year overall survival of 68%.[130]

Large-scale genomic approaches have identified somatic mutations in addition to MYD88 L265P important for prognosis in LPL/WM.[3,61,86] For example, patients whose tumors harbor both MYD88 L265P and CXCR4 nonsense mutations show a more aggressive disease course, with significantly greater bone marrow involvement, higher serum IgM levels, more symptomatic disease (including hyperviscosity syndrome) with shorter time to treatment, lower response and shorter progression-free survival on the BTK inhibitor ibrutinib, and shorter overall survival compared with patients with *MYD88* L265P and wild-type *CXCR4*.[61,132,133] The type of *CXCR4* mutation (nonsense versus frameshift) affects prognosis, as patients with *CXCR4* frameshift mutations have similar outcomes to those with wild-type *CXCR4*.[61,132] Patients with both *MYD88* L265P and *ARID1A* mutations have a significantly greater degree of bone marrow involvement, anemia, and thrombocytopenia than patients with *MYD88* L265P alone.[3] Patients with *MYD88* wild-type tumors have a lower degree of bone marrow involvement but shorter overall survival, decreased response/progression-free survival on ibrutinib, and higher risk of transformation to DLBCL compared with patients with *MYD88* L265P–mutated tumors; these associations appear to be related to the presence of multiple somatic mutations that activate NF-κB signaling downstream of BTK and IRAK and that overlap with somatic alterations in DLBCL.[61,134] Besides *CXCR4* nonsense mutations and wild-type *MYD88*, other alterations associated with diminished response to ibrutinib include mutations involving *PLCG2* and *BTK*, including acquired *BTK* mutations in patients with disease progression on ibrutinib.[62,133-135] Conversely, though *TP53* mutations in LPL/WM are strongly associated with 17p deletion, higher genomic complexity, and shorter overall survival, tumors with *TP53* alterations remain responsive to ibrutinib.[129,136] Patients with high-risk or ibrutinib-resistant mutations may be candidates for novel treatment approaches, including second-generation BTK inhibitors and BCL2 antagonists (see discussion regarding therapy).

Other pathologic characteristics important in determining prognosis include presence of complex karyotype or cytogenetic 6q deletion, each associated with adverse prognosis in various reports,[90,137] whereas some studies have not found a worse outcome in cases harboring a 6q deletion.[92,93] Transformation to DLBCL has been reported in 13% of cases in one series and is associated with an aggressive clinical course and poor prognosis.[46,90]

Current consensus criteria for initiation of therapy and treatment recommendations are based on a number of International Workshops on WM (IWWM) that have convened over the last two decades.[122,138-141] These guidelines were updated in 2020 based on results of several phase 2 studies.[123] Initiation of therapy is appropriate in patients with constitutional symptoms, progressive symptomatic lymphadenopathy or splenomegaly, severe cytopenias secondary to marrow infiltration, or symptomatic complications of disease, such as hyperviscosity, peripheral neuropathy, amyloidosis, renal insufficiency, or cryoglobulinemia.[138] The decision to initiate therapy is not based solely on serum IgM level, which may not correlate with symptom severity.[16] Besides the patient's symptoms, choice of therapy is guided by their neoplasm's genetic profile and drug availability. The updated consensus guidelines endorse use of alkylating agents such as bendamustine or cyclophosphamide, and proteasome inhibitors such as bortezomib, carfilzomib, or ixazomib, in combination with rituximab, and the BTK inhibitor ibrutinib, alone or in combination with rituximab, as preferred first-line treatment options for symptomatic WM patients.[123] Emerging treatment strategies include novel BTK inhibitors, such as acalabrutinib, zanubrutinib, and tirabrutinib, and the BCL2 antagonist venetoclax. Limiting exposure to alkylating agents is recommended in younger patients because of complications of myelosuppression and increased risk for secondary therapy-related myeloid neoplasms.[16,142]

DIFFERENTIAL DIAGNOSIS

Neoplastic Conditions

The main neoplastic entities in the differential diagnosis of LPL include other small B-cell lymphomas with plasmacytic differentiation, particularly the various subtypes of marginal zone lymphoma that, like LPL, lack a distinct immunophenotype (Box 14-2). EMZL and SMZL have clinical presentations and disease distributions different from LPL/WM and can usually be distinguished from LPL on this basis. In addition, LPL has been shown to lack translocations involving *MALT1* and *BCL10* that are frequently detected in EMZL involving the stomach and lung.[30] The distinction between NMZL and nodal involvement by LPL is perhaps the most challenging, particularly on small biopsy specimens. NMZL may exhibit significant plasmacytic differentiation, whereas some LPL cases contain focal monocytoid or marginal zone cytology and prominent follicular colonization.[4,45] The presence of increased mast cells and dilated sinuses has traditionally been thought to favor LPL, but these features are not present in all cases.[45] Studies of nodal LPL have highlighted the utility of *MYD88* L265P mutation analysis performed on formalin-fixed, paraffin-embedded tissue in helping to establish the diagnosis of LPL in nodal biopsy specimens.[4,45] Because the presence of this mutation is neither entirely sensitive nor specific to LPL, correlation with other clinical, laboratory, and pathologic features is still necessary to help establish a diagnosis of LPL. In cases lacking *MYD88* L265P or other LPL-associated mutations for which supporting clinical and laboratory data are limited (e.g., cases without a recent or concurrent bone marrow biopsy, corroborating serum immunoglobulin levels, or serum protein and immunofixation electrophoresis studies), a diagnosis of small B-cell lymphoma with plasmacytic differentiation with provision of a differential diagnosis is most appropriate.

Another neoplastic entity that may enter into the differential diagnosis of LPL is gamma heavy chain disease, a very rare B-cell lymphoproliferative disorder characterized by secretion of an abnormal truncated gamma heavy chain that is unable to bind light chains.[143] The median age of presentation ranges from 51 to 68 years, and a substantial proportion of patients have an underlying autoimmune disease, most commonly rheumatoid arthritis, which may precede the onset of lymphoma by several years.[144] The associated lymphoma typically involves bone marrow, lymph nodes, and spleen, but patients may also present with localized extranodal disease involving the skin, thyroid, salivary glands, gastrointestinal tract, and conjunctiva. Examination of involved tissues usually demonstrates a mixed population of lymphocytes, plasmacytic lymphocytes, and plasma cells that may resemble LPL, though some cases demonstrate clinicopathologic features of other small B-cell neoplasms, including EMZL, SMZL, or other splenic lymphomas.[145] Because of the clinical and morphologic overlap with LPL in many cases, gamma heavy chain disease was previously considered a variant of LPL but has since been shown to lack the *MYD88* L265P mutation.[146]

Other Small B-Cell Lymphomas With Plasmacytic Differentiation (i.e., Marginal Zone Lymphomas)
- No or rare *MYD88* mutations.
- Monocytoid or marginal zone morphology more common.
- Increased mast cells not typically seen.
- Clinical features: Localized extranodal, splenic, or nodal disease.
- Laboratory findings: Lower serum IgM and paraproteinemia.

IgM Monoclonal Gammopathy of Undetermined Significance (MGUS), Not Otherwise Specified (NOS)
- IgM monoclonal paraproteinemia without abnormal bone marrow lymphoplasmacytic infiltrates diagnostic of LPL.
- High prevalence of *MYD88* L265P and *CXCR4* mutations; therefore, these cannot be used to distinguish IgM MGUS from LPL/WM. However, presence of these mutations is helpful in making early or minimal marrow involvement by another small B-cell neoplasm unlikely.
- Monotypic or monoclonal B-cell population may be detectable by flow cytometry or IGH gene rearrangement studies.

IgM Multiple Myeloma
- Typical clinical presentation of multiple myeloma despite rarity of IgM heavy chain subtype (i.e., hypercalcemia, lytic bone lesions); no peripheral lymphadenopathy or splenomegaly. (Note: Anemia and renal insufficiency may be seen with both IgM multiple myeloma and LPL/WM, so cannot be used as clinically distinguishing features.)
- Monoclonal plasma cell component *without* monoclonal B-cell component. Plasma cell immunophenotype similar to IgG or IgA multiple myeloma, including negative staining for CD19 and strong staining for CD56.
- Multiple myeloma–associated cytogenetic abnormalities, including IGH rearrangements and hyperdiploidy of odd-numbered chromosomes; no *MYD88* L265P mutation.

Primary Cold Agglutinin Disease
- Hemolytic anemia associated with the presence of monoclonal IgM kappa paraprotein and cold agglutinins.
- Absence of overt lymphoma by clinical or radiologic evaluation.
- Limited bone marrow lymphoid infiltrates may show B-cell clonality; however, they are often positive for CD5 (approximately 40% of cases), lack plasmacytic differentiation and expression of IRF4/MUM1, and are not associated with increased mast cells.
- Frequent *KMT2D* and *CARD11* mutations and trisomy 3, 12, or 18; no *MYD88* L265P mutation.

Gamma Heavy Chain Disease
- Polymorphous neoplastic infiltrate that includes small lymphocytes and plasma cells, but also immunoblasts, eosinophils, histiocytes, and background hypervascularity.
- Positivity for IgG heavy chain usually with negative staining for kappa or lambda immunoglobulin light chains by immunohistochemistry/in situ hybridization of tissue sections or by flow cytometry.
- Serum or urine immunofixation electrophoresis shows monoclonal IgG heavy chain without associated light chain; however, rare cases may have monotypic light chain secretion.
- Negative for *MYD88* L265P mutation.

It can usually be readily distinguished from LPL on the basis of its immunophenotype, demonstrating positivity for IgG heavy chain with absent staining for light chains by immunohistochemistry or in situ hybridization. Moreover, the neoplastic infiltrate of gamma heavy chain disease is often more polymorphous than that typically seen in LPL, with variable numbers of immunoblasts, including occasional Reed-Sternberg–like forms, eosinophils, histiocytes, and background hypervascularity.[145]

IgM Monoclonal Gammopathy of Undetermined Significance

The differential diagnosis of LPL/WM includes disorders in which the presence of a serum IgM paraprotein is a key disease manifestation, including IgM MGUS. Such patients have less than 10% bone marrow plasma cells and absent or equivocal lymphoplasmacytic infiltrates that are insufficient for a diagnosis of LPL.[1] The 2022 International Consensus Classification recognizes two subtypes of IgM MGUS: plasma cell type and not otherwise specified (NOS).[1]

IgM MGUS, Plasma Cell Type and IgM Multiple Myeloma

IgM MGUS, plasma cell type represents a precursor of IgM-secreting multiple myeloma; both are exceedingly rare. The diagnosis of IgM MGUS, plasma cell type can be established in the absence of findings diagnostic of myeloma and in the presence of clonal IgM-expressing plasma cells without a detectable B-cell component and with wild-type *MYD88*. This diagnosis is also warranted in the setting of t(11;14)(q13;q32) or other cytogenetic abnormalities characteristic of multiple myeloma.[1]

IgM multiple myeloma accounts for approximately 1% of multiple myeloma cases, and affected patients often present with hypercalcemia and lytic bone lesions, symptoms typical of non-IgM multiple myeloma and not seen in LPL/WM.[147] However, because not all patients with multiple myeloma have these symptoms at presentation and because multiple myeloma and LPL/WM share some clinical features, such as anemia and renal insufficiency, the diagnosis of IgM-expressing multiple myeloma should be made only after carefully excluding the presence of peripheral lymphadenopathy, splenomegaly, or a monoclonal B-cell component by histopathologic examination or by flow cytometry.[147] The CD19-negative, CD56-positive immunophenotype of clonal plasma cells in myeloma may be an additional clue to the diagnosis, as the plasmacytic component of LPL should show the opposite pattern of staining.

IgM MGUS, Not Otherwise Specified

Most patients with IgM MGUS fall into this category, defined by the presence of *MYD88* mutation or detectable B-cell clonality by flow cytometry or clonal IGH gene rearrangement studies, but without abnormal bone marrow lymphoplasmacytic infiltrates sufficient for a diagnosis of LPL.[1] As previously discussed, the diagnosis of LPL may now be made in the setting of less than 10% bone marrow lymphoplasmacytic infiltrates (see criteria in "Morphology: Bone Marrow"), so that some cases previously considered IgM MGUS are now to be diagnosed as LPL.[39] The diagnosis requires exclusion of minimal or early marrow involvement by other small B-cell neoplasms. *MYD88* mutational analysis, FISH studies, and targeted sequencing studies can help identify cases more likely to progress to multiple myeloma or a small B-cell lymphoma other than LPL.

The presence or absence of a *MYD88* L265P mutation analysis is not helpful in the distinction between IgM MGUS, NOS and LPL/WM because the mutation has been identified in more than half of IgM MGUS, NOS cases.[57,58,60,64,66-68] IgM MGUS, NOS patients with the *MYD88* L265P mutation have a higher risk for progression to LPL/WM independent of serum M protein concentration, pointing to the importance of *MYD88* L265P as a marker of prognosis and disease progression in patients with IgM MGUS.[66] *CXCR4* mutations have also been identified in 10% to 20% of IgM MGUS, NOS patients.[57,64,148,149] Patients with smoldering or asymptomatic WM have histopathologic evidence of marrow involvement by LPL, but lack symptoms of WM or evidence of end organ damage (i.e., anemia, constitutional symptoms, hyperviscosity, lymphadenopathy, or hepatosplenomegaly).[121,150] Therefore, the distinction between asymptomatic and symptomatic LPL/WM requires clinical correlation. IgM MGUS and asymptomatic WM patients need to be followed but do not require treatment until symptoms develop.[122,150] IgM MGUS patients have an elevated long-term risk for progression to LPL/WM or, to a lesser extent, CLL or primary AL amyloidosis over time, with a cumulative incidence of progression of 10% at 5 years, whereas the risk for progression to symptomatic disease is significantly greater for asymptomatic WM patients, the majority of whom develop symptoms requiring treatment at 5 years or more of follow-up.[150,151]

Primary Cold Agglutinin Disease

Primary cold agglutinin disease, recognized by the 2022 International Consensus Classification as a new diagnostic entity distinct from LPL/WM and IgM MGUS, is an autoimmune hemolytic anemia mediated by the binding of complement-fixing monoclonal IgM kappa cold agglutinins to the I antigen on the surfaces of red blood cells.[152,153] Diagnostic criteria are based on clinical and laboratory findings of chronic hemolysis, the cold agglutinin titer, characteristic abnormalities on direct Coombs testing, and the absence of overt lymphoma by clinical or radiologic assessment.[152] Despite the latter feature, lymphoid aggregates are frequently identified on pathologic examination of bone marrow specimens, and clonal B cells may be detected by flow cytometry of peripheral blood or bone marrow, leading to a diagnosis of an associated B-cell lymphoma in approximately 75% of cases that has often been classified as LPL/WM in prior studies.[152] However, detailed analyses of bone marrow and molecular findings in patients with primary cold agglutinin disease have revealed several key differences from LPL/WM, including relatively limited bone marrow infiltration by monomorphic B cells without lymphoplasmacytic morphology or increased mast cells, expression of CD5 in a significant subset of cases, lack of expression of plasma cell–associated markers such as IRF4/

MUM1, frequent mutations in *KMT2D* and *CARD11* and trisomies of chromosomes 3, 12, and 18, and absence of the *MYD88* L265P mutation.[153-155]

Rare IgM-Secreting Disorders

Rare cases of primary AL amyloidosis associated with a monoclonal IgM paraprotein have been described. These patients appear to have distinct clinicopathologic features, including older age at diagnosis, more frequent kappa light chain production, and less severe organ dysfunction.[156]

Mu heavy chain disease, the rarest of the three heavy chain diseases with only 30 to 40 cases described in the literature, is a lymphoid neoplasm often reported to resemble CLL/SLL and associated with splenomegaly, lymphadenopathy, lytic bone lesions, and kappa Bence Jones proteinuria.[143] Review of the literature, however, indicates that unlike CLL, most cases lack a significant lymphocytosis.[157] Serum immunofixation studies show monoclonal IgM without associated light chains, and examination of bone marrow aspirate specimens reveals small, round lymphocytes and admixed plasma cells containing prominent cytoplasmic vacuoles.[143] Several cases have been reported to harbor *MYD88* L265P mutations, which, along with the lymphoplasmacytic morphology, suggests that at least a subset of mu heavy chain disease is biologically related to LPL and that rare cases of LPL manifest clinically as mu heavy chain disease.[157,158]

Other Conditions

The presence of residual reactive follicles, patent sinuses, and a significant interfollicular plasma cell component in nodal LPL may give rise to the differential diagnosis of the plasma cell variant of Castleman disease. The distinction may be challenging, as some cases of plasma cell Castleman disease, particularly those associated with POEMS syndrome (polyneuropathy, organomegaly, endocrinopathy, monoclonal plasma cell disorder, and skin changes), may contain clonal plasma cells. The diagnosis of LPL can usually be established on the basis of clinical and laboratory features supporting LPL/WM, as well as the immunophenotype of the plasmacytic component, because the clonal plasma cells in POEMS syndrome-associated Castleman disease, when present, are almost always IgG or IgA lambda restricted.[159,160]

Among non-neoplastic conditions, the findings of nodal LPL may mimic lymph nodes biopsied in the setting of rheumatoid arthritis or syphilitic (luetic) lymphadenitis because of overlapping features of follicular hyperplasia and increased interfollicular plasma cells.[161] In addition, lymphadenopathy associated with IgG4-related disease may show features that overlap with LPL.[162-164] The diagnosis of rheumatoid arthritis, syphilis, or IgG4-related disease can be readily established on the basis of clinical and laboratory features and by demonstration of polytypia of the plasmacytic component by stains for immunoglobulin light chains. In addition, LPL lacks the inflamed vasculature seen in syphilis, in which spirochetes can be identified with special histochemical stains or antitreponemal immunohistochemistry.[165]

Pearls and Pitfalls

Pearls

- The diagnosis of LPL/WM requires integration of morphologic, immunophenotypic, molecular, laboratory, and clinical features, with genetic features playing an imperative role in supporting the diagnosis, particularly in cases that show morphologic and immunophenotypic overlap with other small B-cell lymphomas with plasmacytic differentiation.
- The *MYD88* L265P mutation is the most frequent somatic change in LPL/WM, present in up to 95% to 97% of cases, and it is uncommon in other small B-cell lymphomas, including those exhibiting plasmacytic differentiation.
- Other genetic markers of importance in LPL/WM include *CXCR4* loss-of-function mutations, wild type *MYD88*, *TP53* mutations, *BTK* mutations (which may be acquired on BTK inhibitors), and certain cytogenetic abnormalities including deletion 6q, deletion 17p, and complex karyotype.
- The histopathologic diagnosis of LPL is most often established on a bone marrow specimen, in which interstitial and nodular lymphoplasmacytic infiltrates are most common. Patterns of marrow involvement seen in other small B-cell lymphomas, including intrasinusoidal, pure paratrabecular, or diffuse patterns, are rare.
- In classic cases of nodal involvement by LPL, there is subtotal architectural effacement with preservation of sinuses and follicles and an interfollicular lymphoplasmacytic infiltrate, without evidence of proliferation centers. However, many cases show more extensive nodal involvement with complete architectural effacement and obliteration of sinuses; colonization of underlying reactive follicles may be present and does not exclude the diagnosis.

Pitfalls

- The *MYD88* L265P mutation is neither sensitive nor specific for LPL/WM, as up to 10% of cases lack the mutation. It is relatively common in certain subtypes of DLBCL and has been reported at lower frequency in cases of CLL and marginal zone lymphoma of all three types.
- Cases of nodal LPL may show variable morphology with complete architectural effacement, colonization of follicles, or focal monocytoid or marginal zone morphology.
- The diagnosis of LPL outside the bone marrow or lymph nodes, where the histopathology is less well-known, requires correlation with clinical features, laboratory features, and *MYD88* mutation status.
- *MYD88* wild-type cases that lack supporting clinical and laboratory data for the diagnosis of LPL are best classified as small B-cell lymphoma with plasmacytic differentiation with a differential diagnosis given, until further clinical and laboratory supporting data are available to establish a more specific diagnosis.
- The differential diagnosis of LPL/WM includes other IgM-secreting disorders, such as IgM MGUS, rare cases of IgM-positive multiple myeloma, primary AL amyloidosis, primary cold agglutinin disease, and occasional non-neoplastic inflammatory conditions. These can usually be resolved on the basis of immunophenotypic analyses and correlation with other laboratory and clinical data.

KEY REFERENCES

3. Treon SP, Xu L, Yang G, et al. *MYD88* L265P somatic mutation in Waldenström's macroglobulinemia. *N Engl J Med.* 2012;367:826–833.
4. Hamadeh F, MacNamara SP, Aguilera NS, Swerdlow SH, Cook JR. MYD88 L265P mutation analysis helps define nodal lymphoplasmacytic lymphoma. *Mod Pathol.* 2015;28:564–574.
5. Ondrejka SL, Lin JJ, Warden DW, Durkin L, Cook JR, Hsi ED. MYD88 L265P somatic mutation: its usefulness in the differential diagnosis of bone marrow involvement by B-cell lymphoproliferative disorders. *Am J Clin Pathol.* 2013;140:387–394.
28. Lin P, Bueso-Ramos C, Wilson CS, Mansoor A, Medeiros LJ. Waldenström macroglobulinemia involving extramedullary sites: morphologic and immunophenotypic findings in 44 patients. *Am J Surg Pathol.* 2003;27:1104–1113.
39. Owen RG, Treon SP, Al-Katib A, et al. Clinicopathological definition of Waldenstrom's macroglobulinemia: consensus panel recommendations from the Second International Workshop on Waldenstrom's Macroglobulinemia. *Semin Oncol.* 2003;30:110–115.
46. Lin P, Mansoor A, Bueso-Ramos C, Hao S, Lai R, Medeiros LJ. Diffuse large B-cell lymphoma occurring in patients with lymphoplasmacytic lymphoma/Waldenström macroglobulinemia. Clinicopathologic features of 12 cases. *Am J Clin Pathol.* 2003;120:246–253.
58. Xu L, Hunter ZR, Yang G, et al. MYD88 L265P in Waldenström macroglobulinemia, immunoglobulin M monoclonal gammopathy, and other B-cell lymphoproliferative disorders using conventional and quantitative allele-specific polymerase chain reaction. *Blood.* 2013;121:2051–2058.
62. Treon SP, Xu L, Guerrera ML, et al. Genomic landscape of Waldenström macroglobulinemia and its impact on treatment strategies. *J Clin Oncol.* 2020;38:1198–1208.
86. Hunter Z, Xu L, Yang G, et al. The genomic landscape of Waldenström's macroglobulinemia is characterized by highly recurring MYD88 and WHIM-like CXCR4 mutations, and small somatic deletions associated with B-cell lymphomagenesis. *Blood.* 2013;123:1637–1646.
123. Castillo JJ, Advani RH, Branagan AR, et al. Consensus treatment recommendations from the tenth International Workshop for Waldenström macroglobulinaemia. *Lancet Haematol.* 2020;7:e827–e837.

Visit Elsevier eBooks+ for the complete set of references.

Chapter 15

Hairy Cell Leukemia

Robert P. Hasserjian

DEFINITION OF DISEASE AND NOMENCLATURE

Hairy cell leukemia (HCL) is a mature B-cell neoplasm that involves primarily the blood, bone marrow, and splenic red pulp.[1] The neoplastic lymphocytes have surface "hairy" projections and express the B-cell–associated antigens CD19, CD20, and CD22; characteristically, they are also positive for CD103, CD25, CD11c, CD200, CD123, and annexin A1. The vast majority of HCL cases have a recurrent activating point mutation in the *BRAF* oncogene.[2] The long, slender cell surface projections identified on smear preparations and shown most exquisitely by scanning and electron microscopy gave the disease its vivid descriptive name.[3,4]

EPIDEMIOLOGY

HCL is rare, with only about 600 to 1000 cases per year diagnosed in the United States and accounting for only 2% of all leukemias.[5] It affects predominantly middle-aged men and does not occur in children. In the largest published series on HCL patients, the mean age was 54 years (range 23 to 85 years) and the male-to-female ratio was 4:1.[6]

ETIOLOGY

HCL is not associated with Epstein-Barr virus or other infectious pathogens.[7] Several reports of HCL occurring in family members have raised the possibility of a genetic predisposition for the disease.[8-10] In many families, the cases were linked to an HLA A1, B7 haplotype, and association with other HLA haplotypes such as HLA-DRB*11 has also been reported.[9-11] Some studies have suggested exposure to organic solvents and petroleum products as risk factors.[12] Nevertheless, the vast majority of HCL cases appear to be sporadic, arising from an activated memory B cell via acquisition of a somatic *BRAF* V600E mutation.[2]

CLINICAL FEATURES

Symptoms and Signs

Patients with HCL present most often with clinical sequelae related to one or more cytopenias. In one large series, infections (29%) and weakness or fatigue (27%) were the most common initial symptoms. In about one quarter of patients, HCL is diagnosed incidentally as a result of routine hematologic screening in patients lacking symptoms attributable to HCL.[13]

Abnormalities found on physical examination and in laboratory studies in HCL patients at presentation are summarized in Table 15-1.[6,14-16] HCL is characterized by a leukopenic rather than a leukemic presentation: about half of patients are markedly neutropenic at diagnosis (absolute neutrophil count $<0.5 \times 10^9/L$), and half are pancytopenic.[17] An elevated white blood cell count ($>10 \times 10^9/L$) characterizes only 10% to 15% of cases.[6] Marked leukocytosis with numerous circulating neoplastic cells is rare in HCL and, if present, raises the possibility of the so-called *HCL variant* (HCLv, see the section on variants) or another lymphoma subtype showing a leukemic spread. Notably, monocytopenia is seen in almost all HCL cases and is considered to be one of the most sensitive markers of disease. Leukoerythroblastosis is usually not seen, despite the common presence of bone marrow fibrosis (see the

Table 15-1 Clinical and Laboratory Findings of Hairy Cell Leukemia at Presentation

Finding	% of Patients With Finding	Comments
Splenomegaly	86–96	Massive in 25% of patients
Hepatomegaly	73	If biopsied at presentation, the liver is nearly always involved[12]
Lymphadenopathy	13	Mostly abdominal and retroperitoneal; peripheral lymphadenopathy is uncommon[13,14]
Anemia (hemoglobin <12.0 g/dL)	77	
Neutropenia (<1.5 × 10⁹/L)	79	
Monocytopenia (<0.15 × 10⁹/L)	90	
Thrombocytopenia (<100 × 10⁹/L)	73	
Hairy cells detected on peripheral smear examination	85	Often few in number; identification may require careful examination by an experienced observer

Table 15-2 Major Diagnostic Features of Hairy Cell Leukemia

Study	Findings
Morphology of hairy cells	Oval or indented nuclei and abundant pale blue cytoplasm. Absent or inconspicuous nucleoli. Circumferential cell surface "ruffled" projections
Bone marrow biopsy morphology	Diffuse or interstitial bone marrow infiltration, without discrete nodular aggregates. Clear cells with "fried egg" or spindled appearance. Reticulin fibrosis
Flow cytometry	Clonal B cells expressing CD103, CD25, CD200, and CD11c and lacking CD5 expression
Immunohistochemistry	Positive for DBA.44, TRAP, annexin A1, and BRAF V600E
Molecular genetics	*BRAF* V600E mutation

stage HCL.[15,33] However, CT imaging to stage HCL is not common practice in the current era. Skeletal involvement is rare (3% of cases), occurs mostly in advanced disease, and most commonly manifests as lytic lesions of the femoral head and neck.[34]

Diagnostic Procedures

Although a diagnosis of HCL can be based on peripheral blood morphology and immunophenotype, examination of bone marrow is recommended in all newly diagnosed cases to assess the extent of marrow involvement and provide a baseline for assessing response to treatment. The pattern of HCL in bone marrow is highly characteristic and is distinct from other small B-cell lymphomas.[35] The key diagnostic features of HCL are summarized in Table 15-2. A good-quality bone marrow core biopsy is essential, because the bone marrow aspirate is often poorly cellular or unobtainable because of marrow fibrosis.[36] If an aspirate cannot be obtained, the diagnostic HCL immunophenotype can usually be demonstrated by flow cytometry of the peripheral blood, as circulating neoplastic cells are present in almost all patients, even when they are difficult to identify on smears.[12]

MORPHOLOGY

Cell Morphology on Smear Preparations

HCL morphology is ideally represented on well-prepared Wright-Giemsa–stained peripheral blood smears. Hairy cells are 1.5 to 2 times the size of small lymphocytes and are characterized by oval to bean-shaped nuclei, dispersed granular chromatin with features intermediate between a mature lymphocyte and a blast, and absent or inconspicuous, small nucleoli. Hairy cell cytoplasm is moderately abundant, pale blue, and often flocculent, with ill-defined or ruffled borders exhibiting thin circumferential surface projections (Fig. 15-1A–C).[37,38] Occasional cytoplasmic granules or small rod-shaped structures may be evident. These correspond to the ribosome-lamellar complexes frequently seen in hairy cells by electron microscopy.[39] Hairy projections are best seen in thin areas of the smears and, when well demonstrated, are present all around the cell membrane. Poorly prepared or

Morphology section below).[18] Palpable splenomegaly is present at diagnosis in 72% to 90% of patients, whereas peripheral lymphadenopathy is uncommon.[6,13,19] Polyclonal hypergammaglobulinemia may be present in about 20% of patients, but a monoclonal paraprotein is usually not seen.[13]

Infections represent a major cause of morbidity in HCL patients[20,21] and include both bacterial infections and infections by opportunistic organisms such as *Pneumocystis* species and fungi. This striking susceptibility to infections likely reflects both the reduced number of circulating granulocytes and monocytes and disrupted function of immune effector cells, including defective interferon gamma production.[22,23] Uncommon disease manifestations include lytic bone lesions; involvement of extranodal organs such as lung, stomach, and esophagus; and bulky abdominal lymphadenopathy.[24-26] Autoimmune manifestations, including arthritis, vasculitis, and antibody-mediated hemolysis or thrombocytopenia have been reported to occur in up to 25% of HCL patients.[27-30] HCL also appears to have an association with concurrent or subsequent other B-cell lymphomas or plasma cell myeloma that is greater than would be expected by chance, being seen in about 5% of patients.[31] When HCL co-occurs with chronic lymphocytic leukemia (CLL), it often is the predominant population in the bone marrow biopsy despite the prevalence of CLL cells in the blood.[32]

Imaging Studies

Retroperitoneal lymphadenopathy is detected by computed tomography (CT) in about 15% of patients at presentation and in up to 56% of patients later during the course of the disease.[15,33] Massive abdominal lymphadenopathy has been associated with a poorer response to therapy, leading some to suggest the use of abdominal CT scans to

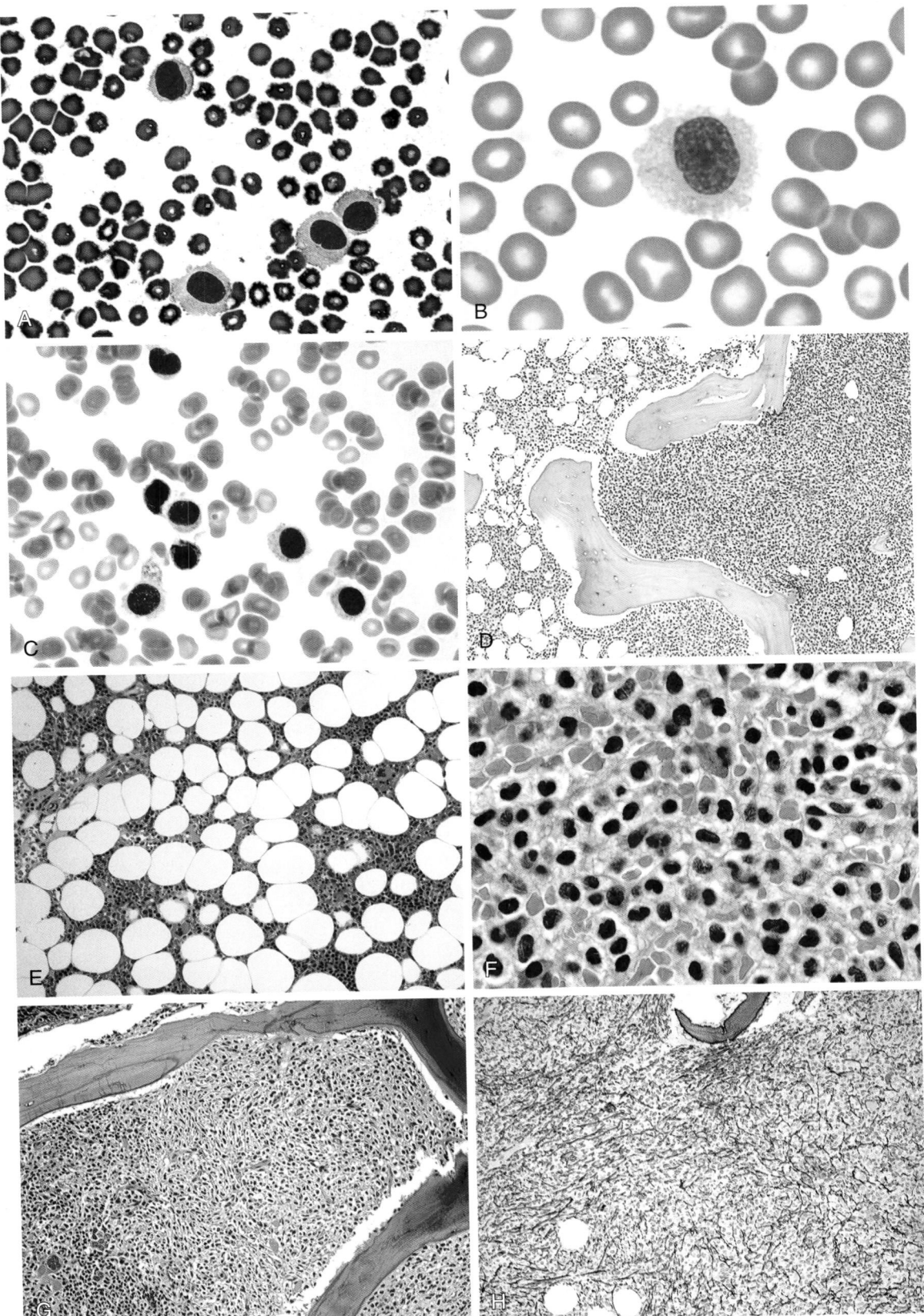

Figure 15-1. A, Hairy cells on peripheral blood smear. The nuclei are oval to indented (kidney- or bean-shaped), with slightly dispersed chromatin, and the cytoplasm is pale blue with a ruffled border showing discrete hairy projections. **B,** Hairy cell on peripheral blood smear. The cytoplasmic border may appear ragged with hard-to-appreciate surface projections. Small nucleoli may be present. **C,** Hairy cells are often poorly preserved in bone marrow aspirate smears, with stripped or relatively scant cytoplasm. **D,** Hairy cell leukemia (HCL) in bone marrow biopsy section (low power), illustrating characteristic diffuse and interstitial infiltration patterns. **E,** Early subtle involvement by HCL in bone marrow biopsy section, in which hairy cells insinuating between the hematopoietic elements are difficult to appreciate and may be easily missed. **F,** HCL in bone marrow biopsy section (high power), illustrating wide spacing of the folded and bean-shaped nuclei. Depending on the fixation and processing method, the cytoplasm may appear clear or pale pink. **G,** Extensive bone marrow involvement in some HCL cases may exhibit a spindled appearance, potentially mimicking a non-hematologic neoplasm. **H,** HCL in bone marrow biopsy (reticulin silver stain). Reticulin is increased in almost all HCL cases, often resulting in a poor or failed aspirate.

thick smears (particularly from bone marrow aspirations) may cause artifactual hairlike projections or cytoplasmic ruffling in other cell types, mimicking hairy cells. Moreover, the cell trauma associated with preparing the bone marrow aspirate renders the characteristic hairy cell cytomorphology more difficult to appreciate in aspirate smears or touch preparations than in peripheral smears.[18]

Cell Morphology and Histologic Features in Bone Marrow Sections

At low power, the bone marrow infiltrate in HCL is interstitial or diffuse and does not form well-defined nodular aggregates that characterize most other small B-cell lymphomas (see Fig. 15-1D). At diagnosis, the bone marrow is hypercellular in most cases, with diffuse sheets of hairy cells.[37] However, in early stages of the disease the bone marrow may be hypocellular or may have a subtle interstitial infiltrate that is not readily apparent on routine histologic stains (Fig. 15-1E).[40] At higher power, the hairy cells appear round and monotonous, with oval to indented and occasionally convoluted nuclei set in an abundant clear cytoplasm that holds the nuclei equidistant and imparts the characteristic "fried egg" appearance; large lymphoid cells are virtually absent.[18,41] Depending on the fixation and processing method, the cytoplasm may appear clear, uniformly pale pink, or flocculent on hematoxylin and eosin (H&E) stain (see Fig. 15-1F). The spaced appearance of hairy cells in tissue sections appears to be caused by pericellular deposition of fibronectin.[42] The hairy projections are usually not evident on routine histologic stains, although these may be visualized with DBA.44 immunohistochemistry.[43] Immunohistochemical stains for CD20 or DBA.44 reveal an intrasinusoidal component to the infiltrate in up to 70% of cases.[44,45] In some cases, particularly when there is extensive involvement, the neoplastic cell infiltrate may appear spindled (Fig. 15-1G).[41] The so-called hairy cell index, representing the proportion of bone marrow space occupied by hairy cells,[46] can be useful in comparing bone marrow samples before and after treatment.

The amount of residual hematopoiesis is variable, but there is often a reduction in normal hematopoietic cells, particularly of the myeloid lineage.[47,48] Not infrequently, there is a modest increase in the number of plasma cells and mast cells.[49] Hematopoietic elements may manifest morphologic dysplasia, potentially mimicking a myelodysplastic syndrome,[48,50] and in some cases the marrow may appear hypoplastic, mimicking aplastic anemia.[40] These observations have suggested that HCL may actively suppress hematopoiesis beyond a mere space-occupying effect, possibly by disrupting the bone marrow microenvironment and by the abnormal release of cytokines such as transforming growth factor-β.[51,52] However, a study revealing that the *BRAF* V600E mutation is present in primitive hematopoietic stem cells from HCL patients (see the Genetics and Molecular Findings section below) raises the possibility that the cytopenias may result at least in part from an inherent defect in hematopoiesis.[53]

Significant reticulin fibrosis, likely mediated by the deposition of pericellular fibronectin, is found in almost all cases of HCL at diagnosis, and this is the presumed cause

of poor aspirate smears or the inability to aspirate marrow (Fig. 15-1H).[42] Collagen fibrosis demonstrated by trichrome staining is uncommon.[54] The bone marrow fibrosis resolves after effective therapy for HCL.[55]

Spleen and Other Organs

HCL almost always involves the spleen, although splenomegaly may be absent early in the course of disease. In contrast to most other B-cell lymphomas (including splenic marginal zone lymphoma [SMZL]), HCL preferentially involves the splenic red pulp rather than the white pulp. On gross examination, the spleen is massively enlarged (median weight, 1300 g) and exhibits inconspicuous white pulp (Fig. 15-2A).[46] Microscopically, the hairy cells in the spleen appear similar to those in involved bone marrow sections.[41,56] Areas of hemorrhage (so-called pseudosinuses or blood lakes) are characteristic but not specific for HCL and result from hairy cell adhesion and damage to sinus endothelial cells.[41,57] Extramedullary hematopoiesis is infrequently observed.[18] Owing to advances in HCL diagnosis and therapy, pathologists now only rarely encounter splenectomy specimens from HCL patients.

HCL also almost always involves the liver at presentation and commonly causes modest hepatomegaly, although the liver is usually not biopsied. In liver biopsies, the hairy cells are located in small clusters in the sinuses and portal tracts. As in the spleen, there may be associated hemorrhage, which in the liver may mimic peliosis hepatis.[16]

HCL commonly involves abdominal and retroperitoneal lymph nodes, particularly after splenectomy or in patients with long-standing disease. In lymph nodes, HCL shows a paracortical and medullary distribution and may surround germinal centers in a pattern mimicking nodal marginal zone lymphoma (MZL) (see Fig. 15-2B).[35,56] Examination of the peripheral blood and bone marrow (including immunophenotyping) is helpful in accurately separating MZL from HCL involving lymph nodes. In HCL patients with lymphadenopathy, the HCL cells in the involved lymph nodes may appear larger and the disease may be refractory to therapy, suggesting transformation to a higher-grade disease biology.[26,58] However, transformation of HCL to bona fide diffuse large B-cell lymphoma is rare.[56]

Although 10% to 12% of HCL patients may develop cutaneous lesions during the disease course, these are mostly secondary to infectious, autoimmune, or drug manifestations. True cutaneous involvement by HCL is rare; it may present as a localized lesion or as generalized cutaneous involvement and appears to respond to purine analogue therapy.[59]

PHENOTYPE

Flow Cytometry

Flow-cytometric demonstration of the characteristic hairy cell immunophenotype, in combination with morphology, is a cornerstone of HCL diagnosis. HCL expresses CD45 (at bright intensity) and the B-cell markers CD19, CD20 (at bright intensity), FMC-7, CD22 (at bright intensity),

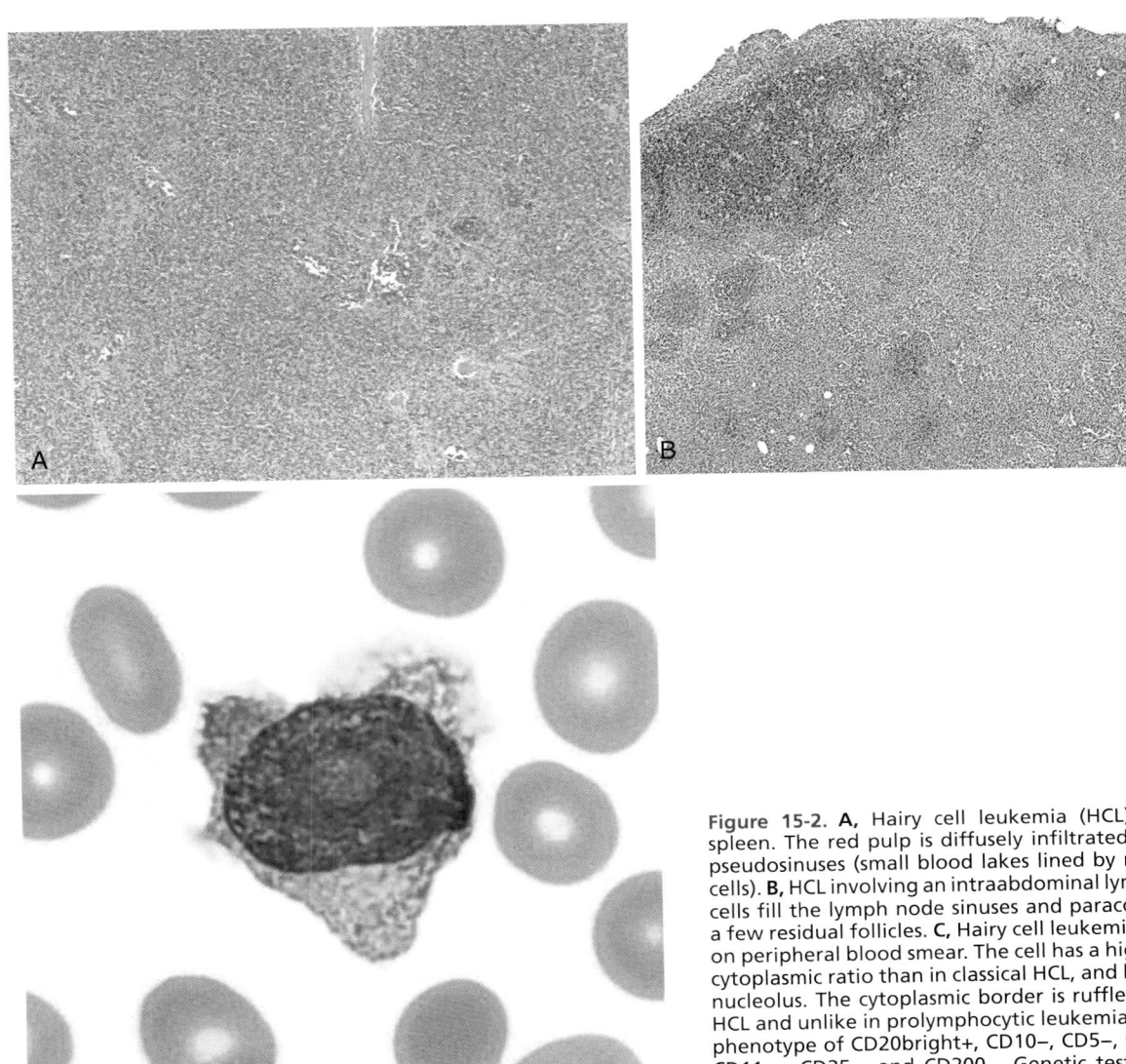

Figure 15-2. A, Hairy cell leukemia (HCL) involving the spleen. The red pulp is diffusely infiltrated with scattered pseudosinuses (small blood lakes lined by neoplastic hairy cells). **B,** HCL involving an intraabdominal lymph node. Hairy cells fill the lymph node sinuses and paracortex, with only a few residual follicles. **C,** Hairy cell leukemia variant (HCLv) on peripheral blood smear. The cell has a higher nuclear-to-cytoplasmic ratio than in classical HCL, and has a prominent nucleolus. The cytoplasmic border is ruffled, as in classical HCL and unlike in prolymphocytic leukemia. The cells had a phenotype of CD20bright+, CD10−, CD5−, CD23−, CD103+, CD11c+, CD25−, and CD200−. Genetic testing showed no *BRAF* mutation, but did show a *CREBBP* mutation.

and CD79a, and it is usually negative for CD5, CD10, and CD79b.[60,61] CD10 can be positive in 10% to 26% of otherwise classical HCL cases and CD23 is positive in 17% to 21% of cases, whereas CD5 is positive in less than 10% of cases.[62-64] HCL expresses monotypic surface immunoglobulin at high intensity in all cases.[65] Bright expression of CD11c, CD25, CD103, and CD200 is characteristic of HCL,[61,65] and these markers are typically included in the flow cytometry immunophenotyping panel when HCL is suspected. In addition, the alpha chain of the IL-3 receptor, CD123, is expressed in 95% of cases of HCL but not in HCLv, SMZL, or most other B-cell lymphomas with the exception of a subset of splenic diffuse red pulp lymphoma.[66-68] Thus CD123 may be helpful in distinguishing other diseases with "hairy" or "villous" morphology from HCL.[69,70] HCL shares with CLL characteristic bright expression of CD200, in contrast to other small B-cell lymphoms, which are dim or negative for CD200.[71] If the characteristic but often elusive hairy cells are

not recognized on examination of the peripheral smear, the typical high forward and side light-scatter qualities of hairy cells on flow cytometry may be helpful clues (Fig. 15-3A). Care must be taken when performing flow-cytometry studies as hairy cells often fall within the monocyte gate, outside of the usual lymphocyte region.[72]

There is no absolutely specific immunophenotypic marker for HCL; the pathologist should evaluate the overall immunophenotype in the context of the morphologic and clinical findings. The vast majority of HCL cases—and only very rare cases of other B-cell lymphomas—express at least three of the four characteristic HCL markers (CD11c, CD103, CD25, and CD123), and most express all four of these markers.[66,73-75] Cases with some atypical immunophenotypic features, such as CD10 or CD5 expression or lack of CD103 or CD25 expression, may still be diagnosed as HCL if the clinical features, marrow infiltration pattern, and cytomorphology are otherwise

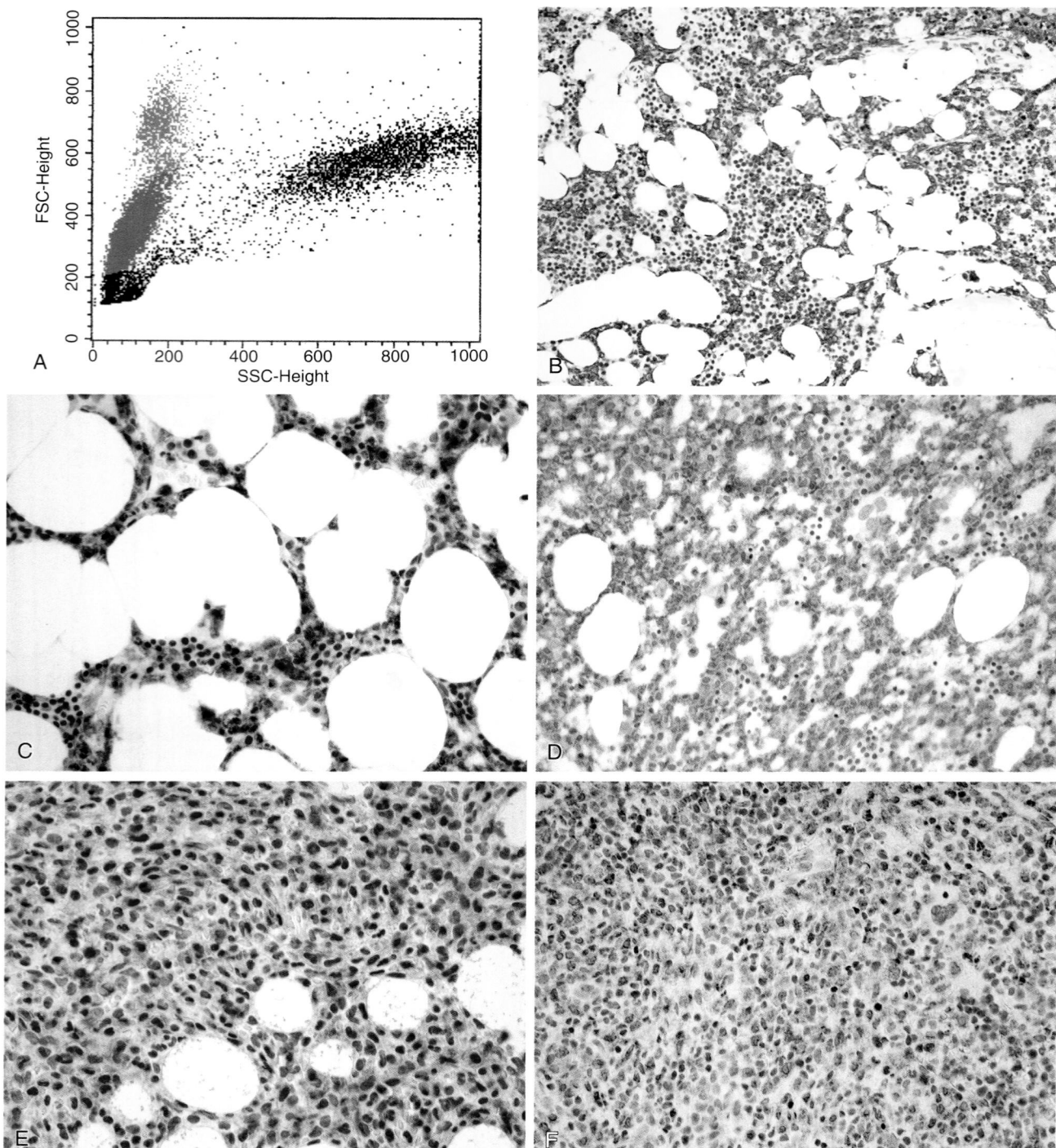

Figure 15-3. A, Light-scatter characteristics of hairy cell leukemia (HCL) in peripheral blood (flow cytometry). The hairy cells *(green)* have higher forward light scatter (FSC, *vertical axis*) and slightly higher side light scatter (SSC, *horizontal axis*) than the normal lymphocytes *(red)*. Also note the absence of monocytes, which would be located between the red lymphocytes and the black granulocytes. **B,** CD20 immunostain of a subtle case of HCL in the bone marrow in which the hairy cells occur in an interstitial pattern and do not form confluent sheets. **C,** CD25 immunostaining of hairy cells in the bone marrow. **D,** Annexin A1 stains hairy cells in the bone marrow. **E,** Cyclin D1 stain shows the weak, variable nuclear expression typically seen in HCL. **F,** Immunostaining of HCL in bone marrow with a mutation-specific antibody to BRAF V600E.

typical, particularly if a *BRAF* V600E mutation is confirmed.[62] In particular, low or absent CD103 expression may rarely occur in about 5% of cases; these patients otherwise have a typical HCL immunophenotype and respond similarly to HCL therapies.[65]

Immunohistochemistry and Cytochemistry

If the characteristic HCL immunophenotype can be demonstrated by flow cytometry of peripheral blood or bone marrow aspirate, paraffin section immunohistochemistry on biopsy samples is usually unnecessary except to help quantify involvement in morphologically subtle or treated cases. Hairy cells can be readily identified in tissue sections by routine B-cell markers such as CD20, PAX5, and CD79a, and these markers often reveal far more hairy cells than are suspected on routine stains (see Fig. 15-3B–C). DBA.44 is a widely used marker, but it does not stain all the neoplastic cells and is expressed in other neoplasms.[76] Hairy cells are nearly unique among lymphocytes in that their acid phosphatase enzyme maintains its function after the addition of tartrate (tartrate-resistant acid phosphatase [TRAP]). This feature can be used to detect HCL relatively specifically in air-dried smears with cytochemical staining for TRAP, but this is now seldom used in HCL diagnosis. Immunohistochemistry for the TRAP enzyme is available[77] but it stains other B-cell neoplasms and is less specific than TRAP cytochemistry.[78] An antibody to a fixation-resistant epitope of CD11c (5D11) is a sensitive marker for HCL in paraffin-embedded bone marrow sections.[79] The annexin A1 gene (*ANXA1*) is markedly upregulated in HCL, and antibody to annexin A1 is a sensitive and specific marker for HCL, being expressed in a cell membrane pattern in 74% to 97% of HCL and uniformly negative in other B-cell lymphomas (see Fig. 15-3D).[35,80,81] However, annexin A1 also stains myeloid elements, macrophages, and T cells and is thus not optimal for the detection of small amounts of bone marrow disease after therapy.[82] By immunohistochemistry, CD123 is expressed in over half of HCL cases (and in 95% by flow cytometry) and is not expressed in most other B-cell lymphomas, but is expressed in some myeloid leukemias, plasmacytoid dendritic cells, and neoplastic mast cells.[35] Cyclin D1 is overexpressed in most HCL cases and can be detected by immunohistochemistry in paraffin sections; the staining is weaker and more variable in intensity compared with the strong, diffuse staining seen in mantle cell lymphoma (see Fig. 15-3E).[35,83] Of note, SOX11 can also be expressed in a subset of HCL cases,[84] and thus the combination of SOX11 and cyclin D1 positivity does not necessarily prove a diagnosis of mantle cell lymphoma. Although small subsets of HCL show expression of CD10 and, to a lesser extent, CD5 by flow cytometry, these stains are almost always negative by immunostaining of HCL in tissue sections.[35]

A monoclonal antibody that recognizes the mutated protein product of *BRAF* V600E (VE1) is applicable to paraffin-embedded decalcified bone marrow material (see Fig. 15-3F). The BRAF V600E antibody is a highly sensitive and specific marker of HCL in bone marrow trephine sections[85] and correlates with the presence of the *BRAF* V600E mutation detected by molecular genetic methods.[86] Table 15-3 summarizes key immunophenotypic, flow cytometric, and cytochemical findings commonly used to diagnose HCL.[43,64,75,77,87-92]

Table 15-3 Useful Immunophenotypic Markers in Hairy Cell Leukemia

Marker	Modality	Sensitivity (%)	Also May Be Positive In
TRAP (CC)	Air-dried smear	99	SMZL (rarely), B-PLL, other lymphomas, mast cell disease
TRAP (antibody)	Paraffin IHC	90–100	Various other B-cell lymphomas (21%), AML (rarely)
CD103	FC	92–100	SMZL (15%), HCLv (~50%), T-cell lymphomas
CD25	FC, paraffin IHC	97–99	SMZL (25%), CLL (low intensity)
CD11c	FC, paraffin IHC	69–100	SMZL (47%), HCLv, other B-cell lymphomas
CD123	FC, paraffin IHC	95	HCLv (9%), SMZL (3%)
CD200	FC, paraffin IHC	100	CLL (95–100%)
DBA.44	Paraffin IHC	99–100	Various other B-cell lymphomas (15%)
Annexin A1 (*ANXA1*)	Paraffin IHC	97	Hematopoietic cells; not reported to be expressed in other B-cell lymphomas
BRAF V600E	Paraffin IHC	91–99	CLL (<1%)
T-bet	Paraffin IHC	100	CLL (20%), marginal zone lymphomas (50%)

AML, Acute myeloid leukemia; *B-PLL,* B-cell prolymphocytic leukemia; *CC,* cytochemical stain; *CLL,* chronic lymphocytic leukemia; *FC,* flow cytometry; *HCLv,* hairy cell leukemia variant; *IHC,* immunohistochemistry; *SMZL,* splenic marginal zone lymphoma; *TRAP,* tartrate-resistant acid phosphatase.

GENETICS AND MOLECULAR FINDINGS

The identification in 2011 of a *BRAF* point mutation in the vast majority of HCL and its negativity in other small B-cell lymphomas has validated HCL as a discrete and unique entity. *BRAF* is a proto-oncogene located at chromosome 7q24. In HCL, a point mutation occurs in exon 15 at codon 600, leading to a substitution of glutamate (E) for valine (V), termed the *V600E mutation.*[2] The *BRAF* V600E mutation can be detected in bone marrow aspirates or peripheral blood by Sanger sequencing, allele-specific polymerase chain reaction (PCR), or next-generation sequencing technologies. Rarely, alternative *BRAF* mutations may occur in exon 11.[93] Cases of bona fide HCL that express IGH VH4-34 (about 10% of cases; see the Variants section below) lack *BRAF* mutations altogether. The *BRAF* V600E mutation causes constitutive activation of the MAP kinase signaling pathway, a hallmark of HCL.[94] Additional gene mutations are found in about one-third of HCL cases, and include *CDKN1B, KLF2, KMT2C, NOTCH1,* and *ARID1B.*[95,96] Interestingly, although the *BRAF* V600E mutation in HCL is thought to originate in a hematopoietic stem cell and is shared with histiocytic/

dendritic cell–derived neoplasms such as Langerhans cell histiocytosis and Erdheim-Chester disease, in HCL the V600E mutation is restricted to the B-cell compartment in mature cells, while in histiocytic/dendritic neoplasms it occurs in myeloid cells and monocytes.[53,97]

Routine cytogenetic analysis of HCL is generally not indicated; the low proliferation of HCL renders karyotyping difficult, the diagnosis can usually be made on morphologic and immunophenotypic grounds, and no prognostic cytogenetic markers have been identified.[98] Karyotypes obtained by stimulation with mitogens or cytokines have revealed clonal abnormalities in up to 67% of cases.[98] These include trisomy 5 and inversions and interstitial deletions involving 5q13 (which are only rarely seen in other B-cell lymphomas), and structural and numerical aberrations of chromosomes 7 and 14, including loss of the wild-type *BRAF* allele at the 7q34 locus through del(7q).[94,95,98-100] Notably, despite the fact that HCL cells express activation-induced cytidine deaminase that has been implicated in the chromosomal translocations of B-cell neoplasms, recurrent chromosomal translocations involving immunoglobulin genes are lacking in HCL.[101,102] Although cyclin D1 expression is detected by immunohistochemistry in a high proportion of HCL cases,[83] translocations involving the *CCND1* locus do not occur in HCL.[103,104]

HCL has a homogeneous gene-expression profile.[82] The expression profile for genes regulating proliferation and apoptosis is similar to that of normal B cells, but exhibits deficient expression of genes related to lymph node homing (*CCR7* and *CXCR5*); overexpression of genes whose products interact with actins (*GAS7*) and promote B-cell adhesion to fibronectin (*IL3RA* and *FLT3*); and marked upregulation of *ANXA1,* the gene encoding annexin A1. These findings help explain the disease distribution, cellular morphology, and bone marrow fibrosis characteristic of HCL.[82] Interestingly, BRAF and MEK inhibitors that induce MEK/ERK dephosphorylation specifically in HCL cells (but not HCL-like normal B cells) were shown to cause silencing of the BRAF-MEK-ERK pathway transcriptional output and loss of the HCL-specific gene-expression signature.[105] These changes were also associated with smoothing of the surface of the hairy cells and, ultimately, apoptosis.

POSTULATED CELL OF ORIGIN AND NORMAL COUNTERPART

Analysis of HCL immunoglobulin gene mutational status has revealed that HCL cells have experienced immunoglobulin heavy chain variable region (IGHV) somatic hypermutation but do not display ongoing mutation, features typically associated with the post–germinal-center B cell.[106] Gene-expression profiling has shown that HCL cells are closely related to memory B cells[82] and that they additionally express the junctional adhesion-molecule C protein that is found in post–germinal-center circulating memory B cells.[107] In spite of these similarities, HCL cells display notable differences from normal memory B cells in terms of their gene-expression profile of cytokines, chemokine receptors, and adhesion molecules; in addition, unlike most memory B cells, HCL cells are CD27 negative.[101,102] The identification of the *BRAF* V600E mutation in hematopoietic stems cells in HCL patients intriguingly suggests that the initial steps of HCL development may occur in a hematopoietic precursor cell; presumably,

the acquisition of additional (as yet unidentified) mutations during differentiation create the full HCL disease phenotype that manifests in post–germinal-center B cells.[53] Such a stem cell origin may explain the increased risk for other B-cell and plasma-cell malignancies observed in HCL patients.

VARIANTS

About 10% of patients with otherwise typical HCL have IGH gene rearrangement using the VH4-34 region. These cases tend to have more advanced disease at presentation, poorer response to purine analogue therapy, and shorter survival compared with other HCL cases. VH4-34-positive HCLs have been reported to lack the *BRAF* V600E mutation,[108] and a subset have been reported to harbor *MAP2K1* gene mutations,[96,109] a feature shared with HCLv. The nature of these HCL cases and their relationship to HCLv and splenic diffuse red pulp small B-cell lymphoma still remains controversial.[108]

The disease known as hairy cell variant (HCLv) is rare, and it is only about 10% as frequent as HCL, which is already a rare disease. These cases display significant morphologic, immunophenotypic, and clinical differences from HCL and also show a profile of genetic aberrations that is distinct from HCL.[110] HCLv is not actually considered as a "true variant" of HCL, but is rather a separate provisional disease entity in the revised WHO 4th ed. and in the 2022 International Consensus Classification (ICC) of Mature Lymphoid Neoplasms.[44,102,111-113] In the proposed WHO 5th ed.,[114] HCLv has been renamed *splenic B-cell lymphoma/leukemia with prominent nucleoli,* a designation that also includes some cases of B-cell prolymphocytic leukemia (a disease no longer recognized by the proposed WHO 5th ed.).

HCLv patients tend to be older than HCL patients, with a median age of 71 years. In contrast to HCL, there is usually marked leukocytosis with a white blood cell count that is greater than 30×10^9/L because of the presence of numerous circulating leukemic cells.[89,115] These resemble hairy cells in terms of having abundant cytoplasm and surface projections, but also have prominent central nucleoli that are not typically seen in HCL and are reminiscent of prolymphocytes (see Fig. 15-2C).[89] Unlike in classical HCL, monocytopenia does not occur. The pattern of bone marrow and splenic red pulp infiltration is largely similar in the two entities, although HCLv often shows sinusoidal infiltration of marrow, which is typically not as prominent in classical HCL. Moreover, in HCLv bone marrow fibrosis, if present at all, tends to be patchy.[89] Immunophenotypically, HCLv shares some similarities with HCL in that it expresses CD11c, DBA.44 (by immunohistochemistry), and often CD103, but it is negative for CD123, cyclin D1, CD200, annexin A1, and CD25.[35,69,115,116] CD43 expression is brighter in HCL compared with HCLv, while CD81 expression is brighter in HCLv.[116] More than half of HCLv cases express immunoglobulin G (IgG) heavy chain, often in combination with other heavy chains—an unusual feature shared with HCL.[89] But unlike HCL, the IGHV gene status is unmutated. HCLv lacks *BRAF* mutations and about 40% show VH4-34 family usage, similar to a small subset of classical HCL as discussed above. It has been shown that 30% to 50% of HCLv cases bear activating mutations in the mitogen-activated protein kinase 1 (*MAP2K1*) gene.[109,117] Activating *ARID1A, KMD6A, CREBBP, CCND3,* and *U2AF1* mutations have also been reported.[95,96] A high proportion of

HCLv cases show 17p *TP53* locus deletion by fluorescence in situ hybridization (FISH),[118] and *TP53* mutations are seen in up to 38% of cases.[95,119] Like HCL, chromosome 7q deletions may also be present.

The clinical course of HCLv is more aggressive than that of HCL, with a median survival of 7 to 9 years in one study, significantly shorter than that of HCL; about 50% of patients are resistant to treatment with purine analogues[89,115,120-124] and the responses are of shorter duration than seen in HCL. HCLv may respond to ibrutinib and some reports suggest that adding rituximab to purine analogue regimens or using anti-CD22 immunotoxin improves outcome.[125-130]

DIFFERENTIAL DIAGNOSIS

The clinical differential diagnosis of pancytopenia, splenomegaly, and a poor or dry aspirate because of bone marrow fibrosis includes myeloid disorders such as myelodysplastic syndromes, myelodysplastic/myeloproliferative neoplasms, primary myelofibrosis, acute myeloid leukemia, and systemic mast cell disease. The spindled appearance of the HCL cells may mimic a sarcoma involving the bone marrow. Diligent review of smear material to identify hairy cells is helpful to exclude these entities and elicit appropriate immunophenotypic studies to confirm the HCL diagnosis; monocytopenia is an additional clue that points to the possibility of HCL in such cases. The relative erythroid hyperplasia and reactive dysplastic changes in hematopoietic elements in bone marrow subtly involved by HCL may lead to an erroneous diagnosis of myelodysplastic syndrome or, in hypoplastic cases, aplastic anemia.[40] Immunostaining on bone marrow biopsy with a B-cell marker such as CD20 is recommended when myelodysplastic syndrome or aplastic anemia is considered but HCL remains a possibility. Mastocytosis and monocytic leukemias on biopsy sections, and large granular lymphocytic leukemia on smear preparations, may morphologically mimic HCL, but can readily be distinguished by their expression of lineage-specific markers and negativity for B-cell markers. In difficult cases, evaluation for the presence of a *BRAF* V600E mutation with molecular genetic techniques or immunostaining may be helpful.

Upon identification of a clonal B-cell population in bone marrow or blood, the unique therapy for HCL requires that this entity be correctly classified; a diagnosis of "low-grade B-cell lymphoma," although appropriate in some instances, should not be rendered if HCL remains a diagnostic possibility. SMZL is the most common differential diagnostic consideration. A nodular and intrasinusoidal (rather than interstitial and diffuse) bone marrow infiltration pattern is a helpful morphologic clue to SMZL. In the peripheral blood, circulating SMZL cells have less prominent and blunter hairy projections that are often "polarized" to one aspect of the cell surface, unlike the encircling hairy projections of HCL.[131] Immunophenotypically, although SMZL cells are also negative for CD5 and CD10, they do not typically manifest the CD103-positive, CD25-positive, CD11c-positive, CD200-bright phenotype characteristic of HCL. In addition, they are CD123 negative and are negative for annexin A1 and cyclin D1 by immunohistochemistry. Splenic diffuse red pulp small B-cell lymphoma (SDRPSBL) is a provisional entity recognized in the revised WHO 4th ed. and in the ICC and is also an entity in the proposed WHO 5th ed. It displays a splenic infiltration pattern similar to HCL and bone marrow intrasinusoidal involvement similar to SMZL. The immunophenotype appears to be more similar to SMZL, although it shares with HCL the expression of DBA.44 and in some cases, expression of CD11c, CD123, and CD103.[111,132-134] There is also some overlap between this entity and HCLv in that they both lack CD25 expression.[44] Useful features in the differential diagnosis of HCL and other lymphoproliferative disorders are summarized in Table 15-4.[61,133-137]

CLINICAL COURSE AND TREATMENT

About 90% of HCL patients will require treatment for symptoms related to recurrent infections, symptomatic splenomegaly, progressive fatigue, or cytopenia (hemoglobin <11 g/dL, platelets <100 × 10⁹/L, or absolute neutrophil count <1.0 × 10⁹/L).[138,139] The clinical course of HCL has changed dramatically owing to major advances in therapy.[140] The purine analogues 2-chlorodeoxyadenosine (2-CdA) and deoxycoformycin (pentostatin, DCF) represent highly effective therapies for HCL, with similar efficacies, and have replaced interferon-α and splenectomy as the first-line therapy.[141-143] The long-term survival of HCL treated with 2-CdA is excellent (96% at 13 years), and death caused by HCL is now uncommon; patients can be expected to experience a normal or near-normal life expectancy.[141,144,145] Although late relapses are relatively common (ranging from 24% at 5 years to nearly 50% at 10 years), relapsed disease usually responds to retreatment with purine analogues.[146] Monoclonal antibodies such as rituximab and anti-CD22 immunotoxin (moxetumomab pasudotox) have proved effective in purine analogue–resistant HCL; rituximab also may be used in combination with purine analogues as first-line therapy.[147-151]

Vemurafenib, a low–molecular-weight inhibitor of BRAF, has been used as a single agent or combined with rituximab to effectively treat HCL cases that are resistant to other therapies.[152-155] Of note, purine analogues and rituximab have been associated with profound immunosuppression and increased risk for severe COVID infection; thus active surveillance or less immunosuppressive agents were used more frequently in HCL patients during the COVID pandemic.[156]

Conventional chemotherapies used to treat other B-cell neoplasms are less helpful in HCL. Splenectomy, which is helpful in the management of SMZL, alleviates symptoms and palliates HCL but does not alter the disease course.[138,157] Thus accurate diagnosis of HCL and distinction from other types of B-cell lymphoma (especially SMZL) are critical in ensuring that patients receive disease-appropriate therapy.

PROGNOSTIC AND PREDICTIVE FACTORS

There are no known morphologic, immunophenotypic, or genetic markers of disease behavior in HCL. Unusual immunophenotypic features such as CD23 or CD10 expression in cases otherwise classic for HCL do not appear to confer an adverse prognosis.[62] The subset of cases using the VH4-34 IGH region and lacking somatic IGHV hypermutation has an inferior prognosis.

Patients are considered to achieve complete remission (CR) if there is near normalization of blood counts (hemoglobin >11 g/dL, platelets >100 × 10⁹/L, absolute

Table 15-4 Differential Diagnosis of Classical Hairy Cell Leukemia

Feature	HCL	SMZL	SDRPSBL	HCLv	CLL	LGL
Morphology						
Nuclei	Oval, indented (bean-shaped)	Round	Round to oval, sometimes eccentric	Round to oval	Round	Round to oval
Chromatin	Finely stippled	Clumped	Clumped	Variable	Clumped	Clumped
Nucleoli	Absent	Small to absent	Small to absent	Present	Small to absent	Absent
Cytoplasm*	Abundant, pale blue	Moderately abundant, basophilic, may be plasmacytoid	Variably abundant, moderately basophilic, may be plasmacytoid	Abundant	Scant, pale	Abundant, blue-gray, granules
Surface*	Circumferential projections	Polar projections	Broad, polar projections	Circumferential projections in a proportion of the cells	Smooth	Smooth
Marrow infiltration pattern	Diffuse and interstitial	Nodular and intrasinusoidal	Intrasinusoidal, interstitial, and nodular	Diffuse, interstitial, and intrasinusoidal	Nodular, interstitial, and/or diffuse	Interstitial and intrasinusoidal
Spleen infiltration pattern	Red pulp	White pulp	Diffuse (red pulp and white pulp)	Red pulp	White pulp	Red pulp
Immunophenotype and Genetics						
Markers	CD20br+ FMC7+ CD5– CD10– CD23– CD103+ CD25+ CD11c+ CD123+ CD200br+ DBA.44+ Annexin A1+ BRAF V600E+	CD20+ FMC7+ CD5– CD10– CD23– CD103– CD25–/+ CD11c+/– CD123– CD200dim+ DBA.44+ Annexin A1– BRAF V600E–	CD20br+ FMC7+ CD5–/+ CD10– CD23– CD103–/+ CD25– CD11c–/+ CD123– Unknown DBA.44+ Annexin A1– BRAF V600E–	CD20br+ FMC7+ CD5– CD10– CD23– CD103+ CD25– CD11c+ CD123– CD200dim DBA.44+ Annexin A1– BRAF V600E–	CD20dim+ FMC7– CD5+ CD10– CD23+ CD103– CD25– CD11c–/+ CD123– CD200br+ BRAF V600E–	CD20– CD3+ BRAF V600E–
Genetics	*BRAF* V600E mutation, may have del(7q) by FISH	del(7q) in about 40%, *NOTCH2* mutation in about 25%	Usually lack del(7q)	*MAP2K1* mutation in 30%–50% 17p *(TP53)* deletion in about 30%	Trisomy 12, del(11q), del(13q), del(17p), rare *BRAF* mutation	*STAT3* and *STAT5B* mutations

*In Wright-Giemsa–stained smear preparations.

br, Bright; *CLL,* chronic lymphocytic leukemia; *FISH,* fluorescence in situ hybridization; *HCL,* hairy cell leukemia; *HCLv,* hairy cell leukemia variant; *LGL,* large granular lymphocytic leukemia; *SDRPSBL,* splenic diffuse red pulp small B-cell lymphoma; *SMZL,* splenic marginal zone lymphoma.

neutrophil count >1.5 × 10⁹/L) without transfusion, regression of any splenomegaly on physical exam, and absence of morphologic evidence of HCL on both peripheral blood and bone marrow examination.[139] Measurable residual disease (MRD) after therapy can be detected by in a subset of patients who are in CR. A consensus opinion suggested that MRD in HCL can be established by identifying hairy cells by bone marrow immunostaining, flow cytometry, or molecular assays to detect a clonal IGH rearrangement or *BRAF* V600E mutation.[158] Immunohistochemical detection of HCL cells in the bone marrow biopsy specimen is particularly valuable given the often hemodilute nature of the aspirate smears in HCL. One study suggested that the presence of low-level HCL in the biopsy can be confirmed by any of the following: CD20-positive cells being more frequent than CD3-positive T cells; more than 50% of CD20 positive cells showing HCL morphology; or the presence of any TRAP-positive cells with HCL morphology.[159] Other investigators have used immunohistochemistry for DBA.44,[20,43,88] CD11c, or an antibody to the T-cell–associated transcription factor T-bet to detect MRD.[78,160] The mutation-specific BRAF V600E

antibody is also a sensitive method to reveal MRD in bone marrow trephine sections, and it effectively detects small amounts of disease after therapy.[86,161]

Flow cytometry[162,163] and molecular genetic methods that detect a specific IGH gene rearrangement[164] or quantitative real-time PCR that detects the *BRAF* V600E mutation[165,166] can also be used to identify MRD in HCL. Flow cytometry can be used to quantify very low levels of HCL cells in the peripheral blood and to follow changes in these levels with therapy.[167,168] Most studies have shown that detectable MRD correlates with disease relapse in HCL after purine analogue therapy,[20,146,169] whereas patients with no detectable MRD (to the level of 10⁻⁴) have a much lower risk for relapse.[170] However, patients with detectable MRD may remain in clinical remission for several years,[88] and MRD detection does not generally guide therapy for HCL patients in clinical remission.[18] Conversely, highly sensitive droplet digital PCR (ddPCR) for the *BRAF* V600E mutation can be used to detect MRD in HCL patients in morphologic remission, and patients with undetectable *BRAF* V600E mutation can be considered to have a complete molecular response.

Pearls and Pitfalls

- Consider performing CD20 immunohistochemistry on bone marrow biopsies to evaluate for subtle hairy cell leukemia (HCL) in patients presenting with an unusual myelodysplastic syndrome–like picture, unexplained infections or fever, or aplastic anemia.
- Look carefully for characteristic HCL morphology in thin areas of well-prepared blood smears to avoid missing hairy cells or overcalling hairy cells owing to smear artifact.
- Consider adding CD103, CD25, CD11c, and CD200 to the flow-cytometry workup of cytopenic patients if any of the following is present:
  - Monocytopenia
  - Splenomegaly (which is unusual in myelodysplastic syndrome)
  - Cells that are suspicious for HCL are detected on review of the peripheral blood or bone marrow smears (especially if lymphocytes with high forward and side scatter on flow cytometry are present).
- Avoid making a general diagnosis of "low-grade B-cell lymphoma" if HCL remains in the differential diagnosis.

KEY REFERENCES

2. Tiacci E, Trifonov V, Schiavoni G, et al. BRAF mutations in hairy-cell leukemia. *N Engl J Med.* 2011;364:2305–2315.
53. Chung SS, Kim E, Park JH, et al. Hematopoietic stem cell origin of BRAFV600E mutations in hairy cell leukemia. *Sci Transl Med.* 2014;6:238ra71.
69. Shao H, Calvo KR, Gronborg M, et al. Distinguishing hairy cell leukemia variant from hairy cell leukemia: development and validation of diagnostic criteria. *Leuk Res.* 2013;37:401–409.
85. Andrulis M, Penzel R, Weichert W, et al. Application of a BRAF V600E mutation-specific antibody for the diagnosis of hairy cell leukemia. *Am J Surg Pathol.* 2012;36:1796–1800.
95. Durham BH, Getta B, Dietrich S, et al. Genomic analysis of hairy cell leukemia identifies novel recurrent genetic alterations. *Blood.* 2017;130(14):1644–1648.
96. Maitre E, Bertrand P, Maingonnat C, et al. New generation sequencing of targeted genes in the classical and the variant form of hairy cell leukemia highlights mutations in epigenetic regulation genes. *Oncotarget.* 2018;9(48):28866–28876.
105. Pettirossi V, Santi A, Imperi E, et al. BRAF inhibitors reverse the unique molecular signature and phenotype of hairy cell leukemia and exert potent antileukemic activity. *Blood.* 2015;125:1207–1216.
109. Waterfall JJ, Arons E, Walker RL, et al. High prevalence of MAP2K1 mutations in variant and IGHV4-34-expressing hairy-cell leukemias. *Nat Genet.* 2014;46:8–10.
139. Grever MR, Abdel-Wahab O, Andritsos LA, et al. Consensus guidelines for the diagnosis and management of patients with classic hairy cell leukemia. *Blood.* 2017;129(5):553–560.
166. Tiacci E, Schiavoni G, Forconi F, et al. Simple genetic diagnosis of hairy cell leukemia by sensitive detection of the BRAF-V600E mutation. *Blood.* 2012;119:192–195.

Visit Elsevier eBooks+ for the complete set of references.

Chapter 16

Splenic Marginal Zone Lymphoma and Other Small B-Cell Neoplasms in the Spleen

Miguel A. Piris and Manuela Mollejo

DEFINITION

The term *splenic marginal zone lymphoma* (SMZL) was coined by Schmid and colleagues[1] in 1992 for a B-cell lymphoma involving the spleen and bone marrow characterized by a micronodular tumoral infiltration that replaces the preexisting lymphoid follicles and shows marginal zone differentiation as a characteristic finding. SMZL is defined in the *World Health Organization (WHO) Classification of Tumours of Haematopoietic and Lymphoid Tissues* as a B-cell neoplasm comprising small lymphocytes that surround and replace the splenic white pulp germinal centers, efface the follicle mantle, and merge with a peripheral (marginal) zone of larger cells, including scattered transformed blasts; both small and larger cells infiltrate the red pulp.[1,2]

A large majority of the cases have a fairly typical clinical presentation characterized by prominent splenomegaly and bone marrow and peripheral blood infiltration. Cells in peripheral blood can frequently be recognized by the villous cytology; this and other findings confirm that SMZL and splenic lymphoma with villous lymphocytes are the same entity.[3,4]

The term splenic marginal zone B-cell lymphoma has prevailed to emphasize the morphologic and molecular features supporting marginal zone differentiation. Despite the name, the clinical, immunophenotypic, and molecular features of SMZL differ from those found in other marginal zone lymphomas (MZLs), indicating SMZL is a distinct clinicopathologic entity unrelated to mucosa-associated lymphoid tissue (MALT) or nodal MZL.

Nowadays, splenectomy is rarely performed, because the diagnosis of splenic low-grade B-cell lymphoma is usually established with the morphologic, immunophenotypic, and molecular findings of bone marrow and peripheral blood samples, integrated with clinical findings.

SYNONYMS AND RELATED TERMS

The WHO 5th edition uses the same terms, with the only exception the hairy cell leukemia variant (HCL$_v$), for which the term *splenic B-cell lymphoma/leukemia with prominent nucleoli* has been proposed.

The term *splenic lymphoma with villous lymphocytes* is quite generic and includes different disorders.

EPIDEMIOLOGY

The incidence of SMZL may be underestimated because, until recently, the diagnosis was typically made on splenectomy specimens; because splenectomy is not performed in many cases of low-grade lymphoma, it is difficult to compare the incidence of this disease with that of other B-cell lymphomas. Nevertheless, SMZL appears to account for about 1% to 2% of all lymphomas.[2,4,5]

The median age at diagnosis is around 65 years, with a range from 30 to 90 years. A female predominance has been found in different series.[6,7]

ETIOLOGY

Analysis of the immunoglobulin (Ig) genes in SMZL shows biased use of selected VH1 genes (*VH1.2*), suggesting a role of unknown antigens in the promotion of tumor cell growth.[8] Interestingly, a small fraction of patients with SMZL harbor hepatitis C virus, and the therapy directed against hepatitis C seems to influence control of the tumor load in these patients, suggesting infectious agents play a role in the pathogenesis of SMZL.[9] This role of infectious agents is supported by the similarities between SMZL and so-called "hyperreactive malarial splenomegaly."[10]

CLINICAL FEATURES

SMZL is a disorder of older adults, with a median age of around 65 years. Most patients are asymptomatic, and usually the disease runs an indolent course. Splenomegaly is the most common sign, observed in 75% of patients; anemia, thrombocytopenia, or leukocytosis is reported in 25% of patients. Autoimmune hemolytic anemia is found in 10% to 15% of patients.[5,11,12] SMZL is infrequently diagnosed incidentally on routine examination, but monoclonal B-lymphocytosis with a marginal zone phenotype has been recognized and could precede some of these marginal zone lymphomas.[13]

Almost without exception, SMZL involves the bone marrow at diagnosis, and roughly 33% of patients have liver involvement. Tumor involvement of peripheral blood (defined as the presence of absolute lymphocytosis or >5% tumor lymphocytes in peripheral blood) was detected in 68% of cases by Chacon's group[11] and in 57% by Berger's.[12] Abdominal lymphadenopathy was observed in 25%; peripheral lymphadenopathy was observed more rarely (17%). Because of the high frequency of bone marrow or liver involvement, most patients are diagnosed at Ann Arbor stage IV at diagnosis. Serum paraproteinemia (usually a small monoclonal IgM) band is observed in 10% to 28% of cases.[5,11,12]

Although the diagnostic criteria were initially based on splenic morphology, the conjunction of clinical features, immunophenotype, and morphology allows a diagnosis with a reasonably high level of confidence on bone marrow biopsy specimens.

MORPHOLOGY

Splenic involvement in SMZL is the rule, and some cases may even show a massive splenomegaly, rarely seen in other B-cell lymphoma disorders, with the exception of HCL. Histologic studies display a micronodular lymphoid infiltrate in which white pulp follicles are increased in both size and number, with a variable degree of red pulp involvement always present (Fig. 16-1). The neoplastic follicles typically have a biphasic appearance, with the presence of both a small-cell and a peripheral marginal cell component. The cells in the center of the follicles are small lymphocytes with generally round nuclei and scant cytoplasm, and the cells in the marginal zones have irregular nuclear contours and moderately abundant pale cytoplasm. In addition, most cases contain scattered proliferating large B cells resembling centroblasts or immunoblasts; in the spleen, these appear in the marginal zone and red pulp, but they can also be seen in the bone marrow and lymph nodes.[14] Residual or colonized germinal centers may be seen in the centers of some nodules (as in the bone marrow), sometimes highlighted by follicular dendritic cell staining. Neoplastic plasma cells may be present within the germinal centers, forming clusters in rare cases, and in the splenic red pulp, surrounding small arterioles. The cellular composition of the tumor follicles may plausibly reflect the capacity of marginal zone B cells to induce germinal-center development through the transport of immune complexes to the follicular dendritic cells[15]; thus, tissue infiltration by SMZL in the bone marrow or other locations is frequently accompanied by the presence of induced lymphoid follicles with reactive/colonized germinal centers.

In contrast with the organoid pattern of involvement of the white pulp, mimicking the architecture of normal splenic lymphoid follicles, the red pulp more frequently shows a diffuse pattern of involvement, with infiltration of both the cords and the sinuses. The cells in the red pulp include both small lymphocytes and large centroblasts or immunoblasts. Epithelioid histiocytes may be present in some cases, sometimes surrounding neoplastic follicles.

Splenic hilar lymph nodes are commonly involved in SMZL (Fig. 16-2), but peripheral lymph node involvement is rarely seen at diagnosis. In these SMZL-involved lymph nodes, a marginal zone pattern is only rarely observed. The pattern is typically micronodular, and the cells are predominantly small; sinuses may be dilated.[16] The variability of the cellular composition of the tumor in various sites suggests the microenvironment is relevant to the pattern of tumor growth.[1,2]

Bone marrow infiltration is the rule in SMZL, although it may be difficult to recognize on routine morphologic sections (Fig. 16-3). CD20 staining helps reveal the presence of intertrabecular lymphoid aggregates and intrasinusoidal small tumor cells. The intertrabecular nodules mimic the architecture and cell composition of tumor nodules in the spleen, with occasional reactive germinal centers surrounded by tumor cells. Characteristically, CD20 staining reveals the presence of linear aggregates of intrasinusoidal B cells.[17,18] The intrasinusoidal pattern can be observed in other B-cell lymphomas, including follicular lymphoma (FL), mantle cell lymphoma (MCL), chronic lymphocytic leukemia (CLL), and HCL, but the combination of intertrabecular nodules with intrasinusoidal infiltration is quite characteristic of SMZL. In contrast with lymphoplasmacytic lymphoma (LPL), bone marrow infiltration in SMZL lacks the prominent mast cell component. Differential diagnosis for FL is facilitated by the staining of SMZL cells with antibodies for MNDA or T-bet, negative in the vast majority of FL cases. Also, although SMZL nodules in the bone marrow may show some peritrabecular arrangement, they lack the characteristic paratrabecular pattern (surrounding bone marrow trabeculae) typical in FL cases and occasionally observed in LPL.

Peripheral blood involvement is less frequent than bone marrow infiltration. However, it is relatively common to find a small number of neoplastic B cells in the blood, some of which may have a villous morphology. This usually takes the form of small cytoplasmic projections at one pole of the rather abundant cytoplasm (Fig. 16-4). There are cases that present clinically with monoclonal lymphocytosis, with morphology, phenotype, and molecular findings compatible with SMZL, and that later develop splenomegaly.[13]

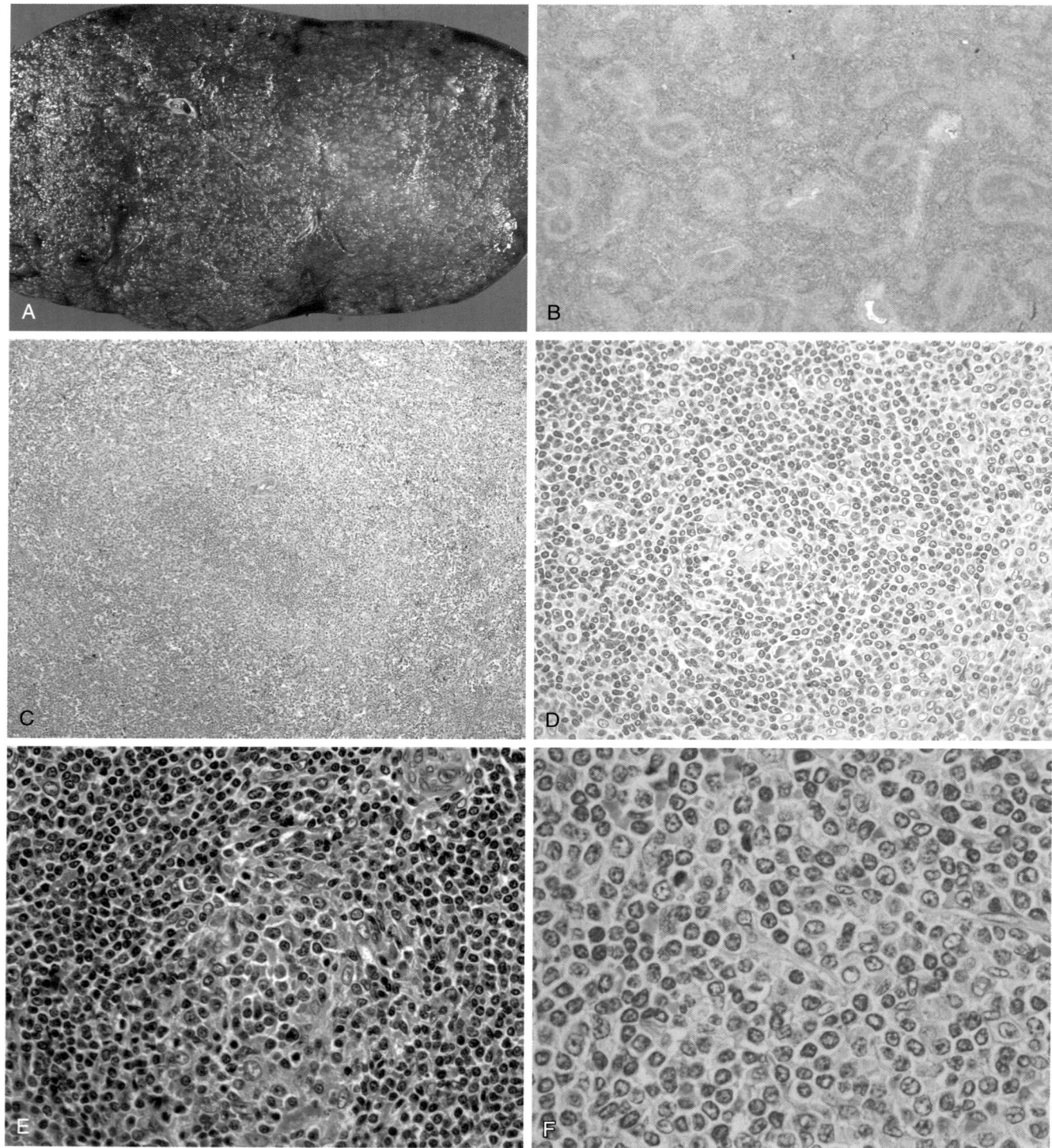

Figure 16-1. Splenic marginal zone lymphoma morphology in the spleen. A, Gross photograph shows a micronodular homogeneous pattern. **B,** Low magnification shows marginal zone differentiation and biphasic cytology, with pale-staining cells in the marginal zone, darker cells in the interior of the follicle, and occasional pale central areas, indicating residual reactive germinal centers. **C** and **D,** Replacement of lymphoid follicles by neoplastic cells (Giemsa stain). **E,** Germinal center infiltration by neoplastic cells at a higher magnification; this case shows plasmacytic differentiation within the germinal center. **F,** Cytologic features. Cells in the marginal zone component have slightly enlarged nuclei and abundant pale cytoplasm, which is in contrast to the neoplastic small-cell component in the center of the nodules (Giemsa stain).

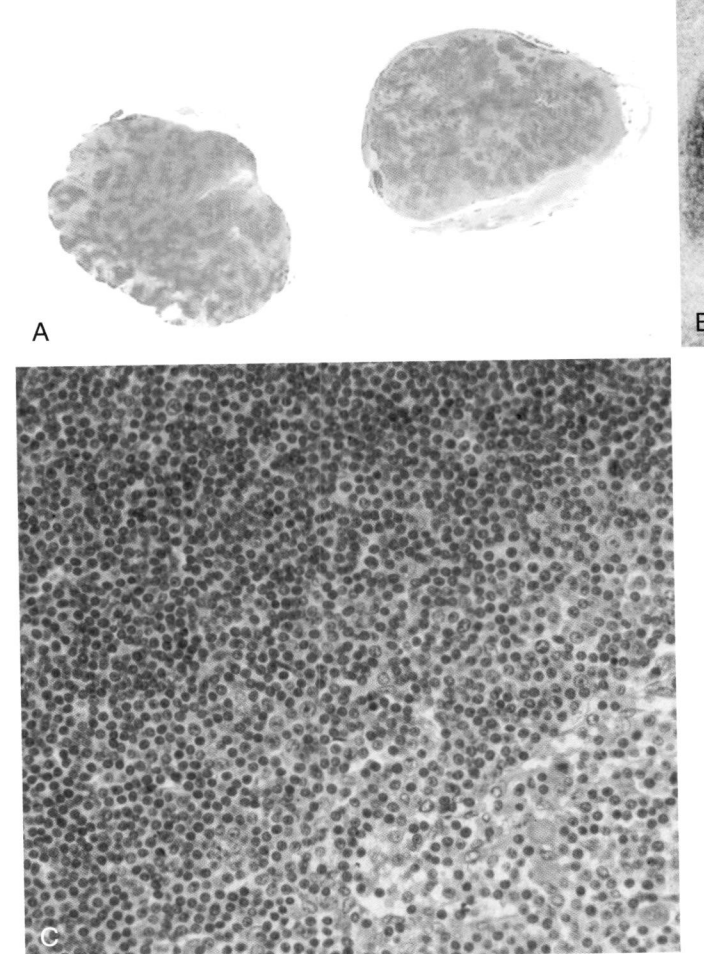

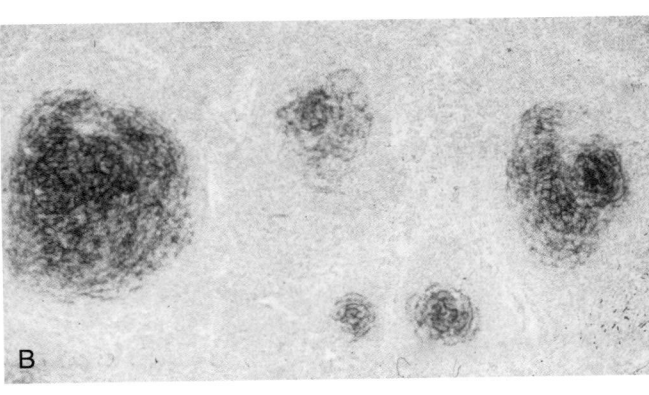

Figure 16-2. Lymph node involvement by splenic marginal zone lymphoma. A, Low magnification of a splenic hilar lymph node with a micronodular pattern and prominent sinusoidal dilation. **B,** Tumor is centered in lymphoid follicles, highlighted by staining for follicular dendritic cells (immunoperoxidase stain for CD23). **C,** Higher magnification shows small tumor cells in the lymph node, with scant cytoplasm and clumped chromatin and lacking marginal zone differentiation.

An increase in the number of large cells can be seen within the marginal zone rings of the spleen and is definitely associated with large cell transformation,[14,19,20] but a reproducible way of counting these large cells and a threshold associated with increased risk of large cell transformation has not been defined.

IMMUNOPHENOTYPE

Immunophenotypic features are summarized in Box 16-1 and shown in Figure 16-5. SMZL cells usually express B-cell markers such as CD20, Pax5, and CD79a and IgD and marginal zone markers such as MNDA and T-bet, with staining for DBA44 in at least a proportion of the neoplastic cells.

SMZL lacks the expression of CLL markers (LEF1, CD5, CD23), although CD5 is expressed in 25%[20,21] of SMZL cases and associated with a more tumoral clinical presentation. SMZL cells are negative for FL markers (BCL6, CD10), MCL markers (SOX11, CyclinD1), and HCL markers (AnnexinA1, CyclinD1).

MIB-1 staining shows a distinctive annular pattern, indicating the presence of an increased growth fraction in both the germinal centers and the marginal zones. BCL2 staining helps to distinguish the reactive germinal centers, occasionally infiltrated by BCL2-positive neoplastic cells. MNDA and T-bet staining are definitely useful in the differential diagnosis for FL.[21]

Flow cytometry is also useful in the recognition of SMZL. According to the Matutes CLL score, most SMZL cases have scores ranging from 0 to 2.[3] In the majority of patients, the immunophenotype is CD20+, CD22+, CD24+, CD27+, FMC7+, IgD+, IgM+, and CD79b+, and some of them are DBA44+ (75%), CD11c+ (50%), CD23+ (30%), CD103+ (<10%), CD25+ (25%), and CD5+ (20%).[3]

An inflamed phenotype of splenic marginal zone B-cell lymphomas, with expression of PD-L1 by intratumoral monocytes/macrophages and dendritic cells, has been demonstrated, a finding that could have important conceptual and therapeutic implications.[22]

GENETICS
Genetic Abnormalities

The analysis of chromosome region 7q22-36 demonstrated allelic loss in up to 40% of cases, a frequency higher than that observed in other B-cell neoplasms (8%).[23] A minimal common deleted region has been mapped to a 3-Mb region at 7q32.1-32.2.[24] This region has been shown to contain some potentially relevant genes[25-27] and a cluster of micro-RNA.[25,28]

Other clonal chromosome abnormalities detected in SMZL are gain of 3q (10% to 20%) and involvement of chromosomes 1, 8, and 14. No t(11;14)(q13;q32) or t(14;18)(q21;q32) are seen. Occasional cytogenetic abnormalities involving 14q32,

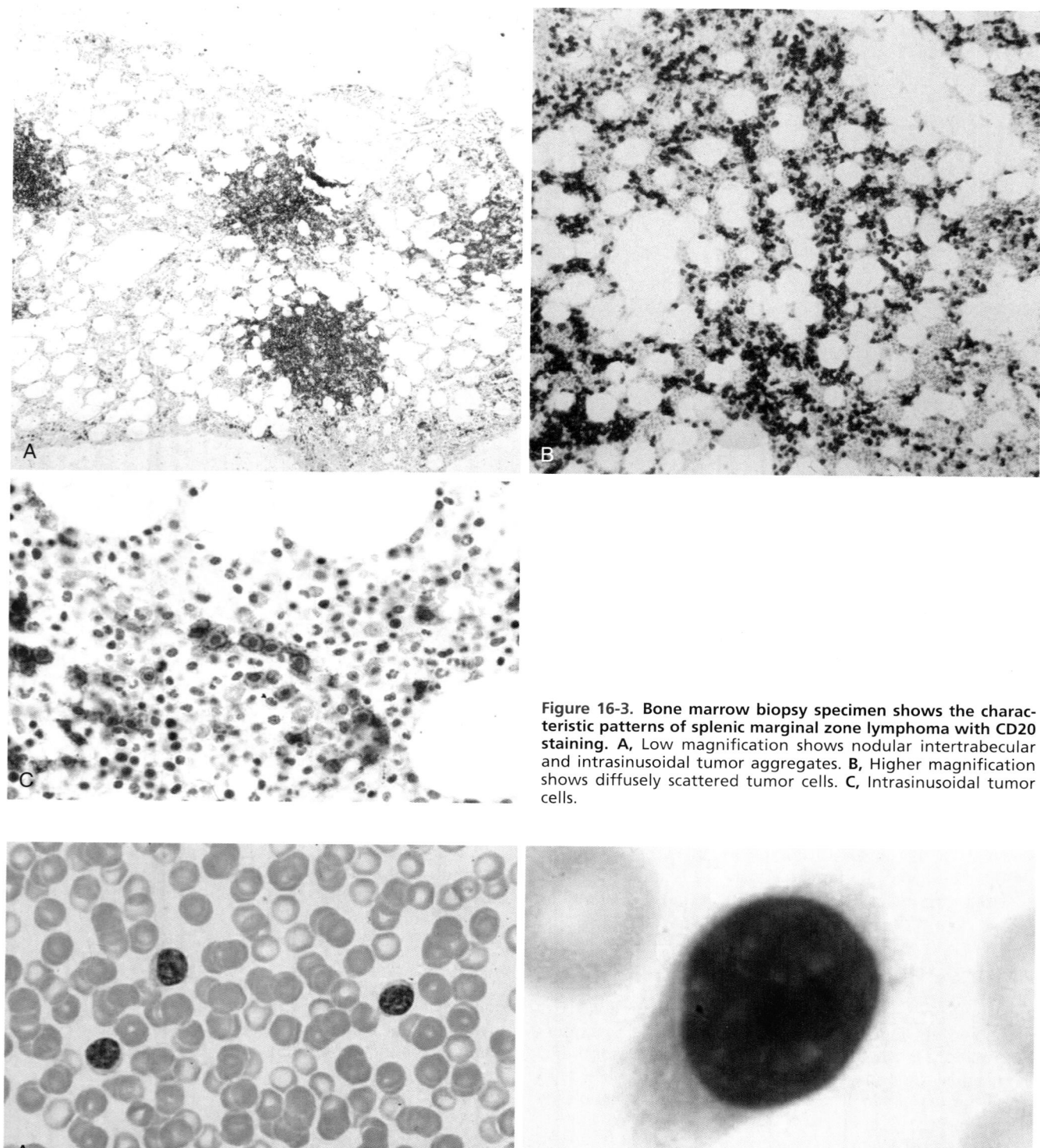

Figure 16-3. Bone marrow biopsy specimen shows the characteristic patterns of splenic marginal zone lymphoma with CD20 staining. A, Low magnification shows nodular intertrabecular and intrasinusoidal tumor aggregates. B, Higher magnification shows diffusely scattered tumor cells. C, Intrasinusoidal tumor cells.

Figure 16-4. A and B, Peripheral blood morphology shows villous lymphocytes. Villi are typically short and are described as polar—that is, they are concentrated at one pole of the cytoplasm, in contrast to the longer, circumferential villi typically seen in hairy cell leukemia. Villi are usually seen in only a subset of cells.

such as t(6;14)(p12;q32) and t(10;14)(q24;q32), or 7q21 (with deregulation of cyclin-dependent kinase 6) are rarely found, but they may distinguish specific clinicopathological variants.[29] Deletion of 17p13 (TP53) has been observed in 3% to 17% of cases.[30-33]

Whole-exome sequencing in SMZL reveals mutations in genes involved in marginal zone differentiation, NOTCH2 and others. The most frequently mutated gene is KLF2, a transcription factor important for B-cell differentiation and NF-κB activation, found in 20% to 42% of SMZL cases.[34,35]

All SMZL genetic studies coincide in showing high frequency of mutations in NF-κB pathway genes; specifically, *TNFAIP3, MYD88, TRAF3, CARD11, IKBKB,* and *BIRC3.*[34-38]

The *MYD88* L265P mutation can be found in otherwise typical SMZL cases (4% to 15%)[39,40]; nevertheless, SMZL cases with the *MYD88* mutation should be investigated for the presence of serum paraproteinemia and other findings suggesting LPL.[40,41]

Published data has confirmed the results of previous molecular studies, disclosing two main genetic clusters in SMZL, one termed NNK (58% of cases, harboring NF-κB, NOTCH, and KLF2 modules) and the second denominated

---

Box 16-1 *Major Diagnostic Features of Splenic Marginal Zone Lymphoma*

Clinical Features
• Splenomegaly
• Bone marrow involvement
• Lymphocytosis with or without villous cells

Morphologic Features
• Spleen: micronodular pattern; biphasic cytology; follicular replacement; marginal zone differentiation; diffuse, micronodular infiltration of red pulp
• Peripheral blood: villous cells, small lymphocytes
• Bone marrow: intertrabecular nodules, occasionally with a marginal zone pattern and follicular dendritic cell remnants
• Lymph nodes: micronodular pattern, small lymphocytes, scattered blasts, rare marginal zone differentiation

Immunophenotypic Features
• CD20+, IgD+, BCL2+, MNDA+, CD3−, CD23−, CD43−, CD5−, CD10−, cyclin D1−, BCL6−, annexin A_1−
• Ki-67 (MIB-1) low (target pattern with higher proliferation in germinal center and marginal zone); residual germinal centers may be BCL2−, BCL6+

Genetic Features
• 7q deletion: 40%
• *TP53* gene alterations: 0% to 20%[32]
• Somatic mutation in *NOTCH2/KLF2* and other marginal zone genes[34,36,38]
• *IgVH* gene somatic mutations: frequent VH1.2 use, low mutational load

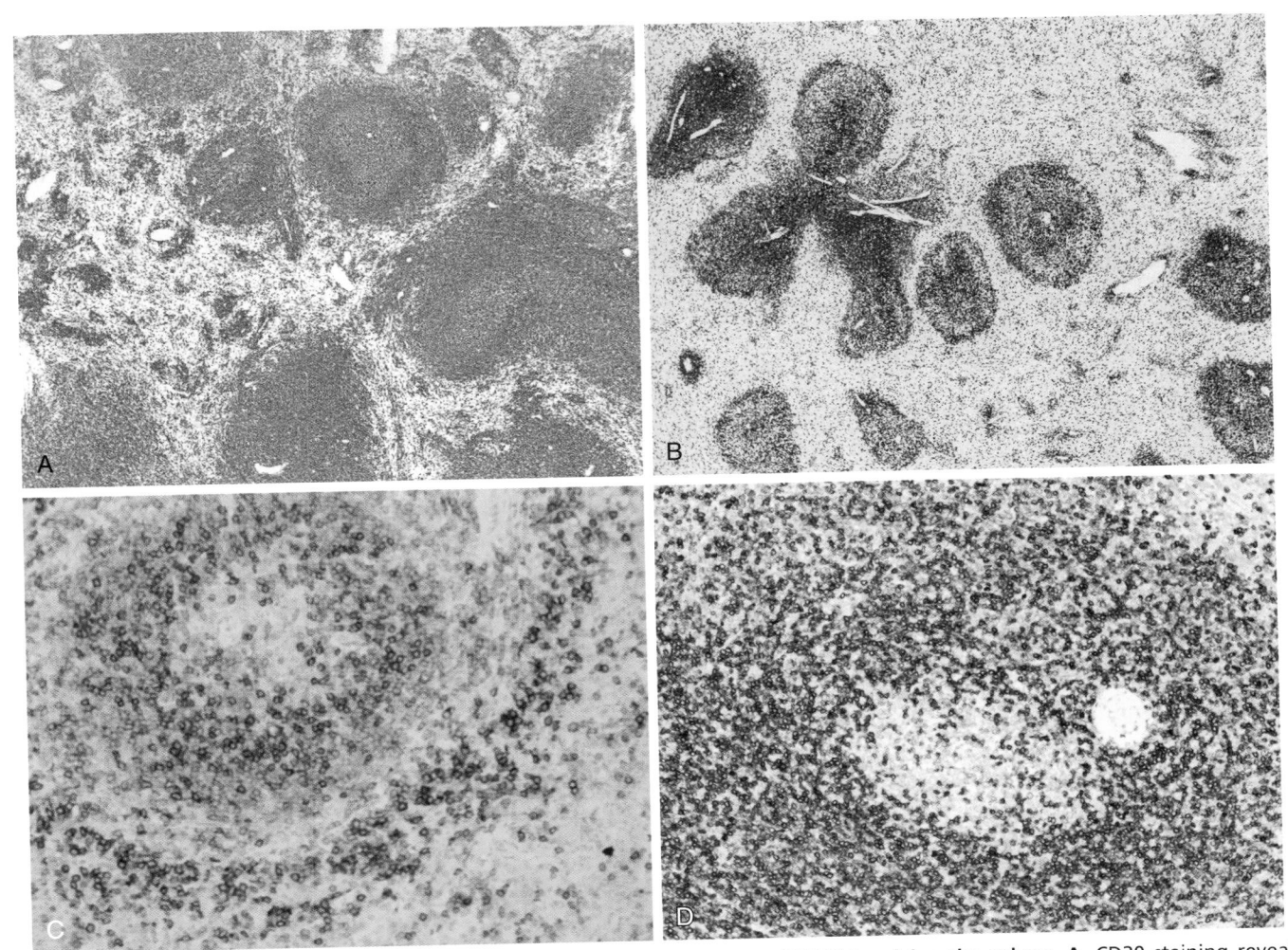

Figure 16-5. Immunophenotypic features of splenic marginal zone lymphoma (SMZL) involving the spleen. A, CD20 staining reveals prominent red pulp infiltration. **B,** CD3-positive T cells in the follicle centers and red pulp, highlighting the micronodular pattern. **C,** Immunoglobulin D staining in the tumor cells. **D,** BCL2 staining shows a BCL2-negative germinal center surrounded and partially replaced by tumor cells.

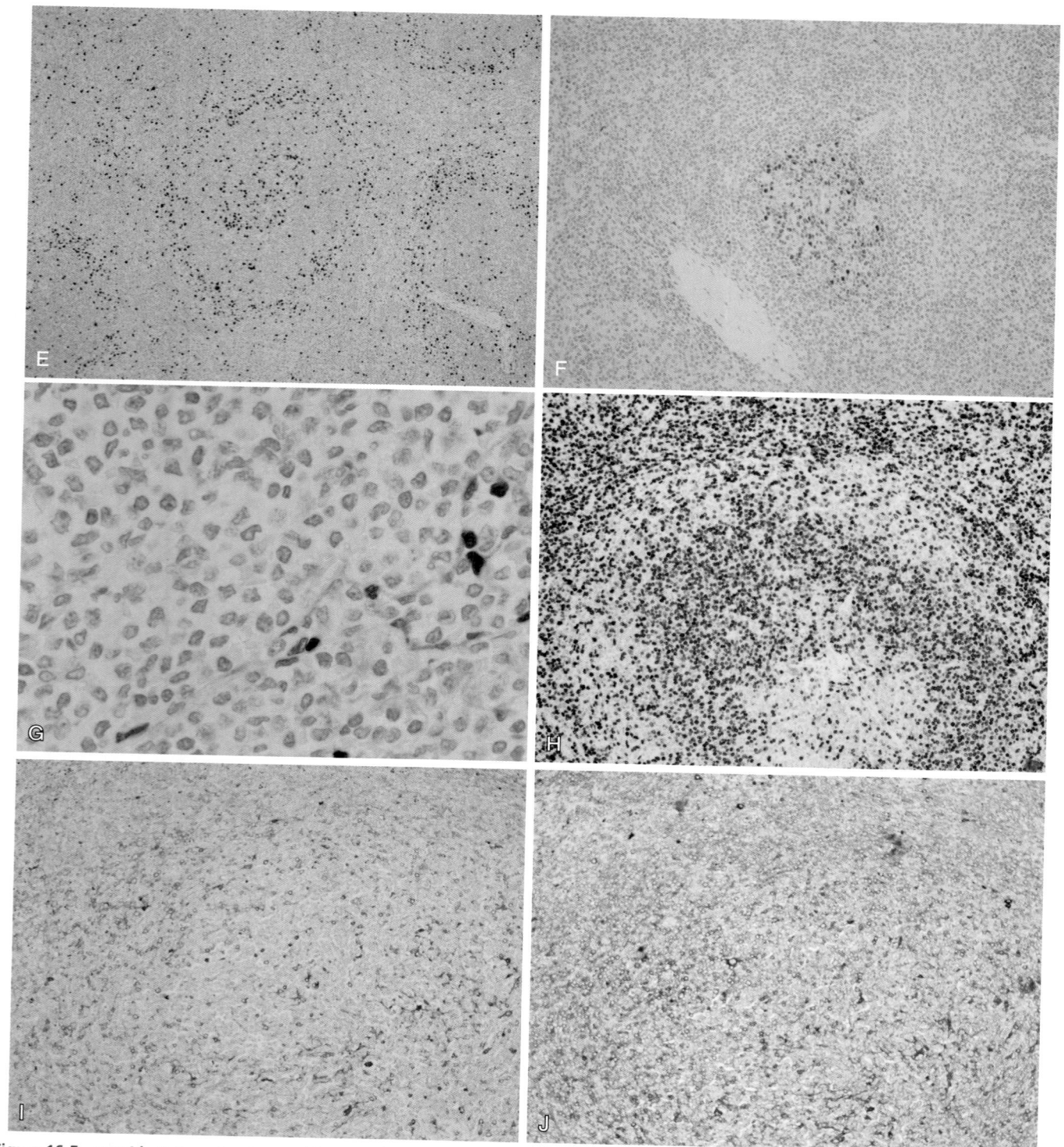

Figure 16-5—cont'd. **E,** Target pattern with MIB-1 (Ki-67) staining; there are proliferating cells in the germinal center and in the peripheral marginal zone. **F,** BCL6 staining outlines the reactive germinal center cells. **G,** Cyclin D1 negativity. **H,** MNDA-positive staining outlines SMZL patterns of infiltration. Light-chain restriction is revealed by **(I)** the negative cytoplasmic staining for lambda and **(J)** positivity for kappa.

as DMT (32% of cases, with DNA-damage response, MAPK, and TLR modules). Both genetic types also differ in survival probability, with inferior survival in NNK-SMZLs. The study also revealed variations in the SMZL immune microenvironments, with two main types denominated as immune-suppressive SMZL (50% of cases, associated with inflammatory cells and immune checkpoint activation) and immune-silent SMZL (50% of cases, associated with an immune-excluded phenotype) with distinct mutational and clinical correlations.[42]

Antigen Receptor Genes

The frequency of Ig heavy-chain variable region (IgVH) somatic mutations has also been investigated in SMZL. The frequency of IGHV1-2 use has been shown to oscillate from 25% to 44% of cases. Most (95%) of these rearrangements were mutated; however, they mostly carried a low mutational load (97% to 99.9% germline identity) of conservative nature and restricted distribution, which supports the presence of antigenic selection in the pathogenesis of SMZL.[8,43-45] Although antigen selection and biased use of Ig genes has been found in different B-cell lymphomas, such as FL, CLL, LPL, and others, the use of IGHV1-2 in SMZL has been confirmed in multiple studies and has allowed the proposition that some SMZL subtypes could derive from B-cell progenitor populations adapted to specific antigenic challenges through selection of VH domain specificities.[43]

Gene-Expression Profiling

Gene-expression profiling studies have revealed potential diagnostic markers and pathogenetic pathways involved in tumor cell survival. Thus, the signature obtained in different studies coincides with upregulation of the following families of genes:

- Genes involved in apoptosis regulation, B-cell receptor and tumor necrosis factor signaling, and nuclear factor-κB activation, such as *SYK, BTK, BIRC3, TRAF3, TRAF5, CD40,* and *LTB.*
- Genes associated with the splenic microenvironment, such as *SELL* and *LPXN.*
- Lymphoma oncogenes such as *ARHH* and *TCL1.*[46] Increased *TCL1* expression is linked with *AKT1* activation in SMZL, as proposed by Thieblemont and colleagues.[47]
- *AP-1* and *NOTCH2* transcription factors.[48]

Cell of Origin

The debate over the cellular origin of SMZL has been fueled by conflicting morphologic and molecular findings. A large proportion of tumor cells in SMZL are IgD-positive small lymphocytes in which marginal zone differentiation is produced only in the microenvironment provided by the splenic marginal zone. The presence of somatic mutations in genes (*NOTCH2, KLF2,* and others) involved in marginal zone differentiation supports the relationship of the neoplastic cells with the normal marginal zone. Alternatively, the low mutational load of the *IgVH* genes in SMZL cases does not support a close relationship with normal marginal zone B cells, which typically have somatic mutations, indicating passage through the germinal center.[49] These findings favor the existence of a subpopulation of small B cells in the primary lymphoid follicles of the spleen with the potential capacity to differentiate into marginal zone B cells in the appropriate environment and to acquire somatic mutations after exposure to antigens present in the germinal center.

Clinical Course

SMZL is a low-grade tumor with a survival probability of 5 years that varies from 65% (for patients diagnosed with SMZL after splenectomy) to 78% (for patients diagnosed with splenic lymphoma with villous lymphocytes [SLVL] in peripheral blood).[5,11] A large SMZL study found 68.5% overall survival after 10 years follow-up.[42]

The few studies performed on relatively large series show that adverse clinical prognostic factors are related to high tumor burden and poor performance status. The biological parameters associated with adverse outcome are *TP53* mutation or overexpression, 7q deletion, and the absence of somatic mutation in *IgVH* genes. SMZL therefore seems to behave similarly to CLL, in which an unfavorable clinical course is associated with *TP53* inactivation and unmutated (naïve) *IgVH* genes. Massive high-throughput studies have shown *NOTCH2* and *TP53* gene mutations are independent markers of reduced treatment-free and overall survival.[34,42,50]

Although little information about SMZL is available from clinical trials, some clear points have emerged. These include the lack of efficacy of 2-chlorodeoxyadenoside typically used in HCL,[51] the relatively favorable course for patients treated with splenectomy,[5,52] and the potential efficacy of fludarabine for patients who relapse after splenectomy or are resistant to chlorambucil.[51] Rituximab, with or without splenectomy, has been found to be a very good option for the treatment of SMZL,[53,54] and rituximab monotherapy has been shown to induce prolonged responses.[54] The BRISMA trial has shown that a combination of bendamustine with rituximab is a good option when a chemotherapy combination with rituximab is deemed necessary for symptomatic patients with SMZL.[55] Consistent with the data generated in gene expression profiling studies demonstrating an activated B-cell receptor signaling pathway in SMZL, durable ibrutinib responses have been shown in relapsed/refractory marginal zone lymphoma cases.[56] Hepatitis C–positive patients seem to benefit from antiviral therapy.[9] Specific recommendations for therapy have been published.[3,57] A simple staging system has also been published and validated, using hemoglobin concentration, platelet count, lactate dehydrogenase (LDH) level, and the presence of extrahilar lymphadenopathy.[58]

Patients with SMZL appear to have a greater frequency of transformation to large B-cell lymphoma (13% of cases with adequate follow-up) than those with CLL (1% to 10%), although the incidence of large cell transformation in SMZL is lower than in follicular lymphoma (25% to 60%). In the cases studied to date, it seems that progression in SMZL could depend on multiple factors, including *TP53* mutations and Epstein-Barr virus (EBV) presence, and is more frequently associated with 7q loss.[14,33,50,59]

Differential Diagnosis

The differential diagnosis of SMZL and other small B-cell lymphomas requires the integration of clinical, morphologic, immunophenotypic, and genetic information (Table 16-1). A micronodular pattern of splenic involvement with villous cells in the peripheral blood can be observed in other conditions, particularly in FL, but also in MCL (Figs. 16-6 and 16-7). Immunophenotyping and genetic features are usually diagnostic; FL is typically CD10 and/or BCL6 positive, though MCL expresses SOX11 and Cyclin D1. The absence of t(14;18)(q32;q21) and t(11;14)(q13;q32) is also helpful in ruling out these entities, respectively.[60] Particularly helpful features are the intrasinusoidal pattern of involvement in the bone marrow[17,18] and IgD expression by tumor cells. Differential diagnosis with FL is also facilitated by the common expression of MNDA and T-bet by SMZL cells.[21,61]

Distinguishing LPL may be problematic, because SMZL has shown some degree of plasmacytic differentiation with serum monoclonal paraproteinemia in up to 28% of cases

Table 16-1　Differential Diagnosis of Splenic Marginal Zone Lymphoma

Feature	SMZL	CLL	MCL	FL	LPL	MALT MZL (Noncutaneous)
Morphology						
Pattern	Micronodular + Marginal zone	Micronodular/Diffuse	Micronodular/Diffuse	Micronodular +/− Marginal zone	Micronodular/Red pulp	Marginal Zone
Cytologic composition	Small lymphocytes, Large B cells, Marginal zone cells	Small lymphocytes, Prolymphocytes, Paraimmunoblasts	Monomorphous centrocytes	Centrocytes, Centroblasts	Small cells, Plasmacytoid cells, Plasma cells	Small lymphocytes, Blast cells, Marginal zone cells
Marginal zone pattern in spleen	+ (not in LN)	−	−/+	+/−	−	+ in all sites
Immunophenotype						
IgD	+	+	+	−	−	−
LEF1	−	+	−	−	−/+	−
CD5	−	+	+	−	−	−
CD23	−	+	−	−	−	−
CD10	−	−	−	+	−	−
Cyclin D1/SOX11	−	−	+	−	−	−
MNDA/T-bet	+/−	−/+	−/+	−/+	−	−
BCL6	−	−	−	+	−/+	+
MIB-1	Target pattern	Low	Low-medium	Low	Low	Low
Genetic Features						
Trisomy 3 (%)	17	3	−	−	−	50-85
Trisomy 12 (%)	10-50	20	5-15	−	−	5-15
7q− (%)	40	−	−	−	−	−
t(11;14)(q13;q32)(%)	−	−	98	−	−	−
t(14;18)(q21;q32)(%)	−	−	−	90	−	−
t(11;18)(q21;q21)(%)	−	−	−	−	−	40-60
IgVH somatic mutations (>2%)	51	54	25	90	100	100
MYD88 L265P	5-15%	4%	−	−	95%	15%
Clinical Findings						
Splenomegaly	+	+	+	+	+	−
BM involvement	+	+	25%	+	+	+
PB involvement	+	+	20%-58%	9%	+	20%
M-component	10%-40%	20%	−	−	95%	20%
Peripheral LN	Rare	Rare	+	10%-20%	+	Rare
Non-hematopoietic extranodal sites	Rare	−	GI, Waldeyer's ring	GI	Rare	+

BM, Bone marrow; CLL, chronic lymphocytic leukemia; FL, follicular lymphoma; GI, gastrointestinal; Ig, immunoglobulin; LN, lymph node; LPL, lymphoplasmacytic lymphoma; MALT MZL, mucosa-associated lymphoid tissue marginal zone lymphoma; MCL, mantle cell lymphoma; PB, peripheral blood; SMZL, splenic marginal zone lymphoma.

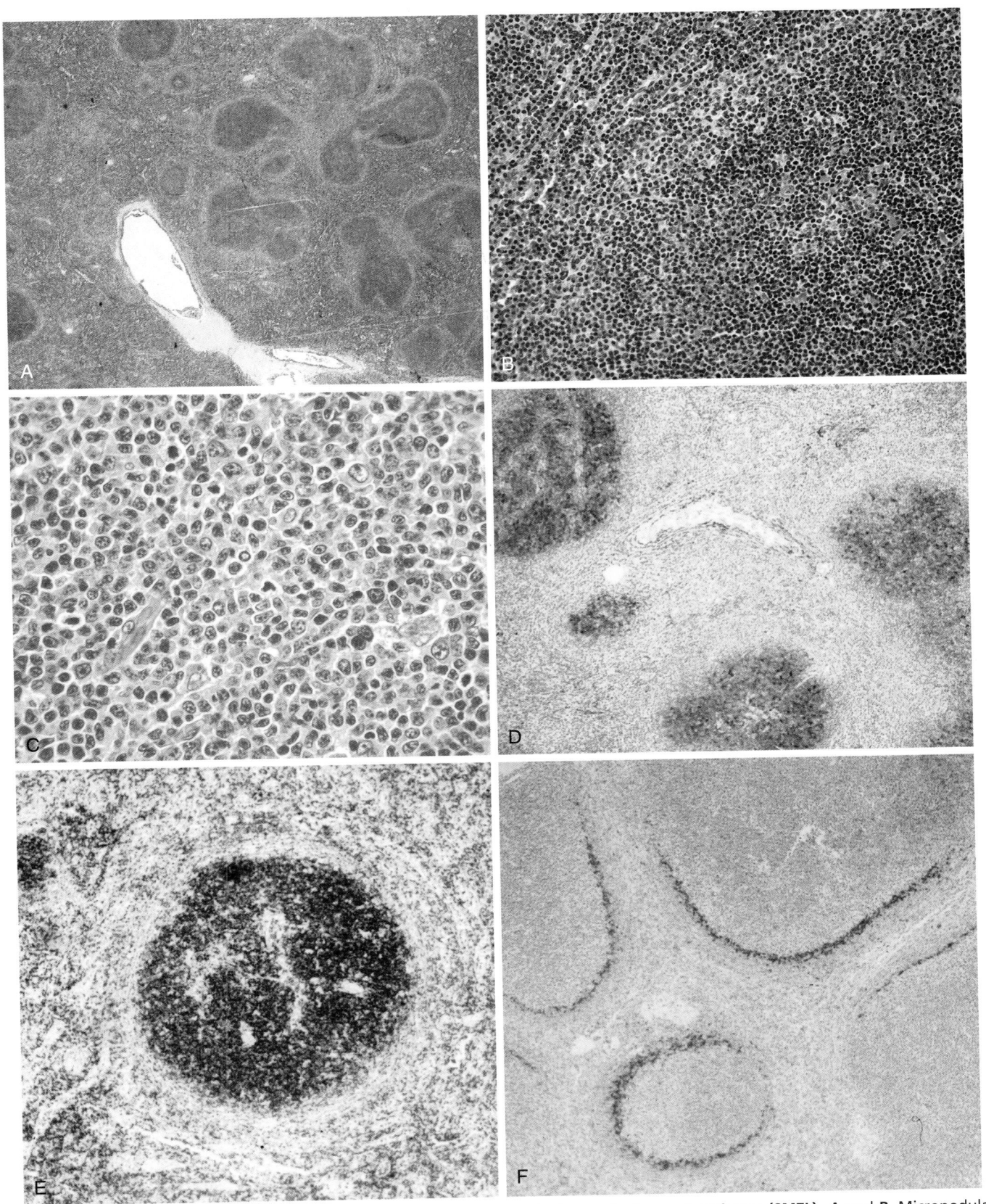

Figure 16-6. Follicular lymphoma with splenic infiltration, mimicking splenic marginal zone lymphoma (SMZL). A and **B,** Micronodular pattern with marginal zone differentiation. **C,** On higher magnification, the cells in the follicles are a mixture of centrocytes and centroblasts, typical of germinal-center cells (Giemsa stain). **D,** CD10 staining highlights the entire follicle rather than just a residual germinal center, as would be seen in SMZL. **E,** Homogeneous BCL2 expression within the follicle. **F,** Characteristic immunoglobulin D staining of residual mantle cells; the neoplastic cells are negative.

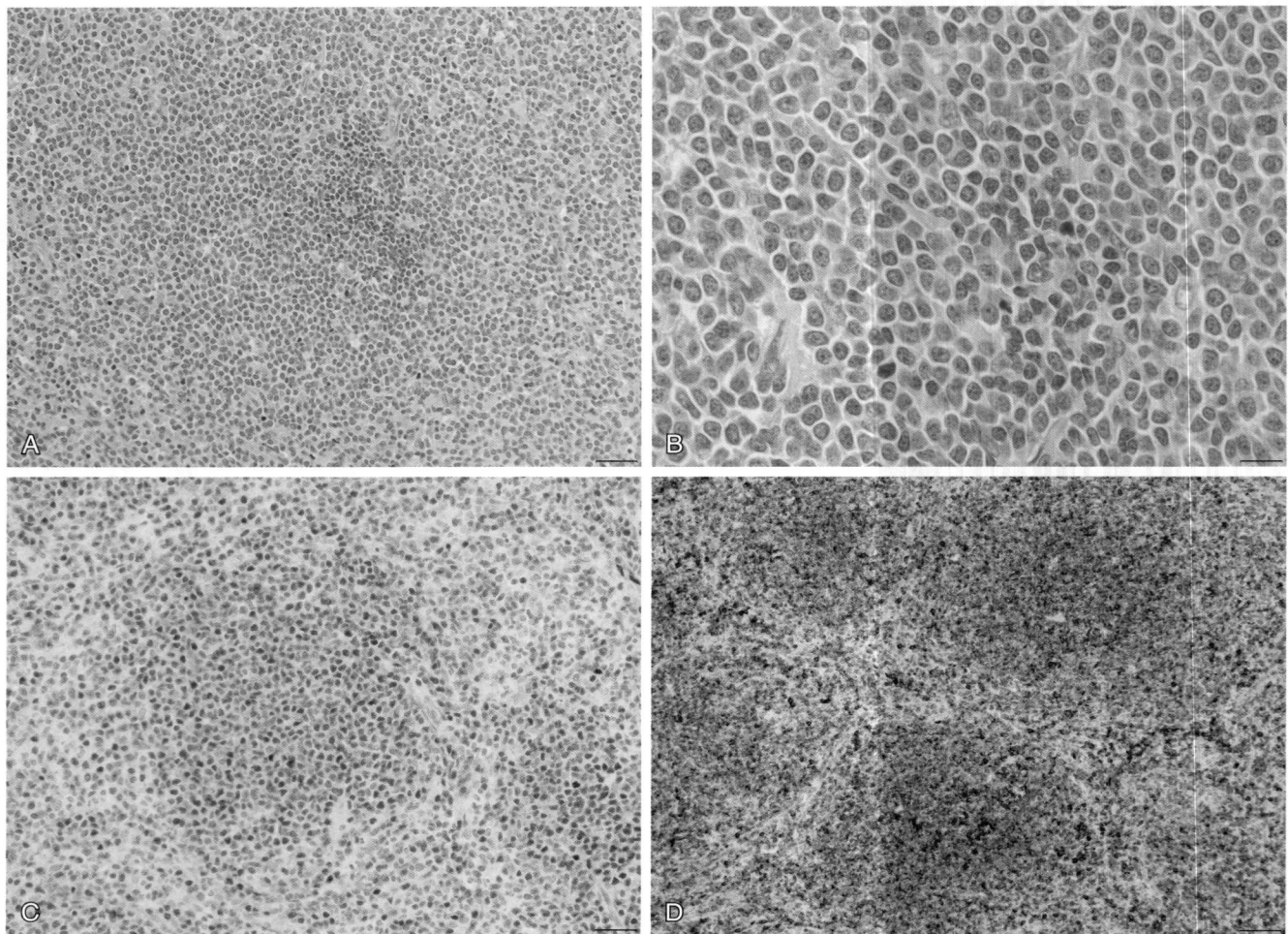

Figure 16-7. Mantle cell lymphoma splenic infiltration. Micronodular pattern **(A)**, with monomorphous cytology **(B)**. Tumor cells are Cyclin D1 positive **(C)** and CD5 positive **(D)**.

in some series. There are no specific immunophenotypic features that distinguish these disorders; however, detection of the characteristic 7q abnormalities favors SMZL. Patients with SMZL rarely have a sufficient serum IgM concentration to result in hyperviscosity syndromes. Bone marrow trephine examination may be useful, because LPL typically produces a subtle, diffuse (sometimes paratrabecular) lymphoplasmacytic infiltrate with striking increase in the proportion of mast cells; if intertrabecular lymphoid aggregates with a marginal zone pattern or intrasinusoidal involvement are recognized, a diagnosis of SMZL should be suspected. Finally, on splenectomy specimens, the pattern of infiltration in LPL is typically diffuse red pulp involvement, in contrast to the nodular involvement of both white and red pulp in SMZL.[62] The presence of a *MYD88* L265P mutation should lead to consideration of a possible LDL diagnosis.[41,63]

Rarely, MALT-type MZL may infiltrate the spleen with a micronodular pattern, characteristically involving the splenic marginal zone and thus causing diagnostic problems. Useful distinguishing features are the absence of t(11;18)(q21;q21) typical of MALT-type MZL in SMZL,[64] the presence of 7q abnormalities in SMZL, and the characteristic IgD expression in SMZL, which is only rarely observed in MALT-type MZL.

OTHER SPLENIC B-CELL LYMPHOMAS
Splenic Diffuse Red Pulp Small B-Cell Lymphoma

This lymphoma presents clinically with splenomegaly, bone marrow, and peripheral blood involvement, similar to SMZL. Villous cells and clonal expansions of B cells in peripheral blood with marginal zone phenotype may precede both entities,[13] although they may be more frequent in splenic diffuse red pulp small B-cell lymphoma (SRPL) (Fig. 16-8).[65] However, the histopathological findings in the splenectomy specimen are quite different. Instead of the micronodular pattern with biphasic cytology composition presented in SMZL, the spleen features in SRPL show diffuse involvement of the red pulp with infiltration of cords and sinuses, effacement of the white pulp, and monomorphous population of small cells resembling marginal zone B cells. Both SMZL and SRPL show intrasinusoidal infiltration in the bone marrow, but it is usually more striking in SRPL cases, where a pure intrasinusoidal pattern may be frequently observed. The expression of cyclin D3, CD180, and DBA44 is more frequent in SRPL than in SMZL.[66-69]

Cytogenetic findings and molecular data such as 7q deletion, trisomies of chromosomes 3 and 18, and mutations

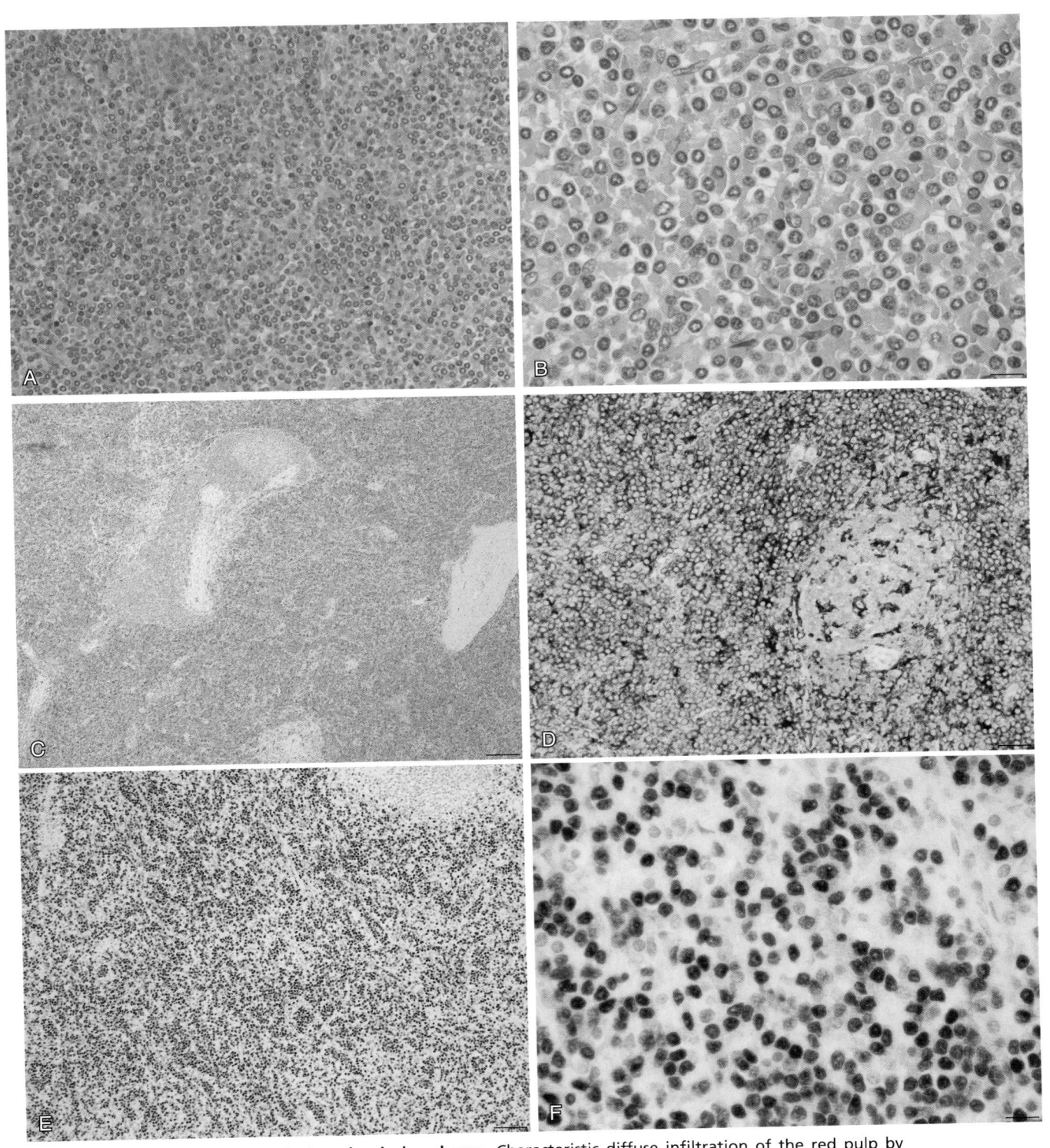

Figure 16-8. Splenic red pulp lymphoma. Characteristic diffuse infiltration of the red pulp by small lymphocytes, with sinusoidal infiltration (**A** and **B**). The diffuse occupation of the red pulp is emphasized by staining with DBA44 (**C**), CD11c (**D**), CYCLIND3 (**E** and **F**), and

Continued

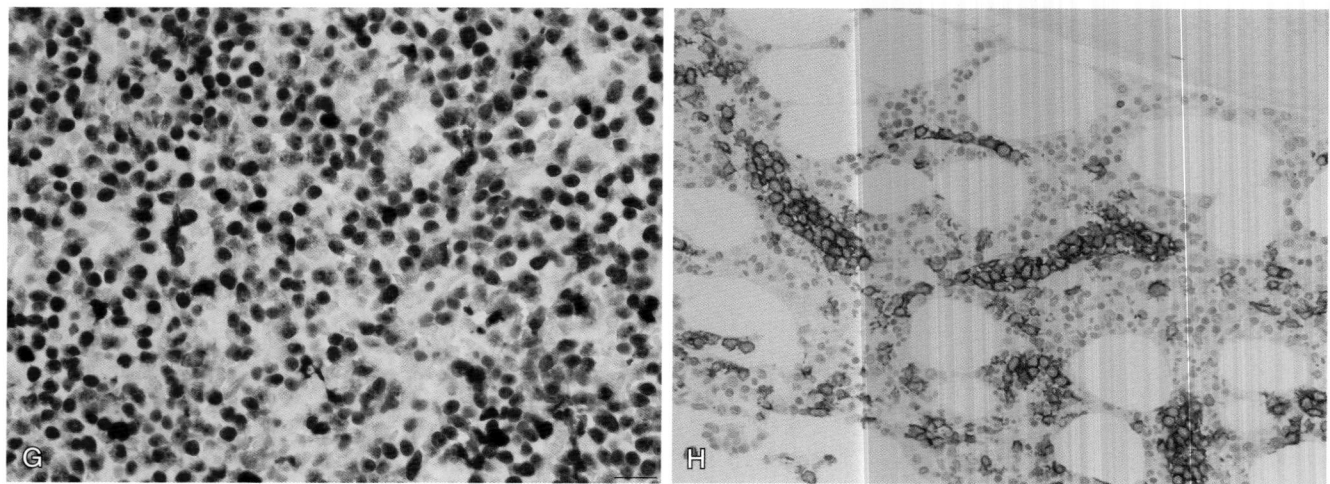

Figure 16-8—cont'd. T-bet **(G)**. The sinusoidal pattern of infiltration of the bone marrow is outlined after CD20 staining **(H)**.

of *KLF2* or *NOTCH2* genes are present in SMZL and rare in SRPL. On the other hand, sequencing studies have shown recurrent mutations in *CCND3* in SRPL.[69]

Hairy Cell Leukemia Variant

Despite its name, this very unusual low-grade B-cell lymphoma bears no relation to HCL in terms of morphology, immunophenotype, or response to therapy. Cases are characterized by large, prolymphocyte-like cells with prominent nucleoli; absence of annexin A_1, CD25, and CD103; and resistance to conventional HCL therapy.[70] Consequently, the next WHO lymphoma book is proposing the term *splenic B-cell lymphoma/leukemia with prominent nucleoli*. Quite interestingly, HCL_v cases seem to lack the *BRAF* V600 mutation typical of HCL, but activating mutations in the *MAP2K1* gene (encoding MEK1) have been found in 50% of these cases.[71] Some degree of overlap has been found between HCLv and SRPL.[68]

Pearls and Pitfalls

Feature	Comments
Follicular replacement	SMZL grows around preexistent follicles, replacing them. MIB-1/BCL2/MNDA/CD21/CD23 stains illustrate this phenomenon.
IgD staining	IgD is expressed in most SMZL cases. Residual mantle cells are absent from this lymphoma. In FL and MALT-type MZL, preserved IgD-positive mantle cells may be observed.
Bone marrow infiltration	Bone marrow histology is quite characteristic in SMZL, with intertrabecular nodules of small lymphocytes surrounding residual/replaced germinal centers. Intrasinusoidal involvement (demonstrated by CD20 staining) is useful, albeit not diagnostic.
Splenic hilar lymph node morphology	Lymph node involvement by SMZL displays characteristic histologic and immunohistochemical features, with frequent loss of marginal zone differentiation.
7q deletion	7q31-32 loss is a relatively specific genetic marker of SMZL, present in 40% of cases.
IgVH somatic mutations	Stereotyped use of Ig genes indicates the role of antigens in SMZL cell survival.
Marginal zone pattern	A marginal zone pattern can be observed in other small B-cell lymphomas involving the spleen. Marginal zone differentiation in bone marrow and lymph node involvement by SMZL are usually absent.
Monoclonal B-cell lymphocytosis	Monoclonal B-cell lymphocytosis, non-CLL phenotype may precede both SRPL and SMZL.
Villous cells in peripheral blood	Villous lymphocytes may also be present in SRPL, MCL, FL, B-CLL, and lymphoplasmacytic lymphoma.
MNDA and T-bet	SMZL cells are usually positive for both, in contrast with FL.

KEY REFERENCES

1. Schmid C, Kirkham N, Diss T, et al. Splenic marginal zone cell lymphoma. *Am J Surg Pathol*. 1992;16:455–466.
3. Matutes E, Oscier D, Montalban C, et al. Splenic marginal zone lymphoma proposals for a revision of diagnostic, staging and therapeutic criteria. *Leukemia*. 2008;22:487–495.
31. Salido M, Baro C, Oscier D, et al. Cytogenetic aberrations and their prognostic value in a series of 330 splenic marginal zone B-cell lymphomas: a multicenter study of the splenic B-Cell Lymphoma Group. *Blood*. 2010;116:1479–1488.
38. Rossi D, Trifonov V, Fangazio M, et al. The coding genome of splenic marginal zone lymphoma: activation of NOTCH2 and other pathways regulating marginal zone development. *J Exp Med*. 2012;209:1537–1551.
41. Hamadeh F, MacNamara SP, Aguilera NS, et al. MYD88 L265P mutation analysis helps define nodal lymphoplasmacytic lymphoma. *Mod Pathol*. 2015;28:564–574.
42. Bonfiglio F, Bruscaggin A, Guidetti F, et al. Genetic and phenotypic attributes of splenic marginal zone lymphoma. *Blood*. 2022;139(5):732–747.
43. Bikos V, Darzentas N, Hadzidimitriou A, et al. Over 30% of patients with splenic marginal zone lymphoma express

the same immunoglobulin heavy variable gene: ontogenetic implications. *Leukemia.* 2012;26:1638–1646.

55. Iannitto E, Bellei M, Amorim S, et al. Efficacy of bendamustine and rituximab in splenic marginal zone lymphoma: results from the phase II BRISMA/IELSG36 study. *Br J Haematol.* 2018;183(5):755–765.

56. Noy A, de Vos S, Coleman M, et al. Durable ibrutinib responses in relapsed/refractory marginal zone lymphoma: long-term follow-up and biomarker analysis. *Blood Adv.* 2020;4(22):5773–5784.

57. Zucca E, Arcaini L, Buske C, et al. Marginal zone lymphomas: ESMO Clinical Practice Guidelines for diagnosis, treatment and follow-up. *Ann Oncol: Official Journal of the European Society for Medical Oncology/ESMO.* 2020;31(1):17–29.

58. Montalban C, Abraira V, Arcaini L, et al. Simplification of risk stratification for splenic marginal zone lymphoma: a point-based score for practical use. *Leuk Lymphoma.* 2014;55:929–931.

66. Kanellis G, Mollejo M, Montes-Moreno S, et al. Splenic diffuse red pulp small B-cell lymphoma: revision of a series of cases reveals characteristic clinico-pathological features. *Haematologica.* 2010;95:1122–1129.

67. Traverse-Glehen A, Baseggio L, Bauchu EC, et al. Splenic red pulp lymphoma with numerous basophilic villous lymphocytes: a distinct clinicopathologic and molecular entity? *Blood.* 2008;111:2253–2260.

Visit Elsevier eBooks+ for the complete set of references.

Chapter 17

Follicular Lymphoma

Abner Louissaint, Jr. and Judith A. Ferry

DEFINITION

Follicular lymphoma (FL) is defined as a neoplasm composed of follicle center (germinal-center) B cells (typically both centrocytes and centroblasts) that usually has at least a partially follicular pattern.[1,2] If diffuse areas composed predominantly of large cells are present in any case of FL, a diagnosis of diffuse large B-cell lymphoma (DLBCL) is also made. Lymphomas composed of centrocytes and centroblasts with an entirely diffuse pattern in the sampled tissue may be included in the category of FL. FL is generally clinically indolent and characteristically harbors a translocation between the *BCL2* and immunoglobulin heavy chain (IGH) genes, leading to the characteristic strong overexpression of the BCL2 protein. The major features of FL are listed in Table 17-1. Several FL variants that have distinctive clinicopathologic features are defined in the International Consensus Classification (ICC) and World Health Organization (WHO) classifications (Table 17-2).

Synonyms and Related Terms

FL has been a distinct entity with classic morphologic and genetic features since the Revised European and American Lymphoma

classification in 1998[3] and WHO Classification of Tumours of the Haematopoietic and Lymphoid Tissues, 2nd edition, in 2002. Increasingly, the diversity of clinical presentations and genetic and mutational variability has been recognized, leading to several subtypes and distinct entities. In particular, FL cases presenting in the pediatric age group; confined to the testes, duodenum, or skin; confined to lymphoid follicles (in situ); and those with *IRF4* rearrangements were described in the WHO 4th edition. A provisional entity including cases lacking *BCL2* gene rearrangements and expressing CD23 has also been described.[1] In addition, new broader groupings of cases based on morphologic features have emerged.[2] These include classic FL (cFL), follicular large B-cell lymphoma (FLBCL), FL with unusual cytologic features (uFL), and FL with predominantly diffuse growth pattern (dFL). See Table 17-2 on Synonyms and Related Terms. These variants and entities will be further discussed throughout this chapter.

EPIDEMIOLOGY

FL predominantly affects adults, with a median age of 65 years (Table 17-1).[3] In contrast to most other hematologic malignancies, it is equally common in women and men. In the

Table 17-1 Major Features of Follicular Lymphoma

Feature	Description
Definition	A lymphoma of germinal-center B cells (centrocytes and centroblasts) with typically at least a partially follicular pattern
Frequency	40% of adult lymphomas in the United States; 20% worldwide
Age	Median, 65 years
Sex	Male = female
Clinical features at presentation	Generalized lymphadenopathy, frequent splenomegaly, often asymptomatic; bone marrow positive in 40%; rare stage I, extranodal or pediatric
Morphology	Pattern: follicular with or without diffuse areas or interfollicular involvement, extracapsular extension, sclerosis, vascular invasion
	Cytology: centroblasts and centrocytes, follicular dendritic cells, reactive T cells
Usual immunophenotype	Ig+, CD19+, CD20+, CD22+, CD79a+, PAX5+, CD10+, BCL2+, BCL6+, CD43−, CD5−; nodular meshworks of CD21+, CD23+ follicular dendritic cells
Genetic features	Immunoglobulin genes rearranged, mutated, intraclonal heterogeneity t(14;18)(q23;q32)/*BCL2::IGH*
Postulated normal counterpart	Germinal-center B cells
Clinical course	Indolent, incurable: prognosis based on histologic grade (grade 1 to 2 indolent, grade 3 aggressive), Follicular Lymphoma International Prognostic Index
Treatment	Symptomatic for grade 1 to 2, aggressive for grade 3

Table 17-2 Synonyms and Related Terms

WHO, 4th Edition	ICC	WHO, Proposed 5th Edition
FL, grade 1 to 2, follicular +/− diffuse pattern	FL, grade 1 to 2, follicular +/− diffuse pattern	Classic FL
FL, grade 3A	FL, grade 3A	Classic FL
FL, grade 3B	FL, grade 3B	Follicular large B-cell lymphoma
FL, grade 1 to 2, diffuse pattern	FL, grade 1 to 2, diffuse pattern*	FL with predominantly diffuse growth pattern
N/A	N/A, see text for the ICC approach to these cases	FL with unusual cytologic features, uFL
In situ follicular neoplasia	In situ follicular neoplasia	In situ follicular B-cell neoplasm
Pediatric-type FL	Pediatric-type FL	Pediatric-type FL
Testicular FL	Primary testicular FL	Subtype of cFL
Duodenal-type FL		Duodenal-type FL
	BCL2-R(neg), CD23(+), follicle center cell lymphoma	Cases with diffuse architecture fall into FL with predominantly diffuse growth pattern
Large B-cell lymphoma with *IRF4*-R	Large B-cell lymphoma with *IRF4*-R	Large B-cell lymphoma with *IRF4*-R

*Many of these cases fulfill criteria for BCL2-R-negative, CD23-positive follicle center lymphoma—see text for ICC criteria for these cases.
cFL, Classic FL; *FL*, follicular lymphoma; *ICC*, International Consensus Classification; *neg*, negative; *R*, rearrangement.

United States, it is two-to-three times more common in Whites than in Black and Asian populations.[4] FL is the second most common lymphoma worldwide (after DLBCL), accounting for 20% of all non-Hodgkin lymphomas.[5] It constitutes almost 40% of non-Hodgkin lymphomas in the United States and up to 70% of "low-grade" lymphomas reported in American clinical trials.[5,6] It is less common in other parts of the world, including eastern and southern Europe, Asia, and nonindustrialized countries.[7]

The incidence of FL in the United States in the past 20 years has been estimated at 2.7 to 3.0 per 100,000 for White men and women and 0.9 to 1.3 per 100,000 for Black men and women.[5] The annual incidence of FL in Asian countries has been estimated at 0.15 to 0.38 per 100,000—less than 10% that in industrialized Western countries.[8,9]

Ethnic susceptibilities have not been extensively evaluated and are difficult to dissect from socioeconomic factors. In one report from Malaysia, FL accounted for only 12% of 158 adult non-Hodgkin lymphomas; lymphomas in Indian patients were more likely to be follicular (31%) than they were in Malaysian (16%) or Chinese (6%) patients.[10] In a study of Chinese and Japanese residents of the United States, the relative risk of FL was low among those born in Asia (relative risk 0.11 to 0.15 compared to White Americans) and higher among those born in America (relative risk 0.36 to 0.84),[11] suggesting environmental factors may be more important than race.

CLINICAL FEATURES

Sites of Involvement

Most patients with FL have widespread nodal disease at the time of diagnosis, even though they may feel relatively well.[6] In most studies, up to two-thirds of the patients are in stage III or IV. They infrequently have systemic "B" symptoms (28%); 44% are in the low-risk group (category 0/1) of the International Prognostic Index, and 48% are in the low-intermediate–risk group (category 2/3).

Peripheral, mediastinal, and retroperitoneal nodes are often involved. Large mediastinal masses are rare, but large retroperitoneal and mesenteric masses often occur and may cause ureteral obstruction. Pure extranodal presentations are uncommon—9% in one survey[5]—and extranodal involvement (other than bone marrow) was seen in 20% of cases in another study.[6] The most common sites of stage IV disease are the bone marrow and liver, with 42% of patients having bone marrow involvement.[6] The majority of patients probably have circulating neoplastic cells, and a small proportion are frankly leukemic.[12]

Non-nodal presentations usually involve the spleen, Waldeyer's ring, skin, or gastrointestinal (GI) tract. Within the GI tract, the small bowel and particularly the duodenum are most often involved (see "Related B-Cell Lymphomas and Follicular Proliferations," later).[13,14] Rare cases of FL presenting as lymphomatous polyposis of the intestinal tract have been reported.[15] Primary cutaneous lymphoma of the follicle center type is an important subset of cutaneous B-cell lymphoma and is discussed in Chapter 19.[16-20]

Clinical Evaluation and Staging

The diagnosis of FL is best made on an excisional lymph node biopsy, which provides the best opportunity to assess histology and architectural pattern. Patients with peripheral lymph nodes that are accessible for open biopsy should have this procedure done. For patients with deeper, less accessible lymph nodes, FL can be diagnosed on core needle biopsies if adequate material is available for morphologic evaluation and for immunophenotyping (flow cytometry or immunohistochemistry) to document clonality and confirm germinal-center origin.[21] Appropriate grading or subclassification of FL may not be possible with these specimens, and in such cases, excision may be considered. In addition, grade 3B cases may not be distinguishable from DLBCL, but this distinction may not be clinically relevant.

Patients typically undergo abdominal and pelvic computed tomography scanning and bone marrow biopsy for staging, in addition to measurement of serum lactate dehydrogenase for stratification within the Follicular Lymphoma International Prognostic Index (FLIPI).[22,23]

MORPHOLOGIC FEATURES

Architectural Patterns

Lymph nodes are typically enlarged, with complete architectural effacement by neoplastic follicles. Follicles are typically uniform in size, closely packed, and evenly distributed throughout the lymph node, obliterating sinuses and extending outside the capsule (Fig. 17-1A). Neoplastic follicles typically lack a starry-sky pattern and polarization. They may range in size from no larger than a primary follicle to much larger than the average reactive follicle; although usually round, they may be irregular and serpiginous (Fig. 17-1B), mimicking floridly reactive hyperplastic follicles. Within a given tumor, the follicles are likely to be relatively uniform and monotonous, but in some cases there is marked variation in size from one follicle to another. In other cases, the follicles may appear irregularly mottled, resembling progressively transformed germinal centers; this usually occurs in cases with increased large cells and has been called the *floral variant* of FL (Fig. 17-1C).[24,25]

Neoplastic follicles usually lack mantle zones, but in some cases, partial or complete mantle zones may be present around all or some of the follicles (Fig. 17-1B).[26] In some FLs, the outer cells of the follicles may resemble marginal zone or monocytoid B cells with nuclei similar to those of centrocytes but with more abundant, pale cytoplasm (Fig. 17-2). These cells may form partial or complete "marginal zones" around some or most of the follicles in a given case, and they may have an interfollicular and perisinusoidal distribution, resembling nodal involvement by extranodal marginal zone lymphoma of mucosa-associated lymphoid tissue or nodal marginal zone lymphoma. This phenomenon should not be regarded as a "composite lymphoma" with follicular and monocytoid B-cell lymphoma, as has been suggested by some authors[27,28]; rather, it should be considered evidence of intratumoral differentiation.[29] Marginal zone B cells in cases of FL with marginal zone differentiation share the same genetic abnormalities as the neoplastic follicles.[30] In one study, the presence of significant marginal zone or monocytoid B-cell

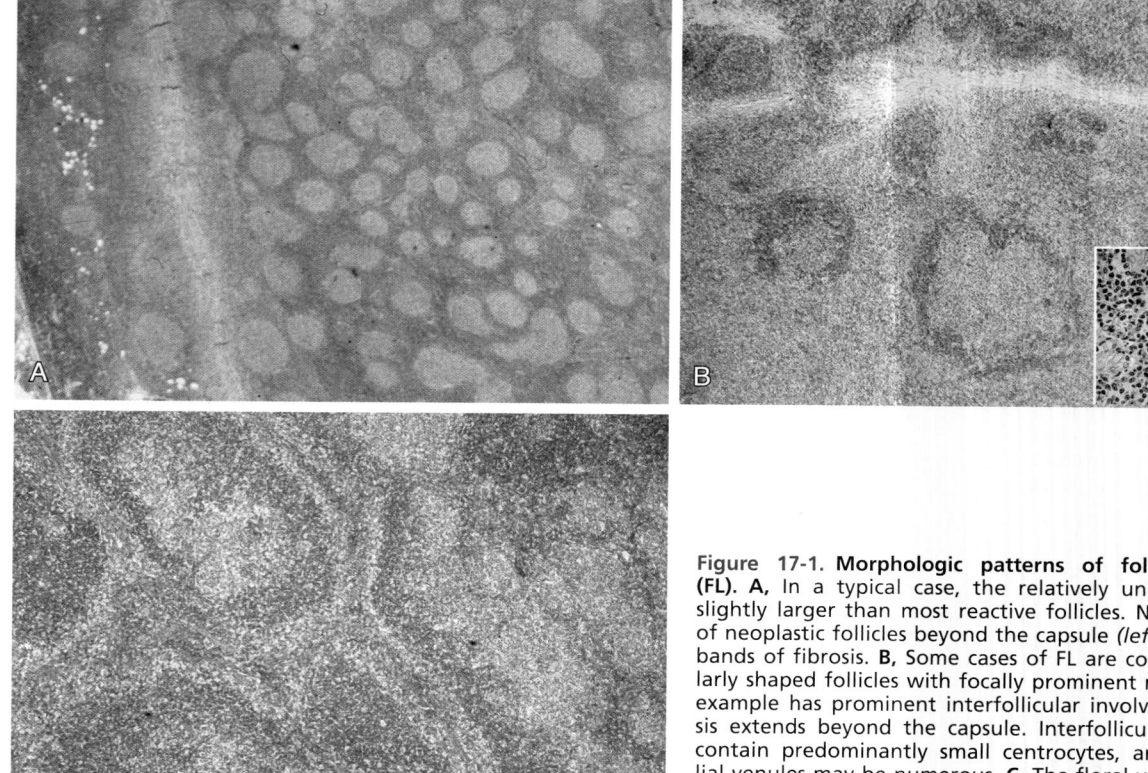

Figure 17-1. Morphologic patterns of follicular lymphoma (FL). A, In a typical case, the relatively uniform follicles are slightly larger than most reactive follicles. Note the extension of neoplastic follicles beyond the capsule *(left)*, with concentric bands of fibrosis. **B,** Some cases of FL are composed of irregularly shaped follicles with focally prominent mantle zones. This example has prominent interfollicular involvement, and fibrosis extends beyond the capsule. Interfollicular regions *(inset)* contain predominantly small centrocytes, and high endothelial venules may be numerous. **C,** The floral variant of FL shows broken-up follicles within a mantle zone of small lymphocytes, resembling progressively transformed germinal centers or nodular lymphocyte-predominant Hodgkin lymphoma.

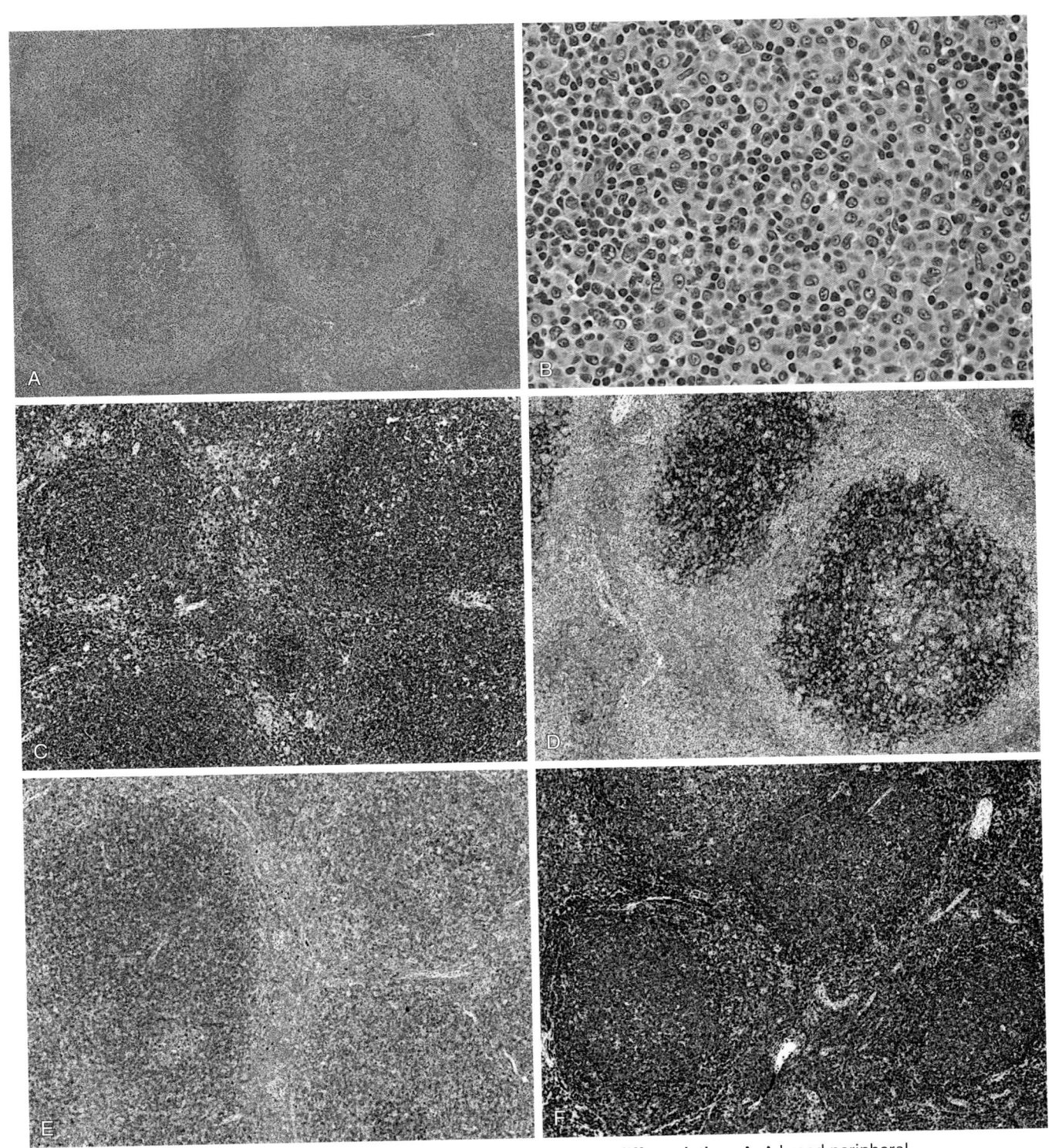

Figure 17-2. Follicular lymphoma (FL) with marginal zone differentiation. A, A broad peripheral band of pale-staining cells outside the mantle zone surrounds the follicles, forming a marginal zone. **B,** The cells in the marginal zone have centrocyte-like nuclei but more abundant cytoplasm. The neoplastic follicles are CD20 positive **(C)** and are associated with CD23-positive FDC meshworks **(D).** Follicles but not marginal zones are CD10 positive **(E).** BCL2 **(F)** stains the follicles, including the marginal zones.

areas in FL was associated with a significantly poorer prognosis compared with cases lacking this feature.[31]

Subcapsular and medullary sinuses are typically obliterated, but sinuses may be partially or completely preserved.

Extracapsular extension is common but not universal; when it occurs, the capsule may be visible as a band of fibrous tissue within the tumor. Successive levels of extracapsular extension may appear as concentric parallel bands of fibrosis in the

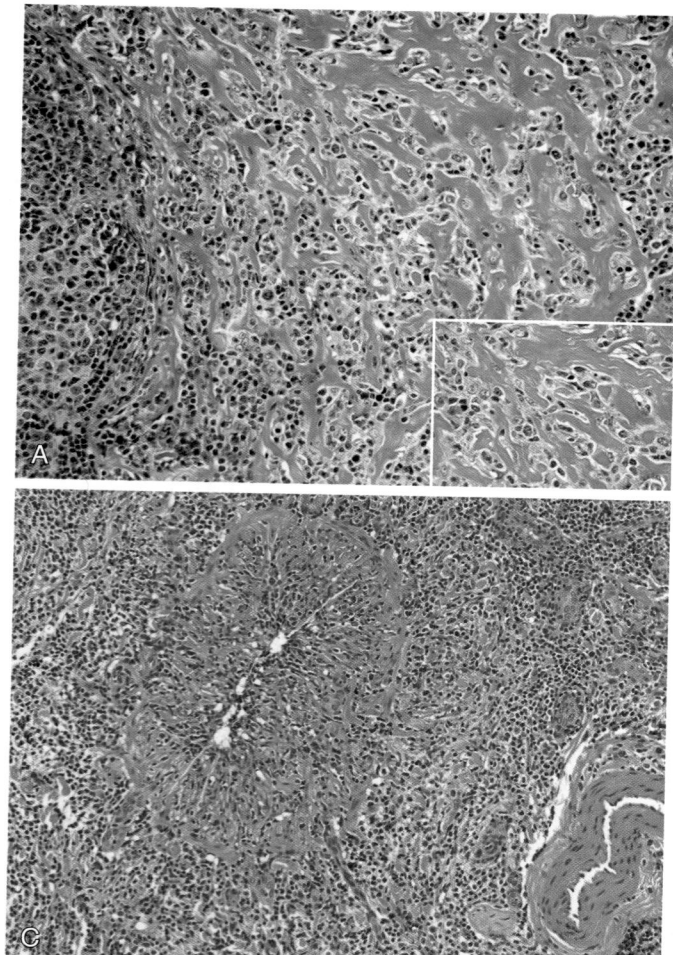

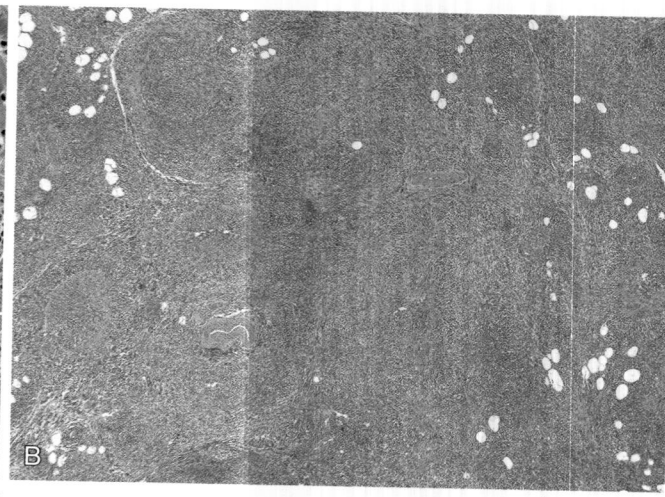

Figure 17-3. Additional morphologic patterns of follicular lymphoma (FL). A, The diffuse area in low-grade FL contains prominent sclerosis; the follicle is at *left*. The inset shows a predominance of centrocytes with distorted, elongated nuclei. B, prominent infiltration of hilar vessel walls is shown in a lymph node involved by FL. C, The neoplastic lymphoid cells infiltrate the wall of a small vein, resulting in obliteration of the lumen; note an intact arteriole *(right)*.

extranodal tissue (Fig. 17-1A). In most cases, the follicles are closely packed, with absence of the normal T zones. The interfollicular region may contain numerous small blood vessels of the high endothelial venule (HEV) type but is poor in transformed lymphocytes and plasma cells and usually contains neoplastic centrocytes.[26,32] In occasional cases, interfollicular involvement is prominent, leading to widely spaced follicles (Fig. 17-1B). This interfollicular involvement is not considered to constitute a diffuse area: a diffuse area is defined as an area completely lacking follicles.

Sclerosis is common and may be present surrounding the follicles, in diffuse areas, or less often, within the follicles.[33] It is more marked in areas in which the infiltrate is diffuse, which can be a useful feature in distinguishing FL from follicular or diffuse lymphoid hyperplasia. In diffuse areas with sclerosis, the neoplastic centrocytes may be spindle shaped, resembling fibroblasts (Fig. 17-3A). Centrocytes are often more numerous in sclerotic areas than in other areas; thus, in difficult cases, careful examination of the cells in areas of sclerosis is useful in establishing the diagnosis.

Occasional cases of FL may have amorphous, eosinophilic, extracellular, periodic acid-Schiff–positive material deposited in an irregular fashion within the follicle centers.[34,35] The nature of this material is not clear; Chittal and colleagues[35] found that, ultrastructurally, it contained membrane fragments, and on immunohistochemistry, it contained many antigens found

in and on the neoplastic cells (CD45, CD22, immunoglobulin [Ig]). Others have speculated that it represents the deposition of antigen-antibody complexes on the processes of follicular dendritic cells (FDCs), analogous to the deposits often seen in reactive follicles.[34] However, in reactive follicles, extracellular Ig deposition is rarely massive enough to be conspicuous by light microscopy, whereas in the few lymphomas that exhibit this phenomenon, it may be impressive. Thus, although uncommon and by no means diagnostic, massive extracellular deposition of amorphous material within follicles should raise the question of lymphoma.

Vascular invasion is surprisingly common in FL, both within involved lymph nodes and in pericapsular veins.[36] Centrocytes infiltrate through the walls of small and even larger veins, accumulating within the intima (Fig. 17-3B and C). Vascular invasion may be useful in distinguishing FL from hyperplasia. Perhaps as a consequence of this invasion, total infarction of the lymph node may occur.[36] The diagnosis can be suspected in totally infarcted nodes by careful evaluation of the cells preserved in the extranodal tissue and by reticulin stains, which demonstrate the follicular pattern throughout the infarcted area; molecular genetic analysis can occasionally demonstrate Ig gene rearrangement in infarcted tissue, and immunohistochemistry may be used to document that the cells are CD45 positive and CD20 positive, although non-specific staining of necrotic tissue by these antibodies can be a problem.[37-39]

Diffuse Areas in Follicular Lymphoma

A diffuse area in FL is defined as an area that lacks evidence of neoplastic follicles and contains a mixture of centrocytes and centroblasts similar to those seen within the neoplastic follicles (Fig. 17-3A). Involvement of the interfollicular region by neoplastic cells is not considered evidence of a diffuse pattern. Although the prognostic importance of diffuse areas is debatable, the WHO classification has historically recognized three patterns of grade 1 to 2 FL: follicular (>75% follicular), follicular and diffuse (25% to 75% follicular), predominantly diffuse (>25% follicular), and diffuse (0% follicular) (Table 17-3). Diffuse areas in low-grade (grade 1 to 2) FL are not prognostically significant. However, diffuse areas composed predominantly of centroblasts (grade 3) are diagnosed as DLBCL (Table 17-3).

Diffuse Follicular Lymphoma

Rare lymphomas composed of both centrocytes and centroblasts have a purely diffuse pattern. In some core biopsy samples, it is likely that focal follicular areas are present in the lymphoma and that the purely diffuse pattern seen in the biopsy is the result of limited sampling. In the ICC classification, diffuse FL is defined as a diffuse lymphoma composed of both centrocytes and centroblasts in which centrocytes predominate (grade 1 to 2, low grade). In the WHO 5th edition classification, these cases are referred to as FL with predominantly diffuse growth pattern (Table 17-2). A significant subset of diffuse FL may fall under the new provisional entity defined in the ICC classification as "BCL2-R-negative, CD23+ follicle center lymphoma" that characteristically has CD23 expression, *STAT6* mutations, and absent *BCL2* rearrangement (see section titled "BCL2-R-Negative, CD23-Positive Follicle Center Lymphoma").

The diagnosis of diffuse FL should be made with caution after other diffuse lymphomas have been excluded and when sufficient tissue is available to exclude FL with follicular pattern. Immunophenotyping studies are essential to show that both small and large cells are B cells (to exclude T-cell/histiocyte–rich large B-cell lymphoma [LBCL]) and that the immunophenotype is consistent with FL (CD10⁺, BCL6⁺, CD5⁻, CD43⁻, cyclin D1⁻). Molecular genetic or cytogenetic analysis for evidence of *BCL2* rearrangement may be useful to confirm this diagnosis. However, the possibility of BCL2-R-negative, CD23-positive follicle center lymphoma should be considered.[40]

BCL2-R-Negative, CD23-Positive Follicle Center Lymphoma

BCL2-R-negative, CD23-positive follicle center lymphoma is a provisional entity described in the ICC classification characterized by a predominance of centrocytes expressing germinal-center markers (CD10 and BCL6), usually with CD23 co-expression, the presence of *CREBBP* and *STAT6* or *SOCS1* mutations, recurrent deletions of 1p36 and/or 16p, and characteristic absence of *BCL2* gene rearrangements (Fig. 17-4). The majority of cases are associated with purely diffuse growth pattern with scattered microfollicles and interstitial sclerosis (as originally described by Katzenberger et al.[40]), but some cases have been found to retain follicular architecture. Clinically, patients with this disease often present with painless

Table 17-3 International Consensus Classification Grading of Follicular Lymphoma*

Grade	Definition
Grade 1 to 2 (low grade)†	0-15 centroblasts/hpf‡
Grade 1	0-5 centroblasts/hpf‡
Grade 2	6-15 centroblasts/hpf‡
Grade 3	>15 centroblasts/hpf‡
Grade 3A	Centrocytes present
Grade 3B	Solid sheets of centroblasts

Reporting of Pattern	Proportion Follicular (%)
Follicular	>75
Follicular and diffuse	25–75§
Focally follicular	<25§
Diffuse	0¶

Diffuse areas containing >15 centroblasts/hpf are reported as diffuse large B-cell lymphoma§ with follicular lymphoma (grade 1 to 2, 3A, or 3B)

*Grading of FL is considered optional in the 5th edition of World Health Organization classification, and, if performed, the recommended grading system is as described in this table, with the exception of FL grade 3B, which goes under the name of Follicular Large B Cell Lymphoma.
†Among cases of grade 1 to 2 follicular lymphoma with a proliferation fraction, >40% may be reported as "follicular lymphoma grade 1 to 2 with a high proliferation fraction."
‡High-power field (hpf) of 0.159 mm² (40× objective). If using an 18-mm field-of-view ocular, count 10 hpf and divide by 10; if using a 20-mm field-of-view ocular, count 8 hpf; if using a 22-mm field-of-view ocular, count 7 hpf for an equivalent area and divide by 10 to get the number of centroblasts/0.159 mm² hpf.
§Give approximate percentages in report.
¶If the biopsy specimen is small, a note should be added that the absence of follicles may reflect sampling error.

localized (stage I-II) lymphadenopathy, most commonly in the inguinal area (more than 75% of cases), but noninguinal sites can also be involved. This type of FL generally has an excellent prognosis.

Partial Nodal Involvement

In some cases of FL, the nodal architecture may be largely or partially preserved, with residual reactive germinal centers; this phenomenon is reportedly associated with a lower stage at diagnosis.[41] In other cases, there may be widely spaced, monomorphous follicles surrounded by a relatively normal-appearing interfollicular region, without evidence of extrafollicular neoplastic cells (Fig. 17-5). This pattern appears to reflect the homing of neoplastic cells to preexisting reactive follicles, with follicular colonization by tumor cells.[42] This phenomenon may occur in lymph nodes with obvious FL elsewhere in the node, in adjacent nodes, or rarely, in patients without evidence of overt lymphoma (see section titled "In Situ Follicular Neoplasia").[43,44]

Cellular Composition

The centrocytes and centroblasts of most cases of FL are morphologically similar to those of normal germinal centers (Fig. 17-6A–F). The nuclei of centrocytes (Fig. 17-6C and D) are usually less than twice the size of small lymphocytes, but they may be almost as large as the nuclei of tissue histiocytes or centroblasts. The nuclei appear irregular or angulated in tissue sections; although the term *cleaved* is used, a distinct nuclear cleft is seldom seen in tissue sections. The chromatin is paler than that of small lymphocytes and is evenly dispersed, giving the nucleus a gray-blue appearance. One or more small

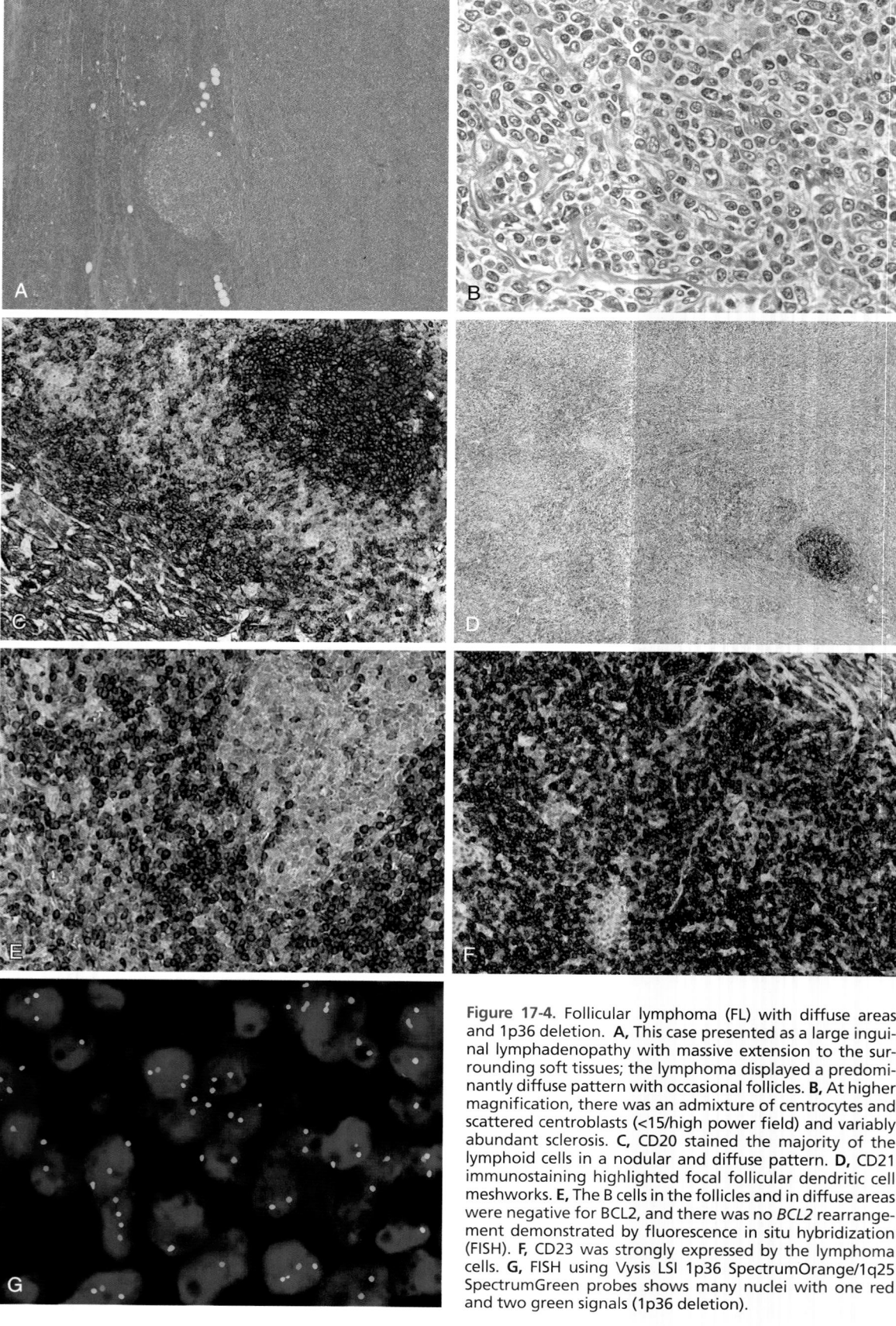

Figure 17-4. Follicular lymphoma (FL) with diffuse areas and 1p36 deletion. **A,** This case presented as a large inguinal lymphadenopathy with massive extension to the surrounding soft tissues; the lymphoma displayed a predominantly diffuse pattern with occasional follicles. **B,** At higher magnification, there was an admixture of centrocytes and scattered centroblasts (<15/high power field) and variably abundant sclerosis. **C,** CD20 stained the majority of the lymphoid cells in a nodular and diffuse pattern. **D,** CD21 immunostaining highlighted focal follicular dendritic cell meshworks. **E,** The B cells in the follicles and in diffuse areas were negative for BCL2, and there was no *BCL2* rearrangement demonstrated by fluorescence in situ hybridization (FISH). **F,** CD23 was strongly expressed by the lymphoma cells. **G,** FISH using Vysis LSI 1p36 SpectrumOrange/1q25 SpectrumGreen probes shows many nuclei with one red and two green signals (1p36 deletion).

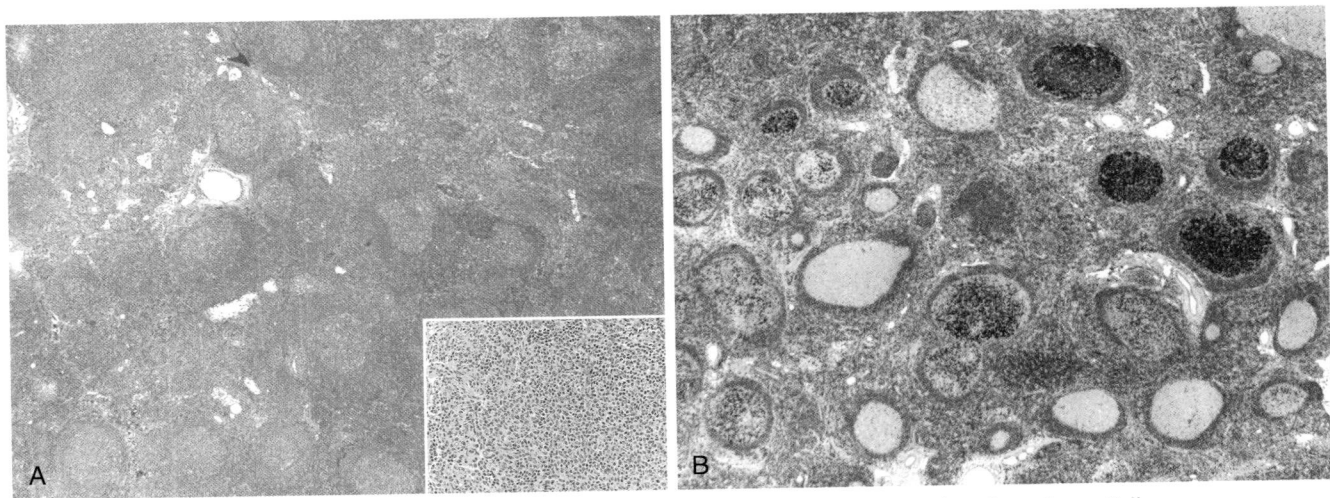

Figure 17-5. Partial nodal involvement by follicular lymphoma (FL). A, A lymph node partially involved by FL contains scattered monomorphous-appearing follicles among other typical reactive follicles with preserved mantle zones. A neoplastic follicle at higher magnification shows a monotonous cellular composition *(inset).* **B,** BCL2 stain shows strongly positive cells in some follicles.

nucleoli may be present. The cytoplasm is scant and pale and is usually not visible on H&E (hematoxylin and eosin)-stained or Giemsa-stained sections. In most cases, the centrocytes appear more monomorphous than those of normal follicles, with the majority approximately the same size. The nuclei of centroblasts (Fig. 17-6B, D–F) are usually three-to-four times the size of small lymphocytes, similar to or larger than the nuclei of tissue histiocytes; the nuclei are round or oval but may be irregular, indented, or multilobated or may even have a cleft. The nucleus is vesicular, with a clear center and some peripheral condensation of chromatin; there are one-to-three basophilic nucleoli, usually apposed to the nuclear membrane. Centroblasts have a narrow rim of cytoplasm that is intensely basophilic on Giemsa staining. The proportion of centroblasts may vary somewhat among follicles in a given case; an extreme example is shown in Figure 17-6G. Areas of DLBCL may be encountered in FL of any grade (Fig. 17-6H). In cases with ill-defined neoplastic follicles, an immunostain for FDCs can be useful in distinguishing follicular and diffuse areas (Fig. 17-6I).

In most cases of FL, the centrocytes are relatively small, and the few centroblasts stand out sharply against the monotonous background of centrocytes. In some cases, however, the centrocytes are larger and may be almost as large as centroblasts. In these cases, the centrocytes may appear more pleomorphic, with more deeply indented or multilobated-appearing nuclei. Centroblasts may also appear atypical, with variable nuclear size and shape, increased heterochromatin, and binucleate or multinucleated forms.

Mitotic activity is low in most cases of FL, and a starry-sky pattern, with phagocytic histiocytes, is absent. However, in cases with increased numbers of centroblasts, mitoses are more numerous, and rarely, phagocytosis of nuclear debris may be seen. Polarization, as seen in reactive follicles, is rare in FL, although in some cases, centroblasts may be more numerous in one area of the follicle than another, creating an impression of polarization.

In addition to clonal B cells, neoplastic follicles contain FDCs; their nuclei are similar in size to centroblast nuclei but have delicate nuclear membranes and are central, small, and

eosinophilic. FDCs are often binucleate, and the two nuclei are typically apposed to each other, with flattening of the adjacent nuclear membranes (Fig. 17-6C and E). In contrast to centroblasts, their cytoplasm does not stain blue with Giemsa stain. Small T cells are also present in neoplastic follicles; these are usually less numerous than in reactive germinal centers, but occasionally they may be numerous.

FL rarely contains an appreciable number of plasma cells, which can be useful in its differentiation from reactive hyperplasia; however, a small proportion of FLs have variably extensive plasmacytic differentiation (Fig. 17-7).[45] FL of any grade may have plasmacytic differentiation.[45,46] The plasma cells may be found predominantly in the interfollicular area or in an intrafollicular distribution. In cases with interfollicular plasma cells, the plasma cells express class-switched Ig; these cases are CD10 positive and harbor *BCL2* gene rearrangements, *BCL6* gene rearrangements (subset), and mutations in chromatin remodelling genes (e.g., *KMT2D, CREBBP, EZH2*). In contrast, cases with intrafollicular plasma cells often lack CD10 expression, feature IgM-positive plasma cells, have less frequent mutations in chromatin remodeling genes, and lack *BCL2* rearrangements, though they often have extra copies of *BCL2* and *BCL6*. The latter group often lacks the usual composition of centrocytes and centroblasts and can have features that overlap with nodal marginal zone lymphoma.[47] In rare cases of FL, the neoplastic centrocytes have large cytoplasmic vacuoles, either clear or eosinophilic, giving them the appearance of signet ring cells (Fig. 17-8A).[48] In most of these cases, cytoplasmic Ig can be demonstrated in the signet ring cells. Cases with clear cytoplasm typically express cytoplasmic IgG, with a predominance of lambda light chain, whereas those with periodic acid-Schiff–positive eosinophilic globules in the cytoplasm or nucleus more commonly express IgM.[48,49] On ultrastructural examination, the clear inclusions are large, membrane-bound vacuoles containing multiple tiny, coated vesicles, whereas the eosinophilic inclusions consist of dilated rough endoplasmic reticulum filled with electron-dense material, presumably Ig.[50] Clinically, FL with a signet ring cell morphology does not differ from typical FL.

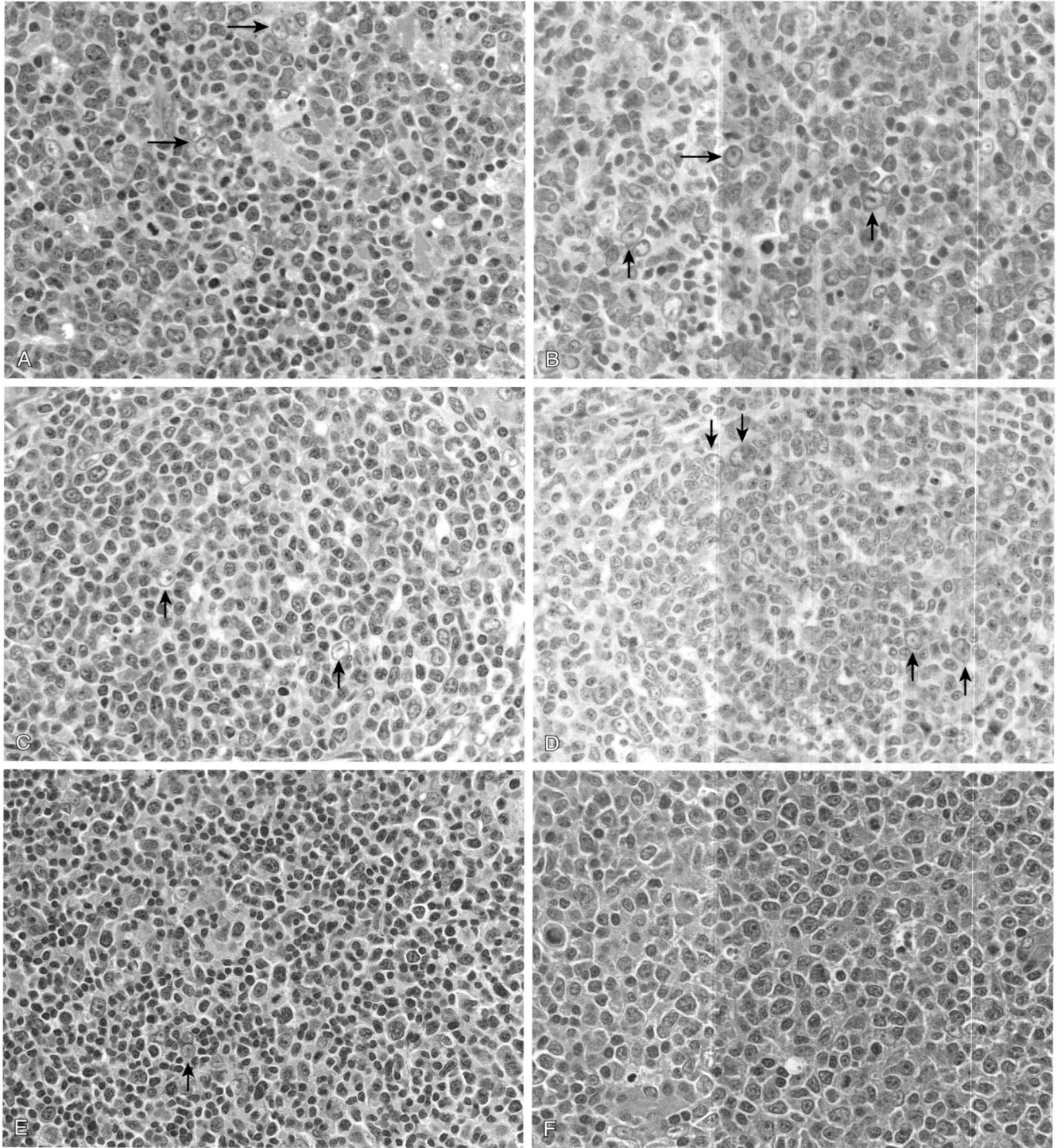

Figure 17-6. Cellular composition and grading of follicular lymphoma (FL). A, This reactive germinal center contains normal centrocytes and centroblasts; follicular dendritic cells are often binucleate and identified by their oval-to-round nuclei with pale chromatin and small distinct eosinophilic nucleoli *(arrows)*. **B,** On a Giemsa stain of a reactive germinal center, the centroblasts show a rim of basophilic cytoplasm *(arrows)*. **C,** A neoplastic follicle in low-grade FL contains centroblasts and centrocytes, similar to those in the reactive germinal centers; however, the follicles have a more monomorphous appearance because of the predominance of centrocytes. *Arrows* indicate follicular dendritic cells. **D,** Scattered centroblasts are best demonstrated by a Giemsa stain in low-grade FL *(arrows)*. **E,** In FL grade 3A, centroblasts are numerous, but centrocytes are still present; note the persistence of follicular dendritic cells *(arrow)*. **F,** In FL grade 3B, there are solid aggregates of centroblasts.

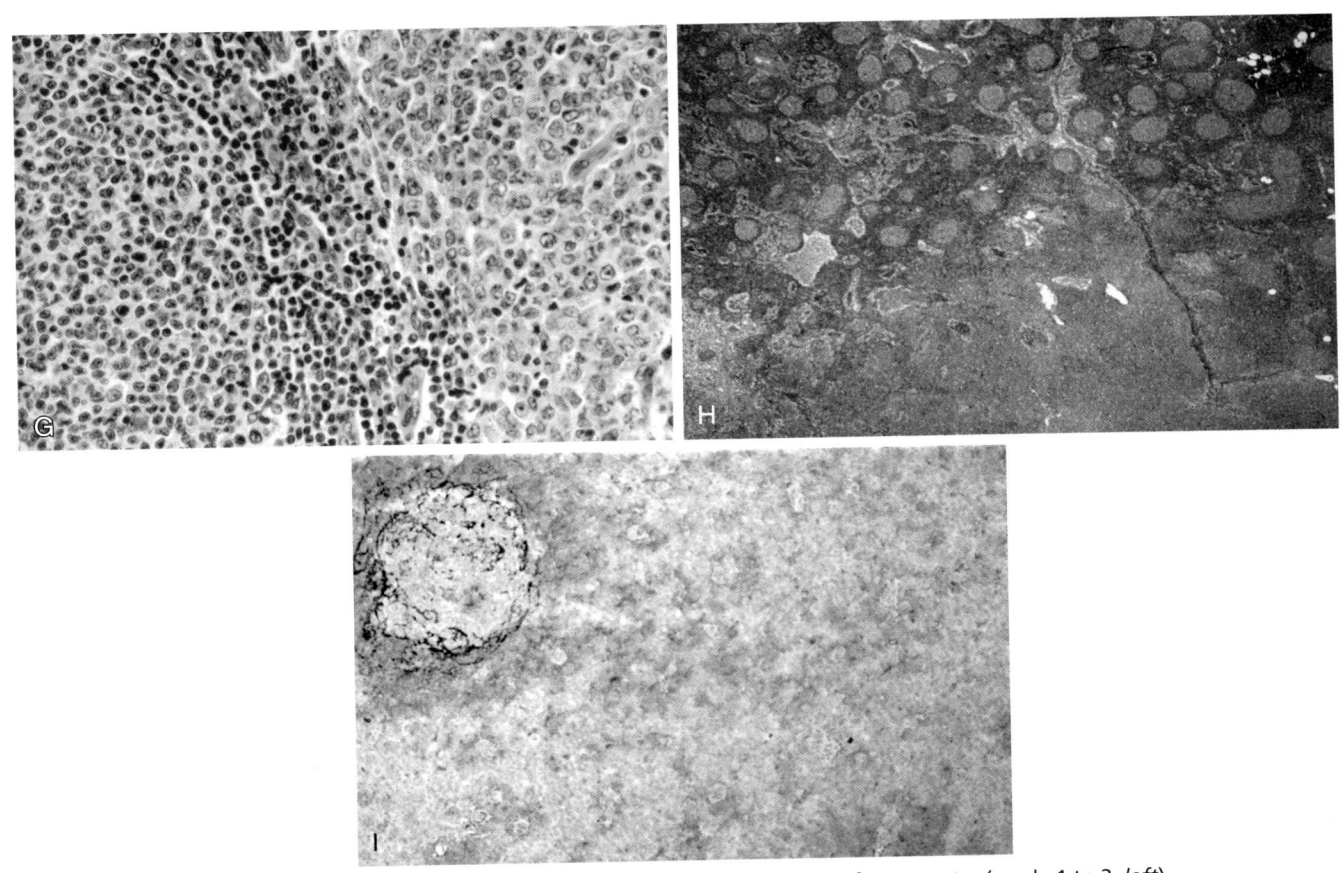

Figure 17-6, cont'd. G, In this FL, a follicle with a predominance of centrocytes (grade 1 to 2, *left*) is adjacent to a follicle with a predominance of centroblasts (grade 3B, *right*). **H,** The bottom of the image shows an area of diffuse large B-cell lymphoma, present in association with a low-grade FL. **I,** CD21 highlights a follicular dendritic cell meshwork associated with a neoplastic follicle *(upper left)*; diffuse areas lack follicular dendritic staining (immunoperoxidase stain for CD21).

Grading and Terminology

The establishment of FL grading was based on the idea that clinical aggressiveness of the lymphoma increased with the number of centroblasts. In particular, early studies had suggested the "cell counting" method of Mann and Berard was more reproducible and better at predicting prognosis than other methods of grading FL.[51-53] In this method, the centroblasts (large nucleolated cells) per 40× microscopic high-power field (hpf) are counted (10 to 20 hpf in different randomly selected follicles). A case with up to five centroblasts/hpf is grade 1, 6 to 15 centroblasts is grade 2, and greater than 15 centroblasts is grade 3 (Fig. 17-6C–F).[54] Using a standard 0.159 mm² hpf, the international study of the REAL classification found that a cutoff of 15 centroblasts/hpf significantly predicted overall and disease-free survival in FL.[55] Approximately 80% of FLs are grade 1 (40% to 60%) or grade 2 (25% to 35%). However, interobserver reliability has been questionable, and the prognostic significance of grading has not been reproducible in studies with more current therapies. In fact, because there is no appreciable difference in clinical behavior between grades 1 and 2, the 4th edition of the WHO classification combined them into a "low-grade" category (Table 17-3).

Using these numerical cutoffs, the spectrum of grade 3 FL ranges from cases with 16 large cells/hpf to those in which the majority of cells in the follicle are centroblasts.[56]

Some studies suggest that cases with solid sheets of centroblasts are biologically distinct from those with a mixture of centrocytes and centroblasts.[46] For this reason, classifications have traditionally recommended subdividing grade 3 FL: grade 3A, with more than 15 centroblasts/hpf, but centrocytes are still present; and grade 3B, with solid sheets of centroblasts (Fig. 17-6E and F). Grade 3B cases are often associated with areas of DLBCL. The relative proportion of centrocytes and centroblasts may vary from one follicle to another in a given case. Examination of multiple sections is often required. The proportion of large cells is estimated based on a representative sample of follicles. Rarely, individual follicles or parts of the node may show an abrupt transition from a predominance of centrocytes (grade 1 to 2) to a predominance of centroblasts (grade 3) (Fig. 17-6G). In such cases, it is appropriate to give the predominant grade (grade 1 to 2) with a separate diagnosis of grade 3 (A or B), giving the relative proportions of each. For some higher-grade lesions, it is difficult to make the critical distinction between grades 3A and 3B. The ICC proposed that the presence of *BCL2* rearrangements (*BCL2*-R) and CD10 positivity (detectable by fluorescence in situ hybridization [FISH]) favor FL 3A.

Areas of DLBCL may also be found in lymph nodes showing FL (Fig. 17-6H); this is more common in grade 3B cases but can occur in other grades. Although there

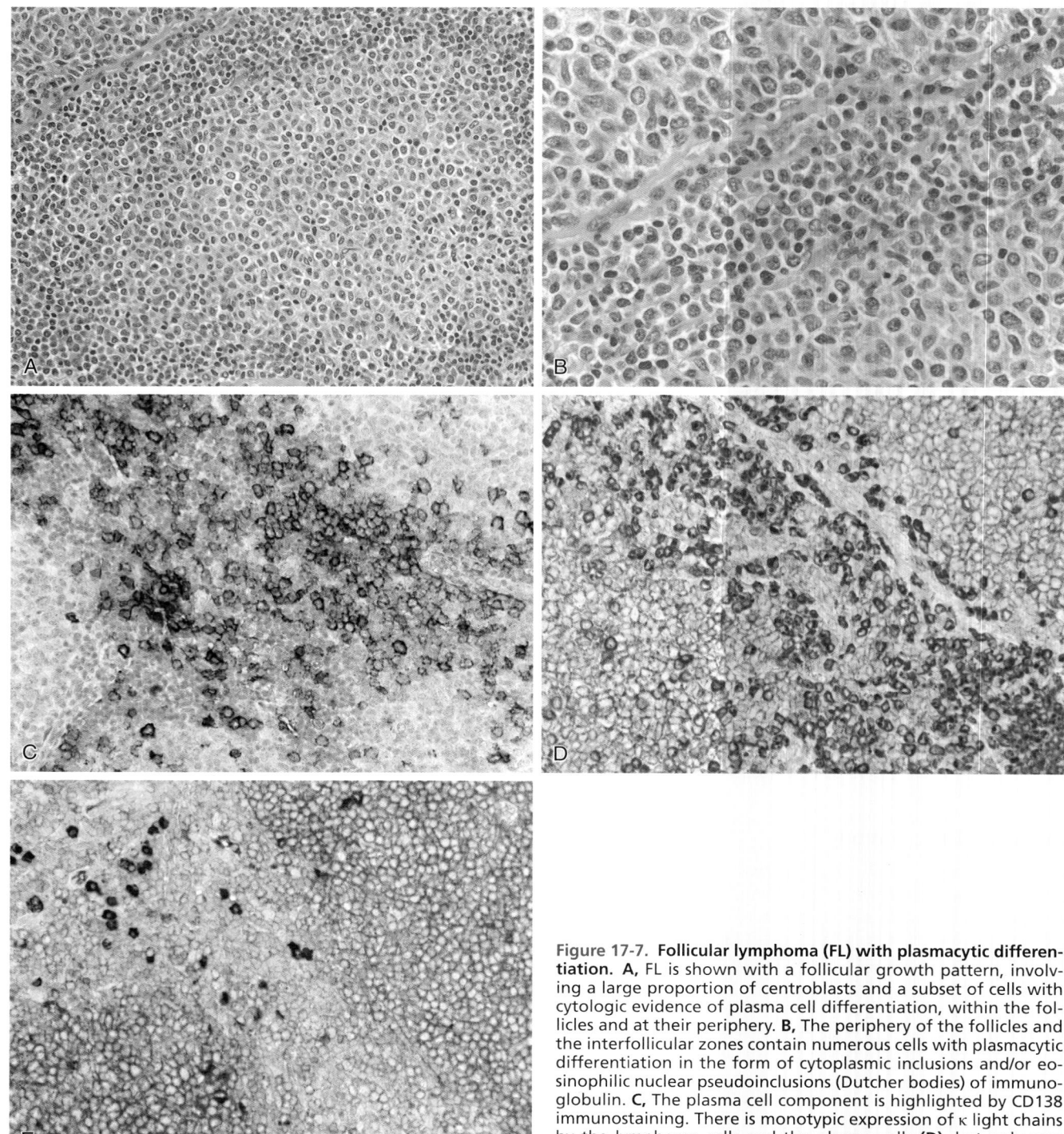

Figure 17-7. Follicular lymphoma (FL) with plasmacytic differentiation. A, FL is shown with a follicular growth pattern, involving a large proportion of centroblasts and a subset of cells with cytologic evidence of plasma cell differentiation, within the follicles and at their periphery. **B,** The periphery of the follicles and the interfollicular zones contain numerous cells with plasmacytic differentiation in the form of cytoplasmic inclusions and/or eosinophilic nuclear pseudoinclusions (Dutcher bodies) of immunoglobulin. **C,** The plasma cell component is highlighted by CD138 immunostaining. There is monotypic expression of κ light chains by the lymphoma cells and the plasma cells **(D),** but only rare plasma cells appear to express γ light chains **(E).**

are no established quantitative criteria, the presence of large confluent sheets of large cells is usually accepted as representative of transformation. In such cases, the primary diagnosis of DLBCL should be reported, followed by addition of the term "transformed from follicular lymphoma" (Table 17-2). An estimate of the proportion of DLBCL and FL can be included. Occasional patients with FL have divergent histologic features in lymph nodes taken simultaneously from different sites, showing variation in grade or progression to DLBCL.[57]

Infrequently, FL is composed predominantly of large centrocytes (large, cleaved cells). Grading of such cases is controversial. According to the ICC classification, such cases would still be considered low grade (grade 1 to 2 of 3)[1]; others, however, have reported that FL, large cleaved cell type, has a prognosis similar to that of FL grade 3, so

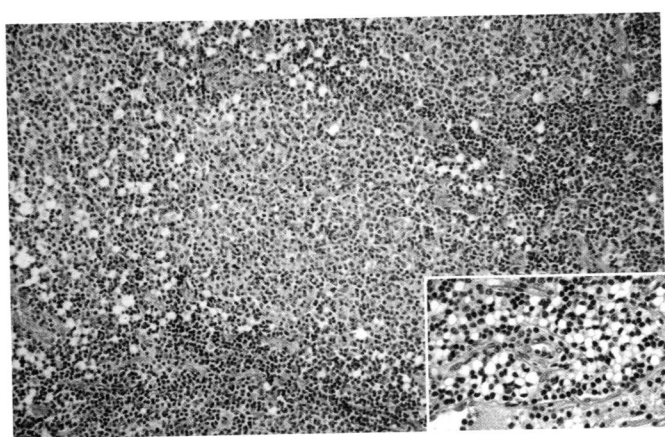

Figure 17-8. Follicular lymphoma (FL) with signet ring cells. In this case of FL with signet ring cells, many of the atypical lymphoid cells contain a large, clear cytoplasmic vacuole *(inset)*, simulating carcinoma cells of the signet ring type.

assigning a designation of grade 3 to such cases may be more appropriate.[58] For this reason, the WHO 5th edition consensus was to include these cases in the distinct uFL subgroup.

The proliferation fraction using immunohistochemical staining for Ki-67 typically mirrors grade, with grade 1 to 2 cases having a proliferation fraction of less than 20% and grade 3 greater than 30%. One study suggested that the Ki-67 fraction was less useful than the histologic grade in predicting outcome.[59] Occasional histologically low-grade cases have a high proliferation fraction.[60,61] In one study, patients with a high proliferation fraction (>40%) had a survival more similar to that of grade 3 FL than that of typical grade 1 to 2 FL.[61] Proliferation index using Ki-67 staining can be performed as an adjunct to grading, but it is has uncertain significance in isolation and is not required for grading. The presence of a high Ki-67 fraction should not change the histologic grade.

Morphology in Sites Other Than Lymph Nodes

Spleen

Splenic involvement by FL typically produces uniform enlargement of white pulp, resembling reactive hyperplasia both on gross examination and at low magnification.[57] This phenomenon has been postulated to reflect the neoplastic cells' ability to "home" to normal B-cell regions (Fig. 17-9A). The white-pulp follicles in FL are increased in number and size and show a monomorphous infiltrate of centrocytes and centroblasts, similar to that in lymph nodes. The marginal zone may be preserved, making it difficult to differentiate FL from splenic marginal zone lymphoma (Fig. 17-9B). The red pulp typically contains numerous small follicles, but diffuse red pulp involvement is uncommon.

Bone Marrow

Bone marrow involvement by FL is seen as large, usually circumscribed nodules adjacent to bony trabeculae (Fig. 17-9C–E).[57] This feature is useful in distinguishing nodules of lymphoma from benign lymphoid aggregates, which are usually central within marrow spaces rather than paratrabecular; however, occasional paratrabecular lymphoid aggregates can

be seen in apparently healthy individuals.[57] Infiltrates that appear to hug or wrap around bony trabeculae are highly suspicious for FL, in contrast to those that simply touch the trabeculae. Marrow aggregates of FL are typically composed predominantly of small centrocytes (Fig. 17-9D), with only rare centroblasts; the cellular composition may not reflect that of the lymph node, which may contain larger centrocytes and more centroblasts. Marrow involvement by centrocytes can be seen in cases of DLBCL—so-called "discordant" bone marrow histology.[62] Thus, lymphomas cannot be accurately subclassified based on their appearance in the bone marrow, as this may not reflect the appearance of a nodal tumor.

Peripheral Blood

Most patients with FL have small numbers of circulating neoplastic cells without an elevated lymphocyte count, which can be detected by flow cytometry or molecular genetic analysis to detect the t(14;18).[63-65] Rare patients with FL have an elevated lymphocyte count with circulating centrocytes, which are usually slightly larger than small lymphocytes and have a nuclear cleft (Fig. 17-9F). Absolute lymphocyte count ranges from 1000 to >200,000/µL.[12,66] Patients with FL presenting with a leukemic phase often have a high-risk FLIPI score (see section titled "Prognosis and Predictive Factors").[12] FLs with a leukemic phase appear to behave in a more aggressive manner than those without,[12,66] with shorter progression-free survival and overall survival (OS).[66] The morphology of the circulating cells is similar in follicular and mantle cell lymphoma, and some cleaved cells may be seen in occasional patients with chronic lymphocytic leukemia. Immunophenotyping by flow cytometry and often lymph node biopsy is typically necessary for correct subclassification.

RELATED B-CELL LYMPHOMAS AND FOLLICULAR PROLIFERATIONS

See Box 17-1.

Pediatric-Type Follicular Lymphoma

When FL occurs in children and adolescents, it often has clinical and pathologic features distinct from those of FL in adults. Although rare, germinal-center derived lymphomas occurring in the pediatric age group appear to be composed of several entities. Among these is pediatric-type nodal FL, designated as a variant of FL in both the ICC and WHO 5th edition classifications.[1]

Pediatric-type FL (PTFL) is a localized neoplasm of germinal-center B-cells with an entirely follicular pattern that occurs in the lymph nodes of children and young adults (Fig. 17-10). PTFL mainly affects young patients with a median age of onset of 15 to 17 years.[67,68] There is no upper age cut-off for diagnosis; the majority of patients range in age from 5 to 30 years.[67-70] Cases with features of PTFL have been identified in patients older than 40 years of age, but these are rare.[70] PTFL predominantly affects male patients (M:F = 10:1).[67-69] PTFL is virtually always localized (stage I) and most commonly presents in the lymph nodes of the head and neck.[67-69] Cases have an entirely follicular pattern with expansile and/or serpiginous follicles that, at least partially, efface the nodal architecture. Evidence of marginal zone differentiation is common, and may be the predominant component in some cases (see Chapter 20). There is often

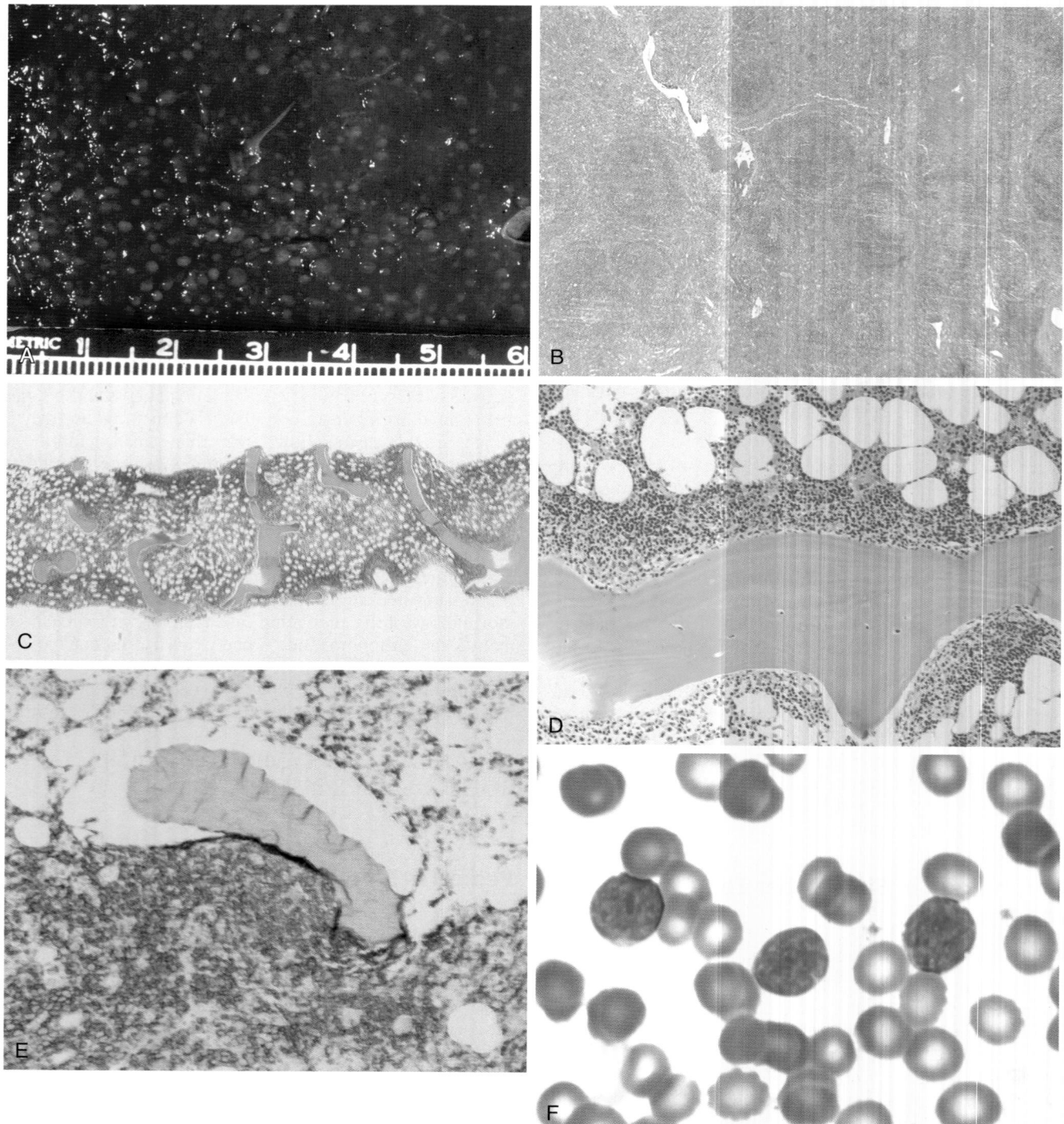

Figure 17-9. Appearance of follicular lymphoma (FL) in the spleen, bone marrow, and peripheral blood. A, In this gross photograph of a spleen involved by FL, nodules of white pulp are increased in size and number, and most are relatively round. **B,** In a low-power photomicrograph of FL in the spleen, white-pulp follicles are enlarged and increased in number; preserved marginal zones are present around some of the neoplastic follicles. **C,** In this bone marrow trephine biopsy, a broad cuff of neoplastic lymphoid cells surrounds many bony trabeculae. Residual normal hematopoietic marrow is present, away from the bone, and is recognizable as areas with a normal distribution of fat. **D,** At higher magnification, there is a predominance of centrocytes. **E,** Immunoperoxidase stain for CD20 confirms that they are B cells. **F,** A peripheral blood smear from a patient with FL shows circulating centrocytes with prominent nuclear clefts (Wright's stain).

a rim of residual normal lymph node architecture at the periphery of the involved node, imparting a "node in node" appearance. As seen in usual FL of older adults, follicles often have attenuated mantle zones. Follicles often consist of a monotonous population of intermediate-sized blastoid cells that are distinct from both centrocytes and centroblasts.[68] Tingible body macrophages are often present. The neoplastic

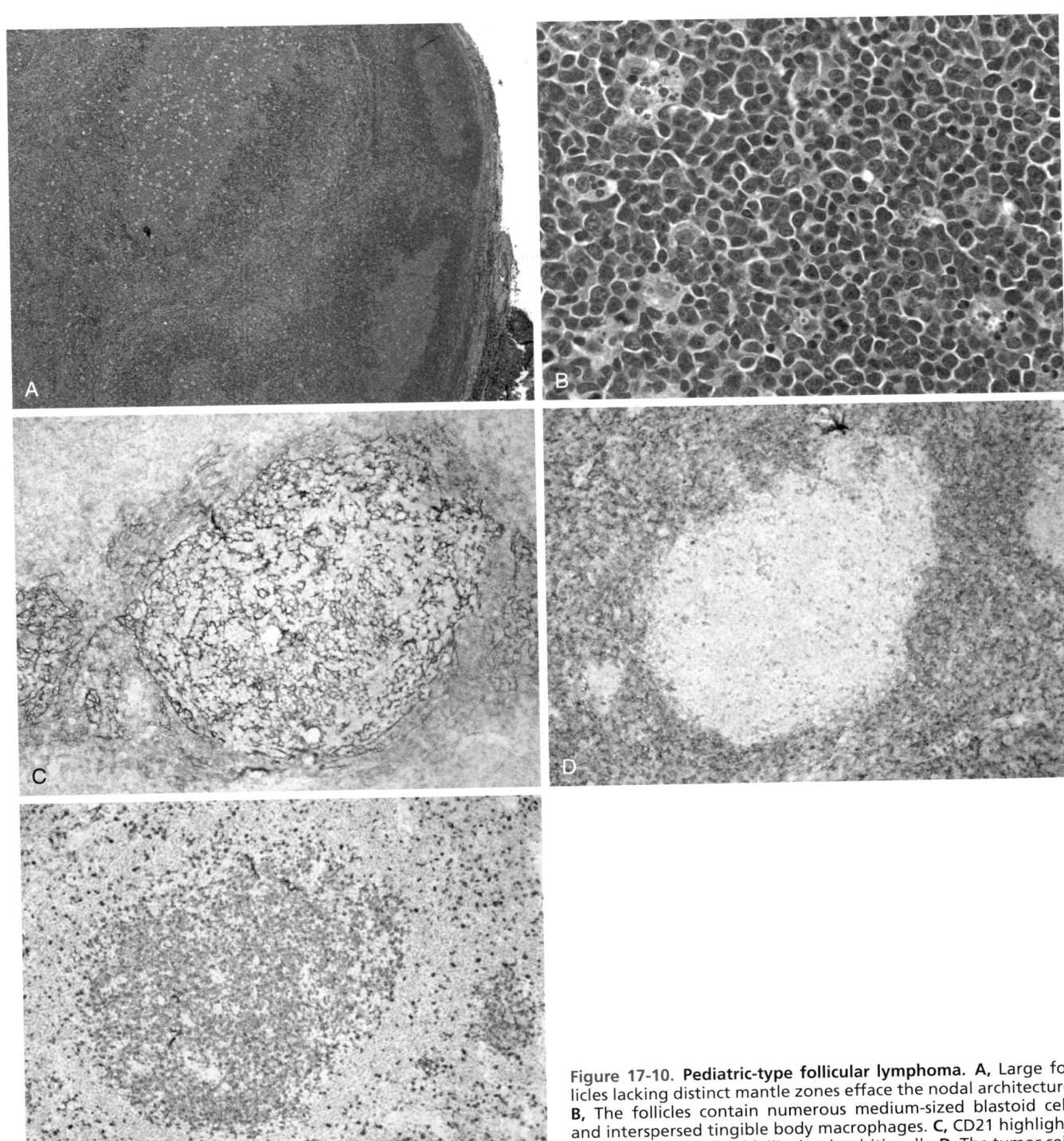

Figure 17-10. Pediatric-type follicular lymphoma. A, Large follicles lacking distinct mantle zones efface the nodal architecture. **B,** The follicles contain numerous medium-sized blastoid cells and interspersed tingible body macrophages. **C,** CD21 highlights nodular meshworks of follicular dendritic cells. **D,** The tumor cells are negative for BCL2. **E,** They have a high proliferation fraction.

cells are CD20-positive CD79a-positive PAX5-positive B cells with consistent expression of BCL6, and a high proliferation fraction of >30% by staining for Ki-67. Cases usually are mostly positive for CD10 and usually do not express BCL2, but they sometimes show faint BCL2 staining in a subset of neoplastic B cells.[67-69] Staining for IRF4/MUM1 is usually negative. Follicles are associated with CD21-positive and CD23-positive FDC meshworks. Cases of PTFL do not show rearrangements or amplification of *BCL2, BCL6, IRF4,* or Ig loci. FISH for these gene rearrangements should be routinely performed, as the presence of any of these rearrangements rules out the diagnosis of PTFL. Approximately 60% of PTFL cases harbor mutations in *MAPK* pathway genes (including *MAPK1*), which are not present in classic FL. In addition, PTFL shows recurrent deletions and copy-neutral loss of heterozygosity at 1p36 in addition to *IRF8* mutations in a subset of cases. PTFL lacks mutations in chromatin-modifying genes and other genes commonly mutated in classic FL, such as *CREBBP, KTM2D, EP300,* and *ARID1A.* Both PTFL and classic FL harbor mutations in *TNFRSF14* in less than 50% of cases.[71] PTFL, when diagnosed according to the criteria listed in Table 17-4, has an excellent prognosis with a 5-year survival of over 95%. There is growing evidence that local excision of PTFL diagnosed in children may be sufficient treatment, with no evidence of subsequent progression or relapse. Retrospective studies have shown that young adults diagnosed with PTFL have a similar excellent prognosis irrespective of therapy, though the majority of adult patients reported have received systemic chemotherapy or radiation therapy.[67,68]

Lymphomas with *IRF4* rearrangement (discussed separately) often affect children and may have a follicular pattern[72]; however, lymphomas with *IRF4* rearrangement represent a different entity and are excluded from the category of PTFL.

Extranodal Follicular Lymphomas

In addition to primary cutaneous follicle center lymphoma[73] and duodenal-type FL,[74] other extranodal sites of FL presentation include Waldeyer's ring,[75] testis,[76,77] ocular adnexa,[78] salivary glands,[79] thyroid,[80] gallbladder and extrahepatic biliary tract,[81] female genital tract,[75] and others. A minority of FLs show primary extranodal involvement without systemic disease. Primary testicular FL is rare and shares many pathologic and clinical features with pediatric-type FL. Testicular FL typically affects young boys, presents with localized disease with BCL2-negative neoplastic germinal center cells, lacks *BCL2* rearrangement and has an excellent prognosis.[76,77,82] On this basis, the 2022 ICC has designated primary testicular FL as a provisional entity. Primary extranodal FL arising in the thyroid, conjunctiva, ovary, and lower female genital tract often lacks BCL2 expression and mutations in chromatin-modifying genes frequently mutated in classic nodal FL. Several cases of primary conjunctival FL reminiscent of pediatric-type FL have been described in the literature. These cases show an expansile follicular proliferation, lack *BCL2* rearrangements and conventional chromatin-modifying genes, harbor *MAP2K1* mutations, and remain localized to this site of presentation. Taken together, extranodal FL tends to present with localized disease, expresses BCL2 less often, has a translocation involving *BCL2* [t(14;18)] less often, and tends to have better survival than nodal FL.[75] However, the

Table 17-4 Diagnostic Features of Pediatric-Type Follicular Lymphoma

	Primary Diagnostic Criteria
Morphology	• At least partial effacement of nodal architecture (required) • Pure follicular proliferation (required)† • Expansile follicles* • Intermediate-sized "blastoid" cells (not centrocytes)*
Immunohistochemistry (required)	• BCL6+ • BCL2–/weak • High proliferation fraction (>30%)
Genomics (required)	• No *BCL2, BCL6, IRF4,* or Ig rearrangement • No amplification of *BCL2*
Clinical	• Nodal disease (required) • Stage I-II (required) • Age <40* • Male >> Female*

*Common features of PTFL, but not required
†Any component of diffuse large B-cell lymphoma (DLBCL) or presence of advanced stage disease excludes pediatric-type follicular lymphoma.

characteristics of FL appear to vary somewhat from one site to another.[70,72,76,82,83]

Large B-Cell Lymphoma With *IRF4* Translocation

A small proportion of all LBCLs have a translocation involving *IRF4* and an Ig gene (Fig. 17-11). LBCL with *IRF4* gene rearrangement is currently considered a definite entity in both the ICC and WHO 5th edition. LBCL-IRF4 most commonly occurs in children and young adults (median age 12 years). These lymphomas usually have at least a partial follicular pattern, but may be entirely diffuse.[72] Therefore, patients with high-grade FL expressing IRF4/MUM1 should be evaluated for IRF4 alterations.

LBCL-IRF4 shows a predilection for head and neck sites, including Waldeyer's ring, and often present with limited-stage disease.[70,72,83a] Immunophenotyping shows that neoplastic cells are CD5–/+, CD10+/–, BCL6+, BCL2+/–, and MUM1+. In contrast to the vast majority of FLs, they lack *BCL2* rearrangement. They often harbor *BCL6* rearrangements. They appear to be associated with a favorable outcome, even if predominantly diffuse. Aggressive B-cell lymphomas with *IRF4* rearrangements associated with *BCL2* or *MYC* rearrangements are excluded from this category. LBCL-IRF4 translocation is a distinct entity from pediatric-type FL, which has previously been discussed.

Duodenal-Type Follicular Lymphoma

Duodenal-type FL is a distinct and uncommon clinicopathologic entity, comprising fewer than 4% of all primary GI lymphomas.[13] In one study of 222 GI lymphomas, 13 duodenal lymphomas and 8 FLs were identified: five of the eight FLs arose in the duodenum, all in its second portion, in the vicinity of the ampulla of Vater.[13] This and subsequent studies have revealed that patients with duodenal-type FL are mostly middle-aged adults with a mean or median age in the fifties[14,74,84] and a female preponderance in most series.[74,85,86]

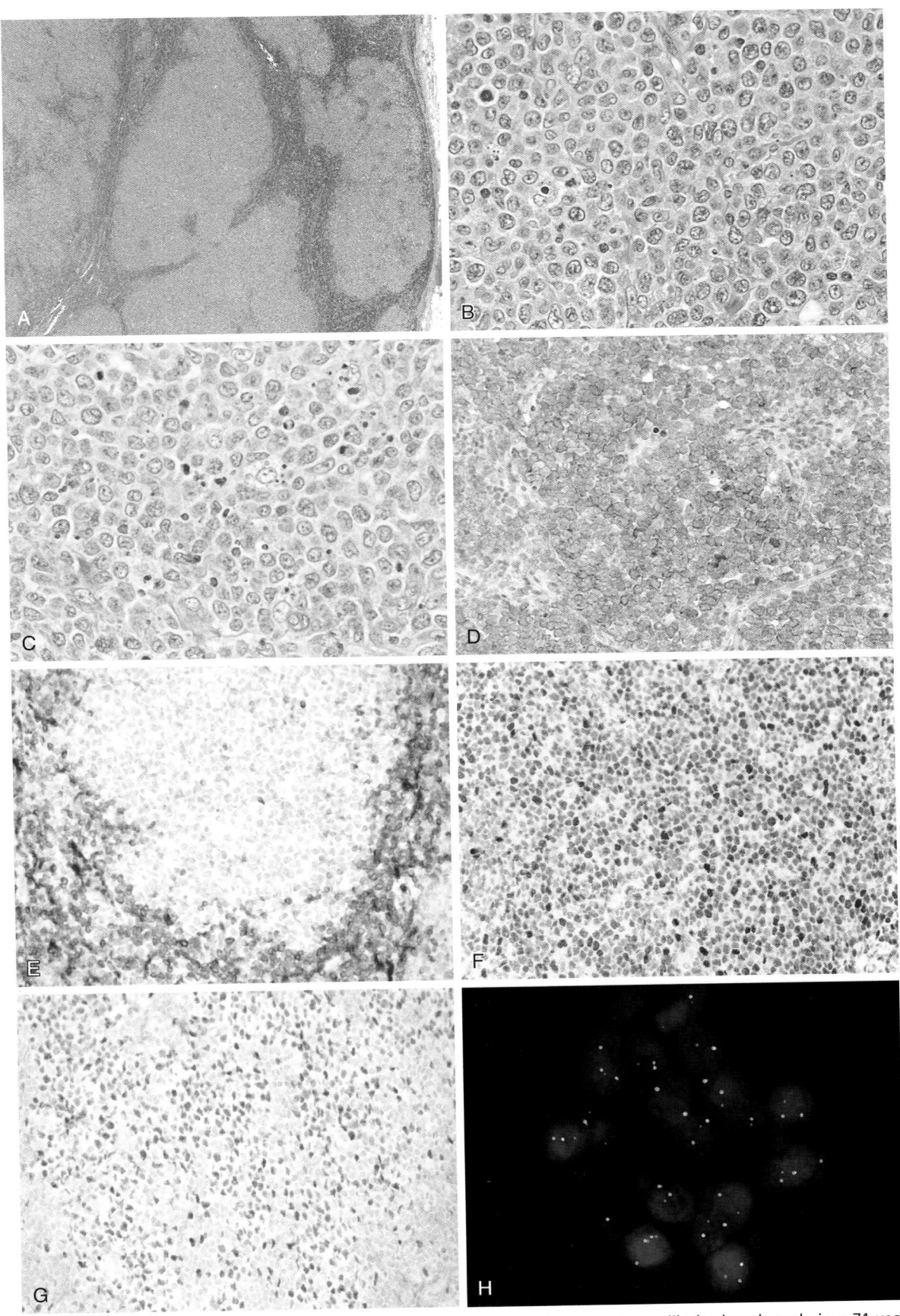

Figure 17-11. Follicular lymphoma with translocation involving IRF4. A, An enlarged submandibular lymph node in a 71-year-old male patient shows a lymphoid proliferation with a jigsaw-like pattern. **B,** The lymphoma involves large centroblastic cells with both mitoses and apoptotic bodies. **C–F,** The lymphoma cells were CD20 positive *(not shown)*, CD10 positive **(D)**, BCL2 negative **(E)** and positive for both MUM1 and BCL6 **(F** and **G)**. **H,** Fluorescence in situ hybridization (FISH) studies demonstrate an *IRF4* (6p25) break (homemade probe, telomeric BAC probe SpectrumOrange CTD-2308G5, centromeric BAC probe SpectrumGreen CTD-3139L20), though no breaks were detected for *BCL2, BCL6* or *MYC (not shown)*.

The small intestine is most often involved; the duodenum is the portion most commonly involved,[74,86] although the stomach and colorectum may be affected. On endoscopy, nodularity of the mucosa is the most common finding; cases with the appearance of multiple lymphomatous polyposis have also been described.[74,87] Taken together, the results of these studies suggest that a high proportion of duodenal lymphomas are FL and that a high proportion of GI FLs arise in the duodenum. Duodenal-type FL is typically localized and associated with excellent prognosis. At last follow-up, nearly all patients are alive, with the majority free of disease.[74,87,88]

On microscopic examination (Fig. 17-12), the vast majority of duodenal-type FL is low grade (Fig. 17-12A and B). The cases typically have an immunophenotype similar to that found in nodal FLs occurring in adults (CD20+, CD10+, BCL2+, BCL6+) (Fig. 17-12C and D).[14,74,85,86] IGH and Ig light-chain genes are clonally rearranged, and *BCL2* rearrangement is identified in most cases.[85,89,90] In-depth evaluation of these lymphomas does reveal some pathologic features that diverge from those of lymph nodal FL, however. GI FL frequently expresses α4β7, the mucosal homing receptor, suggesting an origin from antigen responsive B cells residing in intestinal mucosa.[91] One study described that, in contrast to lymph nodal FLs, intestinal FLs are associated with "hollowed out," rather than intact, FDC meshworks (Fig. 17-12E).[90] The proliferation index is typically low (Fig. 17-12F). Intestinal FLs are reported to lack expression of activation-induced cytidine deaminase *(AID)*.[90] Biased usage of IGH variable region genes (IGHV) has been described, with disproportionate use of *VH4*, in particular *VH4-34*.[84,90] These observations suggest subtle differences in the pathologic features of intestinal and lymph nodal FL; they also suggest an antigen-driven component in the pathogenesis of intestinal FL.[84,90]

Other Extranodal Follicular Lymphomas

In Situ Follicular Neoplasia (ICC)

In situ follicular neoplasia (ISFN) ("in situ follicular B-cell neoplasm", see Table 17-2) designates an unusual condition in which follicles containing abnormal, clonal, BCL2 brightly positive cells are present on a background of architecturally normal lymphoid tissue.[43] Relatively few cases have been reported, but patients have been mostly middle-aged or older adults, with men and women both affected.[43,92-94]

On microscopic examination (Fig. 17-13), affected lymph nodes closely resemble reactive lymph nodes, except that some follicles may have monotonous-appearing follicle centers composed predominantly of centrocytes within mantles that are typically intact. These monotonous follicles have an immunophenotype like that of other FLs, except that BCL2 is almost always very bright (considerably brighter than the aberrant BCL2 expression found in typical FLs). Occasionally, the abnormal follicles histologically resemble reactive follicles and are only recognizable as abnormal because of the strong BCL2 expression.[43,92-94] The number of abnormal follicles varies from case to case, but typically, not all follicles in the involved lymph nodes are abnormal. In addition, some follicles are only partially replaced by abnormal follicle center cells. Flow cytometry detects a clonal population in about half of all cases.[93]

Clonal IGH rearrangement and *BCL2* rearrangement are present in most cases, although detection using microdissected tissue or combined immunohistochemistry and FISH appears to be more sensitive than detection using whole sections of tissue, as the abnormal cells are present in relatively small numbers.[43,92,95] In patients with both ISFN and overt FL, the two share common IGH rearrangements and *BCL2* breakpoints, indicating they are clonally related.[95] However, ISFN has few or no copy number alterations when evaluated by comparative genomic hybridization (CGH), which is in contrast to overt FL.[95] *EZH2* mutations are also identified in a subset of ISFN, supporting the concept that *EZH2* mutations are an early change in the development of FL in at least some cases.[95] ISFN must be distinguished from partial involvement by FL (pFL), in which there is architectural distortion but only partial nodal involvement by lymphoma and some residual reactive follicles. Compared with other FLs, pFL usually presents with localized disease,[94,95] but it is more likely to be associated with progressive disease than ISFN.[94,95]

A subset of patients has a prior history of FL.[93-95] An additional subset has concurrent FL or another lymphoid neoplasm, sometimes in the form of a composite lymphoma.[43,92-95] Most patients with isolated ISFN remain well on follow-up without further therapy.[93,94] It is possible that ISFN represents a preneoplastic change or a very early stage in the development of FL that may or may not progress to clinically evident lymphoma. In cases of ISFN, an outright diagnosis of FL should not be made; the pathology report should indicate that the significance of the finding is unknown and that clinical evaluation for evidence of overt FL elsewhere is suggested.

Florid Follicular Hyperplasia With Clonal B Cells

Rare cases of florid follicular hyperplasia, particularly in young boys, may have clonal populations of CD10-positive B cells detected by flow cytometry and molecular genetic analysis; a diagnosis of lymphoma should not be made in the absence of morphologic features of malignancy.[96] There may be a morphologic overlap between so-called follicular hyperplasia with clonal B cells and PTFL.[96] In the context of this overlap, architectural effacement supports a diagnosis of PTFL.

IMMUNOPHENOTYPE

FL B cells express pan-B antigens (CD19, CD20, CD22, CD79a, PAX5) and surface Ig with light-chain restriction. Flow cytometry is usually required to demonstrate Ig expression; occasionally, it can be detected by immunohistochemistry (Fig. 17-14A–E). In more than 50% of cases, the surface Ig is μ heavy chain, with a minority also expressing δ; a large minority express γ heavy chain, and rare cases express α heavy chain.[97] The frequency of IGH class switching is higher in FL than in other low-grade lymphomas, consistent with the observation that IGH class switching normally occurs in the germinal center. Most cases express the germinal-center–associated protein CD10 (Fig. 17-14F); CD10 expression is often stronger in neoplastic follicles than in reactive germinal centers.[32,97,98] FL also invariably expresses nuclear BCL6 protein in at least a proportion of the tumor cells.[99] In normal germinal centers, virtually all cells are BCL6 positive, whereas a variable proportion of cells are BCL6 positive in FL (Fig. 17-14G). Both CD10 and BCL6 may be downregulated in interfollicular neoplastic cells and

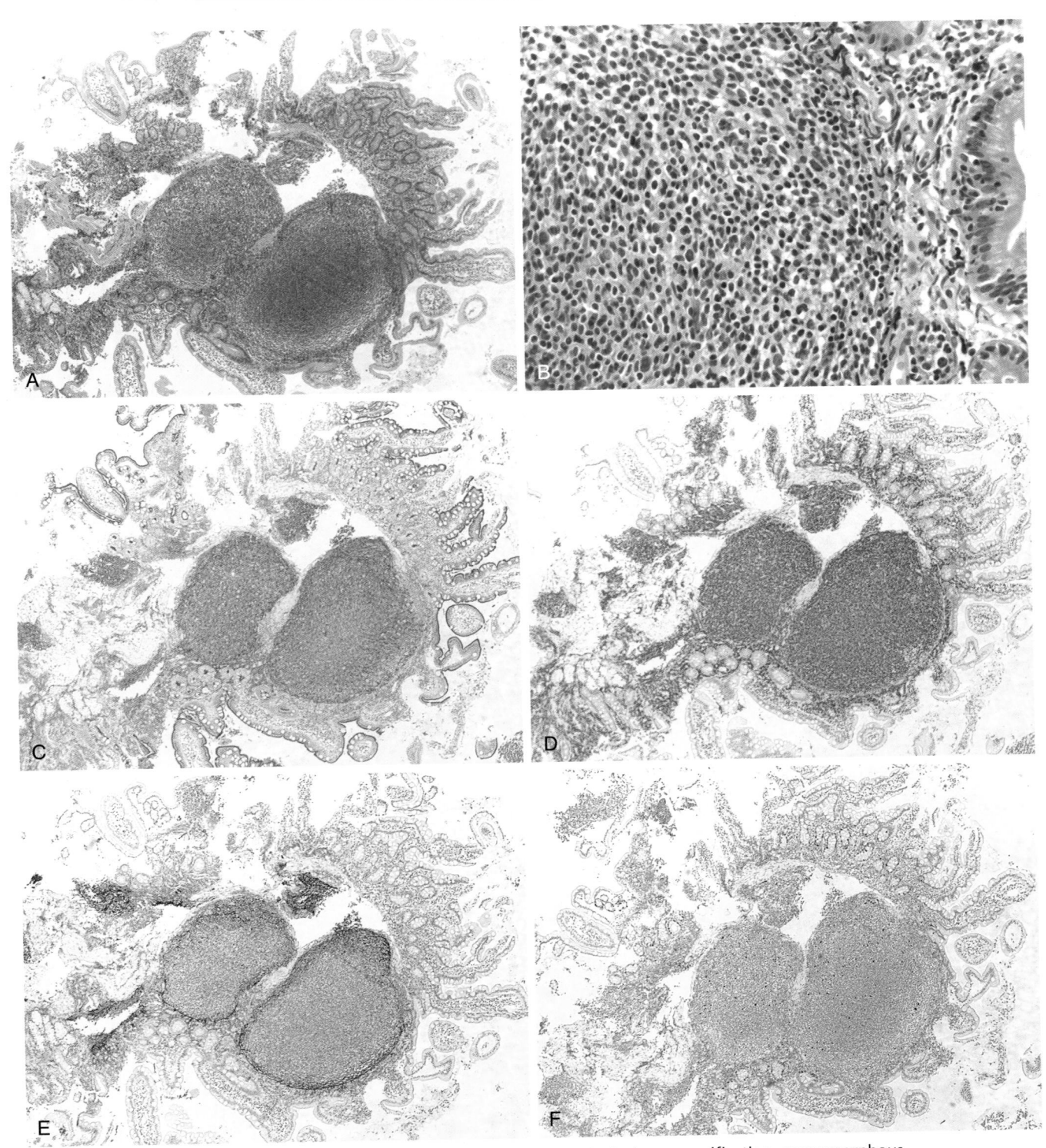

Figure 17-12. Follicular lymphoma of the duodenum. A, At low magnification, monomorphous follicles lacking mantle zones are present in the lamina propria. **B,** At higher magnification, there is a monotonous population of centrocytes. The cells are positive for CD10 **(C)** and BCL2 **(D)**. **E,** CD21 highlights a follicular dendritic cell meshwork concentrated at the periphery of the follicles *(hollowed out pattern)*. **F,** The proliferation fraction highlighted by Ki67 immunostaining is very low.

in areas of marginal zone differentiation (Fig. 17-2E).[32,97,98] A novel marker of germinal-center cells—GCET-1, also known as *centerin*—was discovered by gene expression analysis; it is consistently detected in FL and other lymphomas of germinal-center B-cell derivation.[100]

FL is typically CD5 negative and CD43 negative.[101-103] Rare cases of CD5-positive FL have been reported.[104] Most CD43-positive cases are grade 3, with areas of DLBCL.[103] MUM1/IRF4 is typically not expressed, although occasional cases of grade 3 FL that lack CD10 and BCL2 and express

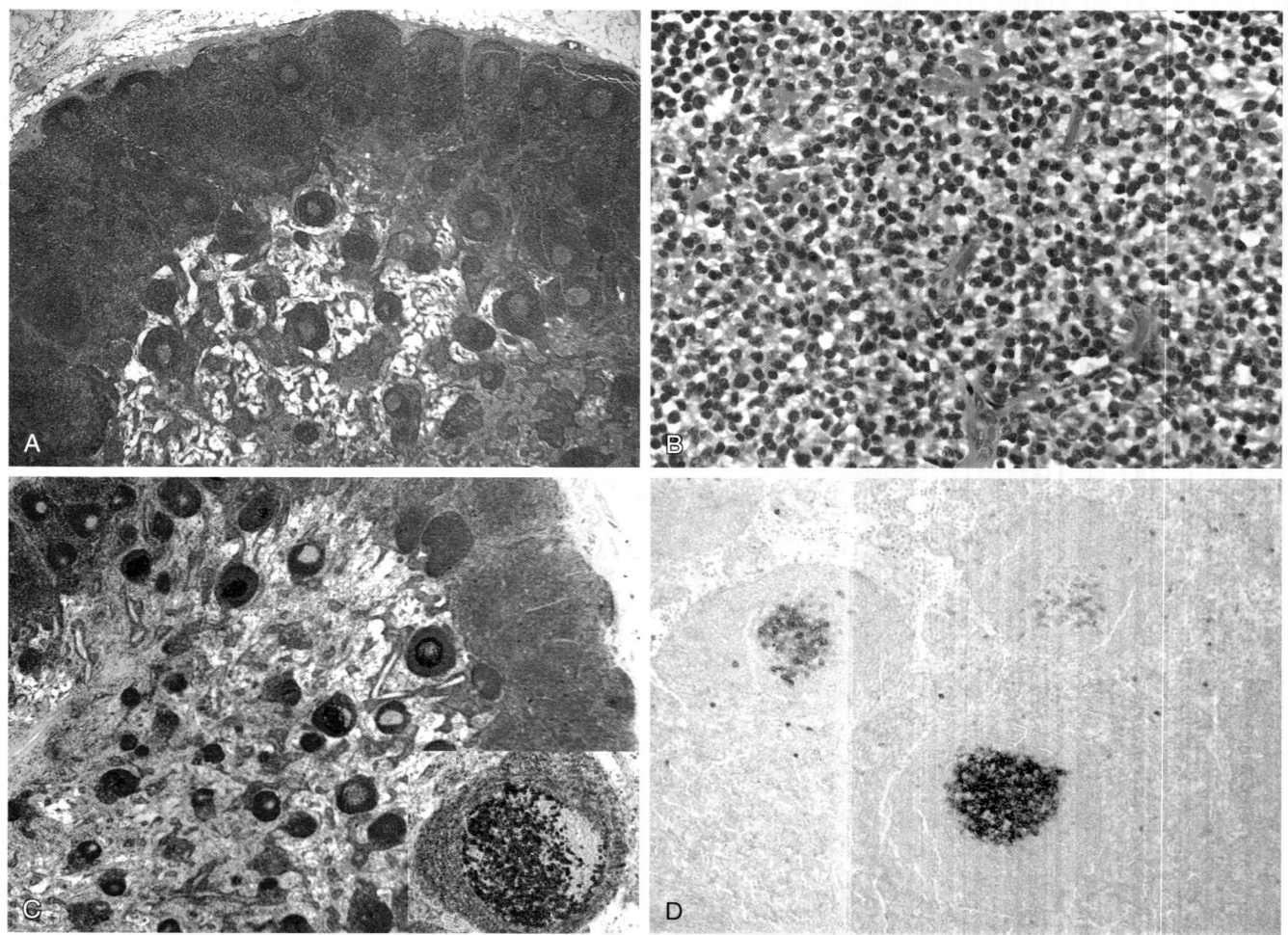

Figure 17-13. In situ follicular neoplasia (in situ follicular B-cell neoplasm, WHO 5th edition). The lymph node architecture is preserved **(A)**, with reactive-appearing follicles **(B)**. **C,** Immunohisto-chemistry for BCL2 reveals occasional follicles containing strongly positive cells. The *inset* shows that some follicles are only partially involved. **D,** The BCL2-positive follicles tend to express CD10 more strongly than ordinary reactive follicles.

MUM1/IRF4 have been reported.[105,106] FL typically expresses the CD95/Fas protein.[107] FL also expresses costimulatory molecules CD80, CD86, and CD40.[32,108] Expression of these antigens is weak compared with that of normal germinal-center B cells.[108]

About 75% of cases express BCL2 protein (Fig. 17-14H)[109]; the frequency is highest (85% to 97%) in grade 1 to 2 cases and as low as 50% to 75% in grade 3 cases.[110,111] Expression of BCL2 protein is highly predictive of the presence of a *BCL2* translocation; however, some cases of FL with *BCL2* rearrangement have mutations in the *BCL2* gene that affect detection of the protein by the commonly used antibody, resulting in a false-negative result (Fig. 17-14I).[112]

Neoplastic follicles contain many elements of the germinal-center microenvironment.[113] Nodular aggregates of FDCs outline the neoplastic follicles, demonstrated by antibodies to CD21 or CD23 (Fig. 17-14J). Expression of CD21 and CD23 is variable, and some FLs may express one and not the other; thus, staining for both may be necessary. In diffuse areas of FL, FDCs are absent (Fig. 17-6I); this may be useful in distinguishing

diffuse FL from mantle cell and marginal zone lymphomas, in which large, irregular aggregates of FDCs are present, even in areas that appear diffuse on routine staining.[17,97] Neoplastic follicles also contain T follicular helper cells (positive for CD3, CD4, CD57, PD1, ICOS, and CXCL13), which are usually less numerous in neoplastic follicles than reactive follicles (Fig. 17-14K) and are randomly distributed; this contrasts with the crescentic arrangement at the junction with the mantle zone that characterizes reactive follicles.[114,115] Varying numbers of FoxP3-positive T-regulatory cells and CD68-positive histiocytes are present, and the number and/or distribution of tumor-infiltrating T-regulatory cells, PD1-positive T follicular helper cells, and CD68-positive macrophages have been reported to predict clinical prognosis in multiples studies,[116-126] although results are not uniform.[127]

Most cases of low-grade FL have a proliferation fraction with Ki-67 of less than 15% (Fig. 17-14L); however, rare cases have a high (>40%) proliferation fraction (Fig. 17-14M and N) and may behave more like grade 3 FL (see the section "Grading and Terminology").[61]

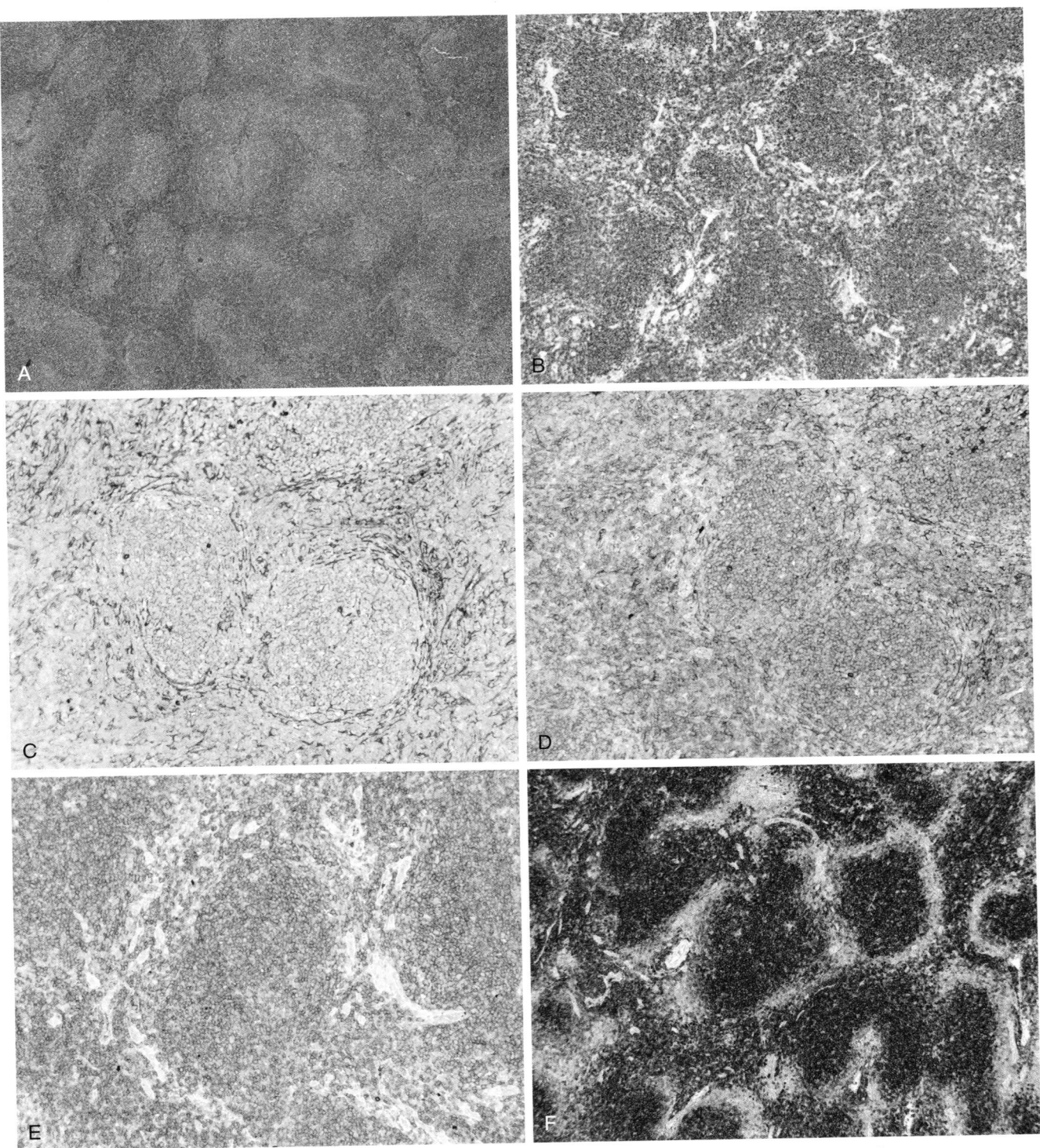

Figure 17-14. Immunohistochemistry of follicular lymphoma (FL) using immunoperoxidase stains in paraffin sections. A, A view at low magnification shows a lymphoproliferation with a nodular pattern. **B,** FL stained for CD20 shows that CD20-positive B cells are present both within and between follicles. Immunostains for immunoglobulin light and heavy chains demonstrate faint interstitial staining for kappa **(C)** and monotypic expression of lambda light chain **(D)** and IgM **(E)** at the membrane of the lymphoma cells. **F,** FL immunostained for CD10 shows strongly positive cells largely confined to follicles.

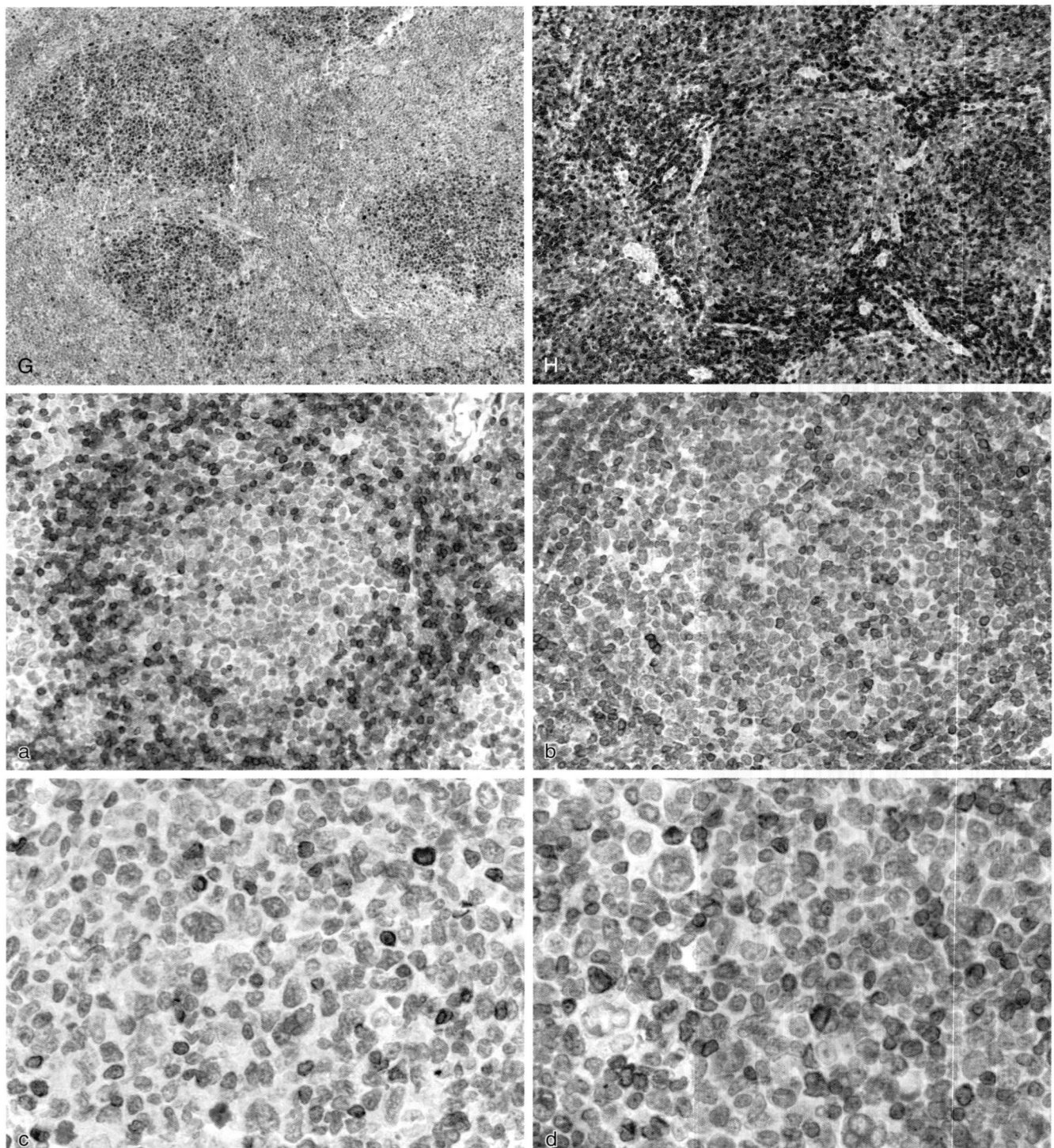

Figure 17-14, cont'd. G, FL stained for BCL6 shows brightly positive cells essentially within the follicles, while a few interfollicular cells show fainter BCL6 staining. **H,** Immunoperoxidase stain for BCL2 in FL shows strong, uniform positivity within follicles. **a-d,** Immunoperoxidase stains show differential results with Dako and Epitomics antibcl2 antibodies in a case of grade 3A FL with *BCL2* rearrangement. The neoplastic follicles are negative for BCL2 with the Dako antibody (**a** and **c**), and positive for BCL2 when using the Epitomics antibody (**b** and **d**).

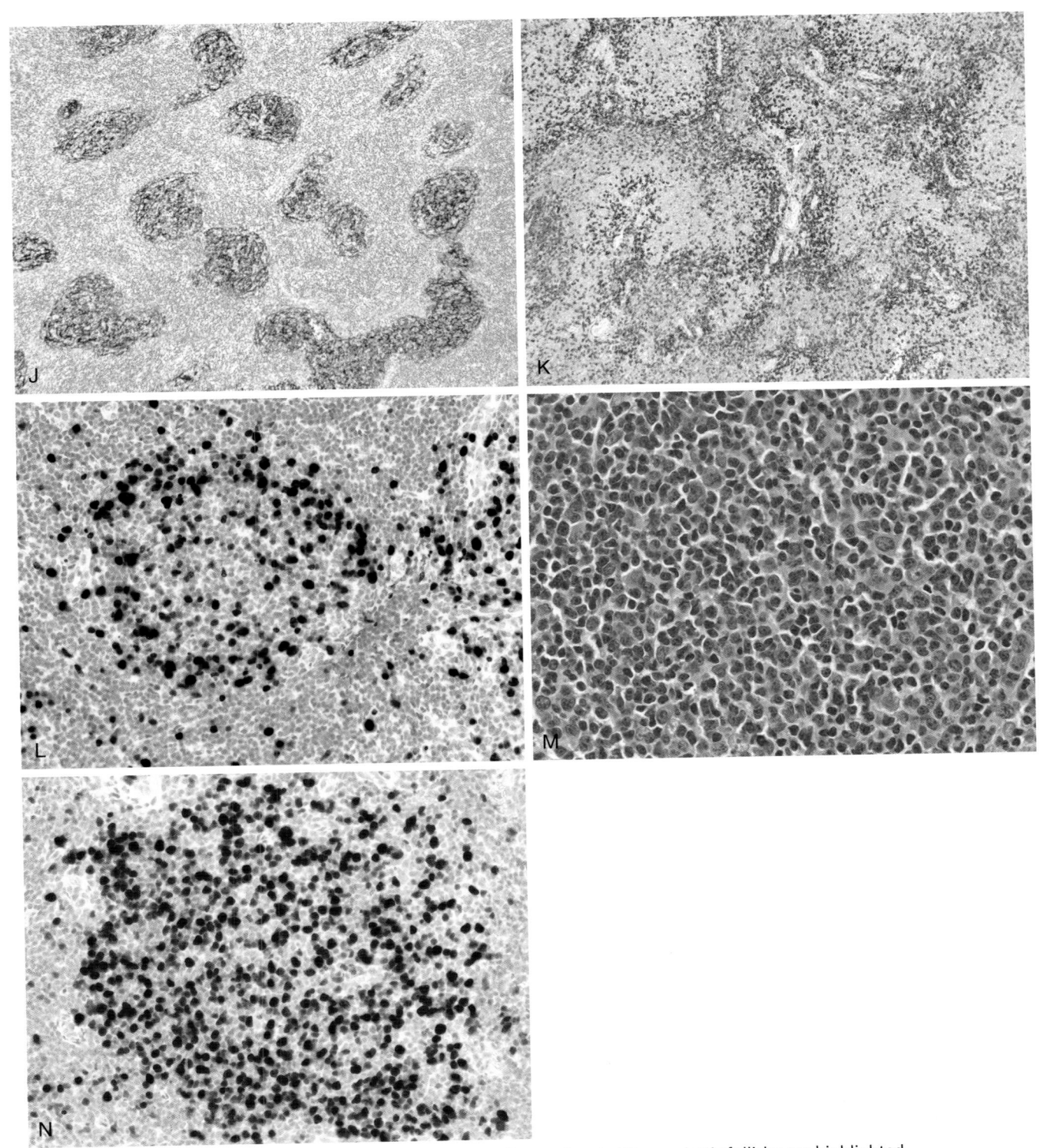

Figure 17-14, cont'd. J, Follicular dendritic cells associated with neoplastic follicles are highlighted by CD21. **K,** Immunostaining of FL for CD5 shows that neoplastic follicles contain few T cells, whereas numerous T cells are present in the interfollicular region. **L, The proliferation fraction with Ki67 is typically low.** Rare cases of low-grade FL **(M)** have a high proliferation fraction with Ki-67 (>40%) **(N).**

CYTOGENETIC AND GENETIC FEATURES

Antigen Receptor Genes

The IGH and Ig light-chain genes are clonally rearranged and, like normal germinal-center B cells, have somatic hypermutation in the variable regions.[128-131] In most cases studied, there is intraclonal variation in the pattern of somatic hypermutation, which has been interpreted to mean that the mutation process is ongoing in these cells—again, similar to normal germinal-center B cells.[132,133] Studies of the frequency of replacement to silent mutations in the framework and complementarity-determining regions have indicated a role for antigen selection.[128] As would be expected from normal germinal-center cells, IGH class switching occurs in approximately 40% of cases.[130] Some cases have evidence of both IgM and class-switched IgG clones in the same tumor; this finding has led to speculation that the class-switch mechanism, like the somatic mutation mechanism, remains active in lymphomas.[135] However, studies of sequential biopsies from the same patient indicate that the same clones persist over years, with some becoming dominant and others receding, but with no increase in the somatic mutation load, more consistent with clonal selection than with clonal evolution.[136,137] In addition, evaluation of microdissected cells from multiple follicles in a single case showed that multiple subclones were present within a single follicle, and a single clone may be found in multiple distant follicles.[138] These observations suggest that the hypermutation and class-switching mechanisms may be active very early in the development of lymphoma, leading to multiple subclones, but by the time the lymphoma is established, additional mutations and switching do not occur with any frequency.

In FLs that transform to LBCL, the Ig genes show identical VDJ rearrangements. In several reported cases, the transformed lymphoma involved a single clone, without intraclonal diversity.[135,139]

Cytogenetic Abnormalities

Virtually all FLs have cytogenetic abnormalities (Table 17-5).[140] Seventy-five percent to 90% have translocations involving the long arms of chromosomes 14 and 18 (t[14;18][q32;q21]), which places the BCL2 gene on chromosome 18 under the influence of the IGH promoter on chromosome 14.[141,142] Rare cases have a t(2;18)(p12;q21), which places the BCL2 gene with the light-chain gene on chromosome 2. In those with t(14;18) translocations, this is the sole abnormality in only 10% of cases; the remainder have additional breaks (a median of six in one study), most commonly involving chromosomes 1, 2, 4, 5, 13, and 17 or additions of X, 7, 12, or 18.[140,143] One study found that the presence of more than six chromosomal breaks was associated with a poor outcome; in addition, breaks at 6q23-26 or 17p conferred a poorer prognosis and a shorter time to transformation.[140,144] Another study found that the addition of X was associated with a worse outcome only in men.[143] The 17p abnormalities may reflect alterations in the TP53 gene at 17p13, which have been associated with a poorer prognosis and with transformation in FL.[145,146] Abnormalities at 6q23-36 are found in 10% to 40% of B-cell lymphomas of all types and are the most common second abnormality in cases with t(14;18). Three distinct deletions have been described at 6q21, 6q23, and 6q25-27, suggesting

Table 17-5 Follicular Lymphoma: Genetic Abnormalities

Abnormality	Approximate % Positive
Cytogenetic Abnormalities	**100**
+7	20
+18	20
t(14;18)(q32;q21)	80
3q27-28 ?rearrangement	15
6q23-26* ?deletion	15
17p* ?deletion	15
1p36 deletion	Uncommon
IRF4 translocation	Uncommon
Oncogene Abnormalities	
BCL2 rearranged	80
BCL6 rearranged	15
BCL6 5′ mutations	40
NOTCH1 and NOTCH2 mutations	6

*Associated with a poor prognosis.[140]

the presence of three distinct tumor-suppressor genes.[147] Deletions and other alterations of chromosome 9p, involving the p15 and p16 gene loci, have been reported in cases of FL that transform to DLBCL.[148,149] Array comparative genomic hybridization studies have demonstrated a large variety of chromosomal gains and losses, some of which are recurrent and have prognostic significance, including increased risk of transformation, particularly at 1p36 and 6q21.[150]

Recurrent Gene Rearrangements

BCL2

Analysis of the t(14;18)(q32;q21) breakpoint revealed a segment of DNA that was clonally rearranged in most FLs and comigrated with the rearranged Ig gene in Southern blots of tumor DNA.[151,152] The gene encoded by this segment was given the name BCL2. BCL2 protein is expressed by resting B and T cells but not by normal germinal-center cells or cortical thymocytes[153]—cell types in which negative selection and apoptosis represent important control mechanisms of immune system development—or by monocytoid B cells.[111] Overexpression of BCL2 protein confers a survival advantage on B cells in vitro by preventing apoptosis under conditions of growth factor deprivation.[154] Lymphocytes with BCL2 rearrangement can be detected by polymerase chain reaction (PCR) in the tonsils and peripheral blood of many healthy individuals.[155,156] Thus, it appears that BCL2 rearrangement by itself is not enough to result in neoplastic transformation. Additional genetic abnormalities, or possibly a proliferative stimulus such as engaging the antigen receptor, are required for lymphoma development.

BCL6

The BCL6 gene is a zinc finger transcriptional repressor gene that was cloned from the breakpoint of the 3q27 translocation found in a subset of DLBCLs.[157,158] It is normally expressed in germinal-center B cells[159,160] and in rare intrafollicular and interfollicular CD4-positive T cells; its presence is required for germinal-center formation.[161] The translocation, which involves a variety of partners, always involves the 5′ noncoding region of the BCL6 gene, which is replaced by the promoter of the partner gene. It is presumed that these translocations prevent downregulation of BCL6 and prevent the cell from progressing past the germinal-center stage, thus facilitating neoplastic transformation.[159] The *BCL6* gene undergoes mutations in the 5′ noncoding region in normal germinal-center B cells,[162-164] and a relationship between this process and Ig gene mutation has been suggested. Abnormalities of 3q27 or *BCL6* rearrangements are found in about 15% of FLs, whereas 5′ mutations of the *BCL6* gene are found in approximately 40%.[164]

MYC

Rare cases of FL studied at the time of diagnosis have both *BCL2* and *MYC* rearrangements ("double hit"); others acquire *MYC* rearrangement at the time of transformation to high-grade lymphoma.[165] Although concurrent *BCL2* and *MYC* rearrangements are typically associated with diffuse, high-grade B-cell lymphomas, rare FLs have concurrent *MYC* and *BCL2* and/or *BCL6* rearrangements (double-hit or "triple-hit" FLs).[166,167] Patients with double-hit or triple-hit FLs are usually middle-aged or older adults, and there is a female preponderance, most with advanced clinical stage. Most cases are grade 2 or grade 3A. In one study, most cases showed >50% of cells expressing MYC protein, and the proliferation index was elevated in most cases (range, 1%–90%; median, 70%),[167] although MYC expression and elevation of proliferation index has not been uniformly as striking.[160] The immunophenotype is otherwise similar to that of conventional FL. In one study of 10 cases, 8 had concurrent *MYC* and *BCL2* rearrangements, one had *MYC* and *BCL6* rearrangements, and one had rearrangements of *MYC*, *BCL2* and *BCL6* (triple-hit FL).[167] Compared with FLs without *MYC* rearrangement, double-hit and triple-hit FLs affect similar patient populations, but they are more often grade 3 and may show more expression of MYC and have a higher proliferation index.[166-168] The behavior of double-hit/triple-hit FL is more indolent than that of high-grade double-hit or triple-hit B-cell lymphomas[168]; however, some investigators report more aggressive behavior than conventional low-grade FL and suggest that patients with double-hit FL may benefit from more aggressive therapy.[168]

Other cytogenetic abnormalities associated with distinctive features include deletions of 1p36 and *IRF4* translocation, discussed separately in this chapter (Table 17-5).

Mutational Landscape

Recurrent mutations in a number of epigenetic regulators are present in most cases of FL, demonstrating that FL is a disease of the epigenome and of the genome. These mutations include recurrent mutations in histone methyltransferases *MLL2* and *EZH2* and histone acetylases *CREBBP*, *EP300*, and *MEF2B*.[169-171] *EZH2* is the best characterized. *EZH2* is a histone methyltransferase catalyzing trimethylation of lysine on histone H3 (H3K27me3). *EZH2* mutations lead to gain of function with enhanced trimethylation. They are relatively frequent, being identified in 27% of FLs in one published series.[172] Another series documented *EZH2* mutations in 22% of all FLs and in 28% of FLs with *BCL2* rearrangement.[173] Mutations in *MLL2* occur most frequently, with approximately 90% of cases having one or more mutations within this gene.

CREBBP is a histone acetyl transferase, mutations of which occur in 33% to 75% of FL cases.[174] Mutations in *CREBBP* may contribute to the pathogenesis of FL by decreasing acetylation

of *BCL6*, leading to altered expression of *BCL6* target genes[174] MEF2B may also deregulate BCL6 transcriptional activity.[175]

Other genes with recurrent mutations in FL include histone linker genes histone *H1 B, C, D,* and *E*; transcription factors *OCT2* and *STAT6*; *TNFRSF14*; and *IRF8* and *ARIDA*.[176,177] Mutations in *NOTCH1* and *NOTCH2* (Table 17-5) are occasionally present.

Gene Expression Profiles

The gene expression profile of FL by DNA microarray analysis shows many similarities to normal germinal-center cells.[178,179] Genes upregulated in FL include *BCL2*; genes involved in cell cycle regulation, including *CDK10*, *p21CIP1*, and *p16INK4A*; transcription factors involved in B-cell differentiation such as *PAX5*; and some genes involved in cell-cell interactions such as *IL4R*. Others are downregulated, including *MRP8* and *MRP14*, which are involved in the inhibition of cell migration, and *CD40*, which is important in interactions with T cells.[178,179] Genes associated with the germinal-center microenvironment (T cells, dendritic cells, macrophages) are also expressed in FL, and differential expression of these genes is associated with clinical aggressiveness.[116-125]

POSTULATED NORMAL COUNTERPART AND PATHOGENESIS

FL is a tumor of germinal-center B cells in which centrocytes fail to undergo apoptosis because they have a chromosomal rearrangement, t(14;18), that prevents the normal switching off of the antiapoptosis gene *BCL2*.[109,153] They retain their ability to interact with T cells and FDCs to form neoplastic follicles. It is likely that cases negative for *BCL2* rearrangement have alternative mechanisms for cell survival, such as decreased expression of proapoptotic proteins.[180]

ETIOLOGY

The cause of FL is unknown. Some case-control studies have found slightly higher risk of FL among individuals exposed to pesticides or hair dye and in meatpackers and smokers, but these risks are small and inconsistent.[5] There are no known links with suspected lymphoma-associated viruses such as human herpesvirus 8 or hepatitis C virus or with immune deficiency states. Rare FLs, usually grade 3, harbor Epstein-Barr virus, which may play a role in lymphomagenesis and/or disease progression.[181,182]

Many, if not most, healthy adults have memory B cells with rearranged *BCL2* genes, detectable by PCR or FISH in peripheral blood, tonsils, bone marrow, or lymph nodes.[156,183] The frequency of these translocations does not appear to vary across populations with differing incidences of FL. However, several studies suggest an increase in such cells with age, and one with exposure to cigarette smoke.[9] It has been postulated that a second genetic "hit" or even simple exposure to antigen in a cell with a *BCL2* translocation could result in the development of lymphoma, because once it begins proliferating in response to antigen, it does not respond to the usual stimuli for apoptosis.

FL cells have somatic hypermutations in the variable regions of their Ig genes, and there is intraclonal variation within most tumors, similar to normal germinal-center B cells.

These features suggest that antigen may be important in either the pathogenesis or the persistence of the neoplastic clone.[133]

As previously noted, numerous genes are mutated in FL. In addition, there is prominent intratumoral clonal diversity with respect to mutations affecting some genes. Dominant clones of FL and later transformation events arise by divergent evolution from a common mutated precursor through acquisition of distinct genetic events.[184] Those mutations that are nearly uniformly present likely represent early events, and those present only in a subset of tumor subclones are likely acquired later.[175] The BCL2 translocation can be considered a founder mutation, enabling cells to live long enough to acquire additional mutations, but it is not sufficient by itself to result in overt lymphoma.[175] The clone may then acquire secondary, driver mutations, such as mutations of CREBBP and EZH2, which, when present, are found in a high proportion of clonal cells. Over time, some clonal cells may acquire tertiary accelerator mutations of genes such as MLL2 or TNFRSF14, further promoting growth of the neoplastic clone.[175]

CLINICAL COURSE

Natural History

FL is usually a disseminated, indolent neoplasm; the median survival of patients treated palliatively is more than 10 years.[185] With current therapies, including the use of monoclonal antibodies in combination with chemotherapy, the median OS is 15 to 20 years. The natural history of FL is characterized by a protracted relapse-remitting course, with eventual treatment refractoriness. This is considered incurable, but there is significant clinical heterogeneity among patients. Of patients who require chemotherapy, 10% to 20% show progression of disease within 24 months of immunochemotherapy (POD24), an event associated with poor outcomes, with 50% of patients alive after 5 years. Histologic transformation of FL to DLBCL occurs at a risk of 1% to 3% per year,[186-189] with a median time to transformation of 2.5 to 4.1 years, also associated with poor outcomes.

Treatment

There are no clearly agreed upon treatment algorithms for patients with FL. As there is no data demonstrating benefit of treating patients early in their course without problematic symptoms or suspicion of high-risk disease, a "watch and wait" approach is often taken for advanced stage low-grade FL. Indications for therapy include symptomatic disease, bulky lymphadenopathy, marrow compromise and rapid progression of disease. Treatment for grade 1 to 2 FL is generally directed at relief of symptoms rather than cure. Patients with localized disease (stage I) may have prolonged disease-free survival after excision or local radiation therapy.[190,191] Patients with more typical advanced-stage disease may be followed clinically until symptoms require treatment.[185] The standard of care for the first-line treatment of patients with advanced stage FL is chemotherapy with rituximab (an anti-CD20 monoclonal antibody). Rituximab is often used in combination with CHOP (cyclophosphamide, doxorubicin, vincristine, and prednisone), CVP (cyclophosphamide, vincristine, and prednisone), fludarabine and cyclophosphamide, or bendamustine. The use of rituximab is more effective than chemotherapy alone and has contributed to better outcomes.[192-196] Of these

chemotherapeutic regimens, studies have provided some evidence of increased progression-free survival and fewer toxic effects with bendamustine plus rituximab (BR), suggesting BR may be considered the preferred first-line treatment.[197,198] High-dose therapies with autologous or allogeneic stem-cell rescue are often used after the first or subsequent chemosensitive relapse; some studies show evidence of improved survival.[199,200] Chimeric antigen receptor (CAR) T cells are now licensed for treatment of multiply relapsed FL.

Prognosis and Predictive Factors

Clinical Factors

Though it is clear that progression of disease by 24 months (POD24) is associated with poor outcomes, there is a need for prognostic markers that can be applied at the time of diagnosis to identify patients who have a good or poor prognosis. There are no clinical predictors or biomarkers yet available to predict who will experience POD24 prior to therapy initiation. Over the years, several prognostic scoring systems have been developed to stratify those patients who will have a good or bad prognosis, including the follicular lymphoma international prognostic index (FLIPI)[201] (based on age, stage, number of involved nodal sites, hemoglobin, and lactate dehydrogenase [LDH] level) and FLIPI2[202] (incorporating β_2-microglobulin, the diameter of the largest lymph node, bone marrow involvement, and hemoglobin level). The FLIPI and FLIPI2 each define three prognostic risk groups, with the latter system discriminating low-risk patients with 96% 5-year OS, intermediate-risk patients with 80% 5-year OS, and high-risk patients with 50% OS. An m7-FLIPI score was also created that incorporates clinical features and mutational status of seven genes (EZH2, ARID1A, MEF2B, EP300, FOXO1, CREBBP, CARD11), which was validated on patients receiving RCHOP or CVP chemotherapy.[203] Histologic transformation is associated with poor prognosis. Biomarkers have yet to be identified that can be used to detect patients at increased risk for histologic transformation.[5,22]

Histologic Grade

The prognostic value of grading FL has been debated for years. Traditionally, the clinical aggressiveness of FL has been thought to increase with the number of centroblasts. For decades, cell counting methods based on the original "Mann and Berard" method have been used to determine FL grade.[52,54] However, the prognostic significance of FL grading has been a matter of debate and considered in each of the past editions of WHO classification. In the 2017 WHO classification (revised 4th edition or WHO-HAEM4R), grade 1 and grade 2 FL were combined into a low-grade FL category (e.g., grade 1 to 2 FL) based on the realization that there is no prognostic significance between grade 1 and grade 2. Several studies conducted in the pre-rituximab era of the 1970s to the 1990s suggested a significantly more aggressive clinical course for grade 3 FL cases.[56,59,204,205] However, more recent studies focusing on genetic features and clinical behavior of cases using this grading system have provided some evidence that grade 3A FL may be more indolent and more closely related to low-grade FL.[206-208] In addition, several clinical trials performed for new targeted therapies have shown no differences in outcome between grade 1 to

2 and grade 3A FL.[209-214] Of all patients receiving first-line therapy, approximately 20% progress within 24 months (POD24 group) with a 5-year survival of 50%, in contrast to the non-POD24 group with a 5-year OS of 90%. POD24 status has shown no correlation with histologic grade.[211,215] Of note, there has been one paper studying genetic alterations predictive of transformation that showed 40% of grade 3A cases displayed subsequent high-grade transformation versus only 10% of FL grade 1 to 2 cases,[211] suggesting grade 3A FL cases are enriched for more aggressive cases. Several studies have shown the frequent association of FL grade 3B with areas of DLBCL and that FL grade 3B is genetically and behaviorally more related to DLBCL.[46,58,216-218]

The 2022 ICC classification continues to recommend morphologic grading of FL (grades 1 to 2, 3A, and 3B) as previously described. In contrast, because of the continued debate over FL grading, the proposal for the WHO 5th edition consensus removed the requirement to grade FL and proposed a new system of subclassification using four subgroups: (1) cFL, having at least a partial follicular pattern and composed of both centrocytes and centroblasts. This subgroup includes grade 1 to 2 and 3A FL as defined by the ICC; (2) FLBCL, having a purely follicular pattern and composed of sheets of centroblasts. These cases are analogous to grade 3B FL as defined by ICC; (3) uFL, having an at least partially follicular pattern and composed of medium-sized cells with blastoid/immature chromatin or large cells with cleaved/irregular nuclei (e.g., large centrocytes), and (4) dFL, having an entirely diffuse pattern (no follicles) and a mixture of centrocytes and centroblasts. This is analogous to diffuse FL as defined by ICC and includes a large subset of the cases with absence of BCL2 gene rearrangement, microfollicles, STAT6 mutations, 1p36 deletions, and frequent inguinal lymph node involvement, designated "BCL2-R-negative, CD23+ FL" by the ICC. Because of these differences (summarized in Table 17-2, Synonyms and Related Terms), for routine clinical diagnosis, it is recommended to provide both the ICC and proposed WHO 5th edition nomenclature for clarity.

Diffuse Areas

The effect of diffuse areas on survival in patients with grade 1 to 2 FL is controversial. Some studies have found that the presence of even very large diffuse areas in FL grade 1 or 2 (small, cleaved cell type or mixed small and large cell type) did not significantly alter the prognosis[219]; others have suggested that the proportion of follicular pattern does affect survival.[220,221] Diffuse areas with sufficient large cells for a diagnosis of DLBCL are more common in grade 3 FL than in grade 1 and grade 2 cases. Most observers believe this finding is clinically significant,[56,58,219] conferring a poorer prognosis, although results have not been uniform.[53,222]

Histologic Transformation

Progression to DLBCL or high-grade B-cell lymphoma (not otherwise specified [NOS] or with concurrent rearrangements of MYC and BCL2 +/− BCL6) is usually associated with a rapidly progressive clinical course and may result in death from a tumor that is refractory to treatment (Fig. 17-15).[185,186,223-226] Of note, rare cases of TdT-positive pre-B-lymphoblastic leukemias/lymphomas (pB-ALL/LBL) have MYC and BCL2 dual translocations and are seen particularly in children and young adults.[227,228] These can be challenging to distinguish from high-grade B-cell lymphomas with BCL2 and MYC gene rearrangements, but flow cytometric characterization to distinguish a precursor versus mature B-cell state and molecular studies (NRAS/KRAS mutations in preB-ALL/LBL) may be helpful.[228]

DIFFERENTIAL DIAGNOSIS

See Box 17-2.

Follicular Hyperplasia

Reactive follicular hyperplasia is the major differential diagnosis in cases of FL. In the vast majority of cases, typical architectural and cytologic features permit the diagnosis of FL based on morphologic criteria alone.[229,230] In difficult cases, immunophenotyping and, occasionally, molecular genetic studies can be helpful in establishing a diagnosis.

Morphologic Criteria

Pattern

Effacement of the normal architecture by closely packed, relatively uniform follicles that lack a mantle zone and extend outside the nodal capsule is characteristic of FL (Table 17-6). Close packing of follicles, even focally—particularly if the follicles are small and uniform—is highly suggestive of lymphoma. If the follicles are widely spaced, the interfollicular region should be examined at high magnification for the presence of centrocytes. Although transformed cells (immunoblasts and occasionally centroblasts) can be seen in the interfollicular regions of reactive nodes, centrocytes are virtually never found outside germinal centers in normal lymph nodes. Extension of follicles outside the capsule in association with concentric bands of sclerosis is a helpful feature supporting FL (Fig. 17-1A). Capsular fibrosis often occurs in lymphadenitis, with small lymphocytes and plasma cells present in perinodal fat, but follicles with germinal centers are rarely seen outside the capsule. Sclerosis within the lymph node, particularly in diffuse areas, is also suggestive of lymphoma; areas of sclerosis should be scrutinized at high magnification for the presence of centrocytes. Finally, transmural invasion of the walls of small or medium-sized veins by centrocytes, either within the node or in perinodal tissue, is highly suggestive of lymphoma (Fig. 17-3B and C).

Cytology

Cases that are difficult to diagnose are typically grade 3, in which the increased number of centroblasts more closely approximates the normal germinal center. In these cases, the absence of phagocytic tingible body macrophages, relatively low mitotic rate, lack of polarization, crowding of follicles, and lack of a mantle zone are helpful features. In some FLs, the centroblasts or large centrocytes have a cytologically atypical appearance, with hyperchromatic or abnormally shaped nuclei. The cytology of the interfollicular, extranodal, and diffuse areas in these cases can be essential in establishing the diagnosis.

Immunophenotyping

In distinguishing benign from malignant lymphoid infiltrates, the most reliable criterion is Ig light-chain restriction, which

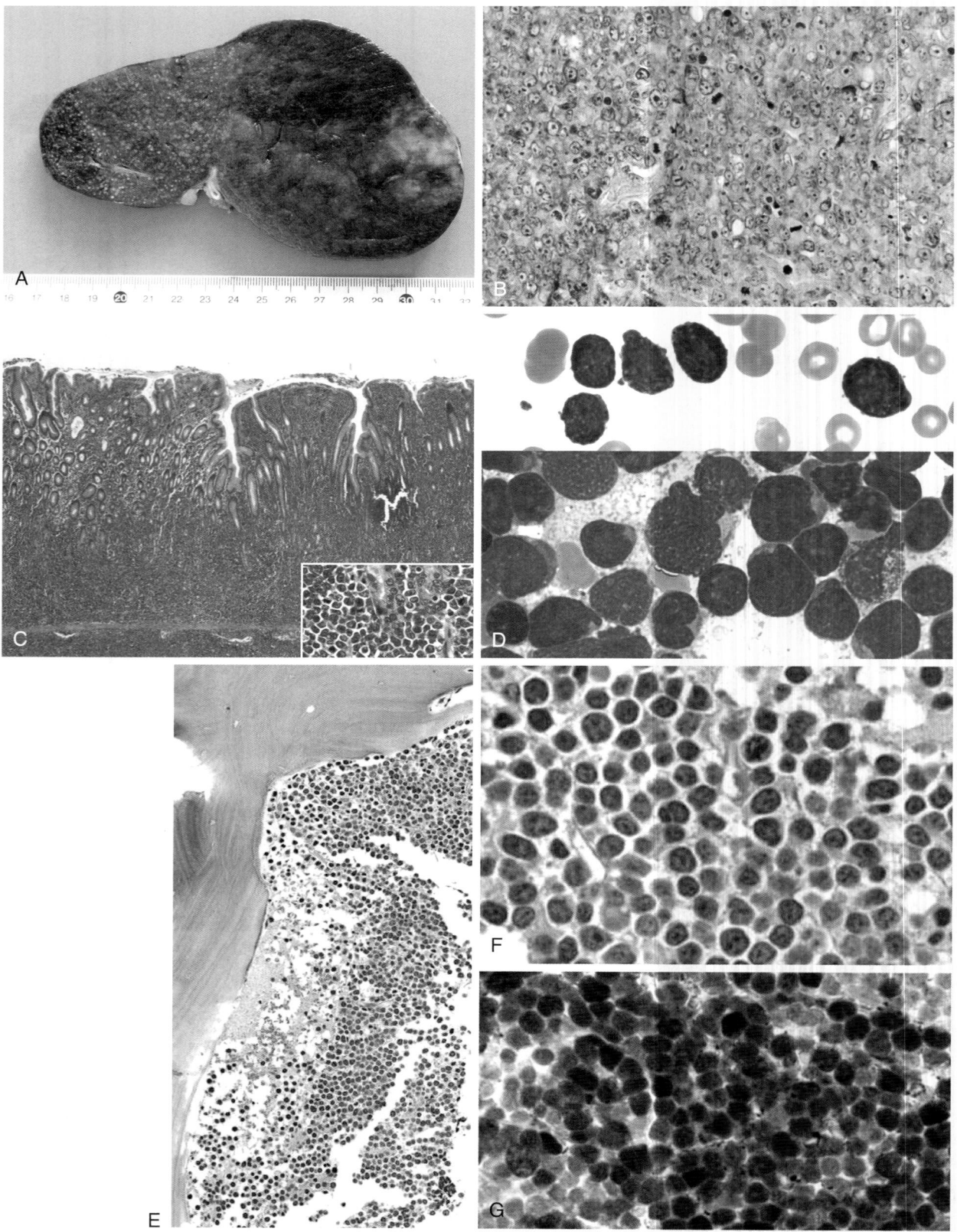

Figure 17-15. Transformed follicular lymphoma (FL). A, Splenic involvement by FL (micronodular pattern, *left*) transformed to diffuse large B-cell lymphoma (macronodular tumor mass, *right*). **B,** Most cases of transformed FL are diffuse large B-cell lymphoma (DLBCL); in this case, the cells resemble centroblasts and immunoblasts (Giemsa stain). **C,** Occasional cases of FL transform to high-grade B-cell lymphoma. This patient with a history of FL grade 1 to 2 developed a gastric mass; resection showed a diffuse lymphoma extending from the lamina propria to the serosa. At higher magnification *(inset)*, the cells are monotonous, of medium size, and resemble Burkitt lymphoma. **D,** Peripheral blood and bone marrow aspirate of a transformed follicular lymphoma with *BCL2* and *MYC* double hit is shown manifesting with leukemia *(upper panel)* and massive bone marrow involvement by medium-sized blastoid cells with irregular nuclei *(lower panel)*; in this case, the leukemic cells were positive for B-cell antigens, CD10 and BCL2, and were TdT negative. **E,** High-grade B-cell lymphoma is shown with rearranged *MYC* and *BCL2*, TdT positive, representing transformation of FL in a 64 year-old male patient who presented with pancytopenia and widespread lymphadenopathy; he underwent a lymph node biopsy involved by grade 1 FL and a bone marrow biopsy, which was heavily infiltrated by medium-sized lymphoid cells with blastic features **(F)** positive for TdT **(G)**. Fluorescence in situ hybridization (FISH) studies demonstrated a *BCL2* rearrangement in FL and a dual rearrangement of *BCL2* and *MYC* in the bone marrow.

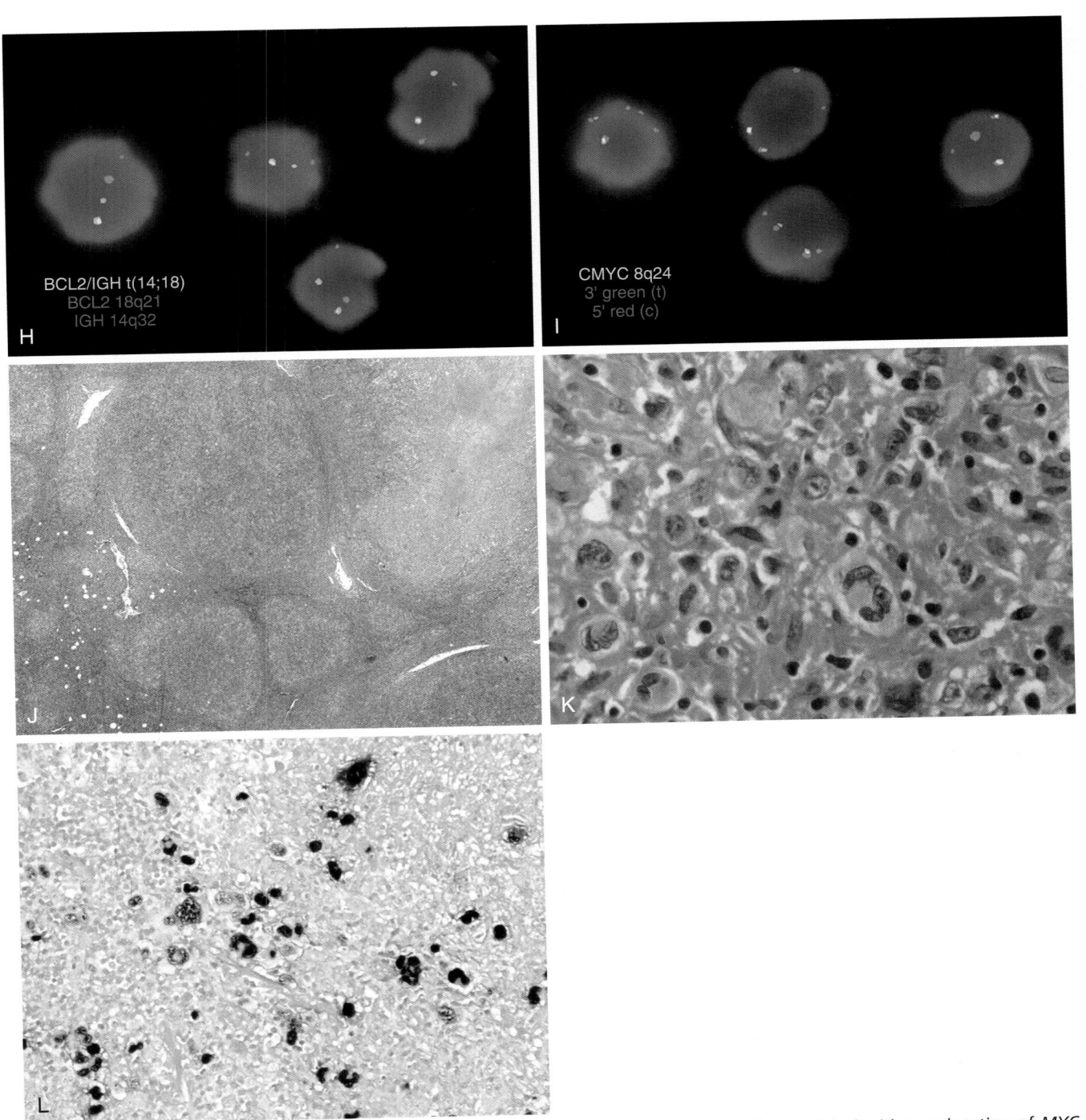

BCL2/IGH t(14;18)
BCL2 18q21
IGH 14q32

H

CMYC 8q24
3' green (t)
5' red (c)

I

J

K

L

Figure 17-15, cont'd. H and **I,** High-grade B-cell lymphoma as seen in C, D, and E are typically associated with translocation of *MYC* in addition to *BCL2.* **J,** Classic Hodgkin lymphoma arising in FL shows FL on the *left* and a pale area of histiocytes and necrosis on the *upper right.* **K,** At higher magnification, Reed-Sternberg cells are seen. **L,** The Reed-Sternberg cells were positive for CD15 and CD30 *(not shown)* and for Epstein-Barr virus–encoded RNA (EBER). *(H and I, Courtesy of Dr. Paola dal Cin, Cytogenetics Laboratory, Massachusetts General Hospital and Brigham and Women's Hospital.)*

is best evaluated by flow cytometry. Evidence of light-chain restriction (kappa or lambda) is usually diagnostic of lymphoma. However, clonal B cells have been reported within some follicles in cases of apparent reactive hyperplasia,[231] and clonal CD10-positive B cells may be detected by flow cytometry in cases of florid follicular hyperplasia in children.[96] Thus, these results must be analyzed in the context of the morphologic appearance.

Immunohistochemical staining for BCL2 protein is the most useful technique for distinguishing FL from follicular hyperplasia on paraffin sections. Sections must be examined together with sections stained for CD20 and CD3, because numerous BCL2-positive T cells may be present in both reactive and neoplastic follicles; staining of these cells should not be misinterpreted as BCL2 expression by neoplastic cells.

- Follicular hyperplasia
- Progressive transformation of germinal centers
- Other small B-cell lymphomas
  - Small lymphocytic lymphoma
  - Mantle cell lymphoma
  - Marginal zone lymphoma
- Hodgkin lymphoma
  - Nodular lymphocyte-predominant Hodgkin lymphoma
  - Nodular sclerosis classic Hodgkin lymphoma

Table 17-6 Histologic Features Useful in Distinguishing Follicular Lymphoma (FL) From Follicular Hyperplasia

Characteristic	Specificity for FL	Frequency in FL
Centrocytes predominate in follicles	Diagnostic	High
Centrocytes present between follicles	Diagnostic	High
Vascular invasion by centrocytes	Diagnostic	Moderate
Close packing of follicles	Highly suggestive	High
Diffuse areas or sclerosis	Highly suggestive	Moderate
Follicles extend beyond nodal capsule	Highly suggestive	High
Mantle zone absent	Suggestive	High
Starry-sky cells absent in follicles	Suggestive	High
Mantle zone present	Not helpful	Low
Some reactive follicles present	Not helpful	Low
Size, shape, uniformity of follicles	Not helpful	—
"Cracking" artifact or compression of reticulin	Not helpful	—

In many cases, the neoplastic follicle center cells express BCL2 more strongly than do the surrounding mantle zone or interfollicular cells; in some cases, however, staining of FL cells may be faint and restricted to a subset of centrocytes. BCL2 staining should be interpreted together with BCL6, CD10, or FDC staining, because expression of BCL2 by non–germinal center B cells is not indicative of lymphoma. Unfortunately, BCL2 positivity is less common in grade 3 FL, making it difficult to differentiate it from reactive hyperplasia, so the absence of BCL2 does not exclude lymphoma.[110] It is important to remember that some BCL2-negative cases have alterations related to somatic hypermutation involving the BCL2 epitope that can prevent standard BCL2 antibodies form binding, resulting in a falsely negative BCL2 staining. In these cases, alternative BCL2 antibodies may be used to show BCL2 expression.

Expression of CD10 or BCL6 by follicles is not a criterion for malignancy, because it is also expressed by normal germinal-center cells.[97] CD10 is typically expressed more strongly in neoplastic than reactive germinal centers, and BCL6 may be expressed by fewer cells in FL than in follicular hyperplasia. Detection of CD10-positive or BCL6-positive cells in the interfollicular region is suggestive of FL. However, rare normal interfollicular cells may be BCL6 positive, and interfollicular neoplastic cells may lack CD10 or express it

more weakly than those within the follicles.[32,97] Assessment of the proliferation fraction using Ki-67 may be helpful, because in reactive follicles, the vast majority of the cells are in cycle, whereas even in grade 3 FL, the proliferation fraction is rarely greater than 60%.

Molecular Genetic Analysis

PCR analysis for clonal Ig rearrangement can be more sensitive for detecting small clonal populations than conventional immunophenotyping and may also prove clonality in Ig-negative or BCL2 protein–negative tumors.[142] This assay may be subject to false negative results in some cases, as extensive somatic hypermutation may result in poor binding of PCR primers.[232] FISH analysis for translocation of BCL2 or BCL6 can also be helpful in establishing a diagnosis of FL in difficult cases.[233]

Other Small B-Cell Lymphomas

Other lymphomas with a nodular or follicular pattern may resemble FL. These include mantle cell lymphoma, marginal zone lymphoma, occasionally small lymphocytic lymphoma, and rarely, Hodgkin lymphoma.

Morphologic Features

The morphologic features of small B-cell lymphomas are summarized in Table 17-7. Chronic lymphocytic leukemia–small lymphocytic lymphoma (CLL/SLL) typically has a pseudofollicular pattern in lymph nodes related to the presence of proliferation centers; this can be mistaken for a true follicular pattern, resulting in confusion with FL. In general, proliferation centers are poorly demarcated from the surrounding infiltrate, so they seem to "disappear" at progressively higher magnifications. They are slightly paler than surrounding small dark lymphocytes, imparting a "cloudy sky" pattern. They contain cells with predominantly round nuclei and show a subtle gradation from small lymphocytes to prolymphocytes to paraimmunoblasts, in contrast to the sharp dichotomy between centrocytes and centroblasts in FL. Sclerosis and extranodal extension are uncommon in CLL/SLL.

Cases of mantle cell lymphoma may have a vaguely nodular or, rarely, a true follicular pattern. In most cases, the follicular pattern is only focal, with large diffuse areas. In contrast to FL, which always contains a mixture of neoplastic centroblasts and centrocytes, mantle cell lymphoma typically contains a monotonous population of small cells that resemble centrocytes, with virtually no blast cells. Occasional centroblasts can be seen in areas of partially overrun follicles. In many cases, foci of preserved germinal centers surrounded by a mantle zone of atypical cells can be found; this appearance would be unusual in FL. Many cases of mantle cell lymphoma contain single epithelioid histiocytes. Mantle cell lymphoma often has a higher mitotic rate than FL. The character of the blood vessels may also provide a clue to the diagnosis. In mantle cell lymphoma, the small vessels usually are not high endothelial venules; they have flat endothelial cells and often have eosinophilic sclerosis of their walls. In contrast, in diffuse areas of FL, the small vessels usually are high endothelial venules and do not show prominent sclerosis. Compartmentalizing fibrosis, which is commonly seen at least focally in diffuse FL, is rare in mantle cell lymphoma. Finally, diffuse areas of FL frequently contain large numbers of small, reactive T lymphocytes, whereas mantle cell lymphoma may show frequent scattered epithelioid histiocytes and fewer other reactive cells.

Marginal zone lymphomas may have a partially follicular pattern owing to the presence of follicles that have been "colonized" by neoplastic marginal zone cells. Typically, these follicles are widely spaced on a background of interfollicular marginal zone cells, but occasionally they may be numerous and mimic FL. In addition, FL may have marginal zone differentiation, mimicking marginal zone lymphoma (Fig. 17-2). Marginal zone B cells have centrocyte-like nuclei but more abundant cytoplasm; however, occasional FLs may have cells with relatively abundant cytoplasm. Marginal zone lymphoma also enters the differential diagnosis of diffuse FL, because both contain a mixture of small cells with irregular nuclei and large centroblasts or immunoblasts. Problems can also arise when biopsy specimens are small and a mixed population of centrocyte-like and centroblast-like cells is present without an obvious pattern. Features favoring marginal zone lymphoma include a predominant interfollicular infiltrate, irregular follicles, foci of reactive-appearing follicles, abundant cytoplasm, and plasmacytoid differentiation. Features favoring FL include monomorphism;

round, uniform, and closely packed follicles; sclerosis; and vascular invasion.

Immunophenotype

The immunophenotypic and genetic features of small B-cell lymphomas are summarized in Table 17-8. Mantle cell lymphoma and CLL/SLL characteristically express IgM, IgD, CD5, and CD43; most cases are CD10 negative. In contrast, FL is usually IgD negative, IgG positive, or IgM positive and CD5 negative; 50% to 80% of cases are CD10 positive.[101] With antibodies to FDCs, follicular areas in FL are highlighted by concentric aggregates of FDCs, whereas diffuse areas show few, if any, FDCs; in contrast, both mantle cell lymphomas and many marginal zone lymphomas contain large, irregular FDC aggregates, even in areas that are diffuse on routine sections.[97,234] Staining for BCL2 may highlight residual negative reactive follicles in mantle cell lymphoma and marginal zone lymphoma, whereas follicle centers are typically positive in FL. BCL2 staining of the extrafollicular neoplastic cells is not helpful in the differential diagnosis of small B-cell lymphomas because all can be positive. Finally, staining for cyclin D1 and/or SOX11 is positive in almost all mantle cell lymphomas but is negative in FL.[235] This is

Table 17-7 Small B-Cell Neoplasms: Histologic Features Useful in the Differential Diagnosis

Neoplasm	Pattern	Small Cells	Transformed Cells
Follicular lymphoma	Follicular ± diffuse areas, rarely diffuse	Centrocytes (cleaved)	Centroblasts
Mantle cell lymphoma	Diffuse, vaguely nodular, mantle zone, rarely follicular	Similar to centrocytes (cleaved, rarely round or oval, may be large); some cases may have blastoid cytology (e.g., blastoid variant)	None
Marginal zone B-cell lymphoma	Diffuse, interfollicular, marginal zone, follicular colonization	Heterogeneous: round (small lymphocytes), cleaved (centrocyte-like, marginal zone, monocytoid B cells), plasma cells	Centroblasts Immunoblasts
CLL/SLL	Diffuse with pseudofollicles	Round (occasionally cleaved)	Prolymphocytes Paraimmunoblasts
Lymphoplasmacytic lymphoma	Diffuse; no pseudofollicles	Round (may be cleaved) Plasma cells	Centroblasts Immunoblasts

CLL/SLL, Chronic lymphocytic leukemia–small lymphocytic lymphoma.

Table 17-8 Small B-Cell Neoplasms: Immunophenotypic and Genetic Features

Neoplasm	sIg; cIg	CD5	CD10	CD23	CD43	Cyclin D1	BCL6	IGV-Region Genes	Genetic Abnormality
Follicular lymphoma	+; −	−	+/−	−/+	−	−	+	Mutated, IH	t(14;18); BCL2R
Mantle cell lymphoma	+; −	+	−	−	+	+	−	70% unmutated, 30% mutated	t(11;14); CCND1R
Extranodal and nodal marginal zone lymphoma	+; +/−	−	−	−/+	−/+	−	−	Mutated, IH?	Trisomy 3; t(11;18) (extranodal)
CLL/SLL	+; −/+	+	−	+	+	−*	−	50% unmutated, 50% mutated	Trisomy 12; 13q deletions, others
Lymphoplasmacytic lymphoma	+; +	−	−	−	−/+	−	−	Mutated	MYD88 L265P
Splenic marginal zone lymphoma	+; −/+	−	−	−	−/+	−	−	50% mutated, 50% unmutated	7q31-32 deletions, subset

*In occasional cases, there may be a few cyclin D1-positive cells in proliferation centers.
cIg, Cytoplasmic immunoglobulin; *CLL/SLL,* chronic lymphocytic leukemia–small lymphocytic lymphoma; *IGV,* immunoglobulin variable region; *IH,* intraclonal heterogeneity; *R,* rearranged; *sIg,* surface immunoglobulin.

particularly useful in the rare cases of CD5-negative mantle cell lymphoma.[236]

Immunophenotyping can be useful in the differential diagnosis between FL and marginal zone lymphoma with follicular colonization, but it requires careful interpretation because of the complex architecture of these neoplasms. The most useful antigens are CD10, BCL6, and BCL2; all must be assessed with respect to CD21-positive or CD23-positive FDC aggregates, which define the follicular areas. In FL, most of the cells within the FDC aggregates should be BCL2 positive, CD10 positive, and BCL6 positive, whereas in marginal zone lymphoma they are heterogeneous. Noncolonized follicles are BCL2 negative, CD10 positive, and BCL6 positive; partially colonized follicles have an admixture of BCL2-positive, CD10-negative, and BCL6-negative neoplastic cells and BCL2-negative, CD10-positive, and BCL6-positive reactive follicle center cells; and completely colonized follicles are typically BCL2 positive, CD10 negative, and BCL6 negative. Expression of CD10 or BCL6 by extrafollicular B cells (away from FDC aggregates) supports follicle center lymphoma, whereas CD10-negative, BCL6-negative extrafollicular B cells favor marginal zone lymphoma.[99,234,237] MUM1/IRF4 is helpful if positive, because most FLs are MUM1/IRF4 negative and some marginal zone lymphomas are positive. The presence of light-chain–restricted plasma cells and aberrant expression of CD43 also favor a diagnosis of marginal zone lymphoma.

Genetic Analysis

The *BCL2* rearrangement characteristic of FL is rare or absent in mantle cell, small lymphocytic, and marginal zone lymphoma. The *CCND1* gene rearrangement is detectable in most cases by FISH and by PCR in about 40% of mantle cell lymphomas but not in FL (Table 17-8).

Pearls and Pitfalls

- FL is a distinctive tumor that reproduces most of the morphologic, immunophenotypic, and genetic features of the lymphoid germinal center. Clinically, FL is usually an indolent lymphoma with a long median survival.
- The majority of FL cases are characterized by follicular architecture, predominantly centrocytic composition and BCL2 expression by germinal center B cells, secondary to *BCL2* gene rearrangements resulting activation of a gene, *BCL2,* that confers a survival advantage on nonproliferating neoplastic cells.
- Several FL variants have been described that present as localized nodal (pediatric-type FL) or extranodal disease, lack *BCL2* gene rearrangements, and have generally excellent prognosis.
- BCL2-R-negative and CD23-positive follicle center lymphoma is a unique variant of FL characterized by the absence of *BCL2* gene rearrangements, often localized lymphadenopathy, most commonly in the inguinal area, and often growing in an architecturally diffuse pattern, though some cases can show follicular architecture. These cases are usually positive for CD23 and have recurrent deletions of 1p36 and *STAT6* or *SOCS1* mutations.

KEY REFERENCES

40. Katzenberger T, Kalla J, Leich E, et al. A distinctive subtype of t(14;18)-negative nodal follicular non-Hodgkin lymphoma characterized by a predominantly diffuse growth pattern and deletions in the chromosomal region 1p36. *Blood.* 2009;113:1053–1061.
67. Louissaint Jr A, Ackerman AM, Dias-Santagata D, et al. Pediatric-type nodal follicular lymphoma: an indolent clonal proliferation in children and adults with high proliferation index and no BCL2 rearrangement. *Blood.* 2012;120:2395–2404.
68. Liu Q, Salaverria I, Pittaluga S, et al. Follicular lymphomas in children and young adults: a comparison of the pediatric variant with usual follicular lymphoma. *Am J Surg Pathol.* 2013;37:333–343.
72. Salaverria I, Philipp C, Oschlies I, et al. Translocations activating IRF4 identify a subtype of germinal center-derived B-cell lymphoma affecting predominantly children and young adults. *Blood.* 2011;118:139–147.
74. Misdraji J, Harris NL, Hasserjian RP, et al. Primary follicular lymphoma of the gastrointestinal tract. *Am J Surg Pathol.* 2011;35:1255–1263.
94. Jegalian AG, Eberle FC, Pack SD, et al. Follicular lymphoma in situ: clinical implications and comparisons with partial involvement by follicular lymphoma. *Blood.* 2011;118:2976–2984.
95. Schmidt J, Salaverria I, Haake A, et al. Increasing genomic and epigenomic complexity in the clonal evolution from in situ to manifest t(14;18)-positive follicular lymphoma. *Leukemia.* 2014;28:1103–1112.
173. Ryan RJ, Nitta M, Borger D, et al. EZH2 codon 641 mutations are common in BCL2-rearranged germinal center B cell lymphomas. *PLoS One.* 2011;6:e28585.
225. Geyer JT, Subramaniyam S, Jiang Y, et al. Lymphoblastic transformation of follicular lymphoma: a clinicopathologic and molecular analysis of seven patients. *Hum Pathol.* 2015;46:260–271.

Visit Elsevier eBooks+ for the complete set of references.

Extranodal Marginal Zone Lymphoma: MALT Lymphoma

James R. Cook and Sarah E. Gibson

In classifying non-Hodgkin lymphomas, considerable attention has been paid to architectural, cytologic, and functional similarities among the various lymphomas and normal lymphoid tissue, exemplified by the peripheral lymph node. However, studies of extranodal lymphomas, particularly gastrointestinal lymphomas (accounting for the majority), suggest that in many cases their clinicopathologic features are related not to lymph nodes but to the structure and function of mucosa-associated lymphoid tissue (MALT).[1,2]

The anatomic distribution and structure of lymph nodes are adapted to deal with antigens carried to the node in afferent lymphatics, which drain sites at various distances from the node. Permeable mucosal sites, such as the gastrointestinal tract, are particularly vulnerable to pathogens and antigens because they are in direct contact with the external environment, and specialized lymphoid tissue—MALT—has evolved to protect them. MALT includes gut-associated lymphoid tissue, nasopharyngeal lymphoid tissue (tonsils), and other less well-characterized aggregates of lymphoid tissue related to other mucosae. Gut-associated lymphoid tissue serves as the paradigm for MALT (Fig. 18-1).

DEFINITION

Extranodal marginal zone lymphoma (MALT lymphoma) is an extranodal lymphoma composed of morphologically heterogeneous small B cells, including marginal zone (centrocyte-like) cells, cells resembling monocytoid cells, small lymphocytes, and scattered immunoblast and centroblast-like cells. There is plasma cell differentiation in a proportion of cases. The infiltrate expands the marginal zone of reactive B-cell follicles and extends into the interfollicular region. In epithelial tissues, the neoplastic cells typically infiltrate the epithelium, forming lymphoepithelial lesions.[3,4]

MALT lymphomas arise in a wide variety of extranodal sites (Boxes 18-1 and 18-2), but curiously, most of these are not sites where MALT is normally present, such as the terminal ileum or the tonsils. One could question whether the term *MALT* is appropriate for lymphomas, such as those of the orbit, that do not arise in mucosal or epithelial tissues; however, their close association with mucosal tissue, together with their histology, immunophenotype, and genetic and clinical properties, tend to support their classification as MALT lymphomas. In the revised 4th edition WHO classification, cases arising at all anatomic sites were

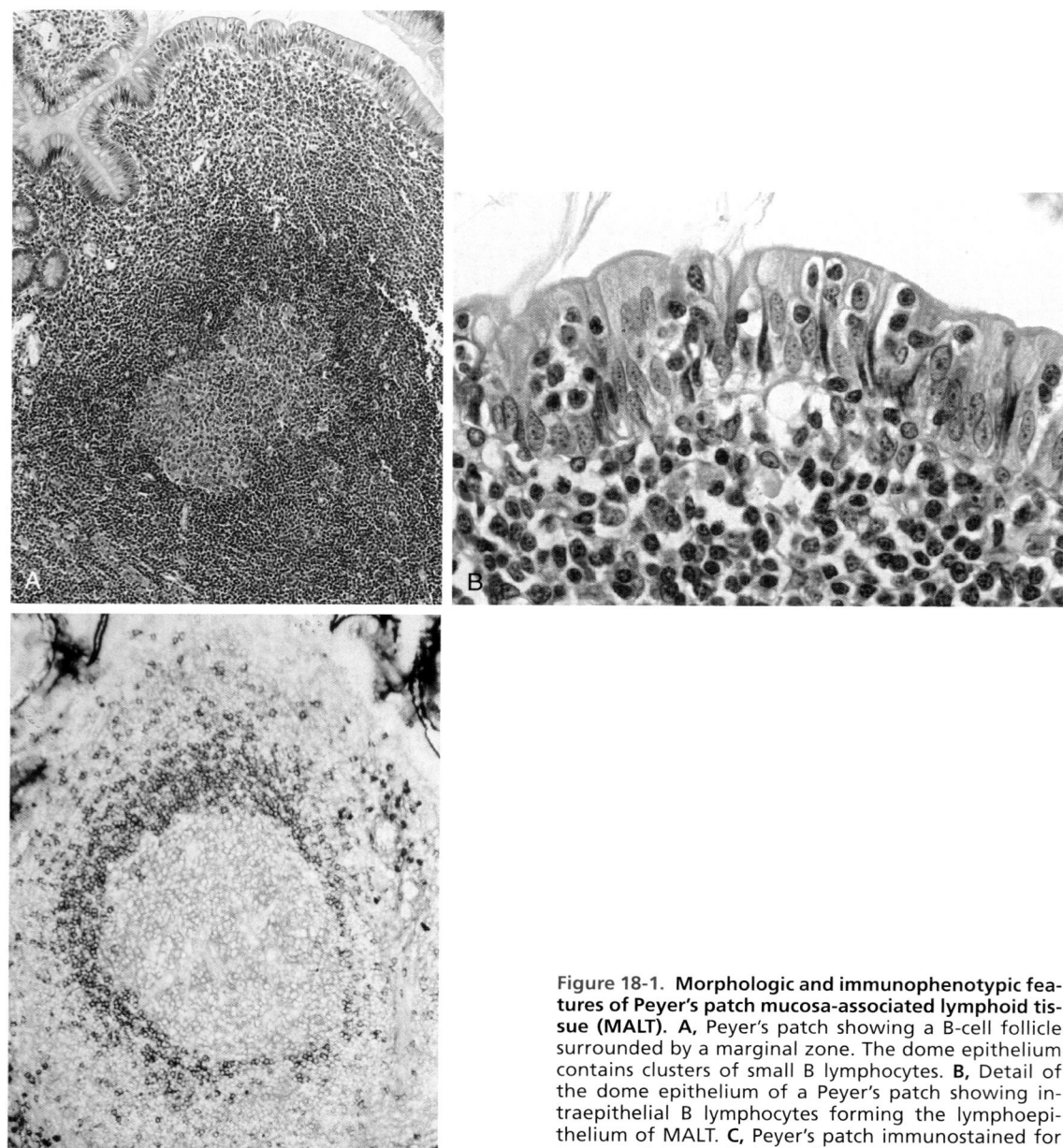

Figure 18-1. Morphologic and immunophenotypic features of Peyer's patch mucosa-associated lymphoid tissue (MALT). A, Peyer's patch showing a B-cell follicle surrounded by a marginal zone. The dome epithelium contains clusters of small B lymphocytes. **B,** Detail of the dome epithelium of a Peyer's patch showing intraepithelial B lymphocytes forming the lymphoepithelium of MALT. **C,** Peyer's patch immunostained for immunoglobulin D (IgD) *(brown)* and CD20 *(blue)*. The IgD-positive mantle zone is surrounded by an IgD-negative (IgM-positive), CD20-positive marginal zone.

classified under the term extranodal marginal zone lymphoma. In the 2022 International Consensus Classification (ICC), primary cutaneous cases are designated as primary cutaneous marginal zone lymphoproliferative disorders in recognition of their very indolent behavior (see Chapter 19). They are also separately designated in the proposed WHO 5th ed.

SYNONYMS AND RELATED TERMS

WHO revised 4th ed. (for all anatomic sites): Extranodal marginal zone lymphoma (MALT lymphoma)
WHO proposed 5th ed. (for cutaneous cases): Primary cutaneous marginal zone lymphoma

WHO proposed 5th ed. (noncutaneous sites): Extranodal marginal zone lymphoma

EPIDEMIOLOGY

MALT lymphomas account for 5% to 8% of all B-cell lymphomas and at least 50% of primary gastric lymphomas.[5-8] The incidence of MALT lymphoma has increased over the past three decades, reflecting at least in part improved pathologic diagnosis during this time period.[6,9-16] Although MALT lymphoma is described in almost all extranodal tissues, the stomach is the most common site (30% of cases), followed by ocular adnexa

Box 18-1 *Localization of MALT Lymphoma*

Box 18-1 *Localization of MALT Lymphoma*

- Gastrointestinal tract
  - Stomach
  - Intestine (including immunoproliferative small intestinal disease)
- Salivary glands
- Respiratory tract
  - Lung, pharynx, trachea
- Ocular adnexa
  - Conjunctiva, lacrimal gland, orbit
- Skin
- Thyroid gland
- Liver
- Genitourinary tract
  - Bladder, prostate gland, kidney
- Breast
- Thymus
- Rare sites

Box 18-2 *Major Diagnostic Features*

- Tumors arise at extranodal locations, usually sites of acquired MALT.
- The neoplastic cells include variable numbers of small lymphocytes, marginal zone–like cells, and scattered large cells; a subset show plasmacytic differentiation.
- Neoplastic cells surround and colonize germinal centers and lymphoepithelial lesions are common at many, but not all, anatomic sites.
- The B cells typically lack expression of CD5, CD10, and CD23. A subset shows co-expression of CD43.
- Translocations including *BIRC3::MALT1, IGH::MALT1,* and *IGH::BCL10* occur in a minority of cases.

(12%), skin (10%), lung (9%), salivary gland (7%), other gastrointestinal sites (7%), breast (3%), and thyroid (2%).[12,16] Several studies have reported a decreasing incidence of gastric MALT lymphomas over time, most likely reflecting a decreasing prevalence of *Helicobacter pylori* infection and widespread early treatment of patients with peptic disease symptoms.[12,17,18] Most MALT lymphomas occur in adults, with a median age in the seventh decade of life.[12,17] Overall, males and females show a largely similar incidence, although gender disparities are found at specific anatomic sites.[12,16] For example, there is a female predominance in salivary gland, thyroid, and breast MALT lymphomas, whereas primary cutaneous marginal zone lymphoproliferative disorder shows a male predominance.[12,16] Although a higher incidence of gastric MALT lymphoma was previously noted in northeastern Italy, probably related to a high prevalence of *H. pylori*–associated gastritis in that region, an incidence on par with other Western countries has been observed more recently.[12,17-19] Immunoproliferative small intestinal disease (IPSID), previously also known as α-heavy chain disease or Mediterranean lymphoma, is a special subtype of MALT lymphoma that most commonly occurs in developing countries, and is linked to factors associated with low socioeconomic status, including poor hygiene, malnutrition, and frequent intestinal infections.[20-22]

ETIOLOGY

MALT lymphomas only rarely arise from native MALT; they usually arise from MALT that has been acquired as a result of a chronic inflammatory disorder at sites normally devoid of MALT, such as the stomach, salivary gland, lung, thyroid gland, and ocular adnexa. MALT lymphomas of the salivary gland and thyroid gland, organs normally containing no lymphoid tissue, are preceded by lymphoepithelial (myoepithelial) sialadenitis (LESA) or lymphocytic thyroiditis,[23-25] usually associated with Sjögren syndrome and Hashimoto's disease, respectively. Histologic and immunohistochemical studies of the heavy lymphoid infiltrate that characterizes these two conditions have shown a remarkable resemblance to Peyer's patches.[23-25] This is most graphically illustrated with reference to LESA. In this condition, lymphoid tissue accumulates around dilated salivary gland ducts and forms, in effect, small Peyer's patches, complete with a germinal center, mantle, small marginal zone, and, significantly, lymphoepithelium comprising collections of intraepithelial B cells (Fig. 18-2).[23,25] This lymphoid tissue, known as acquired MALT, is also a feature of Hashimoto's disease, and it has been identified in fetal and neonatal lung from infants with pulmonary infections of an undetermined nature.[26] It is also seen in a condition termed *follicular bronchiolitis*, which is associated with various autoimmune disorders, including Sjögren syndrome, and immunodeficiency.[27,28] It is worth emphasizing that native MALT, in the form of bronchus-associated lymphoid tissue, is not present in the normal lung. Likewise, lymphoid tissue is not present in the normal stomach, the most common site of MALT lymphoma; here too, MALT is commonly acquired, most frequently subsequent to infection with *H. pylori.*[29] Other infectious organisms have been implicated as etiologic agents of MALT lymphoma at other sites.

Certain common factors relating to the acquisition of MALT may be relevant to the development of lymphoma at these sites. Chronic antigenic stimulation, related to the underlying infection or autoimmune disorder, plays an important role in the underlying disease. MALT accumulates in relation to columnar epithelium and appears to receive antigenic stimuli either from the epithelium itself or, like physiologic MALT, from antigens that enter the lymphoid tissue across the epithelium, rather than from antigens carried in afferent lymphatics.[20,30] The functional characteristics of this acquired MALT and the degree to which it resembles normal MALT remains unclear. Studies of *H. pylori*–associated gastric MALT lymphoma offer insights into the mechanisms that underlie the transition from reactive to neoplastic marginal zone B cells. It is thought that the immune response elicited by *H. pylori* initially supports expansion of polyclonal B cells that have the ability to recognize cross-reactive autoantigens present in the gastric mucosa via their B-cell receptor.[31,32] Several studies have shown that MALT lymphomas from different anatomic sites show biased usage of IGHV genes, lending support to the concept that the B-cell expansion is driven by autoantigens or alloantigens specific to the tissue microenvironment in which the lymphoma develops.[32-35] Persistent activation by autoantigens, *H. pylori*–specific T cells, and potentially direct stimulation by *H. pylori* cytotoxin-associated gene A (CagA) protein encourage polyclonal B-cell expansion and selection, which eventually results in the emergence of an antigen-dependent B-cell clone.[31,32,36,37] Acquisition of additional

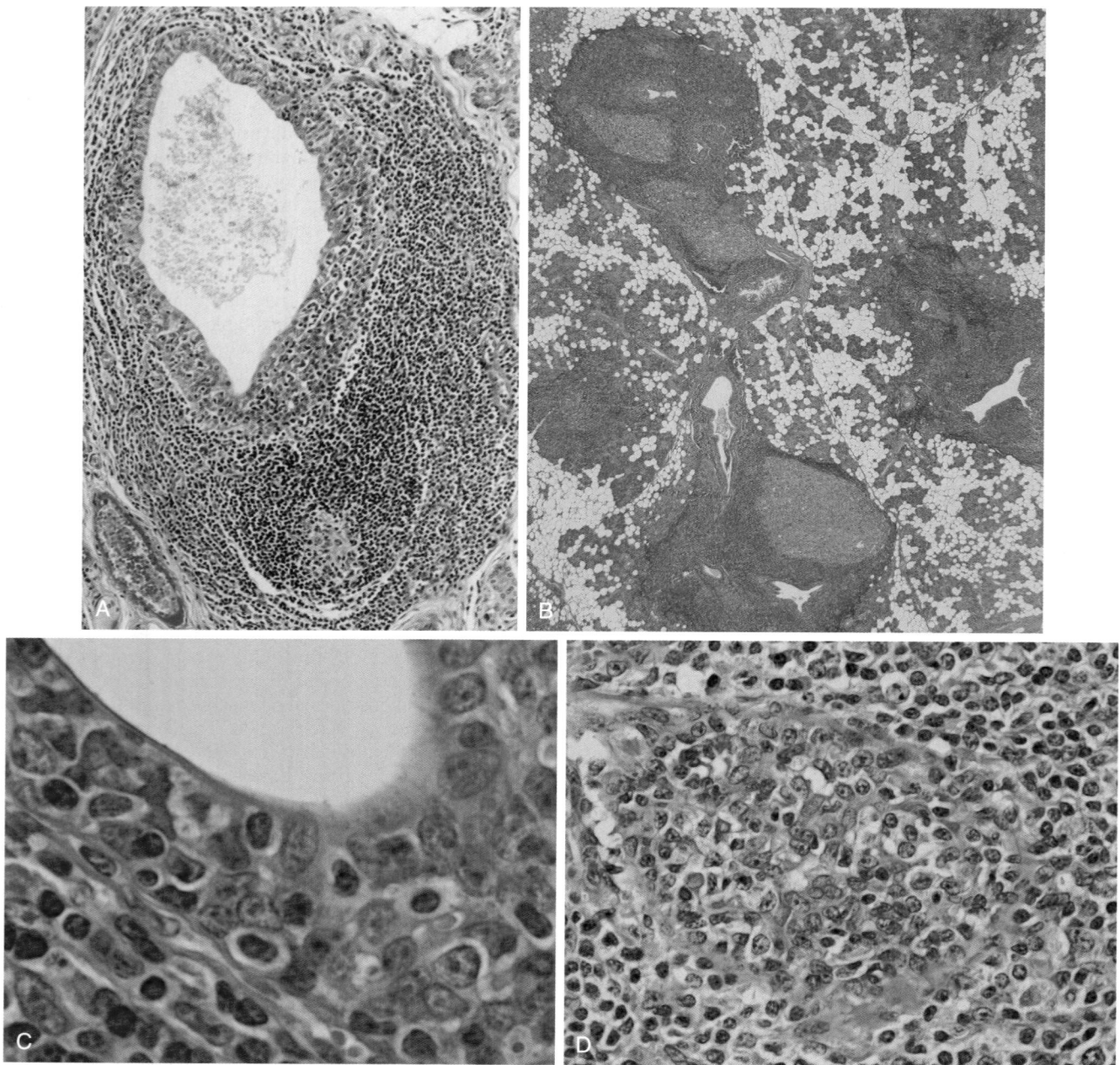

Figure 18-2. Lymphoepithelial sialadenitis (LESA)–acquired MALT. A, Peyer's patch–like lymphoid infiltrate in LESA. **B,** LESA of the parotid gland. Multiple Peyer's patch–like lymphoid infiltrates surround dilated ducts. **C,** High magnification of the lymphoepithelium in LESA. The lymphocytes have pale-staining cytoplasm and slightly irregularly shaped nuclei. **D,** Fully developed lymphoepithelial lesion in LESA.

genetic abnormalities promoting constitutive activation of pathways intrinsic to the chronic inflammatory response, particularly the NF-κB pathway, allows the B-cell clone to progress toward *H. pylori*–independent proliferation and malignant transformation.[30-32]

Infectious Agents

Helicobacter pylori and Gastric MALT Lymphoma

Several lines of evidence suggest that gastric MALT lymphoma arises from MALT acquired as a consequence of *H. pylori* infection. The first study in which this association was examined showed that the organism was present in more than 90% of cases.[38] A subsequent case-control study showed an association between previous *H. pylori* infection and the development of primary gastric lymphoma.[39] More compelling evidence confirming the role of *H. pylori* in the pathogenesis of gastric lymphoma has been obtained from studies that detected the neoplastic B-cell clone in the chronic gastritis that preceded the lymphoma,[40] as well as from a series of in vitro studies showing that lymphoma growth could be stimulated in culture by *H. pylori* strain-specific T cells when crude lymphoma cultures were exposed to the organism.[41] Studies have also shown that *H. pylori* CagA protein can enter B cells, potentially directly promoting cell proliferation and the upregulation of antiapoptotic molecules BCL2 and BCXL.[31,36,37] Finally, after the initial study by Wotherspoon and colleagues,[42] several groups have confirmed that eradication of *H. pylori* with antibiotics results in regression of gastric MALT lymphoma in 75% of cases. More recent studies have shown that in the era of widespread use of antibiotic therapy and treatment of patients with peptic disease symptoms, the incidence of gastric MALT lymphoma, and the percentage of gastric MALT lymphomas containing *H. pylori*, is declining.[12,17,18,43,44]

Campylobacter jejuni and Immunoproliferative Small Intestinal Disease

IPSID is a variant of MALT lymphoma involving the small intestine that is often associated with secretion of an abnormally truncated immunoglobulin alpha heavy chain without accompanying light chains (alpha heavy chain disease).[20,21,31] IPSID has a restricted geographic and socioeconomic distribution, supporting the role of environmental factors in its pathogenesis. An infectious etiology has long been suspected, and it is recognized that the early stages of IPSID may respond to antibiotic treatment (tetracycline or metronidazole and ampicillin), with durable remissions.[20,45-47] In 2004, Lecuit and associates reported detection of *Campylobacter jejuni* DNA in five of seven patients with IPSID and resolution of symptoms in one index patient after antibiotic therapy against *Campylobacter*.[48] A subsequent case report also described resolution after antibiotic therapy.[49] Although these findings suggested that *C. jejuni* may play the same role in IPSID as *H. pylori* does in gastric MALT lymphoma, there is only limited additional evidence supporting this hypothesis. In a polymerase chain reaction (PCR) study published in abstract format, Diss and colleagues confirmed the presence of *C. jejuni* 16s rDNA in one-half of IPSID samples, but also detected the organism in other small intestinal lymphomas.[50] It is also documented that other microbes and parasites, including *Campylobacter coli*, may be isolated from the stool of patients with IPSID.[51,52] *C. jejuni* and *C. coli* are foodborne pathogens that commonly cause an acute enteritis that resolves within 1 to 2 weeks, although in developing countries infection with these organisms is hyperendemic, with repeated exposures from a young age.[53] *Campylobacter* infection is also known to occasionally precipitate reactive (aseptic) arthritis and Guillain-Barré syndrome.[53] In most individuals, excretion of the bacteria resolves within a matter of weeks, but prolonged colonization may occur in patients with underlying immunodeficiency.[53,54] This finding has led to a current hypothesis that IPSID develops in individuals with an impaired gastrointestinal immune response, either from previous infections or an underlying genetic predisposition, who have difficulty clearing *C. jejuni*. This chronic small bowel infection may then produce the chronic antigenic stimulation required for MALT lymphoma development.[55,56] However, additional studies are required to further clarify the role of *Campylobacter* in the development of IPSID.

Borrelia burgdorferi and Primary Cutaneous Marginal Zone Lymphoproliferative Disorder

Borrelia burgdorferi is an *Ixodes* tick-borne spirochete associated with several dermatologic conditions including erythema migrans, lymphadenosis benigna cutis (pseudolymphoma), and acrodermatitis chronica atrophicans.[31,53] In 1991, Garbe and colleagues[57] first described four cases of cutaneous lymphoma, later characterized as primary cutaneous marginal zone lymphoproliferative disorder (pcMZLPD), associated with *B. burgdorferi* infection. In 1997, Kutting and associates[58] reported clinical cures of two cases of pcMZLPD after eradication of *B. burgdorferi* with the antibiotic cefotaxime. Several additional reports have followed from Europe, including one study describing *B. burgdorferi* infection in up to 42% of patients with pcMZLPD from the Scottish Highlands.[59,60] However, there is substantial geographic variability, and other studies of pcMZLPD that include patients from Europe, Asia, and the United States have not found an association with *B. burgdorferi*.[61,62] One large Scandinavian case-control study also found no association of tick bite or the presence of anti-*Borrelia* antibodies with overall risk of marginal zone lymphoma, although specific results for pcMZLPD were not reported.[63]

Chlamydia psittaci and Ocular Adnexal MALT Lymphoma

Chlamydia psittaci, an organism that infects a wide range of birds, is the etiologic agent of psittacosis in humans, which may manifest as an influenza-like syndrome, bronchopneumonia, or more severe illness.[53] In 2004, Yeung and coworkers described a single case of association between a chlamydial organism and a conjunctival MALT lymphoma.[64] Later that year, Ferreri and colleagues,[65] in a PCR study, reported an association between *C. psittaci* and ocular adnexal MALT lymphoma in 80% of cases and went on to demonstrate the complete response of four cases after eradication of *C. psittaci* with doxycycline.[66] In 2008, Ferreri and associates reported the in vitro isolation and growth of *C. psittaci* from patients with ocular MALT lymphoma but not healthy controls.[67] A further study suggested that viable *C. psittaci* resided within the intratumoral monocytes/macrophages of these lymphomas.[68] In addition, *C. psittaci* DNA has been identified in MALT lymphomas at other sites, including lung, thyroid gland, salivary gland, and skin.[69,70] A patient who developed multiple *C. psittaci*–related ocular adnexal MALT lymphomas and pulmonary diffuse large B-cell lymphoma after prolonged exposure to an infected animal has also been reported.[71] Although all of this provides evidence that would support a pathogenic association between *C. psittaci* and MALT lymphoma, there is substantial geographic variability, with high prevalence rates of *C. psittaci* infection in ocular adnexal MALT lymphomas reported from Italy, Austria, and South Korea, and a much lower incidence in the United States, Japan, and China.[72-75]

Achromobacter xylosoxidans and Pulmonary MALT Lymphoma

Achromobacter xylosoxidans is a gram-negative bacterium that is widely distributed in moist environments and soil, and is a well-known opportunistic pathogen that is recurrently isolated from the sputum of patients with cystic fibrosis.[76,77] *A. xylosoxidans* DNA was first described in pulmonary MALT lymphomas in 2008,[78] with a subsequent study in 2014 demonstrating its DNA in 46% of pulmonary MALT lymphomas from six European countries.[76] This was significantly different than the rate of *A. xylosoxidans* infection in control lung tissues (18%). Although data is very limited, there appear to be regional differences in the prevalence of *A. xylosoxidans* infection, ranging from 67% of pulmonary MALT lymphomas in Italy to 2% of cases in Japan.[76,79] There are currently no additional studies definitively demonstrating a causal relationship between *A. xylosoxidans* and pulmonary MALT lymphoma.

Hepatitis C Virus

Hepatitis C virus (HCV) is a hepatotropic and lymphotropic RNA virus that is associated with the development of B-cell non-Hodgkin lymphomas.[80] Multiple studies have shown an increased risk of MALT lymphoma in individuals who are HCV seropositive, and a study from Italy documented HCV infection in 35% of patients with nongastric MALT lymphomas.[81-83] However, there are well-recognized geographic variations in the prevalence of HCV infection, which affect the prevalence of HCV-associated lymphoma.[82,84,85] MALT lymphomas arising in HCV-positive individuals are most common at nongastric sites, most frequently involving skin, salivary glands, and ocular adnexal sites.[81] The biological mechanisms underlying HCV-associated lymphomagenesis are not clarified. Studies have shown that antiviral therapy may result in complete or partial remission of B-cell non-Hodgkin lymphomas, including MALT lymphomas, in HCV-positive patients, while this response is not observed in HCV-negative patients.[86-89] A systematic review documented complete responses to antiviral therapy in 75% of HCV-positive patients with lymphoma.[86] In addition, viral elimination induced by interferon therapy has been associated with a reduced incidence of lymphoma in one study.[90]

Epstein-Barr Virus

In recent years, rare MALT lymphomas associated with Epstein-Barr virus (EBV) have been described in patients with an underlying immunodeficiency. Although initially described in posttransplant patients, with subcutaneous and soft tissue localization,[91] additional reports have recognized these lymphomas at other extranodal sites and in other settings, including iatrogenic immunosuppression for autoimmune disease, prior chemotherapy, congenital immunodeficiency, and increased age.[92,93] An EBV latency pattern I or II has been documented in the cases studied.[91,93] These EBV-positive MALT lymphomas generally follow an indolent clinical course, with a response to immune reconstitution documented in a subset of cases.[91,93]

Autoimmune Disorders

Individuals with B-cell activating autoimmune diseases, such as Sjögren syndrome, Hashimoto's disease, and systemic lupus erythematosus, are at an increased risk for the development of MALT lymphoma.[83,94-96] Although it is impossible to entirely parse out the exact contributions of the underlying autoimmune disease, treatments, and other host factors, it is thought that the level of disease severity and inflammation is the main driver of lymphomagenesis.[16,97] Acquired MALT is a feature of both Sjögren syndrome and Hashimoto's disease.[24,25] A study proposed a model whereby the lymphoepithelial lesions of LESA provide paracrine stimulation to neoplastic B cells via GPR34, a member of the class A G-protein-coupled receptor superfamily.[98] *GPR34* alterations (mutations or translocations) are enriched in salivary gland MALT lymphomas (19% of cases).[99] Sjögren syndrome is strongly associated with

salivary gland lymphoma, and a pooled analysis of almost 30,000 individuals in Europe, North America, and Australia found a 1000-fold increased risk of parotid gland MALT lymphomas.[83,94,96] Similarly, patients with Hashimoto's disease have a 67-fold increased risk of thyroid lymphoma, most commonly as a MALT lymphoma or transformed MALT lymphoma.[95,100] Individuals with systemic lupus erythematosus have about a 3-fold increased risk of developing non-Hodgkin lymphoma, and in particular diffuse large B-cell lymphomas and MALT lymphomas.[83,94,96,101] Although there is an approximately 2-fold increased risk of lymphoma in patients with rheumatoid arthritis, these are frequently diffuse large B-cell lymphomas, and a definite association with MALT lymphomas is not established.[102-104] T-cell activating autoimmune conditions, such as inflammatory bowel disease, multiple sclerosis, sarcoidosis, psoriasis, and type 1 diabetes, are generally not associated with the development of MALT lymphoma.[83,94,96]

HISTOPATHOLOGY OF ACQUIRED MALT

Tissues in which MALT lymphomas occur seem to mount a stereotypic response to certain known and unknown agents with the accumulation of lymphoid tissue that forms Peyer's patch–like structures. The two sites in which this is best illustrated are the salivary gland and the stomach.

Salivary Gland Acquired MALT (Lymphoepithelial Sialadenitis)

Apart from the intrasalivary gland lymph nodes, especially in the parotid glands, normal salivary glands contain no organized lymphoid tissue. Lymphoid tissue may accumulate in the salivary glands as a result of chronic inflammation of varying causes. Chronic inflammation after long-standing sialolithiasis is one example in which numerous lymphoid follicles may be present around dilated ducts that often contain a purulent exudate. This appearance is quite different from the chronic inflammation associated with established Sjögren syndrome. In the earlier phase of this condition, isolated salivary ducts are dilated and surrounded by a lymphoid infiltrate that contains lymphoid follicles and recapitulates the structure of Peyer's patches (see Fig. 18-2B). Small, focal B-cell aggregates are characteristically seen in the duct epithelium, reminiscent of the dome epithelium of the Peyer's patch. These B cells are slightly larger than typical small lymphocytes of the mantle zone; they often have more abundant pale-staining cytoplasm and nuclei with an irregular outline (see Fig. 18-2C). The cytologic appearance and immunophenotype of these cells suggest that they are marginal zone B cells. Plasma cells are also present and tend to concentrate around the duct. As the disease progresses, the ducts condense, with partial or complete loss of their lumens, and form lymphoepithelial lesions that consist of cohesive aggregates of duct epithelium containing variable numbers of marginal zone B lymphocytes (see Fig. 18-2D),[25,105] often associated with atrophy or, not infrequently, fatty replacement of acinar tissue. These Peyer's patch–like lesions may fuse to form larger islands of lymphoid tissue, and some of the lymphoepithelial islands may develop into cystic structures, resulting in a multicystic gland. Not all patients with this pattern of lymphoid infiltration in salivary glands are necessarily suffering from Sjögren syndrome. Identical changes have been described in patients with a variety of other autoimmune diseases and sometimes in those with no evidence of an associated disorder. Hence the generic terms *benign lymphoepithelial lesion* and *myoepithelial sialadenitis* are now more appropriately termed *lymphoepithelial sialadenitis (LESA)*.[106]

Immunohistochemistry shows that the germinal centers are immunophenotypically identical to those in the Peyer's patches and lymph nodes. They are surrounded by CD20-positive, IgM-positive, IgD-positive mantle zone cells that express polytypic light chains. The infiltrate of small lymphocytes present between the follicles is composed principally of CD3-positive T cells, which tend to concentrate around the B-cell follicles and are often accompanied by polytypic plasma cells. In some cases, large numbers of T cells are present and may even outnumber the B cells.

Overall, the border between LESA and lymphoma is blurred, and it can be difficult to differentiate between them in some cases. Immunoglobulin gene rearrangement studies, which demonstrate clonal B cells in MALT lymphoma, may also show clonal B cells in some cases of LESA.[107,108] Whenever a diagnosis of LESA is made, the question of lymphoma remains open, to a certain extent.

Helicobacter pylori Gastritis

Because of its ability to withstand a low pH, *H. pylori* is the one organism, apart from some other rare *Helicobacter* species, that can survive in the human gastric mucosa. The prevalence of *H. pylori* gastritis in any given population varies from 20% to 100%, depending on the locality and the age cohort.[44,109] With some exceptions, the prevalence of gastric MALT lymphoma is related to that of *H. pylori* gastritis. Typically, infection results in active chronic inflammation with B-cell follicles and the formation of a lymphoepithelium by B-cell infiltration of glands immediately adjacent to the follicles—features of acquired MALT. Between the follicles, the gastric mucosa is infiltrated by T lymphocytes, plasma cells, macrophages, and occasional collections of neutrophils. The lymphoid infiltrate may be extremely florid and is sometimes difficult to distinguish from MALT lymphoma, especially when there are large, fused sheets of mantle zone cells in biopsy fragments.

Immunohistochemistry is useful in delineating the B-cell follicles and distinguishing the IgM-positive, IgD-positive mantle zone cells from the IgM-positive, IgD-negative MALT lymphoma cells. Staining for immunoglobulin light chains can be useful in detecting monotypic B cells and plasma cells in some cases of MALT lymphoma; however, the presence of polyclonal plasma cells does not exclude the diagnosis. PCR clonality studies of small endoscopic biopsies present particular technical challenges, and performing analysis in duplicate is critical to eliminate false-positive (so-called "pseudoclonal") results.[110,111] Though some studies have reported clonal results in gastric biopsies from patients with *H. pylori* gastritis,[112,113] when PCR is performed in duplicate and properly interpreted, clonal B-cell populations are extremely uncommon.[114,115] It is noteworthy that in patients with clonal gastritis who later developed overt MALT lymphoma, the identical monoclonal B-cell population has been detected in both lesions.[40]

PATHOLOGY OF MALT LYMPHOMA

Macroscopic Appearance

Macroscopically, MALT lymphomas are quite variable, sometimes forming distinct tumoral masses, and other times grossly resembling the inflammatory lesions that may give rise to MALT lymphoma. Gastric MALT lymphoma, for example, may form a single dominant mass but often results in only slightly raised congested mucosa, with superficial erosions indistinguishable at endoscopy from chronic gastritis.[116] MALT lymphomas are often multifocal, with small, even microscopic foci of clonally identical lymphoma scattered throughout the organ involved.[117]

Histopathology

Although there are some site-specific morphologic differences, the histologic findings in MALT lymphoma are generally similar in that the lymphoma recapitulates the organization of normal Peyer's patches, especially in the early stages of disease.[118,119] The neoplastic B cells proliferate around reactive B-cell follicles, usually external to a preserved follicular mantle, in a marginal zone distribution; they spread out to form larger confluent areas that eventually may overrun some or most of the follicles (see Fig. 18-3). Like benign marginal zone B cells, the neoplastic cells have pale cytoplasm with small-to-medium-sized, slightly irregularly shaped nuclei containing moderately dispersed chromatin and inconspicuous nucleoli. These cells have historically been called centrocyte-like because of their resemblance to germinal center centrocytes. The accumulation of more abundant pale-staining cytoplasm may lead to a monocytoid appearance of the lymphoma cells, especially in some anatomic sites such as the parotid gland where a very monocytoid appearance is the norm. In some cases, the cells more closely resemble small lymphocytes. Scattered large cells resembling centroblasts or immunoblasts are usually present, but these are in the minority and do not form confluent clusters or sheets. Plasma cell differentiation is present in up to one-third of cases[120] and in gastric lymphomas tends to be maximal beneath the surface gastric epithelium.

At many extranodal sites, glandular epithelium is often invaded and destroyed by discrete aggregates of lymphoma cells, resulting in the so-called lymphoepithelial lesions. These are defined as aggregates of three or more neoplastic marginal zone lymphocytes within glandular epithelium, preferably associated with distortion or necrosis of the epithelium. In gastric MALT lymphoma, these lesions are often accompanied by eosinophilic degeneration of the epithelium. Lymphoepithelial lesions, although highly characteristic of MALT lymphoma, especially gastric lymphoma, are not pathognomonic. In benign chronic gastritis, for example, small lymphoepithelial lesions may be present, often directly overlying reactive germinal centers. Lymphoepithelial lesions may be difficult to find or even absent in some MALT lymphomas, such as those of the small intestine and large intestine. In gastric MALT lymphoma, a histologic scoring system that incorporates the typical morphologic features (Table 18-1)[42] has been widely used in research studies; though providing a useful framework to gauge the degree of suspicion for MALT lymphoma on routine H&E (hematoxylin and eosin) sections, establishing a diagnosis in clinical

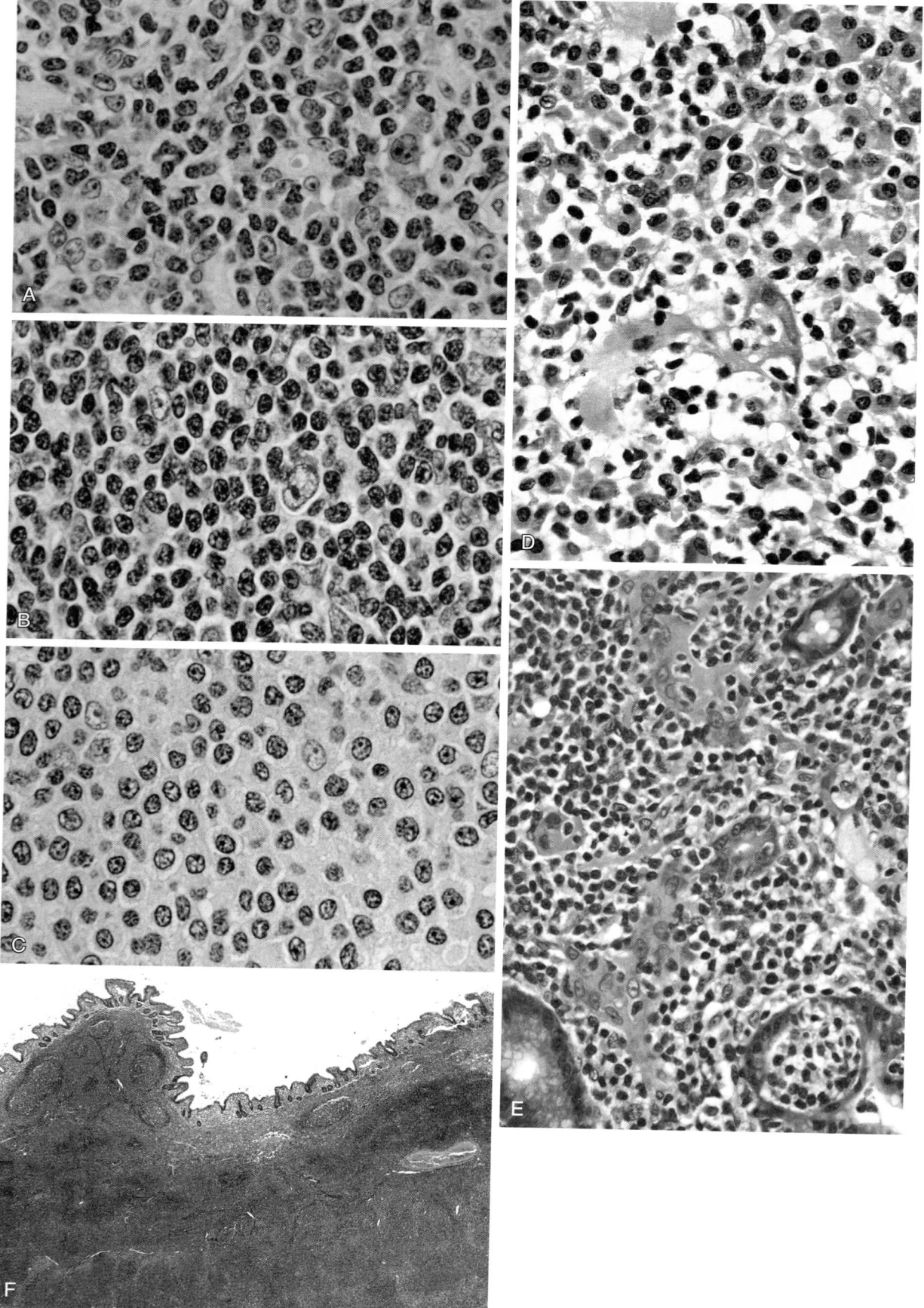

Figure 18-3. Morphology of B cells in gastric MALT lymphoma. **A,** The cells of gastric MALT lymphoma have a centrocyte-like appearance, with irregularly shaped nuclei. **B,** The tumor cells in this MALT lymphoma more closely resemble small lymphocytes. Note the presence of occasional transformed cells. **C,** The neoplastic cells in this MALT lymphoma have acquired more abundant pale-staining cytoplasm, leading to a monocytoid appearance. **D,** Plasma cell differentiation in a case of gastric MALT lymphoma. A lymphoepithelial lesion is present *below.* **E,** The tumor cells in this gastric MALT lymphoma form prominent lymphoepithelial lesions, with distortion and eosinophilic degeneration of gastric glandular epithelium. **F,** The neoplastic cells in this MALT lymphoma encircle reactive B-cell follicles *(upper left)* and have replaced follicles, leading to a nodular appearance *below.*

practice requires immunophenotyping in addition to the H&E morphology.[121,122]

Table 18-1 Use of Histology Score to Differentiate Gastric MALT Lymphoma From Chronic Gastritis

Score	Interpretation	Histology
0	Normal	Scattered plasma cells in lamina propria. No lymphoid follicles.
1	Chronic active gastritis	Small clusters of lymphocytes in lamina propria. No lymphoid follicles. No LELs.
2	Follicular gastritis	Prominent lymphoid follicles with surrounding mantle zone and plasma cells. No LELs.
3	Suspicious, probably reactive	Lymphoid follicles surrounded by small lymphocytes that infiltrate diffusely in the lamina propria and occasionally into epithelium.
4	Suspicious, probably lymphoma	Lymphoid follicles surrounded by marginal zone cells that infiltrate diffusely in the lamina propria and into epithelium in small groups.
5	MALT lymphoma	Presence of dense, diffuse infiltrate of marginal zone cells in lamina propria with prominent LELs.

LEL, Lymphoepithelial lesion; *MALT,* mucosa-associated lymphoid tissue.
Modified from Wotherspoon, et al.[42]

Lymphoma cells sometimes specifically colonize germinal centers of the reactive follicles (see Fig. 18-4).[123] Usually this results in a vaguely nodular or follicular pattern. In some cases, the lymphoma cells specifically target germinal centers, where they may undergo large cell transformation or plasma cell differentiation. Importantly, the presence of large cells confined to preexisting germinal centers is not considered evidence of transformation to large B-cell lymphoma.

As with other small B-cell neoplasms, MALT lymphoma may undergo transformation to diffuse large B-cell lymphoma.[32,121,124] Most studies report large cell transformation in <10% of cases, a lower incidence than in many other small B-cell neoplasms. The diagnosis of large cell transformation requires the presence of solid or sheetlike proliferations of large transformed cells. This transformation may or may not result in complete overgrowth of the preceding MALT lymphoma. In the latter cases, the diagnosis of both diffuse large B-cell lymphoma and concurrent MALT lymphoma should be rendered, and the relative proportions of both should be documented.[121]

Morphology of Gastric MALT Lymphoma Following Eradication of *Helicobacter pylori*

Approximately 75% of gastric MALT lymphomas respond to the eradication of *H. pylori,* with regression of the tumor over a period of up to 18 months.[42,125] Repeated endoscopy

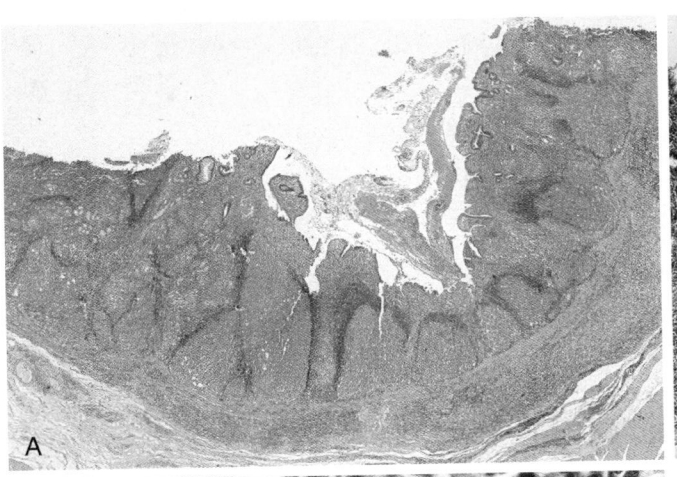
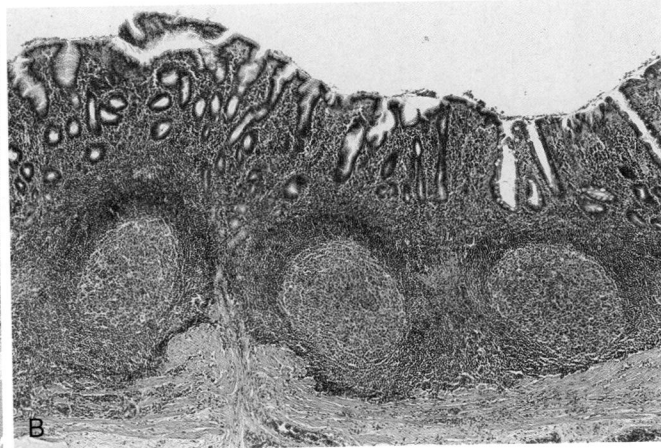
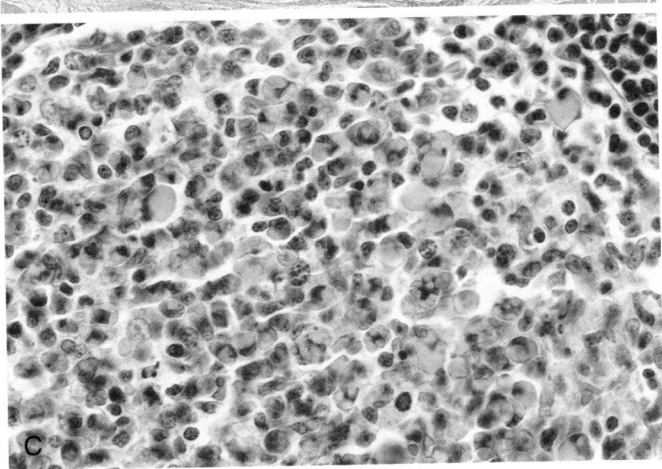

Figure 18-4. MALT lymphoma: relationship to B-cell follicles. A, The germinal centers of reactive B-cell follicles are colonized by transformed MALT lymphoma cells, resulting in an appearance simulating follicular lymphoma. **B,** The germinal centers of these reactive follicles are colonized by MALT lymphoma cells that have undergone plasmacytoid differentiation. **C,** Higher magnification of the germinal centers showing the cells stuffed with eosinophilic immunoglobulin.

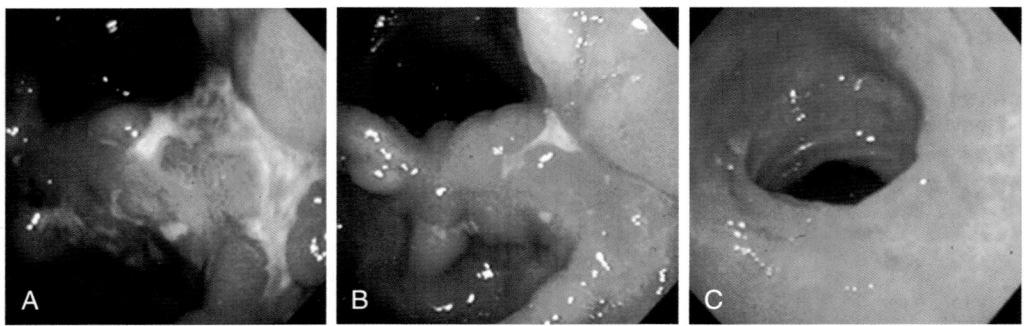

Figure 18-5. Serial endoscopic images of a gastric MALT lymphoma before **(A)**, 2 weeks after **(B)**, and 10 months after **(C)** eradication of *Helicobacter pylori* with antibiotics. The lymphoma has regressed completely after 10 months. *(Courtesy Dr. Naomi Uemara, Hiroshima, Japan.)*

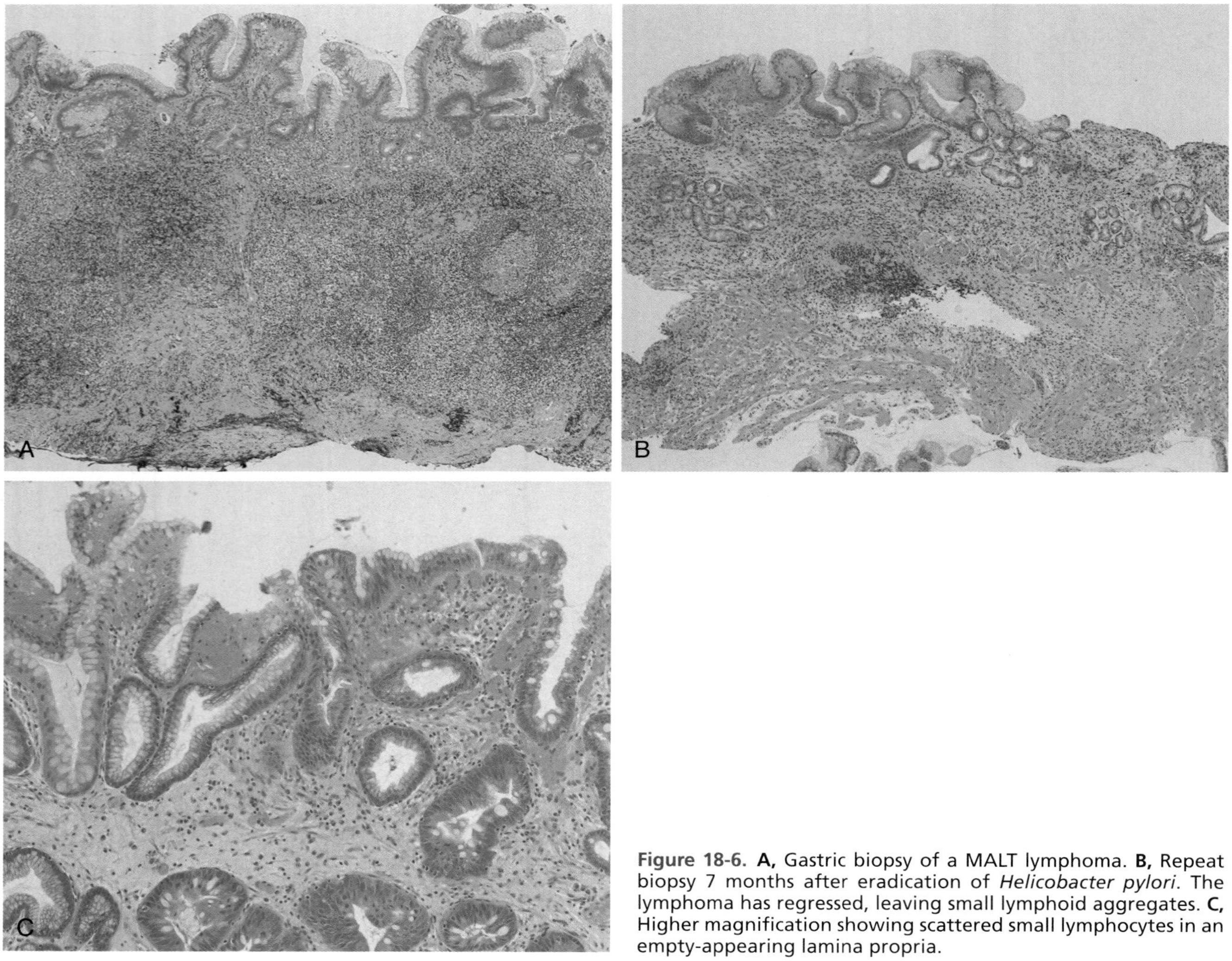

Figure 18-6. A, Gastric biopsy of a MALT lymphoma. **B,** Repeat biopsy 7 months after eradication of *Helicobacter pylori*. The lymphoma has regressed, leaving small lymphoid aggregates. **C,** Higher magnification showing scattered small lymphocytes in an empty-appearing lamina propria.

with biopsy is necessary to determine whether the lymphoma is responding (Fig. 18-5). The endoscopic appearance may revert to normal within 6 months of the eradication of *H. pylori*. There is often a noticeable change in the histologic appearance of the biopsy within a few weeks, with gradual clearance of the lymphoma in the following months. Initially, the inflammatory infiltrate accompanying the lymphoma disappears, with an empty-appearing eosinophilic lamina propria that may contain lymphoid aggregates (Fig. 18-6). These aggregates are composed of small B lymphocytes without significant numbers of large cells and gradually become smaller over time. Immunohistochemistry shows that they contain few accompanying T cells and have a low proliferation fraction. Such aggregates may not disappear altogether and may persist for long periods at the base of the mucosa or in the submucosa. The Groupe d'Etude des

Lymphomes de l'Adulte (GELA) has proposed a histologic scoring system that defines four categories for posttreatment evaluation: complete histologic remission, probable minimal residual disease, responding residual disease, and no change (Table 18-2).[126,127] Although this schema is employed in many research studies, it is not widely used in routine clinical practice.

Despite histologic regression, a persistent neoplastic clone may be detected by PCR in the majority of patients after *Helicobacter* eradication.[128] Persistent clones in the absence of histologic disease have also been reported in some studies after radiation or chemotherapy.[129-131] Such cases suggest that the neoplastic clone can remain quiescent in the absence of antigenic stimulation provided by *Helicobacter* infection.

Dissemination

The frequency and pattern of dissemination of MALT lymphoma vary with the site of disease, and involvement of more than one extranodal site has been reported in 20% to 30% of cases.[132,133] Most gastric MALT lymphomas are stage I when they present, but between 4% and 35% have disseminated to regional lymph nodes, and approximately 5% have disseminated to the bone marrow at the time of diagnosis.[134-136] More than 90% of salivary gland MALT lymphomas present at stage I, whereas 44% of pulmonary MALT lymphomas have disseminated to mediastinal lymph nodes at the time of diagnosis.[137] Approximately 20% of lymphomas of the ocular adnexa are beyond stage I at diagnosis.[138] In one study that grouped all MALT lymphomas together regardless of the site of origin, the disease had disseminated beyond the site of origin in 34% of cases.[139] MALT lymphomas also appear to disseminate to other sites where MALT lymphomas occur. Gastric MALT lymphomas, for example, tend to disseminate to the small intestine, salivary gland, and lung. Interestingly, molecular studies in patients with MALT lymphomas involving more than one MALT site have reported that some cases may represent two independent, clonally unrelated lymphomas rather than true dissemination of one lymphoma.[140]

When MALT lymphomas disseminate to lymphoid tissue, including lymph nodes and spleen, they specifically invade the marginal zone (Fig. 18-7). This can lead to a deceptively benign or reactive appearance, especially in mesenteric lymph nodes, where a marginal zone is normally present. Immunohistochemistry for immunoglobulin light chains can be very helpful in discriminating normal marginal zone from disseminated MALT lymphoma. Subsequently, the lymphoma in the marginal zones expands to form more obvious sheets of interfollicular lymphoma. Occasionally, follicular colonization in involved lymph nodes can lead to an appearance that simulates follicular lymphoma (FL).

IMMUNOHISTOCHEMISTRY

The immunophenotype of MALT lymphoma essentially recapitulates that of marginal zone B cells. The B cells are CD20+, PAX5+, CD79a+, CD21+, CD35+, CD5–, CD10–, CD23–, cyclin D1–, and SOX11–.[141,142] CD43 is aberrantly expressed in approximately 50% of cases, and expression of CD11c is variable. The tumor cells typically express IgM, less often express IgA or IgG, are IgD-negative, and show immunoglobulin light chain restriction. A significant intratumoral population of CD3-positive, predominantly CD4-positive T cells is frequently present. Expanded meshworks of follicular dendritic cells are typically detected with antibodies CD21 and CD23, corresponding to follicles that are colonized or overrun by the lymphoma cells. Variable numbers of BCL6-positive, CD10-positive follicle center cells may be seen in these areas, whereas the neoplastic cells outside of germinal centers are negative for these antigens.

Newer markers proposed as diagnostically useful in the workup of suspected marginal zone lymphomas include MNDA and IRTA1.[32,143] MNDA expression has been reported in 68% to 95% of MALT lymphomas, 5% to 21% of FLs, and 37% to 100% of various other small B-cell lymphomas.[144,145] The demonstration of MNDA expression may therefore be useful in the specific differential diagnosis of MALT lymphoma versus FL. IRTA1 expression has been reported in 52% to 93% of MALT lymphomas versus <10% of other small B-cell neoplasms.[145,146]

GENETIC FEATURES OF MALT LYMPHOMA

Antigen Receptor Genes

In MALT lymphomas, immunoglobulin heavy and light chain genes are clonally rearranged and show evidence of somatic hypermutation in their variable regions, consistent with a postgerminal center memory B-cell origin.[147] Ongoing

Table 18-2 GELA Histologic Scoring System for Posttreatment Evaluation of Gastric MALT Lymphoma

Score (Grade)	Lymphoid Infiltrate	Lymphoepithelial Lesions	Stromal Changes
Complete response (CR)	Absent or scattered plasma cells and small lymphoid cells in the lamina propria	Absent	Normal or empty lamina propria and/or fibrosis
Probable minimal residual disease (pMRD)	Aggregates of lymphoid cells or lymphoid nodules in the lamina propria, muscularis mucosa, and/or submucosa	Absent	Empty lamina propria and/or fibrosis
Responding residual disease (rRD)	Dense, diffuse, or nodular extending around glands in the lamina propria	Focal lymphoepithelial lesions or absent	Focal empty lamina propria and/or fibrosis
No change (NC)	Dense, diffuse, or nodular	Present or "may be absent"	No changes

GELA, Groupe d'Etude des Lymphomes de l'Adulte.

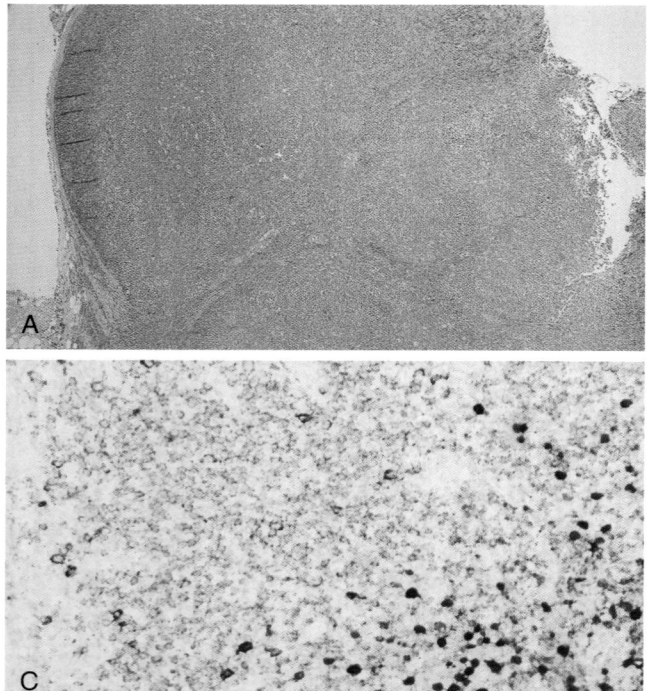

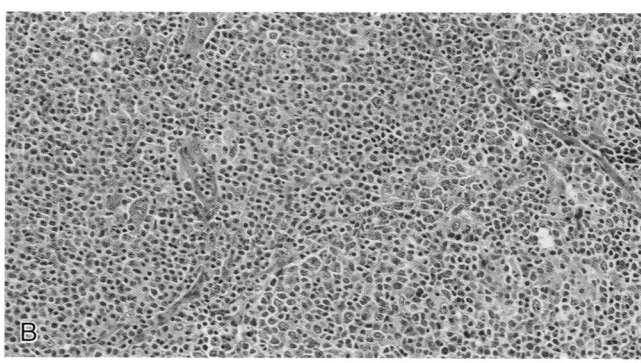

Figure 18-7. A, Gastric lymph node from a case of MALT lymphoma showing a vaguely nodular growth pattern. **B,** At higher magnification, the neoplastic marginal zone cells *(upper left)* surround a residual germinal center *(right)*. **C,** Ultrasensitive in situ hybridization stain for kappa *(brown)* and lambda *(red)* shows kappa monotypic lymphoma cells surrounding a polytypic germinal center.

mutations are thought to occur in most cases.[148] As it is frequently challenging to distinguish between hyperplastic proliferations of acquired MALT versus extranodal MALT lymphoma, especially in small biopsy specimens, molecular analysis is frequently employed during diagnostic evaluation. When testing is performed with BIOMED-2/EuroClonality primer sets targeting IGH and IGK following consensus guidelines,[111] the frequency of false negative results appears to be low (<5%). However, assays employing IGH primers alone may miss monoclonality in up to 15% of cases of overt lymphoma.[149] Monoclonal results may also be seen as a spurious finding (a false positive result) in some samples of reactive MALT tissue, such as in chronic gastritis. The frequency of false positive results varies widely across laboratories, suggesting that variations in technique may be a factor. For these reasons, a diagnosis of MALT lymphoma should never be diagnosed based upon clonal PCR results alone in the absence of histopathologic abnormalities. Similarly, clonal rearrangements may remain detectable by PCR after eradication of *H. pylori* for the treatment of MALT lymphoma, and this finding appears to lack clinical significance in the absence of histologic features of persistent lymphoma.[127]

Sequencing studies of the immunoglobulin genes in MALT lymphomas have shown that cases arising at a given anatomic site show characteristic bias in the usage of specific IGVH gene segments. For example, cases of gastric MALT lymphoma show overrepresentation of IGHV3-7 and IGHV1-69, while cases arising in the salivary gland are biased toward IGHV1-69 and those in the ocular adnexa toward IGHV4-34.[150,151] Comparisons of the resulting amino acid sequences have shown evidence of positive and negative selection for replacement mutations, consistent with antigen-driven selection. These findings emphasize the role of an antigen-directed response in the evolution of the neoplastic clone. In some cases this antigen may represent an underlying

infectious agent, such as *H. pylori* in gastric MALT lymphoma, and in other cases the initial response may be against an autoantigen.[152]

Genetic Abnormalities

A number of genetic abnormalities are recurrent in MALT lymphoma, including trisomies of chromosomes 3, 12, and 18, which also occur in primary nodal marginal zone lymphomas and splenic marginal zone lymphomas. Balanced translocations specifically associated with extranodal MALT lymphoma include t(11;18)(q21;q21) *BIRC3::MALT1*, t(14;18) (q32;q21) *IGH::MALT1*, t(1;14)(p22;q32) *BCL10::IGH*, and t(3;14)(p14;q32) *FOXP1::IGH*. Next-generation sequencing studies have shown a large number of recurrent mutations including *TNFAIP3 (A20)*, *CREBBP, KMT2C, TET2, SPEN, KMT2D, LRP1B,* and *PRDM1*.[151] Many of these genetic abnormalities result in activation of the NF-κB signaling pathway, which is thought to represent a major mechanism of oncogenesis in MALT lymphoma. Notably, the frequency of these various cytogenetic and molecular abnormalities varies with the anatomic site of origin (Table 18-3). Details of the most common abnormalities are discussed further.

t(11;18)(q21;q21) *BIRC3::MALT1* is the most frequent translocation in MALT lymphoma, being found in approximately 40% of pulmonary cases and 30% of gastric MALT lymphomas, with a lower incidence elsewhere.[150,153] This translocation produces a functional *BIRC3::MALT1* fusion protein that leads to constitutive activation of NF-κB signaling. In gastric MALT lymphoma, the *BIRC3::MALT1* fusion is associated with advanced stage disease and decreased response to antibiotic therapy against *H. pylori*. Routine testing for *BIRC3::MALT1* is therefore widely performed in the setting of newly diagnosed gastric MALT lymphoma. This abnormality may be detected from formalin-fixed paraffin embedded

Table 18-3 Molecular/Cytogenetic Abnormalities in Extranodal MALT Lymphomas

Site	Translocations/Trisomies	Mutations
Stomach	BIRC3::MALT1 (6%–23%) IGH::MALT1 (1%–5%) +3 (11%) +18 (6%)	NOTCH1 (17%) NF1 (16%) TNFAIP3 (15%) ATM (13%) TRAF3 (13%)
Ocular adnexa/orbit	IGH::MALT1 (0%–25%) FOXP1::IGH (0%–20%) BIRC3::MALT1 (0%–10%) +3 (38%) +18 (13%)	TNFAIP3 (39%) KMT2D (15%) CREBBP (10%) LRP1B (10%) MYD88 (10%)
Salivary gland	IGH::MALT1 (0%–16%) BIRC3::MALT1 (0%–5%) BCL10::IGH (0%–2%) +3 (55%) +18 (19%)	TBL1XR1 (24%) GRP34 (16%) NOTCH2 (11%) SPEN (11%) KMT2C (11%)
Lung	BIRC3::MALT1 (31%–53%) IGH::MALT1 (6%–10%) BCL10::IGH (2%–7%) +3 (20%) +18 (4%)	KMT2D (25%) TNFAIP3 (18%) PRDM1 (12%) NOTCH1 (12%) EP300 (11%)
Thyroid	FOXP1::IGH (0%–50%) BIRC3::MALT1 (0%–17%) +3 (17%)	TET2 (61%) TNFRSF14 (44%) PIK3CD (23%) SPEN (17%) CREBBP (8%)

Summarized from Vela et al,[198] Streubal et al,[156] and Remstein et al.[199]

tissues using RT-PCR assays or through fluorescence in situ hybridization (FISH) studies with either BIR3::MALT1 fusion probes or MALT1 break-apart probes.

The t(14;18)(q32;q21) IGH::MALT1 translocation has been reported to be the second-most common translocation in extranodal MALT lymphoma.[150,153,154] This abnormality places the intact MALT1 gene under the IGH enhancer region, resulting in overexpression of the MALT1 protein and enhanced NF-κB activity. It should be noted that this translocation involves the same chromosomal breakpoints as the much more common t(14;18)(q32;q21) IGH::BCL2 associated with FL and diffuse large B-cell lymphoma.[154] Definitive recognition of this translocation therefore requires the use of FISH or other molecular methods.

t(1;14)(p22;q32) BCL10::IGH places the BCL10 gene under control of the IGH enhancer and leads to overexpression of the BCL10 protein.[150,153,155,156] BCL10 serves to link signaling from the B-cell antigen receptors to the canonical NF-κB signaling pathway, and the t(1;14) therefore results in constitutive activation of this pathway. The t(1;14) is rare, being reported in 1% to 2% of MALT lymphomas.[153,156] The clinical effect of this translocation in MALT lymphoma is not well characterized to date because of its rarity; however, nuclear overexpression of the BCL10 protein, which may occur either as a result of the t(1;14) or through other mechanisms, has been associated with decreased response to antibiotic therapy in gastric MALT lymphoma.[157-160]

TNFAIP3 (previously known as A20), which is located on chromosome 6q23, is recurrently mutated or deleted in extranodal MALT lymphomas.[150,151] TNFAIP3 serves as a negative regulator of the NF-κB pathway, and deletion of this locus or the presence of inactivating mutations leads to enhanced activation of this signaling pathway. Abnormalities of TNFAIP3 have been reported most frequently in cases lacking

any of the translocations described, with highest frequencies reported in ocular adnexa, salivary gland, and thyroid.

POSTULATED CELL OF ORIGIN

The architectural features of MALT lymphoma, particularly early cases, show quite clearly that the neoplastic cells are infiltrating the marginal zone around B-cell follicles. In non-neoplastic lymphoid tissue, a prominent marginal zone is present in the spleen, Peyer's patches, and mesenteric lymph nodes. This allows a comparison of the cytology and immunophenotype of normal marginal zone cells with those of MALT lymphoma (Fig. 18-8). Cytologically, MALT lymphoma cells bear a close resemblance to marginal zone cells. Both are slightly larger than small lymphocytes and have a slightly irregular nuclear outline and moderate amounts of pale-staining cytoplasm. Interestingly, in both Peyer's patches and LESA, collections of marginal zone cells are found within the dome and ductal epithelium, respectively. The immunophenotypes of cells of the marginal zone and MALT lymphoma are virtually identical, with both expressing CD20 and other pan–B-cell antigens, CD21, CD35, and IgM, but not IgD.[161,162]

CLINICAL COURSE

MALT lymphomas are among the most indolent of all lymphomas and have a good prognosis, regardless of stage. Five-year and ten-year overall survival rates exceeding 80% are the rule, although progression-free survival may be somewhat lower.[139,163] Patients with primary cutaneous disease, despite frequent cutaneous relapses, have an extremely indolent clinical course with 5-year disease-specific survival approaching 100% in most large studies.[164,165] Given this extremely indolent behavior, primary cutaneous marginal zone (MALT) lymphoma is now recognized as primary cutaneous marginal zone lymphoproliferative disorder (pcMZLPD) rather than an overt lymphoma in the 2022 ICC.[4] Although most patients present with localized disease, involvement of multiple mucosal sites at initial presentation or during the disease course is not uncommon in noncutaneous MALT lymphomas, and is not associated with a poorer outcome.[133,139,163,166] The presence of lymph node or bone marrow involvement at diagnosis has been associated with a worse prognosis in some studies, but not in others.[139,163,166] Patients with pcMZLPD by definition do not have extracutaneous disease at initial presentation, and dissemination to noncutaneous sites during the course of disease is rare.[165,167-169] Transformation to diffuse large B-cell lymphoma is reported in <10% of MALT lymphomas, and is associated with an adverse outcome.[139,166,170,171] Preferred treatment modalities differ according to the site of origin and vary from "watch and wait" to surgery, antibiotic or antiviral therapy, radiotherapy, and immunochemotherapy.[32,142,172,173]

The treatment of gastric MALT lymphoma has attracted considerable attention since the initial published report that the lymphoma may regress after eradication of H. pylori with antibiotics. The most recent recommended staging systems for gastric MALT lymphoma include endoscopy with multiple biopsy specimens from the stomach, duodenum, and gastroesophageal junction, and from each site with an abnormal appearance.[142,172] Endoscopic ultrasound is helpful for

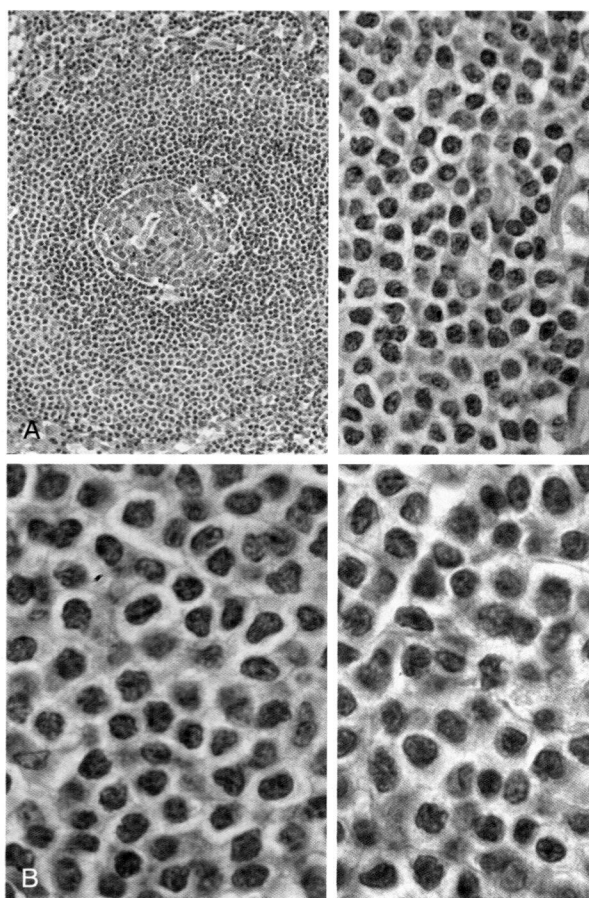

Figure 18-8. A, Reactive mesenteric lymph node with a prominent marginal zone *(left)* and illustrated at higher magnification *(right).* **B,** Marginal zone cells from the mesenteric lymph node *(left)* compared with the cells of a gastric MALT lymphoma *(right).*

identifying dissemination to perigastric lymph nodes and to assess the depth of gastric wall infiltration; studies have shown that the lymphoma is less likely to respond to eradication of *H. pylori* if it has invaded beyond the submucosa.[127,174,175] The follow-up of MALT lymphoma patients after eradication of *H. pylori* is rather complex, requiring repeated gastroscopy with biopsy. Cases that have transformed to a diffuse large B-cell lymphoma are unlikely to respond to *H. pylori* treatment, although there are reports of complete regression in such cases.[176,177] The presence of t(11;18)(q21;q21) *BIRC3::MALT1* in gastric MALT lymphomas is associated with more advanced disease, a lack of associated *H. pylori* infection, and failure to respond to eradication of *H. pylori* when present.[32,178] Recent National Comprehensive Cancer Network guidelines suggest evaluation of t(11;18)(q21;q21) *BIRC3::MALT1* with FISH or PCR in cases that are *H. pylori* positive.[173] Antibiotic treatment with involved-site radiotherapy (preferred) or rituximab is recommended for *H. pylori*–positive patients who harbor the translocation.

DIFFERENTIAL DIAGNOSIS

Reactive Versus Neoplastic MALT

The distinction between acquired MALT, the precursor of MALT lymphoma, and MALT lymphoma in the early stages of evolution often gives rise to diagnostic difficulty.

This is particularly true of gastric and salivary gland MALT lymphomas. Though acquired MALT in the stomach may harbor a lymphoepithelium adjacent to follicles mimicking the lymphoepithelial lesion characteristic of MALT lymphoma (Fig. 18-9), there should not be an extensive infiltrate of B cells external to the IgD-positive, IgM-positive mantle zones or an associated monotypic plasma-cell population; an expanded B-cell infiltrate in the lamina propria outside of follicles is more indicative of a MALT lymphoma (see Table 18-1).[42,179] The earliest sign of lymphoma in salivary glands is an extension of the intraepithelial B cells around the duct, the lumen of which is often partly obliterated by epithelial cells, to form halo-like infiltrates of monocytoid or centrocyte-like B cells around the duct (Fig. 18-10).[180] The cells constituting the halos are immunoglobulin light chain restricted and generally IgM-positive.[25] As the MALT lymphoma further develops, the halos surrounding lymphoepithelial lesions expand and become confluent. A diagnosis of overt MALT lymphoma is not warranted in lymphoproliferations that lack confluent, broad swaths of monocytoid- or centrocyte-like cells, or associated monotypic plasma cells.[105,107,181]

In the distinction between acquired MALT and MALT lymphoma, demonstration of clonality by virtue of light chain restriction of B cells or plasma cells, either by immunohistochemistry/in situ hybridization (paraffin sections) or by flow cytometry, can be diagnostic. Co-expression of CD43 by B cells is a useful hint that the B-cell population is neoplastic, although CD43 co-expression on B cells has also been described in some cases of LESA, and on subsets of reactive B cells and plasma cells.[107,182-184] Use of PCR for IGH and IGK rearrangements to discriminate reactive lymphoid infiltrates from MALT lymphoma is somewhat controversial. Although a positive PCR result is strong evidence of lymphoma in a case with suspicious morphologic and immunophenotypic features, it is well recognized that clonal B-cell populations may be detected in reactive lymphoproliferations at extranodal sites, including in over 50% of LESA.[107,108,181,185] The detection of a clonal cytogenetic abnormality by FISH may be helpful to confirm the diagnosis of MALT lymphoma, although the presence of these alterations is quite variable based on anatomic site (see Table 18-3).

MALT Lymphoma Versus Atypical Marginal Zone Hyperplasia

There are rare atypical marginal zone hyperplasias that may mimic MALT lymphoma.[186-191] Primarily reported in children, these atypical hyperplasias involve sites of native MALT (tonsils, adenoids, and appendix), anatomic locations infrequently involved by MALT lymphoma. First described in 2004 by Attygalle and colleagues,[186] these lymphoproliferations consist of a follicular hyperplasia with expansion of the marginal zones by centrocyte-like B cells admixed with variable numbers of large, transformed cells. Some follicles have a moth-eaten appearance consistent with follicular colonization, and most cases show a component of intraepithelial B cells reminiscent of lymphoepithelial lesions. The marginal zone and intraepithelial B cells in these lymphoproliferations also generally demonstrate lambda light chain restriction by immunohistochemistry/ in situ hybridization or flow cytometry, and may express

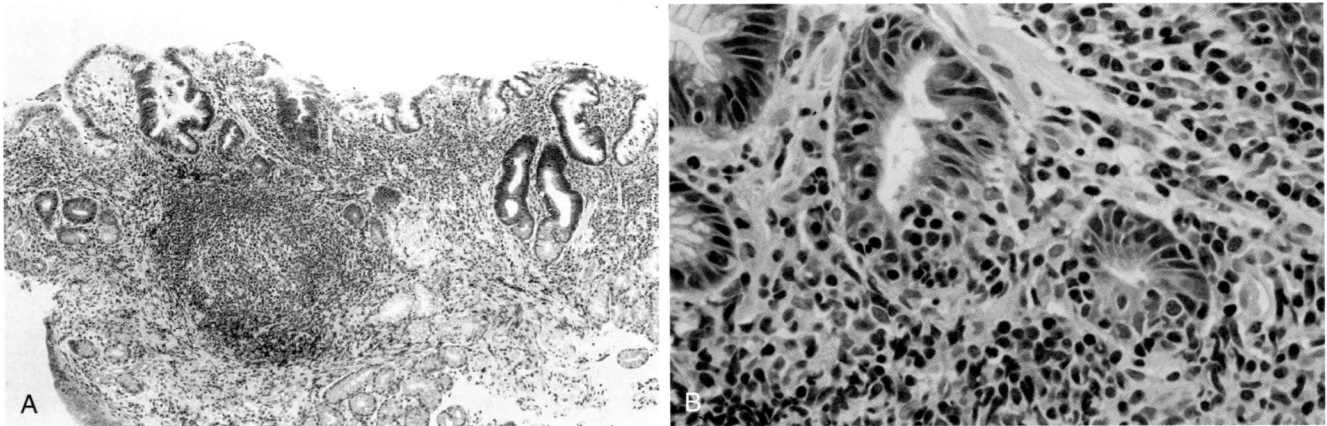

Figure 18-9. A, *Helicobacter pylori* gastritis with a prominent follicle adjacent to gastric glands. **B,** High magnification of gastric glands adjacent to the follicle shows infiltration of glandular epithelium by small lymphocytes, mimicking a lymphoepithelial lesion.

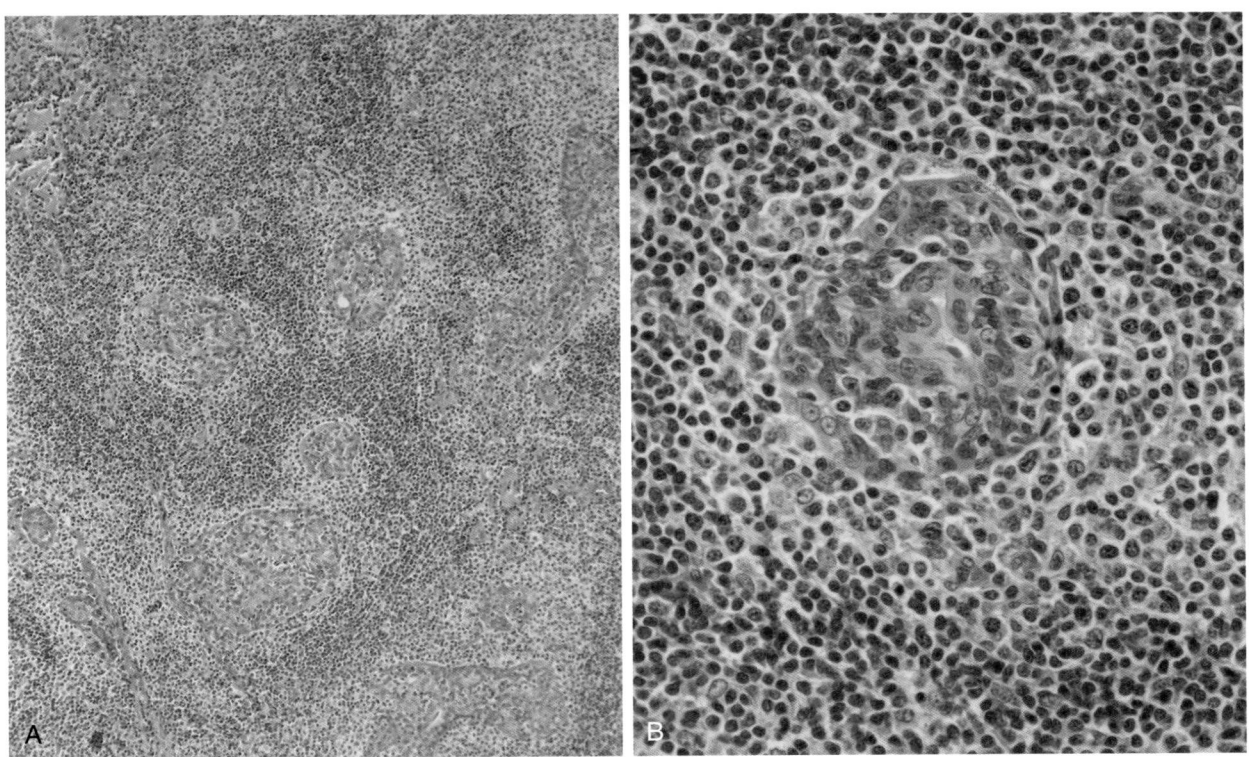

Figure 18-10. An early MALT lymphoma of the parotid gland evolving from lymphoepithelial sialadenitis. A, Lymphoma cells form halos around lymphoepithelial lesions and begin to become confluent. **B,** High magnification of the lymphoma cells constituting the halos.

CD43.[186,187,190,191] Although these histologic and immunophenotypic features raise suspicion for a MALT lymphoma, atypical marginal zone hyperplasias are differentiated by the lack of B-cell clonality with PCR studies for IGH, IGK, and IGL.[186,190,191] The benign nature of these atypical hyperplasias is further supported by clinical outcomes, with patients remaining alive with no evidence of disease, without lymphoma-directed treatment, at a median follow-up of 39 months.[186,190,191]

MALT Versus Other Small B-Cell Lymphomas

Because of differences in clinical behavior and management, it is important to differentiate MALT lymphoma from the other small B-cell lymphomas that may present in or involve extranodal sites (Table 18-4). These include mantle cell lymphoma, chronic lymphocytic leukemia/small lymphocytic lymphoma, and FL. The need to distinguish between MALT

Table 18-4 Differential Diagnosis of MALT Lymphoma and Other Small B-Cell Lymphomas Involving Mucosal Sites*

	MALT	Mantle Cell	Follicular	CLL
Follicles	+	+	+	±
LELs	+	–/+	–/+	–/+
Cytology	CCL	CCL	CC, CB	Occasional CCL
Ig	M+, D–	M+, D+	M±, D±	M+, D+
CD20	+	+	+	+
CD5	–	+	–	+
CD10	–	–	+	–
Cyclin D1	–	+	–	–

*Table highlights typical immunophenotypic features; exceptions may occur in some cases.

CB, Centroblast; *CC,* centrocyte; *CCL,* centrocyte-like; *CLL,* chronic lymphocytic leukemia; *Ig,* immunoglobulin; *LEL,* lymphoepithelial lesion; *MALT,* mucosa-associated lymphoid tissue.

Pearls and Pitfalls

- Antigen drive plays a key role in most MALT lymphomas, although in some cases the initiating antigen has not been identified.
- PCR studies for IGH and IGK rearrangements may be useful for the distinction of reactive hyperplasia from MALT lymphoma; however, both false-positive and false-negative results may occur.
- Demonstration of light chain restriction in a MALT lesion is useful in the distinction of acquired MALT and MALT lymphoma.
- Rare atypical marginal zone hyperplasias, primarily arising at native MALT sites in children, may show lambda light chain restriction and should not be diagnosed as MALT lymphomas in the absence of definitive B-cell clonality by molecular methods.
- Gastric MALT lymphomas with a t(1;14) *BCL10::IGH* or t(11;18) *BIRC3::MALT1* translocation fail to respond to antibiotics as the sole therapeutic modality.
- MALT lymphomas may disseminate late to lymph nodes, and in many cases the distinction between primary and secondary marginal zone lymphomas in lymph nodes is difficult. A careful clinical history is key.

lymphoma and lymphoplasmacytic lymphoma involving extranodal sites can also arise.

The cytologic features of mantle cell lymphoma can closely simulate those of MALT lymphoma, to the extent that occasional lymphoepithelial lesions may be present. However, the absence of transformed lymphoid cells, together with expression of CD5, cyclin D1, a consequence of the t(11;14)(q13;q32) *CCND1::IGH* translocation, and SOX11 can distinguish mantle cell lymphoma.[192] Chronic lymphocytic leukemia/small lymphocytic lymphoma is characterized by small, round lymphocytes, usually with peripheral blood lymphocytosis and often with proliferation centers, although these may be difficult to appreciate in extranodal sites. Expression of CD5, CD23, and LEF1, without cyclin D1, provides further distinction from MALT lymphoma.[193] FL, which may arise extranodally, can be difficult to distinguish from MALT lymphoma with prominent follicular colonization. The transformed MALT lymphoma cells within the follicles may closely resemble centroblasts, but are typically negative for CD10 and BCL6, in contrast to the cells of FL, which usually express both antigens, both within and between follicles. Assessment of these antigens, together with stains for follicular dendritic cells such as CD21 or CD23, is useful. Evaluation of other germinal center–associated markers, such as LMO2, HGAL, GCET and MEF2B, and stains for IRTA1 and MNDA, which show selective expression in marginal zone lymphomas, may provide additional help in selected cases.[145,146,194,195] Cytogenetic and molecular genetic analysis to detect *MALT1* and *BCL2* rearrangements is also useful. Finally, MALT lymphoma with plasmacytic differentiation can be distinguished from lymphoplasmacytic lymphoma if the characteristic architecture is identified and marginal zone/monocytoid B cells are present. In cases lacking such features, the clinical picture—evidence of bone marrow involvement or a paraprotein—may aid in the diagnosis. Furthermore, PCR studies for the *MYD88* L265P point mutation may be helpful, as this abnormality has been demonstrated in the vast majority of lymphoplasmacytic lymphomas, but has been reported in only a minority of cases diagnosed as extranodal MALT lymphoma.[196,197]

KEY REFERENCES

1. Isaacson P, Wright DH. Extranodal malignant lymphoma arising from mucosa-associated lymphoid tissue. *Cancer.* 1984;53:2515–2524.
2. Isaacson P, Wright DH. Malignant lymphoma of mucosa-associated lymphoid tissue. A distinctive type of B-cell lymphoma. *Cancer.* 1983;52:1410–1416.
18. Luminari S, Cesaretti M, Marcheselli L, et al. Decreasing incidence of gastric MALT lymphomas in the era of anti-Helicobacter pylori interventions: results from a population-based study on extranodal marginal zone lymphomas. *Ann Oncol.* 2010;21:855–859.
32. Rossi D, Bertoni F, Zucca E. Marginal-zone lymphomas. *N Engl J Med.* 2022;386:568–581.
38. Wotherspoon AC, Ortiz-Hidalgo C, Falzon MR, Isaacson PG. Helicobacter pylori-associated gastritis and primary B-cell gastric lymphoma. *Lancet (London, England).* 1991;338:1175–1176.
42. Wotherspoon AC, Doglioni C, Diss TC, et al. Regression of primary low-grade B-cell gastric lymphoma of mucosa-associated lymphoid tissue type after eradication of Helicobacter pylori. *Lancet.* 1993;342:575–577.
91. Gibson SE, Swerdlow SH, Craig FE, et al. EBV-positive extranodal marginal zone lymphoma of mucosa-associated lymphoid tissue in the posttransplant setting: a distinct type of posttransplant lymphoproliferative disorder? *Am J Surg Pathol.* 2011;35:807–815.
150. Du M-QQ. MALT lymphoma: a paradigm of NF-κB dysregulation. *Semin Cancer Biol.* 2016;39:49–60.
156. Streubel B, Simonitsch-Klupp I, Mullauer L, et al. Variable frequencies of MALT lymphoma-associated genetic aberrations in MALT lymphomas of different sites. *Leukemia.* 2004;18:1722–1726.
199. Remstein ED, Dogan A, Einerson RR, et al. The incidence and anatomic site specificity of chromosomal translocations in primary extranodal marginal zone B-cell lymphoma of mucosa-associated lymphoid tissue (MALT lymphoma) in North America. *Am J Surg Pathol.* 2006;30:1546–1553.

Visit Elsevier eBooks+ for the complete set of references.

Primary Cutaneous B-Cell Lymphomas

Rein Willemze, Anne M.R. Schrader, and Patty M. Jansen

Primary cutaneous B-cell lymphomas (CBCLs) are a heterogeneous group of B-cell lymphomas that present in the skin without evidence of extracutaneous disease at the time of diagnosis.[1] CBCLs are much less common than primary cutaneous T-cell lymphomas (CTCLs). In Western countries, CBCLs constitute approximately 25% of all primary cutaneous lymphomas, and their overall annual incidence rate is estimated at 3.1 cases per 1 million individuals.[1,2] However, CBCL appears to be much less common in Asian countries.[3,4] It is important to differentiate CBCLs from systemic B-cell lymphomas secondarily involving the skin. Compared with their nodal counterparts, CBCLs often have a completely different clinical behavior and prognosis and require a different therapeutic approach; they are therefore classified separately. For this purpose, in every patient with a diagnosis of B-cell lymphoma in the skin, careful physical examination, routine blood examination, and appropriate imaging studies (computed tomography [CT] or positron emission tomography [PET]-CT) are required to exclude secondary cutaneous disease. Bone marrow examination is mandatory in high-grade malignant CBCL, but it is optional in low-grade malignant CBCL.[5,6]

HISTORICAL BACKGROUND

The history of CBCL dates back to the 1980s after the introduction of immunohistochemistry in the diagnosis and classification of malignant lymphomas.[7] At that time, it was still firmly believed that skin localizations of malignant lymphomas other than mycosis fungoides (MF) and Sézary syndrome (SS) were manifestations of a systemic lymphoma, even if staging procedures failed to demonstrate extracutaneous disease, and patients were treated accordingly.

A major advantage of cutaneous lymphomas compared with malignant lymphomas arising at other sites is that the former can be seen by the naked eye and biopsied easily. This offers the unique opportunity to correlate the clinical appearance and clinical behavior with the histologic, immunophenotypic, and genetic features of these conditions. Clinicopathologic correlation is often essential to make a definite diagnosis. Such an approach contributed significantly to the diagnosis and classification of primary cutaneous lymphomas and resulted in the recognition of new types of CTCL and CBCL. These new types of CTCL and CBCL were found to have highly characteristic clinical and histologic features and often had a completely different clinical behavior and prognosis than morphologically similar nodal lymphomas and required a different type of treatment.[7] Primary cutaneous lymphomas were therefore included as distinct entities in lymphoma classifications, initially in a separate classification for primary cutaneous lymphomas (EORTC classification of cutaneous lymphomas),[8] but after the WHO-EORTC consensus classification in 2005,[9] they were incorporated in the 4th edition of the WHO classification of hematopoietic neoplasms and its updates, including the 2022 International Consensus Classification (ICC).[10-12] In the 2018 update of the WHO-EORTC classification for primary cutaneous lymphomas, the 2022 ICC, and the 5th edition of the WHO classification for hematolymphoid tumors, three main types of CBCL are recognized: primary cutaneous marginal zone lymphoma (PCMZL) considered a lymphoproliferative disorder in the 2022 ICC (PCMZLPD), primary cutaneous follicle center lymphoma (PCFCL), and primary cutaneous diffuse large B-cell lymphoma, leg type (PCDLBCL, LT).[1,11,12] In addition, Epstein-Barr virus (EBV)-positive mucocutaneous ulcer has been included as a distinct entity. Intravascular large B-cell lymphoma and B-lymphoblastic lymphoma can also manifest in the skin first, but these conditions are not considered "primary cutaneous lymphoma." They are considered manifestations of systemic disease and should be treated accordingly, even in those rare cases where initial staging is negative.

PRIMARY CUTANEOUS MARGINAL ZONE LYMPHOPROLIFERATIVE DISORDER

Definition

PCMZLPD is an indolent lymphoma composed of small B cells, plasma cells, and a variable number of reactive T cells. It includes cases previously designated as primary cutaneous immunocytoma,[13] cutaneous follicular lymphoid hyperplasia with monotypic plasma cells,[14] and primary cutaneous plasmacytoma without underlying multiple myeloma (extramedullary plasmacytoma of the skin).[15] In the 4th edition of the WHO classification and revised 4th edition, PCMZLPD was not yet listed separately but included in the broad group of extranodal marginal zone lymphomas of mucosa-associated lymphoid tissue (MALT lymphoma). However, in the 2022 ICC and 5th edition of the WHO classification, PCMZLPD is recognized as a distinct entity, separate from other MALT lymphomas, although still termed PCMZL in the latter classification.[11,12] The 2022 ICC introduced the term lymphoproliferative disorder (LPD) for this entity rather than *lymphoma* because of the extremely indolent clinical behavior with disease-specific survival rates approaching 100%.[12]

Synonyms and Related Terms

WHO Revised 4th edition: Extranodal marginal zone lymphoma of mucosa-associated lymphoid tissue (MALT lymphoma)

WHO Proposed 5th edition: Primary cutaneous marginal zone lymphoma

PCMZLPD was not segregated from other MALT lymphomas in the WHO revised 4th edition.

Epidemiology

PCMZLPDs make up about 9% of all cutaneous lymphomas and about 40% of primary CBCLs.[1] They most commonly affect (young) adults, and a male predominance has been reported.[16-18]

Etiology

PCMZLPDs have been described in relation to tattoo pigments, tick bites, and antigen injection, suggesting they may develop from chronic antigenic stimulation by intradermally applied antigens.[19,20] However, in most cases, the cause is unknown. An association with *Borrelia burgdorferi* infection has been reported in a minority of European cases of PCMZLPD, but not in cases from Asia or the United States.[21-24] One report described a high incidence of gastrointestinal disorders and autoimmune diseases in patients with PCMZLPD.[25]

Clinical Features

PCMZLPD presents with red-to-violaceous papules, plaques, or nodules localized preferentially on the trunk and upper arms (Fig. 19-1A). In contrast to PCFCL, patients more often present with multifocal skin lesions (Table 19-1). Ulceration is uncommon. Cutaneous relapses occur frequently, particularly in patients presenting with multifocal skin lesions.[18,26,27] However, extracutaneous dissemination is uncommon and is reported in only 4% to 8% of the patients.[16-18] Bone marrow involvement is exceedingly rare, and a bone marrow biopsy is therefore not required unless indicated by other staging procedures.[5,6]

Histopathology

These lymphomas show patchy, nodular, or diffuse dermal infiltrates with sparing of the epidermis (Fig. 19-1B). The infiltrates are composed of small B cells, plasma cells, often follicles with reactive germinal centers, and in most cases, an abundant T-cell infiltrate. Monotypic plasma cells are often located at the periphery of the infiltrates and in the subepidermal compartment.[13,28,29] Unlike marginal zone lymphoma (MZL) occurring at other sites, PCMZLPD does not or rarely shows colonization of reactive germinal centers by neoplastic B cells, lymphoepithelial lesions, or transformation into a diffuse large B-cell lymphoma. Diffuse infiltrates of small B cells with a monocytoid appearance should raise suspicion of a systemic lymphoma. In rare cases, a pure population of neoplastic plasma cells, formerly classified as *primary cutaneous plasmacytoma,* can be observed. Reports suggest that amyloid light chain (AL) amyloidoma, which refers to cases showing amyloid deposits in combination with monotypic plasma cells, should be considered a rare variant of PCMZLPD.[30,31]

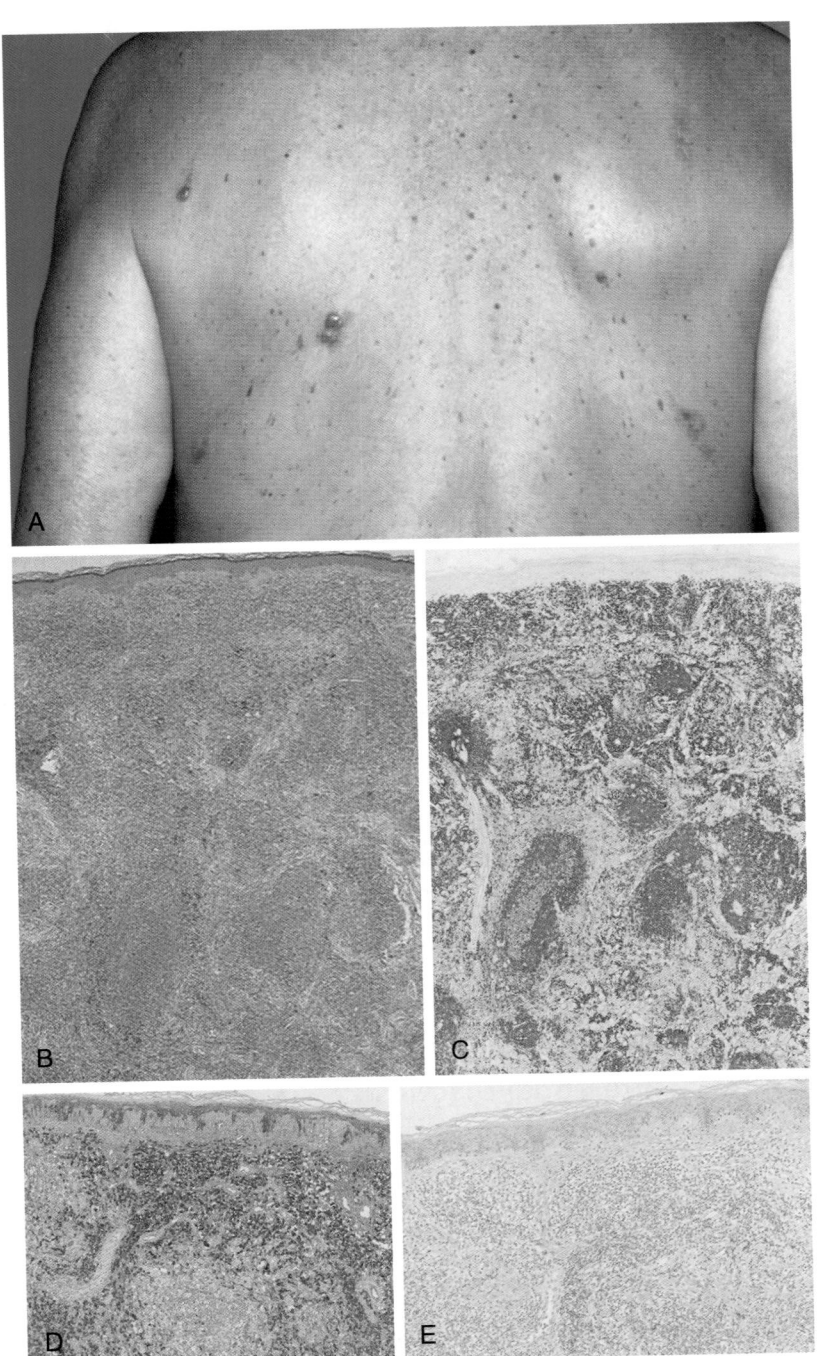

Figure 19-1. Primary cutaneous marginal zone lymphoproliferative disorder. A, Typical clinical presentation with multiple nodules on the back. **B,** Dense infiltrates throughout the dermis are shown. **C,** CD79a staining shows a predominance of B cells and reactive germinal centers. **D,** Monotypic immunoglobulin G, kappa-positive plasma cells in the superficial dermis (kappa staining). **E,** Negative staining for lambda light chains.

Immunophenotype

Tumor cells express CD20, CD79a, and BCL2, but are negative for CD5, CD10, and BCL6, which may be useful in distinction from PCFCL (Table 19-2).[32,33] Reactive germinal centers are typically positive for BCL6 and CD10 and negative for BCL2. Plasma cells express CD138, IRF4/MUM1, and CD79a, but generally not CD20, and show monotypic cytoplasmic immunoglobulin light chain expression on paraffin sections (Fig. 19-1C–E). In some cases, biclonal expression of kappa and lambda light chain–restricted B cells has been reported.[34,35] Studies describe the existence of two types of PCMZLPD.[36-38]

Unlike most other MALT lymphomas, the vast majority of PCMZLPD expresses class-switched immunoglobulins, including immunoglobulin (Ig)G, IgA, and IgE; do not express the chemokine receptor CXCR3, which has been suggested to play a role in homing of the malignant B cells to mucosa-associated malignant tissue; and have a Th2 inflammatory background. These cases show a predominance of T cells and often contain reactive follicles and only a small proportion of small B cells. PD-1 is expressed by variable numbers of T cells, and in some cases, these PD-1–positive T cells even form rosettes, considered characteristic of primary cutaneous CD4-positive small/medium T-cell lymphoproliferative disorders

Table 19-1 Clinical Characteristics of the Main Three Types of Primary Cutaneous B-Cell Lymphomas

	PCMZLPD	PCFCL	PCDLBCL, LT
Age group	Young adults	Middle-aged adults	Older adults, especially females
Clinical presentation	Solitary or multifocal plaques or tumors mainly on the trunk and upper arms	Solitary or localized plaques or tumors on the head (scalp) or trunk. Multifocal lesions in rare cases	Skin tumors on the (lower) leg(s). Uncommonly, lesions at sites other than the leg (20%)
First-choice treatment	Solitary: radiotherapy; excision. Multifocal: wait and see; intralesional steroids, interferon or rituximab; low-dose radiotherapy	Localized: radiotherapy. Multifocal: wait and see; intravenous rituximab	R-CHOP
Cutaneous relapse	50%	30%	65%
Nodal/visceral dissemination	Extremely rare	10%	35%
5-year disease-specific survival rate	99%	95%	50% (→70%)*

*Better survival in patients treated with R-CHOP.
PCDLBCL, LT, Primary cutaneous diffuse large B-cell lymphoma, leg type; *PCFCL,* primary cutaneous follicle center lymphoma; *PCMZLPD,* primary cutaneous marginal zone lymphoproliferative disorder; *R-CHOP,* cyclophosphamide, doxorubicin, vincristine, and prednisone in combination with rituximab.

Table 19-2 Differential Diagnostic Markers in Primary Cutaneous Marginal Zone Lymphoproliferative Disorder and Other Cutaneous B-Cell Lymphoproliferations

	CD20	BCL6	BCL2	CD10	CD5	Cyclin D1
CLH (pseudo–B-cell lymphoma with reactive germinal centers)	+	+	−	+	−	−
PCMZLPD	+	−	+	−	−	−
PCFCL	+	+	−/+	−/+	−	−
Secondary cutaneous follicular lymphoma	+	+	+	+	−	−
Secondary cutaneous mantle cell lymphoma	+	−	+	−	+	+
Secondary cutaneous CLL/SLL	+	−	+	−	+	−

Phenotypic markers refer to the neoplastic cells except in CLH where BCL6, CD10, and BCL2 refer to the reactive germinal centers.
CLH, Cutaneous lymphoid hyperplasia; *CLL/SLL,* chronic lymphocytic leukemia/small lymphocytic lymphoma; *PCFCL,* primary cutaneous follicle center lymphoma; *PCMZLPD,* primary cutaneous marginal zone lymphoproliferative disorder.

(PCSM-TCLPDs).[38,39] As some cases of PCSM-TCLPD may contain monotypic plasma cells, differentiation between the two conditions is sometimes difficult.[38,39] Clusters of CD123-positive plasmacytoid dendritic cells are typically found in the periphery of the infiltrates.[40] IgG4 is expressed in up to 40% of PCMZLPD cases with plasmacytic differentiation, whereas IgG4 is rarely expressed in non-cutaneous MZL.[41,42] There is no evidence of systemic IgG4 disease in these cases, pointing to a localized immunologic IgG4-driven process. The second type, consisting of a small subset of (P)CMZLPD, shows large nodules or sheets of small B-cells, including monocytoid B cells, which express IgM and often CXCR3 and IRTA1.[43] These cases contain a much lower number of admixed T cells and are more likely have extracutaneous disease.[37]

Genetic Features

Clonal rearrangements of the immunoglobulin heavy chain (IGH) gene are found in approximately 80% of cases. The presence of the t(14;18)(q32;q21) translocation involving the IGH gene on chromosome 14, the *MALT* gene on chromosome 18, and the t(3;14)(p14.1;q32) translocation involving the IGH and *FOXP1* genes has been reported in a proportion of PCMZLPDs.[44-46] In one of these studies, the t(14;18)(q32;q21) translocation was only found in cases with a (partly) monocytoid appearance, as often seen in MZL in other organs.[46] Other translocations observed in MALT lymphomas at other sites, such as t(11;18)(q21;q21) and t(1;14)(p22;q32), are not or rarely found in PCMZLPD.[24,46-48] Mutations in the *FAS* gene affecting the functionally relevant death domain of the apoptosis-regulating FAS/CD95 protein were found in more than 60% of PCMZLPD cases, a feature distinct from other MALT lymphomas.[49] Highly recurrent mutations were also found in *SLAMF1, SPEN,* and *NCOR2.*[49] MYD88 L265P mutations have been identified in some cases of non-class-switched (IgM-positive) PCMZLPD, but not in common class-switched (IgG-positive) cases.[50]

Differential Diagnosis

The differential diagnosis of PCMZLPD includes cutaneous lymphoid hyperplasia (CLH) (pseudo–B-cell lymphoma; lymphocytoma cutis), PCFCL with a follicular growth pattern, skin localizations of systemic small B-cell lymphomas/leukemias, and primary cutaneous small/medium T cell lymphoproliferative disorder (PCSM-TCLPD).

Differentiation between the common class-switched form of PCMZLPD and CLH can be challenging. Apart from clinical and histologic similarities, clonal B-cell receptor rearrangements have not only been found in approximately 80% of PCMZLPDs, but also in a small subset of CLH.[19,20] Demonstration of monotypic plasma cells expressing either kappa or lambda light chain by immunohistochemistry or in situ hybridization on paraffin sections is generally used as a decisive criterion for PCMZLPD. However, monotypic plasma cells may be minimal, and when evaluating recurrent lesions, they can be undetectable in some of these lesions. The observation that both PCMZLPDs and CLH may develop from chronic stimulation by intradermally applied antigens (e.g., tattoo pigments, tick bites, and antigen injections) suggests they represent a continuous spectrum of cutaneous B-cell proliferations with a stepwise progression from a reactive to a neoplastic state.[19,20] These observations have also resulted in discussions about whether what has traditionally been considered PCMZL, or at least a major subset of those cases, should be considered a clonal lymphoproliferative disorder rather than an overt malignant lymphoma.[12,38,51] The ICC adopted this new terminology, although the proposed WHO 5th edition classification did not.

The clinical and histologic features of MZL arising at noncutaneous sites and involving the skin secondarily may resemble those of PCMZLPD. Histologic features suggesting secondary cutaneous involvement include the presence of a predominant B-cell infiltrate and expression of IgM by the neoplastic B cells.[37] Colonization of follicular structures by neoplastic marginal zone cells and the presence of lymphoepithelial lesions are common in MALT lymphomas at other sites but are rarely seen in PCMZLPD and should therefore raise suspicion of secondary cutaneous involvement. In particular in such cases, staging is necessary to rule out extracutaneous disease. Differentiation between PCMZLPD and skin localizations of other systemic small B-cell lymphomas (e.g., mantle cell lymphoma, chronic lymphocytic leukemia/small lymphocytic lymphoma) may sometimes be difficult based on histology alone.[52] Staining for CD5 and cyclin D1 may be useful to differentiate PCMZLPD (CD5 negative, cyclin D1 negative) from mantle cell lymphoma (CD5 positive, cyclin D1 positive) and skin localizations of chronic lymphocytic leukemia/small lymphocytic lymphoma (CD5 positive, cyclin D1 negative) (Table 19-2). In cases with a predominance of plasma cells, multiple myeloma should be excluded by appropriate staging, which should include a bone marrow biopsy and serum electrophoresis. Differentiation between PCMZLPD and PCFCL is discussed in this chapter's section on PCFCL.

PCMZLPD shows overlapping clinicopathologic features with PCSM-TCLPD.[39] Clinically, both conditions present with a solitary or multiple papules or plaques and show an indolent clinical course. Histologically, they both show polymorphous dermal infiltrates with mixed populations of B cells and T cells. Some cases of PCSM-TCLPD may show monotypic plasma cells and clonal IGH gene rearrangements characteristic of PCMZLPD, and PCMZLPD often contains clusters or rosettes of CD279/PD-1–positive T-cells considered characteristic of PCSM-TCLPD.[39]

Prognosis and Predictive Factors

PCMZL has an indolent clinical course. The prognosis is excellent, with a 5-year disease-specific survival rate close to 100%.[16-18,27]

Therapy

After EORTC/ISCL consensus recommendations, patients with a solitary tumor can be treated with radiotherapy or surgical excision.[53] In patients with associated *B. burgdorferi* infection, systemic antibiotics should be tried before more aggressive therapies are used. For patients presenting with multifocal skin lesions, a wait-and-see strategy can be adopted. Symptomatic lesions can be treated with topical or intralesional steroids, intralesional interferon α or rituximab, or low-dose radiotherapy. Systemic multiagent chemotherapy is rarely needed and should be reserved for patients who develop extracutaneous disease.

PRIMARY CUTANEOUS FOLLICLE CENTER LYMPHOMA

Definition

PCFCL is a tumor of neoplastic follicle center cells with a predominance of large centrocytes (large cleaved cells) admixed with variable numbers of centroblasts (large noncleaved/transformed cells with prominent and, usually, paracentral nucleoli) that may display a follicular, a follicular and diffuse, or a diffuse growth pattern and generally presents on the head or trunk.[1,11] Lymphomas with a diffuse growth pattern and a monotonous proliferation of centroblasts and immunoblasts are, irrespective of site, excluded and classified as PCDLBCL, LT.

Epidemiology

PCFCLs make up about 10% of all cutaneous lymphomas and about 50% of primary CBCLs. They most commonly affect middle-aged adults, with a slight male predominance.[1,16,17]

Clinical Features

PCFCL has a characteristic clinical presentation, with solitary or grouped plaques and tumors preferentially located on the scalp and forehead or on the trunk, but uncommonly on the legs (Fig. 19-2; Table 19-1).[16,17,54] Particularly on the trunk, these tumors may be surrounded by erythematous papules and slightly indurated plaques, which may precede the development of tumorous lesions for months or even many years. In the past, PCFCL with such a typical presentation on the back was referred to as *reticulohistiocytoma of the dorsum* or *Crosti's lymphoma*.[55] Presentation with multifocal skin lesions is observed in approximately 15% of patients but is not associated with a poor prognosis.[16,17,56,57] If left untreated, the skin lesions gradually increase in size over years, but dissemination to extracutaneous sites is uncommon.[16,17]

Histopathology

PCFCL shows perivascular and periadnexal, nodular or diffuse infiltrates with almost constant sparing of the epidermis. The infiltrates may show a follicular, a follicular and diffuse, or a diffuse growth pattern. Cases with a follicular growth pattern show nodular infiltrates throughout the entire dermis, often extending into the subcutaneous fat (Fig. 19-3). In contrast to reactive follicles in CLHs, the neoplastic follicles in PCFCLs are ill-defined, show a monotonous infiltration of generally medium-sized to large centrocytes enmeshed in a network of CD21-positive follicular dendritic cells, lack tingible body macrophages, generally have a reduced or absent mantle zone, and show a variably high proliferation rate with lack of polarization (Fig. 19-3B).[58,59] Reactive T cells may be numerous, and a stromal component is usually present. Cases with a diffuse growth pattern are characterized by a proliferation of medium-sized to large centrocytes, part of which may have a multilobated or spindle-shaped appearance, and variable numbers of admixed centroblasts (Fig. 19-4A). In rare cases, a predominance of centrocytes with a spindle-shaped appearance can be present (Fig. 19-5).[60-62]

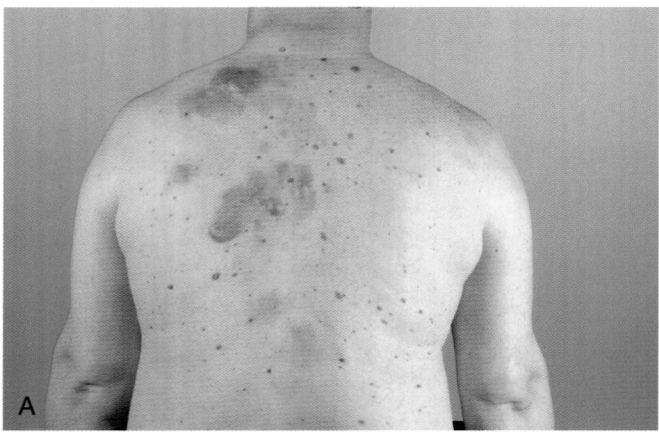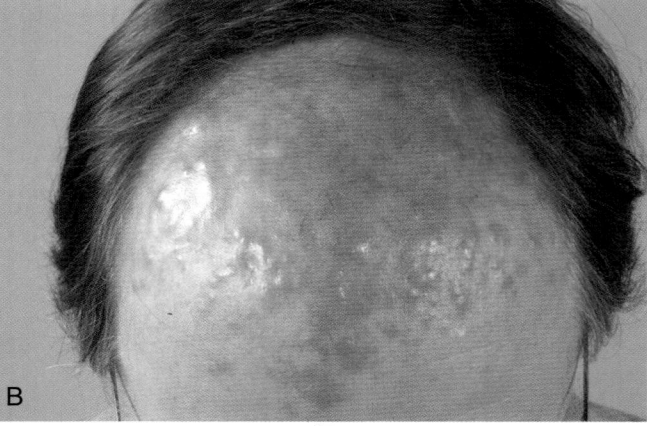

Figure 19-2. Primary cutaneous follicle center lymphoma. Characteristic clinical presentation with localized skin lesions **(A)** on the back (Crosti's lymphoma) and **(B)** on the scalp.

Immunophenotype

The neoplastic cells express the B-cell–associated antigens CD20 and CD79a but are usually Ig negative. PCFCL consistently expresses BCL6, whereas CD10 is often positive in cases with a follicular growth pattern and generally negative in cases with a diffuse growth pattern (Fig. 19-4B).[17,32,33,63-65] Unlike nodal and secondary cutaneous follicular lymphomas, most PCFCLs do not express BCL2 protein or show faint BCL2 staining in a minority of neoplastic B cells (Figs. 19-3 and 19-5).[17,54,58,66-68] However, other studies report BCL2 expression in a significant minority of PCFCL with a (partially) follicular growth pattern.[64,65,69] Notwithstanding, strong and diffuse expression of BCL6, BCL2, and CD10 by the neoplastic B cells should always raise suspicion of a systemic lymphoma secondarily involving the skin (Table 19-1). Staining for IRF4/MUM1, FOXP1, MYC, and IgM is negative in most cases, whereas staining for CD5 and CD43 is always negative.[17,54] In some cases with a diffuse growth pattern, foci of CD21-positive follicular dendritic cells may still be present, though in other cases they may be completely lacking.

Genetic Features

Clonally rearranged immunoglobulin genes are present in most cases. Somatic hypermutation of variable heavy chain and light chain genes has been demonstrated, which further supports the follicle center cell origin of these lymphomas.[70,71] However, another study reported that PCFCL generally lacks ongoing somatic mutation and has low or absent activation-induced cytidine deaminase (AID), both unlike other follicular lymphomas.[72] In many studies, PCFCLs, including cases with a follicular growth pattern, do not or rarely show *BCL2* rearrangements, which is characteristically found in most nodal follicular lymphomas.[58,59,66-68,73] However, other studies report *BCL2* rearrangements using polymerase chain reaction (PCR) and/or fluorescence in situ hybridization (FISH) in about 10% of PCFCL with a follicular growth pattern and in some completely diffuse cases.[65,74-76] Gene expression studies demonstrated that PCFCL has a gene expression profile of germinal-center B-cell (GCB)–type DLBCL.[62,77] Genotypic studies found amplifications of the *REL* gene (63% of cases), as seen in GCB-type DLBCL, deletion of 14q32.33 containing the IGH gene locus (68% of

cases), which may account for the lack of surface Ig in cases of PCFCL, and aberrant somatic hypermutation of certain proto-oncogenes.[78,79] Genes frequently mutated in follicular lymphomas in lymph nodes (e.g., *CREBBP, KTM2D* and *BCL2*) are significantly less commonly mutated in PCFCL.[80,81] Similar to classic follicular lymphomas, but in contrast to PCDLBCL, LT, B-cell receptor genes in PCFCL appear to acquire N-linked glycosylation motifs, although they are mostly at different positions than in other follicular lymphomas.[72] In contrast to PCDLBCL, LT, *MYD88* L265P mutations and inactivation of *CDKN2A* and *CDKN2B* gene loci on chromosome 9p21.3 by deletion or promotor hypermethylation are not or rarely found in PCFCL.[78,82]

Differential Diagnosis

PCFCL with a follicular growth pattern should be differentiated from CLH (pseudo–B-cell lymphoma), PCMZLPD, and systemic follicular lymphomas with secondary cutaneous involvement. In contrast to reactive follicles in pseudo–B-cell lymphomas and PCMZLPDs, neoplastic follicles are ill-defined and show a reduced or absent mantle zone, no or few tingible body macrophages, and a monotonous population of medium-sized to large centrocytes with variable numbers of admixed centroblasts.[58,59] However, distinction between reactive and neoplastic follicles can sometimes be difficult. The presence of clusters of CD10-positive and/or BCL6-positive B cells outside the neoplastic follicles strongly suggests a diagnosis of PCFCL. Demonstration of B-cell clonality supports a diagnosis of CBCL but is by itself insufficient to make a definitive diagnosis. Differentiation between PCFCL and PCMZLPD is generally not difficult and is based on a different clinical presentation and a different morphology and phenotype of the neoplastic B cells (Table 19-2). PCFCL is characterized by the presence of large centrocytes with a BCL6-positive, commonly BCL2-negative, and CD10-positive or CD10-negative phenotype, whereas the neoplastic cells in PCMZLPD have a BCL6-negative, BCL2-positive, and CD10-negative phenotype.[32,33] Moreover, monotypic light chain expression by lymphoplasmacytoid and plasma cells is a hallmark of PCMZLPD and is rarely observed in PCFCL. Distinction between rare cases of PCFCL showing a follicular growth pattern and strong expression of CD10 and BCL2,

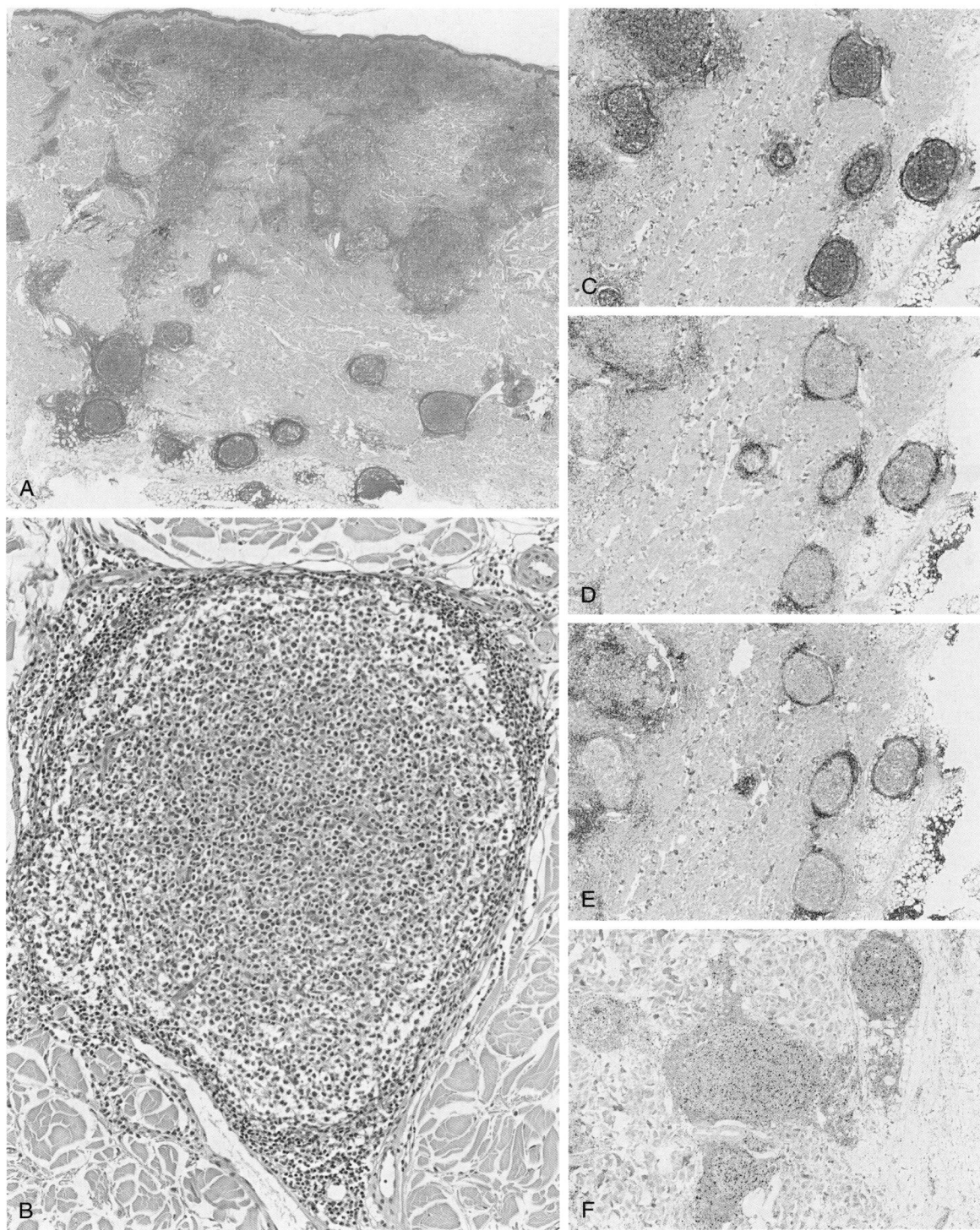

Figure 19-3. Primary cutaneous follicle center lymphoma, follicular and diffuse growth pattern. A, Histology of a skin tumor showing a diffuse infiltrate of neoplastic B cells in the superficial dermis and neoplastic follicles in the deep dermis. **B,** Detail of neoplastic follicles showing a monotonous proliferation of B cells (no polarization), reduced mantle zone, and absence of tingible body macrophages. **C,** Positive staining of neoplastic B cells for CD79a. **D,** CD3-positive T cells at the periphery of the neoplastic follicles. **E,** BCL2 stains T cells, but not intrafollicular neoplastic B cells. **F,** Ki-67 staining shows only few proliferating cells in neoplastic follicles.

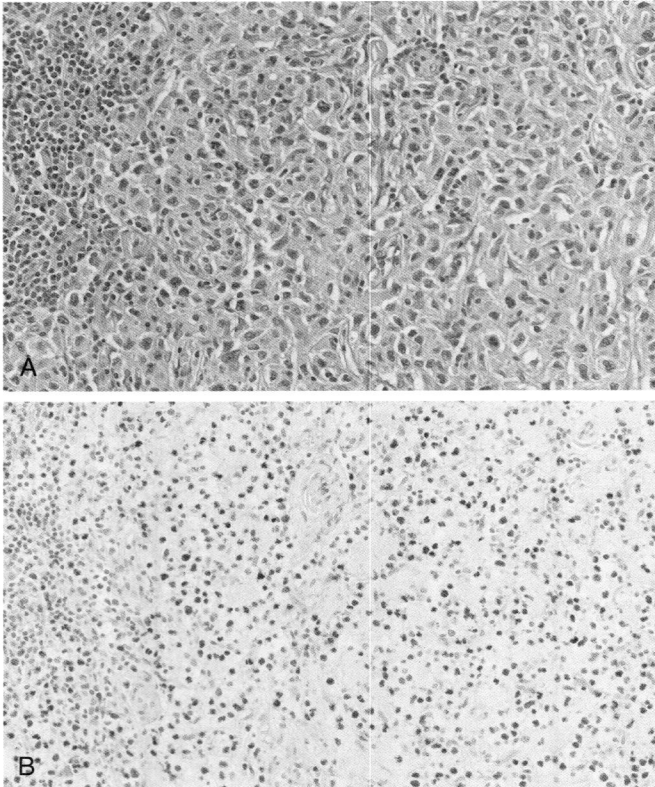

Figure 19-4. Primary cutaneous follicle center lymphoma, diffuse growth pattern. A, Diffuse infiltrate of large centrocytes (large, cleaved cells), partly with a multilobated appearance. **B,** BCL6 expression by neoplastic B cells.

with or without *BCL2* rearrangement, and skin localizations of nodal follicular lymphoma can sometimes be impossible and can only be made after appropriate staging.[64]

PCFCL with a diffuse growth pattern, previously often classified as diffuse large B-cell lymphoma, should be differentiated from PCDLBCL, LT. Clinical, histologic, immunophenotypical, and genetic differences between the conditions are summarized in Table 19-3 and mostly suffice to make a correct diagnosis.

Prognosis and Predictive Factors

PCFCLs have an indolent clinical course. Cutaneous relapses after initial treatment occur in approximately 30% of patients, whereas extracutaneous dissemination is reported in approximately 10% of patients.[16,17] PCFCLs have an excellent prognosis with a 5-year disease-specific survival rate of 95%, irrespective of the growth pattern (follicular, follicular and diffuse, or diffuse), the number of blast cells, the presence or absence of BCL2 expression or *BCL2* rearrangements, or the presence of either localized or generalized skin lesions.[1,16,17,83] Rare cases of PCFCL presenting on the leg are reported to have a poor prognosis, similar to that of patients with PCDLBCL, LT.[17,54]

Therapy

In patients with localized skin lesions, radiotherapy is the preferred mode of treatment.[53] Solitary lesions that are small and well-demarcated can be treated with surgical excision. Cutaneous relapses do not indicate progressive disease and can be treated with radiotherapy as well. For relapses,

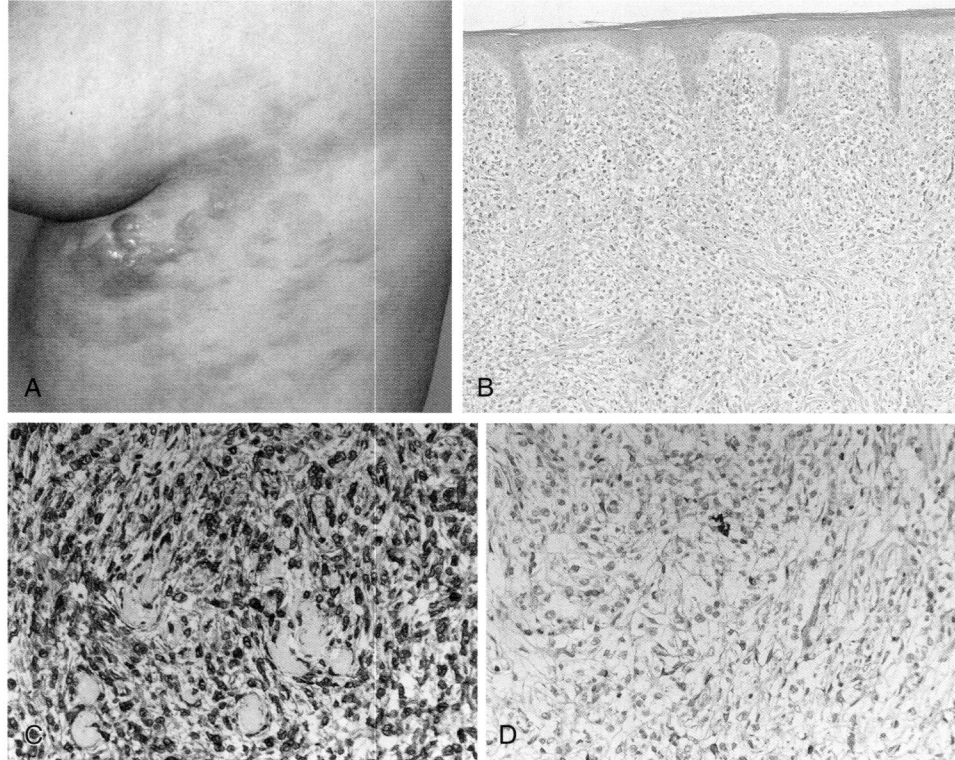

Figure 19-5. Primary cutaneous follicle center lymphoma, spindle-cells. A, Clinical presentation with tumors and plaques on a localized area on the trunk. **B,** Diffuse proliferation of centrocytes with a spindle-cell morphology. **C,** Positive staining for CD79a. **D,** Neoplastic B cells do not stain for BCL2.

Table 19-3 Characteristic Features of PCFCL With a Diffuse Proliferation of Large Cells and PCDLBCL, LT

	PCFCL, Diffuse Large Cell	PCDLBCL, LT
Clinical presentation	Localized skin lesions on head or trunk	Skin tumors on (lower) leg(s); uncommon at other sites
Histopathology		
Morphology tumor cells	Predominance of large centrocytes, including multilobated and spindle cells; centroblasts may be present but not in confluent sheets	Predominance or confluent sheets of medium-sized to large centroblasts and/or immunoblasts
Admixed T cells	Often abundant	Sparse, mainly perivascular
Immunohistochemistry		
B-cell lineage markers	CD20+, CD79a+, PAX5+ IgM−, IgD−	CD20+, CD79a+, PAX5+ IgM+, IgD+/−; monotypic light chain expression
Germinal-center markers	BCL6+, BCL2−/+, CD10−/+	BCL6+/−, BCL2+, CD10−
Post–germinal-center markers	IRF4/MUM1−, FOXP1−	IRF4/MUM1+, FOXP1+
MYC expression	Negative	Positive
CD21: (remnants of) FDC networks	May be present	Absent
Molecular Genetics		
Translocations MYC, BCL6, BCL2	BCL2 (10%)	MYC (30%), BCL6 (30%), IGH (50%); no BCL2 breaks
Copy number variations	Amplification 2p16.1 region, deletion 14q11.2-q12 region	Deletion 6q arm Deletion 9p21.3 region (CDKN2A; 67%)
NF-κB pathway mutations	No MYD88 mutations	MYD88 (70%), CD79B (20%)

FDC, Follicular dendritic cell; IgD, immunoglobulin D; IgM, immunoglobulin M; LT, leg type; PCDLBCL, primary cutaneous diffuse large B-cell lymphoma; PCFCL, primary cutaneous follicle center lymphoma; PCMZLPD, primary cutaneous marginal zone lymphoproliferative disorder.
From Willemze R, Cerroni L, Kempf W, et al. The 2018 update of the WHO-EORTC classification for primary cutaneous lymphomas. *Blood.* 2019;133:1703-1714.

a palliative dose of 4 Gy can be used, which will result in effective local control in 90% of cases.[84] In patients with few scattered lesions, both low-dose radiotherapy and a wait-and-see policy with treatment of only symptomatic lesions can be considered, similar to the recommendations for PCMZLPD. Systemic or intralesional administration of rituximab is a safe and effective treatment for patients with generalized skin lesions, but cutaneous relapses are frequently observed.[85,86] Multiagent chemotherapy (CHOP [cyclophosphamide, doxorubicin, vincristine, and prednisone] in combination with rituximab [R-CHOP]) should be reserved for patients who develop extracutaneous disease and only for exceptional patients with generalized skin lesions that do not respond to other treatment modalities. Patients with a PCFCL presenting on the leg(s) have a similar prognosis as those with PCDLBCL, LT and should be treated as such.[17,54]

PRIMARY CUTANEOUS DIFFUSE LARGE B-CELL LYMPHOMA, LEG TYPE

Definition

PCDLBCL, LT is characterized by tumors with a predominance or confluent sheets of centroblasts and immunoblasts, most commonly arising on the legs. Uncommonly, skin lesions with a similar morphology and phenotype can arise at sites other than the legs. Initially, these lymphomas, classified as centroblastic and/or B-immunoblastic lymphomas according to the Kiel classification, were included in the group of PCFCLs and recognized as a subgroup with an inferior prognosis.[87] Because of their characteristic clinical presentation, morphology, immunophenotype, and clinical behavior that were all different from PCFCL with a diffuse proliferation of large centrocytes, these lymphomas were included as a separate entity in the EORTC classification and, later on, with slight modifications, in the WHO-EORTC, WHO, and ICC classifications.[1,9-11,12]

Epidemiology

PCDLBCL, LTs account for about 4% of all cutaneous lymphomas and about 15% to 20% of primary CBCLs.[1] It typically occurs in elderly patients with a median age of around 75 years and is more frequent in women.[54,72]

Clinical Features

Patients present with generally rapidly growing red or bluish-red tumors on one or both (lower) legs or in approximately 20% at sites other than the legs (Fig. 19-6A).[17,54,88] In contrast to PCFCLs, these lymphomas more often disseminate to extracutaneous sites and have a poor prognosis (Table 19-1).[17,54,89]

Histopathology

These lymphomas show diffuse non-epidermotropic infiltrates, which often extend into the subcutaneous tissue. The infiltrates are composed of a monotonous population or confluent sheets of large B cells with round nuclei and prominent nucleoli; in general, a mixed population of centroblasts and immunoblasts is seen (Fig. 19-6B).[17,63,89] Mitotic figures are frequently observed. Small B cells and (remnants of) CD21-positive follicular dendritic cell networks are lacking, and reactive T cells are relatively few and often confined to perivascular areas.

Immunophenotype

The neoplastic cells express the B-cell–associated antigens CD20 and CD79a and, unlike PCFCLs, are strongly positive for BCL2, IRF4/MUM1, FOXP1, MYC, and cytoplasmic IgM with monotypic light chain expression and co-expression of IgD in 50% of cases (Fig. 19-6C–E). BCL6 is expressed in most cases, whereas CD10 staining is generally absent.[17,63,90-92] However, in approximately 10% of cases, deviations of this typical immunophenotype (e.g., BCL2 or IRF4/MUM1 negativity and weak CD10 positivity) may be found. Such cases might still be diagnosed as PCDLBCL, LT if the other diagnostic features

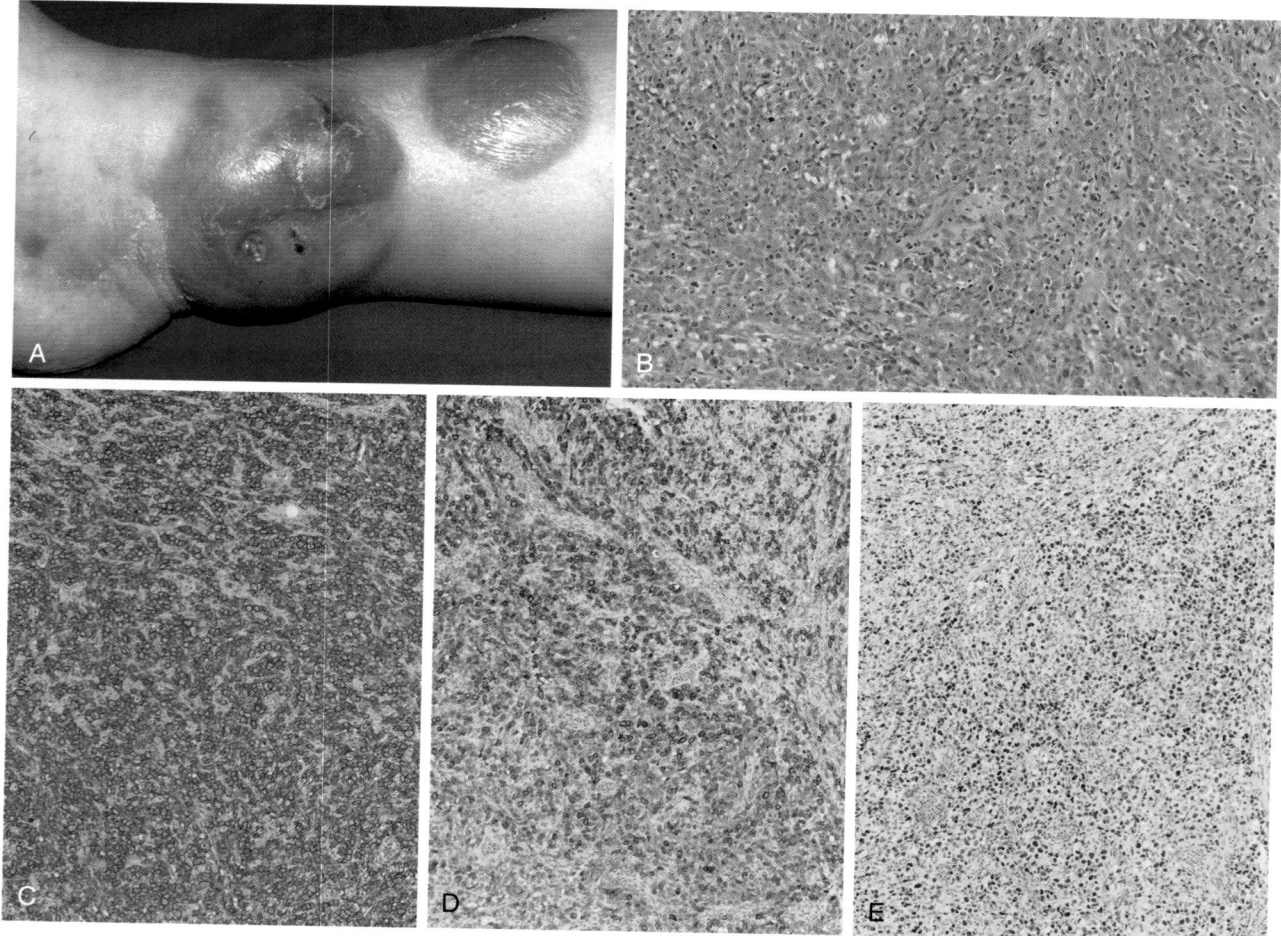

Figure 19-6. Primary cutaneous diffuse large B-cell lymphoma, leg type. A, Clinical presentation with large tumors on the right lower leg. **B,** Diffuse proliferation of centroblasts and immunoblasts. Tumor cells show strong reactivity for CD20 **(C),** immunoglobulin M **(D),** and MYC **(E).**

of the entity are present (Table 19-3).[17,54,93] Ki-67 generally stains more than 75% of the neoplastic cells.

Genetic Features

Genetic studies showed marked differences between PCDLBCL, LT and PCFCL with a diffuse proliferation of large B cells.[62,77,82] Chromosomal translocations involving *BCL6, MYC,* and *IGH* are frequently found in PCDLBCL, LT, but *BCL2* translocations are exceptional.[92,94-96] The strong BCL2 expression in PCDLBCL, LT may be explained by high-level amplifications of the *BCL2* gene reported in 67% of cases.[78] Loss of *CDKN2A* and *CDKN2B* either by gene deletion or promoter methylation has been reported in 67% to 75% of cases and correlates with a poor prognosis.[78,97,98] PCDLBCL, LTs show highly recurrent *MYD88* L265P mutations (70%–75%), frequent mutations in *PIM1,* and mutations in other genes affecting the NF-κB and B-cell receptor signaling pathways, including *CD79B, CARD11,* and *TNFAIP3/A20.*[96,99,100] Genetic alterations in immune evasion pathways, such as deletions of the *MHCI/II* loci and the MHC regulator *CIITA* and translocations of the *PD-L1/2* loci have been described.[98,101] The mutational profile of PCDLBCL, LT resembles that of lymphomas arising in immune-privileged sites, as in primary DLBCL of the central nervous system (CNS) and testis[93,96,98,101] and DLBCL of the MCD/C5 type.[102,103]

Differential Diagnosis

PCDLBCL, LT should be differentiated from PCFCL with a diffuse proliferation of large centrocytes, systemic DLBCL secondarily involving the skin, and several other specific types of large B-cell lymphomas. Differentiation between PCDLBCL, LT and PCFCL is extremely important, because the conditions have different prognoses and require different therapeutic approaches. Distinguishing features are summarized in Table 19-3. In rare cases that cannot be classified as either PCDLBCL, LT or PCFCL, PCDLBCL, NOS might be diagnosed, which should, however, not be considered as a specific entity. Distinction between PCDLBCL, LT and systemic DLBCL with secondary cutaneous involvement requires adequate staging. Plasmablastic lymphomas are seen almost exclusively in the setting of HIV infection or other immune deficiencies, including in the elderly with immune senescence.[104-106] Some of these cases have only skin lesions at presentation.[107] Rare cases of primary cutaneous T-cell/histiocyte–rich B-cell lymphoma, characterized by the presence of large scattered B cells on a background of numerous reactive T cells and histiocytes, have been reported.[108,109] Clinically, these lymphomas commonly present with a solitary skin tumor on the head or on the trunk and show similarities with the group of PCFCLs. Unlike their nodal counterparts, they appear to have an excellent prognosis.[110]

Other specific types of DLBCL that can present with only skin lesions, such as intravascular large B-cell lymphoma, immunodeficiency-related B-cell neoplasms, and B-lymphoblastic lymphoma (B-LBL), are discussed later in this chapter.

Prognosis, Predictive Factors, and Treatment

These lymphomas have a much more aggressive clinical behavior and poorer prognosis than PCFCL and PCMZLPD. Previous studies reported a disease-specific 5-year survival rate of approximately 50%.[17,83,89] More recent studies reported a significantly better clinical outcome for patients treated with a combination of multiagent chemotherapy (CHOP or CHOP-like) and rituximab than for patients treated with multiagent chemotherapy regimens alone.[88,111] The presence of multiple skin lesions at diagnosis, inactivation of *CDKN2A* either by deletion or hypermethylation, and presence of *MYC* translocations have been reported to be associated with an inferior prognosis.[78,83,92,95,112]

INTRAVASCULAR LARGE B-CELL LYMPHOMA

Intravascular large B-cell lymphoma is a large B-cell lymphoma, defined by an accumulation of large neoplastic B cells within blood vessels. These lymphomas preferentially affect the CNS, lungs, and skin and are generally associated with a poor prognosis. Patients often have widely disseminated disease, but cases with only skin involvement may occur. This so-called "cutaneous variant" predominantly affects females and is more frequent in the Western world.[113] Clinically, patients may present with violaceous patches and plaques or telangiectatic skin lesions, usually on the (lower) legs or the trunk (Fig. 19-7A).[113] Patients presenting with only skin lesions appear to have a significantly better survival rate than patients with other clinical presentations.[113] In rare cases, intravascular B-cell lymphomas develop within the capillaries of cutaneous hemangiomas.[114,115] Histologically, blood vessels in the dermis and subcutis are filled and often dilated by a proliferation of large neoplastic B cells (Fig. 19-7B). The tumor cells express the B-cell–associated antigens, BCL2, IRF4/MUM1, IgM, and MYC; CD5 and PD-L1 (CD274) expression is seen in about half of the cases.[116-118] Tumor cells may cause vascular occlusion of venules, capillaries, and arterioles. In some cases, small numbers of tumor cells can also be observed around blood vessels. These lymphomas show recurrent mutations in *MYD88* L265P and *CD79B* Y196 and rearrangements of *PD-L1* and *PD-L2* genes, similar to those observed in PCDLBCL, LT and lymphomas arising in immune-privileged sites such as primary DLBCL of the CNS and testis.[117-119] Multiagent chemotherapy in combination with rituximab is the preferred mode of treatment, also in patients presenting with skin-limited disease.[120,121]

B-LYMPHOBLASTIC LYMPHOMA

B-LBL particularly affects children and young adults and often involves extracutaneous sites, most often the skin. Characteristically, patients present with a solitary tumor in the head and neck region, which can be the only manifestation of the disease.[122-125] Histologically, they show a diffuse monotonous infiltrate of medium-sized blast cells with often round nuclei, finely dispersed chromatin, inconspicuous nucleoli, and scant cytoplasm. A starry-sky pattern may be present. The neoplastic cells usually express CD79a, PAX5, CD10, and TdT, whereas CD20 expression may be weak or absent. CD99 is expressed in a proportion of cases. Patients should be treated with aggressive multiagent chemotherapy analogous to that designed for B-acute lymphoblastic leukemia, even when presenting with a solitary skin tumor. With this approach, the prognosis is often good.[126]

EBV-POSITIVE MUCOCUTANEOUS ULCER AND OTHER CUTANEOUS IMMUNODEFICIENCY-ASSOCIATED B-CELL LYMPHOPROLIFERATIVE DISORDERS

EBV-positive mucocutaneous ulcer (EBVMCU) is defined as a solitary, sharply demarcated ulcerating lesion involving the skin, oropharyngeal mucosa, or gastrointestinal tract in patients with age-related or iatrogenic immunosuppression (e.g., methotrexate [MTX], azathioprine, cyclosporine, TNF inhibitors).[1,11,12] Histologically, the lesions contain large Hodgkin-like EBV-positive B cells on a mixed inflammatory background. These large, transformed cells are PAX5 positive, show variable expression of CD20, display a non–germinal-center phenotype (IRF4/MUM1+, CD10–, BCL6–), and typically express CD30 with co-expression of CD15 in almost half of the cases.[127] EBVMCU usually runs a self-limited, indolent course. In iatrogenic cases, reduction of

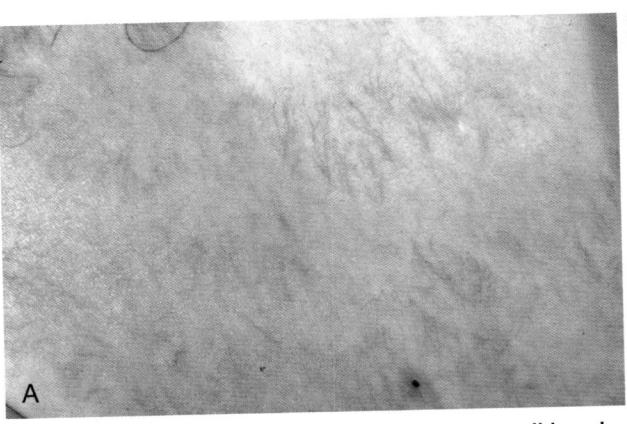
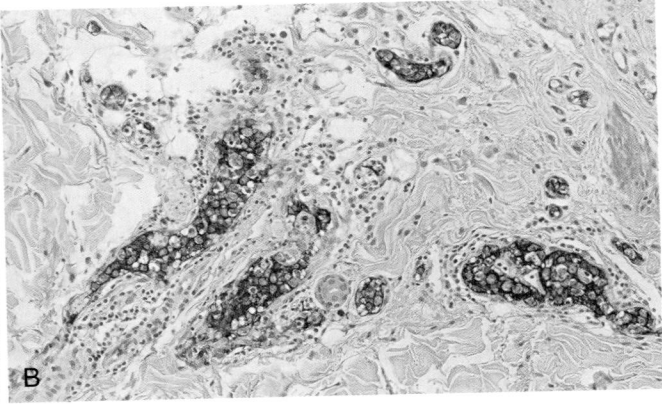

Figure 19-7. Intravascular large B-cell lymphoma. A, Clinical presentation with telangiectatic lesions on the trunk and legs. **B,** Intravascular population of CD20-positive large neoplastic B cells.

immunosuppressive therapy without additional chemotherapy or radiotherapy may result in complete remission.[127]

Apart from EBVMCU, there are other cutaneous manifestations of B-cell LPD occurring in the setting of iatrogenic immunosuppression: skin lesions may be EBV positive or negative and both can be solitary or generalized, with or without ulceration.[128] MTX-associated B-cell LPD usually shows the histology of DLBCL or has Hodgkin-like features. The latter is particularly seen in EBV-positive cases,

which account for 40% to 50% of all cases. Recognition of these iatrogenic immunodeficiency-associated lesions is important, as in all cases reduction or cessation of immunosuppressive treatment may result in (complete) remissions and should be attempted before more aggressive therapy is considered.[128,129]

Other EBV-positive conditions, such as EBV-positive DLBCL of the elderly and lymphomatoid granulomatosis, can occasionally present in the skin but are generally a manifestation of systemic disease (see Chapter 28).[130-132]

Pearls and Pitfalls

- Analogous to the term *CTCL* for primary cutaneous T-cell lymphomas, the term *CBCL* is preferably used only for B-cell lymphomas that present in the skin without evidence of extracutaneous disease at the time of diagnosis (primary CBCL). It is important to differentiate these CBCLs from systemic B-cell lymphomas secondarily involving the skin.
- Although histologic features may suggest a diagnosis of CBCL, a definitive diagnosis of CBCL can only be made if extracutaneous disease has been ruled out by adequate staging procedures.
- The localization of the presenting skin lesions in CBCL provides important diagnostic information: PCFCL preferentially presents with localized skin lesions on the head (mainly the scalp) or trunk, PCMZLPD on the trunk and/or upper arms, and PCDLBCL, LT on the (lower) legs.
- The presence of monotypic plasma cells at the periphery of dermal infiltrates and in the superficial dermis beneath the epidermis is a characteristic feature of PCMZLPD.
- The presence of a diffuse proliferation of small neoplastic B cells, expression of IgM, colonization of reactive germinal centers, and the presence of lymphoepithelial lesions are uncommon in PCMZLPD and should raise suspicion of secondary cutaneous involvement of systemic MZL.
- Distinction between low-grade malignant CBCL (i.e., PCMZLPD and PCFCL) and CLH (pseudo–B-cell lymphoma) may sometimes be extremely difficult. Demonstration of B-cell clonality supports a diagnosis of CBCL but is by itself insufficient evidence for a definitive diagnosis.
- The observation that both PCMZLPD and CLH (pseudo–B-cell lymphoma) may develop from chronic stimulation by intradermally applied antigens, such as tattoo pigments, tick bites, and antigen injections, suggests they represent a continuous spectrum of cutaneous B-cell proliferations.
- PCFCL may show a follicular, a follicular and diffuse, or a completely diffuse growth pattern, with a predominance of large centrocytes with varying proportions of admixed centroblasts (CBs). Neither the growth pattern nor the proportion of CBs affects prognosis.
- Presence of BCL2 expression or a *BCL2* translocation in a cutaneous B-cell lymphoma with a follicular growth pattern should raise the possibility of systemic follicular lymphoma with secondary cutaneous involvement but does not exclude a diagnosis of PCFCL. In case of BCL2 expression or a *BCL2* translocation in PCFCL, prognosis is not affected.
- Distinction between PCFCL, diffuse type and PCDLBCL, LT is primarily based on morphologic criteria: PCFCL shows a predominance of large centrocytes, and PCDLBCL, LT is composed of centroblasts and immunoblasts. Additional immunophenotypic criteria include strong expression of BCL2, IRF4/MUM1, MYC, and cytoplasmic IgM, which is observed in most cases of PCDLBCL, LT but uncommon in PCFCL.
- The mutational profile of PCDLBCL, LT resembles that of B-cell lymphomas arising in immune-privileged sites, such as primary DLBCL of the CNS and testis, and shares similarities with the genetic signatures described in MCD/C5 DLBCL.
- In cases of cutaneous DLBCL with polymorphous or Hodgkin-like B cells, additional CD30 staining and in situ hybridization for EBV (EBER) should be performed and a diagnosis of immunodeficiency-associated lymphoproliferative disorder should be considered.
- B-lymphoblastic lymphoma sometimes presents with a solitary skin tumor in the head and neck region as the only manifestation of the disease. These patients should be treated with aggressive multiagent chemotherapy designed for B-acute lymphoblastic leukemia and may have a good prognosis.

KEY REFERENCES

1. Willemze R, Cerroni L, Kempf W, et al. The 2018 update of the WHO-EORTC classification for primary cutaneous lymphomas. *Blood.* 2019;133:1703–1714.
11. Alaggio R, Amador C, Anagnostopoulos I, et al. The 5th edition of the World Health Organization Classification of Haematolymphoid Tumours: lymphoid neoplasms. *Leukemia.* 2022;36:1720–1748.
12. Campo E, Jaffe ES, Cook JR, et al. The International Consensus Classification of Mature Lymphoid Neoplasms: A Report From the Clinical Advisory Committee. *Blood.* 2022;140:1229–1253.
38. Swerdlow SH. Cutaneous marginal zone lymphomas. *Semin Diagn Pathol.* 2017;34:76–84.
53. Senff NJ, Noordijk EM, Kim YH, et al. European Organization for Research and Treatment of Cancer (EORTC) and International Society for Cutaneous Lymphoma (ISCL) consensus recommendations for the management of cutaneous B-cell lymphomas. *Blood.* 2008;112:1600–1609.

72. Koning MT, Quinten E, Zoutman WH, et al. Acquired N-linked glycosylation motifs in B-cell receptors of primary cutaneous B-cell lymphoma and the normal B-cell repertoire. *J Invest Dermatol.* 2019;139:2195–2203.
80. Barasch NJK, Liu YC, Ho J, et al. The molecular landscape and other distinctive features of primary cutaneous follicle center lymphoma. *Hum Pathol.* 2020;106:93–105.
81. Zhou XA, Yang J, Ringbloom KG, et al. Genomic landscape of cutaneous follicular lymphomas reveals 2 subgroups with clinically predictive molecular features. *Blood Adv.* 2021;5:649–661.
93. Schrader AMR, de Groen RAL, Willemze R, et al. Cell-of-origin classification using the Hans and Lymph2Cx algorithms in primary cutaneous large B-cell lymphomas. *Virchows Arch.* 2022;480:667–675.
101. Zhou XA, Louissaint A, Wenzel A, et al. Genomic analyses identify recurrent alterations in immune evasion genes in diffuse large B-cell lymphoma, leg type. *J Invest Dermatol.* 2018;138:2365–2376.

118. Shimada K, Yoshida K, Suzuki Y, et al. Frequent genetic alterations in immune checkpoint-related genes in intravascular large B-cell lymphoma. *Blood.* 2021;137:1491–1502.

128. Koens L, Senff NJ, Vermeer MH, Willemze R, Jansen PM. Methotrexate-associated B-cell lymphoproliferative disorders presenting in the skin: a clinicopathologic and immunophenotypical study of 10 cases. *Am J Surg Pathol.* 2014;38:999–1006.

Visit Elsevier eBooks+ for the complete set of references.

Chapter 20

Nodal Marginal Zone Lymphoma

Elaine S. Jaffe

DEFINITION

Nodal marginal zone lymphoma (NMZL) is a primary nodal B-cell neoplasm derived from post–germinal-center B cells. This lymphoma shares morphologic and immunophenotypic similarities with other marginal zone lymphomas, particularly extranodal marginal zone lymphoma (EMZL) of mucosa-associated lymphoid tissue (MALT) type and splenic marginal zone lymphoma (SMZL). Thus, secondary lymph node involvement by EMZL and SMZL should be excluded to establish the diagnosis with certainty. NMZL may show some evidence of plasmacytic differentiation, but it is generally less than that seen in lymphoplasmacytic lymphoma (LPL), which is often included in the differential diagnosis.

EPIDEMIOLOGY, ETIOLOGY, AND COFACTORS

NMZL is a relatively uncommon lymphoma, accounting for 1.5% to 1.8% of all lymphoid neoplasms.[1,2] It is primarily a lymphoma of adults. The median age of patients is between 50 and 60 years, with a female predominance in some, but not all, series.[3-6] An association with hepatitis C infection has been suggested in some studies[6,7] but not in others.[3] These discrepant results may relate to overlap among a variety of B-cell neoplasms and different diagnostic criteria. The distinctions among NMZL, EMZL, and SMZL can be difficult, and hepatitis C has been linked to both EMZL and SMZL.[8-11] Alternatively, these differences could relate to different risk factors in different populations of patients or geographic regions.

Underlying autoimmune disease has been implicated in a variety of EMZLs, including Sjögren syndrome and Hashimoto's thyroiditis.[12] However, a history of autoimmune disease is lacking in most patients with NMZL. Nodal involvement may be prominent in many patients with salivary gland MALT lymphoma, with a predominance of monocytoid B cells.[13] Therefore, a careful clinical history is important in the evaluation of these cases. Both autoimmune hemolytic anemia and cryoglobulinemia have been reported in a subset of patients with NMZL.[3,14] However, the incidence is much less than that seen with LPL. Molecular studies have identified a high incidence of mutations in *MYD88* at L265P in Waldenström macroglobulinemia and LPL but only rarely in NMZL, facilitating this distinction.[15,16]

CLINICAL FEATURES

The majority of patients have generalized peripheral lymphadenopathy,[2,3,6] although two series found a higher proportion of localized stage I or stage II disease.[4,5,17]

B symptoms are present in a minority.[18] Clinical evaluation should be undertaken to rule out secondary nodal involvement by EMZL or SMZL, given the significant overlap in the morphologic features in lymph nodes.[17] Most investigators require the absence of extranodal sites of disease (other than bone marrow, liver, or spleen) in making the diagnosis.[4] Similarly, patients presenting with marked splenomegaly and bone marrow involvement with only minimal lymphadenopathy most likely fall into the category of SMZL. These imprecise diagnostic criteria make it difficult to compare clinical features and outcomes.

Bone marrow involvement is relatively uncommon in most series, occurring in less than half of the patients.[6] Peripheral blood involvement is generally rare, and the presence of circulating cells should at least raise the suspicion of other forms of B-cell neoplasia, including SMZL and atypical chronic lymphocytic leukemia (CLL). According to the International Prognostic Index (IPI) or the modified Follicular Lymphoma IPI (FLIPI), most patients are in the low or low-intermediate risk groups.[6] Elevations in lactate dehydrogenase are common but are usually modest.[18]

Although plasmacytoid differentiation can be observed histologically, it is uncommon to find monoclonal gammopathy in the serum.[14] One exception was the French series reported by Traverse-Glehen and colleagues[3] in which 33% of patients had an M component or monoclonal spike. These distinctions may relate to differences in diagnostic criteria and the overlap between NMZL and LPL in tissue biopsies.

MORPHOLOGY

Cytologic Features

The neoplastic cells in NMZL are heterogeneous in appearance and have been described as monocytoid, centrocyte-like, and plasmacytoid.[3,17] These smaller cells are usually admixed with a variable number of transformed cells or blasts. Monocytoid cells have round-to-irregular nuclei with condensed nuclear chromatin, inconspicuous nucleoli, and abundant pale cytoplasm with distinct cytoplasmic membranes (Fig. 20-1). A monocytoid appearance is even more pronounced with secondary lymph node involvement by MALT lymphoma (Fig. 20-2). This histologic pattern should prompt a clinical evaluation for EMZL either concurrently or in the possibly distant past. Late relapses of EMZL have been described, sometimes many years after the primary diagnosis.[12,17] Centrocyte-like cells can be numerous in some cases. These small to medium-sized cells have coarsely clumped chromatin, irregular nuclei, and sparse cytoplasm. Plasmacytoid cells exhibit varying degrees of plasmacytoid differentiation. They are often slightly larger than the other cell types present, with an ample rim of basophilic cytoplasm. The nuclear chromatin is generally more dispersed than that of mature plasma cells, and small nucleoli may be present. Dutcher bodies may be seen but are generally less common than in LPL. Larger lymphoid cells or blasts, reminiscent of centroblasts, are present in variable proportions but should not constitute the

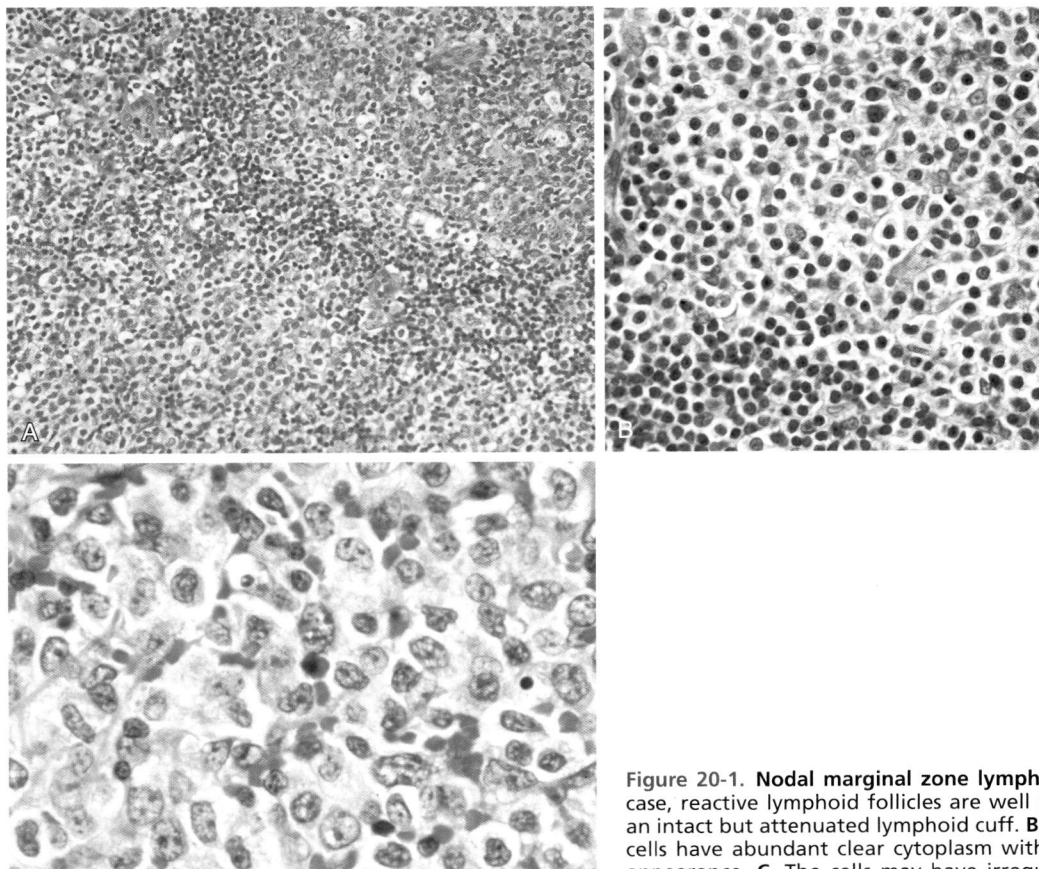

Figure 20-1. **Nodal marginal zone lymphoma. A,** In this case, reactive lymphoid follicles are well preserved, with an intact but attenuated lymphoid cuff. **B,** The neoplastic cells have abundant clear cytoplasm with a monocytoid appearance. **C,** The cells may have irregular nuclei, and admixed blasts are few.

majority of cells present. The overall impression is that of a heterogeneous population of cells that are medium in size, generally round but irregular, and lacking the monotony seen in some other B-cell lymphomas such as CLL or mantle cell lymphoma.

Other inflammatory cells, particularly epithelioid histiocytes, may be present. However, well-formed granulomas are usually absent. Eosinophils may be noted, particularly in cases with plasmacytoid differentiation.[19]

Architectural Features

Varied architectural patterns are seen in NMZL.[3,17,20] In many instances, the infiltrate is diffuse.[20] However, often there is some semblance of residual follicles that can be expanded, regressed, or, in some instances, colonized by neoplastic cells. In most cases, the follicles are regressed, with absence of well-formed germinal centers. The regressed follicles may be better appreciated by stains for CD21, which highlight tight FDC meshworks (Figs. 20-2 and 20-3).

The mantle cuff might be present but is usually attenuated. The neoplastic cells may be weakly immunoglobulin (Ig)D positive, but expression of IgD is dimmer than that seen in residual mantle cuffs.

Follicular colonization can be a prominent feature in NMZL, and extensive infiltration of residual follicles may impart a nodular or follicular growth pattern, mimicking follicular lymphoma (FL).[21] Follicular colonization also has been described in EMZL.[22] In some cases, the cytology of the cells within the colonized follicles may be different from that of the cells in the perifollicular zone and may show evidence of plasmacytoid differentiation. A higher proportion of blastic cells is sometimes noted within the colonized follicles. Finally, in some cases, the follicles contain a high content of small lymphocytes of T-cell lineage,[23] which may be associated with residual FDCs.

Cases that have been referred to as the pediatric variant of NMZL have distinctive features and will be discussed separately.[24]

Other Anatomic Sites

The appearance of NMZL in other anatomic sites is not well described. The incidence of bone marrow involvement has varied in different series, with most centers reporting a range of 20% to 40%.[18] Bone marrow infiltration generally consists of loose non-paratrabecular aggregates or, in some cases, interstitial infiltration.[25] One study also noted paratrabecular aggregates in some cases.[3] As previously noted, peripheral blood involvement is rare. Involvement of other extranodal sites usually leads to consideration of the diagnosis of EMZL.

Grading

There is no established grading system for NMZL, although considerable variation in the proportion of blastic cells or proliferating cells (as measured by Ki67) may be seen. In general, the proportion of blastic cells is less than 20% of the total cell population[14] (Fig. 20-4). Some authors have reported cases with foci of large cell transformation, but the clinical significance of these foci has not been shown.[1] In a subsequent study, the Lyon group noted that a number of cases contained more than 20% blastic cells and suggested that this feature might account for the more aggressive clinical course in that series.[3] However, the investigators were unable to relate outcome to the proportion of large cells or histologic progression. Specifically, there was no difference in survival between the groups with greater than 20% and less than 20% large cells. Nathwani and coworkers[2] reported a relatively high frequency (20%) of transformation to diffuse large B-cell lymphoma in NMZL, but the criteria for transformation were not delineated. Moreover, no difference in survival for those patients who had "transformed" was shown. One study from Japan found a poorer overall survival for cases of NMZL containing a component of diffuse large B-cell lymphoma, but overall, there was no difference in survival for the four histologic subtypes identified: splenic type, floral type, MALT type, and MALT type plus diffuse large B-cell lymphoma.[26] Our practice is to perform Ki67/MIB1 staining in cases of NMZL and to note in the report if the proliferation

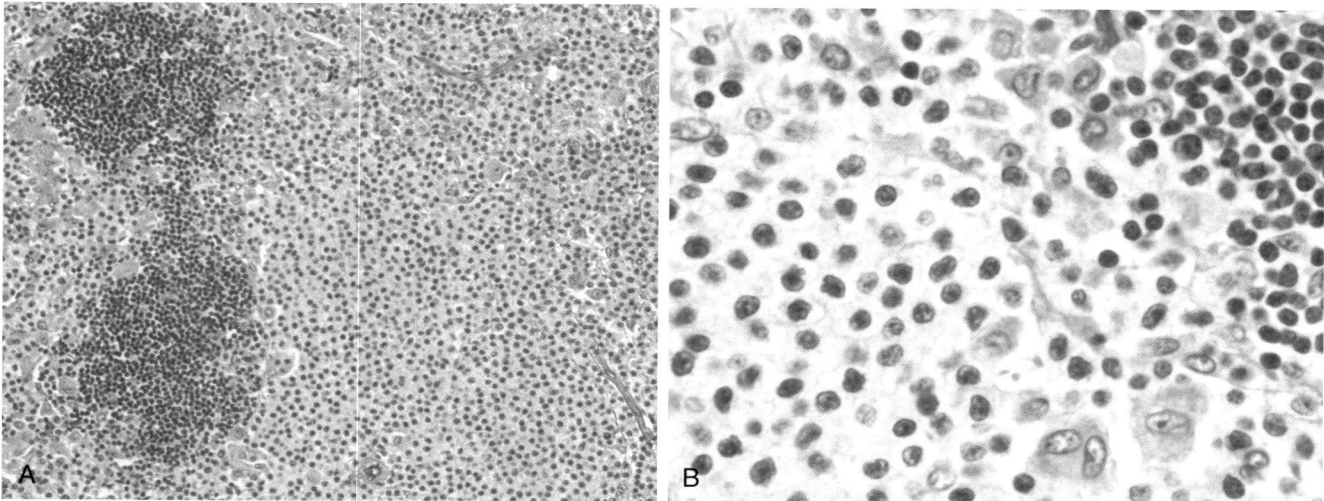

Figure 20-2. Secondary extranodal marginal zone lymphoma in the lymph node of a patient with Sjögren syndrome. A, Atypical monocytoid cells surround residual follicular structures. **B,** The cells have abundant clear cytoplasm and distinct cytoplasmic membranes.

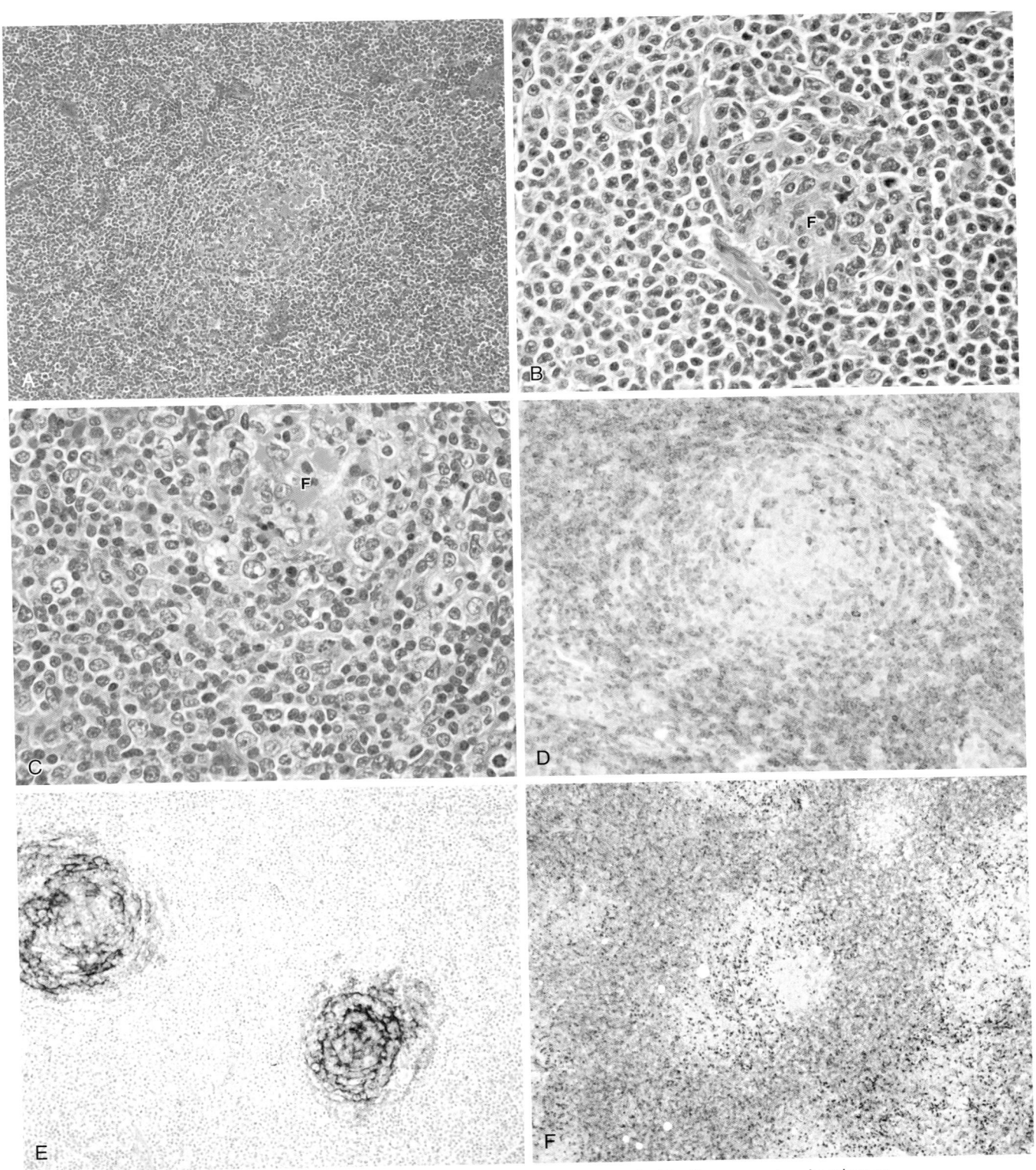

Figure 20-3. Nodal marginal zone lymphoma. A, Atypical lymphoid cells surround and replace regressed germinal centers. **B,** A small, regressed follicle is present in the center (F). The surrounding cells are slightly irregular, with a rim of pale cytoplasm. **C,** In this example, a higher proportion of blastic cells is present. A regressed follicle is shown (F). **D,** With BCL2 immunostain, the neoplastic marginal zone cells are weakly BCL2 positive, whereas the regressed follicle is negative. **E,** CD21 immunostain highlights follicular dendritic cells in the regressed follicle center. **F,** With IgD immunostain, the neoplastic cells are weakly IgD positive, and the disrupted mantle cells are strongly IgD positive.

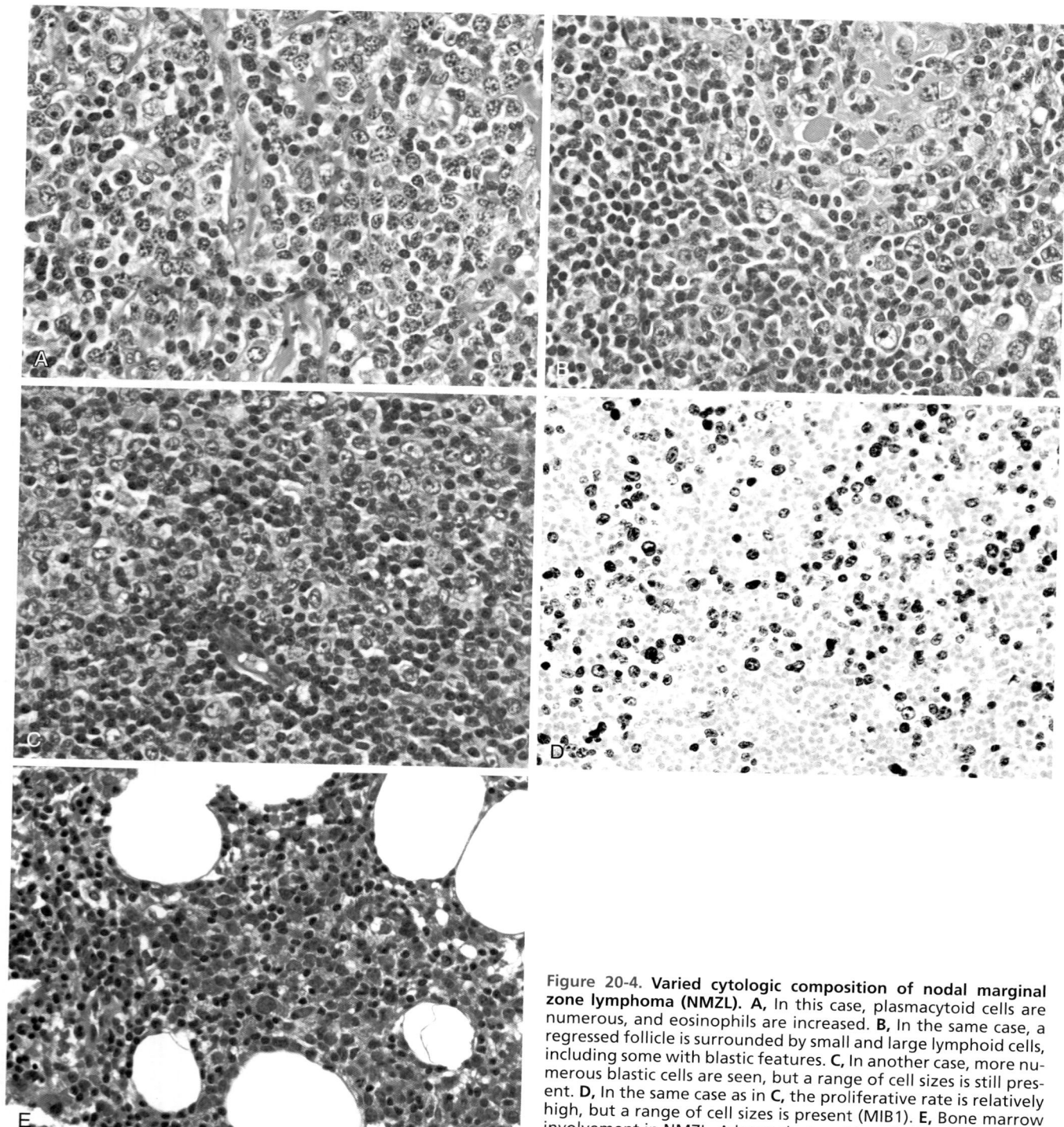

Figure 20-4. Varied cytologic composition of nodal marginal zone lymphoma (NMZL). A, In this case, plasmacytoid cells are numerous, and eosinophils are increased. **B,** In the same case, a regressed follicle is surrounded by small and large lymphoid cells, including some with blastic features. **C,** In another case, more numerous blastic cells are seen, but a range of cell sizes is still present. **D,** In the same case as in C, the proliferative rate is relatively high, but a range of cell sizes is present (MIB1). **E,** Bone marrow involvement in NMZL. A large cluster of lymphoid cells is present in a non-paratrabecular localization.

rate is especially high (>50% of the nucleated cells), but it is not clear whether different therapeutic approaches benefit this subset.[14]

IMMUNOPHENOTYPE

NMZLs are mature B-cell lymphomas that express CD20, CD19, and CD79a but, in most cases, lack CD5, CD23, CD10, and BCL6. CD43 is positive in up to 50% of cases.[17,18] BCL2 protein is generally weakly positive. IgD is a helpful marker in highlighting the presence of a residual mantle cuff, which often illuminates the pattern of infiltration by the neoplastic cells. The neoplastic cells in MALT lymphomas are almost invariably negative for IgD, whereas variable-to-weak expression of IgD can be observed in 25% to 50% of NMZLs overall.[3,5,17]

Plasmacytoid differentiation is seen in approximately 50% of NMZL cases. When present, the plasmacytoid cells may express MUM1/IRF4, but usually only a subset of the cells with plasmacytoid features, either morphologically or immunophenotypically, are MUM1/IRF4 positive.[5,27] Overall, 25% to 50% of cases express this marker by immunohistochemistry, which first appears in late centrocytes and is thought to indicate commitment to the post–germinal center program.[28] CD38, another marker associated with plasmacytoid differentiation, was positive in 41% of cases in one study.[5] MNDA is an antigen found on myelomonocytic cells but, interestingly, also expressed in a high proportion of NMZL cases; however, it is absent in FL.[29] Some tumors have a minor cellular component resembling monocytoid B cells, and IRTA may be expressed focally in those cases.[30]

Cytoplasmic Ig expression can be detected in cells exhibiting morphologic evidence of plasmacytoid differentiation and often in the blastic cells, which display a rim of basophilic cytoplasm. In most cases, the cells are IgM positive, but IgG and IgA expression, indicative of heavy chain class switching, has been reported in a small minority.[3] There is a strong bias toward the expression of kappa light chain over lambda light chain; in contrast, in EMZL, kappa and lambda are expressed in a ratio similar to that of normal B cells.[3,5] The distribution of plasmacytoid cells varies within lymph nodes. The plasmacytoid component is usually admixed with other cell types, but in some cases, plasmacytoid cells preferentially colonize germinal centers (Fig. 20-5).

The neoplastic cells are generally negative for CD21 and CD23 by immunohistochemistry. However, these markers are useful in highlighting the distribution of residual follicular dendritic cell (FDC) meshworks. In contrast to FLs, in which FDCs highlight the expanded follicular structures, the FDCs in NMZL are typically present in tight clusters, indicative of regressed follicles.[17]

The regressed germinal centers may contain a high content of T cells, giving rise to an inverse follicular pattern in which the neoplastic B cells surround nodules of T cells. Overall, NZML has a relatively high content of infiltrating mature T cells, most of which have a T-follicular helper (TFH) phenotype, positive for PD1.[23] Two main patterns of increased TFH infiltration were observed: follicular and diffuse. In cases with a dominant follicular pattern, the T cells were either central (replacing the germinal-center compartment), or more peripheral with remnants of residual germinal centers. However, the T-cell infiltrate often extended into the interfollicular region (Fig. 20-6). The polymorphous cellular composition, in conjunction with a heavy T-cell infiltrate, led to a suspected diagnosis of peripheral T-cell lymphoma in many of these cases. In this setting, evaluation of T-cell and B-cell clonality by polymerase chain reaction (PCR) analysis may be essential for accurate diagnosis. In about one-third of NMZL cases, T cells were not significantly increased.[23]

In exceptional cases with marked follicular colonization, the FDC meshworks may be expanded.[21] The colonizing cells are negative for the germinal-center–associated markers CD10 and BCL6. There are limited data concerning other prognostic markers in NMZL. As previously noted, staining for Ki67/MIB1 usually stains 20% or fewer of the neoplastic cells. However, clinical data correlating a higher proliferative rate with differences in clinical outcome do not exist.[3] Many low-grade B-cell lymphomas have alterations in the apoptosis pathway, leading to prolonged survival of the neoplastic cells. One study identified strong expression of survivin in approximately 40% of cases, with those patients having considerably decreased survival.[5] The same authors identified loss of active caspase E and increased expression of cyclin E as negative prognostic factors. Activation of the nuclear factor κB (NF-κB) pathway has been implicated in most cases of EMZL.[31] However, NMZLs often lack nuclear expression of BCL10, implying a lack of NF-κB activation in such cases.

GENETICS AND MOLECULAR FINDINGS

NMZLs show clonal rearrangement of the Ig heavy-chain (IGH) genes, as expected for any clonal B-cell neoplasm. During B-cell development, and as part of the maturation of the high-affinity antibody response, most B cells enter the germinal center and undergo somatic hypermutation (SHM) of the Ig variable region genes.[32] The detection of mutations in these genes is taken as evidence of transit through the germinal center, and germinal-center neoplasms show evidence of ongoing mutations. NMZLs are heterogeneous with respect to SHM frequency. Most studies have shown evidence of SHM,[3,5,33-36] but rare cases are unmutated.[3,33] The B-cell receptors of selected B-cell lymphomas were shown to bind the hepatitis C viral envelope protein, implicating the virus in lymphoma pathogenesis, including NMZL.[37]

Consistent cytogenetic aberrations have not been identified in NMZL.[14] Numerical abnormalities are most common, with reports of +3, +7, +12, and +18 being most frequent.[14,38,39] Both duplication of chromosome 3 and gains in several regions, as identified by comparative genomic hybridization, have been reported.[40,41] Notably, the genetic and genomic changes in NMZL differ from those reported in EMZL and LPL, providing additional evidence for a distinction among these disorders.[41,42] Mutations in MYD88L265P are uncommon in NMZL but are found in more than 90% of cases of Waldenström macroglobulinemia and LPL.[15,16] Although the genomic profile differs from that of EMZL and LPL, NMZL does show evidence of constitutive NF-κB activation in most instances.[43] Gene expression profiling studies showed a pattern resembling normal marginal zone B cells and memory B cells and differing significantly from that of FL.[44]

High throughput sequencing has identified some recurrent mutations in NZMZL. Notch pathway genes, in particular NOTCH2, are mutated in 10% to 20% of cases of NMZL, but also NOTCH1, SPEN,[45] and NF-κB genes (TNFAIP3, BIRC3, and TRAF3). KLF2 a master regulator of both NOTCH and NF-κB signaling is often mutated in this disease. One study identified KMT2D as the most commonly mutated gene in NMZL, found in 20% of cases.[46] An unexpected finding was mutations in BRAF, found in nearly 10% of cases.[46] Genomic profiling of diffuse large B-cell lymphoma (DLBL) has shown similarities to that of NMZL with the BN2 cluster of DLBCL, as demonstrated by mutations in NOTCH2 and BCL6.[47] This finding suggests a subset of cases of DLBCL in the BN2 cluster may represent transformed marginal zone lymphoma.

POSTULATED CELL OF ORIGIN

NMZLs are heterogeneous and are thought to be related to different subsets of marginal zone or memory B cells.[33] The

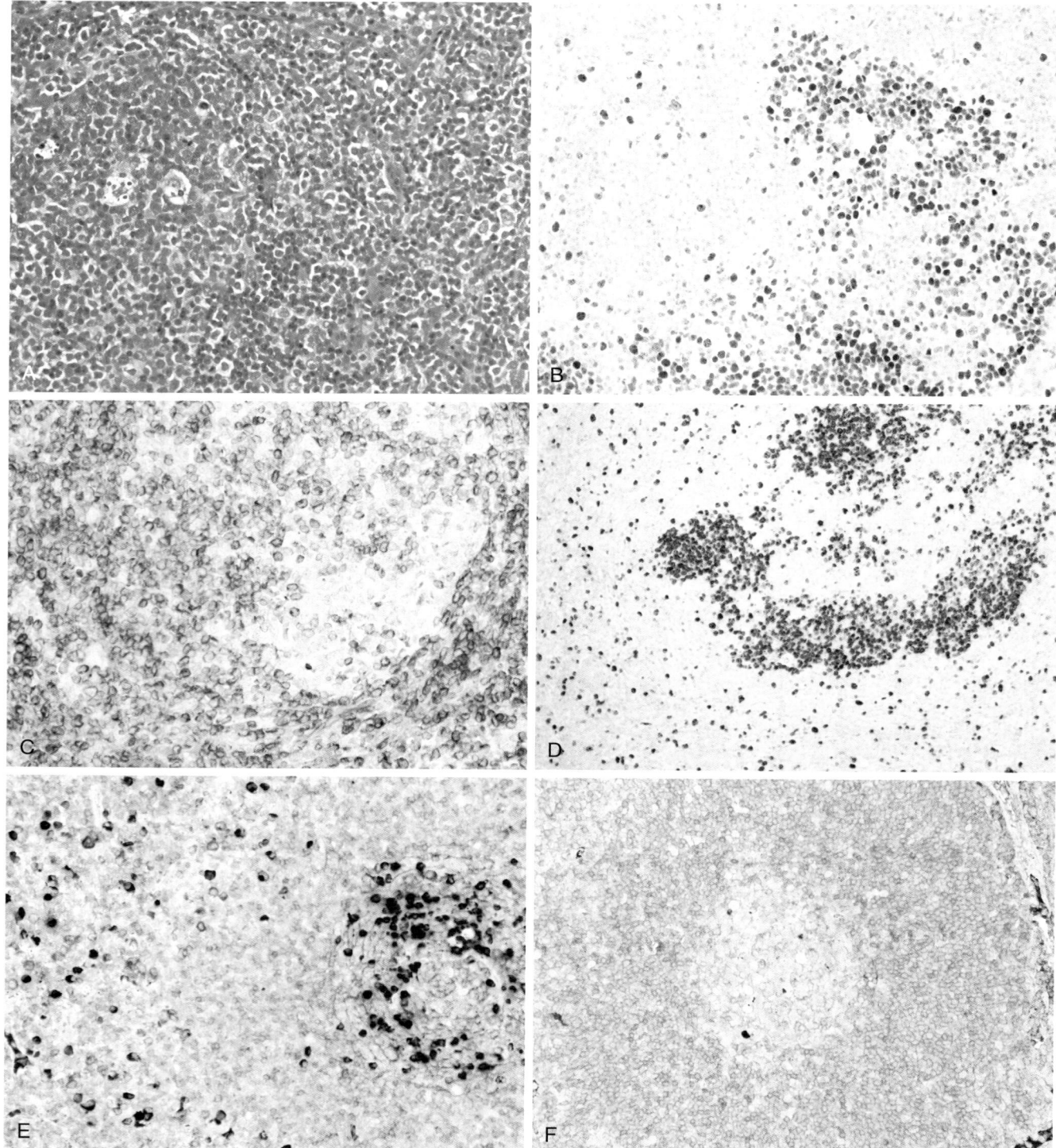

Figure 20-5. Follicular colonization in nodal marginal zone lymphoma (NMZL). A, Germinal center at left is partially infiltrated and replaced by neoplastic cells. Starry-sky macrophages are noted within the disrupted germinal center. **B,** With BCL6 immunostain, the residual germinal-center cells are BCL6 positive, whereas infiltrating NMZL cells are BCL6 negative. **C,** With BCL2 immunostain, the infiltrating NMZL cells are BCL2 positive, whereas normal germinal-center cells are BCL2 negative. **D,** Residual germinal center is highlighted by a high proliferation rate with MIB1. The surrounding neoplastic cells have a low proliferation rate. **E,** In another case, the cells colonizing the germinal center show plasmacytoid differentiation and are lambda light chain restricted. Cells outside the germinal center also show light chain restriction. **F,** Kappa is negative in corresponding areas.

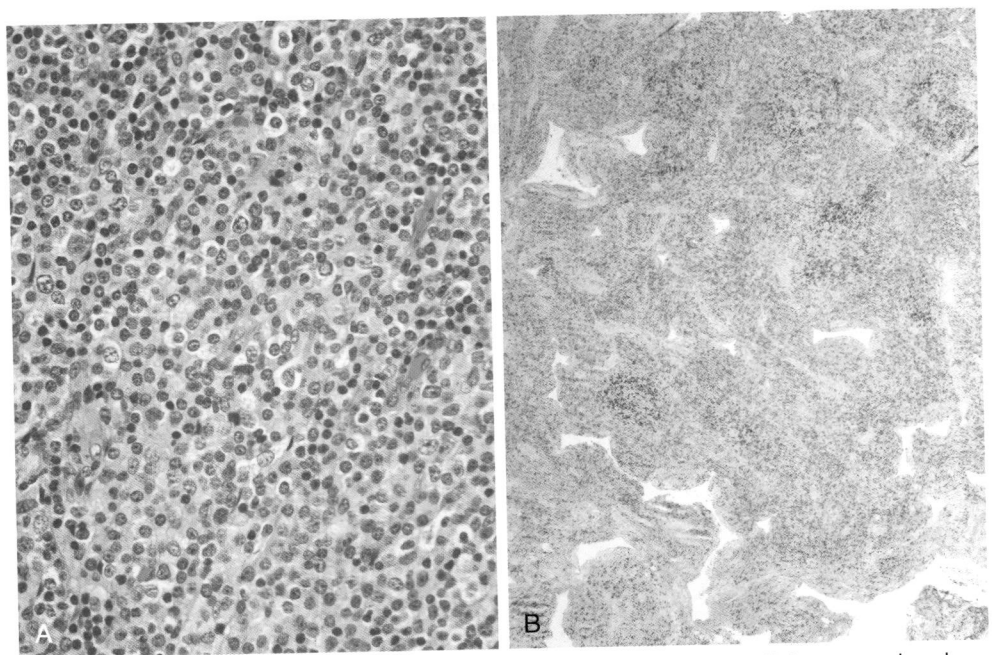

Figure 20-6. A, Nodal marginal zone lymphoma. Cytologic composition is polymorphic. Most cells have round nuclear contours and ample cytoplasm. Small lymphocytes are appreciated in the background. **B,** Same case is stained for PD1 and shows a marked increase in PD1-positive cells, both in residual regressed follicles and in the interfollicular region. The abundance of PD1-positive lymphocytes may raise concern for peripheral T-cell lymphoma.

morphologic, immunophenotypic, and genetic heterogeneity of these lymphomas is likely a reflection of the involvement of different B-cell subsets found within the marginal zone.[10] Marginal zone B cells can be both IgD positive and negative. They can show low levels of SHM, indicative of a pre–germinal-center stage of maturation, or high levels of SHM.[48] In animal models, a variety of cell types populate the marginal zone, including recirculating virgin B cells that can expand by a T-independent mechanism and memory B cells generated in germinal centers. A direct relationship of NMZL to the parasinusoidal monocytoid B cells seen in *Toxoplasma* lymphadenitis has not been suggested in most studies.

CLINICAL COURSE AND PROGNOSTIC FACTORS

NMZL is considered an indolent or "low-grade" B-cell lymphoma. However, the 5-year overall survival is somewhat less than that seen for FL and CLL, two of the most common low-grade B-cell neoplasms. Most studies have reported 5-year overall survival in the range of 55% to 75%, with better outcomes in more recent series, possibly reflecting the increased use of rituximab.[3,5,14,26] The complete remission rate is approximately 50%, with progression-free or event-free survival at 5 years generally between 30% and 40%.[14] Because most patients are in the low or low-intermediate IPI risk groups, the IPI has not been especially useful as a prognostic marker; however, the FLIPI appears to be more predictive.[4,6]

PEDIATRIC-TYPE NODAL MARGINAL ZONE LYMPHOMA (PT-NMZL)

Synonym (proposed): Pediatric-type follicular lymphoma with marginal zone differentiation.

Morphology and Immunophenotype

Cases resembling NMZL presenting in the pediatric age group have distinctive morphologic and clinical features, and in the 2016 update of the World Health Organization classification, these lesions were delineated as a provisional entity.[49,50] In affected lymph nodes, the atypical cells have a predominantly interfollicular distribution, with marked expansion of the marginal zone (Fig. 20-7). The infiltrate is polymorphic, composed of monocytoid cells, centrocyte-like cells, and plasma cells.[24,51] Blasts are usually present but few in number—no more than two or three per high-power field. A characteristic feature, seen in most pediatric cases (70%), is follicular expansion, sharing some features with progressive transformation of germinal centers. The appearance of these atypical follicles is similar to that of the floral variant of FL and shows overlap with the atypical follicles seen in the pediatric type of FL (PTFL).[52,53] In contrast to typical progressive transformation of germinal centers, the peripheral rims of the follicles are irregular, with blurring and disruption by the atypical proliferation in the marginal zone. The overall size of the follicles is expanded; the fragmented and irregular mantle zones are best visualized with stains for IgD. Early reports noted difficulties in the differential diagnosis with PTFL (see Chapter 17). In fact, more recent studies have shown more marked overlap, with 69% of cases showing remarkably similar features and a continuum in the involvement of the follicular versus marginal zone component.[54,55] Moreover, in subsequent genomic studies, it was shown that "pediatric NZML" and PTFL share a common profile and are likely part of the same biological and clinical entity.[54] As will be discussed, they also share a similar clinical profile. In some cases, plasmacytoid differentiation is best documented by stains for cytoplasmic Ig, and small numbers of atypical cells may show light chain restriction in both the interfollicular and follicular components. However, marked

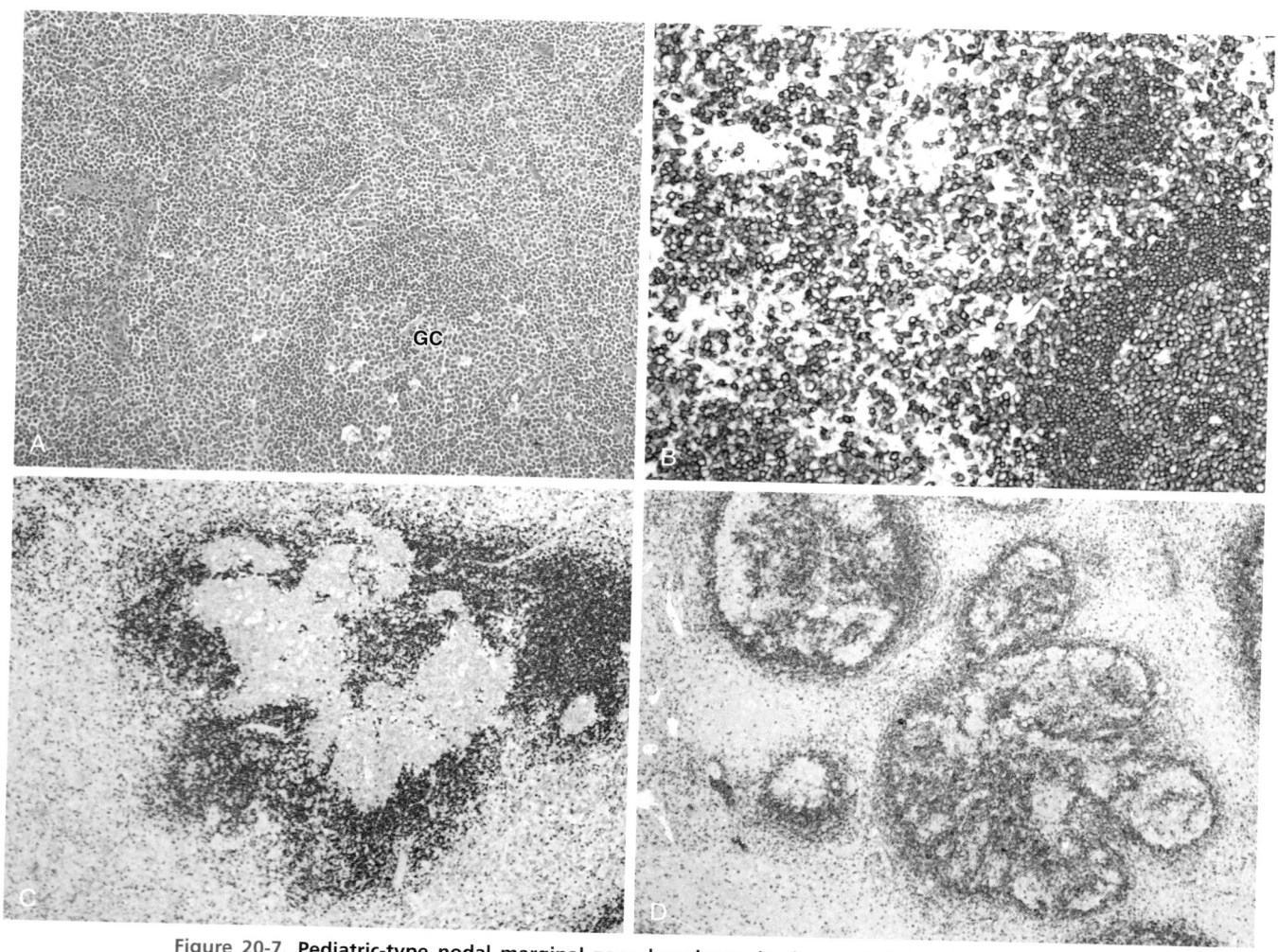

Figure 20-7. Pediatric-type nodal marginal zone lymphoma in the cervical lymph node of an 11-year-old girl. A, Atypical cells expand in the marginal zone and focally infiltrate a follicle (GC). **B,** CD20 staining of the same case shows numerous B cells in the marginal zone. **C,** Immunoglobulin (Ig)D highlights the expanded mantle zone around some of the follicles. The germinal center is partially disrupted and fragmented by the IgD mantle cells, a feature resembling progressive transformation of germinal centers. **D,** The patient received no treatment after surgical excision of the lymph node. Recurrence developed 4 years later, showing similar follicular disruption resembling progressive transformation of germinal centers (IgD immunostain).

plasmacytoid differentiation is rare. The current view is that PT-NMZL and PTFL are a single disease entity with variation in the histologic pattern and expansion of B-cells in both the marginal zone and follicular compartment. Early reports of PTFL noted evidence of marginal zone differentiation surrounding the atypical follicles.[52,53]

The differential diagnosis of PT-NMZL, especially in children, includes atypical marginal zone hyperplasia, which can present in MALT in Waldeyer's ring or the small intestine. In the report by Attygalle and coworkers,[56] these cases all showed lambda light chain restriction but failed to show evidence of clonality at the genetic level by PCR analysis for IGH gene rearrangement. This novel form of marginal zone hyperplasia has been linked to a response to *Haemophilus influenzae*.[57]

Genetic Features

Clonality is best confirmed by PCR studies for clonal rearrangement of the IG genes, which yield a positive result in more than 80% of cases tested.[58] Molecular analysis revealed

that PT-NMZL shows a low level of genetic complexity similar to PTFL.[54] The mutational profile of PT-NMZL was also found to be distinct from adult-type NMZL. Mutations in *MAP2K1*, *TNFRSF14*, and *IRF8* were most commonly found, similar to PTFL. This mutational profile was seen in 78% of cases with morphologic overlap with PTFL, but also in cases lacking significant overlap (61%). One difference with PTFL was that 1p36 CNN loss of heterozygosity (LOH) or deletion was uncommon in cases classified as PT-NMZL.

Clinical Features

The median age at presentation for PT-NMZL is 16 years. There is a striking male predominance, with a 20:1 male-to-female ratio for patients younger than 20 years of age, similar to PTFL. The most common presentation of PT-NMZL is asymptomatic lymphadenopathy involving the head and neck region, most commonly the cervical nodes. The majority of patients have localized stage I disease and show a low rate of recurrence after conservative treatment. This clinical behavior contrasts with that of NMZL in adults. For these reasons, conservative management consisting of clinical observation after surgical excision is recommended for patients with disease in a single lymph node. This is comparable to the management of PTFL.

DIFFERENTIAL DIAGNOSIS

Extranodal Marginal Zone Lymphoma

Patients with EMZL can have lymph node involvement, sometimes many years after the initial diagnosis (see Chapter 18). Therefore, a careful clinical history is most important in distinguishing lymph node involvement by EMZL from that of NMZL. Histologic features more common in EMZL include well-preserved reactive follicles with intact mantle cuffs and a prominent component of monocytoid B cells.[17] EMZLs are nearly always negative for IgD, whereas primary NMZL may be positive (Table 20-1).

Lymphoplasmacytic Lymphoma

One of the more challenging and difficult differential diagnoses is between LPL and NMZL (see Chapter 14). In LPL, the lymph node sinuses are often preserved, whereas in NMZL,

Table 20-1 Differential Diagnosis of Nodal Marginal Zone Lymphoma

Feature	NMZL	LPL	Secondary EMZL	Follicular Lymphoma	CLL/ SLL
Follicular pattern	−/+	−	−	+	−*
Plasmacytoid differentiation	+	++	+	−/+	−/+
Lymph node sinuses effaced	+	−	+/−	+	+
Paraprotein spike	−	+	−	−	−†
Dutcher bodies	−/+	+	+	−	−
Monocytoid cells	+	−	++	−/+	−/+
CD43	+	+	+	−	+
CD3+ (non-neoplastic)	++	−	−	+	−/+
CD5	−†	−†	−†	−†	+
IgD	+/−	−	−	−/+	+
CD23	−	−	−	−/+	+
BCL6/CD10	−	−	−	+	−
MYD88L265P mutation	−†	+	−	−	−†

*Pseudofollicular growth centers.
†Reported in rare cases.
CLL/SLL, Chronic lymphocytic leukemia/small lymphocytic lymphoma; *EMZL,* extranodal marginal zone lymphoma; *Ig,* immunoglobulin; *LPL,* lymphoplasmacytic lymphoma; *NMZL,* nodal marginal zone lymphoma.

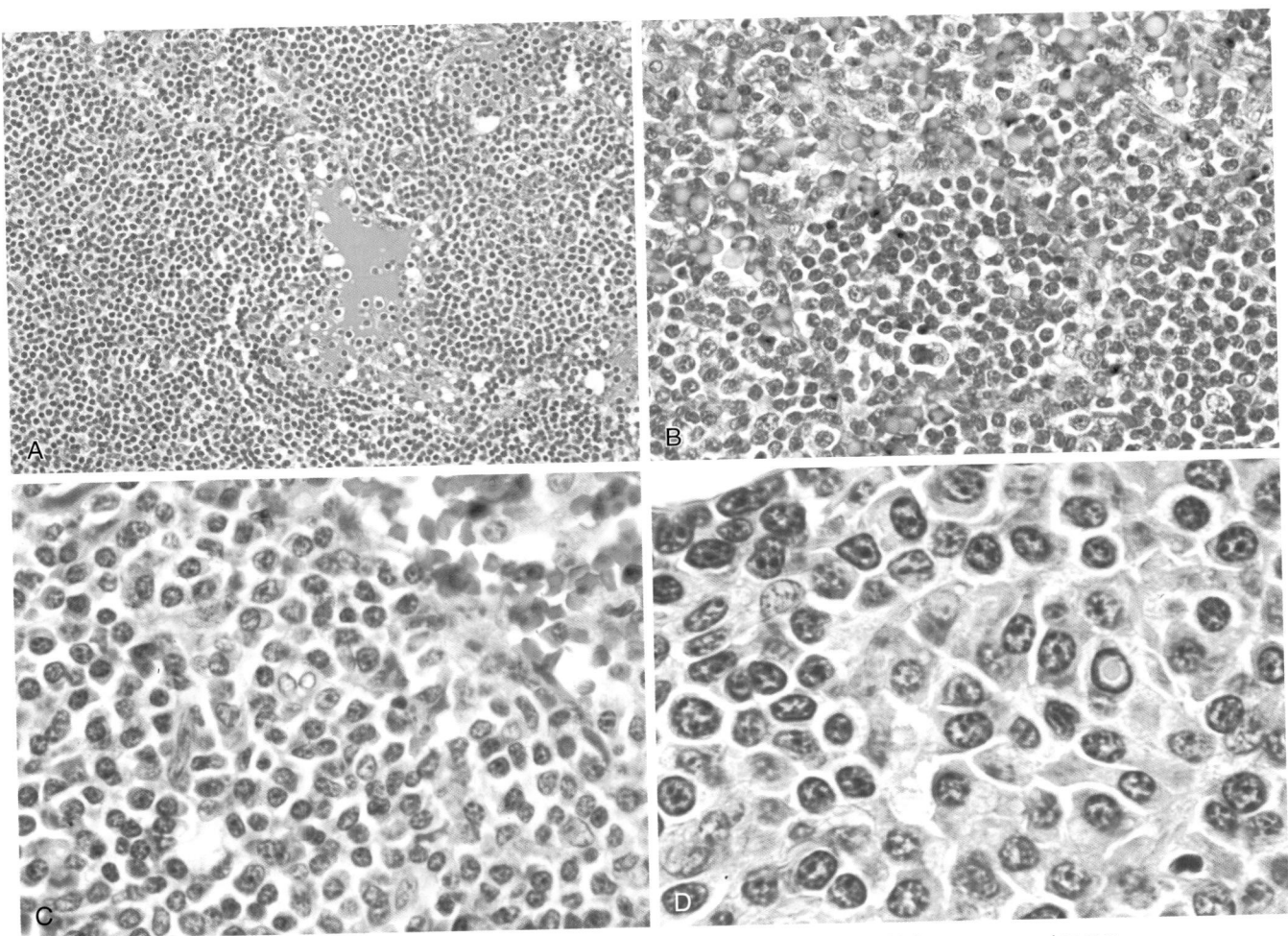

Figure 20-8. Lymphoplasmacytic lymphoma (LPL). A, The infiltrate in LPL is more monotonous than that in nodal marginal zone lymphoma (NMZL). Sinuses are intact and often dilated. **B,** Numerous Mott cells with cytoplasmic globular inclusions are present. Surrounding cells show plasmacytoid features. **C,** Plasmacytoid lymphocytes are usually most conspicuous adjacent to sinuses. **D,** Dutcher bodies are more common in LPL than in NMZL but can be seen in either disease.

the architecture is generally more effaced (Fig. 20-8). The infiltrate in LPL is more uniform, with a relatively monotonous infiltrate of small lymphoid cells with plasmacytoid features. The plasmacytoid cells are usually most prominent adjacent to the lymph node sinuses, and diffuse architectural effacement may be seen in some cases. Dutcher bodies are present in most cases, and increased mast cells can be documented with Giemsa stain. Lymphoid follicles, if present, are usually regressed. It should also be noted that the genetic aberrations in LPL associated with Waldenström macroglobulinemia differ from those seen in NMZL.[15,16,59] The characteristic *MYD88* L265P mutation can be readily detected by PCR analysis of DNA extracted from formalin-fixed paraffin-embedded sections and is useful in borderline cases. Notably, the MYD88L265P mutation has been reported only rarely in NMZL, but of course, it is known to occur in diffuse large B-cell lymphoma of the ABC subtype.[60] Therefore, presence of the mutation does not automatically exclude a diagnosis of NMZL.

Marginal Zone Hyperplasia and Related Reactive Conditions

The normal marginal zone is much less conspicuous in the lymph nodes than it is in the spleen. In peripheral lymph nodes, it is difficult to identify this region under normal circumstances.[61] Mesenteric lymph nodes usually have a more well-developed marginal zone. This region can be distinguished from primary follicles or mantle cuffs because the cells are negative for IgD by immunohistochemistry. Normal marginal zone B cells can express BCL2; therefore, BCL2 reactivity is not helpful in distinguishing benign from malignant marginal zone expansions.[62] The marginal zone can be expanded in some reactive conditions, placing NMZL in the differential diagnosis.[63] Identification of light chain restriction by immunohistochemistry or flow cytometry favors NMZL. However, some cases of marginal zone hyperplasia, particularly in children, can show restricted expression of lambda light chain.[56] Molecular studies for clonal rearrangement of the IG genes are recommended because clonal rearrangements should be absent in marginal zone hyperplasia.

Another process that may mimic the follicular colonization seen in some NMZLs is atypical hyperplasia with monotypic plasma cells found in the germinal centers.[64] These cases usually lack evidence of a monoclonal process at the molecular level, although in a minority, evidence of monoclonality can be found in the microdissected lesions. This form of hyperplasia is more common in women and may be associated with a background of autoimmune disease. Thus, it may be related pathogenetically to the development of some marginal zone neoplasms.

Monocytoid B-Cell Hyperplasia

Marginal zone hyperplasia should be distinguished from monocytoid B-cell hyperplasia, although historically, these cell types have been confused. A prominent monocytoid B-cell reaction is classically seen in acute acquired toxoplasmosis but can also occur in a variety of other reactive conditions,

including reaction to cytomegalovirus infection and the lymphadenopathy associated with human immunodeficiency virus infection.[65,66] Normal monocytoid B cells are found in a parasinusoidal distribution adjacent to the subcapsular and medullary sinuses in lymph nodes and may be significantly expanded in this region. They are usually associated with admixed polymorphonuclear lymphocytes. In contrast to normal marginal zone B cells, monocytoid B cells are negative for BCL2.

Follicular Lymphoma

Some cases of FL may show marginal zone differentiation, mimicking NMZL.[67] In such cases, the atypical follicles usually have an attenuated or ill-defined lymphoid cuff surrounded by a polymorphic infiltrate of cells with more abundant cytoplasm than the follicle center cells (Fig. 20-9). Blastic cells and cells with monocytoid features are usually present. The marginal zone component may differ immunophenotypically from the follicle center cells and often shows downregulation of CD10. BCL6 may be weakly expressed. The follicle center cells are positive for BCL6 and, in most cases, positive for BCL2 and CD10. However, some higher-grade FLs are negative for CD10 and show increased expression of MUM1/IRF4.[68] The diagnosis is more challenging in such cases because MUM1/IRF4 is expressed in post–germinal-center B cells and may be expressed in NMZL. Further complicating the matter is the frequent absence of *BCL2::IGH* translocations in these FL variants.[69] Amplifications of *BCL6* may be present, favoring a follicle center derivation.

The principal differential diagnosis is NMZL with follicular colonization, in which the colonizing cells should be negative for the germinal-center–associated markers BCL6 and CD10 but may express BCL2 protein in the absence of the *BCL2::IGH* translocation. Evidence of plasmacytoid differentiation, in either the intrafollicular or extrafollicular compartment, favors NMZL but can be seen rarely in FL.[70]

It is important to note that NMZL is negative for CD23, but CD23 is highly expressed in certain variants of FL that are negative for *BCL2* rearrangement.[71] This FL variant often presents with localized inguinal involvement and may have a largely diffuse growth pattern, raising the differential diagnosis of NMZL.

Chronic Lymphocytic Leukemia/ Small Lymphocytic Lymphoma With a Parafollicular Pattern

Some cases of chronic lymphocytic leukemia/small lymphocytic lymphoma (CLL/SLL) have a parafollicular pattern of involvement in lymph nodes that superficially resembles NMZL (Fig. 20-10).[72] The infiltrate is usually monotonous, typical of CLL/SLL, and contains pseudofollicular growth centers. Attenuated lymphoid cuffs may be seen and are more readily identified with stains for IgD. With immunohistochemical studies, the typical CLL/SLL phenotype is present: CD5-positive, CD23-positive, LEF1-positive B cells with dim CD20 expression.

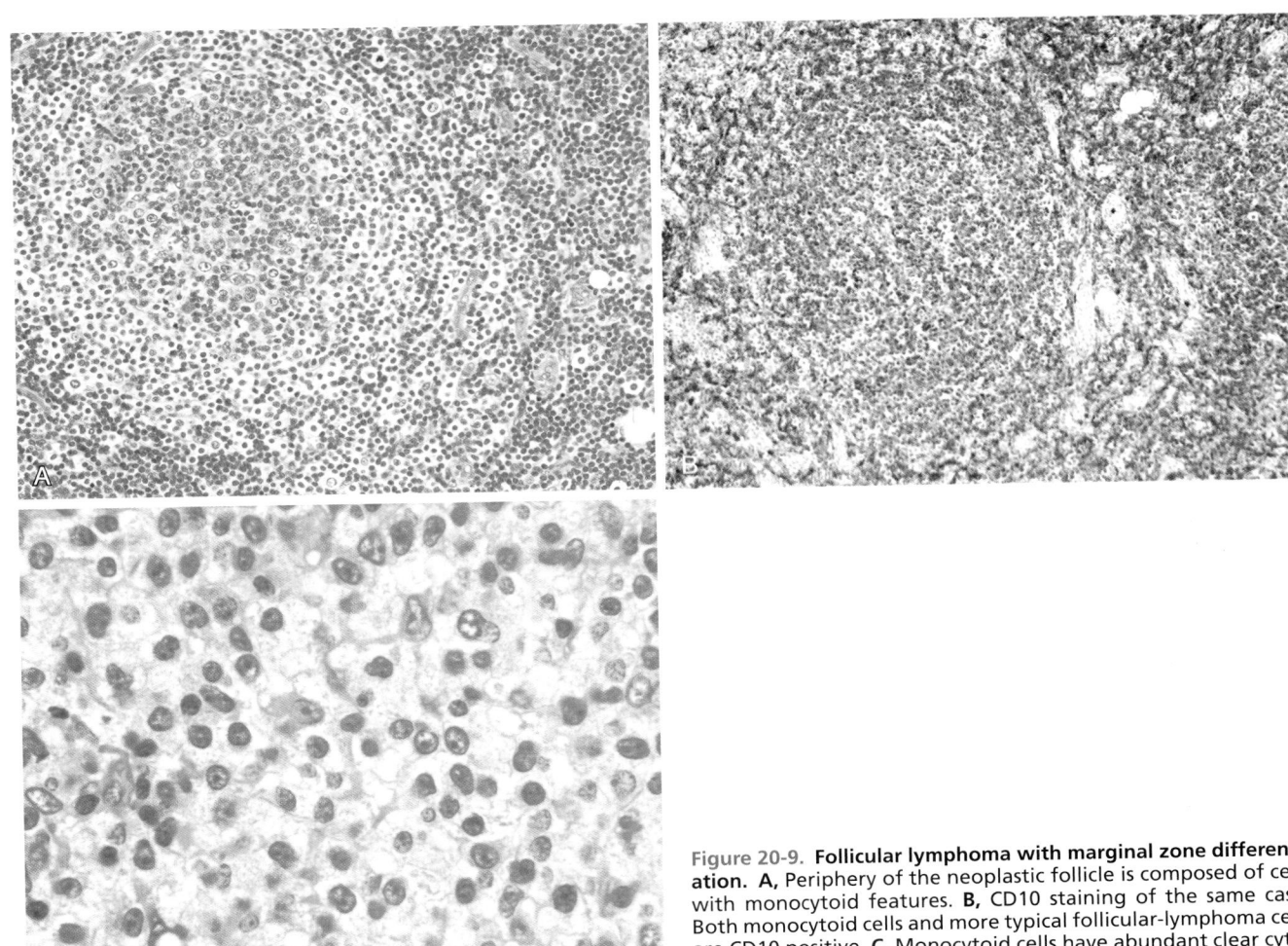

Figure 20-9. Follicular lymphoma with marginal zone differentiation. A, Periphery of the neoplastic follicle is composed of cells with monocytoid features. **B,** CD10 staining of the same case. Both monocytoid cells and more typical follicular-lymphoma cells are CD10 positive. **C,** Monocytoid cells have abundant clear cytoplasm and distinct cytoplasmic membranes.

Splenic Marginal Zone Lymphoma

SMZL usually presents with marked splenomegaly and bone marrow involvement without significant peripheral lymphadenopathy. Splenic hilar lymph nodes usually show intact sinuses with a small lymphocytic infiltrate that replaces preexistent structures, including follicles.[73,74] Interestingly, the cells in splenic hilar lymph nodes usually do not show monocytoid or marginal differentiation and have relatively sparse cytoplasm. However, lymph node involvement can also occur during the course of SMZL and may resemble NMZL (Fig. 20-11).

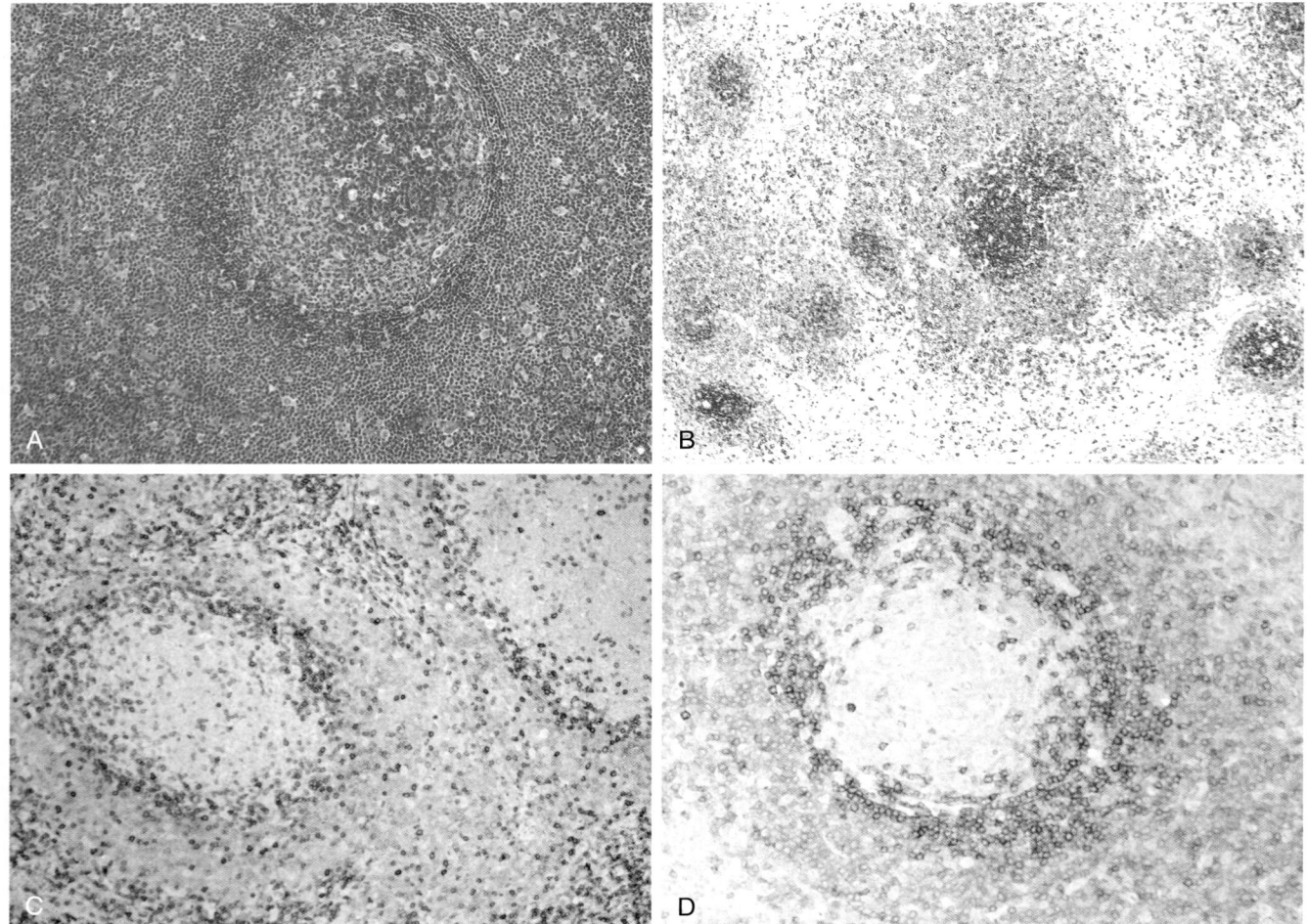

Figure 20-10. **Chronic lymphocytic leukemia/small lymphocytic lymphoma (CLL/SLL) with a para-follicular marginal zone pattern.** **A,** Reactive follicle is surrounded by a rim of CLL cells, resembling an expanded marginal zone. **B,** CLL cells show dim CD20 expression, contrasting with more intense staining of follicular B cells. **C,** CLL cells show dim CD5 expression. There is a thin rim of CD5-positive T cells at the periphery of the germinal center. **D,** The thin mantle cuff is strongly IgD positive, whereas the CLL cells are dimly IgD positive.

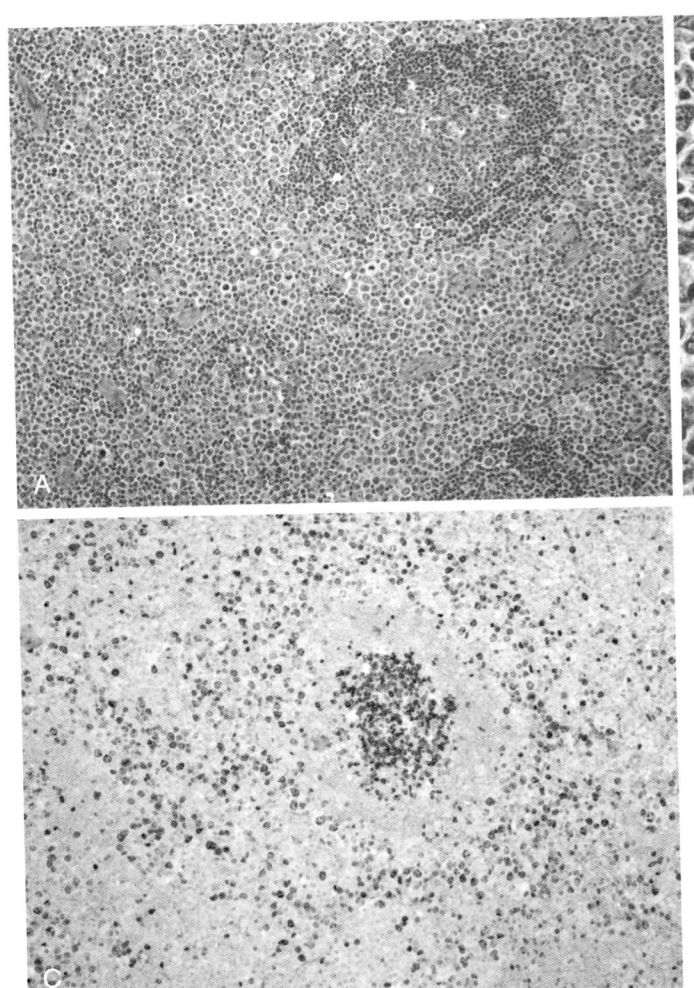
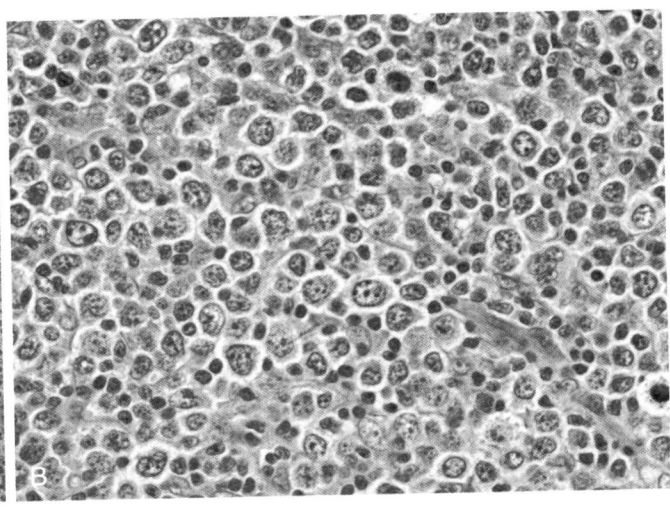

Figure 20-11. Splenic marginal zone lymphoma recurrence in a lymph node. A, Medium-to-large lymphoid cells surround the residual reactive follicle. **B,** At high power, cells show a spectrum of sizes. **C,** Overall, the proliferation rate of the lymphoma is low, although cells abutting the reactive follicle show a somewhat higher proliferation rate (MIB1/Ki67).

Pearls and Pitfalls

- NMZL is most often a diagnosis of exclusion, after other low-grade B-cell lymphoma subtypes have been ruled out.
- In NMZL with prominent monocytoid B cells (MALT type), the diagnosis of secondary EMZL should be considered and ruled out clinically.
- Both NMZL and LPL may show plasmacytoid differentiation.
  - NMZL contains many different cell types—polymorphic cytology.
  - LPL contains few cell types—monomorphic cytology.
- NMZL with follicular colonization may closely mimic FL.
- The proportion of "blastic" or transformed cells varies widely, but no grading of NMZL is required or recommended.
- The pediatric type of NMZL usually presents with localized, stage I disease and is currently considered part of the spectrum of PTFL.

KEY REFERENCES

6. Arcaini L, Paulli M, Burcheri S, et al. Primary nodal marginal zone B-cell lymphoma: clinical features and prognostic assessment of a rare disease. *Br J Haematol.* 2007;136:301–304.

18. van den Brand M, van Krieken JH. Recognizing nodal marginal zone lymphoma: recent advances and pitfalls. A systematic review. *Haematologica.* 2013;98:1003–1013.
19. Zhou T, Wang HW, Ng SB, et al. Tissue eosinophilia in B-cell lymphoma: an underrecognized phenomenon. *Am J Surg Pathol.* In press.
20. Salama ME, Lossos IS, Warnke RA, Natkunam Y. Immunoarchitectural patterns in nodal marginal zone B-cell lymphoma: a study of 51 cases. *Am J Clin Pathol.* 2009;132:39–49.
23. Egan C, Laurent C, Alejo JC, et al. Expansion of PD1-positive T cells in nodal marginal zone lymphoma: a potential diagnostic pitfall. *Am J Surg Pathol.* 2020;44(5):657–664.
39. Krijgsman O, Gonzalez P, Ponz OB, et al. Dissecting the gray zone between follicular lymphoma and marginal zone lymphoma using morphological and genetic features. *Haematologica.* 2013;98:1921–1929.
45. Spina V, Rossi D. Molecular pathogenesis of splenic and nodal marginal zone lymphoma. *Best Pract Res Clin Haematol.* 2017;30(1–2):5–12.

46. Vela V, Juskevicius D, Dirnhofer S, Menter T, Tzankov A. Mutational landscape of marginal zone B-cell lymphomas of various origin: organotypic alterations and diagnostic potential for assignment of organ origin. *Virchows Arch.* 2021.

54. Salmeron-Villalobos J, Egan C, Borgmann V, et al. A unifying hypothesis for PNMZL and PTFL: morphological variants with a common molecular profile. *Blood Adv.* 2022;6(16):4661–4674.

55. Laurent CJ, Cook R, Yoshino T, et al. Follicular lymphoma and marginal zone lymphoma: how many diseases? *Virchows Archiv.* 2023;482:149–162.

57. Kluin PM, Langerak AW, Beverdam-Vincent J, et al. Paediatric nodal marginal zone B-cell lymphadenopathy of the neck: a *Haemophilus influenzae*–driven immune disorder? *J Pathol.* 2015;236:302–314.

Visit Elsevier eBooks+ for the complete set of references.

Chapter 21

Mantle Cell Lymphoma

Elias Campo and Pedro Jares

DEFINITION

Mantle cell lymphoma (MCL) is a mature B-cell neoplasm generally composed of monomorphic small-to-medium-sized lymphoid cells with irregular nuclei that frequently express CD5 and carry *CCND1* rearrangements with immunoglobulin (IG) genes, leading to overexpression of cyclin D1. Some tumors with similar morphology and phenotype have instead *CCND2* or *CCND3* translocations and are also considered as conventional MCL (cMCL).[1] Neoplastic transformed cells (centroblasts), paraimmunoblasts, and pseudofollicles are absent.[2]

Historically MCL was initially recognized as *centrocytic lymphoma* in the Kiel classification,[3] and different subtypes of B-cell lymphomas in the American literature under the terms *lymphocytic lymphoma of intermediate differentiation,*[4] *intermediate lymphocytic lymphoma,*[5] and *mantle zone lymphoma.*[6] The characterization of the t(11;14) translocation targeting *CCND1* as the genetic hallmark of all these tumors and the identification of mantle cells as the normal counterpart led to a better definition and recognition of the broad clinical and pathologic spectrum of the disease.[7,8] The biological behavior of most MCLs is very aggressive although the outcome of the patients is improving with novel therapeutic strategies. In contrast with this cMCL, a different biological and clinical subtype of the disease with an indolent behavior has been recognized and named *leukemic non-nodal MCL* (nnMCL). These patients usually present with leukemic phase, frequent splenomegaly, but no or minimal nodal involvement in the initial phases of the disease.[9,10]

Synonyms and Related Terms

Revised WHO 4th ed.: Mantle cell lymphoma
Proposed WHO 5th ed.: Mantle cell lymphoma

EPIDEMIOLOGY

MCL represents 2.5% to 10% of all lymphoid neoplasms and occurs predominantly in older adult men (male-to-female ratio, 2.1 to 3.9:1) with a median age of approximately 65 years (range, 23 to 96 years) (Table 21-1). The mean annual incidence of this lymphoma estimated from population-based studies is 0.71 per 100,000 (range, 0.42 to 1.01), with a mean of 0.97 for men and 0.44 for women.[11-16] Recent estimation of familial relative cancer risk (FRR) has shown that MCL displayed one of the highest FRR for the same tumor type among hematological malignancies.[17] Previously, epidemiologic studies had reported twofold significant increase of hematological neoplasms among first-degree relatives of patients with MCL.[18-20] In occasional patients, germline mutations in ATM and CHK2 have been reported, but like chronic lymphocytic leukemia (CLL), these genes are not involved in the few studied families with lymphoid neoplasms and MCL.[21] Germline variants in DNA repair genes have been described in early onset MCL.[22]

CLINICAL MANIFESTATIONS

More than 70% of patients present with stage IV disease, generalized lymphadenopathy, and bone marrow involvement; bulky disease and B symptoms are less common (see Table 21-1).[2,11,12,14-16,23,24] Hepatosplenomegaly is relatively frequent, and massive splenomegaly is observed in 30% to 60% of cases, particularly in the nnMCL subtype.[15,25,26] Some patients have prominent splenomegaly with minimal or absent peripheral lymphadenopathy. This presentation is usually associated with peripheral blood involvement, and the differential diagnosis with other lymphoid leukemias may be difficult.[27,28]

Extranodal involvement is frequent in MCL with more than two sites occurring in 30% to 50% of patients. However, an extranodal presentation without apparent nodal involvement occurs in 4% to 15% of cases.[29] Gastrointestinal (GI) infiltration has been reported in 10% to 25% of patients, either at presentation or during the course of the disease. A peculiar manifestation of this involvement is lymphomatoid polyposis, in which multiple lymphoid polyps are identified in the small and large bowel. These patients may present with abdominal pain and melena.[30,31] Isolated involvement of the GI tract has

been associated with a more favorable outcome than cases presenting with lymphadenopathy.[29] Central nervous system involvement occurs in 1% of patients at diagnosis, but it may appear late in the clinical course in 4% of the patients and has an ominous significance.[32,33] These patients frequently have blastoid morphology, high lactate dehydrogenase (LDH), high MCL International Prognostic Index (MIPI), extensive infiltration in other extranodal localizations, and a leukemic phase.[32,33] Other extranodal sites commonly involved are Waldeyer's ring, lung, and pleura (5%–20%). Less common localizations are skin, breast, soft tissue, thyroid, salivary gland, peripheral nerve, conjunctiva, and orbit.[15,25,26,34-38]

Peripheral blood involvement at diagnosis varies among studies, depending in part on the disease definition. Conventional examination may detect leukemic involvement at diagnosis in 20% to 70% of patients. Atypical lymphoid cells may be observed in the peripheral blood in the absence of lymphocytosis,[39] and they may be detected by flow cytometry in virtually all patients.[40] Leukemic involvement may also appear during the evolution of the disease and may represent a manifestation of disease progression.[41,42] Some patients present with a very aggressive leukemic form mimicking acute leukemia. These cases have blastoid morphology; complex karyotypes, occasionally with 8q24 anomalies and MYC rearrangements, and a very rapid evolution, with a median survival of 3 months.[43-47]

nnMCL usually presents with a leukemic phase and no or minimal lymph node involvement.[27,28,48-50] The patients may have a long period of an asymptomatic atypical lymphocytosis, followed by the development of splenomegaly without nodal dissemination. The disease may be controlled with splenectomy without chemotherapy for long periods. Some of these patients may eventually progress with an aggressive disease with or without nodal dissemination.

Anemia and thrombocytopenia occur in 10% to 40% of patients, and high LDH and β_2-microglobulin levels are detected in approximately 50% of cases. A monoclonal serum component, usually at low levels, has been reported in 10% to 30% of patients.[35,51,52] However, the immunoglobulin isotype is different in the serum and tumor cell surface in some cases. A significant increase of second neoplasm associated with MCL has been reported in around 10% of patients, with a predominance of skin, thyroid, CLL, and other lymphoid neoplasms and solid tumors.[53]

MORPHOLOGY

The pathologic characteristics of MCL are relatively distinctive, but the similarities between some morphologic variants and other lymphoid neoplasms require the use of ancillary studies to clarify the differential diagnosis (Table 21-2).

Architectural Patterns

Nodal involvement by MCL usually effaces the architecture with three growth patterns: mantle zone, nodular, or diffuse (Fig. 21-1). The mantle zone pattern is characterized by expansion of the follicle mantle area by tumor cells surrounding a reactive "naked" germinal center. This pattern may be associated with partial preservation of the nodal architecture and may be difficult to distinguish from follicular or mantle cell hyperplasias.[54] Transitional areas between

Table 21-1 Clinical Characteristics of Mantle Cell Lymphoma at Presentation

Characteristic	Percentage of Patients (Range)
Median age:	≈65 years (range, 23–96)
Male-to-female ratio:	3:1 (range 2.15–3.9:1)
Sites of involvement	
Generalized lymphadenopathy	80 (75–87)
Bone marrow	71 (53–82)
Spleen (splenomegaly)	51 (27–59)
Liver (hepatomegaly)	20 (11–35)
Gastrointestinal tract	16 (9–24)
Waldeyer's ring	9 (2–18)
Lung/pleura	9 (2–17)
Peripheral blood	39 (24–53)
Bulky disease (≥10 cm)	18 (5–22)
Poor performance status	24 (6–51)
B symptoms	28 (14–50)
Elevated lactate dehydrogenase	37 (16–55)
Elevated β_2-microglobulin	52 (50–55)
Stage III–IV	81 (72–89)

nodular and diffuse patterns are common, but in rare cases, nodularity is prominent, leading to a misinterpretation of follicular lymphoma.[41] However, some nodules may be solid, without evidence of residual germinal centers, representing the malignant counterpart of primary follicles. Alternatively, the nodular pattern may be caused by a massive infiltration and obliteration of the original germinal center by tumor cells. In some cases, cyclin D1 staining may help identify initial infiltration or colonization of reactive germinal centers, which

may correspond to early stages of a nodular pattern (Fig. 21-2). Residual germinal centers can also be seen in tumors with a more diffuse pattern, although in these cases, they may be identified only focally.

Cytologic Variants

Classic (common or typical) MCLs are characterized by a monotonous proliferation of small-to-medium-sized lymphoid cells with scant cytoplasm, variably irregular nuclei, evenly distributed condensed chromatin, and inconspicuous nucleoli (Fig. 21-3). Large cells with abundant cytoplasm or prominent nucleoli are rare or absent; when present, they may correspond to reactive centroblasts of residual germinal centers overrun by lymphoma cells. Occasional cases may show a predominance of small lymphocytes with round nuclei (Fig. 21-3). This small cell variant may be difficult to distinguish from CLL/small lymphocytic lymphoma (CLL/SLL). However, proliferation centers or isolated prolymphocytes and paraimmunoblasts are absent in MCL. Proliferative activity in classic and small-cell MCL varies from case to case but is usually lower than one to two mitoses per high-power field. However, some tumors with a classic morphology may show a high mitotic index, similar to the blastoid variants, and these patients may have an aggressive

Table 21-2 Major Diagnostic Features in Mantle Cell Lymphoma

Morphology	Description
Architectural pattern	Mantle zone, nodular, or diffuse
Cytologic variants	
Classic	Monotonous proliferation of small-to-intermediate-sized lymphoid cells Nucleus with slightly cleaved contour and absence of nucleolus
Blastoid	Intermediate-sized cells Round nuclei with finely dispersed chromatin Inconspicuous nucleoli Very high mitotic index
Pleomorphic	Intermediate-to-large-sized cells Irregular nuclei with dispersed chromatin and possible small nucleoli High mitotic index
Small cell	Small, round lymphocytes with more clumped chromatin Absence of prolymphocytes, paraimmunoblasts, and proliferation growth centers
Marginal zone–like	Tumor cells with broad, pale cytoplasm Nucleus may have typical or blastoid morphology
Other features	Dispersed pink histiocytes without apoptotic bodies (occasional classic starry-sky pattern in blastoid variants) Hyalinized small vessels
Immunophenotype	B-cell markers with co-expression of CD5 and CD43 Cyclin D1 and SOX11 expression Usually negative for LEF1, CD10, BCL6, and CD23
Genetic	t(11;14)(q13;q32) translocation Complex karyotypes in blastoid variants Tetraploid clones in pleomorphic and blastic variants

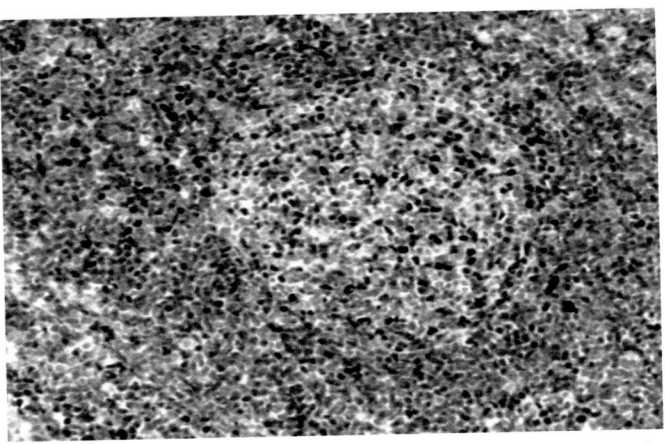

Figure 21-2. Cyclin D1 expression. Tumor cells expand the mantle and infiltrate a reactive germinal center.

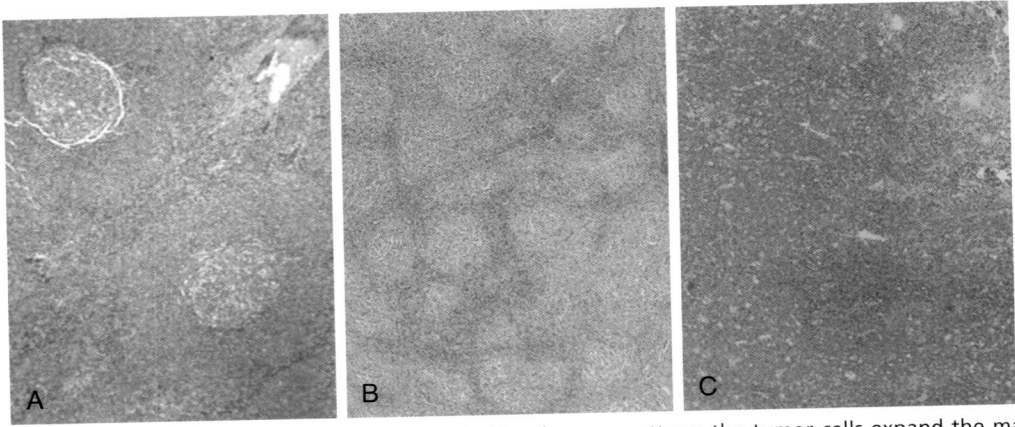

Figure 21-1. Architectural patterns in mantle cell lymphoma. A, Mantle zone pattern: the tumor cells expand the mantle cell cuff surrounding a reactive germinal center. **B,** Nodular pattern. **C,** Diffuse pattern.

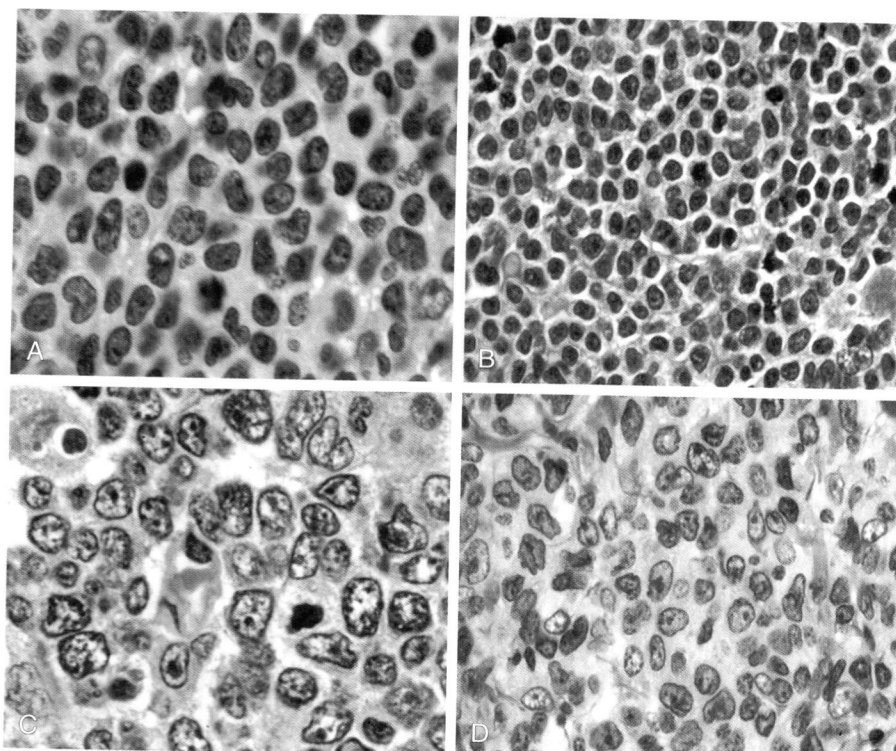

Figure 21-3. Cytologic variants of mantle cell lymphoma. A, Typical or classic mantle cell lymphoma (MCL) is characterized by small-to-medium-sized lymphocytes with irregular nuclei, condensed chromatin, and scant cytoplasm. **B,** The small-cell variant is composed of small lymphocytes with round nuclei. **C,** The blastoid variant has round nuclei, finely distributed chromatin, inconspicuous or very small nucleoli, and a high mitotic index. **D,** The pleomorphic variant with large cells and very irregular nuclei.

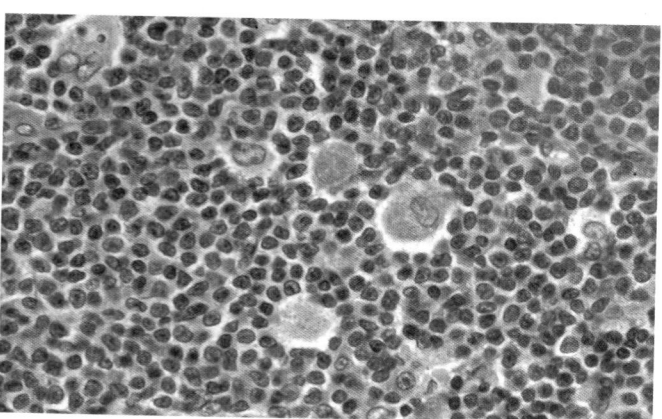

Figure 21-4. Classic variant of mantle cell lymphoma with scattered histiocytes with eosinophilic cytoplasm.

clinical course.[55,56] Scattered epithelioid histiocytes with eosinophilic cytoplasm are relatively common, but well-formed microgranulomas are not usually seen (Fig. 21-4). These histiocytes generally do not contain phagocytosed apoptotic bodies. Nuclei of follicular dendritic cells with the typical features of overlapping nuclei, delicate nuclear membranes, and an "empty" chromatin appearance are frequently identified. In some cases, hyalinized small vessels may be seen scattered throughout the tumor.

More aggressive variants of MCL may have a morphology that ranges from a monotonous population of cells resembling lymphoblasts (blastoid variant) to a more pleomorphic appearance with larger irregular cells resembling diffuse large B-cell lymphoma (Fig. 21-3).[36,57-60] Blastoid MCL are characterized by a monotonous proliferation

of intermediate-sized cells with round nuclei and fine dispersed chromatin. Pleomorphic MCL are composed of a heterogeneous population of large cells with ovoid or irregular, cleaved nuclei; finely dispersed chromatin; and small, distinct nucleoli (Fig. 21-3). The mitotic index is high but usually lower than in blastic cases.[59,61] In some cases, mitotic figures may show a striking hyperchromatic staining, with an apparently high number of chromosomes, usually associated with the presence of tetraploid clones.[62] This pleomorphic variant may be difficult to distinguish from large-cell lymphomas. However, the nuclear characteristics of cleaved contours, finely dispersed chromatin, and discordance between the large nuclei and relatively small nucleoli may suggest a mantle cell origin. Some leukemic MCLs, described as *prolymphocytic variants* of MCL, may in fact represent leukemic forms of the pleomorphic subtype of MCL.[63-66]

Some cases may have a variable number of cells with more abundant pale cytoplasm, mimicking monocytoid B cells (Fig. 21-5).[67] The nucleus of these cells may have blastoid or classic morphology, but the peculiar cytoplasm may raise the possibility of marginal zone lymphomas or hairy cell leukemia (HCL). In some cases, these monocytoid-like cells may even expand to the marginal zone of lymphoid follicles, outside an apparently preserved mantle zone. CD5 and cyclin D1 positivity is crucial in the diagnosis of this variant.

Some occasional MCLs have a clonally related plasma cell component or a subpopulation of cells with lymphoplasmacytic differentiation including the presence of Dutcher bodies that may be confused with lymphoplasmacytic lymphoma (Fig. 21-6).[68-70] These tumors are cyclin D1 and t(11;14) positive but are SOX11 negative and seem to have a more indolent disease.

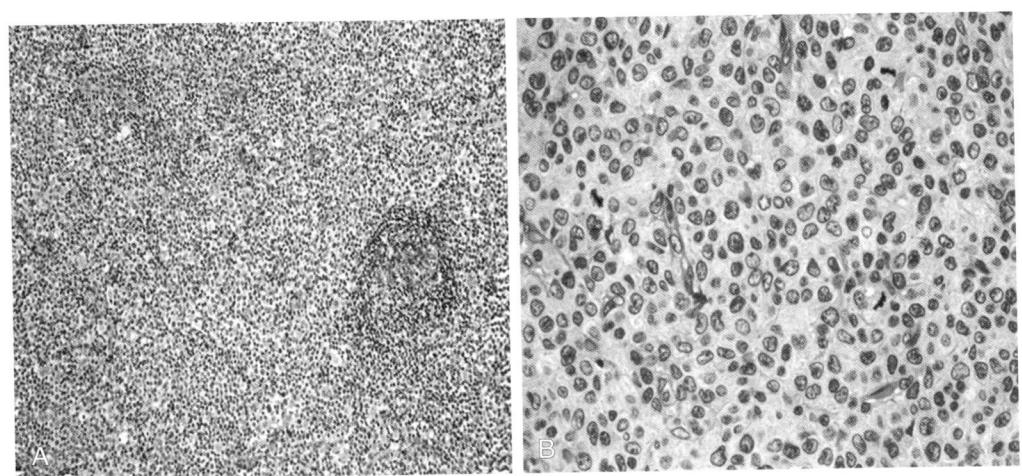

Figure 21-5. Mantle cell lymphoma with a marginal zone pattern. A, Tumor cells expand the marginal zone area outside an apparent preserved mantle cuff. **B,** Tumor cells in the marginal zone area have abundant pale cytoplasm, resembling monocytoid cells.

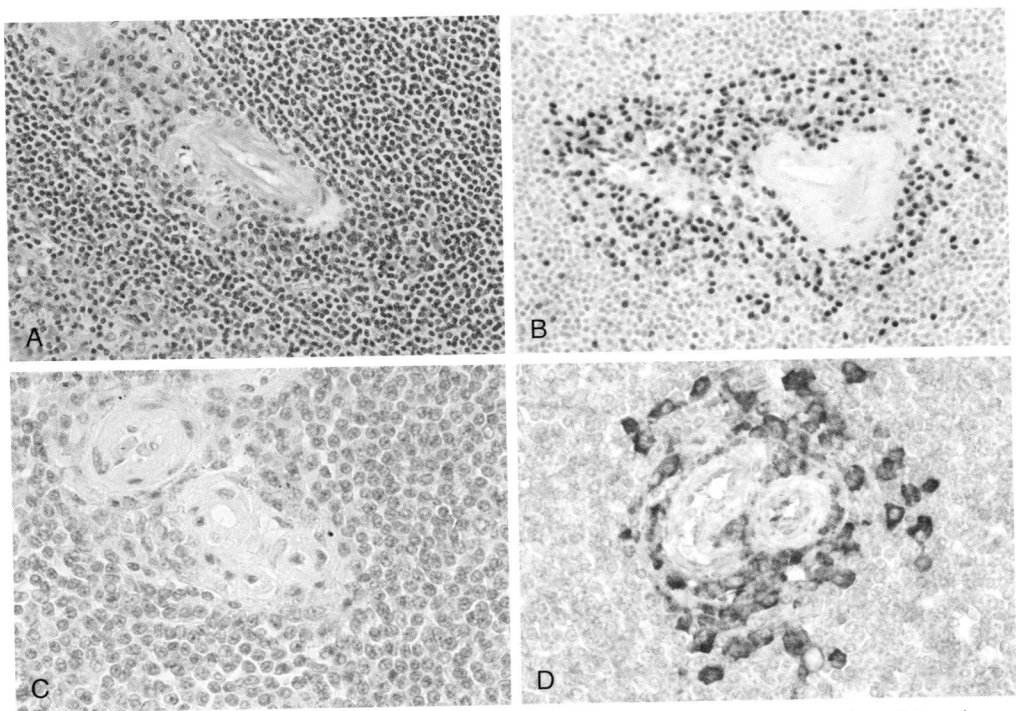

Figure 21-6. Mantle cell lymphoma with clonally related plasma cell differentiation. A, Splenic mantle cell lymphoma with perivascular plasma cell differentiation. **B,** Cyclin D1 is expressed both in the plasma cell component and in the small-cell component. The intensity of the staining is stronger in the plasma cells than in the atypical lymphoid cells. The plasma cells are negative for lambda **(C),** but positive for kappa **(D).** *(Case courtesy Dr. S. Serrano, Hospital del Mar, Barcelona, Spain.)*

Bone Marrow and Peripheral Blood

Bone marrow infiltration, independent of peripheral blood involvement, occurs in 50% to 91% of patients[15,25,26,29,36,39,71,72] and is detected more frequently in core biopsies than in aspirates.[73] The pattern of infiltration may be nodular, interstitial, or paratrabecular, with most biopsies exhibiting a combination of these. Isolated paratrabecular aggregates are rare. In some cases, diffuse infiltration of the bone marrow may be seen. An intrasinusoidal pattern may be seen in some cases, mainly nnMCL (Fig. 21-7). The degree of infiltration does not seem to correlate with the histologic variants of MCL identified in lymph node biopsies, architectural patterns, or patient survival.[73] Immunohistochemical stains, including cyclin D1, can be used in the differential diagnosis of bone marrow biopsies to distinguish MCL from other small-cell lymphomas.[72,74] Dual staining of cyclin D1/CD79a and PAX5/CD5 may be useful for the detection of MCL in the marrow, particularly when there is a low-level or focal involvement.[75]

The cytologic appearance of tumor cells in peripheral blood and bone marrow aspirates is similar to the spectrum seen in tissues (Fig. 21-8). Circulating cells in most MCLs usually show a mixture of small-to-medium-sized cells with scant cytoplasm, prominent nuclear irregularities, and reticular chromatin.

Some cells may have round nuclei, but the chromatin does not have the clumped appearance seen in CLL. Leukemic blastoid MCL may mimic acute leukemia, with medium-to-large-sized cells, a high nuclear-to-cytoplasmic ratio, finely dispersed chromatin, and relatively small or inconspicuous nucleoli.[42,44,76] These cases may have *MYC* rearrangements in addition to the *CCND1* translocation.[46,47,77,78] Some cases of leukemic MCL have very large atypical cells with prominent nucleoli that correspond to a leukemic phase of the pleomorphic variant with similar morphology in the lymph nodes.[63-66] Cases previously diagnosed as B-prolymphocytic leukemia carrying the t(11;14) translocation and cyclin D1 overexpression are now considered leukemic MCL.[79]

Spleen

Macroscopically, splenic involvement by MCL shows a generalized micronodular pattern that is occasionally associated with perivascular infiltration. Histologically, the differential diagnosis of MCL and other small-cell lymphomas in the spleen may be difficult.[80-82] White pulp nodules are enlarged, with variable involvement of the red pulp. Residual "naked" germinal centers are found in 50% of cases. Tumor cells show a similar monotonous morphology as in other locations. Interestingly, some cases may exhibit a marginal zone–like area at the periphery of the nodules, comprising cells with more abundant pale cytoplasm.[81]

Gastrointestinal Tract

A common manifestation of GI disease is lymphomatoid polyposis, in which multiple lymphoid polyps are identified in the small and large bowel (Fig. 21-9). These may be associated with large tumor masses, usually ileocecal, and regional lymphadenopathy.[30,31,83-86] Although this clinicopathologic presentation is relatively characteristic of MCL, it can also be caused by other lymphomas, particularly follicular lymphoma and marginal zone lymphoma of the mucosa-associated lymphoid tissue (MALT).[84,87] Cyclin D1 expression is useful for the differential diagnosis of these tumors.[83] GI involvement without the macroscopic appearance of polyposis may also occur.[88] In these cases, superficial ulcers, large tumor masses, and diffuse thickening of the mucosa are common macroscopic findings. Routine gastroscopy and colonoscopy have identified MCL infiltration in up to 92% of patients.[85,89,90] Asymptomatic

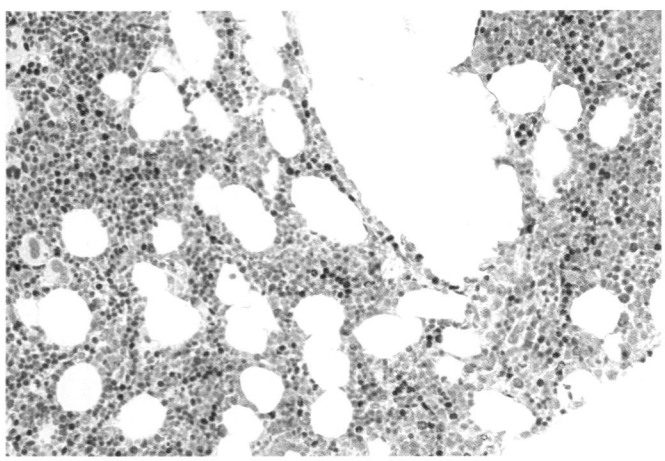

Figure 21-7. Cyclin D1 staining in a bone marrow biopsy highlights the intrasinusoidal infiltration by tumor cells of a leukemic non-nodal MCL.

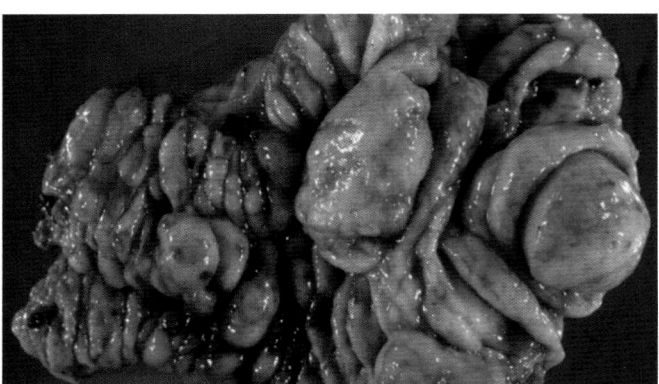

Figure 21-9. Mantle cell lymphoma involving the intestine with multiple lymphomatous polyposis. *(Courtesy Dr. T. Alvaro, Hospital Verge de la Cinta, Tortosa, Spain.)*

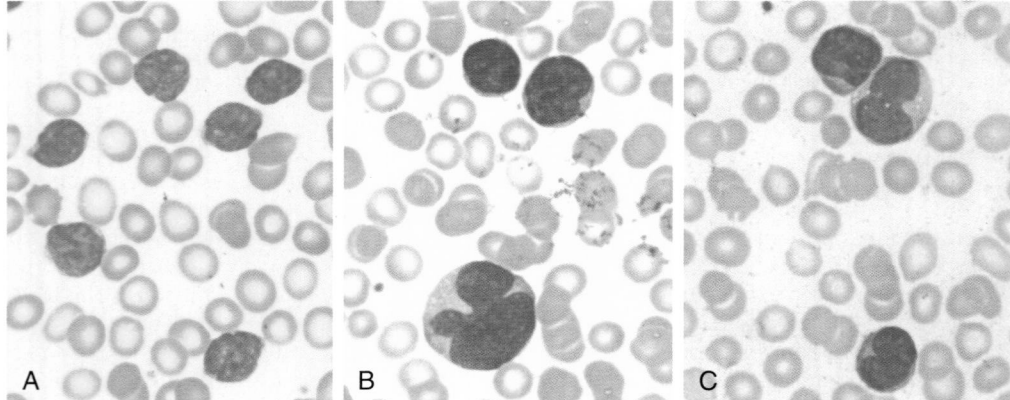

Figure 21-8. **Cytologic spectrum of tumor cells in peripheral blood smears of leukemic mantle cell lymphoma. A,** Classic variant with small lymphocytes, slightly indented or cleaved nuclei, condensed chromatin, and scant cytoplasm. **B,** Blastoid variant may show a mixture of small atypical cells and larger pleomorphic tumor cells with irregular nuclei. **C,** In other cases, all atypical cells have a more blastic morphology, with finely dispersed chromatin and inconspicuous nucleoli (Giemsa stain).

involvement of the GI tract with GI microscopic infiltration of endoscopically normal mucosa is very common (above 80%). However, these findings do not usually change the management decision.[85,89,90] In some cases, glandular infiltration by tumor cells may mimic lymphoepithelial lesions, making the distinction between MCL and marginal zone lymphomas difficult. However, the scarcity of these lesions and the monotonous character of the lymphoid infiltrate should suggest a diagnosis of MCL.[88] Interestingly, MCLs, and other lymphomas involving GI mucosa, express $\alpha_4\beta_7$-integrin, a homing receptor that binds to mucosal vascular addressin cell adhesion molecule 1 (MAdCAM-1), which is selectively expressed in endothelial cells of mucosa.[91]

Histologic Progression

Sequential biopsies have shown that the histologic pattern of MCL remains relatively stable but progression from nodular to diffuse pattern and increased proliferation may be observed in serial biopsies.[34,57,92,93] Some cases may show an oscillating course, with changing patterns during the evolution of the disease.[94] Although most blastoid MCLs are detected already at diagnosis, around 20% to 35% of classic/small-cell variants may progress to a blastoid morphology in subsequent relapses and may be more common at autopsy than at diagnosis.[34,93-95] A clonal relationship has been demonstrated in the progression from classic to blastoid MCL.[96] Transformed blastoid MCLs display significant higher degree of aneuploidy and poor outcomes compared with de novo blastoid variants.[97] On the other hand, 50% of MCLs with blastoid or pleomorphic cytology at primary diagnosis may relapse as a classic variant. In some cases, tumor progression is associated with the development of an overt leukemic phase.[41,42,44,76]

Composite Mantle Cell Lymphoma

MCL may be occasionally associated with a second lymphoid neoplasm at the same site, particularly follicular lymphoma, CLL/SLL, splenic and nodal marginal zone lymphomas, plasma cell neoplasms, and Hodgkin lymphoma.[93,98] Molecular studies have identified unrelated clonal rearrangements in most of these tumors, indicating distinct clonal origins but also the presence of common clone-specific IGH rearrangement in the MCL and the second lymphoma, suggesting the unusual evolution of a single malignant clone resulting in two morphologically, phenotypically, and molecularly distinct lymphomas.[99]

IMMUNOPHENOTYPE

MCL is a mature B-cell neoplasm expressing the B-cell markers CD19, CD20, CD21, PAX5, and CD79a (Fig. 21-10; Table 21-3). Surface immunoglobulins are usually of moderate to strong intensity, with frequent co-expression of immunoglobulin (Ig)M and IgD and a tendency to express lambda more frequently than kappa light chain (Table 21-3). The residual germinal centers seen in these tumors are always polyclonal. A peculiar characteristic of MCL is co-expression of the T cell–associated antigen CD5 in most cases (Fig. 21-10). However, CD5 negativity may be seen in MCL mainly with small-cell morphology and SOX11 negativity.[100-102] CD43 is also frequently expressed, but other T-cell antigens are usually negative. CD8[103] and CD7[104] positivity by flow cytometry have been reported in isolated cases of MCL. Contrary to CLL, CD23 is usually negative but may be seen in indolent nnMCL[105,106] and rare cases of blastoid MCL.[105] CD200, an antigen usually expressed in CLL, is negative in most MCL,[106-108] although it may be positive in a subset of nnMCL.[49,50,109] CD10 and BCL6, two germinal-center cell markers, are usually negative, although occasional positive cases have been documented.[110-112] MCL with co-expression of CD10 and BCL6 are more likely to have bone marrow involvement, blastoid/pleomorphic morphology, higher Ki67 index, and complex cytogenetics with poor prognosis.[109,113] In these cases the differential diagnosis with diffuse large B-cell lymphoma carrying *CCND1* rearrangement as a secondary event has to be considered. LEF1, a transcription factor related to the WNT pathway, is expressed in the nucleus of CLL but not in other mature small B-cell lymphomas, including MCL, although some rare cases may be positive, particularly with blastoid or pleomorphic morphology.[114] LEF1 is also expressed in T cells and some large B-cell lymphomas including those transformed from small cells.[115,116] IRF4/MUM1 may be detected in around 50% of the tumors in at least a minor subset of cells.[69] The plasma cell–associated transcription factors BLIMP1 and XBP1 may be seen in around 50% and 30% of the cases, respectively, but they are significantly more frequently expressed in SOX11-negative MCL.[69] Some blastoid/pleomorphic MCL carrying *MYC* translocations may express terminal deoxynucleotidyl transferase (TdT). These cases are usually SOX11-positive.[47]

Table 21-3 Immunophenotype of Small-Cell Malignant Lymphomas

Diagnosis	Ig*	CD20	CD3	CD5	CD43	CD23	CD10	BCL6	Cyclin D1	LEF1	SOX11	IRF4/ MUM1	Annexin A1
CLL	M/D	+	–	+	+	+	–	–	–	+	–	–/+†	–
MCL	M/D/λ	++	–	+	+	–	–	–/+	++	–	+§	–/+	–
FL	M/G	++	–	–	–	–/+	+	+	–	–	–	–	–
LPL	M	++	–	–/+	+	–	–/+	–	–	–	–	–/+‡	–
MALT	M	++	–	–/+	–/+	–	–	–	–	–	–	–/+‡	–
SMZL	M/D	++	–	–	–	–	–	–	–	–	–	–	–
HCL	G/λ	++	–	–	–	–	–	–	+	–	–/+	–	+

*Kappa more commonly expressed than lambda, except as indicated.
†Positivity in occasional prolymphocytes and paraimmunoblasts.
‡Positivity in cells with plasmacytoid differentiation.
§Some MCLs are SOX11 negative and have particular clinical and biological features.
CLL, Chronic lymphocytic leukemia; *FL,* follicular lymphoma; *HCL,* hairy cell leukemia; *Ig,* immunoglobulin; *LPL,* lymphoplasmacytic lymphoma; *MALT,* marginal zone B-cell lymphoma of mucosa-associated lymphoid tissue; *MCL,* mantle cell lymphoma; *SMZL,* splenic marginal zone lymphoma.

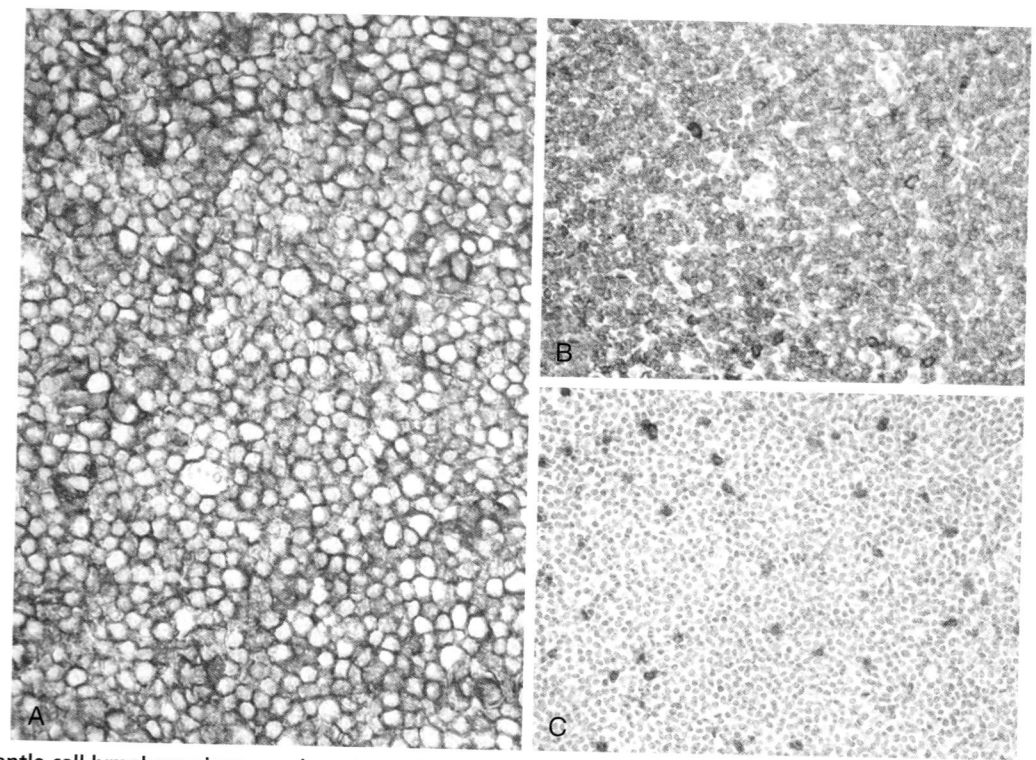

Figure 21-10. Mantle cell lymphoma immunophenotype. A, Tumor cells strongly positive for CD20. **B,** CD5-positive tumor cells. **C,** CD3 is positive only in scattered reactive T cells.

Overexpression of cyclin D1 is a constant and highly specific phenomenon in MCL that is very useful for the diagnosis (Fig. 21-2).[72,117,118] Current available antibodies, including rabbit monoclonal, provide consistent cyclin D1 staining.[119] In addition to immunohistochemistry, cyclin D1 overexpression may be detected by quantitative reverse transcription polymerase chain reaction that may be useful when routine immunohistochemistry cannot be easily applied, such as in leukemic lymphoproliferative disorders or fine-needle aspirates.[120,121] Cyclin D1 is always detected in the cell nucleus, although the intensity may vary from cell to cell and case to case, probably reflecting parameters such as messenger RNA (mRNA) and protein stability. In some cases, extension to the cytoplasm may be seen. Cyclin D1 is also detected in the nuclei of histiocytes, endothelial cells, and epithelial cells, providing an important internal positive control. In addition to MCL, cyclin D1 is expressed in 25% of multiple myelomas with the t(11;14) translocation, amplification of the gene, or without apparent structural alterations of the gene.[122] Low levels of cyclin D1 are also detected in HCL,[123,124] and in cells of the proliferation centers in CLL, but this expression is not associated with the t(11;14) translocation in any of the two entities.[125] However, SOX11 may be expressed in HCL but not in the CLL proliferation centers.[126,127] Cyclin D1 expression has been identified in up to 15% of diffuse large B-cell lymphomas (DLBCLs) in which up to 80% of the cells may be positive. However, these cases are SOX11 negative and usually do not carry the t(11,14) translocation.[128-130] However, occasional DLBCL may express cyclin D1 with *CCND1* rearrangements.[131-133] The differential diagnosis of these cases may require additional genetic and molecular studies. The expression of cyclin D1 associated with copy number gains has been reported in mediastinal large B-cell lymphoma.[134]

Immunohistochemical detection of the cyclin-dependent kinase (CDK) inhibitor p27 is also useful in the differential diagnosis of MCL. Expression of p27 in lymphomas is usually inversely related to the proliferation activity of the cells. Thus it is strongly expressed in CLL, follicular lymphomas, and marginal zone lymphomas, but it is negative or weakly expressed in large-cell lymphomas. In MCL, p27 staining is independent of the proliferative rate and is usually negative or weaker than in the associated T cells in classic MCL and positive in blastoid variants.[135,136] HCL is also negative or very weakly positive.[74]

SOX11 is a neural transcription factor expressed in the nucleus of most MCLs, including blastoid and pleomorphic variants and cyclin D1–negative MCL (Fig. 21-11), but not in other mature B-cell lymphomas apart from weak expression in some Burkitt lymphomas. It is also expressed in T-lymphoblastic and B-lymphoblastic leukemias/lymphomas.[137,138] SOX11 is not expressed or very weak in the nnMCL subtype.[139] New monoclonal antibodies are useful for the recognition of this marker, although they have slightly different specificity and sensitivity. The monoclonal SOX11 antibody clone MRQ-58 (Cell Marque, Rocklin, CA) is highly specific but does not recognize cases with very low SOX11 expression. A meta-analysis evidenced that the MRQ-58 clone shows a robust performance to study SOX11 expression.[140] On the other hand, clone CLO143 (Atlas Antibodies) is more sensitive but cross-reacts with SOX4 and may be seen in some non-MCL cases.[141,142] The definition of guidelines in interlaboratory studies confirms that SOX11 status can reliably be assessed by IHC, also on

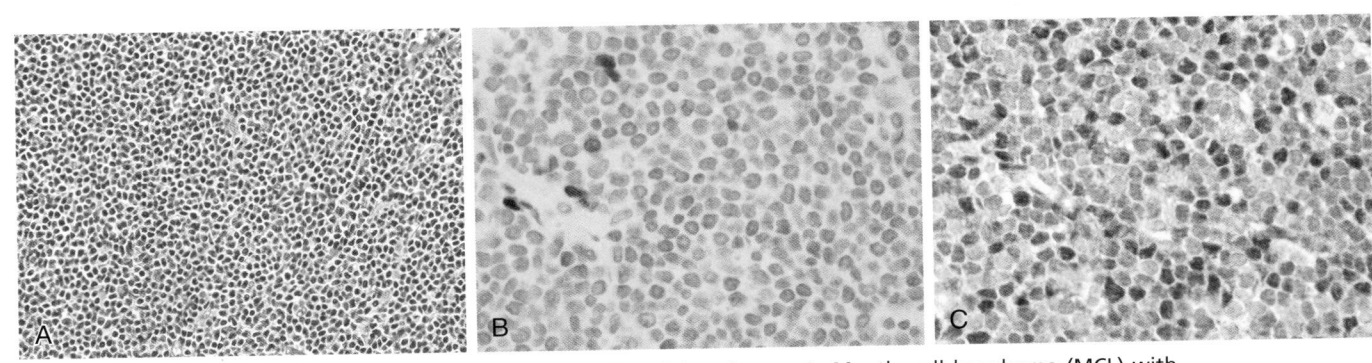

Figure 21-11. Cyclin D1–negative mantle cell lymphoma. A, Mantle cell lymphoma (MCL) with classic variant morphology. **B,** Cyclin D1–negative tumor cells. **C,** SOX11 is strongly positive in the nucleus of the tumor cells.

decalcified tissue, either formalin or B5 fixed.[143,144] The measurement of SOX11 mRNA expression using RNAscope in situ hybridization is also a reliable method to detect SOX11 expression in MCL.[145]

Ki67 staining is very relevant to define prognosis in MCL with a proposed cutoff of 30% defining more aggressive behavior.[143,146,147]

MCL usually contains a prominent meshwork of follicular dendritic cells, which are more variable in frequency and distribution in diffuse than in nodular cases. In nodular cases, two different patterns of follicular dendritic cells have been recognized. A dense and concentric meshwork of cells may represent colonization of preexisting follicular centers by tumor cells, whereas a loose and irregular pattern may correspond to expansion of primary follicles.[148] Cyclin D1 staining may identify early infiltration of germinal centers by tumor cells.

MANTLE CELL LYMPHOMA VARIANTS

Early Alterations and In Situ Mantle Cell Neoplasia

Cells carrying the t(11;14) translocation have been detected at very low levels with sensitive techniques in the blood of healthy individuals (8%).[149] These clones can persist for long periods, but their potential to evolve into an overt lymphoma seems extremely low. However, the observation of a simultaneous MCL with the same clonal origin in recipients and donors many years after an allogenic bone marrow transplantation indicates that these clones may eventually progress to a full-blown tumor, and it may require a long latency period of up to 10 years.[150-152]

Cyclin D1–positive cells carrying the t(11;14) translocation have been incidentally found in the mantle zones of otherwise reactive lymphoid tissue in healthy individuals (Fig. 21-12).[153] These lesions were termed *in situ MCL*, but their malignant potential seems very limited, and the alternative term of *in situ mantle cell neoplasia (isMCN)* was proposed to avoid overtreatment. The cells are seen predominantly within the inner layers of the mantle cuffs of normal-appearing follicles with preserved lymph node architecture. In some cases, the cyclin D1–positive cells may occupy the mantle zone, but they are usually intermingled with negative lymphocytes, and the mantle is not expanded. In some cases, the positive cells may be seen in the center of the follicle. These lesions

are uncommon and were not identified in more than 100 consecutive reactive lesions in two different studies.[153,154] The potential evolution to overt MCL has not been well studied but seems low. In one study, 1 of 12 of these lesions developed an overt MCL 4 years after its detection.[153] Retrospective analyses of reactive biopsies obtained in patients who subsequently developed MCL have identified isMCN or small extranodal MCL infiltrates antedating the diagnosis of MCL from 2 to 15 years, suggesting that MCL might have a long latency period.[154] In some patients, in situ lesions may be seen in different distant lymph nodes.[153,155] Also, some patients with nodal isMCN may have clonal lymphocytosis with cyclin D1 expression.[153,156] None of these findings has been associated with progressive disease, and patients should be managed conservatively. Intriguingly, isMCN has also been found in association with other lymphoid neoplasias.[153] Most in situ lesions express SOX11, whereas few are SOX11 negative, suggesting that the in situ stage may be a common step in both SOX11-negative and SOX11-positive MCL subtypes.[153,157] By immunohistochemistry, these neoplastic cells are also positive for pan-B-cell markers, IgD, and BCL2. However, compared with cMCL, which usually expresses CD5 and CD43, isMCN is more frequently negative for these markers. Incidental in situ lesions have also been found in patients who are apparently in complete remission after treatment, suggesting that this microenvironment may sustain residual tumor cells resistant to chemotherapy.[153]

In situ MCN must be differentiated from early involvement by overt MCL with a mantle zone growth pattern. In these cases, the mantles are usually expanded and densely occupied by cyclin D1–positive cells that may focally extend to interfollicular areas. Images of back-to-back cyclin D1–positive mantle zones are commonly seen. This pattern correlates with progression to disseminated disease more frequently than in situ lesions.[153,154]

Leukemic Non-nodal Mantle Cell Lymphoma

Early studies identified a subset of MCL patients with a more indolent clinical behavior that presented clinically with a leukemic non-nodal disease associated in some cases with splenomegaly.[27,28] Subsequent studies have suggested that these tumors may correspond to a specific subtype of MCL named nnMCL that is characterized by a leukemic phase with asymptomatic lymphocytosis persisting for a long time

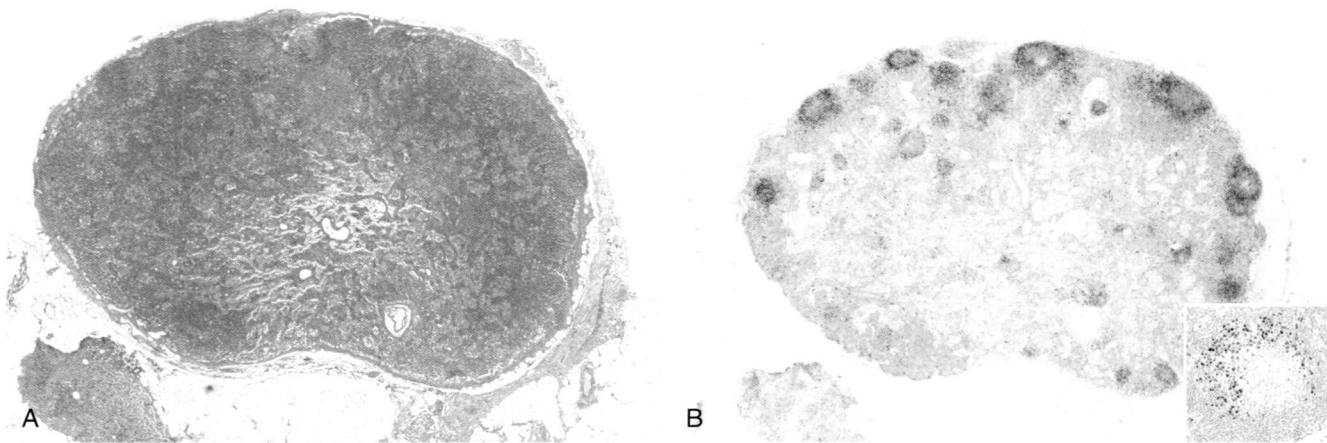

Figure 21-12. In situ mantle cell neoplasia. A, Reactive lymph node without morphologic evidence of mantle cell expansion. **B,** Cyclin D1 staining highlights the infiltration of the mantles of reactive lymphoid follicles by cyclin D1–positive cells. The positive cells are mainly present in the inner layers of the mantle, interspersed with negative lymphoid cells *(inset).*

without requiring treatment. These patients may develop splenomegaly, and splenectomy may temporarily control the disease.[48,49,158-160]

nnMCL frequently has a small-cell morphology, which makes differential diagnosis with CLL or other small B-cell lymphomas difficult. Phenotypically they may express CD200 and CD23, and around one-third are CD5 negative.[49,100,106] Contrary to cMCL, most of these tumors have mutated immunoglobulin heavy chain variable region genes (IGHV) and have simple karyotypes with no or very few chromosomal alterations in addition to the t(11;14) translocation.[48,139] nnMCL and cMCL have marked differences in the gene expression of certain programs and they may be reliably distinguished by the expression of a 16-gene signature.[161] Among the differentially expressed genes is *SOX11* that is negative or very low in nnMCL.[48-50,109,139,158,162] cMCLs have a gene-expression profile closer to that of naïve B cells, whereas the profile of nnMCL is more similar to memory cells. Some SOX11-negative cases show morphologic and phenotypic plasmacytic differentiation (see Fig. 21-6).[69,70,163] Genome-wide sequencing studies have also shown some differences in the mutational landscape of cMCL and nnMCL. Some SOX11-negative MCLs have a blastoid/pleomorphic morphology, *TP53* mutations, and complex karyotypes, suggesting that they correspond to a progression of this disease.

Cyclin D1–Negative Mantle Cell Lymphoma

Some tumors with identical morphologic and phenotypic features as MCL are negative for cyclin D1 and the t(11;14) translocation. Some cases may show a mantle zone pattern or blastoid morphology.[164,165] SOX11 is highly expressed in cyclin D1–negative MCL and is a reliable tool to identify these tumors in clinical practice (Fig. 21-11).[137,140,144,145,164] The expression profile of these MCL is indistinguishable from that of cMCL.[166] These cases carry *CCND2* or *CCND3* translocations with IG genes, sometimes cryptic, including only the enhancer region of kappa or lambda genes inserted in the vicinity of these cyclin genes and can be detected by fluorescence in situ hybridization (FISH) probes.[164,167] Overexpression of these cyclins can be demonstrated by reverse-transcription

quantitative PCR (RT-qPCR).[167,168] Immunohistochemistry is not useful in routine practice because it is not discriminative enough to distinguish the high levels of these cyclins in MCL from their expression in other lymphoid neoplasms without the translocations.[137,164,167] Cyclin D1–negative MCLs have a clinical presentation similar to cyclin D1–positive cases, with frequent nodal and extranodal involvement and aggressive clinical behavior. The Ki67 proliferative index is also of prognostic significance. Genetic studies have detected a similar profile of secondary genetic alterations.[164] Rare MCLs may be cyclin D1 negative by immunohistochemistry but still carry the t(11;14). The negativity in these cases seems to be secondary to mutations or splicing alterations that eliminate the epitope recognized by common antibodies used in the clinics.[169]

CYTOGENETIC FINDINGS

The characteristic cytogenetic alteration in MCL is the t(11;14) (q13;q32) translocation but occasional translocation of 11q13 with the kappa and lambda loci in chromosomes 2 and 22 have also been reported.[170] These translocation are detected by conventional cytogenetics in up to 65% of MCLs. However, with FISH, they can be found in virtually all cases.[171-173] Break-apart probes for *CCND1* may detect cases in which this gene is not translocated to the IGH and they are recommended for routine practice.[70] The t(11;14) translocation has been identified in 20% of multiple myelomas.[8,174] In addition, cyclin D1 gene amplification without translocation has been documented in cases of multiple myeloma and DLBCL but not in MCL.[122,131,132] *CCND1* rearrangement can be seen in occasional DLBCL and in the progression of small B-cell neoplasms as a secondary event.[133,175]

Cytogenetic studies, including conventional analysis, FISH, comparative genomic hybridization, and array-based analysis, have revealed a high number of secondary chromosomal alterations in MCL that target genes involved in proliferation, DNA damage, and cell survival pathways (Table 21-4).[77] The most common secondary alterations are losses of chromosomes 1p, 6q, 8p, 9p, 10p, 11q, 13q, and 17p and gains in 3q, 7p, 8q, 12q, and 18q. Blastoid variants have

Table 21-4 Commonly Altered Chromosomal Regions in Mantle Cell Lymphoma Detected by Comparative Genomic Hybridization and Array-Based Genomic Analysis

Chromosome Region*	Frequency (%)	Suggested Target Genes[†]	Functional Process
Gains			
3q26.1-q26.32	28–50	?	?
7p22.1-p22.3	8–31	?	?
8q24.21	6–32	**MYC**	Cell growth, proliferation, apoptosis
10p12.2-p12.31	6–12	**BMI1**	Cell cycle, DNA damage response
11q13.3-q21	4–14	**CCND1**	Cell cycle
12q14	3–7	**CDK4, MDM2**	Cell cycle, DNA damage response, apoptosis
13q31.3	5–11	**MIR17HG**	Cell cycle, apoptosis
18q21.33	18–55	**BCL2**	Apoptosis
Losses			
1p32.3-p33	18–52	CDKN2C, FAF1	Cell cycle, apoptosis
2q13	3–17	BCL2L11[‡]	Pro-apoptosis
2q37.1	15–33	SP100-SP140	DNA damage response
6q23.3	19–36	TNFAIP3	NF-κB inhibitor
6q25	19–36	LATS1	Hippo signaling pathway
8p21.3	17–34	MCPH1	DNA damage response
9p21.2	10–36	MOBKL2B	Hippo signaling pathway
9p21.3	10–36	**CDKN2A, ARF1[‡]**	Cell cycle, DNA damage response
9q22.2-q22.31	17–31	CDC14B, FANCC, GAS1	?
10p14-p13	18–28		
11q22.3	11–57	**ATM**	DNA damage response
13q13.3-q34	25–70	DLEU1, DLEU2, RB1	Cell cycle, apoptosis
13q34	16–54	CUL4A, ING1	Cell cycle, DNA damage response
17p13	21–45	**TP53**	Cell cycle, DNA damage response
19P13.3	10–24	MOBKL2A	Hippo signaling pathway

*Minimal altered regions vary slightly among different studies.
[†]Confirmed target genes are in boldface.
[‡]Homozygous deletions have been identified.
Modified from Royo C, Salaverria I, Hartmann EM, et al. The complex landscape of genetic alterations in mantle cell lymphoma. *Semin Cancer Biol.* 2011;21:322-334.

more complex karyotypes and high-level DNA amplifications than classic variants.[43-45,61,62,97,176] In addition, certain chromosomal imbalances such as gains of 3q, 7p, and 12q and losses of 17p are significantly more frequent in blastoid than classic variants. Tetraploidy is more frequent in pleomorphic (80%) and blastoid (36%) variants than in classic MCLs (8%).[62] Chromosome 8q24 alterations, including the t(8;14) (q24;q32) translocation and variants, have been identified in occasional blastoid MCLs with a very aggressive clinical course.[45,46,177] Copy neutral loss of heterozygosity is an alternative mechanism for the inactivation of mutated tumor suppressor genes such as *TP53* at 17p13.[178] Complex genome alterations including chromoplexy, chromothripsis, and breakage-fusion-bridge (BFB) cycles are more frequently in aggressive cMCL variants.[61,179]

MOLECULAR CHARACTERISTICS

Translocation (11;14) and Cyclin D1 Expression

The t(11;14) translocation juxtaposes the immunoglobulin heavy chain joining region in chromosome 14 to a broad region on 11q13 designated B-cell lymphoma/leukemia 1 (BCL1). Most rearrangements (30% to 55%) occur in a region known as the *major translocation cluster (MTC)*, whereas up to 10% to 20% of cases may have breakpoints in other distal regions. The MTC breakpoints occur within a relatively small region of around 80 base pairs on chromosome 11 and in the 5′ area of one of the Ig JH regions on chromosome 14, making it possible to detect by PCR techniques.[180]

The target gene of this translocation is *CCND1*, located approximately 120 kb downstream of the BCL1 translocation locus. This translocation occurs at the pro-B stage of differentiation during the recombination of the V(D) J segments of the IGH variable region in the bone marrow. IG breaks are mediated by recombination-activating genes (RAG enzymes) and mainly occur in IGHD and IGHJ genes, likely during the initial D-J recombination. However, in a small subset of cases the t(11;14) seems to occur in mature B stage during somatic hypermutation or class switch recombination mediated by activation-induced cytidine deaminase (AID) machinery.[179] *CCND1* translocation to the immunoglobulin light chain genes are uncommon.[77] Cryptic translocations of IG, particularly insertions of IGK and IGL enhancers near *CCND1*, have been reported.[181,182]

Cyclin D1 is not normally expressed in lymphocytes or myeloid cells, but it is constantly expressed in MCLs.[117,118,120,121] Tumor cells express two major mRNA transcripts of 4.5 and 1.5 kb that contain the whole coding region of the gene and differ only in the length of the 3′ untranslated region. Some MCLs express truncated transcripts at the 3′ untranslated region that are more stable and show very high levels of expression caused by the loss of AUUUA destabilizing sequences of the 3′ region.[117,118] These truncated messages are generated by second chromosomal rearrangements or point mutations at the 3′ region of the gene.[170,174,183-186] These secondary events in the 3′ region of *CCND1* may be important in disease progression. Gains and amplifications of the translocated allele have been observed in some tumors that also have high levels of cyclin D1 expression.[178] A frequent polymorphism of exon 4 may generate a splicing isoform (cyclin D1b) missing exon 5 that may be differentially expressed but does not seem to be relevant in MCL pathogenesis.[187-190]

In addition to the truncations of the 3′ UTR, *CCND1* is frequently mutated in the 5′ region, particularly in nnMCL, because of the activity of AID.[97,179,191-194] Recurrent coding mutations in the first exon of cyclin D1 have been associated with the stabilization of cyclin D1 protein and increased resistance of MCL cell lines to ibrutinib.[195] These mutations seem to be caused by AID. The adoption of all these different mechanisms by MCL cells to increase the levels of cyclin D1 mRNA expression reinforces the relevance of *CCND1* in MCL lymphomagenesis and suggests a dose-dependent oncogenic effect.

Cyclin D1 Oncogenic Mechanisms

Cyclin D1 functions as a weak oncogene in animal models, cooperating with other oncogenes, generally *MYC* and *RAS*, or with frequent deregulated tumor suppressor genes (TSGs), including *ATM* and *BIM*, although their transforming mechanisms are not well understood.[196-198] Cyclin D1 participates in the control of the G_1 phase by binding to CDK4 and CDK6. The complexes phosphorylate retinoblastoma protein, leading to the inactivation of its suppressor effect on cell cycle progression and the release of important transcription factors, such as E2F, that participate in the regulation of other genes involved in cell cycle.[199] *RB1* may be inactivated by truncating mutations in occasional MCL, reinforcing the role of this checkpoint in the pathogenesis of these tumors.[200]

MCL may also have impaired control of late G_1 phase and G_1 phase to S phase transition. This step is regulated by the cyclin E–CDK2 complex and the cyclin kinase inhibitor p27 (*CDKN1B*). In classic MCL, p27 immunohistochemical detection is negative or weak, but it is paradoxically positive in blastic variants. No structural alterations of the *CDKN1B* gene have been found, and low detection of the protein may be caused by increased protein degradation by the proteasome pathway[201] or sequestration by the overexpressed cyclin D1, rendering it inaccessible to antibody detection.[202] p27 inhibits the complexes between CDK2 and cyclin E at the end of the G_1 phase. Increased degradation or blocking of p27 by cyclin D1 releases the activation of these complexes and allows the cell to progress to the following cell-cycle phases.[135] All these observations indicate that cyclin D1 deregulation plays an important role in the development of MCL, probably overcoming the suppressive effect of retinoblastoma protein and p27 (Fig. 21-13). Besides these mechanisms, cyclin D1 may have an important oncogenic potential independent of its catalytic function by acting as a transcriptional modulator of multiple genes or participating in the DNA damage response pathway.[203-207] However, whether these mechanisms participate in the MCL pathogenesis is not yet known.

SOX11 Oncogenic Mechanisms

SOX11 is a transcriptional factor physiologically involved in neural organogenesis and is highly expressed in cMCL, including cyclin D1 negative variants, but not in nnMCL.[137,164,208] SOX11 promotes tumor growth of MCL cells in vivo and regulates a broad transcriptional program that includes B-cell differentiation, proliferation, apoptosis, angiogenesis, motility, invasion, and BCR signaling (Fig. 21-13).[209] SOX11 may contribute to MCL pathogenesis blocking B-cell differentiation forcing PAX5 expression and impairing its necessary downmodulation for B cells to differentiate to plasma cells.[163] SOX11 also represses BCL6 expression that may prevent cells from entering the germinal center.[210] SOX11 may increase cell survival by enhancing BCR signaling.[211] SOX11 also promotes the aggressiveness of MCL cells regulating their interactions with the microenvironment inducing angiogenesis through PDGFA, tumor cell migration, adhesion, and cell proliferation by CXCR4 and FAK, and modulating an immunosuppressive microenvironment characterized by CD70 overexpression in tumor cells and increased Treg cell infiltration. The lack of SOX11 in nnMCL may explain the long period of these cases with a leukemic phase without nodal involvement because they have less angiogenic and tumor invasion capacity.[49,139,158,212-215]

Despite the relevant role of SOX11 in MCL, the mechanisms leading to its specific upregulation in this lymphoma are not well understood. Studies have identified an active distant super enhancer that interacts with the promoter in SOX11 expressing tumors.[216,217] Some evidence suggests that *STAT3* and *CCND1* may act as a transcriptional repressor and positive regulator of SOX11, respectively.[218]

Molecular and Genomic Profile

In addition to cyclin D1 deregulation as the primary oncogenic event, genetic and molecular studies have identified other alterations that are important mechanisms in disease progression. These gene alterations particularly involve cell cycle, DNA damage response, and cell survival pathways, among others.[219-221] Whole-genome/whole-exome sequencing (WGS/WES) studies have confirmed the relevance of these pathways and identified new mutated genes that might be clinically and biologically relevant (Table 21-5).[97,179,191-194,222]

Cell Cycle Deregulation

Highly proliferative and clinically aggressive MCLs carry oncogenic alterations in two major regulatory pathways that are involved in cell-cycle control and senescence: CDKN2A-CDK4-RB1 and ARF-MDM2-TP53. Homozygous deletions of the *CDKN2A* locus on 9p21 have been detected in 20% to 30% of blastoid variants but in less than 5% of typical cases.[56,223,224] Inactivation of other members of the *CDKN2* family, such as *CDKN1B*, *CDKN2B*, and *CDKN2C*, are less frequent.[178,179] *CDK4* amplification and inactivating mutations of *RB1* in some aggressive blastoid MCLs strengthens the significance of the deregulation of the G_1-to-S transition in MCL progression.[200,225] *TP53* mutations are rarely observed in classic low-proliferative MCL, but they are identified in approximately 30% of highly proliferative blastoid MCL, usually associated with a 17p deletion.[61,179] Concomitant alterations in *TP53* and *CDKN2A-CDK4-RB1* may have an additive prognostic effect independent of the Ki67 index.[223-225]

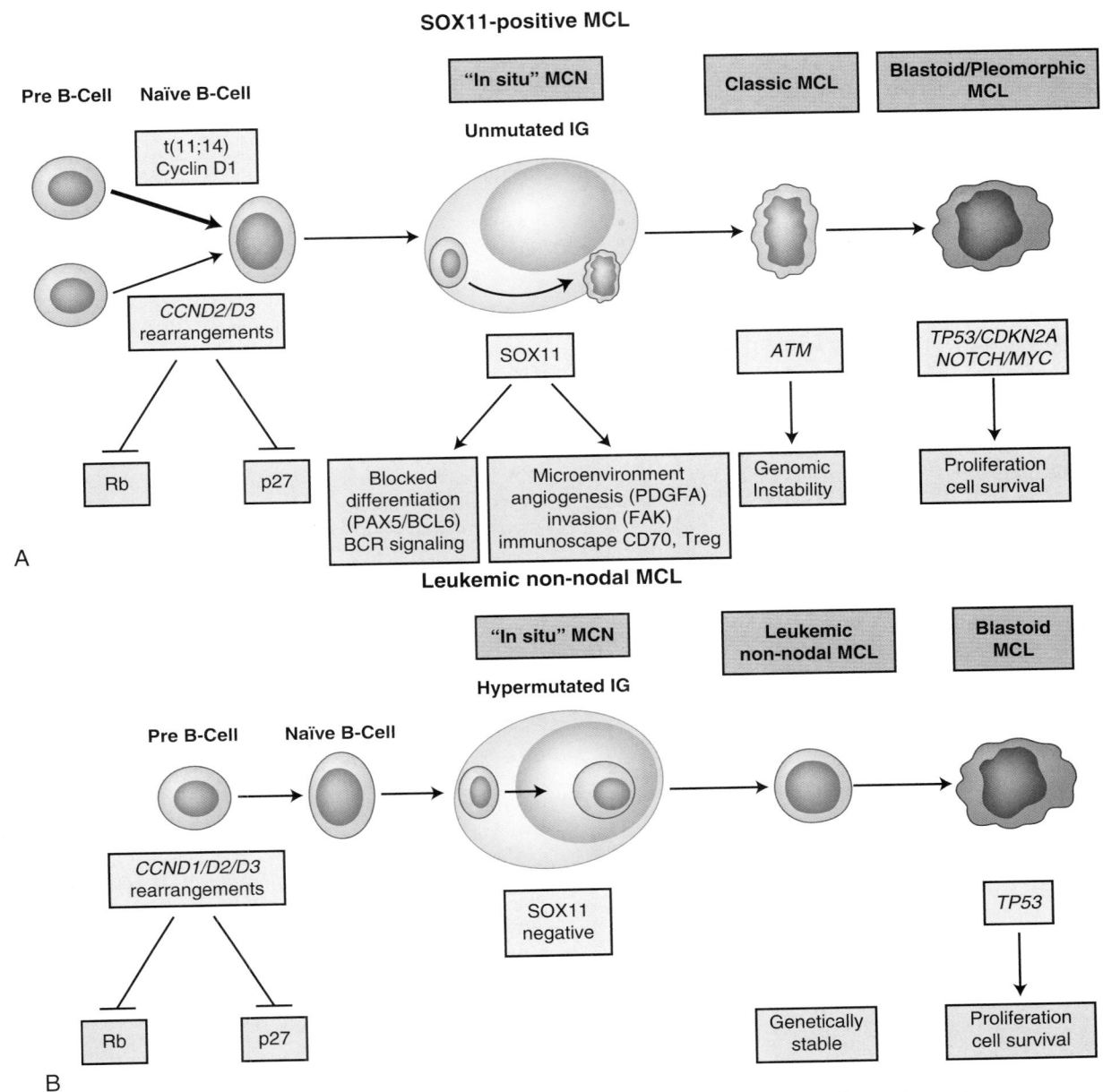

Figure 21-13. Proposed model of molecular pathogenesis of two subtypes of mantle cell lymphoma (MCL), SOX11-positive MCL **(A)** and leukemic non-nodal SOX11-negative subtypes **(B)**. **A,** The t(11;14) translocation occurs in an immature B cell and leads to the constitutive deregulation of cyclin D1 and early expansion of tumor B cells in the mantle zone areas of lymphoid follicles in both subtypes. Rare cases that are negative for the t(11;14) translocation carry *CCND2* or *CCND3* rearrangements and are SOX11 positive. SOX11-positive MCLs usually have unmutated immunoglobulin variable region heavy chain (IGHV) and may be derived from cells with no influence of the germinal-center microenvironment. These tumors acquire frequent ataxia-telangiectasia mutated *(ATM)* mutations that may facilitate the development of additional genetic alterations and expansion of MCL cells with a classic morphology. Increased genomic instability may target genes in the cell-cycle and cell-survival pathways that lead to more aggressive variants. **B,** Leukemic non-nodal MCLs carry hypermutated IGHV and may be derived from a cell with germinal-center experience. These tumors are genetically stable, persist with a leukemic phase for long periods, and may develop splenomegaly. Subsequent acquisition of additional genetic alterations may lead to transformation of the disease. *MCN,* Mantle cell neoplasia.

DNA Damage Response Pathway

One of the most frequent genetic aberrations in MCL is the deletion of 11q22.3, including the *ATM* gene, which plays an important role in the DNA damage response pathway. *ATM* mutations have been detected in 34% to 48% of MCLs (Fig. 21-13).[226-229] WES analysis has confirmed *ATM* as the most frequently mutated gene in MCL and present exclusively in cMCL, in which it may be found in more than 70% of the cases, but is absent in nnMCL.[97,179,191] Occasional patients carry an *ATM* mutation in the germline.[228,229] *CHK2,* a putative tumor suppressor gene located downstream of *ATM,* also may be involved in MCL pathogenesis by protein downregulation and occasional germline mutations. Recently *SAMHD1,* involved in DNA replication and DNA damage response, has been described as a new driver gene in MCL[179] and associated with in vitro resistance to nucleoside analogues in patient-derived MCL cells.[230]

Cell Survival and Other Pathways

Additional molecular events that deregulate survival and apoptosis mechanisms seem to contribute to MCL oncogenesis. Particularly, amplification and overexpression of BCL2 and homozygous deletion of the pro-apoptotic *BIM* gene have been described in MCL cell lines and primary tumors.[178,231] In addition, cyclin D1 itself seems to sequester the pro-apoptotic protein BAX, facilitating the anti-apoptotic effect of BCL2.[232]

Activating mutations in different genes of the nuclear factor-κB (NF-κB) and BCR pathways has been observed including *TRAF2* (5%), *NFKBIE* (5%), *BIRC3* (5%–10%), *BCOR* (5%), and *CARD11* (5%) and have been related to ibrutinib resistance.[179,191,194,233] Activating mutations of *NOTCH1* and *NOTCH2* are seen in 4% to 14% of MCLs, usually with blastoid morphology and aggressive behavior.[97,179,191,222,234] Mutations affecting chromatin modifier genes such as *KMT2D* (14%–23%), *NSD2* (7%–8%), and *MEF2B* (5%–8%) also occur frequently in MCL. Other recurrent mutations occur in

Table 21-5 Driver Genes Reported With Frequency >5% in at Least Two Out of Four Genome-Wide MCL Studies or >10% in a Single Study[179,192,194,222]

Driver Genes	Frequency	Cell Pathway
CCND1[†]	14%–44%	Proliferation
*RB1**	23%	
*CDKN2A**	21%	
*CDKN1B**	12%	
*MYC**	15%	
ATM	34%–48%	DNA damage response
TP53[†]	16%–31%	
SAMHD1	10%	
KMTD2	14%–23%	Chromatin remodeling
NSD2 (WSCH1)	7%–18%	
SP140	8%–13%	
SMARCA4	7%–14%	
*BMI1**	11%	
BIRC3	5%–22%	B-cell regulation
CARD11	4%–5%	
BCOR	5%	
TERT1[†]	15%	Telomere maintenance
NOTCH1	7%–14%	NOTCH pathway
NOTCH2	4%–11%	
HNRNPH1	5%–10%	RNA regulation
DAZAP1	4%–5%	
CARD11	4%–5%	B-cell regulation
MEF2B	5%–8%	Other
S1PRI	4%–6%	
UBR5	5%–10%	

*Targeted mainly by deletion or amplifications.
[†]More frequently reported in nnMCL.

HNRNPH1 (5%–10%), involved in RNA regulation, and *UBR5* (5%–10%) in ubiquitination mechanisms.[179,194]

Mutations in Mantle Cell Lymphoma Subgroups

Sequencing analysis of specific subgroups has shown frequent mutations of *NOTCH2, NOTCH3,* and *UBR5* in blastoid/pleomorphic MCL (Fig. 21-13).[97] *MYC* translocations have been rarely reported in MCL, but almost all cases had blastoid or pleomorphic morphology, leukemic expression, complex karyotypes, and a very aggressive clinical course with a short survival of 2 to 10 months.[46,47,77,235] In one study, relapsed MCLs carry more frequent 9p21 deletions (64%) than tumors at diagnosis (38%). Comparison of the genomic profile between cMCL and nnMCL is still limited.[179,191] cMCLs carry significantly higher numbers of structured variants, copy number alterations, and driver alterations than nnMCLs. Most mutated genes are more common in cMCL than nnMCL, with the exception of TP53 alterations that are more frequent in nnMCL (35%–70% versus 15%–20%).[145,179] *CCND1* 5′ mutations, *TERT* alterations, and activating *TLR2* mutations have been predominantly found in SOX11-negative tumors.[179,191]

POSTULATED CELL OF ORIGIN

The normal counterpart of MCL may be heterogeneous corresponding to different subsets of mature B-cell expressing CD5. Owing to the distribution of tumor cells in the mantle cuff and the positivity for alkaline phosphatase, early studies suggested a relationship between this tumor and cells of the primary lymphoid follicle or the mantle cells of secondary follicles.[236] CD5 expression in MCL is very high, resembling the intensity observed in fetal B cells, in contrast to the low levels detected in the subset of adult follicular mantle cells.[237] In that sense, the CD5-positive fetal-derived lymphocytes B1a have been postulated as putative cell of origin for MCL.[238] The presence of few or no somatic mutations in IGHV genes in most MCL supports a relationship to cells that have not experienced the follicular germinal-center cells. Intermediate cells between naïve and germinal-center cells, or transitional B cells already expressing AID, have been suggested as the cell of origin of cMCL.[239,240] However, somatic hypermutations are detected in 15% to 40% of MCLs, indicating that some tumors originate in cells that have passed through the germinal center. The load of IGHV mutations is related to the molecular subtype of MCL since most cMCLs have no or few mutations, whereas nnMCLs carry hypermutated IGHV, suggesting that they may originate in different subpopulations of B cells.[27,100] This idea was confirmed by DNA methylation studies that show the relationship of cMCL with naïve-like B cells, whereas nnMCL seemed derived from memory-like cells.[216] A biased use of the IGHV4-34, IGHV3-21, IGHV1-8, and IGHV3-23 genes has been detected in MCL. Around 10% of all MCLs have stereotyped heavy complementary-determining region 3 (VH CDR3) sequences. These findings strongly suggest that antigen selection plays an important role in the pathogenesis of at least a subset of MCL.[241-243]

MULTISTEP DEVELOPMENT OF MANTLE CELL LYMPHOMA

The development of MCL may follow different steps, which are important to understand in order to adjust the

management of the patients to the biological significance of these alterations.[244] The identification of the nnMCL subtype clinically and biologically different from the conventional SOX11-positive MCL suggests two major genetic and molecular pathways in the pathogenesis of these tumors (see Fig. 21-13). In both subtypes, the t(11;14) translocation occurs in an immature B cell in the bone marrow, which leads to the constitutive deregulation of cyclin D1 and early expansion of tumor B cells in the mantle zone areas of lymphoid follicles. Rare cases that are negative for the t(11;14) translocation carry *CCND2* or *CCND3* translocations and are SOX11 positive. Overexpression of these G1 cyclins may initiate the development of MCL by overcoming the cell-cycle suppressor effect of retinoblastoma and p27. SOX11-positive MCL usually has unmutated IGHV and may be derived from cells that have not experienced the influence of the germinal-center microenvironment. SOX11 overexpression may contribute to the subsequent development of the tumors by blocking the terminal B-cell differentiation forcing the expression of PAX5 and preventing its downregulation required for the plasma cell differentiation. In addition, SOX11 promotes the expression of the angiogenic factor PDGFA, facilitating the infiltration of tissues by tumor cells. The frequent *ATM* mutations facilitate the development of additional genetic alterations, increased genomic instability, and further alterations in cell-cycle and cell-survival regulatory genes, which leads to more aggressive variants of MCL.

nnMCLs carry hypermutated IGHV and may derive from a cell with germinal-center experience. These tumors are genetically stable, persist with a leukemic phase for long periods, and may develop splenomegaly. Subsequent acquisition of additional genetic alterations such as *TP53* inactivation may lead to transformation of the disease.

CLINICAL COURSE

The clinical behavior of MCL is very heterogeneous, with some patients following a very rapid fatal evolution in less than 1 year, whereas approximately 10% may survive over 10 years. This variability may be in part explained by the two MCL subtypes, with cMCL being more aggressive than nnMCL, and cytologic variants in which blastoid/pleomorphic MCL confer a dismal prognosis.[10,59] The survival of MCL patients is improving over the years, particularly with new therapeutic strategies. Median overall survival (OS) has expanded from less than 3 to more than 6 years (Fig. 21-14).[245,246] Most patients with cMCL have complete initial responses but they are relative short with conventional therapeutic regimens, although maintenance strategies after induction are improving outcomes. After relapse, patients may experience a relatively slow course for several months, with enlargement of lymph nodes and increased resistance to chemotherapy; this is followed by a more rapid and progressive evolution in a final accelerated phase. Although the initial clinical presentation of blastoid/pleomorphic

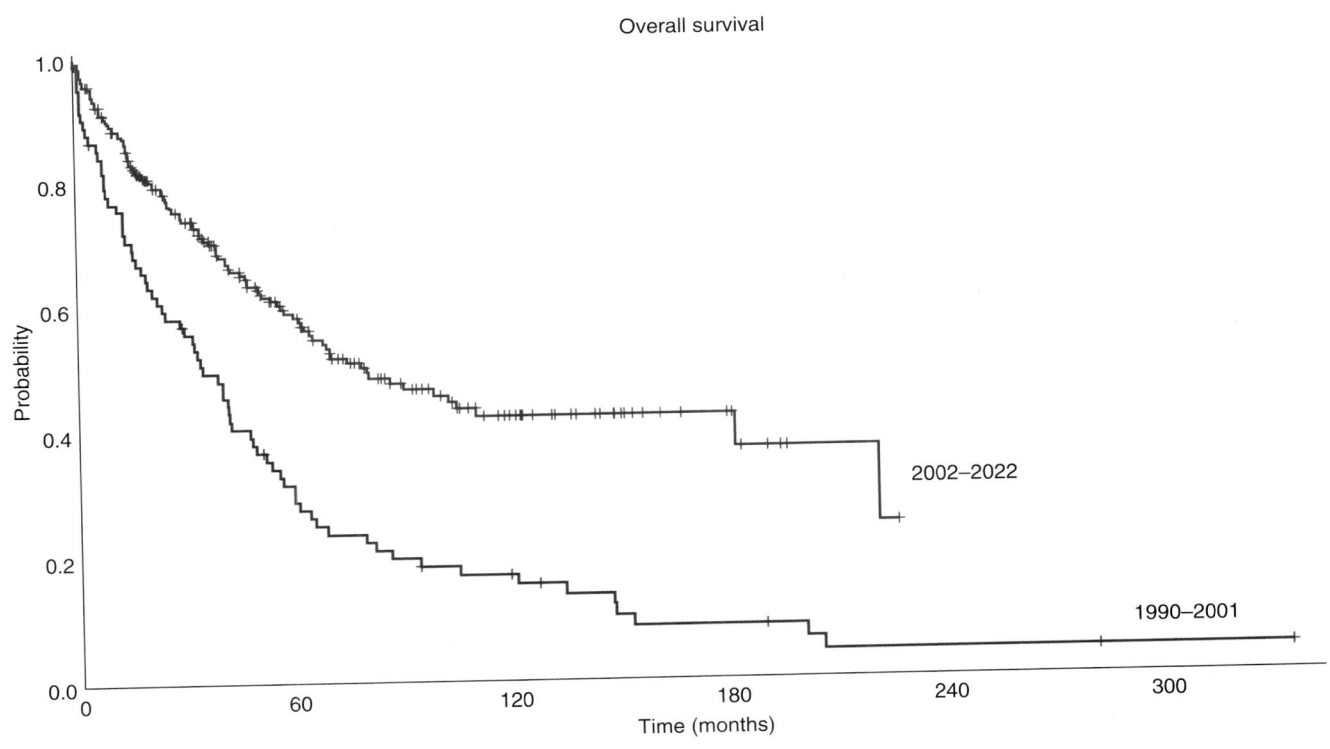

Median OS
1990–2001: 34.5 months (CI95%: 23–45)
2002–2002: 79.8 months (CI95%: 53–106)

Figure 21-14. Overall survival of patients with mantle cell lymphoma has improved, with a median increase from 3 to more than 6 years. Although some long-survival patients have been identified, there is no survival plateau in this type of lymphoma. *(Courtesy Dr. E. Gine and Dr. A. Lopez-Guillermo, Hospital Clinic de Barcelona, Barcelona, Spain.)*

variants is relatively like that of classic MCL, the clinical evolution is much more aggressive. Patients have a poor response to therapy and usually fail to obtain complete remission, which is associated with a rapid clinical course and death from progressive disease. In patients with complete remission, the duration of the response is usually short, and virtually all patients relapse in less than 1 year.[59,97]

Indolent Mantle Cell Lymphoma

Different studies have recognized a subset of MCL patients who do not require treatment at diagnosis and may be maintained under a "watch and wait" approach for long periods without detriment to their OS.[247,248] These patients with deferral treatment usually have stable disease for several months, stage I/II, good performance status, no B symptoms, normal LDH levels, and no or limited nodal presentation than patients receiving early treatment.[249-251] Intriguingly, the proliferation index, one of the best biological indicators of aggressive behavior in MCL, was not able to predict the time to the need of treatment in one of these studies.[251] Interestingly, p53 protein overexpression and non-nodal presentation were associated with shorter and longer time, respectively, to the need of treatment.[249-251]

The pathologic and biological substrates of these clinically indolent MCL are not well known. Some patients may have an early stage or initial MCL characterized by an in situ neoplasm or MCL with a mantle zone pattern.[252] Some cases may correspond to cMCL with a very low proliferative index[253] or they may correspond to the nnMCL subtype. In a clinical trial designed to treat patients with an indolent MCL (stable disease for at least 3 months, no or limited lymphadenopathy <3 cm, good performance status, Ki67 <30%, and no blastoid/pleomorphic morphology), 45% of cases were biologically cMCL and 55% nnMCL. TP53 mutations and complex karyotypes (≥3) were detected in 15% and 41% of the patients, respectively, suggesting that these biological factors are not sufficient to explain initial indolent behavior of the disease, although the disease progressed earlier in patients with TP53 mutations.[254] There are no biological markers validated that may help differentiate between those patients who would benefit by immediate treatment and those who could be expectantly observed. Therefore pathology information should be combined with clinical features of the patients to decide the best management strategy.

PROGNOSTIC PARAMETERS

Clinical and analytical prognostic parameters of adverse evolution currently used in the clinics are older age, poor performance status, advanced stage of disease (Ann Arbor Stage III or IV), splenomegaly, anemia, and high serum levels of b2-microglobulin and LDH.[255]

The proliferative activity is the most important biological prognostic factor in MCL, independent of the method used for its evaluation, mitosis, Ki67 immunostaining, proliferation signature by gene expression profiling, or others.[253] A high proliferative index recognized by Ki67 immunostaining (≥30% of positive tumor cells) has adverse prognosis, and has been validated in randomized trials (Fig. 21-15).[147] Although high proliferation is associated with blastoid morphology, tumors with classic cytology may also have high proliferative activity and a rapid clinical course. Reproducibility among pathologists

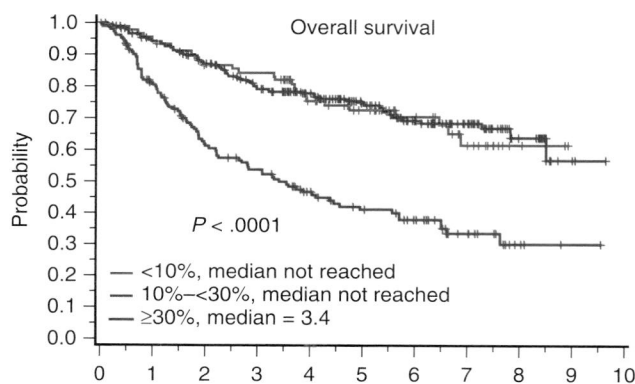

Figure 21-15. Overall survival and Ki67 proliferative index in mantle cell lymphoma. Highly proliferative tumors (>30%) had a worse prognosis than those with a lower proliferative index in the context of randomized clinical trials with high-dose immunochemotherapy. *(From Hoster E, Rosenwald A, Berger F, et al. Prognostic value of Ki-67 index, cytology, and growth pattern in mantle-cell lymphoma: results from randomized trials of the European Mantle Cell Lymphoma Network. J Clin Oncol. 2016;34:1386-1394.)*

of Ki67 assessment has difficulties. Recommendations have been proposed that include assessment of a minimum count of five independent high-power fields or two manual counts of 100 cells each in separated representative areas, avoidance of residual germinal centers, hot spots of proliferation, and proliferating T cells, among others.[143,146] However, the concordance between different labs defining low and high Ki67 index with the 30% cutoff was 65% in one study.[143] A limitation of the Ki67 index is the need of tissue and it cannot be performed in purely leukemic patients. A gene signature composed of 17 genes associated with proliferation (MCL35 assay) stratifies patients in high-risk (26%), standard-risk (29%), and low-risk (45%) groups, with median OS of 1.1, 2.6, and 8.6 years, respectively. This assay can use RNA extracted from routine formalin fixed paraffin embedded tissue, is highly reproducibly among laboratories, and its prognostic value has been confirmed in different clinical trials.[256-259] Morphologic prognostic parameters associated with worse outcome are the diffuse pattern and blastoid/pleomorphic variants, but they are not independent of the Ki67 index.[147]

The MIPI is based on four independent prognostic factors (age, Eastern Cooperative Oncology Group [ECOG] performance, LDH count, and leukocyte count) that stratify MCL patients into three groups with low-risk (44% of patients, median OS not reached), intermediate-risk (35%, 51 months), and high-risk groups (21%, 29 months), and its value has been confirmed in randomized trials.[260] The incorporation of the Ki67 index in the MIPI as a biological parameter (MIPIb)[253] or combining MIPI and Ki67 (MIPIc) improves the power of its prediction stratifying patients in four prognostic groups of low, low-intermediate, high-intermediate, and high risk with median OS of 9.4, 4.9, 3.2, and 1.8 years.[147]

The main prognostic genetic alterations are TP53, CDKN2A inactivation, and MYC amplification/rearrangement. The value of TP53 and CDKN2A have been confirmed in clinical trials.[161,224,261,262] Tumors with complex karyotypes (≥3 alterations) have a more aggressive course.[176,263] TP53 and MYC alterations may have prognostic value independent of genomic complexity.[179] A DNA methylation-based mitotic clock, named epiCMIT (epigenetically determined cumulative mitoses), able to capture the proliferative history of B-cell tumor samples has shown independent prognostic value in MCL.[179]

The minimum residual disease (MRD) analysis, based in the evaluation of circulating residual lymphoma cells, using high sensitivity and specificity methods, has shown prognosis value in MCL and may be a parameter that may guide therapy, particularly with new agents.[254] A meta-analysis has confirmed the use of MRD levels as a prognostic marker during the treatment and management of MCL patients.[264]

THERAPY

The management of MCL has changed owing to stratification of the patients according to stage, age, and, particularly, the fitness of the patients.[255] Some patients may be eligible for a "wait and see" policy for a long period.[249,250] In localized cases without additional risk factors, a shortened immunochemotherapy followed by a consolidating radiotherapy is considered appropriate. For young, fit patients with advanced disease requiring treatment, the introduction of immunotherapy with cytarabine-based regimens in different strategies (and usually consolidated with autologous transplant) has produced a remarkable improvement in survival, with a progression-free survival rate of 70% at 6 years. Rituximab maintenance after this treatment is currently considered for younger patients. Lenalidomide is also of benefit but only in patients not eligible for rituximab.[255] Less-intense regimens are proposed for patients that cannot tolerate these regimens, including immunotherapy combined with different chemotherapy regimens and rituximab maintenance.[255] No standard therapies have been proposed after relapse. Molecular targeted therapies are increasingly used, including Bruton tyrosine kinase inhibitors, BCL2 inhibitors, and lenalidomide among other options, whereas new molecular-targeted combinations and immunotherapeutic approaches are being explored in different trials, opening new perspectives for these patients. Allogenic stem cell transplant could be considered, but the introduction of chimeric antigen receptor T-cell (CART) therapy with very remarkable results in relapsed and refractory MCL patients will probably displace it to further lines in the therapeutic algorithm. On the other side of the spectrum, a clinical trial in patients with indolent MCL has shown that a non-chemotherapy regimen with ibrutinib and rituximab may obtain complete clinical and molecular (minimal residual disease) responses in more than 80% of the patients and 69% of the patients could discontinue ibrutinib after 2 years because of undetectable MRD. *TP53* mutations were associated with progression of the disease.[254]

DIFFERENTIAL DIAGNOSIS

Benign Disorders

Several lymphoid hyperplastic conditions may resemble MCL. In particular, expanded primary lymphoid follicles and mantle zone hyperplasias seen in reactive lymph nodes or associated with Castleman disease may suggest MCL with nodular or mantle zone patterns, respectively.[54,265] In these reactive conditions, lymphoid cells usually lack the nuclear irregularities observed in MCL, the nodal architecture is relatively preserved, and the clinical presentation is localized

lymphadenopathy in a young patient. Although CD5 may be positive in some Castleman disease cases,[266] in most other situations its negativity together with SOX11 and cyclin D1 negativity, as well as lack of monoclonality, rules out the diagnosis of MCL.

Cyclin D1–Negative Mantle Cell Lymphoma

In the case of a small B-cell lymphoma that resembles MCL but in which cyclin D1 is negative, the differential diagnosis is difficult and may encompass three situations: (1) cMCL in which the apparent cyclin D1 negativity is caused by technical immunohistochemical failure or to mutations in *CCND1*, rendering the protein inaccessible to antibodies, (2) true cyclin D1–negative MCL, and (3) other small B-cell lymphomas morphologically and phenotypically mimicking MCL. To rule out the first situation, it is important to investigate the presence of *CCND1* rearrangements by FISH or assess the cyclin D1 expression by other methods such as RT-qPCR. Recognition of the cyclin D1–negative MCL is facilitated by SOX11 expression. SOX11 should be studied in small B-cell lymphomas with monotonous atypical cells, particularly if they are CD5 positive.[137] Given the important clinical effect of the diagnosis of MCL, these cyclin D1–negative MCLs must be identified with great caution. When both cyclin D1 and SOX11 are negative, other small B-cell lymphomas must be considered. However, rare cases of small B-cell lymphomas that mimic MCL and are negative for these two markers and *CCND1/D2/D3* translocations are occasionally seen and are difficult to classify. In these cases, a diagnosis of small B-cell lymphoma, unclassifiable, may be justified.

Atypical Leukemic Lymphoid Neoplasms

Some cases of MCL may present with atypical lymphocytosis without the morphology (round cells) or phenotype (CD5 negative, CD23 positive) suggestive of MCL. Some of these patients may have splenomegaly without peripheral lymphadenopathy, and they may be difficult to diagnose if cytogenetic or molecular studies of the peripheral blood are not performed.[27] Cyclin D1 and SOX11 expression by RT-qPCR should be performed to rule out MCL. Previous cases defined as B-prolymphocytic leukemia with the t(11;14) translocation are now considered MCL, particularly pleomorphic variants.[79,267]

Chronic Lymphocytic Leukemia–Small Lymphocytic Lymphoma

Some CLLs may have a high number of lymphocytes with "cleaved," irregular nuclei, mimicking MCL.[268] In addition, CLL/SLL in lymph nodes may present with a predominant interfollicular pattern surrounding reactive secondary follicles. The tumor cells may even infiltrate the mantle zone, creating "naked" germinal centers without an apparent mantle cuff, as is frequently seen in MCL. The predominance of small cells with round nuclei and the presence of prolymphocytes and paraimmunoblasts with central nucleoli, either isolated or in small aggregates, help in the diagnosis of CLL/SLL because these features are always absent in MCL (Table 21-6). Cyclin D1 and SOX11 expression should facilitate the diagnosis of

Table 21-6 Differential Diagnosis in Mantle Cell Lymphoma

Entity	Confusing Feature	MCL Variant	Features Suggestive of MCL*
CLL/SLL	Interfollicular growth pattern "Naked" germinal centers Cells with cleaved, irregular nuclei	Classic or small, round cell	Absence of prolymphocytes and paraimmunoblasts LEF1 negativity
FL	Nodular pattern Diffuse FL	Nodular Diffuse	Monotonous cell population Less nuclear irregularity Absence of centroblasts CD10, BCL6, LMO2, and CD23 negativity Absence of STAT6 mutations
MZL	Clear cytoplasm Marginal zone pattern	MZL-like	Absence of mantle cell cuff Monotonous cell population No immunoblasts or plasma cells Finely dispersed chromatin
DLBCL	CD5 and cyclin D1 positivity Occasional CCND1 rearrangement	Pleomorphic	Irregular nuclei Finely dispersed chromatin Small nucleoli Mutational profile of MCL rather than DLBCL
Acute leukemia	Blastic nuclei Acute leukemic presentation	Blastoid	In some cases, immunophenotype is the only essential distinguishing feature TdT negativity (some cases may be positive) CD34 negativity

*Immunophenotype, cyclin D1, and SOX11 expression are major differential characteristics.
CLL/SLL, Chronic lymphocytic leukemia–small lymphocytic lymphoma; DLBCL, diffuse large B-cell lymphoma; FL, follicular lymphoma; MCL, mantle cell lymphoma; MZL, marginal zone lymphoma, TdT, terminal deoxynucleotidyl transferase.

MCL, whereas LEF1 positivity would support the diagnosis of CLL/SLL (Table 21-3).

Follicular Lymphoma

Differentiating nodular MCL from follicular lymphoma is one of the most common problems (Table 21-6). Some cases of MCL have a striking nodular pattern, suggestive of follicular lymphoma. The monotonous cell population, with a lack of centroblasts and slightly fewer nuclear irregularities, should raise the possibility of MCL. However, occasional centroblasts representing cells from residual germinal centers may render the diagnosis of MCL difficult. Immunohistochemical staining for CD5, cyclin D1, SOX11, CD10, and BCL6 typically provides the diagnosis (Table 21-3). The differential diagnosis between follicular lymphoma with a diffuse pattern and diffuse MCL may also be difficult on histologic grounds, but it should be resolved by immunophenotyping. The diagnosis of follicular lymphoma with a diffuse pattern requires the presence of a minority of centroblasts and a typical follicular center cell phenotype with expression of CD10, BCL2, and BCL6. These cases usually are CD23 positive and carry STAT6 mutations not seen in MCL.[269]

Marginal Zone Lymphoma

Some cases of MCL may have tumor cells with relatively abundant pale cytoplasm, which, coupled with the presence of residual germinal centers, may suggest a diagnosis of marginal zone lymphoma.[67] The identification of areas of classic MCL and the absence of a mantle cell corona surrounding reactive germinal centers would suggest a diagnosis of MCL (see Table 21-6). However, in some blastoid MCLs with pale cytoplasm, the tumor cells surrounding the germinal centers may be smaller, mimicking a residual mantle cell cuff. The immunophenotype and

molecular characteristics of MCL, with CD5 cyclin D1 and SOX11 expression, should confirm the diagnosis of MCL. It is important to recognize these tumors as MCL because their behavior is aggressive, with extensive dissemination and a rapid clinical course. Some previously described cases of aggressive CD5-positive marginal zone lymphoma may correspond to these MCL variants.[270] Mutational profile may be of help in the differential diagnosis.

Diffuse Large B-Cell Lymphoma

Pleomorphic MCL is sometimes confused with large B-cell lymphoma (Fig. 21-16; Table 21-6). The large size of the cells and the occasional presence of a nucleolus may suggest this diagnosis. CD5, SOX11, and cyclin D1 detection facilitates the diagnosis of MCL. However, CD5 and cyclin D1 may be expressed in some DLBCLs. These cases usually are SOX11 negative and do not carry CCND1 rearrangement,[128] but some cases also carry this CCND1 rearrangement. In these cases the presence of BCL2 translocations or detection of a mutational profile of diffuse large B-cell lymphoma may assist in the differential diagnosis with true MCL.[133]

Acute Leukemias

Blastoid MCL may present as a leukemic disorder with a very aggressive clinical course, mimicking acute myeloid or lymphoblastic leukemia (Table 21-6). Clinically, these cases may represent evolution of a preexisting nodal disease,[271] or the leukemic expression may be the initial manifestation of disease.[44] These cases express the typical MCL phenotype with strong mature B-cell markers, surface immunoglobulins, cyclin D1, and CD5. Terminal deoxynucleotidyl transferase may be positive in some of these cases although CD34 should be negative.[47] Cytogenetics and molecular studies may demonstrate the t(11;14) translocation.

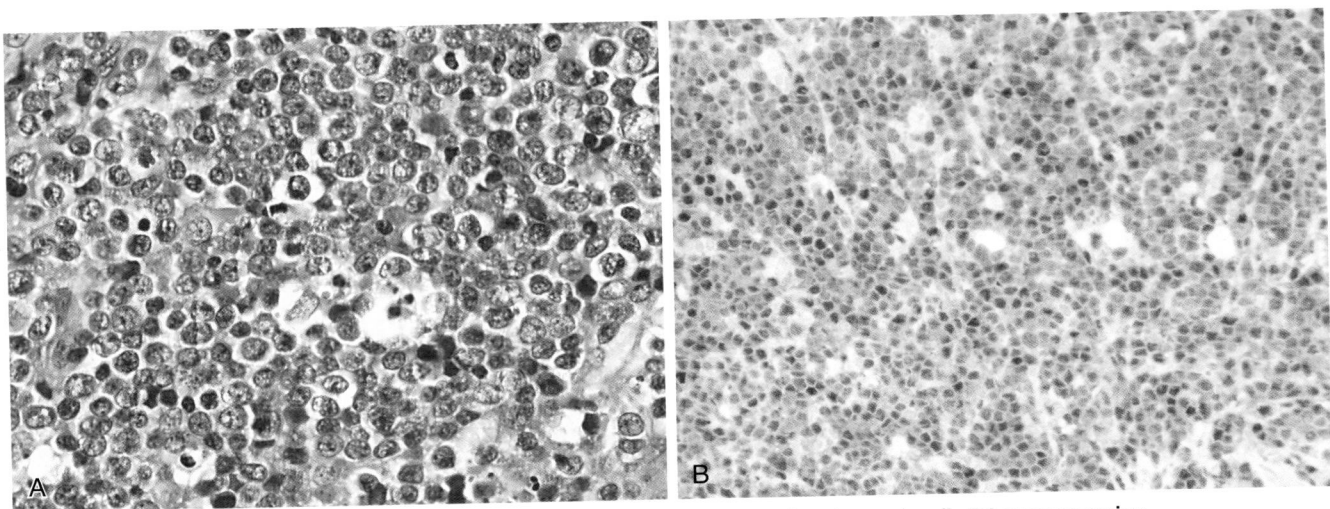

Figure 21-16. Diffuse large B-cell lymphoma with t(11;14) translocation and cyclin D1 overexpression. **A,** Diffuse large B-cell lymphoma. **B,** Cyclin D1 staining shows strong staining in virtually all tumor cells. The tumor was negative for CD5 and SOX11, but carried *CCND1* rearrangements detected by fluorescence in situ hybridization. Genomic sequencing detected a profile of mutations uncommon in mantle cell lymphoma and frequent in diffuse large B-cell lymphoma.

Pearls and Pitfalls

- Mantle cell lymphoma (MCL) is characterized by a monotonous proliferation of small-to-intermediate-sized lymphoid cells with irregular nuclei, a mature B-cell phenotype co-expressing CD5, and the genetic t(11;14) translocation leading to the overexpression of cyclin D1.
- Some tumors may present with small-cell, blastoid, pleomorphic, or marginal zone–like morphologic variants, mimicking other mature B-cell neoplasms such as chronic lymphocytic leukemia, acute leukemia, diffuse large B-cell lymphoma, or marginal zone lymphoma, respectively.
- The phenotype of MCL—expressing mature B-cell markers, SOX11, and CD5, but negative for CD23, BCL6, and CD10—is highly suggestive of the disease. However, some cases may have aberrant phenotypes lacking CD5 or expressing CD23, CD200, CD10, or BCL6. Cyclin D1 overexpression and the presence of the t(11;14) translocation are key elements in the diagnosis.
- Leukemic non-nodal MCL is a distinct molecular and clinical subtype of MCL that also has *CCDN1* rearrangement and overexpression. Cells may express CD23, CD200, and be negative for CD5. These cases may have a stable disease for a long period.
- Occasional cyclin D1–negative MCLs have been recognized. The transcription factor SOX11 is a useful marker for the diagnosis of MCL, including the cyclin D1–negative variant.
- The clinical behavior of MCL is usually aggressive. The tumor's proliferation is considered the most important biological parameter for predicting tumor behavior.
- MCL patients with a relatively indolent clinical course in whom the prognosis is not impaired by deferring initial treatment have been recognized. These patients are usually asymptomatic and present with leukemic non-nodal disease.

KEY REFERENCES

9. Jares P, Colomer D, Campo E. Molecular pathogenesis of mantle cell lymphoma. *J Clin Invest.* 2012;122:3416–3423.
70. Sander B, Quintanilla-Martinez L, Ott G, et al. Mantle cell lymphoma—a spectrum of indolent to aggressive disease. *Virchows Arch.* 2016;468:245–257.

147. Hoster E, Rosenwald A, Berger F, et al. Prognostic value of ki-67 index, cytology, and growth pattern in mantle-cell lymphoma: results from randomized trials of the European mantle cell lymphoma Network. *J Clin Oncol.* 2016;34(12):1386–1394.
161. Clot G, Jares P, Giné E, et al. A gene signature that distinguishes conventional and leukemic nonnodal mantle cell lymphoma helps predict outcome. *Blood.* 2018;132(4):413–422.
167. Martín-Garcia D, Navarro A, Valdés-Mas R, et al. CCND2 and CCND3 hijack immunoglobulin light-chain enhancers in cyclin D1(-) mantle cell lymphoma. *Blood.* 2019;133(9):940–951.
179. Nadeu F, Martin-Garcia D, Clot G, et al. Genomic and epigenomic insights into the origin, pathogenesis, and clinical behavior of mantle cell lymphoma subtypes. *Blood.* 2020;136(12):1419–1432.
209. Beekman R, Amador V, Campo E, et al. SOX11, a key oncogenic factor in mantle cell lymphoma. *Curr Opin Hematol.* 2018;25(4):299–306.
250. Abrisqueta P, Scott DW, Slack GW, et al. Observation as the initial management strategy in patients with mantle cell lymphoma. *Ann Oncol.* 2017;28(10):2489–2495.
255. Silkenstedt E, Linton K, Dreyling M. Mantle cell lymphoma—advances in molecular biology, prognostication and treatment approaches. *Br J Haematol.* 2021;195(2):162–173.
256. Scott DW, Abrisqueta P, Wright GW, et al. New molecular assay for the proliferation signature in mantle cell lymphoma applicable to formalin-fixed paraffin-embedded biopsies. *J Clin Oncol.* 2017;35(15):1668–1677.

Visit Elsevier eBooks+ for the complete set of references.

Chapter **22**

Aggressive B-Cell Lymphomas Including Diffuse Large B-Cell Lymphoma, Not Otherwise Specified and Other Nodal and Extranodal Large B-Cell Lymphomas

David W. Scott and Lisa M. Rimsza

INTRODUCTION

Diffuse large B-cell lymphoma (DLBCL) is a mature aggressive B-cell lymphoma, which has been progressively split into more discrete large B-cell lymphoma entities. The main group, DLBCL, not otherwise specified (DLBCL, NOS) has been further subdivided based on phenotypic and genotypic features. This chapter will cover DLBCL, NOS, its subtypes, and the other distinct large B-cell lymphomas with stricter definitions (Box 22-1). Most likely additional studies will continue to identify specific subgroups within DLBCL, NOS, which will become distinct diseases in future classification systems. In this chapter, terminology use includes both the International Consensus Classification of Mature Lymphoid Neoplasms (ICC) and the proposed 5th edition of the World Health Organization Classification of Tumours of Haematopoietic and Lymphoid Tissues (WHO HAEM5). Where terminology or diagnostic criteria diverge, these differences are briefly explained.

DEFINITIONS, SYNONYMS, AND TERMS

In the most basic sense, DLBCL, NOS and other large B-cell lymphomas (LBCL) consist of diffuse proliferations of large-or-medium-sized neoplastic, immunophenotypically mature, monoclonal B cells with a nuclear size greater than or equal to that of a histiocyte nucleus, or more than twice the size of a small lymphocyte (Fig. 22-1).[1] DLBCL, NOS is the name given to cases not conforming to one of the more specifically defined subtypes covered in this chapter and elsewhere.[2] Table 22-1 contains a list of synonyms and terms of the various entities discussed in this chapter. High-grade B-cell lymphomas (HGBLs), viral-associated lymphomas, and lymphoproliferative disorders associated with immunodeficiency (including posttransplant lymphoproliferative disorders) are discussed in detail in their respective chapters.

DIFFUSE LARGE B-CELL LYMPHOMA, NOT OTHERWISE SPECIFIED

Definition

DLBCL, NOS is a lymphoma composed of large-sized B cells in a diffuse growth pattern. By definition a diagnosis of exclusion, the defining features of other entities specified within the ICC and WHO HAEM5 need to be sought before arriving at this diagnosis. This includes consideration of the anatomic site of disease (DLBCL of the central nervous system [CNS], DLBCL of the testis, Chapter 59, and DLBCL of the skin, leg type, Chapter 19), Epstein-Barr virus (EBV) status of the tumor cells (EBV+ DLBCL, Chapter 28), the clinical history (immune deficiency and dysregulation, including history of transplant, Chapter 54), and presence of concurrent chromosomal rearrangements (HGBL-*MYC/BCL2* and HGBL-*MYC/BCL6*, Chapter 23).

Epidemiology

DLBCL, NOS is the most common type of non-Hodgkin lymphoma, accounting for 31% of all cases according to an international multicenter study.[3] A United States–based

---

Box 22-1 *Diffuse Large B-Cell Lymphoma, Not Otherwise Specified, Variants, Subtypes, and Other Large B-Cell Lymphomas*

DLBCL, Not Otherwise Specified
- Morphologic variants
  - Centroblastic
  - Immunoblastic
  - Anaplastic
  - Other rare variants
- Gene expression (cell-of-origin) subtypes
  - Germinal center B-cell–like (GCB)
  - Activated B-cell–like (ABC)

Other Lymphomas of Large B-Cells
- T-cell/histiocyte–rich large B-cell lymphoma
- Large B-cell lymphomas of immune-privileged sites including primary DLBCL of the central nervous system or primary DLBCL of the testis (see Chapter 59)
- Primary cutaneous DLBCL, leg type (see Chapter 19)
- EBV+ DLBCL, NOS (see Chapter 28)
- Large B-cell lymphoma with *IRF4* rearrangement (see Chapter 17)
- Primary mediastinal large B-cell lymphoma
- Intravascular large B-cell lymphoma
- DLBCL associated with chronic inflammation (see Chapter 28)
- HHV-8 and EBV-negative primary effusion-based lymphoma (ICC) also known as fluid overload-associated B-cell lymphoma (WHO-HAEM5)
- Lymphomatoid granulomatosis (see Chapter 28)
- ALK+ large B-cell lymphoma (see Chapter 24)
- Plasmablastic lymphoma (see Chapter 24)
- HHV-8–positive diffuse large B-cell lymphoma (see Chapter 28)
- Primary effusion lymphoma (see Chapter 28)

High-Grade B-Cell Lymphoma
- Diffuse large/high-grade B-cell lymphoma, with *MYC* and *BCL2* rearrangements (see Chapter 23)
- High-grade B-cell lymphoma, with *MYC* and *BCL6* rearrangements (provisional, see Chapter 23)
- High-grade B-cell lymphoma, NOS (see Chapter 23)

Mediastinal Gray-Zone Lymphoma (see Chapter 27)

ALK, Anaplastic lymphoma kinase; *EBV,* Epstein-Barr virus; *HHV-8,* human herpesvirus 8.

---

evaluation of lymphoma epidemiology confirmed DLBCL, NOS as the most frequent lymphoid neoplasm overall at an incidence of 6.9 cases per 100,000.[4] Non-Hispanic Whites and males have a higher incidence of DLBCL, NOS compared with other racial, ethnic, and sex groupings. The slight male predominance over females is estimated at 1.49:1.[3,4] In Asians, DLBCL, NOS accounts for a higher percentage of all non-Hodgkin lymphomas than in the United States and Western Europe (>40%), most likely explained by a lower incidence of follicular lymphoma (FL) in these populations.[4-6] Any age can be affected; however, DLBCL is much more common in adults.[4,7,8] The median age of the patients is 64 years.[3] The overall trend in incidence for DLBCL, NOS has been fairly stable since 2001 in both men and women.[4]

Etiology

Suspected risk factors in adults with DLBCL, NOS and other LBCL include autoimmune diseases that involve B-cell

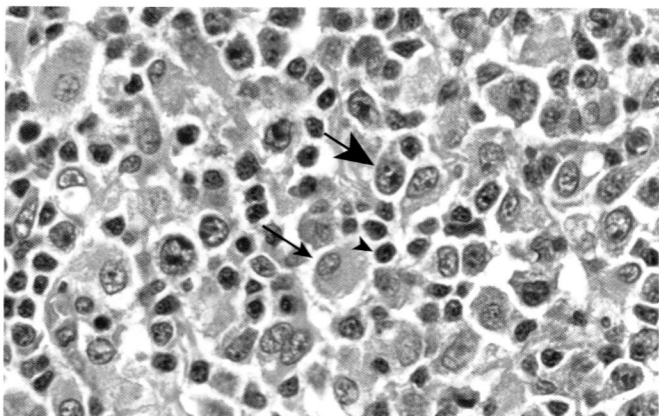

Figure 22-1. Diffuse large B-cell lymphoma: nuclear size assessment. In this example with numerous admixed histiocytes and lymphocytes, the interspersed histiocytes (with abundant eosinophilic cytoplasm) can conveniently be used as internal biological "rulers" for measuring the size of lymphoma cells. The lymphoma cells *(large arrow)* are considered large because their nuclei are slightly larger than those of the histiocytes *(small arrow)*. The neoplastic cells are more than twice the size of the small lymphocytes *(arrowhead)*.

activation, hepatitis C virus seropositivity, farming occupation, and higher body mass index as a young adult.[4]

A minority of cases occur in the setting of congenital, acquired, or iatrogenic immunodeficiency or immune perturbation (such as in angioimmunoblastic T-cell lymphoma).[9,10] EBV-positive DLBCL, NOS (formerly EBV-positive DLBCL of the elderly), which occurs in patients without evidence of overt immunodeficiency, is believed to result from the subtle immunologic deterioration that occurs as part of the aging process.[11,12] Rare extranodal LBCL are associated with chronic inflammation or irritation, such as postmastectomy lymphedema,[13] chronic suppurative inflammation in bone and skin,[14] previous surgery and metallic implants,[15,16] juxta-articular soft tissues in long-standing rheumatoid arthritis,[17] and long-standing pyothorax.[18] Many of these cases are associated with EBV and are covered in the chapter on virally associated B-cell lymphoproliferative disease (see Chapter 28).[19] A rare, but newly defined, entity is the human herpesvirus 8 (HHV-8) and EBV-negative primary effusion-based lymphoma, which overlaps with fluid overload–associated lymphoma. The latter terminology allows for a minority of cases which are HHV-8 negative but EBV positive.[20,21] These lymphomas occur in

Table 22-1 Synonyms and Terms for Large B-Cell Lymphomas

WHO 4th Edition	WHO 5th Edition	ICC

Diffuse large B-cell lymphoma, NOS
  Germinal center B-cell subtype
  Activated B-cell subtype
	Diffuse large B-cell lymphoma, NOS
	  Germinal center B-cell subtype
	  Activated B-cell subtype
		Diffuse large B-cell lymphoma, NOS
		  Germinal center B-cell subtype
		  Activated B-cell subtype

T-cell/histiocyte–rich large B-cell lymphoma	T-cell/histiocyte–rich large B-cell lymphoma	T-cell/histiocyte–rich large B-cell lymphoma
Primary mediastinal (thymic) large B-cell lymphoma	Primary mediastinal large B-cell lymphoma	Primary mediastinal large B-cell lymphoma
Intravascular large B-cell lymphoma	Intravascular large B-cell lymphoma	Intravascular large B-cell lymphoma
Lymphomatoid granulomatosis	Lymphomatoid granulomatosis	Lymphomatoid granulomatosis
EBV-positive diffuse large B-cell lymphoma, NOS	EBV-positive diffuse large B-cell lymphoma	EBV-positive diffuse large B-cell lymphoma, NOS
Diffuse large B-cell lymphoma associated with chronic inflammation	Diffuse large B-cell lymphoma associated with chronic inflammation	Diffuse large B-cell lymphoma associated with chronic inflammation
Not previously recognized	Fibrin-associated large B-cell lymphoma	Subtype of DLBCL associated with chronic inflammation
Not previously recognized	Fluid overload associated large B-cell lymphoma	HHV-8 and EBV-negative primary effusion-based lymphoma
Primary DLBCL of the central nervous system	Primary large B-cell lymphoma of immune-privileged sites (including central nervous system, testis, vitreoretinal)	Primary DLBCL of the central nervous system Primary DLBCL of the testis
Primary cutaneous DLBCL, leg type	Primary cutaneous DLBCL, leg type	Primary cutaneous DLBCL, leg type
ALK-positive large B-cell lymphoma	ALK-positive large B-cell lymphoma	ALK-positive large B-cell lymphoma
Large B-cell lymphoma with *IRF4* rearrangement	Large B-cell lymphoma with *IRF4* rearrangement	Large B-cell lymphoma with *IRF4* rearrangement*
Diffuse large B-cell lymphoma with *MYC* and *BCL2* and/or *BCL6* rearrangements	Diffuse large B-cell lymphoma/high grade B-cell lymphoma with *MYC* and *BCL2* rearrangements	High-grade B-cell lymphoma with *MYC* and *BCL2* rearrangements
		Provisional: High-grade B-cell lymphoma with *MYC* and *BCL6* rearrangements
High-grade B-cell lymphoma, NOS	High-grade B-cell lymphoma, NOS	High-grade B-cell lymphoma, NOS
Burkitt-like lymphoma with 11q aberration	High-grade B-cell lymphoma with 11q aberration	Large B-cell lymphoma with 11q aberration
B-cell lymphoma, unclassifiable, with features intermediate between DLBCL and classic Hodgkin lymphoma	Mediastinal gray-zone lymphoma	Mediastinal gray-zone lymphoma

*Discussed in follicular lymphoma chapter.
ALK, Anaplastic lymphoma kinase; *DLBCL,* diffuse large B-cell lymphoma, *EBV,* Epstein-Barr virus; *HHV-8,* human herpesvirus 8; *ICC,* International Consensus Classification; *NOS,* not otherwise specified; *WHO,* World Health Organization.

older patients who are generally human immunodeficiency virus (HIV) negative, may have hepatitis C, and have a medical condition leading to fluid overload, such as renal, cardiac, or liver disease.[22,23]

Most DLBCL, NOS and LBCL arise de novo, but some cases transform from an underlying low-grade lymphoma such as FL (which may harbor *BCL2* and *MYC* rearrangements), chronic lymphocytic leukemia/small lymphocytic lymphoma (CLL/SLL), lymphoplasmacytic lymphoma (LPL), marginal zone lymphoma (MZL), extranodal marginal zone lymphoma of mucosa-associated lymphoid tissue (MALT) lymphoma, or nodular lymphocyte–predominant B-cell lymphoma (NLPBL). Rare cases of DLBCL, NOS occur synchronously or metachronously with classic Hodgkin lymphoma (CHL).[1]

Clinical Features

Most patients present with rapidly enlarging lymph nodes or tumor masses in extranodal sites. About 30% of cases present in extranodal sites, and 71% have extranodal involvement during the course of the disease.[1] Common primary extranodal sites include the gastrointestinal tract (especially the stomach) and Waldeyer's ring, but practically any organ can be involved, including the skin, CNS, mediastinum, and bone.[1] Extranodal lymphomas of specific sites, especially of the skin, CNS, and testes, show distinctive clinical and biological features (see Chapters 19 and 59).

Approximately 30% of patients present with limited-stage (nonbulky and anatomically localized stage I to II without systemic symptoms) disease,[24] and one-third have B symptoms.[25] Bone marrow involvement occurs in 16%,[25,26] with concordant or discordant histology observed in equal proportions.

Morphology

Involved lymph nodes or tissues show complete or partial effacement of architecture by diffuse infiltrates of lymphoma cells, often with coagulative necrosis and permeation into the surrounding tissues (Fig. 22-2). Uncommonly, the lymphoma shows an interfollicular or sinusoidal pattern of nodal involvement (see Fig. 22-2; Box 22-2). More rarely, tumor cells may form deceptively cohesive nodules, mimicking carcinoma (see Fig. 22-3). There may be necrosis, cell debris, and frequent mitoses, particularly in cases with high proliferation rates. However, these findings do not automatically place a case into the HGBL category (Fig. 22-4). In highly proliferative cases of DLBCL, NOS, close microscopic inspection is needed to determine that one of the typical DLBCL cytologies is present and there is no evidence of a genetic "double hit" (see Chapter 23). Background sclerosis may be present, especially in mediastinal and retroperitoneal tumors (Fig. 22-5). In the case of transformation, the lymph nodes may show evidence of the preexisting low-grade lymphoma (Fig. 22-6).

At extranodal sites, in addition to forming tumor masses, the lymphoma cells commonly infiltrate in an interstitial pattern, resulting in wide separation and loss of the normal specialized structures, such as between gastric glands, salivary acini, seminiferous tubules, thyroid follicles, connective tissue, or epithelium (causing mucosal ulceration) (Fig. 22-7). An

---

Box 22-2 *Differential Diagnoses of Large-Cell Neoplasms With a Prominent Sinusoidal Pattern of Nodal Involvement*

- DLBCL
  - ALK-positive large B-cell lymphoma
  - DLBCL, NOS (uncommon)
- ALK-positive anaplastic large cell lymphoma
- ALK-negative anaplastic large cell lymphoma
- Histiocytic neoplasms or tumor like conditions
  - Langerhans cell histiocytosis
  - Rosai-Dorfman-Destombes disease
  - Histiocytic sarcoma (uncommon)
- Metastatic non-hematolymphoid malignancies (e.g., melanoma, carcinoma, germ-cell tumor)

ALK, Anaplastic lymphoma kinase; *DLBCL,* diffuse large B-cell lymphoma; *NOS,* not otherwise specified.

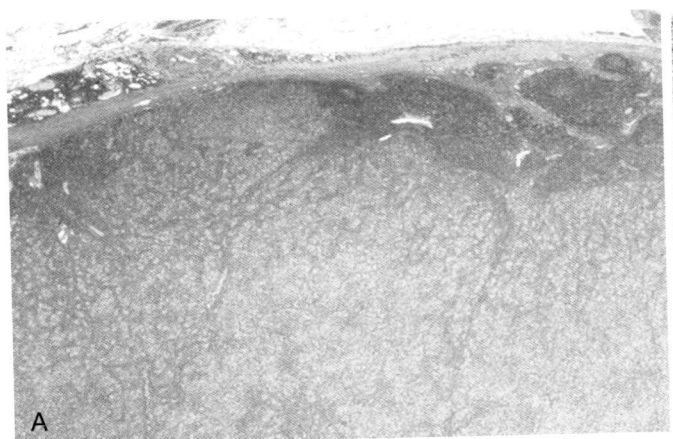
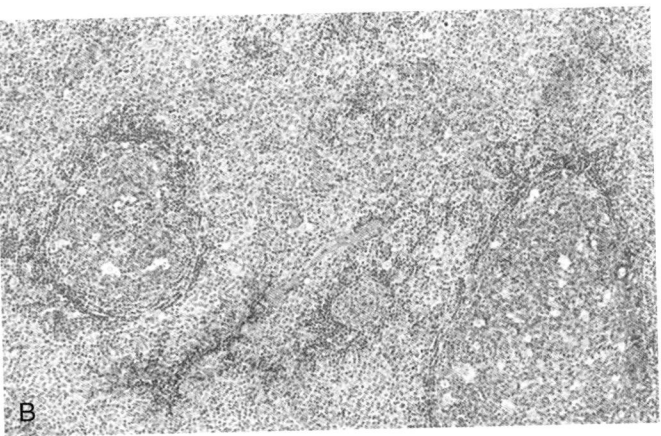

Figure 22-2. Nodal diffuse large B-cell lymphoma. A, The lymph node architecture is effaced by a diffuse lymphomatous infiltrate, with spillover into the perinodal tissue *(upper-left field).* Some residual lymph node tissue is seen *(upper right field).* **B,** In this example, the lymphoma selectively involves the interfollicular zone, mimicking reactive lymphoid hyperplasia. Features supportive of a diagnosis of lymphoma include erosion of the mantles of the reactive follicles and a monotonous interfollicular cellular infiltrate.

intravascular pattern should raise the differential of intravascular large B-cell lymphoma (IVLBCL).

Cytologically, DLBCL, NOS is most commonly comprised of large-to-medium-sized lymphoid cells with the morphologic features of centroblasts (large noncleaved cells) or immunoblasts. Centroblasts have round to oval vesicular nuclei, multiple membrane-bound small basophilic nucleoli, and a thin rim of amphophilic cytoplasm (Fig. 22-8). Immunoblasts have round or oval vesicular nuclei, a single large, centrally located, usually eosinophilic nucleolus, and a broad rim of basophilic cytoplasm (Fig. 22-9). The immunoblasts sometimes exhibit plasmacytoid features, with eccentrically located nuclei and paranuclear hofs. The lymphoma cells may not always conform to these classic cell types, exhibiting hybrid features of centroblasts and immunoblasts (see Fig. 22-9).[1] Lymphomas with greater than 90% immunoblasts are considered the *immunoblastic variant,* whereas those with less than 90% immunoblasts are considered the *centroblastic variant.*[27] Cytologic subclassification of DLBCL, NOS into centroblastic or immunoblastic subtypes is optional for current diagnosis. Rarely, DLBCL, NOS and LBCL can appear anaplastic with bizarre pleomorphic nuclei in at

least a subset of cells often with multinucleated forms, and abundant cytoplasm (Fig. 22-10),[1] or may mimic metastatic carcinoma because of the cellular pleomorphism, cohesive growth, or sinusoidal infiltration. Other rare cytologic variants include spindle cell, signet ring cells, and others. Occasional cases of DLBCL, NOS and LBCL show plasmacytic maturation, with lymphoma cells admixed with variable numbers of neoplastic mature-looking plasma cells (Figs. 22-11 and 22-12). These cases should continue to express a mature B-cell immunophenotype. If B-cell markers are missing and plasma-cell markers are present, the separate plasmablastic entities should be considered.

Predominantly medium-sized cells with multiple nucleoli (reminiscent of Burkitt lymphoma [BL]—"intermediate" morphology) or fine chromatin with inconspicuous nucleoli (reminiscent of acute lymphoblastic leukemia/lymphoma—"blastoid" morphology) suggest a diagnosis of HGBL, NOS, HGBL-*MYC/BCL2,* or the provisional entity HGBL-*MYC/BCL6* (Fig. 22-13 and Table 22-2) (covered in Chapter 23).

In DLBCL, NOS and other LBCL, there can be variable numbers of reactive cells in the background, such as small lymphocytes (mostly T cells), plasma cells, histiocytes, and

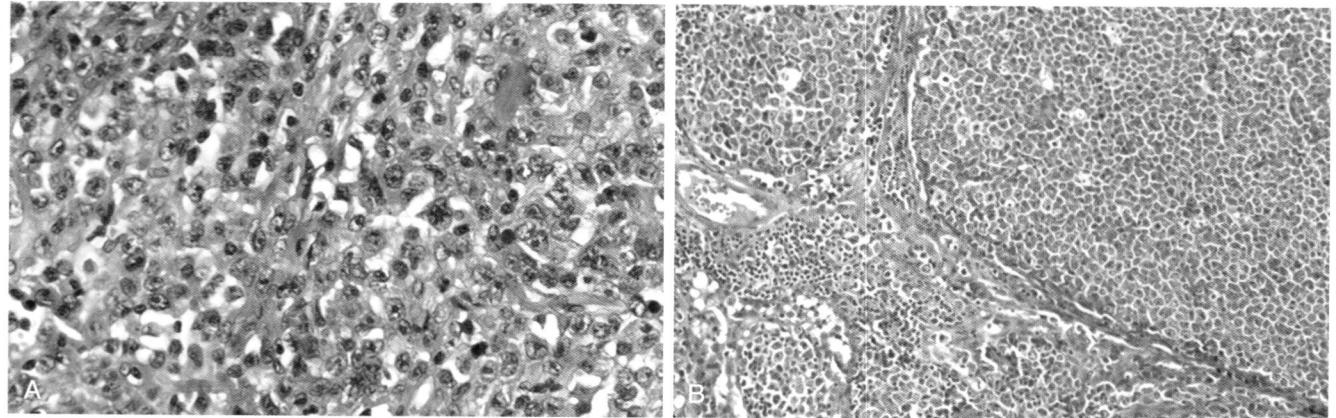

Figure 22-3. Nodal diffuse large B-cell lymphoma. A, In most cases, the infiltrate comprises non-cohesive neoplastic cells growing in a diffuse pattern. **B,** Sometimes the lymphoma cells form nodules or islands that exhibit a sharp interface with the stroma, mimicking carcinoma because of the pseudocohesive appearance or a grade 3 follicular lymphoma because of a pseudonodular appearance. Immunostains for cytokeratins or follicular dendritic cells could be helpful, respectively.

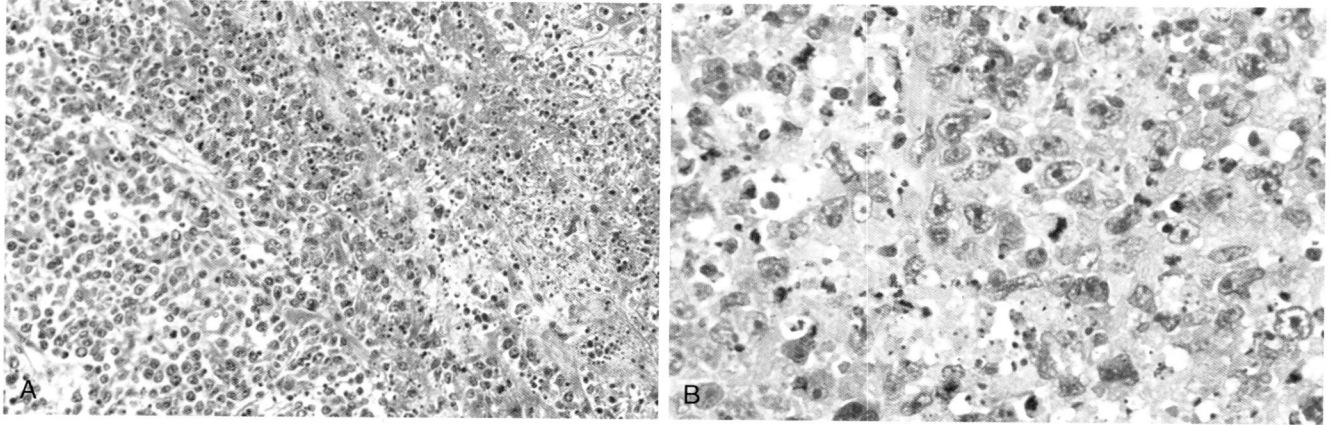

Figure 22-4. Diffuse large B-cell lymphoma. A, Coagulative necrosis *(upper right portion of the field)* is a fairly common finding and may be extensive. **B,** There may be abundant karyorrhectic debris among the lymphoma cells, mimicking reactive Kikuchi lymphadenitis.

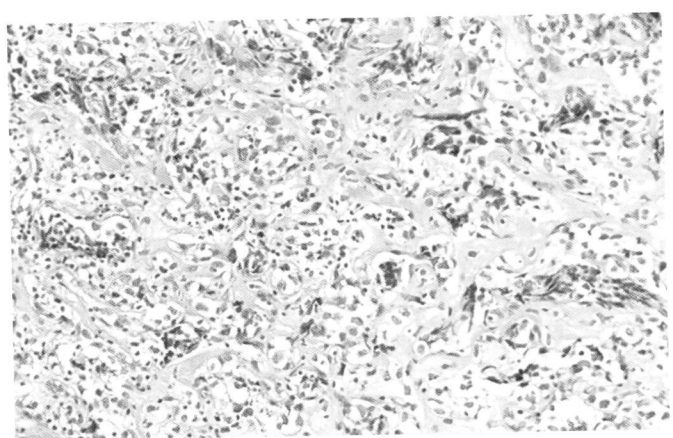

Figure 22-5. Diffuse large B-cell lymphoma with sclerosis. Thin sclerotic bands delineate the tumor into irregular packets. Lymphoma cells entrapped in the sclerotic areas often exhibit retracted cytoplasm or crush artifacts.

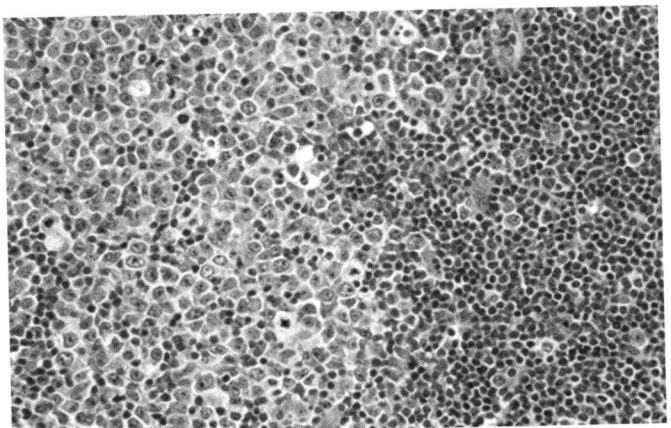

Figure 22-6. Diffuse large B-cell lymphoma arising in chronic lymphocytic leukemia (Richter transformation). The *left side* of the field shows diffuse sheets of large lymphoma cells. The *right side* of the field shows the preexisting chronic lymphocytic leukemia, comprising monotonous small lymphocytes; these small cells are confirmed as neoplastic by a CD20-positive, CD5-positive, and CD23-positive immunophenotype *(not shown).*

neutrophils. Cases with a prominent component of reactive T cells, usually with histiocytes, are categorized as T-cell/histiocyte–rich large B-cell lymphoma (THRLBCL) when no more than 10% of cells are the malignant B cells.[20,21] In rare cases, coalescing small clusters of epithelioid histiocytes are present, mimicking lymphoepithelioid T-cell lymphoma (Lennert lymphoma) (Fig. 22-14).[28] Occasional cases may present initially with lymph node infarction or extensive necrosis.[29] Some uncommon or histologically deceptive morphologic variants are listed in Table 22-3 (Figs. 22-15–22-17).[1,30] A summary of the clinical, morphologic, immunophenotypic, and genetic features of DLBCL, NOS is presented in Box 22-3.

Immunophenotype

DLBCL, NOS expresses a mature B-cell immunophenotype including CD45, CD20, CD22, CD19, CD79a, and PAX5 along with surface or cytoplasmic immunoglobulin. Posttherapy, CD20 expression can be lost in tissues from patients previously treated with rituximab (anti-CD20 chimeric antibody or similar products).[31] Terminal deoxynucleotidyl transferase (TdT) has been reported on DLBCL; however, it is generally weak to variable in intensity and most often focal (with occasional cases showing 60%–70% staining).[32] A study evaluating cases with greater than 10% TdT-positive cells confirmed lack of CD34 expression and the presence of *MYC* rearrangements, including tumors with concurrent *MYC* and *BCL2* rearrangements, indicating that these TdT-positive DLBCL, NOS are sometimes transformational events in DLBCL rather than bona fide B-lymphoblastic lymphomas.[32] Pan–T-cell markers are negative, although CD3 is very rarely expressed (Fig. 22-18).[33]

CD10 expression occurs in 20% to 40% of cases.[34-41] CD10 expression on at least 30% of cells is useful in identifying the subset of DLBCL with a germinal-center B-cell–like gene expression profile (GCB-DLBCL).[42,43] The reported positivity rate for the BCL6 protein is highly variable because the criteria for positive staining vary greatly from study to study.[34,39,44-49] Overall, approximately 70% of cases are BCL6 positive when cases with large aggregates of positively stained tumor cells are considered (Fig. 22-18C).[49] Some DLBCLs express

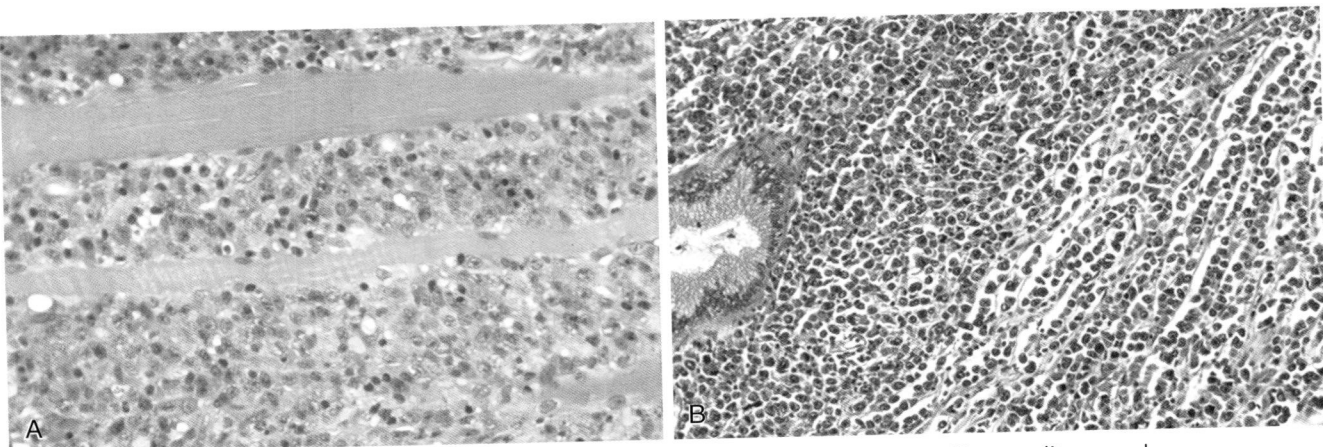

Figure 22-7. Extranodal diffuse large B-cell lymphoma. A, The interstitial infiltrate splits up and destroys the skeletal muscle fibers. **B,** In the fibrous stroma (uterine cervix in this example), a single-file pattern of infiltration can be seen.

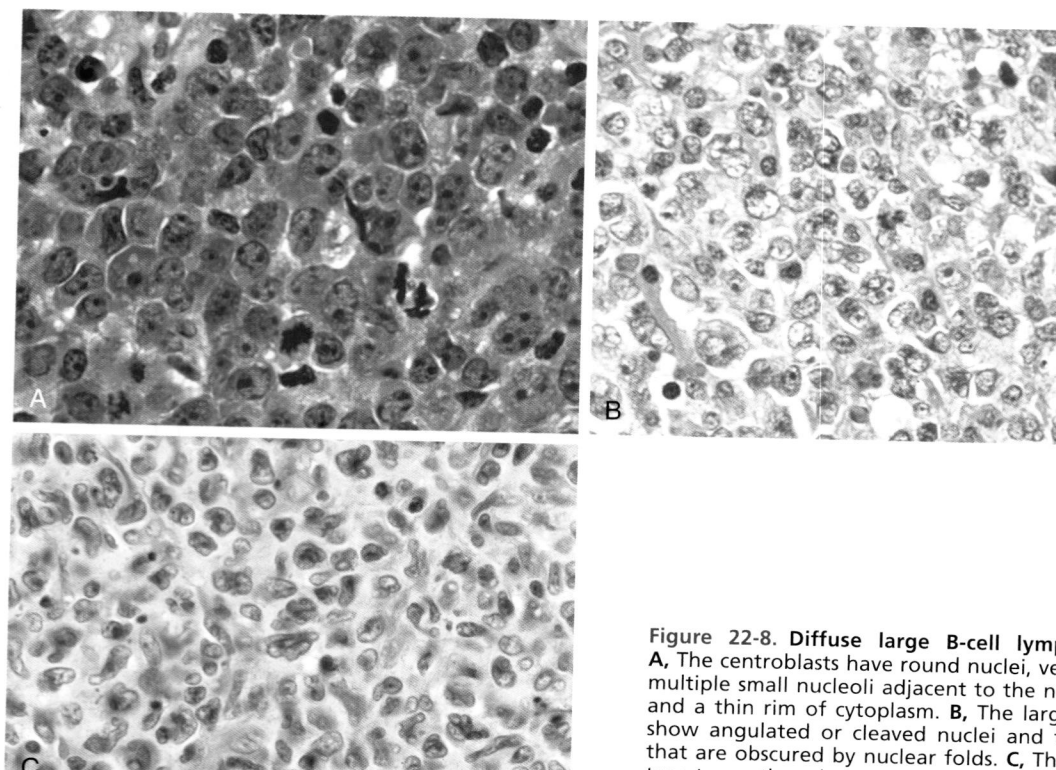

Figure 22-8. Diffuse large B-cell lymphoma, cytology. A, The centroblasts have round nuclei, vesicular chromatin, multiple small nucleoli adjacent to the nuclear membrane, and a thin rim of cytoplasm. **B,** The large lymphoma cells show angulated or cleaved nuclei and the small nucleoli that are obscured by nuclear folds. **C,** These are large centrocytes, rather than centroblasts, so follicular lymphoma should be considered.

post–germinal center or plasma cell–associated markers such as CD38, VS38, and IRF4/MUM-1. However, CD138 expression is seen almost exclusively in tumors showing morphologic evidence of plasmacytic differentiation, such as plasmablastic lymphomas (see Chapter 24).[39,50]

The reported positivity rate for MYC protein expression in DLBCLs varies widely from 12% to 65% (~50% overall),[51-59] attributable to the different cutoff values used (≥40% being the most popular for prognostic purposes; however, other studies have used 70%).[51,60,61] Tumor heterogeneity and whether very weakly stained cells are included in the count also contribute to the variation in cases considered positive.[62] MYC protein expression does not necessarily correlate with MYC rearrangement with a false negative rate of up to 25%[63-65]; thus its possible role as a screening test to predict presence of MYC rearrangement by fluorescence in situ hybridization (FISH) may be limited.[53,66,67] Mechanisms of false MYC IHC negativity for MYC locus rearrangement include low MYC expression and presence of the MYC N11S polymorphism.[65]

About 70% of cases express the BCL2 protein,[39-41,68-70] with a higher frequency observed in nodal than extranodal tumors.[71] The variations in reported BCL2 positivity rate in DLBCL can be explained by the different cutoff values and antibodies used in different series.[72] BCL2 expression in DLBCLs is associated with BCL2 translocation or copy number alterations but there are discrepancies between BCL2

translocation and BCL2 expression, which may be related to mutation of the BCL2 gene at the antibody epitope binding site, type of antibody used, and phosphorylation of the BCL2 protein.[72,73]

CD5 is expressed in approximately 5% to 10% of cases of DLBCL (Box 22-4),[44,74-79] and it is unclear whether de novo CD5-positive DLBCL represents a distinct clinicopathologic entity or merely an immunophenotypic variant of DLBCL, lacking relationship with CLL or mantle cell lymphoma (MCL), and associated with adverse prognostic features. The median age of patients with CD5-positive DLBCL, NOS is in the seventh decade. Four different morphologic variants of CD5-positive DLBCL, NOS have been described.[74,79,80] CD5-positive DLBCL, NOS may show aggressive clinical features.[76,81,82]

The activation marker CD30 is expressed in at least some degree in 14% to 25% of cases, which may be important because CD30 is a potential target for therapy.[83-86] A small proportion of DLBCLs (~2% overall) express cyclin D1 protein, often in only a proportion of tumor cells, with weak to moderate intensity.[87-90] However, in contrast to MCL, cyclin D1-positive DLBCL, NOS do not express CD5 and SOX11 and lack the CCND1 gene translocation (with rare exceptions).[87-93]

Ki67 staining in DLBCL usually shows a high proliferation index (>30%, but often <80%), and some cases may show an index approaching 100%.[94-97]

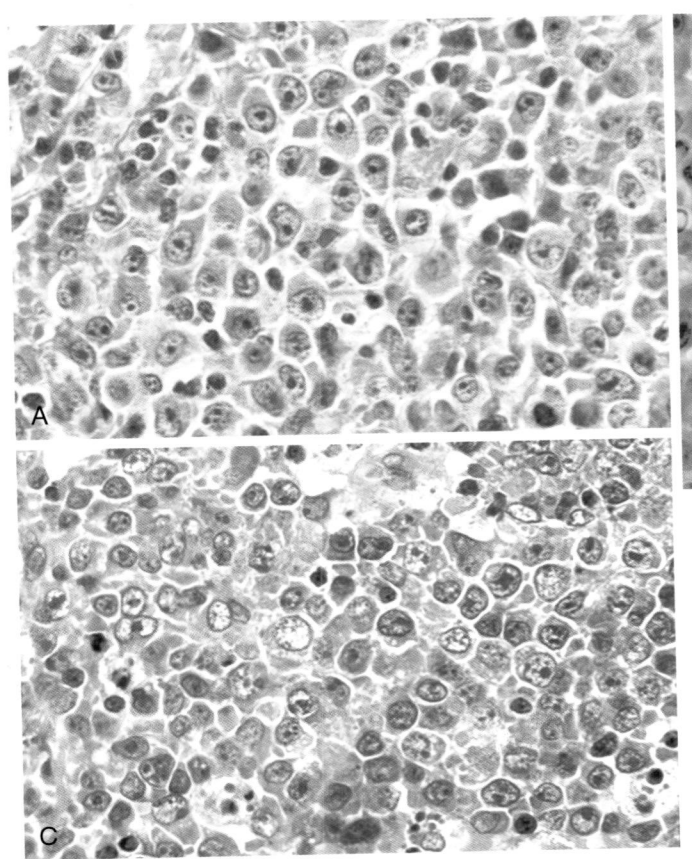

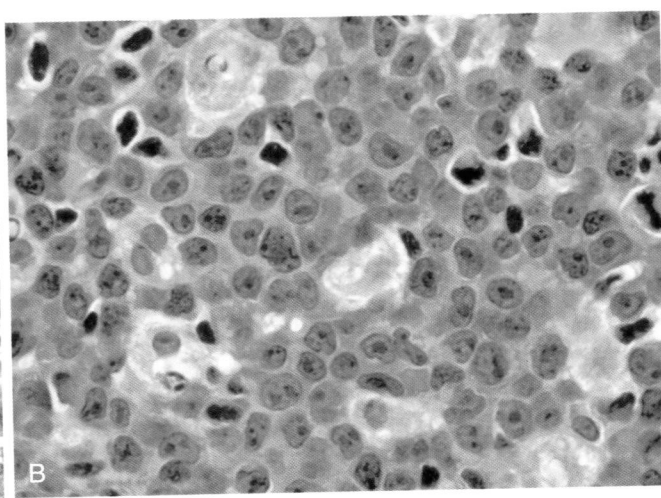

Figure 22-9. **Diffuse large B-cell lymphoma, immunoblastic subtype. A** and **B,** Nearly all of the large lymphoma cells show round or oval nuclei, prominent central nucleoli, and a broad rim of amphophilic cytoplasm (immunoblasts). **C,** This case shows immunoblasts mixed with centroblasts; there are also many cells with an indeterminate appearance between the two cell types and, strictly speaking, would not meet criteria for immunoblastic subtype.

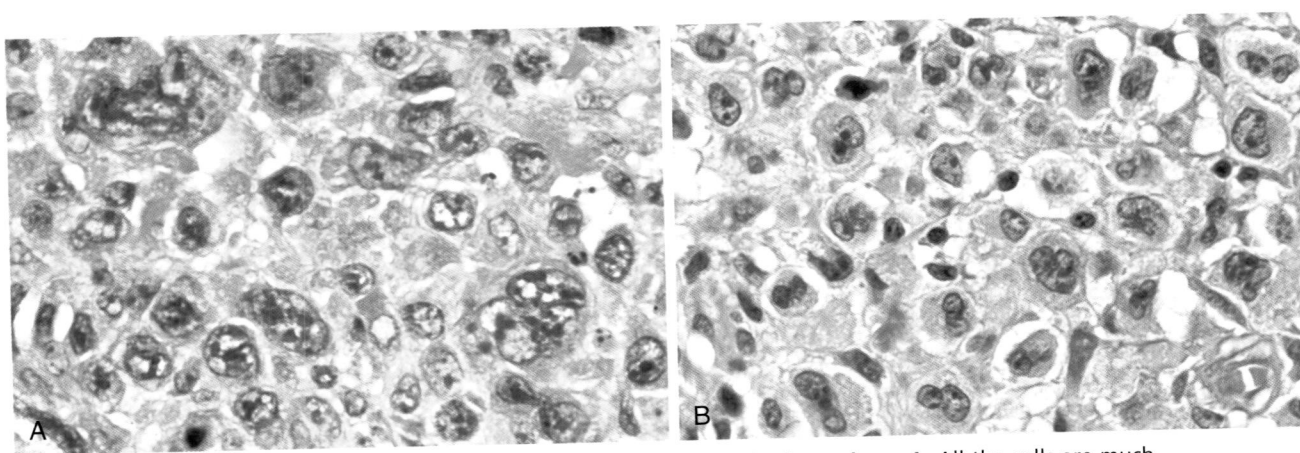

Figure 22-10. **Diffuse large B-cell lymphoma with anaplastic cytology. A,** All the cells are much larger than the usual immunoblasts or centroblasts, and some cells are huge and bizarre. **B,** The lymphoma cells are very large, with indented or irregularly folded nuclei and abundant cytoplasm, resembling those seen in anaplastic large cell lymphoma.

Genetics

DLBCLs have clonally rearranged immunoglobulin heavy chain and light chain genes (IGH, IGK, and IGL) and germline T-cell receptor (TR) genes. The immunoglobulin heavy chain variable region gene (IGHV) is usually hypermutated, with some cases showing ongoing somatic mutations.[98,99] In addition to the mechanisms of mutations observed in other tumors, mutations arise in DLBCL and LBCLs through aberrant activity of the mechanisms by which IG loci undergo V(D)J recombination and somatic hypermutation.[100] Errors in V(D)J recombination and class switch recombination are the origin of many of the observed recurrent chromosomal rearrangements. In aggregate, these genetic aberrations give rise to inappropriate cell proliferation and survival, blocks to terminal B-cell differentiation, and immune evasion, among others.

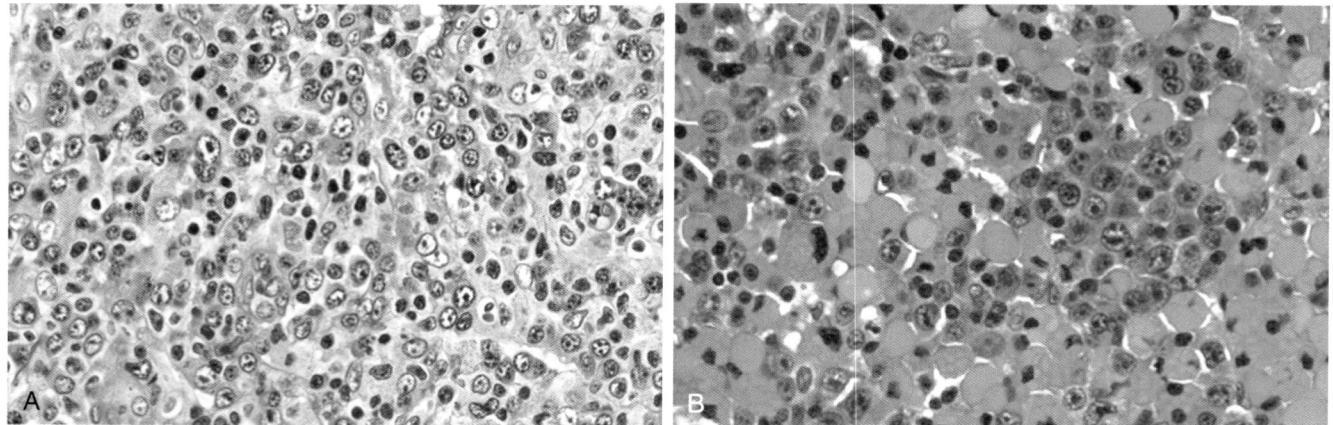

Figure 22-11. Diffuse large B-cell lymphoma with plasma-cell differentiation. A, In this example, the large lymphoma cells show a gradual morphologic transition to plasmablasts and atypical plasma cells. This appearance is similar to that seen in the polymorphic type of posttransplant lymphoproliferative disorder. **B,** In this example, the large lymphoma cells show an abrupt transition to plasma cells, which are engorged with brightly eosinophilic globules of immunoglobulin, giving a signet ring–style appearance.

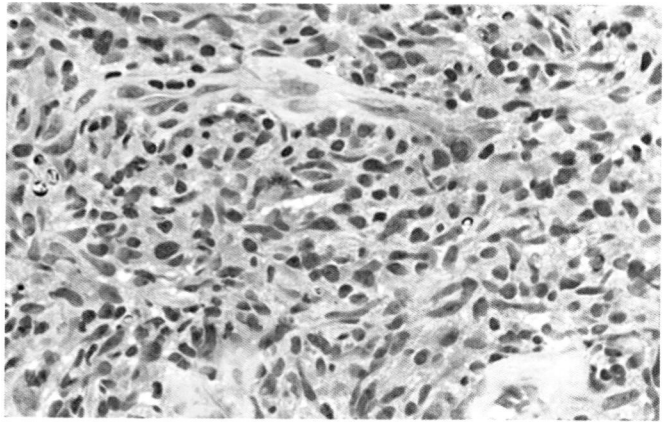

Figure 22-12. Diffuse large B-cell lymphoma with spindly lymphoma cells. Nucleoli are usually not obvious unless the cells are examined under high magnification.

The pathogenesis of DLBCL, NOS is complex and appears to involve at least two different pathways: a transformation pathway and a de novo pathway. The genetics-based subtypes of DLBCL, NOS share core mutations with indolent lymphomas, including FL, nodular lymphocyte predominant B-cell lymphoma (NLPBL), MZL, CLL/SLL, and LPL.[101-104]

Recurrent genomic rearrangements are commonly observed in tumors of DLBCL morphology, including BCL2, BCL6, and MYC. The partners in these rearrangements are typically genes constitutively active in the germinal center, with the resulting promoter or enhancer substitution leading to aberrant expression of these genes. Approximately 20% of tumors harbor t(14;18)(q32;q21) IGH::BCL2 translocation—a hallmark of FL.[53,55,105-113] These translocations arise during VDJ recombination of the IGH locus in the bone marrow through aberrant activity of recombination-activating genes (RAGs) and, thus, represent a very early event in lymphomagenesis.[114] In DLBCL, NOS, these rearrangements occur almost exclusively in the GCB subtype.[115,116]

BCL6 (3q27) rearrangement occurs in about 30% of DLBCL.[55,107-109,113] The translocation partner can be the IG loci, most commonly in the form of t(3;14)(q27;q32) BCL6::IGH, or other genes. Somatic mutations of BCL6, when coding and noncoding regions are considered, is a common event in DLBCL (73% of cases) and is unrelated to the presence or absence of BCL6 rearrangement.[117,118] Persistent expression of the BCL6 protein as a result of BCL6 translocation or mutation inhibits differentiation and apoptosis, resulting in cellular proliferation.[119]

Rearrangement of the MYC locus is observed in about 12% of tumors with DLBCL morphology, being more common in HIV-infected patients, pediatric patients, and extranodal lymphomas.[53,55,58,60,65,106-109,113,120-129] In tumors with DLBCL morphology, about 40% to 60% of cases with MYC rearrangement represent double-hit or triple-hit lymphoma with coexisting BCL2 or BCL6 rearrangement, and such cases are reclassified as HGBL with MYC and BCL2 and/or BCL6 rearrangements in the 2016 WHO classification (see further discussion of MYC rearranged tumor classification updates in Chapter 23 and Table 22-1).[53,55,60,106,107,109,113,123,124] In contrast to BL, MYC rearrangements in other aggressive B-cell lymphomas commonly occur as part of a landscape of complex genomic alterations; while the partner gene, similarly, can be an IG locus, occurring during class switch recombination, approximately half of the rearrangements in HGBL with MYC and BCL2 rearrangements (HGBL-MYC/BCL2) are with non-IG genes.[129,130] Within DLBCL, NOS, MYC rearrangement (sole by definition) occurs in 2% to 4% of tumors and IG partnership is more common than in HGBL-MYC/BCL2.[65,131,132] Other than translocation, increased copy number of MYC has been reported in 7% to 38% of cases.[55,125,133,134] Copy number alterations are not considered in the definition of HGBL-MYC/BCL2 (or HGBL with MYC and BCL6 rearrangements) and MYC copy number changes are not consistently associated with increased MYC mRNA expression.[135]

Mutation of TP53 and immunoreactivity for TP53 protein occur in 22% and 40% of DLBCLs, respectively.[105,136] TP53

IHC positivity correlates with the presence of *TP53* missense mutations with sensitivity of 70% to 80%; however, the specificity is lower with a broad range being reported.[137,138] The role of *TP53* in the genesis of DLBCL is unknown, but it may be associated with histologic transformation from an underlying low-grade lymphoma in some cases.[139,140]

A variety of genetic mechanisms contribute to immune evasion in DLBCL. Reduced or absent expression of major histocompatibility complex (MHC) molecules is facilitated through deletion or mutation of *B2M*,[141] deletion of the MHC genes, translocations and mutation of *CIITA*,[142] and mutations that block differentiation in B-cell stages characterized by low

MHC expression.[143-145] Mutations in *CD58* allow tumors cells that have lost MHC class I to escape elimination by natural killer (NK) cells.[141] Increased expression of PD-L1 and PD-L2 is observed with copy number gains,[146] rearrangements[147] and disruption of the 3′UTR of *CD274*.[148]

The availability of next-generation sequencing technology in recent studies has helped unravel the genetic landscape of DLBCL.[101,102,104,149-152] The coding genome contains on average 50 gene alterations per case,[149,150] with an estimated median of 17 genetic driver alterations.[101] These studies have resulted in an evolving definition of genetics-based subtypes within DLBCL, NOS (see Fig. 22-19).

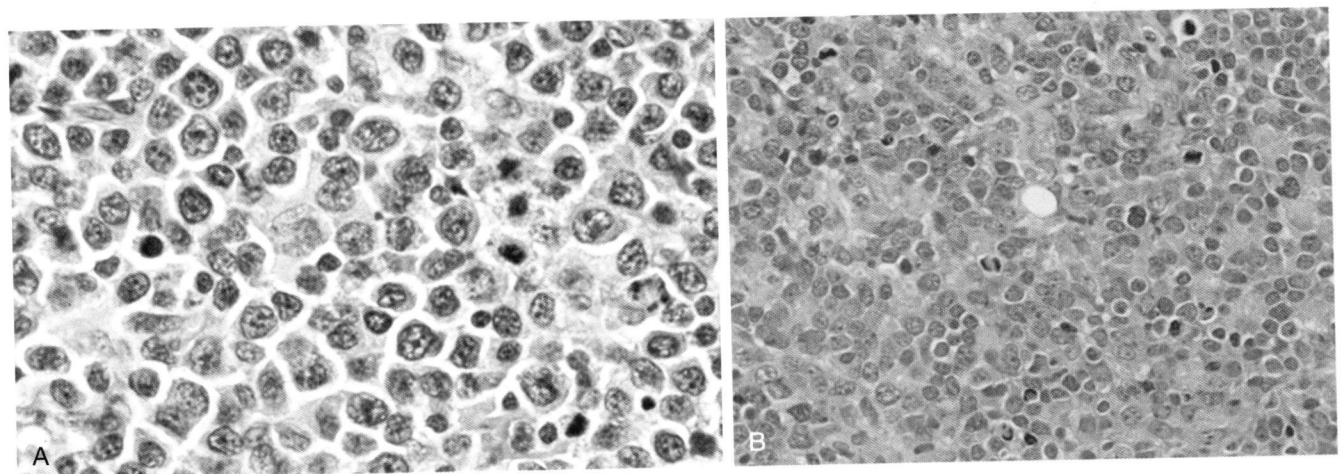

Figure 22-13. Intermediate and blastoid cytology. A, In this case, medium-sized lymphoma cells with finely clumped chromatin, two to five nucleoli, and minimal cytoplasm are identified showing an intermediate cytology between diffuse large B-cell lymphoma, not otherwise specified (DLBCL, NOS) and Burkitt lymphoma. Because this case did not fulfill the current diagnostic criteria for Burkitt lymphoma, it best fit into the high-grade B-cell lymphoma (HGBL), NOS diagnostic category (see Chapter 24). **B,** Another HGBL, NOS shows blastoid cytology with fine chromatin, inconspicuous nucleoli, and minimal cytoplasm. Genetically, there was a *BCL2* rearrangement with *MYC* amplification.

Table 22-2 Cytologic Features of Diffuse Large B-Cell Lymphoma, Not Otherwise Specified Compared With Types of Cytologies Found in Other Aggressive B-Cell Lymphomas

Type of Cytology		DLBCL, NOS	Blastoid	LBL/ALL	DLBCL/BL (Intermediate)	BL
Features						
Low power	Starry sky	Sometimes	Sometimes	No	Usually	Always
Cells	Size	Large	Medium	Small to medium	Mixed large and medium	Medium
	Size uniformity	Uniform to mixed	Uniform	Uniform	Mixed	Uniform
	Shape	Round, oval, irregular, spindled, anaplastic, signet ring, plasmacytoid	Round to oval	Round to oval to convoluted	Round to slightly irregular	Round or plasmacytoid
Nucleus	Chromatin	Vesicular	Fine	Fine	Finely clumped or LBL-like	Finely clumped
Nucleoli	Number	2–4 (CB) 1 (IB)	0–2	0–2	2–5	3–5
	Size	Medium or large (IB)	Small	Small	Medium or large	Small to medium
	Location	Nuclear membrane or central	Variable	Variable	Nuclear membrane	Paracentral
Cytoplasm	Amount	Scant to moderate	Minimal	Minimal to moderate, vacuoles	Minimal to moderate	Minimal, squared, basophilic, vacuoles
Variability in biopsy		Often	Sometimes	Minimal	Often	Minimal

BL, Burkitt lymphoma; *CB,* centroblastic; *DLBCL, NOS,* diffuse large B-cell lymphoma, not otherwise specified; *IB,* immunoblastic; *LBL/ALL,* lymphoblastic lymphoma/acute lymphoblastic leukemia.

Molecular Subtypes: Germinal-Center B-Cell–Like and Activated B-Cell–Like Subtypes

Using DNA microarrays to study gene-expression profiles, two groups of DLBCLs corresponding to different stages of B-cell differentiation (cell-of-origin [COO]) can be identified.[153] One group expresses genes characteristic of germinal center B cells (germinal center B-cell–like [GCB] subtype), and the other expresses genes normally induced during in vitro activation of peripheral blood B cells—the activated B-cell–like (ABC) type. The Bayesian model used to assign tumors to the binary ABC and GCB subtypes result in 10% to 20% of tumors being unable to be assigned to either group with sufficient confidence ("unclassified").[154] The GCB, ABC, and unclassifiable groups account for approximately 50% to 60%, 30% to 40%, and 10% to 20% of all DLBCLs, respectively.[115,155] The proportion of ABC subtype is higher in Asian countries, representing 60% of tumors,[156] although this may be because of the higher incidence of DLBCL EBV positive in these countries. The proportion of ABC may increase with patient age.[157]

Because of issues of tissue requirement (fresh or frozen tissue), complexity, and low reproducibility of gene expression profiling using the microarray platform, various molecular methods adaptable to formalin-fixed paraffin-embedded tissues have been developed, analyzing a limited panel of genes based on data from gene expression studies to distinguish the GCB and ABC subtypes.[158-163] The most promising method appears to be the Lymph2Cx assay of 20 genes using the NanoString platform, which is robust and shows excellent interlaboratory agreement.[164-166] Though these methods have not entered routine clinical practice at this time, they have been applied in prospective clinical trials[167,168] and retrospectively to completed trials.[169-171]

Various immunophenotyping algorithms have also been developed to determine the COO for DLBCLs: GCB subtype

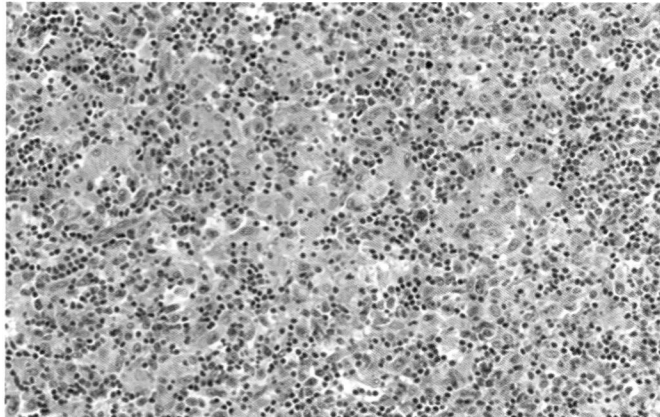

Figure 22-14. Diffuse large B-cell lymphoma with many interspersed small clusters of epithelioid histiocytes, reminiscent of Lennert (lymphoepithelioid) lymphoma, a morphological variant of PTCL, NOS.

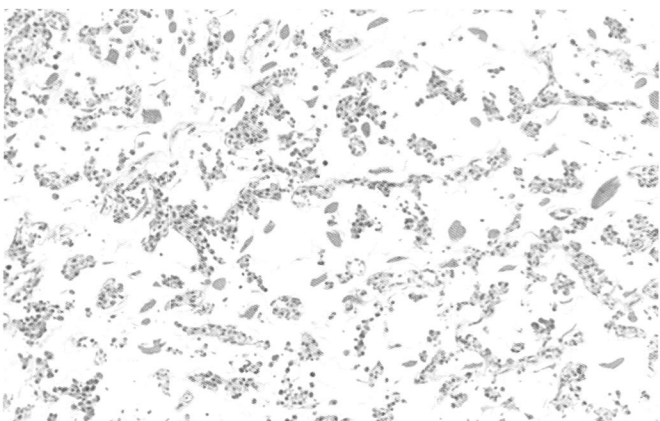

Figure 22-15. Diffuse large B-cell lymphoma with abundant myxoid stroma, mimicking extraskeletal myxoid chondrosarcoma.

Table 22-3 Rare Morphologic Variants of Diffuse Large B-Cell Lymphoma, Not Otherwise Specified

Morphologic Variant	Main Pathologic Features	Tumors With Which It Might Be Confused
Myxoid stroma[519,520]	Sheets, cords, or single lymphoma cells suspended in abundant myxoid stroma	Various types of myxoid sarcomas, such as extraskeletal myxoid chondrosarcoma, myxofibrosarcoma
Spindle-cell morphology[521,522]	Lymphoma cells have a spindly appearance caused by spontaneous cellular spindling or molding by collagen; predilection for skin	Various types of spindle-cell sarcomas, spindle-cell carcinoma, desmoplastic melanoma
Signet ring–cell morphology[523,524]	Lymphoma cells have cytoplasmic vacuoles, which may be caused by immunoglobulin accumulation or aberrant membrane recycling	Signet ring–cell carcinoma, liposarcoma
Fibrillary matrix or rosette formation[525,526]	Lymphoma cells associated with a prominent fibrillary matrix or rosette formation; because the fibrillary material is formed by interdigitating cytoplasmic processes (hence rich in cell membrane materials), it typically shows strong staining for leukocyte markers	Neural tumors, such as neuroblastoma, primitive neuroectodermal tumor
Abundant crystal-storing histiocytes[527]	Lymphoma cells intermixed with histiocytes having ingested crystallized immunoglobulin	Rhabdomyoma
Marked tissue eosinophilia[528]	Lymphoma cells intermixed with numerous eosinophils	Hodgkin lymphoma, peripheral T-cell lymphoma
Microvillous DLBCL[529,530]	Presence of numerous microvillous projections on ultrastructural examination; may show prominent sinusoidal growth pattern (see Box 22-2); CD20+, CD30−, EMA−, CD56+/−	Anaplastic large cell lymphoma (CD20−, CD3+/−, CD30+, EMA+/−, ALK+/−, CD56−/+); IVLBCL
Sinusoidal CD30+ DLBCL[30]	Sinusoidal growth pattern (see Box 22-2); CD20+, CD30+, EMA−/+, ALK−	Anaplastic large cell lymphoma (CD20−, CD3+/−, EMA+/−, ALK+/−); microvillous DLBCL (CD30−); ALK+ DLBCL (CD30−, ALK+); IVLBCL; metastatic carcinoma (cytokeratin +); metastatic melanoma (S100+)

ALK, Anaplastic lymphoma kinase; *DLBCL,* diffuse large B-cell lymphoma; *EMA,* epithelial membrane antigen.

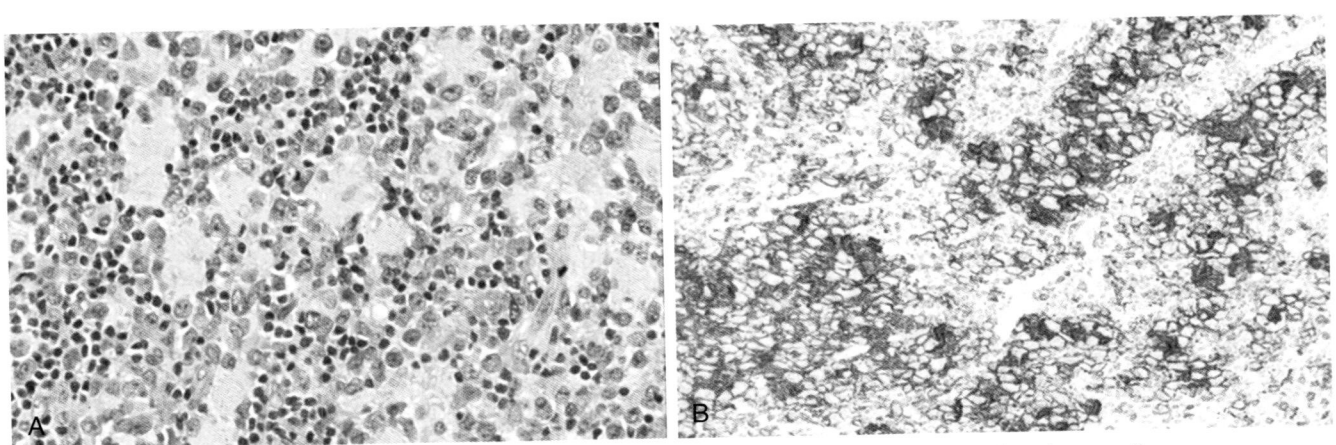

Figure 22-16. Diffuse large B-cell lymphoma with fibrillary matrix. A, The large lymphoma cells are associated with abundant eosinophilic fibrillary matrix. **B,** The matrix is actually formed by cell membrane materials from the lymphoma cells, as attested to by positive CD20 immunostaining.

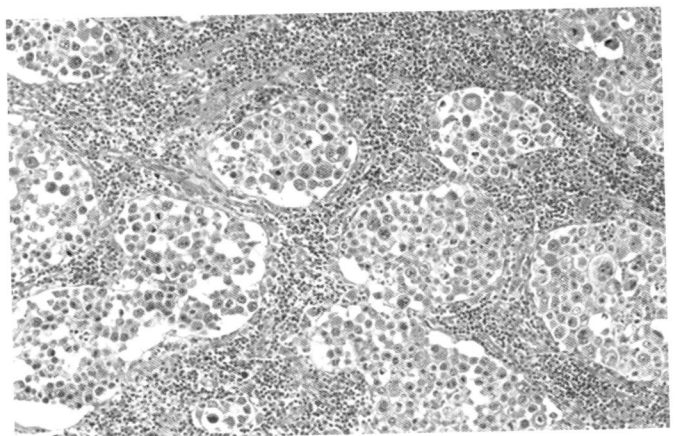

Figure 22-17. Sinusoidal CD30-positive diffuse large B-cell lymphoma. The lymphoma cells are confined within the distended sinuses of the lymph node. Care should be taken to exclude an intravascular large B-cell lymphoma.

versus ABC or non-GCB subtype (Fig. 22-20).[43,172-174] However, the correlation with gene expression profiling results is imperfect, with concordance rate of 75% to 90%.[163,165,173] There is also questionable interalgorithm concordance.[175-177] Because the unclassifiable group cannot be recognized by immunophenotyping, such cases will be forced into either the GCB or ABC/non-GCB group. At least in some studies, DLBCLs classified by immunophenotypic algorithms have failed to show prognostic differences between GCB and non-GCB subtypes.[163,175]

The COO subtypes of DLBCL, NOS were first recognized in the WHO revised 4th ed. (2016) on the weight of differences in prognosis and molecular features[178] and are retained in the ICC[21] and WHO HAEM5.[20] In comparison with GCB-DLBCL, patients with ABC-DLBCL typically present with higher Ann Arbor stage and International Prognostic Index (IPI) category.[155] Progression-free survival (PFS) at 2 years for ABC-DLBCL has been reported to be 50% to 70% compared with 75% to 85% in GCB-DLBCL in population-based registry[155] and clinical trials,[167,168,179-181] after R-CHOP (rituximab, cyclophosphamide, doxorubicin, vincristine, prednisone). Patients with ABC-DLBCL have a higher risk of relapse within the CNS (9% versus 2% in GCB-DLBCL); however, this was not significant in multivariate analysis when CNS-IPI and MYC/BCL2 dual expression was included.[182] ABC-DLBCLs make up a higher proportion of tumor involving specific extranodal sites, including testicular, breast, and adrenal gland.[183]

The molecular pathogenesis of the ABC and GCB subtypes are distinct and are potentially therapeutically targetable. ABC-DLBCL is characterized by genetic alterations leading to chronic active B-cell receptor (BcR) signaling combined with blockade of differentiation to the plasmablastic stage of differentiation.[150,184] Frequent mutations are observed in the pathway from the BcR to NF-κB, including *CD79B*, *CARD11*,[185] and *BCL10* and the negative regulator of this pathway, *TNFAIP3*.[186] In addition, frequent mutations are seen in *MYD88* (primarily L265P),[187] which is downstream of toll-like receptors. MYD88 and CD79B have been shown to interact to form a complex, leading to NF-κB signaling.[188] Rearrangements of *BCL6* and mutations and deletions of *PRDM1* are key events resulting in differentiation blockade.[189] Rearrangements of *BCL2* are rare in ABC-DLBCL,[115] while copy number gains are common[116] and result in similar elevation in *BCL2* mRNA.[135] *MYC* rearrangements are also uncommon (2%–4% of tumors)[65] with a predominance of IG loci partners within the IGH locus consistent with these occurring during class switch recombination.[131]

The genetic landscape of GCB-DLBCL is characterized by the PI3K/Akt/mTOR pathway, chromatin mutations affecting differentiation blockade, and *BCL2* modifiers providing differentiation blockade, and *BCL2* rearrangements. Mutations are observed in *GNA13*, *S1PR2*, and *FOXO1* along with the negative regulator of the PI3K/Akt/ mTOR pathway, *PTEN*. Frequent mutations are seen in *EZH2*, *CREBBP* and, less commonly, *EP300*, with functional studies showing their effect on chromatin. *BCL2* rearrangements are detected in 30% to 40% of GCB-DLBCL, when DLBCL/ HGBL-*MYC/BCL2* are excluded, while *MYC* rearrangements are rare (2%–4%).[65]

The efficacy of targeting COO specific biology has been tested in a number of large clinical trials, with novel agents added to R-CHOP in order to improve the outcomes of the ABC subtype. Initial reports from these trials have not shown improved outcomes,[167,168,181] with the dominant

Box 22-3 *Major Diagnostic Features of Diffuse Large B-Cell Lymphoma*

Clinical Features
- Median age: 64 years
- Slight male predominance
- Presents with rapidly growing nodal (70%) or extranodal (30%) tumor
- B symptoms in one third of cases
- Stage distribution: I, 25%; II, 29%; III, 13%; IV, 33%
- Potentially curable even when widely disseminated; when treated by standard immunochemotherapy, ~70% achieve long-term remission

Morphology
- Diffuse proliferation of large-to-medium-sized lymphoid cells, which can be indistinguishable from normal centroblasts or immunoblasts or can exhibit overt atypia such as irregular nuclear foldings, coarse chromatin, giant size, or bizarre nuclei
- May be associated with an underlying low-grade lymphoma
- Optional cytologic subclassification into centroblastic, immunoblastic, and anaplastic subtypes
- Uncommonly, can show a variety of deceptive growth patterns (e.g., myxoid change, fibrillary matrix, spindle cells); see Table 22-1

Immunophenotype
- Positive for pan–B-cell markers (e.g., CD20, CD22, CD79a, PAX5)
- Positive for surface or cytoplasmic immunoglobulin
- BCL6 positive in ~80%
- CD10 positive in ~40%
- CD5 positive in ~5% to 10%
- CD30 positive in ~15%
- CD43 positive in ~25%
- BCL2 positive in ~60%
- Ki67 index: >20% (mean, 55%)
- MYC positive in ~50%

Molecular Features
- Clonally rearranged immunoglobulin genes
- *BCL2* rearranged in ~20%
- *BCL6* rearranged in ~30%
- *BCL6* mutated in ~70%
- *MYC* rearranged in ~12%
- Usually EBV negative, except in the setting of immunodeficiency and the uncommon cases of EBV-positive DLBCL, NOS

Molecular Variants (Cell of Origin)
- GCB subtype: Expresses genes characteristic of GCBs, and accounts for ~50% to 60% of all DLBCLs. More favorable prognosis than ABC type. Common genetic changes: *BCL2* translocation, *REL* amplification, *EZH2* mutation, mutations of genes in the Gα13 pathway.
- ABC subtype: Expresses genes highly expressed during in vitro activation of peripheral blood B cells, and accounts for ~30% to 40% of all DLBCLs. Common genetic changes: Chronic activation of B-cell receptor pathway, NF-κB pathway activation through mutations in regulator genes of the NF-κB pathway and *MYD88* mutation.
- Unclassified: Unable to be assigned to ABC or GCB subtype with sufficient confidence based on patterns of gene expression.

ABC, Activated B cell; *DLBCL,* diffuse large B-cell lymphoma; *EBV,* Epstein-Barr virus; *GCB,* germinal-center B cells; *NOS,* not otherwise specified.

---

interpretation being that the binary COO classification of DLBCL, NOS is not sufficiently granular to support precision medicine in this lymphoma. However, recent follow-up of REMoDL-B (testing the efficacy of the addition of a proteosome inhibitor) demonstrates significant improvement in patient PFS and overall survival (OS),[190] while a planned subgroup analysis of PHOENIX (testing the efficacy of the addition of a BTK inhibitor) shows improved outcomes in patients under age 60.[181]

Genetic Subtypes

Genetics-based classification schema have emerged from three independent studies,[101,102,104] converging on five to seven subtypes based on patterns of co-occurrence of genetic aberrations, encompassing single nucleotide variants (SNVs)/indels, copy number alterations, and structural variants (*BCL2* and *BCL6* rearrangements). The subtypes are prognostic in R-CHOP treated cohorts and the inferred biology underlying the individual subtypes predict response to currently available targeted agents, providing a framework for precision medicine trials and future drug development. A feature across the studies is that most of the defined subtypes share core mutations with indolent B-cell lymphomas. While this may suggest that apparently de novo DLBCLs arise from clinically occult indolent lymphomas, an alternative is that the evolutionary paths to DLBCL and indolent lymphomas share early key genetic driver events. The latter is supported by the study of late relapse of DLBCL, where the diagnostic and relapse tumors demonstrate branched evolution consistent with a common precursor cell.[191] This is further supported by studies of "transformation" of indolent lymphoma to DLBCL.[192]

At this time, the one publicly available approach to assign tumors to genetics-based subtype is a probabilistic classification tool—the LymphGen algorithm.[103] This tool assigns tumors into seven subtypes. While the schema of the three groups have not been formally harmonized, the described subtypes have significant biological similarity (Fig. 22-21). In the explanatory section, the LymphGen labels will be used, unless otherwise stated, with the labels from Chapuy et al.[101] and Lacy et al.[104] in brackets after.

The EZB (Cluster C3/BCL2) subtype is characterized by *BCL2* rearrangements and mutations in *EZH2* along with other chromatin modifying genes (*CREBBP*), *TNFRSF14* loss of function, and *PTEN* inactivation. These tumors are typically GCB-DLBCL. This subtype shares a number of core mutations with FL. EZB is further subdivided into EZB-MYC positive and EZB-MYC negative based on presence or absence of the DHITsig gene expression signature (see prognostic molecular biology features). EZB-MYC negative is associated with good prognosis, while EZB-MYC positive is associated with poor prognosis, emphasizing an ongoing need for gene expression profiling.

The C4 cluster described by Chapuy et al. comprises tumors that are predominantly GCB-DLBCL and have favorable prognosis. It is possible that this cluster is composed of two subgroups. The first is ST2 (TET2/SGK1) with *SGK1* and *TET2* as the hallmark mutations. These tumors share core mutations with NLPBL. The second, labeled SOCS1/SGK1, was described by Lacy et al. and is not represented in LymphGen. Primary mediastinal large B-cell lymphomas (PMBL) mostly fell into the SOCS1/SGK1 group when classified with their schema.[104]

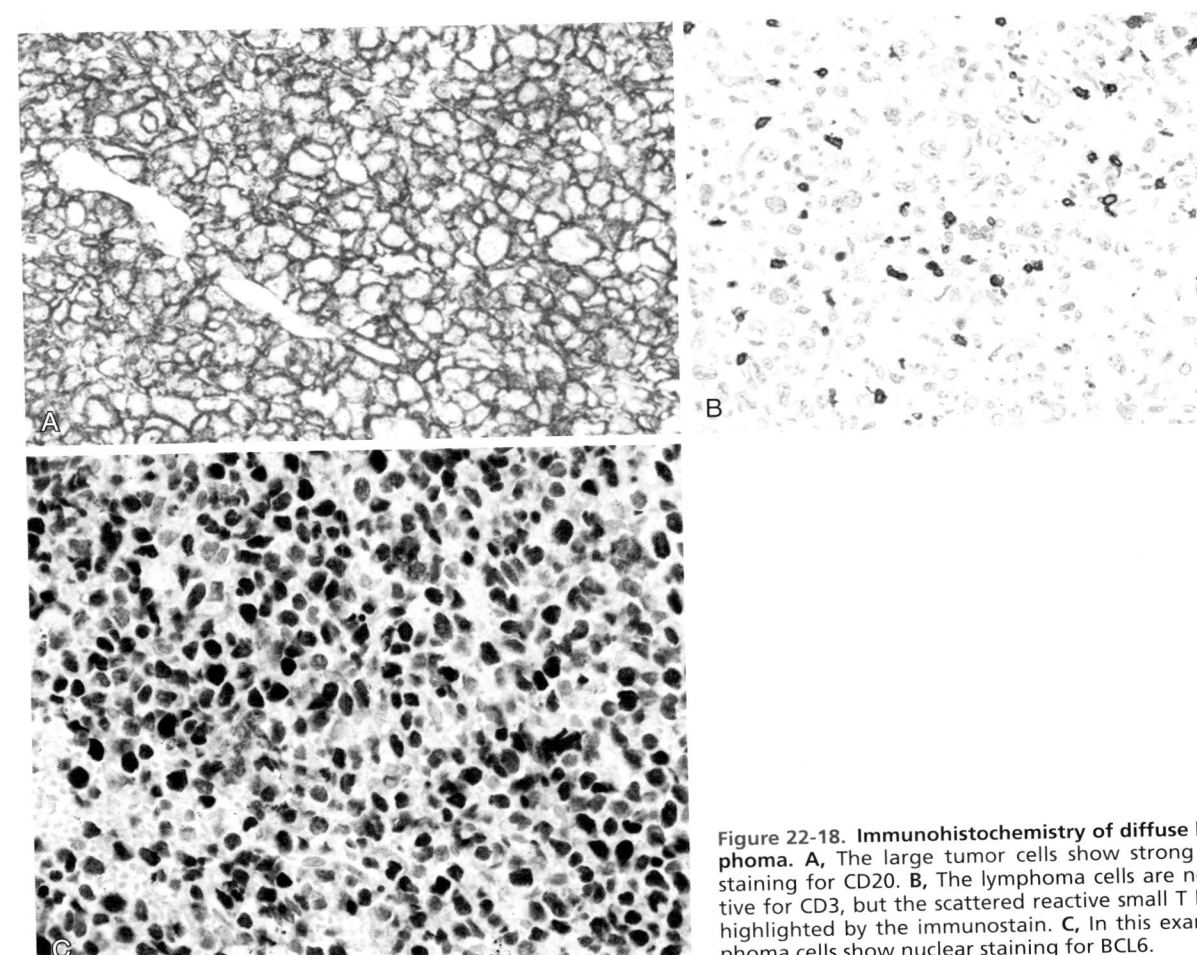

Figure 22-18. **Immunohistochemistry of diffuse large B-cell lymphoma. A,** The large tumor cells show strong cell membrane staining for CD20. **B,** The lymphoma cells are not immunoreactive for CD3, but the scattered reactive small T lymphocytes are highlighted by the immunostain. **C,** In this example, most lymphoma cells show nuclear staining for BCL6.

Box 22-4 *Major Differential Diagnoses of Diffuse Large B-Cell Lymphoma With CD5 Expression*

- Mantle cell lymphoma, blastoid or pleomorphic variant
- Paraimmunoblastic variant of chronic lymphocytic leukemia
- DLBCL arising in chronic lymphocytic leukemia (Richter transformation)
- Intravascular large B-cell lymphoma
- Splenic DLBCL
- De novo CD5-positive DLBCL

DLBCL, Diffuse large B-cell lymphoma.

BN2 (cluster C1/NOTCH2) is characterized by *BCL6* rearrangements and *NOTCH2* mutations. The core mutations are shared with MZL. These tumors make up the majority of DLBCL that are unclassified COO. BN2 is generally associated with favorable outcome.

N1 is a rare subtype characterized by *NOTCH1* mutations, sharing genetic features with CLL/SLL. These tumors are usually ABC-DLBCL and are associated with poor prognosis.

The hallmark mutations in the MCD (cluster C5/MYD88) subtype are *MYD88*^{L265P} and *CD79B*. By COO, they are ABC-DLBCL and typically have poor prognosis. DLBCL of the CNS and DLBCL of the testis are predominantly MCD subtype as

are DLBCL that involve the breast. The core mutations of the MCD subtype are shared with LPL.

The A53 (cluster C2) subtype is defined by *TP53* mutations and complex copy number states. This subtype is associated with poor prognosis and these tumors span the COO groups.

Ongoing refinement is needed to harmonize the three existing schema and to reduce the proportion of tumors (35%) that currently are not assigned with sufficient confidence to any of the seven LymphGen subtypes. For these reasons, the incorporation of the genetics-based classification into either ICC or WHO HAEM5 was deferred to future classifications. However, the promising results emerging from retrospective application to clinical trials[171] and the intention to design prospective precision medicine trials around these schema[191] highlight the future importance of this classification system.

Postulated Cell of Origin

The postulated COO of DLBCL, NOS is the germinal center or post–germinal center B cell for the GCB and ABC subtypes, respectively.

Clinical Course

Although DLBCL is an aggressive tumor, usually resulting in death within 1 or 2 years if left untreated, it is a potentially

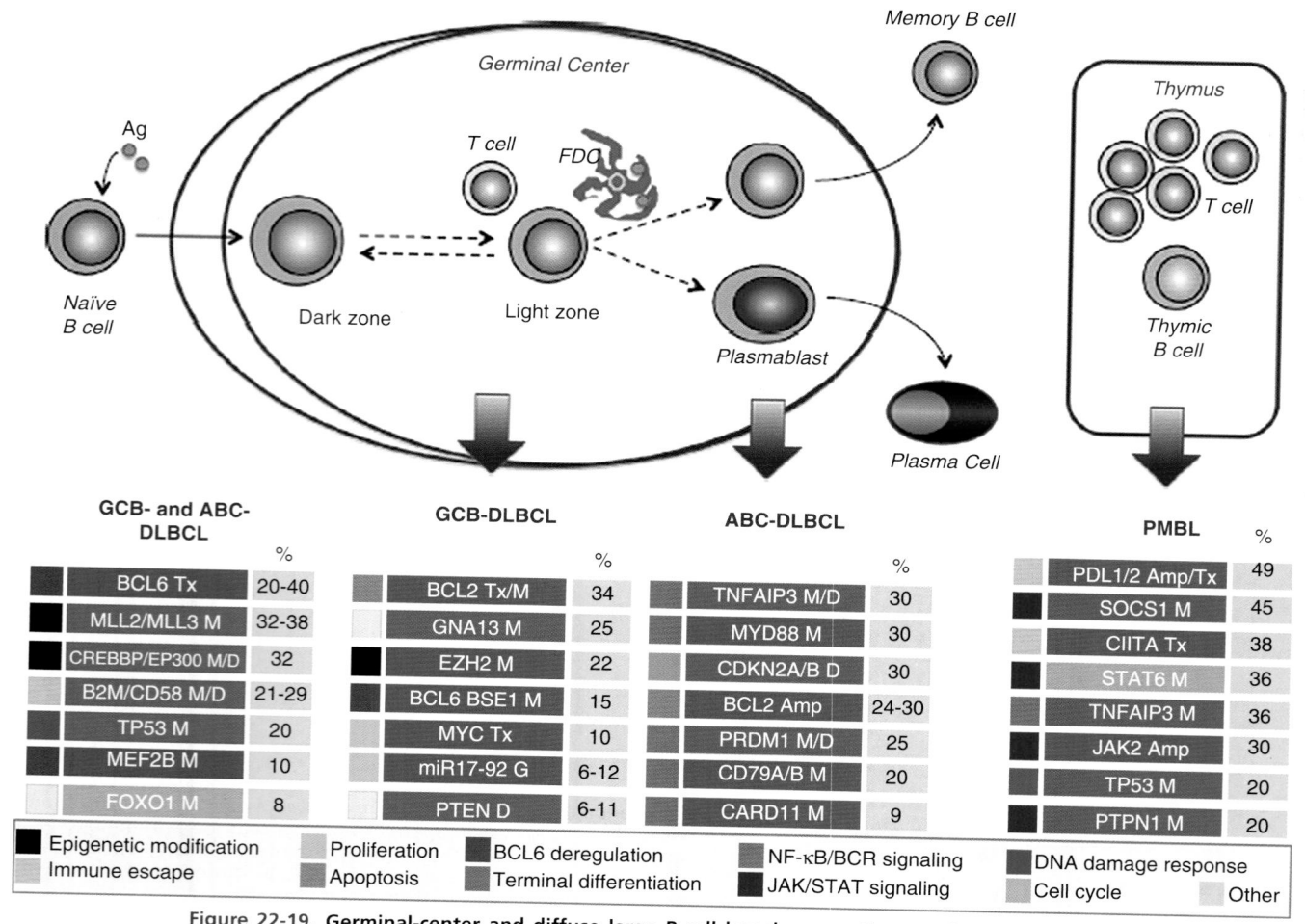

Figure 22-19. Germinal-center and diffuse large B-cell lymphoma pathogenesis. Schematics of the germinal-center reaction and its relationship with major molecular subtypes of diffuse large B-cell lymphoma. The most common shared and subtype-specific genetic alterations are shown, with color codes indicating the involved biological pathway. Loss of function *(blue)* and gain of function *(red)* are shown. *ABC,* Activated B cell; *Ag,* antigen; *Amp,* amplification; *D,* deletion; *DLBCL,* diffuse large B-cell lymphoma; *FDC,* follicular dendritic cell; *G,* gain; *GCB,* germinal-center B cell; *M,* mutation; *PMBL,* primary mediastinal large B-cell lymphoma; *Tx,* translocation. *(From Pasqualucci L, Dalla-Favera R. The genetic landscape of diffuse large B-cell lymphoma. Semin Hematol. 2015;52:67-76, © Elsevier Inc., Figure 1.)*

curable disease even when widely disseminated.[24] The vast majority of relapses occur in the first 2 years after diagnosis and OS for patients event-free at 24 months are reported to be equivalent to that of the age- and sex-matched general population (see Fig. 22-22).[193] R-CHOP was established as the standard of care over 2 decades ago when the addition of the anti-CD20 antibody to CHOP was shown to provide superior outcomes.[194,195] R-CHOP (with or without radiotherapy) results in long-term remission in 60% to 70% of patients.[24] Recently the addition of polatuzumab (an antibody drug conjugate) to R-CHP (without vincristine) has been shown to improve outcomes over R-CHOP.[170] Outcomes of patients that experience relapse or progressive disease have been poor, particularly if the relapse occurs within the first 12 months.[196] Historically, fit, younger patients have been treated with intensive chemotherapy followed by autologous stem cell transplantation, achieving long-term remission in 20% to 30% of patients.[197] The recent advent of chimeric antigen receptor T-cell (CAR-T)

therapy and bispecific antibodies improve the outcomes of patients with relapsed disease, either used in those patients ineligible for transplant (or experiencing disease relapse after transplant) or in those with disease that relapses within 12 months of first-line therapy.[198-201]

Pediatric patients with DLBCL have better outcome (3-year/5-year event-free survival of ~90%) compared with adult patients, and they used to be treated with aggressive chemotherapy regimens similar to those for patients with Burkitt lymphoma.[202,203] The difference in clinical behavior is at least partly related to the different biological features of DLBCL in children: more commonly of the GCB group (~80%),[204,205] lack of *BCL2* translocation,[203] frequent *MYC* rearrangement (33%, associated with a more complex karyotype),[126] and molecular signature of Burkitt lymphoma in ~30% of cases.[206] The use of strict age cutoff to determine treatment protocol has been challenged because this cannot be defined for the age-related biological characteristics.[207] It has only recently been demonstrated that the addition

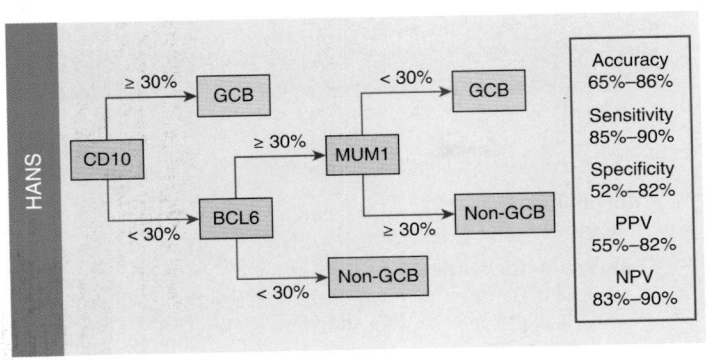

Figure 22-20. Subclassification of diffuse large B-cell lymphoma, not otherwise specified into germinal center B-cell–like (GCB) subtype and non-GCB subtype using immunohistochemistry. The "Hans" algorithm is shown with test characteristics using gene expression profiling as the gold standard.

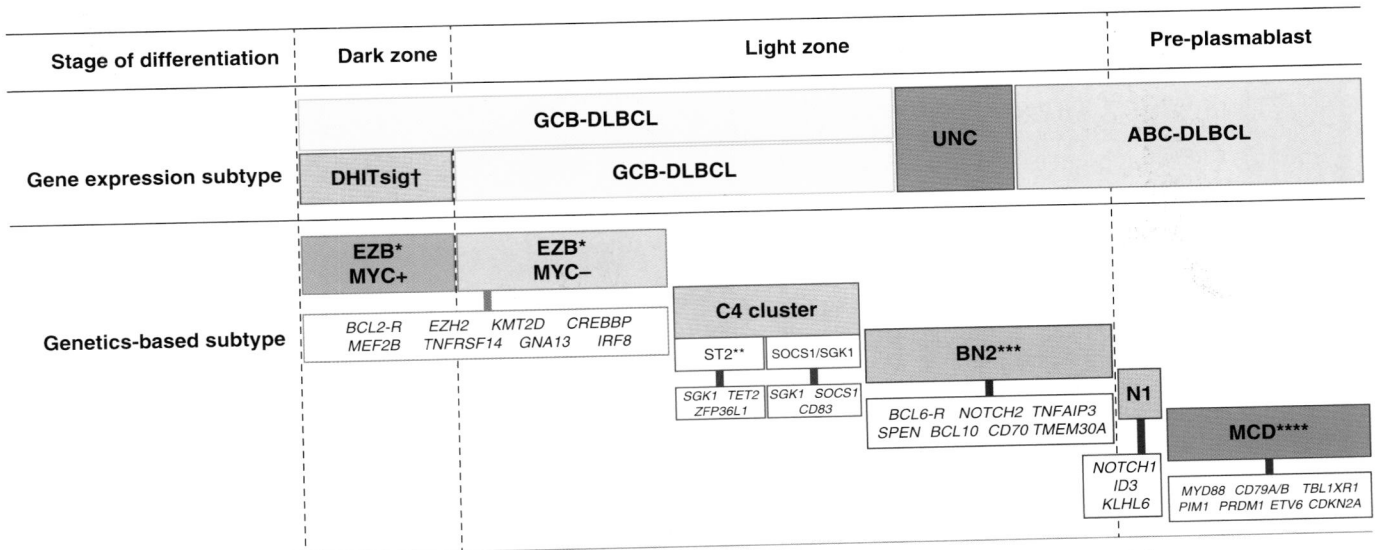

Figure 22-21. Schematic showing the relationship between the cell of origin subtypes and the genetics-based subtypes. The stage of B-cell differentiation most similar to the tumor cells, based on gene expression profiling, is shown at the top. The characteristic genetic mutations and rearrangements are shown below each genetics-based subtype. The A53 (cluster C2) is not shown. †DHITsig or MHG (molecular high grade) signature; *aligned with cluster C3 and BCL2; **aligned with TET2/SGK1; ***aligned with C1 and NOTCH2; ****aligned with C5 and MYD88. *ABC*, Activated B-cell-like subtype; *DHITsig*, double-hit signature; *DLBCL*, diffuse large B-cell lymphoma; *GCB*, germinal center B-cell-like subtype; *UNC*, unclassified.

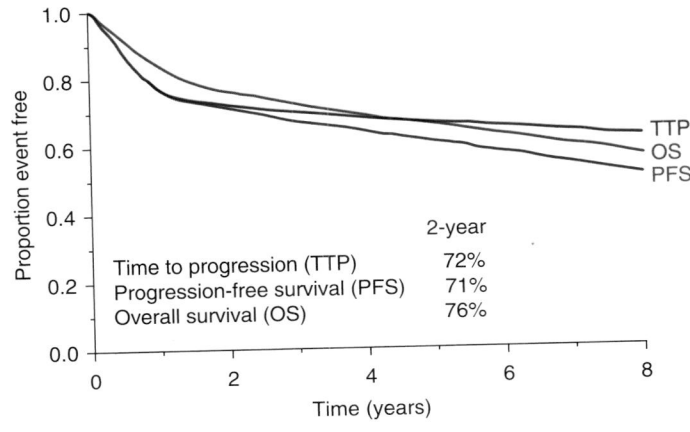

Figure 22-22. Outcome curve of patients with diffuse large B-cell lymphoma after treatment with rituximab, cyclophosphamide, doxorubicin, vincristine, and prednisone (R-CHOP). The data shown are from 3264 patients diagnosed between 2001 and 2022 in British Columbia, Canada. *OS*, Overall survival (events are death from any cause); *TTP*, time to progression (events are progression, relapse, or death from lymphoma or toxicity of lymphoma treatment); *PFS*, progression-free survival (events as per TTP but also including death from any cause).

of rituximab to these regimens improves outcomes in this population.[208]

Prognostic Factors

The adverse prognostic factors in DLBCL are listed in Box 22-5.

Prognostic Clinical Features

The IPI, first defined in 1992, remains a reliable predictor of outcome (Table 22-4).[209] The revised IPI, based on redistribution of the individual IPI factors, has been reported to provide a better prediction of outcome in patients treated with R-CHOP.[210] Finally, the recently described NCCN-IPI further refines prognostication.[211] A clinical model, the CNS-IPI, has been developed and validated to identify patient groups with different risk of relapse of DLBCL within the CNS.[212] Short interval, particularly 2 weeks or less, between diagnosis and treatment has been associated with poor prognosis.[213] This patient group had significantly higher proportions of recognized poor prognosis factors.

Prognostic Morphology and Bone Marrow Involvement

Some but not all studies have shown a slightly poorer outcome for immunoblastic lymphoma compared with centroblastic lymphoma.[128,214-216] The greatest problem with most of these studies is that reproducibility in the subclassification is not addressed. The plasmablastic variant is associated with poor outcome (see Chapter 24).

In DLBCL cases with discordant bone marrow histology (i.e., bone marrow involved by indolent lymphoma instead of DLBCL), survival is better than in cases with concordant bone marrow histology (i.e., involvement by DLBCL). In fact, the survival of the former group is similar to that of patients with negative bone marrow,[26,217] although there is a higher risk for late relapse.[218]

Prognostic Immunohistochemistry

Many studies have shown that immunohistochemistry (IHC) markers, alone or in combination, have prognostic effects in the R-CHOP era. It should be noted that these are not predictive of response to particular therapies at this time and so are not widely used to dictate treatment. COO, as determined by IHC-based algorithms, has been shown to be prognostic in a number of studies,[172-174,219] although this association has been inconsistent and a meta-analysis did not confirm this finding.[220] This may be partly explained by the limitation in reproducibility and accuracy of the IHC-based assays.[165,175]

Dual protein expression of MYC and BCL2 (double-expressor lymphoma) has been established as a strong prognostic biomarker,[51,53,59] with the usual thresholds being ≥40% and ≥50% of malignant cells, respectively. Importantly, dual protein expression does not define a biologically homogeneous group, with ABC-DLBCL (the majority of these tumors) and GCB-DLBCL arriving at this immunophenotype through different mechanisms.[116] This dual expression of MYC and BCL2 protein is prognostic for DLBCL, NOS and is distinctly different from double-hit rearrangements of *MYC* and *BCL2*, which together define a separate disease.

Box 22-5 *Poor Prognostic Indicators in Diffuse Large B-Cell Lymphoma, Not Otherwise Specified*

Clinical
- High IPI score
- Short time from diagnosis to treatment

Morphologic
- Immunoblastic or plasmablastic morphology

Immunohistochemical
- Lack of germinal-center cell phenotype (Hans algorithm)
- Double expression of MYC and BCL2
- CD5 expression
- High proliferation (Ki67) index (controversial)
- Lack of CD30 expression
- TP53 protein expression
- Lack of HLA-DR expression
- Poor tumor-infiltrating T-cell response, especially CD4-positive or FOXP3-positive T cells
- High numbers of granzyme B-positive or TIA-1-positive tumor-infiltrating T cells

Molecular
- ABC subtype by gene-expression profiling or IHC algorithm
- Double-hit or molecular high-grade gene expression signature
- TP53 mutation

ABC, Activated B-cell–like; *IHC,* immunohistochemistry; *IPI,* International Prognostic Index.

Table 22-4 International Prognostic Index Scoring System

Prognostic Factors (1 Point Each)
Age >60 years
Elevated serum lactate dehydrogenase
ECOG Performance Status ≥2
High stage (III–IV)
>1 Extranodal site

Risk Score			
0–1	2	3	4–5
Low	Low-intermediate	High-intermediate	High

De novo CD5-positive DLBCL is associated with a poorer outcome compared with CD5-negative DLBCL,[44,74,80] and is prone to CNS recurrence.[79,80] In the R-CHOP era, CD5 expression remains a significant poor prognostic factor (40%–50% 2-year OS for CD5 positive versus 75%–90% for CD5 negative).[79,221] CD30 expression has been shown to be associated with favorable clinical outcome, especially in GCB subtype and EBV-negative cases.[83,84]

The prognostic significance of the proliferation index as measured by Ki67 immunostaining or other techniques is conflicting. The Southwest Oncology Group and two other groups reported that a high proliferation index (>60%–80%) is associated with poor prognosis.[94,222-225] In contrast, at least two studies have reported the reverse finding.[226,227] The prognostic significance of the proliferative index remains inconsistent in the rituximab era.[54,228,229] Positivity for TP53 by IHC has been associated with poor outcomes, independent of IPI and COO.[137,230]

Signaling the importance of tumor microenvironment, absent MHC class II expression,[144,222,231,232] low tumor-infiltrating T-cell response (especially CD4-positive T cells or FOXP3-positive regulatory T cells),[233-237] and high numbers of granzyme B or TIA-1–positive tumor-infiltrating T cells[238-240] are associated with poor clinical outcome.

Prognostic Molecular Biology Features

COO, assigned using gene expression methods, has been reported in most[155,163,169,241] but not all[179] studies to be prognostic of outcomes after R-CHOP. Recently the COO model has been further refined, recognizing subgroups within the GCB subtype. Anatomically and functionally, the germinal center can be divided into the dark zone, where proliferation and somatic hypermutation of the IGV regions occur, and the light zone, where the B cells undergo selection through interactions with T$_{FH}$ cells in the presence of follicular dendritic cells. Studies have indicated that GCB-DLBCL can be further divided into tumors with gene-expression patterns reminiscent of the dark or light zone.[242-244] The molecular high-grade (MHG) signature[244] was directly derived from the gene expression signatures that were previously shown to distinguish between Burkitt lymphoma (BL—the prototypical dark zone lymphoma) and DLBCL.[130,245] The double-hit signature (DHITsig) defined as the gene-expression pattern that distinguishes HGBL-*MYC/BCL2* from GCB-DLBCL[243] is a misnomer, as all BLs also express this signature, leading to the pattern being renamed the *dark-zone signature*.[246] These signatures are functionally very similar and 30% to 50% of tumors of DLBCL morphology that express these dark-zone signatures are HGBL-*MYC/BCL2*, while a small proportion that are not assigned to HGBL-*MYC/BCL2* by FISH harbor cryptic rearrangements.[247] GCB-DLBCLs (i.e., not HGBL-*MYC/BCL2*) that express DHITsig/MHG have similarly poor outcomes to HGBL-*MYC/BCL2*, but it is not clear whether these patients benefit from the treatment escalation used by many centers for HGBL-*MYC/BCL2*. Patients with "light-zone" GCB-DLBCL have excellent outcomes, even with advanced stage disease.[243]

Gene-expression studies have identified a number of prognostic biomarkers for DLBCL, NOS, beyond the COO subtypes. The tumor microenvironment, as determined in gene expression, is also prognostic.[241] These signatures, stromal-1 and stromal-2, have been refined and developed into an assay applicable to formalin-fixed paraffin embedded biopsies—the lymphoma-associated macrophage interaction signature (LAMIS).[248] A number of other studies have identified further prognostic microenvironment signatures.[249-251] Kotlov et al. identified four groups (GC-like, mesenchymal, inflammatory, and depleted) with distinct outcomes. Meanwhile, Steen et al. developed EcoTyper, a bioinformatic tool that deconvolutes bulk RNA-sequencing to infer the abundance of states of the malignant B cells alongside tumor microenvironment composition.[251] They identified 9 main clusters of B cell state and microenvironment compositions, labeled lymphoma ecosystems, that have distinct outcomes.

In the absence of *MYC* rearrangement, most, but not all, series show no prognostic significance of *BCL2* or *BCL6* rearrangement in DLBCL.[53,55,68,106-113,252-255] The presence of *BCL6* gene mutation is suggested to be a favorable prognostic factor.[255,256] High levels of *BCL6* mRNA

expression are associated with a favorable prognosis.[255,257] Sole *MYC* rearrangement, in the absence of concurrent *BCL2* or *BCL6* rearrangement, is variably associated with poor outcomes,[129] with the largest series finding no association.[132]

TP53 mutation generally correlates with poor prognosis on multivariate analysis, and the effect may depend on the types of mutations.[258-261] Deletion of *CDKN2A* has also been reported to be associated with poor prognosis.[262] The prognostic significance of clusters of mutations are discussed in the section on the genetics-based subtypes of DLBCL.

Differential Diagnosis

In general, the diagnosis of DLBCL is straightforward and established by clinical history, radiologic and laboratory findings, appropriate histology and cytology, immunohistochemistry revealing a mature B-cell immunophenotype, and demonstration of monoclonality of the immunoglobulin heavy or light chains via expression patterns or genetic analysis (Table 22-5). Most important, a benign lymphoid proliferation should be excluded. In addition, the more specific entities in this and other chapters (virally associated LBCL, immunodeficiency associated, etc.) should be excluded as far as possible.

Benign

Reactive B-cell proliferations can be tricky, particularly in small biopsies and in children. In florid reactive immunoblastic proliferations, such as infectious mononucleosis, other viral infections (including cytomegalovirus infection), drug reactions, and postvaccination reactions, the lymph node shows partial effacement of nodal architecture and infiltration by many large lymphoid cells, closely mimicking DLBCL (Fig. 22-23).[263] The subtotal effacement of the lymph node in infectious mononucleosis and other viral and reactive cases can be difficult to detect in core needle biopsies in which the nodal architecture cannot be appreciated, warranting caution. In addition, necrosis is common and Reed-Sternberg–like cells are occasionally found, especially around the necrotic foci. In contrast to DLBCL, the large, activated cells in reactive proliferations often show transition and maturation into plasmablasts and plasma cells, and they usually do not show significant nuclear atypia such as irregular or twisted nuclear outlines. By immunophenotyping, the large cells in infectious mononucleosis consist of a mixture of B cells and T cells, and the B cells are polytypic.[264] Because there is a mixture of B cells at various stages of maturation toward plasma cells, CD20 staining is heterogeneous (with staining lost in late plasmablasts and plasma cells) (Fig. 22-24). Many cells are immunoreactive for EBV-LMP1. Correlation with clinical findings and serology can assist in arriving at the correct diagnosis.

Another diagnostic dilemma is that of Kikuchi (histiocytic necrotizing) lymphadenitis. The lymph nodes show subtotal effacement by patchy, karyorrhectic foci commonly associated with many large lymphoid cells, which may initially mimic DLBCL. In contrast to DLBCL, the proliferating cells in Kikuchi lymphadenitis consist of histiocytes (CD68 positive, myeloperoxidase positive), plasmacytoid dendritic cells (CD68 positive, CD123 positive, myeloperoxidase negative), and cytotoxic CD8-positive T cells, with very few CD20-positive B cells. Some of the histiocytes are typically packed

Table 22-5 Differential Diagnosis of Diffuse Large B-Cell Lymphoma, Not Otherwise Specified

Entity	Features Favoring Diagnosis of Entity	Features Favoring Diagnosis of DLBCL, NOS
Florid-reactive immunoblastic proliferation (including infectious mononucleosis)	At least partial preservation of tissue architecture Polymorphic cellular composition: spectrum of cellular differentiation from immunoblasts to plasmablasts and plasma cells Large cells do not show overt nuclear atypia Large cells usually include CD20-positive B cells and CD3-positive T cells CD20-positive cells often show a range of staining intensity caused by presence of cells in different stages of maturation Large lymphoid cells show polytypic immunoglobulin	Large cells often appear monotonous, without maturation toward plasma cells Large cells commonly but not invariably exhibit atypia (e.g., very large cell size, irregular nuclear folds, granular chromatin pattern) Large cells usually show uniform strong staining for CD20 May show immunoglobulin light-chain restriction
Kikuchi lymphadenitis	Small lymph node (<2 cm) Patchy karyorrhectic foci containing crescentic histiocytes Infiltrate consists of CD68-positive histiocytes and plasmacytoid dendritic cells, as well as CD8-positive T cells, but very few CD20-positive B cells	Large cells are uniformly CD20 positive
Paraimmunoblastic variant of chronic lymphocytic leukemia	Paraimmunoblasts are medium-sized cells, smaller and less pleomorphic than DLBCL Intermixed prolymphocytes and small lymphocytes often present CD5 positive (usually)	Lymphoma cells are usually larger and more pleomorphic
Pleomorphic variant of mantle cell lymphoma	Nucleoli generally inconspicuous, although some cells may have prominent nucleoli Usually chromatin rich Cytoplasm usually scanty Areas of classic mantle cell lymphoma commonly present CD5 positive, cyclin D1 positive, SOX11 positive Presence of t(11;14)(q13;q32)	Nucleoli usually prominent Chromatin pattern commonly vesicular CD5 negative, cyclin D1 negative, SOX11 negative Lack of characteristic translocation
T-cell/histiocyte–rich large B-cell lymphoma	Less than 10% large B cells in a background of CD8-positive, TIA1-positive lymphocytes, see Box 22-6	Greater than 10% large B cells in clusters or sheets
Primary mediastinal large B-cell lymphoma	Young female patients with bulky mediastinal mass and primarily local involvement, fine compartmentalizing sclerosis, clear cell change, expression of MAL, PD-L2, CD30, CD23, BCL6, lacking surface Ig, see Box 22-7 and Table 22-6	Cases lacking features of PMBL
High-grade B-cell lymphoma, NOS	Low power appearance of starry-sky pattern composed of mixed medium-to-large-sized cells with coarse chromatin, two to five nucleoli; however, with more pleomorphism or atypical immunophenotype than is typical of Burkitt lymphoma (intermediate cytology); or medium-sized cells with fine chromatin and zero to two inconspicuous nucleoli (blastoid cytology)	Classical DLBCL, NOS cytology including centroblastic, immunoblastic, anaplastic, or other rare variants as listed in Table 22-1
DLBCL/HGBL with *MYC* and *BCL2* rearrangements	Any cytology, however, with documented evidence of the defining translocations	DLBCL, NOS without features of other entities and lacking the *MYC* and *BCL2,* or *MYC* and *BCL2* and *BCL6* translocations
Burkitt lymphoma	More common in children and young adults Starry-sky pattern Lymphoma cells medium-sized, monotonous, with "squaring" of nuclei and cell borders CD10 positive (commonly) BCL2 negative (usually) Ki67 index ~100% *MYC* gene rearranged *BCL2* and *BCL6* genes not rearranged	More common in adults Starry-sky pattern uncommon Lymphoma cells large- or medium-sized, often with more variation in nuclear size and greater amount of cytoplasm CD10 positive in ~40% BCL2 positive in ~50% Ki67 index often <80% (although rare cases may reach ~100%) *MYC* gene rearrangement uncommon *BCL2* and *BCL6* genes rearranged in a proportion of cases
Anaplastic plasmacytoma	Possible history of multiple myeloma Neoplastic plasma cells of smaller size frequently admixed CD20 negative, CD138 positive	Almost always CD20 positive
Plasmablastic lymphoma	History of immunosuppression or HIV infection Large cells with eccentric nuclei, coarse chromatin, prominent nucleoli, abundant amphophilic cytoplasm with peri-nuclear hof, plasmacytic features, mixed immunoblasts CD20 negative, CD138 positive, EBV positive	Lack of plasmablastic, cytologic, or immunophenotypic features Strong uniform CD20
Intravascular large B-cell lymphoma	Lack of definable mass Frequent central nervous system, bone marrow, or skin involvement Hemophagocytosis in "Asian" variant Mature B-cell phenotype	Identifiable predominant nodal or extranodal mass

Continued

Table 22-5 Differential Diagnosis of Diffuse Large B-Cell Lymphoma, Not Otherwise Specified—cont'd

Entity	Features Favoring Diagnosis of Entity	Features Favoring Diagnosis of DLBCL, NOS
Virally associated lymphomas	History of immunosuppression Nodal, extranodal, or cavitary EBV positive or HHV-8 positive tumor cells	Large B-cell lymphoma lacking characteristic features
Immunodeficiency associated lymphomas	History of primary immune disorder, HIV, prior transplant, or other iatrogenic immunodeficiency Often EBV positive	Lack pertinent clinical history
Lymphocyte predominant B-cell lymphoma	Localized disease Infrequent, individual, typical L&H or popcorn cells Small background B cells Follicular dendritic cell meshworks Rimming of atypical cells by CD57-positive/PD1-positive T cells	Uniformly large B cells with one of the typical DLBCL, NOS cytologies Lack of follicular dendritic-cell meshworks
Classic Hodgkin lymphoma: syncytial variant of nodular sclerosis or lymphocyte depleted	Usual prominence of eosinophils CD30+, CD15+/– CD20– or heterogeneously CD20+ OCT-2–, BOB.1– EBV+ in >35%	CD20+, immunoglobulin+, CD30–/+, CD15– OCT-2+, BOB.1+ EBV rarely positive except in setting of immunosuppression
T-cell or NK-cell lymphomas	CD3+, CD20– CD56+ for NK-cell lymphoma CD30+, ALK+/– for anaplastic large cell lymphoma	CD20 positive, CD3 negative
Histiocytic sarcoma	Tumor cells often larger, with abundant eosinophilic cytoplasm CD68 positive, CD163 positive, CD20 negative, CD3 negative	Lymphoma cells have amphophilic or basophilic cytoplasm CD20 positive, CD68 negative, CD163 negative
Myeloid sarcoma	Neoplastic cells often medium-sized and show blastic nuclear features Cytoplasm often eosinophilic; may have eosinophilic granules May have admixed eosinophilic myelocytes Myeloperoxidase positive, CD20 negative	Cytoplasm usually amphophilic or basophilic rather than eosinophilic CD20 positive, myeloperoxidase negative
Extramedullary hematopoietic tumor	Large cells are megakaryocytes and not neoplastic cells Presence of clusters of erythroid normoblasts	Large cells are CD20 positive
Non-hematolymphoid malignancies	Usually cohesive growth; but melanoma often shows cellular dehiscence within cell clusters Cytoplasm often eosinophilic CD45 negative Expression of specific immunohistochemical markers (e.g., cytokeratin in carcinoma, S-100 protein and HMB45 in melanoma, OCT-3/4 and CD117 in seminoma)	Usually noncohesive and permeative growth Cytoplasm often amphophilic to basophilic Prominent nuclear lobation favors a diagnosis of lymphoma over non-hematolymphoid neoplasm CD45 positive, CD20 positive

ALK, Anaplastic lymphoma kinase; *DLBCL, NOS,* diffuse large B-cell lymphoma, not otherwise specified; *EBV,* Epstein-Barr virus; *HHV-8,* human herpesvirus 8; *L&H,* lymphocytic and histiocytic; *NK,* natural killer.

with phagocytosed materials, compressing the nuclei into a thin crescent (crescentic histiocytes).[265-267]

B-Cell Lymphomas

Cases of DLBCL, especially those accompanied by many apoptotic bodies and a starry-sky pattern, can be difficult to distinguish from BL. Examination of such cases should demonstrate one of the DLBCL cytologies (most commonly centroblastic features) that are distinct from the neoplastic cells in BL, which are usually more monotonous and often exhibit molding of the nuclei and cytoplasmic borders. Immunophenotyping can also be helpful because BL will show expression of germinal center markers (CD10, BCL6) and lack, or have only weak, BCL2 expression. In addition, Burkitt lymphoma should show an extremely high proliferation (Ki67) index, approaching 100%; this is much higher than DLBCLs as an overall group, although occasional examples of DLBCL can show proliferation in this range. *MYC* rearrangement, a characteristic of Burkitt lymphoma, is uncommon in DLBCLs (~10%) and usually occurs as part of a complex genetic aberration.[130] Importantly, DLBCLs with sole *MYC* rearrangement do not typically show the gene expression profile of Burkitt lymphoma; instead, they are similar to DLBCL without *MYC* rearrangement.[130,245] The categories of

HGBL, NOS or HGBL-*MYC/BCL2* should be considered and excluded (see Chapter 24).[20,21]

The pleomorphic and blastoid variants of MCL, which are comprised of large pleomorphic cells with irregularly folded nuclei or moderately sized cells with fine chromatin, respectively, can be difficult to distinguish from DLBCL, NOS (Fig. 22-25).[268-272] However, in these variants, there are often foci with features of classic MCL, including naked germinal centers lacking organized mantle zones or foci with the more usual mantle cell cytology. Evaluation for expression of cyclin D1, SOX11, and CD5 along with FISH for the *CCND1* gene translocation can be helpful to distinguish the two entities.[87-93]

The paraimmunoblastic type of CLL/SLL is an aggressive variant characterized by diffuse infiltration of paraimmunoblasts—the cell type commonly found in proliferation centers.[273,274] Paraimmunoblasts, which are medium-sized cells, are slightly smaller than the lymphoma cells seen in DLBCL. They have vesicular nuclei, single central nucleoli, and a moderate amount of weakly eosinophilic rather than amphophilic cytoplasm (Fig. 22-26). Furthermore, intermixed prolymphocytes and small lymphocytes are often seen, the lymph node capsule is often preserved, and CD5 is positive.[273]

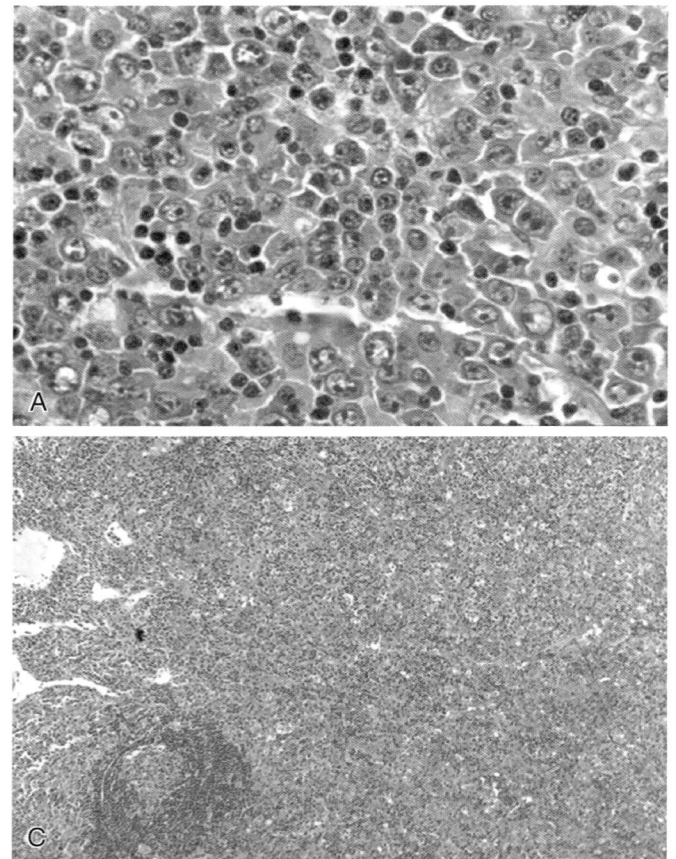

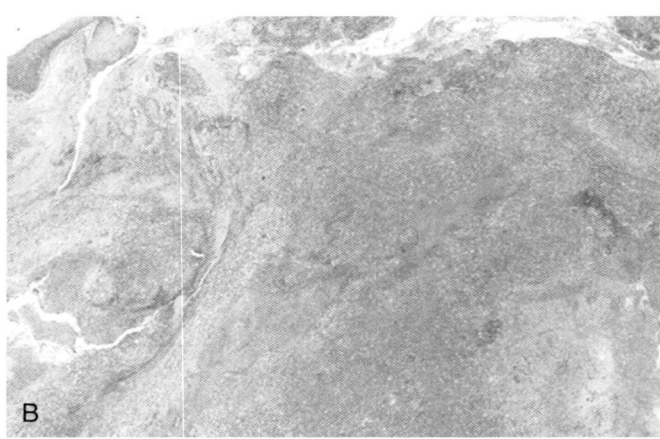

Figure 22-23. Infectious mononucleosis. A, Large lymphoid cells are present in an alarming number, raising the serious consideration of large-cell lymphoma. Usually, the large cells do not exhibit frank atypia and show a transition into recognizable plasmablasts and plasma cells. **B,** The tonsil is commonly involved and usually exhibits ulceration and necrosis. **C,** An important clue to the correct diagnosis of infectious mononucleosis is partial preservation of the normal lymph node architecture. Sinuses and lymphoid follicles are seen in the *left side of the field*.

If CD5 expression is detected on an LBCL, consideration should be given to pleomorphic variant of MCL, paraimmunoblastic variant of CLL/SLL, or DLBCL complicating CLL (Richter transformation), which can closely resemble de novo CD5-positive DLBCL. Distinguishing features of the first two entities are described in the preceding paragraph, while Richter transformation is characterized by a known history of CLL or evidence of CLL infiltrate in the biopsy in the form of monotonous small lymphocytes admixed with prolymphocytes and paraimmunoblasts, along with co-expression of CD5 with CD23.

Large B-cell lymphomas with *IRF4* rearrangement and FL, grade 3, are both discussed in the chapter on FL and other germinal center B-cell lymphomas (Chapter 17). Both of these entities show a predominance of large B cells with expression of germinal center markers and can be confused with DLBCL, NOS. Small biopsies may be problematic because diffuse areas in *IRF4*-rearranged cases and expanded follicles in FL grade 3B can look misleadingly diffuse when only a small amount of tissue is available for review. A high level of suspicion is needed to exclude these entities. While IRF4/MUM1 expression can be seen in both nongerminal center DLBCL and in LBCL with *IRF4*-rearrangement, asymmetric tonsil involvement in children is typical of the latter entity.[275] Staining for follicular dendritic cell markers (CD21, CD23) can be helpful to evaluate for the meshworks typical of FL grade 3.

Plasmablastic or anaplastic plasmacytomas with large neoplastic cells may morphologically resemble DLBCL. Helpfully, the tumor cells in plasmacytomas are usually CD20 negative, whereas DLBCLs are almost always CD20 positive at presentation. A prior history of multiple myeloma or other myeloma-associated clinical and laboratory features can also be used to aid in diagnosis.[276] Other plasmablastic neoplasms such as plasmablastic lymphoma (usually EBV-associated), anaplastic lymphoma kinase (ALK)-positive LBCL, and other entities should be excluded (see Chapter 28 for more complete discussion).

CHL, such as the syncytial variant of nodular sclerosis or lymphocyte-depleted subtypes, and NLPBL can be difficult to distinguish from DLBCL particularly when the expected expression pattern of CD30 and CD15 are not seen. The presence of background eosinophils favors CHL, and syncytial nodular sclerosis CHL almost always shows prominent coagulative necrosis and polarizable sclerosis. Uniform strong CD20 immunoreactivity and immunoglobulin expression favor a diagnosis of DLBCL, whereas negative or heterogeneous staining for CD20 and positive EBV-LMP1 expression favor a diagnosis of CHL. Staining for the B-cell transcription factors OCT2 (POU2F2) and BOB.1 (POU2AF1) can be useful since one or the other is often lacking in classic Hodgkin lymphoma, even when CD20 is expressed, whereas both are usually expressed in DLBCL. Cases with intermediate features (gray-zone lymphoma) presenting with a mediastinal mass are classified as mediastinal gray-zone lymphoma (MGZL).

T-Cell Lymphomas

T-cell or NK-cell lymphomas are comprised of large neoplastic lymphoid cells that may be morphologically indistinguishable from DLBCL, but the distinction can

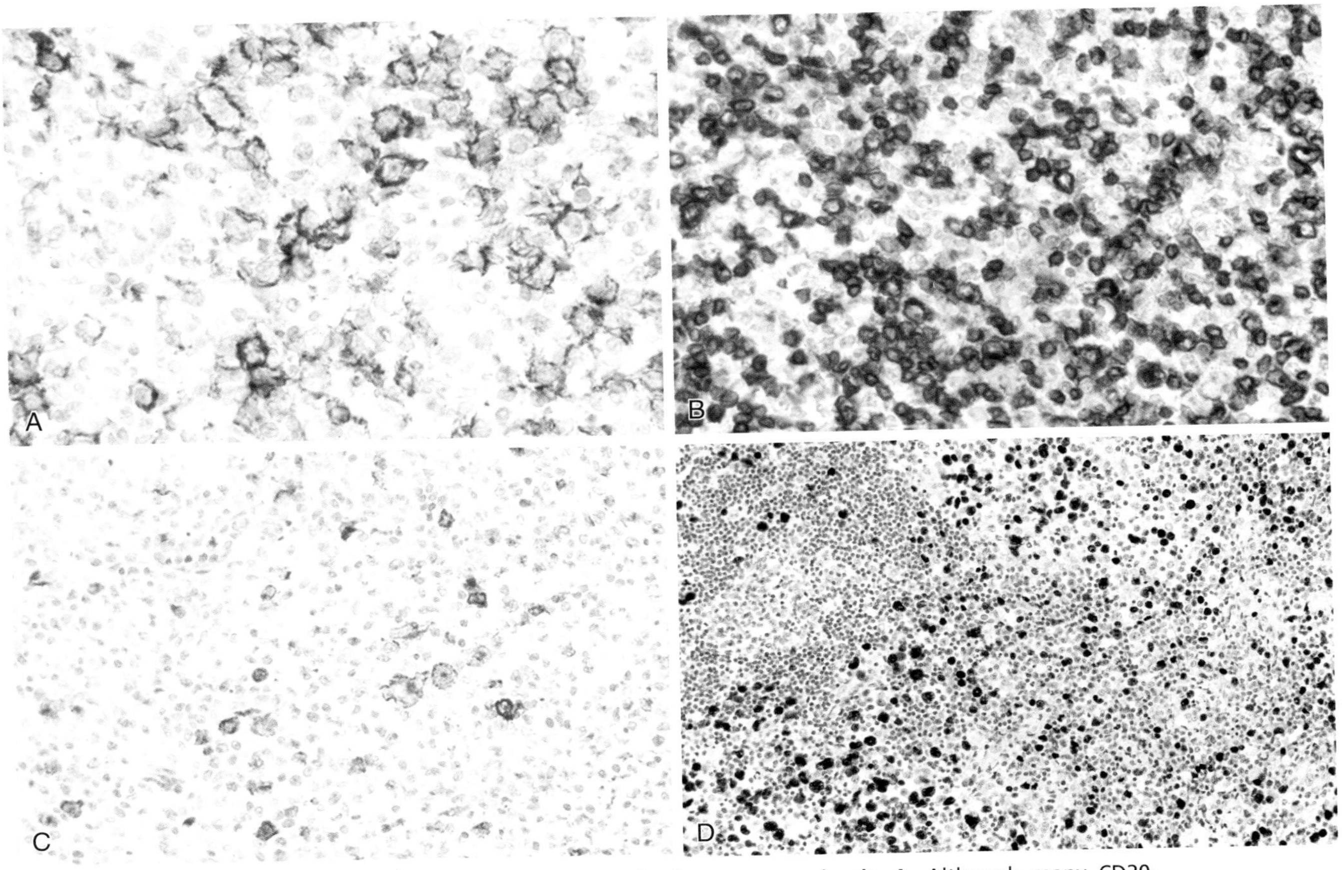

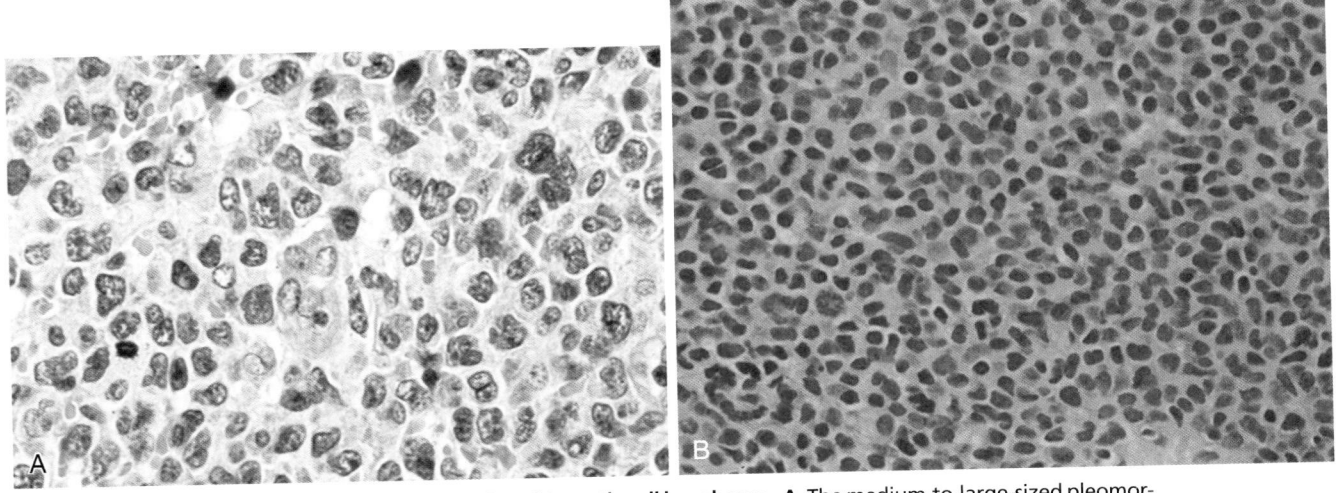

Figure 22-24. Immunohistochemistry of infectious mononucleosis. A, Although many CD20-positive cells are often present, the intensity of staining in the large cells is usually heterogeneous, indicating that some large cells are plasmablasts (weak or negative for CD20). The B cells are polytypic on staining for immunoglobulin *(not shown)*. **B,** There are often many CD3-positive cells, including some large ones. **C,** A proportion of cells stain for EBV-LMP1. **D,** A greater number show nuclear labeling for Epstein-Barr virus–encoded RNA (EBER) on in situ hybridization.

Figure 22-25. Pleomorphic or blastoid mantle cell lymphoma. A, The medium-to-large-sized pleomorphic lymphoma cells can lead to a misdiagnosis of diffuse large B-cell lymphoma. **B,** These medium-sized, irregularly shaped cells with powdery chromatin and barely discernable nucleoli are from a case of blastoid mantle cell lymphoma. Staining for CD5 and cyclin D1 are essential in such cases.

usually be made by applying multiple lineage-associated markers. ALK-negative anaplastic large cell lymphoma can be particularly problematic because of lack of many T-cell markers and co-expression of other nonlineage markers.

Conversely, lymphomas with plasmacytic differentiation may aberrantly co-express T-cell markers or cytokeratins. Thus a large immunophenotyping panel is sometimes needed. Genotyping by studying immunoglobulin and TR

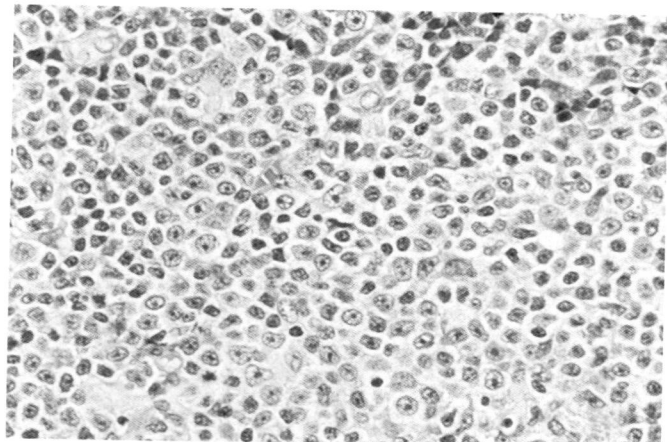

Figure 22-26. Paraimmunoblastic variant of chronic lymphocytic leukemia. The paraimmunoblasts differ from immunoblasts by being smaller and having paler cytoplasm. In addition, there are often admixed small lymphocytes and prolymphocytes, as characteristically seen in chronic lymphocytic leukemia.

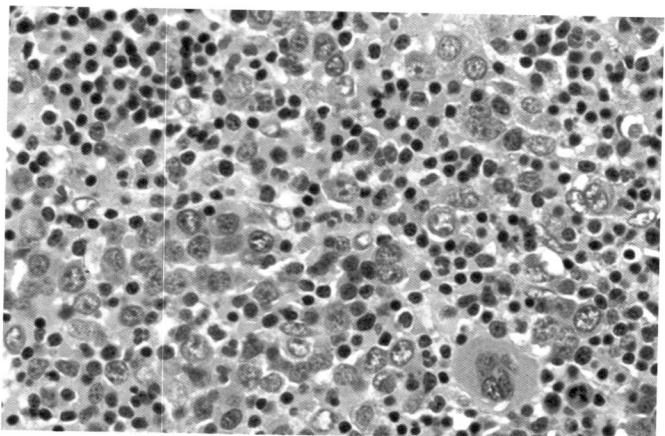

Figure 22-27. Extramedullary hematopoietic tumors. The histologic appearance of extramedullary myelopoiesis can lead to a misdiagnosis of diffuse large B-cell lymphoma. Clues to the correct diagnosis include the finding of megakaryocytes *(lower-right field)* and islands of erythroblasts, which can look superficially like lymphocytes *(upper-left field)*. The large cells are, in fact, immature cells of the myeloid and erythroid series.

gene rearrangement may be necessary to resolve the lineage in some cases.[33]

Myeloid Neoplasm

A diagnosis of myeloid sarcoma should be suspected if there are cytoplasmic eosinophilic granules or interspersed eosinophilic myelocytes in the infiltrate. This diagnosis can be confirmed by immunostaining for myeloperoxidase, lysozyme, CD33, CD34, and CD117. Evaluation of the bone marrow may also be useful. Extramedullary hematopoietic tumors other than myeloid sarcomas can also be mistaken for DLBCL because of the number of large cells. Clues to the correct diagnosis include the identification of megakaryocytes and erythroid normoblasts (Fig. 22-27).

Histiocytic sarcoma is a rare neoplasm that is sometimes part of the differential with DLBCL. The cells of histiocytic sarcoma are usually larger than those of DLBCL; most important, the cytoplasm is eosinophilic rather than amphophilic or basophilic. The diagnosis requires the demonstration of histiocytic markers (e.g., CD68, CD163) and the lack of pan–B-cell markers, pan–T-cell markers, and dendritic cell markers.

Miscellaneous

Non-hematolymphoid malignancies (e.g., carcinoma, melanoma, seminoma) may be confused with DLBCL because of diffuse growth, and conversely because lymphoma can exhibit a deceptively cohesive or packeted growth pattern. Histologic features suggestive of lymphoma include highly permeative growth, amphophilic or basophilic cytoplasm, and marked folding of the nuclear membranes. Non-hematolymphoid neoplasms are consistently negative for CD45 and express their respective specific markers. However, rare cases of DLBCL have been shown to express the epithelial markers cytokeratin and epithelial membrane antigen (EMA). In addition, the "plasma cell" marker CD138 (syndecan-1) is expressed in epithelium and numerous epithelial tumors.[277] It is therefore essential to interpret the findings in context of a complete phenotype.[278,279]

T-CELL/HISTIOCYTE–RICH LARGE B-CELL LYMPHOMA

Definition

THRLBCL is associated with a prominent component of reactive T cells and usually histiocytes.[20,21] By definition, less than 10% of cells in a biopsy should consist of large atypical B cells.[280,281] THRLBCL may arise de novo. Alternatively, THRLBCL may have a close relationship to progression of NLPBL in that NLPBL may include subtotal or total areas indistinguishable from THRLBCL. In addition to morphologic and immunophenotypic overlap, similarities between these two entities have been studied by gene-expression profiling and array comparative genomic hybridization, which support a relationship between the two entities.[282,283] This distinction is discussed further under "Differential Diagnosis."

Epidemiology

The median age of patients with THRLBCL is in the 6th to 7th decades, but children may also be affected.[284] There is a male predominance (male-to-female ratio of 1.7:1).[285,286]

Etiology

No etiologic factors have been identified. The tumor microenvironment is likely engaged in cross talk with the neoplastic cells.[287] The rich T-cell infiltrate and macrophages may both contribute to the characteristic features.[288,289] Tumor-cell apoptosis, perhaps mediated by cytotoxic CD8-positive T cells, may partly explain the relatively low number of neoplastic cells.[290]

At least a proportion of cases are pathogenetically related to NLPBL[291-293] (also see "Genetics"). Some patients may have a prior history of NLPBL,[294] but such cases are often interpreted as the diffuse growth of NLPBL signaling progression of disease rather than de novo THRLBCL.

Clinical Features

THRLBCL is predominantly a nodal disease, but extranodal sites can also be involved.[286] Compared with DLBCL, NOS, THRLBCL more frequently presents with high-stage disease (about two-thirds in stage III to IV),[286,295] and bone marrow involvement is more common (32%–62% versus 16% in DLBCL, NOS) (Box 22-6).[286,296,297] Liver lesions and splenomegaly are more frequent (25%).[25]

Morphology

The lymph node usually shows complete effacement of architecture by a diffuse polymorphic cellular population. The large neoplastic B cells, which should account for less than 10% of the cellular population, are dispersed singly, without the formation of discrete aggregates or sheets, in a background of small lymphocytes. The presence of even a focal component of NLPBL on morphologic or immunohistochemical assessment excludes a diagnosis of THRLBCL.

In THRLBCL, the large cells show variable cytology, including centroblasts, immunoblasts, pleomorphic large cells with irregularly folded nuclei (reminiscent of lymphocytic and histiocytic [L&H] cells of NLPBL) or even Reed-Sternberg-like cells (Fig. 22-28).[298] The small lymphocytes in the background are predominantly reactive T cells and are either cytologically unremarkable or mildly atypical, with a slightly larger cell size and mild nuclear folds (see Fig. 22-28). In addition, variable numbers of histiocytes, epithelioid histiocytes, eosinophils, and plasma cells may be present. Fine trabecular fibrosis is common in the background.[281] In cases rich in nonepithelioid histiocytes, plasma cells and eosinophils are usually scanty.[299,300] Splenic involvement is characterized by a micronodular pattern, with the micronodules showing a cellular composition similar to that of other sites of involvement and lacking follicular dendritic cell meshworks.[298,301] A summary of THRLBCL is presented in Box 22-6.

Immunophenotype

The scattered large neoplastic cells express pan–B-cell markers CD19, CD20, and CD79a, and the germinal center marker BCL6. Light chain restriction is demonstrable in some cases (Fig. 22-29).[285,302,303] The cells should be usually negative for Hodgkin markers CD15 and CD30.[294,298,303-305] CD5 and CD10 are usually negative.[300,302] BCL2 is expressed in 40% of cases, and BCL6 in 40% to 60%.[291,300] EMA expression is variable, ranging from 3% to 100% of cases, with an overall rate of about 30%.[285,294,298,300,303,304,306]

The small cells in the background are overwhelmingly T cells (CD3-positive), predominantly the CD8-positive, TIA-1–positive, cytotoxic type (see Fig. 22-29).[290] In contrast to NLPBL, there are no rosettes of follicular T cells (CD57, PD-1, CXCL13, or ICOS positive) around the large neoplastic cells.[307,308] Cases of THRLBCL reported to have many T-follicular helper lymphocytes in the background may represent the diffuse variant of NLPBL.[291,300] Small reactive B cells should be rare.[300] In contrast to NLPBL, there are no meshworks of CD21-positive follicular dendritic cells among the neoplastic large B cells.

Box 22-6 Major Diagnostic Features of T-Cell/Histiocyte–Rich Large B-Cell Lymphoma

Definition
- Neoplastic large B cells dispersed singly, without forming aggregates or sheets, in a background of abundant reactive T cells and usually histiocytes
- Absence of known or a recognizable component of NLPBL (which can be focal or subtle)

Clinical Features
- Age: older adults (6th to 7th decades)
- Male-to-female ratio 1.7:1
- Nodal or extranodal involvement
- Usually advanced stage at presentation (two-thirds stage III and IV)
- Bone marrow involvement very common (60%)
- Prognosis: no difference compared with comparable-stage conventional DLBCL

Morphology
- Diffuse infiltrate of scattered large neoplastic B cells that may resemble centroblasts, immunoblasts, L&H cells, or Reed-Sternberg cells
- Background cells include small T cells (which can show mild atypia), often with histiocytes, plasma cells, and eosinophils

Immunophenotype
- Large cells: pan–B-cell+, CD30-, CD15-, EMA+/-, BCL6+/-
- Background small cells: CD3+, CD8+, TIA-1+
- There should be no large neoplastic B cells residing within nodules of small B cells or meshworks of follicular dendritic cells, which would otherwise indicate a diagnosis of NLPBL

Molecular Features
- Clonally rearranged immunoglobulin genes
- Germline TCR genes
- EBV negative

DLBCL, Diffuse large B-cell lymphoma; *EBV,* Epstein-Barr virus; *EMA,* epithelial membrane antigen; *NLPBL,* nodular lymphocyte-predominant B-cell (Hodgkin) lymphoma; *TCR,* T-cell receptor.

The neoplastic cells are negative for EBV. The small number of cases reported to be EBV positive[281,304,309-311] are more appropriately reclassified as EBV-positive lymphomas or lymphoproliferative disorders.[20,21,312]

Genetics

THRLBCL has clonally rearranged immunoglobulin genes and germline TCR genes.[303,313-315] Hypermutated IGHV genes and ongoing somatic mutations can be demonstrated in some cases.[316,317] BCL2 gene rearrangement is present in about 25% of cases.[285,294] Mutations in JUNB, DUSP2, SGK1, SOCS1, and CREBBP have been found in these tumors similar to NLPBL, reinforcing the relationship of both entities.[318]

Earlier comparative genomic hybridization of microdissected tumor cells showed similarities and differences in THRLBCL and NLPBL.[319] More recently, array comparative genomic hybridization analysis demonstrated that gains of 2p16.1 and losses of 2p11.2 and 9p11.2 are commonly observed in both THRLBCL and NLPBL[283] while gene expression profiling of microdissected tumor cells of THRLBCL and NLPBL do not show clear-cut differences.[293] These combined molecular findings support a link, but not

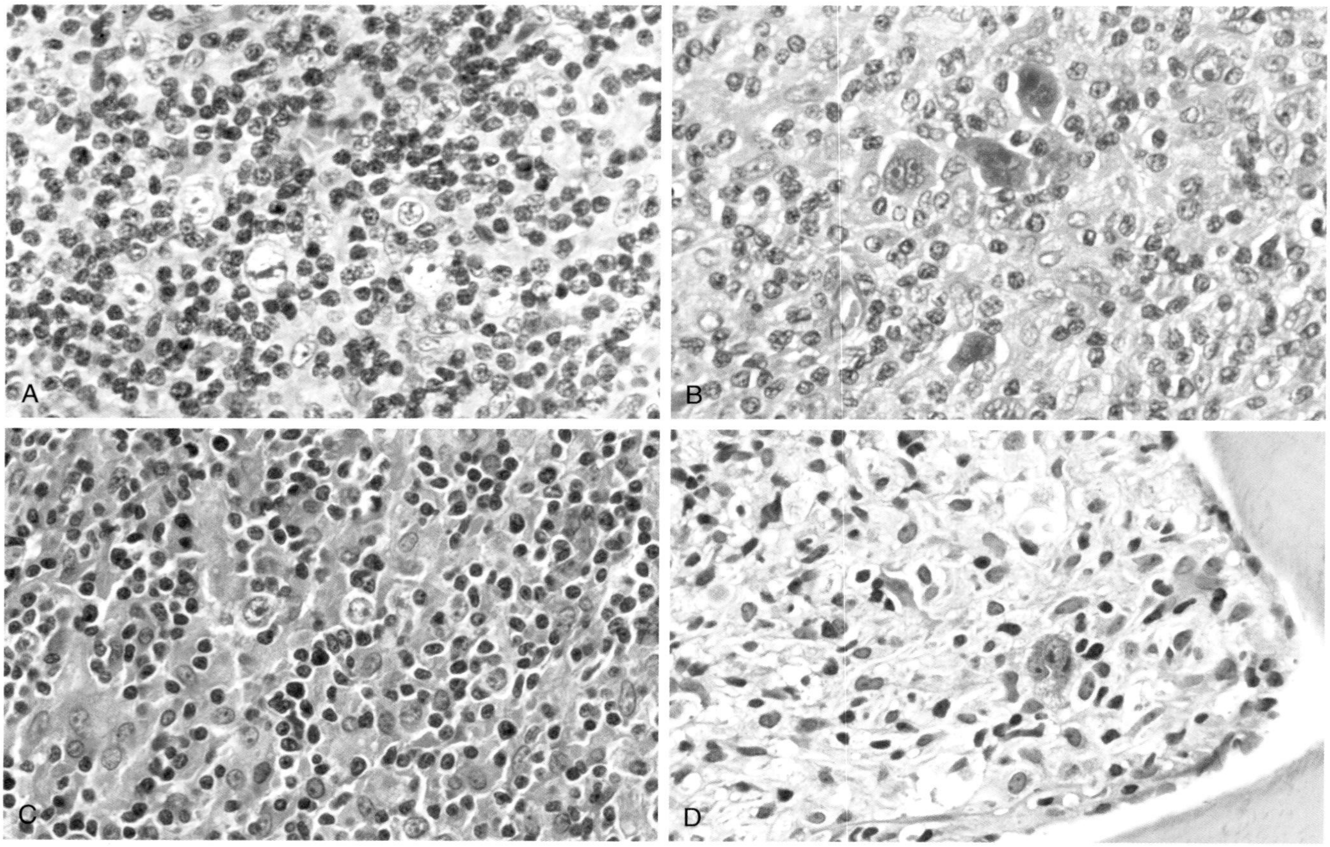

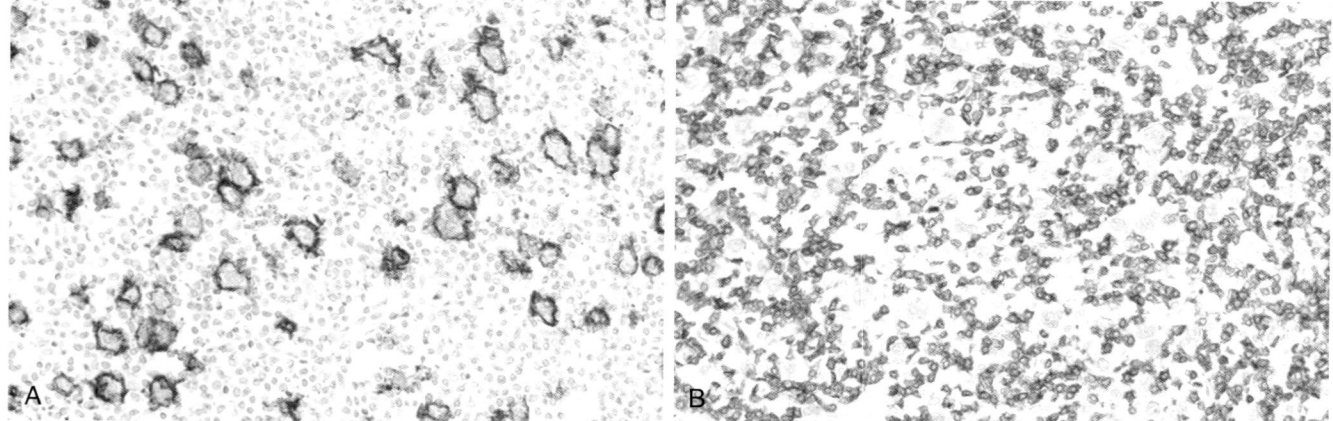

Figure 22-28. T-cell/histiocyte–rich large B-cell lymphoma. A, Large lymphoid cells are scattered singly among small lymphocytes. **B,** Large cells, some resembling Reed-Sternberg cells, occur in a background of slightly activated small lymphoid cells. **C,** This example is rich in small T lymphocytes and histiocytes in the background. **D,** T-cell/histiocyte–rich large B-cell lymphoma with bone marrow involvement. Note the scattered large atypical cells in a background of small cytologically unremarkable lymphoid cells and histiocytes.

Figure 22-29. Immunohistochemistry of T-cell/histiocyte–rich large B-cell lymphoma. A, CD20 immunostain selectively highlights the dispersed large cells. **B,** Numerous small CD3-positive T lymphocytes are present in the background.

complete overlap, between the two entities. Currently, it is thought that THRLBCL and NLPBL likely represent part of a disease spectrum with different clinical behavior, which may be influenced by the differences in the microenvironment of the lymphomas, possibly related to the immune status of the patients.[283,293]

Postulated Cell of Origin

Demonstration of a hypermutated immunoglobulin gene with ongoing somatic mutations and *BCL2* rearrangement in some cases, and expression of BCL6, altogether support a germinal-center stage of differentiation.[20,21,316,317]

Clinical Course

In an examination of US cases from 2010 to 2015, the 5-year OS using rituximab-based immunochemotherapy was 66%; adjusting for socioeconomic variables, THRLBCL was associated with a better survival than DLBCL, NOS (adjusted hazard ratio, 0.80). Prognostic features included age, comorbidity index, and extranodal primary site, but not stage. Adjusted odds of prior NLPBL were 18.2 times higher for THRLBCL than DLBCL, NOS.[320] Clinical outcomes for THRLBCL similar to DLBCL, NOS were also reported from Asia.[321] Cases rich in histiocytes may have a poorer prognosis,[297] and a primary cutaneous counterpart with a more favorable outcome has been reported.[322]

Differential Diagnosis

The main differential diagnoses and their distinguishing features are listed in Table 22-6. In some examples of THRLBCL, the large cells resemble reactive immunoblasts, making it difficult to distinguish from reactive lymphoid hyperplasia. In THRLBCL, definite atypia (e.g., enlarged nuclei, irregular nuclear folding) can usually be recognized in at least a small proportion of the large cells after a careful search, and the pattern of uniform scattering of solitary large cells in a small lymphoid cell background is very unusual for a reactive process. Furthermore, in reactive lymphoid hyperplasia, the large lymphoid cells more often occur in patchy aggregates, show transition to plasmablasts and plasma cells, exhibit heterogeneous staining for CD20 owing to the presence of B cells in different stages of maturation, and show polytypic staining for immunoglobulin light chains.

In NLPBL with an extensive diffuse component, the presence of scattered large LP cells with a B-cell phenotype in a background of small T lymphocytes is indistinguishable from THRLBCL.[304] Patients with NLPBL are younger (30–50 years), and most patients (80%–95%) present with early-stage (I–II) disease.[323] Histologically, a nodular pattern is usually identified at least focally and if not morphologically obvious can sometimes be detected using stains for follicular dendritic cell markers (such as CD21 or CD23). Often, follicular T-cell rosettes around the L&H tumor cells can be demonstrated by

Table 22-6 Comparison of T-Cell/Histiocyte–Rich Large B-Cell Lymphoma, Nodular Lymphocyte Predominant B-Cell Lymphoma, Classic Hodgkin Lymphoma, and Peripheral T-Cell Lymphoma

Feature	T-Cell/Histiocyte–Rich Large B-Cell Lymphoma	Nodular Lymphocyte-Predominant B-Cell Lymphoma	Classic Hodgkin Lymphoma	Peripheral T-Cell Lymphoma
Most commonly affected age group	6th–7th decades	4th–5th decades	Bimodal age distribution: 2nd to 3rd decade and 6th decade onward	7th decade
Site of disease	Nodal or extranodal	Predominantly nodal	Predominantly nodal	Nodal or extranodal; extranodal involvement common
Stage	Advanced stage (III to IV) in 67% of cases	Usually low stage	Advanced stage (III to IV) in 50% of cases	Advanced stage (III to IV) in 80% of cases
Morphology of large atypical cells	Variable appearance	L&H cells with popcorn like nuclei, often occurring within nodules of small lymphocytes	Reed-Sternberg cells and variants	Variable appearance: nuclei often show irregular folds
Background cells	Reactive T cells appear as small lymphocytes or mildly activated cells, histiocytes	Mostly nonactivated small B lymphocytes, or T cells in nonclassical variants, CD21-positive follicular dendritic cell meshworks	Mostly nonactivated small lymphocytes, eosinophils, plasma cells, histiocytes	Often atypical lymphocytes that commonly show a continuum through medium-to-large-sized cells
Immunophenotype	Large cells: CD20+, CD30−/+, CD15−, OCT-2+, BOB.1+ Small cells: CD3+ (many TIA-1+) Absence of CD21+ follicular dendritic cell meshworks among neoplastic cells	Large cells: CD20+, CD30−, CD15−, OCT-2+, BOB.1+ Small cells: CD20+ B-cells in nodular areas (IgM+, IgD+), with CD57+ PD1+/CD57+ CD3+ T cells rosetting around L&H cells; many CD3+ small cells in diffuse areas, but sometimes also abundant within nodules, and usually TIA-1− Meshworks of CD21+ follicular dendritic cells typically present in nodules	Large cells: CD30+, CD15+/−, CD20−/+ (heterogeneous staining if positive), CD45−, weak PAX5+, OCT-2−, BOB.1− Small cells: CD3+	Large and smaller cells: CD3+, but some EBV+ large B cells may be scattered
Genotype	Clonally rearranged immunoglobulin genes; germline TCR genes	Immunoglobulin and TCR genes frequently germline (caused by infrequency of atypical cells in preparations from whole-tissue DNA)	Immunoglobulin genes clonally rearranged or germline; TCR genes germline (whole-tissue DNA)	Clonally rearranged TCR genes; immunoglobulin genes usually germline
EBV association	Absent	Very rare	Common (~40%; higher in non-White populations)	Uncommon, but EBV-positive B cells can be found in some cases, especially angioimmunoblastic T-cell lymphoma

EBV, Epstein-Barr virus; *L&H,* lymphocytic and histiocytic; *TCR,* T-cell receptor.

CD57 or PD-1.[293,307] Although the small lymphocytes within the nodules of NLPBL are mostly B cells, those in the diffuse areas are mostly T cells. The T cells in NLPBL infrequently express the cytotoxic marker TIA-1.[304]

The lymphocyte-rich and mixed cellularity types of CHL can simulate THRLBCL.[309,324,325] Reed-Sternberg cells are either negative for pan–B-cell markers or show heterogeneous staining if positive, are frequently CD30 positive and CD15 positive, and are more likely to harbor EBV.

Lymphomatoid granulomatosis also features large, atypical B cells in a background of reactive T cells, but it always presents in extranodal sites (most commonly lung and skin), and EBV is almost always positive (see Chapter 28).

THRLBCL may also be confused with peripheral T-cell lymphoma (PTCL) because the activated T cells in the background of THRLBCL can show mild atypia. In PTCL, the T cells show a more prominent degree of cytologic atypia, and the atypia involves lymphoid cells of various sizes. The larger PTCL cells within the infiltrate do not stand out distinctly as a separate population, as the large B cells do in THRLBCL, and there is a transition with the smaller atypical cells. Immunophenotypically, the large, atypical cells of PTCL express pan–T-cell rather than pan–B-cell markers. Nonetheless, confusion can arise because some PTCLs, especially angioimmunoblastic T-cell lymphoma, can be accompanied by a reactive large B cell proliferation, which is often EBV driven.[326-329] Careful correlation between immunostaining and morphology reveals that although some large, atypical cells are CD20 positive, most of the atypical medium-sized and large cells are CD20 negative and CD3 positive. Genotyping is confirmatory in difficult cases because THRLBCL has rearranged immunoglobulin genes,[303,313-315,330] whereas PTCL has rearranged TCR genes.

PRIMARY MEDIASTINAL LARGE B-CELL LYMPHOMA

Definition

PMBL is a distinct subtype of DLBCL of putative thymic B-cell origin. By definition, the major bulk of tumor is confined to the anterior superior mediastinum at presentation.[331,332]

Epidemiology

PMBL accounts for 2.4% of all non-Hodgkin lymphomas.[3,333] Most patients are young adults (median age, 37 years),[3,334-336] but children can also be affected.[337] There is a female predominance,[3,334-336] with a female-to-male ratio of 2:1.

Clinical Features

Patients present with symptoms related to the large anterior mediastinal mass, such as superior vena cava obstruction, dyspnea, and chest discomfort.[338-341] Most patients present with early-stage disease (70%–80% stages I and II).[342] The tumor can invade the chest wall, sternum, pericardium, pleura, and lung.[340,343-346] There can sometimes be supraclavicular lymphadenopathy. Involvement outside of the thorax is observed in ~10% of patients, with sites including the kidneys, adrenal glands, and bone marrow.[342,346] These sites, along with the CNS, can be involved at the time of relapse.

Morphology

The tumor exhibits a diffuse infiltrate of large- or medium-sized lymphoma cells with a highly variable appearance. The lymphoma cells can have a centroblastic, immunoblastic, anaplastic, unclassifiable, or Reed-Sternberg–like appearance. The nuclei are round or multilobated. Cytoplasm is often abundant and not uncommonly (40% of cases) shows clearing (Figs. 22-30 and 22-31).[324,325,338,340,344,346,347] Sometimes the lymphoma cells assume a spindly morphology (see Fig. 22-31). Rare cases exhibit a marked tropism for preexisting GCs.[348]

Sclerosis is common, ranging from delicate collagen fibers surrounding individual or groups of lymphoma cells ("compartmentalizing" or "alveolar") to broad septa of dense collagen (Fig. 22-32).[338,343,346] Occasionally there is identifiable remnant thymic epithelium, which can show atrophy, hyperplasia, or cystic change (Fig. 22-33).[344,349] A summary of PMBL is presented in Box 22-7.

Immunophenotype

PMBL expresses pan–B-cell markers.[343,347,350-352] However, most cases do not express surface or cytoplasmic immunoglobulin, despite expression of CD79a (a component of a heterodimer associated with surface immunoglobulin) and the immunoglobulin transactivating factors OCT-2 and BOB.1.[325,350,352-355] Because messenger RNA transcripts of switched immunoglobulin heavy chain can be detected in PMBL,[356] the reason behind the immunoglobulin-negative immunophenotype remains unclear, but may involve downregulation of intronic heavy chain enhancer.[357] The tumor also shows low or absent expression of MHC class I and II molecules.[358,359]

PMBL is negative for CD21 and frequently expresses CD23 (70% of cases), similar to the asteroid B cells normally found in the medulla of the thymus.[351-353,360-363] CD10, BCL6, and CD30 are expressed in ~25%, ~60%, and ~70% of cases, respectively.[355,364-366] Rare cases expressing human chorionic gonadotropin, which could cause confusion with mediastinal germ cell tumors, have been reported.[367]

MAL gene (on chromosome 2q) expression, which can be demonstrated by molecular methods or immunohistochemistry, occurs in 70% of cases but is extremely rare in other DLBCLs (Fig. 22-34).[368,369] Other immunohistochemical markers that have been reported to show preferential expression in PMBL compared with DLBCL, NOS include CD200 (94% versus 7%),[370] TNFAIP2 (87% versus 4%),[371] PD-L2 (CD273) (72% versus 3%),[372] and combined nuclear REL expression and cytoplasmic TRAF1 expression (53% versus 2%).[373]

Genetics

PMBL shows clonally rearranged immunoglobulin heavy chain and light chain genes and germline TCR genes.[374] There is no CCND1 rearrangement and BCL2 rearrangement is rare; BCL6 rearrangement occurs in only ~5% of cases, whereas BCL6 mutations are reported in up to 70% of cases.[255,355,375-377] Rearrangements or point mutations in MYC have been detected in occasional cases.[376,378] EBV is almost always negative.[344,376,378] For the rare occurrence of familial clustering PMBL, KMT2A may be a candidate predisposition gene.[379]

PMBL shows a unique gene-expression profile that is much closer to that of CHL than DLBCL, NOS.[380,381] With PMBL

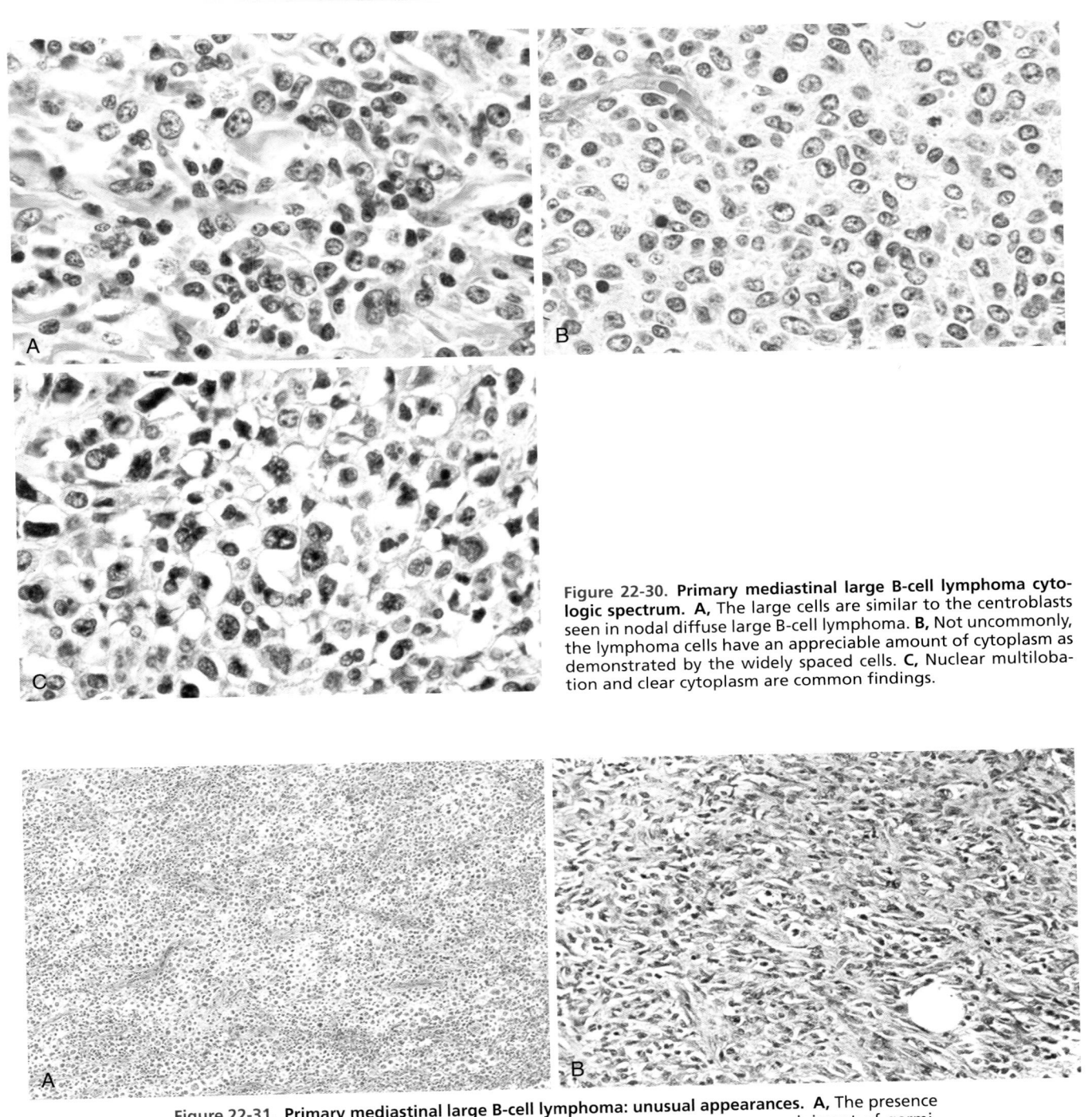

Figure 22-30. Primary mediastinal large B-cell cytologic spectrum. A, The large cells are similar to the centroblasts seen in nodal diffuse large B-cell lymphoma. **B,** Not uncommonly, the lymphoma cells have an appreciable amount of cytoplasm as demonstrated by the widely spaced cells. **C,** Nuclear multilobation and clear cytoplasm are common findings.

Figure 22-31. Primary mediastinal large B-cell lymphoma: unusual appearances. A, The presence of clear cells demarcated by fibrovascular septa produces an appearance reminiscent of germinoma. **B,** Spindly lymphoma cells are sometimes prominent.

being a clinicopathologic diagnosis, these gene expression signatures may be useful in the differential with DLBCL, NOS where the anterior mediastinum is involved.[382] The hallmarks of PMBL are JAK/STAT signaling, activation of NF-κB, and immune evasion.[359,383]

The JAK-STAT pathway is activated as a result of *JAK2* (9q24) amplification, activating mutation of *STAT6*, loss-of-function mutation of *SOCS1* (which normally inhibits JAK phosphorylation and targets phosphorylated JAK for degradation), activating mutations of *IL4R,* and inactivating

mutation of *PTPN1* (negative regulator).[377,384-387] The NF-κB pathway is constitutively activated as a result of *REL* (2p16) amplification, destructive and biallelic mutations in *TNFAIP3* (encoding A20, a tumor-suppressor gene that inhibits NF-κB signaling), and mutation of *NFKBIE.*[365,377,387-390] Immune privilege is mediated by *CIITA* gene (master transcriptional regulator of MHC class II expression) rearrangement with various gene partners causing reduction of MHC class II expression, mutations in *B2M,* deletions of MHC class I and II loci, mutations in

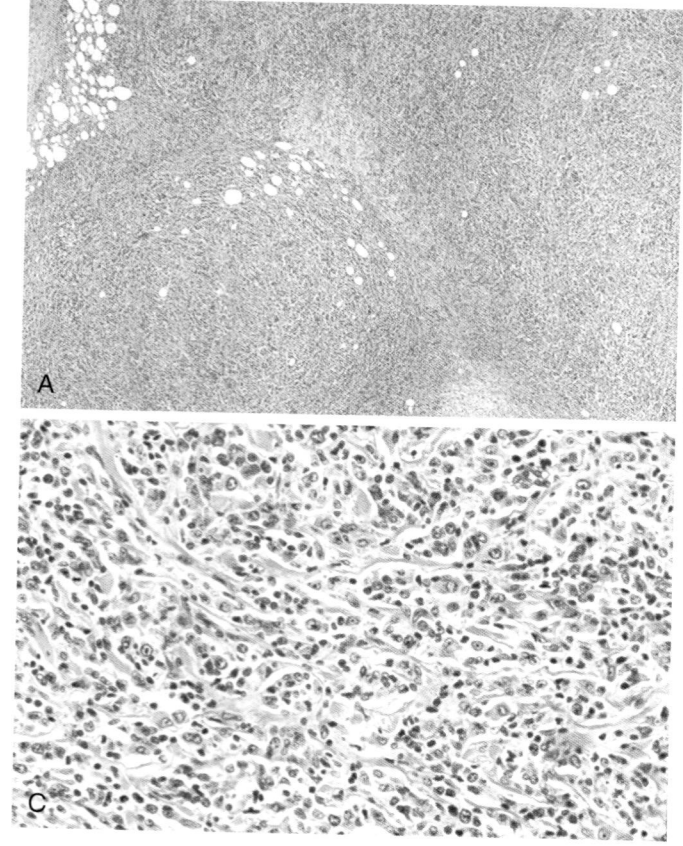

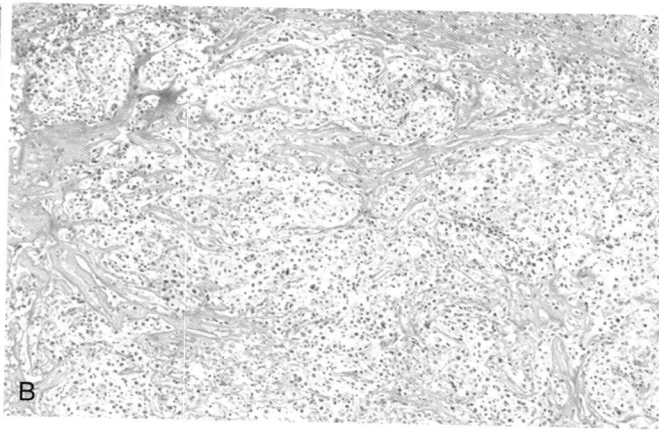

Figure 22-32. Primary mediastinal large B-cell lymphoma: patterns of sclerosis. A, Broad sclerotic bands traverse the tumor to produce large tumor nodules. **B,** Thinner sclerotic bands demarcate the tumor into packets. **C,** Delicate collagen fibrils are found within the tumor.

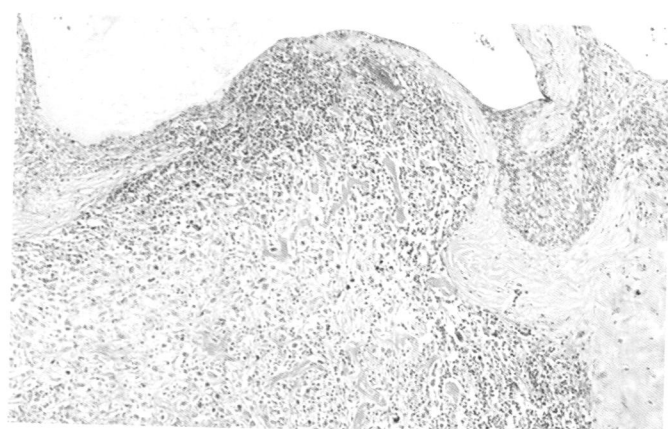

Figure 22-33. Primary mediastinal large B-cell lymphoma. In this example, there is proliferation of the residual thymic epithelium and formation of cysts lined by thymic epithelium.

CD58, and amplification and translocation of *CD274* and *PDCD1LG2* genes (resulting in overexpression of PD-L1 and PD-L2, which interact with PD1 on T lymphocytes to cause T-cell anergy).[147,377,387]

Postulated Cell of Origin

Addis and Isaacson first suggested a thymic B-cell origin for PMBL based on the tumor location, frequent lack of nodal involvement, and presence of residual thymic tissue in some

cases.[343] Subsequently, a distinctive population of CD21-negative thymic B cells was identified in the normal thymus, and these cells (particularly the population with asteroid morphology) are considered the normal counterpart for PMBL.[360,361,363]

Clinical Course

The standard treatment is multiagent chemotherapy and rituximab, with or without radiotherapy, resulting in a 2-year PFS of ~80% or greater (reviewed by Savage[342]). In the 10% to 20% of patients that experience treatment failure, outcomes are poor. At relapse, PD1 inhibitors (alone or in combination with brentuximab vedotin) and CAR-T therapy have shown promising results.[198,200,391-393]

Reported poor prognostic indicators include pleural effusion, pericardial effusion, increased number of involved extranodal sites, high serum lactate dehydrogenase level, low performance score, and high IPI score,[345,394-397] though not confirmed in more recent studies.[398,399] Loss of the MHC class II gene and protein expression is a poor prognostic indicator.[400] Results of the end-of-treatment PET scan are strongly prognostic, with Deauville 5 being associated with very poor PFS (20%–30% at 2 years).[401-403]

At the time of recurrence, PMBL cases have a tendency to spread to unusual extranodal sites, such as the kidney, CNS, adrenal gland, liver, pancreas, gastrointestinal tract, and ovary,[334,336,404,405] and the extranodal predilection may be partly explained by its chemokine receptor profile, which differs from DLBCL, NOS and CHL.[406]

Box 22-7 Major Diagnostic Features of Primary Mediastinal Large B-Cell Lymphoma

Distinctive Clinical Features (Versus DLBCL, NOS)
- Young adult: median age 37 years (versus 64 years)
- Female predominance: male-to-female ratio 1:2 (versus 1.2:1)
- Symptoms related to anterior mediastinal mass (e.g., superior vena cava obstruction, dyspnea)
- Bulky disease (>10 cm) in 52% of cases (versus 30%)
- Early stage (I and II) disease in 66% of cases (versus 54%)
- Marrow involvement very rare (3% versus 16%)
- Relapse tends to occur more frequently in extranodal sites compared with time of diagnosis (e.g., gastrointestinal tract, kidney, adrenal gland, ovary, central nervous system)

Morphology
- Large- or medium-sized lymphoma cells
- Clear cell change, compartmentalizing sclerosis more common than in DLBCL, NOS

Immunophenotype
- Pan-B positive, CD3 negative
- Surface immunoglobulin frequently negative
- BCL6 positive in ~60%
- CD10 positive in ~25%
- CD23 positive in ~70%
- CD30 positive in ~70%
- MAL in ~70%
- PD-L1/2 in ~70%
- EBV negative
- Deficient MHC molecule expression

Molecular Features
- Clonally rearranged immunoglobulin genes
- BCL2 and BCL6 genes usually not rearranged
- Unique gene-expression profile closer to that of classic Hodgkin lymphoma than DLBCL, NOS
- Activation of JAK-STAT pathway (JAK2 amplification, STAT6 and IL4R mutations, inactivating mutation of SOCS1 and PTPN1)
- Activation of NF-κB pathway (REL amplification at 2p16.1, loss of TNFAIP3, mutations in NFKBIE)
- Immune privilege (CIITA gene translocation leading to loss of MHC class II expression, mutations in B2M and CD58, CD274 and PDCD1LG2 [encoding for PD-L1 and PD-L2, respectively] amplification and translocation)

DLBCL, NOS, Diffuse large B-cell lymphoma, not otherwise specified; EBV, Epstein-Barr virus; MHC, major histocompatibility complex.

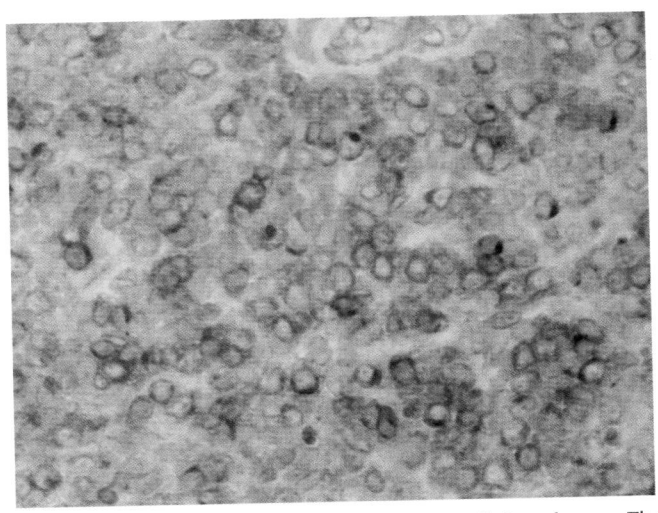

Figure 22-34. Primary mediastinal large B-cell lymphoma. The tumor cells show strong cytoplasmic and membrane staining for MAL, a marker frequently expressed in this entity.

Differential Diagnosis

By definition, the tumor bulk in PMBL is in the anterior mediastinum, thus excluding other nodal or extranodal DLBCLs (DLBCL, NOS) that secondarily involve the mediastinum. In some PMBL cases, the presenting lymph node may be outside the mediastinum. In these cases, characteristic histologic (cytology, fine compartmentalizing sclerosis) and immunophenotypic features of PMBL (MAL, PDL2) should be evaluated in comparison to DLBCL. In addition, a gene expression profiling assay to distinguish DLBCL from PMBL has been described and is in clinical use in select centers.[382] The main differential diagnoses are listed in Table 22-7 (see also "Pearls and Pitfalls").

Another important differential diagnosis for PMBL is nodular sclerosis CHL. Similarities include occurrence in young patients, predominant anterior mediastinal location, large tumor cells, and sclerosis. The problem in differential diagnosis is compounded by the fact that some PMBLs express CD30, and some cases of nodular sclerosis CHL can express pan–B-cell markers. Nodular sclerosis CHL is associated with an inflammatory background, often rich in eosinophils, and the tumor cells express CD30 and CD15 but not CD45. Although pan–B-cell markers may be expressed in Reed-Sternberg cells, the expression is usually heterogeneous, in contrast to the uniformly strong staining in PMBL. Reed-Sternberg cells are usually negative for the immunoglobulin transactivating factors OCT-2 and BOB.1, contrasting with their consistent expression in PMBL.[355,407] EBV, when present, would favor a diagnosis of CHL over PMBL.[332] Composite or metachronous cases of PMBL and nodular sclerosis CHL have been described,[334,408-410] with demonstration of the same clone in the two different components in at least some cases.[410] The link between PMBL and CHL is further supported by similarities in the gene-expression profiles of the two entities[380,381] and the existence of occasional cases of MAL-expressing nodular sclerosis CHL.[369,411]

Cases with overlapping histologic features or transitional immunophenotype that lie between PMBL and CHL are currently categorized as MGZL and are fully discussed in the chapter on Hodgkin lymphoma (Chapter 28).[20,21,410,412,413]

Tumors with the gene expression of PMBL have been observed that present without evidence of mediastinal involvement.[414,415] While these tumors share the expression and sometimes histologic features of PMBL, the genetic mechanisms by which they arrive at these are distinct and a diagnosis of DLBCL, NOS is usually favored.[416]

Anaplastic large cell lymphoma shares similarities with PMBL, including the presence of many large lymphoid cells and CD30 immunoreactivity. However, the former has a T-cell phenotype (PAX5 negative), often with expression of cytotoxic markers, and may express ALK.[417]

PMBL can mimic mediastinal seminoma when there is tumor packeting and the presence of clear cells. However, seminoma occurs exclusively in males, shows round but not multilobated nuclei, and expresses CD117 and OCT3/4, but not CD45 and pan–B-cell markers.

Table 22-7 Differential Diagnosis of Primary Mediastinal Large B-Cell Lymphoma (PMBL)

Entity	Features Favoring Diagnosis of That Entity	Features Favoring Diagnosis of PMBL
DLBCL, NOS	Accompanied by disease in sites other than anterior mediastinum	Predominant mass in anterior mediastinum at presentation CD23 or MAL expression Surface immunoglobulin expression commonly absent
Nodular sclerosis Hodgkin lymphoma, syncytial variant	Many eosinophils, histiocytes, and neutrophils in background Necrosis common within dense sheets of large tumor cells Broad bands of polarizable sclerosis CD45⁻, CD30⁺, CD15⁺/⁻, pan–B-cell⁻/⁺ (heterogeneous if positive), OCT-2⁻, BOB.1⁻ EBV⁺ in >35%	Clear cell change common Fine sclerosis CD45⁺, pan–B-cell⁺, CD30⁺/⁻, CD15⁻, OCT-2⁺, BOB.1⁺ EBV almost always negative
Anaplastic large cell lymphoma	Hallmark cells Pan–B-cell⁻, pan–T-cell⁺/⁻ EMA⁺/⁻, ALK⁺/⁻ Cytotoxic markers⁺/⁻	Sclerosis much more common Pan–B-cell⁺, pan–T-cell⁻ EMA⁻
Mediastinal seminoma	Almost exclusively male Nuclei often round CD45⁻, OCT-3/4⁺, CD117⁺	Although cells may have clear cytoplasm, nuclei are often lobated or folded CD45⁺, pan–B-cell⁺, CD117⁻
Thymic carcinoma	Cohesive growth; sharp interface with desmoplastic stroma May exhibit squamous or squamoid features Cytokeratin +	Although tumor may show packeting pattern, diffuse permeative growth in at least some areas Cytokeratin −, CD20⁺
Thymic carcinoid	Nests of tumor cells separated by rich vasculature May form rosettes Cytokeratin +, neuroendocrine markers +	Although tumor may show packeting pattern, sclerotic septa are relatively avascular Cytokeratin −, CD45⁺, neuroendocrine markers −

ALK, Anaplastic lymphoma kinase; *DLBCL, NOS,* diffuse large B-cell lymphoma, not otherwise specified; *EBV,* Epstein-Barr virus; *EMA,* epithelial membrane antigen.

Thymic carcinoma and neuroendocrine tumors may enter into the differential diagnosis in small biopsy samples. Both express cytokeratin and are negative for CD45 and pan–B-cell markers.

INTRAVASCULAR LARGE B-CELL LYMPHOMA

Definition

IVLBCL is an aggressive disease in which the lymphoma cells reside predominantly or exclusively within the lumens of small blood vessels, with no or few circulating neoplastic cells in the peripheral blood.[418,419] Occasional cases show extravascular involvement. The degree to which extravascular involvement is allowed into the diagnostic category of IVLBCL and when cases should be classified as DLBCL, NOS with significant intravascular involvement is currently under consideration.[420,421] DLBCL, NOS with intravascular involvement has been reported as a poor prognostic factor, but is not considered IVLBCL at this time.[422-424] Three variants of IVLBCL are recognized: classic, hemophagocytic, and primary cutaneous.[425] Although classical and hemophagocytic variants are seen more frequently in Western and Asian countries, respectively, they can be seen in patients from both geographic regions.[425-427]

Epidemiology

IVLBCL is a rare lymphoma occurring predominantly in older patients in the 6th to 7th decades.[428] In Asian countries, the frequency of IVLBCL among all non-Hodgkin lymphomas ranges from 0.24% in Japan to 0.9% in Thailand.[429] A population-based study in North America indicated an incidence of 0.095 (case/1,000,000) with a median age of 70 years. The median 1-year OS was 66.2%, the 3-year OS was

51.8%, and the 5-year OS was 46.3%, which was comparable to DLBCL, NOS.[430]

Etiology

There is no known etiologic factor for IVLBCL. The lymphoma cells' propensity to be localized in the lumens of blood vessels may be partly explained by the lack of expression of CD29 (β_1-integrin) and CD54 (ICAM-1), both of which are important for transvascular lymphocyte migration, and the CD40-CD40L activation of B cells.[431,432]

Clinical Features

IVLBCL can involve any organ, but most commonly involves the CNS, skin, kidney, lung, adrenal glands, and liver.[428,433,434] Patients commonly present with fever; non-specific, nonlocalizing neurologic symptoms; or skin lesions. The neurologic symptoms are often bizarre, owing to the presence of multiple sites of infarct resulting from vascular occlusion. Patients may have multifocal cerebrovascular events, spinal cord and roots lesions, subacute encephalopathy, and peripheral or cranial neuropathy.[435] The cutaneous manifestations are non-specific, most commonly consisting of nodular, subcutaneous, firm masses or plaques, with or without hemorrhage. Overlying telangiectasia may be prominent, and there may be ulceration. The trunk and extremities are frequently involved sites. The rare patients who have disease limited to the skin (cutaneous variant) seem to have a better outcome.[434]

Uncommon presentations include interstitial lung disease,[436] pulmonary small vessel disease,[437] adrenal insufficiency,[438,439] minimal change disease of the kidney,[440] thrombotic microangiopathy,[441] and epididymal mass.[442] IVLBCL may be diagnosed by renal biopsy,[443,444] testicular biopsy,[445] bone marrow aspiration and biopsy,[82] nerve and muscle biopsy,[446] or lacrimal gland biopsy,[447] and it may be an incidental finding in the prostate.[448,449] Association with autoimmune diseases has been observed in some patients,[433] as has acquired immunodeficiency syndrome (AIDS), methotrexate treatment association, or silicone breast implant association.[450-453] IVLBCL may involve preexisting tumors, such as hemangioma,[454] lymphangioma,[455] angiolipoma,[456] meningioma,[457] renal cell carcinoma,[458] and Kaposi sarcoma,[451] or may occur as a clonally related Richter transformation from a preexisting CLL.[459] A rare case of transmission from a solid-organ transplant donor to multiple recipients has been reported.[460]

Histologic bone marrow involvement is reported as 61.5% in a small case series.[461] More frequent demonstration of immunoglobulin gene rearrangement by polymerase chain reaction in histologically negative bone marrow samples has been described, suggesting that subtle bone marrow involvement is common.[462]

The hemophagocytic syndrome–associated variant occurs mostly in Asians (most commonly Japanese),[426,463-467] and is uncommon in Western countries.[468-471] These patients are older adults and present with fever, hepatosplenomegaly, hemophagocytic syndrome with anemia and thrombocytopenia, bone marrow involvement, and disseminated intravascular coagulation. They usually lack lymphadenopathy, mass lesions, or skin lesions. There is no association with EBV or human T-lymphotropic virus-1.[463,466]

Morphology

Histologically, large- or medium-sized lymphoma cells are found within the lumens of small or intermediate-sized blood vessels (Fig. 22-35).[433,472] They can have a centroblastic, immunoblastic, or unclassifiable appearance. They often fill up the vascular lumens, but can sometimes palisade along the luminal side, mimicking angiosarcoma (Fig. 22-36). The cells can appear deceptively cohesive, resembling islands of carcinoma (Fig. 22-37). The lymphoma cells may be entrapped within organized fibrin thrombi, and there may be superimposed florid endothelial hyperplasia. The vascular occlusion can result in tissue infarction and hemorrhage (Fig. 22-38). Some cases may have an extravascular component.[421,428,433,472]

The lymphomatous involvement is usually obvious morphologically but can be so focal and subtle that the neoplastic cells become evident only on immunostaining for B-cell and endothelial markers.

Immunophenotype

The lymphoma cells express CD45 and pan–B-cell markers (Fig. 22-39).[428,472] A small proportion of cases express CD5, CD10, and BCL6 (22% each).[81,82,428,455] Most cases are non-GCB by immunohistochemistry or gene-expression profiling studies.[461,473,474] Expression of the oncofetal protein insulin-like growth factor 2 mRNA binding protein-3 (IMP3) is enriched in IVLBCL and was reported as a potentially useful adjunct test in diagnosis.[475]

CD5 expression is not associated with any specific clinical features. Exceptional cases reportedly express myeloperoxidase or cytokeratin.[476,477] The immunophenotype of the hemophagocytic syndrome–associated variant is similar to that of the usual IVLBCL.[426] PD-L1 is frequently expressed, is associated with a poor prognosis, and may have therapeutic implications with regard to targeted immunotherapy.[478,479] Loss of major histocompatibility class I and II protein expression may be another strategy related to immune escape.[480] Both MYC and BCL2 protein expression have been described.[481]

Genetics

IVLBCL shows clonal immunoglobulin gene rearrangements.[482,483] The BCL2 gene is not translocated,[428] but occasional cases with BCL6, IRF4 or IGH::CCND1 translocation have been described.[421,484,485] Cytogenetic structural abnormalities involving most frequently 6q13 and 8p11.2, and 19q13, 14q32, and chromosome 18 have been reported. On average 4.4 chromosomal gains and losses were detected per case; some cases have complex (more than three clonal aberrations) karyotypes, and some have normal karyotypes. Marker chromosomes were also identified.[426,465,486] Frequent genetic alterations in immune checkpoint-related genes and MYD88 and CD79B mutations (these two latter genes also mutated in ABC-DLBCL) have been reported.[148,480,487] Rearrangements of CD274/PDCD1LG2 involving the 3′UTR are frequently observed and result in PD-L1/PD-L2 overexpression.[148]

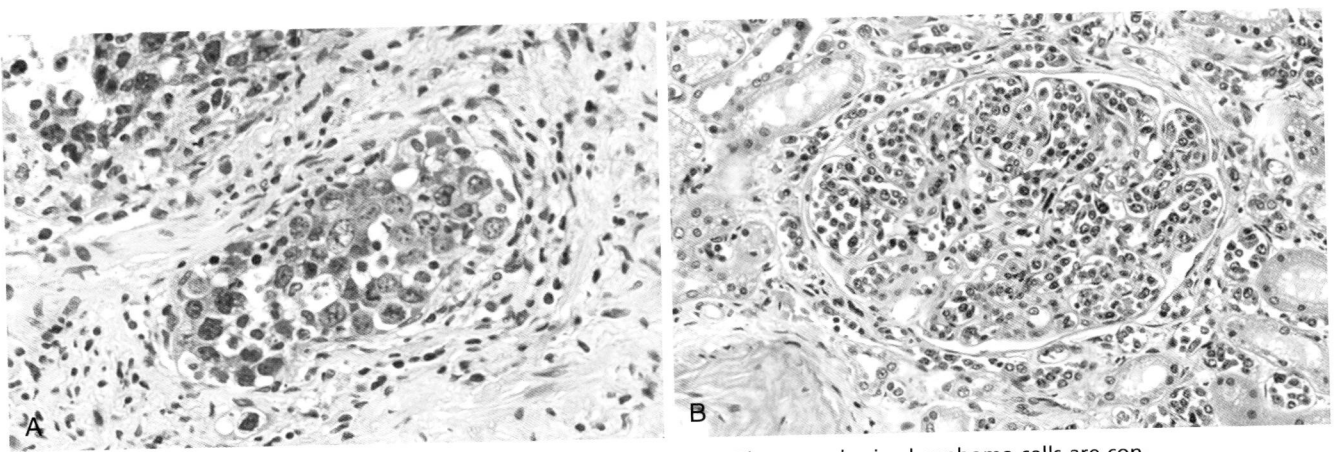

Figure 22-35. Intravascular large B-cell lymphoma. A, The noncohesive lymphoma cells are confined within medium-sized blood vessels. **B,** Lymphoma cells distend the capillaries of the glomeruli and the renal parenchyma.

EBV is negative,[428] except in patients living with AIDS.[451] While those cases with coinfection by HHV-8 probably represent unusual presentation of primary effusion lymphoma,[488,489] rare HHV-8–positive EBV-negative cases have also been described.[490]

Postulated Cell of Origin

IVLBCLs are derived from peripheral B cells, with the majority showing a non–germinal-center immunophenotype according to the Hans algorithm.[43] This most likely reflects origin from a post–germinal center cell, which is blocked from full plasma differentiation.[491,492]

Clinical Course

The poor outcome of IVLBCL in the older literature is related in part to the failure to make a correct antemortem diagnosis.[433] The extended time interval from onset of symptoms to diagnosis significantly contributes to poor outcome in these patients.[473] Combination immunochemotherapy including rituximab has significantly improved the clinical outcome of IVLBCL in both recent Western and Asian series.[493-495] A retrospective study

including patients treated before and after the use of rituximab demonstrated that while the majority of patients will die of their lymphoma, there were many other causes of death.[496] CNS recurrence can be detected in up to 18% of cases, even if not initially involved. Inclusion of high-dose methotrexate and intrathecal chemotherapy was recently reported (including patients without evidence of CNS involvement) with a 2-year PFS of 76%.[497,498] Rare cutaneous variant cases with a protracted clinical course have also been reported.[434,499] The hemophagocytic syndrome–associated variant is aggressive and has a median survival of 7 months.[426,491]

Differential Diagnosis

The most difficult part of diagnosing IVLBCL lies in initially including this disease in the differential diagnosis for patients with an extremely wide variety of presentations involving multiple organ systems and then deciding on a location to biopsy when no masses are present. Numerous case reports exist in the literature describing patients with highly unusual presentations in which the diagnosis of IVLBCL was not initially

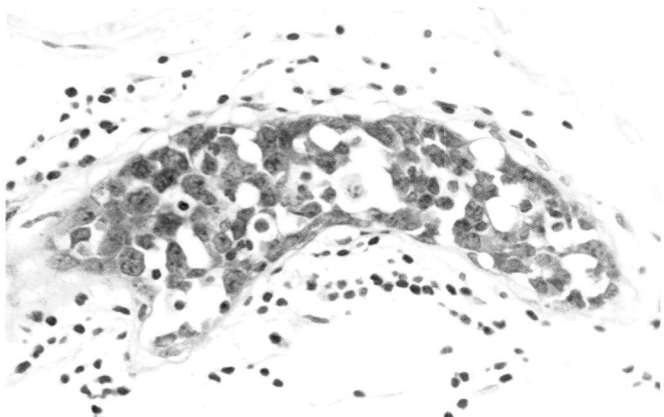

Figure 22-36. Intravascular large B-cell lymphoma involving subcutaneous tissue. Palisading of tumor cells along the luminal side of the blood vessel results in an angiosarcoma-like appearance.

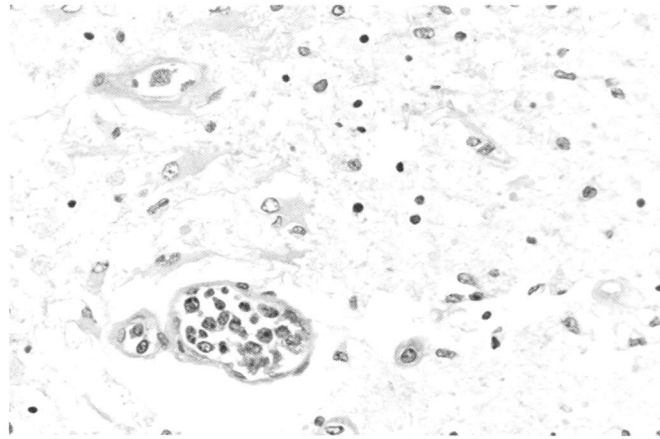

Figure 22-38. Intravascular large B-cell lymphoma involving the brain. The blood vessels are filled with large lymphoma cells. The surrounding brain parenchyma shows rarefaction caused by ischemia from the vascular occlusion.

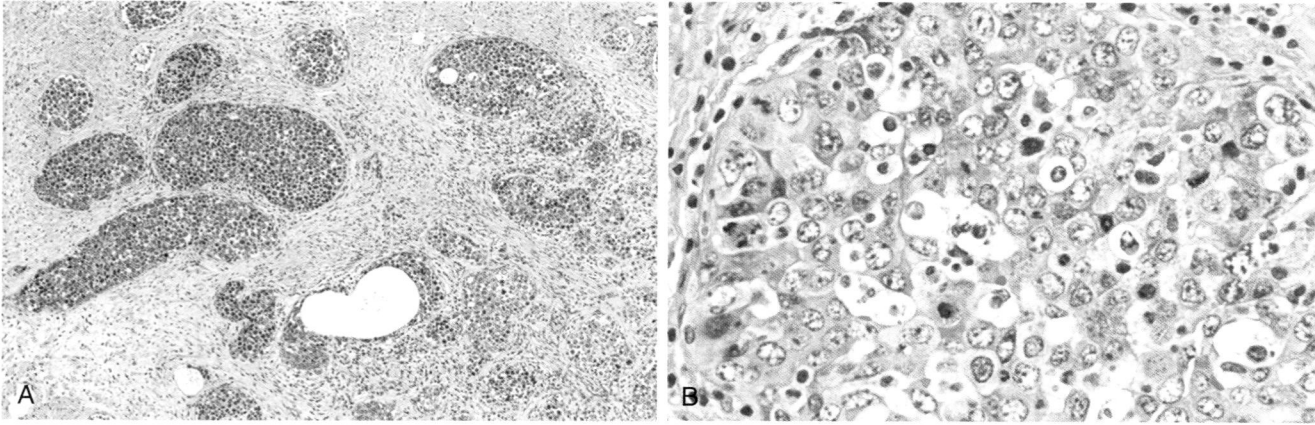

Figure 22-37. Intravascular large B-cell lymphoma mimicking carcinoma. A, In the prostate, plugging of the blood vessels by tumor cells results in a pattern reminiscent of islands of carcinoma. **B,** This island resembles high-grade carcinoma because of the apparently cohesive growth and the presence of glandlike spaces.

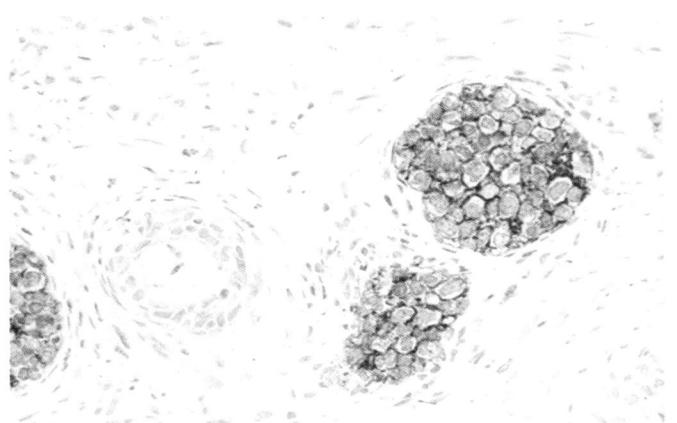

Figure 22-39. Immunohistochemistry of intravascular large B-cell lymphoma. The neoplastic cells within the blood vessels are selectively highlighted by CD20 immunostain.

considered. Many patients are only diagnosed at the time of autopsy.[500] Once the possibility of IVLBCL is considered, there are several studies supporting the use of random skin biopsies of normal-appearing skin (with a preference for incisional over punch biopsies so as to reach the middle adipose tissue) as a first approach to obtaining diagnostic tissue in patients with or without CNS involvement.[501-506] Should skin biopsy be negative, bone marrow biopsy or biopsy of an accessible organ with dysfunction might be considered next. Brain biopsy, in the case of patients with neurologic symptoms, is sometimes the last choice. Recently molecular evaluation for typical IVLBCL gene mutations have been described using cell-free DNA techniques in serum/plasma or cerebrospinal fluid, which may allow for a less invasive diagnosis.[492] Mutated genes investigated in this way for diagnostic use have included *CD79B, PIM1, MYD88, PRDM1,* and *BTG2.*[492,507]

The differential diagnosis with reactive/inflammatory processes can sometimes be confused with IVLBCL when the lumens of the lymphatic channels adjacent to inflamed tissue (e.g., acute appendicitis) are sometimes packed with reactive lymphoid cells.[508] However, these lymphoid cells are smaller, do not have the atypical nuclear features of IVLBCL, and are usually made up of T lymphocytes.

Occasionally, lymphatic spread by a nodal or extranodal large B-cell lymphoma (such as DLBCL, NOS) can be confused with IVLBCL. In this case, clinical features including the overall anatomic pattern of disease and biopsy of any other masses may be helpful.[425] Rare cases of IVLBCL are of T-cell or NK-cell lineage.[509-514] Such cases often show association with EBV.[509,512-515] Cases with a T-cell phenotype may include intravascular ALK-positive anaplastic large-cell lymphoma or the more indolent intralymphatic primary cutaneous anaplastic large cell lymphoma/lymphomatoid papulosis (CD30-positive lymphoproliferative disorders of skin).[516] Intravascular lymphoma of true histiocytic lineage has also been described.[517,518] None of these cases should be classified as IVLBCL.

In acute leukemia, intravascular collections of blast cells can be seen. The blasts usually have fine chromatin, and cytoplasmic granules may be present in the myeloid type. Blasts in acute myeloid leukemia usually express myeloperoxidase but not pan–B-cell or pan–T-cell markers, whereas those in

acute lymphoblastic leukemia express TdT with pan–B-cell or pan–T-cell markers. IVLBCL is always TdT negative.

In patients with carcinomatosis, clusters of carcinoma cells may be lodged in the small lymphovascular channels and initially appear to be IVLBCL. However, the tumor cells are generally cohesive, and they are cytokeratin positive and CD45 negative. Alternatively, "collisions" of incidental IVLBCL with other epithelial and nonepithelial tumors (in which two neoplasms are present) have been described and recently summarized. The low-power appearance of small-to-medium-sized vascular lumens expanded by dyscohesive cells with follow-up immunophenotyping are the key to the diagnosis of IVLBCL.[425]

Pearls and Pitfalls

Diffuse Large B-Cell Lymphoma, Not Otherwise Specified

- Although a diagnosis of DLBCL, NOS can be suspected by morphology, immunohistochemical confirmation is necessary because many types of lymphoma, leukemia, and non-hematolymphoid neoplasms can mimic DLBCL. In most circumstances, a simple immunohistochemical panel of CD20 and CD3 is sufficient to delineate the lineage.
- Detection of rearrangements of *MYC* and *BCL2* (and *BCL6*) should be performed in all cases, where resources allow, to exclude HGBL-*MYC/BCL2*. This can be done sequentially (testing for other rearrangements only when *MYC* is rearranged) or concurrently, per institutional protocol.
- The cell of origin (germinal-center B-cell type versus activated B-cell/non–germinal-center B-cell type) should be determined, either by molecular or immunohistochemical method (specifying methodology being used).
- In young patients, reactive conditions must be seriously considered in the differential diagnosis. Reactive conditions (in particular infectious mononucleosis) have to be suspected when the large cells show heterogeneous staining for CD20, there are many admixed large T cells, and Waldeyer's ring is involved.
- When bone marrow is involved, it is important to distinguish between involvement by large B-cell lymphoma and small-cell or follicular lymphoma (discordant lymphoma). The former is associated with a poorer prognosis.
- If DLBCL, NOS is EBV positive, it should be reclassified as EBV-positive DLBCL with investigation into potential causes of underlying immunosuppression (e.g., posttransplant lymphoproliferative disorder, HIV-associated lymphoma, methotrexate-associated lymphoproliferative disorder).
- If DLBCL is suspected but CD20 is negative, consider the possibility of prior rituximab therapy, ALK-positive large B-cell lymphoma, plasmablastic lymphoma, and anaplastic plasmacytoma. Apply additional B-lineage markers such as CD79a, PAX5, CD22, immunoglobulin, OCT-2, and BOB.1.

Primary Mediastinal Large B-Cell Lymphoma

- A superior-anterior mediastinal mass in a young adult woman is most commonly caused by PMBL or nodular sclerosis Hodgkin lymphoma. DLBCL, NOS, mediastinal germ-cell tumor and T-lymphoblastic lymphoma are additional considerations, particularly in young male patients.
- CD30 expression is not helpful in distinguishing nodular sclerosis CHL from PMBL. The histologic features and immunoprofile must be taken into consideration to make the distinction. If the findings are indeterminate (e.g., CD30 positive, CD15 negative, CD20 positive), lack of OCT-2 and BOB.1 staining and positive staining for EBV-LMP1 favor a diagnosis of nodular sclerosis CHL. Cases with intermediate features are categorized as mediastinal gray-zone lymphoma.

CHL, Classic Hodgkin lymphoma; *DLBCL, NOS,* diffuse large B-cell lymphoma; *EBV,* Epstein-Barr virus; *HGBL,* high-grade B-cell lymphoma; *PMBL,* primary mediastinal large B-cell lymphoma.

KEY REFERENCES

20. Alaggio R, et al. The 5th edition of the World Health Organization classification of haematolymphoid tumours: lymphoid neoplasms. *Leukemia*. 2022;36:1720–1748.

21. Campo E, et al. The International Consensus Classification of mature lymphoid neoplasms: a report from the clinical advisory committee. *Blood*. 2022;140:1229–1253.

24. Sehn LH, Salles G. Diffuse large B-cell lymphoma. *N Engl J Med*. 2021;384:842–858.

43. Hans CP, et al. Confirmation of the molecular classification of diffuse large B-cell lymphoma by immunohistochemistry using a tissue microarray. *Blood*. 2004;103:275–282.

51. Johnson NA, et al. Concurrent expression of MYC and BCL2 in diffuse large B-cell lymphoma treated with rituximab plus cyclophosphamide, doxorubicin, vincristine, and prednisone. *J Clin Oncol*. 2012;30:3452–3459.

101. Chapuy B, et al. Molecular subtypes of diffuse large B cell lymphoma are associated with distinct pathogenic mechanisms and outcomes. *Nat Med*. 2018;24:679–690.

102. Schmitz R, et al. Genetics and pathogenesis of diffuse large B-cell lymphoma. *N Engl J Med*. 2018;378:1396–1407.

103. Wright GW, et al. A probabilistic classification tool for genetic subtypes of diffuse large B cell lymphoma with therapeutic implications. *Cancer Cell*. 2020;37:551–568 e514.

146. Green MR, et al. Integrative analysis reveals selective 9p24.1 amplification, increased PD-1 ligand expression, and further induction via JAK2 in nodular sclerosing Hodgkin lymphoma and primary mediastinal large B-cell lymphoma. *Blood*. 2010;116:3268–3277.

153. Alizadeh AA, et al. Distinct types of diffuse large B-cell lymphoma identified by gene expression profiling. *Nature*. 2000;403:503–511.

164. Scott DW, et al. Determining cell-of-origin subtypes of diffuse large B-cell lymphoma using gene expression in formalin-fixed paraffin-embedded tissue. *Blood*. 2014;123:1214–1217.

281. Lim MS, et al. T-cell/histiocyte-rich large B-cell lymphoma: a heterogeneous entity with derivation from germinal center B cells. *Am J Surg Pathol*. 2002;26:1458–1466.

387. Mottok A, et al. Integrative genomic analysis identifies key pathogenic mechanisms in primary mediastinal large B-cell lymphoma. *Blood*. 2019;134:802–813.

418. Ponzoni M, Campo E, Nakamura S. Intravascular large B-cell lymphoma: a chameleon with multiple faces and many masks. *Blood*. 2018;132:1561–1567.

Visit Elsevier eBooks+ for the complete set of references.

Burkitt Lymphoma, High-Grade B-Cell Lymphoma Not Otherwise Specified, High-Grade B-Cell Lymphoma With *MYC* and *BCL2/BCL6* Rearrangements, Large B-Cell Lymphoma With 11q Aberration, and Provisional Entity High-Grade B-Cell Lymphoma With *MYC* and *BCL6* Rearrangements

Wolfram Klapper and Ilske Oschlies

WHY THESE FOUR ENTITIES IN ONE CHAPTER? A HISTORICAL PERSPECTIVE ON THE DEVELOPMENT OF DISEASE CONCEPTS

This chapter combines several distinct entities of mature aggressive B-cell lymphoma: Burkitt lymphoma, high-grade/large B-cell lymphoma with 11q aberration, diffuse large B-cell lymphoma/high-grade B-cell lymphoma with *MYC* and *BCL2* rearrangements, provisional entity diffuse large B-cell lymphoma/high-grade B-cell lymphoma with *MYC* and *BCL6* rearrangements, and high-grade B-cell lymphoma not otherwise specified (NOS). While the entities differ strikingly in their clinical and molecular features, they share overlapping morphology and phenotype. Thus differential diagnosis is a common and challenging task for diagnostic pathologists in their daily practice. Moreover, these entities are historically linked to each other as they have either not been distinguished from each other in the past or considered more closely related than they are at the present time.

Burkitt lymphoma (BL) is a rather "old" entity, described by Denis Burkitt in 1958 in African children. Soon after the description it was recognized that a disease with identical histopathologic picture also occurred outside Africa but differed in some clinical features. Uncertainty regarding morphologic variability of the disease in elderly patients and the relevance of translocations of the *MYC* gene as possibly the disease-defining alteration led to multiple molecular studies primarily using gene-expression profiling to shape the disease definition and delineate typical BL from other B-cell lymphomas with similar histopathology.[1,2] In these molecular studies, an initially small group of lymphomas were shown to carry a Burkitt signature by gene expression but lacked translocations involving the *MYC* gene. As this group of lymphomas showed considerable morphologic and immunophenotypic similarities with BL, it was initially named *Burkitt-like lymphoma with 11q aberration* in the update of the World Health Organization (WHO) 4th ed. After the genetic landscape of this lymphoma was described and found to be distinct from BL, the name was changed to *large cell* or *high-grade B-cell lymphoma with 11q aberration* in the International Consensus Classification (ICC) and WHO 5th ed., respectively (Table 23-1).[3,4]

Diffuse large B-cell lymphoma/high-grade B-cell lymphoma with *MYC* and *BCL2* rearrangements and high-grade B-cell lymphoma, not otherwise specified (NOS) took a similar route of development. The gene expression studies on BL were mainly intended to define BL molecularly and to provide a better diagnostic distinction from other large B-cell lymphomas especially from diffuse large B-cell lymphoma, NOS (DLBCL, NOS). The gene expression approach used at that time assigned mature aggressive B-cell lymphomas either to the Burkitt group (molecularly defined BL) or to a less well-defined group of lymphomas that were heterogeneous but unified in the fact that they were definitely not BL. The bioinformatic approach of these studies indicated a group of lymphomas that statistically neither fulfilled the criteria of molecularly defined BL nor allowed them to be assigned to the "non-molecular Burkitt" group. The lymphomas of this group were "intermediate" between molecularly defined BL and non-BL in their gene-expression profiles and were enriched for lymphomas with blastoid morphology or synchronous translocations involving *MYC* and *BCL2* or *BCL6*. Soon it became evident that this group of lymphomas differed clinically and molecularly from BL and were subsequently termed *B-cell lymphoma, unclassified, with features intermediate between Burkitt and diffuse large B-cell lymphoma* (used in the WHO 4th ed. in 2008). Subsequently, in the revised WHO 4th ed. in 2017, this category was further subdivided into two groups. The first group, including cases defined by their "intermediate" morphology but lacking specific diagnostic molecular features (except frequent *MYC* translocations), was termed *high-grade B-cell lymphoma, NOS*. Because high-grade B-cell lymphoma, NOS is mainly separated from DLBCL by morphologic features, which can be subjective, this remains a poorly defined entity. Examining the remaining "intermediate" cases, the presence of double-hit (a *MYC* and *BCL2* or *BCL6* rearrangement in the sense of a rearrangement representing a "hit") was associated with unfavorable prognosis. Thus in the revised WHO 4th ed., lymphomas with double-hit or triple-hit (presence of all three—*MYC*, *BLC2*, and *BCL6*—rearrangements in the same lymphoma) were introduced as *high-grade B-cell lymphoma with MYC and BCL2 and/or BCL6 rearrangements* (Table 23-1). Within this group, lymphomas with *MYC* and *BCL2* rearrangements represent a molecularly more homogeneous group sharing mutational features for follicular lymphoma (FL). In contrast, lymphomas with *MYC* and *BCL6* translocations are heterogenous with respect to genetic alterations. Moreover, lymphomas with *MYC* and *BCL6* translocations are less well defined by fluorescence in situ hybridization (FISH) because of the fact that *MYC* and *BCL6* may fuse as chromosomal translocations rather than presenting two independent genetic lesions. Thus in the proposal for the

Table 23-1 Synonyms and Related Terms

4th Ed. WHO 2008	Updated 4th Ed. WHO 2016	ICC	5th Ed. WHO 2022
Burkitt lymphoma	Burkitt lymphoma	Burkitt lymphoma	Burkitt lymphoma
	Burkitt-like lymphoma with 11q aberration	Large B-cell lymphoma with 11q aberration	High-grade B-cell lymphoma with 11q aberration
B-cell lymphoma, unclassified, intermediate between Burkitt and diffuse large B-cell lymphoma	High-grade B-cell lymphoma with *MYC* and *BCL2* and/or *BCL6* rearrangements	High-grade B-cell lymphoma with *MYC* and *BCL2* rearrangements	Diffuse large B-cell lymphoma/high-grade B-cell lymphoma with *MYC* and *BCL2* rearrangements
		Provisional: High-grade B-cell lymphoma with *MYC* and *BCL6* rearrangements	Diffuse large B-cell lymphoma, not otherwise specified
	High-grade B-cell lymphoma, not otherwise specified	High-grade B-cell lymphoma, not otherwise specified	High-grade B-cell lymphoma, not otherwise specified

ICC, International Consensus Classification; *WHO*, World Health Organization.

WHO 5th ed. published in 2022, the entity *double-/triple-hit* was more strictly defined and named as *diffuse large B-cell lymphoma/high-grade B-cell lymphoma with MYC and BCL2 rearrangements*. Of note, these cases may also harbor a *BCL6* translocation and be triple-hit; however, cases with just *MYC* and *BCL6* translocations are no longer considered double-hit by the WHO 5th ed., but are maintained as a "provisional" entity by the ICC in order to promote further study.[4]

Recent molecular studies identified lymphomas that were molecularly similar to large B-cell lymphoma with MYC and BCL2 rearrangements but without detectable *MYC* or *BCL2* translocation by conventional diagnostic methods using FISH technology.[5,6] These lymphomas were characterized by a clinically aggressive course and histologically mostly seemed to fall into the category of DLBCL, NOS or high-grade B-cell lymphoma, NOS. It is foreseeable that these "high-grade" molecular signature assays could be technologically incorporated into the daily practice of diagnostic pathology so that "high-grade" B-cell lymphomas will be expanded to also include some lymphomas that had been previously classified as DLBCL by morphology. Conversely, we can speculate that a subset of lymphomas with blastoid morphology currently classified as high-grade B-cell lymphoma, NOS will be identified as DLBCL by future gene expression, genetic, or even machine learning or artificial intelligence-based methods. However, novel methods are unlikely to replace conventional diagnostics based on morphology, immunophenotype, and FISH since these molecular high-grade signatures are also detected in true BL, reflecting features of B-cells from germinal center dark zones. Thus, as technology continues to evolve, so will the classification.

BURKITT LYMPHOMA

Definition

BL is B-cell neoplasm composed of monomorphic, medium-sized cells with basophilic cytoplasm, multiple small and often inconspicuous nucleoli, forming dense cohesive sheets sparse in microenvironment except for prominent tingible body macrophages. The lymphoma is characterized by a mature germinal-center B cell (GCB) phenotype with high proliferation index and genetics including immunoglobulin (IG) heavy or light chain juxtaposition to the *MYC* gene. See Table 23-1.

The eponym honors the contributions of Denis Burkitt for the pioneering work that led to the first description of the clinical features of this tumor in 1958. But it was not only the description of the disease but also the association with a certain geographic distribution that fostered the discovery of the Epstein-Barr virus (EBV) within the lymphoma cells and the development of novel therapies that made Dennis Burkitt's work a masterpiece of medical science.[7,8] Burkitt described the disease as a rapidly growing tumor in the jaws of children residing in the "malarial belt" of equatorial Africa and New Guinea.[9,10] Since the first description, the concept of an inflammation driving lymphomagenesis was born, and only a few years later the EBV was first described in a tumor specimen of a BL.[11] BL remained a further source of inspiration for lymphoma researchers as it became the entity in which *MYC* gene locus was mapped to chromosome 8 as one of the first chromosomal rearrangements detected in lymphoma.[12]

The nomenclature for this lymphoma entity has changed over the years. Terms like *lymphoma, Burkitt type,* and *Burkitt's lymphoma* are not recommended any more, and the previous and current ICC and WHO classifications use the term *Burkitt lymphoma.* It is important to mention that the nomenclature has developed differently over time in leukemic diseases. The French American-British classification of acute leukemia included a category of B-cell acute lymphoblastic leukemia (ALL) with vacuoles in the cytoplasm, also known as L3-morphology.[5,13] Nowadays, it is widely accepted that most cases of acute leukemia with L3-morphology reflect BL in its leukemic presentation when immunophenotype and genetics are taken into account.

Epidemiology

Three subtypes of BL have been recognized and designated as "endemic," "sporadic," and "immunodeficiency associated."[14] "Endemic" BL refers to the disease originally described by Denis Burkitt in African children in the region characterized by high incidence of malaria, which was long considered to be virtually always EBV positive. However, recent data suggest that not the clinical or geographic context, but rather the presence or absence of EBV in the lymphoma cells, determines the molecular biology of the disease. Moreover, current epidemiologic studies showed that EBV-positive and EBV-negative BLs occur virtually everywhere in the world, even the "endemic" regions in Africa.[3]

The "endemic" BL refers to Denis Burkitt's description of the disease and its distribution as the most common childhood cancer in equatorial Africa and Papua New Guinea. Given the high incidence of this disease in a certain geographic region and characteristic presentation as a tumor for the jaws, the disease was considered "endemic." The high percentage of tumors with EBV in the lymphoma cells and the close association with malaria infection in the same areas seemed to confirm that BL shared features with an infectious "endemic" disease. Current studies confirm a high incidence of BL of 1.09/100,000 in East Africa in children <15 years of age and a close association with the presence/incidence of malaria.[15] However, the age-adjusted incidence of BL in children of the same age in central Europe seems to come close to the incidence reported for Africa, and BL is the most frequent childhood tumor in central Europe too (https://www.kind erkrebsregister.de/). Certainly the incidence of the disease in Africa is underestimated by the registry data[15] since, in countries with a medium-to-low human development index, registration coverage and histopathologic diagnostics of diseases is likely incomplete.[16] Mathematical models in fact suggest a much higher incidence of BL in this region of the world.[16] Moreover, the age composition of populations in Africa and central Europe/Northern America differs strikingly. The United Nations International Children's Emergency Fund estimates Africa's child population will reach 1 billion by the year 2055, making it the largest child population among all continents (https://data.unicef.org/) and consequently making BL in pediatric patients a challenge for health care in this region of the world.

The vast majority of BL from Africa are EBV positive, whereas the EBV occurs less frequently in BL in other geographic regions (e.g., central Europe is about 20%).[17] In certain regions of the world such as southeastern Brazil, the EBV-association of BL seems to be intermediate between Africa and central Europe/Northern America.[18] Even within Brazil, the EBV-association of the disease varies regionally.[19] The picture becomes even more complex once age of patients is considered. Although larger age-overarching cohorts of BL tested for EBV of patients residing in African "endemic" regions are missing so far, in "sporadic" BL in central Europe, the EBV-association increases with age.[17,20] The presence of EBV is also associated with mutational features of BL—independent of the geographic region or age of the patient.[17,21] In immunodeficiency-associated BL, the rate of EBV up to 55% in cohorts of PLWH has been reported.[22]

Regardless of the geographic region, BL rates are 2 to 4 times higher in males than females[23] and the male-to-female ratio is highest at younger ages, generally before puberty. In adults, the male-to-female ratio is nearly equal.[23] The adult and elderly BL cases represent about 1% to 2% of all non-Hodgkin lymphomas in adults or the elderly.[24] The clinical presentation differs between BL occurring in young patients with "endemic" and "sporadic" BL, as "endemic" BL mostly presents as tumors of the face or head (often jaws) whereas "sporadic" BL of the same age group frequently forms masses in the abdomen or involves lymph nodes.[25] In immunodeficiency-associated BL, nodal presentation dominates the clinical picture and bone marrow involvement is frequently detected.[26]

In summary, BL worldwide shares features such as a male predominance in young patients and a high relative incidence among childhood cancers. In a global view, BL differs worldwide in respect to the extent of EBV-association, the anatomic distribution of tumors, and association with other diseases such as malaria infection or immunosuppression. Given this complex picture, the designation of individual cases of BL to the "endemic" or "sporadic" BL subtypes can be problematic. Currently there is no pathologic, clinical, or molecular definition of each of these historical subtypes that would allow identification of "sporadic" BL occurring in "endemic" areas of the world and vice versa.[27] Recent molecular studies indicate that EBV-association is a strong determinant of molecular biology of BL, such that in the future, BL classification may emphasize EBV status rather than the traditional subtypes.[17,21,28]

Etiology and Pathogenesis

Plasmodium falciparum Malaria and Epstein-Barr Virus Infection in "Endemic" Burkitt Lymphoma

Risk factors of BL have been characterized best for BL falling into the historical category of "endemic" disease and include *Plasmodium falciparum* malaria and EBV infection. Whereas EBV can be detected within the neoplastic cells and proteins encoded by the virus may directly contribute to transformation of B cells, the effect of *P. falciparum* to the pathogenesis of the disease may be more indirect since the parasite is not detectable within the lymphoma cells nor within the tumor tissue. Infection by *P. falciparum* malaria may occur repeatedly and may chronically stimulate B cells and suppress T-cell immunity.[29] The infection activates germinal center reactions and activation-induced cytidine deaminase (AID). The enzyme AID is required for somatic hypermutation and class-switch of the IG genes during the germinal center reaction.[30] Unwanted errors of these physiologic genetic processes contribute to the development of *MYC* translocations.[31] The hypothesis

that conditions leading to increased AID activity in germinal centers may favor development of BL seems to be supported by findings in EBV-positive BL that show evidence of antigen selection[32] and AID-typical point mutations, suggesting that they arose from germinal center cells with AID activity.[21]

Understanding the role of EBV in the pathogenesis of BL is challenging. As discussed, the rate of EBV detection in BL varies greatly by age, geographic region, and immune status. EBV is virtually ubiquitously present in the population at risk and over 90% of children in all regions of the world have long been exposed to EBV infection before the age peak of BL, and most children never suffer from BL. A possible explanation may be found in the age when children are EBV-infected. The infection by EBV usually occurs at less than 1 year in sub-Saharan Africa[33] but later in other areas of the world.[34] Early infection has been associated with a high viral burden in infected children—a condition that potentially increases the risk for transformation of B cells.[33] EBV itself encodes for several proteins that have transforming capacity, but only one, the Epstein-Barr nuclear antigen (EBNA)-1, is consistently detected in EBV-positive BL.[35] EBV also likely plays an important role in the early pathogenesis of BL by providing anti-apoptotic signals to B cells, allowing them to avoid cell death during the occurrence of the *MYC* translocation.[36] Indeed, the presence of EBV in the neoplastic cells is associated with various differences in microRNA and gene expression compared with BL negative for EBV.[37,38]

A Role of Epstein-Barr Virus in "Sporadic" Burkitt Lymphoma?

The factors associated with risk of "sporadic" BL in Europe, Asia, and South/North America are not well understood. EBV is detected in only approximately 20% of "sporadic" BL.[39] However, recent data suggest that EBV may also play a role in the pathogenesis of "sporadic" BL. Children suffering from BL in central Europe show significantly more frequent seropositivity (59%) indicating preceding EBV infection compared with patients with other lymphomas (44% in the age group 0.5–5.9 years).[40] However, the BL cells themselves harbor EBV by EBV-encoded RNAs (EBER) in situ hybridization at similar frequencies (about 20% in this geographic region).[17,20] Of note, the incidence of EBV-positive BL increases with patient age in central Europe and Japan.[17,41] The mutational features of EBV-positive and EBV-negative BL differ independent of whether these lymphomas are "endemic" or "sporadic."[21,28] Thus, the EBV-positive BL arising in "non-endemic" patients may present a molecular counterpart of the "endemic" BL observed in central Africa.[17,42]

How Is Epstein-Barr Virus–Positivity of Burkitt Lymphoma Defined?

The role of EBV in BL requires assessment of EBV infection of the host detected serologically by antibody titers against EBV proteins and presence of EBV in the lymphoma cells. In "endemic" BL, most patients show both serologic features of a previous infection by EBV and EBV within the lymphoma cells. In "sporadic" BL, patients may not have been exposed to EBV prior to the time when BL manifests and the lymphoma cells are thus negative for the virus. However, most patients in countries outside "endemic" areas of the world have been exposed to EBV long before the onset of the disease and the lymphoma cells may either be negative or positive for EBV.

The most sensitive technique for assessing the tumor cells of BL specimen at diagnosis is the in-situ hybridization for EBER and the majority of data on the incidence of EBV association are based on this technique. However, a subset of BL may appear negative in EBER in situ hybridization but nevertheless harbor single cells carrying traces of EBV DNA.[43] As EBV is usually maintained in cells in an episomal manner, it may be lost to various extents during pathogenesis and become undetectable by EBER in situ hybridization.[43] The role of EBV in the pathogenesis of BL may thus be a "hit-and-run" mechanism—a hypothesis that supports the relevance of EBV in early pathogenesis of the disease. Interestingly, this observation also allows the conclusion that EBV may be less relevant for the maintenance of the fully neoplastic clone and its expansion. Using EBER in situ hybridization, EBV is found in most of the lymphoma cells. Subclones lacking EBV have not been reported in BL yet and in most cases the occurrence of EBER-negative cells within an otherwise EBR-positive BL may be best explained by technical artifacts such as by poor tissue preservation.

Immunodeficiency

Persons living with HIV (PLWH) show a high incidence of BL. A survey in the United States between 1980 and 2005 showed a crude incidence of 22.0/100,000.[44] Interestingly, the risk of BL is higher in PLWH with CD4 cell counts above, rather than below, the level defining AIDS and BL is frequently the first presentation of HIV infection.[44] These data suggest that an intact CD4 immune response is required for the pathogenesis of BL (e.g., by supporting germinal center reactions rather than an "immune-escape" of EBV-infected cells). This hypothesis is further supported by the fact that introduction of combined antiretroviral therapy has had little effect on the incidence of BL.[45] Similar findings have been reported for Hodgkin lymphoma. In contrast, the incidence of DLBCL has declined under combined antiretroviral therapy.[46] BL in PLWH is positive for EBV in an age-dependent manner, showing the highest rates of positivity of 55% in age group 20 to 34 years and with a significant higher positivity rate in Blacks/Hispanics.[22] In addition to HIV, other types of immunodeficiency are associated with an increased risk for BL. For example, after solid organ transplantation, BL is frequently EBV positive and presents as aggressive disease.[47]

Hereditary Burkitt Lymphoma

The high male-to-female ratio in younger patients suggests a genetic basis for susceptibility in BL.[48] Moreover, rare cases of familial BL have been reported, including families with germline variants in *TCF4* and *CHD8*.[49] In addition, rare inherited disorders have been associated with increased risk of BL, including Purtillo/Duncan Syndrome/XLP (OMIM: 308240), XMEN disease (OMIM: 300853), ataxia telangiectasia (OMIM: 615919), and Williams-Beuren Syndrome (WBS; OMIM: 194050).

Clinical Features and Staging

BL frequently presents at extranodal sites, but the localization of these tumors differs between historical subtypes. In "endemic" BL, the facial bones, especially the jaws, are often involved,[50] but more recently, abdominal masses have been described more frequently[51]—a pattern that is otherwise typical for "sporadic" BL. The latter subtype occurs as an abdominal mass mostly in the ileocecal region. In this region, the tumor forms transmural masses of the intestinal wall but mostly spares lymph nodes even when they are localized immediately adjacent to the tumor (Fig. 23-1). Other sites frequently involved are the orbit, Waldeyer's ring, gingiva, thyroid gland, ovaries, and testis.[52-54] Involvement of the breast seems to be rather uncommon but may rarely occur in lactating women.[55] The clinical presentation of immunodeficiency-associated BL seems to be more heterogeneous with more nodal involvement and combinations of extranodal and nodal presentation.[56] Involvement of the central nervous system (CNS) is rather frequent in BL of all subtypes compared with other mature aggressive B-cell lymphomas. The frequency of CNS involvement differs between reports from population-based[25] and clinical studies from Malawi[57] for "endemic" BL. Data for "sporadic" BL in pediatric patients in the United States and Germany suggest a frequency of CNS involvement between 9% for pediatric[58] and 30% for adult BL.[59]

The clinical picture of patients suffering from BL is characterized by fast-growing masses because of the short doubling time of BL cells. Thus most patients have a high tumor burden and widely disseminated disease at initial presentation. Systemic symptoms are related to the high tumor cell turnover in a subset of patients. Most symptoms are site-specific and reflect organ dysfunction caused by masses, pain, obstruction, or bone destruction. A leukemic presentation occurs in a variable proportion of patients and is formally defined as >25% blasts in the bone marrow independent of the presence of tissue masses and may be associated with spontaneous tumor lysis syndrome. Leukemic presentation seems rarer in "endemic" BL compared with the immunodeficiency-associated BL (~61%)[60] and "sporadic" BL (~26% in pediatric patients).[54] However, bone marrow involvement may be underestimated in limited resource settings. Because of the frequent presentation of BL in extranodal sites, the Ann Arbor staging system is suboptimal to assess tumor dissemination. Therefore, a revised staging according to Murphy is commonly

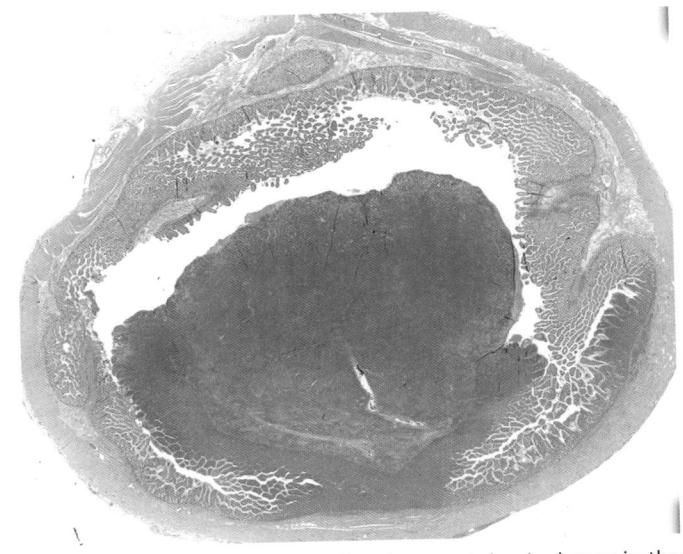

Figure 23-1. Burkitt lymphoma forming an abdominal mass in the small intestine and obstruction of the lumen (H&E).

used for children, the group of patients in which the disease is most frequent.[61]

Morphology

BL infiltration of affected tissue is virtually always obvious and partial infiltration (e.g., of lymph nodes) is rare. The lymphoma grows diffusely, although there are rare cases with a follicular-appearing pattern. Tumor cells are so densely packed that the narrow rim of cytoplasm appears angular, giving the low-power impression of cohesive growth (Fig. 23-2). Scattered macrophages containing apoptotic debris (tingible-body–type macrophages) produce the so-called starry-sky pattern, in which the dense cohesive sheets of blasts appear as the dark sky and the macrophages with bright cytoplasm as the stars (Fig. 23-2).

It is important to keep in mind that the starry-sky picture can be lost because of suboptimal tissue quality (late fixation, early necrosis). A subset of cases can display a true granulomatous reaction and this phenomenon has been linked to good prognosis and even spontaneous remissions in single case reports.[62,63] Reactive T-cells are infrequent. Despite the high proliferation, coagulative necrosis is surprisingly rare. The neoplastic cells show round nuclei with clumped chromatin. The nucleoli are small and often paracentrally located (Fig. 23-3). Overall, there is little cytologic variability, and the vast majority of BL are quite homogenous in their histologic appearance. However, morphologic variability such as more prominent nucleoli or plasmacytoid differentiation with more basophilic cytoplasm may be observed, especially in immunocompromised patients.

In cytologic preparations, such as imprints and smears, the morphology differs because the dense packing of the cells is lost during preparation. The medium-sized lymphoid cells have deeply basophilic roundish cytoplasm that shows lipid vacuoles (designated as L3 morphology in historical classifications,[13] Fig. 23-4). The nuclei appear as round as in histology slides and show multiple basophilic small nucleoli.[64-66] Box 23-1 summarizes the diagnostic features of BL.

Immunophenotype

The immunophenotype of BL is characterized as a mature B-cell phenotype with germinal center markers, absent or weak *BCL2,* and a very high Ki67. BL shows a mature lymphoid phenotype and is thus virtually always terminal deoxynucleotidyl transferase (TdT) negative (Fig. 23-5). BL is characterized by expression of B-cell antigens found in mature B cells (CD19, CD20, CD79a, CD22, and PAX5). Lack of one of these markers is uncommon at initial diagnosis (before treatment). In daily practice, CD20 is often the marker of choice (Fig. 23-5). Immunoglobulin (Ig) M is usually positive on BL cells but immunohistochemistry for IgM is prone to staining artifacts. BL expresses germinal center markers such as CD10, BCL6, CD38, HGAL, GCET1, and MEF2B, of which strong and abundant expression of CD10 seems to be the most helpful (Fig. 23-5). CD10-negative BLs are exceedingly rare, if they exist at all. Expression of markers that are often considered T-cell antigens such as CD43, TCL1, and LEF1 may be found in BL,[67-70] but truly lineage-specific T-cell antigens such as CD3 are absent. MYC expression by immunohistochemistry is high (usually >80% of tumor cells). Rarely, BL lacks positivity

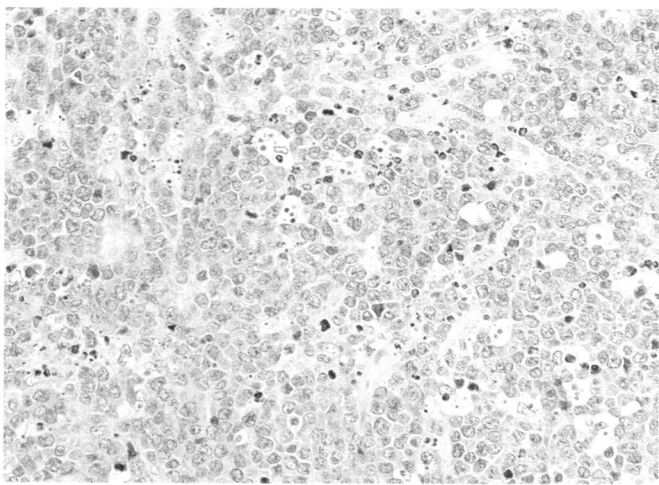

Figure 23-2. Burkitt lymphoma with starry-sky appearance (H&E).

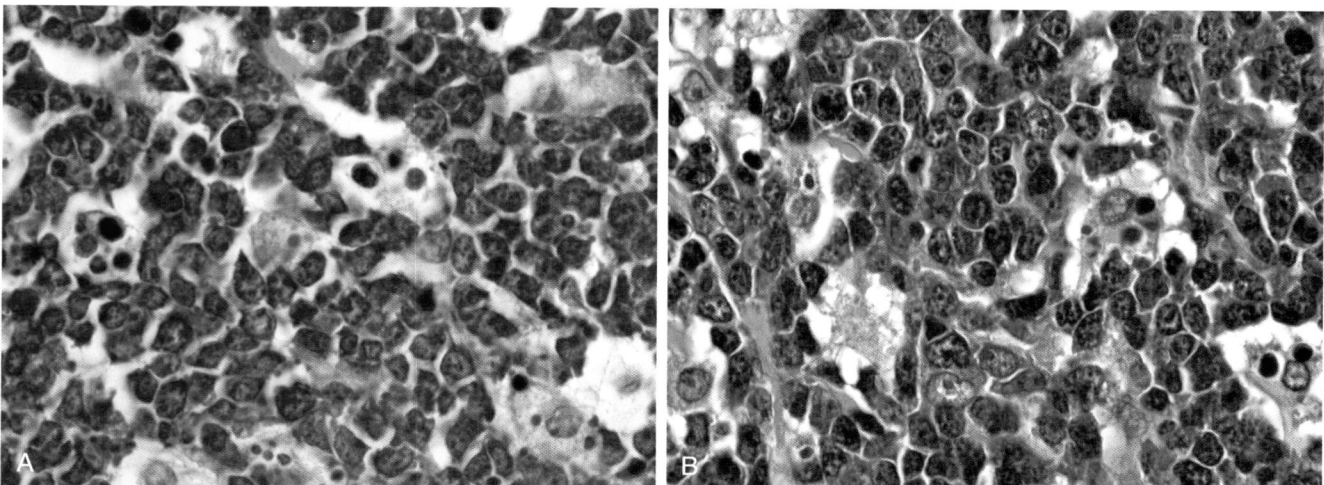

Figure 23-3. High magnification of Burkitt lymphoma stained with Giemsa **(A)** and H&E **(B)**.

for MYC by immunohistochemistry because of mutations and alternative mechanisms of MYC regulation.[71,72] It should be noted that MYC immunohistochemistry requires optimal fixation and tissue processing, and interpretation of MYC staining results needs to be scored in well-preserved

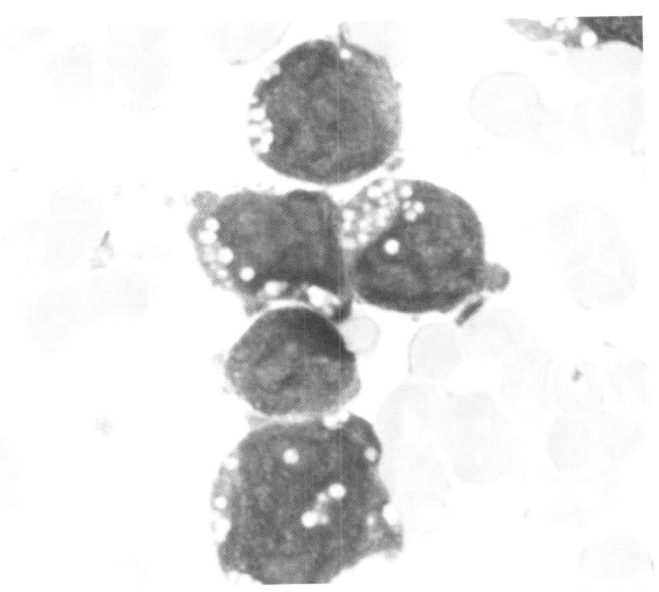

Figure 23-4. Cytology of Burkitt lymphoma with a so-called L3-morphology (May-Grünwald-Giemsa stain).

Box 23-1 *Diagnostic Criteria for Burkitt Lymphoma*

Key Features

Medium-sized, monomorphic lymphoma cells with basophilic cytoplasm and multiple small nucleoli

CD20 and CD10 positivity; absence or weak expression of *BCL2*; Ki67 index >95%

High expression of MYC (>80%) or demonstration of MYC breakage or *IG*::MYC translocation

Additional

Starry-sky pattern, "cohesive" growth pattern

BCL6 positivity, terminal deoxynucleotidyl transferase (TdT) negativity, CD38 positivity

Absence of *BCL2* and *BCL6* translocations (mainly required in adult patients)

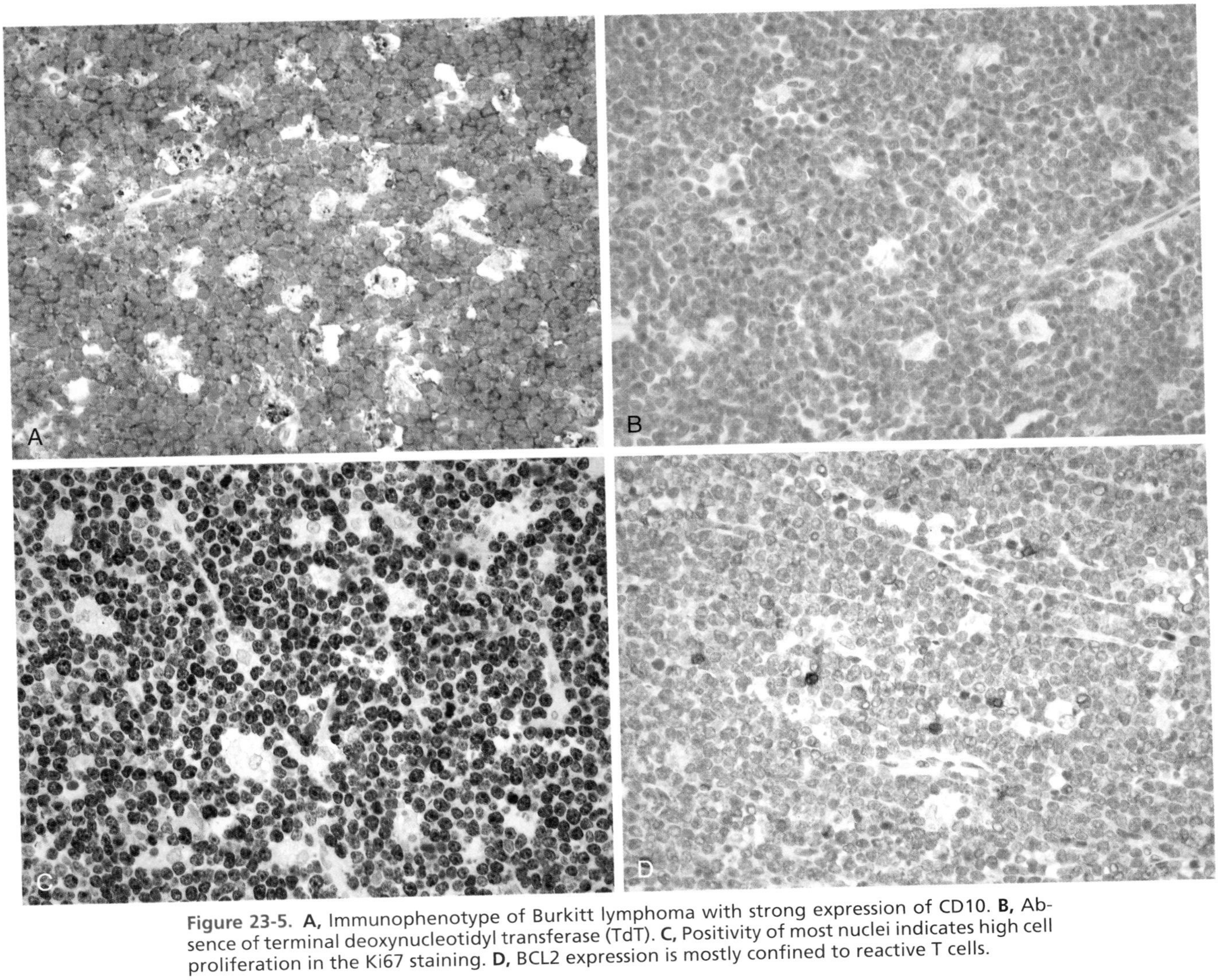

Figure 23-5. A, Immunophenotype of Burkitt lymphoma with strong expression of CD10. **B,** Absence of terminal deoxynucleotidyl transferase (TdT). **C,** Positivity of most nuclei indicates high cell proliferation in the Ki67 staining. **D,** BCL2 expression is mostly confined to reactive T cells.

areas of the tissue only. Immunohistochemistry may replace FISH for *MYC* in a resource limited setting. However, the gold standard to detect MYC rearrangements, as a part of the diagnostic criteria, would still be the detection of the translocation by cytogenetics, FISH, or any other molecular technique. The high proliferation of BL is reflected by a Ki-67 expression in typically >95% of neoplastic cells (Fig. 23-5). In fact, in well-preserved tissue areas, virtually only non-neoplastic cells (macrophages, T cells) will be Ki67-negative upon close examination. Therefore, it is recommended to assess the Ki67 staining in well-preserved areas at a high magnification. Absence of BCL2 staining is a characteristic feature of BL (Fig. 23-5). If BCL2 is positive, it is usually only weakly expressed and appears weaker than the reactive T cells in the same tissue specimen (Fig. 23-5).[73]

Flow Cytometry

Flow cytometric analysis of BL tumor cells usually shows a low expression of CD45, but abundant B-cell markers and CD10. Bright expression of CD38 is a typical feature of BL and more often used in diagnostic algorithms of flow cytometry compared with immunohistochemistry. Also, by flow cytometry, BL cells lack expression of BCL2, CD44, and TdT.[74-76]

Genetics/Molecular Findings

Immunoglobulin Genes

The immunoglobulin (IG) genes of BL cells are clonally rearranged. The breakpoints within the IG genes vary between historical subtypes of BL (Table 23-2) and may be associated with outcome.[77] In addition, the intact allele that is not involved in the *IG::MYC* translocation shows evidence of activity of AID as detected by somatic hypermutations. Interestingly, the level of somatic hypermutation in the IG genes is higher in EBV-positive compared with EBV-negative BL,[21,32] suggesting that a pathogen-driven, germinal center-activating and AID-dependent role is more prominent in EBV-positive BL compared with EBV-negative BL.

Table 23-2 Characteristic Genetic Features of Burkitt Lymphoma

Feature	Endemic BL	Sporadic BL	BL in PLWH
Predominant *MYC* breakpoint in t(8;14) (q24;q32)	Far 5′ (centromeric) of *MYC* (class III)	Exon and intron 1 (class I) and 5′ (centromeric) of *MYC* (class II)	Exon and intron 1 (class I)
Predominant IGH breakpoint in t(8;14) (q24;q32)	VDJ region	Switch region*	Switch region
Somatic IGH mutations	Yes	Yes	Yes
EBV positivity in tumor cells	>90%	5%–30%	25%–55%

*Latest data suggest interdependence of EBV and localization of IGH breakpoints.[42]
BL, Burkitt lymphoma; *EBV*, Epstein-Barr virus; *PLWH*, patients living with HIV.

MYC Translocations

The molecular genetic hallmark of BL is a translocation juxtaposing the *MYC* oncogene on 8q24 next to one IG loci, which is the IG heavy chain locus [*IGH::MYC*, t(8;14) (q24;q32)] in most cases followed by the kappa [*IGK::MYC*, t(8;22)(q24;q11)] and the lambda [*IGL::MYC*, t(2;8) (p12;q24)] light chains.[78] The localization of the breakpoints in the IG genes suggest that they result from AID-mediated somatic hypermutations or class-switch recombinations of the IG genes and AID-induced mutations or breakpoints in *MYC*.[42,79] The *IGH::MYC* and variants lead to juxtaposition of the intact *MYC* gene to IG enhancers, resulting in constitutive expression of *MYC*, compared with the dynamic expression in normal GCB, where it is restricted to a limited number of cells and short periods of time.[80,81] *MYC* encodes a transcription factor that has multiple, complex, and cell context-dependent functions (e.g., MYC is considered to be an amplifier of gene expression, meaning that MYC promotes expression of many genes that are specifically transcribed in a particular cell).[82] In the pathogenesis of BL, the *IGH::MYC* translocation and consequent MYC overexpression is assumed to first occur in a germinal center B cell. Several potential functions of MYC during pathogenesis can be envisioned, such as (1) enhancement of apoptosis, proliferation, metabolism, and angiogenesis; (2) alteration of apoptosis; and (3) genesis of DNA damage and the disruption of double-stranded DNA repair, potentially leading to increased chromosomal abnormalities (Fig. 23-6).[83]

The position of the *MYC* breakpoints depends on the IG partner gene. In the case of t(8;14) involving the IG heavy chain, breakpoints typically lie within the centromeric (5′) part of the *MYC* locus. However, structural differences exist between the three epidemiologic subsets of BL: In "sporadic" and immunodeficiency-associated BL, most breakpoints are nearby or within *MYC*, whereas in endemic cases, most breakpoints are dispersed over several hundred kilobases further upstream of (centromeric to) the gene (Box 23-1).[84-86] This variable distribution may explain why breakpoints are missed in some break-apart FISH assays. In endemic BL, the breakpoints in the IGH locus at 14q32 usually occur 5′ of the intron enhancer in a joining (J) or diversity (D) segment; but in "sporadic" and HIV-associated BL, they mostly occur within or nearby one of the switch regions (Box 23-1).[84-86] Of note, recently cases with cryptic insertion of *MYC* into the IGH locus have been reported. These cases, and lymphomas with widely dispersed *MYC* breakpoints, may escape detection by FISH.[87] Of note, when the partner is IGL or IGK, the breaks in the *MYC* locus are typically downstream of (telomeric to) the *MYC* gene[88] and this genetic constellation has been reported to be associated with unfavorable prognosis in advanced-stage pediatric BL.[77]

Other Mutations and Pathways in Burkitt Lymphoma

Translocations involving *MYC* and the IG genes are considered primary oncogenic events in BL. They usually are part of a simple karyotype, which means that no or very few additional chromosomal aberrations are detectable.[89] The most common secondary aberrations (occurring in 44% of cases) are copy number gains involving 1q, 7, and 12 and losses involving 6q, 13q32-34, and 17p. Gain of 1q seems to be associated with a lack of other recurrent abnormalities. Interestingly, in cases of BL that relapse after therapy, a condition associated with poor outcome, an increase of chromosomal complexity has been observed.[90] The low frequency of chromosomal imbalances identified by conventional cytogenetic studies was confirmed by molecular studies using array comparative genomic hybridization[91] and whole genome sequencing.[92] Chromosomal gains and losses show an identical pattern in pediatric and adult typical BL,[93,94] albeit the mutational profile differs with age and EBV status.

BL harbors mutations in genes that control cell proliferation, growth, and survival, but none of these molecular genetic alterations is as consistently found as the IG::MYC translocations. The most frequently mutated genes are the transcription factor TCF3 (previously called E2A) or its repressor ID3, which supposedly result in tonic activation of B-cell receptor (BCR) signaling.[95-97] Another gene frequently mutated in BL is CCND3, which shows activating mutations often in combination with loss of function mutation of its inhibitor CDKN2A. These mutations are thought to promote G_1-S phase transition and contribute to the very short cell cycle with a 24-hour doubling time characteristic for BL. Other recurrent mutations in BL affect MYC itself, TP53,

GNA13, and SMARCA4. Pathways that are commonly affected by mutations are BCR and PI3K signaling, apoptosis, SWI/SNF complex, and G-protein coupled receptor signaling.[92,98]

Recently the frequency of these mutations in BL was shown to be dependent on the EBV status of the lymphoma cells (EBER positive versus negative). Presence of EBV and mutations in TCF3/ID3 were virtually exclusive in these studies, suggesting that these somatic mutations and EBV may have similar functions during lymphomagenesis.[17,21,28] Thus, a dual mechanism of BL pathogenesis—mutational versus viral driven—has been suggested[17,21,28] and may replace the historical subtyping of BL in the future.[42,99]

Postulated Cell of Origin

Germinal center B cell.

Clinical Course

The prognosis of BL treated with optimized immunochemotherapy, including anti-CD20 antibodies, is generally excellent with

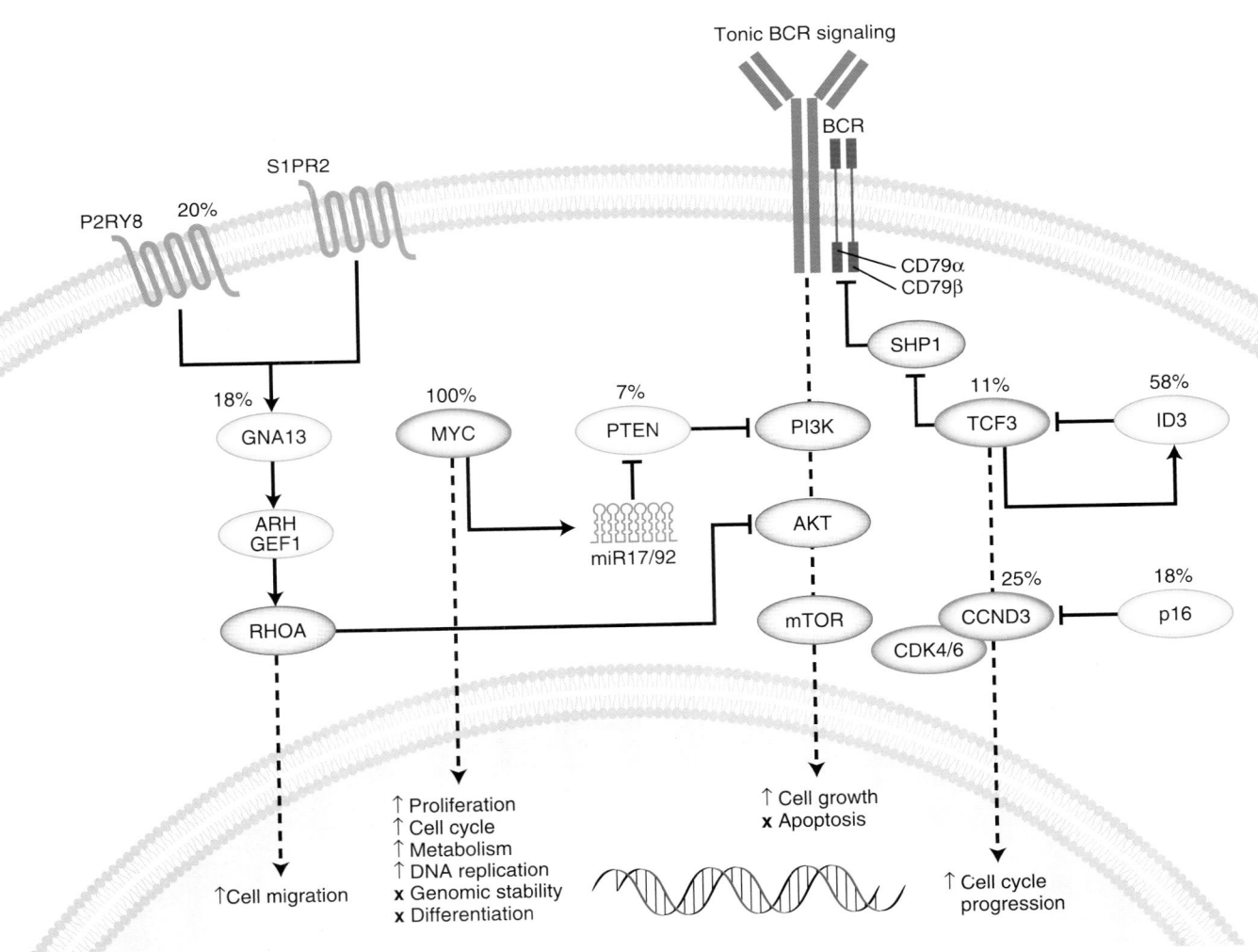

Figure 23-6. Pathogenetic pathways and mutations in Burkitt lymphoma. *(Modified from Fangazio M, Pasqualucci L, Dalla-Favera R. Chromosomal translocations in B cell lymphoma. In: Rowley JD, et al, eds. Chromosomal Translocations and Genome Rearrangements in Cancer. Switzerland: Springer International Publishing; 2015.)*

event-free survival reaching 90% in children[100,101] and 75% in adults.[102] A BL International Prognostic Index is used to assign patients to a low-risk, intermediate-risk, or high-risk group with overall survival rates of 96%, 76%, and 59%, respectively.[79,103-105] The outcome of patients with "endemic" BL is less good and depends on the resources for diagnosis and treatment,[51,106] but has improved with the introduction of polychemotherapy developed for "sporadic" BL.[107] Thus, it seems reasonable to assume that "endemic" and "sporadic" BL do not differ in outcome because of the aggressiveness of the disease but rather because of the health care provided to patients. Additionally, patient outcomes from EBV-positive BL occurring in a "sporadic" setting do not differ from EBV-negative lymphomas when treated similarly.[20] Involvement of the CNS is a risk factor for relapse.[58,108] Once BL relapses after first-line therapy, the outcome is dramatically worse compared with the initial diagnosis,[109,110] but salvage therapy can also be effective.[59,110]

Differential Diagnosis

Most BL can be diagnosed by morphology and a limited number of immunohistochemical stains with sufficient certainty. The differential diagnosis of BL is principally the same in all patients (Table 23-3). However, the clinical context can guide the selection of diagnostic testing. Since BL is the most frequent neoplasia in children and adolescents but rare in adults, the diagnostic strategy in adult patients may be oriented toward diagnoses more common in this age group. In children, the differential diagnosis should include careful exclusion of precursor B-cell lymphomas/leukemias. For countries with limited resources for laboratory testing, simplified diagnostic criteria have been proposed.[111]

The immunophenotype of BL is particularly consistent and should be CD20 positive, CD10 positive, BCL2 negative or partial and weak, and KI67 >90%. In children it may be wise to exclude a precursor B-cell lymphoma by demonstrating absence of TdT. Confirmation of the diagnosis is optimally achieved by demonstrating IG::MYC translocation juxtaposing MYC to either the IGH locus by t(8;14) (q24;q32) (80% of the cases) or, less commonly, to the IGL or the IGK locus by t(8;22)(q24;q11) and t(2;8)(p12;q24) translocations by FISH or cytogenetics. However, in cases with typical morphology and immunophenotype, the use of a break-apart probe for MYC is commonly accepted to prove the diagnosis. In adults and any cases with morphologic or immunophenotypical deviation from the expected, breaks in BCL2 and BCL6 should be excluded and IG::MYC should be demonstrated to achieve a high specificity of diagnosis. Whether a BCL6::MYC translocation can substitute for an IG::MYC translocation is currently uncertain. MYC translocations partnering with other non-IG genes are not typical for BL and should warrant further testing to exclude DLBCL.[7] Similarly, a complex karyotype or multiple chromosomal imbalances are uncommon in BL at first presentation and may lead to additional testing. Of note, mature aggressive B-cell lymphomas with a typical phenotype of BL (CD20 positive, CD10 positive, BCL6 positive, BCL2 negative, Ki67>95%), an IG::MYC, and no BCL2 or BCL6

Table 23-3 Differential Diagnosis of High-Grade B-Cell Lymphomas

Diagnosis	Morphology	Immunophenotype/Immunohistochemistry	Genetics
Burkitt lymphoma	Cohesive monomorphic, medium-sized cells with multiple small nucleoli and basophilic cytoplasm	B cells positive for CD20, CD10, and MYC protein; Ki67 >95%; negative for BCL2, TdT.	MYC translocation, most often IGH::MYC; absence of BCL2 or BCL6 translocation/s
B-lymphoblastic leukemia/lymphoma	Finer nuclear chromatin; nucleoli often less conspicuous	Uniform expression of TdT in most cases; CD34 expression in a subset of cases. Frequently reduced expression of CD20 and strong BCL2. CD10 negative in a subset.	MYC translocations rare; presence of other key defining rearrangements/translocations
High-grade B-cell lymphoma with MYC and BCL2 rearrangements	Variable—intermediate between BL and DLBCL; DLBCL; or blastoid	Most express BCL2 (strong, abundant); occasional cases show subset of cells expressing TdT.	BCL2 translocation in addition to MYC translocation
Provisional: High-grade B-cell lymphoma with MYC and BCL6 rearrangements	Variable—intermediate between BL and DLBCL; DLBCL; or blastoid	Most cases express BCL6. Variable MYC expression dependent on MYC abnormalities. Minority express BCL2.	BCL6 translocation in addition to MYC translocation
High-grade B-cell lymphoma, NOS	Medium-to-large-sized cells; variation in nuclear size and nucleolar content; cohesive growth is usually absent	Most express BCL2 (strong, abundant); variable MYC expression dependent on MYC abnormalities.	Can show isolated MYC, isolated BCL2, or BCL2 and BCL6 translocation/s; do not show BCL2 and MYC translocations
High-grade/large B-cell lymphoma with 11q aberration	Morphologic resemblance to BL, but more pleomorphism with some variation in nuclear shape/size and presence of larger nucleoli in some cases	Variable MYC expression.	Gain in 11q23.3 and the minimal region of loss at 11q24.1-qter*; lack of MYC translocation
Diffuse large B-cell lymphoma, NOS	Larger cells; nucleoli more prominent; peripherally located nucleoli; centroblasts, immunoblasts, pleomorphism	Majority express BCL2; can lack CD10, BCL6, or MYC expression; can show expression of CD44.	Majority lack MYC translocation; variable presence of BCL2 or BCL6 translocation/s

*Region of loss is the terminal end of the long arm of chromosome 11.
BL, Burkitt lymphoma; DLBCL, diffuse large B-cell lymphoma; NOS, not otherwise specified; TdT, terminal deoxynucleotidyl transferase.

translocation, are similar to BL in their mutational pattern even if their morphology deviates from typical cases of BL.[112]

Although genetic testing for *MYC* is the gold standard to confirm the diagnosis of BL, there are certainly limitations of this concept. First, conventional cytogenetic or molecular methods may miss some *IG::MYC* translocations[9] and biologically equivalent alterations leading to MYC deregulation such as cryptic insertions of *MYC* into IGH.[8] However, testing for these alterations depends on sequencing technology, which is currently not available for routine diagnostic testing. Testing for recurrent mutations in BL may guide the diagnosis but its value has not yet been demonstrated for clinical decision making. Second, genetic analyses such as FISH studies on FFPE sections or cytologic smears are currently not available in all parts of the world. To address this, an alternative algorithm for the diagnosis of BL has been proposed that includes immunohistochemistry for MYC instead of testing for *MYC* translocations.[111]

LARGE/HIGH-GRADE B-CELL LYMPHOMA WITH 11Q ABERRATION

Definition

Large/high-grade B-cell lymphoma with 11q aberration (L/HGBL-11q), formerly known as a *Burkitt-like lymphoma with 11q aberration*, is a mature aggressive B-cell lymphoma with a characteristic chromosome 11q-gain/loss pattern often morphologically and immunophenotypically similar to BL. See Table 23-1 with synonyms and related terms and Box 23-2 for diagnostic criteria.

Epidemiology

Systematic analyses of the incidence of L/HGBL-11q have not been published yet; however, the entity is likely rare. Most cases reported so far have been diagnosed in children/adolescents and patients under the age of 60 years.[113-116]

Etiology and Pathogenesis

The etiology of L/HGBL-11q is unknown. Despite morphologic and clinical similarity to BL, a geographic distribution like BL has not been documented yet. Given the fact that L/HGBL-11q resembles BL morphologically and immunophenotypically and may only be identified by genetic testing for *MYC* and

> **Box 23-2** *Diagnostic Criteria for L/HGBL-11q*
>
> **Key Features**
> Characteristic intermediate/blastoid or Burkitt-like morphology in concert with the typical immunophenotype (CD10 positive, BCL6 positive, BCL2 negative)
> Chromosome 11q-gain/loss, telomeric loss or telomeric loss of heterozygosity pattern
> Absence of a MYC translocation
>
> **Additional**
> Expression of CD56 in the absence of CD38^high by flow cytometry

11q aberrations, this entity might frequently be missed diagnostically, and its incidence underestimated.

Clinical Features

Most patients present with symptoms related to the tumor masses. Generalized symptoms like B-symptoms seem to be rare.[113-115] Immunocompromised patients have been reported to suffer from L/HGBL-11q.[117] In pediatric patients, an association with immunodeficiency has not been established.[113] Staging is performed similar to BL in pediatric patients.[61] Based on the limited data available, the outcome seems to be favorable in pediatric patients treated according to BL protocols, with almost no relapses reported so far.[113,114] The clinical experience with adult patients is more limited. However, patients treated according to protocols developed for adult DLBCL may relapse.[114,115,118]

Morphology

A characteristic feature of L/HGBL-11q is the morphologic and immunophenotypical similarity to BL. Most cases show dense diffuse sheets of cells and a starry-sky pattern with strikingly coarse apoptotic debris within starry-sky macrophages.[119] The neoplastic cells are medium-sized with chromatin similar to that observed for BL. Variation in nuclear size and nucleoli can be seen (Fig. 23-7).[116] However, this may not be a distinguishing feature since BL also shows some morphologic variation. Cases with a pure morphology of DLBCL have been observed, prompting the ICC to choose the term *large B-cell lymphoma with 11q aberration* for this entity.[4] The typical "L3-morphology" in smears/imprints as described for BL is not observed.

Immunophenotype

L/HGBL-11q are mature aggressive B-cell lymphomas (TdT negative) that express abundant B-cell markers such as CD20, CD19, and CD79a (Fig. 23-8). In fact, cases lacking expression of CD20 at initial diagnosis have not been observed to the best of our knowledge. The other characteristic features of BL are

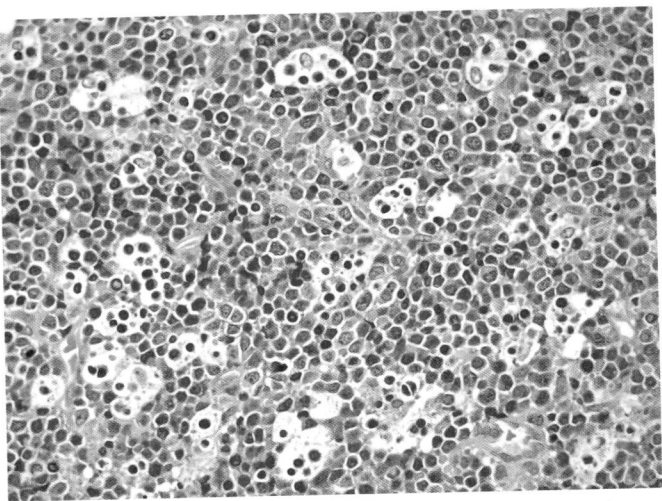

Figure 23-7. Morphology of large/high-grade B-cell lymphoma with 11q aberration (H&E).

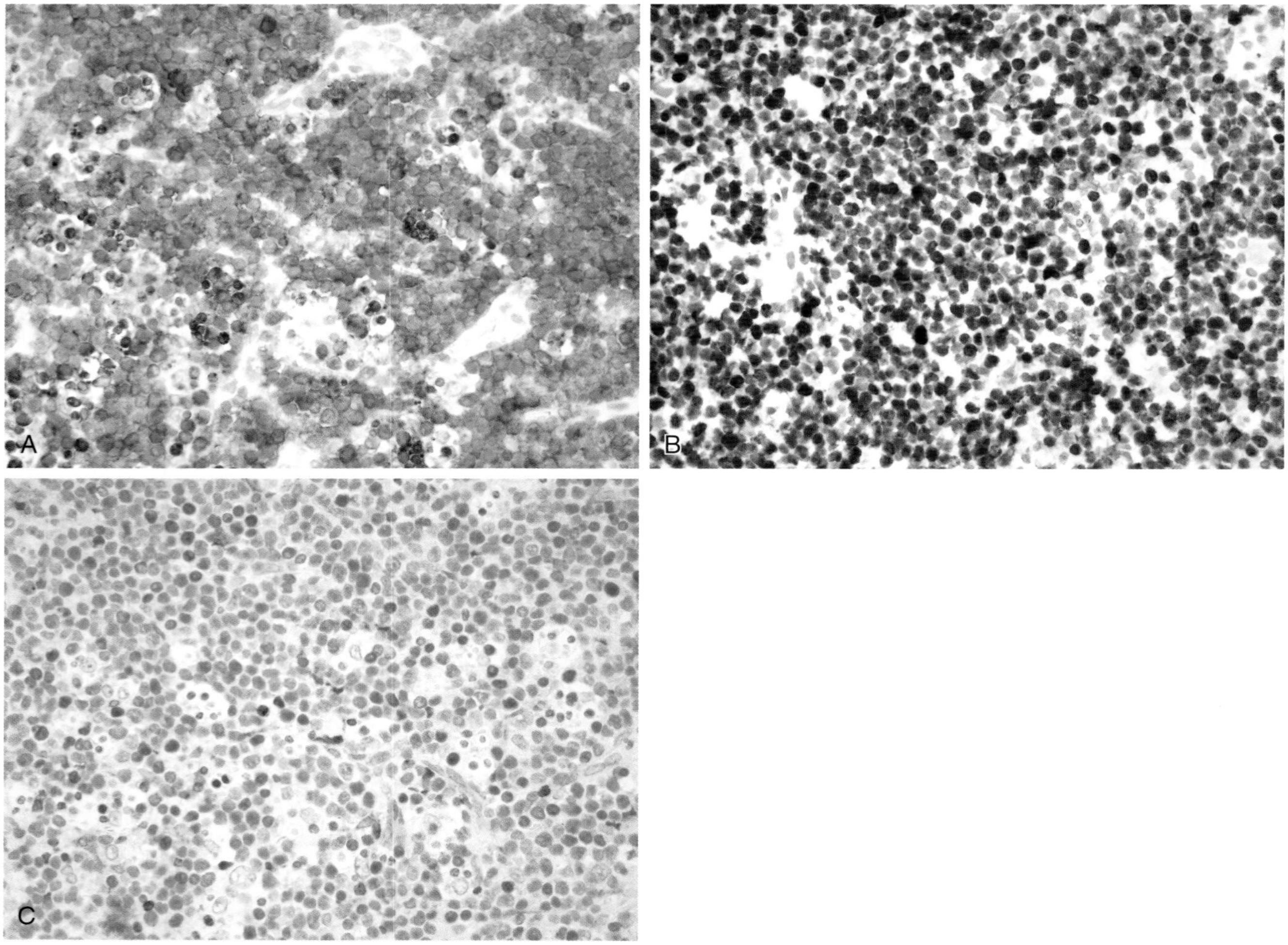

Figure 23-8. Immunophenotype of large/high-grade B-cell lymphoma with 11q aberration with expression of CD10 **(A)**, high Ki67 **(B)**, and absence or weak BCL2 **(C)**.

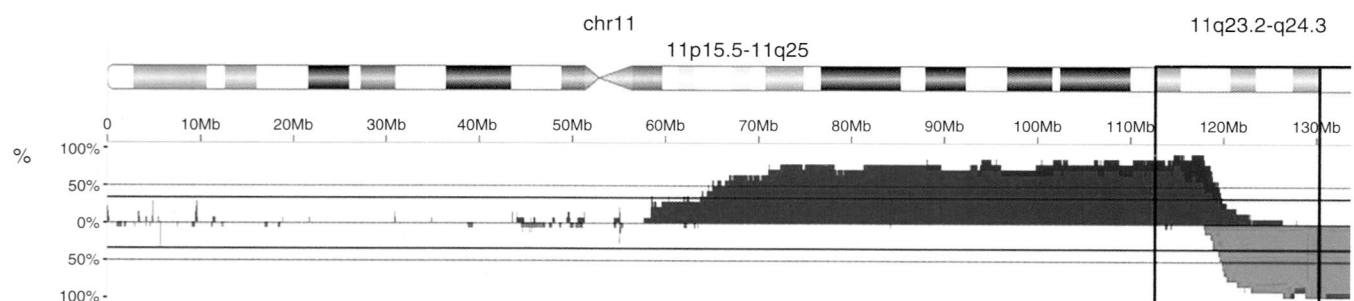

Figure 23-9. **Chromosomal 11q-gain/loss pattern of large/high-grade B-cell lymphoma with 11q aberration.** *(Modified from Itziar S, Martin-Guerrero I, Wagener R, et al. for the Molecular Mechanisms in Malignant Lymphoma Network Project and Berlin-Frankfurt-Münster Non-Hodgkin Lymphoma Group. A recurrent 11q aberration pattern characterizes a subset of MYC-negative high-grade B-cell lymphomas resembling Burkitt lymphoma. Blood. 2014;123(8):1187-1198.)*

observed in this entity too: expression of CD10, KI67>90%, and no or only partial or weak positivity for BCL2 (Fig. 23-9).[116] Of note, in flow cytometry distinguishing features have been described as expression of CD16, CD56, and CD8, and lack of CD38-high but lineage-specific myeloid or T-cell antigens are not detected.[118]

Genetics/Molecular Findings

Gene-expression profiling shows similarities between BL and L/HGBL-11q,[116] probably reflecting the cell of origin or the frozen state of differentiation of the neoplastic cells—a feature which can, to some extent, be captured by morphology and phenotype. Despite the morphologic similarity, the molecular genetic pathways affected in L/HGBL-11q seem to differ strikingly from BL. In L/HGBL-11q, *MYC* translocations are absent. Genes recurrently mutated in BL, such as those in the ID3-TCF3 pathway, are rarely affected in L/HGBL-11q. However, mutations in other genes such as *KMT2D, SWI/SNF, CREBBP*, and *GNA13*, which are commonly found in DLBCL, have been detected in L/HGBL-11q.[114,120] The characteristic genetic feature of this lymphoma is a complex aberration involving chromosome 11 (11q) with a minimal region of gain in 11q23.3 and a minimal region of loss at 11q24.1-qter.[116] Some cases solely harbor the telomeric loss, but without the centromeric gain, and may show combinations with a loss of heterozygosity (Fig. 23-9).[116] To what extent and how the genetic lesion on 11q contributes to the pathogenesis is still uncertain. Of note, L/HGBL-11q does not harbor EBV virus and thus a role for EBV in the pathogenesis is unlikely. Diagnostic criteria are listed in Box 23-2.

Postulated Cell of Origin

Germinal center B cell.

Differential Diagnosis

Since morphology and immunophenotype are not sufficient to distinguish BL from L/HGBL-11q, cases with the morphology and immunophenotype of BL need to be tested for *MYC* translocations. In the absence of *MYC* translocations, testing for the typical gain/loss pattern on 11q is required to confirm the diagnosis of L/HGBL-11q. Testing for MYC expression may be applied when FISH for *MYC* is not available. However, this testing strategy requires a MYC immunohistochemistry protocol and scoring that allows distinction of *MYC* translocation positive and negative lymphomas with sufficient certainty, which can be challenging. In adults, FISH testing for *BCL2* and *BCL6* translocations may be advisable because these do not usually occur in L/HGBL-11q and indicate DLBCL.[116]

The question of how to detect the typical aberration on 11q is a matter of what technology is available. Next-generation sequencing or high-resolution array-based comparative genomic hybridization are certainly the most reliable techniques to identify 11q aberrations because they also detect copy number-balanced lesions (telomeric loss or solely telomeric loss of heterozygosity [LOH] in the absence of gains).[116] However, most labs used FISH as the diagnostic test in daily practice, knowing FISH will miss approximately 10% of cases with LOH at 11q.[115,118] It is important to keep in mind that our current understanding of this entity considers an isolated 11q gain less specific for the entity than a telomeric loss without a gain by FISH. 11q gains without loss have been observed in other entities, making it a less specific finding, whereas the telomeric loss is rarely observed in other entities but may be missed by FISH in cases that show LOH in the respective chromosomal region.[113,115,119,121] For a diagnostic testing strategy, we currently recommend to test only lymphomas with the appropriate morphology and immunophenotype (similar to BL) and absence of *MYC* translocations for this aberration.[119]

DIFFUSE LARGE B-CELL LYMPHOMA/HIGH-GRADE B-CELL LYMPHOMA WITH *MYC* AND *BCL2* REARRANGEMENTS

Definition

Diffuse large B-cell lymphoma/high-grade B-cell lymphoma with *MYC* and *BCL2* rearrangements (HGBL-DH-*BCL2*) is a mature aggressive B-cell lymphoma defined by coincident chromosomal translocations of *MYC* and *BCL2* (double-hit, DH) and thus shares features with transformed FL even in the absence of preceding or concurrent FL. Concurrent *BCL6* translocations may occur along with *MYC* and *BCL2*, creating a triple-hit. Lymphomas solely harboring *MYC* and *BCL6* translocations can also occur.[122] The ICC considers these as a "provisional entity" requiring further study. These lymphomas are described further at the end of this section.[4] In contrast, the WHO 5th ed. proposal does not currently recognize the *MYC* and *BCL6* translocated cases as a distinct entity.[122] See Table 23-1 for synonyms and related terms.

Epidemiology

So far, published data on the incidence of HGBL-DH-*BCL2* are based on cohorts from North America and Europe of DLBCL, NOS screened for *MYC* translocations. About 10% of lymphomas morphologically compatible with DLBCL, NOS harbor *MYC* translocations and about half of those carry additional rearrangements of *BCL2*, with or without additional *BCL6* translocations.[123] Thus, about 5% of all lymphomas with the morphology of DLBCL, NOS fulfill the criteria of HGBL-DH-*BCL2*.[123-125] Since L/HGBL-DH is thought to often originate from transformed FL, which is virtually absent in patients under the age of 18 years, L/HGBL-DH is rare in young adults. Thus the true incidence is likely strongly age dependent.

Etiology and Pathogenesis

Formally, the etiology is unknown. However, because the molecular features of HGBL-DH-*BCL2* overlap with transformed FL, it seems reasonable to assume that the etiology should also be similar to FL. However, preceding or coincident FL is detectable in only about one-third of cases by histopathologic analysis.[124,126,127] One might speculate that the true incidence of association with FL is higher as the association is solely defined by histology and thus dependent on biopsy size and sampling. HGBL-DH-*BCL2* carries, by definition, translocations of *MYC* and *BCL2*.

Clinical Features and Staging

Usually DLBCL/HGBL-*MYC/BCL2* presents at an advanced clinical stage and additional features, such as elevated lactate dehydrogenase, leading to a high International Prognostic Index (IPI) score. Extranodal involvement including CNS infiltration seem to be a frequent finding. Staging is currently performed analogous to DLBCL, NOS.[123,128-132]

Morphology

The morphologic spectrum covers a broad range of what may be found in mature aggressive B-cell lymphomas: (1) typical morphology of DLBCL, NOS with centroblasts and immunoblasts to a variable extent; (2) blastoid morphology reminiscent of precursor cell lymphomas or blastic mantle cell lymphoma; and (3) morphology "intermediate" between BL and DLBCL, NOS with small centroblasts and occasionally a starry-sky pattern (Fig. 23-9). Most likely, cases with blastoid or "intermediate" morphology are enriched for HGBL-DH-*BCL2*.

Immunophenotype

B-cell markers such as CD20 and CD19 are commonly expressed, and proliferation rate, as assessed by Ki67, is usually high. The vast majority of HGBL-DH-*BCL2*s are positive for CD10[124] and are thus classified as GCB-subtype according to the commonly used cell-of-origin classification developed for DLBCL, NOS.[133] BCL2 is commonly positive too and since the MYC translocations usually lead to MYC overexpression, about 80% HGBL-DH-*BCL2* fall into the category of "double expressors."[134] TdT expression in HGBL-DH-*BCL2* is rare and affects probably far less than 10% of cases. Often only a few cells are TdT positive, but cases with abundant expression of TdT have been reported too.[135-137]

Genetics/Molecular Findings

The translocation partner of *MYC* is mostly the IG heavy chain gene (~60%). The remaining cases show rearrangement of *MYC* to the lambda light chain, *BCL6*, *PAX5*, or other non-IG genes.[124] The entity is characterized by a complex karyotype and a mutational pattern that overlaps with FL and involves *BCL2*, *KMT2D*, *CREBBP*, *EZH2*, and *TNRSF14*. As a consequence there is considerable overlap of mutational features with transformed FL.[126,138] Most HGBL-DH-*BCL2* fall into the molecular genetic subtypes of DLBCL associated with FL pathogenesis (referred to as EZB,[139] C3,[140] or BCL2 clusters).[141] Diagnostic features are summarized in Box 23-3.

What Is, and What Is Not, a Double-Hit?

The current definition of the entity HGBL-DH-*BCL2* does not include cases with *MYC* translocations and translocations of other genes such as *CCND1*.[142] Cases with gains or

---

Box 23-3 *Diagnostic Criteria for Diffuse Large B-Cell Lymphoma/High-Grade B-Cell Lymphoma With* MYC *and* BCL2 *Rearrangements*

Key Features
Morphology and phenotype consistent with aggressive B-cell lymphoma
Evidence of concurrent *MYC* and *BCL2* translocations (with or without *BCL6* translocation)

Additional
Germinal-center B cell phenotype
Minimal terminal deoxynucleotidyl transferase protein expression
Determination of *MYC* translocation partner

---

amplifications of the *MYC* gene locus without a break/translocation are not considered DLBCL/HGBL-*MYC*/*BCL2*.[143,144] Of note, sole co-expression of *MYC* and *BCL2* protein, commonly referred to as "double expressor," is far more common than concurrent *MYC* and *BCL2* translocations and does not justify classification as DLBCL/HGBL-MYC/BCL2.

How to Use Immunohistochemistry to Screen for DLBCL/HGBL-*MYC/BCL2*

Multiple strategies have been discussed about how to prescreen mature aggressive B-cell lymphomas for those that require FISH testing for *MYC*/*BCL2* DH. Using immunohistochemistry for MYC and a cutoff of 70% strongly stained nuclei, most cases with underlying *MYC* translocations are detected.[145] However, a considerable number of cases with MYC rearrangements are missed by immunohistochemistry staining. Staining for GCB-type cell of origin may be an alternative to narrow down mature aggressive B-cell lymphomas to those requiring FISH for *MYC*. A recent detailed report describes the performance of each prescreening approach.[125] Focusing on lymphomas with a GCB phenotype would potentially reduce the number of cases that require FISH to approximately 50% in an age-mixed cohort but would potentially detect almost all HGBL-DH-*BCL2* when tested for *MYC* and *BCL2* translocations.[125] Using *MYC*/*BCL2* "double expressors" as a prescreen may further reduce the number of cases requiring FISH, but for the price of a lower positive predictive value.[125] Given the fact that prospective studies of systematic prescreening by immunohistochemistry has not been yet published, applying FISH for *MYC* to all mature aggressive B-cell lymphomas seems to currently be the most reliable approach for daily practice, followed by reflex testing for *BCL2* rearrangement. Very recent developments of deep learning on digitalized H&E (hematoxylin and eosin)-stained slides raise hope that widely available tools for prescreening may become available in the future.[146,147]

What Is the Role of Gene-Expression Profiling to Identify DLBCL/HGBL-*MYC/BCL2*?

As discussed in the introduction of this chapter, the definition of the disease entity DLBCL/HGBL-*MYC/BCL2* has changed over the last years and is very likely to be further modified in the future. Two independent approaches identified a gene-expression signature that characterizes DLBCL/HGBL-*MYC/BCL2* (referred to as DH[125] or molecular high-grade signatures).[5] Of note, these gene-expression signatures identify a subset of cases in which *MYC* rearrangements are not identified by FISH, which may be caused by alternate (genetic) mechanisms of MYC activation or alternative mechanism to achieve dark-zone biology.[125] Thus, gene-expression profiling or next-generation sequencing will extend the group of mature aggressive B-cell lymphomas with the biological and clinical features shared with DLBCL/HGBL-*MYC/BCL2* when introduced into the daily practice. It is important to stress that gene-expression profiling also identifies BL as positive for the high-grade signatures.[148] Thus, an independent diagnostic confirmation of the diagnosis is required.

Postulated Cell of Origin

Germinal center B cell.

Clinical Course

The outcome for DLBCL/HGBL-*MYC/BCL2* (40%–50% 5-year overall survival) is reportedly poor compared with DLBCL, NOS.[123] However, most data on survival were collected retrospectively and the outcome may be better in young patients or patients with a low IPI.[129,130] Moreover, a standard treatment has not been defined, although most oncologists tend to treat more intensively than DLBCL, NOS.[131,132]

Does the Translocation Partner of *MYC* Need to Be Determined?

In one study, the poor outcome of DLBCL/HGBL-*MYC/BCL2* is a feature restricted to lymphomas in which *IG::MYC* rearrangement is detectable, whereas DH lymphomas in which *MYC* is partnered to non-IG genes do not substantially differ in outcome from DLBCL, NOS with single *MYC* rearrangements or without any *MYC* rearrangements at all.[123] However, others did not find that translocation partner was associated with outcome.[149] Although the definition of the entity does not require determining the *MYC* translocation partner, the necessity for testing may arise in certain clinical contexts (e.g., when the choice of therapy is discussed in individual patients).

Differential Diagnosis

The most frequent differential diagnoses are outlined in Table 23-4. As a genetically defined entity, the differential diagnosis is predominantly based on the detection of a concurrent *MYC* and *BCL2* rearrangement. However, there are several practical considerations helpful to consider in daily practice that will be discussed. Of note, transformed lymphomas should be reported according to their aggressive lymphoma entity followed by adding the term *transformed from* and the denominator of the indolent lymphoma from which it has evolved (e.g., HGBL-DH-*BCL2 transformed from FL* in cases with history or concurrent FL). Other well-defined entities with a DH genetics are also recommended to stay in their original category.

PROVISIONAL ENTITY: HIGH-GRADE B-CELL LYMPHOMA WITH *MYC* AND *BCL6* REARRANGEMENTS

The current definition of HGBL-DH-*BCL2* exclusively includes lymphomas in which translocations of *MYC* and

BCL2 are detected in the same mature aggressive B-cell lymphoma with or without *BCL6* translocation. Lymphomas with translocations of *MYC* and *BCL6* (without *BCL2*) were also previously included in the revised WHO 4th ed. as "high-grade B-cell lymphoma with *MYC* and *BCL2* and/or *BCL6* rearrangements"; however, they are now relocated to a provisional entity by the ICC or classified as DLBCL, NOS or HGBL, NOS (depending on the tumor cell morphology), by the WHO 5th ed. proposal.[4] See Table 23-1 for synonyms and related terms. These *MYC* and *BCL6* translocated cases differ from HGBL-DH-*BCL2* as they (1) mostly show a non-GCB phenotype and activated B cell (ABC)-like gene expression by cell-of-origin classification,[126] and (2) lack a mutational profile reminiscent of FL but carry mutations (*CD79B, PIM1*) frequently found in ABC-type DLBCL.[140] However, like HGBL-DH-*BCL2* lymphomas, cases with *MYC* and *BCL6* rearrangements show an inferior outcome compared with common DLBCL, NOS.[123] Lymphomas with *MYC* and *BCL6* translocations and morphology not compatible with DLBCL (such as blastoid morphology) may fall into the category of HGBL, NOS.

HIGH-GRADE B-CELL LYMPHOMA, NOT OTHERWISE SPECIFIED

Definition

High-grade B-cell lymphoma, not otherwise specified (HGBL, NOS) is a poorly defined heterogeneous group of mature aggressive B-cell lymphomas that do not fit into other better-defined categories. Its distinction from DLBCL, NOS is predominantly based on a medium-sized blastoid appearance rather than centroblasts and immunoblasts found in DLBCL, NOS and lacks DH genetic features. Cases with features intermediate between DLBCL and BL may be assigned to HGBL, NOS if phenotypic features argue against BL as the diagnosis. See Table 23-1 for synonyms and related terms.

Epidemiology

As the disease is poorly defined and subjected to changing definitions, the incidence is not known.[112,125,144,148,150]

Table 23-4 Differential Diagnosis of Diffuse Large B-Cell Lymphoma/High-Grade B-Cell Lymphoma With *MYC* and *BCL2* Rearrangements

Entity	Distinguishing Feature
DLBCL, NOS	No difference in morphology or immunophenotype, but by definition, no DH *MYC/BCL2*.
Burkitt lymphoma	*MYC* translocations, but no *BCL2* translocations detected.
High-grade B-cell lymphoma, NOS	No difference in morphology or immunophenotype, but by definition, no DH *MYC/BCL2*.
Precursor B-cell neoplasia	TdT expression usually abundant. Immunophenotypical features of precursor cell neoplasm such as absence/reduction of CD20, expression of CD34, and multilineage phenotype (e.g., with expression of MPO). Molecular analysis may be required in a subset of cases for definite distinction by mutational profile.
Transformed lymphoma	Lymphomas transformed from FL or other low-grade B-cell lymphoma are considered HGBL-DH-*BCL2* when the respective genetic constellation with *MYC* and *BCL2* translocations is identified, but the information "transformed from FL" should be included in the diagnosis.
Localization specific subtype of LBCL (e.g., CNS or leg-type)	No difference in morphology or immunophenotype, but GCB-phenotype rare in certain entities (cutaneous, CNS, etc.) and DH is rare in any other entity of LBCL. However, if the respective genetic constellation (*MYC* and *BCL2* translocations) is detected, disease is considered DLBCL/HGBL-*MYC/BCL2* irrespective of its clinical presentation.
Classic follicular lymphoma	Follicular growth and cytology with centroblasts and centrocytes (classic FL). Even if DH occurs, these lymphomas appear to clinically behave like typical FL,[157] but additional studies are required to determine the prognostic relevance of MYC in FL.

CNS, Central nervous system; *DH*, double-hit; *FL*, follicular lymphoma; *GCB*, germinal-center B cell; *HGBL*, high-grade B-cell lymphoma; *LBCL*, large B-cell lymphoma; *NOS*, not otherwise specified; *TdT*, terminal deoxynucleotidyl transferase.

Etiology

The etiology of HGBL, NOS is unknown.

Clinical Features and Staging

Clinical features are similar to DLBCL, NOS with a high-intermediate or high International Prognostic Index score. However, most data on the clinical presentation and outcome are based on retrospective analyses and there is considerable uncertainty regarding generalizability.[151,152] Staging is performed analogous to DLBCL, NOS.[128,152]

Morphology

HGBL, NOS is characterized by a diffuse growth of intermediate-to-small-sized blastoid cells with a narrow rim of cytoplasm. These cells do not show features of typical centroblasts and immunoblasts found in DLBCL, NOS (Fig. 23-10). Nucleoli are inconspicuous or even absent, similar to cells observed in precursor cell neoplasms or blastoid mantle cell lymphoma.[153] Cases with features intermediate between DLBL and BL may be assigned to HGBL, NOS too if phenotypic features argue against BL as the diagnosis (Fig. 23-11).

Immunophenotype

The lymphoma cells show a mature B-cell phenotype with expression of CD20 and CD19 but lack of TdT. When applying the cell-of-origin classification by immunohistochemistry, the majority of HGBL, NOS cases show a GCB-phenotype.[152] Ki67 is variable but usually lower than seen in BL. Since MYC translocations occur frequently in this rare subtype of mature aggressive B-cell lymphomas, expression of MYC can be detected in a substantial number of cases.[150,154,155]

Genetics/Molecular Findings

As a poorly defined entity, it is not surprising that the molecular features are heterogeneous. The mutational profile of these lymphomas, for example, identifies cases with more GCB-like and others with more ABC-like mutational profiles.[148]

However, three features are rather consistent and may also be helpful for diagnosis and management. First, HGBL, NOS is characterized by a high rate of KMT2D (43) and TP53 mutations (30%).[144] Second, MYC translocations (by definition without concurrent BCL2 translocations) and MYC amplifications are frequent (~8%–58% reported).[112,144,150] Third, gene-expression analysis assigns a large number of cases (54%) to the group with a DH signature.[125] A summary of the diagnostic features are located in Box 23-4.

Postulated Cell of Origin

Germinal center B cell.

Clinical Course

Treatment guidelines have not been defined. Some physicians treat according to DLBCL, NOS whereas others prefer to use intensified regimens.[152] Overexpression of both MYC and BCL2 ("double expresser") has been linked to inferior outcome.[155]

Differential Diagnosis

HGBL, NOS is a diagnosis of exclusion. In any case with blastoid or intermediate cell morphology, a DLBCL/HGBL-DH-MYC/BCL2 should be excluded by FISH for MYC and BCL2. Expression of CD10, Ki67 of more than 90%, absence of BCL2 expression, and the presence of a MYC translocation should raise suspicion of BL. It has been shown that lymphomas with

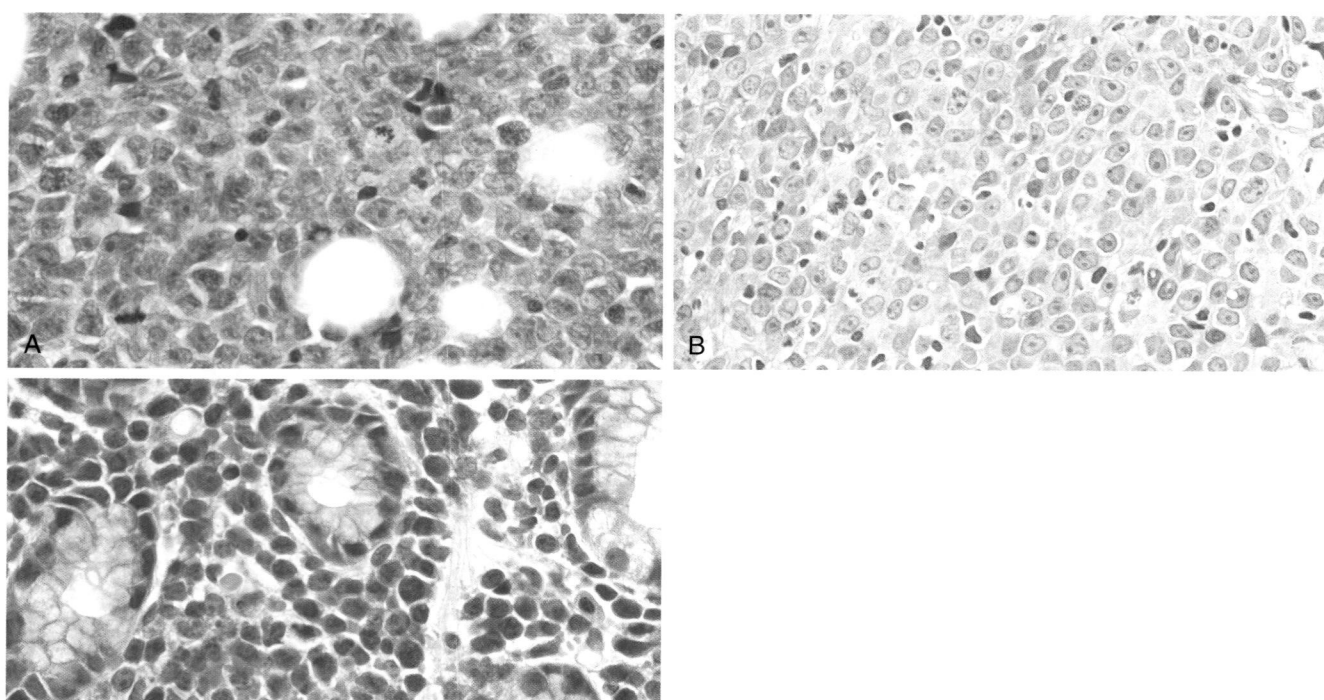

Figure 23-10. Morphologic variability of HGBL-DH-*BCL2* with multiple examples showing a range of differentiation with centroblastic **(A)**, immunoblastic **(B)**, or blastoid morphology **(C)** (H&E). All lymphomas were shown to harbor *MYC* and *BCL2* translocations.

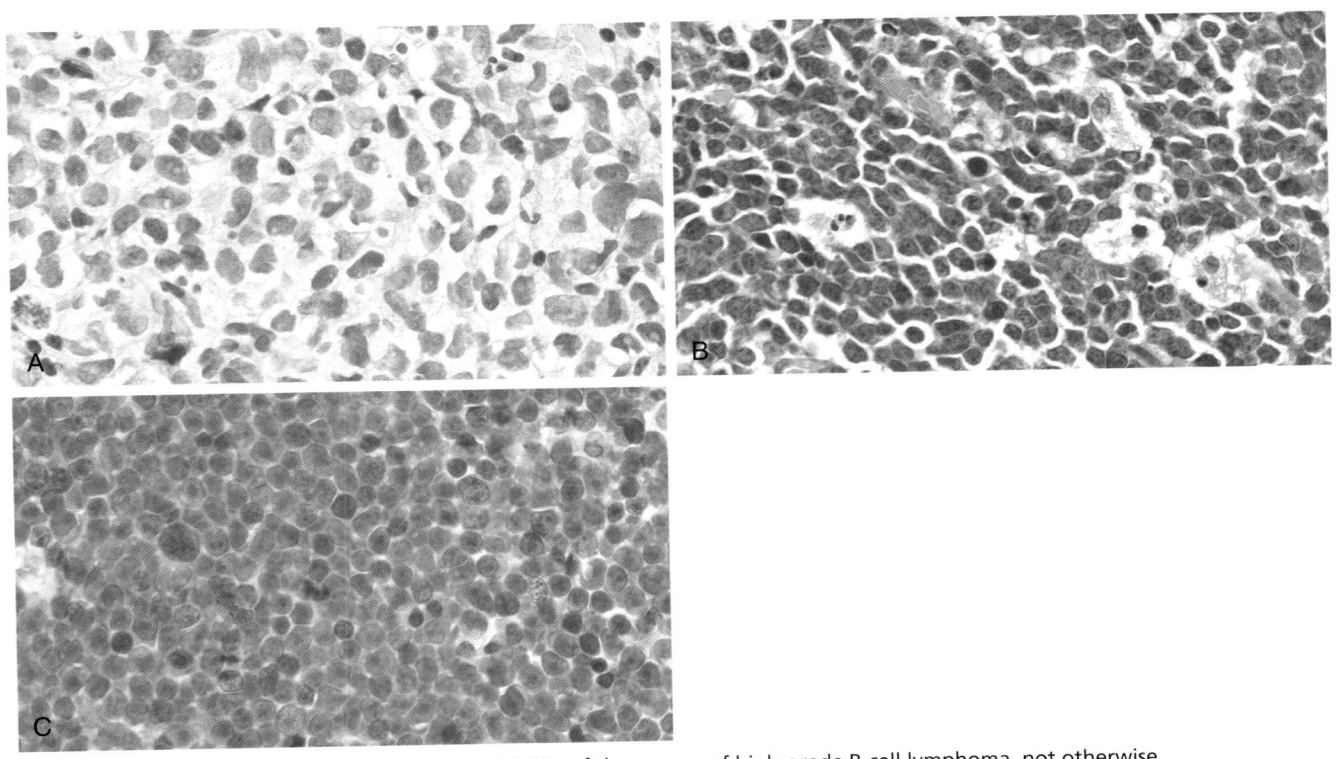

Figure 23-11. Morphologic variability of three cases of high-grade B-cell lymphoma, not otherwise specified (H&E). Polymorphic large cells with abundant cytoplasm **(A)**, dense sheets of medium-sized blasts reminiscent of Burkitt lymphoma **(B)**, and small blasts with very narrow rim of cytoplasm similar to lymphoblastic lymphoma **(C)**.

Box 23-4 *Diagnostic Criteria for High-Grade B-Cell Lymphoma, Not Otherwise Specified*

Key Features

Intermediate or blastoid cytomorphology not consistent with either diffuse large B-cell lymphoma or Burkitt lymphoma

Lack of TdT, CD34 to exclude lymphoblastic lymphoma; lack of cyclin D1 to exclude blastoid MCL

Absence of a dual translocation (DH) involving *MYC* and *BCL2*

Absence of the 11q gain/loss pattern of HGBL-11q

Additional Features

DH B-cell lymphoma gene expression signature
KMT2D and *TP53* mutations

DH, Double-hit; *HGBL-11q,* high-grade B-cell lymphoma with 11q aberration; *MCL,* mantle cell lymphoma; *TdT,* terminal deoxynucleotidyl transferase.

---

the phenotype of BL but absence of typical BL morphology molecularly resemble BL. Absence of BCL2 expression is typical of HGBL, NOS.[112] It is noteworthy to mention that morphologic features of BL, such as the starry-sky pattern, disappear when tissue processing is suboptimal, which might lead to an overdiagnosis of HGBL, NOS, especially in young patients. Differential diagnosis features for these cases are summarized in Table 23-3.

Cases with blastoid morphology and follicular growth should be diagnosed as one of the unusual variants of FL.[156] To identify follicular growth pattern, detection of follicular dendritic cells by staining for CD21 or CD23 can be helpful. Blastoid variants of mantle cell lymphoma need to be distinguished from HGBL, NOS by staining for cyclin D1 and SOX11. Precursor cell lymphoma needs to be excluded by staining for TdT and CD34.

Pearls and Pitfalls

- Be aware that slightly nuclear irregularity and variation in cell size and shape may be caused by fixation or processing artifacts and do not preclude a diagnosis of Burkitt lymphoma (BL). The starry-sky pattern is particularly prone to vanish in poor tissue quality. B5 fixation tends to make cells appear smaller with a single, central nucleolus.

- Weak BCL2 protein expression may be encountered in BL. However, in all cases with any doubt, in particular in non-pediatric patients, the diagnosis should be further substantiated with molecular additional techniques in addition to morphology and immunophenotype.

- Have a low threshold for performing fluorescence in situ hybridization (FISH).

- If a diagnosis of BL is being considered and the results of the cytogenetic studies are available, they should show either a t(8;14) or a variant translocation. Three-way translocations and cryptic translocations that need additional FISH analysis can incidentally be observed in BL.

- If all other criteria of classic BL are met but *MYC* FISH is negative, testing for 11q aberrations is strongly suggested.

- Variant *MYC* translocations require cytogenetic analysis or the use of locus-specific FISH studies. A *MYC* break-apart assay may be negative despite presence of *MYC* translocations.

- The most commonly encountered de novo lymphoma (outside of endemic BL areas) with *MYC* translocation are high-grade B-cell lymphoma (HGBL) and diffuse large B-cell lymphoma (DLBCL) (5%–15% of de novo DLBCL). More than half of those are HGBL with double-hit (DH) with *MYC* and *BCL2* translocations.

- HGBL-DH is strictly defined by rearrangements of both *MYC* and *BCL2* or *BCL6* and includes cases with DLBCL morphology. Cases with other molecular abnormalities (mutations, gain, or amplification without a concomitant breakpoint) of these genes or rearrangements of other genes such as *CCND1* should not be included.

- Although they also have a poor prognosis, the more common DLBCL with double expression of MYC and BCL2 protein (DLBCL "double expressers") should not be mixed up with HGBL-DH.

- DH in follicular lymphoma without any clinical and pathology evidence of transformation and precursor lymphoma blastic lymphoma/leukemia are excluded from HGBL-DH.

KEY REFERENCES

3. WHO, WHO Classification of Hematolymphoid Tumors, 5th edition ed. WHO Classification of Tumors, 5th ed. I.A. Cree. 2022, Lyon (France): International Agency for Research on Cancer (IARC).
4. Campo E, et al. The International Consensus Classification of Mature Lymphoid Neoplasms: A Report from the Clinical Advisory Committee. *Blood.* 2022;140(11):1229–1253.
17. Richter J, et al. Epstein-Barr virus status of sporadic Burkitt lymphoma is associated with patient age and mutational features. *Br J Haematol.* 2022;196(3):681–689.
23. Mbulaiteye SM, et al. Trimodal age-specific incidence patterns for Burkitt lymphoma in the United States, 1973-2005. *Int J Cancer.* 2010;126(7):1732–1739.
42. Thomas N, et al. Genetic subgroups inform on pathobiology in adult and pediatric Burkitt lymphoma. *Blood.* 2023;141(8):904–916.
43. Mundo L, et al. Frequent traces of EBV infection in Hodgkin and non-Hodgkin lymphomas classified as EBV-negative by routine methods: expanding the landscape of EBV-related lymphomas. *Mod Pathol.* 2020;33(12):2407–2421.
95. Schmitz R, et al. Burkitt lymphoma pathogenesis and therapeutic targets from structural and functional genomics. *Nature.* 2012;490(7418):116–120.
96. Richter J, et al. Recurrent mutation of the ID3 gene in Burkitt lymphoma identified by integrated genome, exome and transcriptome sequencing. *Nat Genet.* 2012;44(12):1316–1320.
112. Hüttl KS, et al. The "Burkitt-like" immunophenotype and genotype is rarely encountered in diffuse large B cell lymphoma and high-grade B cell lymphoma, NOS. *Virchows Arch.* 2021;479(3):575–583.
113. Au-Yeung RKH, et al. Experience with provisional WHO-entities large B-cell lymphoma with IRF4-rearrangement and Burkitt-like lymphoma with 11q aberration in paediatric patients of the NHL-BFM group. *Br J Haematol.* 2020;190(5):753–763.
116. Salaverria I, et al. A recurrent 11q aberration pattern characterizes a subset of MYC-negative high-grade B-cell lymphomas resembling Burkitt lymphoma. *Blood.* 2014;123(8):1187–1198.
120. Wagener R, et al. The mutational landscape of Burkitt-like lymphoma with 11q aberration is distinct from that of Burkitt lymphoma. *Blood.* 2019;133(9):962–966.
122. Alaggio R, et al. The 5th edition of the World Health Organization classification of haematolymphoid tumours: lymphoid neoplasms. *Leukemia.* 2022;36(7):1720–1748.

Visit Elsevier eBooks+ for the complete set of references.

Plasmablastic Neoplasms Other Than Plasma Cell Myeloma

Blanca Gonzalez-Farré and Elias Campo

This chapter reviews two aggressive large B-cell lymphomas composed of large cells with a predominant immunoblastic or plasmablastic morphology and the immunophenotype of plasma cells. Despite sharing these morphologic and immunophenotypical features, plasmablastic lymphoma (PBL) occurs in patients with immunodeficiency or advanced age, and most cases are related to Epstein-Barr virus (EBV) infection. Conversely, ALK-positive large B-cell lymphoma occurs in immunocompetent patients, and it is caused by the activation of ALK by different translocations. The morphologic and immunophenotypical features of these lymphomas are also shared by human herpesvirus 8 (HHV-8)–related aggressive lymphomas, which are reviewed in Chapter 29. The recognition of all these entities may raise differential diagnoses with related tumors on both sides of the spectrum, such as diffuse large B-cell lymphomas (DLBCLs) and plasma cell neoplasms. The distinction is important because the clinical context and management of these patients may differ.

PLASMABLASTIC LYMPHOMA

Definition

PBL is a diffuse lymphoma composed of large B cells with a predominant morphology of immunoblasts or plasmablasts that express plasma cell differentiation antigens.[1] PBL may also occur as a transformation from low-grade B-cell lymphomas.[2,3] Other subtypes of large B-cell lymphoma with a plasmablastic immunophenotype, such as ALK-positive large B-cell lymphomas and HHV-8–associated lymphoproliferative disorders, are not included in this category.

The term *plasmablastic lymphoma (PBL)* was introduced by Delecluse and colleagues in 1997 to describe a group of DLBCLs presenting in the oral cavity and jaws of individuals infected with HIV.[4] These tumors showed immunoblastic morphology with an immunophenotype characteristic of plasma cells. Subsequently, PBL has been described in other localizations, mostly in gastrointestinal mucosa, and has been associated with other immunodeficiency states and advanced age.[5-7]

Synonyms

None.

Epidemiology

This lymphoma occurs predominantly in adults with immunodeficiency and is most commonly caused by HIV infection, but it is also associated with iatrogenic immunosuppression (transplant and autoimmune diseases). Some cases arise in older adult patients without an apparent cause of immunodeficiency other than possible immunosenescence, and in children with immunodeficiency, mainly HIV infection.[4,5,7,8] Patients who are HIV positive tend to be younger than those with other types of immunosuppression.[8]

Clinical Features

The clinical presentation is frequently as a tumor mass in extranodal regions of the head and neck, in particular the oral cavity, and less frequently in the nasal cavity or respiratory sinuses. Other sites commonly involved are the gastrointestinal tract, soft tissues, skin, bone, lung, and less frequently, the lymph nodes.[5-8] Nodal presentation is more frequent in posttransplant-associated PBL (30%) than in patients infected with HIV or older adult patients (<10%).[5] Computerized image exploration may detect disseminated bone lesions in 30% of patients.[9] Paraprotein may be detected in some cases.[10] Disseminated stage III/IV disease at presentation, including bone marrow involvement, occurs in 75% of patients who are HIV positive and 50% of patients with posttransplant disease, but only in 25% of patients without apparent immunodeficiency.[5,7]

The prognosis is generally poor, with more than three-quarters of patients dying of the disease at a median interval of 6 to 7 months.[4,5,7,11] Some reports observed patients with longer survival related to new antiretroviral treatments, better immunologic status, and improvements in supportive care and delivery of chemotherapy. However, these results are not consistent among studies.[5] Evaluation of prognostic parameters have not yielded consistent results. However, the presence of the *MYC* translocation has been associated with poorer outcomes in two studies.[5]

Pathology

Histologically, two variants have been recognized: monomorphic PBL and PBL with plasmacytic differentiation. Monomorphic PBL is composed of a diffuse and cohesive proliferation of immunoblasts or large cells with minimal or no morphologic plasma cell differentiation. Cases with plasmacytic differentiation have cells with rounder and eccentric nuclei, coarse chromatin, abundant basophilic cytoplasm, and paranuclear hof (Fig. 24-1). Intermediate features between these monomorphic and plasmacytic variants may be seen in some cases. Monotypic maturing plasma cells may be occasionally present. A starry sky pattern is common in monomorphic cases with high mitotic activity and abundant apoptotic bodies. The border of the tumor infiltration is sometimes relatively well delimited, and areas of geographic necrosis are not uncommon (Fig. 24-2).

The immunophenotype is similar to that of plasma cells with negative expression of CD45, CD20, and PAX5. A variable expression of CD79 may be seen in approximately 40% of the tumors. On the contrary, the tumor cells express plasma cell–associated markers and transcription factors such as CD38, CD138, VS38c, IRF4/MUM-1, BLIMP1, and XBP1[12] (Fig. 24-3). Variable expression of cytoplasmic immunoglobulin (Ig) may be seen. BCL2 and BCL6 expression is usually negative, whereas CD10 is expressed in 20% of cases. Epithelial membrane antigen (EMA) and CD30 are frequently

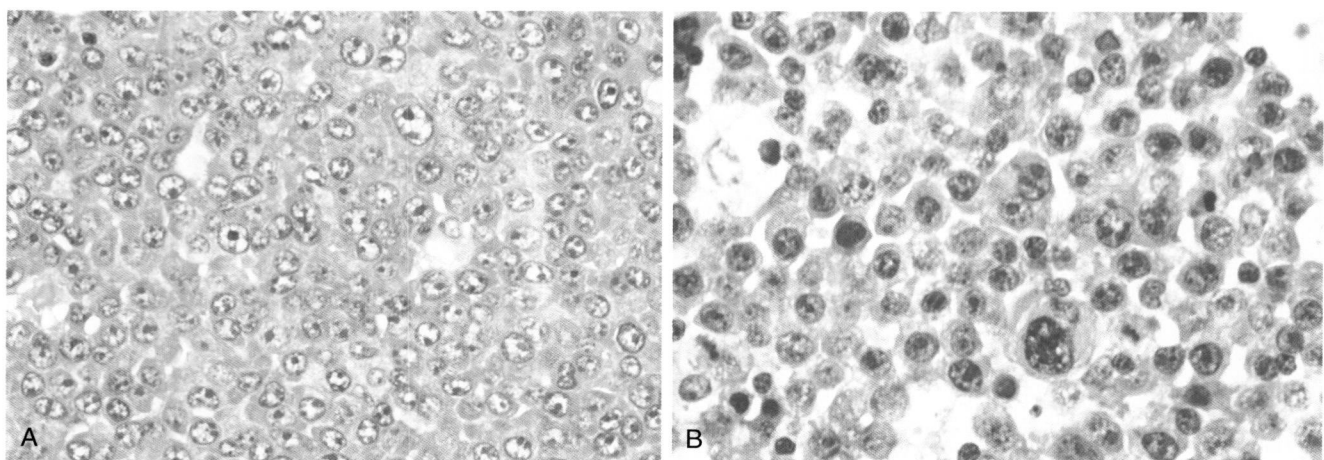

Figure 24-1. Plasmablastic lymphoma, cytologic variants. A, Monomorphic variant with large cohesive immunoblastic cells. **B,** Plasmacytic variant composed of large cells with round eccentric nuclei and coarser chromatin.

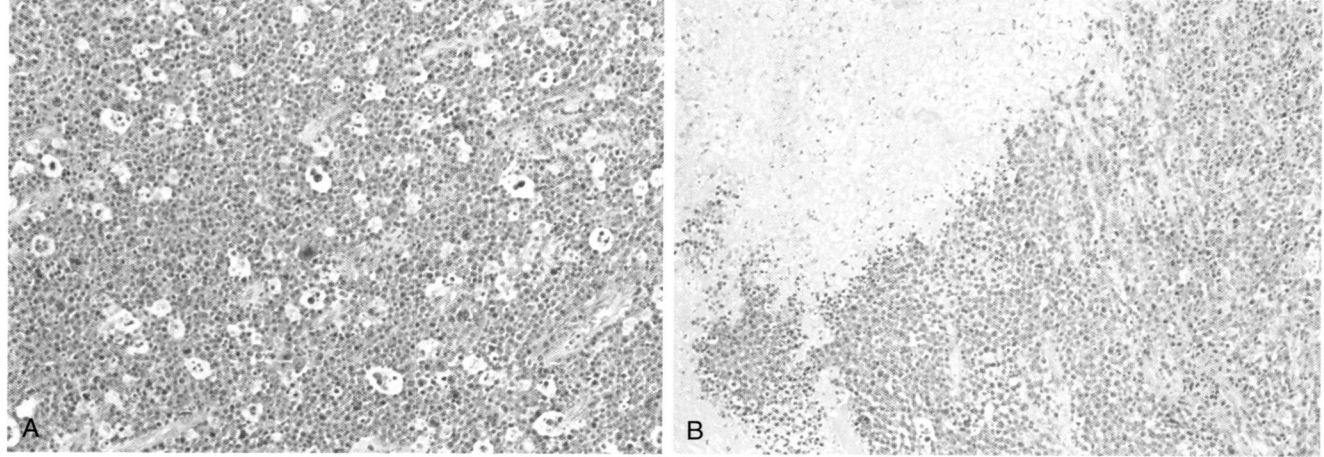

Figure 24-2. Plasmablastic lymphoma. A, A starry-sky pattern at low power may suggest Burkitt lymphoma. **B,** Areas of geographic necrosis may be seen in some cases.

expressed, and CD56 is detected in 25% of cases. MYC is usually overexpressed, even in cases without rearrangement.[13] The tumors have a high proliferation (Ki-67) index (>90%). Reactive infiltrating T cells are usually very scarce.[4,5,7,11,14] Some PBL might aberrantly express T-cell markers, mainly CD3 or CD4, a pitfall that should be considered. This feature is also described in occasional plasmablastic multiple myelomas.[14-16]

Genetic Features

EBV is positive in 70% of cases, usually with latency type I, although occasional cells may express LMP1 (Fig. 24-4). PBL in HIV-positive and posttransplant cases is more frequently EBV positive than in HIV-negative cases.[5,8] HHV-8 is always negative.[4,7,11,17]

Genetic studies have revealed frequent complex karyotypes and specific alterations, such as gains of 12p and 16q11.2-q24.3 CNN-LOH, which may be used in the differential diagnosis with other entities.[18] MYC translocations have been identified in approximately 50% of cases, more in EBV-positive (74%) than EBV-negative tumors (43%), and they are associated with MYC protein expression.[19] The rearrangement usually occurs with IG genes. MYC amplification occurs in some cases.[13] MYC expression in

normal terminal B-cell differentiated cells is suppressed by BLIMP1, a transcription factor required for plasma cell differentiation.[20] Therefore, the activation of MYC by an oncogenic mechanism may be important for the pathogenesis of the disease to overcome the repressor effect of BLIMP1 and provide the tumor cells with a proliferative and survival advantage (Fig. 24-5).[19]

Genomic studies have revealed genetic alterations activating the MAPK and JAK-STAT pathways as the predominant drivers of PBL lymphomagenesis.[18,21-23] The genetic profiles in these tumors are slightly different in relation to EBV and HIV infections. Specifically, EBV-negative PBL harbors a higher mutational and copy number load with more mutations affecting epigenome/chromatin modifiers and more frequent TP53, CARD11, and MYC mutations. Conversely, EBV-positive PBL tends to have more STAT3 and SOCS1 mutations. HIV-negative cases seem to carry STAT3 and LNP1 mutations less frequently but TP53, PRDM1, and IRS4 mutations more frequency, in addition to alterations involving the MAPK pathway. The genomic profile of PBL is different from those of activated B-cell-like (ABC)-DLBCL and multiple myeloma; therefore, sequencing analysis may assist in the differential diagnosis. Particularly, STAT3, NRAS, and EP300 mutations are frequently seen in PBL, whereas STAT3 and EP300 are rare

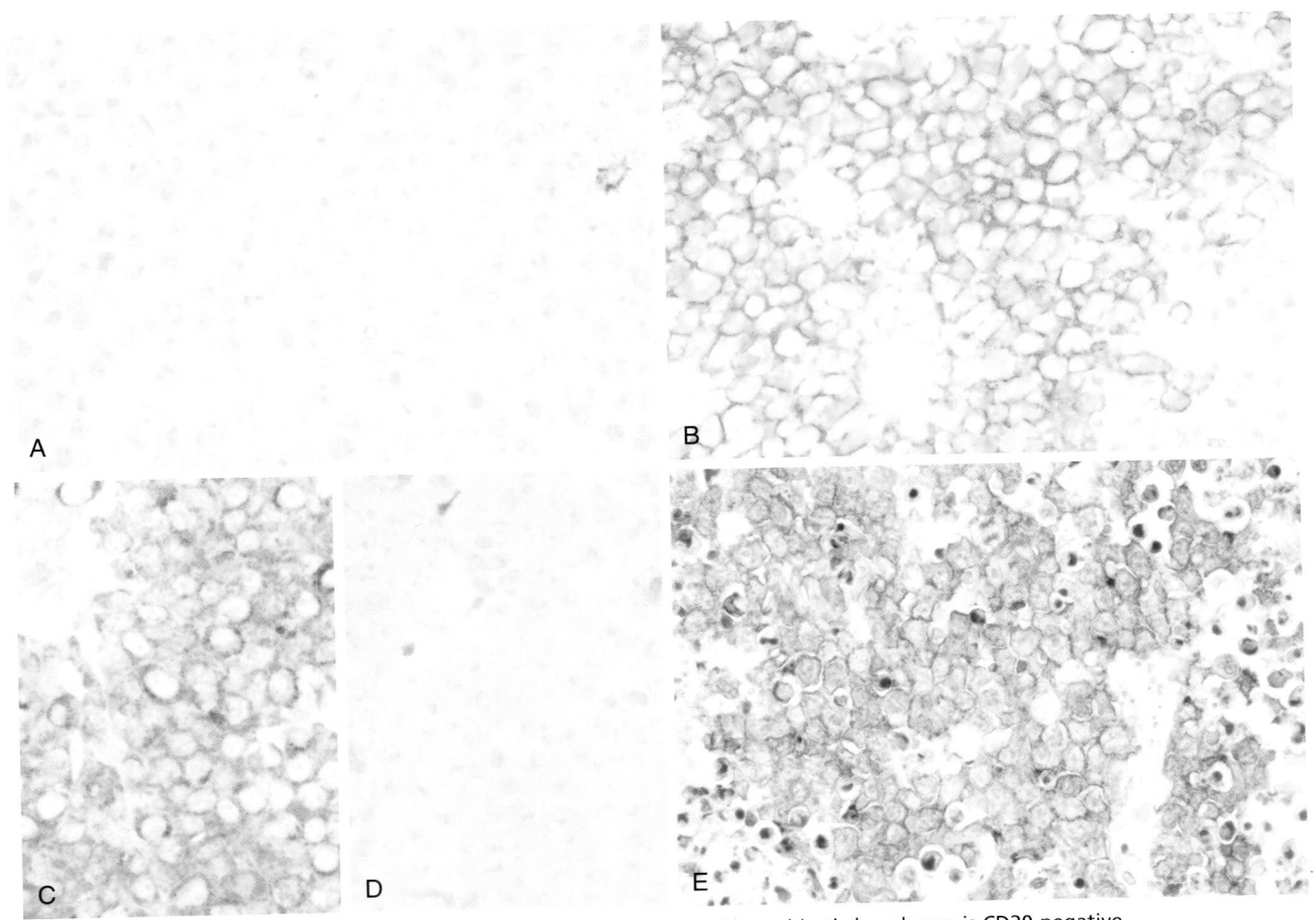

Figure 24-3. Plasmablastic lymphoma phenotype. A, Plasmablastic lymphoma is CD20 negative. **B,** Tumor cells expressed the plasma cell–associated marker CD138. Kappa **(C)** but not lambda **(D)** expression. **E,** Epithelial membrane antigen is often positive.

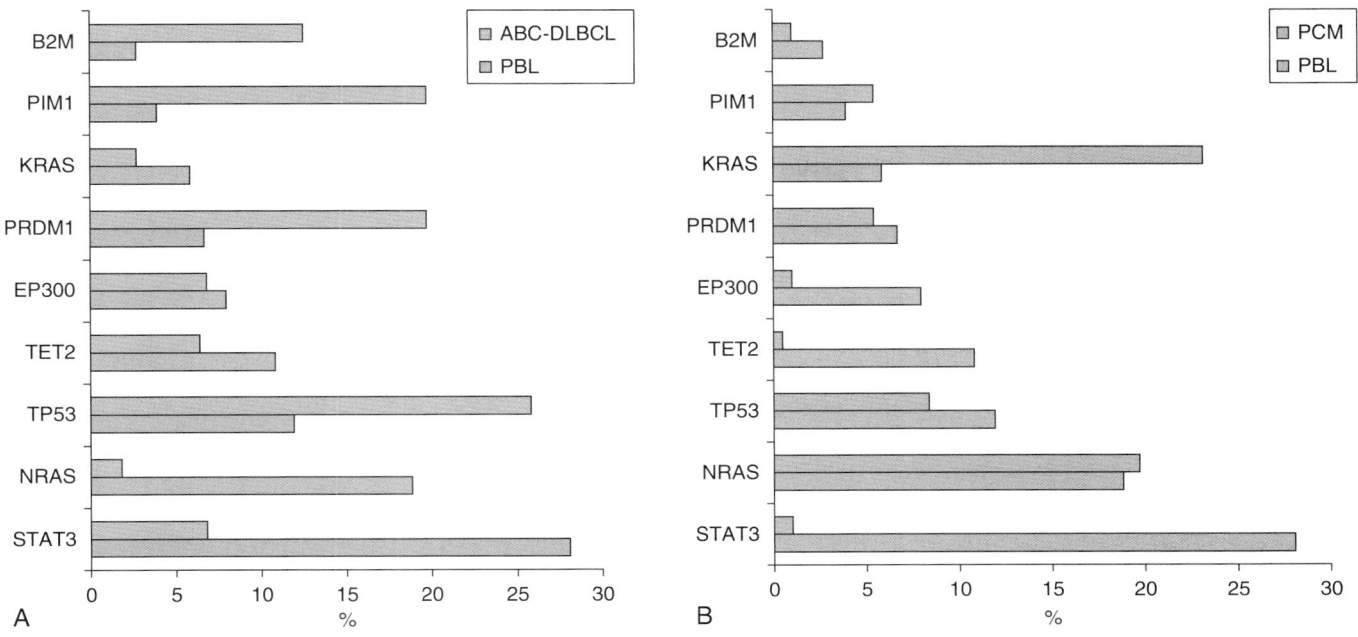

Figure 24-4. EBV in plasmablastic lymphoma. A, Epstein-Barr encoding small RNA (EBER) in situ hybridization shows the presence of Epstein-Barr virus (EBV) in virtually all tumor cells. **B,** Immunostaining of LMP1 is usually negative or only positive in very few cells.

Figure 24-5. Molecular pathogenesis in plasmablastic lymphoma. Plasmablastic lymphomas express the transcription factor BLIMP1 required for plasma cell differentiation. However, BLIMP1 represses *MYC.* The activation of *MYC* by the oncogenic translocation t(8;14) may be important to overcome the repressor effect of BLIMP1 and provide the tumor cells with a proliferative and survival advantage.

in multiple myeloma, and *NRAS* and *STAT3* mutations are uncommon in ABC-DLBCL (Fig. 24-6).[24-26]

Differential Diagnosis

The differential diagnosis of PBL must be established with other large B-cell lymphomas with terminal B-cell differentiation and anaplastic/plasmablastic plasma cell neoplasms that share similar morphology and overlapping phenotypic features. The absence of smaller neoplastic cells with plasmacytic differentiation was originally thought to be a feature that could distinguish PBL from plasmacytoma,[4] but it is now recognized that these cells are present in some cases.[7,11] CD56 expression tends to occur more frequently in plasma cell neoplasms, but it also occurs in some PBLs and therefore cannot be used as a definitive criterion.[7,14] Cyclin D1 is negative in PBL but positive in a subgroup of patients with multiple myeloma. The clinical presentation (immunodeficiency, oral involvement, absence of multiple myeloma), high proliferation index, and frequent EBV association are features supporting a diagnosis of PBL over anaplastic/plasmablastic plasma cell neoplasms. However, some cases occurring in patients who are HIV positive have overlapping features with multiple myelomas such as lytic bone lesions and monoclonal serum immunoglobulins.[7,14] Identification of *STAT3, TET2,* or *EP300* mutations may favor PBL over multiple myeloma (Fig. 24-6).[26] In some cases, a firm distinction cannot be made, and a descriptive diagnosis such as *plasmablastic neoplasm, indeterminate between PBL and anaplastic plasmacytoma* may be acceptable.

The starry-sky pattern and the high proliferation index may suggest a diagnosis of Burkitt lymphoma. However, the cells in PBL are larger and do not express CD20, whereas the cells in Burkitt lymphoma are negative for plasma cell–associated markers. The presence of EBV may raise the differential diagnosis of EBV-positive DLBCL, not otherwise specified (NOS).[27] However, mature B-cell markers (although weak or negative in some cells) are still extensively expressed in these cases, and contrary to PBL, tumor-infiltrating T cells are abundant.

Some cases of DLBCL, NOS may have morphologic features similar to PBL, with eccentric nuclei, basophilic cytoplasm, and strong immunoglobulin cytoplasmic expression.[28] However, contrary to PBL, the tumor cells express strong CD20, CD79a, and PAX5 and have frequent *TP53* alterations. Clinically, the patients do not have immunodeficiency, but the prognosis is also poor. The mutational profile may assist in the differential diagnosis, as *NRAS* and *STAT3* mutations are common in PBL and infrequent in ABC-DLBCL (Fig. 24-6).[25] Large B-cell lymphomas related to HHV-8 infection usually have plasmablastic features.[29-31] However, these tumors are caused by different diseases that must not be confused with PBL (see Chapter 29).

Large B-cell lymphomas with plasmablastic features may occur as a rare transformation of small B-cell lymphoid neoplasms, mainly chronic lymphocytic leukemia and

Figure 24-6. Comparison between mutations in plasmablastic lymphomas and other related lymphoid neoplasms. Percentage of mutated cases in PBL from five different series[19,22-24,42] compared with **(A)** 295 cases of activated B-cell diffuse large B-cell lymphoma (ABC-DLBCL)[43] and **(B)** 203 cases of multiple myeloma[44] including the most frequently mutated genes interrogated in those series.

follicular lymphoma.[2,3] These cases may occur as a relapse or may be detected at diagnosis simultaneously with the small-cell lymphoma component. A clonal relationship may be confirmed either by IGHV rearrangement analysis or the identification of similar genetic alterations in both components. These cases are similar to conventional PBL, but immunodeficiency does not seem to play a role, and EBV infection or *MYC* translocation are only rarely seen.[3]

ALK-POSITIVE LARGE B-CELL LYMPHOMA

Definition

ALK-positive large B-cell lymphoma (ALK-positive LBCL) was initially described by Delsol and colleagues in 1997[32] as an uncommon and aggressive subtype of DLBCL with frequent immunoblastic morphology that expressed a plasma cell immunophenotype and the ALK protein.

Synonyms

None.

Epidemiology

This tumor is very uncommon (<1% of DLBCLs) and occurs predominantly in young adults (median age approximately 40 years) but may present in patients with a broad range of age (9 to 90 years). Around 30% of these lymphomas are diagnosed in childhood. The male-to-female ratio is 5:1.[1,33]

Clinical Features

Most patients present with generalized lymphadenopathy, although occasional cases have been reported in extranodal sites including the nasal cavity, gastrointestinal tract, liver, spleen, soft tissues, skin, and bone. There is no association with immunosuppression. Bone marrow may be infiltrated in 33% of cases. The majority of patients (61%) have high-stage (III to IV) disease. The evolution is aggressive, and the outcome poor, with around half of the patients dying within the first year after diagnosis. Five-year overall survival is only 28%. Patients presenting with localized disease (stage I to II) had a significantly longer survival.[33]

Pathology

The tumor is composed of a diffuse and very monotonous proliferation of large cells with immunoblastic or plasmablastic appearance. The nuclei are vesicular and usually have a large central nucleolus. The cytoplasm is abundant and basophilic. Multinucleated cells may be present (Fig. 24-7). The lymph nodes are usually massively infiltrated, and a more or less prominent sinusoidal growth pattern is seen in most cases (Fig. 24-8). The tumor cells may appear very cohesive and thus may be misinterpreted as carcinoma cells. Focal necrosis can be seen.[34]

These cells are negative or only occasionally positive in very few cells for the mature B-cell markers CD20, CD79, and PAX5. However, they express CD45 (80%), although usually weak, EMA (100%), IRF4 (73%), and kappa or lambda light chain (90%), most often associated with IgA (Fig. 25-7).[34] The plasma cell–related antigens CD138, BLIMP1, and XBP1 are diffusely expressed in virtually all cases (Fig. 24-7). CD30 is usually negative or only weak and focal (6%). CD4 expression may be seen in 40% of tumors and CD57 in some cases. Other T-cell markers are negative. Cytokeratin expression has rarely been described, adding to the possible confusion with metastatic carcinoma,

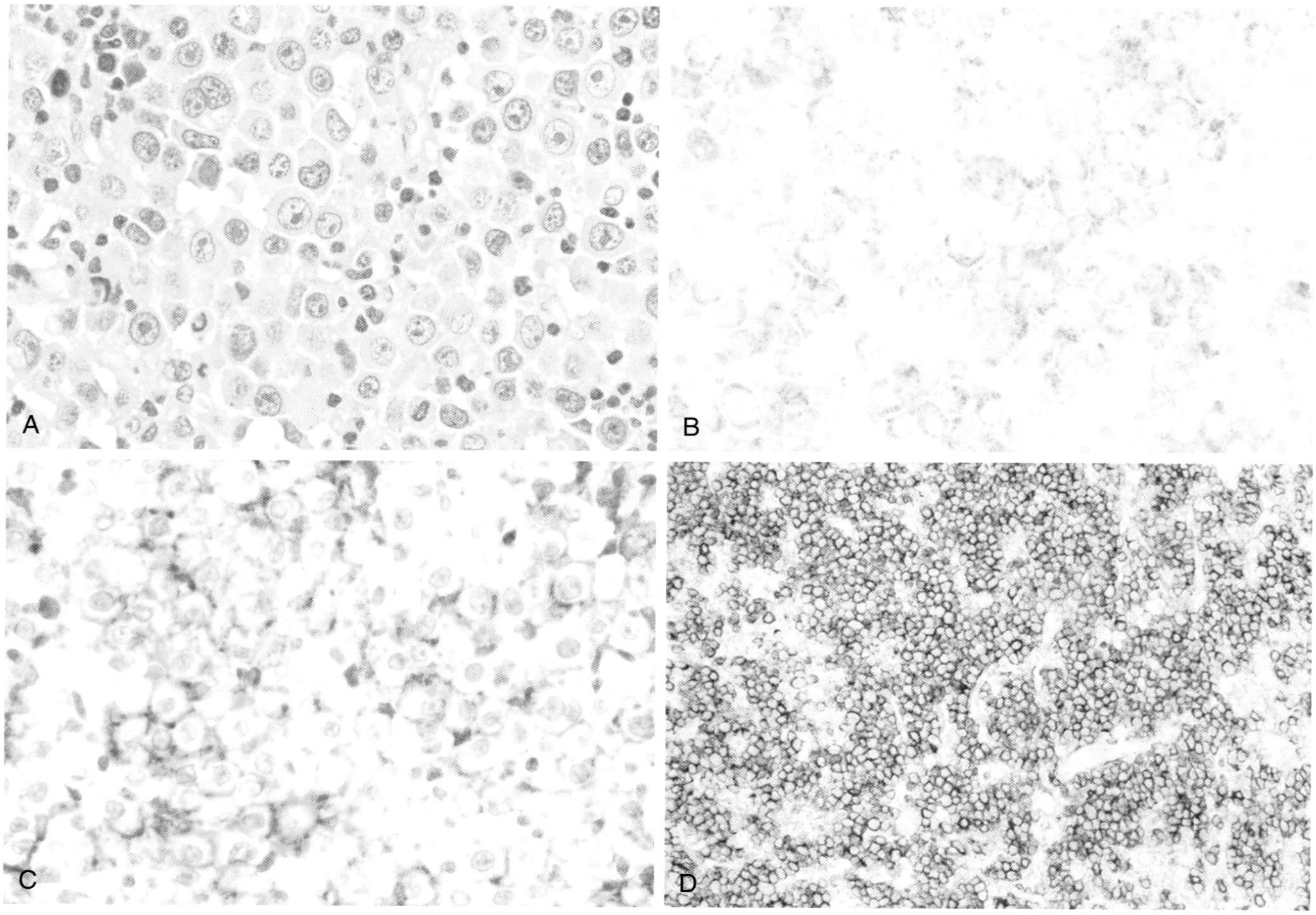

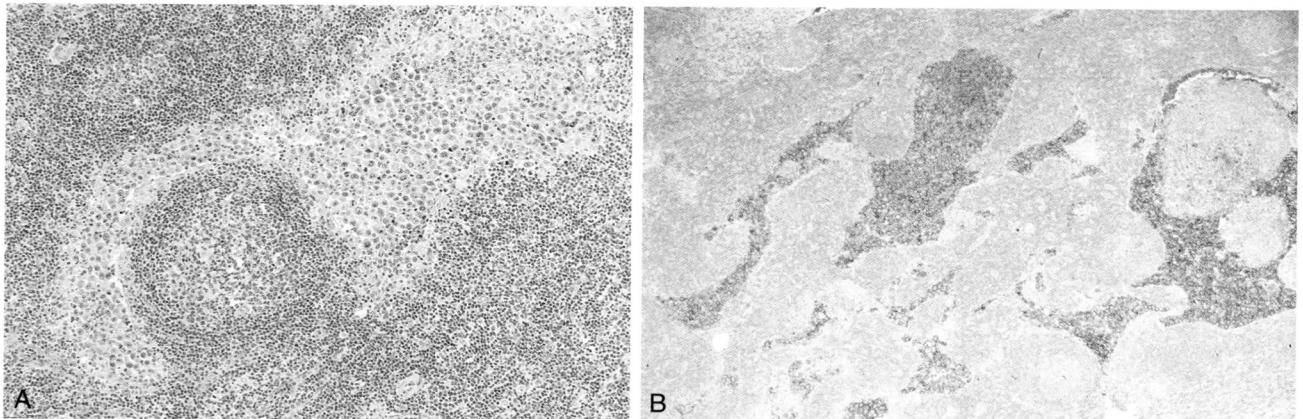

Figure 24-7. **ALK-positive large B-cell lymphoma. A,** This tumor is composed of large cohesive cells with immunoblastic features. **B,** ALK is expressed with a granular cytoplasmic pattern suggestive of the t(2;17)(p23;q23) translocation, which leads to the fusion of *ALK* with *CLTC* (clathrin). **C,** The plasma cell–associated marker CD138 is expressed in tumor cells. **D,** Epithelial membrane antigen is strongly positive in tumor cells.

Figure 24-8. **ALK-positive large B-cell lymphoma. A,** Sinusoidal infiltration. **B,** Epithelial membrane antigen expression in intrasinusoidal tumor cells. *(Courtesy NL Harris)*

especially in combination with EMA positivity.[35] All cases are EBV and HHV-8 negative.[34]

By definition, this lymphoma expresses ALK, with staining frequently confined to the cytoplasm with a granular pattern that is associated with the *ALK-CLTC* (clathrin) translocation (Fig.

24-7). In cases with the *ALK-NPM* translocation, ALK staining is nuclear and cytoplasmic. Homogeneous cytoplasmic staining may be seen with other less common *ALK* translocations. These different immunohistochemical ALK patterns result from the normal distribution of the fusion partner protein. Thus, clathrin

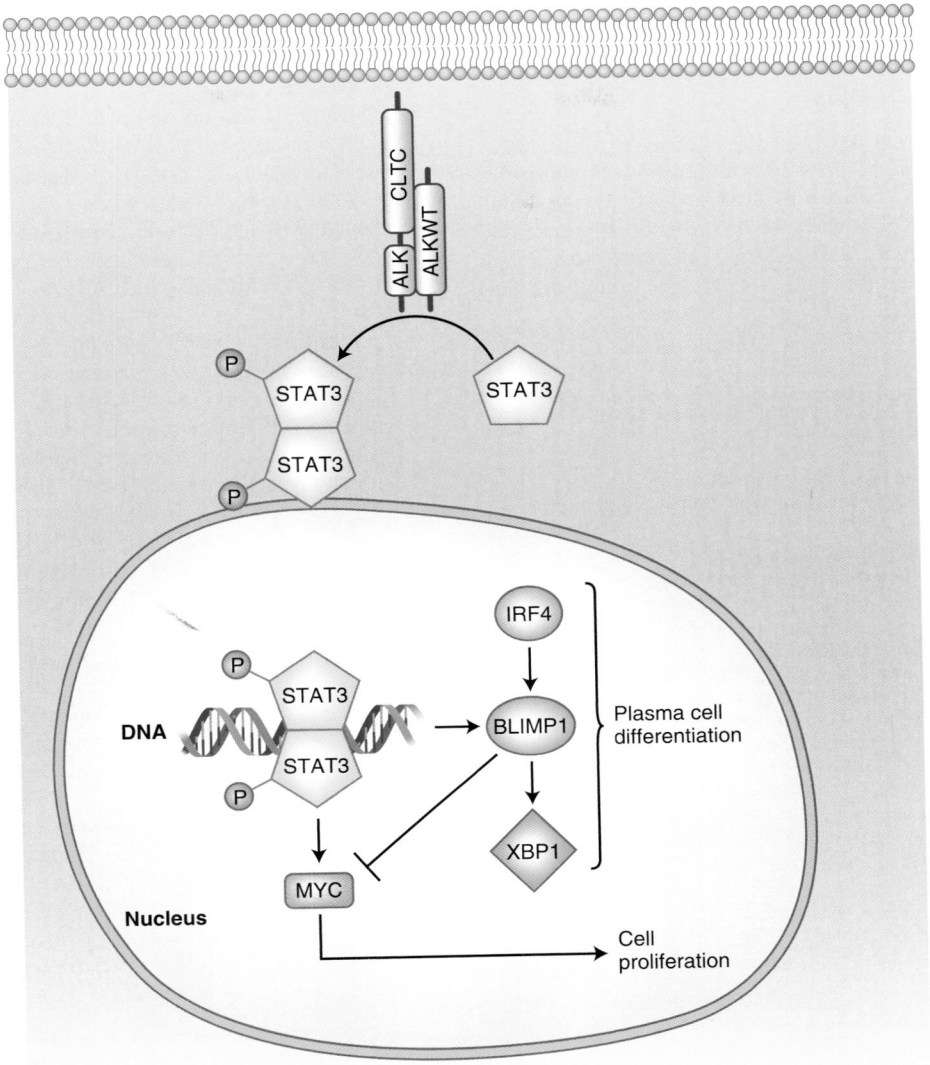

Figure 24-9. ALK-positive large B-cell lymphoma pathogenesis. ALK expression in these lymphomas is activated by translocations that, in turn, activate STAT3. A downstream effector of STAT3 is BLIMP1, which promotes the plasma cell differentiation process, and MYC, which is normally repressed by BLIMP1. MYC is also expressed in ALK-positive large B-cell lymphoma pathogenesis in the absence of gene translocations or amplifications.

is a protein of the membrane of cytoplasmic vesicles, whereas NPM shuttles proteins between the cytoplasm and nucleus.[34]

Genetic Features

These tumors are genetically characterized by *ALK* translocations that activate gene expression. The most common is the t(2;17)(p23;q23) translocation, which leads to fusion of *CLTC* (clathrin) with *ALK*.[36,37] Rare cases with the t(2;5)(p23;q35) (*NPM-ALK*) translocation have also been reported.[38,39] Other uncommon fused genes to *ALK* are *SQSTM1, SEC31A,* and others.[34,40-43] These translocations are detected in the context of complex karyotypes.

ALK is a tyrosine kinase receptor that is not normally expressed in B lymphocytes or T lymphocytes. *ALK*

rearrangements upregulate the expression of oncogenic fusion genes, in which the ALK fragment contains the catalytic domain and the fused partner provides a dimerization domain that activates the receptor without the need of the ligand. ALK oncogenic mechanisms include activation of the STAT3 pathway and, concordant with these experimental observations, ALK-positive LBCLs express high phospho-STAT3.[40] A downstream effector of STAT3 is BLIMP1, which promotes the plasma cell differentiation process, and it is also always expressed in these tumors. On the other hand, STAT3 also upregulates MYC, which is normally repressed by BLIMP1. Concordant with these mechanisms, MYC is also expressed in ALK-positive LBCL in the absence of gene translocations or amplifications (Fig. 24-9).[40] Experimental studies in a murine model have shown that forced expression of ALK in B cells generates large B-cell tumors with plasmablastic features that may correspond to an experimental counterpart of this human tumor.[44]

Differential Diagnosis

ALK-positive LBCL should be distinguished from ALK-positive anaplastic large-cell lymphoma (of T-cell/null-cell phenotype), PBL, and DLBCL-NOS with a sinusoidal growth pattern. The cohesive pattern of the cells, sinusoidal infiltration, lack of mature B-cell markers, and occasional expression of cytokeratins may raise the diagnosis of melanoma or carcinoma.

Pearls and Pitfalls

- B-cell lymphomas with large-cell morphology and expressing plasma cell markers encompass a diverse group of entities. Differential diagnosis requires a combination of pathologic and clinical information and the detection of specific markers such as EBV, HHV-8, or ALK. The mutational profile may assist in the differential diagnosis.

- PBL is frequently associated with a background of immunodeficiency caused by different mechanisms, but it can also be detected in apparently immunocompetent patients, usually of advanced age.

- The differential diagnosis between PBLs and plasma cell neoplasms with anaplastic/plasmablastic features relies on the clinical history of immunodeficiency, previous evidence of other manifestations of plasma cell tumors, or EBV infection. The different mutational profile may also orient the differential diagnosis. However, there are cases with overlapping features, and a clear distinction is not always possible.

- DLBCL with morphologic plasma cell differentiation and expression of mature B-cell markers such as CD20 or PAX5 and strong cytoplasmic immunoglobulin expression should not be considered PBL.

- ALK-positive LBCL should be considered in the differential diagnosis of large-cell tumor with sinusoidal infiltration in a lymph node in the absence of a clear primary solid tumor.

KEY REFERENCES

5. Castillo JJ, Bibas M, Miranda RN. The biology and treatment of plasmablastic lymphoma. *Blood*. 2015;125:2323–2330.
7. Colomo L, Loong F, Rives S, et al. Diffuse large B-cell lymphomas with plasmablastic differentiation represent a heterogeneous group of disease entities. *Am J Surg Pathol*. 2004;28:736–747.
8. Morscio J, Dierickx D, Nijs J, et al. Clinicopathologic comparison of plasmablastic lymphoma in HIV-positive, immunocompetent, and posttransplant patients: single-center series of 25 cases and meta-analysis of 277 reported cases. *Am J Surg Pathol*. 2014;38:875–886.
12. Montes-Moreno S, Gonzalez-Medina AR, Rodriguez-Pinilla SM, et al. Aggressive large B-cell lymphoma with plasma cell differentiation: immunohistochemical characterization of plasmablastic lymphoma and diffuse large B-cell lymphoma with partial plasmablastic phenotype. *Haematologica*. 2010;95:1342–1349.
18. Ramis-Zaldivar JE, Gonzalez-Farre b, Nicolae A, et al. MAPK and JAK-STAT pathways dysregulation in plasmablastic lymphoma. *Haematologica*. 2021;106:2682–2693.
19. Valera A, Balagué O, Colomo L, et al. IG/MYC rearrangements are the main cytogenetic alteration in plasmablastic lymphomas. *Am J Surg Pathol*. 2010;34:1686–1694.
20. Ott G, Rosenwald A, Campo E. Understanding MYC-driven aggressive B-cell lymphomas: pathogenesis and classification. *Blood*. 2013;122:3884–3891.
33. Chen BJ, Chuang SS. Lymphoid neoplasms with plasmablastic differentiation: a comprehensive review and diagnostic approaches. *Adv Anat Pathol*. 2020;27:61–74.
34. Laurent C, Do C, Gascoyne RD, Lamant L, et al. Anaplastic lymphoma kinase-positive diffuse large B-cell lymphoma: a rare clinicopathologic entity with poor prognosis. *J Clin Oncol*. 2009;27:4211–4216.

Visit Elsevier eBooks+ for the complete set of references.

Plasma Cell Neoplasms

Michael A. Linden and Robert B. Lorsbach

CLASSIFICATION OF PLASMA CELL NEOPLASMS

Definition

Plasma cell neoplasms (PCNs) and related disorders are clonal proliferations of immunoglobulin (Ig)-producing plasma cells (PCs) or lymphocytes that make and secrete a single class of Ig or a polypeptide subunit of a single Ig that is usually detectable as a monoclonal protein (M protein) by serum or urine protein electrophoresis. These immunosecretory disorders may consist exclusively of PCs or a mixture of PCs and lymphocytes. The latter are generally categorized as lymphomas and are discussed elsewhere in this book. PCNs are the subject of this chapter. Most of these are bone marrow–based neoplasms, but they occasionally develop in extramedullary sites.

Classification

The categories of PCNs recognized in the published International Consensus Classification (ICC) and the proposed 5th edition of the World Health Organization (WHO) Classification of Tumours of Haematopoietic and Lymphoid Tissues are indicated in Boxes 25-1 and 25-2, respectively.[1,2] ICC nomenclature will be used in this chapter.

PATHOGENESIS OF PLASMA CELL NEOPLASMS

Clinical studies in the 1970s led to the proposal of a pathogenetic pathway in which multiple myeloma (MM) evolves from the precursor state, monoclonal gammopathy of undetermined significance (MGUS), with progression to a "smoldering" phase, ultimately culminating in development of symptomatic MM and necessitating therapeutic intervention.[3] Disease progression of MGUS occurs at a low frequency in affected individuals, whereas some 10% of patients with smoldering MM (SMM) progress each year to symptomatic disease. MGUS was established as an obligatory precursor state in MM through the retrospective analyses of biorepository samples, which confirmed the presence of serum M protein years prior to the development of clinically overt disease in virtually all patients with MM.[4,5]

Box 25-1 *International Consensus Classification of Plasma Cell Neoplasms*

- Monoclonal gammopathy of undetermined significance (MGUS)
  - Non-IgM MGUS
  - IgM MGUS, plasma cell type
- Multiple myeloma (plasma cell myeloma)
  - Multiple myeloma, not otherwise specified (NOS)
  - Multiple myeloma with recurrent genetic abnormality
- Multiple myeloma with *CCND* family translocation
- Multiple myeloma with *MAF* family translocation
- Multiple myeloma with *NSD2* translocation
- Multiple myeloma with hyperdiploidy
- Solitary bone plasmacytoma (SBP)
  - SBP without bone marrow involvement
  - SBP with minimal bone marrow involvement (<10%)
- Solitary extraosseous plasmacytoma
- Monoclonal immunoglobulin deposition diseases
  - Immunoglobulin light chain amyloidosis (AL)
  - Localized AL amyloidosis
  - Light chain and heavy chain deposition

Box 25-2 *World Health Organization Classification (Proposed 5th Edition) of Plasma Cell Neoplasms*

Monoclonal Gammopathies
- Cold agglutinin disease
- IgM monoclonal gammopathy of undetermined significance (MGUS)
- Non-IgM MGUS
- Monoclonal gammopathy of renal significance

Plasma Cell Neoplasms
- Plasma cell myeloma
- Solitary plasmacytoma of bone (SPB)
  - SBP without bone marrow involvement
  - SBP with minimal bone marrow involvement (<10%)
- Extramedullary plasmacytoma (EMP)
- Plasma cell neoplasms with associated paraneoplastic syndrome
  - POEMS syndrome
  - TEMPI syndrome
  - AESOP syndrome

Diseases With Monoclonal Immunoglobulin Deposition
- Immunoglobulin-related (AL) amyloidosis
- Localized AL amyloidosis
- Monoclonal immunoglobulin deposition disease

Heavy Chain Diseases
- μ heavy chain disease
- γ heavy chain disease
- α heavy chain disease

Table 25-1 Frequency of Genetic Subtypes of Multiple Myeloma (MM)

Subtype	Frequency (%)
MM, not otherwise specified	**10**
MM with recurrent genetic abnormality	**90**
MM with CCND family translocation	20
t(11;14) *CCND1::IGH*	16
t(12;14) *CCND2::IGH*	Rare
t(6;14) *CCND3::IGH*	4
MM with *MAF* family translocation	**8**
t(14;16) *IGH::MAF*	4
t(8;14) *MAFA::IGH*	1
t(14;20) *IGH::MAFB*	2
MM with *NSD2* translocation t(4;14)	**14**
MM with hyperdiploidy	**45**

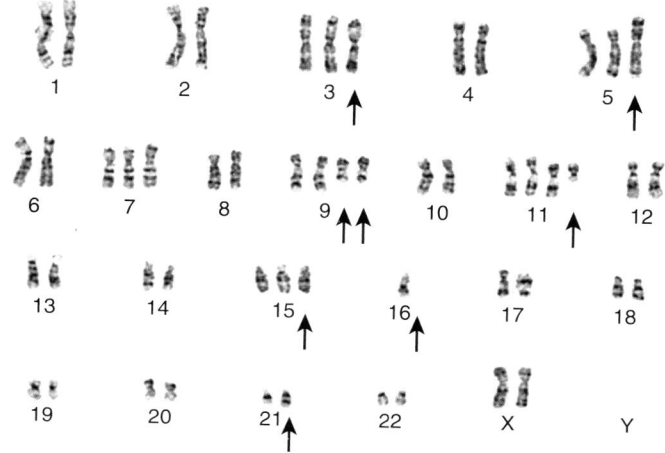

Figure 25-1. Metaphase cytogenetic analysis of hyperdiploid multiple myeloma (MM). There are gains of multiple odd-numbered chromosomes (3, 5, 7, 9, 11, and 15), characteristic karyotypic findings in hyperdiploid MM; other abnormalities are present as well, including t(5;9)(p14;q21), +add(11)(q13), and loss of chromosome 16. *(Courtesy Dr. Teresa Smolarek.)*

The genetics of PC neoplasms have been extensively studied in the past 2 to 3 decades, and the overarching pathogenetic feature that has emerged is that of progressive genomic instability. The initiating genetic lesions, mostly identified using conventional cytogenetic approaches, define two major subtypes of MM, namely hyperdiploidy and Ig heavy chain (IGH) gene translocation-associated (Table 25-1).[6-8] The hyperdiploid group accounts for about 60% of cases and is characterized by trisomies of odd-numbered chromosomes: 3, 5, 7, 9, 11, 15, 19 and 21 (Fig. 25-1).[6,9-11] The *IGH* translocation group in which the IGH locus on chromosome 14q32 is targeted accounts for 40% of myelomas. *IGH* translocations have been identified that target one of several recurrent partner genes, including the cyclin D genes (*CCND1*, 11q13, 15% of cases; *CCND2*, 12p13, <1% of cases; and *CCND3*, 6p21, 2% of cases); *NSD2/FGFR3* (4p16.3, 15% of cases); and *MAF* genes (*CMAF*, 16q23, 5% of cases; *MAFB*, 20q11, 2% of cases; and *MAFA*, 8q24, <1% of cases).[6,8,11-13] Hyperdiploidy and *IGH* translocations are largely mutually exclusive, but some hyperdiploid cases do harbor secondary nonrecurrent translocations involving 14q32. Because they are initiating genetic lesions, hyperdiploidy and *IGH* translocations are detected in both MGUS and MM. The MM subtypes defined by these cytogenetic abnormalities have subsequently been confirmed as distinctive entities through gene expression profiling (GEP) and other genetic analyses.[14,15]

Overexpression of one of the cyclin D genes (*CCND1*, *CCND2*, *CCND3*) is the unifying feature of MM, irrespective of the initiating genetic lesion.[7,8] In MMs harboring the t(11;14), dysregulation is a direct consequence of proximity of *CCND1* to the IGH enhancer, whereas in other subtypes such as those involving *NSD2/FGFR3* or *MAF* loci, which have a high level of *CCND2* expression, upregulation of cyclin D gene expression is indirect. Hyperdiploid myelomas with trisomy, or less commonly, tetrasomy 11, overexpress *CCND1* or *CCND1* and *CCND2*.

Since the identification of these initiating genetic lesions, major strides have been made toward a more comprehensive understanding of the origin of MM and the genetic basis for disease progression. Several secondary genetic lesions are associated with disease progression, including deletion or mutation of *TP53* (17p13), IGH or Ig light chain (IGL) gene translocations, *MYC* or *MYCN* translocations, chromosome 1p deletion or 1q amplification, inactivation of *CDKN2C* or *RB1*, and activating mutations of *KRAS* or *NRAS*.[16] Some of these mutations, e.g., *TP53* deletion and 1q21 amplification, are incorporated into currently used clinical risk stratification schema.[17,18] Because their presence is indicative of disease progression, most of these genetic lesions are significantly less common in MGUS than in symptomatic MM. For example, *KRAS* and *NRAS* mutations are detected in 30% to 40% of myelomas but only in about 5% of MGUSs.[8,19]

The determinants of disease progression in MGUS or SMM are incompletely understood, and risk of progression is influenced by several factors, including family history, gender, ethnicity, age, and tumor burden. Though the risk for progression of SMM, for example, is typically estimated at approximately 10%, the actual risk for progression is not constant over time.[20] In patients newly diagnosed with SMM, some 50% will progress to symptomatic MM within the first 5 years after diagnosis. The risk of progression drops significantly thereafter, with only an additional 20% progressing after 5 to 10 years. Significantly, 25% to 30% of patients will never progress to symptomatic MM. MGUS shows similar heterogeneity in its propensity for disease progression.[21]

Various risk stratification models have been developed to identify those individuals at higher risk for disease progression. It is important to remember that these risk stratification models reflect average risk and do not indicate the actual risk for a given patient.[22] In years past, myeloma therapy was toxic and not always associated with significant improvement in survival. However, with the advent of less toxic and more effective therapies, there is now significant interest in assessing whether early therapeutic intervention before the onset of end organ damage results in improved clinical outcomes in patients with SMM, and possibly MGUS. Obviously, such preemptive therapy is predicated on the accurate identification of patients who are at high risk for disease progression. Analyses have demonstrated that significant differences exist between the spectrum and number of mutations in clonal PCs from patients with MGUS and SMM with stable disease and those who ultimately manifest disease progression, with a significantly higher mutation burden in the latter.[22,23] It is important to note that myeloma driver mutations such as *MYC* abnormalities, chromothripsis, templated insertions, and APOBEC activity were detected only in clonal PCs of patients who developed progressive disease. Though such provocative findings need to be confirmed in large, prospective clinical trials, these findings indicate that the early, prospective identification of patients with MGUS/SMM who will develop disease progression is potentially feasible.

Factors involving the bone marrow microenvironment may also play a key role in disease progression. Extracellular matrix proteins, cytokines, growth factors, and the functional consequences of interaction of bone marrow stromal cells with the neoplastic plasma cells all seem to influence the pathophysiology of myeloma.[24]

The mutation spectrum within a patient often shows significant intrapatient heterogeneity. Next-generation sequencing (NGS) analyses of paired aspirate specimens from iliac crest marrow and from focal lesions have shown that, though driver mutations are present in both paired samples, high-risk genetic abnormalities, such as *TP53* mutations or inactivation of *CDKN2C*, are often detected only in focal lesions.[25] These findings suggest that myeloma cells in physically distinct anatomic locations may pursue independent mutational trajectories, likely influenced in part by distinctive aspects of the microenvironment in which these clones evolve. Such findings add further complexity to the genetic analysis of MM and suggest that the standard sampling of routine iliac crest bone marrow may be insufficient for mutation-based prognostication in many patients with myeloma.

MULTIPLE MYELOMA

MM is a bone marrow–based, multifocal PCN usually associated with M protein in serum and/or urine.[1,2] The bone marrow is the site of origin of nearly all myelomas, and disseminated marrow involvement is typical. Other organs may be secondarily involved. The diagnosis of MM relies on the integration of clinical, morphologic, immunologic, and radiographic information. The neoplasm spans a clinical spectrum from asymptomatic to highly aggressive. The pathologic manifestations of the tissue deposition of abnormal Ig molecules are a major clinical finding in a subset of patients with myeloma.[26]

Diagnostic Criteria

The usual findings in MM are increased and abnormal bone marrow PCs or a plasmacytoma together with M protein in serum or urine. Bone lesions are frequently present. The International Myeloma Working Group (IMWG) diagnostic criteria for MM are indicated in Box 25-3.[27,28]

Epidemiology

MM (and its variants) is the predominant type of malignant immunosecretory disorder. Myeloma accounts for about 1% of malignant tumors and 10% to 15% of hematopoietic neoplasms.[29] Approximately 35,000 new cases of MM will be diagnosed in the United States in 2022, with an estimated 12,600 disease-related deaths.[30] It is more common in men than women (1.2 to 1) and occurs twice as frequently in African Americans as in Whites.[30] The risk for MM is 3.7-fold higher for individuals with a first-degree relative with the disease.[31] Myeloma is extraordinarily rare in children and is uncommon in adults younger than 35 years; the incidence increases progressively with age thereafter, with approximately 90% of cases occurring in individuals older than 50 years. The median age at diagnosis is 68 to 70 years.[29]

Clinical Features

Bone pain in the back or extremities resulting from lytic lesions or osteoporosis is the most common presenting symptom in MM.[28] In advanced cases, vertebral collapse may cause loss of height. Weakness and fatigue, often related to anemia, are common complaints. Some patients present with infections, bleeding, or symptoms related to renal failure or hypercalcemia. Rarely, neurologic manifestations caused by spinal cord compression or peripheral neuropathy are the reason for seeking medical attention.[28] MM is occasionally diagnosed in asymptomatic individuals in whom serum M protein is incidentally detected during evaluation for an unrelated medical condition. These patients often present with elevated total protein levels, which upon further investigation are the result of an M spike.

Physical findings are often non-specific or lacking. Pallor is most common, followed by organomegaly. Palpable plasmacytomas are rare, but tenderness and swelling over the site of a pathologic fracture or plasmacytoma may be encountered. Tissue masses and organomegaly caused by PC infiltration or amyloidosis are occasionally encountered. Skin lesions caused by PC infiltrates or purpura are observed in rare cases.[28]

Laboratory Findings

The diagnostic studies recommended by the IMWG for the evaluation of suspected MM are indicated in Box 25-4.[28,32,33]

The data obtained from these studies form the basis for clinicopathologic criteria for diagnosis of MM and provide important prognostic information.

Assessment of serum and urine for M protein is an essential component of the diagnostic workup of a patient with suspected MM. Capillary electrophoresis is the most commonly used methodology. M protein is evident by serum protein electrophoresis (SPE) in most patients with myeloma, although the sensitivity of detection of monoclonal free light chains (FLCs) by SPE is low (Fig. 25-2).[34] The total Ig is usually increased as a result of the M protein. However, normal polyclonal Igs are commonly decreased, and absolute hypogammaglobulinemia may be present because of the suppressed synthesis of normal serum Ig, or immunoparesis, that is common in myeloma.[29] M protein may be undetectable by SPE in cases with low levels of monoclonal Ig, as is common in IgD, IgE, and light chain (LC) myeloma; hypogammaglobulinemia may be the only abnormal SPE finding in such cases. Urine protein electrophoresis (UPE) performed on a concentrated urine specimen and Ig quantification on a 24-hour urine collection should also be obtained (Fig. 25-3). A monoclonal LC (Bence-Jones protein) is found in some patients without serum M protein. Serum and urine immunofixation electrophoresis (IFE) is the gold standard for the characterization of HCs and LCs and for detecting low-quantity M protein, as may be seen in patients with LC amyloidosis, plasmacytoma, and after treatment for myeloma (Figs. 25-2 and 25-3). IFE can detect an M protein level of 0.02 g/dL in serum and 0.004 g/dL in urine.[32] M protein is identified in the serum or urine by IFE in about 97% of myeloma cases.[29,32] Monoclonal LCs are detected in the urine in 75% of cases, the majority of which are kappa type. The presence of detectable urinary LC is a reflection, in part, of the patient's renal function, as LCs are reabsorbed in the proximal renal tubule.

The serum FLC (SFLC) immunoassay provides a highly sensitive method for detecting very small quantities of monoclonal LCs and is more sensitive than IFE.[35] The SFLC quantity and the kappa-to-lambda ratio are powerful

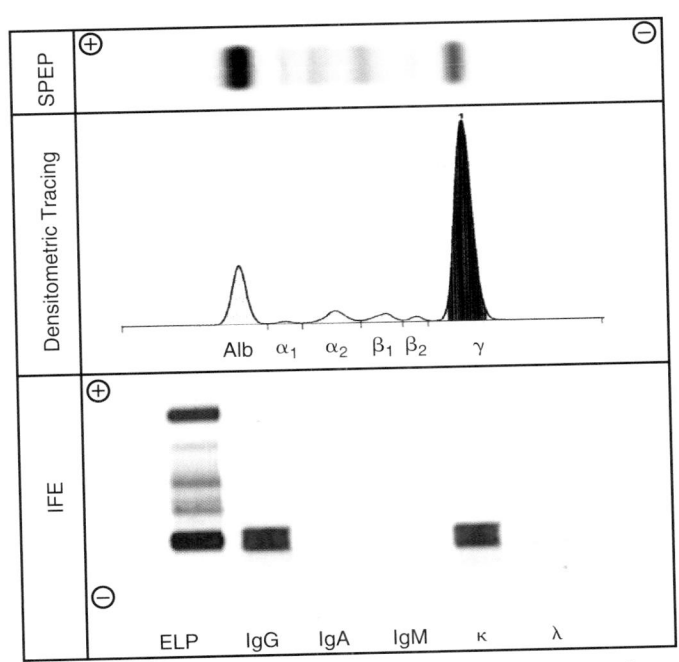

Figure 25-2. Serum electrophoreses study in multiple myeloma (MM). A single, large (8.1 g/dL) M-protein peak (shaded area 1 on densitometric tracing in middle panel) is detected by serum protein electrophoresis located in the γ region of the electrophoretogram. M protein is identified by immunofixation electrophoresis (IFE) as IgG kappa. *(Courtesy Drs. Frank H. Wians Jr. and Dennis C. Wooten.)*

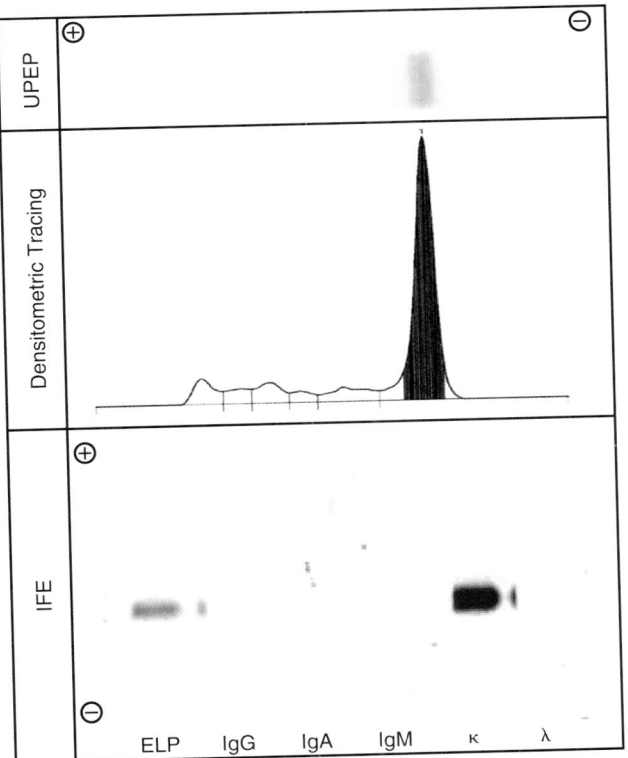

Figure 25-3. Urine protein electrophoreses in light-chain-only multiple myeloma (MM). Analysis of a concentrated 24-hour urine specimen demonstrated a single M-protein peak (140 mg/24 hr) *(shaded area 1 on densitometric tracing in middle panel)* in the γ region of the gel. M protein is identified by immunofixation electrophoresis (IFE) as free kappa light chain. No M protein is detected by serum protein electrophoresis. *(Courtesy Drs. Frank H. Wians Jr. and Dennis C. Wooten.)*

determinants of disease activity.[36] SFLC analysis is important in screening and monitoring patients with PCNs, especially oligosecretory ones such as some LC-chain-only myelomas, amyloidosis, solitary plasmacytoma, and a majority of those previously considered nonsecretory myeloma.[36-38] The baseline SFLC quantity and ratio are important indicators of prognosis for every category of PCN, including MGUS.[37] A normal SFLC ratio is a criterion of stringent complete response for treated PCNs, together with absence of M protein by IFE and absence of clonal PC in the bone marrow.[38] FLCs exist as monomers, dimers, and oligomers, with lambda FLC having a particular propensity to form higher-order complexes. Currently, several SFLC assays are commercially available, each of which uses different assay methodologies and unique antibodies for FLC detection that differ in their capacity to recognize monomeric versus dimeric forms of the FLCs.[39,40] As such, these SFLC platforms are not harmonized. Therefore, initial and subsequent clinical monitoring of SFLC levels in a given patient should be performed using the same SFLC analytic platform.[39,41]

An IgG is the most common M protein in myeloma and is detected in about 50% of cases, followed by IgA and monoclonal LC only, each present in approximately 20% of cases.[29] IgD, IgE, IgM, or biclonal M protein is present in the remaining 5% to 10% of cases. Nonsecretory myeloma, as assessed by IFE, accounts for less than 3% of cases; however, low quantities of monoclonal LC are detectable in most of these "nonsecretory" cases by SFLC analysis.[37,42] Kappa LC is more common than lambda LC for all Ig types of myeloma except IgD.[43-45] The quantity of serum M protein varies considerably from undetectable to more than 10 g/dL, with median levels of approximately 5 g/dL for IgG myeloma and 3.5 g/dL for IgA. Approximately 40% of patients with symptomatic myeloma have an M protein level less than 3 g/dL.[32] The serum M protein level may be very low or undetectable in cases of LC-only myeloma; the 24-hour urine protein is usually mildly-to-markedly elevated.

Anemia is present at diagnosis in about two-thirds of patients.[29,32] Red blood cell indices are usually normocytic and normochromic. Leukopenia and thrombocytopenia are found in less than 20% of patients but frequently worsen as the disease progresses.[29] Leukocytosis or thrombocytosis is occasionally present. The erythrocyte sedimentation rate is variably increased and roughly related to the level of M protein.

Hypercalcemia is present in approximately 20% of patients, and creatinine is elevated in 20% to 35%.[32] Hyperuricemia is detected in over 50% of patients.[29,32] Hypoalbuminemia is observed in patients with advanced disease.

Genetic Studies

Conventional karyotyping was the standard for detecting genomic abnormalities and outcome discrimination in MM for many years. This technique remains an important component of genetic assessment but has a relatively low sensitivity. Only 30% to 40% of MMs have identifiable abnormalities by karyotype analysis, due in part to the low in vitro proliferation and lack of analyzable metaphases of many myelomas and the cryptic nature of several common chromosomal rearrangements. Despite its relatively low sensitivity, conventional cytogenetic analysis should be performed at

Box 25-5 Recommended Genetic Studies for Multiple Myeloma

Fluorescence in situ hybridization (FISH) should be performed on enriched plasma cell (PC) fraction (most commonly used) or combined with cyIg staining.

Minimal FISH Panel:
- t(4;14)(p16;q32)
- t(14;16)(q32;q23)
- del(17p13) [TP53]
- chromosome 1 abnormalities (1q21 gain and 1p32 deletion)
- odd numbered chromosomes

Expanded FISH Panel:
- t(11;14)(q13;q32)
- del(13)

  Include gene expression profiling (GEP) data for risk stratification/prognostication in clinical trials.

Table 25-2 The International Myeloma Working Group (IMWG) Risk Stratification of Multiple Myeloma

Low Risk (50%)	Intermediate Risk (30%)	High Risk (20%)
ISS I/II	ISS III with no adverse FISH*	ISS II/III
No adverse FISH*	ISS I and adverse FISH*	Adverse FISH*
OS: 76% at 4 years	OS: 45% at 4 years	OS: 33% at 4 years

*Adverse FISH includes the presence of either the t(4;14) or 17p13 (TP53) deletion.
FISH, Fluorescence in situ hybridization; ISS, International Staging System; OS, overall survival.

Table 25-3 Revised International Staging System for Multiple Myeloma

R-ISS Stage I	R-ISS Stage II	R-ISS Stage III
ISS I	Not R-ISS stage I or III	ISS III
Normal LDH		
Standard risk CA by FISH*		High-risk CA by FISH, or High LDH
OS: 82% at 5 years	OS: 62% at 5 years	OS: 40% at 5 years

*High-risk CA defined as the presence of either the t(4;14), t(14;16), or 17p13 (TP53) deletion
CA, Chromosomal abnormalities; FISH, fluorescence in situ hybridization; OS, overall survival; R-ISS, revised International Staging System.

diagnosis of MM. Conventional karyotyping readily detects several complex abnormalities in MM, some of which would not be identified by fluorescence in situ hybridization (FISH) studies. For example, patients with important prognostic karyotypic changes, such as hypodiploidy, may not have FISH-defined risk abnormalities.

FISH contributes significantly to current risk stratification models for MM, and as such, should be performed in all cases at initial diagnosis (Box 25-5).[17,18,46] Because it does not depend on the in vitro proliferation of neoplastic PCs, myeloma-associated genetic alterations are readily detected by interphase FISH in more than 90% of cases. FISH also detects important cryptic genetic abnormalities, such as the t(4;14)(p16;q32) NSD2::IGH, that are undetectable by conventional karyotyping. An important technical caveat on FISH analysis is that the PC percentage in a bone marrow specimen may be below the sensitivity threshold of most FISH assays, particularly in MGUS or SMM. In such cases, FISH should be performed on samples in which the PCs have been enriched by either CD138 magnetic bead purification or flow cytometry-based cell sorting or stained for cytoplasmic Ig.[47,48]

Although gene expression profiling and other NGS-based analytic techniques with prognostic discrimination have been reported, most are not widely used in the clinical setting.

Several risk stratification schemes have been published.[46] The revised International Staging System (R-ISS) and that of the IMWG are widely used clinically (Tables 25-2 and 25-3).[17,18,46] Risk stratification in both the R-ISS and IMWG is based in part on the findings of FISH studies.[17,18]

Radiographic Studies

Radiographic skeletal surveys reveal lytic lesions, osteoporosis, or fractures in 70% to 85% of cases of myeloma at diagnosis, all of which are present in some patients.[29,32,49] The vertebrae, pelvis, skull, ribs, femur, and proximal humerus are most often affected.[50]

Computed tomography (CT) and other imaging modalities are more sensitive than the conventional skeletal survey and can detect small osteolytic lesions in areas not well visualized by conventional techniques.[33,50] Consequently, low-dose whole-body CT or FDG positron emission tomography-CT (PET-CT) is now recommended in the diagnostic workup of suspected

MM whenever possible.[33] PET-CT is superior in detection of the extent of myelomatous involvement, including soft-tissue disease.[50] The presence of multiple osseous focal lesions or extramedullary disease by PET-CT and magnetic resonance imaging (MRI) has adverse prognostic significance in patients with symptomatic myeloma.[51-53]

Blood Findings

Rouleaux formation is usually the most striking feature on blood smears and is related to the quantity and type of M protein (Fig. 25-4). Circulating nucleated red cells or a leukoerythroblastic reaction is present in some cases. PCs are found on blood smears in approximately 15% of cases, usually in small numbers. They are more commonly observed in the advanced stages of disease. Cases in which there is significant plasmacytosis may satisfy diagnostic criteria for plasma cell leukemia (discussed subsequently).

Bone Marrow Morphologic Findings

Bone marrow examination is the most important component of the diagnostic workup of MM and is nearly always required to confirm the diagnosis, even when there is substantial clinical, laboratory, and radiographic evidence to suggest a diagnosis of myeloma. Bone marrow evaluation also provides prognostic information and is useful in evaluating the response to therapy or identifying recurrent disease. Because they have complementary roles in the diagnostic workup, both a bone marrow aspirate and biopsy should be obtained if possible.

The bone marrow aspirate affords optimal evaluation of the cytologic features of the neoplastic cells and provides material for flow cytometric, cytogenetic, and molecular studies. The frequency of neoplastic PCs in the bone marrow aspirate smear is widely variable but averages about 20% to 36%.[29,54] PCs account for less than 10% of the marrow cellularity in about 5% of cases of symptomatic myeloma, which likely reflects the patchy marrow involvement that is common in MM.[32,54]

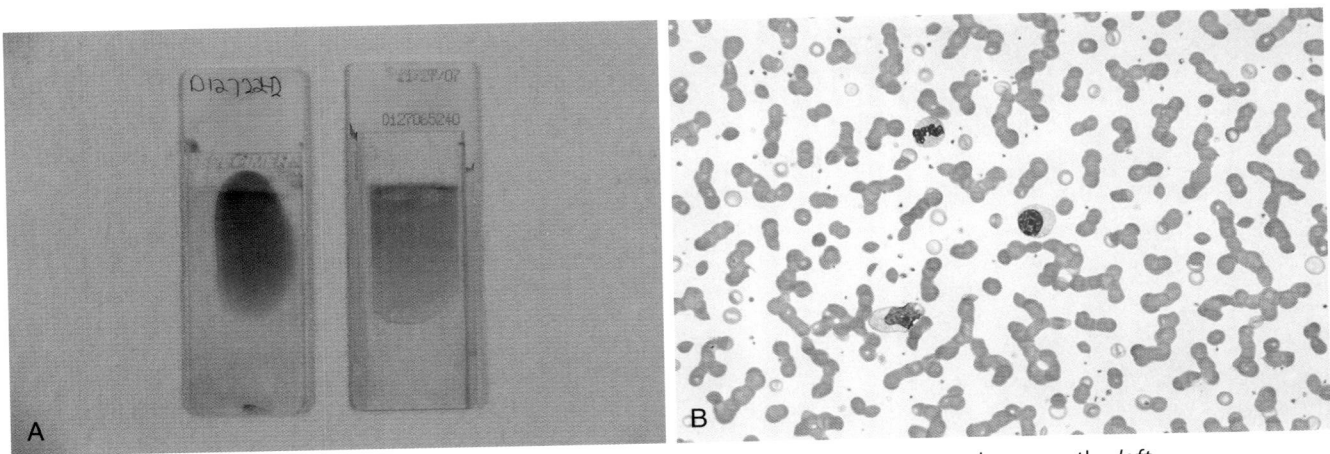

Figure 25-4. Blood smear findings in multiple myeloma (MM). A, The smear shown on the *left* is from a patient with myeloma with a large M-spike *(a normal smear is shown on the right for comparison).* The smear has a distinctly violaceous hue from the paraproteinemia and an abnormal oval shape reflecting altered spreading of red blood cells during slide preparation because of the presence of rouleaux. **B,** There is prominent rouleaux formation in this blood smear from a patient with a high M-protein level. Although rouleaux are an important diagnostic clue to an underlying plasma cell neoplasm (PCN), they may be present in other conditions, including inflammatory states (Wright-Giemsa stain).

An extreme example of this is so-called macrofocal myeloma in which the bulk of the neoplastic PCs reside within focal lesions with only low-level disease present in the intervening bone marrow, including that typically sampled by random marrow aspiration and biopsy.[55,56]

The biopsy usually provides a more accurate assessment of the extent of myelomatous marrow involvement. This is particularly true for myelomas with associated reticulin or collagen fibrosis, as neoplastic PCs are grossly underrepresented in the aspirate smear in such cases. Myelofibrosis is present in approximately 10% of cases, may be extensive, and is associated with diffuse bone marrow involvement and aggressive disease in some studies.[54,57-59] A disproportionately high number of myelofibrotic myelomas produce monoclonal LCs only.[57] Bone marrow biopsies are also useful in post-therapy evaluation, as persistent myelomatous deposits may have significant associated fibrosis. In addition, amyloid deposits and other considerations in the clinical differential diagnosis of MM, such as metastatic carcinoma or disseminated Hodgkin lymphoma, are optimally evaluated in the bone marrow biopsy.

Neoplastic myeloma cells show overt evidence of plasmacytic differentiation in most cases and do not usually pose a diagnostic challenge. Though neoplastic PCs may sometimes closely resemble their benign counterparts (Fig. 25-5), they often manifest one or more cytologic abnormalities. Benign PCs are small and contain single nuclei with smooth, round contours, peripherally clumped chromatin, and indistinct nucleoli. By contrast, neoplastic myeloma cells are often larger than benign PCs. The chromatin may be less condensed in some myelomas, and there may be distinct or prominent nucleoli (Figs. 25-6 to 25-9). Nuclear abnormalities may also be present, including nuclear lobation and convolution (Fig. 25-10).[54,60] In some cases, these cells are mixed with other easily recognizable PCs, but in other cases they make up a relatively uniform population and may be difficult to recognize as myeloma cells (Fig. 25-10).

Myelomas with atypical PC morphology may be difficult to recognize as such in bone marrow biopsies (Figs. 25-11 to 25-13).

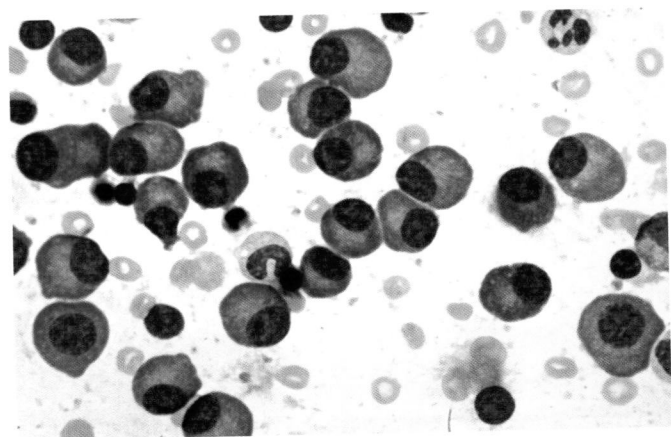

Figure 25-5. Mature-type myeloma. In this case, the myeloma cells have cytologic features approximating those of mature PCs (bone marrow aspirate; Wright-Giemsa stain). *(Courtesy Dr. Patrick C.J. Ward.)*

Myelomas with plasmablastic, lymphoplasmacytic, or anaplastic morphology are particularly problematic. Cytologic examination of the cells in the aspirate smears and immunohistochemistry (IHC) may be essential for diagnosis in these cases.

Myelomas with so-called lymphoplasmacytic morphology may be especially challenging because of their morphologic similarity to mature B-cell neoplasms such as chronic lymphocytic leukemia (CLL). In this variant, which accounts for about 5% of myelomas, the neoplastic PCs have relatively scant cytoplasm and may resemble the mature lymphocytes of CLL and low-grade lymphomas with plasmacytic differentiation (Fig. 25-14). These myelomas usually harbor t(11;14) and frequently co-express CD20 and other B-lineage antigens, including PAX5.[61-64] Positivity for CD138 and cyclin D1 by IHC readily distinguishes lymphoplasmacytic myeloma from these other low-grade B-cell lymphomas. Flow cytometry is also useful, as the myeloma cells usually lack CD19 and often express CD56, which is not seen in other B-cell lymphomas.

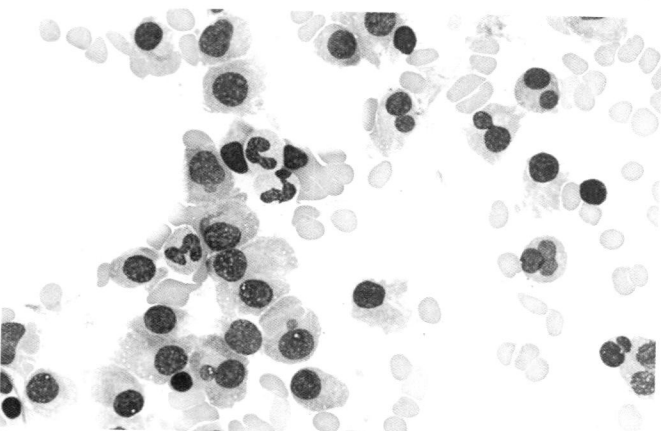

Figure 25-6. Intermediate-type myeloma. The neoplastic plasma cells exhibit features intermediate between mature and immature types of myeloma. They have moderately dispersed chromatin and occasional small nucleoli; several have lobated nuclei, and two are binucleate (bone marrow aspirate; Wright-Giemsa stain).

Various grading schemes have been proposed based on the morphologic features of the neoplastic PCs or frequency of plasmablasts in either the biopsy or aspirate, some of which were predictive of clinical outcome.[59,65-67] All of these were developed 30 to 40 years ago, and it is uncertain whether they retain any prognostic relevance with the advent of novel antimyeloma chemotherapeutics. Though myeloma grading is not mandated in the ICC, it is appropriate to make note of the presence of high-grade cytologic features in the clinical hematopathology report.

The degree of bone marrow involvement in myeloma is best assessed in the bone marrow biopsy. The pattern of the PC infiltrate may be interstitial, focal, or diffuse, and the extent of marrow involvement varies from an apparently small increase in PCs to complete replacement (Fig. 25-15).[54,59] The pattern of marrow involvement is usually directly related to the overall burden of neoplastic PCs. There is often considerable marrow sparing and preservation of normal hematopoiesis

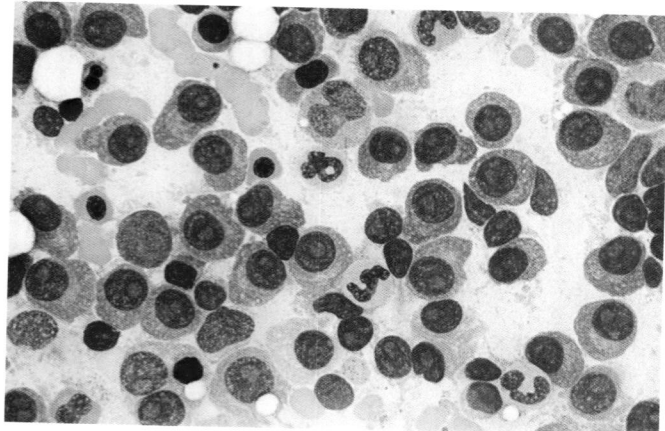

Figure 25-7. Immature-type myeloma. The neoplastic plasma cells contain prominent nucleoli and more dispersed chromatin than those in Figure 25-6. The marrow is extensively replaced with myeloma (bone marrow aspirate; Wright-Giemsa stain).

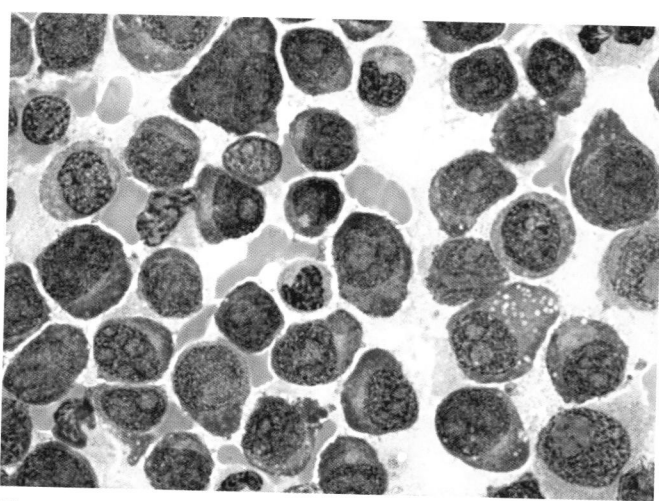

Figure 25-9. Myeloma with high-grade cytologic features. The neoplastic cells in this case are large with dispersed chromatin. Many contain prominent nucleoli and relatively scant cytoplasm, cytologic features of plasmablasts (Wright-Giemsa stain).

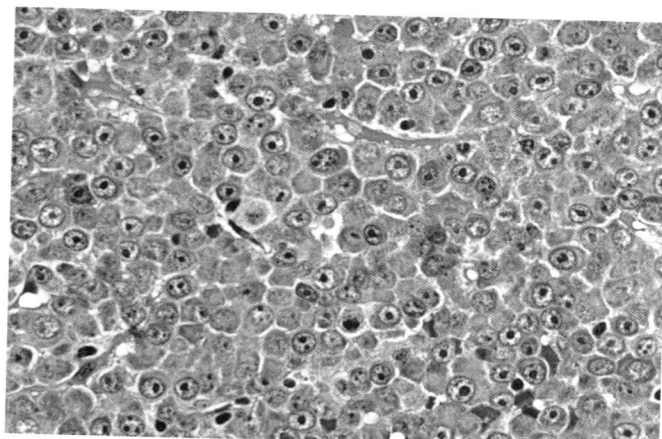

Figure 25-8. Immature-type multiple myeloma (MM). In this case, the myeloma cells are large and contain vesicular nuclei, prominent eosinophilic nucleoli, and a moderate amount of eosinophilic cytoplasm. The corresponding bone marrow aspirate smear is shown in Figure 25-7 (bone marrow biopsy; H&E stain).

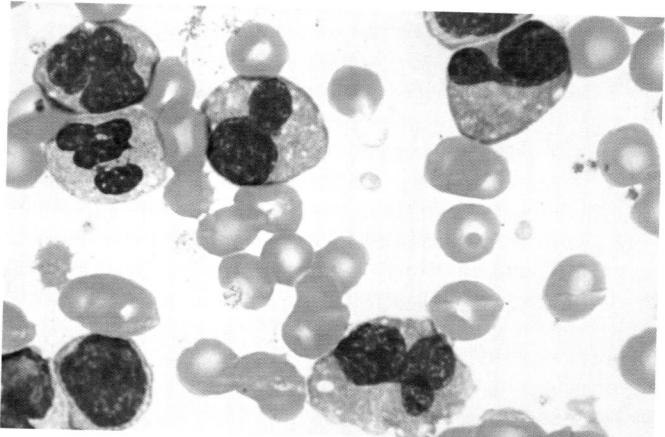

Figure 25-10. Myeloma with nuclear lobulation. Most of the neoplastic plasma cells (PCs) in this case show striking nuclear irregularity and convolution. The neoplastic cells in myelomas of this type may be difficult to recognize as PCs (bone marrow aspirate; Wright-Giemsa stain).

with interstitial and focal involvement. By contrast, diffuse involvement results in extensive replacement of the marrow and suppression of normal hematopoiesis, which may manifest as cytopenias in the complete blood count. Osteolytic lesions may develop in areas of diffuse myelomatous involvement (Fig. 25-16). There is typically progression from interstitial and focal disease in early myeloma to diffuse involvement in advanced stages of the disease.[59]

Myeloma cells may manifest one of several peculiar nuclear and cytoplasmic findings that result mostly from either the synthesis of an abnormal Ig molecule or perturbation of Ig secretion. Many of these are best appreciated in the aspirate smear. Dutcher bodies are occasionally encountered, most commonly in IgA myelomas, where they are present in about 20% of cases.[54] These are pale staining, single, and generally large nuclear pseudoinclusions that result from cytoplasmic invagination into the nucleus (Fig. 25-17).

Cytoplasmic vacuoles are commonly encountered in myeloma. The size and frequency of the vacuoles is quite variable. In some cases, single large vacuoles in myeloma cells peripherally displace the nucleus, imparting a signet ring cell appearance that may resemble that of a metastatic gastrointestinal carcinoma (Fig. 25-18). Cytoplasmic inclusions are also encountered, the most common of which are Russell bodies (Fig. 25-18). In some cases, cytoplasmic inclusions are present that impart a Gaucher cell-like appearance to the neoplastic PCs (Fig. 25-19). Myelomas containing rhomboid or needle-like cytoplasmic crystals are

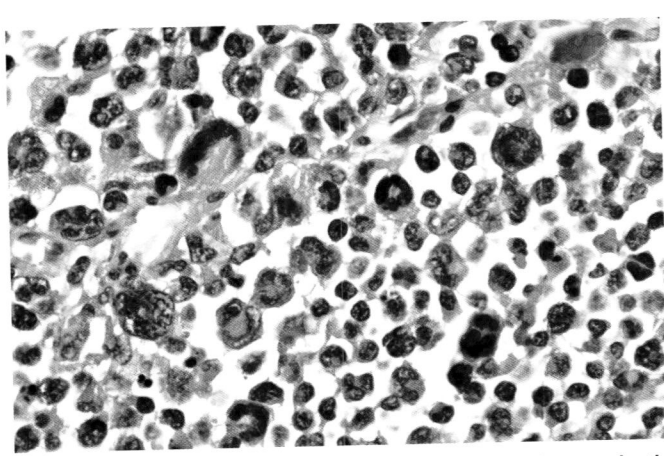

Figure 25-11. Poorly differentiated myeloma with anaplastic cells. A dense infiltrate of anaplastic neoplastic cells is present, most of which lack obvious plasmacytic differentiation. The cells were positive for CD138 kappa light chain restriction by immunohistochemistry. This type of myeloma must be differentiated from anaplastic large cell lymphoma and metastatic tumors such as anaplastic carcinoma and melanoma (bone marrow biopsy; H&E stain). *(Courtesy Dr. Patrick C.J. Ward.)*

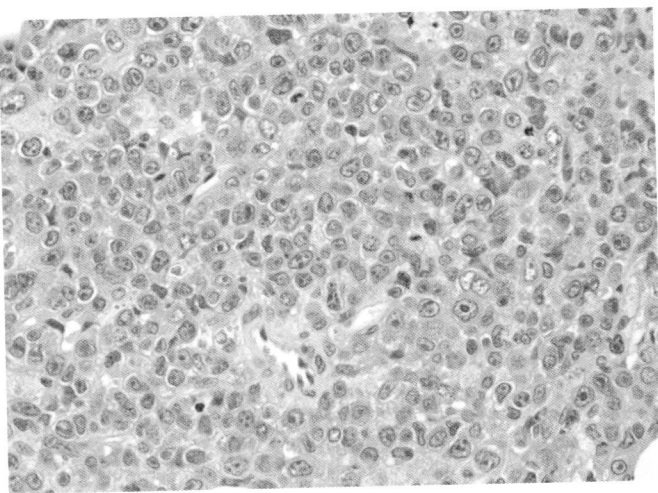

Figure 25-13. Plasmablastic-type multiple myeloma. There is heavy interstitial involvement with myeloma. The neoplastic plasma cells are poorly differentiated with a high nuclear-to-cytoplasmic ratio, dispersed chromatin, and prominent nucleoli. Such high-grade cytologic features raise a differential diagnosis that includes large cell lymphoma and small blue-cell tumors.

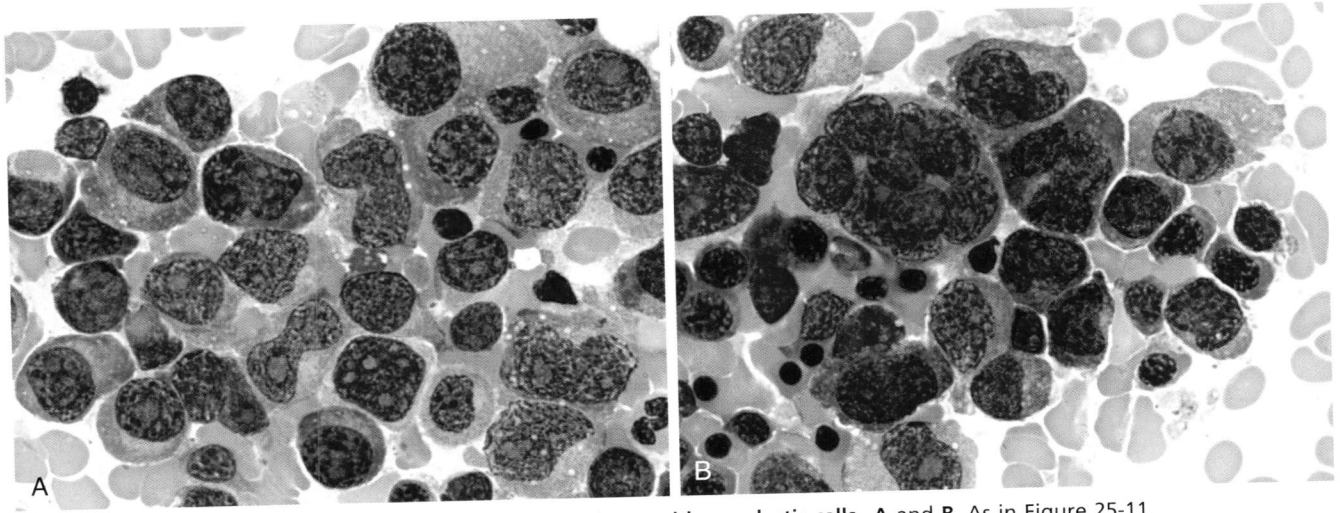

Figure 25-12. Poorly differentiated myeloma with anaplastic cells. A and **B,** As in Figure 25-11, frequent anaplastic cells are present. The plasmacytic features of the neoplastic cells in such cases are often more apparent in the aspirate than in the biopsy. Anaplastic myeloma cells should be distinguished from megakaryocytes and other malignancies (bone marrow aspirate; Wright-Giemsa stain).

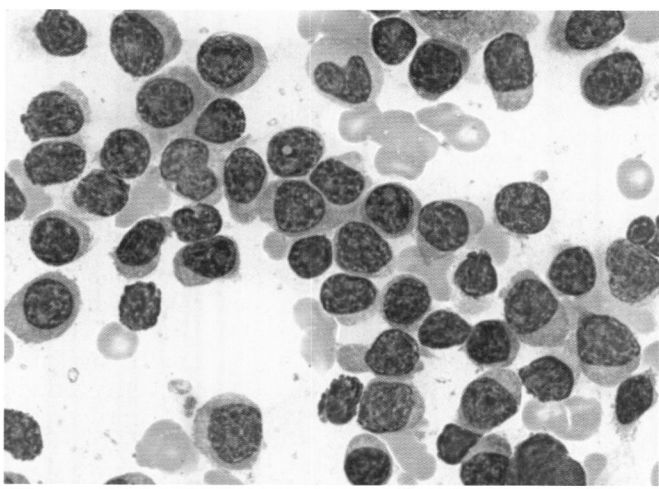

Figure 25-14. Small lymphocyte-like myeloma. The neoplastic plasma cells contain more scant cytoplasm than is typical of most myelomas, cytologically resembling plasmacytoid lymphocytes (bone marrow aspirate; Wright-Giemsa stain).

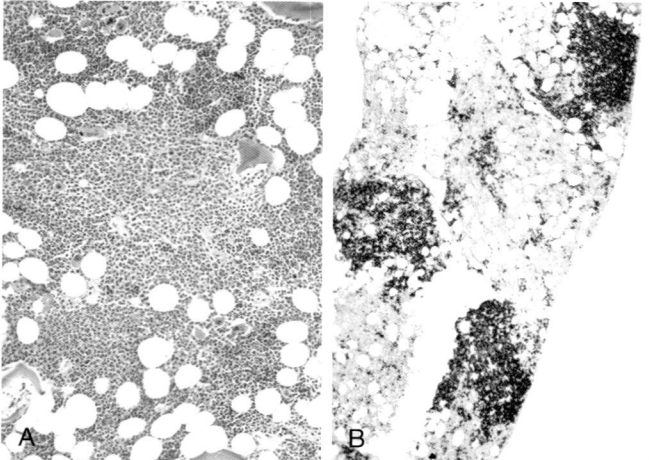

Figure 25-15. Focal bone marrow involvement by myeloma. A, Focal myeloma infiltrates are scattered throughout the bone marrow with mostly normal intervening hematopoietic tissue (H&E stain). **B,** Lambda light chain immunohistochemistry highlights the predominantly focal pattern.

rare and are predominantly kappa-LC restricted (Figs. 25-20 and 25-21). The neoplastic PCs may resemble promyelocytes when needle-like inclusions are abundant (Fig. 25-21). Inclusions may also be present in proximal tubular cells in the kidney and are associated with Fanconi syndrome.[68] Cytoplasmic crystals within clonal neoplastic PCs can be associated with corneal disease and have rarely been reported in a case of polychromatic crystalline keratopathy.[69] Crystal storing histiocytosis (CSH) is a rare reactive proliferation that may develop in association with crystal-containing myelomas and occasionally other lymphomas showing plasmacytic differentiation.[70-72] This histiocytic proliferation may be florid in some cases and obscure the underlying myeloma (Fig. 25-22). The histiocytes in CSH bear some resemblance to those of storage disorders such as Gaucher disease, although the refractile quality of the crystals in CSH is distinctive. PCs with pale, frayed, and fragmented cytoplasm and so-called flaming

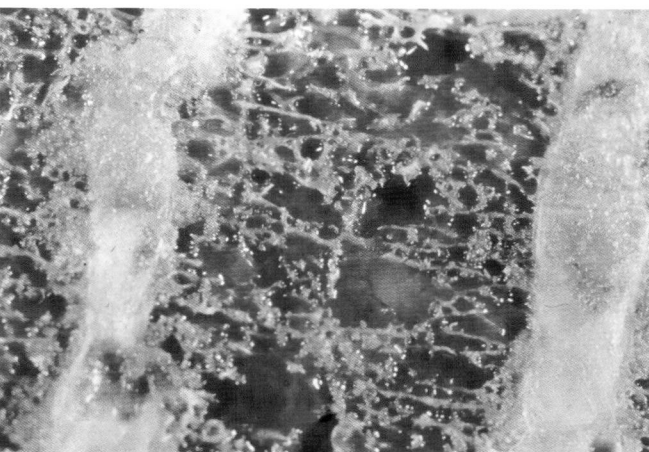

Figure 25-16. Myelomatous involvement of vertebral body. Osteolytic lesions in which there is destruction of trabecular bone are present and filled with an infiltrate of neoplastic plasma cells that has a gelatinous gross appearance.

PCs are more common in IgA myeloma (Fig. 25-23). Finally, phagocytic PCs may rarely be present in myeloma.[73,74]

Multiple Myeloma—Clinical Variants

Smoldering MM (SMM; Asymptomatic MM)

About 8% to 14% of patients with MM are asymptomatic at the time of diagnosis.[20,75] These patients have 10% or more bone marrow PCs and/or M protein at myeloma levels but lack related end-organ impairment (Box 25-3).[28,76]

The median level of serum M protein in patients with SMM is 2 g/dL, and the median bone marrow clonal PCs burden is approximately 20%.[77] Approximately 70% of patients have monoclonal LCs in urine, and polyclonal Igs are decreased in more than 80% of patients.[20,29,78] PCs are cytologically atypical in bone marrow aspirate smears, and focal aggregates of PCs, interstitial infiltration, or both are found in biopsy sections.[20]

Although most patients with SMM remain clinically stable for a long time, they are much more likely to progress to symptomatic MM than are individuals with MGUS.[20,79,80] However, the risk of progression is not static.[81] Rather, the likelihood of disease progression is highest during the first 5 years after diagnosis, approximately 10% per year. The rate of progression then drops significantly to 3% annually during the subsequent 5 to 10 years, and finally to 1% per year in patients 10 or more years out from their initial diagnosis of SMM, a rate of disease progression comparable to that of MGUS. These kinetics are a reflection of the significant heterogeneity of SMM, in which three patient groups exist, including those with MGUS-like disease, patients in whom slow progression to symptomatic MM will occur, and finally, patients whose disease is in evolution to symptomatic MM at the time of presentation with SMM and who will manifest overt disease progression in less than 2 years.[20,81] It should be noted that 25% to 30% of patients with SMM never develop symptomatic disease.

In the past, patients with SMM were rarely treated until the onset of myeloma-related symptoms, as earlier therapeutic intervention showed no clinical benefit. With

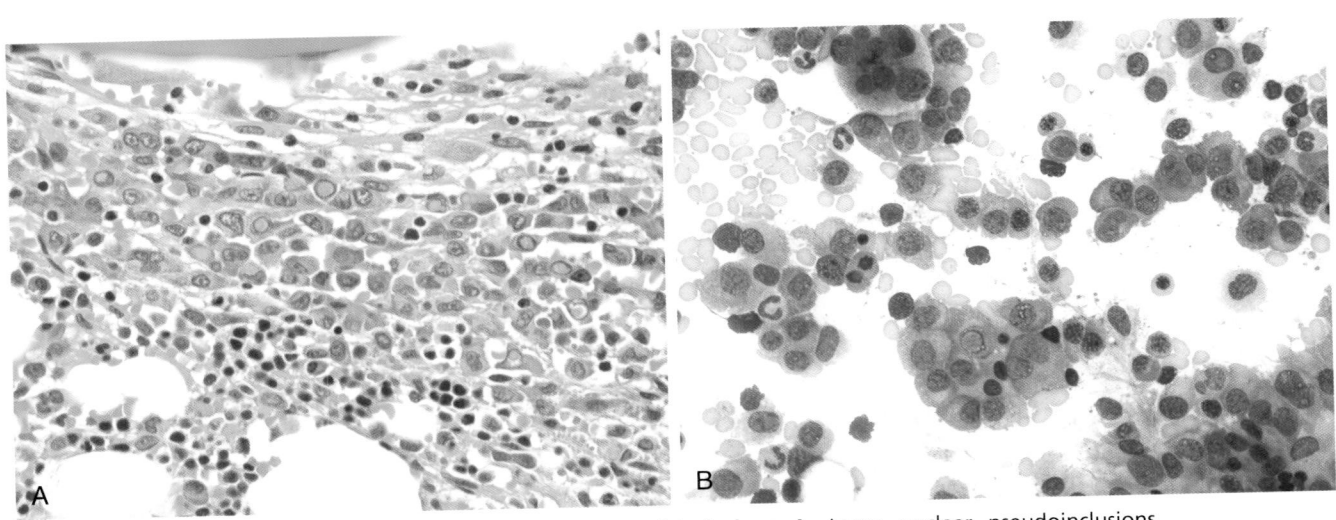

Figure 25-17. Myeloma with nuclear pseudoinclusions. A, Large nuclear pseudoinclusions (Dutcher bodies) are present in many neoplastic plasma cells. **B,** A myeloma cell containing a prominent Dutcher body (bone marrow biopsy and aspirate; H&E and Wright-Giemsa stains).

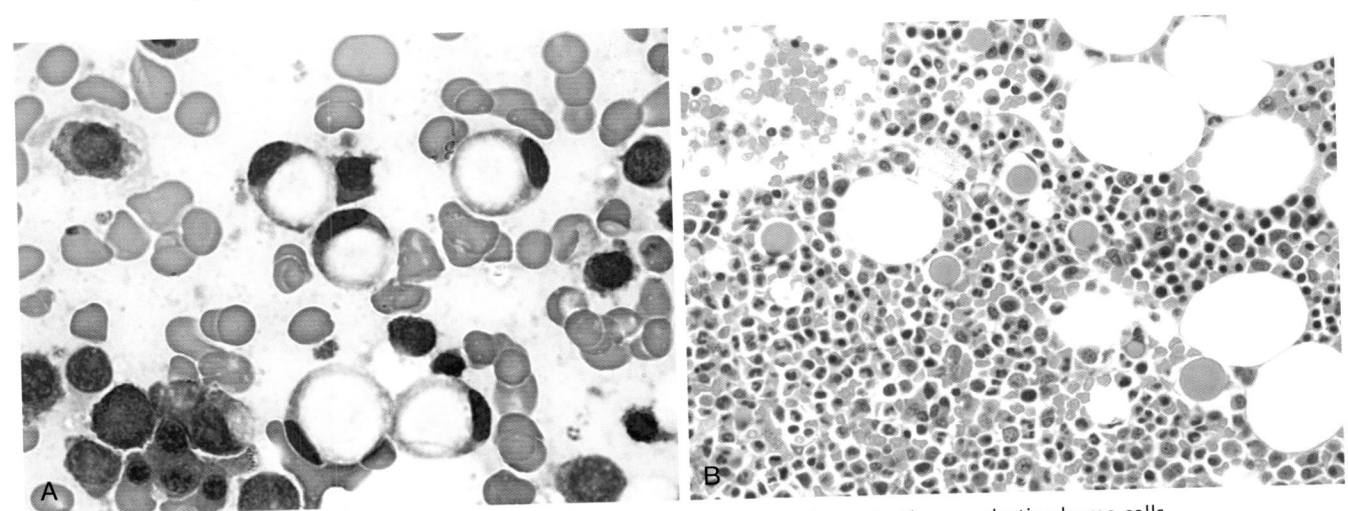

Figure 25-18. Myeloma with cytoplasmic vacuoles and inclusions. A, The neoplastic plasma cells (PCs) in this case contain single large cytoplasmic vacuoles, imparting a signet ring cell appearance. **B,** In this case, single large Russell bodies are present in several neoplastic PCs, distorting and obscuring the plasmacytic features of the cells (bone marrow aspirate and biopsy; Wright-Giemsa and H&E stains).

the advent of more effective and less toxic therapeutics, there is now considerable interest in assessing whether early therapy might improve clinical outcomes in patients with SMM who are at high risk for disease progression. Several risk stratification models have been developed that rely on various parameters, including the bone marrow PC burden, M-protein level, SFLC ratio, predominance within the PC compartment of phenotypically aberrant cells, and presence of immunoparesis.[77,82,83] Such models are imperfect, as there is low concordance among them in the identification of patients with SMM who are at high risk. Moreover, the decision to treat in the context of most clinical trials in which these models are used is made on a single, static assessment based on factors that may lack reproducibility. To date, only one clinical trial has shown improved overall survival in high-risk patients with SMM receiving therapy compared with observation alone.[84] The decision to treat otherwise asymptomatic patients is a complicated one in an overall elderly patient population.

Though less toxic than historical therapy, current myeloma therapeutics nevertheless involve toxicities and may have a significant negative effect on quality of life, to say nothing of the financial and psychological burden of preemptive treatment.[81]

Plasma Cell Leukemia (PCL)

PCL is a myeloma variant in which circulating neoplastic PCs are present in the blood. The neoplastic PCs also commonly infiltrate extramedullary sites, including liver and spleen, the central nervous system, and the pleural and peritoneal cavities. Primary PCL is, by definition, present at the time of initial diagnosis, whereas secondary cases develop during the disease course in patients with relapsed or refractory myeloma; primary PCL accounts for approximately 60% to 70% of cases.[85] Primary PCL is a distinctive type of MM with characteristic cytogenetic and molecular findings and an aggressive clinical course with short remissions and survival.[27]

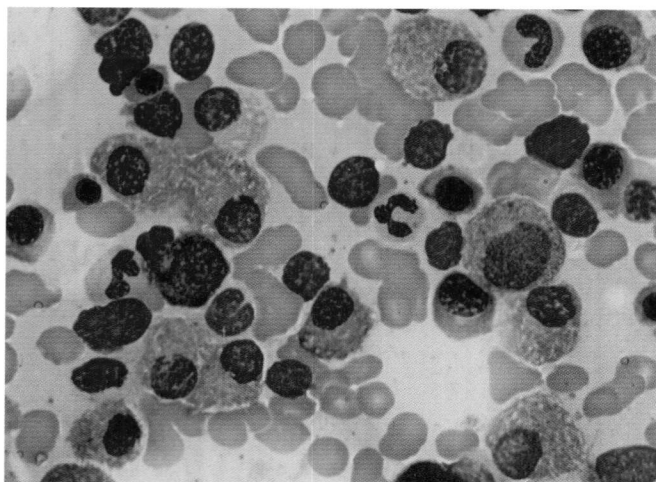

Figure 25-19. Myeloma with cytoplasmic inclusions. The neoplastic plasma cells contain abundant irregular cytoplasmic inclusions that impart an appearance reminiscent of Gaucher-type storage histiocytes (bone marrow aspirate; Wright-Giemsa stain).

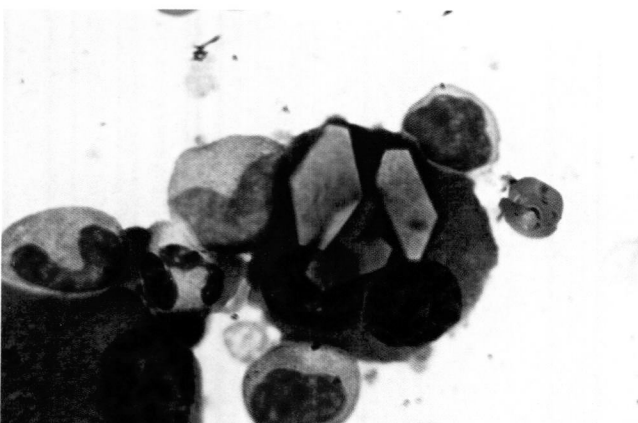

Figure 25-20. Myeloma with cytoplasmic crystals. Large binucleate plasma cell containing prominent cytoplasmic crystals (bone marrow aspirate; Wright-Giemsa stain).

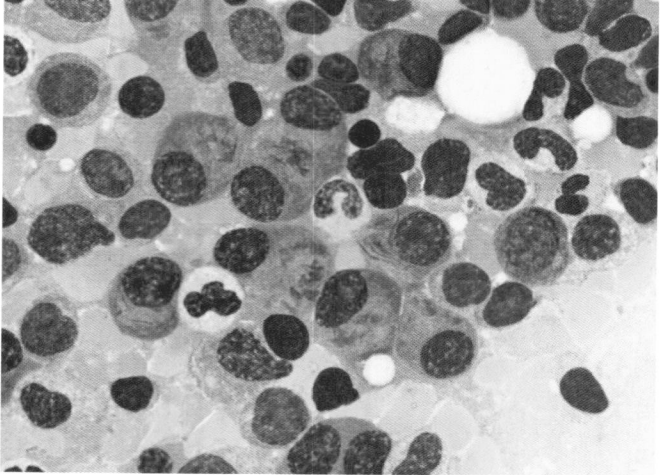

Figure 25-21. Multiple myeloma (MM) with cytoplasmic crystals. The neoplastic PCs contain abundant needle-like immunoglobulin inclusions that resemble Auer rods (bone marrow aspirate; Wright-Giemsa stain).

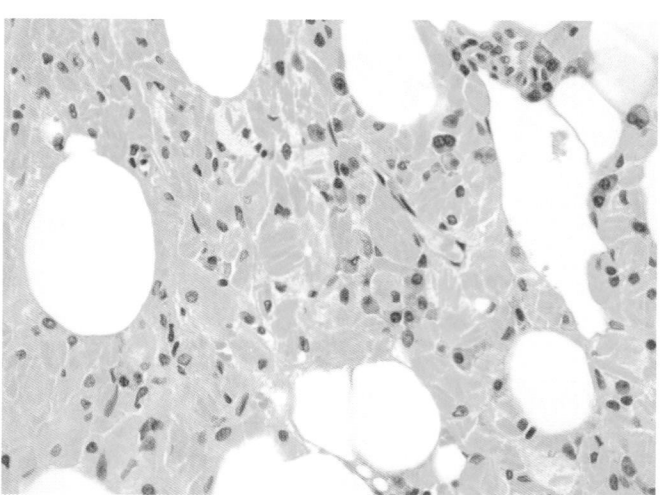

Figure 25-22. Myeloma with crystal-storing histiocytosis. In this case, much of the marrow is filled with large histiocytic cells containing refractile crystals that overshadow the admixed myeloma cells that are present singly and in small aggregates. Crystal-storing histiocytes superficially resemble storage-type histiocytes (bone marrow biopsy; H&E stain).

Primary PCL is found in approximately 2% to 4% of myeloma cases.[85-88] Secondary PCL is detected in approximately 1% of previously diagnosed MM cases.[89]

Circulating clonal PCs are detected at low levels in a significant fraction of patients with PCNs, depending on the sensitivity of the analytic methodology used. Historically, the diagnosis of primary PCL was based on the arbitrarily defined criteria of clonal PCs comprising >20% of total leukocytes or an absolute PC count $>2 \times 10^9/L$.[85] However, more recent studies indicate that the clinical outcome in patients with myeloma with significantly lower levels of circulating PCs is indistinguishable from that of patients with primary PCL.[90,91] In light of this, the IMWG now recommends that patients newly diagnosed with myeloma in whom circulating PCs account for ≥5% of leukocytes based on morphologic enumeration in the blood smear be considered primary PCL.[1,27]

Many of the same clinical and laboratory abnormalities are present in both PCL and typical myeloma. However, PCL is associated with a younger median age at diagnosis. Lymphadenopathy, organomegaly, and renal failure are significantly more common in PCL, and lytic bone lesions and bone pain are less common.[88] Anemia is present in 80% of cases and thrombocytopenia in 50%.[88] Nucleated red cells are often present in blood smears. The leukocyte count is variable but is usually elevated, sometimes markedly so. All types of M proteins have been reported in PCL; however, LC only and IgD myelomas are overrepresented among PCL cases. PCL develops in approximately 20% of IgE MM, a rarely encountered myeloma subtype.[88,92]

The cytologic spectrum of leukemic PCs is similar to that of other myelomas, although anaplastic cells are uncommon in PCL. Though the neoplastic cells typically show overt plasmacytic features, the neoplastic PCs in some cases are larger and may resemble myeloid blasts or peripheralized large cell lymphoma cells (Fig. 25-24). The most challenging are PCLs in which the neoplastic cells contain scant cytoplasm and thus resemble small lymphocytes or plasmacytoid lymphocytes. Recognition and accurate enumeration of neoplastic PCs in

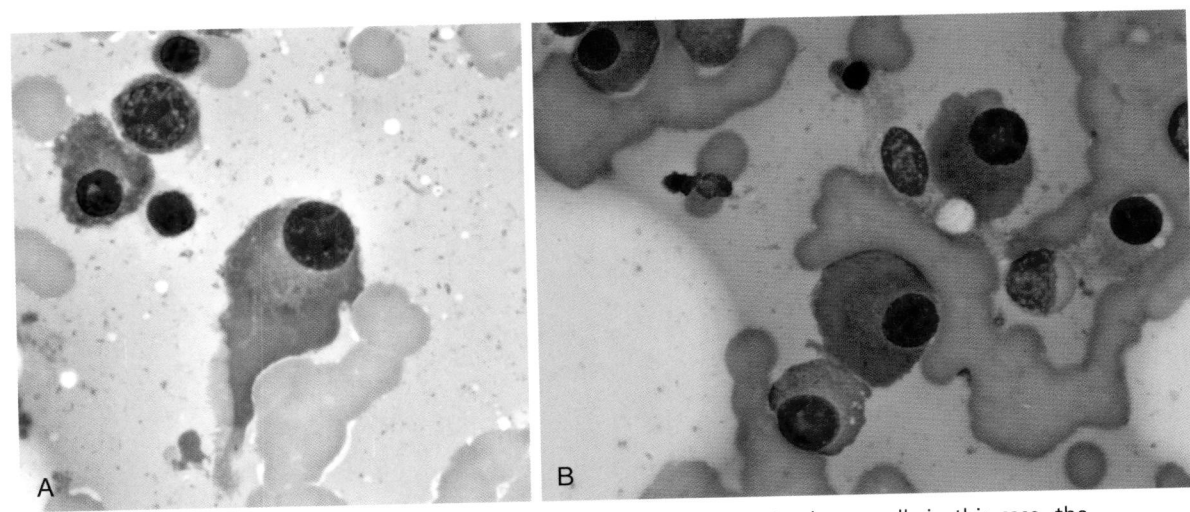

Figure 25-23. IgA myeloma. A and **B,** In many of the neoplastic plasma cells in this case, the periphery of the cytoplasm is distinctly eosinophilic. Such cells have been termed *flame cells* and are most common in IgA myeloma. This appearance is thought to reflect the higher carbohydrate content of IgA compared with other immunoglobulin (Ig) isotypes (bone marrow aspirate; Wright-Giemsa stain).

such cases may be difficult, particularly when the white blood cell count or PC frequency is low, because of their similarity to normal lymphocytes. Flow cytometry permits unequivocal distinction between PCL and CLL or peripheralized lymphoplasmacytic lymphoma (LPL) (previously discussed). Recognition of circulating PCs with variant morphology is most challenging in the initial diagnostic workup of primary PCL, when blood smear evaluation may occur prior to bone marrow examination or serum protein analysis. The presence of rouleaux provides an important clue to the underlying diagnosis.

An abnormal karyotype is more frequently obtained in PCL than in other myelomas, and there is a higher incidence of high-risk genetics in both primary and secondary PCL.[86] These include hypodiploidy, del(13q), del(17p) t(14;16), 1q amplification, and 1p losses.[86,93,94] Although usually associated with a favorable prognosis in MM, t(11;14) is overrepresented in primary PCL.[86,94]

Treatment is similar to that for other advanced myelomas. Even with the advent of therapies incorporating bortezomib and immunomodulatory agents, PCL continues to be an aggressive disease, with a poorer response to therapy and significantly shorter survival than those of typical myeloma.[27,95-97] Patients with secondary PCL have a shorter survival than those with primary PCL, 1.3 months versus 11.2 months, respectively.[94] The high frequency of unfavorable genetic abnormalities only partially explains the poor prognosis of PCL.[86,93,98]

Nonsecretory Multiple Myeloma

Nonsecretory multiple myeloma (NS-MM) is defined as MM with no evidence of M protein as assessed by serum or urine IFE analysis and accounts for about 3% of all myelomas.[29,99-102] Myelomas lacking a detectable M protein by IFE are further subdivided by some investigators using additional analytic tools.[103] Oligosecretory MM has a clonal LC detectable by SFLC analysis and accounts for approximately two-thirds of NS-MM cases.[42] SFLC-negative cases in which the clonal PCs express detectable Ig expression as assessed by IHC or intracytoplasmic staining by flow cytometry represent bona

fide NS-MM. Finally, rare SFLC-negative, Ig IHC-negative myelomas are designated as nonproducer MM.[32] Acquired mutations of the Ig LC variable genes or alteration of the constant region account for the nonsecretory state in these cases.[104,105] Patients with secretory myeloma at the time of diagnosis may occasionally become NS or oligosecretory at relapse. NS-MM should be distinguished from rare IgD and IgE myelomas that generally have low-level paraproteinemia and may not be routinely screened for by immunofixation. The cytologic and histologic features and immunophenotype of NS-MM are similar to those of other myelomas. Other than overrepresentation of t(11;14), the spectrum of genetic abnormalities in NS-MM is similar to that of typical myeloma.[101]

The clinical features of NS-MM are generally similar to those of secretory myeloma, except for a lower incidence of renal insufficiency and hypercalcemia and less suppression of normal polyclonal Ig.[29,106] The presence of osteolytic lesions, absence of an M protein, and lower incidence of renal failure in NS-MM often raises clinical suspicion of metastatic carcinoma or other solid tumor. Treatment of NS-MM is the same as that for other MMs. The effect of the NS state on clinical outcome is unclear, as studies have shown variable survival differences between patients with NS and secretory MM.[100-102] Similar to other myelomas, the prognosis of NS-MM has improved significantly in the past decade.

Differential Diagnosis

The most common differential diagnosis among the PC neoplasms is that of early myeloma versus MGUS or a reactive bone marrow plasmacytosis. In most cases, this is not difficult because the composite clinical and pathologic findings required for a diagnosis of myeloma are lacking in MGUS and in reactive PC proliferations. Only when the M protein or percentage of bone marrow PCs are at the high extreme for MGUS is the distinction from asymptomatic myeloma problematic. In some patients, differentiation of early myeloma and MGUS is not possible at the time of initial

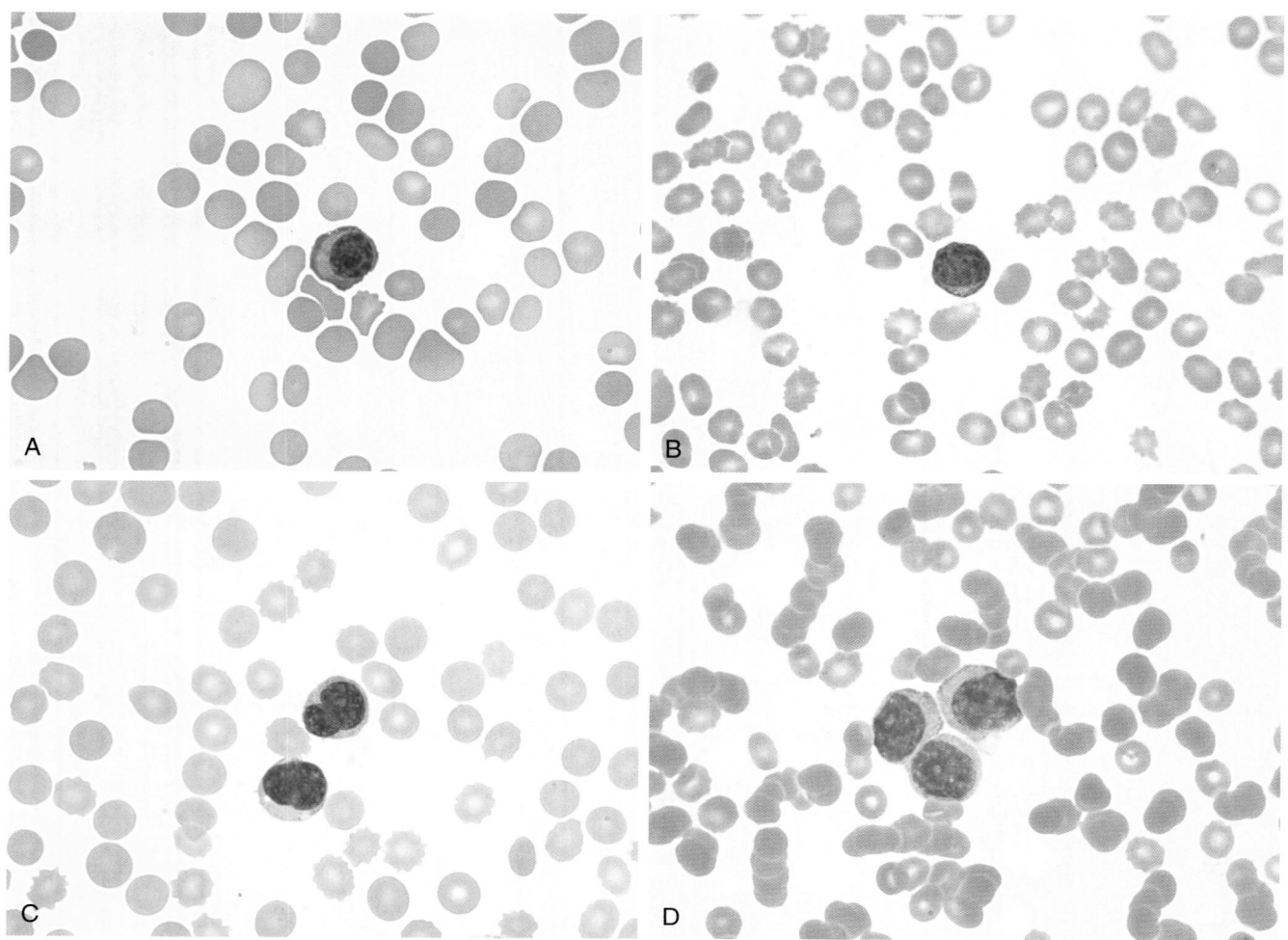

Figure 25-24. Cytologic heterogeneity in plasma cell leukemia. A, The circulating neoplastic cells usually show overt plasmacytic features. **B,** In some cases, the neoplastic cells resemble small lymphocytes with more subtle evidence of plasmacytic differentiation. Such cases may be mistaken for chronic lymphocytic leukemia or peripheralized lymphoplasmacytic lymphoma. **C,** Leukemic plasma cells (PCs) in this case show nuclear irregularity and lobation. **D,** Leukemic PCs are large, in some cases raising a differential diagnosis that includes acute myeloid leukemia and peripheralized large cell lymphoma (Wright-Giemsa stain).

evaluation. Close observation and monitoring for evidence of progression to overt malignancy must be continued indefinitely.

Reactive bone marrow plasmacytosis of 10% or more may occur in several conditions, including viral infections, immune reactions to drugs, autoimmune disorders such as rheumatoid arthritis and lupus, and HIV/AIDS. Reactive plasmacytosis is distinguished from myeloma by the lack of M protein in the serum or urine in most instances. The PCs are generally mature appearing and show polytypic LC expression by IHC (Fig. 25-25).

The rare systemic polyclonal immunoblastic proliferations are among the most difficult reactive plasma cell proliferations to differentiate from myeloma.[107] The disorder usually presents as an acute systemic illness with fever, lymphadenopathy, hepatosplenomegaly, and frequently autoimmune manifestations; anemia and thrombocytopenia are present in most patients. Leukocytosis is typical and includes large numbers of PCs, immunoblasts, and reactive lymphocytes, with eosinophilia and neutrophilia in some cases (Fig. 25-26).

The bone marrow is heavily infiltrated by immunoblasts, PCs, and reactive lymphocytes (Fig. 25-26). Lymph nodes and other organs may also be involved. Marked polyclonal hypergammaglobulinemia is usually present, but an M protein and bone lesions are absent. These polyclonal immunoblastic proliferations usually undergo complete resolution after steroid therapy alone.

Occasionally, myeloma must be distinguished from a lymphoma with extreme PC differentiation such as LPL, marginal zone lymphoma, immunoblastic large-cell lymphoma, plasmablastic lymphoma, or ALK-positive large B-cell lymphoma (Fig. 25-27). Any of these may show morphologic similarities to myeloma and be associated with M protein. In most cases, lymphomas with PC differentiation present with extramedullary disease, and at least some of the diagnostic criteria for myeloma are lacking. Thorough morphologic, immunophenotypic, and genetic characterization will usually distinguish these tumors from myeloma. The identification of a clonally related B-cell population aids in the distinction of myeloma

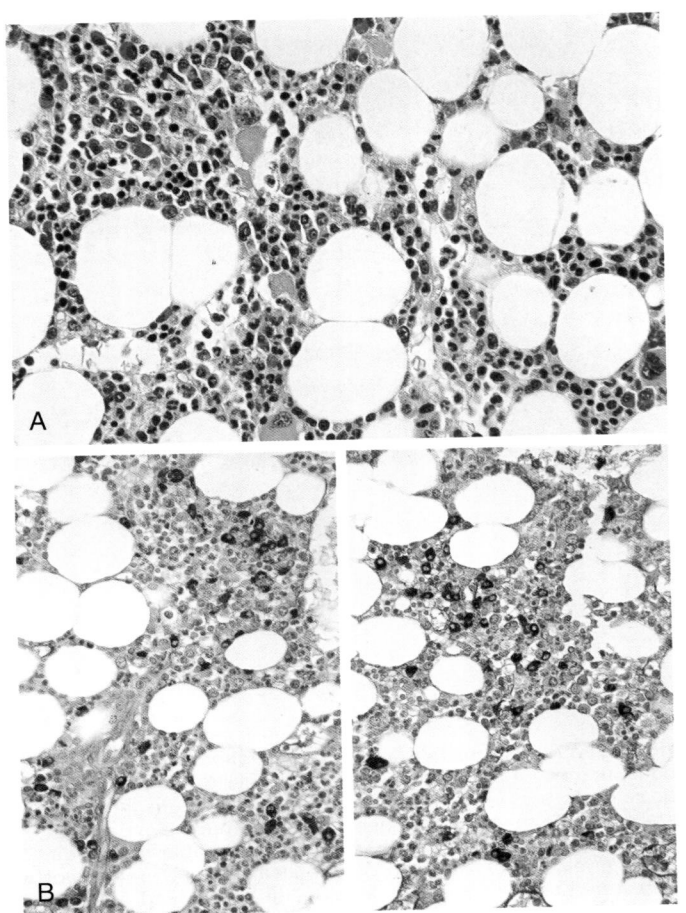

Figure 25-25. **Reactive bone marrow plasmacytosis. A,** In this case, plasma cells are increased but mostly scattered in an interstitial pattern with a few small clusters (H&E stain). Immunohistochemistry (IHC) for kappa **(B)** and lambda **(C)** light chains showed a polyclonal staining pattern, consistent with a reactive plasmacytosis (kappa and lambda IHC).

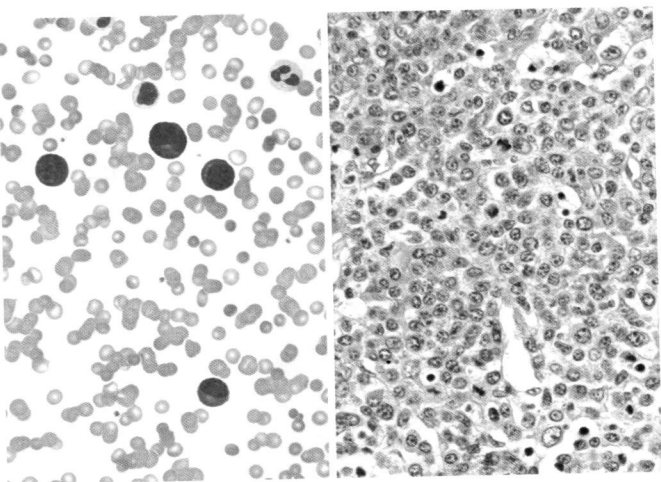

Figure 25-26. **Systemic polyclonal immunoblastic reaction.** Blood smear and bone marrow section from a middle-aged female patient with recent-onset renal failure and hypergammaglobulinemia. The blood smear contains numerous plasma cells (PCs), immunoblasts, and reactive lymphocytes **(A)**. The marrow is hypercellular, with clusters of immature PCs and immunoblasts **(B)**. The hypergammaglobulinemia is polyclonal. Light chain immunohistochemistry (IHC) performed on the bone marrow biopsy confirms a polyclonal PC and immunoblast proliferation. The patient is diagnosed with lupus. The polyclonal immunoblastic reaction promptly resolved with corticosteroid therapy (Wright-Giemsa and H&E stains).

Immunophenotypic Features of Normal and Neoplastic Plasma Cells

Normal Plasma Cells

PCs are generally defined immunophenotypically by bright CD38 expression. CD38 expression is not specific to PCs, as it is seen at various levels on virtually all other nucleated marrow subsets, but normal PCs express higher levels of CD38 than any other normal hematolymphoid cell population.[112-115] PCs also express CD138, and this antigen is essentially specific to PCs among hematolymphoid cells.[116-118] Normal bone marrow PCs usually express CD19 and CD45 and are negative for CD20 and CD56.[113,117,119-123] However, minor subsets of normal bone marrow PCs deviate from each of these prototypic features.[124-127] Notably, some antigens are modulated on the basis of the maturational stage; as they mature, PCs show decreasing intensity of CD45 and CD19 and increasing CD138.[117,128,129] A normal CD19-negative, CD56-positive PC population has been detected in bone marrow, and it is postulated to represent a terminally differentiated, long-lived subset.[127] A typical example of normal bone marrow PCs is shown in Figure 25-28. Additional immunophenotypic findings in normal PCs include bright expression of CD27 and CD81 and lack of CD28, CD117, and CD200.[117,125,126,130,131] These markers are useful to compare normal and abnormal PCs (Table 25-4). Normal PCs express polytypic cytoplasmic Ig, with kappa-to-lambda ratios in the range of 1 to 2:1, but occasionally as high as 4:1. It is important to recall that an elevated kappa-to-lambda or lambda-to-kappa ratio does not always indicate clonality; aberrant surface antigen expression should be evaluated in conjunction with cytoplasmic LCs.

from low-grade B-cell lymphomas, including LPL and marginal zone lymphoma.[108,109]

Myelomas composed of small lymphoid-appearing PCs often express CD20 and may mimic an LPL or marginal zone lymphoma with extreme PC differentiation. They are readily distinguished from lymphoma by cyclin D1 positivity and identification of t(11;14) by FISH.[61,63] Plasmablastic lymphoma usually differs from plasmablastic myeloma in clinical presentation, including its frequent association with HIV and Epstein-Barr virus (EBV). In clinically atypical cases, especially when the bone marrow is involved at presentation, there may be no defining features that distinguish the two disorders.[110,111]

PCL in which the neoplastic PCs are small with lymphoid features may be especially difficult to differentiate from CLL or a peripheralized LPL. The combination of clinical findings, type of M protein, bone marrow examination, immunophenotype, and genetics usually leads to the appropriate diagnosis.

Several metastatic tumors may present with lytic bone lesions and bear morphologic resemblance to myeloma. Thorough IHC evaluation is key to distinguishing metastatic neoplasms from myeloma.

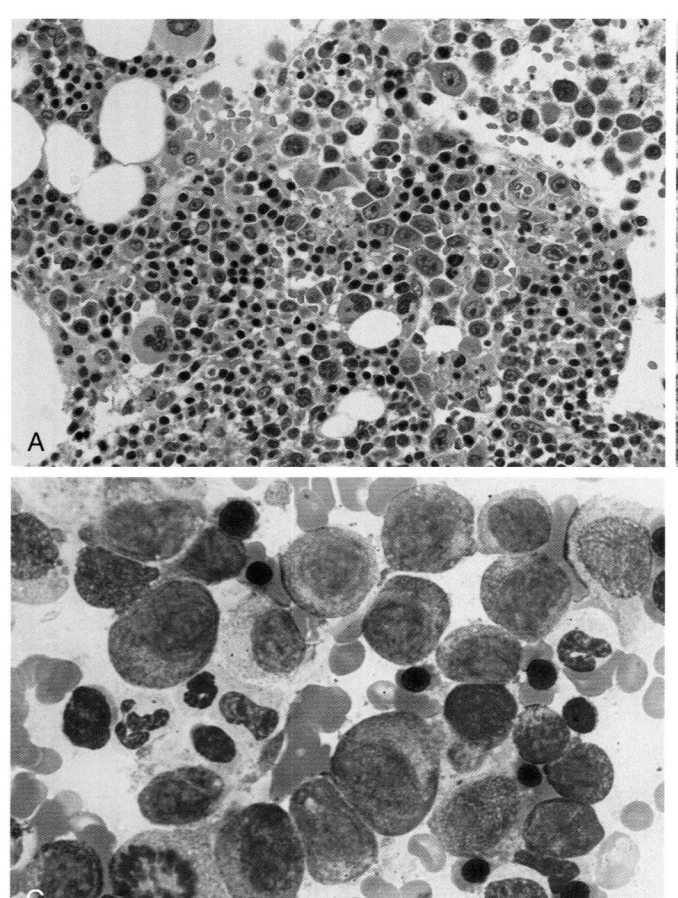

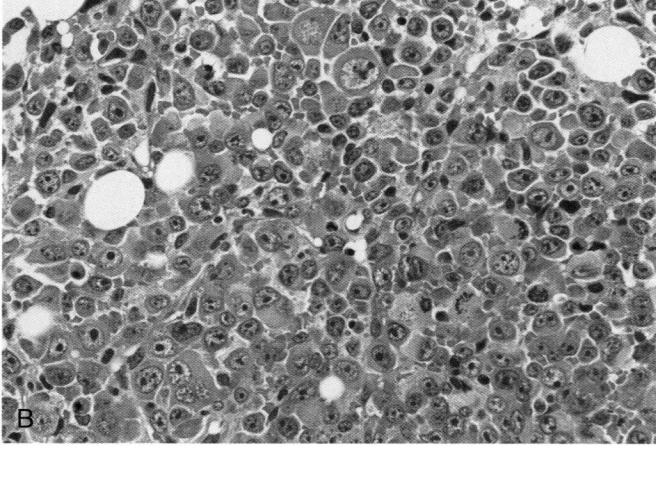

Figure 25-27. ALK-positive large B-cell lymphoma involving the bone marrow. A and **B,** In some areas, small clusters of neoplastic cells are present, whereas diffuse lymphomatous infiltrates are present elsewhere. The neoplastic cells have plasmablastic features and are morphologically indistinguishable from high-grade myeloma **(C)** (H&E and Wright-Giemsa stains). The tumor cells were positive for CD138, lambda light chain, and ALK (not shown).

Neoplastic Plasma Cells

Myeloma cells deviate immunophenotypically from their benign counterparts in virtually all cases (Table 25-4). Like their normal counterparts, myeloma cells express CD38 and CD138, but CD38 can be dimmer than that in normal PCs.[117,124] CD138 is used in most flow cytometry assays, but its expression can be biologically variable.[132] Moreover, the CD138 antigen is sensitive to the typical preanalytic specimen processing used in flow cytometry, including permeabilization and washes, which may compromise its subsequent detection. Thus, CD38 is often a more robust marker than CD138, except in those instances where it is used as a drug target (discussed later in this chapter). CD38 intensity in MM usually exceeds that of other marrow populations, but occasionally there is significant overlap with other cell types. CD19 is absent in about 95% of myelomas, whereas CD56 is expressed in 60% to 80%. The reported percentage of myelomas that express CD45 varies widely, ranging from 18% to 75%. These differences likely result from both technical issues and biological issues. Regarding the latter, as previously described, CD45 decreases with maturation of PCs, and variability of CD45 expression is a common feature in myeloma; the PCs with the brightest CD45 represent the proliferative compartment.[122,128,133] Therefore, it would not be surprising to find variation in CD45 expression depending on disease stage or as a consequence of therapy. Reported variability of CD45 in MM cases during the course of disease supports this notion.[134]

Abnormal PCs can be found both in monoclonal gammopathy of undetermined significance (Fig. 25-29) and newly diagnosed MM (Fig. 25-30). The percentage of PCs by flow cytometry should not be used for disease categorization (morphology is the gold standard), but one should note the proportion of clonal and nonclonal PCs within the marrow. In many cases of MGUS, there is a mix of clonal and polyclonal PCs. The percentage of clonal PCs may predict disease progression in MGUS and SMM.[83]

Technical Issues

General Technical Issues

Several technical issues can be encountered in the flow cytometric evaluation of myeloma that may complicate analysis. First, myeloma cells do not show predictable forward scatter/side scatter and CD45/side scatter patterns and often do not cluster tightly; instead, they require gating that is based on antigen fluorescence parameters, such as CD38 and/ or CD138. Next, depending on the details of the processing protocol, myeloma cells tend to adhere to other cell types, particularly granulocytes, creating potentially confusing light scatter and antigen expression, e.g., CD45 and CD10. This phenomenon may be partly responsible for the widely varying reports of the prevalence of CD45 expression in MM. PC-granulocyte doublets should be excluded based on CD45/SS

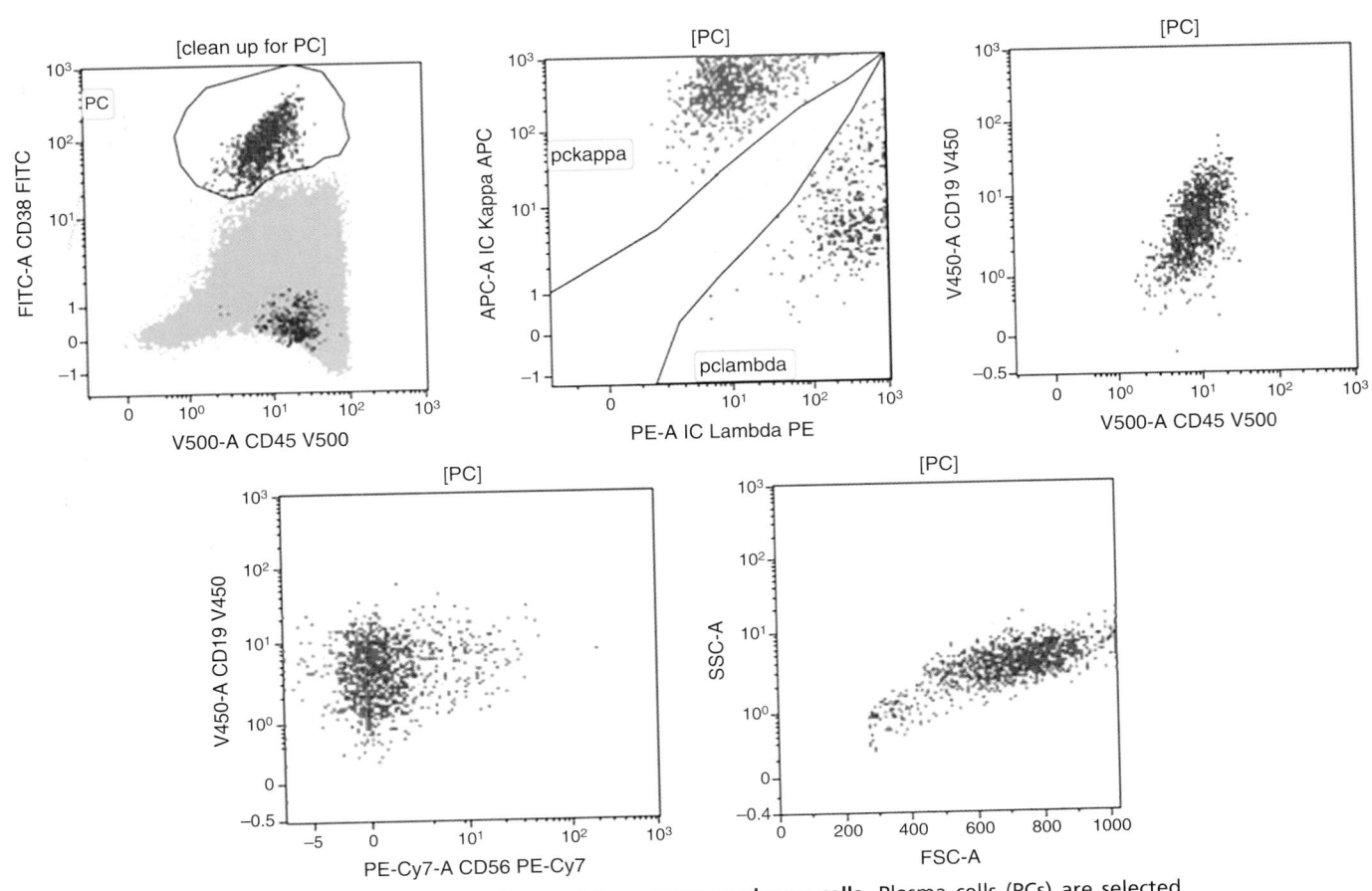

Figure 25-28. Phenotype of normal bone marrow plasma cells. Plasma cells (PCs) are selected based on their bright CD38 and slightly dim CD45 expression. They are composed of a mix of PCs that express either cytoplasmic kappa or cytoplasmic lambda LCs, with a normal ratio of ~ 2:1. The PCs express CD19 and CD45, but they lack CD56. They have variably increased size based on forward scatter (FSC) criteria. The cell populations are indicated as follows: magenta, kappa-expressing B cells; blue, lambda-expressing B cells; red, normal kappa-expressing PCs; green, normal lambda-expressing PCs; black, abnormal PC population; and gray, remainder of non-B, non-PC viable singlet mononuclear cells.

Table 25-4 Expression of Cluster of Differentiation Markers on Normal and Abnormal (Neoplastic) Plasma Cells

CD Marker	Normal PC	Abnormal PC
CD19	Positive	Dim to absent
CD20	Negative	Positive (~1/3 of cases)
CD27	Positive	Dim to absent
CD28	Negative	Positive (~1/2 of cases)
CD33	Negative	Positive in a minority of cases
CD38	Bright	Usually bright, but can be dim in some cases even without targeted therapy
CD45	Slightly dim	Variable, can be increased or decreased
CD56	Negative	Positive on a majority of cases (~2/3)
CD81	Positive	Dim to absent
CD117	Negative	Positive in some cases
CD200	Negative	Positive (~3/4 of patients)

CD, Cluster of differentiation; PC, plasma cell.
Adapted from Paiva B, Almeida J, Pérez-Andrés M, et al. Utility of flow cytometry immunophenotyping in multiple myeloma and other clonal plasma cell-related disorders. *Cytometry B Clin Cytom.* 2010;78:239-252.

patterns. PCs often show high levels of autofluorescence, greater than other cell populations in the bone marrow.[124] Thus, studies that use internal cell populations (e.g., lymphocytes) as negative controls can overestimate the level of antigen expression. Because of this, some labs have recommended the use of an isotype control tube containing CD38 for the accurate determination of a threshold for positivity specifically for the PC population. Finally, it is well established that myeloma cells are generally underrepresented in flow cytometric analysis when compared with morphologic aspirate smear evaluation, on average by 60% to 70%.[135-138] The decrement is frequently attributed to hemodilution in a "second pull" bone marrow aspirate.[139] However, PCs often appear to be disproportionately depleted compared with other cell types expected to be affected similarly by hemodilution (e.g., blasts). One explanation is that PCs may be differentially distributed in the liquid versus particle portions of the bone marrow aspirate, and thus may be disproportionately depleted relative to other cellular elements in less particle-rich aspirate specimens.[135] It is also possible that other physical or biological factors of MM affect flow cytometry recovery.[138]

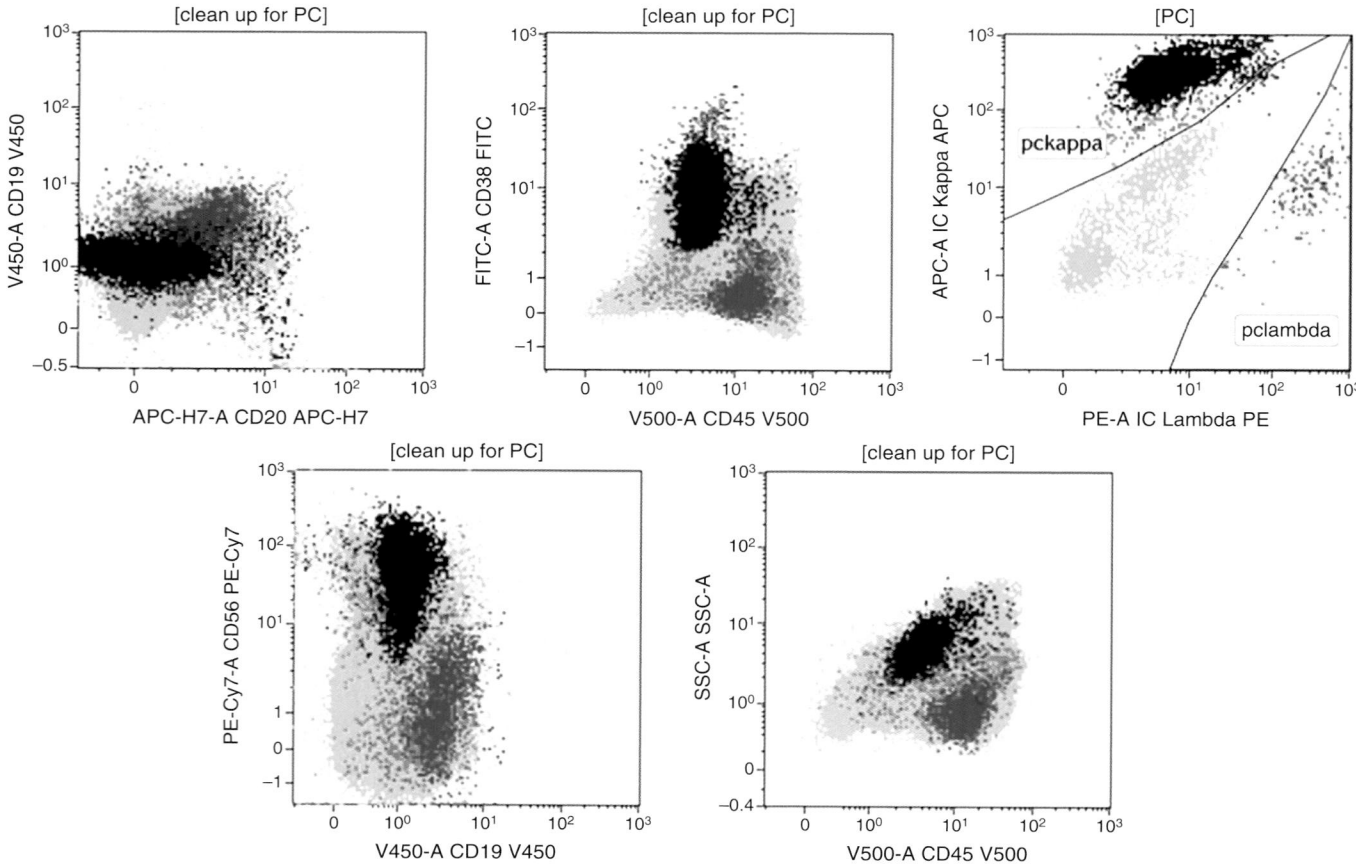

Figure 25-29. Monoclonal gammopathy of undetermined significance (MGUS). This example of a non-IgM MGUS demonstrates typical features in that the bone marrow contains both polyclonal and clonal plasma cells (PCs). The abnormal PC population expresses CD19 (dim to absent), CD20 (partial dim), CD38 (slightly dimmer than the normal PCs), CD45, monotypic cytoplasmic kappa immunoglobulin light chains, and bright CD56. Based on CD45 versus side scatter (SSC) plots, the PCs have increased SSC compared with lymphocytes, with slightly dimmer CD45 (overlapping with the traditional "blast gate"). Cell populations are identified as indicated in Figure 25-28.

Technical Issues Related to Minimal Residual Disease Analysis

Minimal residual disease (MRD) analysis is becoming increasingly important when following patients with MM, and flow cytometry has emerged as the method of choice for MRD detection.[140,141] Because of the wide variability in CD45 expression and light scatter characteristics in myeloma, gating requires the use of specific antigens. Gating on bright CD38-positive events is the most widely used approach to myeloma, and this generally suffices at diagnosis. However, in the setting of MRD analysis, bright CD38 gating alone is insufficiently sensitive or specific because of the dimmer CD38 expression in MM and the potential co-occurrence of non-PC events, aggregates, and debris in the bright CD38 region. In addition, CD38-targeted therapy will alter the approach (see subsequent section). Consequently, MRD analysis in myeloma requires gating on more than one marker. Because of its 100% specificity and sensitivity for PCs, CD138 has emerged as a favored marker by some for MRD gating. However, optimization of CD138 assessment may be hampered by technical issues, including clone choice, lyse reagent, and refrigeration.[116] CD38 and CD138 in tandem can be an effective gating strategy, capturing the vast majority

of cases.[121,139] If feasible, a three-parameter gate with CD38, CD138, and CD45 appears to be maximally sensitive.[121,139]

The detection of MRD in MM depends on the identification of immunophenotypic aberrancy on the PCs. Simply incorporating CD19 and CD56 has been suggested to capture more than 90% of myeloma MRD.[139] An example of a laboratory-developed MRD assay is shown in Figure 25-31. However, the detection of normal CD19-negative, CD56-positive PC populations raises some concerns about the use of these as the sole criteria for MRD.[125,127,142] It appears that assessment of combinations of multiple antigens with aberrant expression patterns (discussed previously) is required for optimal MRD assessment.[139] The EuroFlow group in 2012 recommended CD19 and CD56 as first-tier makers, followed by assessment of CD27, CD28, CD81, and CD117 as follow-up markers if necessary.[143] Assessment of CD200 also appears promising, but it bears further investigation.[131,144] Because of the need for multiparameter gating and the need to assess multiple aberrantly expressed antigens, high-color flow cytometry (≥6 colors) seems to be optimal for MRD analysis of MM.[122,127,130,145,146] It is worth noting that minor immunophenotypic modulations can occur over time in patients treated for MM, but these are unlikely to

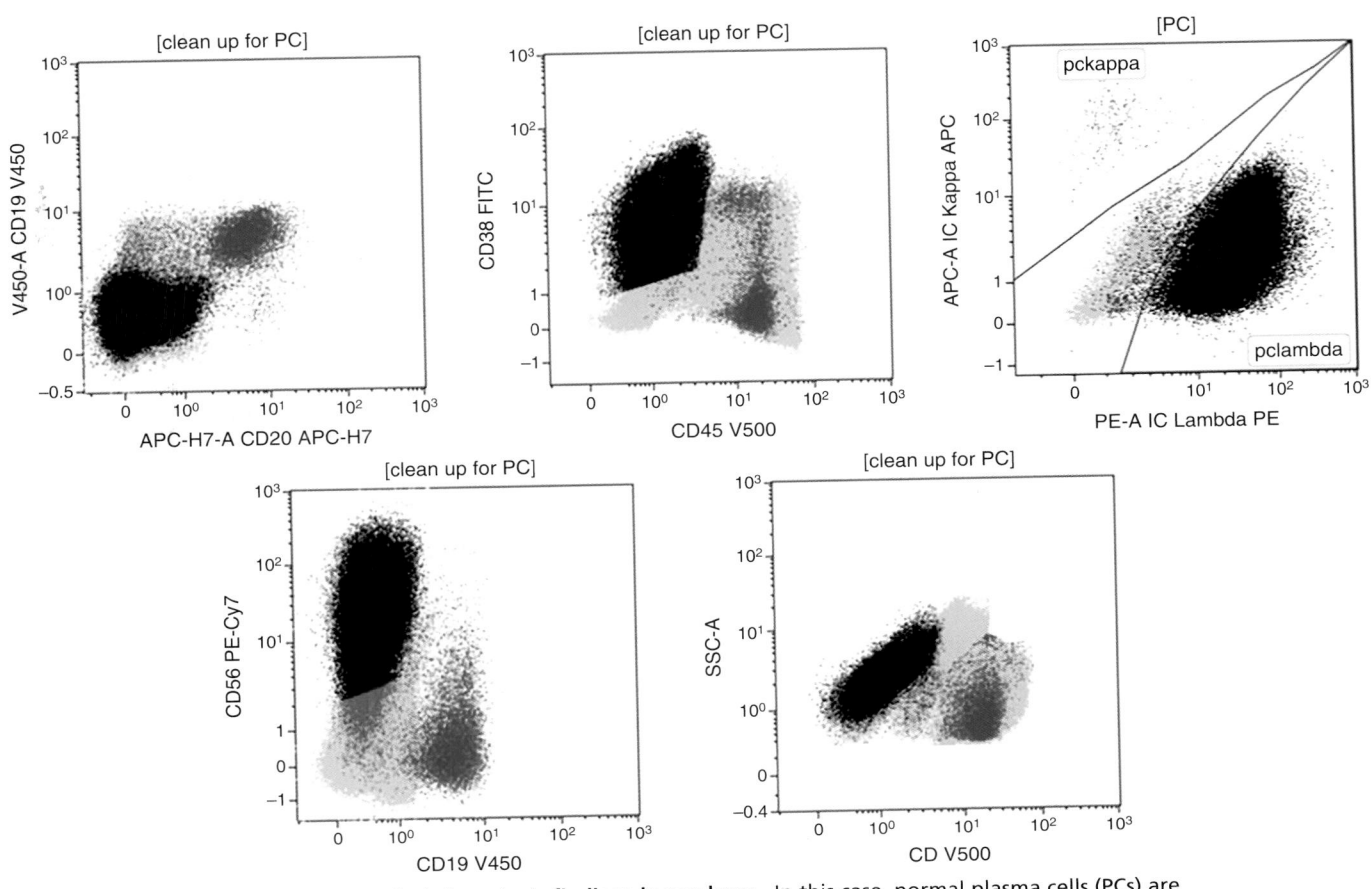

Figure 25-30. Typical phenotypic findings in myeloma. In this case, normal plasma cells (PCs) are rare to absent. The abnormal PCs lack CD19 and CD20. CD38 is brighter than the background B cells but dimmer than what is seen in typical polyclonal PCs. The myeloma cells express monotypic cytoplasmic lambda immunoglobulin light chain. CD45 is dim to absent. Cell populations are identified as indicated in Figure 25-28.

compromise a robust analysis that is based on assessment of multiple antigens.[134]

In general, a sensitivity of 10^{-4} is considered to be the minimal requirement for a standard sensitivity MRD detection method. The European Myeloma Network Report[139] recommended a minimum of 100 aberrant PC events to make a diagnosis of MRD. Thus, to achieve a sensitivity of 10^{-4}, a total of 1 million events needs to be acquired in a single-tube analysis. Note that this group does not require all 100 events to be present in the same tube, just that the aberrant PC events across tubes totals at least 100. If one is using a multitube analysis, fewer events need to be acquired per tube to satisfy the European Myeloma Network recommendation.

As molecular diagnostic testing for MRD in myeloma has become more available, there has been simultaneous development of more sensitive flow cytometry assays.[147] Sometimes termed *next generation flow cytometry*, the new assays target a sensitivity down to 10^{-5}. One of the most common methods to do this testing is EuroFlow.[148] The EuroFlow assay uses two 8-color tubes—after bulk-lysing marrow samples, 5 to 10 million cells are stained so that enough events can be collected to achieve the 10^{-5} sensitivity. As this takes a lot of instrument time, 10-color single tube methods have been developed and show similar performance but require much less acquisition time.[148] Regardless of which method a lab chooses for its MRD assay, a careful validation

with dilutional studies is critical to make sure the MRD assay works as expected.[149] If a lab is accredited by the College of American Pathologists' Laboratory Accreditation Program, the lower limit of detection must appear in the diagnostic report[150,151]; this will provide greater transparency to ordering providers so that they may discern standard from high (next-generation) flow cytometry myeloma MRD assays.

Technical Issues Related to Therapy Targeting CD38

Daratumumab is a highly effective monoclonal antibody that is widely used to treat patients with myeloma at diagnosis, at relapse, and during maintenance therapy. As CD38 has high antigen density on the surface of PCs, it is useful for a therapeutic target in addition to being useful for flow cytometric analysis. Daratumumab remains bound to CD38 on PCs for 4 to 6 months, masking the epitopes recognized by most CD38 antibodies used for the identification of PCs by flow cytometry.[152] As a result, novel approaches for the detection of PCs by flow cytometry must be used in the post-daratumumab setting. Multiple cell surface and cytoplasmic PC markers have been evaluated. The EuroFlow tubes use a "multiepitope" or "polyspecific" antibody that seems to detect CD38 to some degree, even in the context of bound daratumumab.[153] Cytoplasmic staining of PCs for CD38 using a monoclonal antibody

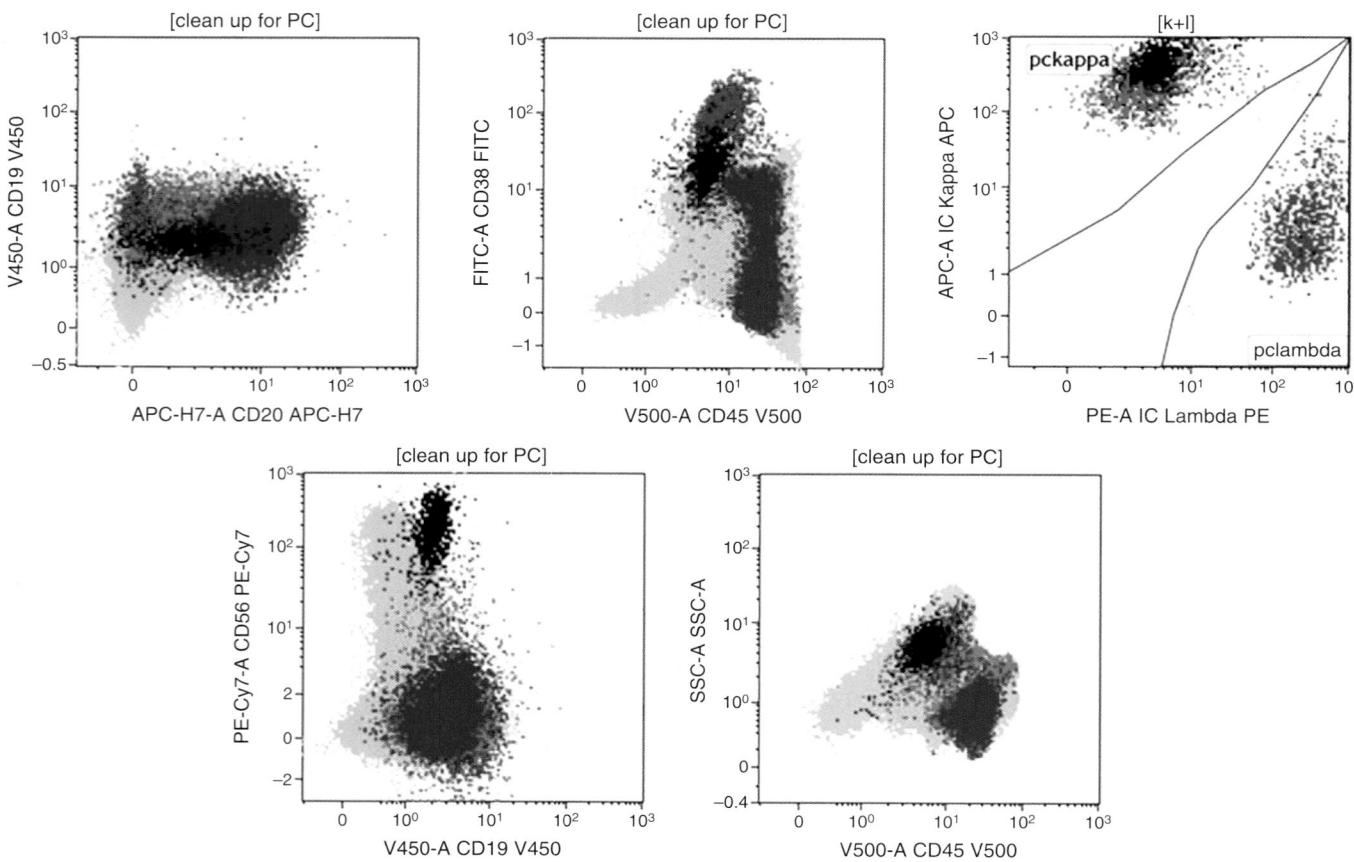

Figure 25-31. Minimal residual disease (MRD) detection in myeloma. This laboratory-developed MRD assay demonstrates how multiple antigens can have a population of abnormal plasma cells (PCs) that has an immunophenotype that is different from normal plasma cells in the background. The abnormal PC population is kappa monotypic and expresses CD38 (dim), CD45 (slightly dim), and CD56 but lacks CD19 and CD20. Though this population is relatively easy to detect by flow cytometry, bone marrow biopsy sections and immunohistochemistry are negative for clusters of clonal PCs. Cell populations are identified as indicated in Figure 25-28.

Table 25-5 Alternative Plasma Cell Flow Cytometry Antigens for Patients Exposed to Anti-CD38 Therapy (Daratumumab)

Marker	Surface or Cytoplasmic
CD38-multiepitope	Surface
CD38-monoclonal	Cytoplasmic
p63 (VS38c or VS38)	Cytoplasmic
CD319 (SLAMF7)	Surface
CD54	Surface
CD229	Surface

has been reported and may afford better PC detection than surface staining with the multiepitope CD38 antibody.[153] Multiple other cell surface markers have been tested, including CD54, CD229, and CD319; one study suggests that CD319 (SLAMF7) is superior for the identification of PCs (Table 25-5).[154] In addition, p63 (VS38 or VS38c) is a rough endoplasmic reticulum protein and is strongly expressed in PCs. Although one lab reported difficulty in using cytoplasmic p63/VS38 in its assay,[155] three other studies have demonstrated that analysis of p63/VS38 expression is highly sensitive for the detection of PCs after daratumumab therapy (Fig. 25-32).[156-158]

Diagnostic Utility of Flow Cytometry

Flow cytometry contributes to the diagnosis of MM by identification of clonal and phenotypically aberrant PCs. Although the diagnosis of MM is generally not dependent on the findings of flow cytometry, it may play a decisive role in the differential diagnosis in some cases, as discussed later in this chapter. The following examples show how flow cytometry can be used in conjunction with data collected from bone marrow morphology, IHC, and protein electrophoresis/immunofixation, etc. to arrive at the correct diagnosis.

Unusual Morphologic and Immunophenotypic Variants of Myeloma

CD20-Positive Plasma Cell Myeloma

Occasionally, myelomas are encountered that are difficult to recognize by morphologic evaluation, especially anaplastic myelomas and those with striking lymphoid or lymphoplasmacytoid cytologic features. Detection of a characteristic immunophenotype by flow cytometry will help discriminate these from other neoplasms. It is worth mentioning that expression of CD20 in MM is often associated

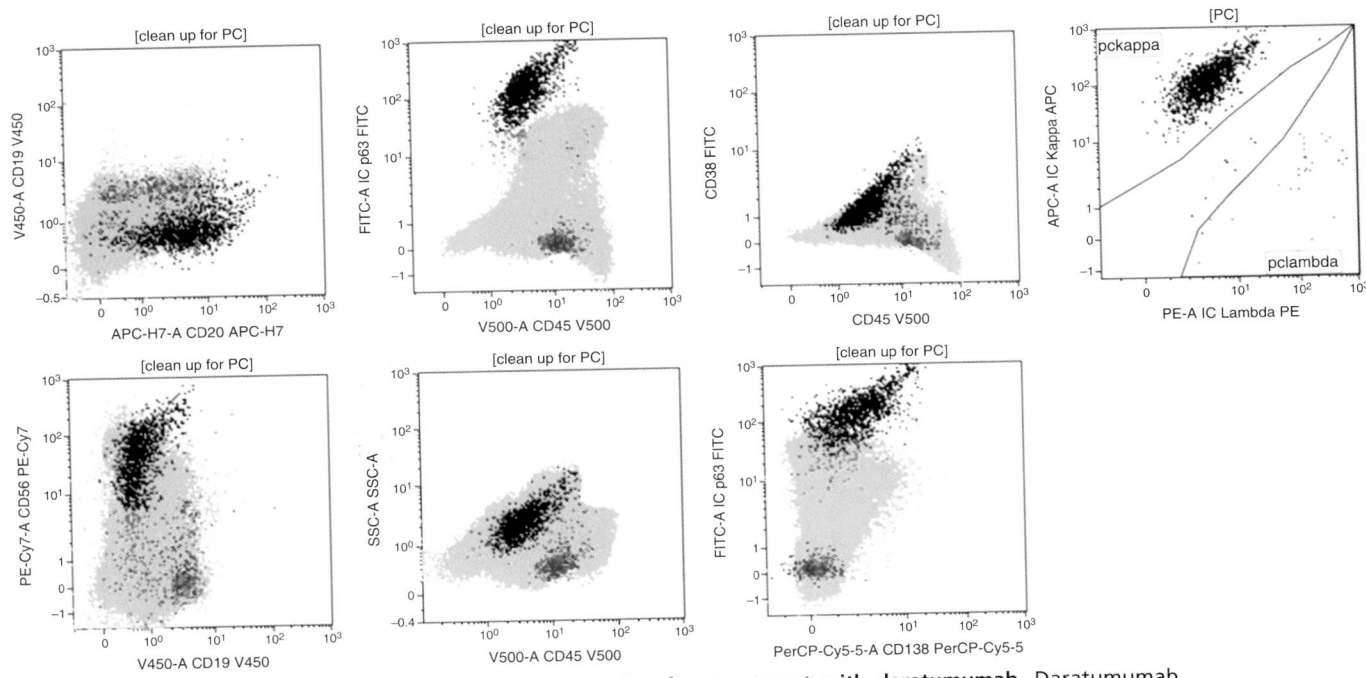

Figure 25-32. Detection of myeloma cells after treatment with daratumumab. Daratumumab binds to CD38 and interferes with flow cytometric detection for 4 to 6 months. As seen in the CD38 versus CD45 dot plot, all mononuclear cells, including plasma cells (PCs), have dim-to-absent CD38 expression. As CD138 can have variable expression (does not discriminate the population well in this example), this laboratory developed test stains for cytoplasmic p63 (VS38). All PCs in the sample (clonal and polyclonal) clearly separate based on CD45 versus intracytoplasmic p63. The abnormal PC population is kappa monotypic and expresses CD20 and CD56 but lacks CD19 and CD45. Cell populations are identified as indicated in Figure 25-28.

with lymphoplasmacytoid morphology, creating an additional diagnostic challenge (Fig. 25-33).[63] Notably, however, co-expression of CD19 and CD20 in MM is extremely rare; thus, when one sees a B-lineage neoplasm expressing CD20 but lacking CD19, it is more likely to represent a PC neoplasm than B-cell non-Hodgkin lymphoma.

Unusual Expression of Cytoplasmic Light Chains in Myeloma

There are a variety of reagent antibodies that can be used to detect cytoplasmic LCs in PCs by flow cytometry and IHC. Reagent antibodies can be either polyclonal or monoclonal, and they are conjugated to a variety of different fluorochromes. Clonal LC proteins in neoplastic myeloma cells may be abnormal because of truncation or antigenic variation resulting from somatic hypermutation. Such variant LCs may not be well recognized by the reagent antibodies routinely used for LC analysis (Fig. 25-34).

In rare instances, PC neoplasms may express both kappa and lambda LCs (Fig. 25-35). Rarely, no demonstrable expression of either kappa or lambda LCs is detected; such myelomas are termed *nonproducers* (Fig. 25-36). Such cases are distinguished from nonsecretory MM in which LC restriction is readily demonstrated by either flow cytometry or IHC despite the absence of a detectable urine or serum M protein by IFE and a normal SFLC ratio.

Plasma Cell Leukemia

The clinical features of newly diagnosed MM may be unusual in some patients and may, as a result, mimic other hematolymphoid neoplasms. Primary PCL is a notorious

example. As discussed previously, hematopathologists may encounter cases of PCL prior to bone marrow examination and with no knowledge of laboratory or radiologic findings. Moreover, PCL may morphologically resemble other hematolymphoid malignancies, including CLL, AML, or even peripheralized large cell lymphoma, depending on the cytologic features of the circulating PCs. Flow cytometry is often essential for demonstrating the plasmacytic differentiation of the neoplastic cells and confirming the diagnosis of PCL (Fig. 25-37). The immunophenotypic features of PCL are generally similar to those of conventional MM, except for more frequent expression of CD20 in PCL and the less frequent expression of CD56, which is lacking in approximately 80% of cases (Fig. 25-24), CD117, and HLA-DR.[85,88,159,160]

MONOCLONAL GAMMOPATHY OF UNDETERMINED SIGNIFICANCE

Definition

MGUS is the designation for a monoclonal Ig in the serum or urine of a patient in whom there is no evidence of MM, amyloidosis, Waldenström macroglobulinemia or other lymphoproliferative disorders, or any other disease known to produce monoclonal Igs. In most instances, the patient will not develop a malignant PC neoplasm during their lifetime, but there is eventual progression to one in a significant minority of cases.

There are two distinctive categories of MGUS: IgM MGUS and non-IgM MGUS (Box 25-6). Non-IgM MGUS accounts for approximately 85% of cases, is caused by an underlying

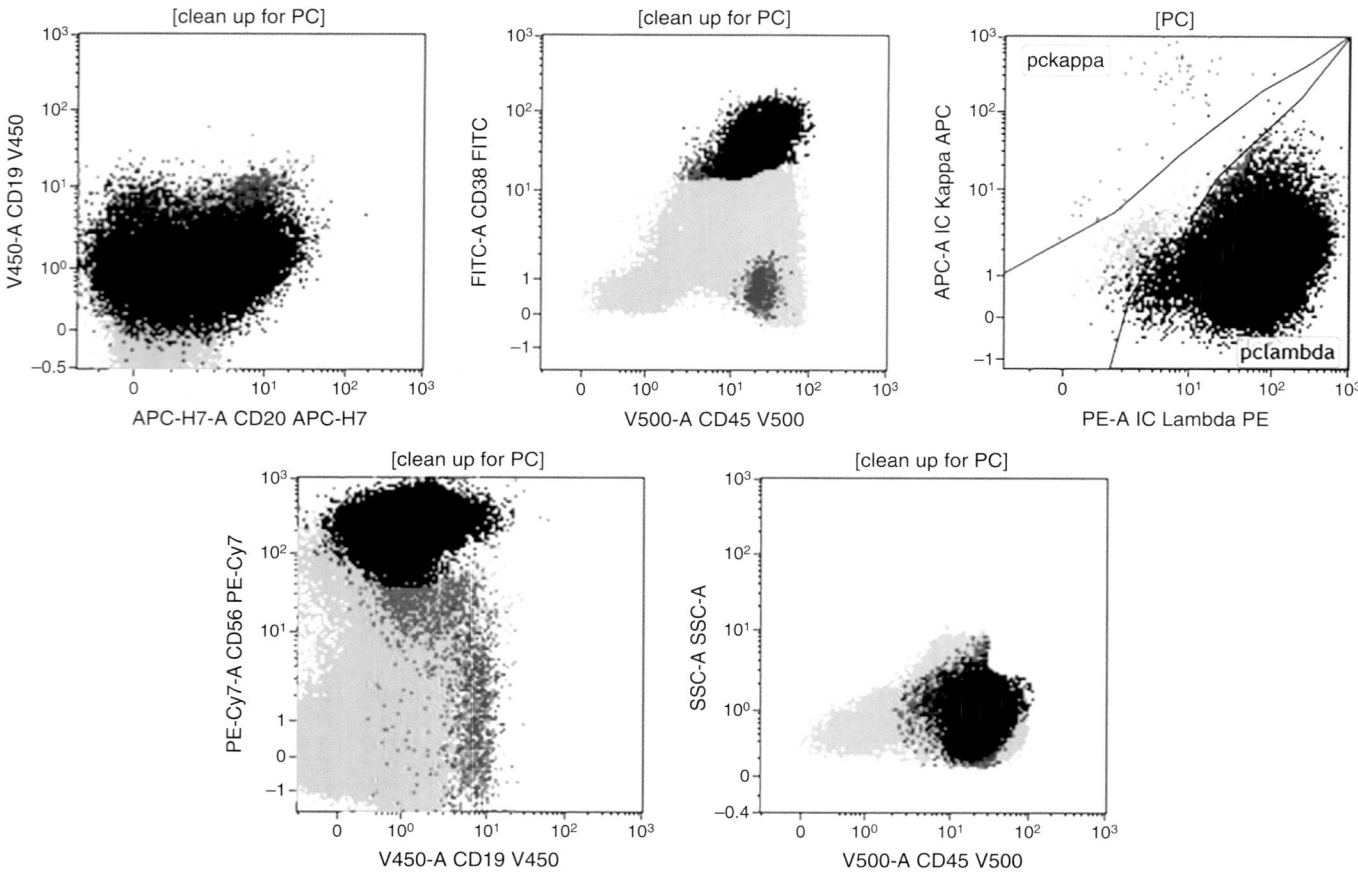

Figure 25-33. Distinction of CD20-positive myeloma from B-cell lymphoma. The neoplastic plasma cells (PCs) in this case have plasmacytoid morphology and express CD138, PAX5, CD20, cyclin D1, and monotypic lambda light chain by immunohistochemistry (not shown). Fluorescence in situ hybridization (FISH) confirmed t(11;14). By flow cytometry, the PCs express CD45 at a level comparable to mature B cells. They express CD20, lack CD19, express increased CD38, are lambda monotypic, and express bright CD56; this immunophenotype argues against B-cell lymphoma and supports the diagnosis of myeloma. Cell populations are identified as indicated in Figure 25-28.

clonal PC population, and may progress to a malignant PC neoplasm, including MM or amyloidosis. In contrast to previous WHO classifications, the ICC recognizes two subtypes of IgM MGUS: IgM MGUS PC type and IgM MGUS, not otherwise specified (NOS). The latter usually has lymphoplasmacytic features and may progress to lymphoma, Waldenström macroglobulinemia, or occasionally to LC amyloidosis; IgM MGUS, NOS is discussed in the chapter on LPL. By contrast, IgM MGUS PC type is defined by the presence of a clonal PC population, typical myeloma IGH rearrangements in many cases, and the absence of both a clonal B-cell component and an *MYD88* mutation. This subtype of IgM MGUS may give rise in a minority of cases to IgM MM.

Epidemiology and Etiology

MGUS is the most common monoclonal gammopathy and is found in about 3% of individuals older than 50 years and in more than 5% of those older than 70 years. The incidence of MGUS is twice as high in African Americans as in Whites, roughly paralleling the difference in incidence of MM. At least 60% of individuals with MGUS are male.

Other than advanced age and ethnicity differences, the development of MGUS has not been associated with any specific disease or predisposing clinical disorder. MGUS is typically discovered incidentally during the evaluation for an unrelated medical disorder. Transient oligoclonal and monoclonal gammopathies have been described in young patients after renal and allogeneic bone marrow transplants; there is a correlation with graft-versus-host disease in bone marrow transplant recipients.

Clinical and Laboratory Features

Other than M protein and mild increase in bone marrow PCs, there are no consistent or specific clinical findings. Abnormal laboratory studies in individuals with MGUS are usually attributable to a co-existing disease. Myeloma-associated laboratory and radiographic abnormalities are absent in MGUS by definition. M protein is found via SPE in most cases (Fig. 25-38). The quantity of M protein is less than 3 g/dL; the median is about 0.5 g/dL. In patients with very low-level paraproteinemia, immunofixation electrophoresis is required for detection of M protein (Fig. 25-38). Normal serum polyclonal Igs are decreased in about 30% of cases, and

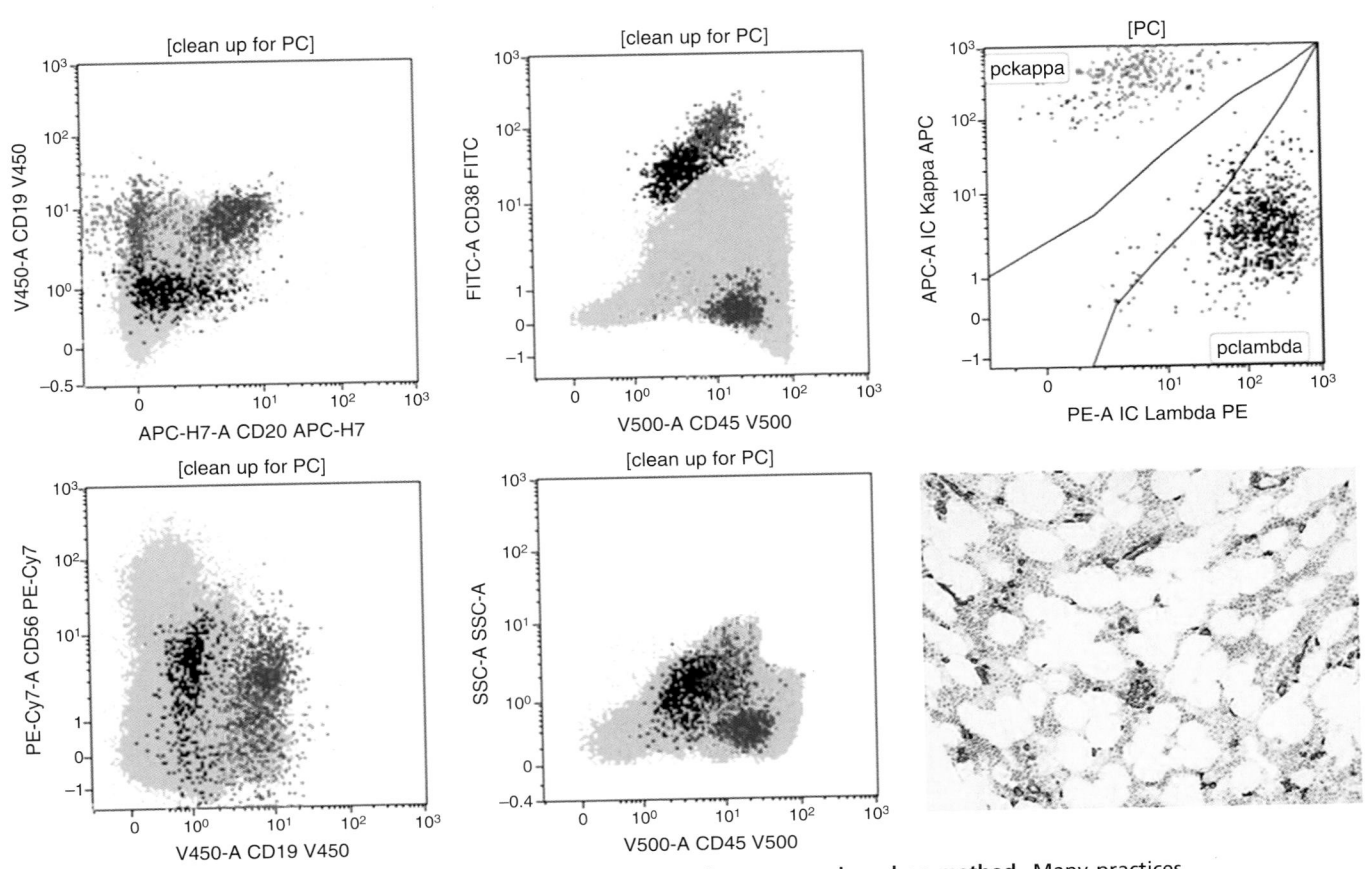

Figure 25-34. Light chain (LC) expression detection can vary based on method. Many practices immunophenotypically approach bone marrow diagnoses with both flow cytometry and immunohistochemistry. The patient presented for a follow-up bone marrow examination 2 years after transplant for myeloma. He had a measurable IgG-lambda M-spike. Immunohistochemistry on the bone marrow showed clusters of CD138-positive PCs, but kappa and lambda immunostains were mostly negative within the clusters (not shown). Flow cytometry showed a lambda monotypic plasma cell (PC) population that expressed CD38 (dim) and CD45 (dim), but it was mostly negative for CD19, CD20, and CD56. The t(11;14) was detected by fluorescence in situ hybridization (FISH) in a subset of CD138-enriched PCs. The flow cytometry kappa and lambda antibodies were polyclonal, and the immunohistochemical kappa and lambda antibodies used were monoclonal. Although rare, mutated or truncated LCs in myeloma cells sometimes react unexpectedly with reagent antibodies, and combinations of polyclonal and monoclonal antibodies can be helpful in such cases. Cell populations are identified as indicated in Figure 25-28.

LCs (Bence-Jones protein) are present in the urine in small quantities in up to 28% of cases; in most cases, the quantity of urinary protein is less than 1 g/24 hr. In 67% to 75% of cases, the monoclonal heavy chain (HC) is IgG. IgM is found in about 15% of cases, IgA in 10% to 14%, and 2% to 3% are biclonal gammopathies; only rare cases of IgD MGUS have been reported. The LC is kappa in 54% to 63% of cases. An isolated LC is present in up to 20% of MGUS cases, which may be detected only with a serum free LC assay (see criteria for LC MGUS in Box 25-6).

Blood and Bone Marrow Findings

There are no specific blood findings associated with MGUS. Rouleaux formation may be increased in patients with M-protein levels approaching a myeloma-defining level of 3 g/dL. Any blood count or other smear abnormalities are usually related to a co-existing disease.

Clonal PCs account for <10% of bone marrow cells (median, 3%), with a mild plasmacytosis in only about 50% of cases.[32,54] Morphologically, the clonal PCs usually appear mature, although mild atypia may be evident, including cytoplasmic inclusions and nucleoli. In biopsy sections, the bone marrow is usually normocellular. PCs are evenly scattered throughout the marrow or found in small clusters. Clustering of PCs is most common in cases with an increased percentage of PCs.

Immunophenotype

CD138 IHC facilitates assessment of PC number and distribution in the bone marrow biopsy. Confirmation of a monoclonal PC population with kappa and lambda stains is feasible in many cases of MGUS. However, detection of LC restriction by kappa and lambda IHC or in situ hybridization (ISH) on biopsy sections may be difficult in cases in which the clone is small or admixed with a prominent background population of normal PCs. The ratio of LC excess is less than that in MM.[161-163] When performing CD138 and LC stains, it is important they be performed on serial sections. Using

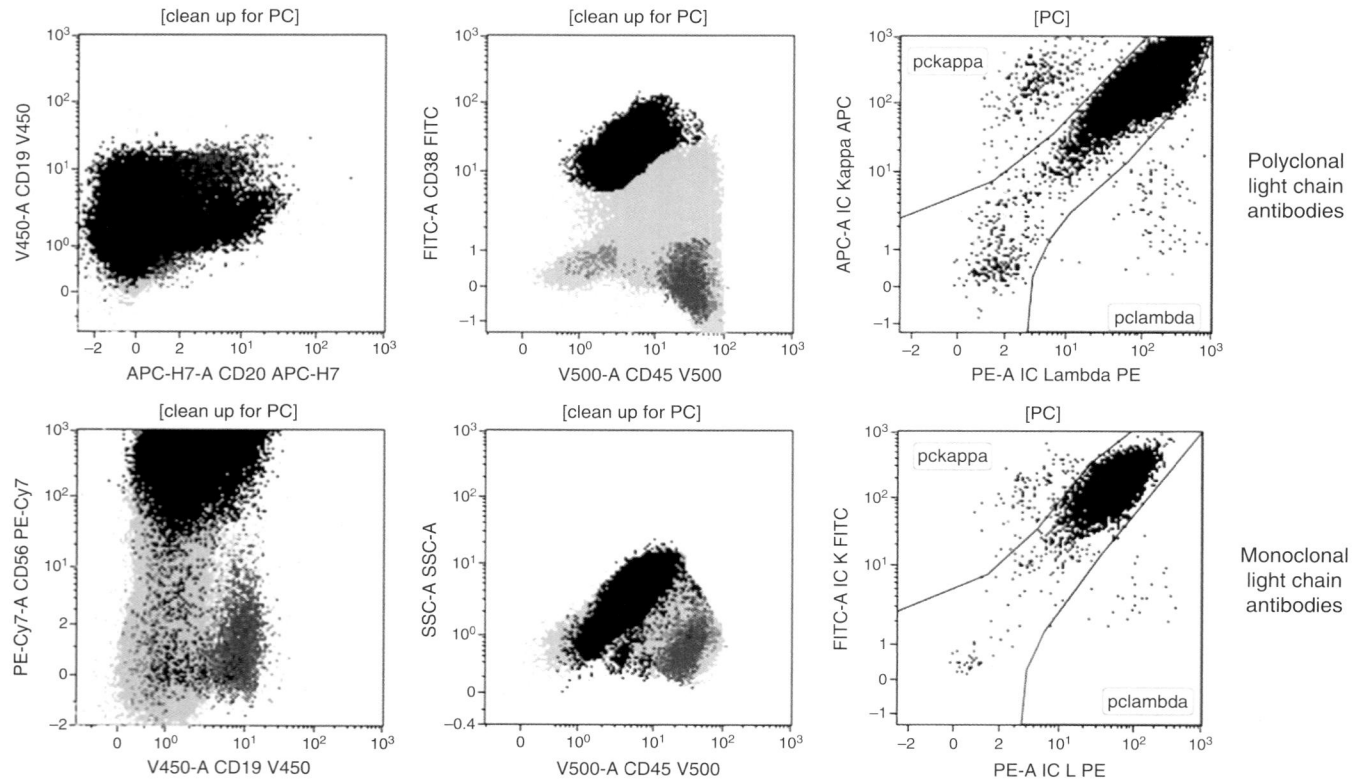

Figure 25-35. Dual-expressing (biphenotypic) multiple myeloma (MM). This patient presented with a lytic lesion and a large IgG-kappa M-spike. Flow cytometry identified an abnormal plasma cell (PC) population that expresses CD45 (dim), CD38, and CD56, with dim-to-absent CD19 and CD20. Using standard polyclonal cytoplasmic kappa and lambda immunoglobulin antibodies, there is poor discrimination (the PCs fall right along the diagonal of the light chain dot plot). A repeat study with monoclonal cytoplasmic kappa and lambda immunoglobulin antibodies showed similar results. On the targeted lytic lesion and bone marrow biopsy sections, kappa and lambda expression is confirmed by both in situ hybridization and immunohistochemistry. Cell populations are identified as indicated in Figure 25-28.

inferential reasoning, one can often detect clusters of LC-restricted PCs among background polyclonal PCs in MGUS and treated MM.

Genetics

Abnormal karyotypes are rarely observed in MGUS by conventional cytogenetic studies, but numeric and/or structural abnormalities are detected by FISH in most cases of non-IgM MGUS.[10,11,13,164] The abnormalities are similar to those in myeloma, but the relative frequencies of specific aberrancies differ. Hyperdiploidy is detected in about 40% of patients with trisomies similar to that observed in myeloma.[10] Translocations targeting *IGH* (14q32) are found in nearly half of patients; the t(11;14) (q23;q32) translocation is present in 15% to 25%, t(4;14) (p16.3;q32) in 2% to 9%, and t(14;16)(q34q23) in 1% to 5%.[13,164] Deletions of 13q are present in 40% to 50% of cases.[11,164-167] Aneuploidy has been observed by image analysis in greater than 60% of MGUS cases, and most of these had numeric abnormalities by FISH analysis.[168] *KRAS* and *NRAS* mutations are less frequent in MGUS (~5%) than in myeloma (~30% to 40%), consistent with their role in disease progression.[169] Currently, no clinical correlates with chromosome abnormalities are recognized in MGUS.

PLASMACYTOMA

Solitary Bone Plasmacytoma

Definition and Diagnostic Criteria

Solitary bone plasmacytoma (SBP) is a localized tumor composed of clonal PCs that are cytologically, immunophenotypically, and genetically similar to those of MM.[26,170] There is no evidence of bone marrow involvement at other sites, and clinical features of MM are lacking. The criteria for diagnosis of SBP are listed in Box 25-7.[2,76,79,170]

Epidemiology

SBP accounts for less than 5% of PC neoplasms.[32,171] The median age is 50 to 55 years (about 10 years younger than that for MM), and 65% to 70% of patients are male.[32,79]

Clinical Features

Most patients with SBP present with a single painful bone lesion or pathologic fracture. Soft tissue extension may result in a palpable mass.[32] Although any bone may be involved, SBP most commonly develops in bones with active hematopoiesis, particularly those of the skull, spine, pelvis, ribs, clavicle, scapula, and femur.[79,172] Involvement of long bones distal to the knee or elbow is rare.[173,174] The most common site is the

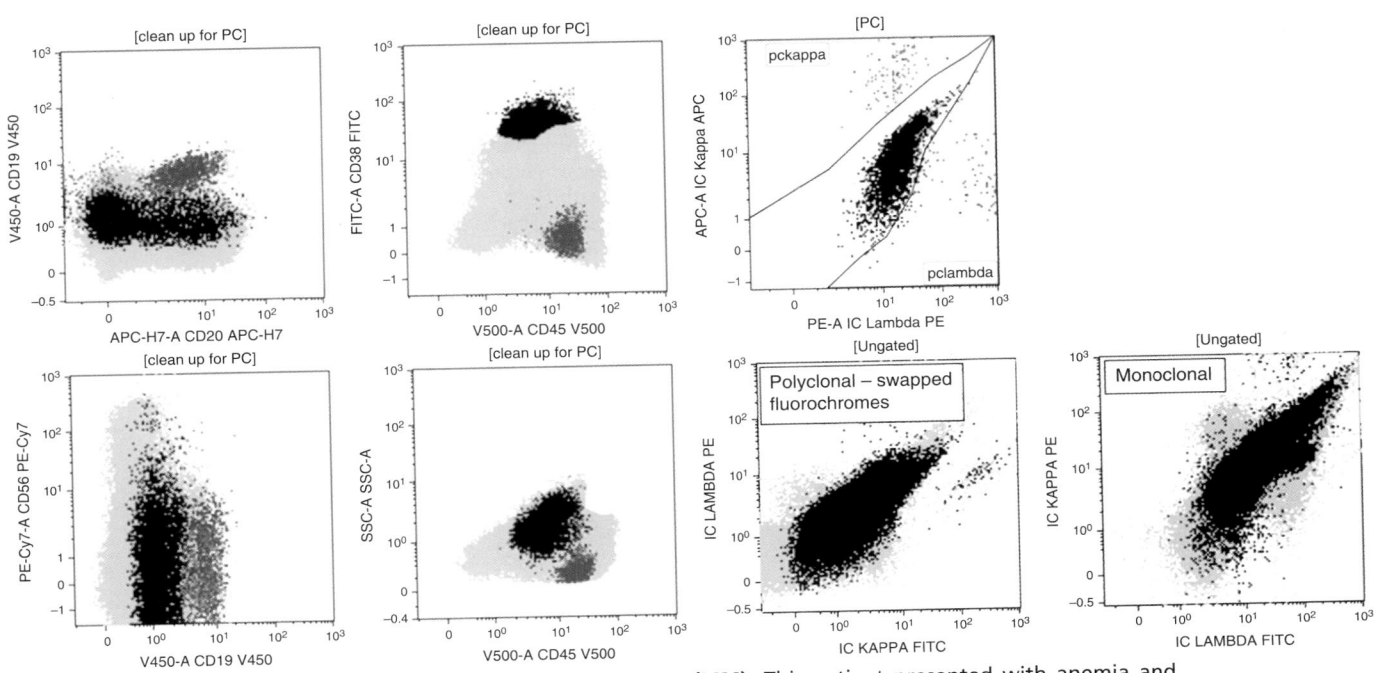

Figure 25-36. Nonproducer multiple myeloma (MM). This patient presented with anemia and had no detectable M protein in either the serum or urine by immunofixation; the SFLC ratio was normal. Sheets of CD138-positive plasma cells (PCs) are present in the bone marrow biopsy that lacks light chain (LC) expression by both in situ hybridization and immunohistochemistry. By flow cytometry, the PCs express CD38 with dim CD45, but they lack expression of CD19 and LC. They mostly lack CD20 and CD56. Repeat analyses using different pairs of LC antibodies (polyclonal, polyclonal with swapped fluorochromes, and monoclonal) yielded similar results. Cell populations are identified as indicated in Figure 25-28.

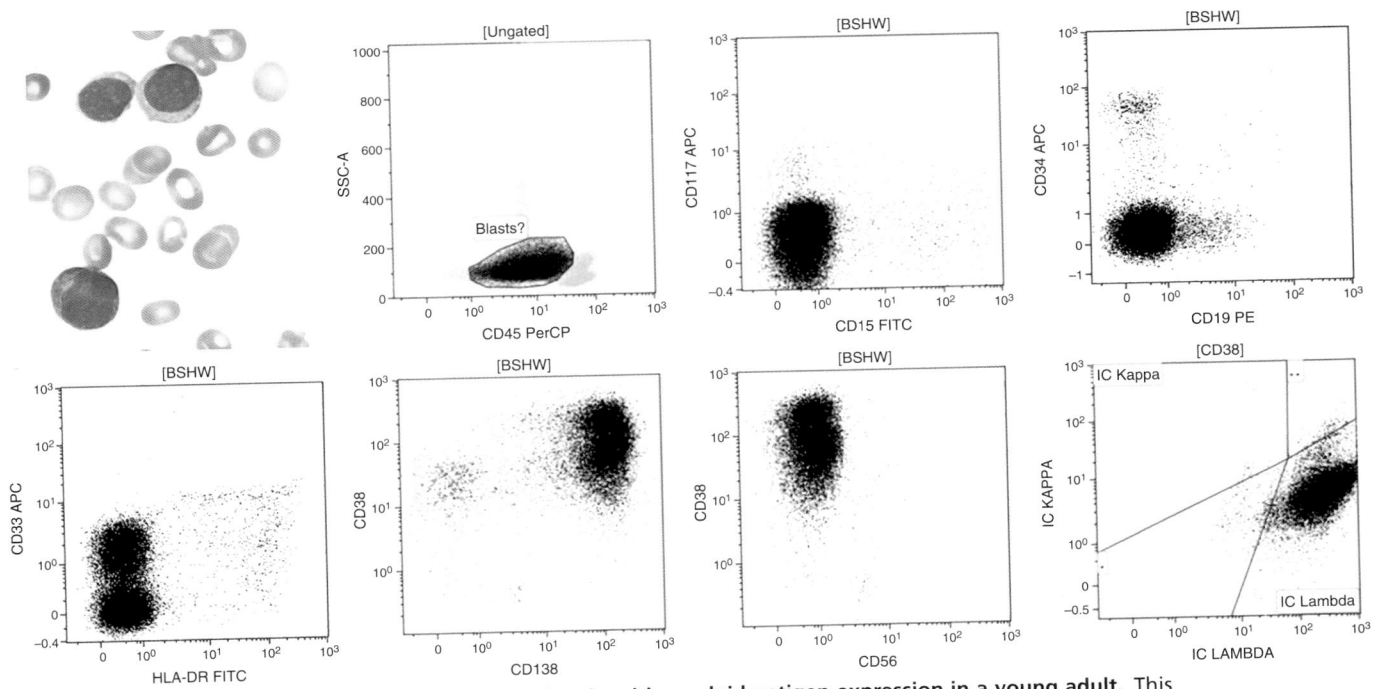

Figure 25-37. Plasma cell (PC) leukemia with myeloid antigen expression in a young adult. This young adult patient presented with circulating blast-like cells, and acute leukemia was suspected clinically. The neoplastic cells fall into the traditional "blast gate" in the CD45 versus SSC plot. Although the "blasts" show partial expression of the myeloid antigen CD33, they lack CD15, CD19, CD34, and CD117. The expression of CD38 and cytoplasmic CD79a without cytoplasmic MPO or CD3 prompts additional workup for PC neoplasm. The expression of bright CD38, CD138, and monotypic cytoplasmic lambda immunoglobulin light chain is confirmed; they are CD56 negative. Cell populations are identified as indicated in Figure 25-28.

Box 25-6 *Diagnostic Criteria for MGUS*

Intact Non-IgM M-Protein Monoclonal Gammopathy of Undetermined Significance (MGUS)

• IgG, IgA, or IgD M protein in serum, <3 g/dL
• Clonal bone marrow plasma cells (PCs) <10%
• No end organ damage (CRAB) or amyloidosis

Light Chain MGUS

• Presence of isolated free light chain with no associated heavy chain by immunofixation electrophoresis (IFE)
• Increased serum level of involved free light chain
• Abnormal serum free light chain ratio (<0.26 or >1.65)
• Urinary light chain excretion is <500 mg/24 hours
• Clonal bone marrow PCs <10%
• No end organ damage (CRAB) or amyloidosis

IgM MGUS, PC Type

• Satisfy intact non-IgM MGUS criteria
• Genetic and phenotypic studies to:
  • Identify clonal PC population with typical multiple myeloma (MM) cytogenetic abnormality
  OR
  • Identify clonal PC population without typical MM cytogenetic abnormality and lacking:
    • *MYD88* mutation
    • Clonal B-cell population

Box 25-7 *Diagnostic Criteria for Solitary Plasmacytoma*

Bone or Extraosseous Plasmacytoma

• Biopsy-proven solitary lesion of bone or soft tissue consisting of clonal plasma cells (PCs)
• Normal random bone marrow biopsy with no evidence of clonal PCs
• Normal skeletal survey and CT or MRI except for the solitary lesion
• Absence of end organ damage (CRAB) attributable to a PC proliferative disorder
• No evidence of a clonal B-cell population or *MYD88* mutation

Solitary Bone Plasmacytoma With Minimal Bone Marrow Involvement

• Satisfy previously described criteria
• Clonal PCs account for <10% of bone marrow cells in random bone marrow biopsy (usually identified by flow cytometry)

spine (40% to 50%); the thoracic spine is more often involved than the lumbar or cervical spine.[32] Vertebral involvement may cause spinal cord or nerve root compression. The radiographic lesions on plain radiographs are lytic, similar to those of MM. Modern imaging techniques, such as MRI and PET-CT, are far more sensitive for the detection of bone lesions in PC neoplasms. Additional bone lesions on MRI are detected in about 30% of presumptive SBPs defined by the traditional skeletal survey.[33,175,176] As such, the diagnosis of SBP requires an MRI or CT study to confirm the solitary nature of the plasmacytoma and exclude the presence of additional osseous lesions.[33,175]

Serum or urine M protein is detected in approximately half of patients, and the SFLC ratio is also abnormal in about half.[32,79,177,178] The magnitude of the paraproteinemia is significantly lower than that in MM, reflecting the relatively smaller burden of clonal PCs in SBP. Because small M-protein levels may be missed by routine electrophoresis, patients should have immunofixation studies of serum and urine to detect minimal M protein. Uninvolved Igs are quantitatively normal in most cases.[79] Blood counts, renal function studies, and serum calcium levels are normal.[32]

Morphology, Immunophenotype, and Genetics

The morphologic features, immunophenotype, and genetics of SBP are similar to those of MM (Fig. 25-39).

Differential Diagnosis

SBP must be distinguished from other diseases that may present with isolated lytic bone lesions. These include many types of metastatic tumors, occasional lymphomas, and other lesions of hematopoietic origin such as Langerhans cell histiocytosis and rare primary bone lesions. Biopsy of the lesion is necessary for diagnosis. SBP is not usually a diagnostic challenge, except in cases in which the neoplastic PCs have plasmablastic or anaplastic morphology and may not be recognized as plasmacytic. Rigorous IHC evaluation is critical in such cases, especially confirmation of monotypic LC expression. Solitary plasmacytoma of bone is distinguished from MM by virtue of its unifocality and absence of the clinical, laboratory, or radiographic findings typical of MM.

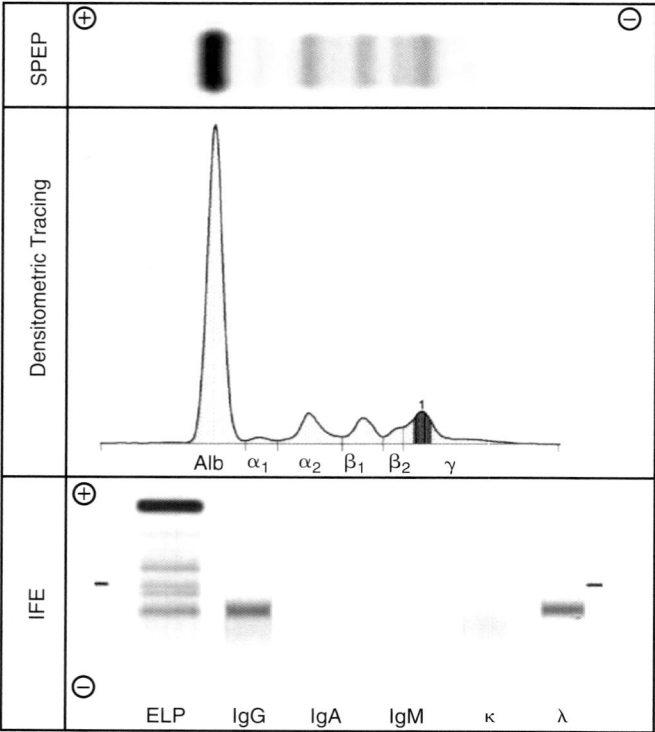

Figure 25-38. Serum electrophoresis in monoclonal gammopathy of undetermined significance (MGUS). The patient has no clinical, hematologic, or radiologic evidence of a PC neoplasm except a persistent, modest (0.4 g/dL), single M-protein peak *(shaded area 1 on densitometric tracing in middle panel)* by serum protein electrophoresis pattern. The M protein was identified by immunofixation electrophoresis as IgG lambda located in the β₂-region of the electrophoretogram. *(Courtesy Drs. Frank H. Wians Jr. and Dennis C. Wooten.)*

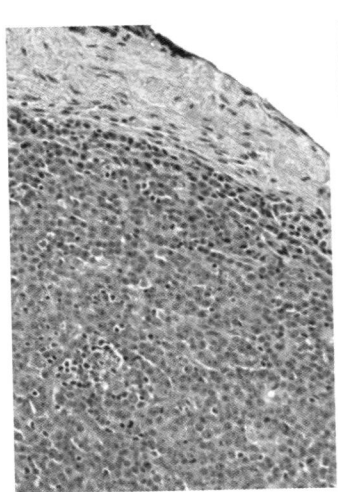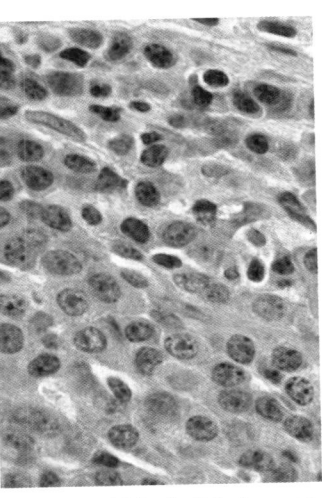

Figure 25-39. Solitary bone plasmacytoma. This skull lesion consists of a plasmacytoma with a fibrous border. The neoplastic cells have a somewhat immature appearance with less dense chromatin than normal PCs, and some contain nucleoli. A radiographic bone survey shows no other lesions, and a routine iliac crest bone marrow examination shows no evidence of a PC neoplasm. A minute serum IgG lambda M protein was detected by serum immunofixation electrophoresis (H&E stain).

Treatment, Clinical Course, and Prognosis

The treatment of choice for SBP is involved-field radiation, which affords long-term local disease control in 90% of cases and symptomatic relief in most cases.[178,179] M protein usually diminishes significantly after radiotherapy, and it disappears altogether in a substantial minority of patients.[180]

One-half to two-thirds of patients develop additional plasmacytomas or MM within 2 to 10 years.[32,177,178,181,182] New bone lesions, generalized marrow plasmacytosis, and increasing M protein are present with disease progression.[32,79,178,183,184] Approximately one-third of patients remain disease free for more than 10 years.[185] Many of the patients with MM have a relatively indolent course.[32]

High-risk factors for progression of SBP to MM include the presence of clonal bone marrow PCs (<10%), persistence of M protein for more than 1 year after radiotherapy, an abnormal SFLC ratio, monoclonal urinary free LCs, and flow cytometric detection of clonal PCs in morphologically disease-free bone marrow.[177,178,186,187] Patients with plasmacytoma in whom clinically occult bone marrow disease is identified by MRI are at a greater risk for progression to MM.[180,188] This finding supports the requirement for negative MRI or CT as a prerequisite for diagnosis of solitary plasmacytoma.[33,175]

Extraosseous Plasmacytoma

Definition

Solitary extraosseous/extramedullary plasmacytomas (SEPs) are localized PC tumors that arise in tissues other than bone marrow. Most appear to be biologically distinct from SBP and MM. Although a precise origin has not been clearly defined, evidence suggests commonality between some cases of SEP and marginal zone lymphoma.[189]

Epidemiology

SEPs account for less than 5% of PC neoplasms.[76,190] The median age at diagnosis is about 55 to 60 years, and two-thirds of patients are male.[190,191]

Clinical Features

SEPs present as a localized mass lesion. About 75% of them occur in the upper respiratory tract, including the nasal passages, sinuses, oropharynx, and larynx, but they may also occur in a variety of anatomic sites including lymph nodes, parotid and thyroid gland, breast, gastrointestinal tract, central nervous system, and several other organs.[170,190,191] SEPs of the upper respiratory tract spread to cervical lymph nodes in about 15% of cases.[192]

Symptoms are usually related to the tumor mass. Patients with SEPs in the upper respiratory tract may experience rhinorrhea, nasal obstruction, and epistaxis as presenting symptoms. Approximately 20% of patients have a detectable low quantity of M protein that is most commonly IgA. Hypercalcemia, renal failure, and anemia are not present, and radiographic and morphologic assessment shows no evidence of bone marrow involvement.

Morphology

The morphologic features are similar to those of other PC neoplasms (Fig. 25-40).[191] A rare type of SEP has been reported that occurs in children and younger adults, is predominantly nodal, and exclusively expresses IgA.[193] The PCs in these IgA SEPs grow in an interfollicular or diffuse pattern and are mature appearing. Bone marrow examination is recommended for adult patients with SEP to rule out overt myeloma or low-level involvement.

Immunophenotype and Genetics

The immunophenotype is similar to that of other PC neoplasms.[76,191] The PCs are clonal and exhibit LC restriction by IHC staining for kappa and lambda LCs (Fig. 25-40). Flow cytometric analysis on bone marrow should be performed in newly diagnosed SEP to evaluate for the presence of a low-level phenotypically aberrant PC population, as such patients appear to be at higher risk for progression to MM.[187] The genetics of SEP is similar to those of MM and include odd chromosome trisomies and *IGH* translocations, with the exception of t(11;14), which is uncommon in SEP, and possible overrepresentation of t(4;14).[76,194]

Differential Diagnosis

The differential diagnosis of SEP includes exuberant reactive PC proliferations and mature B-cell lymphomas with extreme plasmacytic differentiation, especially LPL and marginal zone lymphoma.[76,189] Exuberant reactive PC lesions are easily distinguished from SEPs in most instances by demonstrating a polytypic PC proliferation by IHC staining or flow cytometry. Distinction from lymphoma is often more difficult.

LPL consists of a mixture of clonally related PCs and lymphocytes, usually with lymphocytes predominating. In most cases, they are readily distinguished from a primary PC neoplasm, which has no lymphocyte component. However, in some LPLs, PCs are abundant and/or the lymphocytes have an unusually plasmacytoid morphology that mimics PCs. However, there are a few features that

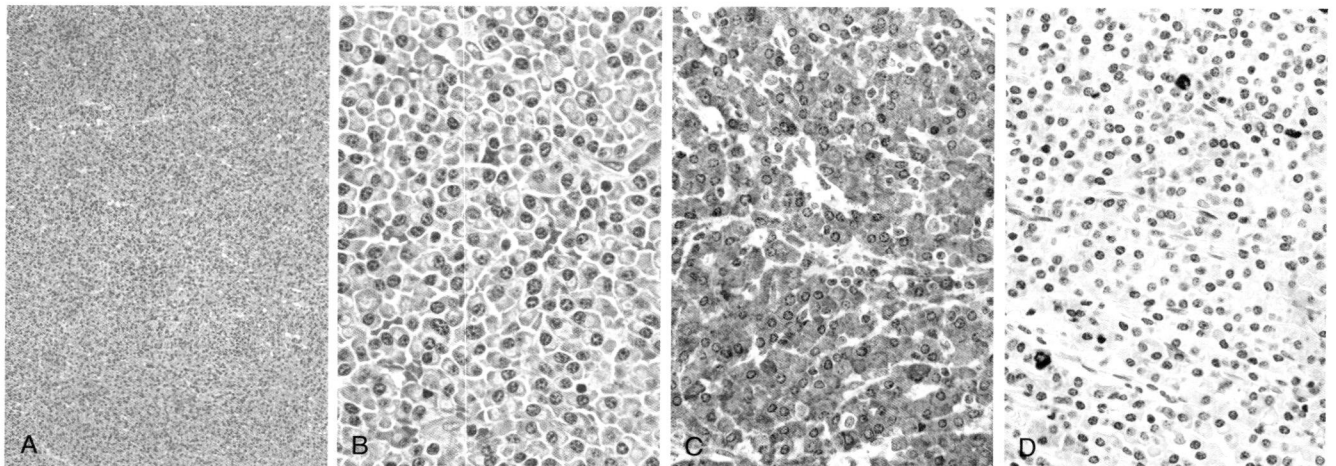

Figure 25-40. Extraosseous (extramedullary) plasmacytoma. A, In a 14-year-old girl with lupus and left cervical lymphadenopathy, the lymph node architecture is diffusely effaced by plasma cell (PC) proliferation. **B,** On higher magnification, the PCs are mature appearing. Lambda **(C)** and kappa **(D)** immunostains of the lymph node illustrated in Figure 25-36 show monotypic lambda light chain expression with only rare kappa positive cells (H&E stain; lambda and kappa light chain immunohistochemistry).

aid in the distinction between these two lesions. In LPL, the PCs express IgM and an associated IgM M protein is present in most cases, whereas the PCs in plasmacytoma usually express IgA or IgG. More precise distinction is made by analysis for the *MYD88* L265P mutation, which is present in approximately 90% of LPL cases but absent in plasmacytoma.[195,196]

Marginal zone lymphoma with extreme PC differentiation may mimic SEP in lymph nodes or extranodal tissue. Careful morphologic examination for areas with features typical of marginal zone lymphocytes and flow-cytometric identification of clonal lymphocytes with a marginal zone immunophenotype are helpful in making the distinction.[109,189] The flow cytometric immunophenotype of the PCs may also contribute. The clonal PCs in lymphoma more frequently express CD19 (95% vs. 10%) and CD45 (91% vs. 41%) and lack CD56 (33% vs. 71%) than do those in a primary PC neoplasm.[109] In some instances, SEP and marginal zone lymphoma with extreme PC differentiation cannot be distinguished with certainty.

Treatment, Clinical Course, and Prognosis

The mainstay of therapy for SEP is surgical excision and local radiotherapy. There is local recurrence or spread to regional lymph nodes in 15% to 25% of patients.[190,197] Occasionally, there is metastasis to distant sites, and 10% to 15% progress to symptomatic MM.[190,197,198] Ten-year disease-free survival ranges from 70% to 90%.[190,197,199]

IMMUNOGLOBULIN DEPOSITION DISEASES

There are two major types of Ig deposition disease: (1) primary amyloidosis and systemic LC (2) and HC deposition disease. These diseases are attributable to the synthesis and deposition of monoclonal Igs in various tissues and organs, eventually leading to organ dysfunction. This process is responsible for the frequently aggressive clinical behavior of these disorders despite the low burden of clonal PCs.

Light Chain Amyloidosis

Systemic amyloidosis consists of three major subtypes: primary or LC (AL) amyloidosis, secondary (AA) amyloidosis, and familial (AF) amyloidosis. The latter two forms of amyloidosis consist of several variants, none of which is associated with PC dyscrasias or IGLs. Neither these nor the local amyloidoses associated with aging, endocrine amyloidosis, or the β_2-microglobulin amyloidosis of hemodialysis patients will be discussed; interested readers are referred to the review by Merlini et al., "Systemic immunoglobulin light chain amyloidosis."[200]

Definition

AL amyloidosis is a PC dyscrasia in which the clonal PCs produce a misfolded LC protein that is deposited in the viscera and ultimately results in end organ damage and dysfunction.

Pathogenesis

The synthesis of an abnormal LC by a typically small clonal PC population in the bone marrow is the defining event in AL amyloidosis. AL amyloid is composed of intact LC or fragments thereof that include the amino-terminal variable (V) region and part of the constant region.[201] Both intact LCs and fragments are present in some cases. Although all LC V-region subgroups are potentially amyloidogenic, several are notably pathogenic, including IGLV1-44, IGLV1-51, IGLV2-14, IGLV3-1, IGLV6-57, IGKV1-33, and IGKV4-1.[201,202] Several physicochemical factors may promote or inhibit the formation of AL fibrils by influencing the aggregation of soluble LC, including polarity and charge complementarity dictated by the LC amino acid sequence, pH, and temperature.[201] Once formed, these fibrils are deposited and accumulate in tissues. AL amyloid deposition causes architectural distortion of the affected organ and toxic effects, including oxidative stress and apoptosis, all of which contributes to the end organ dysfunction that clinically defines the disease.[203] The underlying AL subtype influences, to some extent, the tissue tropism of amyloid deposition. For example, IGLV1-44 AL amyloid is associated with cardiac deposition, whereas deposition of IGLV6-57 amyloid tends to occur in the kidney.[204,205]

Epidemiology

AL amyloidosis is a rare disease, with an incidence of approximately 12 cases per million person-years in the United States[206]; however, the actual incidence of AL amyloidosis in the United States may be somewhat higher because of the underrepresentation in some clinical studies of African Americans, in whom AL amyloidosis is more common. The median age at diagnosis is 63 years, and more than 95% of patients are older than 40 years when diagnosed.[206,207] There is a slight male predominance. In most cases, only a low level of serum M protein and mild-to-moderate clonal plasmacytosis in the bone marrow are present, precluding a diagnosis of myeloma. However, concurrent AL amyloidosis and MM is found in approximately 20% of patients with AL amyloidosis.[208-210]

Clinical Features

AL amyloidosis has protean clinical manifestations, reflecting the underlying variability in tissue tropism for amyloid deposition. This clinical heterogeneity often results in prolonged intervals between presentation and diagnosis, during which time patients experience ongoing worsening of cardiac function, and ultimately poorer clinical outcomes.[211] Patients typically present with non-specific symptoms such as fatigue and weight loss.[203,212] Bone pain, peripheral neuropathy, and carpal tunnel syndrome are the first signs of disease in some cases. Hemorrhagic manifestations (acquired factor X deficiency) and symptoms associated with congestive heart failure, nephrotic syndrome, or malabsorption are all relatively common.[212,213] Physical findings include hepatomegaly in 25% to 30% of patients and, frequently, purpura.[212] Periorbital purpura and macroglossia are classic signs associated with AL amyloidosis; however, they are present in only a small minority of patients. Edema is often present in patients with congestive heart failure or nephrotic syndrome. Splenomegaly and lymphadenopathy are uncommon.[212]

Laboratory Findings

M protein is found in the serum by protein electrophoresis in about 50% of patients, by immunofixation in more than 80%, and by a combination of immunofixation and SFLC ratio analysis in up to 99%.[212,214] IgG is most common, followed by LC only, IgA, IgM, and IgD.[202] The LC is lambda in about 70% of these.[212] The median serum M-protein level is approximately 1.4 g/dL in large clinical studies.[212,215] About 20% of patients have hypogammaglobulinemia.[212] Free LCs detected in AL amyloidosis are significantly more likely to be N-glycosylated than in other PC neoplasms, particularly in cases of kappa AL amyloidosis, suggesting posttranslational modifications may enhance the toxicity of AL amyloid.[203,216]

Proteinuria is present at diagnosis by routine urinalysis in more than 80% of cases, and nephrotic syndrome or renal failure is found in approximately 30%; serum creatinine is >2 mg/dL in 20% to 25% of cases.[212] Hypercalcemia is occasionally present, almost always in patients with myeloma. Abnormal liver function studies are uncommon.

Hemorrhagic manifestations may result from factor X deficiency caused by the binding of factor X to amyloid

proteins.[213] Hemorrhage may also be caused by deficiency of vitamin K–dependent clotting factors, fibrinolysis, disseminated intravascular coagulation, and loss of vascular integrity caused by amyloid deposition.[212,213]

Radiographic studies of bones are normal in most patients with amyloidosis. Osseous lesions are restricted to patients with co-existing myeloma and amyloidosis.

Diagnosis

A diagnosis of amyloidosis is established by detection of amyloid tissue deposits. These deposits are most often evident within blood vessel walls and along basement membranes. These may expand over time to form space-occupying lesions that impinge on or disrupt the architecture of the involved tissue. Amyloid is eosinophilic in hematoxylin and eosin (H&E)-stained sections and has an amorphous, waxy appearance, often with a characteristic cracking artifact; amyloid is weakly positive with periodic acid–Schiff (PAS) stain. Macrophages and foreign body-type giant cells may sometimes be present at the periphery of amyloid deposits. The Congo red stain is the most commonly used technique for confirmation of amyloid in a tissue biopsy. The Congo red dye binds to the amyloid protein and produces a characteristic apple-green birefringence when evaluated under polarized light (Fig. 25-41).[201] Electron microscopy is rarely used today for diagnostic purposes; however, the ultrastructural findings are specific and can be confirmatory of the diagnosis. Amyloid protein consists of rigid, linear, nonbranching aggregated fibrils. The fibrils vary from 7 to 10 nm in width, have hollow cores, and are of indeterminate length.[217-219]

The frequency of amyloid deposition varies by tissue type. Bone marrow and fat pad aspirates each show positive Congo red staining in about 70% of AL amyloidosis cases; the likelihood of a positive Congo red stain increases to nearly 90% for a given patient when both tissues are evaluated.[203,212,220] Although the incidence of amyloid deposition is higher in renal and cardiac biopsies, sampling of these organs is associated with greater morbidity. Thus, the combined evaluation of bone marrow and fat pad is an appropriate first step for diagnostic confirmation in nearly all patients with AL amyloidosis.[203,220] Should these prove negative, renal or endomyocardial biopsy can be pursued in patients for whom amyloidosis is clinically suspected.

Though a positive Congo red stain indicates the presence of amyloid, confirmation of the amyloid subtype should be undertaken. In the past, this was usually achieved by IHC using antibodies that recognized the various amyloid fibril proteins, a technique that suffers from low sensitivity and specificity. Laser microdissection of the amyloid followed by liquid chromatography–tandem mass spectrometry (LC-MS/MS) has largely supplanted IHC for amyloid typing.[221] This technique affords the unequivocal identification of the amyloidogenic protein with nearly 100% sensitivity and specificity and circumvents many of the technical issues that may be encountered with IHC-based amyloid subtyping.[214,221]

It is essential to confirm the presence of LC in the amyloid deposits in any patient with presumptive AL amyloidosis, including those in whom associated serum or urine M protein is present. AA, AF, or other types of amyloid may be incidentally present in patients with MGUS or other PC proliferative disorders.[222-224] Because the treatment of amyloidosis is directed at the underlying cause, the

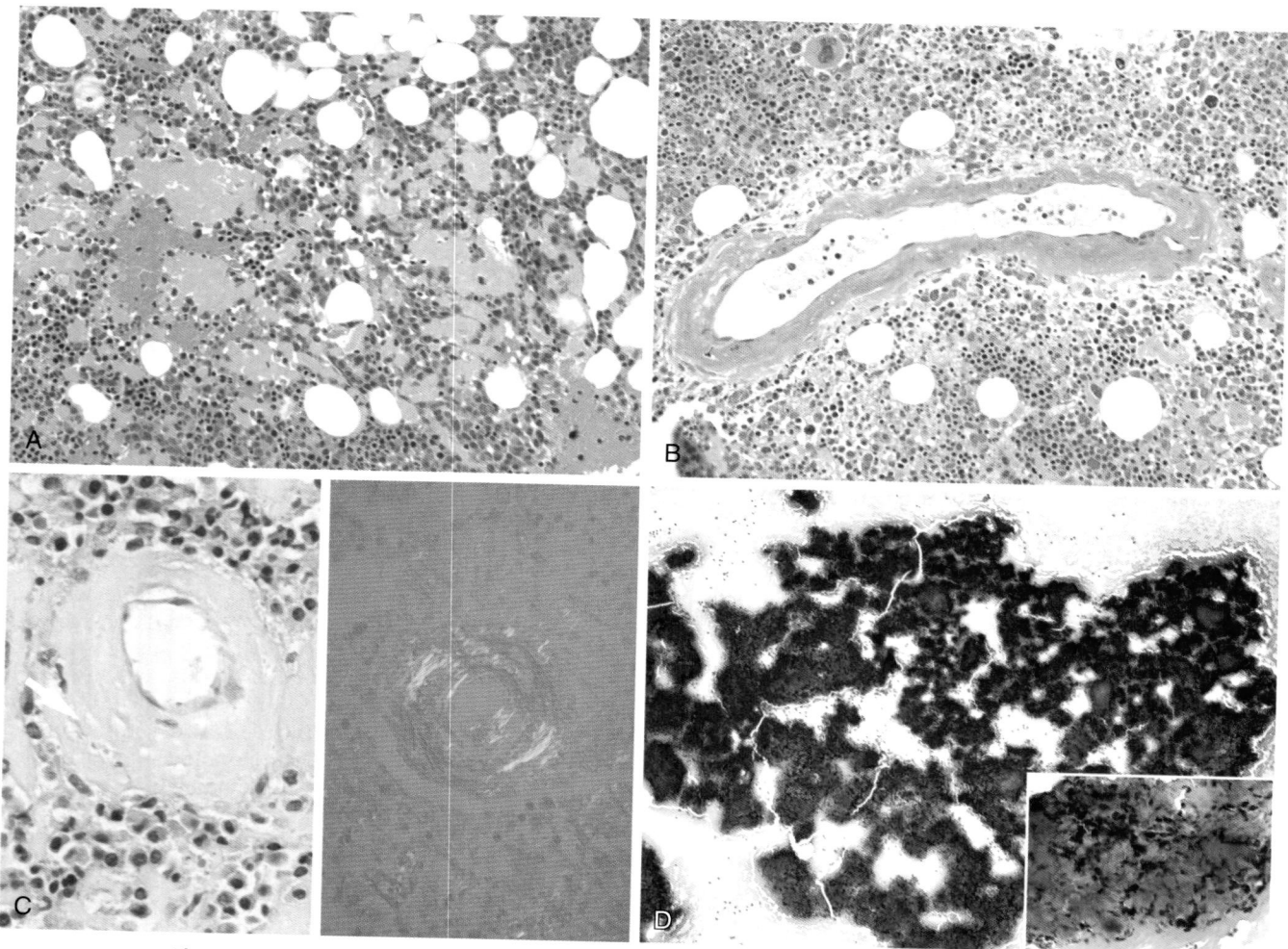

Figure 25-41. Primary (AL) amyloidosis involving bone marrow. A, Amorphous eosinophilic deposits of amyloid are present in the interstitium of the bone and may form space-occupying lesions when extensive. **B,** Blood vessel wall markedly thickened by amyloid deposits that are weakly PAS positive. **C,** Amyloid has a smudgy appearance in H&E stains *(left)* and shows typical birefringence in Congo red–stained sections examined using polarized light *(right)*. **D,** Amyloid deposits may be evident in the bone marrow aspirate and often have an angulated, geometric appearance; amorphous basophilic amyloid deposits are evident at higher magnification *(inset)* (H&E, periodic acid–Schiff, and Wright-Giemsa stains).

management of AL amyloidosis differs dramatically from that of other amyloidoses. Thus, the accurate amyloid subtyping is of paramount importance to appropriate clinical management.

Blood and Bone Marrow Findings

Blood counts are frequently normal at the time of diagnosis, but about 10% of patients present with hemoglobin levels below 10 g/dL. Leukopenia and thrombocytopenia are rare at diagnosis; about 10% of patients have thrombocytosis.[212] Abnormal blood counts are more frequent in patients with co-existing amyloidosis and myeloma. Blood smear findings are usually non-specific; rouleaux may be present in cases with a high M-protein level. Circulating PCs are observed in occasional cases, but substantial numbers of PCs are found only in the rare cases of amyloidosis associated with PCL.

Bone marrow examination should be performed in all cases of suspected AL amyloidosis. In most cases, PCs make up less than 10% of bone marrow cells in the aspirate

smear at diagnosis.[212] However, PCs account for more than 20% of cells in the minority of cases in which there is concurrent amyloid deposition and myeloma. The clonal PCs may appear morphologically mature or manifest the cytologic atypia typical of MM. Vacuolated PCs resembling those seen in μ-HC disease are present in some cases.[54] With extensive amyloid deposition in the bone marrow, variably sized clumps of lightly eosinophilic-to-basophilic proteinaceous material may be evident in the aspirate smears (Fig. 25-41).

The bone marrow biopsy findings are variable, ranging from no identifiable abnormalities to extensive deposition of amyloid or overt myelomatous involvement. A mild plasmacytosis composed of mature-appearing PCs is the most common finding. Amyloid may be evident in a thickened vessel wall if sufficiently large vessels are present in the biopsy or associated periosteum and soft tissue. Perivascular or interstitial amyloid deposition may be evident in the setting of more extensive involvement

(Fig. 25-41). Occasionally, most of the bone marrow biopsy is replaced with amyloid.

Immunophenotype

The immunophenotypic abnormalities of the clonal PCs in AL amyloidosis are identical to those seen in MM and MGUS. The pathogenic PCs in AL amyloidosis show lambda LC restriction in most cases. However, assessment of LC restriction by IHC or ISH performed on the bone marrow biopsy may be problematic in those cases in which normal PCs are abundant and may outnumber the amyloidogenic PC clone.[217,225,226] Phenotypic evaluation by flow cytometry, including confirmation of LC restriction, is preferable in such cases.

Genetics

The karyotypic aberrations in AL amyloidosis are similar to those of MM, with some differences in the relative frequency of specific lesions.[227-229] It should be noted that t(11;14) is present in 40% to 60% of AL amyloidosis cases, a frequency two to three times higher than in MM.[228-230] Other common chromosomal abnormalities include deletion of chromosome 13 or 13q14, trisomy of single chromosomes, and gain of chromosome 1q21. Some of these have adverse prognostic effects. For example, t(11;14) is predictive of a poor response to bortezomib-based chemotherapy and as such is a negative prognostic factor in AL amyloidosis.[231] However, patients with t(11;14) AL amyloid appear to respond well to therapies that incorporate newer agents such as daratumumab and venetoclax.[232]

Differential Diagnosis

The differential diagnosis of AL amyloidosis includes MM with amyloidosis, other types of amyloidosis (e.g., AA, AF, and LC and HC deposition diseases), and rarely, other disorders. MM with amyloidosis is distinguished from amyloidosis by the frequency of PCs in the bone marrow, the clinical findings, and the results of laboratory and imaging studies. Clinical findings and history are important in the distinction of AL amyloidosis from the other types. However, the diagnosis of any amyloidosis is predicated on the detection and subtyping of amyloid deposits by LC-MS/MS, as previously described.[214,221]

A Congo red stain or electron microscopic studies will differentiate AL amyloid from LC and HC deposition diseases. Finally, prominent serous fat atrophy in the bone marrow, sometimes referred to as gelatinous transformation, may histologically resemble extravascular amyloid deposition (Fig. 25-42). A Congo red stain, the clinical history, and laboratory findings readily distinguish between these two processes.

Treatment and Prognosis

Modern therapy for AL amyloidosis is predicated on elimination of the amyloid-producing PC clone, thereby abrogating further production of LC and tissue deposition of amyloid. Early diagnosis is critical, as it increases the likelihood the patient will tolerate subsequent therapy and improves the odds of reversing end organ damage.[233] The appropriate diagnosis of amyloidosis is unfortunately often delayed months or even years because of its rarity and non-specific clinical features. As a result, most patients with AL amyloidosis present with some degree of cardiac and renal impairment, and some 80% are

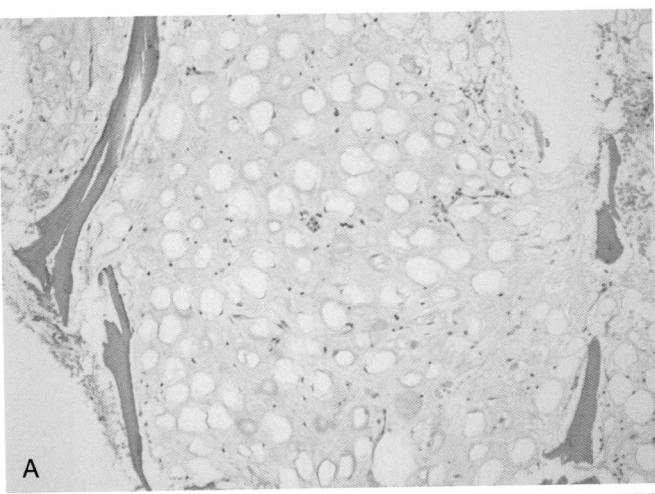

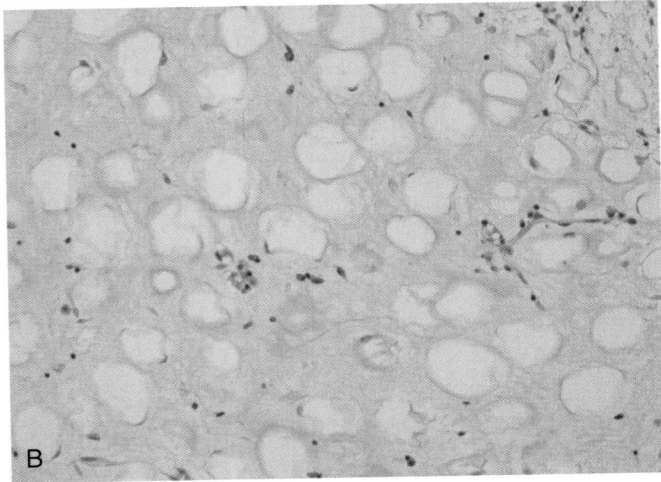

Figure 25-42. Bone marrow with serous atrophy of fat resembling amyloid. A and **B,** When extensive, the amorphous appearance of serous atrophy of fat may mimic amyloid deposition. Most cases of serous fat atrophy occur in individuals with severe malnutrition (bone marrow biopsy; H&E stain).

not suitable candidates, at least initially, for some of the more aggressive therapies such as autologous hematopoietic stem cell transplantation (HSCT).[234]

The advent of new, less toxic agents, including the proteasome inhibitor bortezomib and daratumumab, which targets CD38, has had a profound effect on therapy for AL amyloidosis. Dara-CyBorD (daratumumab, cyclophosphamide, bortezomib, dexamethasone) induces excellent rates of hematologic response, very good partial/complete responses, and significantly higher renal and cardiac response rates than regimens lacking daratumumab; it is now the frontline therapy for eligible patients.[232,235] A rapid and deep response to therapy is an important predictor of survival. It is important to note that inclusion of daratumumab overcomes the negative prognostic effect of t(11;14) in AL amyloidosis treated with previous bortezomib-based regimens.[235] The role of autologous HSCT is evolving and is now primarily reserved for patients who achieve suboptimal hematologic or organ responses to these newer therapeutics.[232] The safety profile of immunomodulatory agents, such as thalidomide and lenalidomide, has limited their use in patients with AL amyloidosis.[236]

Despite these therapeutic advances, prognosis in AL amyloidosis is still largely dictated by the extent of organ dysfunction at presentation. After initiation of therapy, improvement in cardiac, renal, and hepatic function typically lags several months to a year or more behind the hematologic response, highlighting the critical need for ongoing supportive care in patients with AL amyloidosis.[213,237,238] The role of solid organ transplantation in patients with irreversible cardiac or renal damage is controversial, but it may be appropriate in select patients.[236]

The SFLC level combined with two cardiac biomarkers, cardiac troponin-T and N-terminal pro-B-type natriuretic peptide (NT-proBNP), are the basis of the widely used Mayo staging system for AL amyloidosis.[239] Elevation of none or one or more of these parameters delineates four stages, which has prognostic effects. Patients with stage I and stage II disease have median overall survivals of 94 and 40 months, respectively, which is far superior to those of patients with stage III and stage IV disease, in whom the median survival is 14 and 6 months, respectively.[239] Present therapies have improved survival and quality of life for patients with AL amyloidosis, especially those diagnosed early with low-stage disease. For patients with high-stage disease, however, the prognosis remains poor, with significant cardiac involvement being the major determinant of outcome. However, within an advanced cardiac stage III cohort, evaluation of NT-proBNP and blood pressure may identify patients with significantly better outcomes.[233] Other factors associated with poor outcome are clonal PCs at myeloma levels (>10%), high baseline free LC levels, and elevated β_2 microglobulin.[219,239]

Systemic Light Chain and Heavy Chain Deposition Diseases

Definition

The monoclonal Ig deposition diseases (MIDDs) are PC or, rarely, lymphoplasmacytic neoplasms characterized by the secretion and deposition of an abnormal LC or HC chain, or both, in tissues, causing organ dysfunction.[2,26] The abnormal LC deposits neither form amyloid β-pleated sheets nor bind Congo red, and they lack an amyloid P-component. This group of disorders includes LC deposition disease (LCDD), HC deposition disease (HCDD), and LC and HC deposition disease (LHCDD), of which LCDD is the most common.[240-246]

Epidemiology

These are very rare diseases. Most patients are middle aged or elderly, and there is a variable male predominance.[241-243,245,247,248] LCDD often develops in association with MM (40% to 65% of cases) or MGUS.[243,245,249] Some cases are idiopathic or occur in association with a lymphoid neoplasm.[242,243,245]

Pathophysiology

The synthesis and deposition of a structurally altered LC or HC, resulting from either point mutations or deletions, is the central pathogenetic event in MIDDs. The primary defect in LCDD is the acquisition of mutations of the variable region of the IGL gene, with kappa LC of Vκ4 type overrepresented.[242,243,250] These mutations may result in replacement of polar amino acid residues by hydrophobic ones or aberrant N-glycosylation, thereby altering the solubility of the resulting LC, which ultimately results in its tissue deposition.[243,251] Deletion of the first constant domain, CH1, is a consistent finding in HCDD, a mutation that disrupts the association of the resulting IGH to the Ig binding protein, BiP, leading to premature secretion.[243,252] The variable regions in HCDD also contain amino acid substitutions, which result in an increased propensity for tissue deposition.[240,243,247,251]

Clinical and Laboratory Findings

Patients manifest symptoms of organ dysfunction resulting from systemic Ig deposition. The deposition of the aberrant Ig is most prominent on basement membranes and elastic and collagen fibers. Kidneys are most frequently affected. Nearly all patients with LCDD present with renal manifestations, most commonly nephrotic syndrome and/or renal failure.[245,248] Symptomatic extrarenal deposition occurs less frequently in LCDD, most commonly involving the heart, liver, and peripheral nerves, but is rare in HCDD.[243,245,253] Diffuse or nodular pulmonary involvement has also been reported.[254-256] Γ HC deposition is most common in HCDD, but rare cases of α, μ, and δ HCDD have been reported.[257-260] HCDD of IgG3 or IgG1 isotypes is associated with hypocomplementemia, as these subclasses most readily fix complement.[241,261] M protein is detected by SPE or IFE in approximately 85% of cases. An abnormal FLC level is present in virtually all LCDD cases.[243,249]

Morphology

The bone marrow burden of clonal PCs in LCDD and HCDD ranges from that of MGUS to symptomatic MM[243,245,249]; co-existent MM is less common in HCDD.[241,243] LPL, marginal zone lymphoma, and chronic lymphocytic leukemia are rarely encountered.[243,262]

Deposition of LC or HC is mostly found in renal biopsies but can be observed in bone marrow and other tissues in some cases. The Ig deposits consist of amorphous eosinophilic material that is neither amyloid nor fibrillar and stains negatively with Congo red. LCDD is diagnosed in renal biopsies via fluorescent anti-LC antibodies and electron microscopy.[243-245,261] Light microscopic evaluation of the renal biopsy typically shows nodular sclerosing glomerulonephritis. LC deposits in the glomerular and tubular basement membranes have a refractile eosinophilic appearance and are most frequently kappa type. Confirmation of LC deposition is usually achieved by immunofluorescence, which reveals the characteristic smooth, ribbon-like linear peritubular deposits of monotypic Ig along the outer edge of the tubular basement membrane. These deposits are nonfibrillar, powdery, and electron-dense on ultrastructural examination, with absence of a β-pleated sheet structure by radiographic diffraction.[244,245,261] Although uncommon, PCs are found in the vicinity of Ig deposition within visceral organs in some cases.[242,254]

Immunophenotype and Genetics

Kappa LC is expressed in 68% to 80% of LCDD cases, with overrepresentation of IGKV4-1, in contrast to AL amyloidosis, in which lambda LC expression predominates.[243,245,249] Depending on their frequency, the clonal PCs may exhibit an aberrant kappa-to-lambda ratio by LC IHC on bone marrow sections.

The underlying genetic abnormalities in LCDD and HCDD are poorly characterized, but those with co-existent MM presumably have aberrancies similar to those of other myelomas.

Differential Diagnosis

Amyloidosis is the main consideration in the differential diagnosis of LCDD and HCDD. These disorders are distinguished from one another based on their clinical features, Congo red and immunofluorescence staining, and ultrastructural and mass spectrometric analysis of the aberrant Ig deposits (see previous discussion in this chapter's section on the diagnosis of AL amyloidosis).

Treatment and Prognosis

Therapy is predicated on elimination or reduction of the clonal Ig-producing PCs to control deposition of the aberrant Ig in tissues, similar to the approach used for AL amyloidosis. The addition of daratumumab to drug regimens appears to have significant benefit in the few reported cases.[263,264] Supportive measures to preserve organ function, especially renal function, are important components of patient management.[245,253] Autologous HSCT is effective for controlling the disease and reversing renal dysfunction in some patients with LCDD.[265] The reported median overall survival for patients with LCDD varies widely, ranging from 4 years in older studies to 14 years in more recent reports,[245,248] a difference that likely reflects the effects of newer therapeutic agents such as bortezomib and daratumumab and improvements in supportive care. Deep hematologic responses to therapy are critical to preserving renal function and preventing disease recurrence in renal allografts.[248] Response to therapy can be monitored by evaluation of the SFLC levels.

PLASMA CELL NEOPLASMS WITH ASSOCIATED PARANEOPLASTIC SYNDROME

POEMS Syndrome

Definition

Polyneuropathy, **o**rganomegaly, **e**ndocrinopathy, **m**onoclonal gammopathy, and **s**kin lesions (POEMS) syndrome is a paraneoplastic disorder usually associated with an osteosclerotic PC neoplasm.[266-269] Several other features are frequently present that are not included in the POEMS acronym. These include Castleman disease, papilledema, edema and serous effusions, thrombocytosis, erythrocytosis, and elevated serum vascular endothelial growth factor (VEGF).[270] Most patients do not present with all of the manifestations. The diagnostic criteria are indicated in Box 25-8.[270]

Epidemiology, Etiology, and Pathogenesis

POEMS syndrome is a rare disease, accounting for 1% to 2% of PC neoplasms. Men are affected slightly more commonly than women (1.4:1 male-to-female ratio). The median age at diagnosis is about 50 years.[266] Many cases have been reported in Asia.[268]

The pathogenesis of POEMS syndrome is not well defined, but the dysregulated expression of proinflammatory cytokines, in particular VEGF, is a consistent feature of this disorder.[271-273] Despite this, VEGF-targeted therapy has shown

---

Box 25-8 *Criteria for the Diagnosis of POEMS Syndrome*

Mandatory
- Polyneuropathy
- Monoclonal plasma cell (PC) proliferative disorder

Major (One Required)
- Castleman disease
- Sclerotic bone lesions
- Elevated serum vascular endothelial growth factor (VEGF)

Minor (One Required)
- Organomegaly (splenomegaly, hepatomegaly, or lymphadenopathy)
- Extravascular volume overload
- Endocrinopathy
- Skin changes
- Papilledema
- Thrombocytosis

---

variable efficacy in POEMS syndrome, raising questions about its pathologic role in this disorder.[274-276] Although VEGF may influence localized paracrine effects that are not easily targeted therapeutically, this cytokine may instead simply represent a marker of disease rather than a central pathologic driver of it. The pathophysiologic connection among POEMS syndrome, osteosclerotic myeloma, and Castleman disease is not well understood.

Although the serum level of VEGF is elevated in POEMS syndrome in nearly all cases, the origin of VEGF remains controversial. VEGF is produced by both the clonal PCs and the background polyclonal PCs in POEMs. However, the clonal PCs in MGUS and MM express comparable levels of *VEGFA* mRNA; VEGF protein production was not assessed.[277] Because of the high frequency of certain motifs in the lambda variable-joining (VJ) segments in POEMS syndrome, it has been speculated that the aberrant autocrine/paracrine secretion of VEGF may be triggered by the clonal lambda LC through a molecular mimicry mechanism involving the chaperonin HSP90α.[278]

Clinical Features

The diagnosis of POEMS syndrome is often delayed as a result of its rarity and the complexity of clinical findings. The diagnosis of POEMS syndrome relies on fulfillment of mandatory, major, and minor criteria (Box 25-8).[270] The mandatory criteria include polyneuropathy and a monoclonal PC proliferation associated with M protein. The neuropathy is demyelinating, ascending, and symmetric and affects both sensory and motor function. The M protein is usually either IgA or IgG with a lambda LC in more than 95% of cases and is present at low levels (median 1.1 g/dL).[266] In addition to the mandatory criteria, at least one of three major criteria and one of six minor criteria are required for diagnosis. Several of these are usually fulfilled. The serum VEGF level is markedly elevated in most cases and correlates with disease activity.[279] Sclerotic bone lesions are present in approximately 95% of cases.[266,270] Single sclerotic lesions are detected by radiographic studies in about half of cases, and more than three lesions in one-third.[266] Two-thirds of patients with lymphadenopathy have the PC variant of Castleman disease, and most of these have a clonal PC proliferative disorder.[266] A rare Castleman variant of POEMS syndrome that lacks an associated clonal PC proliferation, but with many of the other paraneoplastic features, has been described.[270,280]

Three of the original pathologic findings in the POEMS acronym are presently considered minor criteria for diagnosis, but each is found in at least half of cases. Endocrinopathy, most frequently hypogonadism or thyroid disease, is found in more than two-thirds of patients. Skin changes, mostly hyperpigmentation and hypertrichosis, also occur in more than two-thirds of cases, whereas organomegaly is present in about 50% of patients.[270] Other minor criteria include extravascular volume overload manifesting as peripheral edema, ascites, or pleural effusion (30% to 85%), papilledema (~40%), thrombocytosis (~75%), or polycythemia (~15%). Other common but non-specific clinical findings include weight loss, fatigue, clubbing, bone pain, and arthralgias. Hypercalcemia, renal insufficiency, and pathologic fractures, all relatively common in MM, are rare in patients with POEMS syndrome.

Morphology

There are no specific morphologic changes in blood smears from patients with POEMS syndrome. Blood count abnormalities include thrombocytosis in about 75% of patients and polycythemia/erythrocytosis in 12% to 19%.[266,269,270] Blood counts are normal in some patients, and overall, cytopenias are less frequent in patients with POEMS syndrome than in those with MM.

An osteosclerotic plasmacytoma, either as a single lesion or multiple lesions, is the typical pathologic finding in POEMS syndrome. Directed bone biopsies are often required for diagnosis because of the focal nature of the lesions. The presence of bone trabeculae with marked osteosclerosis is a characteristic feature of these plasmacytomas (Figs. 25-43 to 25-45). Paratrabecular fibrosis is common with entrapped PCs that may appear elongated as a result of distortion by bands of connective tissue.[26] In random bone marrow biopsies away from the plasmacytoma, the marrow is usually normocellular, and the median number of PCs is usually less than 5% but may exceed 50% in patients with extensive marrow disease.[269,281] In patients with disseminated disease, the PCs are interstitially distributed or present in variably sized clusters. Lymphoid aggregates rimmed by monotypic or polytypic PCs may be evident in the bone marrow biopsy. Megakaryocyte hyperplasia is frequently present, often with atypical cytologic features and clustering similar to those in myeloproliferative neoplasms; reticulin fibrosis is absent.[281]

Immunophenotype

A monoclonal PC population is detected in most cases either by flow cytometry or IHC.[281] The clonal PCs are identified in a background of polytypic PCs in most cases. The clonal PCs in POEMS syndrome show the same immunophenotypic aberrancies as observed in other PCNs.[281] The clonal PCs are lambda LC restricted in approximately 95% of cases and express IgA or, less frequently, IgG by IHC.[266,269,281]

Genetics

From the few published analyses, the cytogenetic findings in POEMS syndrome are similar to those of myeloma, albeit

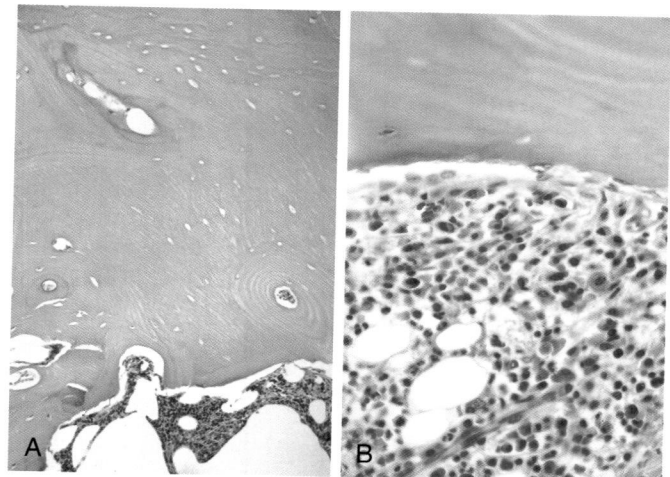

Figure 25-43. Osteosclerotic lesion in POEMS syndrome. Biopsy of an osteosclerotic vertebral lesion in a patient with polyneuropathy and serum IgA lambda M protein. **A,** Low magnification shows markedly thickened bone. **B,** A plasma cell proliferation adjacent to the bone is appreciated at higher magnification, and osteoblasts line the bony surface (bone marrow biopsy; H&E stain).

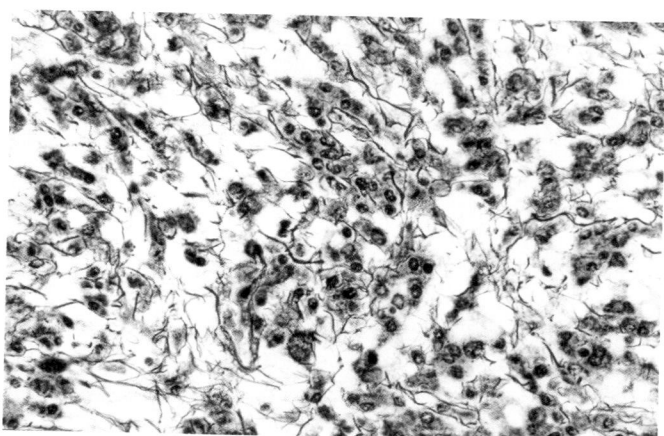

Figure 25-44. Reticulin stain of a PC lesion in POEMS syndrome. There is a moderate increase in reticulin with fibers weaving around clusters of PCs (Wilder's reticulin stain).

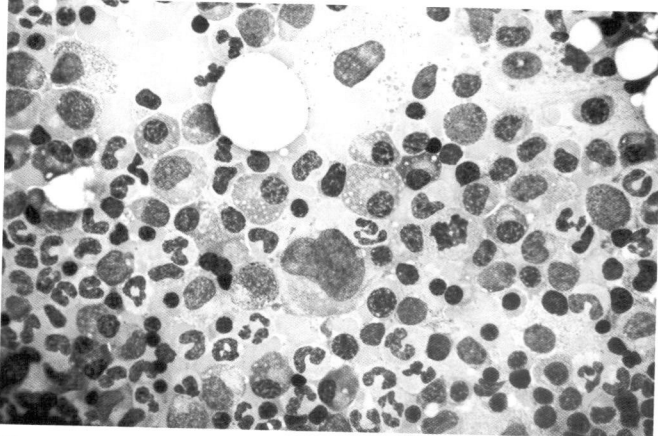

Figure 25-45. POEMS syndrome with multiple osteosclerotic bone lesions. There are increased plasma cells, which appear relatively mature; many contain cytoplasmic vacuoles (bone marrow aspirate; Wright-Giemsa stain).

with different frequencies of individual abnormalities.[282,283] IGH rearrangements are present in 22% to 45% of cases, mostly commonly t(11;14). The frequency of hyperdiploidy is variable in the few reported analyses.[277,282] Monosomy 13/deletion of 13q occurs at a frequency similar to that of myeloma.[282,283] No significant correlation between cytogenetic aberrancies and clinical features has been defined.[283]

As previously mentioned, the PCs in nearly all POEMS syndrome cases show lambda LC restriction. In such cases, there is very restricted use of lambda variable domains, with the clonal lambda sequence containing IGLV1-40 or IGLV1-44 in 83% of cases and rearranged to the IGLJ3*02 segment in 100% of cases.[278,284,285] Further, sequencing analysis has revealed distinctive mutational patterns in the VJ segment in POEMS syndrome, e.g., replacement of the threonine 38 residue in 100% of cases using an IGLV1-44 segment.[278] These restricted lambda variable domain and mutational patterns have obvious potential as diagnostic molecular markers in POEMS syndrome.

Differential Diagnosis

The diagnosis of POEMS syndrome is often problematic because of its rarity and protean clinical manifestations. Diagnosis requires the integration of biopsy findings with clinical data and the results of laboratory and imaging studies. If the primary focus is on any single paraneoplastic manifestation to the exclusion of the larger clinical picture, diagnosis can be delayed. In the early stages of disease, other polyneuropathies and clonal PCNs must be excluded, especially MGUS, asymptomatic myeloma, and solitary plasmacytoma. When POEMS syndrome is considered according to clinical findings, it can be confirmed by radiographic assessment, VEGF testing, and directed or random bone marrow biopsy.[270] Familiarity with the bone marrow changes in POEMS syndrome is important. The findings in random bone marrow biopsies can mimic a myeloproliferative neoplasm in some cases.[281]

Treatment and Prognosis

Radiotherapy is appropriate for patients with isolated bone lesions and no evidence of clonal PCs in the routine bone marrow examination, a therapeutic approach similar to that for solitary bone plasmacytoma. Improvement or resolution of the paraneoplastic symptoms occurs over several months, and in some cases, apparent cure can be achieved.[270] For patients with disseminated disease, systemic therapy is required with adjuvant radiotherapy to reduce any large bone lesions. The same agents used to treat MM are used in POEMS syndrome. Autologous HSCT is also an option.[270]

Overall, POEMS syndrome has a more favorable prognosis than MM or AL amyloidosis. The course is generally chronic and progressive but with a median overall survival up to 165 months, and 60% to 90% of patients survive 5 years or more.[270,286] Patients with localized disease and candidates for radiation therapy fare best. Clinical factors associated with shorter survival include older age, pulmonary hypertension, extravascular fluid overload, fingernail clubbing, and respiratory symptoms.[270,286] The most common causes of death are cardiorespiratory failure and infection.[266]

TEMPI Syndrome

Definition

The telangiectasias, elevated erythropoietin/erythrocytosis, monoclonal gammopathy, perinephric fluid collection, and intrapulmonary shunting (TEMPI) syndrome is a rare PC neoplasm with prominent paraneoplastic features with about 30 cases reported to date.[287,288] Like POEMS syndrome, the manifestations of TEMPI syndrome appear to be related to a clonal PC proliferation and its M protein. The specific clinical and laboratory findings, however, are mostly distinct from those of POEMS syndrome.

Etiology, Epidemiology, and Genetics

The etiology, pathogenesis, and prevalence of TEMPI syndrome are largely unknown. Most patients present in their 30s or 40s—both males and females, with no obvious ethnic or geographic skewing of cases.[287] Because of some degree of clinical overlap with other disorders, TEMPI syndrome may be somewhat more common than is suggested by the few reported cases.

The pathogenesis of TEMPI syndrome is poorly understood. Whole genome sequencing in a single case showed the absence of typical myeloma-associated initiator and driver mutations, including *IGH* translocations, hyperdiploidy, chromosome 13 deletion, and *RAS* gene mutations.[289] Interestingly, duplication of chromosome 22q11.23 was detected, which encompasses the *MIF* gene, which encodes a proinflammatory cytokine with angiogenic biological activity. Analysis of *MIF* mRNA and MIF protein levels in serum and bone marrow revealed significant elevations of MIF in TEMPI syndrome compared with control and MM cases, suggesting a possible pathophysiologic role for dysregulated MIF expression in TEMPI syndrome. In addition, the consistent elevation of serum erythropoietin (EPO) levels suggests the possibility of perturbation of the HIF1-α mediated oxygen sensing pathway in TEMPI syndrome, although the mechanism for this is unknown.[287]

Clinical and Laboratory Features

The onset of TEMPI syndrome is insidious, with slowly progressive symptoms. Most patients present with erythrocytosis and telangiectasias and subsequently develop intrapulmonary shunting and hypoxia. The erythrocytosis is driven by a progressive and marked increase in serum EPO levels. The telangiectasias are usually most prominent on the face, upper back, chest, and arms; the lower extremities are generally spared. The perinephric fluid collects between the kidney and renal capsule, is clear and acellular, and has a composition similar to serum. Venous thrombosis or intracranial hemorrhage is reported in some patients.[288,290,291] M protein is detected in all patients, but there is no clear association with a particular antibody isotype or LC.[288,292-295] The SFLC ratio and absolute levels are within normal limits in many patients.[291] Unlike POEMS syndrome, VEGF levels are not increased.[294]

Morphology

Bone marrow examination is often performed for unexplained erythrocytosis or an abnormal protein electrophoresis. There does not appear to be any specific blood or bone marrow morphologic finding in TEMPI syndrome, but erythrocytosis and marrow hypercellularity caused by erythroid hyperplasia are recurrent findings.[294] In one patient, erythroid and megakaryocytic atypia was described, and reactive lymphoid lesions were present in another.[294] Bone marrow clonal PCs are usually present at MGUS levels (<10%).[291,294] However, mild-moderate plasmacytosis with more than 10% PCs has been reported in a few patients, one of whom was diagnosed with SMM. No patient reported to date has fulfilled the criteria for symptomatic MM. Mildly atypical PCs are usually present, including ones with cytoplasmic vacuolization.[292,294]

Immunophenotypic Features

The immunophenotypic features for only a few TEMPI syndrome cases have been reported; the clonal PCs appear to manifest the same immunophenotypic aberrancies found in other PCNs.[287,289] In most cases, the PCs are IgG kappa restricted.[291]

Differential Diagnosis

Differential diagnosis considerations for TEMPI syndrome include other causes of erythrocytosis, mostly polycythemia vera, and POEMS syndrome. The marked elevation of EPO and lack of a *JAK2* V617F mutation largely exclude polycythemia vera. Secondary erythrocytosis is rarely associated with EPO levels as high as in TEMPI syndrome and can usually be distinguished by associated clinical manifestations. POEMS syndrome with erythrocytosis and skin changes may partially mimic TEMPI syndrome. VEGF levels are characteristically elevated in POEMS syndrome but are not increased in TEMPI syndrome.[294]

Treatment and Prognosis

In the limited reported cases, the main therapeutic approach in TEMPI syndrome has been directed at reduction of the clonal PCs and M protein. Complete or partial resolution of symptoms has been achieved with the proteasome inhibitor bortezomib or a bortezomib-based regimen followed by autologous HSCT.[292,294,296] Complete resolution of symptoms with single-agent daratumumab has been reported in two patients who had partial response or disease recurrence after bortezomib-based therapy.[295] The serum EPO level also provides a good index of therapeutic response in patients with TEMPI syndrome.[287,294] The efficacy of therapy aimed at ablation of the neoplastic PC clone substantiates the central role that the clonal PCs and M protein play in the pathogenesis of this paraneoplastic syndrome. Timely recognition of the disease and prompt initiation of treatment before development of advanced symptoms is key to a good clinical outcome.

Pearls and Pitfalls

Pearls

- Diagnosis of PCNs requires integration of clinical, morphologic, radiographic, and laboratory findings.
- Serum and urine immunofixation electrophoresis is the gold standard for characterizing the HCs and LCs of monoclonal Ig and for detection of small quantities of M protein.
- FLC analysis is highly sensitive for detecting minute quantities of M protein. It is important in monitoring patients and a prognostic indicator in all categories of PCN.
- IHC stains are valuable for quantitative assessment of plasma cells in bone marrow biopsies, for identification of a monoclonal plasma cell proliferation, and in distinguishing myeloma from other neoplasms.
- Flow cytometry should be performed for initial characterization of the neoplastic PC clone and to monitor for MRD.
- Cytogenetic and molecular genetic findings are the strongest predictor of prognosis for MM and should be performed in all cases for risk stratification.
- Patients with MGUS must be monitored indefinitely for evolution to a malignant PCN. The type and size of M protein and FLC ratio are significant predictors of MGUS disease progression.
- The diagnosis of SBP is predicated on sensitive imaging techniques, such as MRI or PET-CT, to exclude MM from the differential diagnosis.
- A high index of suspicion is necessary to avoid missing bone marrow involvement by AL amyloidosis, as amyloid deposits may be subtle, the extent of plasmacytosis is typically low, and the clonal PCs are often cytologically indistinguishable from normal PCs.
- AL amyloidosis can often be diagnosed based on the findings in a bone marrow biopsy and fat pad aspirate, obviating the need in most patients for endomyocardial or renal biopsies, procedures associated with greater risk of morbidity.
- Laser microdissection of the amyloid followed by liquid chromatography–tandem mass spectrometry is now the gold standard for molecular typing of amyloid deposits.

Pitfalls

- Low levels of monoclonal Ig, as commonly seen in IgD, IgE, and LC-only myeloma, may be undetectable by SPE. These can be missed if FLC analysis is not performed.
- Focal myelomatous bone marrow lesions may be missed in random biopsies. In patients with macrofocal myeloma, the extent of plasmacytosis in intervening marrow may be similar to that of MGUS.
- Low-level disease may go undetected if immunophenotyping by flow cytometry or IHC is not performed.
- Myeloma/MGUS-related cytogenetic changes may be undetectable by FISH performed on routine bone marrow specimens unless combined with cytoplasmic Ig staining to highlight PCs for analysis or by performing FISH on PC-enriched samples.
- SEP may be difficult to distinguish from lymphoplasmacytic and MALT lymphoma with extreme plasmacytic differentiation.
- Failure to perform amyloid typing may lead to a misdiagnosis of AL amyloidosis in a patient with unrelated MGUS and lead to inappropriate treatment.
- PCNs with a paraneoplastic syndrome may be deceptive, causing delayed diagnosis. Familiarity with the manifestations of POEMS and TEMPI syndromes is necessary for an appropriate index of suspicion.

KEY REFERENCES

1. Alaggio R, Amador C, Anagnostopoulos I, et al. The 5th edition of the World Health Organization classification of haematolymphoid Tumours: lymphoid neoplasms. *Leukemia.* 2022;36(7):1720–1748.
4. Landgren O, Kyle RA, Pfeiffer RM, et al. Monoclonal gammopathy of undetermined significance (MGUS) consistently precedes multiple myeloma: a prospective study. *Blood.* 2009;113(22):5412–5417.
5. Weiss BM, Abadie J, Verma P, Howard RS, Kuehl WM. A monoclonal gammopathy precedes multiple myeloma in most patients. *Blood.* 2009;113(22):5418–5422.
17. Chng WJ, Dispenzieri A, Chim CS, et al. IMWG consensus on risk stratification in multiple myeloma. *Leukemia.* 2014;28(2):269–277.

18. Palumbo A, Avet-Loiseau H, Oliva S, et al. Revised International Staging System for multiple myeloma: a report from International Myeloma Working Group. *J Clin Oncol.* 2015;33(26):2863–2869.

27. Fernández de Larrea C, Kyle R, Rosiñol L, et al. Primary plasma cell leukemia: consensus definition by the International Myeloma Working Group according to peripheral blood plasma cell percentage. *Blood Cancer J.* 2021;11(12):192.

28. Rajkumar SV, Dimopoulos MA, Palumbo A, et al. International Myeloma Working Group updated criteria for the diagnosis of multiple myeloma. *Lancet Oncol.* 2014;15(12):e538–e548.

76. Fend F, Dogan A, Cook JR. Plasma cell neoplasms and related entities-evolution in diagnosis and classification. *Virchows Arch.* 2023;482(1):163–177.

81. Vaxman I, Gertz MA. How I approach smoldering multiple myeloma. *Blood.* 2022;140(8):828–838.

220. Muchtar E, Dispenzieri A, Lacy MQ, et al. Overuse of organ biopsies in immunoglobulin light chain amyloidosis (AL): the consequence of failure of early recognition. *Ann Med.* 2017;49(7):545–551.

Visit Elsevier eBooks+ for the complete set of references.

Chapter 26

Nodular Lymphocyte-Predominant B-Cell Lymphoma

Andrew L. Feldman and Sylvia Hartmann

DEFINITION

Nodular lymphocyte-predominant B-cell lymphoma (NLPBL), also known as nodular lymphocyte-predominant Hodgkin lymphoma (NLPHL), is an indolent germinal-center (GC) B-cell neoplasm, usually with a nodular growth pattern, comprising a minority of large neoplastic cells with multilobated nuclei, the so-called "popcorn" or lymphocyte-predominant (LP) cells (formerly called *L&H cells [lymphocytic and/or histiocytic Reed-Sternberg cell variants]*), and a majority of reactive lymphocytes and histiocytes. Though previously considered a form of Hodgkin lymphoma, it has long been recognized that NLPBL shows clear and consistent histologic, epidemiologic, immunologic, and genetic differences from classic Hodgkin lymphoma (CHL). Molecular data have confirmed these differences and shown greater similarity to B-cell non-Hodgkin lymphomas (NHL). The Clinical Advisory Committee (CAC) for Lymphoid Malignancies recommended the term NLPBL to reflect this in the 2022 International Consensus Classification (ICC).[1]

SYNONYMS AND RELATED TERMS

The 5th edition of the World Health Organization (WHO) Classification[2] retains the term nodular lymphocyte-predominant Hodgkin lymphoma (NLPHL) as in the revised 4th edition, and this term can be used when needed so as not to interfere with ongoing clinical trials.

HISTORICAL BACKGROUND

The original classification of NLPBL as a Hodgkin lymphoma was in 1947, when Jackson and Parker identified a subtype termed *Hodgkin's paragranuloma*.[3] After describing a nodular variant of paragranuloma,[4] the so-called "Rye classification" combined lymphohistiocytic nodular and diffuse types into one class designated LP.[5,6] Work by Poppema and coworkers on the histology, immunophenotype, and epidemiology of these cases indicated that they represented an entity separate from CHL.[7-9] A more formal distinction from CHL was proposed by the International Lymphoma Study Group in the Revised European American Lymphoma (REAL) classification[10] and adopted by the WHO[11] under the term NLPHL. In 2021, the CAC introduced the term NLPBL and grouped this entity with B-cell NHLs based on molecular findings including data suggesting a pathologic and biological continuum between NLPBL and T-cell/histiocyte-rich large B-cell lymphoma (THRLBCL).[1]

EPIDEMIOLOGY

NLPBL accounts for 3% to 8% of Hodgkin lymphomas in Western countries.[12-14] In older series, one-third to half of the cases may in fact have been lymphocyte-rich (LR) CHL. NLPBL occurs in all age groups, with a peak incidence in the fourth decade, in contrast to a peak incidence in the third decade for the nodular sclerosis subtype of CHL (Fig. 26-1).[9,15] NLPBL shows a male predominance of 2.4:1, different from the slight female predominance in nodular sclerosis CHL. There are no significant differences between the epidemiologic features of cases that are exclusively nodular and those with prominent diffuse areas.

Familial cases of NLPBL have been reported.[16,17] A Finnish population-based study indicated a high familial risk in families with *NPAT* or *TET2* germline alterations.[18-20] First-degree relatives of NLPBL patients had a standardized incidence ratio for NLPBL of 19, compared with 5.3 for CHL and 1.9 for NHL. Familial NLPBL affected males and females equally, in contrast to the male predominance of NLPBL overall. The reasons underlying the familial risk for NLPBL are unknown but may include both genetic and environmental factors, including infectious etiologies.

Immune responses also distinguish NLPBL from CHL. Variants in the *KLHDC8B* gene have been found in familial CHL but were not definitely associated with familial NLPHL.[21] Conversely, NLPBL has been reported in two children with Hermansky-Pudlak type 2 syndrome, a primary immune deficiency associated with *AP3B1* mutations.[22] These patients were found to have reduced NK and NK T-cell subsets, suggesting a possible role of effector cell defects in NLPBL. The risk of Hodgkin lymphoma in young adults decreases with an increasing number of C alleles at position −174 in the interleukin-6 promoter.[23] A significant excess of G alleles at this position was observed in young adults with NLPBL.[24] A truncating germline mutation in *NPAT*, a gene adjacent to *ATM* that encodes a nuclear protein associated with cell-cycle regulation, has been shown to segregate with NLPBL in an affected Finnish family; another germline variant in *NPAT* was found in several other patients with NLPBL or CHL.[25]

There are several indications that Hodgkin lymphoma may have an infectious cause,[26,27] and there is extensive evidence that Epstein-Barr virus (EBV) plays a role in a major subset of CHL.[28,29] Some studies have found evidence of EBV-positive NLPBLs, especially in developing countries,[30-34] whereas other studies found only negative cases.[35,36] Though inclusion of lymphocyte-rich classic Hodgkin lymphoma (LRCHL) cases in older reports[37] and early EBV infection as seen in developing countries[33] might explain rare EBV-positive NLPBL in some series, two North American studies have confirmed the existence of true EBV-positive NLPBLs.[38,39] Data suggest little geographic difference in clinicopathologic features, including EBV positivity.[40] EBV-positive LP cells typically co-express CD30 and demonstrate latency type II. In some cases, the LP cells are only partially EBV positive and/or EBV positivity is also seen in occasional bystander lymphocytes, suggesting EBV may not be a primary driver of NLPBL lymphomagenesis.[41] A possible role of other viruses, including human herpesvirus 6, has been studied[42] but has not been demonstrated to date. Although CHL is seen with increased frequency in patients infected with human immunodeficiency virus (HIV), a risk for NLPBL has not been observed.[43] An antigen screen approach identified an RNA polymerase, RpoC, derived from *Moraxella catarrhalis* as a frequent antigenic target of the B-cell receptor of IgD-positive LP cells; activation induced by RpoC was additive with the *Moraxella* superantigen MID/hag.[44] These patients frequently presented with HLA haplotypes HLA-DRB1*04 and HLA-DRB1*07, indicating a role for cognate T-cell help.[45]

CLINICAL FEATURES

Patients usually present with isolated lymphadenopathy of long duration. There is frequent involvement of cervical and axillary nodes, with less frequent inguinal or femoral nodal involvement. Mediastinal NLPBL is an unusual finding (7%).[15,46] The most frequently involved primary extranodal sites include the tonsil, parotid gland, and soft tissue. The liver and spleen are common extranodal sites of high-stage node-based disease. Splenic involvement is associated with variant histologic patterns and has an increased risk for transformation to DLBCL.[47,48] B symptoms are uncommon and are found in only 10% of patients.[46] Bone marrow involvement by NLPBL is extremely rare (2.5%) and is associated with aggressive clinical behavior and poor prognosis; the frequency of bone marrow involvement is increased in NLPBL with variant histologic patterns.[49,50]

NLPBL typically presents as early-stage disease, with slow progression and an excellent outcome with standard therapy. Approximately 20% of patients have advanced disease at the time of presentation.[15] Recurrences develop in a relatively high percentage (~21%), regardless of original clinical stage, and multiple recurrences (27%) are not uncommon.[15] In 65% of cases, the recurrence is local or regional; in 23%, the recurrence is in a different region; and in 12%, the disease is generalized. Frequently (in 67%), the histopathologic growth pattern at relapse remains identical to that at initial diagnosis, and the time to relapse is related to the growth pattern, with nodular cases relapsing up to 16 years after initial diagnosis.[51]

NLPBL is not known to transform to CHL, though clonally related NLPBL and CHL have been reported.[7,52] In contrast, transformation to DLBCL has been reported to occur in 3% to 14% of cases[7,47,53] and is associated with variant histologic patterns of NLPBL.[54] Less commonly, NLPBL and DLBCL

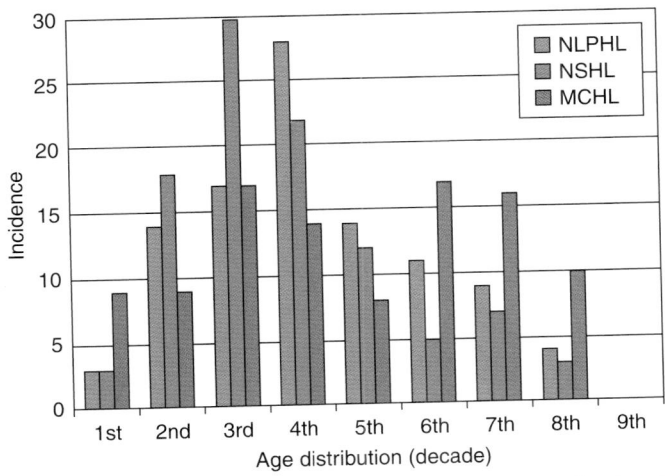

Figure 26-1. Age distribution of nodular lymphocyte-predominant B-cell lymphoma (NLPBL, denoted in the figure as NLPHL; n = 206), nodular sclerosis classic Hodgkin lymphoma (NSHL; n = 398), and mixed cellularity classic Hodgkin lymphoma (MCHL; n = 293) in a case series from the lymph node registry in Kiel, Germany, 1978. Note the peak incidence of NLPBL in the fourth decade versus the peak incidence of NSHL in the third decade.

are seen in the same site as composite lymphoma.[55,56] Transformation to DLBCL and the relationship between NLPBL and THRLBCL are discussed later in this chapter.

MORPHOLOGY

Histologic Patterns

At low magnification, complete obliteration of the lymph node architecture is usually evident. In some cases, a compressed rim of normal lymphoid tissue with reactive follicles is present in the periphery of the node, usually sharply demarcated from the tumor tissue. Fan and associates[57] described six immunoarchitectural patterns of NLPBL, given letter designations A-F: (A) "classic" nodular pattern, B-cell-rich; (B) serpiginous/interconnected nodular pattern; (C) nodular with prominent extranodular LP cells; (D) nodular with T-cell–rich background; (E) diffuse pattern (THRLBCL-like); and (F) diffuse, "moth-eaten," with B-cell–rich background. The histologic pattern, particularly in cases with variant patterns, should be reported. A mixture of patterns in a single biopsy is more commonly observed than a single, pure pattern. At the 2021 CAC conference, it was recommended that the immunoarchitectural patterns be segregated into two groups for clinical purposes because of the prognostic effect of variant histology.[1,58] Grade 1 would include typical cases (Fan patterns A, B, and C). These patterns show retained nodular architecture and prominent small B cells. Grade 2 would include variant patterns (patterns D, E, and F). Cases with grade 2 histology might benefit from treatment similar to those of DLBCL, though clinical features also influence treatment decisions, and additional study is needed. Of note, a study found that pattern C cases were associated with an intermediate clinical stage between patterns A/B (mostly early/intermediate stage) and patterns D/E (mostly advanced stage)[59]; additional study of the prognostic significance of pattern C is warranted.

Neoplastic cells are found both within and outside the macronodules (Fig. 26-2).[7,8] The nodularity created by loose aggregates of follicular dendritic cells (FDCs) is generally easily appreciated in routine H&E (hematoxylin and eosin) slides, but it may be visualized by immunohistochemistry.

The nodules vary in size, but they are mostly large. A diffuse growth pattern can be seen focally; rarely, it may predominate.

The predominant cell population in the nodules is small lymphocytes. The presence of histiocytes and LP cells leads to a "moth-eaten" appearance (Fig. 26-3). In some cases, groups of epithelioid cells may form a ring in a circular pattern around the nodules (Fig. 26-4).

Scattered FDC nuclei can be identified; in some cases, multinucleated, Warthin-Finkeldey–type giant cells are seen. These are most likely FDC multinucleated variants (Fig. 26-5). The cellular composition of the nodules may vary within the same lymph node: nodules with a predominance of lymphocytes can be seen together with nodules showing a large proportion of epithelioid histiocytes.

Occasionally, only a small number of LP cells are present; more often, they can be found with little difficulty. In rare cases, they form large clusters and are the most conspicuous cell type within some nodules[60]; the few published cases with nodules of syncytial LP cells had good outcomes.[60,61] Although typical LP cells have characteristic cytologic features, neoplastic cells

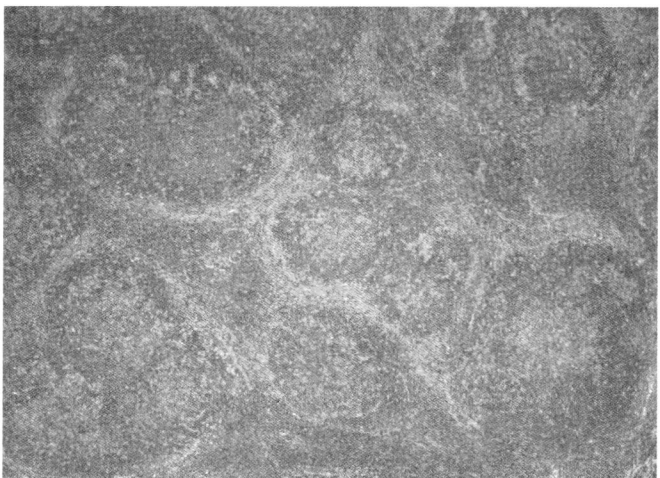

Figure 26-2. Nodular lymphocyte-predominant B-cell lymphoma. The normal lymph node architecture is replaced by nodules containing predominantly small lymphocytes.

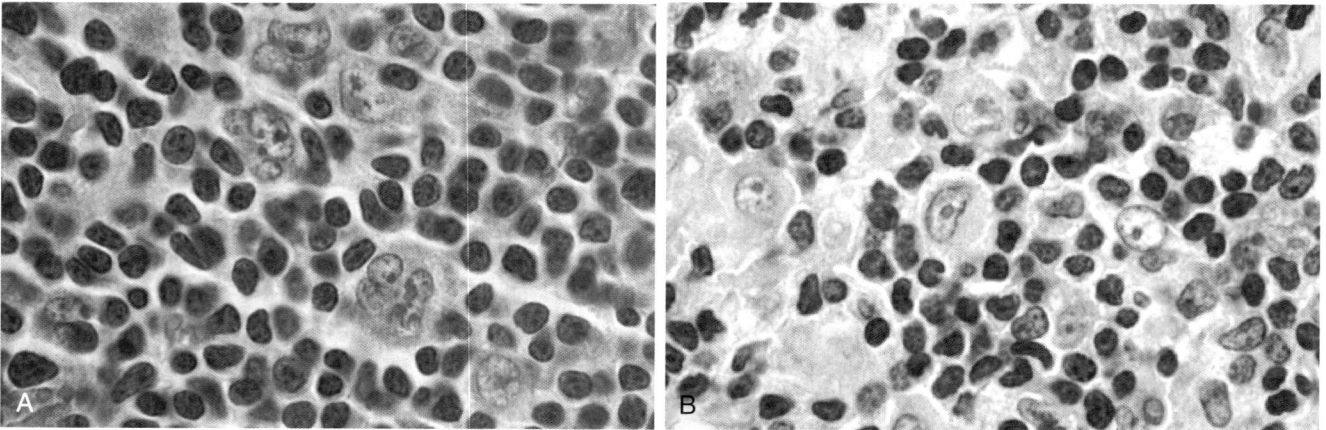

Figure 26-3. A, Several lymphocyte-predominant cells with multilobated nuclei and a small rim of cytoplasm can be seen. **B,** Several histiocytes with prominent cytoplasm are present. Both cell types are surrounded by small lymphocytes.

Figure 26-4. The nodules of nodular lymphocyte-predominant B-cell lymphoma may be surrounded by clusters of epithelioid histiocytes.

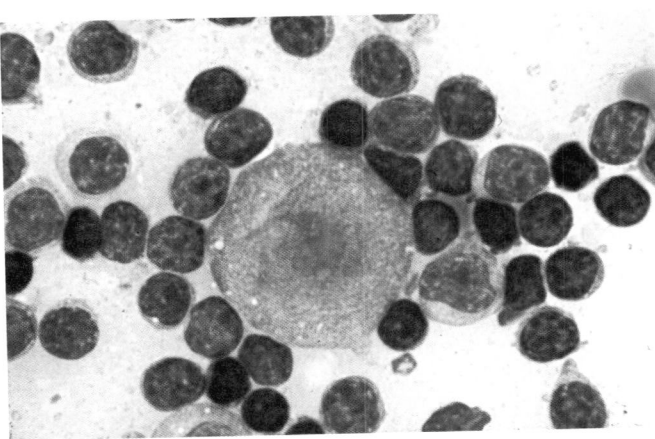

Figure 26-5. Imprint of a lymph node with nodular lymphocyte-predominant B-cell lymphoma showing an LP cell surrounded by rosetting activated lymphocytes.

resembling classical Hodgkin and Reed-Sternberg (HRS) cells also may be seen.[7,37] The identification of classical HRS cells should always prompt careful immunohistochemical evaluation to exclude the possibility of LRCHL with a nodular pattern. However, in some cases of NLPBL, the LP cells may mimic classical HRS cells while retaining the immunophenotype of LP cells. Conversely, cases of otherwise typical NLPBL may express CD30 and/or CD15.[62-64]

The compressed internodular areas contain small lymphocytes and high endothelial venules. Plasma cells and eosinophils are characteristically scarce or absent. In some cases of NLPBL, there is a nodular sclerotic stromal reaction, particularly in large nodal masses. Because a documented history of long-term nodal enlargement is available in some of these cases, it is possible that this represents a chronic-phase tissue reaction to the NLPBL.

Distinction of the diffuse (THRLBCL-like) pattern of NLPBL (Fan pattern E[57]) from THRLBCL has led to some controversy over whether these are actually distinct processes[58]; they likely reside within the same spectrum. An argument in favor of retaining the pattern E terminology is that pattern E may co-exist with other histologic patterns in the same case. In a review

Table 26-1 Major Diagnostic Features of Nodular Lymphocyte-Predominant B-Cell Lymphoma

Feature	LP Cells	Background Cells
Morphology	Nuclei larger than centroblasts, hyperlobated nuclei, medium-sized nucleoli, sparse basophilic cytoplasm	Follicles with predominantly small lymphocytes, together with histiocytes and LP cells; "moth-eaten" appearance
Immunophenotypic features	CD45+, CD20+, CD15−, CD30−, BCL6+, AID+, BSAP+, OCT2+, BOB.1+, PU.1+/−, MUM1+/−, T-bet+/−, HGAL+, BCL2−, p53−, CD10−, CD138−, EBV−	Predominantly CD4+ T cells; CD4+, c-MAF+, CD57+, PD1+ T-cell rosettes around LP cells are present; low ratio of TIA-1+ to CD57+ T cells
Genetic and molecular findings	Clonal immunoglobulin gene rearrangements; ongoing mutations; *BCL6* rearrangements in half of cases; *BCL2* translocation usually not detected	Polyclonal B cells and T cells

AID, Activation-induced cytidine deaminase; *EBV,* Epstein-Barr virus; *HGAL,* human germinal-center–associated lymphoma protein; *LP,* lymphocyte predominant.

of a large case series by the European Task Force on Lymphoma, only 2% lacked nodular areas.[65] In the largest series of NLPBL cases reviewed, only 7 cases out of 219 (3%) closely resembled THRLBCL.[37] Recurrence of NLPBL with a purely diffuse pattern has been described[66] and has been designated THRLBCL-like transformation of NLPBL. The presence of numerous LP cells outside the nodules may predict progression to a THRLBCL-like pattern.[57] This pattern is also encountered as nodular aggregates involving the white pulp of the spleen.

The major diagnostic features of NLPHL are summarized in Table 26-1.

Lymphocyte-Predominant Cells

LP cells are large cells, with nuclei larger than those of normal centroblasts (Fig. 26-5). Owing to their complex lobation, the term *popcorn cells* has been widely used. The nucleoli are medium-sized, generally basophilic, and smaller than those of classical HRS cells. The cytoplasm of LP cells is relatively sparse. In Giemsa-stained tissue sections and in Wright-stained imprints or smears, the cytoplasm may be moderately basophilic.

IMMUNOPHENOTYPE

Lymphocyte-Predominant Cells

Lymphocyte-Signaling Molecules

LP cells stain with antibodies to CD45, in contrast to most classical HRS cells (Table 26-2).[67,68] There is consistent staining for pan–B-cell markers such as CD20 (Fig. 26-6A), CD22, and CDw75.[69-74] This profile differs

Table 26-2 **Antigen Expression of Lymphocyte-Predominant Cells**

Antigen	Significance	Findings
Lymphocyte-Signaling Molecules		
CD45 (LCA)	All leukocytes Tyrosine phosphatase activity	Positive[248]
CD45RA (KIB3)	B cells, T-cell subsets, monocytes	Positive[248]
CD45RB	Thymocytes, T cells	Positive
CD45RC	B cells, CD8-positive T cells	Positive
CD45RO (UCHL1)	Thymocytes, monocytes, macrophages, granulocytes	Negative
CD20 (L26)	B cells (not plasma cells)	~100% positive[68-73]
CDw75 (LN1)	GC cells	Positive[68-73]
CD79A (MB1)	Pan-B cells	Positive, but lower than CD20[37]
CD19	B cells (not plasma cells)	Negative[78]
CD40	B cells, dendritic cells, macrophages	Positive[79]
CD70	Activated B cells and T cells, receptor for CD26	Positive[79]
CD80	GC blasts and APC, receptor for CD28 and CTLA-4	Positive[79]
CD86	GC blasts and APC, receptor for CD28 and CTLA-4	Positive[79]
MHC II (TAL1B5)	Control of immune responses through presentation of peptide antigens to T cells	Positive
CD74 (LN2)	B cells, invariant chain of MHC II	Positive
CD30 (Ki1/Ber H2)	Activated T cells and B cells	Generally negative[37]
CD15 (Leu M1)	Myeloid cells	Negative[37]
J chain	B cells	~60% positive[86,87]
IgG, IgM, IgA, IgD	B cells	Variably positive
Igκ, Igλ	B cells	Variably positive
FREB	Leukocyte Fc receptor family, GC B cells	Positive[89]
AID	Essential for SHM and CSR in GC B cells	Positive[90]
GCET1	GC B cells	Positive[91]
HGAL (GCET2)	GC B cells	Positive[92]
SWAP70	B cells, specificity for the switch regions upstream of the constant region IG genes	Positive[93]
CD10	GC B cells	Negative[81,94]
Signaling Intermediates		
NTAL	Adapter protein, linker for activation of B cells	Positive[95]
CD138 (SDC1)	Post-GC terminal B cells, epithelial cells	Negative[98]
LYN kinase	B-cell intracellular signaling molecule	Usually negative[249]
JAK2	B-cell intracellular nonreceptor tyrosine kinase	Positive[100]
Transcription Factors and Regulators		
OCT1	IG gene TF	Positive[101]
OCT2	IG gene TF	Positive[101]
BOB.1	Essential for response of B cells to antigens and formation of GCs	Positive[101]
BSAP/PAX5	B-cell development and differentiation	Positive[101]
ID2	Negative regulation of E2A and PAX5	Positive[102]
PU.1	IG gene TF	Variably positive[103,104]
MUM1	Subset of GC B cells, plasma cells	Inconsistently positive[250]
BCL6	TF expressed in GC cells	Positive[149]
BLIMP1	GC B cells showing plasma cell differentiation, plasma cells	Negative[107]
FOXP1	Mantle zone, some GC B cells	Negative[111]
T-bet	Th1 cell development, role in Ig class switching	Half of cases positive[115]
GATA3	Th2 cell development	Negative[115]
GATA2	Development of hematopoiesis	Negative[251]
c-MAF	Th2 cells, responsible for tissue-specific expression of IL-4	Negative[115]
NFATc1	Normal homeostasis and differentiation	Usually cytoplasmic positive[119]
REL (c-Rel)	NF-κB family member, antiapoptotic activity, function in lymphopoiesis	Negative ≫ positive[122]
RELA	NF-κB family member, antiapoptotic activity, function in lymphopoiesis	Positive[123]
BAFF-R (TNFRSF13C)	Mantle zone B cells, subset of GC B cells	Weakly positive or negative[125]
JUNB	Component of AP1 transcription complex involved in cell proliferation and apoptosis	Negative[128]

Table 26-2 Antigen Expression of Lymphocyte-Predominant Cells—cont'd

Antigen	Significance	Findings
Cell-Cycle Proteins		
Ki-67 (MKI67)	Marker of proliferation	Positive
PCNA	Proliferating cells	Positive[252]
TOP2A	Cell proliferation marker	Positive[131]
Tumor Suppressors and Apoptosis-Related Proteins		
CASP3	CD95-mediated apoptosis	Negative[132,133]
c-FLIP	Competitive negative regulator of Fas-induced death	Negative ≫ positive[134]
p53	Apoptosis-related protein	Negative[135]
TP73L (p63)	Subset of GC B cells	Positive[138]
BCL2	Represses cell death by apoptosis	Negative[35]
BAX	Promotes cell death by apoptosis	Positive[140]
A20	Inhibits cell death by apoptosis induced by TNF	Variably positive[141]
TRAF1	Downstream component in CD30 signaling pathway	Negative[122]
Structural Proteins and Adhesion Molecules		
Vimentin	Intermediate filament	Negative[143]
Fascin	Actin-bundling protein, dendritic cell marker	Negative[144]
CD44H	Mediates adhesion of leukocytes	Negative[145]
EMA	Epithelial cells, plasma cells	Variably positive[146,68]

AID, Activation-induced cytidine deaminase; *APC,* antigen presenting cell; *AP1,* activator protein-1; *BAFF-R,* B-cell–activating factor receptor; *CSR,* class-switch recombination; *EMA,* epithelial membrane antigen; *FREB,* Fc receptor homologue expressed in B cells; *GC,* germinal center; *GCET,* germinal-center B-cell–expressed transcript; *HGAL,* human germinal-center–associated lymphoma protein; *IG,* immunoglobulin; *IL,* interleukin; *MHC,* major histocompatibility complex; *NFAT,* nuclear factor of activated T cells; *NF-κB,* nuclear factor-κB; *NTAL,* non–T-cell activation linker; *PCNA,* proliferating cell nuclear antigen; *SHM,* somatic hypermutation; *SWAP70,* switch-associated protein-70; *TF,* transcription factor; *TNF,* tumor necrosis factor; *TOP2A,* topoisomerase II alpha enzyme.

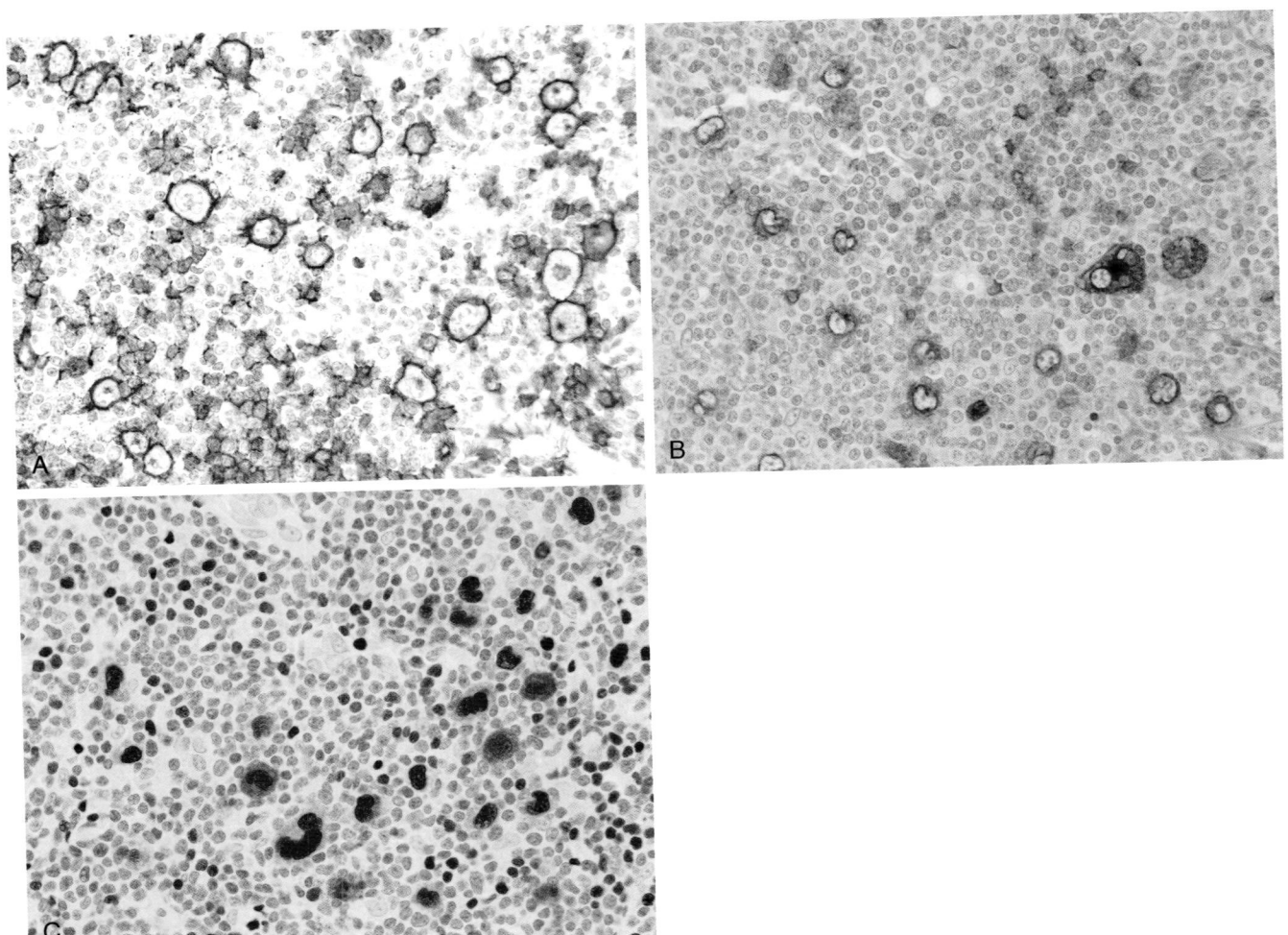

Figure 26-6. A, Immunostain for CD20 showing membrane staining of several lymphocyte-predominant (LP) cells and background small B-cells. **B,** This case involving a 7-year-old male child was positive for IgD. **C,** OCT2 is strongly positive in the neoplastic cells, a finding that facilitates their recognition.

from that of HRS cells in CHL, which typically show CD20 expression in only a subset of neoplastic cells and cases.[75,76] CD79a is usually positive but varies in intensity.[37] LP cells commonly lack CD19.[77,78] LP cells also stain for CD40, CD70, CD80, CD86, HLA class II, and CD74 (the invariant chain of HLA class II).[79,80] All of these are also expressed in normal GC blasts, with the exception of CD70, which is the receptor for CD27. In normal GCs, CD70 expression appears to be confined to GC blasts expressing only IgD, which can be seen sporadically in clusters in GCs of the tonsil.

CD30 staining is usually negative.[81-83] In a few cases, weak, usually cytoplasmic staining of LP cells can be discernible. The NLPBL-derived cell line DEV also expresses CD30, albeit less intensely than CHL-derived cell lines.[84] Thus, expression of CD30 should not totally exclude a diagnosis of NLPHL.[30,63] In contrast, CD30-positive parafollicular immunoblasts located outside the B-cell nodules are commonly identified and represent a potential diagnostic pitfall.[81] LP cells are typically negative for CD15, but CD15 may be expressed in a subset of neoplastic cells in otherwise typical cases.[30,37,62]

LP cells, in contrast to classical HRS cells, produce J chain, a 15-kD polypeptide essential for linking to the tailpieces of multimeric immunoglobulin molecules.[85-87] LP cells infrequently express demonstrable cytoplasmic IgG, IgM, and IgA. However, strong expression for only IgD is identified in a subset of cases, most often in young males with cervical lymph node involvement (Fig. 26-6B).[88] Fc receptor homologue expressed in B cells (FREB), a member of the family of Fc receptors for IgG, is expressed in normal GC B cells, mantle zone cells, and most NLPBLs.[89] Activation-induced cytidine deaminase (AID) is indispensable for class-switch recombination and somatic hypermutation of immunoglobulin genes. In keeping with the notion that LP cells represent transformed GC B cells showing evidence of somatic hypermutation, AID is consistently expressed in LP cells.[90] Other markers of GC derivation, such as GC B-cell expressed transcript 1 (GCET1),[91] human GC-associated lymphoma protein (HGAL),[92] and switch-associated protein-70 (SWAP70),[93] are also expressed in most NLPBLs. CD10 is negative.[94]

Signaling Intermediates

Among transmembrane adapter proteins studied to date, LP cells express only the non–T-cell activation linker (NTAL) that is also expressed in most B cells and B-cell neoplasms.[95] This linker functions as a negative regulator of early stages of B-cell receptor signaling. Syndecans (SDCs) are transmembrane proteoglycans that play an important role in cell-matrix and cell-cell interactions and in modulating receptor activation.[96] In hematopoietic cells, SDC1 (CD138) is expressed only in B cells at pre-B and plasma cell differentiation stages.[97] LP cells are SDC1 negative, in accordance with their derivation from GC B cells.[94,98]

In most CHL cases, several receptor tyrosine kinases are expressed, whereas none are detected in 50% of NLPHL cases. Receptor tyrosine kinase A, which is essential for the survival of memory B cells, was expressed in only 30% of NLPHLs in one study.[99] JAK2, an intracellular non-receptor tyrosine kinase that transduces cytokine-mediated signals via the JAK2/STAT pathway, is expressed in most NLPHLs.[100]

Transcription Factors and Regulators

B-cell transcription factors such as PAX5, OCT1, OCT2, and BOB.1 are consistently expressed in LP cells (Fig. 26-6C).[101] ID2, which is uniformly expressed in the HRS cells of CHL and likely represses B-cell–specific gene expression, is also aberrantly expressed in LP cells and might contribute to the reduced expression of some B-cell genes.[102] PU.1 is variably expressed in NLPBL but absent in both CHL and THRLBCL.[103,104] IRF4 (MUM1) cooperates with PU.1 as a transcriptional regulator in lymphoid cells.[105] In LP cells, BCL6 is consistently present, and IRF4 is inconsistently expressed.[94,98] BLIMP1 (PRDM1), a transcriptional repressor that induces plasmacytic differentiation in B cells,[106] is negative in both CHL and NLPBL.[107]

FOXP1 is expressed in normal activated B cells[108,109] and in DLBCL of the activated B-cell type[110] but is absent in both CHL and NLPBL.[111] T-bet (TBX21) is expressed in Th1 CD4-positive T lymphocytes[112] and a subset of T-cell NHLs, and it may participate in immunoglobulin class switching during B-cell development.[113] In reactive lymphoid tissues, the vast majority of B cells do not express T-bet,[114] whereas the neoplastic cells of NLPHL and CHL are positive.[115] Other T-cell transcription factors such as GATA3, c-MAF, and GATA2 are not expressed in LP cells,[115,116] which is in keeping with the known ability of PU.1 to inhibit expression of GATA transcription factors.[117] Nuclear factor of activated T cells (NFAT) is required for effector differentiation in T cells and normal homeostasis and differentiation in B cells.[118] NFATc1 normally resides in the cytoplasm but relocates to the nucleus when activation of the pathway leads to its dephosphorylation. LP cells show cytoplasmic NFATc1 staining in most cases and nuclear NFATc1 staining in some cases, whereas NFATc1 is expressed in only a minority of CHLs.[119]

Nuclear factor-κB (NF-κB) plays a key role in the regulation of immune and inflammatory responses, functions as a potent inhibitor of apoptosis, and is involved in the malignant transformation of different cell types.[120] The NF-κB family members p50, p52, p65 (RELA), RELB, and REL (c-Rel) form different homodimers or heterodimers in a highly context-dependent manner. Constitutive NF-κB activation promotes proliferation and survival of HRS cells in CHL.[121] REL generally is not expressed in NLPBL,[122] but p65 is expressed in all cases.[123] Most B-cell lymphoproliferative disorders (78%) express B-cell–activating factor receptor (BAFF-R), which is required to activate the alternative NF-κB pathway.[124] NLPBL exhibits weak-to-negative BAFF-R staining,[125] which may imply that the alternative NF-κB pathway is inactive in LP cells. The activator protein-1 (AP1) family of transcription factors has been implicated in the control of proliferation, apoptosis, and malignant transformation. The AP1 family member JUNB binds to the *TNFRSF8* (CD30) promoter and promotes CD30 expression in classical HRS cells,[126] whereas LP cells are typically weakly positive for JUNB and often negative for CD30.[127,128] LP cells also consistently express myocyte enhancer factor 2B (MEF2B) but lack nuclear staining for STAT6, in contrast to CHL.[30,85,129]

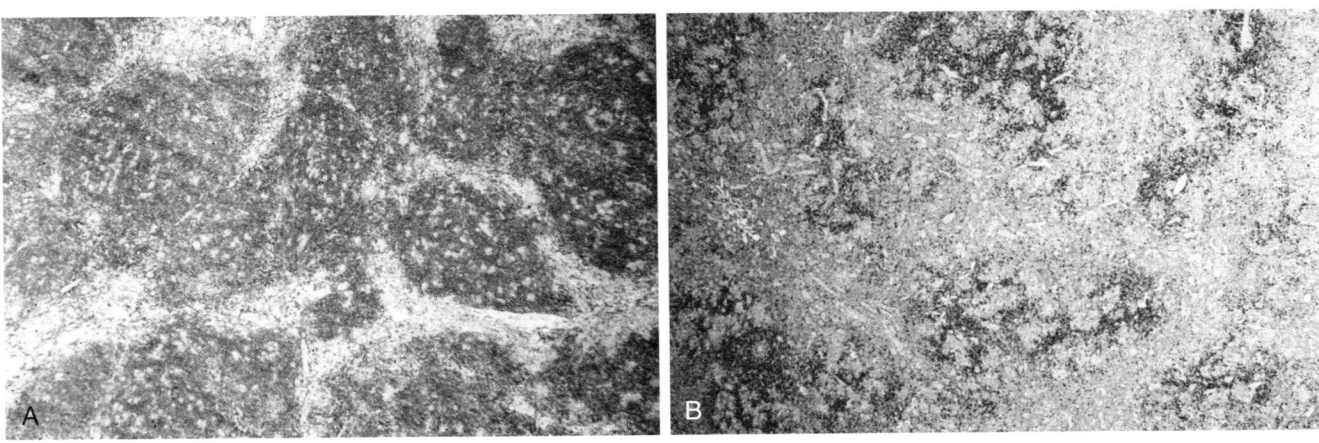

Figure 26-7. Immunostains for CD20 show a large majority of positive-staining small B lymphocytes in the nodules of one case of NLPBL **(A)** and a minority of CD20-positive small B cells in another case **(B)**.

Cell Cycle Proteins

Immunostains for proliferation-associated nuclear proteins such as Ki-67 or proliferating cell nuclear antigen are positive in LP cells, indicating they are in cycle.[130] The topoisomerase II alpha enzyme (TOP2A), which controls and alters the topologic states of DNA during transcription and is the target for several chemotherapeutic agents, is highly expressed in LP cells.[131] High TOP2A expression in LP cells might correlate with a favorable outcome in patients with NLPBL treated with TOP2A inhibitors such as doxorubicin or epirubicin.

Tumor Suppressors and Apoptosis-Related Proteins

Caspase 3, which is important for CD95/Fas-mediated apoptosis, is not expressed at detectable levels in NLPBL, similar to low-grade NHL.[132,133] The competitive negative regulator of Fas-induced apoptosis, c-FLIP, is expressed in fewer NLPBLs (32%) than CHLs (81%) or DLBCLs (93%).[134] In contrast to CHL, p53 is not expressed in NLPBL.[135] However, the p53 family member p63, which has both developmental and putative tumor-suppressor functions,[136,137] is expressed in a subset of GC B cells and in NLPBL, but not in CHL.[138] The balance between antiapoptotic BCL2 and proapoptotic BAX is important for the induction of programmed cell death[139]; though BCL2 is not expressed in LP cells,[35] BAX is expressed in all cases.[140] A20 and TRAF1 are two antiapoptotic components of the tumor necrosis factor receptor (TNFR) family signaling pathway induced by CD30 stimulation.[141] A20 (but not TRAF1) is expressed in NLPBL, although it is expressed in variable numbers of LP cells.[122,141] Because most NLPBLs are CD30 negative, stimulation of another TNFR family member, such as CD40, might control A20 expression in LP cells.[142]

Structural Proteins and Adhesion Molecules

Vimentin[143] and fascin,[144] usually positive in classical HRS cells, are not expressed by LP cells. Staining for CD44H shows variable membranous and Golgi-area reactivity in the neoplastic cells of all CHLs but is negative in NLPBL.[145] Epithelial membrane antigen may be expressed by LP cells[68,146] but is often identified in only a small proportion

of neoplastic cells and is negative in many cases, limiting its diagnostic utility.

Background Cells

LP cells usually reside in a background of small B cells, most of which derive from the follicular mantle and express IgM and IgD.[147,148] These lymphocytes also express CD20, CD21, CD22, and CD45RA, but not CD45RB (Fig. 26-7; Table 26-3).[7,69,71,73,114,148-153] The expression of CD23 is relatively strong, which has also been noted in PTGC. Over time, the proportion of small background B cells tends to decrease, and in multiple-relapse cases, B cells may be few in number.

The number of T cells in the nodules of NLPBL is highly variable, ranging from a minority to a vast majority of cells.[69] In one study, flow-cytometric analysis identified a mean of 61% T cells in five NLPBL cases.[154] The proportion of T cells in the nodules appears to increase over time, and a high proportion of T cells can be found in recurrences. Occasionally, the background T cells may be cytologically atypical, mimicking peripheral T-cell lymphoma (PTCL), but they are nonclonal and retain a normal T-cell phenotype.[155]

A significant proportion of the T cells in NLPBL has a distinctive immunophenotype: c-MAF+, CD2+, CD3+, CD4+, PD1+, CD57+.[69,114,148,151,156,157] Even if few, the T cells usually directly surround the LP cells in rosettes or collarettes (Fig. 26-8).[73] CD4-positive CD57-positive T cells are normally present exclusively in GCs and are mostly confined to the light zones (Fig. 26-9).[158] They are not present in the early phases of GC reactions, when proliferating small centroblasts predominate, nor are they in the population of CD4-positive T cells that can be identified in a sharp rim at the border of the GC and mantle zone. These "rim cells" are CD40L positive and are absent in the nodules of NLPBL and PTGCs. CD4-positive CD57-positive T cells in reactive GCs express the chemokine receptor CXCR5, similar to the small B lymphocytes, and are attracted by the chemokine CXCL13 produced by FDCs. CD4-positive CD57-positive T cells themselves also produce high amounts of CXCL13 upon activation, in contrast to extrafollicular T cells,[159] and have a gene expression profile consistent with T-regulatory-1

Table 26-3 Antigen Expression of Background Cells in Nodular Lymphocyte-Predominant Hodgkin Lymphoma

Antigen	Significance	Findings
Background T Lymphocytes		
CD2	T cells, thymocytes, NK cells	Positive[69,148]
CD3	T cells, thymocytes	Positive[69,148]
CD4	Th and Tr cells	Positive[73]
CD45RA	B cells, naïve T cells, monocytes	Negative[73]
CD45RO	B-cell subsets, T-cell subsets	Positive[73]
CD57	NK cells, GC Th cells	Positive[73]
PD1	GC T cells	Positive[151]
CD69	Early activation marker	Positive[69,73]
CD134	Early activation marker	Positive
CD38	Persistent activation marker	Negative
MHC II	Control of immune responses through presentation of peptide antigens to T cells	Negative[73]
CD25	Activated T cells and B cells and monocytes IL-2R	Negative[73]
CD71	Activated leukocytes, function as transferrin receptor	Negative[73]
CD40L	Activated T-cell subset ligand for CD40	Negative[149]
TIA-1	Cytotoxic T cells and NK cells	Negative or few cells positive[152]
BCL6	GC Th cells	Positive[153]
c-MAF	Th2 cells, responsible for tissue-specific expression of IL-4	Positive[114]
T-bet	Th2 cell development, role in Ig class switching	Predominantly negative[114]
GATA3	Th2 cell development	Predominantly negative[114]
MUM-1	Subset of GC B cells, plasma cells	Positive
Background B Lymphocytes		
CD20 (L26)	B cells (not plasma cells)	Positive[69]
CD21	Mature B cells, FDCs	Positive
CD22	B cells (not plasma cells)	Positive
CD23	Mantle zone B cells, T cells, macrophages, platelets, eosinophils	Positive
CD45RA (KIB3)	B cells, T-cell subsets, monocytes	Positive[150]
CD45RB(MT3)	Thymocytes, T cells	Negative[150]
IgM	Bright on B cells in mantle and marginal zone	Positive[7,69,71]
Follicular Dendritic Cell Meshwork		
IgD	Bright on mantle zone B cells	Positive[7,69,71]
CD21	Mature B cells, FDCs	Positive[7,69]
CD35	FDC marker, C3b rec	Positive[7,69]
FDC	FDC marker	Positive[7,69]
CD23	Mantle zone B cells, T cells, macrophages, platelets, eosinophils	Negative[7,69]
CD21L (R4/23)	FDC marker	Positive[7,69]

FDC, Follicular dendritic cell; *GC,* germinal center; *Ig,* immunoglobulin; *IL,* interleukin; *MHC,* major histocompatibility complex; *NK,* natural killer.

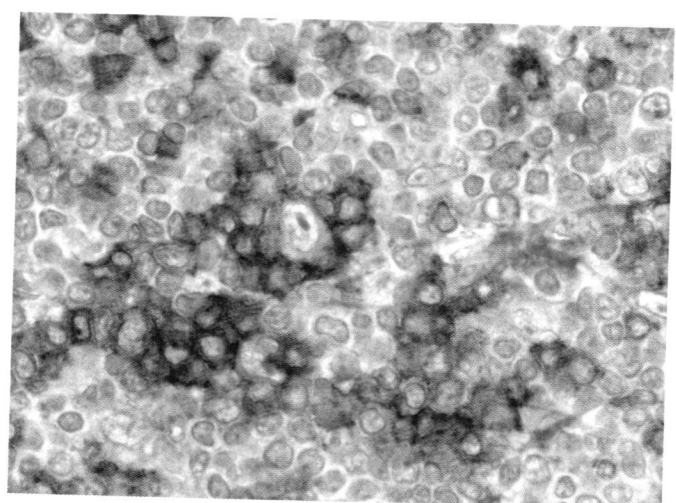

Figure 26-8. LP cell surrounded by an almost complete rosette of PD1 (CD279)-positive lymphocytes.

cells.[154] Data indicate that the rosetting T cells in NLPBL also express CD69 and have TCR proteins that interact directly with class II MHC proteins on the LP cells, suggesting their participation in an immunologic synapse that might represent a therapeutic target.[160] Live cell imaging analyses have demonstrated the dynamic nature of these immunologic synapses.[161]

Most NLPBLs contain a nonneoplastic mature T-cell population co-expressing CD4 and CD8, constituting 10% to 38% of T cells; these may reflect an activated or reactive T-cell subset and should not lead to a misdiagnosis of PTCL.[162] NLPBLs bearing this population do not differ from other NLPHLs in terms of clinical, histologic, or immunohistochemical features.

The FDCs predominant within the macronodules are CD21 positive and CD35 positive but CD23 negative, thus resembling the FDCs of the mantle zone and not those of the GC (Fig. 26-10). They do not carry immunoglobulin complexes. The major interaction between FDCs and

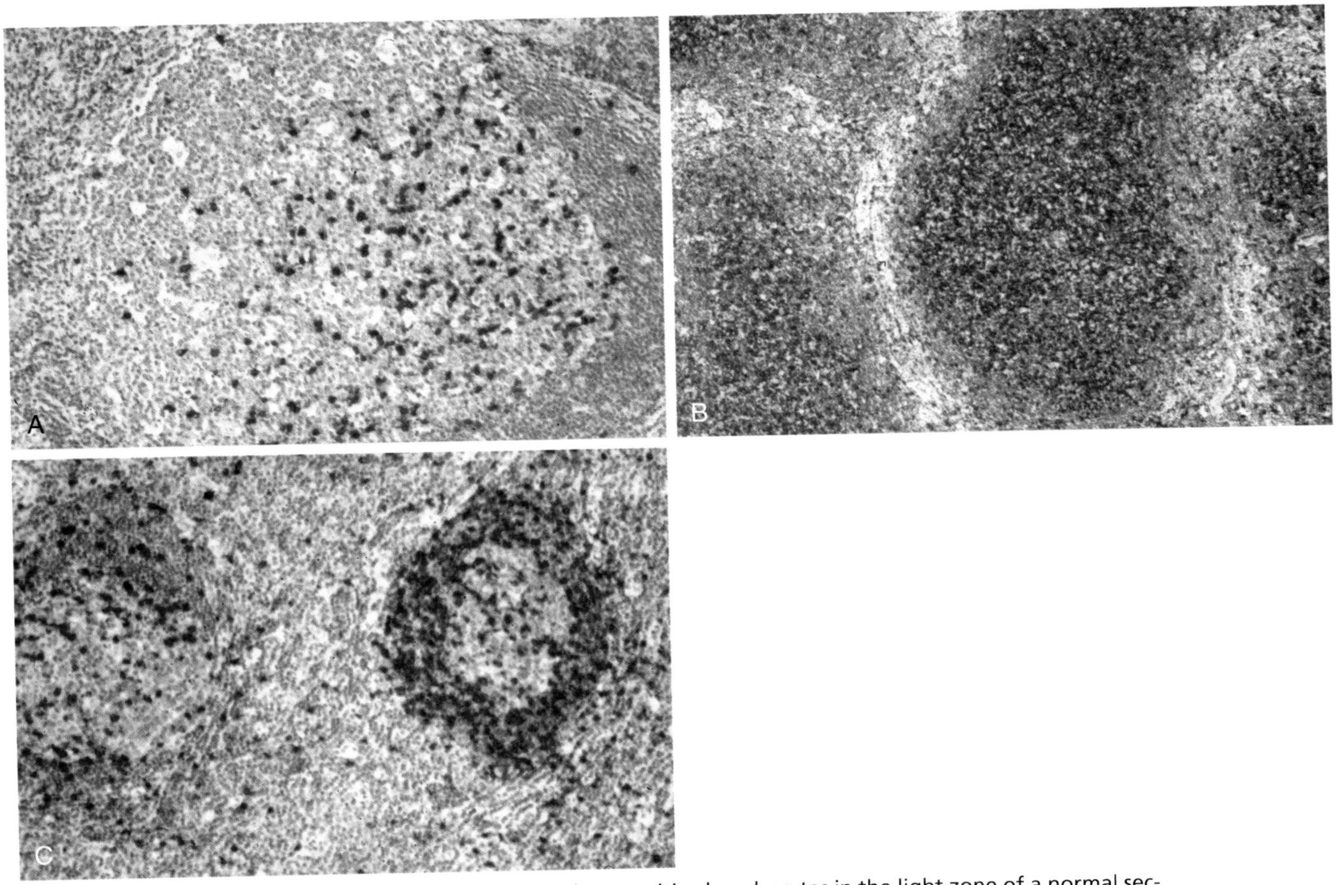

Figure 26-9. Immunostains for CD57 show positive lymphocytes in the light zone of a normal secondary follicle **(A)** and an increased number of positive lymphocytes in progressively transformed germinal centers **(B)** and in the mantle zone of a morphologically normal secondary follicle **(C)** in a case of follicular hyperplasia with progressively transformed germinal centers.

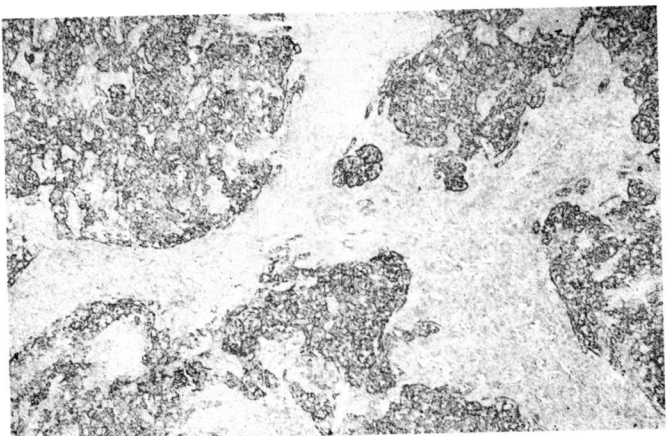

Figure 26-10. Immunostain for CD21 demonstrates loose nodular aggregates of follicular dendritic cells in nodular lymphocyte-predominant B-cell lymphoma.

B cells appears to be mediated by the CD11a/CD18 (LFA1) and CD54 (ICAM-1) pathway.[163] LP cells also express the adhesion molecules CD50 (ICAM-3) and CD54 (ICAM-1) and thus interact with rosetting T cells.[164] Both FDCs and the rosetting CD57-positive/PD1-positive T cells tend to be lost in pattern E NLPBL.[57]

GENETICS AND MOLECULAR FINDINGS

Cytogenetic Findings

Few cytogenetic data on NLPBL are available. All cases studied have a complex karyotype with more than three numerical or structural abnormalities, but most are in the diploid range (46 to 49 chromosomes); tetraploidy, often seen in CHL, is rare.[165,166] With conventional cytogenetics, significant imbalances involve chromosomes 1, 4, 7, 9, and 13.[166] In contrast, comparative genomic hybridization has shown a high number of genomic imbalances (average 10.8 per case) involving all chromosomes except 19, 22, and Y.[167] Gains of 1, 2q, 3, 4q, 5q, 6, 8q, 11q, 12q, and X and loss of chromosome 17 were identified in 36.8% to 68.4% of the analyzed cases. There was frequent overrepresentation of chromosome arm 6q, a region frequently deleted in DLBCL. Cytogenetic analysis of the NLPBL-derived cell line DEV revealed a 48,XY,+X,t(3;7)(q13;p21),der(3)t(3;14)(p14;q32),t(3;22)(q27;q11.2),+12,der(14)t(3;14)(p14;q32),der(22)t(3;22)(q27;q11.2) karyotype.[76] Array comparative genomic hybridization (aCGH) identified a 3-Mb homozygous deletion was in the 17q24 region,[84,167] though this finding was not confirmed by immunofluorescence for CD20 and fluorescence in situ hybridization (FICTION). An additional aCGH study identified similar copy number abnormalities in NLPBL and

THRLBCL, particularly gains of 2p16.1 (including *REL*) and losses of 2p11.2 and 9p11.2.[168]

Recurrent rearrangements of the *BCL6* gene are detected in approximately 50% of NLPBL cases analyzed by interphase fluorescence in situ hybridization[169] and by FICTION.[170,171] *BCL6* aberrations in NLPBL target immunoglobulin and nonimmunoglobulin loci, similar to those found in DLBCL.[170,172] The NLPBL-derived cell line DEV shows a *BCL6* rearrangement with a break in the *BCL6* alternative breakpoint region.[84] FICTION analysis revealed no breaks in the *BCL6* alternative breakpoint region in 12 NLPBL cases, suggesting such breaks may not be common in primary cases of NLPBL.[84] A study demonstrated multiple copies of *BCL6* in the LP cells of some NLPBLs that lack *BCL6* rearrangements.[171] *BCL2* gene rearrangements have been investigated and detected in a small number of cases.[173,174] It is not clear whether the rearrangement was present in LP cells or, more likely, in bystander B cells. Because LP cells generally do not express BCL2 protein, *BCL2* translocation probably does not play a role in the pathogenesis of NLPBL.

Immunoglobulin and T-Cell Receptor Gene Rearrangement Studies

The relative paucity of LP cells in NLPBL has made clonality studies difficult. Though early studies using in situ hybridization (ISH) to detect Igκ or Igλ messenger RNA yielded variable results,[175-178] ultrasensitive ISH demonstrated light chain restriction in all NLPBLs tested.[179] Southern blot studies were of limited use in showing immunoglobulin gene rearrangement, given their relatively low sensitivity and the rarity of LP cells in involved tissues.[173,180] Polymerase chain reaction (PCR) studies on total tissues also yielded conflicting results.[181-183] These discrepancies result from PCR's limited sensitivity owing to the large numbers of reactive B cells present in NLPBL. The most recent PCR-based studies of multiple microdissected LP cells from individual patients have demonstrated the presence of monoclonal immunoglobulin gene rearrangements.[184-186] The same clone has been shown in multiple nodules, multiple paraffin blocks, and multiple lymph nodes from the same patient. NLPBL exhibited ongoing mutations within clonally rearranged gene segments, with intraclonal diversity in the majority of cases. Ongoing mutations are normally confined to GC B cells. This agrees with the finding that the immunoglobulin gene sequences are translated into functional membrane immunoglobulin expression and are therefore subject to antigen selection.

The T-cell receptor (TCR) V-beta chain gene repertoire of rosetting T cells was studied in two cases of NLPBL.[187] There was no evidence of clonal restriction or selection of V-beta receptor gene expression. Trumper and associates[188] examined rosetting complexes of a single NLPBL case by single-cell analysis for the TCR-γ gene. They found clonal TCR-γ sequences in two independent experiments analyzing 7 and 10 different rosetting complexes. These findings have not yet been confirmed by other studies, although rare cases of PTCL have been seen in patients with NLPBL.[56]

Mutation and Gene-Expression Studies

Similar to DLBCL and CHL, the tumor cells of NLPBL are targeted by aberrant somatic hypermutation in at least one of four proto-oncogenes encoding signal transducers and transcription factors involved in B-cell development, differentiation, and lymphomagenesis (*PIM1*, *PAX5*, *RHOH*, and *MYC*).[189] Also similar to CHL, mutations of the suppressor of cytokine signaling *SOCS1*, which is involved in cytokine-induced JAK/STAT activation, are seen in 40% to 50% of NLPBL.[100,190] Unlike CHL, however, mutations and copy number alterations in other genes involved in JAK/STAT activation, including *JAK2*, *STAT6*, *PTPN1*, and *CSF2RB*, are rarely observed in NLPBL.[100,190] Other than gains of *REL*, other events implicated in NF-κB activation in CHL, including gains of *MAP3K14* and *BCL3* and mutations in *NFKBIA*, *NFKBIA*, and *TNFAIP3*, are rare in NLPBL.[190,191] Furthermore, genetic alterations associated with immune evasion in CHL, including those involving *B2M*, *CIITA*, *CD274* (PD-L1) and *PDCD1LG2* (PD-L2), are not characteristic of NLPBL.[190] Conversely, in addition to *BCL6* rearrangements, mutations in *SGK1*, *JUNB*, and *DUSP2* each occur in about 50% of NLPBL but are not typically seen in CHL.[127,190,192]

Gene-expression profiling of microdissected LP cells has shown similarities to both CHL and THRLBCL, including evidence of constitutive NF-κB activation.[193] The proto-oncogene *BIC* (B-cell integration cluster or pre–miR-155) and mature miR-155, which is now considered an onco–micro-RNA,[194] are highly expressed in NLPHL and CHL.[195,196] LP cells also show expression of the *SGK1* kinase gene, and an SGK1 inhibitor induced apoptosis in NLPBL cell line DEV.[127] Hartmann and colleagues compared the gene-expression signatures of microdissected tumor cells from NLPBL, THRLBCL-like NLPBL, and THRLBCL.[197] It is significant that no striking differences in the gene signatures among these entities were identified. The tumor cells in all three groups expressed several markers, most notably HIGD1A and BAT3, and this was confirmed by immunohistochemistry validation. The authors concluded that NLPBL and THRLBCL may represent a spectrum of the same disease and that differences between the distinct clinical and pathologic presentations may be related to microenvironment and immune status rather than differences in the tumor cells themselves. This hypothesis is supported by gene-expression profiling studies on nonmicrodissected samples, which have found a signature suggesting a tolerogenic host immune response in THRLBCL, including genes encoding interferon-γ, toll-like receptors, CCL8, and indoleamine 2,3-dioxygenase (IDO).[198] In contrast, NLPBL showed a microenvironmental signature more similar to follicular hyperplasia.

Paschold et al. used next-generation sequencing (NGS) of the immunoglobulin heavy chain (IGH) gene to map clonal trajectories of NLPBL evolution and transformation.[199] Transformation was associated with the presence of marked intraclonal diversity, suggesting NGS at diagnosis might help identify cases most at risk of transformation. This diversity also suggests a role for antigenic drive in the events leading to transformation, underscoring the need for further study of the role of B-cell receptor antigens in NLPBL lymphomagenesis.[200]

RELATIONSHIP WITH PROGRESSIVELY TRANSFORMED GERMINAL CENTERS

Follicular hyperplasia with progressively transformed germinal centers (PTGCs) is a benign disorder of unknown

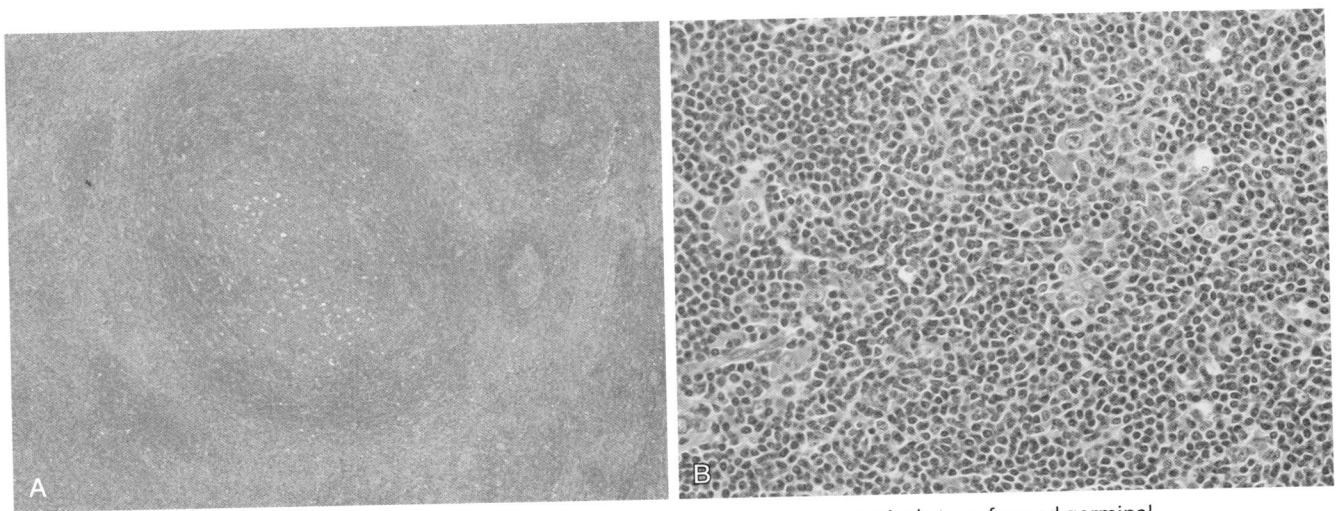

Figure 26-11. A, Lymph node with follicular hyperplasia and a progressively transformed germinal center. **B,** At higher magnification, a predominance of small lymphocytes and a few centroblasts can be identified.

pathogenesis. It is diagnosed most often in the second decade of life, with a male predominance. Patients present with an asymptomatic, solitary enlarged lymph node in the cervical region.[201] Histologically, PTGC follicles are much larger than normal follicles and have expanded mantles, which intrude on the GC. The PTGC follicles are scattered in a background of follicular hyperplasia (Fig. 26-11A). They share with NLPBL the nodular motif of disrupted GCs with increased numbers of small B lymphocytes and dispersed centroblasts; thus, they may mimic NLPBL both cytologically and by the presence of large numbers of T cells, including CD4-positive CD57-positive cells. However, in PTGC, the T cells are dispersed, whereas in NLPBL, the T cells are in clusters surrounding the LP cells.[68] Prominent FDCs and multinucleated Warthin-Finkeldey–type giant cells can also be seen in PTGC. Immunophenotypic studies of PTGC show polyclonal IgM-positive, IgD-positive lymphocytes; FDCs; and increased numbers of CD4+, CD57+, c-MAF+, and CD4+/CD8+ T cells.[114,162] A key difference between PTGC and the nodules of NLPBL is the absence of LP cells and the persistence of normal GC cells, including centroblasts (Fig. 26-11B).

Early studies suggest an association between PTGC and NLPBL.[7] All possible combinations were encountered, with PTGC preceding or following NLPBL or occurring in separate lymph nodes at the same time. Many other studies have confirmed this association.[202,203] The frequent association and the structural similarity between PTGC and the nodules of NLPBL suggested PTGC is a precursor of NLPBL or, alternatively, that PTGC and NLPBL are manifestations of an abnormal follicular-center reaction based on B-cell or T-cell defects. Patients with concurrent PTGC and different types of immunodeficiencies have been reported.[204] Of note, no study has convincingly shown that the presence of a few PTGCs in a case of reactive follicular hyperplasia carries an increased risk for development of NLPBL. Moreover, PTGC is not a clonal process.[205] However, confluent areas of PTGCs should raise the index of suspicion and mandate careful sectioning of the entire lymph node biopsy to rule out focal NLPBL. When the absence of LP cells precludes a diagnosis of NLPBL, a high incidence of NLPBL is found in subsequent biopsies.

Differential Diagnosis

PTGC differs histologically from NLPBL in that LP variants are absent. Epithelioid histiocytes are absent in the expanded follicles but may form a necklace-like reaction around them, as sometimes seen in NLPBL. In contrast to NLPBL, in which complete obliteration of the lymph node is generally observed with only a rim of displaced normal tissue, the lymph node is not totally involved in PTGCs. There is virtually always associated florid follicular hyperplasia. A combination of pan-B and pan-T antigens can be a useful adjunct to morphology in distinguishing NLPBL from PTGCs.[68] Immunostains for CD20, BOB.1, and especially OCT2 may be useful in highlighting the LP cells. Stains for CD3, CD57, and PD1 may highlight rosettes around LP cells, which are not seen in PTGCs. PTGCs may be associated with increased polyclonal IgG4-positive plasma cells, a finding not seen in NLPBL.[206]

Association With Autoimmune Lymphoproliferative Syndrome

Autoimmune lymphoproliferative syndrome (ALPS) is generally caused by a mutation in genes associated with apoptosis, such as *FAS*, *FASL*, *CASP8*, and *CASP10*. As a result, the normal homeostasis of T and B lymphocytes is disturbed, and proliferation of polyclonal T lymphocytes occurs. The proliferating T cells are positive for TCRαβ or TCRγδ, or both, but they lack both CD4 and CD8 (double-negative T cells). Individuals with germline mutations in the *FAS* gene are at high risk for developing non-Hodgkin (14×) and Hodgkin (51×) lymphomas, particularly NLPBL.[207] NLPBL has been reported in two families with ALPS. Moreover, the reactive lymph nodes of patients with ALPS may show PTGC.[204] The common link may be the CD57-positive T cells that are increased in the nodules of NLPHL and PTGC and that are also the proliferative cell population in ALPS.

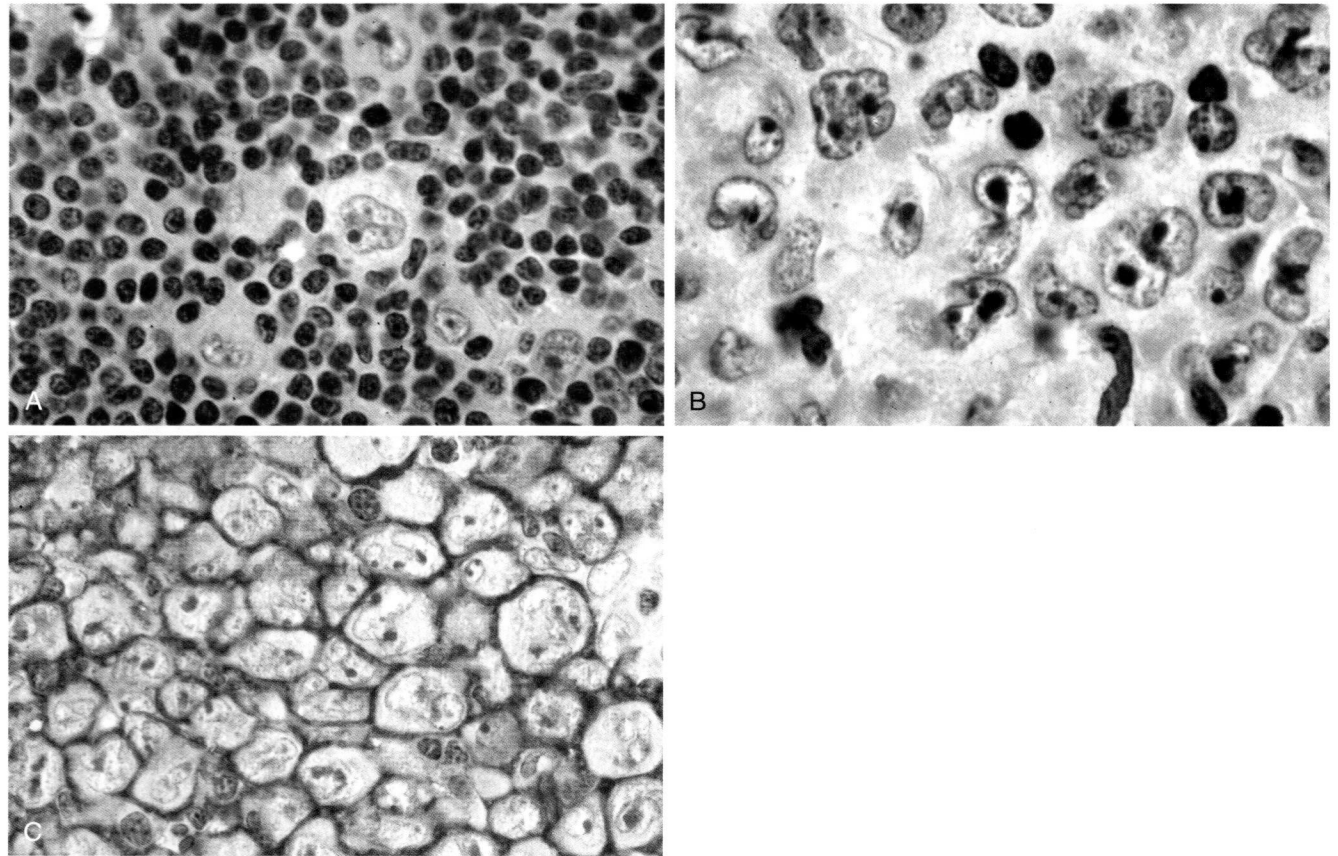

Figure 26-12. Composite lymphoma. Transformation of nodular lymphocyte-predominant B-cell lymphoma **(A)** to diffuse large B-cell lymphoma **(B). C,** The diffuse large B-cell lymphoma cells stain for CD20.

TRANSFORMATION TO DIFFUSE LARGE B-CELL LYMPHOMA

Between 3% and 14% of patients with NLPBL develop DLBCL, suggesting an underlying B-cell clone that can further transform to DLBCL, most likely the LP cells (Fig. 26-12).[7,47,55,208-211] Nodules with an almost pure population of LP cells can be seen in otherwise classical cases of NLPBL, suggesting an intermediate stage in histologic progression. In other cases, NLPBL can be accompanied by histologically typical DLBCL at the same anatomic site.[212,213] The DLBCL component can have either a GC-like or non–GC-like B-cell phenotype by standard immunohistochemical classifiers. LP cells and DLBCL cells expressed the same type of immunoglobulin light-chain mRNA,[214] and PCR studies and sequence analysis of IgH CDRIII supported a clonal relationship.[214-216] Both NLPBL and NLPBL-related DLBCL typically lack EBV. Al-Mansour and associates found a transformation rate of 14%, higher than that identified in previous studies.[53] Although the clonal relationship of NLPBL and DLBCL was not assessed, transformation occurred as late as 20 years after NLPBL (median time to transformation, 8 years), indicating the need for prolonged follow-up. Older age, IgD negativity, splenic involvement, variant histologic pattern, involvement of >2 sites, and high intraclonal diversity have all been associated with transformation risk.[47,54,199,208]

The prognosis of DLBCL arising in NLPBL is controversial. The studies reported in the literature have too few cases,

limited follow-up, and treatment heterogeneity, precluding a firm conclusion. In the study of Ohno and associates,[216] two cases of NLPBL with associated DLBCL showed aggressive behavior, in contrast to the previously published findings that patients with DLBCL arising from NLPBL had a good prognosis, with overall and event-free survivals similar to those of de novo NLPBL.[55,217] Publications have suggested that DLBCL arising in NLPBL has a prognosis similar to that of de novo DLBCL and should be treated as such.[216,218]

Although progression from NLPBL to DLBCL has been well established, fewer cases with an initial presentation of DLBCL before NLPBL have been reported.[57,219] It is uncertain whether the DLBCL and NLPBL in these cases are clonally related. These DLBCLs had an indolent course, and subsequent NLPBL developed at the same site, suggesting the two processes may be related. Rare cases of concurrent NLPBL and therapy-unrelated PTCLs have been reported.[56,220] These two diseases are probably not clonally related, but the PTCL may be related to the initiating role of T cells in the disturbed GC reaction of NLPBL.

RELATIONSHIP WITH T-CELL/HISTIOCYTE-RICH LARGE B-CELL LYMPHOMA

Malignant lymphoma with features of THRLBCL is the most common histologic pattern that develops in the evolution of NLPBL.[219] THRLBCL is characterized by a neoplastic population of large B cells scattered in a reactive background

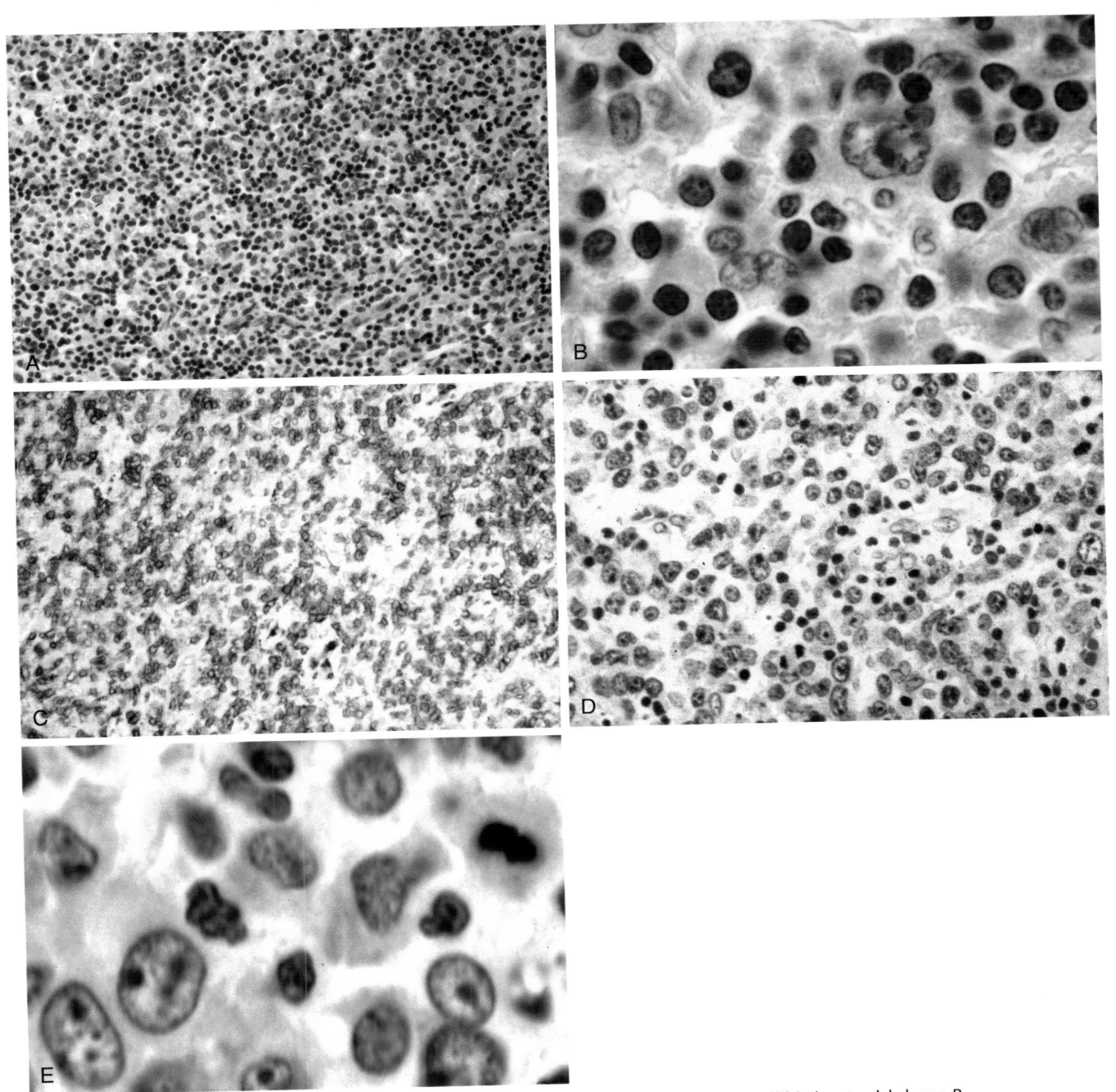

Figure 26-13. T-cell/histiocyte-rich large B-cell lymphoma. A and **B,** T-cell/histiocyte-rich B-cell lymphoma showing a predominance of small lymphocytes **(A)** and large neoplastic cells **(B). C,** The small lymphocytes stain for CD8. **D** and **E,** After 3 months, the lymphoma recurred as diffuse large B-cell lymphoma.

of T lymphocytes and histiocytes.[221] An identical pattern may be seen involving the splenic white pulp in a multifocal pattern. In the WHO and ICC classifications, THRLBCL is a subtype of DLBCL and may represent more than one disease entity (see Chapter 22). However, THRLBCL is largely similar to pattern E NLPBL, and NLPBL and THRLBCL may be the two extremes of a single spectrum of disease[197]; alternatively, THRLBCL could represent transformation of NLPBL. It is still unresolved whether primary and secondary THRLBCL can be distinguished. Early studies suggested that THRLBCL with LP-type tumor cells might be related

to NLPBL (so-called "paragranuloma-like" THRLBCL) (Fig. 26-13).[61,219,222] Moreover, NLPBL and THRLBCL can be seen as composite lymphomas, metachronous lymphomas, or multiple members of the same family.[219] Nevertheless, some THRLBCLs diagnosed after NLPBL lack LP-type cells. Although several morphologic features of THRLBCL are identical to those of NLPBL, most patients with THRLBCL have clinically advanced disease.[221,222] Single-cell studies revealed ongoing mutations in THRLBCL similar to those in NLPBL.[223] A mutational landscape study by Schuhmacher et al. provided additional support for the relationship between

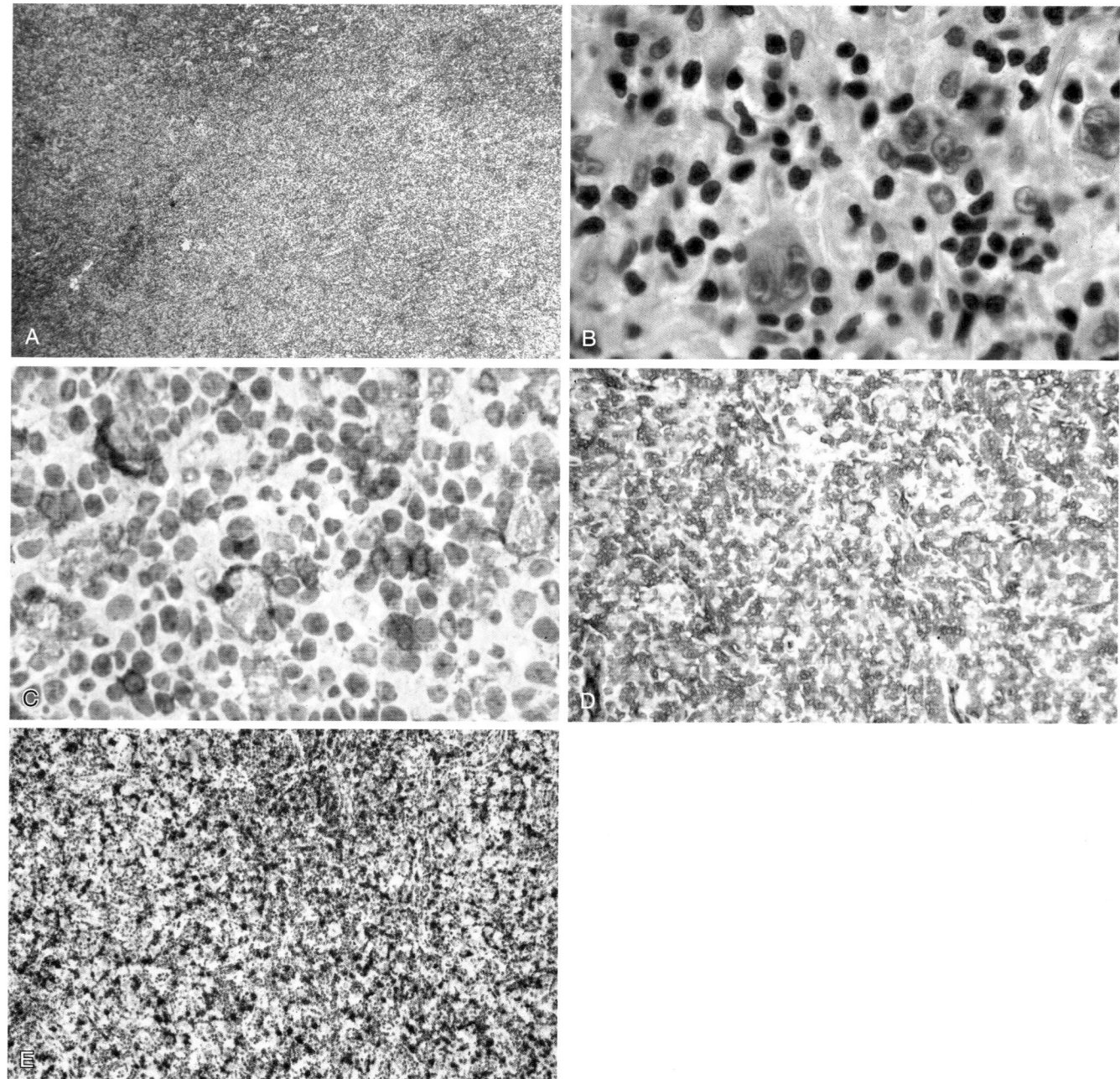

Figure 26-14. Diffuse area of nodular lymphocyte-predominant B-cell lymphoma with a predominance of small lymphocytes **(A)** and LP cells **(B)** that stain for CD22 **(C)**. The small lymphocytes are mostly CD4-positive T cells **(D)**, and many of them, including rosetting cells, also stain for CD57 **(E)**.

NLPBL and THRLBCL.[192] Specifically, recurrent mutations in *JUNB, DUSP2, SGK1, SOCS1,* and *CREBBP* were most frequent in THRLBCL and NLPBL with variant histology. Mutations in *JUNB, DUSP2, SGK1,* and *SOCS1* tended to occur at aberrant somatic hypermutation hotspots, further proving the role of somatic hypermutation in the pathogenesis of NLPBL and THRLBCL.

The BCL6 protein, which is normally present in GC cells, is frequently expressed in LP cells and also in the tumor cells of THRLBCL. It has been proposed that the distinction between NLPBL and THRLBCL can be made in difficult cases by demonstrating IGH or IGK clonality.[224] However, because

NLPBL can progress to diffuse NLPBL or transform to DLBCL, the distinction between these entities remains imprecise. Both CD79a and BCL2 are more frequently expressed in THRLBCL than in NLPBL.[35,225] The neoplastic cells of THRLBCL are leukocyte-specific phosphoprotein (LSP1) positive and generally PU.1 negative,[61,103,104] with some exceptions[226]; in contrast, LP cells are mostly LSP1 negative with variable PU.1 expression.[104] Although the T-cell rosettes typical of NLPHL are less commonly seen in THRLBCL (Fig. 26-14),[114,151] this feature is not a reliable criterion to distinguish the two entities. Likewise, expanded FDC meshworks may be useful in diagnosing NLPBL, but diffuse areas of NLPBL often lack

FDC meshworks. It has been suggested that a high TIA-1–positive or granzyme B-positive–to–CD57-positive ratio supports a diagnosis of THRLBCL, and a low ratio supports a diagnosis of NLPBL[61,152]; however, strict criteria for using this ratio have not been defined. Similarly, though early data suggested the presence of PD1-positive T-cell rosettes could distinguish NLPBL from THRLBCL, more recent findings suggest this is not a reliably criterion.[227,228] Of note, though 2-dimensional images did not show significant differences in the T-cell infiltrates, reconstructed 3-dimensional images have demonstrated that the T cells in THRLBCL have increased nuclear volume and increased CD8-positive T cell:tumor cell contacts than those in NLPBL.[229]

The question remains whether NLPBL can transform into THRLBCL. Loss of the nodular growth pattern and of CD57-positive T cells may be epiphenomena, with the significant change being increased malignant potential of the neoplastic B-cell clone. LP cells might undergo further transformation, or LP cells and the neoplastic cells of THRLBCL might have a common precursor, which undergoes a distinct transforming event. Comparative genomic hybridization after single-cell microdissection has revealed overall similarities between NLPBL and THRLBCL, but with more aberrations in pattern E NLPBL and THRLBCL than in typical NLPBL.[168] Other data, however, has shown significantly fewer genomic imbalances in THRLBCL than in NLPBL.[167,230] Thus, the biological nature of NLPBL that progresses or recurs with features indistinguishable from THRLBCL remains unclear. The preferred nomenclature for this situation remains THRLBCL-like transformation of NLPBL.[231]

OTHER DIFFERENTIAL DIAGNOSES

Other Non-Hodgkin Lymphoma

NLPBL may be architecturally and cytologically similar the floral type of follicular lymphoma, which also has very large nodules. In low-grade follicular lymphoma, centrocytes are admixed with varying numbers of centroblasts that are CD45 positive and CD20 positive and resemble LP cells in some cases. However, the presence of characteristic LP cells with polylobated nuclei, delicate nuclear membranes, and inconspicuous nucleoli helps distinguish NLPBL from follicular lymphoma. In grade 1 follicular lymphoma, all cells have irregular cleaved nuclear outlines and condensed nuclear chromatin, whereas the nuclei of the background cells in NLPBL are mostly round (but also may include some irregular nuclei). Immunophenotyping shows that the neoplastic cells of follicular lymphoma are CD10-positive monoclonal B cells, unlike the small B cells in NLPBL.

Occasional NLPBLs may demonstrate a background of cytologically atypical T lymphocytes, raising the differential diagnosis of PTCL, not otherwise specified (NOS).[155] Reported cases have shown younger age and more frequent cervical lymph node involvement than those of NLPBLs lacking this finding. Despite the cytologic atypia, T cells from cases tested did not show aberrant loss of pan–T-cell antigens or molecular evidence of clonality. These cases should be differentiated from true cases of composite NLPHL and PTCL, NOS.[56,220]

Lymphocyte-Rich Classic Hodgkin Lymphoma

LRCHL is the major morphologic mimic of NLPBL.[64] In a study of 426 cases that were morphologically interpreted as NLPBL, 115 (27%) were reclassified as LRCHL.[15,232,233] On H&E stains, the presence of regressed GCs is a characteristic feature of LRCHL, distinct from the expanded macrofollicles of NLPBL. In addition, in LRCHL, the HRS cells are mainly seen in the periphery of the nodules, in the marginal zone, whereas LP cells are usually clustered centrally within the nodules. Patients with NLPBL and those with LRCHL have similar clinical characteristics,[233] except that patients with LRCHL tend to be older.[234] Immunohistochemical stains are essential for the distinction of LRCHL from NLPBL (Table 26-4). The most important difference is the phenotype of the tumor cells (Fig. 26-15). In LRCHL, these are classical HRS cells, expressing CD30 consistently, CD15 frequently, and

Table 26-4 Differential Diagnosis of Nodular Lymphocyte-Predominant B-Cell Lymphoma

Disease	Morphologic Features		Immunophenotypic and Molecular Features	
	Tumor Cells	Background	Tumor Cells	Background
PTGCs	No LP cells, but centroblasts are present	Nodules with broken-down interface between mantle zone and GCs Lymph node is usually not totally replaced in PTGCs; association with florid follicular hyperplasia	Absent; no reactivity with EMA	CD20+ or CD30+ immunoblasts, irregular broken-up CD20+ nodules; CD57+, PD1+, c-MAF+ T cells, but no prominent T-cell rosettes
LRCHL	Classical HRS cells	Diffuse or nodular variant	CD15+, CD30+, CD45−, CD20+/−, EMA−, EBV+ (~50%)	CD57−, PD1+, loose CD21+ FDC meshwork
FL	Small, cleaved cells together with large centroblasts	Generally smaller nodules Lymphocytes in nodules are atypical	CD20+, CD10+ (60%), BCL2+	BCL2 gene rearrangement is usually present
THRLBCL	Centroblasts, immunoblasts, or popcorn cells	Diffuse pattern	CD20+, EMA+, CD15−, CD30−, LSP+, FREB−	Few background B cells; infrequent CD57+, PD1+, c-MAF+ T-cell rosettes; high TIA-1+-to-CD57+ ratio

EBV, Epstein-Barr virus; *EMA,* epithelial membrane antigen; *FDC,* follicular dendritic cell; *FL,* follicular lymphoma; *GC,* germinal center; *HRS,* Hodgkin and Reed-Sternberg; *LP,* lymphocyte predominant; *LRCHL,* lymphocyte-rich classic Hodgkin lymphoma; *LSP,* leukocyte-specific phosphoprotein; *PTGC,* progressively transformed germinal center; *THRLBCL,* T-cell/histiocyte-rich large B-cell lymphoma.

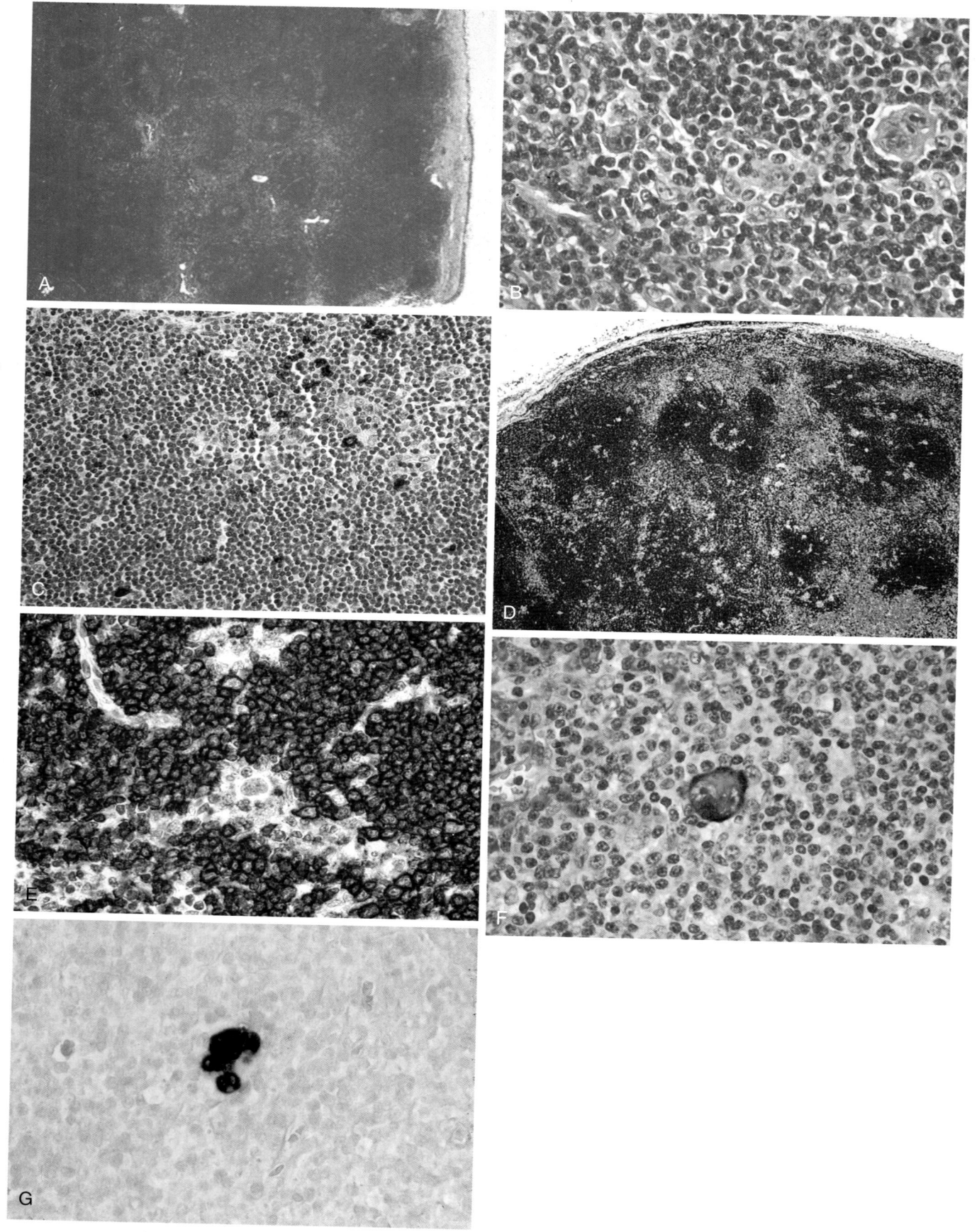

Figure 26-15. A, Lymphocyte-rich classic Hodgkin lymphoma in the tonsil, with a nodular pattern.
B, Typical Reed-Sternberg (RS) cells are present. **C,** There are a few CD57-positive cells that are not
rosetting the RS cells. **D,** The small lymphocytes are CD20 positive, whereas the RS cells are CD20
negative **(E),** CD30 positive **(F),** and EBV-encoded RNA positive by in situ hybridization **(G).**

EBV-encoded RNA (EBER) in approximately 40% of cases; they express CD20 in only some cases,[233] and then typically in only a subset of HRS cells. Bhargava and colleagues reported that staining for both fascin and JUNB was highly sensitive and specific for LRCHL and was not seen in NLPBL.[235] PD1-positive T-cell rosettes may be seen surrounding the HRS cells of LRCHL, and they are not specific for NLPBL.[227,228] Of note, clonally related NLPBL and CHL in the same patient has been reported, providing evidence in addition to gene-expression data that these entities may be more closely related than previously thought.[52]

TREATMENT

Though the optimal treatment for NLPBL remains controversial, treatment approaches for patients with early-stage disease parallel those for low-grade B-cell NHLs more than those for CHL. Some patients in stage IA remain in complete remission after lymphadenectomy alone, and despite previous concerns,[236] data suggest a watch-and-wait approach can be used for selected patients with NLPBL without significantly affecting outcome.[237] Involved-field radiotherapy is effective and is regarded as standard in stage IA NLPBL, with no significant benefit identified from the addition of chemotherapy.[238,239] Rituximab also has excellent activity in previously untreated and relapsed NLPBL,[240] although rituximab alone is associated with a relapse rate of up to 25% in stage IA disease[238,241] and may select CD20-negative subclones, leading to relapse.[242] Even in the relapsed setting, patients with NLPBL may not require high-dose chemotherapy and transplant.[243] For advanced-stage NLPBL, regimens currently used in B-cell NHL, including R-CVP (rituximab, cyclophosphamide, vincristine, prednisone) or R-CHOP (rituximab, cyclophosphamide, doxorubicin, vincristine, prednisone) are reasonable options. Eichenauer et al. have reported that the adverse prognostic effect of variant histology in NLPBL can be diminished using PET-2-guided escalated BEACOPP (bleomycin, etoposide phosphate, doxorubicin hydrochloride (Adriamycin), cyclophosphamide, vincristine sulfate (Oncovin), procarbazine hydrochloride, and prednisone).[48] ABVD (doxorubicin, bleomycin, vinblastine, dacarbazine), highly effective in CHL, is less effective in advanced-stage NLPBL, and spleen involvement has been associated with development of transformation after ABVD-like regimens.[244] Hodgkin-directed therapies have also been associated with ongoing relapses and treatment-related morbidity and mortality[245]—providing a further rationale to distinguish NLPBL from CHL. In summary, for treatment purposes, NLPBL should be considered closer to B-cell NHL than to CHL.

PROGNOSIS

With pathologic staging and standard treatment, mortality from NLPBL is low; nearly all deaths are cardiac related or due to a secondary tumor.[15,246] The prognosis of NLPBL is related primarily to stage and patient age at diagnosis, and survival ranges from 40% to 99%.[219] Life expectancy of patients with stage I NLPBL is about the same as that of the general population. Patients with splenic involvement (stage IIIS)

or with stage IV disease have a poor prognosis with current therapies.

Regula and coworkers[66] compared the clinical course of nodular and diffuse variants in 73 patients. Diffuse cases had few relapses and only two disease-specific deaths. Nodular cases showed significantly more relapses, which occurred independent of stage or treatment and were evenly distributed temporally up to 10 years after initial therapy. Because these cases were diagnosed before the recognition of LRCHL, the results may reflect inclusion of some CHLs. The THRLBCL-like diffuse pattern (pattern E) described by Fan and coworkers was an independent predictor of recurrent disease[57]; however, this result was limited by a short follow-up period for patients without recurrent disease. Hartmann and colleagues studied 423 NLPBLs and found variant histopathologic patterns to be associated with more advanced disease and higher relapse rate than NLPBL with typical histology.[51,58,247] In addition, histologic patterns C to F have been associated with increased frequency of bone marrow involvement in NLPBL.[49,50] Binkley et al. found that variant histology was associated with both inferior progression-free survival and a significantly higher transformation rate.[54] In a report from the German Hodgkin Study Group, Eichenauer et al. reported that variant histology was associated with both stage IV disease and splenic involvement; of note, the adverse prognostic effect was diminished by PET-2-guided escalated BEACOPP chemotherapy.[48] A prognostic score based on a multivariate model, variant histologic pattern, low serum albumin, and male gender could effectively stratify patients into risk groups that predict progression-free and overall survival. Histologically, the majority of relapsed patients have persistence of NLPBL. It is notable that, despite relatively frequent late relapses, NLPBL still maintains an indolent course. The main risk factor related to poor outcome is advanced stage.

CONCLUSION

NLPBL is a rare B-cell lymphoma of GC derivation that differs from CHL in histology, immunophenotype, molecular features, and clinical presentation. Nevertheless, NLPBL and CHL share the key characteristic of a majority of reactive lymphocytes with a minority of transformed lymphoid cells. Although isolated PTGCs may not be a true risk factor for NLPBL, they are associated with NLPBL in many cases. NLPBL transforms relatively frequently to DLBCL; nodules with increased numbers of LP cells may represent a transitional phase. In some cases of NLPBL with co-existent DLBCL, a clonal relationship has been demonstrated by immunoglobulin gene analysis. Clinically, NLPBL has a good prognosis despite frequent relapses, including relapses in distant sites. However, cases that involve the spleen and bone marrow typically have a poor outcome.

Several questions remain unanswered. What is the functional significance of the CD4-positive CD57-positive T cells in the pathogenesis of NLPBL and PTGC? What are the mechanisms of transformation to DLBCL? Is THRLBCL a biologically distinct disease, or does it represent progression of NLPBL? What molecular genetic abnormalities underlie the spectrum from NLPBL to THRLBCL? Long-term studies are needed to answer these questions.

Pearls and Pitfalls

- Evolving clinicopathologic and molecular data suggest NLPBL is related more closely to B-cell NHL than to CHL, reflected in new terminology and grouping within the lymphoma classification.
- The histologic pattern is of clinical importance, and the pattern should be reported as grade 1 (typical histology; Fan patterns A, B, or C) or grade 2 (variant histology; Fan patterns D, E, or F).
- LP cells may show classical HRS cell morphology, and immunohistochemistry is paramount in distinguishing NLPBL from CHL, particularly the lymphocyte-rich subtype.
- Eosinophils, plasma cells, and neutrophils are rarely observed in the background of NLPBL.
- CD20-positive centroblasts must be distinguished from LP cells in the differential diagnosis of PTGC and NLPBL. These centroblasts are not surrounded by CD57-positive rosettes.
- The most useful markers for diagnosis of NLPBL are CD20, OCT2, IgD, CD3, and PD1 (CD279); CD30 and EBV are typically negative.
- The presence of CD4-positive/CD8-positive T cells should not lead to a misdiagnosis of T-cell lymphoma.
- The preferred nomenclature for NLPBL recurring with features resembling THRLBCL is THRLBCL-like transformation of NLPBL.

KEY REFERENCES

7. Poppema S, Kaiserling E, Lennert K. Hodgkin's disease with lymphocytic predominance, nodular type (nodular paragranuloma) and progressively transformed germinal centres—a cytohistological study. *Histopathology.* 1979;3:295–308.
20. Saarinen S, et al. High familial risk in nodular lymphocyte-predominant Hodgkin lymphoma. *J Clin Oncol.* 2013;31:938–943.
53. Al-Mansour M, et al. Transformation to aggressive lymphoma in nodular lymphocyte–predominant Hodgkin's lymphoma. *J Clin Oncol.* 2010;28:793–799.
57. Fan Z, Natkunam Y, Bair E, et al. Characterization of variant patterns of nodular lymphocyte predominant Hodgkin lymphoma with immunohistologic and clinical correlation. *Am J Surg Pathol.* 2003;27:1346–1356.
59. Hartmann S, Soltani AS, Bankov K, et al. Tumour cell characteristics and microenvironment composition correspond to clinical presentation in newly diagnosed nodular lymphocyte-predominant Hodgkin lymphoma. *Br J Haematol.* 2022.
169. Wlodarska I, Nooyen P, Maes B, et al. Frequent occurrence of BCL6 rearrangements in nodular lymphocyte predominance Hodgkin lymphoma but not in classical Hodgkin lymphoma. *Blood.* 2003;101:706–710.
193. Brune V, et al. Origin and pathogenesis of nodular lymphocyte-predominant Hodgkin lymphoma as revealed by global gene expression analysis. *J Exp Med.* 2008;205:2251–2268.
197. Hartmann S, et al. Nodular lymphocyte predominant Hodgkin lymphoma and T cell/histiocyte rich large B cell lymphoma—endpoints of a spectrum of one disease? *PLoS One.* 2013;8:e78812.
227. Nam-Cha SH, et al. PD-1, a follicular T-cell marker useful for recognizing nodular lymphocyte-predominant Hodgkin lymphoma. *Am J Surg Pathol.* 2008;32:1252–1257.
239. Chen RC, et al. Early-stage, lymphocyte-predominant Hodgkin's lymphoma: patient outcomes from a large, single-institution series with long follow-up. *J Clin Oncol.* 2010;28:136–141.

Visit Elsevier eBooks+ for the complete set of references.

Classic Hodgkin Lymphoma

Falko Fend

DEFINITION

Classic Hodgkin lymphoma (CHL) is a clonal, malignant lymphoproliferation originating from germinal-center B cells. In contrast to most other lymphomas, the malignant cells usually represent only a small minority, between 0.1% and 2%, of the total cellular population of involved tissues. A histopathologic diagnosis of CHL is based on the identification of diagnostic Hodgkin and Reed-Sternberg (HRS) cells in an appropriate inflammatory background. Although many cases of CHL can, in principle, be diagnosed or at least suspected on the basis of morphology alone, current diagnostic criteria include the characteristic immunophenotype of the neoplastic population to separate CHL from morphologic mimics. HRS cells express CD30 and CD15 antigens in the majority of cases, lack the common leukocyte antigen CD45, and show an inconsistent and heterogeneous expression of B-lineage–specific lymphoid markers.

Classification of Classic Hodgkin Lymphoma and Its Evolution

The classification of CHL has remained remarkably constant over the years (Box 27-1). Notwithstanding the significant progress in delineating the cell of origin of CHL, the majority of cases are classified much as they were more than 50 years ago, after the development of the Rye classification.[1,2] This underlines the paramount importance of morphology for the correct diagnosis of this neoplasm. The change in terminology from *Hodgkin disease* to *Hodgkin lymphoma* (HL) was first proposed in the Revised European

American Lymphoma (REAL) classification[3] and reflected our better understanding of the nature and histogenesis of this lymphoma. The molecular analysis of single isolated HRS cells firmly established the clonality and B-cell origin of CHL and its derivation from germinal-center B cells, which, together with the establishment of Hodgkin cell lines, brought significant insights into the pathogenesis of the disease.[4-9]

Although it has been argued that the dichotomy between HL and non-Hodgkin lymphoma (NHL) is obsolete in the light of our increased understanding of CHL biology, current classifications retain the term "classic Hodgkin lymphoma" for practical reasons and to highlight the distinct biology of the disease.[10]

In diagnostic terms, the last years have led to refinements in the separation of CHL from mediastinal gray-zone lymphoma (MGZL), EBV-positive diffuse large B-cell lymphoma (DLBCL), and EBV-associated lymphoproliferations both in immunocompetent and immunosuppressed individuals. This also led to the recognition that a diagnosis of primary extranodal CHL should be made with utmost caution, as most of these cases would nowadays be considered different entities, including EBV-positive DLBCL, not otherwise specified (NOS); EBV-positive mucocutaneous ulcer; or others. The renaming of nodular lymphocyte-predominant Hodgkin lymphoma (NLPHL) to nodular lymphocyte-predominant B-cell lymphoma (NLPBL) in the 2022 International Consensus Classification (ICC) based on its preserved B-cell program emphasizes the separation from CHL.[11] CHL, in contrast, shows an extensive loss of the B-cell transcriptional program in the neoplastic cells, resulting in the loss or downregulation of most B-cell specific transcription factors and surface antigens, as a defining feature.[9,12,13]

SYNONYMS AND RELATED TERMS

Hodgkin disease.

EPIDEMIOLOGY

Incidence

HL, including NLPHL (now renamed NLPBL), accounts for approximately 15% to 25% of all malignant lymphomas. With current diagnostic criteria, approximately 95% of HLs fall into the CHL category; the remaining cases are NLPBL. The age-adjusted annual incidence rate of CHL in Western countries is approximately 2 to 4 per 100,000 population. In recent decades, a decrease in incidence has been observed among older adults; however, this can be attributed mainly to the misdiagnosis of NHL as CHL in previous years. In contrast, there has been a slight increase of the nodular sclerosis subtype in young adults. The incidence of CHL is higher in affluent, industrialized nations than in developing countries.[14,15]

Age and Sex Distribution

In industrialized countries, CHL shows a bimodal age distribution: the first, higher peak occurs in early adulthood (15 to 35 years), with a second peak in those older than 55 years. CHL is rare in children and is an exceptional occurrence in those younger than 3 years.[16] The overall male-to-female ratio is approximately 1.5:1. Although males predominate in childhood cases and among older adults, the male-to-female ratio is balanced or even slightly reversed in the early adulthood peak. The distribution of histologic subtypes varies with age. Although the nodular sclerosis subtype predominates in young adults, especially in females, there is a higher percentage of the mixed cellularity subtype in children and older patients. Developing countries show a distinct epidemiologic pattern: the first incidence peak occurs in childhood, with a predominance of the mixed cellularity subtype, and there is no peak in young adulthood.[14,17]

Nodular sclerosis CHL in young adults is associated with a higher socioeconomic status and smaller family size, factors thought to favor a delayed exposure to common childhood viruses.[18,19] Paradoxically, the early adulthood cases show the lowest frequency of Epstein-Barr virus (EBV) positivity, the only infectious agent so far shown to be associated with CHL. EBV is most often identified in CHL in children and older adults and in association with infection with human immunodeficiency virus (HIV).[20-24]

Familial cases of CHL have been reported frequently, and siblings of CHL patients have an increased risk of developing the disease.[19,25] There is a weak but consistent increase in the relative risk of CHL among certain human leukocyte antigen (HLA) types, and association studies have shown that genetic variants associated with CHL are typically in genes regulating the immune system.[26] Interestingly, carriers of HLA-A*01 and HLA-A*02, known to be involved in the cytotoxic response to latency proteins of EBV, show an increased versus decreased incidence of EBV-positive CHL, respectively.[27]

Association With Immunodeficiency Disorders

The risk for developing CHL is increased in patients with some types of immunodeficiency. HIV-infected persons have a 6-fold to 20-fold increased risk of developing CHL.[28,29] In the setting of acquired immunodeficiency syndrome (AIDS), CHL shows a predominance of unfavorable histologies (mixed cellularity and lymphocyte depleted) and advanced-stage disease, and it is almost universally associated with EBV.[30-32] Of note, the risk for CHL is increased in patients undergoing highly active antiretroviral therapy, possibly as result of the reconstitution of the immune system necessary for the inflammatory background of CHL, together with a shift to nodular sclerosis subtype.[24,28,33,34]

A significantly increased risk of CHL has been described in recipients of solid organs and allogeneic bone marrow grafts.[35,36] In either setting, CHL occurs late after transplantation, is almost always EBV positive, and is mainly of the mixed cellularity subtype. The clinical presentation and outcome of CHL in allograft recipients is similar to those in nonimmunocompromised patients.

ETIOLOGY

The cause of CHL is still an open question, but owing to the unique epidemiologic and clinical features of the disease, an infectious cause has long been suspected. Detection of EBV in the neoplastic cells of a significant proportion of CHLs has confirmed the involvement of an infectious agent. However, as evidenced by EBV-negative cases, EBV is not mandatory for the development of the disease but probably contributes to the pathogenesis in positive cases.[37]

Individuals with a history of infectious mononucleosis have an approximately 3-fold increased risk of developing CHL, and increased antibody titers or an altered antibody pattern in response to EBV infection has been demonstrated in patients with CHL.[38-40] The detection of clonal EBV in tissues involved by CHL using Southern blot analysis[41] and the subsequent demonstration of EBV nucleic acids in HRS cells by DNA in situ hybridization (ISH) have confirmed the association between CHL and EBV in a significant proportion of cases.[42] EBV-positive CHL shows a strict latency type II pattern of viral gene expression. In addition to EBV-encoded early RNAs (EBERs), short nontranslated RNA molecules that are abundantly expressed in viral latency (approximately 10^6 to 10^7 copies/cell) and EBV latent membrane protein-1 (LMP-1), the neoplastic cells express EBNA1 and LMP-2A and B but lack EBNA2.[37,43-50] Both immunohistochemistry for LMP-1 and nonradioactive ISH for EBERs are reliable methods for the detection of EBV, as they allow localization of EBV to the neoplastic cells, in contrast to in vitro techniques such as polymerase chain reaction (PCR), which may pick up the presence of latently infected B cells, so-called "bystander" cells present in all seropositive individuals.[45] Although EBER ISH is regarded as the most sensitive method, LMP-1 immunohistochemistry, which shows virtually universal expression by HRS cells in positive cases, helps to separate CHL from other EBV-positive lymphoproliferations. Latency in CHL is tightly controlled, and even in immunosuppressed individuals, there is usually no evidence of lytic infection.[51,52] Expression of EBNA-2, indicative of latency type III, is incompatible with a diagnosis of CHL.[53] EBV is clonal in the neoplastic cells of HL, as shown by Southern blot analysis of the terminal repeat region of the EBV genome.[54] This indicates that the infection takes place before clonal expansion and implicates a direct role for EBV in the transformation process. The EBV genome is present in episomal (nonintegrated) form, and each infected cell contains multiple copies. In EBV-associated HL, tumor cells in multiple involved anatomic sites contain the virus, as do true tumor recurrences.[55-57]

Functional Consequences of Epstein-Barr Virus Infection

LMP-1, which is strongly expressed by the neoplastic cells in HL, is the only viral protein with proven oncogenic properties.[58] LMP-1 induces an array of phenotypic changes in infected cells, including upregulation of activation antigens and antiapoptotic genes and induction of various cytokines; it can also induce an HRS-like phenotype in

germinal-center B cells.[59,60] LMP-1 is a constitutively active CD40 receptor homolog and induces a variety of downstream effects, such as constitutive activation of nuclear factor-κB (NF-κB) and JAK/STAT signaling pathways and upregulation of antiapoptotic genes.[37,59] Of note, virtually all cases of CHL with so-called "crippling" immunoglobulin heavy chain (IGH) mutations are EBV positive, emphasizing the importance of EBV-related genes for rescuing CHL precursor cells from apoptosis.[13] However, there is no clear-cut correlation between EBV positivity and tissue expression of genes known to be regulated by LMP-1 in vitro, and the expression profiles of HRS cells are very similar irrespective of EBV status, indicating the main effect of EBV infection on CHL pathogenesis may lie in the early stage of disease development and in the interaction with the immune system.[61,62]

Epstein-Barr Virus Strains and Variants

Two common strains of EBV, types A and B (or 1 and 2), mainly defined by EBNA-2 and EBNA-3, exist in a worldwide distribution. EBV type A transforms lymphocytes more efficiently and is found in the majority of cases of CHL in nonimmunosuppressed patients. Type B is encountered more often in HIV-associated CHL but has also been found in a higher proportion of cases from Latin America, indicating geographic variations in the prevalence of viral strains can influence their distribution in EBV-associated lymphomas.[37,59,63-65]

In addition to these two viral strains, a number of variations of the EBV genome have been described. Among these, deletions in the carboxy-terminal part of the *LMP-1* gene have received the greatest attention. The deletion variant is not associated with any specific histologic or prognostic features; its frequency in EBV-associated CHL reflects its prevalence in healthy carriers from the same geographic region, with the possible exception of higher frequencies of deletion variants in HIV-associated CHL.[65-68] Of note, CHL cases with EBV type B contain the *LMP-1* deletion very frequently, indicating this deletion may be necessary for the transforming capacity of this less virulent strain.[64,65]

Epidemiology of EBV-Associated Classic Hodgkin Lymphoma

The frequency of the association between EBV and CHL in nonimmunosuppressed patients is influenced by histologic subtype, age at presentation, geographic and ethnic origins, and possibly socioeconomic factors.[12,20,22,59,69] Mixed cellularity CHL is EBV positive in approximately 75% of cases, whereas EBV positivity in the nodular sclerosis subtype ranges from 10% to 25%. Reported rates for both lymphocyte-depleted and lymphocyte-rich CHL (LRCHL) are variable, probably reflecting differences in diagnostic criteria. However, when stringent criteria are used, lymphocyte-depleted CHL is usually EBV positive. Children and older adults are more likely to have EBV-positive CHL, as are males.[20] Developing countries generally show a higher incidence of EBV-associated disease, reaching almost 100% in childhood cases.[22,65] A history of infectious mononucleosis and atypical prediagnosis EBV serology are associated with an increased risk of EBV-positive, but not EBV-negative CHL, further supporting the pathogenetic role of EBV.[27,40,70]

Etiology of EBV-Negative Classic Hodgkin Lymphoma

Based on observations in EBV-positive Burkitt lymphoma cell lines, it has been proposed that the virus might be lost during the malignant progression of CHL once it is no longer required for propagation of the malignant clone. Although some studies reported detection of defective, rearranged EBV in a fraction of CHL negative for EBERs, results from other groups have not provided evidence for this "hit and run" theory.[71-73] Searches for other candidate viruses, such as human herpesvirus 6 or 8, have failed to provide evidence for their involvement in the pathogenesis of CHL.

CLINICAL FEATURES

Clinically, CHL manifests first in the lymph nodes in >90% of cases, usually as a slowly growing, painless mass. Cervical (75%), axillary, and inguinal nodes are the most frequently involved sites. Asymptomatic patients are occasionally diagnosed with mediastinal disease detected on a routine chest radiograph. Symptoms related to specific organ involvement, such as superior vena cava syndrome, bone pain, or neurologic symptoms, can occur. Retroperitoneal lymphadenopathy and splenic involvement are frequent, whereas extra-axial lymph nodes (mesenteric, perigastric, epitrochlear, preauricular, popliteal nodes) are rarely involved. CHL seems to spread in an orderly fashion to contiguous lymph nodes.[74] Bone marrow involvement is relatively rare in CHL, occurring in approximately 5% of nonimmunosuppressed patients. Disease manifestations on both sides of the diaphragm and B symptoms indicate a higher risk of bone marrow involvement.[75]

The distribution of disease correlates with histologic subtype. The nodular sclerosis type typically occurs above the diaphragm, most frequently involving the lower cervical, supraclavicular, and mediastinal nodes and contiguous structures. Patients frequently show an enlarged mediastinal silhouette and present with bulky mediastinal disease (greater than one-third of the intrathoracic diameter) in approximately 50% of cases. The spleen and bone marrow are involved in 10% and 3% of cases, respectively.[12,17,76] The mixed cellularity subtype of CHL presents more frequently in stages III and IV and with B symptoms. It occurs more often below or on both sides of the diaphragm; there is splenic involvement in 30% of cases and bone marrow infiltration in 10%. Bulky mediastinal disease is uncommon. Owing to the change in delineation to an independent subtype, relatively few clinical data are available for LRCHL. It has similarities with NLPBL in terms of clinical symptoms and disease distribution. Seventy percent of patients with LRCHL present with stages I and II, and bulky disease and B symptoms are infrequent.[77-79] Because of its rarity and changes in diagnostic criteria, clinical features of lymphocyte-depleted CHL are not well described. A predominance of elderly patients with higher-stage disease and predominant involvement of abdominal organs and bone marrow has been reported.[80,81] CHL in patients with HIV infection frequently presents as advanced disease and involves unusual sites.[32,82,83] The bone marrow is frequently infiltrated and occasionally represents the primary diagnostic manifestation of the disease.[82,84]

Approximately 30% to 40% of patients with CHL present with B symptoms. Although B symptoms are more frequent in advanced stages of disease, they can also occur in early stages, possibly as a result of inflammatory cytokines produced by the tumor. The so-called "cyclic Pel-Ebstein" type of fever is rare. Other symptoms include generalized pruritus and occasionally pain in involved nodes upon alcohol ingestion.

Laboratory Findings

Laboratory findings are mostly non-specific and include leukocytosis, elevated erythrocyte sedimentation rate, and increased lactate dehydrogenase. Eosinophilia can be observed in approximately 20% of patients, and lymphopenia is present in advanced disease stages. However, most patients with CHL exhibit demonstrable defects in cell-mediated immunity, regardless of stage.[12] A decrease in CD4-positive cells in the peripheral blood is already detectable at an early stage. T lymphocytes from patients with HL show a weaker response to T-cell mitogens and a decrease in cytokine production upon stimulation. Clinically, this anergy can manifest as an increased susceptibility to infections and a lack of reactivity in the tuberculin skin test. It is still unclear whether these immune abnormalities are preexistent; they may contribute to disease development or may be secondary phenomena, possibly caused by immunosuppressive cytokines secreted by the neoplastic population.[85,86]

Extranodal Manifestations

Although CHL is almost always a node-based lymphoma, practically any site and organ of the body can be involved during the course of the disease. Although the spleen, bone marrow, and liver are frequently involved in advanced disease, isolated involvement of these organs is rare.[87] Thymic involvement is frequent in mediastinal disease. Rarely, if lymph node involvement is not apparent, CHL can radiologically simulate other neoplasms of the thymus, prompting surgical removal of the thymic mass.[88] The affected thymus frequently shows cystic degeneration. Bona fide CHL is rare in mucosa-associated lymphoid tissue but can occur in the tonsils and Waldeyer's ring.[89,90] Apart from the liver, the lung is probably the most frequently involved nonlymphoid organ, usually as an extension of mediastinal disease. Interestingly, primary CHL of the gastrointestinal tract was initially reported in association with a history of inflammatory bowel disease or immunosuppression.[91] These cases would today probably be classified as EBV-associated lymphoproliferation with Hodgkin-like features, specifically as EBV-associated mucocutaneous ulcer.[92,93] Many other extranodal primary sites of CHL have been reported, mainly in anecdotal form in older literature. In the skin, CHL may be suspected as a result of the morphologic and phenotypic overlap with CD30-positive lymphoproliferative disorders (LPDs) of the skin, including cutaneous anaplastic large cell lymphoma (ALCL) and lymphomatoid papulosis. Cases of apparently primary cutaneous CHL need to be evaluated with extended phenotyping.[94,95] Central nervous system involvement with CHL is very rare but may exceptionally occur as primary disease.[96] In summary, any diagnosis of primary extranodal CHL, especially in patients without concurrent nodal or systemic disease, should be made with utmost caution and requires extended immunohistochemical studies to rule out morphologic mimics, including EBV-associated LPDs.

Staging

Staging of CHL is performed according to the Ann Arbor staging classification, as last modified in the Lugano meeting.[97] It provides important prognostic information and forms the basis for certain therapeutic decisions. The accuracy of staging in CHL relies on the fact that HL disseminates in a highly predictable manner through lymphatic channels, involving contiguous lymph node stations and other organs in a stepwise fashion.[74,98]

In addition to a detailed clinical history, physical examination, and laboratory studies, staging of HL requires detailed imaging studies, including chest x-ray and contrast-enhanced computed tomography (CT)-scan. Fluorodeoxyglucose positron emission tomography (FDG-PET) in combination with CT (PET/CT) offers greater sensitivity and a higher specificity and is the method of choice for initial staging and during follow-up.[97,99,100] Trephine bone marrow biopsy is not indicated in asymptomatic early-stage and PET/CT-negative cases owing to the very low rate of bone marrow involvement in these groups.[101,102]

MORPHOLOGY

Reed-Sternberg Cells and Variants

The diagnostic cell of CHL is the *Reed-Sternberg* (RS) cell. The classic RS cell is large (up to 100 μm) and contains two to multiple nuclei or a large lobated nucleus, rendering the impression of multinucleation on sectioning. The nuclei show an accentuated membrane, pale chromatin, and a single large, eosinophilic, viral-inclusion–like nucleolus (Fig. 27-1A, C, and D). The cytoplasm is ample and amphophilic. They can also be identified in cytology specimens, e.g., fine needle aspirates (Fig. 27-2E). Mononuclear variants are called *Hodgkin cells* (Fig. 27-1F). They can usually be distinguished from immunoblasts by virtue of their larger size; their huge, eosinophilic nucleolus, frequently surrounded by a clear halo; and their more eosinophilic cytoplasm. In many instances, the classic diagnostic RS cells make up only a minority of the neoplastic population, and mononuclear cells and other variants predominate. Frequently, degenerated HRS cells with condensed, darkly stained cytoplasm and condensed nuclear chromatin can be observed—so-called "mummified" cells (Fig. 27-1E). However, HRS-like cells and variants can be identified in a range of different disorders and are therefore not sufficient for a diagnosis of CHL.[103,104]

The typical cell of the nodular sclerosis subtype is the lacunar variant of the HRS cell. Lacunar cells show abundant clear to slightly eosinophilic cytoplasm and sharply defined, round cellular borders. The nuclei are frequently more lobated, with coarse chromatin. The nucleoli are smaller than those in classic HRS cells. Owing to a shrinkage artifact, the cytoplasm is frequently condensed in the perinuclear area, with spider-web–like extensions to the cell membrane leaving lacuna-like spaces, characteristic of this cell type (Fig. 27-1B). The lymphocyte-predominant (LP; formerly L&H) variant of the RS cell (or "popcorn" cell) is the characteristic cell type of NLPBL, although morphologic mimics can be seen in LRCHL.[77]

Histologic Subtypes

Based on the morphology of the neoplastic cells, the tissue architecture, and the characteristics of the reactive infiltrate, four subtypes of CHL are currently recognized (Table 27-1).[11,105] Although the two most common subtypes, nodular sclerosis and mixed cellularity, are well defined and usually easily recognizable, the two other subtypes, lymphocyte-rich and the rare lymphocyte-depleted, frequently require more extensive immunohistochemical confirmation.

Based on novel insights into disease epidemiology, biology, and genetics, it is currently thought that nodular sclerosis CHL represents a disease entity distinct from the other subtypes of CHL, with a close relationship to MGZL and primary mediastinal large B-cell lymphoma (PMBL).[12,106]

Nodular Sclerosis Classic Hodgkin Lymphoma

This is the most frequent subtype of CHL, accounting for 60% to 80% of cases in most series from Western countries.[12,17,78] Macroscopically, a diagnosis of nodular sclerosis CHL can be suspected in typical cases with advanced fibrosis. The node is firm, and the cut surface reveals distinct white or yellowish nodules separated by bands of connective tissue. Microscopically, the diagnosis can be suspected at low power because of the presence of cellular nodules surrounded by concentrically arranged collagen bands that show birefringence in polarized light (Fig. 27-2A). The nodules frequently show an irregular, mottled appearance resulting from the presence of numerous lacunar cells and may contain areas of frank necrosis and abscess formation (Fig. 27-2B).

The presence of fibrosis is a defining feature of nodular sclerosis, but the amount can be quite variable. A discrete thickening of the lymph node capsule and perivascular adventitial structures may be the only clear sign of increased collagen synthesis. At the other extreme, nodular sclerosis can show almost complete obliterative fibrosis of the node, with a paucity of both tumor cells and reactive inflammatory cells. These cases can present significant diagnostic difficulties, especially when only small biopsy specimens are available, such as cutting needle biopsies of mediastinal masses, which frequently show crush artifacts because of the high fiber content. (Fig. 27-2F-H)

On high power, lacunar cells are easily recognized (Fig. 27-2B). They can be sprinkled throughout the cellular nodules or occur in clusters or compact sheets of cells; the latter is especially true of grade II nodular sclerosis. Classic RS cells are less frequent in nodular sclerosis and may be difficult to identify.

The cellular composition of the reactive background can vary from case to case and from nodule to nodule. Some cases show a predominance of small lymphocytes; more often, a mixed population of lymphocytes, neutrophils, frequent eosinophils, plasma cells, and macrophages can be found. Fibroblasts are especially frequent in the fibrotic pattern of the disease. Eosinophilic or neutrophilic abscesses are common. Sheets of neoplastic cells and histiocytes often rim foci of necrosis, sometimes raising the possibility of a necrotizing granulomatous process.

Owing to its extreme morphologic variability, subclassification of nodular sclerosis CHL into grades I and II based on histologic features had been proposed for prognostic purposes according to the British National

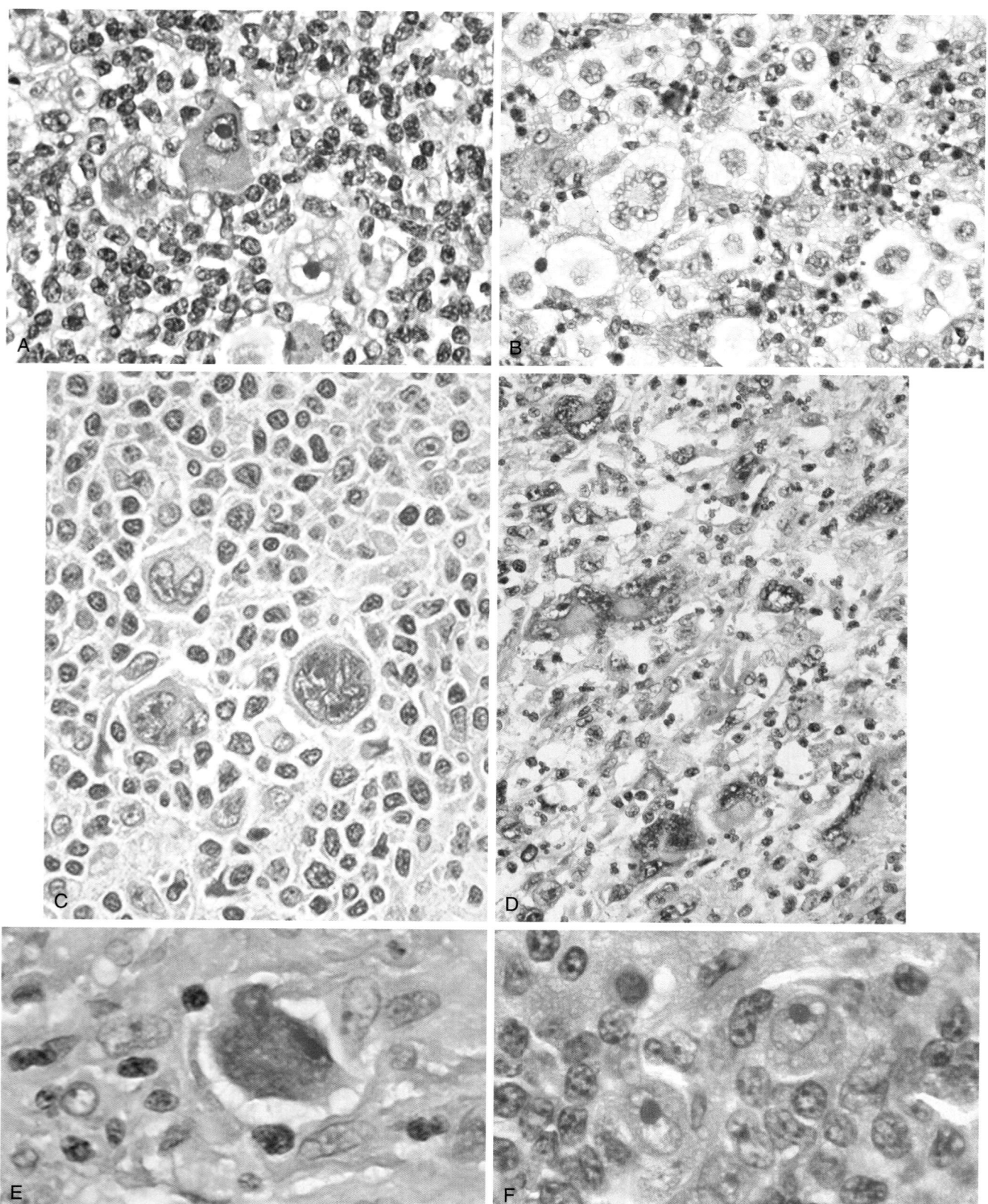

Figure 27-1. Cytologic features of Reed-Sternberg (RS) cells and Hodgkin cells. A, Classic RS cells and variants in mixed cellularity classic Hodgkin lymphoma (CHL) with amphophilic cytoplasm, large nuclei with clear karyoplasm, and huge, viral inclusion-like nucleoli. **B,** Typical lacunar cells in a case of nodular sclerosis CHL. Note the delicate, folded nuclear membranes; less conspicuous nucleoli; and ample, clear cytoplasm with thread-like protrusions. **C,** Typical RS cells, including a binuclear variant, in mixed cellularity CHL. **D,** Abundant, sometimes bizarre multinucleated tumor cells in a case of nodular sclerosis grade II. **E,** So-called "mummified" RS cell with condensed, deeply basophilic cytoplasm. **F,** Two classic mononuclear Hodgkin cells in a case of mixed cellularity CHL.

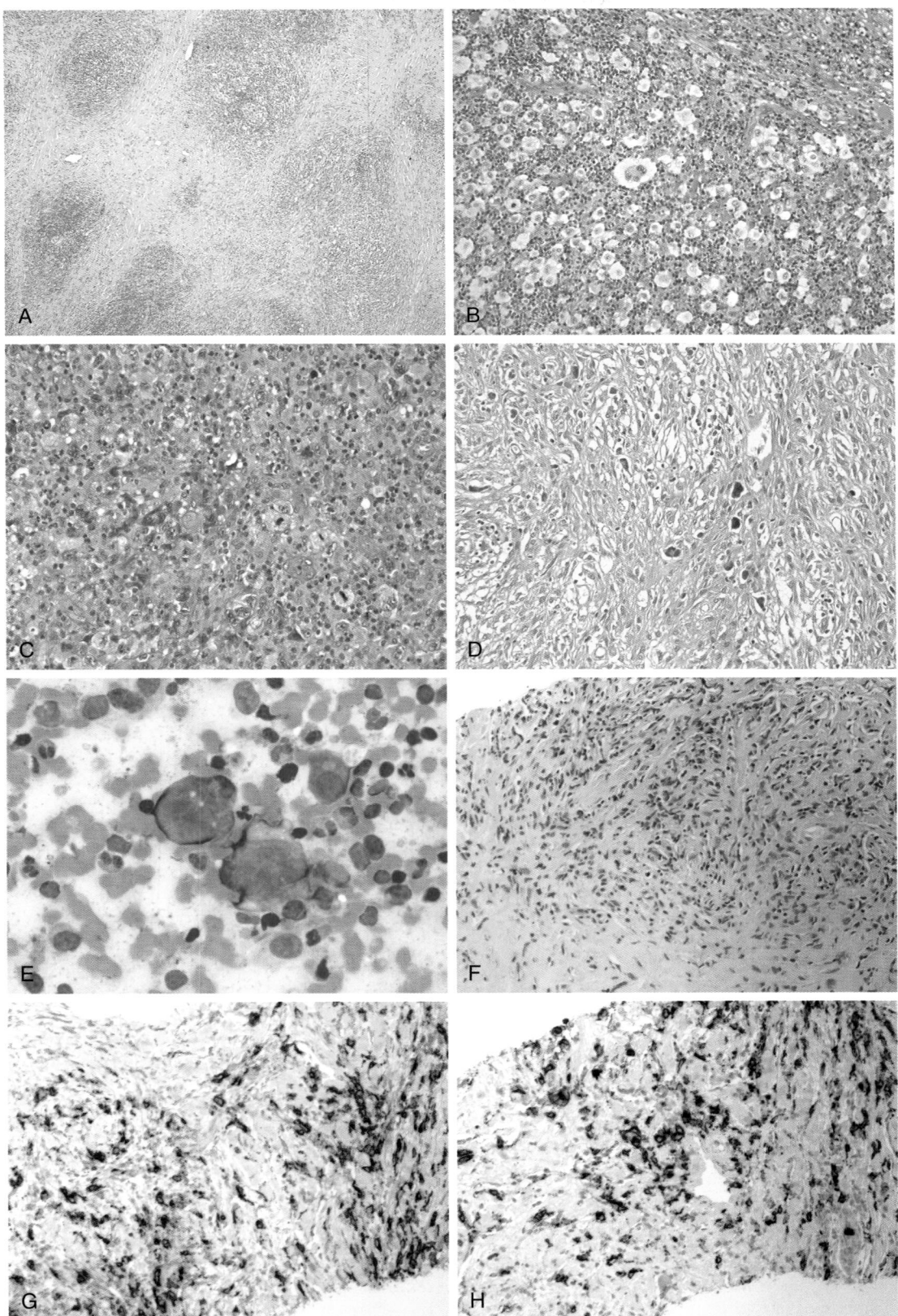

Figure 27-2. **Morphology of classic Hodgkin lymphoma (CHL). A,** Nodular sclerosis CHL (NSCHL). Cellular nodules are separated by concentric bands of mature collagen. **B,** Close-up of cellular nodule shows numerous lacunar cells with clear cytoplasm intermingled with lymphocytes, neutrophils, and eosinophils. Note collagen bands rimming the nodule. **C,** NSCHL grade II. Confluent sheets of neoplastic cells with partly anaplastic features, intermingled with a minority of inflammatory cells. This morphology is consistent with the so-called "syncytial" variant of CHL. **D,** Lymphocyte-depleted CHL, diffuse fibrosis subtype. Neoplastic Hodgkin and Reed-Sternberg (HRS) cells in a hypocellular background with histiocytes and fibroblasts. This case lacks nodularity and ordered collagen bands. **E,** Fine needle aspirate of a mediastinal lymph node with CHL. Two large, atypical cells with large nuclei and prominent nucleoli are accompanied by eosinophils and lymphocytes. **F,** Mediastinal core needle biopsy of NSCHL with significant fibrosis and occasional large mononuclear cells. Immunostaining for CD30 **(G)** and CD15 **(H)** highlights the neoplastic HRS cells.

Table 27-1 Major Diagnostic Features: Histology

Subtype	Tissue Architecture	Neoplastic Cells	Background Cells
Nodular sclerosis	Nodular, concentric collagen fibers, necrosis and microabscesses frequent	Lacunar cells with clear cytoplasm, hyperlobated nuclei; classic RS cells often rare	Frequent eosinophils and neutrophils, CD4+ T cells, macrophages, fibroblasts
Mixed cellularity	Diffuse, rare follicle remnants; frequent epithelioid cell granulomas	Classic binucleated or multinucleated RS cells and Hodgkin cells, lacunar cells absent	Lymphocytes, eosinophils, plasma cells, histiocytes
Lymphocyte depleted	Diffuse reticulin fibrosis or diffuse sheets of neoplastic cells	Variable number of RS cells; frequently sheets of bizarre, anaplastic tumor cells	Reduced background infiltrate, fibroblasts
Lymphocyte rich	Mostly nodular, with atrophic germinal centers; rare cases diffuse or interfollicular	Small numbers of classic RS cells and variants, LP-like cells may occur	Mostly small lymphocytes (B cells in nodular pattern), epithelioid histiocytes

LP, Lymphocyte predominant; *RS,* Reed-Sternberg.

Lymphoma Investigation (BNLI). Nodular sclerosis CHL is classified as grade II if (1) more than 25% of the nodules show pleomorphic or reticular lymphocyte depletion, (2) more than 80% of the nodules show the fibrohistiocytic variant of lymphocyte depletion, or (3) more than 25% of the nodules show numerous bizarre, anaplastic-appearing RS cells. If these criteria are followed, approximately 15% to 25% of cases are classified as grade II.[107-109] This subtyping has lost importance because of improved therapies, which tend to abolish these previously observed prognostic differences.[110] Nodular sclerosis cases with high numbers of tumor cells should be separated from lymphocyte-depleted CHL. By convention, any nodularity of the infiltrate will put a case into the nodular sclerosis category.[111,112] In some cases of CHL with typical lacunar cells, fibrosis is minimal or absent, and there is a prominent nodular pattern with a predominance of lymphocytes. These cases have been designated the cellular phase of nodular sclerosis. Nowadays, some of these cases fall into the lymphocyte-rich category of CHL.[113] A fibroblastic variant of nodular sclerosis with diagnostic importance was observed in the BNLI studies. It is characterized by a diffuse proliferation of fibroblasts, without the heavy collagen deposition characteristic of conventional nodular sclerosis.[109] These cases can be misclassified as mesenchymal tumor, such as malignant fibrous histiocytoma.

Cases described as syncytial variant of nodular sclerosis show sheets of neoplastic cells frequently associated with areas of necrosis and increased pleomorphism of the neoplastic cells (Fig. 27-2C).[114,115] The main importance of this variant is the potential for misdiagnosis as ALCL or nonlymphoid neoplasm.

Mixed Cellularity Classic Hodgkin Lymphoma

This is the second most frequent subtype of CHL, accounting for 20% to 30% of cases in Western countries. The lymph node architecture is usually diffusely obliterated, although early involvement may show an interfollicular growth pattern or residual, sometimes atrophic germinal centers. Classic HRS cells are frequent, easily identifiable, and usually evenly dispersed throughout the node (Fig. 27-3A). The presence of clusters of lacunar cells should raise the possibility of the cellular phase of nodular sclerosis. The background infiltrate consists of a heterogeneous population of small lymphocytes, eosinophils, plasma cells, and histiocytes. The lymphocytes may show some nuclear pleomorphism, but frank background atypia should immediately raise the

differential diagnosis of NHL, especially peripheral T-cell lymphoma. In some cases, sometimes termed the *histiocyte-rich variant of mixed cellularity CHL*, clusters of epithelioid histiocytes are present in abundance (Fig. 27-3B). These cases need to be separated from various subtypes of histiocyte-rich NHL. Rare cases of CHL show an excessive, sometimes granulomatous proliferation of histiocytes, which can obscure both lymphocytes and the neoplastic cells.[116,117] These cases may resemble histiocyte storage disorders or inflammatory conditions and require immunohistochemical stains for identification of the neoplastic cells. Phenomena that should not be confused with infiltration by histiocyte-rich mixed cellularity CHL is the presence of noncaseating, sarcoid-type granulomas in lymph nodes or other tissues in the vicinity of involved nodes or abundant histiocytes in nodes excised after treatment for CHL. Although appropriate stains may show a diffuse increase in reticulin fibers, the presence of collagen fibrosis precludes a diagnosis of mixed cellularity CHL. Similarly, necrosis is not a feature of this subtype.

Although mixed cellularity CHL as initially defined in the Rye classification incorporated all cases that could not be included in any other categories, it is now regarded as a true entity, and cases that cannot be classified properly owing to unusual histologic features or limited material should be termed *CHL, unclassifiable*.[111]

Lymphocyte-Rich Classic Hodgkin Lymphoma

This rare subtype of CHL is characterized by the presence of a small minority of HRS cells of the classic type in a background dominated by small lymphocytes.[77,111,113,118,119] Most cases show prominent nodularity, and a diffuse pattern is rare.[77]

Typical LRCHL shows partially preserved lymph node architecture with an easily discernible nodularity. The nodules consist of small B cells and often contain a regressed, eccentrically placed germinal center, sometimes reminiscent of Castleman disease (Fig. 27-4A and B). Progressively transformed germinal centers are not a feature of LRCHL. Groups of epithelioid cells, sometimes in a concentric arrangement, can occur, closely simulating the appearance of NLPBL. Other inflammatory cells, such as eosinophils, are usually rare. The neoplastic cells are present in the expanded mantle zones in a dispersed pattern, and groups or clusters of tumor cells are infrequent. The peculiar location of the neoplastic cells in the mantles of B-cell follicles led to the initial description

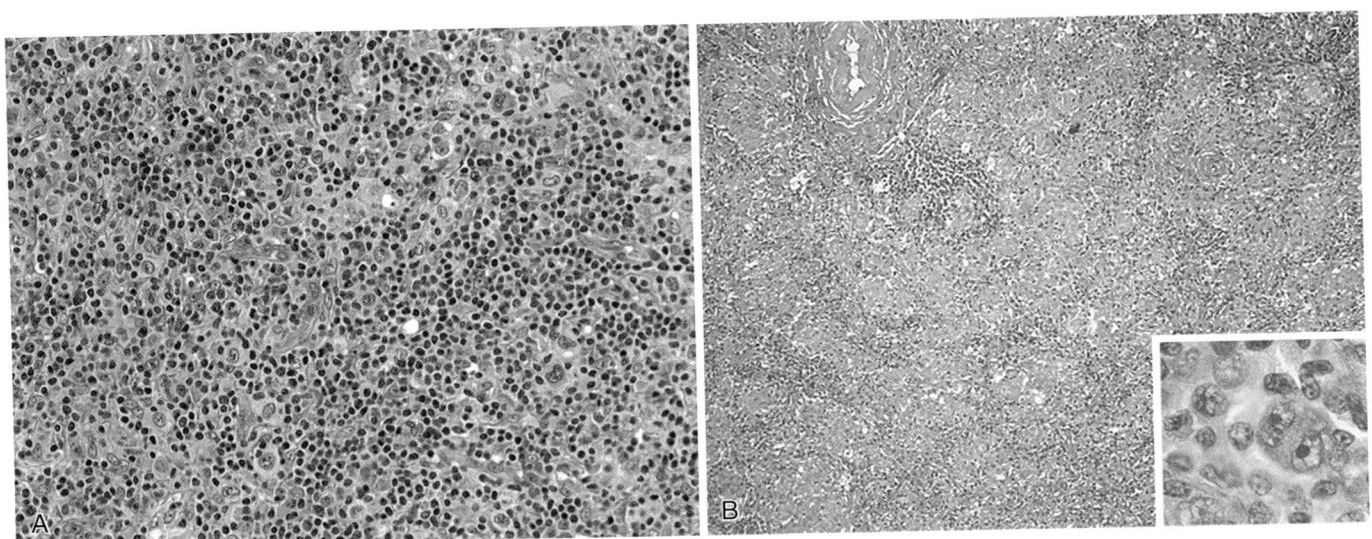

Figure 27-3. Mixed cellularity classic Hodgkin lymphoma (CHL). A, The lymph node contains a mixed population of lymphocytes, plasma cells, eosinophils, histiocytes, and easily recognizable Reed-Sternberg (RS) cells and variants. **B,** Histiocyte-rich mixed cellularity CHL containing confluent sheets of epithelioid cell granulomas with rare, interspersed RS cells *(inset)*. If areas of more typical mixed cellularity CHL are missing, non-Hodgkin lymphoma with epithelioid cell granulomas (e.g., so-called "Lennert" lymphoma) or even reactive conditions may be considered.

of this variant as *follicular Hodgkin disease*.[120,121] Classic HRS cells occur in the majority of cases but may be rare (Fig. 27-4E). Of note, cells with the cytologic features of LP cells typical for NLPBL, with folded or lobated nuclei and less prominent nucleoli, occur also in LRCHL (Fig. 27-4C and D).[77] Therefore, the immunophenotype of neoplastic cells with expression of CD30 and CD15 is crucial for the distinction from NLPBL (Fig. 27-4F).[77,112,113,119] The reactive background consists of small immunoglobulin (Ig) M-positive and IgD-positive B cells, typical for the mantle zone (Fig. 27-4B). Appropriate stains reveal a fine, expanded meshwork of follicular dendritic cells and highlight the nodular architecture of the infiltrate. The neoplastic cells are frequently rimmed by CD3-positive T cells that may show CD57 and/or PD-1 (CD279) expression, markers of follicular T-helper cells.[77,104,112,113,119]

The second, rare variant of LRCHL shows an interfollicular or diffuse growth pattern with classic RS cells in a background of small lymphocytes that, in contrast to those in the nodular pattern, are predominantly of a T-cell phenotype. B-cell follicles are either pushed aside or, rarely, absent.

Overall, LRCHL shows some clinical, morphologic, and immunophenotypical features overlapping those of NLPBL, with more frequent expression of B-cell transcription factors and a follicular T-cell environment, supporting its place as a specific subtype of CHL, although this has been challenged by some authors.[118]

Lymphocyte-Depleted Classic Hodgkin Lymphoma

This is the least frequently diagnosed subtype of CHL, constituting about 1% of patients in recent series.[81] Many cases from earlier series probably represented aggressive NHL or would today be classified as nodular sclerosis CHL grade II.[122] Two types of lymphocyte depletion can be recognized: diffuse fibrosis and reticular variants. The diffuse fibrosis type shows a hypocellular infiltrate with disordered, diffuse reticulin fibrosis and atypical cells, including HRS cells and a sparse,

heterogeneous background population (Fig. 27-2D). The presence of organized collagen bands mandates a diagnosis of nodular sclerosis CHL. The reticular variant is characterized by sheets of atypical cells, including many bizarre, anaplastic RS cells. Immunohistochemical demonstration of a characteristic CHL phenotype is required for the exclusion of large cell lymphomas, especially ALCL.[104,112,123,124]

Classic Hodgkin Lymphoma, Unclassified, and Unusual Morphologic Patterns

All cases that cannot be confidently placed in any of the four categories described should be designated CHL, unclassified. Small biopsy specimens or biopsies from extranodal sites, partial lymph node involvement, unusual histologic features, or poor technical quality may preclude subtyping. Partial involvement by CHL is frequently found, especially if a smaller node from the periphery of a lymph node conglomerate is removed. The infiltrate usually resides in the interfollicular area in a background of T cells, with preserved or regressed germinal centers. This interfollicular pattern may fall into the LRCHL category. RS cells of CHL may occur in monocytoid B-cell clusters, and an accompanying monocytoid B-cell reaction can be observed in a small minority of cases.[125-127] Rarely, sinusoidal involvement by HRS cells and variants can mimic ALCL.

Relapsed CHL usually retains the initial histologic subtype but may show morphologic progression, especially at previously treated sites, with an increase in the number and pleomorphism of tumor cells.[76] These cases are sometimes designated the lymphocyte-depleted subtype, but assignment of the histologic subtype should be based on initial pretherapy biopsies. In patients with suspected relapses of CHL, the possibility of a secondary neoplasm should always be considered if the morphologic and phenotypic criteria for a diagnosis of CHL are not met. Similarly, persistent mass lesions after treatment for CHL may occasionally prompt a biopsy, especially if there is residual PET-positivity.[128] Frequently,

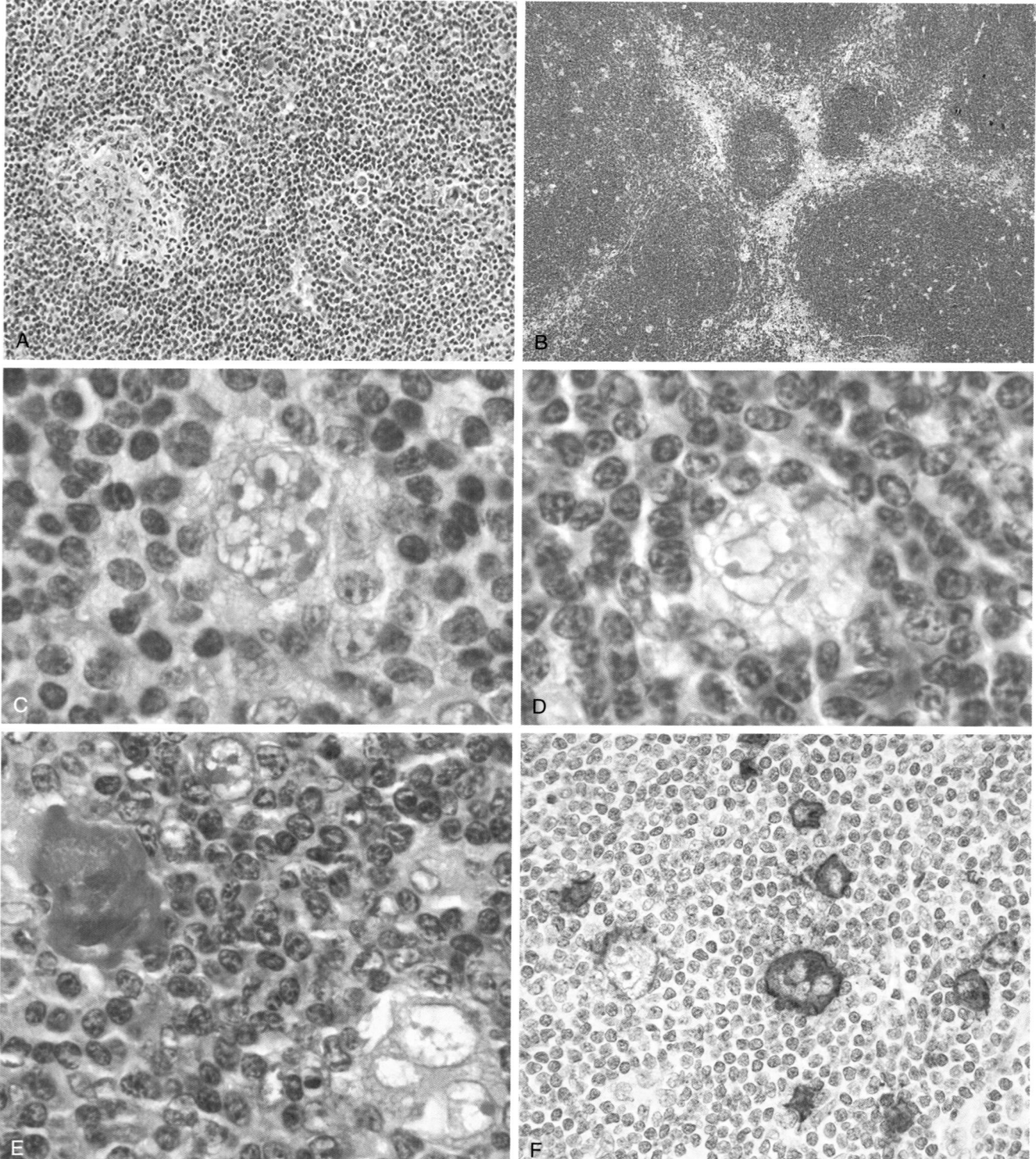

Figure 27-4. Lymphocyte-rich classic Hodgkin lymphoma (CHL), nodular variant. A, The lymph node is dominated by small lymphocytes arranged in a nodular pattern, frequently with atrophic germinal centers. The tumor cells are found in the expanded mantle zones of these B-cell nodules. **B,** Immunohistochemistry for CD20 highlights the nodular pattern with a predominance of B cells. **C** to **E,** the morphologic spectrum of neoplastic cells in lymphocyte-rich CHL varies from classic Reed-Sternberg (RS) cells **(E)** to cells resembling the LP cells of nodular lymphocyte-predominant B-cell lymphoma **(C** and **D). F,** Immunohistochemistry for CD15 reveals strong positivity of the neoplastic cells, including a classic binucleate RS cell.

only hyalinized scar tissue or histiocyte accumulations can be identified. A diagnosis of residual CHL should be made only if HRS cells can be identified unequivocally by morphology and immunophenotype.

Diagnostic Criteria for Extranodal Sites

The criteria for a diagnosis of CHL in an extranodal organ strongly depend on whether the patient has an established diagnosis of CHL at a nodal site. In liver and bone marrow biopsies obtained for staging purposes in patients with CHL, identification of a mixed cellular infiltrate with occasional atypical mononuclear cells with appropriate phenotype is regarded as sufficient for a diagnosis of involvement by CHL, because diagnostic RS cells are lacking in most small tumor foci. In the liver, the infiltrate usually involves the portal triads. In the bone marrow, focal fibrosis detected by reticulin stains is an ominous sign and should prompt further examinations such as step sectioning and immunohistochemistry.[84,129]

As mentioned earlier, the thymus is frequently involved in mediastinal disease, which is almost always of the nodular sclerosis subtype. Thymic CHL can be associated with a prominent reactive proliferation of thymic epithelium intermingled with neoplastic cells and the development of epithelial cysts, sometimes leading to a misdiagnosis of thymoma or multilocular inflammatory thymic cyst unless generous sampling of the lesion and appropriate immunohistochemical studies are performed.[88]

In contrast to patients with known CHL as described in this chapter, a *primary* diagnosis of CHL in an extranodal site should be performed with utmost caution; most cases from previous series nowadays would be classified as B-cell lymphomas or EBV-associated lymphoproliferations.

IMMUNOPHENOTYPE

Owing to the unique features of CHL, both the phenotype of the neoplastic cells and the antigenic profile of the reactive background population are of diagnostic importance. Despite the significant morphologic variability among the four subtypes of CHL, the immunophenotype of the neoplastic cells is quite constant, and minimal sets of markers have been proposed, including CD3, CD20, CD30, CD15, and PAX5, usually complemented by MUM1/IRF4 and detection of EBV by EBER ISH or LMP1 immunostaining.[11,130] The most important antigens of diagnostic relevance are summarized in Table 27-2. HRS cells express various activation-associated antigens, including CD30,[131,132] CD25 (interleukin [IL]-2 receptor α chain),[133] CD40,[134] CD71 (transferrin receptor), CD80, HLA-DR, and antigens normally found on such diverse cell types as T-lymphocytes, granulocytes, and follicular dendritic cells.[12,112,135-137] They characteristically lack the common leukocyte antigen CD45 and show inconstant and heterogeneous expression of some B-cell or, rarely, T-cell markers.[138,139] The immunophenotype of CHL may be difficult to assess owing to the immersion of the neoplastic RS cells in an abundant reactive infiltrate, especially for markers expressed by most or all nonneoplastic cells in the immediate vicinity, such as CD45 or T-cell markers. Another potential source of confusion is the cytoplasmic uptake of serum proteins, such as Igs, by HRS cells.

Table 27-2 Major Diagnostic Features: Phenotype and Molecular Features

	Positive	Negative
Immunophenotype	CD30 CD15 (75%-85%) PAX5 (weak) IRF4/MUM-1 PD-L1 CD25 CD20 −/+ LMP-1 (20%-50%) Fascin Vimentin	CD45 CD43 EMA Cytokeratin ALK1 CD79a (rarely +) J chain BOB.1 Oct-2 −/+ MEF2B BCL6 T-cell markers (rarely +) TIA-1, granzyme B −/+
Genotype and genetic profile	Clonally rearranged immunoglobulin genes detectable by single-cell PCR in >95% of cases, but inconsistently in bulk tissue analysis Clonal EBV infection in 20%-50% or more of cases (MC > NS) Absence of t(14;18), t(2;5) and variants, and other NHL-specific translocations Complex, hyperdiploid karyotype Recurrent amplification of 2p13 *(REL)*, 9p24 *(JAK2, PD-L1/PD-L2)* Mutations/deletions of IκBα, IκBε and A20 *(TNFAIP3), SOCS1, PTPN1, STAT6*, and others Translocations of *CIITA*	

ALK, Anaplastic lymphoma kinase; *EBV,* Epstein-Barr virus; *EMA,* epithelial membrane antigen; *MC,* mixed cellularity; *NHL,* non-Hodgkin lymphoma; *NS,* nodular sclerosis; *PCR,* polymerase chain reaction.

The most reliable and most frequently used markers for CHL are the CD30 and CD15 antigens. CD30 is a member of the TNF-nerve growth factor (NGF) receptor superfamily of cytokine receptors.[140] CD30 is expressed in HRS cells in all cases of CHL.[104,112,135,141] Staining is membranous and cytoplasmic, with frequent dot-like accentuation in the perinuclear area, corresponding to the Golgi field (Fig. 27-5A). In contrast, the LP cells of NLPBL usually lack CD30 staining, with rare cases showing usually weak and heterogeneous positivity.[142,143] CD30 is expressed in a variety of NHLs, most notably ALCL,[104,112,135,144] but also in a subset of peripheral T-cell lymphoma,[145] NOS, lymphomatoid papulosis and in some large B-cell lymphomas, including PMBL, MGZL, and EBV-positive DLBCL.[146-149] Some non-hematopoietic neoplasms, such as embryonal carcinoma, frequently express the CD30 antigen.[150] Perifollicular blasts in reactive lymph nodes are often positive for CD30 and should not be interpreted as interfollicular HL; their positivity is characteristically more variable than in HRS cells.[151,152]

CD15, detected by LeuM1 or other antibodies, is an antigen of late granulopoiesis and is found in 75% to 85% of CHL cases, although staining may be weaker than CD30 and restricted to a subset of the neoplastic cells (Figs. 27-4F and 27-5B).[112,135,137,153] The staining pattern is otherwise similar to that of CD30. The reactivity in RS cells is occasionally obscured by large numbers of granulocytes in cases of nodular sclerosis (Fig. 27-5B). The expression of CD15 is useful for differentiating HRS cells from CD30-positive reactive blasts or HRS-like cells in conditions such as infectious mononucleosis, which usually are CD15

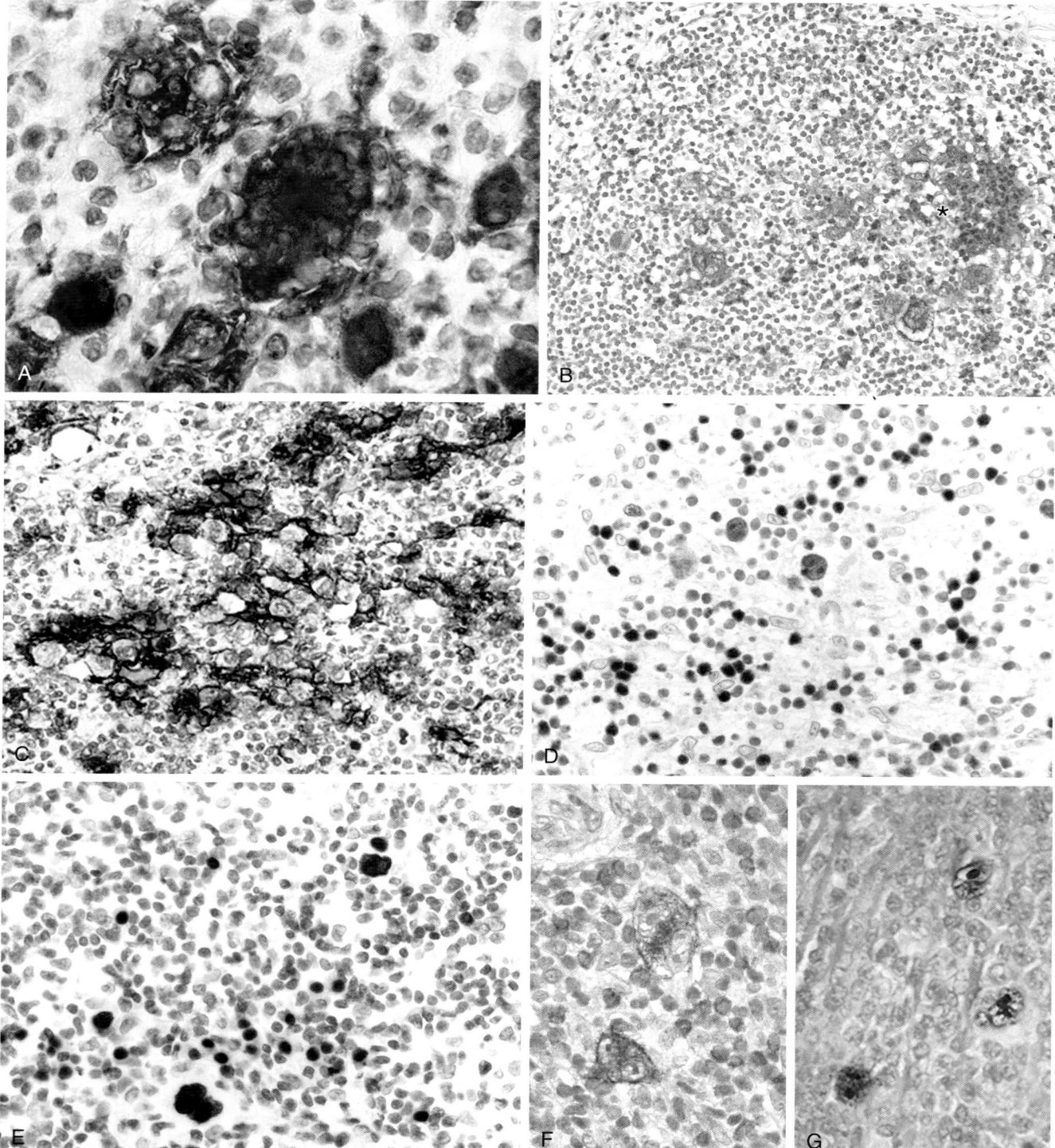

Figure 27-5. Immunophenotype of classic Hodgkin lymphoma (CHL). A, Strong expression of CD30 in Hodgkin and Reed-Sternberg (HRS) cells and variants in nodular sclerosis CHL. **B,** Expression of CD15 in nodular sclerosis CHL. Note the positivity of neutrophils *(asterisk).* **C,** CD20 expression in a case of typical nodular sclerosis CHL. Note the variable and incomplete membranous staining pattern. **D,** PAX5 expression in CHL. The nuclei of the HRS cells typically are weaker than those of the adjacent reactive B cells. **E,** Strong nuclear MUM1/IRF4 expression in HRS cells, equal to that of neighboring plasma cells. **F,** Expression of latent membrane protein-1 (LMP-1) of Epstein-Barr virus (EBV) in mixed cellularity CHL. **G,** RNA in situ hybridization for EBV-encoded RNAs (EBERs) in a case of EBV-positive CHL, with strong nuclear staining restricted to the neoplastic large cells.

negative. A notable exception are cytomegalovirus-infected cells, which show CD15 expression and may simulate Hodgkin cells by virtue of their eosinophilic nuclear inclusions.[154] In lymphomas and lymphoproliferations other than CHL, co-expression of CD15 and CD30 is infrequent and mainly observed in MGZL,[149,155-157] some peripheral T-cell lymphomas,[145,158,159] and EBV-associated lymphoproliferations.[92,93,160-162] Not surprising in light of the B-cell derivation of CHL, expression of pan–B-cell markers—mainly CD20—can be found in a percentage of cases of CHL.[77,136,137,163,164] CD20 positivity of RS cells has been reported in <20% to 80% of cases[163] (the difference probably related to technical factors), with the majority of reports being in the 20% to 40% range. In contrast to most B-cell lymphomas, notably T-cell/histiocyte-rich large B-cell lymphoma (THRLBCL) and NLPBL, CHL usually shows weaker staining restricted to a subpopulation of neoplastic cells (Fig. 27-5C). CD79a is detected infrequently in CHL,[165] and J chain is always absent.[166,167] The only B-cell–restricted antigen found in the neoplastic cells of virtually all CHLs is PAX5/B-cell–specific activator protein (BSAP), whereas in other B-cell transcription factors, including BCL6, MEF2B, Oct2, BOB.1, and PU.1 are either lacking or only partially expressed.[119,166,168-172] The expression profile of B-cell transcription factors and B-cell antigens is helpful in the differential diagnosis.[136,173] Nuclear PAX5 (Fig. 27-5D) is usually weaker than in reactive B cells, and strong expression of both BOB.1 and Oct-2 is very unusual for CHL and should prompt the consideration of MGZL or DLBCL with CHL-like features in extramediastinal cases.[148,149,157,174] The transcription factor IRF4/MUM-1, a marker of late B-cell differentiation, is usually strongly expressed in CHL in a nuclear fashion (Fig. 27-5E) but is also found in ALCL and a subset of DLBCL.[112,130,175] Expression of the germinal-center cell markers "lim domain only 2" (LMO2) and human germinal-center associated lymphoma protein (HGAL) has been found in a subset of CHL cases.[176-178]

Programmed death ligands 1 and 2 (PD-L1/2) are strongly expressed in most cases of CHL through a variety of mechanisms and represent not only an immunohistochemical marker but an important target for immune checkpoint inhibition.[179-182]

Several antigens related to follicular dendritic cells are expressed by HRS cells in varying percentages of cases, among them CD21 and the intermediate filaments restin and fascin.[183-185] The latter is always strongly positive in CHL but lacks specificity.[186]

Positivity of HRS cells for diverse T-cell antigens such as CD2, CD3, CD4, CD45RO, and CD43 has been described in a minority of otherwise typical cases but should not cause concern unless there is absence of PAX5 staining.[138,139] Cytoplasmic staining for the cytotoxic granule-associated proteins TIA-1, granzyme B, or perforin, antigens expressed by activated cytotoxic T cells and natural killer cells and neoplasms derived thereof, is present in approximately 10% to 20% of CHL cases.[187,188] Staining is usually weak and heterogeneous. However, rare cases with the morphologic features of CHL but that lack PAX5 expression and have variable, sometimes strong expression of cytotoxic molecules are difficult to classify[189]; they, at least in part, more likely represent unusual examples of peripheral T-cell lymphoma or ALCL.[190,191] The T-cell transcription factor GATA3 is

expressed in most cases of CHL.[192,193] Epithelial membrane antigen (EMA) and the anaplastic lymphoma kinase (ALK)-1 protein are consistently absent from true CHL.[144,194,195] Absence of the common leukocyte antigen CD45 is a useful diagnostic hallmark of CHL and helps separate it from various NHL mimics and NLPBL.[136,196] The absence of expression of HLA class I antigens, a potential mechanism of immune evasion, is mostly found in EBV-negative CHL.[197]

The LMP-1 protein of EBV is expressed in approximately 25% to 50% of CHLs, depending on histologic subtype and patient characteristics.[12,37,137] The staining is membranous and cytoplasmic, and usually all or most neoplastic cells are positive (Fig. 27-5F). ISH for EBERs shows concordance with LMP-1 immunohistochemistry if the nuclear reactivity of HRS cells (and not of rare small lymphocytes) is considered positive (Fig. 27-5G).[45] The phenotype of HRS cells is usually constant during the course of the disease. Major variations in antigen expression among multiple biopsy sites or recurrences from the same patient are infrequent.[198]

The reactive background lymphocytes of CHL, with the exception of the nodular pattern of LRCHL, are predominantly T cells. The majority express CD4, belong to the memory compartment, and show signs of activation.[12,13,136,199] The T cells surrounding the neoplastic cells express costimulatory molecules and CD30 and CD40 ligands, possibly contributing to the survival of the HRS cells.[200] Numbers of CD8-positive cytotoxic T cells are low in CHL, except in patients with HIV infection. A helpful diagnostic criterion is the rarity of CD57-positive T cells in CHL (with some limitation for the nodular variant of LRCHL), in contrast to NLPBL.[77,119] The nodular pattern of LRCHL is characterized by a predominance of B-cell follicles with expanded mantle zones, containing a fine meshwork of dendritic cells. Residual B-cell follicles and follicular dendritic cells can also be identified in a significant percentage of other subtypes, mainly nodular sclerosis CHL.[201]

GENETICS AND MOLECULAR FINDINGS

Immunoglobulin and T-Cell Receptor Genes

With optimized techniques of single-cell procurement and analysis, HRS cells virtually always contain somatically hypermutated, class-switched, clonally rearranged IGH genes as evidence of their B-cell origin, independent of the expression of B-cell markers.[4,9,202-204] Only rare cases of CHL, even among cases preselected for T-antigen expression, have been shown to contain clonally rearranged T-cell receptor genes.[205,206] As some peripheral T-cell lymphomas may mimic CHL both morphologically and immunophenotypically, attributing cases with rearrangements of the T-cell receptor genes to CHL is controversial. Somehow surprising in light of the molecular findings in primary cases, some of the bona fide CHL-derived cell lines with appropriate gene expression pattern have a T-cell genotype.[7]

Despite the presence of rearranged IG genes and in contrast to NLPBL, CHL lacks BCR and Ig expression on the mRNA and protein level.[9,13] Several reasons for this lack of Ig transcription have been described. Using single-cell PCR, both so-called "crippling" mutations of the rearranged IGH genes leading to a premature stop codon and mutations of the IG promoter regions have been found, aborting Ig transcription.[207] Interestingly, most cases with crippling mutations are EBV positive, indicating EBV's role in the survival of these cells. The lack of B-cell surface markers, of the B-cell transcription factors Oct-2 and PU.1, and of the coactivator BOB.1/OBF.1, which are indispensable for IG gene transcription,[171,208] is probably caused by a combination of promoter hypermethylation, epigenetic silencing, and upregulation of ID2 and NOTCH1.[12,13] The lack of Ig transcription indicates a breakdown of the normal regulatory mechanisms of apoptosis in CHL, as Ig expression is a prerogative for the survival of B cells under normal circumstances.

Despite the progress concerning the histogenesis and clonality of CHL, clonality detection only plays a minor role in its practical diagnosis. Although more sensitive techniques such as the BIOMED-2 primer sets can detect B-cell clonality in a significant subset of CHL cases, clonality studies are of limited use in separating CHL from histologic mimics.[209-211] Nevertheless, the presence of a major clonal B-cell or T-cell population, as evidenced by a strong clonal band in PCR, favors a diagnosis of NHL over CHL and can be useful for NHL cases that simulate CHL morphologically, especially some peripheral T-cell NHLs, including ALCL and follicular T-helper cell lymphoma or low-grade B-cell NHL with RS-like cells.[212-214] Next-generation sequencing (NGS)-based detection of B-cell clonality is more sensitive than conventional techniques and may be useful for the detection of recurrences.[215]

Cytogenetics and Molecular Genetics

Because of the unique cellular composition of CHL and the difficulties in growing HRS cells in culture, cytogenetic examination and molecular studies of CHL using whole tissue extracts have proved difficult until recently. Combining immunophenotypic identification of RS cells and molecular cytogenetics by fluorescence ISH (FISH), chromosomal aberrations and aneuploidy are present in 100% of CHL cases.[216] Although the IGH locus at 14q32 is sometimes involved in translocations in CHL, recurrent translocations typical for NHL are generally absent.[217] Comparative genomic hybridization of isolated HRS cells after random genomic amplification has been used to quantify gains and losses of chromosomal material, leading to the identification of regions of recurrent gains in chromosomes 2p, 7p, 9p, and 11q and losses of 4q and 11q.[218-223] The amplified region on 2p13 contains the REL oncogene, which encodes a part of the Rel-A/NF-κB complex, which is constitutively activated in CHL. Further studies revealed common involvement of other chromosomal regions also harboring genes encoding for positive or negative regulators of the NF-κB pathway, including BCL3 and MAP3K14.[223] In addition, the NF-κB inhibitors IκBα, IκBε, and A20 (TNFAIP3), among others, are commonly mutated in CHL, especially in EBV-negative cases.[224-228] The 9p24 region, which is commonly amplified in HRS cells, contains JAK2 gene and the programmed-death 1 ligand genes PD1L1 and PD1L2, resulting in consistent expression of PD-L1/2.[179,221] In addition, SOCS1 and PTPN1, negative regulators of the JAK/STAT pathway, are inactivated by mutations in subsets of CHL, and gains and activating mutations in STAT6 are common.[229,230] In addition to PD-L1/2 overexpression, recurrent translocations involving the MHC class II transactivator CIITA resulting in downregulation of MHC class II expression and deletions and inactivating

mutations in B2M and CD58 support immune evasion by the neoplastic cells.[182] Although p53 protein is frequently expressed by RS cells, mutations of the TP53 gene are rare, and the same seems true for other examined tumor suppressor genes.[9,12,13]

Studies using comprehensive NGS either on tissue samples, enriched or flow-sorted cells, or cell-free DNA have further elucidated the mutational spectrum of CHL; they have confirmed the importance of genetic alterations leading to activation of NF-κB and JAK/STAT signaling pathways and immune evasion and identified additional recurrent alterations affecting GNA13, involved in the PI3K/AKT pathway and also resulting in impaired cytokinesis, likely leading to the formation of RS giant cells, epigenetic regulators (ARID1A, KMT2D, CREBBP, and EP300), and NOTCH pathway members.[231-233]

Despite the increase in knowledge regarding CHL genetics, mutational analysis does not currently play a role in tissue diagnostics. It remains to be seen which role molecular profiling either of tissue biopsies or cell-free DNA will play in the future for diagnosis and follow-up.[234]

Gene Expression Profile and Activated Signaling Pathways

Large-scale screening strategies have been used to study the expression profile of CHL-derived cell lines or primary HRS cells.[62,235] Despite the presence of clonal IGH gene rearrangements in CHL, the downregulation of most B-cell antigens and the virtual lack of a B-cell–specific gene expression profile justify the separation of CHL from B-cell lymphoma.[235-237] In part, this phenotype is caused by epigenetic silencing of B-cell–specific master transcription factors through promoter region methylation.[238] Furthermore, deregulated expression of genes involved in T-cell differentiation such as NOTCH1 and GATA3 further contribute to loss of the B-cell signature.[12,192,239,240] The survival of the neoplastic cells of CHL despite the lack of a functional B-cell receptor and B-cell program indicates a profound deregulation of apoptotic pathways, which is also evidenced by the constitutive expression of antiapoptotic proteins such as BCL2, BCLxL, and c-FLIP.[9,241] The current hypothesis on CHL pathogenesis postulates that HRS cells are rescued by constitutive activation of diverse signaling pathways through somatic mutations, EBV, and microenvironmental signals.[12,137] Therefore, not surprisingly, expression profiling of CHL shows significant differences with most B-cell neoplasms, with the exception of PMBL and MGZL, entities exhibiting both morphologic, phenotypic, and genotypic overlap with CHL.[242-245] Of interest, gene expression profiling of microdissected HRS cells not only confirmed the profound differences between CHL and other B-cell neoplasms, but it also demonstrated that bona fide Hodgkin cell lines and microdissected HRS cells are very similar in their hallmark features but nevertheless show significant transcriptional differences, probably reflecting the importance of the inflammatory microenvironment in primary cases.[62]

A central feature of CHL is the constitutive activation of the NF-κB pathway.[13,246-248] Signaling through members of the TNF-NGF receptor superfamily expressed by RS cells, such as CD30, CD40, and LMP-1, activates a complex intracellular signaling cascade involving TRAF1 and 2 (among other molecules), ultimately leading to NF-κB activation. The constitutively activated Rel-A/NF-κB complex induces transcription of various genes thought to play an important role in the evasion of apoptosis, survival, and proliferation of HRS cells.[8,13] Of note, constitutive NF-κB activation is achieved through different pathways in EBV-positive and EBV-negative cases, as evidenced by the much higher frequency of genetic alterations affecting NF-κB pathway genes such as A20/TNFAIP3 in the latter group.[12,224,228]

In addition to the genetic lesions described herein, constitutive activation of the JAK/STAT pathway with downstream phosphorylation of STATs is caused also by autocrine and paracrine stimulation and the aberrant activation of a variety of receptor tyrosine kinases. Further signaling cascades with deregulated activity include the NOTCH-1, PI3K/AKT, and MAPK/ERK pathways.[9,13,248]

Role of the Microenvironment in Classic Hodgkin Lymphoma

The intense inflammatory response typical of CHL points to the involvement of disturbed immunologic pathways in disease pathogenesis and underlines the importance of the tumor microenvironment (TME).[199,249-251] As lymphoid cells in a constant state of activation, the neoplastic cells of CHL influence their surroundings with a wide range of secreted cytokines and chemokines; however, they themselves also depend on the crosstalk with reactive cell populations.[252] Among the substances produced by HRS cells, or in part by the accompanying reactive infiltrate, are TNF-α, transforming growth factor-β (TGF-β), interferon-γ, IL-2, IL-5, IL-6, IL-8, IL-9, IL-10, IL-12, and IL-13, in addition to the chemokines eotaxin, thymus and activation-regulated chemokine (TARC), macrophage inflammatory protein (MIP1α), and others.[12,199,252] The majority of factors attract and activate TH2 cells and may contribute to a local suppression of cytotoxic T cells. IL-5 and eotaxin are likely responsible for tissue eosinophilia.[199,253] TGF-β, found predominantly in nodular sclerosis CHL, is immunosuppressive and induces fibroblast proliferation and collagen formation, characteristic of this subtype.[254] The expression of some cytokines, such as IL-10, correlates with the EBV status of the disease.[255] In addition to attracting and modulating the inflammatory infiltrate and providing growth and survival stimuli to the neoplastic cells, the secreted cytokines are probably one of the reasons for the frequent presence of systemic symptoms. In addition to secreting cytokines favoring an immunosuppressive microenvironment and downregulation of HLA class I and II molecules, HRS cells exhibit additional mechanisms of immune evasion, including overexpression of FAS ligand (CD95L), Galectin-1, and the coinhibitory PD1/PD-L1/PD-L2 axis, all of which result in T-cell exhaustion, abrogating an efficient T-cell response.[199,248] Although previously thought to be dominated by CD4-positive TH2 cells, studies have identified CD4-positive/LAG3-positive type-I regulatory T cells and PD1-positive TH1 cells as major immunosuppressive TME components characteristic of CHL.[249-251] As evident from morphology, the TME varies greatly with subtype, with implications for its prognostic role, but is also likely influenced by the genetic profile and the host immune system.

POSTULATED CELL OF ORIGIN

For most cases of CHL studied by single-cell analysis, the presence of clonally rearranged, somatically mutated IG genes indicates a derivation from germinal-center B cells incapable of Ig transcription. However, the virtual lack of a B-cell expression profile underlines that the sum of genetic alterations of a neoplastic cell rather than its origin shapes its phenotype and clinical behavior.

CLINICAL COURSE AND PROGNOSTIC FACTORS

The clinical course and prognosis of CHL have changed dramatically since the introduction of radiotherapy and multimodal chemotherapy. The natural history of the disease is characterized by slow but relentless tumor progression with extensive organ involvement, and in the past, many patients succumbed to infectious complications. Today, the overall cure rate for all patients is around 80% for advanced stages and >90% for limited disease. Current therapeutic approaches combine less toxic, abbreviated chemotherapy regimens with involved field radiotherapy for early-stage disease.[17,256,257] The rationale of this approach is to reduce the frequency of late complications of radiotherapy without compromising the excellent cure rates.[17,99,258] FDG PET/CT is increasingly used to avoid radiotherapy in patients with complete metabolic response. Multiagent chemotherapies such as ABVD (Adriamycin [doxorubicin], bleomycin, vinblastine, dacarbazine) or newer regimens are the mainstay of treatment for advanced-stage HL. High-dose chemotherapy with autologous stem-cell transplantation can be administered successfully to patients with primary progressive disease or early relapse who have an extremely poor prognosis with conventional chemotherapy.[17] New drugs, especially the anti-CD30 antibody-conjugate brentuximab vedotin and blockade of PD-1 signaling with nivolumab or pembrolizumab, show significant activity also in refractory patients and herald a new era for targeted therapy in CHL.[259,260]

Given the high cure rate, complications of therapy, especially second malignancies, have gained importance. Patients cured of CHL have a significantly increased risk of secondary cancers, which are the main cause of death in long-term survivors.[261-263] Although common solid tumors are the most frequently encountered malignancies, the greatest increase in incidence is observed for acute nonlymphocytic leukemias, mainly as a result of alkylating agents. The cumulative incidence of secondary NHL after CHL is approximately 1% according to recent results—a lower rate than in earlier studies. The majority of cases are DLBCLs, frequently at extranodal sites.[264,265] In general, the prognosis of secondary malignancies is poor.

In the last decades, a vast number of clinical features and serum and tissue biomarkers associated with clinical outcome have been described. Stage is the most important single prognostic factor in CHL, with Ann Arbor stages I and II designated as limited stage disease (without or with risk factors) and III and IV as advanced stage disease. Nevertheless, in more than half the patients with stage IV disease, complete remission can be achieved and is durable in a significant fraction of them.[99,258] Other clinical parameters of adverse prognostic significance include age, male sex, bulky mediastinal disease, liver involvement, anemia, leukocytosis, lymphopenia, hypoalbuminemia, and elevated lactate dehydrogenase.[266-268] For advanced disease, the International Prognostic Factor Project has developed a prognostic scoring based on these parameters that identifies patients at high risk of progression.[266] Bone marrow involvement per se does not confer a worse prognosis compared with other patients with advanced disease.[75] Serum surrogates of disease activity, such as increased levels of TARC, soluble CD30, IL-2, and IL-6 have prognostic relevance, with serum TARC always increased at baseline and correlated with treatment response.[199,269] An important new prognostic factor is the use of PET/CT to evaluate the response to chemotherapy.[270] In contrast, the effect of histologic subtype and histologic grade in nodular sclerosis CHL has diminished.

A number of tissue-based features have been analyzed for their potential prognostic relevance, including expression of CD15, CD20, and BCL2 and EBV status of the neoplastic cells, with often conflicting results.[136,199] PD-L1 expression on HRS cells predicts response to checkpoint inhibition in relapsed/refractory CHL.[181] The composition of the background infiltrate, including T-cell subsets, macrophages and their polarization, eosinophils, mast cells, follicular dendritic cells, and B cells, has been scrutinized in many studies. Although the presence of increased numbers of macrophages and activated cytotoxic T cells has been most consistently associated with a worse prognosis, the best way to assess the microenvironment and its relevance is an unresolved issue.[136,199] Other approaches for separating prognostic groups, such as gene expression profiling, which has identified a macrophage signature associated with adverse treatment outcome, microRNA profiling or proteomic analysis have not entered into clinical decision making.[99,136,271]

RELATED LESIONS AND DIFFERENTIAL DIAGNOSES

Although most cases of CHL can be safely classified on the basis of morphology and immunohistochemical features, distinction from various subtypes of NHL, reactive disorders, or even non-hematopoietic neoplasms can prove difficult. Some lymphoid neoplasms show a significant morphologic and phenotypic overlap with CHL, occasionally making a clear distinction impossible. A fraction of these lesions represents true borderline cases between CHL and NHL, namely MGZLs,[148,149,157,174,272] whereas others are mere morphologic and/or phenotypic mimics. A broader group of NHLs may contain HRS-like cells and may exhibit a pattern reminiscent of the reactive inflammatory background of CHL. However, immunohistochemical stains usually make the neoplastic character of the background population in these cases readily apparent. Furthermore, HRS-like cells can occur in reactive disorders or even neoplasms of nonlymphoid origin and may lead to diagnostic difficulties, especially in small biopsy specimens.

Mediastinal (Thymic Niche) Gray-Zone Lymphoma

Given the B-cell origin of CHL, it is not surprising that cases with hybrid features between large B-cell lymphoma and CHL can be observed.[148,149,155,156,273] Since the introduction of the concept of "B-cell lymphoma unclassifiable, with features intermediate between DLBCL and CHL (gray zone lymphoma)" in the 2008 World Health Organization (WHO) classification, the definition of gray-zone lymphoma has evolved significantly in the light of new genetic information documenting that MGZLs occupy a truly intermediate position between PMBL and NSCHL, whereas extramediastinal cases with overlapping morphology and immunophenotype are more similar to conventional DLBCL or EBV-positive DLBCL, NOS, respectively. Therefore, both the ICC and the 5th edition of the WHO classification have now accepted the entity MGZL, excluding extramediastinal cases.[11,105]

Clinical Features

MGZL most commonly affects males in the 3rd to 4th decades of life and presents with bulky disease and occasional involvement of supraclavicular lymph nodes. It can spread to supraclavicular nodes and the lung, spleen, and bone marrow, whereas involvement of unusual extranodal sites as in PMBL is rare. MGZL shows a worse clinical outcome than both CHL and PMBL.[146,174] Regimens for aggressive B-cell lymphomas have been used successfully in MGZL.[274]

Morphology and Immunophenotype

MGZL usually shows asynchrony between morphology and immunophenotype, which may present in two ways: Some cases show morphology of CHL of nodular sclerosis type but have a preserved B-cell program with increased expression of a variety of B-cell markers, including strong and homogeneous expression of CD20 and/or CD79a, frequent positivity for the transcription factors BOB.1 and Oct-2, variable BCL6 reactivity, and common loss of CD15 (Fig. 27-6). The second group of cases exhibit a diffuse proliferation of large cells, which in addition to B-cell marker expression show strong and homogeneous CD30 positivity and often CD15 positivity.[148,155,157,273,275,276] Overall, most cases of MGZL have evidence of a clear B-cell phenotype with expression of more than one B-cell marker. Aberrant expression of single markers normally does not justify inclusion in the MGZL category. Of note, rare EBV-positive cases of MGZL with otherwise typical phenotypic and molecular features have been observed.[157,277] The intermediate position of MGZL between PMBL and CHL is also evident on the molecular level. Translocations involving the MHC class transactivator CIITA and amplifications of REL (2p15) and JAK2 (9p24) oncogenes and mutations of SOCS1, B2M, TNFAIP3, GNA13, STAT6, and NFKBIA are commonly observed in all three entities.[275,277,278] Comparative gene expression profiling demonstrated an intermediate score for MGZL, with cell cycle and extracellular matrix-related genes reflecting cell density and microenvironment.[243,279] Similarly, the methylation profile of MGZL is intermediate between CHL and PMBL, further documenting that it represents a related but distinct lymphoma subtype.[278]

Patients with features of a composite lymphoma, with both morphologically and immunologically typical nodular sclerosis CHL and PMBL in different areas of the same biopsy, must be diagnosed as such, indicating both histologic components, and should not be diagnosed as MGZL.[280] These two components may also be diagnosed sequentially at different times, suggesting phenotypic plasticity of the neoplastic clone.

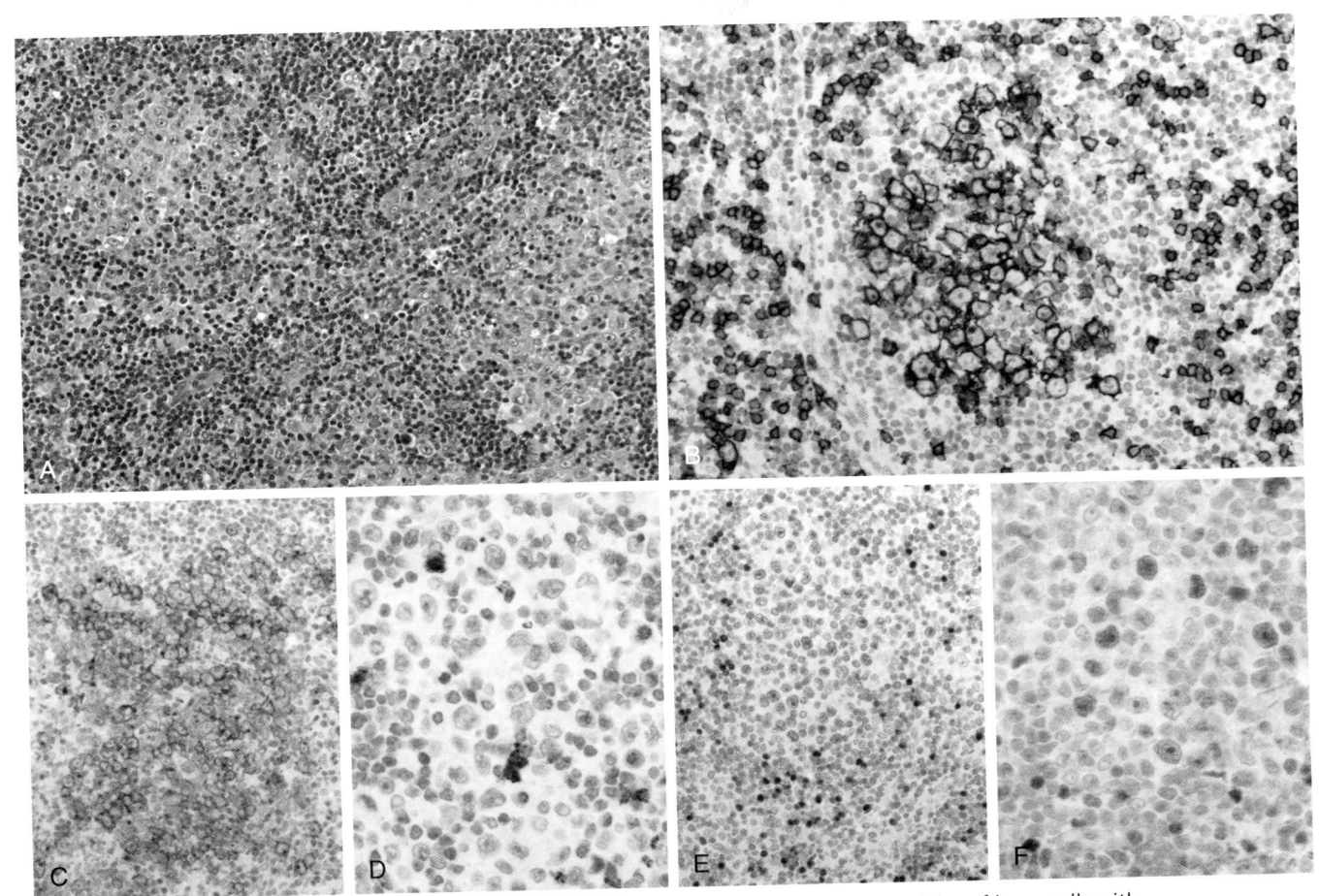

Figure 27-6. Mediastinal gray-zone lymphoma. A, Relatively compact nodules of large cells with prominent nucleoli, resembling Hodgkin cells admixed with occasional Reed-Sternberg (RS)-cells and many eosinophils and small lymphocytes. **B,** Strong and homogeneous expression of CD20 and **(C),** CD30. **D,** CD15 is heterogeneously, but distinctly expressed in a perinuclear fashion. **E,** PAX5 expression is attenuated. **F,** Oct-2 is heterogeneously positive in the neoplastic cells.

Diffuse Large B-Cell Lymphoma, Not Otherwise Specified

The differentiation of CHL from conventional extramediastinal DLBCL is usually straightforward by morphology and is easily confirmed by immunohistochemistry, even in cases with occasional HRS-like giant cells in a background of more conventional immunoblasts or centroblasts. However, some subtypes of DLBCL may occasionally exhibit close morphologic and phenotypic overlap with CHL but are not considered to be biologically related to CHL, in contrast to MGZL.[11,104,157] Genetic studies have shown that extramediastinal large B-cell lymphomas with Hodgkin-like features are distinct from MGZL and PMBL, with occurrence of *BCL2* and *BCL6* translocations and mutations frequently encountered in conventional DLBCL and a gene expression profile more closely related to DLBCL.[277,279]

Although these cases may show abundant HRS-like cells and an inflammatory background simulating CHL, they usually exhibit a broader cytologic range of atypical large cells with positivity for several B-cell markers, including strong CD20 and/or PAX5 expression.

T-cell and histiocyte-rich large B-cell lymphoma (THRLBCL) is a DLBCL characterized by a minority of large blasts of B-cell origin in a background of reactive T cells and histiocytes and is thought to be related to NLPBL. THRLBCL usually exhibits a diffuse growth pattern. Sometimes, the tumor cells may resemble classic HRS cells, but a resemblance to LP cells is more common (Fig. 27-7A). The neoplastic cells of this tumor usually stain strongly for CD20 and other B-cell markers, in addition to BCL6 (Fig. 27-7B); they frequently express EMA but usually lack CD30 and CD15 (Table 27-3).[104,281-283]

EBV-Associated B-Cell Lymphoproliferations and Lymphomas

EBV-Positive Diffuse Large B-Cell Lymphoma, Not Otherwise Specified

EBV-positive DLBCL, NOS may closely simulate CHL but usually shows a broad cytologic spectrum with more abundant neoplastic cells. They show variable, frequently strong expression of B-cell markers, with common positivity for CD30 and CD15 expression in 23% to 68% of cases. LMP1 expression in EBV-positive DLBCL can be heterogeneous and lacks the clear dichotomy between LMP1-positive HRS cells and a negative inflammatory background of EBV-positive CHL.[160,284-287] EBNA-2 expression, which occurs in a minority of EBV-positive DLBCL, rules out a diagnosis

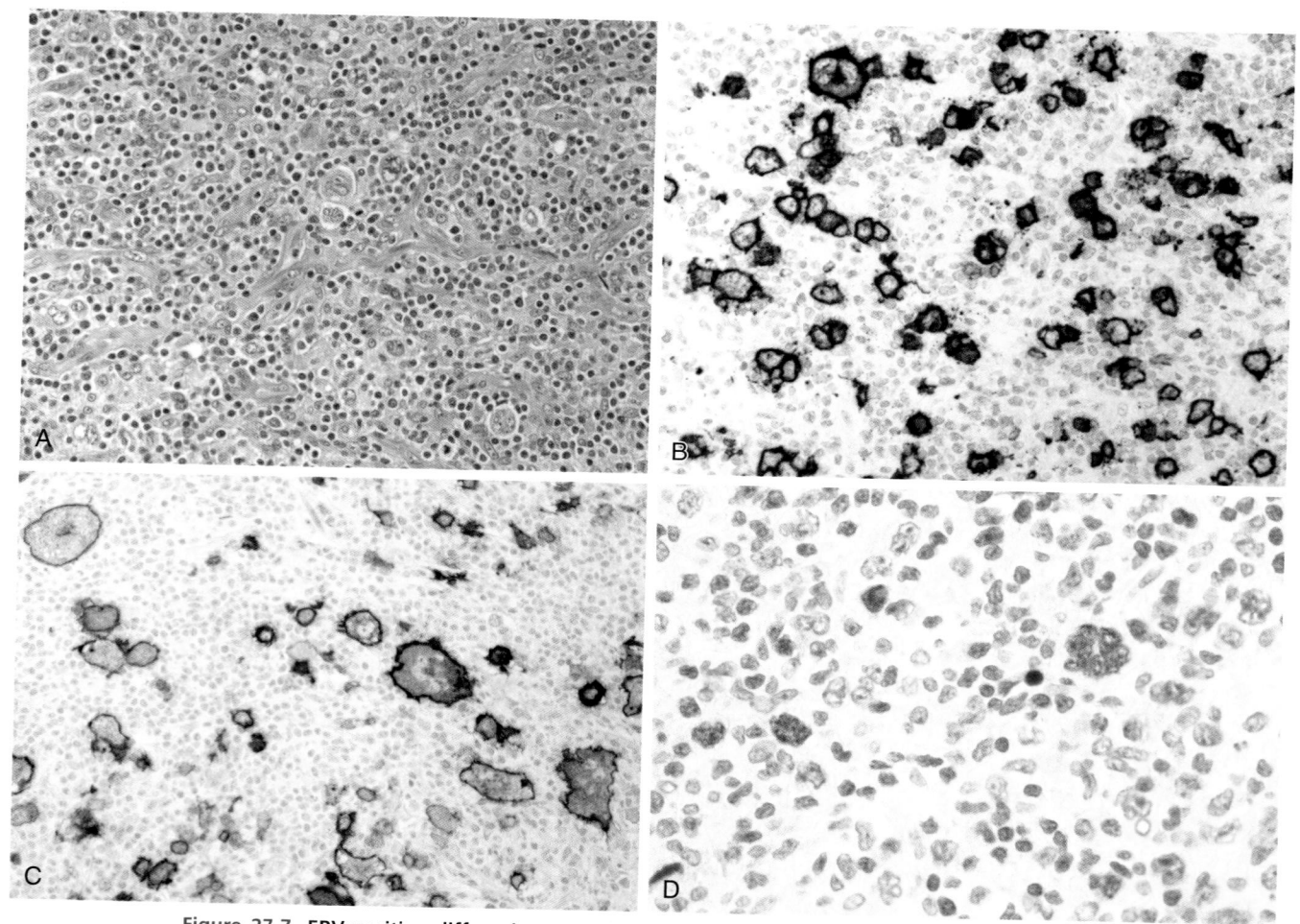

Figure 27-7. EBV-positive diffuse large B-cell lymphoma, not otherwise specified. A, HRS-like cells and mononuclear large cells are intermingled with small lymphocytes and occasional eosinophils. The atypical cells stain strongly and homogeneously for CD20 **(B)** and CD30 **(C)**. Some tumor cells express the EBNA2 antigen of EBV **(D)**, indicative of latency pattern III, which is incompatible with a diagnosis of CHL.

of CHL. The genetic profile of EBV-positive DLBCL, NOS is distinct both from CHL and conventional DLBCL.[277] Clinically, isolated extranodal presentation of an EBV-positive lymphoproliferation with Hodgkin-like features argues strongly against a CHL diagnosis.

Other EBV-Associated Lymphoproliferative Disorders

EBV-associated LPDs arise most frequently in the setting of immunodeficiency or iatrogenic immunosuppression or immunosenescence but may also occur without evident immune defects. They show a broad clinical and morphologic spectrum and may simulate CHL morphologically and phenotypically. CHL-like EBV-positive LPDs consist of a polymorphous proliferation of small-to-large lymphoid cells with frequent RS-like cells. Morphologically, RS-like cells in CHL-like posttransplant LPD or iatrogenic LPD are part of a continuum of lymphoid cells in various stages of transformation rather than embedded in a reactive background of small lymphocytes (Fig. 27-7D).[288] They usually co-express CD30 and CD20 but are CD15 negative and show EBV positivity frequently with latency type III expressing EBNA2, in contrast to CHL.[93,289-291] True CHL can

also occur in the posttransplant setting and simulates sporadic CHL morphologically and phenotypically; it occurs late after transplantation and usually does not respond to a reduction in immunosuppression.

Mucocutaneous Ulcer

EBV-associated mucocutaneous ulcers also frequently show presence of HRS-like cells but can be separated from CHL based on its primary extranodal manifestation, the presence of a polymorphic background population, the common co-expression of B-cell antigens in the HRS-like cells, and the demarcation of the lesion by a cuff of T cells.[92,93]

Nodular Lymphocyte-Predominant B-Cell Lymphoma

Separation of NLPBL and LRCHL may sometimes be difficult (also addressed in this chapter's section on LRCHL). NLPBL is characterized by nodular structures reminiscent of progressively transformed germinal centers, whereas the nodules in LRCHL consist of expanded follicle mantles with atrophic or residual germinal-center remnants.[77,282,283,292,293] The morphology of the neoplastic cells is of limited value because tumor cells with LP

Table 27-3 Differential Diagnosis: Nodular Sclerosis Classic Hodgkin Lymphoma (NSCHL), Mediastinal Gray-Zone Lymphoma (MGZL), and Primary Mediastinal Large B-Cell Lymphoma (PMBL)

	NSCHL	MGZL	PMBL
Architecture	Nodular, fibrous bands, inflammatory background	Nodular or diffuse, variable inflammation	Diffuse, reticular fibrosis, little inflammation
Neoplastic cells	Lacunar cells, HRS cells	Spectrum of HRS-like cells to monotonous large cells	Monotonous proliferation of large cells with clear cytoplasm, occasional HRS-like cells
Phenotype	CD30+, CD15+/–, CD20–/+, CD45–, EMA–, PAX5+ (weak), CD79a–, Oct-2–/+, EBV–/+	CD20+/–, CD79a+/–, PAX5+, Oct-2+/–, BOB.1+/–, CD45+/–, CD30+, CD15+/–, EBV–* ≥2 B-cell markers	CD20+, CD79a+, CD45+, PAX5+, Oct-2+, BCL6+, BOB.1+, CD23+/–, MAL+, CD30+/–, CD15–, EBV–

*Rare positive cases described.
HRS, Hodgkin and Reed-Sternberg.

Table 27-4 Differential Diagnosis: Classic Hodgkin Lymphoma (CHL), Nodular Lymphocyte-Predominant B-Cell Lymphoma (NLPBL), and T-Cell/Histiocyte-Rich Large B-Cell Lymphoma (THRLBCL)

	CHL	NLPBL	THRLBCL
Architecture	Nodular (NS and LR) Diffuse (MC)	Nodular	Diffuse
Neoplastic cells	Classic RS and lacunar cells (NS), occasional LP cells in LRCHL	LP cells	Atypical large blasts, RS-like cells may occur
Phenotype	CD15+, CD30+, CD20–/+, CD45–, EMA–, PAX5+ (weak), CD79a–, J chain–, Oct-2–/+, EBV+/–	CD20+, CD79a+, Oct-2+, J chain+, CD45+, EMA+/–, CD30–*, CD15–*, BOB.1+, EBV–*	CD20+, CD79a+, EMA+/–, CD45+, light chain restriction, CD30–, CD15–, EBV–
Background	T cells (NS and MC) Small B cells and rosetting T cells (LR nodular) FDC+/– (LR, some NS)	B cells, CD57/PD-1+ rosetting T-cells, FDC+	T cells, no small B cells, no FDCs, rare CD57/PD-1+ cells
Genotype (whole tissue)	Usually polyclonal (B- and T-cells), minority B-cell clone	Polyclonal	Often monoclonal (B-cell)

*Rare cases of NLPBL with expression of CD30, CD15, or EBV positivity described.
EBV, Epstein-Barr virus; *EMA,* epithelial membrane antigen; *FDC,* follicular dendritic cell; *LP,* lymphocyte predominant; *LR,* lymphocyte rich; *MC,* mixed cellularity; *NS,* nodular sclerosis; *RS,* Reed-Sternberg.

morphology can occur in both entities, so immunophenotyping is of paramount importance for the differential diagnosis. Strong and homogeneous expression of CD20, CD79a, J chain, and B-cell transcription factors Oct-2, BOB.1, BCL-6, and myocyte enhancer factor 2B (MEF2B), in addition to expression of EMA and CD45, supports a diagnosis of NLPHL, whereas the neoplastic cells of LRCHL are usually positive for CD30 and CD15 and may be infected with EBV.[166,293] The small numbers of CD30-positive blasts frequently observable in NLPHL more commonly represent non-neoplastic perifollicular immunoblasts rather than LP cells, but a fraction of otherwise classic NLPHLs show CD30-positive tumor cells.[142,143] Of note, rare cases of otherwise classic NLPBL showing EBV positivity or CD15 expression of the neoplastic cells have been described.[119,294,295] In these cases, preservation of the B-cell program is the clue to the correct diagnosis. Of note, LRCHL shows a higher incidence of expression of B-cell transcription factors than other CHL subtypes.[119] Both entities usually show a predominance of B cells in the background population and contain follicular dendritic cell networks. Although increased numbers of CD57-positive/PD1-positive T cells forming rosettes are characteristic of NLPBL, they may also be observed in LRCHL, potentially suggesting a relationship between these two entities (Table 27-4).[77,104,112,119]

Anaplastic Large Cell Lymphoma

ALCL, initially identified by virtue of its strong reactivity with antibodies against CD30, shows some morphologic and

phenotypic similarities to CHL.[144,296,297] Tumor cells of ALCL may resemble RS cells or mononuclear variants, but they are usually smaller than the neoplastic cells of CHL and often show bean-shaped or horseshoe-shaped nuclei ("hallmark" cells). Furthermore, ALCL usually grows in cohesive sheets and frequently involves lymph node sinuses—rare features in CHL. Immunophenotypically, expression of T-cell antigens, cytotoxic molecules, EMA, ALK-1 protein, and CD45 supports a diagnosis of ALCL, whereas expression of CD15, CD20, and PAX5 suggests CHL (Table 27-5). MUM1/IRF4 expression is not contributory, because it occurs in both entities. Of note, rare cases of ALK-negative ALCL with PAX5 expression and extra copies of the *PAX5* locus have been described.[298] The presence of a prominent clonal T-cell rearrangement or t(2;5) excludes CHL.[296,297] Rare cases of ALK-positive ALCL with a nodular growth pattern strongly resemble nodular sclerosis CHL, and they are readily diagnosed with immunohistochemical studies because they lack PAX5 and CD15 but may express T-cell markers.[299]

CHL PAX5-Negative With Expression of Cytotoxic T-Cell Markers Versus CHL-Like ALK-Negative ALCL

Although expression of T-cell markers can occasionally be encountered in otherwise typical CHL,[138,139] rare lymphoma cases with CHL morphology and strong CD30 and CD15 positivity may show strong expression of one or several cytotoxic granule markers, including TIA-1, granzyme B, and perforin, usually associated with complete absence of PAX5

Table 27-5 Differential Diagnosis: Classic Hodgkin Lymphoma (CHL) and Anaplastic Large Cell Lymphoma (ALCL)

	CHL	ALCL
Architecture	Nodular or diffuse	Mostly diffuse, dominance of large cells, sinus involvement
Neoplastic cells	Classic HRS cells, lacunar cells,	Mononuclear cells predominate, "hallmark" cells, some RS-like cells
Phenotype	CD30+, CD15+, CD20−/+, LMP-1+/−, PAX5+ (weak), T-cell markers usually negative, ALK1−, EMA−	CD30+, CD15−/+, CD20−, CD4+, CD45+/−, LMP-1−, PAX5−*, T-cell markers often positive, ALK1+/−, EMA+, cytotoxic markers
Genotype	Usually polyclonal (B and T cells), minority shows B-cell clonality	Clonal T-cell rearrangement (80%-90%)

*Rare cases positive.
ALK, Anaplastic lymphoma kinase; *EMA,* epithelial membrane antigen; *LMP,* latent membrane protein; *RS,* Reed-Sternberg

expression.[189] Some of these cases were found to relapse as conventional peripheral T-cell lymphomas,[191] indicating some of these cases might represent PTCL with Hodgkin-like features. Furthermore, cases of CHL-like CD30-positive PTCL harboring *JAK2* rearrangements have been described.[190]

Other Subtypes of Non-Hodgkin Lymphoma and Composite Lymphomas

RS-like cells can occur in a wide range of NHLs of both B-cell and T-cell types. Among B-cell lymphoid neoplasms, this phenomenon is most frequently encountered in chronic lymphocytic leukemia (CLL). In most cases, RS-like cells are present singly or in small clusters in the background of morphologically and phenotypically classic CLL (CD5+, CD20+, CD23+). They frequently express CD30 and sometimes CD15, may co-express CD20, and are usually infected by EBV (EBER+, LMP-1+).[300-302] These cases may represent precursor lesions for CHL, which has an increased incidence in patients with CLL and occasionally presents as a composite lymphoma.[303] A clonal relationship between the two populations has been shown for some, but not all, cases studied by single-cell PCR.[304,305] These cases arise more commonly from CLL with mutated IG genes and seem to carry a better prognosis than conventional Richter transformation but similar to CHL arising in CLL.[300,303] Some of the EBV-positive cases have been observed under fludarabine treatment, thus showing resemblance to EBV-associated CHL-like B-cell LPD in immunosuppressed patients.[306]

Transformed B cells with RS-like morphology and true composite lymphomas with separate areas of both CHL and B-cell NHL have also been observed in other B-cell NHL subtypes, most frequently follicular lymphoma.[202,307] In some cases, a common clonal origin has been demonstrated by molecular studies.[308]

Peripheral T-cell lymphomas frequently show a polymorphic inflammatory background with eosinophils, neutrophils, plasma cells, and histiocytes and may contain RS-like giant cells (Fig. 27-8). In some neoplasms, such as nodal peripheral T-cell

lymphoma, NOS, transformed mycosis fungoides, and nodal involvement by CD30-positive LPDs of the skin, RS-like cells show co-expression of CD30, CD15, and T-cell markers and probably represent transformed cells of the malignant clone. Usually, they form part of a continuum of small to medium-sized and large blasts.[145,158] In contrast, RS-like cells in follicular T-helper cell lymphomas and adult T-cell lymphoma/leukemia are commonly, but not always, EBV transformed, nonclonal B cells and are probably the result of an underlying local immune dysregulation (Fig. 27-8C).[213,214,309,310] Because the background population of neoplastic T cells in cases of T-cell NHL with RS-like giant cells can sometimes show only minimal cytologic atypia, as in cases of follicular T-helper cell lymphomas, detailed immunophenotyping and molecular studies may be necessary for distinction from CHL.[212] Another pitfall is the occurrence of HRS-like cells with CD30 and sometimes CD15 expression in draining lymph nodes of patients with CD30-positive cutaneous LPDs or mycosis fungoides.[158,311]

Reactive Disorders

Reactive lymphadenopathies with a wide range of both infectious and noninfectious causes can exhibit HRS-like cells. Infectious mononucleosis typically shows florid interfollicular hyperplasia, with at least partial preservation of the lymph node architecture. The paracortical proliferation may be dominated by variously sized immunoblasts or show a mixed cytology, with small lymphocytes and interspersed, frequently binucleate blasts closely resembling RS cells. Necrosis may be present. The clinical picture and serologic findings are crucial in avoiding a misdiagnosis of CHL in such cases. Morphologically, the range of cell sizes and the marked cytoplasmic basophilia of many blasts are indicators of a reactive disorder.[312] HRS-like cells in infectious mononucleosis can express CD30, LMP-1, and partly EBNA-2, but they lack CD15 and frequently show CD20 expression.

Other lymphadenitis forms of viral or unknown cause may occasionally mimic CHL, especially the interfollicular growth pattern. As in infectious mononucleosis, these cases can show prominent expression of CD30 with variable downregulation of B-cell transcription factors such as PAX5, but they lack CD15 expression—with the exception of cytomegalovirus lymphadenitis—and express polyclonal Ig light chains.[152,154]

Neoplasms of Nonlymphoid Origin

A large number of nonlymphoid neoplasms may resemble CHL morphologically, especially if only small biopsy specimens are available. In most instances, immunohistochemical studies resolve these cases. However, one should be aware of the potential pitfalls of a limited antibody panel. Both CD15 and CD30 can be expressed by a range of non-hematopoietic neoplasms. Lymph node metastasis of large cell undifferentiated carcinoma or melanoma may resemble the syncytial variant of nodular sclerosis CHL (Fig. 27-8E), but it is usually easily differentiated by appropriate immunostainings for cytokeratins or S-100 protein and melanoma antigens, respectively. Undifferentiated nasopharyngeal carcinoma can resemble CHL both morphologically and clinically because the tumor frequently presents with cervical lymph node metastasis, whereas the primary tumor is often clinically unapparent. Extragonadal germ-cell tumors can simulate NSCHL with a mass lesion in the anterior mediastinum. The

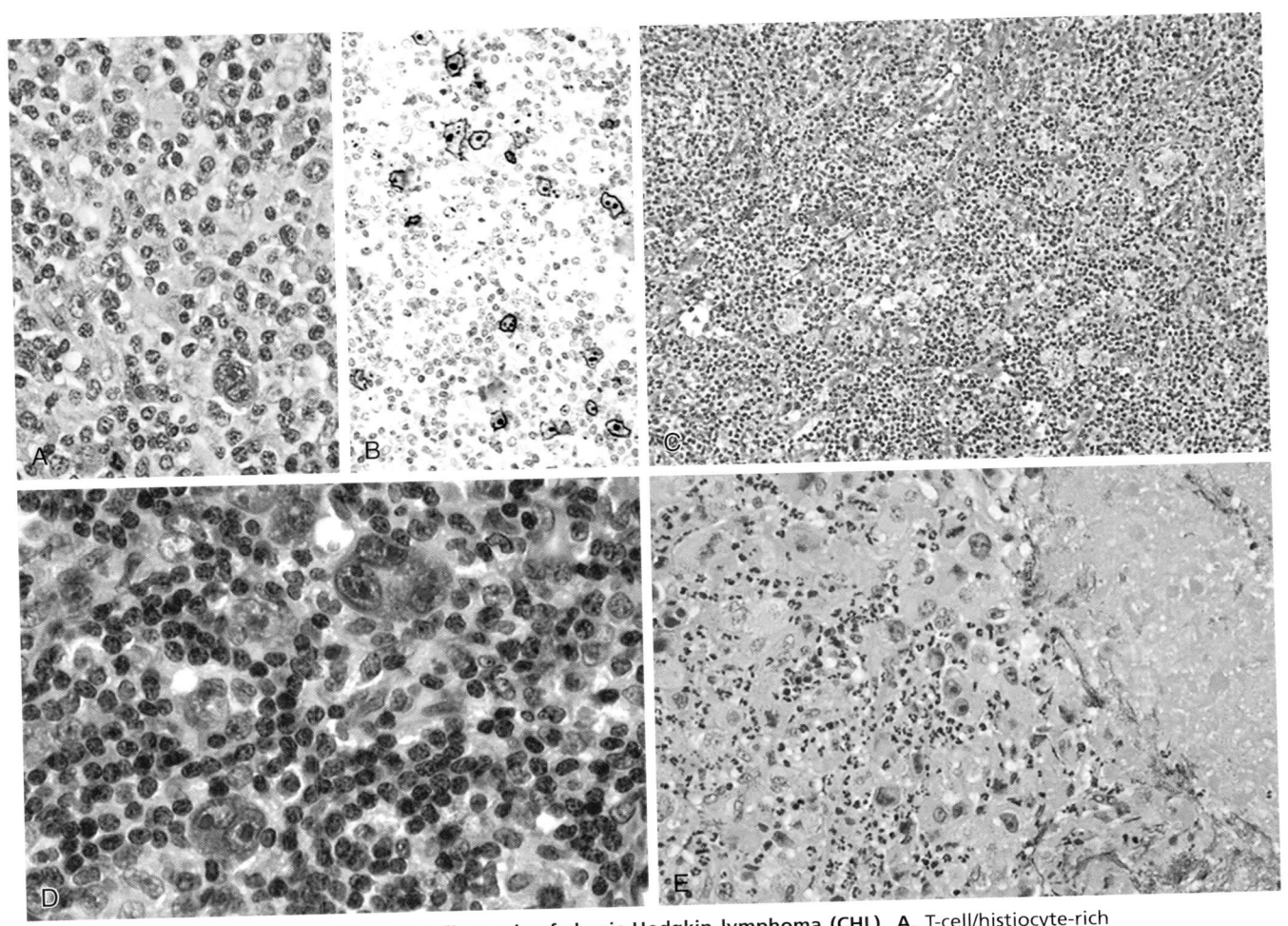

Figure 27-8. Differential diagnosis of classic Hodgkin lymphoma (CHL). A, T-cell/histiocyte-rich large B-cell lymphoma with Reed-Sternberg (RS)–like cells. **B,** Tumor cells show strong and homogeneous staining for CD20 and lack CD30 and CD15. **C,** Follicular helper T-cell lymphoma angioimmunoblastic type, with occasional Epstein-Barr virus (EBV)-positive RS-like cells *(arrows)* of B-cell phenotype (CD20⁺, CD30⁺). **D,** Hodgkin-like posttransplant lymphoproliferative disorder with occasional RS cells in a polymorphous B-cell proliferation. **E,** Mediastinal lymph node biopsy of anaplastic large cell carcinoma with occasional RS-like cells.

neoplastic cells of seminoma may resemble lacunar cells and sometimes exhibit a nodular growth pattern with concentric fibrosis, but demonstration of PLAP (placenta-like alkaline phosphatase), OCT-4, and CD117 positivity resolves these cases. Inflammatory variants of sarcomas may contain RS-like cells, but these usually do not pose major diagnostic problems.

Pearls and Pitfalls

- Diagnosis of CHL requires the presence of HRS cells in the appropriate cellular background. Many reactive and neoplastic disorders can mimic CHL.
- Joint expression of CD30 and CD15, although highly characteristic of CHL, can rarely be seen in other neoplasms, including both aggressive B-cell and T-cell lymphomas and EBV-associated LPDs.
- Nodular sclerosis CHL is distinct from other forms of CHL in terms of its demographics and epidemiology, whereas the mixed cellularity and lymphocyte-depleted subtypes show similar features.
- LRCHL most often has a nodular growth pattern and may show morphologic and immunophenotypical overlap with NLPBL.
- CHL is a B-cell neoplasm in which the B-cell program is highly suppressed. In cases with CHL-like morphology but strong, homogeneous expression of B-cell markers, alternative diagnoses need to be considered, depending on location and EBV status. These include MGZL, EBV-positive DLBCL, DLBCL, NOS, and EBV-positive LPD.

KEY REFERENCES

6. Kanzler H, Kuppers R, Hansmann ML, Rajewsky K. Hodgkin and Reed-Sternberg cells in Hodgkin's disease represent the outgrowth of a dominant tumor clone derived from (crippled) germinal center B cells. *J Exp Med.* 1996;184(4):1495–1505.

12. Connors JM, Cozen W, Steidl C, et al. Hodgkin lymphoma. *Nat Rev Dis Primers.* 2020;6(1):61.

37. Murray PG, Young LS. An etiological role for the Epstein-Barr virus in the pathogenesis of classical Hodgkin lymphoma. *Blood.* 2019;134(7):591–596.

77. Anagnostopoulos I, Hansmann ML, Franssila K, et al. European Task Force on Lymphoma project on lymphocyte predominance Hodgkin disease: histologic and immunohistologic analysis of submitted cases reveals 2 types of Hodgkin disease with a nodular growth pattern and abundant lymphocytes. *Blood.* 2000;96(5):1889–1899.

104. Tousseyn TA, King RL, Fend F, Feldman AL, Brousset P, Jaffe ES. Evolution in the definition and diagnosis of the Hodgkin lymphomas and related entities. *Virchows Arch.* 2023;482(1):207–226.

112. Wang HW, Balakrishna JP, Pittaluga S, Jaffe ES. Diagnosis of Hodgkin lymphoma in the modern era. *Br J Haematol.* 2019;184(1):45–59.

149. Traverse-Glehen A, Pittaluga S, Gaulard P, et al. Mediastinal gray zone lymphoma: the missing link between classic Hodgkin's lymphoma and mediastinal large B-cell lymphoma. *Am J Surg Pathol.* 2005;29(11):1411–1421.

199. Steidl C, Connors JM, Gascoyne RD. Molecular pathogenesis of Hodgkin's lymphoma: increasing evidence of the importance of the microenvironment. *J Clin Oncol.* 2011;29(14):1812–1826.

202. Kuppers R, Duhrsen U, Hansmann ML. Pathogenesis, diagnosis, and treatment of composite lymphomas. *Lancet Oncol.* 2014;15(10):e435–e446.

248. Liu WR, Shipp MA. Signaling pathways and immune evasion mechanisms in classical Hodgkin lymphoma. *Blood.* 2017;130(21):2265–2270.

277. Sarkozy C, Hung SS, Chavez EA, et al. Mutational landscape of gray zone lymphoma. *Blood.* 2021;137(13):1765–1776.

Visit Elsevier eBooks+ for the complete set of references.

Chapter 28

Virally Associated B-Cell Lymphoproliferative Disease

Alina Nicolae, Stefania Pittaluga, and Jonathan W. Said

Epstein-Barr virus (EBV) and Kaposi sarcoma-associated herpesvirus/human herpesvirus 8 (KSHV/HHV-8) are gamma herpesviruses that can infect B lymphocytes. Both establish a latent infection in which no viral progeny is usually produced and only a limited number of genes are expressed. Despite their tumorigenicity, most infected individuals carry a persistent silent infection. In certain settings, mainly of immune deficiency/dysregulation (e.g., inborn error of immunity, iatrogenic/therapy-related, posttransplant, HIV infection, autoimmune disease, or immune senescence), an increased risk for developing EBV or HHV-8-related lymphoproliferative disorders (LPDs) is observed. These LPDs show significant morphologic similarities and, to a certain extent, biological overlap across various immune impairment backgrounds. The pathologic spectrum of virally associated B-LPD is broad, ranging from benign lymphoid hyperplasia to aggressive lymphomas. Their defining feature consists in the identification of EBV or HHV-8 in most atypical lymphoid cells in tissue sections. Often, the virally associated reactive processes can mimic lymphomas, given the clinicopathologic changes mediated by the virus itself and the immune reaction generated. In such situations, a multidisciplinary approach is essential to achieve an accurate diagnosis and to establish the optimal therapy.

This chapter focuses mostly on the EBV- or HHV-8-associated LPDs in noniatrogenic settings. The EBV-related lymphoid proliferations and lymphomas associated with inborn and iatrogenic immune deficiency/dysregulation are further addressed in Chapters 53 and 54. In addition, well-defined B-cell lymphoma entities associated with EBV such as Burkitt lymphoma, plasmablastic lymphoma, and classic Hodgkin lymphoma are discussed in Chapters 23, 24, and 27, respectively. Finally, Chapter 29 expands on EBV-associated T- and NK-cell lymphoid proliferations.

EBV-ASSOCIATED LYMPHOPROLIFERATIVE DISORDERS

Epstein-Barr Virus Life Cycle and Pathogenesis

EBV Life Cycle

EBV, also known as human herpesvirus 4 (HHV-4), is a double-stranded DNA γ-herpesvirus. It was the first tumor virus identified in humans, within Burkitt lymphoma cells, by Epstein et al. in 1964.[1] There are two EBV genotypes (types 1 and 2) encompassing 71 strains (60 type 1 and 11 type 2) with variation mainly in the latent genes.[2-4] EBV is ubiquitous, with approximately 95% of the world's population sustaining a lifelong asymptomatic infection.[5,6] The virus is orally transmitted via saliva exchange and reaches the submucosal secondary lymphoid tissues (i.e., tonsils) through epithelial transcytosis. It commonly infects B lymphocytes, and less commonly epithelial, mesenchymal, T, and NK cells. In healthy carriers, the EBV life cycle is mostly confined to the B cells and it is biphasic, with phases of lytic replication and latency, which can go from III to II to 0 to I (Fig. 28-1).[7,8] The

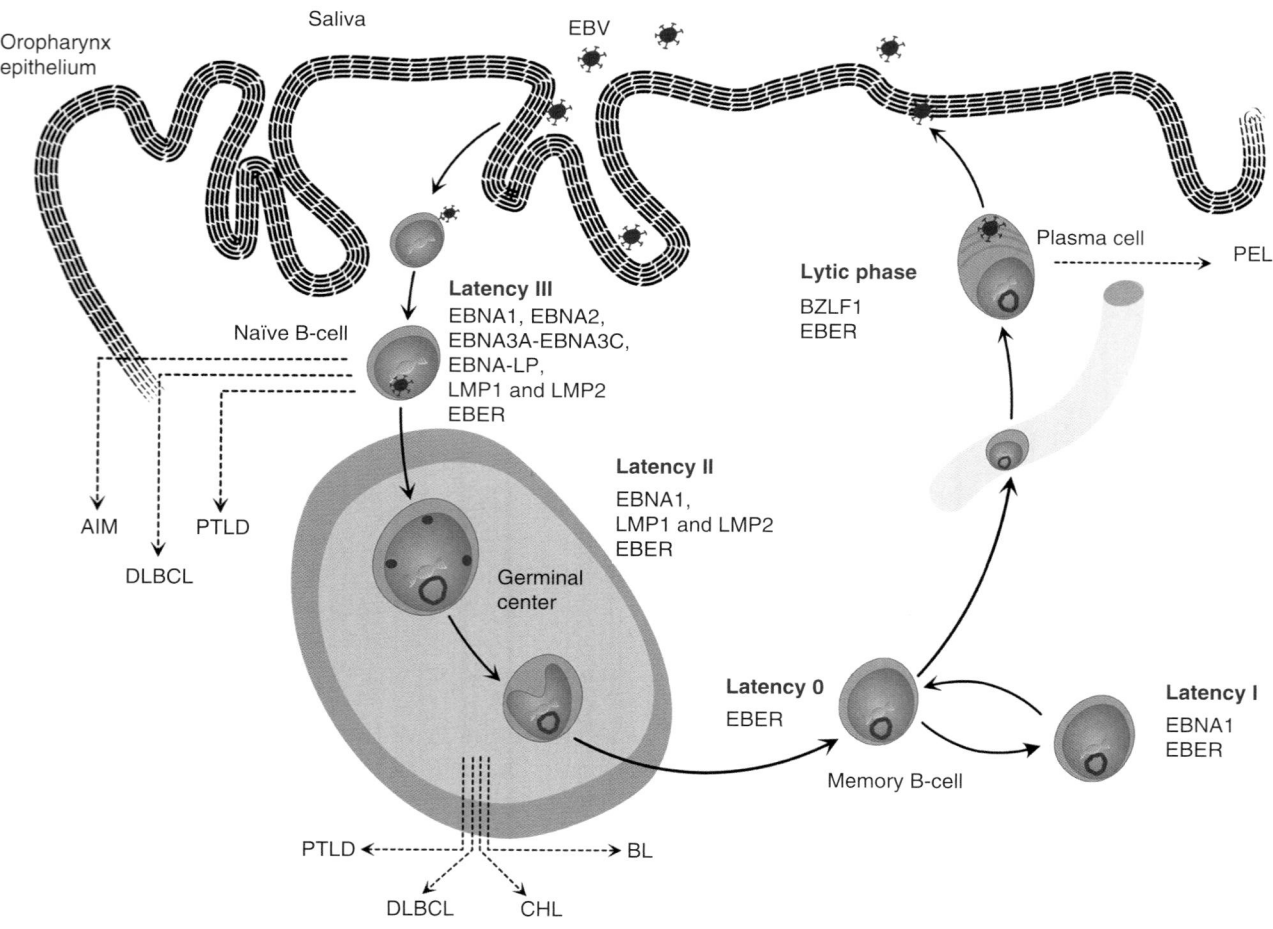

Figure 28-1. Model of Epstein-Barr virus infection and persistence. Epstein-Barr virus (EBV) is orally transmitted via saliva exchange. It infects naïve B lymphocytes of oropharyngeal submucosal lymphoid tissue. It forms extrachromosomal circularized episomes in the latency phases. Upon infection, the EBV enters latency III, in which all latency genes, EBV-encoded RNAs (EBERs), and viral microRNAs are expressed. This "growth program," despite being highly immunogenic, contributes to activation, proliferation, and resistance to cell death of infected cells that may enter into the germinal center reaction. Here, the virus restricts its gene expression to latency II, in which EBNA1, LMP1, LMP2, and EBERs are expressed. This "default program" mediates survival and differentiation. EBV-positive B cells exit the germinal center as EBV-infected memory B cells, where all viral antigens except EBERs are silenced (latency 0). These cells may transiently express EBNA1 (latency I) during homeostatic proliferation. Circulating memory B cells with latency 0 or I may home back to oropharyngeal mucosa. Their activation leads to plasma cell differentiation and the EBV switch to lytic cycle (i.e., *BZLF1*), with virus replication and production of new virions that shed into saliva, allowing virus transmission. An EBV latency type III is found in acute infectious mononucleosis (AIM), in a small subset of EBV-positive diffuse large B-cell lymphoma (DLBCL), and EBV-lymphoproliferative disorders in immunosuppressed individuals, such as posttransplant (PTLD). The germinal center differentiation pathway of EBV-infected B cells likely provides precursors of most EBV-associated DLBCL, PTLD, classic Hodgkin lymphoma (CHL), and Burkitt lymphoma (BL). Although derived from the germinal-center B cells, BL manifests an EBV latency I. As a reflection of plasmacytic differentiation, an increased lytic EBV replication can be found in primary effusion lymphoma (PEL).

EBV genome does not integrate into the host genome and it is linear during replication while forming extrachromosomal circularized episomes in the latency phases. EBV remodels its gene expression during the life cycle to ensure viral replication, immune evasion, and persistence into the memory B-cell pool.[9,10] It infects oropharyngeal naïve B cells via ligation of viral envelope glycoproteins gp350 and gp42, gH and gL complex to CD21/CD3d, and MHC class II coreceptor, respectively, on B cells.[6,7,11] Upon infection, the virus gene-expression program is fully expressed and is referred as latency III. It encodes for six EBV nuclear antigens (EBNA1, -2,

-3A, -3B, -3C, -LP), three latent membrane proteins (LMP1, LMP2A, LMP2B), and 46 viral untranslated RNAs, including two EBV-encoded small RNAs (*EBER1* and *EBER2*) and 44 viral microRNAs (e.g., BART and BHRF1).[7] This "growth program" drives activation, proliferation, and resistance to cell death of infected cells. However, it is also highly immunogenic, triggering a strong cytotoxic T-cell response with clearing of most infected B cells. The surviving ones may enter the germinal-center reaction. Here, the virus restricts its gene repertoire to latency II characterized by expression of EBNA1, LMP proteins and a subset of viral noncoding RNA including

EBERs. This "default program" mediates survival of infected B cells in the germinal center, their differentiation and which exit as memory B cells. To achieve viral persistence into the long-lived memory B-cell pool and avoid immune recognition, all viral antigens are silenced (latency 0). As an alternative route, EBV may directly reach resting memory B cells, bypassing the germinal center.[7,12] During homeostatic proliferation, infected memory B cells may transiently express EBNA1 (latency I), which anchors the viral episome to chromosomal DNA, passing the infection to daughter cells. Activation of memory B cells with latency 0 or I in oropharyngeal mucosa may lead to differentiation into plasma cells with the switch to the EBV lytic cycle (i.e., *BZLF1, BRLF1*), virus replication and production of new virions.[8] In this site, CD4+ and CD8+ T cells specific to EBV lytic cell proteins effectively control virus periodic reactivation.

EBV Transformation and Oncogenesis

EBV is an oncogenic virus, considered a class I carcinogen by the World Health Organization (WHO)[13] with capacity to transform human B cells into indefinitely growing lymphoblastoid cell lines in culture.[14] Its pathogenicity relies on coordinated expression of latency genes, early lytic proteins, and viral noncoding RNAs. EBV-encoded genes hijack important cellular signaling pathways of cellular proliferation (LMP1 and EBNA2) and apoptosis (LMP1, LMP2, EBNA3A, EBNA3C, EBERs, lytic genes [BHRF1 and BALF1-BCL2 viral homologues]). They may induce genetic instability (EBNA1, lytic genes), deregulate the epigenome (EBNA1, EBNA2, LMP1, EBERs), and interfere with immune control (lytic genes *[BZLF1, BILF1]*, microRNAs [miRNA; BHRF1, BART], and viral cytokines [IL10, CCL5]).[6,7,15,16] LMP1 is a major oncogene. It mimics CD4-positive T-cell help in the germinal center, serving as surrogate ligand for the CD40 receptor on B cells with downstream activation of NF-κB, PI3K/AKT, MAPK, and JAK-STAT signaling pathways.[17] LMP2 simulates antigen engagement on B-cell receptors (BCRs), proving a strong survival signal and rescue from apoptosis of infected B cells.[18] EBNA2 induces the transcription of the cellular oncogene *MYC* and imitates a constitutively activated NOTCH receptor.[19] Furthermore, lytic EBV antigens and viral miRNAs contribute to an immune evasive tumor microenvironment. Early lytic EBV replication allows for high levels of IL10 and CCL5 production, with suppression of cytotoxic T-cell response and recruitment of immunosuppressive myeloid cells, respectively.[7] EBV miRNAs promote immune escape at multiple levels. They control EBV latency programs allowing for virus persistence, downregulate MHC-restricted antigen presentation, interfere with CD8-positive T-cell recruitment, alter type I IFN response, and blunt immune sensing via Toll-like receptors.[20,21] Moreover, EBV-infected B cells involved in the germinal-center differentiation are exposed to activation-induced deaminase (AID) machinery with acquisition of additional mutations or chromosomal translocations.[22]

Despite EBV's high tumorigenicity, the finely tuned balance between pathogen and host allows most individuals to carry the virus as a persistent, silent infection. Thus primary infection is usually asymptomatic in children. It may lead to acute infectious mononucleosis (AIM) in 35% to 70% of infected adolescents/young adults in developed countries.[23,24] AIM is a self-limited condition characterized by a complex of symptoms mostly generated by the hyperactive T-cell response to control viral replication and proliferation of infected EBV B cells. Most cases resolve without sequelae within a few weeks, but some patients have a more protracted clinical course.

In cases of host immune impairments, EBV reactivation occurs and, left unchecked, may lead to autoimmune diseases (i.e., multiple sclerosis) or malignancies.[25-27] Defective immune surveillance may be linked to either primary immune defects or secondary to infection (HIV, *Plasmodium falciparum*), immunomodulatory drug use (transplant settings, autoimmune diseases), or related to age. In addition, environmental exposure and hormonal and genetic factors related to racial/ethnic variation are important players to alter and increase susceptibility to develop EBV-related diseases. Hence, EBV contributes to 1% to 2% of human malignancies, with epithelial cancers (nasopharyngeal and gastric carcinomas) outnumbering lymphoproliferative disorders/lymphomas.[28]

EBV+ B-lymphoproliferations have a worldwide distribution and their clinicobiological characteristics are heterogeneous, ranging from benign proliferative lesions to aggressive lymphomas. Their latency pattern is also diverse and depends at least partly on the B-cell differentiation stage from which they arise. An EBV latency III is found not only in naïve infected B cells of healthy carriers and most tonsillar B cells in AIM, but also in severe immunosuppressed patients with posttransplant lymphoproliferative disorders (PTLD). Classic Hodgkin lymphoma (CHL) and most EBV-positive large B-cell lymphomas will manifest an EBV latency II and Burkitt lymphomas show a latency I (Fig. 28-1). Given EBERs constant and high expression in all latency phases, in situ hybridization using EBERs probes represents the gold standard and the most sensitive approach to detect EBV-infected cells in tissue specimens.

Our enhanced understanding of the EBV life cycle, its mechanisms of cellular transformation, and immune control provide opportunities for early diagnostic tool development (i.e., detection of EBV miRNAs) and novel therapeutic interventions. Prophylactic or therapeutic EBV vaccines, adoptive transfer of EBV-specific T cells, immune checkpoint inhibitors, cytolytic virus activation therapy, or poly (ADP-ribose) polymerase 1 (PARP1) inhibitors are among the promising strategies to control EBV pathologies.[29-33]

Epstein-Barr Virus–Positive Mucocutaneous Ulcer

Definition of the Disease

EBV-positive mucocutaneous ulcer (EBVMCU) is a self-limited LPD that usually presents as a solitary, painful, well-circumscribed mucosal or cutaneous ulcer, in the absence of systemic symptoms or lymphadenopathy. In patients with two or more skin lesions, the term *EBV-positive B-cell polymorphic LPD* is preferred, or when the infiltrate is more extensive beyond the ulcer bed, *EBV-positive diffuse large B-cell lymphoma, not otherwise specified (DLBCL, NOS)* or other more specific type of EBV-positive lymphoma or LPD should be considered.[34,35]

Synonyms and Related Terms

None.

Epidemiology and Clinical Features

EBVMCU often affects elderly patients with immune senescence or immunocompromised individuals in settings of organ transplantation, or iatrogenic immunosuppression (e.g., methotrexate, azathioprine, and cyclosporine), HIV infection, or inborn immune disorders. The median age of patients thus affected is 71 (range 0.5–101), with a slight female predominance. It mainly involves the oropharyngeal mucosa (70%, including tonsils), skin, and gastrointestinal tract. The latter are usually associated with iatrogenic immunosuppression.[34] In EBVMCU, a solitary lesion is often encountered, although multifocal ulcers restricted to a single anatomic site have been described.[35,36] It follows an indolent clinical course with a high rate of remission either after reduction/withdrawal of immunosuppression or spontaneously, and rarely recurs.[35-42]

Pathology

Histologically, the mucosal or cutaneous ulcer is shallow or deep and often sharply demarcated by a rim of small lymphocytes (Fig. 28-2). The ulcer bed consists of a polymorphous infiltrate with scattered or clustered large, atypical cells, often with immunoblastic and Hodgkin and Reed-Sternberg (HRS)–like features. Variable numbers of eosinophils, plasma cells, histiocytes, and small lymphocytes are admixed. Based on the density and cytologic features of the atypical lymphocytes, four morphologic patterns have been described: polymorphous, large cell-rich (DLBCL-like), CHL-like, and mucosa-associated lymphoid tissue lymphoma-like (MALT-like). Angioinvasion and focal necrosis are often seen. The adjacent epithelium may be hyperplastic or show reactive atypia.

Phenotypically, the large atypical lymphoid cells are variably positive for B-cell markers (CD20, CD79a, PAX5, OCT2) and BCL6, and commonly express IRF4/MUM1 and CD30, with CD15 staining observed in up to half of cases.[36,38,39,41] They typically show EBV latency type II or III and EBER highlights the wide size range of the atypical B cells. A large number of small T cells delimit the ulcer bed, contributing to its sharp demarcation. Less than 50% of EBVMCU cases show a clonal immunoglobulin gene rearrangement and up to 30% may also demonstrate a clonal T-receptor gene rearrangement.[35,36,39] So far, no recurrent gene mutations have been identified.[43]

Distinction of EBVMCU from EBV-positive DLBCL, NOS usually requires an excisional biopsy and meticulous clinical assessment. In contrast to EBV-positive DLBCL, NOS, the EBV viral load, soluble interleukin 2 receptor (sIL-2R), and LDH are not increased in most patients with EBVMCU, supporting its localized nature.[35,36,38] Decreased immune surveillance by cytotoxic T cells with impaired function or restricted repertoire and further exposure to a site-specific trigger (i.e., tooth extraction) are likely involved in EBV-positive B-cell expansion in EBVMCU.[36,39]

Epstein-Barr Virus–Positive Diffuse Large B-Cell Lymphoma, NOS

Definition of the Disease

EBV-positive DLBCL, NOS is a B-cell malignancy in which most atypical cells (>80%) are EBV infected. By definition, no case of EBV-positive B-cell lymphoma with known underlying primary or acquired immune deficiency/dysregulation should be classified in this category. Furthermore, other well-defined EBV-associated disorders (e.g., Burkitt lymphoma, lymphomatoid granulomatosis [LyG], CHL, primary effusion lymphoma, plasmablastic lymphoma, or DLBCL associated with chronic inflammation) should be excluded.

It was originally described as *senile EBV-associated B-cell lymphoproliferative disorder* or *EBV-positive DLBCL of the elderly* given its occurrence in patients older than 50 years without any known immunodeficiency or prior lymphoma.[44] Its pathobiology was attributed to immunesenescence inherent to physiologic aging. In the original description by Oyama and colleagues, EBV-positive LPD in the elderly showed striking similarities with PTLDs, frequent extranodal presentation, and an overall survival inferior to the EBV-negative DLBCL.[45,46] However, subsequent studies have shown that EBV-positive DLBCL was not restricted to the elderly and also occurred in younger patients, in the absence of an underlying immune impairment.[47-56] To reflect these observations, it is now designated as *EBV-positive diffuse large B-cell lymphoma, NOS*.[34,57]

Synonyms and Related Terms

WHO revised 4th ed.: EBV-positive DLBCL, NOS
WHO proposed 5th ed.: EBV-positive DLBCL
In the ICC and revised WHO 4th ed., NOS was added to indicate that it did not fit any of the other more specific types of EBV-positive large B-cell lymphoma.

Epidemiology

The precise incidence of EBV-positive DLBCL is unknown, as no large population-based studies have been performed to date and it is likely underestimated, as EBV testing is not routinely performed. Based on case series, it accounts for 2% to 5% of all DLBCLs in Western countries[47,48,51,56,58-60] with a higher prevalence (9%–28%) in Asia and Latin America.[46,48,53,61-66] Its incidence increases with age, with a peak in the seventh and eight decades of life, and a smaller peak observed in the third decade of life.[56,67] Among younger patients (<50 years), EBV positivity in DLBCL ranges from 6.7% to 8%.[51,52,54] Males are more commonly affected than women (male-to-female ratio of 1.5–3.6:1).

Clinical Features

Patients commonly present with B-symptoms and nodal disease. Extranodal involvement is frequently observed in the elderly (50%–70%)[37,45,53,56,62,68] and occasionally found in younger individuals.[54,55] The extranodal sites include skin, lung, gastrointestinal tract, and bone marrow. Thus the symptoms are variable. A subset of patients develops hemophagocytic lymphohistiocytosis (HLH).[56] EBV DNA is detectable in the serum or blood of most patients and the viral load seems to correlate with disease burden.[69] Based on retrospective studies, the clinical outcome of elderly patients is poor, with a median overall survival of 24 to 36 months.[46,62] The prognostic effect of EBV status remains controversial in DLBCL treated with immunochemotherapy.[37,53,56,59,60,63,70-75] The response to therapy of younger patients is significantly higher, and most achieve long-term survival.[51,52,54]

Pathology

EBV-positive DLBCL shows a broad histologic spectrum, with geographic necrosis and angiocentric/angiodestructive lesions frequently observed. The lymph node or the extranodal site show architectural effacement by an abnormal lymphoid infiltrate comprising large cells resembling centroblasts,

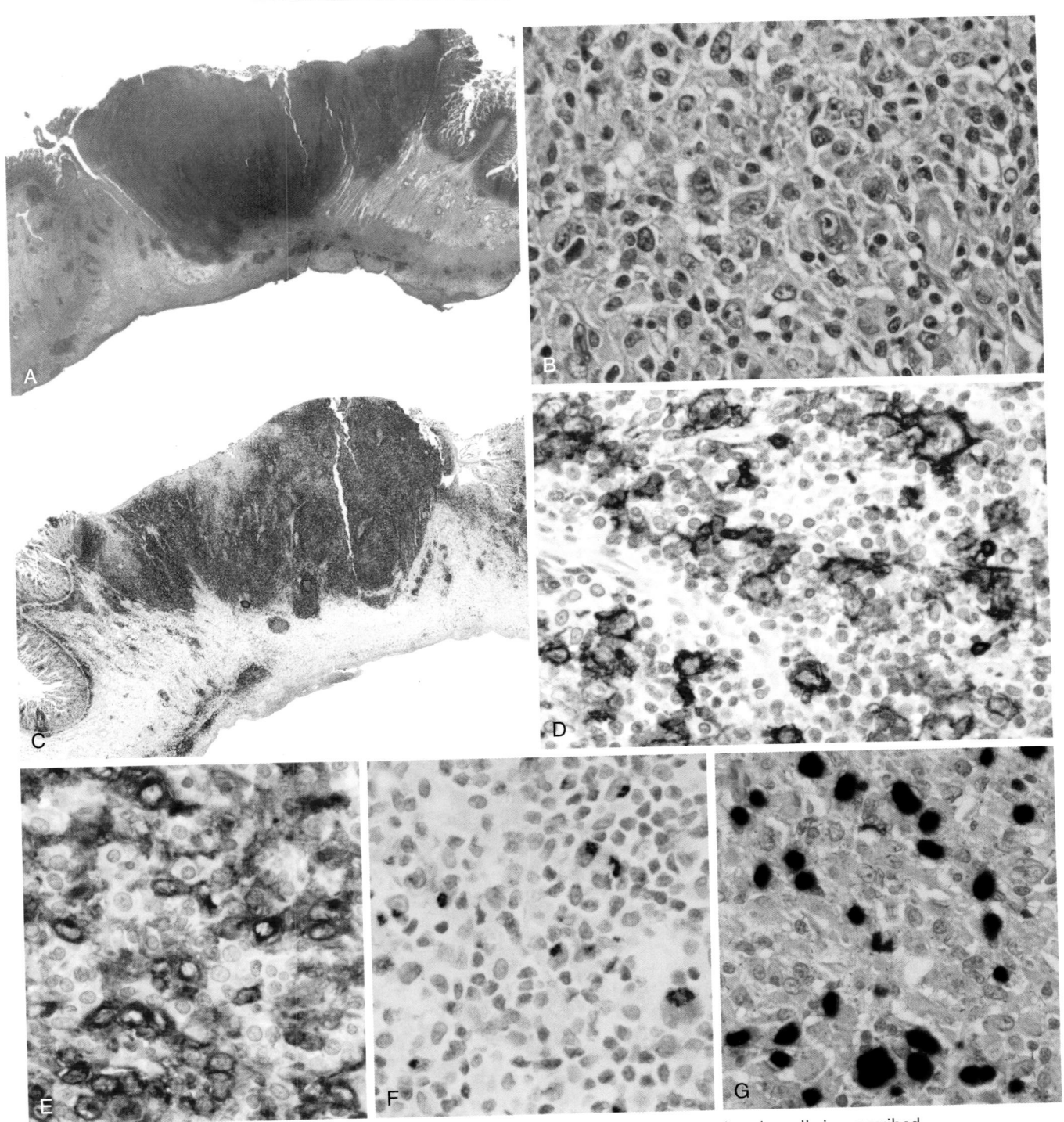

Figure 28-2. Epstein-Barr virus–positive mucocutaneous ulcer. A, Isolated, well-circumscribed small bowel ulcer. **B,** The lesion consists of a polymorphous infiltrate with scattered large, atypical cells, sometimes with Reed-Sternberg–like features in a rich histiocytic background. **C,** The ulcer bed is sharply demarcated by small, CD3-positive T-lymphocytes. **D,** The atypical cells strongly express CD20 and CD30 **(E)** and are focally positive for CD15 with a dot-like pattern **(F). G,** EBV-encoded RNA (EBER) highlights a range of cell sizes, including the large pleomorphic lymphocytes.

immunoblasts, HRS-like cells, lymphocyte predominant (LP)-like cells, and occasional highly pleomorphic cells. Several morphologic variants are recognized based on the density and amount/type of inflammatory background and cytologic appearance of the neoplastic cells.[37,46,56,68,70,76] Most commonly, EBV-positive DLBCL is characterized by a variable number of large cells in a background rich in small lymphocytes, histiocytes, plasma cells, and occasional eosinophils. This histologic pattern, originally referred to as the polymorphic subtype by Oyama et al.,[61] may resemble T-cell/histiocyte–rich large B-cell lymphoma (Fig. 28-3) or CHL (Fig. 28-4). Other cases show a monomorphic appearance with sheets of large cells indistinguishable from EBV-negative DLBCL, NOS (Fig. 28-5). Rarely, the full

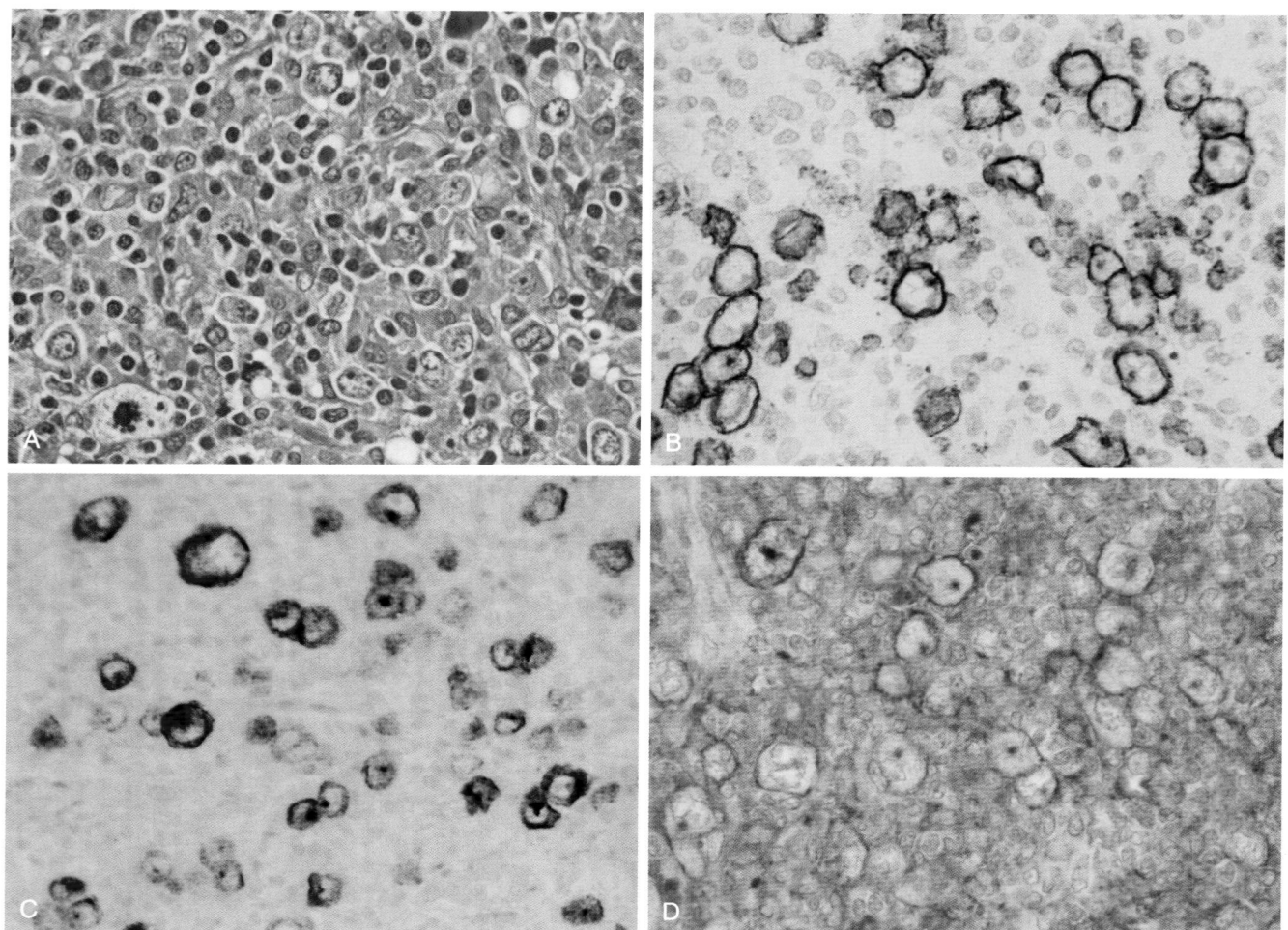

Figure 28-3. Epstein-Barr virus–positive diffuse large B-cell lymphoma, not otherwise specified resembling T-cell/histiocyte–rich large B-cell lymphoma. A, Scattered large, atypical cells with vesicular nuclei are seen in a background rich in histiocytes and small lymphocytes. **B,** The atypical cells are strongly CD20 positive and no small B cells are noted in the background. They also express LMP1 **(C)** and PD-L1 **(D).**

spectrum of B-cell maturation stages with plasmacytoid differentiation and abundant immunoblasts resembling a polymorphic posttransplant lymphoproliferative disorder is encountered (Fig. 28-6). These morphologic patterns do not seem to have prognostic significance.[37,56,70]

Immunophenotypically, the large cells usually express pan–B-cell markers and even in the absence of CD20 expression, they still conserve a strong B-cell program (positivity for CD19, CD79a, PAX5, OCT2, and BOB-1) (Figs. 28-3 to 28-6). They often have a post–germinal-center/activated B-cell phenotype with IRF4/MUM-1 positivity, and variable expression of CD10. Most cases show focal or diffuse staining for CD30 with CD15 expression observed in a small subset.[37,53,54,56,59,68,70,75] The neoplastic cells frequently express PD-L1 and PD-L2.[54,56,74,77,78] By definition, the atypical cells are EBV positive using in situ hybridization, with EBER demonstrated in the majority of tumor cells (>80%). The low cutoffs (between 10% and 20%) of EBV-positive B cells used in several studies raise doubts about the pathogenic role of EBV in such instances.[47,48,62] LMP-1 is expressed in most cases (>90%), with EBNA-2 detected in up to one-third of patients (7%–36%), consistent with a predominant EBV latency type II.[46,54,56,59]

EBV-positive DLBCL showing HRS–like cells in a reactive inflammatory background is particularly challenging to distinguish from mixed cellularity CHL. In contrast to CHL, EBV-positive DLBCL may involve extranodal sites, show a preserved B-cell program, and lack CD15 in most cases.[37,46] In addition, EBER highlights a wider variation in nuclear size of atypical cells in comparison to CHL, where the positivity is more restricted to the HRS cells. In extranodal sites, the differential diagnosis includes EBVMCU and LyG. Notably, EBV-positive DLBCL shows overlapping pathologic features with other EBV-driven LPD in immune dysregulation settings. This distinction can only be made based on clinical context.

Genetics and Pathogenesis

Clonal immunoglobulin gene rearrangement is often demonstrated (60%).[37,54,70] Approximately half of tested cases show a "restricted" or oligoclonal T-cell receptor gene rearrangement, as reflection of reduced T-cell repertoire (senescence) or expanded EBV-specific CD8 cytotoxic T cells.[37]

The pathogenesis of EBV-positive DLBCL is complex and not fully elucidated. It involves disruption of the finely tuned balance between latently EBV-infected B cells and the host

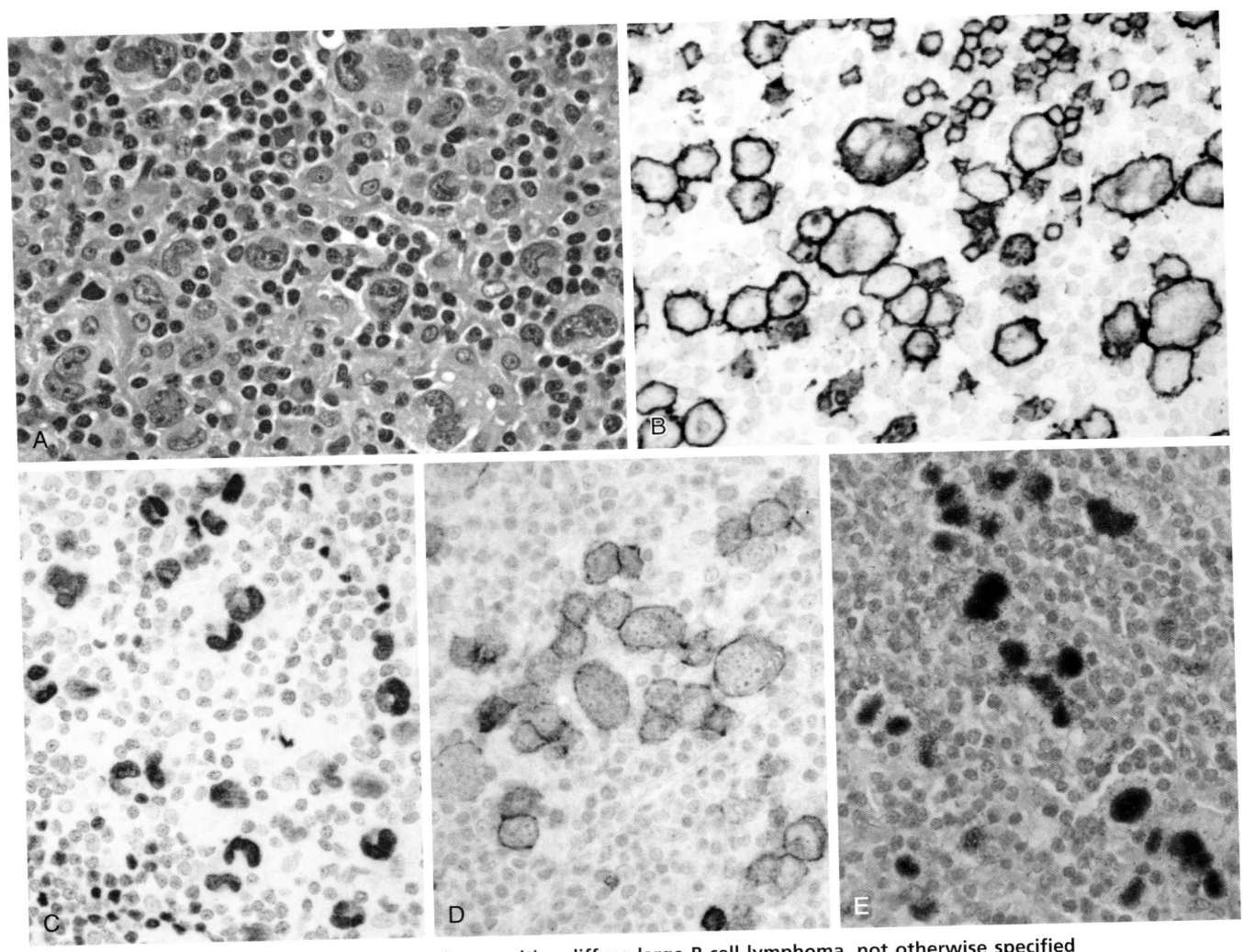

Figure 28-4. Epstein-Barr virus–positive diffuse large B-cell lymphoma, not otherwise specified resembling classic Hodgkin lymphoma. A, Large, atypical cells with Reed-Sternberg–like features are noted in a background rich in histiocytes and small lymphocytes. These cells are strongly and uniformly positive for CD20 **(B)** and OCT2 **(C)**. They also express CD30 **(D)** and Epstein-Barr virus (EBV)-encoded RNA **(E)**. Note the range in size of atypical EBV-infected lymphocytes.

immune system, as well as genomic alterations intrinsic to the neoplastic cells. The immunosenescence or the physiologic decay of the immune system with aging is thought to underlie the biology of this neoplasm in elderly patients (>70 years). Both innate and acquired immunity are remodeled with age, although changes in the T-cell compartment reflect the reduced generation of lymphoid precursors, thymic atrophy with diminished output of naïve T cells, restricted T-cell receptor repertoire, anergic memory cells, and accumulation of viral-specific CD8 T cells, often CMV specific.[79,80] These changes in the T-cell compartment allow latently EBV-infected B cells to expand. The oncogenic driver mechanisms elicited by EBV products exceed other genomic events, explaining the low mutational burden and scarce recurrent abnormalities observed in EBV-positive DLBCL.[78,81] However, they display a broad intratumor heterogeneity with different subclonal populations.[82] Among the genes involved, there is a significant enrichment in alterations in NF-κB, WNT, and IL6/JAK/STAT pathways, as well as in epigenetic modifiers.[81,83,84] An enhanced activity of these pathways and of genes involved in Toll-like receptor signaling and antiviral response have

been documented by gene-expression profile studies.[59,78,85] Of note, *CCR6, DAPK1, TNFRSF21,* and *CCR7* mutations, observed in approximately 15% of cases, appear to be specific for EBV-positive DLBCL. In addition, 6q deletion that encompasses *PRDM1* and *A20/TNFAIP3* is a recurrent feature (44%) of this neoplasm.[81] Interestingly, a mutual exclusivity has been observed between EBV positivity and *MYD88/CD79B* mutations and *MYC, BCL2,* and *BCL6* rearrangements in DLBCL.[86]

Immune tolerance of EBV-infected B cells is another crucial mechanism involved in the pathobiology of this neoplasm, mainly in younger patients.[54,87] The neoplastic EBV-positive B cells overexpress immune checkpoint ligands PD-L1 and PD-L2. The mechanisms involved are multifactorial and related to EBV proteins and cytokine milieu (IFN-γ). EBV-LMP1 upregulates PD-L1/L2 through JAK/STAT, AP-1, and NF-κB pathways and this is finely regulated by EBV miR-BHRF1-2-5p.[70,88,89] In addition, EBNA2 downregulates miR-34a and alters PD-L1 expression in cases with EBV latency type III.[90] Furthermore, genetic abnormalities at the 9p24.1 (PDL1/PDL2) locus have been detected in 19% of cases.[78,83]

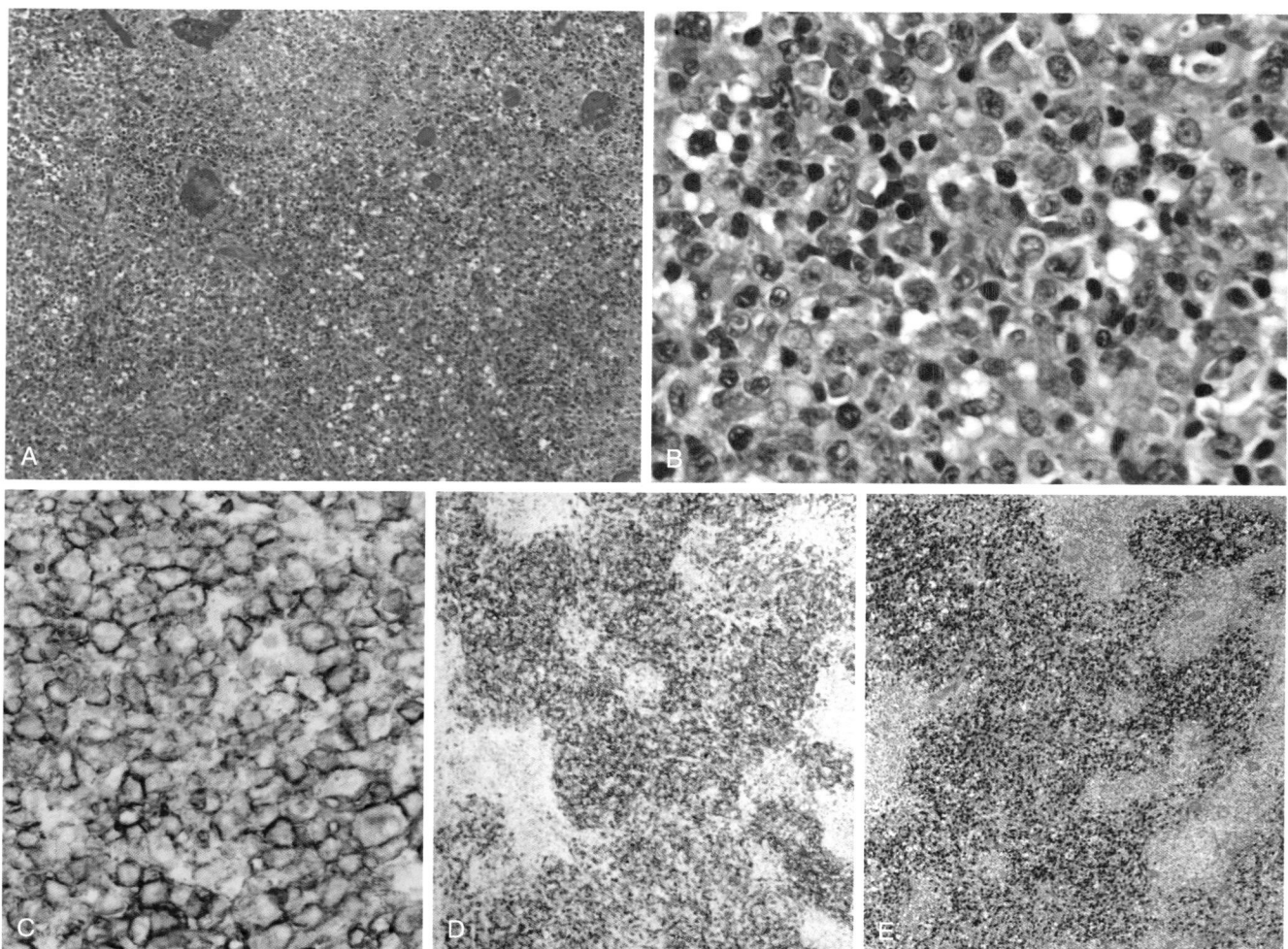

Figure 28-5. Epstein-Barr virus (EBV)-positive diffuse large B-cell lymphoma, not otherwise specified indistinguishable from EBV negative diffuse large B-cell lymphoma, not otherwise specified. A and B, Sheets of large atypical lymphoid cells with extensive areas of necrosis. The large cells are strongly and uniformly positive for CD20 **(C)**, CD30 **(D)**, and EBV by in situ hybridization **(E)**.

Altogether, this makes EBV-positive DLBCL an attractive target for PD-1/PD-L1/PD-L2 inhibitors.[74,91]

Diffuse Large B-Cell Lymphoma Associated With Chronic Inflammation

Definition of the Disease

DLBCL associated with chronic inflammation (DLBCL-CI) is a rare form of EBV-positive lymphoma that occurs in context of long-standing chronic inflammation. Originally called pyothorax-associated lymphoma (PAL), it is characterized by a mass-forming lesion, usually involving the pleural cavity.

Synonyms and Related Terms

Pyothorax-associated lymphoma (subset).

Epidemiology and Clinical Features

Most cases are reported in patients with chronic pyothorax after pleurodesis used to treat pulmonary tuberculosis.[92-95] It is more common in Japan, where therapeutical pneumothorax was a popular practice, and rare in Western populations.

Cases subsequent to chronic empyema after trauma or pneumonectomy have also been described. The mean latency time from infection to lymphoma development was 37 years (range 20–60 years).[92,93,95] DLBCL-CI may rarely occur decades after chronic osteomyelitis and venous skin ulcers or it may arise subsequent to metallic joint prosthesis and surgical mesh implants.[39,96-98] Patients with PAL are commonly in their 70s and there is a marked male predominance (male-to-female ratio >9:1).[92,95,99]

Most patients with PAL are immunocompetent and have a long history of chronic pyothorax. They often present with back or chest pain, fever, cough, dyspnea, or chest tumor mass. The imaging studies usually reveal a large (>10 cm) lenticular or crescent-shaped mass at the margin of the empyema cavity, often at the lateral costal pleura or costophrenic angle.[100] Despite the localized stage of disease at presentation, the outcome of PAL is poor, with an overall survival rate at 5 years of 20% to 35%.[92,95]

Pathology

Typically, there is a diffuse proliferation of large lymphoid cells involving pleura and adjacent structures. The atypical

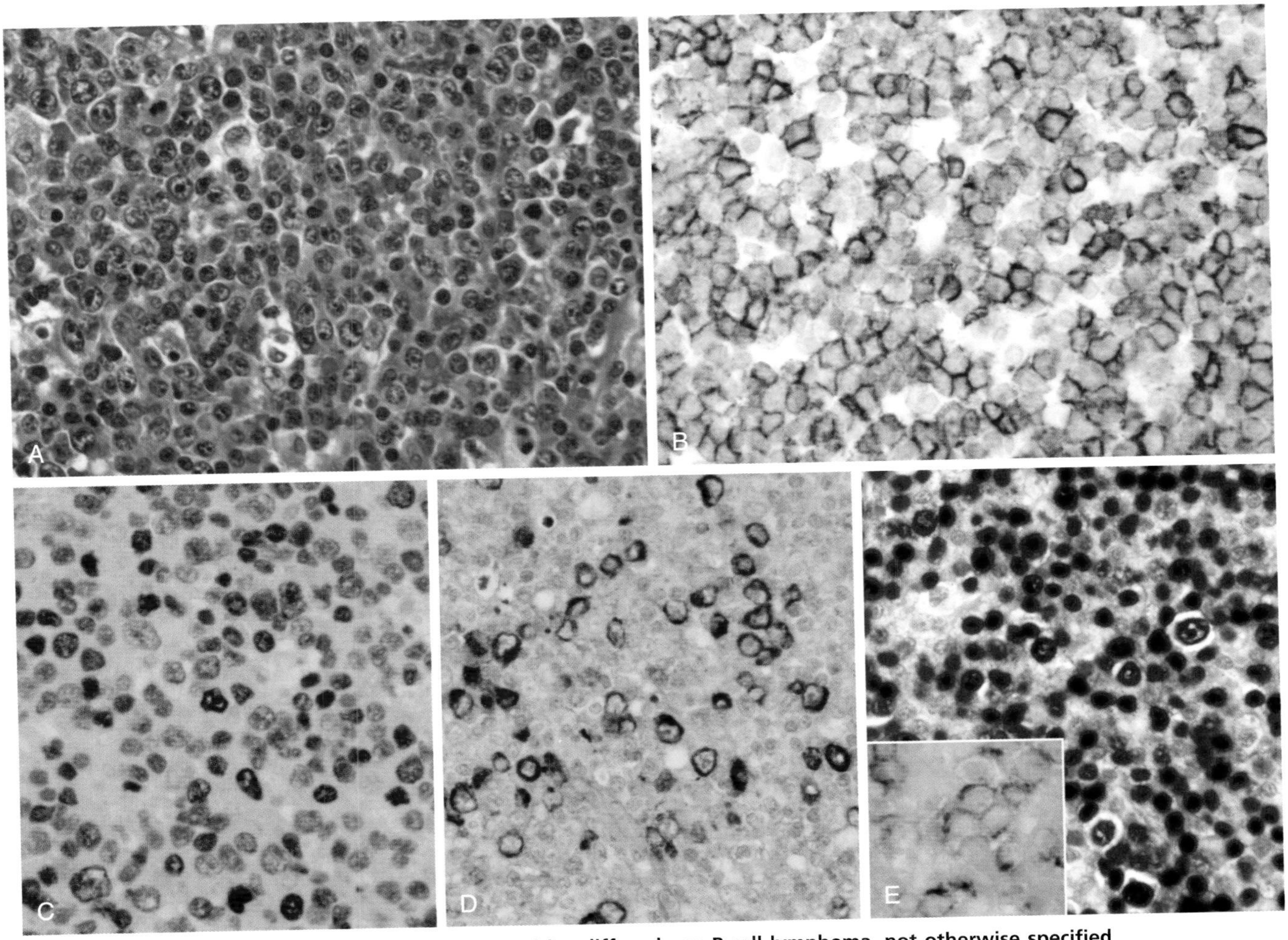

Figure 28-6. Epstein-Barr virus–positive diffuse large B-cell lymphoma, not otherwise specified resembling a polymorphic posttransplant lymphoproliferative disorder. A, The neoplastic infiltrate consists of a polymorphic atypical lymphoid proliferation with plasmacytic differentiation. **B,** The atypical cells are variably positive for CD20, and show diffuse expression of IRF4/MUM1 **(C)** and IgA heavy chain restriction **(D).** Epstein-Barr virus (EBV) is present in more than 90% of atypical cells by in situ hybridization with EBV-encoded RNA probe **(E),** whereas a subset of cells is positive for LMP1 *(inset).*

cells show immunoblastic, centroblastic, or less frequent plasmablastic features (Fig. 28-7).[92,93,95] Necrosis and angiocentricity are commonly seen, as well as various degrees of fibrosis and chronic inflammation. By immunohistochemistry, the neoplastic cells express CD45 and usually pan–B-cell markers. They are frequently positive for IRF4/MUM1 and CD43 (75%), while lacking CD10 and BCL6, in keeping with a post–germinal-center phenotype.[93] The neoplastic cells may stain for CD30 and show aberrant expression of T-cell markers (CD2, CD3, or CD4).[92,93] They manifest an EBV latency type III (positivity for EBER, LMP1, and EBNA2) and are HHV-8 negative.

Pathogenesis and Genetics

DLBCL-CI is consistently EBV positive.[92,93,101,102] The putative cell of origin is considered a crippled B-cell that has passed through the germinal-center reaction.[103] Local chronic inflammation via cytokines (IL6, IL10), chemokines (CCL17,

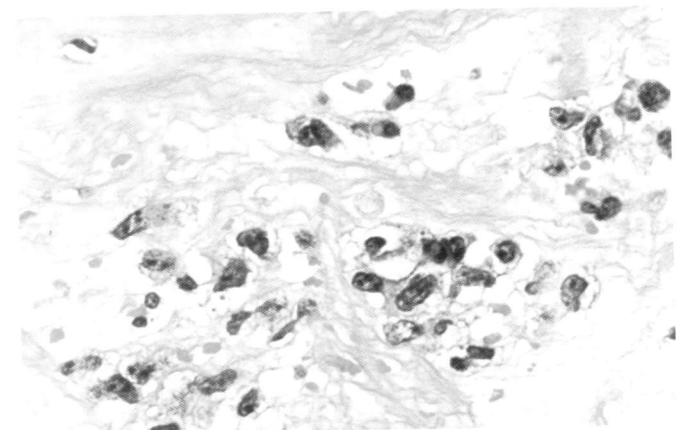

Figure 28-7. Pyothorax-associated lymphoma (diffuse large B-cell lymphoma with chronic inflammation). The large, atypical cells are embedded in a sclerotic stroma and fibrin. *(Courtesy John K.C. Chan.)*

CCL22), and reactive oxygen species likely contributes to the tolerogenic microenvironment, proliferation, and slow progression of EBV-transformed B cells that escaped the host immune surveillance in the enclosed space.[39,94,101,104] There is no association with HHV-8 in contrast to primary effusion lymphoma.[93]

PAL shows clonal rearrangements of immunoglobulin genes without evidence of ongoing somatic mutations.[101,103] It features genomic instability.[105,106] *TP53* mutations, most commonly at dipyrimidine sites, and *MYC* amplification are detected in 70% of cases[94,107,108] and one-third show *A20* (*TNFAIP3*) deletion.[109] The gene-expression profile is distinct from nodal DLBCLs and is characterized, besides an EBV-related signature, by high expression of interferon-inducible genes (i.e., *IFI27*), a feature of chronic inflammation.[110]

Fibrin-Associated Diffuse Large B-Cell Lymphoma

Definition of the Disease

Fibrin-associated DLBCL (FA-DLBCL) is rare, with only case reports and small series described so far. It is characterized by microscopic foci of neoplastic B cells admixed with fibrin exudate in confined anatomic spaces. It follows an indolent clinical course, with no mass formation or infiltrative growth pattern, as opposed to DLBCL-CI.

Synonyms and Related Terms

WHO revised 4th ed.: Fibrin-associated DLBCL
WHO proposed 5th ed.: Fibrin-associated large B-cell lymphoma

Epidemiology and Clinical Features

FA-DLBCL is often incidentally found in surgical specimens removed for various conditions that predispose to fibrin accumulation. Some patients may present with thromboembolic events. It has been seen most commonly lining the surface of cardiac myxomas (32%, frequently of left atrium), in association with prosthetic cardiac valves or endovascular grafts. It also involves pseudocysts (18%), hydrocele, chronic subdural hematoma, or relates to orthopedic devices.[111-116] FA-DLBCL has also been documented in settings of breast implants.[117-119] The time from graft/device placement to lymphoma diagnosis ranges from 1 to more than 20 years. Patients are usually immunocompetent adults (median age 60, range 25–96 years) with male predominance (male-to-female ratio of 2.5:1). They show localized stage IE disease (Lugano classification),[120] with lymphoma restricted to a single extranodal site and have an excellent prognosis. Although no therapeutic guidelines are available so far, early FA-DLBCL diagnosis, complete lesion excision, and close follow-up are likely the optimal strategy.[113,121]

Pathology

FA-DLBCL presents as microscopic aggregates of large lymphoid cells embedded within an abundant fibrinous background (Fig. 28-8). There is no extension to the adjacent normal tissue, although focal infiltration of cardiac myxoma or fibrous capsule may be seen. The atypical cells frequently show irregular nuclei, ≥1 conspicuous nucleoli, and moderate amount of cytoplasm, sometimes with plasmacytic differentiation. Mitotic figures and apoptotic bodies are numerous. Scattered macrophages and chronic inflammation may be associated.

Immunophenotypically, the neoplastic B lymphocytes are CD79a and PAX5 positive, variably express CD20 and CD30, and are seldomly CD138 positive. They frequently have a nongerminal-center B-cell phenotype with IRF4/MUM1 expression and a high Ki67 proliferation index (>90%). Most cases are EBV positive, notably with latency type III (expression of LMP1 and EBNA2). HHV-8 is negative. A monoclonal immunoglobulin gene rearrangement is often detected, but *MYC, BCL6,* or *BCL2* rearrangements or amplifications are usually absent by fluorescence in situ hybridization (FISH) studies.[113]

Given its rarity, FA-DLBCL pathogenesis is largely unknown with no genetic study published so far. It has been suggested that acquired local immunosuppression and restricted environment provided by the dense fibrin strands are contributing to immune evasion and malignant transformation of EBV-infected B cells.[113,122]

Lymphomatoid Granulomatosis

Definition of the Disease

LyG is a rare, progressive, angiocentric, and angiodestructive EBV-associated B-cell LPD that typically involves extranodal sites. Lung involvement is required for the diagnosis.[34,124] The infiltrate characteristically contains scattered EBV-positive B cells and a predominant T-cell background.[125-127] The term was coined by Liebow and colleagues in 1972 to distinguish it from Wegener's granulomatosis (WG), which shares similar clinical and pulmonary radiologic findings.[128]

Synonyms and Related Terms

None.

Epidemiology

LyG occurs in otherwise healthy individuals, although most of them have some degree of quantitative or qualitative impairment of cellular (CD8-positive T cells) or humoral immune response to EBV.[124,127,129] It has been sporadically described in patients with both inborn (i.e., Wiskott-Aldrich syndrome, *DOCK8* deficiency) and acquired immune deficiency (autoimmune diseases, HIV infection, or iatrogenic immunosuppression).[130-134] However, these latter cases are likely distinct from classic LyG and require designation as LPD associated with immune deficiency and dysregulation.[34] LyG presents in adulthood, between the fourth and sixth decade of life, and rarely occurs in children. The male-to-female ratio is approximately 2:1 and there is no racial predisposition.[132,133,135-138]

Clinical Features

LyG is virtually always an extranodal disease, with nearly all patients presenting with bilateral lung involvement. Other common sites include central nervous system (CNS; 40%), skin (34%), kidneys (19%), and liver (17%).[132,133,136,138] Lymph node, spleen, and bone marrow are spared at diagnosis and thus, LyG diagnosis should be questioned if lymph nodes are involved.[133] Presenting symptoms are often insidious (i.e., fever, cough, dyspnea, or chest pain) and the lung lesions may wax and wane, leading to delay in diagnosis. Pulmonary imaging usually shows multiple bilateral lung nodules, frequently in the middle and lower

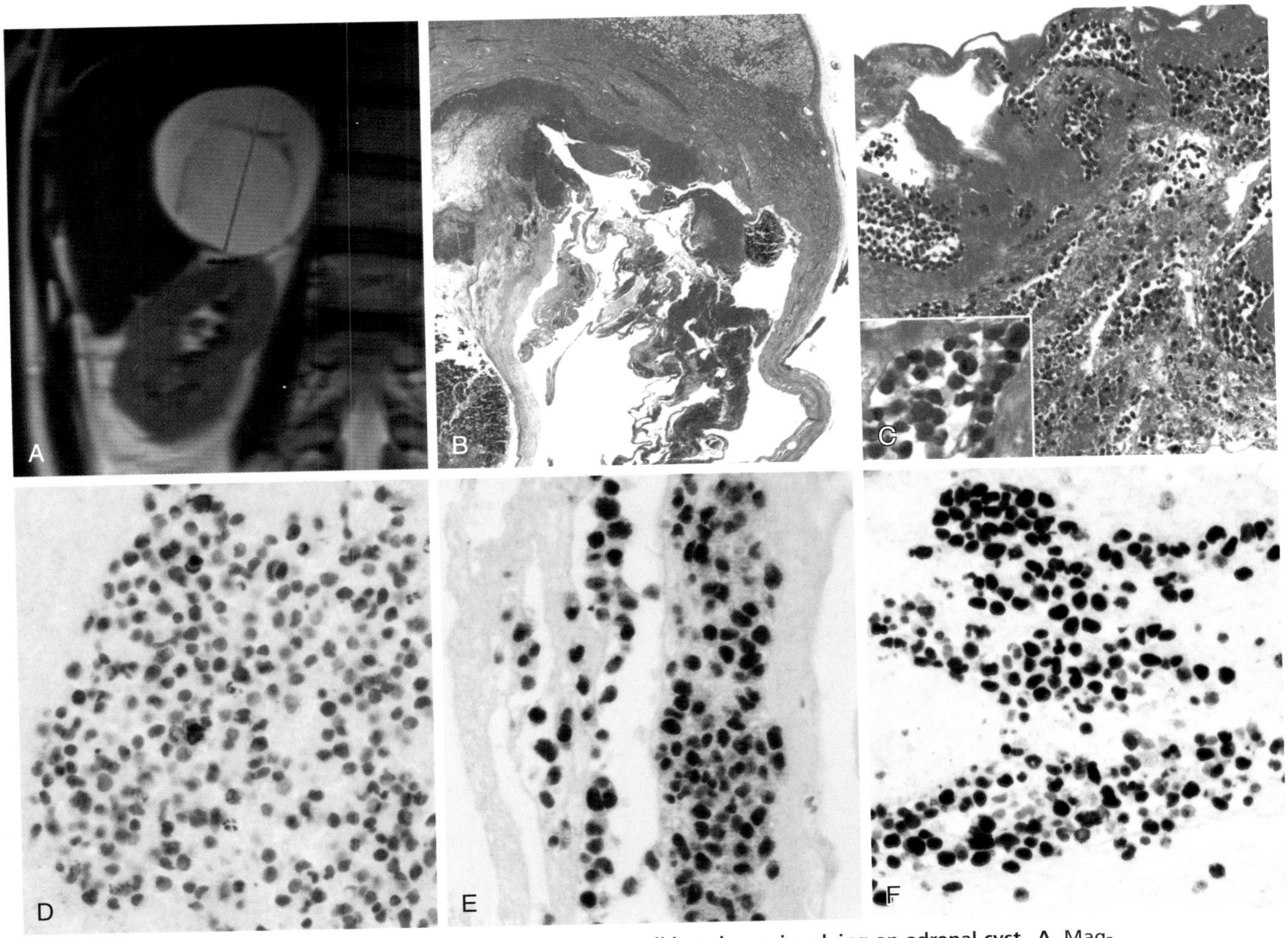

Figure 28-8. Fibrin-associated diffuse large B-cell lymphoma involving an adrenal cyst. A, Magnetic resonance image identified a 10-cm cyst with false membranes and no other associated lesion. **B,** Thick, hyalinized fibrous wall with no luminal lining and entrapped adrenal cortical cells. The lumen of the pseudocyst was filled with fibrin, blood, necrotic debris, and degenerative calcification. **C,** Nests of atypical medium-sized lymphocytes, with round nuclei, dense chromatin, and scant cytoplasm *(inset)* embedded in an abundant fibrinous background, with no infiltration of the fibrous wall. **D,** They were negative for CD20, but strongly expressed PAX5 **(E). F,** The atypical lymphocytes showed an EBV latency III, with expression of EBNA2.

lobes. The nodular lesions are variable in size, usually with peribronchial and vascular distribution, and may display necrosis or cavitation (Fig. 28-9).[132,133,136] CNS involvement on magnetic resonance imaging may show mass lesions or multiple cortical infarcts and has been associated with a poor prognosis.[133,135,136] Though these patients may initially be asymptomatic, confusion, dementia, ataxia, hemiparesis, and seizures or cranial nerve–related signs are likely to develop over time. Cutaneous manifestations are heterogeneous and rarely precede the lung lesions. They present often as disseminated erythematous papules or subcutaneous nodules or, less frequently, as indurated plaques (Fig. 28-10).[124,133,135,139,140] Patients show evidence of prior EBV exposure by serology and an often low level of viremia, in contrast to other EBV-driven lymphoproliferative disorders.[133] The clinical behavior is heterogeneous and depends on histologic grade. Although spontaneous regression can be seen, 60% of patients died of disease, with a median overall survival of 14 months.[124]

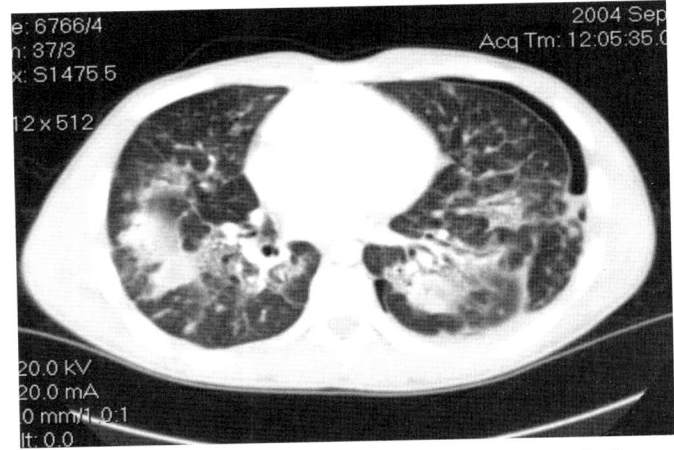

Figure 28-9. Lymphomatoid granulomatosis involving the lungs. Computed tomographic scan shows pulmonary nodules, sometimes with central necrosis, that are seen most often in the lower lung fields.

in a subset of patients. EBV-positive atypical B cells are usually absent in this site.

LyG is divided in three histologic grades based on density of EBV-positive B cells.[127,142] This has prognostic and therapeutic implications, since strategies to improve the host's immune system are usually used for grade 1 and 2 lesions, whereas chemotherapy (DLBCL-like regimens) is required for grade 3 disease.[124] Of note, the number of atypical EBV-positive B cells may vary over time and between sites. Grade 1 lesions are characterized by a polymorphous lymphohistiocytic infiltrate with <5% of large, atypical EBER-positive cells. Focal necrosis is observed in one-third of cases.[133] CD20 stain is useful to highlight the large B-cells. For cases lacking EBV-positive cells, a LyG diagnosis should be made with caution and supported by a high clinical and radiologic suspicion and dense angiocentric T-cell infiltrate. Grade 2 and 3 lesions are morphologically less challenging, as large atypical EBV-positive cells are readily identified. They are usually 5 to 50 cells/high-power field (HPF) in grade 2 and >50 cells/HPF with clusters or aggregates formation in grade 3 (Fig. 28-12).[133] An inflammatory background rich in T cells is always associated and necrosis is common. A uniform population of large atypical EBV-positive cells without a polymorphous inflammatory background should be classified as EBV-positive DLBCL, NOS and is beyond the spectrum of LyG as currently defined.

Phenotypically, the large atypical EBV-positive cells express pan–B-cell markers (CD20, PAX5, or CD79a), are commonly CD30 positive, and lack CD15, which helps in the distinction from CHL. The majority of small lymphocytes are CD3-positive T cells, with a predominance of regulatory CD4+ T cells over CD8+. The EBV latency is type III with expression of LMP-1, EBNA-2, and ZEBRA in most cases.[133] Clonal immunoglobulin gene rearrangement is more commonly demonstrated in grade 2 (50%) and 3 lesions (70%) than in grade 1 LyG (<10%), likely because of the paucity of EBV-positive B cells in the latter.[133] The differential diagnosis of LyG includes other lymphomas and inflammatory and infectious disorders affecting the lung (Box 28-1).

Pathogenesis

LyG pathogenesis is likely the result of local defective immune surveillance by CD8+ cytotoxic T cells and abnormal immune reaction toward EBV. The vasculitic changes and tissue necrosis are related to direct invasion of vessels by inflammatory cells in response to EBV and chemokine mediated (CXCL9 and CXCL10).[124,129] Conversely, a systemic immune response toward EBV likely accounts for the cutaneous manifestations in LyG based on the paucity of EBV-positive B-cells and granuloma formation.

Epstein-Barr Virus–Positive Polymorphic B-Cell Lymphoproliferative Disorder, NOS

The use of this term should be limited to the B-cell proliferations that do not fulfill the criteria of a well-defined EBV-positive lymphoma entity and show altered tissue architecture. Most of these cases will fall between EBV reactivation (i.e., a reactive node with preserved architecture and focal EBV positive B cells) and EBV-positive DLBCL, NOS. Some of the cases previously diagnosed as chronic active EBV disease of B-cell type may also fall in this category. This term may also apply

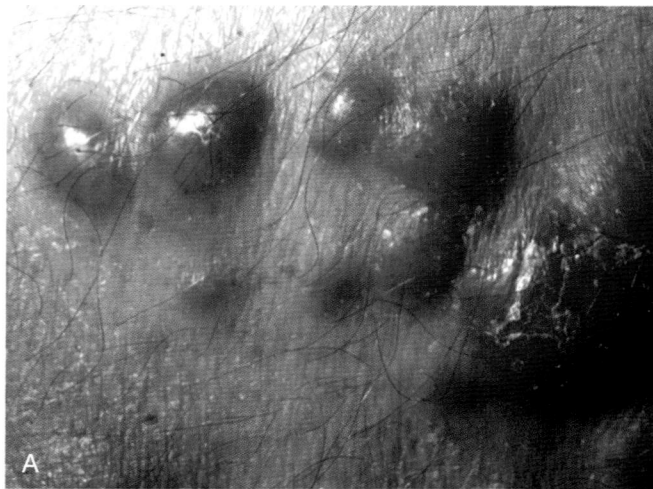

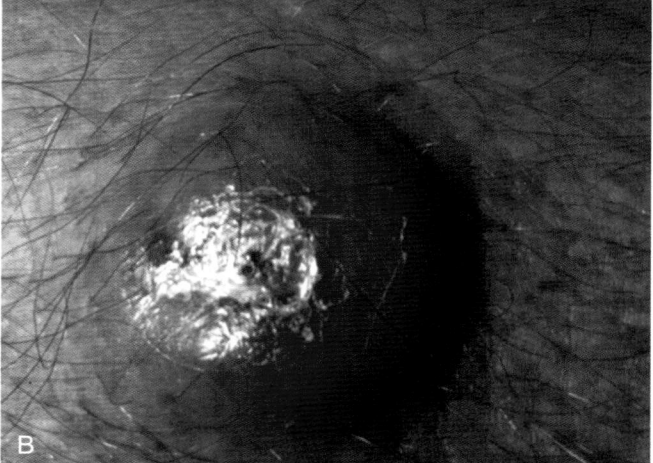

Figure 28-10. Cutaneous manifestations of lymphomatoid granulomatosis. A, Papulonodular lesions are common. **B,** Larger nodules may show ulceration.

Pathology

An adequate, usually excisional biopsy is required for an accurate diagnosis and grading of LyG. The most typical histologic features are observed in the lung nodules. All lesions are angiocentric, with various degrees of angioinvasion and angiodestruction of small-to-medium caliber vessels. The infiltrate is polymorphous with admixture of small lymphocytes, histiocytes, and variable numbers of large atypical lymphoid cells. Plasma cells, when present, are not prominent; neutrophils, eosinophils, multinucleated giant cells, and well-formed granulomas are not seen. Necrosis is common and varies in extent. It is coagulative, often centered on vessels, and contains nuclear debris, but no neutrophils as opposed to necrotizing lesions of WG (Fig. 28-11).[141] The EBV-positive B cells, the hallmark of LyG, are medium-to-large in size, and may resemble immunoblasts and occasionally HRS cells. Similar findings are seen in the brain, kidney, and liver lesions.[140] In the skin, the subcutaneous lesions resemble a lymphohistiocytic panniculitis with or without multinucleated giant cells, granulomas, and foci of necrosis. Nonspecific plaquelike lesions with a sparse, superficial dermal periadnexal and perivascular lymphoid infiltrate reminiscent of lichen sclerosus et atrophicus can be observed

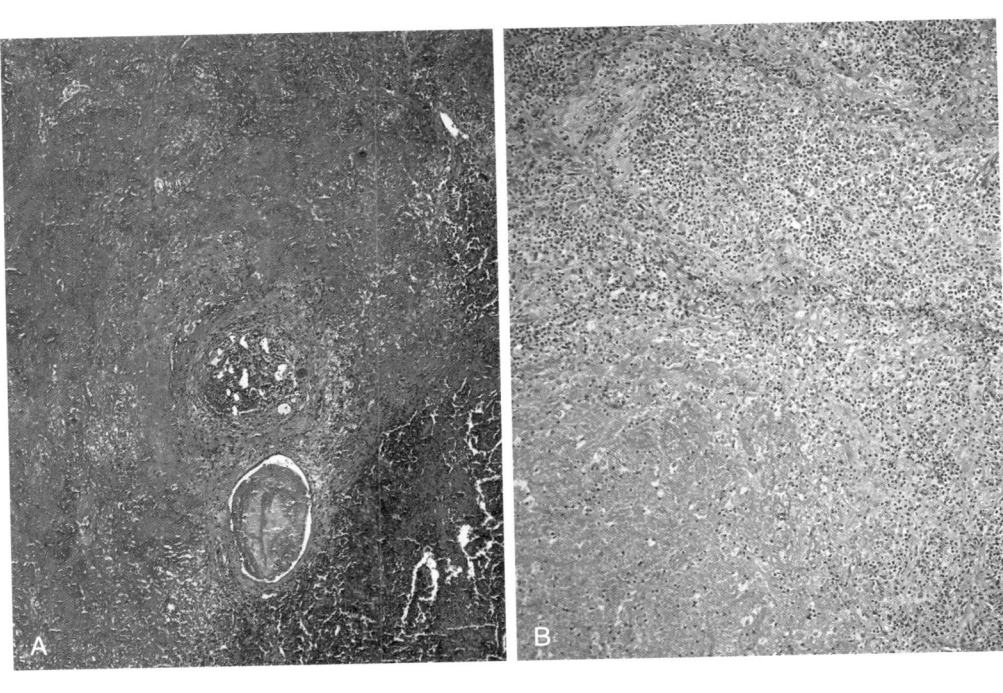

Figure 28-11. Vascular involvement in lymphomatoid granulomatosis. A, Necrotic nodules often contain occluded or damaged blood vessels surrounded by a dense lymphoid infiltrate. **B,** Vessels show medial and intimal infiltration by lymphocytes. Adjacent lung parenchyma is necrotic.

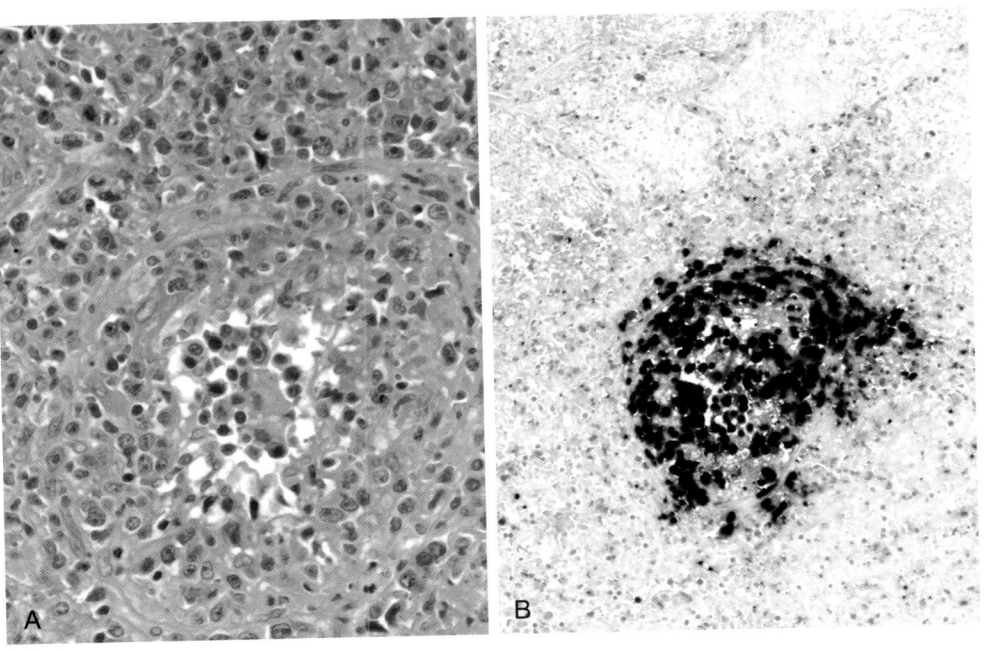

Figure 28-12. Grade 3 lymphomatoid granulomatosis. A, Numerous large lymphoid cells admixed with some histiocytes infiltrating the blood vessels. **B,** Epstein-Barr virus (EBV)–encoded RNA in situ hybridization from the same case. Viable atypical cells are uniformly positive for EBV. Large necrotic areas are nonreactive owing to poor RNA preservation.

to situations when there is uncertainty about the diagnosis because of limited and poor-quality material.

Table 28-1 summarizes the key features of EBV-related B-cell lymphoproliferations including EBVMCU, EBV-positive DLBCL, NOS, DLBCL-CI, LyG, FA-DLBCL, and plasmablastic lymphoma (detailed in Chapter 24).

HHV-8-ASSOCIATED LYMPHOPROLIFERATIVE DISORDERS

HHV-8 Life Cycle and Pathogenesis

KSHV, also known as HHV-8, is endemic in sub-Saharan Africa, the Mediterranean basin, and parts of South America.[143] It was identified in 1994 in AIDS patients with Kaposi sarcoma

by representational difference analysis (RDA), which allowed recognition of two DNA sequences (KS330 Bam and KS631 Bam) unique to this virus.[144,145] HHV-8 is transmitted by saliva, and mainly acquired during childhood and sexual intercourse (predominantly between men). Similar to EBV, it has latency and lytic replication phases, defined by different viral gene expression. During the latency phase, HHV-8 genome (165 kB double-stranded DNA) persists as a circular episome in the host CD19-positive B-cell nuclei.[146,147] It expresses proteins, some homologous to human, that hijack host mechanisms of viral detection and elimination, allowing for asymptomatic lifelong persistence in immune competent individuals. The lytic cycle enables virion production, with the entire HHV-8 genome transcribed. This state facilitates not only virus transmission but also its exposure to host

Posttransplant Lymphoproliferative Disorder
- B-cell rich rather than B-cell poor
- T-cell presence is variable
- Pattern of coagulative necrosis may be similar
- History of iatrogenic immunosuppression

Classic Hodgkin Lymphoma
- HRS cells in a background of lymphocytes, histiocytes, plasma cells, and eosinophils
- HRS cells may be EBER positive or EBER negative
- HRS cells CD30+, CD15+, CD20−/+, PAX5+, CD79a−

DLBCL Associated With Chronic Inflammation (Pyothorax-Associated Lymphoma)
- Pleura-based lesion without primary pulmonary involvement
- EBV-positive large B cells with minimal inflammatory background
- History of tuberculosis or other cause of chronic fibrosing infection

Extranodal NK/T-Cell Lymphoma, Nasal Type
- Lymphoid infiltrate with prominent necrosis may resemble lymphomatoid granulomatosis
- EBV positive, but lacks B-cell markers
- Cells express CD3, CD56, and cytotoxic markers

Peripheral T-Cell Lymphoma, NOS
- Atypical mature T-cell infiltrate, either CD4 positive or CD8 positive
- T cells show cytologic atypia

- Clonal T-cell receptor gene rearrangement positive
- EBER-positive cells absent or rare
- Lymph node involvement or other evidence of systemic disease often present

Inflammatory Pseudotumor of the Lung
- Usually a single pulmonary lesion
- Mixed inflammatory infiltrate without atypia
- Polyclonal plasma cells abundant
- Fibrosis common, but necrosis absent

Wegener's Granulomatosis
- Areas of geographic necrosis surrounded by palisading granulomas
- Inflammatory infiltrate contains abundant neutrophils, including neutrophilic microabscesses
- Fibrinoid vascular necrosis is uncommon
- Capillaritis is a helpful diagnostic feature

Allergic Angiitis and Granulomatosis (Churg-Strauss Syndrome)
- Necrotizing vasculitis with eosinophilic pneumonia
- Granulomatous inflammation with giant cells
- Lymphocytes relatively sparse
- Changes of chronic asthma in bronchioles

Interstitial Pneumonia
- Underlying lung architecture intact without nodular lesions
- Interstitial infiltrate of lymphocytes, histiocytes, and fibroblasts; varies according to type of primary pathology

DLBCL, Diffuse large B-cell lymphoma; *EBER,* Epstein-Barr virus–encoded RNA; *EBV,* Epstein-Barr virus; *HRS,* Hodgkin and Reed-Sternberg; *NK,* natural killer; *NOS,* not otherwise specified.

immune detection. Both latent and lytic gene products are involved in HHV-8 pathogenesis. Latency-associated nuclear antigen (LANA/ORF73), viral cyclin (vCyclin), viral FLICE inhibitory protein (vFLIP), Kaposins (K12), viral miRNA, and viral interferon regularity factor 3 (vIRF3/LANA2) are essential for maintenance of HHV-8 latent infection, cell survival, proliferation, and angiogenesis.[148] Moreover, latently infected cells produce extracellular vesicles that shape the phenotype of adjacent uninfected cells.[149] Lytic-infected cells generate viral IL-6 (vIL-6; a homolog of human IL-6), viral G protein–coupled receptor (vGPCR), and viral interferon regulatory factor 1 (vIRF1). These products enhance B-cell proliferation and differentiation, aberrant angiogenesis, differentiation of blood to lymphatic endothelial cells, and immune evasion.[148,150,151]

Although HHV-8 continuous presence is required for tumor growth, infection alone is insufficient to induce tumorigenesis and other cofactors are needed. These mostly include iatrogenic immune suppression, coinfections (HIV), and genetic predisposition, which lead to inadequate T-cell surveillance and inflammation. Polymorphisms in specific HLA subtypes or in genes regulating immune responses might contribute to the susceptibility to develop this disease.[152,153] Therefore, HHV-8 causes a spectrum of lymphoid proliferations only in a small subset of individuals, ranging from reactive lymphoid hyperplasia to overt lymphoma. These include HHV-8-positive germinotropic lymphoproliferative disorder (GLPD), primary effusion/extracavitary lymphoma (PEL/EC-PEL), and HHV-8-positive diffuse large B-cell lymphoma, NOS (HHV-8+DLBCL). Most, except GLPD, occur in

severely immunocompromised individuals. HHV-8 can also trigger Kaposi sarcoma inflammatory cytokine syndrome, bone marrow failure, and hepatitis. It has become apparent that the morphologic spectrum of HHV-8-related lymphoid proliferations is broader than previously recognized, and there may be considerable overlap between these entities.[34,57,154,155] For example, it may be difficult to differentiate between EC-PEL and HHV-8-positive DLBCL, NOS. An accurate diagnosis of each HHV-8-related LPD is reached by correlation with clinical and pathologic findings, including virus identification in formalin-fixed paraffin embedded (FFPE) tissue sections using an antibody to LANA.

Multicentric Castleman Disease

Definition of the Disease

HHV-8-associated multicentric Castleman disease (HHV-8-MCD) is a tumor-like lesion with B-cell predominance[57] with similar morphology to idiopathic MCD (discussed in more detail in Chapter 8). Likewise, it may manifest inflammatory symptoms caused by hypercytokinemia. A characteristic feature is the presence of HHV-8-infected plasmablasts demonstrated by staining for HHV-8 LANA. Particularly important are IL-6 produced by the virus (vIL-6), in addition to human interleukin-6 (huIL-6) and IL10.[150,156-158] Viral IL-6 promotes cell proliferation, angiogenesis, and human IL-6 secretion.[154] Linked to elevated HHV-8 viral load and cytokine levels, patients present with recurrent flares of inflammatory symptoms, widespread lymphadenopathy (axillary, abdominal,

Table 28-1 Key Features and Phenotype in EBV-Related B-Cell Lymphoproliferative Diseases

Condition	Plasmablastic Lymphoma*	EBV+ DLBCL, NOS	DLBCL-CI	Lymphomatoid Granulomatosis	EBVMCU	FA-DLBCL
Gender/Age	Male-to-female ratio of 3:1, median age 42 years (55 years in HIV negative)	Male-to-female ratio of 1.5–3.6:1; peak seventh to eighth decade, smaller peak third decade	Male-to-female ratio of >9:1; seventh decade	Male-to-female ratio of 2:1; fourth to sixth decade	Male-to-female ratio of 1:1.6; median age 71 years (range 0.5–101 years)	Male-to-female ratio of 2.5:1; median age 60 (range 25–96 years)
Clinical	Symptoms dependent on location	B symptoms common	History of TB related pyothorax, chest pain, fever, cough, dyspnea, chest wall mass; or chronic osteomyelitis, venous ulcers, metallic joint prostheses, and surgical mesh implants	Respiratory symptoms (cough, dyspnea, chest pain), skin lesions, or neurologic symptoms; no LAD	Solitary, well-circumscribed, painful ulcer at mucosal or cutaneous sites, no LAD nor systemic symptoms	Incidental finding, no mass formation
Anatomic site	Extranodal (head and neck, GI), <10% nodal	LN and extranodal (lung, GI, skin, BM)	Pleural cavity, acquired tissue spaces (bone, joints, skin)	Extranodal (lung, CNS, skin, liver, or kidney)	Oropharynx (70%), GI tract, and skin	Sites of chronic fibrin deposition associated with cardiac myxoma, valves, thrombi, cyst walls, implants
Morphology	Diffuse proliferation of large, immunoblastic or plasmablastic cells, starry-sky pattern	Broad spectrum, diffuse proliferation of large centroblasts, immunoblasts, or HRS-like cells, variably abundant microenvironment (THRBCL-like, CHL-like), angioinvasion and necrosis	Diffuse proliferation of centroblastic or immunoblastic cells; may show plasmacytoid differentiation	Angiocentric and angiodestructive polymorphous infiltrate; variable amount of large cells with centroblastic, immunoblastic, or HRS-like features; reactive background rich in T-cell and histiocytes; necrosis	Circumscribed shallow ulcer demarcated by rim of small T-lymphocytes, polymorphous infiltrate with variable number of large immunoblastic or HRS-like cells; some DLBCL-like; angioinvasion and necrosis	Microscopic foci of large cells with immunoblastic or plasmablastic features in a fibrin exudate; no mass formation and no infiltration of adjacent tissue
Phenotype	CD45⁻/⁺ CD20⁻, CD19⁻, CD79a⁺/⁻, PAX5⁻ CD10⁻/⁺, BCL6⁻, IRF4/MUM1⁺ CD138⁺, CD38⁺ CD30⁻/⁺ Ig light chain+ (often cIgG)	CD45⁺/⁻ Pan–B-cell markers usually + (may show downregulation of ≥1 B-cell antigen) CD10⁻, BCL6⁺/⁻, IRF4/MUM1⁺ (~70%) CD138⁻ CD30⁺, CD15⁻/⁺ Ig light chain –/+	CD45⁺ CD20⁺/⁻, CD19⁺, CD79a⁺/⁻, PAX5⁺ CD10⁻, BCL6⁻/⁺, IRF4/MUM1⁺ CD138⁻/⁺ CD30⁺/⁻ Ig light chain +/–	CD45⁺ Pan–B-cell markers + CD10⁻, BCL6⁺/⁻, IRF4/MUM1⁺ CD138⁻ CD30⁺, CD15⁻ Ig light chain –	CD45⁺ Pan–B-cell markers usually + (may show downregulation of ≥1 B-cell antigen) CD10⁻, BCL6⁺/⁻, IRF4/MUM1⁺ CD138⁻ CD30⁺, CD15⁻/⁺ (up to 50%) Ig light chain –	CD45⁺ Pan–B-cell markers usually + (decreased expression in cases with plasmablastic features) CD10⁻, BCL6⁺/⁻, IRF4/MUM1⁺ CD138⁻/⁺ CD30⁺/⁻ Ig light chain –/+
EBV % and latency type	50–75%; latency I, rare II	100%; latency II or III (7%–36%)	70%; latency III, less often II	100%; latency III, less often II	100%, latency II or III	~100%, latency III
Ig gene rearrangements	Monoclonal	Monoclonal (60%)	Monoclonal	Monoclonal (grade II and III)	Monoclonal (<50%)	Monoclonal

Continued

Table 28-1 Key Features and Phenotype in EBV-Related B-Cell Lymphoproliferative Diseases—cont'd

Condition	Plasmablastic Lymphoma*	EBV+ DLBCL, NOS	DLBCL-CI	Lymphomatoid Granulomatosis	EBVMCU	FA-DLBCL
Genetic alterations	Complex karyotypes; *MYC* rearrangement (>50%); recurrent mutations JAK-STAT, MAPK/ERK, and NOTCH pathways, *TP53*	Recurrent alteration in NFκB, WNT, and IL6/JAK/STAT pathways; 6q deletion (*PRDM1*, *TNFAIP3*); PD-L1/L2 overexpression	High genetic complexity; common *TP53* mutation, *MYC* amplification and *TNFAIP3* deletion	Not identified	Not known	Rare *MYC* rearrangement, mutational landscape not known
HIV	Often (up 60%)	Negative	Negative	Negative	Rare	Negative
Prognosis	Poor	Variable	Poor	Variable, dependent on morphologic grade	Favorable	Favorable

*Detailed in Chapter 24.
BM, Bone marrow; *CHL,* classic Hodgkin lymphoma; *CNS,* central nervous system; *DLBCL,* diffuse large B-cell lymphoma; *DLBCL-CI,* diffuse large B-cell lymphoma associated with chronic inflammation; *EBV,* Epstein-Barr virus; *EBVMCU,* Epstein-Barr virus–positive mucocutaneous ulcer; *FA-DLBCL,* fibrin-associated diffuse large B-cell lymphoma; *GI,* gastrointestinal; *HIV,* human immunodeficiency virus; *HRS,* Hodgkin and Reed-Stenberg; *LAD,* lymphadenopathy; *LN,* lymph node; *TB,* tuberculosis; *THRBCL,* T-cell/histiocyte–rich B-cell lymphoma.

pelvic, mediastinal, cervical), and splenomegaly. Bone marrow involvement occurs in a significant proportion of cases.[159] Common laboratory abnormalities include cytopenias, hypoalbuminemia, hypergammaglobulinemia, and elevated C-reactive protein.[150,154,158]

HHV-8-positive MCD occurs most commonly (~90%) in HIV-infected males (median age of 42 years), who may also manifest Kaposi sarcoma or non-Hodgkin lymphoma.[155,160-163] Its incidence appears to increase in HIV settings, affecting older individuals more frequently, with well-preserved immune function, low HIV viral load, and median CD4-positive T-cell count of 150 to 300 cells/mL.[164] Left untreated, the median survival is 2 years, but improved outcomes are seen with newer therapies including rituximab, anti-IL6, and antiretroviral therapy in HIV-positive patients.[163,165] A subset of these individuals will meet the criteria for TAFRO syndrome, characterized by thrombocytopenia, ascites, fever, reticulin fibrosis in bone marrow, organomegaly, and normal amounts of γ-globulin.[166,167]

Synonyms and Related Terms

WHO revised 4th ed.: Multicentric Castleman disease (with HHV8-positive specified when present)
WHO proposed 5th ed.: KSHV/HHV8-associated multicentric Castleman disease

Pathology

Histology in lymph node and spleen is similar to that seen in idiopathic MCD (see Chapter 8), usually with mixed or plasmacytic patterns. The lymph nodes are variably hypertrophic or atrophic and show hyalinized follicles, interfollicular vascular proliferation, and prominent mature plasma cells in the interfollicular zones (Fig. 28-13A–D), which may contain cytoplasmic inclusions (Russell bodies) or crystalline forms. Follicles may demonstrate "onion-skinning" of mantle cuffs, and prominent penetrating venules typical of Castleman disease. Characteristic plasmablasts are present either singly, in small clusters, or larger aggregates formerly called "microlymphomas." They are located mostly in or close

to the mantle zones of germinal centers, but may be seen in intrafollicular or perifollicular locations.[168,169] Occasionally, foci of Kaposi sarcoma can be seen in the same lymph node. The malignant cells infected with HHV-8 correspond to IgM-producing B cells without somatic hypermutations. The malignant cells of extracavitary PEL may appear similar in appearance, but in that lymphoma, EBV is usually positive, and the immunoglobulin genes are hypermutated. Bone marrow usually show polytypic plasmacytosis, with a variable number of scattered interstitial HHV-8-positive plasmablasts.[159]

Phenotypically, the plasmablasts are LANA positive and monotypic IgM lambda (Fig. 28-13E–F). They usually express CD19, OCT2, CD38, and IRF4/MUM1 and are negative for CD20, PAX5, CD79a, BCL6, CD138, CD30, and EBER. A subset is positive for vIL-6.[170,171] Despite infection of Igκ naïve B cells, HHV-8 induces a BCR revision and phenotypic shift to Igλ expression.[172] The infected cells proliferate and acquire a plasmablastic phenotype mainly in response to IL-6.[169,173] These plasmablasts, although monotypic IgMλ, are polyclonal and do not harbor somatic mutations in the rearranged immunoglobulin genes.[169] Follicles show usually a tight, concentric CD21-positive or CD23-positive follicular dendritic cell meshwork (Fig. 28-13G). The interfollicular plasmacytosis is polytypic for immunoglobulin light chains.

With disease progression, the HHV-8-positive plasmablasts may expand to form clusters or aggregates, within or outside the follicles, which are always λ-restricted (Fig. 28-14) but polyclonal or oligoclonal by PCR analysis.

HHV-8-Positive Germinotropic Lymphoproliferative Disorder

Definition of the Disease and Clinical Features

HHV-8-positive germinotropic lymphoproliferative disorder (GLPD) is a rare lymphoproliferation characterized by colonization of germinal centers by large atypical lymphoid cells positive for HHV-8, and often coinfected with EBV. It usually presents with slow-growing localized

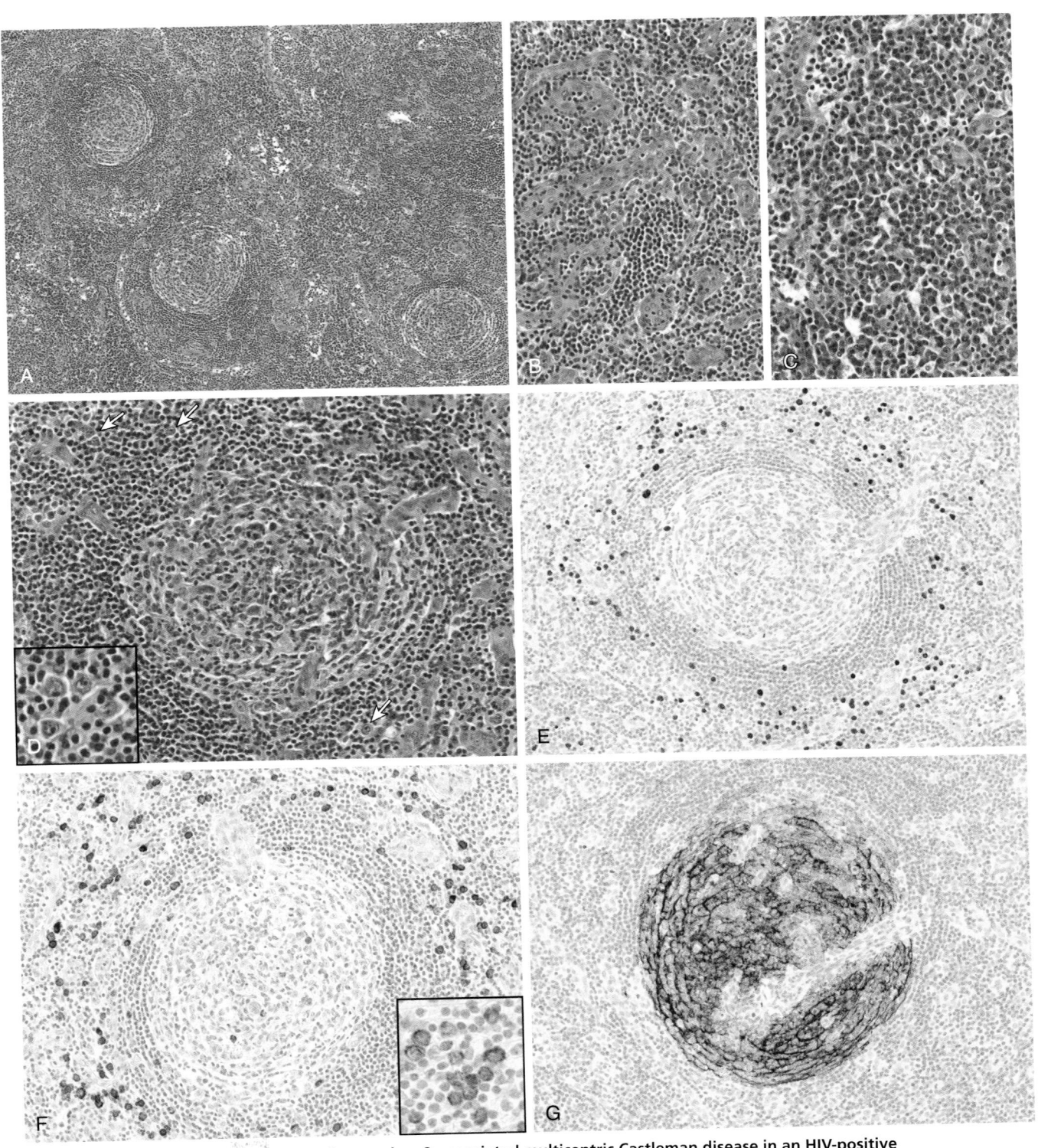

Figure 28-13. Human herpesvirus 8–associated multicentric Castleman disease in an HIV-positive patient. A, The lymph node shows variable atrophic follicles, interfollicular plasmacytosis, and vascular proliferation. **B,** Prominent vascular hyperplasia. **C,** Sheets of mature plasma cells in the medullary cords. **D,** Typical hyaline vascular follicle with a penetrating venule and scattered plasmablasts in the outer part of the mantle zone (*arrows* and *inset*). **E,** Numerous scattered latency-associated nuclear antigen (LANA)–positive plasmablasts close to the mantle cuff. **F,** They are monotypic for IgM heavy chain and lambda light chain *(inset)*. **G,** Follicle with tight concentric CD23-positive follicular dendritic cell meshwork.

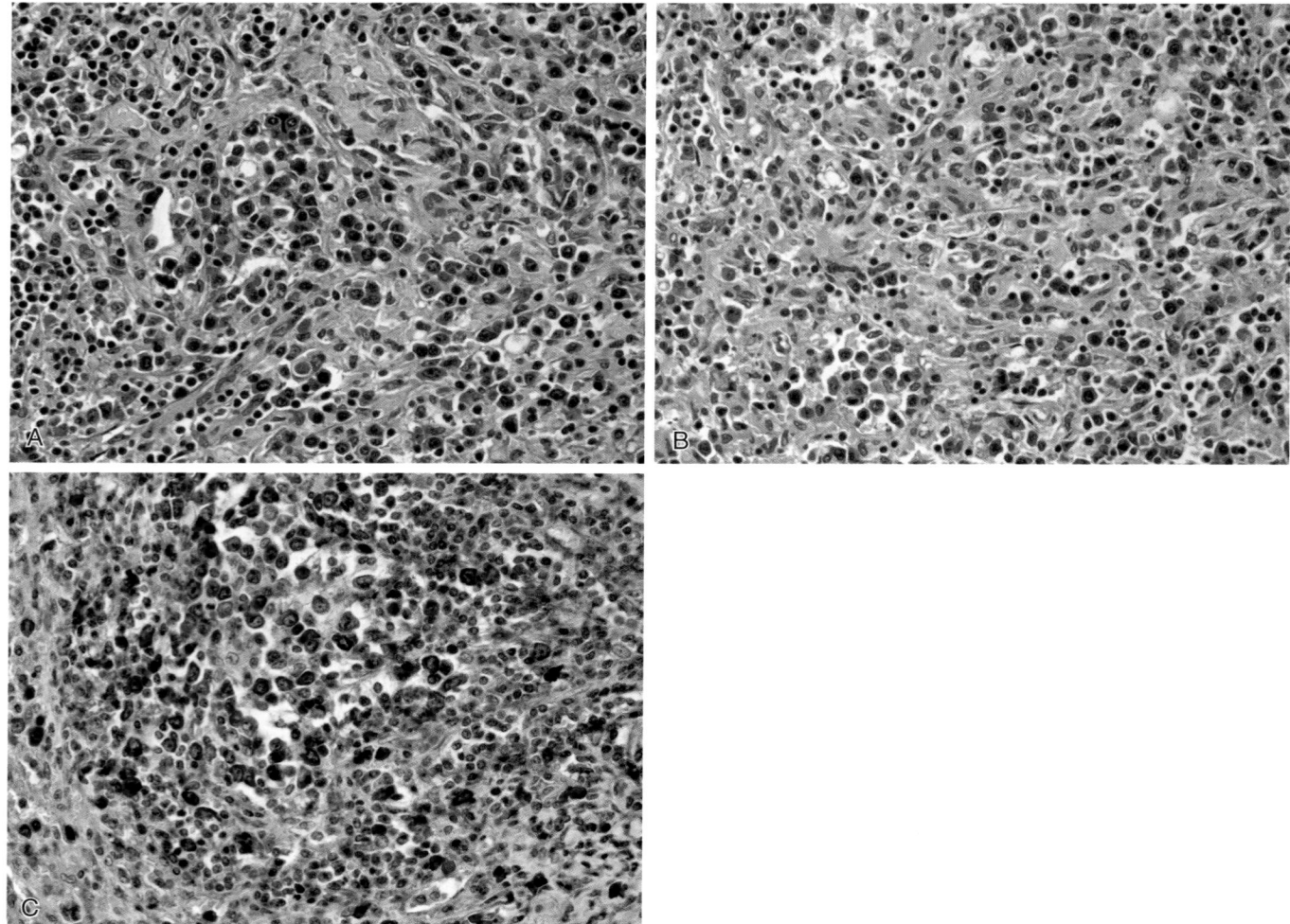

Figure 28-14. Splenic and nodal involvement in a patient with human herpesvirus 8–associated multicentric Castleman disease. Frequent plasmablasts occur in clusters in the spleen **(A)** and infiltrate the lymph node **(B)**. These plasma cells show lambda light-chain restriction but are polyclonal **(C)**.

cervical lymphadenopathy in elderly, immunocompetent patients.[162,171,174-178] It may involve multiple sites without bone marrow disease. Rare cases have been reported in association with HIV, usually in younger males.[176] HHV-8-GLPD follows an indolent course with favorable response and stable disease either untreated or subsequent to radiation, rituximab, or chemotherapy.[178] Rare cases have developed HHV-8-positive or EBV-positive DLBCL, NOS.[176,179]

Synonyms and Related Terms

WHO revised 4th ed.: HHV8-positive germinotropic LPD
WHO proposed 5th ed.: KSHV/HHV8-positive germinotropic LPD

Pathology

Morphologically, the overall lymph node architecture is retained. The germinal centers are variably expanded by large cells with plasmablastic, immunoblastic, or anaplastic features (Fig. 28-15), which may extend into mantle zones, interfollicular areas, and sinuses. Marked interfollicular polytypic plasmacytosis and Castleman-like changes may be observed. The atypical cells are negative for CD45, B-cell antigens (CD19, CD20,

CD79a, PAX5), germinal-center markers, CD138, and CD30. They are usually positive for IRF4/MUM1 and variably express CD38 and EMA. Aberrant CD3 immunostaining can be seen and PD-L1 expression has been reported.[162,176,180] The large cells are enmeshed in CD21-positive follicular dendritic cell meshworks. They show monotypic light chain in most cases, despite common demonstration of a polyclonal pattern of immunoglobulin gene rearrangement with rare monoclonal cases reported in HIV-positive individuals.[162,174,176,178] The atypical cells are coinfected with both HHV-8 and EBV (latency type I) and have somatic hypermutations indicating germinal-center origin. Their genomic alterations are not currently known given the rarity.

HHV-8-Positive Diffuse Large B-Cell Lymphoma, NOS

Definition of the Disease

HHV-8-positive DLBCL, NOS is a large B-cell lymphoma that is HHV-8 positive and does not fulfill the criteria for a primary effusion lymphoma.

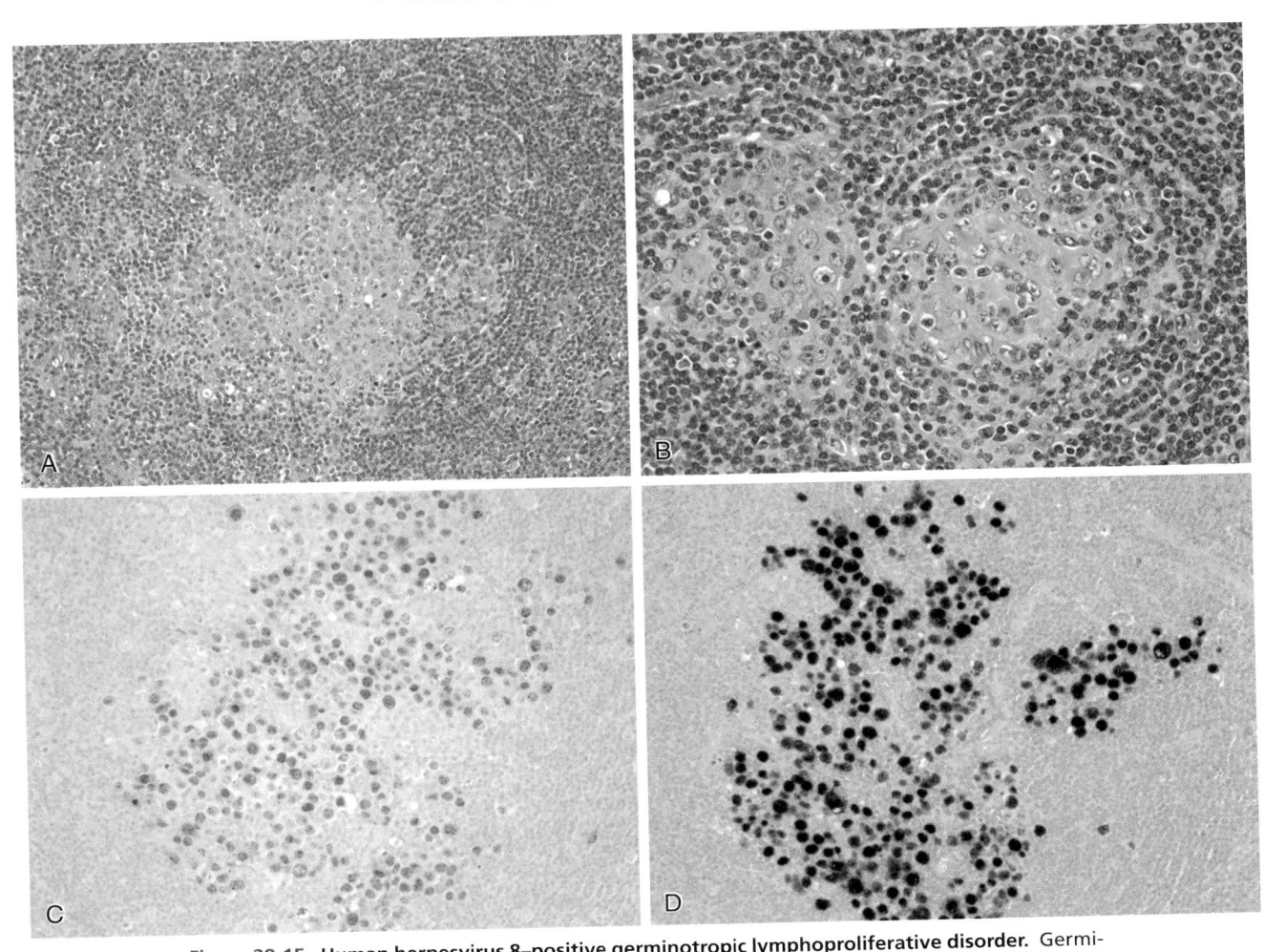

Figure 28-15. Human herpesvirus 8–positive germinotropic lymphoproliferative disorder. Germinal centers and mantle cuff contain large blastic cells (**A** and **B**) that are positive for HHV-8 and EBV (**C** and **D**).

Synonyms and Related Terms

WHO revised 4th ed.: HHV8-positive DLBCL, NOS
WHO proposed 5th ed.: KSHV/HHV8-positive DLBCL

Clinical Features and Pathology

This aggressive neoplasm mainly occurs in HIV-positive males aged 30 to 40 years. It is frequently associated with Kaposi sarcoma or HHV-8-associated MCD. It involves lymph nodes and spleen, and occasionally spreads to extranodal sites including bone marrow and peripheral blood.[160,162,168,171,179] The architecture is effaced by sheets or confluent clusters of plasmablasts or immunoblasts, which are HHV-8-positive (Fig. 28-16). EBER is usually negative, but positive cases have been reported.[162,181] The malignant cells resemble immunoblasts or plasmablasts, and have vesicular nuclei, one or more prominent nucleoli, and amphophilic cytoplasm. Rare cases mimic intravascular or Hodgkin lymphoma.[179,182]

The phenotype is similar to the HHV-8 positive plasmablasts in MCD, but they are monoclonal B-cells and express IRF4/MUM1, IgM, and λ light chain. They are variably positive for CD45, B-cell markers (CD20, CD79a), and CD30, and lack PAX5, CD138, and CD38.[162,171,179] Unlike MCD, the plasmablasts demonstrate monoclonal IGH rearrangement, but lack somatic hypermutations. This lymphoma is thought

to arise from naïve B cells (IgM positive, CD27 negative, and CD138 negative) with nonmutated Ig variable region genes.[183] It may be challenging to distinguish HHV-8-positive DLBCL from extracavitary PEL. However, the neoplastic cells in PEL are hypermutated, usually EBV positive and CD138 positive, and lack cytoplasmic immunoglobulin expression.

Primary Effusion Lymphoma

Definition of the Disease

Primary effusion lymphoma (PEL) is a B-cell neoplasm characterized by malignant effusions, usually involving pleural, peritoneal, or pericardial cavities, without a detectable tumor mass. In some cases, a mass may be present directly related to the body cavity such as a pleural-based mass. PEL is always positive for HHV-8, and usually coinfected with EBV. EC-PEL is a related entity presenting with a tumor mass in the absence of effusion. The association between HHV-8 and PEL was first demonstrated by screening a large group of HIV-related lymphomas with molecular techniques.[184] HHV-8 sequences are present in greater copy number compared with Kaposi sarcoma cases. By electron microscopy, viral

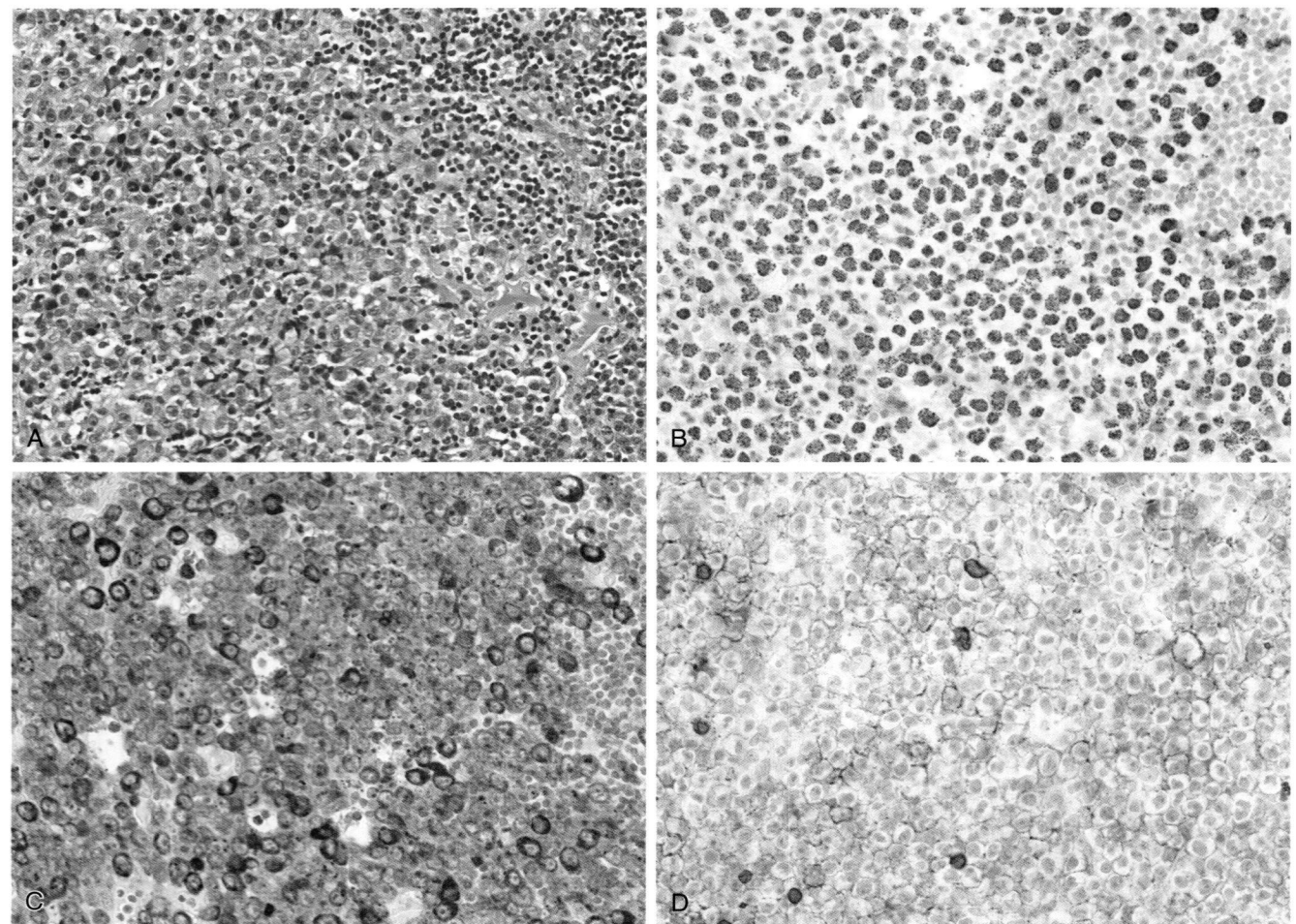

Figure 28-16. Human herpesvirus 8–positive diffuse large B-cell lymphoma, not otherwise specified in a patient with multicentric Castleman disease. A, Sheets of large immunoblasts and plasmablasts with amphophilic cytoplasm and frequent mitoses are shown. Residual nonatypical lymphocytes and mature plasma cell expansion are also noted. **B,** Large malignant B cells are uniformly infected with HHV-8 as demonstrated by the latency-associated nuclear antigen (LANA) stain. **C,** Lymphoma cells demonstrate monoclonal cytoplasmic IgM staining. **D,** They show focal and weak expression of CD20.

particles (100- to 115-nm capsids with central cores) can readily be identified within the nucleus and cytoplasm of the neoplastic cells (Fig. 28-17A).[185-187] The virus is demonstrated by immunohistochemistry in FFPE tissue sections with an antibody to LANA (Fig. 28-17B).

Synonyms and Related Terms

None.

Epidemiology and Clinical Features

Most cases occur in immunocompromised individuals with HIV infection, and PEL accounts for 1% to 4% of HIV-related lymphomas. Male homosexual contact and IV drug use are among the most common risk factors.[188,189] It has also been documented after bone marrow or solid organ transplantation.[171,190-194] Rare cases occurred in elderly patients (median age 73 years) without a setting of immunosuppression other than age, most often originating from regions endemic for HHV-8, such as the Mediterranean and sub-Saharan Africa.[195-198] It is more prevalent in men (90%), with a median age of 55 years. Patients are usually severely immunosuppressed (CD4-positive T cells ≤200 × 10⁶/L) and most have prior AIDS manifestations, including opportunistic infections.[199,200] At presentation, 30% to 50% of patients may have Kaposi sarcoma or MCD.[155,199,201,202]

Neoplastic effusions are usually localized to a single body cavity (pleural, pericardial, or peritoneal), without a contiguous or extracavitary tumor mass.[201,203-205] Symptoms vary from dyspnea and chest pain to heart failure and abdominal distension caused by ascites. Extension to adjacent organs (lung, soft tissues, and regional nodes) or to bone marrow may occur in advanced disease.[206] A subset of patients experiences KSHV inflammatory cytokine syndrome (KICS) with increased KSHV/HHV-8 viral load, IL-6, vIL-6, IL-10, hypoalbuminemia, and thrombocytopenia.[155,207] The prognosis is poor, but chemotherapy and antiretroviral therapy have resulted in improved outcome.[155,188,199,200,208,209] EBV positivity has been associated with better survival in HIV patients with PEL.[155]

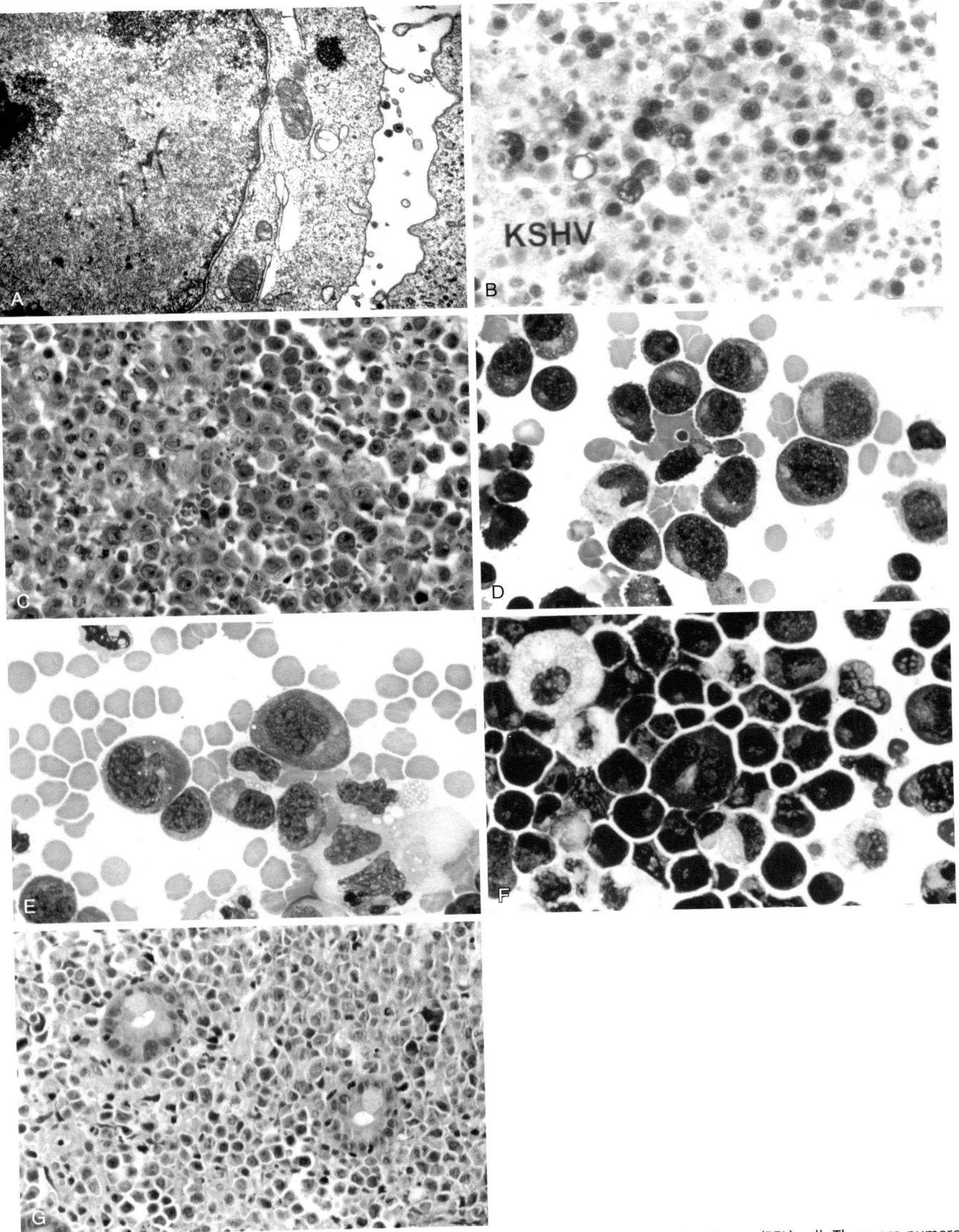

Figure 28-17. Primary effusion lymphoma. A, Ultrastructural appearance of primary effusion lymphoma (PEL) cell. There are numerous herpesvirus particles in the nucleus and cytoplasm, with complete virions being shed from the cell surface (uranyl acetate, lead citrate). **B,** Kaposi sarcoma-associated herpesvirus (KSHV) label on image indicates PEL cells stained for human herpesvirus 8 (HHV-8) latency-associated nuclear antigen (LANA-1/ORF-73) by immunoperoxidase technique in a cell button from pleural fluid (hematoxylin counter-stain). **C,** Cell button shows large pleomorphic cells with prominent nucleoli. **D,** Effusion shows plasmacytoid cells with large blastic nuclei (Giemsa stain). **E,** Effusion shows cells with features of plasmacytoid immunoblasts and anaplastic large cell lymphoma. **F,** PEL exhibits anaplastic and Reed-Sternberg–like cells (Giemsa stain). **G,** HHV-8-positive extracavitary primary effusion lymphoma of the bowel is shown.

Pathology

PEL is typically diagnosed by cytologic examination of effusion fluid. Cells are large or display a marked variation in cell size and range from immunoblastic or plasmablastic to more anaplastic morphology. They show polyploid and lobated nuclei, prominent nucleoli, and abundant basophilic cytoplasm, sometimes with paranuclear Golgi hof and vacuoles (Fig. 28-17C–E). Occasional multinucleated Reed-Sternberg–like cells may be seen (Fig. 28-17F). Phagocytic macrophages and mitotic figures are numerous. Similar morphologic features are observed in the associated solid-tumor masses, but the marked polymorphism seen in cytology may be less evident in the tissue sections.[210]

Immunophenotypically, the neoplastic cells are usually CD45 positive, but lack surface and cytoplasmic immunoglobulins. CD45-negative cases may be mistaken for carcinoma. As reflection of post–germinal-center B-cell origin and plasmablastic differentiation, PEL cells usually express CD38, CD138, VS38c, IRF4/MUM1, and BLIMP1 and lack pan–B-cell antigens (CD20, CD19, CD79a, OCT2, BOB.1, and PAX5).[162,171,201,210-212] They commonly express activation-associated antigens, such as HLA-DR and CD30 (70%), and variably EMA.[213] Rare cases of PEL may show aberrant expression of T-cell markers or focal positivity for keratins.[187,199,214-216] They are usually BCL6 negative and have a high Ki67 proliferation index. By definition, the neoplastic cells are LANA positive, with a subset of cells labeled by vIL-6. In HIV patients, EBV-infected tumor cells disclose a latency type I pattern (EBER⁺EBNA1⁺LMP1⁻EBNA2⁻). Flow cytometry analysis may suggest PEL diagnosis, but a definitive diagnosis requires demonstration of HHV-8.[217]

Pathogenesis

HHV-8 is the etiologic agent in PEL and most tumor cells express a latent viral pattern, with a subset showing lytic phase genes.[218] The viral latent proteins LANA-1, LANA-2 (vIRF3), vCyclin D1, vFLIP, Kaposin B, and v-IL6 are considered to play important roles in oncogenesis.[154,189,219,220] In addition, the neoplastic cells show strong genetic dependency on cellular *IRF4, MDM2, CCND2, MCL1*, and *CFLAR* (c-FLIP).[221] However, HHV-8 alone is not able to transform mature B cells in culture and abnormalities of host immunity are critical pathogenetic players.[155,199,222-224] There is evidence that PEL may be poorly controlled in vivo because of inefficient recognition and killing by the T cells.[225] In addition, LANA-2 and PD-L1 expression contribute to neoplastic cells immune evasion.[77,226] Furthermore, proteins specifically involved in the inflammatory/immune response were enriched in the PEL secretome (cell-conditioning media) by proteomic analysis.[227,228] In HIV-positive patients, PEL is almost invariably associated with EBV, but EBV is not required for its pathogenesis.[221,229,230] Interestingly, despite the EBV genetic variability, individual PEL cases harbor a single EBV strain, consistent with monoclonality of infection, and suggesting that EBV infection preceded clonal expansion.[231]

Genetics

Immunoglobulin genes are clonally rearranged in most cases.[187,218] Cytogenetic studies reveal complex chromosomal abnormalities, with recurrent trisomy 7, trisomy 12, and aberrations in the proximal long arm of chromosome 1 (1q), but no *MYC* or *BCL6* gene rearrangements.[199,201,232,233] The gene-expression signature in PEL is closely related to plasmablastic differentiation and shows overexpression of genes involved in inflammation, cell adhesion, or invasion.[234-236] A downregulation of tumor suppressor miRNAs such as miR-155, miR-220/221, or let-7 family has been reported.[237] The mutational signature of PEL cell lines is dominated by the overactivity of the *APOBEC* gene family (APOBEC3B and APOBEC3B3C) engaged in innate immune defense against viruses.[238] In addition, PEL tumor cells show recurrent interleukin 1 receptor-associated kinase 1 (IRAK1) Phe196Ser mutation, which is essential for PEL survival in vitro and provides reasoning for therapeutic use of IRAK1/4 inhibitors.[239,240] Furthermore, strong dependency on cyclin D2 and MCL1 render PEL cell lines sensitive to specific inhibitors.[221]

Differential Diagnosis

Lymphomas presenting as effusions in the absence of a tumor mass are unusual, and only PEL is associated with HHV-8. PALs typically present as a pleural-based mass in elderly males who are HIV negative. Despite the plasmacytoid differentiation, PAL cells express B-markers; most are EBV positive but HHV-8 negative. HHV-8-negative and EBV-negative primary effusion-based lymphoma (WHO proposed 5th ed. *fluid overload-associated large B-cell lymphoma*) is not associated with HHV-8 and occurs in HIV-negative elderly patients (median age 70 years) with fluid overload states such as cirrhosis secondary to hepatitis C infection or cardiac disease.[241-243] It has a better prognosis than PEL. This neoplasm expresses B-cell–associated antigens and, using more loosely defined criteria, a subset of cases have been reported to be EBV positive or demonstrate *MYC* abnormalities.[242,244] Occasionally, plasmablastic lymphoma and Burkitt lymphoma in HIV patients may involve body cavities. PBL may be indistinguishable morphologically and immunophenotypically from PEL, but usually has cytoplasmic immunoglobulin expression and lacks HHV-8. Burkitt lymphoma show a characteristic phenotype, *MYC* gene rearrangement, and is not associated with HHV-8. Distinction of PEL from other cytologic mimickers such as undifferentiated carcinoma, anaplastic large cell lymphoma, plasmablastic myeloma, or ALK-positive large B-cell lymphoma is facilitated by the clinical presentation and immunophenotype. To accurately diagnose PEL, a combination of clinical, morphologic, and phenotypic studies is required, together with confirmation of HHV-8 either by polymerase chain reaction (PCR) or with LANA antibody.

Extracavitary Primary Effusion Lymphoma

EC-PEL manifests as a tumor mass without an effusion. It most often involves lymph nodes, gastrointestinal tract (Fig. 28-17G), skin, and lung, with rare cases described in the CNS and bone marrow.[162,171,183,199,214,242,245-249] It may also localize in intravascular spaces, mimicking a metastatic carcinoma, anaplastic large-cell lymphoma, or intravascular large B-cell lymphoma.[171,179,183,250,251] The demographic and epidemiologic features of extracavitary lesions closely resemble those of PEL, but they appear to affect less-immunosuppressed HIV-infected patients and have a higher

Table 28-2 Key Features and Phenotype in HHV-8-Related B-Cell Lymphoproliferative Diseases

Diagnosis	HHV-8-Associated MCD	HHV-8+ DLBCL, NOS	PEL and EC-PEL	HHV-8+ GLPD
Gender/age	Male-to-female ratio of 2:1; median age 42 years (65 years for HIV−)	Usually males aged 30–50 years	Male predominance; median age 45 years	Male-to-female ratio of 2:1, median age 59 years
Clinical	Generalized lymphadenopathy, splenomegaly, systemic symptoms	Usually patients with HHV-8-associated-MCD; generalized lymphadenopathy, splenomegaly, occasionally extranodal	PEL: effusions body cavities, usually without mass formation EC-PEL: solid tumors (gastrointestinal tract, skin, lungs, lymph nodes), B symptoms	Localized, slow-growing lymphadenopathy
HIV	Most (~90%)	Positive	Most but not all	Most negative
Morphology	Atrophic to hyperplastic follicles; interfollicular vascular proliferation and plasmacytosis, scattered plasmablasts in the mantle zones	Effacement of architecture; sheets of large cells with plasmablastic or immunoblastic morphology	PEL: effusion rich in large pleomorphic cells with plasmablastic, immunoblastic, or anaplastic morphology; EC-PEL: effacement of architecture; sheets of large cells	Conserved architecture; variable expansion of germinal center by large cells with plasmablastic, immunoblastic, or anaplastic morphology
Phenotype	CD20$^{-/+}$, CD79a$^{-/+}$, PAX5$^-$	CD20$^{-/+}$, CD79a$^{-/+}$, PAX5$^-$	Pan–B-cell antigens negative; may be present in EC-PEL	Pan–B-cell antigens usually −
	BCL6$^-$, CD10$^-$	BCL6$^-$, CD10$^-$	BCL6$^-$, CD10$^-$	BCL6$^-$, CD10$^-$
	IRF4/MUM1$^+$, PRDM1/BLIMP1$^+$, CD38$^+$, CD138$^-$	IRF4/MUM1$^+$, PRDM1/BLIMP1$^+$, CD38$^-$, CD138$^-$	IRF4/MUM1$^+$, PRDM1/BLIMP1$^+$, CD38$^{+/-}$, CD138$^{+/-}$	IRF4/MUM1$^+$, PRDM1/BLIMP1$^+$, CD38$^{+/-}$, CD138$^-$
	IgM lambda	IgM lambda	Ig$^-$ in PEL, Ig$^{-/+}$ (25%) EC-PEL	Monotypic kappa or lambda; any heavy chain
	vIL6$^+$ (subset of cells), CD30$^-$	vIL6$^+$ (subset of cells), CD30$^{-/+}$	vIL6$^+$ (subset), CD30$^+$	vIL6$^+$, CD30$^-$
EBER	Negative	Negative	Positive (>80%)	Positive
Ig gene rearrangements	Polyclonal or oligoclonal	Monoclonal	Monoclonal	Polyclonal or oligoclonal
Cell of origin	Naïve B cells/extrafollicular plasmablasts that lack somatic hypermutations	Naïve B cells/extrafollicular plasmablasts that lack somatic hypermutations	Preterminally differentiated B cells with somatic hypermutations	Germinal-center B cells/germinal-center–associated plasmablasts with somatic hypermutations
Prognosis	Variable	Poor	Poor	Favorable

EBER, Epstein-Barr virus–encoded RNA; *EC-PEL*, extracavitary primary effusion lymphoma; *GLPD*, germinotropic lymphoproliferative disorder; *HHV-8*, human herpesvirus 8; *HIV*, human immunodeficiency virus; *Ig*, immunoglobulin; *KSHV*, Kaposi sarcoma-associated herpesvirus; *MCD*, multicentric Castleman disease; *PEL*, primary effusion lymphoma; *vIL6*, viral interleukin 6.

disease-free survival.[199,212] Cells of EC-PEL are similar to PEL but occur in sheets. Lymph node architecture is usually effaced, but involvement may be partial or sinusoidal. The neoplastic cells may lack CD45 and express B-cell antigens (CD20, CD79a) and immunoglobulin more often than the typical PEL.[212,214,249] Similarly, it may show an aberrant expression of T-cell markers, which can lead to misdiagnosis.[199] Overlap may occur between EC-PEL and HHV-8-positive DLBCL, NOS. Unlike other plasmablastic-appearing lymphomas, it contains both EBV and HHV-8.

Table 28-2 contrasts the key features of HHV-8-related lymphoid proliferations including MCD, HHV-8-positive GLPD, HHV-8-positive DLBCL, NOS, PEL, and EC-PEL.

Kaposi Sarcoma Involving Lymph Nodes

Kaposi sarcoma may involve the lymph nodes, even in the absence of skin lesions. This is discussed further in Chapter 57.

Pearls and Pitfalls

- When diagnosing an Epstein-Barr virus (EBV)–related lymphoproliferative disorder, EBV should be expressed by a majority of the atypical cells and not by the background infiltrate.
- Hodgkin/Reed-Sternberg–like cells are commonly present in EBV-related lymphoproliferative disorders, and the differential diagnosis from classic Hodgkin lymphoma may be challenging.
- Chronic active EBV disease is restricted to the T/natural killer (NK)-cell–derived cases.
- EBV-positive diffuse large B-cell lymphoma, not otherwise specified (DLBCL, NOS) can occur at any age, including young patients, without apparent features of immunodeficiency.
- EBV-positive mucocutaneous ulcer should be considered in the differential diagnosis of any solitary EBV-positive lymphoproliferative disorder involving cutaneous or mucosal sites.
- Lymphomatoid granulomatosis requires lung involvement.
- EBV-positive lymphoproliferative disorders may have an aberrant phenotype with expression of T-cell antigens or CD15.
- EBV-positive polymorphic B-cell lymphoproliferative disorder, NOS can be used for EBV related B-cell proliferations that do not fulfill the criteria of a well-defined lymphoma. It should not be used for cases of EBV reactivation or typical cases of infectious mononucleosis. It can be used in cases with insufficient or low-quality material that prevent a more definitive diagnosis.
- HHV-8-positive lymphoproliferative disorders include a spectrum of disorders which may show overlapping features and their differential diagnosis may be difficult.
- Plasmablasts in HHV-8-associated MCD are light-chain restricted and express IgM lambda in all cases, but they are polyclonal.
- Staining for HHV-8 latency-associated nuclear antigen (LANA) is essential to identify primary effusion lymphoma (PEL) and extracavitary PEL cases given that similar morphology may be encountered in other lymphomas, including some that may also present with effusions.
- HHV-8-positive germinotropic lymphoproliferative disorder shares some features with extracavitary PEL, but lacks immunoglobulin gene rearrangements.

KEY REFERENCES

6. Young LS, Yap LF, Murray PG. Epstein-Barr virus: more than 50 years old and still providing surprises. *Nat Rev Cancer.* 2016;16:789–802.
7. Münz C. Latency and lytic replication in Epstein-Barr virus-associated oncogenesis. *Nat Rev Microbiol.* 2019;17:691–700.
27. Cesarman E. Gammaherpesviruses and lymphoproliferative disorders. *Annu Rev Pathol.* 2014;9:349–372.
34. Campo E, Jaffe ES, Cook JR, et al. The International Consensus Classification of Mature Lymphoid Neoplasms: a report from the Clinical Advisory Committee. *Blood.* 2022;140:1229–1253.
36. Dojcinov SD, Venkataraman G, Raffeld M, Pittaluga S, Jaffe ES. EBV positive mucocutaneous ulcer—a study of 26 cases associated with various sources of immunosuppression. *Am J Surg Pathol.* 2010;34:405–417.
54. Nicolae A, Pittaluga S, Abdullah S, et al. EBV-positive large B-cell lymphomas in young patients: a nodal lymphoma with evidence for a tolerogenic immune environment. *Blood.* 2015;126:863–872.
56. Bourbon E, Maucort-Boulch D, Fontaine J, et al. Clinicopathological features and survival in EBV-positive diffuse large B-cell lymphoma not otherwise specified. *Blood Adv.* 2021;5:3227–3239.
57. Alaggio R, Amador C, Anagnostopoulos I, et al. The 5th edition of the World Health Organization classification of haematolymphoid tumours: lymphoid neoplasms. *Leukemia.* 2022;36:1720–1748.
75. Witte HM, Merz H, Biersack H, et al. Impact of treatment variability and clinicopathological characteristics on survival in patients with Epstein-Barr-Virus positive diffuse large B cell lymphoma. *Br J Haematol.* 2020;189:257–268.
113. Boyer DF, McKelvie PA, de Leval L, et al. Fibrin-associated EBV-positive large B-cell lymphoma: an indolent neoplasm with features distinct from diffuse large B-cell lymphoma associated with chronic inflammation. *Am J Surg Pathol.* 2017;41:299–312.
133. Song JY, Pittaluga S, Dunleavy K, et al. Lymphomatoid granulomatosis—a single institute experience: pathologic findings and clinical correlations. *Am J Surg Pathol.* 2015;39:141–156.
155. Lurain K, Polizzotto MN, Aleman K, et al. Viral, immunologic, and clinical features of primary effusion lymphoma. *Blood.* 2019;133:1753–1761.
171. Chadburn A, Said J, Gratzinger D, et al. HHV8/KSHV-positive lymphoproliferative disorders and the spectrum of plasmablastic and plasma cell neoplasms: 2015 SH/EAHP workshop report—part 3. *Am J Clin Pathol.* 2017;147:171–187.
199. Guillet S, Gérard L, Meignin V, et al. Classic and extracavitary primary effusion lymphoma in 51 HIV-infected patients from a single institution. *Am J Hematol.* 2016;91:233–237.
227. Carbone A, Volpi CC, Caccia D, et al. Extracavitary KSHV-positive solid lymphoma: a large B-cell lymphoma within the spectrum of primary effusion lymphoma. *Am J Surg Pathol.* 2013;37:1460–1461.
241. Alexanian S, Said J, Lones M, Pullarkat ST. KSHV/HHV8-negative effusion-based lymphoma, a distinct entity associated with fluid overload states. *Am J Surg Pathol.* 2013;37:241–249.

Visit Elsevier eBooks+ for the complete set of references.

Epstein-Barr Virus–Associated T-Cell and Natural Killer–Cell Lymphoproliferative Disorders

Young Hyeh Ko, John K.C. Chan, and Leticia Quintanilla-Martinez

INTRODUCTION

Epstein-Barr virus (EBV) is a ubiquitous herpesvirus with tropism for B cells. More than 90% of humans are infected with EBV, and the infection persists for life. Usually primary infection is asymptomatic and occurs early in life, and when symptomatic is usually a self-limited disease occurring in adolescents or young adults manifested as acute infectious mononucleosis (AIM). AIM is characterized by a polyclonal expansion of infected B cells and a cytotoxic T-cell response composed of a transient, antigen-driven oligoclonal expansion of CD8-positive T cells. Both the quantity and quality of the CD8-positive T-cell response to EBV are critical to control the infection. In vivo EBV is capable of infecting, in addition to B cells, T cells and natural killer (NK) cells, as well as epithelial and mesenchymal cells. The infection of T cells and NK cells may lead to several EBV-related lymphoproliferative diseases, with disease manifestations generally depending on the type of EBV-infected cells and the state of host immunity.

EBV-positive T-cell and NK-cell lymphoproliferative disorders encompass disease entities with a broad clinicopathologic spectrum. The term *T/NK-cell chronic active EBV infection* has been used in the literature to encompass a broad spectrum of diseases comprising a systemic polyclonal or monoclonal form (T cells; $\alpha\beta$ or $\gamma\delta$ cells, and NK-cells) and a cutaneous form, including hydroa vacciniforme–like lymphoproliferative disorder (usually of T-cell origin) and severe mosquito bite allergy (usually of NK-cell origin).[1-3] The systemic form was termed *chronic active EBV infection* in the early literature and in the 4th and the revised 4th editions of the *WHO Classification of Tumours of Haematopoietic and Lymphoid Tissues* (WHO 4th ed., revised WHO 4th ed.)[4,5] and renamed as *chronic active EBV disease (CAEBVD)* in the *International Consensus Classification* (ICC)[6] and the 5th edition of the *WHO Classification of Tumours of Haematopoietic and Lymphoid Tissues* (WHO 5th ed.)[7]; because around 95% of the world population are chronically, latently infected, but only few acquire the disease, the term *CAEBVD* is preferred.[6]

Hydroa vacciniform lymphoproliferative disease (HVLPD) replaced the term *hydroa vacciniforme-like LPD* of the revised WHO 4th ed.[5] New studies have shown that "classic" HV in Western countries is also associated with EBV, and therefore, all HV cases belong within the spectrum of the same disease.[8-10] In the ICC and WHO 5th ed., HVLPD is divided into a classic and a systemic form based on the presence or absence of severe systemic symptoms.[6,7] Systemic HVLPD eventually might require similar treatment as CAEBVD.

Systemic EBV-positive T-cell lymphoma represents the fulminant form of a clonal EBV-infected T-cell proliferative disease occurring after primary EBV infection or, less often, after CAEBVD. The WHO 4th ed. recognized systemic T-cell lymphoproliferative disorder of childhood as a neoplasm; to clarify the aggressive nature of this disease, the term was changed to *systemic EBV-positive T-cell lymphoma* in the revised WHO 4th ed.[5]

Systemic EBV-positive T-cell lymphoma shares clinical and pathologic features with aggressive NK-cell leukemia, but they differ in the lineage; the former is of T-cell origin, whereas the latter is of NK-cell origin. A rather difficult differential diagnosis and often overlapping disease is EBV-associated hemophagocytic lymphohistiocytosis (HLH) in childhood, which is a hyperinflammatory syndrome induced by dysregulated immune reaction secondary to EBV infection. Although clonal EBV-infected T cells have been demonstrated in some cases, patients usually respond to treatment, which can be limited in some cases, and recover completely after the acute disease.

Aggressive NK-cell leukemia and extranodal NK/T-cell lymphoma, nasal type (ENKTL-NT) are recognized as the prototypes of EBV-positive T-cell or NK-cell lymphoma/leukemia in the WHO 4th ed.[11] ENKTL-NT primarily involves extranodal sites, mainly the upper aerodigestive tract. Primary nodal EBV-positive T/NK-cell lymphoma is an EBV-positive cytotoxic T-cell or NK-cell lymphoma primarily involving the lymph nodes. It is an uncommon disease, now introduced as a provisional entity in the ICC, and as a definitive entity in the WHO 5th ed.[6,7] This chapter details the clinicopathologic features of all these disease entities (Box 29-1).

EPSTEIN-BARR VIRUS–ASSOCIATED HEMOPHAGOCYTIC LYMPHOHISTIOCYTOSIS

Definition

HLH is a clinicopathologic syndrome encompassing a markedly dysregulated immune response and hypercytokinemia. HLH is characterized clinically by fever, splenomegaly, and cytopenias, and is accompanied by histologic evidence of hemophagocytosis, which causes extremely high serum levels of ferritin, lactate dehydrogenase, and soluble CD25.[12,13] (Capsule summary in Box 29-2.) The disease is classified into a primary (genetic) form and a secondary (acquired) form. Secondary HLH occurs in the setting of infection or underlying autoimmune disorders or malignancy. EBV-associated HLH (EBV-HLH) accounts for 36% to 44% of all HLHs and the most common infection-associated HLH.[14-16] The diagnosis is established when EBV is documented in the blood or tissue in addition to fulfilling the criteria in the HLH-2004 guidelines.[12] EBV infection can be associated with primary HLH, CAEBVD, T/NK-cell lymphoma/leukemia, or B-cell lymphoma, which should be excluded by genetic test and pathologic examination (Box 29-2).

Epidemiology

EBV-HLH is a rare disease. In an observational study in Japan, where HLH is common, annual incidence of HLH is 1 in 800,000 and EBV-HLH accounts for 35% of cases of all HLH.[14] EBV is the most common triggering factor for HLH in children.[16] The median age of children with EBV-HLH is 2.6 years and the male-to-female ratio is equal.[17] In adults, EBV accounts for 15.7% to 40% of the triggering factor in HLH.[18,19] Median age of patients is 49 years with male predominance.[19,20]

Most reports of EBV-HLH in children are from East Asian countries[14-16] and in indigenous populations of Mexico and South America.[21-23] It has also been reported in Western countries, but at a much lower frequency.[24,25]

Specific geographic distribution of adult EBV-HLH is similar to that of childhood EBV-HLH. This ethnic and geographic distribution indicates that similar genetic factors

are involved in the development of secondary EBV-HLH as in other EBV-positive T/NK-cell LPDs.

Pathophysiology

EBV-HLH is primarily a CD8-positive T-cell/macrophage-mediated hyperinflammatory immune reaction driven by EBV infection in the absence of appropriate cytotoxic activity.[26] Primary EBV infection is mostly asymptomatic except for AIM, in which EBV infection in B cells leads to polyclonal B-cell expansion accompanied by antigen-driven proliferation of CD8-positive cytotoxic T cells. In EBV-HLH, EBV ectopically infects CD8-positive T cells[27-29] through the CD21 receptor that can be expressed in mature T cells.[30] In normal individuals with EBV-protective immunity, an expanded EBV-specific CD8-positive T-cell pool is contracted concomitant with the fall in circulating virus loads and back to its normal size.[31,32] In patients with EBV-HLH, deficiencies with impaired T-cell cytotoxicity activity/killing of EBV-infected target cells lead to uncontrolled activation and proliferation of antigen-driven CD8-positive T cells.[33] These activated T cells release excessive IFN-gamma, which leads to continual expansion of CD8-positive T cells, histiocytes, and macrophages.[34] Activated T cells and macrophages infiltrate multiple organs and secrete high levels of inflammatory cytokines, including IL1, IL6, tumor necrosis factor (TNF)-α, and IFN-γ, leading to secondary activation of histiocytes and macrophages.[35,36] This cytokine storm leads to cardinal clinical and laboratory features of HLH. The mechanism leading to impaired protective immunity of EBV and uncontrolled proliferation of T cells in secondary HLH is not well understood. The particular prevalence of EBV-HLH in Asian children suggests that underlying genetic factors contribute to the EBV-related dysregulated immune responses. Studies for primary immunodeficiency-mediated EBV-HLH disclose mutations involving T-cell activation or the costimulatory pathway, as well as genetic defects in the component of the lytic granule exocytosis pathway, which leads to impaired elimination of EBV-infected target cells and protracted T-cell expansion and activation.[26,33] Monoallelic or missense mutation of genes involved in lymphocyte cytotoxicity has been observed in 60% of nonimmunosuppressed EBV-HLH in the Chinese population.[37] Cytokine gene polymorphisms involving TGF-beta1, IL2RA, and IL10 are highly associated with susceptibility to EBV-HLH.[38,39]

Clinical Features

EBV-HLH is a systemic illness that is usually first detected as a persistent fever that is unresponsive to antibiotics. Patients with EBV-HLH exhibit cytopenias, liver dysfunction, hepatosplenomegaly, and hemophagocytosis in the bone marrow, lymph node, liver, or spleen. Coagulopathy, pleural effusions/ascites, and central nervous system (CNS) disease can also occur. Elevated triglyceride or ferritin levels, low fibrinogen level,

low or absent NK-cell cytotoxicity, and elevated soluble CD25 are sometimes seen. EBV viral load in peripheral blood is high and correlates well with disease activity. Serologic study shows that young children with EBV-HLH have elevated VCA-IgM, indicating primary EBV infection,[12-14,35] while adult patients have viral antibodies indicative of past infection or reactivation.[20,40]

Morphology

In patients with EBV-HLH, the bone marrow shows hemophagocytic histiocytes and a variable number of EBV-positive T cells in addition to myeloid and erythroid cells (Fig. 29-1). The liver biopsy shows Kupffer cell hyperplasia, mild infiltration of small T cells in the portal tract and sinusoids, and intrasinusoidal infiltration of hemophagocytic histiocytes. Because of minimal histologic changes in the early stage, diagnostic abnormalities may not be detected with hematoxylin and eosin (H&E) stains. EBV-encoded RNA (EBER) in situ hybridization highlights EBER-positive cells in the bone marrow and hepatic sinusoids.

Immunophenotype and Genetics

Cells infiltrating the bone marrow and liver are cytotoxic T cells that express CD8 and granzyme B or, uncommonly, NK cells.[41,42] In peripheral blood, flow-cytometric analysis may show a significant increase in a subpopulation of CD8-positive T cells that exhibit downregulation of CD5.[29] EBV is best

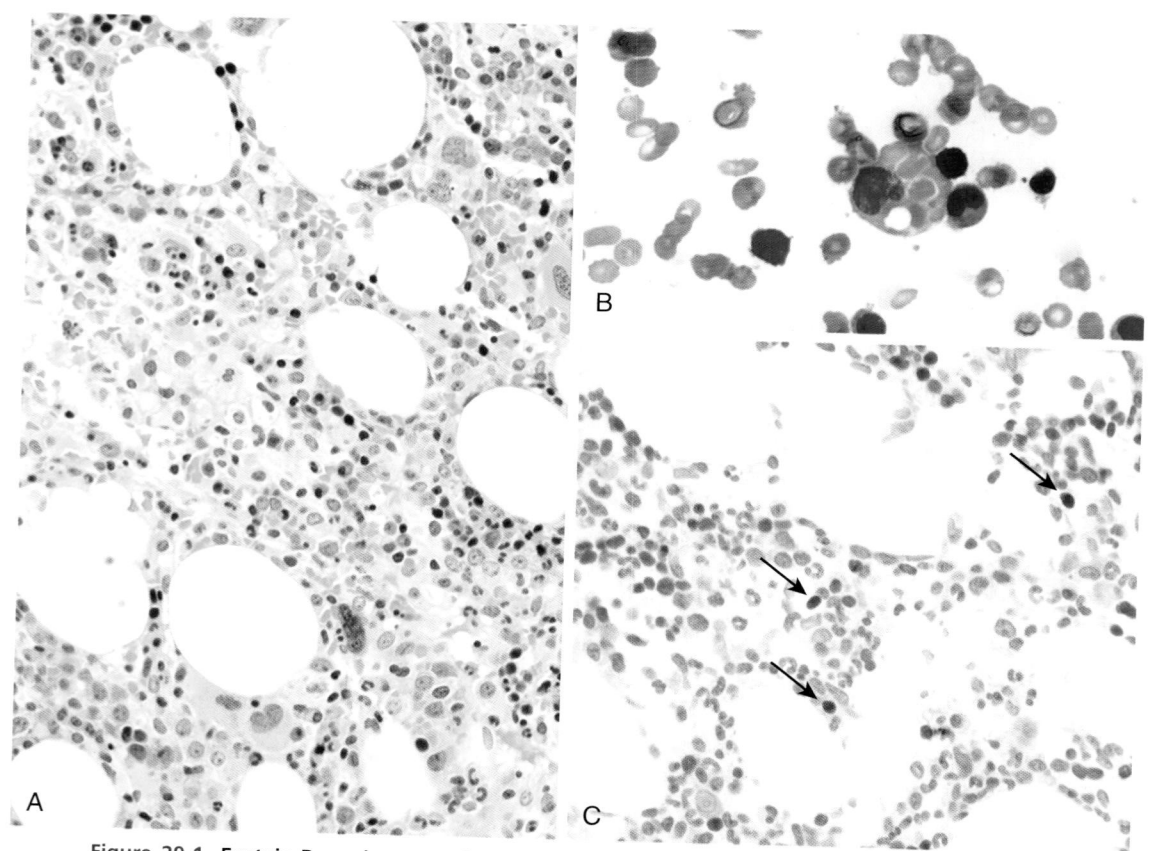

Figure 29-1. Epstein-Barr virus–associated hemophagocytic lymphohistiocytosis. A, Bone marrow shows increased cellularity with normal hematopoietic cells and many histiocytes. **B,** Aspiration smear shows erythrophagocytosis. **C,** Epstein-Barr virus (EBV)–encoded RNA in situ hybridization reveals a few EBV-positive small lymphocytes without atypia.

determined by molecular methods that can detect the presence of EBV genomic DNA or EBER in biological specimens such as serum, bone marrow, or lymph nodes. Antigen-driven CD8-positive T cells in EBV-HLH are commonly monoclonal and can regress with immunoregulatory therapy.[29,43,44]

Postulated Cell of Origin

The postulated cells of origin are EBV-infected CD8-positive cytotoxic T cells and, rarely, NK cells.

Clinical Course and Prognostic Factors

EBV-HLH is a heterogeneous disorder with various symptoms that can range from mild to severe. In the past, a significant proportion of patients died because of cytokine storm or disease progression to CAEBVD or EBV-positive systemic T-cell lymphoma of childhood.[15,45] With the HLH-94/2004 combination treatment including etoposide, dexamethasone, and cyclosporine A, EBV-HLH in children without underlying disease can be effectively controlled in more than 90% of patients. However, the other 10% often die of fulminant disease.[42] Patients with hyperbilirubinemia, hyperferritinemia, renal failure, or CNS hemorrhage at diagnosis, or cytogenetic abnormality, have significantly poorer outcomes. The presence of clonality at the time of diagnosis is not associated with a poor outcome, but a change in clonality may be a good marker of disease activity in childhood EBV-HLH.[42,46] Despite appropriate patient management, the outcome of the adult patients is significantly poorer than the pediatric disease and 46% of patients respond to the HLH-94/2004 regimen.[19,47]

Differential Diagnosis

T/NK-cell leukemia/lymphomas can be complicated with EBV-HLH, but show obvious atypia of infiltrating EBV-positive cells. CAEBVD can present with EBV-HLH. A long clinical history compatible with CAEBVD is helpful in the differential diagnosis. EBV-HLH and systemic EBV-positive T-cell lymphoma of childhood share a significant overlap in clinical presentation and pathologic changes.[48] Because EBV-HLH is frequently associated with clonal T-cell populations, the distinction between these two diseases is challenging. Cytogenetic abnormality may be the only useful marker for distinction.[48,49] Primary HLH that is associated with EBV infection can be excluded by genetic testing and family history.

CHRONIC ACTIVE EPSTEIN-BARR VIRUS DISEASE

Synonyms and Related Terms

WHO revised 4th edition: Chronic active EBV infection of T- and NK-cell type, systemic form
WHO proposed 5th edition: Systemic chronic active EBV disease

Definition

Chronic active EBV disease (CAEBVD) is a systemic EBV-positive polyclonal or monoclonal T-cell or NK-cell lymphoproliferative disorder with a wide range of clinical severity and characterized by intermittent or chronic infectious mononucleosis-like symptoms lasting more than 3 months in patients with no known immunodeficiency.[5] (Capsule summary in Box 29-3.)

CAEBVD was initially proposed by Straus[50] as a severe illness of greater than 6 months duration that (1) begins as a primary EBV infection or is associated with markedly abnormal EBV antibody titers (e.g., anti-EBV viral capsid antigen [VCA] immunoglobulin [Ig]G ≥5120, anti-EBV early antigen IgG ≥640, or anti–Epstein-Barr nuclear antigen [EBNA] <2); (2) shows histologic evidence of major organ involvement, such as interstitial pneumonia, hypoplasia of the bone marrow, uveitis, lymphadenitis, persistent hepatitis, or splenomegaly; and (3) exhibits increased EBV RNA or proteins in affected tissues. Later, Kimura and colleagues proposed modified diagnostic criteria for CAEBVD stipulating that patients should have an EBV-related illness or symptoms lasting more than 3 months' duration and increased EBV DNA ($>10^{2.5}$ copies/µg EBV DNA) in peripheral blood mononuclear cells or RNA in the tissue, or grossly abnormal levels of EBV antibodies.[51] In the initial description, it was always thought that CAEBV was a disorder of B cells, but since then, the cases reported in Japan and East Asia have almost always been associated with a proliferation

---

Box 29-3 *Major Diagnostic Features of Chronic Active Epstein-Barr Virus Disease*

Definition
- CAEBVD is a systemic EBV-positive polyclonal or monoclonal T-cell or NK-cell lymphoproliferative disorder

Diagnostic Criteria
- High viral load in peripheral blood or tissues
- Intermittent or persistent infectious mononucleosis–like symptoms such as fever, lymphadenopathy, and hepatosplenomegaly for at least 3 months
- No known immunodeficiency

Clinical Features and Behavior
- Prevalent in Asia and Latin America
- Most patients are children or young adults (median age, 11.3 years; range, 9 months–53 years); adult patients are not uncommon
- Often accompanied by hydroa vacciniforme LPD or severe mosquito bite allergy
- High antibody titers against EBV VCA and early antigen
- Poor prognostic factors: late onset of disease (older than 8 years), thrombocytopenia, EBV infection in T cells
- Cause of death: hemophagocytic syndrome, multiple organ failure, T-cell or NK-cell malignancy

Morphology
- Polymorphic infiltrates of inflammatory cells with or without granuloma and focal necrosis
- No significant atypia in infiltrating lymphocytes
- Sinusoidal infiltration by small lymphocytes without atypia in liver

Immunophenotype and Genotype
- EBV found mainly in T cells and NK cells
- EBV terminal repeat: polyclonal, oligoclonal, or monoclonal
- TR gene rearrangement: polyclonal, oligoclonal, or often monoclonal

CAEBVD, Chronic active EBV disease; *EBV,* Epstein-Barr virus; *Ig,* immunoglobulin; *LPD,* lymphoproliferative disorder; *NK,* natural killer; *VCA,* viral capsid antigen.

of EBV-infected T cells or NK cells.[52,53] CAEBVD-B lineage has been reported mainly in Western countries[54] and usually a manifestation of underlying primary immunodeficiency[55]; therefore, CAEBVD in the WHO and ICC excludes B-cell lineage and only includes T- or NK-cell disease.[5,6]

Epidemiology

As with other EBV-associated T/NK-cell diseases, CAEBVD has a strong racial predisposition, with most cases reported from East Asia, including Japan, Korea, and China, and Latin America. It occurs uncommonly in Whites and Blacks.[54,56,57]

Pathophysiology

In the primary infection, EBV infects B cells via the cell surface receptor CD21 and EBV-infected B-cell proliferation is normally controlled by an EBV-specific cytotoxic T-lymphocyte (CTL) response. In CAEBVD, T cells or NK cells are the main targets of EBV. T cells and NK cells usually lack the EBV receptor CD21, but normal peripheral T cells express CD21 at low levels,[58] and NK cells can acquire CD21 by synaptic transfer from B cells,[59] allowing EBV to bind to T cell or NK cells during the primary infection. On the other hand, a study showed that EBV can infect human NK cells by direct transfer of viral episome independent of EBV-positive B cells.[60] Unlike classic infectious mononucleosis, EBV-infected T/NK cells are not removed but proliferate to involve multiple organ systems because of defective cellular immunity. Although most patients with CAEBVD have no consistent immunologic abnormality and the diagnostic criteria include the absence of known immunodeficiency, patients with CAEBVD show minor defects in cellular immunity against EBV. Reduced NK-cell cytotoxicity and impaired EBV-specific CTL activity have been reported in some patients with CAEBVD. This defective T-cell function is not limited to EBV, but low numbers of cytomegalovirus-specific CTLs, and an overall T-cell dysfunction, have also been observed.

In addition, EBV-infected T cells and NK cells evade the immune system through decreased antigen presentation and possibly other immunomodulatory factors. EBV-infected T cells or NK cells in CAEBVD express a limited number of EBV-related antigens, including EBNA1, latent membrane protein-1 (LMP1), and LMP2, but not EBNA2, 3A, 3B, or LP. EBNA1 and LMP1 are less antigenic than other EBNA proteins.

EBV-infected T/NK cells in CAEBVD show constitutive activation of NF-κB and STAT3, which contribute to prolonged cell survival of EBV-positive T/NK cells.[61] EBV genome in CAEBVD patients harbored frequent intragenic deletions that were also common in various EBV-associated neoplastic disorders. The deletion of one of the essential genes, BALF5, resulted in upregulation of the lytic cycle and the promotion of lymphomagenesis in a xenograft model. Mutations of DDX3X and other driver genes contribute to clonal evolution of EBV-positive T/NK cells and transformation to lymphoma/leukemia.[62]

Clinical Features

CAEBVD was initially recognized as a disease of children, but according to the recent Japanese nationwide CAEBVD survey, more than half of patients were adults. The median age of

disease onset is 21 years, with a range of 1 to 73 years, and the male-to-female ratio is 1.1:1.[63] The symptoms generally consist of prolonged or intermittent fever (93% of patients), hepatomegaly (79%), splenomegaly (73%), thrombocytopenia (45%), anemia (44%), and lymphadenopathy (40%). Cutaneous manifestations are common and include severe mosquito bite allergy (33%), rash (26%), and HV (10%).[51,64,65] Some patients in South America present with periorbital and facial edema, high levels of EBV DNA, and systemic symptoms. The ICC decided to classify these cases as CAEBVD because of its aggressive clinical course and lack of typical HV lesions.[6,66] Life-threatening complications include hemophagocytic syndrome, interstitial pneumonia, malignant lymphoma, coronary aneurysm, CNS involvement, and bowel perforation.[51,64] Most patients have high antibody titers of EBV VCA IgG and early antigen IgG, and they often have IgA antibodies against VCA and early antigen.[52] All patients have elevated levels of EBV DNA in their blood, which is well correlated with clinical severity.[64]

Morphology

In general, patients with CAEBVD do not exhibit changes suggestive of a neoplastic lymphoproliferative process in affected tissues (Fig. 29-2). The lymph nodes show variable histologic changes with paracortical hyperplasia, a polymorphic and polyclonal lymphoid proliferation, large numbers of EBER-positive cells, and infiltration with many other inflammatory cells, including plasma cells and histiocytes. Granulomas associated with necrosis may be present. The liver shows portal or sinusoidal infiltration by small lymphocytes without atypia.[52] In cases complicated by hemophagocytic syndrome, histiocytic hyperplasia with erythrophagocytosis can be seen in the bone marrow, liver, and skin. In cases with monoclonal CAEBVD, the infiltrating cells tend to have slight cytologic atypia and include a higher proportion of EBV-positive cells.

Immunophenotype

The immunophenotype of the EBV-positive cells infiltrating the tissue and circulating in the peripheral blood varies from case to case and includes αβT cells, γδT cells, CD4-positive T cells, CD8-positive T cells, NK cells, or mixtures of these cells (Fig. 29-2). Many cells express cytotoxic molecules such as perforin, TIA-1, and granzyme B. Rarely, EBV-infected B cells are also present.

Genetics

EBV is polyclonal, oligoclonal, or monoclonal, as confirmed by terminal repeat analysis. T-cell receptor gene rearrangement is also polyclonal, oligoclonal, or monoclonal. Clonality confirmed by the presence of somatic mutations can be detected in about 30% of CAEBVD cases at diagnosis.[62] CAEBVD is largely accompanied by DDX3X mutations, and recurrent mutations also involved other genes, including KMT2D, BCOR, BCORL1, TET2, and KDM6A, which recapitulate the mutation pattern reported in extranodal NK/T-cell lymphoma. Identical driver mutations are shared by different cell lineages, including T, B, and NK cells.[62] No specific chromosomal abnormality has consistently been shown in CAEBVD to

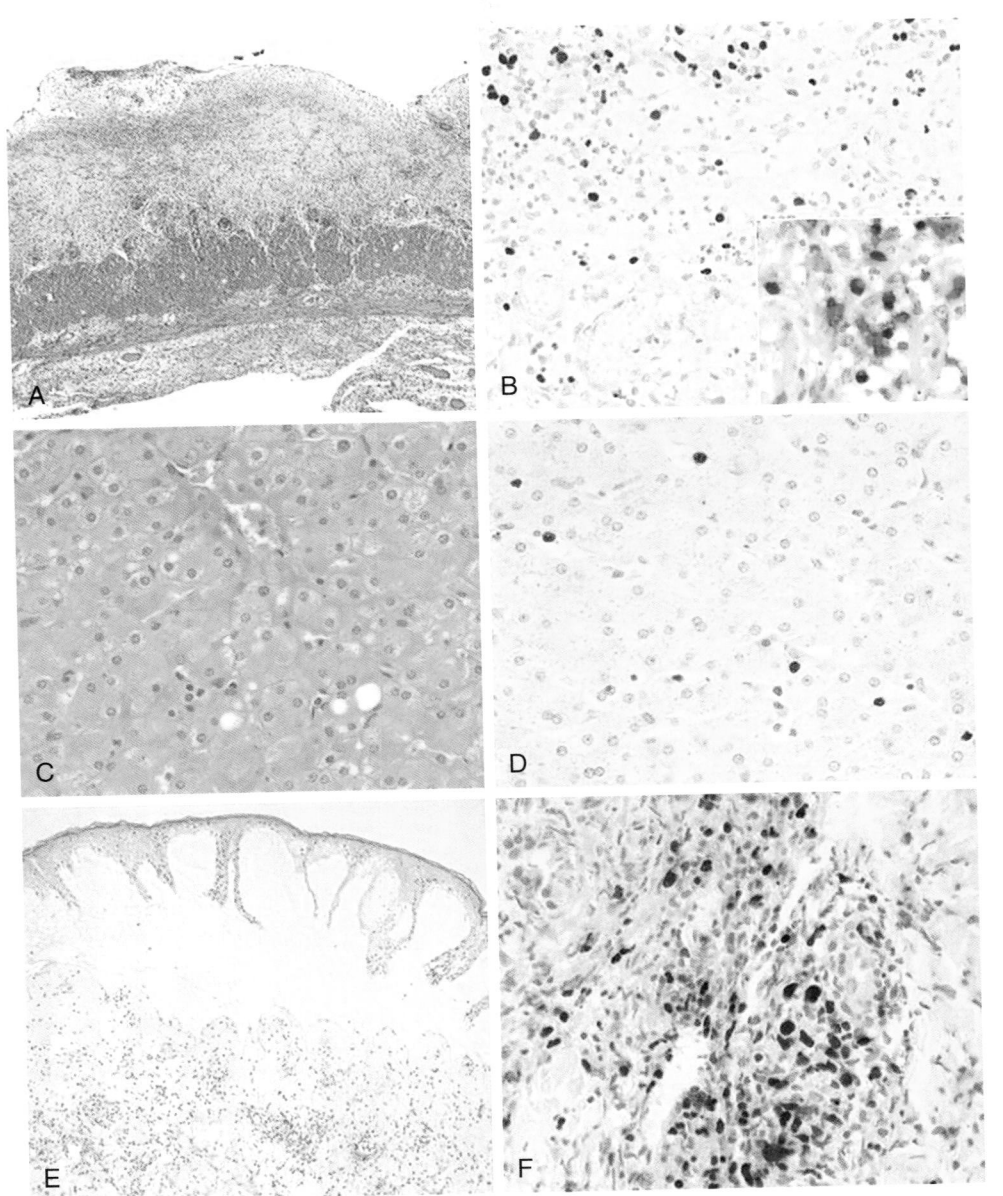

Figure 29-2. Chronic active Epstein-Barr virus disease. A, This 5-year-old boy was admitted because of fever, recurrent bowel perforation, abnormal liver function, skin rashes of the face and neck, and natural killer (NK) lymphocytosis for 2 years. Resected bowel shows granulation tissue infiltrated by small lymphocytes and neutrophils. **B,** Epstein-Barr virus (EBV)–encoded RNA (EBER) in situ hybridization highlights EBV-positive lymphocytes, which are also positive for CD3 *(inset)*. **C,** Liver biopsy of the patient shows minimal histologic change. **D,** EBER in situ hybridization highlights EBV-positive small lymphocytes in hepatic sinusoids. **E,** Skin biopsy reveals suprabasal bulla and perivascular inflammatory infiltration. **F,** EBER is positive in many perivascular lymphocytes.

date, but cases with progression to monoclonal T- or NK-cell lymphoproliferative disorders show complex chromosomal aberrations.[64]

Grading

The proliferating cells in cases of CAEBVD frequently lack histologic evidence of malignancy and can be polyclonal, oligoclonal, or monoclonal according to the stage of transformation. Ohshima and colleagues proposed a three-tier classification for CAEBVD.[52] Category A1 is polymorphic lymphoproliferative disorder with polyclonal proliferation of EBV-infected T cells or NK cells. Category A2 is polymorphic lymphoproliferative disorder with proliferation of monoclonal T cells or NK cells. Category A3 is monomorphic lymphoproliferative disorder of monoclonal T cells or NK cells. Categories A1, A2, and A3 constitute continuous stages in clonal evolution of CAEBVD. Category A3 corresponds to lymphoma/leukemia, including EBV-positive systemic T-cell lymphoma, extranodal NK/T-cell lymphoma, or aggressive NK-cell leukemia.

Postulated Cell of Origin

The postulated cells of origin are cytotoxic T cells or NK cells.

Prognosis and Predictive Factors

The prognosis of CAEBVD is variable. Some patients experience an indolent clinical course, but many patients die of the disease. The process may evolve from a polyclonal to a monoclonal proliferation of T cells or NK cells and eventually progresses to overt lymphoid malignancy. The main causes of death are hemophagocytic syndrome, multiple organ failure, and T-cell or NK-cell malignancy. The median survival is 78 months. In children, patients with a late onset of CAEBVD (older than 8 years), thrombocytopenia, and T-cell infection have poorer outcomes.[51,64,65] Adult-onset disease has poorer outcome compared with disease of children.[67] The monoclonality of EBV alone does not correlate with an increased risk for mortality.[51] Patients with T-cell CAEBVD often present with high fever, lymphadenopathy, hepatosplenomegaly, and high titers of EBV-specific antibodies, and they experience rapid disease progression. Patients with NK-cell disease, in contrast, often have hypersensitivity to mosquito bites, rash, and high levels of IgE but do not necessarily have elevated EBV-specific antibody titers.[68] The 5-year survival rate of patients with T-cell CAEBVD is 59%, whereas that for NK-cell disease is 87%.[51] Hodgkin lymphoma–like lymphoproliferative disease can occur rarely.[69-71]

Differential Diagnosis

Because the infiltrating cells in CAEBVD are bland looking without overt atypia, it is easy to overlook the diagnosis. In situ hybridization for EBER is a valuable tool for recognizing the disease in the appropriate clinical setting. Systemic EBV-positive T-cell lymphoma or other EBV-positive T-cell and NK-cell lymphomas must be distinguished from CAEBVD. Systemic EBV-positive T-cell lymphoma is an acute and fulminant disease while CAEBVD is usually a protracted disease in which patients are diagnosed after months and years of EBV-related symptoms. Clinical history is important for the differential diagnosis (Box 29-4).

SEVERE MOSQUITO BITE ALLERGY

Synonyms and Related Terms

WHO revised 4th ed.: Severe mosquito bite allergy
WHO proposed 5th ed.: Severe mosquito bite allergy

Definition

Severe mosquito bite allergy is a cutaneous manifestation of EBV-positive NK-cell lymphoproliferative disease characterized by intense local skin reactions, including erythema, bullae, and ulcers healing with scar formation, and accompanied by systemic symptoms such as fever, general malaise, and liver dysfunction after mosquito bites, vaccination, or injection.[5] It has a close association with CAEBVD and aggressive NK-cell leukemia occurring in children (capsule summary in Box 29-5).

Epidemiology

Epidemiology of the disease is same as that of other EBV-associated T/NK-cell lymphoproliferative disorder. It is an uncommon disease. Most cases have been reported from Japan, with a few cases from Taiwan, Korea, and Mexico.

Pathophysiology

Severe mosquito bite allergy is not a simple allergic disease but a cutaneous reaction of underlying EBV-positive NK-cell lymphoproliferation induced by mosquito bites.[72] Peripheral blood analysis of patients shows increased CD4-positive T cells and NK cells. NK cells are infected by monoclonal EBV.[73] CD4-positive T cells are mosquito antigen–specific and proliferate in response to mosquito salivary gland extract.[74] When mosquito antigen–specific CD4-positive cells are cocultured with

---

> **Box 29-4 Recommended Tests to Diagnose Chronic Active EBV and Related Diseases**
>
> - In situ hybridization for EBER
> - Immunostains for CD3, CD20, CD4, CD8, and CD56
> - Double stains for EBER with CD3, CD79a, and CD56 to identify cell lineage of EBV-positive cells
> - Immunostains for cytotoxic markers: TIA-1, granzyme B, perforin
> - Viral load in peripheral blood
> - EBV antibody titers
> - EBV terminal repeat analysis (if available)
> - TR gene rearrangement
>
> *EBER,* EBV-encoded RNA; *EBV,* Epstein-Barr virus; *NK,* natural killer.

> **Box 29-5 Major Diagnostic Features of Severe Mosquito Bite Allergy**
>
> **Definition**
> - Cutaneous manifestation of underlying EBV-associated NK-cell lymphoproliferative disorder activated by mosquito bite or injection
>
> **Diagnostic Criteria**
> - Intense local skin symptoms, including erythema, bulla, ulcer, and scar formation, associated with systemic symptoms such as fever, lymphadenopathy, and liver dysfunction after mosquito bites
>
> **Clinical Features**
> - Most patients are in the first two decades of life, with a median age of 6.7 years
> - Often high EBV load and NK-cell lymphocytosis
> - Variable clinical course; some patients may develop HVLPD, systemic symptoms of CAEBVD, or NK-cell lymphoma/leukemia
>
> **Morphology**
> - Necrosis and ulceration of epidermis, with infiltration of neutrophils and small lymphocytes and fibrinoid necrosis of small blood vessels
>
> **Immunophenotype**
> - Cutaneous infiltration by CD4-positive T cells, CD8-positive T cells, and NK cells expressing cytotoxic molecules
> - NK cells containing EBV in peripheral blood
>
> *CAEBVD,* Chronic active EBV disease; *EBV,* Epstein-Barr virus; *HVLPD,* hydroa vacciniforme lymphoproliferative disorder; *NK,* natural killer.

EBV-carrying NK cells, EBV is activated, and NK cells express EBV lytic cycle antigens. The activation of NK cells latently infected by EBV and the subsequent CTL response seem to play a key role in the pathogenesis of the skin lesions and systemic symptoms of patients with severe mosquito bite allergy.[75,76] EBV-carrying NK cells are clonal and preneoplastic cells, with a risk for subsequent development of overt NK-cell lymphoma/leukemia through the oncogenic influence of latent EBV genes.

Clinical Features

Most patients are in the first two decades of life, with a median age of 6.7 years.[77] Skin lesions at the site of the mosquito bite typically demonstrate erythema and bullae that subsequently become necrotic with ulceration and eventually heal with scarring (Fig. 29-3). Systemic symptoms, including fever and malaise, are common. Hematuria, proteinuria, and bloody

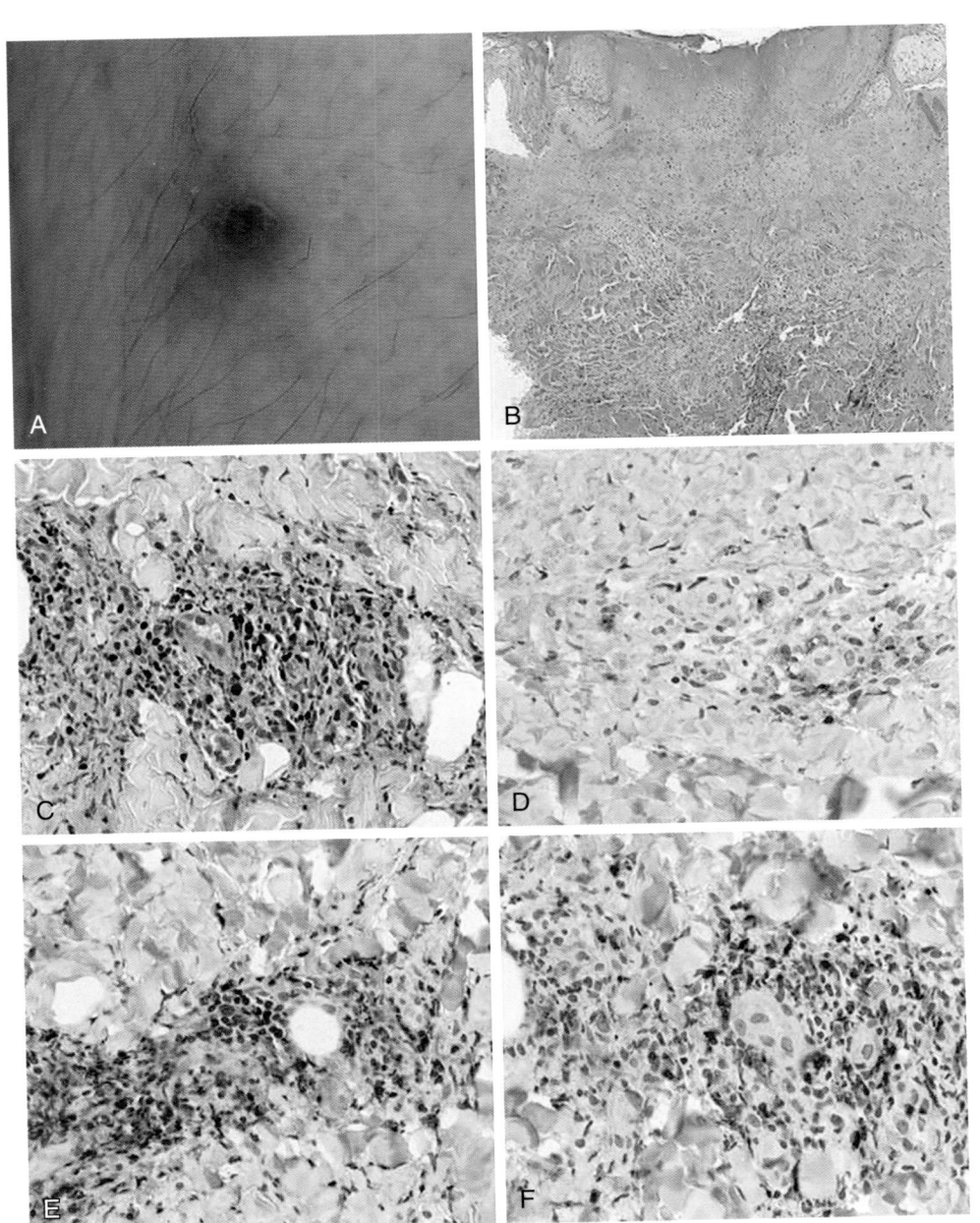

Figure 29-3. **Severe mosquito bite allergy. A,** Skin at the mosquito bite site shows epidermal necrosis and ulceration. **B,** Skin shows necrosis of the epidermis. Blood vessels in the deep dermis exhibit vasculitic changes, with fibrinoid necrosis and fibrin thrombi. **C,** Many perivascular cells are Epstein-Barr virus–encoded RNA (EBER) positive. **D,** CD56 stains scattered perivascular cells. **E,** Many perivascular cells are CD4 positive. **F,** Some cells are CD8 positive. *(A, Courtesy Professor H. S. Kim, Chonnam National University.)*

stool may be seen, with laboratory evidence of anemia or hypoproteinemia. After recovery from the general symptoms, patients are symptom free until the next mosquito bite. Vaccination may cause a similar skin reaction at the injection site in some patients.[77] Patients show a high level of serum IgE, a high EBV load in the peripheral blood, and peripheral NK lymphocytosis (80% of patients).[73]

Patients with CAEBVD can show severe mosquito bite allergy. Complications in patients with severe mosquito bite allergy commonly include NK-cell lymphoma/leukemia and hemophagocytic syndrome.

Morphology

The skin at the mosquito bite site exhibits epidermal necrosis and ulceration. The dermis shows edema and infiltration of polymorphonuclear leukocytes, nuclear debris, and extravasated red blood cells, with fibrinoid necrosis of small

blood vessels in the center of the lesion (see Fig. 29-3). The infiltrate of small lymphoid cells extends from the dermis to subcutaneous tissue in an angiocentric pattern.

Immunophenotype and Genetics

The infiltrating lymphoid cells in the skin are CD4-positive T cells, CD8-positive T cells, and NK cells that express cytotoxic molecules. EBV-positive cells constitute a minor population, accounting for 3% to 10% of infiltrating lymphocytes. Peripheral blood mononuclear cells in patients with NK lymphocytosis typically contain 30% to 70% of NK cells. Blood NK cells are infected with monoclonal EBV or occasionally with biclonal EBV, indicating clonal NK cell proliferation.[73]

Postulated Cell of Origin

NK cells are the postulated cells of origin.

Prognosis

The clinical course is variable. Some patients have a prolonged and indolent disease course that may be complicated with CAEBVD or HVLPD. More than half of the patients die. Half the fatal patients die of hemophagocytic syndrome and other 30% to 40% of patients die of NK-cell lymphoma/leukemia.[77,78]

HYDROA VACCINIFORME LYMPHOPROLIFERATIVE DISORDER

Synonyms and Related Terms

WHO revised 4th ed.: Hydroa vacciniform–like lymphoproliferative disorder

WHO proposed 5th ed.: Hydroa vacciniform lymphoproliferative disorder

Definition

Hydroa vacciniforme lymphoproliferative disorder (HVLPD) is a cutaneous EBV-positive lymphoproliferative disease characterized by recurrent papulovesicular and necrotic eruptions of the skin.[5] This condition is divided into two types based on the clinical features, classic and systemic; classic HVLPD is an indolent and self-limited disease involving only the skin and accounts for the majority of HVLPD occurring in Whites. Systemic HVLPD more commonly affects Asians and Latin Americans and is characterized by skin lesions accompanied by systemic symptoms such as fever, lymphadenopathy, and hepatosplenomegaly during the acute episode (Table 29-1).[6,7]

Previously, similar cutaneous lesions corresponding to systemic HVLPD were reported under various names, including hydroa-like cutaneous T-cell lymphoma, edematous scarring vasculitic panniculitis, EBV-associated lymphoproliferative lesions presenting as recurrent necrotic papulovesicles of the face, and angiocentric cutaneous T-cell lymphoma (hydroa-like lymphoma) of childhood.

Epidemiology

Classic HVLPD occurs worldwide, independent of race.[79] Usually the disease is sporadic, but familial cases have been reported in identical twins and siblings.[80,81] Systemic HVLPD has been described mainly in Asia and Latin America, including Japan,[2] Korea,[82,83] Taiwan,[84] China,[85-87] Mexico,[88-89] Peru,[90] and Guatemala,[91] and rarely in Western countries.[10]

Pathophysiology

EBV is found in both classic HVLPD and systemic HVLPD. In classic HVLPD, even though the lesions are confined to the skin, slightly elevated levels of EBV DNA showed in peripheral blood mononuclear cells compared with normal healthy persons, whereas systemic HVLPD has markedly increased levels of EBV DNA and can be associated with other complications.[92]

The patients with HVLPD have increased $\gamma\delta$T cells in both peripheral blood and skin, and the $\gamma\delta$T-cells in blood contain larger amounts of EBV DNA than non-$\gamma\delta$T cells.[93,94] Although

Table 29-1 Major Diagnostic Features of Hydroa Vacciniforme Lymphoproliferative Disorder

| Feature | HVLPD | |
	Classic HVLPD	Systemic HVLPD
Epidemiology	Worldwide	Asia and Latin America
Skin lesions	Sun exposed	Sun exposed or unexposed
	Vesiculopapular	Vesiculopapular and ulcerative; facial edema
Photoprovocation	Usually positive	Variable
Histopathology	Epidermal vesicles Superficial or deep dermal infiltrates	Epidermal vesicles and ulcers Deeper dermal and subcutaneous infiltrates Variable cytologic atypia
Phenotype	Cytotoxic CD4-positive or CD8-positive T cells	Cytotoxic CD8-positive or CD4-positive T cells or NK cells
EBER-positive cells	5%–50% of lymphocytes	5%–50% of lymphocytes
TR gene	Polyclonal/monoclonal	Monoclonal
Systemic symptoms*	Absent	Present
Anti-EBV antibody profile	Usually normal	Often abnormal
EBV DNA load in peripheral blood	Slightly high	High
Associated conditions	Absent	CAEBVD Severe mosquito bite allergy HPS (rare)
Prognosis	Remission with photoprotection Often recurrent but systemic progression or fatality is rare	Remissions and recurrences Progression to cutaneous or systemic T-cell lymphoma in some patients

*Fever, increased liver enzymes, lymphadenopathy.
CAEBVD, Chronic active EBV disease; *EBER,* EBV-encoded small RNA; *EBV,* Epstein-Barr virus; *HPS,* hemophagocytic syndrome; *HVLPD,* hydroa vacciniforme lymphoproliferative disorder; *LPD,* lymphoproliferative disorder; *NK,* natural killer.

the exact mechanism inducing cutaneous homing of these EBV-positive $\gamma\delta$T cells is unknown, ultraviolet (UV) is one of the triggering factors. EBV-containing $\gamma\delta$T cells homing to the skin admixed with EBV-negative cytotoxic T cells induce an inflammatory reaction and attack the epidermis. The keratinocytes of the epidermis undergo reticular degeneration, leading to the formation of vesicles. An HVLPD skin lesion compared with normal skin showed increased expression of interferon-γ and chemokines that attract T cells and NK cells.[80] Blister fluids from the patients had much higher levels of TNF-α.[95]

Clinical Features

Classic HVLPD

HVLPD usually presents in children younger than 10 years, but occurrence in adults is not uncommon.[83,87,96] The eruption is seasonal, usually occurring in spring or summer. The skin lesions are characterized by recurrent vesicles and crust formation on the face and arms after sun exposure, and they typically heal with vacciniform scarring (Fig. 29-4). Lesions are inducible by sunlight exposure and, less commonly, by repeated exposure to broad-spectrum UVA or, less reliably, UVB irradiation.[97-99]

Systemic HVLPD

Unlike classic HVLPD, the cutaneous lesions can occur in exposed and unexposed sites and are frequently refractory to the wearing of sun protection. Cutaneous lesions might be severe and disfiguring (Fig. 29-5). Patients show necrotic papulovesicles or nodules, which can recur for years.[82,88,90,98,100]

Patients present with systemic symptoms during the acute episode such as fever and malaise, which is accompanied by lymphadenopathy, hepatosplenomegaly, increased liver enzymes and lactate dehydrogenase, and large granular lymphocytosis in the peripheral blood.[101,102] A seasonal variation in eruptions is characteristic, being worse in spring and summer and remitting in autumn and winter. During the remission phase, the patients are asymptomatic. Some patients have hypersensitivity to insect or mosquito bites (Table 29-1).[88] As the disease progresses, there are more extensive and more severe skin lesions and systemic symptoms. Patients who initially respond to steroids or immunomodulating therapies, however, eventually will require similar treatment as CAEBVD.

Morphology

The characteristic histologic features of HVLPD are epidermal reticular degeneration leading to spongiotic vesiculation. The dermis contains perivascular and periappendageal lymphocytic infiltration. There is no cytologic atypia of infiltrating cells in classic HVLPD. The histologic changes of systemic HVLPD are similar to those of classic HVLPD, but the dermal infiltrates may be more extensive and deeper, reaching to the subcutaneous tissue. The infiltrates show variable atypia and are often composed of atypical lymphocytes with enlarged and hyperchromatic nuclei, frequently with an angiocentric and periadnexal arrangement and septal or lobular panniculitis. Reactive histiocytes may be admixed.

Immunophenotype and Genetics

In classic HVLPD, the majority of the T-cell population in the skin is composed of EBV-positive CD4-negative or CD8-negative $\gamma\delta$T cells and reactive EBV-negative CD4-positive or CD8-positive cytotoxic T cells. NK cells are rare.[93] EBV-positive $\gamma\delta$T cells are increased in the peripheral blood.[10,92-94,103] In systemic HVLPD, infiltrating cells in the skin are composed of EBV-positive or EBV-negative T cells that are predominantly CD8-positive CTLs,[90,104] with a minority of CD4-positive cells and some CD56-positive cells.[84,86] A variable number of CD30-positive cells can be seen.[91] EBV-infected cells in peripheral blood are either $\gamma\delta$T cells or, less commonly, $\alpha\beta$T-cells.[105] TR gene rearrangements of infiltrating cells in the skin may be polyclonal,[98] but more frequently monoclonal.[86]

The number of EBV-positive lymphocytes in the skin varies[98,106] and increases in spring and summer; during periods of remission in autumn and winter, very few EBV-positive cells are present. EBV-containing cells do not express LMP1.

Postulated Cell of Origin

The postulated cells of origin are $\gamma\delta$T cells; less commonly, $\alpha\beta$T cells; and rarely, NK cells, homing to the skin.

Prognosis

Patients with classic HVLPD show spontaneous remission; some are cured after protection from sunlight, but other patients experience recurrent eruptions that do not spread systemically. Fatalities are uncommon.[79,107] About half the

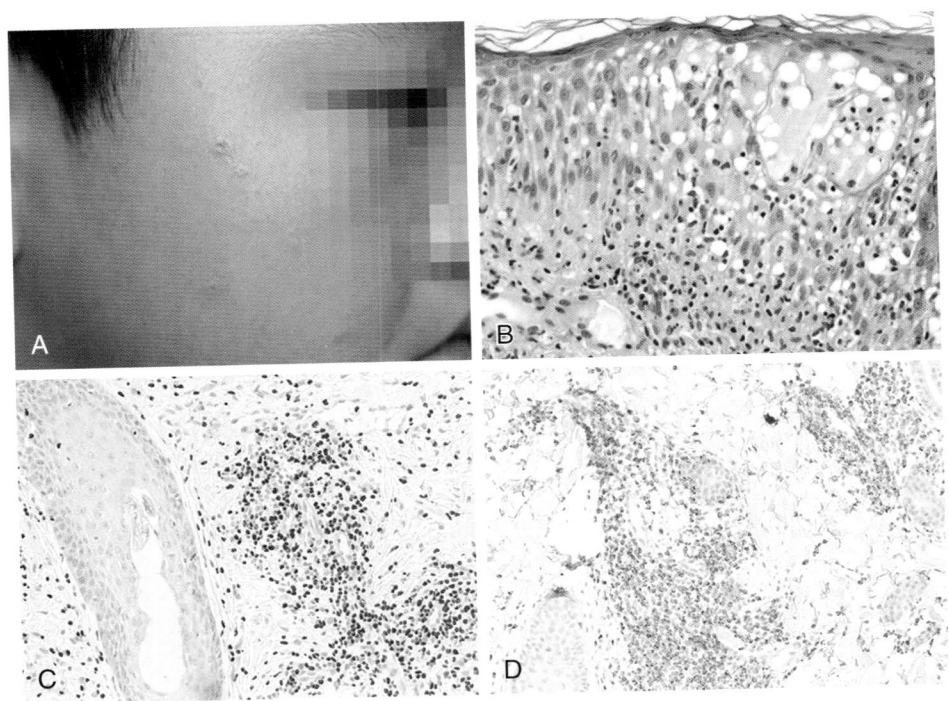

Figure 29-4. Classic hydroa vacciniforme lymphoproliferative disorder. A, This 4-year-old boy has a papulovesicular eruption with vacciniform scarring of the face. **B,** Skin shows epidermal reticular degeneration, leading to spongiotic vesiculation. The dermis contains a perivascular and periappendageal lymphocytic infiltrate. **C,** Perivascular infiltrates are Epstein-Barr virus–positive cells. **D,** Majority of lymphocytes are TIA-1 positive. *(A, Courtesy Dr. J. E. Kwon, Dankook University.)*

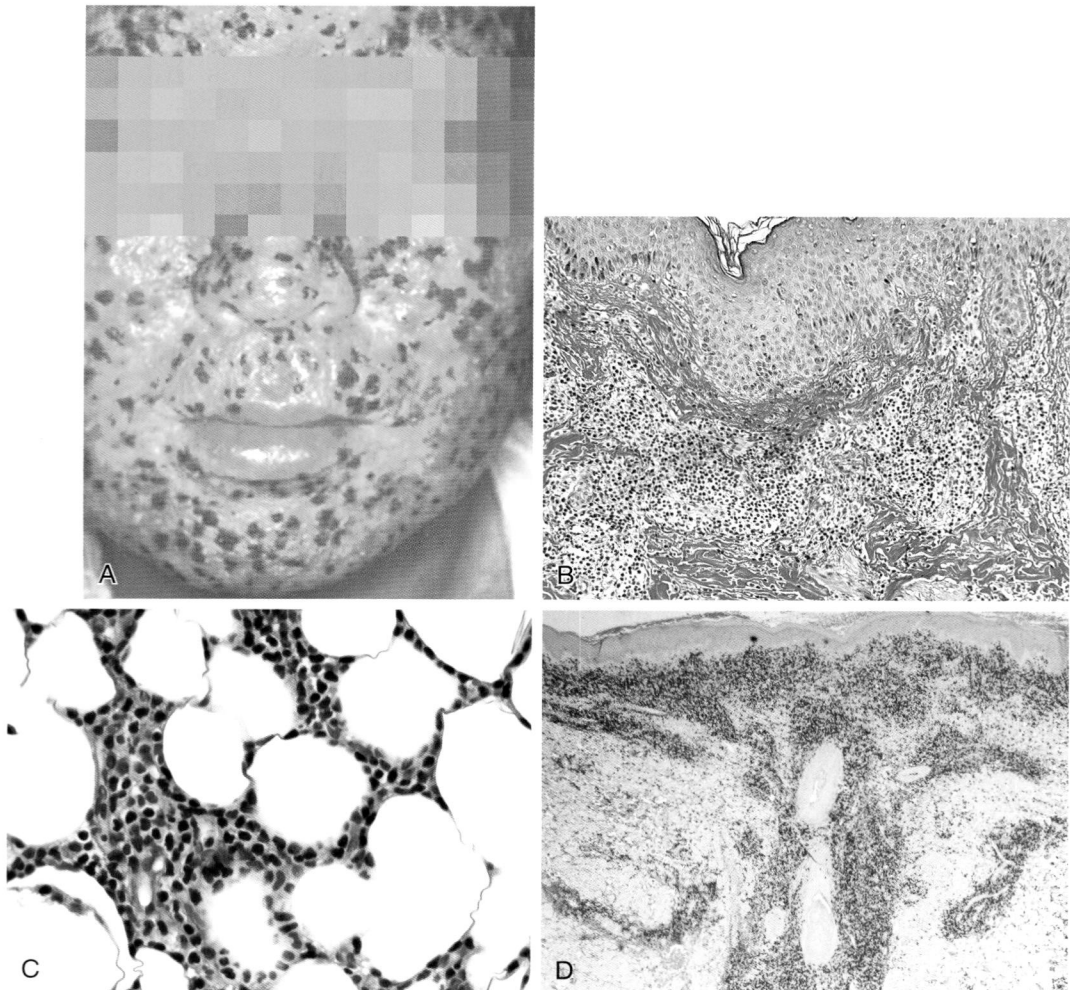

Figure 29-5. Systemic hydroa vacciniforme lymphoproliferative disorder. A, This 24-year-old man with recurrent necrotic papulovesicles on the face for 6 years eventually developed systemic Epstein-Barr virus (EBV)–positive T-cell lymphoma. **B,** Small-to-medium-sized lymphoid cells infiltrate the dermis. **C,** Infiltrate extends into subcutaneous tissue. **D,** Nearly all lymphoid cells are EBV-encoded RNA (EBER) positive (EBER in situ hybridization). *(A, Courtesy Professor K.H. Cho, Seoul National University.)*

patients with systemic HVLPD can be alive with recurrent disease while another half develop EBV-associated NK/T-cell lymphoma in the skin or other organs 2 to 14 years after onset.[2,4,65,82,86,101,102] Prognosis of classic HVLPD and γδT-cell-dominant systemic HVLPD is favorable, but αβT-cell-dominant systemic HVLPD has a poor prognosis with mortality rates of 11.5 per 100 person-years.[105] Prognosis of patients with adult-onset HVLPD is worse compared with HVLPD of children.[83]

Differential Diagnosis

The main differential diagnoses for systemic HVLPD are cutaneous NK/T-cell lymphoma and subcutaneous panniculitis-like T-cell lymphoma. Distinguishing extranodal NK/T-cell lymphoma may be problematic in some cases based only on morphology. Clinical information is essential in these cases. Characteristic recurrent papulovesicular skin lesions favor a diagnosis of HVLPD over ENKTL-NT.

Subcutaneous panniculitis-like T-cell lymphoma presents with deep subcutaneous nodules rather than vesiculopapular skin eruptions and is invariably negative for EBV. Primary cutaneous γδT-cell lymphoma may appear clinically similar, and there may be dermal, epidermal, and subcutaneous involvement; the epidermis may be ulcerated. Primary cutaneous γδT-cell lymphoma is also negative for EBV.

SYSTEMIC EPSTEIN-BARR VIRUS–POSITIVE T-CELL LYMPHOMA OF CHILDHOOD

Synonyms and Related Terms

WHO revised 4th ed.: Systemic Epstein-Barr virus–positive T-cell lymphoma of childhood

WHO proposed 5th ed.: Systemic Epstein-Barr virus–positive T-cell lymphoma of childhood

Definition

Systemic EBV-positive T-cell lymphoma of childhood and young adults is a rare but life-threatening fulminant illness characterized by a clonal proliferation of EBV-infected T cells, usually CD8 positive, with an activated cytotoxic phenotype. It occurs shortly after primary acute EBV infection or rarely develops in the clinical setting of CAEBVD. It is usually characterized by a rapid clinical progression with organ failure, sepsis, and death. A hemophagocytic syndrome is nearly always present.

Epidemiology

Systemic EBV-positive T-cell lymphoma of childhood, which is most prevalent in Asia and Latin America, is nearly always accompanied by a fulminant hemophagocytic syndrome. It has been described under a variety of names, including *fatal EBV-associated hemophagocytic syndrome*,[108] *fulminant EBV-positive T-cell lymphoma*,[109] *fulminant childhood hemophagocytic syndrome mimicking histiocytic medullary reticulosis*,[110] and *fatal hemophagocytic lymphohistiocytosis*.[111] In recognition of the aggressive clinical behavior, the term *systemic EBV-positive T-cell lymphoma* was adopted in the revised WHO 4th ed., a change from the prior term of *systemic EBV-positive lymphoproliferative disorder*.[5] The term *systemic EBV-positive T-cell lymphoma of childhood* has been retained in the WHO 5th ed.[7] and in the ICC.[6] Cases have been reported primarily from Taiwan[110,112,113] and Japan,[108,114] with a few cases from Korea[115] and Mexico.[109] The disease occurs most often in young children[116] and young adults.[117]

Systemic EBV-positive T-cell lymphoma developing during the clinical course of CAEBVD has been described mainly in Japan,[1,118] with a few reports from Korea[117] and Western countries.[119] It occurs mainly in teenagers,[1,117] young children, and adults.[1] There is no sex predilection.

Pathophysiology

Hemophagocytic syndrome with a fulminant clinical course is the characteristic clinical picture of systemic EBV-positive T-cell lymphoma of childhood. The infection of T cells by EBV activates T cells to secrete Th1 cytokines such as TNF-α and interferon-γ, which subsequently activate macrophages.[120] EBV LMP1 activates the transcription factors NF-κB and JNK (c-Jun N-terminal kinase); this not only provides the molecular mechanism for LMP1–induced cell proliferation and transformation but also confers resistance to TNF-α–mediated apoptosis via downregulation of TNF-α receptor 1 in the cytokine milieu of hemophagocytic syndrome.[45,121]

Clinical Features

Patients with systemic EBV-positive T-cell lymphoma developing after primary EBV infection usually present with acute onset of fever and general malaise suggestive of an acute viral respiratory illness. Within a period of 1 to 3 weeks, patients develop hepatosplenomegaly, liver dysfunction, pancytopenia, rash, and CNS symptoms. Lymphadenopathy is not common. The disease is usually complicated by hemophagocytic syndrome, coagulopathy, sepsis, and multiorgan failure.[112,122]

EBV serology is often abnormal with positive anti-VCA IgG titers but low or absent anti-VCA IgM antibodies.[48,109] EBV serology in these cases is misleading in that it does not suggest acute primary or active infection, which can delay the diagnosis.

A related disorder but presenting mainly with lymphadenopathy and high lactate dehydrogenase (LDH) levels was reported in children from Peru.[123] In addition to a history of acute onset with fever, weight loss, and hepatosplenomegaly, these children had peripheral, mediastinal, and intraabdominal lymphadenopathy. The disease progressed rapidly, causing the death of the patient in all cases with a median survival of 7 months (1–13 months). This rare presentation is recognized within the spectrum of EBV-positive T-cell lymphoma of childhood.[124]

Systemic EBV-positive T-cell lymphoma arising in patients with a history of CAEBVD develops at a median of 35 months (range, 3–264 months) after the onset of CAEBVD. Before the development of T-cell lymphoma, patients experience intermittent or persistent fever of unknown origin, lymphadenopathy, or liver dysfunction over months or years, or HV-like skin eruptions occurring over months or several years.[1,115] The clinical course in these patients is somewhat more variable than that in patients with primary disease, but most patients eventually die of the disease.

Morphology

Hyperplasia of histiocytes and marked hemophagocytosis with increased numbers of small T lymphocytes are the most striking histologic changes in the bone marrow, spleen, and liver of patients with systemic EBV-positive T-cell lymphoma. The liver exhibits mild to prominent portal and sinusoidal infiltrates of small lymphocytes with intracellular and intracanalicular cholestasis, steatosis, and focal necrosis, which might be extensive. The spleen shows depleted white pulp and prominent sinusoidal small lymphoid infiltrates. The lymph nodes show preserved architecture with open sinuses. The B-cell areas are depleted, whereas the paracortical areas might be expanded and show a subtle to striking infiltration with relatively homogeneous small, medium, or large lymphocytes with hyperchromatic nuclei and irregular nuclear contours. The more advanced the disease is, the more depleted the lymph nodes look. Epithelioid histiocytes, small granulomas, or necrosis may be present. The degree of cytologic atypia in the EBV-positive lymphocytes is variable, and in many cases the cytology is surprisingly bland (Fig. 29-6); however, some cases show atypical lymphoid infiltrates composed of pleomorphic medium-to-large-sized cells and frequent mitosis. In cases presenting predominantly with lymphadenopathy, the lymph node shows partial or total replacement by a diffuse infiltration of atypical cells. Lymph node excision is required for the diagnosis; core needle biopsies, because of the high content in histiocytes and small lymphocytes, might erroneously suggest a reactive condition. The severe clinical manifestations and the presence of hemophagocytosis usually alert one to the serious nature of the lymphoid proliferation.

EBV-positive systemic T-cell lymphomas that develop after a diagnosis of CAEBVD exhibit variable cytologic atypia; however, it is similar to the systemic disease after primary EBV infection.

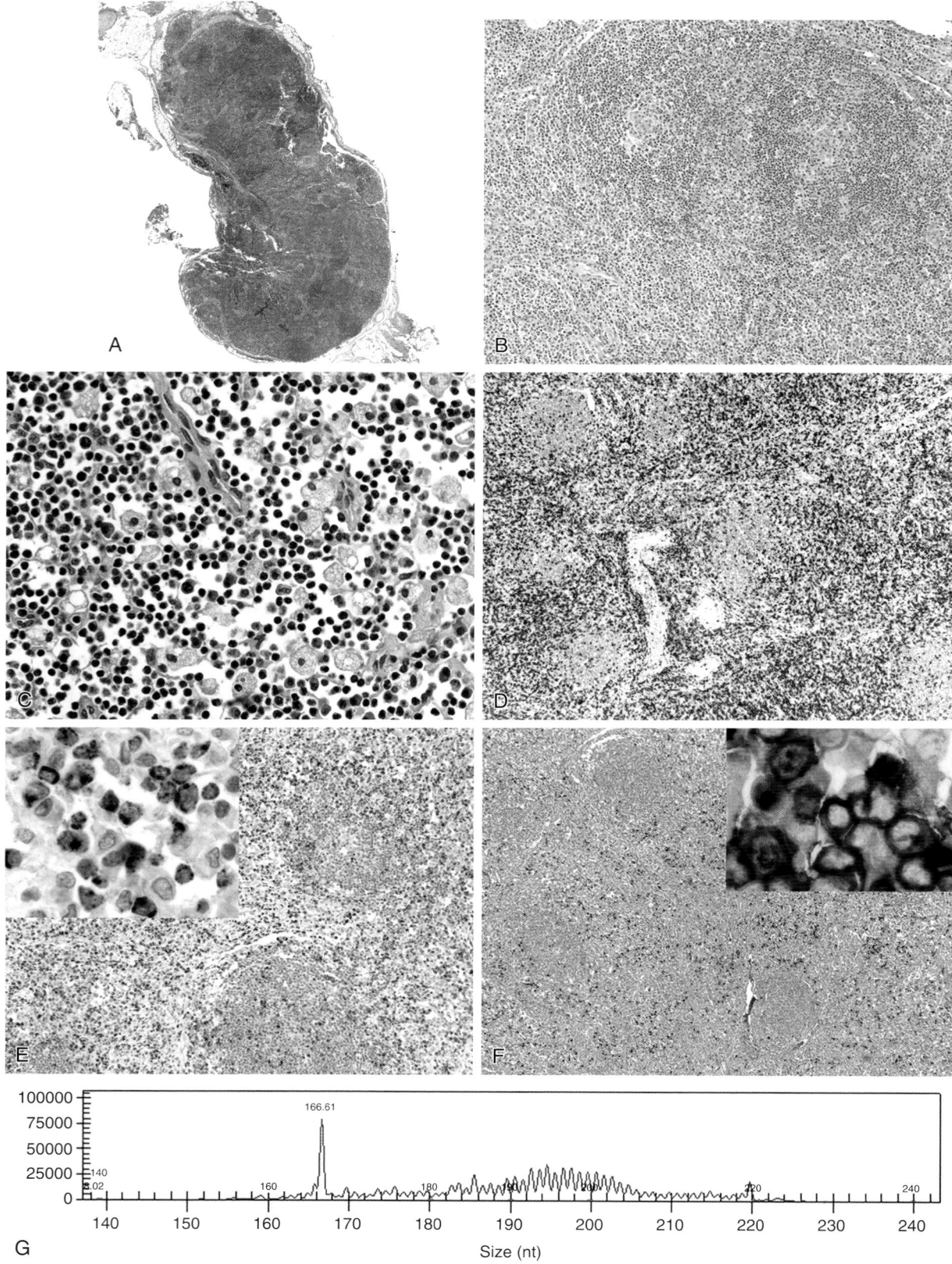

Figure 29-6. Systemic Epstein-Barr virus–positive T-cell lymphoma of childhood. A, Small lymph node with relatively well-preserved architecture. **B,** Depleted germinal centers with expansion of the interfollicular area. **C,** Abundant histiocytes with erythrophagocytosis intermingled with small lymphocytes lacking atypia. **D,** CD8 staining highlights the interfollicular small lymphoid infiltrate. **E** and **F,** The CD8-positive cells are also TIA1 positive and Epstein-Barr virus (EBV)–encoded RNA (EBER) positive. Note that in the double staining only a proportion of CD8-positive cells *(brown)* is also EBER positive *(black) (inset).***G,** TRG gene rearrangement shows a dominant monoclonal peak of 166 base pairs.

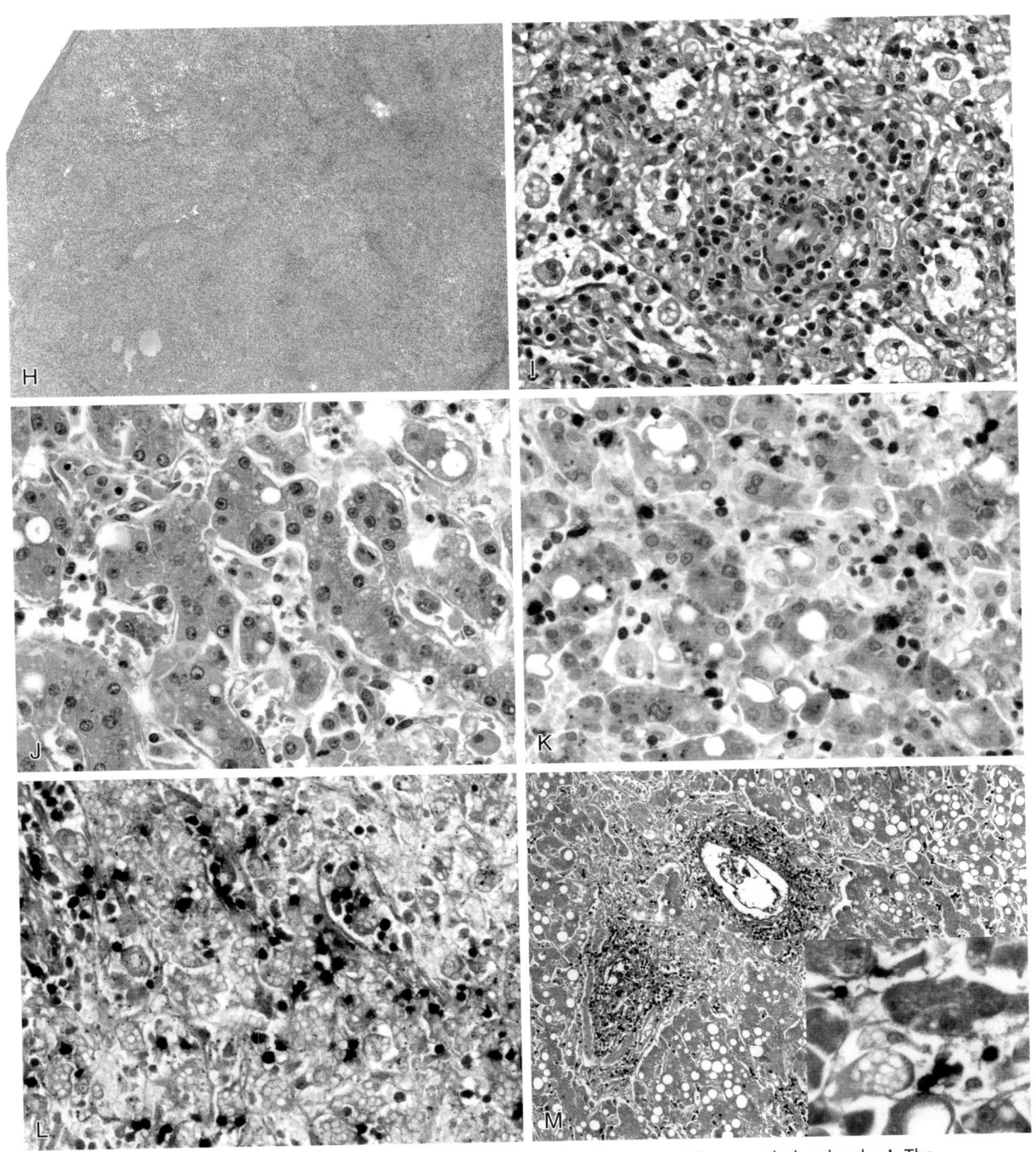

Figure 29-6, cont'd. **H,** The spleen shows a depleted white pulp with expanded red pulp. **I,** The spleen shows striking hemophagocytosis with few lymphoid cells lacking cytologic atypia. **J,** The liver shows a subtle lymphoid infiltrate in the sinusoids with hemophagocytosis. **K,** The lymphoid infiltrate is CD8 positive. **L** and **M,** EBER-positive cells are found both in the spleen and liver.

Immunophenotype and Genetics

The infiltrating cells in primary systemic EBV-positive T-cell lymphoma are predominantly CD8-positive cytotoxic $\alpha\beta$T cells.[109,115] They are CD2 positive, CD3 positive, TIA-1 positive, granzyme B positive, and CD56 negative. Cases after CAEBVD show a more heterogeneous phenotype, mostly CD4 positive,[109,118,119] CD4 positive and CD8 positive, or CD8 positive.[1]

EBV is clonal by terminal repeat analysis.[118] In situ hybridization for EBER is positive in the small lymphoid cells that show minimal cytologic atypia, and in the obviously atypical cells. In general, EBER-positive cells are less than the infiltrating CD8-positive cells. In situ hybridization for EBER and immunohistochemistry (double-staining EBER/CD8 and EBER/CD4) confirm EBV infection in T lymphocytes and the cell derivation. Although EBV-positive T- and NK-cell LPDs carry

EBV latency II, LMP1 is often negative by immunohistochemistry and EBNA2 is always negative. Molecular analysis of the TCRG gene shows a monoclonal T-cell proliferation.[109]

Postulated Cell of Origin

The postulated cell of origin in most cases is proliferation of a cytotoxic CD8 lymphocyte with rare cases being of CD4 T-cell origin.

Clinical Course and Prognostic Factors

Patients with systemic EBV-positive T-cell lymphoma after primary EBV infection have a fulminant clinical course, with all patients dying within a few days to months of diagnosis. The rapidly progressive clinical course is similar to that of aggressive NK-cell leukemia. The optimal therapeutic approach for this disease is not currently standardized. Data suggest that HLH-94 protocol has advantages over the HLH-2004 protocol.[125,126] The goal is to stop the hyperinflammatory process characteristic of HLH and continue with the therapy to prepare the patient for allogeneic hematopoietic stem cell transplantation (alloHSCT), which is the only definitive curative therapy for this disease.[125]

Patients with systemic EBV-positive T-cell lymphoma that develops after CAEBVD may have a more prolonged clinical course, but most patients die of the disease within 1 year. The cause of death is usually disseminated intravascular coagulation, multiorgan failure, and sepsis.[1]

Differential Diagnosis

The differential diagnosis of systemic EBV-positive T-cell lymphoma includes both benign and malignant proliferations of T- and NK-cell derivation. The most challenging differential diagnosis is non-neoplastic EBV-HLH, which shows a relatively favorable outcome with 90% of patients achieving remission with HLH-directed therapy.[42] Importantly, 62% of non-neoplastic EBV-HLH cases show clonal T-cell expansions that do not help in the differential diagnosis.[42,122] Attempts to determine criteria that discern between these two entities have been unsuccessful. Severe hyperbilirubinemia, hyperferritinemia, younger age, higher levels of EBV DNA, and cytologic atypia with extensive architectural effacement are parameters that favor the diagnosis of systemic EBV-positive T-cell lymphoma. The most useful parameter is cytogenetic abnormalities, but these are not always present.[48,49] Systemic EBV-positive T-cell lymphoma, arising either de novo or in the setting of CAEBVD, may show absent or minimal cytologic atypia. Such cases cause diagnostic problems, and the distinction from systemic CAEBVD may be difficult on morphologic grounds alone. In situ hybridization for EBER and clonality analysis does not always help in the differential diagnosis because systemic CAEBVD cases may show a clonal T-cell proliferation.[127,128] The clinical information is necessary to avoid misdiagnosis. The clinical course of systemic CAEBVD is usually protracted, with some patients surviving for many years without disease progression.[51,127]

Aggressive NK-cell leukemia is very similar to systemic EBV-positive T-cell lymphoma arising in young children in terms of the fulminant clinical manifestations, presence of EBV in proliferating cells, and systemic hemophagocytosis. However, aggressive NK-cell leukemia is more common in adults (typically young adults), and the tumor cells express NK-cell markers, including CD56, and do not show clonal T-cell receptor gene rearrangement.[129,130]

EXTRANODAL NK/T-CELL LYMPHOMA, NASAL TYPE

Synonyms and Related Terms

WHO revised 4th ed.: Extranodal NK/T cell lymphoma, nasal-type

WHO proposed 5th ed.: Extranodal NK/T cell lymphoma

Definition

Extranodal NK/T-cell lymphoma, nasal type (ENKTL-NT), is an extranodal lymphoma of NK- or T-cell lineage, characterized by a broad cytologic spectrum, prominent necrosis, angiocentric-angiodestructive growth, cytotoxic phenotype, and association with EBV (capsule summary in Box 29-6).[131] The qualifier "nasal-type" is retained in the ICC to stress the fact that cases presenting outside the nasal region have the same morphologic features; namely, a tumor characterized by vascular damage and destruction, prominent necrosis, cytotoxic phenotype, and association with EBV.[6,9,11,132] Cases with primary nodal presentation are classified as *primary nodal EBV-positive T/NK-cell lymphoma*.[6]

Epidemiology

ENKTL-NT occurs with a higher prevalence among Asians, Mexicans, and South Americans, accounting for 6% to 13% of all non-Hodgkin lymphomas in these populations, compared with less than 1.5% in Western populations.[133-137] Among mature T-cell and NK-cell lymphomas, it constitutes 22.4% of cases in Asia (up to 44%, excluding Japan), compared with 4.3% to 5.1% in North America and Europe.[138] It is the commonest type of primary nasal lymphoma in Asian and Southern American populations.[134,139-142]

This tumor occurs almost exclusively in adults, with a median age of 44 to 58 years. The male-to-female ratio is 2–3:1.[139,143-148]

Etiology

EBV plays an important role in the genesis of ENKTL-NT and EBV is, by definition, present.[11] Cases that are EBV negative are excluded from this category.[149] The EBV exists in a clonal episomal form in the tumor cells, and usually shows type II latency pattern (EBNA1 positive, LMP1 positive, EBNA2 negative) (Box 29-6).[145,150,151] It is usually of subtype A, with a high frequency of 30-base pair deletion of the *LMP1* gene.[145,150,151]

Racial factors appear to be significant as evidenced by marked differences in the incidence of ENKTL-NT in different populations. Genome-wide association studies have identified susceptibility loci at HLA-DPB1 (6p21.32), HLA-DRB1 (6p21.32), and IL18RAP (2q12.1).[152,153]

Some examples occur in organ transplant recipients, suggesting that iatrogenic immunosuppression may facilitate the development of this lymphoma type.[154,155] Exposure to pesticides and chemical solvents has been found to be a risk factor for development of ENKTL-NT.[156] There are isolated reports of occurrence of extranodal NK/T-cell lymphoma in breast implant,[157] by transplacental transmission,[158] and in familial settings, possibly related to pesticide exposure.[159]

ENKTL-NT arising in children or young adults can be preceded by CAEBVD of T or NK type, including severe mosquito bite allergy.[52,160]

Clinical Features

Nasal NK/T-cell lymphomas arise in the nasal cavity, nasopharynx, or upper aerodigestive tract, causing progressive destructive and ulcerative lesions (so-called "midfacial destructive disease") with bleeding and discharge or obstructive symptoms caused by mass lesions. The tumor frequently spreads to the adjacent anatomic structures such as the paranasal sinuses, orbit, oral cavity, palate, and oropharynx, and is typically associated with bone erosion.[161,162] Most patients have early stage disease (~70% stage I and II) at presentation.[139,143,144] Bone marrow involvement occurs in 10% to 16% of patients.[146,163]

EXTRANASAL NK/T-CELL LYMPHOMA

Extranasal (non-nasal) NK/T-cell lymphoma is much less common than nasal NK/T-cell lymphoma.[145,164] The most frequently involved sites are the skin, gastrointestinal tract, testis, and soft tissues, which are the same sites that nasal NK/T-cell lymphoma tends to disseminate to during the course of the disease.[143,144,165-170]

The patients often present at high stage (stage III or IV), with involvement of multiple anatomic sites.[143,147,166] Systemic symptoms such as fever, malaise, and weight loss may occur. Serum lactate dehydrogenase is often raised, and anemia is not uncommon.[143] The performance status is often poor.[143,166] The skin lesions take the form of multiple nodules, which commonly ulcerate with a necrotic center. They most often occur in the limbs.[167] Intestinal lesions commonly manifest as perforation or gastrointestinal bleeding, and sepsis is a common complication.[170,171] Involvement of the testis or soft tissue usually manifests as mass lesion.

Rare cases of intravascular NK/T-cell lymphoma have been reported, usually involving skin and CNS.[172-177] Almost all cases harbor EBV, and the disease is highly aggressive. It is currently unclear whether this represents a distinct entity or an unusual subtype of extranodal NK/T-cell lymphoma or aggressive NK-cell leukemia.

Morphology

General Features

The affected tissue is frequently but not invariably ulcerated and necrotic (Fig. 29-7). It is diffusely infiltrated by closely packed lymphoma cells (Fig. 29-7B).[132] The cytologic composition varies from case to case, ranging from predominantly small-sized cells, medium-sized cells, or large-sized cells to a mixture, with medium-sized cells being the most common. The small cells usually have irregularly folded, angulated, or serpentine-shaped nuclei with dense chromatin, inconspicuous nucleoli, and a narrow-to-moderate rim of pale cytoplasm (Fig. 29-8), but they can sometimes resemble small lymphocytes (Fig. 29-8C).[178,179] The medium-sized cells possess round or irregularly folded nuclei, granular chromatin, small nucleoli, and a moderate amount of pale-to-clear cytoplasm (Fig. 29-9). The large cells have round or folded nuclei, vesicular or granular chromatin, and distinct nucleoli (Fig. 29-10), and occasionally appear anaplastic. Azurophilic cytoplasmic granules are often detectable in Giemsa-stained cytologic preparations (Fig. 29-11), while cytoplasmic granules are usually not seen in H&E-stained histologic sections. Mitotic figures are readily found, even in small-cell-predominant lesions. There are frequently interspersed apoptotic bodies, lying free or ingested by macrophages (Fig. 29-12A). Zonal geographic necrosis is common, comprising ghost shadows of necrotic cells and karyorrhectic debris admixed with fibrinoid exudate and blood (Fig. 29-12B).

Angiocentric growth, defined as accentuation of tumor cells around blood vessels, with infiltration and destruction of the walls (Fig. 29-13), is reported in 25% to 100% of cases.[144,145,147] The lower figure probably results from limited sampling in small biopsies. Even in the absence of lymphoma infiltration, the blood vessels commonly show fibrinoid necrosis, fragmentation of the elastic lamina, and thrombosis (Fig. 29-13C). The necrosis and vascular damage are reminiscent of those observed in other EBV-associated lymphoproliferative disorders such as lymphomatoid granulomatosis; these features have been postulated to be mediated by EBV-induced monokines and chemokines such as Mig and IP-10.[180]

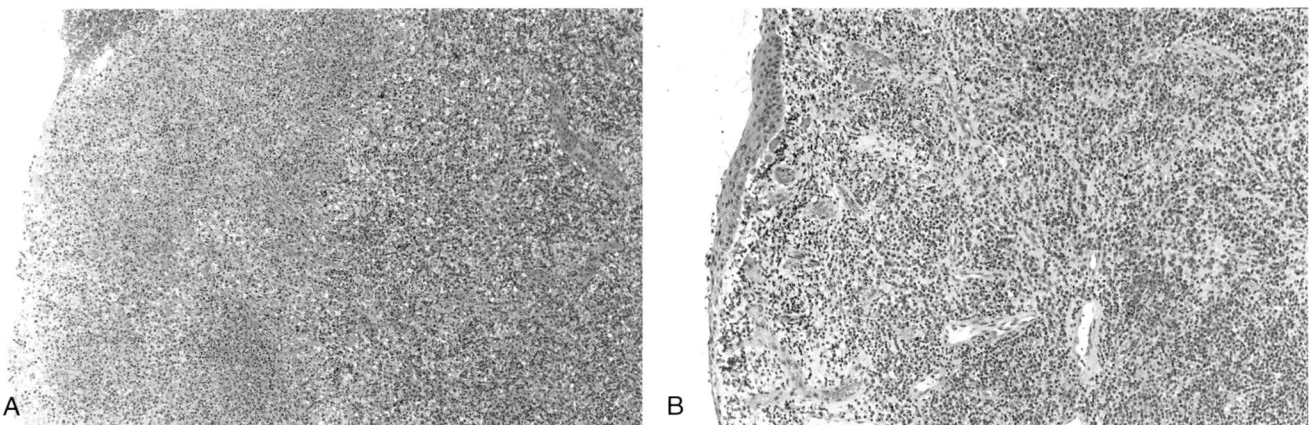

Figure 29-7. **Nasal NK/T-cell lymphoma. A,** The mucosa shows extensive ulceration and necrosis *(left field).* **B,** In this example, the mucosa is intact and densely infiltrated by lymphoma cells.

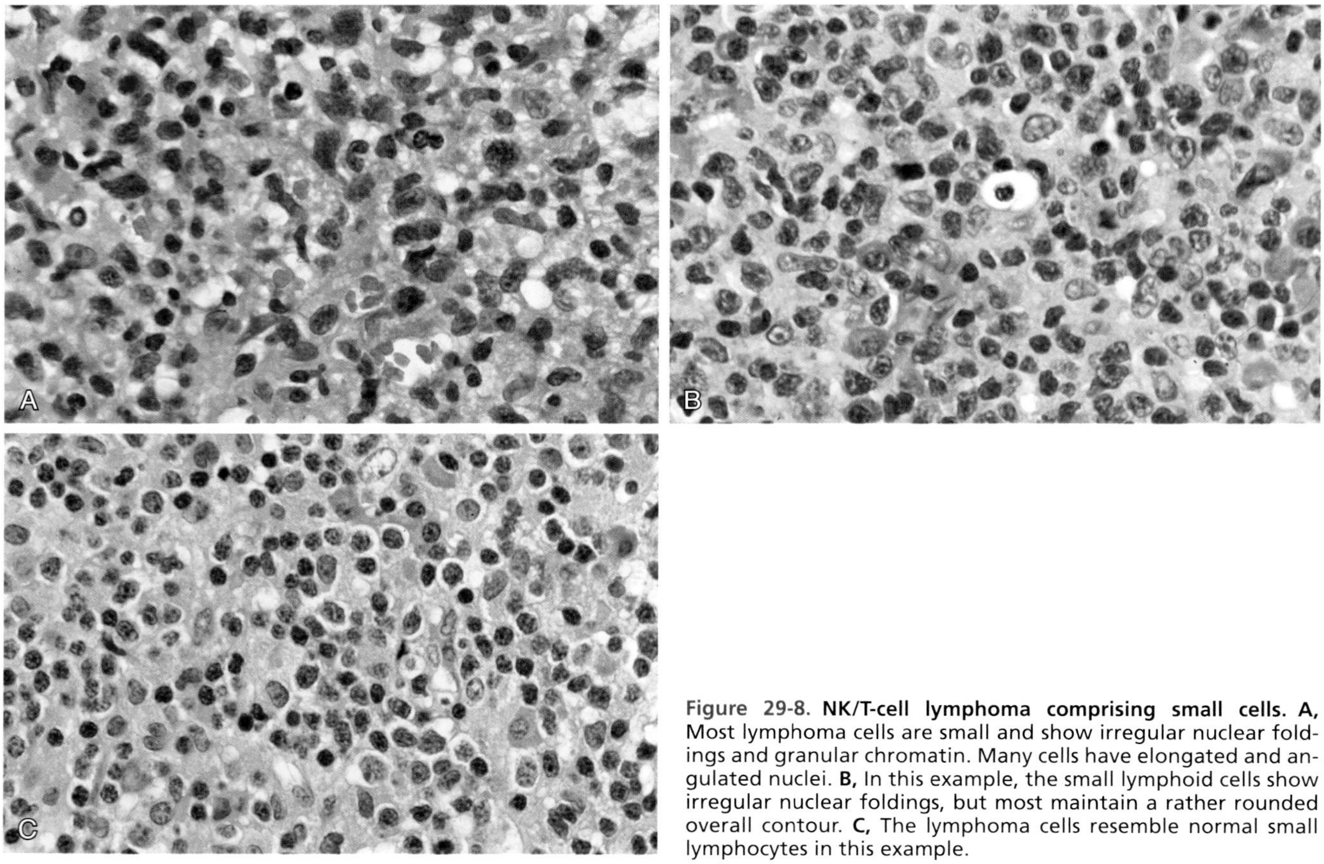

Figure 29-8. **NK/T-cell lymphoma comprising small cells. A,** Most lymphoma cells are small and show irregular nuclear foldings and granular chromatin. Many cells have elongated and angulated nuclei. **B,** In this example, the small lymphoid cells show irregular nuclear foldings, but most maintain a rather rounded overall contour. **C,** The lymphoma cells resemble normal small lymphocytes in this example.

In some cases, the background is rich in inflammatory cells, including small lymphocytes, plasma cells, histiocytes, and neutrophils, overshadowing the lymphoma cells (Fig. 29-14). Eosinophils are, however, uncommon.

Site-Specific Features

In the upper aerodigestive tract, the mucosal glands are often pushed apart and destroyed by the lymphoma cells. Some mucosal glands can exhibit cytoplasmic clearing as a form of cell injury (Fig. 29-15). The surface epithelium can be infiltrated by lymphoma cells, or may undergo squamous

metaplasia and florid pseudoepitheliomatous hyperplasia, with irregular downgrowth and nuclear atypia, mimicking squamous cell carcinoma (Fig. 29-16).[132,181]

In the skin, there is a perivascular, periadnexal, or diffuse infiltrate of lymphoma cells in the mid and deep dermis, with or without subcutaneous involvement (Fig. 29-17). Coagulative necrosis and ulceration are common. Invasion of the epithelial structures is more frequently seen in nasal NK/T-cell lymphoma disseminating to skin than primary cutaneous NK/T-cell lymphoma.[182,183] In the subcutaneous tissue, the lymphoma cells percolate among the adipocytes, producing a

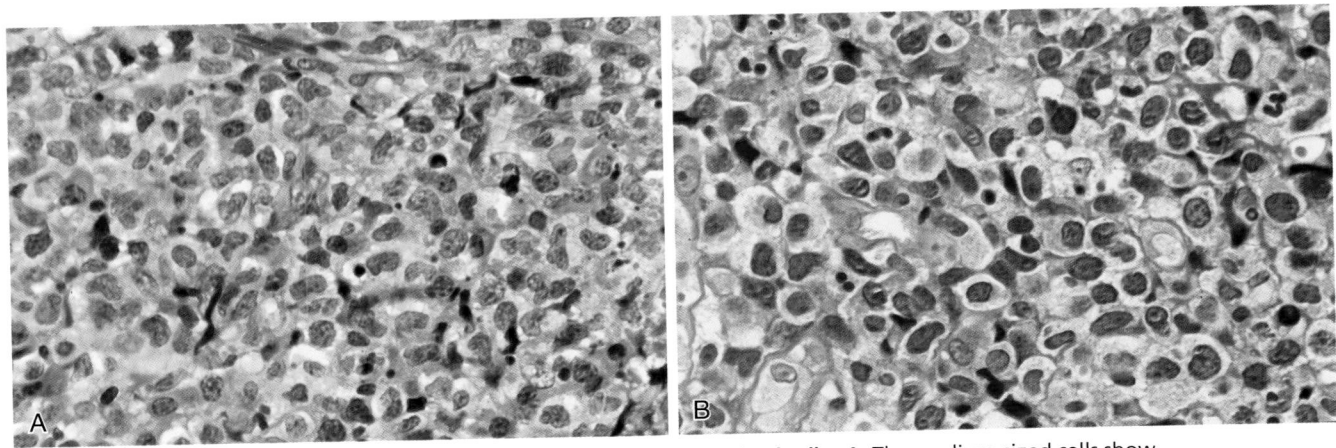

Figure 29-9. NK/T-cell lymphoma comprising medium-sized cells. A, The medium-sized cells show irregular nuclear foldings and scanty cytoplasm. Note the admixed apoptotic bodies. **B,** In this example, the medium-sized lymphoma cells possess a moderate amount of clear cytoplasm.

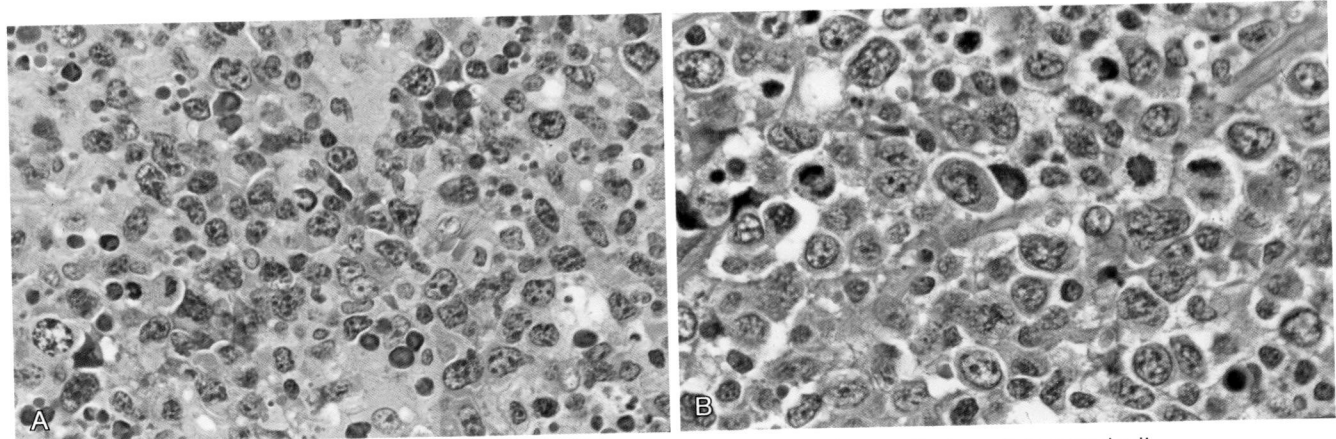

Figure 29-10. NK/T-cell lymphoma comprising large cells. A, The large cells show distinct nucleoli, and there are many intermingled apoptotic bodies. **B,** The cells are even larger in this example. Distinction from a diffuse large B-cell lymphoma cannot be made on morphologic grounds alone.

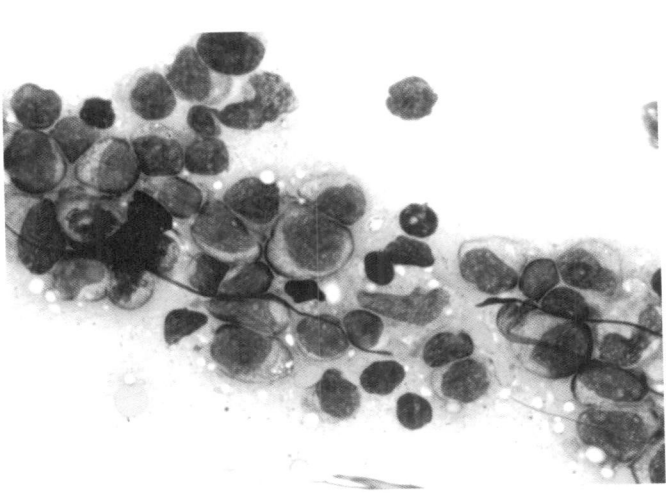

Figure 29-11. Nasal NK/T-cell lymphoma. A Giemsa-stained touch preparation reveals medium-sized cells with pale cytoplasm. Some cells contain fine azurophilic granules (where cytotoxic molecules are stored).

panniculitis-like picture (Fig. 29-18). The lymphoma cells can palisade around fat vacuoles, and fat necrosis is common.[167]

In the gastrointestinal tract, there is usually transmural lymphoma infiltration. Extensive coagulative necrosis, deep ulcers, and perforation are common (Fig. 29-19).[165,170,171,184]

In the testis, there is infiltration of the interstitium by dense sheets of lymphoma cells, often accompanied by angiodestruction and necrosis.[169] The seminiferous tubules are lost, atrophic, or infiltrated by lymphoma cells (Fig. 29-20).

In the soft tissues, there is a permeative growth, prominent destruction of skeletal muscle fibers, and invasion of the nerves (Fig. 29-21). The muscle fibers may show flocculent necrosis, invasion of the cytoplasm by lymphoma cells, or dropout of individual cells, leaving behind empty spaces.

Grading

Cytologic grading of NK/T-cell lymphoma is optional, because of lack of definite prognostic significance.[139,146,147,185] The

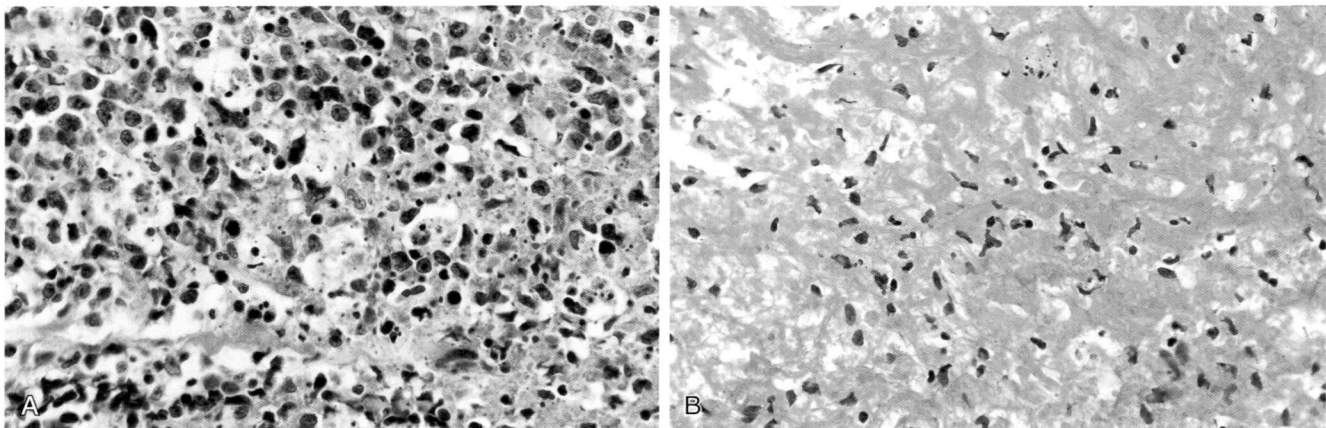

Figure 29-12. Extranodal NK/T-cell lymphoma. A, Numerous apoptotic bodies (karyorrhectic debris) are found among the lymphoma cells. **B,** Extensive necrosis with fibrin deposition is a common finding.

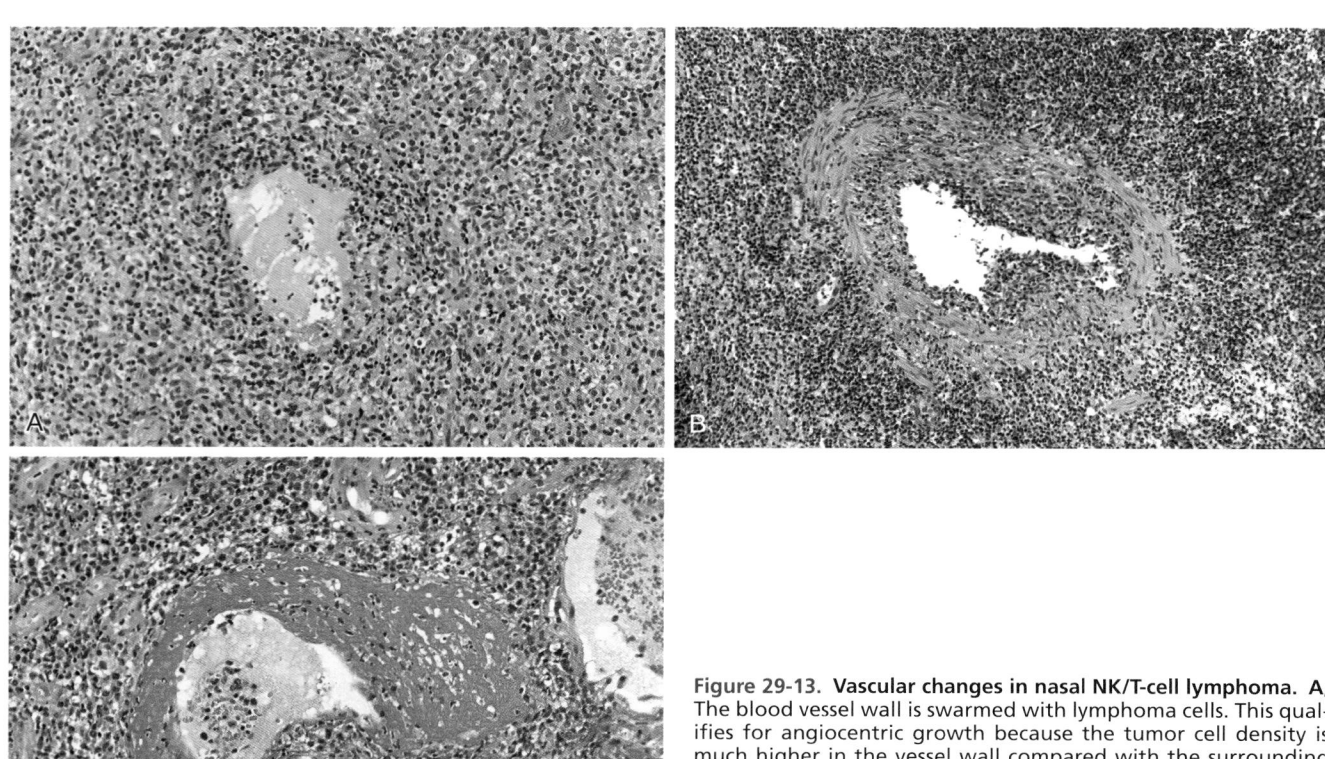

Figure 29-13. Vascular changes in nasal NK/T-cell lymphoma. A, The blood vessel wall is swarmed with lymphoma cells. This qualifies for angiocentric growth because the tumor cell density is much higher in the vessel wall compared with the surrounding involved tissue. **B,** Not only is there concentration of lymphoma cells around and in the wall of this blood vessel, but there is also infiltration of the intima. This qualifies for angiocentric growth. **C,** There is deposition of fibrinoid material in the blood vessel wall.

International Peripheral T-Cell Lymphoma Project reports the presence of >40% transformed cells to predict a worse overall survival in the nasal cases, but not the extranasal cases.[143]

Immunophenotype

The prototypic immunophenotype of NK/T-cell lymphoma is: CD2+, surface CD3−, cytoplasmic CD3ε+, CD5−, and CD56+, although occasional cases may show minor deviations, such as lack of cytoplasmic CD3ε or CD56 expression

(Table 29-2, Box 29-6) (Fig. 29-22).[143-147,149] CD43 and CD45RO are commonly positive, and CD7 is variably expressed. CD4 and CD8 are uncommonly expressed (Table 29-2).[143,186,187] A small percentage of cases express αβ-TCR or γδ-TCR.[144,147,188] Rare cases can exhibit aberrant expression of CD20.[189,190]

The only NK marker that is consistently expressed is CD56, while CD16 and CD57 are usually negative (Table 29-2) (Fig. 29-22C). Although the expression of CD56 is usually consistent in the various sites of involvement and in relapses, a

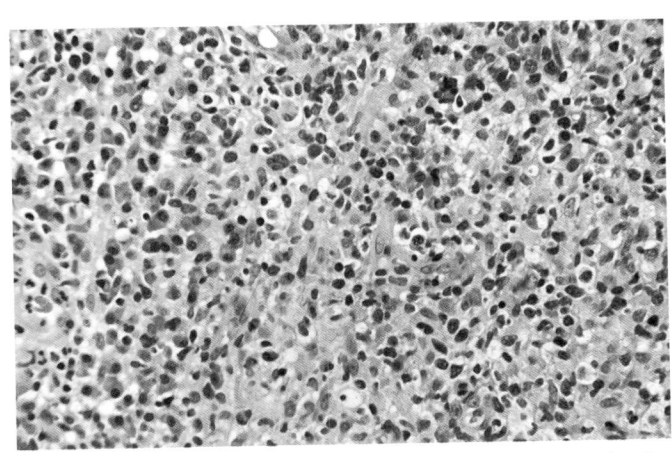

Figure 29-14. Nasal NK/T-cell lymphoma. Not uncommonly, the cellular infiltrate is polymorphous, with many intermingled acute and chronic inflammatory cells.

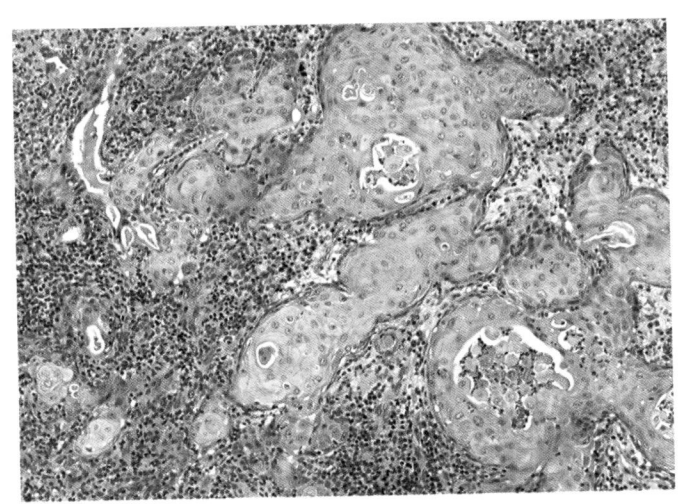

Figure 29-16. Nasal NK/T-cell lymphoma with florid pseudoepitheliomatous hyperplasia, mimicking squamous cell carcinoma.

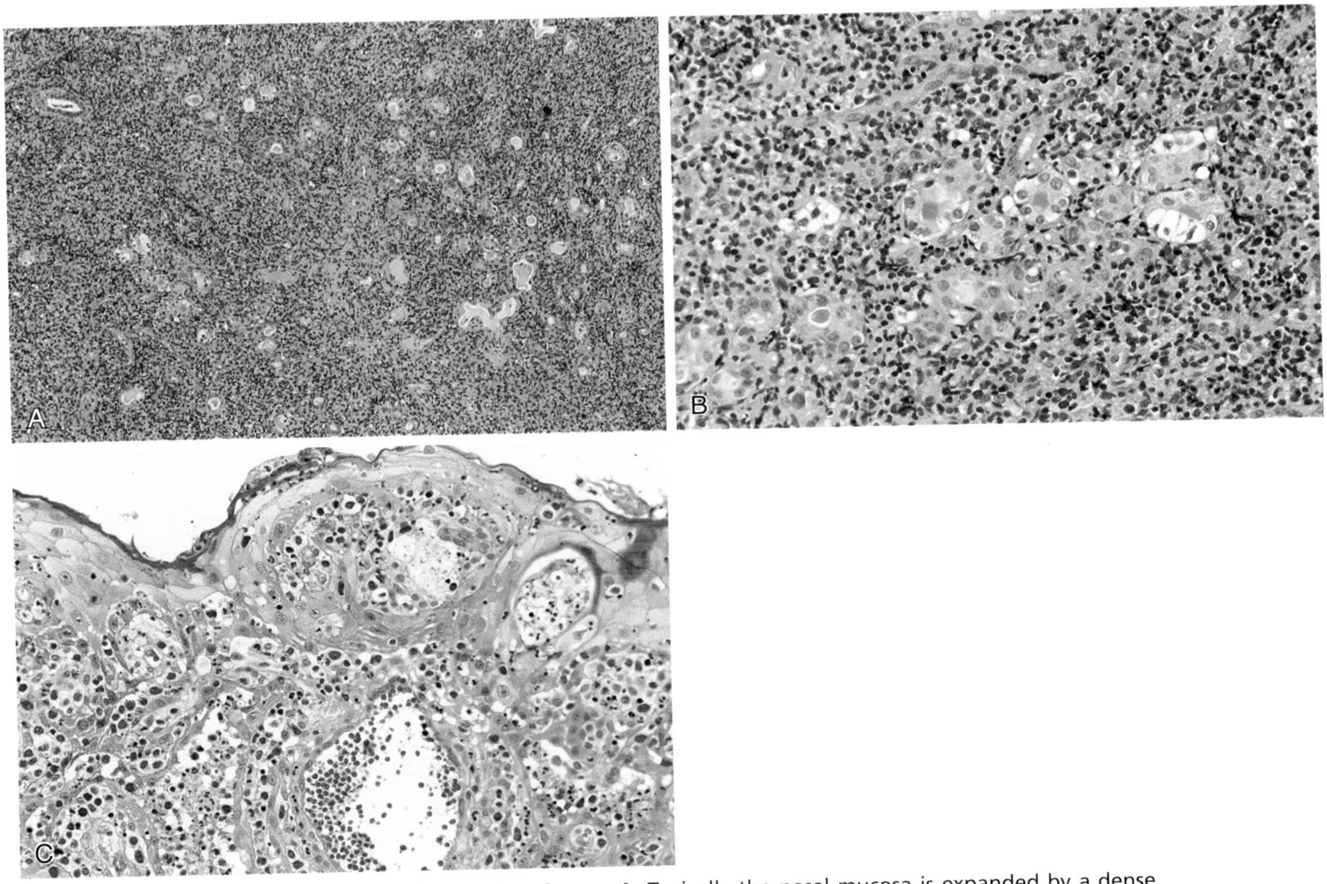

Figure 29-15. Nasal NK/T-cell lymphoma. A, Typically the nasal mucosa is expanded by a dense lymphoid infiltrate. The mucosal glands, which normally occur as discrete lobules, are pushed apart by the lymphomatous infiltrate. **B,** The interstitial lymphomatous infiltrate causes separation of the mucosal glands, which commonly exhibit clear cell change. **C,** In this example, the surface epithelium shows squamous metaplasia and infiltration by lymphoma cells.

CD56-positive tumor may relapse as a CD56-negative tumor, or vice versa. Cytotoxic molecules such as TIA-1, granzyme B, and perforin are usually positive and they may mediate the tissue injury and cell death commonly observed in this lymphoma type.[191]

Similar to normal NK cells, both Fas (CD95) and Fas ligand (CD178) are frequently expressed,[192,193] and the Fas-Fas ligand system has been postulated to play a role in tumor apoptosis and vascular injury. A proportion of cases express HLA-DR (~40%) and CD25 (15-35%).[147] CD30 is positive in

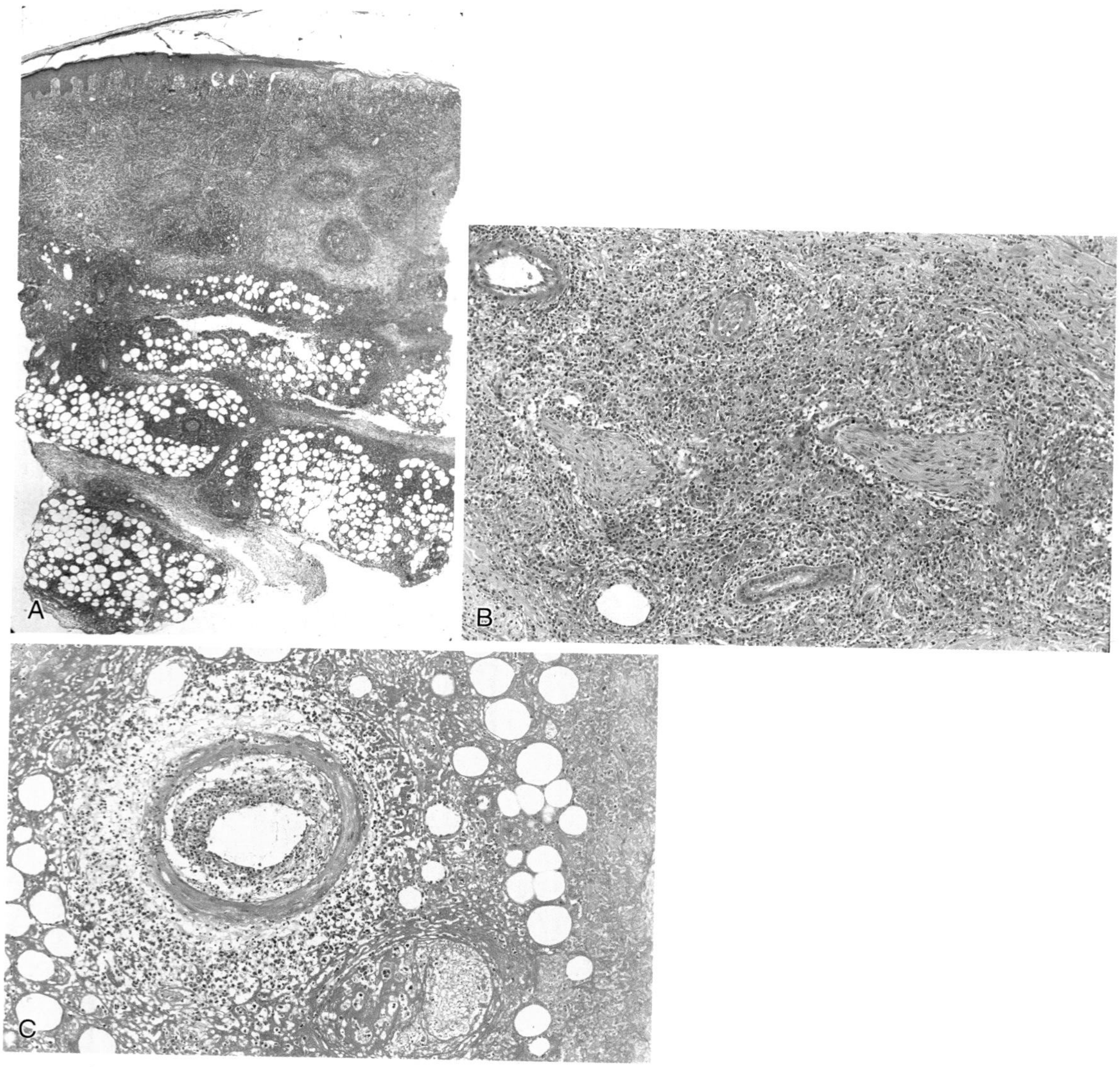

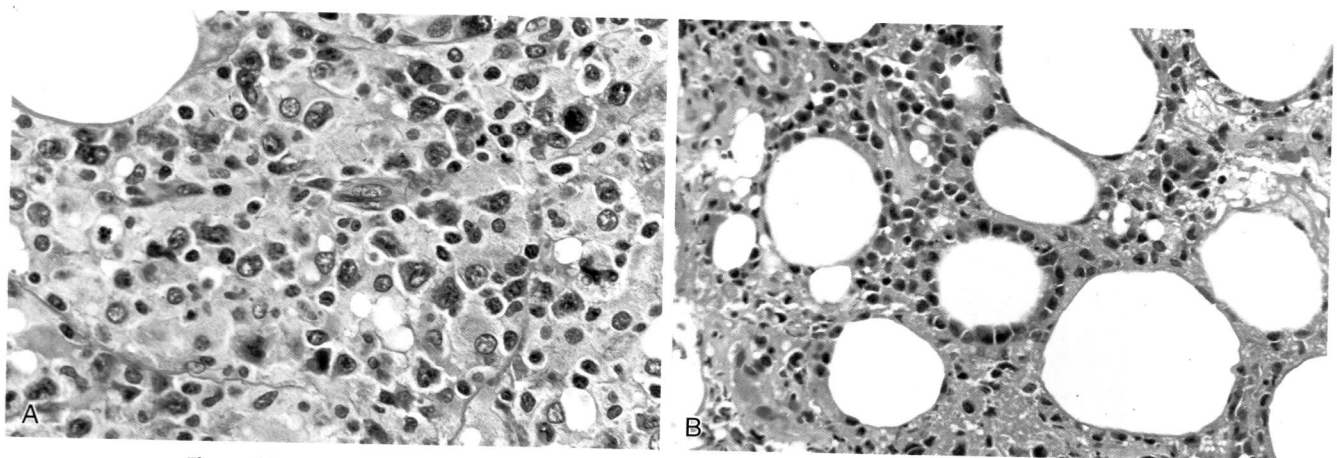

Figure 29-17. Cutaneous NK/T-cell lymphoma. A, Both the dermis and subcutaneous tissue are involved, and there are characteristically necrotic foci *(right upper field).* **B,** The dermis is heavily infiltrated by lymphoma cells, and nerves are also invaded. **C,** The subcutaneous tissue shows prominent necrosis and angiocentric-angiodestructive growth.

Figure 29-18. Cutaneous NK/T-cell lymphoma with involvement of subcutaneous tissue. A, The subcutaneous tissue shows infiltration by a mixture of atypical small-sized, medium-sized and large-sized lymphoid cells. **B,** The lacelike infiltrate and rimming of fat vacuoles by lymphoma cells simulate subcutaneous panniculitis-like T-cell lymphoma.

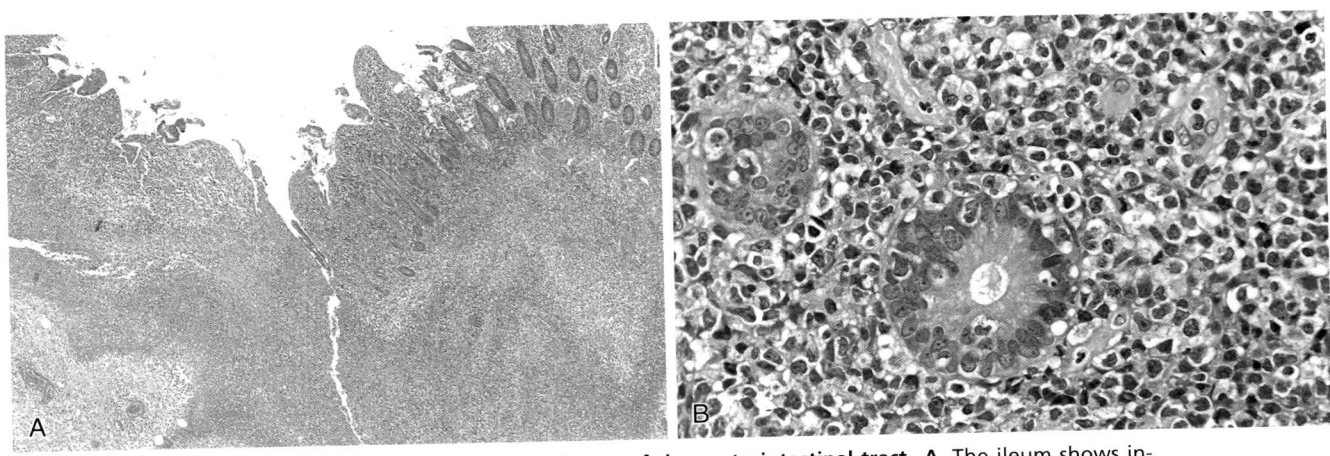

Figure 29-19. Primary NK/T-cell lymphoma of the gastrointestinal tract. A, The ileum shows infiltration by lymphoma, necrosis, deep ulceration, and perforation. **B,** The rectal mucosa shows dense interstitial infiltration by lymphoma cells with clear cytoplasm. There is also invasion of the crypt epithelium.

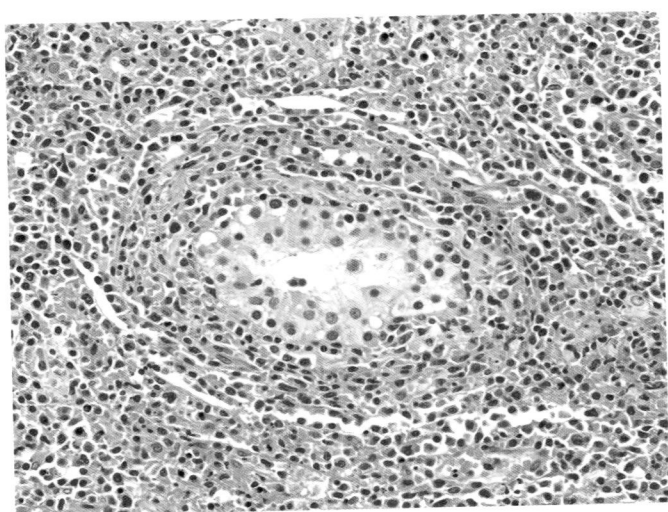

Figure 29-20. Primary testicular NK/T-cell lymphoma. The dense lymphomatous infiltration is accompanied by a striking loss of seminiferous tubules. The tubule in the *center field* shows multilayering of the basement membrane caused by infiltration by lymphoma cells.

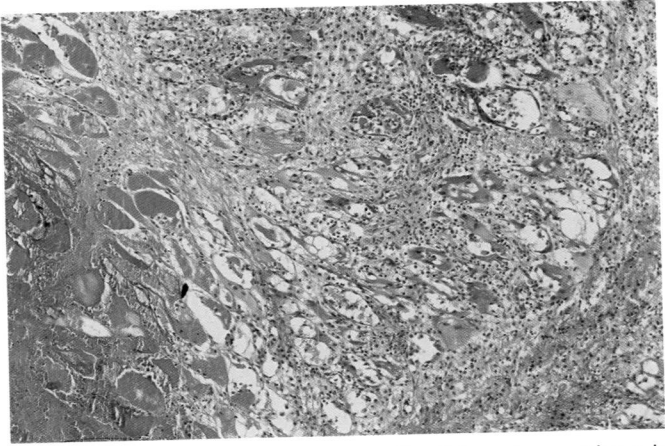

Figure 29-21. Primary soft tissue NK/T-cell lymphoma. There is interstitial infiltration of lymphoma, accompanied by prominent necrosis and destruction of skeletal muscle fibers.

Table 29-2 Immunophenotypic Profiles of Normal NK Cells and NK/T-Cell Neoplasms

	NK Cells (% of Cells Positive for the Marker)*	ENKTL-NT (% Positive Cases)[†]	Aggressive NK-Cell Leukemia (% Positive Cases)[‡]
T-lineage associated markers			
CD2	70%–90%	80%–96%	97%
Surface CD3	0%	0%	0%
Cytoplasmic CD3ε	>95%	71%–100%	64%
CD4	0%	0%–29%	0%
CD5	0%	0%–27%[§]	2%
CD7	80%–90%	14%–63%	59%
CD8	30%–40%	3%–33%	15%
NK-associated markers			
CD16	80%–90%	0%–68%	44%
CD56	>90%	58%–100%	98%
CD57	50%–60%	0%–1%	6%
Cytotoxic markers			
TIA-1, granzyme B, perforin	>95%	78%–100%	100%
NK-cell receptors			
CD94-NKG2	>95%	75%	100%
KIRs	>95%	25%–43%	33%–100%
CD161	>95%	0%	17%

ENKTL-NT, Extranodal NK/T-cell lymphoma, nasal type; *NK,* natural killer.
*References 270,314.
[†]References 143-146,149,186,187.
[‡]References 186,216,268,271,272,277.
[§]CD5 is usually negative for those of NK lineage, but may be expressed in those of cytotoxic T lineage.

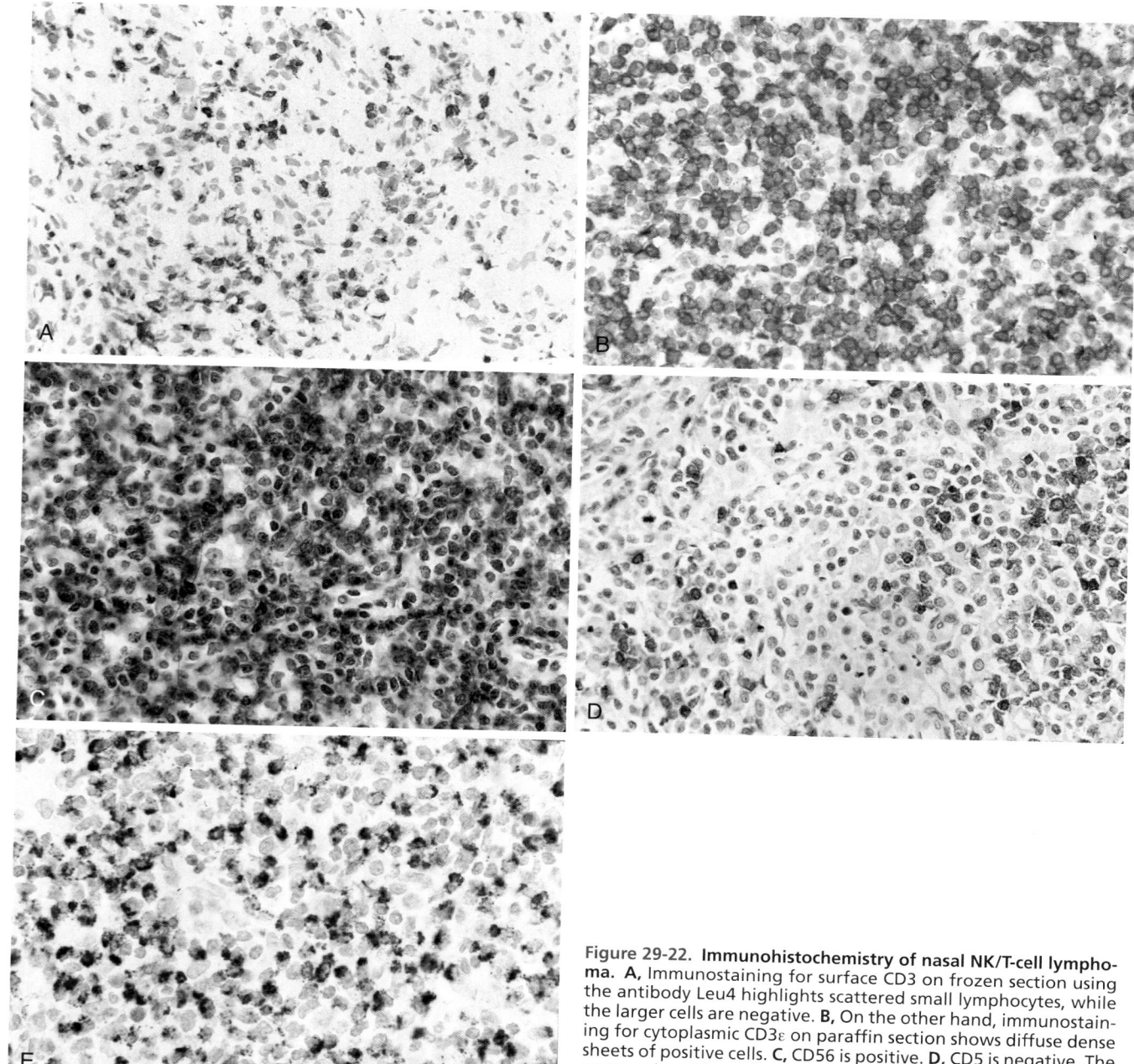

Figure 29-22. Immunohistochemistry of nasal NK/T-cell lymphoma. A, Immunostaining for surface CD3 on frozen section using the antibody Leu4 highlights scattered small lymphocytes, while the larger cells are negative. **B,** On the other hand, immunostaining for cytoplasmic CD3ε on paraffin section shows diffuse dense sheets of positive cells. **C,** CD56 is positive. **D,** CD5 is negative. The scattered positive cells are admixed reactive T cells. **E,** Numerous cells show granular staining for the cytotoxic marker TIA-1.

20% to 57% of cases, especially in those rich in large cells, but the staining is usually focal and not intense,[145,146,149,194,195] and the prognostic significance is controversial.[194-196] Nuclear expression of MATK is common.[147,197]

The proliferative fraction as demonstrated by Ki67 immunostaining is usually high (>50%), even for small-cell-predominant lesions.[144] Some studies suggest that a high Ki67 index (using cutoffs ranging from 60%–70%) is associated with a worse prognosis, and one study reports a Ki67 index of >50% to predict worse overall survival for nasal but not extranasal cases.[146,198-200]

Most NK/T-cell lymphomas express the NK-cell receptor CD94/NGK2, but only some express KIRs.[186,187] NK-cell receptors are not specific for NK/T-cell lymphomas, but are also

expressed by some cytotoxic T-cell lymphomas and hepatosplenic T-cell lymphomas. However, demonstration of a skewed NK-cell repertoire by flow cytometry using antibodies against KIRs, CD94, and NKG2A may imply a monoclonal NK-cell proliferation.[201]

CD56-Negative Subset

Nasal lymphomas that are CD56 negative but demonstrate a CD3ε-positive, cytotoxic molecule–positive, EBV-positive phenotype are also included within the category of nasal NK/T-cell lymphoma.[132] Some of them are probably NK-cell lymphomas that have lost CD56 expression, while others are cytotoxic T-cell lymphomas.[193,202] The clinical features and morphology of the CD56-negative group are indistinguishable from the CD56-positive group.[143] Those nasal lymphomas that show a CD3ε-positive, CD56-negative, cytotoxic molecule–negative, EBV-negative phenotype should be diagnosed instead as peripheral T-cell lymphoma, not otherwise specified (NOS).

Genetics and Molecular Findings

The TR and IG genes are in germline configuration in most cases. Clonal rearrangements of TR genes are reported in 10% to 40% of cases; the positive cases presumably represent neoplasms of cytotoxic T cells rather than NK cells.[141,143-147]

There is, by definition, consistent association with EBV, and in situ hybridization for EBER typically labels virtually all tumor cells (Fig. 29-23).[149] Demonstration of EBV may aid in diagnosis, because the many types of peripheral T-cell lymphomas that show morphologic and immunophenotypic overlap with NK/T-cell lymphoma are almost always negative for EBV.[203] Circulating whole blood or plasma EBV DNA level is often elevated, and a high titer is correlated with extensive disease, unfavorable response to treatment, and poor survival.[204-206] Decline of EBV DNA to undetectable level after treatment is associated with a favorable prognosis.[205,207]

The gene-expression profiles of all extranodal NK/T-cell lymphomas cluster together irrespective of NK- or cytotoxic T-cell lineage, supporting the current classification to include tumors of these two lineages in the same lymphoma category.[208,209] Interestingly, non-hepatosplenic γδT-cell lymphoma also shows very similar gene-expression profiles.[208,209]

Complex chromosomal abnormalities have been found in extranodal NK/T-cell lymphomas.[179,210-213] The most common changes are 6q21-q25 deletion (about 50%), 1q21-q44 gain (about 50%), and 17p11.2-p13.3 deletion (about 40%).[208,209,214-216] Specific chromosomal translocations have not been identified. In the commonly deleted region on 6q21, several candidate tumor suppressor genes (PRDM1, ATG5, AIM1, PTPRK, HACE1, and FOXO3) with low-level transcripts have been identified.[214,217,218] Nonsense mutation and promoter hypermethylation have been reported in PRMD1 (which plays an important role in NK-cell homeostasis),[218-220] and missense mutation in FOXO3.[217] Underexpression of PTPRK may lead to STAT3 activation, since PTPRK normally dephosphorylates phospho-STAT3.[221] The pathogenetic role of HACE1 is controversial.[222-224]

Activation of the JAK-STAT signaling pathway through mutations (JAK23, STAT3, and STAT5B mutations in a low percentage of cases) and phosphorylation appears to play a key role in the pathogenesis of extranodal NK/T-cell lymphoma.[209,225-231] Recurrent mutations are found in RNA helicase (DDX3X, DHX58), epigenetic regulators (KMT2D, BCOR, ARID1A, EP300), and tumor suppressor genes (TP53, MGA).[232-236] There is also activation of NF-κB pathway and overexpression of MYC and EZH2.[237,238] PDL1 expression is upregulated, postulated to be driven by LMP1 or STAT3.[239,240]

Three molecular subtypes of extranodal NK/T-cell lymphoma have been proposed.[236] The TSIM subtype (most common subtype: 55%) is characterized by JAK/STAT activation, TP53 mutation, del6q21, overexpression of PLD1, type II EBV latency with expression of lytic gene BALF3, and NK-cell origin. The MB subtype is characterized by MGA mutation, 1p22.1/BRDT loss of heterozygosity, MYC overexpression, type I EBV latency, T-cell origin, and poor outcome. The HEA subtype is characterized by aberrant

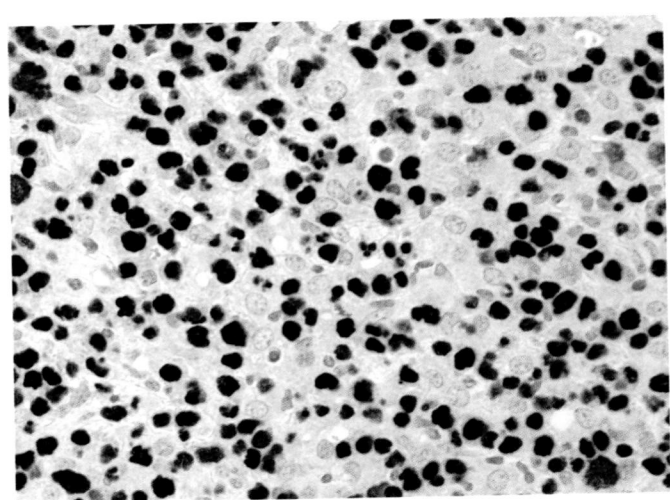

Figure 29-23. Nasal NK/T-cell lymphoma. In situ hybridization for EBER labels the nuclei of most lymphoma cells.

histone acetylation, mutations in HDAC9, EP300, and ARID1A, overexpression of DAXX and MEF2C, NF-κB activation, type II EBV latency with expression of lytic gene BNFR1, T-cell origin, and best outcome. Further studies are needed to validate the significance of this molecular subtyping.

Postulated Cell of Origin

The likely normal counterpart is an activated mature NK cell in most cases, and an cytotoxic T lymphocyte in others.[186,209]

There are no criteria which can absolutely distinguish true NK-cell lineage from cytotoxic T-cell lineage among lymphomas. One approach is to use a combination of TCR expression and TR gene rearrangement to assign lineage.[144] Lack of expression of αβ and γδ TCR proteins, together with lack of clonal TR gene rearrangements, suggests NK lineage. Expression of TCR protein (irrespective of TR gene rearrangement status), or lack of TCR protein expression but presence of clonal TR gene rearrangement, will suggest T-cell lineage. The caveats of the approach are limitations in sensitivity of TCR immunohistochemistry,[203] possible loss of TCR expression in some T-cell lymphomas,[203] and possible false negative results of TR gene rearrangement studies by polymerase chain reaction (PCR). Overall, about 85% of nasal NK/T-cell lymphomas are considered to be of NK lineage, while about 50% of extranasal NK/T-cell lymphomas are considered to be of NK lineage.[144,167,188] The distinction between NK and cytotoxic T cell lineage, however, is not of prognostic importance.[144]

Clinical Course

Although patients with nasal NK/T-cell lymphoma usually present with localized disease; dissemination to various sites frequently occurs either early or late during the clinical course.[139,241] Chemoradiotherapy with nonanthracycline-containing regimens is the single most important key to successful outcome, with 5-year overall survival rate of about 70% being achievable.[242-246]

For patients with advanced stage nasal or extranasal NK/T-cell lymphoma, chemotherapy with anthracycline-based regimens such as CHOP have produced disappointing results, with overall 5-year survival rate of only approximately 10%,[139,143,247,248] which may be attributable to frequent expression of multidrug resistance gene (P-glycoprotein).[249] Favorable overall response has been reported with regimens including L-asparaginase, with response around 80% being reported.[246,250-253]

Immune checkpoint inhibitors hold promise in treatment of patients with relapsed or refractory disease, being able to achieve complete remission in a proportion of these patients.[254-256]

Rare cases of nasal or extranasal (particularly cutaneous) NK/T-cell lymphoma may pursue an indolent or self-regressing clinical course,[257] but it is currently not possible to predict which cases will behave in this fashion.

Differential Diagnosis

The main differential diagnoses are listed in Table 29-3. For lesions composed mostly of large lymphoid cells, it is easy to recognize their neoplastic nature, but the problem is distinction from diffuse large B-cell lymphoma and non-hematolymphoid malignancies. This problem can usually be readily solved by immunohistochemistry.

For lesions composed predominantly of small-sized or mixed cells, distinction from reactive or inflammatory conditions can be very difficult (Table 29-3). In extranodal sites, the normal small lymphocytes often appear mildly atypical, with slightly enlarged and irregularly folded nuclei, and thus morphologically overlap with the small neoplastic cells seen in extranodal NK/T-cell lymphoma (Figs. 29-24 and 29-25). Presence of some or all of the following morphologic features would favor a diagnosis of lymphoma: (1) dense infiltrate causing separation or destruction of the mucosal glands, (2) prominent tissue necrosis and ulceration, (3) angioinvasion, (4) presence of mitotic figures in a small-cell-predominant lymphoid infiltrate, (5) clear cells, and (6) a significant population of atypical medium-sized cells with irregular nuclei (Fig. 29-26). The diagnosis can be confirmed by immunohistochemical demonstration of sheets of CD3ε-positive CD56-positive cells. If the infiltrate is CD3ε positive CD56 negative, positive immunostaining for TIA-1 and in situ hybridization for EBER will support the diagnosis. See Pearls and Pitfalls for assessment of posttreatment biopsies (Fig. 29-27).

Acute EBV-positive cytotoxic T-cell lymphoid hyperplasia of the upper aerodigestive tract, a rare self-limiting condition, can mimic nasal NK/T-cell lymphoma.[258] The patients are young, with a median age of 16 years. They present with acute onset of mass lesion in the upper aerodigestive tract, commonly accompanied by cervical lymphadenopathy and fever. Biopsy shows infiltration of atypical small-to-medium-sized lymphoid cells that represent cytotoxic T cells (CD3 positive, CD5 positive, cytotoxic marker positive, CD56 negative) and express EBER. This condition differs from the usual acute EBV infections (infectious mononucleosis) in implicating T cells rather than B cells, thus showing significant morphologic and immunophenotypic overlap with extranodal NK/T-cell lymphoma. Features suggesting this diagnosis over the latter include young patient age, acute onset of symptoms, presence of cervical lymphadenopathy and fever, CD5 positive lymphoid cells, and CD56 negative.

Wegener's granulomatosis, a destructive lesion of the upper respiratory tract, shares many morphologic features with nasal NK/T-cell lymphoma in the form of mixed inflammatory infiltrate, ulceration, necrosis, and vasculitis or vasculitis-like lesions. The same features helpful for distinction between extranodal NK/T-cell lymphoma and reactive/inflammatory also apply.

Lymphomatoid granulomatosis represents a distinct form of T-cell-rich large B cell lymphoproliferative disorder showing a strong association with EBV.[186-188,259] The atypical cells express B lineage markers rather than NK/T cell markers.

Primary cutaneous γδT-cell lymphoma shows morphologic and immunophenotypic overlap with extranodal NK/T-cell lymphoma (including frequent expression of cytotoxic markers and CD56), but can be distinguished by a usual lack of EBV.[203] Dilemma in classification, however, may arise when a cutaneous T-cell lymphoma is shown to be γδ TCR positive and EBV positive, raising the possibilities of extranodal NK/T-cell lymphoma and the rare occurrence of EBV in primary cutaneous γδT-cell lymphoma.[203,260,261]

Herpes simplex infection can simulate nasal NK/T-cell lymphoma because of the presence of a mass lesion, a dense lymphoid infiltrate with necrosis, and CD56 expression by the lymphoid cells.[262] The presence of scattered herpesvirus inclusions, lack of angioinvasion, expression of CD4 by the T-cell infiltrate, and absence of EBV support this diagnosis over extranodal NK/T-cell lymphoma.

Indolent NK-cell lymphoproliferative disorder of the gastrointestinal tract (formerly known as *NK-cell enteropathy* or *lymphomatoid gastropathy*) is a self-limiting NK-cell proliferation affecting single or multiple sites in the gastrointestinal tract.[6,7,263-265] The patients are asymptomatic or present with vague gastrointestinal symptoms. Endoscopy reveals a superficial small elevated lesion (~1 cm) or ulcer, often with hemorrhage and edema. The lesion shows spontaneous resolution, persistence, or recurrence. Biopsy shows mucosa expanded by atypical medium-sized lymphoid cells with indented or irregularly folded nuclei. Some lymphoid cells contain brightly eosinophilic granules. The atypical lymphoid cells show an NK-cell immunophenotype (CD3 positive, CD5 negative, CD56 positive, cytotoxic markers positive). Features favoring the diagnosis of indolent NK-cell lymphoproliferative disorder over extranodal NK/T-cell lymphoma are as follows: (1) small, relatively circumscribed and superficial lesion; (2) lack of angioinvasion or necrosis; and (3) negative for EBER.

AGGRESSIVE NK-CELL LEUKEMIA

Synonyms and Related Terms

WHO revised 4th ed.: Aggressive NK-cell leukemia
WHO proposed 5th ed.: Aggressive NK-cell leukemia

Definition

Aggressive NK-cell leukemia is a systemic neoplasm of NK cells with primary involvement of peripheral blood and bone marrow and a fulminant clinical course, and frequent association with EBV (capsule summary in Box 29-7).[266,267] In contrast to the usual leukemias, neoplastic cells can be sparse in the peripheral blood and bone marrow.

Table 29-3 Differential Diagnosis for Extranodal NK/T-Cell Lymphoma, Nasal Type

Entity	Features Favoring Diagnosis of the Entity	Features Favoring Diagnosis of ENKTL-NT
Reactive lymphoid hyperplasia	• Non-expansile and non-destructive infiltrate of mixed lymphoid cells • No definite cytologic atypia • Nodular aggregates of CD20-positive B cells are separated by many CD3-positive T cells that are CD56 negative • EBER negative	• Dense expansile infiltrate causing distortion or destruction of mucosal glands • Ulceration and tissue necrosis • Presence of atypical cells—medium-sized cells, clear cells, or cells with significant nuclear irregularities • More than occasional mitotic figures in a small lymphoid cell predominant lesion • Angiocentric and angioinvasive growth • CD3ε⁺, CD56⁺ or CD3ε⁺, CD56⁻, TIA1⁺, EBER⁺
Acute EBV-positive cytotoxic T-cell lymphoid hyperplasia of the upper aerodigestive tract	• Typically affects children and young adults • Usually acute onset of symptoms, accompanied by cervical lymphadenopathy and fever • Lymphoid infiltrate shows cytotoxic T-cell phenotype and is CD56 negative	• Usually occurs in middle-aged to older adults • Usually more gradual onset of symptoms; cervical lymphadenopathy and fever are uncommon in nasal NK/T-cell lymphoma • Lymphoid infiltrate more commonly, but not always, shows NK-cell phenotype, and is often CD56 positive
Wegener's granulomatosis	• Antineutrophil cytoplasmic antibody positive • Involvement of kidney and lung • No definite cytologic atypia • Granuloma formation with multinucleated giant cells • Microabscesses or eosinophils in areas away from necrosis • EBER negative	• Presence of atypical lymphoid cells • Usually no granuloma • Acute inflammatory cells usually confined to the vicinity of ulcers • EBER positive
Lymphomatoid granulomatosis	• Predominantly affects lung; sometimes brain, skin, and kidney • Large atypical tumor cells are B cells (CD20 positive, EBER positive); background rich in reactive T cells	• Most commonly affects sinonasal areas; lung involvement extremely rare • CD3ε positive, CD20 negative
Subcutaneous panniculitis-like T-cell lymphoma	• Clinically subcutaneous nodules alone • Almost exclusively subcutaneous involvement, with at most minimal dermal involvement • Angiocentric growth less common • Usually sCD3 positive, CD8 positive, CD56 negative; αβ-TCR positive • EBER negative	• Skin nodules, often in multiple sites, and commonly accompanied by other sites of disease • Dermal involvement almost always present in additional to subcutaneous involvement • Frequent angiocentric and angioinvasive growth • Usually CD3 negative, CD8 negative, CD56 positive; αβ-TCR often negative • EBER positive
Primary cutaneous γδT-cell lymphoma	• γδ-TCR positive (by definition) • Clonal TR gene rearrangement in almost all cases • EBER negative (with rare exceptions)	• Expression of γδ-TCR uncommon • Clonal TR rearrangement uncommon • EBV positive
Indolent NK-cell lymphoproliferative disorder of the gastrointestinal tract	• Small and superficial lesion • Usually presence of brightly eosinophilic cytoplasmic granules in H&E-stained section • EBER negative	• Usually large and deep (transmural) lesion • Prominent necrosis in most cases • Extremely rare to find eosinophilic cytoplasmic granules in H&E-stained section • EBER positive
Blastic plasmacytoid dendritic cell neoplasm	• Monotonous infiltrate of medium-sized blastic cells with thin nuclear membrane and fine chromatin, morphologically reminiscent of leukemic infiltrate; nuclei commonly round or oval • Angioinvasion and necrosis uncommon • CD56⁺, CD4⁺, CD123⁺, TCF4⁺, TCL1⁺, TdT⁺/⁻, CD3ε usually − • EBER negative	• Monotonous or mixed infiltrate of lymphoma cells of variable sizes; nuclei often irregularly folded and more chromatin-rich • Angioinvasion and necrosis often prominent • CD56 usually +, CD4⁻, CD123⁻, TdT⁻, CD3ε usually + • EBER positive
Squamous cell carcinoma	• Often shows deep invasion • Dysplastic or carcinoma-in-situ changes in the surface epithelium	• Squamous proliferation (pseudoepitheliomatous hyperplasia) limited to the superficial zone of the mucosa • Lack of desmoplastic reaction • Presence of atypical lymphoid cells between the tongues of atypical squamous epithelium

EBER, EBV-encoded RNA; *EBV,* Epstein-Barr virus; *ENKTL-NT,* extranodal NK/T-cell lymphoma, nasal type; *H&E,* hematoxylin and eosin; *NK,* natural killer; *TdT,* terminal deoxynucleotidyl transferase.

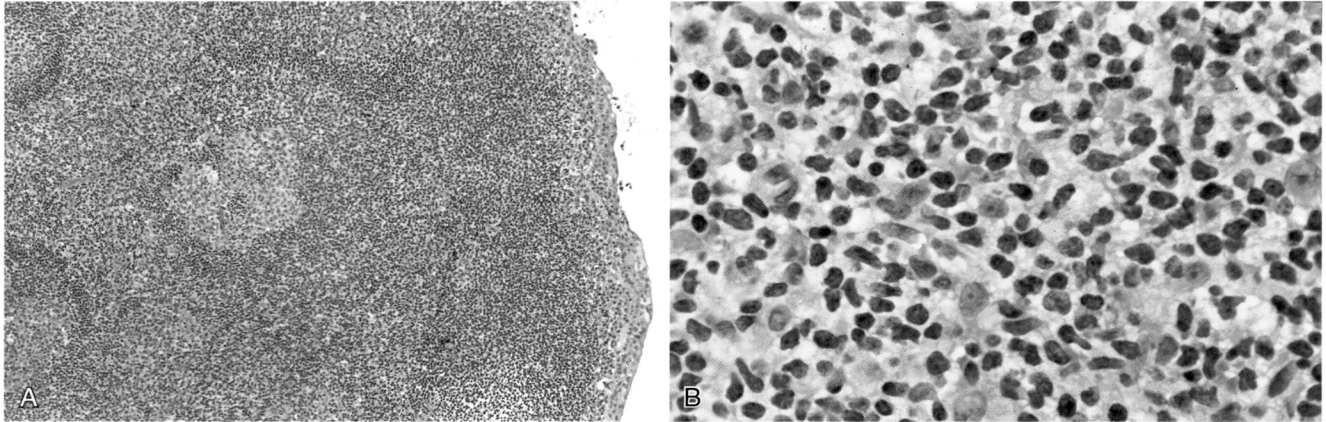

Figure 29-24. Nasopharyngeal mucosa with reactive lymphoid hyperplasia. A, The mucosa is rich in lymphoid cells, and reactive lymphoid follicles are present. **B,** Closer examination of the inter-follicular zone shows that the small lymphoid cells are often slightly larger than small lymphocytes and can exhibit nuclear foldings. Thus there is cytologic overlap of mucosal reactive lymphoid cells and NK/T-cell lymphoma cells (compare with Fig. 29-8).

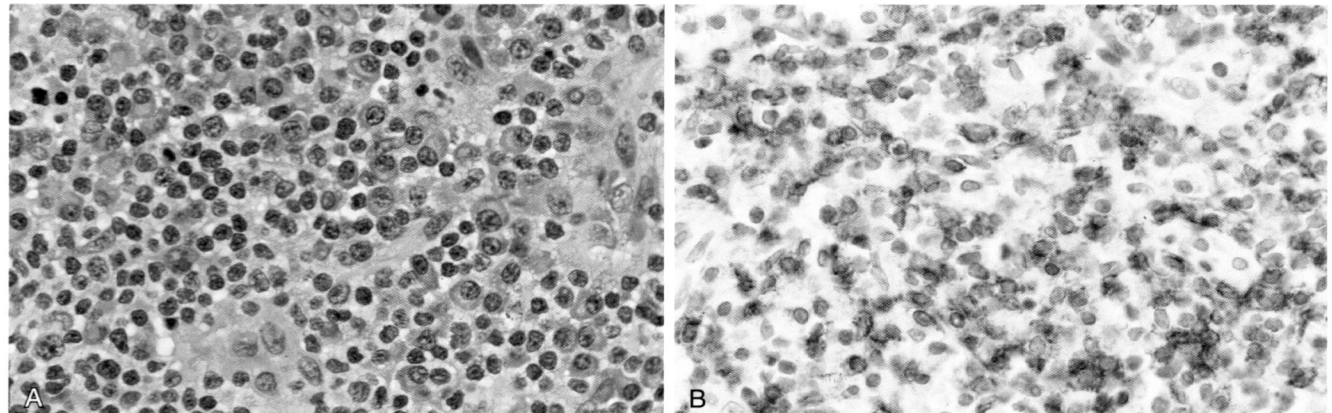

Figure 29-25. Nasal NK/T-cell lymphoma: difficult-to-diagnose case. A, The predominance of small lymphoid cells with round nuclei and admixed plasma cells suggests a benign lymphoid infiltrate. Nonetheless, there are features suggestive of lymphoma such as ulceration and loss of mucosal glands (not shown). **B,** Immunostaining shows many CD56-positive cells (which are also CD3ε positive), supporting a diagnosis of nasal NK/T-cell lymphoma. In the normal or reactive mucosa, CD56-positive cells are not present in such large numbers.

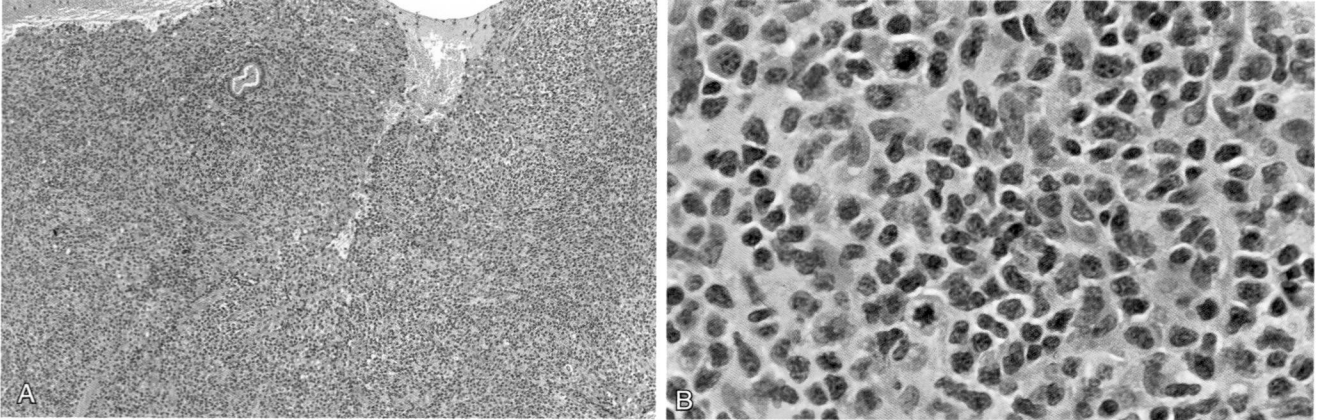

Figure 29-26. Nasal NK/T-cell lymphoma: histologic features supporting a diagnosis of lymphoma over reactive lymphoid hyperplasia. A, An extensive and dense lymphoid infiltrate with loss of mucosal glands. **B,** Definite cytologic atypia in the lymphoid cells, if present, supports a diagnosis of lymphoma. Compared with Fig. 29-24, the cells are slightly larger and show more irregular nuclear foldings. Readily found mitotic figures in a small lymphoid infiltrate are another feature suggestive of lymphoma.

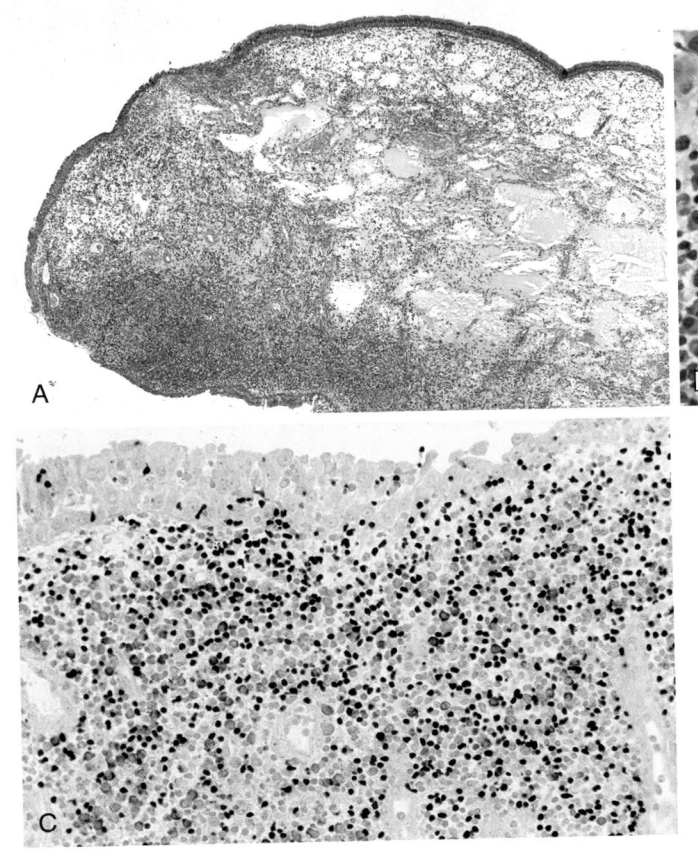

Figure 29-27. Nasal NK/T-cell lymphoma: posttreatment biopsy. A, The nasal mucosa appears hypocellular in most areas. **B,** In the more cellular areas, plasma cells are admixed with small lymphoid cells, suggesting a benign lymphoid infiltrate. **C,** Surprisingly, numerous Epstein-Barr virus–encoded RNA (EBER)–positive cells are present, indicating that there is still residual disease.

Box 29-7 *Major Diagnostic Features of Aggressive NK-Cell Leukemia*

Clinical Features and Behavior
- More prevalent in Asians
- Age: Teenage to middle age (median 40 years)
- Sex: M = F
- Presentation: Ill patient with fever, constitutional symptoms, hepatosplenomegaly, generalized lymphadenopathy, and sometimes bleeding tendency
- Fulminant clinical course with cytopenia, coagulopathy, and multiorgan failure, often resulting in death within a few weeks

Morphology
- Peripheral blood or marrow smear: Few to numerous large granular lymphocytes, many of which are atypical (such as irregular nuclear foldings or very large size) or immature (such as open chromatin or distinct nucleoli).
- Involved tissues: Usually dense, permeative, and monotonous infiltrate of medium-sized lymphoid cells with prominent apoptosis. Angiocentric growth and necrosis common.

Immunophenotype and Genotype
- CD3ε+, surface CD3−, CD5−, CD56+, CD16+/−, cytotoxic molecule+
- EBV positive in majority of cases
- TR genes germline

Epidemiology and Etiology

The disease occurs with a much higher frequency in Asians compared with Whites, and thus ethnic factors may play a role in disease susceptibility. It is strongly associated with EBV, which is present in approximately 90% of cases.[268-273] Rare cases may evolve from CAEBVD of T or NK type,[72,73,103] nasal NK/T-cell lymphoma,[274] or chronic lymphoproliferative disorder of NK cell (NK large granular lymphocytic leukemia)[275]; aggressive NK-cell leukemia arising in the latter setting is EBV negative.

The patients are typically adolescents or young adults, but older patients can also be affected. The median age is 40 years.[186,266,268,271,272,276-279] There is no sex predilection.

Clinical Features

The typical presentations are fever, hepatosplenomegaly, and a leukemic blood picture.[186,266,268,271,272,276,277] Lymphadenopathy may be present. Skin nodules are uncommon, but some patients may have nonspecific skin rash. The patients are often very ill and are commonly complicated by hemophagocytic syndrome.[276,278] Serum lactate dehydrogenase level is often markedly elevated, as is circulating Fas ligand.[280,281] It has been postulated that the systemic shedding of large quantities of Fas ligand from the tumor cells may contribute to the multiorgan failure commonly seen in aggressive NK-cell leukemia—binding of Fas ligand to Fas, which is normally expressed in many different types of normal cells, results in apoptosis of the Fas-bearing cells.

Morphology

Circulating leukemic cells account for <5% to >80% of lymphocytes. They often exhibit a range of appearances in an individual case, from normal-looking to immature or pleomorphic large granular lymphocytes (Fig. 29-28). They have round nuclei with condensed chromatin, or larger nuclei with irregular foldings. Nucleoli can be prominent in some cases. The cytoplasm is moderate to abundant in amount, and is lightly basophilic, with variable numbers of fine and occasionally coarse azurophilic granules. In the bone marrow, the neoplastic cells constitute 6% to 92% of all nucleated cells,[277] with the pattern of involvement ranging from diffuse interstitial to subtle and patchy (Fig. 29-29).[277]

In histologic sections, there is a diffuse, destructive, and permeative infiltrate consisting of cells with round or irregular nuclei, fairly condensed chromatin, and a thin-to-moderate rim of pale or amphophilic cytoplasm. Interspersed apoptotic bodies and zonal cell death are common (Fig. 29-30). Angioinvasive-angiodestructive growth is also frequently noted.[272]

Immunophenotype and Molecular Findings

The typical immunophenotype is CD2+, surface CD3−, cytoplasm CD3ε+, TCR−, CD5−, CD56+, CD16+, and cytotoxic markers+ (Fig. 29-31). CD57 is often negative (Table 29-2).[143,186,216,268,271,272]

The TR genes are typically not rearranged. EBV is reported in about 90% of cases.[268-271,276,277,282] The EBV-negative subset shows clinicopathologic features similar to the EBV-positive cases.[208,283-286]

Although previous comparative genomic hybridization studies suggest similar genetic changes in aggressive NK-cell leukemia and extranodal NK/T-cell lymphoma, such as 3p positive, 6q negative, 11q negative, 12q positive,[179,210] an array-based comparative genomic hybridization study reveals significant differences between the two.[213] For instance, 7p negative, 17p negative, and 1q positive are frequent in aggressive NK-cell leukemia but not in extranodal NK/T-cell lymphoma, while the 6q negative is much more common in the latter.

Molecular studies indicate prominent STAT3 activation and MYC expression.[287] Mutations are commonly found in genes of the JAK-STAT and RAS-MAPK pathways, histone modifying genes (*TET2, CREBBP,* and *KMT2D*), *DDX3X,* and *TP53.*[279,287-289]

Clinical Course

Aggressive NK-cell leukemia pursues an acute fulminant course, frequently complicated by bleeding, coagulopathy, hemophagocytic syndrome, and multiorgan failure. The median survival is 2 months.[277,279] Response to conventional chemotherapy is usually poor,[282] but L-asparaginase-based chemotherapy may produce favorable response in some cases.[279,286,290] alloHSCT is currently the only available treatment that may effect a cure, albeit in only a small fraction of patients, particularly those in complete remission at the time of transplantation.[279,291,292]

Differential Diagnosis

Aggressive NK-cell leukemia must be distinguished from the more common T-cell large granular lymphocytic leukemia, which is EBV negative and frequently pursues an indolent clinical course.[293] Patients with T-cell large granular lymphocytic leukemia are generally older (mean 55–65 years), and commonly present with infection, pure red cell aplasia, or neutropenia, and may be associated with rheumatoid arthritis. The circulating lymphoid cells do not exhibit atypia or immature appearance as commonly observed in aggressive NK-cell leukemia. The leukemia cells show a surface CD3-positive, CD4-negative, CD8-positive phenotype and clonally rearranged TR genes; CD56 is usually negative.

Chronic lymphoproliferative disorder of NK cells (NK-large granular lymphocytic leukemia) is clinically and morphologically similar to T-cell large granular lymphocytic leukemia, but differs in showing surface CD3 negative, CD56 positive or negative, and germline TR genes.[6,7,270,293-297] It differs from aggressive NK-cell leukemia in the following features: (1) indolent clinical course, (2) lack of hepatosplenomegaly, (3) lack of atypia in the large granular lymphocytes, (4) frequent expression of CD16 and CD57, and (5) lack of association with EBV.[270,298-301]

Aggressive NK-cell leukemia shows many similarities with ENKTL-NT, but the clinical features are different. It affects younger patients with acute fulminant presentation, and lacks nasal involvement. Admittedly, in some circumstances,

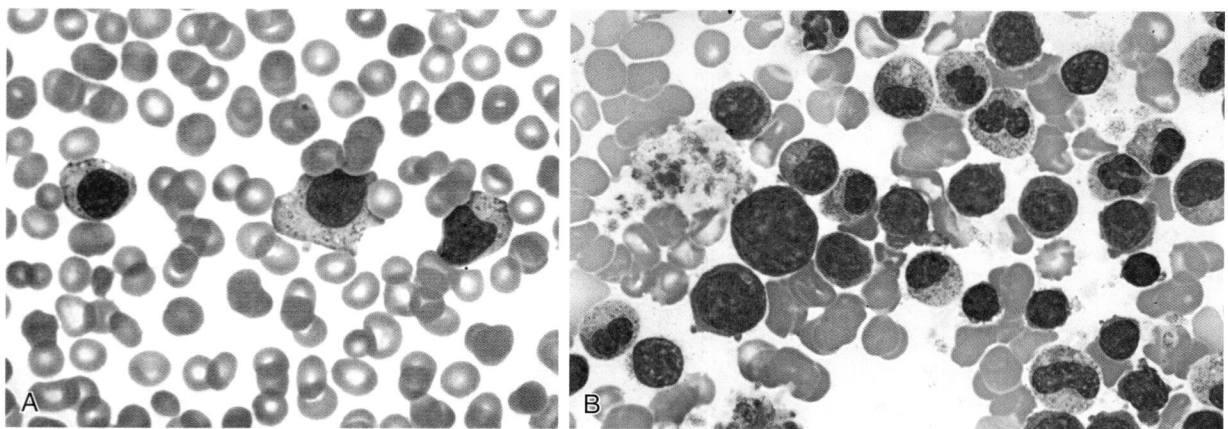

Figure 29-28. Aggressive NK-cell leukemia: peripheral blood or buffy coat findings. A, In the peripheral smear, there are large granular lymphocytes with atypia. Nucleolus is seen in the cell in the *center field.* **B,** Buffy coat smear shows many lymphoid cells with immature nuclear chromatin, distinct nucleoli, and cytoplasmic granules. There are admixed immature cells of the granulocytic series.

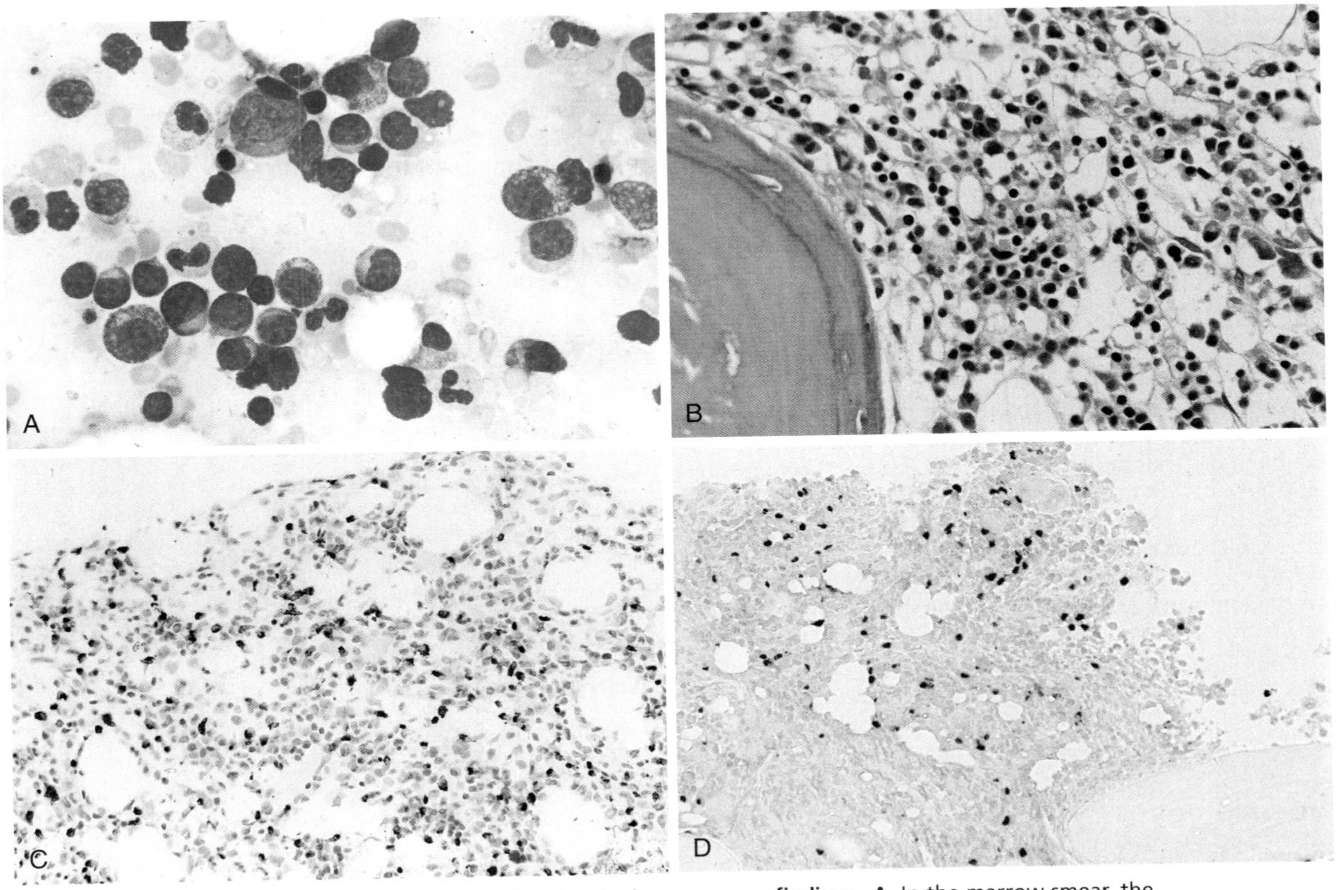

Figure 29-29. **Aggressive NK-cell leukemia: bone marrow findings. A,** In the marrow smear, the leukemic cells have round nuclei, lightly basophilic cytoplasm, and fine azurophilic granules. They occur singly or in small groups among the myeloid cells. **B,** In bone marrow biopsy, the subtle interstitial infiltrate of leukemic cells is often difficult to recognize. **C,** The scattered leukemic cells are much easier to appreciate by immunostaining for cytotoxic molecule such as TIA-1. **D,** These cells can similarly highlighted on in situ hybridization for EBER.

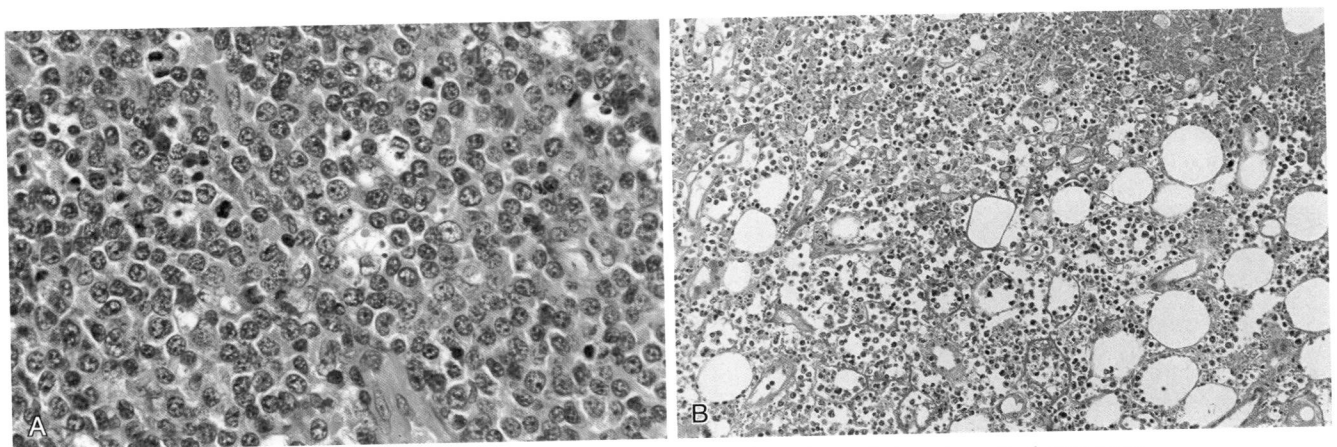

Figure 29-30. **Aggressive NK-cell leukemia: tissue manifestations. A,** Lymph node shows a monotonous infiltrate of medium-sized cells with round nuclei. There are many admixed apoptotic bodies. Because of histologic resemblance to plasmacytoid dendritic cells, the differential diagnosis of Kikuchi-Fujimoto lymphadenitis may be raised. **B,** The pericardial tissue is infiltrated by neoplastic cells, with necrosis and many apoptotic bodies.

their distinction can be very difficult, and may be a matter of semantics.

Aggressive NK-cell leukemia shows many similarities with systemic T-cell lymphoproliferative disorder of childhood clinically and pathologically, except that it rarely occurs in children, it is not always accompanied by fulminant hemophagocytic syndrome, CD56 is usually positive, and TR genes are not rearranged.

PRIMARY NODAL EPSTEIN-BARR VIRUS–POSITIVE T/NK-CELL LYMPHOMA

Synonyms and Related Terms

WHO revised 4th ed.: Subgroup within peripheral T-cell lymphomas

WHO proposed 5th ed.: EBV-positive nodal T- and NK-cell lymphoma

Definition

Primary nodal EBV-positive T/NK-cell lymphoma is, by definition, a nodal EBV-positive cytotoxic T-cell or NK-cell lymphoma. It presents more commonly in elderly or immunodeficient patients, lacks nasal involvement, and is more often of T-cell rather than NK-cell lineage. This was not a separate entity in the revised WHO 4th ed. and included as an EBV-positive variant of peripheral T-cell lymphoma, NOS, but recognized as a distinct entity in the WHO 5th ed.[7] and as a provisional entity in the ICC.[6] It is a primarily nodal disease with predominantly nodal involvement, although the tumor may involve a limited number of extranodal organs except the nasal cavity. ENKTL-NT, aggressive NK-cell leukemia, and transformed lymphoma from EBV-negative mature T-cell lymphoma should be excluded (capsule summary in Box 29-8).

Epidemiology

Primary nodal EBV-positive T/NK-cell lymphoma is very rare. The regional distribution is similar to that of other types of EBV-associated T/NK-cell lymphoma/leukemia. So far, fewer than 100 cases have been reported, mainly from Japan,[302,303] Hong Kong,[304] and Korea.[305,306]

Pathophysiology

EBV can infect virtually all neoplastic cells and appears to play an important role in the pathogenesis of primary EBV-positive nodal T/NK-cell lymphoma. Although they have no definite evidence of immune deficiency, patients are often older adults with a history of other associated viral infections such as

hepatitis B and hepatitis C or diabetes mellitus,[305] suggesting that these patients have impaired immune function that allows viral persistence. Gene-expression analysis revealed upregulation of immune response genes and activation of IFNγ, IL6/JAKL/STAT3, and NFκB with upregulation of PDL1 that allows immune evasion of EBV-infected cells.[305,307] Sustained EBV infection in T cells or NK cells and altered immune responses in immunocompromised older adult patients can lead to oncogenic transformation of EBV-infected cells with the aid of driver mutation.

Clinical Features

The median age of patients is 62 years, but 31% of patients are younger than 50 years. The male-to-female ratio is 2:1. Patients present in stage III or IV in 88% of cases. Patients may have anemia (64%), thrombocytopenia (50%), elevated LDH (77%), or hemophagocytosis (22%). B symptoms are seen in 77% of patients.[305-309] Patients present primarily with nodal disease, and there are no nasal lesions. There may be limited extranodal involvement including the liver in 35%, spleen in 46%, and bone marrow in 27% of patients.[308,309]

Morphology

Lymph nodes show diffuse infiltration of pleomorphic small-to-medium-sized and often medium-to-large-sized cells. The cytomorphology of these cells is variable—more commonly centroblastic, often anaplastic, or plasmacytoid (Fig. 29-32).[306-309]

Box 29-8 *Major Diagnostic Features of Primary Nodal EBV-Positive T/NK-Cell Lymphoma*

Definition
- Primary nodal EBV-positive cytotoxic T- or NK-cell lymphoma

Diagnostic Criteria
- Cytotoxic T-cell or NK-cell lymphoma presenting in the lymph node
- EBV positive in virtually all neoplastic cells
- No nasal lesion
- May involve a limited number of extranodal organs

Clinical Features and Behavior
- Most patients are older adults (median age, 62 years)
- Present with high clinical stage (stage III/IV in 88% of cases)
- Aggressive clinical course (median survival, 4 months)
- Cause of death: Septic shock or disease progression

Morphology
- Variable cytomorphology
- More commonly centroblastic, often anaplastic, or plasmacytoid
- RS cell–like large binucleated or multinucleated giant cells can be observed

Immunophenotype and Genotype
- Mainly composed of cytotoxic T cells or rarely NK cells
- Usually CD3 positive, CD8 positive, betaF-1 positive, cytotoxic granule positive
- A minority of cases show γδT-cell phenotype
- EBER-positive in vast majority of neoplastic cells
- T-cell receptor gene rearrangement: Usually monoclonal

EBER, EBV-encoded RNA; *EBV,* Epstein-Barr virus; *NK,* natural killer; *RS,* Reed-Sternberg.

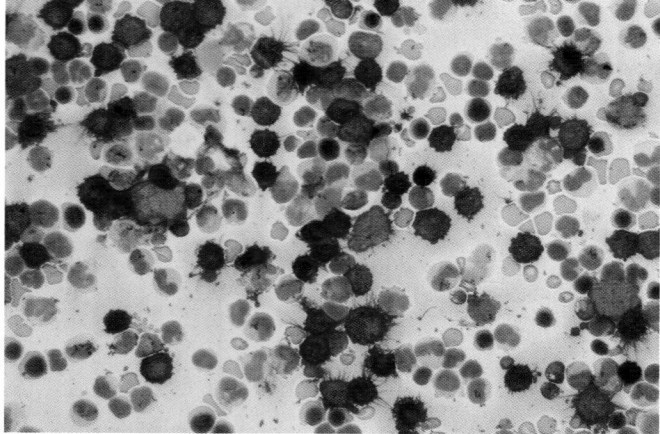

Figure 29-31. Immunocytochemistry of aggressive NK-cell leukemia. In the marrow smear, the atypical cells show cell membrane staining for the NK-cell marker CD56.

Tumor cells have a round or irregular nucleus with hyperchromasia and often prominent nucleoli. Polymorphic lymphoid cells with Reed-Sternberg (RS) cell–like large binucleated or multinucleated giant cells are often found.[305] Some cases show extensive necrosis, many apoptotic bodies, and angiocentric growth patterns as seen in extranodal NK/T-cell lymphomas. An associated inflammatory infiltrate comprising small lymphocytes, plasma cells, and granulomas is often found.[305]

Immunophenotype and Genetics

Based on the TR gene rearrangement and expression of the TCR protein, most cases of primary EBV-positive nodal T/NK-cell lymphoma comprise cytotoxic T cells.[305,308] NK-cell forms are uncommon.[303,304,307] The typical immunophenotype of primary EBV-positive nodal T/NK-cell lymphoma is CD3-positive, CD8-positive, TIA-1-positive, and granzyme B–positive, although CD4 is expressed in a minority cases. Unlike extranodal NK/T-cell lymphoma, expression of CD56 is infrequent. TCR staining reveals expression of TCR βF1 in 58%, TCR-γ in 13%, and TCR-silent in 29% of patients.[309] The TCR-silent type is characterized by high CD30 positivity. As in extranodal T/NK-cell lymphoma, virtually all tumor cells are positive for EBER in situ hybridization.[305-309]

Analysis of viral latency genes revealed a type 3 EBV latency in one-third of cases and type 2 latency in the remainder.[307] Compared with cytotoxic PTCL, NOS, primary nodal EBV-positive T/NK cell lymphoma is a genomically stable disease. Genetic analysis revealed frequent mutation involving *TET2*, *PIK3CD*, *STAT3*, *DDX3X*, and *PTPRD*.[307]

Prognosis

Primary nodal EBV-positive T/NK-cell lymphoma exhibits an aggressive clinical course, with a median survival of 4 months.[305,308,309] The prognosis is similar to that of extranasal lymphoma of ENKTL-NT[308,309] and poorer than cytotoxic PTCL, NOS.[307] The cause of death includes septic shock or disease progression.[305]

Differential Diagnosis

ENKTL-NT can show nodal involvement of a tumor at the time of the initial presentation in 30% of nasal lymphoma cases and 70% of extranasal lymphoma cases.[310] Primary nodal EBV-positive T/NK-cell lymphoma tends to show centroblastic cytology and RS cell–like binucleated or multinucleated giant cells, which are uncommon findings in ENKTL-NT.[308,309]

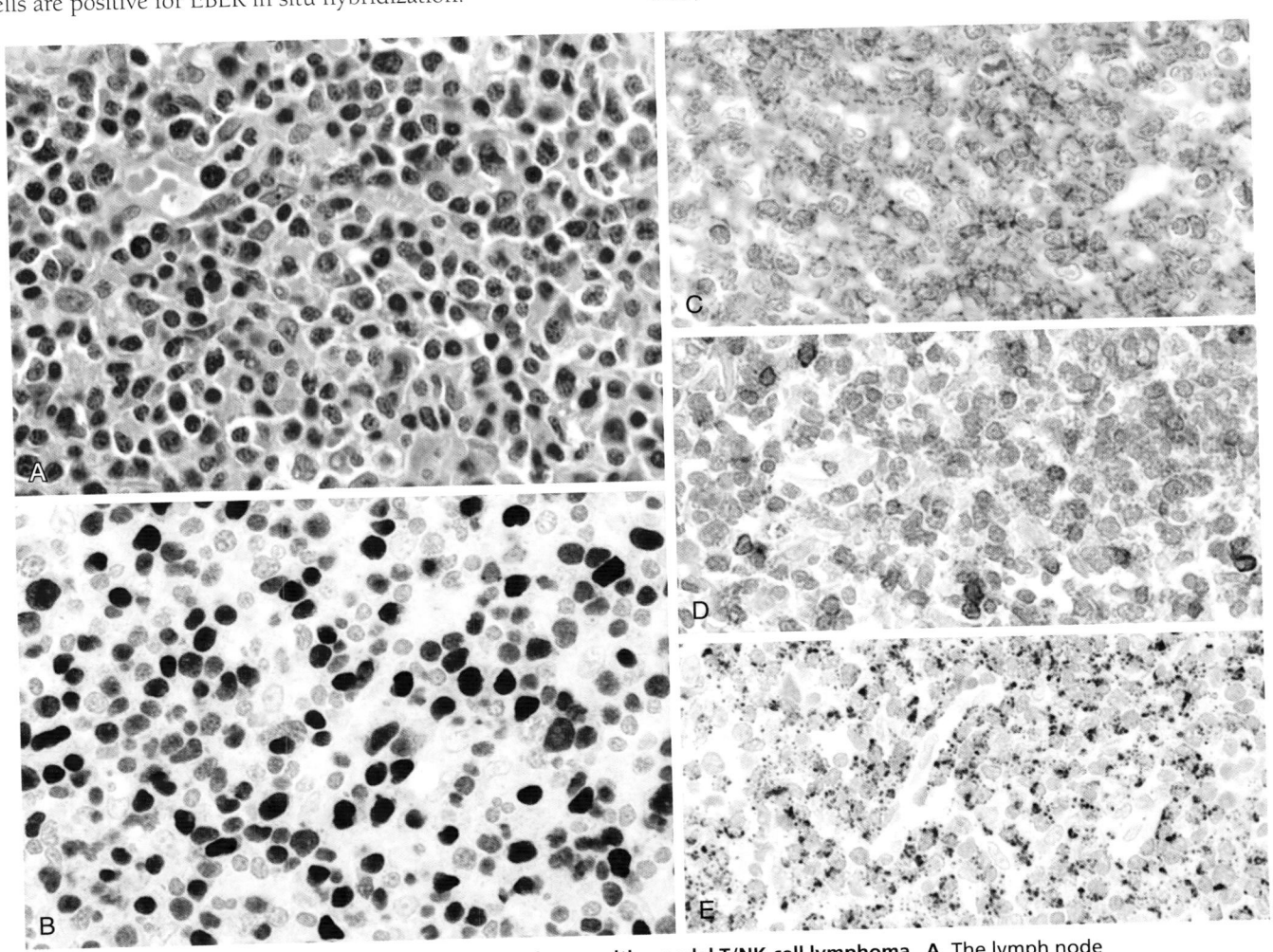

Figure 29-32. Primary Epstein-Barr virus–positive nodal T/NK-cell lymphoma. A, The lymph node is infiltrated by relatively monotonous medium-to-large-sized pleomorphic neoplastic cells. **B,** The vast majority of neoplastic cells are positive for Epstein-Barr virus–encoded RNA (EBER) in situ hybridization. Neoplastic cells are positive for CD8 **(C)**, betaF-1 **(D)**, and TIA-1 **(E)**.

The CD4-negative, CD8-negative, CD56-positive immunophenotype is found most frequently in ENKTL-NT, whereas primary nodal EBV-positive T/NK-cell lymphoma usually expresses CD8 but not CD4 and CD56.[305,308,309] Despite these differences, the two diseases show significant overlap in their histology and immunophenotype. Clinical correlation and examination of the nasal cavity are necessary to exclude ENKTL-NT.

Aggressive NK-cell leukemia and primary nodal EBV-positive T/NK-cell lymphoma of NK-cell lineage may show pathologic and clinical similarities. Aggressive NK-cell leukemia is characterized by systemic proliferation of malignant NK cells with involvement of the bone marrow, spleen, and liver. Nodal involvement at the time of presentation is reported in 20% to 26% of cases,[283,286] although lymphomatous features involving predominantly lymph nodes are uncommon.[304] Rare cases of nodal EBV-positive NK-cell lymphoma have been reported under the term *aggressive NK-cell lymphoma* or *lymphomatous features of aggressive NK-cell leukemia.*[272] Previously, these cases were believed to be a nonleukemic counterpart of aggressive NK-cell leukemia, but they seemed to correspond to primary nodal EBV-positive T/NK-cell lymphoma of NK-lineage.

EBV infection in T-cell lymphoma is also found in other mature T-cell lymphomas including angioimmunoblastic T-cell lymphoma and peripheral T-cell lymphoma, unspecified (PTCL-NOS). Unlike primary nodal EBV-positive T/NK-cell lymphoma, in which EBV infects neoplastic T cells, the EBV genome is found mainly in non-neoplastic B cells, although it may also be identified in T cells or null cells.[311] EBV-positive PTCL can originate from the secondary transformation of low-grade EBV-negative T-cell lymphomas.[312] Secondary EBV infection of an established malignant T-cell clone can occur in vivo and may contribute to its aggressive transformation.[313] Primary nodal EBV-positive T/NK-cell lymphoma is diagnosed after exclusion of such transformed lymphomas.

Pearls and Pitfalls

EBV-Positive Lymphoproliferative Diseases of Childhood

- Correct diagnosis of Epstein-Barr virus (EBV)–positive lymphoproliferative diseases of childhood requires the integration of clinical, immunophenotypic, genotypic, and morphologic features.
- EBV-associated hemophagocytic lymphohistiocytosis (EBV-HLH) is a hyperinflammatory syndrome caused by dysregulated immune response and hypercytokinemia secondary to EBV infection. EBV-HLH and systemic EBV-positive T-cell lymphoma of childhood share a significant overlap in clinical presentation and pathologic changes. The distinction between these two diseases is often challenging.
- Chronic active EBV disease (CAEBVD) includes a constellation of clinical syndromes that vary in their aggressiveness. Elevated EBV load in blood and tissue with clinical symptoms lasting more than 3 months is mandatory for making a diagnosis. Histologic changes in CAEBVD are nonspecific and appear to be inflammation or reactive lymphoid hyperplasia. Double procedure for EBV–encoded RNA (EBER) in situ hybridization with immunohistochemistry for CD3 or CD56 is important to recognize EBV-infected T or NK cells in tissue biopsy.
- Hydroa vacciniforme lymphoproliferative disorder (HVLPD) and severe mosquito bite allergy are cutaneous EBV-associated proliferations of T cells and NK cells in which cytokines and chemokines contribute to the homing of EBV-infected cells to sites of inflammation, leading to the characteristic symptoms.
- HVLPD is divided into classic and systemic forms based on the clinical features.
  - Classic HVLPD is an indolent and self-limited disease involving only the skin.
  - Systemic HVLPD shows systemic symptoms during the acute phase of the disease and might progress to lymphoma. In severe cases, similar treatment as CAEBVD is required.
- Systemic EBV-positive T-cell lymphoproliferative disorder of childhood may appear deceptively benign cytologically, but it pursues an aggressive clinical course.

Extranodal NK/T-Cell Lymphoma, Nasal Type

- The discrepancy between surface CD3 staining (negative) and cytoplasmic CD3ε staining (positive) in extranodal NK/T-cell lymphoma, nasal type (ENKTL-NT) is explainable by the presence of only subunits of CD3 in the cytoplasm but not the completely assembled CD3 molecule that is recognized by the surface CD3 antibodies such as Leu4 and T3.

Specificity of CD56 for NK/T-Cell Lymphoma

- CD56 expression is not specific for NK/T-cell lymphoma, but it is also expressed in some peripheral T-cell lymphomas (particularly those expressing γδ TCR), acute myeloid leukemia, myeloma, small-cell neuroendocrine carcinoma, rhabdomyosarcoma, and some other tumors.
- Thus a diagnosis of ENKTL-NT should not be based on CD56 expression alone, but should be supplemented by positive immunostaining with other leukocyte markers (such as CD3ε and CD2).

Method of Choice for Detection of EBV in Extranodal NK/T-Cell Lymphoma, Nasal Type

- The preferred and most sensitive method for demonstration of EBV in ENKTL-NT is in situ hybridization for EBER.
- Immunostaining for EBV LMP-1 may be weak or negative, and thus cannot be relied on for demonstration of EBV in this lymphoma type.
- Southern blot technique is of limited sensitivity, and furthermore requires fresh or frozen tissue.
- Polymerase chain reaction (PCR) for EBV is highly sensitive but is of limited value because even presence of rare bystander EBV-positive lymphocytes can give rise to a positive result.

Assessment of Posttreatment Biopsies for Nasal NK/T-Cell Lymphoma

- Since the nasal cavity is readily accessible for biopsy, it is fairly common practice to take posttreatment biopsies in patients with nasal NK/T-cell lymphoma to determine whether there is residual lymphoma.
- Residual tumor is easy to recognize for lymphomas comprising predominantly large cells or if dense sheets of atypical lymphoid cells are evident.
- In most cases, the mucosa becomes hypocellular. Scattered residual lymphoma cells hiding among small lymphocytes or residual lymphoma comprising small cells are very difficult, if not impossible, to recognize by morphologic assessment alone. Therefore it is prudent to perform immunostaining for CD56 and in situ hybridization for EBER to look for residual tumor cells. Positive cells must be present at least in aggregates or correlated with atypical cytology to be considered indicative of residual lymphoma. The presence of only isolated or groups of three to four positive cells is considered inconclusive, because low numbers of positive cells can be observed in the normal nasal or nasopharyngeal mucosa.
- With relapse, the cytologic features of the original lymphoma are usually maintained, but may sometimes change, such as from small-sized or medium-sized cells to large-sized cells, or vice versa. Occasionally CD56 expression is diminished or even lost in treated or relapsed lymphoma.

KEY REFERENCES

9. Quintanilla-Martinez L, Swerdlow SH, Tousseyn T, Barrionuevo C, Nakamura S, Jaffe ES. New concepts in EBV-associated B, T, and NK cell lymphoproliferative disorders. *Virchows Arch.* 2023;482(1):227–244.

12. Henter JI, Horne A, Arico M, et al. HLH-2004: diagnostic and therapeutic guidelines for hemophagocytic lymphohistiocytosis. *Pediatr Blood Cancer.* 2007;48:124–131.

14. Ishii E, Ohga S, Imashuku S, et al. Nationwide survey of hemophagocytic lymphohistiocytosis in Japan. *Int J Hematol.* 2007;86:58–65.

17. Yanagisawa R, Nakazawa Y, Matsuda K, et al. Outcomes in children with hemophagocytic lymphohistiocytosis treated using HLH-2004 protocol in Japan. *Int J Hematol.* 2019;109:206–213.

50. Straus SE. The chronic mononucleosis syndrome. *J Infect Dis.* 1988;157:405–412.

52. Ohshima K, Kimura H, Yoshino T, et al. Proposed categorization of pathological states of EBV-associated T/natural killer-cell lymphoproliferative disorder (LPD) in children and young-adults: overlap with chronic active EBV infection and infantile fulminant EBV T-LPD. *Pathol Int.* 2008;58:209–217.

54. Cohen JI, Jaffe ES, Dale JK, et al. Characterization and treatment of chronic active Epstein-Barr virus disease: a 28-year experience in the United States. *Blood.* 2011;117:5835–5849.

64. Kimura H, Hoshino Y, Kanegane H, et al. Clinical and virologic characteristics of chronic active Epstein-Barr virus infection. *Blood.* 2001;98:280–286.

65. Cohen JI, Kimura H, Nakamura S, et al. Epstein-Barr virus associated lymphoproliferative disease in non-immunocompromised hosts: Status report and summary of an international meeting. Bethesda: NIH; September 8–9, 2008. *Ann Oncol.* 2009;20:1472–1482.

72. Ishihara S, Yabuta R, Tokura Y, Ohshima K, Tagawa S. Hypersensitivity to mosquito bites is not an allergic disease, but an Epstein-Barr virus-associated lymphoproliferative disease. *Int J Hematol.* 2000;72:223–228.

79. Gupta G, Man I, Kemmett D. Hydroa vacciniforme: a clinical and follow-up study of 17 cases. *J Am Acad Dermatol.* 2000;42(2 Pt 1):208–213.

80. Lyapichev KA, Sukswai N, Wang XI, Khoury JD, Medeiros LJ. Hydroa vacciniforme-like lymphoproliferative disorder with progression to EBV+ cytotoxic peripheral T-cell lymphoma. *Am J Dermatopathol.* 2020;42:714–716.

94. Kimura H, Miyake K, Yamauchi Y, et al. Identification of Epstein-Barr virus (EBV)-infected lymphocyte subtypes by flow cytometric in situ hybridization in EBV-associated lymphoproliferative diseases. *J Infect Dis.* 2009;200:1078–1087.

102. Cohen JI, Iwatsuki K, Ko YH, et al. Epstein-Barr virus NK and T cell lymphoproliferative disease: report of a 2018 international meeting. *Leuk Lymphoma.* 2020;61:808–819.

103. Kimura H, Ito Y, Kawabe S, et al. EBV-associated T/NK-cell lymphoproliferative diseases in nonimmunocompromised hosts: prospective analysis of 108 cases. *Blood.* 2012;119:673–686.

109. Quintanilla-Martinez L, Kumar S, Fend F, et al. Fulminant EBV+ T-cell lymphoproliferative disorder following acute/chronic EBV infection: a distinct clinicopathologic syndrome. *Blood.* 2000;96:443–451.

209. Huang Y, de Reynies A, de Leval L, et al. Gene expression profiling identifies emerging oncogenic pathways operating in extranodal NK/T-cell lymphoma, nasal type. *Blood.* 2010;115:1226–1237.

234. Jiang L, Gu ZH, Yan ZX, et al. Exome sequencing identifies somatic mutations of DDX3X in natural killer/T-cell lymphoma. *Nat Genet.* 2015;47:1061–1066.

236. Xiong J, Cui BW, Wang N, et al. Genomic and transcriptomic characterization of natural killer T cell lymphoma. *Cancer Cell.* 2020;37:403–419.e406.

288. Dufva O, Kankainen M, Kelkka T, et al. Aggressive natural killer-cell leukemia mutational landscape and drug profiling highlight JAK-STAT signaling as therapeutic target. *Nat Commun.* 2018;9:1567.

306. Jeon YK, Kim JH, Sung JY, Han JH, Ko YH. Hematopathology study group of the Korean Society of pathologists. Epstein-Barr virus–positive nodal T/NK-cell lymphoma: an analysis of 15 cases with distinct clinicopathological features. *Hum Pathol.* 2015;46:981–990.

307. Wai CMM, Chen S, Phyu T, et al. Immune pathway upregulation and lower genomic instability distinguish EBV-positive nodal T/NK-cell lymphoma from ENKTL and PTCL-NOS. *Haematologica.* 2022;107:1864–1879.

309. Kato S, Nakamura S. T-cell receptor (TCR) phenotype of nodal Epstein-Barr virus (EBV)-positive cytotoxic T-cell lymphoma (CTL): a clinicopathologic study of 39 cases. *Am J Surg Pathol.* 2015;39:462–471.

Visit Elsevier eBooks+ for the complete set of references.

Chapter 30

T-Cell and NK-Cell Large Granular Lymphocyte Proliferations

William G. Morice, II, Dragan Jevremovic, and Min Shi

HISTORY AND CLASSIFICATION

The first detailed studies of what is now recognized as T-cell large granular lymphocytic leukemia (T-LGLL) were published in the 1970s and early 1980s.[1-3] These manuscripts described a disorder characterized by neutropenia or anemia that was associated with a proportionate and absolute increase in circulating granular lymphocytes that normally constituted only 10% to 20% of the peripheral blood lymphocytes. These studies also documented that the cytoplasmic granules of these lymphocytes were identical in ultrastructure to those of their normal counterpart (parallel microtubular arrays); formed sheep erythrocyte rosettes consistent with T-cell origin (now recognized as CD2 positivity); and expressed Fc receptors. Based on these attributes, the moniker *large granular lymphocytic leukemia* was coined. It should be noted, however, that this disorder was ascribed a number of different names in the early literature, including *CD8-positive T-cell chronic lymphocytic leukemia* and *T-gamma lymphoproliferative disorder.*

Our understanding of leukemias of large granular lymphocytes (LGLs) greatly advanced in the late 1980s and 1990s with the recognition of cytotoxic T cells and natural killer (NK) cells as discrete lymphocyte subsets and the advent of multicolor flow-cytometric immunophenotyping, which allowed these cell types to be distinguished and characterized in clinical specimens.[4] During this period, T-LGLL became the widely accepted nomenclature, with the fundamental defining attributes being an increase in granular lymphocytes with a CD8-positive T-cell phenotype, aberrant expression of the NK-cell lineage–associated antigens CD16 and CD57, and T-cell clonality as documented by the presence of clonal T-cell receptor (TCR) gene rearrangements. Cases fulfilling these criteria often were associated with neutropenia and

typically had an indolent clinical course. Also recognized during this time period were cases in which the increased granular lymphocytes had a CD3-negative, CD16-positive, CD56-positive NK-cell immunophenotype. Rendering a diagnosis of large granular lymphocytic leukemia in such cases was more problematic, however, as there were few methods to establish NK-cell immunophenotypic aberrancy and NK-cell clonality could not be readily assessed; these cells, by definition, lack TCR gene rearrangement. For these reasons, during this period, the diagnosis of *large granular lymphocytic leukemia of NK-cell lineage (NK-LGLL)* required a greater degree of clinical morbidity to confidently distinguish such cases from a potential reactive NK-cell lymphocytosis. Therefore, NK-LGLL was considered more aggressive than its T-cell counterpart in these earlier reports.[5]

More recently, further advances have improved our ability to identify chronic lymphoproliferative disorders of cytotoxic T cells and NK cells and provided potential insights into pathogenesis, including the identification of novel families of receptors for MHC-I and related proteins that are expressed by NK cells and a subset of cytotoxic T cells (collectively referred to as *natural cytotoxicity receptors, NCRs*).[6] Through the application of these tools, T-LGLL is now recognized as a disorder of memory cytotoxic T cells variably associated with cytopenias that typically has an indolent clinical course.[7] An NK-cell–derived counterpart to T-LGLL with similar clinical and laboratory features, including surrogate markers of clonality, has also been elucidated with the application of these new diagnostic tools. This is now referred to as *chronic lymphoproliferative disorder of NK cells (CLPD-NK)* to distinguish it from the earlier NK-LGLL descriptions, which likely included more aggressive NK-cell malignancies that are described elsewhere in this text. However, it is noteworthy that, in the 5th edition of the World Health Organization (WHO) classification, the NK-LGLL nomenclature was reconsidered, as this terminology does reflect the close clinical relatedness between the T-cell and NK-cell forms of these disorders.

DEFINITIONS

T-LGLL is defined as a clonal or oligoclonal increase in peripheral blood cytotoxic T cells with granular lymphocyte morphology. Cytopenias are usually associated, yet they are not universally present and are not a defining attribute per se. Although increased circulating granular lymphocytes is the quintessential feature of T-LGLL, the use of an absolute LGL count as a diagnostic criterion has changed over time. In early disease definitions, an absolute LGL count of 2×10^9/L was used.[4] However, subsequently, bona fide T-LGLL not reaching this threshold were identified and, over time, it has come to be recognized that up to one-third of cases may have a count lower than 1×10^9/L.[8] For this reason, an absolute LGL count is no longer included as a disease-defining feature, although granular lymphocytes have an absolute count of greater than 0.5×10^9/L or account for more than 50% of the circulating lymphoid cells in most cases.

The T cells of T-LGLL are typically CD8-positive, $\alpha\beta$ type, although cases that are either CD4 positive or of $\gamma\delta$ lineage may uncommonly be encountered.[9,10] In virtually all cases, phenotypic abnormalities are present, with co-expression of NK-associated antigens CD16 and/or CD57 considered pathognomic but not disease-specific.[11] In the vast majority of T-LGLLs, T-cell clonality can be detected through molecular analysis of TCR gene rearrangements, V-β flow cytometry, or TCR β constant 1 (TRBC1) flow cytometry.[12,13] Despite the presence of demonstrable T-cell clonality in T-LGLL on detailed molecular analysis, many cases appear oligoclonal. Therefore, clonality may not be demonstrated in all cases. In such instances, it is prudent to document persistence of the process by repeat studies after a period of 6 months to 1 year before rendering an unequivocal diagnosis.

CLPD-NK (or NK-LGLL) is also defined by an increase in peripheral blood granular lymphocytes (also associated with cytopenias in some instances); however, in this disorder, the lymphocytes are of NK-cell lineage, as documented by flow cytometry.[14] As in T-LGLL, in CLPD-NK, LGLs compose the majority of the peripheral blood lymphocytes, and, although the elevation in the absolute count is usually mild, it tends to be slightly higher than that seen in T-LGLL.[15] NK-cell immunophenotypic aberrancy is variably attributed as a feature of CLPD-NK. This variability likely reflects the limited NK-cell phenotyping, which is routinely used in many clinical laboratories, as aberrancy can be demonstrated in all cases when extensive NK-cell immunophenotyping (including antibodies to NCRs) is performed.[11,16] Because NK cells lack TCR gene rearrangements, evaluation of these genes is not part of the routine diagnostic evaluation or disease definition. The lack of a readily assessed marker of clonality in CLPD-NK places a greater emphasis on documenting the persistence of the process for 6 months to 1 year. As in T-LGLL, cytopenias are frequently associated but not part of the disease definition.

Bone marrow immunohistochemistry revealing intrasinusoidal cytotoxic marrow infiltrates is detected in 75% or more of T-LGLL and CLPD-NK cases.[17,18] Likewise, studies have demonstrated that *STAT3* mutation is present in approximately 40% of both T-LGLLs and CLPD-NKs.[19] Therefore, these features are coming to be accepted as defining characteristics of these conditions, although neither is specific to T-LGLL or CLPD-NK.

SYNONYMS AND RELATED TERMS

T-cell large granular lymphocytic leukemia (International Consensus Classification [ICC] 2022)

T-cell large granular lymphocytic leukemia; chronic lymphoproliferative disorder of NK cells (WHO revised 4th edition)

T-cell large granular lymphocytic leukemia; NK-large granular lymphocytic leukemia (WHO proposed 5th edition)

Others: T-cell large granular lymphocytosis; CD8-positive T-cell chronic lymphocytic leukemia; T-cell lymphoproliferative disease of granular lymphocytes; chronic NK-cell lymphocytosis; chronic NK large granular lymphocyte lymphoproliferative disorder; NK-cell large granular lymphocyte lymphocytosis; indolent large granular NK-cell lymphoproliferative disorder; indolent leukemia of NK cells

ETIOLOGY AND EPIDEMIOLOGY

Antigenic stimulation is considered a primary etiologic event in both T-LGLL and CLPD-NK, although no singular causative agent or predisposing factors have been identified for either condition. Serologic studies have demonstrated that, in 30% or more of T-LGLLs and CLPD-NKs, antibodies to HTLV-1 envelope proteins p21 and p24 are present in the absence of detectable HTLV-1 or HTLV-2 viral DNA. These findings suggest a role of infection by an HTLV-related virus in the development of some cases.[20,21] In T-LGLL, analysis of TCR β-chain variable region gene usage has revealed similar clonotypes among cases and within the oligoclonal expansions of individual cases and also disproportionate use of the TCR V-β 13.1, which is physiologically expanded in response to cytomegalovirus (CMV) infection. These data further implicate viral infection as a potential etiologic agent in T-LGLL.[22-24] CMV infection has also been shown to cause oligoclonal expansion of killer-cell immunoglobulin-like receptor (KIR)-expressing NK cells, and the activating form of the KIR appears important in physiologic responses to viral infection.[25] In CLPD-NK, a disproportionate number have KIR haplotypes that are rich in activating isoforms, and there is frequent expression of these activating KIRs and epigenetic inactivation of the inhibitory *KIR* genes.[26] These data suggest that viral infection may also be an important etiologic factor in the development of CLPD-NK.

T-LGLL after solid organ or hematopoietic stem cell transplantation could also be attributable to chronic viral stimulation. Alternatively, recipient cytotoxic T cells could undergo an uncontrolled clonal proliferation in the setting of solid organ transplantation caused by alloantigen stimulation or donor cytotoxic T cells could clonally expand to self-antigen stimulation in patients with hematopoietic stem cell transplantation.[27] Other stimulants of cytotoxic T cells or NK cells may also play a role in T-LGLL and CLPD-NK development, as demonstrated by the association of these disorders with a variety of autoimmune diseases and other hematolymphoid neoplasms.[28,29]

T-LGLL and CLPD-NK are epidemiologically similar, representing less than 5% and less than 1% of all mature lymphoid leukemias, respectively.[30-33] These figures may not be indicative of the true prevalence of these diseases, however, as these diagnoses require both a high level of clinical suspicion and comprehensive laboratory evaluation; therefore, both may be underrecognized.

T-LGLL and CLPD-NK are diseases of adulthood, both with a median age of 60 years. Only sporadic cases are encountered in adolescents and young adults. Neither shows a predilection for gender, and neither is associated with Epstein-Barr virus (EBV) infection. Although some studies suggest that T-LGLL may be slightly more common in Asian populations, neither shows a strong geographic or ethnic predisposition.[28,34]

CLINICAL FEATURES

Typically, patients present with signs or symptoms related to the disease-associated cytopenias (neutropenic infection or anemia-associated fatigue and dyspnea on exertion), and oftentimes the diagnosis is made during evaluation of asymptomatic lymphocytosis. Over time, more than 70% of patients with T-LGLL develop moderate-to-severe cytopenia(s) requiring treatment. Neutropenia is the most common cytopenia, followed by anemia; transfusion-dependent anemia occurs in 10% to 30% of patients with T-LGLL. At diagnosis, anemia is often associated with neutropenia and/or thrombocytopenia. However, isolated anemia could be seen in a small subset of patients.[35] Less than 25% of patients have thrombocytopenia, almost always associated with other cytopenias.[29] Cytopenias are less frequent in CLPD-NK; therefore, treatment is less frequently required than in T-LGLL.[15,19,29,30,33,36,37]

In general, neither T-LGLL nor CLPD-NK is associated with B symptoms or significant clinical morbidity.[29,37] The most commonly encountered clinical sign in these disorders is organomegaly, particularly splenomegaly, which is present in approximately 20% to 30% of LGLLs.[30,32,36] Hepatomegaly has also been described in approximately 10% of T-LGL and CLPD-NK cases.[30,38,39] In these LGLL disorders, the organomegaly is presumably caused by organ infiltration, although when hepatomegaly is present, it is not usually associated with hepatic dysfunction. Mild lymphadenopathy may be seen in isolated cases. Prominent lymphadenopathy or involvement of extramedullary tissue sites is not typical, however, and, if present, should lead to the consideration of other possible diagnoses.

T-LGLL and CKPD-NK are strongly associated with both autoimmune phenomena and autoimmune disorders. Although the estimates vary among studies, it can be reliably stated that 30% of T-LGLLs and CLPD-NKs have abnormal serologic studies associated with immune activation such as polyclonal hypergammaglobulinemia, the presence of detectable rheumatoid factor, or a positive antinuclear antibody (ANA). Approximately 20% of patients with T-LGLL have clinically diagnosed rheumatoid arthritis, but the association is less evident in patients with CLPD-NK.[36] A number of other autoimmune diseases are also associated with T-LGLL and CLPD-NK with lesser frequency, including systemic lupus erythematosus, chronic inflammatory bowel disease, and Sjögren syndrome.[28,29,36,40,41]

In addition to being associated with autoimmune disorders, T-LGLL and CLPD-NK also have the somewhat unusual feature of being associated with other clonal hematologic disorders, which are present in approximately 10% to 20% of cases. B-cell lymphoproliferative disorders and plasma cell proliferative disorders are most commonly described in this context.[42,43] Among the other hematologic diseases that have been identified in association with T-LGLL are myelodysplastic syndrome, acute myeloid leukemia, aplastic anemia, and paroxysmal nocturnal hemoglobinuria.[29,36,40,41,44,45]

Lastly, case reports have described T-LGLL being diagnosed in the setting of allogeneic renal and bone marrow transplantation.[27,46-48] As reactive CD8-positive T-cell expansions with limited clonal diversity and phenotypically similarities to T-LGLL have been reported after allogeneic transplantation,[49] it could be difficult to determine whether these cases represent bona fide lymphoproliferative disorders or distinct reactive processes of limited clonal diversity driven by interactions between host immunity and the allografted organ.

MORPHOLOGY

T-LGLL and CLPD-NK have identical cytologic features in the peripheral blood, characteristically having small, minimally irregular nuclei and abundant pale-staining cytoplasm containing variably prominent azurophilic granules. In clinical practice, however, the degree of cytoplasmic enlargement and granulation in these LGL disorders varies considerably, and granulation of the lymphoid cells can be difficult to appreciate in some instances. For this reason, absolute granular lymphocyte counts are no longer included in the diagnostic criteria, although making the diagnosis without an obvious increase in granular lymphocytes requires both a high degree of clinical suspicion and comprehensive flow-cytometric immunophenotyping analysis[7] (Table 30-1).

T-LGLL and CLPD-NK cannot be distinguished from each other on cytologic grounds. Likewise, there is no singular morphologic feature in the peripheral blood that enables one to discriminate these disorders from an expansion of normal cytotoxic lymphocytes, although observing granular lymphocytes as part of a cytologic spectrum favors a reactive process. It should be noted that pronounced cytologic atypia and malignant cytology are not seen in either T-LGLL or CLPD-NK and, if present, should lead one to strongly consider the possibility of a leukemic phase of another more aggressive malignancy of cytotoxic lymphocytes, such as aggressive NK-cell leukemia.

In T-LGLL and CLPD-NK, it is difficult to recognize the abnormal lymphocytes in both bone marrow aspirate and biopsy.[17,18,50] In bone marrow aspirate, the cytoplasm is often contracted, obscuring the presence of granules. In hematoxylin and eosin (H&E) stained bone marrow clot sections and biopsies, the cytoplasmic granules are not seen, which, in combination with the bland nuclear features of the cells and the characteristic interstitial pattern of infiltration, renders the cells virtually unidentifiable. For these reasons, histologic screening of bone marrow aspirates and biopsies is not useful when assessing for a potential T-LGLL or CLPD-NK diagnosis.

Table 30-1 Major and Minor Diagnostic Criteria for T-Cell Large Granular Lymphocytic Leukemia and Chronic Lymphoproliferative Disorder of NK Cells

T-Cell Large Granular Lymphocytic Leukemia	
Major criteria	• Flow-cytometric immunophenotyping revealing >50% of the total peripheral blood or bone marrow surface CD3-positive T cells to have two or more of the following*:
	• Uniform expression of CD16 or CD57 (>75% of cells positive)
	• Loss of CD5 or CD7 expression (partial or complete)
	• Uniform expression of one or more of the KIRs CD158a, CD158b, or CD158e[†]
	• Intrasinusoidal bone marrow or splenic infiltration by cytotoxic lymphocytes positive for CD8 and one or more of the cytotoxic markers TIA-1, granzyme B, granzyme M, or perforin[†]
	• T-cell clonality by flow-cytometric analysis of TRBC1, TCR V-β expression or molecular genetic analysis of T-cell–receptor (TCR) gene rearrangements
	• *STAT-3* gene mutation in exons 20 or 21
Minor criteria	• Peripheral blood granular lymphocytes (morphology) or CD8-positive T cells (flow cytometry) either >2 × 10^9/L or >80% of total lymphocytes
	• Unexplained persistence of cell population for longer than 6 months
	• Positive rheumatoid factor, antinuclear antibody (ANA), or polyclonal hypergammaglobulinemia
	• Unexplained neutropenia (<1.8 × 10^9/L) and/or anemia (<10 g/dL)
	• Peripheral blood absolute natural killer (NK)-cell count <0.1 × 10^9/L or <5% of total lymphocytes
	• *STAT-5B* gene mutation in exons encoding the SH2 domain
Chronic Lymphoproliferative Disorder of NK Cells	
Major criteria	• Flow-cytometric immunophenotyping revealing CD16-positive, CD3-negative NK cells accounting for >50% of the total peripheral blood or bone marrow lymphocytes and one or more of the following*:
	• Loss of CD56 expression
	• Uniform CD8 expression (>75% of cells positive), may be dim
	• Loss of CD2 expression
	• Bright, uniform CD94 expression with or without NKG2A
	• Uniform expression of one or more of the KIRs CD158a, CD158b, or CD158e
	• Complete absence of expression of the KIRs CD158a, CD158b, and CD158e
	• Intrasinusoidal bone marrow or splenic infiltration by cytotoxic lymphocytes positive for CD8 and one or more of the cytotoxic markers TIA-1, granzyme B, granzyme M, or perforin[†]
	• *STAT-3* gene mutation in exons 20 or 21
Minor criteria	• Peripheral blood granular lymphocytes (morphology) or NK cells (flow cytometry) either >2 × 10^9/L or >80% of total lymphocytes
	• Unexplained persistence for more than 6 months
	• Unexplained neutropenia (<1.8 × 10^9/L) and/or anemia (<10 g/dL)
	• Diminished CD7 expression

A diagnosis of T-cell large granular lymphocytic leukemia (T-LGLL) or chronic lymphoproliferative disorder of NK cells (CLPD-NK) can be rendered if either three or more major criteria are present *or* at least two major criteria and two or more minor criteria are present.
*Flow-cytometric immunophenotyping is required to distinguish T-LGLL from CLPD-NK. If these studies are not performed and other diagnostic criteria for T-LGLL or CLPD-NK are satisfied, then a diagnosis of large granular lymphocytic (LGL) disorder, not further classifiable should be considered, particularly as the presence of clonal T-cell receptor gene rearrangements does not always demonstrate lineage fidelity. Also note that uniform CD16 expression and absence of CD5 expression can be seen in normal γδ T cells; however, these should not compose greater than 50% of the total T-cell pool. Uniform expression of KIR is *not* seen in normal γδ T cells and is a sign of aberrancy.
[†]The presence of sinusoidal cytotoxic lymphoid infiltrates that distend or disrupt the sinusoidal architecture or the uniform expression of multiple KIR antigens by the abnormal T cells should lead one to consider the possibility of hepatosplenic T-cell lymphoma.

IMMUNOPHENOTYPE

Given the absence of distinctive cytologic or morphologic features, flow-cytometric immunophenotyping is a fundamental element of making a diagnosis of T-LGLL or CLPD-NK, particularly as this is the only way these disorders can be distinguished from each other.[14]

All T-LGLLs are CD3 positive by flow cytometry (usually expressed with TCRαβ heterodimer), and most are CD8 positive (Fig. 30-1A). The majority of T-LGLLs have abnormalities of pan–T-cell antigen expression, with 80% having either diminished expression or partial or complete loss of CD5; diminished or absent expression of CD7 is equally frequent. Diminished expression of CD2 is seen in less than 20% of cases, and abnormalities of CD3 expression are exceedingly rare in this disorder.[11,51]

Although abnormal expression of CD5 and CD7 are frequent in T-LGLL, neither is specific to this disease, and reactive CD8-positive T cells may show decreased expression of one or both.[52,53] For this reason, evaluation for aberrant co-expression of NK-cell–associated antigens, a pathognomic feature of T-LGLL, is critical for the diagnosis. Of the traditionally recognized NK-cell–associated antigens, CD16 and CD57 are most commonly expressed in T-LGLL, with CD16 expressed in 80% of cases and CD57 expressed in over 90% (Fig. 30-1A).[8,40] CD57 is also expressed by normal memory T cells; uniform homogeneous CD57 expression is distinct to T-LGLL, although this pattern is seen in less than half of cases.[11,54] CD56 expression is uncommon in T-LGLL and is present in less than 20% of cases. There are some reports of CD56-positive T-LGLL being associated with

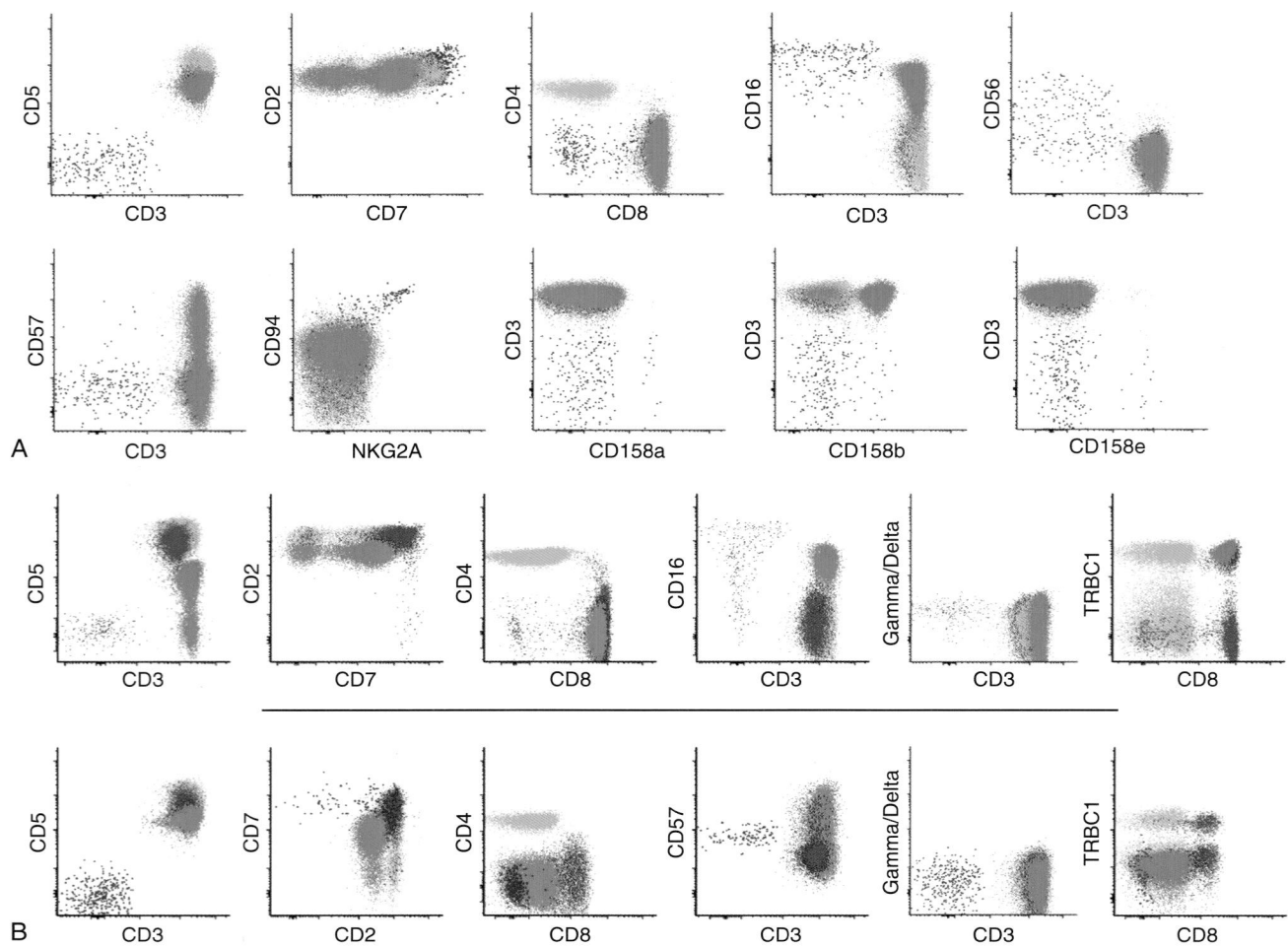

Figure 30-1. Flow cytometric immunophenotype for T-cell large granular lymphocytic leukemia (T-LGLL). The abnormal T cells are in *red*, normal CD4-positive T cells are in *orange*, normal CD8-positive T cells are in *green*, and normal natural killer (NK) cells are in *blue*. **A,** A representative T-LGLL case shows neoplastic cells are CD3-positive, CD2-positive, and CD8-positive T cells, with dim CD5 and partial CD7 expression. They express NK-cell–associated markers, such as CD16 (uniform), CD57 (partial), and CD94 (uniform). They uniformly express CD158b isoform, without CD158a or CD158e expression. **B,** Two T-LGLL cases reveal monotypic TRBC1 expression, characterized by being uniformly TRBC1-positive or TRBC1-negative. The background CD4-positive and CD8-positive T cells show polytypic TRBC1 expression.

STAT5b mutations and aggressive disease, although these may represent peripheral blood involvement by other cytotoxic T-cell malignancies that frequently are CD56 positive, such as hepatosplenic T-cell lymphoma.[55,56] Evaluation of TRBC1 expression by flow cytometry, as a surrogate for clonality, has made identification of a phenotypically aberrant T-cell population more straightforward (see this chapter's section titled Genetics and Molecular Findings).

Assessment of NCR expression by flow cytometry, particularly the KIRs CD158a, CD158b, and CD158e, can be an important aid in the diagnosis of T-LGLL.[11,16,57] Homogeneous expression of one or more KIR by the abnormal T cells is uniformly associated with T-cell clonality and is detected in approximately one-fourth of cases (Fig. 30-1A). Most KIR-positive T-LGLLs express a single isoform, with a strong tendency for CD158b, and in isolated cases (less than 10%), expression of two KIRs is seen. The uniform expression of all three of these KIRs is typical for hepatosplenic T-cell lymphoma, however, which helps distinguish it from T-LGLL in the clinical flow-cytometry laboratory.[58] CD94 is another NCR family member expressed by T-LGLL, often in combination with NKG2A, and is present in half of cases (Fig. 30-1A).

A minor subset of T-LGLL (<10%) are of γδ T-cell lineage.[10,59] Although these have features similar to their CD8-positive αβ counterpart, it should be noted that many of the phenotypic attributes associated with T-LGLL, including diminished CD5 expression and co-expression of CD16, are present in normal γδ T cells, particularly those expressing V-δ2.[60] Given this, evaluation of KIR is of particular utility in establishing an abnormal phenotype of γδ T cells and thereby confirming a γδ T-cell T-LGLL diagnosis. These studies should also be considered in other uncommon T-LGL variants such as CD4-positive, as the patterns of NK-antigen expression can both confirm the diagnosis and exclude other potential considerations such as T-cell prolymphocytic leukemia, HTLV-1–associated lymphoproliferative disease, or other T-cell neoplasms.[9,61]

In clinical flow cytometry, expression of CD2, CD7, CD8, CD16, and CD56 by NK cells are routinely evaluated, and abnormalities of each of these are seen to varying degrees in CLPD-NK.[62] Normal NK cells express CD7 more brightly than normal T cells; in comparison, approximately half of CLPD-NKs have CD7 expression that is dimmer than that in normal T cells. Complete loss of CD7 expression may be seen in some CLPD-NKs, but this is uncommon. In normal peripheral blood, one-third of the NK cells are CD8 positive; in 20% of CLPD-NKs, there is abnormal uniform CD8 positivity. Absence of CD8 expression may also be observed, but given the relatively low level of CD8 expression by normal NK cells, it is difficult to use this as a feature to identify CLPD-NK with confidence. Diminished expression of CD2 is rarely present in CLPD-NK (by definition, these cells lack CD3), though rare CD5-positive CLPD-NKs have been described.[63] A CD5 expression in such a case would make it difficult to discern between a CD5-positive CLPD-NK and a CD3-negative T-LGLL. Cytoplasmic expression of CD3ε by flow cytometry may assist in distinguishing such two entities.[63] In approximately 50% of CLPD-NKs, CD56 expression is either completely or partially lost (Fig. 30-2). Interestingly, the phenotypes of CD56-positive and CD56-negative CLPD-NK cases differ, with the CD56-negative cases having brighter expression of CD16 and a tendency to be KIR positive and CD56-positive cases having slightly dimmer expression of CD16 (compared with CD56-negative cases) and tending to be KIR negative (Fig. 30-2).[64]

Analysis of NCR expression is even more useful in the evaluation of CLPD-NK than it is in the evaluation of T-LGLL. This is largely because, in healthy peripheral blood and bone marrow, the NK cells always express, to some degree, the KIRs CD158a, CD158b, and CD158e.[6,65] Therefore, unlike in T cells (which are not obligate KIR expressers), in NK-cells, both complete absence of KIR expression and homogeneous expression of KIR (single or multiple antigens) are abnormal, and one of these two abnormal patterns is present in almost all CLPD-NK cases.[16,57,66] As previously noted, homogeneous (i.e., restricted) KIR expression is preferentially seen in CD56-negative CLPD-NK, being present in 60% of such cases, whereas the majority of CD56-positive CLPD-NKs (70%) completely lack KIR expression. In 80% of KIR-positive CLPD-NKs, a single KIR is expressed, and most KIR-positive CLPD-NKs express CD158a for reasons that are unclear. In less than 10% of CLPD-NKs, the KIR expression pattern is indeterminate in regard to aberrancy in that it is positive but not with homogeneous expression of a single antigen or multiple antigens. Indeterminate KIR patterns are seen exclusively in cases with some degree of CD56 expression; in such cases, the CLPD-NK diagnosis hinges on other factors. The inhibitory heterodimeric MHC receptor complex CD94/NKG2A is always expressed by a proportion of the normal NK cells in the peripheral blood or bone marrow. Abnormally uniform, bright CD94/NKG2A expression is a distinctive feature of some CLPD-NK (Fig. 30-2).[67] This abnormality is present in nearly all CD56-positive CLPD-NKs and in approximately 50% of CD56-negative CLPD-NKs; it tends to occur in cases lacking KIR expression, although this finding and homogeneous KIR expression are not mutually exclusive.[64]

Because bone marrow involvement by these LGL disorders is not easily seen in routine histologic sections (Fig. 30-3A),

bone marrow immunohistochemistry is required to detect the abnormal cells and is a valuable tool in confirming the diagnosis. The antigens of particular utility in this regard are CD8 and the cytotoxic granule proteins TIA-1 and granzyme B. Bone marrow immunohistochemistry using antibodies to these antigens allows for identification of the cytotoxic lymphocytes. An increase in bone marrow cytotoxic lymphocytes alone, however, is not sufficient to distinguish these disorders from reactive conditions. Rather, the essential diagnostic finding is the presence of linear arrays of cells (causes by intrasinusoidal infiltration) or large interstitial clusters (eight or more cells) (Fig. 30-3A).[17] The frequency with which one or both of these findings is present varies somewhat with the antibody tested, being detected in approximately 80% of cases by CD8 and TIA-1 immunohistochemistry and in approximately 50% of cases by granzyme B immunohistochemistry.[17] This finding may be present even in cases with low peripheral blood absolute granular lymphocyte counts (less than 1.0×10^9/L), although it is seen in only two-thirds of such cases.

When considering the use of immunohistochemistry to render a diagnosis of an LGL disorder, there are some important caveats to remember. Perhaps most important is that this methodology does not allow distinction of CLPD-NK and T-LGLL, as even the former may be CD3 positive by this method, and there is no immunohistochemical stain that is lineage-specific for either cytotoxic T cells or NK cells.[18,68] Furthermore, these stains can be challenging to interpret, as not all cases are CD8 positive or granzyme B positive, and TIA-1 staining of lymphocytes in bone marrow may be difficult to interpret, as normal granulocytes also express this antigen. Therefore, the routine use of TIA-1 immunohistochemistry for this purpose requires bone marrow–specific antibody titration. Lastly, there are other disorders that have similar immunohistochemical features and patterns of bone marrow infiltration, chiefly hepatosplenic T-cell lymphoma.[69,70] Careful observation is helpful in this regard, as hepatosplenic T-cell lymphoma not only infiltrates in a sinusoidal pattern but also frequently distends and distorts the sinusoidal structure, whereas T-LGLL always percolates the sinusoids without causing abnormal distention.

Splenomegaly is attributable to T-LGLL infiltrates, demonstrated by a red pulp expansion of cytotoxic T cells expressing granzyme and TIA-1 (Fig. 30-3B). A focal intrasinusoidal infiltrate of cytotoxic T cells is evident (Fig. 30-3B). It could be challenging to distinguish liver involvement by T-LGLL, especially by γδ T-LGLL, from hepatosplenic T-cell lymphoma, because both have an intrasinusoidal infiltrate pattern. In contrast to highly atypical hepatosplenic T-cell lymphoma, T-LGLL is cytologically bland (Fig. 30-3C). In addition, hepatosplenic T-cell lymphoma has TIA-1 but lacks granzyme B expression, whereas T-LGLL usually expresses granzyme B.[70]

GENETICS AND MOLECULAR FINDINGS

The presence of T-cell clonality is a molecular genetic abnormality universally cited as a disease-defining feature of T-LGLL. T-cell clonality can be assessed by a variety of methods. Traditionally, most commonly used in clinical practice are multiplexed polymerase chain reaction (PCR) amplification of TCR β and γ gene rearrangements (T-PCR) and flow-cytometric assessment of TCR β-chain V-region family usage

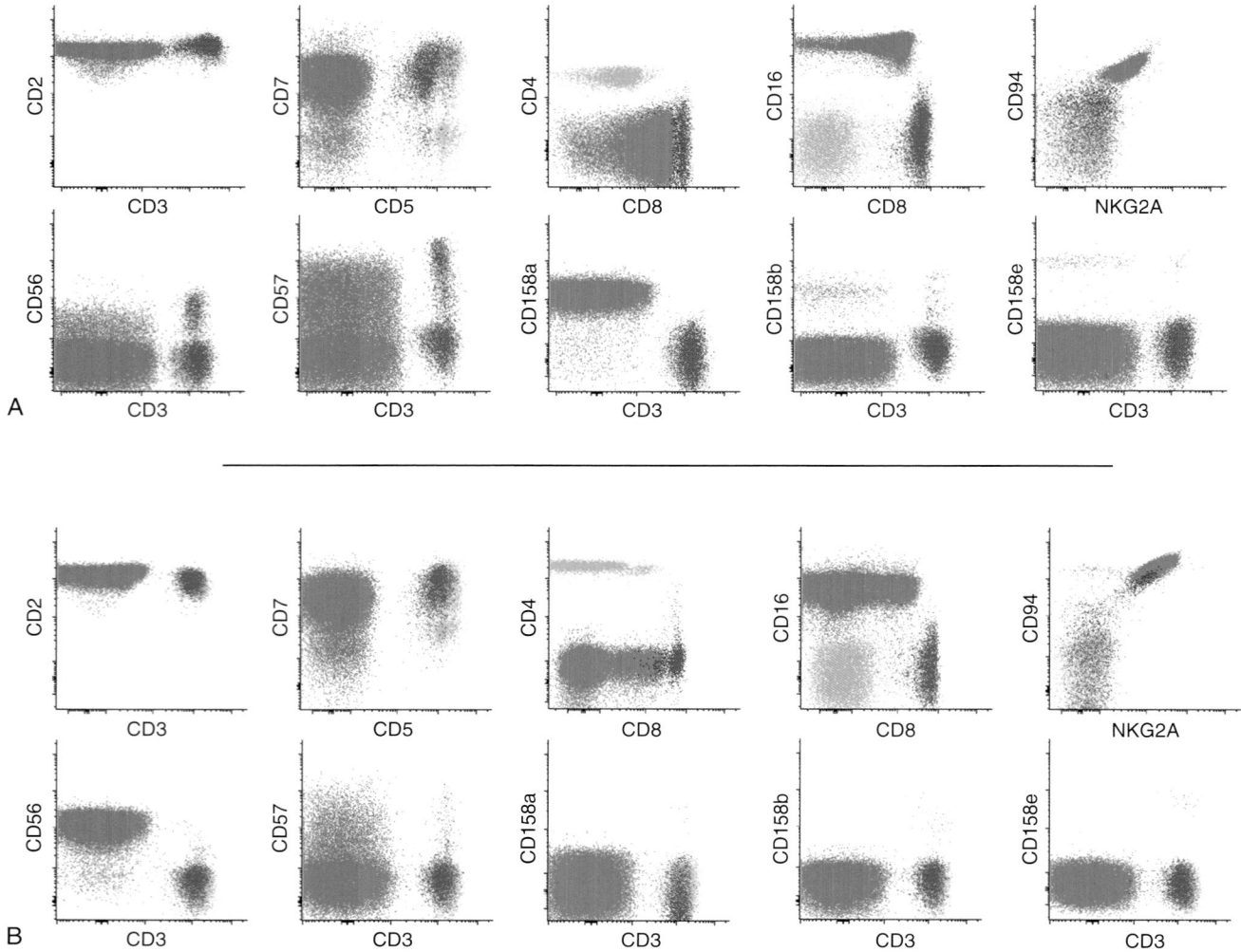

Figure 30-2. Flow cytometric immunophenotype for chronic lymphoproliferative disorder of NK cells (CLPD-NK). The abnormal natural killer (NK) cells are in *red*, normal CD4-positive T cells are in *orange*, and normal CD8-positive T cells are in *green*. **A,** CD56-negative CLPD-NK with brighter CD16 expression and CD158a restriction. **B,** CD56-positive CLPD-NK with dimmer CD16 expression and lack of KIR expression.

(TCR V-β flow). It has been shown that incorporating TRBC1 into flow cytometric T panels provides a rapid, sensitive and cost-effective way to assess clonality of immunophenotypically distinct T-cell populations.[12,71] TRBC1 specifically recognizes one of two mutually exclusive TCR β-chain constant regions; therefore, T-LGLL cells either homogenously express (≥85% of cells) or do not express (≤15% of cells) TRBC1 (Fig. 30-1B). It has been demonstrated that TRBC1 assessment by flow cytometry was comparable to TCGR molecular study and superior to KIR flow cytometric analysis in establishing T-cell clonality in T-LGLL.[71] However, small T-cell clones with a T-LGLL immunophenotype may be detected in up to 20% of patients without other features of this disorder or other T-cell malignancy and therefore, as an isolated laboratory finding, must be interpreted with caution.[72]

Although rare, co-existent T-cell and NK-cell clones or co-existent αβ and γδ T-cell clones have been identified in some LGLL cases.[73] Interestingly, LGLL-directed treatment may alter the proportions of the concurrent clones.[73] Furthermore, serial analysis of individual T-LGLL cases has revealed that the

distribution and proportions of the various "subclones" often change over time.[74] The co-existent clones may result from the emergence of LGLL clones recognizing different epitopes of the same chronic stimulant. Collectively, these data suggest that T-LGLL could be an oligoclonal disorder of cytotoxic T cells, and this may explain the inability to clearly demonstrate clonality in some cases. This oligoclonal nature of T-LGLL is important to keep in mind, as primary differential diagnostic considerations are reactive increases in cytotoxic T cells that may show similarly restricted subclone distributions.

For all of these reasons, practically speaking, a diagnosis of T-LGLL can neither be confirmed nor excluded based on the presence or absence of detectable T-cell clonality alone. TCR gene rearrangements play no role in the evaluation of potential CLPD-NK, as NK cells do not productively rearrange TCR (or other antigen receptor) genes. These limitations of TCR gene rearrangement analysis have spurred investigation of other potential genetic markers of disease clonality in LGL disorders.

Genome-wide mutational analysis has revealed such a marker with detection of an *STAT3* mutation in approximately

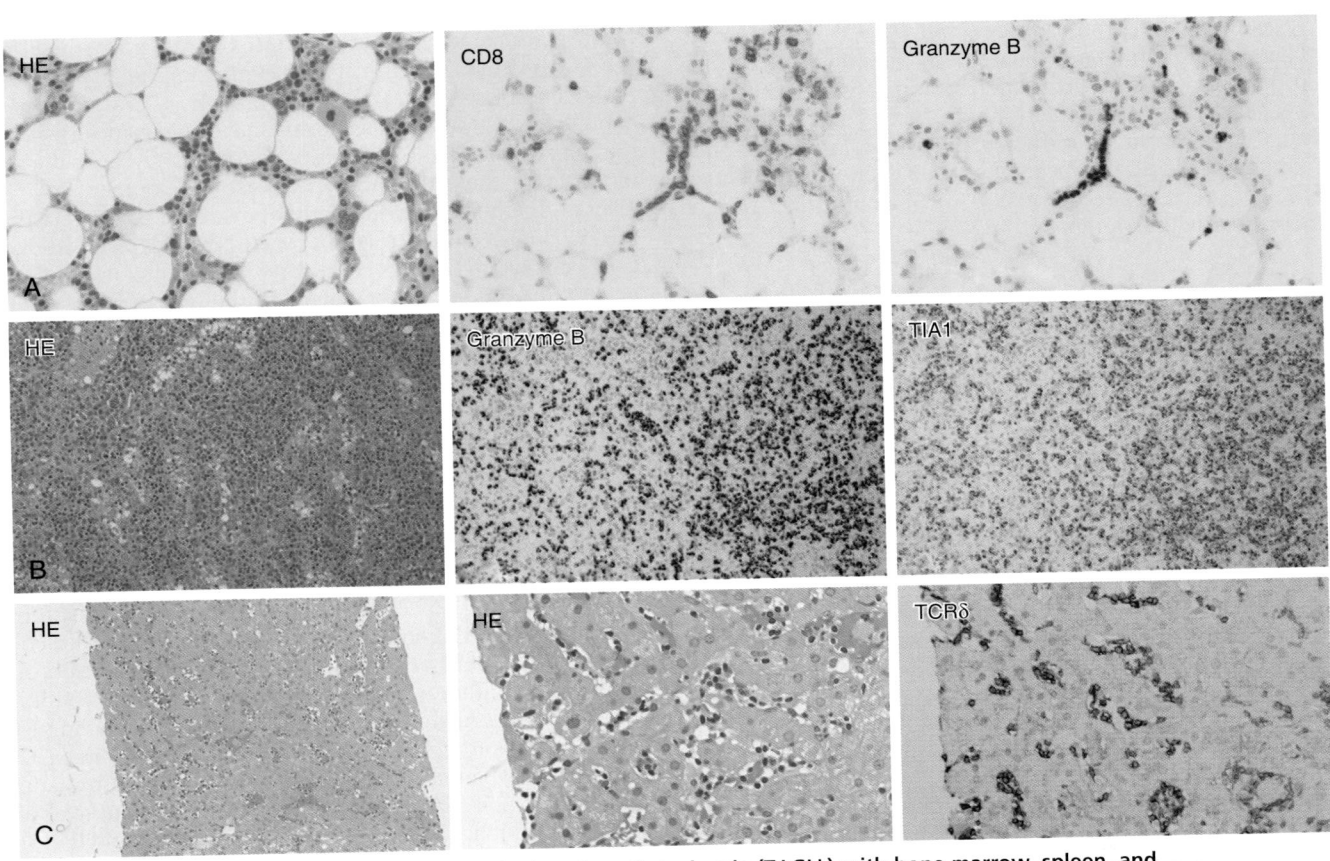

Figure 30-3. T-cell large granular lymphocytic leukemia (T-LGLL) with bone marrow, spleen, and liver involvement. A, Bone marrow histology usually does not reveal evident T-LGLL infiltrates. However, immunohistochemical studies show characteristic intrasinusoidal linear infiltrates of CD8-positive T cells expressing cytotoxic markers, such as granzyme B. **B,** T-LGLL predominantly involves red pulp of the spleen and focally involves intrasinusoidal regions, expressing both granzyme B and TIA1. **C,** T-LGLL infiltrates the liver sinusoids and expresses TCRγδ, making it difficult to distinguish from hepatosplenic T-cell lymphoma. T-LGLL usually has bland cytology and causes minimal architectural distortion.

20% to 70% of both T-LGLL and CLPD-NK cases, depending on the assay sensitivity and the selection criteria.[19,75-83] A number of *STAT3* mutations have been identified in these disorders, preferentially occurring in exons 20 and 21, which encode the SRC homology 2 (SH2) domain of the protein, and also in the DNA-binding or coiled-coil domain.[80] These gain-of-function mutations mediate the constitutive dimerization and activation of STAT3 protein, which raises protein levels of epigenetic regulators, increases global DNA methylation, and upregulates oxidative stress.[84] In T-LGLL, the presence of an *STAT3* mutation is associated with neutropenia, rheumatoid arthritis, a greater need for treatment, and methotrexate responsiveness.[19,75,76] The association of *STAT3* mutations and pure red cell aplasia (PRCA) is controversial: some studies show that *STAT3* mutations are frequent in LGLL with PRCA,[85-87] whereas others reveal *STAT3* mutations are invariably not seen in patients with LGLL and PRCA.[19,76] By multivariate analysis, *STAT3* mutations are independently associated to reduced overall survival in patients with LGLL.[33]

Mutations of the *STAT5b* gene, mainly N642H and Y665F, have been identified in a minor subset of CD8-positive T-LGLL and CLPD-NK cases (<5%). These mutations occur only in cases lacking an *STAT3* mutation, and again effect the SH2 domain.[56,88] Subsequently, it has been found that *STAT5b* mutations are more prevalent in CD4-positive

T-LGLL and γδ T-LGLL.[33,77,89] Although both N642H and Y665F mutations increase the transcriptional activity and tyrosine phosphorylation of *STAT5b*, N642H, but not Y665F, is associated with an aggressive and fatal clinical course in patients with CD8-positive T-LGLL and CLPD-NK. In contrast, patients with *STAT5b*-mutated CD4-positive T-LGLL are mostly asymptomatic with no or mild cytopenia, regardless of the mutation type.[33,56,88,89]

In addition to *STAT3* and *STAT5b* mutations, whole-exome sequencing from untreated patients with LGLL has revealed other recurrent mutations, in particular *TET2* mutations, which appear to be present in approximately 30% of CLPD-NK cases.[90,91] Other genetic abnormalities that have been identified in LGLL by this approach include mutations in transcriptional/epigenetic regulators and tumor suppressor and cell proliferation genes, such as *IGSF3, USH2A, TTN, CCT6P1, IGFN1, MUC4, TYPR1, ARL13B, FAT4, HRNR, KMT2D, NHS, ATN1,* and *PCLO*.[79] Interestingly, most *STAT*-mutation–negative patients harbor at least one of the "STAT-related component" genes, which connect to the MAPK-RAS-ERK pathway or IL-15 pathway, all known to be deregulated in LGLL.[79]

There have been isolated reports of cytogenetic abnormalities in both T-LGLL and CLPD-NK, including reports of abnormalities of chromosome 6 long arm (6q) and inversions and reciprocal translocations involving the

TCR gene loci on chromosomes 7 and 14.[92-94] No recurrent cytogenetic abnormalities have been identified in either disorder, however. Furthermore, cases with abnormal cytogenetics are preferentially found in the older literature, raising the possibility that these may have, in fact, been other conditions. Overall, it appears that cytogenetic abnormalities in what are currently recognized as T-LGLL and CLPD-NK are extraordinarily uncommon.

POSTULATED CELL OF ORIGIN AND PATHOGENESIS

The phenotypes and patterns of gene expression of CD8-positive T-LGLL are all highly similar to normal memory CD8-positive T cells, and T-LGLL is clearly a disorder of this cell type.[22,95] Furthermore, a number of features, including abnormal distribution of TCR β-chain variable region use, are indicative of prior persistent cellular stimulation in T-LGLL.[96] CD4-positive T-LGLL expresses CD56, CD57, and varying levels of CD8 (CD8-negative or CD8-dim), suggesting these cases derive from a distinctive subset of circulating CD4-positive cytotoxic T cells that express NK-associated antigens, variably express CD8, and carry an antitumor/antiviral function.[9,66,89] The γδ T-LGLL co-expresses CD57 and cytotoxic antigens and has gene expression profiling similar to that of effector γδ T cells, indicating the normal effector γδ T cells are its cells of origin.[97]

In considering CLPD-NK, it is important to note that there are two normal mature NK-cell subsets (or types): NK1 cells with bright CD56, dim CD16, and low levels of NCR expression; and NK2 cells with dim CD56, bright CD16, and high levels of NCR expression.[98] The NK1 cells function primarily through cytokine production, whereas the NK2 cells function through cellular cytotoxicity. NK1 cells are converted to NK2 cells through stimulation and exposure to cytokines such as IL-12. In CLPD-NK, it appears that the CD56-positive and CD56-negative cases correspond to the normal NK1 and NK2 NK-cell subsets, respectively. Interestingly, cytopenias and other clinical features typically seen in T-LGLL are much more common in the CD56-negative CLPD-NK compared with CD56-positive cases. Hence, it appears that chronic cellular stimulation is a critical first pathogenetic event in both T-LGLL and CLPD-NK, although the precise nature of the stimuli is still unclear.

If ongoing cellular stimulation with selective enrichment of certain clonotypes is a critical first step in the pathogenesis of these granular lymphocytic disorders, then the equally critical second step is the ability of these clones to survive through circumvention of normal activation-induced cell death and undergo an uncontrolled proliferation. In T-LGLL, the ability of the abnormal cells to survive may be in part attributable to NCR expression. During the course of normal cytotoxic T-cell responses, there is physiologic restriction of the T-cell repertoire and a commensurate increase in NCR expression by the cytotoxic T cells. The NCR expression by these T cells serves a dual purpose, both preventing inappropriate autoreactivity and prolonging cell survival through inhibiting activation-induced cell death.[99,100] T-LGLL, by comparison, appears to be a distortion of this normal immune response, with pronounced oligoclonal or clonal T-cell repertoire restriction and abnormally high levels of NK-associated antigen expression, including NCR. In NK cells, there are varying hypotheses regarding the acquisition of NCR and

how it relates to increased cytotoxic function; therefore, the connection between NCR expression and CLPD-NK pathogenesis is less clear.[6,101] The propensity of CLPD-NK to express the activating KIR isoforms and to epigenetically silence the expression of the inhibitory isoforms may be indicative of a role for these receptors in disease development.[57,102,103] Overall, there is a growing body of evidence suggesting that, in CLPD-NK, the interplay between NK cells and dendritic cells, regulated through NCR and MHC interactions, may be a primary contributing factor to the development of this condition.[104]

There is also a wealth of data indicating that perturbations of cellular signaling cascades are an important facet of the abnormal survivability of the cells in T-LGLL and CLPD-NK. The JAK-STAT pathway appears to be at the center of these perturbations. Constitutive activation of STAT3 appears to play an essential role in the pathogenesis of LGLL, because almost all cases have constitutive activation of the STAT3 pathway, which promotes cell survival and proliferation. The inhibition of STAT3 signaling restores the apoptosis of LGLL cells by reducing BCL2-family protein Mcl-1.[105] Constitutive activation of STAT3 could be caused by the gain of function mutations in STAT3 or somatic mutations in STAT3 responsive genes.[88] In addition, increased proinflammatory cytokine IL-6 or downregulated suppressor of cytokine signaling to 3 (SOCS3) leads to constitutive activation of STAT3 in STAT3-unmutated patients.[106] Similar to STAT3, STAT5b mutation-induced STAT5b activation also promotes cell survival and proliferation. It has been demonstrated that IL-15 and IL-15Rα are elevated in patients with LGLL, inducing the downstream activation of the JAK1/STAT3 and JAK3/STAT5 pathway.[107-109] Abnormalities in other pathways that regulate cell survival, primarily through modulation of BCL2 family proteins, have also been identified in patients with LGLL, including the RAS/MAPK, PI3K/AKT, NF-κB and sphingolipid pathways.[79,110-116]

Lastly, the ability of the abnormal granular lymphocytes to suppress or destroy normal hematopoiesis is the most clinically relevant component of the disease process. In spite of this, the exact mechanism by which this occurs has yet to be defined. There have been a number of studies implicating Fas-Fas ligand interactions through the elevated soluble Fas.[77,117] In addition, there are published cases of both T-LGLL and CLPD-NK in which the ability of the abnormal cells to kill normal human hematopoietic cells has been demonstrated.[118,119] Therefore, it appears that the cytopathic effects of these disorders may be exerted through both humoral and cellular means.

CLINICAL MANAGEMENT AND PROGNOSIS

From a clinical perspective, the same management approach is used for T-LGLL and CLPD-NK; in both disorders, the decision to treat is primarily predicated on the presence or absence of disease-associated cytopenias.[28,29,40] If cytopenias are absent, the disorder may be observed without disease-specific therapeutic intervention. However, therapy is indicated if the patient has moderate-to-profound neutropenia associated with recurrent infections or symptomatic or transfusion-dependent anemia. Therapy typically consists of methotrexate, cyclophosphamide, or cyclosporin, either as single agents or in combination with corticosteroids during the initiation of therapy. Responsiveness to therapy is assessed by improvement of symptoms and complete blood counts, which should occur within the first 6 months of treatment. The overall response rate (complete response and partial response) for the single-agent therapy varies among different studies, ranging from 20% to 80%.[28,30,120,121] It has been reported that patients with LGLL with *STAT3* mutations are more likely to respond to methotrexate treatment.[75,120] In cases of failure of primary therapy, a switch to methotrexate, cyclophosphamide, or cyclosporin should be considered.

Splenectomy may be performed in patients with symptomatic splenomegaly and associated refractory cytopenia, but a proven benefit with a durable response is controversial.[30,122] A small number of studies suggest efficacy of purine analogs (e.g., fludarabine) in the treatment of T-LGLL.[123] Immunotherapy, such as anti-CD52 monoclonal antibody therapy with alemtuzumab and anti-CD20 with rituximab, has been used, although further studies are needed for a clinically demonstrable response.[124-126] Inhibitors for IL-15 or the JAK/STAT pathway could be a good therapeutic option in patients with LGLL.[29,127,128]

The avoidance of therapy-related complications is paramount in T-LGLL and CLPD-NK, as both are indolent disorders typically with a prolonged disease course and minimal morbidity and mortality. The reported proportion of patients requiring therapy at some point for their disease varies, although large series with extended follow-up indicate that the majority of patients with T-LGLL will eventually develop cytopenias requiring treatment. As previously noted, it appears the majority of CD56-negative CLPD-NKs require therapy, whereas the majority of CD56-positive cases do not. Given the paucity of large CLPD-NK studies, however, it is difficult to precisely ascertain how many patients with CLPD-NK will develop the need for treatment over time.

Although the vast majority of cases are indolent, there are sporadic reports of T-LGLL and CLPD-NK exhibiting aggressive clinical behavior, similar to other cytotoxic NK/T-cell malignancies. In T-LGLL, this has been associated with a CD56-positive phenotype, raising the possibility that these may, in fact, be other T-cell disorders that more frequently express this antigen, such as hepatosplenic T-cell lymphoma.[58,70] Likewise, aggressive CLPD-NKs are more common in older adults, suggesting that many were, in fact, other disorders that were subsequently recognized, such as aggressive NK-cell leukemia. Scarcely, transformation of an indolent LGLL to an aggressive T-cell or NK-cell lymphoma/leukemia has been reported.[129-132] It appears that highly malignant T-LGLL and CLPD-NK cases, either at diagnosis or as a feature of disease progression, are extraordinarily rare and difficult to predict based on recognized pathologic features.

DIFFERENTIAL DIAGNOSIS

The primary differential diagnostic considerations for both T-LGLL and CLPD-NK are reactive cytotoxic T-cell and NK-cell expansions at one end of the spectrum and highly aggressive cytotoxic T-cell and NK-cell neoplasms that can involve the peripheral blood, such as hepatosplenic T-cell lymphoma and extranodal NK/T-cell lymphoma, at the other end (Table 30-2). From a clinical perspective, distinguishing these indolent granular lymphoproliferative disorders from these more aggressive diseases is relatively straightforward. From the pathologist's perspective, this distinction can be much more challenging, as the cytology of these malignancies does not always correlate with their clinical aggressiveness. Destructive

Table 30-2 Differential Diagnoses of T-LGLL

	T-CUS	T-LGLL	Hepatosplenic T-Cell Lymphoma
Common locations	PB, BM	PB, BM, spleen, liver	Spleen, liver, BM, PB
Cytologic features	Large granular lymphocytes	Large granular lymphocytes	Highly atypical
Histologic features	Interstitial infiltrates in BM	Linear array infiltrates in BM	Expansile intrasinusoidal infiltrates in BM
Immunophenotyping			
TCR	αβ	αβ	γδ
CD2	+	+	+
CD3	+	+	+
CD4	–	–	–
CD5	Dim/partial	Dim/partial	–
CD7	Dim/partial	Dim/partial	+
CD8	+ (80%)	+ (80%)	–
CD16	+/–	+ (80%)	–
CD56	–/+	–/+ (20%)	+
CD57	+/–	+ (80%)	–
KIR	Could be restricted	Single KIR restriction (25%)	Multiple KIR restriction
Size of Clonal T Cells			
Absolute number	<500 cells/μL	>500 cells/μL	NA
Percentage	<15% of lymphocytes	>50% of lymphocytes	NA

BM, Bone marrow; *PB,* peripheral blood; *T-CUS,* T-cell clones of uncertain significance; *T-LGLL,* T-cell large granular lymphocytic leukemia.

tissue infiltration and clonal cytogenetic abnormalities are not a feature of T-LGLL or CLPD-NK, and, if present, should lead to other diagnostic considerations. Phenotypically, the expression of multiple KIR antigens by the abnormal cells can help distinguish hepatosplenic T-cell lymphoma from T-LGLL. The flow-cytometric immunophenotype of aggressive NK-cell leukemias and lymphomas have not been well characterized, and therefore the phenotypic features that may distinguish these from CLPD-NK are not evident. Assessing for EBV positivity in tissue sections is critical, however, as neither T-LGLL nor CLPD-NK is EBV associated, whereas almost all cases of aggressive NK-cell leukemia and extranodal NK/T-cell lymphoma are.

Distinguishing T-LGLL and CLPD-NK from reactive T-cell and NK-cell expansions is more problematic, as these LGL disorders are derived from cytotoxic immune responses. It has been reported that T-cell clones with uncertain significance (T-CUS) are found in approximately 20% of patients without T-cell neoplasm, indicating T-CUS could be a physiologic expansion of an immunodominant clone. T-CUS is mainly CD8-positive T cells with an immunophenotype closely resembling that of T-LGLL but a much smaller clone size.[72] The natural history of T-CUS is not clear at this point, but the extensive workup of small CD8-positive T-cell clones (<15% of lymphocytes or <500 cells/μL) with an immunophenotype of T-LGLL is likely not warranted.[71] However, in cases with increased granular lymphocytes and unexplained cytopenias, extensive evaluation for, and exclusion of, other potential causes and demonstration of persistence of the clinical features may be required to distinguish between the reactive NK/T-cell expansions and bona fide T-LGLL/CLPD-NK.

Pearls and Pitfalls

Pearls

- T-LGLL and CLPD-NK can only be distinguished from each other by flow-cytometric immunophenotyping. Their peripheral blood and bone marrow morphologies are identical. Both harbor *STAT3/STAT5b* mutations.
- The clinical management of T-LGLL and CLPD-NK are the same; therefore, distinguishing between them is not required for treatment to be initiated.
- Bone marrow immunohistochemistry is required to detect marrow involvement by lymphoproliferative disorders of granular lymphocytes.
- An absolute increase in peripheral blood granular lymphocytes is not present in all cases of T-LGLL or CLPD-NK, although the granular lymphocytes typically account for more than 50% of all lymphoid cells.
- Distention and/or distortion of bone marrow sinusoids and expression of multiple KIRs are not typical of T-LGLL or CLPD-NK and suggest diagnosis of an aggressive disease such as hepatosplenic T-cell lymphoma.

Pitfalls

- A reactive increase in granular lymphocytes can be seen in a number of conditions associated with cytopenias, including myelodysplasia and viral infection.
- Clonal TCR gene rearrangements can be detected in a variety of settings associated with restriction of the T-cell repertoire, including viral infection, after allogeneic organ transplantation, and normal aging. Therefore, these have poor diagnostic specificity in the absence of pathologic features supporting a T-LGLL diagnosis.
- Small T-cell and NK-cell populations with phenotypic attributes similar to those of T-LGLL and CLPD-NK, respectively, can be detected in healthy, asymptomatic adults.
- T-LGLL and hepatosplenic T-cell lymphoma can have similar peripheral blood and bone marrow manifestations.

KEY REFERENCES

17. Morice WG, Kurtin PJ, Tefferi A, Hanson CA. Distinct bone marrow findings in T-cell granular lymphocytic leukemia revealed by paraffin section immunoperoxidase stains for CD8, TIA-1, and granzyme B. *Blood.* 2002;99(1):268–274.

19. Jerez A, Clemente MJ, Makishima H, et al. STAT3 mutations unify the pathogenesis of chronic lymphoproliferative disorders of NK cells and T-cell large granular lymphocyte leukemia. *Blood.* 2012;120(15):3048–3057.

29. Lamy T, Moignet A, Loughran Jr TP. LGL leukemia: from pathogenesis to treatment. *Blood.* 2017;129(9):1082–1094.

36. Poullot E, Zambello R, Leblanc F, et al. Chronic natural killer lymphoproliferative disorders: characteristics of an international cohort of 70 patients. *Ann Oncol.* 2014;25(10):2030–2035.

56. Rajala HL, Eldfors S, Kuusanmaki H, et al. Discovery of somatic STAT5b mutations in large granular lymphocytic leukemia. *Blood.* 2013;121(22):4541–4550.

64. Morice WG, Jevremovic D, Olteanu H, et al. Chronic lymphoproliferative disorder of natural killer cells: a distinct entity with subtypes correlating with normal natural killer cell subsets. *Leukemia.* 2010;24(4):881–884.

74. Clemente MJ, Wlodarski MW, Makishima H, et al. Clonal drift demonstrates unexpected dynamics of the T-cell repertoire in T-large granular lymphocyte leukemia. *Blood.* 2011;118(16):4384–4393.

75. Koskela HL, Eldfors S, Ellonen P, et al. Somatic STAT3 mutations in large granular lymphocytic leukemia. *N Engl J Med.* 2012;366(20):1905–1913.

79. Coppe A, Andersson EI, Binatti A, et al. Genomic landscape characterization of large granular lymphocyte leukemia with a systems genetics approach. *Leukemia.* 2017;31(5):1243–1246.

91. Olson TL, Cheon H, Xing JC, et al. Frequent somatic TET2 mutations in chronic NK-LGL leukemia with distinct patterns of cytopenias. *Blood.* 2021;138(8):662–673.

Visit Elsevier eBooks+ for the complete set of references.

T-Cell Prolymphocytic Leukemia

Anna Porwit

DEFINITION

T-cell prolymphocytic leukemia (T-PLL) is an aggressive disease characterized by a proliferation of small to medium-sized lymphocytes with a postthymic phenotype usually involving the blood, bone marrow, lymph nodes, spleen, and skin.[1-3] This leukemia was first described by Catovsky and colleagues in reference to a patient who presented with cytologic features similar to B-cell prolymphocytic leukemia (B-PLL), but the cells were shown to bind sheep erythrocytes (E-rosette positive).[4] In 1986, Matutes and coworkers published a more detailed report comparing morphologic and clinical characteristics of 29 T-PLL and 33 B-PLL cases and defining the immunophenotype as consistent with mature T cells.[5] In 1987, the same group reported an association of T-PLL with inv(14)(q11q32) and trisomy for 8q.[6]

CONSENSUS CRITERIA FOR DIAGNOSIS

The T-PLL International Study Group published in 2019 standardized criteria for diagnosis, treatment indications, and evaluation of response in patients with T-PLL.[7] Three major and four minor criteria were defined:

Major Criteria

1. $>5 \times 10^9/L$ cells of T-PLL phenotype in peripheral blood or bone marrow
2. T-cell clonality (by polymerase chain reaction [PCR] for TRB/TRG, or by flow cytometry)
3. Abnormalities of 14q32 or Xq28 OR expression of *TCL1A/B* or *MTCP1*

Minor Criteria

1. Abnormalities involving chromosome 11 (11q22.3; *ATM*)
2. Abnormalities in chromosome 8: idic(8)(p11), t(8;8), trisomy 8q
3. Abnormalities in chromosomes 5, 12, 13, or 22 or complex karyotype
4. Involvement of T-PLL specific site (e.g., splenomegaly, effusions)

The T-PLL diagnosis can be established if all major criteria (met in 90% of cases) or two major and one minor criteria (TCL1-family negative T-PLL) are met.

These criteria are generally followed by the published 2022 International Consensus Classification on Mature Lymphoid Neoplasms[8] and proposed World Health Organization (WHO) 5th edition on Hematolymphoid Neoplasms.[9]

EPIDEMIOLOGY

T-PLL represents approximately 2% to 3% of all T-cell disorders but accounts for up to one-third of mature T-cell malignancies with a leukemic presentation.[10,11] This leukemia occurs mainly in older adults (median age 61 years) and more often in men (male-to-female ratio approximately 2:1).[11] An increased frequency has been found in patients with ataxia telangiectasia, an autosomal recessive disorder caused by loss of heterozygosity at 11q22-23 (mutated *ATM* gene).[12] Patients with ataxia telangiectasia develop T-PLL at a younger age (26 to 43 years).[13] A single sporadic pediatric case has been reported.[14]

CLINICAL FEATURES

Most T-PLL patients present with general symptoms: sweating, malaise, weight loss, or fever.[11,15-17] The median duration of symptoms is 2 months before diagnosis. In most patients, a high white blood cell (WBC) count ($>100 \times 10^9/L$ in 72%) is found, sometimes with extreme hyperlymphocytosis, splenomegaly

(79%), lymphadenopathy (46%), and enlarged liver (39%).[15,18-20] Rare aleukemic cases have been described.[21] One-fourth of patients have skin lesions at diagnosis, mainly maculopapular rash, nodules, or (more seldom) erythroderma.[15,22-24] In 15% to 30% of patients, mainly those with high WBC counts, serous effusions are found at diagnosis or may also develop later in the course of the disease.[15,16,18] Central nervous system involvement is rare.[15,18] Thirty percent to 50% of patients present with anemia (hemoglobin <100 g/L), thrombocytopenia (<100 × 10^9/L), or both.[11,15,18] Usually, there is no neutropenia or monocytopenia. Hyperuricemia and increased levels of lactate dehydrogenase are common. Other liver function tests may be mildly elevated, whereas serum immunoglobulin and renal biochemistry are normal.[15,18] Although serum from most Western patients with T-PLL has tested negative for human T-lymphotropic virus (HTLV) types 1 and 2, in some Japanese patients, DNA samples contained an HTLV-1 Tax sequence.[25,26] A single case of T-PLL positive for Epstein-Barr virus has been reported.[27]

MORPHOLOGY

Typical T-PLL cells in the peripheral blood are medium-sized lymphocytes with a high nuclear-to-cytoplasmic ratio and deeply basophilic cytoplasm without granules, often showing protrusions (Box 31-1; Fig. 31-1A). Ultrastructural studies show numerous ribosomes, polyribosomes, and profiles of rough endoplasmic reticulum, accounting for the cytoplasmic basophilia.[5,15,18,23] Nuclei are often irregular, with numerous short indentations, and they have moderately condensed chromatin and prominent nucleoli. Cytochemical staining for α-naphthyl-acetate esterase shows a characteristic dotlike pattern.[28]

In approximately 20% of cases, the leukemic cells are smaller, the nuclei are round, and the nucleoli cannot be readily seen by light microscopy (Fig. 31-1B), although they are easily detected by electron microscopy.[5] In some publications, these cases are called a *small cell variant* of T-PLL. Because the clinical presentation and cytogenetic features are similar, both variants of T-PLL probably belong in the same category.[16,29] Most cases in publications on T-cell chronic lymphocytic leukemia show a typical morphology and immunophenotype and chromosomal changes corresponding to the small cell variant of T-PLL.[30-33] In rare cases, polylobated nuclei are noted, similar to those in adult T-cell leukemia/lymphoma. In other cases, cerebriform nuclei, as seen in Sézary syndrome, are described.[23,34]

In bone marrow trephine biopsies, there is usually increased cellularity, which varies from slightly hypercellular to "packed" bone marrow. Patterns of infiltration may be nodular or interstitial, with leukemic cells constituting only part of the bone marrow cellularity, or diffuse infiltration with a dominance of leukemic cells (Fig. 31-1C).[28] In some cases, there is discordance between the blood and bone marrow involvement, and patients with marked leukocytosis may have a much lower level of marrow involvement. There is often slight fibrosis, shown by an increase in the density of reticulin fibers. On trephine sections, T-PLL cells are small to medium-sized and relatively round, making them difficult to differentiate from the cells of other chronic lymphoproliferative disorders. Characteristic cytologic features are more noticeable on bone marrow imprints or smears that show infiltration of cells like those in peripheral blood.[35]

Lymph nodes show a diffuse infiltration of leukemic cells. These cells are seen mostly in interfollicular areas, but they may also completely replace the normal architecture (Fig. 31-2A). Residual germinal centers may be present.[36] In paraffin sections, leukemic cells are medium-sized and rather monomorphic. Mitotic figures are easily identified, and Ki-67 (MIB-1) staining shows a high fraction of proliferating cells (usually 30%–60%) (Fig. 31-2B). Typical features, including prominent nucleoli and abundant cytoplasm, are more easily appreciated in imprints or fine-needle aspirates from the lymph nodes (Fig. 31-2C).

Osuji and associates described morphologic features of splenic involvement by T-PLL.[37] The spleen is often grossly enlarged. T-PLL cells infiltrate the red pulp—both sinusoids and cords—and the white pulp shows signs of disruption caused by the infiltration of leukemic cells into the follicles (Fig. 31-2D). The sinus pulp cord architecture is not distorted. Angioinvasion and infiltration of fibrous trabeculae are prominent. Leukemic cells infiltrate through the splenic capsule and into perisplenic fat tissue. In the liver, T-PLL infiltrates are usually confined to portal tracts, with variable portal tract expansion and sinusoidal involvement.[36] T-PLL cells can be seen within the blood vessels of portal tracts.

Skin infiltrates are usually confined to the dermis (Fig. 31-2E). The infiltrates sometimes extend into the subcutaneous adipose tissue. Lymphoepidermotropism or a subcutaneous mass may develop.[22,38,39] Infiltrates are usually present around

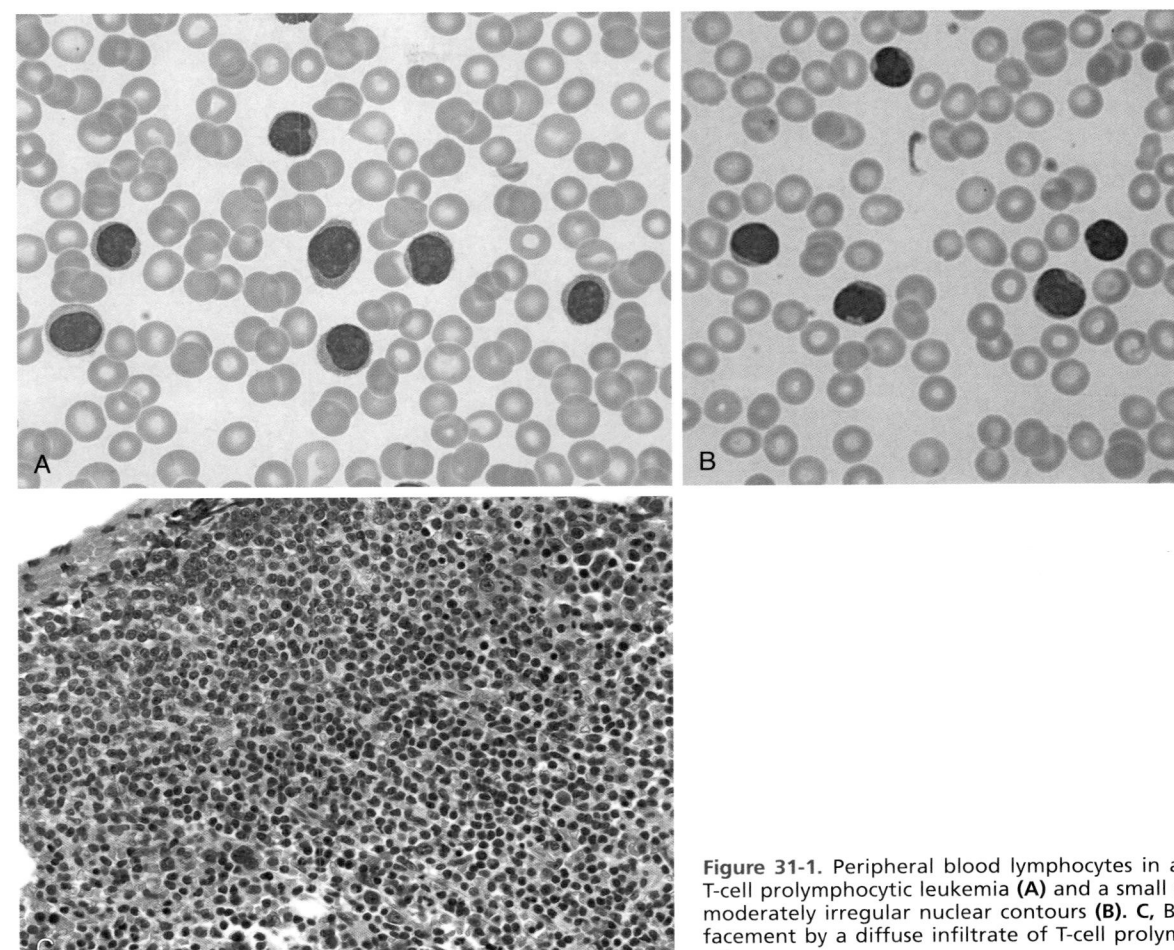

Figure 31-1. Peripheral blood lymphocytes in a typical case of T-cell prolymphocytic leukemia **(A)** and a small cell variant with moderately irregular nuclear contours **(B). C,** Bone marrow effacement by a diffuse infiltrate of T-cell prolymphocytic leukemia.

capillaries and skin appendages. There is a variable degree of stromal edema surrounding the blood vessels, with minimal endothelial damage and few extravasated erythrocytes. In most skin infiltrates, round nuclei are seen. Only rare cases with Sézary-like cells have been found. Progression to high-grade cutaneous CD30-positive large-cell lymphoma, with chromosomal changes identical to those seen in blood T-PLL cells, has been described.[40] Rare cases of ocular involvement have been described presenting with pan-uveitis, retinal detachment, or perivascular conjunctival involvement.[41,42] Reports on the morphology of other extramedullary sites involved by T-PLL are rare in the literature.[36]

IMMUNOPHENOTYPE

By flow cytometry, almost all T-PLL cases are positive for CD7, usually with high intensity. In cases with low or negative CD7, genetic data should be obtained before a diagnosis of T-PLL is considered. Leukemic cells are positive for cytoplasmic CD3, but membrane CD3 is negative in 20% of cases. In most cases, there is a strong expression of CD45, but rare CD45-negative or only weakly CD45-positive cases do occur. The leukemic cells are usually positive for CD2, CD5, CD43, and CD26. Most cases show one homogeneous abnormal population, but several subsets were noted in some cases. Approximately 60% of cases display a CD4-positive CD8-negative phenotype,

but a CD4-positive CD8-positive phenotype (15%–25%) or a CD4-negative CD8-positive phenotype (10%–15%) is also found (Fig. 31-3).[15-18,43] In rare cases, a combination of negative membrane CD3, lower-than-normal CD45, and co-expression of CD4/CD8 may bring a differential diagnosis of T-cell lymphoblastic leukemia-lymphoma. However, T-PLL cases do not express terminal deoxynucleotidyl transferase (TdT), CD1a, CD34, or CD10. CD34 and myeloid markers are not seen, except for CD117, which was noted in rare cases.[43] There is no expression of natural killer (NK)-cell markers (CD56, CD57, CD16) or of the cytotoxic marker TIA-1 (T-cell-restricted intracellular antigen-1), even in CD8-positive cases. However, perforin expression is noted in some cases. T-cell activation markers such as CD25, CD38, and human leukocyte antigen (HLA)-DR are variably expressed.[15-18,43] Two cases of CD103-positive T-PLL have been described, but data on CD103 expression in larger series are not available.[44]

TCL1 protein is detected by immunohistochemistry in 60% to 80% of cases (Fig. 31-4).[36,37,45] CD30, TRAP, anaplastic lymphoma kinase-1 (ALK-1), BCL6, and BCL3 are negative.[17,18,37,46] Data on BCL2 expression are not available in the literature, but our experience suggests that BCL2 is strongly positive (Fig. 31-2F). There are no larger published studies on ZAP-70 expression in T-PLL, but some cases may be positive.[47] In a small studied series of 20 patients with T-PLL, six were found to be positive for S100.[48]

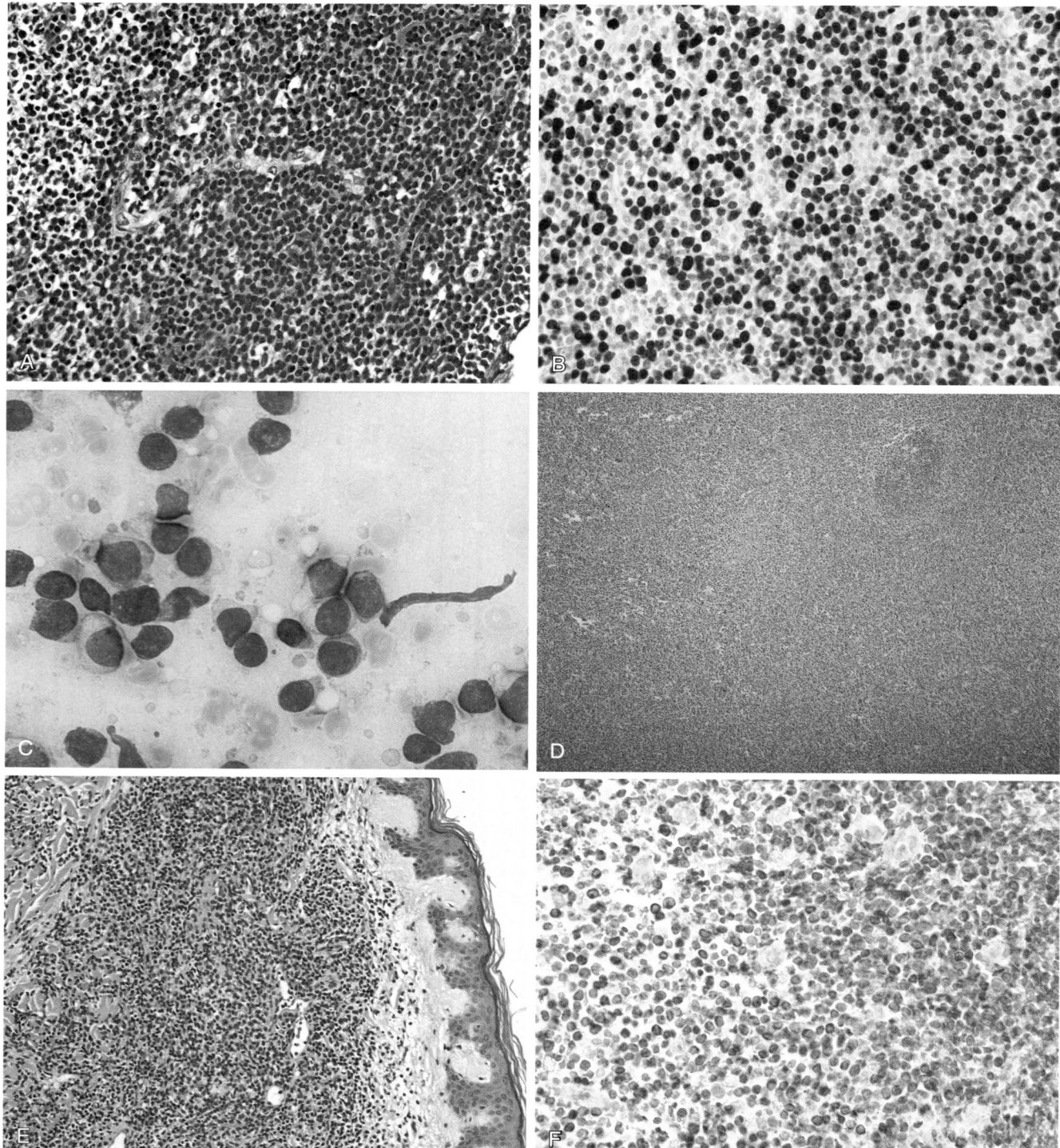

Figure 31-2. A, Core needle biopsy of a lymph node shows a diffuse infiltrate of T-cell prolympho-cytic leukemia (T-PLL). **B,** Ki-67 immunostain shows high proliferative activity of T-PLL (estimated at 60%). **C,** Fine-needle aspirate smear from a lymph node shows prominent nucleoli and abundant cytoplasm of neoplastic cells. **D,** Effacement of splenic red pulp by diffuse T-PLL infiltrate. **E,** Heavy infiltrate in the skin involves primarily the dermis and subcutaneous soft tissues, with characteristic sparing of the epidermal layer. **F,** BCL2 shows uniformly strong expression in neo-plastic cells of T-PLL.

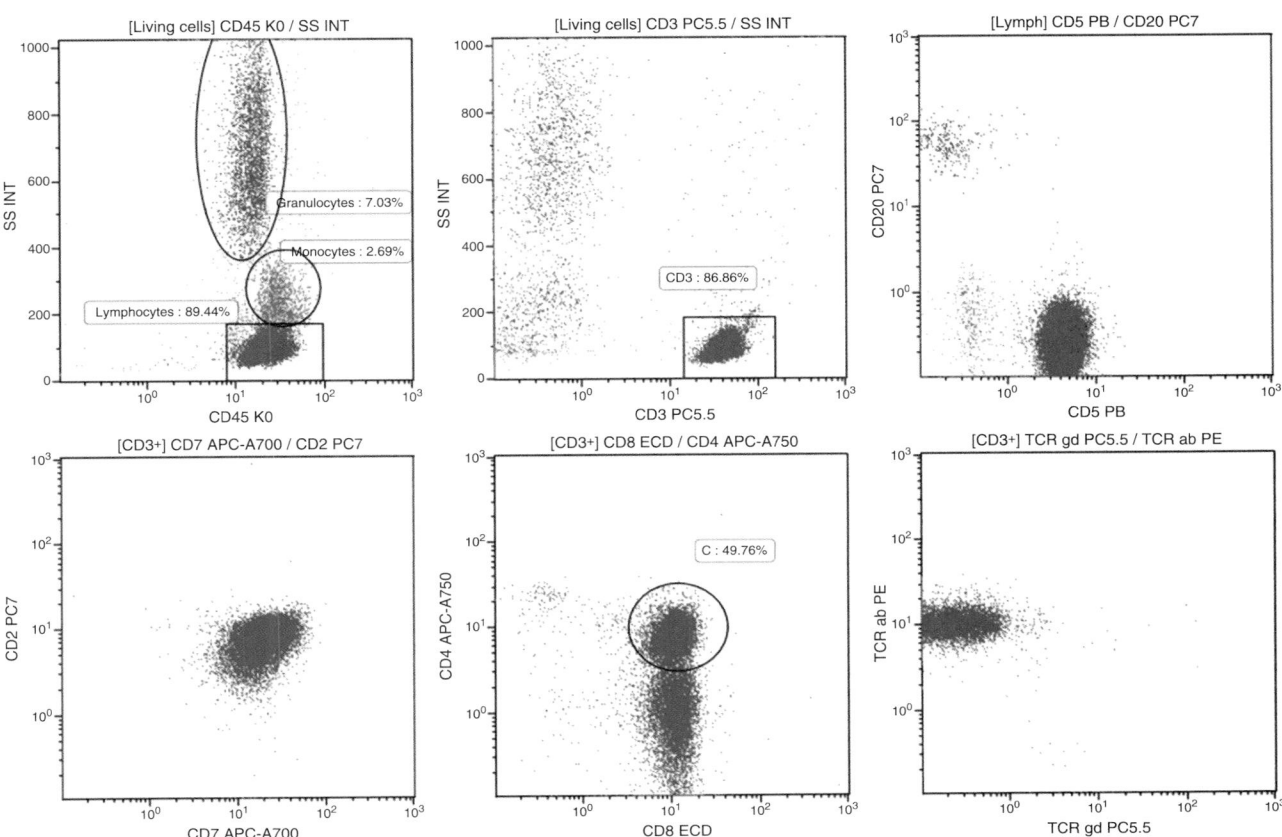

Figure 31-3. Flow cytometry results in T-cell prolymphocytic leukemia (T-PLL). Ten-color flow cytometry was used as described in the literature[91] on a blood sample from a 55-year-old male patient. CD45/SSC plot *(upper-left panel)* shows composition of the sample with 7% granulocytes, 2.7% monocytes, and 89% lymphocytes. The CD3-positive T cells *(violet dots)* account for 89.6% of cells in the blood and are of similar scatter characteristics as B cells (CD20-positive *blue dots*). CD3-positive cells are also positive for CD2, CD7, CD5, CD8, and TCRαβ with an aberrant phenotype of CD8bright+, CD4dim+/− in 49% of cells. CD25, CD56, CD57, CD30, CD1a, and CD10 were negative in the leukemic population *(not shown)*.

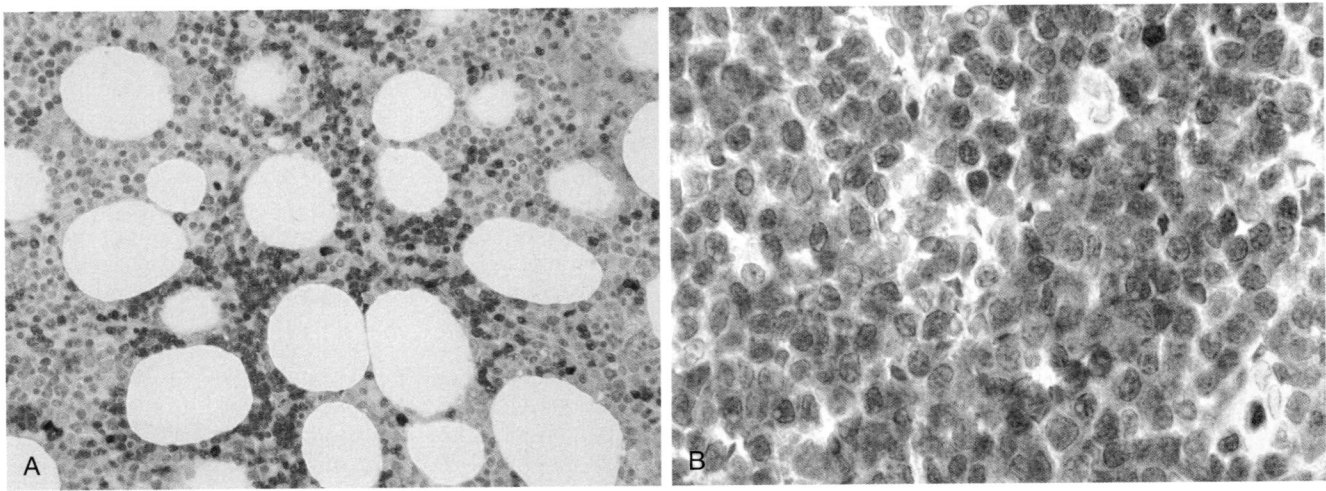

Figure 31-4. Strong nuclear and cytoplasmic staining is seen with anti-TCL1 antibody in bone marrow **(A)** and lymph node **(B)** infiltrated by T-cell prolymphocytic leukemia. *(Courtesy Dr. Elizabeth Hyjek, Department of Pathology, University of Chicago.)*

CD52 is found on T-PLL cells at a higher density than on normal B and T lymphocytes or in B-cell chronic lymphocytic leukemia, which may be the reason for the favorable response to treatment with anti-CD52.[49]

GENETICS AND MOLECULAR FINDINGS

Both TRA and TRB genes are rearranged in most cases.[16,50] However, some cases with only TRG/TRD rearrangement have been described.[36,51,52] Pathologic restriction of the variable (V) region of β-chain use was detected by a broad array of antibodies and flow cytometry.[53]

Cytogenetic studies in T-PLL have found recurrent chromosomal abnormalities. In 90% of cases, the Xq28 (MTCP1) or 14q32.1 (TCL1A and TCL1B) regions were involved in translocations or inversions with TCRA/D at 14q11.[6,54-57] TCL1A and MTCP1 have partial amino acid or nucleotide sequence similarity (41% identical and 61% similar).[58] A third member of this family, TCL1B, located at 14q32.1, also shows similarities to TCL1A in structure and expression.[59] In T-PLL, all three genes are activated and overexpressed by juxtaposition to the αδ locus at 14q11. High-density single-nucleotide polymorphism (SNP)-array analysis detected frequent copy number alterations in TCL oncogenes.[60] TCL1A encodes for a predominantly cytoplasmic protein of 14 kD that is also found in small quantities in the nuclei of lymphoid cells.[61] The TCL1 protein binds to the D_3 phosphoinositide-regulated kinase AKT1, enhancing its activity and promoting its transport to the nucleus.[59] In T-PLL, T-cell receptor (TCR) stimulation leads to the rapid recruitment of TCL1, AKT, and tyrosine kinases to membrane-associated activation complexes.[45]

TCL1 protein expression as shown by immunohisto-chemistry is normally observed in early T-cell progenitors and in the lymphoid cells of B lineage (both progenitors and mature lymphocytes, especially mantle zone cells), but not in mature T lymphocytes.[61,62] In T-PLL, a distinct positivity is found (Fig. 31-4), but other postthymic T-cell lymphomas, including cutaneous T-cell lymphoproliferations, are negative.[17,63]

In most T-PLL cases, changes involving chromosome 14 are accompanied by other complex abnormalities. Unbalanced rearrangements of chromosome 8 have been reported frequently, mainly trisomy 8q; monosomy 8p, such as i(8)(q10); and t(8;8)(p12;q11) or translocations involving 8p and other chromosomal partners.[57,64] Genes commonly affected by breaks on chromosome 8 were PLEKHA2, NBS1, NOV, and MYST3.[60] Although rearrangement of MYC has not been described, overexpression of c-MYC protein has been shown.[65] Thus, additional copies of MYC may represent a secondary abnormality, providing a proliferative advantage.

Abnormalities of chromosome 11, including recurrent losses of the 11q21-q23 regions, have also been detected with fluorescence in situ hybridization (FISH) or loss-of-heterozygosity analysis. Biallelic inactivation (missense mutations) of the ATM gene located at 11q21-q23 was demonstrated in virtually all sporadic cases of T-PLL, suggesting ATM has a tumor-suppressor gene function.[66,67] Truncating mutations in the ATM gene are the main cause of ataxia telangiectasia, a rare familial recessive disorder involving progressive neurologic disease, immunodeficiency syndrome, and chromosomal instability. In patients with ataxia telangiectasia, small clones harboring cytogenetic alterations involving 14q11 (AT clonal proliferations) may be seen several years before the onset of T-PLL.[13] Knockout mice with a complete ataxia telangiectasia–like phenotype consistently produced immature (CD3-negative, CD4-positive, CD8-positive) T-cell thymic lymphomas that arise coincidentally with V(D)J recombination.[68] Development of these malignancies in knockout mice can be prevented by bone marrow transplantation, which replaces the ATM-deficient hematopoiesis.[69]

Other reported abnormalities detected by loss-of-heterozygosity analysis, FISH, or conventional cytogenetics include deletions of 12p13; deletions or translocations involving 5p, 6q, 13q14.3, or 17p; and monosomy 22.[6,57,60,70,71]

Most of the abnormalities were confirmed by comparative genomic hybridization analysis that showed an abnormal profile in virtually all cases, with several recurrent abnormalities present in each T-PLL case.[72,73] The number of chromosomal alterations was not related to morphologic characteristics or the clinical behavior of the disease. Combined SNP-based genomic mapping and global gene-expression profiling showed that several of the upregulated genes in T-PLL are involved in the regulation of transcription, nucleosome assembly, translation, and cell-cycle control (e.g., Nijmegen breakage syndrome 1 [NBS1], TCF7L, CCNB2, CCNB1, CCNG2, PFAS, PAICS, HIST1H2AE, HIST1H2B, HIST1H4G, ELF4EBP1, ELL3). In contrast, various proapoptotic genes, such as FAS, CASP1, CASP4, CASP8, STK17A, and TRAIL, were downmodulated.[74]

Whole-genome sequencing and whole-exome sequencing studies showed largely mutually exclusive mutations of IL2RG, JAK1, JAK3, or STAT5B in 76% of studied T-PLL cases.[75,76] A large meta-analysis of primary data from 275 T-PLL cases from 10 published studies that evaluated genomic lesions involving elements of JAK/STAT signaling identified genomic aberrations potentially leading to constitutive JAK/STAT signaling in approximately 90% of cases.[77]

POSTULATED CELL OF ORIGIN

The cell of origin of T-PLL is unclear, but immunophenotypic and TCR gene rearrangement studies suggest a T cell with a postthymic phenotype. In >95% of T-PLL cases, aberrant constitutive expression of the protooncogenes TCL1A or MTCP1 by inversions or translocations are observed that juxtapose the TCL1A (at 14q32.1) or MTCP1 (at Xq28) loci to the 14q11.2 locus and by that under control of highly active TRA gene enhancer elements. Lack of physiologic downregulation of TCL1A or MTCP1 is considered the initial event of T-PLL's leukemogenesis. The proposed model of clonal evolution of T-PLL cells[78] involves translocations or inversions of chromosome 14q at the double-positive thymocyte stage, resulting in constitutive expression of the protooncogenes TCL1A or MTCP1. These hits impair the genomic stability of the affected T cell by reduced DNA repair capacities of DNA double-stranded breaks or other (oxidative) insults. Deletions and mutations involving ATM lead to a functionally hypomorphic apical regulator of repair, cell fate, and cell-cycle control of the T-PLL precursor. This preleukemic cell becomes unable to execute such safeguarding mechanisms upon genotoxic stress. Subsequently, TCL1A overexpression lowers TCR signaling thresholds, enabling the cell to sustain on low-level input, either by major histocompatibility complex (MHC)-dependent (auto) antigen-presenting cells, by self-MHC drive only, or by autonomous TCR activation. A central distal node is the JAK/STAT transcriptional machinery. Besides major growth pathways such as the TCR and cytokine-mediated cascades feeding into it, there also is a high prevalence of hyperactivating mutations that target *JAK1*, *JAK3*, or *STAT5B* and a high incidence of losses of JAK/STAT negative regulators.

CLINICAL COURSE

The clinical course of T-PLL is usually aggressive, with progressive disease and median survival of 7 to 8 months from diagnosis. There is a poor response to treatment or early relapse after a short remission.[11,15] About one-third of patients in a large French study and several separately described patients had an initially indolent clinical course, lower and stable leukocytosis, no anemia or thrombocytopenia, and no splenomegaly or skin changes.[16,79,80] The morphologic and cytogenetic characteristics of this group were similar to those of patients with aggressive disease. The stable phase had a median duration of 33 months (range, 6 to 103 months), but in seven patients, it was longer than 5 years, and one patient survived for 15 years.[16] At progression, an aggressive clinical course was observed.

TREATMENT

Only rare patients with T-PLL respond to single-agent therapy with alkylating drugs. Approximately 30% of patients achieve short-term remissions with combination chemotherapy, such as CHOP (cyclophosphamide, hydroxydaunomycin, Oncovin [vincristine], prednisone).[15,18,19] Pentostatin treatment produced better results, with 40% overall response and 12% complete remission for a median duration of 6 months.[81] Patients presenting with stable asymptomatic lymphocytosis may be closely monitored until progression. So far, the best treatment response has been achieved in patients treated with humanized anti-CD52 monoclonal antibody (alemtuzumab [Campath-1H]).[11,82-85] Response to alemtuzumab seems to be the most important predictor of outcome.[11] In slow responders, pentostatin may be added to alemtuzumab therapy.[11] Because long-term follow-up showed that all alemtuzumab-treated patients eventually relapsed,[84] all eligible patients who respond to therapy should be considered for consolidation with allo-HSCT.[11,86] Autologous HSCT may also be of benefit but will not result in cure.[87] Induction of apoptosis via reactivation of p53 (e.g., by inhibitors of HDAC or MDM2) and targeting of its downstream pathways (i.e., BCL2 family antagonists, CDK inhibitors) are promising new approaches.[88] Novel strategies also focus on inhibition of the JAK/STAT pathway with the first clinical data.[89] Implementations of immune-checkpoint blockades or CAR-T cell therapy are at the stage of preclinical assessments of activity and feasibility.[90]

DIFFERENTIAL DIAGNOSIS

With modern immunophenotyping by flow cytometry or immunostaining of paraffin tissue sections, the differentiation between B-PLL and T-PLL is rather straightforward owing to the presence of the monoclonal B cell (CD19 and CD20 positivity and light-chain restriction by flow cytometry or PAX5, CD20, and CD79a expression by immunohistochemistry) or T-cell phenotype, respectively. Similarly, T-cell acute lymphocytic leukemia (T-ALL) can be easily distinguished from T-PLL by the expression of TdT or CD1a in T-ALL. The differential diagnosis between T-PLL and other mature T-cell leukemia/lymphomas (e.g., adult T-cell leukemia/lymphoma, mycosis fungoides–Sézary syndrome, large granular lymphocytic leukemia, and hepatosplenic T-cell lymphoma) may be more of a challenge because of highly overlapping morphology and partly overlapping immunophenotypes (especially if a limited panel of markers is applied). The possibility of leukemic presentation of peripheral T-cell lymphoma should also be considered, as cases with blood cytology and immunophenotype findings characteristic of T-PLL but lymph node morphology consistent with large cell T-cell lymphoma have been described.[33] The main differentiating features helpful in obtaining the correct diagnosis are summarized in Table 31-1.

Table 31-1 Differential Diagnosis of T-Cell Prolymphocytic Leukemia

	T-PLL	ATLL	MF-SS	LGLL	HSTCL	PTCL
Lymphocytosis	Marked (usually >100 × 10⁹/L)	Marked	Mild to moderate	Mild (usually <15 × 10⁹/L)	No*	Rare
Peripheral blood morphology	Prolymphocytic (most common), small lymphocytic, cerebriform	Pleomorphic nuclei, multilobated ("flower cell")	Cerebriform nuclei	Large azurophilic granules (cytoplasmic)	Intermediate size	Intermediate-large size
Pattern in bone marrow	Diffuse (common), interstitial, nodular	Patchy, sparse (rarely diffuse)	Uncommon in bone marrow; small focal or interstitial, eosinophilia	Interstitial (small clusters), intrasinusoidal	Intrasinusoidal, interstitial	Interstitial or nodular
Hepatosplenomegaly	Common	Variable	Rare*	Common	Common	Variable
Lymphadenopathy	Variable	Common	Common	Rare	Rare	Common
Skin	Variable (dermal infiltrates)	Common	Common	—	—	Rare
Effusions	>30%, usually pleural	Rare	Rare	Rare	Rare	Rare

Table 31-1 Differential Diagnosis of T-Cell Prolymphocytic Leukemia—cont'd

	T-PLL	ATLL	MF-SS	LGLL	HSTCL	PTCL
Immunophenotype	CD4+/CD8− (common); CD4+/CD8+, CD4−/CD8+	CD4+/CD8−	CD4+/CD8−	CD4−/CD8+ (common); CD4+/CD8−, CD4+/CD8+	CD4−/CD8−	CD4+/CD8− (common); CD4−/CD8−, CD4−/CD8+
	TCRαβ	TCRαβ	TCRαβ	TCRαβ	TCRγδ (common); TCRαβ (rare)	TCRαβ (common)
	CD5+, CD7+	CD5+, usually CD7−	CD5+, usually CD7−	CD7 variable	CD5−, CD7 variable	CD5 and CD7 variable
	CD26+	CD26−, CD25+	CD26−	CD26−	CD26−	CD26− (common)
	NK marker negative, cytotoxic markers negative, TCL1+	Cytotoxic markers negative	Cytotoxic markers negative	CD57+, cytotoxic markers positive, CD56+/−	CD16+, CD56+, TIA-1+, perforin negative	Cytotoxic markers usually negative
Clinical course	Aggressive	Usually aggressive	Chronic	Indolent	Aggressive	Aggressive
Viral etiology	—	HTLV-1	—	—	—	—
Genetics	Rearrangements at 14q32.1 *(TCL1, TCL1β),* Xq28 *(MTCP1),* trisomy 8 or iso8q, 11q23 *(ATM)*	Clonal integration of HTLV-1	Complex karyotypes, no unique abnormalities	No unique abnormalities	iso7q, trisomy 8	Complex karyotypes, no unique abnormalities

*May occur late in disease course.

ATLL, Adult T-cell leukemia/lymphoma; *HSTCL,* hepatosplenic T-cell lymphoma; *HTLV-1,* human T-lymphotropic virus type 1; *LGLL,* large granular lymphocytic leukemia; *MF-SS,* mycosis fungoides–Sézary syndrome; *NK,* natural killer; *PTCL,* peripheral T-cell lymphoma; *TCR,* T-cell receptor; *TIA-1,* T-cell-restricted intracellular antigen; *T-PLL,* T-cell prolymphocytic leukemia.

Pearls and Pitfalls

- Peripheral blood lymphocytosis greater than 100 × 10⁹/L is common, and cases with extreme hyperlymphocytosis occur.
- Different cytomorphologic characteristics of neoplastic cells are described, but in each case, the cells usually show a fairly high degree of cytologic monomorphism.
- Specific genetic abnormalities and immunologic phenotypes do not correlate with morphologic variants.
- Overexpression of TCL1 protein (or its functional homologues) and certain clinical features (e.g., markedly elevated lymphocyte count) provide a higher degree of diagnostic specificity than cytologic characteristics of neoplastic cells, histomorphologic patterns of bone marrow involvement, or immunophenotype. However, TCL1 expression is not mandatory for diagnosis.
- Even in cases with CD8-positive expression, the neoplastic cells do not express cytotoxic granule molecules.
- The characteristic pattern of splenic infiltration involves both red pulp and white pulp, with effacement of normal splenic architecture.

KEY REFERENCES

7. Staber PB, Herling M, Bellido M, et al. Consensus criteria for diagnosis, staging, and treatment response assessment of T-cell prolymphocytic leukemia. *Blood.* 2019;134(14):1132–1143.

15. Matutes E, Brito-Babapulle V, Swansbury J, et al. Clinical and laboratory features of 78 cases of T-prolymphocytic leukemia. *Blood.* 1991;78:3269–3274.
67. Stoppa-Lyonnet D, Soulier J, Lauge A, et al. Inactivation of the ATM gene in T-cell prolymphocytic leukemias. *Blood.* 1998;91:3920–3926.
77. Wahnschaffe L, Braun T, Timonen S, et al. JAK/STAT-Activating genomic alterations are a hallmark of T-PLL. *Cancers (Basel).* 2019;11(12):1833.
78. Braun T, Dechow A, Friedrich G, Seifert M, Stachelscheid J, Herling M. Advanced pathogenetic concepts in T-cell prolymphocytic leukemia and their translational impact. *Front Oncol.* 2021;11:775363.
90. Braun T, von Jan J, Wahnschaffe L, Herling M. Advances and perspectives in the treatment of T-PLL. *Curr Hematol Malig Rep.* 2020;15(2):113–124.

Visit Elsevier eBooks+ for the complete set of references.

Adult T-Cell Leukemia/Lymphoma

Tadashi Yoshino and Elaine S. Jaffe

DEFINITION

Adult T-cell leukemia/lymphoma (ATLL) is a mature T-cell neoplasm pathogenetically linked to human T-lymphotropic virus 1 (HTLV-1; also called *human T-cell leukemia virus*). This is the first retrovirus proved to cause a human neoplasm.[1-3] The disease is derived from mature CD4-positive T cells, and most patients have widely disseminated disease that can be leukemic or lymphomatous in distribution.[4] A characteristic feature is the marked nuclear pleomorphism associated with the neoplastic cells, which have been termed *flower cells*.[5,6] Because of its unique clinical and pathologic features, adult T-cell leukemia was recognized as a disease entity before HTLV-1 was identified as a causal factor.[7]

Synonyms and Related Terms

The term of this entity has been maintained from the International Consensus Classification (ICC) and the 5th edition of the World Health Organization (WHO) Classification of Haematolymphoid Tumours.

EPIDEMIOLOGY

ATLL is endemic in several regions of the world, in particular southwestern Japan, the Caribbean basin, parts of central Africa, and Iran.[8-11] The distribution of the disease is closely linked to the prevalence of HTLV-1 in the population: serologic surveillance has suggested an origin in Africa spread to Austro-Melanesia and the Asian continent, and later North America and South America[12] (Box 32-1; Fig. 32-1). The disease has a long latency, and affected individuals are usually exposed to the virus very early in life. Cord blood lymphocytes are more susceptible to transformation than more fully differentiated and mature lymphocytes.[13] The three major routes of infection are mother-to-infant transmission, mainly in breast milk; sexual transmission; and transmission through blood and blood products. The virus is not transmitted in fresh frozen plasma, and transmission requires the presence of living HTLV-1–infected cells.[14] In Japan, where the disease was first described, seroprevalence in the adult population ranges from 0.2% in some areas to 13% in areas of high endemicity.[10] The cumulative risk for carriers during the adult life span is 2.5%, with an ongoing increased risk until 70 years of age. Most cases present in adulthood (median age, 55 years), with a male-to-female ratio of 1.5:1.

In the Western Hemisphere, most patients come from the Caribbean basin, and the disease is more prevalent among Blacks than Whites.[8] Other areas of prevalence include Central and South America, in particular Brazil and Ecuador. Differences in geographic or ethnic origin correlate with different patterns of disease, with most cases in the Western world presenting as lymphoma rather than leukemia.[15] It is not entirely clear how genetic factors influence the development of ATLL in infected carriers. At least two studies suggest that human leukocyte antigen (HLA) haplotypes correlate with progression to ATLL in infected individuals.[12,16]

The virus has been linked to other disease entities besides ATLL. Young infected children may be immunodeficient and present with superficial cutaneous infections, a pattern termed *infective dermatitis*.[17] HTLV-1–associated myelopathy (HAM), also known as *tropical spastic paralysis* (TSP), is a systemic disease associated with neurologic symptoms and demyelinization.[18] It is thought to be an immune-mediated inflammatory disease with some parallels to multiple sclerosis.[19] Patients with HAM/TSP often acquire the virus later in life through transfusion and rarely develop ATLL. In addition to neurologic symptoms of weakness and muscle

Box 32-1 *Major Diagnostic Features of Adult T-Cell Leukemia/Lymphoma*

Epidemiology
- ATLL is strongly associated with geographic prevalence of HTLV-1.
- ATLL risk is closely linked to HTLV-1 infection in the perinatal period or infancy.

Clinical Features
- Acute and lymphomatous types of ATLL are highly aggressive.
- Chronic and smoldering types of ATLL have a more protracted clinical course.

Morphology
- Appearance of neoplastic cells demonstrates a wide spectrum, including polylobated cells with hyperchromatic nuclei and transformed or blastic cells with round-to-oval nuclei.

Immunophenotype
- CD3[+], CD4[+], CD25[+], CD7[−], $\alpha\beta$ T cells, FOXP3[+/−]
- EBV[+] B cells may be present in the background and may mimic Hodgkin cells in incipient ATLL.

Molecular and Genetic Features
- Clonal T-cell receptor gene rearrangement
- Clonal integration of HTLV-1
- *Tax* gene plays a major role in viral oncogenesis.

ATLL, Adult T-cell leukemia/lymphoma; *EBV,* Epstein-Barr virus; *HTLV-1,* human T-lymphotropic virus 1.

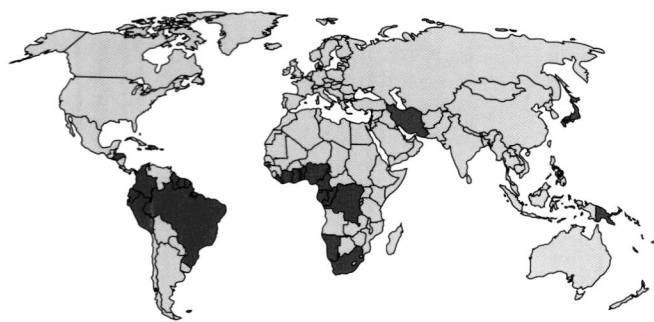

Figure 32-1. Map of the world showing the geographic distribution of HTLV-1 prevalence. Areas in *red* have greater than 2% prevalence in the population.

spasms, patients with HAM/TSP may manifest uveitis, arthritis, polymyositis, keratoconjunctivitis sicca resembling Sjögren syndrome, and pulmonary inflammation.

CLINICAL FEATURES

Several clinical variants are recognized: acute, lymphomatous, chronic, and smoldering (Table 32-1).[6] Because nearly all patients have advanced disease (stage IV) at presentation, Ann Arbor staging is not prognostically useful. The most common acute variant is characterized by a leukemic phase, often with a markedly elevated white blood cell count, rash, and generalized lymphadenopathy. Hypercalcemia, with or without lytic bone lesions, is common (Fig. 32-2). Patients with acute ATLL have systemic disease with hepatosplenomegaly, constitutional symptoms, elevated lactate dehydrogenase,

and marked elevation of soluble interleukin (IL)-2 receptors, which is an independent prognostic factor.[20] Infiltration of any organ system may be evident, including the central nervous system.[21] Leukocytosis and eosinophilia are common. The bone marrow may be hypercellular, with myeloid hyperplasia. Despite stage IV disease and peripheral blood involvement, bone marrow involvement may be absent. Many patients have an associated T-cell immunodeficiency and frequent opportunistic infections, most notably by *Pneumocystis jiroveci* and *Strongyloides stercoralis* (Fig. 32-3).[22] An increased risk for viral infection is also present, including cytomegalovirus and herpes zoster infections.

The lymphomatous variant is characterized by prominent lymphadenopathy without peripheral blood involvement. Most patients have advanced disease, similar to the acute form. However, hypercalcemia is present less often. The lymphomatous variant is seen more often in the Western Hemisphere. Patients presenting with lymphadenopathy may have peripheral blood involvement later in the course of the disease.[23] The lymphomatous and acute forms have comparable survival, usually less than 1 year.

The chronic variant is associated with skin lesions, most commonly an exfoliative rash (Fig. 32-4). Although there may be an absolute lymphocytosis, atypical lymphocytes are not numerous in the blood. Flower cells, if present, are associated with a more aggressive clinical course.[24,25] Hypercalcemia is absent. Patients may have hepatosplenomegaly, but the course is generally indolent, with a median survival of approximately 2 years.

In the smoldering variant, the white blood cell count is normal, with less than 5% circulating neoplastic cells. Patients frequently have skin or pulmonary lesions, but hypercalcemia is not present. Lymphadenopathy should be absent. Patients may progress from chronic or smoldering disease to an acute crisis.

The skin is the most common site of involvement outside of the peripheral blood, with more than 50% of patients having evidence of cutaneous disease.[26-28] The skin lesions are clinically diverse and range from an exfoliative rash to papules and nodules, with the larger nodules showing ulceration (Fig. 32-5).[29] More extensive cutaneous disease, with papules and nodules, appears to correlate with a more aggressive course. The number of circulating neoplastic cells does not correlate with the degree of bone marrow involvement, suggesting that circulating cells are recruited from other organs, such as the skin. Other sites of clinically relevant disease include the gastrointestinal tract, lungs, liver, and central nervous system, all of which may lead to clinical symptoms and morbidity.[21,30] Cardiac involvement may be seen as well, usually as a terminal event.[31]

MORPHOLOGY

The cytologic spectrum of ATLL is extremely diverse. Nevertheless, certain cytologic features are highly characteristic and may suggest the diagnosis, even if studies for HTLV-1 are not performed.[32] These features are best appreciated in the peripheral blood (Fig. 32-6). Most patients are leukemic at some point in the clinical course, although peripheral blood involvement may not be evident at presentation.

The neoplastic cells in the peripheral blood are markedly polylobated and have been termed *flower cells* based on the

Table 32-1 Comparison of Clinical Forms of Adult T-Cell Leukemia/Lymphoma as Defined by the Japanese Lymphoma Study Group[6]

Feature	Smoldering	Chronic	Acute	Lymphomatous
Lymphocytosis	No	Mildly increased, >4 × 10⁹/L	Increased	No
T-cell receptor PCR	Sometimes monoclonal	Monoclonal	Monoclonal	Monoclonal
Elevated LDH	No	Minimal	Yes	Yes
Hypercalcemia	No	No	Yes	Variable
Skin lesions	Erythematous rash	Rash, papules	Variable, >50%	Variable, >50%
Lymphadenopathy	No	Mild	Usually present	Yes
Hepatosplenomegaly	No	Mild	Usually present	Often present
Bone marrow infiltration	No	No	May be present	No
Median survival (yrs)	>2	2	<1	<1
Morphology	Small lymphocytes Minimal atypia	Mild atypia Flower cells sometimes seen	Marked atypia Polylobated and blastic forms	Marked atypia Polylobated and blastic forms

LDH, Lactate dehydrogenase; *PCR,* polymerase chain reaction.

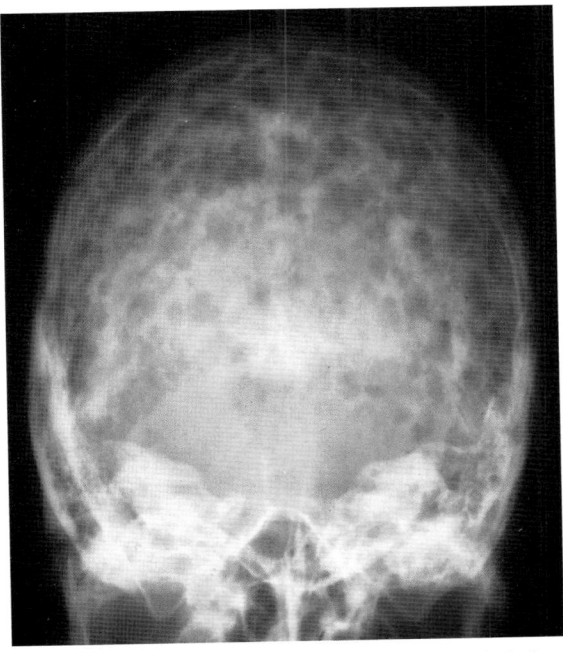

Figure 32-2. Skull radiograph shows multiple osteolytic bone lesions in a patient with acute adult T-cell leukemia/lymphoma.

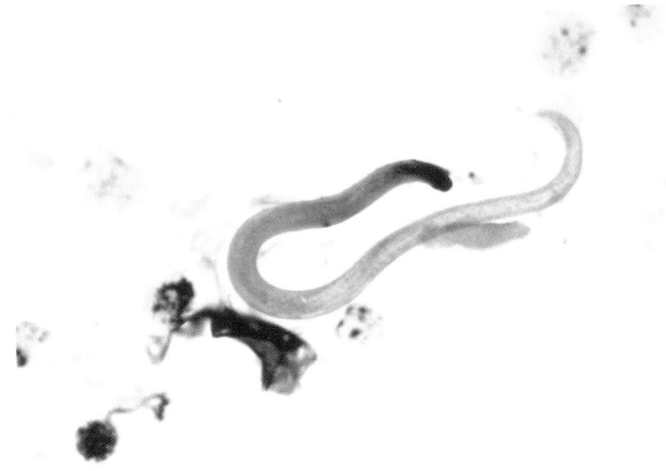

Figure 32-3. Bronchoalveolar lavage specimen shows a larval form in a patient with adult T-cell leukemia/lymphoma and disseminated strongyloidiasis.

petal-like appearance of the nuclear lobes.[5,6,23] The chromatin is condensed and usually hyperchromatic, although the flower cells usually do not manifest prominent nucleoli. The cytoplasm is basophilic, and cytoplasmic vacuoles may be seen. The basophilic cytoplasm and hyperchromasia are useful features in distinguishing ATLL from Sézary syndrome. In addition, the nuclear irregularities in Sézary cells are much subtler, imparting the typical cerebriform appearance without separation into nuclear lobes.

These cytologic features are most evident in the acute type of ATLL. In the chronic and smoldering forms of the disease, atypical cells are relatively sparse in the peripheral blood, and cytologic atypia is less evident.[33,34]

Lymph node involvement is present in most patients. Lymph nodes typically show diffuse architectural effacement. In keeping with a leukemic pattern of involvement, in some instances the sinuses may be preserved or may contain neoplastic cells similar to those in the blood (Fig. 32-7). Preservation of the sinuses is more common in patients with leukemic disease. The cytologic composition of the neoplastic

infiltrate is very diverse. Small pleomorphic lymphoid cells equivalent to the flower cells of the peripheral blood may predominate or may be admixed with larger transformed cells (Fig. 32-8). The transformed cells have vesicular nuclei and usually multiple eosinophilic or basophilic nucleoli. These cells may be relatively uniform in size, with round-to-oval nuclear contours, resembling diffuse large B-cell lymphoma (Fig. 32-9). Alternatively, the transformed cells may have more pleomorphic nuclear features. Giant cells with convoluted or cerebriform nuclear contours may be present. Although it is important for the pathologist to be aware of the diverse cytology that can be encountered in ATLL, the size or shape of the neoplastic cells generally does not affect the clinical course.[23] Some patients with incipient ATLL, such as the smoldering type, may exhibit a Hodgkin lymphoma–like histology in the lymph nodes that is associated with less aggressive disease (Fig. 32-10).[35-38]

Involved lymph nodes show expanded paracortical areas with diffuse infiltrates of small to medium-sized lymphocytes with mild nuclear irregularities, indistinct nucleoli, and scant cytoplasm. There are interspersed Reed-Sternberg–like cells and giant cells with lobulated or convoluted nuclei. These cells are Epstein-Barr virus (EBV)-positive B lymphocytes that express CD30 and CD15. This variant of incipient disease usually progresses to overt disease within months. In its early

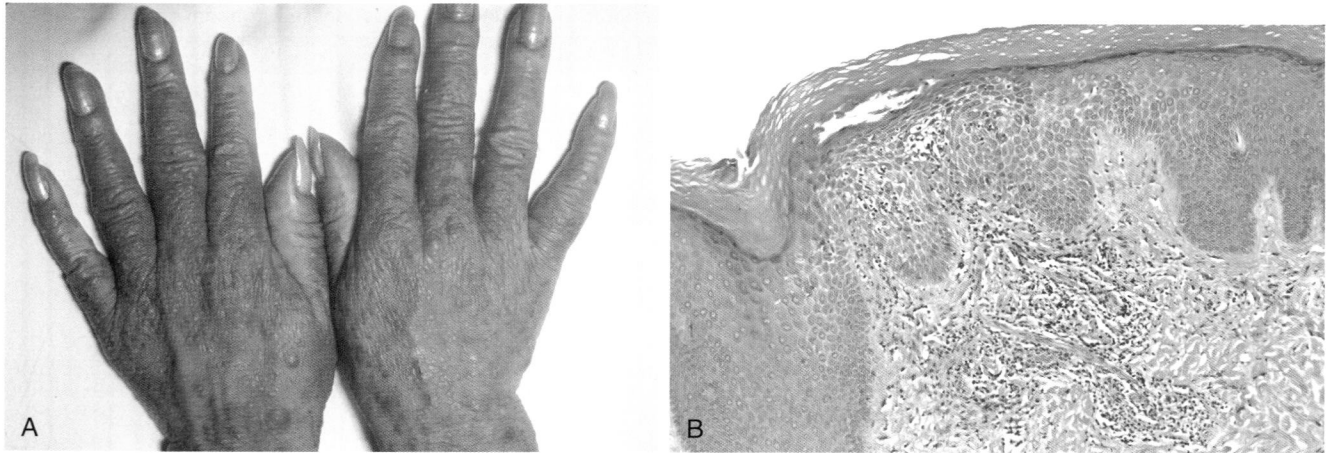

Figure 32-4. Chronic adult T-cell leukemia/lymphoma. A, Skin shows evidence of scaling and hyperkeratosis. **B,** Skin biopsy from the same patient shows a dermal lymphocytic infiltrate composed of small lymphoid cells without significant atypia.

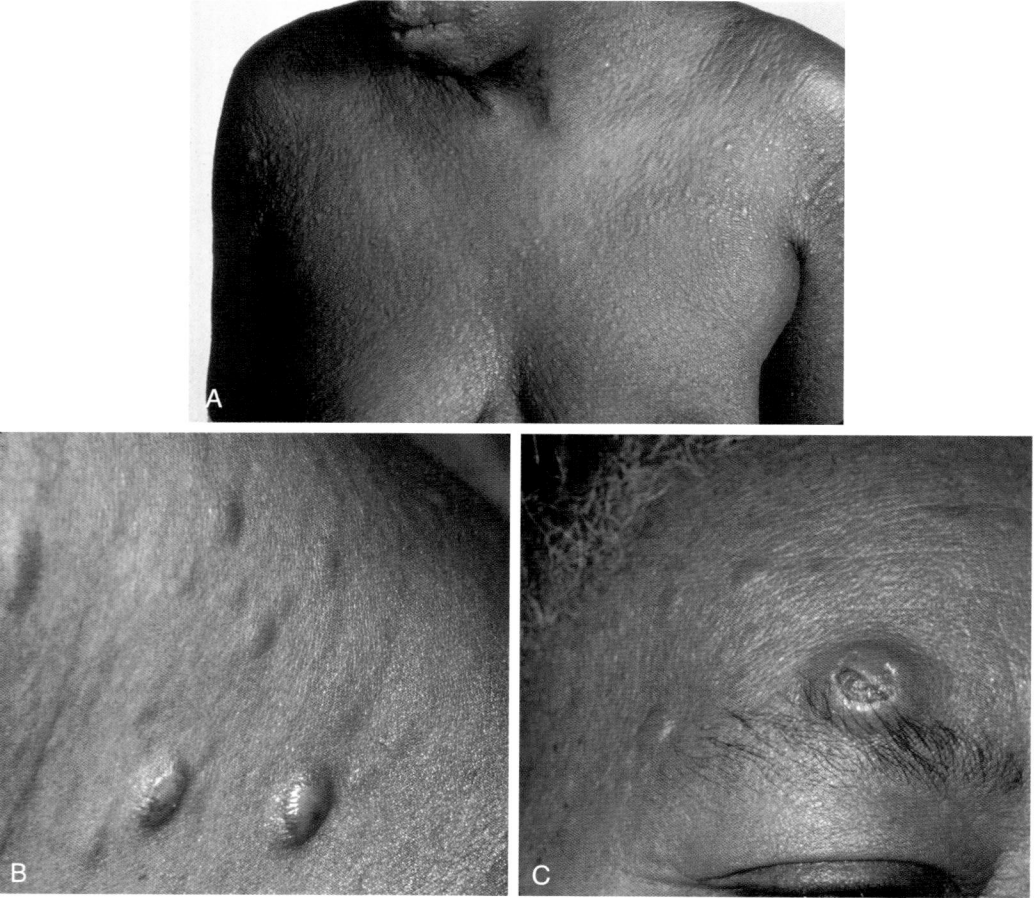

Figure 32-5. Diverse cutaneous manifestations of adult T-cell leukemia/lymphoma range from exfoliative rash **(A)** to papules **(B)** to larger nodules with ulceration **(C).**

stages, neoplastic HTLV-1–positive cells may be few in these lesions, and in fact, the T-cell proliferation may not be clonal. Thus in some respects, this incipient form of ATLL may be preneoplastic. Alternatively, the number of HTLV-1–infected T cells may be beneath the threshold for detection by polymerase chain reaction (PCR) methods for identifying T-cell receptor

gene rearrangement. The expansion of EBV-positive B cells is thought to be secondary to the underlying immunodeficiency in patients with ATLL. Similar Reed-Sternberg–like cells have been described in other forms of peripheral T-cell lymphoma, most commonly angioimmunoblastic T-cell lymphoma.[39] This must be distinguished from HTLV-1–infected cells with

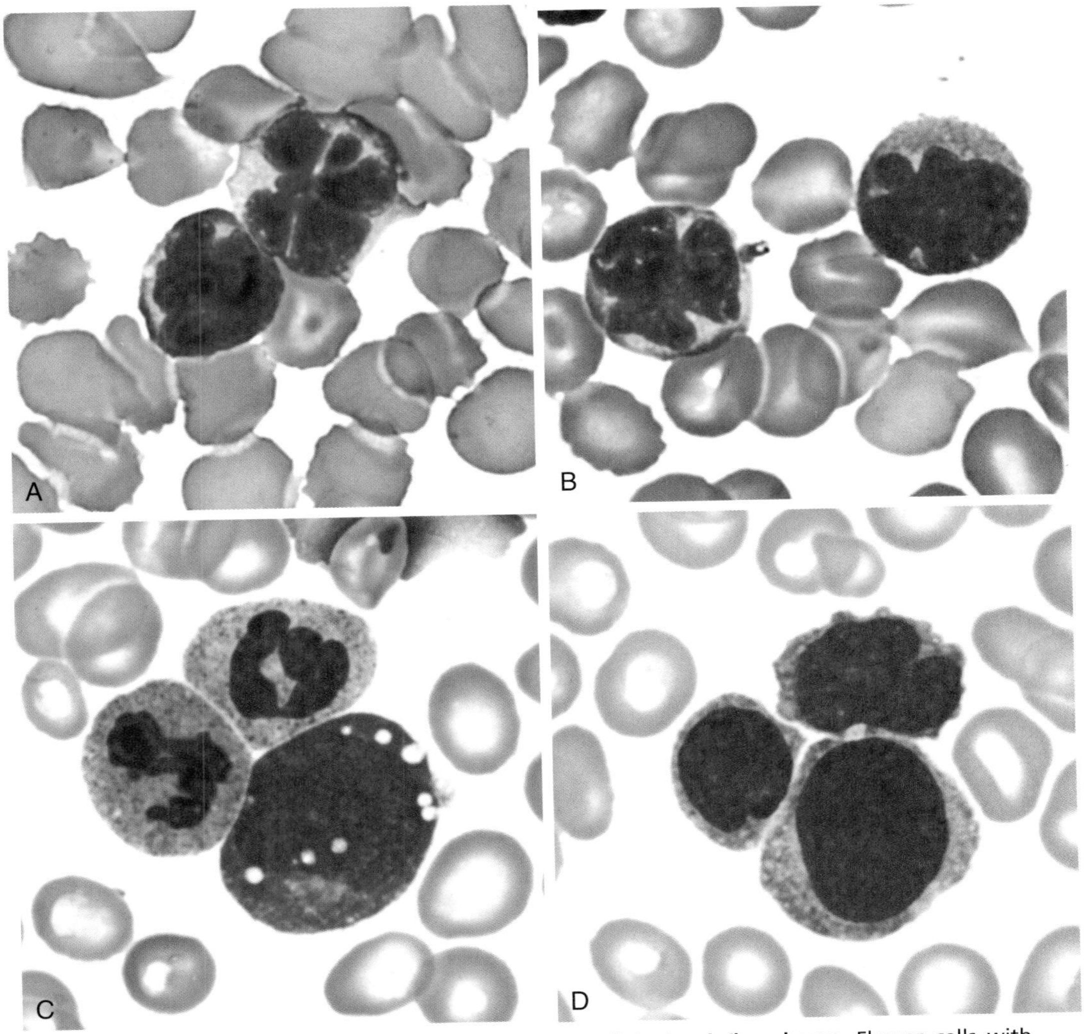

Figure 32-6. **Peripheral blood findings in adult T-cell leukemia/lymphoma.** Flower cells with markedly polylobated nuclei (**A** and **B**) are most common, but one can also see blast-like cells **(C)** and cells with rounder nuclear contours **(D)**.

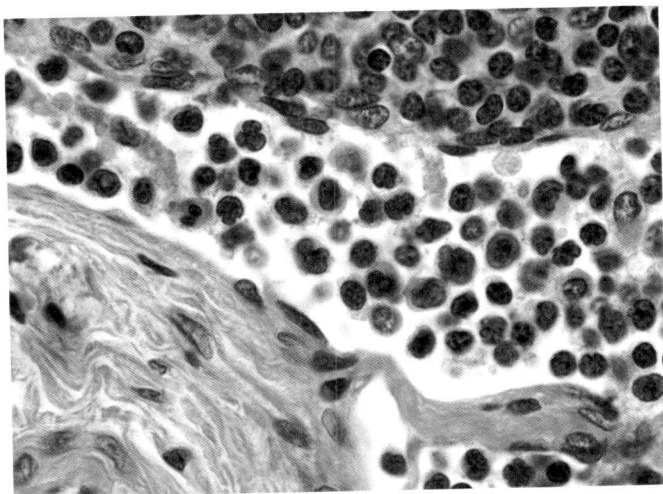

Figure 32-7. Lymph node in a patient with adult T-cell leukemia/ lymphoma. In the leukemic phase, dilated sinuses may contain atypical cells.

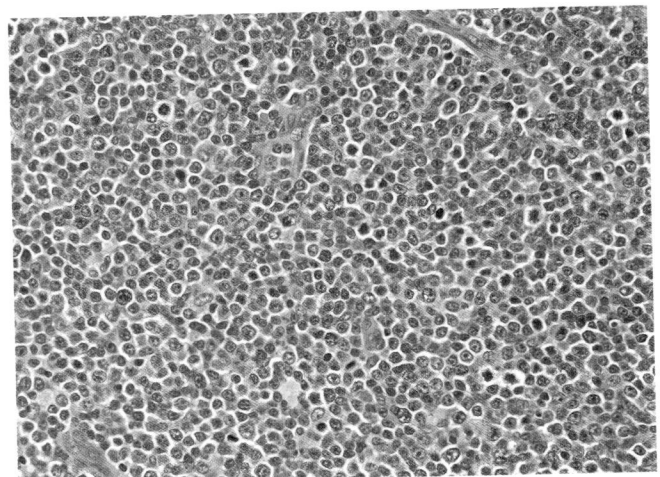

Figure 32-8. Lymph node in a patient with adult T-cell leukemia/ lymphoma. Small pleomorphic lymphoid cells may be admixed with larger blast-like cells with vesicular nuclei and prominent nucleoli.

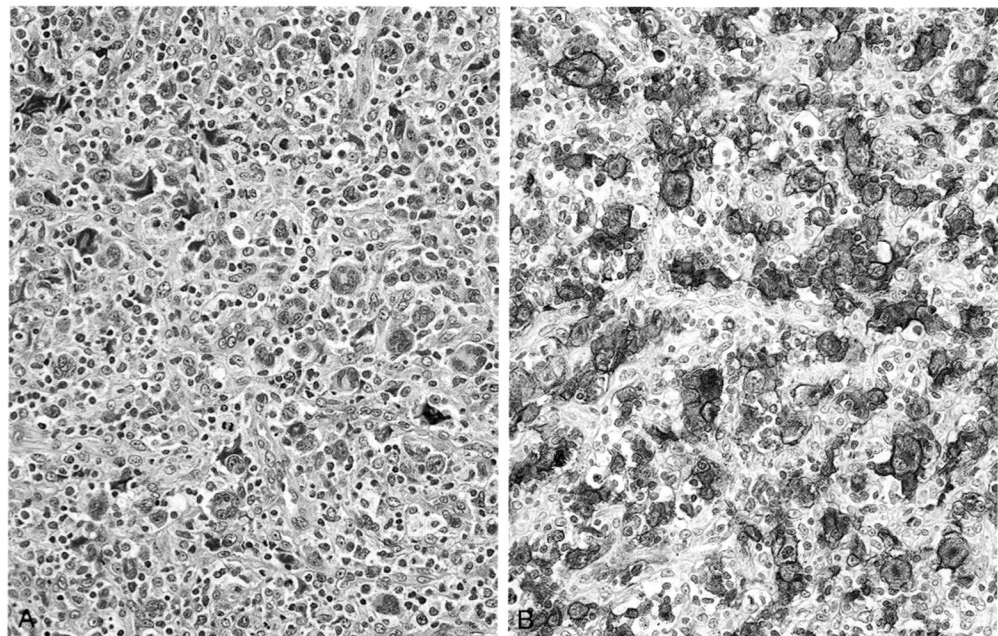

Figure 32-9. Lymph nodes in patients with adult T-cell leukemia/lymphoma. A, In this case, cells with blastic features predominate. The process may mimic a diffuse large B-cell lymphoma if immunohistochemical studies are not performed. **B,** Giant cells with pleomorphic nuclei and CD30 positivity may be present as well (**B:** immunoperoxidase with hematoxylin counterstain).

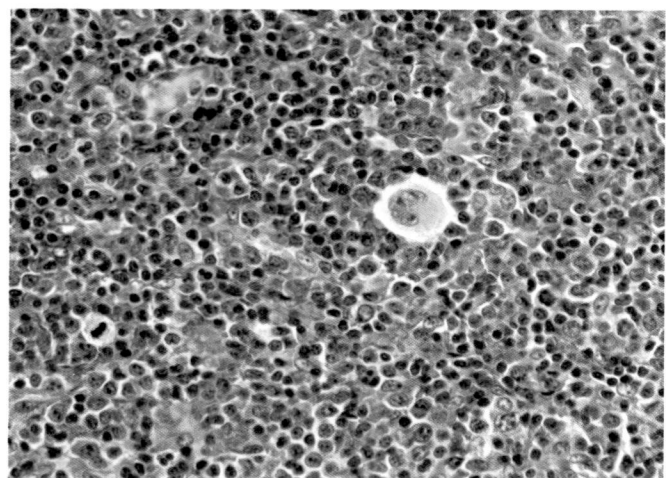

Figure 32-10. Lymph node in a patient with incipient adult T-cell leukemia/lymphoma. Cells resembling Hodgkin and Reed-Sternberg cells may be present, mimicking classic Hodgkin lymphoma. The Hodgkin-like cells are Epstein-Barr virus–positive transformed B cells, and the background contains HTLV-1 T cells.

Hodgkin and Reed-Sternberg morphology that are positive for CD30, CD15, MUM1, CD25, and HTLV-1 and negative for B-cell makers, including PAX5 and EBV.[40]

Skin involvement is seen in more than 50% of patients with the disease. The dermis usually contains a superficial atypical lymphoid infiltrate, often with epidermotropism (Fig. 32-11).[26] Pautrier-like abscesses are common.[23] However, in contrast to Sézary syndrome or mycosis fungoides, the neoplastic infiltrate is usually monomorphic and relatively confluent, without numerous histiocytes or eosinophils. The smaller neoplastic cells usually predominate in the skin. In the smoldering and chronic types, cytologic atypia

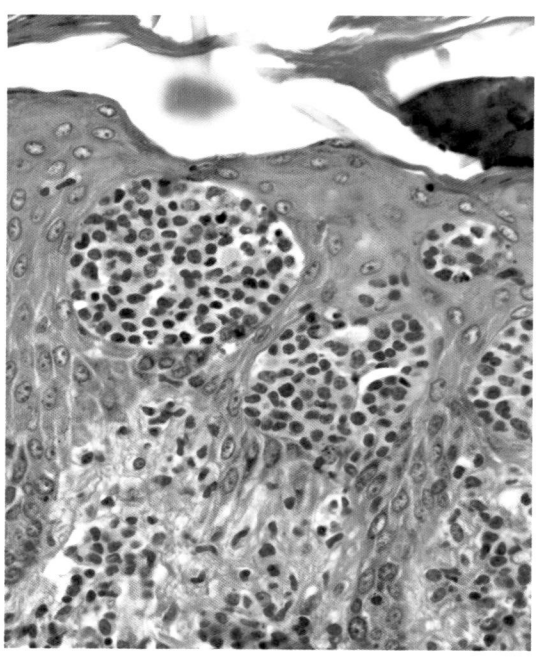

Figure 32-11. Skin biopsy specimen in adult T-cell leukemia/lymphoma. There is marked epidermotropism, with infiltration of the overlying epidermis.

may be minimal. Hyperparakeratosis is variably present in the overlying epidermis. The skin lesions are clinically and histologically diverse and may mimic inflammatory disorders.[41]

Bone marrow involvement is typically not prominent. The marrow may contain patchy atypical lymphoid infiltrates. However, the degree of bone marrow infiltration is less than

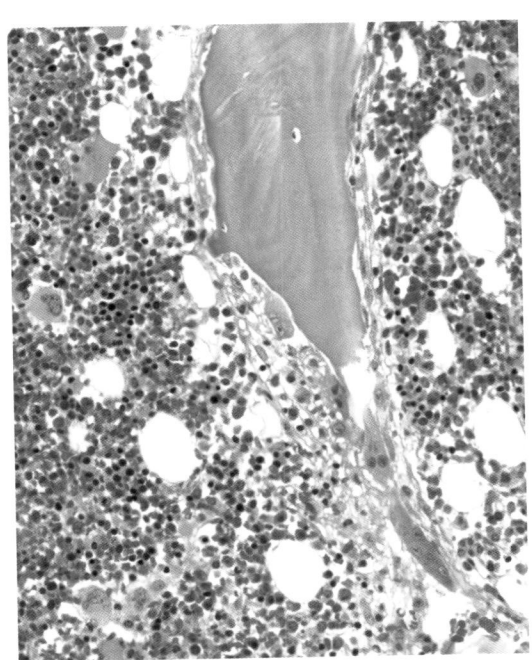

Figure 32-12. Bone marrow core biopsy in adult T-cell leukemia/lymphoma. The bone marrow space shows myeloid hyperplasia without identifiable tumor cells. However, the bone trabeculae show evidence of remodeling and increased osteoclasts.

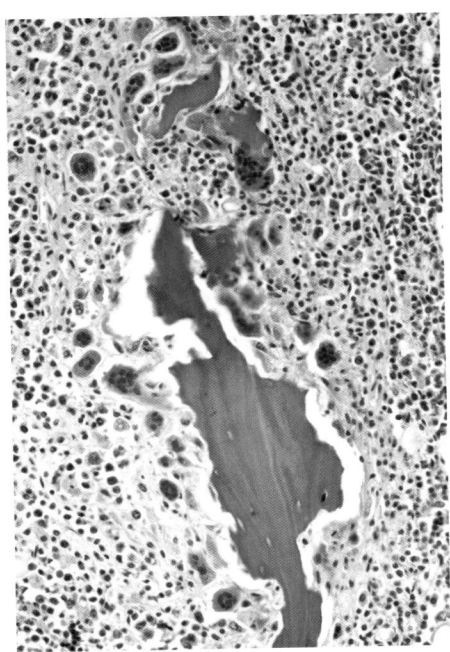

Figure 32-13. Lytic bone lesion in adult T-cell leukemia/lymphoma. Numerous osteoclasts surround bone trabeculae.

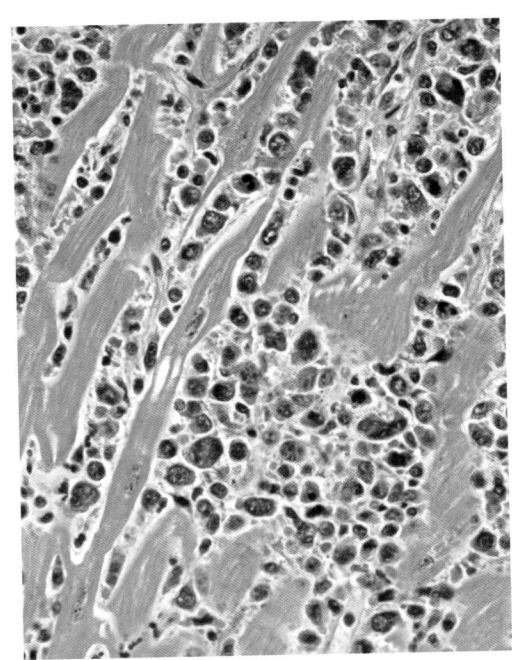

Figure 32-14. Cardiac involvement by adult T-cell leukemia/lymphoma.

expected, given the marked lymphocytosis that may be present. Bone resorption and osteoclastic activity is often seen in patients with hypercalcemia (Fig. 32-12).[42] Bone trabeculae may show evidence of remodeling, and in some patients, lytic bone lesions are present, even in the absence of tumoral bone infiltration (Fig. 32-13).[21]

Other frequent sites of involvement include the lung and cerebrospinal fluid. Correlating with a leukemic phase, the pulmonary infiltrates are generally patchy and interstitial, with no formation of tumor nodules. Cardiac involvement has been reported rarely and is always associated with concomitant pulmonary involvement (Fig. 32-14).[31]

Involvement of the central nervous system usually manifests as meningeal infiltration without nodular parenchymal lesions. Neoplastic cells may be detected in cytologic preparations of cerebrospinal fluid. However, rare cases with parenchymal tumor masses have been reported.[43] Central nervous system involvement is nearly always associated with widespread systemic disease, but rare cases with isolated central nervous system involvement have been reported.[25]

Although there is no formal cytologic grading system for ATLL, the neoplastic cells in the chronic and smoldering variants of the disease usually show minimal cytologic atypia, perhaps in keeping with the more indolent clinical course.

IMMUNOPHENOTYPE

The neoplastic cells, regardless of cytologic subtype, are CD4-positive αβ T cells that strongly express the α chain of the IL-2 receptor (IL-2R) or CD25 (Fig. 32-15).[44] High levels of soluble IL-2R can also be found in the serum and correlate with disease activity.[45] CD7 is nearly always absent, but CD3 and other mature T-cell antigens (CD2, CD5) are usually expressed. CD52 is usually positive, a finding of

clinical relevance for the use of anti-CD52 humanized antibody (alemtuzumab [Campath]) for treatment purposes. CD30 can be expressed in the larger blastic cells, and it is also a target of antibody therapy (brentuximab vedotin). CC chemokine receptor 4 (CCR4) is usually expressed and is closely associated with skin involvement and poor outcome.[46] Anti-CCR4 antibody (mogamulizumab) has been effective therapeutically.[47] Because many peripheral T-cell lymphomas have a CD3-positive, CD4-positive, CD7-negative immunophenotype, the most specific feature of ATLL is strong

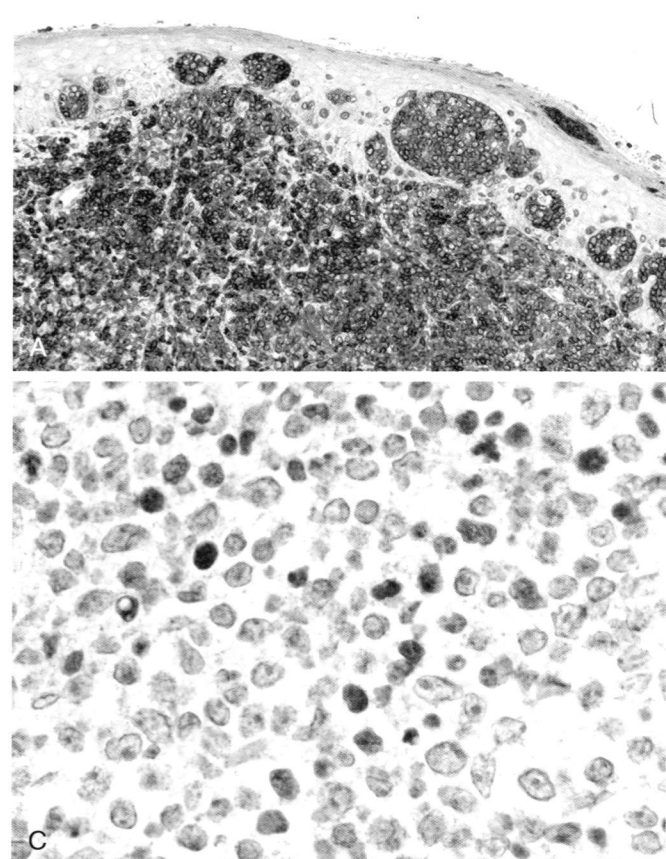

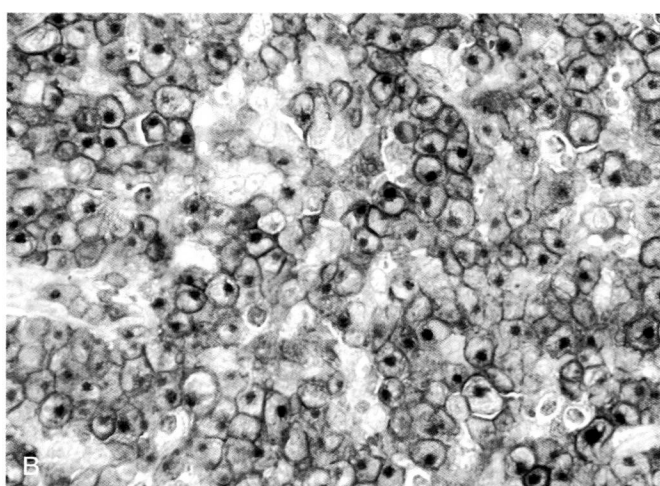

Figure 32-15. Immunohistochemistry of adult T-cell leukemia/lymphoma. A, Skin biopsy shows positive staining for CD3 in epidermal and dermal lymphoid cells. **B,** Tumor cells show strong membrane and Golgi staining for CD25. **C,** A subpopulation of tumor cells is positive for FOXP3, with the larger atypical cells being negative. (**A** to **C,** immunoperoxidase with hematoxylin counterstain.)

CD25 positivity. With enhanced antigen-retrieval techniques, CD25 expression can be detected in formalin-fixed, paraffin-embedded tissue sections.[48] Because of its strong expression, CD25 has become a target of immunotherapy for ATLL.[44] Studies suggest that ATLL cells may be the equivalent of regulatory T (Treg) cells.[49,50] In one study, 68% of the cases tested were positive for the Treg transcription factor FOXP3 in at least some of the neoplastic cells, although usually only a small minority. No other T-cell lymphoma subtype expresses FOXP3 in conjunction with CD25 and CD4. This finding helps explain the immunodeficiency associated with ATLL. FOXP3-positive cases appear to be a lower grade, manifesting fewer cytogenetic abnormalities.[51] TSLC1/CADM1 has been proved to be a marker of neoplastic cells in ATLL that plays a role in tumor growth and organ infiltration of ATLL cells.[52-54]

GENETICS, MOLECULAR FINDINGS, AND ROLE OF HTLV-1

ATLL has clonal rearrangement of the T-cell receptor genes. In patients with acute or lymphomatous ATLL, there is evidence of a single dominant clone in all sites involved by the disease. HTLV-1 carriers do not show a dominant T-cell clone but may have oligoclonal T-cell expansion. The high-density expression of IL-2R renders these cells responsive to growth in response to cytokines both in vitro and in vivo.[55] Similarly, in the early phases of smoldering or chronic ATLL, more than one T-cell clone may be present, with emergence of a dominant clone at the time of progression.[56]

The HTLV-1 proviral DNA is clonally integrated into neoplastic T cells.[35] Patients with incipient ATLL or those with early-stage disease may contain T-cell clones with defective or partial viral integration.[57] Southern blotting techniques are useful to follow the clone, as the unique site of integration produces a distinctive band.[58] PCR techniques for HTLV-1 sequences can be used to quantify the viral load in the peripheral blood.[59,60] Patients with HAM/TSP do not have circulating T cells with clonal integration of the HTLV-1 virus. However, in keeping with the aberrant immune response to HTLV-1 involved in HAM/TSP, clonal and oligoclonal T-cell populations directed against the virus may be identified.[61]

HTLV-1 is the first human retrovirus shown to cause malignant transformation.[1] It contains the structural genes *gag, pol,* and *env* and a pX region at the 3′ end that encodes the regulatory proteins Tax and Rex, among others. The viral gene *Tax* plays a pivotal role in HTLV-1–initiated leukemogenesis. The Tax protein is a transcriptional activator of the viral long-terminal repeat. Tax can act by transactivation to deregulate a variety of cellular genes, leading to activation of signal transduction,[62] deregulation of the cell cycle,[3] and induction of genetic instability, resulting in multiple cytogenetic abnormalities.[63,64] Tax itself is oncogenic and can transform human T cells and rodent fibroblasts.[62]

Tax acts via several signal transduction pathways, including nuclear factor-κB (NF-κB), the CREB/ATF family (leucine zipper protein), serum response factor, and AP-1 families.[65] Tax can bind directly to several members of the NF-κB family of proteins.[66] Tax also binds to proteins that inhibit NF-κB, providing an alternative mechanism for NF-κB activation.

In addition, Tax can inactivate p53. Although many cases of ATLL show p53 mutation or deletion,[67] p53 is inactivated directly by Tax.[68] This promotes destabilization of the genome and the development of other genetic abnormalities. Tax also inhibits the cell-cycle regulator CDKN2A, promoting continuous cellular proliferation of HTLV-1–infected cells.[66]

Tax plays a role in the effects mediated by IL-2 and IL-15. The α chain of IL-2R was the first gene shown to be upregulated by Tax.[69] Tax upregulates the expression of both IL-2 and IL-15, a relative of IL-2, providing a mechanism for an autocrine loop in HTLV-1–infected cells.[70] IL-15 uses the β and γ chains of IL-2R for signaling. Tax also upregulates IL-15Rα in ATLL cells.[70] Other cellular genes may be activated by Tax, such as IL-6; this activity may be responsible for the hypercalcemia characteristic of ATLL by promoting the secretion of parathormone-like substances, leading to osteoclastic activation.[71,72] The hypercalcemia of ATLL can be replicated in Tax-transgenic mice.[73] Activation of NF-κB also appears to play a role in the production of osteoclast-activating factors.[72] Finally, ATLL cells express RANK ligand, which promotes the differentiation of hematopoietic precursors into osteoclasts.[14,74]

Although *Tax* seems to play a crucial role in ATLL leukemogenesis and is present in tumor cells in culture, the gene is not always expressed in primary ATLL cells. Instead, HTLV-1 bZIP factor (HBZ) is consistently detected in primary ATLL cells, and has been shown to affect multiple pathways involved in tumorigenesis.[75] HZB enhances TGF-β signaling, supports proliferation of ATLL cells through suppression of C/EBPα signaling,[76] suppresses apoptosis by attenuating the function of FoxO3a,[77] and dysregulates the Wnt pathways to support proliferation and migration of ATLL cells.[78] The relationship between Tax and HZB is interesting; HBZ is involved in suppression of Tax-mediated viral gene transcription, and HBZ specifically suppresses NF-κB–driven transcription.[79] Findings in HBZ/Tax double transgenic mice further support a role for HBZ in lymphomagenesis.[80]

Accumulation of aberrant DNA hypermethylation at the differentially methylated positions (DMPs) strongly correlates with ATLL development and progression. Region-specific aberrant DNA hypermethylation is mechanistically important for ATL leukemogenesis and an effective therapeutic target.[81,82] Another relevant epigenetic event in ATLL leukemogenesis is Polycomb-mediated aberrant gene expression. Aberrant overexpression of Ezh2, EED and Suz12, which are components of Polycomb repressive complex-2 (PRC2), induce methylation of histone H3 on lysine (K) 27, generating (H3-K27me3), followed by chromatin compaction and various target gene silencing in ATLL.[83-85] Overexpression of Ezh2 mediates down regulation of miR-31 expression, which induces activation of the NIK-dependent NF-κB pathway, contributing to leukemic transformation.[85,86]

ATLL cells show numerous complex structural cytogenetic abnormalities affecting every chromosome pair. There are no recurrent cytogenetic changes, however, that are useful in making the diagnosis.[87,88] Structural abnormalities occur most frequently in chromosome 6, and abnormalities in 6q appear to correlate with a more aggressive clinical course.[87] Translocations are identified in about 10% of cases involving the T-cell receptor-αδ gene locus on 14q11.[89] Comparative genomic hybridization studies have confirmed the diversity and frequency of genetic changes.[90] Different genetic changes were observed in the acute and lymphomatous subtypes, suggesting these two variants may proceed along different molecular pathways. The complexity of the cytogenetic abnormalities is likely mediated by Tax.[62,91,92] Tax impairs DNA repair mechanisms and represses the expression of DNA polymerase-β, an enzyme involved in base excision repair. Tax also represses nucleotide excision repair, which plays a critical role in repairing ultraviolet irradiation–induced damage.

Gene-expression profiling studies have identified overexpression of *BIRC5* (survivin).[93] The antiapoptotic function of *BIRC5* may also play a role in the resistance of ATLL cells to chemotherapy. Somatic alterations characterizing aggressive diseases predict worse prognosis in indolent ATLL, among which *PD-L1* amplifications are a strong genetic predictor for aggressive ATLL.[94] Structural variations (SVs) disrupting the 3′ region of the *PD-L1* gene stabilize and increase the expression of aberrant *PD-L1* transcripts in ATLL (27%).[95]

Thus, although HTLV-1 infection does not lead directly to malignant transformation of T cells, it promotes the development of neoplastic transformation by a variety of mechanisms, including stimulation of T-cell growth, inhibition of T-cell death via apoptosis, deregulation of DNA repair mechanisms and promotion of chromosomal instability, and activation of signal-transduction pathways. The *Tax* gene plays a role in most of these actions. A large-scale genetic study delineated the entire portrait of genetic and epigenetic aberrations in ATLL and identified a large number of novel mutational targets.[67] However, the detailed mechanisms triggering the onset and progression of ATLL remains to be elucidated.[96]

POSTULATED NORMAL COUNTERPART

ATLL cells are αβ T cells that most closely resemble Treg cells. Treg cells play a major role in regulating the immune response, mainly by suppressing it. They require the transcription factor FOXP3 for functional development in the thymus gland[97] and have a CD3-positive, CD4-positive, CD25-positive phenotype. Although FOXP3 is not universally expressed in all cases of ATLL, it is expressed in some instances.[49,50]

CLINICAL COURSE

Acute and lymphomatous forms of ATLL have an aggressive clinical course, with a median survival of less than 1 year and a projected 4-year survival of only 5%.[98] Without treatment, most patients die within weeks to months; even with treatment, most remissions are short-lived.[6,21,99] Major prognostic indicators for acute ATLL include performance status, high lactate dehydrogenase, age (older than 40 years), more than three sites of disease, and hypercalcemia.[100] Other factors that appear to affect prognosis include thrombocytopenia, eosinophilia, and bone marrow involvement. Some molecular alterations are associated with a more aggressive clinical course, including *CDKN2A* gene deletion[101] and *TP53* mutation.[102]

The clinical course is more protracted in patients with chronic or smoldering disease, but median survival is still less than 5 years for these patients. Prognostic factors of predictive value for chronic ATLL include high lactate dehydrogenase, low albumin, and high blood urea nitrogen levels.[100] Deletion of the *CDKN2A* gene in the chronic phase is also a negative prognostic factor, and gene deletion by comparative genomic hybridization correlates with a poor prognosis.[101,103] Genetic alterations also occur during progression from chronic-phase to acute-phase disease.[104]

Conventional chemotherapy regimens (doxorubicin based) have been largely ineffective, prompting the investigation of other agents, such as deoxycoformycin (pentostatin), with limited success.[105] More intensive high-dose chemotherapy and bone marrow transplantation have been used in a limited number of patients. Treatment-related mortality is very high, limiting the utility of this approach.[106] Because ATLL is caused by a retrovirus, there was speculation that drugs active against other retroviruses, such as human immunodeficiency virus (HIV), might show activity. Initial trials using zidovudine (AZT) and α-interferon suggested some efficacy,[107,108] but the initial good outcomes were not reproduced in subsequent studies.[109] However, this regimen may have a role in patients with smoldering or chronic disease.[100] In another study, a combination of arsenic and α-interferon was used, with the suggestion that it might lead to the downregulation of *Tax*.[110] The efficacy of this approach has not been demonstrated in clinical trials. Promising results have been obtained in monoclonal antibody–based therapies directed against IL-2R, which is highly expressed in ATLL; the efficacy of humanized anti-CD25(Tac), either unconjugated or labeled with yttrium-90,[43,111] was highest in patients with chronic or smoldering disease. Other molecular targeted therapies, such as that against CCR4 and allogenic transplantation, are promising.[112,113] Anti-CCR4 antibody (mogamulizumab) and lenalidomide, have been approved for ATLL patients in Japan. The risk of severe, acute, and corticosteroid-refractory graft-versus-host disease was higher in patients who received mogamulizumab before allogeneic hematopoietic cell transplantation (allo-HCT). However, administration of mogamulizumab before allo-HCT tended to improve the survival of patients. Allo-HCT procedures for patients with aggressive ATLL have considerably progressed and have helped improve the prognosis of these patients.[114,115] Because ATLL has such a poor prognosis, clinical efforts to control the disease have been largely directed at preventing infection in susceptible populations.

DIFFERENTIAL DIAGNOSIS

The differential diagnosis of acute and lymphomatous ATLL differs somewhat from that of chronic or smoldering ATLL (Table 32-2). The clinical picture of acute ATLL with hypercalcemia and systemic disease usually prompts consideration of the diagnosis. The diagnosis of ATLL may be less obvious in patients presenting with lymphoma and without hypercalcemia. ATLL cells have an immunophenotype that is relatively specific, so the combination of a T-cell malignancy expressing CD3, CD4, and CD25 is highly suggestive. CD25 is expressed in other B-cell and T-cell malignancies, including hairy cell leukemia,[116] classic Hodgkin lymphoma,[117] and anaplastic lymphoma kinase–positive anaplastic large cell lymphoma[47]; however, demonstration of a B-cell phenotype can readily exclude the diagnosis. Although anaplastic large cell lymphoma is usually positive for CD25, CD3 is often negative in the neoplastic cells. CD30 is strongly expressed

Table 32-2 Differential Diagnosis of Adult T-Cell Leukemia/ Lymphoma

Diagnosis	Clonal TCR	HTLV-1 Integration	CD25	Flower Cells
ATLL	+	+	++	+
Mycosis fungoides	+	–	–	–
T-PLL	+	–	–	–
ALCL	+	–	++	–
PTCL, NOS	+	–	–/+	–

ALCL, Anaplastic large-cell lymphoma; *ATLL,* adult T-cell leukemia/lymphoma; *HTLV-1,* human T-lymphotropic virus 1; *PTCL, NOS,* peripheral T-cell lymphoma, not otherwise specified; *TCR,* T-cell receptor; *T-PLL,* T-cell prolymphocytic leukemia.

in anaplastic large-cell lymphoma, whereas usually only a minority of ATLL cells are CD30 positive. Serologic studies for antibodies to HTLV-1 or PCR studies for HTLV-1 viral sequences can be confirmatory.

To assist in epidemiologic studies of ATLL, a scoring system was proposed.[32] Clinical features counting as 1 point each are hypercalcemia, skin lesions, and a leukemic phase. Laboratory criteria, counting as 2 points each, include a T-cell phenotype, seropositivity for HTLV-1 or HTLV-2, expression of CD25 by tumor cells, and evidence of HTLV-1 or HTLV-2 sequences at the molecular level. A score of 5 or greater is a strong indication for a diagnosis of ATLL. One should bear in mind that patients from endemic areas may be seropositive for HTLV-1 but develop other lymphomas, independent of viral positivity. Thus, demonstration of viral integration in the tumor cells is the strongest indication for a diagnosis of ATLL.

The differential diagnosis of chronic or smoldering ATLL is more diverse and includes mycosis fungoides and other cutaneous T-cell lymphomas, chronic dermatitis, and T-cell prolymphocytic leukemia. ATLL may show marked epidermotropism with Pautrier's microabscesses, mimicking mycosis fungoides. In distinction from mycosis fungoides, ATLL usually lacks an inflammatory background in the cutaneous lesions, with a higher density of neoplastic cells. Indeed, the first patient from which HTLV-1 was isolated was thought to have an aggressive form of mycosis fungoides.[1] In the peripheral blood, Sézary cells have less nuclear hyperchromasia and a cerebriform rather than a polylobated nuclear contour (Fig. 32-16). Further complicating the differential diagnosis was the suggestion in some studies that HTLV-1 sequences might be detected in the blood cells of some cases of otherwise typical cutaneous T-cell lymphomas.[118] Subsequent studies have largely ruled out a role of HTLV-1 in the pathogenesis of mycosis fungoides or Sézary syndrome.[119]

T-cell prolymphocytic leukemia can be CD4 positive or CD8 positive, but CD25 is usually negative. CD7 is usually positive, in contrast to ATLL cells. The cells are typically round or slightly irregular and lack the pronounced nuclear irregularities of ATLL cells. In T-cell prolymphocytic leukemia, the bone marrow biopsy usually shows extensive infiltration, whereas ATLL usually shows less bone marrow involvement than expected, based on the degree of lymphocytosis. The bone marrow does not appear to be a site of proliferation for ATLL cells.

HTLV-2 is a retrovirus related to HTLV-1. It has not been clearly linked to any form of leukemia or lymphoma.[120] The molecular tests for HTLV-1 sequences also detect HTLV-2, so it may be necessary to rule out HTLV-2 infection in some cases.

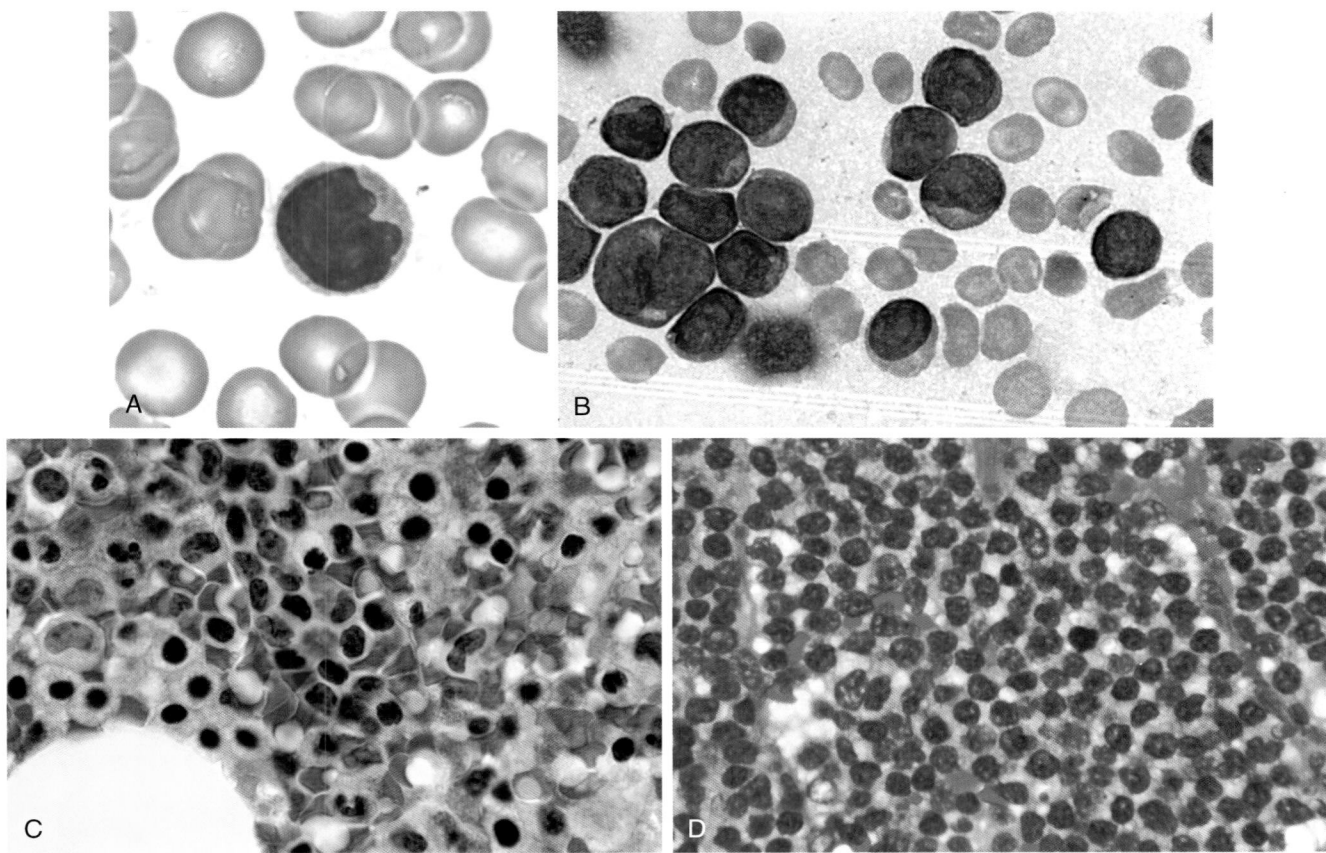

Figure 32-16. Differential diagnosis of adult T-cell leukemia/lymphoma (ATLL). A, Sézary cells show less nuclear hyperchromasia and more subtle nuclear changes. **B,** In T-cell prolymphocytic leukemia, lymphoid cells have round-to-oval nuclear contours and prominent nucleoli. **C,** The bone marrow is diffusely infiltrated, in contrast to ATLL, which typically shows minimal infiltration. **D,** T-cell prolymphocytic leukemia cells in the lymph node are round to slightly irregular, with central small nucleoli.

HTLV-2 has been found most often in intravenous drug users. Its clinical effects have been linked to a HAM/TSP clinical picture.

Pearls and Pitfalls

- HTLV-1 seropositivity does not prove a diagnosis of ATLL. Patients from HTLV-1–endemic areas may have antibodies to HTLV-1.
- ATLL is associated with a broad cytologic spectrum. Most cytologic variants do not have clinical significance.
- The Hodgkin-like form of ATLL may mimic classic Hodgkin lymphoma. It represents an incipient form of ATLL in which HTLV-1–infected cells are sparse. Hodgkin-like cells are EBV-positive B cells.
- Smoldering and chronic forms of ATLL may resemble chronic dermatitis.

KEY REFERENCES

2. Gallo RC, Kalyanaraman VS, Sarngadharan MG, et al. Association of the human type C retrovirus with a subset of adult T-cell cancers. *Cancer Res.* 1983;43:3892–3899.

6. Shimoyama M. Diagnostic criteria and classification of clinical subtypes of adult T-cell leukaemia-lymphoma. A report from the Lymphoma Study Group (1984-87). *Br J Haematol.* 1991;79:428–437.

40. Karube K, Takatori M, Sakihama S, et al. Clinicopathological features of adult T-cell leukemia/lymphoma with HTLV-1-infected Hodgkin and Reed-Sternberg-like cells. *Blood Adv.* 2021;5:198–206.

49. Karube K, Ohshima K, Tsuchiya T, et al. Expression of FoxP3, a key molecule in CD4CD25 regulatory T cells, in adult T-cell leukaemia/lymphoma cells. *Br J Haematol.* 2004;126:81–84.

62. Grassmann R, Aboud M, Jeang KT. Molecular mechanisms of cellular transformation by HTLV-1 Tax. *Oncogene.* 2005;24:5976–5985.

67. Kataoka K, Nagata Y, Kitanaka A, et al. Integrated molecular analysis of adult T cell leukemia/lymphoma. *Nat Genet.* 2015;47:1304–1315.

79. Zhao T, Yasunaga J, Satou Y, et al. Human T-cell leukemia virus type 1 bZIP factor selectively suppresses the classical pathway of NF-kappaB. *Blood.* 2009;113:2755–2764.

82. Watanabe T, Yamashita S, Ureshino H, et al. Targeting aberrant DNA hypermethylation as a driver of ATL leukemogenesis by using the new oral demethylating agent OR-2100. *Blood.* 2020;136(7):871–884.

95. Kataoka K, Shiraishi Y, Takeda Y, et al. Aberrant PD-L1 expression through 3′-UTR disruption in multiple cancers. *Nature.* 2016;534(7607):402–406.

114. Utsunomiya A. Progress in allogeneic hematopoietic cell transplantation in adult T-cell leukemia-lymphoma. *Front Microbiol.* 2019;10:2235.

Visit Elsevier eBooks+ for the complete set of references.

Hepatosplenic T-Cell Lymphoma

Philippe Gaulard and Alina Nicolae

DEFINITION

Hepatosplenic T-cell lymphoma (HSTL) is a rare, aggressive, extranodal lymphoma characterized by hepatosplenic involvement, absence of lymphadenopathy, and poor outcome. It arises from a proliferation of nonactivated, cytotoxic T cells that home to the splenic red pulp. Most cases are derived from the $\gamma\delta$ T cells, with a small subset of $\alpha\beta$ phenotype. The neoplastic lymphocytes are usually monomorphic and medium-sized and exhibit a unique sinusoidal infiltration of the spleen, liver, and bone marrow. Almost 40% of cases occur in settings of immune dysregulation. HSTL shows a recurrent cytogenetic abnormality, the isochromosome 7q, has a distinct molecular signature, and harbors frequent mutations in chromatin modifiers and members of the *JAK/STAT* pathway. The disease follows an aggressive clinical course with common resistance to anthracycline-based chemotherapy regimens.

EPIDEMIOLOGY

HSTL is rare, representing 1.4% to 2% of all T-cell and natural killer (NK)-cell lymphomas.[1-3] This incidence is likely higher given the difficulty to achieve a correct diagnosis because of the various conditions clinically mimicking HSTL. Cases have been reported in both Western and Asian countries.[4-8] It occurs more frequently in men (male-to-female ratio of 2:1), with a median age in the fourth decade of life.[1,4-7,9-12] However, both children and elderly individuals may be affected.[5,13-15]

ETIOLOGY

The pathogenesis of HSTL is complex and not fully understood. More than half of cases occur de novo in the absence of any risk factors. However, up to 40% of patients have underlying chronic immune suppression or immune dysregulation.[5,12,16] HSTL may develop in the setting of solid organ transplantation, and it has been regarded as a late onset posttransplant lymphoproliferative disorder of host origin.[5,10,12,16-18] Cases occur also in patients with autoimmune disorders, most often Crohn's disease and less frequently rheumatoid arthritis, systemic lupus erythematosus, psoriasis, or autoimmune hepatitis. Exposure to thiopurine immunomodulators (azathioprine, 6-mercaptopurine) or tumor necrosis factor α (TNFα) antagonists (infliximab) have been considered to be among the risk factors.[8,16,19-23] Simultaneous use of these drugs dictated by the severity of the underlying disease likely accounts for a higher risk of HSTL development.[8,24] Occasional cases have been observed after acute myeloid leukemia, Epstein-Barr virus (EBV)-positive lymphoproliferative disorders, in patients with *Plasmodium falciparum* infection,[5,25] or during pregnancy.[26] In the view of normal function of $\gamma\delta$ T cells, these observations point toward the role of chronic antigen stimulation in settings of immune dysfunction in HSTL pathogenesis. To further support this rational, expansion and activation of $\gamma\delta$ T cells was observed in the peripheral blood of patients infected with *P. falciparum*[27,28] or renal allograft.[29] Furthermore, an alloreactive response of human γδ T cells to various leukocyte antigen molecules has been documented in vitro.[30]

To date, no association with human T-lymphotropic virus 1 or 2, human immunodeficiency virus, human herpesvirus 8, or hepatitis C virus has been reported. One case each has been linked to hepatitis B,[31] human herpesvirus 6,[32] and parvovirus infection.[33] The vast majority of cases are negative for EBV, with exception of rare instances displaying cytologic features of transformation.[5,9,34]

CLINICAL FEATURES

Patients with HSTL are predominately young adults. They commonly present with constitutional symptoms (i.e., weakness, fever, and weight loss) and abdominal discomfort related to marked splenomegaly and/or hepatomegaly, in the absence of lymphadenopathy. All patients have cytopenias, which is probably multifactorial; related to hypersplenism, bone marrow involvement, or cytokine release; or immune mediated.[4,5,11,16,35-37] Thrombocytopenia is almost always present, and it seems to parallel disease activity.[5,24,35] Anemia is observed in ~75% of patients and neutropenia in about half of them. Seldom, manifestations of idiopathic thrombocytopenic purpura[4,38] or Coombs-negative hemolytic anemia[39] were the first symptoms. Although lymphocytosis is uncommon, a minor population of atypical lymphoid cells can be identified by careful examination of blood smears or by flow cytometry in more than half of patients.[5,24,35,36,40] An overt leukemic picture, rare at presentation, can be seen in advanced disease.[5,40] Hemophagocytic syndrome may occur and is associated with a fulminant clinical course.[5,11,13] Other laboratory findings include elevated levels of lactate dehydrogenase (LDH), β2-microglobulin, and abnormal liver function tests[4,5,11,16,37]

Computed tomography (CT) typically shows hepatosplenomegaly without distinct lesions and absence of lymphadenopathy. ^{18}F-fluorodeoxyglucose positron emission tomography (FDG-PET)/CT may reveal diffuse and intense uptake of spleen, liver, and bone marrow, with normal FDG activity of the lymph nodes.[41]

Virtually all patients have Ann Arbor stage IV disease as a result of bone marrow involvement. They frequently have a performance status >1 and present with two or three adverse risk factors of the age-adjusted International Prognostic Index, which places them in the high-risk group.[5,11]

MORPHOLOGY

The diagnosis of HSTL is based on histopathologic and immunophenotypic evaluation of the involved tissue. The atypical cells are preferentially located in the cords and sinusoids of the splenic red pulp, bone marrow, and liver. Lymph nodes are rarely involved at presentation. In the past, the diagnosis was often made on splenectomy. Currently, bone marrow biopsy is the recommended diagnostic procedure.[42] Although examination of the bone marrow aspirate allows for cytologic, flow cytometry phenotyping, and cytogenetic analysis, it alone does not suffice for the diagnosis.[5,10,40] Though liver biopsy is recommended by the National Comprehensive Cancer Network (NCCN) guidelines,[42] it is less useful in clinical practice given the morphologic finding of HSTL that overlap with other lymphomas or conditions.

Spleen

The spleen is often markedly enlarged (common weight 1000-3500 g), with a homogeneous red-purple cut-surface and no gross lesions identifiable macroscopically. Hilar lymph nodes are not increased in size.

The neoplastic infiltrate diffusely involves and expands the splenic red pulp, without architectural destruction, whereas the white pulp is markedly reduced or lost (Fig. 33-1A). The atypical cells are frequently seen within the sinusoids and, to a variable extent, within the cords of the red pulp. Dilated sinusoids filled with sheets of neoplastic lymphoid cells are the typical features (Fig. 33-1B). The cells are medium-sized, with a monotonous appearance, and they show round or slightly irregular nuclei with loosely condensed chromatin and inconspicuous nucleoli. The cytoplasm is moderately abundant and usually agranular (Fig. 33-1C). Seldom, the atypical lymphocytes range from small to large to pleomorphic.[10,11,43] Mitotic figures are rare. A few small lymphocytes may be admixed, and plasma cells are uncommon. Histiocytes may be numerous and sometimes show erythrophagocytosis either at presentation or during the disease course (Fig. 33-1C).

Although usually not enlarged, splenic hilar lymph nodes commonly manifest some degree of lymphomatous involvement confined to the sinuses or perisinusal areas, without destruction of the normal architecture.[5,35,44]

Liver

Histologic involvement of the liver is fairly constant at presentation. It leads to hepatomegaly, frequently without discrete lesions.[4,5,24,37] The neoplastic lymphoid infiltrate commonly shows a sinusoidal pattern (Fig. 33-1D), which can lead to pseudopeliotic lesions or perisinusoidal fibrosis.[36,45] The atypical lymphocytes may be subtle on slides stained with H&E (hematoxylin and eosin) and may be only highlighted by immunohistochemical stains with T-cell antigens. Marked portal and periportal infiltrate with sinusoidal extension have been uncommonly reported.[11,36]

Bone Marrow

Bone marrow involvement is almost constant when trephine biopsies are carefully investigated by combined histologic and immunohistochemical studies.[5,10,11,40,43,46] At presentation, the bone marrow is usually hypercellular with trilineage hyperplasia (Fig. 33-2A). It may show mild dysmyelopoiesis, which can mislead to diagnosis of myelodysplastic syndrome in settings of peripheral cytopenia. Neoplastic cells selectively involve and expand the bone marrow sinusoids, a feature highly characteristic and thus an essential diagnostic criterion for HSTL. The lymphoid infiltrate is often discrete and subtle and may be difficult to recognize based on morphology. The atypical lymphocytes are small to medium-sized and show an "Indian file" or aggregate-like distribution within variably distended bone marrow sinusoids.[5,10,11,35,40,43,46] This pattern is highlighted by CD3 immunostaining (Fig. 33-2B).

In addition, careful examination of the bone marrow aspirate and peripheral blood smear may identify a minor population of atypical lymphoid cells. They are often intermediate-sized with irregular nuclear contours, dispersed chromatin, inconspicuous nucleoli, and a moderate amount

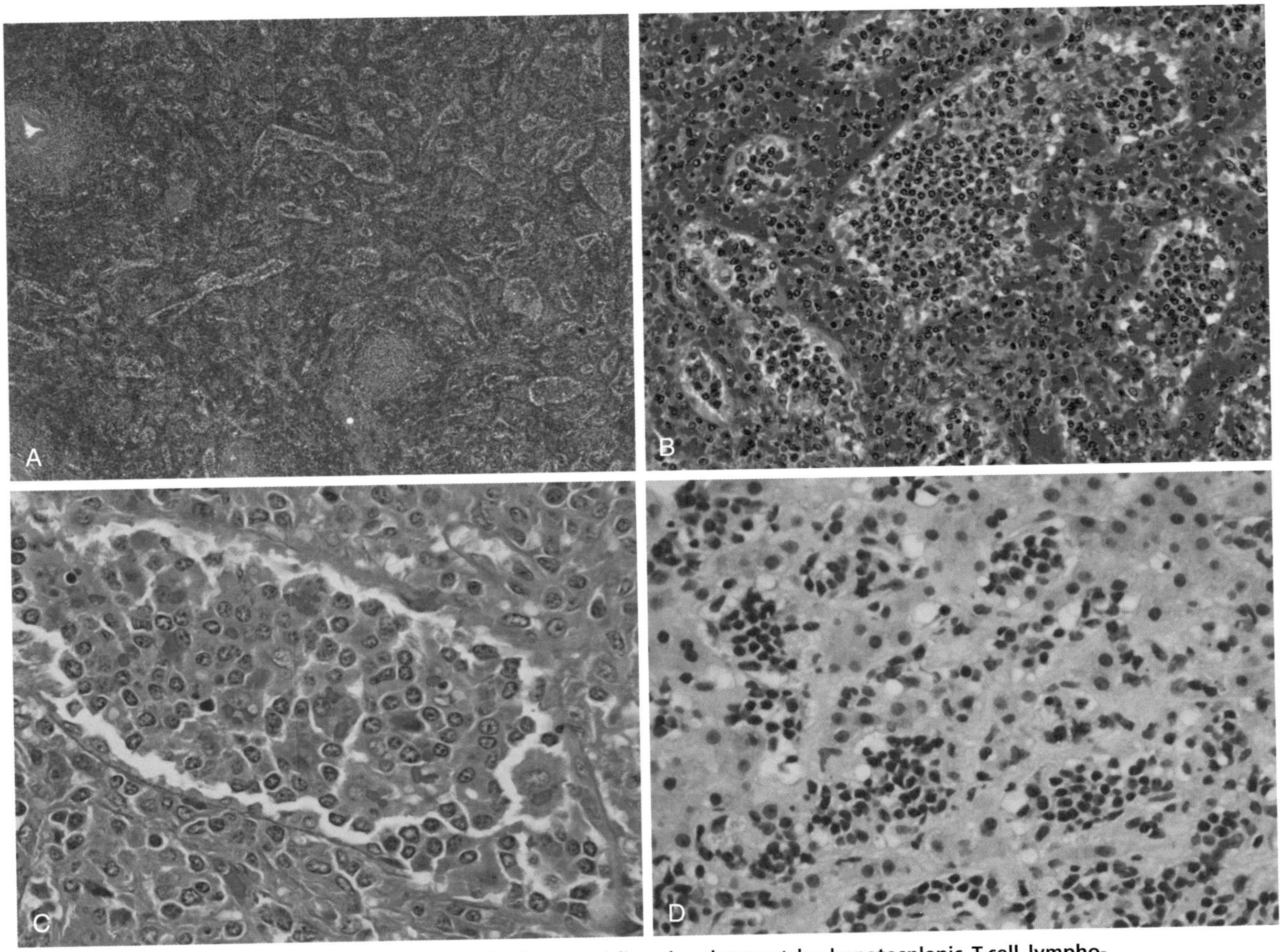

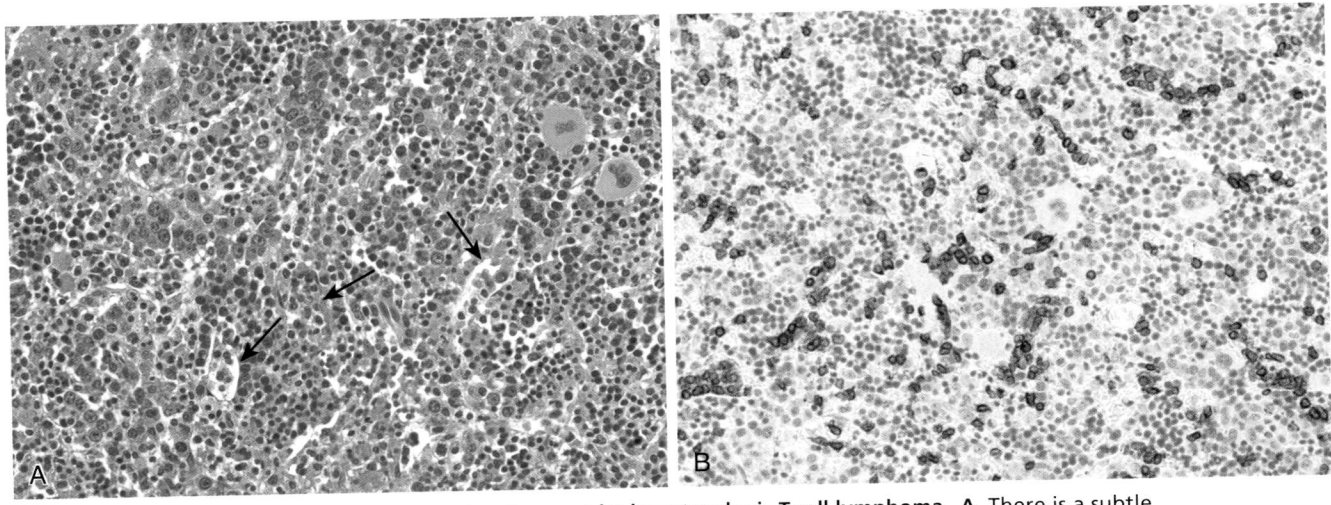

Figure 33-1. Histopathology of spleen and liver involvement by hepatosplenic T-cell lymphoma. A, The spleen shows expansion of the red pulp and atrophic nodules of the white pulp. **B,** The splenic sinusoids are filled and dilated by atypical medium-sized lymphocytes. **C,** They display round nuclei with finely dispersed chromatin and a moderate amount of pale eosinophilic cytoplasm. Hemophagocytic macrophages are also seen. **D,** The neoplastic infiltrate predominantly involves the liver sinusoids.

Figure 33-2. Bone marrow involvement by hepatosplenic T-cell lymphoma. A, There is a subtle atypical lymphoid infiltrate in a hypercellular marrow. The *arrows* indicate the "Indian file" sinusoidal distribution of medium-sized lymphocytes, which are highlighted with CD3 immunostaining **(B).**

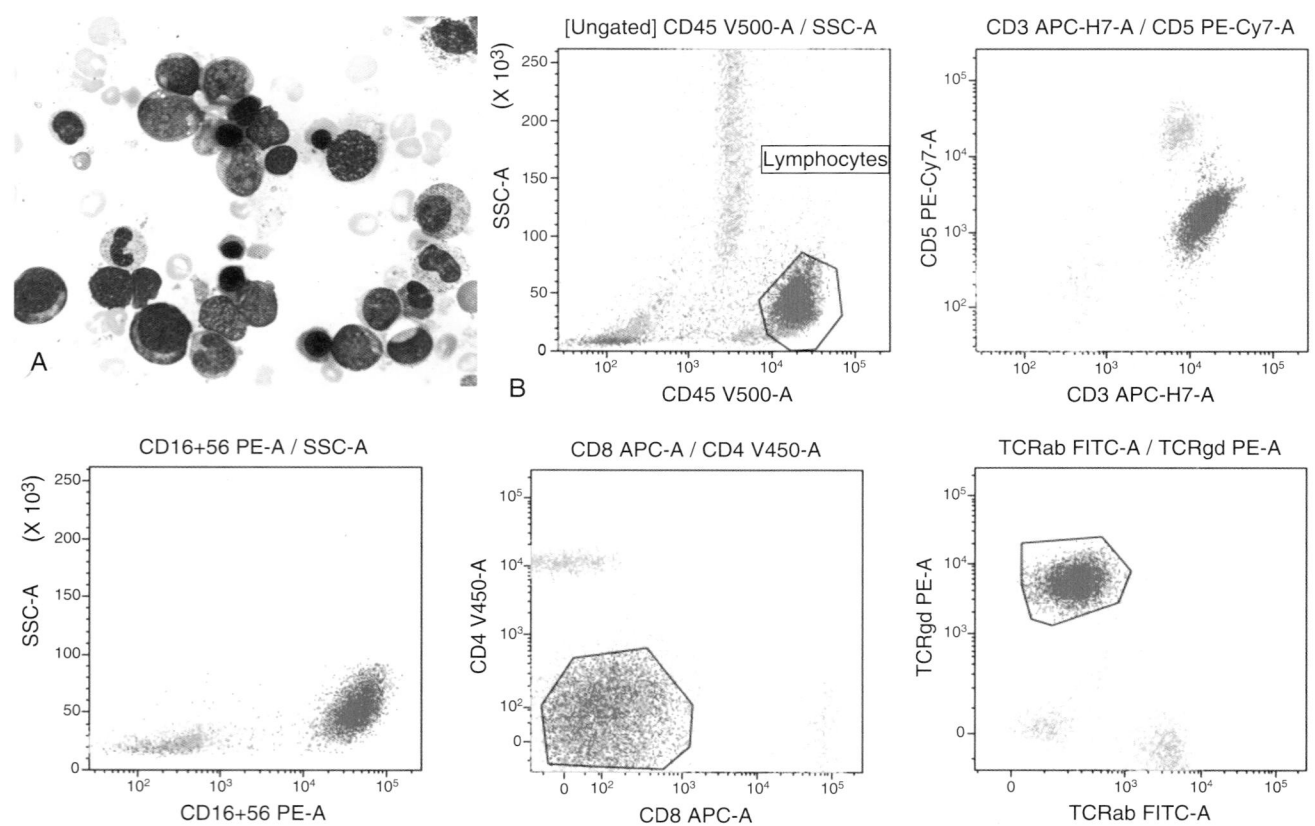

Figure 33-3. Bone marrow aspirate and phenotype of hepatosplenic T-cell lymphoma by flow cytometry. A, Wright-Giemsa–stained smear shows intermediate-sized lymphocytes with irregular nuclear contours, small nucleoli, and a moderate amount of cytoplasm, occasionally showing vacuoles. **B,** By multiparametric flow cytometry, these cells are found in the CD45 lymphocytes gate and show the following phenotype: CD3+, CD5−, CD4−, CD8−, CD16+, CD56+, TCRγδ+. Figs. 33-3 and 33-4 summarize the bone marrow findings in a 5-year-old boy who presented with severe pancytopenia. *(Courtesy of Dr. Caroline Mayeur Rousse and Dr. Anne Galoisy, Hautepierre University Hospital, Strasbourg, France.)*

of light-blue cytoplasm, occasionally showing vacuoles (Fig. 33-3A) or fine azurophilic granules.[47] The atypical cells may resemble hairy cells,[48] lymphoblasts with "hand mirror" cytoplasmic projections,[47] or may even cluster, mimicking a metastasis.[49] Histiocytic cell phagocytosis of red blood cells or other hematopoietic precursors can be observed.

Cytologic Variants

Overall, the cytologic appearance of neoplastic lymphocytes shows little variation among patients at presentation. The cells are usually monomorphic and small to medium-sized. Blastoid or pleomorphic medium-to-large cells have been occasionally observed at diagnosis but more often occur with disease progression.[5,11,40,43,50,51] These cytologic variants manifest a similar tissue distribution in sites involved by HSTL. However, in advanced disease, the bone marrow infiltration may extend beyond the sinuses, resulting in an interstitial (Fig. 33-4A) or diffuse pattern, and the neoplastic cells become larger.

PHENOTYPE

All HSTL cases show immunohistochemical staining with T-cell antigens and are negative for B-cell–associated markers

on formalin-fixed paraffin embedded tissue (FFPE) sections. The neoplastic cells are usually CD2+, CD3+, CD5−, CD7+/−, and CD4−/CD8− (Fig. 33-4C) with a small subset of cases that are CD4−/CD8+.[4,5,11,16,36,37,46,50,52] Among the NK-cell–associated markers, most cases express CD56 (Fig. 33-4D), some are CD16-positive, and CD57 is usually negative. All cases have a cytotoxic phenotype with typical granular cytoplasmic expression of cytotoxic molecule T-cell intracellular antigen 1 (TIA-1) (Fig. 33-4E) and serine protease granzyme M.[53] Most cases of HSTL are negative for granzyme B and perforin, consistent with mature, nonactivated cytotoxic T-cell phenotype.[35,54,55] Cytotoxic activity has been demonstrated in few cases in addition to CD52 positivity.[11,56] Expression of killer immunoglobulin-like receptors (KIRs) and, to a lesser degree, CD94/NKG2A seems to be a common feature.[43,57-59] HSTL is negative for the activation antigens CD25 and CD30. A majority of cases express T-cell receptor (TCR)γδ, as shown by monoclonal antibodies reactive with TCRγ or TCRδ available for routine use on FFPE tissue samples (Fig. 33-4B).[55,60,61] Most γδ HSTLs seem to arise from a subset of γδ T cells of Vδ1 usage, as shown by molecular studies and δTCS-1 antibody expression.[5,16,50,62-64] However, approximately 20% of cases have TCRαβ (βF1+/TCRγ−/δ−) and <5% show a TCR "silent" phenotype (βF1+/TCRγ−/δ−) either at presentation or at relapse.[10,11,36,43,59,60,65] They are classified together with the

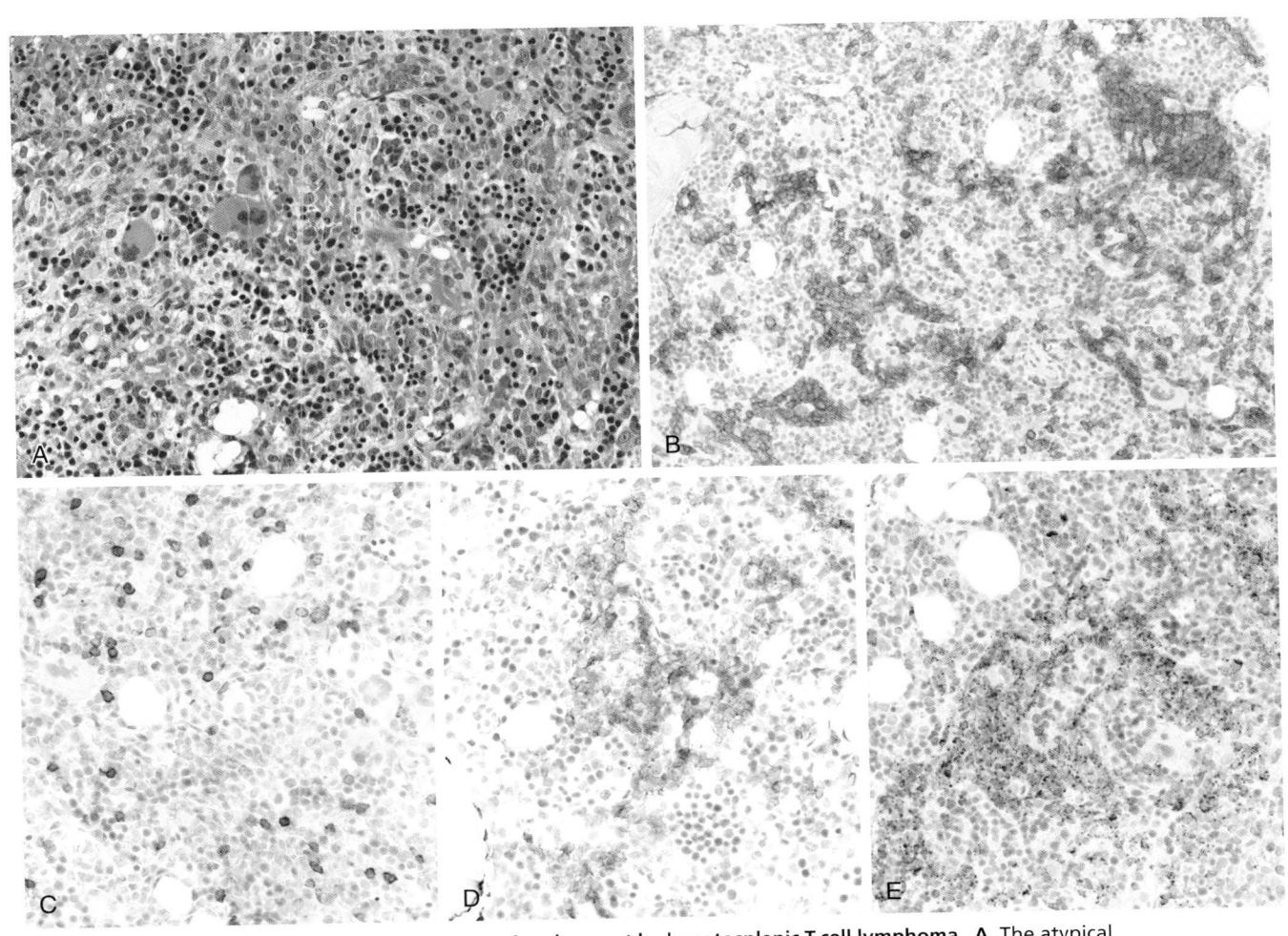

Figure 33-4. Overt bone marrow involvement by hepatosplenic T-cell lymphoma. A, The atypical lymphocytes distend the bone marrow sinusoids and slightly spread in the interstitium. They express TCRδ **(B)** and are CD5⁻ **(C)**, CD56⁺ **(D)**, and TIA-1⁺ **(E)**. Figs. 33-3 and 33-4 summarize the bone marrow findings in a 5-year-old boy who presented with severe pancytopenia.

more common γδ form of the disease based on overlapping clinicopathologic, cytogenetic, and molecular features.[11,59,65]

Although monoclonal antibodies against β, γ, or δ chains of TCR can be used on FFPE tissues, flow cytometric analysis of bone marrow aspirates is highly recommended, enabling not only a complete immunophenotyping of neoplastic cells (Fig. 33-3B), but also access to neoplastic cells for cytogenetic and molecular studies.

CYTOGENETIC AND MOLECULAR FINDINGS

Cytogenetics

Recurrent chromosomal abnormalities have been identified in HSTL, supporting its diagnosis in difficult cases. The most frequent genetic alterations, which frequently co-occur, are isochromosome 7q [i(7)(q10)] and trisomy 8, detected in up to 80% and 50% of γδ HSTL cases, respectively (Fig. 33-5).[4,5,10,11,13,16,36,58,60,66-70] Of note, i(7)(q10) has also been reported in HSTL expressing TCRαβ.[10,36,43,50,60,65,68] Other less common alterations include ring 7 [r(7)], loss of chromosomes Y, 21, 10p, and 11q14, and gain of chromosome 1q.[60,69,71] The relevance of these abnormalities to the HSTL pathogenesis is still unknown. However, i(7)(q10) is regarded as the primary

genetic event, and trisomy 8, r(7), and loss of chromosome Y are likely acquired during disease progression.[67,68] Both i(7)(q10) and r(7) lead to amplification of the 7q22.11q31.1 locus and 7p22.1p14.1 loss. These changes associate an overexpression of *ABCB1, RUNDC3PPP1R9A,* and *CHN2*/β2-chimerin genes, which may be responsible for the intrinsic drug resistance of neoplastic cells and their growth advantages.[69] Although i(7)(q10) characteristically occurs in HSTL, it is not specific for this entity. It has also been reported in acute myeloid and lymphoblastic leukemia, myelodysplastic syndrome, Wilms' tumor, and in rare cases of extranodal NK/T-cell lymphoma, nasal type, and anaplastic large cell lymphoma.[72]

Molecular Features

Irrespective of their γδ-phenotype or αβ-phenotype, HSTLs show a clonal rearrangement of the TCRγ chain gene (TRG) by polymerase chain reaction (PCR)-based study. Often, a biallelic clonal rearrangement of TCRδ chain gene is demonstrated by Southern blot or PCR analysis, in accordance with the γδ-genotype of neoplastic T cells.[5,59,63,64] Unproductive rearrangements of the β chain (TRB) have been reported in some γδ HSTLs, as in the corresponding normal γδ T cells.[63] In addition, the illegitimate somatic rearrangements of both TRG

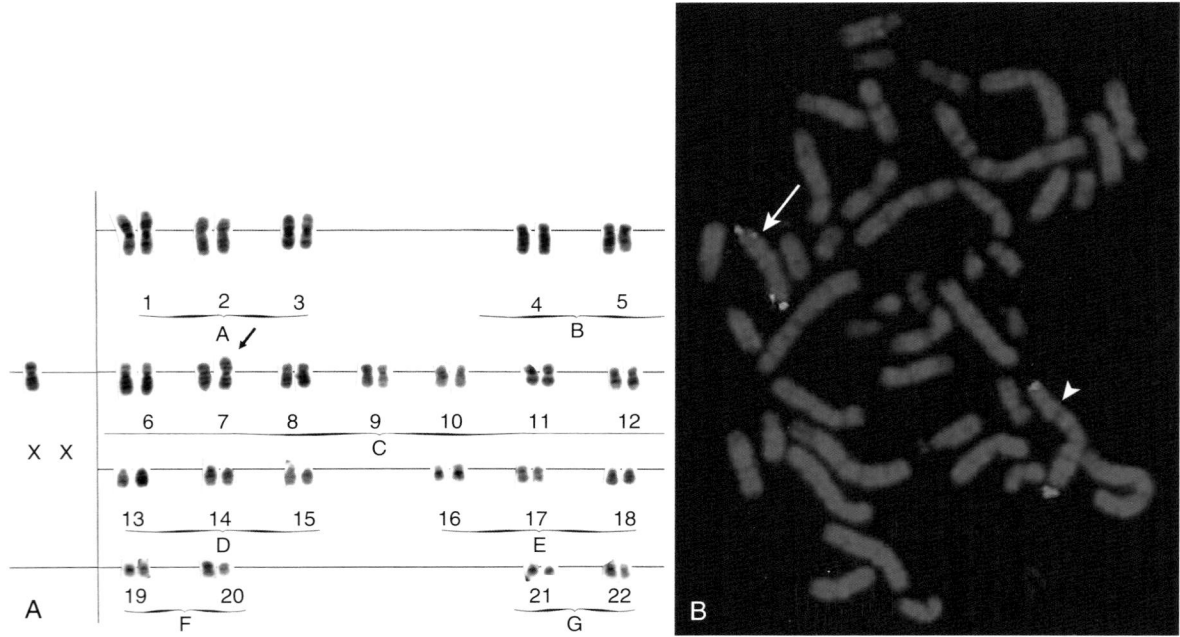

Figure 33-5. Cytogenetics of hepatosplenic T-cell lymphoma. A, Representative karyotype with isochromosome 7q [i(7)(q10)], indicated by the *arrow.* **B,** Example of abnormal metaphase with i(7)(q10) after fluorescence in situ hybridization subtelomeric probes for 7p *(green)* and 7q *(red).* The *arrow* and *arrowhead* show normal chromosome 7 and i(7)(q10), respectively. Note i(7)(q10)-associated loss of the 7p signal and gain of the 7q signal. *(Courtesy of Dr. Iwona Wlodarska, University of Leuven, Belgium.)*

and TRB loci may lead to formation of r(7), as shown by high-resolution array comparative genomic hybridization (CGH) studies.[69] The αβ HSTL cases show a clonal rearrangement of TRB in addition to TRG.[36,39]

HSTL presents a gene expression profile (GEP) signature distinct from other T-cell lymphomas and similar to γδ and αβ HSTL cases. It is characterized by overexpression of genes encoding NK-related antigens, such as *KIRs.*[59,73,74] In addition, a high expression of sphingosine-1-phosphatase receptor 5 (*S1PR5*), involved in cell trafficking, has been reported, which might explain the peculiar sinusoidal pattern with no significant leukemic phase seen in HSTLs.[59] Furthermore, overexpression of *SYK* with sensitivity of HSTL cell lines to Syk inhibitors has been underlined in this entity.[59] Nevertheless, active expression of oncogenes *VAV3, MYBL1,* and multidrug resistance 1 (*MDR-1*) and downregulation of tumor suppressor gene *AIM1* were highlighted as potential players in the pathobiology and aggressiveness of HSTL.[59]

Sequencing studies have revealed highly recurrent mutations in epigenetic regulators and members of the JAK/STAT and PI3K-signaling pathways, proving a framework for innovative therapies in HSTL.[55,60,75] More than 60% of patients manifest genetic changes in chromatin modifying genes such as *SETD2, INO80, TET3,* and *SMARCA2.*[60] In addition, frequent missense mutations in *STAT5B* and, less common, *STAT3* and *PIK3CD* have been reported in 30% and 10% of cases, respectively.[60,70,75] These alterations have been linked to HSTL pathogenesis. Loss of function mutations of tumor suppressor gene *SETD2* and gain-of-function mutations of *STAT5B, STAT3,* and *PIK3CD* genes increase proliferation and activate signalling pathways critical for cell survival in HSTL.[60] However, these mutations are not unique to HSTL and can occur in other mature, cytotoxic T-cell and NK-cell

lymphomas.[52,75-83] Conversely, HSTL lacks *RHOA* mutations and rarely exhibits *CD28* and *CCR4* gene alterations, which are commonly seen in other T-cell neoplasms.[60]

Epstein-Barr Virus Studies

By in situ hybridization with EBV-encoded small RNA (EBER) probes, an association with EBV has been found in exceptional cases of HSTL with cytologic features of transformation, suggesting that EBV might occur as a secondary event.[5,34]

POSTULATED CELL OF ORIGIN

The normal cell counterpart of HSTL has not been clearly identified. It is thought to derive from a subset of cytotoxic T cells, mostly of TCRγδ usage, involved in innate immunity.[84] The γδ T cells are the prototype of "unconventional" T cells, activated in a major histocompatibility complex (MHC)-independent manner. They are derived from CD4-negative CD8-negative (double negative) thymic precursors and represent <5% of mature circulating T cells in healthy adults. These cells are enriched within the intraepithelial regions of the skin and mucosa and in the red pulp of the spleen, serving as first line of defense against pathogens and transformed cells. Although most peripheral-blood γδ T cells express Vδ2 TCR, Vδ1 T cells are higher within tissue, including the spleen.[85,86] This likely explains the Vδ1 TCR detection in most γδ HSTLs.[5,62-64] Furthermore, this lymphoma is thought to arise from cytotoxic T cells of memory phenotype, given the expression of KIR antigens, which are normally encountered on a subset of memory cytotoxic T cells and on NK cells.[58] Of note, KIR-positive normal αβ and γδ cytotoxic T cells typically express a single KIR isoform. However, both γδ and αβ HSTL variants frequently express multiple KIR isoforms.[57-59,73,74] This might link HSTL pathogenesis to chronic antigenic stimulation, which can trigger the expression of multiple KIR isoforms.[5]

CLINICAL COURSE

The disease has an aggressive clinical course, with most patients dying of lymphoma within 2 years of diagnosis.[4,5,11,16,37,87] In a large population-based analysis, HSTL was one of the highest-risk PTCL subtypes.[88] An indolent phase prior to a more aggressive disease has been reported in some patients.[10,89] Male gender, chronic immunosuppression, elevated serum LDH or bilirubin level ($\geq$1.5 mg/dL), and TCR$\alpha\beta$ have been cited as poor prognostic indicators.[4,5,11,16,36,37,87,90] Relapse or disease progression occurs in initially involved sites (i.e., spleen, if splenectomy was not performed, bone marrow, liver) and does not result in lymphadenopathy, thus reinforcing the peculiar homing of the neoplastic cells. In exceptional cases, relapses may occur in skin, mucosa, and meninges. Few patients manifested a significant leukemic phase.[5]

Therapy

Treatment approaches have been highly heterogeneous in HSTLs, and its rarity has hampered prospective clinical trials from being undertaken and standard, effective approaches from being proposed. Disappointing results with early relapses were seen after anthracycline-containing (CHOP [cyclophosphamide, doxorubicin, vincristine, and prednisone] or CHOP-like) regimens.[5,12,16,37] According to the NCCN guidelines, the use of nonanthracycline-based regimens such as ICE (ifosfamide, carboplatin, etoposide) or DHAP (cytosine arabinoside, cisplatin, dexamethasone) is recommended, followed by allogeneic hematopoietic stem cell transplantation (HSCT) when complete remission is achieved.[42] Lower rates of relapse and higher efficacy were seen after allogeneic HSCT compared with autologous HSCT, which is probably related to the graft-versus-lymphoma effect conferred by the former.[91-94] Given its in vitro selective cytotoxic effect on malignant $\gamma\delta$ T cells, 2'deoxycoformycin (pentostatin) has also been suggested as an active agent.[89,95-98]

Novel therapeutic options are needed to improve the outcome of patients with HSTL in the future. Genetic studies have pointed toward recurrent dysregulation of oncogenic pathways such JAK/STAT and *PI3KCD* and chromatin modifying genes, including *SETD2*, which are potentially targetable.[60] *SETD2*-mutated HSTL cells may be sensitive to WEE1 inhibitors.[99,100] Similarly, it is questionable whether Syk inhibitors or hypomethylating agents could be useful to control this disease.[59]

DIFFERENTIAL DIAGNOSIS

The major diagnostic features of HSTL are listed in Box 33-1. The differential diagnosis includes other lymphomas, mainly of T-cell or NK-cell derivation, which present with hepatosplenic disease and infiltration of the splenic red pulp. Particularity challenging is the distinction of HSTL from T-cell large granular lymphocytic leukemia and aggressive NK-cell lymphoma/leukemia. Among the B-cell neoplasms, hairy cell leukemia and splenic diffuse red pulp small B-cell

---

Box 33-1 *Major Diagnostic Features of Hepatosplenic T-Cell Lymphoma*

- Aggressive disease, B symptoms
- Splenomegaly (massive) without nodules
- Hepatomegaly
- No lymphadenopathy
- Thrombocytopenia, frequent anemia, leukopenia
- No lymphocytosis
- Monomorphic small to medium-sized cells
- Sinusoidal pattern of infiltration in the bone marrow, spleen, and liver
- CD3$^+$, CD5$^-$, CD4$^-$/CD8$^-$, CD56$^{+/-}$ phenotype
- Nonactivated cytotoxic profile (TIA-1$^+$, granzyme B$^-$, perforin$^-$)
- Absence of Epstein-Barr virus
- Isochromosome 7q (50%–70%)
- *STAT5B* mutations (30%), *SETD2* mutations (25%)

---

lymphoma must be ruled out. The discriminatory features between these entities are summarized in Table 33-1. HSTL should also be distinguished from benign peripheral-blood $\gamma\delta$ T-cell expansions observed in various benign settings such as infections or autoimmune diseases.[101,102]

Aggressive NK-Cell Lymphoma/Leukemia

Aggressive NK-cell lymphoma/leukemia (ANKL) is a rare systemic NK neoplasm, described commonly in young to middle-aged adults mainly of Asian ethnicity.[103-105] It represents a major differential diagnosis of HSTL given overlapping clinical, cytologic, immunophenotypic, and molecular features. Both entities present with hepatosplenomegaly, B-symptoms, cytopenia, and aggressive behavior. As in HSTL, in ANKL, the splenic red pulp and sinusoids of the liver are infiltrated by atypical lymphocytes CD2$^+$, CD5$^-$, CD56$^+$, CD4$^-$/CD8$^-$, showing JAK/STAT pathway activation, epigenetic dysregulation, and impairment of TP53 and DNA repair.[103-107] However, as opposed to HSTL, the atypical cells in ANKL are more pleomorphic, display prominent cytoplasmic azurophilic granules, and typically show a leukemic spread. In addition, the bone marrow demonstrates a variable degree of interstitial or patchy atypical lymphoid infiltrate, without a sinusoidal predilection. Furthermore, the neoplastic lymphocytes in ANKL are of NK-cell derivation. They are typically negative for *surface* CD3 by flow cytometry, show an activated cytotoxic phenotype, and lack TCR expression and clonal gene rearrangement. Finally, EBV is detected in the neoplastic cells of most patients with ANKL, with only rare exceptions.[108] ANKL is consistently associated with hemophagocytic syndrome and follows a fulminant course with a median survival of approximately 2 months.[103-105,109]

T-Cell Large Granular Lymphocytic Leukemia

T-cell large granular lymphocytic leukemia (T-LGLL) is a chronic, indolent lymphoproliferative disorder with clinical and laboratory manifestations often distinct from those observed in HSTL.[110,111] It usually affects older patients who are either asymptomatic or present with a moderately enlarged spleen and symptoms related to autoimmune disorders or to neutropenia and/or anemia. Dissimilar to HSTL, T-LGLL

Table 33-1 Differential Diagnosis of Hepatosplenic T-Cell Lymphoma: Major Distinguishing Features

Diagnosis	Clinical Features	Cytology	Cell of Origin	Phenotype	Cytotoxic Profile	EBV (EBER)	Bone Marrow	Spleen	Liver	Genetics
Hepatosplenic T-cell lymphoma	B symptoms, splenomegaly, cytopenia, no LAD	Medium-sized, monomorphic Ly, no azurophilic granules	Tγδ (>Tαβ)	CD3+, CD5-, CD4-/CD8-, CD56+, CD57-	Nonactivated (TIA-1+, GrB-, Perf-)	Negative	Sinusoidal, Hypercellular bone marrow	Red pulp (sinusoids and cords), white pulp atrophy	Sinusoidal (predominant)	TR+, i(7q), trisomy 8, STAT5B, epigenetic regulators (SETD2, INO80) mutations
Aggressive NK-cell leukemia	B symptoms, splenomegaly, HPS, leukemic spread, cytopenia, LAD +/-	Medium-to-large Ly, prominent azurophilic granules	NK	sCD3- (cCD3+), CD5-, CD4-/CD8-, CD16+, CD56+, CD57-	Activated (TIA-1+, GrB+, Perf+)	Positive	Interstitial, diffuse, histiocytes + hemophagocytosis	Red pulp (subtle), wall vessels	Sinusoidal and portal	TR-, Del(6q), del(11q) STAT3, DDX3X, TP53, TET2 mutations
T-cell large granular lymphocytic leukemia	Indolent, neutropenia, autoimmune manifestations, leukemic spread, splenomegaly +/-, no LAD	Small-to-medium sized Ly, prominent azurophilic granules	Tαβ (>Tγδ)	CD3+, CD5-, CD4-/CD8+/-, CD16+, CD57+	Activated (TIA-1+, GrB+, Perf+)	Negative	Sinusoidal and interstitial (often subtle) ± nodules, maturation arrest	Red pulp (subtle, cords and sinusoids), white pulp hyperplasia	Sinusoidal and portal	TR+, STAT3, STAT5B mutations
Systemic chronic active EBV disease	B symptoms, cytopenia, splenomegaly, LAD	Small-to-intermediate Ly, no atypia	Tαβ (>NK, Tγδ)	CD4+/CD8-, no phenotypical abnormalities	Activated (TIA-1+, GrB+)	Positive	Sinusoidal and interstitial (subtle)	Red pulp sinusoids (subtle)	Sinusoidal (subtle)	TR+ (>oligoclonal-, polyclonal), DDX3X mutations
Splenic diffuse red pulp small B-cell lymphoma	Splenomegaly, slight lymphocytosis	Small lymphocytes ± villi	B	CD20+, DBA44+/-, cyclin D3+, CD5-, Annexin A1-, CD103-, CD25-, CD11c-	—	Negative	Sinusoidal (predominantly)	Red pulp (sinusoids and cords)	Sinusoidal and portal	Del(7q), trisomy 18 CCND3 mutation, BCOR alterations
Hairy cell leukemia	Splenomegaly, cytopenia	Hairy cells	B	CD20+, Annexin A1+, CD103+, CD11c+, CD25+, CD123+	—	Negative	Interstitial, diffuse, fibrosis	Red pulp (sinusoids and cords), red blood cell lakes	Sinusoidal (predominant)	BRAF mutation

cCD3, Cytoplasmic CD3; del, deletion; EBER, Epstein-Barr virus-encoded RNA; EBV, Epstein-Barr virus; GrB, granzyme B; HPS, hemophagocytic syndrome; i(7q), isochromosome 7q; LAD, lymphadenopathy; Ly, lymphocytes; NK, natural killer; sCD3, surface CD3; TR, T-cell receptor genes rearrangement.

manifests with a leukemic blood picture. The neoplastic cells typically display azurophilic granules within the cytoplasm and show CD3+, CD8+, CD57+, TCRαβ+, CD56⁻, and activated cytotoxic phenotype.[110-112] They exhibit frequent *STAT3* mutations[77,113] and lack i(7q).[114] However, rarely, T-LGLL affects younger patients, shows a CD4-negative CD8-negative and a TCRγδ-positive phenotype.[11,110,114,115] Some cases have *STAT5B* gene mutations and follow an aggressive clinical course,[116] making challenging the distinction from HSTL. Although histopathology is rarely required for T-LGLL diagnosis, the pattern of neoplastic cell distribution within the splenic red pulp and sinusoids of the liver may overlap with that observed in HSTL. However, in T-LGLL, the bone marrow biopsy often demonstrates a mixed interstitial and intrasinusoidal lymphoid infiltrate without notable atypia, blending with hematopoietic cells. In addition, nonneoplastic lymphoid nodules composed of a variable mixture of CD20-positive B lymphocytes and CD4-positive T lymphocytes are frequently associated.[112,117,118]

Other T-Cell Lymphoproliferative Diseases

Other T-cell lymphoproliferations of γδ T-cell derivation or with shared clinical features with HSTL should also be considered in the differential. As previously mentioned, demonstration of γδ T-cell phenotype is not specific to HSTL. Beside T-LGLL and T-lymphoblastic lymphoma/leukemia, a subset of extranodal cytotoxic T-cell lymphomas occurring predominately at mucosal sites such as the nasopharynx, intestine, and skin are also of γδ T-cell derivation.[9,10,61,86,119,120] This is consistent with the normal γδ T-cell distribution,[84] functioning as mature, activated cytotoxic T cells, ensuring the first line of immune defence in the mucosa and skin. Therefore, these non-hepatosplenic γδ T-cell lymphomas constitute a subgroup of activated cytotoxic T-cell neoplasms with mainly extranodal presentation. Despite the shared γδ phenotype, they are classified distinctively as extranodal NK-cell or T-cell lymphoma nasal-type, monomorphic epitheliotropic intestinal T-cell lymphoma, or primary cutaneous γδ T-cell lymphoma.[111] This suggests that their "identity" relies rather upon the site of origin, the functional properties of the corresponding T cells, and the specific pathogenic cues than on their precise γδ T-cell phenotype.[9,61,86,119] Although these lymphomas may show splenic and bone marrow involvement, their distinction from HSTL is less challenging given differences in the clinical and immunophenotypical features.

Patients with chronic active EBV infection or systemic EBV-positive T-cell lymphoma of childhood can present with symptoms mimicking HSTL, such as fever, hepatosplenomegaly, and cytopenia. However, the bone marrow biopsy depicts usually interstitial infiltrate of small to medium-sized EBV-positive T cells or NK cells without significant cytologic atypia.

B-Cell Lymphomas of the Spleen

Among the B-cell neoplasms, certain primary splenic lymphomas are relevant to the differential diagnosis of HSTL given their clinical presentation as hepatosplenic disease and/or pattern of neoplastic cell distribution within the splenic red pulp, liver, or bone marrow. These include hairy cell leukemia, splenic marginal zone lymphoma (SMZL), and splenic diffuse red pulp small B-cell lymphoma. Despite diffuse involvement of splenic red pulp, hairy cell leukemia differs from HSTL by its peculiar cytologic appearance on blood smears, diffuse interstitial bone marrow involvement with notable reticulin fibrosis, B-cell phenotype (typically CD103+, CD25+, CD11c+, Annexin A1+, and CD123+), and *BRAF*-V600E gene mutation.[111,121] As in HSTL, splenic diffuse red pulp small B-cell lymphoma shows splenomegaly with red pulp involvement and usually elective sinusoidal bone marrow spread of small atypical lymphocytes. A sinusoidal bone marrow involvement by small B cells has also been reported in SMZL, but it appears less frequent and is usually associated with an interstitial or nodular bone marrow infiltration. These later lymphomas have a B-cell phenotype and follow an indolent clinical course.[111,122,123]

Overall, the selective sinusoidal bone marrow involvement by the neoplastic lymphocytes is a distinctive feature of HSTL, contrasting with the interstitial and/or nodular pattern of infiltration observed in most B-cell, T-cell, and NK-cell lymphoproliferations. In addition, demonstration of CD3+, CD5–, CD4–/CD8–, CD56+, TIA-1+, granzyme B–, and EBV⁻ phenotype of atypical T-cell infiltrate in the bone marrow specimens provides strong evidence for HSTL diagnosis.

Pearls and Pitfalls

- Clinical presentation of HSTL is not typical for lymphoma. It shares symptoms with many systemic diseases
  - Unexplained weakness with fever and splenomegaly
  - No overt tumoral syndrome with no lymphadenopathy
  - Thrombocytopenia and anemia, occasionally leading to misdiagnosis of idiopathic thrombocytopenic purpura or Coombs-negative hemolytic anemia
- Diagnosis is based on careful examination of the bone marrow biopsy (± aspirate):
  - Look for elective and constant sinusoidal infiltration ("Indian file" or aggregates dilating sinuses)
  - Identification may be difficult in the common context of hypercellular marrow (not to be misinterpreted as myelodysplastic syndrome)
  - CD20 and CD3 immunostainings provide better recognition and are recommended in patients with unexplained splenomegaly
  - Aspirate smears are highly useful for a complete immunophenotypic analysis by flow cytometry, cytogenetic, and molecular studies
- Splenectomy is no longer required for diagnosis.
- Demonstration of a γδ T-cell origin is recommended. Though most HSTL have a γδ phenotype, rare cases with an αβ phenotype have been reported.
- Atypical features in some HSTL cases include an indolent initial phase, a cytologic pleomorphism (medium/large cells), granzyme B staining (partial), and circulating cells in late phase of disease or relapse.
- Integration of clinical, pathologic, and phenotypic data with genetic changes is sometimes needed to distinguish HSTL from ANKL and T-LGLL.

KEY REFERENCES

5. Belhadj K, et al. Hepatosplenic gammadelta T-cell lymphoma is a rare clinicopathologic entity with poor outcome: report on a series of 21 patients. *Blood*. 2003;102:4261–4269.

10. Attygalle AD, et al. Peripheral T-cell and NK-cell lymphomas and their mimics; taking a step forward—report on the lymphoma workshop of the XVIth meeting of the European Association for Haematopathology and the Society for Hematopathology. *Histopathology*. 2014;64:171–199.

19. Deepak P, et al. T-cell non-Hodgkin's lymphomas reported to the FDA AERS with tumor necrosis factor-alpha (TNF-α) inhibitors: results of the REFURBISH study. *Am J Gastroenterol*. 2013;108:99–105.

36. Macon WR, et al. Hepatosplenic alphabeta T-cell lymphomas: a report of 14 cases and comparison with hepatosplenic gammadelta T-cell lymphomas. *Am J Surg Pathol*. 2001;25:285–296.

55. Nicolae A, et al. Frequent STAT5B mutations in γδ hepatosplenic T-cell lymphomas. *Leukemia*. 2014;28:2244–2248.

59. Travert M, et al. Molecular features of hepatosplenic T-cell lymphoma unravels potential novel therapeutic targets. *Blood*. 2012;119:5795–5806.

60. McKinney M, et al. The genetic basis of hepatosplenic T-cell lymphoma. *Cancer Discov*. 2017;7:369–379.

61. Garcia-Herrera A, et al. Nonhepatosplenic γδ T-cell lymphomas represent a spectrum of aggressive cytotoxic T-cell lymphomas with a mainly extranodal presentation. *Am J Surg Pathol*. 2011;35:1214–1225.

67. Alonsozana EL, et al. Isochromosome 7q: the primary cytogenetic abnormality in hepatosplenic gammadelta T cell lymphoma. *Leukemia*. 1997;11:1367–1372.

68. Wlodarska I, et al. Fluorescence in situ hybridization study of chromosome 7 aberrations in hepatosplenic T-cell lymphoma: isochromosome 7q as a common abnormality accumulating in forms with features of cytologic progression. *Genes Chromosomes Cancer*. 2002;33:243–251.

86. Tripodo C, et al. Gamma-delta T-cell lymphomas. *Nat Rev Clin Oncol*. 2009;6:707–717.

Visit Elsevier eBooks+ for the complete set of references.

Chapter 34

Peripheral T-Cell Lymphoma, Not Otherwise Specified

Laurence de Leval

DEFINITION

Peripheral T-cell lymphoma, not otherwise specified (PTCL, NOS) encompasses per definition all mature (peripheral) T-cell neoplasms lacking specific features that qualify for any of the other better defined "specific" entities of postthymic T-cell lymphoma/leukemia.[1-3] The definition is unchanged from the previous World Health Organization (WHO) classifications, and PTCL, NOS remains a diagnosis of exclusion. Importantly, recent advances have led to reclassification of subsets of former PTCL, NOS and have narrowed down the diagnostic criteria. A notion already introduced in the revised 4th ed. of the WHO Classification (2017) is that PTCL, NOS excludes nodal/systemic PTCLs with a follicular helper T-cell (TFH) phenotype, defined by the expression of at least two TFH markers, which are now diagnosed as a TFH lymphoma subtype.[1-3] In addition, primary nodal Epstein-Barr virus (EBV)–positive T/natural killer (NK)-cell lymphoma is no longer a variant of PTCL, NOS, but recognized as an entity in the 2022 International Consensus Classification (ICC) and in the WHO 5th ed. PTCL, NOS is still viewed as a heterogeneous group of neoplasms, which likely do not constitute a single entity, waiting for further individualization of meaningful subgroups and substratification. Although efforts have been made in that direction, and there is growing evidence to substantiate the rationale for molecular or functional subgrouping among PTCL, NOS, neither the ICC nor the revised WHO 5th ed. have yet recognized new diagnostic subtypes.

SYNONYMS AND RELATED TERMS

None.

EPIDEMIOLOGY

PTCL, NOS, formerly PTCL unspecified,[4] has been for decades reported as the most frequent PTCL entity. In the International T-cell Project, which collected PTCL cases from Europe, Asia, and North America between 1990 and 2002, PTCL, NOS was the most prevalent systemic PTCL entity worldwide, accounting for 26% PTCLs,[5] markedly above TFH lymphoma of angioimmunoblastic-type (AITL) (18.5% of the cases). PTCL, NOS was relatively more common in North America and in Europe (34% of the cases) compared with Asia (22%), where other PTCL entities (EBV-associated NK/T-cell neoplasms and human T-cell lymphotropic virus 1 (HTLV1)-associated leukemia/lymphoma) are more prevalent.

In recent years, with the refinement of diagnostic criteria, better knowledge of PTCL entities, and the expansion of the spectrum of TFH lymphomas, the reported prevalence of PTCL, NOS has tended to decrease. In a project conducted by the

North American PTCL study group to evaluate the diagnostic workup of PTCL, based on 336 cases collected from several institutions, PTCL, NOS was the second most common diagnosis (26% of the cases), side by side with AITL (27% of the cases).[6] It is likely that the high prevalence of PTCL, NOS reported in preceding times was caused by incomplete phenotypic characterization, and particularly lack of systematic investigation for TFH markers.[7] Based on an analysis of the French lymphoma registry (Lymphopath) and a review of >32,000 noncutaneous lymphomas between 2010 and 2013, PTCL, NOS accounted for 27% of the cases, and was largely outnumbered by AITL (36% of the cases).[8,9] In a multinational multicentric registry study prospectively conducted in Asia between 2016 and 2019, based on 486 PTCL patients, PTCL, NOS was the third most frequent entity (21% of the cases), after extranodal NK/T-cell lymphoma, nasal type, and AITL.[10]

CLINICAL FEATURES

The disease tends to be diagnosed in middle-aged to older adults at a median age of 60 years, and is very rare in children, adolescents, and young adults.[11] There is a male predominance in most published series.[12,13] PTCL, NOS typically involves lymph nodes, but may primarily present in any extranodal site. Most of the patients (about 70%) have disseminated disease (stage III or IV) at the time of diagnosis with infiltrates in the bone marrow, liver, spleen, gastrointestinal tract, or other extranodal tissues, frequently including the skin. Presentation with bulky disease occurs 10% to 15% of the patients, which is less common than in aggressive B-cell lymphomas.

Constitutional symptoms, a poor performance status, and elevated LDH levels are reported in 40% to 60% of the cases, and approximately 50% to 70% of the patients have an intermediate-risk to high-risk international prognostic index (IPI).[12] Blood eosinophilia, anemia, and thrombocytopenia are present at the time of the diagnosis in a minority of patients. The occurrence of a hematophagocytic syndrome in some patients is often associated with a rapidly fatal course.[14]

The etiology of the disease, or more likely diseases, is unknown. In a minority of cases, associations with other clinical conditions have been reported. For example, patients with the lymphoproliferative variant of the hypereosinophilic syndrome, a condition associated with a clonal proliferation of IL-5 producing T cells, may secondarily develop a T-cell lymphoma most commonly reported, AITL, or PTCL, NOS.[15-20] The occurrence of cutaneous or systemic T-cell neoplasms in patients with chronic lymphocytic leukemia (CLL) has been documented in several case reports and case series; the majority consisted of PTCL, NOS, often with a cytotoxic phenotype, or anaplastic large cell lymphoma (ALCL), anaplastic lymphoma kinase (ALK) positive or ALK negative.[21] The interval between the diagnoses of CLL and PCTL in these patients was on average 5 years.[22-24] Mechanistically, lymphomagenesis has been linked to the accumulation of oligoclonal or monoclonal T-cell populations with abnormal phenotypes or disrupted functional properties commonly observed in CLL patients.[21,22]

Immunocompromised patients in general have an increased risk of developing PTCL, which is more frequently extranodal and develops at a younger age compared with the general population.[25] Among the very rare HIV-associated lymphomas of T-cell phenotype, which tend to occur predominantly in male individuals under combined antiretroviral therapy, PTCL, NOS is the most common type, and a subset of cases are EBV-positive, now classified as primary nodal EBV-positive T/NK-cell lymphoma.[26] PTCL, NOS is also the most frequent type of posttransplant lymphoproliferative disorders of T-cell lineage, the latter representing only a small proportion of all PTCLs, and being EBV negative in less than half of the cases.[27] PTCL, NOS in the posttransplant setting tends to occur late after transplantation and their molecular and genomic alterations appear similar to those found in PTCL, NOS in immunocompetent hosts, suggesting common mechanisms of lymphoma development.[28] The occurrence of nodal T-cell lymphomas has been reported in patients with rheumatoid arthritis under treatment with methotrexate; among the 28 patients described by Satou et al., who were elderly individuals (median 70 years) under methotrexate for 0.5 to 21 years, there were 19 AITL, 8 PTCL, NOS, and 1 case of EBV-positive CD8-positive nodal T-cell lymphoma, consistent of primary nodal EBV-positive T/NK-cell lymphoma following current terminology.[29]

MORPHOLOGY

PTCL, NOS encompasses a broad morphologic spectrum. Most commonly, lymph nodes are involved in a diffuse fashion (Fig. 34-1A). High endothelial venules are usually increased, and arborizing vessels are often abundant (Fig. 34-1B). However, at variance with AITL, an open peripheral sinus and stromal expansion of follicular dendritic cells are not seen (Fig. 34-1C–D). Some cases may present with an interfollicular or paracortical infiltrate sparing persistent follicles, a pattern formerly referred to as "T-zone variant" (Fig. 34-1E–F).[30] However, it has turned out that many cases with a T-zone pattern of involvement correspond to CD4-positive PTCL with a TFH phenotype and are now classified as TFH lymphoma, NOS. Hence, while the term may be used in the histologic description, it is nonspecific and no longer designates a variant of PTCL, NOS. Likewise, follicular PTCL characterized by a nodular growth in association with follicular dendritic cells and variable amounts of small B cells, resembling follicular lymphoma or progressively transformed germinal centers, originally considered as a variant of PTCL, NOS,[31] was later identified as a rare form of nodal TFH-derived lymphoma, and is now classified as TFH lymphoma, follicular type.[1,32,33]

In PTCL, NOS, the neoplastic cells are typically pleomorphic, with most cases containing a mixed population of smaller and larger cells. Many cases consist predominantly of medium-sized or large-sized cells with round, oval, or irregular nuclei containing prominent nucleoli and many mitotic figures (Fig. 34-2A).[4,30,34] Less common, small pleomorphic T-cell lymphomas have a predominance of atypical small cells with irregular nuclei (Fig. 34-2B).[35] Irregularity of nuclear contours may be a helpful hint to suspect the neoplastic nature of infiltrates composed predominantly of small cells. Some cases have atypical cells with clear cytoplasm and irregular or round nuclei. Some tumors contain scattered large, atypical cells resembling Hodgkin or Reed-Sternberg cells (HRS-like cells), which may correspond to the most atypical component of the neoplastic population, or bystander B-cell blasts. With relapse, the tumors tend to retain similar morphologic features and pattern of nodal involvement, or may show histologic progression with increased numbers of large cells.[36] Morphologic grading is not recommended for clinical purposes, but tumors with a predominance of large cells have been found to have a worse outcome.[12]

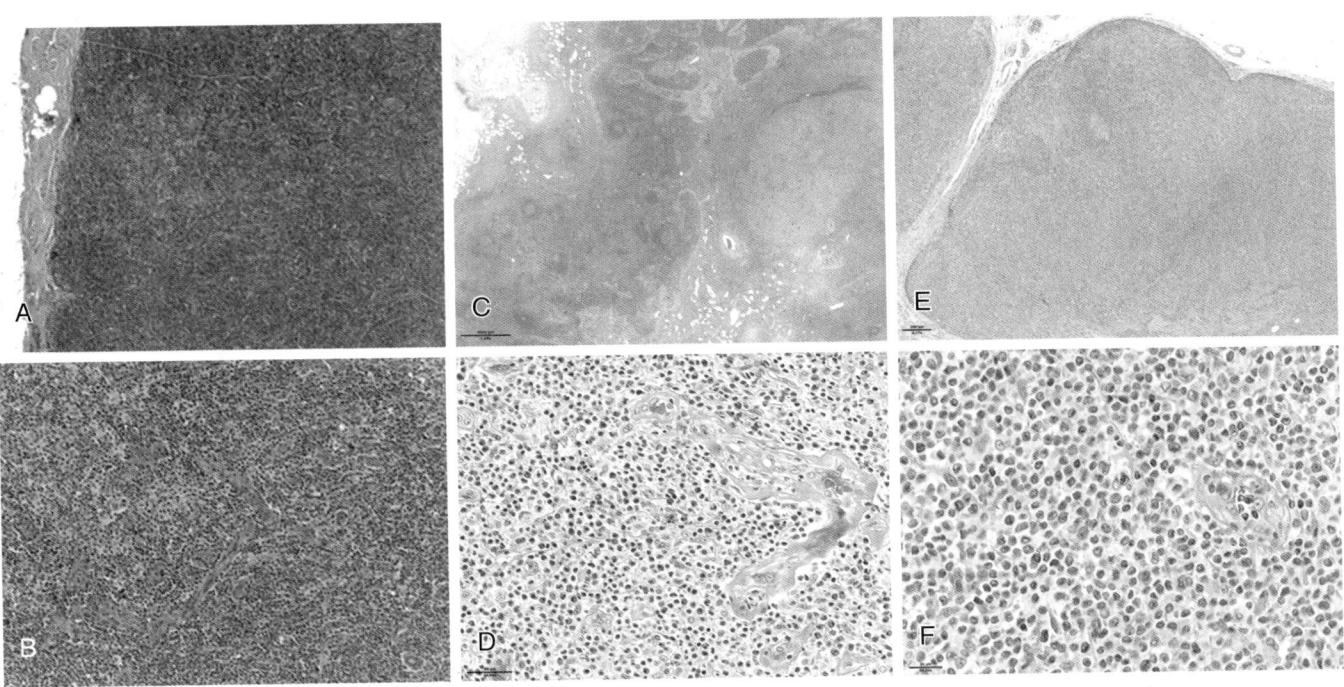

Figure 34-1. Patterns of peripheral T-cell lymphoma, not otherwise specified. A–B, Peripheral T-cell lymphoma, not otherwise specified (PTCL, NOS) with diffuse nodal involvement, and prominent venules. **C–D,** PTCL, NOS extending into the perinodal tissues, without preservation of the sinus; in this case that arose in a patient with a history of lymphocytic variant of hypereosinophilic syndrome, the small-to-medium-sized atypical cells were admixed with numerous eosinophils. **E–F,** PTCL, NOS showing extensive lymph node involvement preserving reactive follicles, and composed of rather monotonous medium-sized atypical cells.

Many cases have a polymorphous cellular composition, with an admixture of reactive cells, including small lymphocytes, eosinophils, histiocytes, B cells, and plasma cells. Any of these bystander cell components can be prominent, obscure the neoplastic cells and represent a compounding factor to establishing a correct diagnosis. The rare cases with a prominent infiltrate of epithelioid histiocytes, referred to as lymphoepithelioid lymphoma (Lennert lymphoma) (Fig. 34-2C–D), may constitute a distinctive subtype.

IMMUNOPHENOTYPE

The common leukocyte antigen (CD45) and T-cell–associated antigens (CD3, CD2, CD5, CD7, CD43) are positive, but aberrant T-cell phenotypes with a lack of one or several of these markers (most commonly CD5 or CD7) are typically encountered (Fig. 34-3).[37,38] Most cases are single positive CD4 positive, or less often CD8-positive T cells, but a significant proportion of tumors are double-negative, or more rarely positive for both antigens.[37-39] Whether the expression of CD4 or CD8 is associated with any prognostic effect is unclear, but there have been suggestions that CD4-positive cases tend to be associated with a better outcome, while conversely a double-negative immunophenotype might be associated with an unfavorable prognosis.[38,39] In >85% of cases the neoplastic cells express the alpha/beta T-cell receptor (TCRβF1+), and a minority cases are either of gamma/delta derivation (positive for TCR gamma or TCR delta), or negative for both (TCR silent).[38,40,41] Loss of BCL2 by the neoplastic T cells, which is observed in 45% to 60% of the cases, can be a useful marker indicative of T-cell malignancy, also applicable to other types of mature T-cell neoplasms.[42,43]

An aberrant immunophenotype is usually interpreted as the phenotypic expression of a neoplastic genotype and represents the main tool available on routine tissue sections to infer clonality/malignancy in T-cell lymphoproliferations. Besides, there are direct means of assessing clonality of T-cell populations by flow cytometry[44] using V-beta analysis with specific antibodies directed to the 24 V-beta families, with a clonal population being defined by expressing one or none of the V-beta families, or by assessment of TRBC1 (T-cell receptor constant beta chain-1) expression. The latter method, recently developed, is based on a single antibody recognizing TRBC1, which is expressed mutually exclusive to TRBC2, a clonal population being defined as positive or negative for TRBC1.[45] This simple assay is unfortunately not applicable for immunohistochemistry on routinely processed tissues.

A subset of PTCL, NOS, ranging from 15% to 30% to 40% of the cases in various series, express one or several cytotoxic granule-associated molecules (T-cell intracellular antigen [TIA], granzyme B, or perforin) indicative of a resting or more commonly activated cytotoxic immunophenotype (Fig. 34-4).[38,39,46]

By definition, the neoplastic cells in PTCL, NOS must lack a TFH immunophenotype. The latter applies to CD4-positive cells expressing two or more key markers of TFH cells. The recommended panel includes five antibodies (BCL6, CD10, CXCL13, PD1, ICOS/CD278),[1,33] but other markers of TFH cells can be taken in consideration as well in this context, for example CD57, CD200, CXCR5, or SAP. Importantly, none of these markers is totally specific for TFH lineage differentiation, and each might be occasionally be expressed in PTCL, NOS, usually in a nonhomogeneous fashion and

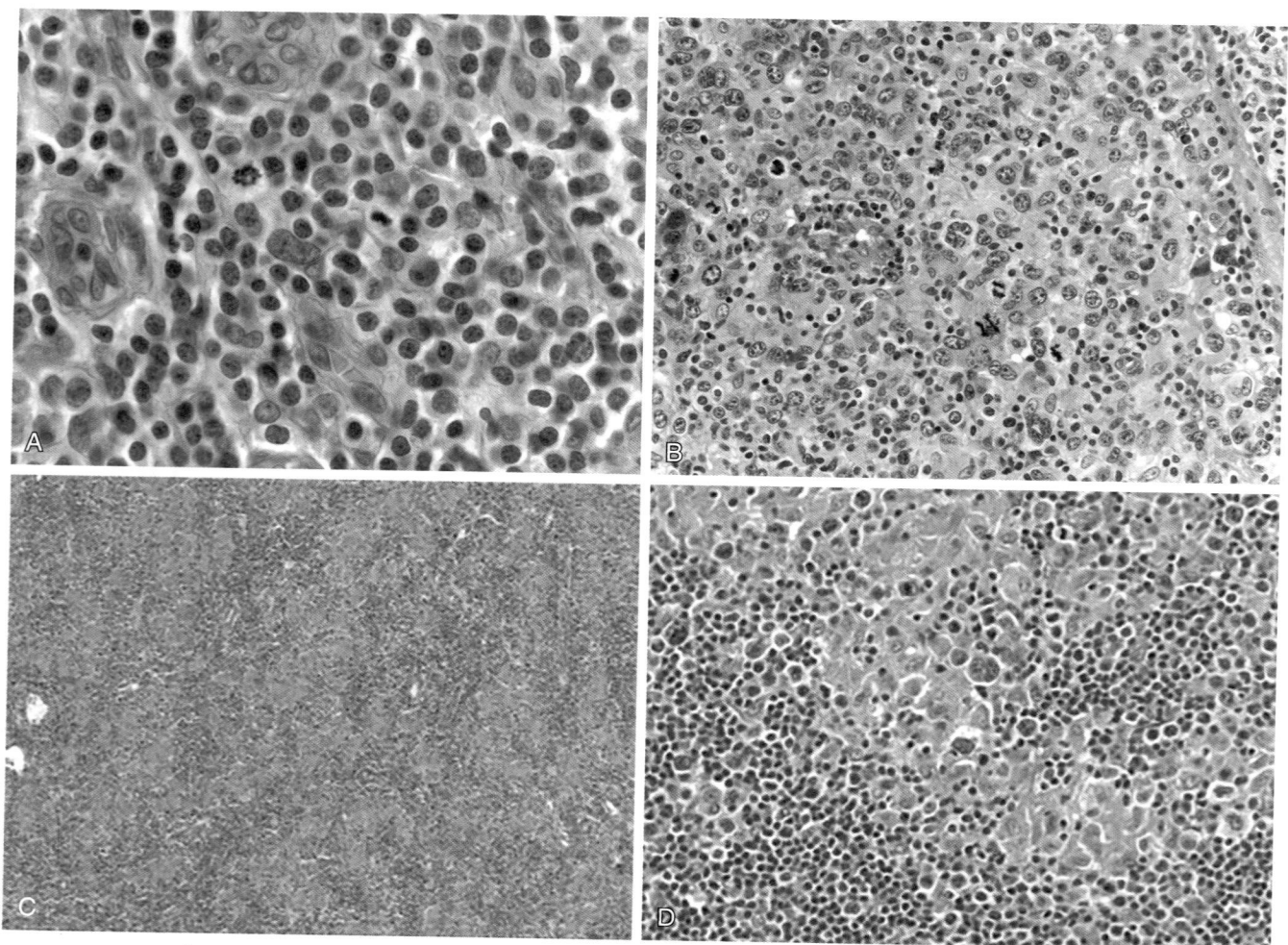

Figure 34-2. Morphologic spectrum of peripheral T-cell lymphoma, not otherwise specified. A, Peripheral T-cell lymphoma, not otherwise specified (PTCL, NOS) composed of pleomorphic medium-to-large-sized cells and occasional Reed-Sternberg (RS)–like cells. **B,** PTCL, NOS composed predominantly of small cells, with scattered large, transformed cells; note the presence of mitotic figures and nuclear irregularities. **C–D,** Lymphoepithelioid variant of PTCL, NOS (Lennert lymphoma) comprising prominent epithelioid histiocytes, imparting a vaguely granulomatous appearance; most lymphoma cells are small, and a few are larger, sometimes with RS-like morphology.

with weaker or heterogeneous intensity than expected in TFH lymphomas (see the cases illustrated in Figs. 34-7 and 34-9).[47] Regarding nuclear markers, PTCL, NOS is usually positive for Lymphoid Enhancer Binding Factor 1 (LEF1)[48] and negative for BCL6, FOXP3, and TCL1 transcription factors, which are, respectively, critical for TFH differentiation and function, related to regulatory T cells, and overexpressed in T-cell prolymphocytic leukemia.[49,50] A few cases of FOXP3-positive PTCL, NOS have been described in patients negative for HTLV1 infection; these cases were composed of large cells, some with EBV reactivation in bystander cells, and the clinical course was aggressive.[51] PTCL, NOS neoplastic cells variably express TBX21 (t-bet), and GATA3, which, in normal lymphoid cells, reflects Th1 and Th2 pathways of differentiation.[52]

CD20 and other B-cell markers usually highlight a small number of reactive B cells. In addition, in rare cases of PTCL, NOS (5% or less) the neoplastic cells co-express CD20 (Fig. 34-4). The intensity of CD20 expression may be dimmer than

that of normal B cells, and its distribution may be restricted to a subset of the neoplastic population that is otherwise positive for pan–T-cell antigen(s). It is unclear whether CD20 expression in PTCL, NOS reflects the derivation from a subset of CD20dim T cells that has undergone transformation, or is a marker of activation and proliferation of neoplastic T cells. There is no correlation with morphologic features and the anatomic sites of disease involvement are variable. CD20-positive PTCL, NOS occurs predominantly in elderly males and pursues an aggressive course in many cases. Expression of other B-cell markers (CD19, CD79a, PAX5) has been documented in rare cases of PTCL, NOS, but co-expression of several of them seems exceptional.[53-56]

The activation marker CD30 is often detected in occasional tumor cells, and can be more extensively expressed.[48,57,58] In a study of 141 PTCL, NOS, we found that 58% of the cases had in at least 5% CD30-positive tumor cells, and more than 20% of the cases were extensively positive (in 50% or more of the tumor cells).[58] Staining extent and intensity tend to

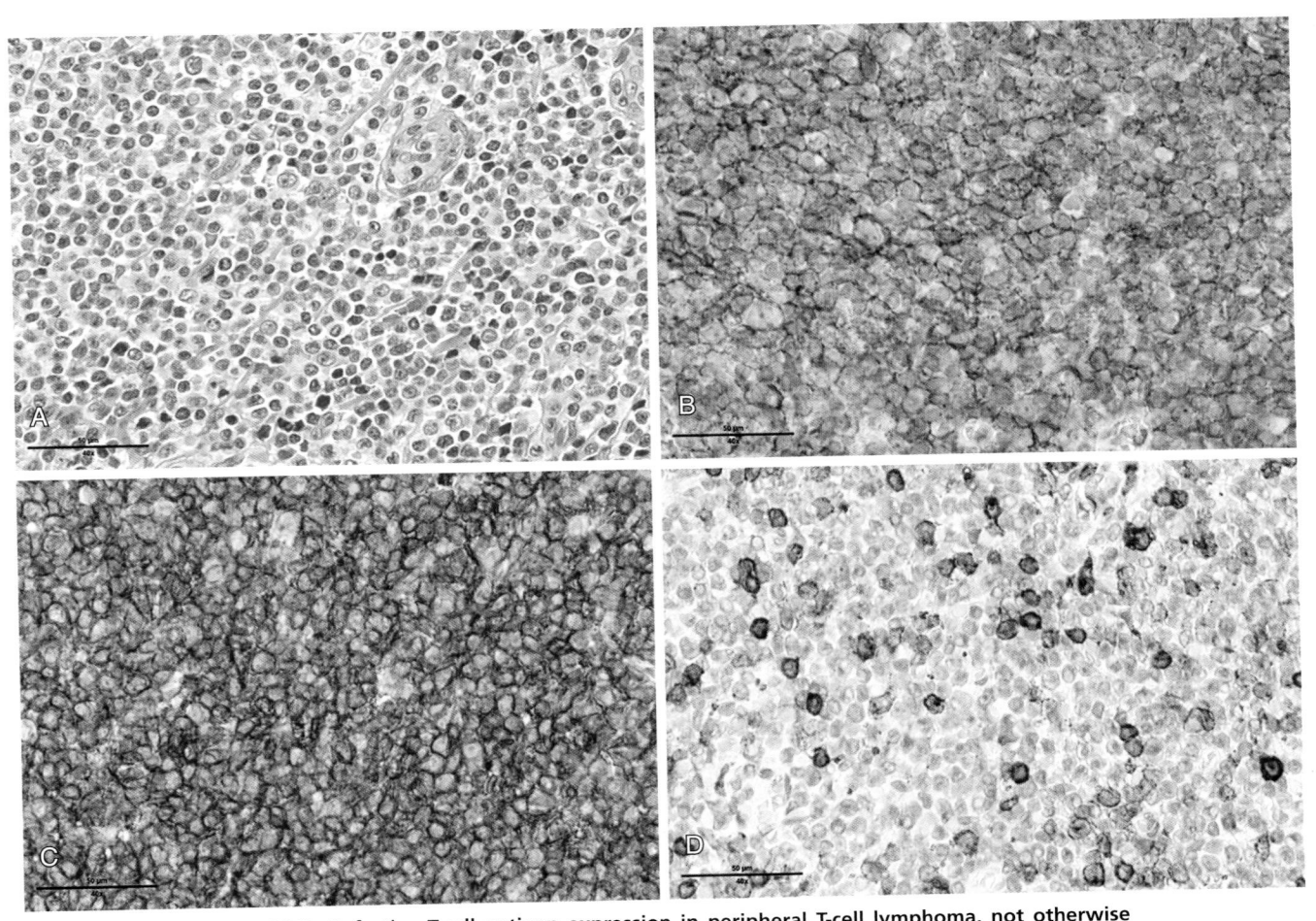

Figure 34-3. Defective T-cell antigen expression in peripheral T-cell lymphoma, not otherwise specified. A, This tumor comprises medium-sized and occasional larger cells. The neoplastic cells are positive for CD4 **(B)**, positive for CD5 **(C)**, and negative for CD7 **(D)**.

correlate, and are higher in cases with large cell morphology. Strong CD30 expression by a majority of the tumor cells is seen occasionally; in these cases, ALK expression must be excluded, and the differential diagnosis consideration is with ALK-negative ALCL. Co-expression of CD30 and CD15 has been reported in some PTCL, NOS, including a subset of cases containing RS–like cells mimicking classic Hodgkin lymphoma (Fig. 34-5), and the expression of CD15 in PTCL, NOS has been reported as an indicator of a poorer prognosis.[38,59] More recently, Fitzpatrick et al. described *JAK2* rearrangements in six cases of CD30-positive nodal T-cell lymphomas with anaplastic morphology and multinucleated cells resembling RS cells in a polymorphous background.[60] Three cases were classified as CD30-positive PTCL, NOS and three as ALK-negative ALCLs, and 4/5 cases were CD15 positive. The presence of *JAK2* fusions defines another genetic variation of ALK-negative ALCL in that context; nevertheless, additional studies are required to confirm these findings.

Besides its diagnostic value, CD30 immunohistochemistry may also inform therapeutic decisions given the availability of CD30 antibody-drug conjugates, which are approved for the treatment of PTCLs. For that purpose, it is recommended to report estimated percent positive expression in tumor cells (or total cells where applicable) and record descriptively if nontumor cells are positive.[61] Any degree of CD30 expression should be reported, and despite the fact that CD30-directed

treatment with brentuximab vedotin is significantly more effective against strongly CD30-positive PTCL, there have been responses observed in patients with very low or undetectable CD30 expression, and therefore, no threshold for positive versus negative expression is established.[62] The interleukin receptor (CD25), another potential target for immunotherapy in PTCL, acted on by a recombinant diphtheria toxin-IL-2 fusion protein, is expressed at significant levels in roughly 40% of PTCL, NOS.[42]

The Epstein-Barr virus (EBV) is detected in up to 50% of the cases, and this finding is correlated with a worse survival.[63,64] In most instances, only a small number of cells are positive by in situ hybridization and mainly represent bystander B cells, although in some cases it cannot be excluded that a fraction of the neoplastic cells may contain the virus.[63] In the rare instances where the majority of the tumor cells harbor EBV, these cases are now classified as a separate entity, namely primary nodal EBV-positive T/NK-cell lymphoma.

The presence of EBV-positive B-blasts or RS-like cells and the occurrence of EBV-negative clonal or monotypic plasma cell or B-cell proliferations with plasma cell differentiation, which are common in PTCLs of TFH origin, have been described less frequently in PTCL, NOS; however, some of these reports antedate the recognition of nodal PTCLs of TFH derivation, and it is uncertain whether they all represent true PTCL, NOS according to the current defining criteria.[65-67]

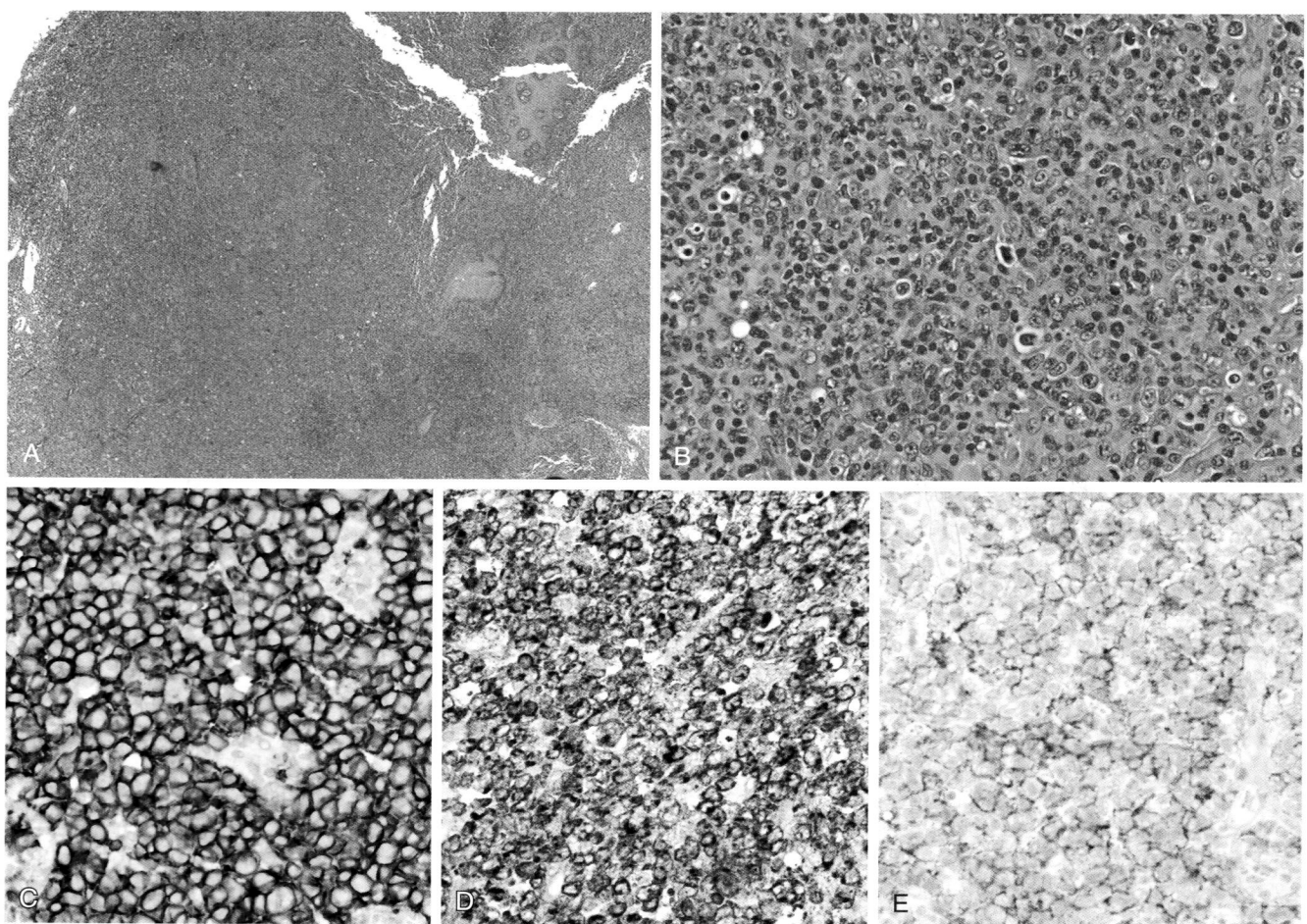

Figure 34-4. Peripheral T-cell lymphoma, not otherwise specified, CD20 positive. A, This case involved the tonsil as an interfollicular and diffuse infiltrate. **B,** The infiltrate was composed of medium-to-large-sized cells with multilobated forms, prominent nucleoli, and focal necrosis. The lymphoma cells are CD8 positive **(C),** show an activated cytotoxic phenotype (granzyme B positive) **(D),** and partially co-express CD20 **(E).** *(Courtesy from Aliyah Sohani and Judith Ferry, Massachusetts General Hospital, Boston, MA.)*

The HRS, which are often EBV positive, may express reduced levels of B-cell antigens, are almost always CD30-positive and also often CD15-positive (at least focally) (Fig. 34-6).[68] EBV-positive HRS-like cells were found almost constantly in cases of methotrexate-associated PTCL.[29] The importance of the B-cell expansion is variable and may be extensive, ranging from isolated or small clusters of activated B cells to confluent sheets of transformed B cells that may even partly obscure the neoplastic population.[65,66] In those instances, a secondary diagnosis of diffuse large B-cell lymphomas might be considered.

GENETIC AND MOLECULAR CHARACTERISTICS

Antigen Receptor Genes

Clonally rearranged TR genes can be demonstrated in most cases. Using the polymerase chain reaction (PCR)–based BIOMED-2 multiplex protocols, the clonality detection rate is >90% for each of both TRB or TRG targets, and reaches 100% when combining both strategies.[69] Simultaneous

detection of a clonal or oligoclonal immunoglobulin (IG) gene rearrangement has been reported in up to one-third of the cases, usually but not always in correlation with the presence of EBV-positive cells or morphologic evidence of a B-cell expansion.[70] The limitations of TR gene clonality assay based on fragment analysis, which encompass low sensitivity and the risk of false-positive results, are overcome by more recent next-generation sequencing (NGS) amplicon-based assays using primer sets targeting various regions of the TRB or TRG genes, which allows more accurate assessment of clonality, with precise identification and quantification of distinct clonal sequences.[71]

Genetic Abnormalities

By conventional cytogenetics, clonal aberrations comprising a vast number of different numerical and structural alterations have been described.[72-74] Complex karyotypes have been reported to correlate with larger cell morphology[73] and with an inferior outcome.[75] Virtually all cases harbor genetic imbalances, with gains outnumbering losses. By CGH,[75-77] recurrent gains have been observed in chromosomes 7q,[78]

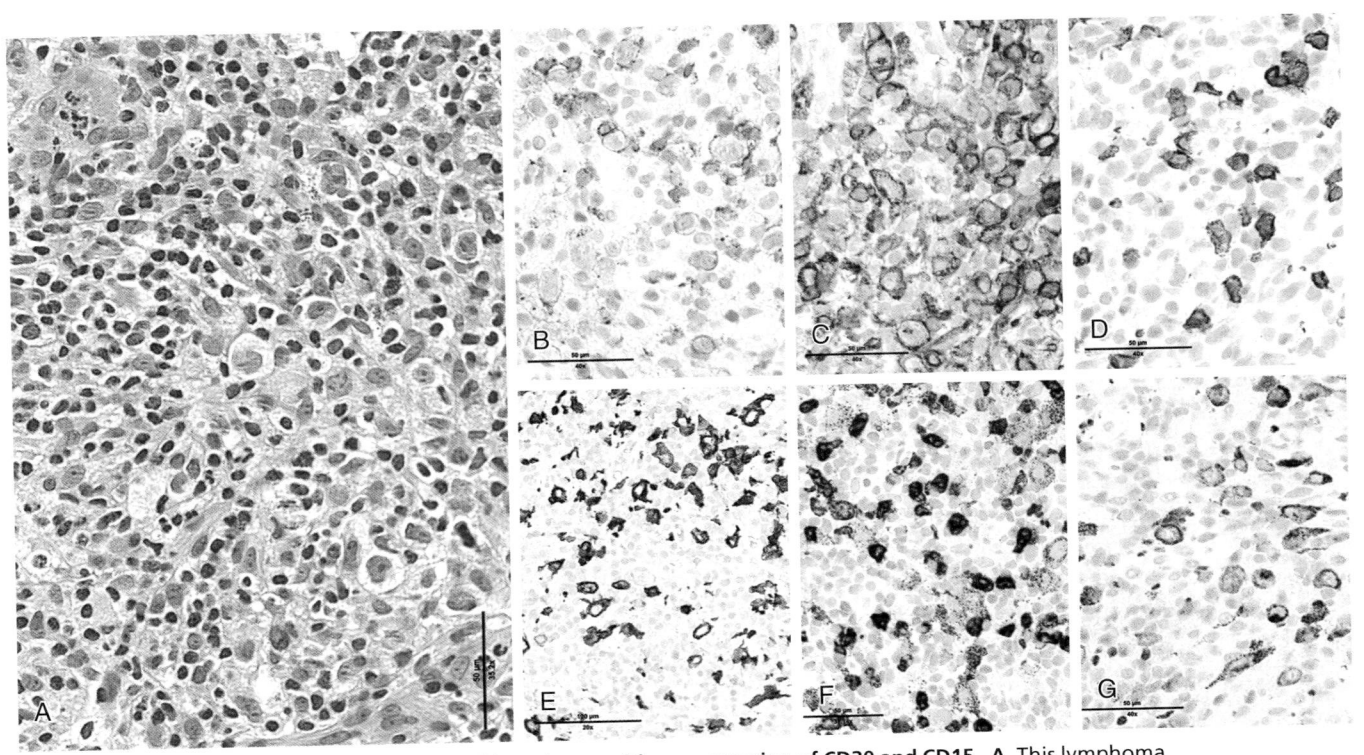

Figure 34-5. Peripheral T-cell lymphoma with co-expression of CD30 and CD15. A, This lymphoma comprises a pleomorphic population of smaller to larger cells including large, atypical cells with prominent nucleoli and abundant cytoplasm. **B,** The neoplastic cells show heterogeneous CD2 expression. They are positive for CD4 **(C)** and negative for CD8, which stains a few reactive cells in the microenvironment **(D).** CD30 is strongly positive in the larger cells **(E),** which are also CD15 positive **(F). G,** A cytotoxic phenotype is demonstrated by perforin expression.

8q,[77] 17q and 22q, and recurrent losses in chromosomes 4q, 5q, 6q, 9p, 10q, 12q, and 13q. In their study, Zettl et al. identified a group of nodal cytotoxic CD5-positive PTCL, NOS, associated with deletions in chromosomes 5q, 10q, and 12q, and with a better prognosis.[76] For a few altered loci, correlation with deregulated gene expression has been demonstrated, and by this approach a few genes of interest have been highlighted. For example, gains at 7q have been found to target cyclin-dependent kinase 6,[78] those at 8q involve the MYC locus,[77] losses at 9p21 associate with a reduced level of expression of two inhibitors of cyclin-dependent kinases, and gains at 7p22 correlate with increased levels of CARMA1, a factor involved in the activation of NF-κB.[79] A whole genome-sequencing study showed that CDKN2A and PTEN deletions are frequent (46% and 26% of the cases, respectively), and may co-occur, this event being specifically associated with PTCL, NOS and never observed in AITL.[80] CDKN2A deletions, which were found associated with shorter survival in that study, are recurrent in the GATA3 molecular subgroup of PTCL, NOS.[81]

Chromosomal breaks involving the TR gene loci (mostly the A/B TR locus at 14q11.2) have been reported in rare cases of PTCL, NOS, but the translocation partner(s) has been identified in only occasional cases.[75,82-84] The t(14;19)(q11;q13) translocation involves the poliovirus receptor-related 2 gene (PVRL2) and induces overexpression of both PVRL2 and BCL3 mRNAs.[85,86] The multiple myeloma oncogene-1/interferon regulatory factor-4 (IRF4) is the gene partner in chromosomal translocations involving the TRA gene in the t(6;14)(p25;q11.2) translocation described in rare

cases of clinically aggressive cytotoxic PTCL, NOS involving the bone marrow and skin or spleen (Fig. 34-7).[87,88]

High-throughput sequencing studies have discovered several recurrent fusion transcripts. Overall, their individual prevalence is low, and they are not specific for PTCL, NOS, as they also occur in other T-cell lymphoma entities, in particular ALK-negative ALCL or TFH lymphomas.[89-92] TP63 rearrangements with TBL1XR1 or other partner genes, encoding fusion proteins homologous to ΔNp63, a dominant-negative p63 isoform that inhibits the p53 pathway, are detected in about 5% of PTCL, NOS. TP63 rearrangements are associated with an aggressive clinical course and bad outcome.[93,94] Fusions involving VAV1 (VAV1::MYOF1, VAV1::THAP4, VAV1::S100A7) result in increased activation of VAV1 effector pathways and the oncogenic properties of VAV1::MYOF1 were demonstrated in mice in vivo.[95,96] The FYN::TRAF3IP2 fusion found in PTCL, NOS and TFH lymphomas activates the NF-κB pathway.[92,97] Fusions involving CD28 (CD28::CTLA4 and CD28::ICOS) occur in PTCL, NOS but are more common in TFH lymphomas and adult T-cell leukemia/lymphoma.[90]

The mutational landscape of PTCL, NOS includes recurrent mutations in epigenetic modifiers, most often TET2 or DNMT3A,[98] less commonly SMARCA4 or KMT2D, in genes related to the TCR signaling pathway, notably activating mutations in PLCG1, CD28 and VAV1.[89,99-101] Mutations in RHOA and IDH2 recurrent in TFH lymphomas, especially of AITL type, are not detected in PTCL, NOS. Alterations in TP53 (mutations or deletions, often biallelic) are detected in 40% of the cases, and portend an adverse prognostic significance.[81,102] One study found that alterations in TP53

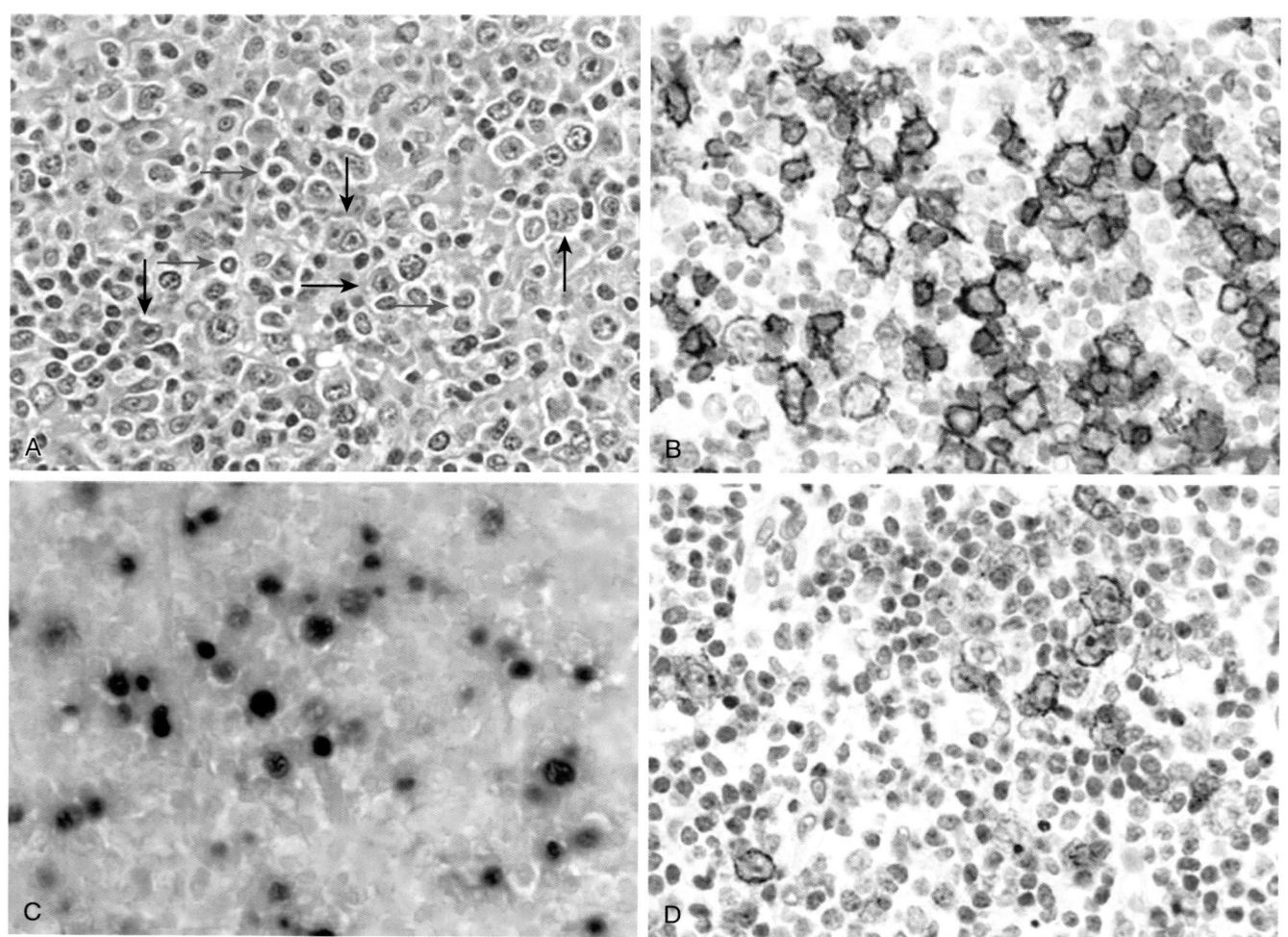

Figure 34-6. Epstein-Barr virus–positive B-cell blasts in peripheral T-cell lymphoma, not otherwise specified. A, Peripheral T-cell lymphoma, not otherwise specified (PTCL, NOS) comprising large atypical blastic cells, sometimes with prominent nucleoli, and sometimes binucleate *(black arrows)*; the neoplastic component is represented by medium-sized lymphoid cells with clear cytoplasm *(blue arrows)*. **B,** CD20 stains the large blastic cells and a few smaller cells. **C,** The B-cell blasts are positive for EBV as shown here by in situ hybridization. **D,** They are positive for CD30.

or *CDKN2A* delineate a group of PTCL, NOS characterized by marked genomic instability, mutations in genes related to immune surveillance and immune evasion *(HLA-A, HLA-B, CIITA, CD58, CD274)*, mutations in transcriptional and posttranscriptional regulators, and a worse outcome.[102]

VARIANTS AND SUBGROUPS

Lymphoepithelioid Variant of PTCL, NOS

The lymphoepithelioid variant of PTCL, NOS, originally described by Professor Karl Lennert in 1952 as a variant of Hodgkin disease, also known by the eponymous *Lennert's lymphoma* or *Lennert lymphoma*, is characterized by a prominent reactive infiltrate of epithelioid histiocytes, consisting mainly of mononucleate cells and distributed singly or more typically in small clusters (Fig. 34-2C–D).[103] The histiocyte cells may be so abundant to mimic a granulomatous reaction and obscure the neoplastic cells, which are small atypical T cells with slight nuclear irregularities.[30] In addition, RS-like cells, eosinophils,

and plasma cells are also commonly seen.[104] The pattern of Lennert lymphoma is usually diffuse but may be interfollicular. Lennert lymphoma is overall rare, accounting for less than 10% of PTCL, NOS in historical series.[12] In addition, in recent years, reassessment of Lennert's own files and other small cohorts of such cases has revealed that many cases of PTCL with a lymphoepithelioid pattern in fact correspond to histiocyte-rich TFH lymphomas of the angioimmunoblastic type or NOS.[105-107] Thus, only a fraction (actually a minority) of lymphoepithelioid T-cell lymphomas remain categorized as PTCL, NOS according to current criteria. These lymphomas tend to mostly involve lymph nodes, are derived from CD8-positive cells in the majority of cases, but may also be CD4 positive, double positive, or double negative, and are characterized by a nonactivated cytotoxic immunophenotype.[39,108,109] Lymphoepithelioid PTCL has been found to be associated with an overall better prognosis than usual PTCL, NOS,[12] and in comparison to patients with lymphoepithelioid lymphoma of TFH derivation, those with lymphoepithelioid PTCL, NOS were found to have a better outcome.[107,109]

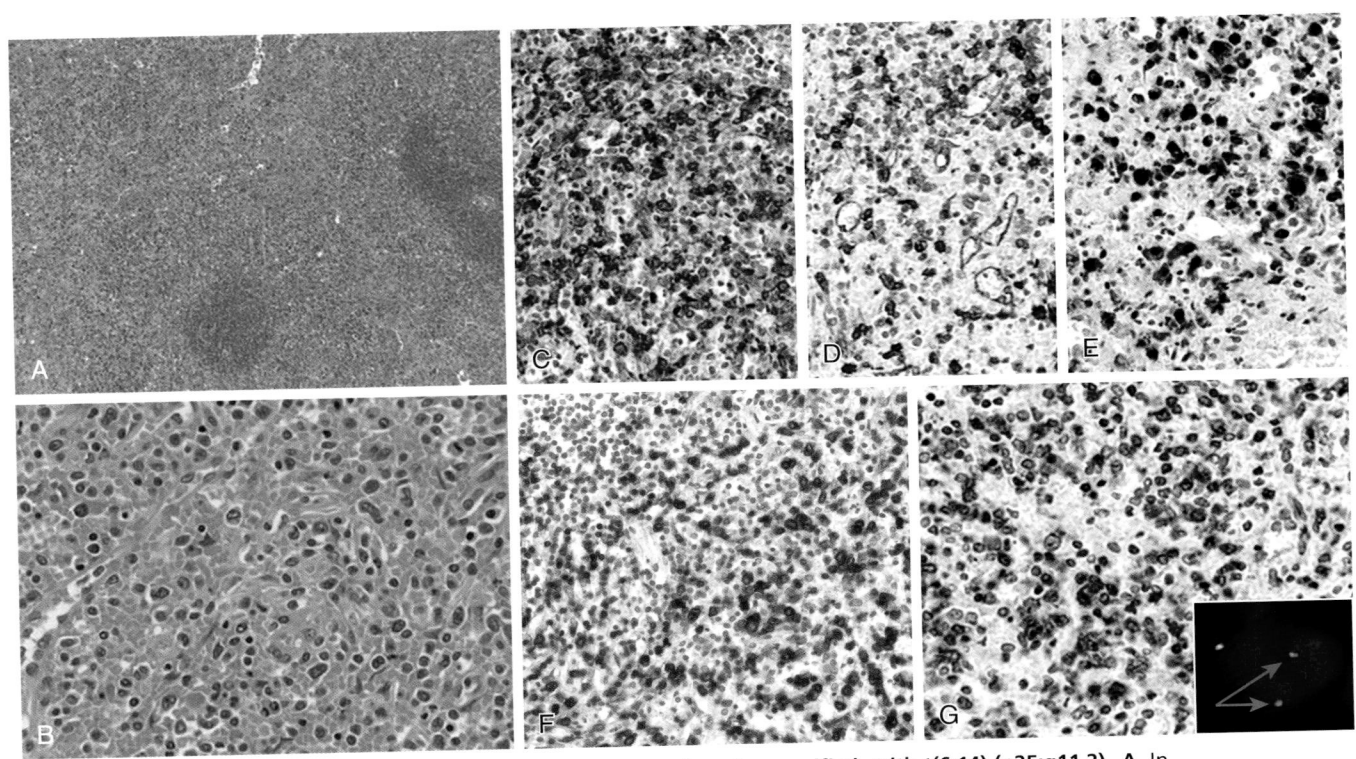

Figure 34-7. Peripheral T-cell lymphoma, not otherwise specified, with t(6;14) (p25;q11.2). A, In this case presenting with splenomegaly, the lymphoma cells diffusely infiltrate the red pulp and colonize the outer layers of the white pulp. **B,** The lymphoma cells are large and pleomorphic. **C,** They express CD4. **D,** A subset are CD8 positive. **E,** They are positive for granzyme B. **F,** They express the alpha/beta TCR isoform (BetaF1 immunostaining). **G,** The lymphoma cells are also positive for PD1 despite being clearly cytotoxic, emphasizing that PD1 expression alone is not specific of a T-cell follicular helper (TFH) immunophenotype. *Inset:* Break-apart fluorescence in situ hybridization (FISH) assay with probes spanning the *IRF4* locus at 6p25, demonstrating one red, one green, and one yellow signal in the large nuclei of the lymphoma cells, indicative of an *IRF4* rearrangement.

Cytotoxic Molecule–Positive PTCL, NOS

Cytotoxic molecule–positive PTCL, NOS, is defined by the expression of one to several cytotoxic granule–associated antigens. Those most routinely tested are T-cell intracellular antigen-1 (TIA-1), which is expressed by both resting and activated cytotoxic T cells, and perforin and granzyme B, considered to be expressed upon activation, and is by definition EBV–negative. Nodal cytotoxic PTCLs composed of EBV-positive neoplastic cells are now classified as a separate entity, namely primary nodal EBV-positive T/NK-cell lymphoma, discussed below.[1,33] Apart from the lymphoepithelioid variant of PTCL, NOS, a subset of PTCL, NOS, estimated to represent between 15% and up to 30% of the cases in different series, have cytotoxic features (Fig. 34-8).[38,39,46,108,110] There is no established cut-off to define the cytotoxic marker positivity, but we recommend positivity in the majority of the neoplastic cells. In most instances an activated cytotoxic phenotype is demonstrated, but some cases may be positive for TIA-1 only, and others may express granzyme B or perforin in the absence of TIA-1. Most case series of cytotoxic PTCL, NOS have been reported from Asia, often admixed with EBV-positive PTCLs. A large European cohort of 45 EBV-negative nodal cytotoxic PTCLs was recently published.[101] In that series, the disease affected predominantly males at a median age of 60 years, primary nodal presentation was associated with extranodal

involvement in the majority of cases, and an association with a previous history of B-cell lymphoma, solid cancer, or underlying immune disorder was noted in one-fifth of the cases. Patients presented with clinical and biological parameters indicative of an aggressive disease and the median survival was 13 months. Comparison with noncytotoxic PTCL, NOS in another study indicates a lower overall survival for cytotoxic PTCL, NOS.[46] Accordingly, a molecular subgroup of PTCL, NOS defined by a cytotoxic signature was also found associated with a poorer survival.[111] Morphology of the tumors is variable, with predominantly medium-to-large-sized neoplastic cells and more or less abundant microenvironment. The neoplastic cells usually express CD2 and CD3, and frequently show partial or complete loss of CD5 or CD7. They are most commonly CD8+ or CD4–CD8–, less commonly CD4+ or CD4+ CD8+, and in most cases TCRβF1+ or TCR-silent, rarely TCR-γδ+.[39,46,101] One study from Japan found that a subset of cases with a CD5+ TCRαβ+ phenotype had a more indolent behavior.[112] CD30 co-expression is frequent and CD56 is expressed in rare cases, more commonly extranodal. Virtually all cases express Th1-associated markers TBX21 or CXCR3. Cytotoxic PTCL, NOS harbors frequent mutations in epigenetic modifiers, notably in *TET2* and *DNMT3A*, recurrent alterations affecting the T-cell receptor and JAK/STAT signaling pathways, including fusions involving *VAV1* and *CD28*, and *TP53* mutations in 18% of the cases.[101]

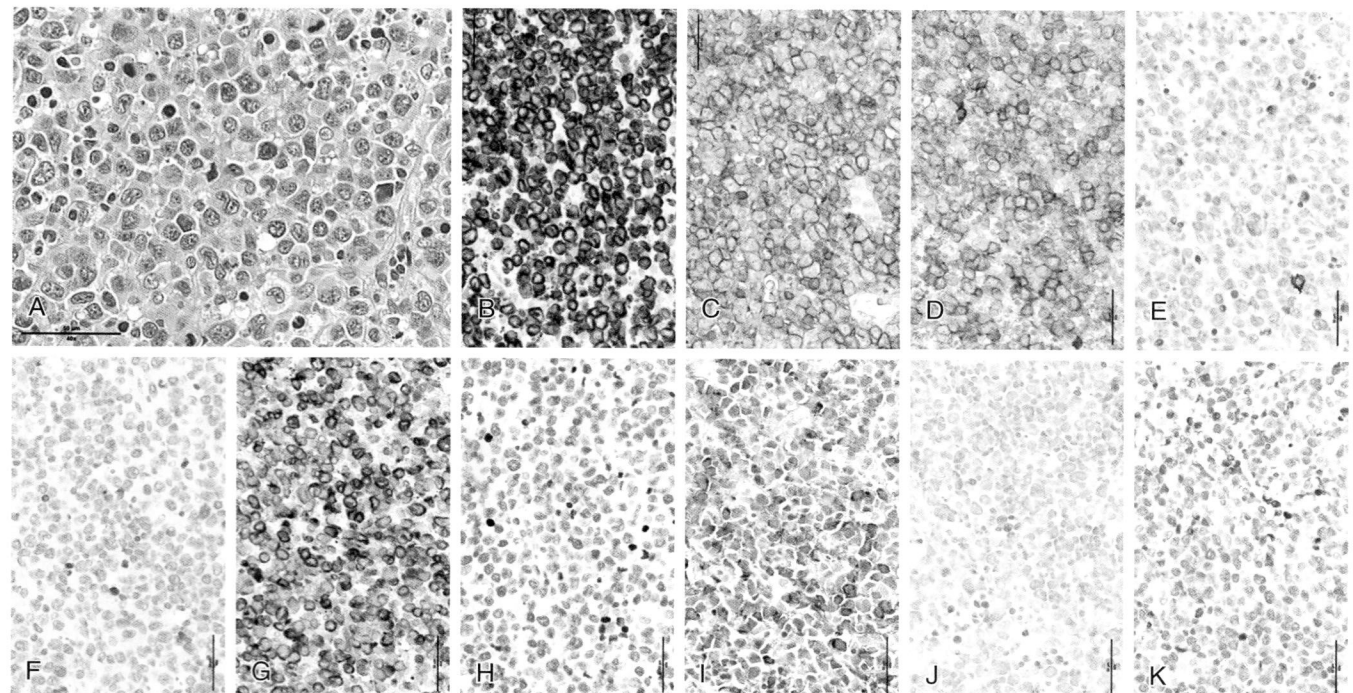

Figure 34-8. Cytotoxic TBX21-peripheral T-cell lymphoma, not otherwise specified. A, This nodal lymphoma is composed of large cells which are: CD3+ **(B)**, CD4+ **(C)**, CD5+ **(D)**, CD8− **(E)**, CD30− **(F)**, and strongly positive for perforin **(G). H,** TBX21 stained a few reactive cells and was negative in the neoplastic cells, which were otherwise positive for the other Th1-associated marker CXCR3 **(I)**, and negative for both Th2-associated markers GATA3 and CCR4 **(J and K)**.

Cell-of-Origin Subgroups

Earlier studies had suggested that subclasses of PTCL, NOS might be delineated by their immunologic profile according to the expression markers associated with Th1 (CXCR3, CCR5, CD134/OX40, CD69 T-bet) or Th2 [CCR4, CXCR4, ST2(L)] differentiation (Table 34-1).[113-117] Cases with expression of CXCR3, CCR5, or ST2(L) were reported to have a more favorable prognosis than those negative for these markers,[116,117] and nonoverlapping subgroups of PTCL, NOS defined by the expression of CCR4, CCR3, or CXCR3 had significantly different outcomes.[117] These classifiers have not been widely applied because of technical difficulty in assessing these markers, which often requires fresh frozen tissue.

By transcriptome profiling, Iqbal et al. have identified two molecular subgroups of PTCL, NOS—PTCL-TBX21 and PTCL-GATA3—based on the similarities of their signatures to those regulated by the transcription factors TBX21 and GATA3, which are master regulators of TH2 and TH1 differentiation pathways, respectively.[111] Hence, the TBX21 subgroup shows high expression of TBX21 and its target genes (*CCL3, CXCR3, EOMES, IFNG, ILR2B*) and enrichment of the NF-κB pathway. Conversely, the GATA3 subgroup is characterized by high expression of GATA3 and its target genes (*CCR4, CXCR7, IL18RA*), high MYC, and proliferation signatures.[111] Histologically, PTCL-TBX21 tends to be polymorphic with a background of reactive inflammatory cells, including cases of Lennert lymphoma, while PTCL-GATA3 tends to lack a prominent inflammatory microenvironment and consists of sheets of medium-sized tumor cells with abundant clear cytoplasm or clusters or sheets of large tumor cells (Fig. 34-9).[52] Further, GATA3-positive PTCL, NOS and cases with cytotoxic phenotype (clustered within the TBX21 subgroup) were found to have a worse outcome than noncytotoxic TBX21-positive tumors.[111,118,119] In addition, subsequent studies showed distinctive genetic features between the subgroups. PTCL-TBX21 has fewer copy number aberrations and a higher frequency of epigenetic-modifying gene mutations, especially those involved in DNA methylation (*TET1, TET3,* and *DNMT3A*). PTCL-GATA3 has greater genomic complexity; frequent losses of *TP53, PTEN, RB1, CDKN2A/B,* and *PRDM1*; gains of *STAT3* and *MYC*; and recurrent mutations of *TP53* and *PRDM1*,[81] probably explaining their worse prognosis. An immunohistochemical algorithm has been developed to distinguish these two groups originally defined by gene-expression profiling–based methods. The algorithm uses four antibodies: TBX21, CXCR3 (a TBX21 transcriptional target), GATA3, and CCR4 (a GATA3 transcriptional target), which are interpreted sequentially.[52] Positivity for TBX21 or CXCR3 in 20% or more of the neoplastic cells defines the TBX21 subgroup. Lymphomas negative or below the threshold for TBX21 markers are classified as GATA3 if they express GATA3 or CCR4 in 50% or more of the neoplastic cells. Other cases remain unclassified. More recently, a simplified transcriptomic assay based on quantification of 153 selected transcripts dedicated for the molecular diagnosis of the major PTCL entities including the two subtypes of PTCL, NOS, has been implemented on a digital gene-expression profiling platform and validated in routinely processed samples.[120] The identification of the

TBX21 and GATA3 subgroups currently has no effect on frontline clinical management of the patients and currently is not yet required or recommended in standard diagnostic practice.

Table 34-1 Comparison of TBX21 and GATA3 Subgroups of Peripheral T-Cell Lymphoma, Not Otherwise Specified

Feature	TBX21	GATA3
Frequency	50%–60% of PTCL, NOS	30%–40% of PTCL, NOS
Defining signature	High expression of TBX21 and its target genes (*CCL3, CXCR3, EOMES, IFNG, ILR2B*)	High expression of GATA3 and its target genes (*CCR4, CXCR7, IL18RA*)
Pathology	Polymorphous Cytotoxic subset	Medium-to-large-sized tumor cells Little inflammatory environment
Immunohisto-chemistry	TBX21 positive or CXCR3 positive	TBX21 negative and CXCR3 negative, GATA3 positive or CCR4 positive
Pathways	Enrichment of the NF-κB pathway	High MYC and proliferation signatures
Genetics	Relatively lower genomic complexity, mutations in epigenetic modifiers frequent	Higher genomic complexity, recurrent *TP53* alterations, *CDKN2A* and *PTEN* deletions
Outcome	Better than GATA3 except for the subset of cytotoxic cases	Worse than TBX21

EXTRANODAL PERIPHERAL T-CELL LYMPHOMA, NOT OTHERWISE SPECIFIED

Bone marrow involvement by PTCL, NOS is detected in 20% to 30% of the staging biopsies. It can be interstitial or diffuse, usually with hypercellularity and extensive replacement of the normal hematopoietic tissue, or focal, usually nonparatrabecular. Mirroring the lymph nodes, the bone marrow infiltrates are often pleomorphic and associated with prominent vascularity, increased reticulin fibrosis, and an admixed reactive inflammatory infiltrate.[121,122] Rarely the bone marrow may be the main presenting site of the disease (Fig. 34-10).[123,124] The few cases of primary bone marrow PTCL, NOS, some of which occurred in children, had an interstitial and diffuse infiltration pattern, with eosinophilia in some cases. The variably sized atypical tumor cells variably express CD4 and CD8, are EBV negative, and expression of cytotoxic granule–associated proteins and PD1 is documented in several cases.

Splenic infiltrates may be in the form of single or multiple discrete lesions, as a micronodular pattern, or as diffuse parenchymal involvement of the red and white pulps (Fig. 34-7). Localization to T-cell–dependent regions, such as the periarteriolar lymphoid sheath (PALS) or marginal zone, may be seen.[125] In the liver, there may be portal, lobular, or sinusoidal infiltrates.

The skin may be the first and main presenting site for PTCL, NOS, and conversely, cutaneous involvement is frequent in cases of systemic PTCL, NOS. While the WHO 5th ed. has created a new category for primary cutaneous

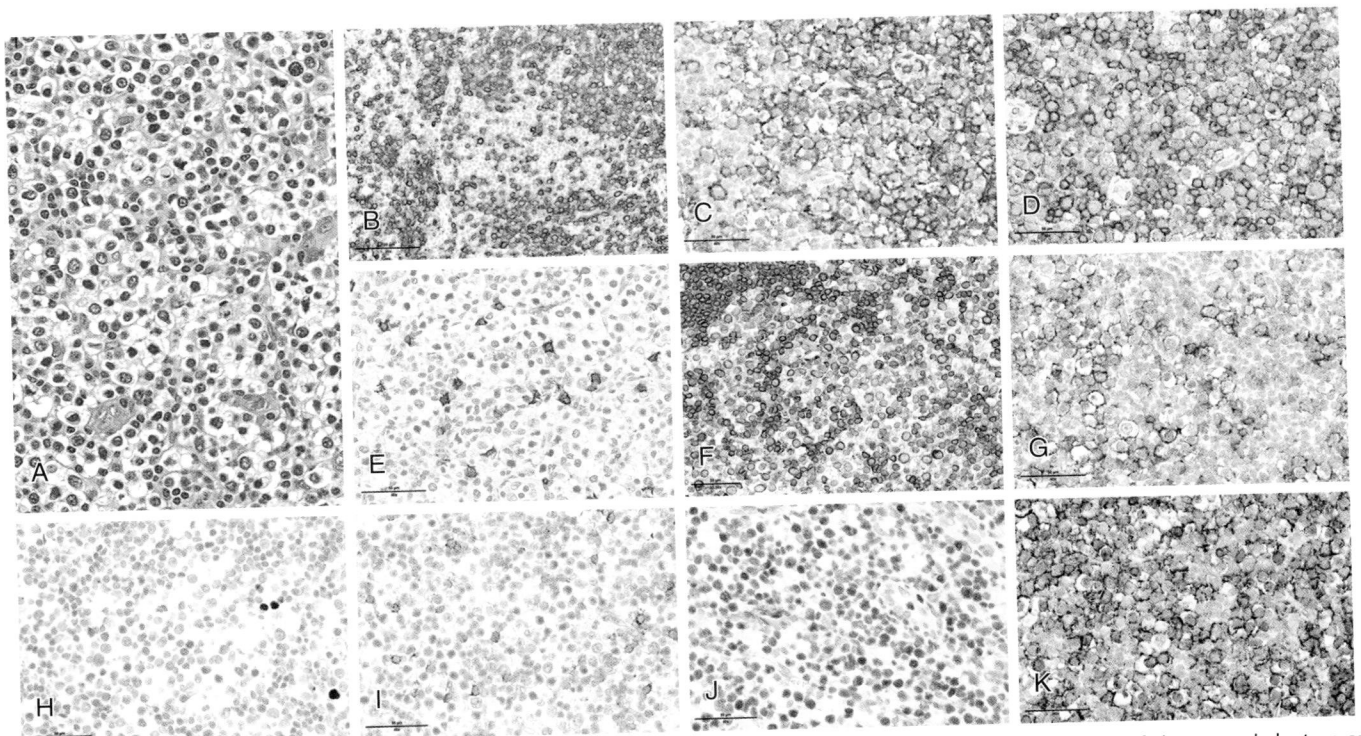

Figure 34-9. GATA3-peripheral T-cell lymphoma, not otherwise specified. A, This nodal lymphoma is composed of sheets and clusters of large cells with abundant clear cytoplasm. The neoplastic cells are CD3 positive **(B),** CD4 positive **(C),** CD5 positive **(D),** and CD8 negative **(E). F,** BCL2 is positive in the neoplastic cells with an intensity of staining weaker than in the reactive small lymphoid cells surrounding the aggregates of clear cells. **G,** The majority lymphoma cells are PD1 positive, but the other T-cell follicular helper (TFH) markers tested (BCL6, CD10, ICOS, and CXCL13) were not detected. The lymphoma cells are negative for TBX21 **(H)** and CXCR3 **(I),** and strongly positive for both GATA3 **(J)** and CCR4 **(K).**

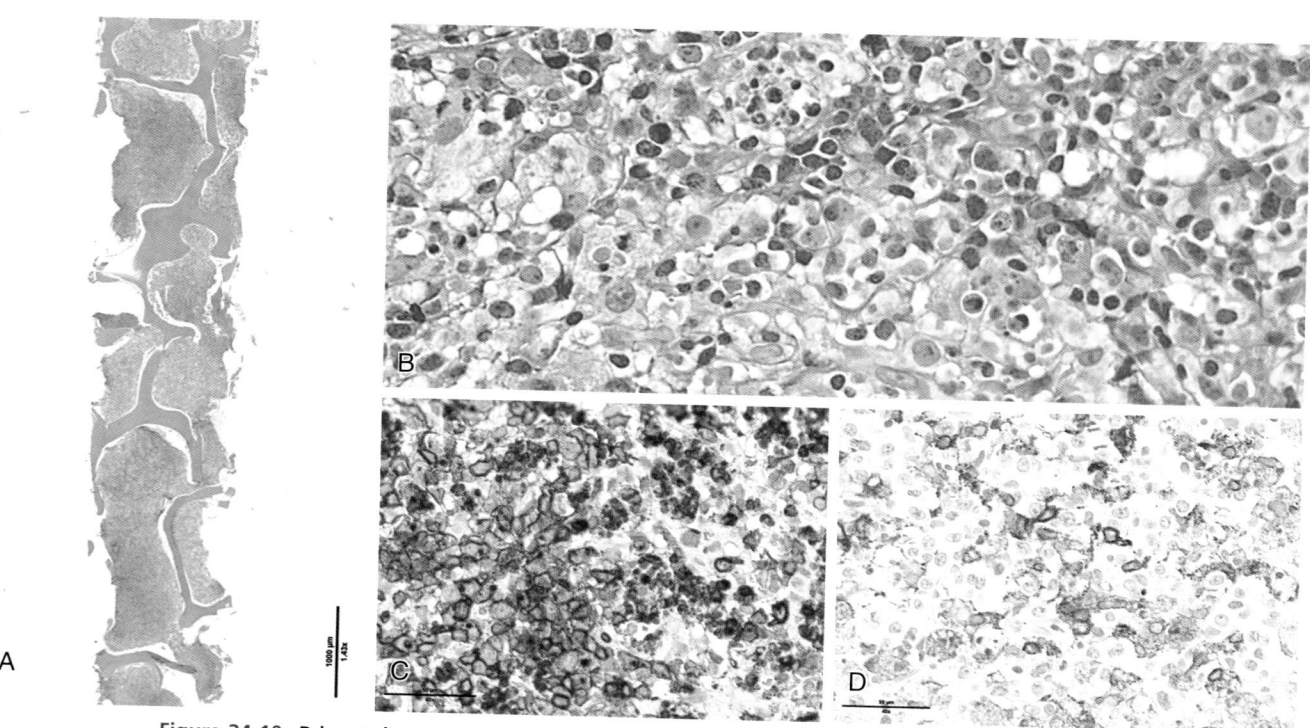

Figure 34-10. Primary bone marrow presentation of peripheral T-cell lymphoma, not otherwise specified. A, Low-power view of the trephine biopsy showing a diffusely, markedly hypercellular bone marrow. **B,** The hematopoietic tissue was replaced by a proliferation of large atypical lymphoid cells; there were numerous nuclear debris and accompanying macrophages. **C,** CD3 highlighted the neoplastic cells. **D,** CD163 stains many histiocytes and macrophages and shows hemophagocytosis.

PTCL, NOS, this entity does not exist in the 2022 ICC. So far, there are no available data to suggest that PTCL, NOS presenting in the skin should be recognized as a separate entity. In principle, PTCL, NOS may present in any extranodal site. The only exception is primary intestinal T-cell lymphoma, NOS, which is individualized from other PTCL, NOS because these cases presenting primarily in the gastrointestinal tract are potentially related to other primary intestinal T-cell lymphomas. Cutaneous infiltrates in PTCL, NOS can be diffuse, nodular, or bandlike; angiocentricity and epidermotropism can be seen.[126]

Primary central nervous system PTCL, NOS is a rare condition accounting for <5% of primary central nervous system lymphomas.[127,128] It affects mostly elderly individuals although a few cases have been reported in younger adults, and manifests with neurologic deficits. The lesions are unique or multiple, usually supratentorial, less often cerebellar. The neoplastic cells are small-to-medium or medium-to-large, and necrosis and perivascular cuffing are frequently observed. They express CD3, CD8, or CD4, often show aberrant T-cell antigen loss, and most of the cases have a cytotoxic phenotype. The few cases analyzed at the genomic level have shown heterogeneous mutations in various genes mutated in other T-cell lymphomas.

PROGNOSIS AND PREDICTIVE FEATURES

PTCL, NOS is usually an aggressive disease, characterized by a poor response to therapy and frequent relapses. The 5-year overall survival of around 30% has not improved over the past years, and stratification of the patients according to the

standard IPI is helpful for prognostication of outcome.[12,13,129] Italian investigators have suggested a novel prognostic index for T-cell lymphomas (PIT) based on four variables (age, performance status, LDH levels, and bone marrow involvement) that might be more appropriate than the IPI for PTCL, NOS patients.[130] Besides clinical factors, selected pathologic and biological prognostic markers are summarized in Table 34-2.

PRIMARY NODAL EPSTEIN-BARR VIRUS–POSITIVE T/NATURAL KILLER–CELL LYMPHOMA

Primary nodal EBV-positive T/NK-cell lymphoma is a new provisional entity in the 2022 ICC of lymphoid neoplasms.[3] It was originally reported and described as *EBV-positive nodal cytotoxic PTCL* in several publications from Asia,[131-134] and it was introduced in the 4th ed. revised WHO classification as a variant of PTCL, NOS (primary EBV-positive nodal peripheral T/NK-cell lymphoma).[2] In 2022, both the ICC and the WHO classification recognized it as a distinct entity, with features different from both PTCL, NOS, and from EBV-associated extranodal NK/T-cell lymphoma, nasal type. The designation in the WHO 5th ed. is *EBV-positive nodal T- and NK-cell lymphoma.*[1] However, the word "primary" used in the ICC stresses one of the main criteria of the disease, namely that it should primarily involve lymph nodes, without nasal involvement.

Primary nodal EBV-positive T/NK-cell lymphoma is a rare disease with most series reported from Asia.[135] It is mostly diagnosed in elderly patients (median 60–65 years) or in a setting of HIV infection or other immunodeficiency conditions, and has a very poor prognosis with a median overall survival inferior to that of extranodal NK/T-cell lymphoma, nasal type (ENKTCL) and EBV-negative PTCL, NOS with a cytotoxic phenotype.[136] Patients tend to present with disseminated disease, generalized lymphadenopathy, frequent liver or spleen involvement, frequent B symptoms, and a high IPI. It is a systemic disease that lacks nasopharyngeal involvement. Such involvement should be investigated and excluded clinically. Involvement of other extranodal sites is variably reported in a small subset of patients.

Table 34-2 Pathologic Features of Peripheral T-Cell Lymphoma, Not Otherwise Specified With Suspected Prognostic Significance

Feature	More Favorable	Unfavorable
Morphology	Lymphoepithelioid variant	Predominance of large cells
Immunophenotype	CD4-positive phenotype Expression of CXCR3, CCR5, or ST2(L) TBX21/T-bet expression	CD8-positive or CD4–CD8-negative phenotype Expression of CCR4 GATA3 expression Cytotoxic phenotype Co-expression of CD20 Expression of p53
Epstein-Barr virus Cytogenetics	Absent	Present Complex karyotypes t(6;14) (p25;q11.2) translocation *TP63* rearrangements, *TP53* mutations, *CDKN2A* alterations
Molecular	NF-κB pathway activation TBX21 signature	Proliferation signature GATA3 signature

The tumors are most commonly monomorphic and composed of large cells with centroblastoid morphology (Fig. 34-11A). Some cases are pleomorphic and may contain tumor cells with horseshoe-like or reniform nuclei. The tumors lack angiocentricity or angioinvasion, and necrosis is usually absent or limited. A subset of cases display massive necrosis or apoptosis, are accompanied by disseminated intravascular coagulation or hematophagocytic syndrome, and pursue a very aggressive or fulminant course.[108,137,138] The neoplastic cells express cytotoxic markers and are usually CD3-positive, CD8-positive, and CD56-negative (Fig. 34-11B–E). The cells might express strong CD30, a pitfall in the diagnosis if EBV-encoded RNA (EBER) in situ hybridization is not performed. Demonstration of EBV in most neoplastic cells is an essential diagnostic feature (Fig. 34-11F). Primary nodal EBV-positive T/NK-cell lymphoma is more often of T-cell rather than NK-cell origin. About 85% of cases carry clonally rearranged TR genes and express TCRαβ more commonly than TCRγδ.[135,139] True NK-cell derivation is inferred from silent TCR expression and lack of monoclonal TR gene rearrangements.

Primary EBV-positive nodal T/NK cell lymphoma is characterized by low genomic instability, upregulation of immune pathways within enhanced expression of proteins related to immune evasion such as the checkpoint protein PD-L1, and downregulation of EBV microRNAs. Few cases have been investigated by high-throughput sequencing and revealed recurrent mutations in *TET2*, *DNMT3A*, *STAT3*, *PIK3CD*, and *DDX3X*.[101,136]

DIAGNOSTIC APPROACH TO PERIPHERAL T-CELL LYMPHOMA, NOT OTHERWISE SPECIFIED AND DIFFERENTIAL DIAGNOSES

The two components of PTCL, NOS diagnosis are, first, establishing a diagnosis of a neoplastic T-cell process, and

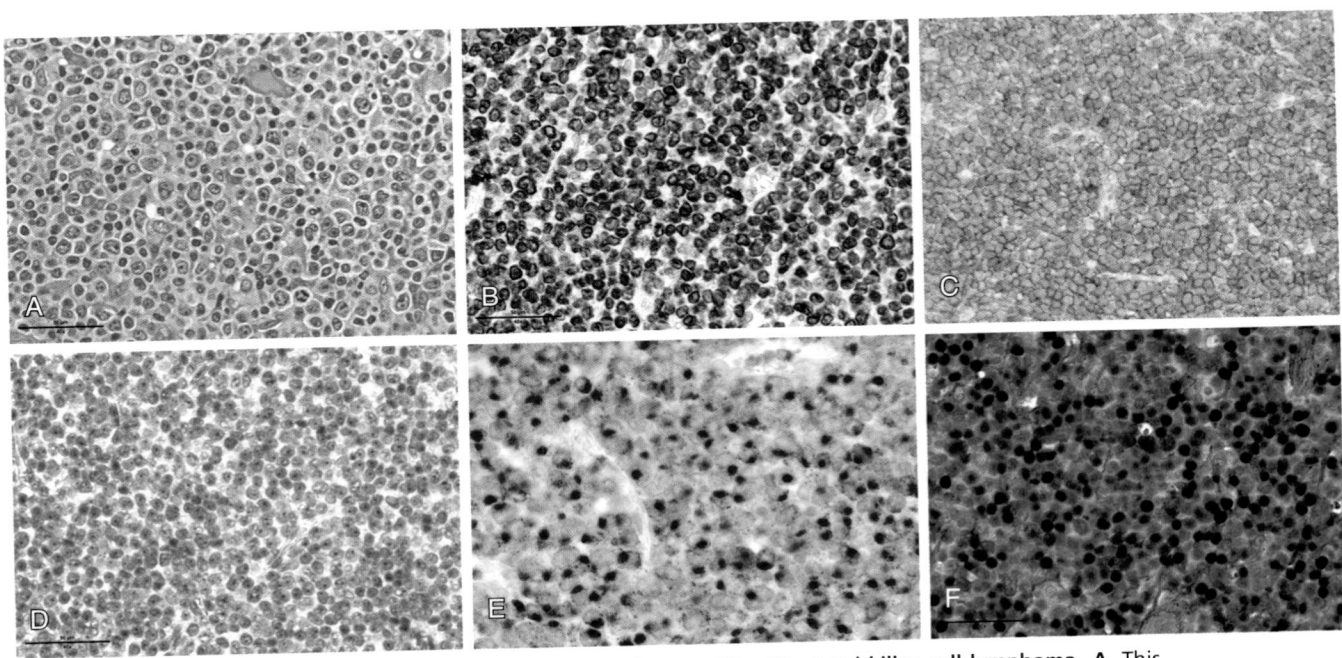

Figure 34-11. Primary nodal Epstein-Barr virus–positive T/natural killer–cell lymphoma. A, This lymphoma comprises diffuse sheets of large centroblastic-like monomorphic cells with no angiotropism or necrosis. The lymphoma cells are CD3 positive **(B)**, CD8 positive **(C)**, negative for CD56 **(D)**, and homogeneously express granzyme B **(E)**. **F,** Most cells are positive for Epstein-Barr virus (EBV), as demonstrated by in situ hybridization with EBV-encoded RNA probes.

second, excluding specific entities, including other nodal or extranodal entities and tissue involvement by leukemic T-cell neoplasms such as T-cell prolymphocytic leukemia. The diagnostic algorithm (Fig. 34-12) requires integration of clinical findings, including site of the disease, potential predisposing conditions like celiac disease, and HTLV1 serology, which should be systematically performed. The work-up characteristically integrates assessment of morphology, immunophenotype, and clonality studies. However, high-throughput sequencing, which is increasingly performed in the diagnostic setting, may provide additional information relevant not only to the diagnosis but potentially to inform therapeutic decisions.[140]

Peripheral T-Cell Lymphoma, Not Otherwise Specified Versus Reactive Lymphoid Hyperplasia

Cases of PTCL, NOS consisting predominantly of small T cells may be confused with a reactive process. This relates particularly to cases showing a preserved architecture with residual, sometimes hyperplastic B-cell follicles, and interfollicular ("T-zone") involvement, and to lymphoepithelioid (Lennert) lymphomas. The correct diagnosis can usually be established by careful morphologic and immunohistologic appraisal: a greater degree of architectural perturbation, extranodal extension of the lymphoproliferation, and cytologic atypia are typically found in cases of lymphoma, as is the demonstration

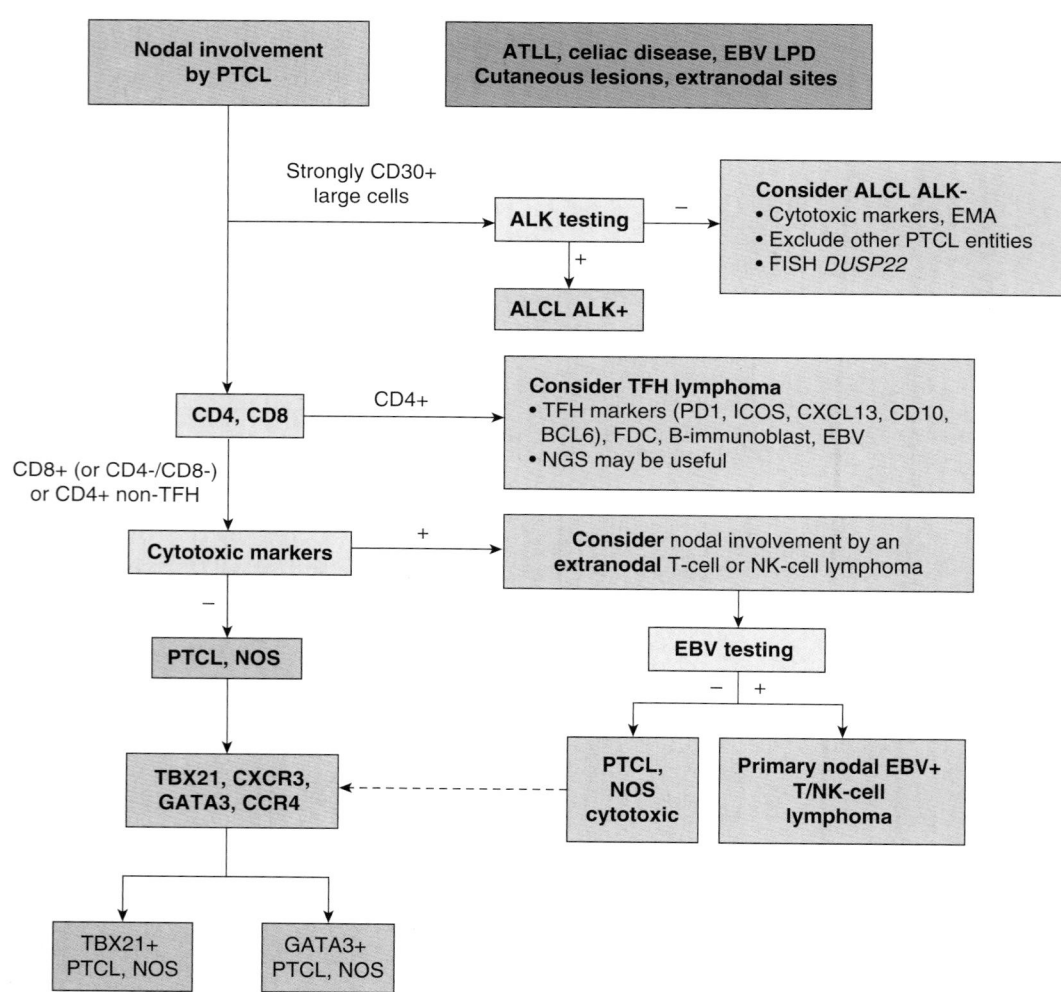

Figure 34-12. Diagnostic work-up of peripheral T-cell lymphoma, not otherwise specified. In cases of suspected nodal involvement by peripheral T-cell lymphoma, not otherwise specified (PTCL, NOS), clinical history and presenting clinical characteristics are important to consider. Adult T-cell leukemia/lymphoma, which is morphologically diverse, is suspected in patients from an endemic area in the presence of a CD4-positive neoplasm with lack of CD7 expression and CD25 positivity and is confirmed by human T lymphotropic virus 1 (HTLV1) infection. Distinction from anaplastic large cell lymphoma (ALCL) largely relies upon morphology and staining for CD30 and ALK. In CD4-positive PTCL, evaluation of T-cell follicular helper (TFH) markers, follicular dendritic cell meshworks, Epstein-Barr virus (EBV), and mutation analyses in some cases, are necessary to exclude TFH PTCL. Many of the cases where morphology raises a differential diagnosis between angioimmunoblastic T-cell lymphoma and PTCL, NOS, are now classified as TFH lymphomas. Cytotoxic marker expression raises the possibility of nodal involvement by an extranodal PTCL or natural killer (NK)/T-cell lymphoma, which requires integration of staging information. In the presence of an EBV-positive cytotoxic lymphoma, either of NK-cell or T-cell derivation, the possibility of secondary localization of extranodal NK/T-cell lymphoma, nasal type (ENKTCL) must be clinically excluded. At present, testing for TBX21 and GATA3 subgroups is not mandatory in routine diagnostic practice. (*Adapted from Campo E, Jaffe ES, Cook JR, et al. The International Consensus Classification of Mature Lymphoid Neoplasms: a report from the Clinical Advisory Committee. Blood. 2022;140(11):1229-1253.*)

of an aberrant T-cell immunophenotype, with loss of T-cell antigen expression. Assessment of clonality is in general desirable to formally confirm the diagnosis. The detection of somatic mutations using high-throughput sequencing may represent a useful adjunct to PCR-based assays for TR clonality testing to establish or, conversely, to exclude the presence of a clonal T-cell population.[141]

In children, the autoimmune lymphoproliferative syndrome (ALPS), a primary immune disorder caused by mutations in the *FAS/FAS-L* leading to defective apoptosis, is characterized by the expansion of a population of double-negative CD4−CD8-mature T cells that enlarges the paracortex of lymph nodes and may mimic PTCL because of its aberrant phenotype.[142] The associated clinical circumstances of autoimmune cytopenias often present, the pediatric age group, and the presence of circulating lymphocytes with the aberrant double-negative immunophenotype with increased CD57-positive T cells are useful hints to the correct diagnosis. Necrotizing lymphohistiocytic lymphadenitis (Kikuchi's disease) comprises a paracortical expansion of activated cytotoxic T cells and histiocytes that is morphologically atypical and may be confused with PTCL.[143,144] The morphologic features and criteria of these diseases are thoroughly described in Chapters 53 and 8, respectively.

Peripheral T-Cell Lymphoma, Not Otherwise Specified With Reed-Sternberg–Like Cells

Large lymphoid cells with RS-like morphology are found frequently in PTCL, NOS. These cells are either part of the neoplastic clone or represent EBV-positive bystander B cells, and by immunohistochemistry may be positive for CD30, or even occasionally positive for both CD30 and CD15. These findings may raise the differential diagnoses with classic Hodgkin lymphoma, reactive EBV-positive lymphoproliferation (infectious mononucleosis), T-cell/histiocyte-rich large B-cell lymphoma, and AITL (Table 34-3).

Lymphoepithelioid Variant of Peripheral T-Cell Lymphoma, Not Otherwise Specified (Lennert Lymphoma)

This variant must be distinguished from other conditions associated with a prominent epithelioid infiltrate: reactive granulomatous conditions, classic Hodgkin lymphoma, mixed cellularity,[145] T-cell/histiocyte–rich large B-cell lymphoma, lymphoplasmacytic lymphoma with a high content of epithelioid cells,[146] and TFH lymphoma with a high content of epithelioid cells (Table 34-3).[147] Indeed, a reappraisal of Lennert's personal collection revealed that many cases previously categorized as lymphoepithelioid/Lennert lymphoma in fact represent examples of histiocyte-rich TFH lymphoma of angioimmunoblastic type or NOS.[105,106]

CD30-Positive Peripheral T-Cell Lymphoma, Not Otherwise Specified

PTCL, NOS occasionally displays strong and homogeneous expression of CD30 in most neoplastic cells, and in those instances, differential diagnosis with ALCL, ALK negative constitutes a major challenge. The distinction is of clinical relevance because ALCL, ALK negative is associated with a better prognosis than PTCL, NOS.[148] *DUSP22* rearrangements recently described in association with ALK-negative ALCL, have not been found in PTCL, NOS, and may represent a useful adjunct to the diagnosis.[149] Another area of confusion is between CD30-positive PTCL, NOS and classic Hodgkin lymphoma, inasmuch as CD30-positive PTCL, NOS occasionally co-expresses CD15. The distinguishing features that are useful to consider in these settings are summarized in Table 34-4.

Table 34-3 Differential Diagnosis of Peripheral T-Cell Lymphoma, Not Otherwise Specified With Reed-Sternberg–Like Cells

	PTCL, NOS With RS-Like Cells		Classic Hodgkin Lymphoma	Reactive EBV⁺ Lymphoproliferation	T-Cell/ Histiocyte–Rich Large B-Cell Lymphoma	TFH Lymphoma
RS-(like) cells	T cells EBV− CD30+/− CD15− Neoplastic	B cells EBV+/− CD30+/− CD15+/− Reactive	B cells EBV+/− CD30+ CD15+/− Neoplastic	B cells EBV+ CD30+ CD15− Reactive	B cells EBV− CD30− CD15− Neoplastic	B cells EBV+ CD30+ CD15−/+ Reactive
T cells	Atypical, often pleomorphic CD4+, CD8+ or other		Small, no atypia CD4+ > CD8+	Small and large, usually no atypia CD8+ > CD4+	Small, no atypia CD4+ and CD8+	Atypical, medium-sized, clear cells TFH phenotype
Epithelioid histiocytes	Variable		Variable	No	Abundant	Variable
Eosinophils, plasma cells	Variable		Present	Usually few	Absent	Present
Follicular dendritic cell meshworks	Not expanded		Not expanded	Not expanded	Not expanded	Expanded in the angioimmunoblastic type
TR genes rearrangement	Monoclonal		Polyclonal	Polyclonal	Polyclonal	Monoclonal
IG genes rearrangement	Sometimes monoclonal		Polyclonal or monoclonal	Polyclonal	Monoclonal	Polyclonal or monoclonal
Somatic mutations	*TET2, DNMT3A* No *RHOA, IDH2* *PLCG1, CD28, VAV1, TP53*, others		Usually not detected on tissue sections	Absent	Usually not detected on tissue sections	*TET2, DNMT3A, RHOA, IDH2*, others

EBV, Epstein-Barr virus; *PTCL, NOS,* peripheral T-cell lymphoma, not otherwise specified; *RS,* Reed-Sternberg; *TFH,* T-follicular helper cell.

Table 34-4 Differential Diagnosis of CD30-Positive Peripheral T-Cell Lymphoma, Not Otherwise Specified

	CD30-Positive PTCL, NOS	Anaplastic Large Cell Lymphoma, ALK-Negative	Classic Hodgkin Lymphoma
Neoplastic cells	Often large cells Monomorphic or polymorphic +/– RS-like cells	Hallmark cells	RS cells
Pattern	Diffuse	Cohesive growth, sinusoidal pattern	Variable
Eosinophils, plasma cells	Variable	Usually absent	Present
CD30	CD30+	CD30+	CD30+
CD15	CD15–/+	CD15–/+	CD15+/–
B-cell antigens	Usually negative, rarely CD20+	Usually negative, rarely PAX5+	CD20–/+, weakly PAX5+
T-cell antigens	+/–	–/+	–/+
T-cell receptor expression	$\alpha\beta > \gamma\delta$	Often negative or reduced	Absent
Cytotoxic molecules	–/+	+	Usually negative, rarely positive
EMA	–/+	+/–	–
EBV in neoplastic cells	Negative	Negative	Negative or positive
TR genes rearrangement	Monoclonal	Monoclonal	Polyclonal
IG genes rearrangement	Polyclonal	Polyclonal	Polyclonal or monoclonal
Somatic mutations	TET2, DNMT3A No RHOA, IDH2 PLCG1, CD28, VAV1, TP53, VAV1, CD28 fusions JAK2 fusions?	JAK/STAT pathway mutations TP53 mutations DUSP22, TP63 fusions JAK2 and other tyrosine kinase gene fusions	Usually not detected on tissue sections

+, Nearly always positive; –/+, usually negative, may be positive; +/–, usually positive, may be negative; *EBV,* Epstein-Barr virus; *EMA,* epithelial membrane antigen; *PTCL, NOS,* peripheral T-cell lymphoma, not otherwise specified; *RS,* Reed-Sternberg.

Pearls and Pitfalls

- Peripheral T-cell lymphoma, not otherwise specified (PTCL, NOS) is a "by default" entity, which requires exclusion of other potential diagnoses. Notably, because the diagnosis of follicular helper T-cell (TFH) lymphoma has been expanding, the prevalence of PTCL, NOS in recent registries is decreasing.
- A T-cell aberrant immunophenotype is indicative of malignancy and present in most cases of PTCL, NOS. High-throughput sequencing is a useful adjunct to other ancillary studies to guide the diagnosis of PTCL, NOS, and potentially to inform therapeutic decisions.
- Two molecular subgroups of PTCL, NOS—TBX21 and GATA3—defined by their gene-expression signature, correspond to distinct pathogenic pathways and outcomes, and can be approached by an immunohistochemistry algorithm.

KEY REFERENCES

43. Siddiqui F, Perez Silos V, Karube K, et al. B-cell lymphoma-2 downregulation is a useful feature supporting a neoplastic phenotype in mature T-cell lymphomas. *Hum Pathol.* 2022;125:48–58.
52. Amador C, Greiner TC, Heavican TB, et al. Reproducing the molecular subclassification of peripheral T-cell lymphoma-NOS by immunohistochemistry. *Blood.* 2019;134(24):2159–2170.
81. Heavican TB, Bouska A, Yu J, et al. Genetic drivers of oncogenic pathways in molecular subgroups of peripheral T-cell lymphoma. *Blood.* 2019;133(15):1664–1676.
101. Nicolae A, Bouilly J, Lara D, et al. Nodal cytotoxic peripheral T-cell lymphoma occurs frequently in the clinical setting of immunodysregulation and is associated with recurrent epigenetic alterations. *Mod Pathol.* 2022;35(8):1126–1136.
102. Watatani Y, Sato Y, Miyoshi H, et al. Molecular heterogeneity in peripheral T-cell lymphoma, not otherwise specified revealed by comprehensive genetic profiling. *Leukemia.* 2019;33(12):2867–2883.
106. Hartmann S, Agostinelli C, Klapper W, et al. Revising the historical collection of epithelioid cell-rich lymphomas of the Kiel Lymph Node Registry: what is Lennert's lymphoma nowadays? *Histopathology.* 2011;59(6):1173–1182.
124. Attygalle AD, Zamo A, Fend F, Johnston P, Arber DA, Laurent C. Challenges and limitations in the primary diagnosis of T-cell and natural killer cell/T-cell lymphoma in bone marrow biopsy. *Histopathology.* 2020;77(1):2–17.
135. Kato S, Yamashita D, Nakamura S. Nodal EBV+ cytotoxic T-cell lymphoma: a literature review based on the 2017 WHO classification. *J Clin Exp Hematop.* 2020;60(2):30–36.
136. Wai CMM, Chen S, Phyu T, et al. Immune pathway upregulation and lower genomic instability distinguish EBV-positive nodal T/NK-cell lymphoma from ENKTL and PTCL-NOS. *Haematologica.* 2022;107(8):1864–1879.
140. de Leval L, Alizadeh AA, Bergsagel PL, et al. Genomic profiling for clinical decision making in lymphoid neoplasms. *Blood.* 2022;140(21):2193–2227.

Visit Elsevier eBooks+ for the complete set of references.

Follicular Helper T-Cell Lymphoma

Leticia Quintanilla-Martinez and German Ott

DEFINITION

Follicular helper T-cell (TFH) lymphomas are nodal, mature T-cell lymphomas that share immunophenotypic features and the gene-expression signature of TFHs,[1] a specialized subset of T cells that constitute a component of secondary lymphoid follicles and that are essential for the formation of germinal centers, affinity maturation, and development of high-affinity antibodies.[2,3] The revised WHO 4th ed. created an umbrella category of "nodal lymphomas of TFH origin" encompassing three entities: angioimmunoblastic T-cell lymphoma (AITL), follicular T-cell lymphoma, and peripheral T-cell lymphoma (PTCL) with TFH phenotype, the latter characterized by a diffuse pattern and lack of follicular dendritic cell (FDC) expansion.[4,5] A TFH phenotype is defined by the expression of two or more TFH-associated immunophenotypic markers including PD1, ICOS, CXCL13, CD10, and BCL6.[6] In addition to these markers, CXCR5, SAP, c-MAF, and CD200 can also be used for diagnostic purposes.[7-10]

TFH lymphomas, in addition to sharing a TFH immunophenotype, are unified by a common gene-expression profile (GEP) and genetic landscape.[11-13] For these reasons, the International Consensus Classification (ICC) proposed to consider all nodal/systemic lymphomas of TFH derivation as a single entity, namely "follicular helper T-cell lymphoma" (TFH lymphoma) with three morphologic subtypes: angioimmunoblastic type (AITL), follicular type, and not otherwise specified (NOS) (Table 35-1).[14] By definition, primary cutaneous small/medium CD4-positive T-cell lymphoproliferative disorder (LPD) or other cutaneous lymphomas with TFH phenotype are excluded.[15] The criteria to discriminate among the three TFH subtypes remain the same as in the revised WHO 4th ed. and are based mainly on morphology, lymph node architecture, microenvironment, and distribution of FDCs.[4,5] Nevertheless, the different subtypes may show considerable plasticity, both within the same patient at diagnosis and between the diagnostic sample and relapses.[16,17] Because the mutational landscape of TFH lymphomas is so characteristic, especially of AITL, mutations in $RHOA^{G17V}$ and $IDH2^{R172}$ are valuable in supporting the diagnosis of TFH lymphoma.[13] Additionally, loss-of-function mutations in $TET2$ or $DNMT3A$ suggest that TFH lymphomas, mainly AITL, in many instances, develop on a background of clonal hematopoiesis.[18]

SYNONYMS AND RELATED TERMS

The revised WHO 4th ed. created an umbrella category of "nodal lymphomas of TFH origin" encompassing three entities: angioimmunoblastic T-cell lymphoma (AITL), follicular T-cell lymphoma, and peripheral T-cell lymphoma (PTCL) with TFH phenotype, the latter characterized by a diffuse pattern and lack of follicular dendritic cell (FDC) expansion.[4,5]

The WHO 5th ed. retained the concept of three, yet closely related, entities under the umbrella term of "nodal T-follicular helper cell lymphomas (nTFHL)": nTFH, angioimmunoblastic lymphoma-type, nTFH, follicular lymphoma type and nTFH, NOS.[19]

EPIDEMIOLOGY

AITL accounts for approximately 1% to 2% of non-Hodgkin lymphomas (NHL). It is the most common specific subtype of PTCL worldwide, representing roughly 36% of noncutaneous PTCL.[20] AITL is most frequently observed in middle-aged

Table 35-1 Morphologic Features of Follicular Helper T-Cell Lymphomas

Feature	Angioimmunoblastic Type	Follicular Type	Not Otherwise Specified
Growth pattern	Diffuse with subcapsular open sinuses	Follicular	Diffuse
FDC proliferation	+++	PTGC-like	No FDC expansion T-zone pattern
	Perifollicular pattern		
EBV-positive B-blasts	Usually present	Often present	Often present
HEVs	+++	+	−/+
Polymorphous environment	+++	−/+	−
TFH immunophenotype	+++	++	++
	Often CD10+/BCL6+		
Molecular features	RHOA, IDH2	RHOA, TET2, DNMT3A,	TET2, DNMT3A,
	TET2, DNMT3A	ITK::SYK	RHOA −/+

EBV, Epstein-Barr virus; FDC, follicular dendritic cell; HEV, high endothelial venules; PTGC, progressive transformation of germinal centers; TFH, T-cell follicular helper.

and older adult patients, with a peak incidence in the 6th and 7th decades of life, although young adults may rarely be affected.[21] It has been reported to be slightly more frequent in males than females and appears to be more prevalent in Europe (29% of PTCL cases)[22] than in North America or Asia, where the prevalence is approximately 16% to 18% of cases.[23]

In contrast, both TFH lymphomas of follicular type and NOS are rare. TFH lymphoma, follicular type accounts for 2% to 2.5% of noncutaneous PTCL.[24] Patients have a median age of onset of 60 to 65 years, and there is a slight male predominance.[16,25-27] Since its definition has changed over the years, no exact data are available regarding the true incidence of TFH lymphoma, NOS, nor is there reliable information on geographic distribution or gender predominance.

ETIOLOGY

The cause of TFH lymphomas is unknown. Originally AITL, the protype of the group, was speculated to be triggered by the administration of drugs, or to occur after an infectious disease, suggesting that AITL represented the manifestation of an abnormal immune reaction.[28] Subsequent work explored the role of Epstein-Barr virus (EBV) in the pathogenesis of AITL. EBV has been detected by in situ hybridization in 80% to 96% of lymph nodes involved by the disease.[29] In most cases, the EBV-infected cells represent transformed B cells. The prevalence of infected B cells in AITL lymph nodes ranges from 1 in 10 to 1 in 500 B cells in lymph nodes.[30] In contrast, in healthy EBV carriers, EBV resides in B cells at a frequency of approximately 1 in 10^6 to 1 in 10^7. Despite the obvious pathogenetic role of EBV in a variety of other lymphomas, the presence of EBV in AITL most likely reflects the underlying immunodeficiency inferred by and characteristic of the neoplastic process.

FOLLICULAR HELPER T CELLS

TFH cells are a distinct functional subset of effector T-helper cells residing in the germinal center that are specialized in providing help to B cells during the germinal center reaction.[31] TFH cells promote B cell survival, formation of germinal centers, immunoglobulin class-switch recombination, and somatic hypermutation, ultimately yielding high-affinity plasma cells and memory B cells.[32] TFH differentiation is dependent on the transcriptional repressor BCL6 and the expression of CXCR5, which are first detectable in T cells at the border between the T-zone and the follicle (T/B zone border) soon after T-cell priming and before germinal-center formation.[33,34]

BCL6 expression in T cells is able to downregulate CCR7 and upregulate CXCR5 inducible costimulator (ICOS), programmed death 1 (PD1), interleukin (IL-)21R, and IL-6R. The expression of ICOS also seems to play an important role in the initial stage of TFH differentiation at the time of T-cell priming by antigen-presenting dendritic cells.[35] These CD4-positive, CXCR5-positive, BCL6-positive T cells, so called "pre-TFH cells," are essential for the initiation of the germinal center and extrafollicular antibody responses.[33] The TFH-specific secretory profile, including IL-21, CXCL13 chemokine, and its receptor CXCR5, are critical to recruit and localize TFH cells in the germinal center. CXCR5 enables the migration of TFH cells into CXCL13-rich areas in B-cell follicles. Once TFH cells are located in the germinal center, they upregulate the expression of PD1, IL-21, CD84, and ICOS. These markers, which are characteristic of TFH cells, can be used in diagnostic practice either by flow cytometry or by immunohistochemistry on routinely formalin-fixed tissue.

CLINICAL FEATURES

The clinical presentation of AITL is unique among malignant lymphomas, and the diagnosis is frequently suspected on clinical grounds. Most patients present with generalized peripheral lymphadenopathy, hepatosplenomegaly, and prominent systemic symptoms including fever, weight loss, and rash, often with pruritus.[36] One-third of patients present with edema, especially in the upper extremities and face; pleural effusion; arthritis; and ascites. A pruritic maculopapular rash can be seen. The bone marrow is commonly involved.[37] Approximately 30% of patients present with eosinophilia, and 10% with plasmacytosis.[38] Polyclonal hypergammaglobulinemia and Coombs-positive hemolytic anemia are frequently present. Laboratory studies may reveal the presence of cold agglutinins, circulating immune complexes, anti–smooth muscle and antinuclear antibodies, positive rheumatoid factor, and cryoglobulins. The evolution of the disease is often complicated by intercurrent infections with conventional and opportunistic microorganisms. There is no consensus regarding the best therapeutic approach to patients with AITL. However, recent studies suggest that TFH lymphomas respond better to histone deacetylase and DNA methyltransferase inhibitors because of the common alterations in epigenetic modifying genes identified in this disease.[39,40]

Patients may respond initially to steroids or mild cytotoxic chemotherapy, but progression usually occurs. Derivation from TFH cells explains many of the distinctive clinical characteristics of AITL, including hypergammaglobulinemia, autoimmune phenomena, and clonal B-cell proliferations, suggesting that the malignant TFH cells, like their normal counterparts, can stimulate B-cell proliferation. Clinical features of TFH lymphoma, follicular type seem to be similar to those of AITL. Advanced stage disease and systemic lymphadenopathy are common, and skin manifestations may occur. Autoimmune phenomena such as polyclonal hypergammaglobulinemia and positive direct Coombs test have been reported.[13,16,25,27,41] Rare data on TFH lymphoma, NOS suggest a similar spectrum of clinical manifestations.[13]

MORPHOLOGY

Follicular Helper T-Cell Lymphoma, Angioimmunoblastic Type

In contrast to the other PTCL, NOS, AITL displays some unique morphologic features in involved lymph nodes (Box 35-1).[42] At low magnification, the lymph node architecture is usually effaced. There is a polymorphic infiltrate of small-to-medium-sized lymphocytes intermingled with granulocytes, eosinophils, plasma cells, fibroblast-like dendritic cells, histiocytes, and epithelioid cells predominantly occupying the paracortical or interfollicular area (Fig. 35-1). Often, the neoplastic T-cell population is obscured by a large number of inflammatory cells, but, occasionally, a neoplastic T-cell population can be readily identified on morphologic grounds. In these cases, there is an infiltration of atypical T cells characterized by round to irregular nuclear contours and sometimes broad, clear cytoplasm with distinct cell membranes (clear cells) (Fig. 35-2A). Cytologic atypia of the lymphoid cells, although frequently observed, is not a prerequisite for the diagnosis (see Fig. 35-2B). The proportion of atypical T cells may vary greatly from small foci to large confluent sheets, sometimes posing problems in the differential diagnosis with TFH lymphoma, NOS or PTCL, NOS. It is noteworthy that medium-to-large-sized basophilic blasts of B-cell phenotype may be present, some of them reminiscent of Hodgkin cells (Fig. 35-3).[42]

The vast majority of AITL cases display a pronounced proliferation of FDCs localized outside the residual follicles, typically abutting the high endothelial venules (HEVs). Occasionally, remnants of follicles with concentrically arranged, onion-shaped FDC meshworks are present, giving them a burned-out appearance (Fig. 35-4). In less obvious cases, FDC proliferation may be recognized only after immunohistochemical staining with antibodies directed against CD21, CD23, or CD35 antigens. Another diagnostic feature of the disease is the extension of the infiltrate beyond the lymph node capsule into the perinodal fat, frequently sparing preserved cortical sinuses that appear to be "jumped over" by the tumor cells (Fig. 35-5). A key feature is the presence of numerous, frequently arborizing, postcapillary HEVs, which are also seen outside the lymph nodes in the perinodal infiltrate. The HEVs are best recognized in silver stains, such as Gomori silver impregnation, or in periodic acid–Schiff stains, highlighting both the conspicuous angioarchitecture and the thickened, hyalinized basement membranes of vessel walls (Fig. 35-6). Three major morphologic patterns are recognized.[43] In pattern 1 (20% of cases), the lymph node architecture is preserved, with hyperplastic germinal centers (Fig. 35-7A). Pattern 2 (30% of cases) is characterized by the

Box 35-1 *Diagnostic Criteria for Follicular Helper T-Cell Lymphoma, Angioimmunoblastic Type (AITL)*

Morphology
- Usually effaced lymph node architecture
- Perinodal extension of infiltrate, with sparing of sinuses
- Polymorphic infiltrate of lymphocytes, granulocytes, plasma cells, and immunoblasts
- T cells with abundant clear cytoplasm (clear cells)
- Proliferation of FDCs
- Proliferation of arborizing high endothelial venules

Immunophenotype
- Demonstration of FDC networks CD21 positive, CD23 positive
- CXCL13+, ICOS+, PD1+, CD10+, BCL6+, CD4+ neoplastic T cells
- CD3 positive, CD5 positive, CD4 ≫ CD8 with no T-cell antigen loss
- EBV-positive B blasts

Molecular Genetics
- TR gene clonally rearranged in 75% of cases (range, 70%–90%)
- IG genes clonally rearranged in 12% of cases (range, 10%–20%)
- TFH molecular signature
- Frequent mutations in *TET2, RHOA, IDH2, DNMT3A* genes
- Rearrangements in *VAV1, ICOS::CD28*
- Cytogenetics
  - Clonal chromosome aberrations in 89%
  - +3, +5, additional X chromosome

EBV Positivity
- 50% to 97% of cases by in situ hybridization
- EBER-positive B cells and rarely T cells

EBER, EBV-encoded small RNA; *EBV*, Epstein-Barr virus; *FDC*, follicular dendritic cell; *IG*, immunoglobulin genes; *TR*, T-cell receptor; *TFH*, follicular helper T cell.

loss of normal architecture and the presence of occasional depleted follicles or "burned-out" germinal centers, sometimes mimicking Castleman disease (see Fig. 35-7B–C). In pattern 3 (50% of cases), the normal architecture of the lymph node is completely effaced, and no B-cell follicles are present. These patterns seem to represent different morphologic stages of the disease, with consecutive biopsies from the same patient showing a transition from pattern 1 to pattern 3, which is thought to represent morphologic evolution rather than clinical progression of the disease.[17]

Pattern 1 is the most difficult to recognize morphologically. The lymph nodes show a largely preserved architecture with hyperplastic follicles mimicking a reactive condition. A clue to the diagnosis is the absence of well-formed mantle cuffs (Fig. 35-7D). There are well-structured (hyperplastic) germinal centers with poorly developed mantle zones and sometimes ill-defined borders, so-called naked germinal centers (see Fig. 35-8A).[44] The specific morphologic alterations are confined to the perifollicular area where a rim of atypical clear cells is observed (Fig. 35-8A). The tumor cells are best recognized upon immunohistochemistry because of their strong CD10 and PD1 reactivity in aberrant localization (Fig. 35-8C). AITL pattern 1 lacks the FDC expansion characteristic of the disease (Fig. 35-8B). The presence of CD4-positive T cells (see Fig. 35-8E) with aberrant expression of TFH markers CD10, BCL6, PD1, CD278, CXCL13, or others in the outer rim of the germinal centers and paracortex has been described as an important diagnostic feature (Fig. 35-8C–E).[43] If this "early" pattern is suspected, evidence of a clonal expansion of T cells by analyzing the T-cell receptor (TR) gene rearrangement configuration or finding characteristic gene mutations should be sought, and clinical features should be compatible with the diagnosis. Despite morphologically "early" involvement, the patients usually have clinically systemic, advanced disease. In subsequent biopsies, some of these cases may show progression to typical AITL with effaced nodal architecture.[17] Pattern 2 is characterized by depleted follicles. In contrast to pattern 1, there is expansion of FDCs as demonstrated by CD21 or CD23 usually extending from the depleted, atrophic follicles. The CD4-positive, PD1-positive, ICOS-positive cells are embedded in the meshworks of FDCs (Fig. 35-9A–D).

Outside of lymph nodes, the most common sites of involvement are bone marrow and skin. Skin biopsies often show mild perivascular or periadnexal lymphoid infiltrates that are difficult to differentiate from inflammatory conditions.[45,46] In some cases, the cutaneous infiltrates may

show the characteristic phenotype of AITL, with aberrant expression of CD10.[17,47] TR rearrangement is identified in more than 80% of the cases and usually is identical to the pattern found in lymph nodes.[45,46] However, it is unlikely that a primary diagnosis can be made based on a skin biopsy alone.

Bone marrow involvement is characterized by single or multiple loose nodular infiltrates with a paratrabecular or interstitial distribution pattern. The infiltrate is usually polymorphic in composition similar to that seen in lymph nodes.[48,49] Aberrant expression of CD10 or strong PD1 expression might be useful in the diagnosis.[50,51] The most frequent aberrations identified in peripheral blood by flow cytometry include loss of surface CD3, CD4 positivity together with altered T-cell receptor expression, and aberrant CD10 expression.[52] AITL may be associated with marked splenomegaly, but splenectomy is not indicated. Because AITL is usually a systemic disease, the characteristic infiltrates may be seen in other sites of involvement, including the liver and lung.

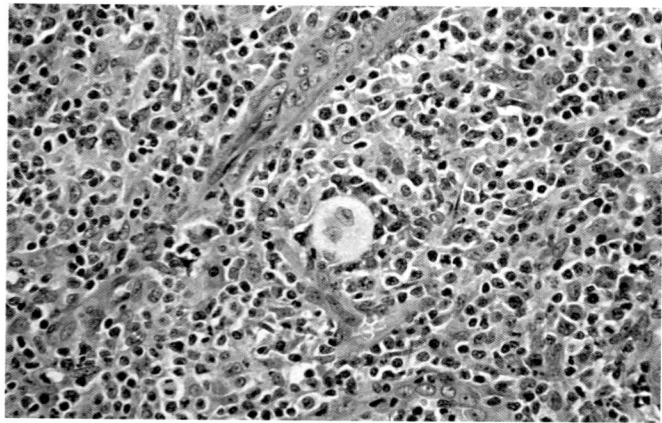

Figure 35-1. Typical morphology of follicular helper T-cell lymphoma, angioimmunoblastic-type (AITL). There is a polymorphic infiltrate of small-to-medium-sized lymphocytes with clear cytoplasm intermingled with eosinophils, plasma cells, fibroblast-like dendritic cells, histiocytes, and epithelioid cells.

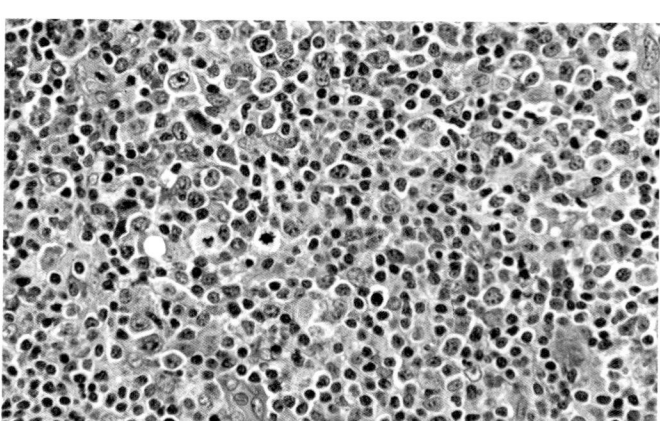

Figure 35-3. Large B-cell blasts. Intermingled with the neoplastic T cells are medium-to-large-sized basophilic blasts of B-cell phenotype, some of them reminiscent of Hodgkin cells.

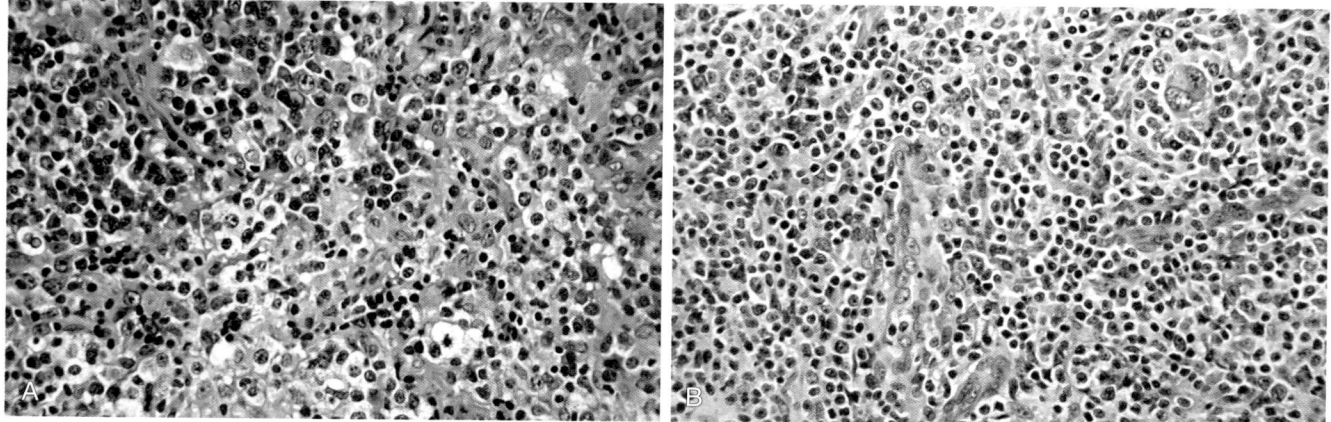

Figure 35-2. Cytologic spectrum of neoplastic T cells in follicular helper T-cell lymphoma. A, The infiltrate is composed of atypical T cells characterized by irregular nuclear contours and broad, clear cytoplasm with distinct cell membranes (clear cells). **B,** The neoplastic T cells are small to intermediate in size, with no atypia and a clear cytoplasm. Note the presence of a Reed-Sternberg–like cell.

Abundant Epithelioid Histiocyte Reaction

Some cases of AITL may show a prominent admixture of epithelioid cells, obscuring the diagnostic morphologic

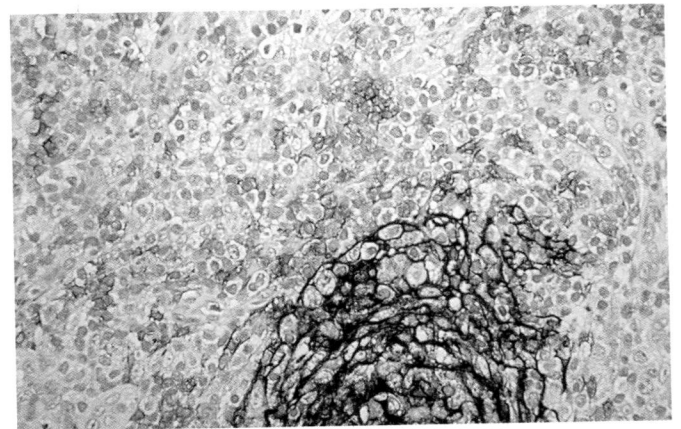

Figure 35-4. Follicular dendritic cells highlighted with CD21 immunostaining. A "burned-out" germinal center with onion-shaped follicular dendritic cell meshworks is depicted. Note the proliferation of CD21-positive dendritic cells beyond the follicles.

features of the disease (Fig. 35-10A). In these cases, the diagnosis relies on the presence of classical criteria such as arborizing HEVs and proliferating FDCs, in contrast to epithelioid cell–rich classic Hodgkin lymphoma (CHL) (containing classic Hodgkin and Reed-Sternberg [HRS] cells) and the lymphoepithelioid variant of PTCL, NOS (Lennert lymphoma), in which these features are lacking.[53]

Sheets of Small-to-Large Neoplastic T Cells ("Tumor Cell Rich")

In some cases, the neoplastic T-cell population becomes unusually predominant, forming sheets of small-sized or medium-to-large-sized cells and obscuring the "inflammatory" background infiltrate commonly present in AITL (see Fig. 35-10B).[54] This pattern may be especially seen at relapse, possibly representing disease progression and sometimes fulfilling criteria of TFH lymphoma, NOS; however, as long as the diagnostic features are still recognizable (e.g., hypervascularity, perinodal extension, and especially FDC proliferation), a diagnosis of tumor cell–rich AITL may still be rendered.[13,54]

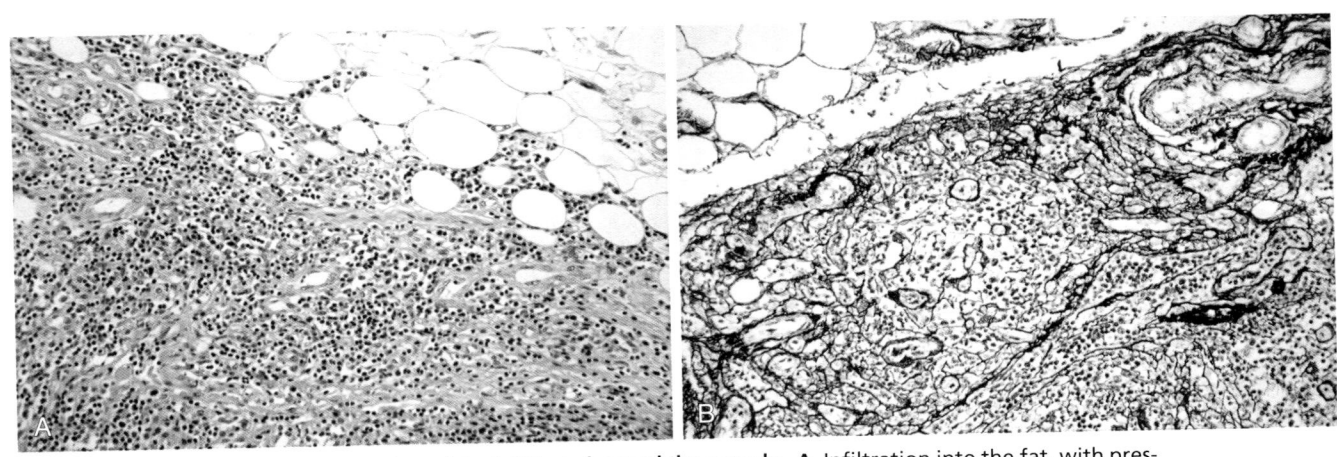

Figure 35-5. Extension of the infiltrate beyond the capsule. A, Infiltration into the fat, with preservation of the cortical sinuses that appear to be "jumped over" by the tumor cells. **B,** Gomori stain highlights the presence of open cortical sinuses, a diagnostic feature of angioimmunoblastic T-cell lymphoma.

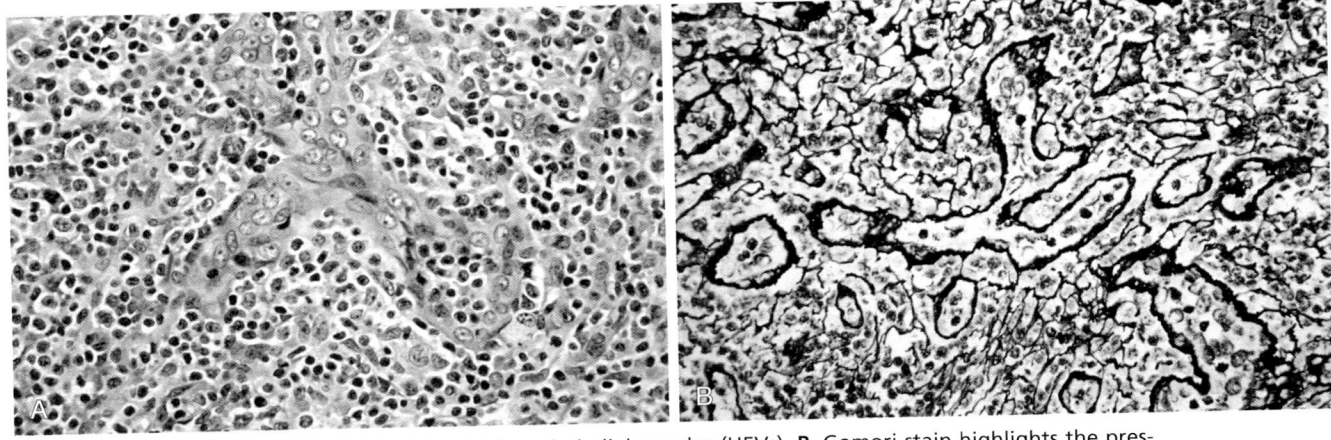

Figure 35-6. A, Arborizing high endothelial venules (HEVs). **B,** Gomori stain highlights the presence of arborizing HEVs, a characteristic finding in angioimmunoblastic T-cell lymphoma.

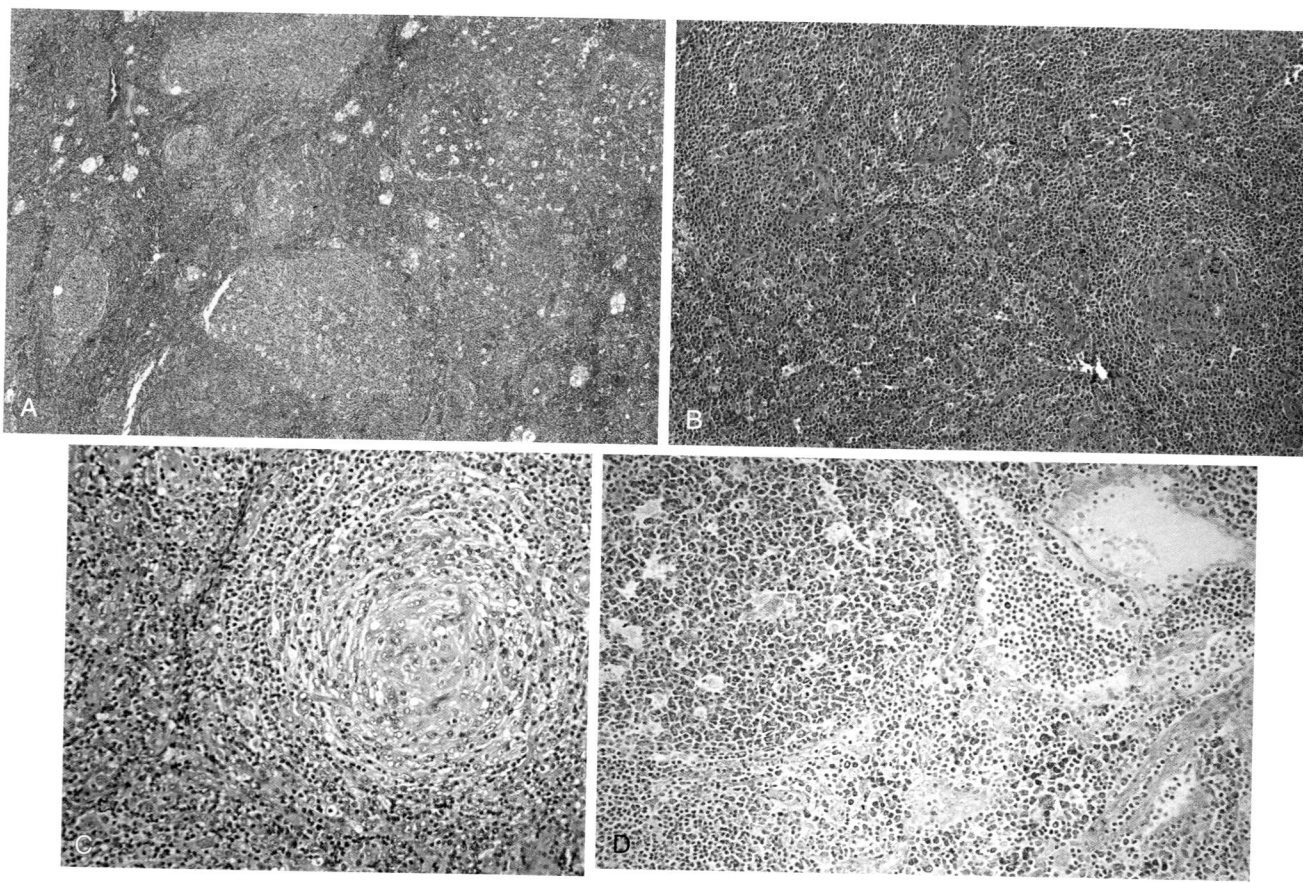

Figure 35-7. Histologic patterns of follicular helper T-cell lymphoma, angioimmunoblastic type. **A,** Early case with hyperplastic follicles without a mantle zone and an expanded paracortical area (pattern 1). **B,** Case with "burned-out" germinal centers, reminiscent of Castleman disease, with paracortical expansion and proliferation of arborizing high endothelial venules (pattern 2). **C,** Higher magnification of a depleted, atrophic follicle with clear proliferation of follicular dendritic cells (pattern 2). **D,** Giemsa stain of a hyperplastic follicle with absence of a mantle zone and an expanded paracortical area (pattern 1).

Follicular Helper T-Cell Lymphoma, Follicular Type

TFH lymphoma, follicular-type shows a proliferation of T cells expressing a TFH phenotype arranged in a follicular growth pattern (Fig. 35-11A–C). HEVs and proliferations of FDCs characteristic of AITL are absent.[14,19,55]

TFH lymphoma, follicular type affects lymph nodes, and systemic disease is common. Extranodal sites of involvement include skin, liver, spleen, and bone marrow. The clinical features of TFH lymphoma, follicular type are similar to those of AITL. TFH lymphoma, follicular type is a rare disease based on few studies available, with a median onset at 60 years and a slight male predominance.[16,25-27]

TFH lymphoma, follicular type shows effacement of the underlying nodal architecture, and a nodular or follicular proliferation of medium-sized tumor cells with often clear cytoplasm and round or slightly irregular nuclei. These neoplastic cells may be organized in well-defined nodules/follicles or in a pattern that is similar to that seen in progressively transformed germinal centers (PTGC), displaying aggregates of neoplastic cells that are surrounded by small lymphocytes of mantle zone type.[16,55] These patterns can also occur simultaneously. In some cases, areas of follicular type overlap

with areas of AITL.[16,41,54] Furthermore, in relapsed disease, patterns may change and follicular type may relapse as AITL morphology or vice versa.[16,17] Scattered large, transformed cells can be interspersed and HRS-like cells are often found in the small cellular background in the PTGC-like pattern.[56]

Staining for FDC markers often discloses slightly expanded FDC meshworks confined to the nodular proliferations seen in conventional morphology. The scattered large cells may be EBV positive.[16] In the PTGC-like pattern, IgD-positive small B cells of mantle zone type encircle clusters of neoplastic T cells.[16] Of note, the HRS-like cells seen in the PTGC-like pattern are often CD30 positive, and show variable expression of CD15, EBV, and B-cell antigens; they are surrounded by neoplastic T cells with a TFH phenotype. These features can lead to an erroneous diagnosis of CHL.[56] The differential diagnoses comprise follicular lymphoma (FL) and CHL in cases with (prominent) admixture with HRS-like cells.

Follicular Helper T-Cell Lymphoma, Not Otherwise Specified

TFH lymphoma, NOS is a primarily node-based PTCL with a TFH immunophenotype, which does not exhibit diagnostic

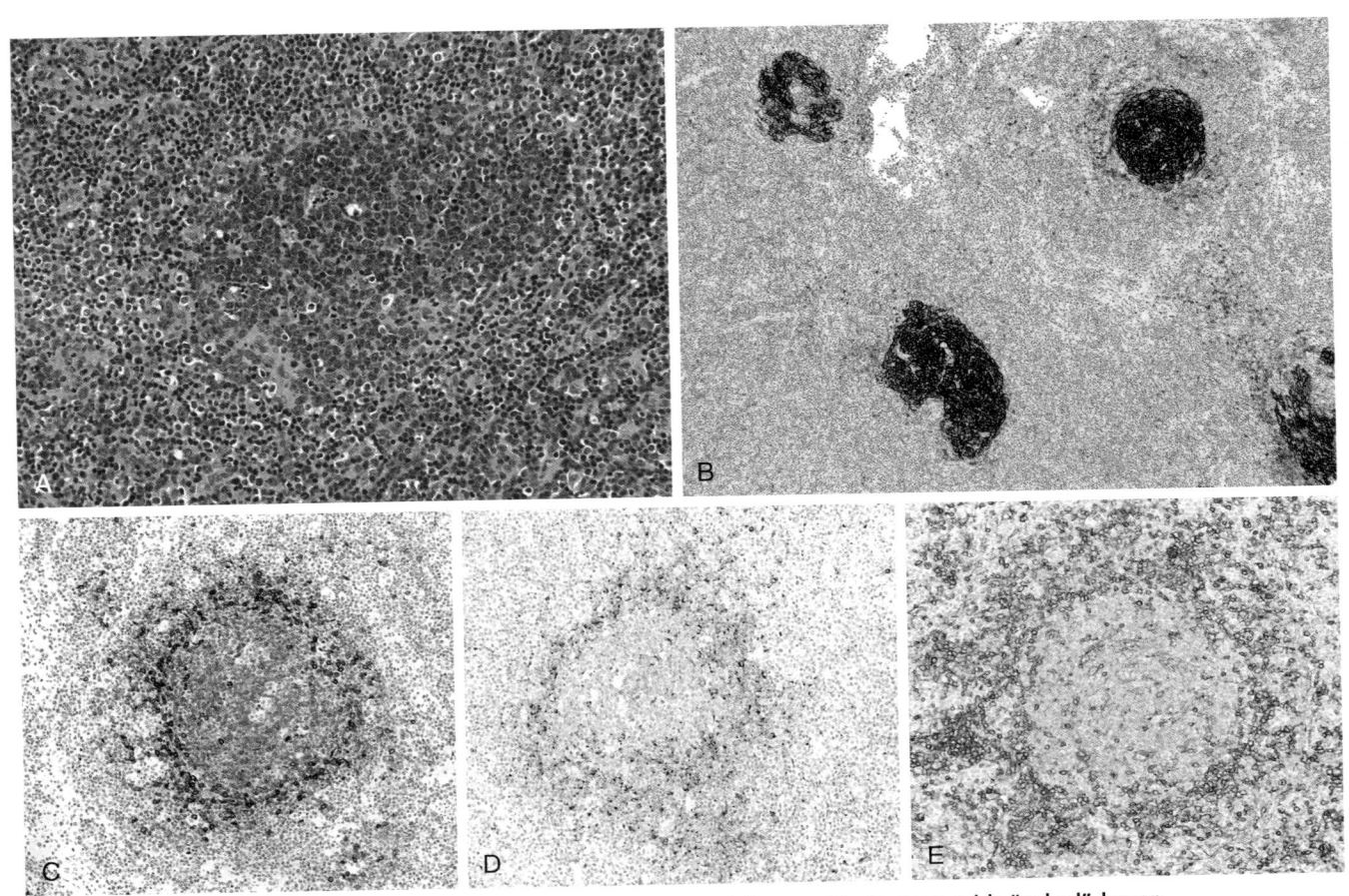

Figure 35-8. Follicular helper T-cell lymphoma, angioimmunoblastic-type with "naked" hyperplastic germinal centers (pattern 1). A, Hyperplastic follicle without a mantle zone and clear cells surrounding the germinal center. **B,** CD23 showing the normal follicular dendritic cells meshwork without expansion. **C,** CD10 is weakly positive in the normal germinal center cells and strongly positive in the tumor cells surrounding the germinal center. CXCL13 **(D)** and CD4 **(E)** are positive in the same cells.

characteristics of AITL or TFH lymphoma, follicular type.[14] Because this morphologic variant was first recognized in the revised 2017 WHO 4th ed., there are no reliable data on the true incidence of this subtype.[5]

Similar to AITL, TFH lymphoma, NOS clinically presents as a systemic nodal disease with autoimmune phenomena such as Coombs-positive hemolytic anemia.[13] Microscopically, the preexisting architecture of the lymph nodes is usually effaced, and there is a diffuse infiltrate of medium-to-large-sized lymphoid cells forming sheets. The inflammatory background, hyperplasia of HEVs, and extrafollicular FDC expansion characteristic of AITL are absent. The latter feature is particularly important because lack of FDC expansion separates TFH lymphoma, NOS from rare cases of AITL with tumor cell–rich or anaplastic features. In some instances, the B-cell follicles are preserved, thus creating a main pattern of involvement in the T zone.[57]

B-Cell Lymphoproliferation or B-Cell Lymphoma

Studies have reported that more than 80% of AITL cases contain a variable number of EBV-positive B cells.[58-61] There is clear evidence that large B-cell lymphomas may arise in TFH lymphomas, mainly described in AITL. These large B-cell

lymphomas may be present at initial diagnosis or develop over time. In the majority of cases, an EBV infection triggers the B-cell lymphoproliferation, which in turn is fostered by the profound immunodeficiency associated with the disease and possibly by the additional immunosuppression induced by chemotherapy.[61] EBV-associated B-cell lymphoproliferations in AITL constitute a spectrum of alterations.[62] The histologic picture in these cases is characterized by the presence of large EBV-positive B blasts in an otherwise typical TFH lymphoma (Fig. 35-12A). These blasts may have the appearance of immunoblasts or bear a resemblance to HRS cells; they may be focally accentuated or diffusely scattered, or they may form confluent sheets indistinguishable from diffuse large B-cell lymphoma.[60] These B-blasts are usually EBV-encoded small RNA (EBER) positive, CD20 positive, CD30 positive, CD15 negative, and latent membrane protein-1 (LMP-1) positive or negative (see Fig. 35-12B–D).[61]

AITL is often associated with polyclonal plasmacytosis and polyclonal hypergammaglobulinemia. AITL cases have been described with a monoclonal plasma cell population. In some cases, the plasma cell expansion can be so extensive as to partially overshadow or extensively obscure the underlying T-cell neoplasm.[63] In addition, clonal proliferations of B-cells with or without plasma cells mimicking nodal or even

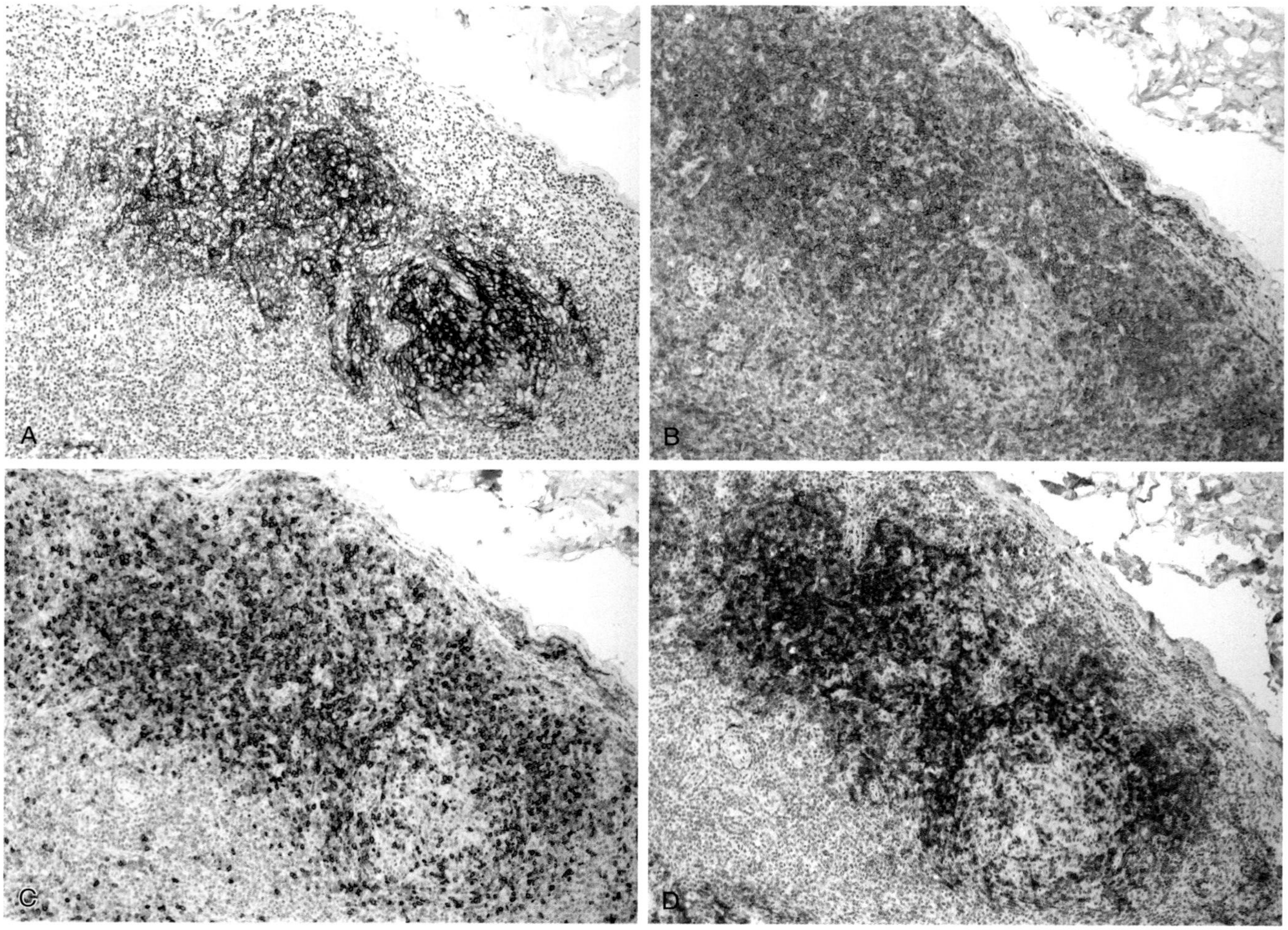

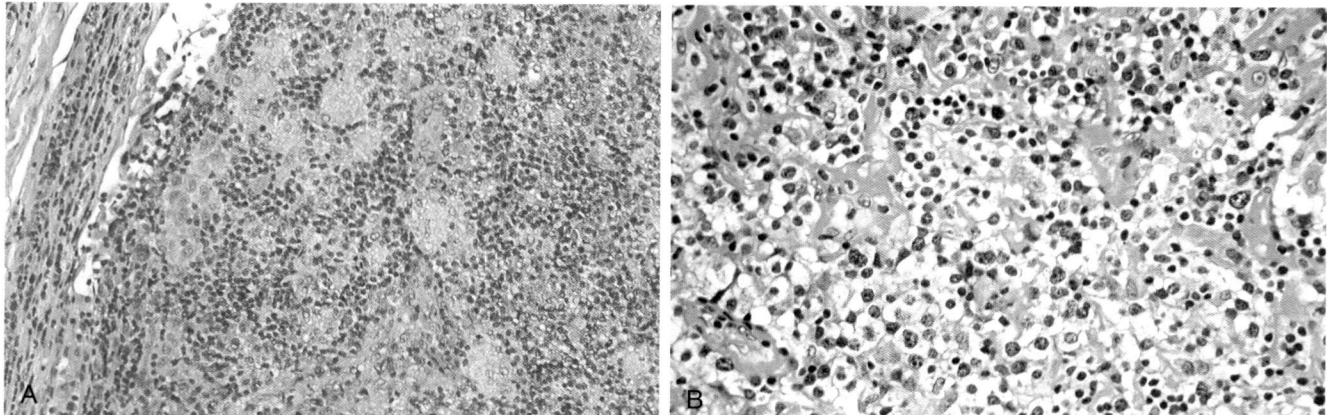

Figure 35-9. Follicular helper T-cell lymphoma, angioimmunoblastic type with depleted follicles (pattern 2). A, Expanded CD21-positive follicular dendritic cell (FDC) meshwork extends from the depleted, atrophic follicle. **B,** CD4-positive T cells surrounding the depleted follicle and embedded in the meshwork of CD21-positive FDCs. **C,** The CD4-positive T cells are strongly positive for CD10. Note the absence of CD10 expression in the depleted follicle. **D,** The same cells are PD1 positive.

Figure 35-10. Pitfalls in the diagnosis of follicular helper T-cell lymphoma, angioimmunoblastic type. A, Follicular helper T-cell lymphoma, angioimmunoblastic type (AITL) with abundant epithelioid histiocytes reaction. Note the open cortical sinus, a characteristic diagnostic feature. **B,** AITL with sheets of large neoplastic T cells.

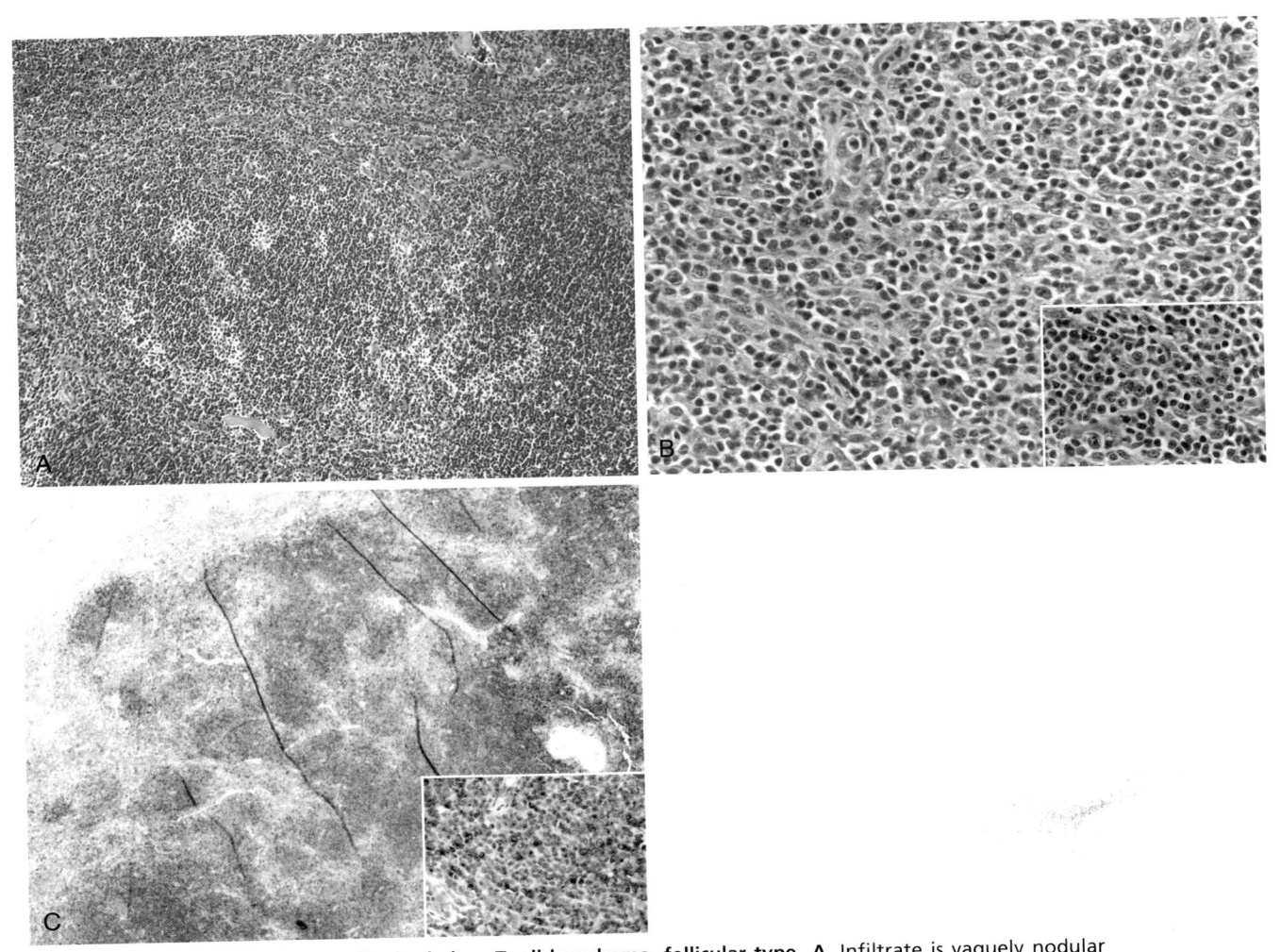

Figure 35-11. Follicular helper T-cell lymphoma, follicular type. A, Infiltrate is vaguely nodular with clusters of atypical clear cells. **B,** The lymphoproliferation comprises small-to-medium-sized lymphocytes with pale cytoplasm. **C,** The neoplastic cells express CXCL13, a marker of TFH cells.

extranodal marginal zone lymphoma have been described in the setting of AITL.[64,65]

Reed-Sternberg–Like Cells

TFH lymphomas may show the presence of typical HRS cells with a classic immunophenotype (CD30 positive, CD15 positive, CD20 positive/negative, EBV positive) (Fig. 35-13).[66] Although these HRS-like cells are EBV positive in most cases, rare EBV-negative cases have been described.[61] In contrast to CHL, molecular studies have revealed clonal rearrangements of TCRG and an oligoclonal pattern of immunoglobulin heavy chain (IGH) gene in the microdissected HRS-like cells. These patients do not seem to be at high risk for progression to CHL.

IMMUNOPHENOTYPE

The infiltrating lymphocytes are predominantly T cells (CD3 positive, CD5 positive), usually with an admixture of CD4 and CD8 cells. The neoplastic population in TFH lymphoma is by definition a T cell with a CD4-positive phenotype (Fig. 35-14A),[43,67] although CD8-positive T cells may constitute the majority of the lymphoid infiltrate in some cases. In contrast to other types of T-cell lymphoma, loss of pan–T-cell antigen expression is an uncommon finding in AITL. Nevertheless, a recent study showed that loss of CD7 expression seems to be a characteristic finding of TFH lymphomas.[67a] However, loss of surface CD3 is commonly seen by flow cytometry and is a clue to the diagnosis.[68] B cells (CD20 positive, CD79a positive) are found in varying numbers and are occasionally present in follicular aggregates. They are usually small cells but may become larger and activated, especially when infected with EBV. Large atypical cells usually express CD30 and EBV LMP1 can be demonstrated in 30% to 50% of cases, although EBER ISH is more sensitive to the virus.[61]

The proliferation of FDCs, a diagnostic hallmark of AITL, can be readily appreciated with immunohistochemical stains. CD21 or CD23 highlight the disorganized and largely expanded meshworks of FDCs, usually surrounding HEVs in the vast majority of cases (see Fig. 35-14B). The exact nature of the CD21-positive cells with dendritic morphology has not been fully resolved. The abnormal proliferation is centered around the HEVs and is often associated with B-cell follicles in early histologic stages of the disease. It has been postulated that the CD21-positive cells are not true FDCs but activated fibroblastic reticulum cells that have upregulated the CD21 antigen; "pre-FDCs."[69] Fibroblastic reticulum cells and FDCs are both derived from mesenchymal cell rather than of hematopoietic origin.[70] TFH lymphomas express

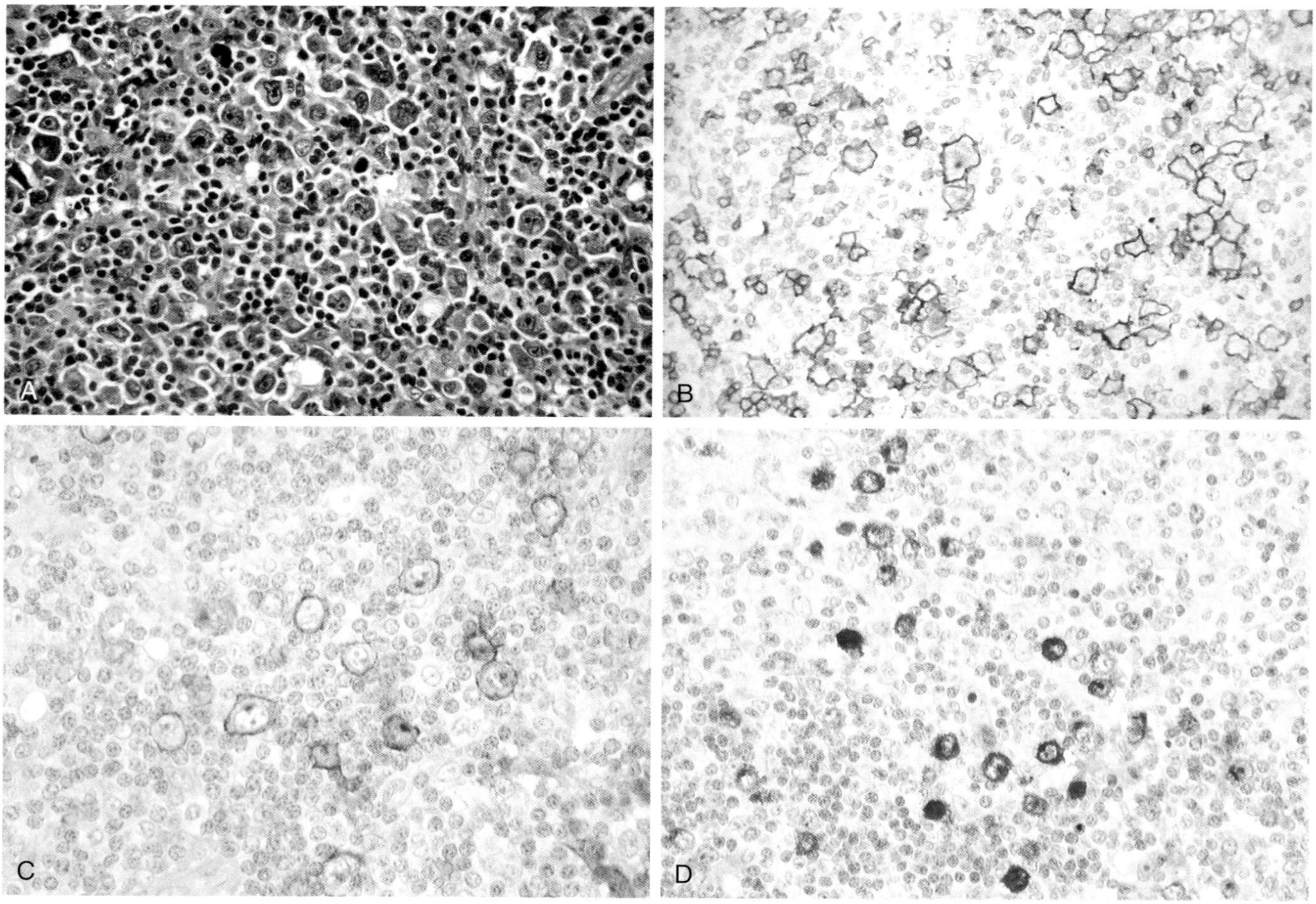

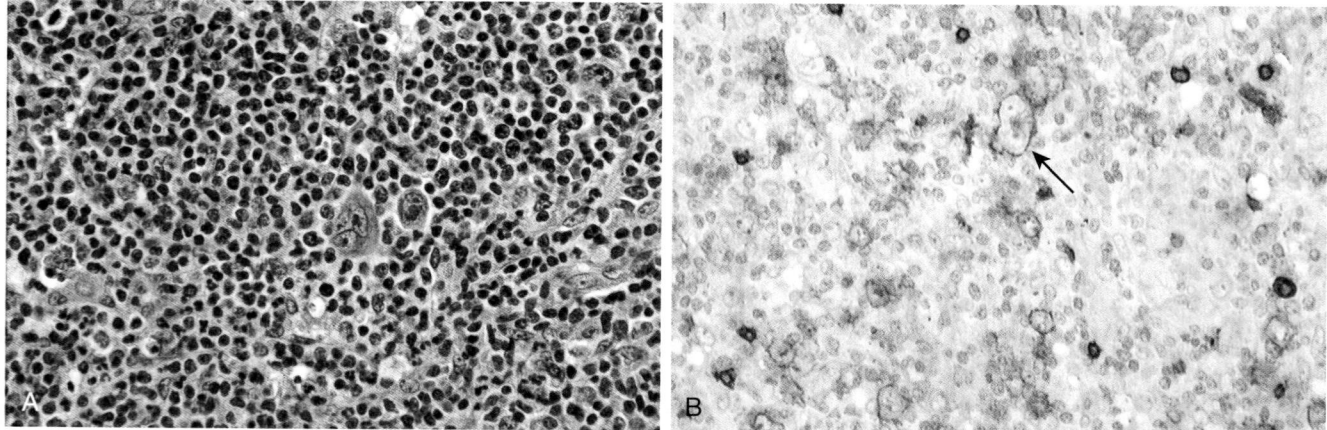

Figure 35-12. Follicular helper T-cell lymphoma, angioimmunoblastic type with B-cell lymphopro-liferation. A, Proliferation of B-cell blasts in an otherwise typical follicular helper T-cell lympho-ma, angioimmunoblastic type (AITL) case. The B cells might resemble centroblasts, immunoblasts, or Hodgkin cells. **B,** CD20 staining highlights the spectrum of B-cell morphology in AITL. **C,** The B cells are positive for CD30. **D,** The B-cell blasts are EBV LMP-1 positive.

Figure 35-13. Follicular helper T-cell lymphoma, angioimmunoblastic type with Reed-Sternberg–like cells. A, Reed-Sternberg (RS)–like cells are depicted. Note the minimal atypia of the surround-ing neoplastic T cells. **B,** The RS-like cells are CD20 positive *(arrow)*.

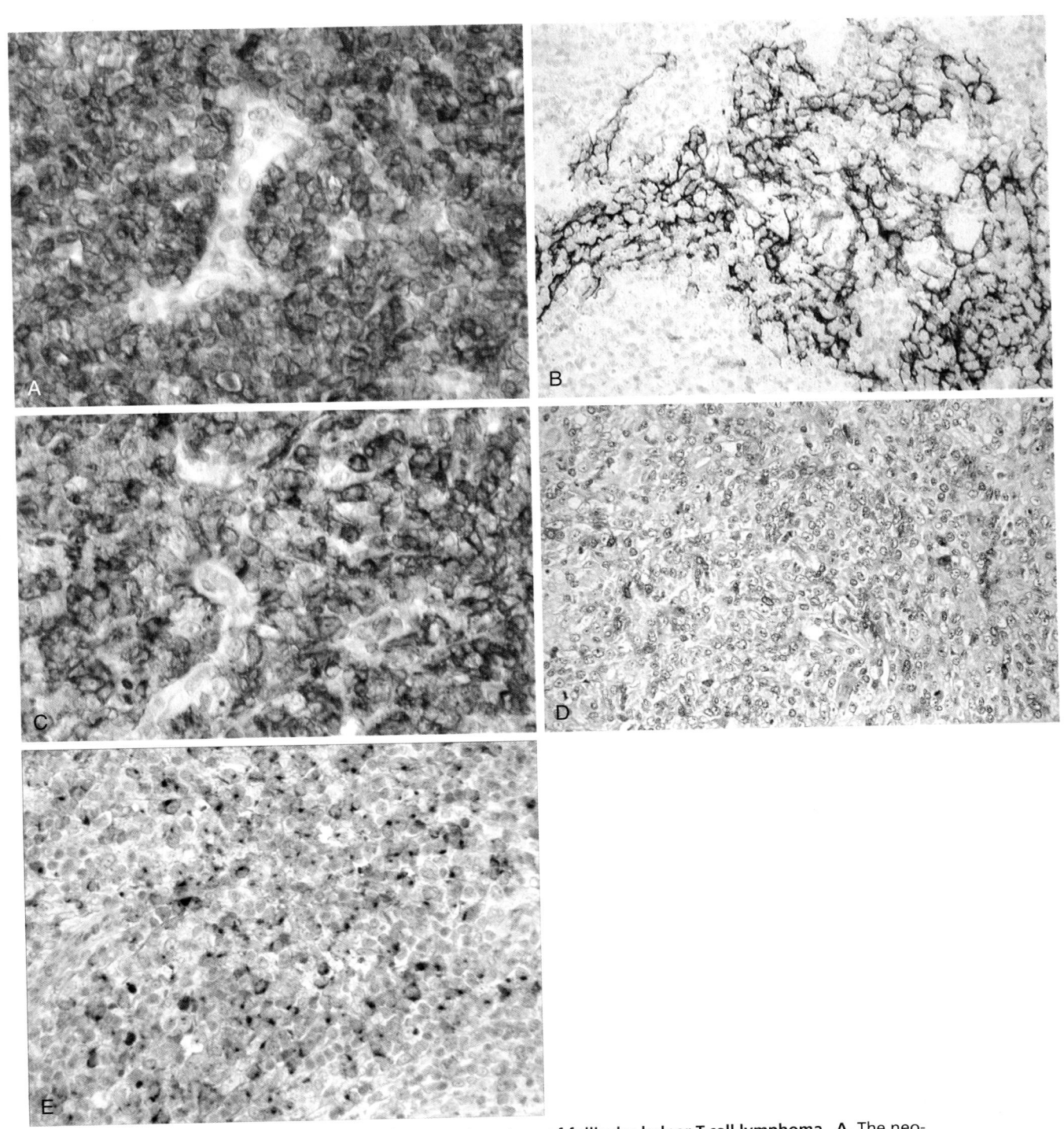

Figure 35-14. Characteristic immunophenotype of follicular helper T-cell lymphoma. A, The neoplastic T cells are CD4 positive. **B,** CD21 highlights the marked follicular dendritic cell proliferation, which envelops high endothelial venules. **C,** A case with strong and uniform CD10 expression in the neoplastic cells. **D,** CD10 expression in only a minority of the tumor cell population. **E,** The neoplastic T cells are strongly CXCL13 positive.

TFH-associated markers CD10, BCL6, PD1 (CD279), ICOS (CD278), and CXCL13 (Fig. 35-14A, C–E), in various numbers and intensities.[6,54,71-73] Overall, PD1 and ICOS are more sensitive than CXCL13, BCL6, or CD10, which in contrast are more specific in identifying the neoplastic TFH cells. By definition, TFH lymphoma derives from a CD4-positive T cell and must express at least two TFH markers.

Strong and homogeneous CD10 expression seems to characterize cases with medium-to-large-sized clear cells harboring the $IDH2^{R172}$ (NP 002159.2) mutation, which can also be detected by IDH2 immunohistochemistry when involving the specific $IDH2^{R172K}$ mutation variant.[74,75] (see Fig. 35-15A–D). AITLs with mutations in $RHOA^{G17V}$ (NP 001655.1) have been shown to often express several TFH

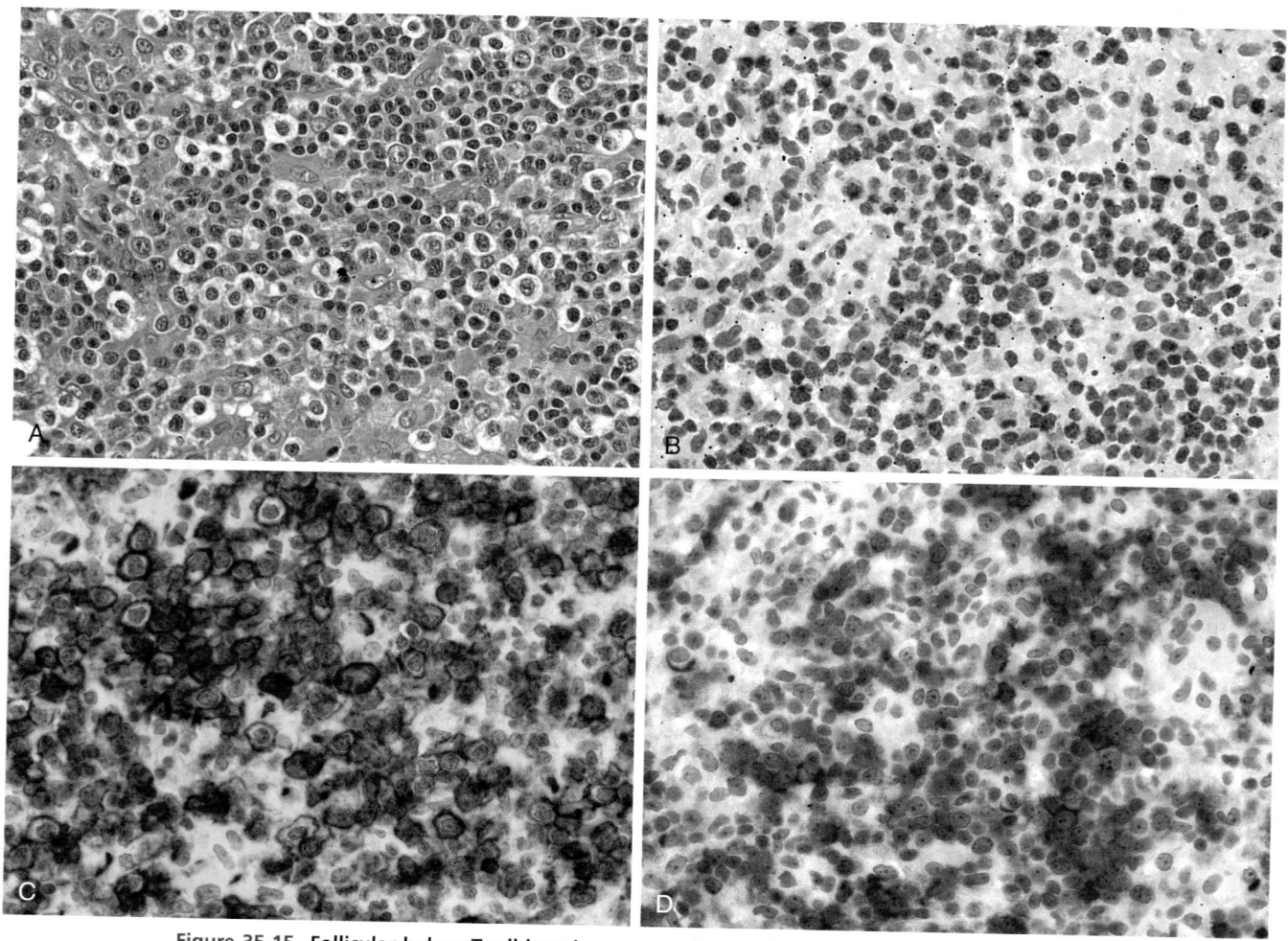

Figure 35-15. Follicular helper T-cell lymphoma, angioimmunoblastic-type with *IDH2*^R172K mutation. A, Medium-to-large-sized clear cells. Note the tumor cells with abundant clear cytoplasm surrounding high endothelial venules and intermingled with small reactive lymphocytes. **B,** The clear cells are positive for the specific antibody against the *IDH2*^R172K mutation. The variant allelic frequency in this case was 17% by next-generation sequencing. The clear cells are strongly positive for ICOS **(C)** and PD1 **(D).**

markers and expanded FDC meshworks.[76] Additional markers of normal TFH cells, including CXCR5, CD154, PD1, and SLAM-associated protein (SAP), have been demonstrated by immunohistochemistry to be expressed in the majority of AITL cases.[8] However, no single marker is diagnostic of AITL or TFH derivation.

GENETICS

A monoclonal expansion of T cells with rearranged TR genes is detectable in 75% of AITL.[77] In up to 50% of cases, monoclonal rearrangements of the IGH or light chain (IGL) genes co-exist with rearrangements of TCRB or TCRG, either at presentation or during the course of the disease.[17,78] A small group of cases (7%) with the morphology of AITL reveal clonal rearrangements of the IGH genes alone. Nodal marginal zone lymphoma (NMZL) rich in PD1-positive T cells should be carefully excluded.[79] The presence of IGH rearrangements in bona fide cases of AITL is thought to be caused by a clonal expansion of EBV-infected B cells that are identified in 80% to 90% of lymph nodes involved by AITL.[29] EBV is found mainly in two types of B cells in AITL: cells resembling

memory B cells, which show relatively little tendency for clonal expansion, and cells resembling germinal-center B cells, which are driven into massive proliferation and acquire somatic mutations during clonal expansion without selection for a functional B-cell receptor (immunoglobulin-deficient or "forbidden" clones).[80]

Cytogenetic studies have demonstrated trisomy 3, trisomy 5, and an additional X chromosome as the most frequent alterations. By combining classic metaphase cytogenetics and interphase cytogenetics, 89% of AITL cases have been found to harbor aberrant chromosomal clones.[81]

GEP studies showed that AITL is derived from TFH cells, and that genes related to cell morphology, intracellular signaling, and promoting angiogenesis such as VEGF are overexpressed in AITL.[1,82-84] Another interesting finding was that 14% to 20% of so-called "PTCL, NOS" cases expressed the characteristic GEP of AITL, now recognized to be TFH lymphomas, NOS.[1]

A key advance in the understanding of TFH lymphoma pathogenesis was the recognition of common molecular features within this group of lymphomas beyond their similar TFH-like gene expression signatures. Frequent recurrent somatic mutations include genes encoding the epigenetic regulators *TET2* (50%–90%), *DNMT3A* (30%–40%), and *IDH2*[R172] (20%–45%), the small GTPase, *RHOA*[G17V] (50%–70%) and components of the TCR signaling pathways such as *PLCG1* (14%), *CD28* (9%–11%), *VAV1* (5%), and *FYN* (3%–4%).[11,85-89] Mutations in *RHOA*[G17V] have been identified in up to 70% of AITL,[11,12,87] in follicular type,[13,41] and TFH lymphoma, NOS (60%), and are considered a hallmark of TFH lymphomas.[11,12,87,89,90] The main function of RHOA is to promote motility and adhesion, and in T cells, RHOA is required for the regulation of transendothelial migration.[91] The mutation enables RHOA to interact with VAV1, a downstream molecule of the TR,[92] and enhances signal transduction by the TR.[93-95] Mutations in *IDH2*[R172] (NP_002159.2) occur almost exclusively in AITL, usually with concurrent *TET2* and *RHOA*[G17V] mutations. This mutation confers increased genome-wide promoter hypermethylation and is associated with characteristic morphologic features including medium-to-large-sized clear tumor cells with strong TFH phenotype.[74,83,88] Recurrent oncogenic fusion genes have been reported, including *ICOS::CD28*, *ITK::SYK*, and *VAV1* fusions.[96] Most of these genomic alterations are seen across the spectrum of TFH lymphomas with the exception of *IDH2*[R172] mutations, which are characteristic of AITL and *ITK::SYK* fusions, which are mostly associated with TFH lymphoma, follicular type.[97]

Loss-of-function mutations in the methylation associated genes *TET2* and *DNMT3A* are likely to occur in a background of clonal hematopoiesis (CH), providing survival advantage to TFH cells.[18,86,98,99] These mutations are not restricted to T cells and have been demonstrated in B cells and hematopoietic stem cells, whereas *RHOA*[G17V] and *IDH2*[R172] mutations appear to be confined to the neoplastic T cells. A scenario of multistep and multilineage tumorigenesis has been suggested, in which the initial mutations in *TET2* or *DNMT3* occur in a hematopoietic stem cell with subsequent acquisition of *RHOA*, *IDH2*, and TCR gene mutations important for T-cell function, leading to TFH lymphoma.[100] CH is also associated with myeloid neoplasms.[101] This explains the frequent association of AITL with myeloid neoplasms, mainly chronic myelomonocytic leukemia, acute myeloid leukemia, and myelodysplastic syndrome, in the same patients. In some patients, it has been demonstrated that the myeloid neoplasm and AITL share common ancestral mutations in *TET2* and *DNMT3A*, suggesting that they arise from divergent evolution of a common CH clone.[18,99] More recently has been shown an increased association of TFH and cytotoxic T-cell lymphomas sharing TET2 and/or DNMT3A mutations suggesting that cytotoxic T-cell lymphomas also develop in a background of CH.[101a]

CLINICAL COURSE AND PROGNOSIS

The clinical course of AITL, which is the prototype of TFH lymphomas, is characterized by rapid progression in most patients; however, spontaneous remissions may occur.[36] The median survival is less than 3 years.[102,103] The majority of deaths are caused by infectious complications rather than progressive lymphoma, which makes AITL particularly difficult to treat with chemotherapy. Owing to the underlying immunodeficiency and abnormalities of T-cell function, in addition to the infectious complications, patients may have expanding EBV-positive B-cell clones that may lead to EBV-positive large B-cell lymphomas in rare cases.[29,62] The clinical course appears to correlate with the extent of systemic symptoms at presentation (i.e., rash, pruritus, edema, ascites). Because 90% of AITL patients have stage III or IV disease at presentation, staging is not very useful in predicting clinical outcome for most patients. Male gender and the presence of mutations in *TET2, DNMT3A,* and *IDH2* have been associated with inferior prognosis.[37,103,104] A prognostic index developed for TFH lymphoma patients has been shown to be more useful than the IPI.[36] A new predictive score that has been developed categorizes patients into three prognostic groups based on beta-2-microglobulin and C-reactive protein levels, age, and ECOG (Eastern Cooperative Oncology group) performance status.[102] The clinical course and the prognosis of TFH lymphomas, follicular type and NOS, is uncertain but may not entirely differ from that of AITL.[6,13,16,27,103,105,106] Two studies have described an overall survival of 50% to 60% for TFH lymphoma, follicular type at 2 years.[16,26] Recent studies suggest that TFH lymphomas respond better to histone deacetylase and DNA methyltransferase inhibitors because of the common alterations in epigenetic modifying genes identified in this disease.[39,40,107]

DIFFERENTIAL DIAGNOSIS

Although the histopathologic features of AITL are well described, there is considerable morphologic overlap with a variety of benign and malignant lymphoid proliferations, including T-zone hyperplasia (paracortical hyperplasia), CHL, and PTCL, NOS (Table 35-2). T-zone hyperplasia is usually associated with viral infections or with a hyperimmune reaction secondary to an autoimmune disease. An important hint to the diagnosis of T-zone or paracortical hyperplasia is preservation of the lymph node architecture, with the presence of follicles and germinal centers and the lack of aberrant FDC proliferation. The paracortical area is expanded with a mixed infiltrate of medium-sized and small-sized lymphoid cells without atypia. Frequently, the numerous plasma cells, immunoblasts, and activated lymphocytes may mimic the cellular composition of AITL. Immunophenotypical analysis reveals a mixed CD4-CD8 population with scattered CD20-positive cells and variable numbers of CD25-positive and CD30-positive cells. No TCR rearrangements are identified. Moreover, CD10-positive cells, if present, are confined to the follicles.

The differential diagnosis between especially tumor-cell–rich variants of AITL and TFH lymphoma, NOS, can be challenging; however, currently there is no effect on clinical management. Morphologic features that favor the diagnosis of AITL are open, usually distended peripheral cortical sinuses; proliferation of FDCs highlighted by CD21/CD23; and prominent arborizing HEVs.[5,54,64,73,108] Occasionally the presence of numerous EBV-positive B cells, some of which acquire HRS-like features, may obscure the underlying TFH lymphoma or mimic CHL.[61,62,66] These cells have the immunophenotype of HRS cells (CD15 positive, CD30 positive, CD20 positive) and harbor EBV in most cases (EBER and LMP-1). Because many AITL cases show minimal cytologic atypia of T cells, the distinction from CHL may be difficult. In contrast to CHL, molecular studies reveal clonal rearrangements of the TCRγ chain gene in TFH lymphomas. Finally, because of the frequent occurrence of randomly scattered B blasts in TFH lymphomas, especially AITL, variant patterns of nodular lymphocyte predominant B-cell (Hodgkin) lymphoma (NLPBL/NLPHL) and T-cell/histiocyte–rich large B-cell lymphoma (THRLBCL) should be included in the differential

Table 35-2 Differential Diagnosis of Follicular Helper T-Cell Lymphoma, Angioimmunoblastic Type

Feature	AITL	T-Zone (Paracortical) Hyperplasia	PTCL, NOS	Classic Hodgkin Lymphoma
Nodal architecture	Usually effaced	Preserved	Usually effaced	Usually effaced
Clear cells	Present	Absent	Frequent	Absent
FDC proliferation	Present	Absent	Absent	Absent
HEVs	Present	Absent	Occasional	Absent
HRS cells	Rare, B-cell phenotype	Absent	Rare, T-cell phenotype	Present, B-cell phenotype −/+, PAX5 weak+
Immunophenotype	CD4+, CD10+, PD1+, ICOS+, CXCL13+, BCL6+ CD21+ FDCs, EBV+, B blasts	Mixed CD4/CD8 Scattered CD20+ Variable CD30+	CD4 > CD8, antigen loss (CD7, CD5)	CD15+, CD30+, CD20−/+, LMP-1+/−
Genotype	TR and IG genes rearranged Oligoclonal pattern Frequent mutations in *TET2, RHOA, DNMT3A,* and *IDH2* genes	No rearrangements No mutations	TR genes rearranged Rare mutations in *TET2, RHOA,* and *DNMT3A* genes in a subgroup	Polyclonal IG genes rearranged in HRS cells

+, Nearly always positive; −/+, may be positive, but usually negative; +/−, may be negative, but usually positive; *AITL,* angioimmunoblastic T-cell lymphoma; *EBV,* Epstein-Barr virus; *FDC,* follicular dendritic cell; *HEV,* high endothelial venule; *HRS,* Hodgkin–Reed-Sternberg; *IG,* immunoglobulin genes; *LMP-1,* latent membrane protein-1; *PTCL, NOS,* peripheral T-cell lymphoma, not otherwise specified; *TR,* T-cell receptor.

diagnosis. In NLPBL and THRLBCL, the background infiltrate is not as polymorphic as in TFH lymphomas and the B blasts are generally CD30 negative and EBV negative. However, in NLPBL, expanded meshworks of FDCs may occur. Molecular analysis may show monoclonal IGH gene rearrangements, and, especially, no TCR gene rearrangements are identified. A recently described pitfall in the differential diagnosis of AITL are cases of NMZL rich in PD1-positive T cells.[79] In these cases, demonstration of IG clonality and lack of typical mutations characteristic of TFH lymphomas support the diagnosis of NMZL.[109]

Pearls and Pitfalls

- The different morphologic subtypes of follicular helper T-cell (TFH) lymphomas have distinctive histologic features, but these features may overlap and the different subtypes may show considerable plasticity within the same patient at diagnosis and between diagnostic samples and relapses.
- Angioimmunoblastic T-cell lymphoma (AITL) is the prototypic form of TFH lymphoma, whereas TFH lymphoma, follicular type and NOS are much rarer.
- The clinical presentation of AITL is an essential diagnostic feature—localized lymphadenopathy is rare.
- B-cell or plasma-cell proliferation, EBV positive or EBV negative, is virtually always present in affected lymph nodes.
- In early phases, reactive follicular hyperplasia may be present, mimicking a reactive process.
- Highly characteristic histologic features of AITL include the following:
  - Extension of the infiltrate beyond the lymph node capsule into the perinodal fat, frequently sparing the preserved cortical sinuses, which are dilated
  - Prominent arborizing postcapillary high endothelial venules
- The most helpful routine immunophenotypical tools for diagnosis are demonstration of expanded FDCs meshworks in AITL with CD21 or CD23 and expression of TFH markers CD10, BCL6, CXCR3, PD1, and ICOS (CD278) in T cells in all forms of TFH lymphomas.
- In "early" pattern 1, the atypical mislocalization of CD10-positive, PD1-positive cells, sometimes with abundant clear cytoplasm surrounding the reactive germinal centers, is a clue to the diagnosis.
- EBV-positive B cells are nearly always present and may evolve to EBV-positive large B-cell lymphoma or a mimic of classic Hodgkin lymphoma.
- Nodal marginal zone lymphoma rich in PD1-positive T-cells might mimic the diagnosis of AITL.

KEY REFERENCES

1. de Leval L, Rickman DS, Thielen C, et al. The gene expression profile of nodal peripheral T-cell lymphoma demonstrates a molecular link between angioimmunoblastic T-cell lymphoma (AITL) and follicular helper T (TFH) cells. *Blood.* 2007;109(11):4952–4963.
11. Palomero T, Couronne L, Khiabanian H, et al. Recurrent mutations in epigenetic regulators, RHOA and FYN kinase in peripheral T cell lymphomas. *Nat Genet.* 2014;46(2):166–170.
13. Dobay MP, Lemonnier F, Missiaglia E, et al. Integrative clinicopathological and molecular analyses of angioimmunoblastic T-cell lymphoma and other nodal lymphomas of follicular helper T-cell origin. *Haematologica.* 2017;102(4):e148–e151.
16. Huang Y, Moreau A, Dupuis J, et al. Peripheral T-cell lymphomas with a follicular growth pattern are derived from follicular helper T cells (TFH) and may show overlapping features with angioimmunoblastic T-cell lymphomas. *Am J Surg Pathol.* 2009;33(5):682–690.
17. Attygalle AD, Kyriakou C, Dupuis J, et al. Histologic evolution of angioimmunoblastic T-cell lymphoma in consecutive biopsies: clinical correlation and insights into natural history and disease progression. *Am J Surg Pathol.* 2007;31(7):1077–1088.
18. Lewis NE, Petrova-Drus K, Huet S, et al. Clonal hematopoiesis in angioimmunoblastic T-cell lymphoma with divergent evolution to myeloid neoplasms. *Blood Adv.* 2020;4(10):2261–2271.
39. Lemonnier F, Dupuis J, Sujobert P, et al. Treatment with 5-azacytidine induces a sustained response in patients with angioimmunoblastic T-cell lymphoma. *Blood.* 2018;132(21):2305–2309.
61. Nicolae A, Pittaluga S, Venkataraman G, et al. Peripheral T-cell lymphomas of follicular T-helper cell derivation with Hodgkin/Reed-Sternberg cells of B-cell lineage: both EBV-positive and EBV-negative variants exist. *Am J Surg Pathol.* 2013;37(6):816–826.
67a. Ondrejka SL, et al. Follicular helper T-cell lymphomas: disease spectrum, relationship with clonal hematopoiesis, and mimics. A report of the 2022 EA4HP/SH lymphoma workshop. *Virchows Arch.* 2023;483:349.

74. Steinhilber J, Mederake M, Bonzheim I, et al. The pathological features of angioimmunoblastic T-cell lymphomas with IDH2(R172) mutations. *Mod Pathol.* 2019;32(8):1123–1134.

88. Wang C, McKeithan TW, Gong Q, et al. IDH2^{R172} mutations define a unique subgroup of patients with angioimmunoblastic T-cell lymphoma. *Blood.* 2015;126(15):1741–1752.

89. Vallois D, Dobay MP, Morin RD, et al. Activating mutations in genes related to TCR signaling in angioimmunoblastic and other follicular helper T-cell-derived lymphomas. *Blood.* 2016;128(11):1490–1502.

Visit Elsevier eBooks+ for the complete set of references.

Chapter 36

Anaplastic Large Cell Lymphoma, ALK Positive and ALK Negative

Laurence Lamant-Rochaix, Andrew L. Feldman, and Camille Laurent

DEFINITION AND BACKGROUND

Among the heterogeneous group of hematopoietic neoplasms with a predominant population of large cells, Stein and coworkers[1] recognized a subgroup of tumors with large cells exhibiting bizarre morphologic features and prominent sinusoidal invasion and expressing the Ki-1 antigen (now referred to as CD30). Based on the strong expression of this molecule, these tumors were designated *Ki-1 lymphoma.*[1] Because of the lack of strict morphologic criteria, some tumors were diagnosed as Ki-1 lymphoma simply because they consisted of large cells positive for the CD30 antigen, whatever their B-, T-, or null-cell phenotype. Later, the term *Ki-1 lymphoma* was replaced by anaplastic large cell lymphoma (ALCL). Although

there was no clear consensus among pathologists with regard to the definition of *anaplastic,* and despite the fact that some of these tumors consist of small-to-medium-sized cells, the term *ALCL* was incorporated into most classifications. Later, it was discovered that a significant proportion of ALCLs are associated with the t(2;5)(p23;q35) translocation.[2] A major advance was made with the cloning of this translocation[3] and the production of antibodies detecting its gene product—fusion of anaplastic lymphoma kinase (ALK).[4] As a consequence, ALCLs were divided in two main categories—those positive for ALK protein and those lacking this marker. In the World Health Organization (WHO) 3rd ed. classification of hematopoietic neoplasms, ALK-positive and ALK-negative ALCLs were considered a single disease entity and were defined as lymphomas consisting of lymphoid cells that are usually large and have abundant cytoplasm and pleomorphic, often horseshoe-shaped nuclei.[5] The cells are CD30 positive, and most cases express cytotoxic granule-associated proteins[6,7] and epithelial membrane antigen (EMA).[8] It became clear that although ALCLs expressing ALK are relatively homogeneous, cases with similar morphology and phenotype but lacking ALK expression are much more heterogeneous. ALCLs lacking ALK also differ from peripheral T-cell lymphomas, not otherwise specified (PTCL, NOS), some of which can be positive for CD30 in a variable number of cells. Current thinking recognizes ALCL, ALK positive, and ALCL, ALK negative as distinct diseases. Breast-implant–associated ALCL, also ALK-negative, is a recently recognized distinct entity and will be discussed. Systemic ALCL, both ALK positive and ALK negative, must be distinguished from primary cutaneous ALCL and from other subtypes of T-cell or B-cell lymphoma with anaplastic features or CD30 expression.[9]

ANAPLASTIC LARGE CELL LYMPHOMA, ALK POSITIVE

Synonyms and Related Terms

WHO revised 4th ed.: Anaplastic large cell lymphoma, ALK-positive

WHO proposed 5th ed.: ALK-positive anaplastic large cell lymphoma

Epidemiology

ALCL accounts for 5% of all non-Hodgkin lymphomas and 10% to 30% of childhood lymphomas.[10] ALK-positive ALCL is most frequent in the first 3 decades of life and shows a slight male predominance.[11,12]

Etiology

No pathogenic factor has been demonstrated. However, in rare cases, an association with recent insect bites has been suggested.[13,14] Occasional cases occur in human immunodeficiency virus (HIV)–positive patients or after solid organ transplantation.[15] It is unlikely that these conditions play a primary etiologic role, but emergence of the disease may be facilitated by abnormal cytokine production.

Clinical Features

Most patients (70%) with ALK-positive ALCL present with advanced stage III to IV disease with peripheral or abdominal lymphadenopathy, often associated with extranodal infiltrates and involvement of the bone marrow.[10,12] Patients often show B symptoms (75%), especially high fever.[10,12,16] Several cases with a leukemic presentation have been reported.[17-19]

Primary systemic ALCL positive for the ALK protein frequently involves both lymph nodes and extranodal sites. Extranodal sites commonly include skin (26%), bone (14%), soft tissues (15%), lung (11%), and liver (8%).[10,12,16] Retinal infiltration responsible for blindness and placental involvement have also been reported.[20] Involvement of the gut and central nervous system is rare. However, occasional cases of ALK-positive ALCL in the stomach, bladder, or central nervous system have been observed (authors' unpublished observations).[21,22] Mediastinal disease is less frequent than in Hodgkin lymphoma. The incidence of bone marrow involvement is approximately 10% when analyzed with hematoxylin and eosin (H&E) but increases significantly (30%) when immunohistochemical stains for CD30, EMA, or ALK are used (Fig. 36-1).[23] This is because bone marrow involvement is often subtle, with only scattered malignant cells that are difficult to detect by routine examination. Most patients have circulating antibodies against nucleophosmin (NPM)-ALK protein, and these antibodies may persist in patients who are apparently in complete remission.[24]

Morphology

The spectrum of morphologic features of ALK-positive ALCL is wider than was initially described,[1,11,25-29] ranging from small cell neoplasms, which pathologists might mistake for PTCL, NOS, to tumors in which very large cells predominate.[11] However, all cases contain a variable proportion of large cells with eccentric horseshoe-shaped or kidney-shaped nuclei, often with an eosinophilic region near the nucleus. These cells have been referred to as *hallmark cells* (Fig. 36-2A) because

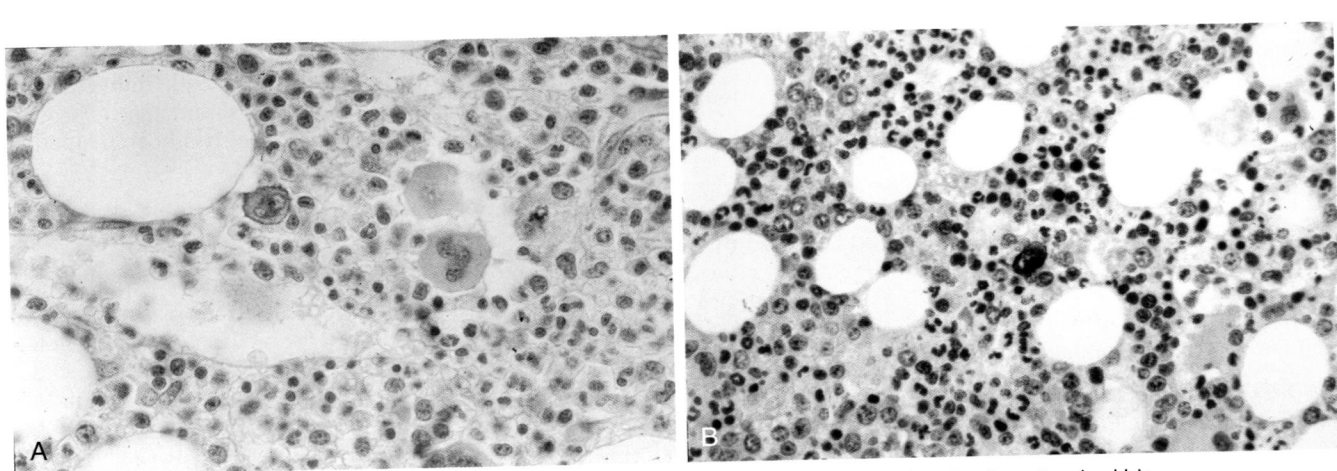

Figure 36-1. Although the bone marrow biopsy was considered to be uninvolved on standard histopathologic examination, immunohistochemistry shows scattered malignant cells strongly positive for CD30/Ber-H2 **(A)** and ALK1 antibody **(B)**.

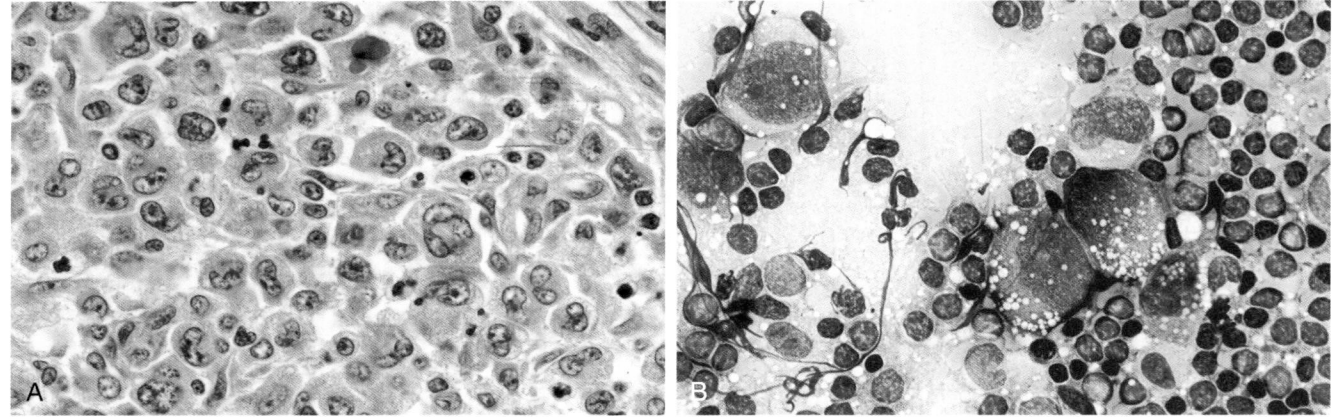

Figure 36-2. Anaplastic large cell lymphoma, common pattern. A, Predominant population of large cells with irregular nuclei. Note the large "hallmark" cells with eccentric kidney-shaped nuclei. One "donut" cell can be seen in this field. **B,** Lymph node imprint preparation shows lymphoma cells with vacuolated cytoplasm.

they are present in all morphologic patterns.[11] Although hallmark cells are typically large, smaller cells with similar cytologic features may be seen and can greatly aid in making the diagnosis.[11] Depending on the plane of the section, some cells may appear to contain cytoplasmic inclusions. These are not true inclusions, however, but invaginations of the nuclear membrane. Cells with these features have been referred to as *donut cells* (see Fig. 36-2A).[30,31] In some cases, the nuclei are round to oval, and the proliferation appears quite monomorphic (see Fig. 36-7A).

The tumor cells have more abundant cytoplasm than most other lymphomas. The cytoplasm may appear clear, basophilic, or eosinophilic. On lymph node imprints these cells show vacuolated cytoplasm (see Fig. 36-2B). Multiple nuclei may occur in a wreathlike pattern, giving rise to cells resembling Reed-Sternberg (RS) cells. The nuclear chromatin is usually finely clumped or dispersed, with multiple small basophilic nucleoli. Prominent inclusion-like nucleoli are relatively uncommon, aiding in the differential diagnosis with classic Hodgkin lymphoma (CHL).[32]

ALCLs exhibit a very broad range of cytologic appearances.[11,32,33] Five morphologic patterns have been recognized since the WHO 4th ed.[34]

Anaplastic Large Cell Lymphoma, Common Pattern

ALCL, common pattern (70%) is composed predominantly of pleomorphic large cells with the hallmark features described earlier. Tumor cells with more monomorphic, rounded nuclei also occur, either as the predominant population or mixed with the more pleomorphic cells. Rarely, erythrophagocytosis by malignant cells may be seen. When the lymph node architecture is only partially effaced, the tumor characteristically grows within the sinuses and thus may resemble a metastatic tumor (Fig. 36-3). Tumor cells may also colonize the paracortex and often grow in a cohesive manner (Fig. 36-4).

Anaplastic Large Cell Lymphoma, Lymphohistiocytic Pattern

ALCL, lymphohistiocytic pattern (10%) is characterized by tumor cells admixed with a large number of histiocytes (Fig. 36-5A–C).[11,27,35,36] The histiocytes may mask the malignant

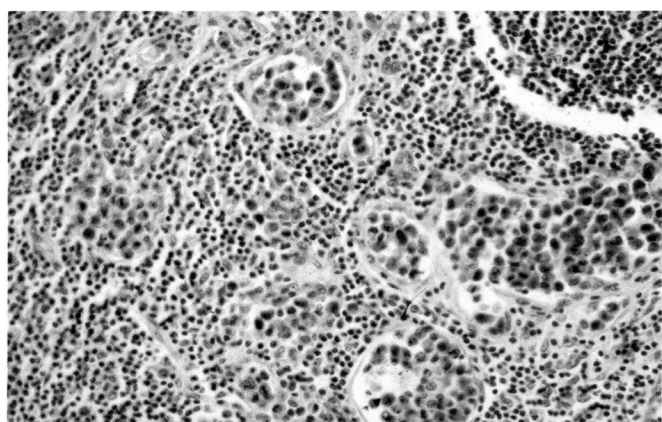

Figure 36-3. General features of anaplastic large cell lymphoma, common pattern. In some cases the predominant sinusoidal growth pattern mimics a metastatic malignancy.

cells, which are often smaller than in the common pattern (see Fig. 36-5D). The neoplastic cells often cluster around blood vessels and can be highlighted by immunostaining using antibodies to CD30 (see Fig. 36-5E–F), ALK, or cytotoxic molecules. Occasionally the histiocytes show signs of erythrophagocytosis. The histiocytes typically have finely granular eosinophilic cytoplasm and small, round uniform nuclei. Well-formed granulomas are absent, and clusters of epithelioid cells (as may be seen in the lymphoepithelioid cell variant of PTCL, NOS) are not seen.

Anaplastic Large Cell Lymphoma, Small Cell Pattern

ALCL, small cell pattern (10%) shows a predominant population of small-to-medium-sized neoplastic cells with irregular nuclei (Fig. 36-6A–C).[11,26,30] However, morphologic features vary from case to case, and cells with round nuclei and clear cytoplasm ("fried egg" cells) may predominate. Hallmark cells are always present and are often concentrated around blood vessels (see Fig. 36-6D).[11] Usually there is massive infiltration of the perinodal connective tissue. This morphologic variant of ALCL is often misdiagnosed as PTCL, NOS by conventional examination. When the blood is

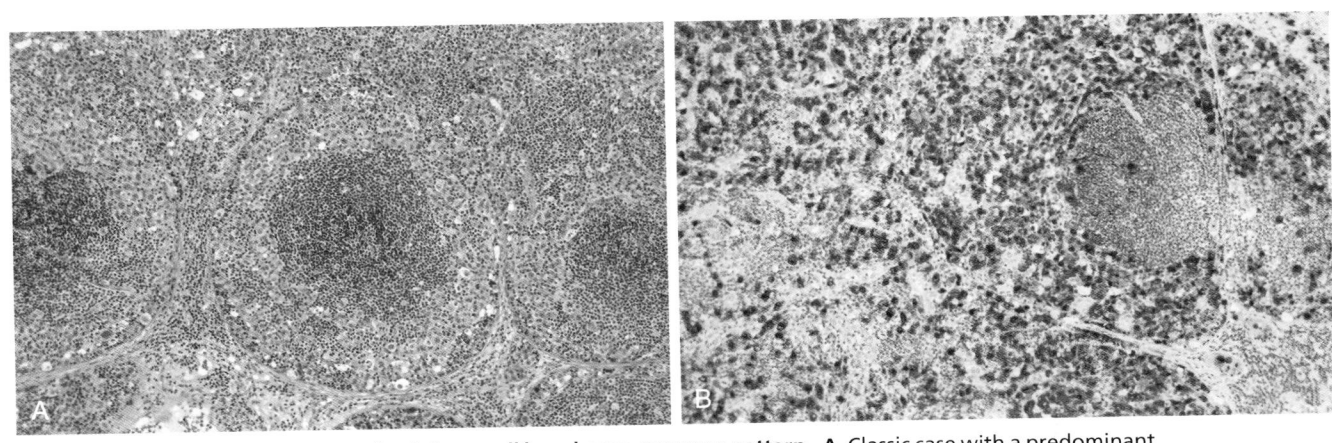

Figure 36-4. Anaplastic large cell lymphoma, common pattern. A, Classic case with a predominant perifollicular and paracortical pattern on hematoxylin and eosin (H&E) stain. **B,** ALK1 staining.

involved, atypical cells reminiscent of flower-like cells may be observed in smear preparations.[17,18] It is likely that the small cell and lymphohistiocytic patterns are closely related.[9,31]

Anaplastic Large Cell Lymphoma, Hodgkin-Like Pattern

ALCL, Hodgkin-like pattern (1%–3%) is characterized by morphologic features mimicking nodular sclerosis CHL.[37] These cases show a vaguely nodular fibrosis associated with capsular thickening and a significant number of tumor cells resembling classic RS cells associated with hallmark cells (see Fig. 36-7E). In the past, many tumors with similar features were referred to as *Hodgkin-like ALCL*. However, most cases designated as such were negative for ALK and were more likely variants of CHL rich in Hodgkin cells or lymphomas with features intermediate between CHL and diffuse large B-cell lymphoma—so-called *gray zone lymphomas*.[31,38] It must be stressed that CD30-positive lymphomas, with or without a sinusoidal growth pattern, should not be diagnosed as ALCL, Hodgkin-like unless they are positive for ALK. In cases negative for ALK protein, additional immunophenotypic and molecular studies usually permit their classification as aggressive B-cell or T-cell lymphomas.

Anaplastic Large Cell Lymphoma, Composite Pattern

ALCL with a composite pattern accounts for 10% to 20% of cases. These cases have features of more than one pattern in a single lymph node biopsy. In addition, in some cases, a repeat biopsy taken at the time of relapse may reveal morphologic features that differ from those seen initially, suggesting that the morphologic patterns of ALCL are simply variations of the same entity.[11,26]

Other Histologic Patterns

Other histologic patterns may be seen, although they are not recognized as distinctive patterns in the WHO classification. They are often responsible for diagnostic difficulties. These include a giant cell–rich pattern (Fig. 36-7B), a sarcomatoid pattern (see Fig. 36-7C), and a "signet ring"–like pattern (see Fig. 36-7D). Some ALCLs may mimic a metastatic malignancy, with cohesive neoplastic cells encased within a dense fibrosis (see Fig. 36-7F). Some ALCLs may show a striking edematous or myxoid background, either focally or throughout the

whole tissue section (see Fig. 36-7G). Tumors with such morphology have been reported as hypocellular ALCL.[39] A starry-sky appearance may also be observed, suggesting Burkitt lymphoma on low-power magnification.

Immunophenotype

By definition, all ALCLs are positive for CD30. In most cases, virtually all neoplastic cells show strong CD30 staining on the cell membrane and in the Golgi region (Fig. 36-8A). In the small cell variant and sometimes in the lymphohistiocytic variant, the strongest immunostaining is seen in the large cells, which often cluster around blood vessels (see Figs. 36-5F and 36-6D)[11]; smaller tumor cells may be only weakly positive or even negative for CD30. The majority of ALCLs are positive for EMA.[8,11] The staining pattern for EMA is usually like that seen with CD30, although in some cases only a proportion of malignant cells is positive (see Fig. 36-8B).

Most ALCLs express one or more T-cell or natural killer (NK)-cell antigens.[10,11,40] However, owing to the loss of several pan–T-cell antigens, some cases may have an apparent null-cell phenotype. Because no other distinctions can be found in ALK-positive ALCLs with a T-cell versus null-cell phenotype, they are considered part of the same entity.[11,41] CD3, the most widely used pan–T-cell marker, is negative in more than 75% of cases.[11] This tendency for loss of CD3 is also seen in ALK-negative ALCL. CD5 and CD7 are often negative as well. CD2 and CD4 are more useful and are positive in a significant proportion of cases. CD43 is expressed in more than two-thirds of cases but lacks lineage specificity (see Fig. 36-8C). Most cases exhibit positivity for the cytotoxic-associated antigens TIA-1, granzyme B, and perforin (see Fig. 36-8D–E).[6,7] CD8 is usually negative, but rare CD8-positive cases exist. Occasional cases are positive for CD68/KP1 but not CD68/PGM1.

Tumor cells are variably positive for CD45 and CD45RO but strongly positive for CD25.[8] Blood group antigens H and Y (detected with antibody BNH.9) have been reported in more than 50% of cases (see Fig. 36-8F).[42] CD15 expression is occasionally observed.[11] ALCLs are consistently negative for Epstein-Barr virus (EBV) (i.e., EBV-encoded small RNA [EBER] and latent membrane protein-1 [LMP-1]).[43] A study employing array technology to detect new genes expressed in ALCL found that clusterin is aberrantly expressed in all cases

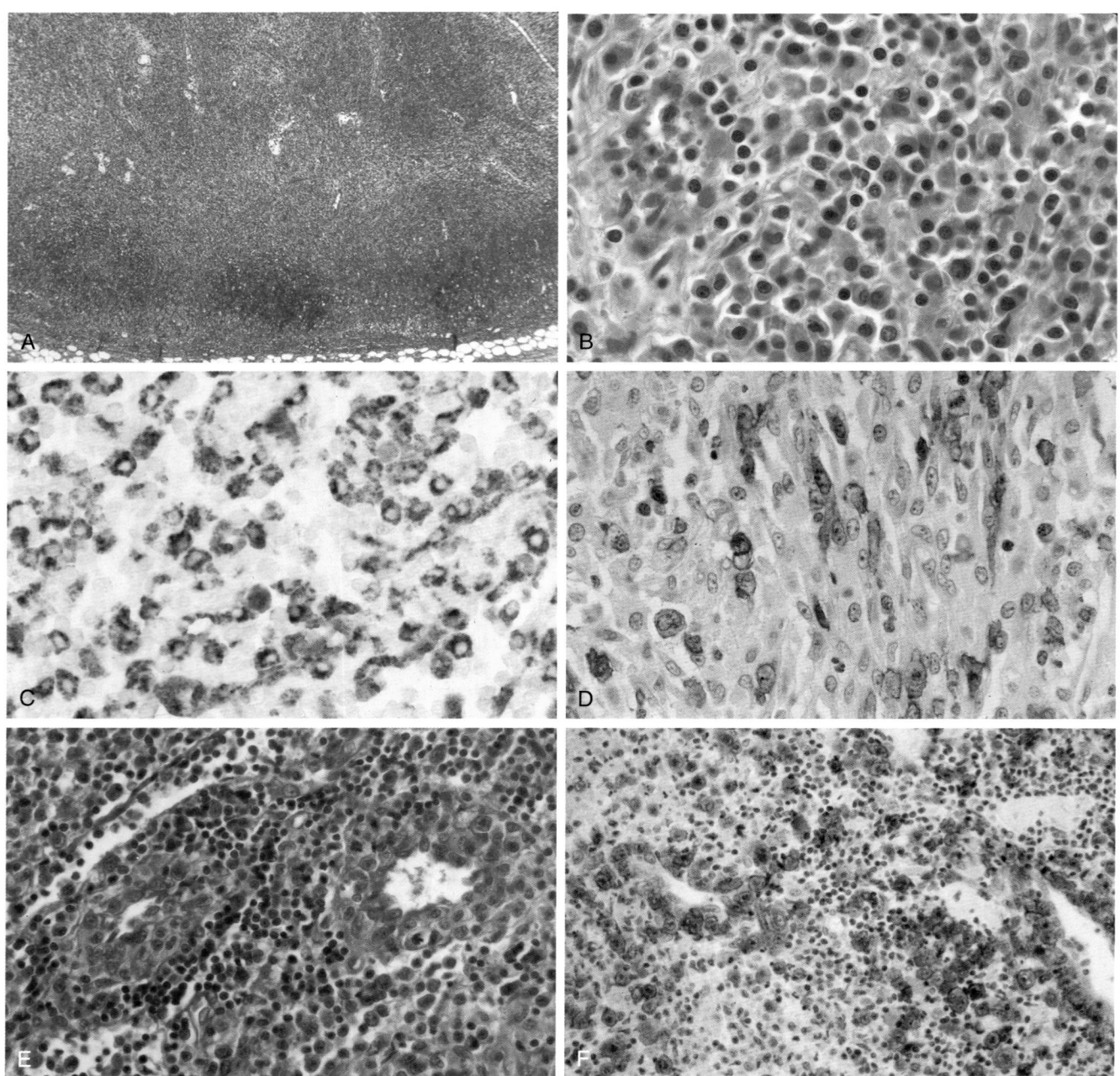

Figure 36-5. Anaplastic large cell lymphoma, lymphohistiocytic pattern. A, At low power, the infiltrate is mainly paracortical in distribution. **B,** On a high-power view, malignant cells are admixed with a predominant population of non-neoplastic histiocytes. The malignant cells may be extremely rare and difficult to detect on hematoxylin and eosin (H&E) stain. **C,** Double immunostaining with CD68/KP1 *(brown)* and ALK1 *(blue)* confirms the paucity of malignant cells (blue nuclear staining). **D,** CD30 staining shows that the malignant cells vary in size, with some exhibiting a fibroblast-like morphology. **E** and **F,** Characteristically, the neoplastic cells often cluster around blood vessels and can be highlighted by immunostaining using antibodies to CD30. Such a perivascular pattern is also observed in anaplastic large cell lymphoma, small cell variant.

of systemic ALCL but not in primary cutaneous ALCL.[44] Most ALK-positive ALCLs are negative for BCL2 (see Fig. 36-8G).[45] A number of other antigens are expressed in ALCL, but they are not of diagnostic value. They include CD56[46-48]; SHP1 phosphatase[49]; BCL6, C/EBPβ, and serpinA1[50,51]; myeloid-associated antigens CD13 and CD33[52]; and p63.[53] Tumor cells express PDL1 via induced expression of STAT3 activity

by NPM-ALK, providing rationale for immune checkpoint inhibitors.[54]

The ALK staining may be cytoplasmic, nuclear, and nucleolar or it may be restricted to either the cytoplasm or, more rarely, the cell membrane (Fig. 36-9). Among hematopoietic neoplasms, ALK expression is virtually specific for ALCL because it is absent from all normal postnatal

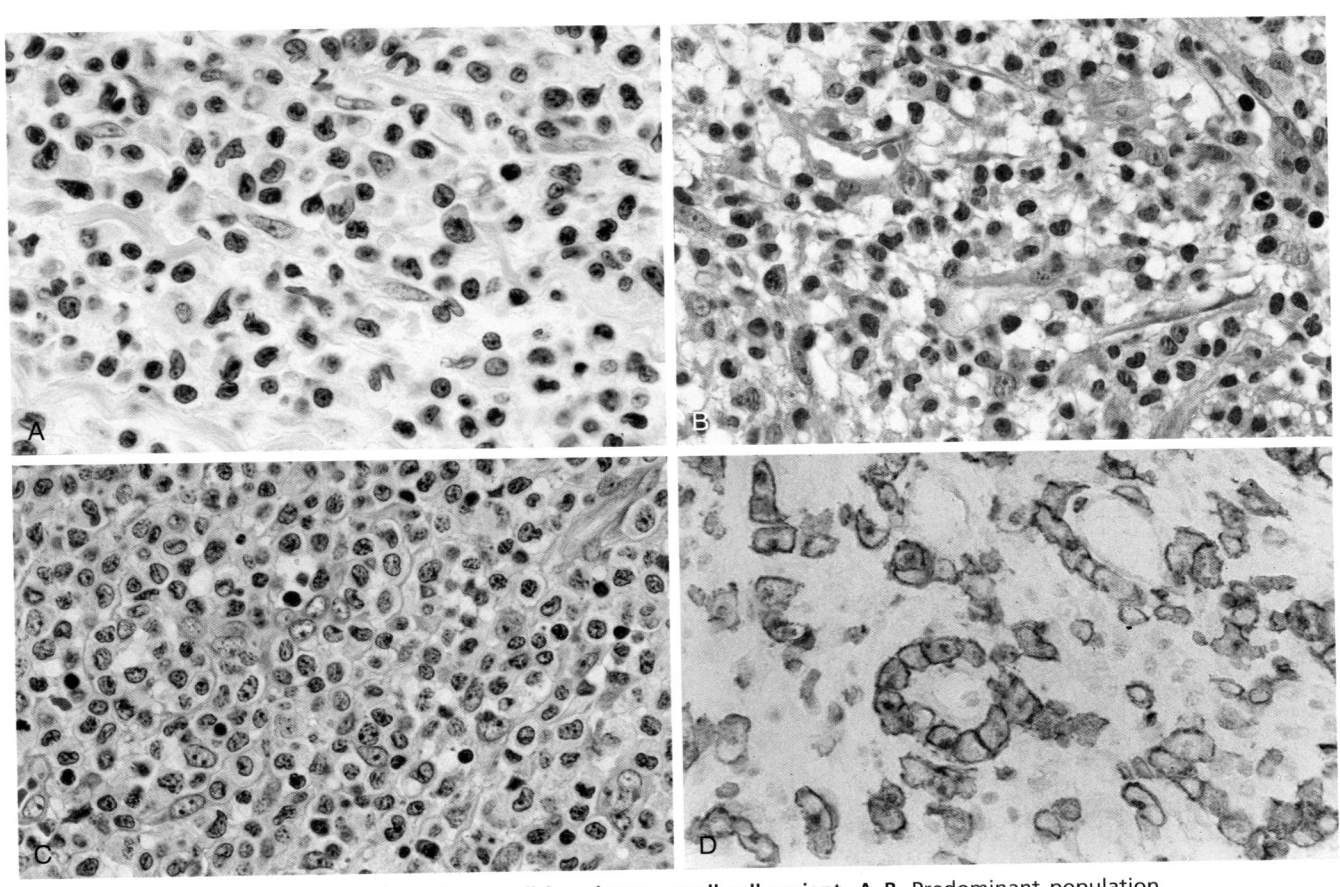

Figure 36-6. Anaplastic large cell lymphoma, small cell variant. A–B, Predominant population of small cells with irregular nuclei associated with scattered hallmark cells with kidney-shaped nuclei. **C,** This case exhibits a monomorphic population of small cells with clear cytoplasm ("fried egg" cells). **D,** In most cases the neoplastic cells are perivascular, a pattern that is highlighted by CD30 staining. Note that the large cells are strongly positive for CD30, whereas the small-sized and medium-sized malignant cells are only weakly stained.

human tissues except for rare cells in the brain[55] and absent from hematopoietic neoplasms other than ALCL, with the exception of ALK-positive large B-cell lymphomas (see Fig. 36-13)[56] and a novel form of ALK-positive histiocytosis seen in infancy.[57] It is important to note that in the small cell pattern and, to a lesser extent, in the lymphohistiocytic pattern, ALK staining may be restricted to scattered large cells. However, ALK staining performed without a nuclear counterstain often reveals small cells showing restricted nuclear staining.

Genetics and Molecular Findings

Approximately 90% of ALCLs show clonal rearrangement of the T-cell receptor (TR) genes, irrespective of whether they express T-cell antigens.[6] The majority of ALCLs are associated with a reciprocal translocation, t(2;5)(p23;q35), which juxtaposes the gene at 5q35 encoding NPM, a nucleolar-associated phosphoprotein, with the gene at 2p23 coding for ALK, a receptor tyrosine kinase.[3,58] Polyclonal and monoclonal antibodies recognizing the intracellular portion of ALK react with both NPM-ALK protein and the full-length ALK protein, but no normal lymphoid cells express full-length ALK; as a consequence, immunostaining with anti-ALK has been used to detect ALCL cases carrying the t(2;5) translocation.[3,55,59] However, variant translocations involving *ALK* and other

partner genes on chromosomes 1, 2, 3, 4, 8, 9, 11, 17, 19, and 22 also occur (Table 36-1).[60-70] All result in the upregulation of *ALK*, but the distribution of the staining varies, depending on the translocation. The classic t(2;5) translocation leads to positive staining for ALK in the nucleolus, nucleus, and cytoplasm (see Fig. 36-9A–B).[71] In the variant translocations, often only cytoplasmic staining is observed (see Fig. 36-9C–E). In t(2;5)(p23;q35) translocation, the particular cytoplasmic, nuclear, and nucleolar staining can be explained by the formation of dimers between wild-type NPM and the fusion NPM-ALK protein. Wild-type NPM provides nuclear localization signals whereby the NPM-ALK protein can enter the nucleus.[71,72] The formation of NPM-ALK homodimers using dimerization sites at the N-terminus of NPM mimics ligand binding and is responsible for activation of the ALK catalytic domain (i.e., autophosphorylation of the tyrosine kinase domain of ALK), which is responsible for its oncogenic properties.

Besides t(2;5) translocation, at least 13 variant translocations involving the *ALK* gene at p23 have been recognized. In all these translocations the *ALK* gene is placed under the control of the promoter of genes that are constitutively expressed in lymphoid cells resulting in expression of an *ALK* fusion gene. The most frequent variant translocation is t(1;2)(q25;p23),[61,62] in which the *TPM3* gene on chromosome 1

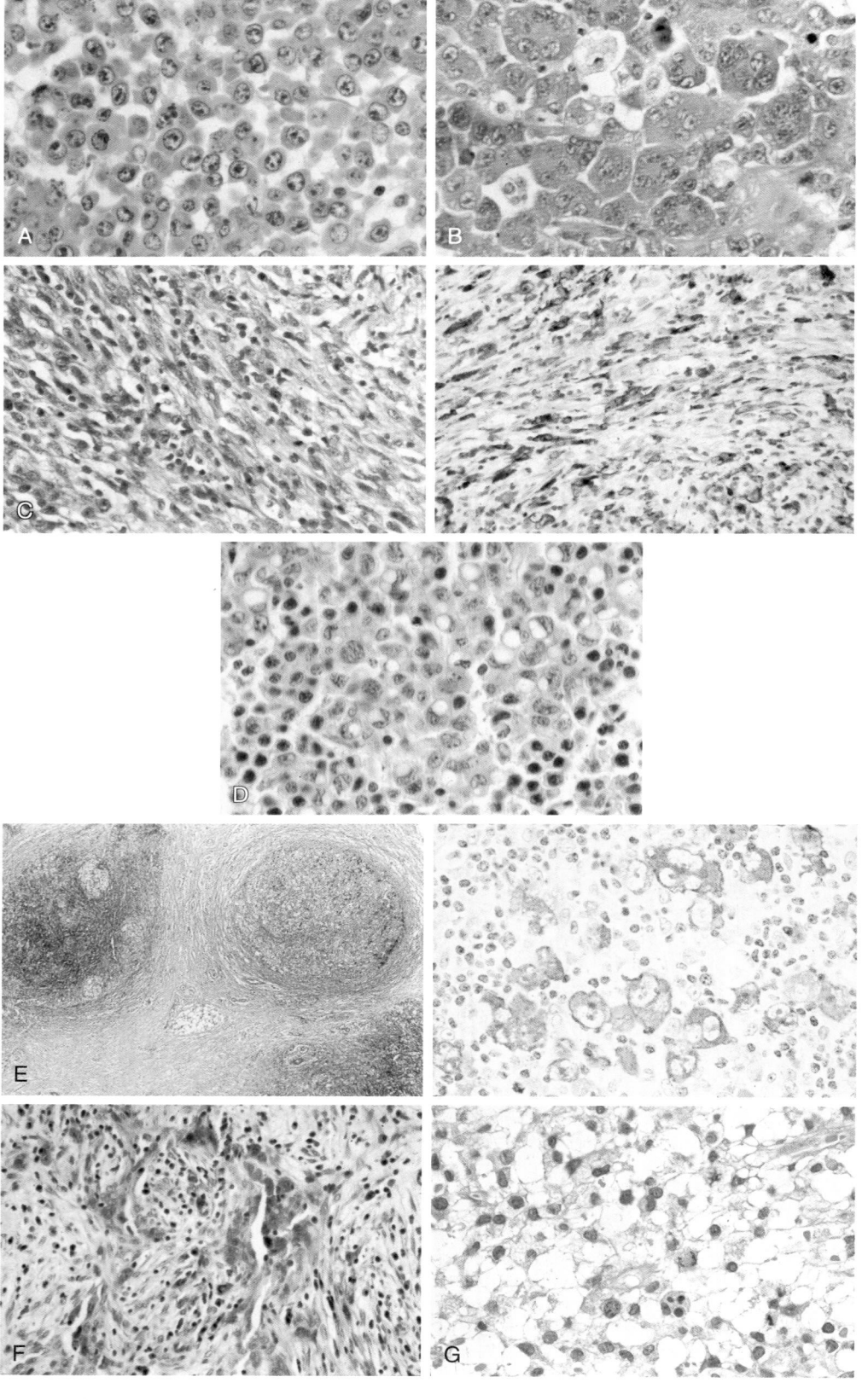

Figure 36-7. Other histologic patterns of anaplastic large cell lymphoma (ALCL). All these cases were positive for anaplastic lymphoma kinase (ALK) protein. **A,** ALCL exhibits monomorphic large cells with round nuclei. **B,** ALCL consisting of pleomorphic giant cells. **C,** ALCL with sarcomatous features (*left:* hematoxylin and eosin; *right:* CD30 staining). **D,** ALCL rich in "signet ring" cells. **E,** ALCL mimicking nodular sclerosis CHL (*left:* hematoxylin and eosin; *right:* ALK staining). Cases of ALCL with this morphology are extremely rare. **F,** ALCL mimicking a metastatic malignancy. **G,** ALCL with edematous stroma. Tumors showing this morphology have been reported as hypocellular ALCL. (**G,** Courtesy of Dr. J. K. C. Chan, Hong Kong.)

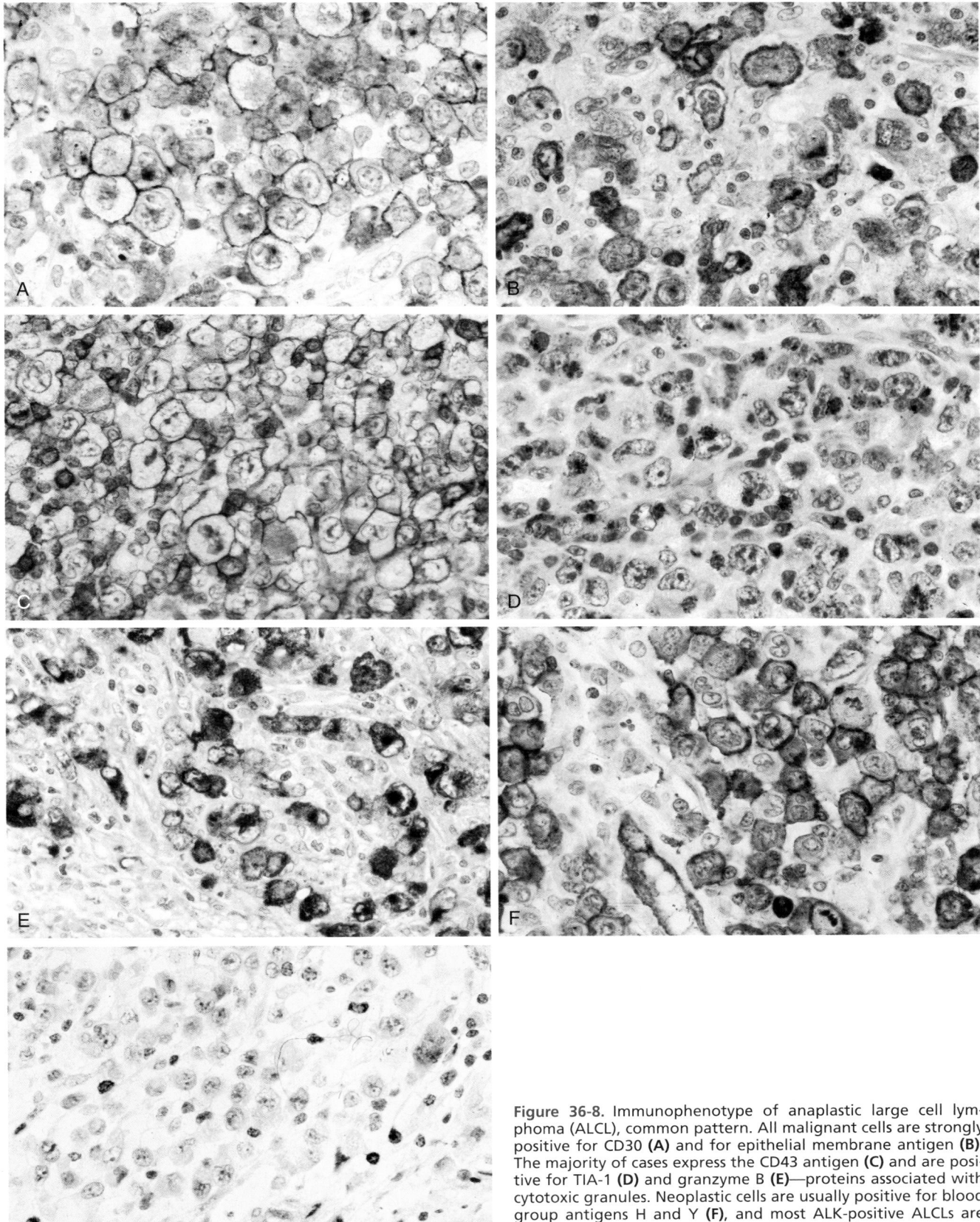

Figure 36-8. Immunophenotype of anaplastic large cell lymphoma (ALCL), common pattern. All malignant cells are strongly positive for CD30 **(A)** and for epithelial membrane antigen **(B)**. The majority of cases express the CD43 antigen **(C)** and are positive for TIA-1 **(D)** and granzyme B **(E)**—proteins associated with cytotoxic granules. Neoplastic cells are usually positive for blood group antigens H and Y **(F)**, and most ALK-positive ALCLs are negative for BCL2 **(G)**. Note the positive small lymphocytes used as internal controls.

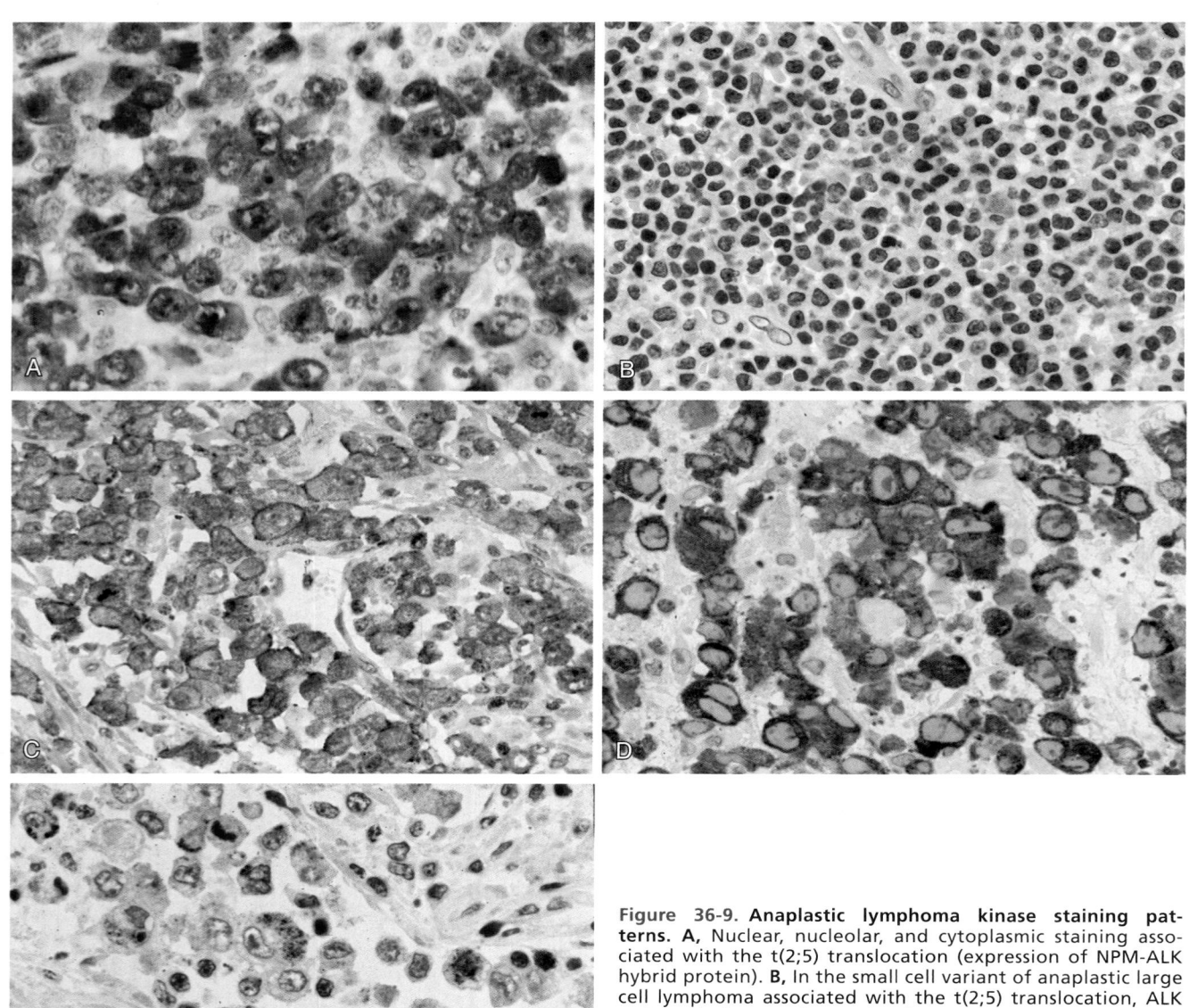

Figure 36-9. Anaplastic lymphoma kinase staining patterns. A, Nuclear, nucleolar, and cytoplasmic staining associated with the t(2;5) translocation (expression of NPM-ALK hybrid protein). **B,** In the small cell variant of anaplastic large cell lymphoma associated with the t(2;5) translocation, ALK staining is frequently restricted to nuclei. **C,** Restricted cytoplasmic staining with enhanced membrane staining in a case associated with the t(1;2) translocation (expression of TPM3-ALK hybrid protein). **D,** Diffuse cytoplasmic staining in a case associated with the inv(2)(p23q35) (expression of ATIC-ALK). **E,** Finely granular cytoplasmic staining associated with the t(2;17) translocation (expression of CLTC-ALK hybrid protein).

(which encodes a nonmuscular tropomyosin protein)[61] is fused to the *ALK* catalytic domain. However, in cases associated with the t(1;2) translocation, which express the TPM3-ALK protein (104 kDa), ALK staining is restricted to the cytoplasm of malignant cells, and in virtually all cases there is stronger staining on the cell membrane (see Fig. 36-9C).[55,61] This staining pattern is found in 15% to 20% of ALK-positive ALCLs. Tropomyosins are known to form dimeric alpha-coiled coil structures that can induce dimerization of the chimeric TPM3-ALK protein and activation of the ALK catalytic domain (i.e., autophosphorylation of ALK protein).[61] The genes fused with *ALK* in t(2;3)(p23;q11)[60,62] and inv(2)(p23q35)[64,65] have been identified (see Fig. 36-9D). Two different fusion proteins of 85 and 97 kDa (TFG-ALK$_{short}$ and TFG-ALK$_{long}$) are associated with t(2;3)(p23;q11) translocation, which involves

TFG (TRK-fused gene).[60] The inv(2)(p23q35) involves the *ATIC* gene (formerly known as *pur-H*), which encodes 5-aminomidazole-4-carboxamide-ribonucleotide transformylase-IMP cyclohydrolase (ATIC), which plays a key role in the de novo purine biosynthesis pathways.[64] In TFG-ALK-positive and ATIC-ALK-positive ALCLs, ALK staining is restricted to the cytoplasm in a diffuse pattern.[60,64]

Rare cases of ALCL show a unique granular ALK cytoplasmic staining pattern (see Fig. 36-9E).[63] In these cases, the *ALK* gene is fused to the *CLTC* gene, which encodes the clathrin heavy polypeptide (CLTC) that is the main structural protein of coated vesicles. The sequence of the fusion gene suggests that these tumors might have reciprocal translocations involving breakpoints at 17q11-qter and 2p23. In *CLTC-ALK*-positive ALCL, the presence of the clathrin heavy polypeptide in

Table 36-1 Genetic Abnormalities in ALK Positive ALCL That Create Fusion Genes

Chromosomal Anomaly	*ALK* Partner	Molecular Weight of ALK Hybrid Protein	ALK Staining Pattern	Percentage*
t(2;5)(p23;q35)	*NPM*	80	Nuclear, diffuse cytoplasmic	84
t(1;2)(q25;p23)	*TPM3*	104	Diffuse cytoplasmic with peripheral intensification	13
inv(2)(p23q35)	*ATIC*	96	Diffuse cytoplasmic	1
t(2;3)(p23;q11)	*TFG*$_{Xlong}$	113	Diffuse cytoplasmic	<1
	TFG$_{long}$	97	Diffuse cytoplasmic	
	TFG$_{short}$	85	Diffuse cytoplasmic	
t(2;17)(p23;q23)	*CLTC*	250	Granular cytoplasmic	<1
t(2; X)(p23;q11-12)	*MSN*	125	Membrane staining	<1
t(2;19)(p23;p13.1)	*TPM4*	95	Diffuse cytoplasmic	<1
t(2;22)(p23;q11.2)	*MYH9*	220	Diffuse cytoplasmic	<1
Dic(2;4)(p23;q33)	*ND*	ND	Cytoplasmic	<1
t(2;17)(p23;q25)	*RNF213*	ND	Diffuse cytoplasmic	<1
t(2;9)(p23;q33)	*TRAF1*	<80	Diffuse cytoplasmic	<1
t(2;11)(p23;q12)	*EEF1G*	ND	Cytoplasmic	<1
t(2;8)(p23;q22)	*PABPC1*	>100	Cytoplasmic	<1

*Percentage of these variants in an unpublished series of 270 cases of ALK-positive ALCL.
ALCL, Anaplastic large cell lymphoma; *ALK,* anaplastic lymphoma kinase; *ND,* not determined.

the hybrid protein accounts for the granular cytoplasmic staining pattern because the CLTC-ALK protein is involved in the formation of the clathrin coat on the surface of vesicles. Moreover, the process of clathrin coat formation mimics ligand binding; this allows the autophosphorylation of the carboxy-terminal domain of ALK protein, which is probably responsible for its oncogenic property.[63] In a single report, the moesin (*MSN*) gene at chromosome Xq11-12 was identified as a new *ALK* fused gene (MSN-ALK fusion protein) in a case of ALCL with a distinct ALK membrane-restricted pattern.[73] The particular membrane staining pattern of ALK is probably caused by the binding properties of the N-terminal domain of moesin to cell membrane–associated proteins. In this case, the *ALK* breakpoint was different from that described in all other translocations and occurred within the exonic sequence coding for the juxtamembrane portion of ALK. The *TRAF1-ALK* fusion encodes part, but not all, of the C-terminal TRAF domain responsible for oligomerization of TRAF1.[68] Thus, the potential dimerization and function of TRAF1-ALK will require further study.[68]

In the translocation of dicentric (2;4)(p23;q33), the *ALK* partner was not identified.[74] *EEF1G* and *PABPC1* genes have been the most recent identified *ALK* gene partners.[69,70]

Whole-exome sequencing of ALK-positive ALCL has shown recurrent mutations in the T-cell receptor and Notch pathways, including potentially targetable, recurrent mutations of *NOTCH1*.[75]

Clinical Course and Prognostic Factors

The overall 5-year survival of ALK-positive ALCL varies from 70% to 80%, in contrast to less than 50% in ALK-negative cases.[76] Relapses are not uncommon (30% of cases), but they often remain sensitive to chemotherapy[77] and, in some cases, ALK small molecular inhibitors.[78] The International Prognostic Index appears to be of some value in predicting outcome, although less so than in other types of lymphoma.[29,79] An important prognostic indicator is ALK positivity, which has been associated with a favorable prognosis in series from North America, Europe, and Japan.[4,79,80] ALK positivity

seems particularly important in patients more than 40 years old, whereas in patients less than 40 years old, ALK has no effect on progression-free survival and overall survival (OS).[81] No differences have been found between NPM-ALK–positive tumors and tumors showing variant translocations involving *ALK* and fusion partners other than *NPM*.[80] In childhood ALK-positive ALCL, small cell or lymphohistiocytic morphologic features are adverse prognostic factors.[82,83] Detection of minimal disseminated disease by qualitative polymerase chain reaction (PCR) for *NPM-ALK* in bone marrow and peripheral blood at diagnosis and an early positive minimal residual disease (MRD) during treatment identify patients at risk of relapse.[84,85] This could be linked to poor immune control of the disease, partly reflected by the anti-ALK antibody titer that is inversely correlated to prognosis.[86] Quantification of early MRD might further improve risk stratification in international clinical studies and patient selection for early clinical trials.[87,88]

ANAPLASTIC LARGE CELL LYMPHOMA, ALK NEGATIVE

Synonyms and Related Terms

WHO revised 4th ed.: Anaplastic large cell lymphoma, ALK-negative

WHO proposed 5th ed.: ALK-negative anaplastic large cell lymphoma

Tumors with morphologic and phenotypic features consistent with ALCL but negative for ALK have been recognized since the initial identification of *ALK* rearrangements and development of ALK immunohistochemistry. A challenge to defining these cases has been the lack of clear phenotypic or molecular markers to form the basis for strict diagnostic criteria. It was recognized, however, that these cases showed distinct clinical features, with OS rates inferior to those of ALK-positive ALCL but superior to those of CD30-positive PTCL, NOS.[72] ALK-negative ALCL was first considered a provisional entity distinct from ALK-positive ALCL in the WHO 4th ed. and upgraded to a definite entity to the revised

WHO 4th ed.[89] Ongoing study of ALK-negative ALCL has revealed additional molecular heterogeneity reflected in part by the recent International Consensus Classification (ICC) of hematopoietic neoplasms.[90]

Definition

ALK-negative ALCL has morphologic and phenotypic features indistinguishable from the common pattern of ALK-positive ALCL, with (1) hallmark cells; (2) a diffuse growth pattern, and (3) strong and uniform expression of CD30.[89] Desirable but not essential features include partial loss of T-cell markers, a cytotoxic phenotype, EMA positivity, and sinusoidal involvement. Unlike ALK-positive ALCL, histologic variants of ALK-negative ALCL are not recognized. ALK-negative ALCL with *DUSP22* rearrangement is now recognized as a genetic subtype of ALK-negative ALCL.

Epidemiology

Unlike ALK-positive ALCL, the incidence of ALK-negative ALCL peaks in adults (40–65 years),[10,82] with a slight male preponderance. The etiology of ALK-negative ALCL remains unclear. Occasional cases positive for EBV or arising in the setting of immunodeficiency have been reported, but most probably do not correspond stricto sensu to ALCL.[91,92] Cases arising in association with breast implants are considered a distinct entity and are discussed separately.

Clinical Features

Patients present with peripheral or abdominal lymphadenopathy or extranodal tumor; however, extranodal involvement is less common than in ALK-positive ALCL.[10] Secondary skin involvement by systemic ALK-negative ALCL must be distinguished from primary cutaneous ALCL, which presents in the skin and in some cases may involve locoregional lymph nodes. Occasional cases involve mucosal sites in the upper aerodigestive tract. Clinical staging is required in these cases as well, because lesions localized to these mucosal sites appear to behave more similarly to primary cutaneous ALCL than to systemic ALCL.[93,94]

Morphology

Morphologically, cases resemble the common pattern of ALK-positive ALCL, including hallmark cells that often grow within sinuses (Fig. 36-10A). Other cases consist of more pleomorphic cells with a high nuclear-to-cytoplasmic ratio (see Fig. 36-10B–C).[5,29,32,89] The classification of cases with morphologic features resembling CHL but of documented T-cell origin is controversial; some of these cases may best be classified as PTCL, NOS.[95] Cases with morphologic features resembling the small cell pattern of ALK-positive ALCL but lacking ALK expression are not included within ALK-negative ALCL because of the lack of phenotypic or molecular markers that allow distinction from CD30-positive PTCL, NOS.

Immunophenotype

CD30 staining should be strong and uniform, and typically shows both a membranous and Golgi pattern. A diagnosis of PTCL, NOS should be considered in cases with variable CD30 expression. An exception is in patients with known ALCL treated with the anti-CD30 immunoconjugate brentuximab vedotin, in which diminished CD30 expression may be seen.[96,97] More than half of cases express one or more T-cell markers.[79] Positive staining for CD3 is more common than in ALK-positive ALCL. CD2 and CD4 are positive in a significant proportion of cases, whereas CD8-positive cases are rare. As in ALK-positive ALCL, the loss of one or more T-cell markers is frequently noted. In cases with a null-cell phenotype, a diagnosis of CHL rich in neoplastic cells must be excluded. PAX5, positive in 95% of CHL cases, is a useful marker in this setting; however, occasional ALCLs express PAX5 and molecular studies should be performed in ambiguous cases.[98] Expression of EMA is variable. The cytotoxic-associated markers TIA-1, granzyme B, and perforin are found in many cases, but are typically negative in the presence of *DUSP22* rearrangements (Fig. 36-11).[99] Almost all ALK-negative ALCL with *DUSP22* rearrangement show a strong expression of LEF1, a transcription factor of the Wnt/β-catenin pathway that may serve as surrogate marker.[100] ALK-negative ALCL is consistently negative for EBV (i.e., EBER and LMP-1).[43]

Genetics and Molecular Findings

TR genes are clonally rearranged in most cases, regardless of whether they express T-cell antigens. ALK-negative ALCL differs from both PTCL, NOS and ALK-positive ALCL in chromosome losses and gains.[101,102] Patients with ALK-negative ALCL and complex chromosomal abnormalities have significantly shorter OS.[103] About two-thirds of ALK-negative ALCLs show activation of the JAK-STAT3 signaling pathway, attributable in some cases to mutations in *JAK1* or *STAT3*, or fusions involving *ROS1*, *TYK2*, or *FRK*.[104,105] Recurrent rearrangements (R) of the *DUSP22-IRF4* locus on 6p25.3 (*DUSP22*-R) (Fig. 36-11F) or the *TP63* locus on 3q28 (*TP63*-R) have been reported in 30% and 8% of ALK-negative ALCLs, respectively.[99,106,107] *DUSP22*-R is associated with decreased expression of the dual-specificity phosphatase gene, *DUSP22*,[106] a putative tumor suppressor that inhibits T-cell receptor signaling.[108] The most common rearrangement, seen in 45% of cases, is t(6;7)(p25.3;q32.3) and is associated with downregulation of microRNAs in the MIR29 cluster on 7q32.3.[109] ALK-negative ALCL with *DUSP22*-R is considered a distinct genetic subtype of ALK-negative ALCL in the new ICC classification based on unique clinicopathologic and molecular features, including characteristic morphologic and phenotypic features, unique transcriptomic profile, DNA hypomethylation, and recurrent mutations of the *MSC* gene.[90,110-112] *TP63*-R occurs most commonly with the *TBL1XR1* gene as inv(3)(q26q28) and leads to expression of fusion proteins sharing homology with oncogenic ΔNp63 isoforms.[107] *DUSP22*-R and *TP63*-R are not specific for ALCL and their utility in diagnosing ALK-negative ALCL has not been established; however, they have significant prognostic associations. Occasional cases may show dual *DUSP22*-R and *TP63*-R.[113] The molecular signature of ALK-negative ALCL includes overexpression of *CCR7*, *CNTFR*, *IL22*, and *IL21* genes but does not identify the underlying oncogenic mechanism associated with these tumors.[50] In addition, these results

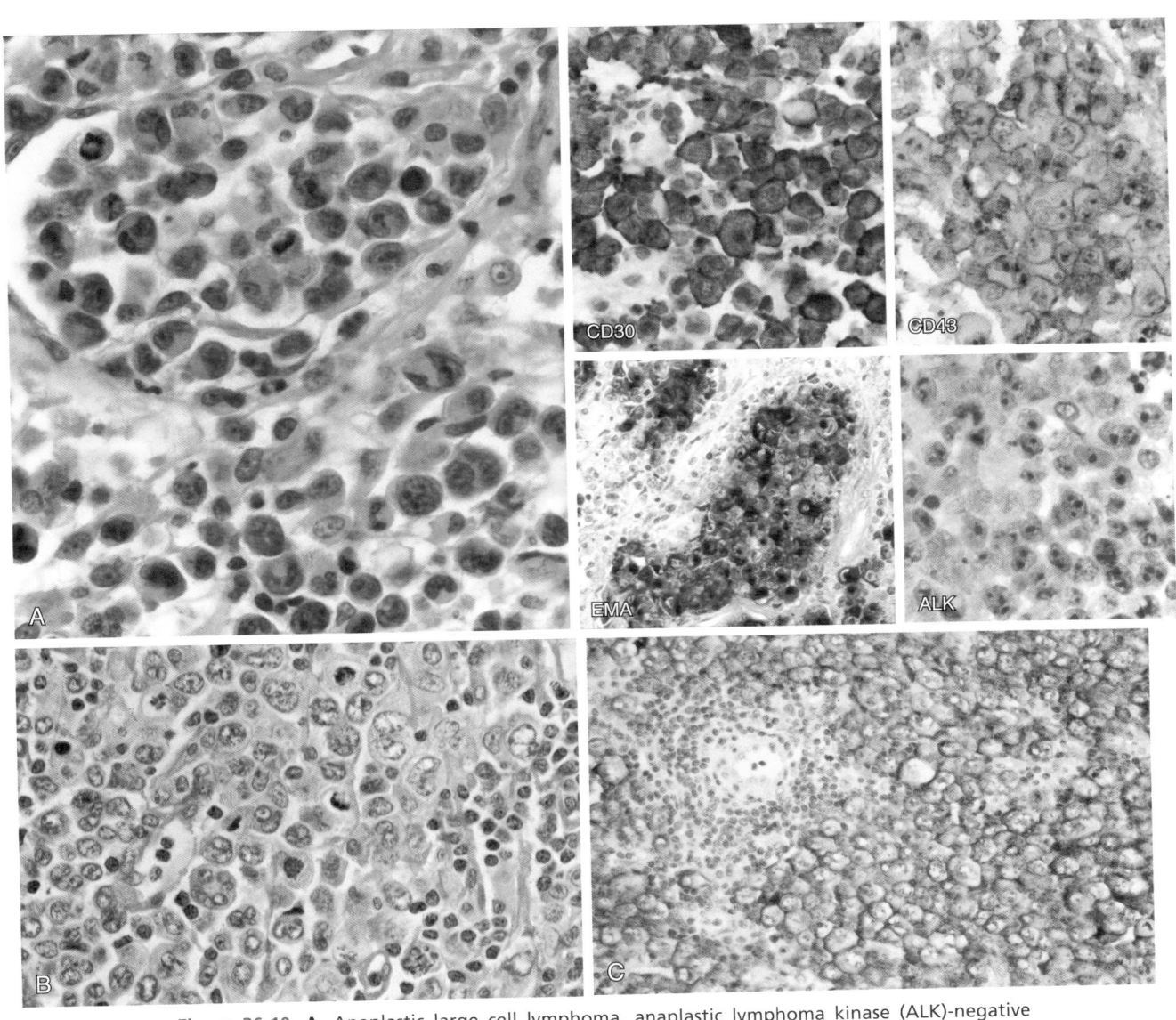

Figure 36-10. A, Anaplastic large cell lymphoma, anaplastic lymphoma kinase (ALK)-negative showing morphologic and phenotypic features closely comparable to those observed in ALK-positive ALCL. ALK staining was repeated twice and proved to be negative. Numerous hallmark cells grow within sinuses. The immunophenotype is similar to that of ALK-positive ALCL in most respects: CD30 positive, epithelial membrane antigen (EMA) positive, perforin positive, CD43 positive, CD2 positive. **B–C,** ALK-negative ALCL consisting of more pleomorphic cells with a high nuclear-to-cytoplasmic ratio, strongly positive for CD30. The case shown in **B** was of T phenotype (CD3 positive and CD4 positive) but negative for EMA.

do not provide definitive evidence of whether ALK-negative ALCL is more closely related to ALK-positive ALCL or to PTCL, NOS.[50,114,115] Recently, gene expression profiling studies have indicated that ALK-negative ALCL and PTCL, NOS have distinct molecular signatures, and may be differentiated by as few as three genes (*TNFRSF8, BATF3,* and *TMOD1*).[116,117]

Clinical Course and Prognostic Factors

Overall, the clinical outcome of conventionally treated ALK-negative ALCL is poorer than that of ALK-positive ALCL.[118] In a study by Savage and coworkers,[79] the 5-year OS of

patients with ALK-negative ALCL was 49% compared with 70% for those with ALK-positive ALCL; PTCL, NOS with high CD30 expression, which can be difficult to differentiate histologically from ALK-negative ALCL, had a poorer prognosis (5-year OS of 19%). Recent data indicate, however, that outcomes of ALK-negative ALCL vary markedly based on genetic subtype.[99,119] In the largest study to date, ALK-negative ALCLs with *DUSP22*-R had a 5-year OS of 90%, similar to that of ALK-positive ALCL. ALK-negative ALCLs with *TP63*-R had a 5-year OS of 17%, while ALK-negative ALCLs lacking *DUSP22*-R, and *TP63*-R had a 5-year OS of 42%. Genomic losses of *TP53* or *PRDM1* also are associated with poor outcomes.[120]

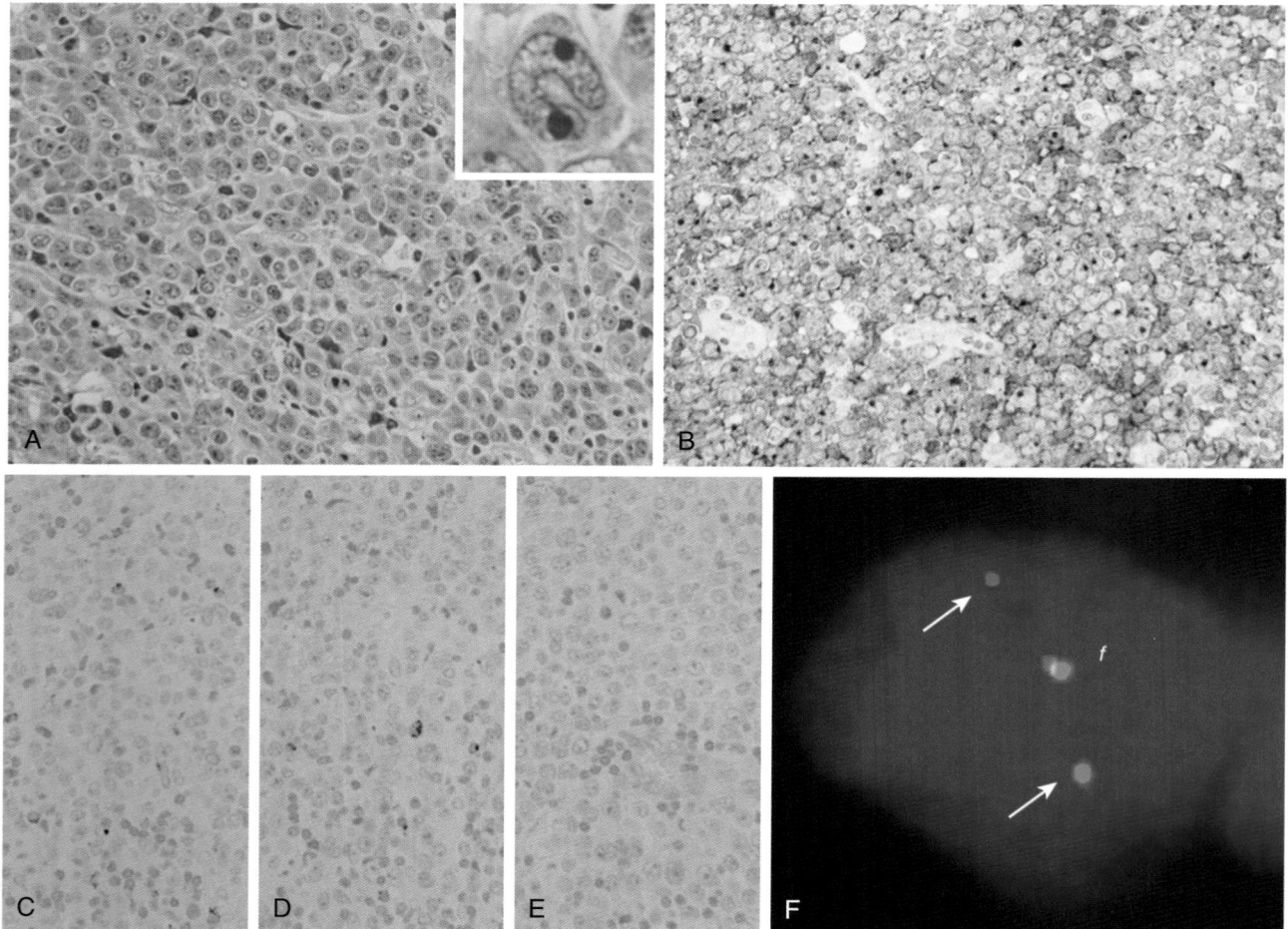

Figure 36-11. Anaplastic large cell lymphoma, ALK negative with *DUSP22* rearrangement. A, Lymph node showing sheets of hallmark cells with characteristic horseshoe-shaped nuclei *(inset).* **B,** Tumor cells show membranous and Golgi staining for CD30. Cases with this rearrangement typically are negative for cytotoxic proteins (**C,** TIA-1; **D,** granzyme B) and ALK (**E**). **F,** Fluorescence in situ hybridization using a break-apart probe for the *DUSP22-IRF4* locus on 6p25.3 shows one allele with a normal fusion signal *(f)* and the other allele with abnormal separation of the *red* and *green* signals *(arrows).*

BREAST IMPLANT–ASSOCIATED ANAPLASTIC LARGE CELL LYMPHOMA

Synonyms and Related Terms

WHO revised 4th ed.: Breast implant-associated anaplastic large cell lymphoma

WHO proposed 5th ed.: Breast implant-associated anaplastic large cell lymphoma

Definition

Breast implant–associated anaplastic large cell lymphoma (BIA-ALCL) is a rare form of ALCL identified as a provisional entity in the revised WHO 4th ed. ICC and the WHO 5th ed. classification has upgraded it to a definite entity.[90] The first case of BIA-ALCL was described in 1997 by Keech and Creech[121] and subsequently, more than 800 cases of BIA-ALCL have been reported in the literature.[122-126]

Etiology

BIA-ALCL is a multifactorial disease, which involves several intrinsic or extrinsic factors.[126] Among them, several studies have implicated high-textured implants and chronic inflammation caused by implant debris and material leached from the bacterial biofilm.[127-129] In addition, an HLA polymorphism (HLA-A*26 antigen) might also increase the risk of BIA-ALCL.[130] Together with the acquisition of mutations or other molecular alterations, these factors are thought to contribute to a clonal expansion of T lymphocytes and lead to BIA-ALCL development.

Epidemiology

The risk of developing BIA-ALCL is very low. The incidence of BIA-ALCL varies from 1/30,000 to 1/1000 women with breast implants, with approximately 660 cases reported to the FDA.[131-133] De Jong D et al. estimated the risk at 0.1 to 0.3

per 100,000 women-years with prostheses.[122] In the French *Lymphopath* network, since 2010, three to four new cases per year have been observed for 340,000 women with prostheses. Interestingly, in the latter series, BIA-ALCL was and still is the most frequent breast T-cell lymphoma.[134]

Clinical Features

The mean age of the patients is 61 years (range 28–87 years) and the mean time elapsed between placement of breast implants and diagnosis of BIA-ALCL is 10 years (range 1–32 years).[123,124,135]

Most BIA-ALCL patients (80%) present with seroma, which is a clinical term used to identify accumulation of fluid around the breast implant.[122,123,135,136] In contrast, a minority of patients (20%) have a palpable tumor mass, generally limited to the breast or associated with axillary lymphadenopathy.[122,135,136] Some patients present with a breast tumor mass associated with seroma.[137]

Morphology

The diagnosis of BIA-ALCL is based on cytologic analysis of a periprosthetic effusion or histologic analysis of capsule

associated with immunohistochemistry panel, including T cell markers and CD30.[138] Histopathologic examination shows two clearly different types of proliferations.

In patients with a seroma, the proliferation is often confined to the luminal surface with early capsular invasion or not. In the latter case, tumor cells are restrained to luminal surface without invading the capsule and defined the so-called *"in situ"* BIA-ALCL form (Fig. 36-12A). However, the distribution of malignant cells on the inner side of the capsule is usually heterogeneous, with some cellular areas and other areas with only fibrous tissue and almost no cells. The proliferation consists of a population of large pleomorphic cells of varying size suggesting a large cell lymphoma, although scattered hallmark-like cells may be observed (Fig. 36-12B). Some neoplastic cells are found to be encased within fibrinoid material. Of note, in seromas, neoplastic cells may be identified in cell suspension.

Patients presenting with a tumor mass show more heterogeneous proliferations, infiltrating surrounding tissues (so-called "tumor-type" BIA-ALCL).[134] They consist of either sheets or clusters of large anaplastic cells accompanied by large numbers of eosinophils. In some cases, the presence of numerous RS-like cells in a background rich in eosinophils may be highly suggestive of CHL (Hodgkin-like feature)

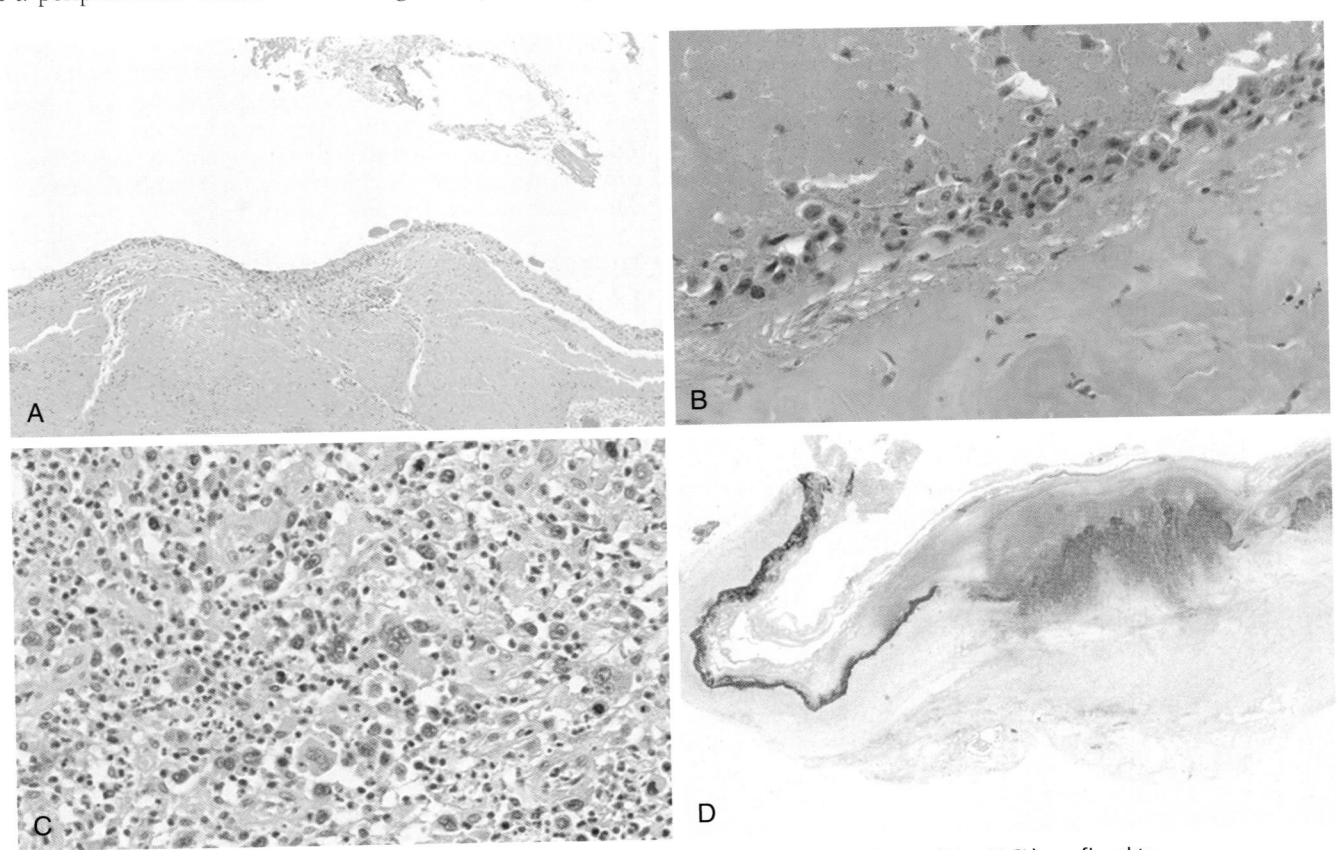

Figure 36-12. A, Breast implant–associated anaplastic large cell lymphoma (BIA-ALCL) confined to the fibrous capsule of a patient who presented with seroma around the implant. **B,** High magnification shows large pleomorphic cells with rare hallmark-like cells. **C,** This tumor mass infiltrated the capsule and the pectoral muscle. On higher magnification, one sees a population of pleomorphic noncohesive cells. As seen in ALCLs, some atypical cells with crown-like or kidney-shaped nuclei are observed. Reed-Sternberg-like cells are also observed, which, in association with large number of eosinophils, may mimic a classic Hodgkin lymphoma. **D,** In occasional cases, the two morphologic patterns (i.e., *in situ* and tumor-mass BIA-ALCLs) are observed. Immunostaining with CD30/Ber-H2 staining highlights a proliferation confined to the fibrous capsule and a focally bulging proliferation that invades the surrounding tissue.

(Fig. 37-12C).[123,135] In tumor-type BIA-ALCL, necrosis or sclerosis may be observed.[135] In occasional cases, the two morphologic patterns (i.e., in situ and tumor-type BIA-ALCL) are observed. In the latter cases, besides a proliferation confined to the fibrous capsule, one sees a focally bulging proliferation that invades the surrounding tissue (Fig. 36-12D). Such an association suggests that lesions confined to the capsule may, with time, evolve to a proliferation invading surrounding tissue.

Immunophenotype

Malignant cells are strongly positive for CD30 and their distribution along the inner side of the capsule is better seen after CD30 staining (Fig. 36-12D).[123] These cells show variable positive staining for EMA.[123,125] In the majority of cases, neoplastic cells are of T-cell phenotype and positive for one or several T-cell markers (i.e., CD2, CD3, CD4, CD43) and cytotoxic-associated markers (TIA-1, granzyme B, or perforin).[123,125,137] CD45/LCA is positive in approximately one-third of cases.[137] BIA-ALCL are consistently negative for EBV (i.e., EBER and LMP1).[123,125] Of note, only one case of breast implant–associated lymphoma was positive for EBV but this particular case was diagnosed as extranodal NK/T-cell lymphoma.[139] In all reported cases, ALK staining was negative. If positive, secondary breast involvement by a systemic ALK-positive ALCL must be suspected (personal observation). Tumor cells frequently express PDL1 and nuclear phospho-STAT3 (p-STAT3) indicative of a role of STAT3 constitutive activation in BIA-ALCL.[134,140,141]

Genetics and Molecular Findings

TR γ genes are clonally rearranged in the majority of cases. However, false negatives can occur, particularly when the number of neoplastic cells is low as frequently observed in the in situ BIA-ALCL subtype.[123,137,142] BIA-ALCLs are negative for ALK, DUSP22, and TP63 gene rearrangements.[141] Copy number aberration (CNA) analysis of BIA-ALCL has identified recurrent alterations including gains on chromosomes 2p, 9p, and 20, and losses on 8p and 20. Interestingly, loss at chromosome 20q13.13 has been considered a specific genomic feature of BIA-ALCL, distinguishing them from other classes of ALCL.[143] Genomic sequencing showed recurrent mutations in the JAK-STAT pathway in up to 60% of BIA-ALCL cases, including activating mutations of STAT3, JAK1, STAT5B, and alterations of negative regulators like SOCS3, SOCS1, and PTPN1.[140,144-146] Whole exome sequencing of the largest series of BIA-ALCL has also reported recurrent mutations of epigenetic modifiers in 74% of cases, involving notably KMT2C, KMT2D, CHD2, and CREBBP genes.[140] Both somatic and germline mutations in TP53 have been found in BIA-ALCL.[140,144-146] Finally, one study reported an increased risk of BIA-ALCL in patients with germline mutations of BRCA1 or BRCA2.[147] Genomic expression profiling showed that BIA-ALCLs exhibit an activated CD4-positive memory T-cell phenotype with upregulation of genes involved in cell motility (CCR6, MET, and CXCL14) and higher expression of RORC1 and IL17A compared with normal CD4-positive T cells.[148] In the same study, the authors also found an overexpression of genes involved in myeloid cell differentiation (e.g., PPARG and JAK2) and genes encoding for ribosomal proteins (RPS10,

RPS19, RPL17, RPL18) in which RPS10 was one of the most differentially expressed genes between BIA-ALCL and other PTCLs.[148]

Finally, though BIA-ALCL and other ALCLs share a common activation of JAK/STAT pathway with downregulation of TCR signaling, BIA-ALCL is more enriched in regulatory T cell–related genes and exhibits a dramatic upregulation of hypoxia signaling genes such as carbonic anhydrase 9 (CA9), VEGFA, VEGFB, and SLC2A3 compared with other ALCLs.[149]

Clinical Course and Prognostic Factors

Capsulectomy with margin evaluation is the optimal treatment for most cases of BIA-ALCL. The use of MD Anderson TNM staging from T1 to T4 is highly recommended.[150] T1 (so-called "in situ" BIA-ALCL) indicates a seroma or tumor cells confined to the luminal capsule only. T2 indicates early capsular invasion. T3 indicates tumor cell aggregates or sheets within the capsule, whereas T4 indicates that tumor cells are beyond the capsule. Nodal involvement refers to the presence of tumor cells in one (N1) or multiple (N2) regional lymph nodes. M1 is notified when the disease spreads to other organs or distant sites. Patients with stage I disease (T1-T3 N0 M0) who are treated with implant removal and total capsulectomy have excellent outcomes.[123-125,135-137] In contrast, patients with II-IV stage disease (T4 N0 M0; T1-T4 N1-2 M0-1) had a more aggressive clinical course.[124,135-137] In the latter cases, systemic therapy with anthracycline-based regimen or brentuximab-vedotin is recommended.[134,135,150,151] Additionally, chest wall radiotherapy should be considered in cases of incomplete resection (even for T1 and T2 stages) or with chest wall infiltration.

DIFFERENTIAL DIAGNOSIS OF ANAPLASTIC LARGE CELL LYMPHOMA

Even if the morphologic features of most ALCLs suggest the diagnosis, a definitive diagnosis cannot be made without immunohistochemistry. A major advance was made with the production of ALK1 and ALKc antibodies.[27,55] They are of critical diagnostic value in some ALK-positive ALCLs with unusual morphologic features. The diagnosis of ALK-negative ALCL is more difficult because of the lack of specific markers. Therefore, all tumors consisting of large cells expressing the CD30 antigen need to be considered in the differential diagnosis (Table 36-2).

Anaplastic Large Cell Lymphoma, Common Pattern

ALCL, common pattern is easy to recognize in children. In adults, the main differential diagnoses are metastatic malignancies because the majority of these ALCL cases exhibit a sinusoidal growth pattern. However, undifferentiated carcinomas usually express cytokeratin and EMA and are negative for the CD30 antigen. We have observed rare cases of carcinomas that are weakly positive for CD30. Conversely, occasional ALCLs may express cytokeratins.[152] Metastasis from a melanoma may simulate ALCL, but most of these tumors are S-100+, HMB45+, PNL2+, EMA-/+, and CD30-; however, rare cases positive for CD30 have also been reported.[153] Embryonal

Table 36-2 Differential Diagnosis of Anaplastic Large Cell Lymphoma

Entity	Phenotype of Neoplastic Cells	Comments
ALCL, common type	CD30+, EMA+, ALK+ (85%), CD45−/+, CD3−/+, CD43+, CD2−/+, CD4−/+, CD5−/+, CD7−/+, CD8−/+, cytotoxic proteins*+/−, BCL2− (most cases)	Sinusoidal growth pattern "Hallmark" cells
Metastatic malignancy		
Carcinoma	Cytokeratin+, EMA+, CD30−, CD45−	Rare cases CD30-positive
Melanoma	S-100+, EMA−/+, HMB45+, PNL2+, CD45−	Weak CD30 staining has been reported
PTCL, NOS with predominantly large cells	CD30−/+, EMA−/+, ALK−, CD3+, CD2−/+, CD4−/+, CD5−/+, CD7−/+, CD8−/+, cytotoxic proteins*+/−, BCL2+	Rare cases with sinusoidal growth pattern and pleomorphic cells
DLBCL		
ALK+ DLBCL	CD30−, EMA+, ALK+, CD20/CD79a−, CD138+, cytoplasmic IgA (most cases)	Sinusoidal growth pattern Immunoblast or plasmablastic cells
DLBCL, anaplastic variant†	CD30−/+, EMA−/+, ALK−, CD20/CD79a+	Some show a sinusoidal growth pattern but are ALK−
Histiocytic sarcoma	CD30−, EMA−, ALK− (most cases), CD68+, CD163+, lysozyme+	
ALCL, lymphohistiocytic	CD30+, EMA+, ALK+, CD68−, CD45−/+, CD3−/+, CD43+, CD2−/+, CD4−/+, CD5−/+, CD7−/+, CD8−/+, cytotoxic proteins*+/−	Sinusoidal growth pattern may be absent, but perivascular pattern is observed in all cases Only reactive histiocytes are CD68+
Lymphadenitis rich in histiocytes	CD30−, EMA−, ALK−	Rare CD30+ immunoblasts No perivascular pattern
ALCL, small cell variant	CD30+, EMA+, ALK+, CD45−/+, CD3+ (most cases), CD43+, CD2+/−, CD4+/−, CD5+/−, CD7+/−, CD8+/−, cytotoxic proteins*+	Sinusoidal growth pattern may be absent, but perivascular pattern is observed in all cases Restricted nuclear ALK staining
PTCL, NOS with small-to-medium-sized cells	CD30−/+, EMA−/+, ALK−, CD45+/−, CD3+ (most cases), CD43+, CD2−/+, CD4−/+, CD5−/+, CD7−/+, CD8−/+, cytotoxic proteins*+/−	Scattered CD30+ cells may be observed, but without perivascular pattern
ALCL, other‡	CD30+, EMA+, ALK+, CD45−/+, CD3−/+, CD43+, CD2−/+, CD4−/+, CD5−/+, CD7−/+, CD8−/+, cytotoxic proteins*+/−, BCL2− (most cases)	Sinusoidal growth pattern "Hallmark" cells Rare cases of ALK+ ALCL may show CD15+ paranuclear staining
Classic Hodgkin lymphoma	CD30+, EMA−, CD15+/−, ALK−, CD45−, CD3−, PAX5+ weak, CD43−, CD20−/+ (heterogeneous staining), EBV/LMP-1+/− (60%), BCL2 variable	Rare sinusoidal growth pattern No perivascular pattern
Inflammatory myofibroblastic tumors	CD30−, EMA−, ALK+ (cyt)	ALCL with sarcomatous morphology is always CD30+, EMA+, and ALK+
Rhabdomyosarcoma	CD30−, EMA−, ALK−/+ (cyt), desmin+	Rare cases of rhabdomyosarcoma may show rare cells positive for CD30 and EMA

*Perforin, TIA-1, granzyme B.
†Rare cases of DLBCL show a predominant sinusoidal growth pattern but are negative for ALK.
‡Includes giant cell, sarcomatous, hypocellular; rare cases may resemble Hodgkin lymphoma at low-power magnification.
ALCL, Anaplastic large cell lymphoma; *ALK,* anaplastic lymphoma kinase; *(cyt),* cytoplasmic; *DLBCL,* diffuse large B-cell lymphoma; *EBV,* Epstein-Barr virus; *EMA,* epithelial membrane antigen; *PTCL, NOS,* peripheral T-cell lymphoma, not otherwise specified.

carcinoma expresses CD30, but morphologically does not resemble ALCL.[154] The most difficult problem in the differential diagnosis is PTCL, NOS with a predominant population of large cells, sometimes infiltrating lymphatic sinuses. Some of these tumors strongly express CD30 and may be positive for EMA.[155] However, the staining for CD30 is typically more variable in intensity or lacks the usual membranous and Golgi pattern characteristic of ALCL. Nevertheless, the distinction between PTCL, NOS and ALK-negative ALCL is not always clear-cut, and it is preferable to diagnose ALK-negative ALCL only if both the morphology and the phenotype are close to those of ALK-positive ALCL.[89] Extranodal nasal-type NK/T-cell lymphoma and enteropathy-associated T-cell lymphoma also may show a varying proportion of tumor cells expressing CD30.[9] Diffuse large B-cell lymphomas with anaplastic morphology may show the morphologic features, including a sinusoidal growth pattern, and the phenotypic features (CD30 positivity) of ALCL. However, these tumors express B-cell antigens, and t(2;5) is absent.[156]

Two additional tumors deserve attention. The first is ALK-positive large B-cell lymphoma, which is now considered a distinct entity.[56] Morphologically, these tumors are composed of monomorphic large plasmablast-like or immunoblast-like cells with large central nucleoli, and often invade lymphatic sinuses (Fig. 36-13A–B). At low magnification, these tumors resemble ALCL, but they lack CD30. These lymphomas strongly express EMA (see Fig. 36-13C), as does ALCL, but they also contain intracytoplasmic immunoglobulin (usually IgA) of a single light chain type. They often lack lineage-associated leukocyte antigens (CD3, CD20, CD79a), except for CD4 and CD57 in some cases. These tumors weakly express or may even be negative for the leukocyte common antigen CD45. Occasional cases are positive for cytokeratin, which, in addition to EMA positivity and weak or negative staining for CD45, may lead to the misdiagnosis of carcinoma. Characteristically, lymphoma cells are strongly positive for ALK. In most cases, the staining is restricted to the cytoplasm and is granular, indicating an association with CLTC-ALK protein.[34,157] ALK-positive diffuse large B-cell lymphoma typically follows an aggressive course. Other lymphomas

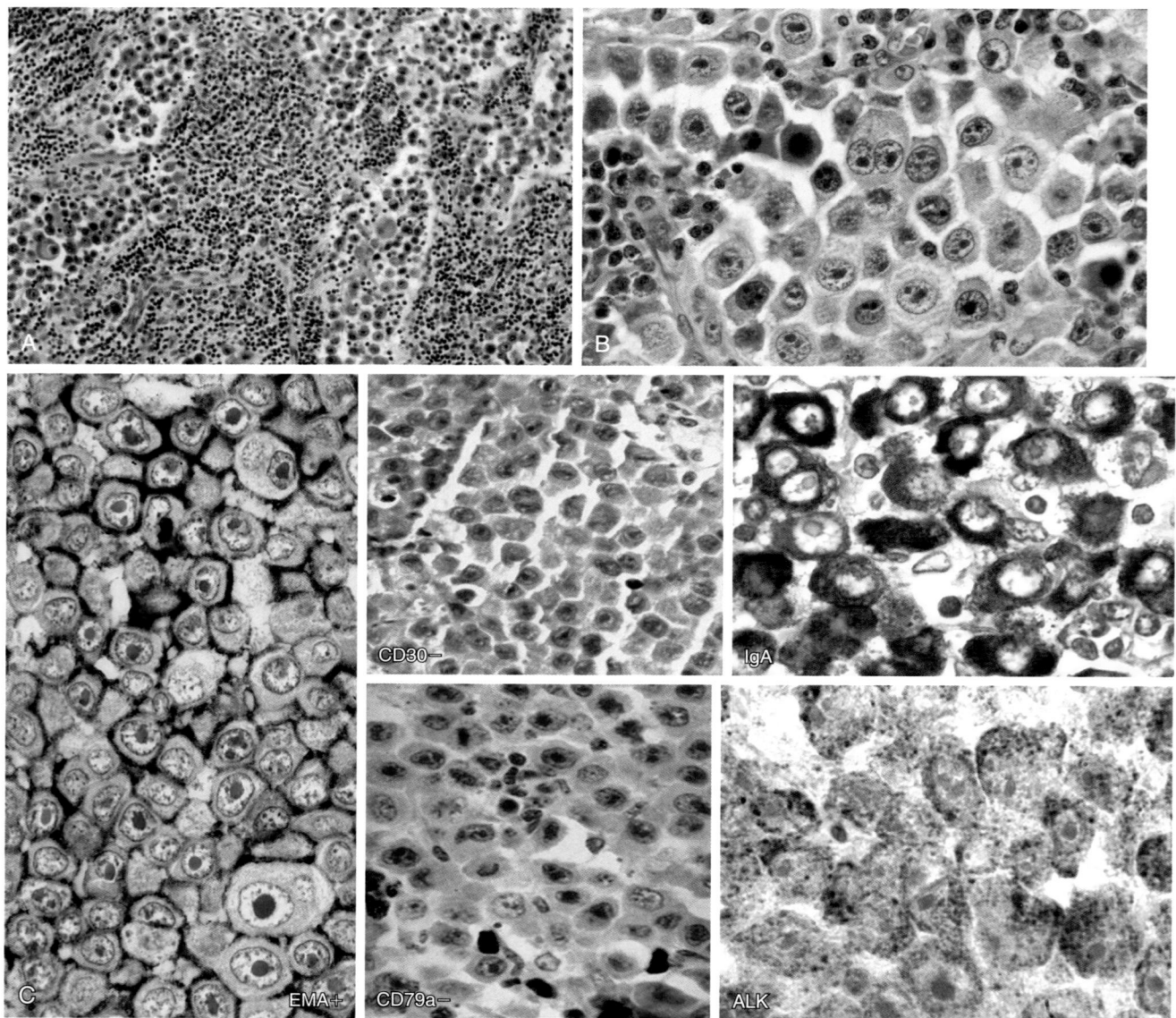

Figure 36-13. Anaplastic lymphoma kinase (ALK)–positive diffuse large B-cell lymphoma exhibiting a sinusoidal growth pattern **(A)** with large immunoblastic or plasmablastic cells **(B)**. The composite figure **(C)** illustrates the phenotype of lymphoma cells that are strongly positive for epithelial membrane antigen (EMA), negative for CD30 and B-cell–associated antigens (including CD79a), and usually immunoglobulin A (IgA) positive and show a cytoplasmic granular ALK staining.

exhibiting a sinusoidal growth pattern, such as so-called "microvillous" lymphomas, may be either negative or positive for CD30.[158,159] However, these tumors are relatively easy to recognize by immunohistochemistry because they express B-cell antigens (CD20 and CD79a) and are negative for ALK.

The second type of tumor deserving attention is the true histiocytic tumor, which is extremely rare. In a report based on the study of more than 900 lymphomas, there were only four true histiocytic tumors.[160] Histiocytic sarcomas usually consist of large cells with moderate or abundant cytoplasm and pleomorphic nuclei with prominent nucleoli. Morphologically malignant-appearing cells are positive for CD68 (KP1 and PGM1) and CD163, macrophage-associated antigens, and for lysozyme. Like normal histiocytes or macrophages, true histiocytic sarcomas react with CD4 but are negative for all other T-cell and B-cell markers. These cells are negative for CD1a and PS100. Recognition of these tumors is important because of their poor prognosis in the majority of cases. Similar morphologic and phenotypic features are seen in monoblastic leukemias, which can be distinguished from histiocytic sarcomas in part by clinical presentation (i.e., bone marrow involvement). Rare cases of aggressive mastocytosis may consist of large cells reminiscent of hallmark cells and express the CD30 antigen. They are positive for CD117, CD4, and CD68 antigens. Acid toluidine blue shows the characteristic metachromatic granules, but in malignant cases, granularity may be sparse. Immunohistochemistry for mast cell tryptase is the preferred diagnostic tool.[161]

Anaplastic Large Cell Lymphoma, Lymphohistiocytic Pattern

ALCL, lymphohistiocytic pattern may be extremely difficult to recognize and is commonly misdiagnosed as histiocyte-rich lymphadenitis. One must keep in mind that the lymph node architecture is obliterated in these lesions, a feature that is rare in reactive processes. As described, malignant cells are difficult to identify because they are obscured by large numbers of reactive histiocytes associated with varying numbers of plasma cells. The key to the diagnosis is immunohistochemistry using CD30 and ALK-reactive antibodies; this highlights the malignant cells scattered among the histiocytes and typically concentrated around blood vessels.[11,162]

Anaplastic Large Cell Lymphoma, Small Cell Pattern

ALCL, small cell pattern is commonly misdiagnosed as PTCL, NOS. Hallmark cells are present but are difficult to detect among small-to-medium-sized cells. Although the majority of small-to-medium-sized lymphoid cells are malignant, they usually express CD30 and EMA weakly, which makes the diagnosis even more difficult. By contrast, large cells strongly express CD30 and ALK and are localized around blood vessels. As noted, a small cell variant of ALK-negative ALCL is not recognized in the revised WHO 4th ed. classification, and T-cell lymphomas showing these morphologic features should be diagnosed as PTCL, NOS.

Anaplastic Large Cell Lymphoma, Hodgkin-Like Pattern

ALCL, Hodgkin-like pattern, mimicking nodular sclerosis CHL, exists but is extremely rare. This diagnosis requires positive staining for ALK.[37] True CHL rich in neoplastic cells must be excluded in ALK-negative cases, bearing in mind that CHL of documented B-cell lineage may express T-cell antigens.[163] Some tumors with Hodgkin-like features, including expression of CD15 and CD30, but of documented T-cell lineage are most appropriately diagnosed as PTCL, NOS rather than ALCL if they are ALK negative.[95] Recently, JAK2-R has been identified in some cases with these features, though it remains unclear whether this finding can be used to aid in the differential diagnosis between ALK-negative ALCL and PTCL, NOS.[164]

Anaplastic Large Cell Lymphoma, Sarcomatous Pattern

ALCL, sarcomatous pattern may simulate lymph node involvement by a soft tissue tumor or even Kaposi sarcoma. However, in the sarcomatous pattern of ALCL, one observes typical features of ALCL in at least some areas. Because ALCL can present as a soft tissue or bone mass, the diagnosis should be considered in a soft tissue sarcoma in a child or young adult. The differential diagnosis is complicated by ALK protein expression in rhabdomyosarcoma and ALK-positive inflammatory myofibroblastic tumor.

ALK-Positive Nonlymphoid Tumors

ALK-positive nonlymphoid tumors may be responsible for diagnostic difficulties. Overall, ALK expression can be considered highly indicative of ALCL. However,

as originally reported by Morris and colleagues,[3] rhabdomyosarcoma occasionally expresses the full-length (200 kDa) ALK protein (Fig. 36-14A–B). Some inflammatory myofibroblastic tumors are associated with ALK gene rearrangement at 2p23 (see Fig. 36-14C–D). Chan and coworkers[57] described a novel form of ALK-positive histiocytosis occurring in infants. The authors concluded that ALK-positive histiocytosis is a distinct histiocytic proliferative disorder that typically resolves slowly but can be life-threatening during the active phase. A more recent study based on 39 cases expanded the clinicopathologic spectrum of ALK-positive histiocytosis.[165] The KIF5B-ALK fusion was the most frequently observed in these tumors. They can occur both in infants and adults, and can present with single-system or multisystemic disease, with frequent neurologic involvement.[165] ALK-positive histiocytosis is now considered a separate histiocytic entity in the ICC classification distinct from Erdheim-Chester disease and juvenile xanthogranuloma.[90]

Some neuroblastomas can also express full-length ALK protein, but in contrast to ALCL, the staining is weak.[166] Somatic and germline mutations of the ALK kinase domain have been reported in familial neuroblastoma.[167] ALK expression is well-known in a subset of non–small cell lung cancers associated with the transforming EML4-ALK fusion gene,[168,169] but also more recently reported in melanocytic tumors,[170] epithelioid fibrous histiocytomas,[171] and rare soft tissue myxoid tumors.[172]

Primary Cutaneous CD30-Positive T-Cell Lymphoproliferative Disorders

Skin involvement by systemic ALCL can cause diagnostic confusion with primary cutaneous CD30-positive T-cell lymphoproliferative disorders (see Chapter 39). Three types of primary cutaneous CD30-positive T-cell lymphoproliferative disorders are distinguished[9]: primary cutaneous ALCL, lymphomatoid papulosis (in which type C shows the most resemblance to ALCL), and borderline lesions. The distinction among these disorders is sometimes difficult and requires the combined assessment of histologic, clinical, and phenotypic features. The expression of EMA is variable. Although ALK protein usually is absent in these lymphoproliferative disorders, rare cases of primary cutaneous ALK-positive ALCL have been reported.[173-175]

ALK-Negative Anaplastic Large Cell Lymphomas Associated With Breast Implants

The diagnosis of BIA-ALCL must be restricted to patients with this distinct clinical context. Secondary breast involvement by a systemic ALK-negative ALCL must be excluded. Breast involvement by PTCL, NOS with a population of CD30-positive large cells may also be responsible for diagnostic difficulties. Some cases reported as ALK-negative BIA-ALCL seem to correspond to the latter entity. In fact, the most difficult differential diagnosis is to rule out the diagnosis of CHL in some cases of BIA-ALCL with RS-like cells, in a background rich in eosinophils. Diagnostic difficulties may be accentuated by the positive staining for CD15 as seen in rare cases of BIA-ALCL (personal observation).[137] However, the clinical context (i.e., breast implant), the rarity (if it

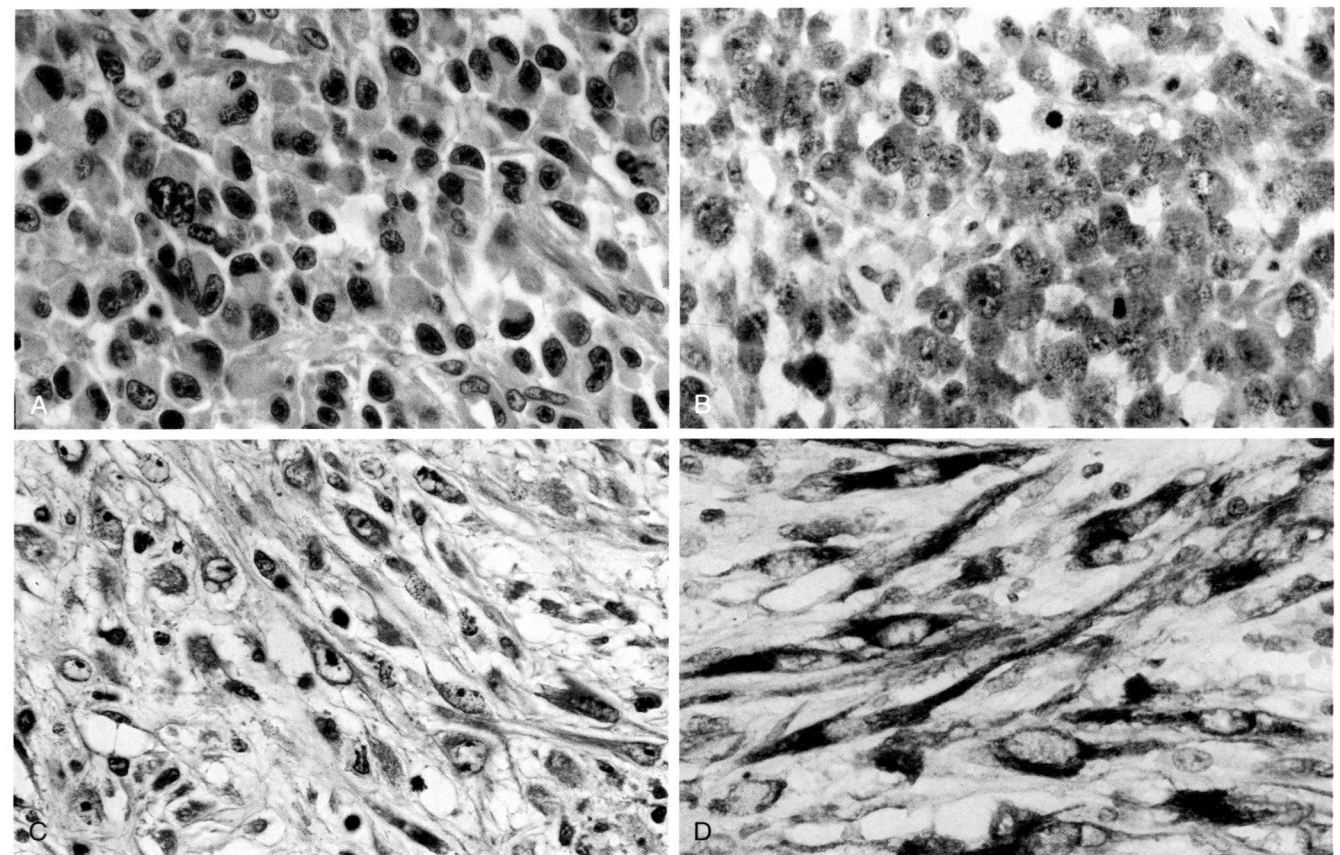

Figure 36-14. Rare soft tissue tumors may express anaplastic lymphoma kinase (ALK) but are negative for CD30 antigen. **A–B,** Rhabdomyosarcoma positive for full-length ALK protein (**A,** hematoxylin and eosin [H&E]; **B,** ALK staining). This tumor was strongly positive for desmin. **C–D,** Inflammatory myofibroblastic tumor strongly positive for ALK protein (**C,** H&E; **D,** ALK staining). Usually this tumor expresses TPM4-ALK protein.

exists) of primary breast CHL, and the phenotype of atypical cells (CD30 positive, EMA positive/negative, T phenotype, and PAX5 negative) allow exclusion of CHL.[123]

Pearls and Pitfalls

- Beware that anaplastic large cell lymphoma (ALCL), anaplastic lymphoma kinase (ALK) postive exhibits a broad spectrum of morphologic features. Do not hesitate to ask for ALK staining.
- Classic Hodgkin lymphoma (CHL) rich in neoplastic cells may be misdiagnosed as ALK-negative ALCL based on negative CD15 staining. Remember that 15% to 25% of CHLs are negative for CD15. CHL also may express T-cell antigens. Additional staining using CD20 and CD79a (which are positive on a proportion of Reed-Sternberg [RS] cells in 30% of cases), PAX5, and Epstein-Barr virus (EBV)–encoded RNA (EBER) in situ hybridization may be useful. ALK-negative ALCL is always negative for EBV.
- In addition to CHL, strong CD30 staining may be observed in peripheral T-cell lymphoma, not otherwise specified (PTCL, NOS); in some extranodal T-cell lymphomas, such as extranodal NK/T-cell lymphoma, nasal type, and enteropathy-associated T-cell lymphoma; in mast cell proliferations; in some diffuse large B-cell lymphomas; and in some nonlymphoid malignancies, such as embryonal carcinoma, melanoma, and some undifferentiated carcinomas.

KEY REFERENCES

3. Morris SW, Kirstein MN, Valentine MB, et al. Fusion of a kinase gene, ALK, to a nucleolar protein gene, NPM, in non-Hodgkin's lymphoma. *Science.* 1994;263:1281–1284.

66. Chiarle R, Voena C, Ambrogio C, et al. The anaplastic lymphoma kinase in the pathogenesis of cancer. *Nat Rev Cancer.* 2008;8:11–23.

82. Lamant L, McCarthy K, d'Amore E, et al. Prognostic impact of morphologic and phenotypic features of childhood ALK-positive anaplastic large-cell lymphoma: results of the ALCL99 study. *J Clin Oncol.* 2011;29:4669–4676.

84. Damm-Welk C, Busch K, Burkhardt B, et al. Prognostic significance of circulating tumor cells in bone marrow or peripheral blood as detected by qualitative and quantitative PCR in pediatric NPM-ALK-positive anaplastic large-cell lymphoma. *Blood.* 2007;110:670–677.

86. Ait-Tahar K, Damm-Welk C, Burkhardt B, et al. Correlation of the autoantibody response to the ALK oncoantigen in pediatric anaplastic lymphoma kinase-positive anaplastic large cell lymphoma with tumor dissemination and relapse risk. *Blood.* 2010;115:3314–3319.

90. Campo E, Jaffe ES, Cook JR, et al. The international consensus classification of mature lymphoid neoplasms: a report from the clinical advisory committee. *Blood.* 2022;140:1229–1253.

99. Parrilla Castellar ER, Jaffe ES, Said JW, et al. ALK-negative anaplastic large cell lymphoma is a genetically

heterogeneous disease with widely disparate clinical outcomes. *Blood*. 2014;124:1473–1480.

106. Feldman AL, Dogan A, Smith DI, et al. Massively parallel mate pair DNA library sequencing for translocation discovery recurrent t(6,7)(p25 3,q32 3) translocations in ALK negative anaplastic large cell lymphomas. *Blood*. 2010;116:278.

134. Laurent C, Delas A, Gaulard P, et al. Breast implant-associated anaplastic large cell lymphoma: two distinct clinicopathological variants with different outcomes. *Ann Oncol*. 2016;27:306–314.

140. Laurent C, Nicolae A, Laurent C, et al. Gene alterations in epigenetic modifiers and JAK-STAT signaling are frequent in breast implant-associated ALCL. *Blood*. 2020;135:360–370.

Visit Elsevier eBooks+ for the complete set of references.

Chapter 37

Enteropathy-Associated T-Cell Lymphoma and Other Primary Intestinal T-Cell Lymphomas

Govind Bhagat

ENTEROPATHY-ASSOCIATED T-CELL LYMPHOMA

An association between malabsorption and intestinal lymphoma was first reported in 1937,[1] at which time lymphoma was considered responsible for the malabsorption. However, in 1962, Gough and coworkers[2] demonstrated that intestinal lymphoma was a complication of celiac disease or gluten-sensitive enteropathy. In 1978, Isaacson and Wright[3] characterized celiac disease–associated lymphoma as a single entity, originally considered a form of malignant histiocytosis. Later, Isaacson and coworkers[4] showed that the neoplastic cells were of T-cell lineage. This lymphoma subtype was categorized in the 2008 World Health Organization (WHO) classification as enteropathy-associated T-cell lymphoma (EATL) type I,[5] or classic EATL. In the revised WHO 4th ed. classification, it was designated simply as *EATL*.[6,7] The 2022 International Consensus classification (ICC)[8] retains the terminology of the revised WHO 4th ed. classification,[6,7] as does the WHO 5th ed. classification.[9]

Definition

EATL is a neoplasm derived from intraepithelial lymphocytes (IELs) showing variable degrees of cellular pleomorphism, often within a polymorphic background.

Synonyms and Related Terms

WHO revised 4th ed., 2017: Enteropathy-associated T-cell lymphoma[7]

WHO 5th ed., 2022: Enteropathy-associated T-cell lymphoma[9]

Epidemiology

EATL is the most common subtype of primary intestinal T-cell lymphoma (66%–80%).[10,11] However, it is a rare lymphoma, accounting for less than 1% of non-Hodgkin lymphomas, less than 5% of primary gastrointestinal lymphomas, and approximately 5% of peripheral T-cell lymphomas (PTCLs) in Western countries.[11,12] EATL characteristically occurs in the 6th and 7th decades of life, although it has been reported in younger adults.[11,13-16] A male predominance (1.04–2.8:1) has been observed in most series.[11,13-16] Most, if not all, patients with EATL have the celiac disease–associated *HLADQA1*0501, DQB1*0201* (HLA-DQ2) genotype.[17] EATL is more common in regions with a high seroprevalence of celiac disease, such as Europe (EATL incidence of 0.05–0.14/100,000)[14,15,18] and the United States (EATL incidence of 0.016/100,000).[19] The reasons for a higher incidence of EATL in individuals of northern European descent (and in certain European countries) despite a similar incidence of celiac disease in most Western countries are unknown. EATL is virtually nonexistent in regions such as the Far East, where most lack the celiac disease susceptibility alleles. There is an increased incidence of EATL in older individuals, 2.92/100,000 in the 60-to-69-year-old age group and 0.05/100,000 in people older than 60 years in Europe and the United States, respectively.[15,19] The incidence of EATL in the celiac population is 0.22 to 1.9/100,000.[20-23] A wide range in the relative risk of non-Hodgkin lymphoma, including EATL, has been reported for celiac disease (and dermatitis herpetiformis) patients (3–100), with population-based studies providing more reliable estimates (at the lower end of the range).[20,24-28]

Etiology

EATL is a recognized complication of celiac disease,[29,30] a common autoimmune disorder (incidence, 1% in most regions of the world) with myriad intestinal and extraintestinal manifestations that occurs in genetically susceptible individuals intolerant to gluten-containing grains (e.g., wheat, barley, and rye).[31] In retrospective studies of patients with EATL, celiac disease has been diagnosed in 38% to 100% of affected patients; this variation is likely a result of incomplete data or inclusion of non-EATL cases.[11,13-16] Evidence for an association between celiac disease and EATL comes from identical human leukocyte antigen (HLA) types in celiac disease patients and those with EATL,[17] the demonstration of gluten sensitivity in EATL patients,[29] and the protective effect of a gluten-free diet against the development of lymphoma[21,24,32]; the risk of lymphoma decreases, albeit gradually, after commencing a gluten-free diet.[26] Homozygosity for HLA-DQ2 alleles, observed in 53% of cases (compared with 21% in uncomplicated celiac disease), is considered a risk factor for development of EATL.[33]

A diagnosis of celiac disease is established in 20% to 73% of cases before the diagnosis of EATL.[13,14,16,34] A short history of "adult-onset" celiac disease usually predates EATL, but it may occur in individuals with long-standing disease, the mean time between diagnosis of celiac disease and EATL ranging from 46.8 months to 10 years.[10,13,24,35] In 10% to 58% of cases, celiac disease and EATL are diagnosed simultaneously, with up to one-third being discovered at surgery for intestinal obstruction or perforation,[13,14,16,36] and the diagnosis of celiac disease is occasionally made at autopsy.[13,14] At times, EATL might occur in patients only manifesting celiac-associated extraintestinal conditions, such as dermatitis herpetiformis.[20,27,28] Gastrointestinal symptoms in celiac disease do not correlate with the degree of small intestinal mucosal damage,[37] and more than 50% of patients may be asymptomatic.[38] Hence, certain individuals with EATL might have had lifelong "silent" or "cryptic" gluten sensitivity because villous atrophy and crypt hyperplasia are found in uninvolved small intestinal mucosa when the tumor is resected. The only manifestation of celiac disease in some cases is an increase in IELs, and in a minority, the jejunum appears nearly normal. Studies showing that the jejunal mucosa can appear normal in "latent" celiac disease[39] might provide an explanation for this finding, which was previously thought to argue against a strict association between EATL and celiac disease.

Clinical Presentation

EATL most commonly presents with abdominal pain (65%–100%) and development of gluten-insensitive malabsorption or diarrhea (40%–70%) in previously well individuals or those with a history of adult-onset (or childhood-onset) celiac disease and a prior response to a gluten-free diet. Other presentations include weight loss (50%–80%), acute abdominal emergency due to intestinal perforation (25%–50%), hemorrhage, anorexia, fatigue, and early satiety or vomiting caused by intestinal obstruction.[11,13,14,16,34,36,40,41] Ichthyotic rash and finger clubbing may be observed. B symptoms, besides weight loss, are present in less than one-third of patients.[16,34,36] The duration of symptoms can range from 1 week to 5 years,[16] and a symptom duration of less than 3 months before EATL diagnosis was observed in 59% of cases in one study.[14]

Small intestinal involvement is detected in 90% to 96% of de novo EATLs,[11,13,14] most commonly in the jejunum.[16] The frequency of small intestinal involvement by EATL with prior refractory celiac disease type II (RCD II) is lower (65%).[13] Multifocal lesions involving different segments of small intestine are seen in 32% to 54%, ulcers or strictures in 51%, and mass lesions in 32% of cases.[13,16] The next most common gastrointestinal sites are the large intestine and stomach.[11] EATL might occasionally present at extraintestinal locations (e.g., skin, lymph nodes, spleen, or central nervous system),[11,13,42,43] usually in cases evolving from RCD II, as the aberrant IELs in RCD II frequently disseminate to extraintestinal sites (Table 37-1).[13,44,45] Common sites of EATL dissemination include intraabdominal lymph nodes (35%), bone marrow (3%–18%), lung and mediastinal lymph nodes (5%–16%), liver (2%–8%), and skin (5%).[11,13,14] Advanced disease at diagnosis has been reported in 43% to 90% of cases, although the staging systems used in different studies have varied.[11,13,14,16] An Eastern Cooperative Oncology Group (ECOG) score >1 is noted in 88%, and many patients have a poor performance status.[14,16] Elevated lactate dehydrogenase levels are observed in 25% to 62%, low serum albumin

Table 37-1 Pathologic, Molecular, and Biological Features of Refractory Celiac Disease (Types I and II) and Enteropathy-Associated T-Cell Lymphoma

	Refractory Celiac Disease Type I	Refractory Celiac Disease Type II	EATL
Mucosa	Villous atrophy and crypt hyperplasia	Villous atrophy and crypt hyperplasia	Villous atrophy and crypt hyperplasia
IEL number	Increased	Increased	Increased
IEL morphology	Normal	Normal	Atypical/pleomorphic
IEL phenotype	sCD3+, cytCD3+, CD8+, sTRαβ+, CD5(variable)+, CD30–	sCD3–, cytCD3+, CD8–/+, sTRαβ–, CD5–, CD30–	sCD3–/+, cytCD3+, CD8–/+, sTRαβ–, CD5–, CD30+/–
Non-neoplastic TRγδ IELs	Increased	Decreased	Decreased
TR rearrangement	Polyclonal	Clonal	Clonal
Genetic alterations/mutated pathways	None	JAK1-STAT3, epigenetic regulators, NF-κB, DNA damage response/repair	JAK1-STAT3, epigenetic regulators, NF-κB, DNA damage response/repair
Lamina propria infiltration by neoplastic cells	No	Yes (up to 50% of cases)	Yes
Peripheral blood involvement	No	Yes (44%–51%)	Yes
Transformation to EATL (4–6 years)	3%–14%	30%–52%	

cyt, Cytoplasmic; *EATL,* enteropathy-associated T-cell lymphoma; *IEL,* intraepithelial lymphocyte; *s,* surface; *TR,* T-cell receptor gene.

concentrations in 76% to 88%, and low hemoglobin levels in 54% to 91% of patients.[11,13,14,16] Abnormalities of the white blood cell count, renal function tests, and erythrocyte sedimentation rate, as well as elevated C-reactive protein and alkaline phosphatase levels, are detected in more than one-third of patients.[11,14,16] A hemophagocytic syndrome may occur in 16% to 40% of cases.[13,46]

Pathology

Macroscopic Appearance

The tumor may form ulcerating nodules, plaques, strictures, or, less commonly, large masses (Fig. 37-1). The adjacent mucosa might appear thin and show loss of mucosal folds. The mesentery is frequently infiltrated, and mesenteric lymph nodes are commonly involved. There is sometimes remarkably little macroscopic evidence of disease in the intestine as opposed to the mesenteric lymph nodes.

Histopathology

The histologic features of EATL show great variation both between cases and within a single case (Fig. 37-2). Generally, a transmural, polymorphic cellular infiltrate is observed, composed of numerous inflammatory cells, particularly eosinophils and plasma cells, which may obscure the scattered or small clusters of pleomorphic, intermediate-to-large-sized neoplastic lymphocytes (Fig. 37-2). Large cells with anaplastic features are seen in 40% of cases.[13] In some cases, the tumor cells can be monomorphic and display prominent central nucleoli (immunoblastic appearance). Angiocentricity and angioinvasion leading to blood vessel destruction is not uncommon, and foci of necrosis are present in a large proportion of cases. Increased numbers of histiocytes are often seen admixed with the neoplastic cells, and granulomas may be present, causing confusion with Crohn's disease. Increased mucosal and submucosal vascularity can occasionally be a prominent feature. Intraepithelial spread of tumor cells may be striking, though in some cases, only rare atypical lymphocytes are observed within the epithelium (Fig. 37-3).

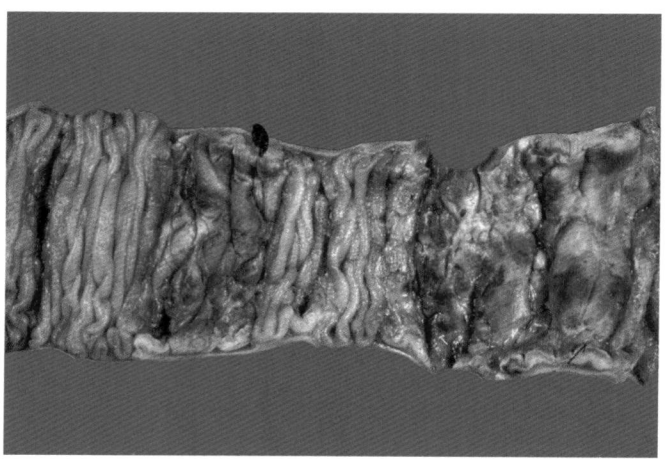

Figure 37-1. Resected jejunum from a patient with enteropathy-associated T-cell lymphoma shows multiple ulcerating tumors.

The histology of the small intestinal mucosa remote from the tumor is an important consideration in the diagnosis of EATL. In most cases, the changes are identical to those of celiac disease, consisting of villous atrophy and crypt hyperplasia, lymphoplasmacytic infiltrates in the lamina propria, and increased IELs (Fig. 37-4). As in uncomplicated celiac disease, the mucosal changes are maximal proximally and improve distally hence the lower jejunum and ileum may be normal. In some cases, the mucosal changes can be subtle.

Numerous shallow ulcers extending into the submucosa are often present remote from the lymphoma. The ulcer bases show granulation tissue and infiltrates of small lymphocytes and plasma cells, and a virtual absence of neoplastic cells (Fig. 37-5). Episodes of ulceration followed by healing lead to scarring with stricture formation and distortion of the mucosal architecture, accompanied by destruction of the muscularis mucosa and the emergence of glands lined by cells of the ulceration-associated cell lineage,[47] previously called *pseudopyloric metaplasia* (Fig. 37-6).

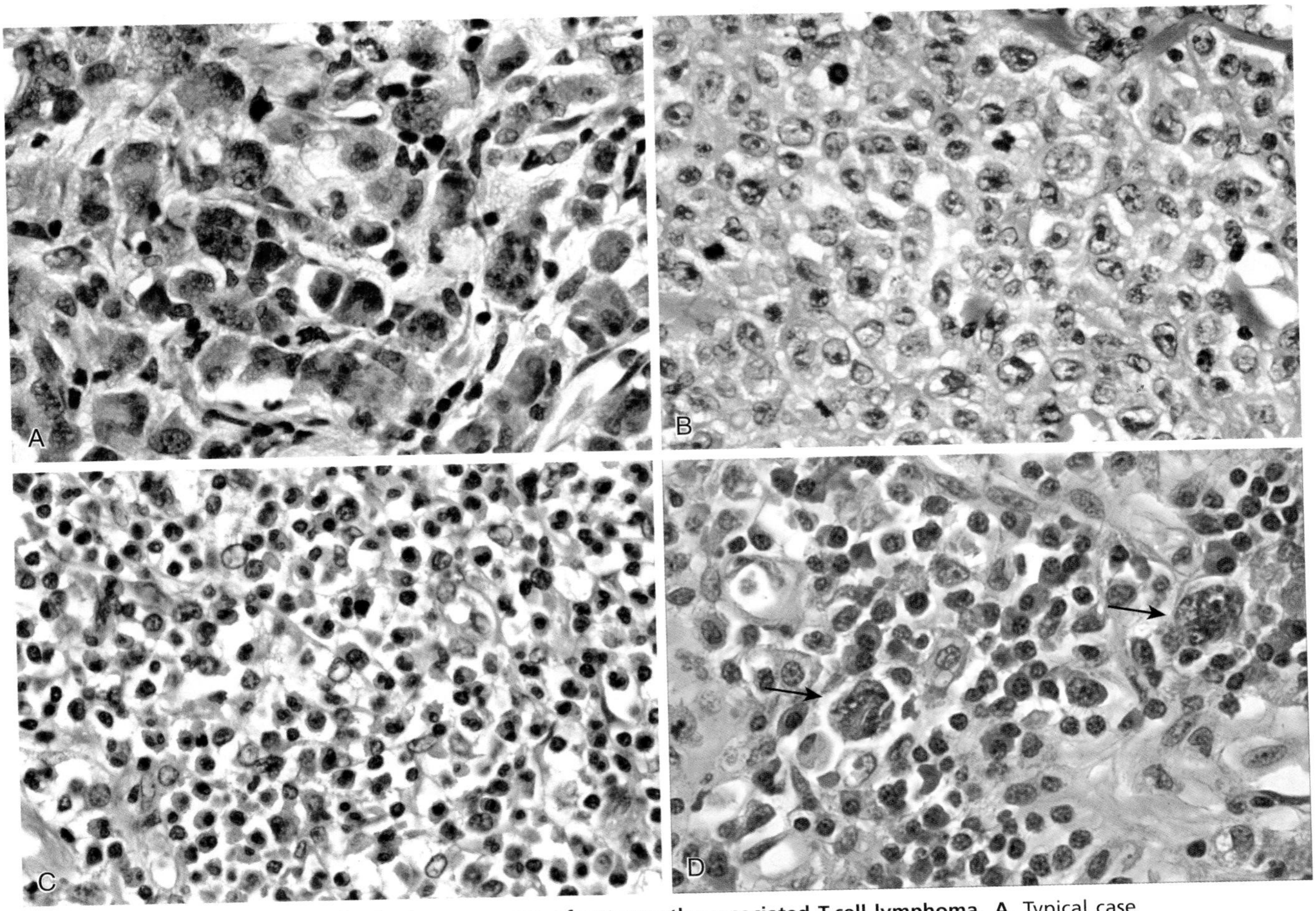

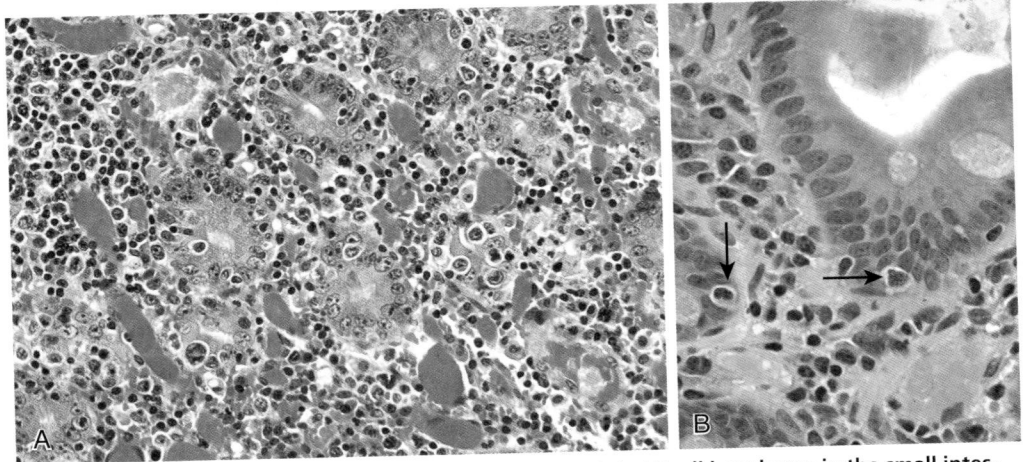

Figure 37-2. Histologic appearance of enteropathy-associated T-cell lymphoma. A, Typical case composed of pleomorphic large cells. **B,** In this case, the tumor cells are immunoblastic. **C,** Heavy inflammatory infiltrate containing principally eosinophils almost obscures the tumor cells. **D,** Scattered large multinucleated tumor cells in a plasma cell–rich inflammatory infiltrate.

Figure 37-3. Intraepithelial spread of enteropathy-associated T-cell lymphoma in the small intestinal mucosa. A, Numerous large intraepithelial neoplastic cells are seen in the epithelium overlying an invasive tumor. **B,** Rare, large, atypical intraepithelial lymphocytes are seen in a duodenal biopsy specimen lacking obvious lymphoma.

Lymph Node Involvement

The pattern of mesenteric (or other) lymph node involvement may be predominantly intrasinusoidal or paracortical, or both compartments may be involved (Fig. 37-7). Lymph nodes

remote from the EATL can show varying degrees of necrosis in the absence of a morphologically recognizable neoplastic cellular infiltrate (Fig. 37-8). Abdominal (and extraabdominal) lymph nodes may show a spectrum of changes ranging from lymphocyte depletion and fibrosis to dissolution of the node and replacement with lymph fluid (Fig. 37-8), referred to as *lymph node cavitation*.[48,49] At times, these lymph nodes can undergo calcification. Similar lymph node alterations can also be observed in individuals with long-standing untreated celiac disease or RCD, often accompanied by splenic atrophy.[49-51] Lymphatic and blood vessel damage by the neoplastic (or non-neoplastic) cytotoxic IELs trafficking to the lymph nodes and bystander killing of nodal constituents possibly contribute to lymph node destruction.

Immunohistochemistry

In most cases of EATL, the neoplastic lymphocytes express CD103, CD3 (cytoplasmic), CD7, T-cell intracellular antigen-1 (TIA-1), perforin, and granzyme B. They are usually negative for CD5, CD4, CD8, and CD56, and similar to RCD II, the majority lack surface and cytoplasmic T-cell receptor (TR) expression (Fig. 37-9). However, these immunophenotypic features are not constant, and the phenotypic profiles of synchronous and metachronous tumors can differ. Cytoplasmic TRβ chain (βF1) expression can been detected in

up to 25% of EATLs.[10,52,53] Some cases may show TRγ chain (or surface TRγδ) expression (Fig. 37-10) and dual TR expression (lineage infidelity) is rarely observed.[54-57] CD8 expression has been described in 19% to 30% of EATLs overall,[10,13,52,53] with a higher frequency (50%) reported in cases not associated with RCD II.[13] In occasional cases, the neoplastic cells fail to express CD3, perforin, or CD103.[13,45,58] CD30 expression varies in the different cytomorphologic variants, but almost all EATLs manifesting large cell morphology are CD30 positive (see Fig. 37-9).[13] Although some tumors resemble anaplastic large cell lymphoma (ALCL), EATLs are anaplastic lymphoma kinase negative except in very rare instances.[59] EATLs are Epstein-Barr virus (EBV)–negative lymphomas, but admixed EBV-positive lymphocytes may be present. Virtually all cases display elevated Ki67 proliferation indices (>50%). Immunohistochemistry is useful in detecting single scattered neoplastic cells in cases lacking a mass lesion and also for discerning increased IELs, as evidence of celiac disease, when small intestinal mucosal architecture in the vicinity of EATLs

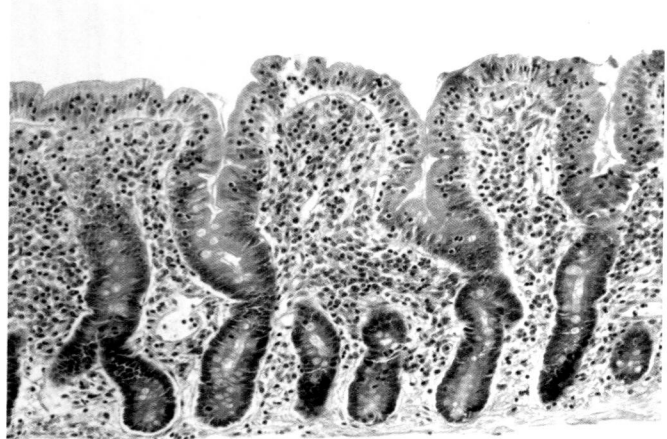

Figure 37-4. Small intestinal mucosa remote from enteropathy-associated T-cell lymphoma shows villous atrophy, crypt hyperplasia, and increased intraepithelial lymphocytes.

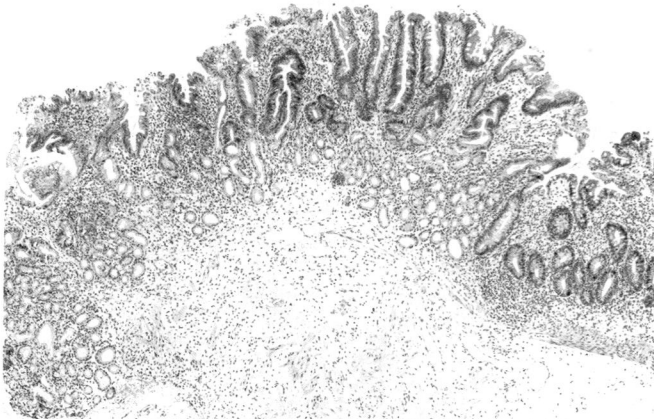

Figure 37-6. Healed ulcer in the nonlymphomatous small intestinal mucosa in a case of enteropathy-associated T-cell lymphoma. There is destruction of the muscularis mucosa, fibrosis of the mucosa and submucosa, and ulceration-associated cell lineage metaplasia of the intestinal crypts.

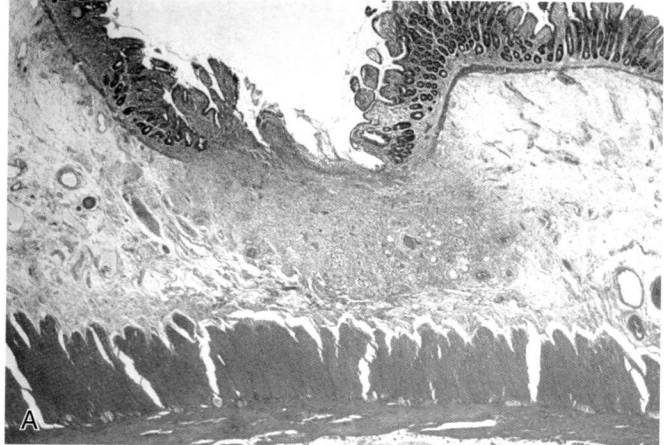

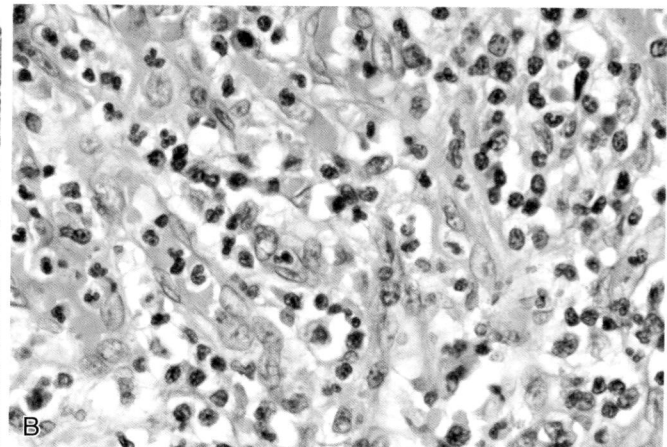

Figure 37-5. A, Shallow mucosal ulcer in a case of enteropathy-associated T-cell lymphoma. Similar changes can also be seen in cases of ulcerative jejunitis. **B,** High magnification of the ulcer base shows granulation tissue and no evidence of lymphoma.

appears normal (Fig. 37-11). The immunophenotype of IELs in the uninvolved small intestinal mucosa is normal in de novo EATLs, but they exhibit an aberrant phenotype in cases preceded by RCD II (see later; see also Table 37-1).

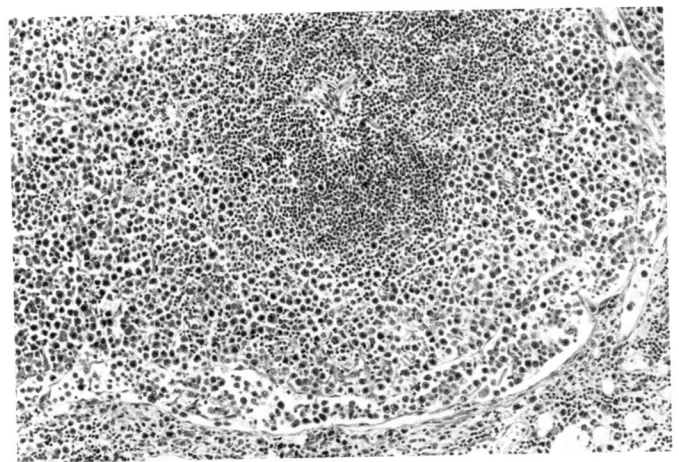

Figure 37-7. Dissemination of enteropathy-associated T-cell lymphoma to a mesenteric lymph node.

Clinical Course

The clinical course of EATL is unfavorable, with median survival ranging from 5 to 10 months and 1-year and 5-year overall survival of 31% to 38.7% and 0% to 58.8%, respectively.[13,14,16,34,36,41,60] Prognostic factors are not well established for this entity. However, the recently developed EATL prognostic index (EPI) has shown better outcome prediction than the International Prognostic Index (IPI) and the prognostic index for PTCL (PIT).[61] Malnutrition, which is common in EATL patients with prior RCD II, is considered responsible for their markedly lower 5-year survival (0%–8%) compared with those with de novo EATL (58.8%).[13,60] Surgical resection is impractical in many cases because of involvement of multiple intestinal segments and dissemination of disease beyond the mesenteric lymph nodes. Although remissions are nondurable, patients receiving chemotherapy with or without surgical resection have higher overall (40%–58%) and complete (27%–43%) response rates and longer survival than those treated with surgery alone.[13,41,62] Better outcomes have been reported for patients treated with intensive chemotherapy followed by autologous stem cell transplantation (4-year and 5-year overall and progression-free survival of 71% and

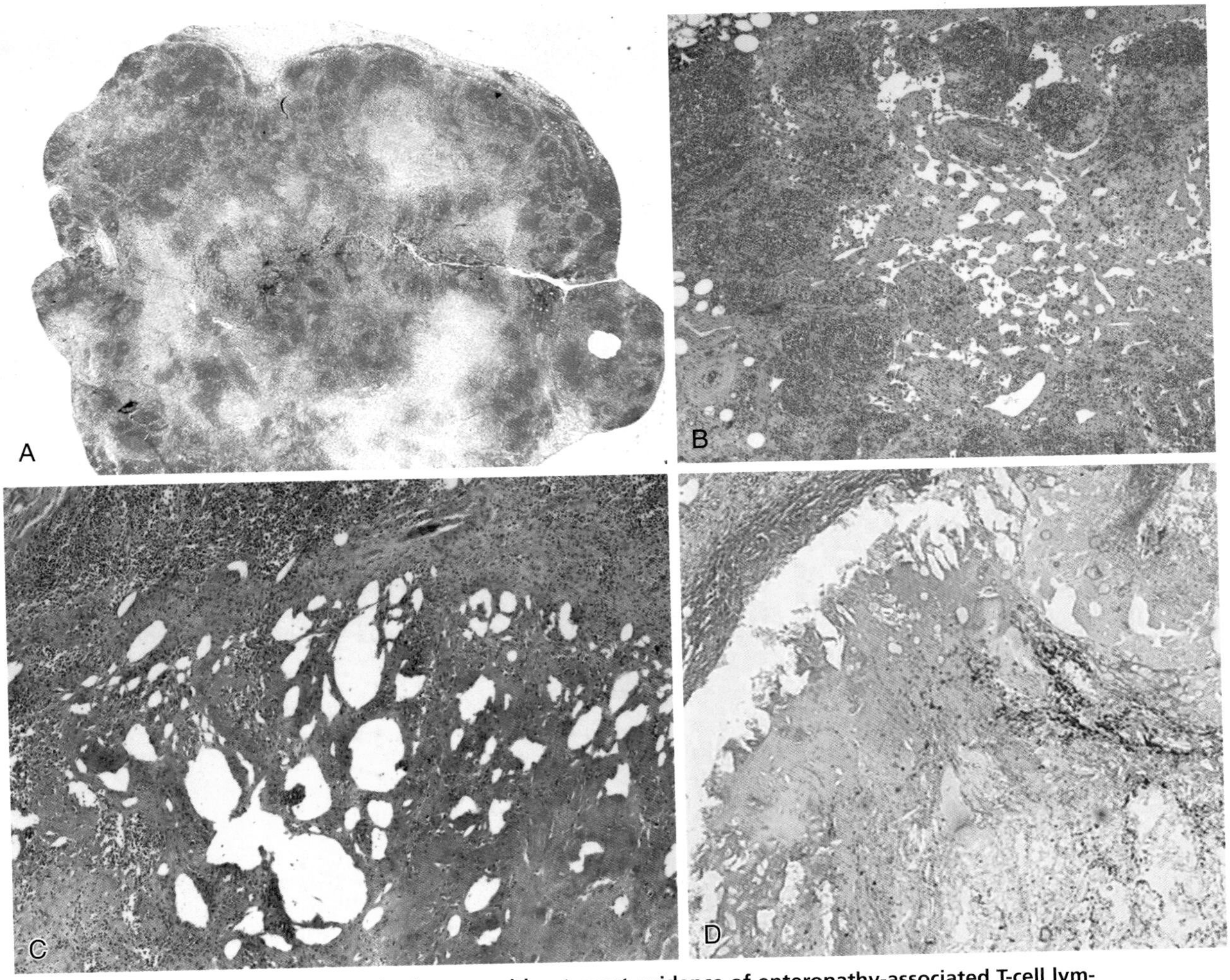

Figure 37-8. **Lymph node changes without overt evidence of enteropathy-associated T-cell lymphoma. A,** Multifocal necrosis in a mesenteric lymph node without evidence of a neoplastic lymphocytic infiltrate. **B,** Depletion of paracortical lymphocytes in an omental lymph node. **C,** Lymph node fibrosis (trichrome stain). **D,** Pseudocyst formation with lymph accumulation—lymph node cavitation (trichrome stain).

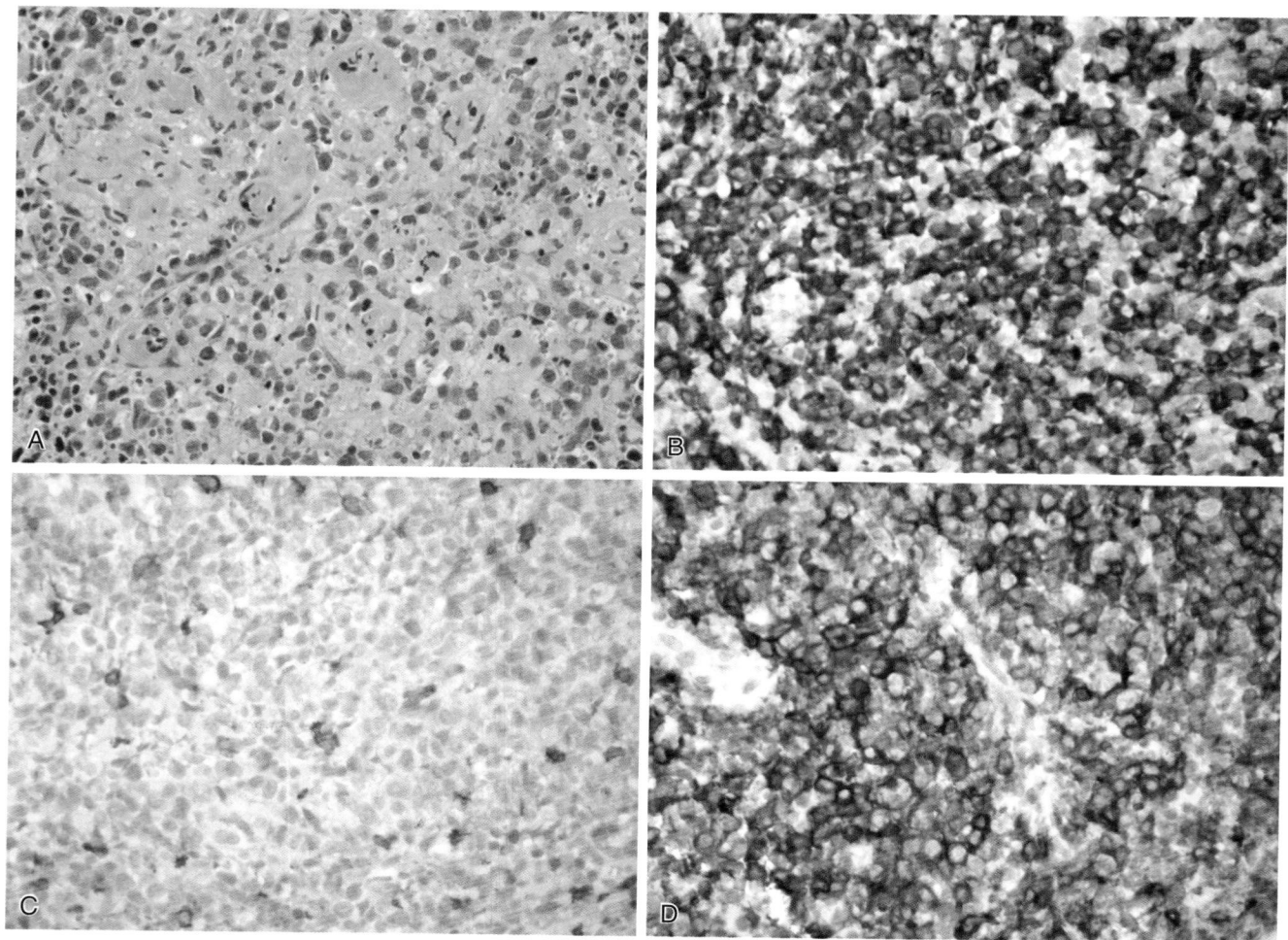

Figure 37-9. A, Enteropathy-associated T-cell lymphoma showing angiocentricity and angiodestruction. **B,** The neoplastic cells express CD3. **C,** They lack CD8 expression. **D,** Virtually all cells show intense CD30 expression.

60% and 71% and 52%, respectively).[14,63] Death is usually attributed to EATL, malnutrition, infections, or complications of therapy.[13,14]

Pathogenesis

Postulated Cell of Origin

EATL is derived from IELs on the basis of shared immunophenotypic features, including integrin $\alpha_E\beta_7$ (HML-1, CD103) expression.[13,64] IELs comprise a phenotypically heterogeneous population of thymus-derived T-cells and bone marrow-derived innate lymphoid cells (ILCs).[65-73] De novo EATLs are thought to arise from the neoplastic transformation of intraepithelial T-cells that have undergone TRA and B rearrangement, express TRαβ and the CD8αβ heterodimer (CD8αβ), and exhibit major histocompatibility complex class I restriction. These lymphocytes, which are referred to as conventional, type a, or induced IELs, account for 80% of all human small intestinal IELs.[74,75] They have latent cytotoxic potential (TIA-1 positive, perforin negative, granzyme B negative)[76,77] and migrate to the intestine in response to antigen stimulation.[78] T-cells that have rearranged TRG and D but not TRB (γδ T-cells)

account for up to 15% of IELs, and the majority display a "double negative" (CD4 and CD8 negative) phenotype.[68,79] The immunophenotypic profile of some EATLs suggests derivation from γδ T-cells; however, the frequency of such cases is presently unknown.[53-57] Since RCD II has been proposed to develop from ILCs, a similar cell of origin is speculated for EATLs evolving from RCD II.

Molecular Analysis and Genetic Abnormalities

Polymerase chain reaction (PCR) analysis for TRB or TRG rearrangement yields clonal TR rearrangements in virtually all EATLs.[13,52,80]

Segmental amplifications of the chromosome 9q31.3-qter region encompassing known proto-oncogenes (e.g., NOTCH1, ABL1, VAV2) or, alternatively, deletions at 16q12.1 have been reported in >80% of EATLs, and a small subset lacking 9q34 amplification exhibits allelic imbalances at 3q27.[81-85] Other common recurrent changes include gains at 1q, 5q, and 7q and losses at 8p, 9p, and 13q, with some studies suggesting gains at 1q and 5q to be more frequent in EATL than in other primary intestinal T-cell lymphomas (Table 37-2).[13,81,84] Although losses involving the 9p21 locus are detected in 10% to 13% of EATLs, loss of heterozygosity (LOH) at 9p21, targeting the cell cycle inhibitors CDKN2A/B, has been observed in up to 56% of

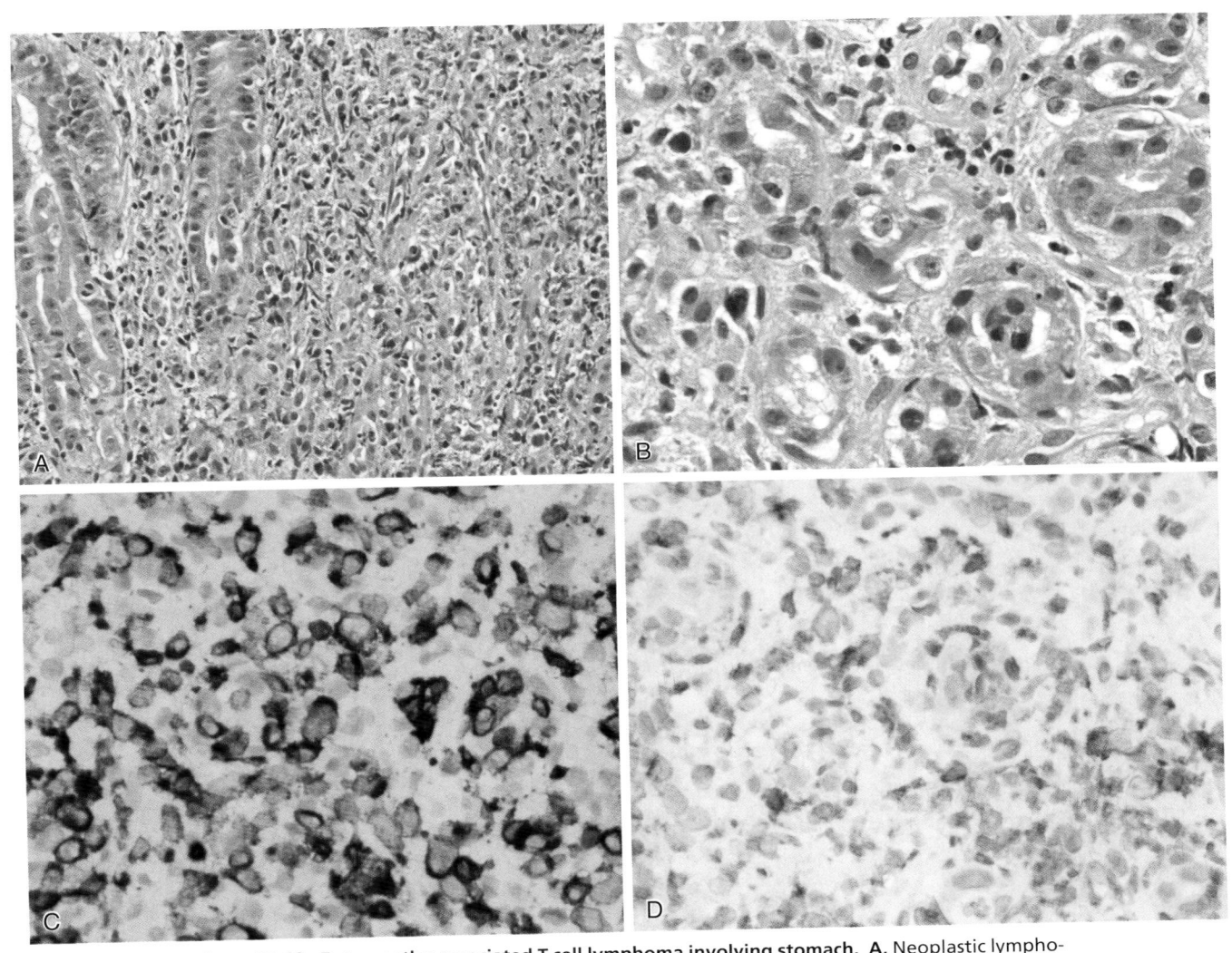

Figure 37-10. Enteropathy-associated T-cell lymphoma involving stomach. A, Neoplastic lymphocytes have destroyed gastric glands. **B,** Large atypical lymphocytes are seen infiltrating glandular epithelium. **C,** Immunohistochemistry for CD3 highlights the pleomorphic large lymphocytic infiltrate. **D,** Immunohistochemistry for TRγ shows weak expression in a subset of neoplastic cells. Flow cytometry showed no CD8 or surface CD3 and TR expression, and polymerase chain reaction (PCR) analysis detected a clonal TRB rearrangement.

cases, with consequent loss of p16 protein expression.[58,81,82] Loss or LOH of the 17p12-p13.2 region, harboring the *TP53* tumor suppressor gene, is noted in 20% and 31% of cases, respectively, but aberrant nuclear p53 expression can be seen in 75% of cases, indicating additional mechanisms of *TP53* deregulation.[58,81,84] EATLs display a significantly higher mean frequency of microsatellite instability, albeit low-level overall, compared with monomorphic epitheliotropic intestinal T-cell lymphomas (MEITLs).[84]

ALK and *DUSP22* rearrangements, characteristic of ALK-positive and ALK-negative ALCLs, have been reported in rare cases of EATL,[59,86,87] with one study documenting secondary acquisition of *DUSP22* rearrangement.[87]

The mutational profiles of de novo and RCD II-associated EATLs overlap with RCD II, but the variant allele frequencies (VAFs) of the somatic alterations are higher in most EATLs and these tumors show emergence of new driver mutations.[88] JAK-STAT pathway mutations are the most pervasive (50%–100%),[85,88-90] commonly involving *JAK1* (20%–74%) and *STAT3* (20%–47%), the vast majority representing activating

JAK1 JH1 kinase and *STAT3* SH2 domain mutations. Multiple *JAK1* or *STAT3* mutations occur in 21% and *JAK1/STAT3* double mutations in approximately one-third of EATLs,[88] while mutations in *JAK3* (0%–10%) and *STAT5B* (0%–10%) are infrequent.[85,88-90] Recurrent mutations are also observed in epigenetic regulators (up to 74%), including *KMT2D* (37%) and *TET2* (15%–32%), members of the NF-κB signaling pathway (33%) including *TNFAIP3* (28%) and *TNIP3* (6%), and DNA damage response and repair pathway (32%) including *POT1* (26%) and *TP53* (5%–10%), and in *DDX3X* (32%), *PRDM1/BLIMP1* (12%–17%), and *BCOR* (16%).[85] *SETD2* mutations (or deletions) are uncommon and RAS-MAPK pathway mutations (≈20%) appear less frequent than in MEITL.[85,88-90] In a limited number of cases evaluated, the mean number and spectrum of mutations detected by targeted sequencing were comparable between de novo and RCD II-associated EATLs.[90] However, *JAK1* mutations, observed in all de novo EATLs, were only seen in 50% of RCD II-associated EATLs, and mutations in *TNFAIP3* were restricted to the latter.

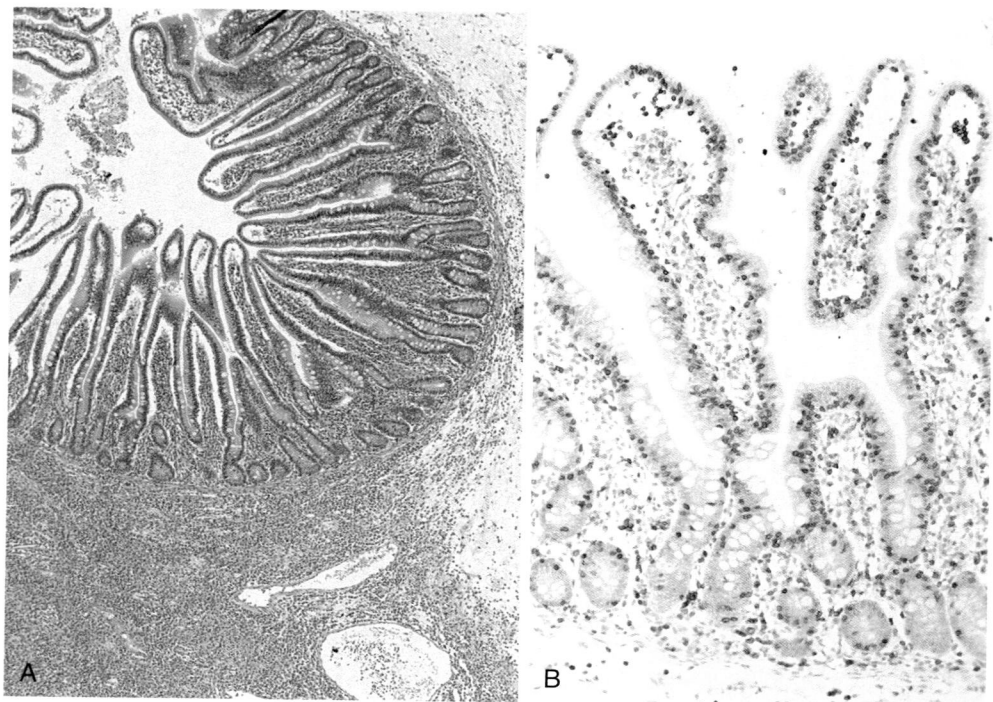

Figure 37-11. A, Enteropathy-associated T-cell lymphoma with overlying mucosa displaying well-formed villi. **B,** Higher magnification of villi immunostained with CD3 shows increased numbers of intraepithelial lymphocytes.

Transcriptome sequencing has shown higher expression of *IRF1/4, STAT3/5A,* and *TGM2* (autoantigen in celiac disease) genes in EATL compared to MEITL, and gene set enrichment analysis has disclosed significant overexpression of the interferon (IFN) γ pathway in EATL, which is a key signaling cascade in celiac disease IELs.[85]

REFRACTORY CELIAC DISEASE

Some individuals with celiac disease may become unresponsive to a gluten-free diet after a variable time or be nonresponsive de novo, a condition associated with heightened morbidity and mortality, referred to as refractory sprue or refractory celiac disease (RCD).[91]

Between 1989 and 2001, a number of investigators demonstrated unique pathologic features of a fraction of adult-onset RCD cases and uncovered an association between such cases and a related disorder, ulcerative jejunitis (see Fig. 37-5),[92] and EATL.[40,52,80,93-96] Although the histologic features of intact mucosa were indistinguishable from untreated celiac disease, the IELs in certain RCD cases displayed an aberrant immunophenotype (see later; see also Table 37-1). TR rearrangement analysis, performed on biopsy specimens or purified IELs, detected clonal products in a high proportion of these cases, and identical clones were observed in ulcerated and intact mucosa and samples of co-existent or subsequent EATLs.[40,52,80,93,95-97] These findings led to the belief that a subset of RCD cases represent low-grade lymphomas of intraepithelial T lymphocytes or cryptic EATL.[94,95,98]

Definition and Classification

RCD is defined as persistent gastrointestinal symptoms and abnormal small intestinal mucosal architecture with increased IELs, despite a strict gluten-free diet for >12 months.[99]

The diagnosis of RCD requires exclusion of certain celiac disease–related conditions (e.g., pancreatic insufficiency, bacterial overgrowth, microscopic colitis, lymphoma) and other small intestinal disorders (e.g., common variable immune deficiency, autoimmune enteropathy, drug-related injury) as causes of the symptoms. RCD may be *primary,* if there is no response to a gluten-free diet at diagnosis, or *secondary,* if refractoriness to gluten-free diet develops after an initial response. Clinicopathologic studies have shown RCD to encompass heterogeneous disorders.[45,60,100,101]

Currently, RCD is categorized into two types based on immunophenotypic and molecular criteria (see Table 37-1): type I, if the IEL phenotype is normal (i.e., they express surface CD3, CD8, and TR) and polyclonal products are detected on TR rearrangement analysis; and type II, if the IEL immunophenotype is aberrant (i.e., surface CD3, CD8, and TR expression is absent) and a clonal T-cell population is identified by TR rearrangement analysis.[99] Although of practical utility, this dichotomous classification has limitations (e.g., lack of consensus for cutoff values for the percentage of abnormal IELs and criteria to define clonality), and it does not capture the full spectrum of RCD II (e.g., surface CD8-positive or CD3-positive/TR-positive cases). The 2022 ICC recognizes RCD II as a precursor lesion to EATL,[8] because 30% to 50% of cases transform to overt EATL within 5 years.[102]

Synonyms and Related Terms

The 2022 ICC recognizes RCDII as a precursor lesion to EATL.

Epidemiology

The true prevalence of RCD and its subtypes is not known as most studies have been conducted at specialized centers and diagnostic criteria have varied. Studies from the United

Table 37-2 Pathologic and Genetic Features of Enteropathy-Associated T-Cell Lymphoma and Monomorphic Epitheliotropic Intestinal T-Cell Lymphoma

	EATL	MEITL
Frequency	66%–80%	20%–34%
Morphology	Variable, usually pleomorphic cells	Usually monomorphic small-to-medium-sized cells
Immunophenotype		
CD8	Negative (19%–30% positive)	Positive (10%–31% negative)
CD56	Negative	Positive (3%–25% negative)
HLA-DQ2/DQ8	90% positive	30%–40% positive
Chromosome/DNA copy number variants		
+9q31.3 or −16q12.1	86%	83%
+1q32.2-q41	73%	27%
+5q34-q35.2	80%	20%
+8q24 (MYC)	27%	13%–73%
Mutations		
JAK/STAT pathway	50%–100% (JAK1>JAK3, STAT3>STAT5B)	75%–89% (JAK3>JAK1, STAT5B>STAT3)
Epigenetic regulators	74% (SETD2 rare)	33%–100% (SETD2 >90%)
NF-κB pathway	33%	Unknown
RAS-MAP kinase pathway	20%	30%–53%
DNA damage response/repair pathway	32%	33%–44%
DDX3X	32%	3%
GNAI2	Unknown	9%–24%

EATL, Enteropathy-associated T-cell lymphoma; MEITL, monomorphic epitheliotropic intestinal T-cell lymphoma.

States and Europe report a wide range in the prevalence of RCD (1.5%–10%) in celiac disease patients.[100,101,103-105] Ulcerative jejunitis, which can be a manifestation of RCD II, was documented in 0.7% of celiac patients in the United Kingdom.[106] An epidemiologic survey from Finland, however, indicates that RCD is a rare complication of celiac disease, with a point prevalence of 0.31% in celiac patients and 0.002% in the general population.[51] Most studies describe a higher frequency of RCD I (68%–80% of all RCD cases),[45,51,60,100,101,107] and although a higher proportion of women are diagnosed with RCD I and II (69%–78% and 58%–60% of all cases, respectively), the frequency of men with RCD II is higher than in uncomplicated celiac disease.

Etiology

Similar to EATL, the duration and dose of gluten exposure appear to be risk factors for RCD, as homozygosity for HLA-DQ2 is observed in 44% to 67% of RCD II and 25% to 40% of RCD I cases,[33,45] and the majority of RCD patients are older than 50 years.[45,51,100] Environmental factors, specifically infections, have been suggested to increase susceptibility to RCD, but conclusive evidence is lacking at present.[45,108,109] The possibility of non-HLA genetic variants predisposing to RCD also exists. A genome-wide association study has reported significant association of a single nucleotide polymorphism on chromosome 7p14.3 with progression of celiac disease to RCD II.[110]

Clinical Presentation

Secondary refractoriness to a gluten-free diet is more common in individuals with RCD I (70%) compared to those with RCD II (50%),[45] while the latter have a higher frequency (and severity) of symptoms (60%–70% versus 30% in RCD I).[45,51,100] RCD II patients are severely malnourished (body mass index <18), with up to 90% presenting with protein-losing enteropathy or low serum albumin levels.[45,51,100] Large mucosal ulcers (>1 cm) are often seen on endoscopy in RCD II but not in RCD I patients.[45] Because the aberrant IELs often disseminate to other gastrointestinal organs (46%–64% of cases) and extragastrointestinal sites (60% of cases), including peripheral blood (44%–51% of cases), RCD II patients may present with extraintestinal symptoms or disorders (e.g., skin lesions; see Table 37-1).[44,45,111]

Histopathology

Small intestinal histologic features of RCD I or II are similar to those observed in untreated celiac disease (Figs. 37-12 and 37-13). At diagnosis, a high proportion of both subtypes manifest severe degrees of villous atrophy (subtotal or total); rare cases of RCD II may only exhibit crypt hyperplasia.[112] Intraepithelial lymphocytosis is evident, but the IELs lack significant cytologic atypia. At times, IELs extend deep within the crypts in RCD II (Fig. 37-13),[113] in contrast to uncomplicated celiac disease and RCD I, where they are mostly confined to the superficial regions of the villous-crypt unit. Although difficult to discern in RCD II, mild patchy lymphocytosis or small aggregates of lymphocytes might be seen in the lamina propria (representing IEL infiltrates), especially adjacent crypts (Fig. 37-13). Moreover, aberrant IELs can be widely distributed throughout the gastrointestinal tract, from the stomach to the anus.[40,44,45] Hence, one needs to recognize that EATLs evolving from prior RCD II may arise at sites besides the small intestine.

Mucosal ulceration associated with granulation tissue and variable degrees of chronic inflammation (ulcerative jejunitis; see Fig. 37-5),[40,45,60,80,93] is more frequently noted in RCD II, and presence of collagenous sprue or collagenous celiac disease has been reported in a subset of RCD I cases.[96,114]

Immunophenotypic and Molecular Analysis

In cases of suspected RCD, the IEL phenotype is best assessed by multiparametric flow cytometry of small intestinal biopsy specimens, as this modality is more sensitive than immunohistochemistry, allows simultaneous interrogation of multiple antigens, and can distinguish between surface (s) and cytoplasmic (cyt) antigen expression. Similar to uncomplicated celiac disease, more than 90% of IELs in RCD express CD103 (HML-1) or $\alpha_E\beta_7$ integrin, which is a receptor for E-cadherin.[115,116]

In RCD I, the majority of IELs are thymus-derived T-cells that express sCD3, sCD8, and sTRαβ (see Fig. 37-12 and Table 37-1).[117] The intensity of CD5 is variable, similar to normal small intestinal intraepithelial T-cells.[118] Upregulation of certain activating natural killer (NK)-cell receptors (e.g.,

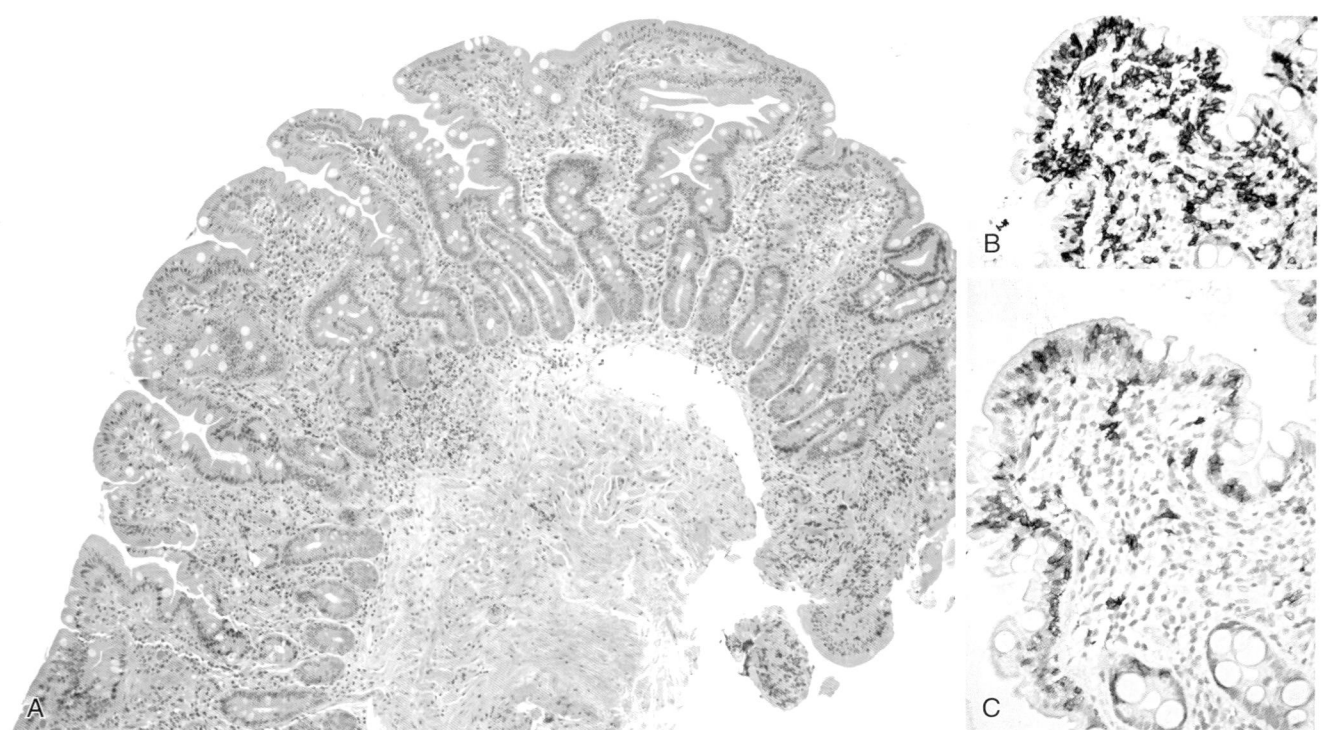

Figure 37-12. Refractory celiac disease type I. A, The small intestinal mucosa shows partial villous atrophy, crypt hyperplasia, and increased intraepithelial lymphocytes. **B,** The intraepithelial lymphocytes express CD3. **C,** Most intraepithelial lymphocytes also express CD8.

CD94/NKG2C) can be observed,[45] and intraepithelial TRγδ-positive T-cells are normally elevated.[119]

In classical cases of RCD II, an increased proportion of IELs (>20% to virtually 100%) are sCD3 negative and sTR negative, but they express intracellular CD3ε. The IELs generally show bright CD7 expression and are CD5 negative, and CD2 expression can vary.[113,117] CD8 expression is usually absent (see Fig. 37-13 and Table 37-1).[40,93] However, cases of RCD II with variant phenotypes, including CD8-positive cases, have been documented in multiple studies.[45,54,113,120-122] The IELs in some RCD II cases display cytTRβ (βF1) expression,[95,96,120,121,123] and rarely may express sCD3 and sTRαβ or sTRγδ, or lack cytCD3 expression.[88,113] Most cases exhibit a spectrum of activating NK-cell receptors (e.g., NKG2D, NKp46),[97,124,125] and a threshold of >25 NKp46-positive IELs per 100 epithelial cells can reliably discriminate RCD II from RCD I.[126] In contrast to EATLs, IELs in RCD II have low proliferation indices, as assessed by Ki67 or proliferating cell nuclear antigen staining.[109,113,118] Presence of CD30-positive IELs should alert one to the possibility of unsampled EATL, as IELs in RCD II do not express CD30.[120] Although aberrant lymphocytes represent a major proportion of IELs, they may account for >20% of lamina propria lymphoid cells in up to 50% of RCD II cases.[111,113]

Immunohistochemical staining of small intestinal biopsy specimens has been used for the evaluation of aberrant IELs and classification of RCD. Most studies have used a cutoff of <50% CD8-positive IELs in formalin-fixed, paraffin embedded biopsy specimens to classify cases as RCD II.[40,44,100,101] Although it is practical, rapid, and cost-effective, immunohistochemistry has limitations and pitfalls. A high interobserver variability

and low sensitivity in detecting cases with low frequencies of aberrant IELs have been reported for this method.[127] Substantial expansions of TRγδ-positive IELs that are mostly CD8 negative are not uncommon in biopsy specimens of celiac disease (and RCD I) patients, which in the absence of TRγ staining may be misinterpreted as "phenotypically aberrant" IELs.[96] Furthermore, CD8-positive RCD II cases will be missed by this approach. Discrepancies in the reported frequencies and clinical outcomes of RCD II patients might relate to the use of different modalities for disease classification. Diagnosis of RCD II by flow cytometry can also be challenging at times because of the presence of other IEL subsets, especially ILCs,[128] which manifest a phenotype similar to aberrant IELs (CD103+, sCD3−, cytCD3ε+, CD5−, CD8−), but these cells typically do not exceed 20% of IELs.[68,70,71]

Clonality assessment is important, yet by itself is inadequate for RCD categorization, as analytical and biological factors can give rise to discordant results. PCR analysis for TRB or G rearrangement generally yields polyclonal products in RCD I (Fig. 37-14; see also Table 37-1) and clonal products in RCD II (Fig. 37-15C; see also Table 37-1).[13,40,45,52,95,96,100,105,122] However, clonal TR rearrangements can occasionally be observed in RCD I,[129] and they may be absent in up to one-third of RCD II cases.[118,129,130] Furthermore, CDR3 sequencing of RCD II cases with clonal rearrangements has revealed incomplete or nonfunctional TRG, D, and B rearrangements in ≈70% of cases.[130] Nonetheless, PCR-based assessment of TR rearrangement is useful in establishing a clonal relationship between RCD II and concomitant or subsequent EATLs (Fig. 37-15C).[13,80,95,96,122]

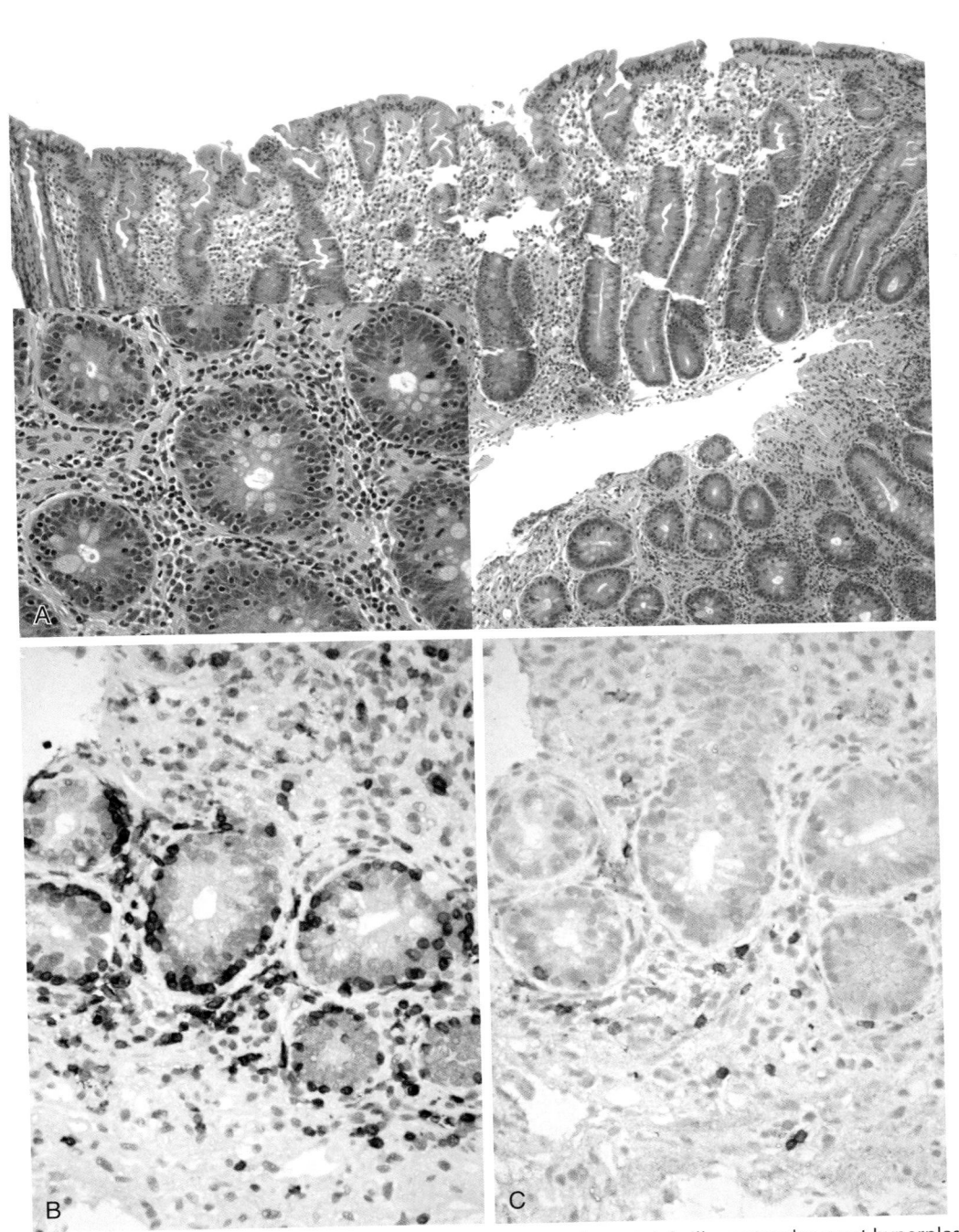

Figure 37-13. Refractory celiac disease type II. A, The small intestinal mucosa shows total villous atrophy, crypt hyperplasia, and increased intraepithelial lymphocytes (*inset:* extension of the lymphocytes into crypt epithelium). **B,** The intraepithelial lymphocytes express CD3 (note small clusters of CD3-positive lymphocytes in lamina propria–adjacent crypts). **C,** Virtually all intraepithelial lymphocytes and most pericryptal, lamina propria lymphocytes are CD8 negative.

Immunophenotypic, genomic, and transcriptional analyses of RCD II cell lines and IELs, as well as functional studies, have suggested an IL-15 responsive subset of bone marrow derived ILCs residing in the small intestinal epithelium to be the normal counterpart of aberrant IELs.[125,130,131] Under physiologic conditions, these cells can differentiate into T-cells and NK-cells, but inactivation of NOTCH1 signaling by IL-15

limits T-cell development in RCD II. The differentiation level of the aberrant IELs varies among cases. An advanced maturation stage of RCD II IELs and a higher intensity of cytCD3 expression (relative to expression of normal IELs) have been associated with an increased risk of progression to EATL.[132,133] Because of the phenotypic heterogeneity of RCD II, an origin of some cases from other subsets of IELs cannot be ruled out.

Clinical Course

The 5-year survival of RCD II patients (44%–58%) is markedly inferior to that of RCD I patients (80%–96%), which is attributed to more severe malnutrition and a higher risk for development of EATL (30%–52% in 4–6 years for RCD II versus 3%–14% for RCD I; see Table 37-1).[45,51,60,100]

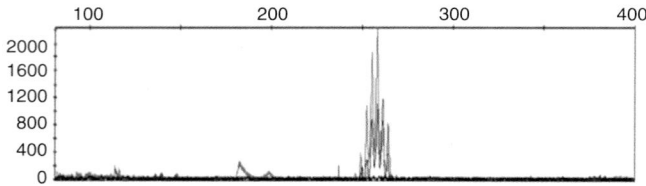

Figure 37-14. Fluorescent polymerase chain reaction (PCR) analysis for TRB rearrangement and capillary gel electrophoresis performed on a small intestinal biopsy sample from a patient with refractory celiac disease type I shows polyclonal products.

RCD I patients in whom surreptitious gluten ingestion has been excluded benefit from immunomodulatory drug (glucocorticoids, azathioprine, and enteric-coated budesonide) therapy.[99,134] Treatment of RCD II patients is challenging. Clinical and pathologic improvement has been documented with open capsule budesonide, which is the preferred first-line therapy.[135] Chemotherapy (e.g., cladribine, alkylating agents) with or without autologous stem cell transplantation, is unable to eradicate the neoplastic cells.[99,136] An improvement in symptoms was reported with use of an anti-IL-15 monoclonal antibody without a significant reduction in aberrant IELs.[137] In vitro studies have demonstrated antiproliferative and cytocidal effects of JAK1-STAT3 pathway inhibitors,[88] but their clinical efficacy remains to be determined.

Pathogenesis

The pathogenesis of RCD I is unclear but appears to be multifactorial. Inadvertent, low-level gluten ingestion is

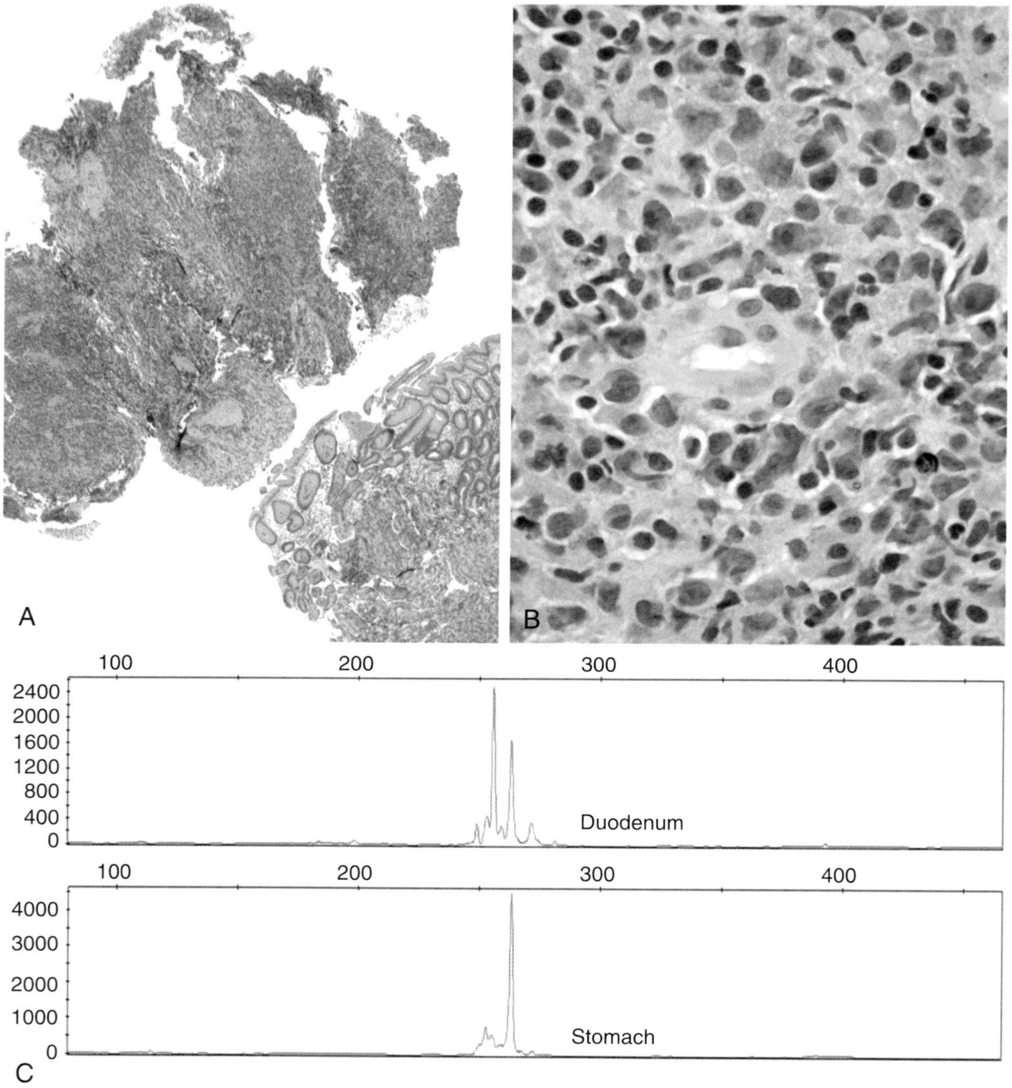

Figure 37-15. Transformation of refractory celiac disease type II to enteropathy-associated T-cell lymphoma in the stomach. A, Gastric mucosa shows a dense and destructive lymphocytic infiltrate. **B,** The neoplastic lymphocytes are large and pleomorphic. **C,** Fluorescent polymerase chain reaction (PCR) analysis for TRB rearrangement and capillary gel electrophoresis show gastric spread and transformation of one of the two duodenal neoplastic T-cell clones.

considered responsible for sustaining intestinal inflammation in at least one-third of patients,[105,138] and transition from a gluten-driven to an autoimmune response is suspected in some cases.[109] No genetic alterations have yet been identified in this subtype.[88] RCD II is a prototypic inflammation-associated lymphoproliferative disorder. Epithelial stress induced by cytotoxic gliadin peptides results in upregulation of IL-15, which augments IFN-γ production and cytotoxicity of aberrant IELs resulting in epithelial damage, and synergizes with cytokines secreted by gliadin-responsive CD4-positive T cells in the lamina propria (e.g., IL-2, TNF-α, IL-21) to stimulate proliferation and enhance the survival of IELs by activating the JAK-STAT signaling cascade.[109,124,139-143]

Somatic mutations have been detected in 80% to 90% of RCD II cases, with mutations in JAK-STAT pathway genes constituting the most frequent alterations (up to 86% of cases) observed in cases displaying classical as well as variant immunophenotypes.[88,113] *JAK1* (36%–48%) and *STAT3* (38%–64%) are the commonly targeted genes. Loss of function mutations in negative regulators of the pathway (*SOCS1, SOCS3, SH2B3*) also occur, albeit at lower frequencies. Other recurrently mutated gene classes and pathways comprise epigenetic regulators (64%), including *TET2* (30%–45%) and *KMT2D* (22%–45%); NF-κB signaling (22%–27%), including *TNFAIP3/A20* (13%–27%) and *TNIP3* (9%); immune escape (20%–36%), including *CD58* (12%–18%) and *FAS* (6%–9%), and DNA damage response/repair (27%), including *POT1* (≈20%) and *TP53* (4%). Mutations in the X-linked RNA helicase *DDX3X* and *BCOR* are seen in 20% and 10% of cases, respectively. The aberrant IELs in virtually all RCD II cases express phospho-STAT3 by immunohistochemistry,[113] and JAK1-STAT3 and NF-κB pathway mutations have been shown to constitutively activate signaling or enhance responsiveness of the IELs to IL-15 and TNF-α, respectively.[88,130] Mutations in *JAK1,* especially the *JAK1* p.G1097 hotspot mutation are present in about half the cases, and *STAT3* and *TNFAIP3* are maintained in RCD II–associated EATL, suggesting driver roles of these alterations.[88,113]

Recurrent trisomies of chromosome 1q22-q44 have been identified on cytogenetic analysis of RCD II cell lines and biopsies.[45,144] Array-based analyses have confirmed 1q gains and also revealed frequent losses at 4q and 6q, including *TNIP3* and *TNFAIP3/A20* loci, respectively.[88,113] Loss of p16 protein, in the absence of LOH at chromosome 9p21, has been reported in 40% of ulcerative jejunitis cases, and aberrant nuclear p53 expression has been detected in 57% of cases in the absence of molecular lesions of *TP53.*[58] Altogether, these observations indicate dysregulated JAK1-STAT3 and NF-κB signaling, disruptions of epigenetic and cell cycle regulators and tumor suppressors, and chromosome 1q gains to be early events in the genesis of RCD II-associated EATL.

MONOMORPHIC EPITHELIOTROPIC INTESTINAL T-CELL LYMPHOMA

Before the era of immunophenotyping, it was assumed that rare primary intestinal lymphomas composed of uniform, small, round lymphocytes represented cytomorphologic variants of EATL, as they were associated with villous atrophy and intraepithelial lymphocytosis of the uninvolved mucosa. In 1992 Chott and colleagues[145] suggested the existence of

at least one subtype of primary intestinal PTCL exhibiting similar architectural and infiltration patterns as EATL but lacking enteropathy. The immunophenotype of the tumor cells of this aggressive variant (CD3 positive, CD8 positive, CD56 positive) was subsequently shown to be different from NK-cell lymphomas and most cases of EATL.[10] Although it shared some clinical features and genetic properties with EATL, there were distinct differences.[10,81] This type of intestinal T-cell lymphoma was categorized as EATL type II in the 2008 WHO 4th ed. classification.[5] Subsequently, studies from Asia confirmed the lack of association between this entity and celiac disease,[146-148] and it was renamed *CD56-positive monomorphic intestinal T-cell lymphoma* in the 2010 4th ed. WHO classification of tumors of the digestive system.[149] Recognition of the not-infrequent variability in phenotype of this neoplasm, especially with regard to CD8 and CD56 expression, as well as its lineage,[55,150-160] led to the designation *monomorphic epitheliotropic intestinal T-cell lymphoma (MEITL)* in the revised WHO 4th ed. classification,[6,7] a term that is maintained in the 2022 ICC and WHO 5th ed. classification.[8,9]

Definition

MEITL is a neoplasm derived from IELs, with most cases characterized by small-to-medium-sized lymphocytes, usually exhibiting minimal cellular pleomorphism.

Synonyms and Related Terms

WHO revised 4th ed., 2017: Monomorphic epitheliotropic intestinal T-cell lymphoma[6,7]

WHO 5th ed., 2022: Monomorphic epitheliotropic intestinal T-cell lymphoma[9]

Epidemiology

MEITL has a wider geographic distribution than EATL, representing up to 34% of primary intestinal T-cell lymphomas in Europe and the United States[10,11] and the majority of primary intestinal T-cell lymphomas in Asia.[150,151,152] Like EATL, it is a rare neoplasm, representing ≈4% of primary intestinal lymphomas in Asia and <5% of Western and 1.9% of Asian PTCL cases.[11,153] It usually occurs in the 5th and 6th decades of life; however, similar to EATL, MEITL has been documented in younger individuals.[55,150-156] Males are affected more frequently than females (male-to-female ratio, 1.8–2.6:1).[55,150,151] The true incidence and prevalence of MEITL is not known at present.

Etiology

The etiology of MEITL is unknown. Although a clinical history of celiac disease or "histologic enteropathy" has been reported in a variable proportion of cases,[10,11,55,150-154] the frequency of HLA-DQ2/DQ8 alleles in Western cases mirrors that of the normal population (30%–40%),[81,85,139] and series of well-characterized cases from Europe and Asia have reported a lack of association with celiac disease i.e., absence of steatorrhea or malabsorption[10,55,150,151,155,156] and negative celiac serology (anti–tissue transglutaminase and anti–endomysial antibodies).[10,151] The occurrence of isolated large intestinal disease in some individuals also supports distinct etiopathogenesis.[150,151,156-158] Expansions of IELs with an aberrant phenotype are not uncommon in the uninvolved small intestinal mucosa of patients with MEITL. However, a prior indolent precursor phase, analogous to RCD II, has not been established in this entity.

Clinical Presentation

An acute presentation has been reported in 40% to 85% of cases. Common symptoms and signs include abdominal pain (31%–89%), perforation (12%–70%), weight loss (28%–63%), diarrhea (21%–45%), obstruction (16%–28%), and bleeding (4%–17%).[10,55,85,150-158] B symptoms are noted in 36% to 48% of patients.[85,150,153,156] The small intestine is the most common primary site of lymphoma (73%–95%),[55,150,151,156,85,155] with jejunal and ileal involvement noted in 50% to 73% and 27% to 45% of cases, respectively.[10,151,156] Concurrent stomach and large bowel disease is detected in 5% and 5% to 28% of cases, respectively,[55,150-152,158] and multifocal disease is observed in 12% to 58% of cases, most often involving the jejunum and ileum.[10,55,150,154,153,156] Individuals with small intestine involvement, with or without large intestine involvement, have more advanced disease, whereas those with isolated large intestinal involvement (10%–18%) seem to have more localized disease.[150,151] Sites of disease dissemination include abdominal or inguinal lymph nodes (27%–44%), omentum or mesentery (22%), abdominal or pelvic organs (5%–11%), lung/pleura (5%–12%), bone marrow (3%–12%), and cervical lymph nodes (6%), and central nervous system involvement may be observed on occasion.[55,105,151,153,155,156] The extent of disease at diagnosis varies between studies, with high-stage disease (Lugano IIE-IV) reported in 33% to 73% of cases.[150-156] The frequency of patients with good performance status (ECOG ≤1) ranges from 43% to 76%, lactate dehydrogenase levels are elevated in 29% to 91%, and analogous to EATL, a high proportion of individuals have hypoalbuminemia (67%–90%).[150,153-156]

Pathology

Macroscopic Appearance

Similar to EATL, MEITL can present as solitary or multiple tumors, which may show central ulceration, at times with exudate. In some instances, the overlying mucosa might appear nodular. Strictures are less common. Mucosal folds adjacent to tumors are often enlarged or swollen, and the muscularis propria is often thin and stretched. Gross involvement of mesenteric and abdominal lymph nodes is not uncommon.

Histopathology

In the majority of cases, the neoplastic lymphocytes are small-to-medium-sized and have small nuclei with fine granular chromatin, inconspicuous or small nucleoli, and scant to moderate pale pink or clear cytoplasm (monocytoid appearance). There is usually little variation in cell size within a given tumor. A variable proportion of cases, however, can be comprised of large lymphocytes with irregular nuclei, vesicular chromatin, and prominent nucleoli, or exhibit significant cellular pleomorphism.[10,151,152,155,157] A subset of

cases may also manifest other atypical morphologic features such as a starry-sky appearance or increased apoptotic activity, angiocentricity or angioinvasion, and coagulative necrosis.[155,157] In contrast to EATLs, chronic inflammatory cells are either absent or sparse in nearly all MEITLs.[55,151,155] Most lymphomas have a central "tumor zone" characterized by a dense and diffuse transmural infiltrate of neoplastic cells and frequent ulceration and perforation (Fig. 37-16); a "peripheral zone" representing lateral, predominantly mucosal infiltration by lymphoma associated with crypt destruction and variable degrees of villous atrophy, which in 68% to 89% of cases displays prominent epitheliotropism by the atypical lymphocytes (Fig. 37-17); and a contiguous or distant "IEL zone" (35%–100% of cases) exhibiting normal villous architecture or mild villous atrophy and increased IELs lacking cytologic atypia (small size and hyperchromatic nuclei).[10,55,150-155,157]

Immunohistochemistry

MEITLs exhibit a distinctive cytotoxic immunophenotype in that the tumor cells express CD3, CD8, CD56 (see Fig. 37-16), and TIA-1, but similar to EATL, most express CD7 and >90% lack CD5 expression (Table 37-3). A minority may express CD4 (3%–11%) or both CD4 and CD8 (3%–19%).[53,150,152,155,158] Of the CD8-positive cases, 77% have been shown to express CD8α homodimers (CD8αα), and the remainder, CD8αβ heterodimers.[151] Studies have highlighted variability in the expression of T-cell antigens by a proportion (or all) of the neoplastic lymphocytes at diagnosis or relapse.[53,55,150-155,157,158,161] Notably, absence of CD8 and CD56 has been described in 10% to 31% and 3% to 25% of cases, respectively (up to 11% lacking both), and 2% to 18% can be TIA-1 negative; granzyme B and perforin expression is heterogeneous and positivity is lower than TIA-1.[55,150-158] Lack of βF1 expression has been reported in 54% to 90% of cases,[10,53,150,151,155,157,161,162] and TRγ or TRδ expression has been documented in 26% to 78% of tumors, indicating TRγδ lineage[55,150,151,155,157]; some of these may lack surface TR expression by flow cytometry but show cytoplasmic TRγ expression (Fig. 37-18). A variable number of cases (6%–34%) are "TR silent," lacking both βF1 and TRγ/δ expression,[53,55,150,151,154,155,157] whereas co-expression of TRβ and TRγ/δ (lineage infidelity) is observed in 3% to 17% of cases.[53,55,151,155,157] A high proportion of cases (91%) express phospho-MEK1/2, evidence of mitogen-activated protein kinase (MAPK) pathway activation.[154] Megakaryocyte-associated tyrosine kinase (MATK) and spleen tyrosine kinase (SYK), expressed by 87% and 95% of cases, respectively, are highly discriminatory for MEITL, as they are not expressed by EATL.[53,151] Aberrant expression of B-cell antigens, usually by a subset of the neoplastic cells and weaker in intensity than normal B-cells, has been recorded in 10% to 24% of cases.[55,151,155,158] Positivity for CD20 is more common than CD79a and occasional tumors can co-express both antigens, but PAX5 is negative. Both CD103-positive and CD103-negative MEITLs exist, the former accounting for 80% of cases in a large series.[155] Epithelial membrane antigen is usually negative and CD30 expression is only noted in rare instances.[6,53,152,155,156] A few studies have reported EBV infection in a minority of cases (≈10%); it is not certain if some (or all) such cases represent

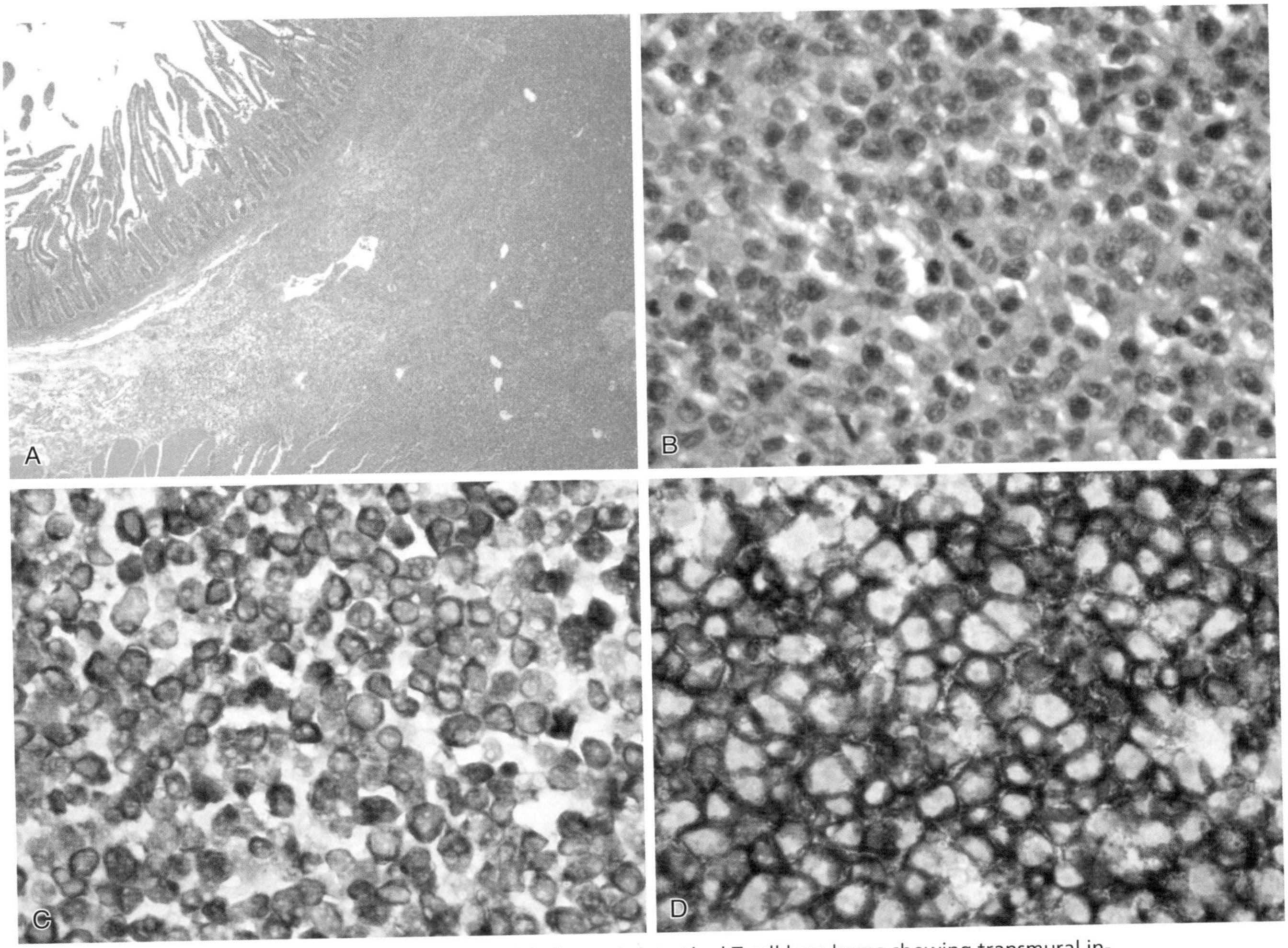

Figure 37-16. **A,** Monomorphic epitheliotropic intestinal T-cell lymphoma showing transmural infiltration by neoplastic lymphocytes ("tumor zone"). **B,** The neoplastic cells are medium sized. **C,** The majority are CD8 positive. **D,** Most show intense CD56 expression.

primary intestinal extranodal NK/T-cell lymphomas, nasal type.[10,150,162] The Ki67 labeling index of the tumor cells is >50% in the majority of cases.[53,55,155] C-MYC overexpression and aberrant P53 expression have both been described in 30% to 40% of MEITLs overall, and in a greater proportion of cases exhibiting atypical morphology.[154,155]

The immunophenotype of the atypical IELs in the peripheral zone is similar to the tumor in the central zone (see Fig. 37-17) or intermediate between that of the tumor and the mature appearing IELs in the distal mucosa.[55,151] The antigen profile of the latter has been shown to be discordant with the tumor in up to 65% of cases (CD56 and MATK expression is usually weak or negative in IELs, while CD2, CD8, and TR are expressed by the IELs, but may be downregulated/absent in the tumor).[55,147,151] In contrast to the mucosal infiltrate, the Ki67 proliferation index of the intraepithelial component is low (<10%).[55]

Clinical Course

Similar to EATLs, the clinical outcome of patients with MEITL is poor, with median survival ranging from 7 to 14.8 months.[85,150,151,154-156,158] One-year and 5-year overall survival rates of 31% to 57% and 32%, respectively, have

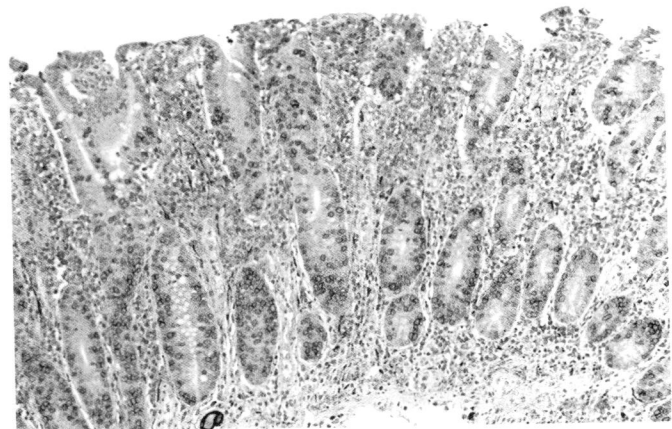

Figure 37-17. The peripheral zone of a monomorphic epitheliotropic intestinal T-cell lymphoma showing villous atrophy and increased numbers of intraepithelial lymphocytes *(brown)*, many expressing CD56 *(blue)*.

been reported.[55,85,150,154-156] Prognostic factors are not well established for this disease. A recent study described independent adverse prognostic effects of *TP53* and *STAT5B* mutations and a favorable prognosis for cases expressing

Table 37-3 Differential Diagnosis of Intestinal T-Cell and Natural Killer–Cell Lymphomas and Lymphoproliferative Disorders

	EATL	MEITL	Indolent Clonal T-Cell Lymphoproliferative Disorder of the Gastrointestinal Tract	Indolent NK-Cell Lymphoproliferative Disorder of the Gastrointestinal Tract	Extranodal NK/T-Cell Lymphoma, Nasal Type	ALCL
Morphology	Pleomorphic large cells	Monomorphic small-to-medium-sized cells	Monomorphic small cells	Medium-to-large-sized cells	Pleomorphic small-to-medium-sized cells	Pleomorphic large cells
Phenotype	CD3+, CD4−/CD8−/+, CD30+/−	CD3+, CD4−, CD8+, CD56+	CD3+, CD4+ or CD8+; rarely CD4−CD8− or CD4+CD8+	CD3+, CD4−, CD8−, CD56+	CD3+/−, CD4−, CD8−, CD56+	CD3−/+, CD8−, CD4+/−, CD30+
TR rearrangement	Clonal	Clonal	Clonal	Germline	Germline	Clonal
Mucosa	Villous atrophy	Villous atrophy	Normal/villous atrophy	Normal	Villous atrophy in involved areas	Normal
IELs	Increased CD4−/8−/+	Increased CD8+	Normal/focally increased CD4+ or CD8+	Normal	Increased in involved areas CD4−/CD8−	Normal
EBV	−	−	−	−	+	−

ALCL, Anaplastic large cell lymphoma; *EATL,* enteropathy-associated T-cell lymphoma; *EBV,* Epstein-Barr virus; *IEL,* intraepithelial lymphocyte; *MEITL,* monomorphic epitheliotropic intestinal T-cell lymphoma; *NK,* natural killer; *TR,* T-cell receptor gene.

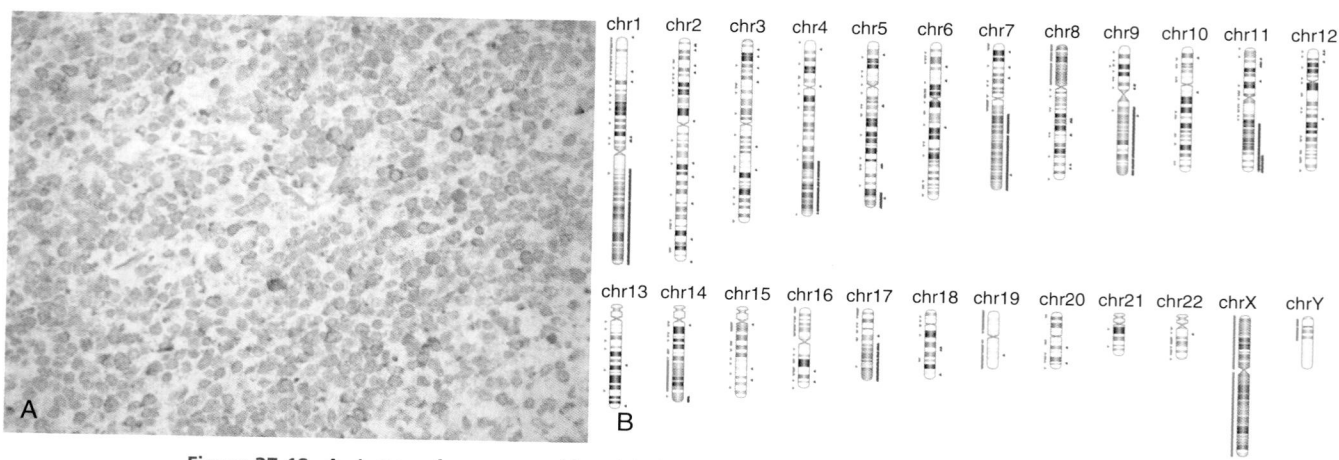

Figure 37-18. A, A case of monomorphic epitheliotropic intestinal T-cell lymphoma, which lacked surface TRαβ and γδ expression, shows variable cytoplasmic TRγ expression; polymerase chain reaction (PCR) analysis detected a clonal TRG rearrangement; no clonal TRB rearrangement was observed. **B,** Single-nucleotide polymorphism array analysis displays complex genomic aberrations, representing gains *(blue)* and losses *(red)* of chromosome regions. Similar changes may also be observed in enteropathy-associated T-cell lymphoma (see Table 37-2).

B-cell antigens.[155] Response to initial therapy is associated with better overall and progression-free survival, and a good performance status (≤1) is associated with better overall survival.[150,155,156] The use of chemotherapy is associated with higher response rates compared with surgery alone. The overall and complete response rate of patients receiving chemotherapy, with or without surgical resection, is 44% to 59% and 16% to 43%, respectively.[150,151,155,156] Limited data regarding autologous bone marrow transplantation after intensive chemotherapy appear promising, with 4-year and 5-year overall survival rates of 45% and 28%.[55,63,150,151,156]

Pathogenesis

Postulated Cell of Origin

MEITL is considered to arise from either intraepithelial TRαβ or TRγδ T-cells, the majority expressing CD8α homodimers

(CD8αα) irrespective of αβ or γδ lineage.[151] The ontogeny of CD8αα-positive TRαβ-positive and CD8αα-positive TRγδ-positive IELs, also referred to as unconventional, type b, or natural IELs, has not been clarified in humans.[74,75] The thymus appears to be the major source of natural IELs in mice. Extrathymic development of a subset of natural IELs, especially TRγδ T-cells, has been suggested,[163] but this remains controversial. Under certain conditions, expression of CD8αα (and CD103) can also be acquired by conventional CD8αβ T-cells ("induced" CD8αα IELs).[164,165] The development or maintenance of CD8ααT-cell subsets is dependent on a variety of transcription factors (TBET, RUNX3, and MYC) and cytokines (IL-15, IL-27, and transforming growth factor β1).[166-169]

Because of the nearly ubiquitous expression of CD56, derivation from an intestinal CD56-positive IEL subset has been speculated for MEITL. In humans, small intestinal

CD3-positive CD56-positive lymphocytes comprise a minor but heterogeneous population, including NK-T cells and invariant NK-T cells, accounting for approximately 10% of all IELs overall.[66,69,71,170,171] However, CD56 can be induced in diverse T-cells upon activation.[172,173] This knowledge, the intertumoral and intratumoral variability in CD56 expression, and CD56 negativity of IELs at a distance from the tumor in a significant proportion of cases, argue against an origin of MEITLs from a specific CD56-positive IEL subset.[55,147,151,155] It is currently believed that intraepithelial CD8-positive T-cells with latent cytotoxic potential upregulate CD56, MATK, and cytotoxic granule proteins upon neoplastic transformation or disease progression.[151] Whether specific infectious, immune, or dietary factors lead to the preferential activation or expansion of select innate IELs and play a role in the initiation of MEITLs remains to be determined.

Molecular Analysis and Genetic Abnormalities

Clonal TR rearrangements are detected in 91% to 95% of MEITLs,[150,151,162] and a clonal relationship between the tumor and distant IELs lacking atypia has been established in the limited number of cases analyzed.[147,151,160]

Genomic changes in MEITLs are similar to those in EATLs (see Fig. 37-18 and Table 37-2), but the frequencies of some aberrations vary.[81,85,90,157,158,174,175] The prevalence of chromosome 9q and 7q gains and losses at 8p and 16q is comparable to that observed in EATL, while gains at 1q and 5q appear less frequent in this disease. In contrast to EATL, losses at 3p21.31/SETD2 locus (27%–33% of cases) and gains at 8q, encompassing 8q24/CMYC locus (13%–73% of cases), are more common in MEITL (Table 37-2),[81,85,90,151,154,155,157,158,161,174] and CMYC translocations are seen in 4% to 7% of cases.[151,155]

The functional gene classes and pathways mutated in MEITL also overlap with EATL; however, some differences are apparent. Genetic alterations of epigenetic regulators are among the most frequent events in MEITL (33%–100%)[85,89,90,152,155,158,174,175a] with SETD2 inactivation by mutation or deletion being a unique feature of this disease, including cases with atypical morphology and immunophenotype, and irrespective of the TR status. SETD2 alterations have been documented in >90% of lymphomas in many, but not all, series (range 22%–100%) and multiple SETD2 aberrations have been detected in 33% to 75% of cases. Additional mutated genes include CREBBP (11%–30%), TET2 (6%–15%), and KMT2D (6%). SETD2, which encodes a histone H3 lysine methyltransferase, orchestrates diverse processes, including DNA damage signaling and repair, chromosome segregation, transcriptional regulation and mRNA processing, and functions as a tumor suppressor.[176] Loss of SETD2 protein expression and decreased/absent H3K36 trimethylation is seen in 70% to 90% and 83% to 95% of cases with SETD2 alterations, respectively,[90,155,175a] and H3K36me3 immunohistochemistry has been shown to be a reliable method for inferring SETD2 abnormalities.[155]

JAK-STAT pathway mutations are observed in 75% to 89% of tumors.[85,89,90,152,155,158,174,175a] As opposed to EATL, mutations in JAK3 (33%–67%) and STAT5B (33%–65%) are more common in MEITL, most representing activating JH2 pseudokinase and SH2 domain mutations, respectively, while JAK1 (2%–44%) and STAT3 (0%–11%) mutations are less prevalent. Multiple JAK3 or STAT5B and dual JAK3/STAT5B

mutations are seen in 12% to 20% and 19% to 27% of cases, respectively.[90,152,155,158,174,175a] STAT5B mutations have been identified in lymphomas of all TR genotypes and more often in CD8αα-positive cases.[90,174] The higher VAFs of STAT5B mutations than of JAK3 (and SETD2) mutations, in part caused by copy-neutral LOH, suggest an important role of mutation dosage in disease pathogenesis.[85,90,155,174]

DNA damage response and repair pathway genes are mutated in 33% to 44% of cases, including ATM (11%) and TP53 (10%–44%).[85,89,90,152,155,158,174,175a] RAS-MAPK pathway mutations (30%–53%), targeting KRAS (10%–24%), NRAS (7%–20%), and BRAF (2%–27%), appear more frequent in this disease than in EATL.[85,89,90,152,155,158,174,175a] Mutations in GNAI2, which encodes the alpha subunit of guanine nucleotide binding proteins, reported in 9% to 24% of cases, have yet to be described in EATL.[152,155,158,174] BCOR mutations (11%) occur at a similar frequency as in EATL, but mutations in DDX3X (3%) are uncommon in MEITL.[155]

Higher transcript levels of SYK, NCAM1 (CD56), FASLG, and TGBR1 genes have been observed in MEITLs compared with EATLs,[85] and gene set enrichment analyses of MEITL transcriptomes have demonstrated enrichment in the NK-like cytotoxicity and JAK-STAT, GPCR, and MAPK signaling pathways,[85,174] in line with the proteomic and genetic alterations in these tumors.

INTESTINAL T-CELL LYMPHOMA, NOT OTHERWISE SPECIFIED

A variety of PTCLs can secondarily involve the gastrointestinal tract and show overlapping histopathologic and immunophenotypic features with specific subtypes of intestinal T-cell lymphomas (see Table 37-3). At times, determining the primary site of these neoplasms can be difficult despite use of sensitive imaging modalities. Rarely, PTCLs characteristically occurring at other extranodal or nodal sites (e.g., extranodal NK/T-cell lymphoma, nasal type, ALCL) may also arise in the gastrointestinal tract (see Table 37-3).[146,162,177] The diagnosis of intestinal T-cell lymphoma, not otherwise specified (ITCL, NOS), in essence, is one of exclusion and should be rendered for aggressive primary intestinal T/NK-cell lymphomas that on the basis of clinical, morphologic, and phenotypic criteria cannot be classified as any of the currently recognized entities.[6,7] The 2022 ICC and WHO 5th ed. classification have retained the term ITCL, NOS.[8] Importantly, this designation should be avoided when the biopsies are limited, precluding adequate morphologic and immunophenotypic evaluation.

Synonyms and Related Terms

WHO revised 4th ed., 2017: Intestinal T-cell lymphoma, not otherwise specified[6,7]

WHO 5th ed., 2022: Intestinal T-cell lymphoma, not otherwise specified[9]

The geographic distribution of ITCL, NOS is wide and this disease has constituted 18% to 44% of primary intestinal T-cell lymphomas in Asian series.[152,153,178] Patient demographics are largely similar to those described for EATL and MEITL, as are the clinical outcomes. ITCL, NOS can present as localized tumors or involve multiple gastrointestinal sites, more often in the colon and small intestine, and dissemination to regional lymph nodes and extragastrointestinal sites may be seen.[54,152,153,179] Symptoms and signs depend on the site and extent of disease. Some studies have reported lower rates of intestinal perforation in this subtype compared with EATL and MEITL.[152,153]

The cytomorphology of ITCL, NOS can vary and epitheliotropism is only observed in a minority of cases (≈20%).[54,179,180] The lymphomas are usually CD4 positive or CD4 negative/CD8 negative and a subset can express CD30. Although many exhibit a cytotoxic phenotype, lineage assignment may not always be possible as these tumors can lack TR expression (TR silent).[54] This entity is characteristically EBV negative and the occasional EBV-positive cases described likely represent gastrointestinal tract involvement by extranodal NK/T-cell lymphoma, nasal type.[180] Similar to other subtypes of primary intestinal T-cell lymphomas, targeted sequencing of a limited number of ITCL, NOS cases has revealed mutations in epigenetic regulators and JAK/STAT and RAS-MAPK pathway genes,[89,152,181] with one study reporting lower frequencies of *SETD2* and *STAT5B* mutations in this disease compared with MEITL.[152] Cases of ITCL, NOS may be reassigned to specific categories of intestinal T-cell lymphomas as our understanding of their clinical, morphologic, phenotypic, and genetic spectrum evolves (e.g., reclassification of primary intestinal TRγδ T-cell lymphomas and a subset of pleomorphic CD8-positive CD56-positive ITCLs as MEITLs).[152,159,182]

INDOLENT NATURAL KILLER–CELL AND T-CELL LYMPHOPROLIFERATIVE DISORDERS OF THE GASTROINTESTINAL TRACT

A mucosal infiltrate of small or intermediate-sized lymphocytes in the gastrointestinal tract should raise the possibility of a primary indolent NK-cell or T-cell lymphoproliferative disorder (LPD) of the gastrointestinal tract (see Table 37-3). These LPDs can be challenging to distinguish from inflammatory diseases, aggressive primary intestinal T-cell lymphomas, and extranodal NK/T-cell lymphoma, nasal type occurring in or involving the gastrointestinal tract (see Table 37-3). A detailed clinical history and knowledge of the clinical presentation are essential for appropriate diagnosis.

Indolent Natural Killer–Cell Lymphoproliferative Disorder of the Gastrointestinal Tract

An indolent NK-cell LPD involving the gastrointestinal tract was first described by Vega and associates in 2006.[183] Subsequently, case series from Japan[184,185] and the United States,[186-188] and isolated reports,[189-192] variably designated lymphomatoid gastropathy or NK-cell enteropathy, clarified the clinical, pathologic, and genetic features of this disease, prompting a change in nomenclature to *indolent NK-cell lymphoproliferative disorder of the gastrointestinal tract* and its inclusion as a distinct entity in the 2022 ICC and WHO 5th ed. classification.[8,9]

Synonyms and Related Terms

Lymphomatoid gastropathy, NK-cell enteropathy (Obsolete)

WHO revised 4th ed., 2017: Not included[6,7]
WHO 5th ed., 2022: Indolent NK-cell lymphoproliferative disorder of the gastrointestinal tract[9]

Most of the indolent NK-cell LPDs have been reported from Asia and the United States.[192] However, recent publications suggest a broad geographic distribution.[86,193] These disorders are most often diagnosed in the 4th and 5th decades (range 14–75 years) and a female preponderance has been noted in a few studies.[184-192] The etiology of indolent NK-cell LPDs is unclear. Patients with intestinal involvement lack evidence of celiac disease or inflammatory bowel disease, but a history of gastric cancer and presence of *Helicobacter pylori* infection has been documented in some patients with gastric disease. Symptoms and signs include abdominal pain or discomfort, diarrhea, rectal bleeding, and weight loss; however, some individuals may be asymptomatic.[191]

The stomach and intestines are commonly involved organs.[184-192] Rare cases have been reported in the gall bladder and cystic duct lymph node and also at extragastrointestinal sites.[187,194,194a] Superficial mucosal ulcers, erosions, or polyps can be observed on endoscopy.

Microscopic examination shows expansion of the lamina propria by an infiltrate of intermediate-to-large-sized cells that have round, oval or irregular nuclei, fine chromatin, inconspicuous or small nucleoli, and moderate pale cytoplasm (histiocytoid appearance) (Fig. 37-19). Eosinophilic cytoplasmic granules may be seen in a variable proportion of cells. Polymorphic infiltrates of histiocytes, plasma cells, and eosinophils and lymphoid aggregates are present at the periphery. Scattered apoptotic cells are observed, but in the absence of ulceration, necrosis is uncommon and angiocentricity or angiodestruction is not seen. Glandular displacement or destruction may be noted, but epitheliotropism is minimal or absent, and crypt hyperplasia and villous atrophy are not apparent when the small intestine is involved.[86,184-188]

The atypical lymphoid cells have an EBV– NK-cell phenotype (cytCD3+, sCD3–, CD5–, CD4–/CD8–, CD56+, TIA-1+, granzyme B+, TR–) (Fig. 37-19; see also Table 37-3), and they do not express markers of T-cell or NK-T-cell subsets (TRαβ, TRγδ, CD161, CD158, TRVα24). Some cases display downregulation or loss of CD2, and expression of CD8 or CD16, and CD56 negativity may be seen occasionally.[185,194b] The Ki67 proliferation index is generally low (<40%).

In keeping with an NK-cell derivation, all cases analyzed have lacked clonal TR rearrangements. It is not known at present if indolent NK-cell LPDs arise from circulating, conventional NK cells or tissue-resident NK cells (or ILCs) in the gastrointestinal mucosa or at other sites.[128] It has been debated whether this disease represents an immune-mediated, reactive (polyclonal) condition or a clonal NK-cell proliferation. The recent identification of somatic genetic variants in 70% of cases, including activating *JAK3* mutations in 30% of cases, supports the latter view.[188] Moreover, detection of phospho-STAT5 expression in all evaluated cases indicates pervasive JAK3-STAT5 pathway activation in indolent NK-cell LPDs. The clinical course can vary, with spontaneous regression in most patients and occasional recurrences. Chemotherapy is not advised for disease management.

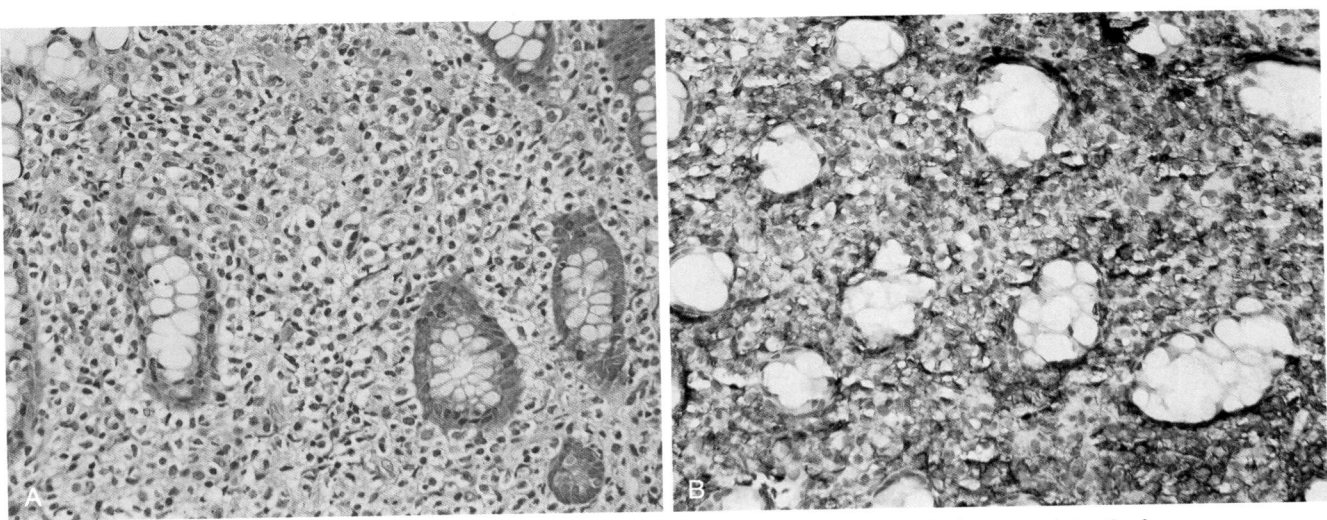

Figure 37-19. Indolent natural killer–cell lymphoproliferative disorder of the gastrointestinal tract. A, The colonic crypts are displaced by an infiltrate of medium-sized to focally large cells in the lamina propria that have ample clear or lightly eosinophilic cytoplasm, oval or irregular nuclei, fine chromatin, and inconspicuous or small nucleoli (histiocytoid appearance). **B,** The cells show variable intensity of CD56 expression.

Indolent Clonal T-Cell Lymphoproliferative Disorder of the Gastrointestinal Tract

Indolent *clonal* T-cell lymphoproliferative disorder (LPD) of the gastrointestinal tract is the new term for indolent T-cell lymphoproliferative disorder of the gastrointestinal tract in the 2022 ICC.[8] This disease, which was a provisional entity in the revised WHO 4th ed. classification,[6,7] was first described in 1994 by Carbonnel and coworkers, who later reported a series of four CD4-positive cases.[195] Subsequent case reports[191,192,194b,196–202] and series[86,203–207] have documented the existence of CD4-positive, CD8-positive, and occasional CD4-negative/CD8-negative and CD4-positive/CD8-positive lymphoid proliferations (Fig. 37-20; see also Table 37-3).

Synonyms and Related Terms

WHO revised 4th ed., 2017: Indolent T-cell lymphoproliferative disorder of the gastrointestinal tract[6,7]

WHO 5th ed., 2022: Indolent T-cell lymphoma of the gastrointestinal tract[9]

Indolent clonal T-cell LPD of the gastrointestinal tract has a wide geographic distribution and a slight male predominance, and similar to indolent NK-cell LPD of the gastrointestinal tract, is more frequently detected in the 4th and 5th decades (range 15–77 years).[195,203–205] The etiologies of the different phenotypic subtypes are not known. Some patients with CD8-positive LPDs have a history of inflammatory bowel disease, including a few having received immunomodulatory therapy, while infections or autoimmune disorders have been described in a subset of patients with CD4-positive LPDs.[194b,204,205,207,209] Chronic diarrhea, abdominal pain, and weight loss are common presentations.[191,192,207]

The small intestine or colon are common sites of disease, but any site in the gastrointestinal tract and multiple organs may be involved. Dissemination outside the gastrointestinal tract (e.g., bone marrow, tonsils, peripheral blood) is infrequent

at diagnosis, however, it can occur at disease progression or transformation.[192,195,203-205] On endoscopy, the small intestinal mucosa can exhibit a mosaic appearance with loss of mucosal folds, nodularity, or scalloping. Erythema, shallow ulcers, erosions, or multiple small polyps may also be seen at this and other locations.[191,192,195,203-205] Thickened intestinal folds, dilated intestinal loops, and enlarged abdominal lymph nodes are at times observed on imaging.[191,192]

On histopathologic evaluation, a mucosal and occasionally submucosal, nondestructive, EBV-negative, clonal lymphocytic infiltrate is seen, composed of mostly small-sized lymphocytes displaying minimal cytologic atypia (Fig. 37-20).[191] Patchy eosinophilia and scattered multinucleated giant cells or epithelioid granulomas may be present.[195,203,205] The mucosal architecture is generally preserved but some cases show villous atrophy or crypt hyperplasia. Intraepithelial lymphocytosis is uncommon; however, infiltration of the crypt epithelium is observed in a proportion of cases.

Indolent clonal T-cell LPD of the gastrointestinal tract is presumed to originate from lamina propria T-cells. CD8-positive cases usually display a type 2 effector and latent cytotoxic phenotype (TIA-1 positive, granzyme B negative, perforin negative),[207] similar to primary cutaneous acral CD8-positive T-cell LPDs,[210] while CD4-positive cases, although bearing some resemblance to primary cutaneous CD4-positive small or medium T-cell LPDs,[211,212] manifest a helper T-cell phenotype and lack evidence of follicular helper or regulatory T-cell derivation.[194b,202,203,207] Expression of CD2 and CD3 is almost universal, but variable downregulation or loss of CD5 or CD7 is seen in approximately 25% of cases, and rarely CD103 or CD20 expression may be observed.[194b] All phenotypic subtypes express surface TRαβ, and they have low Ki67 labeling indices (<5%).

All evaluated cases have displayed clonal TRB or TRG rearrangements. Conventional cytogenetic analysis has revealed non-recurrent chromosomal abnormalities, with

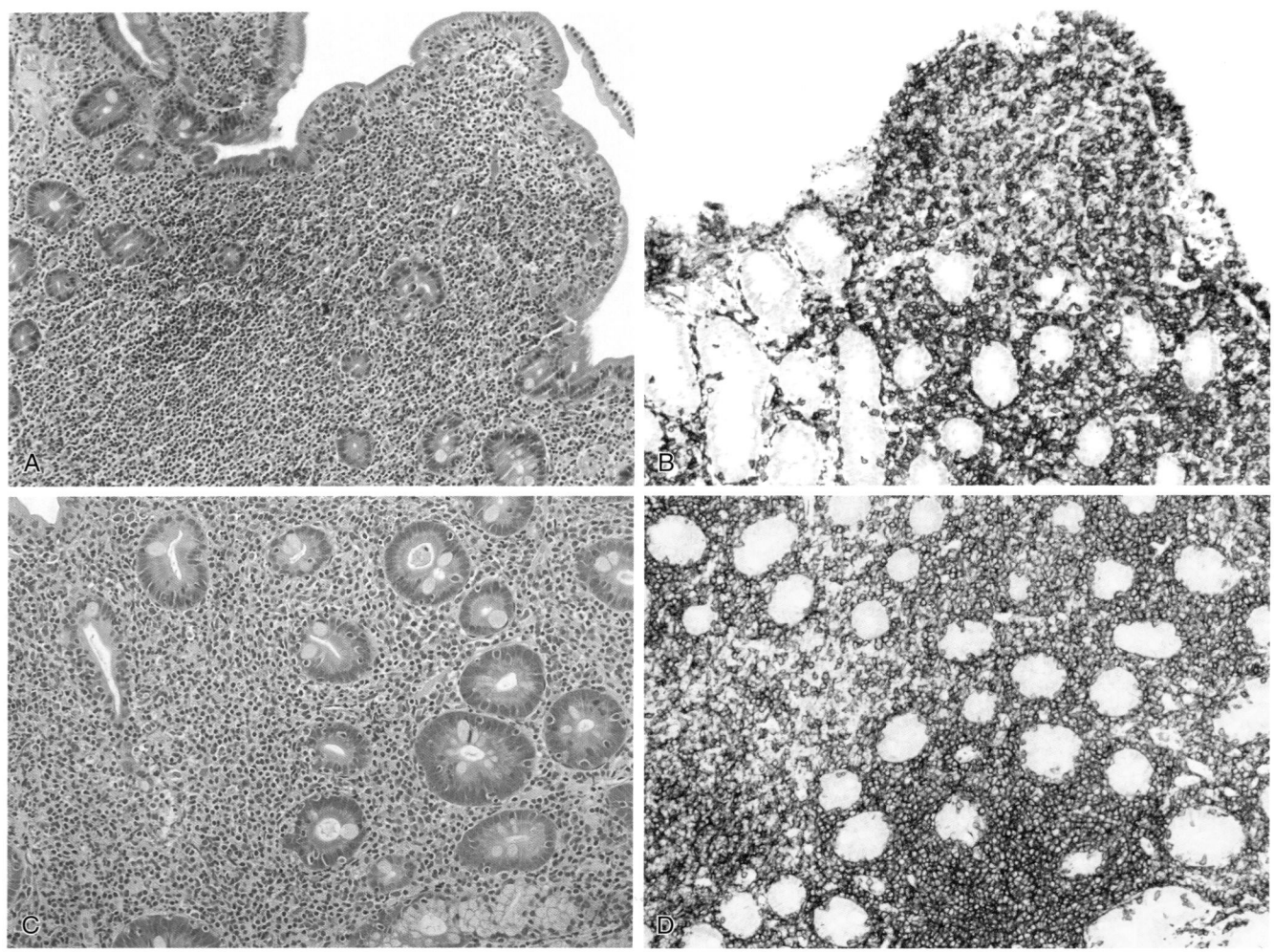

Figure 37-20. Indolent clonal lymphoproliferative disorder of the gastrointestinal tract. A, A dense infiltrate of predominantly small lymphocytes is seen in the jejunal lamina propria with focal infiltration of the villous and crypt epithelium. **B,** The neoplastic lymphocytes express CD8. **C,** Another case showing a small lymphocytic infiltrate in the duodenal lamina propria with infiltration of the crypt epithelium. **D,** The lymphocytes in this case express CD4.

the exception of translocation t(9;17)(p24.1;q21.2) in CD4-positive LPDs that was later shown to represent a *STAT3::JAK2* fusion.[195,206,207,213] Single nucleotide polymorphism microarray investigations of CD4-positive cases have also demonstrated non-recurrent copy number changes[203,205]; however, some altered loci harbor genes of potential relevance to disease pathogenesis (e.g., 1p13/*SOCS1*, 17q21/*STAT3*), and copy number gains of 17q21/*STAT3* have been observed upon large cell transformation in two cases.[203,206] The spectrum of mutations and structural genetic variants differs in distinct phenotypic subtypes of LPDs.[86,206,207] *STAT3::JAK2* fusions have been identified in 45% of CD4-positive cases analyzed. The resultant chimeric protein retains many key functional domains of *STAT3*, including the SH2 domain, and *JAK2*, including the JH1 tyrosine kinase domain, and dimerization of the fusion protein preferentially activates STAT5 (over STAT3) enabling cytokine independent growth.[206,213a] Some CD4-positive LPDs lacking *STAT3::JAK2* fusions have other genetic

alterations in the JAK-STAT signaling pathway (e.g., *STAT3* mutations).[207] Activating *STAT3* mutations have also been detected in CD4-positive/CD8-positive and CD4-negative/CD8-negative cases, but in none of the CD8-positive LPDs assessed thus far.[86,204,207] Mutations in epigenetic regulators (e.g., *TET2, KMT2D*) have been observed in all phenotypic subtypes of disease.[207,215] Structural alterations involving the 3′ untranslated region of the *IL2* gene have been reported in a few CD8-positive LPDs.[207]

Most patients do well with conservative management (e.g., luminal steroids) and have prolonged survival. The LPDs do not respond to chemotherapy and persist or recur after treatment in virtually all cases. Accordingly, the name *LPD* is preferred over *lymphoma* to deter aggressive therapy. Disease progression and, rarely, transformation to aggressive T-cell lymphoma can occur after many years, the latter having been reported in CD4-positive, CD8-positive, and CD4-negative/CD8-negative cases.[195,203,206,207,214,215]

Pearls and Pitfalls

- Enteropathy-associated T-cell lymphoma (EATL) is the most common (but not the only) intestinal T-cell lymphoma in Western countries.
- EATL is a rare complication of celiac disease that appears largely restricted to individuals of northern European origin.
- Monomorphic epitheliotropic intestinal T-cell lymphomas (MEITLs) have a wide geographic distribution and constitute a distinct subtype, unrelated to celiac disease.
- Indolent lymphoproliferative disorders of the gastrointestinal tract are rare clonal disorders that may be confused with inflammatory diseases or other aggressive types of intestinal T-cell lymphomas.
- The appropriate classification of intestinal T-cell lymphomas requires knowledge of their clinical presentation and correlation of the cytomorphologic features with results of comprehensive immunophenotypic and molecular analyses.

KEY REFERENCES

88. Cording S, Lhermitte L, Malamut G, CELAC network, et al. Oncogenetic landscape of lymphomagenesis in coeliac disease. *Gut.* 2022;71(3):497–508.

113. Soderquist CR, Lewis SK, Gru AA, et al. Immunophenotypic spectrum and genomic landscape of refractory celiac disease type II. *Am J Surg Pathol.* 2021;45(7):905–916.

152. Hang JF, Yuan CT, Chang KC, et al. Targeted next-generation sequencing reveals a wide morphologic and immunophenotypic spectrum of monomorphic epitheliotropic intestinal T-cell lymphoma. *Am J Surg Pathol.* 2022;46(9):1207–1218.

155. Veloza L, Cavalieri D, Missiaglia E, et al. Monomorphic epitheliotropic intestinal T-cell lymphoma comprises morphologic and genomic heterogeneity impacting outcome. *Haematologica.* 2022.

174. Nairismägi ML, Tan J, Lim JQ, et al. JAK-STAT and G-protein-coupled receptor signaling pathways are frequently altered in epitheliotropic intestinal T-cell lymphoma. *Leukemia.* 2016;30(6):1311–1319.

184. Takeuchi K, Yokoyama M, Ishizawa S, et al. Lymphomatoid gastropathy: a distinct clinicopathologic entity of self-limited pseudomalignant NK-cell proliferation. *Blood.* 2010;116(25):5631–5637.

186. Mansoor A, Pittaluga S, Beck PL, Wilson WH, Ferry JA, Jaffe ES. NK-cell enteropathy: a benign NK-cell lymphoproliferative disease mimicking intestinal lymphoma: clinicopathologic features and follow-up in a unique case series. *Blood.* 2011;117(5):1447–1452.

188. Xiao W, Gupta GK, Yao J, et al. Recurrent somatic *JAK3* mutations in NK-cell enteropathy. *Blood.* 2019;134(12):986–991.

204. Perry AM, Warnke RA, Hu Q, et al. Indolent T-cell lymphoproliferative disease of the gastrointestinal tract. *Blood.* 2013;122(22):3599–3606.

206. Sharma A, Oishi N, Boddicker RL, et al. Recurrent *STAT3-JAK2* fusions in indolent T-cell lymphoproliferative disorder of the gastrointestinal tract. *Blood.* 2018;131(20):2262–2266.

207. Soderquist CR, Patel N, Murty VV, et al. Genetic and phenotypic characterization of indolent T-cell lymphoproliferative disorders of the gastrointestinal tract. *Haematologica.* 2020;105(7):1895–1906.

Visit Elsevier eBooks+ for the complete set of references.

Chapter 38

Mycosis Fungoides and Sézary Syndrome

Philip E. LeBoit and Laura B. Pincus

Mycosis fungoides and Sézary syndrome are two closely related conditions in which neoplastic T cells infiltrate the skin and circulate in the peripheral blood. Both conditions are neoplasms that typically have a mature helper T-cell phenotype and a propensity to colonize the epidermis. Because individual patients can have discrete cutaneous lesions at one point in time and erythroderma with circulating neoplastic cells at another time, some advocate the term cutaneous T-cell lymphoma to describe what they consider to be a single disease.[1] However, the delineation of a variety of other distinct clinicopathologic entities that are also cutaneous T-cell lymphomas[2] has, in our opinion, rendered this term non-specific. We consider *cutaneous T-cell lymphoma* as an umbrella term that encompasses many different subtypes, including mycosis fungoides and Sézary syndrome. Although Sézary syndrome was formerly considered to be a leukemic counterpart of mycosis fungoides,[3] more recent studies have demonstrated different molecular phenotypes in these two conditions.[4,5] Furthermore, they have very different clinical presentations. Therefore, these conditions are now considered to be different diseases. This chapter covers mycosis fungoides and its many variants and Sézary syndrome.

MYCOSIS FUNGOIDES

Definition

Mycosis fungoides is a T-cell lymphoma in which lymphocytes infiltrate the epidermis in its early stages, resulting in flat, often slightly scaly lesions (patches). In some patients, lymphocytes acquire the ability to proliferate in the dermis, forming plaques and nodules. A small minority of patients will have involvement of internal organs in the course of their disease. The neoplastic cells in mycosis fungoides are skin resident effector memory T-cells.[6] Most cases of mycosis fungoides have a T-helper phenotype, but clinically and histopathologically identical infiltrates can be seen in which the neoplastic cells are CD8 positive or CD20 positive. Our view, which is not shared by all authorities, is that the clinical evolution of patches to plaques and tumors determines whether a patient has the disease mycosis fungoides, not a specific immunophenotype. If a patient has indolent patches in which there are epidermotropic CD8-positive T cells, there is no harm in labeling that mycosis fungoides. Indeed, in many centers, immunophenotypic studies are not routinely performed, and patients are treated with excellent results. The term *mycosis fungoides* does not apply, however, to a disease caused by infection with the retrovirus human T-lymphotropic virus 1 (HTLV-1), despite the clinical and pathologic resemblance of some cases; that condition is referred to as *adult T-cell leukemia/lymphoma*. The major diagnostic features of mycosis fungoides are listed in Box 38-1.

Epidemiology

Mycosis fungoides is largely a disease of middle-aged and older people. However, as clinicians and pathologists have

Box 38-1 *Key Diagnostic Features of Mycosis Fungoides*

Clinical Features

Patch stage: Patches with fine overlying scale, often more than 5 cm in diameter in photoprotected sites

Plaque stage: Same location and size as patches, but lesions are thicker with induration and elevation

Tumor stage: Solid nodules at least 1 cm in diameter that usually develop in patches and plaques

Histopathologic Features

Patch stage: Sparse perivascular to bandlike infiltrate of lymphocytes with variable infiltration of the epidermis and variable cytologic atypia

Plaque stage: Infiltrate denser and extends into reticular dermis

Tumor stage: Diffuse infiltrate extending throughout the reticular dermis

Immunohistochemical Features

βF1-positive, CD3-positive, CD4-positive, CD8-negative immunophenotype is most common, but variations in otherwise typical disease occur and have little meaning

Genotypic Findings

Demonstrable clonality common but not obligatory by polymerase chain reaction (PCR)–based gamma alone or gamma plus beta chain gene rearrangements

---

become more adept at recognizing its early stages, more cases in young adults and even in children have come to light. The incidence of mycosis fungoides in a population is certainly affected by the number of dermatologists in the community, their interest in and awareness of the disease, and their threshold for diagnosis. An interesting observation is that the incidence of mycosis fungoides rose rapidly in the early 1980s,[7] coincident with the delineation of criteria for the diagnosis of patch-stage disease by Sanchez and Ackerman.[8] After the publication of their paper, many pathologists began to diagnose mycosis fungoides on the basis of infiltrates they might have previously regarded as parapsoriasis en plaques or inflammatory conditions, such as spongiotic dermatitis. The increased incidence of mycosis fungoides in the United States seems to reflect a rise in the detection and diagnosis of early patch-stage disease.

Etiology

A number of investigators have tried to link mycosis fungoides to environmental exposures, without success. Studies to determine whether common inflammatory skin diseases, such as atopic dermatitis, chronic allergic contact dermatitis, and psoriasis, give rise to mycosis fungoides are undermined by several factors. Early patches of mycosis fungoides can resemble these diseases clinically, so a patient with a 20-year history of "atopic dermatitis" preceding mycosis fungoides might have had patches of mycosis fungoides that were simply not recognized as such. Early patch-stage lesions of mycosis fungoides can resemble various inflammatory conditions under the microscope, so that even "biopsy-proven" psoriasis may not be that disease at all.

Several studies have sought the presence of a virus in the cells of mycosis fungoides. In the 1970s, interest centered on the identification of viral particles in skin biopsy samples of mycosis fungoides by electron microscopy.[9] Later, interest focused on a possible role for HTLV-1, the retrovirus that causes adult T-cell leukemia/lymphoma, in mycosis fungoides.[10] An initial study seemed to identify partial viral transcripts in the cells of mycosis fungoides, but further investigation has not borne this out in most cases. Another theory related to infection is that mycosis fungoides is an abnormal response to bacterial superantigens, in particular *Staphylococcus aureus.*[11]

Clinical Features

Mycosis fungoides is largely defined by the clinical features of its early stages. Requisite to this definition is an initial presentation as flat, scaly lesions called *patches*. These first appear in areas of the skin that are best protected from sunlight—the buttocks and groins of both sexes and the breasts of women. Subtle wrinkling, slight erythema, telangiectasias, and either hypopigmentation or hyperpigmentation are variable findings. Often, the patches are so subtle that patients do not notice them for some time, and both patients and their physicians may attribute the condition to dry skin or atopic dermatitis. Patches are generally round or oval, although they are sometimes finger shaped or digitate (Fig. 38-1). Their size can range from about 1 cm to more than 15 cm.

Some clinicians use the term *small plaque parapsoriasis* to refer to small patches (smaller than an adult palm) and the term *large plaque parapsoriasis* to refer to larger lesions of patch-stage mycosis fungoides. Those who think that mycosis fungoides begins as an inflammatory condition that may regress often use the term *parapsoriasis*. This usage originated with the work of the French dermatologist Brocq in the late 19th and early 20th centuries. He envisaged a complex relationship among psoriasis, eczema, seborrheic dermatitis, the conditions now known as pityriasis lichenoides acuta and chronica, and mycosis fungoides.[12] In our opinion, the term *parapsoriasis* is invalid scientifically, although it may have some functional utility in that it is shorthand for "I suspect that this is an early patch of mycosis fungoides but am not sure." This dilemma is better expressed in clear language, however. Confounding this already confusing situation is the older use of the term *parapsoriasis lichenoides* to refer to pityriasis lichenoides, an inflammatory disease.

Digitate or finger-shaped patches may occur by themselves in a condition called *digitate dermatosis*. It was initially reported that it should be separated from "true" parapsoriasis and be considered as a benign dermatosis.[13] Later, it was noted that similarly shaped patches can be found alongside conventional lesions of mycosis fungoides. This led some observers to conclude that digitate dermatosis is in fact a form of mycosis fungoides.[14] Because the prognosis of patients with only digitate lesions is excellent and the histopathologic findings are often paltry, others question the usefulness of labeling patients with digitate dermatosis as having mycosis fungoides.[15] There are, however, patients who present with small digitate lesions and develop recognizable mycosis fungoides or even erythroderma.[16,17] Whether these patients truly presented with digitate dermatosis or had digitate lesion of mycosis fungoides from the outset is difficult to know. Many authors regard small plaque parapsoriasis either

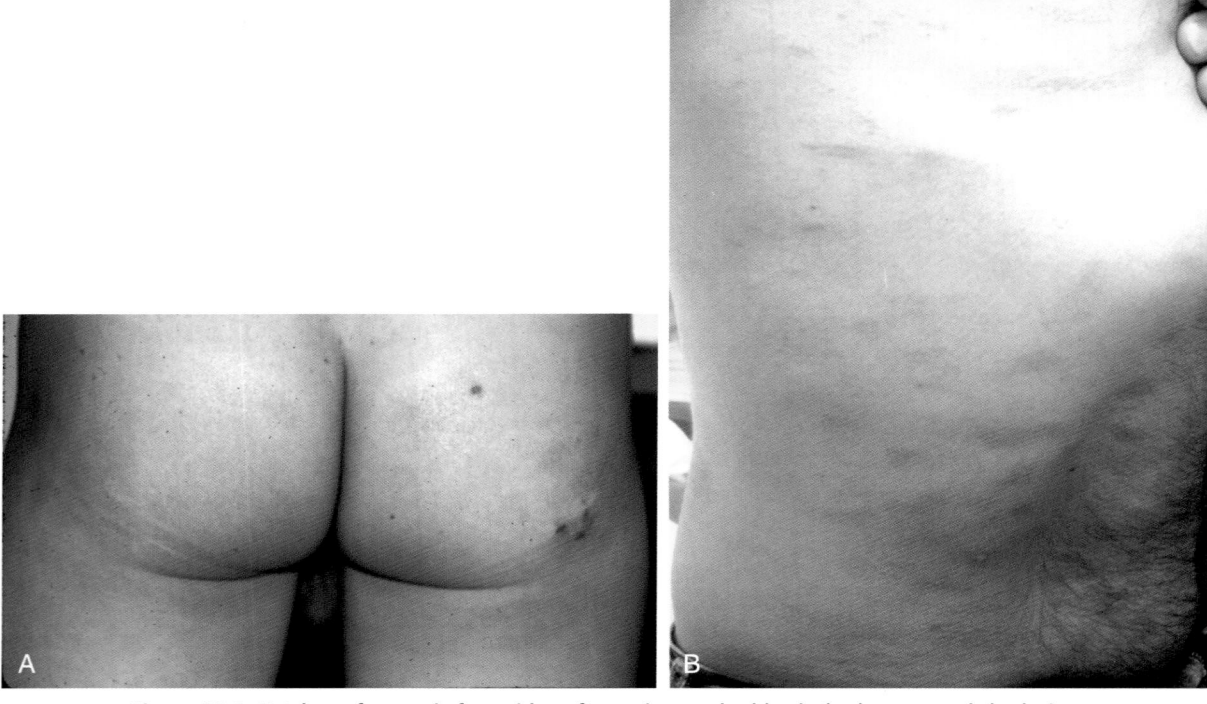

Figure 38-1. Patches of mycosis fungoides often arise on double-clothed areas, and the lesions may recede with light exposure. A, Classic patches are often the size of a palm or larger. **B,** Digitate lesions of mycosis fungoides are so called because they are finger-shaped patches, often aligned along Langer's lines.

as a spongiotic dermatitis or as an "abortive" cutaneous T cell lymphoma, a lymphoproliferative disease that rarely progresses.[18,19]

In some patients with preexisting patches of mycosis fungoides and in others who claim that they never had such patches, areas of the skin can become thin and wrinkled and marked by macules of hypopigmentation and hyperpigmentation, along with telangiectasias. This appearance is known as *poikiloderma* or *poikiloderma vasculare atrophicans*. It appears to be a manifestation of regression of patch-stage mycosis fungoides.

The large majority of patients with mycosis fungoides who have patches over a small area of skin at presentation prove to have an indolent condition that seldom becomes more than a cosmetic problem, even if it is untreated. In a minority of such patients, disseminated patches arise.

Plaques of mycosis fungoides are usually located in the same locations as patches but differ from patches in that they are raised. Plaques are varying shades of red to red-brown and scaly. They are often polycyclic, with clearing in the center (Fig. 38-2A). They sometimes ulcerate, but not as much as nodules or tumors do.

Tumors of mycosis fungoides are raised nodules that are often smooth but frequently ulcerate (Fig. 38-2B). They are clinically indistinguishable from nodules and tumors of other cutaneous lymphomas. However, tumors almost invariably arise within or adjacent to preexisting patches and plaques of mycosis fungoides, and thus a careful clinical examination to assess for concomitant patches and plaques can be helpful to distinguish tumors of mycosis fungoides from other cutaneous

lymphomas. The tumors can sometimes assume a mushroom-like configuration, and this attribute resulted in Alibert giving the condition the name *mycosis fungoides*.[20]

Histopathology

There is vast variability in the histopathologic appearance of mycosis fungoides, especially in patch-stage disease. This reflects the fact that early lesions may be composed largely of non-neoplastic cells, exerting their influence through cytotoxicity and cytokine production and in ways not yet appreciated.

The early patches of mycosis fungoides feature lymphocytes that are not usually morphologically atypical and thus can appear similar to those found in inflammatory skin diseases. In fact, studies have demonstrated that 4% (27 of 745) of biopsy specimens of early mycosis fungoides reviewed had atypical lymphocytes within the epidermis.[21] Therefore, identification of a section as representing early mycosis fungoides, either definitely or possibly, usually requires attention to the histopathologic pattern of the infiltrate rather than the identification of atypical lymphocytes.

The earliest patches of mycosis fungoides feature small lymphocytes around venules of the superficial plexus; some are scattered interstitially in the papillary dermis, with only a few within the epidermis (Fig. 38-3). In some cases, when the cells of mycosis fungoides enter the epidermis, they can elicit spongiosis or edema between keratinocytes. The degree of spongiosis is usually less than that seen when the same number of lymphocytes enter the epidermis in

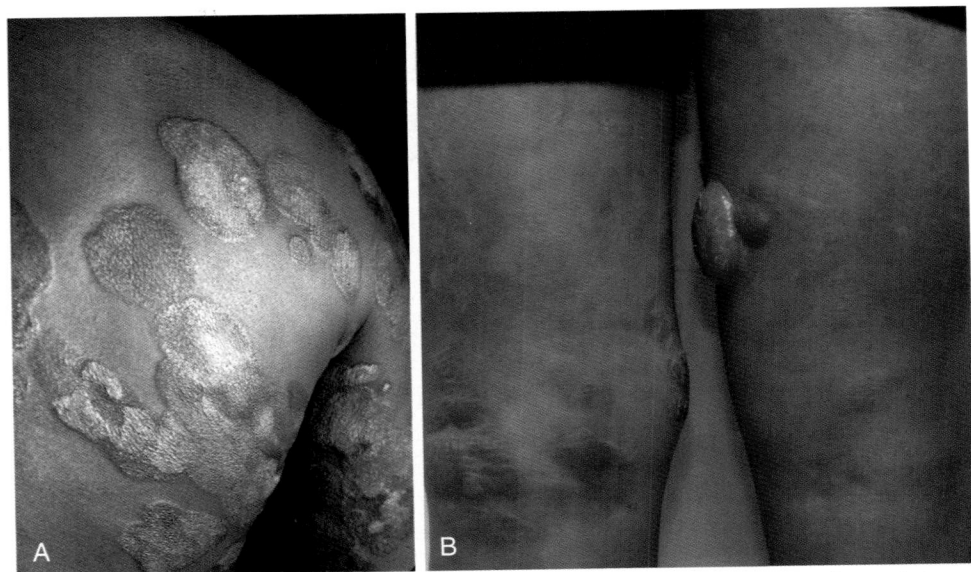

Figure 38-2. A, Plaques of mycosis fungoides often have a polycyclic appearance. **B,** Tumors are more elevated above the skin surface and usually arise within or adjacent to preexisting patches and plaques of mycosis fungoides.

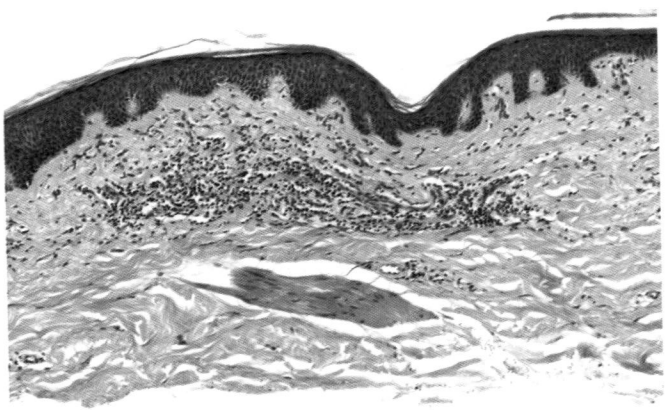

Figure 38-3. Early patch of mycosis fungoides featuring a psoriasiform lichenoid pattern, with small lymphocytes in a band in the papillary dermis and only a few in the epidermis. An unequivocal diagnosis is not possible in this case.

an inflammatory skin disease. The tendency of the cells of mycosis fungoides to colonize the epidermis is referred to as *epidermotropism*. This term is also used to connote that there are areas of the epidermis that have only slight spongiosis and many lymphocytes. *Exocytosis* describes the migration of inflammatory cells into the epidermis and is a more neutral term. Because the term *epidermotropism* presupposes the ultimate diagnosis, it is best avoided if the diagnosis of mycosis fungoides is equivocal.

In early patch-stage disease, mycosis fungoides is often not recognizable with certainty. As the patches develop, the papillary dermis becomes fibrotic. The collagen bundles of the papillary dermis are usually fine and haphazardly oriented. This meshwork changes to one in which there are coarse fibers sometimes likened to "pink fettuccini." At the same time, rete ridges begin to elongate, usually only slightly and very evenly. Their bases remain rounded, unlike in many interface dermatitides. Lymphocytes may lodge in the basal layer of the

epidermis, with only slight vacuolar changes and few necrotic keratinocytes.[22]

The papillary dermal lymphocytic infiltrate often becomes bandlike, at least in foci. The combination of elongated rete ridges with rounded bases and bandlike lymphocytic infiltrates is known as a *psoriasiform lichenoid pattern;* if spongiosis is also present, it is referred to as a *spongiotic psoriasiform lichenoid pattern.* If the lymphocytes engaged as a host response to the neoplasm kill keratinocytes that constitute rete ridges, the epidermis may become thin and flat based—an *atrophic lichenoid pattern.* These three patterns should raise the pathologist's suspicion that he or she may be dealing with a lesion of mycosis fungoides because only a few inflammatory skin diseases share these patterns (Box 38-2).

As the infiltrates of mycosis fungoides become dense and bandlike in the papillary dermis, they also begin to exhibit cells with atypical nuclei (Fig. 38-4). Cells of patch-stage mycosis fungoides have slightly larger nuclei than those of lymphocytes in inflammatory conditions, with an irregular nuclear contour—the so-called "cerebriform lymphocyte" (Fig. 38-5). An important caveat is that if nuclear atypia is used as a criterion for the differential diagnosis between a patch of mycosis fungoides and an inflammatory condition, the atypia must be unmistakable. Many pathologists can convince themselves that the nuclei of lymphocytes are atypical by staring at them for too long under an oil immersion lens.

Some patches of mycosis fungoides feature epidermal atrophy, in concert with a patchy lichenoid lymphocytic infiltrate. The papillary dermis is often markedly fibrotic and contains telangiectasias and melanophages, corresponding to the clinical picture of poikiloderma vasculare atrophicans. In such atrophic patch-stage lesions, it may be difficult to demonstrate a sufficient number of lymphocytes in the epidermis to rule out an inflammatory disease with an atrophic lichenoid pattern (Box 38-2).

In plaques of mycosis fungoides, lymphocytes extend into the reticular dermis, not only around vessels but also

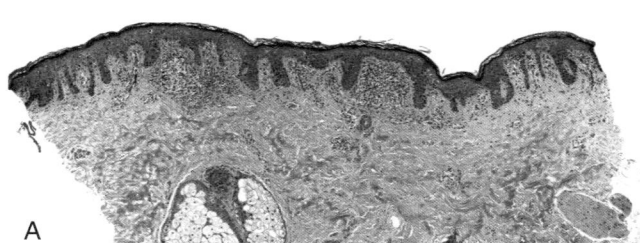

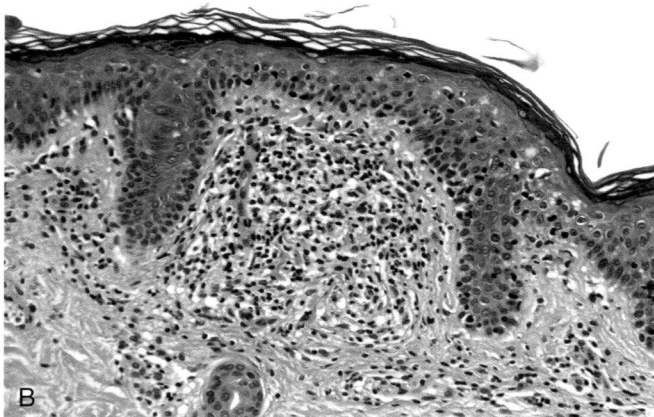

Figure 38-4. A, Later patch of mycosis fungoides, again with a psoriasiform lichenoid pattern. **B,** In this lesion (unlike that in Fig. 38-3), many lymphocytes infiltrate the epidermis, with only scant spongiosis. Those in the epidermis have slightly larger and darker nuclei than those in the dermis.

Box 38-2 *Common Patterns of Patch-Stage Mycosis Fungoides and the Inflammatory Skin Diseases That Share Them*

Psoriasiform Lichenoid Pattern
Mycosis fungoides, patch stage
Secondary syphilis (usually superficial and deep, with many plasma cells and histiocytes)
Lichenoid purpura (extravasated erythrocytes and siderophages)
Lichen striatus (linear eruption of papules in a child or teenager)
Early lesions of lichen sclerosus et atrophicus
Surface of some lesions of morphea
Drug reaction (one pattern among many)

Spongiotic Psoriasiform Lichenoid Pattern
Mycosis fungoides, patch stage
Urticarial stage of bullous pemphigoid
Drug reactions (one pattern among many)
Allergic contact dermatitis (rare; so-called "lichenoid contact dermatitis")
Chronic photoallergic dermatitis (actinic reticuloid)

Atrophic Lichenoid Pattern
Mycosis fungoides, atrophic patch stage
Atrophic lichen planus
Lichenoid purpura
Regression of melanoma, Bowen's disease, superficial basal cell carcinoma
Centers of lesions of porokeratosis (sometimes)
Poikilodermatous lesions of dermatomyositis

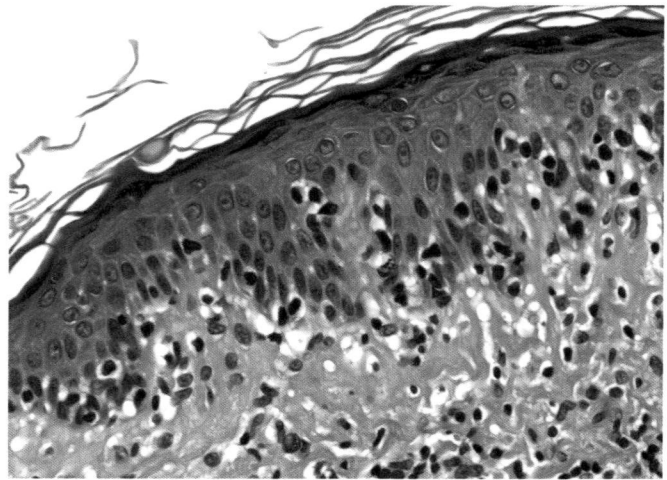

Figure 38-5. Lymphocytes in the epidermis of a patch of mycosis fungoides with scant cytoplasm and large hyperchromatic nuclei. Small halos are present around some of them.

interspersed between reticular dermal collagen bundles (Fig. 38-6). This finding occurs beneath an epidermis and papillary dermis displaying the changes described for fully developed patches of mycosis fungoides. Although lymphocytes with atypical nuclei are few in early patches and more numerous in late ones, they almost always constitute a significant percentage of the infiltrate in plaques. Similarly, aggregations of lymphocytes, termed *Pautrier's microabscesses* or *collections*, are rare in patches but common in plaques. Interestingly, this distinctive clue to the diagnosis of mycosis fungoides was discovered not by Pautrier but by Darier.[23] The atypical lymphocytes of

patches have scant cytoplasm and irregular, sometimes cerebriform lymphocytes. By contrast, in plaques, some of the lesional lymphocytes can have large vesicular nuclei, large nucleoli, and some discernible cytoplasm, and with larger cerebriform cells than are seen in patches. Furthermore, in contrast to patches, which lack eosinophils and plasma cells, plaques and tumors of mycosis fungoides often have many of these cells. This might correlate with a shift from Th1 to Th2-like cytokine production as lesions change from patches to plaques.

Nodules or tumors of mycosis fungoides acquire their clinical features by virtue of lymphocytic infiltrates that are present as nodules or diffusely replace the reticular dermis (Fig. 38-7). Large cell transformation, defined as when more than 25% of the infiltrate is composed of large cells, can occur in tumors of mycosis fungoides.[24] The appearance of the large cells ranges from cells with large round or slightly oval vesicular nuclei and scant cytoplasm to cells with large

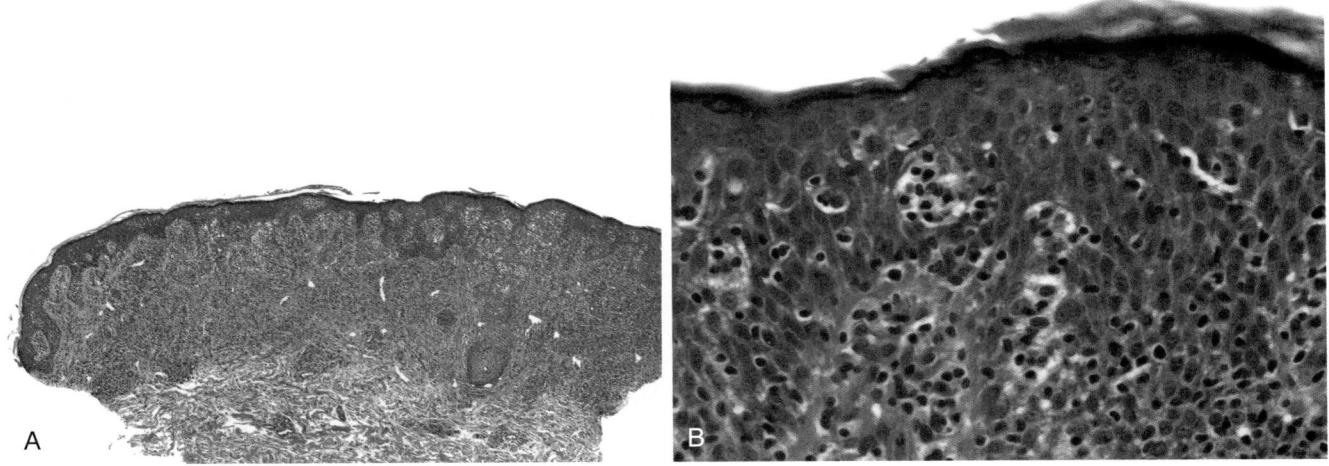

Figure 38-6. A, Plaque-stage mycosis fungoides features infiltration of the superficial reticular dermis. **B,** In this case, there are prominent collections of lymphocytes (Pautrier's microabscesses) in the epidermis as well.

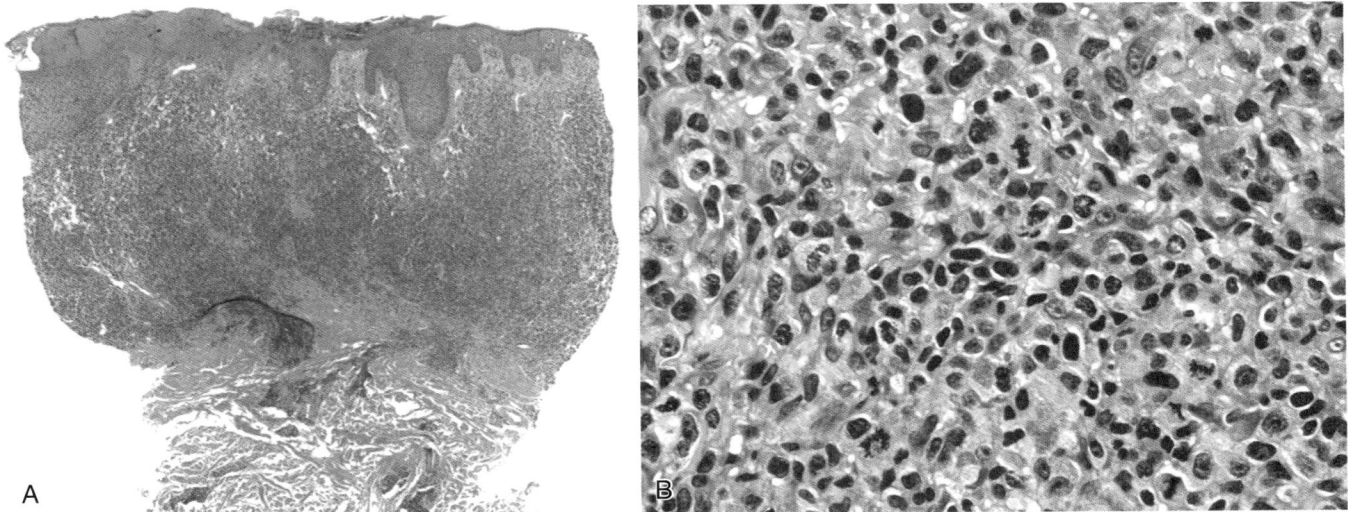

Figure 38-7. A, Mycosis fungoides tumor with diffuse infiltration of the dermis. Tumors sometimes ulcerate, as in this case. There may be a variety of cytomorphologic findings in the lymphocytes of tumor-stage lesions, but large cerebriform cells or cells with large vesicular nuclei usually predominate. **B,** The lesional lymphocytes often are markedly atypical, and numerous mitotic figures are evident among them.

oval vesicular nuclei, large nucleoli, and abundant cytoplasm, similar to the cells of anaplastic large cell lymphoma. This usually occurs in advanced disease and may have an adverse prognostic effect. Nevertheless, large cell transformation can occasionally occur in patches and plaques as well, although less commonly than in tumors (Fig. 38-8).[25,26] While increased expression of CD30 can occur in large cell transformation, the definition of large cell transformation is based on morphology and not on the status of the CD30 on the lesional lymphocytes.

Anaplastic large cells may predominate to such an extent that only the clinical identification of patches or plaques at other sites allows the distinction from anaplastic large cell lymphoma. Although lymphocytes home to the epidermis in patch-stage and plaque-stage lesions, some tumors of mycosis fungoides completely lack intraepidermal lymphocytes. The loss of dependence on an epidermal environment for cellular proliferation in the skin occurs apace with the cells' capacity to lodge in internal organs in mycosis fungoides.

Grading

Although biopsy interpretation is critical in establishing a diagnosis of mycosis fungoides, little prognostic information can be gleaned from histopathologic sections. Whether a patient has patches, plaques, or tumors can be determined clinically (there are a few pitfalls, however, such as mistaking lesions elevated by comedones for nodules). Most studies have demonstrated that the detection of transformed lymphocytes in plaques and tumors of

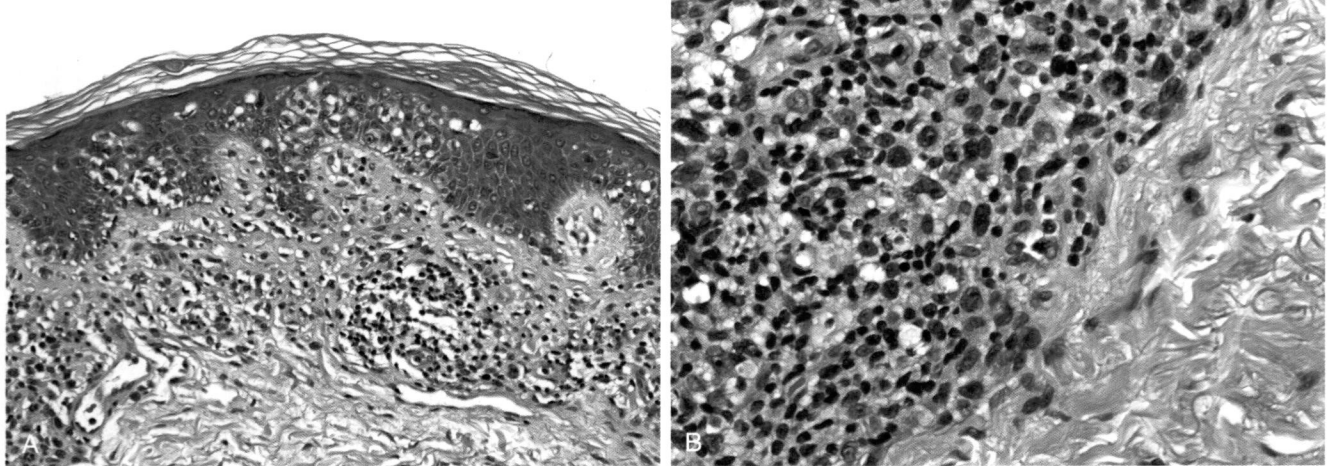

Figure 38-8. A, Thin plaque of mycosis fungoides with large cell transformation. **B,** Although the infiltrate is sparser than that of the plaque in Figure 38-6, many lymphocytes have large, vesicular nuclei with prominent nucleoli.

mycosis fungoides has an adverse effect on survival.[25,26] However, it has been recognized that a subset of patients with histopathologic evidence of transformation has an indolent clinical course.[27]

Immunophenotype

The cells of mycosis fungoides are mature helper T cells in the large majority of cases, with a βF1-positive, CD3-positive, CD4-positive, CD8-negative phenotype. Patches of mycosis fungoides usually have neoplastic cells that express the normal panoply of T-cell antigens, such as CD2 and CD5, but may not express CD7.[28] Some papers refer to a "loss" of CD7, whereas others view mycosis fungoides as a neoplastic expansion of the normally occurring (but minority population) of CD7-negative helper T cells. Whether the finding of large numbers of CD3-positive, CD4-positive, CD7-negative cells in a cutaneous infiltrate is diagnostic of mycosis fungoides is controversial. There are practical impediments to the implementation of this finding as a diagnostic criterion, even if it were a scientifically valid concept. Nevertheless, some groups have published results suggesting that CD7 staining in paraffin embedded sections may be helpful in the diagnosis.[29] Well-developed patches, plaques, and tumors may show a high CD4:CD8 ratio, and loss of pan–T cell antigens. However, in early lesions, there may be more reactive than neoplastic cells, making it difficult to assess the immunophenotype of the putative neoplastic cells. In our experience, only rarely is there enough of an altered CD4:CD8 ratio, enough cells with a double negative (CD4 negative, CD8 negative) immunophenotype or loss of pan–T cell antigens for immunostaining to be decisive in difficult cases.

As noted, a variety of immunophenotypes can occur in patients who, on clinical grounds and by conventional histopathologic examination, seem to have mycosis fungoides. These include CD8-positive and even CD56-positive immunophenotypes. How common this situation is depends on how many cases are tested with these antibodies. CD8-positive cases usually have a cytotoxic immunophenotype.

CD56-positive cases are rarer and can have several different immunophenotypes, including CD4 positive and CD8 positive.[30]

Plaques and tumors of mycosis fungoides often have other aberrations—diminished expression of CD5, CD2, or even CD3—but by the time these findings are present, the diagnosis can be easily established by routine methods. A cytotoxic phenotype with T-cell intracellular antigen-1 and granzyme B expression can occur in later stage lesions.[31]

CD30 is an antigen expressed on the cells of Hodgkin lymphoma and by those of anaplastic large cell lymphoma. Its presence is not specific, and it is also expressed by lymphocytes that have been stimulated by antigen in infectious and inflammatory conditions. CD30-positive cells occur in some plaques of mycosis fungoides, but mostly in tumors that have anaplastic large cells. There seems to be no prognostic significance to CD30 expression in mycosis fungoides when it is detected in patches.[32] However, when CD30 is expressed on lesional lymphocytes that have undergone large cell transformation, it does seem to have prognostic significance as one study demonstrated that CD30 expression is associated with improved survival compared with lack of CD30 expression.[27] Brentuximab vedotin is a relatively new medication that is a monoclonal antibody directed at CD30, and which is used to treat some lymphomas that express CD30. Therefore the CD30 status of an infiltrate of mycosis fungoides may now be relevant to treatment. As such, clinical teams may request staining with this antibody.[33]

Programmed death 1 (PD-1, CD279), a member of the CD28/CTLA-1 receptor family, is thought to play an important role in the inhibition of T-cell activity.[34,35] Studies have demonstrated disparate findings with regard to the expression of PD-1 on the lesional lymphocytes in mycosis fungoides; some reports document relatively high rates of expression of PD-1 (40% of patches and plaques and 60% of tumors),[35] whereas others show low rates of expression (13% of patches and plaques and 14% of tumors).[36] Other antigens associated with T follicular helper cells including ICOS, BCL6, CXCL13, and even CD10 have also been reported in variable proportions in biopsies of mycosis fungoides.[36,37]

Genotypic Features

Mycosis fungoides cells have undergone rearrangement of their T-cell receptor genes, even though this cannot always be documented. It is also important to recognize that T-cell clonality may be demonstrable in inflammatory skin disorders of various kinds, with precise specificity and sensitivity depending on both technical factors and the extent of the neoplastic infiltrate.[38,39] Many laboratories currently use polymerase chain reaction (PCR)–based methods from paraffin embedded tissue for this testing. Depending on how they are analyzed, the addition of probes for T-cell receptor beta genes to those for T-cell receptor gamma genes can lead to an increase in specificity, but at a loss of sensitivity.[39] An increase in sensitivity may be achieved but at some loss of specificity. It is therefore important that PCR be applied judiciously to cases in which mycosis fungoides is compatible clinically and suspected microscopically. An algorithm for how to interpret PCR findings based on pretest probability for mycosis fungoides has been suggested.[39] Next-generation sequencing is currently used at some centers to assess for T-cell clonality and may be a technology that replaces PCR-based assays in the future for T-cell clonality assessment.[40,41]

Much has also been learned about genetic and epigenetic abnormalities in mycosis fungoides using next-generation sequencing and other technologies. This has been recently reviewed.[42]

Postulated Cell of Origin

Mycosis fungoides is considered a neoplasm of skin resident effector memory T-cells (CCR7/L-selectin and CD27 negative, but showing strong expression of CCR4 and CLA).[6] They usually represent activated, mature helper T cells. Attention has been given to the role of T regulatory cells in several inflammatory skin diseases and in mycosis fungoides. It appears that these cells, which are positive for CD25 and FOXP3, may play a role in mycosis fungoides.[31,43]

Clinical Course

Most of the literature written before 1980 applies to patients with plaques and tumors because the patch stage was not widely recognized before that time. Many of these early studies reported a grim prognosis for patients with mycosis fungoides, and the more recent decline in mortality[44] seems to be caused by recognition of the disease at an earlier stage rather than to better treatments.

More current studies have demonstrated that patients with patches of mycosis fungoides often have indolent disease for many years; if the condition is limited to less than 10% of the body surface, lifespan is often unaffected.[45] Those with more extensive patches are more likely to develop plaques, tumors, and internal disease. Patients with disseminated plaques, tumors, or both may develop internal disease. This can take the form of adenopathy, hepatosplenomegaly, or infiltrates in other organs that can be detected only by biopsy or necropsy. The most serious effects are on the immune system, however. Although the peripheral helper T-cell counts of patients with mycosis fungoides may be nearly normal or high, those with advanced disease often have diminished numbers of functional T-helper cells. Those in the blood may be neoplastic cells, which cannot respond effectively to infection. In its terminal stages, mycosis fungoides results in death from immunodeficiency.[46] The 5-year and 10-year overall survival in tumor-stage MF has been reported as 40% to 65% and 20% to 39%, respectively, and the mean survival in tumor-stage MF has been reported at 2.9 to 4.7 years.[46a]

Differential Diagnosis

A number of inflammatory skin conditions simulate mycosis fungoides clinically, pathologically, or both. Knowledge of the differential diagnosis of mycosis fungoides is most critical in these circumstances for recognition of its patch stage.

The skin diseases that simulate the patch stage of mycosis fungoides result in macules or patches of slightly inflamed, scaling skin. These include forms of spongiotic dermatitis, such as allergic contact or nummular dermatitis; pityriasis rosea; and interface dermatitides, such as lichenoid drug eruptions. Spongiotic dermatitis usually has perivascular rather than bandlike infiltrates in the superficial dermis, as well as areas with abundant spongiosis without many lymphocytes. A helpful feature in some cases is the presence of eosinophils. Early patches of mycosis fungoides seldom have more than a few eosinophils.[47] Although spongiotic dermatitides may lack eosinophils entirely, many cases have eosinophils in both the dermis and (if one looks carefully) the epidermis.

One pitfall posed by the spongiotic dermatitides is the presence of collections of pale-staining mononuclear cells in the epidermis (Fig. 38-9). These collections, composed of Langerhans cells and their monocytic precursors, have a heterogeneous composition.[48] Their cells have pale cytoplasm and reniform vesicular nuclei. True Pautrier's microabscesses or collections in mycosis fungoides are compactly arranged aggregations in which lymphocytes predominate. The cells have scant cytoplasm, and the nuclei are darker than in so-called "Langerhans cell pustules." Another clue is the shape of the aggregations. True Pautrier's microabscesses are round, whereas their spongiotic counterparts often have a vaselike shape, with everted lips on the epidermal surface.[48] In the rare case when immunohistochemistry is used to distinguish between Pautrier's microabscesses and Langerhans cell pustules, Pautrier's microabscesses are composed mostly of cells that stain for CD3, and Langerhans cell pustules are composed of cells that

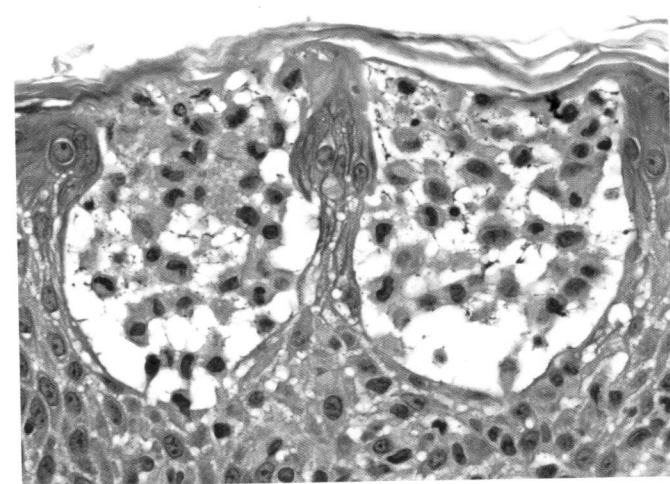

Figure 38-9. Vase-shaped collection of Langerhans cells in spongiotic dermatitis.

stain for either CD1a, langerin, or CD68. A Langerhans cell is usually found at the center of each Pautrier's microabscess.

Interface dermatitides are a clinically diverse group of diseases in which lymphocytes obscure the dermoepidermal junction. The consequences of this infiltration include vacuolar change, an alteration in the shape of rete ridges (they become serrated or recede entirely), and cytotoxic damage to keratinocytes, visible as dyskeratotic cells in the epidermis and as colloid bodies when these descend into the papillary dermis. Small foci with these findings commonly occur in mycosis fungoides. They are seldom the dominant feature in all lesions of a single patient, although there is a rare variant in which such changes occur (Fig. 38-10).[49] It cannot be overemphasized, however, that a single biopsy specimen from a patient with mycosis fungoides can show an interface pattern and that several biopsy specimens must be obtained if mycosis fungoides is suspected clinically.[21] Pathologists unfamiliar with lichen planus, lichenoid drug eruptions, lichenoid keratoses, and even densely infiltrated lesions of lupus erythematosus may mistake these lesions for mycosis fungoides owing to numerous lymphocytes in the lower part of the epidermis in such cases. Lichenoid keratoses may present a particular diagnostic challenge because they can feature many lymphocytes in the epidermis.[50] An important reminder is that mycosis fungoides does not present as a small solitary keratosis (in the solitary variant of mycosis fungoides, the lesions are usually relatively large in size).

There are several inflammatory diseases that cause a psoriasiform lichenoid pattern or a psoriasiform lichenoid spongiotic pattern, the most common patterns in patches of mycosis fungoides. In some cases, lymphocytes even lie in the basal layer of the epidermis in a linear fashion ("beads on a string"), without the same degree of vacuolar change or number of necrotic keratinocytes seen in most interface dermatitides. Luckily, many of these conditions do not simulate mycosis fungoides clinically. Lichen striatus, for example, causes linearly arranged papules along Blaschko's lines in children and adolescents more often than in adults.[51] Lichen sclerosus et atrophicus has an inflammatory phase that can mimic mycosis fungoides, but solitary lesions of mycosis fungoides on the skin of the genitalia essentially do not occur. Extragenital lichen sclerosus may present problems in this regard, especially if it is sampled by a thin shave biopsy.[52]

Among the most treacherous entities with a psoriasiform lichenoid pattern are members of a group of conditions termed *persistent pigmented purpuric dermatitis.*[53,54] These diseases usually affect the skin of the legs, resulting in red to rust or golden-brown macules, papules, and sometimes plaques. They are caused by infiltrates of lymphocytes that somehow induce venules to leak red blood cells into the dermis. Over time, siderophages accumulate. Two forms—lichenoid purpura of Gougerot and Blum and lichen aureus—have dense, bandlike infiltrates of lymphocytes, sometimes in a fibrotic and thickened papillary dermis (Fig. 38-11). Because lesions of mycosis fungoides can become purpuric, it is possible for the lichenoid variants of persistent pigmented purpuric dermatitis to have all the features of purpuric mycosis fungoides except for the striking cytologic atypia or epidermotropism of lymphocytes into the upper spinous layers (in persistent pigmented purpuric dermatitis, lymphocytes can be present within the basal layer but typically do not colonize the upper spinous layers). To the extent that there may be edema of the papillary dermis in persistent pigmented purpuric dermatitis, the conditions can be distinguished histopathologically because the papillary dermis typically is not edematous in mycosis fungoides.

Whether the close histomorphologic similarities between mycosis fungoides and persistent pigmented purpuric dermatitis indicate a biological relationship is an unanswered question. One of the first cases of lichen aureus reported in North America turned out to be mycosis fungoides.[55] Clonality can be present in many cases of persistent pigmented purpuric dermatitis with use of PCR-based methods, making that technique less useful for telling the conditions apart. The clinical picture—whether lesions are mostly on the legs or disseminated—can be more helpful than histopathologic or immunophenotypic findings. Patients with clinically typical lichen aureus show no significant tendency to progress to mycosis fungoides, despite the finding of clonality detected in PCR-based methods in about half the cases.[56] To our knowledge, at the time of writing this, there are no studies using high-throughput sequencing to evaluate for T-cell clonality in persistent pigmented purpuric dermatitis.

Although children only rarely develop mycosis fungoides, there are several pitfalls in diagnosing such cases. Mycosis fungoides in children seems to result in hypopigmentation in a disproportionate number of cases[57]; so-called "hypopigmented

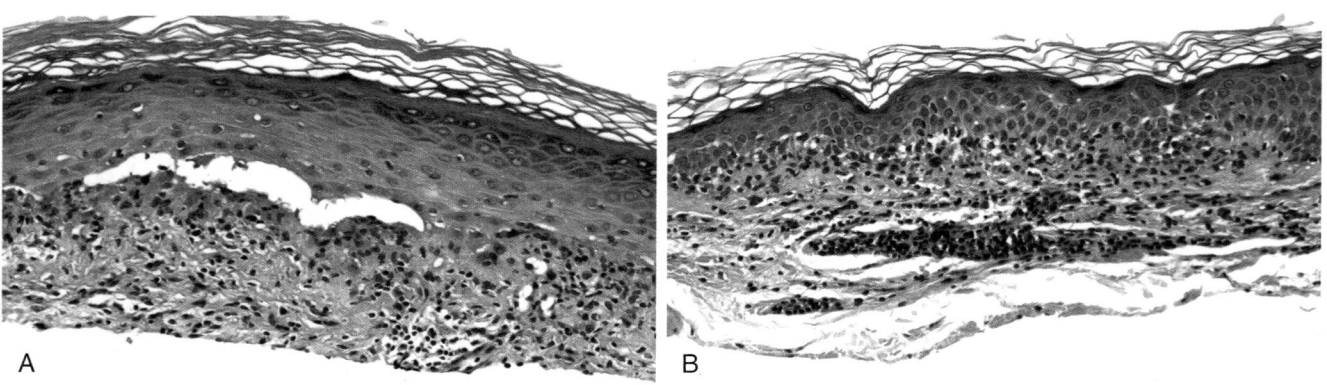

Figure 38-10. A, The lichenoid variant of mycosis fungoides is easily mistaken for an interface dermatitis. Clefts may be present at the dermoepidermal junction, and there may be wedge-shaped foci of hypergranulosis, as in lichen planus. **B,** Another area features a more characteristic pattern.

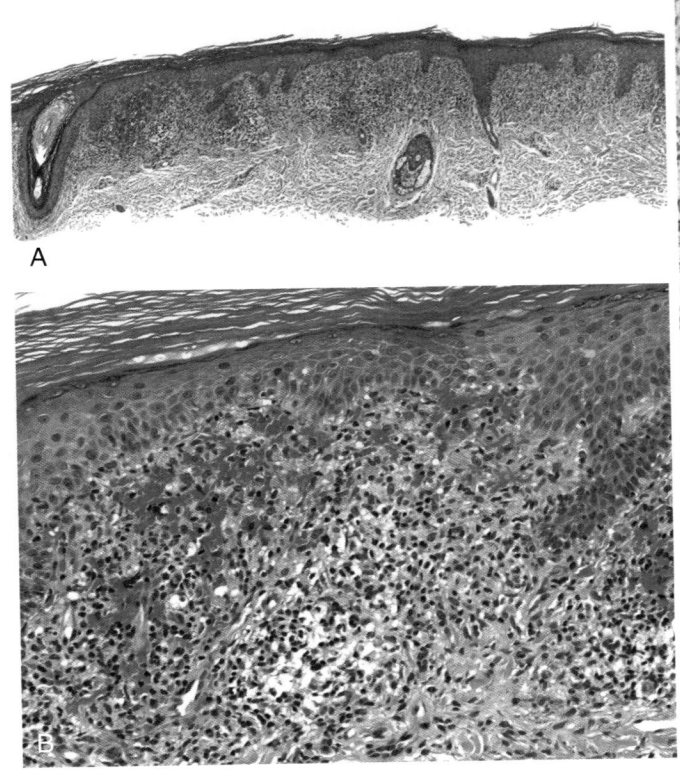

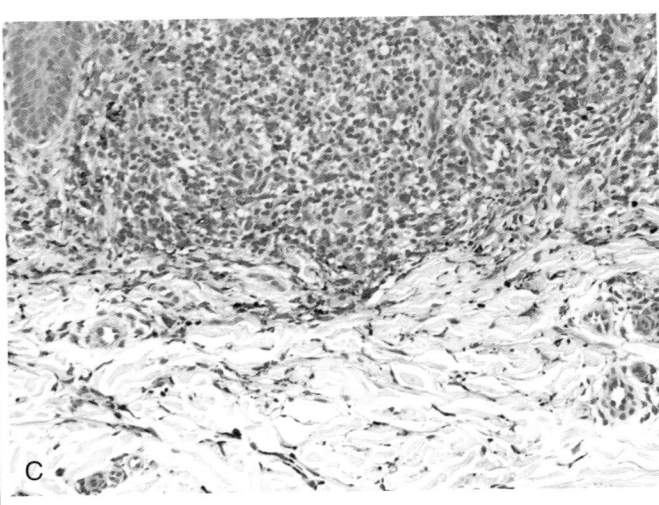

Figure 38-11. A, Lichenoid purpura can simulate mycosis fungoides because of its psoriasiform lichenoid pattern. **B,** Many extravasated erythrocytes are often present, resulting in the deposition of siderophages. **C,** Siderophages can be highlighted by Perls' stain.

mycosis fungoides" can be mistaken for vitiligo, tinea versicolor, pityriasis alba, and pityriasis lichenoides chronica, and vice versa. Vitiligo usually has symmetrically distributed lesions (unlike those of mycosis fungoides), with a tendency to affect flexural skin. One problem is that biopsy specimens from the edge of the lesion, especially in so-called "trichrome vitiligo," can feature many lymphocytes among keratinocytes of the basal layer. Biopsy of the center of the lesion should show a picture devoid of lymphocytes and with a lack of melanocytes. Pityriasis alba is a spongiotic dermatitis that results in pale, slightly scaly lesions. There are superficial lymphocytic infiltrates with a touch of spongiosis. The lymphocytes do not align themselves along the junction and are no larger than their dermal counterparts. The dermal papillae should be edematous, not fibrotic. Pityriasis lichenoides chronica is an interface dermatitis, and vacuolar change coupled with single necrotic keratinocytes at the junction should be present along with a broad overlying tier of parakeratosis.

Annular lichenoid dermatitis of youth[58] may simulate mycosis fungoides by virtue of large, annular lesions and a tendency for lymphocytes to be clustered at the bases of rete ridges. The condition, initially reported in children, can also affect young adults. Although the clusters of lymphocytes can resemble those of mycosis fungoides in terms of size, the shape of some of the rete ridges is distinctive. They can be square based in annular lichenoid dermatitis of youth, and the cells in the basal layer are squamous rather than cuboid. In the only large series to date on this condition, clonal T-cell populations were not present. The immunophenotype is usually CD8 positive and cytotoxic.[59]

The atrophic or poikilodermatous patch stage of mycosis fungoides is imitated by several conditions in which the epidermis is thinned by an interface dermatitis (Fig. 38-12).

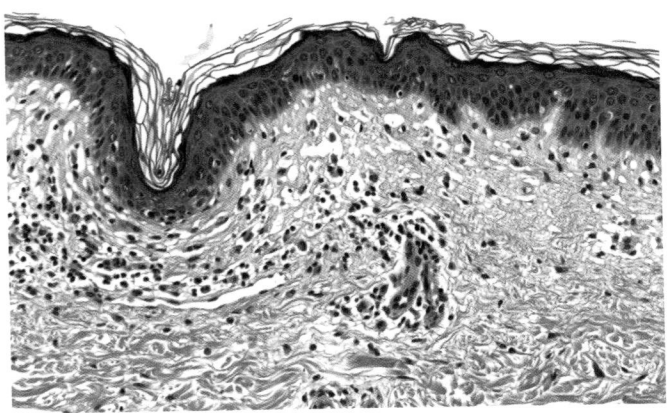

Figure 38-12. In the atrophic patch stage of mycosis fungoides, there are often very few lymphocytes within the epidermis, making a specific diagnosis problematic, especially with small biopsy specimens.

These include the atrophic variant of lichen planus (and, rarely, atrophy from a lichenoid drug eruption), poikilodermic dermatomyositis, atrophic centers of lesions of porokeratosis (a condition in which a clone of abnormal keratinocytes migrates centrifugally, sometimes leaving atrophy in its wake), and, occasionally, atrophic lesions of persistent pigmented purpuric dermatitis. There are other rare forms of poikiloderma, such as the congenital Rothmund-Thomson syndrome[60] and dyskeratosis congenita. Similar histopathologic changes also result from regression of melanoma if little pigment is present and from regression of Bowen's disease, superficial basal cell carcinoma, and solar lentigo (so-called "lichen planus–like keratosis"). In all these conditions, and in atrophic patches of mycosis fungoides, lymphocytes of the host response to a neoplasm destroy the keratinocytes of rete ridges, resulting in epidermal atrophy. It may not be possible to distinguish between atrophic mycosis fungoides and these conditions unless many lymphocytes reside in the basal layer of the epidermis. This may require extensive sampling.

Another important mimic of mycosis fungoides is lymphomatoid allergic contact dermatitis.[61] In this unusual type of allergic contact dermatitis, many more lymphocytes are attracted to the epidermis than normally; sometimes the lymphocytes are cytologically atypical. Although a distinction between conventional spongiotic dermatitis and mycosis fungoides is usually possible without recourse to clinical information, in some cases of lymphomatoid contact dermatitis, the clinical history is key.

Drug eruptions can also simulate the patch stage of mycosis fungoides. Diphenylhydantoin can cause a systemic illness in which adenopathy is accompanied by an eruption resembling mycosis fungoides. This may also occur without any systemic symptoms. The clinical history is one key to making this diagnosis. Other drugs can cause reactions that mimic the patches of mycosis fungoides, even digitate ones.[62] A rash with some clinical and histopathologic similarities to mycosis fungoides can occur in patients treated with mogamulizumab, which is a newer medication that was FDA approved for previously treated advanced-stage mycosis fungoides in 2018. Some potentially helpful discriminatory features that favor a mogamulizumab-associated rash over mycosis fungoides include an inverted or normalized CD4:CD8 ratio and lack of a T-cell clone.[63]

For the most part, the plaque and tumor stages of mycosis fungoides are simulated by other lymphomas, not by inflammatory conditions. One exception is the interstitial type of mycosis fungoides.[64] Interstitial mycosis fungoides usually has scant lymphocytes in the epidermis and papillary dermis in comparison with conventional plaque-stage disease. Its hallmark is the finding of strands of lymphocytes positioned between collagen bundles in the reticular dermis. Clinically, it may resemble some dusky lesions of morphea or granuloma annulare, and it can be very difficult to distinguish it from morphea.

Tumors of mycosis fungoides may be impossible to distinguish from those of other T-cell lymphomas without recourse to clinical examination. The infiltrates of peripheral T-cell lymphomas, not otherwise specified, can present in the skin or with systemic disease.[65] The infiltrates are predominantly dermal. Because some lymphocytes can infiltrate the epidermis in peripheral T-cell lymphomas, a pathologist with no knowledge of the clinical picture cannot differentiate a plaque or tumor of mycosis fungoides from a nodule of peripheral T-cell lymphoma, not otherwise specified. Only the presence of patches elsewhere on the patient's body allows these conditions to be distinguished. A tumor of mycosis fungoides in which anaplastic large lymphocytes predominate and diffusely express CD30 can be an exact replica of anaplastic large cell lymphoma, but the patient has a much worse prognosis. Again, the clinical examination is key.

In some cases, CD4-positive small-to-medium-sized T-cell lymphoproliferative disorder can be particularly problematic to distinguish pathologically from tumor-stage mycosis fungoides. Usually, very few lymphocytes are present in the epidermis. Therefore, the differential diagnosis is a tumor of mycosis fungoides with little epidermal involvement and a predominance of smaller cells. The number of B cells in this condition is substantial and has been attributed to a proliferation of T follicular helper cells.[66-68] Primary cutaneous CD4-positive small-to-medium-sized T-cell lymphoproliferative disorder usually presents as a single plaque or nodule, whereas mycosis fungoides presents with multiple lesions. Therefore, it is imperative to perform a full-body skin examination to assess for clinical evidence of mycosis fungoides before making the diagnosis of CD4-positive small-to-medium-sized T-cell lymphoproliferative disorder. For this reason, we typically render descriptive reports for this condition and include a note that a full-body skin examination needs to be done to assess for mycosis fungoides before an unequivocal diagnosis can be rendered. The prognosis is excellent compared with that of tumor-stage mycosis fungoides.

Variants

The various effects of the cells of mycosis fungoides on the different constituents of the skin, the effects of host inflammatory cells responding to the neoplastic ones, and the disturbed microenvironment of cytokines, chemokines, and the like account for the prodigious differences in the clinical and microscopic appearance of mycosis fungoides lesions. The cells of mycosis fungoides, which are usually home to the epidermis, can also localize in other sites.

Folliculotropic Mycosis Fungoides

The hair follicles can become a magnet for the cells of mycosis fungoides (Fig. 38-13A). On histopathologic evaluation, lesions of folliculotropic mycosis fungoides feature variably dense perifollicular infiltrates of lymphocytes and, notably, eosinophils; lymphocytes within the follicular epithelium; and plugging of follicular ostia by compact hyperkeratosis. The interfollicular epidermis is often spared, and most of the lymphocytes are relatively small, making an outright diagnosis of lymphoma difficult. This reaction is sometimes although not always accompanied by the accumulation of mucopolysaccharides between keratinocytes in the outer root sheath (Fig. 38-13B). The result is the distention of intercellular spaces in the outer root sheath. In well-balanced hematoxylin-eosin–stained sections, the mucin can be detected as tiny basophilic granules. Keratinocytes adjacent to the widened spaces are often elongated, and the spines connecting them appear stretched. In some cases, lymphocytes do not infiltrate the epithelium and are not sufficiently atypical to establish a diagnosis of mycosis fungoides on cytologic grounds alone. Nonetheless, a widespread eruption composed of folliculocentric plaques is probably best classified as folliculotropic mycosis fungoides.

Clinically, this variant presents with a different distribution compared with conventional mycosis fungoides because lesions are typically on the head, neck, and upper trunk rather than on the double-clothed areas. The clinical lesions are often erythematous patches and plaques with follicular prominence that are markedly pruritic and frequently are associated with hair loss. Small follicular-based papules can occur as well. These follicular papules can clinically simulate keratosis pilaris or other follicular diseases, such as follicular lichen planus.

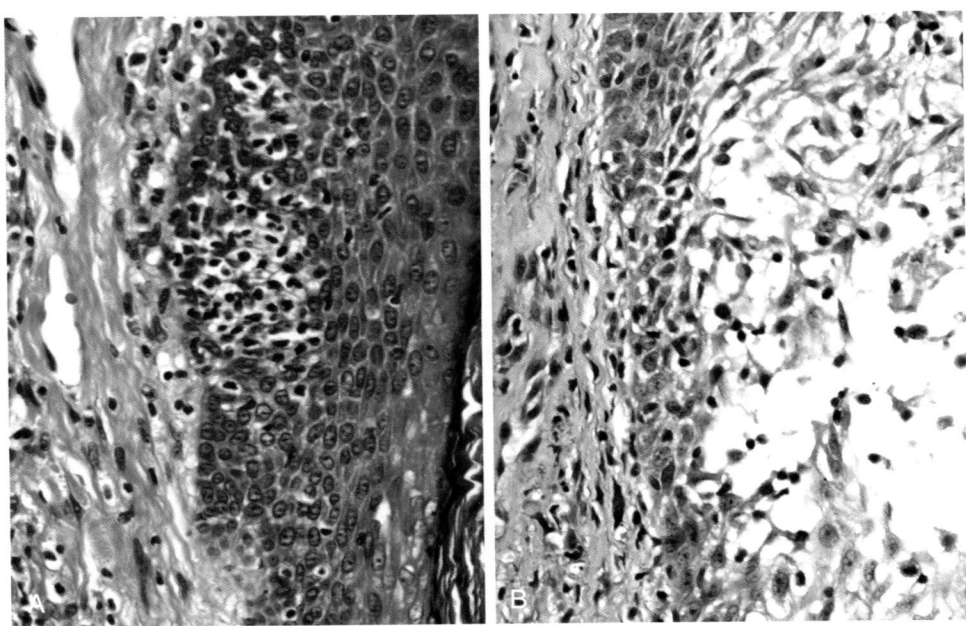

Figure 38-13. A, In folliculotropic mycosis fungoides, lymphocytes may home to the follicular epithelium rather than to the epidermis. **B,** In some cases of folliculotropic mycosis fungoides, spaces between keratinocytes are markedly widened because of the accumulation of mucin.

Although early studies suggested that these patients have a less favorable prognosis than those with conventional mycosis fungoides,[69-71] later series have demonstrated that prognosis is not as poor as the earlier studies suggested.[72]

Although it was mentioned earlier that mucin can be present within the affected follicles, it should be noted that mucin within follicles is not specific for folliculotropic mycosis fungoides and can occur as an incidental finding, in conventional lesions of mycosis fungoides (usually in plaques or tumors) or in a condition termed *alopecia mucinosa*. *Alopecia mucinosa* is a term initially coined to refer to a condition thought to be an inflammatory reaction (i.e., not a lymphoma) in which plaques of alopecia are present on the hair-bearing skin of young persons, with mucin accumulating in the affected follicles. Some studies suggest that the distinction between alopecia mucinosa and folliculotropic mycosis fungoides may not be valid and that alopecia mucinosa may in fact be an indolent form of mycosis fungoides.[73,74] Further, studies of T-cell receptor gene rearrangements have found clonal populations in about the same number of cases of both idiopathic alopecia mucinosa and mycosis fungoides with follicular mucinosis. Nevertheless, the relationship between alopecia mucinosa and mycosis fungoides remains an area of debate.

Mycosis Fungoides With Cysts and Comedones

Some patients with follicular mycosis fungoides, with or without follicular mucinosis, have lesions in which large comedones or even follicular cysts develop.[75,76] This probably results from occlusion of the follicular infundibulum by the infiltrates of mycosis fungoides. This complication is disfiguring but may respond to treatment of the disease. The prognosis is the same as that for follicular mycosis fungoides.

Bullous Mycosis Fungoides

In this rare variant, the cells of mycosis fungoides replace basal keratinocytes to the extent that cohesion between the epidermis and dermis is compromised, and trivial shearing forces result in clinical vesiculation. The diagnosis can usually be made by examining areas that have not vesiculated.[77]

Syringotropic Mycosis Fungoides

Lymphoma cells' tropism for secretory glands is exemplified by the lymphoepithelial lesions formed in some low-grade B-cell lymphomas, such as extranodal marginal zone lymphomas (although not in the skin). Some patients with mycosis fungoides have dense infiltrates of lymphocytes around eccrine secretory coils in addition to infiltrates elsewhere in the dermis and epidermis (Fig. 38-14).[78,79] A more purely syringotropic variant of mycosis fungoides in a patient who also had folliculotropic infiltrates was initially described as *syringolymphoid hyperplasia with alopecia*.[80] The cutaneous lesions are often small papules and may be accompanied by anhidrosis. Most authors accept that this condition is a variant of mycosis fungoides rather than an inflammatory disease.[81] This variant is too rare to know with certainty whether its prognosis is different from that of more common forms, but in a review of 15 cases published before 2004, its behavior seemed unremarkable.[82]

Pagetoid Reticulosis

In contrast to the bullous and syringotropic variants, which have lymphocytes that ignore the epidermis in favor of adnexal epithelium, the lymphocytes' attraction to the epidermis is exaggerated in pagetoid reticulosis. The affected skin is usually on the extremities, so the clinical lesions are warty, hyperkeratotic plaques on the hands and feet (Fig. 38-15). Pagetoid reticulosis was initially described by Woringer and Kolopp in two children; subsequent reports have highlighted that it occurs in younger patients than is usual for mycosis fungoides. It also differs from conventional mycosis fungoides by its failure to disseminate in most cases as it usually presents as a solitary plaque.

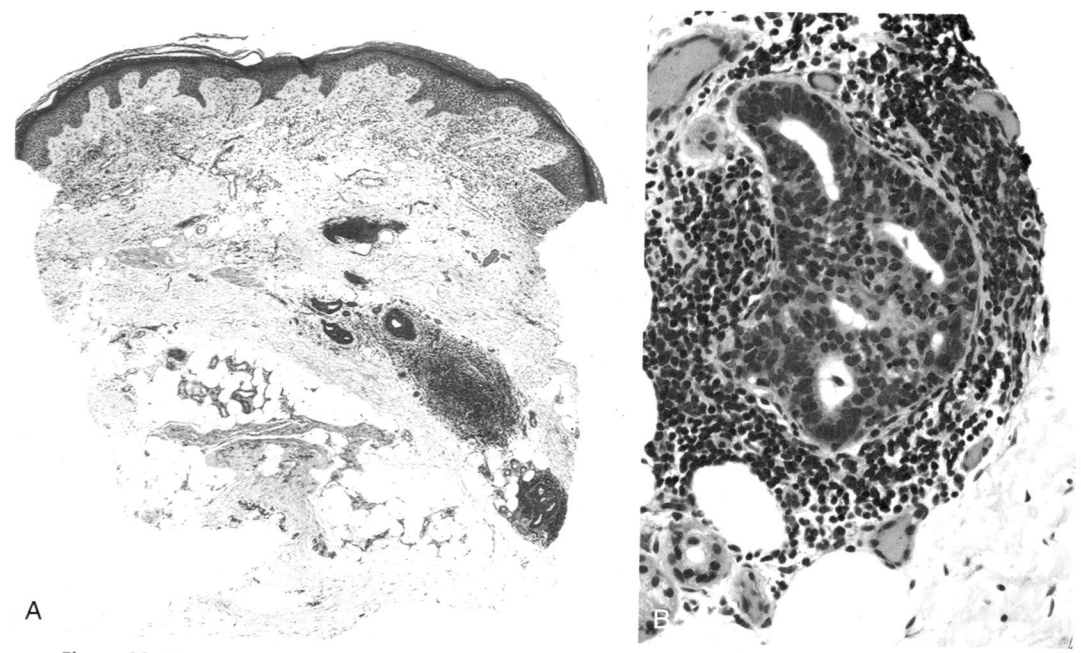

Figure 38-14. A, Syringotropic mycosis fungoides features dense infiltrates of lymphocytes around the eccrine secretory coils. **B,** There may be hyperplasia of the epithelial cells, similar to that in lymphoepithelial lesions.

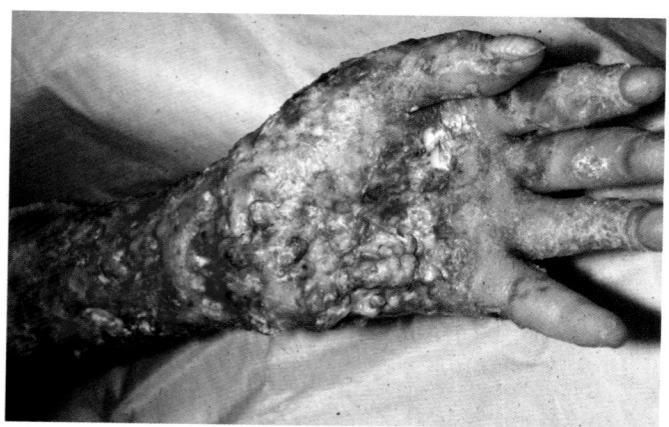

Figure 38-15. Woringer-Kolopp disease, or pagetoid reticulosis, presents as verrucous plaques on acral skin. (*Courtesy Dr. Sabine Kohler, Stanford University.***)**

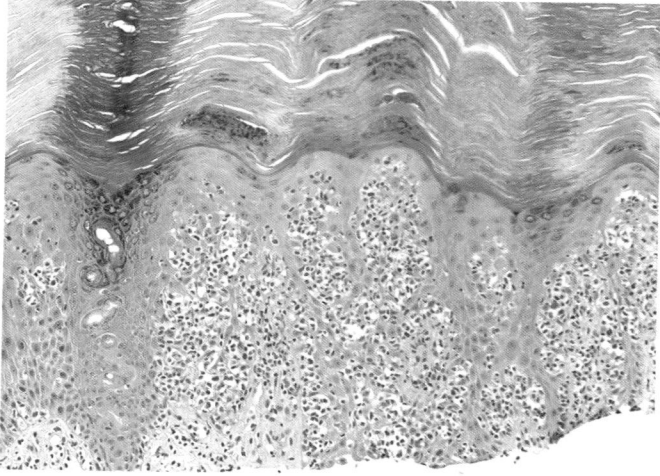

Figure 38-16. Histopathologic findings in pagetoid reticulosis include verrucous epidermal hyperplasia with infiltration of the epidermis, similar to or even more pronounced than that seen in conventional mycosis fungoides.

Its histopathologic hallmark is verrucous epidermal hyperplasia, coupled with infiltrates of lymphocytes that have cytologic atypia and are disproportionately situated in the epidermis (Fig. 38-16).[83] The immunophenotype includes CD4-positive or CD8-positive T cells. Compared with conventional mycosis fungoides, pagetoid reticulosis has a greater propensity to be CD30 positive, although most cases will not label with CD30. In addition, some cases of pagetoid reticulosis lack CD45 expression (leukocyte common antigen).[84] Its prognosis is far better than that of conventional mycosis fungoides. Many patients achieve durable remissions by local therapeutic means, such as excision of lesions or radiation therapy.

Another entity that shares the moniker pagetoid reticulosis is the Ketron-Goodman variant of mycosis fungoides, with striking epidermotropism and disseminated lesions. Some examples of this condition have a CD4-negative, CD8-negative (double negative) phenotype.[85] Most of these cases have now been reclassified as primary cutaneous CD8-positive aggressive epidermotropic T-cell lymphoma, sometimes termed *Berti's lymphoma*.[86]

Solitary Mycosis Fungoides

Whereas pagetoid reticulosis represents a solitary variant of mycosis fungoides that usually develops on acral skin, mycosis fungoides can occasionally present as a solitary lesion in the typical distribution of mycosis fungoides (i.e., the double-clothed areas).[87] Such cases are best regarded as a solitary variant of mycosis fungoides. Most reports have

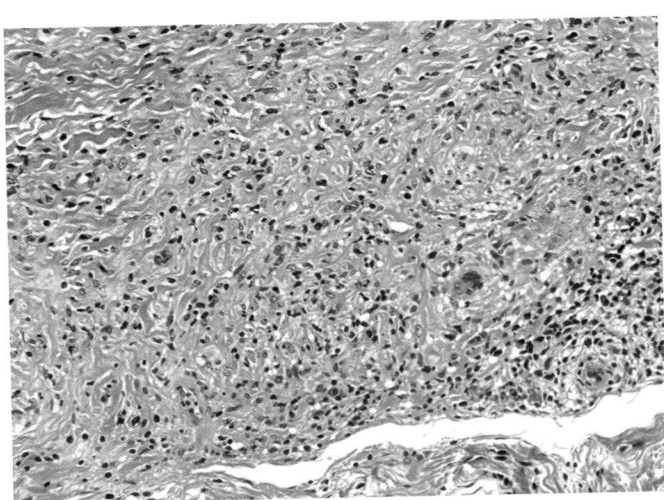

Figure 38-17. Granulomatous mycosis fungoides is not distinctive clinically, but its histopathologic findings include many histiocytes, sometimes multinucleated, interspersed with lymphocytic infiltrates in the dermis.

not demonstrated development of more widespread lesions in such patients.[88] Of note, folliculotropic mycosis fungoides can present with a solitary lesion as well.[89]

Granulomatous Mycosis Fungoides

There are many lymphomas, both cutaneous and nodal, that have foci in which histiocytes predominate. Plaques and tumors of mycosis fungoides can contain such foci in the reticular dermis. The findings can range from loose clusters of histiocytes to scattered giant cells to well-formed granulomatous tubercles (Fig. 38-17). The plaques and tumors of granulomatous mycosis fungoides usually do not have a distinct appearance.

In the initial description of granulomatous mycosis fungoides, the authors noted that their patient had survived longer than expected. Fourteen years later, their patient was still alive and had had granulomatous mycosis fungoides for nearly 3 decades.[90] Their conclusion, that the prognosis of granulomatous mycosis fungoides is more favorable than that of conventional mycosis fungoides, has not been confirmed by other studies.[91,92] There may be a variety of causes of granulomatous infiltrates in mycosis fungoides: lymphocytes may attract histiocytes, giant cells may be moved to phagocytize elastotic fibers (similar to the foci that resemble actinic granuloma in many inflammatory diseases in sun-damaged skin), or keratin or mucin from leaky follicles may incite a granulomatous reaction. A reanalysis of the data seems to be prudent before firm conclusions are reached about the prognosis of this variant.

Granulomatous Slack Skin

Granulomatous slack skin is a peculiar condition in which the cells of an epidermotropic T-cell lymphoma attract histiocytes, which in turn digest elastic tissue and lead to the formation of large saclike skin folds. The disease affects younger patients than is usual for mycosis fungoides, with most cases beginning in young adulthood. The usual sites of involvement are the axilla and groin (Fig. 38-18). Hodgkin lymphoma has reportedly developed in several patients with granulomatous slack skin.[93,94] However, it is uncertain whether the lymphoma that develops

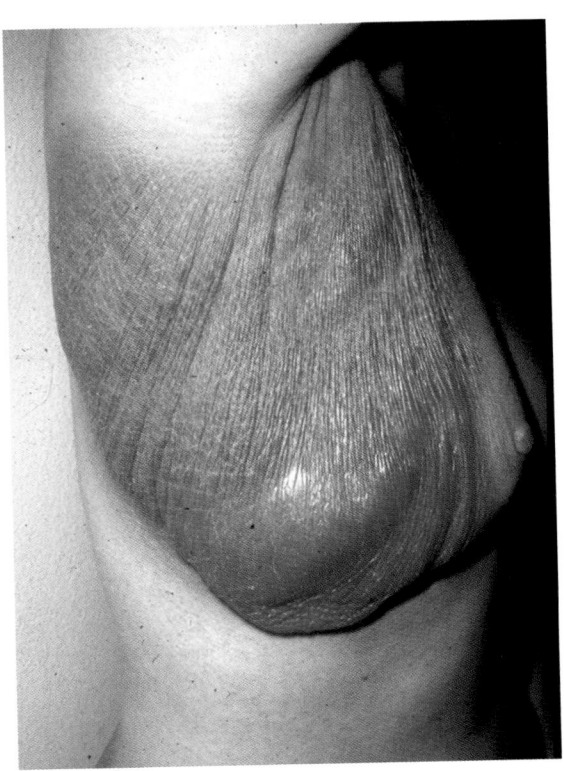

Figure 38-18. Granulomatous slack skin typically presents with pendulous masses in the axilla and groin.

in the internal organs of patients with granulomatous slack skin is truly Hodgkin lymphoma or a large T-cell lymphoma, given that the reported cases were not comprehensively worked up by current standards. In a retrospective multicenter study of patients with granulomatous slack skin, 25% were associated with visceral involvement.[95]

The most striking histopathologic feature of granulomatous slack skin is involvement of the dermis and subcutaneous lobules by tuberculoid granulomas—clusters of histiocytes and giant cells surrounded and infiltrated by small lymphocytes.[96-98] The tubercles tend to be discrete and spaced at regular intervals throughout the infiltrate (Fig. 38-19). The giant cells sometimes contain elastic fibers as seen in specially stained sections, indicating that they are responsible for the profound elastolysis that occurs in this condition and leads to the distinctive pendulous skin folds.

Only when one examines the epidermis and papillary dermis is it evident that granulomatous slack skin is related to mycosis fungoides. Indeed, the changes in the superficial part of the biopsy specimen can be identical to those of mycosis fungoides. Immunophenotypic studies have been performed in only a few cases, but they indicate a CD4-positive, CD7-negative T-cell population, like that of mycosis fungoides. Gene rearrangement studies have shown clonality in almost all cases tested to date.

SÉZARY SYNDROME

Definition

The classic features of Sézary syndrome include Sézary cells in the peripheral blood (lymphocytes with abnormally

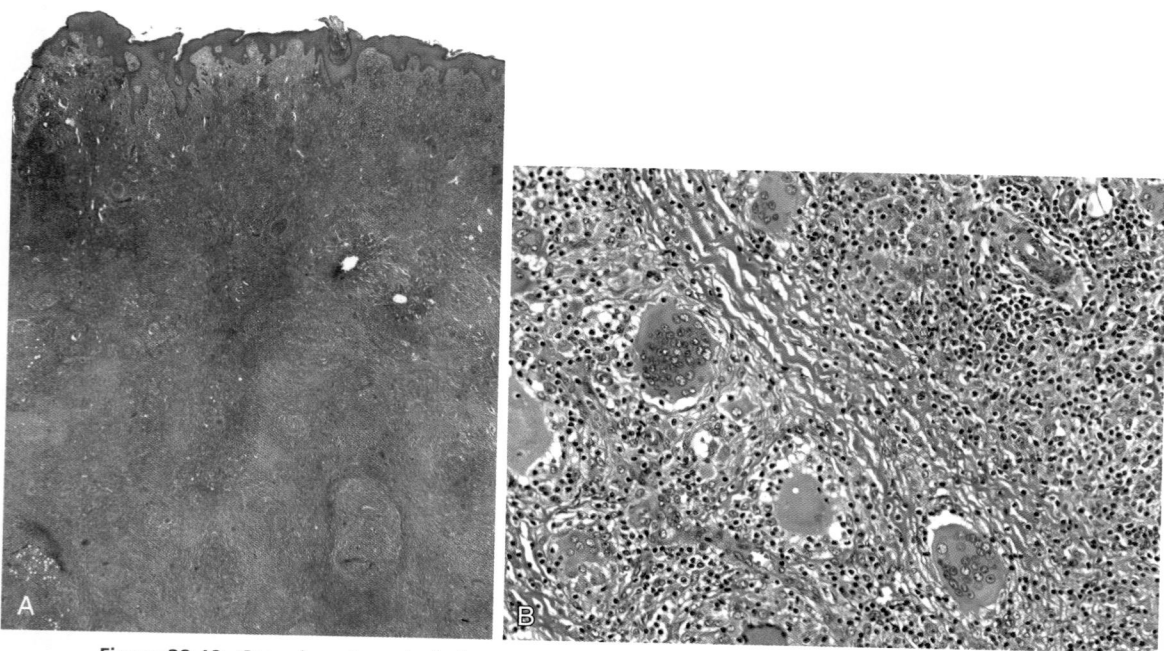

Figure 38-19. Granulomatous slack skin usually shows a dense, diffuse infiltrate of small lymphocytes throughout the dermis **(A)**, with infiltration of the epidermis similar to that seen in mycosis fungoides and large histiocytic giant cells that exhibit elastophagocytosis **(B)**.

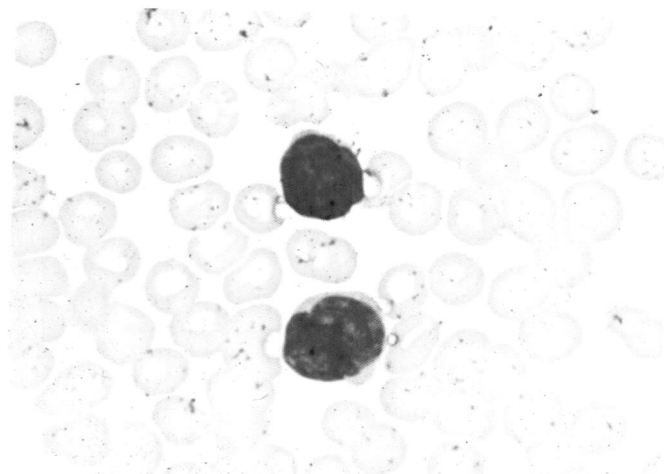

Figure 38-20. Sézary cells in a peripheral blood smear. Recognition of these cells is no longer critical for the diagnosis since the advent of clonality studies and flow cytometry.

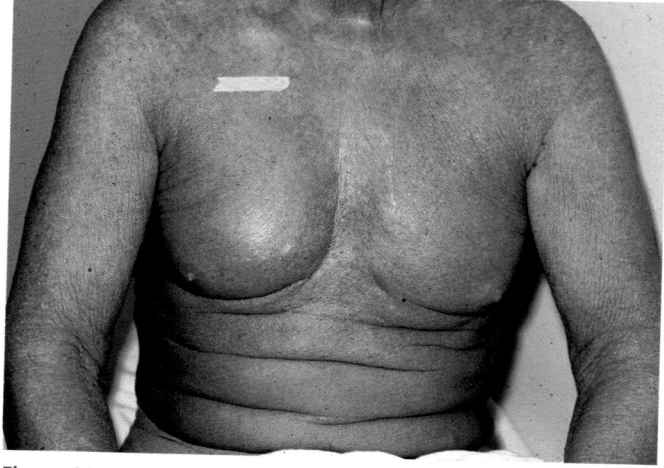

Figure 38-21. Sézary syndrome presents with erythroderma—diffuse red skin. The term *erythroderma* is often overused by clinicians; it should refer to confluent erythema, not just widespread erythematous lesions.

convoluted nuclei; Fig. 38-20), erythroderma (diffuse reddening of the skin; Fig. 38-21), and lymphadenopathy.

Whereas light microscopic evaluation of peripheral blood was used in the past to assess for the presence of Sézary cells in the peripheral blood, studies have since demonstrated limitations to this method. In particular, a small cell variant of the Sézary cell was described that would not have been detected on a peripheral smear.[99] Furthermore, normal resting lymphocytes were demonstrated to be able to acquire a Sézary cell phenotype under experimental conditions.[100] Finally, on occasion, morphologically similar lymphocytes could be detected in benign dermatoses.[101] For these reasons, alternative methods to assess blood involvement in patients with possible Sézary syndrome are now used at most medical

centers. In particular, a combination of flow cytometry with genotypic analysis is used in most centers to assess for the presence of Sézary cells in the blood, and criteria that need to be met to render a diagnosis of Sézary syndrome in the blood have been published. Specifically, these criteria state that there needs to be a T-cell clone in the blood along with flow cytometry showing either a CD4/CD8 ratio of more than 10:1 or loss of either CD7 on more than 40% of the CD4-positive cells or loss of CD26 on more than 30% of the CD4-positive cells.[102] Criteria for "high blood tumor burden" in mycosis fungoides or Sézary Syndrome (B2 in the revised classification of the International Society for Cutaneous Lymphomas and European Organisation of Research and Treatment of Cancer) include finding clonal rearrangement of the TCR in the blood and either 1.0 K/L or more Sézary cells or one of the two following criteria: (1) increased CD4-positive or CD3-positive cells with a CD4/CD8 ratio of 10 or more or (2) increase in CD4-positive cells with an abnormal phenotype (≥40% CD4 positive/CD7 negative or ≥30% CD4 positive/CD26 negative.[102] The major diagnostic features of Sézary syndrome are listed in Box 38-3.

Epidemiology

Like mycosis fungoides, Sézary syndrome is a disease of the middle-aged and elderly, although we have seen occasional cases in younger patients in their early 20s at our center. When strictly defined—requiring true erythroderma rather than just disseminated lesions—it is much less common than mycosis fungoides.

Etiology

There are no widely accepted risk factors for Sézary syndrome. The high level of UV signature mutations in about one-quarter of cases raises the possibility that this exposure could be causative in some patients.[103]

Immunophenotype

The majority of cases of Sézary syndrome are CD3+, CD4+, CD8−, CD7−, CD26− neoplasms consisting of mature helper T cells, similar in these respects to mycosis fungoides. Using the numerical assessments for CD4/CD8, CD4-positive/CD7-negative, and CD4-positive/CD26-negative T cells noted, flow cytometry can be helpful in making the diagnosis of Sézary syndrome from peripheral blood in the presence of the other diagnostic criteria. This phenotypic profile, however, does not exclude a benign disorder, leading to recommended additional phenotypic analyses, such as a more complete analysis looking for other immunophenotypic aberrancies and TRBC1 analysis on T-cell subsets.[104-106] As with mycosis fungoides, the neoplastic cells in Sézary syndrome may also express T follicular helper cell antigens.[36,37] One must also remember that in skin biopsy specimens, an elevated CD4/CD8 ratio is not as specific.[107] The phenotype in a given patient is sufficiently stable that flow cytometry can be used to monitor response to therapy.[108] However, while one or more aberrancies may remain stable, phenotypic variation does occur over time in a subset of patients, so caution is advised.[103]

Genotypic Features

Sézary syndrome has long been known to be a clonal T-cell proliferation.[109] Because a clonal population of T cells cannot be detected in a subset of skin biopsy specimens from patients with Sézary syndrome, and because a clonal population of T cells is present in the blood by definition in Sézary syndrome, the detection of a clonal population of T cells in the blood rather than in the skin can be used to prove clonality in Sézary syndrome. Some criteria do require clonally related neoplastic cells in skin, lymph node, and blood, although this is not a standard part of the required workup. Chromosomal abnormalities, including complex numerical and structural alterations and with recurrent copy number alterations, can be

---

Box 38-3 *Key Diagnostic Features of Sézary Syndrome*

Clinical Features
- Erythroderma caused by atypical lymphocytes in the skin
- Atypical lymphocytes in blood
- Atypical lymphocytes in lymph nodes

Histopathologic Features
- Dense bandlike infiltrate of lymphocytes in the upper dermis, sometimes with lymphocytes in the epidermis (i.e., epidermotropism)
- In some cases, some of the lymphocytes might have somewhat large and hyperchromatic nuclei

Immunohistochemical Features
- βF1-positive, CD3-positive, CD4-positive, CD8-negative immunophenotype

Genotypic Findings
- Demonstrable clonality common but not obligatory by polymerase chain reaction (PCR)–based gamma alone or gamma plus beta chain gene rearrangements

---

identified in Sézary syndrome, but no one abnormality is found in a preponderance of cases.[110] They do highlight the genomic instability in this neoplasm. Next-generation sequencing have revealed frequent mutations in elements of the JAK-STAT (*JAK3, STAT3*) and TCR signaling (*PLCG1, CD28, TNFR1F1B*) pathways, *RHOA, TP53*, and in epigenetic regulators. Some of these alterations are also present in mycosis fungoides.[111-114] The molecular/cytogenetic abnormalities in Sézary syndrome have been recently reviewed.[42]

Postulated Cell of Origin

Sézary syndrome appears to be a malignant disease of central memory CD4-positive T cells based on their expression of CCR7, L-selectin, and CD27.[115]

Clinical Features

The salient clinical features of Sézary syndrome—erythroderma, palmar and plantar hyperkeratosis, and lymphadenopathy—were first noted by Sézary and Bouvrain in their original report (Fig. 38-21). Erythroderma is a clinical sign in which the entire skin becomes red and sometimes scaly. It has also been called the "red man" effect. In erythroderma caused by lymphoma, the skin can become doughy as well in some cases, but not in all. There are many other causes of erythroderma besides Sézary syndrome, but its presence in a middle-aged or older patient should evoke a differential diagnosis that includes lymphoma. Hyperkeratosis of the palms and soles leads to red, scaly, and sometimes fissured skin. The nails may be lost or become dystrophic. Generalized lymphadenopathy is often present in patients with Sézary syndrome. The 5-year disease specific survival in Sézary syndrome is reported at 36%.[115a]

Histopathology

Diagnostic biopsy specimens of Sézary syndrome show identical features to definitive biopsy specimens of late patch-stage or plaque-stage mycosis fungoides. In particular, there is usually a dense bandlike infiltrate of lymphocytes, some of which exhibit epidermotropism. Some of the lesional

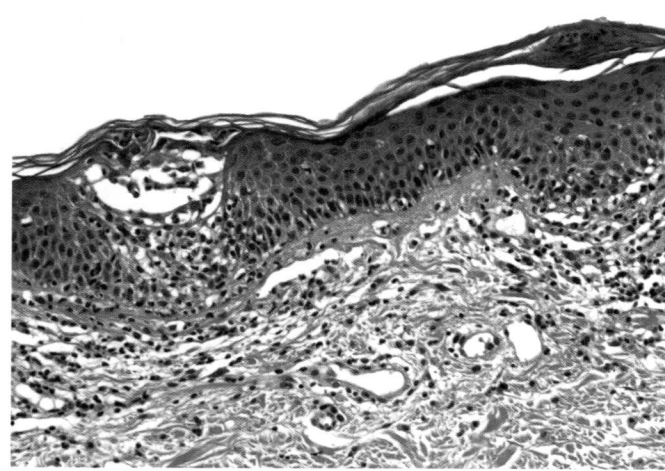

Figure 38-22. The histopathologic findings in Sézary syndrome often fall short of being diagnostic. In this example, there is too much spongiosis for an outright diagnosis without knowing the clinical and peripheral blood findings.

lymphocytes can be large, although the cells will not appear atypical in some cases. Nonetheless, performing skin biopsies as a method to diagnose Sézary syndrome can be a frustrating exercise because spongiosis can be the predominant finding and epidermotropism may be absent (Fig. 38-22). In fact, one study showed that diagnostic findings of Sézary syndrome are present in 60% of cases.[116] Therefore, the lack of a diagnostic biopsy does not exclude Sézary syndrome. As such, if Sézary syndrome is a serious clinical consideration, evaluation of the peripheral blood for the presence of a clone or an abnormal immunophenotype as assessed by flow cytometry should be performed. If these tests show findings that meet the criteria for diagnosis, the patient should be classified as having Sézary syndrome with nondiagnostic skin biopsies.

Differential Diagnosis

Because of the many inflammatory conditions that cause erythroderma and because of the lack of diagnostic changes in the biopsy specimens of many patients with Sézary syndrome, one must approach the differential diagnosis of erythroderma with great caution. The most common causes of erythroderma include psoriasis, pityriasis rubra pilaris, generalized allergic contact dermatitis, and drug eruptions. In some patients the erythroderma resolves spontaneously, and its cause is never determined. In general, the histopathologic features of erythrodermic presentations of inflammatory skin diseases are those of the underlying condition.

The findings in erythrodermic psoriasis resemble those of early patches of psoriasis rather than well-developed plaques. The rete ridges are slightly elongated; keratinocytes have pale cytoplasm; and dilated, tortuous vessels are prominent in edematous dermal papillae and may even appear to touch the undersurface of the epidermis. Small mounds of parakeratosis, both with and without neutrophils, may be present.

Pityriasis rubra pilaris shares many features with psoriasis, but it presents with diffuse orange-red skin. The palms and soles of affected patients are often thickened by cornified material that has been likened to carnauba wax. Biopsy

specimens of pityriasis rubra pilaris often show slight psoriasiform epidermal hyperplasia, an epidermis with a gently undulating surface, and lamellar hyperkeratosis containing scattered parakeratotic nuclei.

Erythrodermic allergic contact dermatitis represents a generalized response to a contactant. Its features are essentially those of a conventional spongiotic dermatitis. There may be more of a tendency for the inflammatory cells in the papillary dermis to have a bandlike pattern than in conventional allergic contact dermatitis.

Erythrodermic drug eruptions have a variety of histopathologic presentations. These include the findings of spongiotic dermatitis, interface dermatitis, and, rarely, psoriasiform dermatitis.

Pearls and Pitfalls

Diagnosing Early Mycosis Fungoides

- Diagnosis during the patch stage is optimal but may not influence survival.
- Overdiagnosis of mycosis fungoides can be emotionally traumatic to patients.
- Immunophenotypic studies are usually not essential for diagnosis and do not provide prognostic information.
- Genotypic studies are useful for confirming the diagnosis only if mycosis fungoides is clinically and pathologically plausible. T-cell clonality is not equivalent to the diagnosis of a lymphoid neoplasm.
- There are myriad inflammatory skin diseases, and many can simulate mycosis fungoides clinically and pathologically. The diagnosis of mycosis fungoides is best established with the collaboration of a knowledgeable clinician, unless the histopathologic findings are unequivocal.

KEY REFERENCES

2. Willemze R, Jaffe E, Burg G, et al. WHO-EORTC classification for primary cutaneous lymphoma. *Blood.* 2005;105:3768–3785.
4. van Doorn R, van Kester MS, Dijkman R, et al. Oncogenomic analysis of mycosis fungoides reveals major differences with Sézary syndrome. *Blood.* 2009;113:127–136.
6. Campbell JJ, Clark RA, Watanabe R, et al. Sezary syndrome and mycosis fungoides arise from distinct T-cell subsets: a biologic rationale for their distinct clinical behaviors. *Blood.* 2010;116(5):767–771.
21. Massone C, Kodama K, Kerl H, Cerroni L. Histopathologic features of early (patch) lesions of mycosis fungoides: a morphologic study on 745 biopsy specimens from 427 patients. *Am J Surg Pathol.* 2005;29:550–560.
22. Nickoloff BJ. Light-microscopic assessment of 100 patients with patch/plaque-stage mycosis fungoides. *Am J Dermatopathol.* 1988;10:469–477.
24. Salhany KE, Cousar JB, Greer JP, et al. Transformation of cutaneous T cell lymphoma to large cell lymphoma. A clinicopathologic and immunologic study. *Am J Pathol.* 1988;132:265–277.
26. Diamandidou E, Colome-Grimmer M, Fayad L, et al. Transformation of mycosis fungoides/Sézary syndrome: clinical characteristics and prognosis. *Blood.* 1998;92:1150–1159.
42. Tensen CP, Quint KD, Vermeer MH. Genetic and epigenetic insights into cutaneous T-cell lymphoma. *Blood.* 2022;139(1):15–33.

45. Kim YH, Liu HL, Mraz-Gernhard S, et al. Long-term outcome of 525 patients with mycosis fungoides and Sézary syndrome: clinical prognostic factors and risk for disease progression. *Arch Dermatol.* 2003;139:857–866.

69. van Doorn R, Scheffer E, Willemze R. Follicular mycosis fungoides, a distinct disease entity with or without associated follicular mucinosis: a clinicopathologic and follow-up study of 51 patients. *Arch Dermatol.* 2002;138:191–198.

102. Olsen E, Vonderheid E, Pimpinelli N, et al. Revisions to the staging and classification of mycosis fungoides and Sézary syndrome: a proposal of the International Society for Cutaneous Lymphomas (ISCL) and the cutaneous lymphoma task force of the European Organization of Research and Treatment of Cancer (EORTC). *Blood.* 2007;1101:1713–1722.

116. Trotter MJ, Whittaker SJ, Orchard GE, et al. Cutaneous histopathology of Sézary syndrome: a study of 41 cases with a proven circulating T-cell clone. *J Cutan Pathol.* 1997;24:286–291.

Visit Elsevier eBooks+ for the complete set of references.

Chapter 39

Primary Cutaneous CD30-Positive T-Cell Lymphoproliferative Disorders

Werner Kempf and Marshall E. Kadin

DEFINITION

Primary cutaneous CD30-positive T-cell lymphoproliferative disorders (CD30+ LPDs) are the second-most-common form of cutaneous T-cell lymphoma (CTCL), accounting for 25% to 30% of CTCLs. Three types of CD30+ LPDs are recognized in the 4th, revised 4th, and proposed 5th editions of the World Health Organization (WHO) classification, the WHO-EORTC classification, and the 2022 International Consensus Classification (ICC): primary cutaneous anaplastic large cell lymphoma (C-ALCL), lymphomatoid papulosis (LyP), and borderline lesions. These entities represent a continuous spectrum with overlapping clinical and histopathological features (Table 39-1).[1-3]

LyP is defined by multiple recurrent, papulonodular lesions up to 2 cm in diameter that may become centrally necrotic and may ulcerate.[4] The individual lesions regress spontaneously, usually in 4 to 6 weeks, occasionally leaving a hyperpigmented or hypopigmented scar.[5,6] C-ALCL commonly presents as one to several tumors greater than 2 cm in diameter and is often solitary or localized, but can present with multifocal lesions in some cases.[4,6] The tumors of primary C-ALCL frequently ulcerate. Partial or complete regression of tumors occurs at diagnosis or relapse in up to 42% of patients.[7] Occasionally LyP and C-ALCL cannot be distinguished even by a clinicopathologic correlation. For these lesions, the term *borderline lesion* can be used. Borderline lesions are intermediate in size, clinical appearance, and histology and usually persist for several months if not treated (Fig. 39-1).[8]

Primary cutaneous CD30-positive T-cell LPDs present in the skin without extranodal manifestations at the time of diagnosis.[4,7] Primary cutaneous CD30-positive T-cell LPDs must be distinguished from secondary cutaneous manifestations of systemic ALCLs and from other CTCLs such as mycosis fungoides (MF) or Sézary syndrome (SS) that may show expression of CD30 by tumor cells, usually in advanced disease. Secondary CD30-positive cutaneous lesions generally have a worse prognosis than primary cutaneous CD30+ LPDs.[7,9]

SYNONYMS AND RELATED TERMS

Lymphomatoid papulosis
Cutaneous anaplastic large cell lymphoma

EPIDEMIOLOGY

LyP has an incidence of 1.2 to 1.9 cases per 1,000,000 people.[7,10-12] The peak incidence is in the 4th and 5th decades (median age 35–45 years), although children younger than 10 years and patients up to 80 years old can be affected.[13,14] The male-to-female ratio for LyP patients from 10 published series is 1.5:1.[7,10-12,15,16]

For primary C-ALCL, the male-to-female ratio is 2.5:1.[7] Primary C-ALCL can occur in children; importantly, not all cases of C-ALCL in children should be considered secondary manifestations of systemic ALCL. Lack of anaplastic lymphoma kinase (ALK) expression favors primary C-ALCL.

The LyP registry data at Beth Israel Deaconess Medical Center in Boston revealed an interesting bimodal distribution of patients at age of diagnosis. Most patients younger than 19 years were male, and most of those aged 19 or older at diagnosis were female.

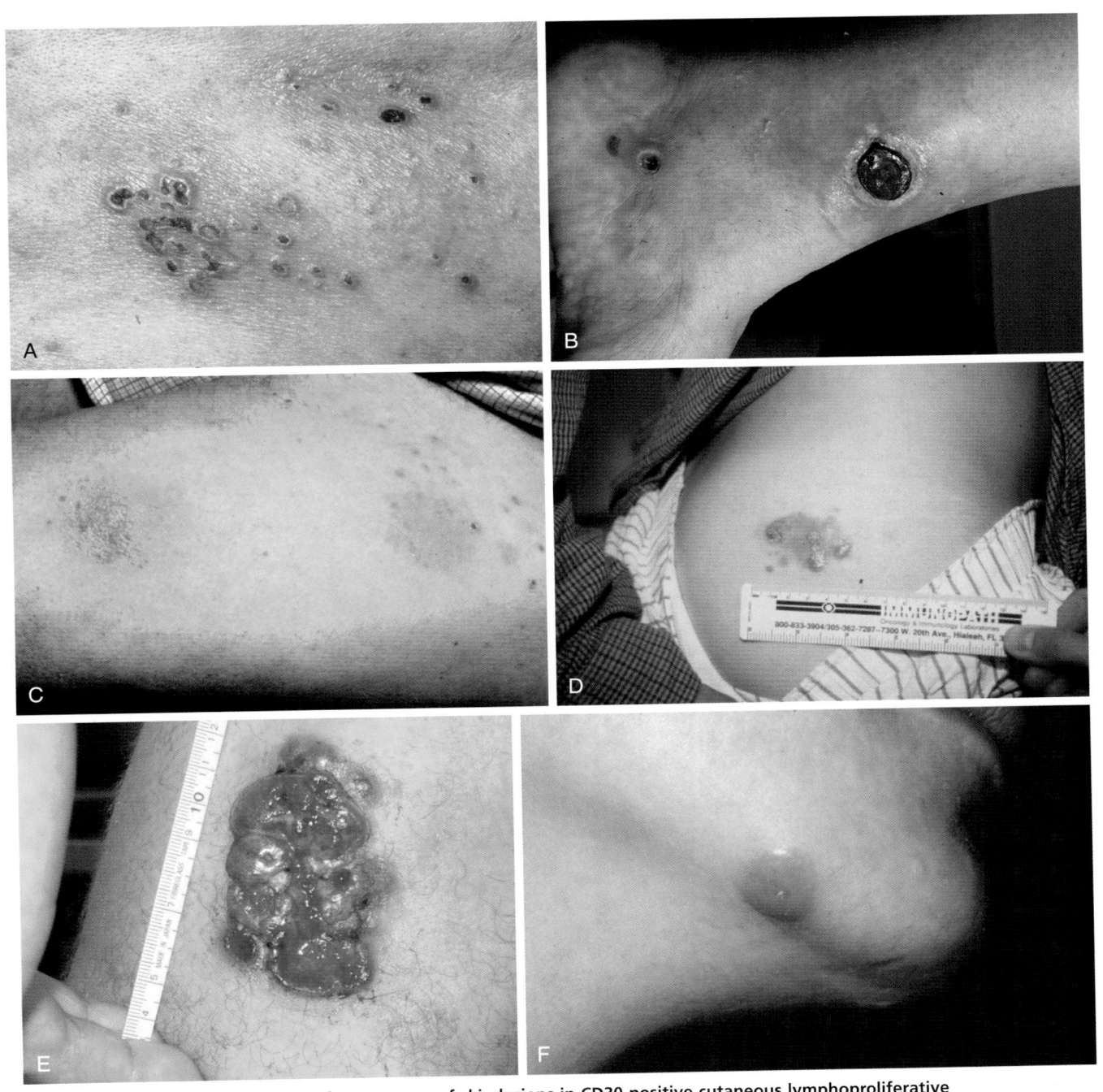

Figure 39-1. Clinical appearance of skin lesions in CD30-positive cutaneous lymphoproliferative diseases. A, Clustered lesions of lymphomatoid papulosis (LyP) with necrotic centers in various stages of spontaneous regression. **B,** Eschar as a result of angioinvasive LyP type E. **C,** Coexistent lesions of LyP and patch-stage mycosis fungoides. **D,** Coalescence of multiple separate lesions to form a cutaneous anaplastic large cell lymphoma (C-ALCL). **E,** Multiple clustered tumors of C-ALCL. **F,** Borderline lesion of intermediate appearance. No regression was observed.

Two-thirds of 35 patients who developed LyP in childhood (younger than 18 years) had atopy, which is significantly more than the expected prevalence (relative risk, 3.1; 95% confidence interval [CI], 2.2–4.3).[14] Fletcher et al. reported four cases of primary cutaneous CD30+ LPDs (one LyP, three C-ALCLs) in young adult patients with active atopic eczema since early childhood.[17] These results from separate medical centers suggest an association between primary cutaneous CD30+ LPDs and atopy.[18]

A remarkable association between LyP and other lymphomas occurs in 10% up to 62% of patients (for details

see Kempf et al. 2014).[19] The most common lymphomas are MF, Hodgkin lymphoma (HL), and ALCL.[7,10,12,15,16,20-26] In addition, the incidence of non-hematologic neoplasms such as breast cancer seems also to be increased in patients with LyP.[22,26] A case-control study revealed that of 57 LyP patients, 3 had HL, 3 had non-HL, 10 had MF, and 4 had nonlymphoid malignancies (1 brain tumor, 2 lung cancers, 1 breast cancer).[15] In addition, four patients had received radiation therapy 8 to 40 years before the onset of LyP. None of 67 age-and-gender-matched controls had any history of radiation or

Table 39-1 Major Distinguishing Features of Primary Cutaneous CD30-Positive T-Cell Lymphoproliferative Disorders

	LyP	C-ALCL	Borderline Lesions
Clinical	Crops of papules with central necrosis; spontaneous regression mostly within a few weeks	One to several, often localized ulcerating nodules or tumors; partial or complete regression (10%–42% of the cases)	Intermediate-size nodules (1–2 cm); tendency for slow regression
Histopathology	Various histologic types (A–E) and one distinct genetic type (DUSP22/IRF4 rearrangement) Early lesions have superficial dermal perivascular infiltrates Atypical large cells scattered and concentrated around blood vessels, surrounded by inflammatory cells (eosinophils, neutrophils, histiocytes) Fully developed lesions show wedge-shaped infiltrate	Dense dermal infiltrate, generally sparing epidermis; some exocytosis of atypical lymphocytes possible; infiltrate extends into and often involves subcutis Confluent sheets of large atypical cells Inflammatory cells confined to periphery, except for numerous PMNs in neutrophil-rich variant	Clusters or sheets of large atypical cells usually confined to dermis, but sometimes extending focally into subcutis Admixture of inflammatory cells Often a spectrum of cerebriform and large RS-like cells
Immunophenotype	CD30+, CD4+, LCA+, TIA-1+ Less frequently CD8+	CD30+, CD4+, LCA+, TIA-1+ Less frequently CD8+	CD30+, CD4+, LCA+, TIA-1+
Genetics	Absence of t(2;5)(p23;q35) Diploid or aneuploid Polyclonal, oligoclonal, or monoclonal by TCR gene analysis IRF4 translocations in a small subset of cases (<5% of the cases)	Absence of t(2;5)(p23;q35) except in rare cases, primarily in children* Complex aneuploid karyotype Clonal by TCR analysis IRF4 translocations in approx. one-third of C-ALCL	Absence of t(2;5)(p23;q35) No data on cytogenetics Clonal by TCR gene analysis

*As an exception, a very small subset of C-ALCL carries t(2;5)(p23;q35) and expresses ALK, but shows a similar biological behavior as ALK-negative C-ALCL.
C-ALCL, Cutaneous anaplastic large cell lymphoma; *LCA,* leukocyte common antigen; *LyP,* lymphomatoid papulosis; *PMN,* polymorphonuclear leukocyte; *RS,* Reed-Sternberg; *TCR,* T-cell receptor.

lymphoid or nonlymphoid malignancy. A Dutch study of 118 LyP patients found that 23 (19%) had lymphomas (11 MF, 10 C-ALCL, 2 HL).[7] In addition to lymphomas, prospective follow-up of our 57 LyP case-control patients revealed a high frequency of nonlymphoid malignancies (10 of 57; 18%). The relative risk of developing lymphoid and nonlymphoid malignancies in this cohort of patients over 8.5 years of follow-up was 13 (95% CI, 2.2–44) and 3.1 (95% CI, 1.206–6.47), respectively.[22] The factors that predispose these patients to develop malignancies are unknown. Possible risk factors based mostly on small case series include age at onset, male gender, histologic subtype, and expression of fascin by CD30-positive cells in LyP.[12,14,27-29] For example, Dutch investigators found that patients with type C LyP have an increased risk of developing malignant lymphoma, whereas none of seven patients with pure type B lesions had or developed a malignant lymphoma.[27] Clinical manifestations of MF or HL can occur before, after, or simultaneously with LyP. In nearly all cases, LyP lesions precede the development of C-ALCL.[27]

ETIOLOGY

The etiology of LyP and C-ALCL is unknown. A viral origin was initially suspected but has not been confirmed.[30-32] Human T-lymphotropic virus 1 (HTLV-1), herpesviruses 6, 7, and 8, and Epstein-Barr virus (EBV) could not be detected in primary skin lesions or in cell lines derived from CD30-positive cutaneous lymphomas.[33-35] Interestingly, sequences of endogenous retroviral elements were identified, but their role still needs to be elucidated.[35]

CD30 expression is a hallmark of LyP and C-ALCL.[36-38] CD30 is a "late" activation antigen maximally expressed 72 hours after lymphocyte activation in vitro.[39] Engagement of CD30 by its natural ligand CD30L (CD156) can lead to sustained proliferation, cell cycle arrest, or apoptosis, depending on the target cell, its state of differentiation, and environmental costimulatory signals.[40-43] CD30

cross-linking of ALCL cell lines clonally derived from LyP causes upregulation of nuclear factor-κB (NF-κB) and ERK/MAP kinases, promoting cell survival and proliferation.[42] CD30 activation also enhances expression of FLICE-like inhibitory protein, which protects lymphocytes from apoptosis induced by Fas/CD95.[44] Our studies suggest that the level of CD30 transcription is genetically determined, rendering some individuals more or less susceptible to CD30+ LPDs, including primary cutaneous LPDs.[45] This might explain LyP patients' increased risk of developing HL and ALCL. Because LyP patients have a significantly increased risk of both lymphoid and nonlymphoid malignancies, an as-yet-undefined genetic defect that is not limited to lymphoid cells is suspected.[22]

CLINICAL FEATURES

LyP lesions appear as self-healing papules, which may develop a necrotic center (Fig. 39-1A).[5] Occasionally, larger eschar-type ulcerated lesions result from angioinvasive LyP (type E) (Fig. 39-1B).[46] Typically, lesions in different evolutionary stages are present at the same time.[7,12] Most lesions are asymptomatic, but patients rarely experience itching. LyP lesions often appear in clusters and recur in the same region of the body. Extremities, trunk, and particularly the buttocks are most commonly affected. Lesions occur infrequently on the face, palms, soles, and anogenital areas and only rarely on mucous membranes.[47,48] These clinical observations raise the possibility that cytokines or chemokines released from epidermal keratinocytes or Langerhans cells may contribute to the development of LyP.

Patients experience the development of new lesions while others are regressing, and lesions may persist for several months.[7,12] LyP lesions occur in crops, often with long lesion-free intervals. LyP lesions often reoccur in the original site. In some women, LyP lesions appear to be modulated by the menstrual cycle or develop during pregnancy.[49] LyP lesions occur in crops, often with long lesion-free intervals. In other patients, one or a few lesions grow progressively to form a primary C-ALCL (Fig. 39-1D). Large lesions often ulcerate centrally and show some degree of spontaneous regression, even after 2 to 3 months. In a few patients, continual eruptions of papulo-nodules histologically typical of LyP occur in a well-circumscribed area, equivalent to limited plaque MF (Fig. 39-1C), which is also referred to as *persistent agminated LyP*.[50] In borderline lesions, the distinction between C-ALCL and LyP cannot be established (Fig. 39-1F); however, in most patients, follow-up clarifies the lesion type.[4]

C-ALCL usually presents as solitary or grouped (localized) rapidly growing tumors reaching several centimeters in diameter or thick plaques (Fig. 39-1E); presentation with multifocal tumors is rare. Tumors tend to undergo ulceration. Spontaneous complete or partial regression was reported in the literature to occur in 10% to 42% of the cases, but in our experience complete regression of C-ALCL is a rare phenomenon.[51] Spontaneous regression is associated with a good prognosis.[9]

Regional lymphadenopathy can develop and likely represents the local spread of tumor cells (Fig. 39-2). The prognosis does not appear to be affected by regional lymphadenopathy.[7,52,53] Regional lymph node enlargement can also represent dermatopathic lymphadenopathy. Staging procedures are generally not warranted for asymptomatic patients with uncomplicated LyP.

The development of systemic symptoms of fatigue, fever, weight loss, night sweats, or bone pain should raise the possibility of systemic lymphoma complicating LyP. In these individuals, more extensive staging with imaging of the chest and abdomen (i.e., PET-CT) should be done. Abdominal or intrathoracic lymphadenopathy should be regarded as highly suspicious for nodal lymphoma. Bone lesions have been observed in some LyP patients who developed systemic CD30-positive ALCL (Fig. 39-3).

Staging procedures are recommended for C-ALCL.[54] Bone marrow examination is not recommended owing to the low frequency of involvement.[55] A Sézary preparation or flow cytometry of the peripheral blood is not necessary in patients with uncomplicated primary cutaneous CD30+ LPDs. A chest radiograph is recommended to exclude asymptomatic mediastinal lymphadenopathy, which can be a presenting feature of nodal ALCL or HL. International consensus recommendations for management and treatment of primary cutaneous CD30-positive lymphoproliferative disorders have been reported in detail by the European Organization for Research and Treatment of Cancer, the International Society for Cutaneous Lymphomas, and the United States Cutaneous Lymphoma Consortium.[54]

Because of overlapping histologic features, CD30+ LPDs need to be differentiated from other cutaneous lymphomas, especially large cell transformation of MF, by a careful clinicopathologic correlation.[54,56] The development of persistent patches, plaques, or scaly erythematous lesions; hair loss; or onychodystrophy is indicative the presence of MF complicating LyP (Fig. 39-1C).

MORPHOLOGY

LyP lesions vary in appearance, depending on their stage of development at the time of biopsy (Fig. 39-4). Early lesions reveal mainly perivascular and superficial dermal accumulations of atypical lymphoid cells surrounded by variable numbers of inflammatory cells (Figs. 39-4A and Fig. 39-4C). Neutrophils within the lumens of blood vessels are a nearly constant feature of LyP (Fig. 39-4B). Neutrophils may percolate through the epidermis, accounting for the pustular appearance of LyP lesions. Histiocyte/macrophages may be numerous. Plasma cells generally are not prominent. Fully developed or late lesions are often wedge-shaped, sometimes extending into the deep dermis with little or no involvement of the subcutis in most cases (Fig. 39-4D). Hair follicles and sweat glands may be infiltrated by atypical cells. Other unusual histopathologic patterns associated with LyP include follicular mucinosis[57]; syringotropic infiltrates and syringosquamous metaplasia[58]; angiocentric/angiodestructive (Fig. 39-5G)[46,59]; and a bandlike rather than wedge-shaped distribution of lymphoid cells.[60] The atypical cells often concentrate around and can be found within the lumina of blood vessels.

LyP comprises six main histologic or genetic types, with some overlapping features (Table 39-2; Figs. 39-4 and 39-5).[6,7,46,61-63] Type A may resemble HL because of the presence of large Reed-Sternberg (RS)–like cells with prominent, often eosinophilic nucleoli (Fig. 39-5A). In some lesions, the atypical cells resemble immunoblasts with amphophilic to basophilic cytoplasm, slightly eccentric nuclei, and conspicuous but usually not huge nucleoli. Surrounding the large atypical cells are variable numbers of neutrophils, eosinophils, histiocytes, and small lymphocytes (Fig. 39-5B). In some cases LyP type A cells have a plasmacytoid appearance (Fig. 39-5C). When large atypical cells are confluent or occur in sheets confined to the dermis, with relatively few inflammatory cells, the lesion is classified as LyP type C (Fig. 39-5D). Type B lesions resemble MF with epidermotropism of small-to-medium-sized atypical lymphocytes (see Fig. 39-5E). The predominant cell is a mononuclear cell with nuclear irregularities, sometimes cerebriform, without prominent nucleoli. Mitoses are infrequent. Epidermotropism is often present. Neutrophils and other inflammatory cells are not abundant. There is some controversy over whether LyP type B lesions represent a papular variant of MF.[64] In contrast to LyP lesions, the papular lesions in MF do not show spontaneous regression. It is not uncommon to find LyP lesions that contain a spectrum of cerebriform cells to larger immunoblasts or RS-like cells with abundant inflammatory cells that makes distinction from inflammatory skin disorders such as arthropod bite reactions, infestation, or drug eruptions challenging in those cases. These lesions can be referred to as type A/B to indicate a hybrid or mixed histology.[6,65-67] Different histologic LyP types can be observed in lesions of the same patient at the same time point.[60]

LyP type D shows a prominent epidermotropism of CD8-positive small-to-medium-sized atypical lymphocytes in a pagetoid pattern (Fig. 39-5F). It must be distinguished from cutaneous CD8-positive aggressive epidermotropic cytotoxic T-cell lymphoma.[62] LyP type E is characterized by angioinvasive infiltrates of mostly medium-sized CD30-positive and often CD8-positive atypical lymphocytes resulting in extensive necrosis and clinically in eschar-like ulcers (Fig. 39-1B and Fig. 39-5G).[46]

LyP with 6p25.3 rearrangement is distinctive for a biphasic pattern with an epidermotropic and a dermal nodular component (Fig. 39-5H). Intraepidermal cells are small-to-medium-sized, whereas dermal cells are larger, but only

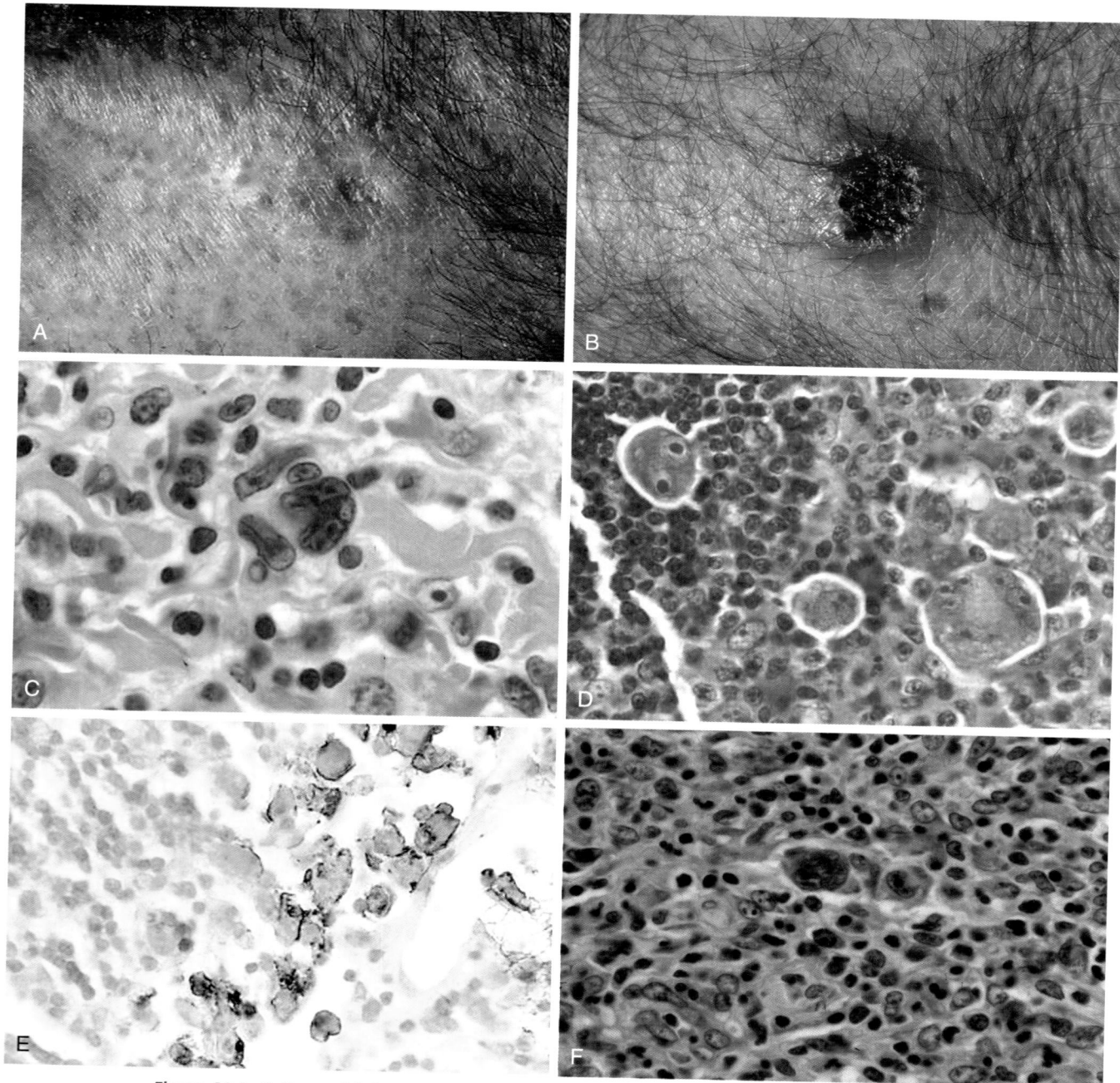

Figure 39-2. Patient with lymphomatoid papulosis, cutaneous anaplastic large cell lymphoma, and nodal lymphoma. A, Cluster of lymphomatoid papulosis (LyP) lesions. **B,** Ulcerated cutaneous anaplastic large cell lymphoma (C-ALCL). **C,** LyP showed anaplastic large cells in skin admixed with small lymphocytes and histiocytes. **D,** Lymph node with Reed-Sternberg (RS) cells and variants possibly representing classic Hodgkin lymphoma (HL) versus an ALCL. **E,** Staining of tumor cells for CD15. **F,** In a different patient with LyP, multinucleated cells are surrounded by eosinophils in a lymph node. Such cases raise the differential diagnosis of HL versus ALCL.

infrequently anaplastic. Dermal cells may infiltrate skin adnexae.[63]

C-ALCL commonly occurs as an extensive nodular dermal infiltrate, usually sparing the epidermis, and is composed almost entirely of large markedly pleomorphic anaplastic cells (Fig. 39-6A–D). The deep part of the lesion usually extends into the subcutis (Fig. 39-6B). Inflammatory cells are less frequent than in LyP; they are often nearly absent or confined to the lesion's periphery. An exception is the neutrophil-rich variant of C-ALCL (Fig. 39-6E), in which a confluence of neutrophils may obscure the appearance of the large atypical cells.[68,69]

Mitoses are common among the large atypical cells in LyP and especially in C-ALCL (Fig. 39-5B and Fig. 39-6D). Several studies indicate a high ratio of apoptotic cells to dividing cells in LyP. A significantly higher apoptotic index is found in LyP (12.5%) than in CD30-positive large T-cell lymphoma (3.1%).[70] The high rate of apoptosis in LyP can be attributed in part to the low expression of BCL2[71,72] and the high expression of the proapoptotic protein BAX.[73] The proportion of CD30-positive cells expressing death receptor apoptosis pathway mediators FADD and cleaved caspase 3 is significantly higher in primary cutaneous CD30-positive LPDs than in systemic ALCL.[74] In regressing LyP lesions, binding of CD30 and its ligand was detected by immunohistochemistry.[75] The tumor microenvironment in LyP and C-ALCL is characterized by the presence of numerous tumor-associated macrophages.[76]

Borderline lesions contain an extensive infiltrate or sheets of atypical cells with focal extension into the subcutis, making them difficult to distinguish from LyP type C or C-ALCL.[54,77]

IMMUNOPHENOTYPE

The usual immunophenotype of the large atypical cells in LyP (Fig. 39-7A) is that of activated helper T lymphocytes expressing CD4 and lymphocyte activation antigens such as CD30 (Fig. 39-7B), CD25, CD71, and HLA-DR.[36-38] Other T-cell antigens (e.g., CD3, CD2, CD5, CD7) are often not expressed, resulting in an aberrant T-cell phenotype (Fig. 39-7C).[78] A natural killer (NK)–cell phenotype for the large atypical cells was noted in 10% to nearly 50% of cases in one study, but in none of 18 cases in another study.[60,79] In one series, one-third of cases had a CD8-positive phenotype.[60] CD8-positive LyP type D can be confused with aggressive epidermotropic CD8-positive cytotoxic T-cell lymphoma.[62,80] LyP type E, which expresses CD8 in 70% of cases, can mimic angioinvasive lymphomas such as extranodal NK/T-cell lymphoma, nasal type and peripheral T-cell lymphoma, not otherwise specified (NOS).[46] LyP with 6p25.3 rearrangement often displays a CD4/CD8 double-negative phenotype.

In most cases, the atypical cells express cytotoxic proteins, including TIA-1, granzyme B, and perforin (Fig. 39-7D).[81] ALK is negative, leukocyte common antigen (LCA; CD45) is characteristically expressed, and CD15 is absent in most LyP

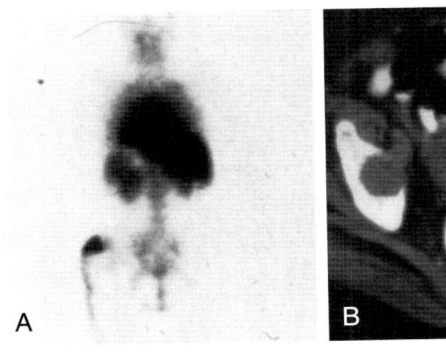
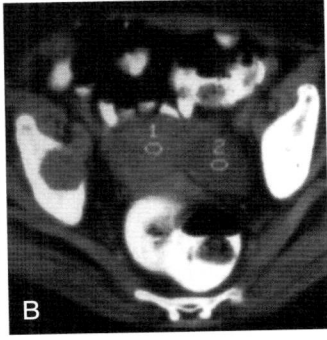

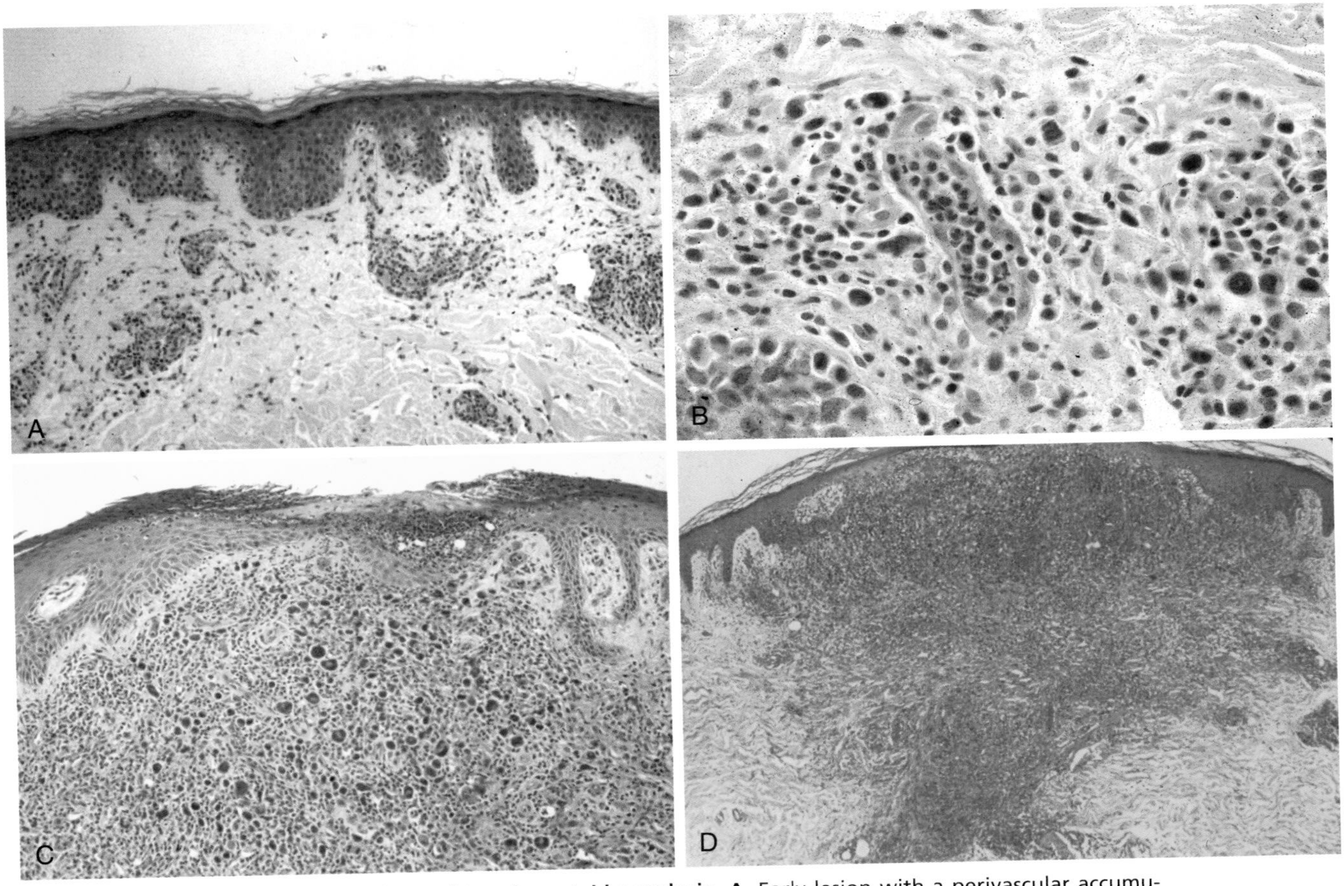

Figure 39-3. Bone lesions in two patients with cutaneous anaplastic large cell lymphoma secondary to lymphomatoid papulosis. A, Bone scan shows an area of increased activity in the right ileum. **B,** Computed tomography scan shows a large, round lytic lesion in the ileum of a second patient.

Figure 39-4. Histology of lymphomatoid papulosis. A, Early lesion with a perivascular accumulation of atypical lymphocytes. **B,** Collection of neutrophils in a dermal venule surrounded by anaplastic cells, characteristic of lymphomatoid papulosis (LyP). **C,** Erosion of the epidermis and scattered anaplastic cells in LyP. **D,** Fully developed wedge-shaped lesion.

cases. EBV (EBER, LMP-1) is not found in LyP and C-ALCL. This profile helps distinguish LyP and ALCL from HL.[82]

C-ALCL also displays an activated T-cell phenotype and expresses CLA, may show loss of T-cell antigens, especially CD3, and frequent expression of cytotoxic molecules.[7,81,83] C-ALCL can exhibit a CD4-positive CD8-negative or CD4-negative CD8-positive phenotype, but double-positive or double-negative cases were also observed.[84] CD30 must be expressed by at least 75% of large cells.[85] Epithelial membrane antigen (EMA) and ALK staining is usually absent in C-ALCL, in contrast to systemic ALCL.[86,87] Rare cases of ALK-positive C-ALCL, however, have been documented (Fig. 39-8) (see also Genetics and Molecular Findings).[88] IRF4/MUM1 encoded by the *IRF4* gene is strongly positive, and CD15 is expressed

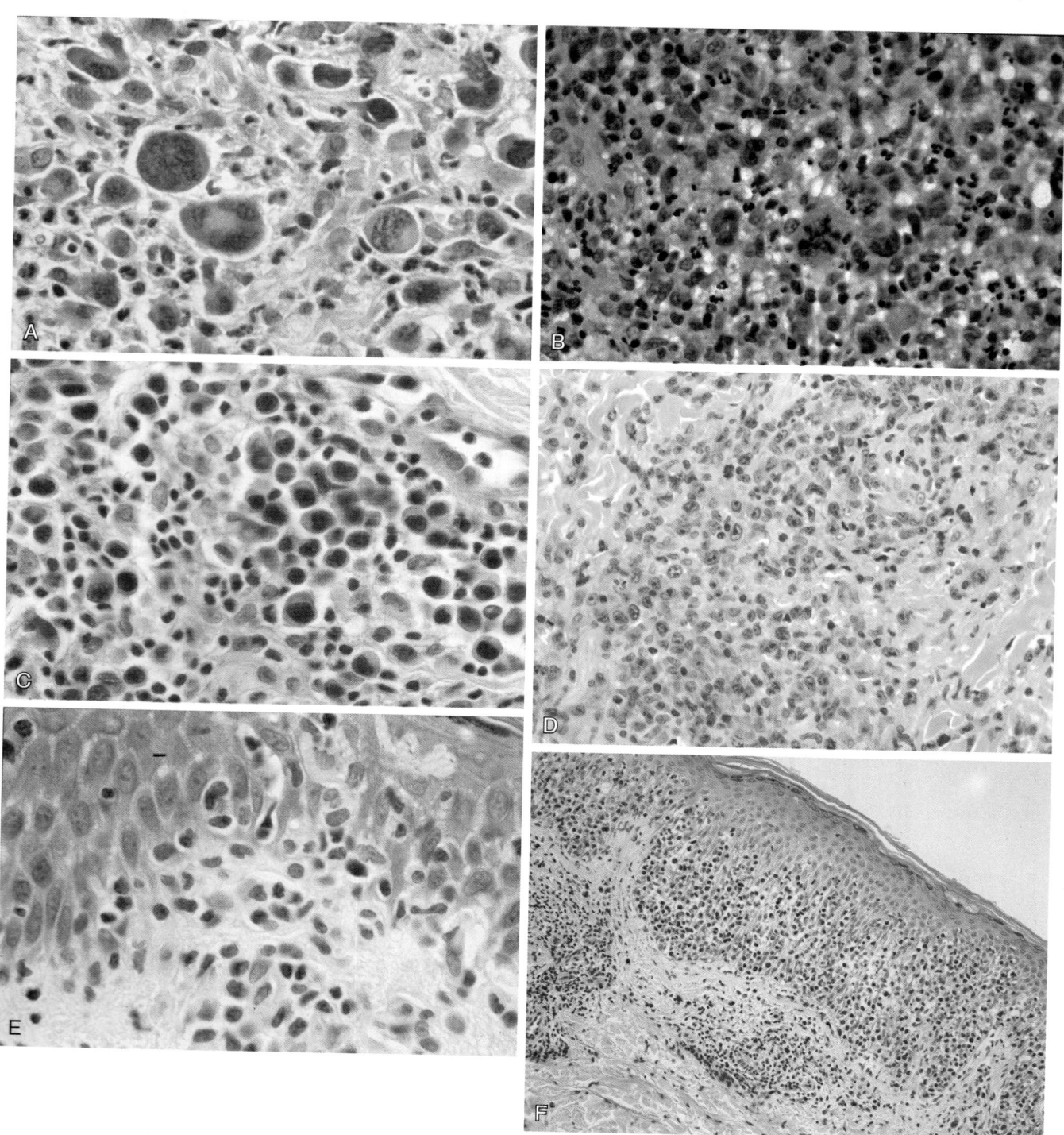

Figure 39-5. A, LyP type A with Reed-Sternberg (RS)–like cells surrounded by inflammatory cells. Apoptotic bodies are present. **B,** Minority of large, atypical cells and abnormal mitosis surrounded by numerous neutrophils and eosinophils in LyP. **C,** LyP cells with plasmacytoid morphology. **D,** LyP type C with sheets of large cells in the dermis. **E,** LyP type B with epidermotropic cerebriform cells. **F,** LyP type D with pagetoid infiltration of the epidermis.

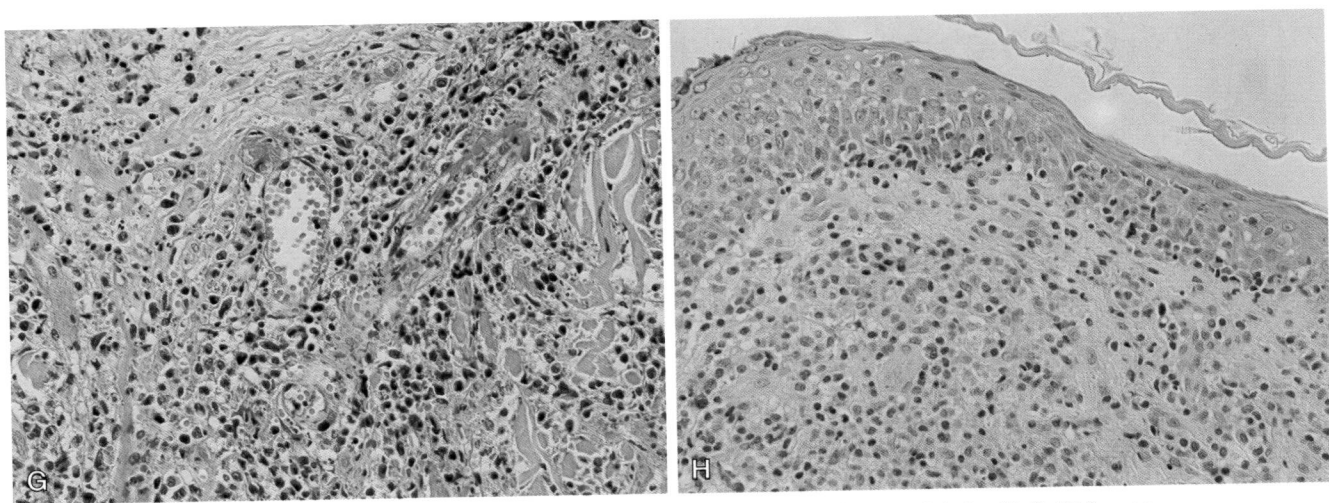

Figure 39-5, cont'd. **G,** LyP type E with angioinvasive lymphoid infiltrate. **H,** LyP with 6p25.3 gene rearrangement. Note biphasic morphology with small irregular epidermotropic lymphocytes and admixture of larger cells with pale nuclei in dermis.

Table 39-2 Comparison of Six Major Subtypes of Lymphomatoid Papulosis

	Type A	Type B	Type C	Type D	Type E	6p25.3 Rearrangement
Growth pattern	Dermal, wedge-shaped infiltrate	Epidermotropic	Dermal, nodular, or wedge shaped	Epidermotropic (pagetoid) and dermal infiltrate	Angioinvasive	Biphasic: Epidermotropic and dermal nodular infiltrate
Cytology	Immunoblasts, sometimes Reed-Sternberg–like cells	Cerebriform cells	Immunoblasts, sometimes a spectrum of cerebriform cells and immunoblasts	Small-to-medium-sized pleomorphic cells	Medium-sized pleomorphic cells	Small-to-medium-sized epidermotropic cells and medium-sized dermal cells
Inflammatory cells	Numerous	Infrequent	Variable	Few to moderate	Variable	Variable
Mitoses	Frequent	Infrequent	Frequent	Infrequent	Frequent	Infrequent
Phenotype	CD4+ > CD8+	CD4+	CD4+ > CD8+	CD8+	CD8+ > CD4+	CD4− CD8−
Differential diagnoses	MF (tumor); C-ALCL Arthropod bite reaction, infestation, viral infections	MF (patch/plaque)	C-ALCL; systemic ALCL; ATLL	Primary cutaneous CD8+ aggressive epidermotropic cytotoxic T-cell lymphoma; cutaneous gamma/delta T-cell lymphoma	Extranodal NK/T-cell lymphoma, nasal type; cutaneous gamma/delta T-cell lymphoma	MF (tumor); C-ALCL

ALCL, Anaplastic large cell lymphoma; *ATLL,* adult T-cell leukemia/lymphoma; *C-ALCL,* cutaneous anaplastic large cell lymphoma; *NK,* natural killer.

in about half of the cases.[89] C-ALCLs commonly express skin-homing molecules such as CCR4, CCR10, and CCR8 as well as homeobox gene *HOXC5* and CD158k.[90-94] SATB1 (special AT-rich sequence-binding protein) is a thymocyte nuclear protein and chromatin organizer that is crucial to T lymphocyte development. It is expressed in most LyP cases with T helper 17 cytokines and repressed T helper genes and is expressed in 40% of C-ALCL.[95]

GENETICS AND MOLECULAR FINDINGS

Clonal rearrangements of the T-cell receptor (TCR) beta or gamma chain genes have been detected in nearly all C-ALCLs and in most individual lesions of LyP.[21,65,96-100] The frequency of clonal rearrangements in LyP varies from 20% to 100%,

depending on the method and the tissue (fresh versus archival tissue, with or without microdissection) used. Weiss and associates reported clonal or oligoclonal T-cell populations detected by Southern blot in LyP.[98] In one patient studied at multiple sites, different clonal populations were detected. Using Southern blot, Whittaker and coworkers reported clones in most type B and mixed type A/B lesions but in no pure type A lesions of LyP.[100] Analyzing archival (i.e., formalin-fixed paraffin embedded) LyP biopsies, Greisser et al. found clonal T-cells in 20% to 70% of LyP lesions.[101] These results demonstrate that the lack of detection of T-cell clonality does not argue against the diagnosis of LyP. Using a more sensitive polymerase chain reaction (PCR) approach with variable region–specific primers, Chott and colleagues found dominant T-cell clones in 9 of 11 LyP patients.[65] In several patients, the

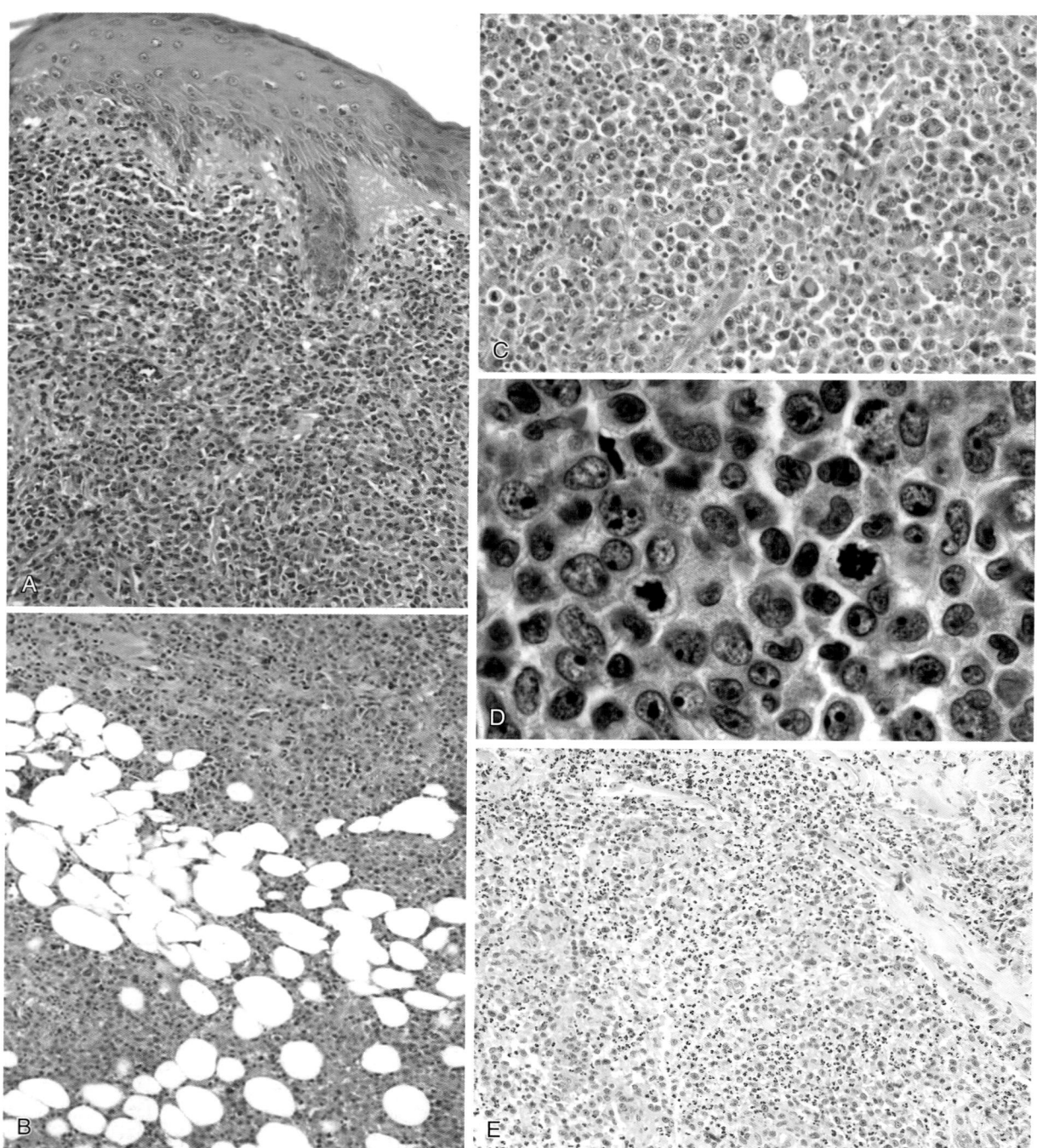

Figure 39-6. Histology of CD30-positive cutaneous anaplastic large cell lymphoma. A, Dense infiltrate of lymphoma cells throughout the dermis. **B,** Extension of lymphoma into the subcutis. **C,** Large anaplastic cells surrounded by neutrophils in cutaneous anaplastic large cell lymphoma (C-ALCL). **D,** Large cells with pleomorphic, anaplastic morphology. **E,** Neutrophil-rich C-ALCL.

same clone was detected in LyP lesions of different histologic types. A single-cell analysis of CD30-positive cells in LyP demonstrated that they were monoclonal in each of the 11 patients evaluated.[102] One patient who had progressed from LyP to C-ALCL had the same dominant clone detected in all lesions. Humme and coworkers performed molecular genetic analysis of skin lesions and blood of LyP patients by combining TCR-PCR and beta-variable complementarity-determining region 3 (CDR3) spectratyping.[103] They were able to detect a clonal T-cell population in 36 of 43 skin samples (84%) and

in 35 of 83 blood samples (42%). Comparison of skin and blood demonstrated different T-cell clones, suggesting the unrelated nature of the clonal T cells in the skin and blood. Moreover, CDR3 spectratyping revealed a restricted T-cell repertoire in the blood, suggesting T-cell stimulation by an unknown antigen. The T-cell clone found in T-cell lymphomas that develop in patients with LyP is often the dominant clone in the LyP lesions.[21,65,96,104-107] Progression of LyP to C-ALCL appears to be associated with an altered response to CD30 signaling. Although CD30 ligand expression is quantitatively

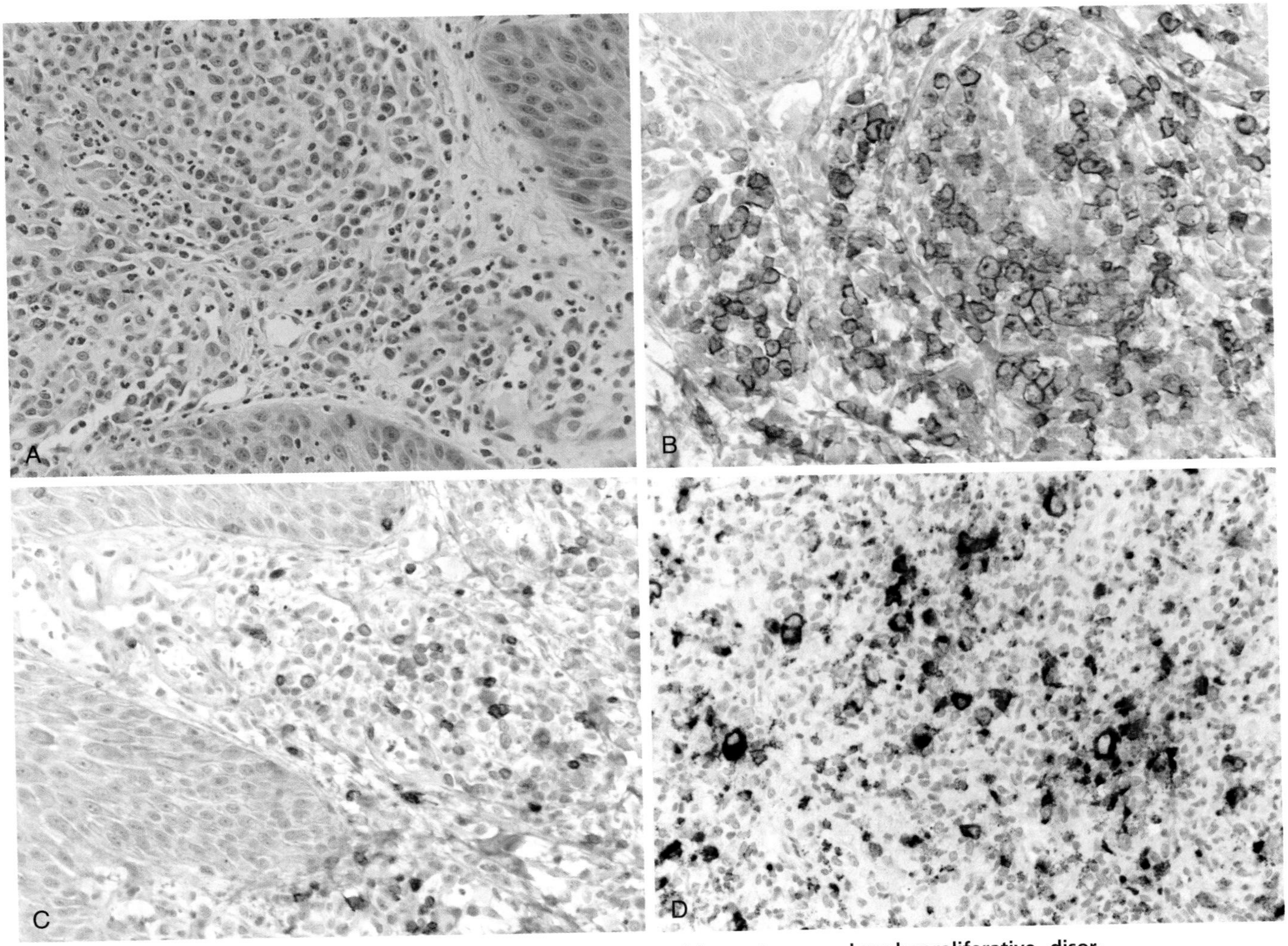

Figure 39-7. Immunohistochemistry of CD30-positive cutaneous lymphoproliferative disorders. A, Hematoxylin and eosin stain of large atypical cells and inflammatory infiltrate in lymphomatoid papulosis (LyP) type A. **B,** CD30 expression on atypical cells in LyP. **C,** CD3 expression on small T lymphocytes but not on atypical cells in LyP. Aberrant expression of T-cell antigens is common on large atypical cells in LyP. **D,** Staining for granzyme B in large atypical cells of LyP.

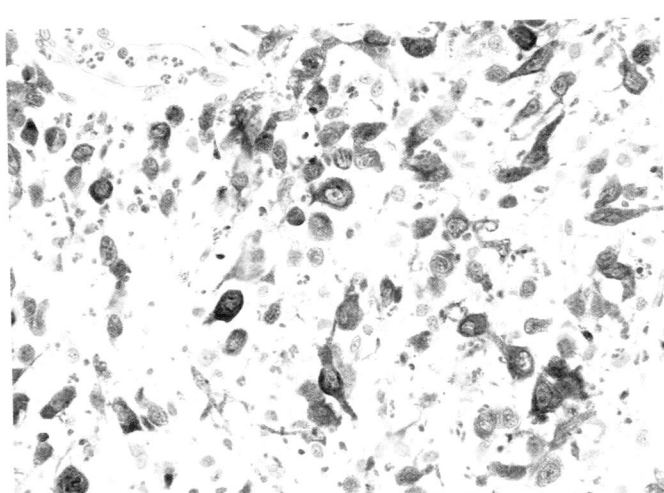

Figure 39-8. Cytoplasmic variant of anaplastic lymphoma kinase (ALK) in cutaneous anaplastic large cell lymphoma. Note the absence of staining over the nuclei of tumor cells. ALK was confirmed to be activated (phosphorylated) in this case.

increased in regressing CD30-positive skin lesions, CD30 ligation in C-ALCL cell lines that have progressed from LyP causes increased cell proliferation, associated with activation of NF κB.[42,75] CD30 ligation of NPM-ALK cell lines (e.g., Karpas 299) causes growth arrest by upregulation of cell cycle inhibitor p21 and accumulation of Rb (retinoblastoma) protein in the unphosphorylated state.[42,43] Thus, CD30 signaling plays an important role in the biology of LyP and ALCL.

DNA cytophotometry has shown that LyP cells may be diploid, hypertetraploid, or aneuploid. Willemze and associates found that aneuploidy is associated with a type A histology.[16,108,109] Cytogenetic studies of regressing lesions in LyP have demonstrated either a normal karyotype or numerical and structural abnormalities of chromosomes 7, 10, and 12.[110]

In contrast to systemic ALCL, the t(2;5)(p23;q35) translocations involving the ALK gene are absent in almost all C-ALCL cases.[110,111] Nevertheless, rare cases of ALK-positive C-ALCL have been reported in children and adults, in some patients after insect bites.[112] Both, cases with nuclear and cytoplasmic staining typical of the t(2;5) chromosomal translocation and cases expressing cytoplasmic ALK protein indicating a variant translocation were found.[88,113-115] Most ALK-positive C-ALCL have an excellent prognosis. In ALK-positive cases, however, staging and close follow-up are essential because the skin lesions could represent the first manifestation of a systemic ALCL.[116,117]

C-ALCLs display multiple complex karyotypic abnormalities.[118] Multiple chromosomal imbalances including gains of 7q31 and losses at 6q16-21 and 13q34 were identified in almost half of C-ALCL cases.[94,119,120] The most common regions of oncogene amplification involved CTSB (8p22), RAF1 (3p25), REL (2p12p12), and JUNB (19p13.2). Immunohistochemical studies support the amplification of JUNB in C-ALCL and LyP.[119,121] Allelic deletion at 9p21-22, causing inactivation of the p16 tumor suppressor gene, has been reported in some C-ALCL.[122] Loss of 9p21.3 harboring the tumor suppressor gene CDKN2A is rarely found in C-ALCL, which contrasts with MF (tumor stage) and peripheral T-cell lymphoma, unspecified/NOS.[123]

IRF4 translocations with DUSP22 rearrangement are found in approximately one-third of all cases.[124] In LyP, IRF4 translocations are present in less than 5% of the cases.[124] The clinical outcome of DUSP22-rearranged C-ALCL and LyP does not differ from that of nonrearranged cases.

Gene rearrangements of TP63 on chromosome 3q28 have been described in C-ALCL and exhibit an aggressive clinical course with unfavorable outcome.[92] Expression of TP63 protein assessed by immunohistochemistry does not necessarily indicate an underlying TP63 translocation which has to be evaluated by FISH analysis.

A novel recurrent NPM::TYK2 gene fusion, resulting in constitutive STAT signaling, has been identified in LyP and C-ALCL.[125] RNA sequencing of C-ALCL revealed overexpression of genes involved in the neurotrophin signaling pathway (NTRK1, NTRK2, NTF3, NGF), which activates the JAK/STAT, PI3K/Akt and MEK/ERK signaling cascades that promote proliferation and survival.[126]

JAK-STAT signaling is a common feature of all ALCL subtypes and is found also in C-ALCL and LyP. Highly recurrent activating hotspot mutations and oncogenic fusion transcripts affecting the JAK and signal transducer and activator of transcription (STAT) signaling pathway (STAT5A and DNMT3A mutations) are reported as common molecular mechanisms of transformation occurring in up to 50% of CD30-positive LPDs.[127] Oncogenic fusions were found in the JAK/signal transducer and activator of transcription signaling pathway, namely NPM::TYK2 in and ILF3::JAK2 in two patients with LyP and clonally related MF.[128] These data suggest that somatic mutations in JAK/STAT genes play a key role in the pathogenesis of CD30-positive LPD.

POSTULATED CELL OF ORIGIN

The cell of origin for LyP and C-ALCL is an activated helper T lymphocyte expressing cytotoxic proteins.[36-38,78] Most cases express TCR alpha/beta, but a small subset of LyP is derived from gamma-delta T cells.[129] In vitro studies of the cytokine profile of the CD30-positive cells point to a predominant Th2 type. The tumor cells secrete interleukin (IL)-4, IL-6, and IL-10 but not interferon (IFN)-gamma or IL-2. This is consistent with the usual functional profile of CD30-positive T lymphocytes.[130] The Th2 profile of LyP cells has justified the use of IFN-gamma in the treatment of primary cutaneous CD30-positive LPDs.[131] Alternatively, the CD30-positive cells in LyP and C-ALCL can have a phenotype (CD4 positive, CD25high, CD45RO positive, surface transforming growth factor-beta [TGF-beta] positive) consistent with induced regulatory T cells that can suppress proliferation and cytokine production of CD25-negative T cells, at least in part by the action of the inhibitory cytokine TGF-beta.[132] The suppressor activity of natural regulatory T cells requires cell contact and is mediated by granzyme B, a property of CD30-positive cells in LyP.[81,133] In contrast to natural regulatory T cells, the CD30-positive cells in LyP and C-ALCL generally lack FOXP3 expression, which, however, is expressed by tumor infiltrating lymphocytes.[134] A subset of primary cutaneous CD30+ LPD associated with pseudoepitheliomatous hyperplasia was shown to be associated with Th17 cytokines IL-17 and IL-22 detected in the cytoplasm of CD30-positive cells.[135]

CLINICAL COURSE

LyP usually follows a chronic course, with intermittent lesion-free periods. In many patients, LyP persists for years and decades; occasionally it is a lifelong disease, but in some patients, particularly children, the disease may spontaneously remit.[136,137] There is often a long delay before the correct diagnosis of LyP is made. Most patients with LyP do not require active treatment, at least not initially. If lesions are numerous, cause unsightly scarring, or occur on the face, hands, or other cosmetically undesirable areas, treatment with UVB narrowband PUVA or low-dose oral methotrexate (starting at 10–25 mg/week) is most effective; 90% of patients treated with methotrexate achieve a significant reduction in lesions, but recurrence after withdrawal is commonly seen.[54,138] Long-term treatment (i.e., maintenance therapy with low-dose MTX) requires monitoring of side effects such as liver fibrosis. PUVA accelerates photoaging of the skin and increases the risk of skin cancer.[139] Bexarotene is an RXR (retinoid X receptor)-selective retinoid that decreases the number or duration of LyP lesions when given orally or applied as a gel.[140] High-potency steroids applied topically have minimal benefit. These treatments suppress LyP, but the lesions are likely to recur when treatment is stopped. X-irradiation is an effective treatment for nonregressing skin lesions complicating LyP.[7,54] An observation period of 2 to 3 months is usually recommended before irradiation, because some lesions regress spontaneously even after months. Multiagent chemotherapy is not recommended for LyP as recurrence is almost always seen. Importantly, treatment is unlikely to prevent the development of LyP-associated lymphomas, particularly MF or HL, but it may inhibit the progression to C-ALCL.[7] No definite risk factors for tumor progression have been identified. However, mutations of receptors for the lymphocyte growth inhibitory cytokine TGF-beta, high expression of BCL2 genes, and expression of the cytoskeletal protein fascin have been associated with progression of LyP to C-ALCL.[29,71,141-143]

C-ALCL has a favorable prognosis with a 10-year-survival rate of 90%.[7,10] Multifocal presentation and involvement of loco-regional lymph nodes is not associated with impaired prognosis, but cases with extensive involvement of the legs and extracutaneous spread have a worse prognosis.[7,8,10,144] Sites of relapse in C-ALCL are unpredictable and may be either local or distant in the skin. Regional lymph nodes in proximity to large skin lesions are most often involved.

Table 39-3 Differential Diagnostic Features of CD30-Positive Primary Cutaneous Lymphoproliferative Disorders

	Systemic ALCL*	Hodgkin Lymphoma	Mycosis Fungoides	Pityriasis Lichenoides	Arthropod Bite	Scabies
Clinical	Generalized lymphadenopathy Lack of spontaneous regression	Advanced disease, generally has multifocal lymphadenopathy, splenomegaly Deep-seated tumors in primary cutaneous Hodgkin lymphoma	Scaling, erythematous patches or plaques; lack of central necrosis	Younger age Papular and scaly lesions Central hemorrhage	History of exposure Distribution of skin lesions Itching	History of exposure Distribution of skin lesions Itching
Histopathology and immunophenotype	Lack of epidermotropism and cerebriform cells	Classic HRS cells, CD15+, EBV+/−	Epidermotropism of cerebriform cells Lack of inflammatory cells and RS-like cells	Interface changes, scattered necrotic of keratinocytes Extravasation of erythrocytes Lack of RS-like cells	Wedge-shaped infiltrate Polymorphic inflammation CD30+ cells may be present Insect parts may be identified	Presence of mite in histologic sections CD30+ cells and B cells present
Genetics	t(2;5)(p23;q35) frequently present Clonal TCR	t(2;5)(p23;q35) absent TCR gene clonality generally absent	t(2;5)(p23;q35) absent TCR clonal in the majority of cases	Clonal TCR in up to 60% of cases	Polyclonal TCR genes	Polyclonal TCR genes

*Refers to ALK-positive and ALK-negative ALCL with *ALK* rearrangement always present in the ALK-positive cases.
ALCL, Anaplastic large cell lymphoma; *EBV,* Epstein-Barr virus; *HRS,* Hodgkin and Reed-Sternberg; *LCA,* leukocyte common antigen; *RS,* Reed-Sternberg; *TCR,* T-cell receptor.

Extracutaneous spread is often to the bony skeleton (see Fig. 39-3).[105] Patients with C-ALCL or HL may relapse with LyP after primary systemic therapy.[21,27,54,66] For solitary and localized C-ALCL lesions, surgical excision or radiation are the first-line treatment. Treatment for multifocal C-ALCL includes MTX and targeted therapy with brentuximab vedotin (BV), an anti-CD30-antibody conjugated to the cytotoxic agent monomethyl auristatin E (MMA).[54,145] Treatment with BV has been shown to be effective in cutaneous CD30+ LPD and in other CTCL with variable expression of CD30.[146,147] It represents a therapeutic alternative for patients with multifocal ALCL, extracutaneous spread, and LyP with disseminated lesions not responsive to other therapies. Treatment with BV is complicated by a sensory neuropathy affecting 40% of patients. Multiagent chemotherapy with CHOP (cyclophosphamide, hydroxydaunorubicin, Oncovin [vincristine], and prednisone or prednisolone) is only indicated for cases with extracutaneous spread and lack of response to BV.[7,9,54] Such aggressive approaches are not curative and should therefore be avoided because they produce unwarranted toxicity and limit future treatment options, particularly if the patient develops an extracutaneous lymphoma.

It is important to note that there is a tendency to treat LyP and C-ALCL too aggressively because of the high-grade histopathology, with many large atypical cells and high mitotic rate; frequent recurrences; and frequent clinicians' lack of familiarity with the natural history of the disease.[54,66] Clinicians may resort to systemic and even high-dose ablative chemotherapy with peripheral stem cell rescue or bone marrow transplantation.

DIFFERENTIAL DIAGNOSIS

Several neoplastic and non-neoplastic lesions may mimic primary cutaneous CD30+ LPDs either clinically or histologically (Table 39-3).

Systemic Anaplastic Large Cell Lymphoma

Systemic ALCL is associated with extranodal disease in 40% of cases, and the skin is the most common extranodal site.[148,149] Secondary skin lesions of systemic ALCL and C-ALCL can be histologically similar or even identical. Clinical features that favor primary C-ALCL are spontaneous regression, localized skin lesions, absence of lymphadenopathy, and age older than 30 years. Pathologic and immunophenotypic features that favor primary C-ALCL are tumor cells in the epidermis, absence of t(2;5) and lack of ALK staining, absence or only partial expression of EMA, and expression of cutaneous lymphocyte antigen.[80,88,150] The distinction between systemic ALCL and C-ALCL, however, has to be based on radiologic staging examination (i.e., PET-CT).

Mycosis Fungoides

MF can occur before, after, or simultaneously with LyP.[65,96,104,151] MF lesions are usually erythematous and scaly patches or plaques that can clinically be readily distinguished from LyP. In rare cases, however, MF can present with small papular lesions (referred to as papular MF) that clinically may closely resemble LyP.[107,152] In contrast to LyP, the papular lesions in MF do not show spontaneous regression.[64] MF lesions can be readily distinguished morphologically from LyP type A by the absence of RS-like cells and neutrophils. Epidermotropic infiltrates typically found in LyP type B are histologically indistinguishable from MF (patch stage). Pagetoid lesions of LyP type D can resemble MF but LyP type D is clinically characterized by papular lesions with spontaneous regression and histologically by predominant expression of CD8 and CD30.[62] Transformed or tumor-stage MF can present with cohesive sheets of large CD30-positive tumor cells that resemble LyP type C and C-ALCL. Clinicopathologic correlation is essential to distinguish MF from LyP.

Systemic Hodgkin Lymphoma

HL can involve the skin as a secondary site. This is usually a consequence of direct obstruction from regional lymph nodes and occurs only in advanced disease, when the diagnosis of HL is obvious.[153-155] Cutaneous lesions of secondary HL most commonly occur on the trunk. HL occurs with increased frequency in LyP patients and can appear before or after the clinical manifestations of LyP.[21,27,153,154] LyP can persist or recur after successful chemotherapy of HL and has no known adverse prognostic significance; therefore, the distinction of LyP from cutaneous HL is clinically important.[153] Clinically, LyP lesions regress, whereas those of secondary HL do not. LyP can be distinguished from HL by the expression of LCA and T-cell antigens and the absence of CD15 and EBV-associated antigens.[36,82,156]

Primary Cutaneous Hodgkin Lymphoma

Primary cutaneous HL is exceedingly rare and usually presents as solitary or multiple deep dermal lesions producing tumors on the extremities or trunk.[156,157] The skin lesions contain classic RS cells that have a CD15-positive, LCA-negative phenotype and may be positive for EBV-associated antigens (e.g., LMP-1).[156] Lesions of primary cutaneous HL do not regress. Patients with primary cutaneous HL appear to have a significant risk of developing nodal HL.[156]

Pityriasis Lichenoides

Pityriasis lichenoides et varioliformis acuta (PLEVA) and chronica (PLC) can be indistinguishable from LyP clinically and histologically (Fig. 39-9).[158-160] PLEVA tends to occur in

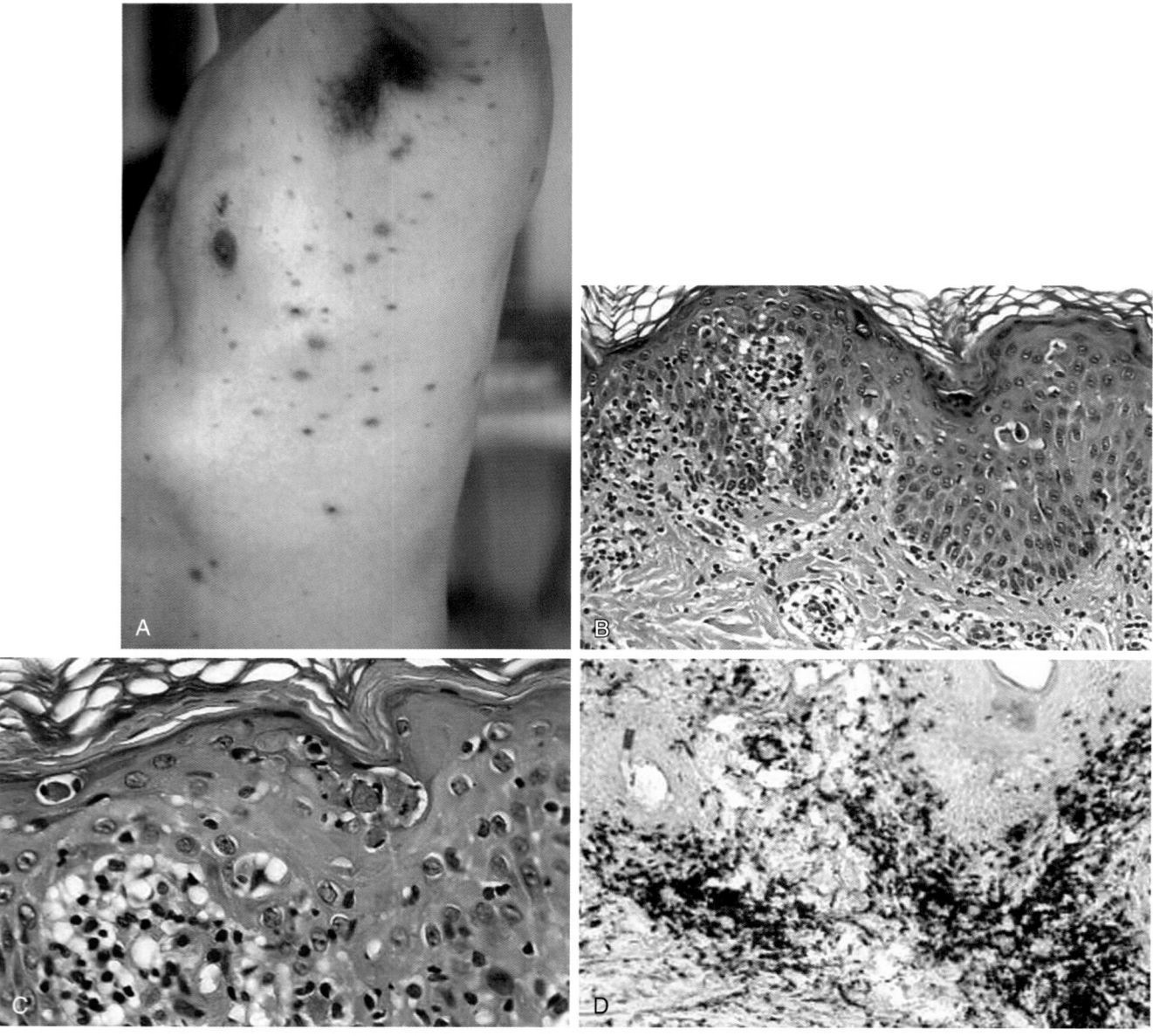

Figure 39-9. Pityriasis lichenoides et varioliformis acuta. A, Clinical photograph of centrally necrotic lesions on the thorax. **B,** Histology showing a lichenoid lymphoid infiltrate. **C,** Necrotic keratinocytes. **D,** Prevalence of CD8-positive cells.

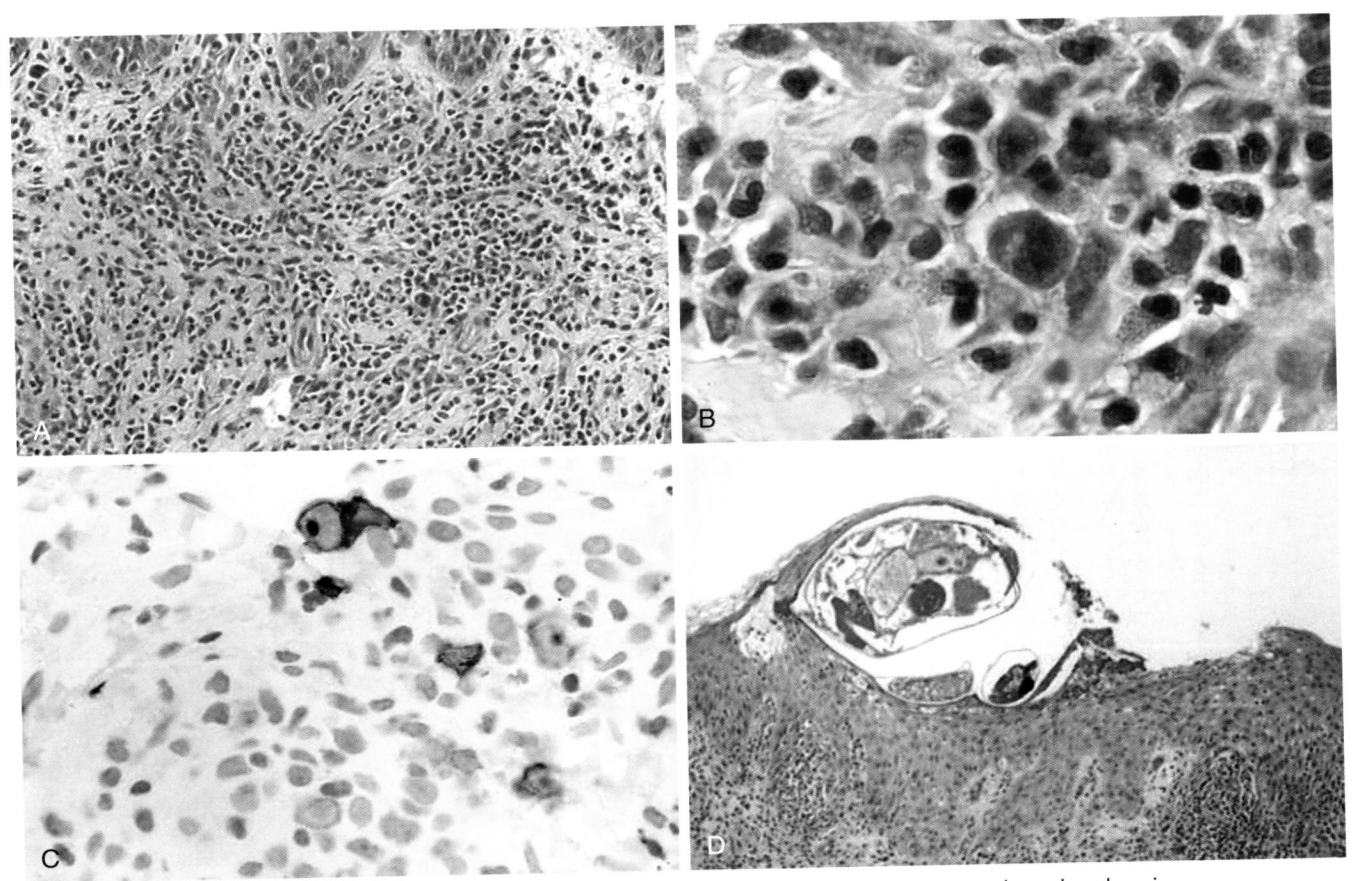

Figure 39-10. Nodular scabies resembling lymphomatoid papulosis. A, Dense dermal and perivascular infiltrate. **B,** Large atypical cell surrounded by eosinophils. **C,** CD30 stain of large atypical cells. **D,** Mite *(Sarcoptes scabiei var. hominis)* embedded in the epidermis.

patients younger than 30 years, is often not recurrent, and is not generally associated with an increased risk of developing malignant lymphoma.[161] However, a French study did report that 29% and 80% of children with LyP and MF, respectively, presented with PLC before onset of their disease.[162] Similar to LyP, clonality of T cells can be found in many PLEVA cases.[163] However, PLEVA usually lacks the large, atypical RS-like cells of LyP type A and has few neutrophils or eosinophils. PLEVA shows apoptotic keratinocytes and extravasation of erythrocytes. Neutrophils in blood vessels characteristic of LyP are lacking in PLEVA. The lichenoid lymphoid infiltrate in PLEVA usually lacks the frequent CD30-positive cells found in LyP and contains a predominance of CD8-positive cells, whereas CD4-positive cells predominate in LyP.[164] However, Kempf et al. reported exceptional cases of PLEVA with numerous CD30-positive cells mimicking LyP.[160] Parvovirus B19 DNA was identified in 4 of 10 cases investigated, suggesting a possible link of parvovirus B19 to this subset of PLEVA cases. Similar cases have been designated as atypical PLEVA.[165]

Arthropod Bite and Infestation

LyP can be confused with arthropod bites clinically and histologically.[166] A clinical history and follow-up may be necessary to exclude arthropod bite from the differential diagnosis of LyP type A.

Nodular scabies can closely resemble LyP clinically and histologically as scabies lesions often contain CD30-positive immunoblasts surrounded by inflammatory cells, usually eosinophils.[167] The key distinction is demonstration of the offending mite in scabies (Fig. 39-10). Detection of clonal T-cells is an argument for LyP and against inflammatory disorders such as arthropod bites and infestation.

Other Skin Conditions With CD30-Positive Large Cells

Several other cutaneous disorders that contain significant numbers of CD30-positive cells can enter into the differential diagnosis of primary cutaneous CD30+ LPDs. These include atopic dermatitis, molluscum contagiosum, herpes simplex infection, herpes varicella-zoster, tuberculosis, Milker's nodule, leishmaniasis, syphilis, lymphomatoid drug eruption, and hydroa vacciniforme lymphoproliferative disorder.[56,168-173] In most cases, the correct diagnosis can be established by clinical history, physical examination, and laboratory tests.

Pearls and Pitfalls

- Primary cutaneous CD30-positive T-cell lymphoproliferative disorder (CD30+ LPD) represents a spectrum including lymphomatoid papulosis (LyP), primary cutaneous anaplastic large cell lymphoma (C-ALCL), and borderline lesions with the expression of CD30 by atypical T-cells as the common denominator.
- LyP and C-ALCL display a phenotype of activated T helper cells, most commonly CD4 or CD8 positive, with frequent expression of cytotoxic markers and variable loss of T-cell antigens, especially CD3. Most cases are T-cell receptor (TCR) alpha/beta positive, but rare gamma/delta positive cases have been documented.
- In contrast to many cases of systemic ALCL, C-ALCL does not express anaplastic lymphoma kinase (ALK), does not harbor a t(2;5), and shows only partial or focal expression of epithelial membrane antigen (EMA).
- Very rare cases of C-ALCL show positivity for ALK without evidence of systemic ALCL at the time of diagnosis. These cases appear to have the same biological behavior as ALK-negative C-ALCL.
- LyP and C-ALCL exhibit overlapping histologic and phenotypic features not only with each other, but also with other cutaneous T-cell lymphomas (CTCLs) such as mycosis fungoides (MF), but also with systemic ALCL or Hodgkin lymphoma (HL). Therefore, clinicopathological correlation is essential to differentiate LyP from other T-cell lymphomas, especially MF, and staging examination is crucial for the distinction from cutaneous involvement by systemic ALCL or HL.
- Certain inflammatory (e.g., pityriasis lichenoides [PL]) or infectious skin diseases (e.g., arthropod bite reaction, infestation, viral infections) may simulate LyP, especially the histologic type A. Except for PL, often harboring a T-cell clone, detection of clonal T-cells can serve as an additional diagnostic clue for LyP.
- LyP has chronic course characterized by recurrent papulo-nodular lesions undergoing spontaneous regression within weeks to few months and an excellent prognosis. Approximately 15% to 20% of LyP patients develop MF, C-ALCL, systemic ALCL, or HL that may precede, occur synchronously, or occur after the diagnosis of LyP. Thus life-long follow-up is recommended.
- Treatment modalities for LyP include UV light (UVB narrow band or PUVA) or low-dose MTX, which is effective and indicated if numerous or socially stigmatizing lesions are present. Nodular lesions that may persist over months can be irradiated. In children, potent topical corticosteroids may be effective. Suppression of LyP during active treatment is usually temporary and does not prevent the development of LyP-associated lymphomas such as MF or HL. Thus a strategy without active intervention can be justified in individual patients.
- C-ALCL in general has a favorable prognosis with a 5-year survival rate of 90%. Loco-regional lymph node involvement in C-ALCL is not associated with impaired prognosis. There is an impaired prognosis (approximately 75%) in patients with extensive leg involvement or extracutaneous spread.
- Surgical excision or radiation are first-line therapies for solitary and localized C-ALCL. Low-dose MTX and CD30-targeting therapy with brentuximab vedotin are effective for multifocal C-ALCL.
- The correct diagnosis of LyP and C-ALCL is essential to avoid overtreatment. Neither LyP nor C-ALCL should be treated with multiagent chemotherapy with the exception of the rare event of extracutaneous spread, if other treatment strategies such as CD30-targeting therapies are not effective.

KEY REFERENCES

7. Bekkenk MW, Geelen FA, van Voorst Vader PC, et al. Primary and secondary cutaneous CD30(+) lymphoproliferative disorders: a report from the Dutch Cutaneous Lymphoma Group on the long-term follow-up data of 219 patients and guidelines for diagnosis and treatment. *Blood*. 2000;95(12):3653–3661.
54. Kempf W, Pfaltz K, Vermeer MH, et al. EORTC, ISCL, and USCLC consensus recommendations for the treatment of primary cutaneous CD30-positive lymphoproliferative disorders: lymphomatoid papulosis and primary cutaneous anaplastic large-cell lymphoma. *Blood*. 2011;118(15):4024–4035.
65. Chott A, Vonderheid EC, Olbricht S, Miao NN, Balk SP, Kadin ME. The dominant T cell clone is present in multiple regressing skin lesions and associated T cell lymphomas of patients with lymphomatoid papulosis. *J Invest Dermatol*. 1996;106(4):696–700.
66. Kadin ME. Current management of primary cutaneous CD30+ T-cell lymphoproliferative disorders. *Oncology (Williston Park)*. 2009;23(13):1158–1164.
102. Steinhoff M, Hummel M, Anagnostopoulos I, et al. Single-cell analysis of CD30+ cells in lymphomatoid papulosis demonstrates a common clonal T-cell origin. *Blood*. 2002;100(2):578–584.
135. Guitart J, Martinez-Escala ME, Deonizio JM, Gerami P, Kadin ME. CD30(+) cutaneous lymphoproliferative disorders with pseudocarcinomatous hyperplasia are associated with a T-helper-17 cytokine profile and infiltrating granulocytes. *J Am Acad Dermatol*. 2015;72(3):508–515.
138. Vonderheid EC, Sajjadian A, Kadin ME. Methotrexate is effective therapy for lymphomatoid papulosis and other primary cutaneous CD30-positive lymphoproliferative disorders. *J Am Acad Dermatol*. 1996;34(3):470–481.
150. DeCoteau JF, Butmarc JR, Kinney MC, Kadin ME. The t(2;5) chromosomal translocation is not a common feature of primary cutaneous CD30+ lymphoproliferative disorders: comparison with anaplastic large-cell lymphoma of nodal origin. *Blood*. 1996;87(8):3437–3441.
160. Kempf W, Kazakov DV, Palmedo G, Fraitag S, Schaerer L, Kutzner H. Pityriasis lichenoides et varioliformis acuta with numerous CD30+ cells: a variant mimicking lymphomatoid papulosis and other cutaneous lymphomas. A clinicopathologic, immunohistochemical, and molecular biological study of 13 cases. *Am J Surg Pathol*. 2012;36(7):1021–1029.

Visit Elsevier eBooks+ for the complete set of references.

Primary Cutaneous T-Cell Lymphomas: Rare Subtypes

Tony Petrella and Elaine S. Jaffe

INTRODUCTION

Cutaneous T-cell lymphomas (CTCLs) include, for the most part, mycosis fungoides (MF) and variants and cutaneous CD30-positive lymphoproliferative disorders, but other rare subtypes may be the source of diagnostic and therapeutic challenges. Some of these rare lymphomas show overlapping clinicopathologic features, and distinction from MF may be difficult or even impossible without proper history and complete clinical information. Despite extensive phenotypic and genotypic studies, a few cases may defy precise classification. In this context, some considerations are necessary.

Epidermotropism is not diagnostic of any type of cutaneous lymphoma. It can be encountered in different variants of CTCL and rarely in cutaneous B-cell lymphomas as well. Prominent epidermotropism of single lymphocytes (pagetoid epidermotropism), on the other hand, is usually observed in some cases of MF (pagetoid reticulosis, cytotoxic variants of MF) and in cutaneous aggressive cytotoxic natural killer (NK)/T-cell lymphomas (primary cutaneous γδ T-cell lymphoma [pcγδTCL], cutaneous aggressive epidermotropic CD8-positive cytotoxic T-cell lymphoma, and cutaneous extranodal NK/T-cell lymphoma, nasal-type [cENKTCL-NT]).

Prominent involvement of the subcutaneous fat with "rimming" of adipocytes is not synonymous with subcutaneous panniculitis-like T-cell lymphoma (SPTCL). It can be encountered in other types of CTCL as well (particularly pcγδTCL and cENKTCL-NT). Although association with Epstein-Barr virus (EBV) is typical of cENKTCL-NT, other T-cell and B-cell neoplasms can be positive for EBV, which may raise challenges for accurate diagnosis.

Many of the rare forms of cutaneous T-cell lymphoma have a cytotoxic phenotype. The histopathologic findings and differential diagnosis of these lesions are summarized in Table 40-1.

PRIMARY CUTANEOUS CD8-POSITIVE AGGRESSIVE EPIDERMOTROPIC CYTOTOXIC T-CELL LYMPHOMA

Definition

This is a cutaneous lymphoma composed of CD8-positive cytotoxic T lymphocytes, characterized morphologically by prominent epidermotropism and clinically by an aggressive clinical course.[1-4] In the past, this lymphoma was classified as either aggressive MF (MF tumeur d'emblée) or generalized pagetoid reticulosis (Ketron-Goodman type).

Synonyms and Related Terms

The same term is used in all contemporary classification systems: the International Consensus Classification (ICC, 2022); the revised World Health Organization (WHO) 4th edition of the Classification of Tumours of Haematopoietic and Lymphoid Tissues (2017), and the proposed WHO 5th edition of the Classification of Tumours of Haematopoietic and Lymphoid Tissues (2022).

Epidemiology

The tumor occurs in adults of both sexes with a slight male predominance. Only one case has been reported in a child.[5]

Etiology

The etiology is not known.

Clinical Features

Patients have localized or, more frequently, generalized patches, plaques, and tumors, almost invariably ulcerated (Fig. 40-1). Involvement of mucosal regions is common. Before a case is classified as primary cutaneous CD8-positive aggressive epidermotropic cytotoxic T-cell lymphoma, it is crucial to exclude a diagnosis of MF or of lymphomatoid papulosis.

Morphology

Histology reveals a plaquelike, nodular, or diffuse proliferation of lymphocytes with marked epidermotropism (Fig. 40-2). Although prominent epidermotropism may confer a so-called "pagetoid" appearance to the infiltrate, it may be less pronounced or even missing in some lesions, particularly in advanced stages; thus, lack of epidermotropic lymphocytes is not sufficient to rule out this entity. Spongiosis

Table 40-1 Histopathologic Differential Diagnostic Features of Cutaneous NK/T-Cell Lymphomas With Cytotoxic Phenotype

	pcγδTCL	cENKTCL-NT	pcAECD8CTCL	SPTCL	MF-C	LyP-D	cALCL	cPTCL-NOS	pcACD8TCLPD
Pagetoid epidermotropism	+/−	− (+)	+	−	+	+	− (+)	−	−
Subcutaneous panniculitis-like pattern	+	+	−	+	−	−	−	−	−
CD4	−	−	−	−	−	−	−	+	−
CD8	−/+	−	+	+	+	+	+/−	−/+	+
CD30	−	−	−	−	−	+	+	−	−
EBV	− (+)	+	−	− (+)	−	−	−	−	−
αβ phenotype	−	−/+	+	+	+	+	+	+	+
γδ phenotype	+	(+)	−	−	− (+)	− (+)	−	−	−
TCR-R monoclonal	+	−/+	+	+	+	+	−	+	+

cALCL, Cutaneous anaplastic large cell lymphoma; *cENKTCL-NT,* cutaneous extranodal NK/T-cell lymphoma, nasal-type; *cPTCL-NOS,* cutaneous peripheral T-cell lymphoma, not otherwise specified; *LyP-D,* lymphomatoid papulosis, type D; *MF-C,* mycosis fungoides, cytotoxic; *pcACD8TCLPD,* primary cutaneous acral CD8-positive T-cell lymphoproliferative disorder; *pcAECD8CTCL,* primary cutaneous aggressive epidermotropic CD8-positive cytotoxic T-cell lymphoma; *pcγδTCL,* primary cutaneous γδ T-cell lymphoma; *SPTCL,* subcutaneous panniculitis-like T-cell lymphoma; *TCR-R,* T-cell receptor gene rearrangement.

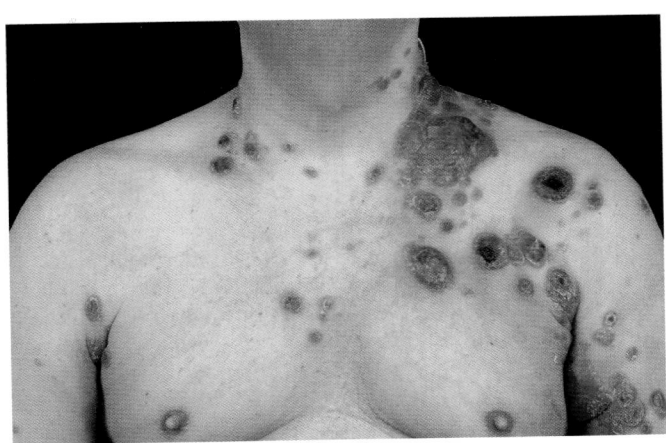

Figure 40-1. Primary cutaneous CD8-positive aggressive epidermotropic cytotoxic T-cell lymphoma. Partly ulcerated papules, plaques, and tumors.

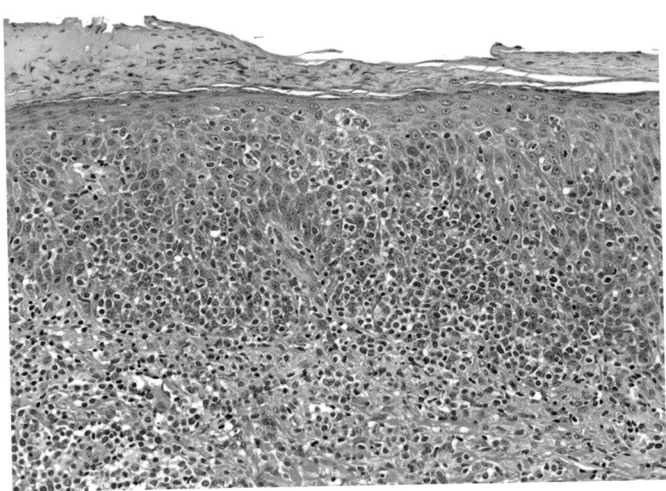

Figure 40-2. Primary cutaneous CD8-positive aggressive epidermotropic cytotoxic T-cell lymphoma. Prominent (pagetoid) epidermotropism of neoplastic lymphocytes.

and intraepidermal or subepidermal vesiculation may be observed. Invasion and destruction of adnexal skin structures are common, but angiocentricity and angiodestruction are infrequent. Cytomorphology is variable and can be characterized by small, medium-sized, or large pleomorphic cells.

Immunophenotype

Immunohistology reveals a characteristic phenotypic profile of neoplastic lymphocytes (βF1$^+$, TCRγ^-, CD2$^{-/+}$, CD3$^+$, CD4$^-$, CD5$^{-/+}$, CD7$^+$, CD8$^+$, TIA-1$^+$, granzyme B$^+$, CD30$^-$, CD45RA$^+$, CD45RO$^-$, CD56$^-$; Fig. 40-3), but pan–T-cell markers may be lost. EBV is not detectable in neoplastic cells.

Genetics

T-cell receptor (TCR) genes are monoclonally rearranged. Array comparative genomic hybridization has shown that gains (particularly in chromosomes 3, 7, 8, 11, 17, 18, and 22) are more frequent than losses (found frequently at 1p, 9p21, suggesting a role of *CDKN2A*, 13q, and 16p).[6-8] One study suggests this lymphoma could be a result of overactivation of the JAK2 signaling pathway via structural changes in *JAK2* and *SH2B3*.[9]

Clinical Course

The prognosis is poor, with an estimated 5-year survival of less than 10%. The disease often disseminates to the lung, testis, and central nervous system.

Differential Diagnoses

Distinction from cases of CD8-positive MF and from lymphomatoid papulosis type D is made mainly based on the clinical presentation and behavior. In contrast to MF, patients with primary cutaneous CD8-positive aggressive epidermotropic cytotoxic T-cell lymphoma present from the beginning with generalized plaques and tumors.

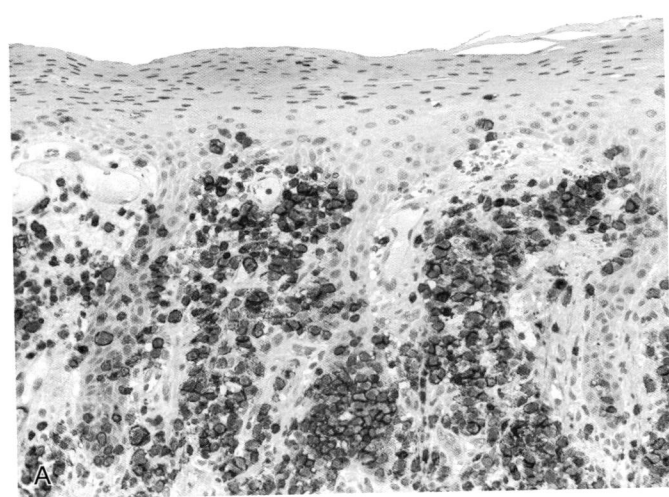
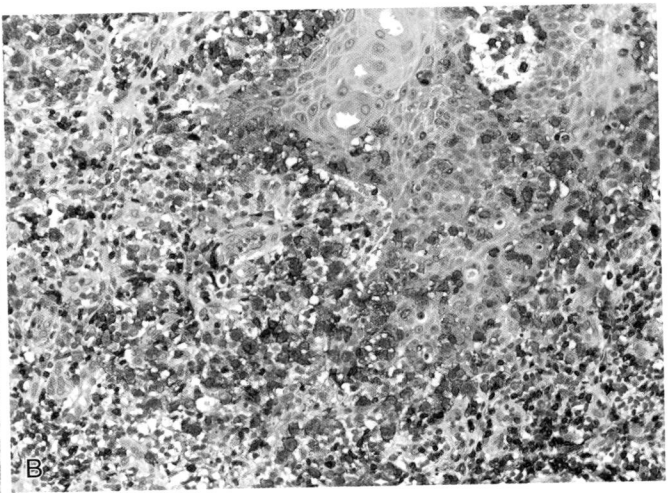

Figure 40-3. Primary cutaneous CD8-positive aggressive epidermotropic cytotoxic T-cell lymphoma. Strong positivity for CD8 **(A)** and βF1 **(B)**.

Lymphomatoid papulosis type D is characterized by the typical "waxing and waning" of papules and small nodules.[10]

Pediatric patients with a clinical presentation associated with sun exposure and positivity for EBV should be classified as hydroa vacciniforme lymphoproliferative disorder (LPD), either classic or systemic (see Chapter 29). Cases of CD8-positive T-cell lymphoma with exclusive involvement of the subcutis with rimming of fat spaces should be classified as SPTCL. Distinction of primary cutaneous CD8-positive aggressive epidermotropic cytotoxic T-cell lymphoma from cutaneous γδ T-cell lymphoma is achieved mainly by demonstration of expression of αβ and negativity for γδ. Primary cutaneous acral CD8-positive LPD is characterized by dermal infiltrates lacking epidermotropism and usually by solitary, nonulcerated lesions (mostly on the ears and face).

PRIMARY CUTANEOUS γδ T-CELL LYMPHOMA

Definition

pcγδTCL is a tumor of cytotoxic γδ T lymphocytes with specific tropism for the skin.[1,2] This lymphoma shows overlapping features with other CTCLs, particularly MF, SPTCL, and primary cutaneous CD8-positive aggressive epidermotropic cytotoxic T-cell lymphoma. Cases of pcγδTCL in the past have been classified as aggressive MF (MF tumeur d'emblée), generalized pagetoid reticulosis (Ketron-Goodman type), or subcutaneous T-cell lymphoma. It is crucial to remember that a γδ phenotype is not unique to pcγδTCL. It can be observed in several cutaneous (and extracutaneous) lymphoma types, including MF.[11,12]

Synonyms and Related Terms

The same term is used in all contemporary classification systems: ICC (2022), revised WHO 4th edition (2017), and proposed WHO 5th edition (2022).

Epidemiology

pcγδTCL occurs in adults, with an equal distribution between men and women. Cases in children have been reported.[13]

Etiology

Etiologic factors are not known.

Clinical Features

Patients have localized or generalized patches, plaques, and tumors, often ulcerated, and the clinical features may be indistinguishable from those of advanced MF (Fig. 40-4). In some patients, lesions are restricted to the lower extremities. Subcutaneous tumors may also be seen. Involvement of the mucosal regions is common. Lactate dehydrogenase is elevated in most patients,[14] whereas bone marrow involvement is uncommon. A hemophagocytic syndrome is a frequent complication. Almost one-fourth of the patients had an associated autoimmune disorder in one study,[14] and onset of pcγδTCL has also been observed during treatment with etanercept for rheumatoid arthritis.[15]

In addition to cutaneous and hepatosplenic cases, γδ T-cell lymphomas can be observed at other nodal or extranodal sites,[16] thus underlying the need for staging investigations.

Morphology

Histology reveals a diffuse proliferation of lymphocytes (Fig. 40-5), usually with prominent involvement of the subcutaneous tissue (Fig. 40-6A). Epidermotropism is variable and may be marked (pagetoid epidermotropism; Fig. 40-6B). Although epidermotropic lesions may resemble those observed in MF, unlike in MF, intraepidermal vesiculation and prominent edema within the papillary dermis are not uncommon in pcγδTCL. Angiocentricity or angiodestruction is a frequent finding (Fig. 40-7), sometimes with necrosis of the overlying epidermis. Cytomorphology is variable (small, medium-sized, or large pleomorphic cells) and is not related to prognosis. The neoplastic cells show frequent apoptosis, and admixed macrophages contain prominent phagocytosis of nuclear debris (Fig. 40-8).

Immunophenotype

Immunohistochemical demonstration of expression of TCRγ or TCRδ is a prerequisite for the diagnosis (Fig. 40-9).[12] In fact, lack of αβ expression is not synonymous with γδ differentiation, as "TCR-silent" (null-cell) cases negative for both αβ and γδ may be observed.[16] Immunohistology reveals a characteristic phenotypic profile of neoplastic lymphocytes (TCRγ+, TCRδ+, βF1−, CD3+, CD4−, CD8−, TIA-1+, CD56+, CD57−).[17] Some pan–T-cell markers may be lost, especially CD5. Almost one-fourth of pcγδTCL has expression of CD4 or CD8.[18] EBV is not present in the neoplastic cells. The classification of rare cases of CTCL with a γδ phenotype and positivity for EBV is ambiguous, as extranodal NK/T-cell lymphomas may exhibit a T-cell phenotype.[14,19,20] As mentioned, cutaneous aggressive

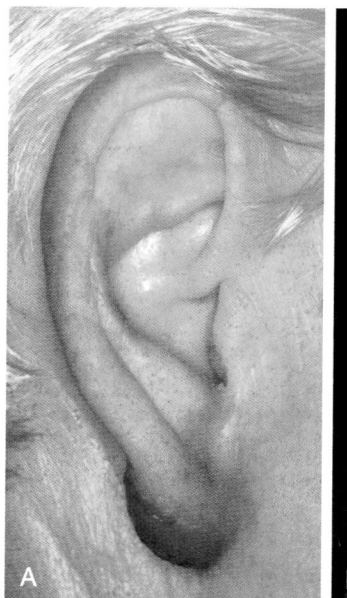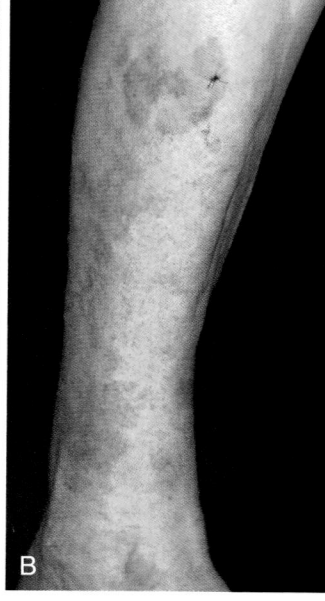

Figure 40-4. Primary cutaneous γδ T-cell lymphoma. Simultaneous occurrence of ulcerated tumor on the ear **(A)** and infiltrated patches and plaques on the leg **(B)**. These last lesions are indistinguishable from mycosis fungoides.

cytotoxic lymphomas present several overlapping features, and classification of a given case may be subjective.

Genetics

Molecular biology shows a monoclonal rearrangement of the TCR genes. γδ T-cell lymphomas (both cutaneous and extracutaneous) have a different molecular profile from αβ T-cell lymphomas, with overexpression of genes of NK-cell–associated molecules, such as killer-cell immunoglobulin-like receptor (*KIR*) genes (*KIR3DL1, KIR2DL2, KIR2DL4*) and killer-cell lectin-like receptor genes (*KLRC1, KLRC2, KLRC4*).[21] Hepatosplenic γδ T-cell lymphoma shows a different molecular profile from γδ T-cell lymphomas arising at other sites, including the skin.[21] Cytogenetic abnormalities including amplifications and deletions, and breakpoints in different chromosomes (1q, 15q, 7 q, 9p, 14 q, and 18q) were found.[22,23] Multiple alterations affecting several oncogenic pathways, including STAT3, STS5B, MYC, JAK/STAT, and MAPK and chromatin mutations have been described.[22-24]

Clinical Course

The prognosis of patients with pcγδTCL is poor, although rare patients may show a prolonged course.[25] As MF can present with a γδ cytotoxic phenotype, at least some of the cases of pcγδTCL reported to have an indolent behavior may in fact

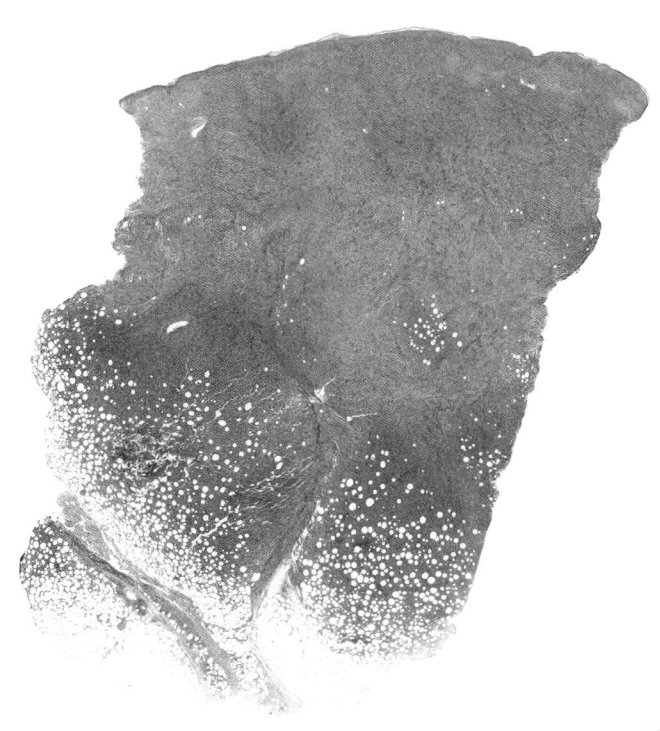

Figure 40-5. Primary cutaneous γδ T-cell lymphoma. Dense, diffuse infiltrates involving the entire dermis and subcutaneous tissue.

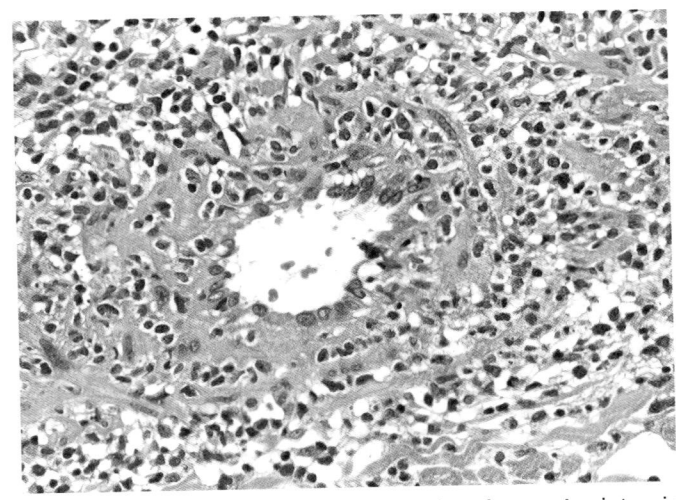

Figure 40-7. Primary cutaneous γδ T-cell lymphoma. Angiotropic lymphocytes with predominantly medium-sized pleomorphic nuclei.

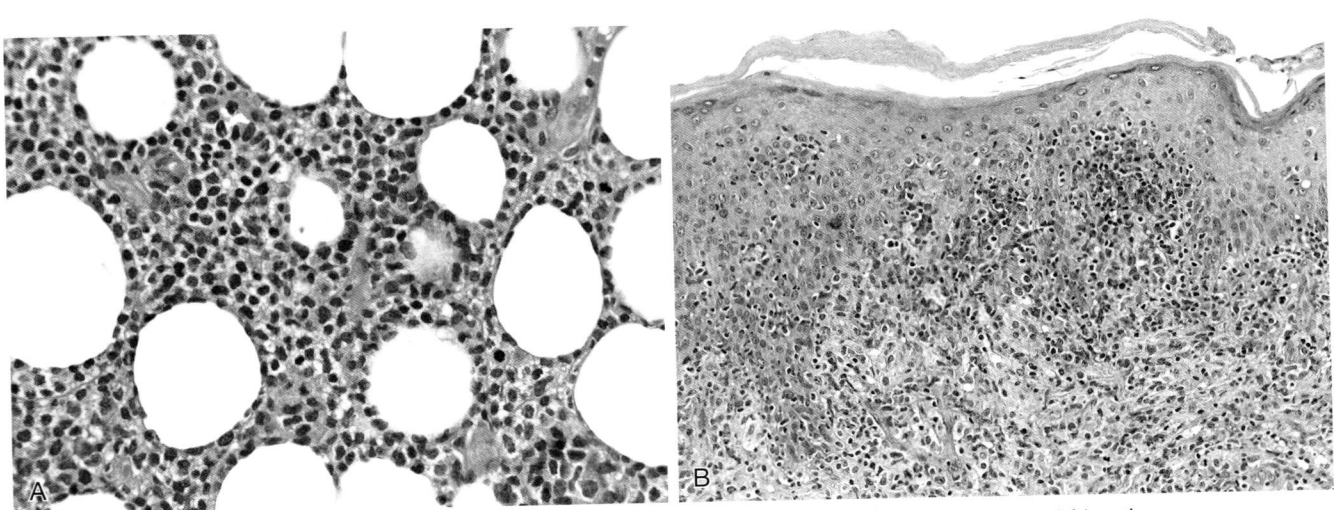

Figure 40-6. Primary cutaneous γδ T-cell lymphoma. A, Subcutaneous involvement mimicking the pattern of subcutaneous panniculitis-like T-cell lymphoma. **B,** Epidermotropism of pleomorphic lymphocytes.

have been examples of MF. The prognostic significance of epidermal involvement by pcγδTCL is unclear.[24,26]

Differential Diagnosis

Involvement of the dermis and epidermis allows a clear morphologic distinction from SPTCL, in which only the subcutaneous tissues are involved. Distinction from rare cases of conventional MF with γδ T-cell phenotype is made exclusively on the basis of the clinical presentation and behavior. In contrast to MF, patients with pcγδTCL show rapidly growing patches, plaques, and tumors already at onset of the disease. The distinction of pcγδTCL from primary cutaneous CD8-positive aggressive epidermotropic cytotoxic T-cell lymphoma is achieved by demonstration of the γδ phenotype of neoplastic cells. Distinction from cutaneous cENKTCL-NT may be impossible on morphology alone, as these two entities may show a similar, prominent involvement of both the epidermis and the subcutis. Demonstration of a γδ phenotype is suggestive of pcγδTCL, and positivity for EBV strongly supports a diagnosis of cENKTCL-NT. CD30

positivity and ALK negativity, along with the presence of hallmark cells, can mimic ALK-negative anaplastic large cell lymphoma. However, the presence of rimming of adipocytes and TCR γδ phenotype favors pcγδTCL.[27]

SUBCUTANEOUS PANNICULITIS-LIKE T-CELL LYMPHOMA

Definition

SPTCL is an αβ CD8-positive cytotoxic T-cell lymphoma restricted to the subcutaneous fat, characterized by histopathologic features that mimic those of a lobular panniculitis.[1,28,29] The association with hemophagocytic syndrome (HPS) in older cases led to misdiagnosis as malignant histiocytosis, termed "histiocytic cytophagic panniculitis." Cases with a γδ T-cell phenotype were formerly included with SPTCL, but based on aggressive behavior are now classified as pcγδTCL. In this context, a positive staining for the αβ receptor is mandatory for the diagnosis of SPTCL. Diagnostic criteria for SPTCL have evolved over the years.

Synonyms and Related Terms

The same term is used in all contemporary classification systems: ICC (2022), revised WHO 4th edition (2017), and proposed WHO 5th edition (2022).

Epidemiology

Patients are adults of both sexes, often with a variably long history of panniculitis (particularly lupus erythematosus panniculitis [LEP]). Reports in children exist, with variation in the clinical behavior.[30,31]

Etiology

The etiology of SPTCL is unknown. Autoimmune disorders, particularly lupus erythematosus, have been reported in a proportion of patients.[32,33] In a patient with lupus, the diagnosis should be made with caution, as lupus profundus can resemble SPTCL. The disease has been observed also in patients receiving immune modulatory drugs[34] and in an immunosuppressed patient after cardiac transplantation.[35]

A study showed that neoplastic lymphocytes express CCL5, a ligand for the C-chemokine receptor 5 expressed by adipocytes, providing a possible explanation for the tropism of neoplastic T lymphocytes for the adipose tissues.[36]

Clinical Features

Patients present clinically with solitary or multiple, infiltrated, subcutaneous (panniculitis-like) plaques or tumors, mostly located on the extremities (Fig. 40-10). Partial or complete spontaneous resolution of individual lesions may be observed, and patients respond well to immunomodulatory therapy in most instances.[37] A history of autoimmune disorders, particularly lupus erythematosus, is present in about 20% to 40% of patients,[33,37] and they may show positivity for antinuclear antibodies and subsets, hematologic changes, renal changes, and positive result of immunofluorescence testing on lesional skin.[32]

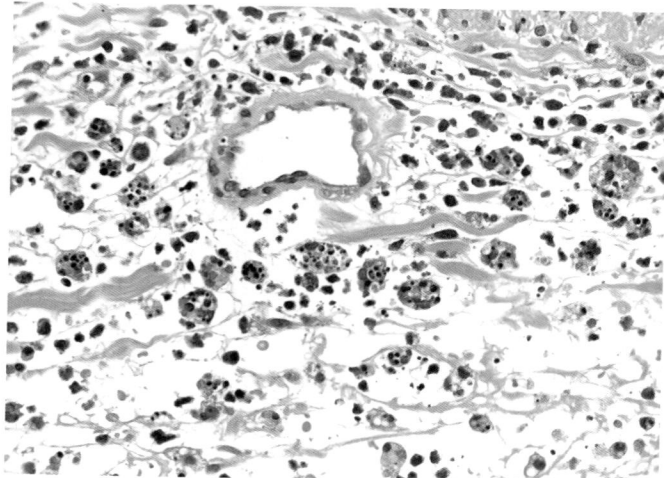

Figure 40-8. Primary cutaneous γδ T-cell lymphoma. Histiocytes showing features of hemophagocytosis.

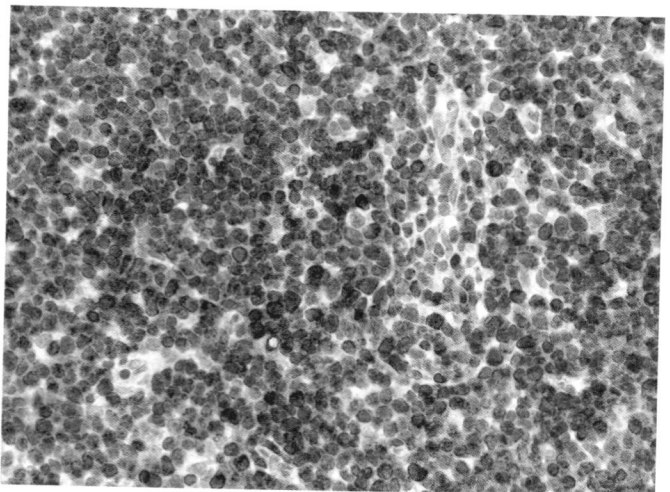

Figure 40-9. Primary cutaneous γδ T-cell lymphoma. Strong positivity for anti-TCRγ antibody.

In a small minority of patients, there are accompanying symptoms such as fever, malaise, fatigue, and weight loss. A hemophagocytic syndrome may be seen in advanced stages or, rarely, at first presentation and can be the cause of death.[32] A hemophagocytic syndrome, however, is more common in pcγδTCL or in cENKTCL-NT.

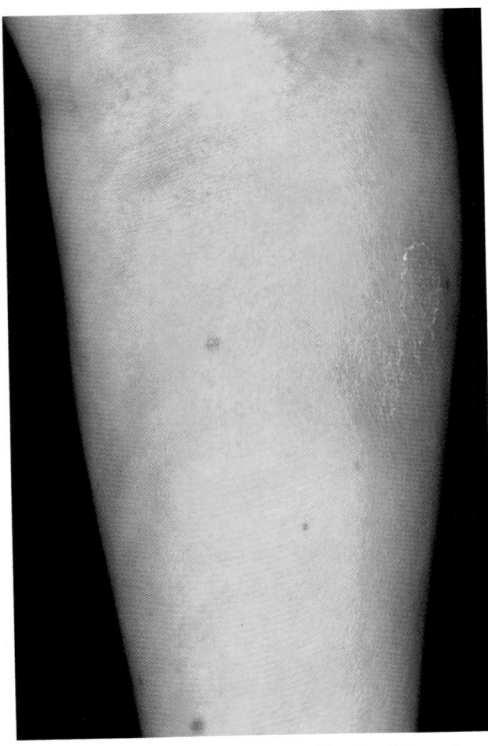

Figure 40-10. Subcutaneous panniculitis-like T-cell lymphoma. Large, ill-defined, infiltrated subcutaneous plaque.

Morphology

Histopathology reveals dense, nodular, or diffuse infiltrates of atypical medium and (rarely) large pleomorphic lymphocytes confined to the subcutaneous fat with the histopathologic pattern of a lobular panniculitis (Fig. 40-11A). Because of morphologic overlap with lobular panniculitis, identification of cytologic atypia is an important diagnostic criterion. Clusters of neoplastic T lymphocytes are almost never observed outside of the subcutaneous tissues, and epidermotropism is never found. Neoplastic cells within the subcutaneous fat are arranged in small clusters or as solitary units around the single adipocytes (so-called "rimming" of the adipocytes; Fig. 40-11B). Fat necrosis is often a prominent feature and is usually combined with a prominent histiocytic infiltrate, often with formation of granulomas. A specific diagnosis may be impossible in cases with prominent necrosis and secondary degenerative changes. Angiocentricity or angiodestruction is uncommon.

Although rimming of adipocytes is a typical histopathologic feature of SPTCL, a similar phenomenon can be observed in virtually all lymphomas with prominent involvement of the subcutaneous fat (both T-cell and B-cell lymphomas) and in reactive subcutaneous infiltrates.[38] SPTCL and LEP may be challenging differentials, with caution warranted in cases with ambiguous histologic features.[39]

Immunophenotype

SPTCL is characterized by an αβ T-suppressor phenotype (βF1+, TCRγ−, CD3+, CD4−, CD8+, TIA-1+, CD30−, CD56−; Fig. 40-12A–C). Particularly in recurrent lesions, βF1 expression may be partially lost by neoplastic cells, but it is usually retained by at least a proportion of them. A negative staining for TCRγ is helpful in these cases. Staining for proliferation markers highlights the pattern of neoplastic cells arranged in small clusters and around the adipocytes (Fig. 40-12D).

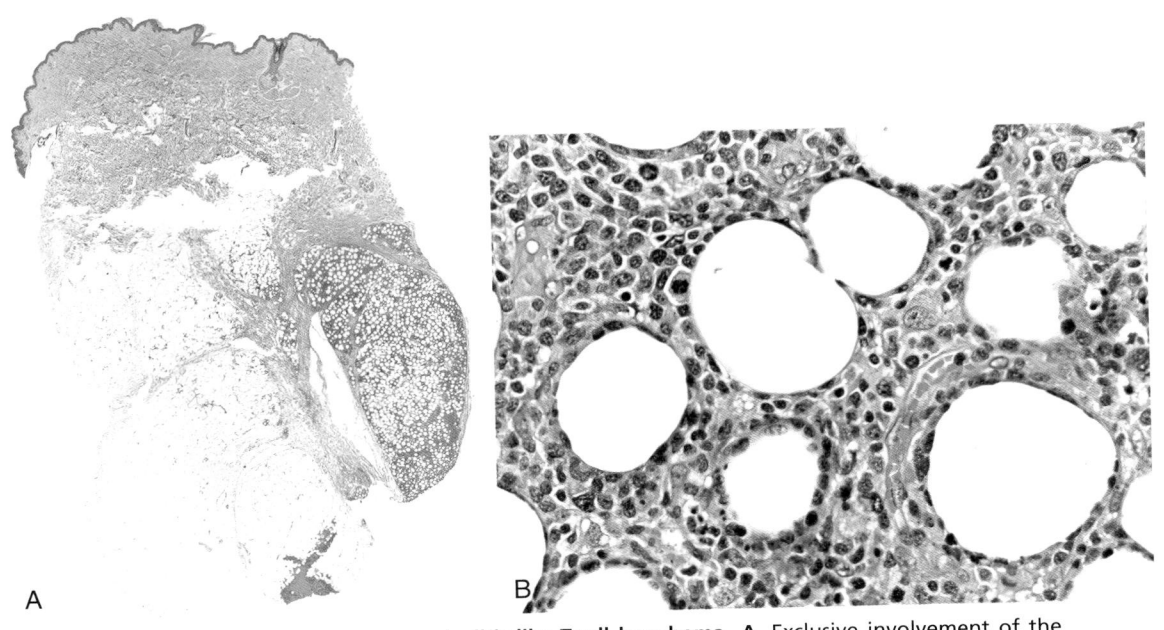

A   B

Figure 40-11. Subcutaneous panniculitis-like T-cell lymphoma. A, Exclusive involvement of the subcutaneous fat with the pattern of a lobular panniculitis. **B,** Pleomorphic lymphocytes showing rimming of adipocytes.

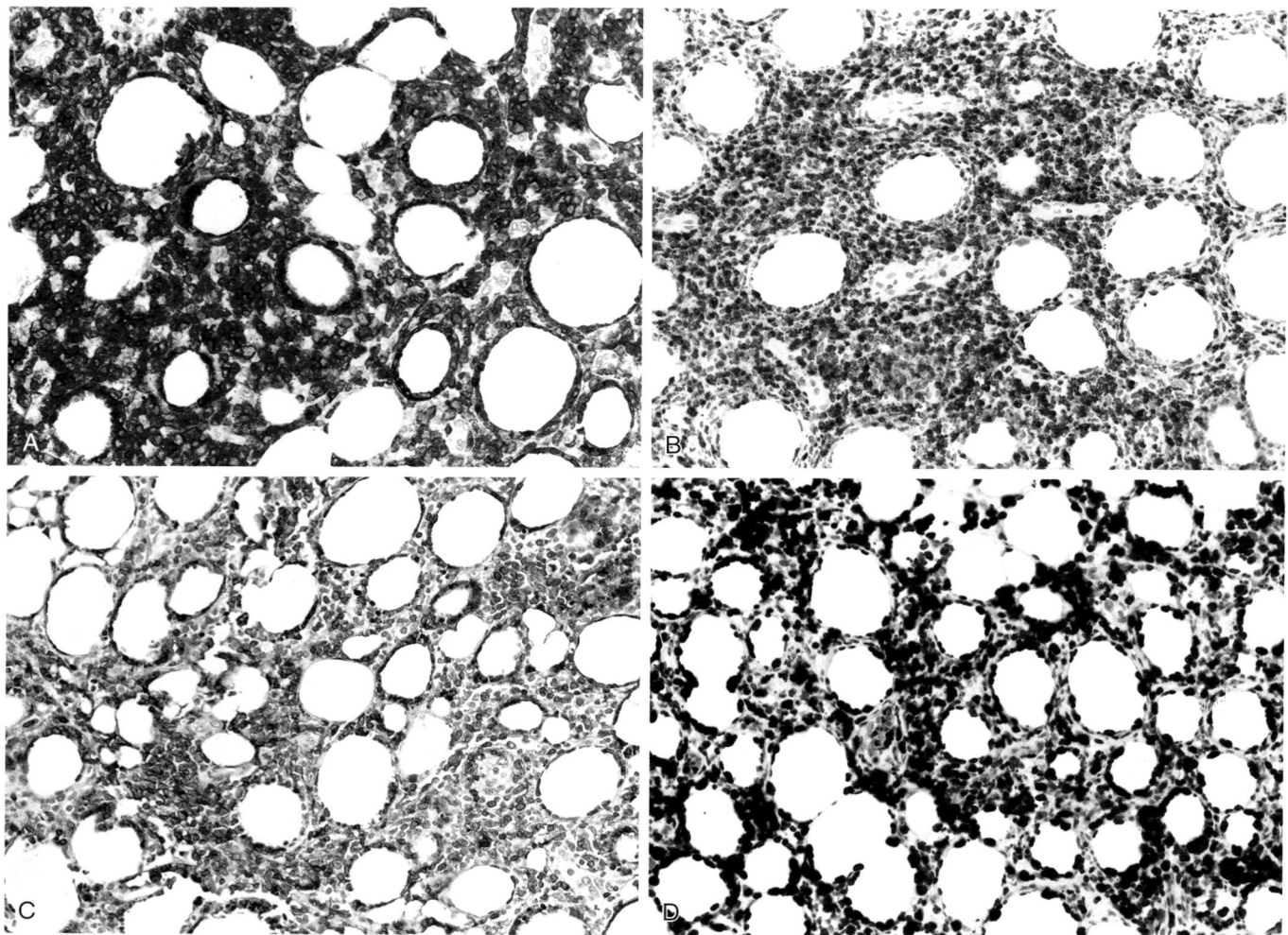

Figure 40-12. Subcutaneous panniculitis-like T-cell lymphoma. Immunohistology reveals positivity for CD8 **(A)**, granzyme B **(B)**, and βF1 **(C)**. Note high proliferation and positivity of lymphocytes around the adipocytes, as detected by Ki67 **(D)**.

Genetics

Molecular analysis of the TCR genes shows a monoclonal rearrangement in most cases. Genetic analyses are hindered by the small number of neoplastic cells, and only limited (and unconfirmed) data are available. Gains of chromosomes 2q and 4q and losses of chromosomes 1pter, 2pter, 10qter, 11qter, 12qter, 16, 19, 20, and 22 have been described in a study of nine patients.[40] In the same study, allelic *NAV3* aberrations were found by loss of heterozygosity and fluorescence in situ hybridization analyses in almost half of the cases.[40] Studies have identified a germline mutation of *HAVCR2,* encoding T-cell immunoglobulin mucin 3 (TIM3) in patients with sporadic tumors.[41,42] This mutation is seen with higher frequency in Asian populations. Various triggers have been proposed for patients without germline mutations, including viral infection and autoimmunity.[43]

Clinical Course

SPTCL is an indolent lymphoma with good prognosis and a 5-year overall survival of more than 80%.[32] Immunosuppressive drugs should be considered as the first-line treatment

instead of polychemotherapy.[33,37] The onset of HPS is a poor prognostic sign.[32] Such cases are significantly associated with *HAVCR2* mutations; therefore, genetic screening should be recommended in such cases. The presence of angiotropism was linked to a worse prognosis in one study.[44]

Differential Diagnoses

Differentiation of SPTCL from LEP (Fig. 40-13) may be impossible in some cases, and it has been proposed that the two diseases represent two ends of a spectrum of panniculitic T-cell dyscrasia.[45] The presence of clusters of CD123-positive plasmacytoid dendritic cells favors the diagnosis of LEP (Fig. 40-13E),[46] whereas the finding of pleomorphic, CD8-positive cytotoxic T lymphocytes with high proliferation favors SPTCL. Plasma cells are often present within the inflammatory infiltrate in LEP (Fig. 40-13D) but not in SPTCL. Nodular aggregates of B cells, sometimes forming small germinal centers, are another typical feature of LEP (Fig. 40-13A and B) but not of SPTCL. The proliferation rate as detected by Ki67 tends to be lower in LEP than in SPTCL. (Fig. 40-13F). Evidence of a clonal rearrangement of the TCR genes supports a diagnosis of SPTCL and should be sought

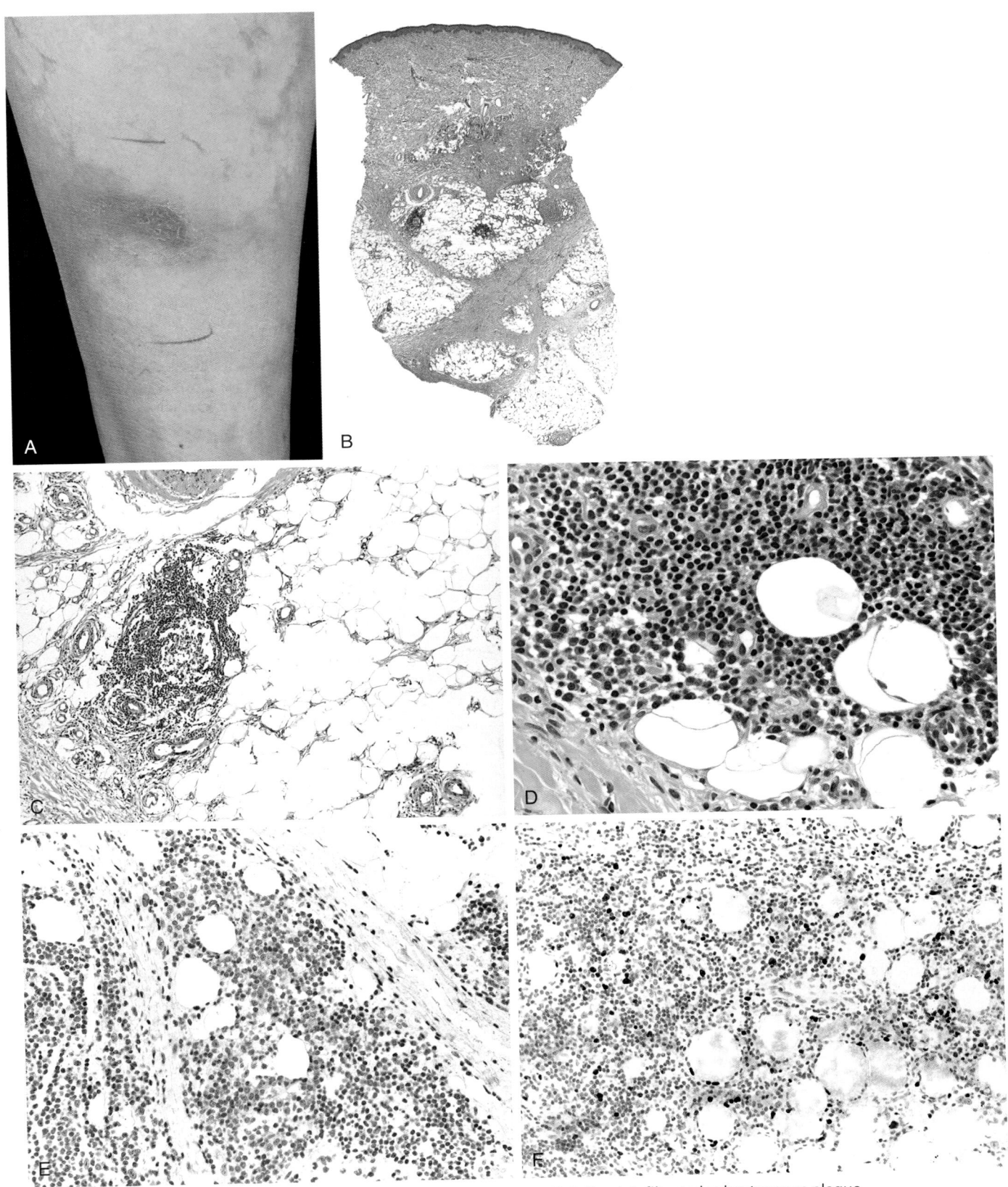

Figure 40-13. Lupus erythematosus panniculitis. A, Ill-defined, infiltrated subcutaneous plaque. **B,** Histology reveals features of a lobular panniculitis. **C,** Note nodules of B lymphocytes with formation of a germinal center. **D,** Several plasma cells admixed within the infiltrate. **E,** Clusters of CD123-positive plasmacytoid dendritic cells. **F,** Low proliferation as detected by Ki67.

Table 40-2 Histopathologic Differential Diagnostic Features of SPTCL and LEP

	SPTCL	LEP
Vacuolar alterations of the basal layer	– (+)	– (+)
Lobular panniculitis-like pattern	+	+
Rimming of adipocytes	+	–/+
Interface dermatitis	–/+	–/+
Dermal involvement	–	+/–
Degenerative changes (fat necrosis, granulomatous reaction)	+	+
Mucin deposition	–/+	+
Clusters of atypical CD8+ cells	+	–
Nodules of B cells	–	+
Plasma cells	–	+
Clusters of plasmacytoid dendritic cells (CD123+)	–	+
High proliferation (Ki67)	+	–

LEP, Lupus erythematosus panniculitis; *SPTCL,* subcutaneous panniculitis-like T-cell lymphoma.

for confirmation in most cases. Histopathologic differential diagnostic features between SPTCL and LEP are summarized in Table 40-2. Rare cases of MF presenting with subcutaneous lesions usually show a CD4-positive phenotype, in contrast to the CD8-positive one of SPTCL. The presence of positivity for EBV as detected by Epstein-Barr encoding region (EBER) in situ hybridization excludes the diagnosis of SPTCL. Similarly, strong expression of CD30 should prompt consideration for anaplastic large cell lymphoma.

PRIMARY CUTANEOUS CD4-POSITIVE SMALL/MEDIUM T-CELL LYMPHOPROLIFERATIVE DISORDER

Definition

This lesion is characterized by a proliferation of small to medium-sized T-cells with a T follicular helper (TFH) phenotype within the dermis, sometimes with involvement of the subcutaneous fat.[1,2] Since the first description by Friedmann and colleagues in 1995,[47] this lymphoproliferative disorder has been the subject of numerous debates and controversial interpretations, and there is still no consensus regarding the underlying biology and pathogenesis of this lesion. Though evidence of T-cell clonality initially suggested that it was a neoplasm, the localized nature of the process and its excellent prognosis has pointed toward an atypical reactive or antigen-driven immune response for most cases.[48-50]

At the present state of knowledge, it is yet unclear whether cutaneous CD4-positive small/medium T-cell lymphoproliferative disorder represents a subtype of CTCL, a lymphoma precursor, or a fully benign, reactive condition (pseudolymphoma). Patients presenting with solitary lesions located on the head and neck area, who represent most of the reported cases, have an invariably good prognosis and the term LPD reflects this benign clinical behavior.

Synonyms and Related Terms

The same term is used in all contemporary classification systems: ICC (2022); revised WHO 4th edition (2017), and proposed WHO 5th edition (2022)

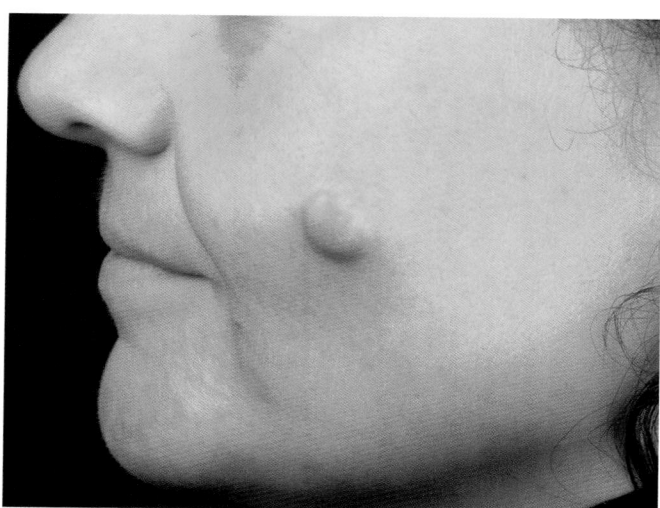

Figure 40-14. Primary cutaneous CD4-positive small/medium T-cell lymphoproliferative disorder. Solitary erythematous tumor on the cheek.

Epidemiology

Patients are adults or elderly individuals, and there is no clear-cut gender predilection. Rarely, children may be affected.[48,49]

Etiology

Etiologic factors are not known, but the absence of recurrent genomic aberrations suggests an abnormal immune reaction rather than a neoplasm.[50]

Clinical Features

Patients present usually with solitary reddish or purple tumors, commonly located on the face and neck or upper trunk (Fig. 40-14). Patients with multiple tumors have been reported in the literature, but many of these cases may represent a different entity (probably peripheral T-cell lymphoma, not otherwise specified [NOS]). Ulceration is uncommon. Spontaneous resolution after incisional biopsy may be observed.

Morphology

Primary cutaneous CD4-positive small/medium T-cell lymphoproliferative disorder is characterized by a dense, lymphoid infiltrate within the entire dermis, often involving the superficial part of the subcutaneous fat (Fig. 40-15A). Cytomorphology shows a predominance of small to medium-sized lymphocytes with mildly pleomorphic nuclei (Fig. 40-15B). Larger immunoblastic cells, when present, are few in number (less than 20%). Epidermotropism is usually absent, and prominent epidermotropism rules out the diagnosis. Many reactive cells are commonly found admixed with the neoplastic ones (lymphocytes, histiocytes, eosinophils, sometimes plasma cells). A granulomatous reaction can be observed in a proportion of the cases. Reactive germinal centers can be present within B-cell nodules.

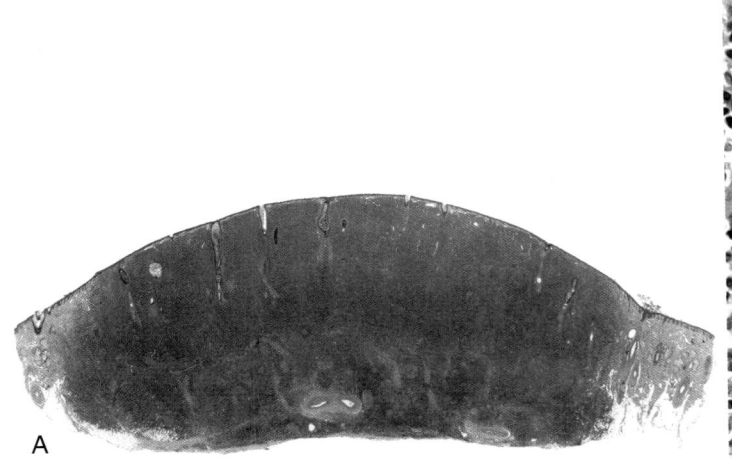
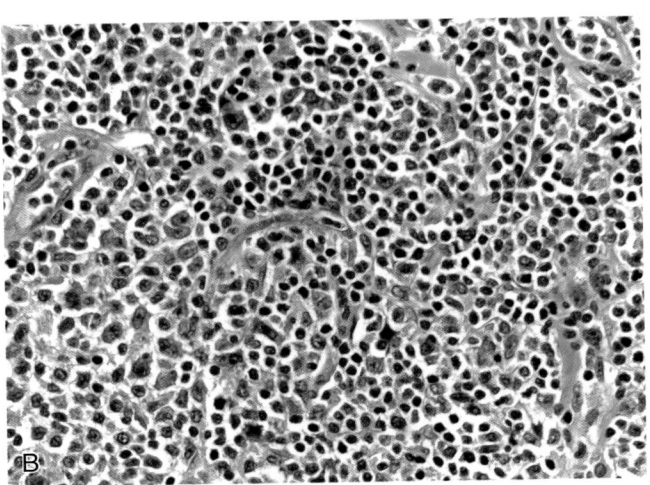

Figure 40-15. Primary cutaneous CD4-positive small/medium T-cell lymphoproliferative disorder. A, Dense, nodular infiltrate of lymphocytes within the dermis and subcutaneous fat. **B,** Small to medium-sized lymphocytes predominate.

Immunophenotype

Neoplastic cells show an αβ T-helper phenotype (CD3+, CD4+, CD5+, CD8−, TIA-1−, βF1+, TCRγ−; Fig. 40-16A and B). Staining for CD30 is negative or limited to a small minority of cells. Admixed reactive B lymphocytes are commonly found (Fig. 40-16C), sometimes in follicular aggregates. Ki-67 is usually moderately expressed (Fig. 40-16D). PD-1 and other TFH markers (CXCL13, ICOS, BCL6, or CD10) are commonly expressed (Fig. 40-16E).[49,51]

Genetics

Molecular analysis of the TCR gene rearrangement shows monoclonality of T lymphocytes in the majority of the cases. To date, at least on unilesional lesions, genetic aberrations are rarely found.[50] Only one case was identified with a *DNMT3A* mutation,[52] a finding that might point toward underlying clonal hematopoiesis in some patients.[53]

Clinical Course

Patients with solitary lesions have an excellent prognosis,[48,54-59] and cases associated with progression are almost invariably those showing multiple lesions at presentation.[60] Patients with lesions confined to the legs or with bulky disease may have a more aggressive course, but they may correspond to other type of lymphomas, e.g., primary cutaneous peripheral T-cell lymphoma, NOS (PTCL, NOS).[61]

Differential Diagnosis

Primary cutaneous acral CD8-positive T-cell lymphoproliferative disorder may be clinically indistinguishable from cutaneous CD4-positive small/medium T-cell lymphoproliferative disorder, but it presents with more monomorphous infiltrates morphologically and with positivity for CD8 and cytotoxic proteins phenotypically. Primary cutaneous PTCL, NOS is usually characterized by multiple lesions and by more profound phenotypic aberrations; in addition, despite CD4 positivity, many cases display expression of cytotoxic markers.

Differentiation of primary cutaneous CD4-positive small/medium T-cell lymphoproliferative disorder from MF may be difficult without correlation with the clinical picture; in general, presence of many reactive cells is uncommon in tumors of MF. The differential diagnosis also includes primary cutaneous marginal zone lymphoma. Some cases even have ambiguous genetic findings with identification of clonal populations of both T cells and B cells by polymerase chain reaction (PCR) of IG and TCR genes.[50,62,63] As previously mentioned, differentiation of cutaneous CD4-positive small/medium T-cell lymphoproliferative disorder from reactive conditions may be impossible. It has been suggested that at least some of these cases (particularly those presenting with solitary lesions on the head and neck area) are an antigen-driven clonal expansion of T cells that is benign in nature.

PRIMARY CUTANEOUS ACRAL CD8-POSITIVE T-CELL LYMPHOPROLIFERATIVE DISORDER

Definition

Primary cutaneous acral CD8-positive T-cell lymphoproliferative disorder (pcACD8TCLPD) is characterized by skin infiltration of atypical clonal medium-sized CD8-positive lymphocytes. Clinically, the tumor was initially described in acral sites,[64] particularly ear and nose localization, and is characterized by a good prognosis.[64-68]

Synonyms and Related Terms

Primary cutaneous acral CD8-positive T-cell LPD (ICC 2022)
Primary cutaneous acral CD8-positive T-cell lymphoma (WHO 4th edition 2017)
Primary cutaneous acral CD8-positive LPD (proposed WHO 5th edition, 2022)

Epidemiology

The disease affects adults, with a male predominance (male-to-female ratio 3.2:1). The median age is around 56 years.[69] Only one suspected case was reported in an adolescent.[70]

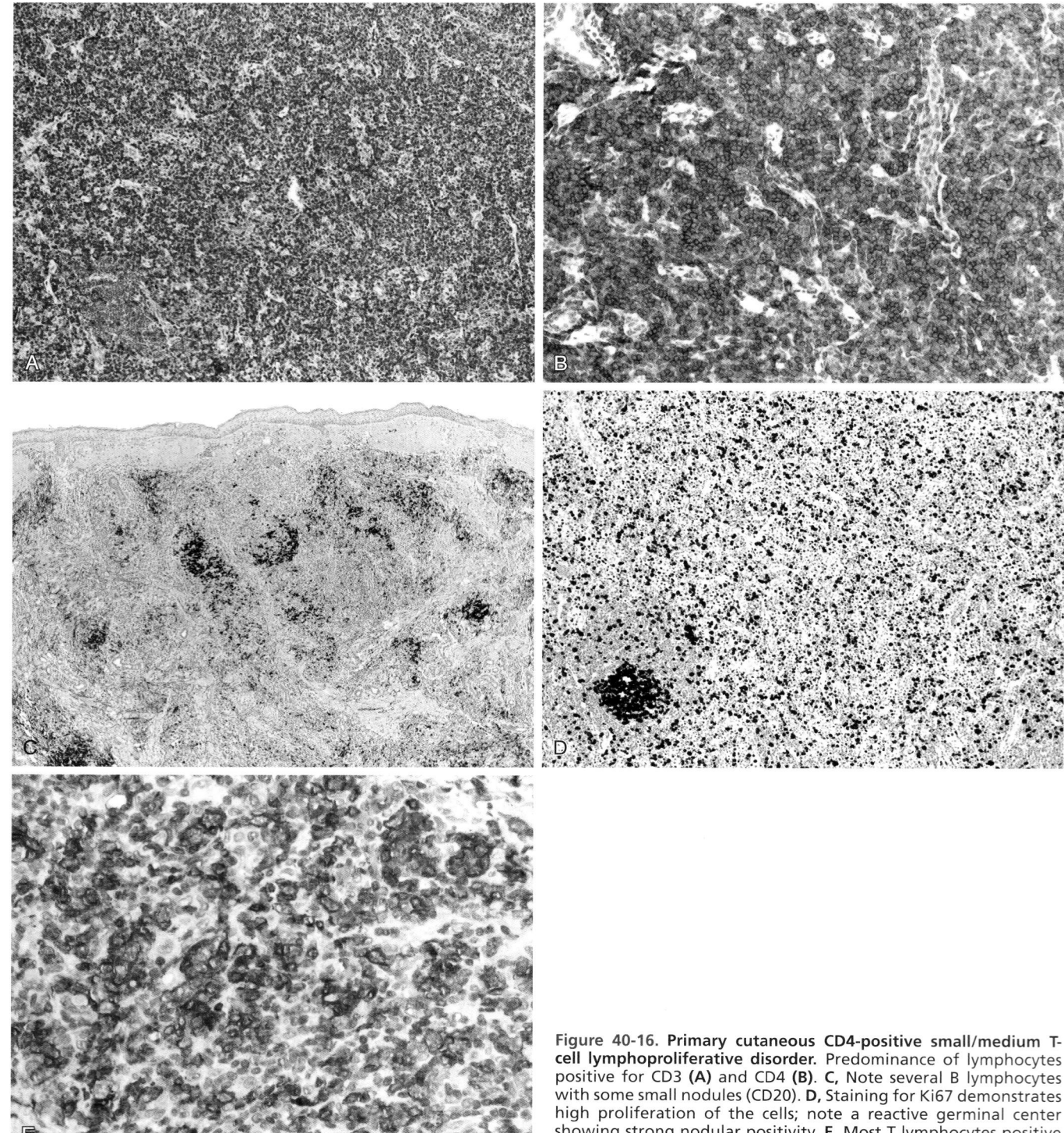

Figure 40-16. Primary cutaneous CD4-positive small/medium T-cell lymphoproliferative disorder. Predominance of lymphocytes positive for CD3 **(A)** and CD4 **(B)**. **C**, Note several B lymphocytes with some small nodules (CD20). **D**, Staining for Ki67 demonstrates high proliferation of the cells; note a reactive germinal center showing strong nodular positivity. **E**, Most T lymphocytes positive for PD-1.

Etiology

It is yet unclear whether this peculiar cutaneous cytotoxic lymphoid proliferation represents a reactive process (pseudolymphoma), a phenotypic variant of cutaneous CD4-positive small/medium T-cell lymphoproliferative disorder, or a distinct entity of CTCL. A local trigger agent may be suspected, but to date, none has been identified. A case presumedly induced by gold earrings has been published.[71] The postulated normal counterpart is a skin-homing CD8-positive T cell. However, similar cases in terms of morphology, phenotype, and clinical outcome have also been described in the gastrointestinal tract (see Chapter 37) and genital tract,[72] suggesting the existence of rare lymphomas arising from tissue-resident CD8-positive memory T cells.

Clinical Features

The skin lesion is most often a unique erythematous nodule or papule of 0.5 to 2 cm in diameter. An erythematous and/or squamous plaque measuring up to 5 cm can be seen, most frequently on the feet. Lesions should not be ulcerated (see differential diagnosis). There is generally a history of slow growth over several weeks or months, with a median duration of 19 months.[69] The most frequent site is the ears (two-thirds of the cases), followed by the nose and feet. Eyelids, hands, arms, and legs are sites that have also been reported. Occasionally, lesions are multiple[68] and particularly bilateral for ears[64,66] and feet.[73] Rare cases have been identified with more disseminated disease (unpublished observation).

Morphology

Histologic features are very typical. The skin biopsies show a dense and diffuse dermal infiltration by very monotonous medium-sized atypical lymphoid cells with irregular and folded nuclei and small nucleoli[64] (Fig. 40-17A). Mitoses and apoptotic figures are absent or very rare. A rare case with signet ring cell morphology has been reported.[74] Some reactive B-cell lymphoid aggregates of follicles may be seen within the atypical infiltrate. Plasma cells, neutrophils, or eosinophils are absent or very rare. Granulomatous reaction is absent. The epidermis is most often spared with a grenz zone, particularly on nodular lesions. Infiltration of superficial dermis, with or without minimal epidermotropism, may be seen, particularly in thicker plaques.[68,75] Skin appendages are always spared. Angiotropism can occasionally be seen, but never angiodestruction or necrosis. The proliferation frequently involves the underlying subcutaneous tissue.

Immunophenotype

By definition, tumor cells express CD8 (Fig. 40-17B), and they always express CD3, TIA-1, and βF1. TIA-1 displays a very characteristic Golgi dot-like staining (Fig. 40-17C). However, Granzyme B and perforin are typically negative. In the large majority of the cases, CD68 is also positive, displaying as does TIA-1 a Golgi dot-like staining (Fig. 40-17D), which is considered by some authors to be helpful in differential diagnosis.[76] CD30 is always negative. Rare co-expression of CD4 may be seen, and CD2, CD5, and CD7 are usually expressed. CD99 is usually positive, but this is not a specific finding (Fig. 40-17E). CD56, CD57, and TdT are negative, as are TFH markers (CD10, BCL6, PD1, CXCL13).[68] Proliferative index with Ki-67 staining is usually low (<10%). If the Ki-67 is greater than 50%, other CD8-positive cutaneous lymphomas should be considered. B cells are generally not abundant, and LMP1 and EBER are negative.

Genetics

The neoplastic T cells show clonal TCR gene rearrangements. Specific genetic abnormalities have not yet been described.

Clinical Course

Most cases do not relapse after treatment. Treatment consists of surgical excision or local radiotherapy. Systemic chemotherapy is not indicated. Spontaneous regression has been noted after biopsy. Recurrences in cutaneous sites occur in around 20% of cases, but extension beyond the skin is very rare.[77]

Differential Diagnosis

The differential diagnosis includes primary cutaneous CD8-positive PTCL, NOS and cutaneous CD8-positive lymphoproliferative disorders associated with congenital or acquired immunodeficiency, usually common variable immune deficiency (CVID).[78] Unlike pcACD8TCLPD, most cutaneous CD8-positive T-cell lymphomas are clinically aggressive with a cytotoxic T-cell phenotype. In addition, a CD8-positive T-cell phenotype can be seen in some cases of MF, particularly in the pediatric age group.[79,80]

OTHER TYPES OF CUTANEOUS T-CELL LYMPHOMA

Besides the four entities mentioned in the preceding sections, other subtypes of CTCL deserve a brief discussion.

Primary Cutaneous T-Follicular Helper–Cell Lymphoma and Cutaneous Angioimmunoblastic T-Cell Lymphoma

Angioimmunoblastic T-cell lymphoma (AITL) is a systemic form of T-cell lymphoma with a TFH phenotype.[49,51] A skin rash is a common finding, and in rare cases, a skin biopsy may be the initial diagnostic procedure.[81] The TFH phenotype is characterized by positivity of at least three markers of TFH lymphocytes (PD1, ICOS, CXCL13, CD10, BCL6). In addition, a TFH phenotype has been observed in conventional types of CTCL such as MF or Sézary syndrome, among others.[82] At present, it is not clear whether a primary cutaneous TFH-cell lymphoma exists as an entity distinct from other types of CTCL.

Cutaneous Intravascular NK/T-Cell Lymphoma

Most cases of intravascular large cell lymphoma have a B-cell phenotype, but T-cell and NK-cell phenotypes have been reported in rare instances.[83-86] In contrast to intravascular large B-cell lymphoma, intravascular large NK/T-cell lymphoma (IVLNKTCL) is commonly associated with EBV infection.[83,84]

Neurologic symptoms as a sign of involvement of the central nervous system are commonly present. Histology shows a proliferation of large lymphocytes confined to dilated blood vessels within the dermis and subcutaneous tissues. Lymphatic vessels are not affected. The malignant cells are large with scant cytoplasm and often with prominent nucleoli. Neoplastic cells in IVLNKTCL express CD2, CD3, and cytotoxic proteins but are commonly negative for CD5. CD56 is positive in the majority of cases, whereas βF1 is usually negative. Molecular analysis of the TCR gene rearrangement reveals monoclonality in approximately one-third of cases

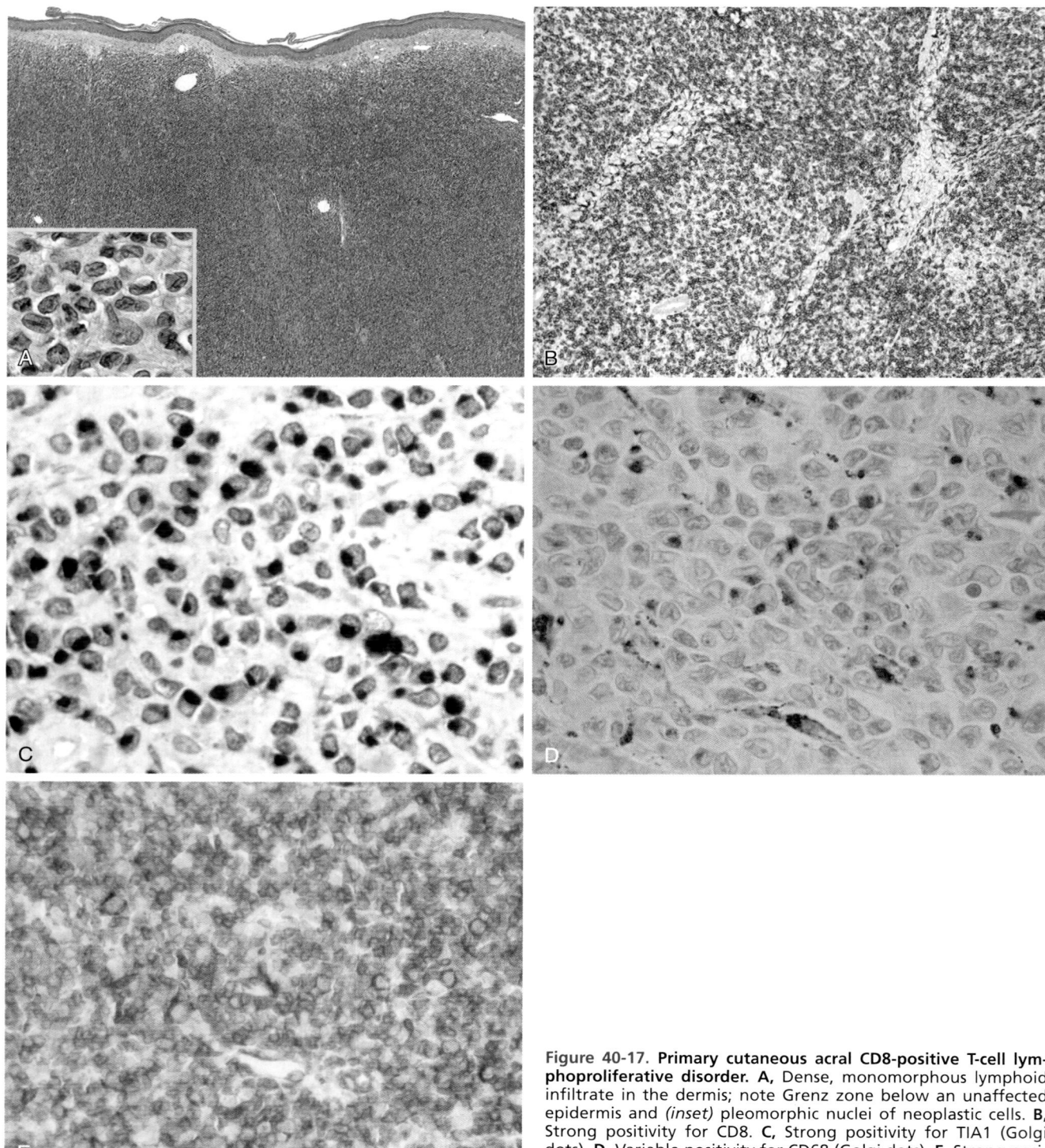

Figure 40-17. Primary cutaneous acral CD8-positive T-cell lymphoproliferative disorder. A, Dense, monomorphous lymphoid infiltrate in the dermis; note Grenz zone below an unaffected epidermis and *(inset)* pleomorphic nuclei of neoplastic cells. **B,** Strong positivity for CD8. **C,** Strong positivity for TIA1 (Golgi dots). **D,** Variable positivity for CD68 (Golgi dots). **E,** Strong positivity for CD99.

(the negative ones possibly representing those with an NK-cell phenotype). The course is very aggressive.

Phenotypic analyses allow the distinction of IVLNKTCL from the more common B-cell variant of intravascular large cell lymphoma. IVLNKTCL should also be differentiated from benign conditions such as intralymphatic histiocytosis and benign intralymphatic proliferation of T-cell lymphoid blasts.

Benign intralymphatic proliferation of T-cell lymphoid blasts has been observed in the skin at sites of previous trauma, within hemangiomas, within endometrial polyps, and in association with appendicitis.[87-92] In contrast to IVLNKTCL, a proliferation of large T lymphocytes in this peculiar condition is observed within lymphatic vessels rather than within blood vessels, and large lymphoid cells are also present outside of the vessels admixed with inflammatory infiltrates. Finally,

IVLNKTCL should be differentiated from intralymphatic CD30-positive ALCL.[93,94]

Three other rare types of cutaneous NK/T-cell lymphoma (hydroa vacciniforme lymphoproliferative disease; cutaneous extranodal NK/T-cell lymphoma, nasal-type; and adult T-cell leukemia/lymphoma) are discussed elsewhere (Chapter 29 and 32).

Primary Cutaneous Peripheral T-Cell Lymphoma, Not Otherwise Specified

All cases of PCTL that do not fit within the definition of a specific PCTL entity are referred to as primary cutaneous PCTL, NOS. To be able to exclude a specific entity, one needs an adequate sampling of the lesion. A punch biopsy may be not enough. In addition, the specimen must be examined in conjunction with a thorough clinical history. By definition, PCTL, NOS is heterogeneous clinically and pathologically.[95] In one study, the majority of patients were male (75%), with a medium age of 66.5 years. Clinical lesions were solitary or multiple. When solitary, they were most frequently located on the legs. Histology was variable in terms of morphology of the tumor cells and the presence of reactive cells such as eosinophils, histiocytes, or plasma cells. Frequent aberrant phenotypes such as CD4-negative/CD8-negative or CD4-positive/CD8-positive were found. An aberrant expression of CD20 by tumor cells was found in 18% of the cases. Globally, the prognosis was very poor independently of age, gender, clinical presentation, and CD4/CD8 phenotype.

Pearls and Pitfalls

- Epidermotropism is a pattern that may be encountered in different types of cutaneous lymphoma.
- A diagnostic biopsy should be sufficient to allow for detailed assessment of the morphology and immunophenotype.
- Sufficient material to allow for assessment of clonality and the genomic profile may be required for accurate diagnosis.
- Involvement of subcutaneous fat may be encountered in different types of cutaneous lymphoma.
- Teach surgeons to avoid putting the biopsy specimens on gauze; drying artifacts occur quickly in skin specimens, particularly in small punch biopsies.

KEY REFERENCES

1. Goodlad JR, Cerroni L, Swerdlow SH. Recent advances in cutaneous lymphoma—implications for current and future classifications. *Virchows Arch.* 2023;482(1):281–298.

3. Berti E, Tomasini D, Vermeer MH, et al. Primary cutaneous CD8-positive epidermotropic cytotoxic T cell lymphomas. A distinct clinicopathological entity with an aggressive clinical behaviour. *Am J Pathol.* 1999;155:483–492.

4. Robson A, Assaf C, Bagot M, et al. Aggressive epidermotropic cutaneous CD8+ lymphoma: a cutaneous lymphoma with distinct clinical and pathological features. Report of an EORTC Cutaneous Lymphoma Task Force Workshop. *Histopathology.* 2015;67:425–441.

10. Saggini A, Gulia A, Argenyi Z, et al. A variant of lymphomatoid papulosis simulating primary cutaneous aggressive epidermotropic CD8+ cytotoxic T-cell lymphoma. Description of 9 cases. *Am J Surg Pathol.* 2010;34:1168–1175.

14. Guitart J, Weisenburger DD, Subtil A, et al. Cutaneous gamma/delta T-cell lymphomas. A spectrum of presentations with overlap with other cytotoxic lymphomas. *Am J Surg Pathol.* 2012;36:1656–1665.

32. Willemze R, Jansen PM, Cerroni L, et al. Subcutaneous panniculitis-like T-cell lymphoma: definition, classification, and prognostic factors: an EORTC Cutaneous Lymphoma Group Study of 83 cases. *Blood.* 2008;111:838–845.

39. Bosisio F, Boi S, Caputo V, et al. Lobular panniculitic infiltrates with overlapping histopathologic features of lupus panniculitis (lupus profundus) and subcutaneous T-cell lymphoma: a conceptual and practical dilemma. *Am J Surg Pathol.* 2015;39:206–211.

55. Beltraminelli H, Leinweber B, Kerl H, Cerroni L. Primary cutaneous CD4+ small/medium-sized pleomorphic T cell lymphoma: a cutaneous nodular proliferation of pleomorphic T lymphocytes of undetermined significance? A study of 136 cases. *Am J Dermatopathol.* 2009;31:317–322.

67. Kempf W, Kazakov DV, Cozzio A, et al. Primary cutaneous CD8+ small- to medium-sized lymphoproliferative disorder in extrafacial sites: clinicopathologic features and concept on their classification. *Am J Dermatopathol.* 2013;35:159–166.

83. Cerroni L, Massone C, Kutzner H, et al. Intravascular large T-cell or NK-cell lymphoma. A rare variant of intravascular large cell lymphoma with frequent cytotoxic phenotype and association with Epstein-Barr virus infection. *Am J Surg Pathol.* 2008;32:891–898.

Visit Elsevier eBooks+ for the complete set of references.

Chapter **41**

Precursor B-Cell and T-Cell Neoplasms

Amy S. Duffield, Frederick Racke, and Michael J. Borowitz

CLASSIFICATION OF PRECURSOR LYMPHOID NEOPLASMS

Precursor lymphoid neoplasms, often referred to as acute lymphoblastic leukemia (ALL) or lymphoblastic lymphoma, are of either B-cell or T-cell origin. Depending on the cell of origin, these neoplasms are subdivided into B-lymphoblastic leukemia/lymphoma (B-ALL) or T-lymphoblastic leukemia/lymphoma (T-ALL), which may also be abbreviated "B-LL" or "T-LL," respectively. The distinction between lymphoma and leukemia is somewhat arbitrary. If there is significant blood or bone marrow involvement, then the term *leukemia* is used. If the tumor primarily presents at an extramedullary site with little or no blood or bone marrow involvement, then the term *lymphoma* is preferred. Conventionally, bone marrow involvement by 25% or more blasts has been used as the cutoff between leukemia and lymphoma. The majority of precursor lymphoid neoplasms that present as leukemia are derived from precursor B cells, and the majority of those that present as tumor masses possess a precursor T-cell phenotype. In practice, the leukemic and lymphomatous presentations of both B-ALL and T-ALL are considered biologically equivalent, and it is generally conceded that this distinction bears little clinical significance. However, distinguishing precursor B-cell from precursor T-cell neoplasms is important because these tumors are biologically and clinically distinct. As such, they are discussed separately.

B-CELL LYMPHOBLASTIC LEUKEMIA/ LYMPHOBLASTIC LYMPHOMA

Definition

B-ALL is a clonal disorder of hematopoietic precursors with evidence of early B-cell differentiation. The disease is characterized by the presence of a proliferating population of blasts, with minimal morphologic evidence of differentiation. Defining these tumors generally requires immunophenotypic demonstration of B-cell lineage antigen expression. For example, more than 95% of cases express CD19 and HLA-DR.[1] Further, nearly all show clonal rearrangement of the immunoglobulin heavy chain (IGH) gene.[2,3] Unlike most acute myeloid leukemias, a specific blast percentage in the marrow is not required for a formal diagnosis of B-ALL. Marrow-based disease with a low blast count is rare, and the diagnosis should be made with caution in specimens with <20% blasts.

Synonyms and Related Terms

None.

Epidemiology

Overall, ALLs are the most common malignancy in children, accounting for about 80% of childhood leukemias but only about 20% of adult acute leukemias. Most cases occur in children younger than 6 years, and the majority are B-ALL.[4] The peak incidence is approximately four to five cases per 100,000 children between 2 and 5 years of age; the incidence decreases thereafter until 50 years of age, when it begins to climb slightly again. B-ALL incidence differs based on self-identified race: it affects Whites and Hispanics more commonly than Blacks, and Hispanic children have a higher incidence of ALL[5,6] and a higher relapse rate than do White children.[7] Lymphomatous presentations of B-ALL (B-LBL) are less common than lymphomatous presentations of T-ALL (T-LBL), with B-LBL accounting for only about 10% of lymphoblastic lymphomas. B-LBL is also a disease of young individuals, with the majority of cases occurring in those younger than 20 years.[8,9]

Etiology

The etiology of B-ALL is unknown. A number of studies have suggested a prenatal origin of the genetic events predisposing to the development of leukemia; others have demonstrated the presence of clone-specific antigen receptor gene rearrangements in infants, consistent with an in utero origin of at least a portion of childhood ALLs.[10,11] Further, identical leukemia-specific translocations and antigen receptor gene rearrangements have been documented in monozygotic twins with B-ALL.[12] However, these findings are thought to represent somatic mutations occurring in one twin and shared via in utero circulation rather than constitutional genetic lesions. Although the specific environmental and genetic factors that predispose to B-ALL are not well defined, several factors, such as exposure to ionizing radiation, germline variants including mutations in PAX5 and ETV6, and certain genetic diseases such as Down syndrome have been associated with the development of B-ALL.[13-15] Studies have also shown that single-nucleotide polymorphisms (SNPs) of several genes, including GATA3, ARID5B, IKZF1, CEBPE, and CDKN2A/B, are associated with susceptibility to B-ALL.[16,17] Disease in these patients has a relatively poor outcome, and a disproportionate percentage are adolescents and young adults. One of these SNPs (rs3824662) is more common in Hispanics[18] and has been suggested to account, in part, for the poorer outcomes seen in this group relative to White patients. However, true familial ALL is rare, with kindreds described having mutations in PAX5, ETV6, and TP53.[19-21]

Also, rare cases of B-ALL after chemotherapy have been documented; these often possess rearrangements or amplification of the homeotic regulator mixed lineage leukemia (MLL) gene (now called KMT2A) on chromosome 11q23.3.[22,23] Interestingly, patients treated with lenalidomide (for plasma cell neoplasms) have an increased risk of secondary B-ALL. Full characterization of lenalidomide-associated B-ALL is ongoing, but this entity tends to present with new-onset cytopenias, low-level marrow involvement, and a relatively favorable prognosis, with some patients reported to respond to withdrawal of lenalidomide alone.[24-26]

Clinical Features

The typical clinical presentation of B-ALL (Box 41-1) relates to the development of cytopenias secondary to the replacement of normal bone marrow by leukemic blasts. Clinical manifestations include weakness and pallor caused by anemia, petechiae, and bruising secondary to thrombocytopenia and fever despite granulocytopenia. It is important to note that patients with B-ALL may present with low, normal, or elevated peripheral white blood cell counts, and circulating blasts may be very rare. Thus, patients with unexplained pancytopenia may warrant a bone marrow examination to exclude leukemia. In addition, hepatosplenomegaly or lymphadenopathy may be present at diagnosis, and there may be organ dysfunction caused by leukemic infiltration. Bone or joint pain is also common, particularly in children, and is a result of intramedullary growth of the leukemic cells. B-LBL typically presents with skin or lymph-node involvement with or without peripheral blood or bone marrow involvement, and has infrequently been reported to present as lytic bone lesions.[8,27] In contrast to T-LBL, B-LBL rarely involves the mediastinum.

Morphology

The morphologic examination of peripheral blood or bone marrow remains an essential part of the initial diagnosis of ALL. Blasts in B-ALL can be heterogeneous. Previous classification schemes attempted to subdivide B-ALL on the basis of cytologic features, including nuclear-to-cytoplasmic ratio, nucleoli, nuclear membrane contours, and cell size. However, subdividing B-ALL on the basis of morphology alone has no significant prognostic value and has been supplanted by cytogenetic and molecular subclassification. Nevertheless, recognition of lymphoblasts is important to initiate the appropriate diagnostic evaluation. On a peripheral blood or bone marrow smear, lymphoblasts range from small, round blasts with high nuclear-to-cytoplasmic ratios, relatively condensed chromatin, and inconspicuous nucleoli to larger cells with an increased amount of blue-gray to blue cytoplasm, irregular nuclei with dispersed chromatin, and variably distinct nucleoli. Cytoplasmic vacuoles may be present and can be seen in MYC-rearranged B-ALL and MEF2D-rearranged B-ALL.[28]

Box 41-1 Major Clinical and Diagnostic Features of Acute Lymphoblastic Leukemia

- Increased lymphoblasts in bone marrow or peripheral blood; no absolute threshold for diagnosis, but rarely <10% in marrow
- Immunophenotypic evidence of either early B (~80%) or early T (~20%) differentiation
- Absence of significant myeloid differentiation
- Anemia, thrombocytopenia, and granulocytopenia (common)
- Clinical features that include fatigue, bleeding, bone pain, fever, lymphadenopathy, organomegaly, and central nervous system involvement

Several morphologic variants of B-ALL have been described. The first, so-called "hand-mirror–cell leukemia," in which blasts display a distinctive morphology characterized by the presence of an asymmetric cytoplasmic projection called a *uropod,* is of historical interest[29] but of no biological or clinical significance. The second and less common morphologic variant is granular B-ALL. Awareness of this variant is important because the lymphoblasts may be confused with myeloid blasts on morphologic evaluation. In this variant, the blasts contain azurophilic cytoplasmic granules that do not contain myeloperoxidase but can contain acid phosphatase or acid esterase activity, suggesting a lysosomal origin.[30] These cases may not show the increased right-angle side scatter that is characteristically seen in flow cytometric analysis of myeloid blasts that contain abundant granules. Rarely, cases of B-ALL may be associated with peripheral blood eosinophilia that is so marked that it virtually obscures the lymphoblasts. This unusual manifestation is often associated with the chromosomal abnormality t(5;14) (discussed later in this chapter). B lymphoblasts in the setting of eosinophilia may also be seen in "myeloid/

lymphoid neoplasms with eosinophilia and tyrosine kinase gene fusions" (see Chapter 50).

The cytomorphology of B-ALL that presents as both leukemia and lymphoma is indistinguishable, and the distinction between the subtypes is based on the distribution of tissue involvement. In B-lymphoblastic leukemia, the bone marrow is almost always hypercellular, with replacement of normal marrow elements by a diffuse infiltrate of immature cells (Fig. 41-1). High-power examination reveals morphologic variability similar to that observed on smear preparations, ranging from small blasts with fine chromatin and inconspicuous nucleoli to more heterogeneous cells with irregular nuclei and more abundant cytoplasm. Occasionally, tingible body macrophages accompany the infiltrate, imparting a starry-sky appearance; however, the tingible body macrophages are usually not as abundant as in Burkitt lymphoma and may occur only focally. With leukemic presentations, there can be significant organ involvement, with the liver, spleen, kidneys, gonads, and central nervous system (CNS) being common sites. B-LBL is diagnosed when there is an extramedullary tumor composed of lymphoblasts, with less than 25% lymphoblasts in the

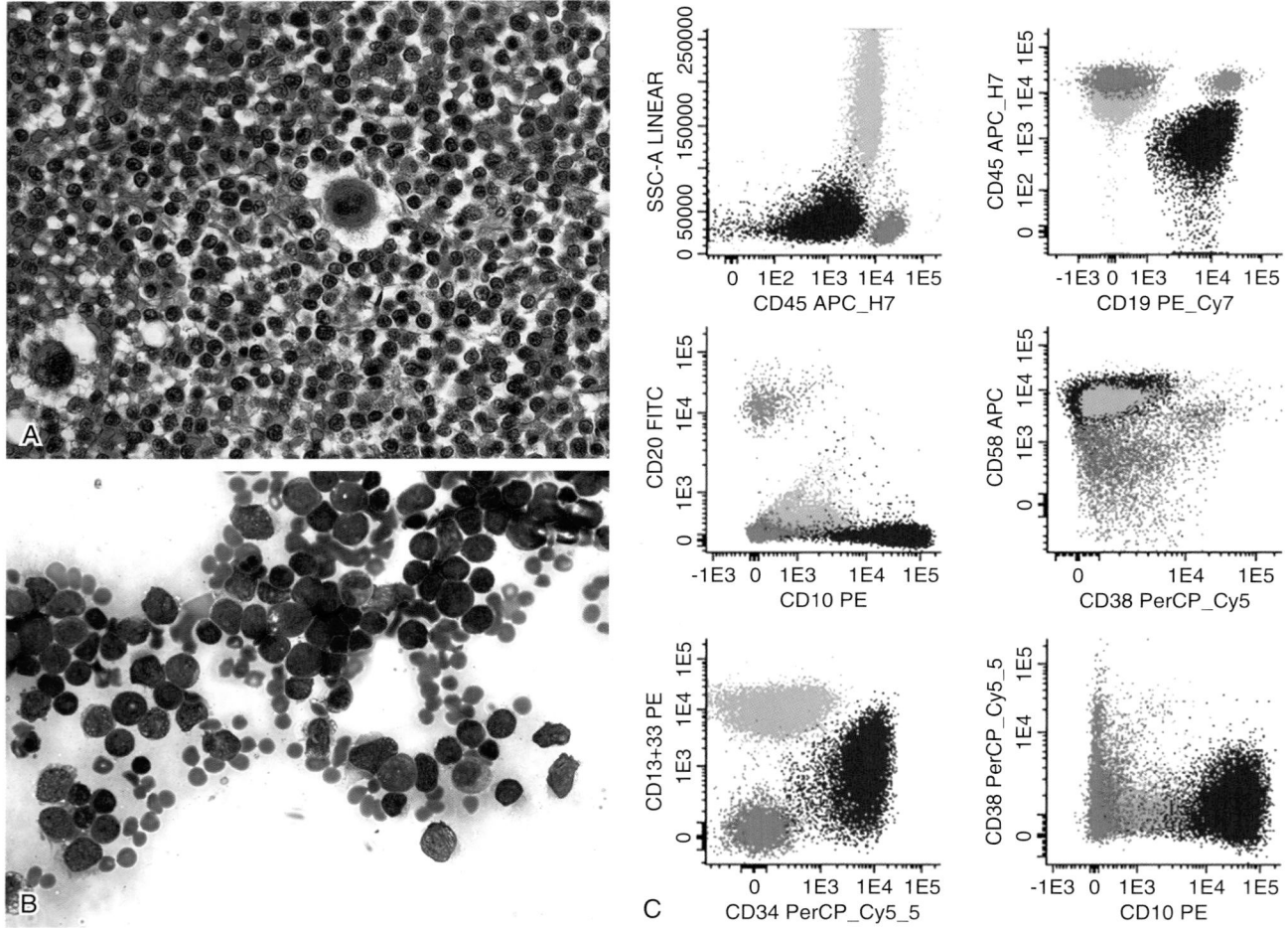

Figure 41-1. B-cell acute lymphoblastic leukemia (ALL). A, Bone marrow infiltrated by an interstitial immature lymphoblast population. **B,** Accompanying bone marrow aspirate shows an increase in immature blasts. **C,** Multiparametric flow cytometry demonstrates the blasts *(dark blue)* to be CD45-dim, CD19+, CD34+, CD10+, CD58-bright, CD38-low, and CD20−, with variable aberrant myeloid antigen expression. Normal granulocytes *(cyan),* B cells *(green),* and T cells *(red)* are also present.

blood or bone marrow. Lymphomatous presentations are found most often in extranodal sites, most commonly skin or bone, and often involve the head and neck in children. Lymph nodes are less commonly involved and may demonstrate a paracortical distribution, with preservation of follicles. Hepatic involvement is typically sinusoidal, and splenic disease involves the red pulp.

Immunophenotype

B-ALL is defined by evidence of B-cell differentiation. (Fig. 41-1C). B lymphoblasts are the neoplastic counterpart of normal precursor B cells (hematogones), which exist in variable numbers in the bone marrow. Hematogones undergo a reproducible pattern of antigen expression during normal B-cell differentiation. In contrast, B-ALL almost always demonstrates an aberrant antigen profile that is incompatible with normal B-cell differentiation, thus permitting a distinction between malignant and reactive precursor B cells.[31] Nearly all cases of B-ALL express CD19, cytoplasmic CD79a, terminal deoxynucleotidyl transferase (TdT), and HLA-DR. CD10 is present in most, but not all, cases. Surface expression of CD22 is often weak but expressed in almost all cases. CD20 is usually variably expressed, although individual cases can range from complete absence of CD20 to moderately intense and uniform expression of this antigen. Cytoplasmic CD22 is a very sensitive marker for B-ALL, but it may also be detected in some cases of acute myeloid leukemia (AML)[32] in conjunction with possible weak expression of CD19 and TdT. CD79a has been suggested as both a sensitive and a specific marker of B-lineage ALL, but it is not specific for B-ALL because it is also seen in a significant fraction of T-ALLs.[33] Outside of AML with t(8;21), which expresses many B-lymphoid markers, PAX5 is highly specific for B-cell lineage.[34] Although IGH gene rearrangements occur relatively early in B-cell development and B-ALLs show clonal rearrangements by molecular analysis, most fail to express surface immunoglobulin. Low levels of surface immunoglobulin are, however, expressed in a minor subset of B-ALL cases.

Additional antigenic markers have been useful in characterizing B-ALL, with an emphasis placed on those that are suitable for distinguishing normal and leukemic precursors. These include CD24, CD34, CD123, CD73, CD304, CD81, CD58, CD38, and CD9, all of which are expressed in a significant fraction of cases, often at abnormal levels.[1,35-37] It should be noted that, among B-cell neoplasms, CD34 is uniquely expressed in lymphoblastic lesions and has particular significance in classifying these lesions as precursor-derived. TdT expression is also characteristic of immature B-lymphoblastic lesions, although it is not always present and has been very rarely reported in high-grade or transformed mature B-cell lymphomas.[38-41] CD45, or the leukocyte common antigen, is not expressed in approximately 10% to 20% of cases of B-ALL, and in the remaining cases, it typically shows lower levels of expression than those found in normal B precursors.[42,43] CD99, more commonly thought of as a marker of Ewing's sarcoma, is also expressed by most hematopoietic tumors that express TdT.[44-46] Thus, expression of CD99 coupled with lack of CD45 expression does not exclude a diagnosis of B-ALL. Finally, expression of myeloid antigens, including CD13, CD33, and CD15, is found in about 10% to 15% of childhood B-ALLs[47] and in

approximately 25% of adult cases.[48,49] However, the myeloid-blast–associated antigen CD117 is only very rarely present in B-cell ALL and should prompt consideration for AML with aberrant expression of B-cell antigens or B/myeloid mixed-phenotype acute leukemia (MPAL).[50] The routine evaluation for myeloperoxidase (MPO) expression in B-ALL can be problematic because otherwise typical cases of B-ALL have occasionally been shown to express low levels of MPO,[51-54] and this should not automatically result in a diagnosis of MPAL in the absence of other criteria.

Genetics and Molecular Findings

Nearly all cases of B-ALL have rearrangement of the IGH gene.[3] However, IGH gene rearrangement can also occur in both T-ALL and AML, limiting the utility of this test as a marker of lineage commitment. Immunoglobulin light chain (IGL) rearrangement can also occur and is thought to be a more specific marker of B-cell differentiation.

B-ALL is increasingly defined by specific genetic abnormalities that are associated with specific phenotypes and clinical behaviors (Table 41-1), many of which are incorporated into the International Consensus Classification (ICC) and the proposed World Health Organization (WHO) 5th edition of the Classification of Tumours of Haematopoietic and Lymphoid Tissues.[55-57] Initially, classical cytogenetic studies were mostly used to subclassify B-ALLs, and this method was subsequently supplemented by fluorescence in situ hybridization (FISH) and targeted polymerase chain reaction (PCR). More recently, large-scale studies that use clustering algorithms to correlate RNA-seq based gene expression (GEX) patterns with genetic findings have enabled the identification of multiple new subtypes of B-ALL. Although detailed discussion of methodology used to identify these lesions is beyond the scope of this chapter, many entities can now be recognized by FISH, multiplex PCR, or standard next-generation sequencing studies, and some have immunohistochemical or flow cytometric surrogates. Whole transcriptome sequencing, or unbiased RNA-seq, is probably the single most robust method that can be used to detect most of these lesions.[58]

The increasingly granular subclassification of B-ALL is significant because some of the identified genetic abnormalities enable targeted therapy. In addition, the prognostic information may be used to identify patients for whom low-intensity therapy will likely be curative, thus avoiding complications of more aggressive treatment. Thus, it is useful to consider these recurrent chromosomal and molecular abnormalities (Box 41-2) individually.

Quantitative Chromosomal Abnormalities

It has long been known that hyperdiploidy with greater than 50 chromosomes (sometimes called *high hyperdiploidy*) is a strong predictor of durable response to therapy in childhood B-ALL; this entity is recognized and defined similarly by both the ICC and the proposed WHO 5th edition. These patients account for about 25% of childhood B-ALL cases and often possess other favorable features, including lower peripheral white blood cell counts and age between 2 and 10 years.[59,60] However, hyperdiploidy confers a good prognosis independent of these other indicators, and it predicts a favorable response, regardless of peripheral white blood cell count.[61] The good

Table 41-1 Characteristics of B-ALL Entities in the ICC

Diagnosis	Frequency and Clinical Features	Comments
B-ALL with t(9;22)(q34.1;q11.2)/BCR::ABL1	~5% of children, ~30% of adults; poor prognosis but much improved with TKI therapy. Multilineage type akin to CML in blast crisis, but no antecedent history and typically no splenomegaly	CD19+10+, often with myeloid antigens or CD25; Divided into lymphoid only and multilineage, depending on cells that have Ph chromosome
B-ALL with t(v;11q23.3)/KMT2A rearranged	Half of infant ALL; uncommon but seen in all age groups. High WBC and CNS involvement, poor prognosis	Multiple partners, AFF1 most common. Blasts typically CD19+, CD22-dim, CD10−, CD24−, CD15/65+, especially with AFF4
B-ALL with t(12;21) (p13.2;q22.1)/ETV6::RUNX1	25% of childhood ALL, good prognosis; 3% of adults	CD19+, CD10+, CD27+, CD44-low/−, CD9−
B-ALL, hyperdiploid	25% of childhood ALL, good prognosis; uncommon to rare in adults	>50 chromosomes (not triploid or tetraploid), typically simple additions without structural abnormalities
B-ALL, low hypodiploid	Rare, poor prognosis	32–39 chromosomes; TP53 and RB1 mutations; TP53 often germline
B-ALL, near haploid	Rare, poor prognosis	24–31 chromosomes; RAS and RTK signaling mutations
B-ALL with t(5;14)(q31.1;q32.3)/IL3::IGH	Rare, poor prognosis	Eosinophilia from upregulation of IL3
B-ALL with t(1;19)(q23.3;p13.3)/TCF3::PBX1	Relatively common, average prognosis if treated appropriately	Pre-B phenotype: CD19+, 10+, CD34− with cytoplasmic mu expression
B-ALL, BCR::ABL1–like, ABL-1 class rearranged	2%–3% of childhood ALL, higher in adults. Poor prognosis but some patients respond very well to TKI therapy	Rearranged genes include ABL1, ABL2, CSF1R, LYN, PDGFRA, PDGFRB
B-ALL, BCR::ABL1–like, JAK-STAT activated	5%–10% of childhood ALL, 25% of adults; poor prognosis	~50% have CRLF2 rearrangements with overexpression of TSLPR, the CRLF2 gene product; JAK mutated or rearranged
B-ALL with iAMP21	~2% of childhood ALL, rare in adults. Poor prognosis but intensive treatment improves outcome	Typically detected by RUNX1 FISH as five or more signals per cell
B-ALL with MYC rearrangement	2%–5%, higher in adults and AYA; poor prognosis	May also have BCL2/6 rearrangements
B-ALL with DUX4 rearrangement	5%–10%, highest in AYA and adult; excellent prognosis	ERG and IKZF1 deletions but still excellent prognosis; CD371 expression an excellent surrogate
B-ALL with MEF2D rearrangement	3%–5%; poor prognosis	CD10 low/−; CD38 high; Multiple partners, most common BCL9
B-ALL with ZNF384 rearrangement	5%–10%; highest in AYA	CD10 low/−, myeloid antigen+; common in B/myeloid MPAL. EP300 most common partner with better prognosis
B-ALL with NUTM1 rearrangement	2% or less, mostly infants; far better prognosis than KMT2A-r	Multiple partners. Can detect with IHC
B-ALL with HLF rearrangement	<<1% children, very poor prognosis	TCF3 most common partner ("t(17;19)"; TCF4 rare but same poor prognosis
B-ALL with UBTF::ATXN7L3/PAN3,CDX2 ("CDX2/UBTF")	<1%; higher in AYA, female predominance, poor prognosis	Two alterations: gene fusion detectable by PCR; deletion on chromosome 13 and 17, resulting in CDX2 deregulation
B-ALL with mutated IKZF1 N159Y	<1%, variable prognosis	Detectable by targeted NGS
B-ALL with mutated PAX5 P80R	2%–5%, more common in adults; good prognosis in adults	Detectable by targeted NGS

ALL, Acute lymphoblastic leukemia; *AYA,* adolescents and young adults; *B-ALL,* B-lymphoblastic leukemia/lymphoma; *CML,* chronic myeloid leukemia; *CNS,* central nervous system; *IHC,* immunohistochemistry; *MPAL,* mixed phenotype acute leukemia; *NGS,* next-generation sequencing; *Ph,* Philadelphia; *RTK,* receptor tyrosine kinase; *TKI,* tyrosine kinase inhibitor; *TSLPR,* thymic stromal lymphopoietin receptor; *WBC,* white blood cell.

prognosis associated with hyperdiploidy appears to be a result of the addition of specific chromosomes, and in some clinical trials, finding trisomies involving chromosomes 4 and 10 have been used as a surrogate for high hyperdiploidy for treatment assignment.[62] Children with B-ALL having hyperdiploidy with 47 to 50 chromosomes account for 10% to 15% of cases, and these patients do not have the same favorable prognosis.[59]

Hypodiploidy also occurs, usually cause by the loss of one or more chromosomes, an unbalanced translocation, or the formation of dicentric chromosomes. Unlike hyperdiploidy,

hypodiploidy is associated with poor prognosis.[63] In the ICC, hypodiploid B-ALL is formally separated into two different entities: "B-ALL, low hypodiploid" (32-39 chromosomes), and "B-ALL, near haploid" (24-31 chromosomes). The low hypodiploid group is associated with loss-of-function mutations in TP53 and RB1,[64] and could be considered a form of Li-Fraumeni syndrome in that subset of patients that are found to have germline TP53 mutations.[65] In contrast, near-haploid B-ALL is associated with a different set of mutations, especially RAS and receptor tyrosine kinase signaling mutations.[65,66]

Box 41-2 *ICC of Acute Lymphoblastic Leukemias*

B-Lymphoblastic Leukemia/Lymphoma (B-ALL)
B-ALL with recurrent genetic abnormalities
   B-ALL with t(9;22)(q34.1;q11.2)/BCR::ABL1
      With lymphoid-only involvement[a]
      With multilineage involvement[a]
   B-ALL with t(v;11q23.3)/KMT2A rearranged
   B-ALL with t(12;21)(p13.2;q22.1)/ETV6::RUNX1
   B-ALL, hyperdiploid[b]
      B-ALL, low hypodiploid[c]
      B-ALL, near haploid[c]
   B-ALL with t(5;14)(q31.1;q32.3)/IL3::IGH
   B-ALL with t(1;19)(q23.3;p13.3)/TCF3::PBX1
   B-ALL, *BCR::ABL1*–like, ABL-1 class rearranged[d]
   B-ALL, *BCR::ABL1*–like, JAK-STAT activated[d]
   B-ALL, BCR::ABL1–like, not otherwise specified[d]
   B-ALL with iAMP21
   B-ALL with *MYC* rearrangement[e]
   B-ALL with *DUX4* rearrangement[e]
   B-ALL with *MEF2D* rearrangement[e]
   B-ALL with *ZNF384* rearrangement[e]
   B-ALL with *NUTM1* rearrangement[e]
   B-ALL with *HLF* rearrangement[f]
   B-ALL with *UBTF::ATXN7L3/PAN3,CDX2* ("CDX2/UBTF")[g]
   B-ALL with mutated *IKZF1* N159Y[e]
   B-ALL with mutated *PAX5* P80R[e]
B-ALL, not otherwise specified

Provisional entity: B-ALL, *ETV6::RUNX1*-like[h]
Provisional entity: B-ALL, with *PAX5* alteration[e]
Provisional entity: B-ALL, with mutated *ZEB2* H1038R/*IGH::CEBPE*[g]
Provisional entity: B-ALL, *ZNF384* rearranged-like[g]
Provisional entity: B-ALL, *KMT2A* rearranged-like[g]

T-Lymphoblastic Leukemia/Lymphoma (T-ALL)
Early T-cell precursor ALL with BCL11B activation[i]
Early T-cell precursor ALL, not otherwise specified[i]
T-ALL, not otherwise specified
   Provisional entity: T-ALL with *TAL1/2* dysregulation[g]
   Provisional entity: T-ALL with *TLX1* rearrangement[g]
   Provisional entity: T-ALL with *TLX3* rearrangement[g]
   Provisional entity: T-ALL with *HOXA* dysregulation[g]
   Provisional entity: T-ALL with *LMO1/2* dysregulation[g]
   Provisional entity: T-ALL with *NKX2* rearrangement[g]
   Provisional entity: T-ALL with *SPI1*-rearrangement[g]
   Provisional entity: T-ALL with other *bHLH* alterations[g]

Provisional entity: natural killer (NK) cell ALL[j]

Entities in **bold** are included in the World Health Organization (WHO) proposed 5th edition of the Classification of Tumours of Haematopoietic and Lymphoid Tissues. The WHO has slightly different terminology, not including the cytogenetic translocation terminology, and uses the term "fusion" rather "rearrangement" in the definition.

[a]Combined as B-lymphoblastic leukemia/lymphoma with *BCR::ABL1* in proposed WHO 5th edition and WHO 4th edition.
[b]B-lymphoblastic leukemia/lymphoma with high hyperdiploidy in proposed WHO 5th edition and WHO 4th edition.
[c]Combined as B-lymphoblastic leukemia/lymphoma with hypodiploidy in proposed WHO 5th edition and WHO 4th edition.
[d]Combined as B-lymphoblastic leukemia/lymphoma with *BCR::ABL1*-like features in proposed WHO 5th edition and WHO 4th edition.
[e]Included with B-lymphoblastic leukemia/lymphoma with other defined genetic abnormalities in proposed WHO 5th edition; not included in WHO 4th edition.
[f]Only B-lymphoblastic leukemia/lymphoma with *TCF3::HLF* fusion in proposed WHO 5th edition; not included in WHO 4th edition.
[g]Not included in proposed WHO 5th edition or WHO 4th edition.
[h]B-lymphoblastic leukemia/lymphoma with *ETV6::RUNX1*-like features in WHO 5th edition; not included in WHO 4th edition.
[i]Combined as early T-cell precursor ALL in proposed WHO 5th edition and WHO revised 4th edition.
[j]Provisional entity in WHO revised 4th edition but deleted from proposed WHO 5th edition.

Another distinct subgroup of B-ALL exhibits intrachromosomal amplification of one copy of chromosome 21 (iAMP21) with at least four copies of *RUNX1* on an abnormal chromosome.[67] iAMP21 is also associated with other characteristic cytogenetic abnormalities, including gain of chromosome X, loss or deletions of chromosome 7, and deletions of *ETV6* and *RB1*. These cases comprise approximately 2% of B-cell ALL cases, tend to affect older children but not adults, are associated with low white blood cell counts at diagnosis, and are commonly associated with CRLF2 overexpression. This abnormality can be most reliably detected by FISH for *RUNX1*, and identification of these patients is critical because iAMP21 has been associated with poor prognosis if intensive chemotherapeutic regimens are not used.[67]

Translocations and Other Molecular Alterations

There are a number of well-characterized chromosomal translocations associated with B-ALL. In children, the most common molecular abnormality is the *ETV6::RUNX1* fusion. It is observed in approximately 25% of childhood B-ALL but in only 3% of adult cases.[68] This translocation produces an abnormal fusion protein between the Ets family transcription factor *ETV6 (TEL)* and the DNA-binding subunit of the core binding factor complex RUNX1 *(AML1)*.

Both these transcription factors appear to be necessary for hematopoiesis,[69,70] and transduction of the *ETV6::RUNX1* fusion protein into mouse hematopoietic stem cells has been shown to induce ALL.[71] It is important to note that detection of this lesion generally requires the use of FISH because there is generally a balanced cryptic t(12;21)(p13.2;q22.1) not apparent when classic karyotyping is used.[72] B-ALLs harboring this translocation often possess a characteristic immunophenotype: expression of CD34, partial expression of CD20, and in particular, little or no expression of CD9.[73] Also, unlike most other ALLs, they are CD27 positive and CD44 negative or low.[74] The presence of *ETV6::RUNX1* confers an improved event-free survival in children,[75] though some have suggested that these patients are at increased risk for late relapse.[76] Although this point remains controversial, the unusual demonstration of clonally identical *ETV6::RUNX1* leukemias arising years apart in monozygotic twins has led to the hypothesis that this fusion is an early event in leukemogenesis,[10] which raises the interesting question of whether late relapses might be new second leukemias derived from a dormant leukemic precursor.

In adults, the most frequently observed chromosomal abnormality is t(9;22)(q34.1;q11.2), or the Philadelphia (Ph) chromosome. This translocation, present in about 25% of adult and up to 5% of childhood B-ALL,[68] involves the *ABL1* oncogene on chromosome 9 and the guanosine triphosphate–binding protein BCR on chromosome 22. The resultant fusion protein has abnormal tyrosine kinase activity, leading to disturbances in cell proliferation, survival, and adhesion.[77] Although the BCR::ABL1 fusion protein is also found in chronic myeloid leukemia (CML), in about 70% of cases of BCR::ABL1-positive ALL, the expressed protein is only 190 kDa rather than the 210 kDa typically seen in CML, reflecting less contribution of the BCR gene to the fusion protein.[78] Ph chromosome positivity is associated with a poor prognosis in both children[79,80] and adults,[81] although the availability of tyrosine kinase inhibitors has improved outcome.[82]

The ICC further divides "BCR::ABL1-positive B-ALL" into two subtypes: "B-ALL with t(9;22)(q34.1;q11.2)/BCR::ABL1 with lymphoid only involvement" (BCR::ABL1-positive ALL-L) and "B-ALL with t(9;22)(q34.1;q11.2)/BCR::ABL1 with multilineage involvement" (BCR::ABL1-positive ALL-M). In BCR::ABL1-positive ALL-M, the target cell for the transformation event is a multipotent progenitor, whereas in BCR::ABL1-positive ALL-L, the target cell is a later progenitor. BCR::ABL1-positive ALL-M is akin to CML presenting in lymphoid blast phase (CML-LBP), but it lacks significant splenomegaly and a history of CML characteristic in CML-LPB. In BCR::ABL1-positive ALL-L, however, the translocation is only seen in blasts. BCR::ABL1-positive ALL-L and ALL-M may be difficult to differentiate at diagnosis when blasts greatly predominate, and cell separation techniques coupled with FISH may be needed to assess which cells harbor the fusion signal.[83] BCR::ABL1-positive ALL-M may also be suspected when the percentage of cells that are Ph positive is significantly greater than the blast percentage or after therapy when there is a discordance between levels of residual leukemia detected by reverse transcription (RT)-PCR compared with flow cytometry or DNA PCR methods.[83]

Recurrent chromosomal abnormalities involving the KMT2A (formerly MLL) gene on the chromosome 11q23.3 locus have been observed in B-ALL and have prognostic significance.[84] The most common of these is the rearrangement t(4;11)(q21;q23)/KMT2A::AFF1. KMT2A-rearranged B-ALL can use a large number of different partner genes, the most common alternative of which is MLLT1 at 19p13. B-ALLs with KMT2A rearrangements, especially t(4;11), tend to occur in infants. They often present with high white blood cell counts, organomegaly, and CNS involvement, and patients have a poor prognosis. These lymphoblastic leukemias have a unique phenotype that distinguishes them from other B-ALLs. They characteristically express CD19 but lack CD10 and CD24.[85] They also have a propensity to co-express the myeloid antigens CD15 and CD65,[86] prompting the mixed lineage leukemia moniker. Although t(4;11) leukemia confers poor prognosis, there is some controversy as to whether leukemias that use alternative fusion partners with KMT2A have an equally poor outcome. B-ALL with KMT2A rearrangements are characterized by lineage ambiguity and may present or recur as either B-ALL or B/myeloid MPAL.

TCF3 (formerly E2A)::PBX1/t(1;19)(q23.3;p13.3) is another well-characterized and relatively common translocation in B-ALL. This leukemia has a characteristic immunophenotype expressing CD19, CD10, homogeneous CD9, and partial CD20 but completely lacking CD34.[87] Although the presence of t(1;19) was once thought to confer poor prognosis, with

current intensive therapies, the outcome in these children is comparable to that of patients with similar risk factors.[88,89]

A distinctive subtype of ALL associated with t(5;14)(q31.1;q22.1) is characterized by a marked eosinophilia. This translocation juxtaposes the interleukin-3 (IL3) gene with the IGH gene on chromosome 14.[90-92] The lymphoblasts themselves are not morphologically distinctive; however, the eosinophils, which are not part of the neoplastic clone, often show morphologic atypia, including areas of cytoplasmic clearing and abnormal nuclear segmentation. Circulating blasts tend to be infrequent and are often obscured by the eosinophilia, but blasts are more numerous in the bone marrow. Patients with this variant often have symptoms related to the toxic effects of eosinophil degranulation, particularly cardiac disease.

Though most of the common translocations in B-ALL were originally detected via karyotype and are now more typically detected by FISH or PCR, GEX profiling was first used to define a number of new entities, including "B-ALL, BCR::ABL1-like." This entity was first recognized based on a GEX profile similar to B-ALL positive for Ph but lacking the BCR::ABL1 translocation.[93] This entity was introduced in the revised WHO 4th edition and is retained in the proposed WHO 5th edition; however, the ICC further subclassifies these "BCR::ABL1-like" cases into three subtypes: ABL1-class rearranged, JAK-STAT activated, and not otherwise specified (NOS). Comprehensive identification of these subtypes requires genomic studies, as none of these entities, apart from rearrangement of CRLF2 in a subset of cases in the JAK-STAT subgroup, shows distinctive immunophenotypic abnormalities.

"B-ALL, BCR::ABL1-like: ABL1-class rearranged" includes fusions between ABL1, ABL2, CSF1R, or PDGFRB and various partner genes. Identification of this group is particularly important because these cases may respond to tyrosine kinase inhibitors (TKIs) that target ABL1.[94] Though PDGFRB-r lymphoid neoplasms are typically included in "myeloid/lymphoid neoplasms with PDGFRB rearrangement," those presenting as B-ALL are best classified as BCR::ABL1-like ALL, ABL1-class rearranged. The second new subclassification in the ICC is the "B-ALL, BCR::ABL1-like: JAK-STAT activated" cases. The most common mutations that result in activation of JAK-STAT pathway signaling are CRLF2 rearrangements to IGH or P2RY8, resulting in overexpression of the gene product TSLPR (thymic stromal lymphopoietin), although this is commonly conventionally referred to as CRLF2 as well. This group also includes cases with JAK translocations or mutations. JAK inhibitors are currently in trials for this entity. The third subclass is "B-ALL, BCR::ABL1-like, NOS," which encompasses heterogeneous alterations of other kinases and cytokine receptors; it should be noted that many have been shown to be responsive to TKIs in preclinical models, particularly kinase rearrangements (FLT3, FGFR1, NTRK3, and PTK2B). Fusions involving NTKR3 may show profound responses to TKIs such as larotrectinib.

BCR::ABL1-like B-ALL has a poor prognosis overall.[94] Further subclassification of this category may allow for the identification of specific targetable lesions and provide novel therapeutic opportunities for these patients.

Several additional entities characterized by gene fusions are included as specific entities in the ICC and most also in the proposed WHO 5th edition, either explicitly or part of a larger group with miscellaneous genetic abnormalities. Many of these have distinct prognoses. With the exception of "B-ALL with *DUX4*-rearrangement" and "B-ALL with *ZNF384*-rearrangement," which each account for about 5% to 10% of cases, the other entities with defining fusion proteins are rare. B-ALL with double homeobox 4 (*DUX4*)-rearrangement is relatively common in adolescents and young adults. This entity is associated with an excellent prognosis in both children and adults, even in the presence of otherwise poor-risk genetic features.[74] The *IGH::DUX4* translocation is inconsistently detected by transcriptome sequencing and is difficult to detect by FISH because of the repetitive nature of both the *DUX4* and IGH loci; however, these cases characteristically show expression of CD371 on flow cytometric analysis.[95] Rearrangements of the transcription factor zinc finger 384 (*ZNF384*) defines a subtype of B-ALL that is most common in children and young adults and has a variable prognosis. Similar to *KMT2A*-rearranged B-ALL, these cases are characterized by lineage ambiguity and may present as either B-ALL or B/myeloid MPAL.[96] *ZNF384* has numerous fusion partners, most commonly *EP300*, *TCF3*, and *TAF15*, and the prognosis depends on the fusion partner.[97]

Though *MYC* translocations are more frequently associated with mature B-cell lymphoma, they are also reported in about 4% of adult B-ALL and, rarely, pediatric B-ALL. *MYC*-r B-ALL and *MYC*-r mature B-cell lymphoma are genetically distinct from one another. *IG::MYC* positive B-ALL cases are characterized by aberrant VDJ joining in a B cell precursor undergoing VDJ recombination, whereas *B-ALLs* with *MYC*-r are characterized by unmutated IGVH genes.[98] Accordingly, these entities may be separable via somatic hypermutation studies, with only *MYC*-rearranged (*MYC*-r) mature large B-cell lymphomas exhibiting somatic hypermutation. The clinical presentations of *MYC*-r mature B-cell lymphomas and *MYC*-r B-ALL are also typically very different, with mass lesions in the former and bone marrow replacement in the latter; however, there is some clinical overlap, and definitive distinction requires laboratory studies. CD34 or TdT expression favors a diagnosis of B-ALL, though transformed or aggressive mature B-cell lymphomas can show TdT expression, and a diagnosis of *MYC*-r B-ALL should be avoided in patients with such a history. *MYC*-r B-ALL is associated with a very poor prognosis.

There are other rare fusions included in the ICC, most of which have a poor prognosis, including B-ALL with myocyte enhancer factor 2D (*MEF2D*) rearrangements[99] and B-ALL with *HLF* rearrangement. Another B-ALL subtype, found only in the ICC and referred to as "*CDX2/UBTF*," harbors two alterations in all cases, namely a fusion oncoprotein-encoding rearrangement *UBTF::ATXN7L3* and a deletion upstream of *FLT3* that results in deregulation of CDX2; both alterations are required to produce leukemia. This subtype also has a poor prognosis. One final B-ALL subtype that is defined by a fusion is NUT midline carcinoma family member 1 (*NUTM1*)-rearranged B-ALL. This subtype typically affects infants and has a relatively favorable prognosis.

Finally, the ICC incorporates two new entities that are defined by point mutations: B-ALL with *PAX5* P80R and B-ALL with *IKZF1* N159Y. B-ALL with a *PAX5* P80R mutation accounts for 2% to 5% of B-ALL cases, is more common in adults, and has a relatively good prognosis. B-ALL with a DNA-binding protein Ikaros (*IKZF1*) N159Y mutation accounts for less than 1% of cases, is more common in adults, and has an intermediate prognosis.

The ICC also includes several provisional entities (Box 41-2), one of which is included in the proposed WHO 5th edition classification: "B-ALL, *ETV6::RUNX1*-like." These cases share the same GEX profile and CD27-positive, CD44-dim/negative phenotype as B-ALL with *ETV6::RUNX1* fusion, but they lack the defining t(12;21)(p13.2;q22.1).

Additional Genetic Lesions

Virtually all cases of ALL harbor additional genetic alterations beyond the driver lesions that define the entity. These are seen across different entities and so are not included in the classification. Many of these, most notably *IKZF1* and *CDKN2A/B* deletions, are commonly associated with poor prognosis; however, as exemplified by the good outcome of patients with *DUX4*-r ALL and *IKZF1* deletions, the significance of specific mutations may be different in different genetic subgroups.[100]

Normal Counterpart

The normal counterpart for the B-lymphoblasts in B-ALL is the normal precursor B cell that resides within the bone marrow. These cells, also known as *hematogones*, are seen with increased frequency in children and tend to decrease with age. However, hematogone content can vary widely, especially during hematopoietic regeneration, and may be significantly increased after umbilical cord blood stem cell transplant.[101] Hematogones possess a very reproducible pattern of antigen acquisition that helps distinguish them from B-ALL. The earliest hematogones express dim CD45 with low right-angle light scatter, CD19, CD10, CD34, CD38, and TdT. These cells lack CD20 and surface immunoglobulin expression and express dim CD22. As the cells mature, CD20 is acquired, and early antigens such as CD34 and CD10 are lost. Because of the reproducible nature of antigen expression on normal precursor B cells, multiparametric flow cytometry can reliably distinguish normal cells from leukemic precursor B cells in most cases.[102] This principle is routinely applied in monitoring patients with B-ALL for the presence of minimal residual disease (MRD).

Clinical Course

In general, B-cell ALL of childhood has become a disease with a high cure rate, whereas adults with B-cell ALL have a poorer prognosis, in part because the good prognosis lesions of hyperdiploidy and *ETV6::RUNX1* are much less common in adults. Use of tyrosine kinase inhibitors to treat *BCR::ABL1*-positive B-ALL in both children and adults has resulted in improved outcomes.[82,103] Other promising therapeutic strategies include the application of pediatric chemotherapy to young adults[104]; the use of improved formulations of standard chemotherapeutics such as PEG-asparaginase; and the use of immunotherapeutics such as rituximab and anti-CD22 monoclonal antibodies,[105] bispecific anti-CD19/CD3 antibody therapy,[106,107] and chimeric antigen receptor (CAR) T-cell therapy.[108,109]

Prognosis, however, hinges on the presence or absence of increasingly well-characterized genetic and molecular abnormalities. Children with leukemias harboring the *ETV6::RUNX1* translocation or possessing more than 50 chromosomes have a long-term event-free survival rate of 90%

or greater. However, those with molecular lesions associated with *BCR::ABL1*-like ALL or those with t(4;11) fare much more poorly, and some children with other high-risk features have a long-term event-free survival rate of less than 50%. As noted, many of the more recently recognized entities also have prognostic significance, and most, with the exception of *DUX4*-rearranged ALL, have a poor prognosis.[99] The reason for the different clinical outcomes in these subtypes remains unknown, but new insights into the molecular and cellular biology of these subtypes may help tailor subgroup-oriented therapies. In addition, it is hoped that use of the refined ICC and proposed WHO 5th edition classification will assist in risk stratification and optimal treatment selection for patients with B-ALL.

Although new prognostically relevant genetic risk factors continue to be discovered, early response to therapy remains the most important prognostic factor. How rapidly a patient clears morphologically evident disease during induction predicts long-term outcome,[110] but the presence of MRD at levels below that of morphologic detection is an even stronger prognostic factor,[111-113] and such measurements play a vital role in risk stratification and management of patients with ALL. MRD may be measured by flow cytometry[111,113] (Fig. 41-2) or by PCR[112] directed against antigen receptor genes, although the latter technique is more cumbersome and expensive because it requires the production of patient-specific probes or primers. Thresholds of 0.01% of blasts detected by flow cytometry at the end of induction therapy are typically used to identify patients in need of enhanced treatment, but other thresholds and other timepoints are used for treatment assignment with PCR-based MRD. Next-generation sequencing[114] strategies are even more sensitive, potentially easier to standardize, and are becoming more routinely used for MRD analysis in ALL. There is some evidence that this enhanced sensitivity can identify additional patients at risk for relapse.[115]

Differential Diagnosis

The differential diagnosis generally includes a number of hematopoietic tumors that may possess blast-like morphology and a small number of undifferentiated or primitive non-hematopoietic tumors (Tables 41-2 and 41-3). Immunophenotypic analysis is typically required to distinguish among these neoplasms.

T-CELL LYMPHOBLASTIC LYMPHOMA/ LYMPHOBLASTIC LEUKEMIA

Definition

Like precursor B-cell tumors, T-cell lymphoblastic lesions are clonal hematopoietic stem cell disorders, but they are characterized by an immature T-cell, rather than B-cell, phenotype. Operationally, identification of T-cell antigen expression is required for the diagnosis of T-cell lymphoblastic tumors, and the phenotypic pattern must be that of an immature T cell. These tumors may have a leukemic presentation (T-ALL), or present as lymphoblastic lymphoma with tissue masses (T-LBL), although commonly blood, marrow, and tissue are all involved. To date, there is no convincing evidence that the leukemic and lymphomatous presentations are different biological entities, but extensive

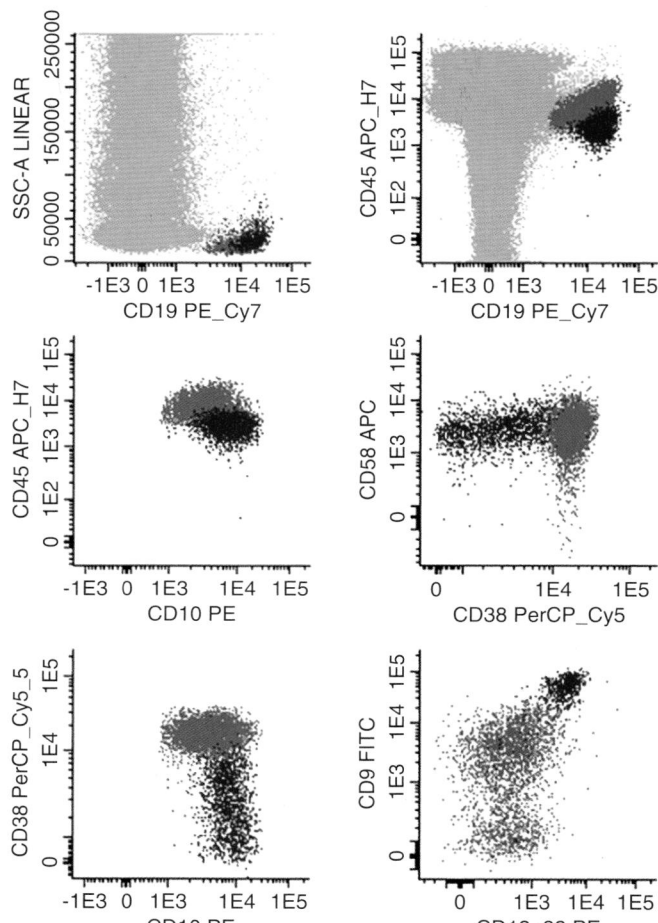

Figure 41-2. Minimal residual disease in B-ALL. Multiparametric flow cytometry showing the distinction between hematogones *(pink)* and residual B-ALL blasts *(blue)*. Blasts have slightly brighter CD19 and CD10 and slightly dimmer CD45 compared with hematogones but hematogones and blasts overlap in these displays. However, blasts have much dimmer CD38 and brighter expression of CD9 and myeloid antigens CD13/33, allowing better separation from hematogones.

genomic investigation comparing T-LBL to T-ALL has not been performed. As noted, many treatment protocols use ≥25% bone marrow blasts as a cut-off for classification as T-ALL.

Synonyms and Related Terms

None.

Epidemiology

Perhaps because the thymus is the major site of normal T-cell development, the majority of T-LBLs are found in the mediastinum. T-lymphoblastic tumors account for only about 15% of childhood acute lymphoblastic leukemias, but nearly 90% of LBLs. LBLs are more common in late childhood and account for about one-third of all pediatric cases of non-Hodgkin lymphoma; they constitute only a small percentage of adult cases. Both leukemia and lymphomatous presentations show a male predominance.

Table 41-2 Differential Diagnosis of Acute Lymphoblastic Leukemia

Tumor	Distinguishing Features
Acute myeloid leukemia with minimal differentiation	Myeloid phenotype
Acute leukemias of ambiguous lineage	Co-expression of myeloid and lymphoid antigens or evidence of both myeloid and lymphoid differentiation
Lymphoid blast crisis of chronic myeloid leukemia (CML)	History of antecedent CML, Ph+
Chronic lymphocytic leukemia	Condensed nuclear chromatin, mature B-cell phenotype
Prolymphocytic leukemia	Lower nuclear-to-cytoplasmic ratio, prominent nucleolus, mature B-cell phenotype
Blastic variant of mantle cell lymphoma	Mature B-cell phenotype, t(11;14), cyclin D1 expression
Large B-cell lymphoma	Larger cells; mature B-cell phenotype
Burkitt lymphoma/leukemia	More prominent nucleoli; prominent basophilic cytoplasm; mature B-cell phenotype, t(8;14)
Small, round, blue cell tumors (including Ewing's sarcoma, neuroblastoma, embryonal rhabdomyosarcoma, medulloblastoma)	Cohesive growth, absence of lymphoid markers
Reactive proliferations of normal precursor B cells (hematogones)	Indistinct or absent nucleoli, normal continuum of B-cell antigen acquisition during differentiation

Table 41-3 Differential Diagnosis of Lymphoblastic Lymphoma

Tumor	Distinguishing Features
Myeloid sarcoma	More distinct cytoplasm, eosinophilic myelocytes, myeloid phenotype
Lymphocytic thymoma	Presence of abnormal cytokeratin+ thymic epithelial cells
Chronic lymphocytic leukemia/small lymphocytic lymphoma	Condensed nuclear chromatin, mature B-cell phenotype
	Smudge cells can be present in both acute lymphoblastic leukemia and chronic lymphocytic leukemia
Blastic variant of mantle cell lymphoma	Mature B-cell phenotype, t(11;14), cyclin D1 and/or Sox11 expression
Large B-cell lymphoma	Large cells, more prominent nucleoli, mature B-cell phenotype/absence of CD34 expression
Burkitt lymphoma	More prominent nucleoli, distinct cytoplasmic rim, mature B-cell phenotype, t(8;14)
Small, round, blue cell tumors (including Ewing's sarcoma, neuroblastoma, embryonal rhabdomyosarcoma, medulloblastoma)	May show cohesive growth, absence of lymphoid markers
Ectopic thymus	Indistinct or absent nucleoli, normal continuum of T-cell antigen acquisition during differentiation, normal epithelium
Indolent T-lymphoblastic proliferation	Extrathymic involvement, preserved architecture with interfollicular expansion, T-cell receptor gene rearrangement studies show polyclonality

Etiology

Although specific genetic disturbances are involved in T-lymphoblastic lesions, the underlying etiologic factors are unknown. Patients with ataxia telangiectasia have an increased risk of developing T-ALL, but only rarely develop B-ALL.[116]

Clinical Features

Patients with T-ALL typically present with high peripheral white blood cell counts (>50,000/µL), organomegaly, and peripheral lymphadenopathy. Children with T-ALL are typically older than those with B-ALL. The presence of a mediastinal mass is highly associated with a T-cell phenotype in ALL. Like patients with B-ALL, those with T-ALL may present with anemia, thrombocytopenia, organomegaly, and bone pain; however, leukopenia is less common in T-ALL than in B-ALL.

Patients with T-LBL also have high tumor burdens, evidenced by advanced stage or bulky disease. In patients with mediastinal involvement, the mass is often quite large, leading to compromise of regional anatomic structures. This may manifest with clinical symptoms such as dyspnea caused by airway obstruction, dysphagia caused by esophageal compromise, or superior vena cava syndrome. Pulmonary and cardiac function may also be compromised by the presence of pleural or pericardial effusions.

Morphology

Like precursor B-cell lesions, leukemic and lymphomatous presentations of T-ALL are morphologically indistinguishable. Moreover, differentiating T-ALL from B-ALL by morphology alone is impossible. Cytologically, lymphoblasts range from small, round blasts with a high nuclear-to-cytoplasmic ratio, relatively condensed chromatin, and inconspicuous nucleoli to larger cells with increased amounts of blue-gray to blue cytoplasm, irregular nuclei with dispersed chromatin, and variable numbers of distinct nucleoli (Fig. 41-3). Cytoplasmic vacuoles are occasionally seen. Typically, T-cell lymphoblasts tend to have more cytologic heterogeneity and more nuclear convolutions than B lymphoblasts; however, no phenotypic, molecular, or clinical differences have been correlated with convoluted nuclear morphology. Histologically, T-LBL is a diffuse infiltrative process that occasionally involves lymph nodes in an interfollicular pattern but more commonly diffusely

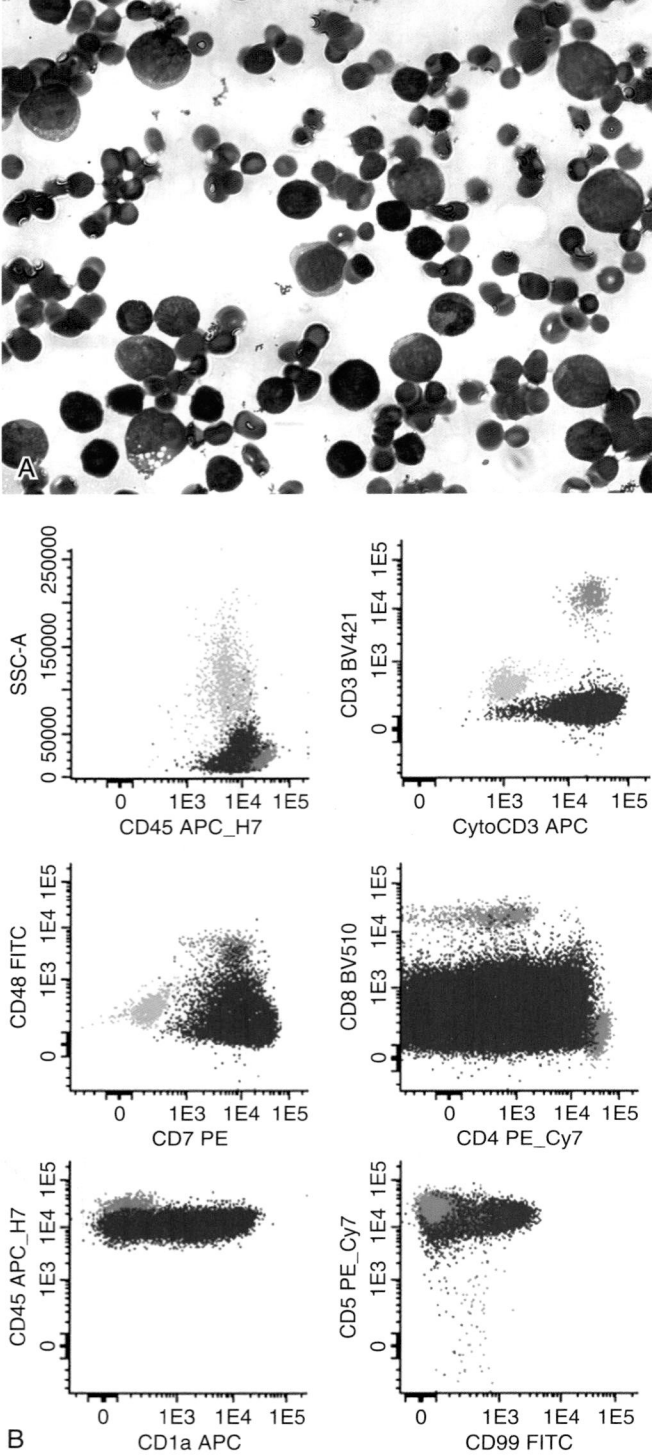

Figure 41-3. T-cell acute lymphoblastic leukemia. A, Bone marrow aspirate shows a predominant population of heterogeneous blasts with a range of sizes. **B,** Multiparametric flow cytometry shows a population of abnormal T-cell blasts with slightly dim CD45 expressing cytoplasmic but not surface CD3, CD5, variable CD4 with limited CD8, partial CD1a, and CD99 with loss of CD48. Color convention as in Figure 42-1.

replaces the nodal architecture (Fig. 41-4). Frequently, the tumor grows in a single-file pattern and can extend through the capsule, infiltrating the perinodal fat. T-cell LBL tends to be a proliferative process with numerous mitotic figures. Rapid cell turnover can give rise to a starry-sky appearance as a result of the presence of tingible body macrophages, but this pattern rarely predominates to the extent seen in Burkitt lymphoma.

Immunophenotype

Precursor T-cell malignancies can express markers associated with T-cell differentiation and maturation in almost any combination (Fig. 41-3B and 41-4), although an understanding of phenotypic changes associated with normal T-cell maturation is helpful in understanding malignant phenotypes. Normal common lymphoid progenitors express TdT, CD34, and HLA-DR. Other early markers in T-cell differentiation include CD7, which can also be expressed on some myeloid precursors,[117] and CD2, which is also on dendritic cell precursors[118]; however, expression of cytoplasmic CD3 is generally considered the first definitive marker of T-cell lineage commitment. Early T-cell precursors first enter the thymus at the corticomedullary junction and proceed to the outer cortex, acquiring CD5 and CD1a and losing HLA-DR. These are the so-called "double-negative" thymocytes, which lack expression of CD4 and CD8. At this stage, the T-cell receptor (TCR) chains remain in a germline configuration. TCR gene rearrangement then occurs, with the sequential rearrangement of the δ, γ, β, and finally α chains. This allows the development of a functional TCR to permit thymic education through both positive and negative selection. The CD4, CD8 double-positive common thymocyte represents the major thymic population. The double-positive thymocytes that successfully engage major histocompatibility complex (MHC)-I are destined to be CD8-positive T cells, and those that engage MHC-II will become CD4-positive T cells. TdT continues to be expressed throughout cortical thymic development and is lost as the thymocytes enter the medullary phase of maturation.

Because precursor T-cell tumors resemble their normal thymic counterparts, knowledge of the normal patterns of antigen expression that highlight the uniqueness of thymocytes can be helpful in the recognition of T-cell ALL. For example, expression of TdT and CD1a on T cells outside the thymus does not normally occur; when seen, this typically indicates an abnormal population, although rare TdT-positive extrathymic cortical thymocytes can normally be seen in the tonsils and cervical lymph nodes. Most T-LBLs have a phenotype resembling a late cortical thymic phenotype, with expression of cytoplasmic CD3, TdT, and both CD4 and CD8. An important point is that virtually all precursor T-cell tumors have aberrant patterns of antigen expression that distinguish them from normal thymocytes. These changes include loss of pan–T-cell markers and aberrant co-expression of B-cell–associated antigens (CD24, CD9, CD21) or myeloid antigens (CD13, CD33), but as with B-ALL, the most common abnormalities represent deviation from the normal pattern of antigen expression with maturation.

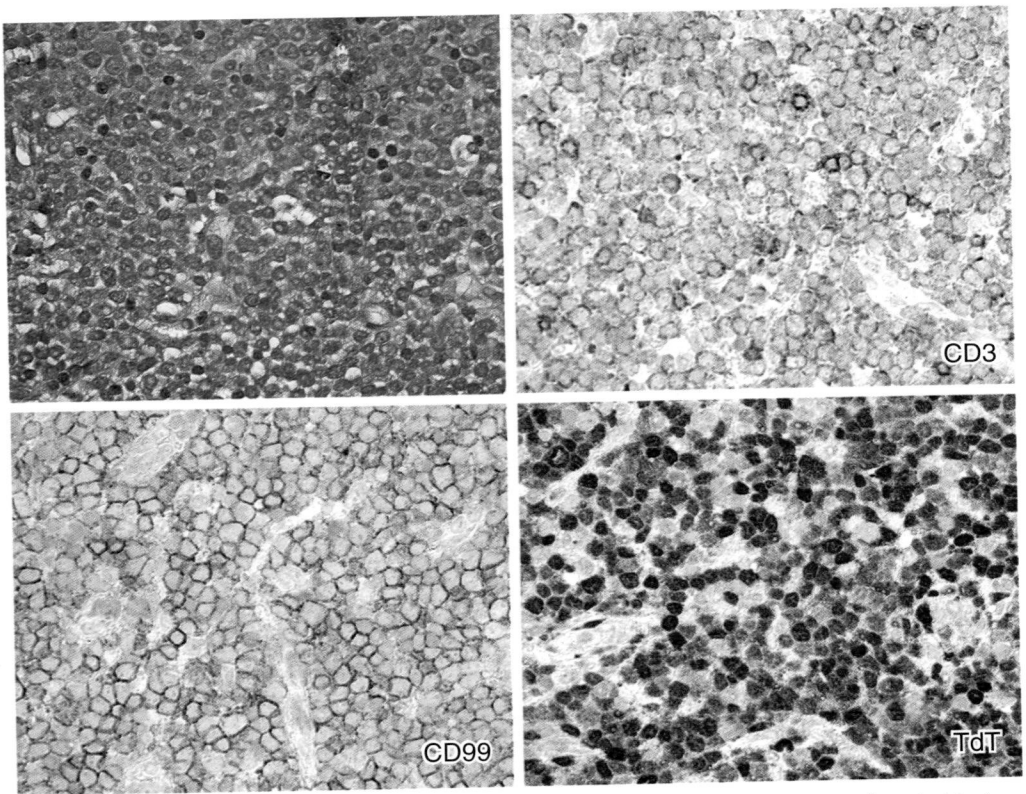

Figure 41-4. T-cell lymphoblastic lymphoma. Mediastinal mass shows malignant lymphoblasts with dispersed chromatin. The tumor expresses CD3, CD99, and terminal deoxynucleotidyl transferase (TdT), as indicated.

In some cases, T-cell ALL has a more primitive immunophenotype than T-cell LBL, perhaps reflecting either an earlier thymocyte precursor or even an earlier bone marrow progenitor. These cases of so-called "early T-cell precursor" (ETP) ALL represent a formal category of T-ALL in both the ICC and the proposed WHO 5th edition. ETP ALL is defined by its distinctive immunophenotype: CD1a negative, CD8 negative, and limited CD5 expression (<75% of blasts), with stem cell or myeloid antigen expression, including CD34, HLADR, CD13, CD33, CD117, CD15 and/or CD65.[119] Most of these cases also express TdT.[120] ETP ALL invariably expresses CD7, which appears to be the most sensitive antigen for T-cell ALL; however, CD7 is also frequently expressed in AML, including some cases of myeloperoxidase-negative AML.[121] Though ETP ALL frequently expresses myeloid antigens, by definition it does not express MPO. Clinical studies of ALL initially suggested that patients with ETP ALL have a particularly poor prognosis[119]; however, more recent studies using intensive therapy showed a slower initial response to therapy in ETP ALL compared with other T-ALLs, but no significant difference in survival.[122]

A subset of T-ALL that otherwise meets criteria for ETP ALL but that shows expression of CD5 on ≥75% blasts is often referred to as "near-ETP ALL".[123] Despite the immunophenotypic similarity to ETP ALL, near-ETP ALL has different genetic lesions than ETP ALL, with enrichment for *TLX3*-rearrangements. Near-ETP ALL also shows minor differences from ETP ALL in clinical presentation and response to therapy and is not included in formal classification systems.

In some cases, definitive distinction between AML and T-ALL may also be difficult. TdT is expressed in over 90% of T-ALL, and although it is present in up to 20% of AML cases, bright expression of TdT favors T-ALL.[124] HLA-DR may be helpful because it is expressed in virtually all CD7-positive AMLs but in only a small portion of T-cell ALLs. T-cell antigens such as CD1a, surface CD3, and CD8 show higher specificity for T-ALL, but they are often not expressed. Of all the markers, cytoplasmic CD3 appears to be the most reliable marker for establishing T-cell lineage and is expressed by virtually all precursor T-cell neoplasms. Cytoplasmic CD3 is brightly positive in most cases of T-ALL but may be dim, in which case distinction from AML may be more difficult.

Genetics and Molecular Findings

As mentioned, during normal T-cell development, there is an ordered rearrangement of TCR chain loci, starting with the δ chain, followed by γ and β, and finally, if γ and δ fail to generate a competent rearrangement, T-cell receptor α (TRA). T-ALLs often show patterns of TCR gene rearrangement that reflect this. As such, the most primitive T-ALL may have no rearranged TCR genes or only show TCR γ (TRG) rearrangement. TRA often remains in a germline configuration, except for tumors with the most mature phenotypes. Although TCR rearrangements are a vital step in T-cell development, there is significant lineage infidelity at the molecular level, and TCR rearrangements are also frequently observed in B-ALL. The rearrangement of IGH loci in precursor T-cell tumors is less frequent, and IGL locus rearrangement is almost never observed in precursor T-cell neoplasms.

In addition to the demonstration of TCR gene rearrangements, a number of nonrandom chromosomal translocations have been consistently observed in precursor T-ALL. Unlike precursor B-cell lesions, which rarely involve the immunoglobulin loci, these translocations frequently involve the TCR loci on chromosomes 7 and 14.[125] Most of the rearrangements involve transcription factors, suggesting disruption or inappropriate regulation of these factors contribute to leukemogenesis. In fact, it has long been recognized that T-ALL could be divided into families based on dysregulation of different transcription factors.[126] More recently, GEX studies similar to those performed in B-ALL have shown distinct clusters of T-ALL cases. Each cluster shares activation of common transcription factors. However, in contrast to B-ALL, where many cases in clusters share a common translocation, the T-ALL entities within each cluster may have various alterations (e.g., TCR rearrangements, chimeric fusion oncoproteins, and enhancer mutations) that deregulate different drivers; thus, comprehensive genomic analysis may be required to classify all cases. Moreover, the identification of a specific translocation in T-ALL may not be sufficient to define an entity, because many different genetic lesions may result in the downstream activation of the same pathways with similar GEX profiles. As a result of the complexity of the mechanisms associated with T-cell leukemogenesis, all members of a class can only be identified by GEX profiling or comprehensive genomic analysis. These methods are not routinely available in a clinical setting, and there is still no formal use of this transcription-based classification in ALL treatment protocols; therefore, entities defined in this manner are considered provisional in the ICC and are not part of the provisional WHO 5th edition (Box 41-2). However, there is evidence of clinical differences among these entities, some of which are summarized in Table 41-4.

An interesting observation from GEX studies of cases of ETP ALL was that a subset, comprising about 30% of cases, formed a distinct cluster separate from all other T-ALL cases. Further investigation into these cases revealed that this cluster had in common activation of the T cell transcription factor gene *BCL11B*. Approximately 80% of cases of ETP ALL with *BCL11B* alterations are associated with interchromosomal rearrangements that result in upregulation of BCL11B protein, and the remaining cases overexpress BCL11B via focal amplifications that generate a neoenhancer distal to the gene; for these reasons, this group has been termed "*BCL11B* activated" (*BCL11B*-a), rather than "*BCL11B* rearranged." Because *BCL11B*-a cases are biologically so different from other cases of ETP ALL, it is considered a new entity in the ICC (Table 41-4). These cases can be recognized by immunohistochemistry for BCL11B.[127] It is, however, important to use immunostaining for BCL11B to subclassify only cases of immunophenotypically proven ETP ALL, because BCL11B can also be upregulated in other types of T-ALL such as *TLX3*-dysregulated T-ALL.

Other Genetic Lesions in T-ALL

As is the case with B-ALL and AML, cases of T-ALL have cooperating mutations that are seen across many different entities. Among the most common, *NOTCH1* gene mutations have been implicated in the pathogenesis of a significant subset of T-ALL.[128,129] Although only rare cases with a (7;9) translocation involving *NOTCH1* have been identified, point mutations, insertions, and deletions in the *NOTCH1* gene, all

Table 41-4 Characteristics of Novel T-ALL Entities in the ICC

Subtype	Frequency and Clinical Features	Maturational Stage
BCL11B-activated	~30% of ETP ALL, prognosis possibly better than other ETP ALL	ETP: CD7+, CD5– (<75%), CD8–, CD1a– with myeloid or stem cell antigens
TAL1/2-dysregulated	30%–40% of T-ALL (TAL2 rare) poor prognosis	Late cortical-medullary thymocyte, often CD3+
TLX1-rearranged	5%–10% children ~30% adults very good prognosis	Cortical thymocyte
TLX3-rearranged	20%–25% children, <5% adult, very good prognosis	Some near-ETP/cortical thymocyte
HOXA-dysregulated	15%–25% variable prognosis	Immature, many ETP
LMO1/2-dysregulated	5%–10% LMO2>LMO1 and has worse prognosis	Immature, some ETP
NKX2-rearranged	<5% children	Late cortical thymocyte
SPI1-rearranged	<5% children, very poor prognosis	Early cortical thymocyte
bHLH, other	<2%	Immature

ETP ALL, Early T-cell precursor acute lymphoblastic leukemia; *T-ALL,* T-lymphoblastic leukemia/lymphoma.

leading to an increase in signaling, have been found in more than half of T-ALL cases, including those in all the molecular subgroups previously noted.[129] This suggests that these mutations play a central role in pathogenesis. Of interest, the increased *NOTCH1* signaling associated with these mutations is dependent on the downstream activity of γ secretase,[128] suggesting that γ secretase inhibitors might play a role in the treatment of T-cell ALL. Also common in T-ALL are deletions in *CDKN2A/B*, seen in about 70% of cases and considered fundamental to T-cell leukemogenesis. Other common mutations affect the JAK-STAT or RAS pathways.[129]

ETP T-ALL, however, characteristically lacks *NOTCH1* mutations, and instead is frequently associated with mutations such as *FLT3* (both ITD and D835), *DNMT3A*, *WT1*, and *RUNX1* that are more typically associated with myeloid disease. In addition, ETP T-ALL has a relatively low frequency of clonal TCR rearrangements[130] and a global transcriptional profile similar to that of normal hematopoietic and myeloid leukemia stem cells,[131] suggesting these neoplasms arise from early hematopoietic progenitors or stem cells. Interestingly, the *BCL11B* activation seen in the ETP ALL subset can also be seen in cases of AML, undifferentiated leukemia, and T/myeloid MPAL, and GEX studies show that all such cases co-cluster.[132,133] Whether the myeloid-related and stem cell related genetic features of ETP ALL are enriched in the *BCL11B*-a subset is as yet unknown.

Normal Counterpart

The normal counterpart of T-cell ALL/LBL is thought to be the precursor T cells that arise from bone marrow–derived hematopoietic stem cells that migrate to the thymus, where they develop. As noted, these precursor cells possess unique antigen-expression patterns that clearly distinguish them from more mature extrathymic T cells.

Clinical Course

Children with T-ALL generally have a more aggressive clinical course than those with B-ALL,[134,135] which is due, in part, to the characteristic presence of higher-risk clinical features. T-ALL tends to occur in older children, and patients have higher white blood cell counts. These patients also have a higher incidence of CNS involvement. Adults with T-ALL are typically treated with intensive therapy. These patients may actually fare better than those with B-ALL, likely reflecting the relatively high incidence of B-ALL with *BCR::ABL1* and *BCR::ABL1*-like B-ALL in adults. Patients with T-LBL with even minimal bone marrow disease at diagnosis have a poorer prognosis than those without it.[136] The majority of patients with T-LBL have advanced disease, evidence of B symptoms, and high lactate dehydrogenase levels. In contrast to leukemic presentations, there is typically preservation of peripheral blood counts, presumably owing to the lack of bone marrow replacement. Bone marrow or testicular involvement by LBL is strongly correlated with CNS disease. Historically, LBL has been an aggressive disease associated with poor survival in response to standard lymphoma therapy.

As a result of the similarities between T-cell ALL and LBL, most LBLs are treated with ALL-like therapy. On the adoption of these ALL-like regimens, dramatic improvements in outcome were seen,[137] particularly for low-stage LBL. Studies in adult patients with T-cell LBL indicated that they too can benefit from ALL-type regimens.[138] Another important therapeutic strategy is CNS prophylaxis, given the high rate of CNS relapse in patients who do not receive it. Because local recurrence is also a major indication of treatment failure, inclusion of mediastinal radiotherapy may play a role in preventing relapse, particularly in adult patients. MRD in T-ALL is also prognostically important; however, available data suggest that T-ALL responds more slowly than B-ALL, so MRD measured at later timepoints is more prognostically relevant than MRD measured at the end of induction therapy.[139]

Although intensified ALL-type therapy has improved outcomes in T-cell LBL, knowledge of biological features that predict remission or survival is still limited, and risk stratification largely depends on disease stage and initial response to therapy.

Differential Diagnosis

The distinction of T-ALL or T-LBL from other neoplasms (Tables 41-2 and 41-3) typically rests on immunophenotypic analysis. Recognition that precursor T-cell tumors have an abnormal immunophenotype can help distinguish these neoplasms from thymic tissue if sent for flow-cytometric analysis, because normal thymocytes and those of thymoma will typically show a normal pattern of T-cell maturation, in contrast to the aberrancies seen in neoplasia.[140] T-LBL occurring in the mediastinum may sometimes be confused with thymomas histologically, especially if a thymic T-cell phenotype demonstrated by immunohistochemistry is misinterpreted. Cytokeratin staining is helpful in avoiding this pitfall, provided attention is paid to the different pattern of cytokeratin expression in thymoma versus residual thymus.

It is also important to distinguish T-ALL from benign entities. In the case of T-LBL, one important condition to consider is an "indolent T-lymphoblastic proliferation."[141,142] This entity often involves head and neck nodes and is remarkable for paracortical expansion by phenotypically normal T-cell precursors without architectural effacement of the node. It can also be seen in nodes involved by carcinoma or lymphoma. As this rare entity requires no or only local therapy, its recognition is critically important.

CONCLUSION

Precursor lymphoid neoplasms are aggressive tumors that require immediate diagnosis and treatment. However, with appropriate intensive therapy, these malignancies may be curable, particularly in the pediatric population. Greater understanding of the biology of lymphoblastic tumors and the enhanced specificity in new classification systems will allow for improved risk stratification and the development of targeted therapeutic agents.

Pearls and Pitfalls

Diagnosis of Acute Lymphoblastic Leukemia (ALL)

Pearls

- Precursor B-cell neoplasms generally present as leukemias, and precursor T-cell neoplasms generally present as lymphomas; if leukemic, the latter are associated with significant tissue involvement. Mediastinal masses in patients with ALL are seen almost exclusively with precursor T-cell neoplasms.
- Precursor lymphoid tumors recapitulate certain aspects of normal precursor lymphoid maturation. However, because of the reproducible nature of antigen acquisition in normal precursors, virtually all neoplastic populations can be reliably distinguished from normal precursors by multiparametric flow cytometry.
- For B-cell ALL, the presence of hyperdiploidy or *ETV6-RUNX1* fusion confers a favorable prognosis in childhood, whereas *BCR::ABL1* fusion or *KMT2A* rearrangement confers a poor prognosis. *BCR::ABL1*-like ALL is also a poor prognosis lesion.
- Bone marrow and testicular involvement by lymphoblastic lymphoma is associated with CNS involvement.

Pitfalls

- Precursor lymphoid tumors may lack common leukocyte antigen (CD45) and express CD99; as such, this profile does not distinguish them from Ewing's sarcoma. Inclusion of other lymphoid markers and TdT may be helpful in distinguishing between these alternatives.
- CD79a, commonly used as a B-cell marker, may be occasionally expressed on T-cell tumors, including precursor T-cell neoplasms.
- Expression of myeloid antigens such as CD13, CD33, and CD15 occurs commonly in B-cell ALL and does not imply that the tumor is biphenotypic (see Chapter 43).
- In the absence of morphology suggestive of Burkitt lymphoma/leukemia or of an *MYC* translocation, expression of clonal surface IGL does not exclude a diagnosis of B-cell ALL.
- The presence of CD19-positive CD10-positive cells in the bone marrow, even in significant numbers, does not necessarily establish a diagnosis of B-cell ALL because these cells must be distinguished from normal B-cell precursors (hematogones).
- Dim MPO expression can be detected by flow cytometry or immunohistochemistry in B-ALL and should not be the sole criterion for a diagnosis of B/myeloid MPAL.
- Patients with ALL with packed marrows may be aleukemic but circulate occasional myeloblasts pushed out from the marrow; thus, a diagnosis of AML should not be made without marrow examination if only a few myeloblasts are identified in peripheral blood by flow cytometry.

KEY REFERENCES

36. Coustan-Smith E, Song G, Clark C, et al. New markers for minimal residual disease detection in acute lymphoblastic leukemia. *Blood*. 2011;117:6267–6276.
56. Duffield AS, Mulligan CG, Borowitz MJ. International Consensus Classification of acute lymphoblastic leukemia/lymphoma. *Virchows Arch*. 2023;482:11–26.
58. Iacobucci I, Kimura S, Mulligan CG. Biologic and therapeutic implications of genomic alterations in acute lymphoblastic leukemia. *J Clin Med*. 2021;10:3792.
75. Schultz KR, Pullen DJ, Sather HN, et al. Risk- and response-based classification of childhood B-precursor acute lymphoblastic leukemia: a combined analysis of prognostic markers from the Pediatric Oncology Group (POG) and Children's Cancer Group (CCG). *Blood*. 2007;109:926–935.
83. Hovorkova L, Zaliova M, Venn NC, et al. Monitoring of childhood ALL using BCR-ABL1 genomic breakpoints identifies a subgroup with CML-like biology. *Blood*. 2017;18:129:2771–2781.

94. Roberts KG, Li Y, Payne-Turner D, et al. Targetable kinase-activating lesions in Ph-like acute lymphoblastic leukemia. *N Engl J Med*. 2014;371:1005–1015.
112. Conter V, Bartram CR, Valsecchi MG, et al. Molecular response to treatment redefines all prognostic factors in children and adolescents with B-cell precursor acute lymphoblastic leukemia: results in 3184 patients of the AIEOP-BFM ALL 2000 study. *Blood*. 2010;115:3206–3214.
113. Borowitz MJ, Devidas M, Hunger SP, et al. Clinical significance of minimal residual disease in childhood acute lymphoblastic leukemia and its relationship to other prognostic factors: a Children's Oncology Group study. *Blood*. 2008;111:5477–5485.
115. Wood B, Wu D, Crossley B, et al. Measurable residual disease detection by high-throughput sequencing improves risk stratification for pediatric B-ALL. *Blood*. 2018;131:1350–1359.

Visit Elsevier eBooks+ for the complete set of references.

Acute Leukemias of Ambiguous Lineage

Olga K. Weinberg

DEFINITIONS

Acute leukemias of ambiguous lineage (ALAL) are those leukemias that either fail to show evidence of myeloid, B-lymphoid, or T-lymphoid lineage commitment or show evidence of commitment to more than one lineage.[1-4] These leukemias include acute undifferentiated leukemia (AUL) and mixed-phenotype acute leukemia (MPAL). MPAL includes both biphenotypic leukemia (a leukemia with more than one lineage-defining marker on a single blast population) and bilineal leukemia (a leukemia composed of two or more single-lineage leukemia populations). AUL is a rare type of acute leukemia that shows no evidence of differentiation along any lineage and is included under ALAL in classifications of acute leukemias.

SYNONYMS AND RELATED TERMS

Initial classification systems of ALAL used a scoring system whereby certain lineage markers were assigned points, with the diagnosis of biphenotypic acute leukemia (BAL) dependent on a final score reached.[5] The first scoring system was described by Catovsky et al. The European Group for the Immunologic Characterization of Leukemias (EGIL) further modified the Catovsky system, primarily by increasing the weight of certain markers and adding and subtracting others[6,7] (Table 42-1); subsequently, the World Health Organization (WHO) 3rd edition of the Classification of Tumours of Haematopoietic and Lymphoid Tissues (2001) included this system.[8] The WHO 4th edition eliminated a scoring system and sought to simplify the diagnosis by reducing the specific markers necessary to ascribe a lineage to biphenotypic leukemias and combined biphenotypic leukemias and bilineal leukemias within the MPAL category;

the revised WHO 4th edition classification kept this approach.[9] Both the proposed WHO 5th edition and the International Consensus Classification (ICC) of acute leukemias continued using lineage-specific markers outlined in the WHO 4th edition and included more genetically defined subtypes[10,10a,11] (Tables 42-2 and 42-3). Based on the markers expressed on the blast cells, BAL/MPAL can also be further divided into B/myeloid, T/myeloid, B/T-cell, and B/T/myeloid subtypes.

EPIDEMIOLOGY

The incidence of MPAL depends on the classification used. Historically, BAL accounted for up to 5% of acute leukemias.[12] The updated WHO classifications led to a decreased number of MPAL cases, and in the two largest case series using the WHO criteria, MPAL cases accounted for between 0.5% and 2.4% of all leukemias.[13] In a study of 7627 pediatric and adult patients with acute leukemia, 2.8% had bilineal acute leukemia using the EGIL classification, and 1.6% had MPAL using the 4th edition of the WHO classification.[14] The incidence of MPAL

Table 42-1 European Group for the Immunologic Characterization of Leukemias (EGIL) Scoring System for Biphenotypic Acute Leukemia

Points	B Lineage	T Lineage	Myeloid Lineage
2	CD79a, cIgM, cCD22	CD3, TCRαβ, TCRγδ	MPO, lysozyme
1	CD19, CD10, CD20	CD2, CD5, CD8, CD10	CD13, CD33, CDw65, CD117
0.5	TdT, CD24	TdT, CD7, CD1a	CD14, CD15, CD64

Table 42-2 Proposed 5th Edition WHO Classification of Acute Leukemia of Ambiguous Lineage Entities

Acute leukemia of ambiguous lineage with defining genetic abnormalities
  Mixed-phenotype acute leukemia with *BCR::ABL1* fusion
  Mixed-phenotype acute leukemia with *KMT2A* rearrangement
  Acute leukemia of ambiguous lineage with other defined genetic alterations
  Mixed-phenotype acute leukemia with *ZNF384* rearrangement
  Acute leukemia of ambiguous lineage with *BCL11B* rearrangement
Acute leukemia of ambiguous lineage, immunophenotypically defined
  Mixed-phenotype acute leukemia, B/myeloid
  Mixed-phenotype acute leukemia, T/myeloid
  Mixed-phenotype acute leukemia, rare types
Acute leukemia of ambiguous lineage, not otherwise specified
Acute undifferentiated leukemia

Table 42-3 International Consensus Classification (ICC) of Acute Leukemia of Ambiguous Lineage

MPAL with defining genetic alterations
  MPAL with *BCR::ABL1*
  MPAL with t(v;11q23.3), *KMT2A* rearrangement
  MPAL with *ZNF384* rearrangement
  MPAL with *BCL11B* activation
MPAL with defining immunophenotypic changes
  B/myeloid MPAL
  T/myeloid MPAL
  B/T/myeloid MPAL
  B/T MPAL
Acute undifferentiated leukemia (AUL)
Acute leukemias of ambiguous lineage, not otherwise specified (ALAL, NOS)

has a bimodal age distribution with peaks observed at 19 and 60 years of age.[15] Because of its rarity, little is known about AUL. Using the SEER database, the age-adjusted AUL incidence rate is reported to be 1.34 per million person-years[16]; however, this appears to have decreased over time, likely the result of better diagnostic tools assigning patients either to the myeloid or lymphoid lineage.

CLINICAL FEATURES

Patients with MPAL generally present with clinical findings that reflect pancytopenia, such as fatigue, weakness, infections, and/or bleeding (e.g., epistaxis, gingival bleeding, ecchymoses). Other findings may relate to accumulation of leukemic cells in peripheral blood, bone marrow, or extramedullary sites (e.g., abdominal fullness from splenomegaly, bone pain). This clinical presentation does not distinguish MPAL from other forms of acute leukemia.

DIAGNOSTIC CRITERIA AND LINEAGE ASSIGNMENT

Blasts in MPAL are morphologically diverse and range from small to intermediate in size with variable cytoplasm, and

in some cases, two separate blasts with distinctive size, morphology, and phenotype can be identified (Fig. 42-1). Extensive immunophenotyping is essential for an accurate diagnosis of ALAL. Lineage assignment is best performed by flow cytometric immunophenotyping to correlate the patterns of antigen expression on one or more cell populations. When evaluating the flow cytometry data and particularly co-expression of markers, it is important to exclude doublets and address compensation (process of correcting for fluorescence spillover) and autofluorescence issues so that dim populations can be differentiated from negative populations. Immunohistochemical stains may be used to show expression of lineage-associated antigens such as MPO, CD3, and PAX5 (Table 42-4). The proposed WHO 5th edition stresses that the assignment of lineage by immunophenotyping is dependent on the strength of association between each antigen and the lineage being assessed. As a general principle, the closer the expression of an antigen is to either the intensity and/or pattern of expression seen on the most similar normal population, the more likely it reflects commitment to that lineage. Unlike the EGIL, the WHO does not clearly provide a threshold for the percentage of cells for lineage-specific antigens, but they recommend a level of expression exceeding 50% of that seen on normal mature T-cells and B-cells or neutrophils. In the most recently proposed WHO classification, the intensity of antigen expression is considered to be more lineage specific.

The diagnosis of ALAL requires the presence of ≥20% blasts in peripheral blood or marrow. In bilineal MPAL cases, each abnormal progenitor population must meet the immunophenotypic criteria for that lineage, but the numerical blast criterion only applies to aggregate. In cases with separate blast populations, each population needs to be classified according to acute myeloid leukemia (AML) and acute lymphoblastic leukemia (ALL) criteria (Fig. 42-1). The ICC proposed that, in cases with small aberrant clones of divergent lineage (>5%), a diagnosis of MPAL could be rendered if clear immunophenotypic aberrancies are identified. Identification of such aberrancies is essential to differentiate a small bilineal blast population from normal myeloid or B-cell precursors. For cases with aberrant clones which represent less than 5% of all cells, a diagnosis should be based on the major leukemic population with a descriptive modifier.

AUL is rare and defined by the absence of both myeloid and lymphoid markers. Little is known about its incidence, survival, and optimal management.

In a multi-institutional study of AUL cases, a significant number of cases were reclassified as AML with myelodysplasia-related changes (AML-MRC) based on cytogenetic findings, and only a small number (24 cases) were qualified as AUL.[17] Of these, only six AUL cases showed no myeloid marker expression (CD117, CD13, or CD33), though 15 showed partial or full expression of one myeloid marker. Restricting the definition of AUL to cases with one or fewer myeloid marker expressions showed no difference in overall survival or relapse-free survival when comparing this group with AML with minimal differentiation. Compared with AML with minimal differentiation, AUL cases were characterized by significantly more frequent mutations in *PHF6*, and this difference was even more significant when reassigning AUL cases with partial expression of a second myeloid marker to the AML with minimal differentiation group.[17]

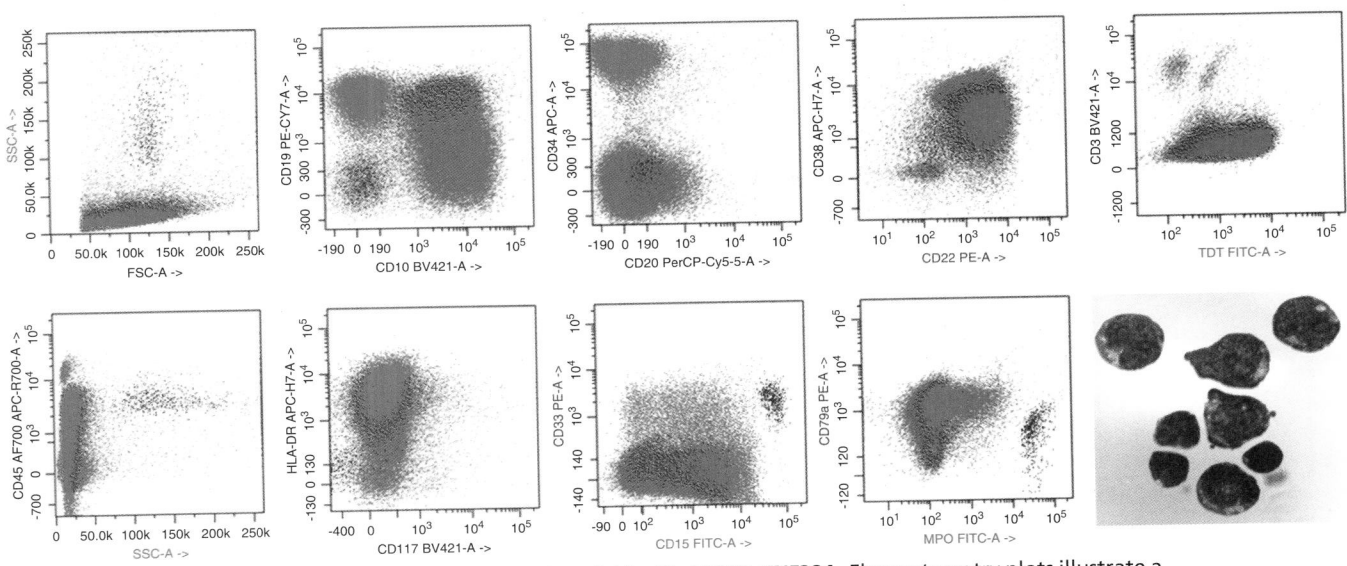

Figure 42-1. Flow plots of MPAL, B/myeloid with *EP300::ZNF384*. Flow cytometry plots illustrate a population of B-lymphoblasts *(green)* accounting for 70% and a B/myeloid population accounting for 24%. The aspirate smears show two separate populations of blasts *(inset)*.

Table 42-4 Markers Used in Lineage Assignment in Both Proposed WHO 5th Edition and ICC Classifications

B Lineage

Strong CD19 *and* one or more marker expression: CD10, CD22, or CD79a

Weak CD19 *and* two more strongly expressed: CD10, CD22, or CD79a

Consider PAX5, OCT2, BOB1 *immunohistochemical stains for B lineage*

T Lineage

CD3 (surface or cytoplasmic)

Myeloid Lineage

MPO

Monocytic differentiation NSE, CD64, CD11c, CD14, or lysozyme

B Lineage

Assignment of B lineage requires strong CD19 expression on blasts in addition to strong expression of at least one other B-lineage marker (Table 42-4) or weak CD19 expression, requiring two additional markers. The most specific marker for B-lineage leukemias is CD19; however, it can be detected in a subset of AML, including t(8;21)(q22;q22.1) rearranged AML, which precludes its use as the sole lineage assignment marker.[18,19] The proposed WHO 5th edition recommends that a level of expression exceeding 50% of that seen on normal mature B cells should be seen on at least a portion of the leukemic cells, though the ICC does not have this requirement. The additional B-lineage marker CD79a is expressed early in B cells and is retained through plasmacytic differentiation; however, its expression is not unique to acute leukemias of B lineage.[20] CD10 is similarly expressed early in B-cell development; however, it is detected in a subset of T-cell acute lymphoblastic leukemia (T-ALL), making it less sensitive and specific than CD19.[21]

Cytoplasmic expression of CD22 is detected in most cases of B-cell acute lymphoblastic leukemia (B-ALL) and not identified in AML or T-ALL, but its expression in basophils and dendritic cells make it less specific for assigning B lineage.[22,23]

T Lineage

For T lineage, blasts must express CD3 on the surface or within the cytoplasm. The proposed WHO 5th edition recommends that a level of expression exceeding 50% of that seen on normal mature T cells should be seen on at least a portion of the leukemic cells, though the ICC does not have this requirement. The WHO also recommends using a bright fluorochrome such as phycoerythrin (PE), allophycocyanin (APC), or Brilliant Violet (BV) dyes to provide an increased dynamic range to aid in this determination. An example of a T/myeloid MPAL is shown in Figure 42-2. Other T-cell markers, including CD2, CD4, CD5, CD7, CD8, and TCR αβ, have been used in prior scoring systems; however, CD2 and CD7 are commonly found expressed on blasts for leukemias that otherwise are consistent with AML, and CD4 is expressed on early granulocytic, monocytic, and dendritic precursors.[22,23]

Myeloid Lineage

Myeloid lineage is assigned when blasts express myeloperoxidase (MPO), or at least two of the following monocytic markers: non-specific esterase, CD11c, CD14, CD64, or lysozyme. MPO has long been considered the most specific marker for myeloid-lineage leukemias.[24] MPO expression by immunohistochemistry, cytochemistry, or flow cytometry or monocytic differentiation is considered a requirement for assigning the myeloid lineage when considering a diagnosis of MPAL. Variable MPO expression with an intensity and pattern similar to that seen in early

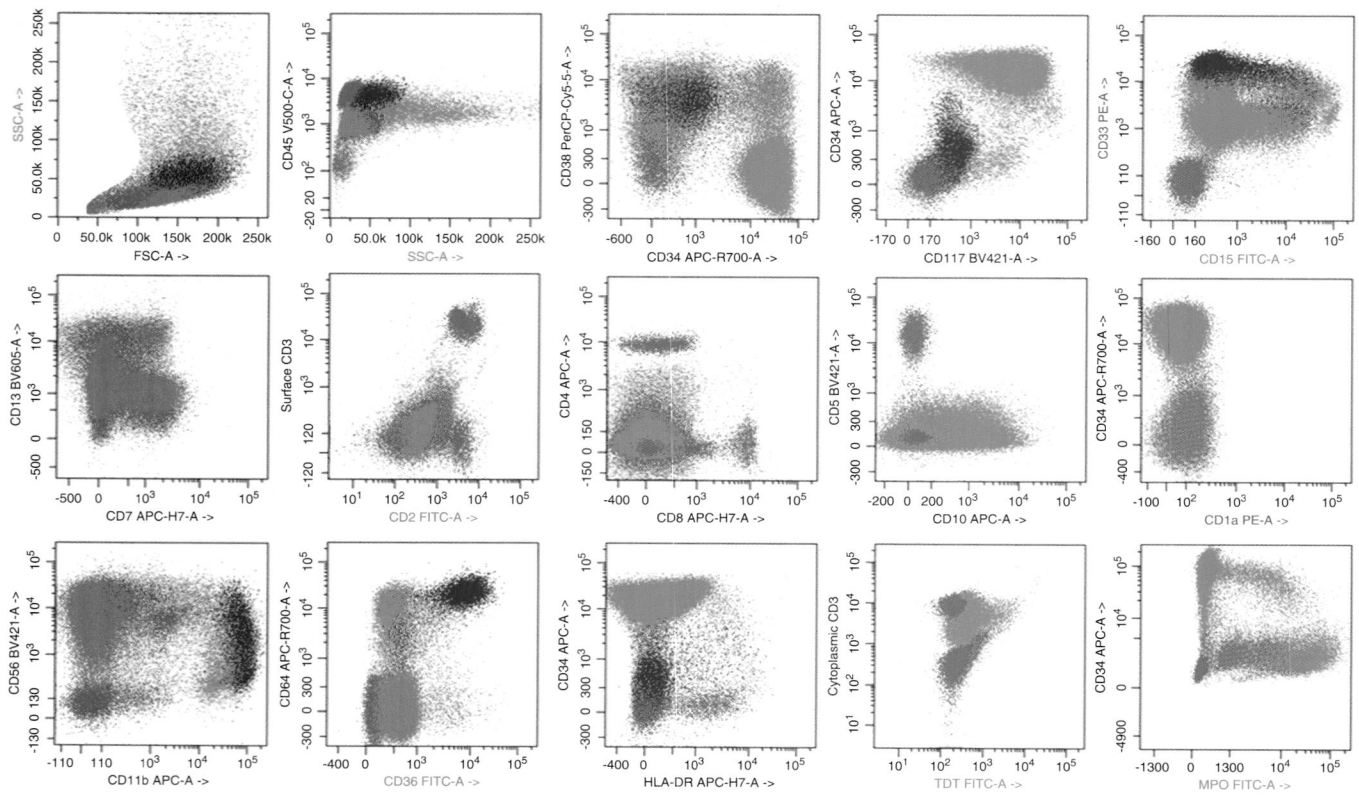

Red: Biphenotypic Blasts   Purple: Lymphocytes   Green: Granulocytes   Blue: Monocytes

Figure 42-2. Flow cytometry plots of MPAL, T/myeloid case. Blast population in red shows expression of CD34 and CD117, variable expression of myeloid markers including CD33, CD13, MPO, and CD15, and T-cell markers including cytoplasmic CD3, CD56, CD7, and CD10.

myeloid maturation is more strongly associated with myeloid lineage than uniform dim MPO expression. Although older studies suggest a cutoff of 3% for cytochemistry based on expert opinion (Table 42-5), no formally established cutoff guidelines exist for immunohistochemistry and flow cytometry.[25-30] The issue is further compounded by the availability of many MPO clones, known non-specific staining patterns, and lack of criteria for evaluating the stains, especially in cases that may contain a significant number of non-blast myeloid cells. To standardize flow cytometric interpretation of MPO based on internal positive and negative control populations, the proposed WHO 5th edition has clarified that the intensity of MPO expression on blasts must exceed 50% of the background mature neutrophils and both the WHO and ICC recommend a 10% cut off.[10,11]

GENETIC AND MOLECULAR FINDINGS

The majority (64%–87%) of MPALs have an abnormal karyotype.[31] The most common abnormalities are rearrangements of t(9;22) and t(v;11q23.3), and these now form specific subgroups of MPAL (WHO and ICC). MPALs with *KMT2A* rearrangement are more common in the pediatric group (infants) and account for about 10% of MPALs. MPAL with *BCR::ABL1* is more common in adults and accounts for about 20% of MPAL cases.[32] In addition to these two widely recognized aberrancies, other cytogenetic abnormalities, particularly observed in the B/myeloid subtype,

Table 42-5 Myeloperoxidase Antibodies Used and the Cutoff Recommended in Various Studies

Study	Antibody	Threshold Recommendations
Van den Ancker et al., 2013	Flow cytometry (clone used not reported)	>10%
Arber et al., 2001	IHC 1:1000 dilution, Dako, Carpinteria, CA), polyclonal and monoclonal MPO antibody (clone MPO-7;1:100 dilution; Dako)	≥5%
Ahuja et al., 2018	IHC: anti-human MPO (Thermo Scientific, United Kingdom)	3% for IHC 10% for cytochemistry
Oberley et al., 2017	Flow cytometry: MPO (clone 8E6; Life Tech, Waltham, MA) IHC (clone 59A5; Leica Biosystems, Newcastle, United Kingdom) plus cytochemistry	>20% for flow cytometry 3% cytochemistry
Guy et al., 2013	Flow cytometry: monoclonal antibody (Dako or Immunotech), FITC	>13% (if using isotype control) >28% (if using internal control: lymphocytes)
Matutes et al., 2011	Flow cytometry: monoclonal MPO (clone used not reported)	>10%

FITC, Fluorescein isothiocyanate; *IHC,* immunohistochemistry.

include del[1](p32), trisomy 4, del(6q), and 12p11.2 abnormalities and near-tetraploidy.

Studies have performed genomic analyses of MPAL cases and have found that gene mutations are a mixture of those commonly seen in both AML and ALL. In 2012, Yan et al. reported deletions of the ALL-associated gene *IKZF1* and mutations of the AML-associated epigenetic modifiers *TET2*, *EZH2*, and *ASXL1* in B/myeloid leukemias.[33] In 2016, Eckstein and colleagues performed whole exome sequencing on 23 cases of MPAL; they found similar mutations and identified AML-associated *DNMT3A* mutations, *WT1* mutations, and frequent *NOTCH* mutations (32%) in cases with a T-lineage component, suggesting genetic overlap with unilineage T-ALL.[34] In a series of 31 cases, Takahashi et al. reported genomic anomalies and methylation patterns in a comparison of T/myeloid and B/myeloid MPALS with AML, T-ALL, and B-ALL.[31] They found both AML-type and ALL-type mutations in MPAL, and more mutations and broader methylation profiles were present in T/myeloid MPALs than in B/myeloid MPALs. B/myeloid MPALs typically presented with *RUNX1* mutations, and T/myeloid MPALs were enriched in *NOTCH1* mutations. It is interesting to note that analysis of the methylome showed T/myeloid MPALs preferentially segregated with T-ALL and B/myeloid MPALs preferentially segregated with AML.[31] T/myeloid MPAL appears to consist of a more heterogeneous group of driver mutations, with fusions that overlap with T-ALL such as *ZEB2::BCL11B* and *NUP214::ABL1* and fusions with *ETV6* involving multiple different partners. In a study of 8 pediatric and 18 adult patients, Xiao and colleagues identified recurrent and largely mutually exclusive alterations in *PHF6*, *DNMT3A*, and *WT1* in MPAL with a T-lineage immunophenotype.[35] A series of B/T MPALs has identified recurrent acquired aberrations, including mutations in the putative transcriptional regulator *PHF6* and the JAK-STAT and Ras signaling pathways.[36]

Whole exome and genome sequencing in a cohort of 115 pediatric MPAL/ALAL cases identified *WT1*, *FLT3*, *RUNX1*, and *PHF6* mutations among the most recurrent alterations in pediatric T/myeloid MPAL.[37] Fusion genes involving the *ZNF384* transcription factor gene were identified in nearly 50% of cases and more prominent in B/myeloid MPAL. *ZNF384* fusions are also common in B-ALL,[17,18] which had an overlapping gene expression profile with *ZNF384*-rearranged B/myeloid MPAL, supporting the notion that genomic alteration, rather than immunophenotype, more accurately classifies certain subtypes of leukemia. An example of a *ZNF384*-rearranged case is shown in Figure 42-1. These fusions were not identified in adult B/myeloid cases, confirming that subsets of pediatric and adult MPAL have distinct genetic origins. ALAL with rearrangements leading to deregulation of *BCL11B* (BCL11B-activated) accounts for 10% to 15% of MPAL and is further enriched in patients with T/myeloid MPAL cases, representing up to one-third of this population.[38-40] Unlike the *BCL11B* alterations described for T-ALL (amino acid substitutions and deletions and rearrangements of the *BCL11B* enhancer to *TLX3*), the 14q32 structural variants identified in ambiguous lineage leukemias usually leave the *BCL11B* coding region intact. These alterations involve juxtaposition of super-enhancers active in hematopoietic stem cells to *BCL11B,* or in 20% of cases, amplification of a 2kb region distal to *BCL11B* resulting in generation of a neo-enhancer that deregulates *BCL11B* expression.

Based on these findings, the proposed WHO 5th edition and ICC systems recognize two new entities with defined genetic alterations, MPAL with *ZNF384* rearrangements and MPAL with *BCL11B* activation.[10,11] Though *ZNF384* rearrangements have been identified in B-ALL, Alexander et al. characterized them in the pediatric setting at a rate of 48% of B/myeloid MPAL.[37] Gene expression profiling suggests *ZNF384*-rearranged MPAL more closely resembles B-ALL than AML, with a maturation profile that is more mature than in most B/myeloid MPAL cases but less mature than in most B-ALL cases. *BCL11B* cases present with absence of CD5 and expression of cCD3 or MPO, resulting in variable classification, and are driven by aberrant allele-specific deregulation of BCL11B, a master transcription factor responsible for thymic T-lineage commitment and specification. Mechanistically, this deregulation was driven by chromosomal rearrangements that juxtapose *BCL11B* to super-enhancers active in hematopoietic progenitors or focal amplifications that generate a super-enhancer from a noncoding element distal to *BCL11B*.[40] Moreover, emerging work is showing that the biology of immature leukemias is explained by diverse genomic alterations converging on a conserved set of stem cell genes, showing phenotypic ambiguity: early T-cell precursor (ETP), MPAL, or neither; this further suggests that genetic alterations rather than phenotypic expression may in the future be a better way of classifying these leukemias.[40]

CLINICAL COURSE

It has been widely recognized that the clinical outcome of ALAL is markedly adverse, and the overall survival (OS) ranges from 9 months to 3.5 years according to published data.[13,41,42] The rarity of MPAL with the capability to switch lineages under pressure (treatment) defines the challenges in treating MPAL. MPAL has a poor prognosis and worse outcomes than standard-risk AML or ALL.[43] A meta-analysis inclusive of international case reports and small case series from a variety of pathology and clinical journals identified over a thousand patients diagnosed with MPAL using either the EGIL or WHO criteria.[44] In this large analysis, patients beginning therapy with an AML-style induction regimen were significantly less likely to achieve a complete remission and nearly twice as likely to die of their disease as those receiving an ALL-style induction. The currently recommended treatment approach for MPAL in both pediatric and adult patients is induction therapy with an ALL regimen.[43,45] Patients with MPAL with *BCR::ABL1* may ultimately benefit from addition of a tyrosine kinase inhibitor.[46] Clinical outcomes of children with MPAL tend to be better compared to those of adults with MPAL, with a higher OS and fewer relapses; however, outcomes for acute leukemia are in general better in children than in adults.[15,47] The debate on the most appropriate induction regimen remains unresolved over the controversy whether initial therapy should be based on immunophenotype, cytogenetics, or molecular biology.

LINEAGE SWITCH

Immunophenotypic properties of MPAL are not stable over time: both variable proportions of different lineages and phenotypic alterations are known as lineage switch. Most cases of lineage transformation involve a switch from ALL to AML, and a retrospective review can often reveal the presence of an unrecognized or underappreciated malignant subclonal

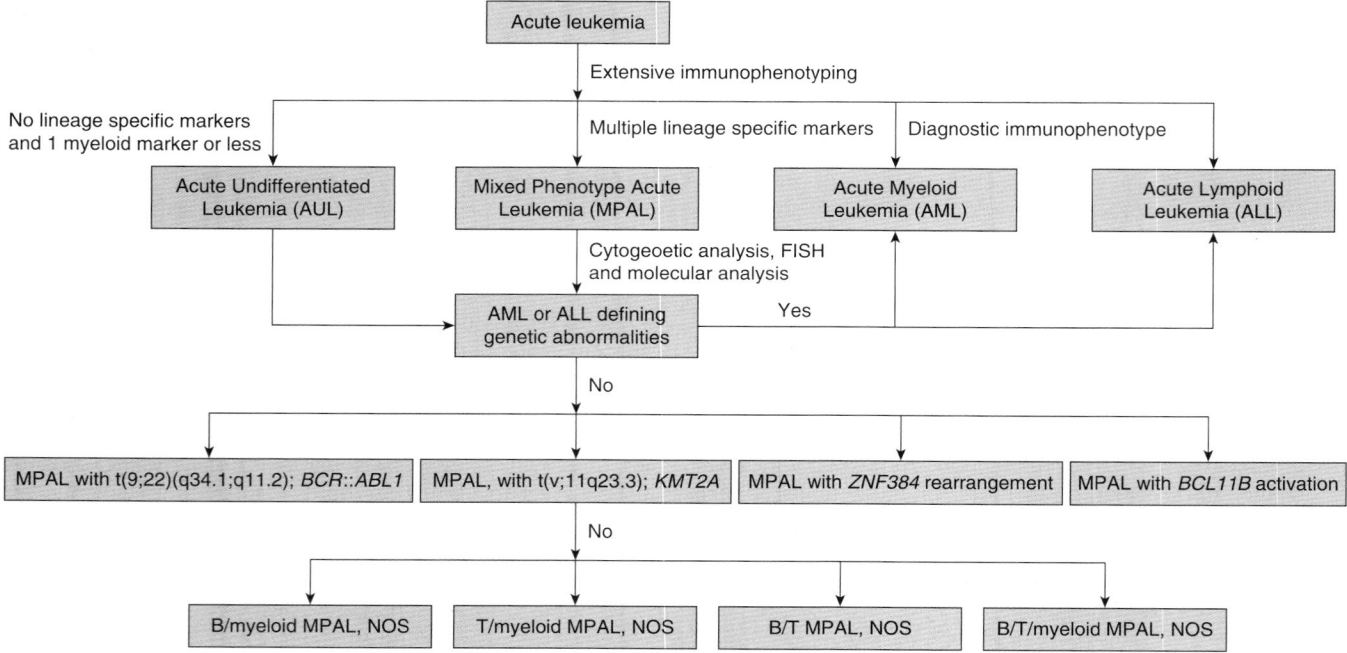

Figure 42-3. Proposed acute leukemias of ambiguous lineage (ALAL) classification scheme.

population present in the initial specimen, which displayed more chemoresistance and emerged after eradication of the chemosensitive dominant clone.[48]

The selective pressure brought on by specific therapies can influence these transformations, especially in MPAL (e.g., resultant AML after the use of B-cell specific therapy such as blinatumomab). However, frank ALL-to-AML lineage switch must be distinguished from the B-monocytic transition commonly seen in ALL with *DUX4*-rearrangements and other alterations early in therapy in which such changes do not affect prognosis with continued ALL therapy.[49]

DIFFERENTIAL DIAGNOSIS

The primary challenge in diagnosing MPAL is ruling out cytogenetically defined neoplasms that demonstrate an MPAL-like immunophenotype (Fig. 42-3). A careful review of patient history is thus essential. For example, patients with a history of chronic myeloid leukemia (CML) who develop blast crisis with mixed phenotype should not be diagnosed as MPAL with t(9;22). Similarly, patients with CML in blast crisis with lineage switch are also excluded from this category. AML with t(8;21)(q22;q22.1) often expresses B-lineage markers, including CD19, PAX5, and CD79a, and care should be taken to not diagnose MPAL in this setting. Cytogenetic abnormalities and molecular findings diagnostic of AML-MRC or AML with myelodysplasia-related mutation[50] also preclude diagnosis of MPAL, but such a diagnosis could be modified in such a way as to highlight the immunophenotype (i.e., AML with myelodysplasia-related gene mutations and a mixed [B/myeloid] immunophenotype). Myeloid/lymphoid neoplasms with eosinophilia and *FGFR1* rearrangement are a group of hematopoietic neoplasms that can present as acute leukemias expressing mixed lineage markers, but they should not be diagnosed as MPAL at initial presentation.

ETP lymphoblastic leukemia is characterized by expression of CD7, weak or absent CD5, one or more myeloid/stem cell markers other than MPO, and cytoplasmic CD3.[51] The co-expression of myeloid markers and CD3 makes distinguishing ETP-ALL from T/myeloid MPAL problematic; molecular data blur the distinction between these entities, and the distinction is increasingly artificial: The *BCL11B* cases have a strict ETP immunophenotype with negativity of CD5 but variable cCD3+/− or MPO+/− resulting in variable classification. Moreover, emerging work is showing the biology of the immature leukemias are explained by diverse genomic alterations converging on a conserved set of stem cell genes: *HOXA9, HOXA13, ETV6, MED12,* and *ZNF36L2.* These cases have homogeneous gene expression but variable ambiguity: ETP, MPAL, or not (i.e., non-ETP T-ALL).

Pearls and Pitfalls

Pearls

- MPAL is a heterogenous group of leukemias that are genetically, immunophenotypically, and clinically diverse.
- ALAL includes biologically diverse leukemias that fail to show commitment to either the myeloid or lymphoid lineages or show evidence of commitment to more than one lineage. Cases in the former group are referred to as AUL, and those in the latter are identified as MPAL.
- A diagnosis of MPAL is based on the presence of two disparate populations of blasts, each of which demonstrates a distinct and lineage-specific phenotype, or a single population of blasts expressing markers specific to more than one lineage.

Pitfalls

- In cases with separate blast populations, each population needs to be classified according to AML and ALL criteria.
- Gene mutations found within MPAL are a mixture of those commonly seen in both AML and ALL and, as such, cannot be used to define a lineage.
- Immunophenotypic properties of MPAL are not stable over time; both variable proportions of different lineages and phenotypic alterations are known as lineage switch.

KEY REFERENCES

10. Arber DA, Orazi A, Hasserjian RP, et al. *International Consensus Classification of Myeloid Neoplasms and Acute Leukemias:* integrating morphologic, clinical, and genomic data. *Blood.* 2022;140(11):1200–1228.

10a. Weinberg OK, Arber DA, Döhner H, et al. The International Consensus Classification of Acute Leukemia of Ambiguous Lineage. *Blood.* 2023;141(18):2275–2277.

11. Khoury JD, Solary E, Abla O, et al. The 5th edition of the *World Health Organization Classification of Haematolymphoid Tumours: Myeloid and Histiocytic/Dendritic Neoplasms. Leukemia.* 2022;36(7):1703–1719.

14. Weinberg OK, Seetharam M, Ren L, Alizadeh A, Arber DA. Mixed phenotype acute leukemia: a study of 61 cases using World Health Organization and European group for the immunological classification of leukaemias criteria. *Am J Clin Pathol.* 2014;142(6):803–808.

15. Matutes E, Pickl WF, Van't Veer M, et al. Mixed-phenotype acute leukemia: clinical and laboratory features and outcome in 100 patients defined according to the WHO 2008 classification. *Blood.* 2011;117(11):3163–3171.

17. Weinberg OK, Hasserjian RP, Baraban E, et al. Clinical, immunophenotypic, and genomic findings of acute undifferentiated leukemia and comparison to acute myeloid leukemia with minimal differentiation: a study from the bone marrow pathology group. *Mod Pathol.* 2019;32(9):1373–1385.

31. Takahashi K, Wang F, Morita K, et al. Integrative genomic analysis of adult mixed phenotype acute leukemia delineates lineage associated molecular subtypes. *Nat Commun.* 2018;9(1):2670.

35. Xiao W, Bharadwaj M, Levine M, et al. PHF6 and DNMT3A mutations are enriched in distinct subgroups of mixed phenotype acute leukemia with T-lineage differentiation. *Blood Adv.* 2018;2(23):3526–3539. Erratum in: *Blood Adv.* 2019 Apr 9;3(7):956.

37. Alexander TB, Gu Z, Iacobucci I, et al. The genetic basis and cell of origin of mixed phenotype acute leukaemia. *Nature.* 2018;562(7727):373–379.

40. Montefiori LE, Bendig S, Gu Z, et al. Enhancer hijacking drives oncogenic BCL11B expression in lineage-ambiguous stem cell leukemia. *Cancer Discov.* 2021;11(11):2846–2867.

46. Orgel E, Alexander TB, Wood BL, et al. *Children's Oncology Group Acute Leukemia of Ambiguous Lineage Task Force.* Mixed-phenotype acute leukemia: a cohort and consensus research strategy from the Children's Oncology Group Acute Leukemia of Ambiguous Lineage Task Force. *Cancer.* 2020;126(3):593–601.

Visit Elsevier eBooks+ for the complete set of references.

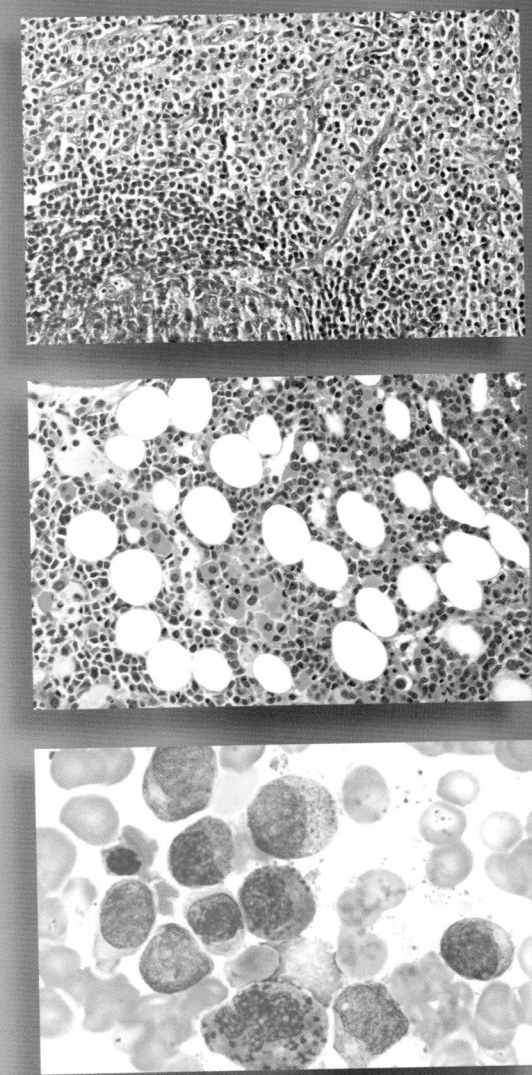

PART **IV**

Myeloid, Histiocytic, and Related Proliferations

Chapter 43

Principles of Classification of Myeloid Neoplasms

Daniel A. Arber and Attilio Orazi

INTRODUCTION

The International Consensus Classification (ICC, 2022) of myeloid neoplasms[1] is primarily used in this book in comparison with the revised 4th edition of the World Health Organization (WHO) Classification of Tumours of Haematopoietic and Lymphoid Tissues first published in 2016.[2] At the time of this writing, a 5th edition of the WHO Classification of Tumours of Haematopoietic and Lymphoid Tissues has been proposed but is not yet final.[3] The principles of the ICC 2022 have been described elsewhere,[4,5] and the process for developing this consensus classification is summarized in Chapter 12. Briefly, the ICC 2022 follows the approach of the 3rd, 4th, and revised 4th editions of the WHO Classification of Tumours of Haematopoietic and Lymphoid Tissues, with changes informed by input from a Clinical Advisory Committee (CAC). This approach relies on a combination of clinical, morphologic, immunophenotypic, genetic, and other biological features to define specific disease entities—a logical approach similar to that followed by a clinician and a pathologist working together to reach a diagnosis in a patient suspected of having a myeloid neoplasm. The relative contribution of each feature varies, depending on the case. Only through familiarity with the classification system and with the criteria for each entity can the appropriate studies be chosen to arrive at an accurate diagnosis in an expeditious manner. Although perhaps overused as an example of the prototype for the classification of myeloid neoplasms, chronic myeloid leukemia (CML) symbolizes the utility of the prior WHO and current ICC 2022 approaches. This leukemia is recognized mainly by its clinical and morphologic features and is consistently associated with a specific genetic abnormality, the BCR::ABL1 fusion gene, which leads to the production of a constitutively activated protein tyrosine kinase that interacts with a number of different cellular pathways to influence the proliferation, survival, and differentiation of neoplastic cells. The protein is sufficient to cause the leukemia, but it also provides a target for therapy that has prolonged the lives of thousands of patients with this disease.[6] The diagnosis of CML, however, is not based on any single parameter. There are other myeloid leukemias that mimic its clinical presentation and morphology, and the BCR::ABL1 fusion is seen not only in CML but also in some cases of de novo acute lymphoblastic leukemia, acute myeloid leukemia (AML), and mixed phenotype acute leukemia (MPAL). Thus, CML is a perfect model for the integration of all pieces of relevant information to define an entity in a classification scheme. Furthermore, there are still mysteries regarding CML, so there is still more to learn (see Chapter 47).

As the focus in all neoplasms turns increasingly to the genetic infrastructure of malignant cells and to molecular abnormalities that may be targets for therapeutic agents, it is only natural that more genetic and molecular data are incorporated into the diagnostic algorithms or nomenclature of classification schemes. The 2001 3rd edition of the WHO classification included, for the first time in any widely used system, genetic information as criteria for the diagnosis of not only CML but also some subtypes of AML.[7] By the time the 2008 4th edition and 2016 revised 4th edition of the WHO classification were published, a number of significant genetic abnormalities were discovered that are associated with subgroups of myeloid neoplasms or with specific disease entities within the subgroups. Since that time, an even larger number of genetic and epigenetic events associated with myeloid neoplasms have been described, making an approach that uses these data for both classification and prognostication more challenging.

In some instances, such as myeloid/lymphoid neoplasms with eosinophilia and tyrosine kinase gene fusions, the genetic defect (coupled with the morphology and clinical findings) is the major criterion for naming the disease and for selecting specific targeted therapy (see Chapter 50). In other instances, such as the *BCR::ABL1*-negative myeloproliferative neoplasms (MPNs) that are often but not invariably associated with the *JAK2* V617F mutation, the presence of the genetic defect is an objective criterion that identifies the myeloid proliferation as neoplastic. Additional criteria are necessary to define the specific disease associated with the mutated *JAK2* and to distinguish it from other MPNs that share the same mutation (see Chapter 47). Therefore, although the ICC 2022 incorporates an increased number of genetic abnormalities, a multidisciplinary approach is still required for the classification of myeloid neoplasms. This multidisciplinary approach succeeds in defining many distinct disease entities that cannot be adequately identified by relying on morphology or clinical features alone. Such a limited approach to myeloid neoplasms is no longer adequate, and a diagnosis is not complete in many cases until the results of all studies have been correlated, often requiring amended pathology reports.

New entities and new diagnostic criteria for old entities in the ICC 2022 are based mainly on published clinical and scientific studies that have been extensively quoted and their significance widely acknowledged. However, to accommodate data that have not yet "matured," the classification continues to have a number of "provisional entities" to include diseases that are clinically or scientifically important and should be considered in the classification but for which additional studies are needed to clarify their significance. Some previous provisional entities have been refined in the current classification and are now incorporated as full entities, and their presence emphasizes that the classification is ever-changing.

EVALUATION OF MYELOID NEOPLASMS

Myeloid neoplasms are serious, often life-threatening disorders, and their diagnosis requires a concerted effort by the clinician and the pathologist to thoroughly and carefully evaluate the clinical, morphologic, immunophenotypic, and genetic data. Too often, a diagnosis is based on insufficient knowledge of the clinical and laboratory information and, particularly, on inadequate diagnostic specimens. Although the proper collection and processing and testing of blood and bone marrow specimens are addressed elsewhere,[8] Box 43-1 emphasizes additional guidelines in assessing specimens from patients suspected of having myeloid neoplasms. One rule of thumb is that morphology is a key criterion in the diagnosis of all myeloid neoplasms, even those in which there is a closely associated genetic defect or characteristic immunophenotypic profile. If the specimen is not adequate to evaluate morphologically, a new specimen should be obtained.

The ICC 2022 and prior WHO criteria apply to initial peripheral blood and bone marrow specimens obtained before any definitive therapy (including growth factor therapy) for the suspected hematologic neoplasm. Morphologic, cytochemical, and immunophenotypic features are used to establish the lineage of the neoplastic cells and to assess their maturation. The blast percentage remains a practical tool

for subcategorizing myeloid neoplasms and judging their progression, but use of the blast percentage has evolved in the ICC 2022. Traditionally, a myeloid neoplasm with 20% or more blasts in the blood or bone marrow is considered AML when it occurs de novo or evolution to AML if it occurs in the setting of a previously diagnosed myelodysplastic syndrome (MDS), MDS/MPN, or blast transformation of a previously diagnosed MPN. For de novo disease, a diagnosis of AML can now be made with blast counts of 10% or more in the setting of most recurring genetic abnormalities. Furthermore, a gradually increasing blast count at any level is usually associated with disease progression. A new category of MDS/AML with blasts between 10% and 19% is introduced in the ICC 2022 based on biological similarities between cases independent of blast cell count.[9] This new category applies to cases that have evolved from MDS and to de novo cases not associated with an AML-defining genetic abnormality, including cases with MDS-related gene mutations, *TP53* mutations, and MDS-related cytogenetic abnormalities. Blast percentages should be derived, when possible, from 200-cell leukocyte differential counts of the peripheral blood smear and 500-cell differential counts of all nucleated bone marrow cells on cellular bone marrow aspirate smears stained with Wright-Giemsa or a similar stain. Blasts are defined with the criteria proposed by the International Working Group on Morphology of Myelodysplastic Syndrome[10] and as outlined in Box 43-1. Determination of the blast percentage by flow cytometry assessment of CD34-positive cells is not recommended as a substitute for visual inspection; not all leukemic blasts express CD34, and hemodilution and other processing artifacts can produce misleading results. The detection of more CD34-positive cells by flow cytometry than expected from the morphologic evaluation, however, requires a reassessment of both specimens to resolve the discrepancy. CD34 immunohistochemistry might also play a valuable role in such circumstances. This reassessment may identify unusually small blasts that were initially confused with lymphocytes, or it may show erythroid hyperplasia that, after red blood cell lysis of the flow cytometry specimen, resulted in a falsely elevated CD34 count.

For acute leukemia, multiparameter flow cytometry (see Chapter 4) with CD45 versus side scatter gating is the method of choice for determining the blast lineage and for detecting aberrant antigenic profiles that may prove useful for disease monitoring. Figure 43-1 demonstrates antigens expressed at various levels of normal myeloid differentiation. These can be detected by flow cytometry or by immunohistochemistry on bone marrow biopsy specimens. However, asynchronous expression of maturation-associated antigens by neoplastic myeloid cells is not uncommon and is best determined by flow cytometric analysis.[11]

Although a bone marrow biopsy is not required for diagnosis in every patient with a myeloid neoplasm (particularly if the patient is frail and there are few treatment options available), an adequate biopsy provides the most accurate assessment of marrow cellularity, topography, stromal changes, and maturation patterns of the various lineages, and it can be invaluable in detecting measurable residual disease after therapy. In addition, the biopsy provides material for the immunohistochemical detection of antigens that can be diagnostically and prognostically useful, particularly if marrow aspirate smears are poorly cellular.[12]

Specimen Requirements
- Peripheral blood and bone marrow specimens obtained before any definitive therapy for the suspected myeloid neoplasm
- Peripheral blood and cellular marrow aspirate smears or touch preparations stained with Wright-Giemsa or similar stains
- Bone marrow biopsy at least 1.5 cm long and at right angles to the cortical bone for all cases, if feasible
- Bone marrow specimens for complete cytogenetic analysis and, when indicated, for flow cytometry, with an additional specimen cryopreserved for molecular genetic studies; the latter studies should be performed on the basis of initial karyotypic, clinical, morphologic, and immunophenotypic findings

Assessment of Blasts in Peripheral Blood and Bone Marrow Specimens
- Determine the blast percentage in peripheral blood and cellular bone marrow aspirate smears by visual inspection.
- Count myeloblasts, monoblasts, promonocytes, and megakaryoblasts (but not dysplastic megakaryocytes) as blasts when determining blast percentage for diagnosis of AML or blast transformation; count abnormal promyelocytes as "blast equivalents" in acute promyelocytic leukemia.
- Proerythroblasts are not counted as blasts except in rare instances of pure erythroleukemia.
- Flow cytometric assessment of CD34-positive cells is not recommended as a substitute for visual inspection; not all blasts express CD34, and artifacts introduced by specimen processing may result in erroneous estimates.
- If the aspirate is poor or marrow fibrosis is present, immunohistochemistry on biopsy sections for CD34 may be informative if blasts are CD34 positive.

Assessment of Blast Lineage
- Multiparameter flow cytometry should be performed; the panel should be sufficient to determine lineage and aberrant antigen profile of the neoplastic population.
- Cytochemistry, such as myeloperoxidase or non-specific esterase, may be helpful, particularly in AML, NOS, but it is not essential in all cases.
- Immunohistochemistry on bone marrow biopsy may be helpful; many antibodies are now available for the recognition of myeloid and lymphoid antigens.

Assessment of Genetic Features
- Complete cytogenetic analysis of bone marrow at initial diagnosis
- Additional studies, such as fluorescence in situ hybridization (FISH) or reverse transcriptase polymerase chain reaction (RT-PCR), should be guided by clinical, laboratory, and morphologic information
- Mutational studies for *JAK2*, followed by *CALR* and *MPL*, if indicated, should be sought in *BCR::ABL1*-negative MPNs
- Mutation panels that include *a broad panel of genes* should be performed on new cases of AML and MDS and should be considered in other case types

Correlation and Reporting of Data
- All data should be assimilated into one report that states the diagnosis and what classification was used.

AML, Acute myeloid leukemia; *MPN*, myeloproliferative neoplasm; *NOS*, not otherwise specified.

A complete cytogenetic analysis of bone marrow cells is essential during the initial evaluation for establishing a baseline karyotype; thereafter, repeated analyses are recommended as needed to judge the response to therapy or to detect genetic evolution. Additional genetic studies should be guided by the results of the initial karyotype and by the suspected diagnosis based on the clinical, morphologic, and immunophenotypic studies. In some cases, reverse transcriptase polymerase chain reaction (RT-PCR), fluorescence in situ hybridization (FISH), or RNA sequencing methods may detect variants of well-recognized cytogenetic abnormalities or submicroscopic abnormalities not detected by routine karyotyping, such as the *FIP1L1::PDGFRA* rearrangement found in some myeloid neoplasms associated with eosinophilia[13] or the *BCR::ABL1* fusion in about 5% to 10% of cases of CML when the Philadelphia (Ph) chromosome is not found by routine cytogenetic studies. Molecular studies may also prove useful in emergency situations while awaiting routine cytogenetic results, such as detection of *PML::RARA* fusion in cases of acute promyelocytic leukemia. In addition, gene mutations are important diagnostic and prognostic markers in myeloid neoplasms (as will become apparent in the chapters that follow). These include mutations of *JAK2*, *CALR*, *MPL*, and *KIT* in MPN[14-21]; *ASXL1*, *TET2*, *NRAS*, *KRAS*, *NF1*, *RUNX1*, and *PTPN11* in MDS/MPN[22-29]; *BCOR*, *CEBPA*, *DNMT3A*, *EZH2*, *FLT3*, *KIT*, *NPM1*, *RUNX1*, *SF3B1*, *SRSF2*, *STAG2*, *TP53*, *U2AF1*, *WT1*, and *ZRSR2*, in AML[1,30-35]; *ASXL1*, *TP53*, *EZH2*, *ETV6*, and *RUNX1* in MDS[36]; and *GATA1*[37] in myeloid proliferations associated with Down syndrome. In many cases, the mutational analysis should be done up front in the evaluation of diagnostic specimens; for example, in suspected cases of *BCR::ABL1*-negative MPNs, detecting the *JAK2* V617F mutation can substantiate the diagnosis of a clonal myeloproliferation. Gene panels are now widely available, and their use up front has become the standard of care for all new leukemia specimens.

INTERNATIONAL CONSENSUS CLASSIFICATION

The ICC 2022 of myeloid neoplasms is shown in Box 43-2. The term *myeloid* includes all cells belonging to the granulocytic (neutrophil, eosinophil, basophil), monocyte/macrophage, erythroid, megakaryocytic, and mast-cell lineages.

In general, the diseases are stratified into neoplasms comprising precursor cells (blasts) with minimal, if any, maturation (i.e., AML) and those in which there is maturation, either effective or ineffective, in the myeloid lineages. Each subgroup includes entities that are clinically or nosologically relevant and defined with ICC 2022 principles. Table 43-1 lists the major subgroups of myeloid neoplasms and their characteristics at diagnosis. Each subgroup is described in detail in the upcoming chapters, but some brief comments regarding the rationale for the classification and the major changes from previous schemes are provided here.

Myeloproliferative Neoplasms

In previous classification schemes used for MPNs,[7] detection of the Ph chromosome or *BCR::ABL1* fusion gene was used to confirm the diagnosis of CML. The remaining subtypes

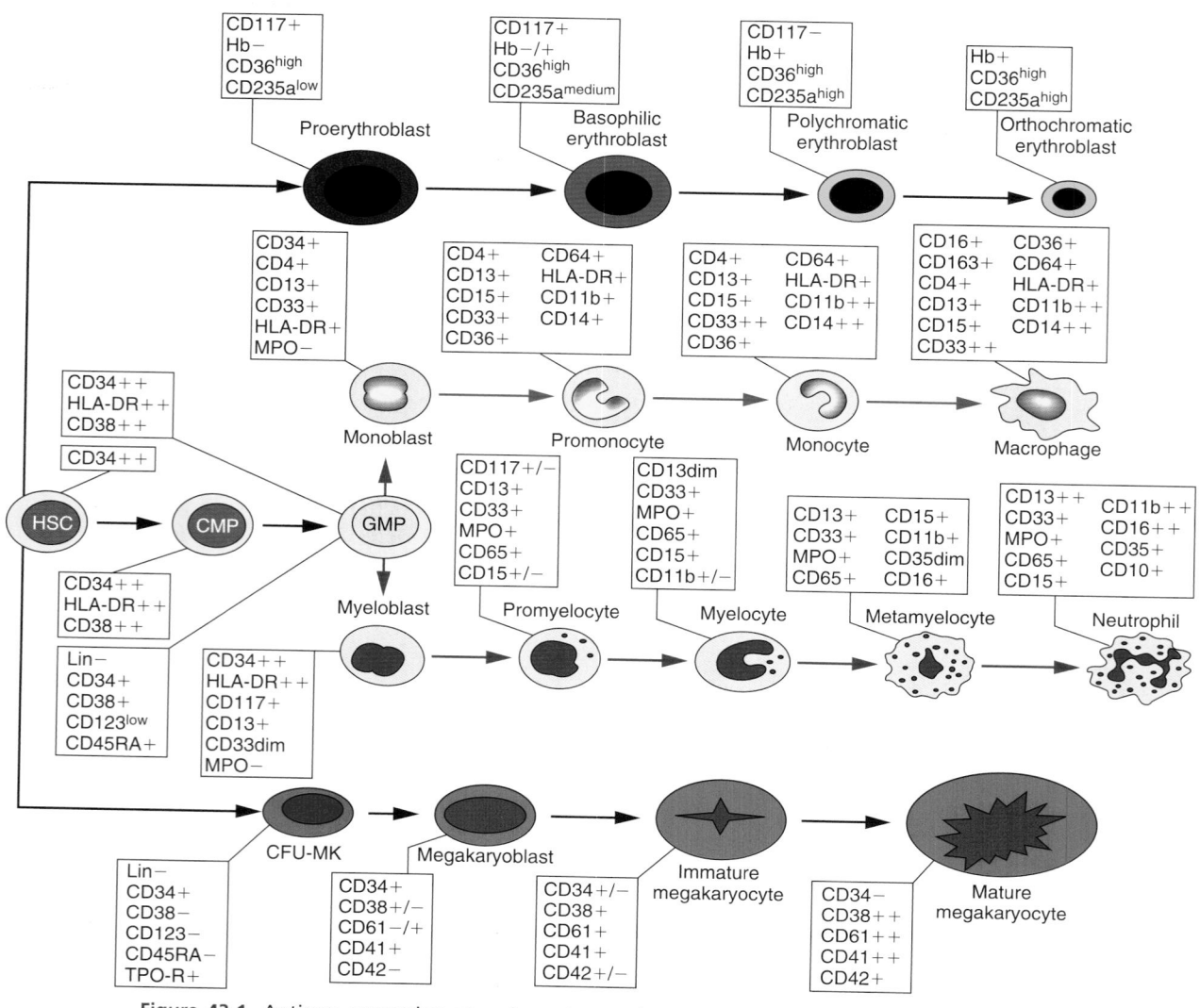

Figure 43-1. Antigen expression at various stages of normal myeloid differentiation. *CFU-MK,* Colony-forming unit–megakaryocyte; *CMP,* common myeloid progenitor; *GMP,* granulocyte-monocyte progenitor; *HSC,* hematopoietic stem cell. *(Courtesy Dr. Anna Porwit, Professor Emerita, Lund University.)*

of *BCR::ABL1*-negative MPNs, including polycythemia vera, primary myelofibrosis, and essential thrombocythemia, were diagnosed by somewhat complicated algorithms that included non-specific clinical and laboratory features intended to distinguish subtypes of MPN from one another and from reactive bone marrow hyperplasia that can mimic MPN.[38] However, the discovery in 2005 of the *JAK2* V617F and similar mutations in virtually all cases of polycythemia vera and in 50% of cases of essential thrombocythemia and primary myelofibrosis revolutionized, yet also simplified, the diagnostic criteria for these neoplasms.[14,15,39-41] Since that time, the detection of mutations in *JAK2* exon 12, *MPL,* and more commonly, *CALR* have been discovered in many cases of *JAK2*-negative MPN.[18,20,21,42] Although not specific for any MPN, detection of one of these activating mutations identifies the case in question as clonal and thus eliminates a number of diagnostic procedures used to distinguish MPNs from reactive hyperplasia. Unfortunately, for the cases of essential thrombocythemia and primary myelofibrosis that

lack a mutation, the distinction between a neoplastic and a reactive process occasionally remains problematic because absence of *JAK2* V617F or a similar activating mutation does not exclude an MPN. In addition, even when a mutation is present, it does not distinguish one MPN from another (except that polycythemia vera is only associated with *JAK2* mutations), so additional criteria are necessary. In previous schemes, histopathology and morphologic features played only a minor role in substantiating the diagnosis of an MPN and distinguishing the various subtypes, and hematologic data or clinical information was more important; but the past decade has brought better characterization and more widespread recognition of the histologic features associated with the MPN subtypes, and specific histopathologic features were included as diagnostic parameters in the prior WHO and current ICC 2022 schemes. Therefore, the diagnostic algorithms for MPNs now include clinical, hematologic, genetic, and histologic data to accurately identify and classify the various subtypes.

Box 43-2 2022 International Consensus Classification of Myeloid Neoplasms

Myeloproliferative Neoplasms
Chronic myeloid leukemia
Polycythemia vera
Essential thrombocythemia
Primary myelofibrosis
Early/prefibrotic primary myelofibrosis
Overt primary myelofibrosis
Chronic neutrophilic leukemia
Chronic eosinophilic, not otherwise specified
Myeloproliferative neoplasm, unclassifiable

Myeloid/Lymphoid Neoplasms With Eosinophilia and Tyrosine Kinase Gene Fusions
Myeloid/lymphoid neoplasm with *PDGFRA* rearrangement
Myeloid/lymphoid neoplasm with *PDGFRB* rearrangement
Myeloid/lymphoid neoplasm with *FGFR1* rearrangement
Myeloid/lymphoid neoplasm with *JAK2* rearrangement
Myeloid/lymphoid neoplasm with *FLT3* rearrangement
Myeloid/lymphoid neoplasm with *ETV6::ABL1*

Mastocytosis

Myelodysplastic/Myeloproliferative Neoplasms
Chronic myelomonocytic leukemia
Clonal cytopenia with monocytosis of undetermined significance
Clonal monocytosis of undetermined significance
Atypical chronic myeloid leukemia
Myelodysplastic/myeloproliferative neoplasm with thrombocytosis and *SF3B1* mutation
Myelodysplastic/myeloproliferative neoplasm with ring sideroblasts and thrombocytosis, not otherwise specified
Myelodysplastic/myeloproliferative neoplasm, not otherwise specified

Premalignant Clonal Cytopenias and Myelodysplastic Syndromes
Clonal cytopenia of undetermined significance
Myelodysplastic syndrome with mutated *SF3B1*
Myelodysplastic syndrome with del(5q)
Myelodysplastic syndrome with mutated *TP53*
Myelodysplastic syndrome, not otherwise specified (MDS, NOS)
  MDS, NOS without dysplasia
  MDS, NOS with single lineage dysplasia
  MDS, NOS with multilineage dysplasia
Myelodysplastic syndrome with excess blasts
Myelodysplastic syndrome/acute myeloid leukemia (MDS/AML)
  MDS/AML with mutated *TP53*
  MDS/AML with myelodysplasia-related gene mutations

MDS/AML with myelodysplasia-related cytogenetic abnormalities
MDS/AML, not otherwise specified

Pediatric and/or Germline Mutation-Associated Disorders
Juvenile myelomonocytic leukemia
Juvenile myelomonocytic leukemia-like neoplasms
Noonan syndrome-associated myeloproliferative disorder
Refractory cytopenia of childhood
Hematologic neoplasms with germline predisposition

Acute Myeloid Leukemias
Acute promyelocytic leukemia (APL) with t(15;17)(q24.1;q21.2)/*PML::RARA*
APL with other *RARA* rearrangements
AML with t(8;21)(q22;q22.1)/*RUNX1::RUNX1T1*
AML with inv(16)(p13.1q22) or t(16;16)(p13.1;q22)/*CBFB::MYH11*
AML with t(9;11)(p21.3;q23.3)/*MLLT3::KMT2A*
AML with other *KMT2A* rearrangements
AML with t(6;9)(p22.3;q34.1)/*DEK::NUP214*
AML with inv(3)(q21.3q26.2) or t(3;3)(q21.3;q26.2)/*GATA2; MECOM(EVI1)*
AML with other *MECOM* rearrangements
AML with other rare recurring translocations
AML with t(9;22)(q34.1;q11.2)/*BCR::ABL1*
AML with mutated *NPM1*
AML with in-frame bZIP *CEBPA* mutations
AML and MDS/AML with mutated *TP53*
AML and MDS/AML with myelodysplasia-related gene mutations
AML and MDS/AML with myelodysplasia-related cytogenetic abnormalities
AML and MDS/AML, not otherwise specified (NOS)
  Myeloid sarcoma
Myeloid sarcoma

Myeloid Proliferations Associated With Down Syndrome

Acute Leukemia of Ambiguous Lineage
Mixed phenotype acute leukemia (MPAL) with defining genetic alterations
  MPAL with *BCR::ABL1*
  MPAL with t(v;11q23.3): *KMT2A* rearranged
  MPAL with *BCL11B* activation
MPAL with defining immunophenotypic changes
B/Myeloid MPAL
T/Myeloid MPAL
B/T MPAL
Acute undifferentiated leukemia
Acute leukemia of ambiguous lineage, NOS

Myeloid/Lymphoid Neoplasms With Eosinophilia and Tyrosine Kinase Gene Fusions

Synonyms and Related Terms

WHO revised 4th edition: Myeloid/Lymphoid Neoplasms with Eosinophilia and Rearrangement of *PDGFRA*, *PDGFRB*, *FGFR1* or with *PCM-JAK2*

WHO proposed 5th edition: Myeloid/Lymphoid Neoplasms with Eosinophilia and Tyrosine Kinase Gene Fusions

Some myeloid neoplasms associated with eosinophilia, including cases formerly designated chronic eosinophilic leukemia (CEL) or hypereosinophilic syndrome, are caused by abnormalities in genes that encode the α or β forms of

platelet-derived growth factor receptor (PDGFR) and result in its constitutive activation. Rearrangements of *PDGFRB* were first recognized in cases variably diagnosed as chronic myelomonocytic leukemia (CMML) with eosinophilia or as CEL,[43-46] whereas rearranged *PDGFRA* was found to be involved in CEL and in cases previously considered hypereosinophilic syndrome.[13] Rearrangements of *FGFR1* have also been implicated in myeloproliferations with prominent eosinophilia, such as 8p11.2 myeloproliferative syndrome.[47] However, patients with *FGFR1* rearrangements may initially have T-lymphoblastic or B-lymphoblastic leukemia/lymphoma associated with prominent tissue eosinophilia that later evolves to a myeloid neoplasm with eosinophilia, or vice versa.[47,48] Rare cases associated

Table 43-1 Myeloid Neoplasms: Major Subgroups and Characteristics at Diagnosis

Disease	Basic Pathogenesis	Blood Counts	BM Cellularity	BM Blasts (%)	Maturation	Morphology of Cells/Dysplasia	Hematopoiesis	Organomegaly
MPN	Constitutive activation of PTKs involved in signal transduction pathways leading to excess proliferation, decreased apoptosis	Variable, one or more myeloid lineages usually increased	Usually increased, but often normal in ET	<10 in chronic phase	Present	Granulocytes and erythroid precursors relatively normal; megakaryocytes abnormal, ranging from small in CML to pleomorphic and bizarre in PMF to very large in ET	Effective	Common
Myeloid/lymphoid neoplasms with eosinophilia and tyrosine kinase gene fusions	Constitutive activation of tyrosine kinase surface receptor leading to activated signal transduction pathways and excess proliferation	Eosinophilia ≥1.5 × 10^9/L	Increased	<20*	Present	Relatively normal in patients who first present with eosinophilia in chronic phase of disease	Effective	Common
MDS	Genetic, epigenetic, and immune abnormalities leading to proliferation with abnormal maturation, early apoptosis	Cytopenia of one or more myeloid lineages	Increased, occasionally normal, rarely hypocellular	<10	Present	Dysplasia in one or more myeloid lineages usually present	Ineffective	Uncommon
MDS/MPN	Constitutive activation of signaling pathways, with additional cooperating lesions that result in MDS-like features	Variable, WBC count often increased, usually anemia, platelets variable	Increased	<20	Present	Usually one or more lineages dysplastic	Varies among lineages	Common
MDS/AML	Genetic, epigenetic, and immune abnormalities leading to proliferation with abnormal maturation, early apoptosis	Variable, but usually with cytopenia of one or more myeloid lineages	Increased, occasionally normal, rarely hypocellular	10%–19%	Present	Dysplasia in one or more myeloid lineages usually present	Ineffective	Uncommon
AML	Genetic abnormalities leading to impaired maturation, plus additional cooperating abnormalities leading to proliferation and survival of neoplastic clone	WBC count variable, usually anemia and decreased platelets	Usually increased	≥20, except in cases with specific cytogenetic or molecular genetic abnormalities	Varies, but usually minimal	Blasts may have features of various myeloid lineages and may be associated with dysplasia in one or more lineages	Ineffective or effective	Uncommon

*Approximately 50% of patients with rearrangements of *FGFR1* initially are seen with a T-lymphoblastic or, less commonly, B-lymphoblastic leukemia/lymphoma. Rare cases of *PDGFRA* rearrangements may initially have lymphoblastic leukemia/lymphoma.

AML, Acute myeloid leukemia; *BM,* bone marrow; *CML,* chronic myeloid leukemia, *BCR::ABL1* positive; *ET,* essential thrombocythemia; *MDS,* myelodysplastic syndrome; *MPN,* myeloproliferative neoplasm; *PMF,* primary myelofibrosis; *PTKs,* protein tyrosine kinases; *WBC,* white blood cell.

with *PDGFRA* rearrangements initially had a lymphoblastic neoplasm associated with eosinophilia.[49] Other gene fusions resulting in similar clinical disorders have been described, most notably involving *JAK2, FLT3, ETV6* and *ABL1*.[50,51] These somewhat varied clinical and morphologic presentations—CMML with eosinophilia, CEL, lymphoblastic leukemia/lymphoma with eosinophilia—argued for the creation of a separate category defined by the genetic lesions rather than dispersing the entities in multiple different subgroups throughout the classification. The creation of this subgroup—previously termed myeloid and lymphoid neoplasms with eosinophilia and rearrangements of *PDGFRA, PDGFRB,* or *FGFR1* or with *PCM1::JAK2* but now updated to myeloid and lymphoid neoplasms with eosinophilia and tyrosine kinase gene fusions—is a practical way to emphasize that patients with these rearrangements may respond to tyrosine kinase inhibitor therapies (see Chapter 50).

Myelodysplastic/Myeloproliferative Neoplasms

The MDS/MPN category was introduced in the WHO 3rd edition to include myeloid neoplasms with clinical, laboratory, and morphologic features that overlap MDS and MPN. Most of the entities included in this category have elevated white blood cell counts, anemia or thrombocytopenia, and variable amounts of morphologic dysplasia. This disease group included CMML, atypical CML, juvenile myelomonocytic leukemia, and a newer entity within the MDS/MPN unclassifiable group: refractory anemia with ring sideroblasts and thrombocytosis (subsequently termed MDS/MPN with ring sideroblasts and thrombocytosis; MDS/MPN-RS-T). Many cases of MDS/MPN-RS-T had mutations of *JAK2* or other MPN-associated genes and mutations of *SF3B1,* common in MDS with ring sideroblasts,[52] supporting the mixed myelodysplastic/myeloproliferative features of the disease. The ICC 2022 further refines this category of MDS/MPN to include (1) myelodysplastic/myeloproliferative neoplasm with *SF3B1* mutation and thrombocytosis and (2) myelodysplastic/myeloproliferative neoplasm with ring sideroblasts and thrombocytosis, not otherwise specified (NOS) (for cases without *SF3B1* mutations). The proposed WHO 5th edition only includes the former disease group, and it is unclear at the time of this writing where cases without *SF3B1* mutations would reside in that classification. A few cases of CMML and atypical CML have been reported to demonstrate *JAK2* V617F mutations,[40,41,53] but when mutations are detected in CMML and atypical CML, they do not occur in isolation, i.e., mutations in other genes are also present.[54-57] In juvenile myelomonocytic leukemia, more than 80% of patients demonstrate mutually exclusive RAS pathway mutations.[22,24,57] Approximately 30% to 40% of cases of CMML and atypical CML also exhibit *NRAS* or *KRAS* mutations.[25-27,58] The ICC 2022 recognizes the unique features of juvenile myelomonocytic leukemia (JMML) and related disorders, often with germline gene mutations, and now groups them in a new section of pediatric disorders and/or germline mutation-associated disorders. The proposed WHO 5th edition moves JMML to the myeloproliferative disorder category, which seems inappropriate for a neoplasm so different from the other adult preponderant MPNs.

Myelodysplastic Syndromes

Synonyms and Related Terms

WHO revised 4th edition: Myelodysplastic Syndromes
WHO proposed 5th edition: Myelodysplastic Neoplasms

Most cases of MDS are readily recognized by the characteristic findings of cytopenia in an older adult associated with morphologic dysplasia in the blood and bone marrow, with or without an increase in the number of blasts in the blood or bone marrow. Nearly 50% of cases have a cytogenetic lesion at the time of diagnosis that is characteristically associated with loss of genetic material, through either chromosomal loss or epigenetic phenomena, and the majority have gene mutations, even when a relatively small mutation panel is used.[36] In most cases, subclassification of MDS is readily achieved by assessing the number of lineages that are dysplastic and accurately counting the number of blasts in the blood and bone marrow—essentially a grading system. Still, MDS remains one of the most challenging of the myeloid neoplasms for diagnosticians. In particular, problems arise when the clinical and laboratory findings suggest MDS but the morphologic findings are inconclusive; when secondary or transient dysplasia caused by nutritional deficiencies, medications, toxins, growth factor therapy, inflammation, or infection mimics the dysplasia of MDS; or when marrow hypocellularity or myelofibrosis obscures the underlying disease process.[12,59-62] The ICC 2022 provides guidelines for the minimal morphologic criteria for the diagnosis of MDS, provides criteria for clonal cytopenia of undetermined significance and other premalignant clonal cytopenias, and has incorporated gene mutation studies into the classification by adding new categories of MDS with mutated *SF3B1* (usually with ring sideroblasts) and MDS with mutated *TP53* (see Chapter 44). The ICC 2022 introduces a category of MDS/AML for some patients with 10% to 19% peripheral blood or bone marrow blasts, which replaces many cases of adult MDS with excess blasts-2. This category does not apply to children with MDS and 10% to 19% blast cells. The WHO 4th edition introduced a new, provisional entity, refractory cytopenia of childhood, for children with MDS who have cytopenia, multilineage dysplasia, less than 2% blasts in the blood, and less than 5% blasts in the bone marrow. This provisional clinicopathologic entity remains in the classification, but it is not currently clear if it actually represents a neoplastic process in most cases; it is now included in the section on pediatric disorders and/or germline mutation-associated disorders. Refractory cytopenia of childhood is renamed childhood MDS with low blasts in the proposed WHO 5th edition.

Acute Myeloid Leukemia

The 2001 WHO 3rd edition opened the door to the formal inclusion of genetic abnormalities in the diagnostic algorithms for AML. The genetic defects included were mainly chromosomal translocations involving transcription factors associated with characteristic morphologic and clinical features, thus forming distinct clinicopathologic-genetic entities. By the WHO 4th edition in 2008, it had become accepted that, in many cases of AML, multiple genetic lesions—including not only microscopically detectable chromosomal rearrangements or numerical abnormalities but also submicroscopic gene mutations—cooperate to establish the leukemic process and influence its morphologic and clinical characteristics. Rearrangements or mutations of genes that normally encode transcription factors important for myeloid differentiation and maturation, such as *RUNX1, RARA,* or *NPM1,* may result in impaired maturation of leukemic cells, whereas mutations of genes involved in signal transduction pathways, such as *FLT3, JAK2, RAS,* or *KIT,* may be required for the proliferation or survival of the neoplastic clone.[63] It is now understood that gene mutations are even more complicated than assumed in that simple two-group approach, and numerous cooperating mutations occur in AML.[35] Often, the combination of these abnormalities leads to a leukemia with distinct clinical and morphologic findings and distinct survival characteristics. Discovery of the role of genetic mutations in leukemia was initially focused on the largest cytogenetic subgroup of patients with AML—those with normal karyotypes—and an entirely new understanding and subclassification of this group emerged.[30] Gene mutations demonstrate importance across other genetic AML types, however, and such studies are now indicated for all AML types.[35,64]

With the ICC 2022, AML classification moves to a more pronounced genetic approach with creation of new categories with recurring genetic abnormalities and gene mutations. AML with *TP53* is a high-risk group, not included in the proposed WHO 5th edition, but it naturally follows the categories of MDS and MDS/AML with this gene mutation. Of note, our understanding of AMLs with myelodysplasia-associated changes has grown over the last 2 decades, and both the ICC 2022 and the proposed WHO 5th edition move toward cytogenetic and molecular genetic definitions of these disorders that no longer include morphologic changes of non-blast cells. The ICC 2022 also clearly defines cases by genetic changes first, with qualifiers used to note prior MDS, MDS/MPN, or cytotoxic therapy and qualifiers to note the presence of germline gene abnormalities.

The subgroup AML, NOS (now termed AML defined by differentiation in the proposed WHO 5th edition), remains largely defined by morphology; no distinct clinical, immunophenotypic, or genetic disease entities are currently recognized in this category. Similar to diffuse large B-cell lymphoma, NOS and peripheral T-cell lymphoma, NOS, AML, NOS represents a heterogeneous group of disorders. The number of cases falling into this group has decreased with the addition of new specific AML genetic entities.

Acute Leukemias of Ambiguous Lineage

Although they are not truly myeloid neoplasms, the diagnostic approach to acute leukemias of ambiguous lineage is similar to that of the myeloid neoplasms, requiring correlation of morphologic features with cytogenetic, molecular, genetic, and immunophenotypic results. In particular, the ICC 2022 and proposed WHO 5th edition define criteria for the diagnosis of acute leukemias of mixed phenotype, which are now termed mixed phenotype acute leukemia, or MPAL. Genetic categories of MPAL are defined to emphasize the biological and clinical importance of *BCR::ABL1* and *KMT2A* translocations and newly added *ZNF384* and *BCL11B* activation[65]; in these disorders, these features probably define clinical disease entities better than immunophenotyping studies alone (see Chapter 42).

Pediatric Disorders and/or Germline Mutation–Associated Disorders

A major addition to the 2016 revised 4th edition of the WHO classification was a section on germline predisposition to myeloid neoplasms (see Chapter 45), which may be identified in patients of all ages. These patients may have thrombocytopenia that progresses to myeloid neoplasms or presents as de novo cases of AML or MDS.[66] Whereas many of the germline mutations in these patients are similar to the ones acquired sporadically in other patients with AML or MDS, the detection of a germline mutation should result in screening of family members for predisposition to these neoplasms. The ICC 2022 expanded the categories of hematologic neoplasms with germline predisposition and also more clearly separated JMML from adult MDS/MPN and refractory cytopenia of childhood from MDS. In addition to JMML, which is now defined by the presence of RAS pathway mutations, the ICC 2022 provides criteria for JMML-like neoplasms that do not have such mutations and criteria for Noonan syndrome–associated myeloproliferative disorder.

CONCLUSION

There will continue to be new information about many of the myeloid neoplasms, even as this text is published, and perhaps even new disease entities will have been proposed during that time. To continue to be useful in practice and in the evaluation of data from clinical trials and laboratory investigations, any classification must be continually reviewed and updated. Conversely, new information needs to "mature" and to be confirmed in large studies by numerous investigators to be widely accepted and integrated into daily practice. Therefore, although we eagerly await new data on the myeloid neoplasms discussed in this volume, it is hoped that the principles of classification exemplified in the CAC approach used for the ICC 2022 will endure.

Acknowledgment

The authors thank James W. Vardiman, a coauthor of the 1st edition of this chapter.

KEY REFERENCES

1. Arber DA, Orazi A, Hasserjian RP, et al. *International Consensus Classification of Myeloid Neoplasms and Acute Leukemias*: integrating morphologic, clinical, and genomic data. *Blood.* 2022;140(11):1200–1228.
8. Arber DA, Borowitz MJ, Cessna M, et al. Initial diagnostic workup of acute leukemia: guideline from the College of American Pathologists and the American Society of Hematology. *Arch Pathol Lab Med.* 2017.
9. Estey E, Hasserjian RP, Dohner H. Distinguishing AML from MDS: a fixed blast percentage may no longer be optimal. *Blood.* 2022;139(3):323–332.

35. Cancer Genome Atlas Research Network. Genomic and epigenomic landscapes of adult de novo acute myeloid leukemia. *N Engl J Med*. 2013;368:2059–2074.

36. Bejar R, et al. Clinical effect of point mutations in myelodysplastic syndromes. *N Engl J Med*. 2011;364:2496–2506.

51. Tzankov A, Reichard KK, Hasserjian RP, Arber DA, Orazi A, Wang SA. Updates on eosinophilic disorders. *Virchows Arch*. 2023;482(1):85–97.

65. Weinberg OK, Arber DA, Dohner H, et al. The international consensus classification of acute leukemias of ambiguous lineage. *Blood*. 2023;141(18):2275–2277.

Visit Elsevier eBooks+ for the complete set of references.

Chapter 44

The Myelodysplastic Syndromes

Robert P. Hasserjian

INCIDENCE

Myelodysplastic syndrome (MDS) is a disease predominantly of the elderly; its incidence increases exponentially with age, with a noticeable rise beginning in the fifth decade and a median age estimated at approximately 76 years.[1-6] MDS is more common in men, with a male-to-female ratio approaching 2:1, although one subtype (**MDS with deletion 5q**) more commonly affects women. Though the incidence of MDS in children and young adults is in the range of only 0.05 to 0.4 cases per 100,000 per year,[7-11] its incidence exceeds 25/100,000 cases per year by the age of 70 years and rises to more than 36/100,000 cases per year in individuals older than 80 years.[2-5,8-11] However, there are several caveats in interpreting these epidemiologic data: (1) MDS may be difficult to diagnose, and some cases may be confused with other diseases.[12] (2) Some elderly patients receive only supportive treatment for presumed MDS, without a diagnostic workup or an explicit diagnosis. (3) In the past, there has been disagreement as to whether MDS is truly neoplastic, and many national cancer epidemiology registries have failed to record cases of MDS. However, according to current concepts, MDS is by definition a myeloid neoplasm.

SYNONYMS AND RELATED TERMS

The proposed 5th edition of the World Health Organization (WHO) Classification of Tumours of Haematopoietic and Lymphoid Tissues changed "myelodysplastic syndrome" to "myelodysplastic neoplasm," while retaining the "MDS" abbreviation.

CLINICAL FEATURES

MDS typically presents with symptoms and signs related to single or multiple peripheral blood cytopenias: anemia (weakness, pallor, fatigue), thrombocytopenia (petechiae, bleeding), or neutropenia (recurrent infections).[13-15] Occasionally, cases are recognized when asymptomatic cytopenias are noted during a routine complete blood count or when increased blasts, dysplastic morphology, or clonal cytogenetic abnormalities are identified in studies of peripheral blood or bone marrow obtained for other purposes.

Granulocytic or myeloid sarcomas (mass-forming collections of myeloblasts) can present as extramedullary tumors in patients with a history of MDS. If confirmed histologically, they are considered to represent transformation to acute myeloid leukemia (AML), even if the bone marrow myeloblast count remains below 20%. Splenomegaly is uncommon in MDS and, if present, tends to suggest an alternate diagnosis. Skin infiltrates of atypical myeloid and/or histiocytoid-looking cells (including Sweet's syndrome and so-called "histiocytoid Sweet's syndrome" or "specific lesions") are described rarely in MDS.[16] Some investigators have proposed the term "myelodysplasia cutis" to encompass cases of perivascular atypical histiocytoid-appearing cells with elongated nuclei, likely representing dysplastic granulocytes, occurring in skin biopsies of patients with MDS.[17,18] Although not equivalent to cutaneous myeloid sarcoma (in which the skin infiltrate contains myeloblasts and/or promonocytes), this finding has been associated with poor outcomes in MDS.

LABORATORY FEATURES

Blood Counts

An important hallmark of MDS is ineffective hematopoiesis resulting in one or more peripheral blood cytopenias; the presence of at least one cytopenia is an absolute requirement for a diagnosis of MDS. The thresholds defining cytopenia for the purposes of establishing a diagnosis of MDS are shown in Table 44-1. Conversely, non-neoplastic causes of cytopenia (particularly anemia) are common, and only a very small minority of patients presenting with cytopenia actually have MDS.[19] Anemia is the most common presenting cytopenia in patients with MDS, and it is usually normocytic or macrocytic (median mean corpuscular volume of 97 fL). Less than 10% of patients with MDS have microcytic anemia, which in some cases represents acquired α-thalassemia.[20] There is frequently an increased red cell distribution width.[14,15] The anemia may be isolated, or it may co-exist with neutropenia and/or thrombocytopenia.[21] Adults with MDS present only rarely with isolated neutropenia or thrombocytopenia; however, this presentation is seen more frequently in pediatric MDS.[21-24] The cytopenias in MDS vary in severity, but they are typically sustained and progressive without treatment. Although reticulocyte production is typically low in MDS, the reticulocyte count may be spuriously elevated in some patients owing to abnormally retained cytoplasmic ribosomal material (basophilic stippling) in circulating red blood cells rather than actual increased red blood cell production.[25,26] This may cause diagnostic confusion with hemolytic anemia.

Though documenting a persistent, unexplained cytopenia is a diagnostic requirement for MDS, blood counts may also play a role in excluding MDS in some instances. An important hallmark of MDS is ineffective hematopoiesis; an elevated blood count (cytosis) is unexpected and tends to exclude a diagnosis of MDS and, if a neoplastic process is confirmed, suggests a diagnosis of MDS/myeloproliferative neoplasm (MPN) or even "pure" MPN. With the exception of MDS cases with an inv(3)/t(3;3) cytogenetic abnormality or fulfilling features of **MDS with del(5q)**, a sustained platelet count of ≥450 × 10⁹/L excludes a diagnosis of MDS, even if other cytopenias are present. A sustained elevated white

blood cell count (≥13 × 10⁹/L, not from lymphocytosis) or absolute and relative monocytosis (≥0.5 × 10⁹/L and ≥10% of all leukocytes) also exclude a diagnosis of MDS and suggest an alternate diagnosis of MDS/MPN (Table 44-1). Finally, if ≥20% of circulating blasts are identified in the blood, even in a patient with leukopenia and <20% marrow blasts, the diagnosis is AML rather than MDS.

In summary, abnormal blood counts (cytopenia) are required to establish an initial diagnosis of MDS. Blood counts also establish the boundaries of MDS with MDS/MPN and AML. Within MDS, blood counts do not affect the current disease classification. However, blood counts play an important role in prognosticating MDS and when monitoring response to therapy (Table 44-2).

Microscopic Features in Peripheral Blood and Bone Marrow

Despite the presence of peripheral cytopenias, the marrow is typically hypercellular for age in MDS.[27] Less commonly, it is normocellular, and in 10% to 15% of cases, it is hypocellular for age (which defines a specific MDS subtype **MDS, hypoplastic** in the proposed 5th edition WHO classification). Hypocellularity is more frequent in pediatric MDS, after prior aplastic anemia, and in therapy-related MDS.[28-31]

The "dysplasia" in the disease name reflects an unusual set of abnormal cytologic features found in hematopoietic cells in the marrow and peripheral blood (Table 44-3; Figs. 44-1–44-3). Although it is not pathognomonic for MDS, dysplastic morphology is a critical feature in establishing the diagnosis, and according to current International Consensus Classification (ICC) and proposed 5th edition WHO criteria, it must be present in at least 10% of cells to designate a lineage as dysplastic. At least one dysplastic lineage must be present to diagnose MDS, with rare exceptions for cases in which the diagnosis is established by increased blasts or specific genetic abnormalities in the absence of dysplasia. Some dysplastic features are best seen in mature cells in the peripheral blood, such as large or abnormally granulated platelets, basophilic stippling and poikilocytosis in red blood cells, and pseudo–Pelger-Huët anomaly and hypogranular cytoplasm in neutrophils. Others occur in immature precursors and are best seen in the bone marrow. Immature hematopoietic precursors (nucleated red blood cells, immature granulocytes, megakaryocyte nuclei, and mononuclear megakaryocytes) may circulate in the peripheral blood of patients with MDS and can show the same anomalies as seen in the marrow. However, nuclear irregularities in circulating erythroid cells are non-specific, as they can occur in non-MDS myeloid neoplasms and even non-neoplastic conditions associated with leukoerythroblastosis. Marrow myeloblasts are increased in higher-grade MDS and may circulate in the peripheral blood, but they are always less than 20% of the bone marrow and peripheral blood nucleated cells. Auer rods are uncommonly seen in MDS; if present in blasts, they indicate highly aggressive disease, even if the actual blast percentages do not reach the designated thresholds.[32-34]

Table 44-1 Defining Cytopenias for Myelodysplastic Syndrome (MDS)

Peripheral Blood Count Abnormality	Threshold	Significance
Anemia	Hemoglobin <13 g/dL (men) or <12 g/dL (women)	Unexplained anemia is a cytopenia that can qualify for a diagnosis of MDS.
Neutropenia	Absolute neutrophil count (ANC) <1.8 × 10⁹/L	Unexplained neutropenia is a cytopenia that can qualify for a diagnosis of MDS. Adjustment should be made for specific patient populations and according to the individual laboratory reference range.
Thrombocytopenia	Platelets <150 × 10⁹/L	Unexplained thrombocytopenia is a cytopenia that can qualify for a diagnosis of MDS. Adjustment should be made according to the individual laboratory reference range.
Monocytosis	Monocytes ≥0.5 × 10⁹/L and comprising ≥10% of all leukocytes	Unexplained persistent monocytosis at the time of initial diagnosis disqualifies a diagnosis of MDS; CMML should be considered.
Leukocytosis	White blood count ≥13 × 10⁹/L	Unexplained persistent leukocytosis (not from a lymphocytosis) at the time of initial diagnosis disqualifies a diagnosis of MDS; an MDS/MPN or MPN should be considered.
Thrombocytosis	Platelets ≥450 × 10⁹/L	Unexplained persistent thrombocytosis at the time of initial diagnosis disqualifies a diagnosis of MDS; an MDS/MPN or MPN should be considered. Exception: MDS diagnosis is allowed if criteria for MDS with del(5q) are present, or if there is inv(3) or t(3;3) cytogenetic abnormality involving *MECOM*.

CMML, Chronic myelomonocytic leukemia; *MDS,* myelodysplastic syndrome; *MDS/MPN,* myelodysplastic/myeloproliferative neoplasm; *MPN,* myeloproliferative neoplasm.

Table 44-2 Comparison of Criteria Used in MDS Classification and Prognostic Schemes

Feature	Classification		Prognostication	
	ICC	Proposed 5th Edition WHO	IPSS-R	IPSS-M
Degree of cytopenias	No	No	Yes: Degree of anemia, neutropenia, thrombocytopenia	Yes: Degree of anemia and thrombocytopenia
Blast % in blood	Yes: <2%, 2%–4%, 5%–9%, 10%–19%	Yes: <2%, 2%–4%, 5%–19%	No	No
Blast % in bone marrow	Yes: <5%, 5%–9%, 10%–19%	Same as ICC	Yes: <2%, 2%–4%, 5%–10%, 11%–19%	Yes: Continuous variable
Degree of dysplasia	Yes: 1 vs. ≥2 lineages	No	No	No
Auer rods	Yes: mandates MDS-EB classification	Yes: Mandates MDS-IB2 classification	No	No
Ring sideroblasts	No	Yes: Used to diagnose MDS-LB-RS	No	No
Bone marrow cellularity	No	Yes: Used to diagnose hypoplastic MDS	No	No
Bone marrow fibrosis	No	Yes: Used to diagnose MDS with fibrosis	No	No
Karyotype	Yes: del(5q)	Same as ICC	Yes: 5 Prognostic groups (CCSS)	Yes: 5 prognostic groups
Gene mutations	Yes: *SF3B1* and multihit *TP53*	Same as ICC	No	Yes: 36 genes
Flow cytometry abnormalities	No	No	No	No

CCSS, Comprehensive Cytogenetic Scoring System; *EB,* excess blasts; *IB,* increased blasts; *ICC,* International Consensus Classification; *IPSS-M,* Molecular International Prognostic Scoring System; *IPSS-R,* Revised International Prognostic Scoring System; *LB,* low blasts; *MDS,* myelodysplastic syndrome; *RS,* ring sideroblasts; *WHO,* World Health Organization.
Data from Arber DA, Orazi A, Hasserjian RP, et al. International Consensus Classification of Myeloid Neoplasms and Acute Leukemia: integrating morphological, clinical, and genomic data. *Blood.* 2022;140(11):1200-1228. Khoury JD, Solary E, Abla O, et al. The 5th edition of the World Health Organization Classification of Haematolymphoid Tumours: myeloid and histiocytic/dendritic neoplasms. *Leukemia.* 2022;36(7):1703-1719. Schanz J, Tuechler H, Sole F, et al. New comprehensive cytogenetic scoring system for primary myelodysplastic syndromes (MDS) and oligoblastic acute myeloid leukemia after MDS derived from an international database merge. *J Clin Oncol.* 2012;30:820-829. Greenberg PL, Tuechler H, Schanz J, et al. Revised international prognostic scoring system for myelodysplastic syndromes. *Blood.* 2012;120:2454-2465. Bernard E, et al. Molecular international prognostic scoring system for myelodysplastic syndromes. *NEJM Evidence.* 2022;1(7):EVIDoa2200008.

Table 44-3 Dysplastic Morphologic Features of Myelodysplastic Syndrome

Cell Lineage	Peripheral Blood	Bone Marrow
Red blood cells and erythroid precursors	Anisocytosis and poikilocytosis* Dual red blood cell populations Basophilic stippling Siderocytes	Cloverleaf nuclei and variations and nuclear budding Megaloblastoid change Multinuclearity Vacuolated erythroblasts Internuclear bridging Pyknotic nuclei Irregular hemoglobinization of precursors Howell-Jolly bodies Ring sideroblasts, or abnormal sideroblasts with large or multiple iron granules
Granulocytes and precursors	Acquired (pseudo) Pelger-Huët anomaly Hypogranularity Nuclear hypersegmentation Ring nuclei	Megaloblastoid change Hypogranularity Myeloperoxidase deficiency Abnormal localization of immature precursors† Nuclear-cytoplasmic asynchrony Pseudo–Chédiak-Higashi granules
Platelets and megakaryocytes	Large, vacuolated, or hypogranular platelets	Small mononuclear megakaryocytes Large megakaryocytes with multiple small nuclei Hypolobated megakaryocytes Large megakaryocytes with large hyperchromic nuclei

*Numerous types of abnormal forms may be seen, including ovalocytes, elliptocytes, teardrops, targets, and fragmented forms.
†In the normal marrow biopsy, CD34-positive myeloid blasts and other immature precursors are mostly located adjacent to bone trabeculae and blood vessels. In myelodysplastic syndrome, CD34-positive blasts may cluster and be abnormally located in the center of marrow spaces, hence the descriptive name "abnormal localization of immature precursors."

Although experienced observers can generally agree on the presence of significant dysplasia and the presence or absence of increased blasts in a bone marrow sample,[35] the quantification of dysplastic features (i.e., involving one versus multiple lineages) is inherently variable among observers for several reasons: (1) the subtlety of some dysplastic features; (2) the observers' experience; (3) differing significance and subjective weighting of individual dysplastic features; and (4) sampling variability in the cells observed on smears by different individuals.[36,37] It is important to emphasize that dysplastic features may be encountered in healthy individuals who do not have MDS and are even more frequently seen in patients with secondary cytopenias caused by non-MDS conditions, as discussed in the Differential Diagnosis section of this chapter.[35,38-40]

In summary, with the exception of rare cases defined by specific cytogenetic abnormalities or mutations (discussed below), the presence of significant morphologic dysplasia of hematopoietic cells in the blood and/or bone marrow is required to diagnose MDS. Morphology also affects disease classification in terms of the blast percentage and presence of any Auer rods (ICC and 5th edition WHO classification), single versus multilineage dysplasia (ICC), marrow cellularity (5th edition WHO classification), ring sideroblasts (5th edition WHO classification), and bone marrow fibrosis (5th edition WHO classification). The only morphologic parameter incorporated into the International Prognostic Scoring System schemes (2012 revised version, IPSS-R and 2022 version incorporating mutations, IPSS-M) is the bone marrow blast percentage (Table 44-2). Bone marrow blast percentage is also important in monitoring MDS response after therapy.[41]

Flow Cytometry

MDS hematopoietic cells exhibit recurring quantitative and qualitative abnormalities in antigen expression and maturation patterns that can be interrogated by multiparameter flow cytometry immunophenotyping. These include abnormalities in the quantity and phenotype of blasts, the phenotype and light scatter qualities of maturing myeloid cells, the phenotype of erythroid cells and monocytes, and the maturation patterns of maturing myeloid cells and monocytes. A list of the main flow cytometry abnormalities observed in the most frequently assessed hematopoietic lineages (blasts, maturing myeloid cells, and monocytes) is shown in Table 44-4. These abnormalities correlate with the types and degrees of morphologic dysplasia and cytogenetic abnormalities, predict prognosis independent of other known risk factors,[42,43] have been shown to predict response to certain therapies (such as growth factors and hypomethylating agents),[44,45] and may provide insight into the biology and pathogenesis of MDS.[46] Although these phenotypic abnormalities have been validated in numerous studies, the way in which flow cytometry should be optimally applied to diagnose MDS remains controversial. Some of the abnormalities in myeloid and monocytic maturation patterns that are typical of MDS may also be seen in reactive conditions such as HIV infection, bone marrow regeneration, or autoimmune conditions.[47] Some aberrant antigen expression patterns have proved difficult to implement in a clinical laboratory setting.[48,49] In contrast, phenotypic aberrations observed in the blast compartment, such as a paucity of CD19-positive hematogones, altered expression of CD45, CD34, CD117, CD33, CD13, or CD38, and aberrant expression of lymphoid antigens (such as CD2, CD5, CD7, or CD56), appear to be more specific to MDS.[50,51]

Implementation of flow cytometry evaluation of MDS in individual laboratories requires sufficient case volume and experience. Ideally, published recommended panels should be used and multiple simultaneous

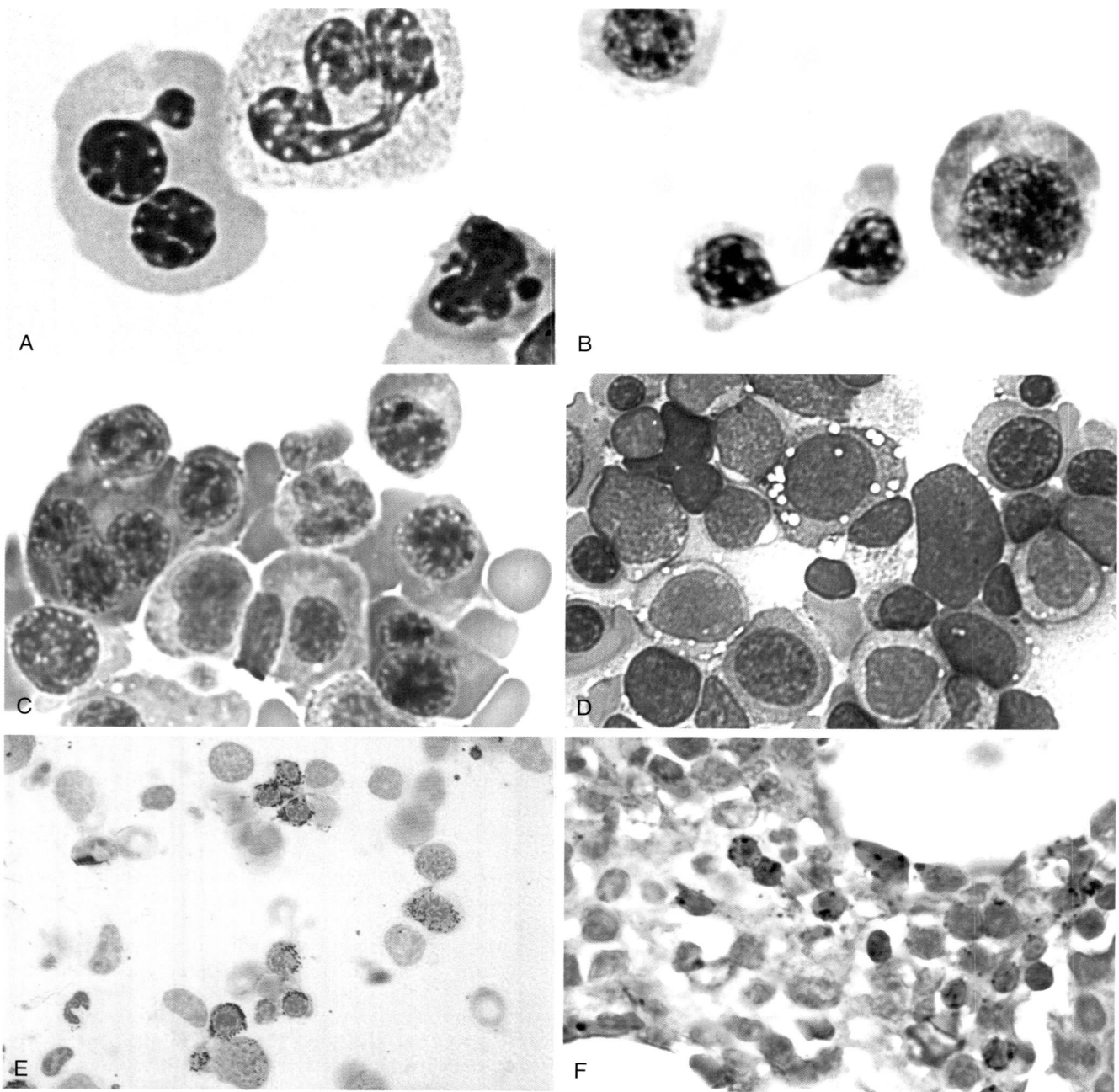

Figure 44-1. Dysplastic features of erythroid precursors in bone marrow aspirate smears in myelodysplastic syndrome. A, Erythroid precursors with abnormal nuclear lobulation. **B,** Internuclear bridge in erythroid precursors (note the pointed nuclei at the base of the bridge). **C,** Multinucleation and megaloblastoid change in erythroid precursors. **D,** Erythroblasts containing cytoplasmic vacuoles. **E and F,** Ring sideroblasts in the bone marrow aspirate smear **(E)** and clot section **(F)** (Prussian blue stain).

abnormalities should be observed to suggest a diagnosis of MDS.[52,53] Updated guidelines put forth by the European LeukemiaNet/International Myelodysplastic Syndrome Flow Cytometry Working Group were published in 2023.[51] These guidelines recommend the use of flow cytometry, including a core set of 17 markers, to evaluate a bone marrow specimen taken for cytopenia and evaluation of the number and immunophenotype of myeloid precursor cells and maturing cell populations.[51] Overall, flow cytometry immunophenotyping in suspected MDS is considered a helpful adjunctive test that can be used to support a diagnosis of MDS suspected on morphology and clinical features, particularly if the morphology is suboptimal or ambiguous.[54-56] Conversely, normal flow cytometry findings can prompt more careful investigations for non-MDS causes of cytopenia. However, flow cytometry

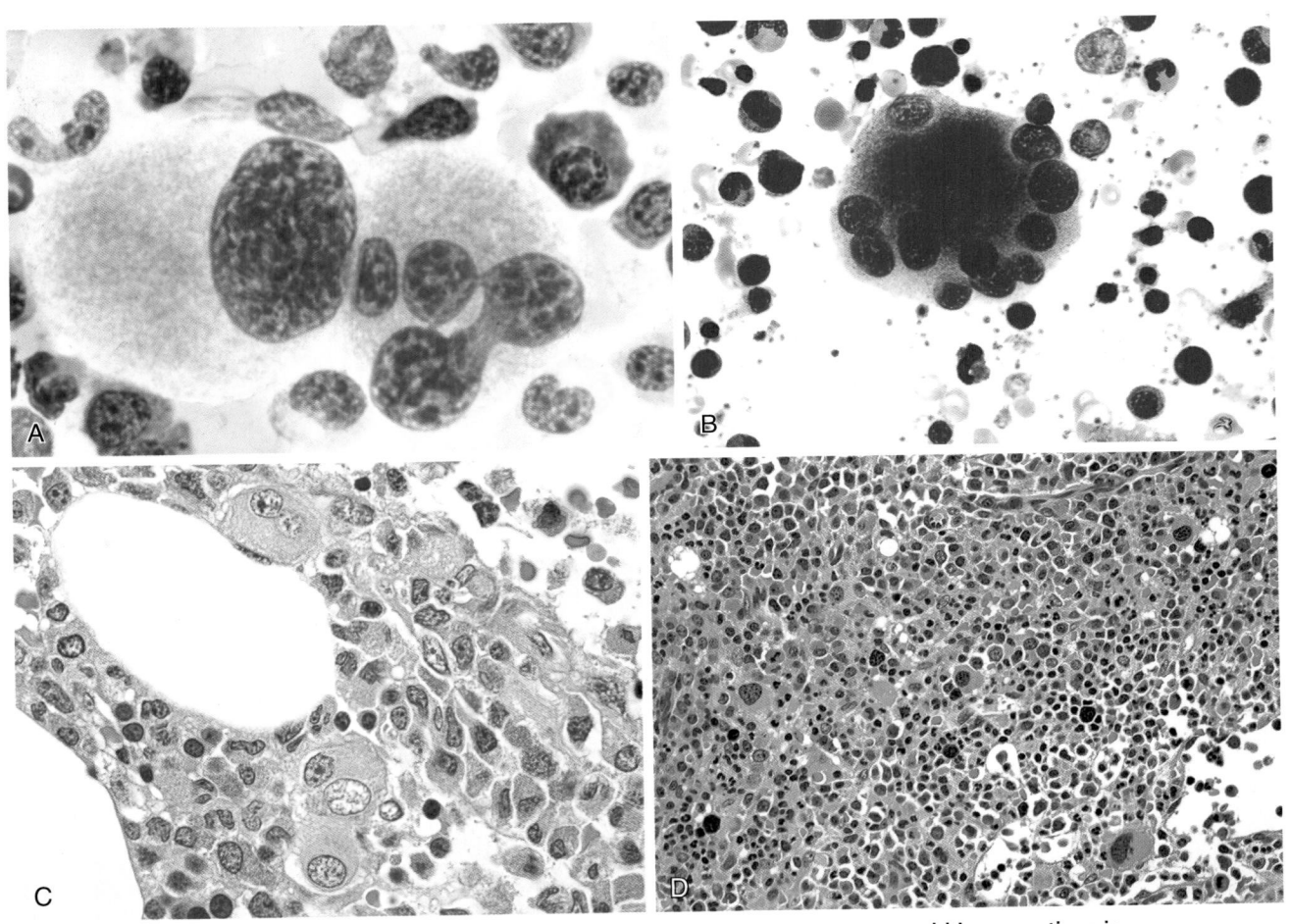

Figure 44-2. Megakaryocytic dysplasia in bone marrow aspirate smears and biopsy sections in myelodysplastic syndrome. A and **B,** Abnormal nuclear features in bone marrow aspirate smears include non-lobated (**A,** cell on left) and multiple separated small nuclei (**B**). **C,** Small non-lobated megakaryocytes in a bone marrow biopsy specimen. **D,** Characteristic megakaryocyte morphology in MDS with del(5q), showing numerous small to medium-sized megakaryocytes with rounded nuclei; there is also relative erythroid hypoplasia.

findings alone should not be used to make a diagnosis of MDS if other criteria are lacking, nor should a negative flow cytometry result be used to unequivocally exclude the possibility of MDS. At the time of this writing, flow cytometry abnormalities do not affect prognostic schemes or MDS disease monitoring posttherapy.

Genetic Abnormalities

MDS is, by definition, a clonal disease, and one of the important hallmarks of abnormal MDS hematopoiesis is the presence of recurrent genetic abnormalities that originate in the MDS stem cell. These genetic abnormalities can be manifested as gross chromosomal alterations (detected by conventional karyotype or fluorescence in situ hybridization [FISH]), smaller chromosomal deletions or gains (detected by single nucleotide polymorphism [SNP] arrays or copy number abnormalities predicted by next-generation sequencing [NGS]), or mutations in specific genes. The recurring genetic abnormalities in MDS have

several important implications: (1) they are often helpful in establishing a diagnosis; (2) certain specific abnormalities define particular disease subtypes within MDS; and (3) many recurring genetic abnormalities provide critical prognostic information, and some may suggest the use of specific targeted therapies.

Cytogenetic abnormalities are present at diagnosis in 50% to 60% of patients with MDS. The typical recurring clonal cytogenetic abnormalities seen in MDS are shown in Table 44-5.[57,58] The large majority of identified abnormalities consist of loss or gain of large segments of chromosomes, the most frequent being −7, del(5q), and +8. Deletions or losses of chromosomal material may also result from unbalanced translocations. It is presumed that these deletions or duplications result in the respective loss or gain of function of critical genes, but most of the genes in question are unknown. Balanced chromosomal translocations, which are common in AML, are infrequent in MDS. Many of the cytogenetic abnormalities in MDS appear to be secondary events that follow initial inciting somatic gene mutations, particularly

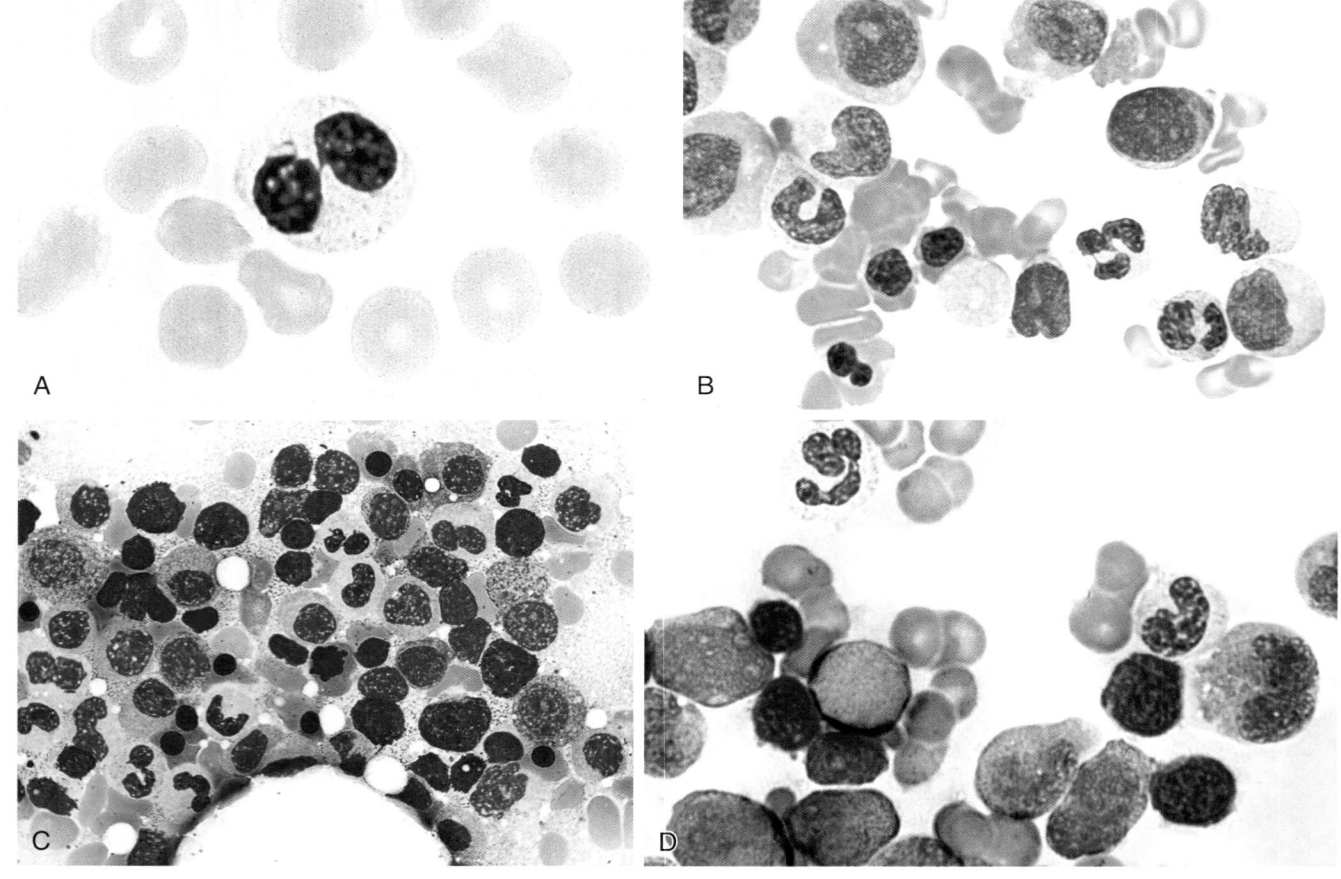

Figure 44-3. Granulocytic dysplasia in peripheral blood and bone marrow aspirate smears in myelodysplastic syndrome. A, Pseudo–Pelger-Huët cell with bilobed nucleus and hypogranular cytoplasm in peripheral blood smear. **B,** Asynchronous maturation of granulocytes with hyposegmented nuclei in bone marrow aspirate smear. **C,** Prominent granulocytic nuclear hyposegmentation and hypogranulation in bone marrow aspirate smear. **D,** Myeloperoxidase-negative granulocytes *(yellow is positive)* in bone marrow aspirate smear (myeloperoxidase stain, Giemsa counterstain).

Table 44-4 **Abnormalities Identified by Flow Cytometry in Blast, Myeloid, and Monocytic Lineages in Myelodysplastic Syndrome**

Cell Population	Abnormalities Seen in Myelodysplastic Syndrome
CD34+ blasts	Increased numbers (≥3%) Decreased proportion of CD19+ hematogones Altered CD45 and side scatter Increased CD13+/CD33− or CD13−/CD33+ subset Increased CD11b expression Increased CD123+ subset Decreased expression of CD38 or HLA-DR Aberrant expression of CD2, CD4, CD5, CD7, or CD56
Maturing myeloids	Decreased side scatter relative to lymphocytes Decreased expression of CD33 Increased expression of CD36, CD117, or HLA-DR Abnormal pattern of CD11b, CD13, CD16 expression Abnormal pattern of CD15 and CD10 expression Aberrant expression of CD34, CD5, CD56, or CD7
Monocytes	Decreased CD45/side scatter Decreased expression of CD13, CD15, CD36, CD64, CD11b, CD11c, HLA-DR, or CD14 Aberrant expression of CD56 (bright) or CD2

Porwit A, et al. Multiparameter flow cytometry in the evaluation of myelodysplasia: analytical issues: recommendations from the European LeukemiaNet/international myelodysplastic syndrome flow cytometry working group. *Cytometry B Clin Cytom.* 2023;104(1):27–50. Westers TM, Ireland R, Kern W, et al. Standardization of flow cytometry in myelodysplastic syndromes: a report from an international consortium and the European LeukemiaNet Working Group. *Leukemia.* 2012;26:1730–1741.

the presence of complex karyotype in the setting of biallelic alteration of the *TP53* gene.[59-61]

Whereas the effect of cytogenetics on MDS diagnosis and prognosis has been known for several decades, the significance of mutations in MDS has only become apparent in the last 10 to 15 years, facilitated by rapid advances in NGS technologies. Recurring somatic (i.e., acquired and residing in the MDS clone, not inherited in the germline) mutations in more than 100 genes have been identified and have fostered the development of NGS panels that cover most or all of these genes. Using such panels, at least one acquired genetic abnormality is found in over 90% of patients with MDS, a significantly higher proportion compared with abnormalities detected by conventional karyotyping alone.[62-64] A list of the most commonly mutated genes in MDS is shown in Table 44-6. These genes fall into several general functional categories. Mutations affecting proteins in the *spliceosome complex*, which controls RNA splicing and thereby affects global gene expression, are among the most common in MDS. Spliceosome complex gene mutations in aggregate are found in more than 50% of MDS cases and tend to be mutually exclusive to one another.[65] Epigenetic regulation of gene expression is also commonly altered in MDS through mutations in genes controlling *DNA methylation* or *histone modification.* Other commonly mutated genes are those encoding hematopoietic *transcription factors, signaling proteins* (such as tyrosine kinases), *tumor suppressors*

Table 44-5 Common Recurrent Cytogenetic Abnormalities in Myelodysplastic Syndrome and Their Significance

Abnormality	Frequency in MDS	Significance
−7 or del(7q)	5%–10%	MDS defining in ICC Poor prognosis in CCSS
Del(5q)	15%	MDS defining in ICC Good prognosis in CCSS (if isolated)
+8	5%–10%	Intermediate prognosis in CCSS
+21	2%	Intermediate prognosis in CCSS
i(17q)	<1%	Intermediate prognosis in CCSS
−17, del(17p), unbalanced translocations at 17p	2%–5%	Indicate multihit/biallelic *TP53* lesion if accompanied by *TP53* mutation
t(3;3)(q21;q26), inv(3)(q21q26), and other 3q translocations involving *MECOM*	<1%	Considered AML-defining in ICC and WHO (≥10% blasts required in ICC). May have thrombocytosis Poor prognosis in CCSS
Complex karyotype (3 or more independent cytogenetic aberrations)	10%	MDS defining in ICC. Poor prognosis in ICC (very poor if >3 abnormalities)
Del(12p)	2%	Good prognosis in CCSS
Del(20q)	3%–5%	Good prognosis in CCSS (if isolated)
Del(11q)	2%	Very good prognosis in CCSS (if isolated)
−Y	5%	Can occur in older males without myeloid malignancy Very good prognosis in CCSS (if isolated)

CCSS, Comprehensive Cytogenetic Scoring System; *ICC,* International Consensus Classification; *MDS,* myelodysplastic syndrome; *WHO,* World Health Organization Classification.

Data from Vallespi T, Imbert M, Mecucci C, Preudhomme C, Fenaux P. Diagnosis, classification, and cytogenetics of myelodysplastic syndromes. *Haematologica.* 1998;83:258-275. Raimondi SC. Cytogenetics in MDS. In: Lopes LF, Hasle H, eds. *Myelodysplastic and Myeloproliferative Disorders in Children.* Sao Paulo: Le Mar; 2003:119-161. Ouseph MM, Hasserjian RP, Dal Cin P, et al. Genomic alterations in patients with somatic loss of the Y chromosome as the sole cytogenetic finding in bone marrow cells. *Haematologica.* 2021;106(2):555-564. Bernard E, Tuechler H, Greenberg PL, et al. Molecular International Prognostic Scoring System for myelodysplastic syndromes. *NEJM Evidence.* 2022;1(7):EVIDoa2200008. Arber DA, Orazi A, Hasserjian RP, et al. International Consensus Classification of myeloid neoplasms and acute leukemia: integrating morphological, clinical, and genomic data. *Blood.* 2022;140(11):1200-1228. Khoury JD, Solary E, Abla O, et al, The 5th edition of the World Health Organization classification of haematolymphoid tumours: myeloid and histiocytic/dendritic neoplasms. *Leukemia.* 2022;36(7):1703-1719.

(typically DNA damage-response genes), and the *cohesin complex,* which controls the cohesion of sister chromatids, DNA repair, and transcriptional regulation.

Several points must be made regarding the interpretation of NGS results in MDS.

1. The mutational landscape of MDS is complex and dynamic: an individual MDS case typically bears multiple mutations (e.g., in a spliceosome gene plus an epigenetic regulator), and in aggregate, MDS-associated mutations show nonrandom associations with one another. Moreover, some mutations may be present in only a subclone of the tumor cells, and the relative proportions of these subclones may shift during the course of the disease, with or without treatment.[66]

2. Mutations identical to those seen in MDS can occur in apparently healthy individuals without cytopenia (termed clonal hematopoiesis of indeterminate potential [CHIP]) or with unexplained cytopenia (termed clonal cytopenia of undetermined significance [CCUS]), neither of which is considered a hematologic neoplasm. Thus, the presence of MDS-associated mutations does not prove the presence of MDS.[67]

3. Even with the combination of conventional karyotype and broad NGS panels designed to pick up somatic mutations associated with MDS, 5% to 10% of bona fide MDS cases lack detectable genetic abnormalities.[62]

4. Some cases of MDS (with or without a family history of hematologic neoplasia) may bear inherited germline mutations in genes that predispose to the development of hematologic malignancy. Such potential germline mutations can be investigated by interrogating non-MDS patient tissue (cultured fibroblasts, hair follicles, or a skin biopsy) by NGS panels that are designed to detect these germline predisposition genes. Moreover, these germline mutations may be associated with dysplastic morphology and cytopenia at baseline in patients with stable counts; thus, caution must be exercised when diagnosing MDS in a patient with a possible germline predisposition mutation.

Although the genes included in NGS panels vary, a list of 39 genes has been proposed to optimally include for mutation testing in adult patients with suspected MDS: *ASXL1, BCOR, BCORL1, CBL, CEBPA, CSF3R, DDX41, DMNT3A, ETV6, ETNK1, EZH2, FLT3, GATA2, GNB1, IDH1, IDH2, JAK2, KIT, KRAS, KMT2A, NF1, NPM1, NRAS, PHF6, PPM1D, PRPF8, PTPN11, RAD21, RUNX1, SETBP1, SF3B1, SRSF2, STAG2, TET2, TP53, U2AF1, UBA1, WT1,* and *ZRSR2.* This list includes mutations that are AML-defining (*NPM1* and *CEBPA*), that establish or exclude specific MDS subtypes (*SF3B1, RUNX1, TP53*), and that influence prognosis or have therapeutic implications.[68]

According to the ICC, the presence of certain somatic genetic abnormalities (Tables 44-5 and 44-6) is sufficient to confirm a diagnosis of MDS in a cytopenic patient, even if significant dysplasia is lacking. A del(5q) cytogenetic abnormality, when isolated or occurring with only one additional abnormality (except for −7 or del[7q]), is associated with a unique disease phenotype, response to a specific therapy, and a generally favorable prognosis (see section on **MDS with del[5q]**). The del(5q) typically occurs in primitive MDS stem cells as a founding event before the acquisition of other genetic aberrations and is associated with a highly differential gene expression profile.[69] Loss of chromosome 7 or del(7q) and complex karyotype (three or more independent cytogenetic abnormalities, seen more frequently in therapy-related MDS) are also considered to be MDS defining in patients with unexplained cytopenia.

Table 44-6 Recurrent Mutations in Hematopoietic Cells From Patients With Myelodysplastic Syndromes

	Mutation Frequency	Significance
Splicing Factor Genes		
SF3B1	15%–33%	MDS-defining (if VAF ≥10%) in ICC. Defines a specific MDS subtype in ICC and 5th edition WHO. In general, a favorable prognosis; adverse prognosis in the setting of del(5q)
SRSF2	10%–19%	More commonly seen in CMML than in MDS. Adverse prognosis
U2AF1	7%–12%	Adverse prognosis
ZRSR2	3%–11%	
PRPF8	1%–4%	Adverse prognosis
DDX41	1%–2%	Somatic mutation often occurs in setting of germline DDX41 mutation. May confer favorable prognosis
DNA Methylation Genes		
TET2	20%–33%	Commonly mutated in non-MDS cytopenias
DNMT3A	5%–16%	Commonly mutated in non-MDS cytopenias; neutral to adverse prognosis.
IDH1/IDH2	4%–10%	Adverse prognosis. Targeted therapies available
KMT2A	3%	Partial tandem duplication in gene (not detected by all NGS assays) associated with adverse prognosis
Histone Modification Genes		
ASXL1	11%–25%	Adverse prognosis
EZH2	5%–12%	Adverse prognosis
PHF6	3%–4%	Adverse prognosis
Transcription Factors		
RUNX1	8%–15%	Adverse prognosis
SETBP1	2%–5%	Adverse prognosis
ETV6	2%–5%	Adverse prognosis
BCOR/BCORL	4%–7%	Adverse prognosis
CUX1	3%	
Cohesin Complex Genes		
STAG2	4%–10%	Adverse prognosis
RAD21	1%–5%	Adverse prognosis
Signaling Genes		
NRAS/KRAS	5%–10%	Adverse prognosis
CBL	2%–5%	Adverse prognosis
JAK2	2%–5%	More commonly seen in MPN than in MDS
FLT3	1%–4%	Adverse prognosis
PTPN11	2%–3%	Adverse prognosis
DNA-Damage Response		
TP53	5%–11%	MDS defining (if biallelic and VAF ≥10%) in ICC. Defines a specific MDS subtype in ICC and 5th edition WHO. Commonly associated with therapy-related disease. Adverse prognosis
PPM1D	1%–3%	Associated with therapy-related disease. Adverse prognosis

CMML, Chronic myelomonocytic leukemia; ICC, International Consensus Classification; MDS, myelodysplastic syndrome; MPN, myeloproliferative neoplasm; NGS, next-generation sequencing; VAF, variant allele frequency; WHO, World Health Organization Classification.

All other cytogenetic abnormalities are not considered sufficient to establish a diagnosis of MDS in the absence of other diagnostic criteria. These include relatively common cytogenetic abnormalities associated with MDS (+8, del[20q], and –Y), which can also be seen in healthy older males (–Y) or in individuals with non-MDS causes of cytopenia, such as aplastic anemia or immune thrombocytopenia.[70-73] Some cytogenetic aberrations may be seen transiently in patients recovering from chemotherapy or receiving tyrosine kinase therapy, and their presence does not necessarily indicate emerging MDS in this setting.[74,75] Cytogenetic abnormalities in aplastic anemia, some of the congenital marrow failure syndromes, and megaloblastic anemia may be transient and recede spontaneously.[76-79] In rare pediatric patients with germline predisposition conditions (particularly germline SAMD9/SAMD9L and SBDS mutations) and an acquired –7, the cytogenetic abnormality may regress spontaneously to a normal karyotype, with no subsequent evidence of MDS or hematologic disease (so-called "somatic rescue").[80,81] Thus, though −7 is considered to be MDS-defining in the ICC, caution is advised in the context of some rare germline conditions.

The MDS clonal precursor lesions CHIP and CCUS refer to the presence of mutated myeloid cells derived from a hematopoietic stem cell clone in individuals without any known hematologic neoplasm and with normal blood counts (CHIP) or with an unexplained cytopenia (CCUS). CCUS is distinguished from MDS only by the presence of significant morphologic dysplasia; thus, a bone marrow biopsy to assess for dysplasia is mandatory to exclude MDS and diagnose CCUS. Given that all humans carry mutated hematopoietic stem cells (which progressively increase with age), a minimum threshold variant allele frequency (VAF) of 2% has been established in both the ICC and 5th edition WHO Classification to define CHIP and CCUS. The mutations seen in CHIP and CCUS affect genes that are frequently mutated in MDS and other myeloid neoplasms (*ASXL1, TP53, JAK2, SF3B1, TET2, DNMT3A*). Compared with MDS, CHIP and CCUS tend to have a smaller number of detectable mutations (typically only a single mutation), and these mutations occur at a lower VAF.[82] However, given the overlap of the types of mutated genes and their VAFs between CCUS and MDS, the identification of MDS-type mutations alone, even in a patient with cytopenia, is not sufficient to establish a diagnosis of MDS in the absence of other diagnostic criteria. The only exceptions are mutations in *SF3B1* and multihit *TP53* lesions (with mutations at minimal VAFs of 10%), which are considered to be MDS-defining in a cytopenic patient in the ICC. Studies have revealed that some mutation patterns in CCUS indicate particularly high risk of progressing to MDS or another myeloid neoplasm; these include a mutant gene with a VAF ≥10%, the presence of a splicing gene mutation, a *TP53* mutation, or comutation of *TET2, ASXL1*, or *DNMT3A* with at least one other gene.[82,83] However, further study is needed to determine whether some CCUS cases can be considered equivalent to true MDS defined by morphologic dysplasia.[67]

It is well established that specific cytogenetic abnormalities strongly influence the prognosis of MDS, and thus the karyotype findings represent a cornerstone of MDS risk stratification schemes (Table 44-7). Not surprisingly, individual mutations also show a strong association with outcome in MDS, and the addition of mutational data enhances the ability of existing risk stratification schemes to predict prognosis in MDS.[59,84-87] Most of the recurring gene mutations in MDS have been associated with an unfavorable prognosis, whereas mutation in *SF3B1* is the only gene definitively associated with a more favorable prognosis (Table 44-6). Emerging data also suggest that *DDX41*, when occurring in the setting of a germline *DDX41* mutation, may also convey favorable prognosis, and MDS cases with mutated *DDX41* may not be effectively risk stratified by current prognostic schemes.[88]

Though several risk stratification schemes that incorporate mutation data have been developed,[59,84] the most comprehensive scheme is the IPSS-M, which incorporates mutations of 36 genes alongside the karyotype, blood counts, and bone marrow blast percentage.[85] It is interesting to note that the context of an individual gene mutation appears to modify its prognostic effect: for

Table 44-7 Comprehensive Cytogenetic Scoring System for MDS

Prognostic Subgroup	Cytogenetic Abnormalities	Median Overall Survival*
Very good	−Y, del(11q)	5.4 years
Good	Normal, del(5q), del(12p), del(20q), double including del(5q)	4.8 years
Intermediate	del(7q), +8, +19, i(17q), any other single or double independent clones	2.7 years
Poor	−7, inv(3)/t(3q)/del(3q), double including −7/ del(7q), complex (3 abnormalities)	1.5 years
Very poor	Complex (>3 abnormalities)	0.7 years

*For patients not receiving disease-altering therapy.
MDS, Myelodysplastic syndrome.
Data from Greenberg PL, Tuechler H, Schanz J, et al. Revised international prognostic scoring system for myelodysplastic syndromes. *Blood*. 2012;120:2454-2465.

example, though *SF3B1* mutation is generally prognostically favorable, it imparts an unfavorable prognosis when it occurs in the setting of a del(5q) cytogenetic abnormality. In addition, evaluation of the *TP53* gene requires a more complex analysis: two lesions affecting the *TP53* gene (so-called "multihit" status or "biallelic inactivation", typically a mutation in one allele in combination with an inactivating mutation or deletion of the other *TP53* allele) impart a dismal prognosis, but a single or monoallelic *TP53* mutation may not confer adverse prognosis in MDS.[89,90] *TP53* mutations in **MDS with del(5q)** (most of which are monoallelic)[90] do predict a poorer response to lenalidomide.[91] It is important to note that bulk sequencing used in clinical practice does not resolve the genetic complexity of individual MDS cases, which could include subclones and low-level mutations not detectable by standard assays. Thus, it is likely that, in the future, more complex genetic analyses (such as single-cell sequencing) may achieve more accuracy in predicting the prognosis of patients with MDS.[92,93]

Aberrant Function of Hematopoietic Cells

A variety of losses of function (or abnormal function) have been described in the hematopoietic cells of patients with MDS. Neutrophil precursors may lose myeloperoxidase function in rare MDS cases, and in the large subset of MDS cases with ring sideroblasts, there is abnormal accumulation of iron in the mitochondria of erythroid precursors. Small paroxysmal nocturnal hemoglobinuria clones,[94,95] reticulocytosis simulating a hemolytic process,[25,26] increased hemoglobin F,[96] changes in blood group antigen expression,[97] and acquired α-thalassemia[98,99] can occur in association with MDS and may cause diagnostic confusion with non-MDS conditions (see this chapter's discussion of Differential Diagnosis).

DIAGNOSIS

There is no single completely sensitive or specific feature or test that can be used to unequivocally diagnose MDS; because of these limitations and the numerous clinical situations that can mimic MDS, clinicopathologic correlation and integration of information from the multiple diagnostic modalities are essential for an accurate and reliable diagnosis. The minimal diagnostic criteria for MDS are listed in Box 44-1. The application of these criteria must take into account the clinical context of each case because many of these abnormalities may be present in non-MDS conditions. Cytopenias should be stable or worsen over several weeks at least; thus, it is of value to seek blood counts prior to those of the bone marrow date to document chronicity. If a subsequent marrow sample is performed at a later time, any dysplastic changes should persist or worsen. If only unilineage dysplasia is present without excess blasts and no cytogenetic or molecular abnormalities are detected, it is reasonable to request the patient be followed, and another marrow sample should be taken at a later date to document persistent dysplasia and cytopenia before MDS is diagnosed outright.[100]

To evaluate a potential case of MDS, the minimal requisite studies are (1) a complete blood count with white blood cell differential and examination of the peripheral smear, (2) a Wright-Giemsa–stained bone marrow aspirate smear, (3) a hematoxylin-eosin–stained biopsy section, (4) an iron stain on a bone marrow aspirate smear to evaluate for ring sideroblasts, (5) a full bone marrow karyotype, and (6) NGS studies to include evaluation of at least *SF3B1* and *TP53* genes. Flow cytometry to identify immunophenotypic aberrancies may be a helpful adjunctive test to support a diagnosis of MDS, although it is not part of the formal diagnostic criteria. Review of a high-quality aspirate smear is paramount, both to accurately identify dysplasia and to establish an accurate blast count. The aspirate should optimally contain spicules with well-preserved, well-stained cellular trails that allow counting of at least 500 cells. If an aspirate is unobtainable because of fibrosis, a touch imprint from the bone marrow core often provides adequate material for evaluation. The bone marrow biopsy is essential to evaluate the cellularity, topography of maturing myeloid and erythroid elements and megakaryocytes, and focal accumulations of blasts that may not be represented in the aspirate smear. The bone marrow biopsy also evaluates for other pathologies that may mimic MDS, such as metastatic carcinoma or lymphoma involving the bone marrow. A reticulin stain should be performed on the biopsy to assess for fibrosis, which is relevant for diagnosis of **MDS with increased blasts and fibrosis** subtype in the proposed 5th edition WHO classification. Reticulin stain is also an independent prognostic factor in MDS.[101]

Though cytogenetic abnormalities in a putative new MDS case should always be evaluated on a conventional karyotype of bone marrow, FISH analysis for the common MDS abnormalities (particularly loss of chromosomes 5 and 7) may be helpful if the karyotype fails or is insufficient (less than 20 metaphases).[102] However, FISH probably does not add meaningful information in the workup of a possible MDS case if 20 normal metaphases are obtained from a bone marrow sample.[103,104] The iron stain should be performed on a bone marrow aspirate smear rather than on the biopsy specimen because decalcification leaches iron from the biopsy sample; in some instances, ring sideroblasts may be identifiable in a nondecalcified paraffin-embedded particle section stained for iron. An immunostain for CD34 in the biopsy section can help corroborate the aspirate blast count and may upgrade the diagnosis if the CD34-positive cells in the core biopsy are greater than the blast count in the aspirate smear (discussed in the section on **MDS-EB**).[105,106] Immunostaining of the

biopsy section with a megakaryocyte marker such as CD61 or CD42b helps reveal small, dysplastic megakaryocytes that can be missed on routine histology. Clinical tests are important in excluding metabolic abnormalities that can cause cytopenias mimicking MDS, including vitamin B_{12}, folate, pyridoxine, and copper deficiencies. Paroxysmal nocturnal hemoglobinuria clones detected by flow cytometry, platelet function abnormalities on coagulation testing, and other acquired functional abnormalities in hematopoietic cells may be seen both in MDS and in non-neoplastic conditions and are not generally used in the diagnosis of MDS.

CLASSIFICATION

Disease Border: Myelodysplastic Syndrome Versus Clonal Hematopoiesis

MDS is a clonal disease that is separated from other clonal hematopoietic proliferations by the presence of significant morphologic dysplasia in at least one lineage or persistent and unexplained increase in bone marrow blasts (below the level required to define AML). The minimal diagnostic criteria for MDS are shown in Box 44-1, and features of non-MDS clonal hematopoietic proliferations are shown in Table 44-8. In evaluating dysplasia in a cytopenic patient, it is critical to consider non-neoplastic causes of dysplasia and cytopenia (discussed in the Differential Diagnosis section). Some data suggests that the distinction between CCUS with high-risk mutations and lower-risk MDS is irrelevant, as these patients may have a similar prognosis.[83] However, until further data is accumulated, the requirement for identifying morphologic dysplasia to diagnose MDS has been retained in both the ICC and proposed 5th edition WHO classification; the only exceptions that are made are for a small group of genetic

---

Box 44-1 *Minimal Criteria for a Diagnosis of Myelodysplastic Syndrome (ICC)*

- Sustained unexplained anemia, neutropenia, or thrombocytopenia in the absence of a sustained unexplained leukocytosis or absolute and relative monocytosis (see Table 44-1 for requisite levels)

AND

- At least one of the following:
  - Dysplastic morphology in erythroid cells, granulocytes, or megakaryocytes, affecting at least 10% of the cells of at least one of these lineages.
  - Increased blasts in bond marrow (at least 5% of marrow cells) or blood (at least 2% of leukocytes) not attributable to exogenous growth factor administration or transient marrow recovery from injury, and in the absence of diagnostic criteria for AML established by ≥20% blood/marrow blasts and/or an AML-defining genetic abnormality
  - Del(5q), −7, del(7q), or complex karyotype detected on bone marrow cytogenetics
  - *SF3B1* mutation at VAF of ≥10%
  - Multihit TP53 mutation defined by a somatic *TP53* mutation at VAF ≥50%
  - Multihit TP53 mutation defined by a somatic *TP53* mutation at VAF of ≥10% and with inactivation of the second *TP53* allele through mutation (VAF of ≥10%), deletion, or copy-neutral loss-of-heterozygosity

AML, Acute myeloid leukemia; *VAF,* variant allele frequency.

Table 44-8 Non-MDS Clonal Myeloid Proliferations*

Designation	Unexplained Cytopenia (See Table 44-1)	Dysplasia (≥10% of Any Lineage)†	MDS-Defining Genetic Abnormality‡	Genetic Lesion
Clonal hematopoiesis of indeterminate potential (CHIP)	No	No	No	Variable
Clonal cytopenia of undetermined significance (CCUS)	Yes	No	No	Variable
Paroxysmal nocturnal hemoglobinuria (PNH)	Yes	Usually not	No	*PIGA* mutation
Aplastic anemia with clonal hematopoiesis	Yes	No	No	Variable
VEXAS syndrome	Yes	No	No	*UBA1* mutation

*Defined as identification of a pathogenic somatic mutation in hematopoietic cells (from blood or bone marrow) in a gene recurrently mutated in myeloid neoplasms, at VAF ≥2%, or a clonal cytogenetic abnormality detected by karyotype.
†Requires bone marrow examination.
‡Del(5q), −7, del(7q), or complex karyotype detected on bone marrow conventional karyotype, or multihit *TP53* mutation (VAF ≥10%) or *SF3B1* mutation (VAF ≥10%).
MDS, Myelodysplastic syndrome; *VEXAS*, vacuoles, E1-enzyme, X-linked, autoinflammatory, somatic.

aberrations that are considered to be MDS-defining in the ICC (Tables 44-5 and 44-6).

Disease Border: Myelodysplastic Syndrome Versus Acute Myeloid Leukemia

An AML-defining threshold of 30% was used in the prior French-American-British (FAB) classification of AML. In this scheme, MDS with 20% to 30% marrow blasts was designated refractory anemia with excess blasts in transformation (RAEB-T).[32] In the 2001 WHO classification, the threshold for separating MDS and AML was decreased to 20%, and the diagnostic category of RAEB-T was thus eliminated and merged into AML. This change generated some discussion and disagreement in the literature[107,108] centered on the ambiguity of distinguishing MDS from AML on the basis of the single parameter of the blast percentage.[109,110] Moreover, in clinical practice, the most biologically relevant distinction is often not the separation of MDS from AML but the separation of de novo AML from MDS and MDS-related AML entities (such as AML progressed from MDS in the ICC, AML with myelodysplasia-related changes [AML-MRC] in the 4th edition WHO classification, and AML, myelodysplasia-related [AML-MR] in the proposed 5th edition WHO classification). The therapeutic approach to MDS with excess blasts is frequently similar to that of AML that has progressed from MDS. In contrast, intensive chemotherapy may induce long-term complete remissions in patients with de novo AML, particularly those with certain specific recurring genetic abnormalities (AML-RGA). Younger patient age and a more rapid clinical presentation without prior cytopenia are clues to de novo AML-RGA rather than MDS-related disease.[111] The AML-RGA cytogenetic aberrations *PML::RARA*, *RUNX1::RUNX1T1*, and *CBFB::MYH11* have been considered to be AML-defining irrespective of the blast count. In the ICC and proposed 5th edition WHO classification, this list of AML-RGA entities has been expanded to include several other genetic aberrations that are now considered to be AML defining, even in cases with <20% blasts, as data suggest that the blast count is not relevant in the presence of these genetic lesions (see Chapter 46).[112-116] In the ICC, a minimum threshold of 10% blasts is applied for any AML diagnosis based on an AML-defining genetic feature. These changes result in some cases previously

categorized as MDS with excess blasts-2 (MDS-EB2) in the revised 4th edition WHO classification to be considered as AML and potentially eligible for AML-type intensive chemotherapy. It should be emphasized that such cases are rare; the vast majority of myeloid neoplasms bearing AML-defining genetic aberrations present with a blast percentage of at least 20%.

MDS is a bone marrow failure syndrome characterized by ineffective hematopoiesis, whereas AML is a dysregulated hyperproliferation of blasts. In this context, some cases with a blast percentage of 20% to 30% (i.e., prior RAEB-T) may behave like MDS, with clinical manifestation as marrow failure and cytopenias, whereas others behave like AML, with rapid accumulation of blasts in the blood and bone marrow. It is often not possible to reliably distinguish between a progressive blast hyperproliferation and a more stable marrow failure syndrome on the basis of a single bone marrow examination, but serial examination may allow this distinction (Fig. 44-4); if the marrow blast percentage remains relatively constant or rises slowly over time to exceed the 20% threshold, the case may continue to behave like MDS, whereas if the blast percentage rises abruptly, the disease process has likely transformed to a proliferative state and may be best considered AML. Overall, de novo AML cases with low blast counts (20% to 29%) that lack AML-RGA abnormalities appear to behave more indolently and generally lack hyperproliferative features, similar to high-grade MDS, an observation that underscores the arbitrary nature of the 20% blast cutoff that has been used to define AML.[117] Conversely, some patients with 10% to 19% blasts may benefit from treatment with more intensive AML-like regimens versus standard MDS-directed therapies.[112,118,119]

In light of these evolving concepts surrounding the MDS versus AML distinction (and increased overlap between AML-directed and MDS-directed therapies), the ICC introduced a category of disease intermediate between MDS and AML to acknowledge the biological continuum between these two myeloid neoplasms. This new disease category, **MDS/AML**, encompasses cases of cytopenic patients exhibiting morphologic features of MDS with 10% to 19% blasts in blood or bone marrow, thus corresponding to most cases of MDS-EB2 in the revised 4th edition WHO classification and **MDS with increased blasts-2 (MDS-IB2)** in the proposed 5th edition WHO classification. This change allows patients

MDS progression

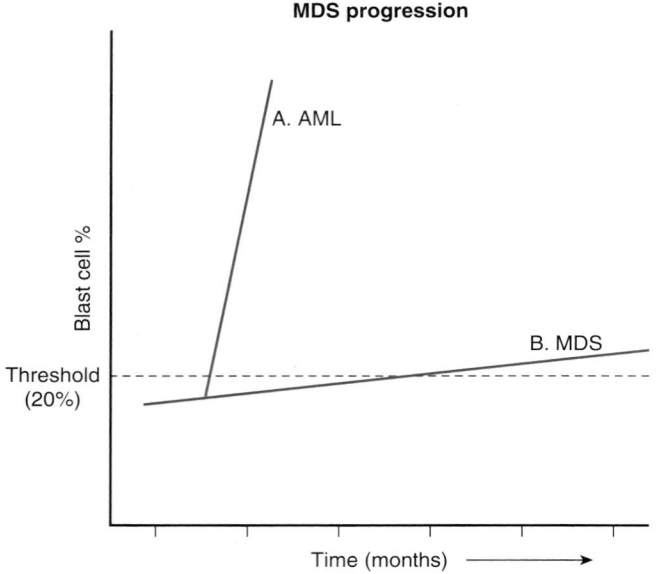

Figure 44-4. Blast progression over time in myelodysplastic syndrome (MDS). If the blast percentage in marrow rises rapidly *(line A)*, the case may be more biologically related to acute myeloid leukemia (AML), even at earlier blast percentages of <20%. In contrast, if the blast percentage rises slowly over several months *(line B)*, the case is likely more biologically akin to MDS, even if the blast percentage exceeds 20%.[109] Despite these differences in disease tempo that suggest different clinical behaviors, MDS and AML continue to be separated largely by a static blast threshold of 20%.

with **MDS/AML** to be potentially eligible for both MDS and AML trials and treatments while accumulating data to optimize the treatment approach to such patients. Rather than basing treatment decisions on an arbitrary blast threshold cutoff, this more nuanced approach takes into account features such as stable versus rapid progression in blast count and cytopenias and the mutation profile, potentially driving more patient-centered therapeutic choices.[118,119] Trials are needed to investigate the effectiveness of novel AML and MDS therapies as applied to this "transitional" MDS/AML group.[120]

Disease Heterogeneity Within Myelodysplastic Syndrome

The biological behavior of MDS is highly variable, ranging from genetically and clinically stable disease to aggressive disease that acquires increasingly complex genetic abnormalities and rapidly progresses to severe marrow failure and cytopenias or AML.[60,61,121] Some subtypes of MDS are associated with a relatively long median survival (6–8 years or longer), a low rate of progression to AML (<10% overall), and a low percentage of blasts in the peripheral blood (<2%) and bone marrow (<5%).[13,32] These lower-risk subtypes include **MDS with del(5q), MDS with mutated *SF3B1*,** and **MDS, not otherwise specified (MDS-NOS).**

More aggressive cases of MDS are often characterized by an increase in blasts; a blast threshold of 5% in the bone marrow or 2% in the blood or the presence of Auer rods in blasts defines the MDS subtype **MDS-EB**. *TP53* mutation in MDS also defines a highly aggressive disease with several unique features and defines a new entity: **MDS with mutated *TP53*.** The distinction between aggressive subtypes of MDS

and AML is often less critical than the distinction between aggressive MDS and lower-risk MDS subtypes for the purpose of determining the general direction of treatment; for these reasons, the ICC introduced the transitional disease category of **MDS/AML**, as discussed above. It should be emphasized that, although different MDS disease categories are associated with different clinical outcomes, risk assessment in MDS for the purpose of clinical management is best assessed by applying the IPSS-M or IPSS-R.

International Consensus Classification and World Health Organization Classification

In 1976, the FAB Working Group proposed that the previously chaotic nomenclature of MDS be standardized and created a classification that was subsequently updated in 1982.[32,109,122] The FAB classification of MDS included five categories: refractory anemia (RA), RA with ring sideroblasts (RARS), RA with excess blasts (RAEB), RAEB in transformation (RAEB-T), and chronic myelomonocytic leukemia (CMML). This classification standardized the reporting of data related to these diseases and allowed the comparison of treatment regimens in defined sets of patients. Subsequent revisions of this classification were incorporated in the 3rd edition of the WHO classification published in 2001 and were retained with relatively minor modifications in the 4th edition of this classification published in 2008. A revised 4th edition of the WHO classification of MDS was issued in 2016 and published in 2017.[123] This update included nomenclature changes enacted to avoid reference to specific cytopenias (such as anemia) in the disease names and included most cases of the prior entity "acute erythroid leukemia, erythroid/myeloid subtype" into MDS-EB by calculating the bone marrow myeloblast percentage from all nucleated cells, irrespective of the percentage of erythroid cells. In 2022, two separate updated classifications of MDS were introduced: the ICC and the 5th edition WHO classification.[124-126] Though the ICC has been published in its final form,[124] the 5th edition WHO classification Blue Book is still pending publication at the time of this writing. This chapter focuses on the ICC scheme, providing information regarding the 5th edition WHO classification approach based on the published proposal[125] with the caveat that there may be differences in the final published 5th edition Blue Book. A comparison of the ICC, revised 4th edition WHO classification, and proposed 5th edition WHO classification is shown in Table 44-9.

Myelodysplastic Syndrome With del(5q) (MDS-del5q)

MDS with del(5q) (MDS-del5q) is a discrete subset of MDS with an excellent prognosis.[127-130] In the proposed WHO 5th edition classification, this entity is named **myelodysplastic neoplasm with low blasts and isolated 5q deletion (MDS-5q).** MDS-del5q also corresponds to the WHO revised 4th edition classification's **myelodysplastic syndrome with isolated del(5q).** The only updates to this entity from the revised 4th edition classification are to allow cases with pancytopenia or 1% peripheral blood blasts (measured on only one occasion) in MDS-del5q; previously, these rare cases were placed into the MDS, unclassifiable category, which has been eliminated in the ICC.

Unlike the majority of MDS, **MDS-del5q** has a female predominance. Patients typically present with macrocytic

Table 44-9 Myelodysplastic Syndromes in Adults (Aged ≥18 Years, Blasts <20%): International Consensus Classification and Comparison to Revised 4th Edition and Proposed 5th Edition WHO Classifications (Adult Patients)

International Consensus Classification	Revised 4th Edition WHO Classification	Proposed 5th Edition WHO Classification
MDS with mutated *SF3B1* (MDS-*SF3B1*)	MDS with ring sideroblasts with single lineage or multilineage dysplasia (MDS-RS-SLD, MDS-RS-MLD) (most cases)	MDS with low blasts and *SF3B1* mutation (MDS-*SF3B1*)
MDS with del(5q)	MDS with isolated del(5q)	MDS with low blasts and isolated 5q deletion (MDS-5q)
MDS with mutated *TP53* (MDS-TP53)	None (distributed across several MDS subtypes)	MDS with biallelic *TP53* inactivation (MDS-biTP53)
MDS/AML with mutated *TP53* (MDS/AML-TP53)	MDS with excess blasts-2 (MDS-EB2)	MDS with biallelic *TP53* inactivation (MDS-biTP53)
MDS-NOS, without dysplasia	MDS, unclassifiable	Clonal cytopenia of undetermined significance (CCUS)
MDS-NOS, with single lineage dysplasia (MDS-NOS-SLD)	MDS with single lineage dysplasia (MDS-SLD, most cases)	MDS with low blasts (MDS-LB), some *SF3B1* wild-type MDS-LB with ring sideroblasts, and some MDS, hypoplastic (MDS-h)
MDS-NOS with multilineage dysplasia (MDS-NOS-MLD)	MDS with multilineage dysplasia (MDS-MLD, most cases)	MDS with low blasts (MDS-LB) most *SF3B1* wild-type MDS-LB with ring sideroblasts, and some MDS, hypoplastic (MDS-h)
MDS with excess blasts (MDS-EB)	MDS with excess blasts-1 (MDS-EB1)	MDS with increased blasts-1 (MDS-IB1) and some MDS with increased blasts and fibrosis (MDS-f)
MDS/AML*	MDS with excess blasts-2 (MDS-EB2)	MDS with increased blasts-2 (MDS-IB2) and some MDS with increased blasts and fibrosis (MDS-f)

*MDS/AML cases (excluding MDS/AML-*TP53*) are further subdivided into MDS/AML with MDS-related gene mutations, MDS/AML with MDS-related cytogenetic abnormalities, and MDS/AML-NOS.

AML, Acute myeloid leukemia; *MDS,* myelodysplastic syndrome; *NOS,* not otherwise specified; *WHO,* World Health Organization.
Data from Arber DA, Orazi A, Hasserjian RP, et al. International Consensus Classification of Myeloid Neoplasms and Acute Leukemia: integrating morphological, clinical, and genomic data. *Blood.* 2022;140(11):1200-1228. Khoury JD, Solary E, Abla O, et al, The 5th edition of the World Health Organization classification of haematolymphoid tumours: myeloid and histiocytic/dendritic neoplasms. *Leukemia.* 2022;36(7):1703-1719.

anemia with megaloblastoid erythropoiesis, normal granulopoiesis and neutrophil count, and normal or increased platelets associated with increased and prominently mononuclear bone marrow megakaryocytes. Ring sideroblasts and/or *SF3B1* mutation may be present and should not lead to misclassification as another MDS subtype if isolated del(5q) is present on karyotype; it is interesting that, in the context of a del(5q) cytogenetic abnormality, *SF3B1* mutation has an adverse prognostic effect.[85] Granulocytic dysplasia is usually minimal or absent, and there must be no excess of blasts in blood or bone marrow.[131,132] MDS-del5q has a favorable prognosis, whether del(5q) is the sole finding on karyotype or if one (but not two or more) additional cytogenetic abnormality is present.[133,134] Thus, one other cytogenetic abnormality (aside from monosomy 7 or del[7q]) is allowed in **MDS-del5q.** Defined as such, survival in **MDS-del5q** is excellent, with a low rate of progression to higher-grade MDS or AML. It should be noted that patients usually have excellent response to the thalidomide analog lenalidomide, and thus this MDS subtype has therapeutic implications.[123,135,136] However, as with other lower-grade MDS subtypes, a small number of cases behave more aggressively and may progress to AML. In particular, *TP53* mutation is present in up to 20% of cases and is associated with increased risk of leukemic progression and poorer lenalidomide response.[91] The *TP53* mutation may be identified by sequencing or by p53 immunohistochemistry and is usually monoallelic.[90,91] According to the ICC, a multihit *TP53* abnormality excludes a diagnosis of **MDS-del5q.** The diagnostic criteria for **MDS-del5q** are shown in Table 44-10.

Myelodysplastic Syndrome With Mutated *SF3B1* (MDS-*SF3B1*)

In the proposed WHO 5th edition classification, this entity corresponds to **myelodysplastic neoplasm with low blasts**

Table 44-10 Diagnostic Criteria for MDS With del(5q)

Feature	Requirements	Exclusions
Blood counts	At least one cytopenia	No leukocytosis or monocytosis.
Morphology	Dysplasia (particularly in the megakaryocytic lineage) is usually present, but not required.	<5% BM blasts, <2% PB blasts No Auer rods in blasts.
Cytogenetics	Del(5q) with up to 1 additional abnormality.	No −7 or del(7q)
Molecular genetics	NA	No multihit *TP53* mutation (VAF ≥10%)
WHO 5th edition differences	None	

BM, Bone marrow; *MDS,* myelodysplastic syndrome; *NA,* not applicable; *PB,* peripheral blood.

and *SF3B1* mutation (MDS-LB-*SF3B1*). It includes most, but not all cases previously classified as **myelodysplastic syndrome with ring sideroblasts (MDS-RS)** in the WHO revised 4th edition classification. The presence of ring sideroblasts in all myeloid neoplasms is closely associated with mutation in the spliceosome gene *SF3B1*, which conveys a favorable prognosis.[102] In most MDS cases bearing an *SF3B1* mutation, ring sideroblasts are frequent and account for at least 15% of the erythroid cells; in a significant minority, they are present but account for less than 15% of all erythroid cells. Only 1% to 2% of MDS cases with *SF3B1* mutation lack ring sideroblasts altogether.[137-139] Unsupervised molecular clustering data have shown that *SF3B1* mutation segregates a major MDS subgroup with a large number of differentially expressed genes.[140,141] In addition, *SF3B1* mutation, rather than the morphologic finding of ring sideroblasts, appears to define a more homogeneous MDS disease entity with respect to favorable patient outcome; MDS cases with ring sideroblasts that lack *SF3B1* mutation have less favorable prognosis, a different mutation profile, and more frequent multilineage dysplasia.[138,142,143] For these reasons, the revised 4th edition classification entity MDS-RS has been replaced in the ICC by **MDS with mutated *SF3B1* (MDS-*SF3B1*)**, and ring sideroblasts no longer affect the classification of MDS in the ICC (except to signify a type of erythroid dysplasia). Though **MDS-*SF3B1*** is not subdivided based on single versus multilineage dysplasia, the presence of excess blood (≥2%) or bone marrow (≥5%) blasts or Auer rods excludes the diagnosis and mandates classification as **MDS-EB**. **MDS-*SF3B1*** frequently has a bimodal red cell distribution in the peripheral blood, with a normocytic or microcytic, hypochromic population and a macrocytic population.[32] The diagnostic criteria for **MDS-*SF3B1*** are shown in Table 44-11.

Myelodysplastic Syndrome, Not Otherwise Specified (MDS-NOS)

The ICC entity **MDS-NOS** corresponds to the proposed WHO 5th edition classification entity **myelodysplastic neoplasm with low blasts (MDS-LB)** and encompasses most cases categorized as **myelodysplastic syndrome with single lineage dysplasia (MDS-SLD), myelodysplastic syndrome with multilineage dysplasia (MDS-MLD), and myelodysplastic syndrome, unclassifiable (MDS-U)** in the revised 4th edition WHO classification.

Table 44-11 Diagnostic Criteria for MDS With Mutated *SF3B1*

Feature	Requirements	Exclusions
Blood counts	At least one cytopenia	No leukocytosis, monocytosis, or thrombocytosis.
Morphology	Dysplasia (particularly in the erythroid lineage) is usually present, but not required. Ring sideroblasts are usually present, but not required.	<5% BM blasts, <2% PB blasts No Auer rods in blasts.
Cytogenetics	NA	No del(5q), −7, del(7q), abnormal 3q26.2, or complex karyotype (3 or more independent cytogenetic abnormalities)
Molecular genetics	*SF3B1* mutation (VAF ≥10%)	No multihit *TP53* mutation (VAF ≥10%) No *RUNX1* mutation
WHO 5th edition differences	Del(7q) is allowed, *RUNX1* mutation is allowed. No VAF cutoff required for *SF3B1* mutation; ≥15% bone marrow ring sideroblasts may substitute for *SF3B1* mutation (MDS with low blasts and ring sideroblasts).	

BM, Bone marrow; *MDS,* myelodysplastic syndrome; *NA,* not applicable; *PB,* peripheral blood; *VAF,* variant allele frequency; *WHO,* World Health Organization.

MDS-NOS includes lower-grade MDS cases that fail to place in the two genetically defined subtypes of **MDS-del5q** or **MDS-*SF3B1*.** Like the revised 4th edition WHO classification, these cases continue to be separated into entities with significant (at least 10%) dysplasia in only one lineage (single lineage dysplasia, **MDS-NOS-SLD**) and those with significant dysplasia involving two or three hematopoietic lineages (multilineage dysplasia, **MDS-NOS-MLD**). It should be noted that the dysplastic lineages often do not coincide with the cytopenic lineage or lineages.[135,136] That being said, most cases of **MDS-NOS-SLD** present with anemia and isolated erythroid lineage dysplasia. Pancytopenia was exclusionary for **MDS-SLD** in the revised 4th edition WHO classification category and mandated categorization as **MDS-U** in an MDS with single lineage dysplasia because of apparently more aggressive behavior.[135,144] In the ICC, pancytopenia is no longer taken into account in MDS classification, as the degree of cytopenias is already taken into account in current MDS prognostic schemes. Though distinction between single and multilineage dysplasia is not perfectly reproducible among pathologists[145] (and has been eliminated as a requirement in **MDS-LB** in the proposed 5th edition WHO classification), it has been retained in the ICC because several studies have shown it to delineate prognostically distinct disease categories. **MDS-NOS-SLD** has an indolent clinical course with a median survival of 5.5 to 6 years, leukemic progression of less than 5%, and survival approaching that of age-matched peers in some series, reflecting a relatively stable disease process.[13,24,121,127,128] Because dysplasia in only one lineage may be borderline and relies on subjective observation, it is reasonable to defer an initial diagnosis of **MDS-NOS-SLD** to ensure cytopenia and dysplasia persist upon follow-up with repeat bone marrow biopsy. Indeed, most data suggest there is no detriment to delaying treatment in lower-grade MDS subtypes such as **MDS-NOS-SLD**.[146,147]

The prognosis of **MDS-NOS-MLD** is substantially worse than that of **MDS-NOS-SLD**, justifying the continued requirement to distinguish these entities.[121,127-129,144,148-150] The median survival of **MDS-NOS-MLD** (as defined in the prior WHO classifications) has been reported to be 2.5 to 3 years and 10% to 11% overall progression to AML[121,127,128]; however, this may change given the creation of the genetic categories **MDS-*SF3B1*** and **MDS-*TP53*,** which alters the makeup of the ICC entity **MDS-NOS-MLD**. Cytogenetic abnormalities are present in approximately 50% of patients with **MDS-NOS** and tend to be more frequent in **MDS-NOS-MLD** than in **MDS-NOS-SLD**, but there are no specific or defining cytogenetic abnormalities.[121,151]

MDS-NOS, without dysplasia encompasses cases previously categorized as **MDS-U** in the revised 4th edition WHO classification because of unexplained cytopenias and MDS-defining cytogenetic abnormalities, but it lacks sufficient dysplasia in any lineage (or increased blasts) to qualify for a morphologic diagnosis of MDS. These cases are very rare; indeed, the failure to identify dysplasia may reflect an inadequate or suboptimal bone marrow sample rather than true absence of dysplasia. As the list of defining genetic abnormalities in the ICC is now different from those defining **MDS-U** in the revised 4th edition WHO classification, the frequency, clinical features, and prognosis of these cases remain to be determined. The proposed 5th edition WHO classification does not allow a diagnosis of MDS without morphologic dysplasia or increased blasts and encompasses **MDS-NOS, without dysplasia** within CCUS. One study has validated the neoplastic nature of MDS-defining cytogenetic abnormalities in cytopenic patients, as they have similar outcomes whether MDS-defining dysplasia is present or absent.[152] The diagnostic criteria for the three **MDS-NOS** subtypes are shown in Table 44-12.

Myelodysplastic Syndrome With Mutated *TP53* (MDS-*TP53*)

MDS with mutated *TP53* (MDS-*TP53*) represents a new genetically-defined MDS entity with highly aggressive clinical behavior. It corresponds to **myelodysplastic neoplasm with biallelic *TP53* inactivation (MDS-bi*TP53*)** in the proposed 5th edition WHO classification. Unlike other MDS cases, blast percentage does not appear to influence prognosis in the setting of a *TP53* mutation,[90,153] even when including cases with sufficient blasts to warrant a diagnosis of AML. Thus, in the ICC, **MDS-*TP53*** is considered within the disease group of *TP53*-mutated myeloid neoplasms together with **MDS/AML with mutated *TP53*** and **AML with mutated *TP53*** (including pure erythroid leukemia).[153,154] In one series of *TP53*-mutated MDS, about half of the cases lacked excess blasts, and the vast majority of these showed multilineage dysplasia.[155] *TP53* mutation can be suspected in MDS based on intense nuclear staining of at least 2% of cells in the bone marrow trephine biopsy,[156,157] although these results should be confirmed by mutation testing. Because cases appear to behave similarly irrespective of the blast count, **MDS-*TP53*** is not subdivided based on the blood and bone marrow blast thresholds of 2% and 5%, respectively. Instead, it encompasses MDS cases with any blast percentage up to 9% in the marrow or blood, with or without Auer rods.

As *TP53* functions as a tumor suppressor gene, both copies of the gene must be inactivated to fully realize the loss of its tumor suppressor function. Supporting this concept, studies have shown that the highly aggressive phenotype conferred by mutated *TP53* in MDS requires multiple hits to the *TP53* gene ("multihit" or "biallelic" status). Multihit *TP53* status in MDS can be confirmed by the presence of two or more distinct *TP53* mutations (each at VAF ≥10%) or a single *TP53* mutation (VAF ≥10%) associated with either deletion involving the *TP53* locus at 17p13.1 or copy-neutral loss of heterozygosity (LOH) at the 17p *TP53* locus; a single *TP53* mutation with VAF ≥50% is also considered to represent presumptive evidence of multihit status caused by loss of the wild-type *TP53* allele.[90,154,158] In the absence of LOH information, the presence of a single *TP53* mutation at VAF ≥10% in the context of any complex karyotype is also considered equivalent to a multihit *TP53* in the ICC, although this is not considered sufficient to confirm biallelic *TP53* according to the proposed 5th edition WHO classification.[90,154] This is based on evidence that multihit *TP53* is strongly associated with complex karyotype, whereas a true monoallelic *TP53* mutation usually displays a noncomplex karyotype; the VAF may be lower than expected as a result of hemodilution or other preanalytic factors.[90] At the time of this writing, any mutation in the *TP53* gene is considered pathogenic, but it remains to be determined whether different mutations convey different disease phenotypes and if these should be incorporated into risk stratification of *TP53*-mutated cases.[155,159] It is emphasized that complex karyotype alone without a *TP53* mutation (even

Table 44-12 Diagnostic Criteria for MDS-NOS

Feature	Requirements	Exclusions
Blood counts	At least one cytopenia	No leukocytosis, monocytosis, or thrombocytosis.
Morphology	≥10% dysplastic cells in one lineage (MDS-NOS-SLD) or 2 or 3 lineages (MDS-NOS-MLD). No dysplasia required in the presence of a cytogenetic abnormality defining MDS-NOS, without dysplasia.	<5% BM blasts, <2% PB blasts No Auer rods in blasts.
Cytogenetics	MDS-NOS, without dysplasia: −7, del(7q), or complex karyotype (3 or more independent cytogenetic abnormalities)	Does not meet criteria for MDS-del5q (Table 44-10).
Molecular genetics	NA	No multihit *TP53* mutation (VAF ≥10%) No *SF3B1* mutation, unless there is a *RUNX1* mutation
WHO 5th edition differences	MDS with low blasts does not require distinction between SLD and MLD. Presence of ≥15% ring sideroblasts mandates classification as MDS with low blasts and ring sideroblasts. Cases with <25% bone marrow cellularity (age-adjusted) are classified as MDS, hypoplastic. Dysplasia is required in all cases, irrespective of cytogenetic findings.	

BM, Bone marrow; *MDS,* myelodysplastic syndrome; *MLD,* multilineage dysplasia; *NA,* not applicable; *NOS,* not otherwise specified; *PB,* peripheral blood; *SLD,* single lineage dysplasia; *VAF,* variant allele frequency; *WHO,* World Health Organization Classification.

if there is deletion of the *TP53* locus at 17p) does not qualify for this category, as these cases have a better prognosis than cases of *TP53*-mutated MDS.[153,160] Monoallelic *TP53* mutations in MDS differ biologically from those of multihit *TP53* cases, and they are not included in the **MDS-*TP53*** category. The diagnostic criteria for **MDS-*TP53*** are shown in Table 44-13.

Myelodysplastic Syndrome With Excess Blasts (MDS-EB)

MDS-EB corresponds to **myelodysplastic neoplasm with increased blasts [MDS-IB1]**, in the proposed WHO 5th edition and **myelodysplastic syndrome with excess blasts-1 (MDS-EB1)** in the revised 4th edition WHO classification. **MDS-EB** can exhibit any degree of morphologic dysplasia and variable cytogenetic abnormalities, but it manifests excess (≥5%) blasts in the bone marrow. Less commonly, blasts may be <5% in the marrow but increased (≥2%) in the blood, or Auer rods may be present in blasts; such cases should also be categorized as MDS-EB, irrespective of the bone marrow blast count.[32,161,162] CD34 immunostaining of the biopsy section helps reveal increased blasts in cases with a hemodilute or poorly stained aspirate smear (particularly in cases with increased bone marrow fibrosis) and may be

Table 44-13 Diagnostic Criteria for MDS With Mutated *TP53*

Feature	Requirements	Exclusions
Blood counts	At least one cytopenia	No leukocytosis, monocytosis, or thrombocytosis.
Morphology	Dysplasia is usually seen, but not required.	<10% BM blasts, <10% PB blasts, with or without Auer Rods
Cytogenetics	If only a single *TP53* mutation with VAF ≥10% but <50% is present and LOH information is not available, a complex karyotype (3 or more independent abnormalities) and/or 17p deletion is required.	NA
Molecular genetics	Multihit *TP53*: Either two or more *TP53* mutations (each with VAF ≥10%) or a single *TP53* mutation with VAF >50%, or a single *TP53* mutation with VAF≥10% and copy-neutral LOH at the 17p *TP53* locus.	NA
WHO 5th edition differences	MDS with biallelic *TP53* inactivation includes cases up to 19% blasts in BM or PB. No minimum VAF level for *TP53* mutation. 17p deletion must be demonstrated if there is a single *TP53* mutation with VAF <50% and no (or unknown) LOH.	

BM, Bone marrow; *LOH*, loss of heterozygosity; *MDS*, myelodysplastic syndrome; *NA*, not applicable; *PB*, peripheral blood; *VAF*, variant allele frequency.

Table 44-14 Diagnostic Criteria for MDS-EB

Feature	Requirements	Exclusions
Blood counts	At least one cytopenia	No leukocytosis, monocytosis, or thrombocytosis.
Morphology	5%–9% BM blasts, or 2%–9% PB blasts, or Auer rods in any blasts. Dysplasia is usually seen, but not required	NA
Cytogenetics	NA	NA
Molecular genetics	NA	No multihit *TP53* mutation (VAF ≥10%)
WHO 5th edition differences	MDS with increased blasts-1 (MDS-IB1) can have up to 4% PB blasts and can not have Auer rods in blasts; cases with AML-defining genetic abnormalities are excluded from this category and classified as AML. Cases with Grade 2-3 (of 3) bone marrow fibrosis are classified as MDS with increased blasts and fibrosis (MDS-f)	

AML, Acute myeloid leukemia; *BM*, bone marrow; *MDS*, myelodysplastic syndrome; *NA*, not applicable; *PB*, peripheral blood; *VAF*, variant allele frequency; *WHO*, World Health Organization Classification.

2% peripheral blood blast threshold for **MDS-EB**, and 1% blood blasts measured on a single occasion is acceptable for lower-grade MDS entities. However, the ICC recommends that these patients be followed closely and be classified as **MDS-EB** if blood blasts at the level of 1% or higher are documented on multiple occasions, even if marrow blasts remain at <5%. The diagnostic features of **MDS-EB** are shown in Table 44-14.

Myelodysplastic Syndrome/Acute Myeloid Leukemia (MDS/AML)

To acknowledge the biological continuum between MDS and AML and some imprecision in counting blasts around the historic 20% threshold, myeloid neoplasms with 10% to 19% blasts in the blood and/or marrow are placed in a new disease entity, **MDS/AML**, in the ICC. The optimal treatment of this group of patients (previously classified as **MDS-EB2** in the revised 4th edition WHO classification and still classified as **myelodysplastic neoplasm with increased blasts-2 [MDS-IB2]** in the proposed 5th edition WHO classification) is still unknown; the future personalized treatment of individual patients in this **MDS/AML** group will likely be dictated by genetic, biological, and patient-related factors rather than an arbitrary blast cutoff.[119,154,166] Studies have shown that mutations in some genes (*NRAS, PTPN11, FLT3, CBL, IDH1,* and *IDH2*) could drive the progression of MDS to AML and thus inform the management of patients with MDS/AML.[167,168] Stable versus rapid progression of the blast percentage and cytopenias during clinical follow-up may also be informative (Fig. 44-4).[169] In the meantime, this change allows patients with **MDS/AML** to be eligible for both MDS and AML trials, providing them more treatment options. Pediatric patients with 10% to 19% blasts (with the exception of those with AML-defining genetic aberrations) continue to be classified as **MDS-EB**, as these patients have features that

useful all MDS cases, even if the aspirate is of high quality. If blasts enumerated from a CD34 immunostain appear to account for at least 5% of the core biopsy cells, it is reasonable to upgrade a case to **MDS-EB** even if the aspirate blast count is <5%.[106,163] CD117 also stains blasts in most MDS cases, but interpretation is more difficult, as this marker also stains early erythroids, promyelocytes, and mast cells, rendering myeloblast enumeration challenging; in general, CD117 staining on myeloblasts is stronger than on early erythroids but weaker than on mast cells. Median survival is approximately 16 months for **MDS-EB**, and approximately 25% of patients progress to AML. Some cases of **MDS-EB** harbor an *SF3B1* mutation, and this mutation does not appear to convey a favorable prognosis in this context as it does for lower-grade MDS subtypes.[142]

Cases with exactly 1% circulating blasts appear to exhibit aggressive behavior similar to those of **MDS-EB**[164,165]; such cases were considered within **MDS-U** in the revised 4th edition WHO classification. Though it was noted in that prior classification that 1% circulating blasts should be documented on two separate occasions, this may be difficult to do in practice; moreover, a blast percentage of exactly 1% is not likely to be reproducible on multiple measurements. For these reasons, both the ICC and WHO have applied a

are distinct from adult **MDS/AML**. AML-defining cytogenetic aberrations or mutations (*NPM1* or in-frame bZIP *CEBPA*) must be excluded in patients presenting with ≥10% bone marrow or blood blasts.

It is recommended that patients with MDS/AML who are treated as AML be subclassified according to the genetic AML categories **MDS/AML with MDS-related cytogenetic abnormalities**, **MDS/AML with MDS-related gene mutations**, **MDS/AML with mutated *TP53***, and **MDS/AML, NOS**[170] (see Chapter 46). It should be noted that, unlike **MDS with mutated *TP53***, which requires multihit *TP53* mutation, a monoallelic *TP53* mutation suffices to classify an **MDS/AML** case with 10% to 19% blasts as **MDS/AML with mutated *TP53***. This is based on evidence that, in cases with increased blasts (≥10%), there appears to be no significant difference in prognosis conveyed by monoallelic versus multihit *TP53*.[154] The diagnostic features of **MDS/AML** are shown in Table 44-15.

Myelodysplastic Syndrome in Children and Refractory Cytopenia of Childhood

MDS is rare in children (<18 years of age), and the disease subtypes and spectrum of mutations differ from those found in adults.[171-174] **MDS-SF3B1** is exceedingly rare in children, and if ring sideroblasts are observed in a pediatric patient, Pearson's syndrome must be excluded.[175] **MDS-del5q** is also very rare in children. When a del(5q) is present, other karyotypic abnormalities are usually present, often in the context of a complex karyotype and therapy-related disease.[176] **Refractory cytopenia of childhood (RCC)** represents cytopenic conditions affecting children that have diagnostic features largely similar to those seen in cases of **MDS-NOS** with hypocellular bone marrow. **RCC** has a lower incidence of somatic mutations and cytogenetic abnormalities than adult MDS, and it more frequently occurs in the setting of a genetic predisposition syndrome (see the separate section in this chapter, Ontogenetic Qualifier to Myelodysplastic Syndrome: Germline Predisposition).[22,177,178] Aside from **RCC** and myeloid leukemia associated with Down syndrome, other MDS cases occurring in children are classified like adult MDS, with the following exceptions: (1) There is no distinction between **MDS-NOS-SLD** and **MDS-NOS-MLD** in pediatric populations, as this is still of uncertain prognostic significance.[179] (2) The ICC entity **MDS/AML** does not apply to pediatric MDS, as pediatric patients with MDS with increased blasts (even those with 20%–30% blasts) may not require intensive induction therapy, but rather are often treated with up-front stem cell transplant. In pediatric patients (<18 years of age), **MDS-EB** extends to up to 19% of bone marrow or blood blasts.[178]

The proposed 5th edition WHO classification eliminates **RCC** and replaces it with **childhood MDS with low blasts,** including hypoplastic cases. This entity corresponds to most cases fulfilling features of **RCC**; however, it is important to note that a subset of **RCC** cases may not be true myeloid neoplasms and thus are not equivalent to bona fide MDS (Table 44-16).[180] As with adult MDS, it is critically important to exclude non-neoplastic mimickers. Because of the frequent hypocellularity in pediatric MDS, distinction from aplastic anemia may be particularly challenging. Although application of the diagnostic criteria of **RCC** usually allows accurate distinction,[28,181] extended observation may be required in some cases to distinguish hypocellular **RCC** cases from aplastic anemia. An important consideration in **RCC** and other MDS cases occurring in pediatric patients is their frequent occurrence on the background of a genetic predisposition

Table 44-15 Diagnostic Criteria for MDS/AML*

Feature	Requirements	Exclusions
Blood counts	At least one cytopenia	No leukocytosis, monocytosis, or thrombocytosis.
Morphology	Dysplasia is usually seen, but not required.	10%–19% BM blasts or 10%–19% PB blasts, with or without Auer Rods
Cytogenetics	NA	No AML-defining abnormality (Chapter 46)
Molecular genetics	NA	No *NPM1* mutation and no in-frame bZIP *CEBPA* mutation
WHO 5th edition differences		MDS with increased blasts-2 (MDS-IB2) also includes 5%–9% PB blasts and any cases with Auer rods in blasts. Cases with Grade 2–3 (of 3) bone marrow fibrosis are classified as MDS with increased blasts and fibrosis (MDS-f). Cases with in-frame bZIP *CEBPA* mutation are included.

*MDS/AML cases are subclassified as MDS/AML with mutated *TP53*, MDS/AML with MDS-related cytogenetic abnormalities, MDS/AML with MDS-related gene mutations, and MDS/AML-NOS (see Chapter 46, Acute Myeloid Leukemia).
AML, Acute myeloid leukemia; *BM,* bone marrow; *MDS,* myelodysplastic syndrome; *NA,* not applicable; *PB,* peripheral blood.

Table 44-16 Myelodysplastic Syndromes in Pediatric Patients (Aged <18 Years, Blasts <20%): International Consensus Classification and Comparison to Revised 4th Edition and Proposed 5th Edition WHO Classifications

International Consensus Classification	Revised 4th Edition WHO Classification	Proposed 5th Edition WHO Classification
Refractory cytopenia of childhood (RCC)	Refractory cytopenia of childhood (RCC) (provisional entity)	Childhood MDS with low blasts, hypocellular
MDS-NOS*	MDS-SLD and MDS-MLD	Childhood MDS with low blasts, NOS
MDS with excess blasts (MDS-EB)	MDS with excess blasts-1 (MDS-EB1) and MDS with excess blasts-2 (MDS-EB2)	Childhood MDS with increased blasts

*Rare pediatric MDS cases that fulfill features of MDS-*SF3B1*, MDS-*TP53*, MDS/AML-*TP53*, or MDS-del5q are classified as for adult MDS (Table 44-9).
MDS, Myelodysplastic syndrome; *NOS,* not otherwise specified; *WHO,* World Health Organization.
Data from Arber DA, Orazi A, Hasserjian RP, et al. International Consensus Classification of Myeloid Neoplasms and Acute Leukemia: integrating morphological, clinical, and genomic data. *Blood.* 2022;140(11):1200-1228. Khoury JD, Solary E, Abla O, et al, The 5th edition of the World Health Organization classification of haematolymphoid tumours: myeloid and histiocytic/dendritic neoplasms. *Leukemia.* 2022;36(7):1703-1719. Rudelius M, Weinberg OK, Niemeyer CM, Shimamura A, Calvo KR. The International Consensus Classification (ICC) of hematologic neoplasms with germline predisposition, pediatric myelodysplastic syndrome, and juvenile myelomonocytic leukemia. *Virchows Arch.* 2023;482(1):113-130.

syndrome (up to 30% of cases, which may increase in the future as more genes predisposing to myeloid malignancies are discovered).[178] Thus, screening for a germline syndrome should be performed in any pediatric patient presenting with RCC or other MDS.

Ontogenetic Qualifier to Myelodysplastic Syndrome: Therapy-Relatedness

In the 4th edition and prior WHO classifications, therapy-related MDS was grouped together with therapy-related AML, as these diseases were felt to have similarly poor prognoses, irrespective of the blast count.[182] Therapy-related MDS occurs principally after exposure to agents that cause damage to DNA (alkylating agents, platinum derivatives, nitrosoureas) or after exposure of the bone marrow to ionizing radiation.[183] The mechanism by which these agents cause disease appears to be through cytotoxic effects on the marrow environment that foster the expansion of preexisting hematopoietic stem cell clones bearing mutations, typically in DNA-damage response genes such as TP53 and PPM1D.[184,185] The onset of clinical disease may begin as early as 6 months or 1 year after initiation of therapy with the causative agent; more characteristically, latency is 2 years or more and peaks at 5 to 6 years. Patients typically present with cytopenias and morphologic dysplasia similar to non–therapy-related disease, but the marrow is more often hypocellular than in non–therapy-related disease. More than 90% of therapy-related MDS cases show an abnormal karyotype. Cytogenetic abnormalities involving deletions of chromosomes 5 and 7 are relatively common.[186]

Although as a whole therapy-related MDS tends to show more rapid progression of cytopenias, progression to AML, and shorter survival compared with de novo disease, data suggest that this is caused by overrepresentation of high-risk genetic lesions (such as TP53 and complex karyotypes) compared with de novo MDS.[187-189] For example, the IPSS-R scheme effectively risk stratifies patients with therapy-related MDS, and the minority of these patients who have low IPSS-R risk scores appear to have a more favorable prognosis.[189] For these reasons, therapy-relatedness is no longer used as a major MDS disease classifier in the ICC. Instead, it is applied as a qualifier to the MDS disease subtype, which is classified the same as for de novo disease (example: **MDS with mutated TP53, therapy-related**, or **MDS-NOS-MLD, therapy-related**). As it is sometimes unclear whether an MDS developing in a patient with cytotoxic exposure is truly related to the prior therapy or is merely coincidental, the proposed 5th edition WHO classification prefers the term "post cytotoxic therapy" in lieu of "therapy-related" to designate such cases.

Ontogenetic Qualifier to Myelodysplastic Syndrome: Germline Predisposition

As mentioned previously, MDS in children frequently occurs in the background of a congenital syndrome. Congenital syndromes associated with pediatric MDS include Fanconi anemia, Down syndrome, severe congenital neutropenia (Kostmann syndrome), Shwachman-Diamond syndrome, dyskeratosis congenita, amegakaryocytic thrombocytopenia, Bloom syndrome, GATA2 deficiency, and others.[190-192] The ICC categorizes germline predisposition states into three categories: (1) germline predisposition without a constitutional

disorder affecting multiple organ systems (which typically have no prodromal phenotype prior to the development of MDS or another myeloid neoplasm); (2) germline predisposition associated with a constitutional platelet disorder (such as germline RUNX1, ANKRD26, or ETV6 mutation); and (3) germline predisposition associated with a constitutional disorder affecting multiple organ systems (such as Fanconi anemia, neurofibromatosis, or dyskeratosis congenita).[178]

MDS evolving from a congenital syndrome often behaves differently from de novo disease. For example, the incidence of MDS and AML in Down syndrome is increased, but the clinical behavior and underlying biology of MDS in young patients (<5 years of age) with Down syndrome differ markedly from MDS in other clinical settings: somatic GATA1 mutations are common, and these patients have a very favorable prognosis. Such cases are considered within a single category of "myeloid leukemia associated with Down syndrome," irrespective of the blast percentage.[193-196] Patients with Fanconi anemia may be particularly sensitive to preparative regimens for allogeneic transplantation.

It is essential in diagnosing pediatric MDS to note whether the MDS is primary or secondary to such an antecedent condition because this may affect treatment decisions and alter outcome. MDS occurring in the background of a familial condition could also influence the choice of family members as donors if stem cell transplantation (SCT) is being considered as a therapeutic option. It is also important to note that some adults presenting with MDS have predisposing constitutional gene mutations that convey increased risk of myeloid malignant neoplasms and are probably under recognized in clinical practice; germline DDX41 mutation is the most common of these and does not have a prodromal phenotype prior to presentation with MDS or AML.[88] Thus, in any patient with MDS, it is important to query carefully to uncover any personal or family history of cytopenias that may be a clue to the presence of an underlying predisposing syndrome, which should stimulate testing using NGS panels targeting the common germline predisposition genes (which overlap only partly with genes that are also somatically mutated in MDS).[197,198] As the germline mutation may be newly acquired in the patient without any family history, more widespread germline testing in older patients and in those without a family history may be warranted.[178]

Prognostic Scoring Systems

In an attempt to improve the ability to predict disease course in individual patients, the International MDS Study Group, composed of clinical experts in the treatment of MDS, developed the IPSS for MDS in 1997.[151] The original proposal, which used a limited number of prognostic variables (marrow blast percentage, three tiers of karyotype abnormalities, and the number of cytopenias), was refined as the IPSS-R in 2012.[199] The IPSS-R was more complex than the IPSS, using a larger number of blast strata, five instead of three categories of karyotype findings, and more detailed assessments of cytopenias in each lineage. This combined information generates five IPSS-R risk groups instead of the previous three risk IPSS groups. An alternative WHO classification–based prognostic scoring system (WPSS) uses karyotype risk, WHO disease subtype, and transfusion requirement to identify five prognostically distinct risk groups.[147]

The IPSS-R has been widely adopted in clinical practice as a basis for treatment decisions and appears to predict outcome both at diagnosis and dynamically in patients being observed at later time points.[200,201] By incorporating the bone marrow blast percentage, the IPSS-R scheme overlaps somewhat with the ICC and WHO classifications. However, the IPSS-R does not incorporate ring sideroblasts, peripheral blood blasts, Auer rods, the number of dysplastic lineages, bone marrow cellularity, or bone marrow fibrosis, which are used as classifiers in the ICC and the proposed 5th edition of the WHO classification.

The IPSS-M was published as an update to the IPSS-R scheme.[85] The IPSS-M differs from the IPSS-R as follows: (1) Neutropenia (absolute neutrophil count $<0.8 \times 10^9$/L) is no longer taken into account, as it was not found to be prognostic when additional genetic information was incorporated. (2) Anemia and thrombocytopenia are incorporated as continuous variables rather than categories with specific cutoff values. (3) Mutations in 36 genes with variable contributions of the prognostic score have been incorporated. (4) Allowance is made for missing values, with a range of uncertainty for the calculated prognostic score. The IPSS-M output is a number score, with 0 representing the median survival of all patients in the cohort and each increase or decrease of 1 representing a doubling or halving of the hazard ratio, respectively, for leukemia-free survival. Based on the score ranges, there are six prognostic categories, ranging from Very Low to Very High. Most MDS patients fall into the lower risk cohorts, but a subset of patients have very high risk, some with a hazard ratio of over 4 compared to the median survival of MDS patients. Compared to the IPSS-R, the IPSS-M more accurately predicts MDS outcome.[85] The IPSS-M risk calculator can be accessed at https://www.mds-risk-model.com.

Additional Considerations in Myelodysplastic Syndrome Diagnosis

Hypoplastic Myelodysplastic Syndrome

Most cases of MDS have hypercellular marrow despite the presence of cytopenias, reflecting the ineffective hematopoiesis that is a hallmark of the disease. However, 10% to 15% of MDS in adults (and a much higher percentage in children) has reduced marrow cellularity for age.[31,202,203] The clinical behavior of these hypoplastic MDS cases tends to reflect the blast percentage, similar to other MDS subtypes. Some studies suggest that hypocellularity in MDS is an independent favorable prognostic variable.[204,205] Because aplastic anemia may manifest mildly dysplastic morphology and even transient clonal cytogenetic abnormalities similar to MDS, distinction between hypoplastic MDS and aplastic anemia, which is a destruction of hematopoietic stem cells usually caused by an autoimmune process, may be difficult (see this chapter's section on Differential Diagnosis).[30,76-78] Hypoplastic MDS is more likely than more cellular MDS to respond favorably to immunosuppression, suggesting a possible etiologic link to aplastic anemia.[206-210] Additionally, the finding of a hypocellular marrow in a younger patient with MDS raises consideration of a genetic predisposition syndrome, and such patients may not benefit from immunosuppressive therapy.[211]

Hypoplastic MDS is not a specific disease subtype in the 4th edition WHO classification or ICC, but it has been added as a specific low-risk MDS subtype in the proposed 5th edition WHO classification. To accurately diagnose this entity, is it important to have an adequate bone marrow biopsy in a newly diagnosed MDS case so that cellularity can be accurately estimated, and the bone marrow cellularity should be specified in the bone marrow report. In patients <70 years of age, hypocellularity is defined as cellularity of <30%; for patients ≥70 years of age, it is defined as cellularity <20%.[206] It is important to note that some cases of AML and MDS with excess blasts may present with a hypocellular marrow, and these cases are not included within this hypoplastic MDS entity. Thus, a careful blast count on the (often paucicellular) aspirate smear must be performed to distinguish hypoplastic **MDS-EB** from **hypoplastic MDS** as defined in the 5th edition WHO classification; CD34 staining of the biopsy section can be helpful in this regard.[30]

Myelodysplastic Syndrome With Fibrosis

Mild-to-moderate and occasionally marked reticulin fibrosis can occur in MDS.[101,212,213] Significant fibrosis (grade 2 or 3 of 3 in the WHO myelofibrosis grading scheme) confers an inferior prognosis to MDS that is independent of the karyotype risk, WHO disease subtype, or IPSS-R score.[101] Classification of MDS cases with fibrosis is based on the same criteria used in other MDS cases, and MDS with fibrosis is not a specific MDS disease subtype in the revised 4th edition WHO classification or the ICC. The proposed 5th edition WHO classification has introduced a new subtype of MDS with increased blasts and increased fibrosis, termed **MDS with increased blasts and fibrosis.** It is important to note that MDS cases that lack increased blasts may also show increased fibrosis, and such cases have a poorer prognosis than their counterparts lacking increased fibrosis: the 5th edition WHO entity **MDS with increased blasts and fibrosis** is specifically limited to cases with increased blood or bone marrow blasts and excludes cases with biallelic *TP53* mutation or any AML-defining genetic abnormalities.[125]

Fibrosis may complicate the diagnosis by interfering with the acquisition of an aspirate (so-called "dry tap"). Thus, quantitation of blasts on smears and by flow cytometry may be significantly hampered and requires careful analysis of the core biopsy sample to estimate the blast count. Immunohistochemical staining with CD34 to highlight possible increased blasts in the bone marrow biopsy sample is essential in fibrotic cases with a compromised aspirate smear. CD61 immunostaining is also helpful to reveal micromegakaryocytes that are commonly seen in fibrotic MDS cases. Wright-Giemsa–stained touch imprints from the bone marrow core should always be made if the bone marrow aspirate is dry or appears aspicular, as accurate blast counts can usually be obtained from well-prepared touch preparations. Fibrotic MDS cases may mimic primary myelofibrosis, other chronic MPNs with fibrosis, and acute megakaryoblastic leukemia. These differential diagnoses are discussed later in this chapter.

Erythroid-Predominant Myelodysplastic Syndromes

Cases of MDS with erythroid predominance (≥50% erythroid elements) accounts for about 15% of all MDS cases and have a higher incidence of high-risk cytogenetic abnormalities than other MDS; they are also more frequently therapy related.[214] Erythroid predominance does not define a specific MDS subtype; cases are most frequently classified as MDS-NOS-MLD,

MDS-NOS-SLD, or MDS-*SF3B1*.[214] It is critical to distinguish erythroid-predominant MDS, in which erythroid elements are increased and dysplastic but exhibit complete maturation, from pure erythroid leukemia, a subtype of acute myeloid leukemia in which erythroid maturation is arrested and there is a proliferation of primitive erythroblasts. Pure erythroid leukemia is a highly aggressive AML subtype with very short survival and nearly universal highly complex karyotypes and multihit *TP53* mutation.[215-218] Some cases of **MDS with mutated *TP53*** are erythroid-rich and may have increased pronormoblasts, yet do not meet criteria for pure erythroid leukemia because of insufficient erythroid elements (<80%) or insufficient pronormoblasts (<30%).[219] Prior studies have suggested that increased pronormoblasts represents an unfavorable prognostic feature in MDS in general.[220] However, enumeration of pronormoblasts in MDS is not part of current classification schemes, in part because pronormoblast numbers and erythroid left shift may be influenced by metabolic deficiencies, treatment, and effects of exogenous growth factors.[221]

DIFFERENTIAL DIAGNOSIS

One of the most challenging aspects of MDS diagnosis confronting both the clinician and the pathologist is its differential diagnosis with non-neoplastic and other neoplastic conditions that may cause cytopenia. Dysplasia—the main and defining morphologic finding of MDS—can be seen in many non-neoplastic cytopenic conditions and in several non-MDS myeloid neoplasms.[40] Navigating this minefield of potential MDS mimickers requires consideration of all available diagnostic information and an open mind in approaching a putative MDS diagnosis. Specific scenarios of differential diagnosis with MDS are presented herein.

Non-Neoplastic Conditions Associated With Morphologic Dysplasia and Cytopenia

Megaloblastic Anemia

Megaloblastic anemia often exhibits dysplastic features in the erythroid lineage that closely mimic MDS. Therefore, it is essential that this readily treatable, non-neoplastic condition be excluded during the diagnostic evaluation for possible MDS. In megaloblastic anemia, overt megaloblastic changes usually predominate over dysplastic features, and conversely, the megaloblastoid changes in MDS are usually milder than those seen in megaloblastic anemia. Megaloblastic changes in the myeloid series (giant band forms and metamyelocytes) are rare in MDS but commonly accompany the prominent erythroid changes of megaloblastic anemia. The differential diagnosis may be complicated by the rare occurrence of transient clonal cytogenetic abnormalities, such as del(7q), in megaloblastic anemias.[79] When the differential diagnosis of a case includes megaloblastic anemia, serum vitamin B_{12} and folate levels should be measured before a diagnosis of MDS is rendered. Measurement of methylmalonic acid levels is a more sensitive indicator of vitamin B_{12} deficiency and may be helpful in borderline cases.

Chemotherapy-Induced Dysplasia and Cytopenias

Many chemotherapy agents induce dysplastic and megaloblastoid morphology and cause peripheral blood cytopenias. This combination may mimic MDS, or even occasionally AML, if neutropenic patients receive granulocyte-colony stimulating factor that transiently increases the blast percentage in bone marrow or blood. The most striking megaloblastic changes are seen with folate antagonists (e.g., methotrexate) and drugs that directly interfere with DNA synthesis (e.g., antimetabolites such as hydroxyurea and 5-fluorouracil). Early recovery from chemotherapy may be manifested as a transient burst of regenerating blasts potentially mimicking MDS with excess blasts.

The type of response to specific chemotherapeutic agents varies among individuals, in part on the basis of polymorphisms of cellular defense genes and drug transport proteins such as MDR1. At least partially for these reasons, in some patients, even standard doses of chemotherapy may lead to prolonged cytopenias, marrow hypocellularity, and morphologic changes mimicking MDS.[222-224] Distinguishing prolonged chemotherapy effects from emerging therapy-related MDS may be difficult or impossible by the examination of a single bone marrow sample; identification of MDS-associated immunophenotypic abnormalities detected by flow cytometry may be helpful in this regard.[225] Cytogenetics may be helpful if MDS-associated clonal abnormalities such as −7 or del(5q) are demonstrated, but mutations found on NGS are less specific, as they can represent clonal hematopoiesis after chemotherapy that may not progress to bona fide MDS.[226] Often, one must resort to clinical follow-up, monitoring of peripheral blood counts, and if necessary, repeated marrow examination to resolve this differential diagnosis. Of particular note in this context, up to 2% of patients with acute promyelocytic leukemia treated with combined all-trans retinoic acid (ATRA)/anthracycline regimens develop therapy-related MDS or AML, with typical dysplastic morphology and MDS-type cytogenetic abnormalities and lacking the *PML::RARA* abnormality of the original leukemia.[227]

Post-Acute Myeloid Leukemia Dysplasia and Clonal Hematopoiesis

After chemotherapy for AML, marrow hematopoiesis may show dysplastic morphology and/or clonal genetic abnormalities, even if the bone marrow blast percentage is less than 5% and the platelet and neutrophil counts have recovered sufficiently to qualify for complete remission. Clonal cytogenetic abnormalities and gene mutations present in the original AML, particularly *DNMT3A*, *TET2*, and *ASXL1* (so-called "DTA" mutations), may persist as a chemotherapy-resistant preleukemic stem cell population.[228,229] If morphologic dysplasia and cytopenias persist and bone marrow blasts are ≥5%, this is considered to represent residual AML,[170] although biologically, the disease may be more related to MDS-EB.[230] In the post-AML treatment setting, dysplastic changes and even clonal genetic abnormalities should be interpreted with caution and described in the report, but not used in isolation to confirm recurrent or residual AML in the absence of increased blasts. Measurable residual AML is detected by flow cytometry and/or sensitive genetic studies that assess for certain AML-specific genetic aberrations: *NPM1* mutation or *PML::RARA*, *RUNX1::RUNX1T1*, *KMT2A::MLLT3*, *DEK::NUP214*, *BCR::ABL1*, or *CBFB::MYH11* rearrangements.[170]

Marrow Recovery After Acute Marrow Injury or Stem Cell Transplantation

After an acute marrow injury (such as an injury induced by chemotherapy, toxin, infection, or occasionally an unknown cause), there may be a transient excess of blasts in blood or marrow accompanying marrow recovery, along with dysplastic changes, especially in the erythroid and occasionally megakaryocytic lineages. Identification of left-shifted myeloid forms and toxic granulation in the blood can be helpful clues to appropriate marrow recovery rather than MDS with circulating blasts; circulating granulocytic forms in MDS are often hypogranulated but only seldom show toxic granulation. Similar changes may be seen at the time of donor marrow engraftment after myeloablative SCT. Macrocytosis and mild megaloblastoid change are also often seen after SCT and may persist for months or years. This phenomenon can complicate the morphologic interpretation of post-SCT bone marrow samples, and megaloblastic changes should not be overinterpreted as evidence of new or persistent MDS in this context. Molecular chimerism studies that assess donor engraftment will usually resolve the interpretation of these morphologic findings. However, rare cases of donor-derived MDS or AML may occur after SCT,[231] particularly in patients with germline predisposition syndromes who receive SCT from a similarly affected sibling.[232] Therapy-related MDS can also occur after autologous stem cell transplant as a result of prior chemotherapy or radiotherapy for the patient's primary malignant disease or preparative regimens for the SCT.[233-235]

Marrow Dysplasia in HIV Infection

Patients with HIV/AIDS may develop peripheral blood cytopenias. Marrow examination in such cases often reveals dysplastic morphologic features, particularly in the erythroid and megakaryocytic lineages, potentially mimicking MDS. Despite such dysplastic morphology, cytogenetic abnormalities of MDS are lacking in cytopenic HIV-infected patients. The cause of the dysplastic morphology in these patients is not always clear. Some antiviral agents used in treating HIV infection may contribute to the cytopenias and the dysplastic morphologic abnormalities, but similar features were observed in patients with HIV/AIDS before the advent of effective therapy for the disease.

Congenital Dyserythropoietic Anemias

MDS may mimic congenital dyserythropoietic anemias (CDAs) by exhibiting internuclear bridging, megaloblastoid hematopoiesis, and multinucleation of erythroid progenitors as manifestations of erythroid lineage dysplasia.[236] This differential diagnosis is critical because the treatment and prognosis of MDS and CDAs differ drastically. Of great practical help is the fact that MDS is a relatively common disease, whereas CDAs are very rare. CDA types I and II typically present in childhood or adolescence, but even in infancy and childhood, MDS predominates in incidence over CDAs and must be assiduously ruled out before CDA is diagnosed. In older patients, this caveat is even more important because CDA becomes progressively less frequent with advancing age. In CDAs, dysplastic morphology and cytopenias are restricted to the erythroid lineage. If neutropenia, thrombocytopenia, or dysplasia in the granulocytic or megakaryocytic lineages is present, a diagnosis of MDS should be strongly considered.

Cytogenetics and sequential clinical observation may be helpful, as progressive disease over time is more suggestive of MDS.

Non-Myelodysplastic Syndrome Sideroblastic Anemias

By far, the most frequent cause of ring sideroblasts in bone marrow is MDS, but other diverse conditions are also associated with ring sideroblasts. Active alcohol abuse inhibits multiple steps of heme synthesis, resulting in the accumulation of mitochondrial iron as ring sideroblasts. Dietary deficiencies associated with alcoholism may result in concomitant megaloblastoid hematopoiesis, and acute alcohol intoxication may cause vacuolization of erythroid precursors, changes shared with MDS.[237,238] Other reversible causes of ring sideroblasts include antituberculosis drugs (especially isoniazid),[239] severe copper deficiency or zinc poisoning,[240,241] and penicillamine therapy.[242]

Congenital causes of sideroblastic anemia are diverse, including X-linked (the most common), autosomal, and mitochondrial inheritance forms.[243,244] In contrast to the typically macrocytic anemia of MDS, anemia in the congenital sideroblastic cases is microcytic and hypochromic and may respond to exogenous pyridoxine; patients may have accompanying iron overload. Pearson's syndrome is a mitochondrial cytopathy characterized by refractory sideroblastic anemia, vacuolated marrow erythroid precursors, and exocrine pancreatic dysfunction. Pearson's syndrome has a mitochondrial inheritance pattern and an onset of disease symptoms in infancy. Variant mitochondrial cytopathies with ring sideroblasts have also been described, and ring sideroblasts may also be seen with erythropoietic protoporphyria. All of these congenital diseases are rare, and in most cases, the cytopenia and morphologic abnormalities are restricted to the erythroid lineage.

Copper Deficiency and Zinc Toxicity

Copper (and selenium) deficiency and zinc toxicity, which itself causes copper deficiency,[241] can present with pancytopenia and dysplastic marrow morphology, closely mimicking MDS.[245] Vacuolization of erythroid precursors may be prominent, in addition to vacuolated granulocyte precursors and neutropenia. Patients are often premature infants; those with prolonged parenteral hyperalimentation, postgastrectomy, or malnourished states; or those undergoing copper chelation therapy.[246] Hematopoietic parameters may improve with folate and vitamin B_{12} treatment, but this does not prevent progression of the neurologic abnormalities. Accurate diagnosis and early treatment are essential to prevent irreversible neurologic damage and to avoid erroneous treatment for misdiagnosed MDS.

Arsenic Exposure

Arsenic trioxide, now frequently used to treat acute promyelocytic leukemia and under investigation for use in other disorders, causes striking dysplastic morphology in marrow, particularly in erythroid progenitors, mimicking the erythroid dysplasia of MDS.[247]

Chronic Viral Infections

Epstein-Barr virus, herpesvirus, and cytomegalovirus infections may present with hypercellular marrow and dysplastic marrow morphology.[248,249] Chronic parvovirus B19 infection can also mimic MDS if the giant pronormoblasts are interpreted as dysplastic cells. Some cases of MDS may present with pure red cell aplasia, and thus both MDS and parvovirus infection must be considered in the differential diagnosis of this condition.[250,251] Morphologic abnormalities in parvovirus infection are usually restricted to the erythroid lineage.

Aplastic Anemia

Aplastic anemia may have dysplastic morphology in hematopoietic progenitors and occasionally has cytogenetic abnormalities similar to those of MDS.[29,31,77,78] The interrelationship of MDS and aplastic anemia is complicated and not completely understood. Some cases of aplastic anemia progress to MDS, and conversely, some cases of MDS have hypocellular marrow; thus, distinction between hypocellular MDS and aplastic anemia may be difficult. Somatic mutations occur in approximately one-third of patients with aplastic anemia, and these genes include those frequently mutated in MDS, such as *BCOR/BCORL*, *DNMT3A*, and *ASXL1*.[252] In MDS, the dysplastic features tend to be more prominent than in aplastic anemia, and the cytopenias are disproportionate to degree of hypocellularity. Persistent clonal cytogenetic abnormalities strongly favor MDS. In some cases, it is not possible to discriminate unequivocally between hypocellular MDS and aplastic anemia, except with clinical follow-up. CD34 immunostaining can be useful in distinguishing MDS from aplastic anemia because CD34 cells are never increased in aplastic anemia, whereas they are increased in a substantial subset of hypocellular MDS.[30] Clonal proliferations of cells with loss of glycosylphosphatidylinositol (GPI)–anchored proteins (characteristic of paroxysmal nocturnal hemoglobinuria [PNH]) may be seen in both MDS and aplastic anemia, although the PNH clone size is usually larger in aplastic anemia than in MDS.

Paroxysmal Nocturnal Hemoglobinuria

PNH is a clonal cytopenic condition associated with a somatic mutation in in the *PIGA* gene (phosphatidylinositol glycan anchor biosynthesis, class A), which is responsible for the first step in the synthesis of the GPI anchor that attaches a subset of proteins to the cell surface. PNH, aplastic anemia, and MDS are interrelated entities. A subset of patients with MDS has marrow hypocellularity (see the section, Hypoplastic Myelodysplastic Syndrome), similar to aplastic anemia and PNH,[31] and a subset of patients with PNH progresses to MDS (up to 5%) or AML (1%).[253,254] It is hypothesized that patients with MDS who acquire a variety of mutations could secondarily acquire homozygous loss of function of *PIGA*.[255] An alternative explanation is that an abnormal clone with the PNH anomaly arises first through selective pressure on stem cells as a result of autoimmune attack and evolves over time to MDS.[256] A diagnosis of PNH established by flow cytometric demonstration of GPI-anchored protein loss does not preclude a diagnosis of MDS if other criteria corroborate the diagnosis, even in the presence of overt clinical PNH and *PIGA* mutation. However, in most cases of MDS, the PNH clone is small (<5%).[94] If a patient with PNH develops significant marrow dysplasia or a clonal cytogenetic abnormality consistent with MDS, evolution to MDS should be strongly considered.

Idiopathic Cytopenia of Undetermined Significance (ICUS)

Patients who have persistent (>6 months), significant, and unexplained cytopenia but lack MDS-defining dysplasia, excess blasts, or an MDS-defining genetic abnormality are considered in the general category of idiopathic cytopenia of undetermined significance (ICUS). A bone marrow examination is required to diagnose ICUS because there must be documented absence of significant dysplasia in any lineage or excess blasts and also absence of an MDS-associated cytogenetic abnormality on a complete bone marrow karyotype.[105,257] It is recommended that patients with ICUS be observed with periodic blood counts, and a repeated marrow examination should be performed if the cytopenias worsen significantly and remain unexplained. Over time, some patients will develop bona fide MDS or another myeloid neoplasm. Flow cytometry aberrations and mutations (see this chapter's section Clonal Hematopoiesis of Indeterminate Potential [CHIP] and Clonal Cytopenia of Undetermined Significance [CCUS]) may help predict the likelihood of ICUS progression to MDS or AML.[258]

Idiopathic Dysplasia of Undetermined Significance (IDUS)

Cytopenia is a sine qua non of MDS, and therefore patients who undergo bone marrow examination for any reason that shows significant dysplasia in one or more lineages but lack any cytopenia (during at least a 6-month period) cannot be diagnosed with MDS, even if an MDS-defining genetic abnormality is found. In such situations, it is important to consider other myeloid and nonmyeloid neoplasms, particularly rare MDS/MPN cases that may manifest dysplasia but lack significant cytopenia. Plasma cell myeloma and some bone marrow lymphomas can produce reactive dysplastic changes in marrow hematopoietic elements. Finally, secondary dysplastic changes in hematopoietic elements can be produced by a variety of non-neoplastic conditions, including infections and autoimmune disease, and by drugs, toxins, and metabolic deficiencies, as discussed previously. Indeed, just as patients with ICUS often progress to MDS or AML on follow-up, patients with idiopathic dysplasia of undermined significance (IDUS) often subsequently are found to have neoplastic conditions. These are often neoplasms other than MDS, such as myeloproliferative neoplasms, AML, or MDS/MPN overlap disease.[259]

Germline Predisposition Conditions

As discussed previously, many MDS cases in children and some MDS cases in adults occur in the background of a germline predisposition syndrome, which may be unknown at the time of MDS diagnosis. Some of these conditions (particularly ones associated with thrombocytopenia, such as *RUNX1*, *ANKRD26*, and *ETV6* mutation) can exhibit dysplasia in the bone marrow, which is typically unilineage and is seen in megakaryocytes. This creates challenges in diagnosing the onset of bona fide MDS, which occurs frequently in patients affected by these germline predisposition conditions. The ICC proposes a set of features that indicate progression to MDS in these conditions: Either increased blasts should be present, or two of the following conditions: (1) a pathogenic somatic genetic aberration (mutation or cytogenetic abnormality);

(2) one of the MDS-defining genetic abnormalities (delineated in Tables 44-5 and 44-6); (3) development of a new cytopenia or progressive cytopenia, particularly in the context of increasing marrow cellularity; or (4) dysplasia seen in ≥10% of cells in two or three hematopoietic lineages.[178] In children, note that cytopenia levels should be age-adjusted based on each institution's reference range.

Non-Neoplastic Clonal Myeloid Proliferations

Clonal Hematopoiesis of Indeterminate Potential (CHIP) and Clonal Cytopenia of Undetermined Significance (CCUS)

Although some specific genetic abnormalities, such as *SF3B1* mutation or multihit *TP53*, are considered sufficient to diagnose MDS in a cytopenic patient, the same does not hold true for other genetic abnormalities. It is tempting to assume that a cytopenic patient with clonal hematopoiesis proven by the presence of MDS-type mutations has MDS. However, MDS-type mutations and gene copy number abnormalities have been found in the blood of healthy individuals who do not have MDS. Every individual has approximately 10,000 self-renewing hematopoietic stem cells, which progressively accumulate mutations as an individual ages (estimated at approximately 1.3 somatic mutations per stem cell per decade).[260] Most of this mutational "baggage" represents nonpathogenic so-called "passenger" mutations, but some affect key genes that confer growth advantage to the stem cell (driver mutations) and allow it to outcompete its unmutated neighbors. Eventually, the differentiating progeny of this expanded, mutated stem cell population are detectable by sequencing peripheral blood leukocytes. CHIP is proposed to encompass such individuals who have identifiable acquired genetic abnormalities but have no known diagnosable hematologic disease and no unexplained cytopenias. A minimal variant allele fraction of 2% is set as an arbitrary threshold for CHIP because it is likely that most, if not all, individuals harbor mutations in a small fraction of hematopoietic cells that will be detectable with increasingly sensitive sequencing technology.[67] The incidence of CHIP is estimated at approximately 5% to 10% of individuals older than 65 or 70 years of age and up to 18.4% of individuals older than 90 years of age; it is rare in those younger than 40 years of age.[261-263] Individuals with CHIP appear to be at modestly increased risk for development of a subsequent hematologic malignant neoplasm compared with age-matched controls without CHIP, but this is only approximately 0.5% to 1% per year. Interestingly, such individuals are also at increased risk of death from causes other than hematologic neoplasms. It is currently unclear how individuals found to have CHIP should be managed, but at the time of this writing, they are not considered to have a neoplasm and do not warrant therapy. The related condition CCUS represents CHIP with the additional feature of a persistent unexplained cytopenia; looked at another way, CCUS can also be defined as ICUS with the additional feature of a myeloid-type somatic mutation or cytogenetic aberration that is not MDS defining.

VEXAS Syndrome

VEXAS (**V**acuoles, **E**1-enzyme, **X**-linked, **A**utoinflammatory, **S**omatic) syndrome is an autoinflammatory syndrome associated with a somatic mutation in the *UBA1* gene in hematopoietic cells. *UBA1*, which resides on the X chromosome, encodes a cytoplasmic E1 enzyme that is deficient when the gene is mutated. Given its presence on the X chromosome, male patients are much more frequently affected with VEXAS. Patients characteristically present with macrocytic anemia and have vacuolation of erythroid and myeloid precursor cells in the bone marrow.[264] Autoimmune diseases, particularly relapsing polychondritis, are a typical feature of the syndrome.[265] As with other non-neoplastic clonal cytopenias, MDS-defining morphologic dysplasia (or an MDS-defining genetic abnormality) is required to diagnose MDS in the setting of VEXAS syndrome; erythroid and myeloid vacuolization should not be taken into account when evaluating these lineages for morphologic dysplasia.[266]

The implications of MDS developing in the setting of VEXAS are uncertain, as these patients rarely develop increased blasts or progress to AML, indicating a uniquely indolent MDS behavior in this setting.[266] Given its relatively recent identification, further study is needed to clarify the relationship between VEXAS and MDS and other myeloid neoplasms and the optimal treatment approach to these patients, who often suffer significant clinical sequelae from their autoimmune diseases.

Other Neoplasms

Acute Myeloid Leukemia With Recurrent Genetic Abnormalities (AML-RGA) and <20% Blasts

Cytogenetic examination of the bone marrow and NGS studies are essential in the evaluation of all MDS and AML. One example of the critical importance of this testing is in identifying AML-RGA with <20% blasts.[267] The ICC mandates a diagnosis of AML in a patient presenting de novo with any AML-defining genetic aberrations, provided the bone marrow or blood blast percentage is at least 10%. Since it is unclear whether patients with AML-type recurrent genetic abnormalities but no increase in blasts benefit from intensive AML-type chemotherapy, further study is warranted to determine the appropriate classification and optimal therapeutic approach to the rare cases with <10% blasts and AML-RGA genetics. Nevertheless, is important to recognize and correctly diagnose AML-RGA in patients with 10% to 19% blasts because a misdiagnosis of MDS may lead to an unnecessary delay in the institution of potentially curative chemotherapy and poor patient outcome.[112] Whereas the incidence of MDS and MDS-related AML increases exponentially with age,[1] most subtypes of AML-RGA have an approximately flat incidence throughout life, and these are often genetically simple, with no or few genetic abnormalities aside from the defining one.

Clues to suspecting a low–blast count AML-RGA versus MDS include frequent promyelocytes with Auer rods in AML with *PML::RARA*; abnormal eosinophils with mixed eosinophilic-basophilic granules and monocytic blast morphology in AML with *CBFB::MYH11*; blasts with "salmon-colored" cytoplasm, fine granules, and Auer rods in AML with *RUNX1::RUNX1T1*; and "cup-shaped" blasts in AML with mutated *NPM1*. These AML-RGA entities tend to occur in a much younger population than MDS but can also affect elderly individuals. Several additional cytogenetic subtypes of AML-RGA have been added in the ICC and proposed 5th edition WHO classification (see Chapter 46, Acute Myeloid Leukemia).[124,125] These include t(3;3) (q21;q26), inv(3)(q21q26), and other 3q26 cytogenetic abnormalities that involve the *MECOM* gene. Such cases tend to have prominent megakaryocytic dysplasia and often an increased platelet count.[113,268] In addition to AML-defining cytogenetic aberrations, two mutations, *NPM1* mutation and in frame mutation in the bZIP domain of *CEBPA*, are also considered to be AML-defining in the ICC, with a minimum blast count of 10%. In the proposed 5th edition WHO classification, *NPM1,* but not *CEPBA,* is considered to be AML-defining.

Primary Myelofibrosis

Mild reticulin fibrosis in marrow is common in MDS, presumably secondary to the release of stromal tissue growth factors from dysplastic precursors, similar to the pathogenesis of primary myelofibrosis (PMF).[212,213] Significant marrow fibrosis in MDS may lead to confusion with PMF. Although both diseases involve an acquired clonal genetic abnormality of a multipotential marrow progenitor, the distinction has important clinical consequence, as the two diseases have different clinical courses and are treated differently. Splenomegaly is unusual in MDS, and the presence of any extramedullary hematopoiesis would tend to favor a diagnosis of PMF over MDS. A leukoerythroblastic peripheral blood smear picture, with numerous circulating nucleated erythroid forms, teardrop erythrocytes, and left-shifted granulocytes, is also more suggestive of PMF, although leukoerythroblastosis can also be seen in MDS with fibrosis. PMF typically has clusters of abnormal megakaryocytes in the marrow that are often enlarged with abnormal patterns of chromatin clumping, including hyperchromatic, bulbous-shaped nuclei. In MDS, the megakaryocytes are usually small with hypolobated, abnormally lobulated, or separated nuclei and rounded rather than scalloped nuclear contours; moreover, intrasinusoidal hematopoiesis is more commonly seen in PMF than MDS.[141] Whereas PMF usually shows an increased myeloid-erythroid ratio as a result of increased granulopoiesis, MDS is more often associated with erythroid predominance that may appear megaloblastoid, left-shifted, and dysplastic. Marked reticulin fibrosis, mature collagen fibrosis (indicated by marrow stromal staining on a trichrome stain), and osteosclerosis are more commonly seen in advanced stages of PMF and are uncommon in MDS. Cytogenetic abnormalities in PMF—including del(13q), del(20q), +8, and abnormalities of chromosomes 1, 5, 7, 9, and 21—largely overlap those of MDS and thus may not be informative in distinguishing these entities.[269] Conversely, *JAK2, MPL,* or *CALR* mutations are found in 80% to 90% of patients with PMF, and these mutations are rare in MDS, even in those cases with fibrosis.[35,270-272] Advanced phases of polycythemia vera and chronic myeloid leukemia may also have marrow fibrosis and can also show dysplastic morphology, but clinical history and genetic studies (*JAK2, MPL, CALR,* and *BCR::ABL1* analyses) can usually reliably separate these entities from MDS.

Myelodysplastic/Myeloproliferative Neoplasms

Although most patients with MDS and neutropenia are unable to mount a significant leukocytotic response to an infection (even when exogenous myeloid growth factors are administered), some patients with MDS with a superimposed infectious or inflammatory process may develop a leukemoid reaction, mimicking MDS/MPN. The leukemoid reaction may include monocytosis mimicking CMML or left-shifted granulocytic elements mimicking atypical CML.[273] Complicating the issue, some patients with MDS subsequently develop monocytosis resembling CMML, which appears to represent a type of disease progression in MDS.[274] It is important to recognize these possibilities because patients with MDS are prone to infectious complications as a result of their neutrophil dysfunction, and the treatment and prognosis of an MDS patient with a leukemoid reaction differ from those of patients with various MDS/MPN entities. The presence of a known infectious or inflammatory clinical process should raise suspicion for a leukemoid reaction, and treatment of the underlying process should result in reversion to peripheral blood counts typical of the underlying MDS.

A spontaneous and persistent development of leukocytosis, thrombocytosis, or monocytosis in a patient previously diagnosed with MDS does not mandate reclassification as MDS/MPN. Instead, these patients should retain the label of MDS, with the elevated counts noted in the report. Such changes in the disease phenotype can be harbingers of disease progression and poorer outcome.[274] Conversely, persistent leukocytosis ($\geq 13 \times 10^9$/L) and/or absolute and relative monocytosis ($\geq 0.5 \times 10^9$/L and 10% of all leukocytes) in any myeloid neoplasm at diagnosis that are not attributable to an underlying infectious or inflammatory process exclude MDS and require classification as MDS/MPN or MPN, even if cytopenias in other lineages are present. Notably, in the ICC and proposed 5th edition WHO classification, the threshold of absolute monocytosis defining CMML has been lowered from 1.0 to 0.5×10^9/L; thus, cases with relative monocytosis and 0.5 to 0.9×10^9/L monocytes (so-called "oligomonocytic" CMML)[275] that would have previously been classified as MDS are now classified as CMML.

Large Granular Lymphocytic Leukemia

As opposed to most lymphoid leukemias, which present with overt lymphocytosis, patients with large granular lymphocytic (LGL) leukemia typically present with cytopenias and minimal or no lymphocytosis, thus potentially mimicking MDS. Compounding the issue, reactive dysplastic changes may be seen in the maturing hematopoietic cells in LGL leukemia, and the neoplastic T-cell infiltrates in the bone marrow biopsy sample may be subtle. Conversely, reactive lymphoid aggregates may be present in MDS. In general, patients with LGL leukemia present predominantly with neutropenia, whereas an anemic presentation is more common in MDS. Flow cytometry identifies an expanded population of immunophenotypically aberrant CD8-positive, CD57-positive T cells, and polymerase chain reaction (PCR) study of blood or marrow discloses a clonal T-cell receptor rearrangement in LGL leukemia.[276] Whereas the neoplastic T cells in LGL leukemia occur in an interstitial and often intrasinusoidal pattern in the bone marrow biopsy sample (best revealed by immunohistochemistry for cytotoxic markers, such as TIA-1, perforin, or granzyme), any increased lymphoid cells in MDS typically form nonparatrabecular aggregates. If *STAT3* or *STAT5B* mutations are identified on NGS of a putative MDS case (particularly if flow cytometry discloses increased large granular lymphocytes with an aberrant immunophenotype), an alternative diagnosis of LGL leukemia as a cause of the cytopenias should be considered.[277] Rarely, MDS and LGL leukemia may occur together, and *STAT3* mutations and small clonal T-cell populations that typify LGL leukemia have been identified in MDS patients.[278,279] Thus, in some cases, it may be difficult to distinguish LGL leukemia from MDS with an expanded clonal T-cell population. Close clinical follow-up may be the most prudent approach in such cases.

ETIOLOGY AND PATHOGENESIS

A variety of agents and diseases are associated with an increased incidence of MDS. Germline predispositions, which have been previously discussed, typically result in MDS in childhood, but they can also present in adulthood.[190] A variety of exposures (ionizing radiation, agents that cause cross-link DNA damage, benzene, other solvents and petrochemicals, agricultural or farming chemicals, smoking, hair dyes) have been linked to an increased incidence of MDS and AML. With some (alkylating agents), the association is strong; in others, the contribution to causation is less definite. Some cytotoxic therapies may not actually initiate the abnormal clone through DNA damage, but rather appear to promote the expansion of a preexisting low-level mutated stem cell clone through selection in the marrow microenvironment.[185,235]

MDS is a clonal proliferation of cells originating from an abnormal hematopoietic stem cell: the stem cell is thought to acquire a founding genetic abnormality (or more often multiple cooperating abnormalities) that gives it a growth advantage, allowing its differentiating progeny to progressively replace normal hematopoiesis. This model is supported by the presence of recurring mutations and karyotype abnormalities in most MDS cases and the fact that these mutations can be traced back to the most primitive, self-renewing multipotent hematopoietic stem cells that bear the original growth-promoting mutations.[69] Ultimately, future MDS therapies should be directed against the MDS stem cells, but these are difficult to target owing to their quiescence and are seldom eradicated with most current therapies.

Most MDS cases bear not one but multiple concurrent genetic abnormalities whose interactions are complex and poorly understood. In **MDS with del(5q)**, there is presumed loss of a tumor suppressor gene or genes in the deleted region. Haploinsufficiency of the *RPS14* gene that encodes a ribosomal structural protein appears to contribute to the disease phenotype, possibly through p53 pathway activation.[280] Deficiency of two micro-RNAs, miR-145 and miR-146a, in the deleted region may also contribute to the megakaryocyte abnormalities and thrombocytosis characteristic of this MDS subtype.[281]

Splicing genes are mutated in over 50% of MDS cases. In MDS cases with mutation in the spliceosome complex gene *SF3B1*, there is evidence that differential splicing of *ABCB7* and other gene products involved in mitochondrial iron metabolism may underlie the formation of ring sideroblasts.[282-284] However, data in mouse models are conflicting as to whether *SF3B1* haploinsufficiency truly creates an MDS phenotype.[285,286] Epigenetic gene regulation through histone modification and DNA methylation is also perturbed in MDS, with recurring somatic mutations in epigenetic regulator genes such as *EZH2, ASXL1, DNMT3A, TET2, IDH1,* and *IDH2*.[287]

There is increasing interest in the role of the bone marrow microenvironment in contributing to MDS pathogenesis. A number of abnormalities have been identified in cytokines (such as tumor necrosis factor-α and interleukin-32) and in stromal cell signaling to CD34-positive stem cells in patients with MDS.[288] There is also evidence that the so-called "niche" (the physical sites where hematopoietic stem cells reside and are supported by surrounding cells, extracellular matrix, and soluble factors) may be altered in myeloid neoplasms such that it fosters the growth and self-renewal of MDS stem cells over normal stem cells.[289,290] The gene mutated in Schwachman-Diamond syndrome, *SBDS*, encodes a protein necessary for creation of the stem cell niche by osteoprogenitor cells.[291,292] In some murine models, manipulation of the osteoblastic stem cell niche has been shown to induce MDS.[293] Abnormal expression of β-catenin in osteoblasts associated with activated Notch signaling has also been implicated in MDS pathogenesis.[294] At the time of this writing, it is unclear how these stromal abnormalities coordinate with the genetic abnormalities in the MDS stem cells to create the disease phenotype; it is tempting to speculate that microenvironmental abnormalities may be particularly important in the approximately 10% of MDS cases that lack demonstrable genetic abnormalities in hematopoietic cells, but this remains to be proven.

CONCLUSION

MDS is a heterogeneous myeloid neoplasm characterized by clonal, mutated hematopoiesis, morphologic dysplasia, and infective hematopoiesis resulting in cytopenia. The role of the mutation profile and bone marrow microenvironment in creating the phenotype of each unique disease is complex and remains elusive. The patient's genetic background (germline predisposition conditions) and extrinsic factors such exposure to cytotoxic chemotherapy also contribute to MDS heterogeneity. Whereas diagnostic tools are rapidly expanding, the diagnosis of MDS is still based on secondary disease features—cytopenias and dysplastic morphology—that are neither completely specific nor pathognomonic. It is nevertheless important that MDS be diagnosed and subclassified accurately because of the prognostic and therapeutic implications of the specific disease subtypes. MDS has an extensive and difficult set of differential diagnoses, some of which can be ruled in or out only by clinical follow-up. It is hoped that further characterization of genetic abnormalities and their role in dictating the disease pathogenesis will result in improved diagnostic capabilities and clarification of important clinical and biological subsets of this intriguing set of diseases.

Pearls and Pitfalls

- A good bone marrow sample (aspirate smear or touch preparation and biopsy section) and a full complement of ancillary tests (complete blood count with differential and peripheral smear review, bone marrow cytogenetics, and NGS studies) are essential for the correct diagnosis and classification of MDS. Flow cytometry to identify recurrent immunophenotypic abnormalities are also helpful.
- Most of the features of MDS (cytopenias, dysplastic morphology, genetic abnormalities, and flow cytometry abnormalities) are neither pathognomonic nor a sine qua non for the diagnosis. Ideally, multiple abnormalities should be present to support the diagnosis. However, at least one (unexplained) cytopenia is an absolute requirement for a diagnosis of MDS.
- The clinical behavior of MDS is highly heterogeneous, ranging from nonprogressive disease with survival approaching that of age-matched peers to rapidly progressive and fatal disease; this heterogeneity is captured in the various MDS disease subtypes and in comprehensive risk-stratification models.
- The differential diagnosis of MDS is extensive, and careful exclusion of other possible non-MDS entities is imperative before a definitive diagnosis is rendered.

KEY REFERENCES

35. Della Porta MG, Travaglino E, Boveri E, et al. Minimal morphological criteria for defining bone marrow dysplasia: a basis for clinical implementation of WHO classification of myelodysplastic syndromes. *Leukemia.* 2014;29:66–75.
40. Steensma DP. Dysplasia has a differential diagnosis: distinguishing genuine myelodysplastic syndromes (MDS) from mimics, imitators, copycats and impostors. *Curr Hematol Malig Rep.* 2012;7:310–320.
51. Porwit A, et al. Multiparameter flow cytometry in the evaluation of myelodysplasia: analytical issues: recommendations from the European LeukemiaNet/international myelodysplastic syndrome flow cytometry working group. *Cytometry B Clin Cytom.* 2023;104(1):27–50.
67. Steensma DP, Bejar R, Jaiswal S, et al. Clonal hematopoiesis of indeterminate potential and its distinction from myelodysplastic syndromes. *Blood.* 2015;126:9–16.
68. Duncavage EJ, et al. Genomic profiling for clinical decision making in myeloid neoplasms and acute leukemia. *Blood.* 2022;140(21):2228–2247.
90. Bernard E, et al. Implications of TP53 allelic state for genome stability, clinical presentation and outcomes in myelodysplastic syndromes. *Nat Med.* 2020;26(10):1549–1556.
119. Estey E, Hasserjian RP, Dohner H. Distinguishing AML from MDS: a fixed blast percentage may no longer be optimal. *Blood.* 2022;139(3):323–332.
124. Arber DA, et al. *International Consensus Classification of Myeloid Neoplasms and Acute Leukemia:* integrating morphological, clinical, and genomic data. *Blood.* 2022.
125. Khoury JD, et al. The 5th edition of the *World Health Organization Classification of Haematolymphoid Tumours: Myeloid and Histiocytic/Dendritic Neoplasms. Leukemia.* 2022;36(7):1703–1719.
199. Greenberg PL, Tuechler H, Schanz J, et al. Revised international prognostic scoring system for myelodysplastic syndromes. *Blood.* 2012;120:2454–2465.

Visit Elsevier eBooks+ for the complete set of references.

Chapter 45

Myeloid and Hematologic Neoplasms With Germline Predisposition

Katherine R. Calvo and Olga K. Weinberg

DEFINITION AND INTRODUCTION

Germline predisposition to hematologic neoplasia occurs in individuals with inherited or de novo mutations in the germline in genes that confer increased risk of developing hematologic malignancy or cancer. Additional acquired genetic alterations cooperate with underlying germline mutations to drive the development of cancer, which often occurs at an earlier age than corresponding sporadic neoplasms. Germline predisposition to cancer was demonstrated as early as early as 1866 when French physician Paul Broca published the *Broca Report* showing four generations of breast cancer, suggesting inherited predisposition. A century later in 1969, Drs. Li and Fraumeni described families with increased incidence of solid tumors and leukemia with an autosomal dominant inheritance pattern, which later was shown to be caused by germline mutations in *TP53*.[1,2] Classical bone marrow failure (BMF)

syndromes, including Fanconi anemia (FA), were known to have increased risk of cancer and myeloid malignancy. In 1999, germline mutations in *RUNX1* (i.e., *CBFA2*) were discovered in six families with familial platelet disorder with propensity to develop myeloid malignancy.[3] Since then the number of genes known to be associated with germline predisposition to myeloid malignancy have grown, largely aided by next-generation sequencing (NGS) technology. There is increased recognition of the contribution of germline mutations to the development of myeloid and other hematologic malignancies, particularly in pediatric, adolescent, and young and middle-aged adults.

Classification

In 2017 the revised WHO 4th ed. devoted a new chapter to myeloid neoplasms with germline predisposition underscoring

Hematologic Neoplasms With Germline Predisposition Without a Constitutional Disorder Affecting Multiple Organ Systems
Myeloid neoplasms with germline *CEBPA* mutation*†
Myeloid or lymphoid neoplasms with germline *DDX41* mutation*†
Myeloid or lymphoid neoplasms with germline *TP53* mutation*

Hematologic Neoplasms With Germline Predisposition Associated With a Constitutional Platelet Disorder
Myeloid or lymphoid neoplasms with germline *RUNX1* mutation*†
Myeloid neoplasms with germline *ANKRD26* mutation*†
Myeloid or lymphoid neoplasms with germline *ETV6* mutation*†

Hematologic Neoplasms With Germline Predisposition Associated With a Constitutional Disorder Affecting Multiple Organ Systems
Myeloid neoplasms with germline *GATA2* mutation*†
Myeloid neoplasms with germline *SAMD9* mutation*
Myeloid neoplasms with germline *SAMD9L* mutation*
Myeloid neoplasms associated with bone marrow failure syndromes*†
  Fanconi anemia*†
  Shwachman-Diamond syndrome*†
  Telomere biology disorders including dyskeratosis congenita*†
  Severe congenital neutropenia*†
  Diamond-Blackfan anemia*†
Juvenile myelomonocytic leukemia associated with neurofibromatosis*†
Juvenile myelomonocytic leukemia associated with Noonan syndrome and Noonan-syndrome-like disorder (CBL-syndrome)*†
Myeloid or lymphoid neoplasms associated with Down syndrome*†

Acute Lymphoblastic Leukemia With Germline Predisposition‡
Acute lymphoblastic leukemia with germline *PAX5* mutation
Acute lymphoblastic leukemia with germline *IKZF1* mutation

*Included in the WHO 5th ed. 2022 classification.
†Included in the revised WHO 4th ed. 2016 classification.
‡Down syndrome, and germline mutations in *ETV6* or *TP53*, also predispose to acute lymphoblastic leukemia.

the importance of properly identifying these patients.[4] The germline mutations were divided into three major categories: (1) myeloid malignancies with germline predisposition without a preexisting disorder (*CEBPA*, *DDX41*); (2) myeloid neoplasms with germline predisposition and preexisting platelet disorders (*RUNX1*, *ANKRD26*, and *ETV6*); and (3) myeloid neoplasms with germline mutation associated with other organ disfunction (*GATA2*, inherited marrow failure syndromes, telomere biology disorders, juvenile myelomonocytic leukemia [JMML] associated with neurofibromatosis and Noonan/Noonan-like disorders, and Down syndrome). In 2022, the International Consensus Classification (ICC)[5,6] and the WHO 5th ed. classification[7] expanded the number of recognized genes associated with germline predisposition (Box 45-1). Both the ICC and the 2022 WHO 5th ed. added *TP53*, *SAMD9*, and *SAMD9L*. The ICC broadened the title to *hematologic neoplasms with germline predisposition*, emphasizing that many germline mutations predisposing to myeloid malignancy also predispose to lymphoid neoplasia. The ICC also added a category of germline predisposition to acute lymphoblastic leukemia (*IKZF1* and *PAX*). The WHO 5th ed. classification incorporated myeloid neoplasms with germline predisposition under a broader

category of secondary myeloid neoplasms. This approach was not taken by the ICC, as many patients with germline predisposition and hematologic neoplasms present to clinicians with primary disease. Both the ICC and WHO 5th ed. classifications allow for incorporation of new germline predisposition genes as they are discovered and compelling evidence emerges.

Recognition of germline predisposition to hematologic malignancy is critical for proper patient management, surveillance of disease progression, genetic counseling, and for screening potential matched related donors for hematopoietic stem cell transplantation (HSCT). Many patients with myeloid malignancies associated with underlying germline mutations require tailored chemotherapy regimens to avoid toxicity or poor outcome. Germline mutations may have variable penetrance and expressivity even within family members harboring the same mutation. Age of onset of disease manifestations or malignancy onset may vary widely. In general, germline predisposition should be considered in patients with a history of multiple cancers, first- or second-degree relative with a hematologic malignancy or solid tumor at a relatively young age (<50), thrombocytopenia or BMF preceding a diagnosis of myelodysplastic syndrome (MDS)/acute myeloid leukemia (AML), immunodeficiency, warts, lymphedema, early graying of hair, pulmonary fibrosis, or other physical stigmata associated with specific germline predisposition syndromes (Box 45-2). It is important to note that some patients with germline mutations in genes that are classically associated with physical stigmata or syndromic features may not have overt stigmata or syndromic features, or they may be subtle on physical exam (i.e., FA).

Recognition of underlying germline mutation is critical for any patient undergoing HSCT who will be transplanted using a related donor. Phenotype is not always an indicator of genotype because of variable penetrance and expressivity. For this reason, all potential related donors should be screened for the patient's germline mutation, regardless of the health of the donor. Multiple reports have shown that inadvertent use of a related donor harboring the same germline mutation as the patient can result in donor-derived MDS/AML, graft failure, or poor outcome.[8-11] Knowledge of a germline mutation also has important implications for offspring and other family members. Genetic counseling plays an important role in patient management.

Types of Germline Mutations and Genetic Testing Considerations

Somatic or acquired mutations occur in specific cells and may give rise to cancer associated with the tissue of the cell of origin. The majority of cancer in older individuals is associated with somatic mutations. In contrast, germline mutations are present in all of the cells of the body, and may be inherited and present in multiple family members. De novo germline mutations are present in the patient but not detected in the parents. In this setting the original mutation may have occurred in a germ cell (i.e., sperm or ova), or in the fertilized egg during embryogenesis.[12] Although de novo germline mutations are not present in parents or siblings, they may be passed on to offspring.

Germline mutations predisposing to cancer may have autosomal dominant, autosomal recessive, or X-linked inheritance patterns. In general, autosomal recessive mutations are homozygous and require two mutated copies of the gene in each cell, which are inherited from both parents who are carriers and may have no evidence of disease. Genes with autosomal

Box 45-2 *Germline Testing Considerations*

1. Consider germline testing for patients with hematologic malignancy (HM) and any of the following:
   - Two or more cancers, including HM
   - Family history of HM, solid tumor, hematologic abnormality within two generations
   - Pediatric patients and young adults (<50 yrs) with HM (caveat: germline mutations in *DDX41* are associated with HM development in similar age range of sporadic HMs)
   - Preceding history of thrombocytopenia, bone marrow failure, immunodeficiency, warts, lymphedema, early graying of hair, pulmonary fibrosis, dystrophic nails, physical stigmata, or other syndromic features associated with germline predisposition syndromes
   - High variant allele frequency (VAF) (30%–60%) of pathogenic mutation in germline predisposition genes detected on next-generation sequencing (NGS) profiling suggestive of possible germline mutation
   - Persistence of pathogenic mutation at high VAF on serial NGS tests before and after chemotherapy treatment
   - Biallelic mutations in genes associated with germline predisposition to HM (e.g., *CEBPA, RUNX1, DDX41*)
   - Plan to undergo hematopoietic stem cell transplantation (HSCT) using related donor—testing to inform donor selection to ensure donor does not harbor same germline mutation as patient, if germline mutation is present
     - Therapy-related myeloid neoplasms (MN)
2. Tissue for germline testing:
   - Gold standard:
     - Cultured fibroblasts from skin biopsy (no contamination from hematopoietic cells)
   - Other possible samples:
     - Skin biopsy with wash-out of peripheral blood
     - Buccal swab—may be contaminated with peripheral blood
     - Hair follicles—may yield low genomic DNA
   - Not recommended:
     - Peripheral blood or bone marrow—cannot reliably differentiate somatic from germline mutations
     - Saliva—contamination with peripheral blood
     - Nail clippings—possible contamination with monocytes
3. Additional testing considerations:
   - Chromosomal breakage assay—informative for Fanconi anemia diagnosis
   - Flow-fluorescence in situ hybridization (FISH) for telomere length—informative for diagnosis of telomeropathies
   - Germline testing for young patients with bone marrow failure (<50 yrs) for early detection of germline mutation to inform surveillance for disease progression and HM

dominant inheritance are associated with heterozygous germline mutations with one mutated copy of the gene that is typically inherited from one parent who may or may not have evidence of disease, and may be associated with a family history of disease. In patients with de novo germline autosomal dominant mutations, they are the first person in their family to have the mutation and it may be passed on to their offspring. X-linked mutations are in genes on the X chromosome and may be recessive or dominant. In diseases with X-linked recessive mutations, males are most often affected; females are typically nonaffected as females have two copies of the gene (one mutated and one wild type), while males have only one mutated copy of the gene. Females may be affected if the female has or develops monosomy X, or via X-inactivation/

lionization. X-linked dominant mutations affect both males and females. The development of hematologic malignancy in the setting of germline predisposition is associated with acquisition of additional genetic alterations that cooperate with the underlying germline mutation(s) to drive oncogenesis.

Given the widespread use of NGS panels on blood or marrow specimens in clinical hematology/oncology practice, many cases of myeloid malignancies with germline predisposition have been initially suspected on NGS panels designed to detect somatic mutations. A high variant allele frequency (VAF) above 30% may suggest germline mutation; however, somatic mutations can also have high VAF and germline testing is recommended for confirmation. Genetic testing of a germline tissue source, such as cultured fibroblasts from a skin biopsy, is the gold standard for confirming germline mutations (Box 45-2). Buccal swabs may contain contamination from blood cells and are not ideal germline tissue sources. Hair follicles have been used by some labs to identify germline mutations; however, the yield of genomic DNA may be low. Nail clippings may contain monocytes and are not ideal. If the same mutation is present in multiple family members, this provides strong evidence for the germline nature of the mutation. Other clues include persistence of a pathogenic mutation at a high VAF after chemotherapy treatment; and HMs with double mutations in certain genes, possibly representing an underlying germline mutation and a somatic hit in the same gene, which is common for some germline predisposition genes (e.g., *CEBBPA, RUNX1,* and *DDX41*).

Germline mutations are often broadly classified as missense, nonsense, or null mutations. Mutations may consist of large deletions or translocations that may be difficult to identify on NGS platforms. Notably, some genes have germline mutations in noncoding regions involving intronic enhancers (e.g., *GATA2*) or 5' promoter regions (e.g., *ANKRD26*).[13,14] Mutations in noncoding regions can be missed by whole exome sequencing or targeted panels that do not cover these regions. Recently there is more awareness of pathogenic synonymous germline mutations that alter RNA sequence affecting RNA splicing sites without altering protein sequence. If regions of a germline mutation are covered on a routine NGS panel designed to identify somatic mutations, the germline mutation may be identified; however, it will not be possible to definitively determine whether the mutation is germline or somatic if hematopoietic cells are used as the source for testing. If suspicion of a germline predisposition gene mutation is high but not found on routine testing, subsequent testing at a specialized laboratory may be considered. Many laboratories specialized in germline testing use enhanced whole exome sequencing (WES) that incorporates probes for noncoding regulatory and intronic regions known to contain hotspot loci for predisposition mutations.[15]

General Considerations Regarding Bone Marrow Morphology and Diagnosis of Myeloid Malignancy in the Setting of Germline Predisposition

There is no specific morphologic or immunophenotypic finding diagnostic of MDS/AML with germline mutation. There are typical pathologic features that are associated with some germline mutations that will be discussed in the genetic sections. The presence of a germline mutation predisposing to MDS/AML

Box 45-3 *Features Associated With Progression to Myelodysplastic Syndrome in Patients With Germline Predisposition**

Two out of three of the following:
- Acquired pathogenic genetic alteration
  - Monosomy 7; monosomy 5; del(7q); del(5q); multihit *TP53* mutations, defined as two or more distinct *TP53* mutations each with VAF ≥ 10%, or a single *TP53* mutation with (1) 17p deletion on cytogenetics, (2) VAF ≥ 50%, or (3) copy neutral LOH at the 17p*TP53* locus; *TP53* mutation (VAF ≥ 10%) and complex karyotype (often with loss of 17p); or *SF3B1* mutation (VAF ≥ 10%) are considered MDS-defining†
- Cytopenia in a new lineage(s) or progressive cytopenia,‡ particularly in the context of increasing marrow cellularity
- Multilineage dysplasia§

Or:
- Increased blasts
  - ≥5% in marrow; ≥2% in peripheral blood

*These are guidelines and are not intended as absolute criteria; clinical judgment must be applied in each case.
†Genetic alterations should be interpreted in the context of the specific germline condition. Progression to acute myeloid leukemia (AML) may occur if AML-defining genetic abnormalities are present or criteria is met for AML. Progression to chronic myelomonocytic leukemia (CMML) or myelodysplastic syndrome (MDS)/myeloproliferative neoplasm (MPN) may also occur.
‡In adults, cytopenias are defined as hemoglobin <12 g/dL in females and <13 g/dL in males, absolute neutrophil count <1.8 × 10⁹/L, or platelets <150 × 10⁹/L. In children, cytopenia is defined according to age-adjusted values for hemoglobin, absolute neutrophil count, and platelet count.
§Baseline marrows in patients with germline predisposition may show evidence of dyspoiesis, hence, care must be made not to overinterpret dysmorphology as criteria for MDS in the absence of additional supporting evidence. Patients with germline mutations in *RUNX1*, *ANKRD26*, and *ETV6* with isolated thrombocytopenia commonly show megakaryocytic atypia at baseline, and as a sole finding this is not sufficient for a diagnosis of MDS. Dysplasia is defined as dysplastic cytologic changes in ≥10% of erythroid cells, ≥10% of granulocytic cells, and/or ≥10% of megakaryocytes.

is not diagnostic of myeloid malignancy until unequivocal features of overt malignancy develop. Importantly, bone marrow of many patients with germline mutations may show at baseline dysplastic features that remain stable and may not progress to MDS or AML for many years or may never progress depending on the inherent risk of malignancy conferred by the specific genetic mutation. Evaluation of bone marrow morphology requires expertise and must be interpreted with caution in order to avoid overdiagnosis of MDS. It is recommended that these cases not be interpreted as MDS unless additional supporting features are present, including frank multilineage dysplasia, increased blasts, increasing cellularity in the setting of worsening cytopenias, or emergence of MDS or AML defining cytogenetic or molecular genetic abnormalities (Box 45-3). This is particularly critical for patients with familial platelet disorders who typically show baseline dysmegakaryopoiesis that is associated with isolated thrombocytopenia caused by mutations in *RUNX1*, *ANKRD26*, or *ETV6* in the absence of MDS. Conversely, some patients may have borderline or minimal evidence of dysplasia in a hypocellular marrow, with emergence of monosomy 7 or other MDS-defining cytogenetic abnormality indicative of progression to MDS. Not all cytogenetic abnormalities warrant a diagnosis of MDS and some may be associated with stable disease. MDS-defining genetic abnormalities include: monosomy 7; monosomy 5; del(7q); del(5q); multihit *TP53* mutations—defined as two or more distinct *TP53* mutations each with VAF ≥10%, or a single *TP53* mutation with (1) 17p deletion on cytogenetics,

(2) VAF of ≥50%, or (3) copy neutral loss of heterozygosity (LOH) at the 17p*TP53* locus; *TP53* mutation (VAF ≥ 10%) and complex karyotype (often with loss of 17p); or *SF3B1* mutation (VAF ≥ 10%).[5] Clonal hematopoiesis is not uncommon in patients with germline predisposition and must be interpreted in the context of the specific germline predisposition and the bone marrow/peripheral blood findings. Of note, monoallelic *TP53* mutations with low VAF are common in patients with Shwachman-Diamond syndrome; but biallelic mutations are associated with myeloid malignancy. The morphologic diagnosis of MDS in patients with germline predisposition may be challenging and requires close collaboration between clinicians and pathologists to arrive at the appropriate diagnosis and treatment. Myeloid neoplasms should be diagnosed with indication of the associated germline mutation or syndrome; for example, AML with germline mutation in *CEBPA*, or JMML associated with Noonan syndrome. If a patient is diagnosed with MDS/AML and a germline mutation is subsequently identified, the diagnosis can be modified to incorporate the underlying germline mutation.

SYNONYMS AND RELATED TERMS

Inherited hematologic neoplasms; familial myelodysplastic syndromes/acute leukemias.

HEMATOLOGIC NEOPLASMS WITH GERMLINE PREDISPOSITION WITHOUT A CONSTITUTIONAL DISORDER AFFECTING MULTIPLE ORGAN SYSTEMS

Myeloid Neoplasm With Germline *CEBPA* Mutation

CEBPA is a single-exon gene located on chromosome 19q13.1 that encodes for CCAAT/enhancer-binding protein-α, a lineage-specific basic leucine zipper (bZIP) transcription factor. The *CEBPA* zipper domain is required for dimerization, and the adjacent basic region is responsible for DNA binding, thereby promoting transcription of target genes.[16-18] The N terminus is unique to *CEBPA*, containing two transactivation domains that regulate transcription control and protein interaction.[17] The mRNA may be translated into either a full-length 42-kDA isoform (p42) or a truncated 30-kDa (p30) isoform, both of which can homodimerize or heterodimerize with other CEBP proteins to regulate genes involved in cell differentiation, survival, metabolism, growth, and inflammation.[19]

The inheritance of a germline *CEBPA* mutation predisposes to the development of AML with autosomal dominant inheritance and was first described in 2004.[20] Germline mutated CEBPA-associated AML is defined as the presence of a heterozygous germline *CEBPA* pathogenic variant in an individual with AML. Progression to AML is frequently associated with an acquired mutation in the remaining wild-type CEBPA allele.[21,22] The germline (often protein-truncating) mutation commonly affects the N terminus, whereas the acquired mutation arises in the C-terminal bZIP region (predominantly missense or in-frame indels).[23] Although numbers are limited, families with germline N-terminal mutations display a higher degree of penetrance (~90%) compared with fewer families harboring germline C-terminal mutations (~50%).[21]

Tawana and colleagues noted a >90% remission rate in patients with CEBPA-associated familial AML but found a 50% cumulative incidence of relapse, with some patients relapsing three or four times.[21] Molecular sequencing of five patients' tumors at the time of relapse revealed that they harbored new C-terminus somatic mutations, representing the development of a second primary AML rather than true disease relapse.[21] This pattern of progression likely underlies the clinical observations that patients with AML and germline CEBPA mutations have a good outcome yet are prone to second leukemias that continue to be sensitive to chemotherapy, unlike true relapsed disease. Up to 11% of presumed sporadic AML with biallelic CEBPA mutations may harbor a germline CEBPA mutation.[24]

Myeloid or Lymphoid Neoplasms With Germline DDX41 Mutation

DDX41 belongs to the DEAD-box helicase family of genes that have been characterized in multiple cellular roles, composed of 17 exons, and is encoded on the distal end of the long arm of chromosome 5.[25] DDX41 encodes a member of the DEAD-box ATP-dependent RNA helicases, which are involved in premRNA splicing, RNA processing, ribosome biogenesis, and small nucleolar RNA processing.[26,27] In addition, DDX41 interacts with intracellular DNA in dendritic cells and macrophages, and activates innate immunity through the stimulator of interferon genes (STING)-interferon pathway.[28,29]

DDX41 germline mutations are clinically associated with an increased lifetime risk of myeloid neoplasms, including the early presentation of idiopathic cytopenia of undetermined significance (ICUS).[30] Other diseases reported to be associated with DDX41 mutations include myeloproliferative neoplasms, chronic myeloid leukemia, multiple myeloma, myelodysplastic syndrome (Fig. 45-1), and acute myeloid leukemia.[27,31,32] Lymphoid neoplasms have also been described but are less common with germline DDX41 mutations. In a recently published study using a multinational cohort, DDX41 germline mutations account for about 80% of patients with myeloid neoplasms with germline predisposition.[33] In contrast to other hereditary hematologic malignancies, DDX41 mutation is associated with late onset

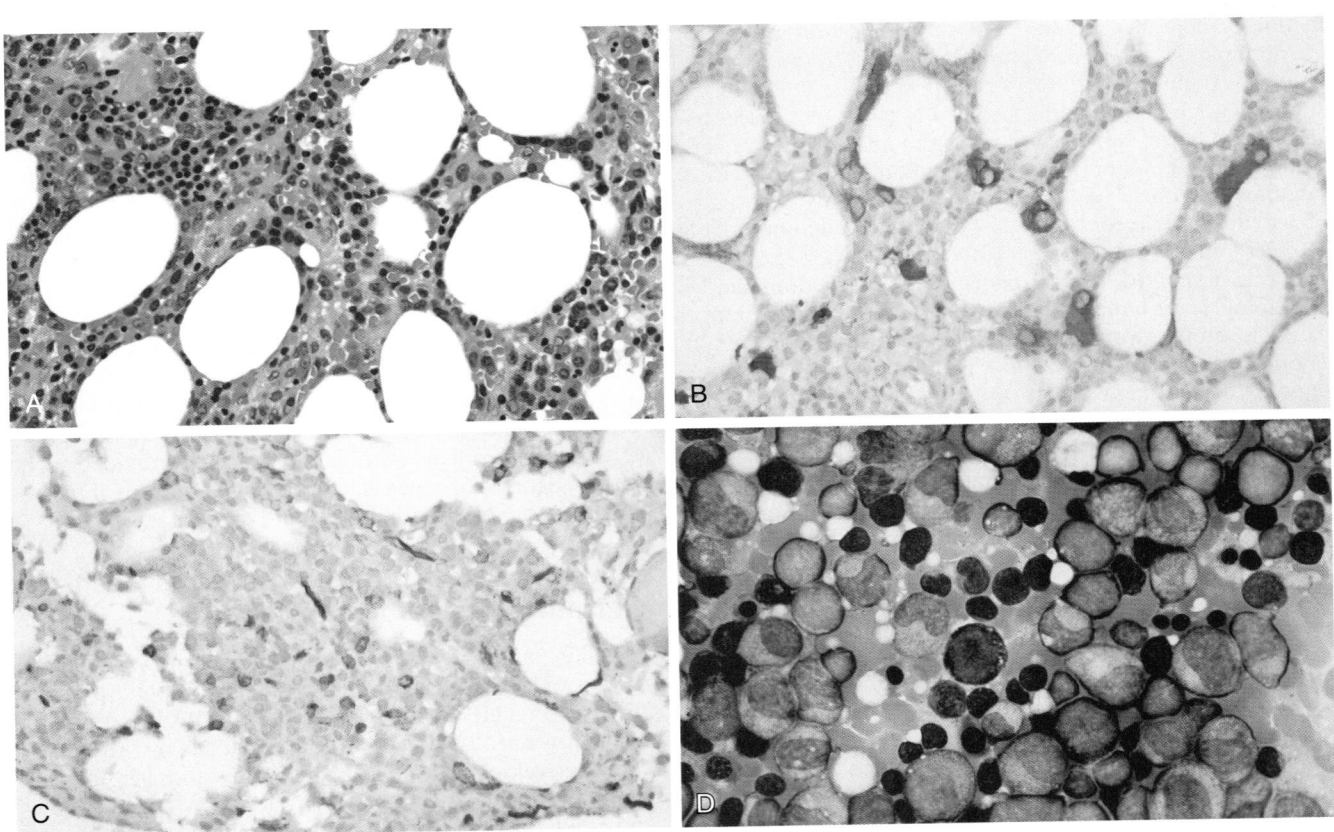

Figure 45-1. Myelodysplastic syndrome with excess blasts (ICC) and germline DDX41 mutation. Bone marrow from a male in his 6th decade with a history of progressive cytopenias and myelodysplastic syndrome (MDS) in at least one other family member. **A,** The bone marrow was normocellular for age with evidence of dysplastic hypolobated megakaryocytes on hematoxylin and eosin (H&E) stain. **B,** CD61 IHC showed multiple dysplastic megakaryocytes with hypobated nuclei and micromegakaryocytes. **C,** CD34 IHC showed 5% to 9% increased positive cells consistent with blasts, confirmed on flow cytometry as aberrant myeloblasts with downregulated expression of CD38. **D,** Bone marrow biopsy touch prep showed left shift in myeloid precursors and increased blasts. Cytogenetic analysis was normal. Next-generation sequencing (NGS) myeloid mutation panel performed on bone marrow detected two DDX41 mutations, one at 50% VAF and the other at 19% VAF. Testing on skin biopsy confirmed presence of a germline DDX41 mutation. This case may also be diagnosed as MDS with increased blasts and germline DDX41 mutation (MDS-IB-1) (WHO 5th ed.).

myeloid neoplasms typically in the 6th decade, often occurring after years of typically mild cytopenia, or macrocytosis. While germline *DDX41* mutations should be considered in patients with a personal or family history of hematologic malignancy, a family history of malignancy is often lacking.[26]

AML with germline *DDX41* mutation is often associated with a second acquired *DDX41* mutation. Bone marrow is often hypocellular with a borderline increase in blasts with mostly normal immunophenotype and with normal karyotype. These features make the initial diagnosis of this inherited AML more challenging than other hereditary hematologic predisposition syndromes. When assessing the frequency of *DDX41*-mutated variants across the spectrum myeloid neoplasms, *DDX41* variants had the highest representation in high-risk MDS and secondary AML.[33]

Myeloid or Lymphoid Neoplasms With Germline *TP53* Mutation

Transcription factor p53, encoded by the *TP53* gene, is a key tumor suppressor gene with protean functions associated with preservation of genomic balance, including regulation of cellular senescence, apoptotic pathways, metabolism functions, and DNA repair.[34] Li-Fraumeni syndrome (LFS) is a dominantly inherited condition caused by pathogenic germline variants in the TP53 tumor suppressor gene.[35,36] Patients with LFS are predisposed to a range of neoplasms such as sarcomas, adrenocortical carcinoma, breast cancer, medulloblastoma, choroid plexus carcinoma, and anaplastic rhabdomyosarcoma.[36] Approximately 50% of individuals with LFS will develop cancer by age 30 years, with a lifetime risk of up to 75% in men and almost 100% in women.[37] Incidence of leukemias in LFS is approximately 4%[38] predominantly hypodiploid acute lymphoblastic leukemia (ALL) and therapy-related myeloid disorders including AML and MDS.[1,39,40] Genome-wide studies suggest that germline variants are more frequent than estimated prevalence of LFS, suggesting that many carriers of potentially pathogenic mutations may not develop the syndrome.[41] Carriers of a germline *TP53* mutation who are detected in a clinical context have a penetrance of 80% at age 70 and penetrance varies according to age, sex, and mutation type. Temporal tumor patterns show distinct phases, with childhood phase (0–15 years, 22% of all cancers) characterized by adrenal cortical carcinoma, choroid plexus carcinoma, rhabdomyosarcoma, and medulloblastoma; early adulthood phase (16–50 years, 51%) including breast cancer, sarcomas, leukemia, astrocytoma, and glioblastoma, colorectal, and lung cancer; and late adulthood phase (51–80 years, 27%) including pancreatic and prostate cancer.[41]

Whereas *TP53* alterations are generally rare in ALL, they are almost universally present in the low hypodiploid subtype of ALL, approximately 50% of which are germline in nature.[42] A recent study involving 3801 children with ALL showed that LFS-associated ALL accounts for less than 1% of ALL cases and was associated with inferior event-free survival as well as overall survival, and higher risk of second malignant neoplasms.[43] Observations show that more than half of *TP53* mutations in low-hypodiploid ALL in children are also present in nontumoral cells, indicating that low-hypodiploid ALL is a manifestation of LFS. *TP53* mutations in AML are associated with older age, lower blast counts (both in the bone marrow and in the peripheral blood), adverse risk karyotypes, and exposure to antecedent

chemotherapy. Therapy-related AML and MDS frequently occur in patients with LFS, likely related to the patients' extensive cancer history and prior myelosuppressive treatments. Cytotoxic agents like alkylating agents and topoisomerase inhibitors, as well as radiation therapy, are known to be associated with therapy-related MDS/therapy-related AML.[44]

HEMATOLOGIC NEOPLASMS WITH GERMLINE PREDISPOSITION ASSOCIATED WITH A CONSTITUTIONAL PLATELET DISORDER

Hematologic neoplasms with germline predisposition associated with constitutional platelet disorders include germline mutations in *RUNX1*, *ANKRD26*, and *ETV6*. There are important baseline morphologic features seen in all three of these disorders that are critical for hematopathologists to recognize. Patients may have isolated thrombocytopenia with normal platelet size and dysmegakaryopoiesis in the marrow in the setting of stable nonmalignant disease for decades. Dysmegakaryopoiesis with small hypolobated megakaryocytes or forms with separated nuclear lobes is often seen in the setting of isolated thrombocytopenia indicative of inherent abnormal megakaryopoiesis with impaired proplatelet formation, and not indicative of MDS in the absence of other criteria supporting a diagnosis of MDS.[45-47] Because of baseline dysmegakaryopoiesis, many patients with germline *RUNX1* and *ANRD26* mutations are overdiagnosed or misdiagnosed with MDS-with single lineage dysplasia.[48] Bona fide progression to MDS or other myeloid malignancy is typically associated with increased marrow cellularity, emergence of new cytopenias (in addition to thrombocytopenia) or cytoses, multilineage dysplasia, increased blasts, cytogenetic abnormalities, or acquired genetic/molecular abnormalities associated with malignancy (Box 45-3).[6,45] Morphologically, the marrow features may also overlap with those seen in immune thrombocytopenic purpura (ITP). Germline mutations in *RUNX1*, *ANKRD26*, or *ETV6* should be considered in patients evaluated for isolated thrombocytopenia with evidence of dysmegakaryopoiesis, particularly if there is a family history of thrombocytopenia or MDS/AML.

Myeloid or Lymphoid Neoplasms With Germline *RUNX1* Mutation

Germline mutations in *RUNX1* (previously known as *CBFA2* or *AML1*) were discovered in patients with FPD with propensity to develop acute myeloid leukemia in 1999.[3] The syndrome is characterized by lifelong thrombocytopenia with increased risk of developing myeloid malignancies and, less frequently, lymphoid malignancy. Platelet studies show normal size with impaired platelet aggregation to epinephrine and collagen, and dense granule storage deficiency. A minority of patients may have near-normal platelet counts; however, platelet function is typically abnormal, leading to increased bleeding risk out of proportion to quantitative platelet count. The overall risk of developing myeloid malignancies is estimated at 30% to 40% with a median age of 34, with a wide age range of 6 to 72 years.[49] The most common malignancies are myeloid including MDS, AML, and chronic myelomonocytic leukemia (CMML), and often show somatic mutations in the second *RUNX1* allele.[50] T lymphoblastic leukemia (T-ALL) is also reported less frequently, and B lymphoblastic leukemia (B-ALL) or other B-lineage neoplasms are rare.

RUNX1 encodes a subunit of core binding transcription factor that is a regulator of hematopoiesis. It is the most commonly targeted gene in chromosomal translocations in sporadic acute leukemia. *RUNX1* is located on chromosome 21q22 and has been shown to be critical for megakaryopoiesis and proplatelet formation.[46] The germline mutations are heterozygous (monoallelic) with an autosomal dominant inheritance pattern. Mutations comprise missense, frameshift, nonsense, deletions, intragenic duplications, or rearrangements and can occur throughout the gene. The prevalence of germline *RUNX1* mutations has not been determined. The penetrance is incomplete with variable expressivity. Cases of donor-derived leukemia have been reported in patients undergoing stem cell transplantation using a healthy related donor who unknowingly carries the same germline *RUNX1* mutation as the recipient.[11]

Typical baseline bone marrow findings in *RUNX1* patients with isolated thrombocytopenia include normocellular or hypocellular marrow for age with evidence of occasional atypical megakaryocytes or frank dysmegakaryopoiesis. The number of megakaryocytes may be normal or slightly increased with small hypolobated forms or forms with separated nuclear lobes (Fig. 45-2). Morphologically, the marrow features may overlap with those seen in ITP. A subset of *RUNX1* patients is misdiagnosed with ITP or "familial ITP" prior to the discovery of germline *RUNX1* mutation. Alternatively, some patients who are stable with isolated thrombocytopenia have been misdiagnosed with MDS solely on the basis of dysmegakaryopoiesis. Dysmegakaryopoiesis is a fundamental feature in RUNX1-FPD that is seen even in asymptomatic family members with the mutation, and should not be considered as a criterion for MDS in the absence of other findings supporting a diagnosis of MDS.[6,45] Marrows may also show a mild increase in eosinophils, which may be related to increased incidence of allergies and atopic symptoms in *RUNX1* patients. As noted, progression to MDS, AML, or CMML is associated with hypercellularity in the setting of new cytopenias, increased blasts, multilineage dysplasia, or cytogenetic/molecular abnormalities (Fig. 45-3). The blasts in AML cases typically are with or without maturation demonstrating myeloid immunophenotype, and often contain Auer rods.

Myeloid Neoplasms With Germline *ANKRD26* Mutation

Germline mutations in *ANKRD26* (chromosome 10p12.1) were identified in multiple families with familial thrombocytopenia 2 (THC2) in 2011.[51,52] THC2 is characterized by moderate thrombocytopenia with normal-sized platelets with reduced alpha granules, and absent or mild bleeding. No consistent defect is seen on platelet aggregation studies. The mutations are heterozygous and have an autosomal dominant inheritance pattern. Germline mutations in *ANKRD26* are located in the 5′ untranslated region. These mutations disrupt binding of corepressors RUNX1 and FLI1 to the promoter and lead to increased *ANKRD26* transcription. The mutations are gain-of-function, resulting in increased signaling in the MPL pathway, impairing proplatelet formation.[14] *ANKRD26* mutations may be missed on standard whole exome sequencing or on NGS panels that do not cover the noncoding 5′UTR. Currently the prevalence of *ANKRD26* germline mutations is unknown. The

risk of developing MDS/AML is estimated to be about 24 times greater than expected in the general population. The onset of MDS/AML ranges from 35 to 70 years of age.[53] Other reported HM include CMML, CML, and CLL. Similar to RUNX1-FPD, dysmegakaryopoiesis is common in the bone marrow in patients with stable disease and without malignancy.[48] The development of MDS/AML is associated with additional cytopenia/cytoses, multilineage dysplasia, increased blasts, and acquired cytogenetic/molecular abnormalities.

Myeloid or Lymphoid Neoplasms With Germline *ETV6* Mutation

ETV6 is located on chromosome 12p13. It is a member of the ETS family of transcription factors and is a transcriptional repressor. *ETV6* is targeted in chromosomal translocations with over 30 partners in sporadic acute myeloid and lymphoblastic leukemia. In 2015, several families with thrombocytopenia and increased hematologic neoplasms were found to have germline mutations in *ETV6*.[54,55] Both myeloid and lymphoid malignancies were reported, including B lymphoblastic leukemia (most common), MDS, AML, CMML, and myeloma. Other cancers were also reported, including breast cancer and colorectal carcinoma. Currently, the prevalence of germline *ETV6* mutations is undefined. A hematologic malignancy has been diagnosed in approximately 30% of all reported carriers. Patients have mild to moderate thrombocytopenia, with normal platelet size, and mild to moderate bleeding tendency. Germline mutations typically involve the ETS DNA binding domain, resulting in impaired nuclear localization and reduced transcriptional repression by ETV6 leading to decreased proplatelet formation. Increased small hypolobated immature megakaryocytes are typically seen in the marrow with decreased mature forms (Fig. 45-4). There may also be prominent dyserythropoiesis.

HEMATOLOGIC NEOPLASMS WITH GERMLINE PREDISPOSITION ASSOCIATED WITH A CONSTITUTIONAL DISORDER AFFECTING MULTIPLE ORGAN SYSTEMS

Myeloid Neoplasms With Germline *GATA2* Mutation

Germline heterozygous mutations in *GATA2* were first reported in 2011 by multiple groups that described four overlapping syndromes, each of which was associated with development of myeloid malignancies. The four syndromes were:

- **MonoMac syndrome** characterized by monocytopenia, severe immunodeficiency with *Mycobacterium avium* complex (MAC) infections, human papillomavirus (HPV), and other viral infections; pulmonary alveolar proteinosis; and hypoplastic MDS and CMML[56-58]
- **Dendritic cell, monocyte, and lymphocyte (DCML) deficiency**, characterized by low monocytes, dendritic cells, B cells, and natural killer (NK) cells with opportunistic infections and high incidence of MDS[59,60]
- **Familial MDS/AML** families with increased incidence of MDS and AML[61]
- **Emberger syndrome** characterized by lymphedema, sensorineural deafness, warts, and MDS[62,63]

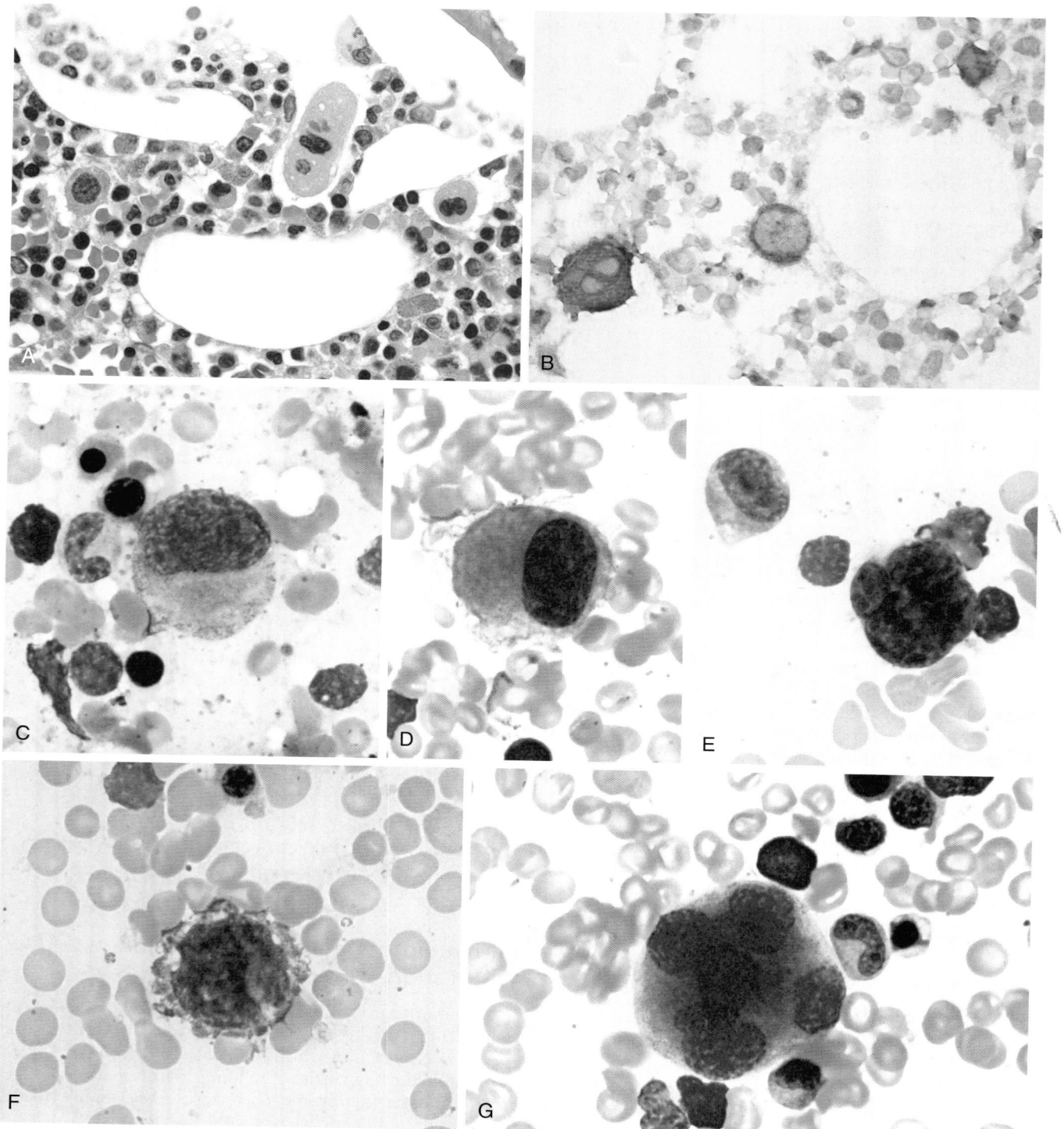

Figure 45-2. **Dysmegakaryopoiesis in RUNX1 familial platelet disorder in the absence of myelodysplastic syndrome (MDS) or myeloid malignancy. A,** Normocellular marrow with dysmegakaryopoiesis (small monolobated or hypolobated megakaryocytes, and megakaryocytes with
separated nuclear lobes) from a female in her 4th decade with a lifelong history of stable isolated
thrombocytopenia and germline *RUNX1* mutation. There were no additional cytopenias or cytoses. Myelopoiesis and erythropoiesis were normal and there was no increase in blasts. Cytogenetics revealed a normal karyotype. Next-generation sequencing (NGS) myeloid mutation analysis
revealed only the known germline *RUNX1* mutation. **B,** CD61 stain demonstrated abnormal small
hypolobated megakaryocytes. **C–G,** Typical baseline abnormal megakaryocytes often seen on aspirate smears of stable pediatric and adult RUNX1 FPD patients with isolated thrombocytopenia and no additional evidence of myelodysplasia. The abnormal megakaryocytes include small
mononuclear forms, forms resembling micromegakaryocytes, naked megakaryocyte nuclei, and
forms with separated nuclear lobes. The baseline abnormal megakaryocytes may represent over
10% of the megakaryocytes in the marrow; however, this finding should not be used as a criterion
for myelodysplasia. The development of MDS is associated with multilineage dysplasia, additional
cytopenia other than thrombocytopenia, increased blasts, or MDS defining genetic abnormalities.

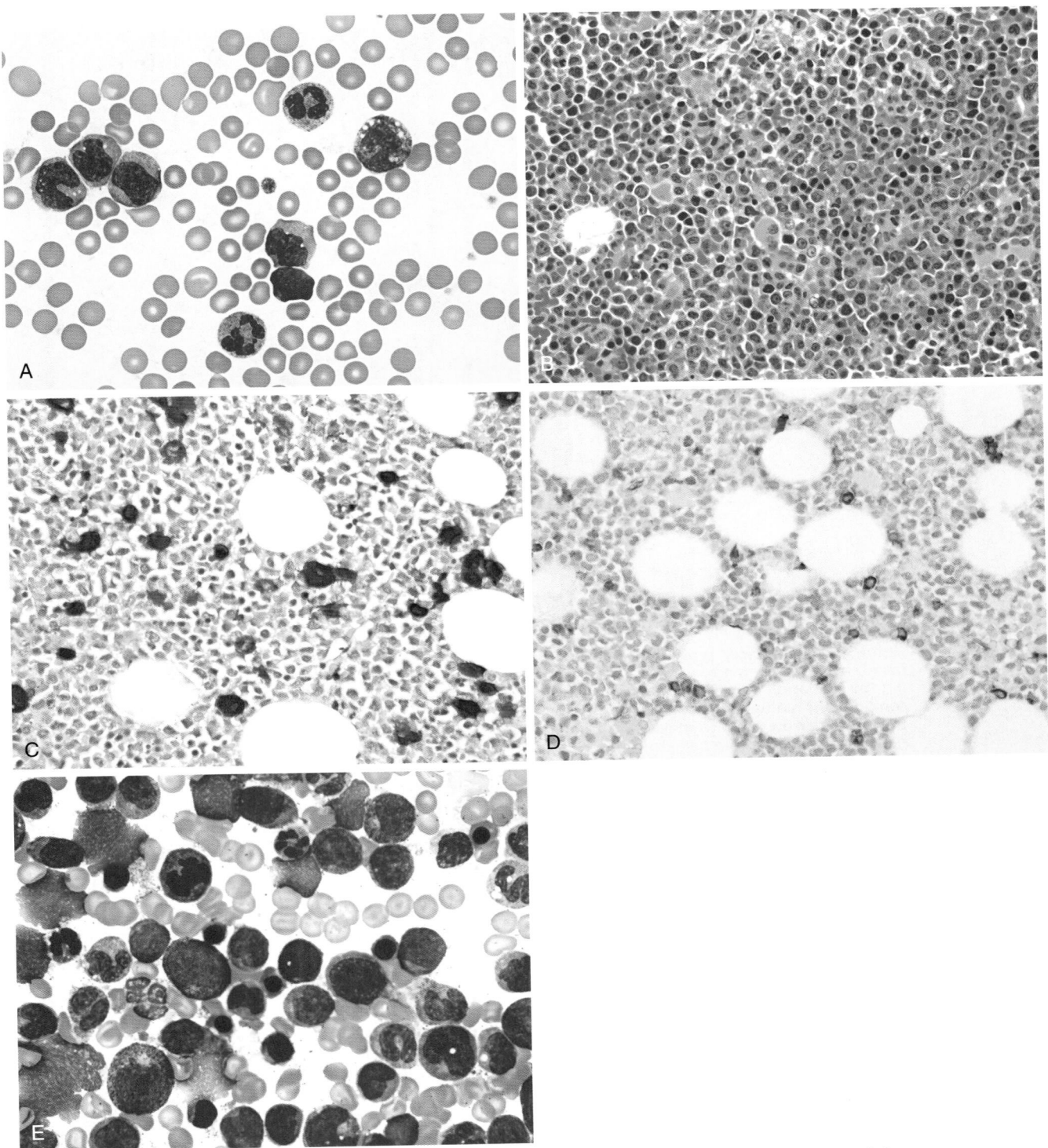

Figure 45-3. RUNX1 FPD and development of myeloid malignancy: chronic myelomonocytic leukemia with germline *RUNX1* mutation. Images from the peripheral blood and marrow of a woman in her 6th decade with a lifelong history of thrombocytopenia, confirmed germline mutation in *RUNX1,* and a more recent diagnosis of myelodysplastic syndrome (MDS) with 5q– in the past several years. At presentation in our institution her white blood cell count (WBC) was markedly elevated with a monocytosis over 8 K/mcL. **A,** Peripheral blood smear showing leukocytosis with increased monocytic cells, left-shifted granulocytes, and circulating blasts. Flow cytometry analysis showed 8% circulating blasts with abnormal myeloid phenotype expressing CD7 *(not shown).* **B,** Bone marrow core biopsy showing markedly hypercellular marrow with dysplastic megakaryocytes and increased immature precursors. **C,** CD61 highlights frequent small monolobated megakaryocytes. **D,** CD34 stain demonstrates increased blasts. **E,** Aspirate smear showing increased blasts, immature monocytic cells, and left-shifted myeloid cells. Flow cytometry analysis of the marrow aspirate showed 13% blasts, half of which were CD34 positive with an abnormal myeloid phenotype (CD7 positive) and half of which were monoblasts expressing CD64, CD36, HLA-DR++, CD33++, with dim to negative CD14 expression *(not shown).* Cytogenetic analysis was normal. Next-generation sequencing (NGS) myeloid panel showed presence of the known *RUNX1* germline mutation and additional new mutations in *NRAS, PHF6,* and *BCOR.*

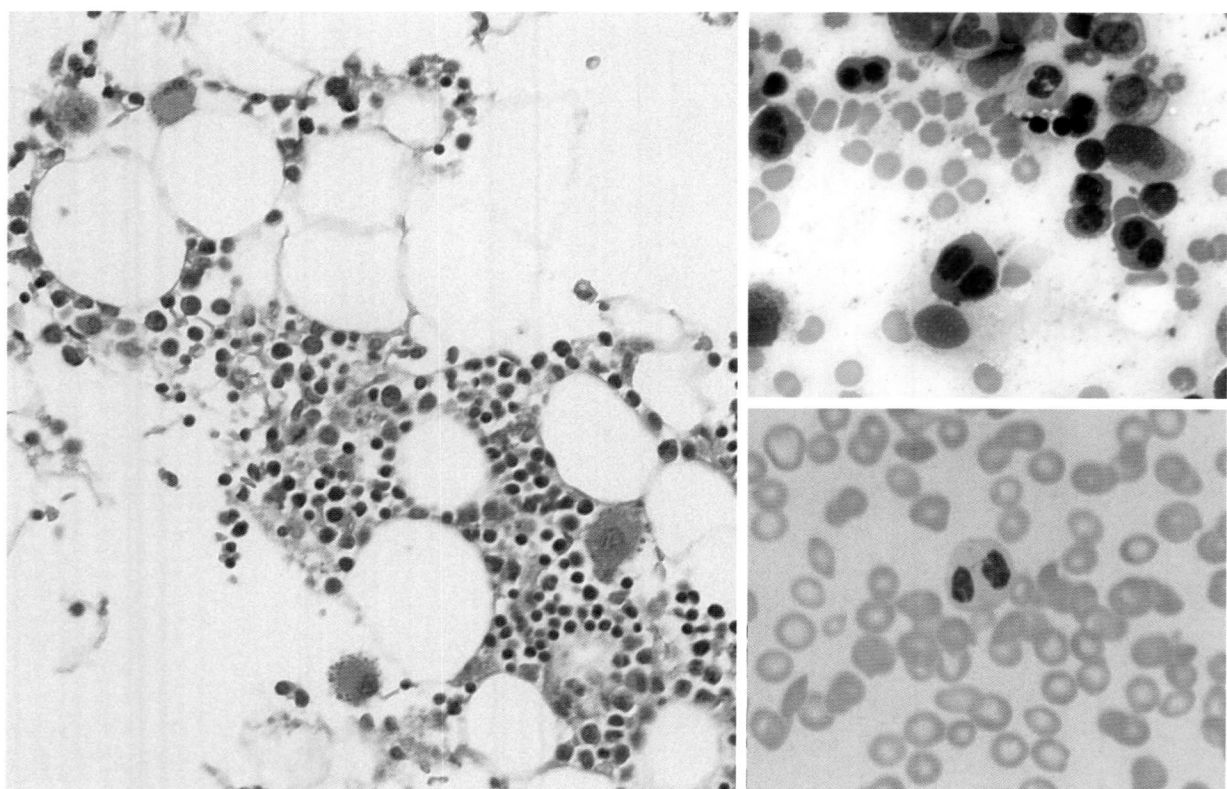

Figure 45-4. Refractory cytopenia of childhood (RCC; ICC) with germline *ETV6* mutation. *Left panel*, hypocellular marrow from a 9-year-old female with thrombocytopenia and easy bruising since infancy. Bone marrow was markedly hypocellular for age with dysmegakaryopoiesis composed of multiple hypolobated megakaryocytes. *Top right*, dyserythropoiesis was evident on the bone marrow aspirate smear with frequent binucleated erythroid precursors. *Bottom right*, peripheral smear showed pelgeroid and hypogranular neutrophils. There was no increase in blasts and cytogenetics revealed a normal karyotype. Several years later, in adolescence, the patient developed myelodysplastic syndrome with excess blasts (MDS-EB) and was transplanted. Other family members were discovered to have thrombocytopenia and germline mutations in *ETV6*. *(Courtesy of Drs. Akiko Shimamura and Keith Loeb.)*

The majority of patients initially described were young or middle-aged adults, with some pediatric representation. Subsequently, a large study of pediatric MDS found germline *GATA2* mutations present in up to 7% of pediatric MDS overall, 37% of pediatric MDS with monosomy 7, and in 75% of adolescents with MDS and monosomy 7.[64] *GATA2* is now recognized as one of the most common germline-mutated genes in pediatric MDS. Approximately two-thirds of the pediatric cases harbor de novo mutations not present in either parent. *GATA2* germline mutations have also been reported in cases of congenital neutropenia, bone marrow failure, and aplastic anemia.[65,66] All disorders with germline *GATA2* mutations have overlapping features and are now known as a single genetic disorder with protean manifestations termed *GATA2 deficiency*.[67,68]

GATA2 is a zinc finger transcription factor that regulates hematopoiesis and is critical for stem cell renewal. Germline mutations in *GATA2* are heterozygous with autosomal dominant inheritance. The mutations lead to loss of function and haploinsufficiency. The mutations are classified as missense, null, and regulatory. More recently, synonymous mutations have been reported.[69] Most mutations involve coding regions affecting one of the two the zinc finger

domains; however, importantly a minority of patients may have mutations in an intronic region containing an enhancer element that will not be detected on standard whole exome sequencing[13] or NGS panels that do not cover this region. Ideally, *GATA2* deficiency is diagnosed by full gene sequencing on non-hematopoietic tissue (e.g., cultured fibroblasts from skin biopsy). However, many cases have been picked up by routine NGS targeted-sequencing panels performed on bone marrow or peripheral blood showing pathogenic *GATA2* mutations with high VAFs that undergo subsequent germline confirmation.

The penetrance and expressivity of germline *GATA2* mutations is variable and may be different among family members harboring the same germline mutation. A subset of GATA2 patients present with severe immunodeficiency characterized by markedly decreased monocytes, dendritic cells, B cells, and NK cells. Though a minority have CD4 T-cell lymphopenia, the majority show preservation of T-cell populations, with or without increased large granular lymphocytes or NK/T-cells. Cases with clonal T-cell LGL populations are reported.[67] Opportunistic infections by nontuberculous mycobacteria, fungal organisms, and viral pathogens are not uncommon. HPV infections can lead to severe genital warts, disseminated warts, cervical dysplasia, and squamous cell carcinomas of the genital/anal region[70] in both females and males. Epstein-Barr virus (EBV) may cause severe primary infection and EBV-associated cancers.[71] Though immunodeficiency is marked in many cases, this phenotype is variable and some GATA2 patients have only mildly decreased immune populations, or no evidence of immunodeficiency at all. Other manifestations may include lymphedema, sensorineural deafness, pulmonary alveolar proteinosis, deep vein thrombosis, and miscarriage.

The most common malignancies in GATA2 deficiency are myeloid and include refractory cytopenia of childhood (RCC) in pediatric patients, MDS, AML, CMML, and MDS/MPN. The overall lifetime risk of myeloid malignancy in GATA2 deficiency has been estimated at 70%.[68] The age of onset of myeloid malignancy is highly variable ranging from 5 months to 78 years, with a median onset ranging from 12 to 35.5 years, depending on the study.[68] In some patients, the development of immunodeficiency precedes the development of myeloid malignancy.[72] However, other patients present with myeloid malignancy without recognition of a preceding immunodeficiency.[61] Progressive BMF with features resembling aplastic anemia can also precede progression to MDS or AML (Fig. 45-5). Solid tumors have also been reported in GATA2 deficiency.[67] Other hematologic malignancies including B lymphoblastic leukemia and T lymphoblastic leukemia have been rarely described.[73,74]

Bone marrow histologic patterns in GATA2 deficiency demonstrate a range pathology.[75] Common patterns include (1) acute myeloid leukemia in a hypercellular or hypocellular marrow; (2) frank hypoplastic MDS with multilineage dysplasia with or without increased blasts (Fig. 45-6); (3) RCC in pediatric patients; (4) hypocellular marrow with mildly dysplastic features approaching but not reaching 10% of cells within lineages, no increase in blasts, and not meeting formal morphologic criteria for MDS called GATA2 bone marrow and immunodeficiency disorder (G2BMID)[76]; or (5) a severely hypocellular marrow resembling aplastic anemia with too few cells to evaluate for dysplastic features (Fig. 45-5A). Some patients may present with disseminated MAC in the bone marrow with or without MDS (Fig. 45-7). Bone marrow flow cytometry analysis may be helpful in demonstrating disproportionate loss of monocytes, dendritic cells, B-cell precursors, mature B-cells, or NK-cells indicative of underlying immunodeficiency (Fig. 45-8), which is typically not seen in aplastic anemia, or sporadic MDS to the degree seen in GATA2 deficiency.[77] Flow cytometry can also be helpful in evaluating dysplastic immunophenotypic changes. MDS in GATA2 deficiency commonly shows multilineage dysplasia. Rarely one may see marked cellular depletion with serous fat atrophy or prominent fibrosis (Fig. 45-9), usually in the setting of pancytopenia without leukoerythroblastosis, and often with clonal cytogenetic abnormalities, and absence of mutations in JAK2, MPL, or CALR. Dysmegakaryopoiesis is present in nearly all cases often with osteoclast-like megakaryocytes displaying separated nuclear lobes (Fig. 45-6A) or micromegakaryocytes (Fig. 45-5F), which can be highlighted by CD61 on core biopsies (Fig. 45-5D).[58] Myeloid cells often show hypogranularity with abnormal granulation patterns and hyposegmentation

(Fig. 45-6B). Frequently, the M:E ratio is inverted, with erythroid predominance. Increased blasts (less than 20%) may or may not be present. Despite reduction or loss of B cells and B-cell precursors in many patients, plasma cells are usually present and may aberrantly express CD56. Likewise, despite the loss of monocytes in many patients, macrophages and histiocytes are readily identified.

The most common cytogenetic abnormalities detected in GATA2 deficiency are monosomy 7, trisomy 8, and unbalanced translocation der(1;7)(q10;p10), which support a diagnosis of MDS.[78] The genetic landscape of MDS in GATA2 deficiency differs from that in de novo MDS. The most common acquired mutations include ASXL1, STAG2, DNMT3A, and SETBP1.[76,79,80] SF3B1 mutations are notably uncommon, as are ring sideroblasts, in contrast to de novo adult MDS.

Cytopenic patients with hypocellular marrows need to be carefully followed as transformation to AML can occur suddenly.[81] Transformation to AML or CMML may be accompanied by increased cellularity in the marrow. A subset of patients present with AML without clinical recognition of syndromic features. AML blasts often demonstrate a myeloid immunophenotype (CD34+, CD117+, CD13+, CD33+, CD64−) but can show evidence of monocytic/monoblastic differentiation (CD34−, CD33 bright+, CD64+, CD14 partial + or −). GATA2 patients may present with CMML or MDS/MPN.[82] CMML may occur after the emergence of malignant monocytes after years of monocytopenia.[67]

HSCT can be curative, not only for myeloid malignancy but also for manifestations related to immunodeficiency.[70,83,84] Some family members with the mutation may be asymptomatic and have normal blood counts throughout life. All potential related donors must be screened for GATA2 mutation to prevent donor-derived MDS/AML, which has developed when healthy mutation-positive donors were inadvertently used as HSCT donors.[8]

Myeloid Neoplasms With Germline *SAMD9* or *SAMD9L* Mutation

In 2016, a syndrome called MIRAGE was reported that was associated with germline mutations in *SAMD9* and characterized by **m**yelodysplasia with monosomy 7, **i**nfection, **r**estriction of growth, **a**drenal hypoplasia, **g**enital phenotypes, and **e**nteropathy.[85] In the same year, ataxia pancytopenia syndrome was described with germline mutations in a related gene, *SAMD9L*, that was associated with BMF and MDS with monosomy 7.[86] Subsequent studies showed that germline mutations in *SAMD9* and *SAMD9L* are among the most common overall in pediatric MDS in patients without syndromic features of MIRAGE or ataxia pancytopenia syndromes, and in patients suspected of having inherited bone marrow failure.[87,88] *SAMD9L* germline mutations have also been identified in children with severe autoinflammatory disease.[89] *SAMD9* and *SAMD9L* are both located on chromosome 7. Germline mutations are gain-of-function and have antiproliferative effects on hematopoietic cells leading to cytopenia and bone marrow failure. There are multiple compensatory genetic outcomes that are not uncommon in these patients that are either adaptive or maladaptive, representing somatic genetic rescue (SGR).[88] Maladaptive mechanisms to rid cells of the germline mutation

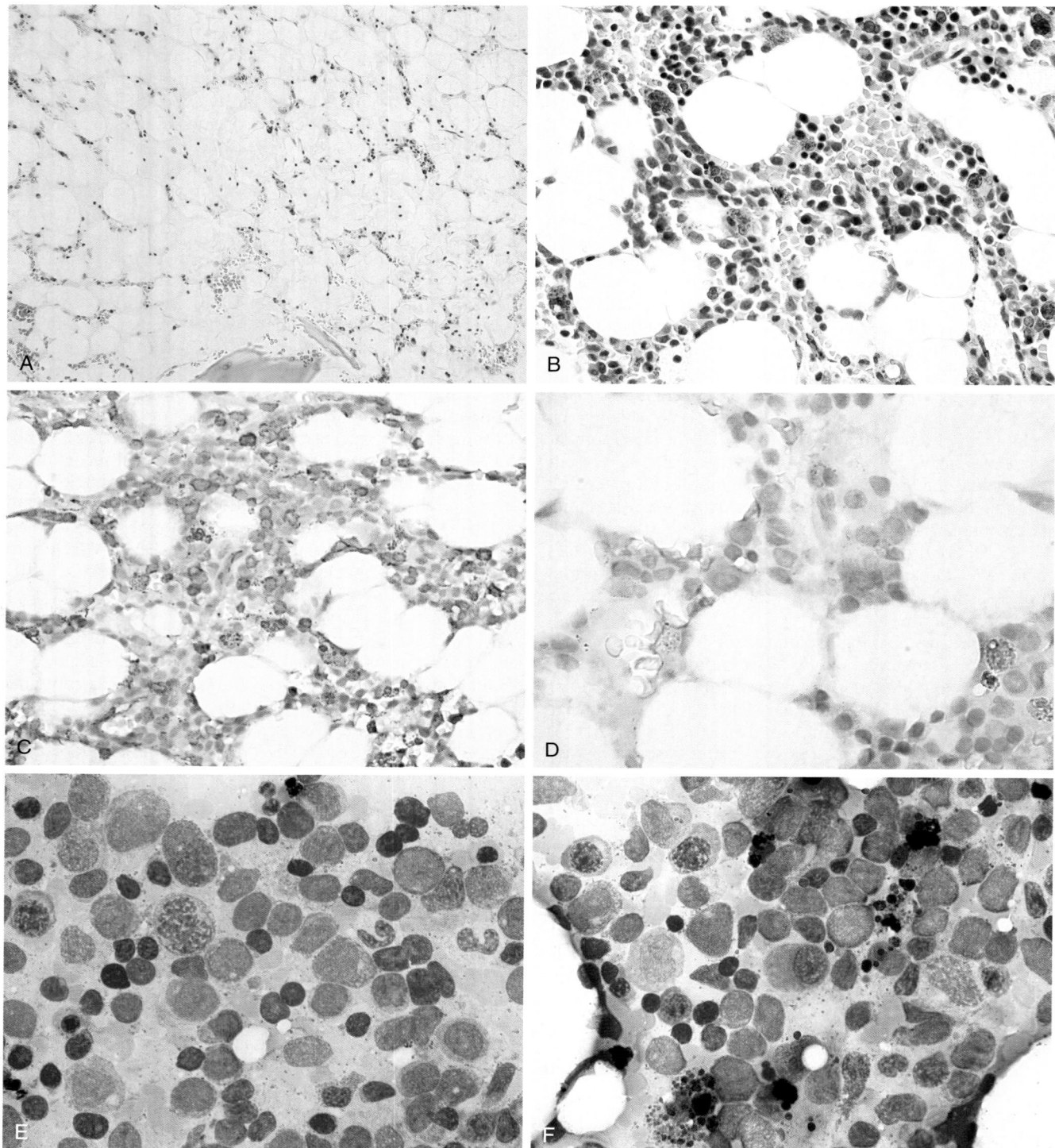

Figure 45-5. Acute myeloid leukemia with germline *GATA2* mutation arising in a patient previously diagnosed with aplastic anemia. A, Hypocellular marrow with trilineage hypoplasia in a late adolescent male with pancytopenia diagnosed with aplastic anemia (×500). There were areas of serous fat atrophy with a few scattered erythroid precursors and lymphocytes. No megakaryocytes were seen. The aspirate was paucicellular. There was no increase in blasts and the karyotype was normal. **B,** Three years later in the beginning of his 3rd decade, the bone marrow was hypocellular for age with increased immature precursors, dysplastic megakaryocytes and hemosiderin-laden macrophages (×500). **C,** CD34 showed increased blasts (overall 30%–40%, ×500) that had a myeloid phenotype on flow cytometry analysis *(not shown)*. **D,** CD61 demonstrated very small mononuclear dysplastic megakaryocytes and micromegakaryocytes (×1000). **E,** Bone marrow aspirate smear showed increased blasts with high N:C ratio and dispersed chromatin (×1000). **F,** Micromegakaryocyte with eccentric nucleus in center of field (×1000). Germline *GATA2* mutation was subsequently identified.

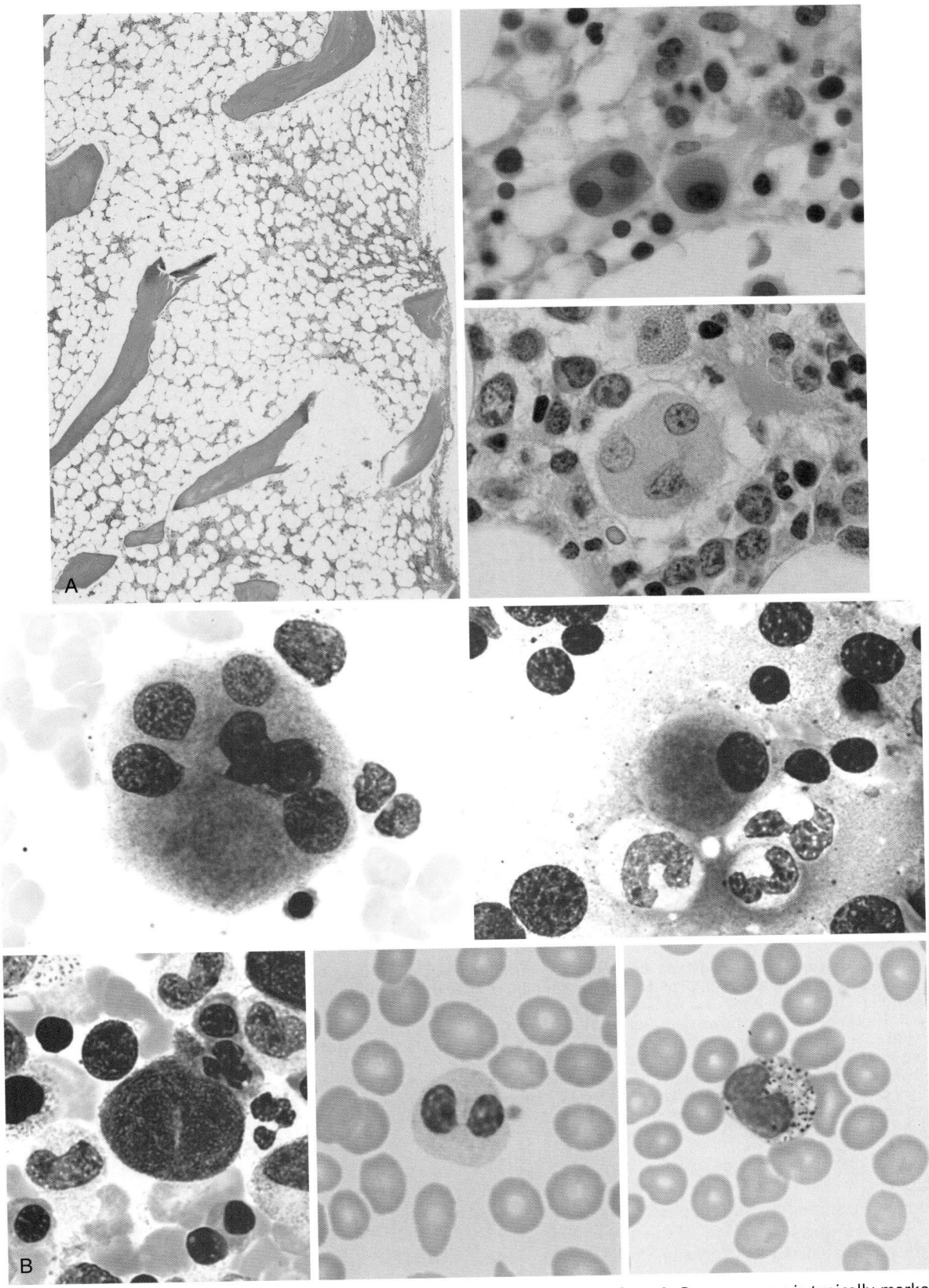

Figure 45-6. Hypoplastic MDS with multilineage dysplasia and germline *GATA2* mutation. A, Bone marrow is typically markedly hypocellular for age in a young/middle-aged adult or pediatric patient (*left panel,* ×100), with dysplastic megakaryocytes, including micromegakaryocytes and megakaryocytes with separated nuclear lobes both small and large (*right panels,* ×1000). **B,** Multilineage dysplasia is typically seen on the aspirate smear and peripheral blood (×1000 images). *Upper images:* large megakaryocyte with separated nuclear lobes *(left)* and micromegakaryocyte *(right),* bone marrow. *Lower images:* dysplastic binucleated erythroid precursor *(left)* bone marrow; dysplastic hyposegmented and hypogranular neutrophil on peripheral smear *(middle);* and hypogranular basophil on peripheral smear *(right).*

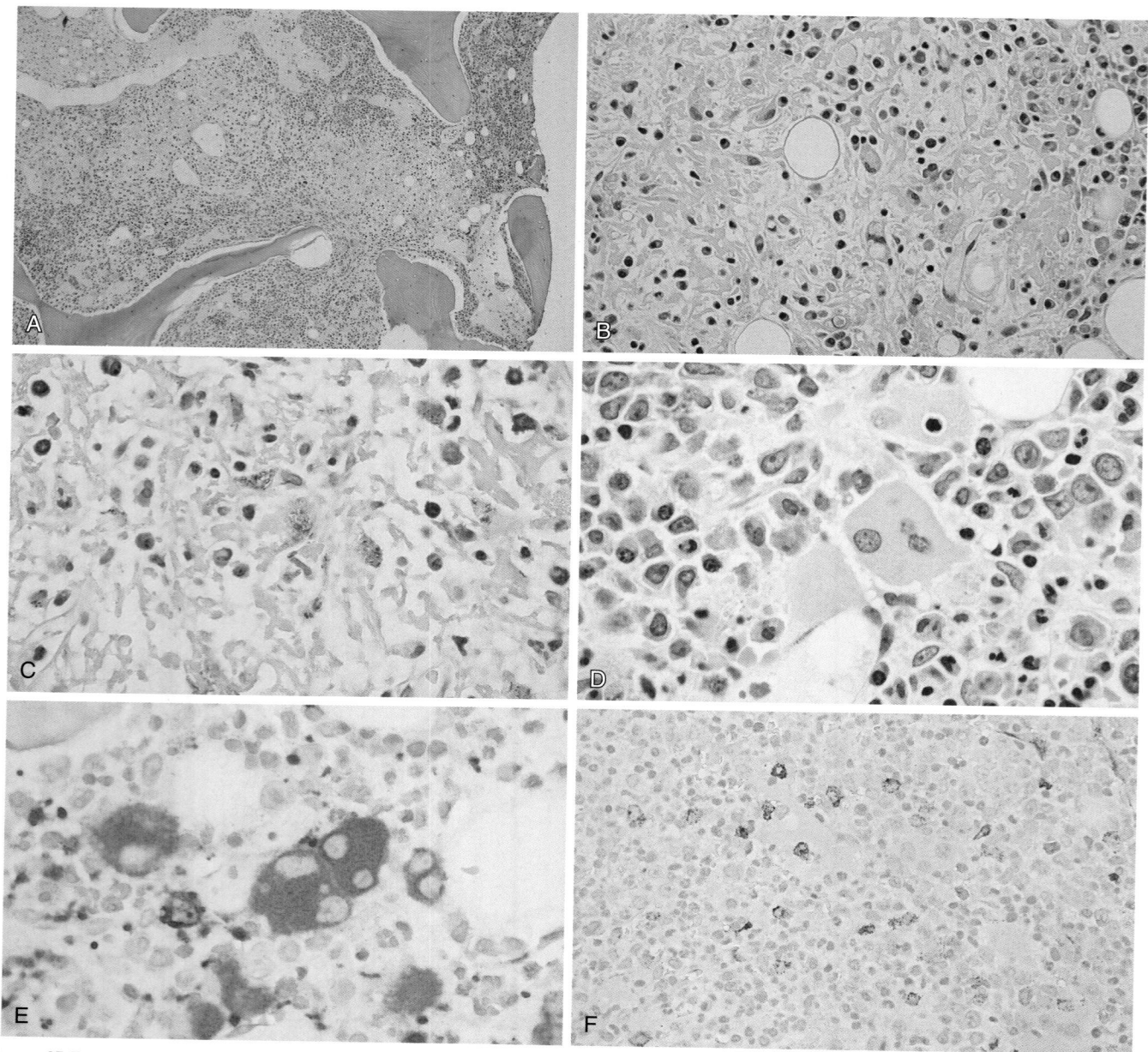

Figure 45-7. Bone marrow with coexistent disseminated nontuberculous mycobacterial infection and myelodysplastic syndrome (MDS) with excess blasts with germline *GATA2* mutation. A, Bone marrow with prominent granulomatous inflammation (×100) from a woman presenting in her 5th decade with disseminated *Mycobacterium avium* complex (MAC) and aspergillus infection diagnosed with *GATA2* deficiency. **B,** High-power view showing presence of dysplastic megakaryocytes, plasma cells, and lymphocytes. **C,** Acid-fast bacilli stain demonstrated AFB-positive organisms (×1000). **D,** Dysplastic megakaryocyte with separated nuclear lobes (×1000). **E,** CD61 immunostain highlighting megakaryocytes with separated nuclear lobes and a small mononuclear form. **F,** CD34 immunostain demonstrated increased CD34 positive cells (×500) that were overall 6% to 8% with a myeloid immunophenotype on flow cytometry analysis that also showed near absence of monocytes, plasmacytoid dendritic cells, natural killer (NK) cells, and B-cell precursors *(not shown)*. Cytogenetic analysis revealed an abnormal karyotype with trisomy 8.

include loss of chromosome 7 associated with MDS. Other more adaptive mechanisms include uniparental disomy of chromosome 7q resulting in wild-type *SAMD9* or *SAMD9L* in affected cells, or acquisition of loss-of-function mutations in *cis* to counteract the effect of the germline mutation. In some cases, monosomy 7 may be transient and associated with hematologic remission. Importantly for interpretation of NGS studies, the VAF of *SAMD9* or *SAMD9L* mutations may be lower than expected for germline mutations in hematopoietic cells because of SGR, and may confound the diagnosis. Bone

marrow evaluation typically shows a hypocellular marrow with or without dysplastic features (Fig. 45-10).

Myeloid Neoplasms Associated With Bone Marrow Failure Syndromes

Fanconi Anemia

FA is a heterogeneous genetic disorder with widely variable presentation including congenital anomalies, bone marrow failure, and nonhematologic symptoms.[90] Congenital

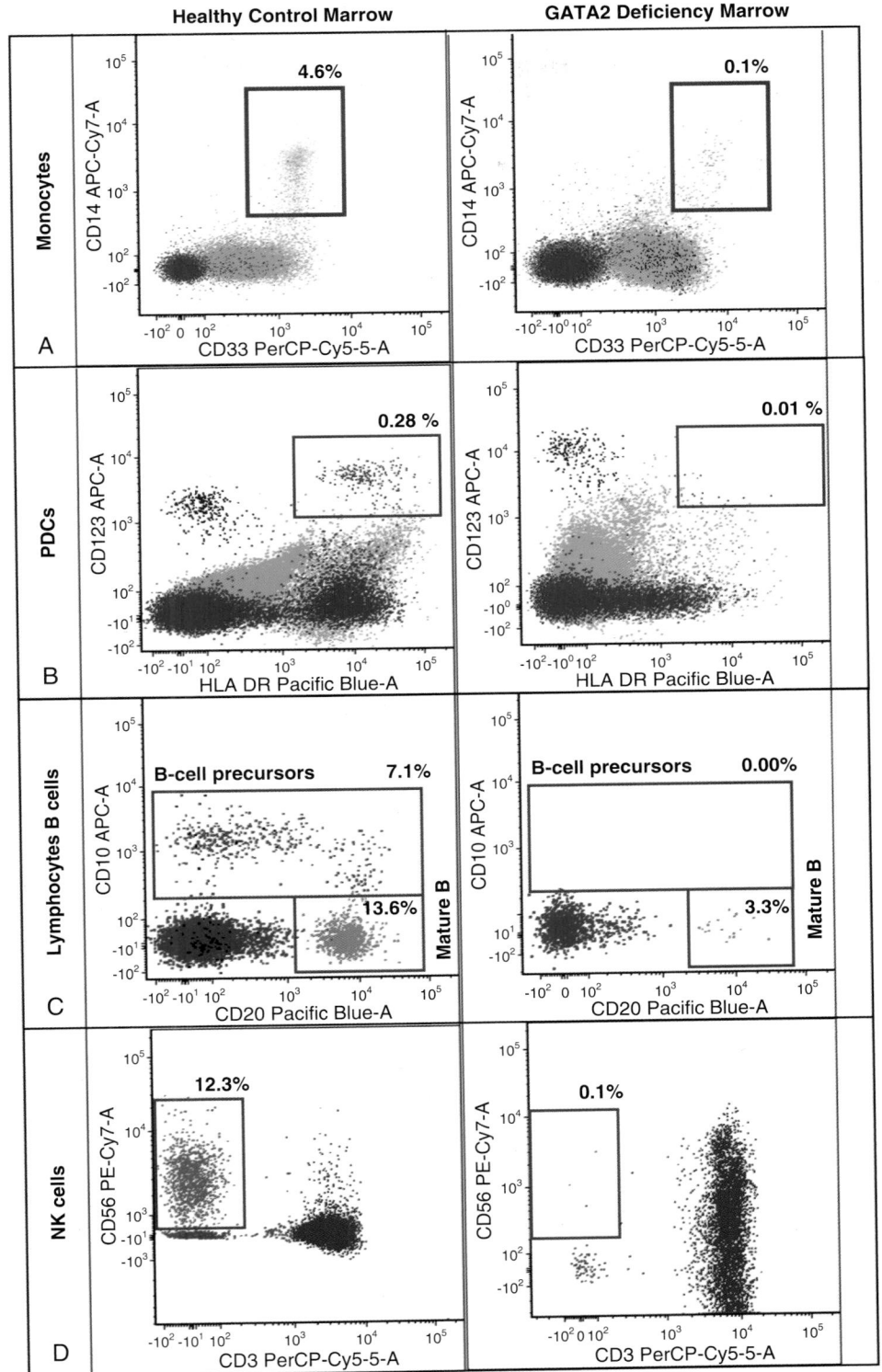

Figure 45-8. Bone marrow flow cytometry analysis may show underlying immunodeficiency in patients with germline *GATA2* mutations and bone marrow failure or myeloid malignancy. Male in his 4th decade with myelodysplastic syndrome (MDS) with multilineage dysplasia and germline *GATA2* mutation. A subset of patients with *GATA2* deficiency *(right panels)* and cytopenias show evidence of disproportionate loss of monocytes (CD14+ and CD33+) **(A)**; plasmacytoid dendritic cells (B, CD123+ and HLA-DR+) **(B)**; B-cell precursors (CD10+ lymphocytes) and mature B-cells (CD20+ and CD10– lymphocytes) **(C)**; natural killer (NK) cells (CD56+ and CD3– lymphocytes) in the bone marrow **(D)** in comparison to healthy control marrow *(left panels)*.

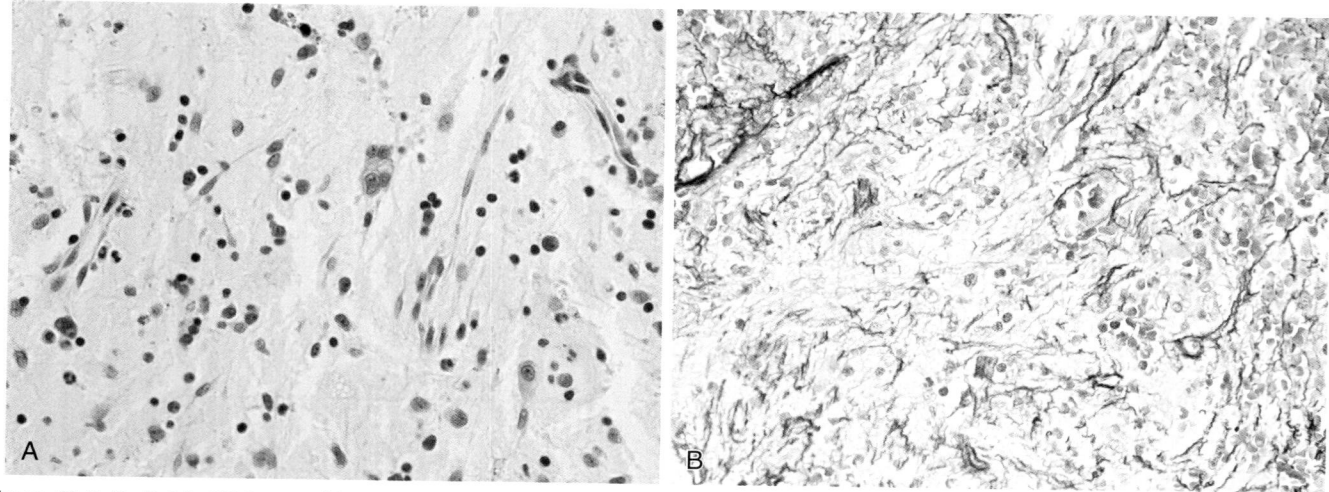

Figure 45-9. Pediatric MDS resembling atypical myelofibrosis in GATA2 deficiency. Bone marrow from pediatric male in first decade of life with history of pancytopenia, warts, and respiratory infections. Family history was significant for a sibling with MDS. **A,** Marrow shows marked cellular depletion in a fibrotic background with a few dysplastic megakaryocytes, scattered lymphocytes, and plasma cells; no increase in blasts. **B,** Reticulin stain showed evidence of reticulin fibrosis. Monosomy 7 detected. Germline *GATA2* mutation identified. The findings were consistent with MDS, not otherwise specified (NOS; ICC) or childhood MDS with low blasts (WHO, 5th ed.), with germline *GATA2* mutation.

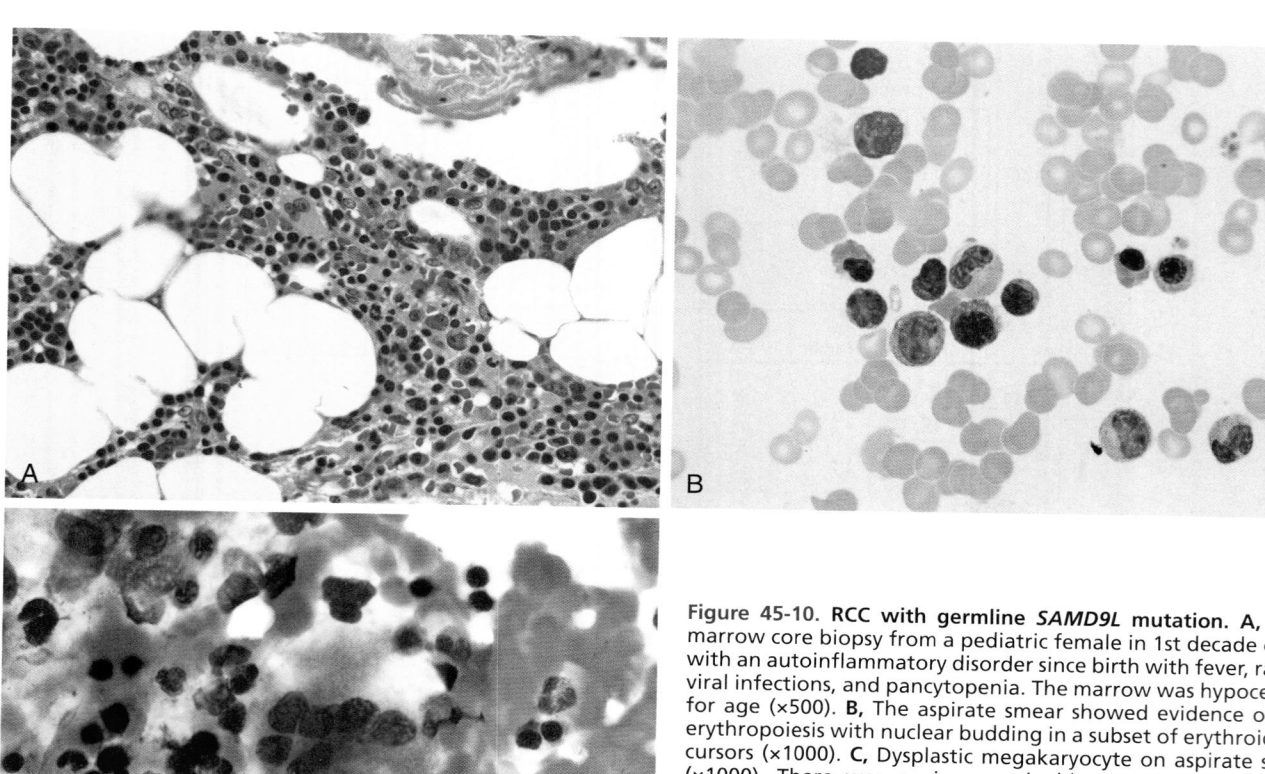

Figure 45-10. RCC with germline *SAMD9L* mutation. A, Bone marrow core biopsy from a pediatric female in 1st decade of life with an autoinflammatory disorder since birth with fever, rashes, viral infections, and pancytopenia. The marrow was hypocellular for age (×500). **B,** The aspirate smear showed evidence of dyserythropoiesis with nuclear budding in a subset of erythroid precursors (×1000). **C,** Dysplastic megakaryocyte on aspirate smear (×1000). There was no increase in blasts. Cytogenetic analysis showed an abnormal karyotype with monosomy 7 and the patient was diagnosed with refractory cytopenia of childhood (RCC; ICC). A de novo germline mutation in *SAMD9L* was identified. Unexpectedly, 6 months later the cytopenias spontaneously improved. The subsequent bone marrow biopsy/aspirate showed no overt evidence of dysplasia and the cytogenetic analysis showed a normal karyotype without monosomy 7. Evaluation of the *SAMD9L* mutation in hematopoietic cells showed evidence of somatic genetic reversion via uniparental disomy of 7q.

anomalies may include thumb and radial ray abnormalities, kidney and urinary tract malformations, café-au-lait spots, and short stature. Patients may present at any age including adulthood, though typical age of presentation is between 5 and 10 years of age. Diagnosing FA requires a high index of suspicion owing to the diversity of symptoms and similarities between FA and other syndromes.[91] FA is likely underdiagnosed; it is occasionally recognized in adults who develop unusual cancers or toxicities upon anticancer treatment. FA is caused by germline mutations in one of multiple FA genes, and mutations may involve any of 23 genes and are mostly autosomal recessive with some rare X-linked recessive or autosomal dominant subtypes. The cumulative incidence of BMF varies from 18% to 83% depending on the risk groups.[92] The cumulative incidence of AML at age 40 years is estimated at 15% to 20%, while the incidence of MDS at age 50 years is 40%.[93] The relative risk of AML is increased 700-fold in comparison with the general population and that of MDS is increased 6000-fold.[94] AML is particularly more frequent in FANCD1/BRCA2 group. Chromosomal aberration involving chromosome 7, including –7/–7q, is significantly correlated with more advanced dysplasia and commonly part of a clone with a more complex karyotype that frequently also shows gain of 3q material.[92] Sequential analysis of clonal progression in FA has revealed that 3q-gains often precede changes involving partial or whole loss of chromosome 7.[92] The emergence of monosomy 7 in FA is associated with poorer prognosis and increased risk of developing MDS and AML.[95] Patients with FA may also present with T-ALL and are also at risk for solid tumors, particularly squamous cell carcinomas of the head, neck, gastrointestinal (GI) tract, vulva, and hepatic tumors. In a family study of FA, heterozygous mutations in *FANCA* or *FANCC* were not associated with increased cancer risk; because of small numbers, other FA genotypes could not be assessed. Microscopic examination of a bone marrow biopsy shows hypoplasia and hypocellularity. Hypocellularity is often out of proportion of cytopenias. In some cases, erythroid hyperplasia and dysplasia are also present. Bone marrow evaluation every year starting in early childhood is used to screen for early evidence of MDS (Fig. 45-11) or AML before clinical symptoms occur. Therapy for AML in FA is challenging given the hypersensitivity of patients' cells to cytotoxic chemotherapeutics used to treat routine de novo AML; reduced-intensity chemotherapy leading to HSCT is recommended.

Shwachman-Diamond Syndrome

Shwachman-Diamond syndrome (SDS) is a multisystem disorder that is characterized by BMF, exocrine pancreatic dysfunction, and predisposition to myeloid malignancies. SDS is caused by biallelic or homozygous variants in the gene *SBDS* encoding Shwachman Bodian-Diamond syndrome protein that account for >90% of cases of SDS.[96] Classically, SDS presents in infancy or early childhood with failure to thrive, steatorrhea, recurrent infections, or growth retardation; nearly all affected children have intermittent or persistent neutropenia at presentation. In a case series that included 129 patients in 116 SDS families who were diagnosed clinically (before the widespread availability of genetic testing), the median age at diagnosis was 1 year (and ranged from 0.1 to 13 years).[97] Although SDS patients typically present with neutropenia as

their initial hematologic finding, other cytopenias may present in any lineage either singly or in combination.[98] Cytopenias may be mild or absent; however, patients remain at risk for myeloid malignancies even if cytopenias were previously asymptomatic.[99] At baseline, the marrow is typically hypocellular even if blood counts are normal. Myeloid dysplasia such as nuclear hyposegmentation and hypogranularity are common, and mild megakaryocytic dysplasia may be present. Erythroid dysplasia is typically absent at baseline.[99]

Clonal cytogenic abnormalities involving i(7q) and del(20q) are reported in patients with SDS but are not associated with progression to malignancy.[100] The risk of worsening cytopenia(s), clonal myeloid evolution, or AML is estimated at 20% and typically occurs by age 18.[101] The Severe Chronic Neutropenia International Registry reported a 1% per year progression rate to MDS/AML in patients with SDS, with a cumulative risk of MDS/AML reaching 36% by 30 years of age.[102] Small stable clones with heterozygous *TP53* mutations are common in patients with SDS; however, biallelic *TP53* mutations were observed in myeloid malignancies and may be present prior to the development of overt malignancy.[103]

Telomere Biology Disorders Including Dyskeratosis Congenita

Dyskeratosis congenita (DC) is an inherited BMF syndrome characterized by abnormal skin pigmentation, nail dystrophy, oral premalignant leukoplakia, BMF, and cancer predisposition, with increased risk for squamous cell carcinoma and hematolymphoid neoplasms. DC and telomere biology disorders (TBD) are a spectrum of disorders caused by pathogenic germline variants in telomere biology genes. Although germline mutations in *DKC1* are classically associated with triad of dysplastic nails, reticular skin pigmentation, and oral leukoplakia, a large subset of patients lack these findings at diagnosis.[104] DC is heterogeneous at the genetic level, depending on the affected gene and can be inherited in X-linked (*DKC1*), autosomal dominant (*TERC, TINF2, ZCCHC8, RPA1, NAF1*), autosomal recessive (*CTC1, NHP2, NOP10, POT1, STN1, WRAP53*), or both autosomal dominant and autosomal recessive patterns (*PARN, RTEL1, TERT*).[105] Mutations in at least 16 telomere- and telomerase-associated genes have been linked to DC, although the genetic basis of the disease is still undetectable in approximately 30% to 40% of DC cases.[106] DC is a disease of defective telomere maintenance, and patients with DC have premature telomere shortening and subsequent replicative senescence, leading to premature stem cell exhaustion and tissue failure. The BM findings in DC are variable and range from normal to different severity of aplasia depending on the stage of the disease. Sometimes it is indistinguishable from aplastic anemia caused by other causes.[107] Fetal hemoglobin levels are increased. NCI cohort of 197 DC patients found a cumulative incidence of cancer of 2% by age 50 years for leukemia and 11% by age 50 years for solid cancers.[108] Patients with autosomal dominant mutations in *TERT* or *TERC* may display variable penetrance and present in adulthood with pulmonary fibrosis, hepatic cirrhosis, and early graying of the hair.[109] Bone marrow is typically hypocellular with diminished hematopoietic progenitors (Fig. 45-12).[109]

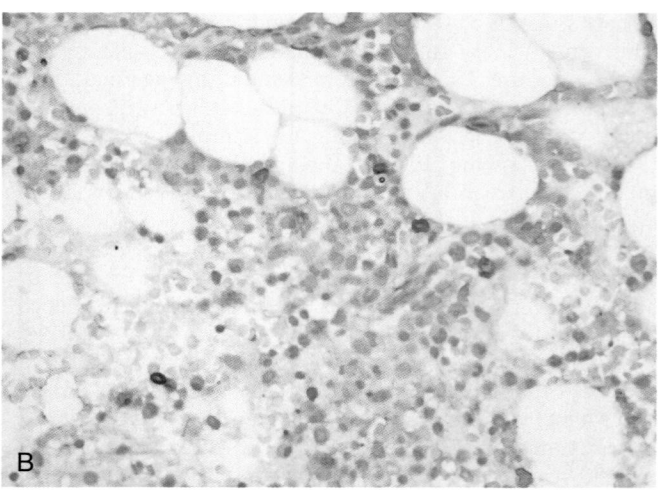

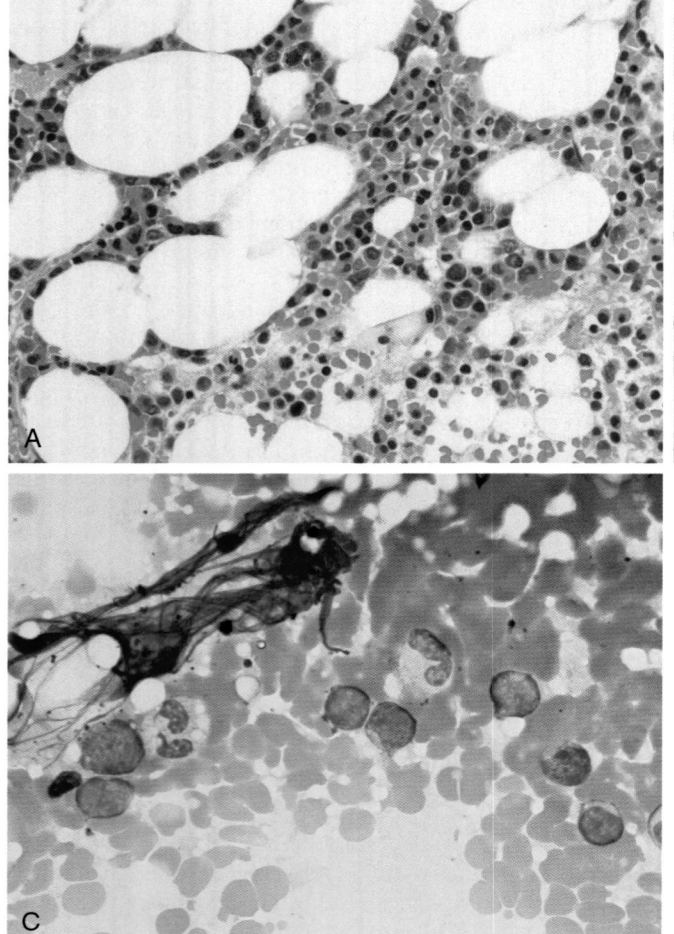

Figure 45-11. Refractory cytopenia of childhood (RCC) with monosomy 7 in Fanconi anemia. A, Bone marrow from young female in 1st decade of life with history of Fanconi anemia. The marrow is hypocellular for age with trilineage hypoplasia and scattered hemosiderin laden macrophages reflecting history of transfusions. Megakaryocytes were essentially absent confirmed by CD61 stain *(not shown)*. **B,** CD34 immunostain showed few scattered positive cells consistent with blasts that were less than 5%. Flow cytometry analysis demonstrated lack of hematogones suggesting that nearly all the CD34-positive cells were myeloid. **C,** Touch prep of the biopsy showed areas with left-shifted myeloid cells and blasts. Cytogenetic analysis revealed an abnormal karyotype with monosomy 7 that was not detected on prior analysis.

Severe Congenital Neutropenia

Severe congenital neutropenia (SCN) is a genetically heterogeneous condition of BMF usually diagnosed in early childhood and characterized by a chronic and severe shortage of neutrophils that manifest early in infancy with absolute neutrophil count (ANC) below 0.5 × 10⁹/L, leading to life-threatening bacterial infections. Patients are highly susceptible to bacterial infections, with infections by *Staphylococcus aureus* and gram-negative bacteria being the most life-threatening. It is now well-established that mutations in autosomal dominant mutations in *ELANE* the gene-encoding neutrophil elastase, as well as *HAX1* and other genes (*CSF3R, GFI1, G6PC3, JAGN1, WAS*), are the most frequently observed genetic defects in SCN patients. At baseline, the marrow for *ELANE*-mutant SCN is mostly normocellular and classically shows early myeloid maturation arrest at the promyelocyte stage.[110]

Up to 40% of patients with SCN may develop clonal hematopoiesis with acquired mutations in *CSF3R*. These clones may persist for months or even years without progressing to malignancy. Importantly, SCN patients have a high risk of developing MDS or AML, with a median incidence of ~20%, 15 years after initiation of granulocyte colony stimulating factor (GCSF) treatment.[111,112] The majority of SCN patients with leukemic progression show the appearance of hematopoietic clones with somatic mutations in *CSF3R*, resulting in a truncated form of CSF3R with defective internalization and aberrant signaling properties,[113] and somatic mutations in *RUNX1*.[110]

Diamond Blackfan Anemia

Diamond-Blackfan anemia (DBA) is inherited pure red blood cell aplasia typically caused by pathogenic autosomal dominant variants in genes encoding ribosomal proteins (*RPS19, RPS17, RPS24, RPL35A, RPL5, RPL11, RPS7, RPS26, RPS10*) and is a genetically and clinically heterogeneous disorder characterized by erythroid failure, congenital anomalies, and a predisposition to cancer. The molecular biology of DBA is being extensively explored and, in more than 50% of cases, the syndrome appears to result from haploinsufficiency of either a small or large subunit-associated ribosomal protein.[114] X-linked mutations in GATA1 also cause a DBA phenotype. DBA is often associated with congenital anomalies, particularly abnormalities of the thumbs, facial features, kidneys, heart, and short stature. The classic presentation of DBA includes a usually macrocytic, or occasionally normocytic, anemia with reticulocytopenia, essentially normal neutrophil and platelet counts, and a normocellular

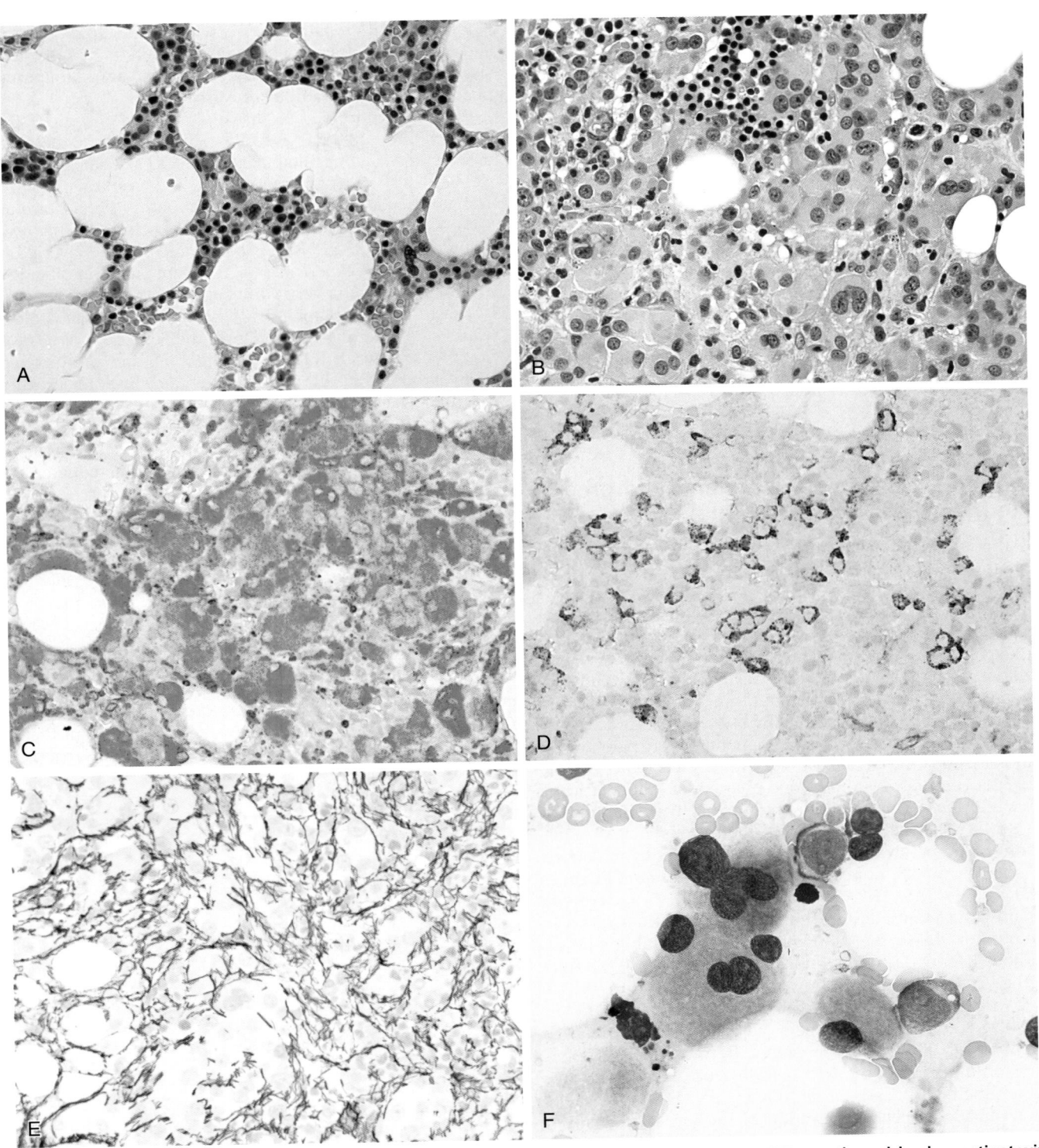

Figure 45-12. Myelodysplastic syndrome (MDS)/acute myeloid leukemia (AML; ICC) with germline *TERT* mutation arising in a patient with prior history of aplastic anemia. A, Bone marrow core biopsy from a male in his 6th decade with a history of pulmonary fibrosis, early graying of the hair, and moderate pancytopenia. The biopsy showed a hypocellular marrow for age with decreased trilineage hematopoiesis with a few small hypolobated megakaryocytes, but without overt dysplasia in more than 10% of cells in any lineage, and no increase in blasts (×500). Cytogenetic analysis revealed a normal karyotype, and the patient was diagnosed with moderately severe aplastic anemia. Flow fluorescence in situ hybridization (FISH) showed very short telomeres. Genetic studies identified a germline *TERT* mutation. **B,** Six years later, there was a significant drop in the patient's peripheral blood counts. Bone marrow biopsy showed a markedly hypercellular marrow with sheets of dysplastic megakaryocytes (×500). **C,** Dysplastic megakaryocytes highlighted by CD61 immunostain. **D,** CD34-stained increased blasts with clustering overall 15% to 19%. The blasts were of myeloid on flow cytometric analysis *(not shown)*. **E,** Reticulin stain showing marked reticulin fibrosis in the areas of dysplastic megakaryocytes. **F,** Aspirate smear showing dysplastic megakaryocytes and a few blasts (×1000). Cytogenetic analysis showed trisomy 8 and duplication of 1q MDS/AML (ICC).

bone marrow with a paucity of erythroid precursors in a child younger than 1 year, but patients may present in adulthood.[115] In addition to macrocytosis, the presence of elevated fetal hemoglobin levels (HbF) and an elevation in erythrocyte adenosine deaminase enzyme (eADA) activity are important supporting features associated with DBA. The presence of macrocytosis and elevated HbF, each felt to be a consequence of "stress erythropoiesis" and skipped erythroid cell divisions, is not unique to DBA but is observed in many incidences of BMF. Patients appear to be at an increased risk of cancer; the two most prevalent solid tumors are colorectal cancer and osteogenic sarcoma.[116] There is also some increased risk of myeloid malignancy.[117] The bone marrow is usually normocellular or slightly hypocellular and shows a characteristic of erythroblastopenia with normal granulocytic and megakaryocytic lineages.[118]

Juvenile Myelomonocytic Leukemia Associated With Neurofibromatosis, Noonan Syndrome, or Noonan-Syndrome-Like Disorders (CBL-Syndrome)

JMML is an MDS/myeloproliferative neoplasm (MPN) overlap syndrome of the pediatric age group characterized by sustained, abnormal, and excessive production of myeloid progenitors and monocytes, aggressive clinical course, and poor outcomes. JMML accounts for 1% of all pediatric leukemias, with an incidence of about 1.2 cases per million persons per year.[119] The median age at which it is diagnosed is 2 years old, and about three-fourths of cases are diagnosed before 3 years of age; by 6 years, 95% of cases are detected. Patients present with splenomegaly, hepatomegaly, lymphadenopathy, enlarged tonsils, interstitial lung disease, and gut infiltrates. About one-quarter of patients have leukemic skin lesions. The common molecular denominator of JMML is the deregulation of the intracellular RAS signal transduction pathway, caused in >90% of cases by mutations in one (or, rarely, more than one) of five primordial genes (PTPN11, NRAS, KRAS, NF1, or CBL).[120] Karyotype abnormalities and additional epigenetic alterations can also be found in JMML. Neoplasms in children resembling JMML without RAS-pathway mutations are classified as JMML-like in the ICC.[5,6]

Two congenital developmental disorders predispose to JMML: Neurofibromatosis type 1 (NF1) and Casitas B-lineage lymphoma (CBL) syndrome caused by monoallelic loss-of-function mutation of the NF1 or CBL gene, which may have been inherited or arisen de novo.[121,122] JMML develops after somatic biallelic inactivation of the respective gene in hematopoietic progenitor cells, predominantly by mitotic gene recombination resulting in uniparental isodisomy.[123,124] Overall, 10% to 15% of JMML cases are driven by NF1, and indicative features in children with JMML/NF1 include presence of ≥6 cutaneous café-au-lait spots or family history, neurofibromas, optic pathway gliomas, bone lesions, and neurologic abnormalities.[125] NF1 functions as a Ras-GAP and thus negatively regulates the RAS pathway.[126] CBL is a E3 ubiquitin ligase mediating the decay of receptor tyrosine kinases in the RAS pathway. Mutations targeting exons 8 or 9 account for ~15% of JMML cases.[127] CBL syndrome, a

Noonan-like RASopathy, has a wide phenotypic spectrum and presenting features including impaired growth, facial anomalies, developmental delay, cryptorchidism, autoimmune phenomena, and notably, neurovasculitis.[124]

Noonan syndrome (NS) has an incidence of 1 in 1000 to 2500 children; patients with NS exhibit a short statue, facial dysmorphism, congenital heart defects, skeletal defects, a webbed neck, mental retardation, and cryptorchidism.[128] The genetic basis is a germline mutation in PTPN11 (around 50% of NS cases), and other members of the RAS pathway include SOS1, RAF1, KRAS, BRAF, and NRAS.[129] Children with NS may experience a transient myeloproliferative disorder (MPD) at a very young age, although the condition is indistinguishable from JMML by clinical and hematologic features.[130] There is an overlap in the landscape of PTPN11 mutations between JMML and NS/MPD, and it is not well understood how the same mutation elicits a transient disorder when present in the germline and a fatal disorder when acquired somatically. The occurrence of germline and somatic RAS pathway mutations in the same clinical context requires analysis of nonhematopoietic to differentiate these conditions.

Diagnostic criteria for JMML is listed in Chapter 48. Leukocytosis is usually present, but occasionally, the WBC is within the normal range.[131] There is monocytosis, often with dysplastic forms, and a monocyte count typically >1 × 10⁹/L. Presence of myeloid and often erythroid precursors is a consistent feature of JMML. Thrombocytopenia is often present with the exception of cases of NF1-associated JMML, who mostly have platelet counts within the normal range.[131] The bone marrow is hypercellular with myeloid cell predominance and reduced megakaryocytes, and the monocytic compartment is generally less prominent than in peripheral blood. The blast percentage must be less than 20%.

Myeloid or Lymphoid Neoplasms Associated With Down Syndrome

Down syndrome (DS) is the most common chromosomal abnormality among live-born infants. DS manifests as a developmental delay with a characteristic spectrum of congenital malformations, which may include the heart, gastrointestinal, musculoskeletal, and complications in other organ systems. Hematologic abnormalities are common in children with DS. Among other hematologic disorders, neonates with DS may exhibit transient abnormal myelopoiesis (TAM), a preleukemic condition that is unique to infants with DS or mosaic trisomy 21. In most cases, TAM regresses spontaneously, however one-quarter of these children will go on to develop acute leukemia or myelodysplastic syndrome. Acute lymphoblastic leukemia in DS shares genetic features with that occurring in non-DS patients, but with a different distribution of genotypes including a lower level of good-risk subtypes.[132] Myeloid leukemia associated with DS (ML-DS) is a unique form of childhood leukemia that arises before age 4 years in a child with DS and is estimated at 3-fold to 400-fold that of AML in the general pediatric population.[133] The clinical presentation, pathogenesis, response to treatment, and excellent prognosis distinguish ML-DS from other acute leukemias in children.[134] ML-DS is usually manifest as acute megakaryocytic leukemia, and diagnosis often follows a MDS-like phase with prolonged cytopenias. ML-DS can arise in a child with a history of TAM, but most cases develop in children who were not documented to have TAM. Blasts in TAM and ML-DS patients have overlapping immunophenotypes, including the presence of CD33, CD36, CD48, and the TPO-R, and frequently the megakaryocytic markers CD41, CD42b, and CD61.[135]

Acquired mutations in megakaryocyte transcription factor gene *GATA1* have recently been reported in DS, TAM, and acute megakaryoblastic leukemia.[136] *GATA1* is an essential regulator of numerous hematopoietic lineages, including red blood cells and megakaryocytes.[137] Recent sequencing studies have demonstrated that TAM is driven by the combination of a *GATA1* mutation and trisomy 21 without the need for additional genetic alterations.[138] However, after TAM has resolved, any remaining disease-driving clones can acquire a third hit that leads to development of ML-DS. The most common additional acquired molecular abnormalities are acquired loss-of-function mutations of cohesin complex or epigenetic regulators and gain-of-function mutations of signal transducers or components of the RAS signaling pathway.[135,138,139]

ACUTE LYMPHOBLASTIC LEUKEMIA WITH GERMLINE PREDISPOSITION

Germline mutations in aforementioned *TP53*, *ETV6*, and Down syndrome predispose to both myeloid neoplasms and B-ALL. Predisposition to B-ALL is also associated with ataxia telangiectasia, Nijmegen breakage syndrome, and constitutional Robertsonian translocation. Two genes that are critical for B-cell development, *PAX5* and *IKZF1*, have been shown to predispose to familial B-ALL when mutated in the germline.

Acute Lymphoblastic Leukemia With Germline *PAX5* Mutation

PAX5 is located on chromosome 9p13 and is required for normal B-cell development.[140] *PAX5* is commonly mutated in sporadic B-ALL via translocations, copy number alterations, or missense variants involving the DNA binding domain, resulting in loss of function and maturation arrest of B-cell progenitors.[141] Several families with increased B-ALL were shown to harbor germline mutations in *PAX5*, primarily involving a conserved residue in the octapeptide domain of the protein p.G183S,[142,143] but other mutations have also been reported, including R38H.[144] Notably, the development of B-ALL in these families was associated with loss of the wild-type copy of *PAX5* via deletion of chromosome 9p, formation of iso or dicentric 9q, or other mechanisms leading to biallelic inactivation of the gene. Not all family members with germline pathogenic *PAX5* mutations develop B-ALL, indicating that penetrance is incomplete. Donor-derived B-ALL has occurred in patients posttransplant who were inadvertently transplanted using healthy related donors who also harbored the germline mutation,[144] underscoring the importance of recognizing patients who may have germline mutations. The bone marrow morphology and immunophenotype of the B-ALL blasts is similar to that seen in sporadic B-ALL. The prevalence of germline *PAX5* mutations is not currently defined.

Acute Lymphoblastic Leukemia With Germline *IKZF1* Mutation

IKZF1 is located on chromosome 7p12.2 and encodes the transcription factor Ikaros, which plays an important role in lymphoid development.[145] Somatic mutations in *IKZF1*, resulting in loss of function, have been identified in sporadic B-ALL, and in particular BCR-ABL+ B-ALL.[146] Germline mutations in *IKZF1* were later found in families with hypogammaglobulinemia and common variable immunodeficiency with B lymphopenia, and were associated with an increased risk of B-ALL.[147,148] The prevalence is not yet known; however, up to 1% of presumed sporadic B-ALL cases have predicted pathogenic germline variants in *IKZF1*.[148]

Pearls and Pitfalls

Germline predisposition to hematologic malignancy (HM) is more common than previously thought and should be considered:

- Patients with a family history of cancer
- Young age at HM diagnosis (<40 years of age); caveat: *DDX41* mutations associated with HM presentation in older age range overlapping with sporadic HM
- Patients with HM and high variant allele frequency (VAF) mutation in a germline predisposition gene detected on next-generation sequencing (NGS) targeted panel
- Persistence of high VAF mutation in a germline predisposition gene after chemotherapy
- Presence of syndromic or unique features:
  - Telomere biology:
    - Early graying of hair, pulmonary/hepatic fibrosis
    - *DKC1*: dystrophic nails, leukoplakia, hypopigmented skin patches
  - GATA2 deficiency
    - Immunodeficiency: loss of monocytes, B cells, natural killer (NK) cells, dendritic cells
    - Lymphedema
    - Monosomy 7, trisomy 8 or der (1;7)(q10;p10), *ASXL1* and *STAG2* mutations
  - *RUNX1, ANKRD26, ETV6*
    - Thrombocytopenia since early age/birth
    - Patients may be misdiagnosed with immune thrombocytopenic purpura (ITP)
    - Dysmegakaryopoiesis is common at baseline in the bone marrow and is not sufficient for a diagnosis of myelodysplastic syndrome (MDS) in the absence of other supporting criteria
  - *SAMD9/SAMD9L*
    - Monosomy 7 is common and may lead to lower VAF of mutation as *SAMD9* and *SAMD9L* are located on chromosome 7
    - Somatic genetic rescue (SGR) via uniparental disomy in hematopoietic cells is common
  - Shwachman-Diamond syndrome
    - *TP53* mutations common, biallelic *TP53* mutations associated with HM
- Syndromic features may not be present
- Penetrance may be highly variable even within family members harboring the same mutation
- Patients with de novo germline mutations typically have no family history of disease
- Gold-standard tissue source for germline testing is cultured skin fibroblasts. Other tissue sources are less optimal. Buccal swabs may contain contamination with hematopoietic cells, making it difficult to distinguish germline mutations from somatic mutations. DNA yield from hair follicles may be low. Nail clippings may be contaminated with monocytes.

KEY REFERENCES

5. Arber DA, Orazi A, Hasserjian RP, et al. International consensus classification of myeloid neoplasms and acute leukemias: integrating morphologic, clinical, and genomic data. *Blood*. 2022;140(11):1200–1228.

6. Rudelius M, Weinberg OK, Niemeyer CM, Shimamura A, Calvo KR. The International Consensus Classification (ICC) of hematologic neoplasms with germline predisposition, pediatric myelodysplastic syndrome, and juvenile myelomonocytic leukemia. *Virchows Arch*. 2023;482(1):113–130.

7. Khoury JD, Solary E, Abla O, et al. The 5th Edition of the World Health Organization Classification of Haematolymphoid Tumours: myeloid and histiocytic/dendritic neoplasms. *Leukemia*. 2022;36(7):1703–1719.

20. Smith ML, Cavenagh JD, Lister TA, Fitzgibbon J. Mutation of CEBPA in familial acute myeloid leukemia. *N Engl J Med*. 2004;351(23):2403–2407.

26. Polprasert C, Schulze I, Sekeres MA, et al. Inherited and somatic defects in DDX41 in myeloid neoplasms. *Cancer Cell*. 2015;27(5):658–670.

35. Malkin D, Li FP, Strong LC, et al. Germ line p53 mutations in a familial syndrome of breast cancer, sarcomas, and other neoplasms. *Science*. 1990;250(4985):1233–1238.

45. Kanagal-Shamanna R, Loghavi S, DiNardo CD, et al. Bone marrow pathologic abnormalities in familial platelet disorder with propensity for myeloid malignancy and germline RUNX1 mutation. *Haematologica*. 2017;102(10):1661–1670.

53. Noris P, Favier R, Alessi MC, et al. ANKRD26-related thrombocytopenia and myeloid malignancies. *Blood*. 2013;122(11):1987–1989.

55. Noetzli L, Lo RW, Lee-Sherick AB, et al. Germline mutations in ETV6 are associated with thrombocytopenia, red cell macrocytosis and predisposition to lymphoblastic leukemia. *Nat Genet*. 2015;47(5):535–538.

67. Spinner MA, Sanchez LA, Hsu AP, et al. GATA2 deficiency: a protean disorder of hematopoiesis, lymphatics, and immunity. *Blood*. 2014;123(6):809–821.

75. Calvo KR, Hickstein DD. The spectrum of GATA2 deficiency syndrome. *Blood*. 2023;141(13):1524–1532.

88. Sahoo SS, Pastor VB, Goodings C, et al. Clinical evolution, genetic landscape and trajectories of clonal hematopoiesis in SAMD9/SAMD9L syndromes. *Nat Med*. 2021;27(10):1806–1817.

Visit Elsevier eBooks+ for the complete set of references.

Acute Myeloid Leukemia

Daniel A. Arber

Acute myeloid leukemia (AML) is a heterogeneous group of diseases representing clonal proliferations of immature, nonlymphoid, bone marrow–derived cells termed *blasts* that most often involve the bone marrow and peripheral blood and may present in extramedullary tissues. If untreated, AML follows an aggressive clinical course. AML has traditionally been differentiated from other myeloid neoplasms on the basis of a minimum blast cell count in bone marrow or peripheral blood. Although this remains the case for some disease types,

several specific AML types are now defined even in the presence of a relatively low blast cell count.

The French American-British Cooperative Group (FAB) described a number of AML subtypes based originally on morphologic and cytochemical features; other studies, including immunophenotyping and electron microscopy, were added later as defining features of some subtypes.[1-4] The FAB classification defined all AML types as proliferations of 30% or more marrow blasts of either all bone marrow cells or all marrow nonerythroid progenitor cells. Although other classification systems were subsequently proposed to incorporate more comprehensive immunophenotyping studies, cytogenetic studies, and combinations of these two ancillary testing methods,[5-8] the FAB classification remained the primary system used by most pathologists and hematologists for many years. The terminology of the FAB classification continues to be used, but this system is now considered obsolete owing to its inability to accurately identify many prognostically significant disease types.

The 2001 3rd ed. World Health Organization (WHO) classification of AML incorporated findings not included in the FAB classification, including the significance of therapy-related disease, the significance of recurring cytogenetic abnormalities, and the possible significance of multilineage dysplasia in non–blast cells in AML.[9] These changes partially addressed the concepts of de novo AML versus myelodysplasia-related AML proposed by Head.[10] The 2016 revised 4th ed. WHO classification of AML further expanded and refined the categories first introduced in 2001 and expanded in 2008.[11] In 2022, the International Consensus Classification (ICC) of AML further expanded genetically defined disease groups (Box 46-1).[12] Though a proposed WHO 5th ed. classification was published in 2022,[13] many details of that classification remain undefined at the time of the update of this chapter. The ICC approach will be the major focus of this chapter with attempts to correlate the disease categories with what appears to be proposed in the upcoming WHO 5th ed. classification.

SYNONYMS AND RELATED TERMS

None.

EPIDEMIOLOGY

The incidence of AML is approximately 3.5 cases per 100,000 per year. The median age at diagnosis is 67 years, and there is a slight male predominance. The frequency of AML increases with age; approximately 6% of cases occur in children and adults younger than 20 years, and more than 50% of cases occur in patients 65 years of age and older.[14]

ETIOLOGY

The cause of many cases of AML is unknown, particularly those arising in children and young adults. A subset of AML arises from a preexisting myelodysplastic syndrome (MDS) or is a secondary leukemia related to prior therapy for a nonleukemic disorder. AML occurs more commonly in patients with preexisting genetic predisposition syndromes or genetic disorders, including Fanconi's anemia and Down syndrome, and familial cases of AML are now increasingly recognized even in the adult population.[15]

CLINICAL FEATURES

Patients with AML usually are seen with symptoms related to anemia and thrombocytopenia, including fatigue and bleeding, and symptoms related to white blood cell dysfunction, especially infections. They may also have extramedullary tumor proliferations, which appear to be more common in childhood AML.

Box 46-1 *Classification of Acute Myeloid Leukemia*

Acute Myeloid Leukemias
Acute promyelocytic leukemia (APL) with t(15;17)
  (q24.1;q21.2)/*PML::RARA*
APL with other *RARA* rearrangements
Acute myeloid leukemia (AML) with t(8;21)(q22;q22.1)/
  RUNX1::RUNX1T1
AML with inv(16)(p13.1q22) or t(16;16)(p13.1;q22)/*CBFB::MYH11*
AML with t(9;11)(p21.3;q23.3)/*MLLT3::KMT2A*
AML with other *KMT2A* rearrangements
AML with t(6;9)(p22.3;q34.1)/*DEK::NUP214*
AML with inv(3)(q21.3q26.2) or t(3;3)(q21.3;q26.2)/*GATA2;*
  MECOM(EVI1)
AML with other *MECOM* rearrangements
AML with other rare recurring translocations
AML with t(9;22)(q34.1;q11.2)/*BCR::ABL1*
AML with mutated *NPM1*
AML with in-frame bZIP *CEBPA* mutations
AML and MDS/AML with mutated *TP53*
AML and MDS/AML with myelodysplasia-related gene mutations
AML and MDS/AML with myelodysplasia-related cytogenetic
  abnormalities
AML and MDS/AML not otherwise specified (NOS)
Myeloid sarcoma

Myeloid Proliferations Associated With Down Syndrome

International Consensus Classification, 2022.

MORPHOLOGY

Most cases of AML have increased bone marrow myeloblasts, which may also be present in the peripheral blood. A variety of blast cell changes may be present, and some are suggestive of specific AML types; however, some general blast cell features occur in most types. For instance, blasts have immature nuclear chromatin, characterized by a lack of chromatin clumping and the presence of nucleoli. Myeloblast nuclei may be round or have nuclear invaginations. Variable numbers of cytoplasmic granules may be present in myeloblasts, but such granules identified on Wright-stained smears are not lineage specific. The presence of coalesced granules that form rod-shaped cytoplasmic bodies (Auer rods) is considered specific for myeloid lineage. Monoblasts may range from cells with round nuclei and moderate basophilic cytoplasm, with or without vacuoles, to more intermediate cells (promonocytes) with similar immature nuclear chromatin but more folded nuclear features, similar to mature monocytes. The morphologic features of non–blast cell elements of the blood and marrow are also markers of potential genetic abnormalities and are discussed in more detail under the specific disease types.

CYTOCHEMISTRY

Cytochemical studies were used extensively in the past to assign lineage to acute leukemias and to subclassify AML in the FAB classification. These studies have now been largely supplanted by immunophenotyping and are no longer necessary for the diagnosis of most cases of AML. However, a limited cytochemical panel of myeloperoxidase (or Sudan black B for older smears) and non-specific esterase can be helpful in selected cases. A very strong myeloperoxidase cytochemical reaction may be useful in distinguishing acute promyelocytic leukemia (APL) from monocytic leukemia, and cytochemical studies can be helpful in subclassifying cases of AML, not otherwise specified (AML, NOS).

IMMUNOPHENOTYPE

Immunophenotyping studies are now performed in all cases of acute leukemia to distinguish myeloid from lymphoblastic lineage and to identify acute leukemias of ambiguous lineage. Multiparameter flow cytometric methods with CD45/side scatter gating are preferred because of the large number of antigens that can be studied quickly with this method.[16,17] Immunophenotyping studies are often helpful in subclassifying the various types of AML.[18] The specific features of each are described later and in Chapter 4. In addition, flow cytometric immunophenotyping studies at diagnosis can identify aberrant patterns of antigen expression on the leukemic cells, which can be useful in searching for minimal residual disease in post-therapy samples.

GENETICS

The role of genetic changes in AML has been the subject of intense study and has been facilitated by the diagnostic use of next-generation sequencing (NGS) techniques. Karyotype analysis is essential in all cases of AML, and these findings play a major role in the proper classification of these leukemias.[19,20]

Initially, the focus on gene mutations in AML was directed toward cases with a normal karyotype,[21,22] but subsequent studies included all AML types and both genetic and epigenetic changes.[23-25] Mutations were initially divided into two types. So-called "type I" (or "class I") mutations impart a proliferation or survival advantage without affecting differentiation.[26] These are often later events in the development of leukemia and are generally viewed as prognostic markers. Receptor tyrosine kinase mutations are common type I mutations in AML. Mutations in FLT3 and KIT are the most common clinically relevant type I abnormalities used in AML stratification. FLT3 is expressed on hematopoietic progenitors. Activation through ligand binding, or constitutive activation from FLT3 mutations, leads to cell proliferation and survival. So-called "type II" (or "class II") mutations impair hematopoietic cell differentiation and subsequent programmed cell death (apoptosis).[26] These are thought to be primary genetic events in the development of AML and are viewed as disease-defining abnormalities rather than simply prognostic factors. Many of the gene fusions involved in the AML with recurring cytogenetic abnormalities described previously fall into this group. In addition, mutations of CCAAT/enhancer binding protein-α (CEBPA), RUNX1, and probably nucleophosmin (NPM1) are type II mutations. As such, mutations in NPM1 and CEBPA tend to occur in cases of AML with normal cytogenetics and define unique clinicobiological entities with favorable prognoses in the absence of FLT3 abnormalities. Class II translocations and mutations defined specific disease categories in the WHO classification. It is now understood, however, that there are more than two classes of mutations in AML,[23] that not all "disease-defining" mutations are the initial genetic event,[27,28] and that most AML cases have more than a single mutation (so-called "cooperating mutations"),[24,25] and some groups of genes may define prognostic AML types when one or more genes in the group are mutated.[29-31]

FLT3, KIT, and many of the other more recently described mutations do not define exclusive categories of AML because they are present in many of the previously described diagnostic categories. FLT3 abnormalities include internal tandem duplications (ITDs) and tyrosine kinase domain point/juxtamembrane domain (TKD) mutations.[32] FLT3-ITD mutations are associated with shorter remission duration and shorter overall survival (OS) for most AML types. The ratio of mutant FLT3 to wild-type allele can identify patients with poor outcomes. KIT mutations appear most commonly and have the most clinical relevance in core binding factor leukemias,[33] especially adults with AML with t(8;21)(q22;q22.1). In contrast, FLT3-ITDs are rare in core binding factor leukemias and in AML with KMT2A translocations. Therefore the various cooperating gene mutations associated with the different AML subtypes are discussed in those sections throughout the chapter.

Although not a discrete AML type in most classifications, detection of FLT3 mutations in AML are important for prognostic reasons and to identify patients that might benefit from targeted therapies directed against the mutation.[34]

An increasing number of targeted therapies have emerged related to gene mutations, and mutation panels are now routinely performed at the time of diagnosis for most AML cases. Some gene mutations associated with AML are germline mutations, and their recognition is important for screening of family members (see Chapter 45).

Mutation analysis for a growing number of genes is also needed to determine the prognosis, and in some cases the diagnosis, of AML types. Evaluation for mutations of FLT3, particularly for ITDs, is indicated in all cases in current guidelines. In addition, most, if not all, AMLs should now be tested with a large gene mutation panel that includes ASXL1, BCOR, CEBPA, EZH2, NPM1, RUNX1, SF3B1, SRSF2, STAG2, TP53, U2AF1, and ZRSR2.[12,29,30] More rapid evaluation of FLT3, IDH1, and IDH2 is becoming necessary because of targeted therapies that are now used in up-front treatment regimens.[35] Evaluation for mutations of KIT are of value in AML with t(8;21)(q22;q22.1) (RUNX1::RUNX1T1) and AML with inv(16)(p13.1q22) or t(16;16)(p13.1;q22) (CBFB::MYH11).[33] Other gene mutations are of emerging prognostic significance in AML and may be also included in NGS mutation panels.[23]

In addition to mutations, overexpression of some genes has prognostic significance. In particular, MECOM (previously known as EVI1) is inappropriately expressed in a variety of AMLs, including AML with inv(3)(q21.3q26.2) or t(3;3)(q21.3;q26.2), and high expression of MECOM is a poor prognostic indicator independent of 3q26.2 translocations.[36] Overexpression of the MECOM (EVI1) gene has also been described in multiple variant translocations of 11q23.3 and is associated with a very poor prognosis.[37] Some data suggest that MECOM-positive AML with KMT2A translocations is biologically different from MECOM-negative cases,[38,39] but in the ICC the presence of a KMT2A translocation trumps a MECOM abnormality in the diagnostic hierarchy.

PROGNOSIS

The overall 5-year survival rate for AML is between 20% and 25%, but it varies by disease type.[14]

ACUTE MYELOID LEUKEMIA DISEASE TYPES

Although many AML types have distinctive morphologic, clinical, and prognostic features in addition to the specific cytogenetic and molecular genetic findings,[18,20] the ICC approach to AML is primarily based on genetics with nongenetically defined disorders placed in the ever-shrinking category of AML, NOS.[12] In addition to a more genetic approach, the ICC also makes major changes related to blast cell counts required for an AML diagnosis. Many of the genetically defined abnormalities in de novo AML types define biologically distinct entities in which the biology does not change based on blast cell count. The best characterized of these is APL with t(15;17)(q24.1;q21.2)/*PML::RARA* and the core binding factor leukemias (AML with t(8;21)(q22;q22.1)/*RUNX1::RUNX1T1* and AML with inv(16)(p13.1q22) or t(16;16)(p13.1;q22)/*CBFB::MYH11*) and prior classifications have allowed for a diagnosis of AML in such cases without regard to blast cell count.[40] The ICC expands the list of de novo type genetic groups, but there is less data on some of these types to be confident that such a finding in the absence of an increase in blasts warrants a diagnosis of AML. Additionally, mutations in *NPM1* may be secondary, such as in the setting of chronic myelomonocytic leukemia (CMML),[41] and such a finding in that context should not automatically trigger a diagnosis of AML. For consistency among disease groups, the ICC requires at least 10% peripheral blood or bone marrow blasts for a diagnosis of AML, understanding that rare cases, especially with features of APL or core binding factor leukemias, may be exceptions to this cutoff. One exception to this approach, however, is AML with (9;22)(q34.1;q11.2)/*BCR::ABL1* for which the 20% blast requirement is retained because of difficulty in distinguishing accelerated phase of CML from AML in cases with less than 20% blast cells. For cases of AML with mutated *TP53*, AML with myelodysplasia-related gene mutations, AML with myelodysplasia-related cytogenetic abnormalities, and AML, NOS, the 20% blast requirement is retained, but a new category of MDS/AML is introduced in which peripheral blood or marrow blasts are 10% to 19%. Such cases should be treated based on their clinical behavior, with some being slowly progressive, similar to MDS, and others progressing quickly, similar to AML.[42]

Acute Promyelocytic Leukemia With t(15;17)(q24.1;q21.2)/*PML::RARA*

APL usually has an abrupt onset, and it constitutes 5% to 8% of AML cases. It is most common in young adults, rarely occurring before 10 years of age and diminishing in incidence after age 60 years. Organomegaly is uncommon. Prompt diagnosis is essential because of the high frequency of life-threatening disseminated intravascular coagulation. The t(15;17)(q24.1;q21.2) results in fusion of the promyelocytic gene *(PML)* on chromosome 15 with the retinoic acid receptor *(RARA)* gene on chromosome 17. The blasts are highly sensitive to anthracycline-based chemotherapy and differentiate in response to all-*trans*retinoic acid (ATRA) and arsenic trioxide treatment.[43,44]

Two morphologic variants are common. Hypergranular or typical APL accounts for 60% to 70% of cases and usually presents with a low white blood cell count (Box 46-2).

Box 46-2 *Key Features of Acute Promyelocytic Leukemia With t(15;17)(q24.1;q21.2)/PML::RARA*

- Hypergranular type exhibits abundant cytoplasmic granules and bundles of Auer rods
- Characteristic myeloid-lineage immunophenotype, with weak or absent HLA-DR and absent CD34
- Hypogranular type exhibits indistinct granules and folded nuclei and is often CD34 positive
- Common association with disseminated intravascular coagulation
- Favorable prognosis in cases that are *FLT3* negative and treated with combination all-*trans*retinoic acid and arsenic trioxide

---

Hypogranular or microgranular APL typically presents with leukocytosis, with numerous circulating abnormal promyelocytes.[45,46] Both forms have abnormal reniform or bilobed nuclei, and recognition of these characteristic nuclear features is an important element of the diagnosis. In hypergranular APL, the abnormal promyelocytes have numerous red to purple cytoplasmic granules (Fig. 46-1A). The granules are often larger and more darkly stained than normal neutrophil granules, and they may be so numerous that they obscure the nuclear borders. In some cases, a high percentage of leukemic cells have deeply basophilic, granular cytoplasm. Cells containing multiple Auer rods are reportedly found in up to 90% of cases of the hypergranular form. The Auer rods may be numerous and intertwined. Large globular inclusions of Auer rod–like material are found in the cytoplasm of occasional cells. Typical myeloblasts are a minor component in most cases, rarely reaching 20%. The abnormal promyelocytes are considered comparable to blasts for the purpose of diagnosing APL. In the microgranular variant of APL, the leukemic cells have sparse or fine granulation and markedly irregular nuclei (Fig. 46-1B). The bilobed or butterfly-shaped nuclei should raise suspicion of the microgranular variant. Cells containing multiple Auer rods are less abundant than in typical hypergranular APL. Myeloperoxidase and Sudan black B reactions are similarly strong in both variants.

The immunophenotype of hypergranular APL displays increased side scatter, lack of expression of HLA-DR and CD34, bright CD33, bright cytoplasmic myeloperoxidase, and variable expression of CD13.[47,48] The microgranular variant shows similar CD13, CD33, and myeloperoxidase expression but may show dim HLA-DR and commonly demonstrates dim CD34. The CD34-negative, HLA-DR-negative immunophenotype is not specific to APL[49]; it is also observed in some cases of cytogenetically normal AML without differentiation. Expression of CD15 is uncommon. CD117 is expressed in both morphologic variants. Many cases exhibit CD64 expression, and caution is warranted to avoid misdiagnosing microgranular APL as AML with monocytic differentiation. Aberrant expression of CD2 is more commonly observed in microgranular APL[50] and has been associated with *FLT3*-ITD mutations.[51] CD56 expression is described in 15% to 20% of patients with APL and has been associated with shorter complete remissions and poorer OS in some studies.[52,53]

Three breakpoint regions are described on the *PML* gene at band q24.1 of chromosome 15.[54] Two lead to long transcripts,

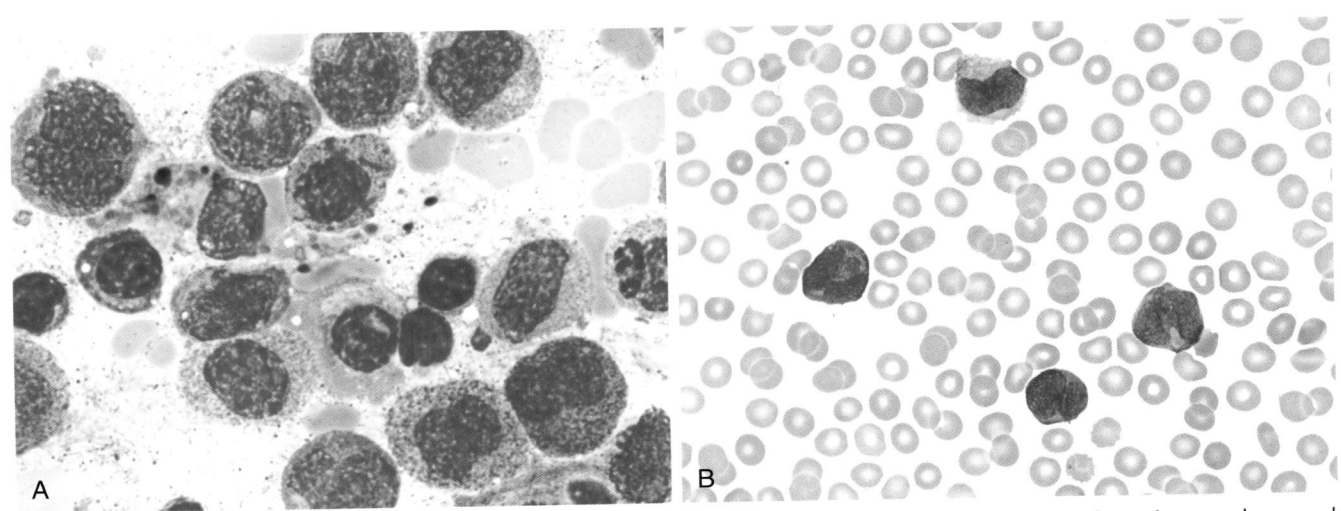

Figure 46-1. Acute promyelocytic leukemia with t(15;17)(q24.1;q21.2)/*PML::RARA*. A, Bone marrow aspirate shows increased promyelocytes and blasts with folded nuclei and numerous cytoplasmic granules, characteristic of the hypergranular type of acute promyelocytic leukemia. Note one blast in the upper center of the panel exhibiting Auer rods. **B,** Peripheral blood from another case shows blasts with bilobed nuclei and less obvious cytoplasmic granules, characteristic of the microgranular variant of acute promyelocytic leukemia.

and the third leads to the short transcript. The short transcript is more common in the microgranular variant. Cytogenetics, fluorescence in situ hybridization (FISH), or reverse transcriptase polymerase chain reaction (RT-PCR) is necessary for genetic confirmation of the *PML::RARA* fusion. FISH, RT-PCR, and immunofluorescence for the microspeckled nuclear distribution of PML protein may facilitate a rapid diagnosis.[55] RT-PCR is the only technique that can identify the *PML::RARA* isoform useful for the monitoring of minimal residual disease.[56] The PML::RARA fusion protein mediates a block in myeloid differentiation, which can be overcome with ATRA or arsenic trioxide therapy. ATRA targets the RARA component of the fusion protein, whereas arsenic trioxide targets PML, causing maturation and apoptosis. In most cases, remission can be achieved with ATRA alone, but relapse invariably occurs. Therefore standard induction chemotherapy with high-dose anthracyclines was generally given with or after ATRA, though more recent combinations of ATRA and arsenic trioxide do not require the addition of standard chemotherapy in most patients.[57] In adult patients who achieve complete remission, the prognosis is better than for any other category of AML. Rapid diagnosis and initiation of therapy are critical in APL. Because of the high risk of early death and the high potential for cure, initiation of therapy should not await genetic confirmation when clinical, morphologic, flow cytometric, and rapid molecular pathology results all suggest a diagnosis of APL.

FLT3 mutations are common in APL[58-60] and occur in approximately 40% of patients, with the majority being ITD mutations. *FLT3*-ITD in APL is strongly associated with the microgranular subtype, high white blood cell counts in peripheral blood, and breakpoint region 3 (short form) in *PML*. In one retrospective study, patients with mutant *FLT3* had a higher rate of death during the induction of chemotherapy but no significant difference in relapse rate or 5-year OS. The significance of the various historic prognostic factors in APL is unclear with current therapies that combine ATRA with arsenic trioxide.

Atypical promyelocytes may persist in the marrow for several weeks after induction chemotherapy, as may the detection of *PML::RARA* by karyotyping, FISH, or RT-PCR. These findings do not necessarily indicate resistant disease. The postinduction detection of *PML::RARA* by RT-PCR does not affect subsequent clinical outcome. However, detection of *PML::RARA* after complete remission is obtained strongly predicts the risk of relapse.

The differential diagnosis of the hypergranular variant of APL includes agranulocytosis with arrested maturation at the promyelocyte stage. With careful assessment, this distinction can usually be made quickly. In cases of agranulocytosis, the platelet count and hemoglobin level are generally normal, the marrow is not hypercellular, the nuclear features of neoplastic promyelocytes are not present, and Auer rods are not observed. The immunophenotypic differential diagnosis includes cases of HLA-DR–negative, CD34-negative AML, usually AML without differentiation or AML with mutated *NPM1*. These cases can be distinguished by the abnormal "butterfly" nuclei and cytoplasmic granulation of APL. Cases of HLA-DR–negative, CD34-negative AML with mutated *NPM1* often shows the "fish-mouth" deformity or cuplike nuclear inclusions (Fig. 46-2). The microgranular variant of APL may mimic AML types with monocytic differentiation, also displaying folded nuclei. Strong myeloperoxidase reactivity by cytochemistry or flow cytometry can resolve this dilemma. In difficult cases, rapid FISH or RT-PCR assessment for the *PML::RARA* fusion can be requested, but in most cases, treatment should not be delayed for molecular genetic confirmation.

Acute Promyelocytic Leukemia With Other *RARA* Rearrangements

Uncommonly, a case with many of the morphologic, immunophenotypic, and clinical features of promyelocytic leukemia has a variant cytogenetic translocation that involves the *RARA* gene on chromosome 17 but not the *PML* gene on chromosome 15.[61-63] Box 46-3 lists the *RARA* fusions included in the ICC. The t(11;17)(q23.1;q21.2) (*ZBTB16::RARA*; formerly known as *PLZF::RARA*) is the best-described translocation. The morphology differs from that of hypergranular or microgranular APL in that the majority

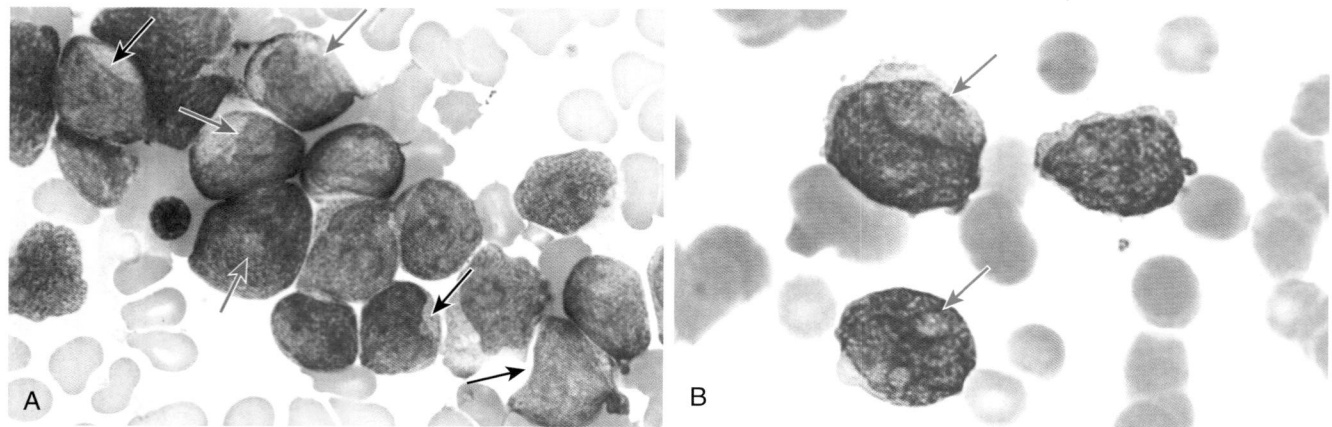

Figure 46-2. Acute myeloid leukemia with mutated *NPM1* displaying cuplike nuclear inclusions. **A** and **B,** Nuclear indentations from the side are most obvious *(black arrows);* from other angles, they may appear as large, pale nucleoli *(green arrows).* These features are reportedly associated with *NPM1* mutations.

Box 46-3 *Acute Promyelocytic Leukemia With Other RARA Rearrangements*

Acute Promyelocytic Leukemias (APLs) With:
t(1;17)(q42.3;q21.2)/*IRF2BP2::RARA*
t(3;17)(q26.3;q21.2)/*TBL1XR1::RARA*
t(4;17)(q12;q21.1)/*FIP1L1::RARA*
t(5;17)(q35.1;q21.2)/*NPM1::RARA*
t(11;17)(q23.2;q21.2)/*ZBTB16::RARA*
inv(17q)* or del(17)(q21.2q21.2)*/*STAT5B::RARA,STAT3::RARA*
t(X;17)(p11.4;q21.1)/*BCOR::RARA*

*Cryptic.

of blast cell nuclei are round to oval (Fig. 46-3), Auer rods are usually absent, and pelgeroid neutrophils may be seen. Patients with variant *RARA* translocations often experience disseminated intravascular coagulation. These cases are important to recognize because although they have many of the features of typical APL, some variants, including those with *ZBTB16::RARA*, do not respond to ATRA therapy.

Acute Myeloid Leukemia With t(8;21)(q22;q22.1)/*RUNX1::RUNX1T1*

AML with t(8;21)(q22;q22.1) has distinctive morphologic and immunophenotypic findings that correlate well with a specific cytogenetic abnormality (Box 46-4).[64-66] This type of leukemia is common in both children and adults, accounting for approximately 8% of AML. Although blasts are common in both blood and bone marrow, the morphologic features are more distinctive in the bone marrow. The blasts in the bone marrow have perinuclear cytoplasmic hoflike clearing, occasional Auer rods, and occasional large, salmon-colored granules (Fig. 46-4). Abundant granules may suggest a promyelocyte proliferation, but these granular cells are the neoplastic cells and should be considered blasts. The maturing neutrophils are usually dysplastic, with nuclear abnormalities; background eosinophilia is often present, without morphologic abnormalities of the eosinophils. The bone marrow biopsy is usually hypercellular, with sheets of immature cells. The abundance of granules and cytoplasm in the cells may give the appearance of a left shift on biopsy

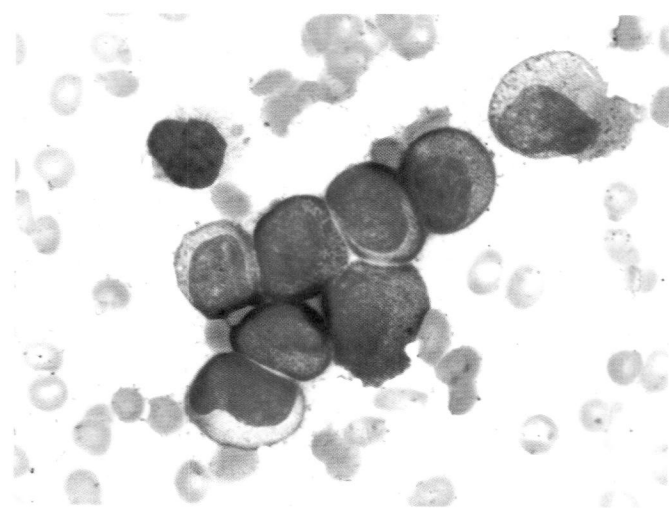

Figure 46-3. Acute promyelocytic leukemia with t(11;17)(q23.2;q 21.2)/*ZBTB16::RARA.* This rare type of acute promyelocytic leukemia is associated with abundant cytoplasmic granules, similar to the more common acute promyelocytic leukemia with *PML::RARA.* However, it has more round to oval blast cell nuclei, rather than the typical bilobed nuclei of the disease with *PML::RARA.*

Box 46-4 *Key Features of Acute Myeloid Leukemia With t(8;21)(q22;q22.1)/RUNX1::RUNX1T1*

- Blasts with perinuclear hofs, abundant granules, and large pink or salmon-colored granules
- Myeloid-lineage blasts expressing CD34 and CD19
- Favorable prognosis when presenting with white blood cell count <20 × 10⁹/L and absence of *KIT* mutations

sections rather than a definite blast cell increase, and the distinctive blast cell features are best identified on aspirate smears. The blasts are large, with a background of myeloid maturation; however, the features are more distinctive than just the myeloid maturation of the heterogeneous group of FAB M2 AML. Cases may also present as extramedullary disease (myeloid sarcoma), especially in children.

Immunophenotypically, cases express CD34, with usually strong expression of CD13 and HLA-DR and more variable

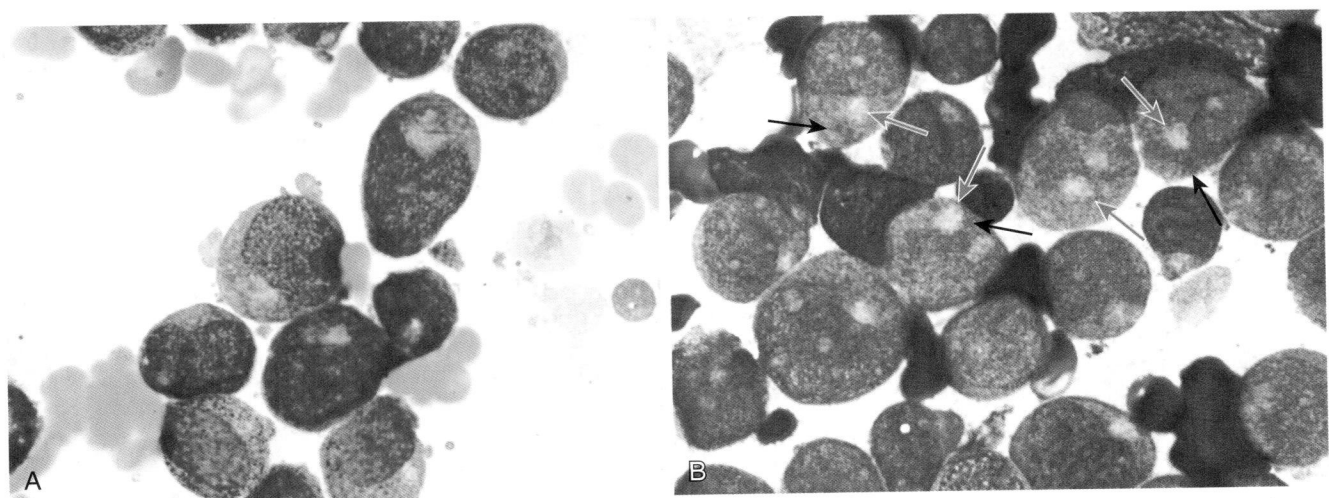

Figure 46-4. Acute myeloid leukemia (AML) with t(8;21)(q22;q22.1)/*RUNX1::RUNX1T1*. A, Blasts show a variable number of granules, suggesting cell maturation. One blast contains thin Auer rods. **B,** Perinuclear hofs *(green arrows)* and large pink granules *(black arrows)* are characteristic features of this type of AML.

expression of CD33. Myeloperoxidase is easily detected by either cytochemistry or flow cytometry. There is aberrant expression of the B-lymphocyte–associated surface antigen CD19 (weak) in the majority of cases, and many cases also express CD56.[64-66] Some studies suggest that CD56 expression is associated with increased relapse in this disease group.[67] PAX5 is frequently expressed when cases are studied by immunohistochemistry, and CD79a may be expressed in some cases.[68]

The t(8;21)(q22;q22.1) is usually easily detected by karyotype analysis and results in the fusion of *RUNX1* (also known as core binding factor-α and *AML1*) on chromosome 21, band q22.1, and *RUNX1T1* (also known as *ETO*) on chromosome 8, band q22. The translocation disrupts function of the core binding factor (which has both alpha and beta subunits) that is normally involved in regulating hematopoiesis.[69] AML with inv(16)(p13.1q22) or t(16;16) (p13.1;q22) (*CBFB::MYH11*) disrupts the beta subunit of the core binding factor, and these two AML types are commonly referred to as the *core binding factor leukemias*. Core binding factor leukemias are associated with a favorable prognosis in children and adults,[70] especially when treated with repetitive cycles of high-dose cytarabine (HiDAC) after remission. Cases of t(8;21) AML with a white blood cell count greater than 20×10^9/L at presentation appear to behave more like intermediate-risk disease, and patients may benefit from allogeneic hematopoietic cell transplantation during the first remission. Mutations of *KIT* in core binding factor AML are common (20%–25%).[33] In adults, *KIT* mutations in exons 8 and 17 appear to be associated with a worse prognosis. It is unclear whether they have a similar prognostic effect in children, or whether t(8;21) AML with *KIT* mutation benefits from allogeneic hematopoietic cell transplantation during the first remission. Mutations in *FLT3* are uncommon in core binding factor leukemia. However, mutations of *KRAS*, *NRAS*, *ASXL1*, and *ASXL2* do occur in subsets of patients with AML with t(8;21)(q22;q22.1).[71,72] Additional cytogenetic abnormalities are present in more than 70% of t(8;21) AML, most commonly loss of a sex chromosome or partial deletion of the long arm of chromosome 9 (del[9q]). In general, the presence of additional cytogenetic abnormalities in this

disease group does not have prognostic significance. After therapy, RT-PCR may detect *RUNX1::RUNX1T1* transcripts in the absence of clinical disease. The messenger RNA can be detected in some stem cells, mature monocytes, and hematopoietic progenitors during remission; detection of low levels of this fusion transcript is of unclear significance. Quantitative RT-PCR for *RUNX1::RUNX1T1* transcripts is more useful for monitoring of minimal residual disease.[73]

The differential diagnosis of AML with t(8;21)(q22;q22.1) includes APL, mixed phenotype acute leukemia, MDS, and regenerative changes that include the effects of growth factors. APL exhibits more folded blast cell nuclei and finer cytoplasmic granules than AML with t(8;21)(q22;q22.1). Immunophenotypic studies can also distinguish between these AML types, with APL usually lacking CD34, HLA-DR, and CD19, markers that are positive in the majority of cases of AML with t(8;21)(q22;q22.1). Despite the common expression of B-cell–associated antigens in AML with t(8;21)(q22;q22.1), these cases should not be diagnosed as mixed phenotype acute leukemias. The distinctive morphologic features of AML with t(8;21)(q22;q22.1), coupled with the characteristic immunophenotype of myeloid antigen expression with CD34 and CD19, warrant investigation for t(8;21) before a diagnosis of mixed phenotype leukemia is considered. On occasion, AML with t(8;21)(q22;q22.1) presents with a blast count less than 20% at diagnosis. Although these cases meet the criteria for MDS with excess blasts or MDS/AML, when treated appropriately, they behave similarly to other cases of AML with t(8;21)(q22;q22.1) and should be diagnosed as such rather than as myelodysplasia. If the abnormal cells with abundant granules of this AML type are counted as blasts, the vast majority will meet the 10% blast requirement of the current ICC. Patients recovering from toxic events or receiving granulocyte or granulocyte-monocyte colony-stimulating factor may show a marrow proliferation of promyelocytes with perinuclear hofs which may partially resemble blasts seen in AML with t(8;21)(q22;q22.1). These reactive proliferations do not contain Auer rods and usually do not exhibit the distinct, large, salmon or pink granules of AML. Investigation of the blood often shows toxic granulation of neutrophils associated with reactive promyelocyte proliferations, which is not usually seen with AML. Finally, reactive promyelocytes are usually CD34 negative and always CD19 negative, features that can help in the differential diagnosis. This differential diagnosis is particularly difficult in post-therapy patients with a history of AML with t(8;21)(q22;q22.1) who are receiving growth factors. In such cases, correlation with cytogenetic studies is helpful. In addition, a repeat bone marrow biopsy 2 weeks after cessation of growth factor should clarify whether the cell proliferation in question represents regenerative promyelocytes (which mature over time) or leukemic cells (which persist).

Acute Myeloid Leukemia With inv(16)(p13.1q22) or t(16;16)(p13.1;q22)/ *CBFB::MYH11*

AML with inv(16)(p13.1q22) or t(16;16)(p13.1;q22) accounts for less than 10% of adult AML and approximately 6% of childhood AML. The inv(16)(p13.1q22) is a pericentric inversion of chromosome 16. The genes at the breakpoint junction are the beta subunit of the core binding factor (*CBFB*) at 16q22 and a gene-encoding smooth muscle myosin heavy chain (*MYH11*) at 16p13.1.[74] AML with inv(16) usually has a characteristic morphology of acute myelomonocytic leukemia with abnormal eosinophils (AML M4Eo in the FAB classification) in the bone marrow (Box 46-5).[75] Typical myeloblasts, monoblasts, promonocytes, and mature monocytes are seen in the peripheral blood and marrow, with increased and dysplastic or abnormal eosinophils in the marrow (Fig. 46-5). The abnormal eosinophils have abundant and large, often irregularly shaped, basophilic-staining granules. These cells, however, may be admixed with normal-appearing eosinophils and are often absent in the peripheral blood. Flow cytometric immunophenotyping typically reveals multiple populations, including an immature blast population expressing CD34 or CD117, or both, as well as groups of cells exhibiting granulocytic (CD13, CD33, CD15, myeloperoxidase) or monocytic (CD4, CD11b, CD11c, CD14, CD64, CD36, lysozyme) differentiation. Aberrant co-expression of CD2 in the blast population occurs in a subset of cases,[76,77] but it is not specific for this type of AML.

The incidence of extramedullary disease in AML with inv(16)(p13.1q22) or t(16;16)(p13.1;q22) is reportedly as high as 50%, higher than for most types of AML. Similarly, lymphadenopathy and hepatomegaly are particularly common. Myeloid sarcoma may precede or present concurrently with bone marrow involvement. Some investigators have reported a high incidence of central nervous system relapse with intracerebral myeloid proliferations. Like AML with t(8;21), this core binding factor leukemia has a generally favorable prognosis.[78,79] *KIT* mutations are present in approximately 30% of cases, and exon 8 mutations in particular reportedly have a negative effect on prognosis in adults.[33] A co-existing trisomy 22 is associated with an improved prognosis, whereas trisomy 8 and tyrosine kinase domain mutations of *FLT3* are associated with a worse prognosis.[71,80] Levels of the *CBFB::MYH11* transcript detected by RT-PCR decrease slowly after therapy, and patients may continue to test positive during early complete remission.[81] Molecular remissions are possible and correlate well with long-term remission.

The differential diagnosis of AML with inv(16)(p13.1q22) or t(16;16)(p13.1;q22) includes myelomonocytic types of AML, NOS; MDS/myeloproliferative neoplasm (MPN); and reactive monocytic proliferations. In a small subset of cases of AML with inv(16)(p13.1q22) or t(16;16)(p13.1;q22), abnormal eosinophils are very scarce or even absent, and the diagnosis can be made only when the karyotype studies are complete. To complicate matters, inv(16)(p13.1q22) is often subtle and may be missed on routine karyotyping. Therefore the laboratory performing the karyotype analysis should be informed if abnormal eosinophils are identified and inv(16)(p13.1q22) is suspected, and other studies, such as FISH, should be performed before a sample with abnormal eosinophils is considered negative for inv(16)(p13.1q22) or

---

Box 46-5 *Key Features of Acute Myeloid Leukemia With inv(16)(p13.1q22) or t(16;16)(p13.1;q22)/CBFB::MYH11*

- Blasts have myelomonocytic features
- Abnormal eosinophils contain large, basophilic granules
- Favorable prognosis in the absence of *KIT* mutations

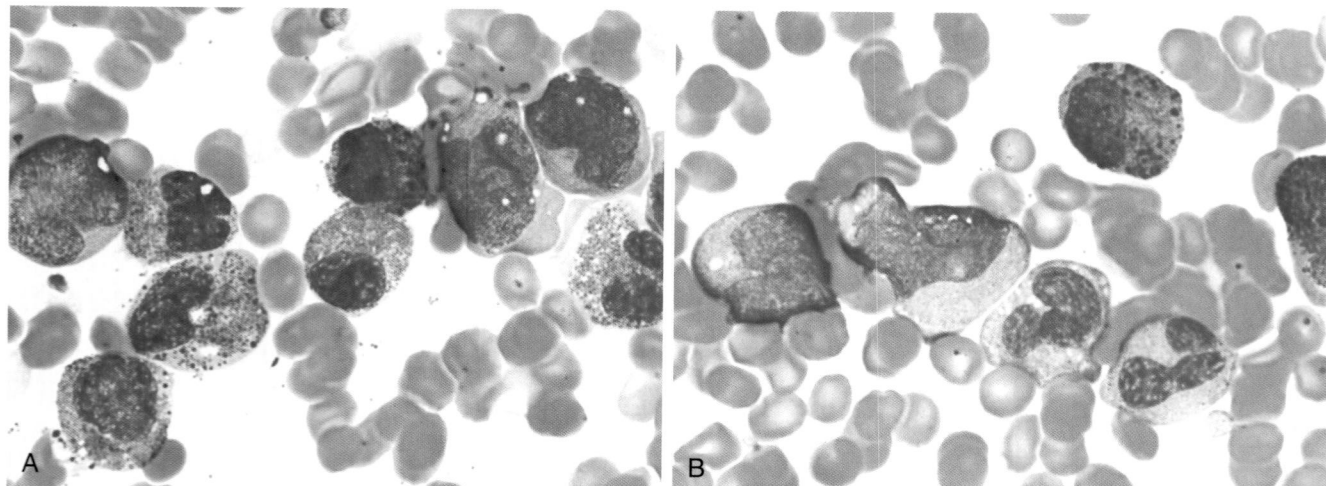

Figure 46-5. Acute myeloid leukemia with inv(16)(p13.1q22) or t(16;16)(p13.1;q22)/*CBFB::MYH11*. Both cases show blasts with monocytoid nuclear features and abundant cytoplasm. One of the cases **(A)** exhibits numerous eosinophil precursors, some of which have the characteristic large basophilic granules. The other one **(B)** shows only a single abnormal eosinophil.

t(16;16)(p13.1;q22). The presence of an increase in normal-appearing eosinophils may occur with other AML types and is not specific for a diagnosis of AML with inv(16)(p13.1q22) or t(16;16)(p13.1;q22). Some patients with this type of AML present with numerous eosinophils, at least some of which are abnormal, as well as numerous monocytes, so that the marrow blast cell count falls below 20%. Such cases should not be considered MDS or CMML but rather AML if inv(16) (p13.1q22) or t(16;16)(p13.1;q22) is detectable. Finally, reactive monocytosis should not demonstrate an increase in blasts and promonocytes or abnormal eosinophils, which, along with detection of the karyotype abnormality, are the most helpful indicators of AML in this differential diagnosis.

Acute Myeloid Leukemia With t(9;11)(p21.3;q23.3)/*MLLT3::KMT2A*

Translocations involving the *KMT2A* gene (previously known as *MLL*) on chromosome 11q23.3 are found in approximately 6% of cases of AML and are associated with more than 100 different partner genes.[82-86] In addition to de novo AML, *KMT2A* rearrangements are common in therapy-related myeloid proliferations, acute lymphoblastic leukemia (ALL), and acute leukemias of ambiguous lineage. AML with t(9;11)(p21.3;q23.3) typically occurs in children and has an intermediate prognosis (Box 46-6).[87] These patients may present with disseminated intravascular coagulation or extramedullary disease involving the gingiva and skin. The blasts typically have monocytic or myelomonocytic morphology, although they occasionally lack differentiation

Box 46-6 *Key Features of Acute Myeloid Leukemia With t(9;11)(p21.3;q23.3)/MLLT3::KMT2A*
• Typically occurs in childhood • Monocytic morphology of blast cells most common • Intermediate prognosis

(Fig. 46-6). Cases composed morphologically of mostly monoblasts and promonocytes are typically myeloperoxidase negative by cytochemistry. In children, AML with t(9;11) (p21.3;q23.3) expresses CD33, CD4, CD65, and HLA-DR, with minimal or no CD13, CD14, and CD34 expression.[88] In adults, AML with 11q23.3 translocations often shows monocytic morphologic differentiation and may express multiple monocytic antigens, including CD14, CD64, CD11b, CD11c, and CD4. CD34 is often negative, with variable CD117 and CD56 reactivity.[89]

Approximately 20% of AML cases with t(9;11) (p21.3;q23.3) have activating loop domain point mutations in *FLT3*, but these are of uncertain prognostic significance. Pediatric AML with t(9;11)(p21.3;q23.3) has an intermediate prognosis, whereas leukemias with an 11q23.3 translocation involving a different partner chromosome generally have a poorer prognosis.

The differential diagnosis of AML with t(9;11) (p21.3;q23.3) includes various categories of AML, NOS and mixed-phenotype acute leukemia. The morphologic and immunophenotypic features cannot resolve the differential diagnosis with AML, NOS; proper classification depends on the cytogenetic findings. Though a history of prior cytotoxic therapy took precedence over this AML category in prior classifications, such therapy-related cases are now diagnosed based on their genetic findings with the prior therapy noted in the diagnosis as a qualifier. Cases that meet immunophenotypic criteria for mixed phenotype acute leukemia with *KMT2A* rearranged may be designated as such, but the presence of t(9;11)(p21.3;q23.3) should be clearly designated because this may be a more important prognostic finding than the mixed phenotype.

Acute Myeloid Leukemia With Other *KMT2A* Rearrangements

AML with balanced translocations of 11q23.3 other than t(9;11)(p21.3;q23.3) are diagnosed separately from AML with t(9;11)(p21.3;q23.3)/*MLLT3::KMT2A*. Box 46-7 lists

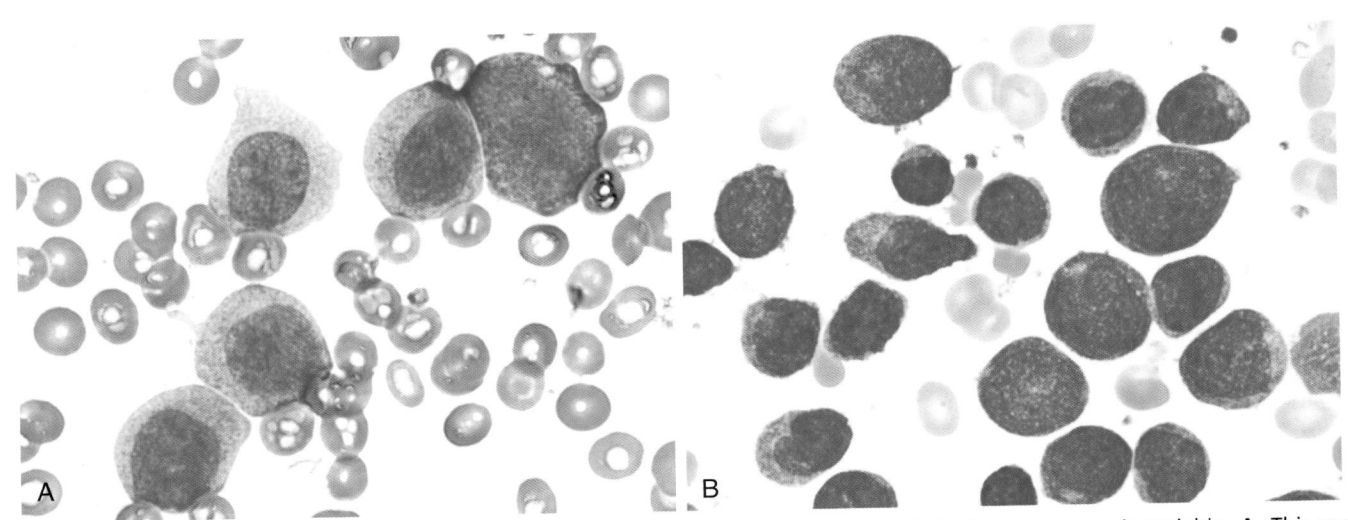

Figure 46-6. Acute myeloid leukemia with t(9;11)(p21.3;q23.3)/*MLLT3::KMT2A*. The morphologic appearance is variable. **A,** This case shows abundant basophilic cytoplasm, suggestive of monocytic differentiation. **B,** This other case shows blasts with a more myeloblastic appearance, including some cells with granules. Although myelomonocytic or monocytic features are most common, there are no specific morphologic features of this translocation.

the other *KMT2A* translocations in AML included in the ICC, although many more are now reported in acute leukemia.[86] Gene mutations in *KIT* or *FLT3*-ITD are uncommon in AML with *KMT2A* translocations.

Acute Myeloid Leukemia With t(6;9)(p22.3;q34.1)/*DEK::NUP214*

AML with t(6;9)(p22.3;q34.1) is a rare subtype accounting for approximately 1% of cases in both children and adults.[90-93] The median age in adults with this subtype of AML is 35 years. The translocation is reported in de novo AML, AML arising from MDS, and, less commonly, postcytotoxic therapy. Most cases would have been classified as AML with multilineage dysplasia in the 2001 3rd ed. WHO classification and meet the criteria for a variety of morphologic AML types, other than APL (Box 46-8). Adults with AML with t(6;9) (p22.3;q34.1) tend to have low white blood cell counts compared with other types of AML. Children may have more profound anemia. The blasts of AML with t(6;9) (p22.3;q34.1) may show occasional Auer rods and may exhibit monocytic features. Anisopoikilocytosis, circulating nucleated red blood cells, hypogranular neutrophils, and hypogranular platelets may be seen on the peripheral blood smear. Residual myeloid maturation is often present in the marrow, with dysplastic-appearing mature forms. Erythroid hyperplasia with dyserythropoiesis is also common, including ring sideroblasts in some cases. Small hypolobated megakaryocytes may be seen (Fig. 46-7). Basophilia (>2%

marrow or blood basophils) is present in roughly half of reported cases, a feature unique to this type of AML. By flow cytometry, blasts typically express CD45, CD13, CD33, HLA-DR, and intracytoplasmic myeloperoxidase, with variable expression of CD34, CD15, and CD11c. Terminal deoxynucleotidyl transferase (TdT) may be positive in some cases by flow cytometry or immunohistochemistry.[93] *FLT3*-ITD mutations are common in this type of AML,[91,93,94] with a reported frequency of 70% to 80%. Although the majority of patients with t(6;9) AML may achieve complete remission, survival rates are very poor with conventional chemotherapy. As in other high-risk categories of AML, patients may benefit from allogeneic hematopoietic cell transplantation. It appears that the poor prognosis of AML with t(6;9) is independent of *FLT3* status.[94] Some studies suggest a role for monitoring of *DEK::NUP214* molecular status in management of the patient.[95]

The differential diagnosis of AML with t(6;9) (p22.3;q34.1) includes blast transformation of chronic myeloid leukemia (CML) and rare AML with t(9;22) (q34.1;q11.2). Although the presence of basophilia is unusual in AML and is one clue to the diagnosis of AML with t(6;9)(p22.3;q34.1), basophilia is common in blast transformation of CML, and a prior history of CML is more suggestive of blast transformation than AML with t(6;9)(p22.3;q34.1). Basophilia may also be seen in the rare de novo AML with t(9;22)(q34.1;q11.2). Multilineage dysplasia appears to be less common in AML with t(9;22) (q34.1;q11.2), but this differential diagnosis is usually clarified only with cytogenetic studies.

Box 46-7 *Acute Myeloid Leukemia With Other KMT2A Rearrangements*

Acute Myeloid Leukemias (AMLs) With:
t(4;11)(q21.3;q23.3)/*AFF1::KMT2A*
t(6;11)(q27;q23.3)/*AFDN::KMT2A*
t(10;11)(p12.3;q23.3)/*MLLT10::KMT2A*
t(10;11)(q21.3;q23.3)/*TET1::KMT2A*
t(11;19)(q23.3;p13.1)/*KMT2A::ELL*
t(11;19)(q23.3;p13.3)/*KMT2A::MLLT1*

Box 46-8 *Key Features of Acute Myeloid Leukemia With t(6;9)(p23;q34.1)/DEK::NUP214*

• No specific blast cell morphology
• Often associated with erythroid hyperplasia and dysplasia
• Basophilia common
• Frequently associated with *FLT3* mutations
• Generally poor prognosis

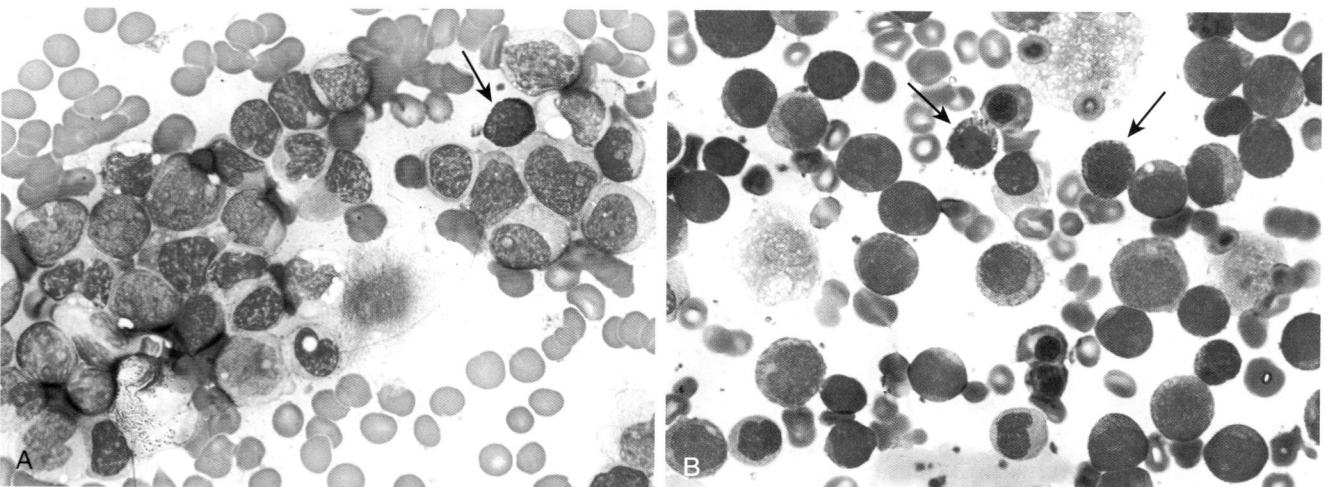

Figure 46-7. Acute myeloid leukemia with t(6;9)(p23;q34.1)/*DEK::NUP214*. Blast cells exhibit variable morphology but are often associated with admixed basophils *(arrows)*. **A,** Blasts with monocytic features. **B,** Myeloblasts without maturation and dysplastic erythroid precursors.

Acute Myeloid Leukemia With inv(3)(q21.3q26.2) or t(3;3) (q21.3;q26.2)/*GATA2; MECOM (EVI1)*

AML with inv(3)(q21.3q26.2) or t(3;3)(q21.3;q26.2) occurs most commonly in adults, with only rare examples of this translocation reported in children, often in association with monosomy 7. The median age at diagnosis is 56 years, younger than the reported average of 63 years for adult AML in general. It represents 1% to 2% of AML in adults and may present de novo or after a history of MDS.[96-98] Most cases would have been classified as AML with multilineage dysplasia in the 2001 3rd ed. WHO classification and meet the criteria for a variety of morphologic AML types, other than APL. Patients typically are seen with anemia, and platelets may be normal or elevated, in contrast to the usual thrombocytopenia associated with other types of AML (Box 46-9). Some patients have hepatosplenomegaly. In addition to blasts, the peripheral blood may show dysplastic features, including hypogranular neutrophils with pseudo–Pelger-Huët nuclear morphology and large hypogranular platelets. Circulating megakaryocyte naked nuclei may be seen. The bone marrow blasts may show multiple morphologies, including myeloid blasts without differentiation, a mixture of myeloid and monocytic morphologies, and blasts with megakaryoblastic differentiation. Myeloperoxidase activity is often low. Megakaryocytes may be normal or increased in number, frequently with small nonlobated and bilobated forms or other dysplastic features. Dyserythropoiesis or dysmyelopoiesis is commonly present (Fig. 46-8). The core

> **Box 46-9 *Key Features of Acute Myeloid Leukemia With inv(3)(q21.3q26.2) or t(3;3)(q21.3;q26.2)/GATA2; MECOM(EVI1)***
>
> - Mixture of blasts and monolobed or bilobed megakaryocytes
> - Often associated with normal or elevated platelet counts
> - Multilineage dysplasia common
> - Generally poor prognosis

biopsy may show decreased cellularity and occasionally fibrosis. Flow cytometric studies in this disease are limited. Expression of CD34, CD13, CD33, and HLA-DR is typically described, with aberrant CD7 expression in some cases.[99-101] Cases with megakaryocytic differentiation may express CD41 and CD61.

Chromosome 3q26.2 rearrangements may be cryptic on routine cytogenetic studies but detectable by FISH. The inv(3)(q21.3q26.2) or t(3;3)(q21.3;q26.2) repositions a distal *GATA2* enhancer to activate *MECOM* expression. High expression of MECOM is a poor prognostic indicator independent of 3q26.2 translocations.[36] The translocation or inversion also simultaneously confers *GATA2* haploinsufficiency.[102,103] Secondary karyotypic abnormalities are reported in 75% of cases.[97] They are most commonly myelodysplasia-associated abnormalities, including −7, −5q, and complex aberrant karyotypes. Mutations of genes activating RAS/receptor tyrosine kinase signaling pathways are reported in 98% of cases with mutations of *NRAS* (27%), *PTPN11* (20%), *FLT3* (13%), *KRAS* (11%), *NF1* (9%), *CBL* (7%), and *KIT* (2%), and mutations of *GATA2* (15%), *RUNX1* (12%), and *SF3B1* (27%, often with *GATA2*) are also common.[104]

Patients with AML with inv(3) or t(3;3) have a poor prognosis, typically with short survival.[105,106] This poor prognosis appears to be independent of *FLT3*-ITD status, although the data are limited by the rarity of this subtype. The presence of a complex karyotype or monosomy 7, however, appears to be associated with an even worse prognosis.[107] Age older than 60 years appears to be an independent risk factor for poor OS. Patients who can tolerate allogeneic hematopoietic cell transplantation may benefit from this therapy, but no survival advantage has been shown in some studies.[97,108] As in some patients with the t(6;9)(p23;q34) abnormality, some patients whose neoplastic cells have inv(3)(q21.3q26.2) or t(3;3)(q21.3;q26.2) may be seen with less than 20% blasts. Such cases have been shown to have a similar prognosis, independent of blast cell count,[106] although response to traditional AML therapy appears to be poor in all groups.

The differential diagnosis of AML with inv(3)(q21.3q26.2) or t(3;3)(q21.3;q26.2) includes the megakaryoblastic type of AML, NOS; AML with t(1;22)(p13.3;q13.1); and myeloid

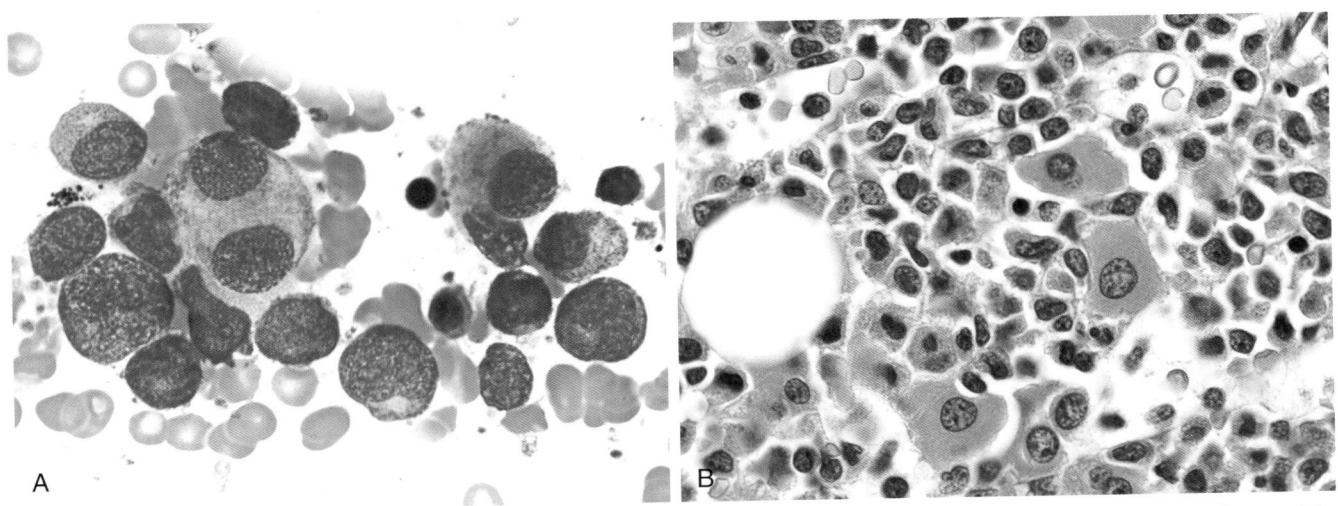

Figure 46-8. Acute myeloid leukemia with inv(3)(q21.3q26.2) or t(3;3)(q21.3;q26.2)/*GATA2; MECOM*. A, Increased blasts with monolobed and bilobed megakaryocytes are typical of this disorder. **B,** Distinctive hypolobated megakaryocytes are apparent on the biopsy specimen.

proliferations of Down syndrome. The absence of Down syndrome obviously excludes the last possibility. The category of AML with inv(3)(q21.3q26.2) or t(3;3)(q21.3;q26.2) takes precedence over AML, NOS, so the karyotype resolves that differential diagnosis. The patient's age and karyotype are helpful in distinguishing AML with t(1;22)(p13.3;q13.1), which occurs in very young children, from AML with inv(3)(q21.3q26.2) or t(3;3)(q21.3;q26.2), which occurs primarily in adults.

Acute Myeloid Leukemia With Other *MECOM* Rearrangements

MECOM is involved in other translocations in AML (see Box 46-10). These nonclassic *MECOM* rearrangements appear to present more commonly as MDS, often therapy-related, but may evolve to AML and have a similarly poor prognosis to the more classic *GATA2, MECOM* abnormalities. Although classic and nonclassic *MECOM* associated AMLs show similar mutation profiles, these nonclassic cases appear to be more commonly associated with complex karyotypes and chromosome 7 abnormalities.[109]

Acute Myeloid Leukemia With Other Rare Recurring Translocations

The ICC now includes a category to capture AML subtypes with rare recurring translocations, some of which were previous specific AML subtypes, such as AML with t(1;22)(p13.3;q13.1), or were captured by the prior category of AML with myelodysplasia-related changes, such as cases with t(3;5)(q25.3;q35.1). Box 46-11 shows the different abnormalities included in this section, with many being more common in infants and children. The proposed WHO 5th ed. lists a similar category, but the specifics of what is included in the category remain unclear at the time that this chapter was prepared. In the ICC, cases in this category should be diagnosed as AML with the specific translocation listed rather than using "AML with rare recurring translocations" as the diagnosis. The specific features of the various types of AML in this category are variably described, but some have fairly distinctive clinical and pathologic features.

AML (megakaryoblastic) with t(1;22)(p13.3;q13.1)/ *RBM15::MRTFA (MRTF1/MKL1)* is a rare form of AML presenting almost exclusively in infants and young children (less than 2.5 years).[110-112] The median age at diagnosis is 4 months, and 80% of cases are diagnosed in the first year of life. Some cases are congenital.[113] AML with t(1;22)(p13.3;q13.1) constitutes 1% or less of childhood AML and appears to be more common in girls. The clinical presentation commonly mimics a solid tumor, with hepatosplenomegaly or skeletal lesions (bilaterally symmetric periostitis and osteolytic lesions). Some cases present as myeloid sarcoma without evidence of

marrow involvement. The complete blood count may show anemia and thrombocytopenia. Blasts in the blood or bone marrow exhibit typical features of megakaryoblasts, with a modest amount of agranular cytoplasm that may show blebs or budding of platelets. The nuclear chromatin may be more condensed than myeloid blasts and is infrequently nucleolated (Fig. 46-9). The bone marrow aspirate may be hemodilute or aparticulate because of marrow fibrosis. Micromegakaryocytes are common, but multilineage dysplasia is not present. The bone marrow biopsy or biopsy of extramedullary involvement may show clumps of megakaryoblasts in fibrosis. Few cases have a reported flow cytometric immunophenotype. CD45 and CD34 may be negative, as in other AML with megakaryoblastic morphology. The myeloid antigens CD13 and CD33 are inconsistently expressed, as is HLA-DR. Immunoreactivity for megakaryocytic antigens CD41 and CD61 is commonly seen, and some cases may express CD56. Immunohistochemically, the cells are often negative for CD45, although they commonly express CD43. Other markers associated with megakaryocytic differentiation such as von Willebrand factor (factor VIII–related antigen) may be positive. Additional complex karyotypic abnormalities are common in "older" patients (older than 6 months). Mutations in *FLT3, NPM1, CEBPA,* and *WT1* are usually absent in AML with t(1;22)(p13.3;q13.1).[112] Although the role of the *RBM15:MRTFA* in leukemogenesis is still unclear, the fusion gene may modulate chromatin organization, *HOX*-induced differentiation, and extracellular signaling pathways, as well as confer an antiproliferative effect.[114,115]

Diagnosis may be delayed in these patients owing to the difficulties described. The prognosis of AML with t(1;22)(p13.3;q13.1) is variable in the literature. Some studies suggested that patients respond well to intensive AML therapy[116]; however, others have found this to be a high-risk disease compared with other pediatric acute megakaryoblastic leukemias.[117,118]

The differential diagnosis of AML with t(1;22)(p13.3;q13.1) includes other AML with megakaryocytic features, including the myeloid proliferations of Down syndrome; these can be distinguished only by clinical history and karyotyping. However, multilineage dysplasia is usually present in other types of megakaryoblastic leukemias and is not seen in AML with t(1;22)(p13.3;q13.1). Though a Children's Oncology Group study found t(1;22)(p13.3q13.1) to be the most

---

Box 46-10 *Acute Myeloid Leukemia With Other* MECOM *Rearrangements*

Acute Myeloid Leukemias (AMLs) With:

- t(2;3)(p11~23;q26.2)/*MECOM*::?
- t(3;8)(q26.2;q24.2)/*MYC, MECOM*
- t(3;12)(q26.2;p13.2)/*ETV6*::*MECOM*
- t(3;21)(q26.2;q22.1)/*MECOM*::*RUNX1*

Box 46-11 *Acute Myeloid Leukemia With Other Rare Recurring Translocations*

- Acute myeloid leukemia (AML) with t(1;3)(p36.3;q21.3)/ *PRDM16*::*RPN1*
- AML with t(3;5)(q25.3;q35.1)/*NPM1*::*MLF1*
- AML with t(8;16)(p11.2;p13.3)/*KAT6A*::*CREBBP*
- AML (megakaryoblastic) with t(1;22)(p13.3;q13.1)/*RBM15*:: *MRTFA**
- AML with t(5;11)(q35.2;p15.4)/*NUP98*::*NSD1**
- AML with t(11;12)(p15.4;p13.3)/*NUP98*::*KMD5A**
- AML with *NUP98* and other partners*
- AML with t(7;12)(q36.3;p13.2)/*ETV6*::*MNX1**
- AML with t(10;11)(p12.3;q14.2)/*PICALM*::*MLLT10*
- AML with t(16;21)(p11.2;q22.2)/*FUS*::*ERG*
- AML with t(16;21)(q24.3;q22.1)/*RUNX1*::*CBFA2T3*
- AML with inv(16)(p13.3q24.3)/*CBFA2T3*::*GLIS2*

*Occurs predominantly in infants and children.

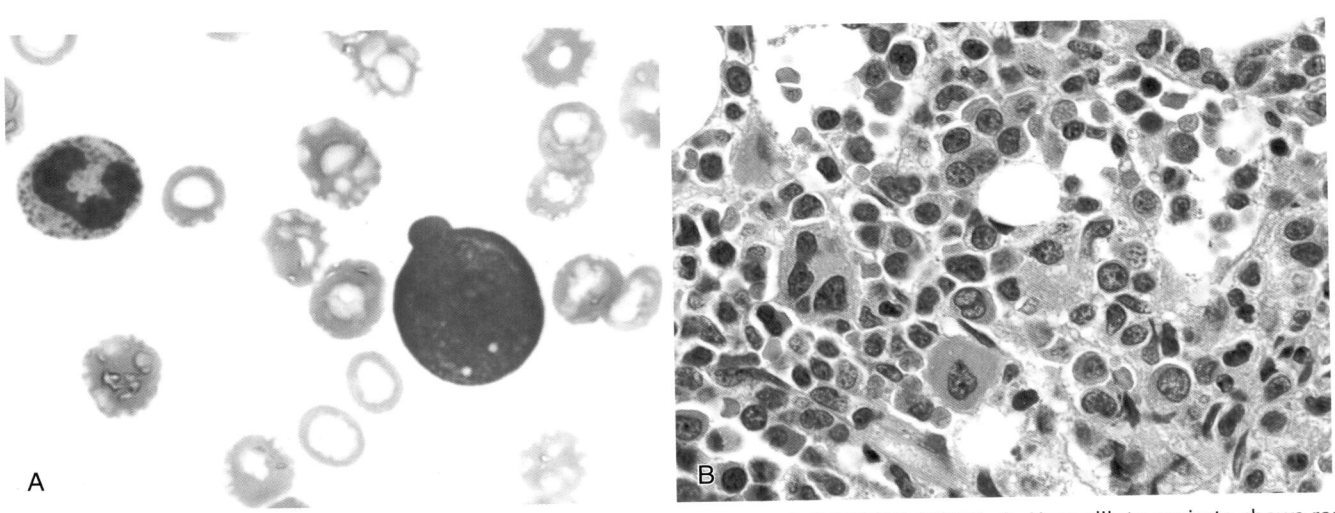

Figure 46-9. Acute myeloid leukemia (megakaryoblastic) with t(1;22)(p13.3;q13.1)/*RBM15::MRTF1*. A, Hemodilute aspirate shows rare blasts with basophilic cytoplasm and blebbing. **B,** Core biopsy shows blasts and atypical megakaryocytes.

common recurring cytogenetic abnormality in pediatric acute megakaryocytic leukemia, the rare AML inv(16) (p13.3q24.3)/*CBFA2T3::GLIS2* and AMLs with *NUP98* translocations may also be of megakaryocytic lineage.[112] The differential diagnosis also includes other pediatric small, blue, round cell tumors. Biopsy of the marrow or extramedullary lesions of AML with t(1;22)(p13.3;q13.1) may show cohesive nests of small, blue, round cells, suggestive of a childhood solid tumor and leading to an erroneous diagnosis of neuroblastoma or hepatoblastoma in some cases. Especially in myeloid sarcoma cases, the diagnosis may not be obvious until cytogenetic studies reveal the presence of t(1;22)(p13.3;q13.1).

AML with t(3;5)(q25.3;q35.1)/*NPM1::MLF1* is also a rare subtype that probably represents less than 1% of AML.[119,120] Myeloid proliferations with this cytogenetic abnormality may present as an MDS or as a number of morphologic AML subtypes. The AML cases were previously included in the category of AML with myelodysplasia-related changes of the revised WHO 4th ed. classification (Fig. 46-10). This AML type appears to be more common in young adult men than are other types of dysplasia-associated AMLs. It most cases, the t(3;5) is the sole cytogenetic abnormality, but very little is known about cooperating mutations in this disease. The translocation appears to result in cytoplasmic expression of the NPM protein, similar to AML with mutated *NPM1*,[121] but is a more aggressive disease. Interestingly, the translocation results in nuclear expression of the MLF1 protein, which is normally cytoplasmic, and this change appears to cause instability in *TP53*, which might explain the more aggressive behavior of these rare cases compared with AML with mutated *NPM1*.[122] Patients tend to relapse early after therapy and may benefit from early hematopoietic cell transplantation.[123]

AML with t(8;16)(p11.2;p13.3)/*KAT6A::CREBBP* is most commonly associated with therapy-related disease, which is now designated separately as a qualifier. This AML type is associated with erythrophagocytosis and usually myelomonocytic or monocytic features (Fig. 46-11).[124-126] It occurs in both adults and children and may be congenital, de novo, or therapy related. Congenital cases are usually limited to the skin and may remit spontaneously during a few days.[127] Approximately 40% of cases are associated with disseminated

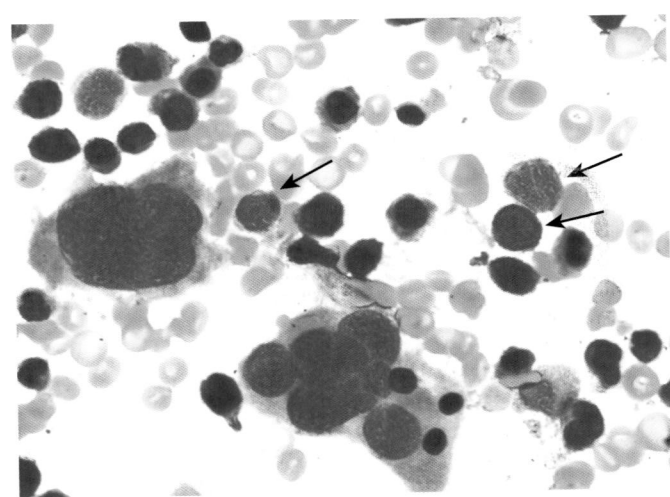

Figure 46-10. Acute myeloid leukemia with t(3;5)(q25.3;q35.1)/ *MLF1::NPM1*. This disease is characterized by multilineage dysplasia. This example shows a florid erythroid hyperplasia constituting more than 50% of cells, with dysplastic megakaryocytes and scattered myeloblasts *(arrows)*. In the 4th ed. WHO classification (2008), the case would have met the criteria for erythroid leukemia (erythroid/myeloid type), with more than 20% of the nonerythroid cells being myeloblasts.

intravascular coagulopathy[126] and may have increased promyelocytes, mimicking APL.[128] AML with t(8;16), therapy related, may occur after either alkylating agent or topoisomerase II inhibitor therapy and usually has a short latency period. Gene-expression profiling and microRNA pattern studies of this leukemia type have shown overexpression of RET and PRL and a unique pattern of HOX gene expression.[129,130] The overall prognosis of AML with t(8;16) is variable, but cases that arise after therapy have a poor prognosis.

Acute Myeloid Leukemia With t(9;22)(q34.1;q11.2)/*BCR::ABL1*

Although most blast proliferations with a *BCR::ABL1* fusion, usually caused by t(9;22)(q34.1;q11.2), represent blast transformation of CML, ALL, or mixed-phenotype acute

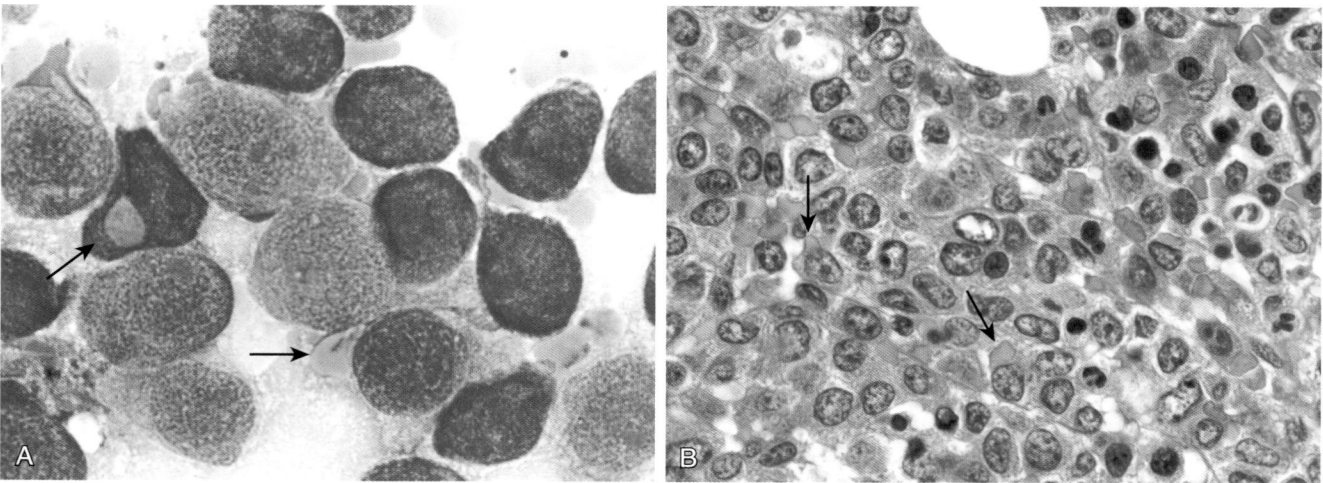

Figure 46-11. Acute myeloid leukemia with t(8;16)(p11.2;p13.3)/*KAT6A::CREBBP.* This disease is characterized by blasts showing erythrophagocytosis *(arrows)*, which can be seen on aspirate smears **(A)** or biopsy sections **(B)**.

leukemia, rare cases of de novo AML with *BCR::ABL1* occur and are included as an entity in current classifications (Box 46-12). This AML type is rare, representing less than 1% of all cases, with a possible male predominance.[131-134] It is difficult to distinguish on an individual basis de novo AML with *BCR::ABL1* from myeloid blast transformation of CML, and exclusion of an occult chronic phase of CML preceding the diagnosis of AML, or after therapy for AML, is essential for diagnosis. Cases of de novo AML with *BCR::ABL1* appear to differ from blast crisis of CML by having less frequent splenomegaly and basophilia and slightly lower marrow cellularity. These cases fall into a variety of morphologic subtypes, other than APL. The average marrow cellularity in de novo cases is reported to be less than that typically seen in blast transformation of CML (80% versus 95%–100%), and dwarf megakaryocytes are reported to be less common in AML with *BCR::ABL1* compared with blast transformation of CML.[131,133,134] The immunophenotype of the blast cells in AML with *BCR::ABL1* is non-specific with expression of CD13, CD33, and CD34. Aberrant expression of CD19, CD7, and TdT is reportedly common.[131,133]

Although most cases demonstrate t(9;22)(q34.1;q11.2), the translocation may be cryptic. The *BCR::ABL1* fusion, usually the p210 transcript, is present in all cases. Most cases have additional cytogenetic abnormalities, including a complex karyotype, monosomy 7, or trisomy 8.[131,133,134] AML-associated mutations, particularly *NPM1* and *FLT3*-ITD, are reported in AML with *BCR::ABL1* but not in blast transformation of CML, but these mutations are relatively uncommon.[134] Loss of *IKZF1* and *CDKN2A* in AML with *BCR::ABL1* and cryptic deletions within the IGH and TRG genes have been described as useful in differentiating de novo AML from myeloid blast transformation of CML, but such testing is not routinely available and has not been validated in multiple laboratories.[135]

Although rare, AML with *BCR::ABL1* appears to demonstrate a poor response to traditional AML therapy or to tyrosine kinase inhibitor therapy alone.[131] However, survival may be improved with tyrosine kinase inhibitor therapy followed by allogeneic hematopoietic cell transplantation.[136-139]

> **Box 46-12** *Key Features of Acute Myeloid Leukemia t(9;22)(q34.1;q11.2)/BCR::ABL1*
>
> • Must be distinguished from myeloid blast crisis of chronic myeloid leukemia
> • May benefit from tyrosine kinase inhibitor therapy and hematopoietic cell transplantation

Acute Myeloid Leukemia With Mutated *NPM1*

AML with mutated *NPM1* shows a female predominance and is found in approximately 50% of adult AML with a normal karyotype and 20% of pediatric AML with a normal karyotype.[140-144] *NPM1* mutations of exon 12 are best detected by PCR or NGS, but identification of cytoplasmic dislocation of *NPM1* by immunohistochemistry may be useful as a surrogate method for detecting this gene mutation. The immunohistochemical approach has been improved in recent years with the development of mutant-specific antibodies that make interpretation easier. Approximately 40% of *NPM1*-mutated patients are also positive for *FLT3*-ITD mutations. In the absence of an *FLT3*-ITD mutation, *NPM1* mutation in cytogenetically normal AML is associated with a favorable prognosis, similar to that of core binding factor leukemias. The presence of *FLT3*-ITD mutations appears to abrogate that effect, and for that reason, mutations of both genes must be studied and the use of large NGS gene panels has become routine for the diagnosis. *NPM1* mutations are only rarely reported in association with other disease-defining recurring cytogenetic abnormalities.

In adults, the majority of *NPM1*-mutated AML cases show monocytic differentiation, often with "cup-shaped" or "fish-mouth" nuclear indentations. In children, *NPM1*-mutated cases most commonly show myeloid blasts with or without differentiation or show myelomonocytic differentiation. Rare cases of erythroleukemia with *NPM1* mutation are described in children. Adult cases of AML with mutated *NPM1* are predominantly CD34 negative. Among cases with nonmonocytic morphology are those demonstrating cuplike nuclear invaginations and lacking CD34 and HLA-DR expression (see Fig. 46-2).[145,146] Approximately one-quarter of cases of de novo AML with mutated *NPM1* demonstrate multilineage dysplasia, despite usually having a normal karyotype. Such cases were considered AML-MRC in the 2008 4th ed. WHO classification, but the presence of dyspoiesis in this setting does not appear to affect prognosis,[147,148] and such findings no longer affect the diagnosis in current classifications. This AML type is characterized by high CD33 expression; common expression of CD117, CD123, and CD110; and often low CD13 expression.[149] HLA-DR is often negative. AML with mutated *NPM1* may have an immature myeloid immunophenotype or a monocytic immunophenotype (positive for CD36, CD64, CD14).[150] Although less common, CD34-positive cases occur and have been associated with worse prognosis.[151,152]

The *NPM1* gene at chromosome 5q35.1 encodes a molecular chaperone, shuttling molecules from the nucleus to the cytoplasm; in addition, it plays multiple other roles, including ribosome biogenesis, centrosomal duplication, and regulation of the ARF-TP53 tumor suppressor pathway.[153,154] Mutations in exon 12 affect the amino acid composition of the nucleophosmin C terminus; this creates a nuclear export motif, with resultant dislocation of nucleophosmin to the cytoplasm. *NPM1* is a chromosomal translocation partner in various types of leukemia and lymphoma in which the aberrantly regulated product appears to be oncogenic. The native product apparently has both oncogenic and tumor suppressor capabilities. *NPM1* is typically located in nucleoli. In patients with *NPM1* mutations, the aberrantly localized mutant nucleophosmin can be identified in the blast cytoplasm by immunohistochemistry. However, the mutation status of *NPM1* with other gene mutations, including *FLT3*-ITD, *DNMT3A*, *IDH1*, *KRAS/NRAS*, and cohesin complex genes are relatively common,[23] and should be assessed. Of AMLs with mutated *NPM1*, 5% to 15% show chromosomal aberrations, including +8 and del(9q).[155] These karyotype abnormalities appear to not affect prognosis.

Whereas *NPM1* mutation is a disease-defining lesion in the appropriate clinical and pathologic setting, it frequently represents a later event in leukemogenesis, commonly secondary to mutations in epigenetic modifiers, such as *DNMT3A*, *TET2*, *IDH1*, and *IDH2*.[27,28,156] AML with mutated *NPM1* shows a distinct gene-expression profile characterized by upregulation of *HOX* genes[157,158] that differs from that of other AML types, including AML with *KMT2A* translocations.[159] *NPM1*-mutated AML is also characterized by a unique microRNA signature.[160]

NPM1 mutations may occur as a late event in CMML and may portend more rapid transformation to acute leukemia,[41] but in the ICC such cases should be diagnosed as CMML whenever they fulfill the diagnostic criteria for such entity. The ICC requires a blast count of at least 10% in an *NPM1* mutated case before diagnosing AML, while the proposed WHO 5th ed. classification does not appear to have a blast cell count requirement for such a diagnosis.

AML with mutated *NPM1* has a generally favorable prognosis in the absence of *FLT3*-ITD mutations. However, the combination of *NPM1*, *FLT3*-ITD, and *DNMT3A* mutations in individual cases is associated with a particularly poor outcome.[161]

Acute Myeloid Leukemia With In-Frame bZIP *CEBPA* Mutations

CEBPA is a tumor suppressor gene located on chromosome 19q13.1 that encodes a differentiation-inducing transcription factor involved in granulocytic differentiation and diverse programs such as lung development, adipogenesis, and glucose metabolism.[162] *CEBPA* may be inactivated through multiple mechanisms, including transcriptional repression by the RUNX1::RUNX1T1 fusion protein of t(8;21) AML and epigenetic modification. Point mutations of *CEBPA* are detected in 13% of cytogenetically normal AML in adults and in 17% to 20% of cytogenetically normal AML in children.[163-165] It was initially thought that any mutation in *CEBPA* and later only biallelic mutations of the gene were prognostically significant.[166-170] More than 100 different nonsilent mutations have been described. This range of mutation sites made routine testing for this mutation more complicated, but the assay has become more widely available. Mutations commonly lead to synthesis of a smaller dominant negative isoform that inhibits wild-type protein function. Unlike the common association between *NPM1* and *FLT3*-ITD mutations, *FLT3* abnormalities are relatively uncommon in AML with *CEBPA* mutations. With more in-depth study, it is now understood that the prognostic significance of *CEBPA* mutations in AML relates to the presence of in-frame bZIP mutations of the gene.[171-173] AML with in-frame bZIP *CEBPA* mutations has a favorable prognosis, and patients are unlikely to benefit from allogeneic hematopoietic cell transplantation.

The morphologic subtypes of myeloblasts in AML with in-frame bZIP *CEBPA* mutations are most commonly AML with or without differentiation. AML with myelomonocytic or monocytic differentiation is less commonly seen, and erythroleukemia or megakaryoblastic leukemia has not been described. *CEBPA* mutations are rarely described in therapy-related AML. Similar to AML with mutated *NPM1*, as many as 26% of AML cases with *CEBPA* mutations may have multilineage dysplasia,[174] which does not affect the prognosis or diagnosis. There is no specific immunophenotype for the blasts in AML with mutations of *CEBPA*, but the myeloblasts frequently show aberrant expression of CD7 without other T-lineage–associated markers.[175,176] More than 70% of AMLs with mutations of *CEBPA* have a normal karyotype. Approximately 10% have a single karyotypic abnormality, and only rare cases have a complex karyotype. *FLT3*-ITD mutations occur in 5% to 9% of cases and *GATA2* mutations in 39% of cases.[177,178]

Germline mutations of *CEBPA* may also occur and are associated with a familial syndrome.[15] For this reason, consideration of screening of germline DNA and family members may be indicated once a diagnosis of AML with in-frame bZIP *CEBPA* mutations is made.

The diagnosis of AML with *CEBPA* mutations differs between the ICC and proposed WHO 5th ed. classification. The ICC allows only in-frame bZIP mutations for the diagnosis and allows for a diagnosis of AML when 10% or more blasts are present in the bone marrow or peripheral blood. The WHO appears to allow for either bZIP or biallelic mutations, and also requires a blast count of 20% or more for a diagnosis of AML.

Acute Myeloid Leukemia and Myelodysplastic Syndrome/Acute Myeloid Leukemia With Mutated *TP53*

The ICC introduced the new category of AML and MDS/AML with mutated TP53 with, as previously mentioned, AML defined by 20% or more peripheral blood or bone marrow blasts and the new category of MDS/AML defined by 10% to 19% peripheral blood or bone marrow blasts. Mutations of *TP53* in AML are usually associated with a complex karyotype and confer an even worse prognosis in such cases compared with AML with a complex karyotype and no *TP53* mutation.[25,179-181] For this reason, the new category was created with most such cases falling in the prior WHO categories of AML with myelodysplasia-related changes, therapy-related myeloid neoplasms, or pure erythroid leukemia. The former two categories are eliminated in the ICC.

Alterations of *TP53* are complex and include gene deletions, loss of heterozygosity, and single nucleotide and insertion/deletion mutations.[182] Most *TP53* mutations in AML are missense mutations that involve the DNA-binding domain (DBD).[183] Mutant premature termination codons and frameshift mutations result in strong disruption of TP53 function, whereas the effect of mutations resulting in a single amino-acid substitution or deletion is dependent on their position within the DBD. The frequency of *TP53* mutations in AML is approximately 10% but is increased in certain subpopulations such as those with AML after MDS or MDS/MPN, therapy-related AML, or pure erythroid leukemia.[184-187] *TP53* mutation is in the adverse prognostic group of the 2022 European LeukemiaNet (ELN) classification[188] with *TP53*-mutated AML having a particularly poor prognosis compared with the rest of the AML in this group.[189] The dismal effect of *TP53* mutations on patient outcome appears to transcend blast count with equally poor outcomes in patients presenting as MDS or AML, and whether the disease is therapy-related or clinically de novo.[190]

The prognosis of AML and MDS with mutated *TP53* varies, somewhat, when monoallelic versus biallelic mutations are compared; biallelic mutations, which are the typical type identified in AML, are associated with a worse prognosis. Despite this, the poor prognosis of AML with monoallelic *TP53* mutations remains significant, and the ICC allows for a case to be classified as AML or MDS/AML with either allelic type if the variant allele frequency is ≥10%. Some studies have found a higher *TP53* VAF (>40%) to be associated with shorter survival in AML, while other studies have not.[179,180]

Immunohistochemistry for TP53 protein expression can be used as a screening test for this category but is not adequate alone. Each laboratory must optimize the stain for decalcified bone marrow biopsies to reduce false negative results, but even with an optimized assay, false positive and false negative results may occur.[191] Therefore, the category is defined by the molecular detection of a *TP53* mutation.

As mentioned, most cases of AML with mutated *TP53* demonstrate features of pure erythroid leukemia, or of the prior categories of AML with myelodysplasia-related changes or therapy-related myeloid neoplasms. Most cases demonstrate multilineage dysplasia (Fig. 46-12). Cases meeting prior criteria for pure erythroid leukemia have at least two *TP53* abnormalities (both mutations and aberrant or deleted chromosome 17p) in over 90% of cases,[186] and these

cases should now be classified as AML with mutated *TP53* with a note that they represent the pure erythroid leukemia type. Cases now diagnosed as MDS/AML with mutated *TP53* based on 10% to 19% blast cells in the blood or marrow would have been previously diagnosed as MDS with excess blasts-2 (MDS-EB-2) or therapy-related myeloid neoplasm in the revised WHO 4th ed. classification. In addition to *TP53* mutations, AML and MDS/AML cases often have co-existing myelodysplasia-related cytogenetic abnormalities, including complex karyotypes. Despite the presence of a category of AML or MDS/AML with myelodysplasia-related cytogenetic abnormalities in the ICC, the presence of a *TP53* mutation takes diagnostic precedence over those cytogenetic abnormalities.

The proposed WHO 5th ed. does not include a category of AML with mutated *TP53* but does include a category of MDS with mutated *TP53* that would overlap with the ICC disease MDS/AML with mutated *TP53*. In the proposed WHO 5th ed. classification, ICC AML with mutated *TP53* cases (having 20% or more blasts) would most commonly fall into the more general category of AML, myelodysplasia-related based on co-existing myelodysplasia-related cytogenetic abnormalities. Such categorization, however, fails to highlight the extremely poor prognosis of the *TP53* mutated group. The diagnostic criteria for the proposed WHO 5th ed. category of MDS with mutated *TP53* differ from the ICC category MDS/AML with mutated *TP53* (having 10%–19% blasts) in that the ICC allows for monoallelic or biallelic mutations while the proposed WHO category requires the mutations be biallelic.

Acute Myeloid Leukemia and Myelodysplastic Syndrome/Acute Myeloid Leukemia With Myelodysplasia-Related Gene Mutations

As mentioned, the prior WHO category of AML with myelodysplasia-related changes has been eliminated in the ICC and replaced by several categories, particularly AML with mutated *TP53*, AML with myelodysplasia-related gene mutations, and AML with myelodysplasia-related cytogenetic abnormalities; similar categories with these features have also been added to the MDS/AML group. The proposed WHO 5th ed. classification also modified the prior category of AML with myelodysplasia-related changes, now renamed AML, myelodysplasia-related, and both ICC and the WHO eliminate cases from these categories based on the presence of morphology (multilineage dysplasia) alone.

Although multilineage dysplasia in AML is associated with a poor prognosis,[20,192] it has become clear that some genetic abnormalities, such as mutated *NPM1*,[148] take precedence over this finding and that other genetic abnormalities are better predictors of prognosis than the morphologic changes.

Several studies have evaluated cases of myelodysplasia-related AML or AML arising after prior MDS or prior therapy and identified clusters of gene mutations associated with those changes.[29-31,193] These genetic abnormalities, which vary somewhat among studies, have been termed "secondary" or "spliceosome" type mutations. When these mutations were found among AML cohorts without recurring genetic abnormalities, prior therapy, or MDS (generally corresponding to cases of AML, NOS in prior classifications), their presence remained predictive of a poor prognosis. For this reason, both the ICC and revised WHO 5th ed. classification adopted

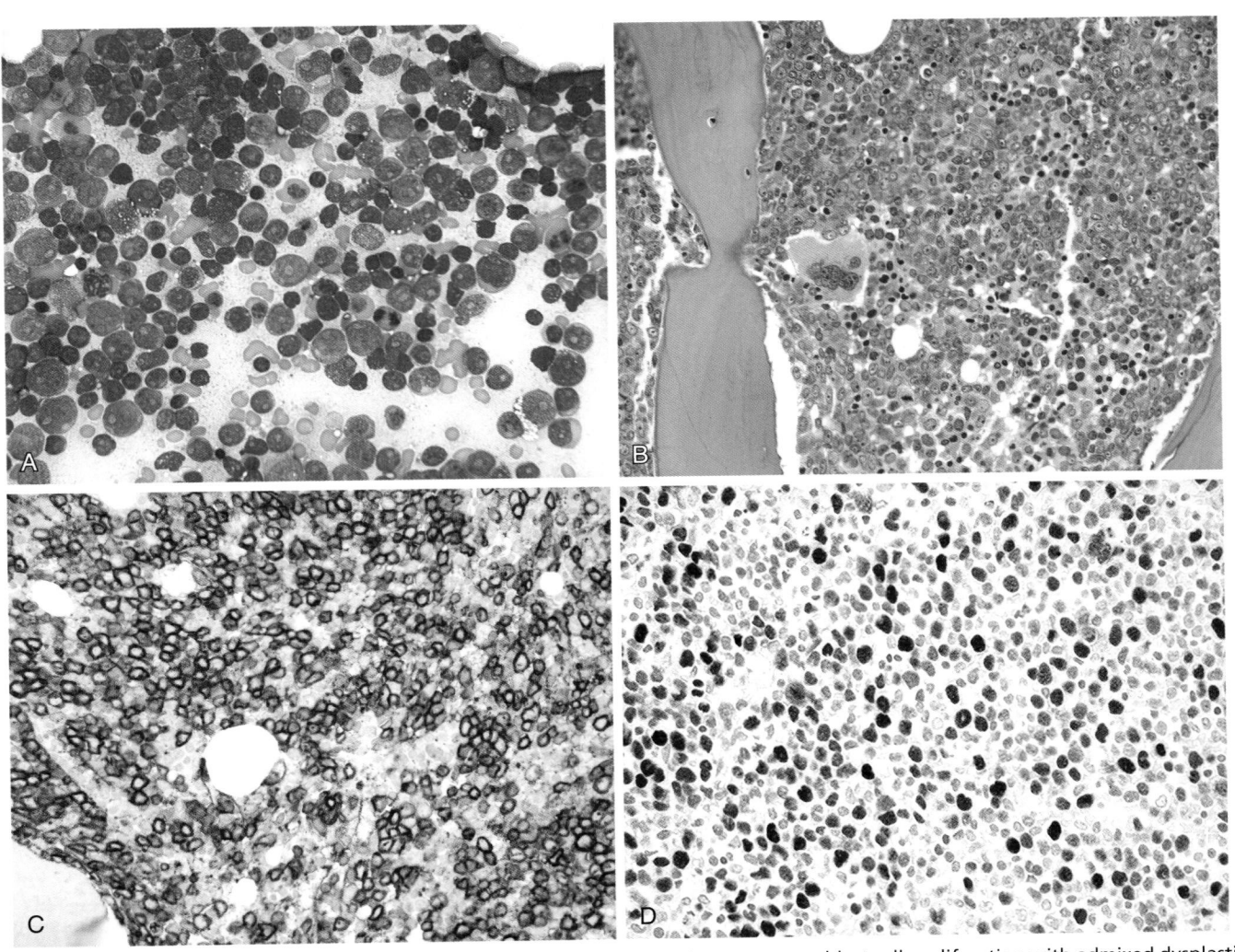

Figure 46-12. Acute myeloid leukemia with mutated *TP53*. A, The aspirate demonstrates a blast cell proliferation with admixed dysplastic erythroid precursors and immature erythroid cells. **B,** The biopsy shows sheets of immature cells with admixed maturing erythroid cells. Atypical megakaryocytes were also present. The cells express CD34 **(C)** with nuclear expression of TP53 **(D)**. The case had a complex karyotype and a *TP53* mutation, meeting criteria for acute myeloid leukemia with mutated *TP53*.

similar, but not identical, gene lists in which the presence of any one of those genes places the case in this new category. In the ICC, a patient with 10% or more peripheral blood or marrow blasts and any one of these gene mutations (*ASXL1, BCOR, EZH2, RUNX1, SF3B1, SRSF2, STAG2, U2AF1,* or *ZRSR2*) is diagnosed as AML or MDS/AML with myelodysplasia-related gene mutations based on the blast cell count (AML if 20% or more and MDS/AML if 10%–19%). Many such cases will have multilineage dysplasia (Fig. 46-13) or myelodysplasia-related cytogenetic abnormalities in addition to the gene mutation, but the new ICC mutation category takes precedence over the morphologic and cytogenetic abnormalities. In addition to overlapping with the prior WHO category of AML with myelodysplasia-related changes, this category replaces the prior provision entity in the revised WHO 4th ed. classification of AML with mutated *RUNX1*. The proposed WHO 5th ed. classification includes a similar gene list as one pathway for the diagnosis of AML, myelodysplasia-related, but the proposed WHO gene mutation list does not include *RUNX1* (Table 46-1). AML with mutated *RUNX1* is entirely eliminated in the proposed WHO 5th ed. classification. Also, cases in

this category diagnosed as MDS/AML with myelodysplasia-related gene mutations by ICC would be classified as MDS with increased blasts 2 (MDS-IB-2) in the proposed WHO 5th ed. classification.

Acute Myeloid Leukemia and Myelodysplastic Syndrome/Acute Myeloid Leukemia With Myelodysplasia-Related Cytogenetic Abnormalities

The final MDS-related AML category of the ICC is AML and MDS/AML with myelodysplasia-related cytogenetic abnormalities. MDS-related cytogenetic abnormalities have been a pathway to making a diagnosis of AML with myelodysplasia-related changes in the WHO 4th ed. and revised 4th ed. classification,[11,40] but the ICC reduces the number of cytogenetic abnormalities that fall into this category (see Table 46-2).[12] Specifically, balance cytogenetic translocations previously listed in this group are largely moved to the category of AML with other rare recurring translocations (see Box 46-11) and monosomy 13 or 13q deletions are no

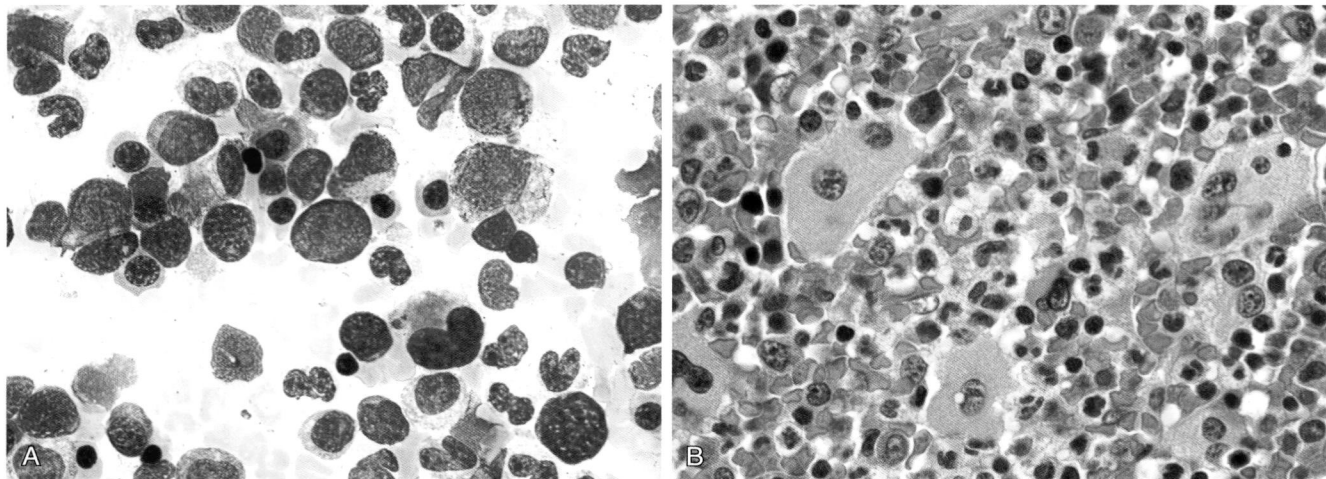

Figure 46-13. Background dysplasia in acute myeloid leukemia. Though multilineage dysplasia is no longer a diagnostic criterion for a specific acute myeloid leukemia (AML) subtype, it is common in AML with mutated *TP53*, AML with myelodysplasia-related gene mutations, AML with myelodysplasia-related cytogenetic abnormalities, and therapy-related AMLs. Dysplastic changes are best seen on aspirate smears **(A)**, but dysplastic megakaryocytes are often apparent on biopsy sections **(B)**. On the aspirate smear **(A)**, note the hypogranular neutrophils with abnormal nuclear lobation, erythroid precursors with irregular nuclear contours, and small hypolobated megakaryocytes with admixed blast cells.

Table 46-1 Definitional Gene Mutations for Acute Myeloid Leukemia and Myelodysplastic Syndrome/Acute Myeloid Leukemia With Myelodysplasia-Related Gene Mutations (ICC) and Acute Myeloid Leukemia, Myelodysplasia Related (Proposed WHO 5th Ed.)

ICC*	Proposed WHO 5th Ed.
ASXL1	*ASXL1*
BCOR	*BCOR*
EZH2	*EZH2*
RUNX1	*SF3B1*
SF3B1	*SRSF2*
SRSF2	*STAG2*
STAG2	*U2AF1*
U2AF1	*ZRSR2*
ZRSR2	

*Considered definitional in the absence of a mutation in *TP53*.
ICC, International Consensus Classification; *WHO,* World Health Organization.

Table 46-2 Definitional Cytogenetic Abnormalities for Acute Myeloid Leukemia and Myelodysplastic Syndrome/ Acute Myeloid Leukemia With Myelodysplasia-Related Cytogenetic Abnormalities (ICC) and Acute Myeloid Leukemia, Myelodysplasia Related (Proposed WHO 5th Ed.)

ICC*	Proposed WHO 5th Ed.
Complex karyotype†	Complex karyotype†
del(5q)/t(5q)/add(5q)	5q deletion or loss of 5q caused by
−7/del(7q)	unbalanced translocation
+8	monosomy 7, 7q deletion, or loss of 7q
del(12p)/t(12p)/add(12p)	caused by unbalanced translocation
i(17q)	11q deletion
−17/add(17p)	12p deletion or loss of 12p caused by
del(17p)	unbalanced translocation
del(20q)	monosomy 13 or 13q deletion
idic(X)(q13)	17p deletion or loss of 17p caused by
	unbalanced translocation
	isochromosome 17q
	idic(X)(q13)

*Considered definitional in the absence of a mutation in *TP53* or a myelodysplasia-related gene mutation (see Table 46-1).
†Three or more unrelated abnormalities, none of which is included as an acute myeloid leukemia specific genetic abnormality in the classifications (such cases should be classified in the appropriate cytogenetic group).
ICC, International Consensus Classification; *WHO,* World Health Organization.

longer included because of a lack of prognostic significance. Though the presence of trisomy 8 or del(20q) are not sufficient to make a diagnosis of MDS without a blast cell increase, their presence in cases with 10% or more blasts (MDS/AML and AML) are predictors of a poor prognosis, and these two abnormalities have been added to the ICC list of MDS-related cytogenetic abnormalities. Like AML and MDS/AML with myelodysplasia-related gene mutations, these cases frequently evolve from prior MDS, may be therapy related and are often associated with multilineage dysplasia (Fig. 46-13). There is also overlap between MDS-related cytogenetic abnormalities, *TP53* mutations, and MDS-related gene mutations, but these later categories take diagnostic priority over the category of AML and MDS/AML with myelodysplasia-related cytogenetic abnormalities.

Most cases of the ICC category of AML with myelodysplasia-related cytogenetic abnormalities (defined as having 20% or more peripheral blood or bone marrow blasts) would be included in the proposed WHO 5th ed. classification as AML, myelodysplasia related, but the WHO continues to include cases with monosomy 13 or 13q deletions in this category and does not include cases with +8 or del(20q). Cases of ICC MDS/AML with myelodysplasia-related cytogenetic abnormalities would be classified as MDS with increased blasts 2 (MDS-IB-2) in the proposed WHO 5th ed. classification.

Acute Myeloid Leukemia and Myelodysplastic Syndrome/Acute Myeloid Leukemia, Not Otherwise Specified

Cases with 10% or more peripheral blood or bone marrow blasts that do not fulfill the definition of AML or MDS/AML in any of the prior categories or myeloid neoplasms of Down syndrome are considered AML or MDS/AML, NOS, with AML used for those with 20% or more blasts and MDS/AML for those with 10% to 19% blasts. There are a number of subtypes of AML, NOS that have been used in prior WHO classifications, but these lack the cytogenetic or clinical features that would warrant calling them specific disease types, and they should be considered morphologic subtypes if the reader wishes to subclassify them.[20,194,195] Morphologic subclassification is not essential. The exceptions to this might include pure erythroid leukemia and acute panmyelosis with myelofibrosis (APMF), which are defined by different criteria, but cases belonging to those categories have become extraordinarily rare because of the larger number of cytogenetic and molecular genetic diagnostic qualifiers that take diagnostic precedence in both settings.

Most of the morphologic subtypes of AML, NOS are defined by previous FAB criteria,[2] but their blast thresholds reflect lower blast cell counts than originally proposed by FAB. Because flow cytometric immunophenotyping is routine in modern practice, cytochemical studies are not required for the subtyping of AML, NOS, although they may provide helpful information in selected cases.

This category continues to shrink in terms of percentage of cases as the genetic categories of AML and MDS/AML expand and there are really no data on the genetic characteristics of this group as genetic disease subtypes fall into the other disease categories in both the ICC and proposed WHO 5th ed. classification.

In general, this ICC category of AML, NOS corresponds to AML, defined by differentiation in the proposed WHO 5th ed., while cases of ICC MDS/AML NOS would generally be diagnosed as MDS-EB-2. These sections describe the historic features of the AML, NOS subtypes. It is difficult to use these criteria for MDS/AML cases, and a diagnosis of MDS/AML, NOS is suggested rather than attempting to subclassify such cases with AML, NOS criteria.

Acute Myeloid Leukemia With Minimal Differentiation

AML with minimal differentiation have 20% or more peripheral blood or marrow blasts that lack definitive cytologic and cytochemical evidence of myeloid lineage but demonstrate immunophenotypic evidence of myeloid lineage. The blasts lack granules or Auer rods and may be confused with lymphoblasts. The blasts are cytochemically negative for myeloperoxidase or Sudan black B (<3% positive) and are non-specific esterase negative (<20%), but they may show immunophenotypic evidence of myeloperoxidase expression. By flow cytometry, blasts express CD34, CD38, and HLA-DR. They commonly express CD13, CD33, or CD117. The blasts usually lack expression of monocytic or myeloid antigens, such as CD15, CD11b, CD14, or CD64. Expression of CD7, CD19, and TdT may be present, but blasts are negative for the more definitive B-lymphoid and T-lymphoid–associated cytoplasmic antigens CD79a, CD22, and CD3.

Acute Myeloid Leukemia Without Maturation

AML without maturation is defined as a peripheral blood or bone marrow blast population of 20% or more that is cytochemically positive for myeloperoxidase or Sudan black B and negative (<20%) for non-specific esterase. In addition, blasts must constitute 90% or more of the nonerythroid marrow cells. Blasts usually have sparse granules and infrequent Auer rods, although the identification of these features does not preclude this diagnosis. Cases may be mistaken for lymphoblastic proliferations without immunophenotyping or cytochemical studies. Blasts express myeloid-associated antigens, but there is no specific immunophenotypic profile.

Acute Myeloid Leukemia With Maturation

AML with maturation is probably the most common morphologic type of AML, NOS. It has cytochemical features identical to those of AML without maturation; however, it differs by having more than 10% of nonerythroid marrow cells showing maturation to the promyelocyte or later stage of differentiation. Blasts more frequently contain cytoplasmic granules or Auer rods but exhibit no specific cytogenetic abnormalities or immunophenotypic profile.

Acute Myelomonocytic Leukemia

In acute myelomonocytic leukemia, the sum of myeloblasts, monoblasts, and promonocytes is 20% or more. Of the leukemic cells, 20% to 79% are of monocyte lineage, often demonstrated by reactivity with the non-specific esterase stain; however, cytochemical studies are not necessary for diagnosis when the morphologic identity of the monocyte lineage is obvious. Numerous monocytes may be present in the peripheral blood and may mimic MDS/MPN, especially CMML. Both granulocytic and monocytic differentiation are observed in varying proportions in the bone marrow. The major criterion distinguishing acute myelomonocytic leukemia from AML with maturation is the proportion of neoplastic cells with monocytic features, which collectively must equal 20% or more of the blasts. The immunophenotype of acute myelomonocytic leukemia generally reflects the dual differentiation pattern of the leukemic cells, with some populations expressing fairly typical myeloid antigens and others expressing more monocytic antigens, including CD14 and CD64.

Careful distinction of promonocytes from abnormal monocytes in the bone marrow is essential to separate acute myelomonocytic leukemia from CMML.[196] Promonocytes retain fine chromatin, indistinct nucleoli, and delicate nuclear folds, reflecting their immaturity. In contrast, abnormal immature-appearing monocytes of CMML have more condensed chromatin and generally more folded or convoluted nuclear contours. In a new diagnosis, the distinction between CMML and acute myelomonocytic leukemia may not be possible with a peripheral blood smear. Correlation with bone marrow findings is essential to resolve the diagnosis because the immature populations of acute myelomonocytic leukemia are more readily identified in marrow. A reliable discriminating immunophenotype is not available because promonocytes typically lack CD34.

Acute Monoblastic and Monocytic Leukemias

Acute monoblastic and monocytic leukemias have 20% or more immature cells (blasts or promonocytes) in peripheral blood or bone marrow, and 80% or more of the marrow cells have monocytic features by morphology (Fig. 46-14), cytochemistry, or immunophenotyping studies. Cases can be further subdivided by the maturity of the monocytic cells. If 80% or more of the blasts are poorly differentiated (monoblasts), the case is considered acute monoblastic leukemia; if the monoblasts are less than 80%

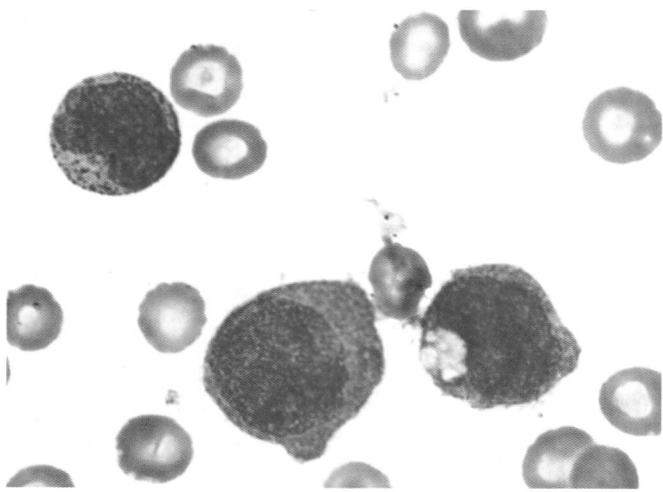

Figure 46-14. Acute monocytic leukemia (AML, NOS). Blasts may have round or more monocytoid folded nuclei and cytoplasmic vacuoles. The leukemia demonstrated no recurring genetic abnormality or defining gene mutations and meets criteria for acute myeloid leukemia, not otherwise specified.

and the cells show promonocytic and monocytic features, it is considered acute monocytic leukemia. Monoblasts are large and have moderately abundant, variably basophilic cytoplasm, which frequently contains delicate peroxidase-negative azurophilic granules or vacuoles. Auer rods are not observed. The nucleus is round, with reticular chromatin and one or more prominent nucleoli. Monoblasts are non-specific esterase positive and myeloperoxidase negative. When the leukemic cells manifest more obvious cytologic evidence of monocytic differentiation and maturation, they are called *promonocytes*. These cells are considered to be blast equivalent and for diagnostic purposes are counted as blasts. Their nucleus has delicate chromatin and a characteristic folded or cerebriform appearance. The cytoplasm is less basophilic than that of monoblasts and contains a variable number of azurophilic granules. The promonocytes are usually non-specific esterase positive; some exhibit weak myeloperoxidase activity.

The immunophenotype of acute monoblastic and monocytic leukemia is characterized by the expression of monocytic differentiation antigens, but the patterns of expression vary. Both subtypes often lack CD34 but may express CD117. They commonly express HLA-DR, CD13, and bright CD33, with CD15 and CD65. Typically, at least two markers of monocytic differentiation are present, including CD14, CD4, CD11b, CD11c, CD64, CD68, CD36, lysozyme, and CD163. Aberrant expression of CD7 and CD56 is not unusual. Myeloperoxidase may be weakly positive in acute monocytic leukemia. Immunohistochemistry may show positivity for CD68 and lysozyme, but these are relatively non-specific. CD163 appears to be a more specific marker for monocyte lineage, but it may be less sensitive.

Monoblastic and monocytic leukemias are associated with a high incidence of organomegaly, lymphadenopathy, and other tissue infiltration. In a significant number of cases, the first clinical manifestations of leukemia result from extramedullary tissue infiltrates. Despite these seemingly unique clinical features, a diagnosis of acute monoblastic or acute monocytic leukemia does not confer prognostic significance.[194]

Pure Erythroid Leukemia

Pure erythroid leukemia is composed predominantly of erythroid cells and differs from other AML types by having no increase in myeloblasts. Two subtypes of erythroid leukemia were historically recognized and were included in the 2008 4th ed. WHO classification, but only one, pure erythroid leukemia, is currently recognized.[197]

The prior erythroid/myeloid leukemia has been eliminated as an AML, NOS subtype; by definition, 50% or more of all nucleated bone marrow cells were erythroid precursors, and 20% or more of the remaining cells (nonerythroid) were myeloblasts. Such cases would now be classified as MDS if blasts are below 10% and most as MDS/AML with mutated *TP53*, MDS/AML with myelodysplasia-related gene mutations, or MDS/AML with myelodysplasia-related cytogenetic abnormalities if blasts are 10% to 19%.

In pure erythroid leukemia, the erythroid lineage is the only obvious component of acute leukemia; no significant myeloblast component is apparent. The neoplastic cells are predominantly or exclusively pronormoblasts and early basophilic normoblasts. These cells must constitute over 80% of the marrow elements, with at least 30% of cells being proerythroblasts. The erythroblasts are commonly CD34 negative and HLA-DR negative by flow cytometry and lack expression of myeloid-associated antigens. The more mature forms express hemoglobin A and glycophorin. The more immature erythroid progenitors may be CD36 positive. Some cases may also express megakaryocytic markers, such as CD41 and CD61, and it may not be possible to distinguish such cases as having an erythroid or a megakaryocytic lineage.[198] E-cadherin staining may be useful to quantitate more immature erythroid cells.[199]

Pure erythroid leukemia is highly associated with *TP53* mutations and complex karyotype and other MDS-related cytogenetic abnormalities.[187] Cases with mutated *TP53* should be classified as AML with mutated *TP53* (Fig. 46-15) in the ICC, and cases without such mutations should be carefully assessed for other causes of erythroid hyperplasia. Pure erythroid leukemias must be distinguished from several non-neoplastic disorders that manifest marked dyserythropoiesis. These include megaloblastic anemia caused by vitamin B_{12} or folate deficiency, heavy metal intoxication from arsenic, drug effects, congenital dyserythropoiesis, and exogenous erythropoietin administration. These possibilities should be considered when the sample lacks *TP53* mutations or MDS-related cytogenetic abnormalities.

Acute Megakaryoblastic Leukemia

Acute megakaryoblastic leukemia is defined by the presence of 20% or more bone marrow blasts, at least 50% of which are megakaryoblasts, in patients who do not meet the criteria for a myeloid neoplasm associated with Down syndrome, AML with t(1;22)(p13.3;q13.1), AML with t(3;3)(q21.3;q26) or inv(3)(q21.3;q6), AML with inv(16)(p13.3q24.3)/*CBFA2T3::GLIS2*, and AMLs with *NUP98* translocations or any of the other AML categories otherwise defined, including those with myelodysplasia-related gene mutations and myelodysplasia-related cytogenetic abnormalities.[116,200] With use of these criteria, the acute megakaryoblastic leukemia type of AML, NOS is uncommon. In blood and bone marrow smears, megakaryoblasts are usually medium-to-large-sized cells with

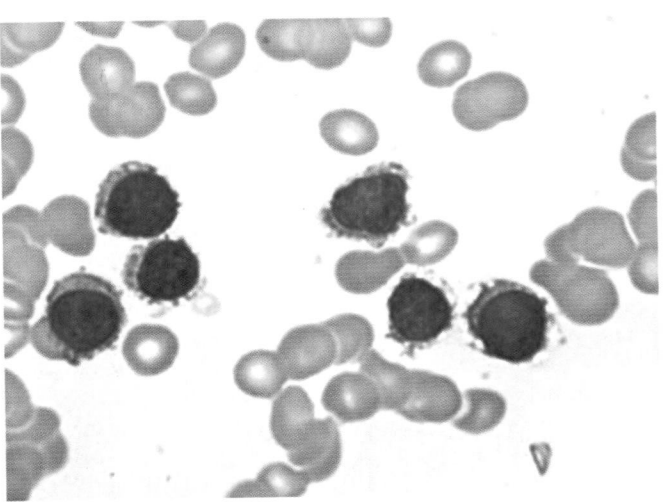

Figure 46-15. Acute myeloid leukemia with mutated *TP53*, pure erythroid leukemia type. This rare leukemia exhibits a pure population of erythroblasts with cytoplasmic vacuoles and no myeloblast proliferation. These cells represent more than 80% of peripheral blood and marrow cells and express erythroid-associated markers of hemoglobin and glycophorin. The vast majority of such cases demonstrate mutations of *TP53*.

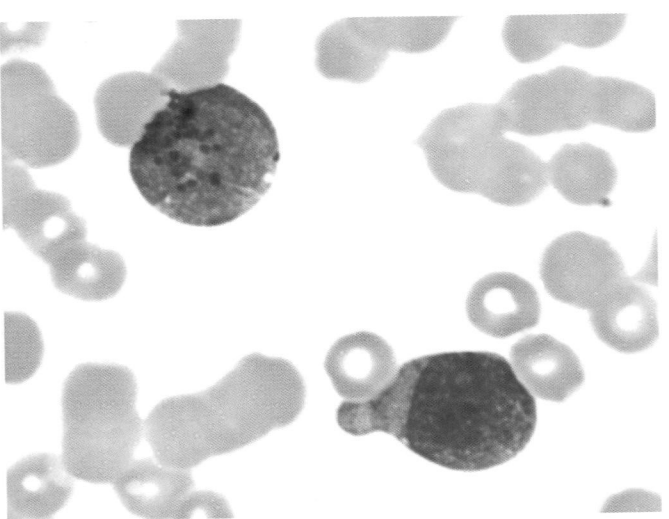

Figure 46-16. Acute basophilic leukemia. Blast cell proliferation in which many of the blasts contain basophilic granules. This patient had no history of chronic myeloid leukemia and did not meet the criteria for another type of acute myeloid leukemia and was therefore diagnosed with acute basophilic leukemia.

a high nuclear-to-cytoplasmic ratio. Nuclear chromatin is dense and homogeneous. Nucleoli are variably prominent. There is scant to moderately abundant cytoplasm, which may be vacuolated. An irregular cytoplasmic border is often noted, and projections resembling budding platelets are occasionally present. Transitional forms between poorly differentiated blasts and recognizable micromegakaryocytes may be observed. In some cases, the majority of the leukemic cells consist of small lymphoid-like blasts. A marrow aspirate may be difficult to obtain because of frequent myelofibrosis. Trephine biopsy sections may reveal morphologic evidence of megakaryocytic differentiation that is not appreciated in the marrow aspirate smears.

Identification of a megakaryocyte lineage cannot be made by morphologic features alone and requires immunophenotyping or electron microscopy and ultracytochemistry.[3] The more differentiated blasts are recognized by the presence of demarcation membranes and "bull's-eye" granules by electron microscopy. Ultrastructural peroxidase activity is found in the nuclear envelope and endoplasmic reticulum and is absent from the granules and Golgi complexes of leukemic megakaryoblasts. This pattern of localization of the ultrastructural peroxidase reaction distinguishes megakaryoblasts from myeloblasts and is the earliest distinctive, recognizable characteristic of megakaryoblasts. By flow cytometry, the megakaryoblasts are myeloperoxidase negative and may be CD45 negative, CD34 negative, and HLA-DR negative, with variable expression of CD13 or CD33. Aberrant CD7 expression may be seen. Immunophenotyping by flow cytometry or immunohistochemistry with antibodies to megakaryocyte-restricted antigens, such as CD41, CD42b, and CD61, is usually diagnostic. Bone marrow cytogenetics may be difficult to obtain owing to the presence of marrow fibrosis.

Acute Basophilic Leukemia

Acute basophilic leukemia is an extremely rare AML with 20% or more bone marrow blast cells and evidence of

basophilic differentiation. Described cases have been defined by morphologic features of basophilic blast cell granules or solely by the ultrastructural detection of basophilic features (Fig. 46-16).[201-203] The latter criterion is problematic because electron microscopy studies are not routinely performed on acute leukemias. The blasts may resemble AML without differentiation, lacking myeloperoxidase or Sudan black B. By flow cytometry, they lack CD117 (excluding mast cell leukemia) and show variable expression of CD34 and HLA-DR. CD13 and CD33 are usually detected, and blasts are usually positive for CD123 and CD11b.[204,205] Expression of CD203c in the absence of CD117 is considered fairly specific for a basophilic lineage.[204] There is no consistent chromosomal abnormality identified in most cases, but a recurring t(X;6)(p11.2;q23.3) *MYB::GATA1* appears to occur in male infants with acute basophilic leukemia.[206,207] Other reported cytogenetic abnormalities in acute basophilic leukemia include t(3;6)(q21;p21) and abnormalities involving 12p.[208,209] Other leukemias with basophilia must be excluded, including AML with t(6;9)(p22.3;q34.1), AML with *BCR::ABL1*, and blast transformation of CML.

Acute Panmyelosis With Myelofibrosis

APMF is an extremely rare disorder that is included as a subtype of AML, NOS. It occurs most commonly in adults with pancytopenia and no splenomegaly.[210-212] The marrow is fibrotic and shows panmyelosis, usually involving immature granulocytic, megakaryocytic, and erythroid cells (Fig. 46-17). Marrow myeloblast counts are usually difficult to perform owing to the inability to aspirate marrow as well as the panmyelosis, but most cases have 20% or more marrow blasts. The differential diagnosis of APMF includes primary myelofibrosis and other MPNs in their later stages, acute megakaryoblastic leukemia, AML with myelodysplasia-related gene mutations and myelodysplasia-related cytogenetic abnormalities, MDS with excess of blasts and myelofibrosis, and other neoplasms

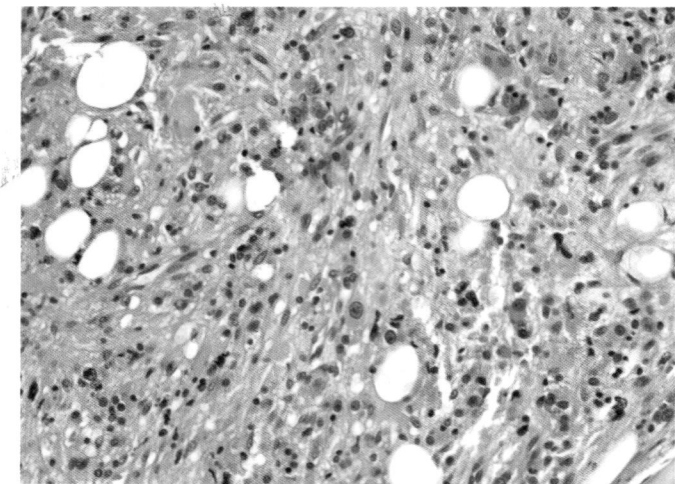

Figure 46-17. Acute panmyelosis with myelofibrosis. The marrow is replaced by fibrosis, with admixed immature cells that include myeloblasts, dysplastic and immature megakaryocytes, and erythroid precursors. The patient lacked splenomegaly and other features of a myeloproliferative neoplasm.

with fibrosis in the marrow, including metastatic tumors. The lack of splenomegaly helps distinguish this disorder from many of the MPNs. Exclusion of the myelodysplasia-related AML types may be difficult owing to poor aspirates for molecular or cytogenetic analysis, but a diagnosis of either AML with myelodysplasia-related gene mutations or AML with myelodysplasia-related cytogenetic abnormalities takes precedence over APMF. APMF can be distinguished from acute megakaryoblastic leukemia by the frequent expression of CD34 on the blasts of APMF and the proliferation of immature cells from all three lineages, not just megakaryoblasts. APMF has an aggressive course and a more abrupt clinical onset, with fever and bone pain, than MDS with increased blasts and myelofibrosis; however, in some cases, it may be impossible to distinguish APMF from myelodysplasia with fibrosis.[213]

MYELOID PROLIFERATIONS OF DOWN SYNDROME

Patients with Down syndrome are at increased risk for both ALL and AML (see also Chapter 45). Infants and children with Down syndrome often have myeloid proliferations in blood and bone marrow that in some cases would meet the criteria for AML.[214] Because of the unique nature of these myeloid proliferations, they were grouped in a separate category in the 2008 4th ed. WHO classification.[215] Approximately 10% of neonates with Down syndrome manifest a transient myeloproliferative disorder indistinguishable from acute leukemia that is called transient abnormal myelopoiesis (TAM). This proliferation spontaneously resolves in most cases. In the first 4 years of life, children with Down syndrome are at high risk for development of acute megakaryoblastic leukemia. This AML most commonly follows TAM and is phenotypically and, in many respects, genetically identical to the blasts of TAM. After the age of 5 years, the ratio of AML to ALL normalizes to that of the general pediatric population, but children with Down syndrome remain at higher risk for development of acute leukemia. Both TAM and the myeloid

leukemia of Down syndrome are associated with mutations in the megakaryocyte transcription factor *GATA1* acquired in utero.[216]

Transient Abnormal Myelopoiesis

TAM presents in the newborn period with a median age at diagnosis of 3 to 7 days.[217,218] Most patients have leukocytosis and increased peripheral blood blasts.[219] The blasts usually show morphologic features similar to megakaryoblasts in other settings, including basophilic cytoplasm with or without coarse basophilic granules and cytoplasmic projections (Fig. 46-18). Red blood cell and platelet indices are variable, with near-normal median values. Dysplastic changes of marrow elements may be present. By flow cytometry, the blasts of TAM commonly express moderate CD45 and HLA-DR; the myeloid antigen CD33 with or without CD13; and CD38, CD117, and CD34.[220-222] They frequently show aberrant CD7 and CD56 expression and evidence of megakaryocytic differentiation, with expression of CD41, CD61, and CD71. Clonal cytogenetic abnormalities are typically limited to trisomy 21, although non-clonal abnormalities are frequently observed. *GATA1* and *JAK3* mutations are both common in TAM.[223-226]

Hepatic dysfunction is a marker for poor outcome in TAM. Patients frequently demonstrate hepatomegaly. Clinically significant liver disease is manifested as hyperbilirubinemia with or without elevated transaminases. Biopsy may demonstrate cholestasis, fibrosis (portal and perisinusoidal), a paucity of bile ducts, variable hepatocellular necrosis, and a variable amount of extramedullary hematopoiesis. Some cases show an abundance of megakaryocyte precursors; others may show only occasional mononuclear cells. This may be a function of their myeloproliferative state and whether the biopsy is performed during TAM, with elevated blast counts, or after the resolution of TAM. Patients with severe perinatal disease may have fibrosis of other organs, including the pancreas and kidneys. Generalized skin involvement by TAM has been reported, including lesions showing perivascular immature cell infiltrates[227] and erythematous maculopapular lesions and indurated subcutaneous nodules.[228]

Only a subset of patients requires intervention because of hyperviscosity, blast counts greater than 100,000/µL, organomegaly with respiratory compromise, renal dysfunction, or disseminated intravascular coagulation. Three risk groups have been described: low risk, with no palpable hepatomegaly or hepatic dysfunction (38% of patients; OS, 92% ± 8%); intermediate risk, with hepatomegaly and non–life-threatening hepatic dysfunction (40% of patients; OS, 82% ± 11%); and high risk, with a white blood cell count greater than 100,000/µL or life-threatening cardiorespiratory compromise because of TAM (21% of patients; OS, 49% ± 20%). The reported median time to TAM resolution is 46 days. A later myeloid proliferation develops in 10% to 30% of patients, including some treated with low-dose chemotherapy.[217,218]

Myeloid Leukemia Associated With Down Syndrome

An AML-like presentation in Down syndrome typically occurs in the first 3 years of life, often after a prolonged

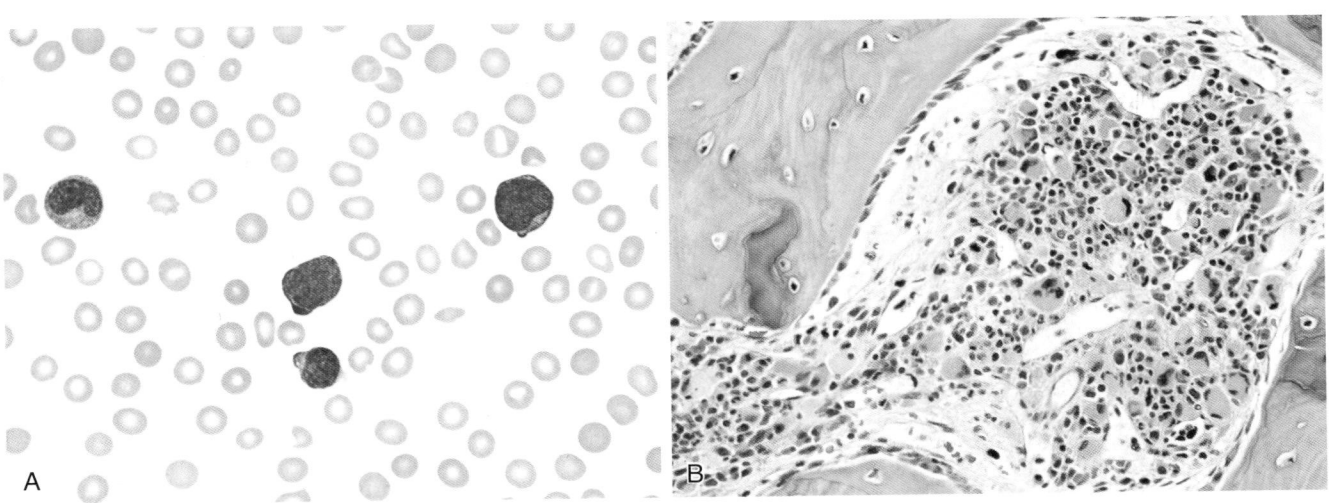

Figure 46-18. Transient abnormal myelopoiesis in an infant with Down syndrome. A, Peripheral blood from an infant with Down syndrome contains blasts with basophilic cytoplasm and shows cytoplasmic blebbing. These blasts express CD41 and CD61, consistent with megakaryoblasts. **B,** Bone marrow biopsy shows a predominance of immature cells and megakaryocytes.

myelodysplasia-like phase.[229] Because cases with 5% to 20% blasts and cases of overt AML are biologically and clinically similar, they are often treated with similar protocols are not separated in MDS and AML types. Acute megakaryoblastic proliferations are the most common. Studies suggest that nearly all myeloid leukemias associated with Down syndrome in children younger than 4 years are megakaryoblastic proliferations.

Blasts in myeloid leukemia associated with Down syndrome can be identified in the blood, bone marrow, liver, and spleen and exhibit features common to megakaryoblasts, as described earlier (Fig. 46-19). Dyserythropoiesis is usually evident in the blood (anisopoikilocytosis) and marrow (megaloblastic changes, nuclear contour abnormalities, multinucleate forms). By flow cytometry, the blasts show a similar immunophenotypic profile to that of TAM, with a few possible differences.[220,222,223] The blasts of AML may show more consistent expression of CD13 and CD11b, with less CD34 (93% of TAM cases compared with 50% of myeloid leukemia associated with Down syndrome) and possibly less HLA-DR. In addition, myeloid leukemia associated with Down syndrome often demonstrates more severe cytopenias, more background dysplasia and marrow fibrosis, and more frequent clonal karyotypic abnormalities other than trisomy 21 (including complete or partial trisomies of chromosomes 1 and 8) compared with TAM.[222] Despite these clonal abnormalities, many of which are considered myelodysplasia related in non–Down syndrome patients, the prognosis of myeloid leukemia associated with Down syndrome is very good compared with that in non–Down syndrome patients, especially when it is treated with HiDAC. However, the prognosis in patients older than 5 years is similar to that in non–Down syndrome patients.[230] Age is a significant predictor of outcome even in younger children. The event-free survival for children aged 0 to 2 years is 86%; for those aged 2 to 4 years, it is 70%; and for those older than 4 years, it is 28%.[230] There is a trend toward more frequent monosomy 7 in older children, but it is not clear whether this significantly affects outcome. Although *GATA1* mutations are present in both TAM and myeloid leukemia associated with Down syndrome, myeloid leukemias in this

setting appear to arise from a *GATA1*-mutated TAM clone that has acquired additional mutations. Implicated additional mutations include *CTCF, EZH2, KANSL1, JAK2, JAK3, MPL, SH2B3,* and RAS pathway genes.[231,232]

MYELOID SARCOMA

Myeloid sarcoma is an extramedullary mass forming proliferation of myeloid blasts that may be associated with a concurrent myeloid neoplasm involving the bone marrow, but such an association is not required.[233-237] In some cases, myeloid sarcoma may herald relapse in a patient with previously treated disease. In others, it may be the first indication of acute leukemia. In adults, roughly one-third of myeloid sarcomas present with concurrent myeloid disease (including AML, MDS, MPN, and MDS/MPN), and one-third have a history of a prior myeloid neoplasm. By definition, the infiltrates efface the underlying tissue architecture. Synonyms include chloroma, granulocytic sarcoma, and extramedullary myeloid tumor. The de novo presence of myeloid sarcoma is diagnostic of AML, regardless of the bone marrow or blood status. The most common site of involvement is the skin, followed by mucous membranes, orbits, central nervous system, lymph nodes, bones, gonads, and other internal organs. Myeloid sarcoma is considered more common in pediatric AML, occurring in approximately 10% of cases,[198] although the true incidence in adults is unknown. The frequency in children may reflect associations with the t(8;21), inv(16), and 11q23.3 translocation subtypes, which are relatively more common in younger patients.

Previously, three subtypes of myeloid sarcoma were described on the basis of the degree of maturation: blastic, immature, and differentiated.[199,237] Such subtyping is no longer considered relevant, but it may be useful in recognizing the morphologic variability of the myeloid blast infiltrate. Myeloid sarcoma should not be considered a type of AML but rather a type of presentation of AML or blast transformation. Every attempt should be made to classify myeloid sarcoma cytogenetically and immunophenotypically, in the same manner as if it were AML in the bone marrow. In patients with

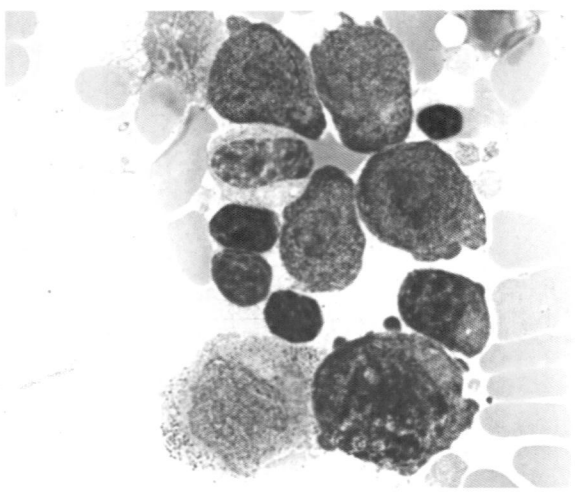

Figure 46-19. Myeloid neoplasm associated with Down syndrome. Bone marrow shows abnormal erythroid precursors and blasts that mark as megakaryoblasts. Although the features are similar to those in Figure 46-18, the diagnosis of myeloid neoplasm associated with Down syndrome rather than transient abnormal myelopoiesis is dependent on the child's age and the clinical features.

concurrent bone marrow or peripheral blood involvement, this classification is straightforward. In patients with de novo disease limited to myeloid sarcoma, precise classification may be difficult. Repeated biopsy or fine-needle aspiration may be necessary to obtain smears and fresh material for flow cytometric immunophenotyping and cytogenetic and molecular genetic studies to properly classify the AML.[238]

The myeloblasts of myeloid sarcoma usually form sheets of mononuclear cells, with an interfollicular pattern common in lymph nodes (Fig. 46-20). The blast cells may have admixed maturing granulocytes, erythroid precursors, or megakaryocytes, which are useful clues to the myeloid lineage of the immature cell population (Fig. 46-20A). Eosinophilic myelocytes are the most easily recognized maturing cell population. Although they are present in only a subset of myeloid sarcomas, their presence is highly associated with a myeloblast cell population. The blasts themselves may have round to folded nuclei, usually with fine nuclear chromatin with a more stippled pattern than that typically seen in large B-cell lymphoma. Flow cytometric immunophenotyping usually demonstrates a lack of lineage-specific B-cell or T-cell markers and expression of myeloid or myelomonocytic markers, such as CD13, CD33, myeloperoxidase, CD14, or CD64. However, as with AML in other sites, aberrant lymphoid antigen expression commonly occurs, and a relatively large panel of antibodies is useful to ensure accurate lineage determination. Fewer antibodies are available for characterization in paraffin sections, but lack of specific B-lineage or T-lineage markers with expression of myeloperoxidase, CD33, or the monocyte-specific marker CD163 is fairly specific for myeloid sarcoma. Other markers that are commonly positive but less lineage-specific are CD43, lysozyme, and CD68. Only about half of cases are CD34 positive, but CD117 expression is apparently more common.[239]

Myeloid sarcoma shows some variability in presentation. Nearly one-quarter of children with AML with t(8;21) (q22;q22.1)/*RUNX1::RUNX1T1* develop myeloid

sarcoma.[240,241] Head and neck localization with orbital, skull, and central nervous system extramedullary involvement is most common in this group. A smaller percentage (approximately 10%) of adults with t(8;21) AML have myeloid sarcoma,[240] without the pattern of head and neck localization. Skin involvement in pediatric patients (leukemia cutis) tends to occur at a younger age (median, 2.6 years), and the skin lesions are most commonly associated with 11q23.3 translocations and with abnormalities of chromosome 16. Myelomonocytic morphology is most common in this setting. A unique and rare subset of skin tumors appears to represent a congenital leukemia, with multiple skin lesions of myeloid sarcoma presenting within the first week after birth (a form of "blueberry muffin" baby). In some of these babies, disease is limited to the skin. Such cases tend to have spontaneous remissions, sometimes during a period of days. The most common AML type in this setting is AML with t(8;16)(p11.2;q13.3)/*KAT6A::CREBBP*,[127] which is frequently associated with erythrophagocytosis, therapy-related disease, and poor prognosis in adults. Because chemotherapy is very toxic to newborns, some reports recommend careful observation for patients with congenital myeloid sarcoma limited to the skin and no systemic manifestations, cytopenias, or lymph node involvement. Some spontaneously remitting cases with t(8;16) recur. Reserving chemotherapy for recurrences in spontaneously remitting cases may be an appropriate course of action,[242] sparing the infant excessive and possibly unnecessary toxicity. In contrast to babies with t(8;16) disease, those with 11q23.3 translocations tend to have a poor prognosis.

The clinical significance of myeloid sarcoma remains unclear, but the site of involvement may affect outcome, with improved survival reported for isolated cases involving the pelvis and genitourinary organs, eyes, gonads, and gastrointestinal mucosa.[243] Other than the self-limited congenital forms, it is not clear whether myeloid sarcoma confers any specific prognosis in the era of HiDAC therapy, particularly when cases are classified according to known risk groups.[240,244] Low-dose radiation therapy may be useful for the emergent treatment of life-threatening or organ-threatening (e.g., orbital) myeloid sarcomas. The use of radiation therapy in the routine management of these patients does not appear to be indicated, however. Hematopoietic cell transplantation may be appropriate, especially if myeloid sarcoma presents early in the patient's disease course.[238,245,246]

The differential diagnosis of myeloid sarcoma versus lymphoma, especially diffuse large B-cell lymphoma, lymphoblastic lymphoma, blastic mantle cell lymphoma, and Burkitt lymphoma, is challenging on morphologic grounds alone. Fine nuclear chromatin with a high mitotic rate is often helpful in differentiating large B-cell lymphoma, which usually shows more distinct nucleoli and chromatin clearing. The presence of admixed erythroid cells, megakaryocytes, or eosinophilic myelocytes is a helpful clue to the possibility of a myeloid tumor. Immunophenotyping, however, is essential to the proper diagnosis of myeloid sarcoma. Cases of suspected lymphoma that lack B-lineage or T-lineage–specific markers, including those with a CD43-only immunophenotype, should be further evaluated for evidence of myeloid sarcoma. Aberrant B-lineage marker expression, particularly CD19 and PAX5, in AML with t(8;21)(q22;q22.1) can lead to an incorrect diagnosis of B-cell lymphoma in a case of myeloid sarcoma. Subsets of APL and AML with inv(16)(p13.1q22)

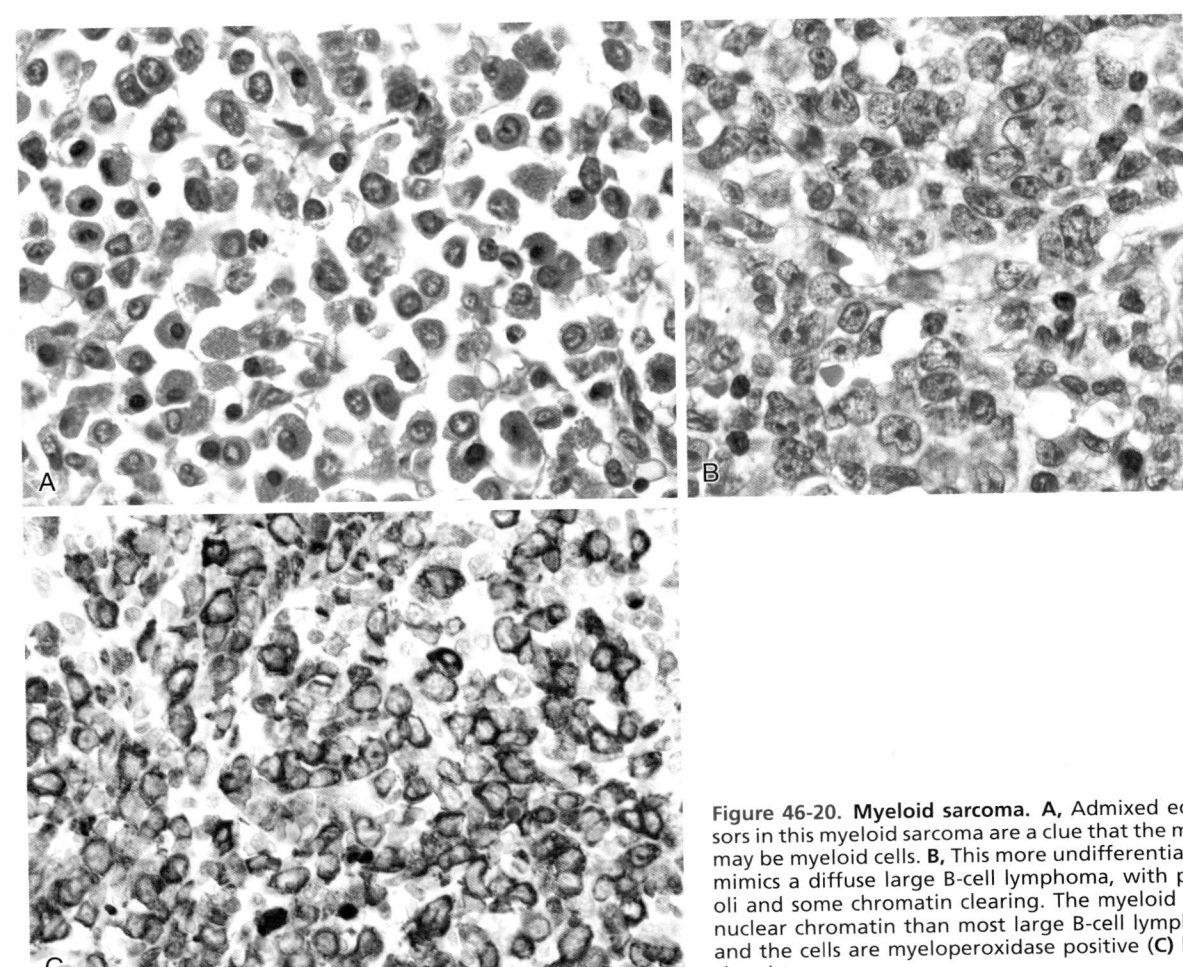

Figure 46-20. Myeloid sarcoma. A, Admixed eosinophil precursors in this myeloid sarcoma are a clue that the mononuclear cells may be myeloid cells. **B,** This more undifferentiated proliferation mimics a diffuse large B-cell lymphoma, with prominent nucleoli and some chromatin clearing. The myeloid blasts have finer nuclear chromatin than most large B-cell lymphomas, however, and the cells are myeloperoxidase positive **(C)** by immunohistochemistry.

or t(16;16)(p13.1;q22)/*CBFB::MYH11* aberrantly express the T-lineage–associated marker CD2 and can be mistaken for T-cell lymphomas. CD7 and CD56 are also frequently expressed in myeloid sarcoma, and neither marker should be used alone to diagnose a T-cell or natural killer cell malignant neoplasm. Rare extramedullary tumors of AML (megakaryocytic) with t(1;22)(p13.3;q13.1)/*RBM15::MRTFA* often show cell clustering in infants and may be mistaken for small, blue, round cell tumors of infancy. Paraffin detection of CD41, CD42b, and CD61 expression is useful in these cases, which are characteristically myeloperoxidase negative. Von Willebrand factor and LAT (linker for activation of T cells) are less-specific markers of megakaryocytic lineage. Without knowledge of this tumor and investigation with megakaryocytic markers, the diagnosis may be missed.

Other aspects of the differential diagnosis include the interpretation of sparse immature myeloid cell infiltrates in extramedullary sites. The diagnosis of myeloid sarcoma should be restricted to tumors that form space-occupying lesions. Patients with AML may have leukemic infiltrates in multiple sites that do not form masses that disrupt normal tissue architecture, and such cases should not be considered myeloid sarcoma. Patients receiving growth factors may have left-shifted granulocytes in various tissues that do not form masses, and these should not be overinterpreted as myeloid sarcoma. Similarly, maturing granulocyte proliferations of the

skin must be distinguished from a dermal myeloid sarcoma. Sweet syndrome,[247] also known as acute febrile neutrophilic dermatosis, may occur in patients with AML, but this does not represent an extramedullary leukemic infiltrate. Sweet syndrome is associated with pronounced dermal edema with a marked mature neutrophilic infiltrate, in contrast to the more immature cell infiltrate of cutaneous myeloid sarcoma. Sweet syndrome often resolves with treatment of the associated AML; the lesions also respond to systemic corticosteroid therapy.

DIAGNOSTIC QUALIFIERS IN ACUTE MYELOID LEUKEMIA

The ICC introduced the use of diagnostic qualifiers that slightly alter the approach to the diagnosis or MDS, AML, and MDS/AML.[12] Diagnostic qualifiers in AML relate to (1) therapy-related disease; (2) progression from MDS or MDS/MPN; and (3) presence of a germline predisposition. In prior classifications, therapy-related myeloid neoplasms were grouped together and not further classified. Though it was understood that some types of prior therapy correlate with genetic abnormalities, such as MDS-related cytogenetic abnormalities or *KMT2A* translocations (see Figs. 46-21 and 46-22), these findings were not used diagnostically. Though a history of prior cytotoxic therapy is a poor prognostic indicator in these disorders, the underlying

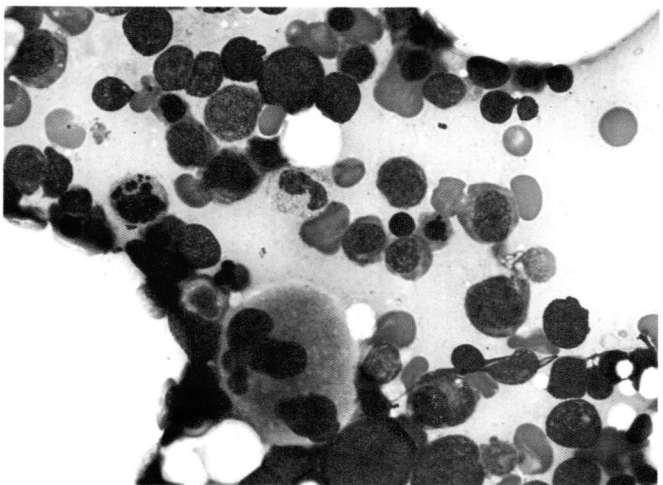

Figure 46-21. Acute myeloid leukemia (AML) with myelodysplasia-related cytogenetic abnormalities (complex karyotype), therapy-related after alkylating agent chemotherapy. Multilineage dysplasia is characteristically present. Such cases are now diagnosed similar to other AML types with "therapy-related" added as a qualifier.

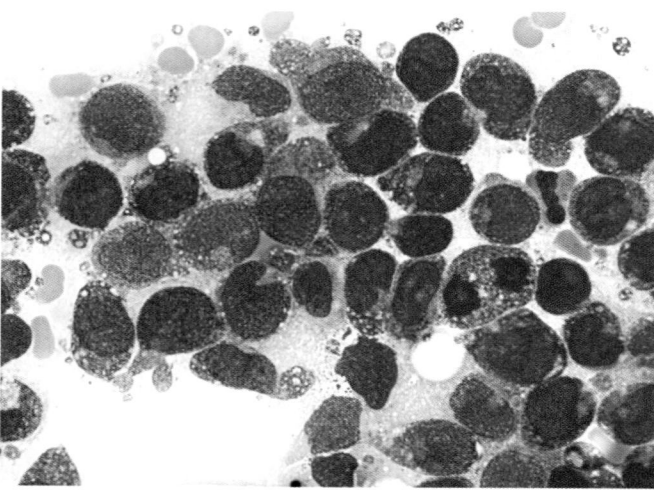

Figure 46-22. Acute myeloid leukemia (AML) with t(9;11)(p21.3;q23.3)/*MLLT3::KMT2A*, therapy-related after topoisomerase II inhibitor therapy. This case shows blasts with monocytic features and no background dysplasia, typical of therapy-related disease with this cytogenetic abnormality.

genetic abnormalities remain prognostically significant. For this reason, such cases should now be diagnosed similar to de novo cases with the qualifier "therapy-related" added after the diagnosis. Cases arising from prior MDS or MDS/MPN should also be diagnosed like de novo disease with a comment that they represent progression of the underlying disorder (i.e., AML with mutated *TP53* progressing from MDS). Finally, many germline gene abnormalities are now recognized (see Chapter 45) that predispose to the development of MDS, AML, and even ALL. Detection of these germline mutations is not sufficient for a diagnosis of AML, MDS, or MDS/AML, but when the clinical features meet criteria for those disorders, the germline abnormality should be noted to clarify the familial risk associated with the neoplasm. The proposed WHO 5th ed. classification appears to take a different approach to these disorders. They retain the category of myeloid neoplasms postcytotoxic therapy but suggest that a recurring genetic abnormality be described in the pathology report. Cases with prior MDS or MDS/MPN that evolve to AML appear to fall into the proposed WHO category of AML, myelodysplasia-related. It is unclear at the time this chapter was prepared how the proposed WHO 5th ed. classification will address germline abnormalities in the setting of AML.

INTEGRATED APPROACH TO THE DIAGNOSIS OF ACUTE MYELOID LEUKEMIA

A complex approach is necessary to diagnose and appropriately classify cases of AML.[248] This requires an integration of morphologic, immunophenotypic, cytogenetic, and molecular genetic data. Such integration is best done in a single, final pathology report. Such reports need to be amended as genetic results become available, and diagnoses will be revised on the basis of those data. Although morphologic and immunophenotypic clues can suggest specific cytogenetic abnormalities, cytogenetic or molecular genetic confirmation is essential. Diagnosis based on any single element of the workup of AML is fraught with difficulty and pitfalls. Some cases with 10% or more peripheral blood or bone marrow blast cells on morphologic examination are now considered acute leukemia if they have specific recurring cytogenetic abnormalities. These cases might be missed if the appropriate cytogenetic studies are not available to the diagnosing pathologist. Similarly, samples with high numbers of marrow red blood cell precursors may result in falsely elevated blast cell counts when such counts are performed only by flow cytometry, and these cases may be overdiagnosed as AML. Cases of AML with specific recurring cytogenetic abnormalities, such as AML with t(8;21)(q22;q22.1)/*RUNX1::RUNX1T1*, may be misdiagnosed as mixed phenotype acute leukemia if only flow cytometry methods are used for diagnosis.

Although the various studies necessary to diagnose AML may be performed in different laboratories, the pathologist must review all the diagnostic data and incorporate them into a final report that explains how the different studies contribute to the diagnosis. Figure 46-23 shows a diagnostic algorithm for the integrated approach to these specimens. This approach adds an extra layer of complexity to pathology reporting, but it also provides the most clinically relevant diagnosis for a given case. Based on that diagnosis, appropriate treatment can be administered, and markers for the detection of residual disease can be identified, resulting in better patient care.

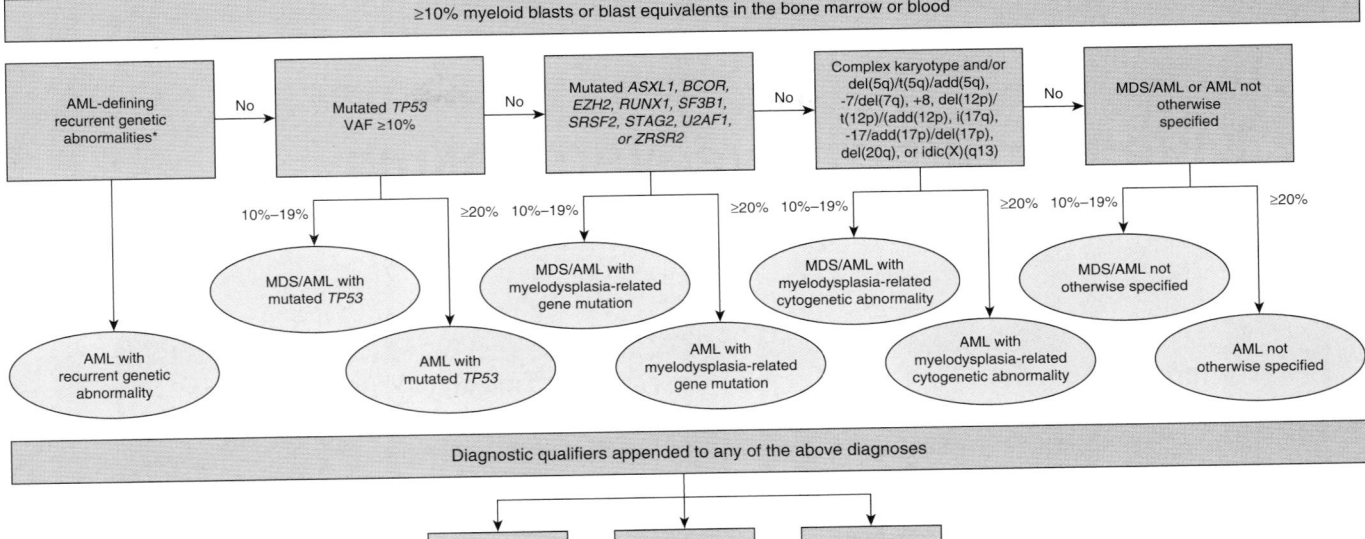

Figure 46-23. Diagnostic hierarchy of acute myeloid leukemia (AML) using the International Consensus Classification (ICC). *AML,* Acute myeloid leukemia; *MDS,* myelodysplastic syndrome; *MPN,* myeloproliferative neoplasm; *VAF,* variant allele frequency. *(Adapted from Dohner H, Wei AH, Appelbaum FR, et al. Diagnosis and management of AML in adults: 2022 recommendations from an international expert panel on behalf of the ELN. Blood. 2022;140(12):1345–1377.)*

Pearls and Pitfalls

- Manual blast cell counts on aspirate smears are still required for classification and take precedence over flow cytometry or other methods of blast cell enumeration.
- Immunohistochemical enumeration of blast cells is useful particularly in the presence of marrow fibrosis or marked hypocellularity (fatty marrows).
- Both flow cytometry and immunohistochemistry may underestimate marrow blast counts because of a variety of factors, including lack of CD34 expression on all blasts.
- Acute myeloid leukemia (AML) with monocytic features may mimic chronic myelomonocytic leukemia in the peripheral blood, so bone marrow examination is required for diagnosis.
- Close communication with the cytogenetics laboratory is essential to alert staff to potentially subtle abnormalities such as inv(16)(p13.1q22).
- Folded blast cell nuclei without other features of monocytic differentiation should raise concern for hypogranular acute promyelocytic leukemia (APL).
- Hypogranular APL often has weak CD34 expression.
- Admixed eosinophilic myelocytes, erythroid precursors, or megakaryocytes in an extramedullary mononuclear cell proliferation should raise concern for myeloid sarcoma.
- A final diagnosis of AML or myelodysplastic syndrome (MDS)/AML cannot usually be made until results of immunophenotyping and genetic studies are complete, requiring amended reports.
- Gene-mutation panels add prognostic significance to an AML or MDS/AML diagnosis even when they do not alter the diagnosis.

KEY REFERENCES

12. Arber DA, Orazi A, Hasserjian RP, et al. International Consensus classification of myeloid neoplasms and acute leukemias: integrating morphologic, clinical, and genomic data. *Blood.* 2022;140(11):1200–1228.

23. Genomic and epigenomic landscapes of adult de novo acute myeloid leukemia. *N Engl J Med.* 2013;368(22):2059–2074.

29. Lindsley RC, Mar BG, Mazzola E, et al. Acute myeloid leukemia ontogeny is defined by distinct somatic mutations. *Blood.* 2015;125(9):1367–1376.

30. Papaemmanuil E, Gerstung M, Bullinger L, et al. Genomic classification and prognosis in acute myeloid leukemia. *N Engl J Med.* 2016;374(23):2209–2221.

42. Estey E, Hasserjian RP, Dohner H. Distinguishing AML from MDS: a fixed blast percentage may no longer be optimal. *Blood.* 2022;139(3):323–332.

171. Tarlock K, Lamble AJ, Wang YC, et al. CEBPA-bZip mutations are associated with favorable prognosis in de novo AML: a report from the Children's Oncology Group. *Blood.* 2021;138(13):1137–1147.

179. Grob T, Al Hinai AS, Sanders MA, et al. Molecular characterization of mutant TP53 acute myeloid leukemia and high-risk myelodysplastic syndrome. *Blood.* 2022.

180. Weinberg OK, Siddon AJ, Madanat Y, et al. TP53 mutation defines a unique subgroup within complex karyotype de novo and therapy-related MDS/AML. *Blood Adv.* 2022.

188. Dohner H, Wei AH, Appelbaum FR, et al. Diagnosis and management of AML in adults: 2022 recommendations from an international expert panel on behalf of the ELN. *Blood.* 2022;140(12):1345–1377.

Visit Elsevier eBooks+ for the complete set of references.

Chapter 47

Myeloproliferative Neoplasms

Sonam Prakash, Attilio Orazi, and Hans Michael Kvasnicka

INTRODUCTION

The myeloproliferative neoplasms (MPNs) are clonal hematopoietic disorders characterized by proliferation of cells of one or more of the myeloid lineages: erythroid, granulocytic, or megakaryocytic. Initially, the proliferation in the bone marrow is effective and associated with maturation of the neoplastic cells that leads to increased numbers of mature granulocytes, red blood cells (RBCs), and platelets in the peripheral blood. Splenomegaly and hepatomegaly are common and caused by the sequestration of excess blood cells, extramedullary hematopoiesis (EMH), or both in these organs. Despite an insidious onset, each MPN entity has the potential to progress to bone marrow failure because of myelofibrosis, ineffective hematopoiesis, transformation to a blast phase (BP), or any combination of these events. Disease progression is usually accompanied by genetic evolution. Entities included in both the International Consensus Classification 2022 (ICC) and proposed World Health Organization classification (proposed WHO 5th edition) of MPNs are listed in Box 47-1 and include chronic myeloid leukemia (CML); chronic neutrophilic leukemia (CNL); essential thrombocythemia (ET); primary myelofibrosis (PMF, including both prefibrotic and overtly fibrotic variants/stages); polycythemia vera (PV); chronic eosinophilic leukemia, not otherwise specified (CEL,

NOS); and MPN, unclassifiable (MPN-U).[1,2] Among these clinicopathologic entities, ET, PV, and PMF share similar genetic and bone marrow morphologic characteristics, especially in regard to their close association with *JAK2/CALR/MPL* mutations, with *JAK2* mutation being the most prevalent in each of these entities. This chapter provides an integrated diagnostic approach to MPNs including hematologic, morphologic, cytogenetic, and molecular genetic findings.

ETIOLOGY AND PATHOGENESIS

The cause of MPNs is not known in most cases. There are reports of CML, PV, and PMF after exposure to ionizing irradiation, but except for cases of CML after the atomic bomb explosions in Hiroshima and Nagasaki, documented instances are rare.[3-6] Most cases of MPN are sporadic, but an inherited susceptibility has been described. Relatives of patients with MPNs have an increased risk for development of PV, ET, or PMF, and many families have been reported with multiple members affected.[7-11] In some, the inheritance pattern is autosomal dominant with incomplete penetrance; in other families, the mode of inheritance is not clear. Single-nucleotide polymorphisms of specific genes in the germline reportedly predispose to acquisition of somatic mutations important in the pathogenesis of MPNs. The best-known predisposing factor for sporadic MPNs associated with the acquired somatic *JAK2* V617F mutation is the germline *JAK2* 46/1 haplotype, which may figure in the familial predisposition for PV, ET, and PMF. However, this haplotype is relatively common, and most individuals who carry it do not develop an MPN.[12] Rare cases of CNL with familial/germline predisposition have been reported.[13,14]

Although a complete understanding of the cellular defects in MPNs is still evolving, there is considerable information about specific genetic abnormalities that contribute to their pathogenesis. A major breakthrough in unraveling the pathogenesis of MPNs occurred in 1960, when Nowell and Hungerford described the chromosomal abnormality in CML, the Philadelphia (Ph) chromosome[15] (Fig. 47-1). Rowley demonstrated that the Ph chromosome results from the reciprocal translocation of genetic material between chromosomes 9 and 22, that is, t(9;22)(q34.1;q11.2).[16] This translocation was subsequently shown to fuse sequences of the *BCR* gene on chromosome 22 and of the *ABL1* gene on chromosome 9, resulting in an abnormal fusion gene, *BCR::ABL1*, that encodes a chimeric BCR::ABL1 protein with a constitutively activated tyrosine kinase (TK) derived

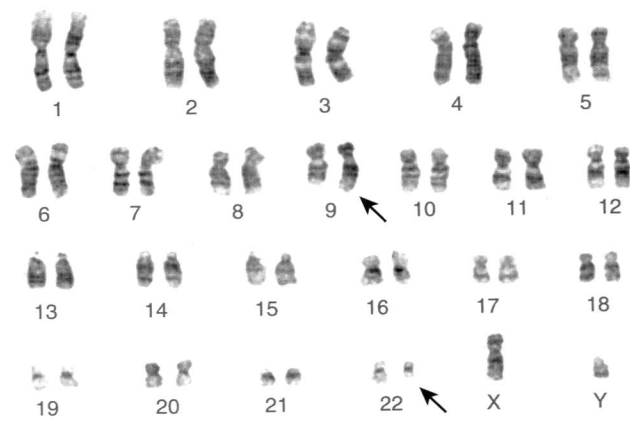

Figure 47-1. Karyotype showing the Philadelphia chromosome, der(22q), which results from the translocation of material between 9q34 and 22q11.2 *(arrows). (Courtesy Dr. Yanming Zhang, University of Chicago.)*

from the translocated *ABL1*[17-20] (Figs. 47-2 and 47-3). Experimental evidence has shown the BCR::ABL1 protein is necessary and sufficient for the initiation of CML.[21,22] The constitutively activated TK leads to autophosphorylation of BCR::ABL1, which in turn autophosphorylates other sites on the protein to activate a network of downstream signaling pathways including JAK/STAT, PI3K/AKT, RAS/MEK, mTOR, Src kinase, and BCL2/BCL-XL, among others (Fig. 47-4), that results in growth factor independence, inhibition of cell death and autophagy, and defects in cellular adhesion.[23-25] In essence, BCR::ABL1 gains control of major cellular pathways to promote the leukemic state. An understanding of the molecular events related to the abnormal signaling pathways in CML led to the design and synthesis of small molecules that target and inhibit the TK activity of BCR::ABL1. Imatinib was the first such TK inhibitor (TKI) to be used clinically. It competes with adenosine triphosphate for binding to the BCR::ABL1 kinase domain and prevents phosphorylation of tyrosine residues on BCR::ABL1 substrates. Its ability to induce remission in most patients provided further proof of the central role of BCR::ABL1 in the pathogenesis of CML.[26] However, evidence suggests that the CML leukemic stem cell, which is largely quiescent, may not rely on BCR::ABL1 kinase activity for survival.[27,28]

Mutations of the Janus 2 kinase gene, *JAK2* V617F and *JAK2* exon 12,[29-32] the myeloproliferative leukemia virus oncogene *MPL*,[33] and the calreticulin gene (*CALR*)[34,35] represent driver mutations in the *BCR::ABL1*-negative MPNs PV, ET, and PMF. Mutations in these genes affect encoding proteins that directly or indirectly activate downstream signaling in the JAK-STAT pathway and lead to myeloproliferation. In addition, activating mutations of the colony-stimulating factor 3 receptor gene (*CSF3R*) have been recognized in chronic neutrophilic leukemia (CNL)[36] (Table 47-1).

The JAK kinases are essential to cytokine signaling and signal transduction through their association with homodimeric type 1 cytokine receptors that lack intrinsic kinase activity. The JAK2 protein is the sole JAK kinase that associates with the erythropoietin (EPO) receptor, EPOR. It also associates with the thrombopoietin (TPO) receptor, MPL, and G-CSFR, the granulocyte colony-stimulating factor (G-CSF) receptor, among others.[37,38] Normally, engagement of the cytokine receptor with its ligand results in receptor dimerization, followed by autophosphorylation and transphosphorylation of the receptor and of JAK2 kinase. The activated JAK2-receptor complex then leads to recruitment and phosphorylation of substrate molecules, including signal transducers and activators of transcription (STAT) proteins, which subsequently leads to target gene transcription in the nucleus.[29-31] The *JAK2* V617F mutation is an acquired somatic

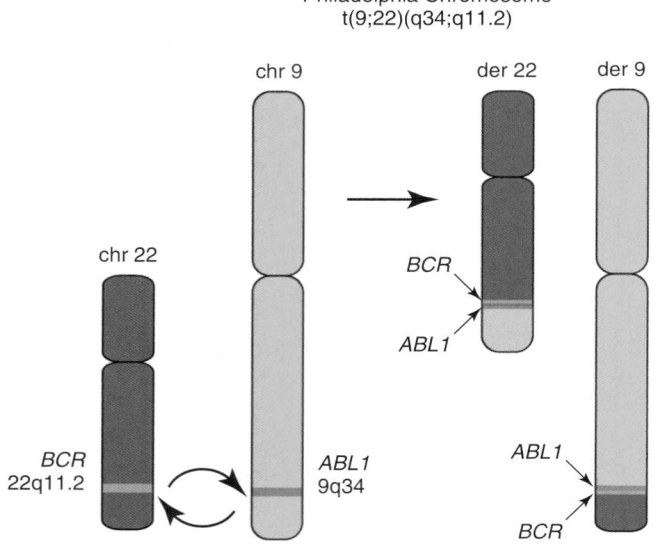

Philadelphia Chromosome
t(9;22)(q34;q11.2)

Figure 47-2. The Philadelphia chromosome, der(22q), results from the reciprocal translocation of a portion of the *ABL1* gene on chromosome 9 at band q34 to the region of the *BCR* gene on chromosome 22 at band q11.2. In turn, a portion of *BCR* is translocated to chromosome 9 to the region of *ABL1*. In 5% to 10% of patients with chronic myeloid leukemia, cryptic or complex rearrangements result in a *BCR::ABL1* fusion gene, even though no Philadelphia chromosome is detected cytogenetically.

mutation found in all myeloid lineages and in some B and T lymphocytes in affected individuals.[39] The V617F mutation occurs in exon 14 of the gene and affects a domain (JH2) that lacks kinase activity but serves instead as a negative regulator of the active JAK2 kinase domain. The V617F mutation leads to loss of function of the inhibitory JH2 domain, resulting in a gain of function of JAK2 TK activity, that is, JAK2 is constitutively activated and continually induces JAK-STAT signaling.[40] The *JAK2* exon 12 mutation reportedly has a similar function.[41] *JAK2* V617F is found in about 96% of cases of PV, 55% to 60% of cases of PMF, and 50% to 60% of ET, in which it can be considered a driver mutation. Mutated *JAK2* exon 12 is found in 3% of patients with PV but rarely in PMF or ET.[42,43]

Megakaryocyte proliferation and maturation are regulated by TPO, which binds to the cytokine receptor MPL to induce signaling through the JAK-STAT pathway. Gain of function mutations of exon 10 of *MPL*, the gene encoding MPL, lead to cytokine-independent growth through activation of JAK-STAT. Mutations of *MPL*, the most frequent of which is *MPL* W515L/K, are present in about 3% of cases of ET and 7% to 10% of cases of PMF but rarely, if at all, in PV.[44,45]

Somatic mutations are found in exon 9 of *CALR*, the gene that encodes calreticulin, a multifunction calcium-binding protein chaperone mostly localized in the endoplasmic reticulum.[34,35] The mutations are base pair insertions or deletions, all of which lead to a frameshift to the same alternative reading frame and a novel C-terminal peptide in the mutant protein. Two major variants represent more than 80% of the *CALR* mutations. The type 1 variant is a 52-base pair deletion, whereas the type 2 variant is a 5-base pair insertion. The mutant protein is thought to enhance JAK-STAT signaling. Approximately 20% to 25% of patients with ET have mutated *CALR*, and a similar incidence is seen in PMF; the mutation is not seen in PV. Evidence suggests that the type of *CALR* mutation may influence the clinical findings in MPNs that carry mutated *CALR*; type 2 mutations, as opposed to

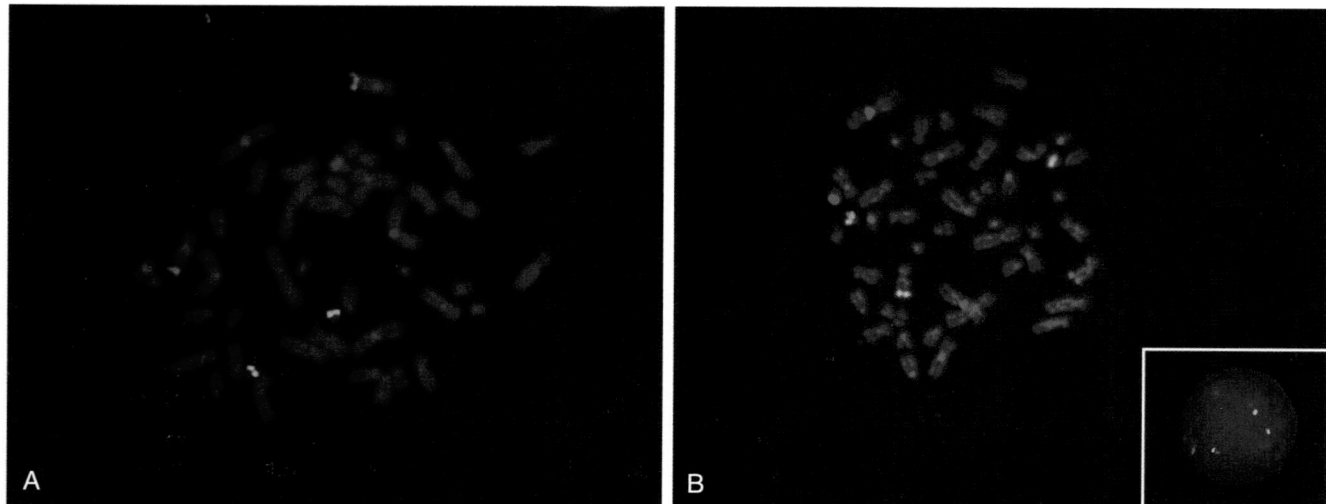

Figure 47-3. Fluorescence in situ hybridization for t(9;22)(q34;q11.2) with dual color and dual fusion probes on a normal metaphase cell **(A)** and a metaphase cell from a patient with chronic myeloid leukemia **(B)**, including an interphase cell *(inset)*. The *ABL1* and *BCR* probes are labeled with SpectrumOrange and SpectrumGreen (Vysis Corporation, Downers Grove, Il.), respectively. In normal cells **(A)**, two orange signals representing *ABL1* at 9q34 and two green signals representing *BCR* at 22q11.2 are seen, whereas in the leukemia cells **(B)**, one orange signal (the normal 9q34), one green signal (the normal 22q11.2), and two orange-green (yellow) fusion signals representing der(9q) and der(22q) are detected. *(Courtesy Dr. Yanming Zhang, University of Chicago.)*

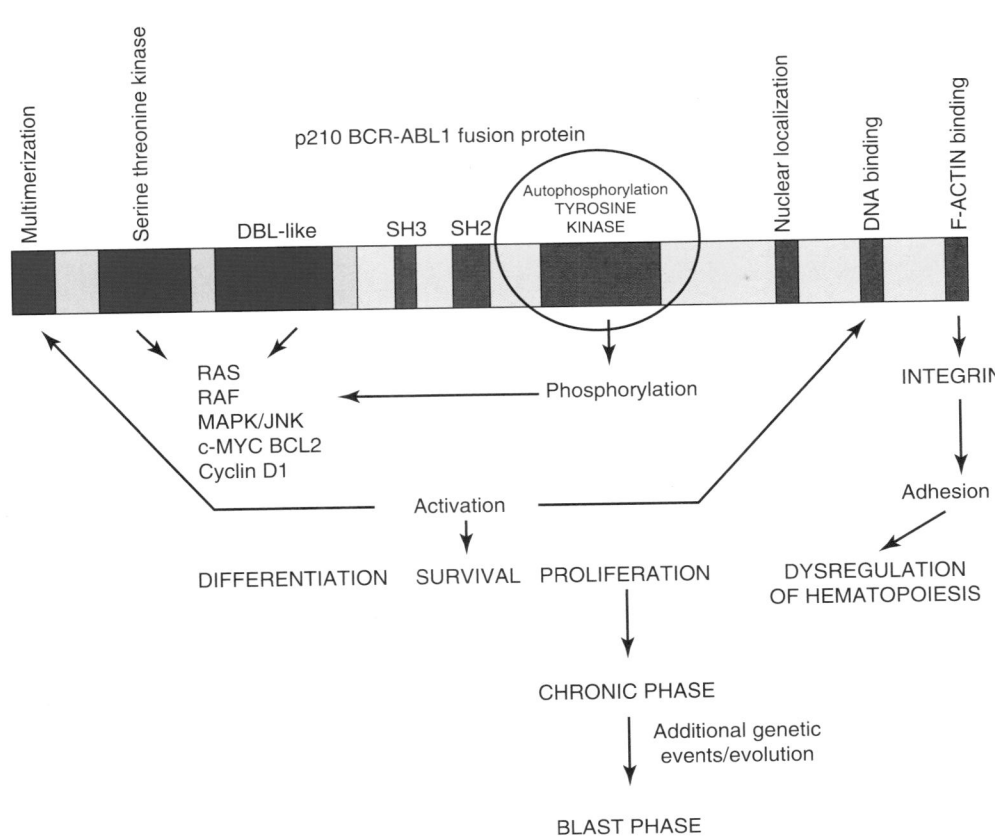

Figure 47-4. *BCR::ABL1* fusion on chromosome 22 leads to a BCR::ABL1 fusion protein with a constitutively activated tyrosine kinase in a domain of the protein encoded by *ABL1*. This tyrosine kinase plays a pivotal role in the pathogenesis of chronic myeloid leukemia and leads to autophosphorylation of other sites on the oncoprotein. These serve as sites of phosphorylation of cellular proteins involved in pathways of differentiation, survival, proliferation, cellular adhesion, and regulation of hematopoiesis.

Table 47-1 Approximate Frequency of Genetic Abnormalities in Myeloproliferative Neoplasms (MPNs)

MPN-Specific "Driver" Abnormality	Chromosome	CML, CP(%)	PV (%)	ET (%)	PMF (%)	CNL (%)
Ph chromosome	t(9;22) (q34.1;q11.2)	95*	0	0	0	0
BCR::ABL1	t(9;22) (q34.1;q11.2)	100	0	0	0	0
JAK2 V617F	9p24	0	95–97	50–60	55–60	Rare
JAK2 exon 12 mutations	9p24	0	2–3	Rare	Rare	0
CALR exon 9 mutations	19p13.2	0	Rare	25	25	0
MPL exon 10 mutations	1p34	0	Rare	3–5	5–10	0
CSF3R T6181	1p35	0	0	0	0	80

*In 5% to 10% of patients with CML, cryptic or complex rearrangements result in *BCR::ABL1* fusion gene, although no Ph chromosome is detected in the karyotype.[43,179,232]

Rare = <3%.

CML, CP, chronic myeloid leukemia, chronic phase; *CNL,* chronic neutrophilic leukemia; *ET,* essential thrombocythemia; *PMF,* primary myelofibrosis; *PV,* polycythemia vera.

type 1, are associated with higher platelet counts in ET and shorter survival times in PMF.[46,47]

An activating mutation of *CSF3R*, located at chromosome 1p34.3, that encodes the CSF3R, has been reported as the driver mutation in CNL and in occasional cases of myelodysplastic/myeloproliferative neoplasm (MDS/MPN) atypical CML (aCML).[36,48,49] The extracellular domain of CSF3R includes a membrane proximal region important for granulocytic proliferation, whereas a cytoplasmic region is important for regulation of granulocytic differentiation and function. The mutation commonly associated with CNL, *CSF3R* T6181, is

an activating mutation in the membrane proximal region that results in dimerization of the receptor with ligand independence and activation of the JAK-STAT pathway.[36,50] Of interest is that mutations encoding the distal cytoplasmic tail of *CSF3R* are found in approximately 40% of cases of severe congenital neutropenia, which does not have an inherent tendency to progress to leukemia. However, patients with severe congenital neutropenia who are treated with the growth factor GCSF are at risk for development of acute myeloid leukemia (AML); if leukemia occurs, it is often associated with a second mutation of *CSF3R* identical to that observed in CNL.[50]

Associated Mutations, Cytogenetic Abnormalities, and Pathogenetic Mechanisms in Myeloproliferative Neoplasms

In addition to the major MPN-related driver genetic abnormalities already listed, whole exome/genome studies have revealed mutations of genes affecting numerous cellular pathways in MPNs. These mutations are not specific for or restricted to MPNs but are likely to be important in cooperating with the driver mutations to influence the disease phenotype and prognosis. The most commonly affected genes are those important in epigenetic regulation (*TET2, ASXL1, EZH2, IDH1, IDH2, DNMT3A*), RNA splicing (*SF3B1, SRSF2, SETBP1*), or transcriptional mechanisms (*TP53, IKZF1, NFE2, CUX1*).[42,43,51-55] These gene mutations are not mutually exclusive, and more than one can exist simultaneously in neoplastic cells. Their frequency depends on the MPN subtype and the stage of disease; they tend to be more common in patients with progressive disease. New karyotypic abnormalities also often emerge in the course of the disease and are predictors of worse prognosis. Finally, many of the *BCR::ABL1*-negative MPNs (particularly PMF) have an inflammatory component resulting from the production and release of numerous cytokines from neoplastic and nonneoplastic cells that contribute to the clinical and pathologic findings, although the reason for this abnormal cytokine milieu is not well understood.[56]

CHRONIC MYELOID LEUKEMIA (CML)

Definition

CML is an MPN harboring the *BCR::ABL1* gene in which granulocytes predominate in the blood and bone marrow. It arises in an abnormal hematopoietic stem cell (leukemic stem cell) and is characterized by the t(9;22)(q34.1;q11.2) chromosomal translocation, which results in the formation of the Ph chromosome that contains the *BCR::ABL1* fusion gene. The fusion gene (invariably present in CML) encodes an abnormal oncoprotein, BCR::ABL1, with constitutively activated TK activity that is central to the pathogenesis of CML.[15,16] Granulocytes are the major proliferative component, but all myeloid lineages and some lymphoid and endothelial cells carry the abnormal gene.[57,58] The natural history of untreated CML is biphasic or triphasic: an initially chronic phase (CP) is followed by an accelerated phase (AP), a BP, or both. Though the ICC retains the three phases of CML, the AP is no longer included in the proposed WHO 5th edition.[2]

The diagnosis of CML requires detection of the Ph chromosome or *BCR::ABL1* fusion gene in the appropriate clinical and laboratory setting. The National Comprehensive Cancer Network (NCCN) practice guidelines recommend that, in addition to a thorough clinical history and physical examination, the workup of CML include a complete blood count with leukocyte differential and chemistry profile.[59] A bone marrow aspiration is necessary to obtain material for a complete karyotype and for morphologic evaluation to assess the phase of disease. A bone marrow trephine biopsy is indicated for patients who meet any of the criteria for AP (CML-AP) or BP (CML-BP) and for patients who have a clinical history suggestive of disease progression (e.g., progressive

splenomegaly).[1] Although not required for diagnosis, a bone marrow biopsy can be helpful to evaluate for the presence and degree of marrow fibrosis. In addition, fluorescence in situ hybridization (FISH) studies to detect the *BCR::ABL1* fusion gene and quantitative reverse transcriptase polymerase chain reaction (RT-PCR) for baseline measurement of *BCR::ABL1* transcripts are necessary for disease monitoring. The major findings of CML-CP are listed in Box 47-2.

Synonyms and Related Terms

Chronic myelogenous leukemia; chronic granulocytic leukemia; chronic myelocytic leukemia

Epidemiology

Although CML has an annual incidence of only 1 or 2 per 100,000 persons,[60,61] it is one of the most thoroughly studied of all hematopoietic neoplasms. The development of TKIs that block the TK activity of *BCR::ABL1* has markedly improved survival, so the prevalence of CML is increasing and predicted to exceed that of chronic lymphocytic leukemia, AML, and lymphoblastic leukemia combined in the next 2 to 3 decades.[62,63]

Box 47-2 *Common Features of the Chronic Phase of Chronic Myeloid Leukemia*

Annual Incidence
- 1 or 2 per 100,000 individuals

Age
- Any, median age about 65 years; pediatric cases rare

Clinical Findings
- Fatigue
- Weight loss
- Fever
- Splenomegaly
- Nearly 50% of patients are asymptomatic at initial diagnosis

Blood Findings
- Leukocytosis
- Platelets normal or increased
- Anemia often present
- Spectrum of maturing granulocytes with a "myelocyte bulge"
- Blasts usually <2% of white blood cells
- Absolute basophilia
- No significant dysplasia

Bone Marrow Findings
- Hypercellularity
- Increased myeloid-to-erythroid ratio
- Blasts usually <5%, always <10%
- Widening of cuff of immature granulocytes around bone trabeculae
- Spectrum of maturing granulocytes with myelocyte bulge but no dysplasia
- Megakaryocytes normal or increased in number, but with "dwarf" morphology
- Reticulin fibers normal to moderately increased

Genetics
- 100% have Philadelphia chromosome or *BCR::ABL1* fusion gene

Clinical Findings

The median age at diagnosis is 65 years, but CML can occur at any age, including childhood.[60,64,65] The age at onset is reportedly lower in regions of lower socioeconomic conditions.[61] There is a slight male predominance. Most patients are diagnosed in CP, which has an insidious onset. Nearly 50% of newly diagnosed patients are asymptomatic and discovered when an abnormal white blood cell (WBC) count is found during a routine medical examination.[60,66] When symptoms are present, they include fatigue, malaise, weight loss, night sweats, and symptoms related to anemia. Palpable splenomegaly is present in about 50% of patients and may be associated with early satiety; hepatomegaly may also be present. Significant lymphadenopathy is uncommon, and if present, a lymph node biopsy should be considered to exclude blastic proliferation in the node. About 5% of patients initially present in AP or BP without a previously recognized CP.[60]

Morphologic Findings

Peripheral Blood, Chronic Phase

In CML-CP, the peripheral blood shows leukocytosis (12–1000 × 10^9/L; median, ≈80 × 10^9/L).[60,66] Children, however, typically have a higher WBC count (median, ≈250 × 10^9/L).[64,65] The leukocytosis is caused by neutrophils in different stages of maturation, with peaks in the percentages of myelocytes and segmented neutrophils (Fig. 47-5). Significant dysplasia is absent. Blasts usually account for less than 2% of the WBCs. Absolute basophilia and eosinophilia are common. Although the absolute monocyte count may be elevated (>1 × 10^9/L), the percentage of monocytes is generally less than 3%.[60,67] In most cases, the platelet count is mildly or moderately elevated; however, in 10% to 15% of patients, it is in excess of 1000 × 10^9/L. Marked thrombocytopenia is unusual. Anemia is common, but hemoglobin values of less than 10 g/dL are initially present in only a minority of cases. Occasional patients are seen with findings that do not fit the classic presentation and that can suggest a different diagnosis, such as a normal or only modestly elevated WBC count but marked thrombocytosis (mimicking ET)[68,69] or leukocytosis composed almost exclusively of segmented neutrophils (resembling CNL).[70] In some cases, monocytes are substantially increased, and the case resembles chronic myelomonocytic leukemia (CMML).[71] These unusual presentations of CML often correlate with variations in the size of the BCR::ABL1 fusion protein caused by varying breakpoints within the *BCR* gene[72] (see the subsection, Cytogenetics/Molecular Findings).

Bone Marrow, Chronic Phase

The peripheral blood findings, when combined with molecular genetic studies (FISH, PCR) to detect *BCR::ABL1*, are often diagnostic, but a bone marrow aspirate is essential to provide adequate material for a complete karyotype and to assess marrow morphology to determine the phase of disease. A bone marrow biopsy is not required for diagnosis in every case but should be obtained if the blood findings are atypical or the bone marrow cannot be aspirated. In addition, bone marrow fibrosis should be evaluated, as even mild fibrosis at diagnosis correlates with a decreased major molecular response (MMR) rate in the first year of TKI therapy.[73]

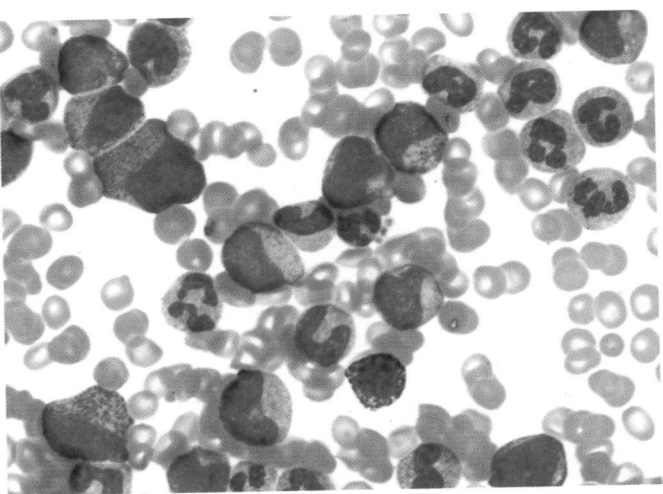

Figure 47-5. Peripheral blood smear of a patient with chronic myeloid leukemia illustrates marked leukocytosis with a spectrum of neutrophil maturation, including a prominence of myelocytes and segmented neutrophils. Basophils are invariably increased in absolute numbers.

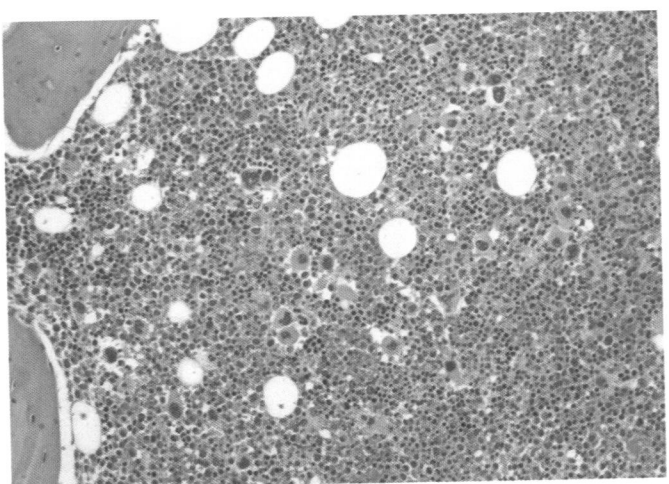

Figure 47-6. The bone marrow in the chronic phase of chronic myeloid leukemia is hypercellular. It shows granulocytic proliferation, with small islands of erythroid precursors interspersed and increased numbers of megakaryocytes, many of which are "dwarf" megakaryocytes.

Bone marrow specimens in untreated CP are hypercellular as a result of marked granulocytic proliferation (Fig. 47-6), which shows a maturation pattern similar to that in the blood with expansion of the myelocyte and segmented neutrophil stages.[74] There is no significant dysplasia[75] (Fig. 47-7). Blasts typically account for less than 5% of the marrow cells; 10% or more blasts indicate disease progression to AP.[76] Erythroid precursors are reduced in percentage but show normal maturation. Basophils and eosinophils are frequently conspicuous. Histiocytes resembling Gaucher cells or "sea blue" histiocytes are commonly observed (Fig. 47-8) and attributed to an excess of phospholipids from the increased cellular burden and cell turnover. These "pseudo-Gaucher" histiocytes carry *BCR::ABL1* because they are progeny of the affected leukemic stem cell.[77] Megakaryocytes may be normal or decreased in number, but 40% to 50% of cases exhibit moderate to marked megakaryocytic proliferation (Fig. 47-9).

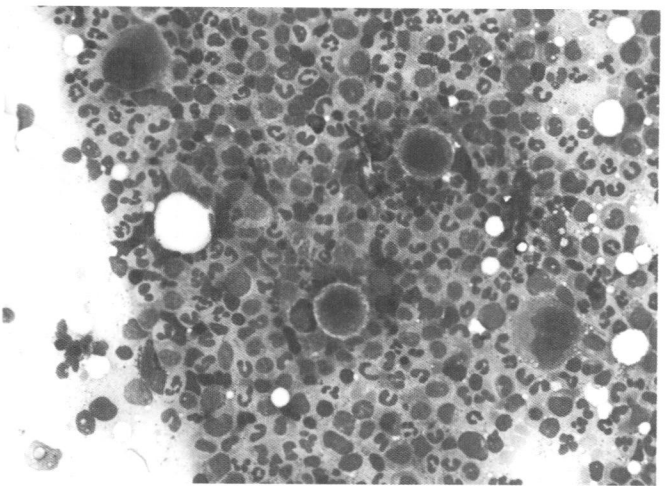

Figure 47-7. Bone marrow aspirate smear from a patient with chronic myeloid leukemia, chronic phase.

In CP, the megakaryocytes are smaller than normal and tend to have hypolobated nuclei (i.e., "dwarf megakaryocytes").[78] However, they are not true "micromegakaryocytes," such as those found in myelodysplastic syndromes (MDS). In CML, the finding of significant numbers of MDS-like micromegakaryocytes should raise concern for disease progression.

In marrow biopsy sections, a 5-cell to 10-cell–thick layer of immature granulocytes is common around bone trabeculae (Fig. 47-10), compared with the 2-cell or 3-cell–thick layer normally present.[74,78] Granulocytic maturation proceeds toward the center of the intertrabecular spaces. A modest number of blasts may be seen immediately adjacent to the bone and scattered among the maturing cells, but sizable clusters of blasts are not present in CP, although focal aggregates of myelocytes are not uncommon. Moderate to marked reticulin fibrosis is seen in 30% to 40% of biopsies at diagnosis, sometimes accompanied by increased numbers of megakaryocytes and splenomegaly.[79]

Extramedullary Tissues

In CP, the spleen is variably enlarged because of infiltration of the red pulp cords by granulocytes. A similar infiltrate is seen in the hepatic sinuses and occasionally in lymph nodes. These extramedullary infiltrates are composed of a mixture of immature and mature granulocytes; any significant shift toward immaturity with an increased percentage of blasts (≥10%) indicates progressing or transformed disease. In BP (≥20% blasts), any extramedullary tissue can be infiltrated, but the spleen, liver, lymph node, skin, and soft tissues are most commonly involved.[74] In CML, regardless of blood and

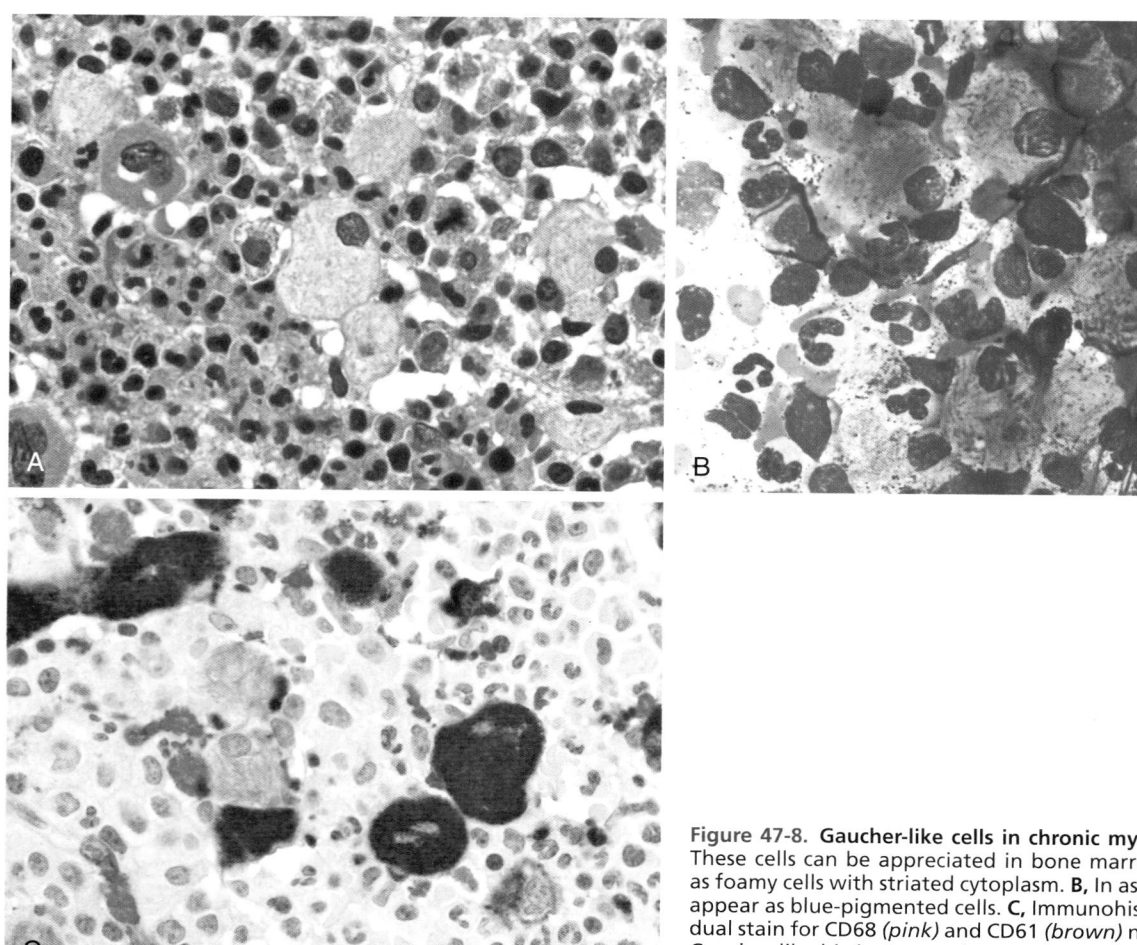

Figure 47-8. Gaucher-like cells in chronic myeloid leukemia. A, These cells can be appreciated in bone marrow biopsy sections as foamy cells with striated cytoplasm. **B,** In aspirate smears, they appear as blue-pigmented cells. **C,** Immunohistochemistry with a dual stain for CD68 *(pink)* and CD61 *(brown)* nicely demonstrates Gaucher-like histiocytes and small megakaryocytes, respectively. *(Courtesy Dr. Elizabeth Hyjek.)*

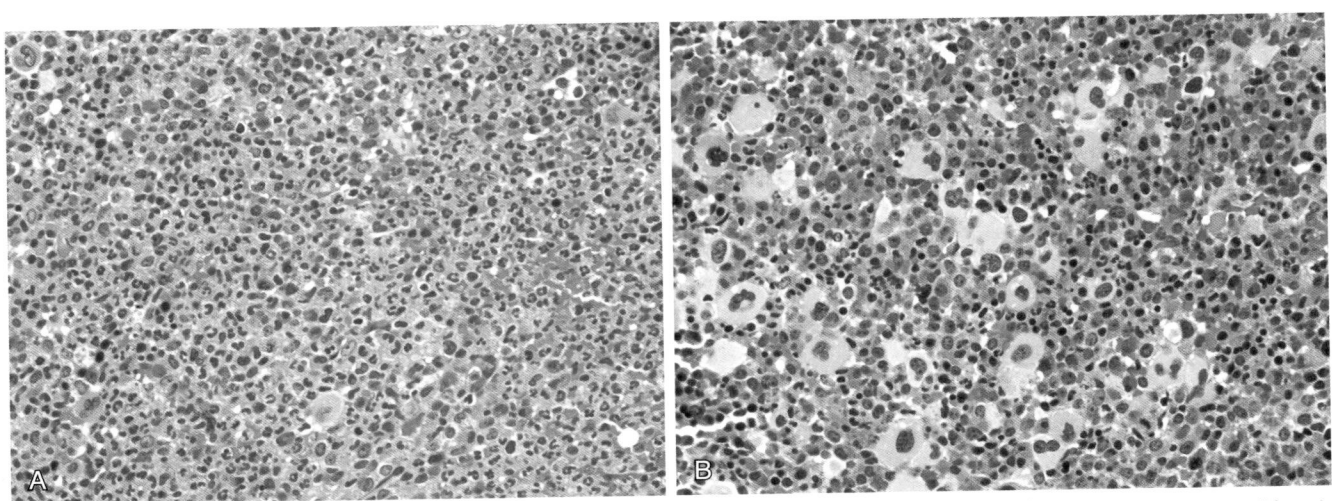

Figure 47-9. The number of megakaryocytes in chronic myeloid leukemia (CML) varies, from cases with mainly granulocytic proliferation and few megakaryocytes **(A)** to cases with substantially increased megakaryocytes **(B)**.

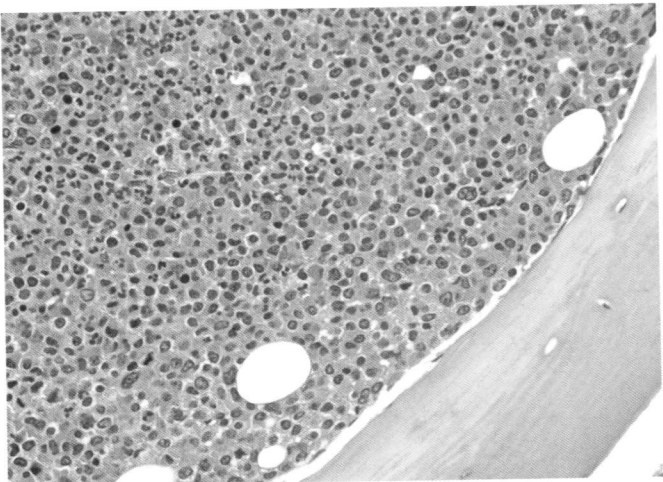

Figure 47-10. In chronic myeloid leukemia, the peritrabecular rim of immature granulocytes is thickened from the normal two-cell or three-cell layer to five or more cells, with mature cells farther from the bone in the intertrabecular region.

marrow findings, clinical evidence of an infiltrative process in any extramedullary site should be investigated to exclude BP.

Immunophenotype

Immunophenotypic analysis of the granulocytes contributes little to the diagnosis of CML-CP, although reportedly, the expression of CD7 on CD34-positive cells in the blood or bone marrow has adverse prognostic significance, whereas a normal CD34-positive stem cell population that lacks any abnormal markers, such as CD7, CD56, or CD11b, predicts a better response to TKI therapy.[80-82]

Cytogenetics/Molecular Findings

All patients with CML have the t(9;22)(q34;q11.2) abnormality, which results in the BCR::ABL1 fusion gene.[16] In 90% to 95% of cases, this reciprocal chromosomal translocation is recognized on routine karyotype as the Ph

chromosome, der(22)t(9;22). In the remaining cases, the rearrangement of genetic material may be complex (involving one or more additional chromosomes) or is cryptic and not identified by routine cytogenetic analysis but detected instead by FISH or RT-PCR analyses.[25] This fusion gene is necessary and sufficient to cause CML through its constitutive activation of multiple signal transduction pathways.

The Ph chromosome is not specific to CML but is also present in 15% to 30% of adults and 5% of children with B-lymphoblastic leukemia, in some cases of mixed phenotype acute leukemia, and in rare cases of AML. The site of the breakpoint in BCR (Fig. 47-11) determines the phenotype of the disease associated with the translocation.[72] In 95% of cases of CML and 25% to 30% of cases of Ph-positive acute lymphoblastic leukemia (ALL), the breakpoint is in the major breakpoint cluster region, spanning exons 12 to 16, and an abnormal fusion protein, p210, is formed. Rarely, the breakpoint in BCR occurs in the mu breakpoint region, spanning exons 17 to 20, and a larger fusion protein, p230, is formed. Patients with the p230 protein usually demonstrate marked peripheral blood neutrophilia or thrombocytosis.[70] Breaks in the minor breakpoint region result in a short fusion protein (p190) that is usually associated with Ph-positive ALL, although small amounts of the p190 transcript can be detected in most patients with CML because of alternative splicing of the BCR gene.[72,83] The short p190 transcript is also found in rare cases of CML with increased numbers of monocytes that resemble CMML.[71] Cases with the p230 or p190 variant breakpoint exhibit other morphologic features of CML, such as basophilia and small megakaryocytes with hypolobated nuclei.

Although the BCR::ABL1 fusion gene may be detected by FISH or PCR in blood or marrow cells, a complete karyotype is mandatory at the time of diagnosis. The Ph chromosome is often the sole cytogenetic abnormality at diagnosis, but additional karyotypic abnormalities may be present in the same clone. If, at diagnosis, any of the "major route" karyotypic abnormalities (+8, +19, isochromosome 17q, extra Ph chromosome) are present in addition to the Ph chromosome, the patient should be considered as presenting in AP. If these or any other additional chromosomal abnormalities appear in subsequent specimens, they indicate disease progression.[84]

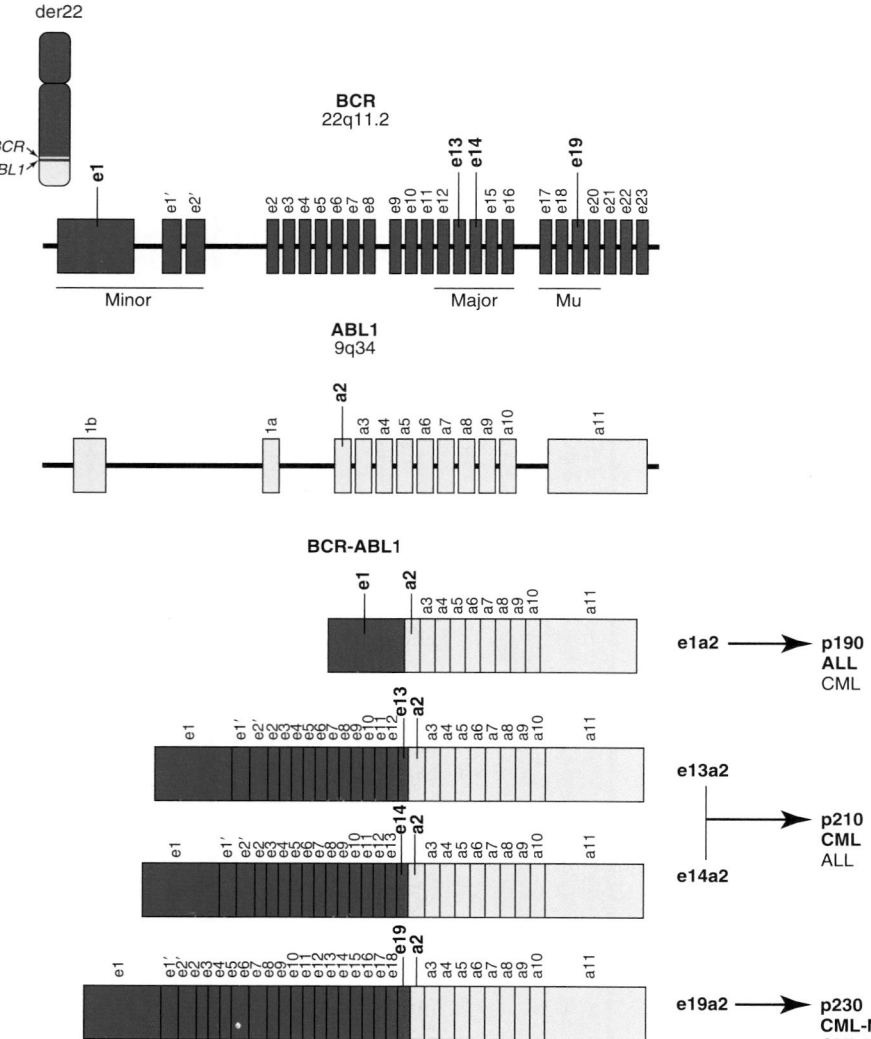

Figure 47-11. Schematic representation of the *BCR* gene *(blue)* and *ABL1* gene *(cream)* and their breakpoints in t(9;22) (q34;q11.2). Breakpoints in *ABL1* generally occur upstream of exon 2a, either between 1b and 1a or between 1a and 2a. The breakpoints in *BCR* are variable and can occur in the minor breakpoint cluster region, giving rise to the e1a2 fusion; the major breakpoint cluster region, fusing either e13 or e14 with a2; or the mu breakpoint region, leading to an e19a2 fusion. These varying breakpoints result in different-sized fusion proteins that correlate with disease phenotype. Almost all cases of chronic myeloid leukemia (CML) are associated with breakpoints in the major breakpoint cluster region that result in the p210 protein, although some cases of Ph-positive acute lymphoblastic leukemia (ALL) exhibit this breakpoint as well. The minor breakpoint, e1a2, gives rise to the p190 protein; it is seen in more than 50% of Ph-positive ALLs and only rarely in CML, in which case it is associated with monocytosis, mimicking chronic myelomonocytic leukemia. Breaks in the mu region lead to the p230 protein, which is associated with CML with excessive neutrophils or excessive thrombocytosis.

The significance of mutations of genes involved in epigenetic regulation, translational mechanisms, or RNA splicing is not yet clear in CML-CP. Mutations of *ASXL1, DNMT3A, RUNX1,* and *TET2* are reportedly present in some newly diagnosed CML patients in the few series reported to date, but their influence on disease features is not yet known. Of interest, in rare cases, mutations have been found in Ph-positive and Ph-negative clones simultaneously, raising the possibility that the mutation preceded the acquisition of *BCR::ABL1*.[51-53]

In patients who progress to AP or BP, the genetic landscape changes remarkably as additional chromosomal and submicroscopic genetic aberrations occur and accumulate to disrupt maturation and to drive uncontrolled proliferation.

Clinical Course

In the absence of effective therapy, patients with CML will invariably demonstrate disease progression. In some, the progression is characterized by gradual but persistent deterioration in hematologic parameters and performance status (i.e., AP), which may result in death or show yet further evolution to overt BP. Other patients progress directly from

CP to BP, which is characterized by 20% or more blasts in the blood or bone marrow or by a proliferation of blasts in an extramedullary site. Disease progression is invariably associated with additional genetic abnormalities.

Recognition of disease progression is important, but the clinical and morphologic boundaries among CP, AP, and BP are not sharp, and the parameters to define these phases vary among different guidelines. Furthermore, gene expression profiles of AP and BP are similar, with changes in the expression profile occurring late in CP or early in AP, before clinical or morphologic evidence of overt progression.[84] It should be noted that 20% to 30% of patients receiving TKI therapy have apparent disease progression caused by acquired mutations in *BCR::ABL1* that affect the TK binding domain and thus affect alterations in the binding site of the oncoprotein, rendering the TKI ineffective.[59,85] To date, more than 90 such mutations have been described that confer TKI resistance. Less commonly, subclones of leukemic cells with amplification of *BCR::ABL1* or mutations in the SH3-SH2 domain result in disease progression, or there may be genetic alterations that occur in the *BCR::ABL1*-independent signaling pathways.[86,87] In patients in CP with TK domain mutations or *BCR::ABL1* amplification, disease progression may be circumvented or reversed by increasing the dosage or switching to a newer-generation TKI. A new class of small molecules targeting the myristoyl pocket of ABL1 has been introduced into the treatment of CML.[88,89]

The genetic events responsible for evolution into AP or BP are largely unknown, although nearly 80% of patients with advanced disease have additional chromosomal abnormalities including +8, i(17q), +19, and an extra Ph chromosome, suggesting that additional genetic "hits" likely induce transformation.[74,84] Though *ASXL1* mutations may be present in CP, patients with *ASXL1* mutations acquire other additional variants during progression to BP, including *RUNX1, TP53, BCOR,* and *SETD1B*.[90]

Accelerated Phase

In accordance with the ICC guidelines, AP is defined by 10% to 19% bone marrow or peripheral blood blasts, peripheral blood basophilia ≥20%, or the identification of additional clonal cytogenetic abnormalities in Ph-positive cells, i.e., second Ph, +8, i(17q), +19, complex karyotype, or abnormalities of 3q26.2.[1] In the proposed WHO 5th edition, however, AP at diagnosis or during treatment has been omitted; only the CP and BP are recognized.[2]

Bone marrow specimens of patients with AP may show variable cellularity, and there may be dysplastic features in the granulocytic and other myeloid lineages.[75] An increase in myeloid lineage blasts (10% to 19%) may be appreciated on aspirate smears or in biopsy sections (Figs. 47-12 and 47-13), in which they can be highlighted with immunohistochemical stains for CD34. Sizable clusters of megakaryocytes are sometimes seen, including true micromegakaryocytes similar to those in MDS, often associated with significant reticulin or collagen fibrosis.[76] Lymphoid blasts may be seen in AP, but any bona fide lymphoblasts in the blood or bone marrow, even during CP, should raise concern of an imminent lymphoblastic crisis, as lymphoblastic BP is reported to sometimes have an abrupt onset and usually lacks a preceding AP.[91,92]

Blast Phase

The ICC guidelines have maintained a blast percentage threshold of at least 20% in the blood or bone marrow to establish a diagnosis of CML-BP.[1] Increasing numbers of lymphoblasts (>5%) in peripheral blood or bone marrow indicate impending lymphoid BP and thus should prompt further laboratory and genetic studies.[91] Of note, other classification and risk stratification systems that include the International Blood and Marrow Transplant Registry, MD Anderson Cancer Center, and European Leukemia Net have defined a higher blast threshold of more than 30% for BP and are frequently used for eligibility criteria in clinical trials.[59,93,94]

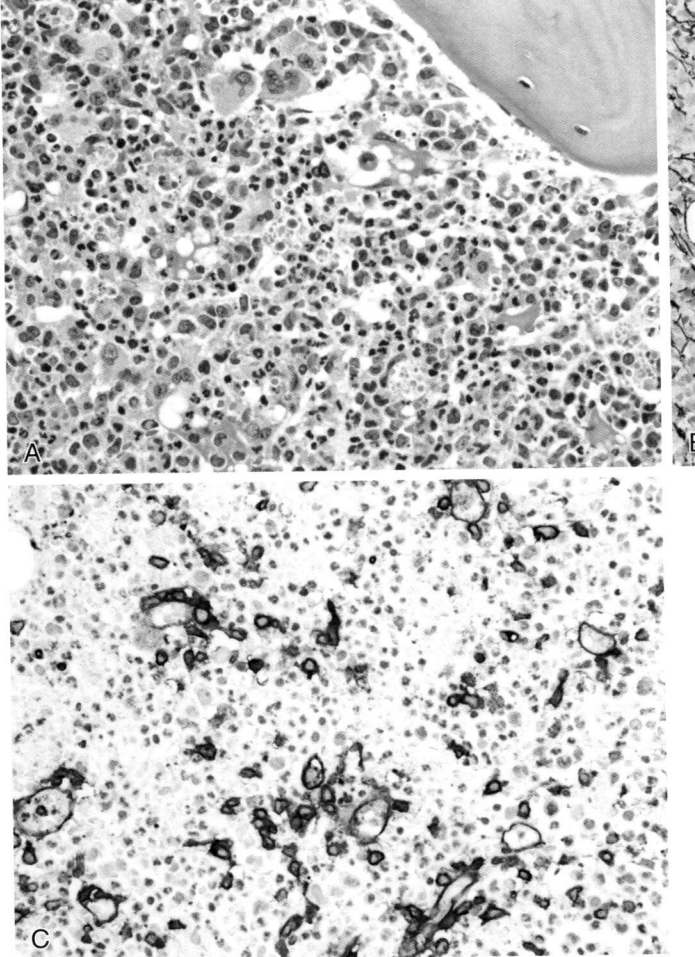

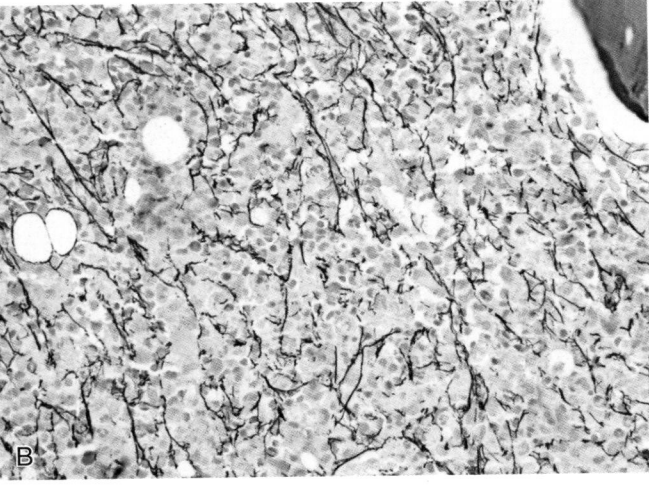

Figure 47-12. CML, accelerated phase. This patient, who had Ph-positive CML for 5 years, developed cytopenia in the blood with 12% blasts. The bone marrow biopsy specimen is hypercellular **(A)**, with reticulin fibrosis **(B)**. An immunohistochemical stain for CD34 **(C)** reveals more blasts than were appreciated in the hematoxylin-eosin–stained section.

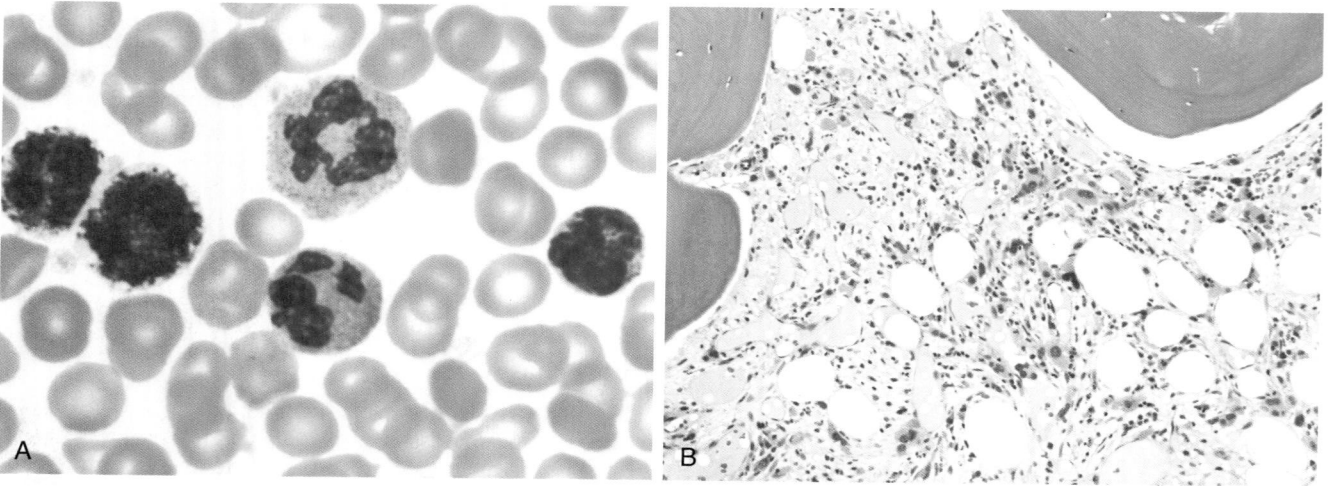

Figure 47-13. CML, accelerated phase. A, This patient with chronic myeloid leukemia had more than 20% basophils in the blood. **B,** The bone marrow biopsy shows marked fibrosis and atypical megakaryocytic proliferation.

The ICC and proposed WHO 5th edition criteria for BP include the finding of 20% or more blasts in the blood or bone marrow and an extramedullary proliferation of blasts that disrupts the architecture of the infiltrated tissue (Box 47-3). In addition, if blasts occupy focal but significant areas of the bone marrow, such as an entire intertrabecular space, a presumptive diagnosis of BP is warranted, even if the remainder of the marrow shows CP.[76]

In the majority of BP cases, the blasts are of myeloid lineage (neutrophilic, monocytic, megakaryocytic, basophilic, eosinophilic, erythroid blasts, or any combination thereof) (Fig. 47-14); but 20% to 30% of cases are composed of lymphoblasts that are usually of B-cell origin, although cases of T-lymphoblastic and NK-cell transformation have been reported[95] (Fig. 47-15). Sequential lymphoblastic and myeloblastic crises may also occur. The origin of the blasts is often morphologically obvious, but sometimes, the blasts are primitive or heterogeneous, and mixed-phenotype cases are common; thus, immunophenotypic analysis, preferably by multiparameter flow cytometry, is recommended. In myeloid BP, the blasts have strong, weak, or no myeloperoxidase activity but express one or more antigens associated with granulocytic, monocytic megakaryocytic, or erythroid differentiation (e.g., CD33, CD13, CD14, CD11c, CD11b, CD117, CD15, CD41, CD61, CD71, glycophorin A or C). However, in many cases of myeloid origin, the blasts also express one or more lymphoid-related antigens. Most lymphoblastic cases are precursor-B in origin and express terminal deoxynucleotidyl transferase in addition to B-related antigens (CD19, CD10, CD79a, PAX5, CD20), but a minority of cases express T-cell–related antigens (CD3, CD2, CD5, CD4, CD8, CD7).[96,97] Expression of one or more myeloid-related antigens is common in B-cell and T-cell–derived BPs. An increased incidence of unusual immunophenotypes and types of blasts (e.g., basophil blasts, megakaryoblasts) has been described in the era of TKIs.[98] Rare cases of myeloid BP have cytogenetic abnormalities in which a specific recurring chromosomal rearrangement associated with AML, such as inv(16)(p13.1q22) or t(16;16)(p13.2;q22), is found in the same cells as the Ph chromosome (Fig. 47-14). In such cases, however, these chromosomal abnormalities, often associated

with favorable outcomes in AML, reportedly have no favorable effect when found with the Ph chromosome.[99]

Therapy, Disease Monitoring, and Prognosis

The development of TKIs that target the constitutively activated TK domain of the BCR::ABL1 fusion protein is a remarkable advance that led to dramatic improvements in survival and quality of life in patients with CML.[100] Now, most patients with newly diagnosed CML can be expected to live a nearly normal life span if treated with TKI therapy.

The key to the success of TKI therapy is regular and continual assessment of the hematologic, cytogenetic, and molecular status of the patient to detect changes indicative of drug failure or resistance. In general, hematologic and genetic monitoring once every 3 months is recommended, depending on the response to the TKI. The morphologic features in blood and bone marrow specimens of patients receiving TKI therapy

---

Box 47-3 *Diagnostic Criteria for Accelerated and Blast Phase Chronic Myeloid Leukemia (CML) According to International Consensus Classification*

Accelerated Phase
- Bone marrow or peripheral blood blasts 10% to 19%
- Peripheral blood basophils ≥20%
- Presence of additional clonal cytogenetic abnormality in Ph-positive cells (ACA)
  - Second Ph, trisomy 8, isochromosome 17q, trisomy 19, complex karyotype, or abnormalities of 3q26.2

Blast Phase
- Bone marrow or peripheral blood blasts ≥20%
- Myeloid sarcoma, extramedullary blast proliferation
- Bone marrow or peripheral blood lymphoid blasts >5% is consistent with lymphoblastic crisis
  - Immunophenotypic analysis is required to confirm lymphoid lineage

ACA, Additional chromosome abnormality; *Ph,* Philadelphia chromosome. Data from Arber DA, Orazi A, Hasserjian RP, et al. International Consensus Classification of myeloid neoplasms and acute leukemias: integrating morphologic, clinical, and genomic data. *Blood.* 2022;140(11):1200-1228.

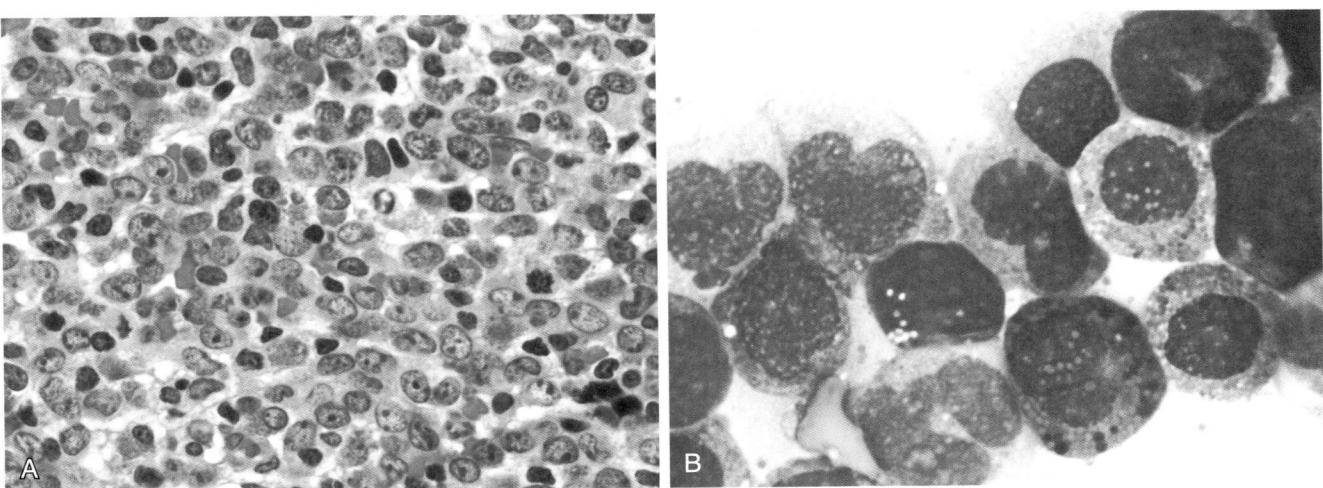

Figure 47-14. Chronic myeloid leukemia, myeloid blast phase. A, Bone marrow biopsy shows sheets of blasts with some eosinophils intermixed. **B,** Marrow aspirate contains abnormal eosinophils and monocytic cells. This patient's leukemic cells showed t(9;22)(q34;q11.2) plus inv(16)(p13.1q22).

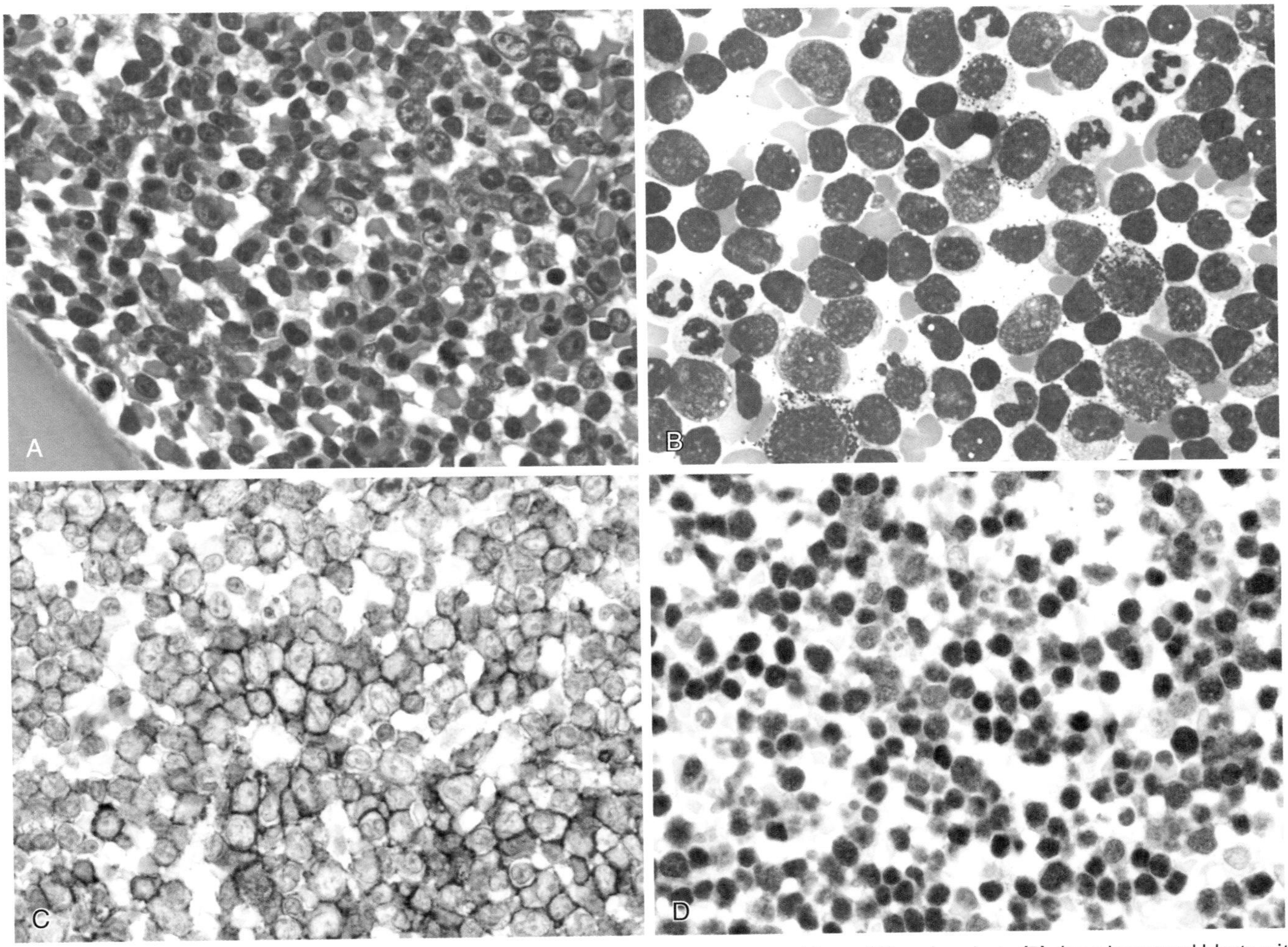

Figure 47-15. Chronic myeloid leukemia (CML), lymphoid blast phase. Bone marrow biopsy **(A)** and aspirate **(B)** show increased blasts with lymphoid morphology in a background of granulocytic cells. The blasts express CD19 **(C)** and terminal deoxynucleotidyl transferase **(D)** in a patient with *BCR::ABL1*-positive CML diagnosed 8 years previously.

reflect the changes in the cytogenetic and molecular events as the patient responds (Fig. 47-16), with normalization of the WBC count and return to a cellular bone marrow with relatively normal morphology, usually during a period of 3 to 6 months.[101] Although morphologic features are not sensitive enough to reflect early increases in the burden of the *BCR::ABL1* transcript that usually indicate drug resistance, the persistence or reappearance of any morphologic features indicative of CML in follow-up specimens of patients receiving TKI therapy should raise concern for drug resistance and prompt further evaluation of the cytogenetic or molecular status. In the current age of TKI therapy, the most important prognostic indicator is the response to therapy at the hematologic, cytogenetic, and molecular levels.

Differential Diagnosis

Chronic Phase

The differential diagnosis of CML-CP includes reactive leukocytosis, myeloid/lymphoid neoplasms with prominent eosinophilia, the MDS/MPNs (including CMML and aCML),

and MPNS (including CNL and the *BCR::ABL1*-negative MPNs). None of these neoplasms has a Ph chromosome or *BCR::ABL1* fusion gene but might be considered an alternative diagnosis if a case thought to be CML is determined to lack the genetic requirement. These myeloid neoplasms have been described in detail elsewhere in this chapter and in Chapters 48 and 50; the features that may overlap with CML, CP are briefly mentioned in Table 47-2.

Reactive Granulocytosis

Reactive granulocytosis and leukemoid reactions can usually be distinguished from CML by the clinical history or evidence of an underlying infection, inflammatory process, or nonmyeloid neoplasm that accounts for the abnormal peripheral blood findings, but careful examination of a blood smear is usually the most valuable tool in distinguishing reactive granulocytosis from CML. Basophilia and the "myelocyte bulge" characteristic of CML are absent in reactive granulocytosis, whereas toxic granulation or cytoplasmic vacuoles commonly observed in reactive neutrophilia are rarely found in CML. However, genetic studies to exclude CML should be performed in

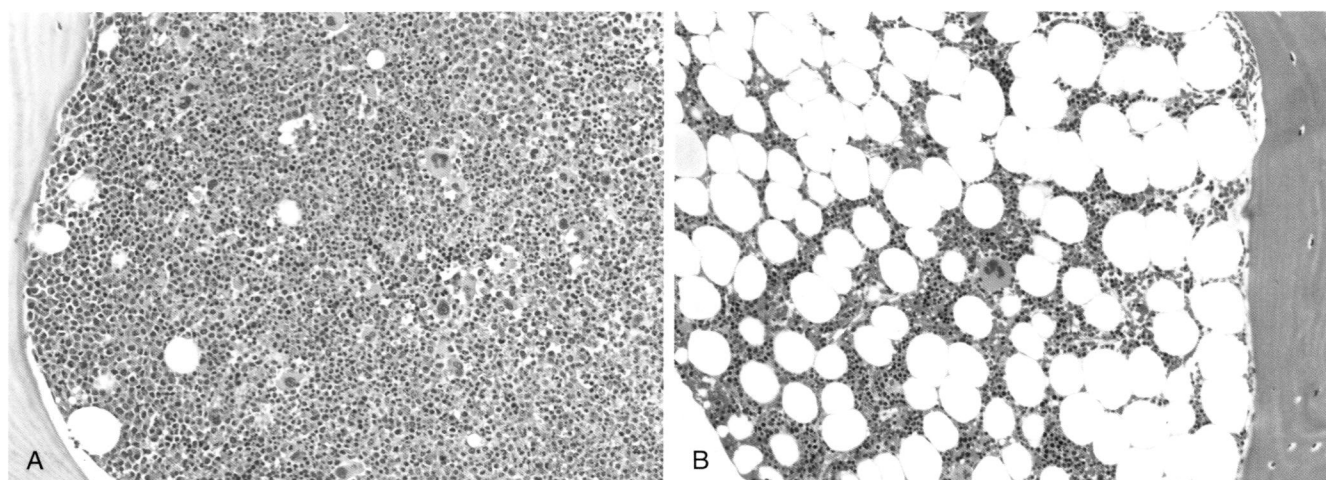

Figure 47-16. Initial bone marrow biopsy **(A)** of a patient with Ph-positive chronic myeloid leukemia and a repeated biopsy 12 months after the institution of imatinib therapy **(B)**, at which time a complete hematologic and cytogenetic remission had been achieved. Notice the small megakaryocytes in the initial marrow and the normal-sized megakaryocytes in the remission marrow.

Table 47-2 Comparison of Major Features of Chronic Myeloid Leukemia and Other Myeloid Neoplasms to Consider in the Differential Diagnosis

Feature	CML, Chronic Phase	CNL	CMML	aCML
Philadelphia chromosome	≈95%	0	0	0
BCR::ABL1 fusion gene	100%	0	0	0
Principal proliferating cells	Granulocytes, megakaryocytes	Granulocytes	Monocytes, granulocytes	Granulocytes
Monocytes	Usually <3%	<1 × 10⁹/L	≥0.5 × 10⁹/L; ≥10%	<1 × 10⁹/L; <10%
Basophils	>2%	<2%	<2%	<2%
Dysplasia	Absent to minimal	Absent, "toxic" changes reported	Usually in one or more lineages	Significant dysgranulopoiesis, often trilineage dysplasia
Immature granulocytes (peripheral blood)	Often >20%	<10%	Usually <20%	≥10%
Megakaryocytes	Usually normal or increased numbers, with "dwarf" morphology; occasionally mildly decreased	Normal or increased numbers, with normal morphology	Decreased, normal, or occasionally increased numbers, with variable but often dysplastic morphology	Normal, decreased, or rarely increased numbers, often with dysplastic morphology

aCML, Atypical chronic myeloid leukemia; *CML,* chronic myeloid leukemia; *CMML,* chronic myelomonocytic leukemia; *CNL,* chronic neutrophilic leukemia.

cases with persistent, unexplained neutrophilia, as CML—particularly those with the variant p230 transcript—may initially present with predominantly mature neutrophils and minimal granulocytic immaturity.[70,72]

Reactive and Neoplastic Disorders Associated With Eosinophilia

Most cases of eosinophilia are secondary to inflammatory diseases (including allergies, hypersensitivity conditions, and collagen vascular diseases), infections (particularly with tissue-invasive parasites), or nonmyeloid neoplasms in which reactive or neoplastic T cells or other inflammatory cells secrete cytokines that promote eosinophil proliferation. However, a number of myeloid disorders are associated with persistent hypereosinophilia (≥1500 eosinophils/µL), in which the eosinophils belong to the neoplastic clone. These include the group of myeloid/lymphoid neoplasms with eosinophilia and tyrosine kinase gene fusions (M/LN-Eo); chronic eosinophilic leukemia, not otherwise specified; and CML.[1,102] The first two conditions are described in detail in Chapter 50, but some cases of CML have an absolute eosinophil count that exceeds 1500 eosinophils/µL and should be included in the differential diagnosis. In any case with unexplained hypereosinophilia, appropriate genetic studies, including BCR::ABL1 analysis, should be performed without delay. Early diagnosis and treatment of hypereosinophilia is essential, as eosinophils release cationic proteins that may lead to extensive tissue damage, particularly in the cardiovascular, pulmonary, or central nervous systems.

Chronic Myelomonocytic Leukemia (CMML)

CMML is characterized by monocytosis in the blood (≥0.5 × 10^9/L and 10% or more monocytes), cytopenia, presence of clonality by cytogenetics or at least one myeloid neoplasm associated mutation, and less than 20% blasts in the blood or bone marrow.[1,103] There is no Ph chromosome or BCR::ABL1 fusion gene. The "≥10% monocytes rule" for the diagnosis of CMML is helpful to distinguish CMML from CML. A patient with CML and a WBC count of 100 × 10^9/L with only 1% monocytes in the blood has an absolute monocyte count of 1000/µL, but rarely do CML patients have 10% or more monocytes in the blood. On the other hand, CMML often has prominent granulocytic proliferation in the marrow and small, dysplastic megakaryocytes that may resemble the dwarf megakaryocytes characteristic of CML. In addition, splenomegaly is common in both disorders. Thus, confusion between CMML and CML is possible. Furthermore, the rare cases of CML that carry the BCR::ABL1 fusion protein p190 have monocytosis and closely mimic CMML. Therefore, the leukemic cells of any patient in whom the diagnosis of CMML is considered should be analyzed by routine karyotyping, FISH, or RT-PCR to exclude the possibility of CML.

Atypical CML (aCML)

Atypical CML is not an atypical form of CML.[1,103] Though aCML is characterized by leukocytosis with neutrophilia and immature circulating neutrophilic precursors, associated with a granulocytic proliferation in the marrow, there is no BCR::ABL1 fusion gene, and in contrast to CML, the granulocytes in aCML are dysplastic, there is no significant basophilia or eosinophilia, and thrombocytopenia is common.

Chronic Neutrophilic Leukemia (CNL)

CNL is an MPN characterized by a proliferation of normal-appearing neutrophils lacking granulocytic dysplasia with only rare (<10%) circulating granulocytic precursors. CNL lacks a BCR::ABL1 fusion gene but has a high prevalence of mutations in CSF3R that activate the receptor, leading to the proliferation of neutrophils. A subset of cases of CML can show marked neutrophilia; however, they are associated with a BCR::ABL1 fusion protein, often p230. A positive BCR::ABL1 FISH result will help in identifying these rare cases.

Myeloid or Lymphoid Blast Phase

The differential diagnosis of CML-BP is not problematic if there is a history of preexisting CML; but occasional patients with CML initially present in BP, in which case it may be nearly impossible to distinguish between CML-BP and de novo Ph-positive ALL, Ph-positive mixed phenotype acute leukemia, or Ph-positive AML. If the blood or bone marrow shows blasts in a background of granulocytes with a left shift, myelocyte bulge, absolute basophilia, or dwarf megakaryocytes, the diagnosis of CML-BP is most likely. However, if these features are absent and blasts constitute the majority of cells in the blood and bone marrow, the diagnosis is sometimes more difficult. If a p190 transcript is present, the diagnosis of Ph-positive ALL de novo is strongly supported.[72] A breakpoint in the major BCR region does not resolve the issue, however, because a minority of cases of apparent Ph-positive ALL de novo demonstrate the p210 transcript. One detailed study that examined the morphology of cells harboring the BCR::ABL1 fusion gene in cases of Ph+ B-ALL in children reported that, in some cases, only the lymphoblasts harbored the fusion gene, whereas in others, the myeloid and lymphoblasts were BCR::ABL1 positive. In the latter group, some patients had a CML-CP picture after therapy, suggesting the lineage of involvement may be more limited in Ph-positive ALL than in CML.[104] Whether de novo Ph-positive AML exists has been a controversial issue, but data suggest that such cases can be recognized by deletions within the TCR and IGH genes, usually accompanied by loss of IKZF1 and CDNK1A/B, which will distinguish the de novo leukemia from CML in myeloid BP.[105,106]

CHRONIC NEUTROPHILIC LEUKEMIA (CNL)

Definition

CNL is a rare MPN characterized by sustained neutrophilia in the peripheral blood and a proliferation of neutrophilic granulocytes in the bone marrow that is shifted toward mature forms.[107] Hepatosplenomegaly is commonly present as a result of leukemic infiltration of the spleen and liver. Most patients with CNL have been shown to have point mutations in the proximal membrane region of CSF3R (exon 14), the gene encoding the CSF3R.[36] These mutations lead to constitutive activation of JAK/STAT signaling and are the drivers of the abnormal granulocytic proliferation. Detection of mutations of CSF3R is a valuable diagnostic tool to distinguish CNL from reactive leukocytosis, which it most closely resembles. There is no Ph chromosome or BCR::ABL1 fusion gene; cases of marked neutrophilia associated with a BCR::ABL1 fusion protein, including p230, are categorized as CML, not CNL.[70,72] The diagnosis of "CSF3R-negative" CNL requires exclusion of reactive neutrophilia and other MPNs and MDS/MPNs.

Synonyms and Related Terms

None.

Diagnosis

The diagnosis of CNL may be problematic because of its rarity and the overlap of its morphologic findings with those of infection, inflammation, and other myeloid neoplasms.[108] Previous criteria for CNL were largely exclusionary to rule out leukemoid reactions, other MPNs, and neutrophilia as a result of abnormal cytokine release by hematopoietic or non-hematopoietic neoplasms. Furthermore, nearly 30% of reported cases of CNL occurred in patients with a concomitant plasma cell neoplasm.[109,110] Most of these latter cases are thought to be reactive neutrophilia caused by release of G-CSF from the neoplastic plasma cells rather than CNL. Still, in a few cases of CNL with associated plasma cell abnormalities, the plasma cells were proven to be clonal; thus, the relation between CNL and plasma cell neoplasms may not be entirely settled.[109,111]

The ICC criteria for the diagnosis of CNL are outlined in Box 47-4. The ICC guidelines lowered the key diagnostic threshold for leukocytosis from ≥25 to ≥13 × 10^9/L in cases with *CSF3R* T618I or other activating *CSF3R* mutations. However, the proposed WHO 5th edition retained a leukocytosis threshold of ≥25 × 10^9/L for all cases.[2] The finding of *CSF3R* T618I or other activating *CSF3R* mutations is a major step in establishing the neutrophil proliferation as clonal; however, these mutations are not present in all cases, and they have been reported in occasional cases of aCML and in AML that arises in a background of congenital neutropenia.[36,48,112] Therefore, correlation of clinical history, hematologic data, morphology of the blood and bone marrow, and cytogenetic and molecular genetic data is necessary to reach a final diagnosis of CNL.

Epidemiology

Epidemiologic data on CNL is limited as a result of challenges in making a diagnosis for reasons cited herein. The true incidence of CNL is unknown. Based on available data, the overall incidence is 0.1 cases/1,000,000 individuals in the United States.[113] Although CNL usually affects adults in their 60s, it has been reported in all age groups with a slight male predominance.[108]

Clinical Findings

Many patients are asymptomatic when a complete blood count performed during a routine medical examination reveals leukocytosis, but others have symptoms of fatigue, bone pain, pruritus, easy bruising, or gout.[110,114] Bleeding diathesis can be seen in some patients. Splenomegaly is the most consistent physical finding and is present in about 36% of cases.[115] Hepatomegaly can also be present, but lymphadenopathy is uncommon.[116]

Morphologic Findings

Peripheral Blood

The WBC count is ≥13 × 10^9/L in patients with *CSF3R* T618I or other activating *CSF3R* mutations and ≥25 × 10^9/L

Box 47-4 *Diagnostic Criteria* for Chronic Neutrophilic Leukemia (CNL) According to International Consensus Classification[1]*

1. Peripheral blood white blood cell count ≥13 × 10^9/L[†]
   Segmented neutrophils plus banded neutrophils constitute ≥80% of the white blood cells.
      Neutrophil precursors (promyelocytes, myelocytes, and metamyelocytes) constitute <10% of the white blood cells
   No significant dysgranulopoiesis
   Circulating blasts only rarely observed[‡]
   Monocyte count <10% of all leukocytes
2. Hypercellular bone marrow with neutrophil granulocytes increased in percentage and absolute number, showing normal maturation
3. *CSF3R* T618I or another activating *CSF3R* mutation
or
Persistent neutrophilia (≥3 months), splenomegaly, and no identifiable cause of reactive neutrophilia including absence of a plasma cell neoplasm
or
If a plasma cell neoplasm is present, demonstration of clonality of myeloid cells by cytogenetic or molecular studies
4. Not meeting diagnostic criteria for *BCR::ABL1*-positive chronic myeloid leukemia, polycythemia vera, essential thrombocythemia, primary myelofibrosis or of a myeloid/lymphoid neoplasm with eosinophilia and tyrosine kinase gene fusions

*The diagnosis of CNL requires all four criteria.
[†]At least 25 × 10^9/L in cases lacking *CSF3R* T618I or another activating *CSF3R* mutation.
[‡]10% to 19% blasts in peripheral blood or bone marrow represent CNL in accelerated phase; ≥20% blasts represents blast phase.
Data from Arber DA, Orazi A, Hasserjian RP, et al. International Consensus Classification of myeloid neoplasms and acute leukemias: integrating morphologic, clinical, and genomic data. *Blood*. 2022;140(11):1200-1228.

---

in patients without *CSF3R* mutations (median, 50 × 10^9/L). Segmented neutrophils and bands account for 80% or more of the WBCs, whereas the sum of promyelocytes, myelocytes, and metamyelocytes is always less than 10% (Fig. 47-17). There is no significant granulocytic dysplasia, but toxic granulation or Döhle bodies may be seen. Myeloblasts are almost never observed in the blood at the time of diagnosis. Monocytes are less than 1 × 10^9/L, and there is no absolute basophilia or eosinophilia.[1,115] Mild to moderate anemia is common. The platelet count is usually normal; severe thrombocytopenia or thrombocytosis is rare. Findings of platelet function studies are reportedly abnormal in some cases, but most patients described in the literature have not been evaluated for platelet defects.

Bone Marrow

The bone marrow biopsy is hypercellular for age and shows marked proliferation of neutrophils. The myeloid-to-erythroid ratio is often 20:1 or more (Fig. 47-17). The percentage of blasts and promyelocytes in the marrow is not increased at the time of diagnosis, but there is an increase in the percentage of myelocytes, metamyelocytes, bands, and segmented neutrophils.[108] The neutrophils in the bone marrow usually resemble those in the blood. It is important to note that there is no significant dysplasia in the granulocytes or any other myeloid lineage. Basophilia and eosinophilia are generally not observed. Erythroid precursors are usually reduced in percentage but are normoblastic. Megakaryocytes

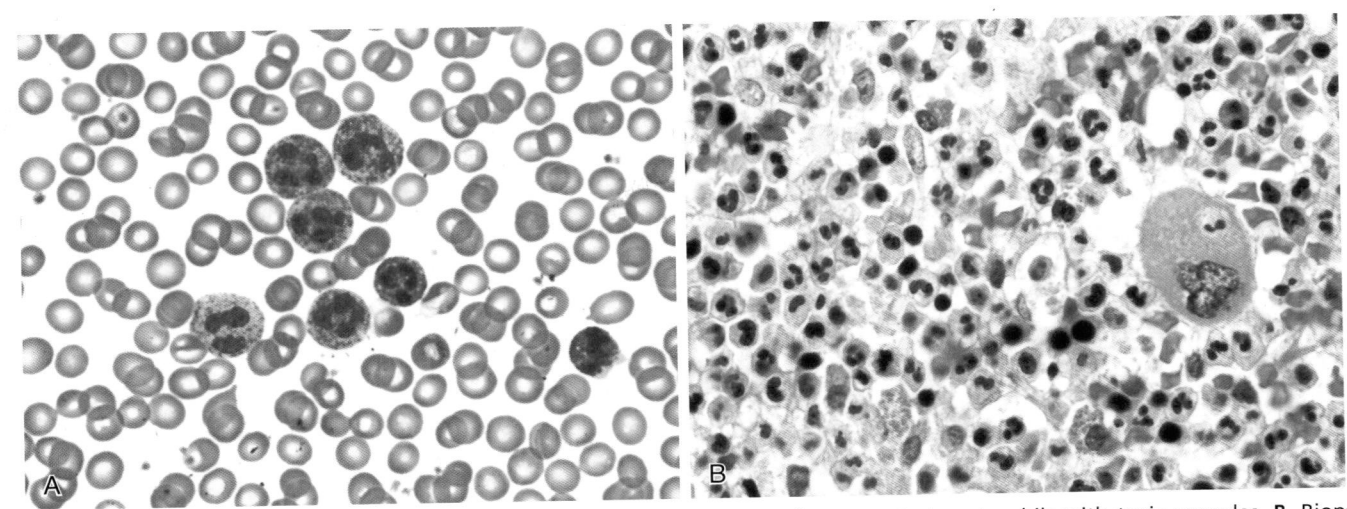

Figure 47-17. Chronic neutrophilic leukemia. A, Peripheral blood shows mainly segmented neutrophils with toxic granules. **B,** Biopsy shows a similar shift toward mature forms. No underlying disease could be found to explain the neutrophilia, and splenomegaly was present.

are also morphologically normal, but mild megakaryocytic proliferation has been reported in some cases. Mild increase of reticulin fibrosis (MF-1) can be seen in a minority of cases.[115] Ten percent to 19% blasts in peripheral blood or bone marrow represent AP of disease, and ≥20% blasts represent BP of CNL. In view of the reported relation between neutrophilia and plasma cell abnormalities, careful attention should be given to the marrow plasma cells in all cases in which a diagnosis of CNL is contemplated. If abnormal or clonal plasma cells are present, clonality of the neutrophils should be demonstrated before a diagnosis of CNL is rendered.

Extramedullary Tissues

Splenomegaly and hepatomegaly are caused by tissue infiltration by neutrophils. In the spleen, the infiltrate assumes a typical leukemic pattern, with infiltration in the red pulp cords and sinuses, whereas in the liver, the sinuses or portal areas, or both, may be infiltrated.[117]

Genetics

Nearly 25% of patients who meet the current criteria for diagnosis of CNL have clonal cytogenetic abnormalities at diagnosis, and in another 10%, cytogenetic abnormalities appear during disease evolution.[116] None are specific for CNL, but their presence confirms the neoplastic nature of the neutrophilia. The most common abnormalities include +8, +9, +21, del(20q), and del(11q). There is no Ph chromosome or *BCR::ABL1* fusion gene and specifically no BCR::ABL1 p230 isoform, which is associated with CML with prominent neutrophilia or thrombocytosis but not with CNL.

The presence of driver mutations in the *CSF3R* is the diagnostic genetic signature of CNL and is seen in 80% of cases. The mutation most strongly associated with CNL is an activating point mutation in *CSF3R* T618I, located on chromosome 1p34.3, which encodes the transmembrane receptor CSF3R.[36,48-50] The absence of a *CSF3R* mutation does not exclude the possibility of CNL. Additional mutations can be seen in many cases, including *SETBP1, ASXL1, SRSF2,* and signaling mutations.[118] Occasional patients with CNL have been described with *JAK2* V617F and mutated *CALR*.[116]

Patients with CNL with *CSF3R* mutations were found to represent two phenotypically and prognostically distinct subsets.[119] The *CSF3R* T618I-mutated individuals clustered with adverse clinical and laboratory features, demonstrating more advanced age at diagnosis, higher white WBC counts, lower hemoglobin values and platelet counts at diagnosis, more frequently with abnormal karyotype, and lower overall survival (OS) than patients harboring other *CSF3R* mutations.

Clinical Course

CNL follows a progressive disease course with a short overall survival of approximately 2 years.[108,113] Causes of death include intracranial hemorrhage, progressive disease, infections, and leukemic transformation.[108] Progression of CNL is often associated with increasing neutrophilia, worsening anemia, and thrombocytopenia. Transformation to AML has been reported to occur in 10% to 15% of cases.[110,117] Intracranial hemorrhage as a cause of death has been reported in a disproportionate number of patients. Although this may be a manifestation of an underlying coagulation or platelet abnormality, it may also be attributed to thrombocytopenia related to progressive disease or to therapy.[114,116]

Differential Diagnosis

The differential diagnosis of CNL includes reactive neutrophilia and other myeloid proliferations with a prominent neutrophil component. Reactive neutrophilia caused by infection and inflammation may be revealed by a thorough clinical history and additional laboratory studies, but inspection of the blood or bone marrow may not reveal any significant morphologic differences between reactive neutrophilia and CNL. Rouleaux formation of RBCs on the blood smear may suggest an underlying plasma cell lesion, in which case the blood should be examined for abnormal immunoglobulins and a bone marrow specimen searched for an abnormal plasma cell population. Epithelial tumors and sarcomas may also secrete cytokines that stimulate neutrophil production. In the presence of either a plasma cell lesion or another underlying neoplasm, a diagnosis of CNL should not be made unless there is convincing evidence of clonality of the neutrophils, such as the presence of mutated *CSF3R*. Other disorders to consider in the differential diagnosis of CNL include CML associated with the p230 BCR::ABL1 isoform[72] and aCML. The distinguishing features of these neoplasms are listed in Table 47-2.

CLASSIC *BCR::ABL1*-NEGATIVE MYELOPROLIFERATIVE NEOPLASMS

This group of MPNs includes ET, PV, and PMF. They share a close association with *JAK2*, *CALR*, and *MPL* mutations, with *JAK2* mutation being the most prevalent in each one of these entities.

An accurate classification of MPNs in this category requires the following: (1) bone marrow aspirate smears and trephine biopsies collected at time of diagnosis, or within a short time frame thereafter, and in the absence of active therapy, especially with cytoreductive drugs; (2) adequate core biopsy specimens that are ≥1.5 cm in length, free of artifact, performed at a right angle to the cortical bone, and accompanied by properly spread particulate bone marrow aspirate smears; and (3) additional peripheral blood and bone marrow samples for cytogenetic and molecular studies, including *JAK2* (both exons 12 and 14), *CALR*, and *MPL* mutations.[120] A carefully processed specimen should allow accurate grading of fibrosis (3-grade scoring system) as shown

in Table 47-3 and assessment of age-adjusted hematopoietic cellularity, both of which are crucial diagnostic features.[121-123] Figure 47-18 demonstrates semiquantitative grading of bone marrow fibrosis. Assessment of bone marrow fibrosis must also include its quality (i.e., reticulin versus collagen).[124]

Table 47-3 Semiquantitative Grading of Bone Marrow Fibrosis

Grade*	Description
MF-0	Scattered linear reticulin fibers with no intersections (crossovers), corresponding to normal bone marrow
MF-1	Loose network of reticulin with many intersections, especially in perivascular areas
MF-2[†]	Diffuse and dense increase in reticulin fibers with extensive intersections, occasionally with focal bundles of thick fibers mostly consistent with collagen or focal osteosclerosis
MF-3[†]	Diffuse and dense increase in reticulin with extensive intersections and coarse bundles of thick fibers consistent with collagen, usually associated with osteosclerosis

*Should be assessed only in hematopoietic areas. If the fibrosis pattern is heterogeneous, the final score is determined by the highest grade present in at least 30% of the marrow area.
[†]In grades MF-2 and MF-3, trichrome staining is recommended.
Data from Thiele J, Kvasnicka HM, Facchetti F, Franco V, van der Walt J, Orazi A. European consensus on grading bone marrow fibrosis and assessment of cellularity. *Haematologica.* 2005;90(8):1128-1132.

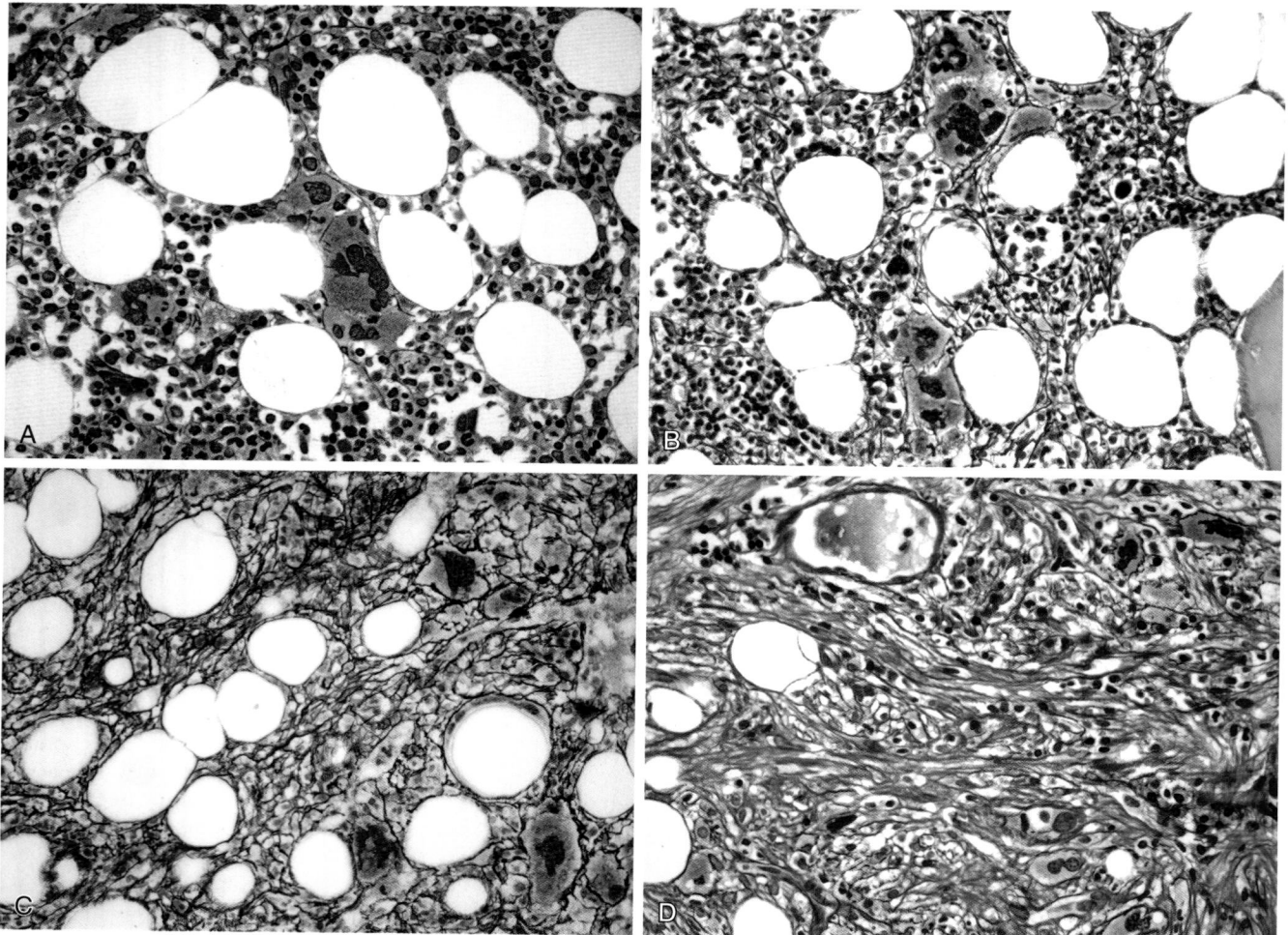

Figure 47-18. Semiquantitative grading of bone marrow fibrosis. A, Grade MF-0. **B,** Grade MF-1. **C,** Grade MF-2. **D,** Grade MF-3. See Table 47-3 for a description of the grades.

A systematic approach integrating evaluation of bone marrow cellularity, relative proportions of the three lineages, spatial distribution/organization of the different hematopoietic cell lineages, and morphologic hallmarks of each lineage provides unique histologic patterns that have significant diagnostic value (Table 47-4).[125]

ESSENTIAL THROMBOCYTHEMIA (ET)

Definition

Essential thrombocythemia (ET) is a CMN characterized by sustained thrombocytosis of 450 × 10⁹/L or more in the peripheral blood; increased numbers of large, mature megakaryocytes in the bone marrow; and episodes of thrombosis or hemorrhage.[126] The ICC diagnostic criteria for ET are listed in Box 47-5.

Synonyms and Related Terms

Idiopathic thrombocythaemia/thrombocytosis; essential hemorrhagicthrombocythaemia; idiopathic hemorrhagicthrombocythaemia; idiopathic thrombocythaemia; megakaryocytic myelosis; hemorrhagic thrombocythaemia; primary thrombocythaemia/thrombocytosis

Epidemiology

Incidence is estimated at 1.2 to 3.0 per 100,000 population per year[127] with a median age at diagnosis of 58 years and a slight female predominance.

Clinical Features

More than 50% of the patients are asymptomatic and discovered incidentally with thrombocytosis (by definition ≥450 × 10⁹/L). It should be noted that reactive etiologies of thrombocytosis including infections, inflammation, recent acute bleeding, postsurgical state, splenectomy, and iron deficiency are more common than clonal thrombocytosis. In addition to ET, clonal thrombocytosis can be seen in PV, PMF, CML, and MDS/MPN with ring sideroblasts and thrombocytosis (MDS/MPN-T-*SF3B1* and MDS/MPN-RS-T, NOS). Diagnosis of ET requires integration of clinical, morphologic, and laboratory features. Symptoms are more frequently associated with thrombosis, ranging from transient ischemic attacks involving small vessels to splanchnic vein thrombosis or hemorrhages, more frequently involving the gastrointestinal and respiratory tracts.[128,129] Splenomegaly is typically absent, but mild splenomegaly can be seen in 15% to 20% of cases; hepatomegaly is rare.

Morphology

Peripheral Blood

Thrombocytosis is the most striking abnormality noted on the hemogram and may range from 450 to more than 2000 × 10⁹/L.[46,130] On microscopic examination, the platelets may show anisocytosis ranging from tiny to markedly enlarged forms. Atypical platelets including hypogranular, enlarged, or bizarrely shaped forms, can be seen but are uncommon (Fig. 47-19). The WBC count and leukocyte differential are usually normal; immature granulocytes are generally not present, and basophilia is minimal, if present at all.[126,130] The RBCs are usually normal unless there has been significant bleeding, in which case they may be hypochromic and microcytic; however, significant anisopoikilocytosis is uncommon, and teardrop-shaped RBCs are not observed. Leukoerythroblastosis is not present. Patients with mutated *CALR* reportedly have a lower Hb level but higher platelet counts than those with mutated *JAK2*.[46]

Bone Marrow

A bone marrow biopsy is essential to diagnose ET and to distinguish it from prefibrotic PMF, PV, other MPNs and myeloid neoplasms associated with thrombocytosis, and reactive thrombocytosis.[126,131,132]

Table 47-4 Differential Morphologic Features of Essential Thrombocythemia (ET), Early/Prefibrotic Primary Myelofibrosis (Pre-PMF), Overt Myelofibrosis (PMF), and Polycythemia Vera (PV)

Feature	ET	Pre-PMF	PMF	PV
Increased cellularity (age matched)	–	+	+	+
Increased granulopoiesis	–	+	+	+
Increased erythropoiesis	–	–	–	+
Increased megakaryopoiesis	+	+	+	+
Megakaryocytes				
Dense large clusters (≥6 megakaryocytes)	–	+	+	–
Size: Small	–	+	+	+
Giant	++	+	+	+
Hyperlobulated nuclei (staghorn)	+	–	–	+
Hypolobulated nuclei (bulbous/cloud-like)	–	+	+	–
Nuclear maturation defects	–	+	+	–
Reticulin fibrosis ≥MF-2	–	–	+	–

ET, Essential thrombocythemia; *PMF,* primary myelofibrosis; *pre-PMF,* early/prefibrotic primary myelofibrosis; *PV,* polycythemia vera.

The bone marrow is normocellular for the patients' age, with only a few cases of mild hypercellularity (Fig. 47-19). Erythropoiesis, granulopoiesis, and the myeloid-to-erythroid ratio do not show significant abnormalities. The most striking abnormality in biopsy sections is an increase in the number and size of the megakaryocytes. They may occur in loose clusters but are more often dispersed throughout the bone marrow. There is a predominance of large-to-giant forms with abundant, mature cytoplasm and deeply lobulated or hyperlobulated nuclei that sometimes assume a staghorn appearance. Dense megakaryocyte clusters, defined as three or more megakaryocytes without other intervening bone marrow cells, are infrequent in ET and usually small (i.e., <6 megakaryocytes).[133] In these cases, differential diagnosis with prefibrotic PMF might be challenging, but lack of atypia of the megakaryocytes (increased nuclear-to-cytoplasmic ratio, irregular chromatin clumping, and bulbous appearance), lack of granulocytic proliferation, and lack of clinical features like increased lactate dehydrogenase (LDH) or splenomegaly are key to distinguishing these cases from prefibrotic PMF.

Myeloblasts are usually less than 5%, and a mild increase in reticulin fibers (MF-1) is rare, being present in less than 5% of patients at initial diagnosis.[125,134,135]

Bone marrow aspirate smears may not be as informative as marrow biopsy. The smears often show large megakaryocytes, frequently associated with large pools of platelets. Emperipolesis of bone marrow cells is sometimes seen; however, this is not specific and can also be seen in megakaryocytes from normal or reactive bone marrow specimens.

Extramedullary Tissues

Splenic enlargement is uncommon at the time of diagnosis; if present, it may be largely because of pooling and sequestration of platelets. Extramedullary hematopoiesis is absent or minimal.

Genetics

Cytogenetics

The majority of cases with ET demonstrate a normal karyotype. According to published data on cytogenetically annotated patients with well-defined ET, 7% had abnormal karyotype, including loss of chromosome Y (2%) and abnormalities other than –Y (4.8%), the most frequent being sole 20q–.[136] The cytogenetic findings were associated with clinical and molecular genetic findings and prognosis. Abnormal karyotype, other than –Y, was associated with older age, higher leukocyte count, and arterial thrombosis history. Normal karyotype/–Y clustered with *ASXL1* mutations, and abnormal karyotype clustered with *TP53* mutations. The OS was significantly shorter in patients with abnormal karyotype or –Y than in those with normal karyotype (medians 12, 10, and 21 years, respectively).

Mutations

Driver mutations for *JAK2* V617F (50%–70%), *CALR* (20%–25%), and *MPL* (3%–8%) are seen in the majority of patients with ET; however, up to 10% of cases can be triple negative.[137,138] Except for PV, in which *CALR* or *MPL* mutations virtually do not occur, the type of driver mutations are not helpful in differentiating ET from other MPNs. However, the type of mutations has functional consequences. *JAK2* V617F is associated with older age, higher hemoglobin level, leukocytosis, lower platelet count, and increased risk of thrombosis.[139-141] Mutant *CALR* (vs. *JAK2*) is associated with younger age, male sex, higher platelet count, lower hemoglobin level, lower leukocyte count, and lower incidence of thrombotic events, and type 2 *CALR* mutations (vs. type 1) are associated with higher platelet count.[141]

By next-generation sequencing (NGS) analysis in patients with confirmed ET, mutations other than *JAK2/CALR/MPL* can be seen in some patients, the most frequent being *TET2* and *ASXL1*.[142] Presence of high molecular risk mutations (e.g., *TP53*, *SF3B1*, *SRSF2*, *U2AF1*) have been shown to affect overall, myelofibrosis-free, and leukemia-free survival rates.[136] In particular, *TP53* mutations have been associated with leukemic transformation.[136]

Clinical Course

The natural history of ET is that of an indolent disorder punctuated by episodes of thrombosis or hemorrhage with long symptom-free intervals. Median survival in ET has been reported to range from approximately 11 to 35 years, with a median of 35 years for patients aged 40 or younger, 22 years for those aged 41 to 60 years, and 11 years for those aged >60 years.[135,137,143] Thrombotic and hemorrhagic complications

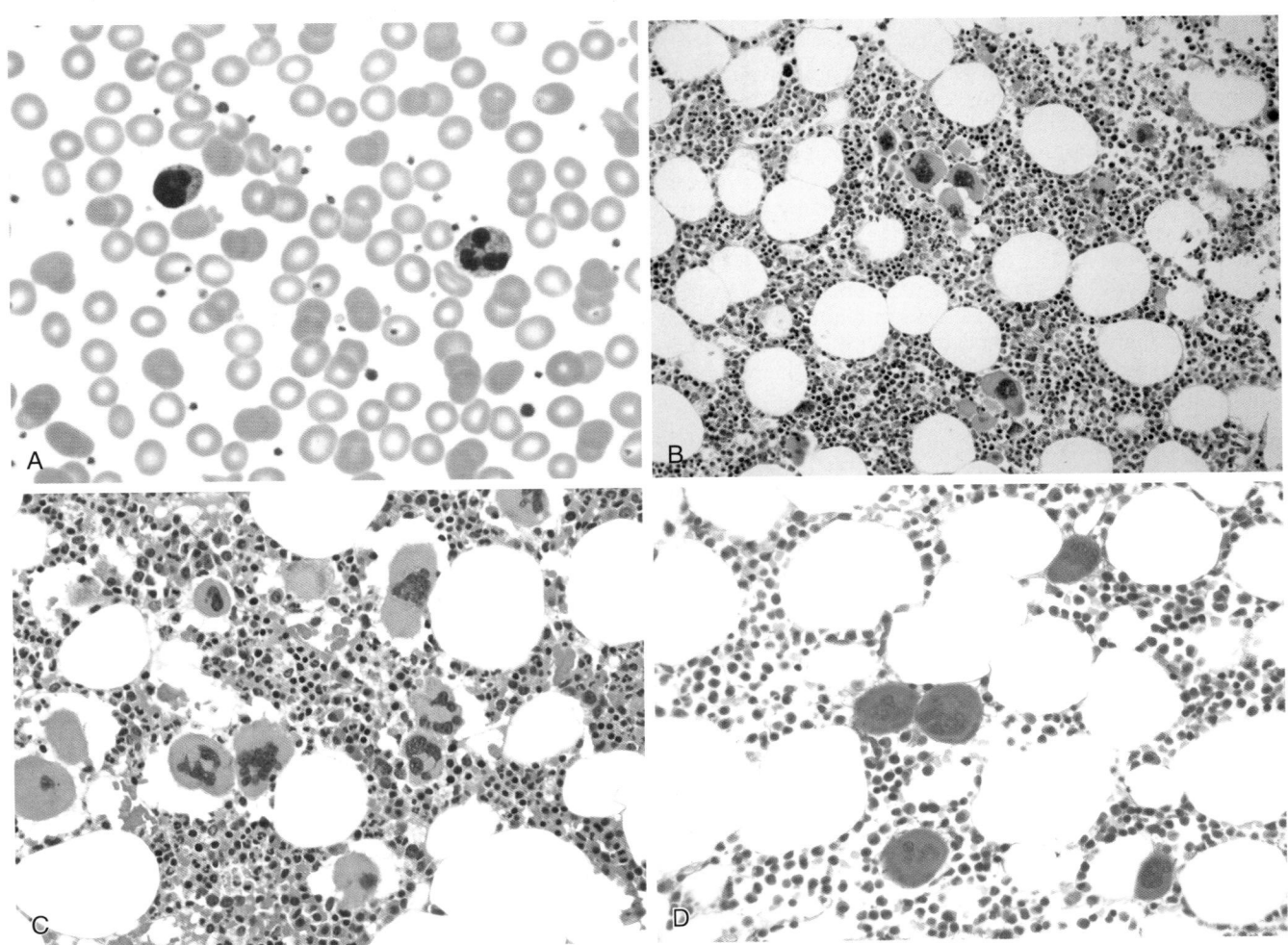

Figure 47-19. Essential thrombocythemia in a 42-year-old woman. A, Peripheral blood is largely unremarkable, except for thrombocytosis (800 × 10⁹/L). **B, C,** Bone marrow biopsy exhibits normal cellularity but increased numbers of large megakaryocytes with hyperlobulated nuclei. **D,** Loose clustering of megakaryocytes can be observed.

represent two of the main causes of morbidity and mortality in patients with ET, and therefore, the main goal of therapy is to prevent this outcome.

Approximately 10% of ET cases can develop bone marrow fibrosis grade 2 to 3 associated with extramedullary hematopoiesis, so-called post-ET myelofibrosis. The diagnostic criteria for post-ET myelofibrosis are listed in Box 47-6. The cumulative probability of post-ET myelofibrosis is about 4% at 10 years and 9% at 15 years. Risk factors for fibrotic transformation reportedly include older age, anemia, bone marrow hypercellularity, and reticulin fibrosis at diagnosis.[144] A large study of 1607 patients with ET from three independent centers showed a higher risk of fibrotic progression in patients with a *JAK2* V617F allele burden >35% and *CALR* type 1/1-like or *MPL* mutations.[145]

The risk of transformation to AP (10%–19% blasts) and BP (≥20% blasts) remains unpredictable, as the transformation may occur in young individuals even without detectable high-risk genomic profiles.[146] In other studies, reported risk factors for transformation to BP in ET included advanced age, extreme thrombocytosis, anemia, leukocytosis, and mutations involving *TP53* and *EZH2*.[147]

Box 47-6 *Diagnostic Criteria* for Post-essential Thrombocythemia Myelofibrosis (post-ET MF)[1]*

Required Criteria
1. Previous established diagnosis of ET
2. Bone marrow fibrosis of grade 2 or 3

Additional Criteria
1. Anemia (i.e., below the reference range given age, sex, and altitude considerations) and a >2 g/dL decrease from baseline hemoglobin concentration
2. Leukoerythroblastosis
3. Increase in palpable splenomegaly of >5 cm from baseline or the development of a newly palpable splenomegaly
4. Elevated lactate dehydrogenase (LDH) level above the reference range
5. Development of any 2 (or all 3) of the following constitutional symptoms: >10% weight loss in 6 months, night sweats, unexplained fever (>37.5 °C)

*The diagnosis of post-ET MF is established by all required criteria and at least two additional criteria.
Data from Arber DA, Orazi A, Hasserjian RP, et al. International Consensus Classification of myeloid neoplasms and acute leukemias: integrating morphologic, clinical, and genomic data. *Blood.* 2022;140(11):1200-1228.

Differential Diagnosis

Thrombocytosis is a common hematologic abnormality and is associated with a wide range of hematopoietic and non-hematopoietic neoplasms, inflammatory and autoimmune conditions, infections, recent bleeding, and iron deficiency (Box 47-7). Even the majority of cases with platelet counts of 1000 × 10⁹/L or more are usually caused by a reactive megakaryocytic proliferation.[148] Of the MPNs that have marked thrombocytosis, ET is the disorder that most clinicians and pathologists associate with a markedly elevated platelet count; however, CML, PV, and prefibrotic PMF also demonstrate marked thrombocytosis, with platelet counts sometimes exceeding 1000 × 10⁹/L, and each of them is more common than ET.

Reactive Thrombocytosis

There may be some clinical urgency to determine the reason for marked thrombocytosis because thrombohemorrhagic complications are more likely in thrombocytosis because of myeloid neoplasms than in reactive thrombocytosis. The clinical history, physical findings, examination of the peripheral blood smear, and a few ancillary laboratory studies are often sufficient to distinguish between reactive and neoplastic thrombocytosis. A history of chronic thrombocytosis, prior bleeding or thrombotic episodes, and the finding of splenomegaly favor MPN, whereas the lack of these plus any clinical or laboratory evidence of an underlying inflammatory disease, such as elevated C-reactive protein, or of a non-hematopoietic neoplasm favors reactive thrombocytosis. Nevertheless, if an underlying cause for the thrombocytosis is not readily apparent, studies for *JAK2* V617F, *CALR,* and *MPL* mutations and a *BCR::ABL1* fusion gene should be performed from the blood or bone marrow specimen, and the bone marrow should be examined for an MPN or any other hematopoietic or non-hematopoietic neoplasm that would explain the thrombocytosis (Box 47-7).

Other Myeloid Neoplasms Associated With Thrombocytosis

The most commonly encountered myeloid neoplasms associated with thrombocytosis other than ET include PV, prefibrotic early/primary myelofibrosis (pre-PMF), and CML. Each of these diseases has been characterized separately in this chapter; the characteristic morphology that distinguishes ET from pre-PMF, which can sometimes be challenging, is summarized in Table 47-5 and illustrated in Fig. 47-20. Some cases of CML, particularly those with the p230 oncoprotein, can initially display marked thrombocytosis and minimal leukocytosis; therefore, cytogenetic or molecular genetic studies should always be performed to exclude a *BCR::ABL1* fusion gene and CML as a cause of thrombocytosis.[72] Yet another diagnostic consideration is the possibility of MDS/MPN-T-*SF3B1* and MDS/MPN-RS-T, NOS. Both may resemble ET in that they are characterized by a platelet count of 450 × 10⁹/L or greater and have a proliferation of megakaryocytes in the bone marrow that morphologically resemble those of an MPN. Furthermore, nearly half of cases carry the *JAK2* V617F mutation. However, MDS/MPN-T-*SF3B1* and MDS/MPN-RS-T, NOS demonstrate anemia and ineffective erythroid proliferation with dyserythropoiesis and ring sideroblasts, features not expected in an MPN. In

---

Box 47-7 *Possible Causes of Thrombocytosis (Platelet Count ≥450 × 10⁹/L)*

Secondary (Reactive) Thrombocytosis
- Infection
- Inflammatory and autoimmune diseases
- Blood loss, hemorrhage
- Chronic iron deficiency
- Postsplenectomy
- Hyposplenism
- Trauma (particularly brain injury)
- Postsurgical procedures
- Neoplasms (nonhematopoietic and nonmyeloid)
- Bone marrow regeneration, rebound after chemotherapy

Myeloid Neoplasm Related
- Myeloproliferative neoplasms
- Chronic myeloid leukemia, *BCR::ABL1*-positive
- Polycythemia vera
- Primary myelofibrosis
- Essential thrombocythemia
- Acute myeloid leukemia or myelodysplastic syndrome with t(3;3)(q21.3;q26.2) or inv(3)(q21.3q26.2)
- Myelodysplastic syndrome with del(5q)
- Myelodysplastic/myeloproliferative neoplasm with ring sideroblasts and thrombocytosis (MDS/MPN-T-*SF3B1* and MDS/MPN-RS-T)

Table 47-5 Main Clinical and Morphologic Differences Between Essential Thrombocythemia (ET) and Early/Prefibrotic Primary Myelofibrosis (Pre-PMF)

	ET	Pre-PMF
Clinical Features		
Splenomegaly	Uncommon	Common (45% cases)
Anemia	Absent	May be present
White blood cell count	Usually normal, occasionally mildly increased	Variable, often increased
Platelet count	Always ≥450 × 10⁹/L	Often ≥450 × 10⁹/L, sometimes >1.000 × 10⁹/L, very rarely decreased
Increased LDH	Absent	Often increased
Morphologic Findings		
Bone marrow cellularity (age-adjusted)	Normal to minimally increased	Increased
Granulocytic-to-erythroid ratio	Normal	Increased because of granulocytic hyperplasia
Megakaryocytic Morphology		
Dense clusters	Very rare (small, <6 megakaryocytes)	Common (often ≥6 megakaryocytes)
Pleomorphism (variability in size and shape)	Absent	Present
Nuclear features	Hyperchromatic and hyperlobulated nuclei, "staghorn nuclei"	Hypolobulated cloud-like, bulbous, bizarre-shaped nuclei, bare or hyperchromatic nuclei

ET, Essential thrombocythemia; *LDH,* lactate dehydrogenase; *pre-PMF,* early/prefibrotic primary myelofibrosis.

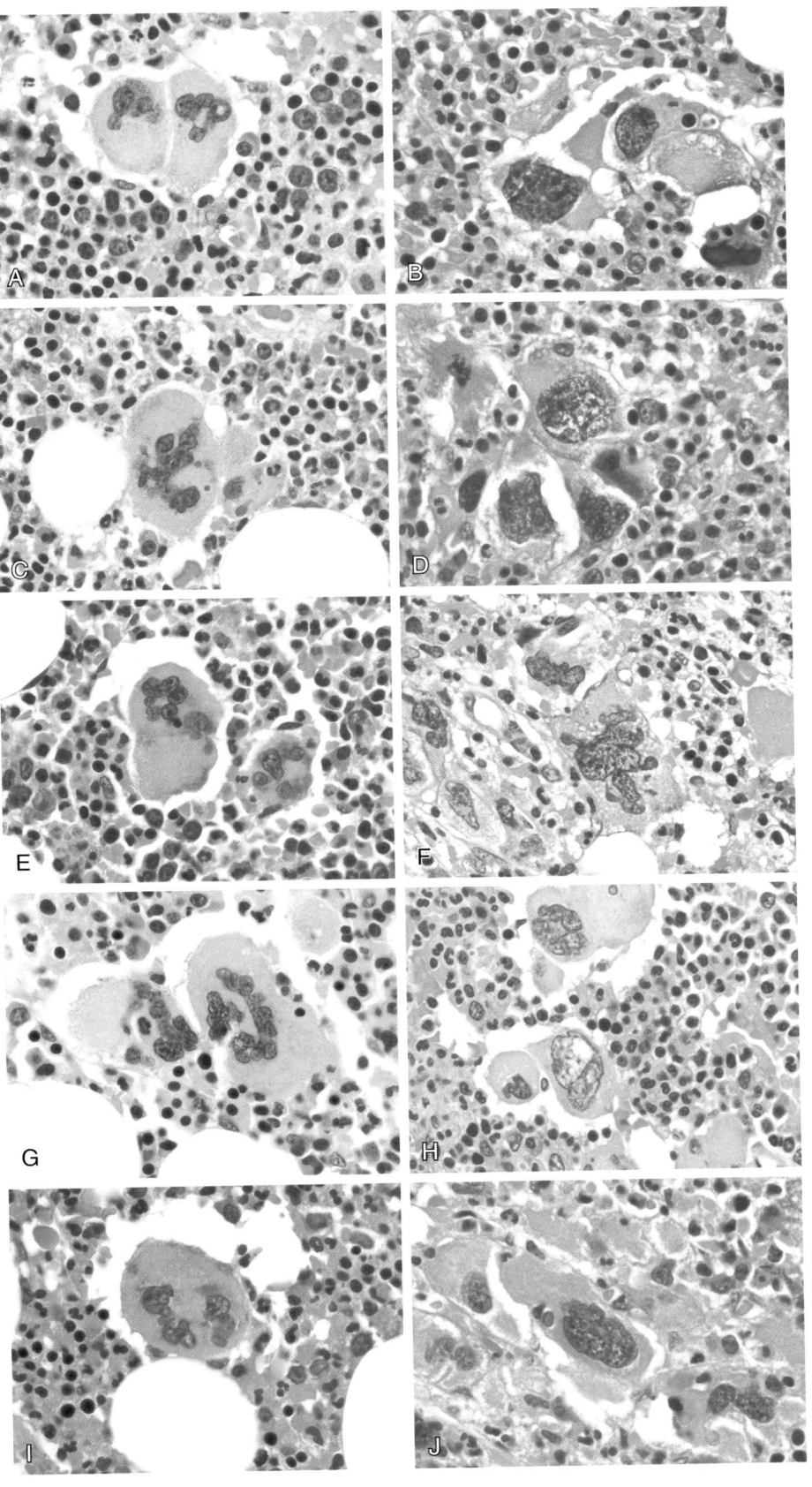

Figure 47-20. **Megakaryocytes in essential thrombocythemia (ET) and prefibrotic/early primary myelofibrosis (pre-PMF).** Although ET and pre-PMF may have overlapping clinical and laboratory features, the megakaryocytes differ morphologically between the two disorders; however, megakaryocyte morphology is not the sole basis for diagnosis. The megakaryocytes illustrated in the *left* column of this figure (**A, C, E, G,** and **I**) are from cases of ET in which the majority (but not all) of the megakaryocytes have hyperlobulated nuclei and voluminous cytoplasm. In contrast, those illustrated in the *right* column (**B, D, F, H,** and **J**) are from cases of pre-PMF, in which the majority of megakaryocytes have an altered nuclear-to-cytoplasmic ratio, bulky, cloudlike nuclei, and an overall bizarre appearance.

the presence of an *SF3B1* mutation (≥10% variant allele frequency), an association with the *JAK2* V617F mutation is common, whereas mutations in *CALR* or *MPL* W515 are less frequent. Elevated platelet counts are uncommon in MDS and AML, but in some specific instances, the platelet count may be markedly elevated. MDS with del(5q) and MDS or AML with t(3;3)(q21.3;q26.2) or inv(3)(q21.3q26.2) are frequently associated with thrombocytosis. Cases of MDS with del(5q) are characterized by megakaryocytes that are usually smaller than normal and have hypolobulated nuclei, in contrast to the large and hyperlobulated nuclei of the megakaryocytes of ET. MDS and AML cases associated with t(3;3) or inv(3) are characterized by the proliferation of micromegakaryocytes.

PRIMARY MYELOFIBROSIS (PMF)

Myelofibrosis is an increase in the amount and density of the discontinuous, linear network of delicate reticulin fibers that provides the structural framework on which hematopoiesis normally occurs. This increase can vary from a focal, loose, yet nearly continuous network of reticulin fibers to dense, diffuse collagen fibrosis and osteosclerosis. Reticulin fibrosis and collagen fibrosis are non-specific, secondary responses to various injuries and diseases that involve the bone marrow and are mediated by cytokines released from marrow stromal cells and hematopoietic cells, including megakaryocytes, T cells, and cells of the monocyte-macrophage lineages.[149,150] Reticulin fibrosis is commonly associated with infections and inflammatory conditions that involve the bone marrow, whereas overt collagen fibrosis more often accompanies neoplastic diseases, such as carcinoma and lymphoma, when they infiltrate the marrow.[149] However, nearly half of all cases of myelofibrosis are associated with myeloid neoplasms, the MPNs in particular. Although any MPN can demonstrate myelofibrosis, particularly during disease progression, PMF stands out as the MPN most commonly linked to this complication.

Definition

PMF is a clonal MPN characterized by a proliferation of abnormal megakaryocytes and granulocytes in the bone marrow, which in fully developed disease, i.e., overt PMF, is associated with significant fibrosis and extramedullary hematopoiesis.

Similar to the 2016 WHO classification, the ICC defines two subtypes of PMF: pre-PMF and overt fibrotic PMF. Several studies have defined the early/prefibrotic stage of PMF as different from ET and overt PMF because of its distinct clinical, morphologic, and molecular features.[137,151-153] Pre-PMF can present with isolated thrombocytosis and develop thrombohemorrhagic complications similar to ET. Cases of pre-PMF may progress to overt fibrotic PMF, and that blurs the distinction of the two "entities." However, the rate of progression is variable, and not all patients with pre-PMF will necessarily develop an overt disease.[153]

Early/Prefibrotic Primary Myelofibrosis (Pre-PMF)

Pre-PMF was formally introduced in the WHO classification of tumors in 2001,[154] confirmed and revised in 2008,[155] and then further defined as its own entity in the WHO

2016 revision.[156] Pre-PMF is a clonal MPN characterized by megakaryocytic proliferation and atypia, without reticulin fibrosis grade >1, accompanied by increased age-adjusted bone marrow cellularity and granulocytic proliferation. The diagnostic criteria for pre-PMF as defined by ICC are listed in Box 47-8.

Synonyms and Related Terms

Early stage myelofibrosis

Epidemiology

There are no registry-based prevalence or incidence data available for pre-PMF, as many of these cases were previously diagnosed as ET. The incidence of pre-PMF may be grossly calculated by referring to results derived from reclassifications of bone marrow biopsies and corresponding clinical data to differentiate patients with "true" ET from those with pre-PMF, ranging between 14% and 18% after centralized evaluations at centers of excellence.[157-159]

Clinical Features

Approximately 30% to 40% of patients with pre-PMF are asymptomatic at diagnosis and present with an abnormal

---

Box 47-8 *Diagnostic Criteria* for Prefibrotic Early/ Primary Myelofibrosis (pre-PMF) According to International Consensus Classification*

Major Criteria
1. Bone marrow biopsy showing megakaryocytic proliferation and atypia,[†] bone marrow fibrosis grade <2, increased age-adjusted bone marrow cellularity, granulocytic proliferation, and (often) decreased erythropoiesis
2. *JAK2, CALR,* or *MPL* mutation[‡]
   or
   presence of another clonal marker[§]
   or
   absence of reactive bone marrow reticulin fibrosis[¶]
3. Diagnostic criteria for *BCR::ABL1*-positive chronic myeloid leukemia, polycythemia vera, essential thrombocythemia, myelodysplastic syndromes, or other myeloid neoplasms are not met

Minor Criteria
1. Anemia not attributed to a comorbid condition
2. Leukocytosis ≥11 × 10⁹/L
3. Palpable splenomegaly
4. Lactate dehydrogenase level above the reference range

*The diagnosis of pre-PMF requires all three major criteria and at least one minor criterion confirmed in two consecutive determinations.
†Morphology of megakaryocytes in pre-PMF demonstrates a high degree of megakaryocytic atypia including small to giant megakaryocytes with a prevalence of severe maturation defects (cloud-like, hypolobulated, and hyperchromatic nuclei) and presence of abnormal large dense clusters (mostly >6 megakaryocytes lying strictly adjacent).
‡Highly sensitive assays for *JAK2* V617F (sensitivity level <1%) and *CALR* and *MPL* (sensitivity level 1% to 3%) are recommended; in negative cases, search for noncanonical *JAK2* and *MPL* mutations should be considered.
§Assessed by cytogenetics or sensitive next-generation sequencing techniques; detection of mutations associated with myeloid neoplasms (e.g., *ASXL1, EZH2, IDH1, IDH2, SF3B1, SRSF2,* and *TET2* mutations) supports the clonal nature of the disease.
¶Minimal reticulin fibrosis (MF-1) secondary to infection, autoimmune disorder or other chronic inflammatory conditions, hairy cell leukemia or another lymphoid neoplasm, metastatic malignancy, or toxic (chronic) myelopathies.
Data from Arber DA, Orazi A, Hasserjian RP, et al. International Consensus Classification of myeloid neoplasms and acute leukemias: integrating morphologic, clinical, and genomic data. *Blood.* 2022;140(11):1200-1228.

CBC, usually from anemia, leukocytosis, thrombocytosis, or more rarely, from splenomegaly. Thrombocytosis clinically mimicking ET is the most common and challenging presentation in pre-PMF. Less commonly, the diagnosis results from discovery of unexplained leukoerythroblastosis or increased LDH level. Compared to those with overt PMF, patients with pre-PMF are younger, with higher hemoglobin, leukocyte, and platelet counts.[152] Symptomatic cases are characterized by constitutional symptoms (fatigue, weight loss, night sweats, dyspnea). The degree of splenomegaly varies depending on the stage and length of the disease, and splenomegaly is seen in approximately 45% of patients with pre-PMF.[152,160]

Morphology

Peripheral Blood

Pre-PMF is typically characterized by borderline anemia, mild leukocytosis, and moderate to marked thrombocytosis (mean platelet count, 962 × 10⁹/L; range, 104–3215 × 10⁹/L).[161,162] In the peripheral blood, the most striking finding is often the marked increase in platelets (Fig. 47-21). Mild neutrophilia with a left shift may be seen, but myeloblasts, nucleated RBCs, and teardrop-shaped RBCs are uncommon.

Bone Marrow

The bone marrow is characteristically hypercellular for the patient's age with a granulocytic proliferation and an increased myeloid-to-erythroid ratio. Megakaryocytes are also increased in number and often form dense clusters. They show pleomorphic features in terms of their size, shape, and nuclear features. Nuclear atypia (increased nuclear-to-cytoplasmic ratio, abnormal chromatin clumping, and bulbous nuclei) is usually pronounced (Fig. 47-22). By definition, reticulin fibrosis is absent (MF-0) or mild (MF-1). Considering dense clusters of megakaryocytes can also rarely be found in ET, diagnosis of pre-PMF and the differential diagnosis with ET should be based on the evaluation of the complete histologic pattern, including the overall cellularity, myeloid-to-erythroid ratio, morphology of megakaryocytes, and size of their clusters, in conjunction with clinical data.

Extramedullary Tissues

Extramedullary hematopoiesis in the spleen is minimal, if any.

Genetic Findings

In pre-PMF, abnormal cytogenetics were found in about 18% of cases and unfavorable karyotypes (complex karyotype or single or two abnormalities, including +8, −7/7q−, i[17q], −5/5q−, 12p−, inv[3], or 11q23 rearrangement) in 4% to 8% of cases. Incidence of *JAK2* V617F mutations in pre-PMF is very similar to that in ET, ranging from 52% to 67% and 54% to 66%, respectively.[137,152]

In a large study comparing pre-PMF and overt-PMF, the three driver mutations (*JAK2* V617F, *MPL*W515x, and *CALR*) were similarly distributed in the two cohorts. *JAK2* V617F mutation was found in 67.2% of pre-PMF cases and in 58.2% of overt PMF cases; *CALR* type 1 and type 2 were found in 12.2% and 5.8% and 17.8% and 4.4%, respectively. Patients with *MPL* W515x mutation accounted for 4.7% and 6.0% in the two cohorts, respectively. The proportions of patients with triple-negative PMF, a prognostically negative

condition, were similar: 10.1% and 13.6% in pre-PMF and overt PMF, respectively. On the contrary, the high mutation risk (HMR) category (any mutations in *ASXL1*, *SRSF2*, *IDH1*, *IDH2*, or *EZH2*) was less common in pre-PMF than in overt PMF.[152]

Clinical Course

Median survival in pre-PMF has been calculated to range between 11 to 17 years, contrasting to only 7 years in overt PMF. Grade 1 reticulin fibrosis and anemia at initial diagnosis have been identified as risk factors for progression from pre-PMF to overt PMF. In the largest study of well-diagnosed pre-PMF cases, the rate of progression to overt PMF at 10 years was 12.3%.[144] Variables associated with BP evolution include age >65 years, leukocytosis (WBC >15 × 10⁹/L), an LDH ratio >1.5 times the normal institutional value, and cytogenetic abnormalities.[163] Thrombohemorrhagic complications occur in pre-PMF. Though the risk of arterial and venous thrombosis is similar to that in ET, major hemorrhages during follow-up are more common in pre-PMF.[127,128,143,164]

Differential Diagnosis

In a significant subset of patients with pre-PMF, the peripheral blood shows marked thrombocytosis, and the differential diagnosis includes other MPNs that present with increased platelet counts. These include CML, PV, ET, MDS/MPN with ring sideroblasts and thrombocytosis (MDS/MPN-T-*SF3B1* and MDS/MPN-RS-T, NOS), and a variety of nonmyeloid neoplasms and inflammatory conditions that provoke thrombocytosis through the release of inflammatory cytokines.

The lack of *BCR::ABL1* gene fusion excludes CML. In addition, in CML, the megakaryocytes can be increased; however, they are small, with hypolobated nuclei, and lack the nuclear atypia seen in pre-PMF.

In contrast to the tightly clustered, highly atypical megakaryocytes of pre-PMF found in a background of mainly neutrophils, the megakaryocytes in PV are usually more dispersed in the bone marrow, have variable sizes but lack nuclear atypia, and are found in a background of mainly erythroid precursors.

In ET, the marrow is normocellular to mildly hypocellular for age and lacks granulocytic hyperplasia that is characteristic of pre-PMF. The megakaryocytes in ET are usually enlarged with deeply lobulated ("staghorn") nuclei, but they are not tightly clustered in most cases. Clinical features of increased LDH or splenomegaly are uncommon in ET. Table 47-5 summarizes the salient clinical and morphologic differences between ET and pre-PMF.

Overt Primary Myelofibrosis

Overt primary myelofibrosis is a clonal MPN characterized by a proliferation of abnormal megakaryocytes and granulocytes in the bone marrow, with significant fibrosis and often extramedullary hematopoiesis. Approximately 10% to 15% of cases of overt PMF represent progression from pre-PMF.[144] About 50% of overt PMF cases are associated with the *JAK2* V617F mutation, 30% with mutated *CALR*, and 5% to 10% with mutated *MPL*. In the remaining 10% to 15% of cases, the driver mutation is not yet known; such cases are referred to as triple-negative PMF.[34,35,165] The diagnostic criteria of overt PMF are listed in Box 47-9.

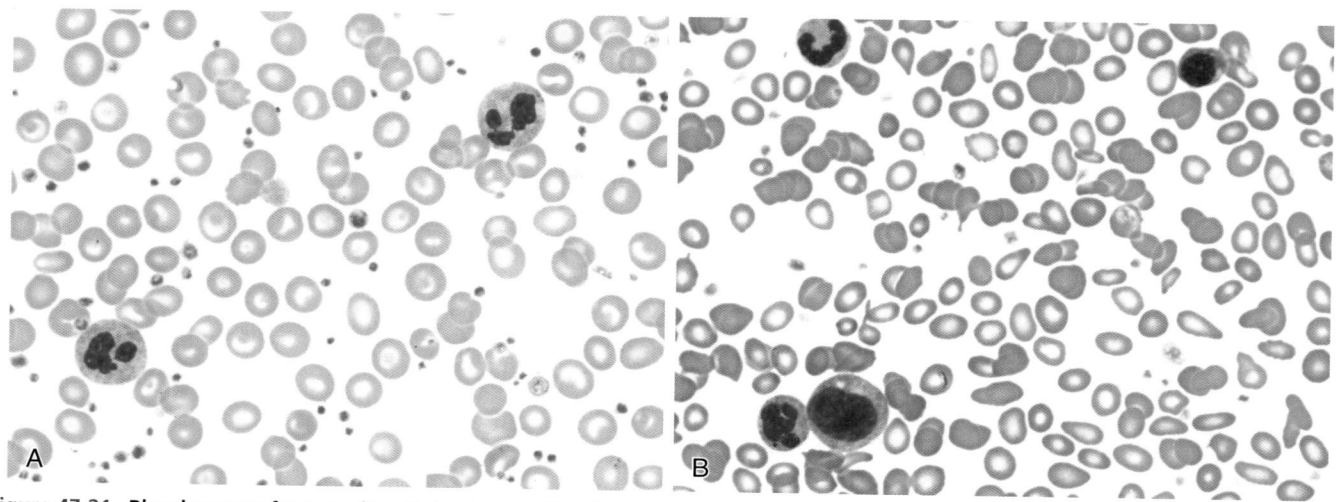

Figure 47-21. Blood smears from prefibrotic/early and fibrotic stages of primary myelofibrosis. A, This smear from the prefibrotic/early stage shows neutrophilia and thrombocytosis but minimal red cell changes (corresponding bone marrow is shown in Fig. 47-23). **B,** This smear from the fibrotic stage shows leukoerythroblastosis with marked red cell abnormalities, including many teardrop forms (corresponding bone marrow is shown in Fig. 47-24).

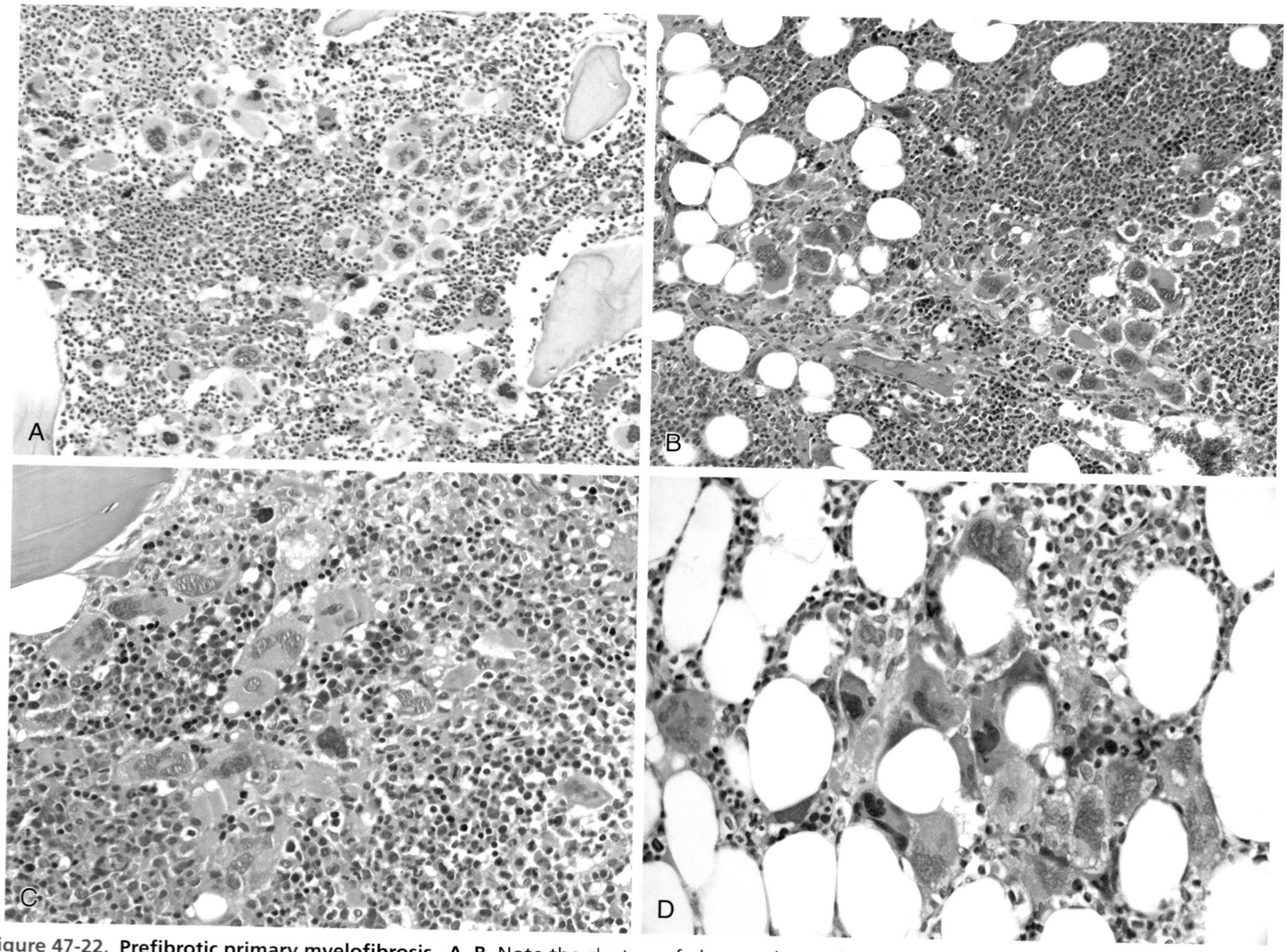

Figure 47-22. Prefibrotic primary myelofibrosis. A, B, Note the clusters of abnormal megakaryocytes in a background of neutrophils. This patient's peripheral blood is illustrated in **(A). C, D,** Dense clusters of often more than six atypical megakaryocytes are a common finding.

Box 47-9 *Diagnostic Criteria* for Primary Myelofibrosis (Overt Fibrotic Stage PMF) According to International Consensus Classification*

Major Criteria

1. Bone marrow biopsy showing megakaryocytic proliferation and atypia,[†] accompanied by reticulin and/or collagen fibrosis grades 2 or 3
2. *JAK2, CALR,* or *MPL* mutation[‡]
   or
   presence of another clonal marker[§]
   or
   absence of reactive bone marrow reticulin fibrosis[||]
3. Diagnostic criteria for *BCR::ABL1*-positive chronic myeloid leukemia, polycythemia vera, essential thrombocythemia, myelodysplastic syndromes, or other myeloid neoplasms[¶] are not met

Minor Criteria

1. Anemia not attributed to a comorbid condition
2. Leukocytosis ≥11 × 10^9/L
3. Palpable splenomegaly
4. Lactate dehydrogenase level above the reference range
5. Leukoerythroblastosis

*The diagnosis of PMF requires all three major criteria and at least one minor criterion confirmed in two consecutive determinations.
[†]Morphology of megakaryocytes in PMF demonstrates a high degree of megakaryocytic atypia including small to giant megakaryocytes with a prevalence of severe maturation defects (cloud-like, hypolobulated, and hyperchromatic nuclei) and presence of abnormal large dense clusters (mostly >6 megakaryocytes lying strictly adjacent).
[‡]Highly sensitive assays for *JAK2* V617F (sensitivity level <1%) and *CALR* and *MPL* (sensitivity level 1% to 3%) are recommended; in negative cases, search for noncanonical *JAK2* and *MPL* mutations should be considered.
[§]Assessed by cytogenetics or sensitive next-generation sequencing techniques; detection of mutations associated with myeloid neoplasms (e.g., *ASXL1, EZH2, IDH1, IDH2, SF3B1, SRSF2,* and *TET2* mutations) supports the clonal nature of the disease.
[||]Reticulin fibrosis secondary to infection, autoimmune disorder or other chronic inflammatory conditions, hairy cell leukemia or another lymphoid neoplasm, metastatic malignancy, or toxic (chronic) myelopathies.
[¶]Monocytosis can be present at diagnosis or develop during the course of PMF; in these cases, a history of myeloproliferative neoplasm (MPN) excludes chronic myelomonocytic leukemia (CMML). Furthermore, a higher variant allelic frequency for MPN-associated driver mutations supports the diagnosis of PMF with monocytosis rather than CMML. In contrast, multihit *TET2* mutations, often in combination with mutated *ASXL1* and *SRSF2,* are very common in CMML.
Data from Arber DA, Orazi A, Hasserjian RP, et al. International Consensus Classification of myeloid neoplasms and acute leukemias: integrating morphologic, clinical, and genomic data. *Blood.* 2022;140(11):1200-1228.

Although granulocytes and megakaryocytes are the major proliferative cells, all myeloid lineages, B lymphocytes, and some T lymphocytes are derived from the neoplastic clone.[166] In contrast, the fibroblasts are not clonal. Rather, the myelofibrosis and osteosclerosis are secondary changes caused by the abnormal release of growth factors and fibrogenic cytokines, including, among others, platelet-derived growth factor and transforming growth factor β, which are synthesized, packaged, and released from abnormal megakaryocytes and platelets.[149,167,168] There is also prominent angiogenesis in the bone marrow and spleen as a result of increased serum levels of vascular endothelial growth factor. Other cytokines that are increased in overt PMF include macrophage inflammatory protein 1β, tissue inhibitor of metalloproteinase, insulin-like growth binding factor 2, and tumor necrosis factor alpha. Therefore, the morphologic and some of the clinical features are related not only to the hematologic effects of the neoplastic cells in the marrow but also to the release of multiple inflammatory cytokines.[168-170]

Synonyms and Related Terms

Chronic idiopathic myelofibrosis; myelofibrosis/sclerosis with myeloid metaplasia; agnogenic myeloid metaplasia; megakaryocytic myelosclerosis; idiopathic myelofibrosis; myelofibrosis with myeloid metaplasia; osteomyelofibrosis; osteomyelosclerosis

Epidemiology

Incidence of overt PMF accounts for 0.5 to 1.5 cases per 100,000 population per year. Both sexes are equally affected. The median age at diagnosis is in the 7th decade; less than 10% are younger than 40 years. Although PMF has been reported in children, it is exceedingly rare, and every effort should be made to exclude other diseases that might mimic PMF in a child.[171,172]

Clinical Features

Clinical manifestations in overt PMF include severe anemia, marked hepatosplenomegaly, constitutional symptoms (e.g., fatigue, night sweats, fever), cachexia, bone pain, splenic infarct, pruritus, thrombosis, and bleeding.[169] Ineffective erythropoiesis and hepatosplenic EMH are the main causes of anemia and organomegaly, respectively. Splenomegaly, caused by EMH, can be massive and may lead to early satiety, abdominal discomfort, or acute abdominal pain caused by splenic infarct.[169] Aberrant cytokine production by clonal cells and host immune reaction are thought to contribute to PMF-associated bone marrow stromal changes, ineffective erythropoiesis, EMH, cachexia, and constitutional symptoms. Causes of death in overt PMF include leukemic progression that occurs in approximately 20% of patients and comorbid conditions, including cardiovascular events and consequences of cytopenias such as infection or bleeding.[173]

Morphology

Peripheral Blood

Leukoerythroblastosis with numerous teardrop-shaped RBCs is common (Fig. 47-21B). Although mild leukocytosis is common in the fibrotic stage, severe leukopenia may occur, as bone marrow failure becomes more prominent as a result of increasing fibrosis. Circulating megakaryocytic nuclei and fragments are frequently observed at this time. Blasts can be seen on the peripheral blood smear during the fibrotic stage and occasionally account for 5% or more of the WBCs. However, when this is the case, the patient should be carefully monitored for further evidence of progression to AP or BP. Absolute monocyte counts above 1 × 10^9/L have also been reported to indicate disease acceleration. Blast percentages of 10% to 19% in the peripheral blood indicate there is progression to AP, and 20% or more blasts is sufficient for the diagnosis of blast transformation.[169,174]

Bone Marrow

A bone marrow biopsy is essential for the diagnosis of overt PMF. An adequate, well-processed biopsy allows assessment of cellularity, the relative number of cells in the various myeloid lineages and their degree of maturation, megakaryocyte morphology, and the amount and grade of fibrosis—all of which are critical for establishing the diagnosis and following disease progression. The stain for reticulin fibers should be performed with a standard, uniform protocol to avoid technical variation, and the reticulin fiber content should be evaluated with a reproducible, semiquantitative grading system (Table 47-3; Fig. 47-18).[175] An immunohistochemical stain for CD34 is helpful to highlight blasts, particularly in cases with a dry tap. If a bone marrow aspirate is obtained, it may provide helpful information about maturation of the neoplastic cells.

In most cases, the bone marrow is hypercellular for age and shows an increased number of neutrophils and atypical megakaryocytes. Erythropoiesis is usually reduced. The megakaryocytes are markedly abnormal in both their topography and cytology and are the key that distinguishes PMF from the other MPNs. Megakaryocytes in PMF are morphologically more atypical than in any other MPN. The megakaryocytes are often present in dense clusters defined as ≥3 megakaryocytes present back-to-back without any cells in between; however, the majority of patients show large clusters with more than six atypical megakaryocytes. The megakaryocytes vary from small to large with an abnormal nuclear-to-cytoplasmic ratio and disorganized, plump, cloud-like, or balloon-like nuclear lobulation. The nuclei are often hyperchromatic, but numerous bare megakaryocytic nuclei

may be seen as well. There is an increase in reticulin fibers, at least grade 2, and a trichrome stain typically shows deposition of collagen (MF-2 or MF-3) (Fig. 47-23).

With disease progression, the marrow cellularity decreases, and at times, the marrow can appear nearly depleted of normal hematopoiesis. Reticulin or even overt collagen fibrosis of the marrow becomes more obvious. Islands of hematopoiesis are separated by regions of loose connective tissue or by fat or dense fibrosis. Dilation of marrow sinuses is usually prominent, and the sinuses may contain megakaryocytes and other immature hematopoietic cells, a feature which is particularly prominent in patients in the advanced stage. New bone formation and osteosclerosis are usually present at this time.[174]

The finding of 10% to 19% blasts in the blood or bone marrow is indicative of PMF in an accelerated disease stage, whereas 20% or more blasts is evidence of transformation to BP.[174]

Extramedullary Tissues

Many of the morphologic abnormalities noted in the peripheral blood in the fibrotic stage, such as teardrop-shaped RBCs and leukoerythroblastosis, are caused by the abnormal release of cells from sites of EMH, particularly the spleen

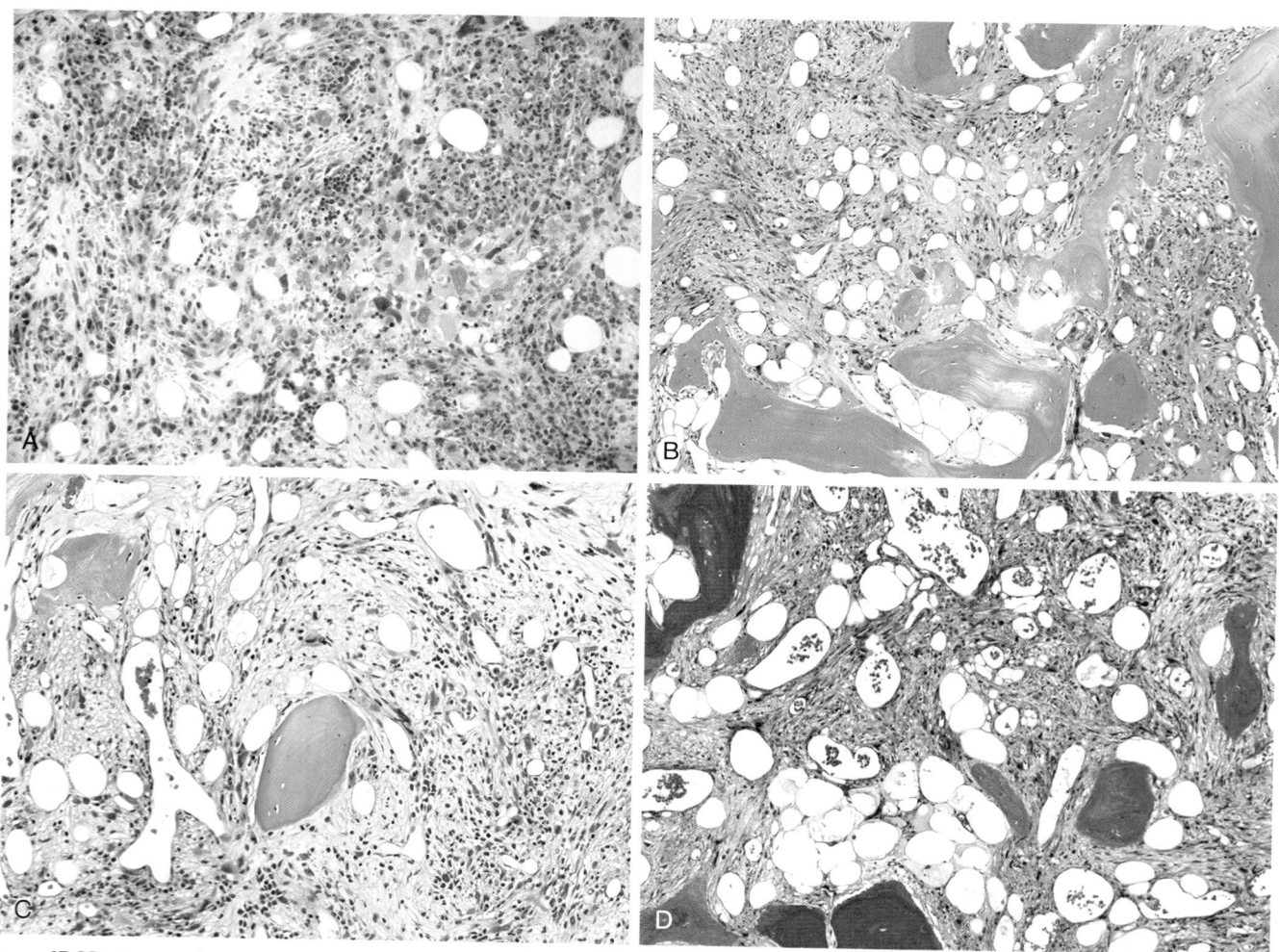

Figure 47-23. Overt primary myelofibrosis. A, Bone marrow shows numerous dense clusters of atypical megakaryocytes (MF-2). This patient's peripheral blood is illustrated in Figure 47-22B. **B,** In more advanced disease stages (MF-3), osteosclerosis can be seen. **C,** Overall cellularity can be significantly reduced in overt fibrotic cases because of the gross accumulation of collagen fibers, as illustrated in **(D)** (Masson's trichrome stain).

and liver, although almost any organ, including the kidney, breast, adrenal gland, lymph node, dura mater, and other soft tissues, can be involved (Fig. 47-24). The EMH seen in various tissues in overt PMF is composed of neoplastic cells, likely derived from hematopoietic stem cells, and precursor cells from the bone marrow.[176] The structure of the marrow sinuses is distorted and compromised by surrounding reticulin fibrosis, which allows immature, proliferative bone marrow cells to gain access to the marrow sinuses and hence to the circulation. CD34-positive cells are markedly increased in the blood of patients with PMF compared with those of patients with other MPNs and normal controls, and an increase in CD34-positive cells can also be demonstrated in the spleen.[177] Morphologically, the EMH in the spleen can be present as nodules or as diffuse involvement of the red pulp. A diffuse granulocytic predominance seems to portend a worse prognosis.[178] In some cases, the spleen may be the site of extramedullary leukemic transformation.

Genetics

No specific genetic marker has been identified for overt PMF. Approximately 50% to 60% of patients have *JAK2* V617F, 25% to 30% have mutated *CALR,* and 5% to 10% carry mutations of *MPL*; these genetic abnormalities are mutually exclusive.[169,179,180] The remaining cases carry none of the currently known MPN driver mutations and are referred to as triple negative. The driver mutations result in constitutive activation of Janus kinase–signal transducers and activators of transcription (JAK-STAT) target genes.[174] *CALR* mutations occur more often in younger patients with a higher platelet count and, in the case of type 1 *CALR* mutations, a more favorable prognosis, whereas the patients with triple-negative PMF have inferior survival.[181,182] Mutations other than *JAK2/ CALR/MPL* that include *ASXL1, SRSF2, IDH1/IDH2, EZH2, SF3B1,* and *TET2,* among others, are also seen in patients with PMF and have been reported in up to 80% of PMF patients in one study.[180] Identification of these mutations is useful in establishing clonality in triple-negative PMF cases. These additional mutations likely affect various phenotypic features of PMF, including prognosis. In addition, some studies have

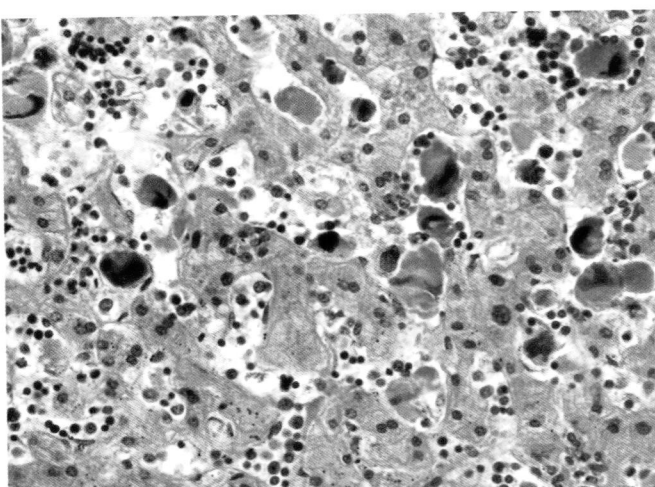

Figure 47-24. Extramedullary hematopoiesis in the liver of a patient with primary myelofibrosis. Note that the sinuses are filled with hematopoietic cells, and megakaryocytes are particularly prominent.

demonstrated the presence of somatic noncanonical variants or germline *MPL* or *JAK2* variants in some patients with triple-negative PMF.[183,184]

Karyotypic abnormalities are present in 40% to 50% of patients with overt PMF. The most frequent abnormalities include del(20q), del(13q), +8, +9, and abnormalities of 1q. Complex karyotypes are found in about 15% of cases.[185] More than 90% of patients who experience a leukemic transformation have cytogenetic abnormalities that are often complex and involve abnormalities of chromosomes 5 and 7.

Knowledge of cytogenetics and somatic mutations not only facilitates a diagnosis of MPN but is also used as a prognostic factor.

Clinical Course

The clinical course of overt PMF includes progressive anemia, often requiring RBC transfusions, marked hepatosplenomegaly, profound constitutional symptoms, and cachexia. The natural evolution of PMF is gradual progression to a markedly fibrotic, often osteosclerotic, bone marrow with cellular depletion, dilated marrow sinuses with intrasinusoidal hematopoiesis composed mainly of abnormal megakaryocytes, osteosclerosis, and eventually, bone marrow failure. The increase in spleen size from EMH contributes to the worsening cytopenias because of splenic sequestration and also leads to portal hypertension and abdominal pain. Myeloid blast transformation occurs in about 5% to 20% of cases at a median of 3 years after the diagnosis of the fibrotic stage of PMF.[169]

The median survival is about 7 years for overt PMF. The survival of patients with PMF depends on the stage in which the diagnosis is made and the number of parameters that are present that have been determined to adversely affect prognosis. Prognostic assessment tools for PMF have evolved over the years. The International Prognostic Scoring System (IPSS) developed in 2009 included clinical and laboratory variables at diagnosis. The Dynamic International Prognostic Scoring System (DIPSS) uses the same clinical and laboratory variables obtained at any time point of disease course. The more recent models incorporate cytogenetic and molecular genetic findings for risk stratification and are used to inform decisions to select patients with PMF for allogeneic transplant.[160,186-188] The genetically inspired prognostic scoring system (GIPSS) is based exclusively on mutations and karyotype, and MIPSS70+ version 2.0 (mutation-enhanced and karyotype-enhanced international prognostic scoring system) uses both genetic and clinical risk factors.[189] Mutations comprising the high mutation risk category for prognosis or leukemia-free survival include those of *ASXL1, SRSF2, IDH1, IDH2,* and *EZH2.* Both the type of mutation and number of mutations have been shown to affect prognosis.[180,190]

Similar to somatic mutations, cytogenetic abnormalities are used for prognostic assessment. The revised cytogenetic risk categories include a three-tiered risk model: "very high risk (VHR)"—single/multiple abnormalities of −7, i(17q), inv(3)/3q21, 12p−/12p11.2, 11q−/11q23, or other autosomal trisomies not including +8 or +9 (e.g., +21, +19); "favorable"—normal karyotype or sole abnormalities of 13q−, +9, 20q−, chromosome 1 translocation/duplication, or sex chromosome abnormality including −Y; "unfavorable"—all other abnormalities.[191] The 5-year survival rates independent of clinically derived prognostic systems, driver and "additional" mutations, range from 8% for VHR to 45% for "favorable" karyotype.

Differential Diagnosis

The differential diagnosis of overt PMF includes post-PV and post-ET myelofibrosis. Whether this distinction can be made with confidence is controversial; some authors have noted that the megakaryocytes in the fibrotic stages of PV, PMF, and ET retain similar morphology as in the proliferative stages of these diseases, but others have not been able to make such a distinction.[192,193] The differentiation of other myeloid neoplasms, metastatic tumors, and even inflammatory diseases associated with thrombocytosis can be challenging.

Other myeloid neoplasms to consider in the differential diagnosis of overt PMF include acute panmyelosis with myelofibrosis (APMF) and myelodysplastic syndrome with fibrosis (MDS-F). Table 47-6 shows a comparison of salient features in PMF, MDS-F, and APMF.

APMF is a subtype of AML with myelofibrosis generally associated with multilineage dysplasia, small dysplastic megakaryocytes, and 20% or more blasts in the blood or bone marrow.[194] The blasts typically express CD34.[194] Patients with APMF usually present with acute onset of severe constitutional symptoms, pancytopenia, no splenomegaly, and increased circulating blasts. Although genetic data is available in only a small number of patients with APMF, no *JAK2* V617F, *MPL*, or *CALR* mutations have been detected.[195]

MDS-F, though not a distinct entity in the ICC, is recognized as a distinct subtype in the proposed WHO 5th edition.[2] It is characterized by peripheral cytopenia, hypercellular marrow with increased dysplastic megakaryocytes and often increased blasts, and significant marrow fibrosis (MF-2 or MF-3). Though megakaryocytic hyperplasia and fibrosis are similar to overt PMF, in MDS-F, the megakaryocytes are small with hypolobated nuclei and often include micromegakaryocytes (Fig. 47-25). Tight clusters of megakaryocytes are uncommon, and nuclear atypia seen in PMF is typically absent.[196-198] The marrow often shows increased blasts. Driver mutations in *JAK2, CALR,* and *MPL* are infrequent but have been identified in 5% to 10% of cases.[199,200] Leukoerythroblastosis and elevated LDH may be seen similar to overt PMF; however, splenomegaly is distinctly uncommon in MDS-F.[196-198,201]

Autoimmune myelofibrosis (AIMF) also needs to be distinguished from PMF. AIMF is a clinicopathological entity that can present as a primary disease known as primary AIMF or secondary to an established systemic autoimmune disorder. The marrow fibrosis of AIMF is usually responsive to steroids or other immunosuppressive therapy and has a generally favorable outcome. AIMF has been reported in association with systemic lupus erythematosus, Sjögren syndrome, Hashimoto thyroiditis, autoimmune hepatitis, and Evans syndrome (secondary AIMF); however, it can also be seen with autoantibodies, only without a defined disorder (primary AIMF).[202] Patients with AIMF commonly present with cytopenia, prompting a bone marrow biopsy for evaluation. The peripheral blood smear typically lacks leukoerythroblastosis or teardrop red cells. The bone marrow is often hypercellular, usually from erythroid hyperplasia. Megakaryocytes may be increased in number and pleomorphic; however, they lack tight clustering and nuclear atypia as seen in PMF (Fig. 47-26). Marrow fibrosis is usually mild (MF-1); however, some cases may show significant fibrosis (≥MF-2), raising the differential diagnosis of overt PMF. Lymphoid aggregates are common and predominantly composed of T cells. Variable plasmacytosis can be observed. AIMF lacks driver mutations (*JAK2, CALR, MPL*) and other clonal markers. Splenomegaly is uncommon in AIMF and, when present, is usually minimal and asymptomatic, although neutropenia and splenomegaly can occur in patients with rheumatoid arthritis (Felty's syndrome). The important clinical and morphologic differences between AIMF and PMF are included in Table 47-7.

POLYCYTHEMIA VERA

Normally, erythropoiesis is fine-tuned to produce just the number of RBCs needed to carry oxygen to the tissues. Tissue hypoxia leads to an increase in production of EPO, the primary regulator of erythropoiesis. When EPO binds to EPOR on erythroid progenitors, there is dimerization of EPOR and phosphorylation of the associated JAK2 kinase, which in turn activates downstream effectors, including the JAK/STAT pathway, and culminates in the proliferation and reduced apoptosis of erythroid precursors.[203,204] Downregulation of EPOR and JAK2 signaling is mediated by protein tyrosine phosphatases such as SHP-1, by suppressors of cytokine signaling, and by other inhibitors of the activated pathways.[205] The synthesis of EPO occurs in peritubular cells in the kidney and is regulated by a family of transcription factors that are produced in response to hypoxia, the hypoxia-inducible factors (HIFs). HIFs undergo degradation through an interaction of HIF, oxygen, prolyl hydroxylase domain (PHD)-containing enzymes, and the von Hippel–Lindau tumor suppressor protein (VHL) as normal oxygen concentrations

Table 47-6 Comparison of Salient Features in Overt Primary Myelofibrosis (PMF), Myelodysplastic Syndrome With Fibrosis (MDS-F) and Acute Panmyelosis With Myelofibrosis (APMF)

Feature	PMF	MDS-F	APMF
Splenomegaly	Usually present	Usually absent	Absent
White blood cell count	Increased, normal, or decreased	Decreased, rarely normal	Decreased
Bone marrow blasts	<20%	<20%	≥20%
Megakaryocyte morphology	Variable size, small to large; dense clusters, atypical morphology; bizarre; altered nuclear-to-cytoplasmic ratio	Small with hypolobated or separated nuclei or micromegakaryocytes; dispersed or in clusters	Mainly small and dysplastic, but few large abnormal forms also seen
Dysgranulopoiesis	Minimal, but may be present as disease transforms	Usually prominent	Usually prominent
Dyserythropoiesis	Minimal	Often prominent	Usually prominent

APMF, Acute panmyelosis with myelofibrosis; *MDS-F,* myelodysplastic syndrome with fibrosis; *PMF,* primary myelofibrosis.

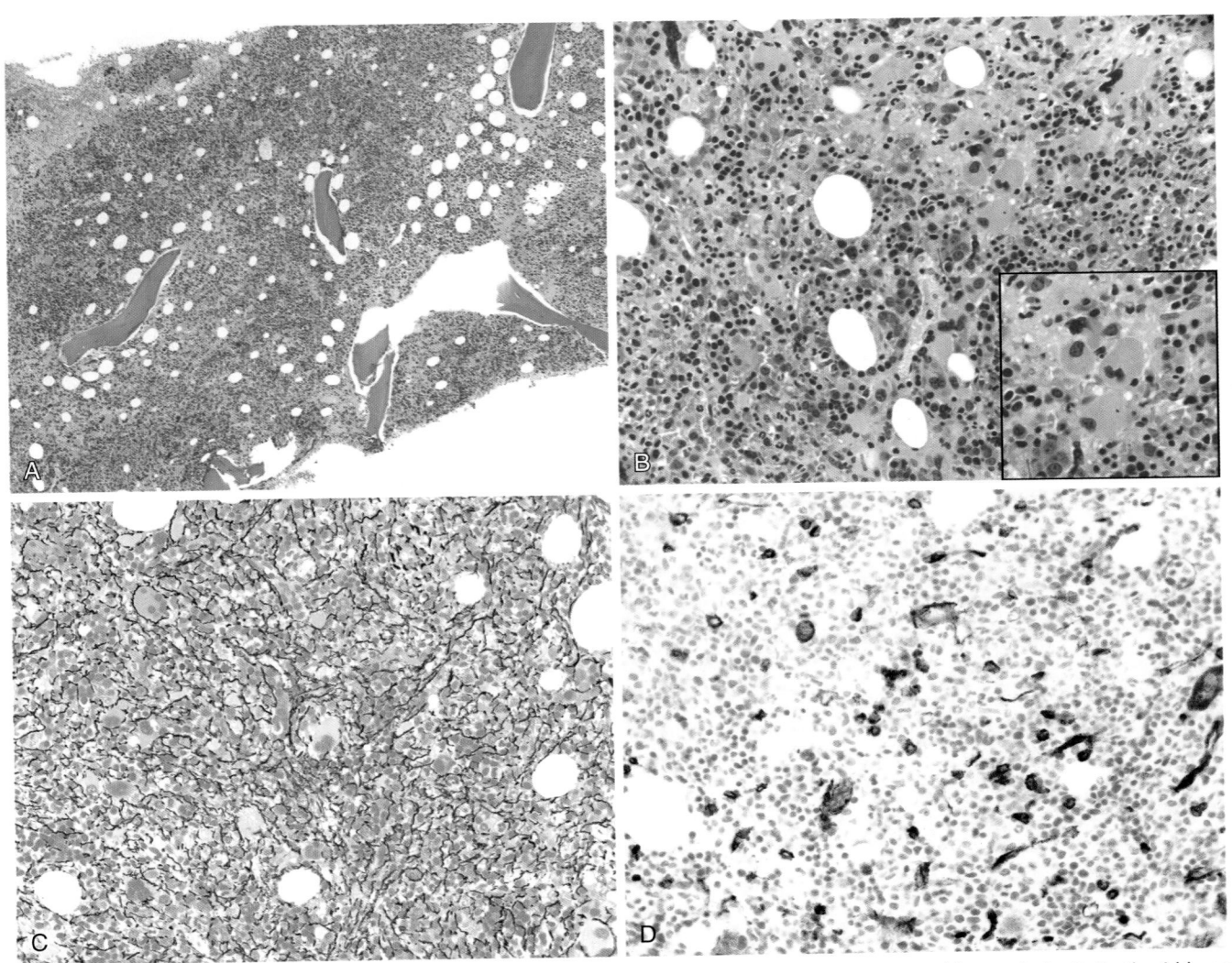

Figure 47-25. Myelodysplastic syndrome with fibrosis (MDS-F). A, Hypercellular marrow with erythroid hyperplasia. **B,** Erythroid hyperplasia and increased megakaryocytes; megakaryocytes are small and dysplastic with hypolobated nuclei *(inset)*. **C,** Reticulin stain demonstrating moderate increase in reticulin fibers, MF2. **D,** CD34 immunohistochemistry demonstrating mildly increased blasts, ~7%.

are reached. Under conditions of hypoxia, HIF degradation is slowed, and EPO synthesis is increased. Any disturbance in the synthesis of EPO or in the JAK/STAT pathway will result in too many or too few RBCs.[204]

Polycythemia is an increase in the number of RBCs per unit volume of blood, usually defined as a greater than two standard deviations increase from the age-adjusted, sex-adjusted, race-adjusted, and altitude-adjusted normal value for hemoglobin (Hb), hematocrit, or RBC mass.[206] There are multiple causes of polycythemia. Polycythemia is usually a "true" increase in the RBC mass, but occasionally, diminished plasma volume leads to hemoconcentration and to "relative polycythemia." True polycythemia may be "primary," in which an intrinsic abnormality of erythroid progenitors renders them hypersensitive to or independent of factors that normally regulate their proliferation. More commonly, however, polycythemia is "secondary," in which case the polycythemia is caused by increased EPO that is caused by an appropriate physiologic response to tissue hypoxia or, occasionally, to inappropriate secretion of EPO by various neoplasms. Primary

and secondary polycythemia may be acquired or congenital (Box 47-10).[204,206]

Definition

PV is an MPN predominantly characterized by increased RBC production independent of the mechanisms that normally regulate erythropoiesis. Almost all patients with PV have an acquired somatic gain of function mutation of the Janus 2 kinase gene, *JAK2* V617F, or less commonly, a functionally similar *JAK2* exon 12 mutation.[29-32] The diagnostic criteria of PV are listed in Box 47-11.

JAK2 mutations in PV encode a constitutively activated JAK2 kinase that binds to and activates non-TK cytokine receptors such as EPOR.[33,37] The *JAK2* mutation originates in a hematopoietic stem cell.[38] Because the JAK2 kinase binds not only with EPOR but with other non-TK receptors, including G-CSFR and MPL, granulocytes and megakaryocytes also carry the mutation and proliferate autonomously, resulting in "panmyelosis" in the blood and marrow.[39]

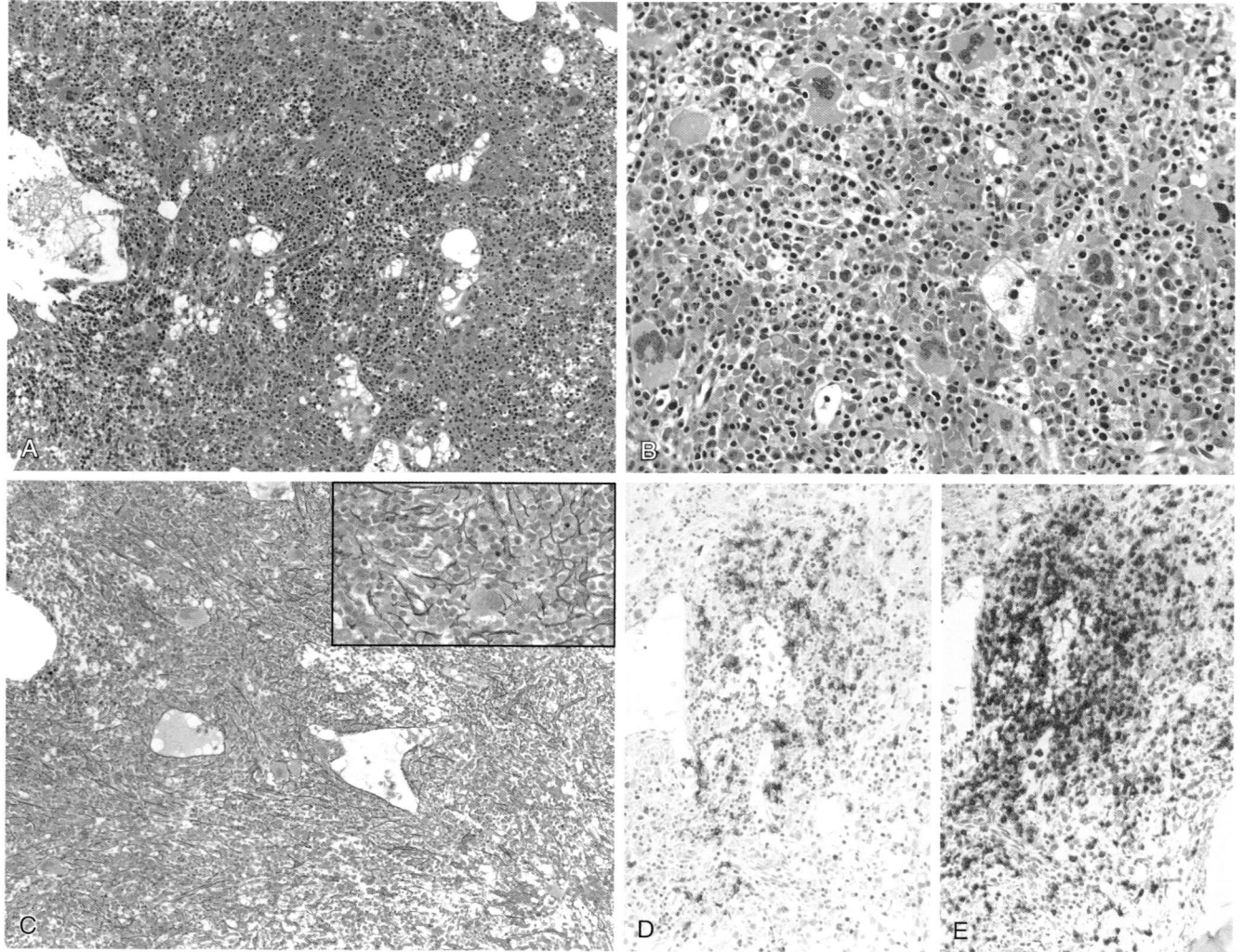

Figure 47-26. Autoimmune myelofibrosis. A, Hypercellular marrow with a few dilated sinusoids. **B,** Erythroid hyperplasia with increased megakaryocytes that are scattered in distribution and normal in morphology. **C,** Diffuse mild increase in reticulin fibers, MF-1. **D,** Lymphoid aggregate with few CD20-positive B cells. **E,** Lymphoid aggregate predominantly composed of CD3-positive T cells.

Synonyms and Related Terms

Polycythemia rubra vera, primary polycythemia

Epidemiology

PV is a rare disease, with an annual incidence of 1 to 3 per 100,000 individuals in the Western world; it is less common in Asia.[207,208] There is a slight male predominance. Most often, PV is encountered in patients in their 60s, and patients younger than 20 years are rarely described.[171]

Clinical Features

The principal symptoms are vascular disturbances caused by the increased RBC mass, including hypertension, thrombosis, and bleeding, which are also the leading causes of morbidity and mortality. Headache, dizziness, paresthesia, scotomas, and erythromelalgia are generally caused by thrombotic events in the microvasculature, but thrombosis involving major arteries or veins also occurs and can pose life-threatening events.[141]

In particular, in case of splanchnic vein thrombosis and Budd-Chiari syndrome, a differential diagnosis of PV should always be considered. Fatigue, aquagenic pruritus, gout, and gastrointestinal complaints are additional symptoms. The most prominent physical findings include plethora in up to 80% of cases, palpable splenomegaly in 70%, and hepatomegaly in 40% to 50%.[209,210]

Morphology

The diagnosis of PV requires integration of clinical and laboratory data with histologic findings in adequate, well-prepared peripheral blood smear and bone marrow biopsy specimens.

Peripheral Blood

The major hematologic finding in the blood is the increase in hemoglobin, hematocrit, and red blood cells.[211] Diagnostic thresholds have not been changed by the ICC, and PV is defined by an acquired increase in hemoglobin/hematocrit level above

Table 47-7 Comparison of Salient Features Between Primary Myelofibrosis and Autoimmune Myelofibrosis

	Primary Myelofibrosis	Autoimmune Myelofibrosis
Clinical Findings		
Splenomegaly	Common	Absent/mild
Laboratory Findings		
CBC	Anemia, leukocytosis, or thrombocytosis; leukoerythroblastosis	Peripheral cytopenias
LDH levels	Often increased	Normal or increased
Autoantibodies	Uncommon	Present
Morphologic Findings		
Marrow cellularity	Hypercellular	Hypercellular
Megakaryocytes	Increased with dense clusters; atypia with nuclear maturation abnormalities	May be increased; no dense clusters; may show pleomorphism but lack atypia
Granulocytic-to-erythroid ratio	Increased	Usually decreased because of erythroid hyperplasia
Lymphocytic infiltration	May be present	Usually present
Fibrosis	≥MF-2 in overt PMF	Often mild, rare cases with reticulin ≥MF-2
Molecular/Genetic Findings		
Driver mutations in *JAK2*, *CALR*, or *MPL*	Present in 90% of cases	Absent
Nondriver mutations associated with myeloid neoplasms or other clonal markers	Often present	Absent

CBC, Complete blood count; *LDH,* lactate dehydrogenase.

16.5 g/dL or 49% in men and 16 g/dL or 48% in women, in the context of a *JAK2* mutation and characteristic bone marrow morphology.[1] The RBC indices are usually normal unless there is concomitant iron deficiency, in which case the mean corpuscular volume and mean corpuscular hemoglobin concentration may be low. Although not commonly measured in clinical practice, the red cell mass is >25% above the mean normal predicted value.[211] Neutrophilia and, rarely, basophilia may be present. Leukoerythroblastosis is not typically seen.

Bone Marrow

The bone marrow biopsy specimens show hypercellularity for age caused by erythroid, granulocytic, and megakaryocytic proliferation (panmyelosis; Fig. 47-27). Erythropoiesis is prominent, often occurs in expanded erythroid islands, and demonstrates normoblastic maturation. Granulopoiesis may show a shift toward immaturity, but there is no increase in the percentage of blasts and no significant dysplasia. Megakaryocytes are increased in number and characteristically show increased pleomorphism with wide variation in their size. Although the megakaryocyte nucleus may be enlarged and/or irregularly folded, they do not demonstrate significant atypia such as presence of bizarre shapes or nuclear maturation

---

Box 47-10 *Causes of Polycythemia*

"True" Primary Polycythemia
- Congenital: primary familial congenital erythrocytosis, including EPOR mutations
- Acquired: polycythemia vera

"True" Secondary Polycythemia
- Congenital
- VHL mutations, including Chuvash polycythemia
- 2,3-Bisphosphoglycerate mutase deficiency
- High-oxygen-affinity hemoglobin
- Congenital methemoglobinemia
- Hypoxia-inducible factor 2α mutations
- Prolyl hydroxylase domain 2 mutations
- Acquired
- Physiologically appropriate response to hypoxia: cardiac, pulmonary, renal, and hepatic diseases; carbon monoxide poisoning; sleep apnea; renal artery stenosis; smoker's polycythemia; after renal transplantation*
- Inappropriate production of erythropoietin: cerebellar hemangioblastoma, uterine leiomyoma, pheochromocytoma, renal cell carcinoma, hepatocellular carcinoma, meningioma, parathyroid adenoma

Relative, "Spurious," or "False" Polycythemia
- Acute, transient hemoconcentration caused by dehydration or other causes of contraction of plasma volume; red cell mass is not increased, so it is not true polycythemia

*The cause of post-renal transplantation polycythemia is not clear; in some cases, it is likely from retained, chronically ischemic native kidney with endogenous erythropoietin production plus increased sensitivity of the erythroid precursors to erythropoietin.

Box 47-11 *Diagnostic Criteria* for Polycythemia Vera (PV) According to International Consensus Classification*

Major Criteria
1. Elevated hemoglobin concentration or elevated hematocrit or increased red blood cell mass[†]
2. Bone marrow biopsy showing age-adjusted hypercellularity with trilineage proliferation (panmyelosis), including prominent erythroid, granulocytic, and increase in pleomorphic, mature megakaryocytes without atypia[‡]
3. Presence of *JAK2* V617F or *JAK2* exon 12 mutation[§]

Minor Criterion
1. Subnormal serum erythropoietin level

*The diagnosis of PV requires either all three major criteria or the first two major criteria plus the minor criterion.
[†]Diagnostic thresholds: hemoglobin: >16.5 g/dL in men and >16.0 g/dL in women; hematocrit: >49% in men and >48% in women; red blood cell mass: >25% above mean normal predicted value.
[‡]A bone marrow biopsy may not be required in patients with sustained absolute erythrocytosis (hemoglobin concentrations of >18.5 g/dL in men or >16.5 g/dL in women and hematocrit values of >55.5% in men or >49.5% in women) and the presence of a *JAK2* V617F or *JAK2* exon 12 mutation
[§]It is recommended to use highly sensitive assays for *JAK2* V617F (sensitivity level <1%); in negative cases, consider searching for noncanonical or atypical *JAK2* mutations in exons 12 to 15.
Data from Arber DA, Orazi A, Hasserjian RP, et al. International Consensus Classification of myeloid neoplasms and acute leukemias: integrating morphologic, clinical, and genomic data. *Blood.* 2022;140(11):1200-1228.

abnormalities. They sometimes form loose clusters close to the bone trabeculae, but large dense clusters, which characterize PMF, are not seen in PV.[78,211] About 20% of patients exhibit a minimal increase in reticulin fibers (MF-1) at presentation, a finding associated with more rapid evolution to post-PV myelofibrosis.[212] A minority of cases show occasional reactive

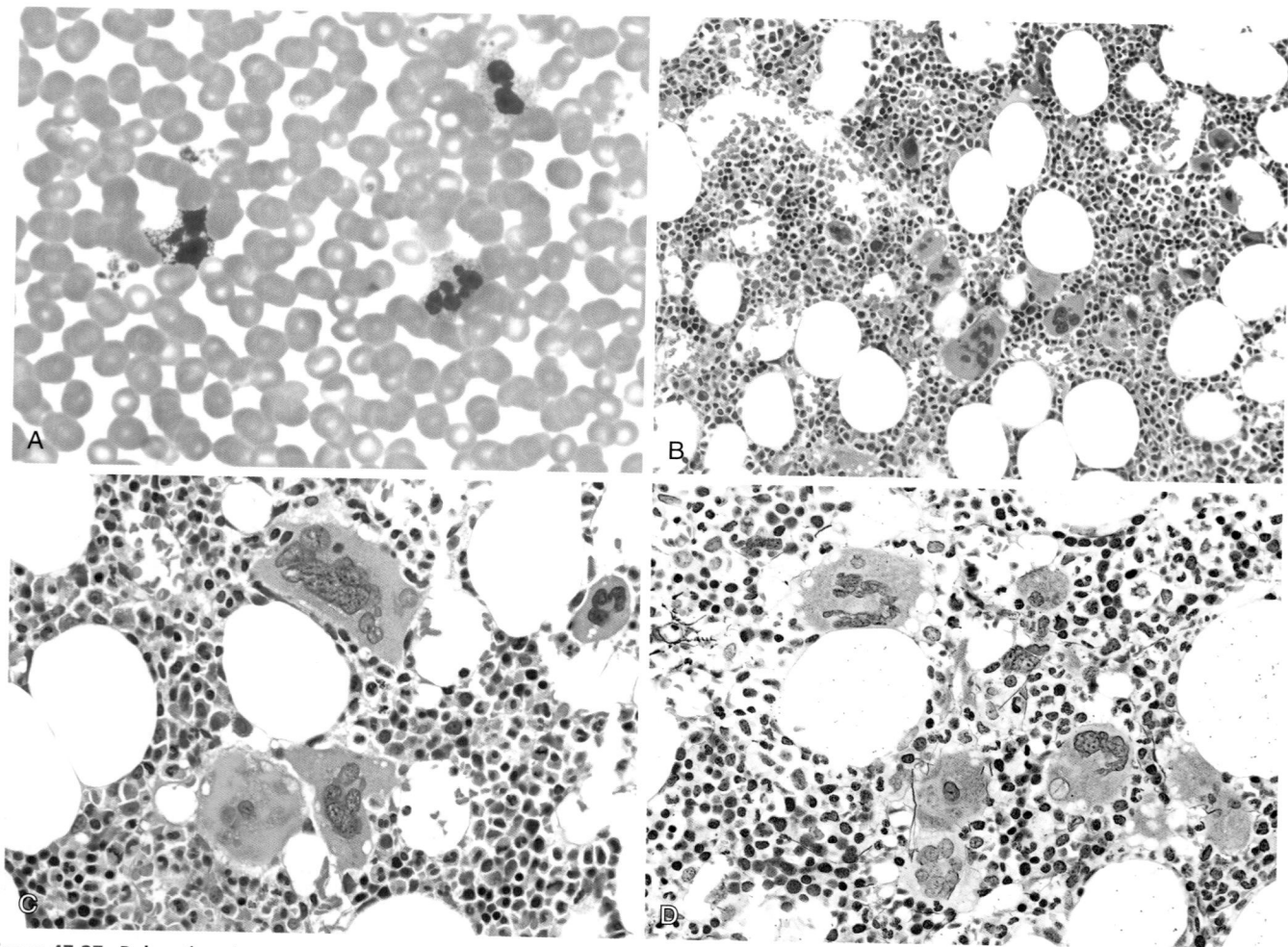

Figure 47-27. Polycythemia vera. A, Peripheral blood is characterized by mild neutrophilia and occasional basophils. **B,** Bone marrow biopsy reveals hypercellularity and panmyelosis. **C,** The megakaryocytes are variable in size and reveal hypersegmented nuclei, but overall, they are not atypical or bizarre. **D,** In the majority of cases diagnosed with PV, there is no significant increase in reticulin fibers.

lymphoid follicles.[213] Marrow aspirate smears generally reflect these changes, but the diagnostic morphologic features are not as readily appreciated on smears as in biopsy sections. Stainable iron is absent in aspirate smears in most cases. Patients with PV and *JAK2* exon 12 mutations show clinical findings similar to those with *JAK2* V617F, although the bone marrow often shows primarily erythroid proliferation with less granulocytic and megakaryocytic expansion than that in patients with *JAK2* V617F.[41]

Extramedullary Tissues

During the polycythemic phase, the splenomegaly is caused by engorgement of the cords and sinuses with RBCs, with minimal, if any, EMH. Similar changes may be seen in the hepatic sinuses.[214]

Genetics

More than 95% of patients with PV have the *JAK2* V617F mutation, and a *JAK2* exon 12 mutation is found in most of the remaining cases. Considering the central role of *JAK2* mutations in PV, it is important to recognize the need for diagnostic assays with <1% sensitivity.[215] Also, the possibility of other noncanonical *JAK2* mutations should be considered

in *JAK2* V617F-negative cases with high suspicion of PV. The *JAK2* V617F mutation is not unique to PV; it is present in 50% to 60% of cases of ET and PMF, occasionally in MDS/MPNs, and in rare cases of AML. It is not clear what determines the disease phenotype in an individual patient, but the genetic background of the host and the dosage of the mutant allele may be important factors. Homozygosity for *JAK2* V617F, which results from mitotic recombination, is more common in PV than in other MPNs that carry the mutation. NGS analysis has revealed the presence of non-*JAK2* concomitant mutations in more than half of patients with PV, with the most frequent being *TET2, ASXL1,* and *SH2B3*.[142] In that particular study, *ASXL1, SRSF2, IDH2,* and *EZH2* mutations were associated with inferior survival.

Approximately 10% to 20% of patients with PV have karyotypic abnormalities at diagnosis, the most common of which are +8, +9, del(20q), and loss of Y.[216] An abnormal karyotype has been associated with inferior OS.[142]

Clinical Course

Thrombohemorrhagic complications represent the most common causes for morbidity and mortality in PV. Phlebotomy combined with aspirin is the most common form of therapy; but if the patient has an increased risk for thrombosis, cytoreductive therapy may also be used.[141] OS in PV exceeds 13 years[141,217-219] and maybe as high as 37 years in younger patients (aged <40 years).[220] Risk factors for survival in PV include advanced age, leukocytosis, abnormal karyotype, *SRSF2* mutation, and treatment with pipobroman, chlorambucil, or 32P.[141,217] A mutation-enhanced prognostic scoring system (MIPSS-PV) includes age >60 years, *SRSF2* mutations, abnormal karyotype, and leukocyte count ≥11 × 10⁹/L for a four-tiered survival model with an estimated median survival range of 5.4 to 25.3 years.[142] Reported rates of fibrotic progression in PV range from 6% to 14% at 15 years.[221] In younger patients (aged ≤40 years) with PV followed for a median of 11.3 years, fibrotic and leukemic progressions were reported in 22% and 4% of patients, respectively.[220]

During the later phases of PV, there is a progressive decrease in erythropoiesis, the RBC mass normalizes, and the panmyelosis in the marrow gives way to marrow failure accompanied by anemia, the so-called "spent phase." Two additional patterns of disease progression are also recognized: post-polycythemia vera myelofibrosis (post-PV MF) and progression to BP.

Post-Polycythemia Vera Myelofibrosis

The progressive and often terminal complication of post-PV MF develops in approximately 15% of patients 10 to 15 years after the initial diagnosis of PV and in approximately 25% or more in those who survive 20 years or more.[222] The presence of marrow reticulin fibrosis at diagnosis predicts a higher incidence of such progression.[212] Post-PV MF is characterized by anemia, a leukoerythroblastic blood smear with RBC poikilocytosis and teardrop-shaped RBCs, grade 2 or 3 fibrosis of the bone marrow, and splenomegaly caused by EMH.[211] The diagnostic criteria for post-PV MF are listed in Box 47-12. Bone marrow specimens are variably cellular but demonstrate overt reticulin and often collagen fibrosis and osteosclerosis (Fig. 47-28). Granulopoiesis and, particularly, erythropoiesis are diminished in quantity, and clusters of abnormal megakaryocytes of variable sizes with hyperchromatic, bizarre nuclei are frequently the predominant marrow component. Marrow sinuses are dilated and filled with hematopoietic precursors and megakaryocytes.[78] In the spleen, EMH in the cords and sinuses contributes to the leukoerythroblastosis in the blood. A similar pattern of EMH is seen in the liver. Nearly 80% to 90% of patients with post-PV MF exhibit an abnormal karyotype.[223]

Blast Phase/Myelodysplastic Phase

A myelodysplastic (MDS)-like phase and leukemic transformation are rare and usually late events in PV. The incidence in patients treated with only phlebotomy is 1% to 2%, which is assumed to be the incidence of MDS or acute leukemia in the natural course of disease.[222] The risk of development of these complications appears to be related to the patient's age (higher risk in older patients) and exposure to certain cytotoxic treatment modalities, such as alkylating agents and 32P, which are now rarely used in therapy for PV. In virtually all cases, the BP is myeloid and may be preceded by an MDS-like phase. The leukemic transformation may occur in the setting of post-PV MF. In such cases, fibrosis may prevent aspiration, and the detection of blasts in the biopsy may be facilitated by staining for CD34. The finding of more than 10% blasts in the blood or marrow or severe myelodysplastic features, particularly in the granulocytic and erythroid

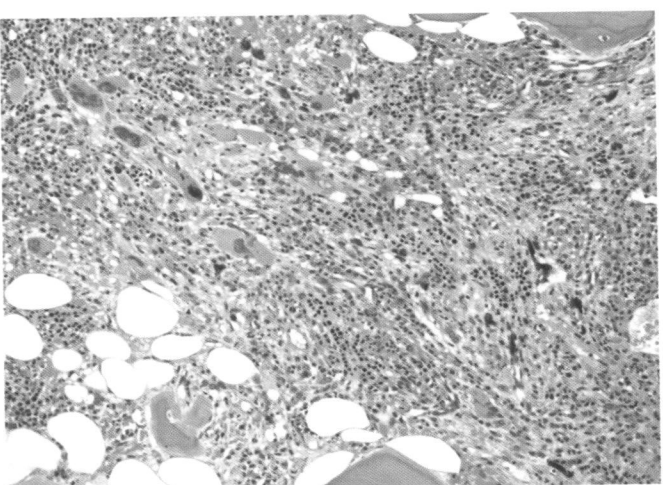

Figure 47-28. Post-polycythemia vera myelofibrosis (Post-PV MF). Bone marrow biopsy from a patient with polycythemia vera for nearly 15 years who then had anemia, leukoerythroblastosis, and increasing splenomegaly. The bone marrow is somewhat depleted, with a background of reticulin fibrosis and atypical megakaryocytes.

lineages, generally supports accelerated or MDS-like phase, respectively, and 20% or more blasts indicates BP, i.e., overt acute leukemia. Almost all patients who have MDS features or leukemic transformation show karyotypic evolution, often with the acquisition of complex chromosomal abnormalities. However, at transformation, the leukemic blasts may not carry the *JAK2* V617F mutation, giving rise to speculation that the transformation arises from an abnormal clone that preceded the *JAK2* mutation.[224]

Differential Diagnosis

The different causes of polycythemia are listed in Box 47-10. Most cases encountered are either primary or secondary acquired polycythemia. Serum EPO levels and genetic testing for *JAK2* V617F should be considered "up-front" tests for the diagnosis of PV and its differentiation from other causes of erythrocytosis.

Primary Polycythemia, Acquired and Congenital

PV is the only acquired primary polycythemia. The only congenital primary polycythemia that has been well characterized is primary familial congenital polycythemia, a rare condition caused by mutations in *EPOR,* usually with an autosomal dominant inheritance pattern.[225,226] These mutations lead to truncation of the cytoplasmic portion of EPOR and loss of the binding site of SHP-1, which normally downregulates EPO-mediated activation of the JAK2/STAT pathway. This results in hypersensitivity of the erythroid precursors to EPO.[204] As a consequence, serum EPO levels are low or normal. There is erythrocytosis but no granulocytosis or thrombocytosis. Patients are often asymptomatic but have a predisposition for development of cardiovascular disease. *EPOR* mutations account for only a small number of cases of primary familial congenital polycythemia; for the majority, the defect is unknown.[226] In some families, there is a predilection to develop PV or other MPNs because of a genetic factor that predisposes them to acquire a somatic *JAK2* mutation. Such cases should not be considered congenital polycythemia but familial primary acquired PV.

Secondary Polycythemia, Acquired and Congenital

The most common case of polycythemia is acquired secondary polycythemia induced by hypoxia. Chronic obstructive lung disease, right-to-left cardiopulmonary shunts, sleep apnea, and renal disease that compromises blood flow to the kidneys are the most frequent causes.[204,206] Individuals living at high altitudes compensate for the lower atmospheric oxygen by increasing their Hb levels as a consequence of tissue hypoxia. Chronic carbon monoxide poisoning causes tissue hypoxia and is responsible, in part, for "smoker's polycythemia"; nicotine also contributes by lowering plasma volume through its diuretic effect.

Inappropriate production of EPO is an often overlooked cause of secondary erythrocytosis. Cerebellar hemangioblastoma, uterine leiomyoma, pheochromocytoma, hepatocellular adenoma, and meningioma are among the tumors reported to be associated with EPO production.[204,206] Exogenous EPO administration to improve sports performance also leads to polycythemia; androgens have a similar effect. Post-renal transplantation polycythemia is a phenomenon of uncertain cause reported in 10% to 15% of renal transplant recipients 6 to 24 months after transplantation. Its incidence is decreasing and has been attributed to improvement in the immunosuppressive agents administered in the posttransplantation period.[227,228]

Congenital secondary polycythemia should be considered in young patients or in those with lifelong polycythemia in whom the serum EPO level is normal or elevated. Two broad groups of defects are found in this category—those associated with abnormal Hb affinity for oxygen and those associated with mutations of genes in the oxygen-sensing–EPO synthesis pathway. More than 90 Hb variants have been described with abnormal Hb-oxygen dissociation curves. Those with increased affinity for oxygen do not readily give up oxygen to tissues, and the oxygen dissociation curve is shifted to the left.

This results in reduced P_{50}, and the resulting tissue hypoxia leads to increased EPO levels and secondary erythrocytosis. Although some of the high-oxygen-affinity Hb variants are detected by electrophoretic techniques, a substantial number are not. Therefore, P_{50} is an appropriate screening test when an Hb variant is suspected. A similar effect is caused by the rare disorder 2,3-bisphosphoglycerate mutase deficiency.[204,227]

Mutations in genes encoding proteins in the oxygen-sensing pathway and in the synthesis of EPO do not result in abnormalities of the oxygen dissociation curve, and patients with these abnormalities have a normal P_{50}. Chuvash polycythemia is the most frequent of these disorders. This inherited form of secondary polycythemia affects individuals in the Chuvash region of Russia and is caused by a mutation in the von Hippel–Lindau *(VHL)* gene that results in inhibition of degradation of HIF-α, thus allowing increased EPO production. Mutations of the genes that encode the PHD-containing enzymes are also important in the degradation of HIF-α *(PHD2)* and of the genes that encode the HIF-α isoforms, which can lead to similar changes. Patients with mutations affecting these genes may have erythrocytosis as a result of increased serum EPO and are thus "secondary."[204,228]

CHRONIC EOSINOPHILIC LEUKEMIA, NOT OTHERWISE SPECIFIED (CEL, NOS)

Considering the strict relationship of CEL, NOS with other myeloid neoplasms with eosinophilia, it has been described in detail in Chapter 50. Box 47-13 lists the ICC criteria for diagnosis of CEL, NOS. A brief summary of CEL, NOS is included herein.

CEL is characterized by persistent eosinophilia not meeting the criteria for other genetically defined entities. The peripheral blood demonstrates an absolute eosinophil count $\geq 1.5 \times 10^9$/L and relative eosinophilia ($\geq$10% of leukocytes). If a chronic myeloid neoplasm shows a relative and absolute eosinophilia without defining genetic lesions, a diagnosis of CEL, NOS supersedes a diagnosis of aCML, MDS/MPN-U, or MPN-U.

Ideally, a diagnosis of CEL, NOS is supported by the presence of clonal molecular genetic abnormalities and abnormal bone marrow findings or increased blasts. Mutations detected by NGS have helped to establish clonality in a significant subset of cases with eosinophilic disorders. Mutations in genes such as *ASXL1, TET2, EZH2, DNMT3A, SRSF2, TP53, SETBP1,* and *STAT5B* N642H have been identified.[229-231] Clonal cytogenetic or molecular alterations may not be demonstrated in all cases of CEL, NOS.

The bone marrow of CEL, NOS typically shows hypercellularity caused by a prominent proliferation of eosinophils and granulocytic cells. Megakaryocytes can show dysplastic features or a mixture of MDS-like and MPN-like features, with or without dysplastic features in other lineages. Significant marrow fibrosis ($\geq$MF-2) is seen in 20% to 30% of cases. Cytologic abnormalities in a significant subset of eosinophils including abnormal granulation (hypogranular, uneven granulation), abnormal nuclear lobation (multilobation, hypolobation, nuclear branching), and large or markedly left-shifted forms are common; however, these findings are not specific to CEL, NOS. These abnormal bone marrow features are helpful in separating CEL, NOS from related entities such as idiopathic hypereosinophilic syndromes (iHES) and hypereosinophilia of unknown significance (HEus) and are

Box 47-13 Diagnostic Criteria* for Chronic Eosinophilic Leukemia, Not Otherwise Specified (CEL, NOS) According to International Consensus Classification

1. Peripheral blood hypereosinophilia (eosinophil count ≥1.5 × 10^9/L and eosinophils ≥10% of white blood cells)
2. Blasts constitute <20% cells in peripheral blood and bone marrow, not meeting other diagnostic criteria for acute myeloid leukemia (AML)[†]
3. No tyrosine kinase gene fusion including *BCR::ABL1*, other *ABL1*, *PDGFRA*, *PDGFRB*, *FGFR1*, *JAK2*, or *FLT3* fusions
4. Not meeting criteria for other well-defined myeloproliferative neoplasms (MPNs); chronic myelomonocytic leukemia, or systemic mastocytosis[‡]
5. Bone marrow shows increased cellularity with dysplastic megakaryocytes with or without dysplastic features in other lineages and often significant fibrosis, associated with an eosinophilic infiltrate or increased blasts ≥5% in the bone marrow and/or ≥2% in the peripheral blood
6. Demonstration of a clonal cytogenetic abnormality and/or somatic mutation(s)[§]

*The diagnosis of CEL requires all six criteria.
[†]AML with recurrent genetic abnormalities with <20% blasts is excluded.
[‡]Eosinophilia can be seen in association with systemic mastocytosis (SM). However, "true" CEL, NOS may occur as SM with an associated myeloid neoplasm (SM-AMN).
[§]In the absence of a clonal cytogenetic abnormality and/or somatic mutation(s) or increased blasts, bone marrow findings supportive of the diagnosis will suffice in the presence of persistent eosinophilia, provided other causes of eosinophilia have been excluded.
Data from Arber DA, Orazi A, Hasserjian RP, et al. International Consensus Classification of myeloid neoplasms and acute leukemias: integrating morphologic, clinical, and genomic data. *Blood.* 2022;140(11):1200-1228.

Box 47-14 Diagnostic Criteria* for Myeloproliferative Neoplasm, Unclassifiable (MPN-U) According to International Consensus Classification

1. Clinical and hematologic features of an MPN are present[†]
2. *JAK2*, *CALR*, or *MPL* mutation[‡] or presence of another clonal marker[§]
3. Diagnostic criteria for any other MPN, MDS, MDS/MPN[¶] or chronic myeloid leukemia are not met

*The diagnosis of MPN-U requires all three criteria.
[†]In cases presenting with bone marrow fibrosis reactive causes must be excluded, in particular fibrosis secondary to infection, autoimmune disorder or another chronic inflammatory condition, hairy cell leukemia or another lymphoid neoplasm, metastatic malignancy, or toxic (chronic) myelopathy.
[‡]It is recommended to use highly sensitive assays for *JAK2* V617F (sensitivity level <1%) and *CALR* and *MPL* (sensitivity level 1% to 3%); in negative cases, consider searching for noncanonical *JAK2* and *MPL* mutations.
[§]Assessed by cytogenetics or sensitive NGS techniques; detection of mutations associated with myeloid neoplasms (e.g., *ASXL1*, *EZH2*, *IDH1*, *IDH2*, *SF3B1*, *SRSF2*, and *TET2* mutations) supports the clonal nature of the disease.
[¶]In cases presenting with myelodysplastic features effects of any previous treatment, severe comorbidity, and changes during the natural progression of the disease process must be carefully excluded.
Data from Arber DA, Orazi A, Hasserjian RP, et al. International Consensus Classification of myeloid neoplasms and acute leukemias: integrating morphologic, clinical, and genomic data. *Blood.* 2022;140(11):1200-1228.

now incorporated into the diagnostic criteria. Except for increased eosinophils, the bone marrow in iHES and HEus is largely morphologically unremarkable.

MYELOPROLIFERATIVE NEOPLASMS, UNCLASSIFIABLE (MPN-U)

The designation MPN-U should be applied only to cases that have definite clinical, laboratory, and morphologic features of an MPN but fail to meet the criteria for any of the specific MPN entities or that present with features that overlap two or more of the MPN categories (Box 47-14).[1] Most cases fall into one of three categories: (1) early stages of PV, PMF, or ET in which the clinical, laboratory, and morphologic manifestations are not yet fully developed. Patients presenting with splanchnic vein thrombosis associated with *JAK2* mutation that fails to meet the diagnostic criteria for any of the specific MPN entities may also be considered to belong in this group; (2) advanced-stage MPN, in which myelofibrosis, osteosclerosis, or transformation to a more aggressive stage obscures the underlying diagnosis; and (3) patients with convincing evidence of MPN in which a concomitant neoplastic or inflammatory process obscures the diagnostic clinical or morphologic classification. The designation MPN-U should not be used if laboratory data necessary for classification are incomplete or were never obtained, the size or quality of the bone marrow specimen is inadequate for complete evaluation, or the patient has received prior growth factor or cytotoxic therapy. In these instances, the morphologic features should be described with the suggestion of additional clinical and laboratory information that is necessary to accurately diagnose and classify the case. The finding of a *BCR::ABL1*

fusion gene or rearrangements of *PDGFRA*, *PDGFRB*, *FGFR1*, or *PCM1::JAK2* precludes the diagnosis of MPN-U. Although *JAK2* V617F, *CALR*, and *CSF3R* mutations are most commonly observed in MPNs, they have been described in other myeloid neoplasms as well and cannot be used as the sole evidence to designate a case MPN-U if other data are not supportive.

If a case does not have features of one of the well-defined MPN entities, the possibility (or probability) that it is not an MPN must be seriously considered. Reactive bone marrow responses to a number of inflammatory and infectious agents must be kept in mind, particularly when considering CNL and chronic eosinophilic leukemia. Marrow fibrosis with osteosclerosis may be found in some inflammatory and neoplastic conditions, including chronic osteomyelitis, Paget's disease, metabolic bone diseases, osteosclerotic myeloma, hairy cell leukemia, metastatic carcinoma, and malignant lymphoma.

When a diagnosis of MPN-U is made, the report should indicate why a more definitive diagnosis is not possible. If one or more specific MPNs can be excluded on the basis of the laboratory, clinical, and morphologic data available, that should be stated as well. Recommendations for additional studies to clarify the diagnosis should be given, even if it is only a suggestion to repeat the same studies after an appropriate time interval. Sharing the case with colleagues, particularly with the clinicians responsible for the patient's care, is important. Sending the case for an expert opinion may help reach a diagnostic conclusion or at least confirm that someone with more experience could not classify the case either.

CONCLUSION

The major categories of MPNs remain unchanged in the ICC and proposed WHO 5th edition. The diagnoses of these entities require an integrated approach incorporating clinical, morphologic, and genetic features. Continuous integration of new molecular data has improved understanding of the morphology and prognosis and have also helped refine the diagnostic criteria.

Acknowledgments

The authors graciously appreciate and acknowledge the work from the prior author, Dr. James Vardiman, who has inspired and contributed significantly to this updated chapter.

Pearls and Pitfalls

- Diagnosis of MPNs requires integration of clinical, laboratory, morphologic, and genetic findings.
- Increased peripheral blood counts are more common in the presence of reactive etiologies than neoplastic ones, and the former should be excluded before performing a bone marrow examination.
- Well-prepared peripheral blood and bone marrow aspirate smears and adequate bone marrow core biopsy specimens are essential for accurate diagnosis.
- Treatment and prognosis of MPNs require an accurate diagnosis. ET, PV, and pre-PMF can share similar presentation (e.g., thrombocytosis) and genetic findings (e.g., *JAK2* mutation). Bone marrow histology is required for reaching a correct diagnosis in *BCR::ABL1*-negative MPNs.
- Though megakaryocytic morphology and topography is important to distinguish between the various *BCR::ABL1*-negative MPNs, other features including cellularity, granulocytic-to-erythroid ratio, bone marrow fibrosis, clinical history, genetics, and laboratory data must be taken into consideration to make an accurate diagnosis.
- In cases of "triple-negative" ET and PMF, cytogenetics or NGS for mutations in genes associated with myeloid neoplasms can be helpful in establishing clonality.
- Although the diagnosis of CML is straightforward in most cases, it can have unusual manifestations that overlap with other myeloid neoplasms and reactive conditions, such as marked neutrophilia resembling CNL, thrombocytosis resembling ET, and monocytosis resembling CMML. Appropriate cytogenetic and molecular testing for *BCR::ABL1* fusion should be obtained in these cases.
- The threshold for leukocytosis in CNL varies depending on the presence or absence of activating *CSF3R* mutations.
- The diagnosis of MPN-U is not intended for cases with insufficient or inadequate diagnostic material, when there is lack of clinical information, or when appropriate preliminary laboratory workup has not been performed. In such cases, the report should specify what additional material or studies are required to render a conclusive diagnosis.

KEY REFERENCES

1. Arber DA, Orazi A, Hasserjian RP, et al. International consensus classification of myeloid neoplasms and acute leukemias: integrating morphologic, clinical, and genomic data. *Blood*. 2022;140(11):1200–1228.
43. Langabeer SE, Andrikovics H, Asp J, et al. Molecular diagnostics of myeloproliferative neoplasms. *Eur J Haematol*. 2015;95(4):270–279.
100. Jabbour E, Kantarjian H. Chronic myeloid leukemia: 2022 update on diagnosis, therapy, and monitoring. *Am J Hematol*. 2022;97(9):1236–1256.
115. Gianelli U, Thiele J, Orazi A, et al. International Consensus Classification of myeloid and lymphoid neoplasms: myeloproliferative neoplasms. *Virchows Arch*. 2023;482(1):53–68.
116. Szuber N, Elliott M, Tefferi A. Chronic neutrophilic leukemia: 2022 update on diagnosis, genomic landscape, prognosis, and management. *Am J Hematol*. 2022;97(4):491–505.
123. Thiele J, Kvasnicka HM, Facchetti F, Franco V, van der Walt J, Orazi A. European consensus on grading bone marrow fibrosis and assessment of cellularity. *Haematologica*. 2005;90(8):1128–1132.
131. Gianelli U, Bossi A, Cortinovis I, et al. Reproducibility of the WHO histological criteria for the diagnosis of Philadelphia chromosome-negative myeloproliferative neoplasms. *Mod Pathol*. 2014;27(6):814–822.
133. Thiele J, Kvasnicka HM, Orazi A, et al. The International Consensus Classification of myeloid neoplasms and acute leukemias: myeloproliferative neoplasms. *Am J Hematol*. 2023;98(1):166–179.
141. Tefferi A, Barbui T. Polycythemia vera and essential thrombocythemia: 2021 update on diagnosis, risk-stratification and management. *Am J Hematol*. 2020;95(12):1599–1613.
144. Barbui T, Thiele J, Passamonti F, et al. Survival and disease progression in essential thrombocythemia are significantly influenced by accurate morphologic diagnosis: an international study. *J Clin Oncol*. 2011;29(23):3179–3184.

Visit Elsevier eBooks+ for the complete set of references.

Chapter 48

Myelodysplastic/Myeloproliferative Neoplasms and Premalignant Conditions

Kaaren K. Reichard, Daniel A. Arber, Sonam Prakash, and Attilio Orazi

INTRODUCTION

The myelodysplastic syndrome/myeloproliferative neoplasm (MDS/MPN) category is a heterogeneous group of diseases characterized by the co-existence of clinicopathologic features of both MDS and MPNs. These disorders are also referred to as hybrid or overlapping myeloid disorders to reflect the fact that they harbor features of both MDS and MPNs.

In the International Consensus Classification (ICC), an update from the previous 2016 World Health Organization (WHO) revised 4th edition classification, neoplasms in

> **Box 48-1** *International Consensus Classification of Myelodysplastic/Myeloproliferative Neoplasms*
>
> Chronic myelomonocytic leukemia
> Atypical chronic myeloid leukemia
> Myelodysplastic/myeloproliferative neoplasm with *SF3B1* mutation and thrombocytosis
> Myelodysplastic/myeloproliferative neoplasm with ring sideroblasts and thrombocytosis, not otherwise specified
> Myelodysplastic/myeloproliferative neoplasm, not otherwise specified
> • Includes the provisional subentity of myelodysplastic/myeloproliferative neoplasm with i(17q)

> **Box 48-2** *International Consensus Classification of Premalignant Clonal Monocytosis*
>
> Clonal monocytosis of undetermined significance
> • Clonal cytopenia with monocytosis of undetermined significance

> **Box 48-3** *Diagnostic Criteria for Chronic Myelomonocytic Leukemia (CMML)*
>
> • Monocytosis defined as monocytes $\geq 0.5 \times 10^9$/L and $\geq 10\%$ of the WBC
> • Cytopenia(s)*—thresholds same as for MDS*
> • Blasts/promonocytes <20% of the cells in peripheral blood and bone marrow
> • Presence of clonality: abnormal cytogenetics and/or detection of at least one myeloid neoplasm–associated mutation of at least 10% variant allele frequency[†]
> • In cases without evidence of clonality, monocytes must be $\geq 1.0 \times 10^9$/L and $\geq 10\%$ of the WBC—AND—at least one of the following:
>   • increased blasts/promonocytes[‡]
>   • morphologic dysplasia
>   • an abnormal immunophenotype consistent with CMML
> • Bone marrow morphologic findings consistent with CMML (hypercellularity caused by a myeloid proliferation often with increased monocytes), and lacking diagnostic features of acute myeloid leukemia, myeloproliferative neoplasm, or other conditions associated with monocytosis[§]
> • No *BCR::ABL1* or genetic abnormalities of myeloid/lymphoid neoplasms with eosinophilia and tyrosine kinase gene fusions
>
> *Occasional cases may show no or borderline cytopenia(s) (usually in the early phase of the disease), but the diagnosis of CMML can still be made; anemia, Hb <13 g/dL [males], <12 g/dL [females]; neutropenia, absolute neutrophil count <1.8 × 10⁹/L; thrombocytopenia, platelets <150 × 10⁹/L.
> [†]Based on International Consensus Group Conference, Vienna, 2018 (Valent et al., 2019).
> [‡]Increased blasts: ≥5% in the bone marrow and/or ≥2% in the peripheral blood.
> [§]For cases lacking bone marrow findings of CMML, a diagnosis of clonal monocytosis of undetermined significance could be considered. If a cytopenia is present, a diagnosis of clonal cytopenia and monocytosis of undetermined significance could be entertained. In these diagnostic settings, however, an alternative cause for the observed monocytosis must be excluded.
> *MDS,* Myelodysplastic syndrome; *WBC,* white blood cell count.
> Data from Arber DA, Orazi A, Hasserjian R, et al. The 2016 revision to the World Health Organization classification of myeloid neoplasms and acute leukemia. *Blood.* 2016;127(20):2391-2405.

the MDS/MPN diagnostic category include the following entities: chronic myelomonocytic leukemia (CMML), atypical chronic myeloid leukemia, MDS/MPN with *SF3B1* mutation and thrombocytosis, MDS/MPN with ring sideroblasts and thrombocytosis, not otherwise specified, and MDS/MPN, not otherwise specified (Box 48-1).[1-4]

Additional related entries in the ICC include the pre-CMML conditions of clonal cytopenia with monocytosis of undetermined significance and clonal monocytosis of undetermined significance (Box 48-2).[3-5] These precursor conditions are somewhat comparable to those occurring in MDS.

The ICC stresses the concept that cases in the MDS/MPN diagnostic category should have at least one cytopenia and one cytosis by complete blood cell (CBC) analysis. The definition of cytopenia is anemia, Hb <13 g/dL (males), <12 g/dL (females); neutropenia, absolute neutrophil count (ANC) <1.8 × 10⁹/L; thrombocytopenia, platelets <150 × 10⁹/L.[6] One exception to requiring a cytopenia is in early stage CMML. A small proportion of these patients may not be cytopenic, but a CMML diagnosis can still be made based on morphology and immunophenotypic and molecular data. As previously established cases of MPN may develop cytopenia(s) or monocytosis in the course of disease progression, it is essential that a diagnosis of MDS/MPN only be made for cases that did not have another preceding myeloid neoplasm.

CHRONIC MYELOMONOCYTIC LEUKEMIA (CMML)

Definition

CMML is a clonal hematopoietic stem cell disorder with monocytosis and features of both MDS and MPN.[3,7,8] It is characterized by the presence of sustained (>3 months) peripheral blood (PB) monocytosis ($\geq 0.5 \times 10^9$/L; monocytes $\geq 10\%$ of white blood cell [WBC] count). Blasts, including promonocytes (which are considered blast equivalents), account for less than 20% of the cells in the PB and less than 20% of the nucleated cells in the bone marrow. The diagnostic criteria for CMML are presented in Box 48-3.

Data, particularly molecular genetics, has demonstrated that there is a similar mutational landscape between oligomonocytic CMML (cases with >10% circulating monocytes but an absolute monocyte count of 0.5 to <1.0 × 10⁹/L) and traditional CMML (absolute monocytes $\geq 1.0 \times 10^9$/L). As such, they should be considered as one disease.[9,10] Consequently, in the presence of clonality, the criteria for diagnosing CMML now has a lower value of required absolute monocytosis, $\geq 0.5 \times 10^9$/L (modified from the 2016 WHO classification); however, monocytes must still account for $\geq 10\%$ of the WBC count.

Based on the WBC count, two distinct subtypes of CMML are recognized; the proliferative subtype (CMML-MP) (WBC $\geq 13 \times 10^9$/L) and the myelodysplastic subtype (CMML-MD).

Though the 2016 revision of the WHO classification introduced a three-tier classification of CMML, it has been shown that there is no clinical significance in separating CMML-0 (<2% blasts in PB and <5% blasts in bone marrow).[11,12] Therefore, based on the percentage of blasts and promonocytes (blast equivalents) in the blood and bone marrow, the ICC reverts to a two-tier system of CMML-1 (<5% blasts in PB, <10% in bone marrow) and CMML-2 (5%–19% blasts in PB, 10%–19% in bone marrow, or presence of Auer rods).

Synonyms and Related Terms

Chronic myelomonocytic leukemia (WHO 5th edition, Khoury 2022)[13]

Epidemiology

The incidence of CMML is not well defined; however, two studies have reported an approximate incidence of CMML as 2 to 4 cases per 100,000 persons/year.[14,15] However, the incidence may be higher because of misclassification (such as MDS or MPN) or bone marrow biopsies not being performed in older individuals.

Etiology

The etiology of CMML is unknown. Occupational exposures, environmental carcinogens, and ionizing radiation have been suggested as possible causes in some cases. Therapy-related CMML has been described and is associated with a poor outcome.[16]

Clinical Features

CMML occurs commonly in older adults, with a median age at diagnosis of 65 to 75 years with a male-to-female ratio of 1.5 to 3.1. The clinical presentation of patients with CMML is highly variable and may manifest differently depending on whether it is the myeloproliferative or myelodysplastic variant. With the myeloproliferative variant (CMML-MP), patients often have "myeloproliferative-like" features such as leukocytosis, hepatosplenomegaly, fever, and night sweats.[17] Patients with high WBC counts are also more likely to have lymphadenopathy and leukemic skin infiltrates. There may be hemorrhagic episodes in up to 30% of patients and thrombotic complications in 10% to 15%; in some patients, early satiety caused by splenomegaly may be an initial complaint.[18] Approximately 30% of patients with CMML can present with manifestations of antecedent or concomitant autoimmune diseases (rheumatoid arthritis, psoriasis, etc.), vasculitic syndromes, classic connective tissue diseases, and poorly defined systemic inflammatory syndromes.

Morphology

Laboratory Findings

The WBC count is usually between 10 and 20 × 10^9/L. Uncommonly, cases may show a range of 2 to 500 × 10^9/L. Patients often have modest thrombocytopenia (80 to 100 × 10^9/L), and this is one of the typical laboratory presentations (Fig. 48-1B). Anemia is usually mild and typically normocytic or macrocytic.

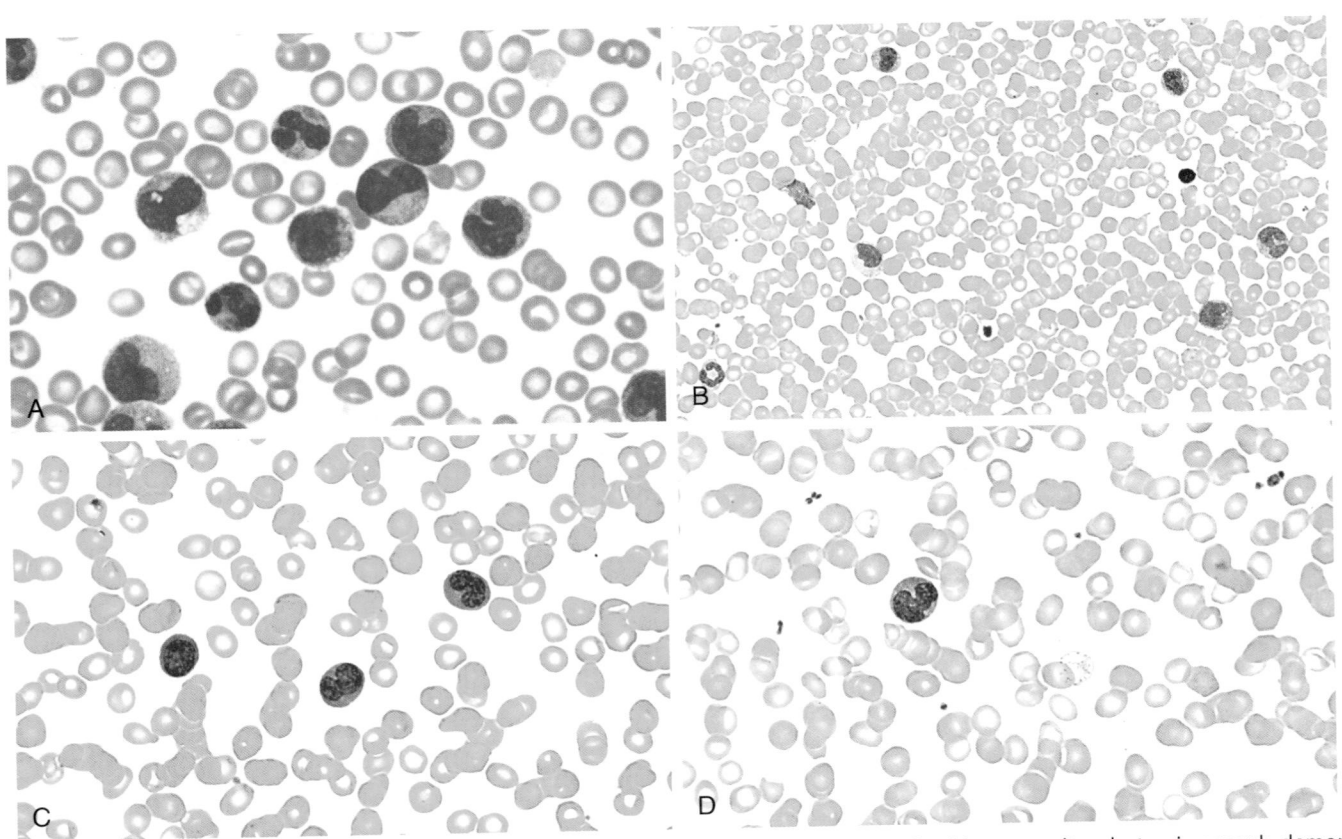

Figure 48-1. Peripheral blood findings in chronic myelomonocytic leukemia (CMML) (A–D). This composite photomicrograph demonstrates some typical peripheral blood features that may be encountered in CMML. **A,** Peripheral blood smear shows slightly elevated white blood cell count with absolute monocytosis and minimal dysplasia in the neutrophil lineage. **B,** Absolute monocytosis with abnormal appearing yet mature monocytes. Thrombocytopenia is notable in the background, which is common in CMML presentation. **C,** Abnormal-appearing monocytes with unusually clumped chromatin. **D,** Coarse basophilic stippling *(center of photographs)* in a case of CMML with ring sideroblasts.

By definition, monocytosis is present. The reported range of absolute monocytosis is impressive, varying from 0.5 to greater than 200×10^9/L, but in a significant majority of patients, monocytes are less than 5×10^9/L. Monocytes must account for 10% or more of the WBCs and are typically in the range of >15%, such that it is not a question as to whether monocytes are truly increased. This percentage is important because, in a number of diseases with elevated WBC counts, there may be only 1% to 2% monocytes in the leukocyte differential, but this can result in a significant so-called "absolute monocytosis."

Peripheral Blood

In CMML, the monocytes in the PB are typically mature, with minimal morphologic abnormality (Fig. 48-1). However, they can exhibit unusual nuclear lobation and delicate nuclear chromatin. When these latter features are present, the cells are best termed abnormal monocytes—this means the monocytes are atypical (Fig. 48-2) but lack the features of promonocytes (aka blast equivalents). Use of the term "immature monocytes" is confusing and, as such, should be avoided. Distinction between abnormal monocytes, promonocytes, and monoblasts is critical to not overestimate the blast percent (Fig. 48-2).

Promonocytes, which are blast equivalents, are cells with more delicately folded nuclei, thin nuclear slits, fine chromatin, small nucleoli, finely granular cytoplasm, and slightly less gray/more light-blue cytoplasm (Wright-Giemsa stain) (Fig. 48-2B and C). An increase in blasts in CMML may also be due to myeloblasts or monoblasts, or both. Monoblasts are large cells with abundant cytoplasm that may contain a few vacuoles or fine granules; they have lacy, delicate nuclear chromatin and one or more nucleoli (Fig. 48-2A). Monoblasts exhibit a morphologic continuum with promonocytes (Fig. 48-2B), from which it may be difficult to distinguish them, but both cell types are considered together in tallying the number of blasts for classification purposes. Distinguishing myeloblasts, monoblasts, and promonocytes from the more mature "abnormal" monocytes and from normal monocytes is extremely important in distinguishing CMML from AML, although at times it may be problematic.[19] When blasts (myeloblasts, monoblasts, and promonocytes) account for 5% to 19% of the WBCs in the blood or 10% to 19% of the nucleated cells in the bone marrow, the diagnosis is CMML-2; if 20% or more are present in either location, the diagnosis is AML. The finding of Auer rods in blood or marrow cells also prompts the diagnosis of CMML-2 if blasts in the blood and marrow are less than 20%.

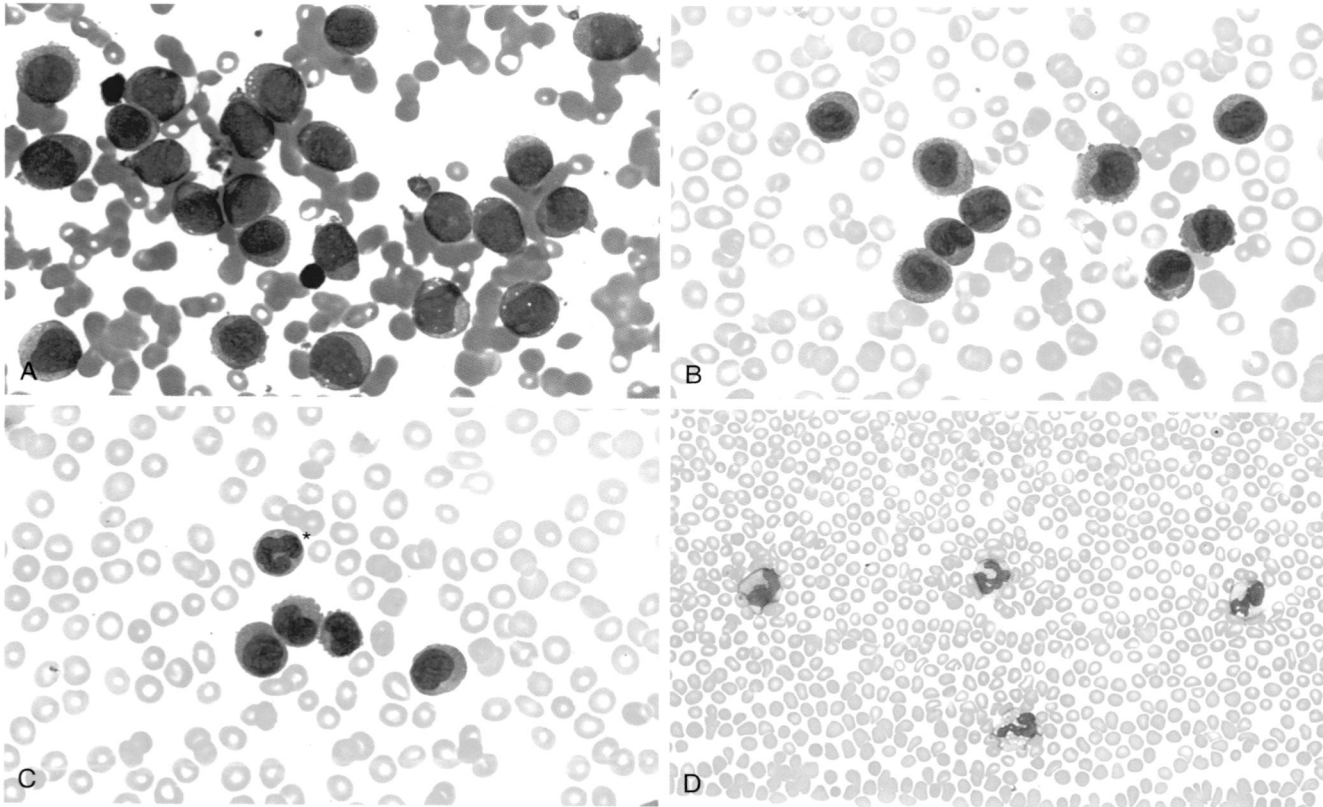

Figure 48-2. Monoblasts, promonocytes, and abnormal monocytes (A–D). A, Monoblasts are large, with round-to-oval nuclei that may be slightly irregular, lacy chromatin, one or more variably prominent nucleoli, and moderate to abundant, often moderately basophilic cytoplasm that may contain a few vacuoles or fine granules. **B and C,** Promonocytes have slightly irregular and slightly folded nuclei with delicate nuclear slits, fine chromatin, indistinct nucleoli, and moderate-to-abundant, light-blue/light-gray, finely granulated cytoplasm that may contain a few vacuoles. Promonocytes may have overlapping features with monoblasts. In some cases, one can appreciate the transition to a monoblast with an increase in overall cell size, increasing blue hue to the cytoplasm, emergence of a nucleolus, and less irregular nuclear contours. In contrast to a promonocyte, an abnormal monocyte *(highlighted with an asterisk in C)* shows more nuclear lobation, less fine chromatin, absence of delicate nuclear slits, and grayer cytoplasm. **D,** Abnormal monocytes in CMML have more condensed chromatin; abnormally shaped, irregular, or folded nuclei; and abundant grayish (minimal blue) cytoplasm, with more cytoplasmic granules and, often, more cytoplasmic vacuoles.

Neutrophil precursors (promyelocytes, myelocytes, and metamyelocytes) typically account for less than 10% of the WBCs in the blood at diagnosis. Dysgranulopoiesis is uncommon and, if present at all, is seen in a substantial minority of cases. It has been suggested that patients with higher WBC counts have less dyspoiesis than those with lower counts, but in the opinion of the authors, there is no significant relationship between severity of dysplasia and the leukocyte count.

Platelets may exhibit dysplastic features such as being large and/or hypogranular. Indeed, in the setting of unexplained prolonged monocytosis and thrombocytopenia, dysplastic-appearing platelets may be the initial PB clue to the presence of a clonal myeloid disorder, including CMML.

Red blood cells may show a range of anisopoikilocytosis. In cases with macrocytic anemia, macrocytes may be present. If ring sideroblasts are present in the bone marrow, a dimorphic appearance and coarse basophilic stippling (Fig. 48-1D) may be seen in circulating erythrocytes.

If a significant granulocytic left shift, granulocytic dysplasia, increased blasts, basophilia, or eosinophilia accompanies the monocytosis, it is incumbent upon the pathologist to exclude an alternative diagnosis (to CMML) such as chronic myeloid leukemia, BCR::ABL1-positive acute myeloid leukemia (AML), progression of an MPN with monocytosis, a myeloid neoplasm with eosinophilia, and a recurring genetic alteration involving a tyrosine kinase gene. These latter considerations are part of the exclusionary criteria in the diagnosis of CMML (Box 48-3).

Bone Marrow

Cellular bone marrow aspirate smears provide the best material for assessing the number of myeloblasts, monoblasts, promonocytes, and monocytes and for appreciating dysplasia in the various lineages (Fig. 48-3A). A granulocytic proliferation often left shifted is typically seen in the aspirate. Monocytes can be hard to identify. Cytochemical staining for alpha-naphthyl acetate esterase or alpha-naphthyl butyrate esterase to detect monocytes—either alone or in combination with naphthol AS-D chloroacetate esterase (CAE), which stains primarily neutrophils—can be very useful when the diagnosis of CMML is being considered (Fig. 48-3B). Dysgranulopoiesis, which is occasionally present, is more often appreciated in aspirate smears than in the PB. Dyserythropoiesis, particularly megaloblastoid changes or ring sideroblasts, is reported in about 25% of cases.

The bone marrow biopsy is hypercellular in more than 75% of cases (Fig. 48-4); rarely, normocellular or even hypocellular specimens may be encountered, but in the authors' opinion, the diagnosis should be questioned in these cases.[20,21] Granulocytic proliferation with left-shift, like the aspirate smears, is the most prominent feature in the biopsy, with a significant increase in the myeloid-to-erythroid ratio (Fig. 48-4). The number of megakaryocytes may be increased, normal, or decreased. Up to 75% of patients are reported to have micromegakaryocytes or megakaryocytes with abnormal nuclear lobation; however, in some cases, enlarged megakaryocytes can be found as well. Clustering of megakaryocytes is distinctly unusual in CMML.

The frequency of monocytes required in the bone marrow for the diagnosis of CMML has never been established, and the percentages reported in the literature vary widely; arguably, this is not relevant. However, in our experience, monocytes accounting for ≥10% of the marrow nucleated cells would indicate clear-cut bone marrow monocytosis. In well-fixed, thinly sectioned, and nicely stained biopsies, a proliferation of monocytes may be appreciated (Fig. 48-4B). Immunohistochemical stains such as CD14, CD68 (PG-M1), and CD163 can help their identification in histology sections (Fig. 48-4). An increase in blasts can be very difficult to appreciate in the biopsy because the granulocytes are left-shifted, and blasts/blast equivalents are often individually distributed and not in clusters, precluding their accurate recognition. In addition, clustering of myelocytes can be a morphologic distraction. In this situation, it is critical that one has a well-stained, well-sampled aspirate smear from which an accurate assessment of the blast count can be made. It can also be difficult in some cases to distinguish hypogranular myelocytes from monocytes. In that regard, immunostains for a monocyte-associated marker such as CD14 is helpful. Staining of the biopsy specimen for CD34 may be useful in estimating the myeloblast percentage, but it is not helpful for assessing the monoblasts or promonocytes because these cell types are almost always CD34 negative.

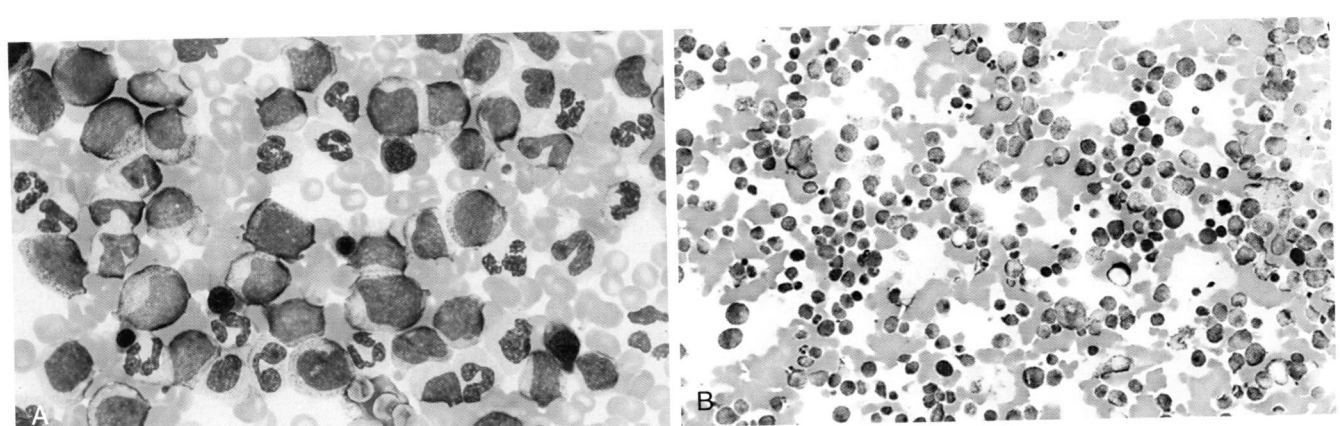

Figure 48-3. Bone marrow aspirate features in chronic myelomonocytic leukemia (CMML) (A, B). A, Well-stained, cellular bone marrow aspirate smears provide the best material for assessing the number of blasts, promonocytes, and monocytes and for appreciating dysplasia in the various lineages. **B,** Monocytic and granulocytic components in the bone marrow can be better appreciated with the combined esterase stains; chloroacetate esterase (CAE) combined with butyrate esterase (BE) *(monocytes are brown; neutrophils are blue)*. One will also notice increased dual esterase positive cells characterized by an admixture of both blue and brown staining.

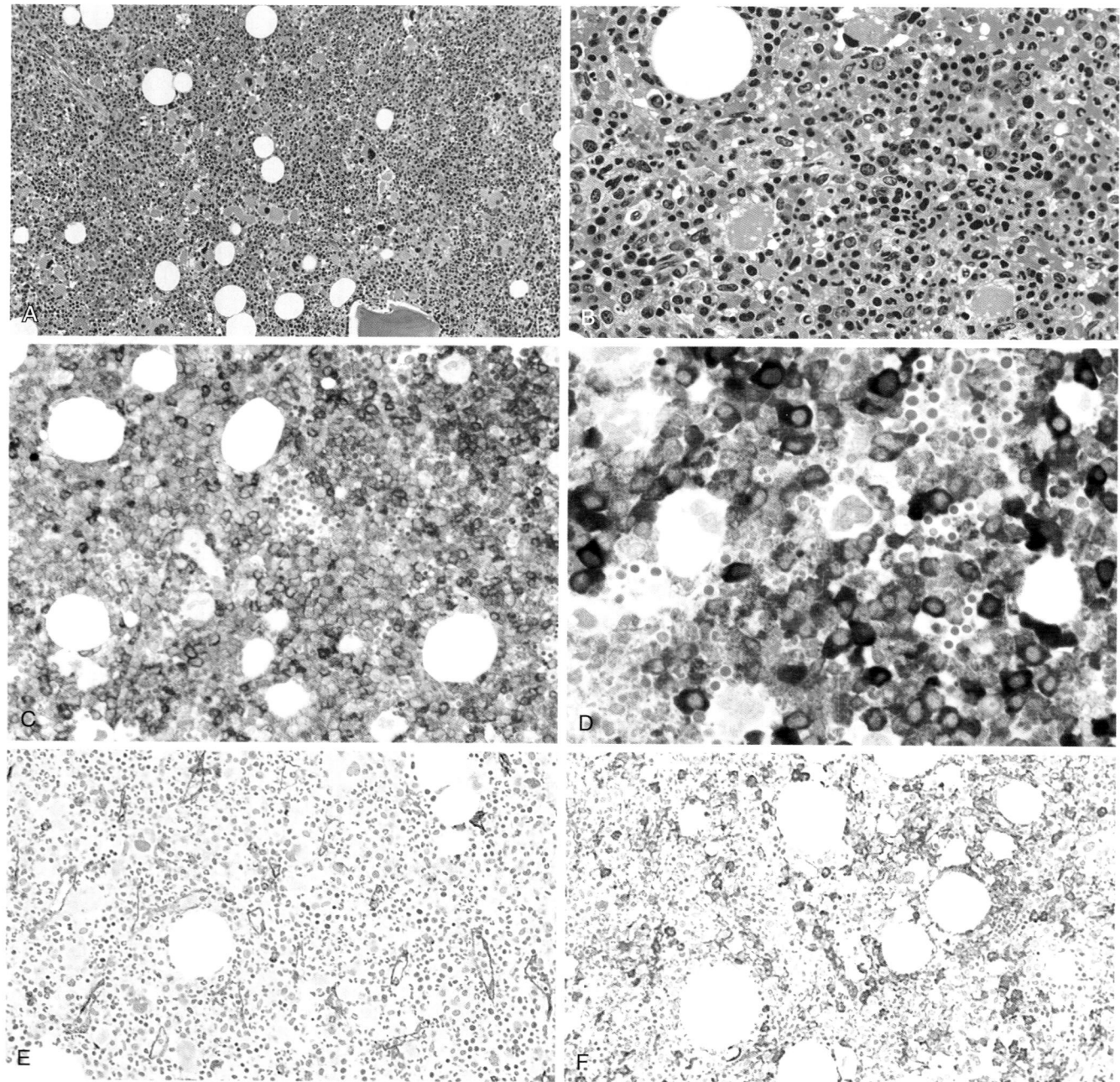

Figure 48-4. Bone marrow core biopsy morphologic and immunohistochemical features in chronic myelomonocytic leukemia (CMML) (A–F). A and B, The bone marrow is typically hypercellular with prominent, often left-shifted, granulocytic components. The increased number of monocytes cannot be appreciated at low magnification. Megakaryocytes may range in appearance from otherwise relatively normal appearing to small dysplastic forms more often noted in the myelodysplastic variant of CMML to larger hyperlobulated forms, which may be seen in the myeloproliferative variant. **B,** On higher magnification, the folded nuclei of monocytes dispersed among the granulocytes can be better appreciated. Immunohistochemical stains for CD33 **(C)** and lysozyme **(D)** highlight the myelomonocytic components. **E,** In most cases of chronic myelomonocytic leukemia, an increase in true myeloblasts is infrequent but can be evaluated using a CD34 immunostain. It should be remembered that not all myeloblasts are CD34 positive. CD34 immunohistochemistry is not helpful in assessing for monoblasts and promonocytes because the cell types are almost always CD34 negative. **F,** Immunohistochemical staining for CD14 is very helpful in elucidating the increased monocytic component in chronic myelomonocytic leukemia. (H&E, 400× and 600× magnification; CD33, lysozyme, CD34 and CD14 immunohistochemistry).

Variably sized nodules of plasmacytoid dendritic cells, which strongly express CD123, can be found in the bone marrow core biopsy in approximately 30% to 40% of cases (Figs. 48-5 and 48-6).[21] These findings are not specific for CMML but are a helpful clue. A proportion of cases may also be associated with systemic mastocytosis (Fig. 48-7), and when diagnosing CMML, immunostaining for CD117 should always be performed to facilitate identifying the mast cells. If mast cells appear abnormally increased, the more specific (but often less sensitive) tryptase should be used to confirm their mast cell nature.

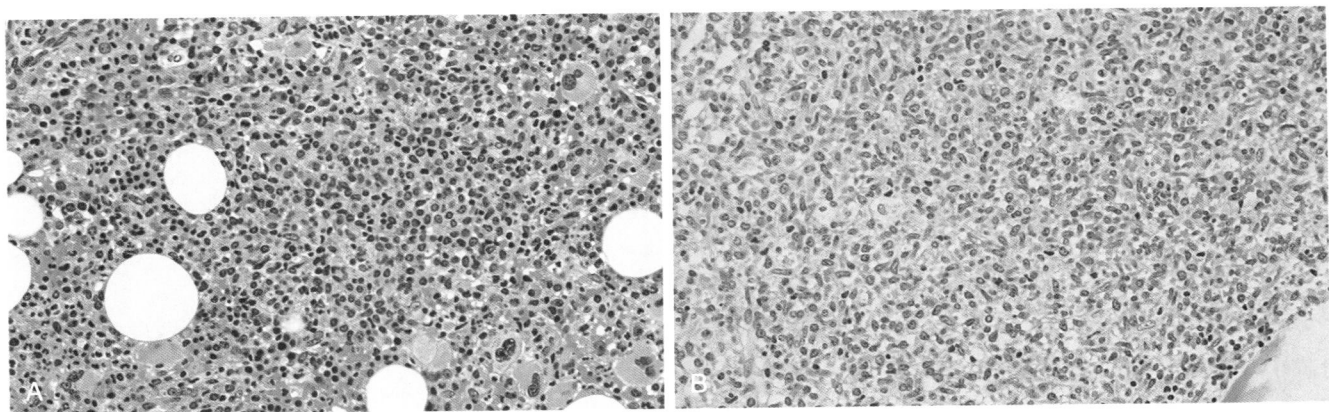

Figure 48-5. Plasmacytoid dendritic cell nodules in chronic myelomonocytic leukemia (CMML) (A, B). Plasmacytoid dendritic cell (pDC) nodules are seen in approximately 30% to 40% of cases of CMML. **A,** PDC nodules may be composed of a predominance of cells with a plasmacytoid type appearance characterized by small to intermediate sized cells with an eccentrically located round nucleus with an occasional small pinpoint nucleolus. **B,** Less commonly, pDC nodules may have a striking admixed spindle type of nuclear appearance characteristic of the dendritic origin of these cells.

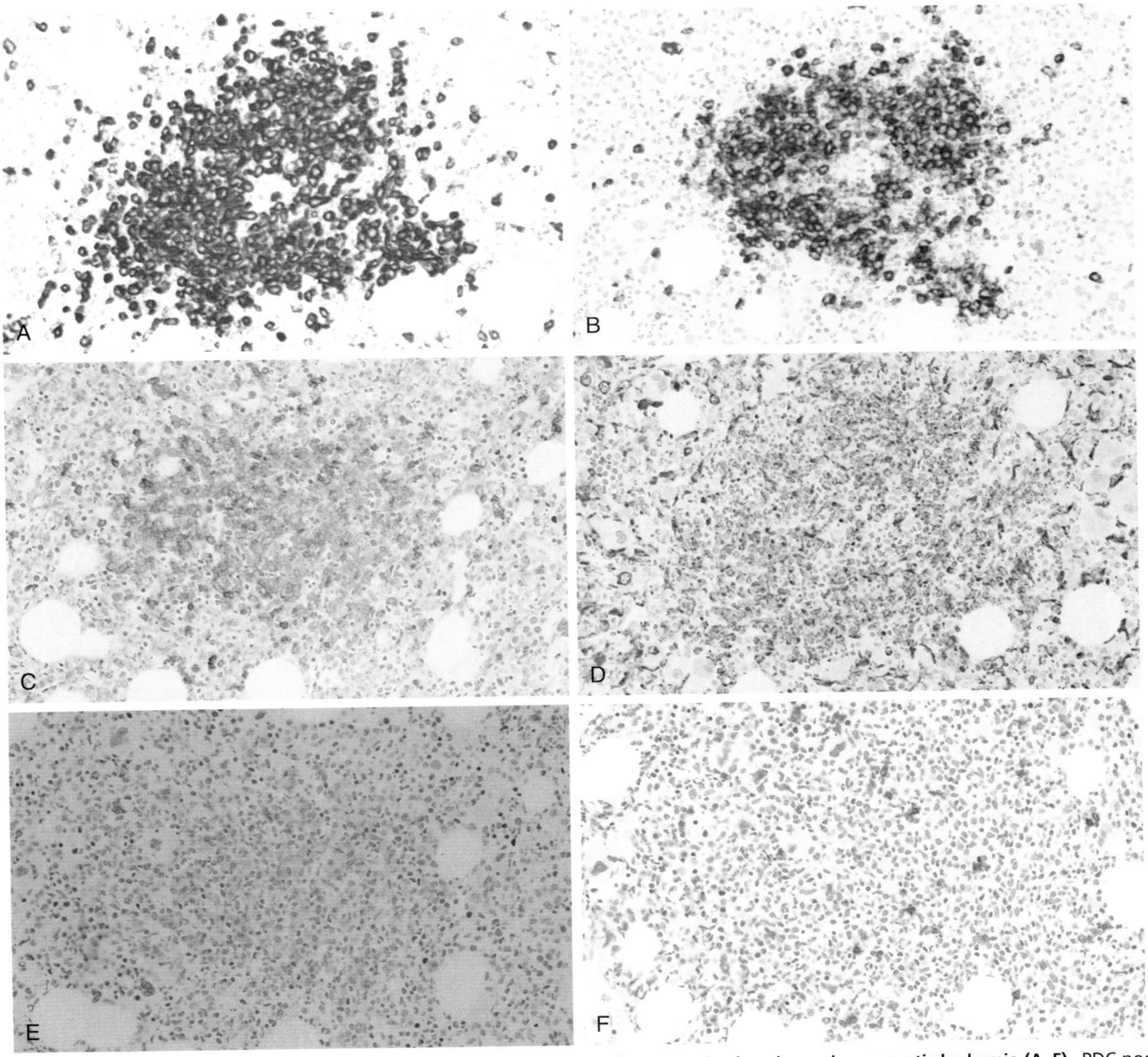

Figure 48-6. Immunohistochemical features of plasmacytoid dendritic cell nodules in chronic myelomonocytic leukemia (A–F). PDC nodules typically show the following immunophenotypic characteristics: Positive for CD123 **(A)**, CD303 **(B)**, CD4 **(C)**, CD68 (PG-M1 clone) **(D)**, TCL1A **(E)** and negative for CD56 **(F)**.

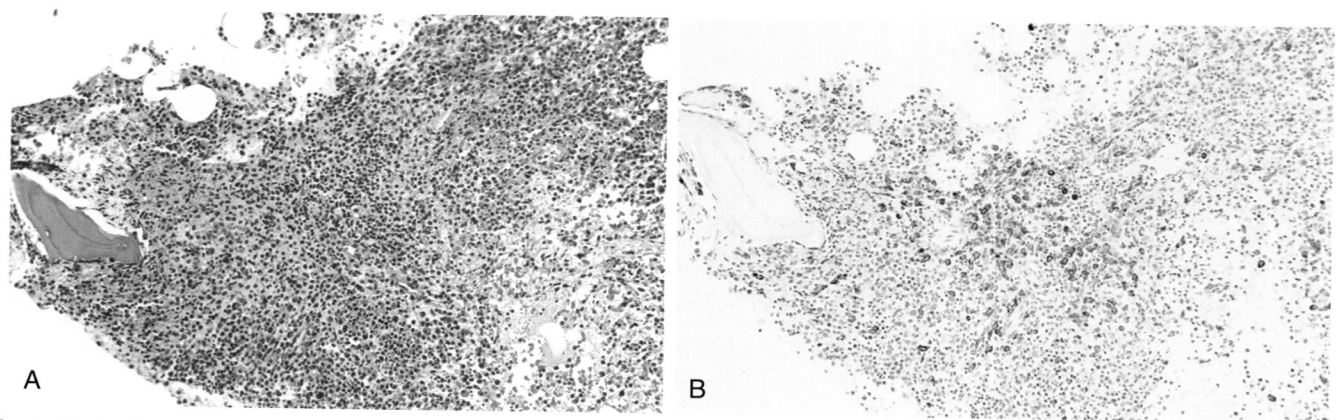

Figure 48-7. Chronic myelomonocytic leukemia (CMML) associated with systemic mastocytosis (A, B). A, A sneaky focus of systemic mastocytosis was seen in this case of CMML. As such, it is suggested to routinely perform a CD117 and/or tryptase immunostain in newly diagnosed cases of CMML to assess for the presence of occult systemic mastocytosis. **B,** A tryptase immunohistochemical stain identifies a focus of systemic mastocytosis in the setting of CMML.

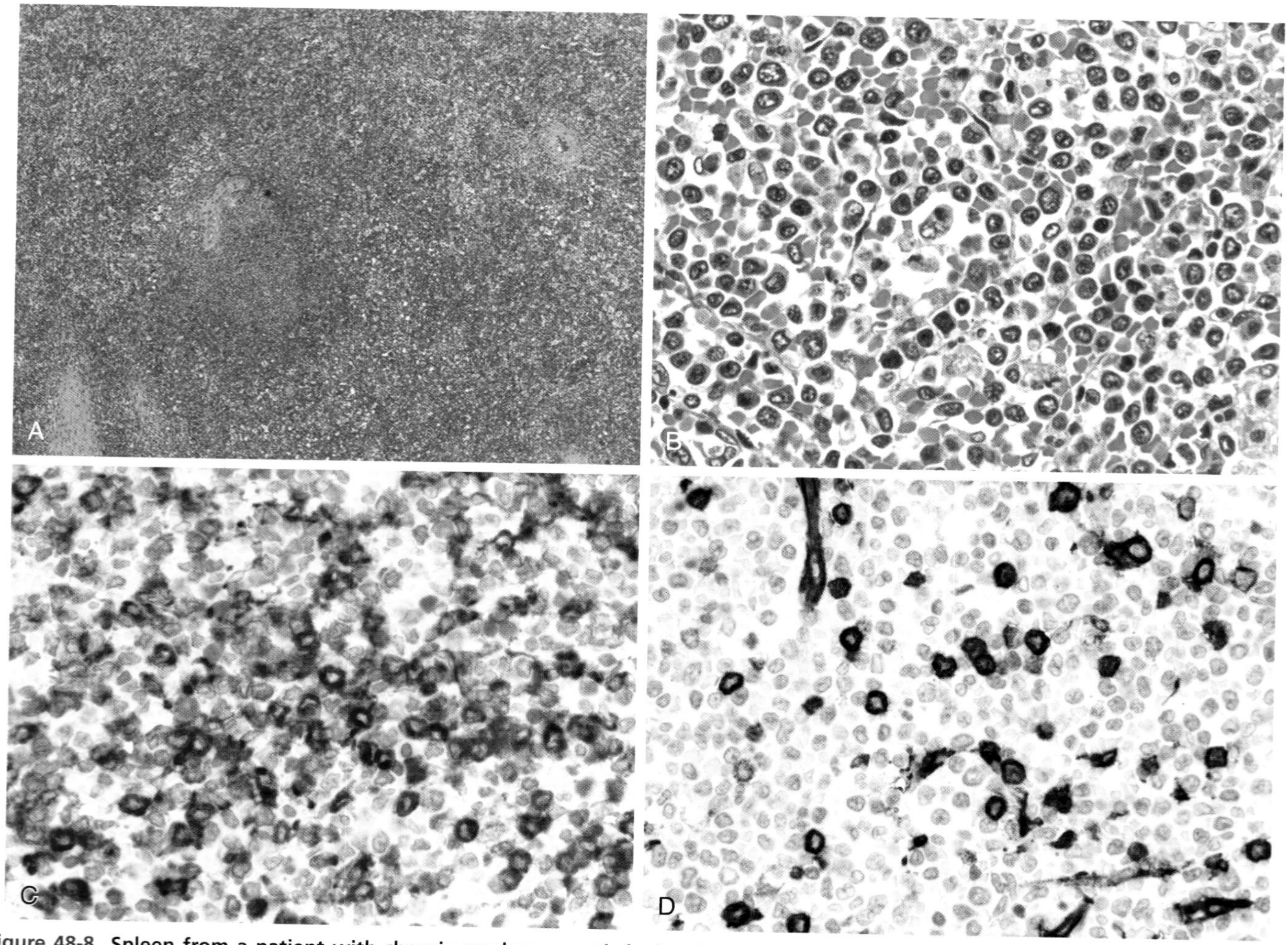

Figure 48-8. Spleen from a patient with chronic myelomonocytic leukemia 2. A, Leukemic infiltrate in the red pulp of the spleen encroaches on the white pulp. **B,** The infiltrate is composed of blasts, immature granulocytes, and monocytes. **C,** Immunohistochemical stain for CD14 highlights the monocytic component of the infiltrate. **D,** Immunohistochemical stain for CD34 demonstrates increased CD34-positive blasts.

Extramedullary Tissues

Splenic enlargement is frequent and is caused by leukemic infiltration of primarily the red pulp by myelomonocytic cells (Fig. 48-8). Trilineage extramedullary hematopoiesis has been reported in some splenectomy specimens from patients with CMML, and numerous foamy macrophages may be seen, particularly when the spleen has been removed as a therapeutic maneuver to relieve thrombocytopenia.[22] Some authors report high mortality and morbidity rates associated with splenectomy in patients with CMML.

Lymphadenopathy is seen in a minority of patients, and a biopsy is recommended in such cases because it may indicate extramedullary transformation to acute leukemia. In rare patients with CMML, tumoral proliferations of plasmacytoid dendritic cells, identical to those described in the bone marrow, may be seen in splenectomy or lymph node specimens.[23,24]

Cutaneous involvement can also be seen in CMML and rarely may be the initial presenting symptom. Plasmacytoid dendritic cells may also be part of abnormal skin proliferation.[25]

Immunophenotype

Immunohistochemistry on tissue sections of bone marrow biopsies is useful for assessing cellular components in their architectural context and may be helpful in distinguishing CMML (Fig. 48-4). Both granulocytes and monocytes, including immature forms and blasts, express CD33, which may be demonstrated in paraffin-embedded specimens (Fig. 48-4C). Immunostaining for lysozyme may help highlight granulocytic and monocytic components, but neither CD33 nor lysozyme can discern between them (Fig. 48-4C and D, respectively). Immunohistochemical staining for CD14 can be incredibly useful in the identification of increased monocytic cells (Fig. 48-4F). CD34 may help in estimating the myeloblast percentage in the core biopsy specimen, but it is not helpful for assessing the monoblasts or promonocytes because these cell types are almost always CD34 negative (Fig. 48-4E). Markers such as CD68R (PG-M1), CD11b, CD11c, CD14, CD16, CD56, CD117, CD163, and HLA-DR are reportedly helpful in assessing the granulocytic and monocytic components of CMML, and some authors have suggested that, when a number of these markers are used in combination, the staining pattern may be useful in the differential diagnosis of CMML, aCML, and CML.[26-29]

Clusters of plasmacytoid dendritic cells associated with CMML can be identified with CD123 (Fig. 48-7).[21] Although seen more often in CMML than in MDS or MPN, these nodules are not specific to CMML. The cells are positive for antigens normally expressed by reactive plasmacytoid dendritic cells, such as CD4, CD68/CD68R, TCL1A, and CD303[30] (Fig. 48-7). In some cases, plasmacytoid dendritic cells may aberrantly express other antigens, such as CD2, CD5, CD7, CD13, or CD33. Recognition of this aberrant immunostaining is important because, in small or fragmented biopsies, an initial misdiagnosis of peripheral T-cell lymphoma is possible.

Multiparametric flow cytometry with carefully designed antibody panels allows for a comprehensive characterization of monocyte lineage maturation stages from early monocytic commitment of CD34-positive precursors to late mature monocytes and of the neutrophil maturation pathway from myeloid blasts to mature polynuclear neutrophilic granulocytes.[31,32] Abnormal antigen expression in blast, monocytic, and granulocytic compartments can be detected in many patients with CMML.[31-34] Comprehensive antibody panels may therefore be helpful in the diagnosis of CMML

and in follow-up by detection of phenotypic aberrancies associated with disease progression and regression of aberrancies in response to therapy.[35] By flow cytometric analysis, the leukemic cells express myelomonocytic antigens such as CD33 and CD13, with variable expression of CD14, CD36, and CD64. The monocytes in CMML often exhibit aberrant expression of two or more antigens, including overexpression of CD56; aberrant expression of CD2; and decreased expression of HLA-DR, CD14, CD11c, CD13, CD15, CD64, or CD36.

Several studies have shown that flow cytometric analysis of monocyte subsets may be useful to confirm the presence of distinct monocyte populations and distinguish reactive monocytic populations from those associated with CMML.[31,36,37] Based on the expression of CD14 and CD16, monocytes can be divided into classical (MO1, CD14 bright/CD16 negative), intermediate (MO2, CD14 bright/CD16 positive) and nonclassical monocytes (MO3, CD14 dim/CD16 positive), differing in phagocytic activities and inflammatory characteristics. By comparing healthy donors and patients with reactive monocytosis, Selimoglu-Buet et al. showed the percentages of classical monocytes in PB are higher, and the percentage of nonclassical monocytes is lower in patients with CMML.[36] Using a cutoff value of ≥94% classical monocytes, CMML cases can be identified by these authors with a sensitivity of 92% and a specificity of 94%. However, false negatives with this approach can be experienced, particularly in patients with CMML with autoimmune diseases, where the intermediate fraction increases (relative decrease in classical monocytes), and in other myeloid malignancies such as CML and atypical CML.[38] A study based on real life experience has called into question the utility of this flow cytometric technique to distinguish the etiology of monocytosis.[39]

Cytogenetics

Clonal cytogenetic abnormalities are seen in approximately 20% to 30% of patients with CMML.[17] Common alterations include trisomy 8, abnormalities of chromosome 7, trisomy 21, deletion 20q, –Y, and complex karyotypes. No specific cytogenetic or genetic abnormalities have yet been identified in CMML, but the type of detected abnormality plays a role in risk stratification. In one study, survival analysis resulted in three cytogenetic risk categories: high (complex and monosomal karyotypes), intermediate (all abnormalities not in the high- or low-risk groups), and low (normal, sole –Y, and sole der [3q]). The overall median survivals in these three groups were 3, 21, and 41 months, respectively.[40]

Rearrangements of *KMT2A* (previously known as *MLL*) at 11q23.3 are not typical of CMML, and in the authors' opinion, detection of such rearrangements should be considered extraordinarily unusual. In such a situation, re-review of the entire case to exclude AML with a monocytic component is absolutely necessary.

Molecular Findings

Detection of pathogenic mutations can be diagnostically helpful in difficult cases of CMML/emerging CMML, particularly in cases with a normal karyotype or minimal/

absent dysplasia. However, the molecular findings should always be integrated with the entirety of the case and not used solely to establish a final diagnosis. This is particularly true when only a single abnormality is detected at a low variant allele frequency (VAF <10%) and in a gene that is associated with clonal hematopoiesis (CH) in normal aging individuals (e.g., *DNMT3A, TET2, ASXL1,* etc.).[41,42]

Somatic mutations are frequently found in patients with CMML.[17] These mutations can be subdivided into categories based on their role in the cell life cycle: histone modification (*EZH2, ASXL1*), DNA methylation (*TET2, DNMT3A*), spliceosome machinery (*SF3B1, SRSF2, U2AF1, ZRSR2*), regulation of cell signaling (*JAK2, KRAS, NRAS, CBL, PTPN11,* and *FLT3*), transcription factors and nucleosome assembly regulators (*RUNX1, SETBP1*), and DNA damage response genes such as *TP53*. Of these, mutations involving *TET2* (60%), *SRSF2* (50%), *ASXL1* (40%), and the *RAS* pathway (30%) are the most frequent. Overall, about 90% of patients with CMML exhibit one or more mutations, and concurrent mutations of *TET2* and *SRSF2* appear to be highly specific to CMML.[43-46] Multiple *TET2* mutations (aka multihit *TET2*) (defined as two or more *TET2* mutations/deletions and/or VAF ≥55%) also appear to be more frequent in CMML (including oligomonocytic CMML) than in MDS or MPN (approximately 50% versus 5%–6%).[47] In addition, the VAF of the first *TET2* hit is similar to the second *TET2* hit, in contrast to patients with MDS or MPN.[47] Though multihit *TET2* may show a higher percentage of peripheral blood/bone marrow monocytes and more dysgranulopoiesis than *TET2* wild-type patients, Garcia-Gisbert et al. did not observe statistically significant differences in OS between these two groups.[47]

Although the acquisition of genetic alterations remains an area of active investigation, it is believed that the initial driver mutation likely involves *TET2*. Second acquired alterations often include another *TET2* and/or *SRSF2* mutation. *ASXL1, DNMT3A, RUNX1, SETBP1,* and *SF3B1* mutations are usually seen in the myelodysplastic subtype of CMML, whereas *RAS* pathway, and *JAK2* V617F mutations tend to occur in the myeloproliferative subtype of CMML.

Frame-shift and nonsense *ASXL1* mutations adversely affect OS in CMML; however, although frequent, *TET2* mutations do not. *ASXL1* mutations have been incorporated into prognostic scoring systems along with karyotype and clinicopathologic parameters.[48]

Mutations in *SF3B1* can be identified in <10% cases of CMML with frequent ring sideroblasts.[49] These cases have low frequency of *ASXL1* mutations and a superior AML-free survival compared with CMML cases lacking the *SF3B1* mutation.[50]

SETBP1 mutations in patients with CMML are associated with elevated WBC counts, more frequent extramedullary disease, more frequent *ASXL1* mutations, less frequent *TET2* mutations, and an adverse prognosis, suggesting distinct cooperative molecular events in *SETBP1*-mutated CMML.

Detection of an *NPM1* mutation is also distinctly unusual and should raise concern for AML. Though it is recognized that *NPM1* mutations may occur in chronic myeloid neoplasms,[51,52] careful scrutinization for an emerging AML is warranted.

Clinical Course

In view of the variable clinical, morphologic, and biological properties of CMML, it is not surprising that reported survival times differ widely. Although a median survival of 20 to 40 months is reported in most series, the range for individual patients is 1 month to more than 120 months. Adverse prognostic factors vary depending on the study but may include thrombocytopenia (<100 × 10⁹/L), transfusion history, severity of anemia, immature granulocytes in the blood (≥1%), serum lactate dehydrogenase greater than 700 U/L, an absolute lymphocyte count of 2.5 × 10⁹/L or greater, bone marrow blasts exceeding 10%, and abnormal karyotype. Transformation of CMML to AML occurs in 20% to 30% of patients; more patients die of other complications, such as infection, without evidence of transformation.

There are several prognostic systems for CMML that facilitate predicting the clinical course for patients. In the Global MD Anderson prognostic system, four tiers of median survival have been identified: 54 months, 25 months, 14 months, and 6 months based on age, performance status, hemoglobin, platelet count, bone marrow myeloblast percentage, karyotype, leukocyte count, and transfusion history. The Mayo Clinic has derived a prognostic scoring system integrating the molecular alterations seen in CMML[53] based on five adverse independent prognostic factors: *ASXL1* mutations, absolute monocyte count >10 × 10⁹/L, hemoglobin <10 g/dL, platelets <100 × 10⁹/L, and circulating immature myeloid cells. In this model, they were able to show four risk categories (low, intermediate-1, intermediate-2, high) with median survivals of 97, 59, 31, and 16 months, respectively. The CMML-specific prognostic scoring system molecular model has also identified four risk groups (low, intermediate-1, intermediate-2, high): median OS not reached, 64, 37, and 18 months. With this stratification, the 4-year leukemic transformation rates of 0%, 3%, 21%, and 48%, respectively, were identified.[54]

Identifying the myelodysplastic versus myeloproliferative variant of CMML remains important. The myeloproliferative variant of CMML is associated with an adverse prognosis as captured by various CMML-specific prognostic scoring systems.[53,54] Also, given the potential difference in clinical behavior based on the different underlying genetic drivers, the separation of the myelodysplastic versus myeloproliferative variant of CMML may be of therapeutic benefit.

Currently, the only curative therapy for CMML is allogeneic stem cell transplantation; however, given that many patients are older and/or have multiple comorbid conditions, such treatment may not be an option. Hypomethylating agents (azacitidine and decitabine) are currently the most commonly used therapies for CMML.[17]

Differential Diagnosis

The diagnosis of CMML is often difficult—particularly when clinical history is minimal, dysplasia is minimal, the degree of monocytosis is slight/borderline, no cytogenetic abnormalities are present, and the duration of the monocytosis is unknown. As such, while one is awaiting the results of next-generation sequencing (NGS) results (if performed), there are multiple non-neoplastic and neoplastic conditions that should be considered in the differential diagnosis of CMML (Box 48-4).

Box 48-4 *Differential Diagnosis of Chronic Myelomonocytic Leukemia*

Infection (tuberculosis, syphilis, subacute bacterial endocarditis)

Autoimmune disease (rheumatoid arthritis, systemic lupus erythematosus, ulcerative colitis, polyarteritis)

Sarcoidosis

Malignant, nonmyeloid, disease (Hodgkin lymphoma, B-cell and T-cell lymphomas, carcinoma)

Myeloid neoplasm with rearrangements of *PDGFRA, PDGFRB, FGFR1, JAK2, FLT3, ABL1* (particularly when eosinophilia is present)

Atypical chronic myeloid leukemia

Acute leukemia with monocytic differentiation

Chronic myeloid leukemia, *BCR::ABL1* positive

BCR::ABL1-negative myeloproliferative neoplasms (e.g., primary myelofibrosis or polycythemia vera with monocytosis)

Myelodysplastic syndrome

Reactive Monocytosis

Reactive monocytosis is far more common than monocytosis occurring as a clonal condition. The hallmark of CMML—absolute monocytosis—is a non-specific finding associated with a wide variety of inflammatory and hematopoietic and non-hematopoietic neoplasms, all of which should be considered and excluded before a diagnosis of CMML is rendered. Viral, fungal, protozoal, rickettsial, and mycobacterial infections are commonly accompanied by monocytosis, as are autoimmune diseases and other chronic inflammatory disorders. Monocytosis is also common in patients with lymphoma, particularly Hodgkin lymphoma, but may be found in other hematopoietic and non-hematopoietic malignant neoplasms as well.

The most important steps in distinguishing reactive monocytosis from CMML are a careful review of the clinical history for evidence of an underlying inflammatory or neoplastic disorder; physical examination to determine whether organomegaly is present (which would favor CMML); and inspection of the blood smear for evidence of dysplasia and morphologically abnormal or immature monocytes and for the absence of findings, such as in lymphoma cells, (which would support a different diagnosis). If, after these steps have been taken, the diagnosis of CMML is still being considered, a bone marrow specimen with appropriate genetic studies should be obtained to corroborate the diagnosis. Flow cytometric studies of the peripheral blood or bone marrow monocytes may provide useful information. The finding of >94% classical monocytes (repartitioning of monocytic subsets) or multiple aberrancies, such as overexpression of CD56 and underexpression of myeloid antigens on monocytes, supports the diagnosis of CMML. Nevertheless, reactive monocytes may also show aberrant phenotypes, and correlation with all the pathologic data is needed.

A prudent approach in all cases is to recognize that reactive monocytosis is more common than CMML. If dysplasia is lacking or minimal in the blood and bone marrow and there is no myeloid-related karyotypic abnormality or other genetic abnormality that clearly defines the process, it is best to give a descriptive diagnosis and to defer a definitive diagnosis until after an observation period of 3 to 6 months to ascertain that the monocytosis is persistent and that no underlying cause has been discovered.

Acute Myeloid Leukemia With Monocytic Differentiation

Acute leukemia must always be considered in the differential diagnosis of CMML, particularly CMML-2. A bone marrow aspirate and biopsy are crucial in distinguishing between these entities because blasts and promonocytes are usually more prominent in the bone marrow than in the blood. Even in bone marrow specimens, the blasts may be irregularly distributed, and inspection of both the biopsy and aspirate together yields the most useful information. Moreover, the distinction between monocytes, abnormal monocytes, promonocytes, and blasts is sometimes difficult,[19] and distinguishing some cases of AML from CMML-2 can be challenging. When the number of blasts plus promonocytes is 20% or more in the blood or bone marrow, the diagnosis is AML rather than CMML. An additional difficulty is the finding of mutated *NPM1* in a case in which the diagnosis of CMML is being considered. In such cases, close follow-up and aggressive clinical intervention are suggested, as mutated *NPM1* is generally regarded as an AML-related mutation.[52]

Chronic Myeloid Leukemia, *BCR::ABL1* Positive

The distinction between CML, *BCR::ABL1* positive and CMML is made on the basis of morphology combined with cytogenetics and molecular genetic studies; the *BCR::ABL1* fusion gene is always present in CML and never present in CMML. In rare cases of CML, the BCR breakpoint is in the minor breakpoint cluster region, which leads to production of the p190 fusion protein, which is smaller than the p210 protein found in almost all cases of CML. The p190 protein is usually associated with Philadelphia (Ph) chromosome–positive acute lymphoblastic leukemia, but rare cases with this breakpoint may initially be CML with a chronic phase that exhibits increased numbers of monocytes, mimicking CMML (Fig. 48-9). Therefore, cytogenetic and genetic testing for the *BCR::ABL1* fusion gene is strongly recommended whenever the diagnosis of CMML is considered.

Myeloid Neoplasms Associated With Eosinophilia and Rearrangements of *PDGFRB*

The initial cases of rearrangement of *PDGFRB* and some subsequently reported cases had features of CMML with eosinophilia. However, the finding of this rearrangement and of rearrangements of *PDGFRA, FGFR1, JAK1, FLT3,* and *ABL1* excludes the diagnosis of CMML; such cases are classified according to the specific gene involved.

Atypical Chronic Myeloid Leukemia

This entity is discussed in detail later in this chapter. Briefly, aCML has many similarities to CMML, but it can be distinguished by the percentage of monocytes in the PB (rarely >2% to 4% and always <10% in aCML) and by the more severe granulocytic dysplasia in aCML. The use of cytochemistry for non-specific esterase to detect monocytes in the blood and bone marrow can be invaluable in difficult cases. Because the prognosis for aCML is particularly poor, its distinction from CMML is of clinical importance.

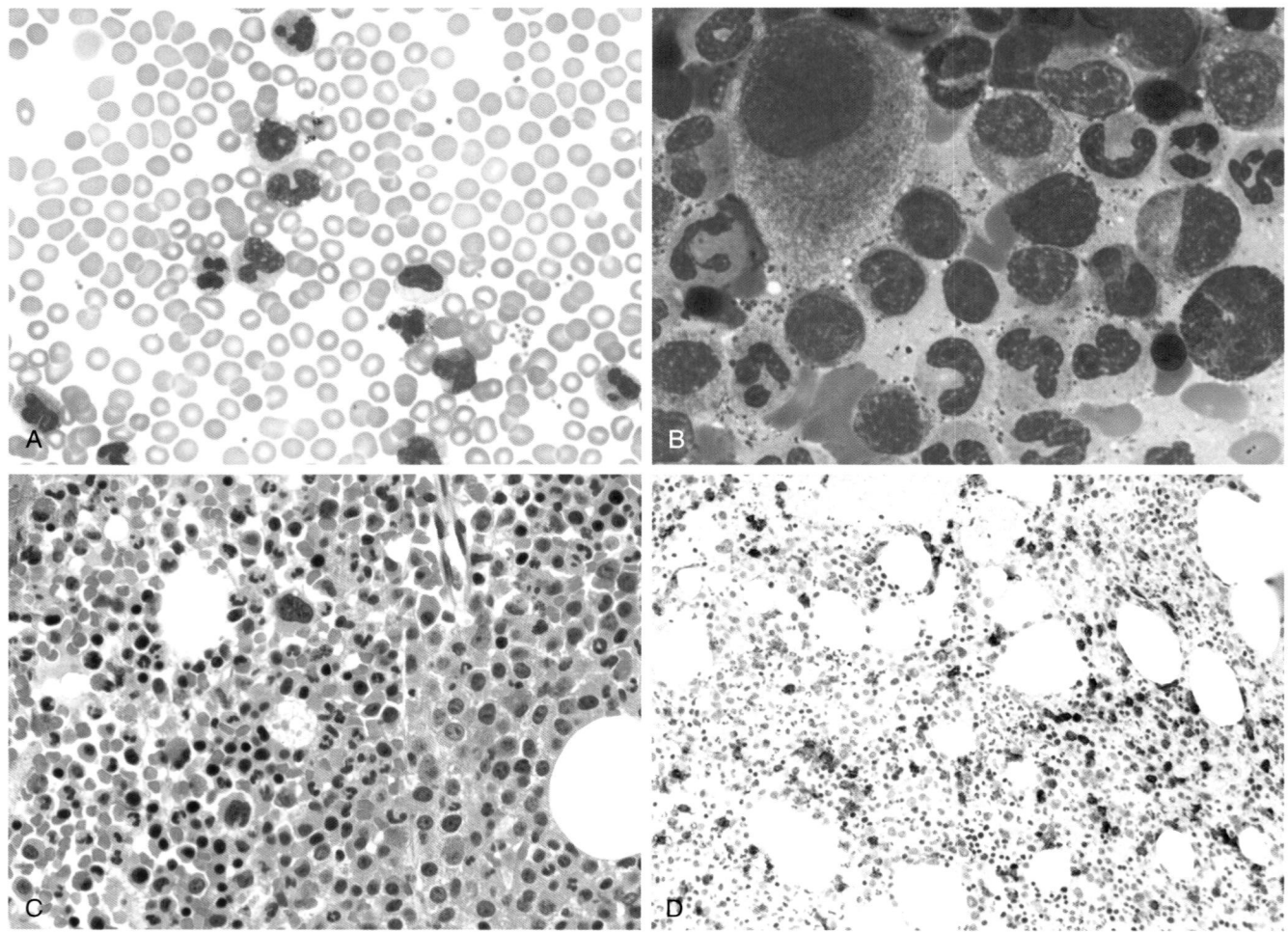

Figure 48-9. Chronic myeloid leukemia, *BCR::ABL1* positive (with p190 fusion protein) mimicking chronic myelomonocytic leukemia. A, Peripheral blood smear demonstrates leukocytosis with monocytosis, circulating granulocytes at all stages of maturation, and basophilia. **B** and **C,** Bone marrow aspirate smear **(B)** and bone marrow biopsy **(C)** demonstrate monocytosis, with granulocytic proliferation and small, hypolobated megakaryocytes. **D,** Immunohistochemical stain for CD14 highlights increased monocytes.

BCR::ABL1-Negative Myeloproliferative Neoplasms Associated With Monocytosis

Monocytosis can occur in *BCR::ABL1*-negative MPNs such as primary myelofibrosis and polycythemia vera; it is considered a form of disease progression and adversely affects survival.[55,56]

Because CMML may be associated with prominent reticulin fibrosis,[57] its differentiation from primary myelofibrosis and other MPNs can be difficult. In such cases, the bone marrow biopsy finding of clusters of pleomorphic, bizarre megakaryocytes that range in size from small to large with abnormal, bulky nuclei may be the most helpful distinguishing feature; tight clusters of such bizarre megakaryocytes are rarely observed in CMML.[58,59] The *JAK2* VAF may also be a useful discriminating factor.[60]

Myelodysplastic Syndrome

Cases of CMML with normal or even low WBC counts and prominent dysplasia may be difficult to distinguish from MDS, particularly at an early stage of presentation. Despite the similarities with MDS, if the ICC criteria are carefully applied, the finding of monocytosis of at least 0.5×10^9/L is sufficient for a diagnosis of CMML rather than MDS, assuming the bone marrow findings and other diagnostic features support such an interpretation. Rarely, MDS cases can transform to "secondary" CMML during the course of disease.[61]

CLONAL CYTOPENIA WITH MONOCYTOSIS OF UNDETERMINED SIGNIFICANCE AND CLONAL MONOCYTOSIS OF UNDETERMINED SIGNIFICANCE

The concept of CH occurring in normal individuals without a hematologic malignancy has its origins in several articles from the last decade.[41,42] Targeted NGS most often reveals single genetic mutations (e.g., *ASXL1, TET2, DNMT3A*) at variant allele frequencies of less than 10% in these individuals. Similarly, these alterations may be detected in some individuals with unexplained cytopenia(s) and no dysplasia—the latter being termed as clonal cytopenia of uncertain significance (CCUS).

It has similarly been noted that some individuals with CH may exhibit persistent unexplained mild monocytosis. These cases do not meet the criteria for CMML, and as such, this raises the distinct possibility that they represent a precursor state to CMML or other MDS/MPD; however, it is likely that only a small subset will develop a true hematologic malignancy (similar to CCUS). In these patients, the types of myeloid mutations, number of mutations, and VAF tend to overlap with CMML, but it is not a perfect correlation. As mentioned, it does appear that these individuals carry a higher risk of developing an overt myeloid malignancy.[62-64]

As a result of these findings, the ICC recognizes that there is a CMML precursor condition of CMUS.[3,4] This is based on the following criteria: absence of cytopenia, persistent monocytosis (monocytes ≥10% and ≥0.5 × 10^9/L of the WBC), presence of myeloid neoplasm–associated mutation(s), and absence of bone marrow morphologic findings of CMML. If cytopenia(s) is also present, then the ICC recommends the terminology of clonal cytopenia and monocytosis of undetermined significance (CCMUS). Box 48-5 delineates the diagnostic criteria for CMUS and CCMUS.

ATYPICAL CHRONIC MYELOID LEUKEMIA (aCML)

Definition

aCML is a clonal hematopoietic stem cell disorder that exhibits myelodysplastic and myeloproliferative features with characteristic granulocytic leukocytosis and dysplastic neutrophils. It is a diagnosis of exclusion, requiring clinical history, especially for possible antecedent myeloid neoplasms or prior chemotherapy, comprehensive genetic testing, exclusion of eosinophilia, and methodical evaluation of leukocytes in the blood and bone marrow.[3,65] The term aCML is quite unfortunate, as it is of no relation to CML, *BCR::ABL1* positive. Diagnostic criteria are shown in Box 48-6.

Synonyms and Related Terms

Atypical chronic myeloid leukemia, *BCR::ABL1* negative; atypical chronic myeloid leukemia, Ph chromosome negative; MDS/MPN with neutrophilia (WHO 5th edition, Khoury 2022)[13]

Epidemiology

The incidence of aCML is unknown. Although a number of reports have described patients with aCML, only a few have adhered to the diagnostic criteria first established by the French-American-British Cooperative Group and later adopted by the WHO.[65-67] Most cases occur in patients in the 7th or 8th decade of life, but younger patients may be affected as well.[67-69] The reported male-to-female ratio varies.

Etiology

The etiology of aCML is unknown.

Clinical Features

Symptoms related to anemia or thrombocytopenia are most frequently mentioned, but the chief complaint may also be related to splenomegaly.[67,69] Patients with aCML tend to be elderly, with the median patient age at diagnosis in the 7th or 8th decade of life.

Box 48-5 *Diagnostic Criteria for Clonal Monocytosis of Undetermined Significance (CMUS)*

- Persistent monocytosis defined as monocytes ≥0.5 × 10^9/L and ≥10% of the WBC
- Absence or presence of cytopenia (thresholds same as for MDS)* (anemia, Hb <13 g/dL [males], <12 g/dL [females]; neutropenia, absolute neutrophil count <1.8 × 10^9/L; thrombocytopenia, platelets <150 × 10^9/L)†
- Presence of at least one myeloid neoplasm-associated mutation of appropriate allele frequency (i.e., ≥2%)*
- No significant dysplasia, increased blasts/promonocytes, or morphologic findings of CMML on bone marrow examination‡
- No criteria for a myeloid or other hematopoietic neoplasm are filled
- No reactive condition that would explain a monocytosis is detected

*Based on International Consensus Group Conference, Vienna, 2018 (Valent et al., 2019).
†If a cytopenia is present, the nomenclature of clonal cytopenia and monocytosis of undetermined significance (CCMUS) is suggested.
‡Bone marrow findings of CMML include hypercellularity with myeloid predominance, often with increased monocytes and in a proportion of cases monoblasts and/or blast equivalents (i.e., promonocytes) and/or dysplasia in at least one lineage.
CMML, Chronic myelomonocytic leukemia; *MDS*, myelodysplastic syndrome; *WBC*, white blood cell count.

Box 48-6 *Diagnostic Criteria for Atypical Chronic Myeloid Leukemia (aCML)*

- Leukocytosis ≥13 × 10^9/L, caused by increased numbers of neutrophils and their precursors (promyelocytes, myelocytes and metamyelocytes), the latter constituting ≥10% of the leukocytes
- Cytopenia(s) (thresholds same as for myelodysplastic syndrome [MDS])* (anemia, Hb <13 g/dL [males], <12 g/dL [females]; neutropenia, absolute neutrophil count <1.8 × 10^9/L; thrombocytopenia, platelets <150 × 10^9/L)
- Blasts <20% of the cells in blood and bone marrow
- Dysgranulopoiesis, including the presence of abnormal hyposegmented and/or hypersegmented neutrophils and abnormal chromatin clumping
- No or minimal absolute monocytosis; monocytes constitute <10% of the peripheral blood leukocytes
- No eosinophilia; eosinophils constitute <10% and <1.5 × 10^9/L of the peripheral blood leukocytes
- Hypercellular bone marrow with granulocytic proliferation and granulocytic dysplasia, with or without dysplasia in the erythroid and megakaryocytic lineages
- No *BCR::ABL1* or genetic abnormalities of myeloid/lymphoid neoplasms with eosinophilia and tyrosine kinase gene fusions. The absence of myeloproliferative neoplasm–associated driver mutations and the presence of a *SETBP1* mutation in association with an *ASXL1* pathogenic variant provide additional support for a diagnosis of aCML.

*Based on International Consensus Group Conference, Vienna, 2018 (Valent et al., 2019).

Morphology

Blood

The WBC count is always greater than 13 × 10^9/L, with median reported values ranging from 32 to 96 × 10^9/L. Occasionally, some patients have WBC counts in excess of 300 × 10^9/L.[68,69] Granulocytic precursors (promyelocytes, myelocytes, and metamyelocytes) constitute ≥10% of the leukocytes. Thrombocytopenia is often present and may be severe, but thrombocytosis can occur as well. Anemia is usually present.

The peripheral blood smear is most remarkable for pronounced dysgranulopoiesis (Fig. 48-10). Neutrophils, many with hypogranular cytoplasm and abnormally lobated nuclei, usually predominate. Prominent nuclear clumping of neutrophils is also a feature (Fig. 48-11).[70-72] Immature neutrophils (promyelocytes, myelocytes, metamyelocytes) account for at least 10% or more of the WBCs, but the percentage of blasts is always less than 20% (usually less than 5%). In most cases, basophils account for 2% or less of the WBCs. It is important to enumerate monocytes carefully because they are a key feature in distinguishing aCML from CMML. In aCML, slight absolute monocytosis may be present, but the monocyte percentage is always less than 10% of the WBCs. Evidence of dyserythropoiesis, such as macroovalocytosis, is commonly observed.

Bone Marrow

The bone marrow is hypercellular and shows a predominantly granulocytic proliferation (Fig. 48-10). Blasts may be modestly increased in number but are always less than 20% of the nucleated bone marrow cells. In cases with a suboptimal aspirate smear or in cytologically difficult cases, blast identification may be facilitated by staining biopsy sections for CD34, being careful to remember that not all blasts are CD34 positive. As in the peripheral blood smear, granulocytic dysplasia is marked and can even be appreciated in the biopsy (Fig. 48-11). Megakaryocytes vary in number, with most cases displaying some degree of megakaryocytic dysplasia similar to that observed in MDS (small megakaryocytes with abnormal, hypolobated nuclei). Dyserythropoiesis is found in more than 50% of cases. Reticulin fibers are increased in some patients at the time of diagnosis and may increase during the course of the disease.

Cytochemical staining of the bone marrow for non-specific esterase, either alone or in combination with CAE, is strongly recommended to assess the percentage of monocytes and to help distinguish aCML from CMML. Immunohistochemical staining of the marrow biopsy specimen can also be helpful, but it is often not as sensitive as cytochemical techniques.

Most cases reported as the syndrome of abnormal chromatin clumping can be considered variants of aCML.[70,71] These

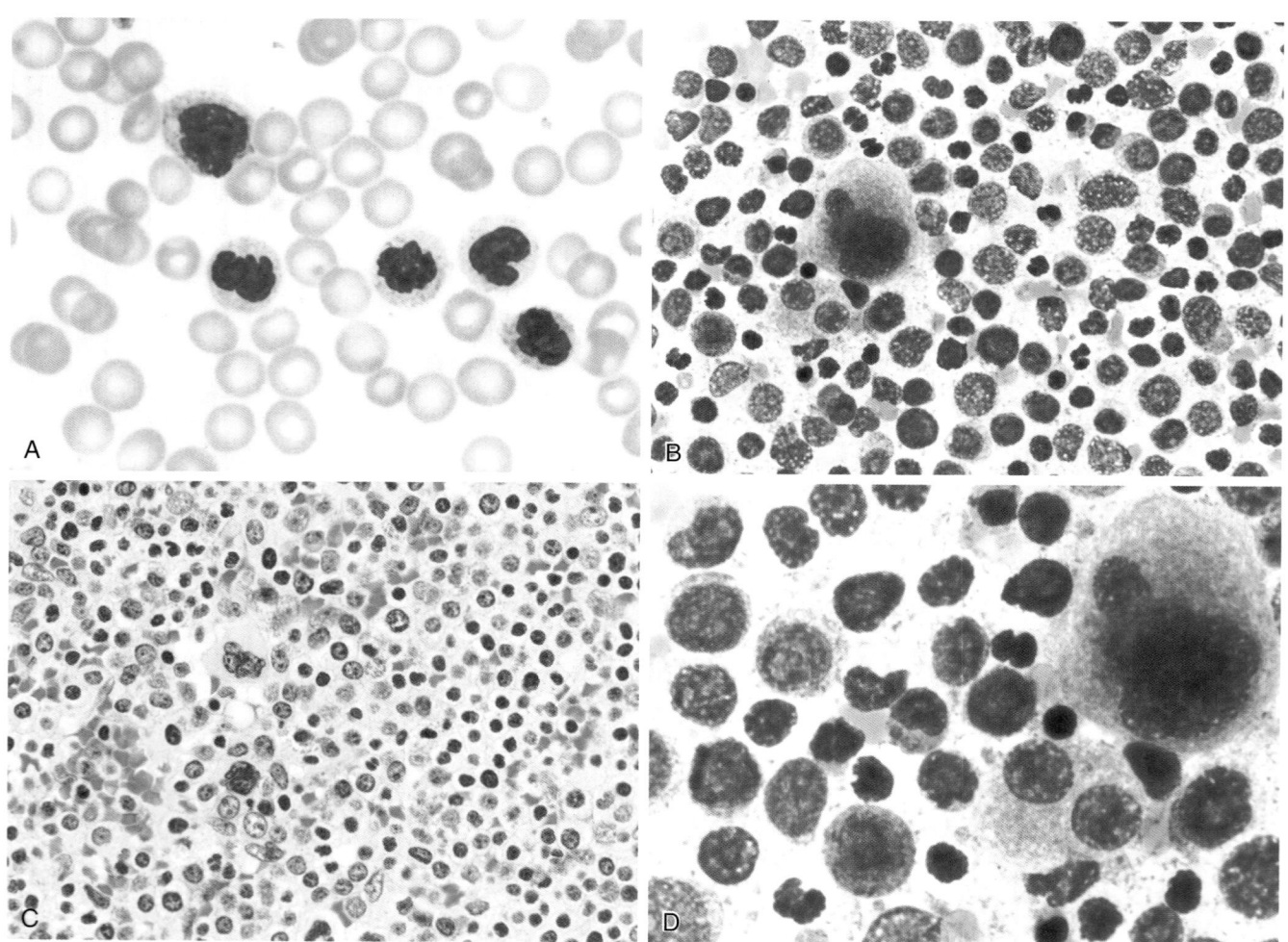

Figure 48-10. Atypical chronic myeloid leukemia. A, Peripheral blood smear shows elevated white blood cell count, with marked granulocytic dysplasia and immature granulocytes. **B,** Bone marrow aspirate smear shows granulocytic and megakaryocytic dysplasia. **C,** Bone marrow biopsy is hypercellular because of granulocytic proliferation with dysplasia and dysmegakaryopoiesis. Cells with clear cytoplasm are dysplastic granulocytes with marked pseudo–Pelger-Huët changes. **D,** On higher magnification, granulocytic and megakaryocytic dysplasia can be better appreciated.

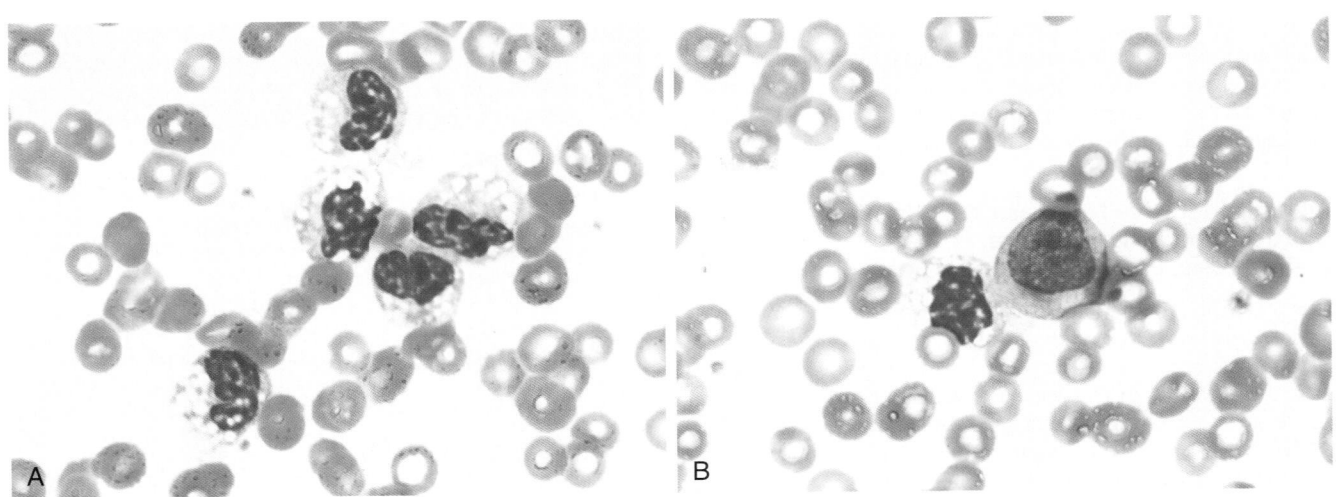

Figure 48-11. Atypical chronic myeloid leukemia: "syndrome of abnormal chromatin clumping" variant. A and **B,** Peripheral blood smear shows marked granulocytic dysplasia, with abnormally lobated nuclei, clumped chromatin, and immature neutrophils.

are characterized in the blood and bone marrow by a high percentage of neutrophils and precursors, with exaggerated clumping of the nuclear chromatin (Fig. 48-11).

Immunophenotype

No specific immunophenotypic characteristics have been reported. By multiparameter flow cytometry, however, asynchronous expression of maturation antigens on the myeloblasts and maturing granulocytes, similar to that reported in MPNs and MDS, would be expected. Similarly, there is abnormal (decreased) side-angle light scatter properties caused by the hypogranular cytoplasm of granulocytes. Immunohistochemistry may be helpful in some cases. CD14 and CD163 may highlight increased monocytic cells, which if present, should call into question an alternative diagnosis such as CMML. CD61 may facilitate recognition of small, dysplastic megakaryocytes.

Cytogenetics/Molecular Findings

Karyotypic abnormalities are reported in up to 80% of patients with aCML.[3] The most common chromosome abnormalities include trisomy 8 and del(20q), but deletions involving chromosomes 12, 13, 14, and 17 are also seen. It is important to note that a recurrent genetic abnormality that implicates a different disease should *not* be seen in aCML. Examples include BCR::ABL1, rearrangements of PDGFRA, PDGFRB, FGFR1, JAK2, FLT3, and ABL1, and rearrangements of KMT2A.

JAK2 mutations are very uncommon and should prompt consideration of an MPN.[1,72,73] Similarly, the detection of a CSF3R mutation should prompt strong consideration of chronic neutrophilic leukemia. Recurrent mutations in genes reported in confirmed cases of aCML include SETBP1, ETNK1,[74-76] ASXL1, TET2, and NRAS; in most cases, there is >1 mutation.[67] The majority of SETBP1 missense mutations in aCML are reported to occur between codons 858 and 871 and are gain-of-function; they co-occur frequently with mutations in ASXL1 and EZH2. Co-mutation of SETBP1 and SRSF2 has also been reported. Whenever a SRSF2 mutation is detected in a case of aCML, it is not found in association with TET2 mutation. EZH2 co-mutated with ASXL1 or RUNX1 can also be observed.

Clinical Course

Most patients seem to fare poorly, with an overall median survival of 11 to 25 months. Age older than 65 years, female sex, WBC counts greater than 50×10^9/L, severe anemia, and thrombocytopenia are generally considered unfavorable prognostic features.[77] Patients who receive bone marrow transplants may have an improved outcome. In 15% to 40% of patients, aCML evolves to AML, whereas the remainder succumb to bone marrow failure. In addition, mutations in ASXL1, SETBP1, and TET2 genes have been associated with a more aggressive disease.[78]

Differential Diagnosis

Chronic Myelomonocytic Leukemia

The major distinguishing features between CMML and aCML are the percentage of monocytes in the blood (≥10% in CMML and <10% in aCML) and the extreme granulocytic dysplasia seen in most cases of aCML. Differences in the morphologic findings, underlying genetic alterations and overall median survival, argue that CMML and aCML are biologically separate entities. However, in clinical practice, occasional cases arise in which the distinction cannot be made with any degree of confidence. In such instances, denoting the two different differential diagnostic possibilities and perhaps assessing how the morphology plays out over time may help further clarify.

Chronic Myeloid Leukemia (CML), *BCR::ABL1* Positive

aCML (despite the unfortunate similar terminology) is easily distinguished from CML, BCR::ABL1 positive, because the latter, by definition, harbors the Ph chromosome and/or BCR::ABL1 fusion gene, which are not present in aCML. Appropriate cytogenetic or molecular genetic studies should always be performed when either diagnosis is suspected. Morphology can usually readily distinguish between these two disorders. Granulocytic dysplasia is essentially absent in the chronic phase of CML but prominent in aCML. Basophilia may be present in both diseases, but it is usually less than 2% of the PB cells in aCML and greater than

2% in CML. Nevertheless, the accelerated phase of CML may be difficult to distinguish from aCML because dysplasia becomes more noticeable when CML progresses beyond the chronic phase. Cytogenetic/molecular genetic studies to exclude the *BCR::ABL1* fusion gene facilitate the correct diagnosis.

Myeloproliferative Neoplasms, *BCR::ABL1* Negative (Polycythemia Vera, Primary Myelofibrosis, Essential Thrombocythemia)

Cases of MPN, particularly those in accelerated phase and postpolycythemic or post–essential thrombocythemic myelofibrosis, may simulate aCML. A previous history of MPN, the presence of classical MPN-associated features in the bone marrow, and MPN-associated mutations (*JAK2, CALR,* or *MPL*) argue against a diagnosis of aCML.[1,3] Conversely, a diagnosis of aCML is supported by the presence of *SETBP1* or *EZH2* mutations.[79] The presence of a *CSF3R* mutation is very uncommon in aCML and should prompt careful morphologic review for an alternative diagnosis of chronic neutrophilic leukemia or other myeloid neoplasm.

Myelodysplastic Syndrome

Although the dysplasia observed in aCML is similar to that in MDS, the leukocytosis observed in aCML would not be expected in MDS. Rarely, an MDS case can transform to "secondary" aCML during the course of disease, a phenomenon that may be associated with the acquisition of novel gene mutations.[80]

Prognosis and Prognostic Factors

The limited number of cases reported in the literature precludes any definitive statement about disease outcome, but most patients seem to fare poorly, with an overall median survival of 11 to 25 months.[65,67] Age older than 65 years, WBC counts greater than 50×10^9/L, severe anemia, and thrombocytopenia are generally considered unfavorable prognostic features. Patients who receive bone marrow transplants may have an improved outcome. In 15% to 40% of patients, aCML evolves to AML, whereas the remainder succumb to bone marrow failure.[67-69]

MYELODYSPLASTIC/MYELOPROLIFERATIVE NEOPLASM WITH *SF3B1* MUTATION AND THROMBOCYTOSIS (MDS/MPN-*SF3B1*-T)

It has been learned that a distinct subset of cases previously categorized as MDS/MPN with ring sideroblasts and thrombocytosis (platelets $\geq450 \times 10^9$/L) frequently shows mutations in *SF3B1* and that these are highly correlated with the presence of ring sideroblasts. Based on these findings, the ICC recognizes MDS/MPN with *SF3B1* mutation and thrombocytosis (MDS/MPN- *SF3B1*-T) as a distinct diagnostic clinicopathologic entity.[1,3,81-84] The diagnostic criteria for this entity are shown in Box 48-7.

Definition

MDS/MPN-*SF3B1*-T is a clonal hematopoietic stem cell disorder characterized by thrombocytosis and ring sideroblasts in the presence of an *SF3B1* mutation.

Box 48-7 *Diagnostic Criteria for Myelodysplastic/ Myeloproliferative Neoplasm With SF3B1 Mutation and Thrombocytosis (MDS/MPN-SF3B1-T)*

- Thrombocytosis, with platelet count $\geq450 \times 10^9$/L
- Anemia (threshold same as for myelodysplastic syndrome)— (Hb <13 g/dL [males], <12 g/dL [females])
- Blasts <1% in blood and <5% in bone marrow
- Presence of *SF3B1* mutation (variant allele frequency ≥10%), isolated or associated with abnormal cytogenetics and/or other myeloid neoplasm associated mutations
- No history of recent cytotoxic or growth factor therapy that could explain the myelodysplastic/myeloproliferative features
- No *BCR::ABL1* or genetic abnormalities of myeloid/lymphoid neoplasms with eosinophilia and tyrosine kinase gene fusions; no t(3;3)(q21.3;q26.2), inv(3)(q21.3q26.2), or del(5q)*
- No history of myeloproliferative neoplasm, myelodysplastic syndrome, or other myelodysplastic/myeloproliferative neoplasm

*In a case that otherwise meets the diagnostic criteria for myelodysplastic syndrome with del(5q).

Synonyms

Refractory anemia with ring sideroblasts associated with marked thrombocytosis; myelodysplastic/myeloproliferative neoplasm with *SF3B1* mutation and thrombocytosis (WHO 5th edition 2022, Khoury 2022)[13]

Epidemiology

The incidence of MDS/MPN-*SF3B1*-T is unknown, but of myelodysplastic/myeloproliferative neoplasm with ring sideroblasts and thrombocytosis, not otherwise specified (MDS/MPN-RS-T, NOS) appears to represent the vast majority of cases. A median age of 74 years at the time of diagnosis has been reported, which is higher than that in MPNs such as essential thrombocythemia, with a slight female prevalence.

Etiology

The etiology is unknown.

Clinical Findings

Patients may present with symptoms related to the refractory anemia, which is often severe, or to excessive thrombocytosis, with bleeding or thrombosis; in many, the symptoms are related to both abnormalities. Splenomegaly has been reported in about 40% cases, and hepatomegaly may also occur.

Morphology

Blood

The WBC count is usually normal to modestly elevated, and there are no circulating blasts, or if present, they represent less than 1% of PB leukocytes.[82] Macrocytic or normocytic anemia is present, and the red blood cells often show a dimorphic pattern (Fig. 48-12A). Dysplasia is lacking in the neutrophils (Fig. 48-12B). Platelets, by definition, are at

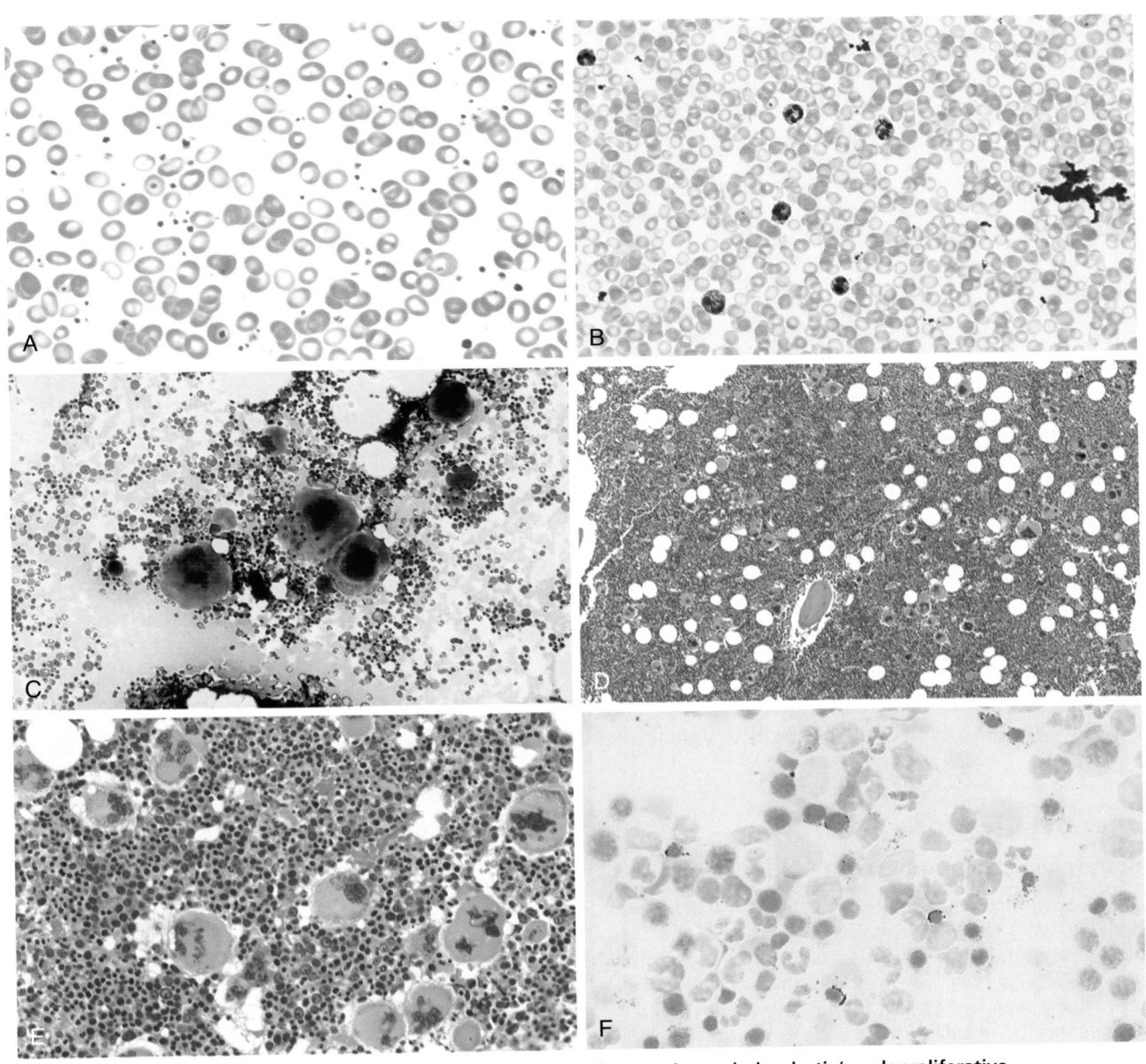

Figure 48-12. Peripheral blood and bone marrow features in myelodysplastic/myeloproliferative neoplasm with *SF3B1* mutation and thrombocytosis (A–F). A, Peripheral blood smear from an 83-year-old man with severe anemia and thrombocytosis of 1048 × 10⁹/L shows abnormal macrocytic hypochromic red cells and a marked increase in platelets, showing anisocytosis. **B,** Peripheral blood smear showing lack of neutrophil dysplasia and marked platelet clumping in the setting of marked thrombocytosis. **C,** Bone marrow aspirate smear demonstrates maturing trilineage hematopoiesis with markedly enlarged megakaryocytes with hyperlobulation with similar morphologic features to those seen in essential thrombocythemia. **D** and **E,** Bone marrow core biopsy shows a hypercellular bone marrow with marked erythroid and megakaryocytic proliferation and megakaryocytes with hyperlobulation and "staghorn-like" nuclei, mimicking essential thrombocythemia. **F,** The majority of sideroblasts are ring sideroblasts.

least 450×10^9/L and may show clumping on the PB smear (Fig. 48-12B).

Bone Marrow

The bone marrow biopsy and aspirate smears are hypercellular and shows increased erythropoiesis often with megaloblastoid features and megakaryopoiesis (Fig. 48-12C–E). The megakaryocytic morphology is distinctive with many enlarged, hyperlobulated, and/or hyperchromatic forms morphologically similar to those seen in ET or primary myelofibrosis (PMF) (Fig. 48-12D and E). Dysplastic-appearing megakaryocytes are unusual and, if present, warrant consideration of an alternative diagnosis such as MDS. Erythropoiesis usually predominates and may be dysplastic, a feature that can best be appreciated in aspirate smears. Though in most cases at least 15% of the erythroid precursors are ring sideroblasts, in the presence of an *SF3B1* mutation ($\geq$10% VAF), the identification of ring sideroblasts is no longer required for the diagnosis (Fig. 48-12F). Blasts represent less than 5% of nucleated cells.

Immunophenotype

There are no specific immunophenotypic features reported.

Cytogenetics and Genetics

No karyotypic abnormality has been specifically associated with this disease, and the overwhelming majority show a normal karyotype. Nearly 50% of patients have the *JAK2* V617F mutation, and a smaller number (<10%) have mutated *MPL* W515K/L or a classic *CALR* mutation.[85-87] By definition, these cases harbor an *SF3B1* mutation, and most also show a co-mutation status with a *JAK2* mutation, which supports this diagnosis.[3,87,88]

Differential Diagnosis

Myelodysplastic Syndrome With *SF3B1* Mutation

In the uncommon instance of MDS-*SF3B1* with thrombocytosis, the morphologic features of the megakaryocytes should be of utility in discriminating these entities. In MDS/MPN-*SF3B1*-T, the megakaryocytes typically resemble those seen in ET or PMF and are not dysplastic as would be expected in MDS-RS. In one study of MDS, *SF3B1* mutated, a significantly higher prevalence of *JAK2* and *MPL* mutations was observed compared with *SF3B1*-unmutated MDS. Though the authors reported that these patients did not fulfill diagnostic criteria for a diagnosis of MDS/MPN-RS-T, it was noted that a significantly higher platelet count was found in patients with *SF3B1*-mutated MDS carrying either *JAK2* or *MPL* mutation compared with those who were co-wild type (P < 0.001).[88] This finding supports consideration of a diagnostic continuum between the two *SF3B1* mutated entities, particularly because cases that initially present as MDS-*SF3B1* but later, upon acquisition of *JAK2* V617F mutation, progress to resemble MDS/MPN-*SF3B1*-T have been documented.[89]

Myeloproliferative Neoplasm With *SF3B1* Mutation

In MPN, *SF3B1* is mutated in approximately 10% of patients with PMF and 3% to 5% with PV or ET.[90,91] It is important for pathologists to recognize that a minor subset of classic *BCR::ABL1*-negative MPNs may harbor this mutation and that ring sideroblasts may also be seen in a subset of cases either at disease presentation or with progression.[91,92] Given that mutations in *JAK2/CALR/MPL* are highly prevalent in MPN, in the rare cases of MPN that harbor a concomitant *SF3B1* mutation, the distinction from MDS/MPN-*SF3B1*-T may be challenging. In the study by Boiocchi et al., the presence of an *SF3B1* mutation in a myeloproliferative neoplasm was not associated with myelodysplastic evolution/progression.[91] Therefore, the absence of a dysplastic component argues in favor of MPN. In addition, the absence or low percentage of ring sideroblasts (<15%) supports a diagnosis of a classic MPN.[92] The presence of anemia, often macrocytic and associated with marrow erythroid predominance in MDS/MPN-*SF3B1*-T, would also argue against a diagnosis of ET with ring sideroblasts.

Prognosis and Prognostic Factors

In general, MDS/MPN-*SF3B1*-T shows an overall better median survival than MDS/MPN-RS-T, NOS (6.9 vs. 3.3 years, P = 0.003, respectively).[93] *JAK2* mutations are also independent factors for better prognosis. It is important to note that patients with MDS/MPN-RS-T do not fare as well as those with ET, who may have a near-normal life span if appropriately managed.[93] Thus, the distinction between these disorders is important from clinical, biological, and prognostic points of view.

MYELODYSPLASTIC/MYELOPROLIFERATIVE NEOPLASM WITH RING SIDEROBLASTS AND THROMBOCYTOSIS, NOT OTHERWISE SPECIFIED (MDS/MPN-RS-T, NOS)

There are less frequent cases of MDS/MPN with thrombocytosis and >15% ring sideroblasts that lack a *SF3B1* mutation. In such cases, the ICC determines that designation as MDS/MPN-RS-T, NOS is appropriate. The diagnostic criteria for this entity are shown in Box 48-8. Both thrombocytosis and anemia must be present at the time of initial diagnosis. In addition, the presence of anemia that is thought to be related to the hematologic malignancy argues against classification as ET with ring sideroblasts. The clinical and morphologic features are apparently similar to MDS/MPN-T-*SF3B1*, although at least 15% ring sideroblasts are required. In terms of prognosis, in a multivariate analysis, age older than 80 years at diagnosis, *SF3B1* wild type, and *JAK2* wild type were independent factors of a worse prognosis.[93] Also, an *SF3B1* wild-type profile is more common in males (23.1%) than in females (5.1%), and mean ring sideroblast counts are lower than in *SF3B1* mutated cases (38% vs. 55%).[93]

Differential Diagnosis

Myeloproliferative Neoplasm With Ring Sideroblasts; *SF3B1* Mutation Negative

In the uncommon scenario of an MPN with ring sideroblasts, the percentage of ring sideroblasts is expected to be low (<15%), and dysplasia would be absent.

> **Box 48-8** *Diagnostic Criteria for Myelodysplastic/Myeloproliferative Neoplasm With Ring Sideroblasts and Thrombocytosis, Not Otherwise Specified (MDS/MPN-RS-T, NOS)*
>
> - Thrombocytosis, with platelet count ≥450 × 10⁹/L
> - Anemia associated with erythroid-lineage dysplasia, with or without multilineage dysplasia, and ≥15% ring sideroblasts
> - Blasts <1% in blood and <5% in bone marrow
> - Presence of clonality: demonstration of a clonal cytogenetic abnormality and/or somatic mutation(s). In their absence, no history of recent cytotoxic or growth factor therapy that could explain the myelodysplastic/myeloproliferative features
> - Absence of *SF3B1* mutation; no *BCR::ABL1* or genetic abnormalities of myeloid/lymphoid neoplasms with eosinophilia and tyrosine kinase gene fusions; no t(3;3) (q21.3;q26.2), inv(3) (q21.3q26.2), or del(5q)*
> - No history of myeloproliferative neoplasm, myelodysplastic syndrome, or other myelodysplastic/myeloproliferative neoplasm
>
> *In a case that otherwise meets the diagnostic criteria for myelodysplastic syndrome with del(5q).

> **Box 48-9** *Diagnostic Criteria for Myelodysplastic/Myeloproliferative Neoplasm, Not Otherwise Specified (MDS/MPN, NOS)*
>
> - Myeloid neoplasm with mixed myeloproliferative and myelodysplastic features, not meeting the International Consensus Classification (ICC) criteria for any other myelodysplastic/myeloproliferative neoplasm, myelodysplastic syndrome, or myeloproliferative neoplasm*
> - Cytopenia (thresholds same as for myelodysplastic syndrome [MDS])†—anemia, Hb <13 g/dL [males], <12 g/dL [females]; neutropenia, absolute neutrophil count <1.8 × 10⁹/L; thrombocytopenia, platelets <150 × 10⁹/L)
> - Blasts <20% of the cells in blood and bone marrow
> - A platelet count of ≥450 × 10⁹/L and/or a white blood cell count of ≥13 × 10⁹/L
> - Presence of clonality: demonstration of a clonal cytogenetic abnormality and/or somatic mutation(s). If clonality cannot be determined, the findings have persisted and all other causes (e.g., history of cytotoxic or growth factor therapy or other primary causes that could explain the myelodysplastic/myeloproliferative features) have been excluded.
> - No *BCR::ABL1* or genetic abnormalities of myeloid/lymphoid neoplasms with eosinophilia and tyrosine kinase gene fusions; absence of t(3;3)(q21.3;q26.2), inv(3) (q21.3q26.2),‡ or del(5q)§
>
> *Myeloproliferative neoplasms, in particular those in accelerated phase and/or post–polycythemia vera or post–essential thrombocythemia myelofibrotic stage, may simulate MDS/MPN, NOS. A history of MPN and/or the presence of MPN-associated mutations (in *JAK2, CALR*, or *MPL*), particularly if associated with a high variant allele frequency, tend to exclude a diagnosis of MDS/MPN, NOS. The presence of hypereosinophilia would favor a diagnosis of chronic eosinophilic leukemia, not otherwise specified.
> †Based on International Consensus Group Conference, Vienna, 2018 (Valent et al., 2019).
> ‡In a case that otherwise meets criteria for myelodysplastic syndrome, not otherwise specified.
> §In a case that otherwise meets the diagnostic criteria for myelodysplastic syndrome with isolated del(5q).

MYELODYSPLASTIC/MYELOPROLIFERATIVE NEOPLASM, NOT OTHERWISE SPECIFIED (MDS/MPN, NOS)

When patients exhibit features that do not easily fit into any existing subcategory of the MDS/MPN disease types or any other myeloid malignancy, subclassification as MDS/MPN, NOS, is justified.[1,94,95] However, the term NOS should *only* be used when the appropriate clinical, morphologic, immunophenotypic, and genetic studies have been performed to determine that the disease truly does not fit a well-defined category. This subcategory is essentially a diagnosis of exclusion, as reflected in the diagnostic criteria (Box 48-9).

In MDS/MPN, NOS, by definition, cases must satisfy criteria for both MDS and MPN, (truly an overlap syndrome), and must not meet criteria for any other MDS/MPN subtype or myeloid malignancy (Box 48-9). As expected, the finding of a *BCR::ABL1* fusion gene or rearrangements of *PDGFRA, PDGFRB, FGFR1, JAK2, FLT3*, or *ABL1* excludes the diagnosis of MDS/MPN, NOS. In addition, the presence of a mutation in *JAK2, CALR*, or *MPL* should raise the possibility of an alternative diagnosis of MPN.

The designation of "NOS" must not be applied to patients with MPNs who have dyspoietic features/cytopenias as a consequence of therapy or disease progression. This category should not be used for advanced-stage MPN or triple-negative MPN cases. If the patient has received any growth factor or cytotoxic therapy before the initial diagnostic evaluation, additional clinical and laboratory studies are essential to prove that the dyspoietic or proliferative features are not related to the therapy.

MYELODYSPLASTIC/MYELOPROLIFERATIVE NEOPLASM WITH ISOLATED ISOCHROMOSOME (17q) (MDS/MPM WITH I[17q]; ICC PROVISIONAL SUBENTITY)

MDS/MPN with i(17q) is a provisional subentity under the category of MDS/MPN, NOS.[3,4] These neoplasms are rare and are often associated with hybrid myelodysplastic/myeloproliferative features, hence their inclusion in this overarching category.

The diagnostic criteria are outlined in Box 48-10.

Definition

MDS/MPN with i(17q) is a clonal hematopoietic stem cell disorder with features of both a myelodysplastic and myeloproliferative neoplasm with a characteristic cytogenetic abnormality of isochromosome 17q and/or one additional chromosomal abnormality, excluding an abnormality of chromosome 7 (del 7q/monosomy 7).

Epidemiology

The incidence of this disease is unknown.

Etiology

The etiology is unknown.

Clinical Findings

The average age at presentation is 67 years with an approximately equal male-to-female distribution. Spleno-megaly is quite frequent at approximately 70%.

Box 48-10 *Diagnostic Criteria for Myelodysplastic/Myeloproliferative Neoplasm With Isolated Isochromosome (17q) [MDS/MPN with i(17q)]**

Fulfills the general criteria for a diagnosis of MDS/MPN, NOS
- Leukocytosis of ≥13 × 10⁹/L
- Cytopenia (thresholds same as for myelodysplastic syndrome [MDS])† —(anemia, Hb <13 g/dL [males], <12 g/dL [females]; neutropenia, absolute neutrophil count <1.8 × 10⁹/L; thrombocytopenia, platelets <150 × 10⁹/L)
- Blasts <20% of the cells in blood and bone marrow
- Dysgranulopoiesis with non-segmented or Pseudo–Pelger-Huët neutrophils
- An i(17q), either isolated or occurring with one other additional abnormality (other than –7/del[7q])
- No BCR::ABL1 or genetic abnormalities of myeloid/lymphoid neoplasms with eosinophilia and tyrosine kinase gene fusions
- Absence of myeloproliferative neoplasm–associated mutations (JAK2, CALR, and MPL)‡
- No history of recent cytotoxic or growth factor therapy that could explain the MDS/MPN features

*MDS/MPN with i(17q) is considered a provisional subentity of MDS/MPN, NOS.
†Based on International Consensus Group Conference, Vienna, 2018 (Valent et al., 2019).
‡Presence of MPN features in the bone marrow and/or MPN-associated mutations (in JAK2, CALR, or MPL) suggests progression of an underlying MPN that was not diagnosed and should be excluded; conversely, in the appropriate clinical context, presence of mutations, particularly co-existent mutation in SRSF2 and SETBP1 genes, further supports this diagnosis.

Morphology

Blood

At initial presentation, leukocytosis and anemia are prevalent. By definition, there is no monocytosis (≤10% monocytes). In one multiinstitutional study, 79% of the patients had leukocytosis (WBC ≥13 × 10⁹/L) and 25% had thrombocytosis (platelet count ≥450 × 10⁹/L). Every patient had anemia (Hgb <12 g/dL). Neutrophils typically show distinctive and prevalent dysplastic features characterized strongly by nonlobated or hypolobated pseudo–Pelger-Huët nuclei and cytoplasmic hypogranulation (Fig. 48-13A and B). There are less than 20% blasts in the PB.

Bone Marrow

The bone marrow is typically hypercellular with abundant pseudo–Pelger-Huët neutrophils in bone marrow, as seen in the PB.[96-98] Dysplastic-appearing megakaryocytes may be seen in some cases, characterized by micromegakaryocytes, hypolobated/monolobated forms, and forms with separate distinct nuclear lobes. Ring sideroblasts are uncommon (Fig. 48-13C–F). There are less than 20% blasts in the bone marrow. Bone marrow fibrosis may be seen but is not more prevalent than in cases of MDS/MPN, NOS without i(17q).

Genetics

By definition, these cases harbor an isochromosome 17q resulting in a TP53 gene deletion. In a study evaluating molecular genetic alterations using NGS technology, this provisional entity was noted to have an increased frequency of mutations in SRSF2, SETBP1, and ASXL1 genes. Double mutations involving SRSF2 and SETBP1 were seen in 44% of cases.[99] The genetic signatures show overlap with aCML and somewhat with CMML—supporting some similarities in their pathogenesis.

One interesting finding is that, although there is a TP53 deletion by cytogenetics, an additional TP53 mutation was not significantly detected in these neoplasms. Thus, these cases appear to be characterized, for the most part, by a monoallelic TP53 mutation state; the remaining TP53 allele is wild type. FISH and array comparative genomic hybridization/single nucleotide polymorphism (aCGH/SNP) studies performed on a subset of cases confirmed the heterozygous nature of the TP53 deletion and absence of copy-neutral loss of heterozygosity, confirming monoallelic TP53 alteration.[99]

Prognosis

The prognosis for patients with chronic myeloid neoplasms with i(17q) is adverse, with an overall median survival of approximately 11 months.[99] There is a high rate of transformation to AML.[98,100,101] Given these findings, it is thought to be important to annotate these cases specifically, such that an ongoing prospective evaluation of these cases may be performed.

Differential Diagnosis

The differential diagnosis, based on clinical, morphology, and laboratory features, could include CMML, MPN, aCML, and MDS/MPN, NOS. Overall, perhaps one of the initial discriminating clues to a homogenous entity is presence of the i(17q) genetic abnormality. There is genetic overlap with the aforementioned disorders (CMML with mutations in TET2, SRSF2, ASXL1, or CBL and aCML with mutations in ASXL1, SETBP1, and SRSF2). CMML should, however, show monocytosis by definition, and although it may occur, striking dysgranulopoiesis is relatively uncommon. Presence of MPN features in the bone marrow and/or MPN-associated mutations (in JAK2, CALR, or MPL) suggests progression of an underlying MPN that was not diagnosed and should be excluded. Though there is definite overlap with aCML, which arguably serves the primary diagnostic challenge, the high frequency of co-mutations in SRSF2 and SETBP1 genes observed in one study may help in supporting a diagnosis MDS/MPN with i(17q).[99] In summary, at the present time, the finding of i(17q) in the otherwise appropriate clinical and morphologic context would favor subclassification as the provisional subentity of MDS/MPN with i(17q).

Acknowledgments

The authors graciously appreciate and acknowledge the work of the prior authors, Drs. James Vardiman and Elizabeth Hyjek, that has inspired and contributed significantly to this updated chapter.

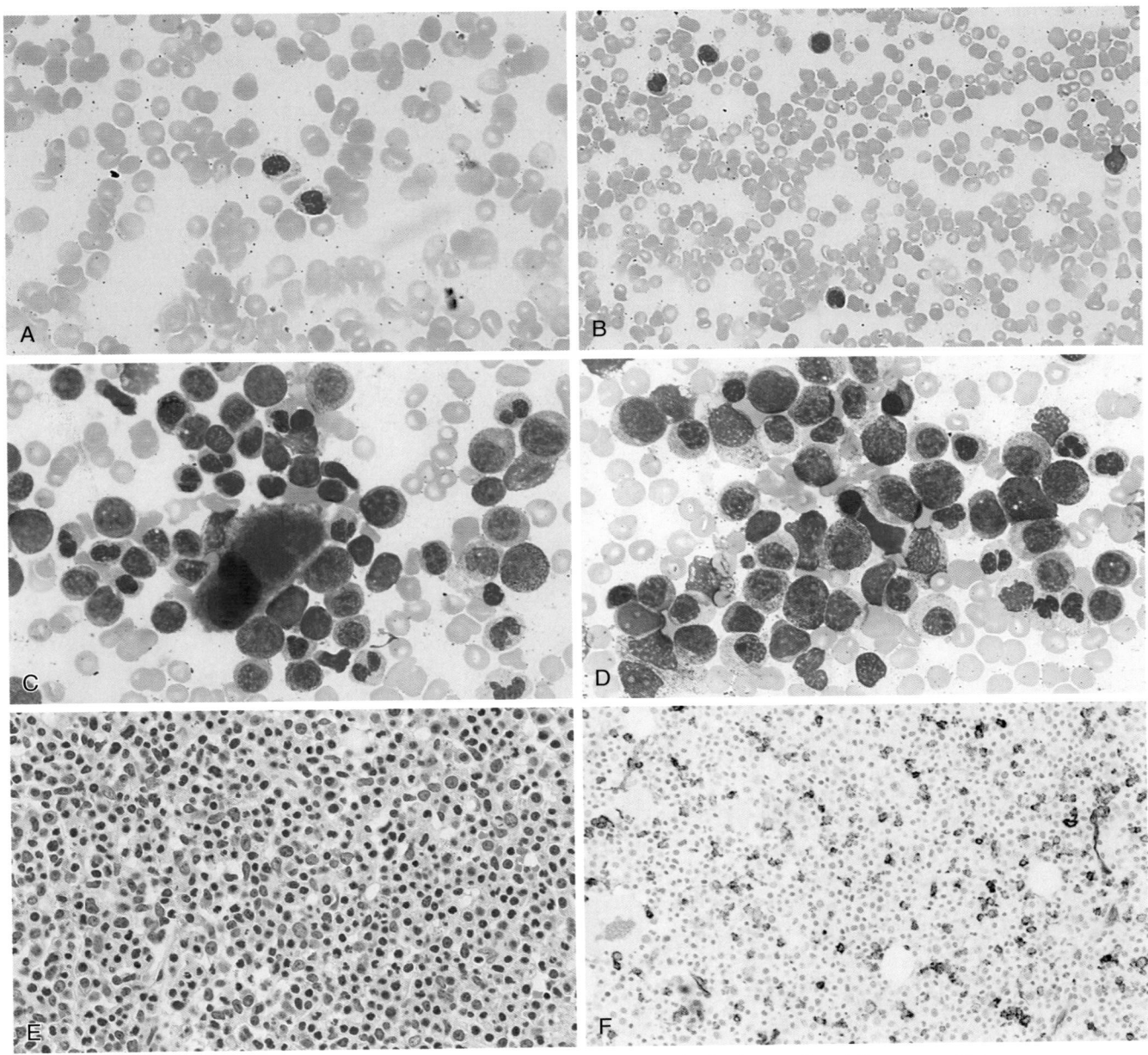

Figure 48-13. Peripheral blood and bone marrow features in the International Consensus Classification (ICC) provisional subentity myelodysplastic/myeloproliferative neoplasm with isochromosome (17q) (A–F). A, Dysplastic granulocytes showing Pelger-Huet-like nuclei with condensed chromatin and hypogranular cytoplasm are common. **B,** Many patients will have absolute monocytosis with abnormal appearing yet mature monocytes. In the illustrated case, a circulating blast can be seen on the *right-hand side* of the photomicrograph. **C** and **D,** Aspirate smears are hypercellular with a granulocytic proliferation and marked dysplasia and dysmegakaryopoiesis. **E,** Bone marrow core biopsy shows granulocytic proliferation; even the dysplasia can be appreciated on the section. **F,** Immunohistochemical staining for CD34 demonstrates an increase in CD34-positive blasts.

Pearls and Pitfalls

- All the MDS/MPN entities and their subtypes are *BCR::ABL1*-negative myeloid neoplasms. Their blast count is less than 20%.
- A diagnosis of MDS/MPN requires, in almost all instances, both proliferative (i.e. cytosis/es) and dysplastic/cytopenic features being present at disease presentation.
- CMML should be subclassified as either the myelodysplastic or myeloproliferative subtype, depending on the WBC count at presentation.
- Distinguishing monoblasts, promonocytes, and abnormal monocytes is essential for the diagnosis of CMML and its (lower) blast count versus AML.
- Reactive monocytosis is much more common than CMML.
- Rearrangement of *KMT2A* or an *NPM1* mutation should prompt rereview of a case thought to be CMML (to exclude AML).
- Cases of CMML are enriched for mutations in the *TET2, ASXL1,* and *SRSF2* genes.
- If there is no significant myeloid dysplasia, no clonal myeloid-related cytogenetic abnormality, no significant increase in blasts, and monocytosis is persistent and unexplained, in the setting of a molecular genetic abnormality, a premalignant condition associated with monocytosis could be considered.
- CMUS is a CMML precursor condition that can be diagnosed in patients with persistent monocytosis (monocytes ≥10% and ≥0.5 × 10^9/L of the WBC), presence of myeloid neoplasm-associated mutation(s) and absence of bone marrow morphologic findings of CMML.
- In cases of CMUS in which a cytopenia(s) is also present, the terminology of CCMUS is suggested.
- Eosinophilia in what looks like an MDS/MPN should always prompt the consideration of rearrangement of *PDGFRA, PDGFRB, FGFR1, JAK2, FLT3,* and *ABL1*.
- aCML is a rare entity characterized by neutrophilic leukocytosis associated with dysgranulopoiesis and circulating immature neutrophilic precursors. Abnormal nuclear chromatin clumping of neutrophils is also a feature.
- It is important to enumerate monocytes and eosinophils carefully because they are a key feature in distinguishing aCML from CMML.
- Eosinophils should not be prominent in aCML and should account for <10% and <1.5 × 10^9/L of the leukocytes.
- In MDS/MPN, NOS, by definition, cases must satisfy criteria for both MDS and MPN (truly an overlap syndrome), and must not meet criteria for any other MDS/MPN subtype or myeloid malignancy. In particular, such cases should not represent accelerated phase and/or post–PV or post–ET myelofibrotic stages. A history of MPN and/or the presence of MPN-associated mutations (in *JAK2, CALR,* or *MPL*), particularly if associated with a high VAF, should call into question a diagnosis of MDS/MPN, NOS.
- MDS/MPN with i(17q) is a provisional subentity under the category of MDS/MPN, NOS. Neutrophils typically show distinctive and prevalent dysplastic features characterized strongly by pseudo–Pelger-Huët nuclei and cytoplasmic hypogranulation. Molecular genetic overlap with CMML with mutations in *TET2, SRSF2, ASXL1,* and aCML with mutations in *ASXL1, SETBP1,* and *SRSF2* can be seen.

KEY REFERENCES

3. Arber DA, Orazi A, Hasserjian RP, et al. International consensus classification of myeloid neoplasms and acute leukemias: integrating morphologic, clinical, and genomic data. *Blood.* 2022;140(11):1200–1228.
4. Prakash S, Arber DA, Bueso-Ramos C, Hasserjian RP, Orazi A. Advances in myelodysplastic/myeloproliferative neoplasms. *Virchows Arch.* 2022;482(1):69–83.
34. van de Loosdrecht AA, Kern W, Porwit A, et al. Clinical application of flow cytometry in patients with unexplained cytopenia and suspected myelodysplastic syndrome: a report of the European LeukemiaNet International MDS-Flow Cytometry Working Group. *Cytometry B Clin Cytom.* 2021.
36. Selimoglu-Buet D, Wagner-Ballon O, Saada V, Francophone Myelodysplasia Group, et al. Characteristic repartition of monocyte subsets as a diagnostic signature of chronic myelomonocytic leukemia. *Blood.* 2015;125(23):3618–3626.
86. Patnaik MM, Lasho TL. Genomics of myelodysplastic syndrome/myeloproliferative neoplasm overlap syndromes. *Hematology Am Soc Hematol Educ Program.* 2020;2020(1):450–459.
91. Boiocchi L, Hasserjian RP, Pozdnyakova O, et al. Clinicopathological and molecular features of SF3B1-mutated myeloproliferative neoplasms. *Hum Pathol.* 2019;86:1–11.
96. McClure RF, Dewald GW, Hoyer JD, et al. Isolated isochromosome 17q: a distinct type of mixed myeloproliferative disorder/myelodysplastic syndrome with an aggressive clinical course. *Br J Haematol.* 1999;106(2):445–454.
99. Kanagal-Shamanna R, Orazi A, Hasserjian RP, et al. Myelodysplastic/myeloproliferative neoplasms-unclassifiable with isolated isochromosome 17q represents a distinct clinico-biologic subset: a multi-institutional collaborative study from the Bone Marrow Pathology Group. *Mod Pathol.* 2022;35(4):470–479.

Visit Elsevier eBooks+ for the complete set of references.

Chapter 49

Mastocytosis

Alexandar Tzankov, Karl Sotlar, Peter Valent,
Hans-Peter Horny, and Tracy I. George

The most common subtype of cutaneous mastocytosis (CM), termed at that time *urticaria pigmentosa* (UP), was first described in the 19th century, a decade before mast cells (MCs) were defined by Paul Ehrlich as metachromatic cells of the connective tissue.[1,2] In 1949, the first histologic proof of involvement of visceral organs by mastocytosis was reported.[3] Since that time, many terms have been introduced to describe mastocytosis. These terms are now obsolete and should no longer be used (e.g., generalized mastocytosis, malignant mastocytosis, aleukemic or subacute basophilic mastocytoma or leukemia, UP with bone involvement or with systemic lesions, and eosinophilic fibrohistiocytic lesion of the bone marrow [BM]).[4-10] Various classification systems for mastocytosis have been proposed and finally established.[11-15] During the past 3 decades, major discoveries have led to both a better understanding of the pathophysiologic processes involved in the evolution of mastocytosis and clarification of the nosology of this group of diseases. Using an animal model, Kitamura and coworkers[16] demonstrated that MCs are of hematopoietic origin. Later, the hematopoietic origin of MCs was confirmed for other species, including humans.[17-22] Evidence has also accumulated from extensive histologic and cytologic studies that the BM and the skin are the preferred sites of involvement in human mastocytosis, that MCs share some histochemical properties with other cells of the myeloid lineage, and that systemic mastocytosis (SM) may be associated with myeloid (non-MC) neoplasms.[23-26] It has also been demonstrated that human MCs differentiate under the influence of stem cell factor, also known as MC growth factor, a cytokine that binds to the KIT (CD117) tyrosine kinase receptor, also known as KIT-ligand, and that MCs arise from a BM-derived CD34-positive, KIT-positive progenitor cell.[19-22] As far as the diagnosis of mastocytosis is concerned, immunohistochemical markers such as tryptase, CD2, CD25, CD30, and KIT/CD117 are well established.[27-32] Finally, recurrent activating somatic point mutations in certain regions of the *KIT* proto-oncogene, especially *KIT* D816V, have been detected in MCs in tissue infiltrates of SM.[33-35] Altogether, these findings clearly indicate that SM is a BM-derived myeloid neoplasm exhibiting an unusually broad clinical and morphologic spectrum of disorders. A consensus classification of mastocytosis was initially proposed at the Year 2000 Working Conference on Mastocytosis in Vienna, Austria.[35] This consensus classification was adopted by the World Health Organization (WHO) classification in 2001 and in 2008 and refined in 2017 in the revised WHO classification.[36-38] In 2022, both the International Consensus Classification (ICC) and the proposed WHO 5th edition further modified diagnostic criteria for SM.[12,13] These updates are essentially based on clinical studies and the outcomes of the Year 2020 Working Conference on Mastocytosis in Vienna, Austria.[39]

DEFINITION

Mastocytosis is characterized by an abnormal accumulation of MCs in various organ systems. Two main categories of disease exist: a) CM, which involves only the skin; and b) SM, which by definition involves at least one extracutaneous organ, most commonly the BM. CM and SM include an array of heterogeneous disorders that nevertheless constitute a discrete group among the hematologic diseases (Box 49-1). These diseases range from benign and regressing solitary mastocytomas in children to aggressive MC leukemias, predominantly in adults. Hence, whereas it is probable that all variants of SM and most adult patients with CM have true neoplasms, it is not clear whether this also holds true for all children with CM, as approximately 40% show spontaneous regression of symptoms at puberty, and not all CM cases present with *KIT* mutations.

SYNONYMS AND RELATED TERMS

None.

GENERAL ASPECTS

Mastocytosis can occur at any age and presents with an unusually broad spectrum of symptoms. Among these, disseminated red-brown macules and papules that become red and swollen on rubbing or scratching (Darier's sign) are almost pathognomonic of maculopapular CM (MPCM; formerly termed UP, which is the most common variant of CM. However, the same skin lesions are also seen frequently in indolent SM (ISM).[40] On the other hand, absence of skin lesions does not exclude the presence of SM. In contrast to patients with CM, most patients with SM have elevated levels of serum tryptase, which is produced almost exclusively by normal and neoplastic MCs and can be used to monitor patients with confirmed SM.[41]

Elevated serum tryptase is thus an important sign of an underlying SM. However, elevated serum tryptase can also be detected in individuals with a recently described autosomal dominant genetic condition, hereditary alpha tryptasemia (HαT), which is characterized by increased copies of the *TPSAB1* gene encoding for α-tryptase and affects 4% to 6% of the general population.[42,43] Interestingly, HαT is two to three times more common in patients with SM than in healthy individuals, and *Hymenoptera* venom hypersensitivity reactions and severe anaphylaxis is by far more frequent in patients with mastocytosis with HαT than in those without HαT.[44,45] An important practical aspect in that consideration is noted in the proposed WHO 5th edition classification,[13] which prescribes serum tryptase to be adjusted in HαT, following the proposal of the 2020 consensus group.[39] Although the optimal adjustment remains to be defined, it is suggested to divide the basal tryptase level by 1 plus the extra copy numbers of the *TPSAB1* gene, e.g. when the tryptase level is 30 and two extra copies of the gene are found in a patient with HαT, the HαT-corrected tryptase level is 10 (30/3 = 10) and thus not a minor SM criterion.[39]

Patients with advanced SM, defined as MC leukemia (MCL), aggressive SM (ASM), or SM with an associated myeloid/hematologic neoplasm (AMN/AHN) may have marked (palpable) hepatosplenomegaly and generalized lymphadenopathy, ascites, weight loss, and/or signs of malabsorption; rarely, they may also have larger (i.e., ≥2 cm) osteolyses.[14,36-39] A significant number of patients with SM, many of them with ASM, have an AHN; most of the AMNs have been proven to be of the same clonal origin as the neoplastic MCs, though those of the lymphoid were not.[46,47] For this reason, the ICC 2022 is not as restrictive and only includes SM with an AMN for this category.[12] A definitive diagnosis of mastocytosis can be made only based on a histopathologic analysis of tissue specimens (particularly BM), including immunostaining with antibodies against tryptase, KIT/CD117, CD25, and CD30; it should not be based on clinical and serologic findings alone.[14,29-32,39,48-50]

Box 49-1 *International Consensus Classification (ICC) and Proposed World Health Organization (WHO) 5th Edition Classification of Mastocytosis*

ICC 2022	Proposed WHO 5th Edition

• Cutaneous mastocytosis
  • Urticaria pigmentosa/maculopapular cutaneous mastocytosis
  • Diffuse cutaneous mastocytosis
  • Mastocytoma of skin
• Systemic mastocytosis
  • Indolent systemic mastocytosis (includes bone marrow mastocytosis)
  • Smoldering systemic mastocytosis
  • Aggressive systemic mastocytosis
  • Mast cell leukemia
  • Systemic mastocytosis with an associated myeloid neoplasm
• Mast cell sarcoma
	• Cutaneous mastocytosis
	  • Urticaria pigmentosa/maculopapular cutaneous mastocytosis
	    • Monomorphic
	    • Polymorphic
	  • Diffuse cutaneous mastocytosis
	  • Cutaneous mastocytoma
	    • Isolated mastocytoma
	    • Multilocalized mastocytoma
	• Systemic mastocytosis
	  • Bone marrow mastocytosis
	  • Indolent systemic mastocytosis
	  • Smoldering systemic mastocytosis
	  • Aggressive systemic mastocytosis
	  • Systemic mastocytosis with an associated hematologic neoplasm
	  • Mast cell leukemia
	  • Mast cell sarcoma

Data from Arber DA, Orazi A, Hasserjian RP, et al. International Consensus Classification of myeloid neoplasms and acute leukemias: integrating morphologic, clinical, and genomic data. *Blood*. 2022;140:1200; Khoury JD, Solary E, Abla O, et al. The 5th edition of the World Health Organization classification of haematolymphoid tumours: myeloid and histiocytic/dendritic neoplasms. *Leukemia*. 2022;36:1703; Valent P, Akin C, Hartmann K, et al. Updated diagnostic criteria and classification of mast cell disorders: a consensus proposal. *HemaSphere*. 2021;5:e646.

EPIDEMIOLOGY AND ETIOLOGY

Mastocytosis is a rare disease, especially the systemic variants. MCL is one of the rarest forms of human leukemia, with a few hundred well-documented cases reported to date.[51-56] The exact incidence of mastocytosis is unknown, and similar to other rare hematologic disorders, the apparent incidence may vary according to the experience of clinicians and pathologists.[57] There is a slight male predominance. Disease onset generally occurs either during the first year of life, when most cases of CM develop, or during adulthood, with a peak in the 5th and 6th decades, accounting for most cases of SM. In many cases with ISM without skin involvement, the disease may not be detected or is detected by chance (occult SM). In many of these cases, (isolated) BM mastocytosis (BMM) may be diagnosed. Whereas BMM has previously been described as a provisional subset of ISM,[14] BMM is recognized in the proposed WHO 5th edition[13] as a distinct variant of SM based on its unique clinical features and a more favorable prognosis than that of ISM.[39,58] BMM is considered a subtype of ISM in the ICC 2022.[12]

The cause of mastocytosis is unknown. Very rare familial cases have been reported, which particularly applies to a distinct morphologic subvariant of SM characterized by early onset, diffuse cutaneous involvement, specific phenotype with absent to low expression of CD2 and CD25, consistent high expression of CD30, a female predominance of 4:1, childhood disease onset in >90% and wild-type *KIT* or *KIT* variant mutations; this subvariant is termed SM with well-differentiated mast cells (WDSM).[59]

POSTULATED CELL OF ORIGIN AND NORMAL COUNTERPART

Normal MCs are phenotypically more closely related to myeloid cells than to lymphoid cells. However, in SM, MCs often display lymphoid marker antigens, such as CD2, CD25, or CD30.[14,29-32,39,48-50] Nevertheless, SM, irrespective of subtype, is considered a myeloid neoplasm that evolves from neoplastic CD34-positive hematopoietic stem cells, which give rise to MC-committed precursor cells and neoplastic MCs.[60] The cell of origin in CM is also considered to be an MC-committed stem and precursor cell, although the exact source organ from which these cells invade the skin remains uncertain. Pointing toward the myeloid origin of MCs in CM, at least in a group of mainly adult patients with CM, BM involvement is demonstrable, even if the full criteria to diagnose SM are not fulfilled.[40]

There is considerable morphologic overlap between basophils and MCs, but these are distinctly different cell types.[17,18] Both are the only myeloid cells that contain intracytoplasmic metachromatic granules and are therefore usually recognizable on certain histochemical stains, such as Giemsa and toluidine blue. Mature MCs do not circulate and are found predominantly in the perivascular connective tissue. The differentiation and maturation of MCs usually occur at extramedullary sites.[17,18,61,62] In contrast to MCs, basophils differentiate in the BM, circulate as mature leukocytes, and finally migrate into the perivascular tissues. Also, basophils have an estimated life span of only a few days, whereas MCs exhibit a life span of several months to years.[61,63] Although mature MCs and basophils can be differentiated from each other on BM smears, neoplastic metachromatic cells (including metachromatic blasts or immature mast cells) may exhibit marked atypia, making it almost impossible to clearly distinguish between basophils and neoplastic MCs by morphologic examination. The metachromatic granules of basophils, unlike those of MCs, are water soluble so that basophils, whether normal, reactive, or neoplastic, are undetectable by the pathologist in routinely processed tissue specimens. However, basophil-specific monoclonal antibodies, namely 2D7 and BB1, are applicable to formalin-fixed, paraffin-embedded tissues, and basophils do not express KIT/CD117.[64,65] A summary of the most important phenotypic differences between MCs and basophils is provided in Table 49-1.

GENETICS AND MOLECULAR FINDINGS

Various mutations of the *KIT* proto-oncogene and other genetic defects have been shown to result in stem cell

Table 49-1 Major Phenotypic Features Distinguishing Between Mast Cells and Basophils*

Marker	Mast Cells	Basophils
Metachromasia/ Giemsa	++/+++	–[†]
CAE	++/+++	–
Tryptase	+++	–/+/+[‡]
Chymase	++/+	–
CD2	++[§]	–
CD9	++	++[¶]
CD25	+++[§]	+[¶]
CD30	+/++[§]	–
CD34	–	–
CD45	+++	+++
CD68	+++	–
CD117 (KIT)	+++/++	–
2D7	–	++/+
BB1	–	++/+

*Histologic distinction in routinely processed (formalin-fixed) tissues, including bone marrow trephine biopsy specimens. Phenotypic expression by flow cytometry is present for the following markers used in routine clinical practice: CD2, CD9, CD25, CD34, CD45, and CD117. CD9 is expressed in normal basophils by flow cytometry, and CD25 is dimly expressed in normal basophils by flow cytometry.
[†]Unlike in smears, basophils contain no metachromatic granules in sections.
[‡]Expression is inconsistent and occurs only in neoplastic states (e.g., in chronic myeloid leukemia).
[§]Expressed in mast cells only in neoplastic states (mastocytosis); CD2 expression by flow cytometry on mast cells is more sensitive than immunohistochemistry.
[¶]CD9 is expressed in normal basophils by flow cytometry, and CD25 is dimly expressed in normal basophils by flow cytometry.
+++, Strong expression (strong staining of virtually all cells); ++, moderate expression (moderate staining of most cells); +, weak expression (weak staining of a minority of cells); –, no specific staining of cells.
CAE, Naphthol AS-D chloroacetate esterase.

factor–independent activation of KIT and KIT-downstream signaling pathways.[66] One of these point mutations, *KIT* D816V, was first described by Furitsu and associates in HMC-1 cells derived from a patient with MCL.[33] Most of the mutations described in patients with mastocytosis cluster in exons 11 and 17. The most frequently detected mutation is *KIT* D816V. In rare cases, mutations in other exons have been described (Table 49-2).[33,34,67-77] The vast majority of mutations described in mastocytosis are somatic. In contrast, germline mutations are extremely rare and have been described in only a few cases of familial mastocytosis.[59,69,72,75,78-80] The K509I *KIT* variant deserves special attention, as it may be either germline or somatic, and in addition to increasing the sensitivity of the affected cells to stem cell factor, the resulting mutant KIT protein it is sensitive to imatinib.[70,81]

The respective *KIT* mutation may be largely confined to MCs and their precursor cells or may be detectable in multiple lineages. Mutational involvement of multiple hematopoietic cell lineages is usually associated with smoldering SM (SSM) or more aggressive (advanced) forms of SM (SM-AMN, ASM, MCL).[74,82] In these patients, an increased variant allele frequency (VAF) of the mutant *KIT* and, notably, *KIT* D816V mutation with VAF ≥10% in BM cells or peripheral blood leukocytes may be detected; in the context of SSM, a VAF ≥10% qualifies as a B finding (diagnostic sign of SSM) according to the proposed WHO 5th edition[13,39] but is not included as such in the ICC 2022.[12] Not only *KIT* D816V but also other *KIT* codon 816 mutations (D816Y, D816H, and D816F, the last representing a combination of D816V and

Table 49-2 KIT-Activating *KIT* Mutations in Mastocytosis

Exon	Mutation	Frequency	Remark
8	Del417–419insF	<3%	
	Del417–419insI	<3%	
	Del417–419insNA	<3%	
	Del417–419insY	<3%	
	Del419	<3%; 15%–20% in children	Also detected in germline configuration
	InsFF419	<3%	
9	ITD501–502	<3%	
	501_502InsAF	<3%	
	ITD502–503	<3%; 3%–7% in children	
	503_504insAY	<3%	
	ITD504	<3%	
	ITD505–508	<3%	
	K509I	<3%	Also detected in germline configuration
10	F522C	<3%	Also detected in germline configuration
11	W557R	<3%	Also detected in germline configuration
	V559A	<3%	Also detected in germline configuration
	V559I	<3%	
	Del559–560	<3%	Also detected in germline configuration
	V560G	<3%	
13	K642E	<3%	
	V654A	<3%	
17	L799F	<3%	
	D816A	<3%	
	D816F	<3%	
	D816H	<3%	
	D816I	<3%	
	D816V	>80%; 20%–30% in children	
	D816Y	<3%	
	D816T	<1%	
	D820G	<3%	
	N822I	<3%	Also detected in germline configuration
	N822K	<3%	

Adapted from Valent P, Akin C, Sperr WR, et al. New insights into the pathogenesis of mastocytosis: emerging concepts in diagnosis and therapy. *Ann Rev Pathol.* 2023;18:361.[18]

D816Y mutations) and mutations in other codons of *KIT* may act as gain-of-function mutations.[34,67,68,75] This is important, as in the ICC 2022, the proposed WHO 5th edition, and the consensus group proposal, any type of activating mutation in *KIT* qualifies as a minor diagnostic criterion of SM.[12,13,39] It is also worth noting that the non-D816V codon 816 mutations are significantly more frequent in CM than in SM, with D816F being detected only in CM so far.[18,75]

KIT mutations can be detected in more than 90% of all patients with SM and in about 40% of those with CM.

Therefore, all SM cases and most pediatric cases with *KIT* mutated (persistent) CM can be regarded as hematopoietic neoplasms.[18,30,74] As mentioned, any activating *KIT* mutation has been promoted as a minor diagnostic criterion for SM in both the ICC 2022 and the proposed WHO 5th edition classifications of mastocytosis (Boxes 49-2 and 49-3).[12,13,36-39] Various techniques have been used to detect *KIT* mutations, including restriction fragment length polymorphism analysis, direct sequencing, peptide nucleic acid–mediated polymerase chain reaction (PCR) clamping and melting point analysis, various allele-specific PCR techniques, and digital droplet PCR (ddPCR).[18,34,67,68,83-87] The sensitivity for the detection of *KIT* mutations is increased when MCs are enriched by cell sorting or by microdissection, which is usually not needed when applying ddPCR. A remarkable aspect is that, although MCs are usually not detectable in the bloodstream, *KIT* D816V can be detected in peripheral blood leukocytes with highly sensitive assays in most patients with SM.[34,67,68,88] Recommendations for *KIT* mutation analysis in MC neoplasms and approaches to both diagnosis and follow-up of patients with SM have been published.[34,67,68]

Detection of *KIT* mutations has prime importance in mastocytosis in general and in SM in particular. This is because such mutations (1) represent a minor diagnostic criterion required by the current classification systems[12,13,39]; (2) are associated with aberrant expression of CD25, CD2, and probably CD30[89]; (3) represent a decisive tool for pathologists to select cases to be specifically tested for myeloid/lymphoid neoplasms with eosinophilia (M/LN-Eo) and tyrosine kinase gene fusions, which are *KIT* wild type[90]; (4) are—if assessed in a quantitative manner—of significant prognostic value; and (5) are a major predictive marker of various targeted drug sensitivities, including the highly selective D816V KIT variant inhibitor avapritinib,[91,92] the less selective tyrosine kinase inhibitor with activity against D816V KIT midostaurin,[93] and imatinib in cases associated with "noncanonical" *KIT* mutations and even rare wild-type instances.[94] Finally, the degree to which non-MC lineages are affected by *KIT* mutations, which is roughly reflected by the respective VAFs, appears to substantially determine the clinical course of mastocytosis; the more MC lineage-restricted progenitors are affected, the more indolent form of disease the patients suffers from, and vice versa, the more undifferentiated progenitor cells and the more hematopoietic lineages are affected, the more aggressive the disease is.[95,96] An exception is SSM, in which multiple lineages and progenitors are affected but the prognosis is excellent and progression to an advanced SM is rather uncommon.[14,39] As mentioned, *KIT* D816V mutation with a VAF ≥10% is regarded as a B finding in the proposed WHO 5th edition classification,[13] which would upgrade ISM to SSM (when a second B finding is also detected) in respective rare instances. Thus, D816 hot-spot and—if wild-type—complete *KIT* gene sequencing should be considered mandatory in SM.

It should be noted that ISM and, to a degree, SSM are typically unimutational diseases, with most cases harboring only a *KIT* mutation.[82,95,96] In contrast, advanced SMs (SM-AMN and ASM) are multimutational diseases, with almost all cases displaying additional non-*KIT* mutations, often more than one.[96-98] Identification of poor-risk non-*KIT* variants (e.g., mutations in *ASXL1, CBL, DNMT3A, EZH2, NRAS,*

Box 49-2 *Systemic Mastocytosis: Diagnostic Criteria*

Major Criterion

Multifocal dense infiltrates of tryptase-positive and/or CD117-positive mast cells (≥15 mast cells in aggregates) detected in sections of bone marrow and/or other extracutaneous organ(s)*

Minor Criteria

In bone marrow biopsy or in section of other extracutaneous organs, >25% of mast cells are spindle shaped or have an atypical immature morphology

Mast cells in bone marrow, peripheral blood, or other extracutaneous organs express CD2, CD25, and/or CD30, in addition to mast cell markers

KIT D816V mutation or other activating *KIT* mutation detected in bone marrow, peripheral blood, or other extracutaneous organs†

Elevated serum tryptase level persistently >20 ng/mL.‡ In cases of SM-AMN, an elevated tryptase does not count as a systemic mastocytosis minor criterion

The diagnosis of systemic mastocytosis can be established when the major criterion is present according to the ICC 2022,[12] the major and one minor criteria are present according to the proposed WHO 5th edition and the 2020 Working Conference on Mast Cell Disorders,[13,39] or three minor criteria are fulfilled[12-14,39]

*In the absence of a *KIT* mutation, particularly in cases with eosinophilia, the presence of tyrosine kinase gene fusions associated with myeloid/lymphoid neoplasm with eosinophilia must be excluded according to the ICC 2022.

†To avoid "false negative" results, use of a high sensitivity polymerase chain reaction assay for detection of *KIT* D816V mutation is recommended. If negative, exclusion of *KIT* mutation variants is strongly recommended in suspected systemic mastocytosis.

‡According to the proposed WHO 5th edition, mast cell tryptase level should be adjusted in the case of hereditary alpha-tryptasemia.[13,39]

ICC, International Consensus Classification; *SM-AMN,* systemic mastocytosis with associated myeloid neoplasm; *WHO,* World Health Organization.

Data from Arber DA, Orazi A, Hasserjian RP, et al. International Consensus Classification of myeloid neoplasms and acute leukemias: integrating morphologic, clinical, and genomic data. *Blood.* 2022;140:1200; Khoury JD, Solary E, Abla O, et al. The 5th edition of the World Health Organization classification of haematolymphoid tumours: myeloid and histiocytic/dendritic neoplasms. *Leukemia.* 2022;36:1703; Valent P, Horny HP, Escribano L, et al. Diagnostic criteria and classification of mastocytosis: a consensus proposal. *Leuk Res.* 2001;25:603; Valent P, Akin C, Hartmann K, et al. Updated diagnostic criteria and classification of mast cell disorders: a consensus proposal. *HemaSphere.* 2021;5:e646.

Box 49-3 *B and C Findings*

B Findings[14,39]

High mast cell burden, ≥30% of infiltration of bone marrow cellularity by mast cell aggregates (assessed on bone marrow biopsy) and/or serum total tryptase ≥200 ng/mL[14,39] and/or *KIT* D816V mutation with VAF ≥10% in bone marrow cells or peripheral blood leukocytes[39]

Cytopenia (not meeting criteria for C findings) or –cytosis; reactive causes are excluded, and criteria for other myeloid neoplasms are not met[14,39]

or

Signs of dysplasia or myeloproliferation in non–mast cell lineages, not meeting criteria for an associated hematologic neoplasm, with normal or only slightly abnormal blood counts[14,39]

Hepatomegaly without impairment of liver function or splenomegaly without features of hypersplenism, including thrombocytopenia, and/or lymphadenopathy (>1 cm size), on palpation or imaging

C Findings[14,39]

Bone marrow dysfunction caused by neoplastic mast cell infiltration, manifested by ≥1 cytopenia: absolute neutrophil count <1.0 × 10⁹/L, hemoglobin level <10 g/dL, and/or platelet count <100 × 10⁹/L

Hepatomegaly with impairment of liver function, ascites, and/or portal hypertension

Skeletal involvement, with large (≥2 cm) osteolytic lesions with or without pathologic fractures

Splenomegaly with hypersplenism

Malabsorption with weight loss caused by gastrointestinal tract mast cell infiltrates

VAF, Variant allele frequency.

RUNX1, and *SRSF2*) aids in the risk stratification of patients and should be actively sought in the latter SM subtypes.[95,97-103]

CYTOLOGIC AND HISTOLOGIC DIAGNOSIS

Cytology

The diagnosis of mastocytosis based on BM smears alone is difficult because of the small number of aspirated MCs, even in patients whose BM trephine biopsy specimens reveal marked MC infiltration. The aspiration of MCs is hampered by the marked reticulin and/or collagen fibrosis accompanying the compact tissue infiltrates and by the fact that infiltration is predominantly focal. Nevertheless, the BM aspirate is of great importance in the diagnosis, staging, and grading of SM. Normally, MCs account for <0.1% of all nucleated BM cells.[29] Larger numbers of MCs are only occasionally seen in smears (Figs. 49-1 and 49-2). In most cases of ISM/SSM, the number of MCs in BM smears is only slightly elevated and ranges from 0.1% to a maximum of about 2%.[104] In most patients with ASM, the percentage

of MCs in BM smears ranges between 1% and 5%. In a small proportion of cases, however, the MC count in BM smears is markedly elevated and correlates with the prognosis and final diagnosis; indeed, ≥20% MCs on aspirates (proposed WHO 5th edition) or ≥20% immature MCs (ICC 2022) define MCL (in instances fulfilling diagnostic criteria of SM).[12,13] In patients with ASM in which MCs account for up to 19%, the prognosis is poor, as many of them progress to MCL. The percentage of MCs in BM smears in ASM correlate with prognosis. In those with ASM with a BM MC count of 5% to 19%, the diagnosis ASM in transformation (ASM-t) applies.[39,105]

The degree of MC atypia varies greatly and is most pronounced in MCL. In general, the following MC types can be recognized in BM smears in patients with SM: metachromatic blast (immature MC); atypical MC type I (spindle shaped); atypical MC type II (promastocyte); and typical mature tissue (well-differentiated) MC, defined as a well-granulated round cell with a round central nucleus.[14,39,105,106]

The following criteria define atypical MCs type I[106]:

1. Hypogranulation with reduction of metachromatic granules. Markedly hypogranulated MCs may even appear nonmetachromatic on staining with basic dyes such as Giemsa and toluidine blue and may only very weakly stain for tryptase on immunohistochemistry.
2. Oval and eccentric nuclei.
3. Spindling. This is typically seen in SM but is occasionally seen in reactive states of MC hyperplasia as well.

If two or three of these criteria are fulfilled, the cells should be called atypical MCs type I.[106] If the MC nuclei are bilobed

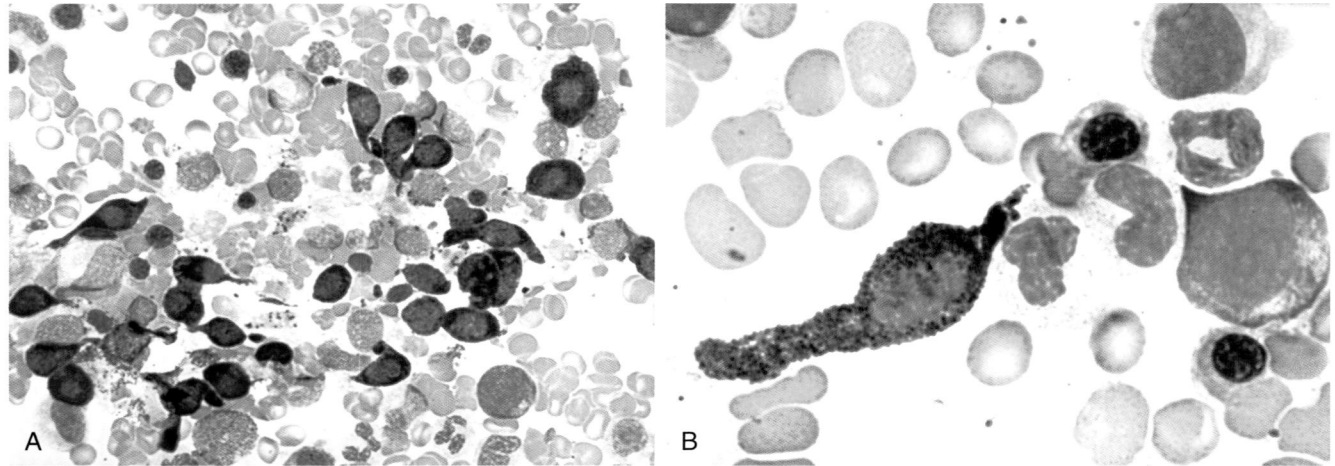

Figure 49-1. Indolent systemic mastocytosis: bone marrow smear. A, This case exhibits unusually large numbers of strongly metachromatic mast cells, which are round or spindle shaped and contain centrally located, slightly pleomorphic nuclei without prominent nucleoli. **B,** On higher magnification, note that the spindle-shaped mast cell is larger than the normal blood cell precursors.

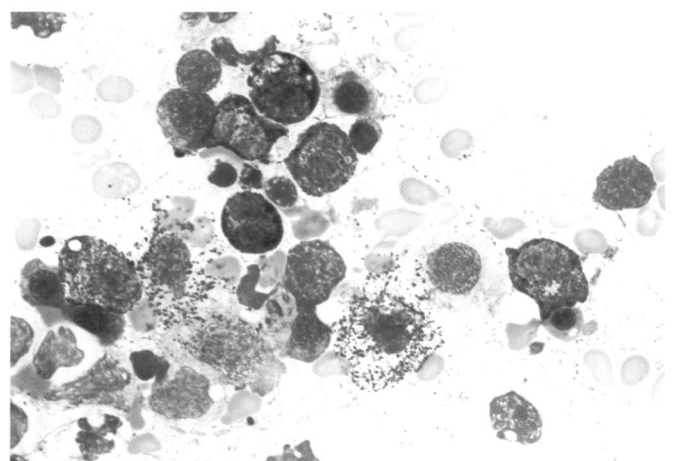

Figure 49-2. Aggressive systemic mastocytosis: bone marrow smear. In this case with a large number of mast cells, note that the mast cells contain fewer granules than those depicted in Figure 49-1.

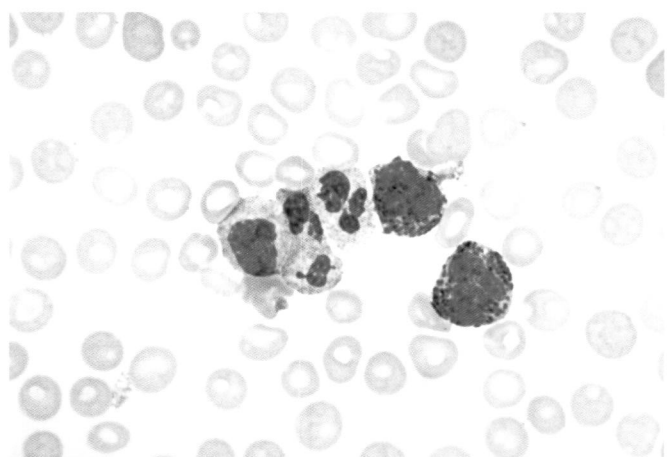

Figure 49-3. Myelomastocytic leukemia: blood smear. Two atypical cells with metachromatic granules are shown. It is not possible to determine the nature of these cells (mast cells or basophils) on the basis of morphology alone. Because bone marrow sections from this case showed a significant increase in tryptase-positive, CD117-positive mast cells (see Fig. 49-14), it can be assumed that these circulating cells are atypical mast cells.

or polylobed, the cells are termed atypical MCs type II or promastocytes.[106]

The rare diagnosis of MCL can sometimes be suspected from blood smears in which circulating MCs are present. In these patients, circulating MCs usually exhibit varying degrees of atypia. MCs may be strongly metachromatic and easily identifiable, or they may be very atypical, with scanty metachromatic granules and, occasionally, a blast-like appearance (Fig. 49-3). A definitive diagnosis of MCL can be made when MCs constitute more than 20% of all nucleated cells in BM smears, though in the presence of suboptimal smears (dry tap), which is unfortunately often the case, diffuse, dense infiltration of atypical immature MCs is considered sufficient to support the diagnosis of MCL in ICC 2022.[12] In classical MCL, circulating MCs represent more than 10% of blood leukocytes (Fig. 49-4). If MCs constitute more than 20% of nucleated BM cells but less than 10% of leukocytes in the peripheral blood, an aleukemic MCL can be diagnosed.[13,14,36-38,39,105] Although the ICC 2022 does not

use the term aleukemic MCL, MCL can be diagnosed in such cases based on 20% or more atypical, immature MC in the BM.[12]

Histology

Histologic investigation is imperative for the diagnosis, subtyping, and grading (confirmation of SM-induced organ damage) of mastocytosis.[36-38] Histologic evaluation of BM trephine biopsy specimens taken from the iliac crest provides the definitive diagnosis of SM in most cases.[15,107] Noticeably, the biopsy may be taken at the exact site of SM involvement (*locus minoris resistentiae*); thus, special attention should be paid to the specimen's ends, edges, and break lines. This investigation should always include immunohistochemistry with antibodies against tryptase, KIT/CD117, CD25, and

CD30.[12,13] In addition, stains for detection or exclusion of an AMN, including CD34, should be applied in all cases. Staining for tryptase and KIT/CD117 not only enables MC numbers to be assessed easily and reliably but also facilitates the assessment of MC infiltration patterns in the BM, allowing the detection of compact MC infiltrates even if they are very small (Figs. 49-5–49-7). It is highly recommended to stain for both tryptase and KIT/CD117 so as not to miss or underestimate tryptase[dim]-positive atypical MCs or overestimate KIT/CD117-positive non-MCs. Expression of CD25 and/or CD30 confirms the neoplastic state of an MC and enables the diagnosis of SM to be established in the setting of the other required criteria, given these are not expressed on normal or reactive MCs. CD2 expression also defines an atypical immunophenotype of MC[108] but is more easily detected by flow cytometry than by immunohistochemistry. CD30 has been promoted as a novel minor criterion of SM, being an aberrant marker regularly expressed on neoplastic MCs.[12,13,31,32,50] Especially in advanced SM, MCs often display strong cytoplasmic expression of CD30 (Fig. 49-8). However, CD30 expression is not specific for ASM or MCL but is also found in ISM and particularly WDSM, the latter usually lacking CD2 and CD25.[59]

Four major types of BM infiltration patterns have been defined based on the number and localization of MCs[109]:

1. Focal, with disseminated or multifocal compact MC infiltrates. This is the most common pattern in ISM and SM-AMN/AHN.
2. Diffuse-interstitial, with an increase in loosely scattered MCs. The exclusive occurrence of a diffuse-interstitial pattern generally indicates the reactive state of MC hyperplasia, but it may also be encountered in the BM of patients with CM or HαT.
3. Diffuse-compact, with complete effacement of preexisting BM. This type of infiltration pattern is usually seen in MCL, but it may also be encountered in advanced stages of SSM and ASM.

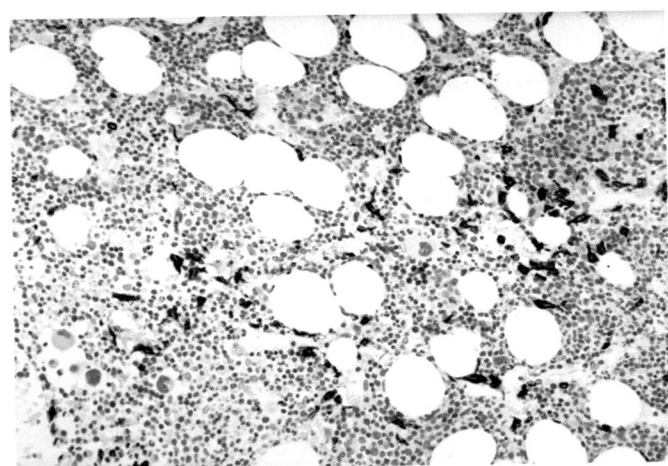

Figure 49-5. Bone marrow from a patient with cutaneous mastocytosis. Immunostaining for tryptase reveals an increase in loosely scattered mast cells within a slightly hypercellular bone marrow. Some small groups of mast cells can be seen, but there are no compact infiltrates. By definition, this is not indolent systemic mastocytosis. This case illustrates the diffuse infiltration pattern (interstitial subtype) that can be seen in reactive states (mast cell hyperplasia) and in systemic mastocytosis.

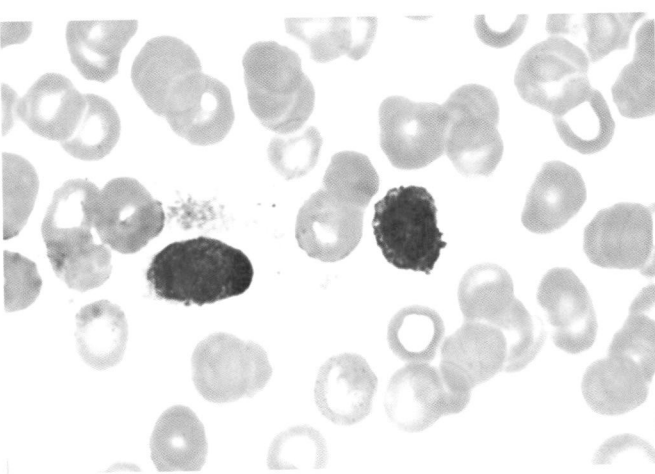

Figure 49-4. Mast cell leukemia: blood smear. Circulating pleomorphic mast cells with many metachromatic granules can be seen. Note the round nuclei, which distinguish these cells from basophils.

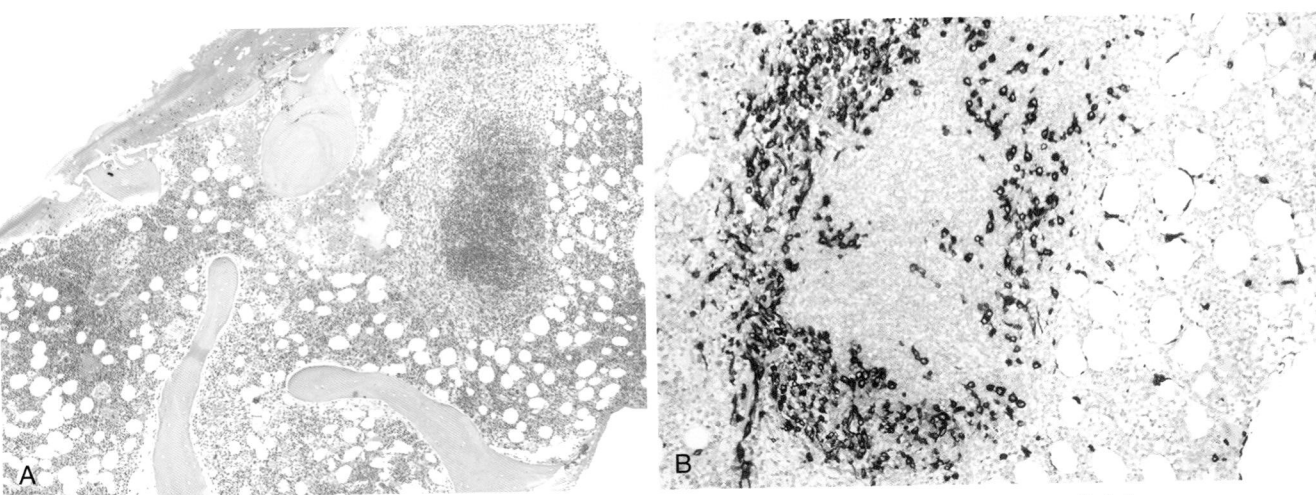

Figure 49-6. Indolent systemic mastocytosis: bone marrow findings. A, The marrow is slightly hypercellular and exhibits intact hematopoiesis and an aggregate of mast cells with admixed lymphocytes. **B,** The mast cells surrounding the lymphocytes show strong expression of tryptase. Note the spindle shape of most of the mast cells and the absence of increased mast cell numbers in the diffuse infiltrate (compare with Fig. 49-5). The patient has also mastocytosis in the skin.

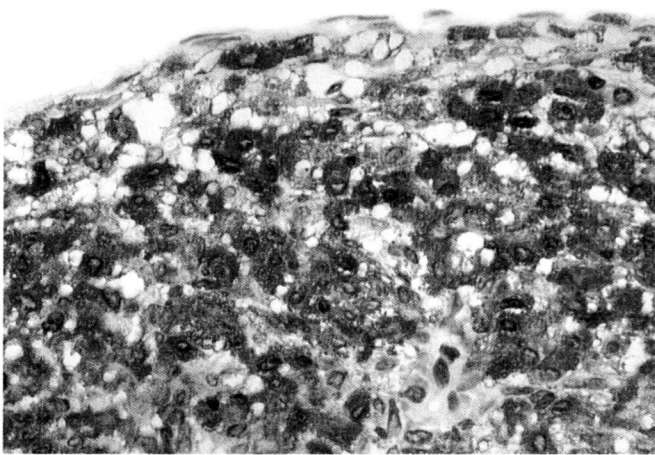

Figure 49-7. Mast cell leukemia: bone marrow findings. The diffuse-compact infiltration pattern on tryptase staining is found almost exclusively in mast cell leukemia (compare with Figs. 49-5 and 49-6). The mast cells exhibit strong expression of tryptase, reflected in the typical granular cytoplasmic staining. Note the absence of spindling of mast cells and the subtotal depletion of fat cells and normal blood cell precursors.

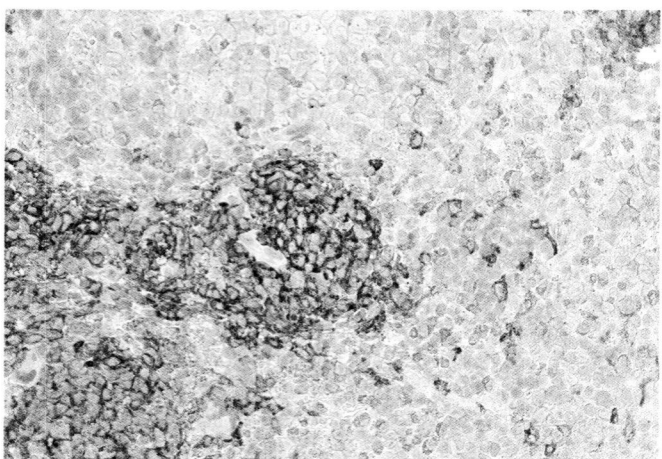

Figure 49-8. Aggressive systemic mastocytosis (same case as Fig. 49-20) positive for CD30 with a typical membrane-accentuated expression pattern.

4. Mixed (focal and diffuse-interstitial). This pattern is typically seen in ASM and MCL and is commonly associated with clinical signs of BM failure, but it also occurs in a subgroup of patients with SSM.

It has been shown by morphometry that the number of MCs in diffuse-interstitial infiltration patterns is usually significantly higher in cases of mastocytosis, irrespective of subtype, than in reactive states.[49] However, it cannot be overemphasized that the demonstration of at least one dense or compact MC infiltrate comprising ≥15 cells is the key finding for a definitive diagnosis of SM.[34] This holds true for the BM and for extramedullary organs such as the spleen, lymph nodes, and gastrointestinal (GI) tract.

Immunophenotype

Virtually all reactive and neoplastic MCs express tryptase, for which staining is granular and intracytoplasmic, and KIT/

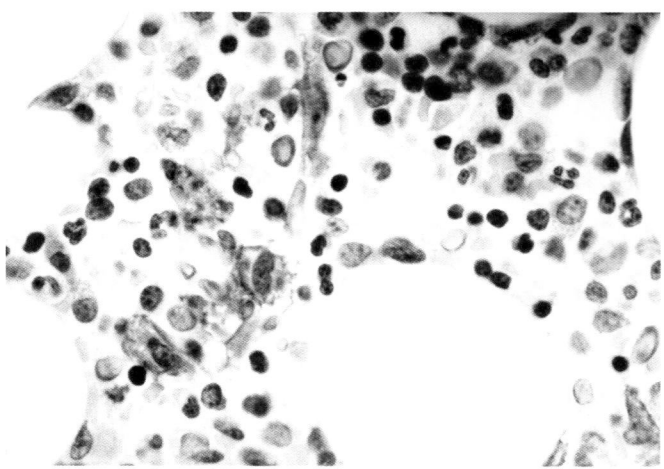

Figure 49-9. Indolent systemic mastocytosis: bone marrow findings. Slightly hypercellular marrow with a significant increase in mast cells that exhibit typical annular membrane-associated staining by an antibody against CD117.

CD117, for which staining is usually annular and membrane associated (but can be also cytoplasmic) (Fig. 49-9).[48,49] An important exception is that SM involving the GI tract typically shows dim to occasionally negative expression of tryptase by immunohistochemistry.[110] Typically, the co-expression of tryptase and KIT enables MCs to be clearly distinguished from basophils. The basophils may produce small amounts of tryptase in neoplastic states, usually chronic myeloid leukemia (CML), but they are usually negative for KIT/CD117 (exception: immature basophil precursor cells).[111] Several studies have shown that neoplastic MCs in SM react with antibodies against CD2, CD25, and CD30, whereas normal and reactive MCs are usually negative for these markers.[30-33,50] In about 50% of ISM cases, MCs in BM infiltrates express CD2, although the membrane-associated reactivity is often relatively weak; in contrast, the surrounding or intermingled T cells are strongly positive for CD2.[108] CD25 staining produces a granular cytoplasmic and membrane-associated positive and clearly diagnostic result in almost all patients with SM. However, there are also cases in which SM cannot be diagnosed but MCs still express CD25. Examples are chronic inflammatory reactions, monoclonal MC activation syndromes (MCAS), M/LN-Eo,[90] and chronic eosinophilic leukemia (CEL). Because lymphoid cells expressing CD25 are rarely found in the normal or reactive BM, and because megakaryocytes, which are often dim CD25-positive, can clearly be distinguished from MCs, the BM is the ideal tissue to confirm or to exclude CD25 expression in (atypical/neoplastic) MCs.[30] Identifying CD25-positive MCs is often difficult at extramedullary sites, especially in samples containing larger amounts of lymphocytes, such as mucosal layers, lymph nodes, and spleen. As mentioned, neoplastic MCs in SM often express CD30 in a moderate to strong granular cytoplasmic and occasionally membranous pattern.[31,32] MCs also may react with some of the routinely used macrophage-associated antibodies, especially those against CD68 and PG-M1/CD68r.[112,113] MCs, particularly neoplastic MCs, also express a variety of other antigens, such as CD4, CD13, CD33, CD43, CD45, CD56, CD123, vascular endothelial growth factor, and chymase, which is another highly specific but less sensitive

MC-associated protease.[114-116] A summary of the markers relevant to the diagnosis of SM is provided in Table 49-3.

In neoplastic states, it is necessary to phenotypically distinguish mastocytosis from myeloid leukemias exhibiting signs of MC differentiation but not fulfilling the diagnostic criteria of mastocytosis, including tryptase-positive acute myeloid leukemia (AML) and myelomastocytic leukemia (MML), but also from primary and secondary basophilic leukemias and accelerated CML with marked basophilia.[117] Discrimination among MCs, immature basophils and metachromatic blasts is hampered by the fact that, in contrast to normal or reactive MCs, atypical MCs may exhibit irregularly contoured and sometimes bilobed nuclei and thus resemble monocytes or granulocytic cells.[109,111] A clear distinction among MCs and basophils and their neoplastic derivatives can be achieved by applying a limited panel of stains such as naphthol AS-D chloroacetate esterase (CAE), tryptase, KIT/CD117, and 2D7 or BB1. Normal and neoplastic MCs express CAE, tryptase, and KIT but only little, if any, 2D7 and BB1; basophils usually lack CAE and KIT but express 2D7 and BB1 and (when immature) may also express small amounts of tryptase, especially in CML.[104,111] MML is a myeloid neoplasm, defined by the presence of increased MCs (typically metachromatic blasts or immature MCs) and increased myeloblasts, not meeting criteria for SM-AMN/AHN (AML) or MCL.[105] MCs in MML comprise at least 10% of all nucleated BM or peripheral blood cells, and myeloblasts are usually >5%. In contrast to MCL and SM-AML, MML lacks MC aggregates, expression of CD25 (rare positive instances being described), and the *KIT* D816V mutation (while other *KIT* mutations can be found in a subset of cases).[118] MML often displays a complex karyotype. About half of patients meeting the definition of MML present with a history of a myeloid neoplasm with increased immature MCs upon progression, while others have a de novo presentation of disease resembling MDS, MPN, or AML.

Histopathologic Findings

The histopathologic findings commonly associated with tissue infiltration by mastocytosis in different organs are provided herein (Box 49-4).

Bone Marrow

Because the BM is involved in almost all cases of SM,[11,15,107,109] the definitive diagnosis is usually based on the histopathologic findings in trephine specimens taken from the iliac crest. The typical histopathologic picture is a multifocal or disseminated, usually perivascular and paratrabecular, granulomatous-appearing infiltrate of mixed cellularity. The cellular composition of these infiltrates varies greatly, but diagnostically, MCs are the most important component. They form cohesive groups of round, epithelioid, or spindle-shaped cells that may be located centrally or peripherally. Lymphoid aggregates adjacent to compact MC infiltrates are commonly seen in BM infiltrates of ISM/SSM but are rarely encountered in ASM and MCL. The reactive lymphocytic component may be so pronounced that a diagnosis of low-grade lymphoma may be suspected.[119] The fact that lymphoplasmacytic lymphoma and some cases of chronic lymphocytic leukemia are associated with increased numbers of reactive MCs may cause some diagnostic

Table 49-3 Sensitivity and Specificity of Markers Used to Diagnose Mastocytosis*

Antigen/ Marker	Specificity		Sensitivity
	For MCs	For SM	
Metachromasia	++	−	++
CAE	++	−	++
Tryptase	++	−	+++
Chymase	+++	−	++
CD2	−	+++[†]	+
CD4	−	−	+
CD9	+	−	+++
CD13/CD33	−	−	+
CD14	−	+	+
CD25	−	+++[†]	+++
CD30	−	+	+
CD43	−	−	++
CD45	−	−	++
CD56	−	−	+
CD68	+	−	+++
CD73	+	+	+
CD117 (KIT)	+	−	+++
CD123	−	+	+
HDC	+	−	+
VEGF	−	−	++

*In routinely processed tissues, including decalcified bone marrow trephine biopsy specimens.
†High specificity for MCs in SM; not expressed in normal or reactive MCs.
+++, High; ++, moderate; +, low; −, absent.
CAE, Naphthol AS-D chloroacetate esterase; *HDC*, histidine decarboxylase; *MCs*, mast cells; *SM*, systemic mastocytosis; *VEGF*, vascular endothelial growth factor.

Box 49-4 *Histopathologic Findings Associated With Tissue Infiltrates of Mastocytosis**

Reticulin fibrosis
Neoangiogenesis
Collagen fibrosis
Osteosclerosis (bone marrow)
Eosinophilia
Lymphocytosis
Plasmacytosis

* Listed in decreasing order of frequency.

---

problems, yet MC clusters would not be observed.[120] There is almost always an increase in eosinophils, plasma cells, histiocytes, and fibroblast-like cells within or around tissue MC infiltrates of SM.

Compact tryptase and/or KIT/CD117-positive MC infiltrates are the histologic hallmark of mastocytosis, representing the major diagnostic SM criterion that is sufficient for the diagnosis of SM according to the consensus group, the WHO, and the ICC 2022,[12,32,39] and contain a dense network of reticulin fibers. In long-standing SM, collagen fibrosis develops. Paratrabecular MC infiltrates almost always produce osteosclerosis, which is predominantly focal. Finally, prominent neoangiogenesis, with an increase in small blood vessels of the capillary type, is almost always seen in compact MC infiltrates.[121] The highly specific microarchitecture of such compact MC infiltrates is related to certain MC mediators, such as fibroblast growth factor, tryptase, chymase, vascular endothelial growth factor, chemokines, and interleukins.[121,122] The number and size of MC infiltrates vary greatly. Compared with ISM, SSM, and ASM usually exhibit more MC infiltrates, which are also larger and sometimes confluent. In SSM, a high MC burden, defined as >30% of infiltration of

BM cellularity by MC aggregates, is a disease-related feature (B finding). Hematopoiesis is largely intact in most cases of ISM but is markedly reduced and often associated with clinical signs of BM failure (cytopenia) in ASM, MCL, and SM-AMN. Most cases of MCL can be easily recognized by the extreme hypercellularity of the marrow because of diffuse-compact infiltration, which leads to pronounced displacement of fat cells and normal hematopoiesis. There is usually only a slight to moderate increase in reticulin fibers. SM-AMN may represent a particular diagnostic challenge because small, compact MC infiltrates may be obscured by the associated hematologic malignant neoplasm and can be detected only in tryptase immunostains.[123] Indeed, it has been shown for AML t(8;21)(q22;q22.1)/*RUNX1::RUNX1T1* that 12.5% of patients had SM when marrow biopsies were stained for tryptase, and 10% to 15% of patients with CMML are expected to also have SM, the prognosis in both instances being worse when associated to SM.[55,124-127] Thus, it is recommended to perform tryptase immunostaining in all cases of AML t(8;21)(q22;q22.1)/*RUNX1::RUNX1T1* and all cases of CMML to capture SM-AMN/AHN.

Spleen

Normal and reactive splenic tissue (except the fibrous capsule) is virtually devoid of MCs; therefore, an increase in metachromatic cells, especially cohesive groups or larger infiltrates of MCs, is almost pathognomonic of mastocytosis.[128-130] The degree of infiltration varies greatly; it may be pronounced and associated with marked splenomegaly (>1000 g). MC infiltrates may be either found predominantly in the red pulp or in the white pulp, but they are more often evenly distributed between the two compartments (Fig. 49-10). As in the BM, MC infiltrates often have a granulomatous appearance; as such, a histiocytic/dendritic or reticulum cell tumor may initially be suspected, especially if the MCs are atypical and metachromatic granules are absent. The correct diagnosis is easily missed in cases of SM-AMN/AHN and may be almost impossible without immunostaining for tryptase. Application of ancillary methods (immunohistochemistry, sequencing) leads to the diagnosis of SM in such cases, even if other organs are not affected. Isolated splenic mastocytosis is a rare diagnosis, although a few cases of mastocytosis with predominant involvement of the spleen associated with splenomegaly and clinical signs of hypersplenism have been reported.[131] In such instances, the degree of BM involvement may be very small and can be assessed definitively only by immunohistochemistry. This underlines the fact that, in mastocytosis, as in other malignant neoplasms, the extent of infiltration of one organ does not allow one to draw definitive conclusions about other tissues. As in the BM, MC infiltrates in the spleen are always accompanied by an increase in reticulin

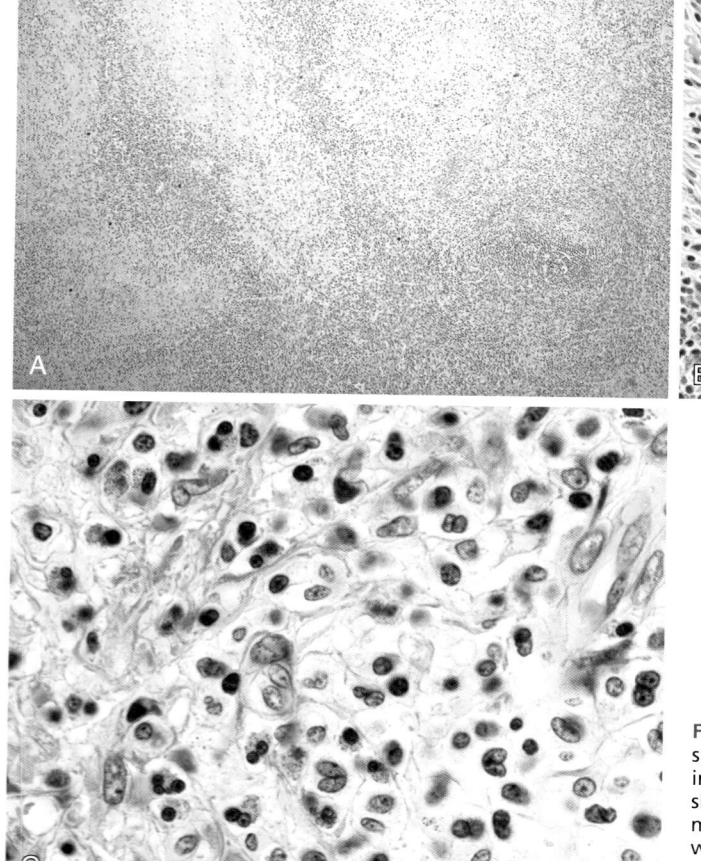

Figure 49-10. Spleen findings in systemic mastocytosis. A, The spleen shows patchy areas of fibrosis and mast cell aggregates in the red pulp and adjacent to the white pulp. **B,** Fibrotic areas show an infiltration of spindled and round mast cells with admixed eosinophils. **C,** Red pulp aggregates of round mast cells with abundant cytoplasm and admixed eosinophils are also present. The mast cell infiltrate is stained for KIT, tryptase, and CD25 (not shown).

and, in later stages of the disease, collagen fibers. A reactive increase in eosinophils and plasma cells is often seen as well.

Liver

It is likely that involvement of the liver is more frequent in SM than would be supposed from clinical findings alone.[132-134] Even in patients without significant hepatomegaly and normal liver enzyme levels, microscopy may reveal small periportal or intrasinusoidal MC infiltrates. Because intrasinusoidal MCs are never encountered in normal or reactive states, such findings can be regarded as proof of involvement by mastocytosis (Fig. 49-11). In almost all cases, the portal triads are the main site of infiltration and show fibrotic enlargement. Accordingly, liver fibrosis is a frequent finding in mastocytosis and may even be associated with clinical signs of portal hypertension,[135] especially in ASM and MCL. Cirrhosis does not develop and therefore should not be regarded as a consequence of MC infiltration. However, in most patients with advanced SM with marked liver involvement (C finding), signs of liver fibrosis, ascites, and elevated liver enzyme levels (especially alkaline phosphatase) will be present. As

in other tissues, immunohistochemical staining for tryptase, KIT/CD117, CD25, and CD30 must always be performed to evaluate the number of infiltrating MCs and supported by sequencing techniques regarding at least the *KIT* gene to establish a definitive diagnosis. Periportal MC infiltrates may be accompanied by large numbers of lymphocytes, so a so-called low-grade lymphoma with liver involvement may initially be suspected in a small number of cases.

Lymph Nodes

Lymph node infiltration is seen in about half of the patients with SM, making it less frequent than involvement of the BM, spleen, and liver.[130,136] Whereas enlargement of abdominal lymph nodes is found in some patients with advanced SM, involvement of peripheral lymph nodes is very rare. On histologic evaluation, the enlarged lymph nodes almost always exhibit MC infiltration, which may be minimal and therefore difficult to detect. Generalized lymphadenopathy is a rare finding in SM and is usually associated with an aggressive clinical course and sometimes with eosinophilia. This particular rare presentation of ASM has previously

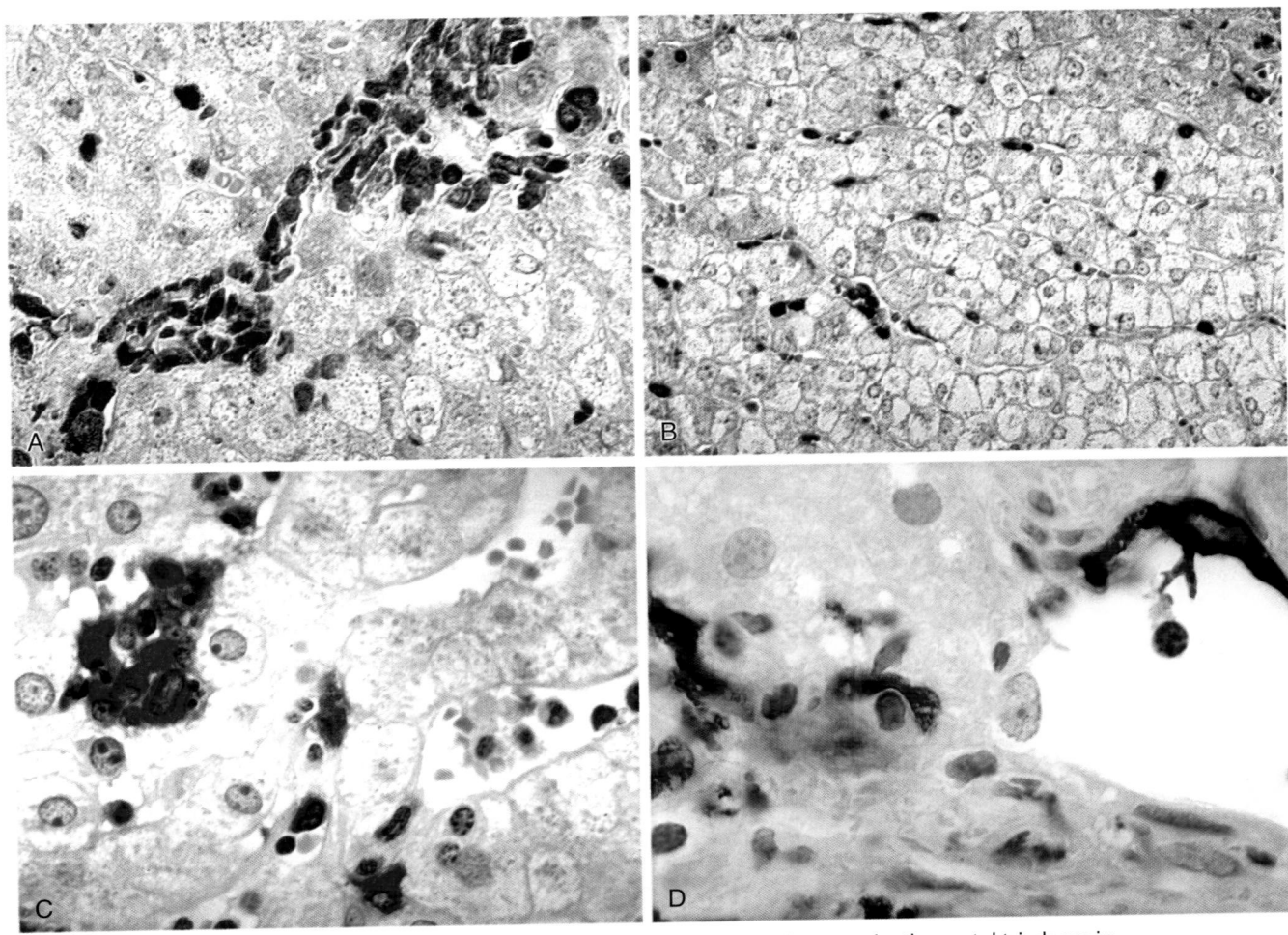

Figure 49-11. Liver findings in systemic mastocytosis. A, On Giemsa stain, the portal triads are infiltrated by strongly metachromatic mast cells in a case of indolent systemic mastocytosis. **B,** In the same case, there are loosely scattered intrasinusoidal mast cells in otherwise normal liver tissue. Although there are no compact infiltrates, such findings are interpreted as involvement by mastocytosis. **C,** At higher magnification, the same case shows pleomorphic mast cells strongly reactive with chloroacetate esterase but negative for myeloperoxidase (not depicted). **D,** Immunostaining for tryptase reveals some unusual stellate mast cells resembling endothelial cells.

been described as lymphadenopathic mastocytosis with eosinophilia.[137] Because lymph nodes in normal and reactive states often contain large numbers of MCs located predominantly in the sinuses, it can be difficult to confirm or to exclude involvement by mastocytosis. The most relevant findings concern the distributional pattern of MCs. Compact MC infiltrates within the paracortical regions or the pulp can be regarded as evidence of nodal involvement by mastocytosis (Fig. 49-12). These infiltrates are often small and are visible only when immunostaining with an antibody against tryptase is performed. Again, CD25 and CD30 stains may be helpful to raise suspicion for the presence of neoplastic MCs and, supported by results of sequencing techniques regarding at least the *KIT* gene, enable establishment of the SM diagnosis. Loosely scattered intrasinusoidal MCs may be numerous in reactive states (e.g., in a node draining an invasive cancer) but may be also observable in mastocytosis. In patients with known mastocytosis, a significant increase in intrasinusoidal MCs should be regarded as specific involvement, even if there are no compact infiltrates. As in other tissues involved by mastocytosis, reticulin or even collagen fibrosis is a consistent finding, but eosinophilia, plasmacytosis, and follicular hyperplasia are not present in all cases.

Gastrointestinal Tract

An increase in loosely distributed reactive MCs (MC hyperplasia) is a common finding in inflammatory processes involving the GI tract mucosa, and GI symptoms are frequent in patients with SM; GI symptoms in SM are mostly caused by MC mediators and not by MC lesions of the GI tract.[138] Thus, it may be difficult to determine whether the GI tract is directly involved by mastocytosis, even if immunohistochemistry is performed.[110,139-141] In these cases, immunohistochemical staining with antibodies against tryptase, KIT/CD117, CD25, and CD30 should be performed to determine the distribution of MCs and to detect small groups or compact infiltrates of MCs. As always, special care must be taken to ensure the proper recognition of CD25-positive MCs because some lymphocytes also express this antigen. Tryptase expression in MCs of SM in the GI tract is often variable and reduced compared with normal MCs.[110] Compact intramucosal MC

infiltrates are relatively rare, but as in the BM and other tissues, these are the histologic hallmark of involvement by mastocytosis (Fig. 49-13). Such dense MC infiltrates are often located in the subepithelial layers of the *lamina propria*.[110] The small and large bowel are more often involved in SM than the stomach. Surprisingly, one study detected a decrease of intramucosal MCs in patients with SM compared with those of patients exhibiting pure CM and normal controls, and expression of CD25 by intramucosal MCs was not seen.[142] There are several different forms of involvement of the GI tract by SM that will allow different levels of diagnostic certainty, especially if supported by sequencing results:

Loosely scattered MCs expressing CD25 or carrying the *KIT* D816V mutation (usually seen in patients with known SM). However, diagnostic criteria of mastocytosis involving the mucosa are not fulfilled, and a preliminary diagnosis of monoclonal MC activation syndrome (MCAS) can be established.

Disseminated nodular (granulomatous) compact MC infiltrates (comparable to findings in other organs, especially the BM). If MCs express CD25 and/or CD30 or carry the mutation *KIT* D816V, the diagnostic criteria of SM (involving the mucosa) are fulfilled.

Bandlike, subepithelial, compact MC infiltrates (detectable only in GI tract mucosa). If MCs express CD25 and/or CD30 and/or carry the mutation *KIT* D816V, the diagnostic criteria of SM are fulfilled.

Diffuse-compact MC infiltrates distorting preexisting cryptal structures and mimicking inflammatory bowel disease. Expression of CD25 and/or CD30 by MCs and/or demonstration of *KIT* D816V mutation allows the diagnosis of SM.

Sarcomatous destructive growth. SM should be excluded by proper study of the recommended diagnostic SM criteria.

Skin

The histopathologic findings in patients with CM vary greatly, irrespective of the age at onset, but there is generally good correlation with the macroscopic appearance of the lesions.[40,143,144] Disseminated perivascular and periadnexal MC infiltrates throughout the dermis is the most common cutaneous pattern and is associated with MPCM. MCs

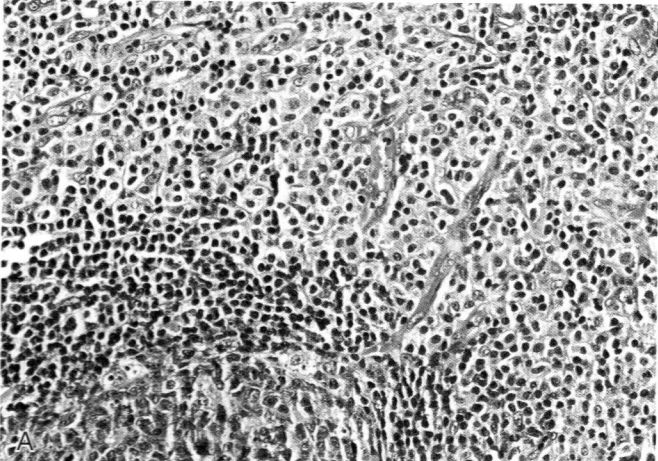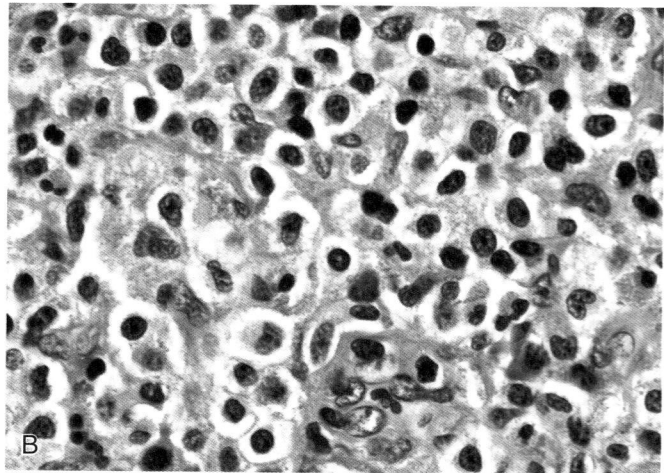

Figure 49-12. Lymph node findings in systemic mastocytosis. A, Diffuse infiltration and partial effacement of the paracortical lymph node architecture by metachromatic mast cells. Such histologic findings are typical of enlarged peripheral lymph nodes in patients with long-standing cutaneous mastocytosis (urticaria pigmentosa) and signify a diagnosis of indolent systemic mastocytosis. **B,** At higher magnification (same case), the mast cells have abundant granular or clear cytoplasm with admixed eosinophils.

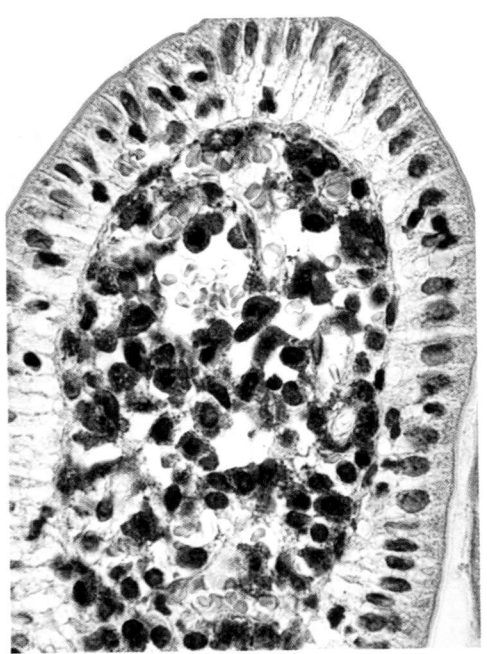

Figure 49-13. Systemic mastocytosis involving the duodenum. The lamina propria of the duodenal mucosa is densely infiltrated by slightly pleomorphic mast cells exhibiting strong reactivity for chloroacetate esterase. The patient had complained of diarrhea. Because there was also mild focal involvement of the bone marrow, this case could be classified as indolent systemic mastocytosis. Note that the epithelium is completely intact and contains no mast cells.

Table 49-4 Differential Diagnosis of Mastocytosis

Diagnosis	Definition
Mast cell hyperplasia	Nonneoplastic, local, or systemic increase in mast cells
Myeloid neoplasm with mast cell differentiation but lacking SM criteria	MDS, MPN, or AML with focal increase in neoplastic atypical mast cells, especially myelomastocytic leukemia
Tryptase-positive AML or AML with KIT D816V mutation	AML with aberrant expression of tryptase but without compact infiltrates or other criteria for SM
Mastocytosis (mast cell neoplasm)	Typical skin lesions of cutaneous mastocytosis and/or fulfilled SM criteria, or localized mast cell tumor

AML, Acute myeloid leukemia; *MDS,* myelodysplastic syndrome/neoplasm; *MPN,* myeloproliferative neoplasm; *SM,* systemic mastocytosis.

Table 49-5 Differential Diagnosis of Subtypes of Mastocytosis

Subtype	Differential Diagnosis
CM	ISM
ISM	MCH, MCAS, BMM, SSM
SM-AMN	Tryptase-positive AML, MML, SSM, ASM
ASM	SSM, aleukemic MCL, lymphoma*
MCL	MML, ASM, chronic basophilic leukemia
MCS	High-grade sarcoma, myeloid/histiocytic sarcoma, melanoma, mastocytoma

*Lymphadenopathic mastocytosis with eosinophilia, a previously described subvariant of SSM, may present with massive (abdominal) lymphadenopathy and thereby mimic a lymphoma.
AML, Acute myeloid leukemia; *ASM,* aggressive systemic mastocytosis; *BMM,* bone marrow mastocytosis; *CM,* cutaneous mastocytosis; *ISM,* indolent systemic mastocytosis; *MCAS,* mast cell activation syndrome; *MCH,* mast cell hyperplasia; *MCL,* mast cell leukemia; *MCS,* mast cell sarcoma; *MML,* myelomastocytic leukemia; *SM-AMN,* systemic mastocytosis with associated myeloid neoplasm; *SSM,* smoldering systemic mastocytosis.

usually show an abundance of intracytoplasmic granules and are therefore strongly metachromatic. In longer-standing lesions, the basal layers of the epidermis show marked hyperpigmentation caused by an increase in melanin, producing the lesions' red-brown color. Only rarely is the number of melanophages in the dermis increased. An increase in reticulin and collagen fibers is almost always seen in CM. The number of eosinophils and lymphocytes is mostly slightly or moderately increased. Although mastocytoma and the rare nodular or plaquelike variants of MPCM exhibit strands and sheets of strongly metachromatic round MCs within a thickened fibrotic dermis, the increase in MCs in patients with what was previously known as the telangiectatic subtype of CM (*telangiectasia macularis eruptiva perstans* [TMEP]) may be minimal and detectable only by immunostaining for tryptase. TMEP is no longer recognized as a specific subtype of CM, as such lesions are included in the MPCM subtype. In this subtype, MCs accumulate in the upper third of the dermis and often assume a spindle shape. A bandlike infiltrate consisting almost exclusively of MCs is seen in the subepidermal connective tissue in the rare erythrodermic subtype of CM. In contrast to other involved tissues, expression of CD2, CD25, or CD30 is variable in cases of clinically and histologically diagnosed CM; therefore, respective negativity is not as useful as in other (extracutaneous) tissues.

DIFFERENTIAL DIAGNOSIS

Tables 49-4 and 49-5 summarize the major conditions that must be considered in the differential diagnosis of mastocytosis. One main problem is the recognition of MC hyperplasia,

which can be pronounced in solid tumors of neurogenic origin and in a few hematologic malignant neoplasms, especially in cases with lymphoplasmacytic lymphoma, and in patients receiving stem cell factor (KIT ligand).[145] However, even if the reactive increase in MCs is massive, compact infiltrates are virtually absent; they have been detected only in a few cases of stem cell factor–induced MC hyperplasia.[146] It is therefore crucial to look carefully for compact or dense MC infiltrates, which should consist of ≥15 cells. The compact infiltrates in many cases of ISM are typically intermingled with many small lymphocytes, which sometimes form follicle-like structures, making it difficult to distinguish this disorder from so-called low-grade lymphoma involving the BM.[119,120] Myeloid neoplasms, especially myelodysplastic and myelodysplastic/myeloproliferative neoplasms, occasionally show a marked increase in atypical, sometimes blast-like MCs in the BM and peripheral blood. Such phenomena are best considered signs of MC differentiation and must be distinguished from "true" mastocytosis in the context of the results of CD25 and CD30 staining and ddPCR for the KIT D816V mutation. If the number of atypical metachromatic cells in the BM smear or peripheral blood is >10% and SM criteria are not met, the designation of MML is appropriate (Fig. 49-14).[105,118,147] MML lacks MC aggregates, expression of CD25 (rare positive instances being described), and the KIT D816V mutation (though other KIT mutations can be found in a subset of cases).[118] The existence of tryptase-expressing blast cells in cases of AML can be designated tryptase-positive AML, which often belongs to AML

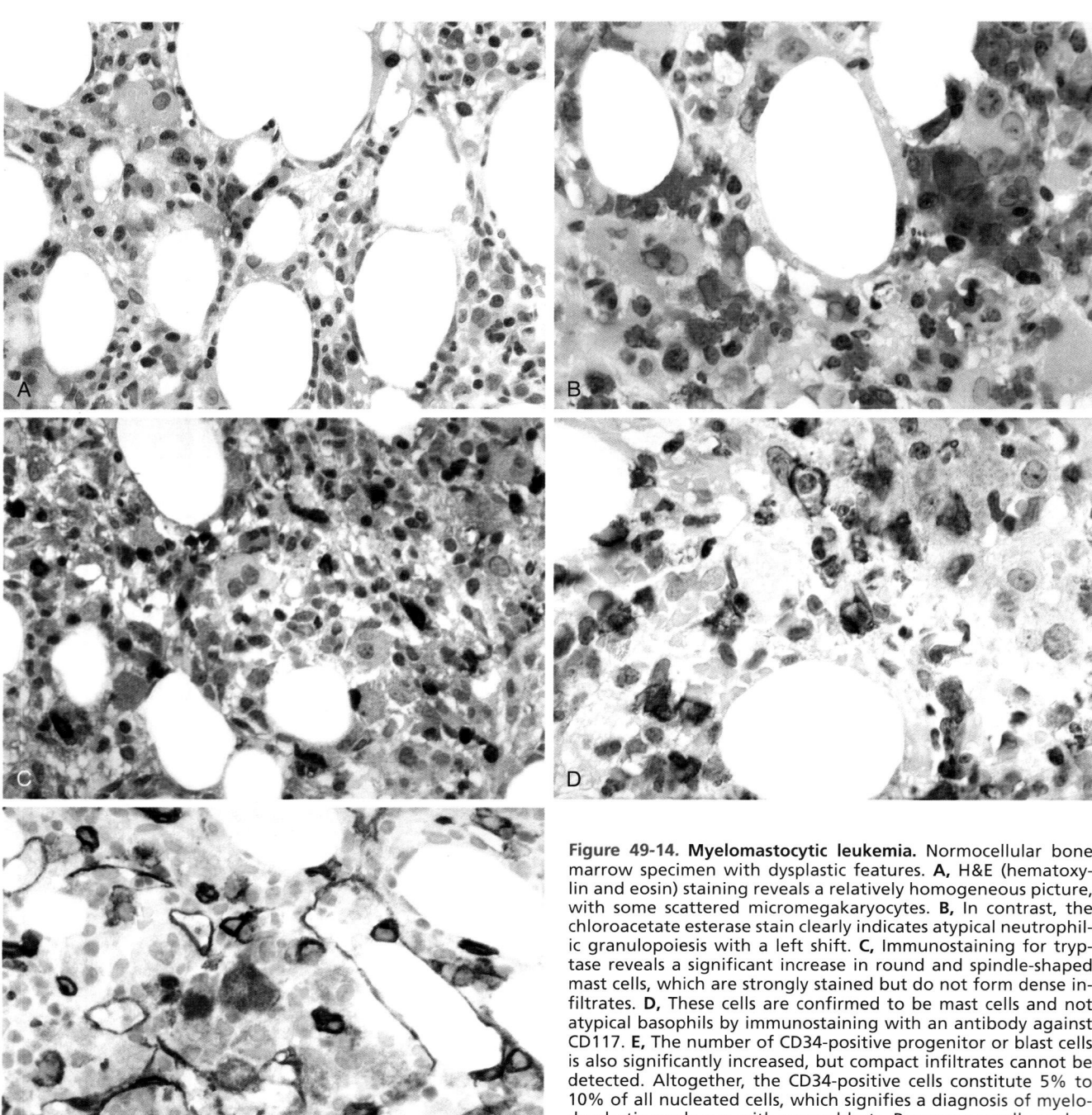

Figure 49-14. Myelomastocytic leukemia. Normocellular bone marrow specimen with dysplastic features. **A,** H&E (hematoxylin and eosin) staining reveals a relatively homogeneous picture, with some scattered micromegakaryocytes. **B,** In contrast, the chloroacetate esterase stain clearly indicates atypical neutrophilic granulopoiesis with a left shift. **C,** Immunostaining for tryptase reveals a significant increase in round and spindle-shaped mast cells, which are strongly stained but do not form dense infiltrates. **D,** These cells are confirmed to be mast cells and not atypical basophils by immunostaining with an antibody against CD117. **E,** The number of CD34-positive progenitor or blast cells is also significantly increased, but compact infiltrates cannot be detected. Altogether, the CD34-positive cells constitute 5% to 10% of all nucleated cells, which signifies a diagnosis of myelodysplastic syndrome with excess blasts. Because a small number of circulating mast cells was also detected, this case shows the typical features of myelomastocytic leukemia and cannot be diagnosed as mastocytosis or mast cell leukemia (compare with Fig. 49-3).

with minimal differentiation or without maturation (Fig. 49-15). Blasts in both MML and tryptase-positive AML will often co-express CD34, though MCs in mastocytosis (and reactive MCs) are negative for CD34. This immunohistochemical finding is reflected in an elevation of the serum tryptase level, which is sometimes extremely high and can exceed levels found in patients with SM.[148] However, such cases should not be classified as mastocytosis unless SM criteria are met (SM-AML). When tryptase immunohistochemistry is routinely used in the workup of BM trephine biopsy specimens, the

described phenomenon termed tryptase-positive compact round cell infiltrate of the BM (TROCI-bm) is an important diagnostic checkpoint. By definition, TROCI-bm may be focal or diffuse and consists exclusively of round (not spindle-shaped) cells forming compact (dense) tissue infiltrates.[149] The differential diagnosis of TROCI-bm includes six distinct but rare hematologic neoplasms (tryptase-positive AML, MCL, SM, MML, and acute and chronic basophilic leukemia) that can be separated only with a panel of antibodies mainly directed against MC-related and basophil-related antigens

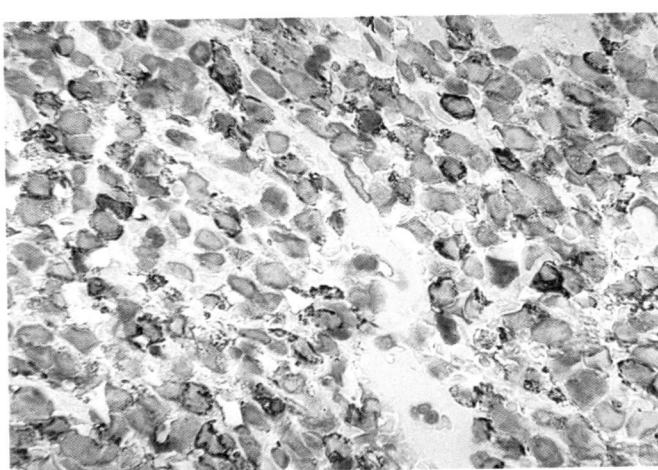

Figure 49-15. Tryptase-positive myeloid blast crisis of myeloid leukemia. Immunostaining for tryptase reveals strong focal cytoplasmic reactivity in most of the blast cells. The blast cells also expressed KIT (CD117).

such as KIT/CD117, CD25, CD30, 2D7, and BB1 and—in equivocal cases—KIT sequencing results applying a sensitive technology. Because the BB1 and 2D7 antigens are expressed preferentially on basophilic granulocytes, respectively positive focal TROCI-bm in the setting of CML indicates secondary basophilic leukemia and therefore disease progression.[64,65] TROCI-bm with co-expression of KIT/CD117, CD25, and/ or CD30 indicates SM, whereas lack of CD25 but positivity for CD30 in this setting is typical of WDSM.[59,71] Finally, co-expression of CD34 by tryptase-positive cells in diffuse TROCI-bm indicates either MML or tryptase-positive AML.

If the diagnostically relevant antibodies against tryptase and KIT/CD117 are not applied, the differential diagnosis includes a much broader range of reactive and neoplastic disorders. In general and considering extramedullary sites, granulomatous diseases, osteodystrophy (also called tunneling fibro-osteoclasia) in chronic renal insufficiency/hyperparathyroidism, histiocytoses, myelofibrosis, angioimmunoblastic and anaplastic large cell T-cell lymphoma, multiple myeloma, Hodgkin lymphoma, seminoma, GI stromal tumor (GIST), sarcomas with spindle cell and epithelioid morphology, and melanoma represent the most important considerations.[55] In cases of SM-AMN, the associated hematologic neoplasm often dominates the histologic picture and may obscure small MCs, which may even become visible upon therapy for the former.[123,124]

The principal key to the diagnosis of mastocytosis in the BM is to be aware that clusters of fibroblast-like spindle cells or epithelioid cells are almost always the primary histologic sign of SM. Spindle cells are extremely rare in other hematopoietic neoplasms but may be seen in reticulum cell sarcoma and multiple myeloma. Infiltrates or metastases of spindle cell sarcomas are also exceedingly rare. GIST with expression of KIT might be the only difficult differential diagnosis; however, GIST involving the BM has not been reported.

Mast Cell Activation Syndrome

Mast cell activation syndrome (MCAS) applies to conditions in which patients experience symptoms caused by the release of an inappropriate amount of MC mediators fulfilling all three of the following criteria: (1) typical clinical signs of severe, recurrent, acute, systemic MC activation (e.g., pruritus, flushing, blistering, urticaria, headache, diarrhea, abdominal pain, vomiting, fainting, respiratory problems, anaphylaxis); (2) involvement of MC demonstrated by biochemical analyses (preferably through an increase in tryptase following the 20% + 2 ng/mL formula, which means event-related transient elevation of the serum tryptase level by at least 20% over the individual baseline plus 2 ng/mL absolute within a 2- to 4-hour window after the anaphylactic reaction); and (3) symptoms respond to treatment with MC-stabilizing agents or drugs targeted against MC mediator production, secretion, or receptor binding.[150-152] Given the definition, it is obvious that MCAS is neither a morphologic diagnosis nor an ICC/WHO subentity of mastocytosis. Nevertheless, and as comprehensible from the list here, at least one variant represents a clonal MC condition.

Five different variants of MCAS are currently recognized[150-152]:
1. Monoclonal (primary or clonal) MCAS; defined by the presence of KIT mutation(s) or the aberrant expression of CD25 on MCs as a surrogate of clonality (irrespective of whether other diagnostic criteria of mastocytosis are met),
2. Secondary MCAS; associated with an underlying nonneoplastic disease (e.g., IgE-dependent allergy or other hypersensitivity reaction),
3. HαT-positive MCAS; in which HαT is detected, all diagnostic MCAS criteria are fulfilled, and no related allergic cause or underlying clonal MC disease is detected,
4. Combined MCAS; in which patients with MCAS have two or more of the following: (a) CM or SM, (b), overt allergy/atopic disease, and (c) a known genetic predisposition such as HαT (in these patients, the risk for severe anaphylaxis is extremely high),
5. Idiopathic MCAS, in which no related reactive disease, IgE-dependent allergy, HαT, or neoplastic/clonal MCs are found.

MCAS is not a histopathological diagnosis, yet there is a clear role for the pathologist in the classification ruling out monoclonal MCAS by high sensitivity and specificity assays to detect KIT mutations (e.g., ddPCR) and/or expression of CD25.

CLASSIFICATION

We describe herein each of the variants of mastocytosis defined in the ICC 2022 and the proposed WHO 5th edition classification (Boxes 49-1–49-3).[12,105,153] Transitions between disease categories may occur, and the exact diagnosis may depend on the accuracy of the investigatory procedures.[90,154] The incidence of transition to a higher disease category is unknown. In advanced SM involving multiple myeloid lineages, the borders between ASM, SM-AMN, and MCL may occasionally be blurred.[155] In addition, the BM smear may sometimes be of poor quality or difficult to examine because of contamination with blood cells or because only a few BM cells are aspirated (dry tap). In regard to ASM/MCL, this has been accounted for by the ICC 2022 recognizing that diffuse, dense infiltration of atypical immature MCs may support the diagnosis of MCL.[12] In adult patients with CM who have not undergone a BM examination, it is recommended to establish the presumptive diagnosis of mastocytosis in the skin (MIS)[156] and prompt an extensive workup—including peripheral blood analysis for mutant KIT by means of a sensitive technique—and perform a BM biopsy later to exclude SM, as it is expected in >90% of adult cases of MIS.[40] Because most pediatric cases are pure

CM,[157] BM biopsy is usually not recommended unless there are clinical or laboratory signs of systemic advanced or aggressive disease variants, such as marked cytopenia, a very high and steadily increasing serum tryptase level, organomegaly and/or mutant *KIT* with high VAF in the peripheral blood.[158,159] Table 49-5 summarizes the defined disease categories and the main diseases and conditions to consider in the differential diagnosis.

Cutaneous Mastocytosis

Definition

CM is an accumulation of MCs within the dermis associated with typical clinical findings, usually disseminated maculopapular lesions of CM. CM can be diagnosed only if there are no signs of systemic disease, i.e., no criteria to diagnose SM. Multifocal compact MC infiltrates (major SM criterion) are not found on histologic evaluation of the BM or in other extracutaneous tissues. However, in patients with CM, one or two minor SM criteria may be detected, and in a proper context, they may fulfill diagnostic criteria for monoclonal MCAS. The skin lesions in the majority of patients with ISM are clinically and histologically indistinguishable from pure CM.

Epidemiology

CM is the most common variant of MC disease, especially in children (juvenile CM), and it reportedly accounts for more than 80% of cases. In children, there is a male predominance (approximately 1.3×), and 90% of the affected present as MPCM (75% of cases) before the age of 2 years, mostly in the first 6 months of life.[157,159] However, if adult patients with mastocytosis are staged—especially with an appropriate investigation of BM trephine specimens, including immunohistochemistry (e.g., tryptase and CD25), and molecular analyses for *KIT* codon 816 mutations—the incidence of SM markedly increases.[40]

Clinical Features

Three major clinical types of CM are recognized[156,160]:

1. MPCM, formerly termed UP, is the most common subtype. It can be further subdivided into two clinical variants: a monomorphic variant that can be seen in children and adults and that is characterized by small, round, brown or red maculopapular lesions and a polymorphic variant that is almost always restricted to children and is characterized by larger lesions of variable size and shape, often accompanied by plaques or nodules.
2. Diffuse CM is very rare and is almost always seen in young children.
3. Mastocytoma of the skin is also rare, usually solitary, rarely multilocalized (i.e., <4 lesions, otherwise MPCM should be diagnosed), occurs almost exclusively in children, and has a tendency to regress spontaneously.

TMEP should not be regarded as a special type of CM and should be included in the MPCM subtype, as it is usually accompanied by lesions typical of MPCM.

MPCM can be detected in childhood (>90% of cases) and less frequently in adulthood (<10% of cases). An important aspect is that children with MPCM can further be divided into those with monomorphic small-sized skin infiltrates and those with polymorphic (smaller and larger) skin lesions, a distinction that is of prognostic significance.[156]

Another important aspect is that adults with CM (MPCM) have a significantly better prognosis concerning progression-free survival than adults with ISM.[160] Therefore, a BM investigation is recommended in all adult patients with MPCM-like skin lesions (suspected SM). If such patients refuse a BM biopsy, the diagnosis CM or SM cannot be established, and the provisional diagnosis should be MIS.[14,39,160]

Morphology

The histologic picture in typical cases of MPCM is one of disseminated aggregates of mature-appearing, strongly metachromatic, mostly round to ovoid MCs found mainly around small blood vessels and adnexal structures within the dermis (Fig. 49-16). Prominent signs of epidermotropism are not seen. Confluent clusters of MCs are rarely found. Some cases may display very subtle changes that will be only appreciated with immunohistochemistry. Diffuse CM can be

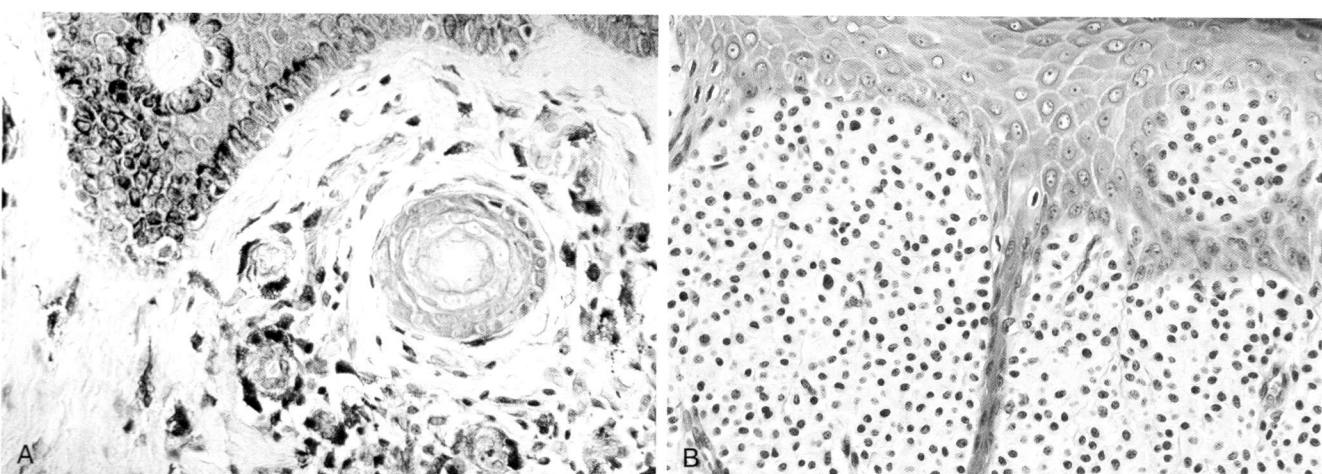

Figure 49-16. Cutaneous mastocytosis. A, Giemsa stain of a skin biopsy specimen from a patient with long-standing maculopapular cutaneous mastocytosis. Note the preferential perivascular and periadnexal localization of the metachromatic mast cells, without the formation of larger infiltrates. Hyperpigmentation of the basal layer of the epidermis is responsible for the typical red-brown macroscopic appearance of the lesions. **B,** H&E (hematoxylin and eosin) staining of a skin biopsy section from a child with mastocytoma. Note the sheets of slightly pleomorphic mast cells within the dermis.

recognized by a diffuse, bandlike, subepidermal infiltrate of MCs often accompanied by edema, whereas mastocytoma shows nodular compact infiltrates, often elevating the overlying intact epidermis.

Immunophenotype and Genetics

Virtually all MCs in all cases of CM express tryptase and KIT/ CD117, whereas co-expression of CD25 and CD30 varies considerably. The MCs in CM, unlike those in SM, usually also express chymase, although this is of little diagnostic relevance. The frequency of expression of CD2 in CM is not known.

The *KIT* D816V mutation in exon 17 is only present in a third of pediatric patients with CM.[161-163] Mutations outside the exon 17, especially in the extracellular domains (exon 8 and 9), are detected in another third of patients, and in another third of patients, *KIT* is wild type. It is important to recall that the presence of a *KIT* mutation only in extracutaneous organs is a criterion for SM. When positive in CM, these mutations are usually detectable within the lesions and not in the peripheral blood; if detected in blood samples, they strongly indicate systemic disease.[164]

Postulated Cell of Origin

The postulated cell of origin is a committed MC precursor.

Clinical Course

The clinical course of CM is usually that of a benign dermatologic disorder, and spontaneous regression after a period of 12 to 13 years occurs in a significant proportion of juvenile cases.[156,157,162,165] So far, it remains unknown what factors predict persistence of CM lesions into adulthood. In patients with CM who present with small monomorphic skin lesions, the disease tends to persist into adulthood, and in some cases, SM is diagnosed later in life.[156] By contrast, in patients with polymorphic (larger and smaller irregular) lesions, the disease often resolves during or before puberty.[156] In line with this observation, this form of lesion is found only in children, whereas almost all adult patients present with small monomorphic lesions. Mastocytoma is often resected under suspicion of a nevus. In patients with diffuse CM, severe mediator-induced symptoms resulting from degranulation of MCs may occur, sometimes in form of life-threatening anaphylaxis. Serum tryptase is normal in children with a mastocytoma and most children with MPCM but generally elevated in DCM, reflecting the high MC burden caused by the extensive skin involvement. Serum tryptase levels, peripheral blood *KIT* mutation status, peripheral blood counts, and other clinical signs should be evaluated in a child with CM to assess risk of systemic involvement.[166] In adults, the vast majority of patients with suspected CM will have ISM. However, as mentioned, CM can sometimes also be detected in adults. If the skin is the only diagnostic specimen and no BM investigation was performed, it is advised to diagnose MIS, not CM, and recommend additional diagnostic procedures (BM biopsy, high sensitivity *KIT* mutational testing of the peripheral blood).[40,55,153,156] It should be noted that adult-onset MIS and CM do not tend to spontaneously regress, and the affected individuals are at a much higher risk of experiencing anaphylaxis than children.[156]

Differential Diagnosis

Because of the typical dermatologic findings, including a positive Darier's sign, the diagnosis of typical MPCM is rarely missed. However, there are several atypical variants of MPCM that can be missed or confused, such as the nodular form, telangiectatic form, or plaque form of MPCM. Histopathologic features are nearly pathognomonic in MPCM. In adult patients with typical skin lesions (MPCM-like), a *KIT* mutation like D816V in peripheral blood leukocytes, and markedly (and persistently) elevated serum tryptase level (>30 ng/mL) without HαT, the diagnosis of ISM is more likely than that of CM. Thus, these findings in an adult require appropriate staging procedures, including histologic investigation of a BM biopsy specimen. Mastocytoma may be misinterpreted as a malignant neoplasm unless appropriate stains (e.g., Giemsa, toluidine blue, tryptase) are performed. Of note, melanocytic tumors may express KIT/CD117, once again pointing toward the importance of always applying both tryptase and KIT/ CD117 staining whenever mastocytosis is suspected.

Indolent Systemic Mastocytosis

Definition

ISM is defined by the presence of a diagnostic minimum of SM criteria (at least the major SM criterion[12] and the major and one minor SM criterion[13] or at least three minor SM criteria[12,13]) and absence of criteria to diagnose a more advanced type of SM. In fact, patients with ISM lack any C findings and have only one or no B findings. In addition, the diagnoses of SM-AMN/AHN and MCL have to be excluded (Boxes 49-1–49-3).[12-14,39,153] From a histopathological point of view, multifocal MC infiltrates are detectable in at least one extracutaneous organ, usually the BM. Most patients have the typical skin lesions of MPCM. However, today, more and more patients with ISM without skin lesions are diagnosed and referred to as having BM mastocytosis (BMM). A clinically relevant involvement of lymph nodes, liver, spleen, or the GI tract mucosa is less frequent than in advanced SM. By definition, signs of organ failure are not present.

Epidemiology

ISM is the most common subtype of SM and is much more frequent than all the other defined SM subtypes put together.

Clinical Features

Because cutaneous involvement is present in most cases of ISM, the clinical picture is usually dominated by the typical skin lesions, signs of MC activation (usually in the form of mild mediator-induced symptoms but sometimes also in the form of severe symptoms), and osteopenia or osteoporosis. In those with an accompanying IgE-dependent allergy and/ or HαT, the risk of anaphylaxis (MCAS) is high. In a subset of patients, osteoporosis with bone pain is a major complaint requiring specific therapy. The serum tryptase level exceeds 20 ng/mL in most patients with ISM. Organomegaly (hepatosplenomegaly or lymphadenopathy) is usually not found and would represent one (of at least two needed) B finding for the diagnosis of SSM.

Morphology

ISM is characterized by a multifocal, often paratrabecular, compact MC infiltrate in the BM (Figs. 49-17 and 49-18). The MCs may sometimes be round, but in most patients with ISM, they are spindle shaped (atypical MC type I). In most cases,

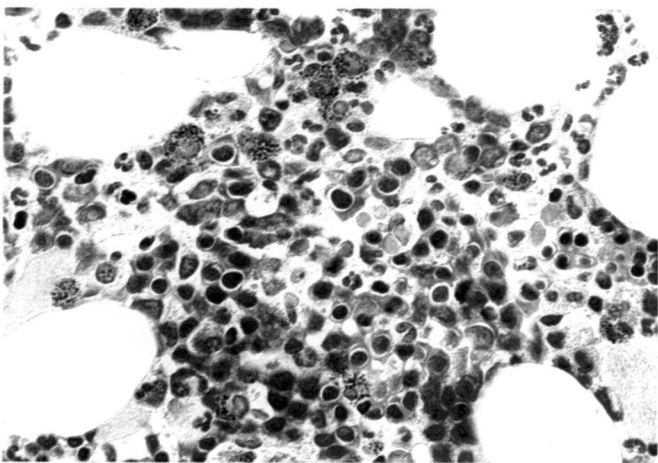

Figure 49-17. Mast cell hyperplasia. Slightly hypercellular bone marrow specimen with prominent erythropoiesis and an increase in loosely scattered metachromatic mast cells. This finding alone does not establish a diagnosis of indolent systemic mastocytosis, even in patients with known cutaneous mastocytosis and elevated serum tryptase levels. Note that the mast cells do not form compact infiltrates. This case illustrates the interstitial type of diffuse infiltration, which is typically seen in hyperplastic states (mast cell hyperplasia).

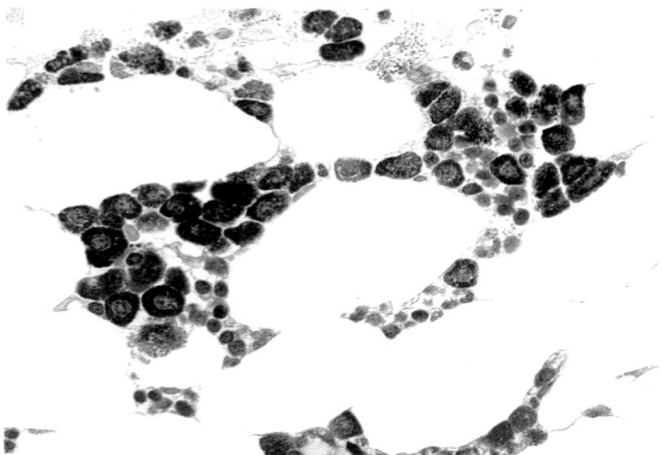

Figure 49-18. Indolent systemic mastocytosis. Hypocellular bone marrow specimen with a focal increase in strongly metachromatic mast cells. Because the patient was known to have mastocytosis in the skin, a diagnosis of indolent systemic mastocytosis was established (compare with Fig. 49-17). The finding of mast cell infiltrates in a hypocellular marrow specimen is uncommon.

the degree of infiltration is low and does not exceed 10% of the section area. In most patients with ISM, the distribution of fat cells is normal, and hematopoiesis is intact in nonaffected BM sites. Mild reactive BM changes, including hemosiderosis, eosinophilia, lymphocytosis, and plasmacytosis, are frequently seen. An increase in reticulin or collagen fibers is confined to the compact MC infiltrates. Thickening of the bone trabeculae is typically found in ISM but is also seen in other SM variants.

Immunophenotype and Genetics

Immunostaining for tryptase and KIT/CD117 is crucial for the diagnosis of ISM to identify even very small compact MC infiltrates. The neoplastic MCs almost always co-express CD25 and often dim (but sometimes strong) CD30; in a subset of cases, CD2 is also present but may be difficult to discern given the accompanying T-cell infiltration. In the rare cases of WDSM, however, expression of CD25 and CD2 is absent, whereas CD30 is brightly expressed in MCs. Focal accumulations of lymphocytes, composed of almost equal proportions of CD20-positive B cells and CD3-positive T cells, are found relatively often in the immediate vicinity of the compact MC infiltrates in ISM, but they are rarely seen in other variants of SM. MCs co-expressing tryptase and chymase (MC_{TC}) are seen relatively frequently in ISM and CM but are relatively rare in ASM and MCL. The latter entities exhibit a majority of MCs that express only tryptase (MC_T type).

The *KIT* D816 mutation is present in >90% of ISM, but >50 other rare *KIT* mutations have been described.[18] *KIT* D816V VAF in serum and BM is usually low (<10%) in ISM, also pointing toward the unilineage involvement.[167] Indeed, the *KIT* D816V mutation in non-MC lineages (multilineage involvement) is only rarely found in ISM compared with advanced SM.[74] The consensus group and the proposed WHO 5th edition account for that and promote *KIT* D816 mutation VAF ≥10% in BM or peripheral blood as a B finding.[13,39] Use of a highly sensitive PCR assay for detection of *KIT* D816V mutation is recommended.[12,153] Other *KIT* mutations and wild-type *KIT* are more frequently encountered in SM with well-differentiated morphology[59] or in advanced SM. If *KIT* D816V is negative, exclusion of *KIT* mutational variants is needed in suspected SM, as any activating *KIT* mutation qualifies as a minor diagnostic criterion.[12,13] If no *KIT* mutation is detected, the presence of M/LN-Eo and tyrosine kinase gene fusion must be excluded.[90] Usually, no other mutations are detected in BM affected by ISM. Yet in elderly patients, characteristic CHIP-mutations with low VAF may be encountered, which may be challenging to interpret.

Postulated Cell of Origin

The postulated cell of origin is a mast cell committed stem/progenitor cell.

Clinical Course

The course of the disease is usually benign. Mediator-related symptoms and/or complications caused by the accompanying osteopathy are often leading. Patients have a slightly increased risk for development of an associated myeloid neoplasm or advanced SM compared with those of adult patients with CM and the general population.

Bone Marrow Mastocytosis and Other (Sub) Variants and Differential Diagnoses

BMM is recognized as a clinicopathologic variant of ISM in the ICC 2022 and as a separate SM entity by the consensus group and in the proposed WHO 5th edition.[12-14,39] BMM is defined by isolated (preferential) BM involvement with mastocytosis in the absence of skin lesions, lack of (any) B findings, and a tryptase level <125 ng/mL.[39] Regarding progression, the prognosis of patients with BMM is favorable compared with other patients with ISM.[168] In addition, patients with BMM have a high risk of developing severe anaphylaxis (>60% of patients) after *Hymenoptera* insect venom exposure (stings), which is much more frequent than in patients with typical ISM (approximately 15%).[168] BMM accounts for the majority of cases formerly designated eosinophilic fibrohistiocytic BM lesions.[9] Compared with typical ISM, BMM shows lower serum tryptase levels, a male predominance, significantly older age at presentation, lower MC burden, and fewer MC-related symptoms between acute episodes.[168,169] Because of the lower MC burden, the major criterion is often not met, so the diagnosis mostly relies on the presence of the three minor SM criteria; therefore, the use of a very sensitive technique to detect a KIT mutation is of importance. Because serum tryptase may not be routinely measured in patients presenting with anaphylaxis, BMM is likely underrecognized. Although patients with BMM have an excellent prognosis in terms of progression, they are at risk for potentially life-threatening allergic reactions and bone fractures. Another important aspect is that most patients with ASM and MCL also lack skin lesions. Therefore, it is of great importance to delineate between advanced SM (ASM/MCL) and BMM. Whereas in BMM no B or C findings and no circulating MCs are seen and serum tryptase levels and KIT mutational VAFs are low, a markedly elevated serum tryptase, C findings, circulating MCs (in MCL) and high KIT mutational VAFs (often accompanied by other mutations) are detected in ASM and/or MCL.

WDSM is characterized by the presence of enlarged, round, well-granulated MCs forming multifocal infiltrates; CD2 and CD25 are usually not expressed, and the KIT D816V mutation is lacking; this constellation is commonly seen in a characteristic clinicopathologic setting.[59] Yet, WDSM morphology is detectable in patients with ISM (often BMM) and SSM and even sometimes in those with MCL. Therefore, it is currently considered a morphologic pattern and not as a separate SM subentity.[12,13]

Smoldering Systemic Mastocytosis

SSM was initially considered a subvariant of ISM, assuming an intermediate position between ISM and ASM, exhibiting at least two B findings but no C findings and no AMN. The patients often display organomegaly without functional impairment (i.e., hepatomegaly and/or splenomegaly and/or >1 cm lymphadenopathy on palpation or imaging without ascites, portal hypertension, or hypersplenism; B finding #3). The degree of BM infiltration is higher than that seen in typical ISM, exceeding 30% of the section area (B finding #1). Cytopenia or cytosis not meeting criteria for C findings and not explained by another reactive process or AMN can be observed and is considered a B finding in the ICC 2022.[12] Signs of mild hematopoietic dysplasia or mild myeloproliferative features may be present in the BM (not meeting the diagnostic criteria for AMN/AHN), which is still considered a B finding by the consensus group and in the proposed WHO 5th edition (but not in the ICC 2022).[13,14,39] A markedly elevated serum tryptase level (>200 ng/mL) is seen in most patients with SSM (B finding #1).[170,171] In 2022, both classifications recognize SSM as a separate variant of SM.

Systemic Mastocytosis With an Associated Myeloid/Hematologic Neoplasm

Definition

The diagnosis of SM-AMN (AHN according to the proposed WHO 5th edition) can be made only when there is clear evidence of both SM and concurrent myeloid neoplasm.[153] SM-AMN/AHN meets the diagnostic criteria of both SM and the associated myeloid neoplasm (ICC 2022) or any hematologic neoplasm (proposed WHO 5th edition), both of which should be classified according to established criteria. As hematologic neoplasms accompanying SM are almost exclusively of myeloid origin—and often of clonality proven to be shared with the SM[46,68]—and co-occurring lymphoid or plasma cell neoplasms are rare and considered to be clonally unrelated,[46,47,126] the latter two groups are excluded as associated neoplasms in the ICC 2022.[12] The diagnosis of SM-AMN/AHN can be difficult to establish because the histologic and cytologic features of SM may be obscured by the associated malignant neoplasm. In some patients, diagnosis and subtyping of the AMN/AHN are possible only in the blood owing to an extensive compact infiltration of the BM, mimicking pure ASM or MCL at first glance. In some patients, the initial BM biopsy specimen enables establishment of a diagnosis of SM-AMN/AHN, whereas in a following biopsy, progression of SM with extensive infiltration of the BM may obscure the AMN. The following diseases have been identified within the setting of SM-AMN: MDS, AML (most commonly AML t[8;21][q22;q22.1]/RUNX1::RUNX1T1), CML, MPN, and MDS/MPN (most commonly CMML); because of the common co-occurrence of SM in CMML and AML t(8;21) (q22;q22.1)/RUNX1::RUNX1T1, active search by means of tryptase staining on a regular basis is advisable in such instances.

Epidemiology

SM-AMN/AHN is the second most common subtype of SM. However, its true incidence is probably underestimated because the SM component is often missed owing to the dominance of the AMN. Cases have been recognized in which the presence of SM was disclosed after therapy for AML, enabling the retrospective diagnosis of SM-AML.[55,124,126,172]

Clinical Features

Clinical features are generally dominated by the non-MC AMN, including significant cytopenia(s) or cytosis, monocytosis and/or eosinophilia, splenomegaly, and elevated LDH.[153] In addition, high KIT D816V VAF (usually much higher than anticipated from the MC numbers in the biopsy), and additional somatic mutations in genes associated with myeloid malignancies (particularly if occurring in combination) should raise a high degree of suspicion for an AMN in SM. The typical skin lesions seen in ISM are present in <50% of patients with SM-AMN/AHN.[173-175]

Morphology

The histologic picture of SM-AMN/AHN in the BM is heterogeneous and largely dependent on the type of AMN/AHN (Fig. 49-19). The BM almost always exhibits marked hypercellularity, with subtotal depletion of fat cells. Both multifocal compact MC infiltrates and the typical morphologic findings of AMN/AHN must be detectable.[12,13] A few cases of pure CM with AMN/AHN have also been reported.[176] We think such cases should not be termed SM (or SM-AMN/AHN) and that they represent coincidental findings.

If eosinophilia is present, the presence of tyrosine kinase gene fusions associated with M/LN-Eo must be excluded.[90] Although usually mutually exclusive, rare cases with both KIT mutation and tyrosine kinase gene fusion have been reported.[177] In such an exceptional instance, the M/LN-Eo would represent the AMN, but such cases should only be diagnosed in the presence of unequivocal molecular evidence of both a KIT mutation and a characteristic M/LN-Eo gene fusion.

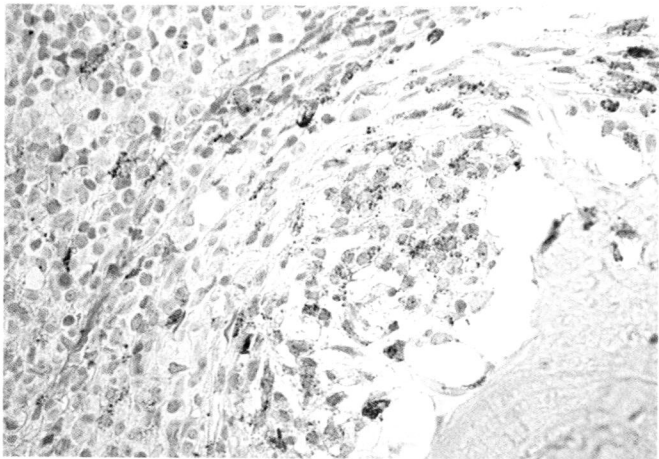

Figure 49-19. Systemic mastocytosis with an associated hematologic neoplasm. Immunostaining for tryptase in this case of acute myeloid leukemia reveals a focal paratrabecular infiltrate of mast cells, diagnostic of concurrent systemic mastocytosis. Sequencing analysis revealed *RUNX1* R162K mutation with a variant allele frequency (VAF) of 81% and a *KIT* D816V mutation with a VAF of 41%, indicating multimutational high VAF-burden disease and suggesting that the *KIT* D816V mutation was acquired after the *RUNX1* R162K mutation and played a role as "phenotype modifier," paving the way to accompanying mast cell differentiation.

Immunophenotype and Genetics

Immunostaining for tryptase, KIT/CD117, CD25, and CD30 is usually sufficient to establish the diagnosis of SM in the setting of SM-AMN/AHN. Regarding the AMN, appropriate immunostainings (e.g., for CD14, CD34, IRF8,[178] and myeloperoxidase, etc.) are indicated.

The *KIT* D816V mutation is found in 60% to 94% of patients and is usually detected in the SM component but also in the AMN component.[12,13] Especially in SM-CMML, *KIT* mutations have been detected in CMML cells in 89% of cases, suggesting a common (MC/monocytic) precursor cell. In SM-AML, except for AML t(8;21)(q22;q22.1)/*RUNX1::RUNX1T1*, and SM-MPN, the frequency of a *KIT* mutation in the AMN component is lower (30% and 20%, respectively).[46,47,126] Non-*KIT* mutations are very frequent in SM-AMN; they are often observable at higher VAFs, indicating the *KIT* D816V mutation may act as a modifier toward MC differentiation of an initially non-*KIT* mutated background precursor cell.[82,96] It should be noted that the mutational profile differs between ISM-AMN and ASM-AMN or MCL-AMN. In the former, non-*KIT* mutations predominantly involve *JAK2, ETV6, U2AF1, EZH2,* and/or *SF3B1*; in ASM-AMN or MCL-AMN, non-*KIT* mutations mainly involve *TET2, SRSF2, ASXL1, RUNX1, N/KRAS,* and *IDH2*.[97]

Postulated Cell of Origin

The postulated cell of origin: pluripotent hematopoietic stem and progenitor cells.

Clinical Course

In most patients, the clinical course and prognosis are dominated by the AMN/AHN, not by the SM. However, if the SM corresponds to ASM or MCL, SM will be prognostically decisive. Both the SM component and the AMN/AHN component of the disease need to be classified accordingly. The presence of an *ASXL1* or *SRSF2* mutation and the number

of mutations in the *SRSF2/ASXL1/RUNX1* panel seem to be independent prognostic factors, negatively affecting overall survival.[12,13] Modern midostaurin, polychemotherapy, stem cell transplantation, and especially avapritinib-based/containing regimens have significantly improved the outcomes in patients with SM-AMN.[56,93,179]

Differential Diagnosis

SM-AMN must be distinguished from non-MC myeloid tumors with signs of MC differentiation (e.g., tryptase-positive AML) and from MDS/AML with prominent involvement of the MC lineage, as seen in MML.[105,118,147,180] MC differentiation in AML is associated with tryptase expression in otherwise morphologically unremarkable blast cells, which sometimes form clusters, without the typical focal MC infiltrates of SM. In MML, there is a diffuse but variable increase in tryptase-expressing metachromatic cells (metachromatic blasts) that are often highly atypical, may express CD34, an antigen never expressed by MCs, and are almost always CD25 negative. As in tryptase-positive AML, focal compact MC infiltrates are not seen in MML.

Aggressive Systemic Mastocytosis

Definition

ASM is a rare subtype of SM that exhibits the clinical characteristics of a high-grade hematologic neoplasm and signs of severe organ damage caused by MC infiltration, usually involving the BM and extramedullary organs, thus displaying ≥1 so-called "C finding."

Epidemiology

ASM is much less common than ISM and SM-AMN/AHN, accounting for about 5% of all SM cases.

Clinical Features

ASM is characterized by an aggressive clinical course with marked MC infiltration of various organs and tissues, including the BM, liver, spleen, GI tract mucosa, lymph nodes and/or skeleton. Skin lesions are present in <50% of cases. The total MC burden is high, with corresponding organomegaly (usually hepatomegaly and/or splenomegaly, occasionally lymphadenopathy) and signs of impaired organ function (e.g., cytopenia, ascites, portal hypertension, hypersplenism, malabsorption caused by GI tract MS infiltration, large osteolysis with or without pathologic fracture) that are all summarized as so-called "C findings" (indicative of organ damage).[55,181,182] Serum tryptase levels are almost always markedly elevated.

Morphology

The BM is hypercellular, with focal and diffuse infiltration by atypical, hypogranular, nonmetachromatic MCs that usually show prominent spindling (Fig. 49-20). However, a subset of these cells may also be quite immature. There may be slight atypia of blood cell precursors or signs of myeloproliferation. An AMN/AHN may be present, which can become more evident after treatment of the ASM, and the disease should be then reclassified accordingly (SM-AMN/AHN). ASM-t, in which progression to MCL is ongoing, will usually display >5% MCs on BM smears, and as soon as the percentage is 20%, the diagnosis of a secondary MCL should be established.[105]

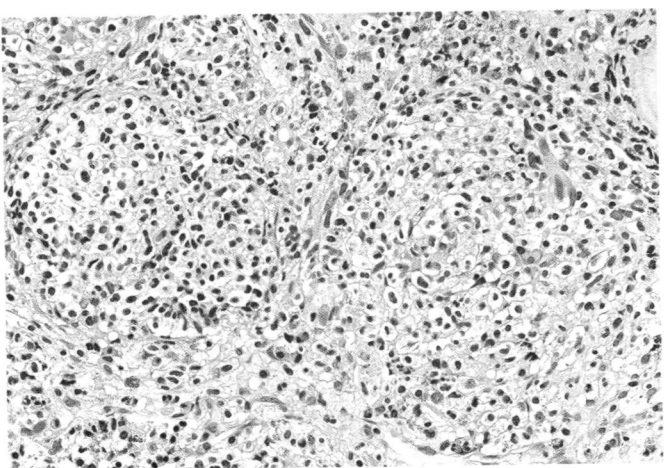

Figure 49-20. Aggressive systemic mastocytosis infiltrating the bone marrow. Note the cytologic atypia of mast cells. Sequencing analysis revealed *ASXL1* S1028fs with a variant allele frequency (VAF) of 17%, CKIT: *KIT* D816V with a VAF of 15%, *RUNX1* S322fs with a VAF of 7%, *SRSF2* P95L with a VAF of 40%, *TET2* H1904R with a VAF of 44%, and Y1245fs with a VAF of 44%, indicating multimutational high VAF-burden disease. This suggests the *TET2* and *SRSF2* mutations were founding, the *ASXL1* mutation was disease progression mutation, and the *CKIT* mutation was a "phenotype modifier" mutation.

A distinct variant of ASM with clinical features mimicking generalized malignant lymphoma has been termed lymphadenopathic mastocytosis with eosinophilia. In contrast to classic ASM, this condition is associated with generalized lymphadenopathy and marked blood eosinophilia.[183]

Immunophenotype and Genetics

The MCs in ASM are always tryptase positive and usually co-express CD25, CD30, and KIT/CD117. In a proportion of cases, the MCs also express CD2, whereas chymase is relatively rarely detected and is usually not expressed by all MCs in a given case.

The *KIT* D816V mutation is detected in approximately 80% of cases. Molecular studies in ASM brought evidence for the presence of multilineage involvement by the *KIT* mutations, often accompanied by the presence of additional "myeloid" mutations.[55,82,153,184,185] Thus, ASM and SM-AMN are genetically very close, being multimutational and high *KIT* mutational burden diseases, ASM not reaching criteria for a straightforward diagnosis of an additional myeloid neoplasm.

Postulated Cell of Origin

The postulated cell of origin is a hematopoietic MC-committed stem cell.

Clinical Course

The prognosis of ASM is worse than that of ISM or SSM. The median overall survival of patients with ASM is approximately 4.5 years.[153] As mentioned, patients with ASM-t have a very poor prognosis.[105] These patients rapidly progress to MCL, which is otherwise generally observable in a sixth of individuals affected by ASM.[105,185,186]

Differential Diagnosis

ASM must be differentiated from SSM (C findings are missing), SM-AMN, and particularly aleukemic MCL (MC count <20% in BM smears excludes MCL and favors ASM).[12]

Mast Cell Leukemia

Definition

MCL is a highly malignant neoplasm meeting the criteria of SM that is accompanied by a significant increase of atypical MCs in the BM smears (>20% of all cells in BM smears). In the ICC 2022,[12] the diagnosis does not solely rely on the aspirate and, in the presence of a suboptimal aspirate (dry tap), a BM biopsy showing a diffuse MC infiltration of immature atypical MCs (e.g., immature bilobed forms and multinucleated or bizarre MCs) in the proper clinical context can be used to support a diagnosis of MCL, which is in contrast to previous WHO proposals and the proposals of the consensus group.[39,105] This is of major practical importance, as especially dry taps apply to many diagnostically challenging cases.

MCL can be divided in a leukemic form, defined by ≥10% MCs of all leukocytes in peripheral blood, and the more frequent aleukemic form with <10% MCs.[39,105] Although it is still recommended to document the presence of circulating MCs, their presence no longer indicates a separate subcategory because data show that any circulating MCs are linked to poorer prognosis of MCL.[56] Finally, MCL can be divided into acute MCL, defined by signs of MCL-induced organ damage, and chronic MCL, in which no signs of MCL-induced organ damage are found.[39,105]

Epidemiology

MCL is extremely uncommon and probably represents the rarest form of leukemia in humans. A few hundred well-documented cases have been reported.[51-56,187]

Clinical Features

Patients with MCL usually present with signs of an acute leukemia, including prominent cytopenia, and often signs of organ damage. If this is not the case and no other signs of SM-related organ damage are noted (i.e., lacking C findings) but the criteria of MCL are fulfilled, the final diagnosis of chronic MCL should be rendered.[39,56,105] The typical skin lesions of MPCM are absent, but disseminated leukemic skin infiltrates have occasionally been described, and signs of MC activation are rarely found. Owing to the large MC burden, serum tryptase levels are markedly or even excessively elevated, and mediator-related symptoms regularly occur. Most patients with MCL die within 1 year of diagnosis unless treated with polychemotherapy and stem cell transplantation. More prolonged survival is observed in the rare form of chronic MCL.[188]

Morphology

As in most cases of acute leukemia, the BM in MCL usually shows a dense, diffuse-compact infiltration pattern, with subtotal displacement of fat cells and normal hematopoiesis (Fig. 49-21). Abundant, highly atypical, often round MCs are seen in BM and blood smears in most cases. These MCs are often hypogranular and exhibit immature blast-like morphology with monocytoid or even lobulated nuclei (metachromatic blasts). Metachromatically granulated blast cells are also recorded in patients with MCL. In rare cases, the MCs exhibit a mature phenotype, with round nuclei and an abundance of metachromatic granules. Fibrosis is typically less than that seen in ASM.

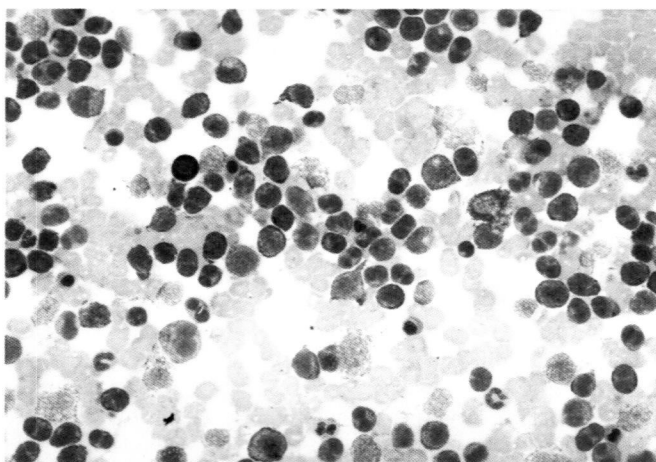

Figure 49-21. Mast cell leukemia. This bone marrow smear shows an extremely pronounced increase in atypical mast cells containing varying amounts of metachromatic granules. The mast cells constitute more than 90% of all the nucleated cells. A large number of circulating mast cells is also present (compare with Fig. 49-4).

Immunophenotype and Genetics

Leukemic cells in MCL express tryptase, CD25, KIT/CD117, and often also CD30.[189] Like the neoplastic MCs in all other types of SM, they may also co-express CD2 but are more frequently CD2 negative.

The *KIT* D816V mutation is found in 50% to 70% of cases. Other *KIT* mutations and wild-type *KIT* are each observable in 10% to 20%. Non-*KIT* mutations are frequent and recurrently involve *TET2, SF3B1, SRSF2, ASXL1, BRAF, KRAS,* and *NRAS*.[55,56,190]

Postulated Cell of Origin

The postulated cell of origin is an MC-committed hematopoietic stem or progenitor cell.[60]

Clinical Course

MCL may occur as primary (de novo) or secondary, evolving from an anteceding MC neoplasm, mainly SM-AMN or ASM.[55,190] MCL almost always behaves aggressively. At the time of this writing, the median survival time was 1.6 years (without intensive therapy). The prognosis seems to be better in the very few examples of chronic MCL, in *KIT* D816V mutated cases, in patients treated with midostaurin or avapritinib, and in patients without abnormal karyotype with primary MCL.[56] Exceptional patients with complete remission and long-term survival after polychemotherapy and allogenic stem cell transplantation have been reported as well.[179] Impressive responses have also been reported with application of the KIT D816V-specific tyrosine kinase inhibitor avapritinib.[92]

Differential Diagnosis

The differential diagnosis includes basophilic leukemia, SM-AMN, and MML. The aleukemic variant of MCL has to be discriminated from ASM and ASM-AHN and is accounted for in the ICC 2022.

Mast Cell Sarcoma

Definition

MCS is even rarer than MCL. It presents as local, sarcomatous, destructive tumor of highly atypical MCs, initially without clinical signs of dissemination or generalization.

Epidemiology

Few well-documented cases of MCS have been described, and 10 more have been more recently reported, summarizing the up-to-date publications.[116,191-194] It is interesting that, in addition to bones (skull, tibia), involved sites were not the lymphoreticular tissues commonly affected by mastocytosis but instead the larynx, colon, dura, uterus, small intestine, inner lip, pelvis, skin/soft tissue of the ankle, spleen, and liver. The sex distribution is nearly equal, and there is a huge variation of age (range 1–77 years, median 39).[116]

Clinical Features

MCS presents with signs of local tumor growth that are largely non-specific, but in all patients reported, an aggressive growth and expansion of the local tumor has been described. As per definition, MCS is a strictly localized tumor, but secondary dissemination and progression to MCL is often seen. When an antecedent or accompanying SM is found, the disease should not be called MCS but should be regarded as MCS-like progression in SM.[55,116,195] It is remarkable that, in three MCS cases, the patients had a history of a germ cell tumor, and in one, the *KIT* D579del mutation was shared between the MCS and the antecedent mediastinal yolk sack tumor.[116,196] Though based on the small number of cases described, it appears that MCS tends to rapidly disseminate and transform to MCL.

Morphology

MCS is one of the most aggressive neoplasms within the spectrum of MC disorders and is characterized by atypical hypogranular tumor cells that often exhibit bizarre nuclei and prominent nucleoli, mimicking a high-grade sarcoma at first glance (Fig. 49-22). The morphology of these cells mostly resembles that seen in MCL.

Immunophenotype and Genetics

The tumor cells express tryptase and KIT/CD117.

The majority of MCSs are *KIT* wild type. The *KIT* D816V mutation is reported in <10% of cases, and a fifth seems to display other *KIT* mutations, including L799F, N822Y, N822K, V560G, D419del, and D579del.[116,196]

Postulated Cell of Origin

The postulated cell of origin is an MC-committed stem/precursor cell.

Clinical Course

MCS follows a highly aggressive course with a median survival of 24 months.[116,191-196] Most patients progress to MCL within a short time. Some may temporally respond to a KIT-targeting drug like imatinib.[197,198] The survival time is very short in almost all cases.

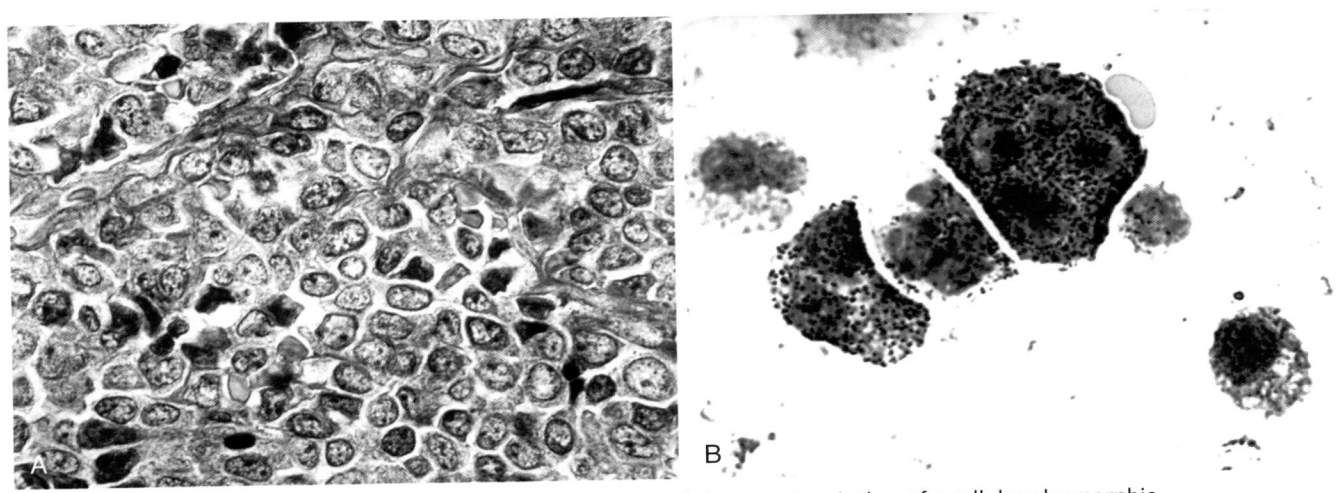

Figure 49-22. Mast cell sarcoma. A, The histopathologic picture is that of a cellular pleomorphic tumor with only a mild desmoplastic reaction. Even with the meticulous evaluation of Giemsa-stained sections, no metachromatic granules can be detected. Because most of the tumor cells strongly expressed chloroacetate esterase, CD117, and tryptase, a diagnosis of mast cell sarcoma was established. **B,** Touch preparations also provide the correct diagnosis. With this technique, the pleomorphic, sometimes multinucleated tumor cells can be seen to contain an abundance of metachromatic granules; these were not detectable in routinely processed specimens, presumably because of water solubility. The granules of normal basophils are water soluble, as may be the case for highly malignant mast cell tumors (mast cell leukemia and mast cell sarcoma).

Differential Diagnosis

The differential diagnosis includes high-grade round cell sarcomas, histiocytic sarcoma, Langerhans cell sarcoma, ALK-negative anaplastic large cell lymphoma, myeloid sarcoma, and melanoma. The expression of tryptase by MCS and its negativity for CD1a, langerin, S100, melanocytic markers, and myeloperoxidase clearly distinguish it from these listed neoplasms.[116,199] A diagnosis of extracutaneous mastocytoma, which exhibits monomorphic, round, well-differentiated, strongly metachromatic tumor cells, is easy to exclude. Fibromastocytic tumors, which are extremely rare, should also be considered in the differential diagnosis.[200]

Extracutaneous Mastocytoma

Definition

Extracutaneous mastocytoma (ECM) is a benign localized tumor consisting of mature-appearing MCs, with no signs of systemic involvement. Although not included in the current classifications, ECM is discussed herein.

Epidemiology

Unlike CM, ECM is extremely rare and has been found predominantly in the lung and occasionally in the head, neck, and stomach.[55,201,202]

Clinical Features

In ECM, the clinical features are those of an organ tumor that may appear intensively yellowish on macroscopic examination,[55] with no specific clinical signs.

Morphology

In contrast to MCS, ECM exhibits relatively monomorphic, strongly metachromatic, round MCs that are easily recognizable when basic dyes such as Giemsa and toluidine blue are applied.

Immunophenotype

The tumor cells express tryptase and KIT/CD117.

Postulated Cell of Origin

The postulated cell of origin is an MC-committed precursor.

Clinical Course

The clinical course is that of a benign tumor, with complete remission after resection. Progression to an aggressive disease has not been reported, yet one patient with gastric ECM was diagnosed with ISM within disease course.[53]

Differential Diagnosis

The major differential diagnosis of ECM is local MC hyperplasia. Another differential diagnosis may be ISM. Therefore, the diagnosis of ECM should be established only after a careful and thorough investigation of the adjacent tissue and definitive exclusion of all other SM criteria. In some instances, the hematopathologist may ask for another organ biopsy (to detect a second infiltrate) before making the final diagnosis of ECM. Because ECM consists of sheets of well-differentiated metachromatic MCs, it can be easily distinguished from MCS and soft tissue sarcomas. In H&E (hematoxylin and eosin) stains, the MCs may have a plasmacytoid appearance, initially suggesting a diagnosis of plasma cell granuloma. GIST, also at extra GI sites, should always be taken into consideration and excluded by staining for tryptase and DOG1.

Pearls and Pitfalls

Pearls

- A multifocal, compact tryptase and/or KIT/CD117-positive mast cell infiltrate in internal organs, such as bone marrow or spleen, is the major diagnostic criterion for SM.
- Mast cells exhibiting a spindle shape, co-expression of CD2, CD25, and/or CD30, or any activating mutation of *KIT* are strongly indicative of SM.
- The most common variants of mastocytosis—CM and ISM—usually have a benign clinical course.
- SM with an associated myeloid neoplasm is distinctive among hematologic neoplasms.
- Indolent mast cell neoplasms are unimutational disorders with single (mast cell) lineage involvement by a driver *KIT* mutation, but advanced mast cell neoplasms are multimutational disorders with multilineage hematopoietic involvement in which *KIT* mutations usually play a role as "phenotype modifier," paving the way to mast cell differentiation.

Pitfalls

- Mastocytosis must be distinguished from a variety of rare hematopoietic and non-hematopoietic disorders, especially myelomastocytic neoplasms (tryptase-positive AML, MML), myeloid/lymphoid neoplasms with eosinophilia and tyrosine kinase gene fusions, chronic eosinophilic and basophilic leukemias, lymphomas, sarcomas, gastrointestinal stromal tumors, and melanomas.
- Mast cells in reactive and neoplastic states usually co-express tryptase and CD117/KIT; cells expressing only tryptase (neoplastic basophils) or only CD117 (hematopoietic progenitor cells and/or others) must not be termed mast cells.
- Detection of *KIT* mutations has prime importance in mastocytosis and must by assessed by sensitive methods, as these mutations represent a minor diagnostic criterion of SM; if assessed in a quantitative manner they are of significant prognostic value and are major predictors of targeted drug sensitivities.

KEY REFERENCES

18. Valent P, Akin C, Sperr WR, et al. New insights into the pathogenesis of mastocytosis: emerging concepts in diagnosis and therapy. *Ann Rev Pathol.* 2023;18:361.
33. Furitsu T, Tsujimura T, Tono T, et al. Identification of mutations in the coding sequence of the proto-oncogene c-kit in a human mast cell leukemia cell line causing ligand-independent activation of c-kit product. *J Clin Invest.* 1993;92:1736.
39. Valent P, Akin C, Hartmann K, et al. Updated diagnostic criteria and classification of mast cell disorders: a consensus proposal. *Hemasphere.* 2021;5:e646.
56. Kennedy VE, Perkins C, Reiter A, et al. Mast cell leukemia: clinical and molecular features and survival outcomes of patients in the ECNM Registry. *Blood Adv.* 2023;7:1713.
67. Hoermann G, Sotlar K, Jawhar M, et al. Standards of genetic testing in the diagnosis and prognostication of systemic mastocytosis in 2022: recommendations of the EU-US Cooperative Group. *J Allergy Clin Immunol Pract.* 2022;10:1953.
82. Jawhar M, Schwaab J, Schnittger S, et al. Molecular profiling of myeloid progenitor cells in multi-mutated advanced systemic mastocytosis identifies KIT D816V as a distinct and late event. *Leukemia.* 2015;29:1115.
105. Valent P, Sotlar K, Sperr WR, et al. Refined diagnostic criteria and classification of mast cell leukemia (MCL) and myelomastocytic leukemia (MML): a consensus proposal. *Ann Oncol.* 2014;25:1691.
116. Matsumoto NP, Yuan J, Wang J, et al. Mast cell sarcoma: clinicopathologic and molecular analysis of 10 new cases and review of literature. *Mod Pathol.* 2022;35:865.
152. Valent P, Hartmann K, Bonadonna P, et al. Global classification of mast cell activation disorders: an ICD-10-CM-adjusted proposal of the ECNM-AIM Consortium. *J Allergy Clin Immunol Pract.* 2022;10:1941.
155. Reiter A, George TI, Gotlib J. New molecular genetics and treatment paradigms in advanced systemic mastocytosis. *Blood.* 2020;135:1365.

Visit Elsevier eBooks+ for the complete set of references.

Chapter 50

Eosinophilia, Chronic Eosinophilic Leukemia, Not Otherwise Specified, and Myeloid/Lymphoid Neoplasms With Eosinophilia and Tyrosine Kinase Gene Fusions

Kaaren K. Reichard, Sa A. Wang, Daniel A. Arber, and Attilio Orazi

OVERVIEW

Eosinophilia encompasses a complex group of disorders of diverse etiology for which there are many tools available for the workup and diagnosis. This chapter addresses the clinical, pathologic, and genetic features of the International Consensus Conference (ICC) category of myeloid/lymphoid neoplasms with eosinophilia and tyrosine kinase gene fusions (M/LN-eo-TK), chronic eosinophilic leukemia, not otherwise specified (CEL, NOS), and idiopathic hypereosinophilia (iHE)/idiopathic hypereosinophilic syndrome (iHES).[1-11]

This chapter focuses on the workup and diagnosis of eosinophilic disorders. First, a reasonable yet comprehensive approach to the initial workup of hypereosinophilic disorders is presented, with specific attention paid to the role of morphologic and laboratory features and proper use of ancillary testing, particularly genetic tools. Second, specific clinicopathologic aspects of the ICC categories of M/LN-eo-TK (e.g., myeloid/lymphoid neoplasms with eosinophilia and *PDGFRA, PDGFRB, FGFR1, JAK2,* or *FLT3* rearrangement or *ETV6::ABL1*), CEL, NOS, and iHE/iHES are discussed.[1-11] It is beyond the scope of this chapter to provide a detailed description of other entities often in the differential diagnosis with eosinophilia, which are covered in other chapters of this book (chronic myeloid leukemia [CML], see Chapter 47; acute myeloid leukemia [AML] with inv[16], see Chapter 46; systemic mastocytosis, see Chapter 49). It should also be mentioned that pediatric/constitutional/immunodeficiency disorders that are associated with eosinophilia are also beyond the scope of this chapter.

INTRODUCTION

Eosinophilia can be caused by or associated with a complex group of disorders. Given the diversity of the underlying etiology, the initial approach is to organize eosinophilic conditions into primary (clonal) and secondary (reactive) categories for further discussion (see Box 50-1 for a non-exhaustive listing of etiologies).[12-15] As can be seen in Box 50-1, the underlying causes of an eosinophilic disorder may range from drug/medication exposure, infection, and autoimmune conditions to a malignancy wherein the eosinophilia is a reactive consequence or a primary clonal proliferation of eosinophils. The cause of eosinophilia is best identified by the patient's history, clinical presentation, and specific laboratory testing. Reactive eosinophils typically demonstrate normal eosinophilic cytology; however, abnormal features such as hypogranulation, eccentric location of granules within the cytoplasm, hyposegmentation, and cytoplasmic vacuoles may be seen in some eosinophils in reactive expansions (Fig. 50-1).

By far, the nonclonal forms of eosinophilia greatly outweigh the clonal forms. For example, allergy, drug/medication, hypersensitivity reactions, and infection are common causes of eosinophilia. Given the breadth of possible causes of eosinophilia, one can appreciate the variety of testing options that should or should not be undertaken depending on the features of an individual case. Depending on the patient's clinical condition, a proper and timely workup of such disorders is crucial because of the clinical potential for eosinophilic organ infiltration with subsequent tissue damage (hypereosinophilic syndrome).[15] iHES can be associated with significant morbidity and mortality, and prompt delineation of a definitive and treatable etiology, if possible, is desired.

Eosinophilia is defined by an absolute eosinophil count (AEC) that exceeds 0.5×10^9/L or relative peripheral blood eosinophilia of >6% eosinophils on the differential count.[15-18] It may further be designated as mild ($0.5–1.49 \times 10^9$/L), moderate ($1.5–5.0 \times 10^9$/L), or severe (>5×10^9/L). The AEC is calculated as follows: white blood cell (WBC) count × 10^9/L × percentage of eosinophils = AEC (eosinophils × 10^9/L).[16,17]

CLASSIFICATION

The classification of eosinophilic diseases should be specific and reference whether it is reactive or clonal, when possible. For example, it should be stated that a patient has reactive eosinophilia in the setting of a known medication, or for clonal eosinophilic disorders, the diagnosis should adhere to the most recent classification scheme such as the International Consensus Conference.[3,5] Box 50-1 lists the ICC entities that may be associated with clonal eosinophilia.

CLINICAL PRESENTATION

It should be noted that the AEC neither predicts the underlying etiology nor the potential clinical severity of the disease. Though an extremely increased AEC (>20–30 × 10^9/L) is uncommon in allergic and asthmatic conditions and may help point toward a neoplastic disorder, this is insufficient, by itself, for a malignant diagnosis. Similarly, the AEC cannot predict the degree, if any, of eosinophil-related end organ damage. For example, a patient with mild eosinophilia may experience significant organ damage/dysfunction. Organ involvement/damage requires clinical, imaging, and laboratory evaluation.

Given the diverse underlying causes of eosinophilia and involvement of various organs/tissues by eosinophilia, patients may present with different symptoms and show different signs, such as constitutional symptoms; skin rash/cutaneous lesions; gastrointestinal, respiratory/pulmonary, cardiac, muscular/joint, endocrine, and/or central nervous system involvement; or newly emerging lymphadenopathy,

---

Box 50-1　*Etiologies Underlying Eosinophilia*

Secondary (Reactive Eosinophilia)
Allergic diseases: Asthma, allergic rhinitis, atopic dermatitis, drug hypersensitivity
Infections: Helminths, parasites, protozoans, fungi, viruses
Neoplastic disorders: Solid tumors, lymphoid malignancies (e.g., lymphoblastic leukemia, classic Hodgkin lymphoma, B-cell and T-cell lymphomas)
Immunologic disorders: Immunodeficiencies, autoimmune and other connective tissue disorders
Eosinophilic disorders: Eosinophilic granulomatosis with polyangiitis, eosinophilic gastrointestinal disorders
Other: Radiation exposure, cholesterol emboli, hypoadrenalism, IL-2 therapy

Primary (Clonal Eosinophilia); International Consensus Classification (ICC)-Recognized Entities
Myeloid/lymphoid neoplasms with eosinophilia and tyrosine kinase gene fusions (myeloid/lymphoid neoplasm with *PDGFRA* rearrangement, myeloid/lymphoid neoplasm with *PDGFRB* rearrangement, myeloid/lymphoid neoplasm with *FGFR1* rearrangement, myeloid/lymphoid neoplasm with *JAK2* rearrangement, myeloid/lymphoid neoplasm with *FLT3* rearrangement, and myeloid/lymphoid neoplasm with *ETV6::ABL1*)
Myeloproliferative neoplasms (particularly chronic eosinophilic leukemia, not otherwise specified; chronic myeloid leukemia with eosinophilia)
Acute myeloid leukemia, particularly AML with inv(16)
Systemic mastocytosis (the eosinophils are not clonal in all cases)
Myelodysplastic syndromes (rare)
Chronic myelomonocytic leukemia (rare)

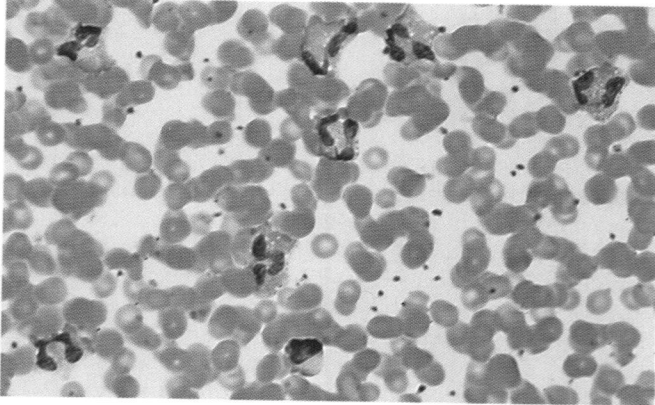

Figure 50-1. Reactive eosinophilia. Peripheral blood smear from a 55-year-old male with an absolute eosinophil count of 10.3 × 10^9/L discovered incidentally after taking antibiotics for an upper respiratory infection. Though many of the eosinophils demonstrate normal cytologic features, several exhibit vacuolization, partial degranulation, and eccentric localization of granules within the cytoplasm (1000× magnification; Wright-Giemsa).

hepatomegaly, or splenomegaly.[6,15-19] Although less common than dermatologic, pulmonary, and gastrointestinal manifestations, cardiac failure due to endocardial damage and subsequent fibrosis and valvular insufficiency may result in significant morbidity and mortality. Similarly, central nervous system involvement is uncommon but associated with a grave outcome. The clinical presentation and prognosis of clonal eosinophilia is very depending on the underlying hematopoietic neoplasm; and patients often have cytopenia(s) and/or cytosis with or without increased blasts. Eosinophilia-associated organ damage may occur in around 30% to 40% of patients with clonal eosinophilia.

APPROACH TO DIAGNOSIS

A reasonable initial approach to the diagnosis in a case of unexplained eosinophilia is to exclude secondary causes, assuming the patient is clinically stable.[13,20-25] Secondary eosinophilia has many causes (Box 50-1) and is much more common than primary eosinophilia. The diagnostic workup often involves consultation with multiple medical specialties including allergy, hematology, pulmonary, infectious disease, rheumatology, and gastroenterology. Specific entities such as drug/medication reactions, hypersensitivity, and pulmonary eosinophilic disorders (e.g., chronic eosinophilic pneumonia, eosinophilic granulomatosis with polyangiitis) are typically diagnosed in the appropriate clinical, radiologic, and pathologic context. Underlying malignancies, such as lymphoma and solid tumor, may also be associated with reactive eosinophilia. In these cases, the eosinophilia results from the production and release of cytokines such as interleukin (IL)-3 and IL-5 by the tumor cells, which promote eosinophil proliferation. Evaluation for underlying infectious conditions or immunologic/immunodeficiency disorders would be predicated on the clinical presentation and history. Depending on the clinical scenario, additional radiologic, laboratory, and/or pathologic testing may be necessary.

If secondary/reactive causes for eosinophilia have been excluded, it is appropriate to begin evaluation for a primary clonal eosinophilia (Fig. 50-2). The pace and/or extent of the diagnostic workup may be influenced by the clinical stability of the patient and where the patient is seeking care. In the community setting, an exhaustive clinical investigation into the etiology of the eosinophilia may not be performed. In contrast, a medical center/institution that specializes in eosinophilic disorders may provide a more in-depth and specialized evaluation. In the case of a clinically unstable patient, a systematic and progressive algorithmic approach will not be possible. In such situations, it is prudent to obtain as many "pretreatment" tests (e.g., laboratory studies, tissue biopsies, peripheral blood, and bone marrow samples) as possible given the effects treatment may have on subsequent diagnostic evaluation.

The workup will vary (less to more extensive) depending on the clinical, laboratory, radiologic, and/or morphologic features.[13-15,20-26] If it is determined from a clinical perspective that a peripheral blood/bone marrow sample should be obtained, the morphology becomes a critical driver for next-step(s) decision making. For example, the workup of a patient with "eosinophilia" but in the context of morphologic features otherwise consistent with CML may not require extensive immunophenotypic and/or genetic testing outside of the context of demonstrating presence of the Philadelphia chromosome/BCR::ABL1 fusion. On the other hand, a patient who lacks features that may be diagnostic of a particular entity may require additional flow cytometric, immunohistochemical, and genetic testing (Fig. 50-2). Several pathology-focused, algorithmic approaches have been published with roughly similar strategies that may very slightly among institutions based on patient case types, clinical trial availability, and access to research.[6,20-25] In general, bone marrow specimens should be submitted for flow cytometry (exclude T-cell lymphoma or lymphocytic variant of hypereosinophilic syndrome), immunohistochemistry for tryptase, CD117, and CD25 to evaluate for mast cells/mastocytosis, fluorescence in situ hybridization (FISH) or reverse transcription polymerase chain reaction (RT-PCR) for the FIP1L1::PDGFRA fusion (typically cytogenetically cryptic), and karyotype to assess for CEL, NOS or detect a possible recurring genetic abnormality (4q12 [PDGFRA], 5q32 [PDGFRB], 8p11.23 [FGFR1], 9p24.1 [JAK2], 13q12.2 [FLT3] or 9q34.12 [ABL]), which can be further proven by FISH and/or molecular studies. Also, given the increasing recognition and prevalence of molecular genetic abnormalities in eosinophilia that are not detected by FISH or cytogenetics, submission of a sample for DNA and RNA extract and hold should be considered. This may be important in the diagnostic workup if the aforementioned studies do not reveal a specific diagnosis and there remains clinical and/or pathologic concern for a clonal eosinophilic disorder. If next generation sequencing (NGS) studies are performed, it is important to remember that specific recurring abnormalities in primary clonal eosinophilia have yet to be unveiled, and one should be careful to distinguish an identified mutation diagnostic of CEL, NOS from one diagnostic of clonal hematopoiesis of indeterminate potential (CHIP)/clonal cytopenias of uncertain significance. In the ICC, bone marrow morphology has been incorporated in the diagnostic criteria for CEL, NOS.

The identification of the specific tyrosine kinase fusion gene is critical for diagnosis and subsequent treatment, as tyrosine kinase inhibitors (TKIs) have significantly improved the treatment and outcome of patients with PDGFRA and PDGFRB gene rearrangements[3-5] and are beneficial for patients with ETV6::ABL1. Other patients with FLT3 and/or JAK2 rearrangements may benefit from FLT3 and JAK2 inhibitors, respectively. See the discussion of that particular entity for more detailed information.

MYELOID/LYMPHOID NEOPLASMS WITH EOSINOPHILIA AND REARRANGEMENTS OF PDGFRA, PDGFRB, FGFR1, FLT3, OR JAK2 OR WITH ETV6::ABL1

Overview

In 2008, the World Health Organization (WHO) classification introduced a new category of primary clonal eosinophilic conditions that result from tyrosine kinase gene fusions. This new category was termed "myeloid/lymphoid neoplasms with eosinophilia and rearrangement of PDGFRA, PDGFRB, or FGFR1." In 2017, the WHO classification was revised to add myeloid/lymphoid neoplasms with PCM1-JAK2 as a provisional entity.[1,2] In the

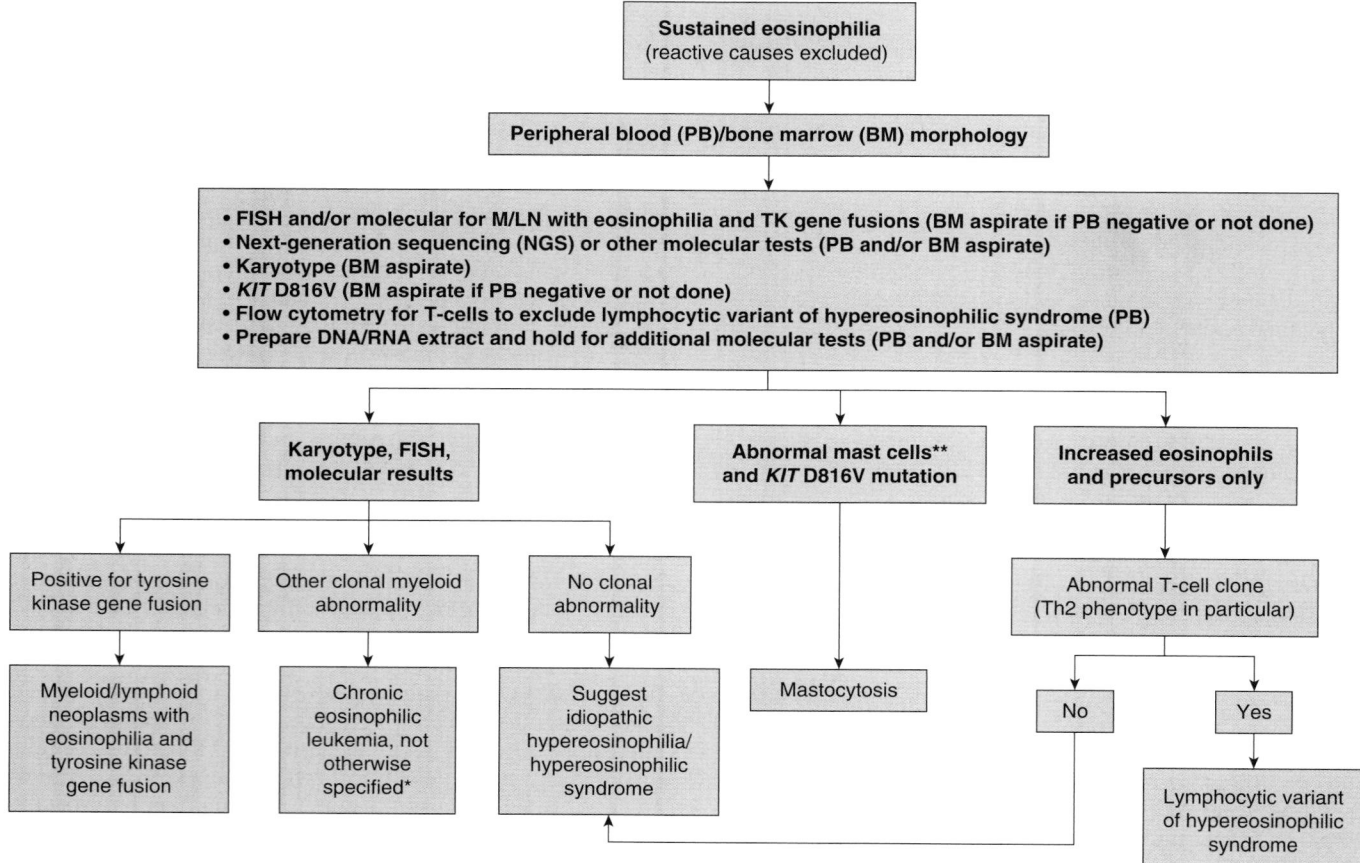

Figure 50-2. An algorithmic approach to the workup and diagnosis of unexplained cases of eosinophilia that undergo bone marrow examination. *BM typically shows additional morphologic abnormalities (e.g., megakaryocytic dysplasia). **Abnormal morphology (mature spindled hypogranular; promastocytes; metachromatic blasts); abnormal immunophenotype (expression of CD2 and/or CD25, CD30). *FISH*, Fluorescence in situ hybridization; *M/LN*, myeloid/lymphoid neoplasm; *TK*, tyrosine kinase.

ICC, additional rearrangements involving other tyrosine kinase fusion genes, *FLT3* and *ETV6::ABL1*, that may present as myeloid/lymphoid neoplasms with eosinophilia have been recognized and are now formally a part of the classification.[3,5,9,11] The 2022 name change to "myeloid/lymphoid neoplasms with eosinophilia and tyrosine kinase gene fusions" reflects the importance of consequent constitutive tyrosine kinase activity and subsequent therapeutic implications.[3] A few cases of rearrangement of *LYN*[27] have been reported to bear features resembling M/LN-eo-TK; however, more data are needed to understand the disease spectrum and response to TKI before being formally included in the category. Other potential members are *FGFR2* and *KIT* rearrangement.

These entities share some clinical similarities, including frequent constitutional symptoms such as fatigue, weight loss, pruritis, and hepatosplenomegaly. Eosinophilic end organ damage/dysfunction has been reported in around 30% to 40% of patients and may involve the heart, lungs, and other organs. It is now well recognized that this group of disorders presents as a variety of different disease phenotypes, including chronic myeloid neoplasm (CMN), blast phase CMN, lymphoblastic lymphoma/myeloid sarcoma in an extramedullary site, complex presentation with CMN in bone marrow, and extramedullary lymphoblastic lymphoma. Eosinophilia is

frequently but not invariably present. These features are further elaborated upon in the individual diagnostic sections. Given the variety of potential presentations, a high index of suspicion and knowledge of the heterogeneity of these disorders is necessary for proper workup, diagnosis, and treatment.[28]

A list of the known partner genes in the fusions involving *PDGFRA*, *PDGFRB*, *FGFR1*, *JAK2*, *FLT3*, and *ABL1* are listed in Box 50-2.

Myeloid/Lymphoid Neoplasms With Eosinophilia and Rearrangement of *PDGFRA*

Definition

A myeloid and/or lymphoid neoplasm that has a demonstrable rearrangement of the *PDGFRA* gene or, less commonly, an activating mutation leading to constitutive activation of tyrosine kinase. In the case of de novo presentation as B-lymphoblastic or T-lymphoblastic leukemia/lymphoma, if the *PDGFRA* rearrangement is not present in background myeloid cells, the best diagnosis is Philadelphia-like B-lymphoblastic leukemia (B-ALL) or de novo T-lymphoblastic leukemia (T-ALL) with *PDGFRA* rearrangement.

Box 50-2 *Fusion Genes in Clonal (Primary) Hypereosinophilia**

PDGFRA(4q12) *FIP1L1*(4q12), *BCR*(22q11), *CDK5RAP2*(9q33), *ETV6*(12p13), *FOXP1*(3p14), *KIF5B*(10p11), *STRN*(2p24), *TNKS2*(10q23), *USP25*(21q21.1)

PDGFRB(5q31-33) *ETV6*(12p13), *BIN2*(12q13), *CCDC6*(10q21), *CCDC88C*(14q32), *CEP85L*(6q22), *CPSF6*(12q15), *DIAPH1*(5q31), *DTD1*(20p11), *ERC1*(12p13), *GIT2*(12q24), *GOLGA4*(3p22), *GOLGB1*(3q12), *GPIAP1*(11p13), *HIP1*(7q11), *KANK1*(9p24), *MPRIP*(17p11), *MYO18A*(17q11), *NDE1*(16p13), *NDEL1*(17p13), *NIN*(14q24), *PDE4DIP*(1q22), *PRKG2*(4q21), *RABEP1*(17p13), *SART3*(12q23), *SPDR*(2q32), *SPECC1*(17p11), *SPTBN1*(2p16), *TNIP1*(5q33), *TP53BP1*(15q22), *TPM3*(1q21), *TRIP11*(14q32), *WDR48*(3p22)

FGFR1(8p11) *ZMYM2*(13q12), *BCR*(22q11), *CNTRL*(9q33), *CPSF6*(12q15), *CUX1*(7q22), *FGFR1OP*(6q27), *FGFR1OP2*(12p11), *HERV-K*(19q13), *LRRFIP1*(2q37), *MYO18A*(17q11), *RANBP2*(2q13), *SQSTM1*(5q35), *TPR1*(1q25), *TRIM24*(7q34), *TFG* (3q12)

JAK2(9p34) *PCM1*(8p22), *BCR*(22q11), *ETV6*(12p13)

FLT3(13q12) *ETV6*(12p13), *GOLGB1*(3q12), *SPTBN1*(2p16), *TRIP11*(14q32), *ZMYM2*(13q12)

ABL1(9q34) *ETV6*(12p13)

*Common fusion gene partners are underlined.

Genetics

The majority of these cases (approximately 90%) present as CMN and carry the *FIP1L1::PDGFRA* fusion. A minority of cases will show alternative gene partners (Box 50-2).

Synonyms and Related Terms

Myeloid and lymphoid neoplasms with *PDGFRA* rearrangement; myeloid and lymphoid neoplasms associated with *PDGFRA* rearrangement; myeloid/lymphoid neoplasm with *PDGFRA* rearrangement.[4]

Epidemiology

There is a marked male predominance with a male-to-female ratio of approximately 17:1. The median age of presentation is in the late 40s. It is the most common rearrangement among M/LN-eo-TK cases.

Etiology

The cause of this disorder is unknown. Rare cases have been reported to occur after cytotoxic chemotherapy.

Clinical Features

There is a marked male predominance with splenomegaly, marked increase in serum vitamin B_{12}, and elevated serum tryptase.[29-31] Extramedullary lesions are very common, in around 40% of patients. End organ damage may occur from the release of enzymes and other proteins by the eosinophils, causing tissue destruction. Various organs may be affected, including the heart, lungs, skin, gastrointestinal tract, and nervous system. Because of bone marrow involvement and/or eosinophil deposition in other tissues, patients may present with anemia or symptoms related to the particular organ involved, such as difficulty breathing/shortness of breath, cardiac failure, and pruritus. Peripheral blood eosinophilia is reported in >90% of patients.

Morphology

Peripheral blood: The majority of cases with *FIP1L1::PDGFRA* fusion present as a CMN with morphologic features resembling CEL, NOS (Fig. 50-3).[1-11,32] The peripheral blood smear typically demonstrates moderate to marked eosinophilia, although this is not invariable,[33] in the majority of cells exhibit mature cytology. There are typically very few or no eosinophilic myelocytes. The eosinophils may show cytologic abnormalities, including cytoplasmic hypogranulation or eccentric localization of granules, nuclear hyposegmentation, nuclear hypersegmentation, and/or cytoplasmic vacuolization. There is typically no monocytosis, circulating blasts, dysplastic platelets, or dysplastic granulocytes. The complete blood cell count may show anemia and/or thrombocytopenia in a subset of cases.

Bone marrow: The bone marrow is often hypercellular from eosinophilic hyperplasia with minimal dysplastic features in the erythroid and granulocytic lineages and no increase in blasts (Fig. 50-3). Megakaryocytes can be decreased, normal, or increased in number; morphologically, they may exhibit myeloproliferative neoplasm (MPN)-like features, dysplastic features, or be unremarkable. In addition, increased, interstitial, individually distributed, spindled mast cells (typically highlighted by immunohistochemical stains such as tryptase, CD117), which show aberrant expression of CD25, are invariably present. These cases are negative for the *KIT* D816V mutation and usually do not show focal compact dense mast cell clusters as seen in systemic mastocytosis (SM), although this can rarely occur.[9,34] In cases that fulfill criteria for SM but are *KIT* negative, these patients should be tested for *PDGFRA*[9] and possibly other tyrosine kinase genes, depending on the case. This constellation of bone marrow findings is often associated with variable degrees of reticulin fibrosis. The majority of cases present as a chronic disease process, and myeloid blasts are not elevated. However, some cases may present in myeloid or lymphoid blast phase (Fig. 50-4). In the event that a population of B- or T-lymphoblasts are detected, thorough evaluation for extramedullary disease and/or concern for a more aggressive disease course is warranted.

Immunophenotype

Given that the majority of cases present as a CMN without an increase in morphologic blasts, an extensive immunophenotypic analysis is typically not necessary except to demonstrate the atypical, spindled mast cells. The mast cells can be revealed by positive staining with CD117 and tryptase and show aberrant expression of CD25. If there is an increase in blasts, flow cytometric immunophenotyping or immunohistochemistry should be used to characterize the blast phenotype.

Genetic/Molecular Findings

By far the most common fusion gene partner for *PDGFRA* in this disorder is *FIP1L1* (80%–85% of cases). It should be noted that this fusion gene is cytogenetically cryptic and therefore requires either FISH or a molecular-based strategy for detection.[32] This fusion is the result of an interstitial deletion on 4q12 whereby the *CHIC2* gene (located in-between *PDGFRA* and *FIP1L1*) is deleted. Because of the *CHIC2* deletion, the FISH strategy used in many laboratories to assess for the presence of this abnormality is often referred to as "CHIC2 FISH or FISH for the *CHIC2* deletion" (Fig. 50-5).

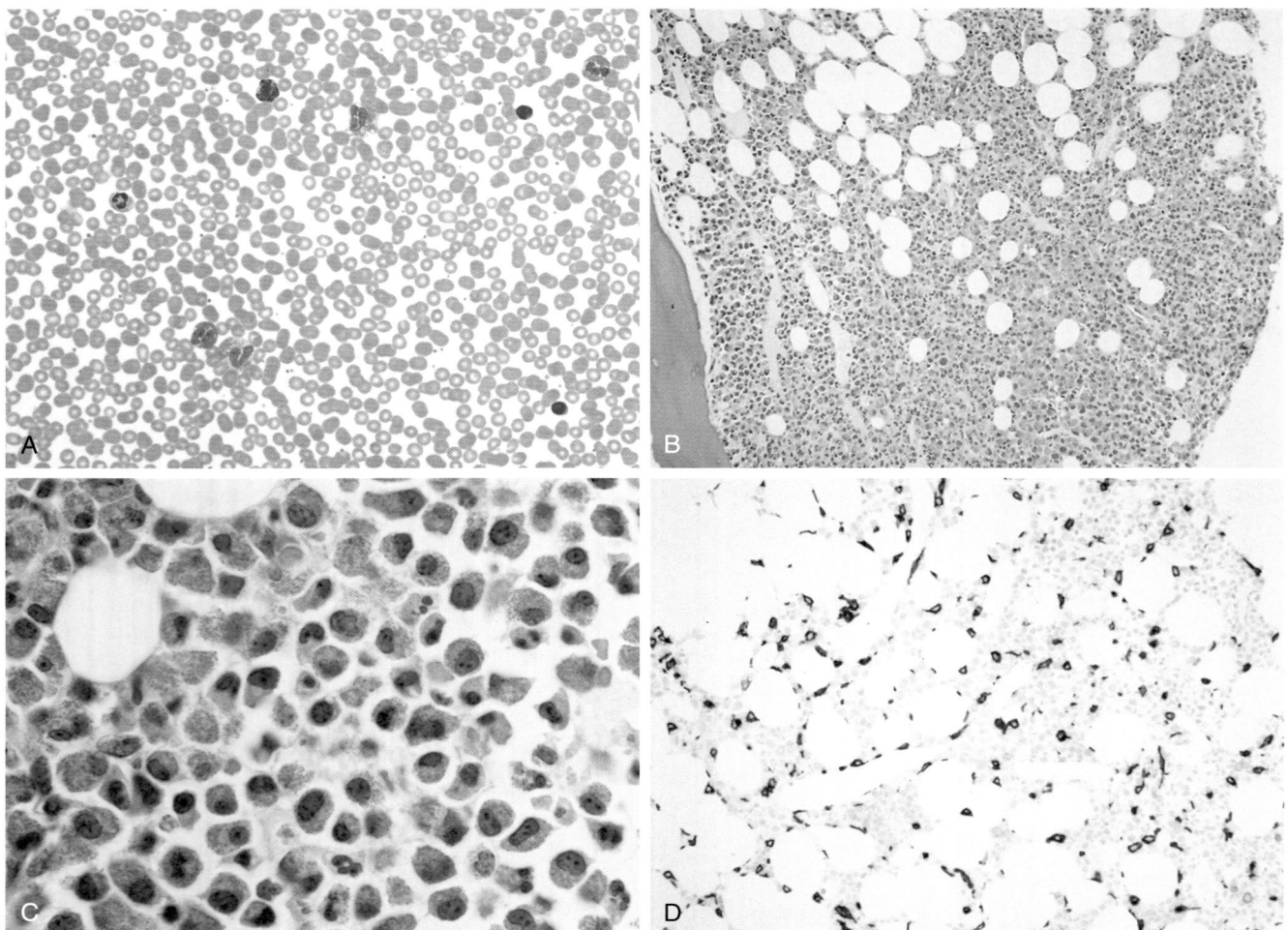

Figure 50-3. Myeloid neoplasm with eosinophilia and *FIP1L1::PDGFRA* rearrangement. A, A peripheral blood smear demonstrates hyper-eosinophilia (absolute eosinophil count of 2.3 × 10⁹/L) without concomitant anemia or thrombocytopenia in a 59-year-old male patient who presented with weight loss. In this image, two of the four eosinophils display atypical cytologic features, including degranulation, vacuolization, and eccentric localization of granules in the cytoplasm. No features of dysplasia in the granulocytic series, circulating blasts, or monocytosis are present. (1000× magnification, Wright-Giemsa). **B,** The bone marrow core biopsy is hypercellular for age (50%–60%) and shows a striking eosinophilic infiltrate. Increased blasts are not present, and mast cells are not obvious (400× magnification, H&E [hematoxylin and eosin]). **C,** High-power magnification of the bone marrow core biopsy reveals striking eosinophilia with numerous eosinophilic precursors. An increased blast population is not present, and there are no abnormal mast cell infiltrates visible by morphology (1000× magnification, H&E [hematoxylin and eosin]). **D,** Mast cells are increased and spindle-shaped (atypical) and demonstrate the typical interstitial, individually distributed infiltration pattern (immunohistochemistry for CD117). When tested, the mast cells show aberrant CD25 expression (not shown). On rare occasion, the mast cells may form focal, compact, dense aggregates mimicking systemic mastocytosis.

Alternative methods to FISH include RT-PCR based assays to specifically detect the fusion gene or RNA sequencing to detect the gene fusions.

In the case of an alternative fusion partner (Box 50-2), conventional cytogenetic studies may reveal an apparently balanced translocation involving the 4q12 locus, which serves as the initial clue to a rearrangement of *PDGFRA*, especially in the presence of eosinophilia. Specific genetic testing for *PDGFRA* rearrangements is needed in such cases to confirm this genetic alteration.

NGS can detect various mutations in myeloid disorder–associated genes in myeloid/lymphoid neoplasms with eosinophilia and rearrangement of *PDGFRA*. These genes are non-specific, have been reported in less than half of cases, and include *ASXL1, BCOR, DNMT3A, ETV6, SRSF2,* and *RUNX1* genes.[5,9]

Postulated Cell of Origin/Normal Counterpart

Pluripotent hematopoietic stem cell that can differentiate into either a myeloid or lymphoid progenitor.

Clinical Course

Patients with the typical CMN or CEL-like presentation and the *FIP1L1::PDGFRA* fusion respond remarkably well to imatinib, the first-generation TKI therapy. Imatinib is highly successful in the treatment of these patients with long-term hematologic and molecular responses.[6,7,28] In situations of presentation in acute blastic phase or disease progression from an initial chronic phase, imatinib may continue to be used; however, induction chemotherapy and/or allogenic hematopoietic stem cell transplant is typically needed to achieve long-term remission. Case reports of variant fusion partners have also reported treatment success with

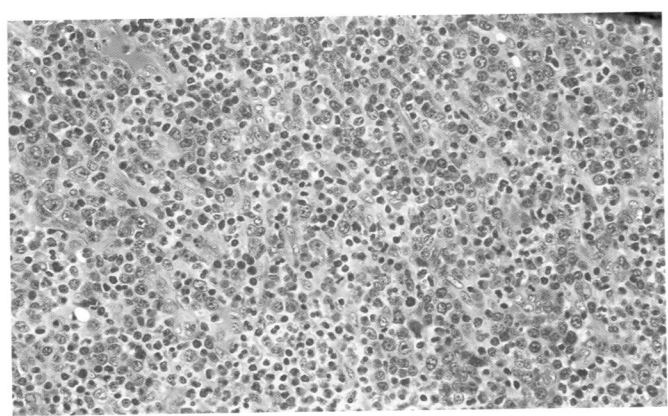

Figure 50-4. Myeloid sarcoma associated with eosinophilia and *FIP1L1::PDGFRA* rearrangement. This left axillary lymph node biopsy is from a 53-year-old male who presented with hypereosinophilia and lymphadenopathy. The lymph node biopsy showed features of a myeloid sarcoma and associated eosinophilia. The peripheral blood and bone marrow showed morphologic features of chronic eosinophilic leukemia. Genetic testing in both the bone marrow and lymph node demonstrated a "*CHIC2* deletion," indicating the presence of *FIP1L1::PDGFRA* rearrangement (1000× magnification, H&E [hematoxylin and eosin]).

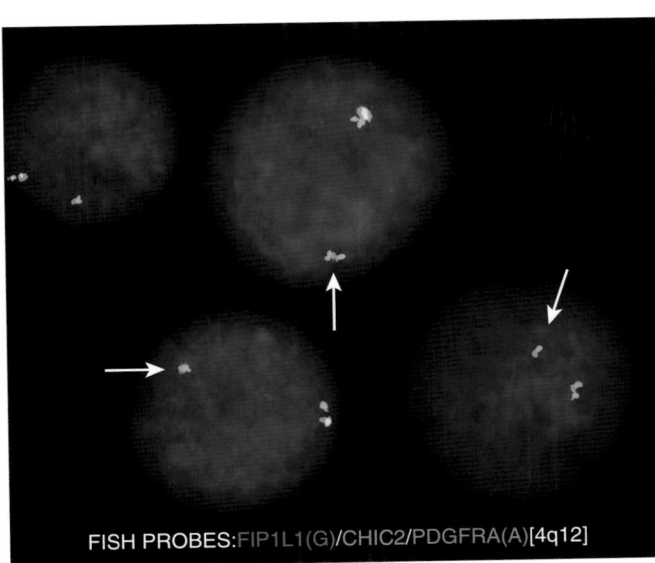

FISH PROBES:FIP1L1(G)/CHIC2/PDGFRA(A)[4q12]

Figure 50-5. Interphase fluorescence in situ hybridization (FISH) demonstrating the *FIP1L1::PDGFRA* fusion via *CHIC2* deletion. On the long arm of chromosome 4 at locus 4q12, the *FIP1L1, CHIC2,* and *PDGFRA* genes reside in a row when moving telomeric. In this assay, the FISH probes are labeled *green* for *FIP1L1,* red for *CHIC2,* and *aqua* for *PDGFRA.* A normal signal pattern is seen as three probes colocalized together. In the situation of *FIP1L1::PDGFRA* fusion, the red signal *(CHIC2)* is deleted (absent), leaving behind just the green and aqua signals *(arrows* show the abnormal signal).

TKI. Several activating point mutations in *PDGFRA* have also been identified that appear to demonstrate a similar sensitivity to TKI treatment.

Treatment resistance is unusual, but resistance to imatinib may be acquired over time in some patients as a result of a T6741 or D842V mutation.[35,36] In these situations, transitioning to a second- or third-generation TKI can be helpful.

Differential Diagnosis

The differential diagnosis is incredibly broad and includes both primary and secondary causes of eosinophilia. As such, following some type of methodical testing algorithm is suggested to arrive at the correct final diagnosis. If a reactive cause or underlying unrelated neoplastic process (e.g., carcinoma, T-cell lymphoma) is not present and/or does not explain the clinical and/or pathologic picture, additional immunophenotypic and genetic testing may be required for further evaluation. In particular, the age (younger) and sex (male) at presentation, along with the eosinophilia and atypical mast cell proliferation in the absence of other well-defined genetic abnormalities such as *BCR::ABL1,* inversion should draw attention to myeloid/lymphoid neoplasms with eosinophilia and *PDGFRA* rearrangement as a possible diagnosis.

In the occasional cases that do not exhibit peripheral blood eosinophilia, in which eosinophilia is minimal, or that present as an acute leukemia, several other clinicopathological features may help raise suspicion for this entity. These features include (1) bone marrow involved by a CMN that is difficult to put in a specific subtype and lack of disease-defining molecular genetic features in a young male patient; (2) increased eosinophils in tissue or bone marrow biopsy despite no peripheral blood eosinophilia; (3) complex disease presentation with extramedullary involvement; (4) persistent myeloproliferative features after achieving remission of acute leukemia—eosinophilia may emerge; and (5) atypical mast cell proliferation with aberrant CD25 expression but *KIT* mutation testing is negative. With respect to the latter, the mast cell proliferation may be quite striking in rare cases, showing focal compact dense aggregate formation, spindled mast cell morphology, and aberrant CD25 expression mimicking SM. The disease biology, treatment implications, and response to treatment are vastly different between myeloid/lymphoid neoplasms with eosinophilia and rearrangement of *PDGFRA* and SM. It is therefore prudent to lower one's threshold for suspicion and discuss performing more in-depth testing (FISH or RNA sequencing) to evaluate for occult, potentially targetable, genetic rearrangements and/or point mutations.

Myeloid/lymphoid neoplasms with eosinophilia can exhibit other clinical presentations, including AML and, rarely, T-ALL or myeloid sarcoma (Table 50-1)[1-11,34,37-39] (Fig. 50-4). In some cases, the presentation is complex with an extramedullary blastic proliferation and CMN in the bone marrow. Alternatively, the extramedullary presentation may precede or succeed the detection of the CMN in the bone marrow. When there is significant eosinophilia in an extramedullary tissue site with a lymphoblastic lymphoma/myeloid sarcoma, molecular testing for a rearrangement of *PDGFRA* (and *PDGFRB, FGFR1, JAK2, FLT3,* and *ABL1*) should be considered.

Myeloid/Lymphoid Neoplasms With Eosinophilia and Rearrangement of *PDGFRB*

Definition

A myeloid or lymphoid neoplasm that frequently but not invariably is associated with eosinophilia that has a

Table 50-1 Myeloid/Lymphoid Neoplasms With Eosinophilia With *PDGFRA, PDGFRB, FGFR1, or JAK2* Rearrangement

Disease Presentation	PDGFRA Rearrangement Heterogeneous	PDGFRB Rearrangement Heterogeneous	FGFR1 Rearrangement Heterogeneous, Complex*	JAK2 Rearrangement Heterogeneous
Peripheral Blood and Bone Marrow				
CEL, NOS	+++	+++	++	++ (+ fibrosis)
CMML		++		
AML	+	+	+	+
B-ALL	+†	+†	+	+†
T-ALL	+	+	+	+
Other	+ (MPN-U, MDS/MPN-U, SM)	+ (MPN-U, MDS, MDS/MPN-U, SM)	++ (MPN, SM, MDS/MPN, MPAL)	+ (MPN-U, MDS/MPN-U, aCML)
Extramedullary	+ (MS, rare T-ALL or B-ALL)	+ (MS, rare T-ALL or B-ALL)	+++ (MS, T-ALL, or B-ALL)	+ (MS, T-ALL, or B-ALL)
Hypereosinophilia	>90%	70–80%	80%	80% (CMN) <10% (LL)
Progression	AML > T-ALL or B-ALL	AML > T-ALL or B-ALL	AML > T-ALL or B-ALL	AML > T-ALL or B-ALL

*A complex presentation is defined as presentation as a chronic myeloid neoplasm in the peripheral blood and bone marrow and a lymphoblastic lymphoma/myeloid sarcoma/mixed phenotype acute leukemia in an extramedullary site.

†If the clinical presentation is typical B-lymphoblastic leukemia/lymphoma without an underlying or associated myeloid neoplasm with eosinophilia, the disease should be classified as Philadelphia-like/*BCR::ABL1*-like B-ALL.

aCML, Atypical chronic myeloid leukemia; *AML,* acute myeloid leukemia; *B-ALL,* B-acute lymphoblastic leukemia; *CEL, NOS,* chronic eosinophilic leukemia, not otherwise specified; *CMML,* chronic myelomonocytic leukemia; *MDS,* myelodysplastic syndrome; *MDS/MPN,* myelodysplastic/myeloproliferative neoplasm; *MPAL,* mixed phenotype acute leukemia; *MPN,* myeloproliferative neoplasm; *MPN, NOS,* myeloproliferative neoplasm, not otherwise specified; *MS,* myeloid sarcoma; *SM,* systemic mastocytosis; *T-ALL,* T-lymphoblastic leukemia.

demonstrable rearrangement of the *PDGFRB* gene.[1-5,9-11,40-43] In the rare case of de novo presentation as B-ALL or T-ALL, if the *PDGFRB* rearrangement is not present in background myeloid cells, the best diagnosis is Philadelphia-like B-ALL or de novo T-ALL with *PDGFRB* rearrangement.

Synonyms and Related Terms

Myeloid and lymphoid neoplasms with *PDGFRB* rearrangement; myeloid and lymphoid neoplasms associated with *PDGFRB* rearrangement; myeloid/lymphoid neoplasm with *PDGFRB* rearrangement; chronic myelomonocytic leukemia (CMML) with eosinophilia and t(5;12).

Epidemiology

This neoplasm shows a slight male predominance with a male-to-female ratio of 2:1. The age range of presentation is quite broad, from children to the elderly; however, like myeloid and lymphoid neoplasms with *PDGFRA* rearrangement, the median age is in the 4th decade of life.

Etiology

The cause of this disorder is unknown. Rare cases have been reported after cytotoxic chemotherapy.

Clinical Features

There is a slight male predominance, and splenomegaly is typical. Hepatomegaly may also be seen but is less common.[2,5,9] Serum tryptase may be elevated but is not typically markedly increased. End organ damage may occur as a result of the release of enzymes and other proteins by the eosinophils. Because of bone marrow involvement and/or eosinophil deposition in various tissues, patients may present with symptoms related to the particular organ involved such as difficulty breathing/shortness of breath (respiratory system), cardiac failure (heart), and pruritus (cutaneous involvement).

Morphology

Similar to the other tyrosine kinase gene rearrangements described in this chapter, myeloid/lymphoid neoplasms with eosinophilia and *PDGFRB* rearrangement show a heterogeneous presentation in the peripheral blood/bone marrow. This may include CMML with eosinophilia (Fig. 50-6), CEL (Fig. 50-7), atypical CML (aCML), a CMN that is difficult to categorize, AML, lymphoblastic leukemia, and SM (rare). In extramedullary tissue sites, transformation to or presentation as myeloid sarcoma or lymphoblastic leukemia/lymphoma may occur. If the presentation is typical B-ALL without an underlying (including preceding or succeeding) or associated myeloid neoplasm with eosinophilia, then the disease should be reclassified as Philadelphia-like/*BCR::ABL1*-like B-ALL according to the ICC.[2,3,5,9]

Peripheral blood: The peripheral blood often demonstrates leukocytosis, including eosinophilia (but not invariable) and associated monocytosis in those cases that resemble CMML (Fig. 50-6). Eosinophil morphology may show abnormal features, such as uneven granulation, cytoplasmic vacuolization, or abnormal nuclear segmentation or lobulation but is not always present. Monocytosis in combination with eosinophilia suggests the presence of and appropriate testing for a *PDGFRB* rearrangement. Only about three-quarters of cases are associated with eosinophilia; therefore, it is imperative that the reviewing pathologist and clinician consider this genetic abnormality, particularly when the karyotype may not be suggestive.

Bone marrow: The bone marrow is hypercellular with a variable admixture and increase in eosinophils (Figs. 50-6 and 50-7), granulocytes, monocytes, and mast cells. Like myeloid/lymphoid neoplasms with eosinophilia and *PDGFRA* rearrangement, the bone marrow, in addition to the features distinctive to the CMN disease presentation, may show increased, interstitial, individually distributed spindled mast cells (typically highlighted by immunohistochemical stains

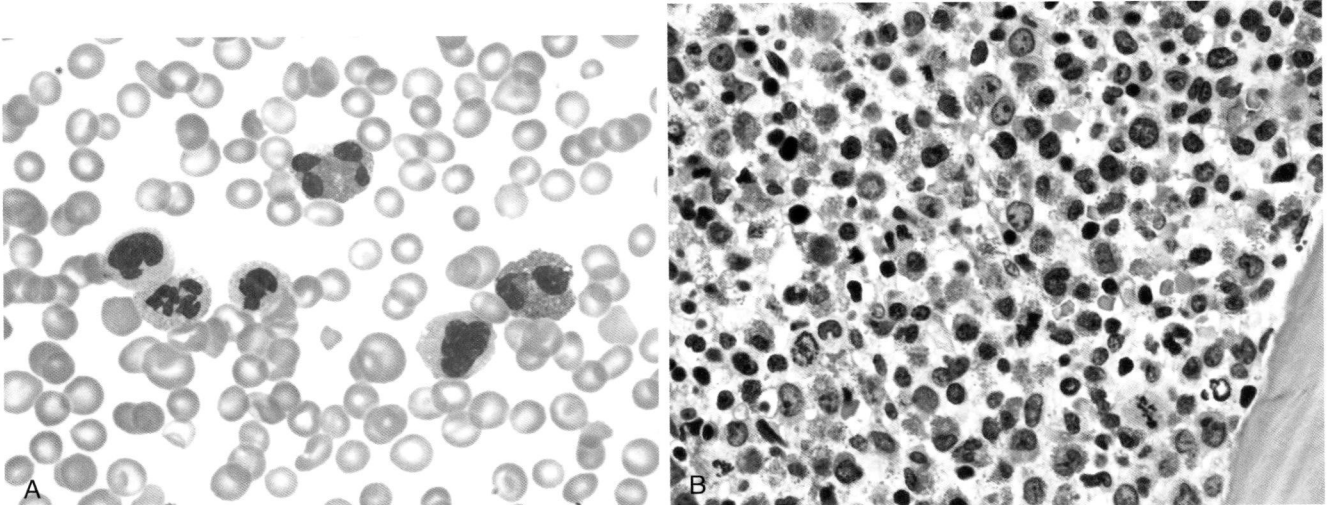

Figure 50-6. Peripheral blood film **(A)** and bone marrow biopsy **(B)** showing marked eosinophilia in a patient with monocytosis, resembling chronic myelomonocytic leukemia. Cytogenetic analysis revealed t(5;12)(q31;p12), *ETV6::PDGFRB*.

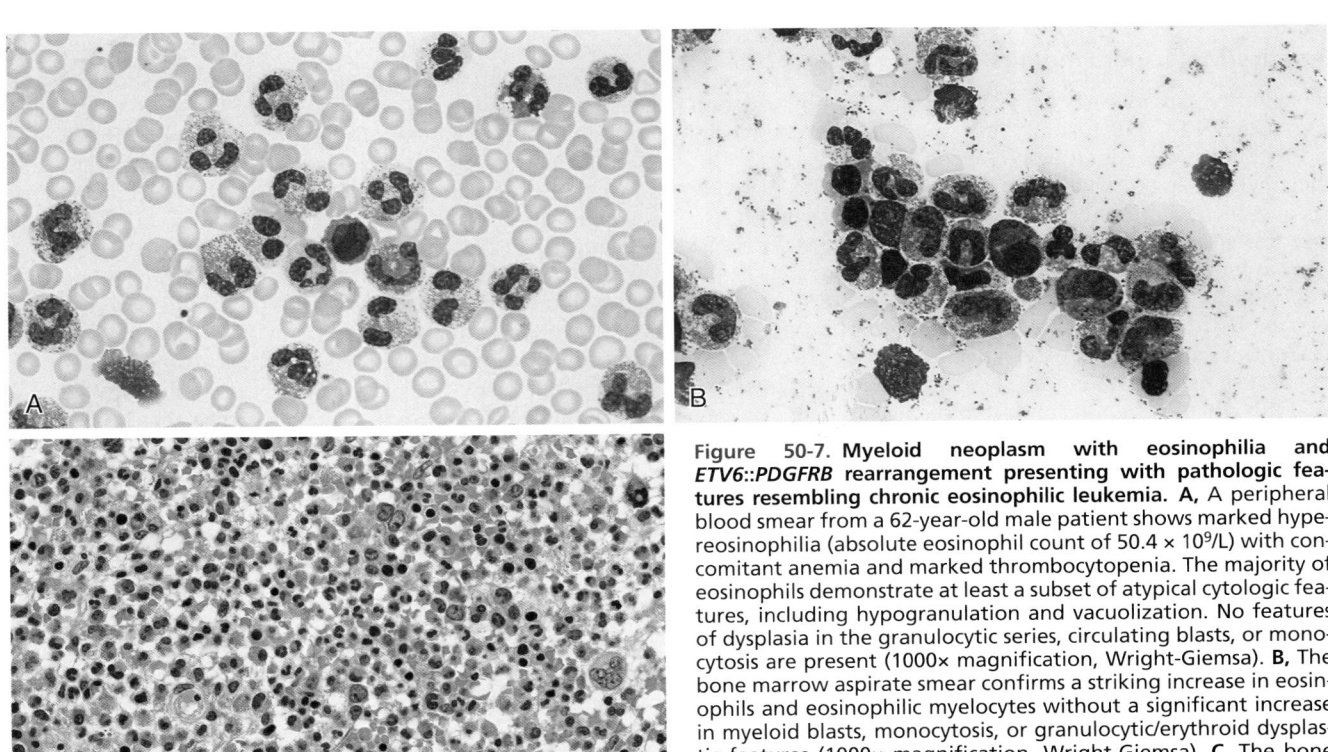

Figure **50-7. Myeloid neoplasm with eosinophilia and *ETV6::PDGFRB* rearrangement presenting with pathologic features resembling chronic eosinophilic leukemia. A,** A peripheral blood smear from a 62-year-old male patient shows marked hypereosinophilia (absolute eosinophil count of 50.4 × 10⁹/L) with concomitant anemia and marked thrombocytopenia. The majority of eosinophils demonstrate at least a subset of atypical cytologic features, including hypogranulation and vacuolization. No features of dysplasia in the granulocytic series, circulating blasts, or monocytosis are present (1000× magnification, Wright-Giemsa). **B,** The bone marrow aspirate smear confirms a striking increase in eosinophils and eosinophilic myelocytes without a significant increase in myeloid blasts, monocytosis, or granulocytic/erythroid dysplastic features (1000× magnification, Wright-Giemsa). **C,** The bone marrow core biopsy is markedly hypercellular for age (100%) and is predominated by eosinophils and eosinophilic precursors with diminished quantities of erythroid precursors and megakaryocytes (600× magnification, H&E [hematoxylin and eosin]).

such as tryptase, CD117) that show aberrant expression of CD25. Rarely, focal compact dense clusters of mast cells may be seen mimicking SM. Megakaryocytes can be unremarkable or show dysplastic features; occasionally, there are myeloproliferative-type megakaryocytes.

In the uncommon situations in which the disease presents as an acute leukemia or a combination of both a chronic myeloid process and an acute leukemia, increased blasts will be seen either in the bone marrow or in an extramedullary tissue site. Demonstration of the *PDGFRB* rearrangement in both the chronic and acute processes is necessary to exclude the possibility of an isolated acute lymphoblastic leukemia presenting as Philadelphia-like/*BCR::ABL1*-like B-ALL.

Immunophenotype

Given that the majority of these cases present as a CMN without an increase in morphologic blasts, an extensive immunophenotypic analysis is typically not necessary except to demonstrate the atypical, spindled mast cells and rule out eosinophilia with a T-cell neoplasm or lymphocyte variant hypereosinophilic syndrome. The mast cells can be revealed by positive staining with CD117 and tryptase and show aberrant expression of CD25. In the cases presenting as an acute leukemia, increased blasts are present. Immunophenotyping in those instances is necessary to determine the acute leukemia lineage.

Genetics/Molecular Findings

The majority of cases carry t(5;12)(q32;p13.2) with formation of an *ETV6::PDGFRB* fusion. This is usually karyotypically evident; however, subsequent genetic testing via FISH or other methodology is mandatory to demonstrate a *PDGFRB* rearrangement. Rarely, the translocation may involve three or more chromosomes; therefore, recognition by the geneticist of the involvement of the genetic location on 5q31-q33 is important to prompt confirmatory FISH or other testing. This has both diagnostic and therapeutic implications given these entities are exquisitely sensitive to imatinib therapy.[6,7,28] Not all instances involving 5q31-5q33 show involvement of *PDGFRB*, which is significant in that the neoplasm would not fall into this diagnostic category and the treatment benefits from a TKI would not be present.

Though the most common partner with *PDGFRB* is *ETV6*, more than 30 alternate genes have been reported (Box 50-2). It is increasingly recognized that *PDGFRB* rearrangements may be cryptic both karyotypically or by FISH, especially in cases where *PDGFRB* is rearranged with other partner genes. Therefore, if there is suspicion of this abnormality at the molecular level and/or that it is involved in complex genetic rearrangements, multiple genetic testing modalities (FISH, RNA sequencing) are often needed to identify the rearrangements.[9,44,45]

PDGFRB rearrangements with alternative partners including, but not limited to, *EBF1*, *SSBP2*, *TNIP1*, *ZEB2*, and *ATF7IP* often present as de novo B-ALL, which is currently classified as Philadelphia-like/*BCR::ABL1*-like B-ALL and not as a myeloid/lymphoid neoplasm with eosinophilia and *PDGFRB* rearrangement. Distinction between myeloid/lymphoid neoplasm with eosinophilia and *PDGFRB* rearrangement and *BCR::ABL1*-like B-ALL, similar to myeloid/lymphoid neoplasm with eosinophilia and *PDGFRA* rearrangement, is determined based on the presence or absence of an underlying myeloid neoplasm with rearrangement of *PDGFRB*.

NGS can detect various mutations in myeloid disorder-associated genes in myeloid/lymphoid neoplasms with eosinophilia and rearrangement of *PDGFRB*. These genes are non-specific, have been reported in less than 50% of cases, and include *ASXL1*, *TET2*, *BCOR*, *ETV6*, *STAG2*, and *RUNX1*.[5,9]

Postulated Cell of Origin/Normal Counterpart

Pluripotent hematopoietic stem cell that can differentiate into either a myeloid or lymphoid progenitor.

Clinical Course

Similar to CMNs with rearrangement of *PDGFRA*, those with *PDGFRB* rearrangement respond remarkably well to imatinib TKI therapy, with long-term hematologic and molecular responses. In situations of presentation in blast phase or disease progression from an initial chronic phase, imatinib may continue to be used; however, induction chemotherapy and/or allogenic hematopoietic stem cell transplant is typically needed for long-term remission.[6]

Differential Diagnosis

Depending on the degree of laboratory and morphologic abnormalities, the initial differential diagnosis for a chronic myeloid process may be broad and include both primary and secondary causes of eosinophilia and a clonal myeloid neoplasm that lacks significant eosinophilia. In particular, those cases with monocytosis and eosinophilia should raise the distinct possibility of t(5;12) involving *PDGFRB*. For the other possibilities, a combination of appropriate immunophenotypic and genetic testing may be needed to distinguish reactive from clonal disorders and to further evaluate for a specific recurring genetic abnormality that would result in a specific ICC diagnosis. In particular, the age (younger) and sex (male) at presentation, along with the eosinophilia and/or monocytosis and atypical mast cell proliferation, should draw attention to "myeloid/lymphoid neoplasms with eosinophilia and rearrangement of *PDGFRB*" as a possible diagnosis.

Though CEL-like or CMML presentations tend to predominate, it is important to recognize that other clinical presentations may include B-ALL and, less commonly, AML, T-ALL, or myeloid sarcoma (Table 50-1).[1-11,34,37-39] In some cases, the presentation is complex, with an extramedullary blastic proliferation and CMN in the bone marrow. Alternatively, the extramedullary presentation may precede or succeed the detection of CMN in the bone marrow. When there is significant eosinophilia in an extramedullary tissue site with a lymphoblastic lymphoma/myeloid sarcoma, molecular testing for a rearrangement of *PDGFRB* (and of *PDGFRA*, *FGFR1*, *JAK2*, *FLT3*, and *ABL1*) should be considered. In these situations, both entities harbor the same genetic alteration.

In the cases with an uncharacteristic presentation such as lack of significant peripheral blood eosinophilia and karyotypically cryptic, the clinicopathological features that help raise a suspicion of the presence of tyrosine kinase (TK) fusion (listed under Myeloid/Lymphoid Neoplasms With Eosinophilia and Rearrangement of *PDGFRA*) are also applicable to cases of *PDGFRB* rearrangement. When approaching these cases, it is important to lower the threshold for eosinophilia (many cases have mild eosinophilia rather than hypereosinophilia) to also consider tissue and bone marrow eosinophilia in addition to peripheral blood eosinophilia, to assess mast cells, to be cautious making a generic diagnosis of a CMN lacking a characteristic genetic alteration in a young patient, and to pay attention to the background bone marrow and complete blood cell count features in patients presenting in blast phase.

Myeloid/Lymphoid Neoplasms With Eosinophilia and Rearrangement of *FGFR1*

Definition

A hematopoietic neoplasm with rearrangement of *FGFR1* that typically shows eosinophilia and may manifest as a CMN or as an acute leukemia (T-cell, B-cell, myeloid, and mixed phenotype).[1-11] This entity is heterogenous in its presentation.

Synonyms and Related Terms

8p11 myeloproliferative syndrome, 8p11 stem cell syndrome, myeloid and lymphoid neoplasms with *FGFR1* abnormalities, stem cell leukemia/lymphoma syndrome.[1-3,46-57]

Epidemiology

There is a slight male predominance with a male-to-female ratio of approximately 1.5:1. The median age at presentation is in the 3rd and 4th decades of life with a wide age range (toddler to octogenarian).[1-3,9,10,52]

Etiology

The etiology is unknown.

Morphology

The disease is well-known for its heterogenous and complex presentations, including CEL, myelodysplastic/myeloproliferative neoplasm (MDN/MPN), AML, T-ALL, or (less often) B-ALL or mixed-phenotype acute leukemia. There is a frequent association with peripheral blood and/or bone marrow eosinophilia (70%–80%), and extramedullary disease presentation is typical (Table 50-1). In fact, acute and chronic disease manifestations may occur concurrently or manifest subsequently (Fig. 50-8). For example, in cases that present as CEL, there may be subsequent transformation to AML (including myeloid sarcoma), T-ALL, B-ALL, or mixed-phenotype acute leukemia. Alternatively, some cases may present as acute leukemia, but it is only after treatment that an underlying *FGFR1*-rearranged CMN is appreciated. T-ALL in the extramedullary site (often lymph node) often shows an immature myeloid component in the periphery or perivascular location.

Like cases with *PDGFRA* or *PDGFRB* rearrangement, scattered spindle mast cells with aberrant CD25 expression are frequent, but only rarely do cases satisfy the diagnostic criteria for SM.[58,59] In the latter scenario, such cases should not be diagnosed as SM with an associated myeloid neoplasm unless it is a legitimate unique occurrence of *FGFR1* rearrangement in the non–mast cells and *KIT* D816V is mutated in the mast cells. Rather, the case should be classified as an *FGFR1*-rearranged myeloid/lymphoid neoplasms with eosinophilia.

The disease phenotype may differ with different partner genes. Cases with *BCR::FGFR1* fusion tend to have hematologic features resembling those of CML with eosinophilia rather than those of CEL.[54,55] An unusual feature of *FGFR10P1::FGFR1* is that five of the reported cases had polycythemia.[56,57]

Immunophenotype

Depending on the morphologic findings, more or less immunophenotypic studies may be needed to clarify the diagnostic process. If the case presents as CMN, assessment for an aberrant mast cell population (e.g., CD117, tryptase, CD25) may be all that is needed. If there is a proliferation of immature-appearing cells/blasts, then a more extensive immunophenotypic analysis is required. In the latter case, flow cytometric immunophenotyping is preferred, particularly when a diagnosis of mixed phenotype acute leukemia is being considered.

Genetics/Molecular Findings

FGFR1 is a tyrosine kinase that plays an essential role in the regulation of cell proliferation, differentiation, and migration and is located on 8p11.23. At the time of this writing, there were at least 14 gene partners reported to fuse with *FGFR1* (Box 50-2). *FGFR1* fusion genes form chimeric proteins that constitutively activate the *FGFR1* tyrosine kinase and associated downstream signalling pathways. The most common partners include *ZMYM2*(13q12) and *CNTRL*(9q33).

FGFR1 rearrangements are not cytogenetically cryptic[2,9,60-68]; however, the reported bands may range from 8p11.2 to 8p21, likely attributable to banding quality, the relatively small size of band 8p11, and the quality of chromosomal morphology. Given this variability in band reporting and the fact that not all cases that involve this chromosomal location will involve the *FGFR1* gene, confirmation of *FGFR1* gene involvement is mandatory.[69] This can be done using a break-apart FISH probe for *FGFR1*. However, ideally, an RNA sequencing methodology would be deployed to identify all fusion products.

These disorders appear to be enriched for *RUNX1* mutations when evaluated by gene sequencing studies.[70] Mutations in *RUNX1* may increase proliferation of the clone with the *FGFR1* fusion and contribute to disease evolution and poor outcome.[46,70]

Postulated Cell of Origin/Normal Counterpart

Pluripotent hematopoietic stem cell.

Clinical Course

The clinical outcome in this disorder is variable, as might be expected, given the diversity of disease presentations. However, many cases follow an aggressive course, terminating in blast phase/blast transformation in less than 3 years.[6] *FGFR1*-rearranged neoplasms do not respond to first-generation TKI (imatinib) therapy. Prognosis is poor for acute leukemias and transformed cases, so aggressive chemotherapy and hematopoietic stem cell transplantation are considered the best curative option. Clinical trials evaluating newer agents, including FGFR1 inhibitors (e.g., pemigatinib) and third generation TKIs such as ponatinib, may provide positive results.[71-73]

Differential Diagnosis

The differential diagnoses include other morphologically similar entities such as MPNs, MDS/MPNs, and acute leukemias/extramedullary disease involvement by acute leukemia. A proper, and often exhaustive, genetic and immunophenotypic workup is required to distinguish these various entities. In situations of a complex presentation, CMN

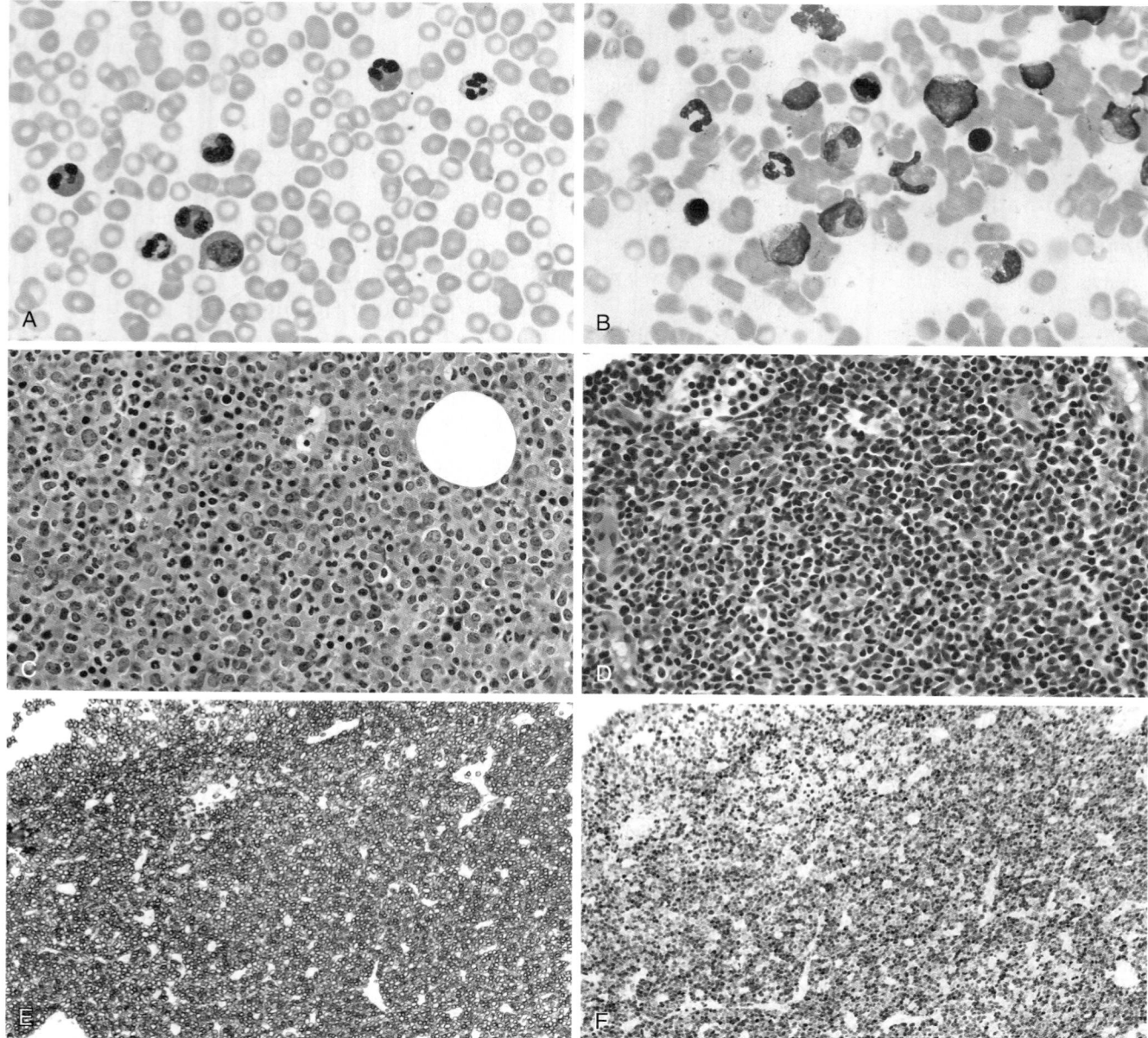

Figure 50-8. Myeloid/lymphoid neoplasm with eosinophilia and *FGFR1*-rearrangement present-ing as chronic myelomonocytic leukemia with eosinophilia in the peripheral blood and bone marrow and concurrent T-lymphoblastic lymphoma in a left cervical lymph node. A, This periph-eral blood smear from a 53-year-old male patient who presented with lymphadenopathy dem-onstrates hypereosinophilia (absolute eosinophil count 1.5 × 10⁹/L) and borderline monocytosis (absolute monocyte count 1.1 × 10⁹/L) (1000× magnification, Wright-Giemsa). **B,** A bone marrow aspirate smear demonstrates maturing trilineage hematopoiesis with an increase in eosinophils and precursors (approximately 40% of bone marrow elements). There was a slight increase in monocytes (12% of bone marrow elements). No significant dysplasia or increase in blasts is pres-ent (1000× magnification, Wright-Giemsa). **C,** The bone marrow core biopsy is packed and es-sentially effaced by an eosinophilic and myelomonocytic proliferation. Megakaryocytes and ery-throid precursors were markedly decreased (600× magnification, H&E [hematoxylin and eosin]). **D,** Left cervical lymph node biopsy demonstrates diffuse effacement of nodal architecture by an intermediate size monotonous population of round to slightly indented cells with blastic chro-matin consistent with an acute leukemic process. Extensive immunohistochemical stain demon-strated an immunophenotypic profile of T-lymphoblastic lymphoma (600× magnification, H&E [hematoxylin and eosin]). **E,** Left cervical lymph node biopsy demonstrates diffuse staining for cy-toplasmic CD3 (immunohistochemistry for CD3). **F,** Left cervical lymph node biopsy demonstrates diffuse staining for the immature marker TdT, confirming a diagnosis of T-lymphoblastic lym-phoma (immunohistochemistry for TdT).

in the peripheral blood/bone marrow, and extramedullary involvement by acute leukemia, *FGFR1* rearrangement testing is needed, regardless of the presence of eosinophilia.

Myeloid/Lymphoid Neoplasms With Eosinophilia and Rearrangement of *JAK2*

Myeloid/lymphoid neoplasms with eosinophilia and *PCM1::JAK2* and two genetic variants *ETV6::JAK2* and *BCR::JAK2*.

Definition

Myeloid and/or lymphoid neoplasms associated with a *JAK2* fusion.[1-5,9,74,75] The most common fusion partner for this entity is *PCM1*. Additional partner genes exist and are included in this diagnostic category, specifically, t(9;12)(p24.1;p13.2)/*ETV6::JAK2* and t(9;22)(p24.1;q11.2)/*BCR::JAK2*.

Synonyms and Related Terms

Myeloid or lymphoid neoplasm with *JAK2* rearrangement; myeloid/lymphoid neoplasms with *PCM1::JAK2* and genetic variants.

Epidemiology

Cases of myeloid/lymphoid neoplasms with eosinophilia and *PCM1::JAK2* fusion currently account for less than 70 total cases in the literature.[1-3,9,11,76-81] The median age at presentation is 50 years, with a wide age range, and there is a male predominance (>3:1 male-to-female ratio).

Etiology

The etiology is unknown.

Clinical Features

These neoplasms show a heterogenous presentation ranging from MPNs and MDS/MPN, most commonly (approximately 60%), to AML and B-ALL; extramedullary disease involvement is common (Table 50-1).[2,3,5,9,79-81] Organomegaly (hepatosplenomegaly) and/or lymphadenopathy are also very common. Rare presentations include manifestation of B-lymphoblastic crisis of an underlying CMN, myeloid sarcoma, pure erythroid leukemia or erythroblastic sarcoma, and T-cell lymphoma.[5,9,82] It has been reported that two cases of mycosis fungoides harbored the *PCM1::JAK2* fusion and that *JAK2* rearrangements may be seen in CD30-positive systemic T-cell lymphomas with anaplastic cytology.[83,84] Neither case exhibited eosinophilia. It remains debatable whether these cases belong to M/LN-eo-TK or T-cell lymphoma with *PCM1::JAK2*.

Morphology

Peripheral blood: Eosinophilia is common in patients with CMNs, ranging from mild to marked. Eosinophil morphology is variable, ranging from morphologically unremarkable forms to abnormal/dysplastic-appearing forms.

Bone marrow: The bone marrow shows the typical histopathologic "triad," which includes hypercellularity with an eosinophilic infiltrate, large aggregates of immature erythroid precursors (pronormoblasts), and myelofibrosis (Fig. 50-9).[2,5,9] The identification of these erythroid "microtumors" in the setting of eosinophilia and MPN features should immediately prompt the pathologist to consider this diagnostic entity and initiate appropriate genetic testing. In some cases, erythroid hyperplasia, dysplasia in the erythroid, and granulocytic and/or megakaryocytic lineage may be seen.

Extramedullary sites: The features of an eosinophilic infiltrate, large aggregates of immature erythroid precursors (pronormoblasts), and myelofibrosis may be seen. If the pronormoblasts form large sheets and efface the extramedullary tissue architecture, this may indicate a diagnosis of erythroblastic sarcoma.[80,82]

Immunophenotype

Similar to other M/LN-eo-TKs, if blasts are not increased, immunophenotyping may serve as a tool to rule out other causes of eosinophilia and identify aberrant mast cells. Erythroid microtumors or extramedullary erythroid nodules can be confirmed by CD71 and E-cadherin. For cases with increased blasts, flow cytometry immunophenotyping and immunohistochemistry will help characterize blast phenotype.

Genetics/Molecular Findings

JAK2 is a cytoplasmic tyrosine kinase that plays an important role in hematopoiesis and cell proliferation. Constitutive activation of the JAK pathway by the gene mutation *JAK2* V617F is common in Philadelphia-negative MPNs (essential thrombocytosis, polycythemia vera, and primary myelofibrosis).

In contrast to the common *JAK2* V617F mutation, chromosomal translocations involving *JAK2* are rare and have been reported in various hematologic malignancies.

JAK2 is located at the terminal band of the short arm of chromosome 9. The vast majority of *PCM::JAK2* cases are not cryptic and demonstrate t(8;9)(p22;p24.1) if sufficient metaphases are obtained. However, a translocation involving *JAK2* has the potential to be cytogenetically cryptic, especially if the partner gene happens to also be located at the terminal end of a chromosome. For extramedullary lesions, when karyotyping is not available, a high index of suspicion for this genetic abnormality is needed in the appropriate morphologic context and complex presentation. FISH or RNA sequencing should be used in clinical practice. Though *PCM1* is the most common partner, several additional partners have been reported (*ETV6* and *BCR*) (Box 50-2). The potential therapeutic benefit of targeted therapy (JAK2 inhibitors) warrants accurate and timely diagnosis of this genetic abnormality.[6,7,76,77,85]

Postulated Cell of Origin/Normal Counterpart

Pluripotent hematopoietic stem cell that can give rise to a proliferation of myeloid, erythroid, or B-lymphoid or T-lymphoid lineage cells.

Clinical Course

The disease course appears to be highly variable, with chronic phase disease showing a longer overall survival and a 5-year survival of approximately 80%.[6,9,74,80] The prognosis is dismal for patients who present with increased blasts or progress to acute leukemia. Targeted therapy with JAK2 inhibitors such as ruxolitinib may offer potential benefit,[76,77] but the response may be limited.[76,77,80,85] The 2024 National Comprehensive Cancer Network (NCCN) guidelines for myeloid/lymphoid neoplasms with eosinophilia and *PCM1::JAK2* fusion state that a clinical trial is the preferred treatment option for

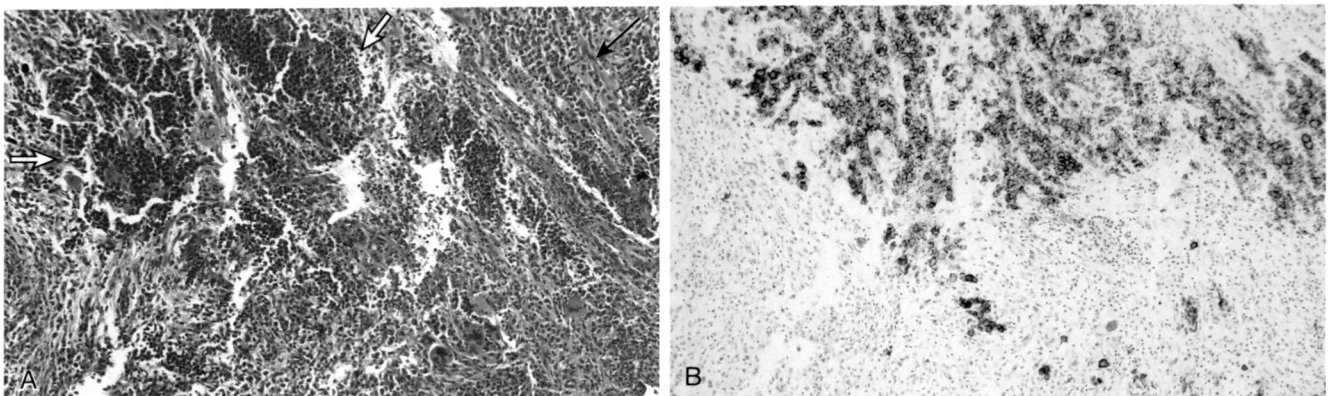

Figure 50-9. Myeloid/lymphoid neoplasm with eosinophilia and *PCM1::JAK2* fusion. A, The bone marrow core biopsy is markedly hypercellular for age (61-year-old patient) and demonstrates the typical "triad" histopathologic features, including clusters of early erythroid precursors/pronormoblasts *(block arrows)*, fibrosis *(lower left and center of image)*, and eosinophilia *(single line arrow)* (400× magnification; H&E [hematoxylin and eosin]). **B,** Clusters of early erythroid precursors/pronormoblasts are nicely highlighted by an immunohistochemical stain for E-cadherin.

patients with chronic phase disease.[7] Allogeneic stem cell transplantation has the promise of disease cure.

Differential Diagnosis

The differential diagnostic considerations include the other morphologically similar entities such as MDS/MPN with eosinophilia, MPNs, CEL, NOS, and acute leukemias/extramedullary disease involvement by acute leukemia. A proper, and often exhaustive, genetic and immunophenotypic workup is required to distinguish among these various entities. In situations of a complex presentation, CMN in the peripheral blood/bone marrow, and extramedullary involvement by acute leukemia, *JAK2* rearrangement testing is needed, regardless of the presence of eosinophilia.

JAK2 rearrangements are common in de novo Philadelphia-like B-ALL. Frequent partners including *SSBP2, PAX5, USP25,* and *ZNF274*. Patients with de novo B-ALL with *PCM1::JAK2* and no apparent myeloid component or eosinophilia may be best classified as Philadelphia-like B-ALL. Demonstration of a *JAK2* rearrangement in the myeloid cells in cases presenting as B-ALL and a prior history of a *JAK2*-rearranged CMN or *JAK2*-rearranged myeloid cells after treatment would support a diagnosis of myeloid/lymphoid neoplasm with *JAK2* rearrangement.

Variants of Myeloid/Lymphoid Neoplasms With Eosinophilia and *JAK2* Rearrangement (Not *PCM1::JAK2*)

BCR::JAK2: t(9;22) (p24;q11.2)

This is a rare myeloid/lymphoid neoplasm with fewer than 20 documented cases reported in the literature.[2,3,5,9,86-88] *BCR::JAK2* cases have a heterogeneous clinical presentation. These neoplasms have been predominantly classified as CML-like MPN, MPN with eosinophilia, and aCML; less often, they are classified as B-ALL, AML, and mixed phenotype acute leukemia. The presence of both myeloid and lymphoid neoplasms in patients with *BCR::JAK2* fusion suggests this genetic alteration occurs in a pluripotent progenitor stem cell. In the cases of B-ALL, the alternate diagnostic possibility

of Philadelphia-like B-ALL should be rendered if there is no evidence of a preceding, concurrent, or subsequent underlying CMN.

The median age at time of presentation is approximately 50 years, although there is a wide range from toddler to the seventh decade of life.[2,5,6,81,83,84] The histologic bone marrow features do not appear, thus far, to show the classic triad features of *PCM1::JAK2* (eosinophilic infiltrate, large aggregates of immature erythroid precursors [pronormoblasts], and myelofibrosis).[9] Myeloid neoplasms with eosinophilia and *BCR::JAK2*/t(9;22) (p24;q11.2) usually do not respond to *BCR-ABL1* TKIs, a therapy that is effective for CML.[85]

ETV6::JAK2: t(9;12)(p24;p13.2)

Less than 15 cases of this entity have been described to date. Of these, the majority present as acute lymphoblastic leukemia (mostly B lineage, but a few T lineage); a minor subset presents as a chronic neoplasm such as CEL, myelodysplasia, or aCML.[2,9,74,89,90] The histologic bone marrow features do not appear, thus far, to show the classic triad features of *PCM1::JAK2* (eosinophilic infiltrate, large aggregates of immature erythroid precursors [pronormoblasts], and myelofibrosis).[9] The cases with B-ALL presentation may belong more appropriately to the ICC category of Philadelphia-like B-ALL if there is no evidence of a preceding, concurrent, or subsequent underlying CMN.

Myeloid/Lymphoid Neoplasms With Eosinophilia and Rearrangement of *FLT3*

Definition

Myeloid/lymphoid neoplasms that harbor an FMS-related receptor tyrosine kinase 3 (*FLT3*) rearrangement that results in the formation of a fusion gene involving *FLT3*.

Synonyms and Related Terms

Myeloid/lymphoid neoplasms with eosinophilia and *FLT3* rearrangement.[4]

Epidemiology

The disease appears to be slightly more common in men, with a male-to-female ratio of approximately 1.4:1.0. There is a broad range of age at presentation, with the median age in the 50s.

Etiology

The etiology is unknown.

Clinical Features

Like the other myeloid/lymphoid neoplasms associated with eosinophilia and a rearrangement of *PDGFRA*, *PDGFRB*, *FGFR1*, and *JAK2*, hematopoietic neoplasms with *FLT3* rearrangement share some clinical and morphologic overlap (Table 50-2).[3,5,9,91,92] Patients typically present with peripheral blood abnormalities, including leukocytosis, occasionally monocytosis, and cytopenias. Eosinophilia is common but not invariably present (or it can be mild). Lymphadenopathy, splenomegaly, and extramedullary mass lesions are common. Clinical features are a manifestation of the disease presentation(s) and may include fatigue, easy bruising, rash, itching, or effects of extramedullary disease involvement.

Morphology

The pathologic presentation is heterogenous, including as a CMN (CEL-like, CMML-like, aCML, myelodysplastic syndromes), a higher grade myeloid disorder with excess blasts, or an acute leukemia (T-ALL, B-ALL, and myeloid sarcoma) or as mixed lineage neoplasm (mixed phenotype acute leukemia) (Fig. 50-10). Extramedullary disease involvement is common and has been described in two-thirds of cases. Two cases of T-cell lymphoma have been reported.

Table 50-2 Myeloid/Lymphoid Neoplasms With Eosinophilia With *FLT3* Rearrangement and *ETV6::ABL1*

Disease Presentation	FLT3 *Rearrangement* Heterogeneous	ETV6::ABL1 Predominantly Chronic Phase, but Not Universal
Peripheral Blood and Bone Marrow		
CEL (MPN-eo)	+++	++
MDS/MPN	+	+++
AML		<+
MDS with increased blasts (<20%)	<+	
T-ALL/ETP	<+	
Hypereosinophilia	Around 70% (PB/BM/tissue)	>95%
Basophilia		+
Extramedullary	+++	+
MS	++	+
T-ALL	+++	+
MPAL	+	
Disease progression	T-ALL > AML	T-ALL, AML

AML, Acute myeloid leukemia; *CEL*, chronic eosinophilic leukemia; *ETP*, early T-cell precursor ALL; *MDS*, myelodysplastic syndrome; *MDS/MPN*, myelodysplastic/myeloproliferative neoplasm; *MPAL*, mixed phenotype acute leukemia; *MPN-eo*, myeloproliferative neoplasm with eosinophilia; *MS*, myeloid sarcoma; *T-ALL*, T-lymphoblastic leukemia/lymphoma.

Peripheral blood/bone marrow: The peripheral blood and bone marrow features vary depending on the type of disease presentation. There is often, but not invariably, eosinophilia. There may be monocytosis in cases with a CMML-like appearance or dysgranulopoiesis in cases with aCML-like presentation. Features resembling SM may be seen, and careful evaluation to distinguish true SM from an associated myeloid neoplasm is critical. If there is a higher-grade myeloid neoplasm, increased myeloid blasts are noted. Variable numbers of lymphoblasts or mixed lineage blasts may be present if there is a concurrent acute leukemia involving an extramedullary site.

Extramedullary sites: Extramedullary disease involvement by T-ALL, mixed phenotype acute leukemia, and myeloid sarcoma is common. Increased eosinophils and/or mast cells may be seen in these lesions.

Immunophenotype

Depending on the morphologic findings, more or less immunophenotypic studies may be needed to clarify the diagnostic process. If the case presents as a CMN, additional testing may not be needed. If there is a proliferation of immature-appearing cells/blasts, then a more extensive immunophenotypic analysis is required. In the latter case, flow cytometric immunophenotyping is preferred, particularly when a diagnosis of mixed phenotype acute leukemia is being considered.

Genetics/Molecular Findings

The *FLT3* gene, located on chromosome 13q12, belongs to the receptor tyrosine kinase family. Unlike *FLT3* mutations (common in AML), *FLT3* rearrangements in hematolymphoid neoplasms are rare, with fewer than 30 cases reported in the published literature.[3,5,9,91,92] The most common partner gene is *ETV6*, located at 12p13.2, accounting for just under half of the reported cases. The fusion of *ETV6::FLT3* is typically not cryptic in conventional chromosomal analysis, and involvement of the *FLT3* gene should be considered in cases of a hematopoietic neoplasm in which 13q12 is rearranged. The presence of the *FLT3* fusion gene should be confirmed using FISH probes for *FLT3*, RT-PCR, or RNA-sequencing methods because not all cases with 13q12 rearrangements involve the *FLT3* gene. Cases that have a chromosomal rearrangement at 13q12 wherein *FLT3* is not rearranged are excluded from this diagnostic category.

Additional partners that have been reported include *ZMYM2*/13q12.11, *BCR*(22q11), *TRIP11*/14q32.12, *SPTBN1*/2p16.2, *GOLGB1*/3q13.33, *CCDC88C*/14q32.11-14q32.12, and *MYO18A*/17q11.2.[91-96] Given that some partners (known or unknown) may be cryptic at the chromosomal level, additional testing with FISH and/or RNA sequencing should be strongly considered when there is a complex disease presentation with both a CMN and an extramedullary acute component, regardless of whether eosinophilia is present.

There is limited information regarding additional genetic mutations detected by NGS. These mutations include variants in *ASXL1*, *PTPN11*, *RUNX1*, *SETBP1*, *SRSF2*, *STAT5B*, *TET2*, *TP53*, and *U2AF1* genes, present in around 50% of cases.[5,9] The prognostic effect of these mutations is not known.

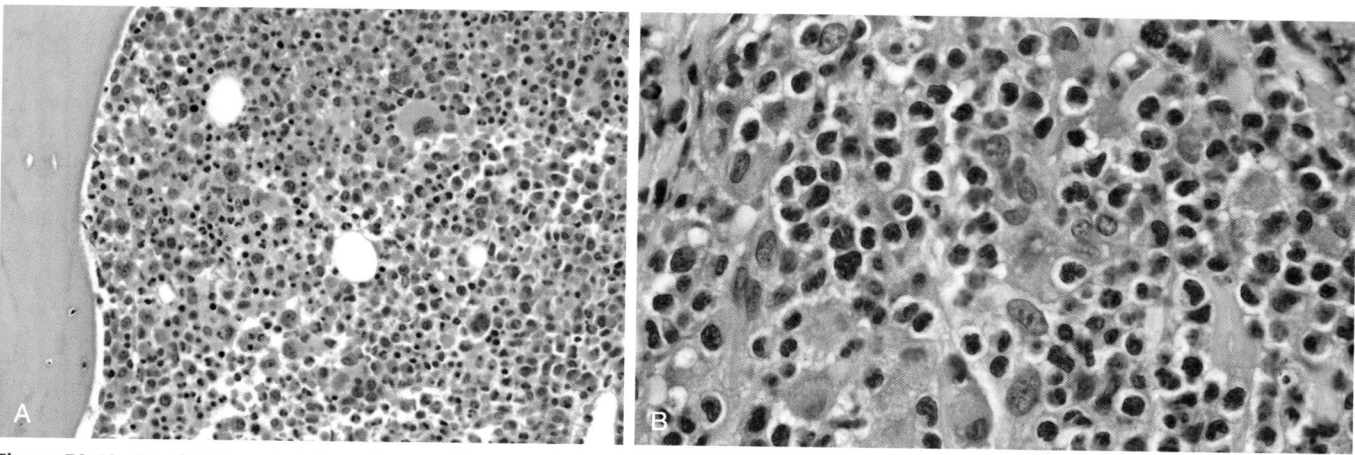

Figure 50-10. Myeloid/lymphoid neoplasm with eosinophilia and *FLT3*-rearrangement. **A,** The bone marrow core biopsy shows hypercellular bone marrow with numerous eosinophils, no overt megakaryocytic dysplasia, and no increase in blasts—very much the appearance of a chronic eosinophilic leukemia, not otherwise specified (1000× magnification; H&E [hematoxylin and eosin]). Cytogenetic studies confirmed by fluorescence in situ hybridization (FISH) indicated a *FLT3*-rearrangement. **B,** This lymph node biopsy from the same patient shows effacement by intermediate size cells with irregular nuclear contours, inconspicuous nucleoli, and somewhat immature-appearing chromatin. Eosinophils are notably absent. Extensive immunohistochemistry demonstrates that this is a T-lymphoblastic lymphoma. FISH identified a *FLT3*-rearrangement, indicating this acute leukemia is genetically related to the chronic myeloid neoplasm with eosinophilia in the bone marrow.

Postulated Cell of Origin/Normal Counterpart

A pluripotent hematopoietic stem cell capable of myeloid and/or lymphoid differentiation.

Clinical Course

These cases tend be associated with an aggressive clinical course or early disease progression. A number of these cases have shown therapeutic benefit from FLT3 inhibitors such as sorafenib, sunitinib, or midostaurin monotherapy, although durability can be short, necessitating consideration of allogeneic hematopoietic stem cell transplantation for an attempt to cure.[7,92,97] Some patients may exhibit a durable clinical response to this therapy, whereas others may require more aggressive chemotherapy and/or allogeneic hematopoietic stem cell transplantation.[7]

Differential Diagnosis

The differential diagnoses include other morphologically similar entities such as aCML, CMML, CEL, NOS, and acute leukemias/extramedullary disease involvement by acute leukemia. The proper, and often exhaustive, genetic and immunophenotypic workup is required to distinguish among these various entities. In situations of a complex presentation as a CMN and as extramedullary involvement by acute leukemia, *FLT3* rearrangement testing is needed, regardless of eosinophilia presence.

Myeloid Neoplasms With Eosinophilia and *ETV6::ABL1*

Definition

This is a hematopoietic stem cell neoplasm of myeloid and/or lymphoid lineage associated with fusion of the *ETV6* and *ABL1* genes.

Epidemiology

There appears to be a slight male predominance, with a male-to-female ratio of 2:1. The median age of presentation is in the 5th decade of life.[3,5]

Etiology

The etiology is unknown.

Clinical Features

Most patients exhibit splenomegaly. The diagnosis is typically made in chronic phase and should be separated from de novo B-ALL with *ETV6::ABL1*, which may be diagnosed as Philadelphia-like/B-ALL.

Morphology

In a review of the literature, it was reported that patients with rearrangement of *ETV6::ABL1* present with a clonal myeloid proliferation and eosinophilia most often in chronic phase[98] (Fig. 50-11). However, like the other myeloid neoplasms with eosinophilia and recurring genetic rearrangements, AML may be seen at presentation, or the chronic cases may transform to AML, T-ALL, or B-ALL (Table 50-2). Patients often present with leukocytosis and anemia; basophilia also may be seen (Fig. 50-11A). There may be thrombocytosis or thrombocytopenia. Eosinophilia is very common in myeloid neoplasm presentation. When presenting in chronic phase, the pathologic appearance may resemble CML, aCML, or MPN. However, the genetic rearrangement of *ABL1* should drive the classification. A subset of cases may exhibit extramedullary disease involvement.

Immunophenotype

Depending on the morphologic findings, immunophenotypic studies may be needed to clarify the diagnostic process. If the case presents as a CMN, minimal phenotyping may be needed. If there is a proliferation of immature-appearing cells/blasts,

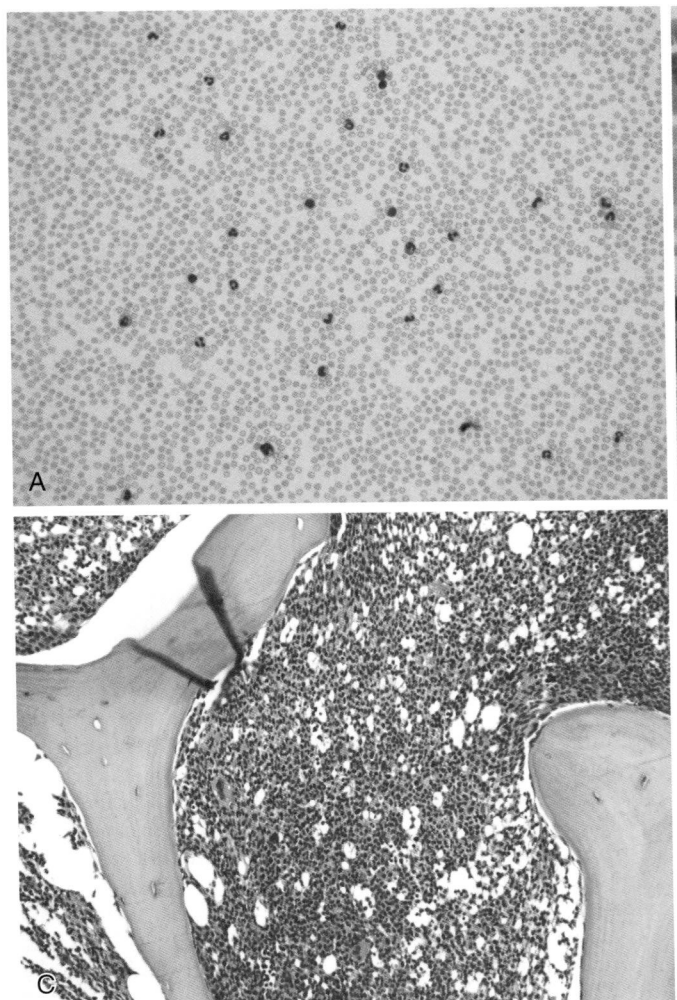
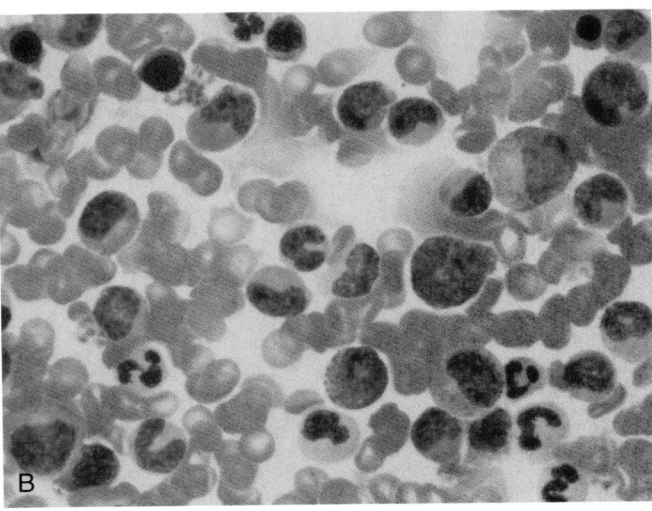

Figure 50-11. Myeloid neoplasm with *ETV6::ABL1*. A, Peripheral blood smear shows marked leukocytosis with eosinophilia, neutrophilia, occasional basophils, and monocytosis (400× magnification, Wright-Giemsa). **B,** Bone marrow aspirate smear reveals increased granulocytes with progressive maturation and unremarkable morphology, increased eosinophils, and relatively decreased erythrocytes (1000× magnification, Wright-Giemsa). **C,** Bone marrow core biopsy reveals hypercellular bone marrow with granulocytic hyperplasia; megakaryocytes are decreased in number with unremarkable changes (600× magnification, H&E [hematoxylin and eosin]).

then a more extensive immunophenotypic analysis is required. In the latter case, flow cytometric immunophenotyping is preferred, particularly when a diagnosis of mixed phenotype acute leukemia is being considered.

Genetics/Molecular Findings

The *ABL1* gene, located on chromosome 9q34.12, is a nonreceptor tyrosine kinase. *ABL1* rearrangements (excluding *BCR::ABL1*) in hematolymphoid neoplasms are rare.[3,5,9,11,98-102] The most common partner gene is *ETV6*, located at 12p13.2. Other partner genes are mostly identified in de novo T-ALL or Philadelphia-like B-ALL.

Postulated Cell of Origin/Normal Counterpart

Pluripotent hematopoietic stem cell

Clinical Course

Most patients present in chronic phase; however, disease progression to blast phase or extramedullary blastic tumor may occur in 30% of cases. Patients in chronic phase show various responses to TKIs.[103]

Differential Diagnosis

Given the known response to TKI treatment, it is absolutely critical to identify the *ETV6::ABL1* fusion or a variant-*ABL1*

fusion and incorporate TKI treatment at an early stage of disease.[7,101] A high index of suspicion is critical to initiate proper testing in patients presenting with signs of myeloproliferative disease and eosinophilia. The differential diagnostic considerations include other morphologically similar entities such as CML, CMML, and CEL, NOS. The proper genetic workup is required to distinguish among these various entities. Cases that present as B-ALL should be diagnosed as Philadelphia-like B-ALL in the absence of an underlying CMN.

CEL, NOS, IHE/IHES, AND OTHER RARE REPORTED GENETIC ALTERATIONS ASSOCIATED WITH CLONAL EOSINOPHILIA

Chronic Eosinophilic Leukemia, Not Otherwise Specified (CEL, NOS)

Definition

CEL, NOS is an MPN in which a clonal proliferation of eosinophils and precursors results in persistent eosinophilia involving the peripheral blood, bone marrow, and other tissues, with the eosinophilia being the dominant pathologic manifestation (Box 50-3). The diagnostic criteria for an

> **Box 50-3** *Diagnostic Criteria for Chronic Eosinophilic Leukemia, Not Otherwise Specified (CEL, NOS)*
>
> Peripheral blood hypereosinophilia (eosinophil count ≥1.5 × 10^9/L and eosinophils ≥10% of white blood cells)
>
> Blasts constitute <20% of the cells in peripheral blood and bone marrow, not meeting any other diagnostic criteria for AML*
>
> No tyrosine kinase gene fusion, including *BCR::ABL1* and other *ABL1*, *PDGFRA*, *PDGFRB*, *FGFR1*, *JAK2*, and *FLT3* fusions
>
> Not meeting criteria for other well-defined MPNs, chronic myelomonocytic leukemia, or systemic mastocytosis†
>
> Bone marrow shows increased cellularity with dysplastic megakaryocytes with or without dysplastic features in other lineages and often significant fibrosis, associated with an eosinophilic infiltrate, **OR** there are increased blasts ≥5% in the bone marrow and/or ≥2% in the peripheral blood
>
> Demonstration of a clonal cytogenetic abnormality and/or somatic mutation(s)‡
>
> *AML,* Acute myeloid leukemia; *MPN,* myeloproliferative neoplasm.
> *AML with recurrent genetic abnormalities and <20% blasts is excluded.
> †CEL, NOS may occur as the associated myeloid neoplasm in cases of systemic mastocytosis with an associated myeloid neoplasm.
> ‡In the absence of a clonal cytogenetic abnormality and/or somatic mutation(s) or increased blasts, bone marrow findings supportive of the diagnosis will suffice in the presence of persistent eosinophilia, provided other causes of eosinophilia having been excluded.

alternative ICC-recognized hematopoietic neoplasm are not met. A diagnosis of CEL, NOS supersedes a diagnosis of aCML, MDS/MPN, NOS, or MPN-unclassified, but not classic MPN with MPN driver mutations or CMML with eosinophilia.

Synonyms and Related Terms

Chronic eosinophilic leukemia.[4]

Epidemiology

Given the longstanding challenges in definitively distinguishing many cases of true CEL, NOS from iHE/iHES, the true incidence of CEL, NOS (rare) is unknown. The range of age at presentation is quite broad (14–92 years) but on average is in the 60s.[104-106] There appears to be a male predominance with a male-to-female ratio of 2 to 3:1.[3,4,106] In one study, CEL, NOS represented 1.2% of patients with peripheral blood eosinophilia.[106]

Etiology

There are no known risk factors or a genetic predisposition to CEL, NOS.

Clinical Features

Though patients may occasionally present without symptoms, many patients appear to present with systemic symptoms. Like patients with other CMNs, those with CEL, NOS present with frequent constitutional symptoms (approximately 50%) such as fatigue, night sweats, fever, weight loss, abnormal complete blood count (including eosinophilia, cytopenia[s], and/or cytosis) in 70% to 80%, organomegaly (around 20%–30%) and elevated lactate

dehydrogenase (approximately 60%). Unlike iHES, organ damage/dysfunction attributed to an eosinophilic infiltrate is not required for diagnosis but may be seen in 50% of patients. The symptoms directly attributable to hypereosinophilia may vary depending on the tissue site(s) involved. The most common sign is skin rash (approximately 30%), but it may involve the gastrointestinal tract and cardiac, pulmonary, and central nervous systems. Depending on the degree of eosinophilic infiltration/end organ damage, endomyocardial fibrosis, scarring of cardiac valves with subsequent cardiac failure, and central nervous system dysfunction may result in serious morbidity and mortality. Thrombotic events are reported in approximately 10% of patients. In contrast to iHES, symptoms of allergy/hypersensitivity and upper respiratory symptoms such as asthma/cough are uncommon.

Morphology

Peripheral blood: The peripheral blood smear, by diagnostic criteria, shows hypereosinophilia (eosinophils ≥1.5 × 10^9/L and eosinophils ≥10% of white blood cells) that is often quite striking[3,5] (Fig. 50-12). There is usually accompanying leukocytosis, but this is not a requirement for the diagnosis. Eosinophils are mostly mature and may show a range of abnormal morphologic features, including abnormal granulation (hypogranulation or uneven granulation), cytoplasmic vacuoles, or abnormal nuclear lobation (Fig. 50-12). Of note, cytologic abnormalities of eosinophils are not specific to CEL, NOS or other neoplastic conditions and can also be seen in reactive conditions, but usually at a mild degree. Though cases of CEL, NOS may show normal eosinophil cytology, the absence of eosinophil cytologic abnormalities generally is more common in a reactive condition.[104] Anemia is present in the majority of patients, and thrombocytopenia may be seen.[104,105] Occasional cases show thrombocytosis. Mild basophilia has also been reported.[1] Some cases exhibit mild monocytosis but do not meet diagnostic criteria for CMML. The peripheral blood blast percentage is typically low.[106]

Bone marrow: Bone marrow aspirate smears and core biopsy sections are generally significantly hypercellular, predominantly from an increase in eosinophils and granulocytic precursors with a resultant increase in the myeloid-to-erythroid ratio (>10) (Fig. 50-12).[26] Eosinophils may display cytologic abnormalities like those described in the peripheral blood, but they are often less striking. Megakaryocytes are essentially always abnormal, exhibiting most commonly myelodysplastic-type forms (hypolobated or small forms with distinctly separate nuclear lobes) (Fig. 50-12). In some cases, there may be a spectrum of megakaryocytic morphology including MDS-like forms and larger, hyperlobulated forms mimicking an MPN. Not infrequently, the proportion of increased eosinophils and granulocytes may render evaluation of megakaryocyte morphology more challenging. Regardless, careful morphologic assessment for abnormal megakaryocytes and/or the use of a megakaryocyte-associated immunohistochemical stain (e.g., CD61) may be helpful in discerning the presence of dysplastic megakaryocytes. Dysgranulopoiesis and dyserythropoiesis may be present and helpful in further supporting a diagnosis of CEL, NOS;

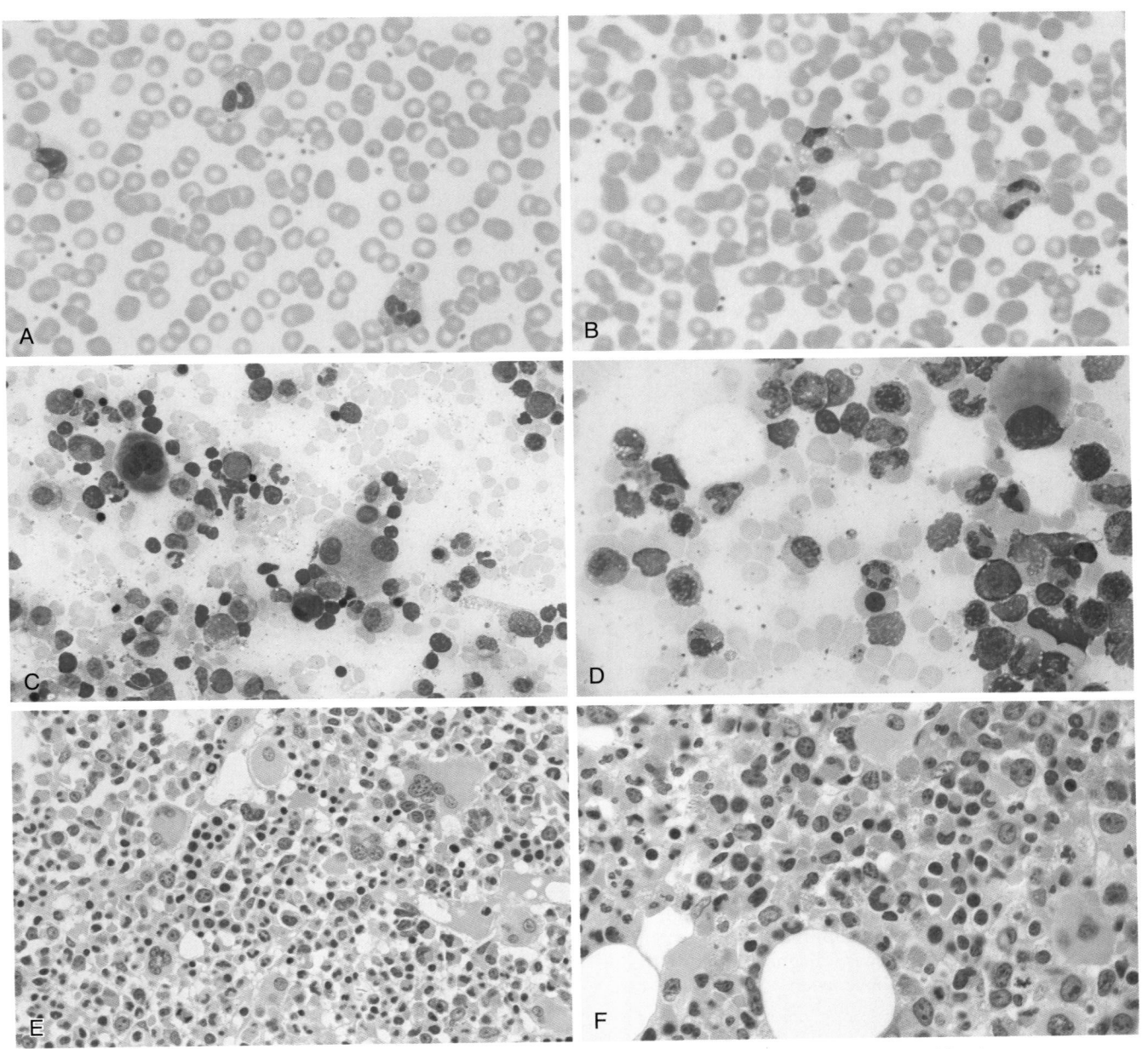

Figure 50-12. Chronic eosinophilic leukemia, not otherwise specified. A, The peripheral blood may show abnormal eosinophils characterized by hypolobated and hypogranular forms (1000× magnification, Wright-Giemsa). **B,** The peripheral blood may show abnormal eosinophils with vacuolization (1000× magnification, Wright-Giemsa). **C,** Bone marrow aspirate smears are spicular and hypercellular with very typical dysplastic-appearing megakaryocytes. In some instances, there may be more of a spectrum of megakaryocyte morphology, including admixed larger (myeloproliferative neoplasm–like) forms. Dysgranulopoiesis and dyserythropoiesis are relatively uncommon. An increase in blasts is uncommon (1000× magnification, Wright-Giemsa). **D,** Bone marrow aspirate smears show a remarkable increase in eosinophils and dysplastic megakaryocytes (1000× magnification, Wright-Giemsa). **E,** The bone marrow core biopsy is essentially always hypercellular with increased eosinophils, resulting in a markedly increased myeloid-to-erythroid ratio. Admixed dysplastic-appearing megakaryocytes may be identified (600× magnification, H&E [hematoxylin and eosin]). **F,** The bone marrow core biopsy shows increased granulocytes and eosinophils with background dysplastic megakaryocytes. There is no overt increase in blasts (1000× magnification, H&E [hematoxylin and eosin]).

however, this is not an invariable finding. Monocytes are not increased. Bone marrow blasts tend to represent, in most cases, less than 5% of the total nucleated cells. Increased reticulin fibrosis (grade 2 and grade 3 of 3) may be observed in approximately 20% to 30% of cases.

Immunophenotype/Genetic Testing

There are no specific immunophenotypic abnormalities in CEL, NOS. Given that CEL, NOS is largely a diagnosis of exclusion, other diagnoses that may exhibit a significant proportion of eosinophils must be excluded (Fig. 50-2). Immunohistochemical studies for CD117, tryptase, and CD25 will help exclude the presence of SM. Caution should be exercised in the latter scenario, particularly if the bone marrow is markedly hypercellular with extensive eosinophilic infiltration, because SM may rarely be associated with CEL, NOS, meeting ICC criteria for SM with associated myeloid neoplasm (SM-AMN). Additional testing via immunohistochemistry and/or flow cytometry to exclude the presence of the lymphocytic variant of hypereosinophilic syndrome and T-cell/B-cell lymphoma is also suggested. The CD34-positive myeloblasts often exhibit immunophenotypic aberrancy if the flow cytometry tests used are designed for myelodysplastic syndromes or AML minimal residual disease detection, supporting a myeloid neoplasm.

Genetics/Molecular Findings

There is no specific cytogenetic or molecular genetic abnormality identified in CEL, NOS. However, the finding of a cytogenetic abnormality that is typically associated with myeloid neoplasms (trisomy 8, monosomy 7, etc.) may be useful in supporting the presence of a myeloid neoplasm best characterized as CEL, NOS.

With the increased availability of NGS panels, novel additional mutations are being identified in cases previously diagnosed as iHE/iHES.[104,107,108] In particular, in the setting of abnormal bone marrow morphology, gene mutations may help solidify a diagnosis of CEL, NOS rather than iHE/iHES. In one study, 11/98 patients with hypereosinophilic syndrome demonstrated a single positive mutation in *TET2, ASXL1, KIT, TP53, IDH2, JAK2,* and *SF3B1*.[107] In another study, 14/51 patients with the diagnosis of hypereosinophilic syndrome showed a single mutated gene in 7 patients and two or more mutated genes in another 7 patients.[104] In this series, the most commonly mutated genes were *ASXL1, TET2, EZH2, SETBP1, CBL,* and *NOTCH. STAT5B* N642H has been reported in a small subset of patients referred with eosinophilia (1.6%), including patients who would be otherwise diagnosed with iHES.[109] Additional mutations that have been identified in other rare cases of clonal eosinophilia include those in *JAK2* exon 13 Leu583-Ala586DelInsSer,[110] *JAK1* R629_S632delinsSA in a patient with CEL,[111] and *CCT6B*.[112]

It is important to emphasize that, when only a single gene is mutated and the involved gene has been associated with clonal hematopoiesis of indeterminate potential (CHIP) and is at relatively low variant allele frequency (e.g. *ASXL1, TET2, JAK2*), it is incumbent upon the multidisciplinary team to discriminate true clonal eosinophilia from CHIP. It is also acknowledged that, like other myeloid neoplasms, occasional cases may not show a molecular genetic alteration with the currently available testing methods. In the presence of persistent hypereosinophilia and the other clinical features mentioned, abnormal bone marrow morphology consistent with a CMN should suffice to make a diagnosis of CEL, NOS.

Genetic testing should include assessment for *KIT* D816V, conventional cytogenetics to exclude a recurring genetic abnormality diagnostic of another entity such as AML with inv(16) or CML, and exclusion of M/LN-eo-TK by appropriate cytogenetic, FISH, RT-PCR, and/or RNA sequencing technologies. In the authors' opinion, it is crucial to perform DNA and RNA extract and hold on to the bone marrow specimen to ensure there is material for NGS or RNA testing that may be necessary to evaluate for additional clonal abnormalities.

Clinical Course

Prognosis in patients with CEL, NOS is largely unfavorable, with median overall survivals reported in the literature of 14.4 months,[104] 16 months (range, 1–49 months),[106] and 22.2 months.[105]

Differential Diagnosis

CEL, NOS is a diagnosis of exclusion, and appropriate morphologic, clinical, laboratory, and genetic testing is necessary to exclude potential differential diagnoses such as iHE/iHES, the lymphocytic variant of hypereosinophilic syndrome, reactive hypereosinophilia (including T-cell/B-cell lymphoma and Hodgkin lymphoma), clonal hypereosinophilia associated with a well-defined hematopoietic neoplasm such as AML with inv(16) or CML, and M/LN-eo-TK.

In particular, with iHES, features that would tend to support the diagnosis of CEL, NOS include older age, higher white blood cell counts and AECs, cytopenia(s) and/or cytosis, frequent constitutional symptoms, hepatosplenomegaly, and high lactate dehydrogenase.[5,13,26,104] In contrast, patients with iHES are significantly younger, with more allergic or rheumatoid symptoms, skin rash, and pulmonary, gastrointestinal, an/or endocrine involvement. Genetic testing may also be helpful, particularly if a convincing myeloid neoplasm–associated cytogenetic abnormality is observed or if multiple myeloid disorder gene mutations are detected by NGS at high variant allele frequencies.

Idiopathic Hypereosinophilia/ Hypereosinophilic Syndrome (iHE/iHES)

Definition

iHES is defined as persistent hypereosinophilia (≥6 months) with associated tissue/organ damage/injury from eosinophil-released cytokines or enzymes when the underlying cause, either a reactive or a clonal myeloid process, cannot be identified (Box 50-4). iHE or hypereosinophilia of unknown significance (HEus) is referred to as persistent hypereosinophilia of unknown etiology without related organ/tissue damage.

A diagnosis of iHE/HEus or iHES requires exclusion of all possible reactive causes and clonal neoplasms (Box 50-2).[6] With the improved recognition of eosinophilia cases that harbor a disease-associated molecular genetic abnormality, if appropriate and proper genetic workup is performed, the number of "idiopathic" cases should be significantly reduced.

Synonyms and Related Terms

Hypereosinophilic syndrome.

Epidemiology

The epidemiology is unknown given the overlap with CEL, NOS and difficulty distinguishing M/LN-eo-TK.

Box 50-4 *Diagnosis of Idiopathic Hypereosinophilia or Idiopathic Hypereosinophilic Syndrome*

Persistent peripheral blood hypereosinophilia (eosinophil count $\geq 1.5 \times 10^9$/L and $\geq 10\%$ eosinophils)*

Organ damage and/or dysfunction attributable to tissue eosinophilic infiltrate†

No evidence of a reactive, well-defined autoimmune disease or neoplastic condition/disorder underlying the hypereosinophilia

Lymphocytic variant of hypereosinophilic syndrome ruled out‡

Bone marrow morphologically within normal limits except for increased eosinophils

No molecular genetic clonal abnormality, with the caveat of clonal hematopoiesis of indeterminate potential (CHIP)

*Preferably a minimal duration of 6 months if documentation is available.
†Hypereosinophilia of uncertain significance/idiopathic hypereosinophilia has no tissue damage; otherwise, should follow the same diagnostic criteria.
‡The abnormal T-cell population needs to be detected immunophenotypically with or without T-cell receptor clonality by polymerase chain reaction.

Etiology

There are no known risk factors or a genetic predisposition to iHE/iHES.

Clinical Features

The average age at presentation is in the high 40s but shows a broad spectrum (range 13.5–90 years). The male-to-female ratio is approximately 1:1. In the study by Wang et al., when comparing hypereosinophilic conditions in morphologically abnormal bone marrow (presumably CEL, NOS) with the conditions in morphologically unremarkable bone marrow (presumably iHE/iHES), iHE/iHES showed fewer constitutional symptoms (approximately 20%), organomegaly (approximately 10%), elevated lactate dehydrogenase (approximately 25%), and thrombotic events (2%) and a greater proportion of allergies/hypersensitivity symptoms (approximately 30%), muscular/fasciitis (approximately 30%), gastrointestinal involvement (approximately 30%), and pulmonary symptoms (approximately 25%).[26] Compared with CEL, NOS, patients with iHE/iHES present with fewer cases of thrombocytopenia (10% vs. 33%), significantly lower AEC (3.9 vs. 11.2), similar degrees of anemia (13.1 vs. 12.2), and an overall normal average white blood cell count (11.5 vs. 29.7). Another study from a single institution demonstrated similar findings when clonal hypereosinophilic cases were excluded from the analysis.[107]

Morphology

Peripheral blood: The most striking peripheral blood feature in iHE/iHES is the hypereosinophilia (Fig. 50-13). Though some cases may exhibit eosinophilic cytologic abnormalities, the majority of these cases will show minimal alterations in eosinophils and are more noticeable in true CEL, NOS. Some cases may present with mild thrombocytopenia and/or anemia, but features suggestive of a myeloid disorder such as dysplasia, circulating blasts, monocytosis, and basophilia should not be observed.

Bone marrow: The bone marrow is normocellular or slightly hypercellular largely because of the eosinophilic infiltrate (Fig. 50-13). Aside from the eosinophils, the bone marrow should otherwise be morphologically unremarkable. Granulopoiesis, erythropoiesis, and megakaryopoiesis should be adequate without dysplastic features. Increased blasts are not observed. Eosinophil cytologic abnormalities tend to not be as prominent as they are described in CEL, NOS.

Immunophenotype

There are no specific immunophenotypic abnormalities. It should be noted that an exhaustive exclusion of all possible primary clonal eosinophilic conditions and secondary reactive conditions is needed. This may include a variety of immunohistochemical and flow cytometry studies, as discussed in the section on CEL, NOS. A T-cell workup to rule out a T-cell lymphoma or Th2 type T-cells associated with lymphocyte variant of HES is essential before assigning a case of HES as idiopathic. Detection of abnormal mast cells should prompt a diligent search of clonal eosinophilia, though a partial/weak expression of one of the markers, either CD25 or CD30, may be observed on reactive mast cells.[113]

Genetics/Molecular Findings

There are no recurring and/or specific genetic findings in iHE/iHES aside from a possible CHIP mutation. As discussed in CEL, NOS, the presence of a convincing chromosomal abnormality and/or mutations by NGS would support a diagnosis of CEL, NOS rather than iHE/iHES.

Clinical Course

In studies in which an overt hematopoietic neoplasm (such as CEL, NOS, hypereosinophilia associated with a myeloid neoplasm, and myeloid/lymphoid neoplasm with a TK gene fusion) is excluded, patients with iHES showed a more benign clinical course with a disease-related mortality rate around 10% to 15% in the long-term follow-up.[26,107,114,115] Mortality is related to an older age (>60 years), cardiac involvement, cytopenia (anemia or thrombocytopenia), a low absolute lymphocyte count, an increased neutrophil-to-lymphocyte ratio,[115] and hepatosplenomegaly.

For patients with iHES, corticosteroids are effective in producing a rapid reduction in eosinophil count or tissue/organ dysfunction in the majority of cases.[116,117] Resistance or intolerance to steroid treatment occurs in about 20% of patients. Long-term treatment with steroids to suppress eosinophilia and organ damage may carry significant side effects. For patients who cannot tolerate or fail corticosteroid treatment, other agents such as an IL-5 antagonist (mepolizumab)[118] have been shown to significantly reduce the occurrences of symptom flares.

Differential Diagnosis

iHE/iHES are diagnoses of exclusion and require a comprehensive morphologic, clinical, laboratory, and genetic testing approach to exclude reactive etiologies and differential diagnoses such as iHE/iHES, the lymphocytic variant of hypereosinophilic syndrome, T-cell/B-cell lymphoma, Hodgkin lymphoma, AML with inv(16) or CML, and M/LN-eo-TK.

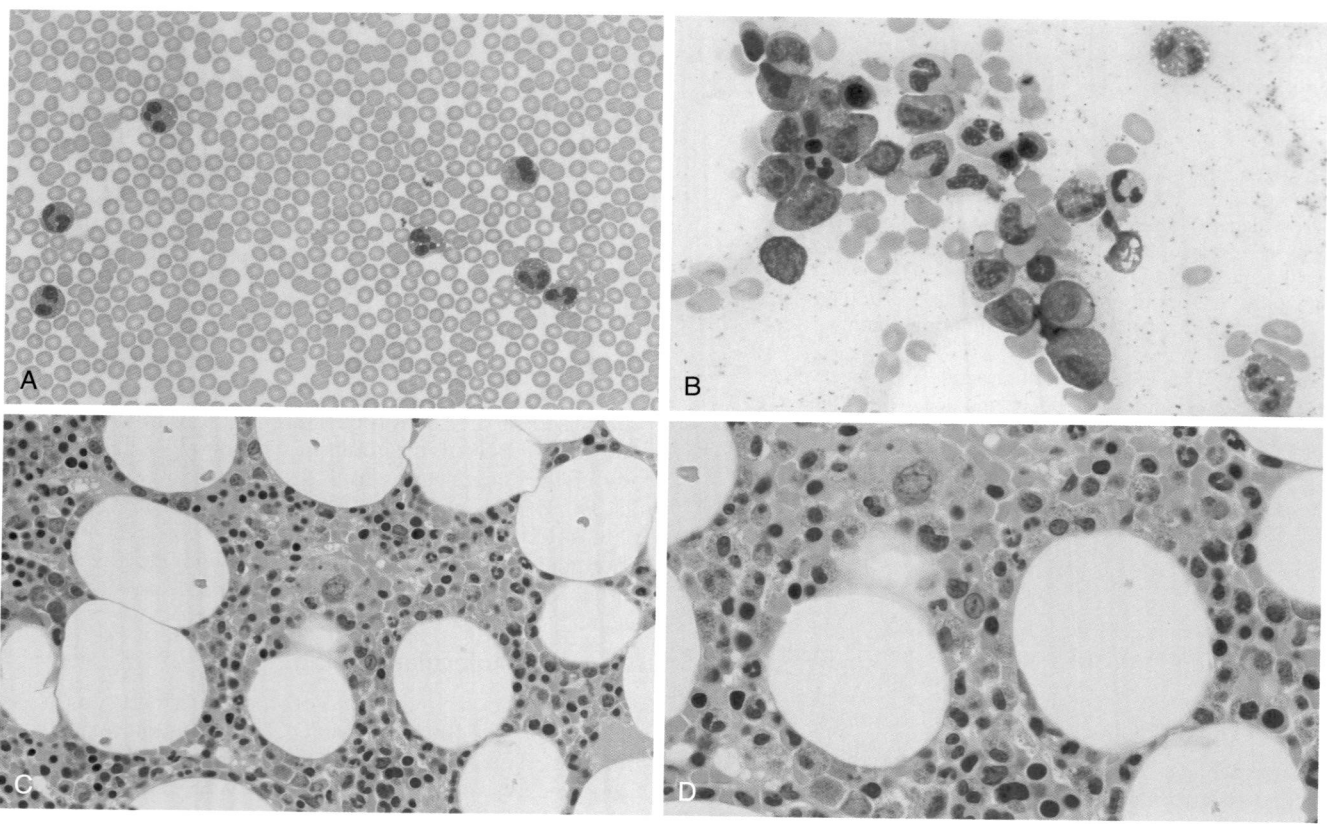

Figure 50-13. Idiopathic hypereosinophilia syndrome. A, The peripheral blood smear, by definition, will demonstrate hypereosinophilia with, most often, only occasional forms showing abnormal eosinophil cytology. As seen here, most of the eosinophils are normally granulated and segmented; occasional vacuolization is seen (1000× magnification, Wright-Giemsa). **B,** Bone marrow aspirate smears are spicular and cellular with predominantly normal-appearing eosinophils, which are increased in number. Dyserythropoiesis, dysgranulopoiesis, and dysmegakaryopoiesis are absent. Monocytes and blasts are not increased (1000× magnification, Wright-Giemsa). **C,** The bone marrow core biopsy is typically normocellular/slightly hypercellular, corresponding to the increase in eosinophils and precursors. The distribution of erythroid and granulocytic precursors is normal, and megakaryocytes exhibit normal morphology (600× magnification, H&E [hematoxylin and eosin]). **D,** The bone marrow core biopsy, on higher power magnification, demonstrates a predominantly interstitial increase in unremarkable-appearing eosinophils (1000× magnification, H&E [hematoxylin and eosin]).

CONCLUSION

The eosinophilic disorders are a complex group of entities of diverse and vastly heterogeneous etiologies. As such, an integrated approach that evaluates clinical, laboratory, morphologic, genetic, and immunophenotypic features may be required in the simultaneous pursuit and exclusion of a specific diagnosis. With the specific diagnosis/cause identified, the case can be managed appropriately. If a specific diagnosis is not identified, the case should be considered as iHE or iHES, depending on the absence or presence of end-organ damage, respectively.

In cases of M/LN-eo-TK (rearrangement of *PDGFRA, PDGFRB, FGFR1, JAK2,* or *FLT3* or with *ETV6::ABL1*), it is important to remember that the clinical presentations are heterogenous and often complex (combined acute and chronic components), extramedullary disease is frequent, eosinophilia is not uniformly present, and the genetic abnormality may be cytogenetically and/or FISH cryptic. As such, a heightened awareness to these distinct entities and their presentations is required of both clinicians and pathologists, and targeted genetic testing should be considered, as appropriate. In addition, if a particular case does not fit or exemplify the typical pathologic or genetic profile of a usual ICC-defined entity (e.g., CMML), these recurring genetic abnormalities should be considered.

CEL, NOS is a diagnosis of exclusion, and appropriate morphologic, clinical, laboratory, and genetic evaluation is necessary to exclude differential diagnostic considerations. In particular, the presence of abnormal bone marrow morphologic findings and/or convincing molecular genetic/cytogenetic mutations allows for a diagnosis more definitive than iHE/iHES.

Acknowledgments

The editors and author would like to gratefully acknowledge the excellent prior work and authorship on this chapter by Dr. Barbara Bain.

Pearls and Pitfalls

- Eosinophilia encompasses a complex group of disorders of diverse etiology for which there are many tools available for the workup and diagnosis.
- The classification of eosinophilic diseases should reference whether they are reactive or clonal and connote the specific etiology, when possible.
- Given the many causes of eosinophilia, presenting signs and symptoms may vary, including weight loss, fever, cytopenia(s)/cytosis, and cutaneous, pulmonary, cardiac, gastrointestinal and/or central nervous system involvement or newly emerging lymphadenopathy, hepatomegaly, or splenomegaly.
- Secondary eosinophilia is much more common than primary eosinophilia, and the diagnostic workup often involves consultation with multiple medical specialties, including allergy, hematology, pulmonary, infectious disease, rheumatology, and gastroenterology.
- In myeloid/lymphoid neoplasms with eosinophilia and rearrangements of *PDGFRA*, there is a marked male predominance with a male-to-female ratio of approximately 17:1. The median age at presentation is in the late 40s. The majority of these cases (approximately 90%) are chronic and myeloid in nature and carry the *FIP1L1::PDGFRA* fusion. Patients with *PDGFRA* fusion respond remarkably well to imatinib TKI therapy.
- Myeloid/lymphoid neoplasms with eosinophilia and rearrangements of *PDGFRB* show a slight male predominance with a male-to-female ratio of 2:1. The median age at presentation is in the 40s. Though CEL-like or CMML presentations tend to predominate, it is important to recognize that there may be other clinical presentations such as B-ALL and, less commonly, AML, T-ALL, or myeloid sarcoma. The majority of cases carry t(5;12)(q32;p13.2) with formation of an *ETV6::PDGFRB* fusion. *PDGFRB* with partner genes other than *ETV6* may be cryptic. Similar to cases of *PDGFRA*, cases with *PDGFRB* respond remarkably well to imatinib TKI therapy, with long-term hematologic and molecular responses.
- In myeloid/lymphoid neoplasms with eosinophilia and rearrangement of *FGFR1*, there is a slight male predominance with a male-to-female ratio of approximately 1.5:1. The median age at presentation is in the 30s to 40s. The disease is well-known for its heterogenous and complex presentations, including CEL, MDS/MPN, AML, T-ALL, or (less often) B-ALL or mixed-phenotype acute leukemia, with frequent eosinophilia and extramedullary disease. *FGFR1* rearrangements are not cytogenetically cryptic. *RUNX1* is highly mutated (>70%). The overall clinical outcome is aggressive. *FGFR1*-rearranged neoplasms do not respond to first-generation TKI therapy but have shown benefit from FGFR inhibitors or third-generation TKI.
- In myeloid/lymphoid neoplasms with eosinophilia and *PCM1::JAK2* and genetic variants, the median age at presentation is 50 years

with a wide age range, and there is a male predominance (>3:1 male-to-female ratio). Patients typically exhibit hepatosplenomegaly. These neoplasms show a heterogenous presentation ranging from MPN and MDS/MPN (approximately 60%) to AML and B-ALL; extramedullary disease involvement is common. The bone marrow in *PCM1::JAK2* shows a typical histopathologic "triad," which includes hypercellularity with an eosinophilic infiltrate, large aggregates of immature erythroid precursors (pronormoblasts), and myelofibrosis. *PCM1::JAK2* is often not cryptic. *ETV6::JAK2* and *BCR::JAK2* have been recognized as two genetic variants. These lesions show limited benefit from JAK2 inhibitor therapy.
- In myeloid/lymphoid neoplasms with eosinophilia and *FLT3*-rearrangement, the disease appears to be slightly more common in men, with a male-to-female ratio of approximately 1.4:1. There is a broad age of presentation, with the median age in the 50s. The pathologic presentation is heterogenous, including as a CMN (CEL-like, CMML-like, aCML, myelodysplastic syndrome), a higher-grade myeloid disorder with excess blasts, an acute leukemia (T-ALL, B-ALL, and myeloid sarcoma), or a mixed lineage neoplasm (mixed phenotype acute leukemia). The genetic alteration *ETV6::FLT3* is typically not cryptic in conventional chromosomal analysis, and involvement of the *FLT3* gene should be considered in cases of a hematopoietic neoplasm in which 13q12 is rearranged. However, alternate partner genes can be cryptic. These cases tend be associated with an aggressive clinical course or early disease progression. Cases, especially those in the chronic phase, often respond to FLT3 inhibitor therapy, though some of the responses may be short-lived.
- In myeloid neoplasms with eosinophilia and *ETV6::ABL1,* there appears to be a slight male predominance, with a male-to-female ratio of 2:1. The median age at presentation is in the 5th decade of life. Patients with *ETV6::ABL1* rearrangement typically present with a clonal myeloid proliferation and eosinophilia (sometimes basophilia), most often in chronic phase. There is a known response to TKI treatment.
- In cases without a clear-cut clonal genetic abnormality diagnostic of CEL, NOS (i.e., negative or possible CHIP), clinical and morphologic features may be helpful to distinguish CEL, NOS from iHE/iHES. The bone marrow in patients with CEL, NOS is dramatically hypercellular because of a proliferation of granulocytes and eosinophils. Megakaryocytes are almost invariably abnormal. In contrast, the bone marrow in patients with iHES is unremarkable except for increased eosinophils.
- A heightened awareness of these distinct entities and their occasional complex presentations is required of both clinicians and pathologists, and targeted genetic testing should be considered, as appropriate.

KEY REFERENCES

1. Arber DA, Orazi A, Hasserjian R, et al. The 2016 revision to the World Health Organization classification of myeloid neoplasms and acute leukemia. *Blood.* 2016;127:2391–2405.
2. Bain BJ, Horny H-P, Arber DA, et al. Myeloid/lymphoid neoplasms with eosinophilia and rearrangements of PDG-FRA, PDGFRB or FGFR1, or with PCM1-JAK2. In: Swerdlow SH, Campo E, Harris NL, et al., eds. *WHO Classification of Tumours of Haematopoietic and Lymphoid Tissues. Rev.* 4th ed. Lyon, France: International Agency for Research on Cancer (IARC); 2017:72–79.
3. Arber DA, Orazi A, Hasserjian RP, et al. International Consensus Classification of myeloid neoplasms and acute leukemias: integrating morphologic, clinical, and genomic data. *Blood.* 2022;140(11):1200–1228.
40. Ondrejka SL, Jegalian AG, Kim AS, et al. PDGFRB-rearranged T-lymphoblastic leukemia/lymphoma occurring with myeloid neoplasms: the missing link supporting a stem cell origin. *Haematologica.* 2014;99:e148–e151.

Visit Elsevier eBooks+ for the complete set of references.

Chapter 51

Blastic Plasmacytoid Dendritic Cell Neoplasm

Fabio Facchetti

DEFINITION

Blastic plasmacytoid dendritic cell neoplasm (BPDCN) is a rare aggressive hematologic malignancy characterized by the clonal proliferation of immature plasmacytoid dendritic cells (pDCs), also known as natural interferon type I–producing cells[1] or their precursors. Nomenclature widely varied over time, reflecting the uncertainty of its histogenesis, including *agranular CD4+ natural killer (NK) cell leukemia, blastic NK cell leukemia/ lymphoma, agranular CD4+, CD56+ hematodermic neoplasm,* and *tumor, blastic NK-cell lymphoma.*[2-6] On the evidence of its relationship to pDCs,[7-11] the term *blastic plasmacytoid dendritic cell neoplasm* was introduced in the 2008 World Health Organization (WHO) classification (4th edition),[12] where it was included within the acute myeloid leukemia (AML)–related precursor neoplasms; in the 2017 WHO 4th updated edition,[13] BPDCN was classified as an entity distinct from AML, as it remains in the 2022 ICC classification.[14] In contrast, the proposed WHO 5th ed. includes BPDCN in the *histiocytic/dendritic cell neoplasms* category.[15]

BPDCN typically occurs in elderly men, in good states of health, with skin lesions associated with involvement of other sites, mainly bone marrow, lymph nodes, and peripheral blood (Box 51-1). Morphologically, the tumor cells show immature features, and immunophenotyping is mandatory for diagnosis. Despite the improvement of knowledge on tumor cell biology and of treatment strategies, prognosis remains poor.

SYNONYMS AND RELATED TERMS

Revised WHO 4th ed.: Blastic Plasmacytoid Dendritic Cell Neoplasm

Proposed WHO 5th ed.: Blastic Plasmacytoid Dendritic Cell Neoplasm

EPIDEMIOLOGY

BPDCN is rare, accounting for <1% of all hematologic malignancies[8,16,17]; according to SEER-18 data, the incidence in the United States is 0.04 cases per 100,000 individuals,[18] with a significantly higher frequency in Caucasians,[18] in contrast to other reports where no ethnic prevalence was found.[8] The male-to-female ratio is about 3 to 4:1, and the median age at diagnosis is 67 years.[18-24] Women are generally 8 to 10 years younger than men and, interestingly, they do not show a significant age peak of occurrence, in contrast to males in which a marked increase from the 5th decade on is observed.[21] About 5% of BPDCN patients are younger than 10 years old[21]; in a survey of 219 cases, 26.9% of patients were less than 20 years old, determining a bimodal pattern of age distribution.[18]

ETIOLOGY

Epstein-Barr virus (EBV) and other lymphotropic viruses (human immunodeficiency virus, hepatitis C virus, human herpesvirus 6 and 8, cytomegalovirus, human T-lymphotropic virus 1 and 2) are negative.[8]

The occurrence of BPDCN as secondary leukemia in patients with other myeloid neoplasms, especially myelodysplastic syndrome (MDS) and chronic myelomonocytic leukemia (CMML) or even solid tumors,[25-29] supports the hypothesis that exposure to therapy may represent a pathogenic factor for BPDCN development, and that BPDCN represents a second event in a context of MDS.[26,30-33] Furthermore, clonal hematopoiesis is highly prevalent in BPDCN patients beyond an associated diagnosis of MDS/CMML,[34,35] suggesting that the earliest events in BPDCN pathogenesis occur in hematopoietic progenitor cells, which subsequently seed peripheral sites during full-blown malignant transformation.[35]

An early pathogenetic event may depend on *ETV6* anomalies, because a high rate of monoallelic and biallelic 12p13/*ETV6* deletions have been found in the bone marrows of BPDCN patients without detectable disease.[36] Ceribelli et al. identified that the E-box transcription factor TCF4 (also known as *E2-2*), a key regulator in the committed development of pDCs from common dendritic cell progenitors,[37] plays a master regulatory role in BPDCN cells and can be regulated by the bromodomain and extraterminal domain (BET) protein BRD4.[38] IKZF1 inactivation was found as a key event in the development of BPDCN.[39]

CLINICAL FEATURES

The clinical features and evolution of BPDCN are rather homogeneous[5,8,9,17,19,22,23,40-44] and consist of two main patterns, one (70%–90% of cases) dominated by skin lesions followed by tumor dissemination, the other (10%–30%) by skin lesions, acute leukemia, and systemic involvement from the beginning. The interval between the onset of lesions and diagnosis is variable, with a mean time of 6.2 months (range 2–18 months), a delay likely depending on the rarity of the disease and poor knowledge by both clinicians and pathologists.[22]

Skin lesions are usually asymptomatic and sometimes last for months.[22,45] Patients are in good general health without systemic symptoms, concealing the aggressive nature of the underlying disease; however, they usually show pancytopenia and leukemic cells in the blood. In about 30% to 50% of cases, skin lesions are the only detectable clinical manifestation.[5,17,22,23,40,41] In a series of 398 patients, the skin was involved at diagnosis in 89% of cases, as unique site (30%) or associated with disseminated disease (57%), while disseminated noncutaneous disease occurred in 13% of cases.[19]

Skin lesions can be single, but usually are multiple; they can involve any body site, appear as reddish to bluish nodules, plaques, or bruiselike areas, with size variability from a few millimeters to several centimeters (Fig. 51-1).[8,22,41,44,46] At presentation, bone marrow involvement occurs in 50% to 90% of cases and it is mostly extensive[47]; when minimal, it invariably increases with disease progression. Localized or disseminated lymphadenopathy occurs in about 40% to 50% of cases, and splenomegaly and hepatomegaly in 9% to 25% and 6% to 17 of cases, respectively.[5,8,19,22,23] Uncommon

affected sites include oral mucosa, lung, tonsils, soft tissue, and eyes.[22,48]

Circulating tumor cells are found in about 50% to 70% of the patients, generally with low counts at presentation.[23,25,42,45,49,50] The "leukemic" BPDCN variant is characterized by an elevated white blood cell count with blasts and massive bone marrow infiltration,[23,25,26,50-52] and it is generally associated with multiple skin lesions as well.[42] Cases showing a "pure" leukemic presentation are rare, occur in individuals with younger age (median, 52 years), and are frequently associated with splenomegaly and lymphadenopathy.[21]

At onset of disease, patients frequently show anemia, thrombocytopenia, and neutropenia,[23] which, in a minority of cases, are severe, indicating bone marrow failure[5,25]; marrow or blood monocytosis can reveal the co-existence of a myeloid neoplasm.[5,23] In about 15% to 20% of patients, BPDCN is associated with CMML, MDS, or AML, which may precede, concur, or follow BPDCN.[5,9,10,17,22,25-29,44,53-57]

The frequency of central nervous system (CNS) involvement is probably underestimated because of the lack of systematic application of cerebrospinal fluid testing in BPDCN patients.[58] At diagnosis, overt or occult CNS involvement has been reported in 8% to 60% of patients, even asymptomatic,[22,23,40,58,59] and frequently occurs at relapse.[25,26,58,59]

MORPHOLOGY

BPDCN tumor cells morphology varies from medium-sized pleomorphic blasts with irregular elongated, twisted nuclei, to small-to-medium-sized cells resembling lymphoblasts; chromatin is finely dispersed and the nucleoli, when present, are small, single, or multiple, except in the immunoblast-like variant associated with *MYC* gene rearrangement.[60] The cytoplasm is scant and difficult to visualize; on Giemsa stain it appears gray-blue and devoid of azurophilic granules. Mitotic activity is markedly variable, as is the Ki-67 expression (20%–80%) (Fig. 51-2A–C).[44,53,61,62]

In skin biopsies, the tumoral infiltrate predominantly involves the dermis, often extending to the subcutaneous fat; epidermis and adnexa are spared, with rare exceptions; angioinvasion and coagulative necrosis are generally absent (Fig. 51-3A).[44] Tumor-associated inflammatory cells are scant and mainly represented by T lymphocytes and scattered macrophages.

Lymph nodes are initially infiltrated in the interfollicular areas and the medulla, sparing B follicles (Fig. 51-3B). The bone marrow is usually involved with high tumor load (Fig. 51-3C); when sparse, it is only detectable by immunohistochemistry,[63,64] although the presence of reactive pDCs may cause false positivity and analysis of the marrow aspirate using flow-cytometry is preferable in these cases.[65]

On blood or marrow smears, tumor cell morphology is quite heterogeneous.[23] Typical blasts are medium sized with round or irregular, often eccentric, nucleus; small nucleoli; and a faintly and irregularly basophilic cytoplasm with variability of coloration. Small vacuoles are frequently found arranged under the cytoplasmic membrane, and cytoplasmic pseudopodia occur in a fraction of cells (Fig. 51-2D). Blasts with a dominant lymphoid-like features or with immature features including high nuclear-to-cytoplasmic ratio, fine

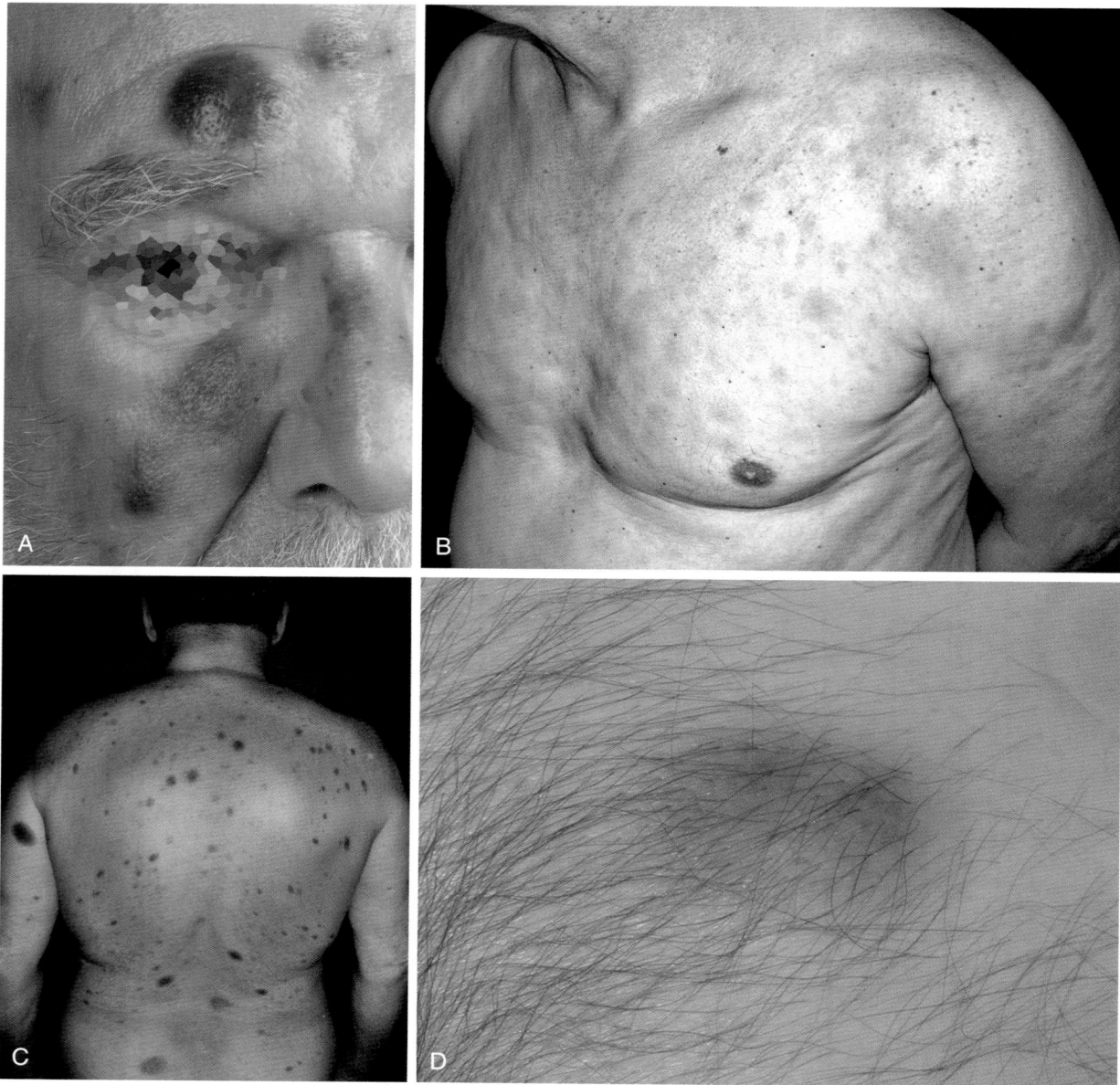

Figure 51-1. A–D, Examples of skin lesions in blastic plasmacytoid dendritic cell neoplasm. Lesions may consist of nodules, plaques, or bruiselike areas, with variable colors. *(Courtesy of Prof. Lorenzo Cerroni, Graz, Austria; Dr. Stefano Corsico, Brescia, Italy; and Prof. Piergia-como Calzavara, Brescia, Italy.)*

chromatin, and large nucleolus can also occur; in addition, a portion or, more rarely, the entire blast population, displays monoblastic-like features. Despite most cells not showing granules or crystals,[23,25] rare cells with azurophilic fine or large granulations have been detected in a minority of blasts.[23]

In about one-third of cases, residual hematopoietic cells show dysplasia in ≥1 lineages, especially in the myeloid cells and megakaryocytes, and numbers of monocytes can be increased.[17,23,66]

IMMUNOPHENOTYPE

The diagnosis of BPDCN is usually made on a skin biopsy or, less frequently, on marrow aspirate and peripheral blood;

it is essentially based on immunohistochemistry and flow cytometry analysis.

In the suspicion of BPDCN, the diagnostic approach should comprise diagnosis-supportive and diagnosis-excluding markers, the former including CD4, CD56, and other pDCs' specific antigens CD123, TCL1, CD303, and TCF4, the latter encompassing CD3, CD19, CD20, CD11c, CD14, CD163, lysozyme, and myeloperoxidase (Table 51-1) (Fig. 51-4A–F).[4,8,10,19,21,23,25,29,38,43,44,57,60-62,67-72]

CD123, recognizing the interleukin-3 receptor alpha chain, is positive in the majority of BPDCN,[4,19,44,62,73] in association with CD4 and CD56 in 87% to 96% of cases.[19,21] High levels of TCL1 are found in 80% to 85% of cases, mostly in association with CD4, CD56, and CD123.[19,44,46,47,54,62,72,74-76]

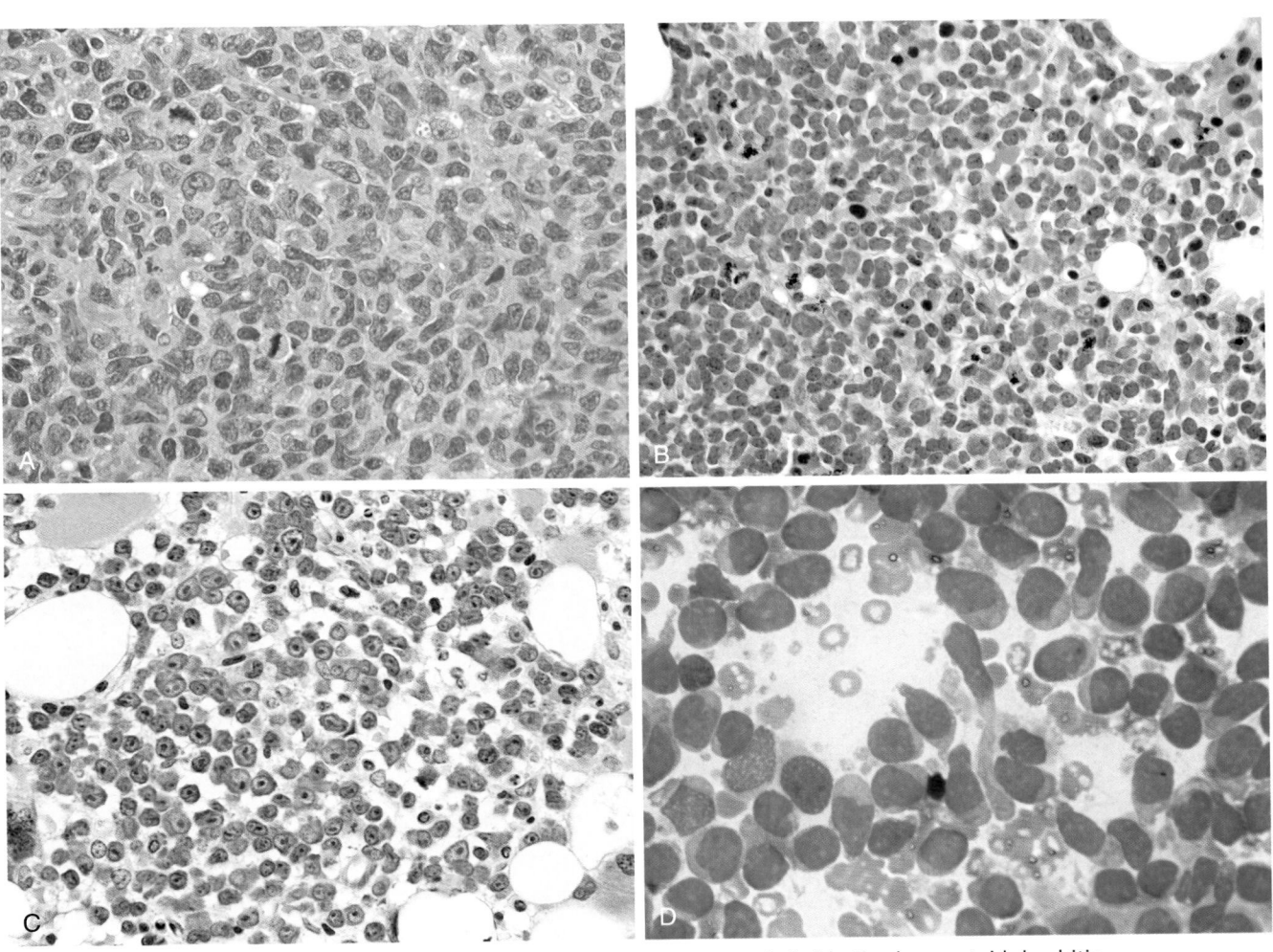

Figure 51-2. The cytomorphology of the immature tumor cells in blastic plasmacytoid dendritic cell neoplasm varies from medium-sized pleomorphic blasts with irregular elongated twisted nuclei **(A)** to lymphoblast-like cells **(B)** to immunoblast-like cells **(C)** (hematoxylin-eosin). In bone marrow aspirate **(D)**, tumor cells show a blastic appearance and pseudopodia-like extensions of the cytoplasm, which may be irregularly basophilic and contain small peripheral vacuoles.

CD303 recognizes the BDCA-2 antigen and represents a high specific marker for BPDCN,[55,70,71] but its sensitivity varies according to series from more than 70% of cases[8,10,19,21,61,70,71] to significantly lower values.[49,57,62,69,72] It cannot be excluded that this variability may depend on the reagent applied, the substrate used (fresh-frozen versus formalin-fixed tissue) or the degree of differentiation or activation of tumor cells.[65]

TCF4 (also known as E2-2) has been shown to have high specificity and sensitivity for BPDCN,[38,46,77] alone or in combination with CD123 (Fig. 51-4E).[72]

Additional markers expressed in normal/reactive pDCs have been found to be useful to support the diagnosis of BPDCN, such as MX1,[10,62,75,77] CD2AP,[73] BCL11a,[78] SPIB,[79] and E-cadherin.[77] In contrast, CD68 and granzyme-B, two molecules usually strongly expressed by pDCs,[80,81] are respectively positive in about half of BPDCN cases with a cytoplasmic dot pattern (Fig. 51-4H),[4,17,19,44,62,67] or completely negative.[4,19,67]

Terminal deoxynucleotidyl transferase (TdT) is expressed in about one-third of cases in 10% to 80% of tumor cells.[3,4,43,67,73] CD117 can be positive, while CD34 has consistently been reported negative (Fig. 51-4F–G).[10,17,50,67]

In addition to CD56, BPDCN can express markers generally lacking in normal pDCs, such as BCL2 (Fig. 51-4I), BCL6, and S100 protein[9,19,55,70]; positivity for myeloid or lymphoid markers, including CD2, CD5, CD7, CD22, CD33, and cCD 79a[19,60,62,82] can make the diagnosis of BPDCN sometimes complex.[66]

A confident BPDCN diagnosis can be made when tumor cells are positive for at least four among CD4, CD56, CD123, CD303, and TCL1,[62] or when positivity for CD4 and CD56 is associated with ≥1 among CD123, TCL1, and BDCA2/ CD303 and negativity of lineage-specific markers for myeloid cells (myeloperoxidase), T cells (CD3), B cells (CD20), and monocytes (CD11c, CD163, lysozyme).[19] According to the proposed WHO 5th ed., immunophenotypic diagnostic criteria include the expression of CD123 and one among the pDC markers TCF4, TCL1, CD303, and CD304, or positivity of any three pDC markers and negativity for all expected negative ones (CD3, CD14, CD19, CD34, lysozyme, and myeloperoxidase).[15]

On flow cytometry, tumor cells occur in the low-side scatter blast-gate with dim expression of CD45.[49,50,83] Comparing 20 cases of BPDCN and 113 lymphoid and myeloid acute

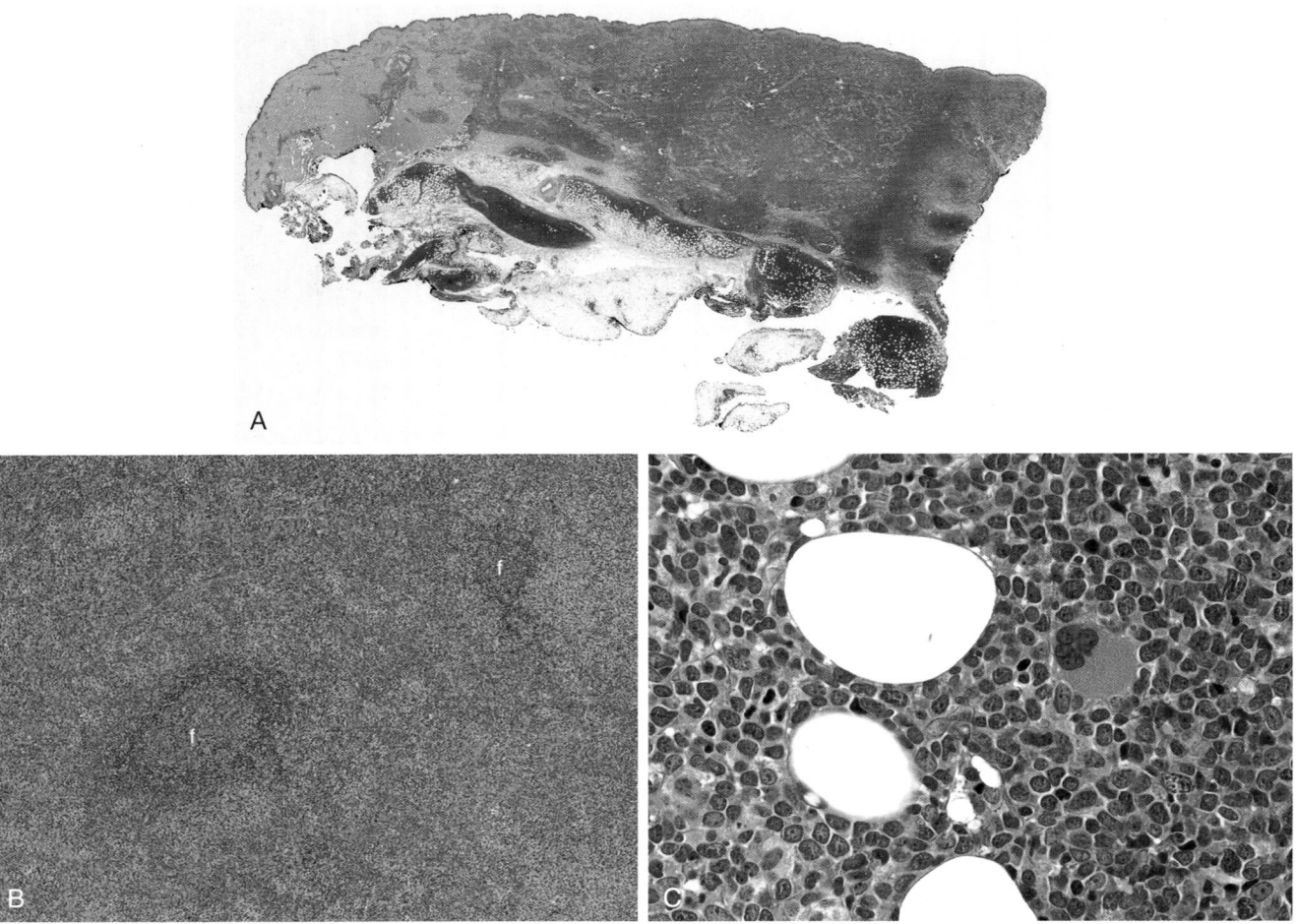

Figure 51-3. Blastic plasmacytoid dendritic cell neoplasm (BPDCN) involving the skin **(A)**, lymph node **(B)**, and bone marrow **(C)**. In the skin **(A)**, the infiltrate spares the papillary dermis and diffusely involves the dermis, extending to the subcutaneous fat. In the lymph node **(B)**, BPDCN obliterates the interfollicular and paracortical areas, sparing follicles *(f)*. Bone marrow **(C)** is usually extensively replaced by tumor cells.

Table 51-1 Comparison of Immunohistochemical Markers Expressed in Paraffin Sections by Normal Plasmacytoid Dendritic Cells and Blastic Plasmacytoid Dendritic Cell Neoplasm Tumor Cells

Expression	Markers
Positive in normal pDCs and in BPDCN	CD4, CD43, CD45RA, CD68,* CD123, CD303, CD2AP, SPIB, TCF4, TCL1, BCL11a, MxA
Negative in normal pDCs and positive in BPDCN	BCL2, CD2, CD7, CD33, CD38, CD56, CD79a, CD117, TdT[S100†]
Negative in normal pDCs and in BPDCN	CD1a, CD3, CD8, CD11c, CD13, CD14, CD16, CD19, CD20, CD21, CD23, CD25, CD30, CD34, CD45R0, CD57, CD138, immunoglobulin (surface and cytoplasmic), Langerin/CD207, lysozyme, myeloperoxidase, MNDA, PAX5, perforin, TCR-AB and TCR-GD, TIA-1

*In normal PDCs, CD68 expression is constantly diffuse in the cytoplasm, while in BPDCN, expression may be negative or positive with dot-lite expression.
†The expression of all these markers except CD56 is variable in BPDCN.
BPDCN, Blastic plasmacytoid dendritic cell neoplasm; *MNDA,* myeloid nuclear differentiation antigen; *pDC,* plasmacytoid dendritic cell; *TCR,* T-cell receptor; *TdT,* terminal deoxynucleotidyl transferase.

leukemias, it has been defined a BPDCN diagnostic score with a minimum value of 3 obtained from four parameters including CD4 positivity (not necessarily CD56) plus negativity of myeloperoxidase, cCD3, cCD79a, and CD11c (score = 1), CD123 positivity (score = 1), CD303 positivity (score = 2), and CD304 positivity (score = 1).[49]

Similarly to immunohistochemistry, cytofluorimetry has highlighted the frequent and even combined expression of markers from myeloid, B-lymphoid, and T-lymphoid lineages, excluding myeloperoxidase, CD14, cCD3, CD19, and cCD22.[23,65] Accordingly, a more detailed BPDCN diagnostic flow chart includes as admission criterion the negativity for specific lineage markers (CD3, CD19, cCD22, myeloperoxidase, CD14, CD11c, and CD64), regardless of expression of isolated or associated less-specific lineage markers (e.g., CD7, CD2, CD33, CD13, CD117, CD22, and cCD79a), followed as supportive criterion by the high expression of CD123 and HLA-DR, plus CD4 and CD56

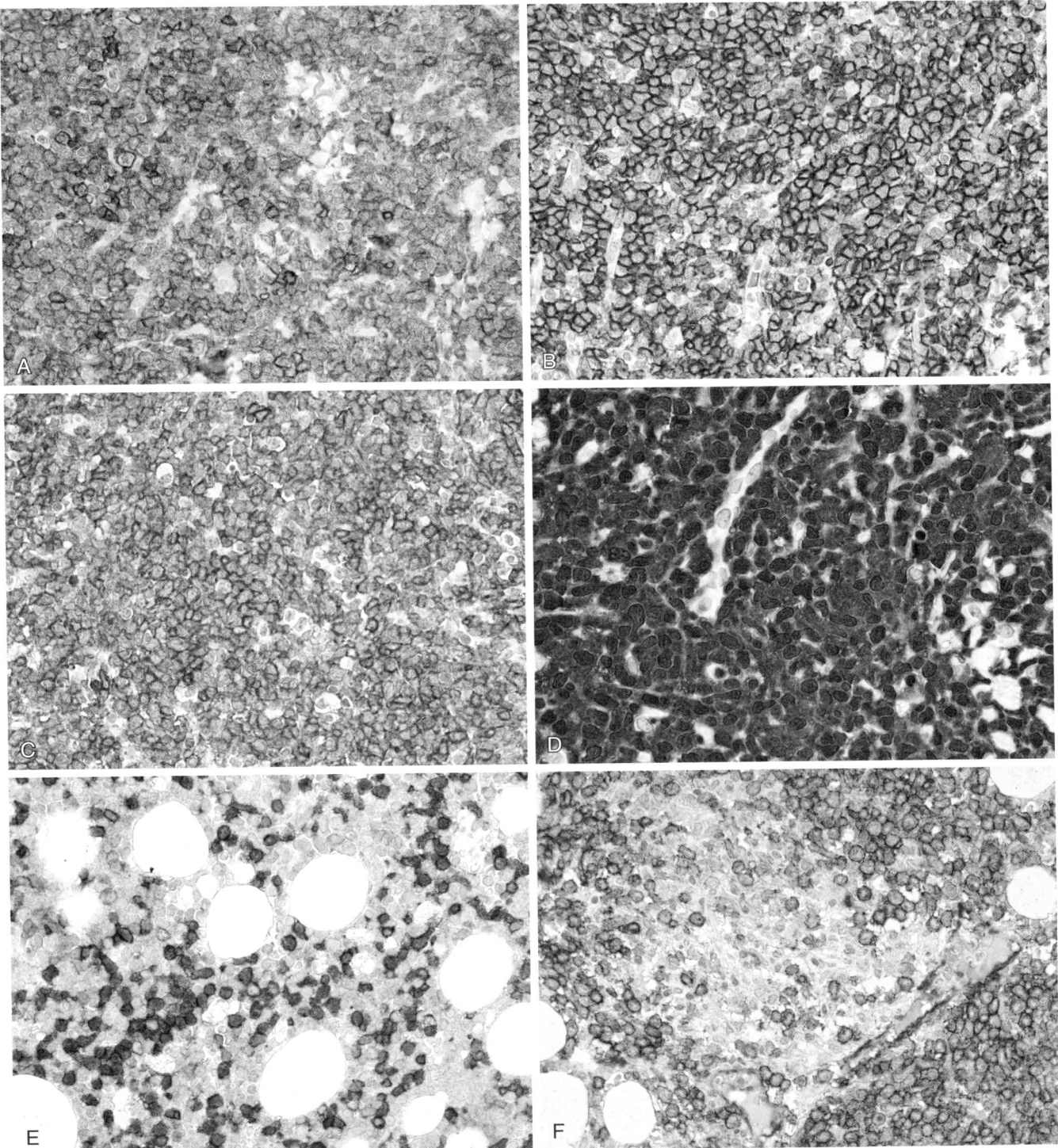

Figure 51-4. Immunohistochemical features of blastic plasmacytoid dendritic cell neoplasm. Positive tumor markers are represented by CD4 **(A)**, CD56 **(B)**, CD123 **(C)**, and TCL1 **(D)**, respectively. Tumor cells in bone marrow biopsies show co-expression of CD123 (cell membrane, *brown*) and TCF4 (nucleus, *blue*) **(E)**; they are CD303-positive (cell membrane, *brown*) and negative for CD34 *(blue)* **(F)**.

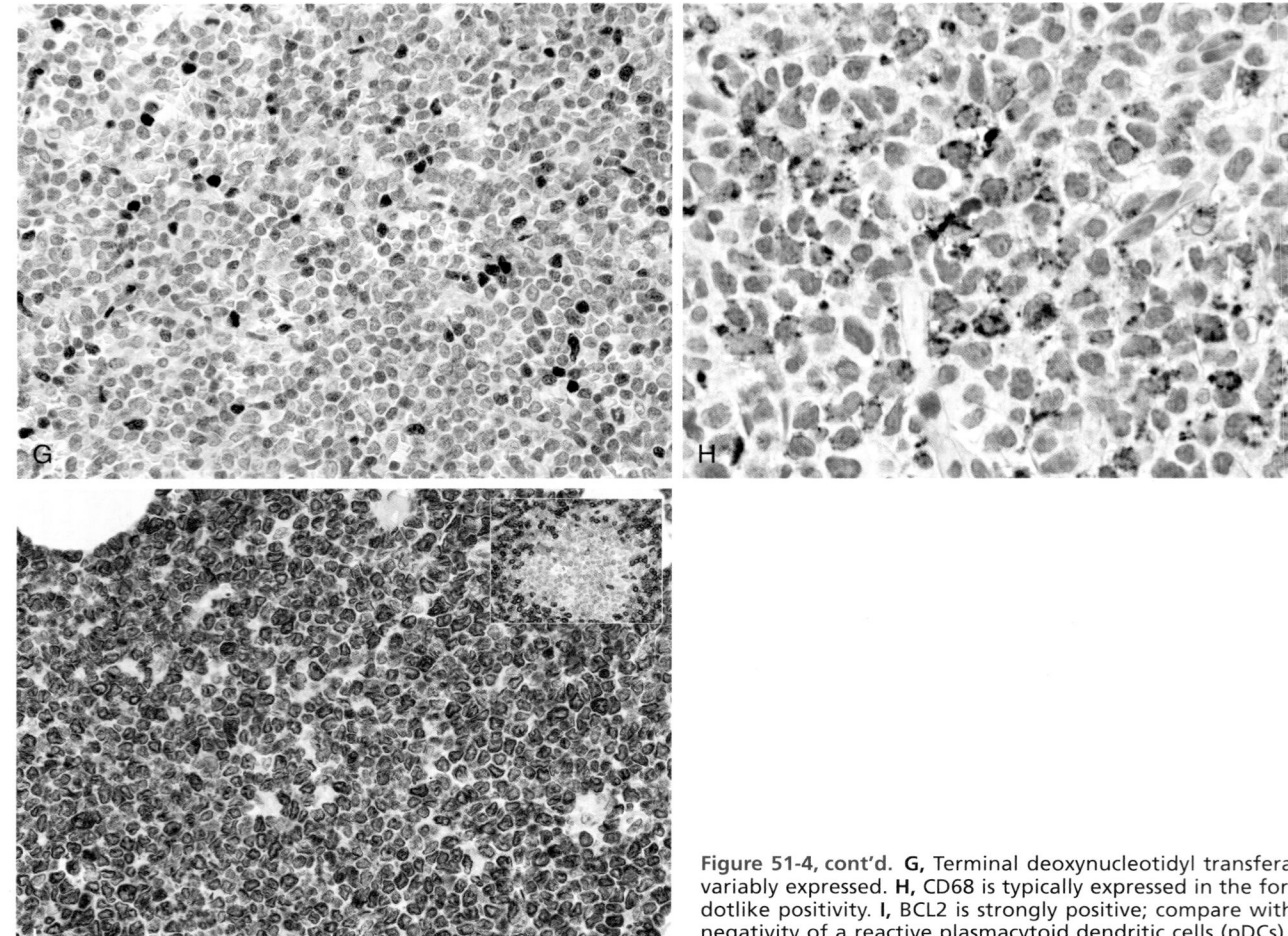

Figure 51-4, cont'd. **G,** Terminal deoxynucleotidyl transferase is variably expressed. **H,** CD68 is typically expressed in the form of dotlike positivity. **I,** BCL2 is strongly positive; compare with the negativity of a reactive plasmacytoid dendritic cells (pDCs) cluster *(inset).*

(which can be negative), and for final confirmation by the positivity for cTCL1, CD303, and CD304.[23] To note, the level of CD4, CD56, and CD303 is frequently lower compared with normal T cells, NK cells, and reactive pDCs.[23,65] Because reactive pDCs may co-exist with BPDCN in the bone marrow, including a small subset positive for CD56, CD2, and CD38,[65] a 10-color flow cytometric panel has been applied to distinguish reactive from neoplastic pDCs and to identify with a sensitivity up to 0.01% BPDCN minimal residual disease in patients under treatment.[65]

CYTOCHEMISTRY

BPDCN tumor cells are nonreactive for alpha-naphthyl butyrate esterase, naphthol AS-D chloroacetate esterase, and peroxidase cytochemical reactions.[9,23,25,53]

GENETICS AND MOLECULAR FINDINGS

T-cell and B-cell receptor gene are usually germline[9,17,43]; the rearrangement of the T-cell receptor gamma observed in few cases[5,17,23,29,84,85] may depend on clonal bystander T cells or T-cell clonotype expansion.[86]

Recurrent and usually multiple (≥3) chromosomal alterations occur in the large majority of cases, especially represented by genomic losses of 5q21 or 5q34 (72%), 12p13 (64%), 13q13-21 (64%), 6q23-qter (50%), 15q (43%), and of the entire chromosome 9 (28%), resulting in the defeat of cell cycle–related and tumor suppressor genes such as *CDKN1B, CDKN2A, CDKN2B, RB1, TP53, LATS2,* and *IKZF1.*[9,29,40,67,87-93] Although none of these recurrent alterations are BPDCN-specific, being detected also in other mostly myeloid malignancies, their co-existence, leading to a combination of deletions of several tumor suppressor genes, represents a peculiar genomic feature of BPDCN.

FISH analysis showed frequent rearrangements of the *ETS* variant gene 6 (*ETV6*),[36] similarly to other myeloid malignancies. *MYC* translocations have been detected in 12% to 38% of cases,[94,95] and are associated with high MYC protein expression, immunoblast-like morphology,[60] and a more aggressive behavior.[60,96] The most prevalent *MYC* rearrangement is t(6;8)(p21;q24),[60,94,96] resulting in a chimeric transcript involving *SUPT3H* (6p21) and *PVT1* 50 kb downstream of *MYC.*[97] Notably, the genomic sequence of *SUPT3H* overlaps with *RUNX2,* a super-enhancer gene highly expressed in BPDCN.[38] Rearrangements of the oncogenic transcription factor *MYB* have been found especially in pediatric or young patients,[60,94,98] with fusions involving different partner genes resulting in the activation of *MYB* target genes. Notably, *MYB* and *MYC* rearrangements do not co-exist in the same tumor, suggesting mutual exclusion of their functions in BPDCN.[60]

On gene expression analysis, BPDCN has a signature distinct from that of acute myeloid and lymphoid leukemias,[82,88,93] with significant enrichment of pDCs-related genes.[82,88,93] A minority of cases, however, have a B-lymphoid origin signature, or signatures of the pDC-like dendritic cells AS-DCs.[99] Compared with normal pDCs, BPDCN downregulates genes encoding type I interferons (IFN), and genes regulating the immune system, signal transduction, and ubiquitination, the most relevant being represented by GZMB, CLEC4C, NPC1, BCL11A, NPC2, IL10RA, CXCR3, UBE2W, and UBE3C[93]; in contrast, top upregulated genes in BPDCN include cell proliferation and division, such as IGLL1, GLUL, CLEC11A, UBE2T, BCL6, TLR2, UBE2C, BCL2, LRMP, UBE2S, and the transcription factor SOX4, the latter involved in pDCs ontogeny and differentiation, and, as upregulator of TCF4[38] appearing crucial for BPDCN oncogenesis.[93] Moreover BPDCN shows overexpression of genes involved in Notch signaling[88] and encoding for cyclin D1 and BCL2, and NF-κB activation.[82,93,100] Cholesterol homeostasis–related genes are downregulated in BPDCN, resulting in cholesterol accumulation within tumor cells, which can be normalized by treatment with LXR agonists, ensuing NF-κB inhibition and tumor cell apoptosis.[101] Haploinsufficiency of the gene encoding the glucocorticoid receptor NR3C1 was found in a subset (13/47, 28%) of cases with a balanced t(3;5)(q21;q31) translocation, resulting in the fusion of NR3C1 with a long noncoding RNA gene (lincRNA-3q) involved in the regulation of leukemia stem cell programs and G1/S transition via E2F. The consequent overexpression of lincRNA-3q consistently present in malignant cells can be abrogated by BET protein inhibition and may explain the high aggressiveness of this subset of tumors.[102] Similarly, tumor aggressiveness may be explained by neural features found in BPDCN, with overexpression of multiple neural receptors that stimulate tumor proliferation and migration.[93,103]

The majority of BPDCN are characterized by multiple but not specific mutations. They most frequently involve TET2 (36%–80%) and ASXL1, often co-existing in the same tumor. Similarly to the cytogenetic landscape, the BPDCN mutational profile is close to that found in myeloid neoplasms, mostly influencing the epigenetic program (TET2, ASXL1, EZH2, ATRX, IDH1, IDH2, DNMT3A, IKAROS family, SUZ12, ARID1A, PHF2, CHD8), the RAS pathway (NRAS, KRAS), splicing (SF3B1, SRSF2, ZRSR2), and tumor suppression control (TP53, RB1, ATM).[29,34,40,91-93,104-107] Loss-of-function mutations of ZRSR2 on X chromosome (Xp22.2) are enriched in BPDCN and nearly all occur in males, which might explain the striking male predominance of BPDCN.[108] Clonal evolution of BPDCN is characterized by additional mutations occurring during disease progression or in different sites.[35,40,109,110] Notably, mutations that are frequently found in AML, like FLT3-ITD and NPM1, have been rarely observed in BPDCN.[19,34,40,92,106,111]

POSTULATED CELL OF ORIGIN AND NORMAL COUNTERPART

On the basis of shared immunophenotypic (Fig. 51-5A–D) and molecular features pDCs precursors have been considered to represent the cell of origin of BPDCN.[4,5,7,8,10,11,23,38,54,61,69,74,82,88,93,112,113] Box 51-2 lists the main morphologic and phenotypical features of pDCs and their involvement in human diseases.

The definition of the nature and functions of pDCs has been a long and controversial process, testified by the heterogeneous terms proposed over time, such as lymphoblast, T-associated plasma cell, plasmacytoid T cell, plasmacytoid monocyte, natural interferon type I–producing cells, and plasmacytoid dendritic cell, the last two likely representing the essential properties of pDCs, the rapid and massive production of type I interferons (IFN-I) in response to viruses, and the ability to differentiate into classical dendritic cells (cDCs).[1,114-116]

A novel subset of dendritic cells has been identified in mice and humans, showing expression of AXL and SIGLEC6 and defined AS-DCs.[99] AS-DCs share with pDCs CD123[high], HLA-DR[high], and CD303 (hence the alternative term pDC-like DCs),[117] and similarly to pDCs, they are absent from normal skin.[118,119] The AS-DCs differ from canonical pDCs by the expression of classical DC markers (e.g., CD2, CD33, CD5, CD86) and some B-cell features (IGLL11, SIGLEC11, CD221, LYZ1).[99,117,119-121] Moreover, they show pDC- and cDC-like enriched signatures, are characterized by low IFN secretion but high ability to stimulate T-cell proliferation, thus having a transition state from pDCs to cDCs. It has been suggested that the T-cell stimulatory capacity of pDCs isolated with standard markers (e.g., CD123 and CD303) may depend on the AS-DCs fraction, thus indicating that pure pDCs correspond more closely to the natural type I interferon-producing cells.[99]

In a recent series of 13 BPDCN cases, about half showed a canonical pDC-like signature, while the remaining revealed expression of SIGLEC6, supporting an AS-DCs origin, as also supposed for the CAL-1 BPDCN cell line.[93] Therefore, BPDCN might have a heterogeneous ontogeny, with derivation either from canonical pDCs or from AS-DCs. Nevertheless, the lack of IFN-I production or defective IFN-I signature reported in BPDCN[82,93,122,123] can be unrelated to the cell of origin, but to oncogenic events, such as IFN-I gene loss,[93] functional status, or inhibitory mechanisms.[77,124]

pDC development can derive from a common myeloid progenitor through a common dendritic cell precursor or from either myeloid or lymphoid progenitors.[117,125-129] The myeloid-like mutational landscape observed in the majority of BPDCN and its association with myeloid neoplasms with shared mutations suggest that a significant percentage of BPDCN originate from a myeloid precursor. Yet a lymphoid-like origin of BPDCN is supported by overexpression of lymphoid-related genes and occurrence of lymphoid-type mutations,[92,93] as well as IKZF1 abnormalities[39] normally absent in myeloid neoplasms. Thence, an evolutionary theory of BPDCN has been proposed, in which in the preleukemic phase pDCs or AS-DC precursors display low-variant allele frequency (VAF) myeloid-type mutations related to clonal hematopoiesis, followed during disease progression by the occurrence of additional oncogenic events, including lymphoid abnormalities and pan-cancer mutations.[93]

CLINICAL COURSE AND PROGNOSIS

Despite the deceptively indolent clinical presentation with initial response to a variety of intensive chemotherapy regimens, the course is almost invariably aggressive, with

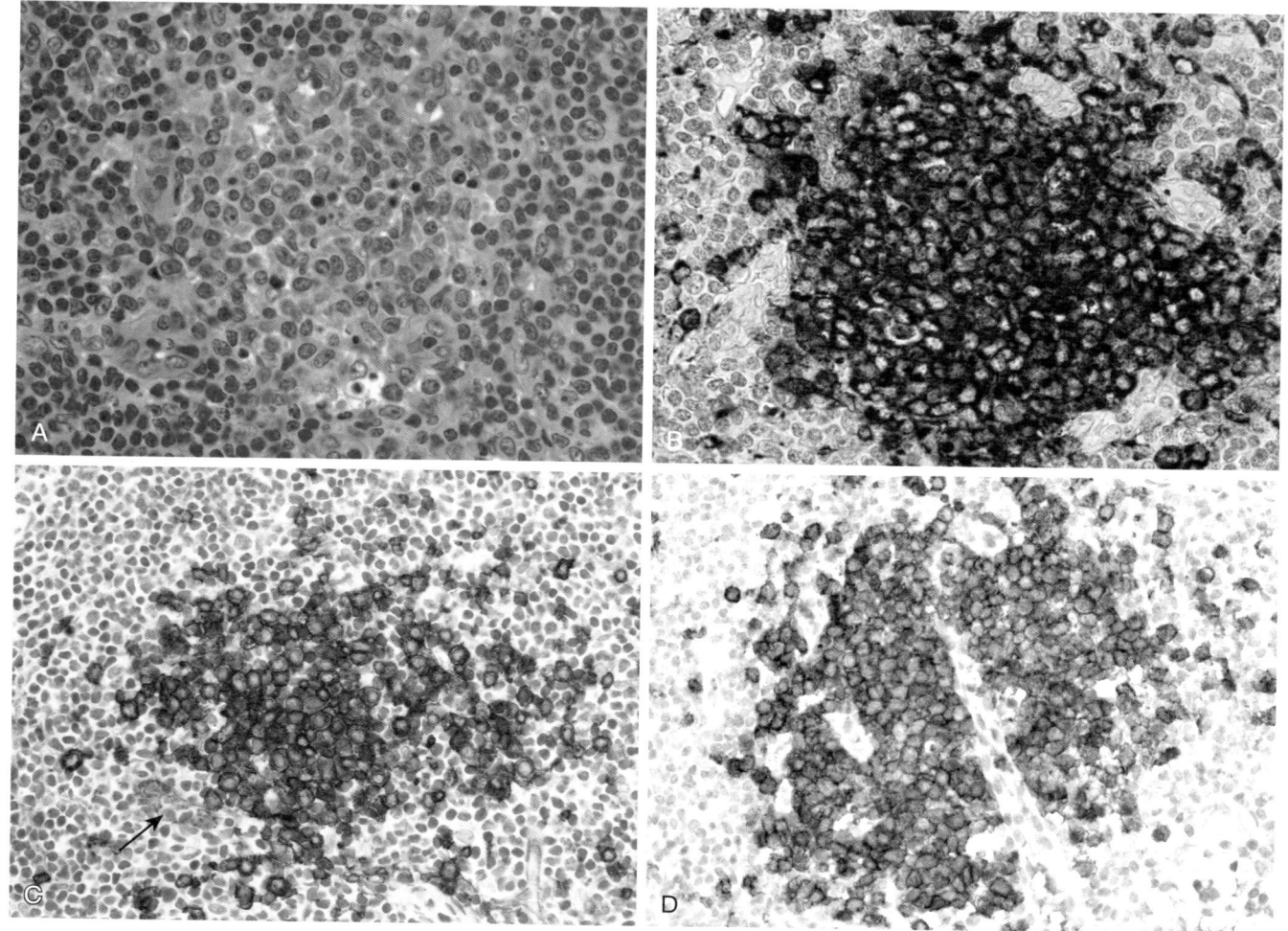

Figure 51-5. Plasmacytoid dendritic cell cluster in a reactive lymph node. The cytomorphology **(A)** and markers typically expressed on plasmacytoid dendritic cells (pDCs) are illustrated: CD68 **(B)**, CD123, which also stains high endothelial venules *(arrow)* **(C)**, and CD303 and TCF4 (CD303 on the cell membrane, *brown*; TCF4 in the nucleus, *blue*) **(D)**.

a median survival of 10 to 24 months, not significantly improved during years.[5,8,17-19,22-26,34,44,45,51]

Negative prognostic factors include older age,[18,19,23,34,40,70,130] disseminated disease at diagnosis,[19,23] and high blast counts in the bone marrow or peripheral blood.[23,34,42] Better outcome occurs in patients who respond to the first line of treatment and receive hematopoietic stem cell transplantation.[19,23,26,34,40,41,131,132]

Among biological parameters, high TdT expression and Ki67 index[19,42,69] have been associated with better survival, whereas positivity for CD303 had contrasting results.[62,69] The presence and the amount of cytogenetic aberrations do not correlate with prognosis,[19,40,92] while a significantly reduced overall survival is related to a high mutation load,[40] to mutations of genes encoding for epigenetic factors or belonging to the *IKAROS* family and DNA methylation pathway,[40,105] loss of the glucocorticoid receptor gene *NR3C1*,[102] *CDKN2A/CDKN2B* deletions,[90] and *MYC* rearrangement.[60]

At present, there is no consensus on the optimal treatment of BPDCN, but all patients should receive systemic therapy, regardless of the extension of the disease at presentation.[133] Intensive induction leukemia-like regimens achieving complete remission followed by hematopoietic,

especially allogenic, stem cell transplantation (allo-HSCT) offers a chance of longer survival.[19,23,25,26,40,131,132,134,135] Unfortunately, only a minority of BPDCN patients are eligible for allo-HSCT and alternative low intensity treatments have been considered, such as single-agent pralatrexate, bendamustine, and gemcitabine/docetaxel combinations, with promising results, though applied in sporadic cases.[136,137]

Differently from adults, in children the current recommendation suggests ALL-type chemotherapy followed by observation, reserving allo-HSCT for relapse and second complete remission.[70,130,138]

In adults and pediatric patients, it has shown frequent CNS involvement and a high rate of CNS relapse of BPDCN, suggesting prophylactic intrathecal chemotherapy.[130,139]

The understanding of the pathophysiology of BPDCN is significantly improved during the last years and prompted to identify and apply novel target-specific agents based on relatively constant biological features of the disease, such as the strong expression of CD123, the extensive epigenetic dysregulation, and the aberrant activation of NF-κB pathway leading to BCL-2 overexpression. For other BPDCN-associated molecular mechanisms (e.g., the highly dependence on TCF4- and BRD4-transcriptional network and the deregulation

data indicate that a single targeted therapy agent is not sufficient to achieve long-term remission, and combination with conventional therapy is necessary.[20] Several clinical trials are ongoing,[139] and they remain the main option for patients not eligible for allo-HSCT or not achieving first-line or second-line complete remission.[133,139]

DIFFERENTIAL DIAGNOSIS

In most of the cases, the differential diagnosis includes immature ("blastoid") hematologic neoplasms, such as ALL, AML, and myeloid sarcoma (MS) (Box 51-3). Notably, all of them can express markers typically used for BPDCN diagnosis. CD4 and CD56 positivity can be found in AML and MS, especially with monocytic differentiation[43,57,74,88]; CD123 is expressed, albeit weakly, in acute B-ALL and T-ALL, and more frequently in AML, even in association with CD4 and CD56.[62,148] TCL1 is expressed in about 20% of AML[43,54,74,149] in addition to mature lymphoid malignancies[150] and T-cell prolymphocytic leukemia.[151]

Thus, as discussed in the immunophenotype section, a panel of markers is required for the definite distinction of BPDCN from mimickers.[21,57,75,76,152] Notably, CD34 is almost never expressed in BPDCN, and E-cadherin has been proven very useful to distinguish BPDCN from leukemia cutis.[77]

BPDCN differential also includes other pDC neoplastic proliferations regularly associated with clonally related myeloid neoplasms, represented by *mature pDC proliferation* (MPDCP)[153-156] and *AML with pDC expansion*.[157-159] In the proposed WHO 5th ed., MPDCP has been recognized as a distinct entity among the pDC neoplasms included in the *histiocytic/dendritic cell neoplasms* category.[15] MPDCP predominantly occurs in elderly males, mostly affected by CMML or, more rarely, by MDS or AML with monocytic differentiation.[57,155,156,160] MPDCP can be accidentally identified on a bone marrow biopsy control, or in patients

cholesterol metabolism, especially inactivation of LXRs target genes), the effectiveness of pharmacologic interventions still refers to preclinical models.

The anti-CD123 immunotoxin tagraxofusp (SL-401) has been specifically approved for the treatment of adult and pediatric BPDCN.[140,141] In addition, various CD123 antibody-based drugs have been developed,[137] such as the humanized anti-CD123 drug-conjugated antibody IMGN632, which has shown to be useful in patients relapsed on prior therapy or after tagraxofusp[139]; the anti-CD123/CD3 bispecific monoclonal antibody XmAb14045, currently being studied in a phase I trial (NCT02730312); and the CD123-specific CAR-T, which has given encouraging results in preclinical and clinical studies.[142] BPDCN treatment using the anti-NF-κB proteasome inhibitor bortezomib, especially in association with other drugs, resulted in discrete but mostly transient responses.[143-145] Similar results have been obtained by using the BCL-2 inhibitor venetoclax,[100] while complete remission even in relapsed/refractory was achieved in BPDCN patients treated with venetoclax and hyper-CVAD regimen[146] or in combinations with hypomethylating agents.[147] The efficacy of hypomethylating agents (e.g., 5-azacitidine) shown in treating BPDCN patients, especially in association with anti-CD123 or anti-BCL2 agents, recently led to a clinical trial with triplet drug combination (NCT03113643).

The treatment of BPDCN remains difficult in obtaining effective and lasting results. Altogether, except for tagraxofusp,

developing lymphadenopathy or skin erythematous macules or papules.[57,161-163] Circulating pDCs are very rarely found in MPDCP,[164] except for cases with high (>5%) pDC counts in the bone marrow, which correlates with increased risk of AML transformation and higher incidence of mutations in the *RAS* pathway.[165] A distinctive histologic feature of MPDCP consists of the occurrence of multiple nodular or irregular aggregates of pDCs, mostly occurring in the bone marrow, skin, or lymph nodes, often admixed with the associated myeloid neoplasm (Fig. 51-6A–D).[57,153,155,156,160,163,166,167] PDCs exhibit a morphology akin to reactive pDCs, with some variability in nuclear size and contour; the phenotype also overlaps that of reactive pDCs,[165,168] except for occasional aberrant expression of CD2, CD5, CD7, CD10, CD13, CD14, CD15, and CD33.[57,73,155,162,163] In contrast to BPDCN, pDCs in MPDCP express CD68 and granzyme B, and are negative for CD56 and BCL2, although weak CD56 expression sometimes occurs.[57,81] The proliferation index is low (<10% Ki-67) and TdT is negative. On gene-expression analysis, the pDCs in MPDCP are close to healthy donors' pDCs,[165] but their neoplastic nature and relatedness to the associated myeloid neoplasm

has been proven by the identification of similar chromosomal abnormalities or mutations.[47,155,162,164,165,167,169-171]

AML-pDC is characterized by AML associated with increased numbers of pDCs in the bone marrow and peripheral blood.[157-159,172] The pDCs show a heterogeneous immunophenotypic profile, including an immature subset expressing CD34, and more mature pDCs with low or no CD56 expression, and frequent negativity or low expression of TCL1.[157,159,172] Notably, a phenotypic continuum has been observed between myeloid blasts and mature pDCs,[157-159,172] and it is likely that the immature subgroup of BPDCN reported by Martín-Martín et al.[83] corresponds to AML-pDCs.[157] Several mutations have been detected in AML-pDCs, with *RUNX1* occurring in 43 of 57 (75%) cases; the mutations are shared by blasts, pDCs, monocytes and cDCs, suggesting a common differentiation pathway.[157,158]

Various features distinguish AML-pDCs from BPDCN: myeloid blasts are >20% in all patients; skin and extramedullary site involvement is infrequent at onset of the disease; pDCs are heterogeneous, including an immature subset expressing CD34, and a more mature one mostly negative for CD56 and

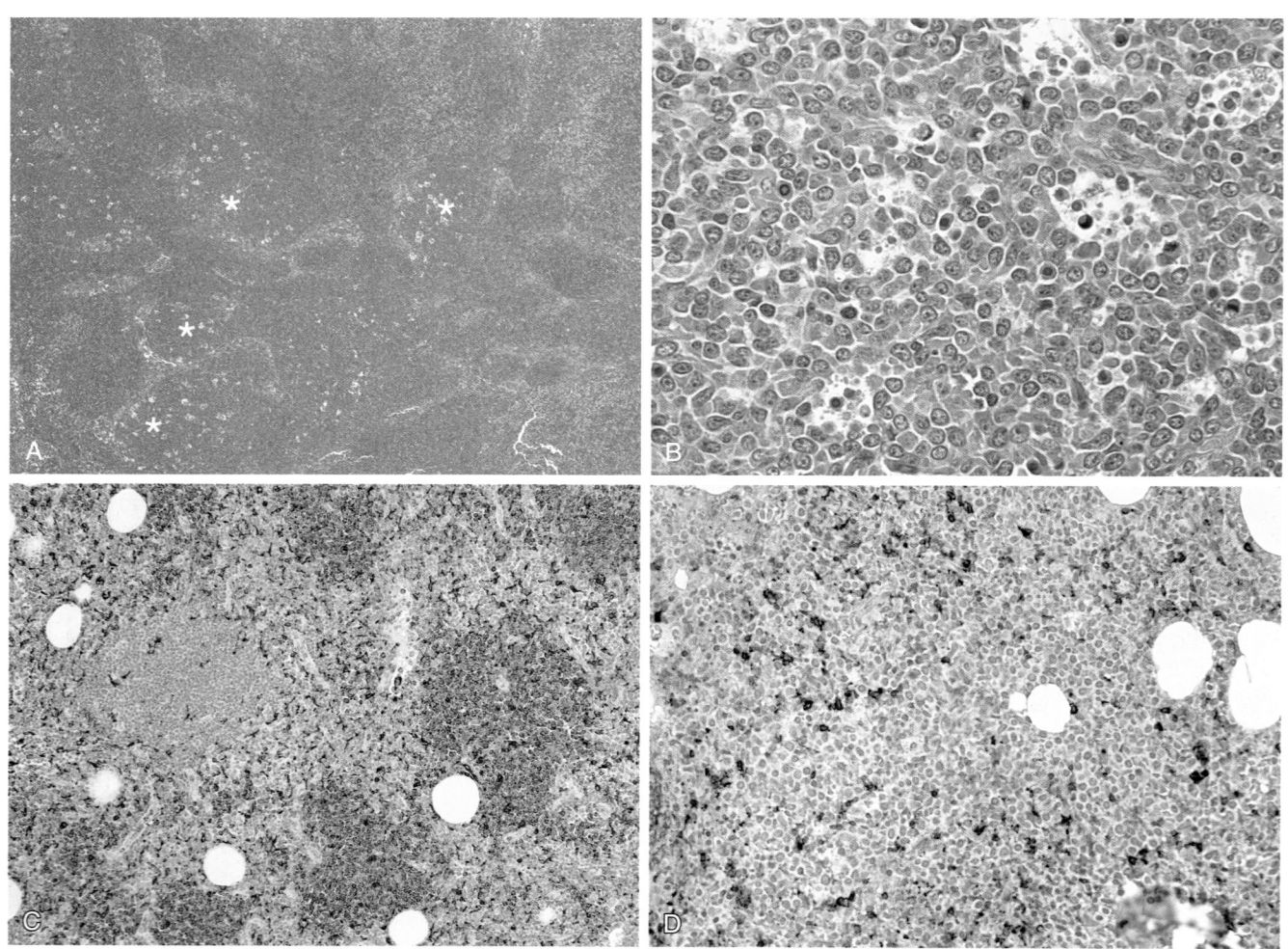

Figure 51-6. Mature plasmacytoid dendritic cell proliferation (MPDCP) involving a lymph node in a patient with chronic myelomonocytic leukemia (CMML), showing numerous nodular aggregates of plasmacytoid dendritic cells *(asterisks)* **(A)**. Note the mature morphology of the plasmacytoid dendritic cells (pDCs) and the numerous apoptotic bodies **(B)**. There is strong expression of CD68 **(C)**, while CD56 is negative **(D)**.

TCL1; and *RUNX1* mutation occurs in the majority of cases, while it has rarely been reported in BPDCN.[105,106]

Pearls and Pitfalls

- There is no single morphologic feature absolutely distinctive for blastic plasmacytoid dendritic cell neoplasm (BPDCN).
- Consider BPDCN in any infiltrate composed of monotonous medium-sized immature cells, especially involving the skin, bone marrow, or lymph nodes.
- Expression of CD4 and CD56 suggests the diagnosis of BPDCN, but it is not specific and must prompt to extend the phenotypic analysis.
- Plasmacytoid dendritic cell (pDC)–specific markers (e.g., CD123, TCL1, CD303, TCF4) are required for a correct diagnosis.
- The indolent clinical presentation contrasts with the systemic dissemination of the disease and might divert from a prompt diagnosis, leading to delayed and inappropriate treatments.

KEY REFERENCES

13. Facchetti F, Petrella T, Pileri SA. Blastic plasmacytoid dendritic cell neoplasm. In: Swerdlow SH, Campo E, Harri NL, et al., eds. *WHO Classification of Tumors of Haematopoietic and Lymphoid Tissues.* IARC; 2017:173–177.
14. Arber DA, Orazi A, Hasserjian RP, et al. International Consensus Classification of myeloid neoplasms and acute leukemias: integrating morphologic, clinical, and genomic data. *Blood.* 2022;140:1200–1228.
15. Khoury JD, Solary E, Abla O, et al. The 5th edition of the World Health Organization classification of haematolymphoid tumours: myeloid and histiocytic/dendritic neoplasms. *Leukemia.* 2022;36:1703–1719.
19. Laribi K, Baugier de Materre A, Sobh M, et al. Blastic plasmacytoid dendritic cell neoplasms: results of an international survey on 398 adult patients. *Blood Adv.* 2020;4:4838–4848.
23. Garnache-Ottou F, Vidal C, Biichlé S, et al. How should we diagnose and treat blastic plasmacytoid dendritic cell neoplasm patients? *Blood Adv.* 2019;3:4238–4251.
66. Deconinck E, Petrella T, Garnache Ottou F. Blastic plasmacytoid dendritic cell neoplasm: clinical presentation and diagnosis. *Hematol Oncol Clin North Am.* 2020;34:491–500.
93. Renosi F, Roggy A, Giguelay A, et al. Transcriptomic and genomic heterogeneity in blastic plasmacytoid dendritic cell neoplasms: from ontogeny to oncogenesis. *Blood Adv.* 2021;5:1540–1551.
141. Pemmaraju N, Lane AA, Sweet KL, et al. Tagraxofusp in blastic plasmacytoid dendritic-cell neoplasm. *N Engl J Med.* 2019;380:1628–1637.
155. Vermi W, Facchetti F, Rosati S, et al. Nodal and extranodal tumor-forming accumulation of plasmacytoid monocytes/interferon-producing cells associated with myeloid disorders. *Am J Surg Pathol.* 2004;28:585–595.
172. Huang Y, Wang Y, Chang Y, et al. Myeloid neoplasms with elevated plasmacytoid dendritic cell differentiation reflect the maturation process of dendritic cells. *Cytometry.* 2020;97:61–69.

Visit Elsevier eBooks+ for the complete set of references.

Chapter 52

Histiocytic and Dendritic Cell Proliferations—Systemic and Neoplastic

Caoimhe Egan, Mark Raffeld, and Fabio Facchetti

NON-NEOPLASTIC HISTIOCYTIC DISORDERS

Hemophagocytic Lymphohistiocytosis

Definition

Hemophagocytic lymphohistiocytosis (HLH)[1] is a rare and often lethal condition characterized by immune dysregulation of T cells or natural killer (NK) cells and persistent hypercytokinemia, leading to an exaggerated activation of macrophages that accumulate in organs and tissues and show hemophagocytosis. In the 2016 revised classification of histiocytoses and neoplasms of the macrophage-dendritic cell lineages,[2] HLH has been classified in the H group, and includes primary or familial HLH (FHLH) arising in the setting of genetic or familial inheritance and accounting for about 25% of cases, and secondary or reactive HLH (SHLH), mostly related to infections, neoplasia, and autoimmunity.

This dichotomous definition of HLH has recently been questioned by the North American Consortium for Histiocytosis (NACHO) because both FHLH and SHLH can be triggered by infections or other immune activating events, and heterozygous or low-penetrance mutations in FHLH-associated genes are involved in the pathogenesis of some forms of SHLH.[3,4]

Epidemiology

HLH is a rare but likely underrecognized disease, occurring in both children and adults, with an increasing incidence. The precise epidemiologic profile of HLH is not well defined. About 25% of cases of HLH are FHLH and typically present in children under 1 year of age. Surveys from Italy, Sweden, and the United States[5-8] have reported an annual incidence of FHLH in 1 to 10 per million children, with a 1:1 male-to-female ratio. In children, genetic defects play a predominant part in the development of HLH, which usually manifests within the first 6 months of life and in rare cases may even develop in utero or at birth. HLH is estimated to occur in the neonatal period at a rate of 1 in 50,000 to 150,000 births.[4] However, cases with late onset up to adulthood have been reported.[5] In about 50% of cases, FHLH occurs in a known familial setting, and in the remaining cases, as a sporadic event.[5] Because of ethnic variations in the causative mutations of FHLH, 47% of White patients have mutations in *UNC13D*, 22% in *STXBP2*, and 20% in *PRF1*, while *PRF1* mutations occur in 71% and 98% of Hispanic and Black patients, respectively, and in 36% of Arabs.[4]

SHLH may occur at any age,[2] and it is frequently associated with an identifiable predisposition or trigger. A countrywide survey in Japan found an annual incidence of HLH of 1 per 800,000 individuals of all ages, with a male-to-female ratio of 0.94. More than 95% of cases were SHLH and 40% of all HLH cases had associated Epstein-Barr virus (EBV) infection.[9] In a revised series of 775 adults with HLH, the mean age at diagnosis was 49 years, with a male-to-female ratio of 1.7:1.[10] HLH occurring in adults has a significant geographic variability, suggesting a specific genetic background or differences in susceptibility to triggering, especially by infectious agents.[10,11] SHLH occurring in children and young adults is mostly associated with EBV infection, followed by cytomegalovirus (CMV) infection. HLH occurs in about 10% of children with systemic juvenile idiopathic arthritis, especially in early stages of the disease.[4] In adults, disease triggers, especially infections and neoplasms, and, less frequently, autoimmunity, are the main causative factors.[10] The occurrence of HLH in adults has been increasingly recognized over the past decades, especially related to hematologic neoplasms,[10,12] and an underlying malignancy occurs in >50% of adult cases.[13] However, nearly one-third of adult HLH has more than one cause.[10]

Etiology and Pathogenesis

The cellular and molecular mechanisms contributing to the development of HLH are only partially understood, and it is thought that instead of representing one definite disease, HLH consists of different conditions characterized by a persistent activation of the immune system through different pathways, depending on individual predispositions and variable environmental triggers.[4]

Clinical observations, genetic analysis, and animal models have shown that HLH is primarily driven by an aberrant immune response that does not appear to target self-antigens and can be eventually triggered by infections.[3] In most FHLH variants, the main anomaly is an uncontrolled activation of T cells (especially CD8-positive cytotoxic T cells), with consequent activation of other immune cells, especially macrophages, resulting in a persistent amplification loop where these cells stimulate each other. Interferon gamma (IFN-γ) is a key mediator of disease development, causing an exaggerated inflammatory response with macrophage activation by T cells and hypersecretion of proinflammatory cytokines (e.g., tumor necrosis factor [TNF]-α, interleukin [IL]-1β, IL-6, IL-10, and IL-18).[3,4,10,14,15] Notably, the reciprocal activation of T cells and macrophages is strongly supported by soluble IL-2 receptor (sIL-2R) and soluble hemoglobin-haptoglobin scavenger receptor (CD163), respectively representing a T cell and a macrophage activation marker.[4,16]

Tissue infiltration by activated immune cells and local and systemic effects of the "cytokine storm" are responsible for the development of the main clinical and laboratory features of HLH and contribute to tissue damage, progressive systemic organ failure, and hemophagocytosis.[17]

Primary or Genetic HLH

There are many genetic causes of predisposition to HLH (Table 52-1). FHLH clusters around genes (PRF1, UNC13D, STX11, and STXBP2) whose related molecules are involved in cell-mediated cytotoxicity and lymphocyte activation/survival.

The cause of FHLH type 1 (FHLH1), accounting for approximately 10% of FHLH cases, remains to be elucidated. FHLH type 2 (FHLH2) is caused by perforin deficiency caused by mutation of PRF1, which was the first gene reported as a cause of FHLH, accounting for about 30% to 35% of cases.[18] During granule-mediated cytotoxicity, perforin is released from the cytotoxic granules of effector T or NK cells within an immunologic synapse and oligomerizes on target cells, causing the formation of pores through which cytotoxic granule contents enter into the target cell, inducing apoptosis. The perforin and the Fas systems are important in the maintenance of dendritic cell homeostasis and in limiting T-cell activation by antigen presentation, thus controlling the inflammatory response.[19] The deficiency of the cytolytic effector perforin, resulting in absent or scarcely detectable cytotoxic granules in cytotoxic lymphocytes, leads to a pathophysiologic setup for HLH.[17,20] In addition, several unusual missense mutations of the perforin gene have been identified, that result in a mutated protein that is not cytotoxic to the target cell, which may be associated with atypical (late-onset) FHLH.[21] Perforin polymorphism c.272C>T (p.A91V) is also frequently found in late-onset FHLH, and homozygosity for this allele appears to be associated with susceptibility to lymphoma and leukemia.[22,23]

FHLH types 3 to 5 are caused by mutations in UNC13D, STX11, and STXBP2, respectively.[24-27] These genes encode for protein products that are critical for normal cytotoxic granule exocytosis, resulting in the lack of granule release into the immunologic synapse and failure to kill target cells. FHLH type 3 accounts for about 30% of FHLH cases[28] and is associated with MUNC13-4 deficiency. In FHLH type 4, patients with mutations in STX11 encoding syntaxin-11[26] have a worldwide distribution, although the vast majority are of Turkish/Arab descent (accounting for 20% of cases) and show late-onset disease.[26] The most recently identified, FHLH type 5, is caused by mutations in the STXBP2 gene resulting in deficiency of syntaxin-binding protein 2, also named MUNC18-2.[27]

Pigmentary disorders (Griscelli syndrome type 2, Chediak-Higashi syndrome, and Hermansky-Pudlak syndrome type 2; respectively associated with mutations of RAB27A, LYST and AP3B1), show widespread compromise of lysosomal granule trafficking that can also affect melanocytes and other cells.[29-31] These disorders share with FHLH the common pathophysiologic mechanism of impaired cytotoxicity responses that lead to the inability of effector lymphocytes to kill infected cells. Remarkably, patients with Hermansky-Pudlak syndrome type 2 have a lower incidence of HLH than other disorders.[20] Because some of the proteins essential for lytic granule secretion by effector lymphocytes are also required for melanocyte trafficking of pigment granules, these disorders are associated with albinism, while their variable involvement in platelet and neutrophil functions also can be responsible for bleeding, neutropenia, and progressive neurodevelopmental abnormalities.[20]

The X-linked lymphoproliferative (XLP) diseases type 1 and 2 are caused by pathologic variants in SH2D1A and XIAP.[32-35] In XLP1, the consequent functional defect of the encoded protein, SLAM-associated protein (SAP), leads to defective 2B4-mediated cytotoxicity, especially toward EBV-infected B-cells, lack of invariant NK/T cell development, and resistance to T-cell restimulation-induced cell death, thus impairing the physiologic mechanism of T-cell response downregulation.[36-39]

The HLH occurring in XLP1 patients is almost exclusively associated with EBV infection and can be associated with malignant lymphoproliferation.[40] In XLP2, XIAP deficiency

Table 52-1 Genetic Conditions Associated With Predisposition to Hemophagocytic Lymphohistiocytosis

Familial HLH		
Disease	**Gene**	**Pathogenetic Mechanism**
FHLH1	Locus on 9q21.3-q22 Gene unknown	Unknown
FHLH2	PRF1	Defective lymphocyte granule–mediated cytotoxicity
FHLH3	UNC13D	Defective lymphocyte granule–mediated cytotoxicity
FHLH4	STX11	Defective lymphocyte granule–mediated cytotoxicity
FHLH5	STXBP2	Defective lymphocyte granule–mediated cytotoxicity
Pigmentary Disorders Associated With HLH		
Disease	**Gene**	**Pathogenetic Mechanism**
Griscelli syndrome type 2	RAB27A	Defective lymphocyte granule–mediated cytotoxicity
Chédiak-Higashi syndrome	LYST	Defective lymphocyte granule–mediated cytotoxicity
Hermansky-Pudlak syndrome 2	AP3B1	Defective lymphocyte granule–mediated cytotoxicity
XLP		
Disease	**Gene**	**Pathogenetic Mechanism**
XLP-type 1	SH2D1A	Defective 2B4-mediated cytotoxicity; defective T-cell restimulation–induced cell death; absent iNKT cells
XLP-type 2	XIAP	Dysregulated NLRP3 inflammasome function; increased effector cell susceptibility to cell death
Other Diseases		
	NLRC4	Constitutively active NLRC4 inflammasome
	CDC42	Defective formation of actin-based structures; defective proliferation, migration, and cytotoxicity; increased IL-1β and IL-18 production
EBV Susceptibility Disorders		
	Gene	**Pathogenetic Mechanism**
	MAGT1	Defective Mg^{2+} transporter, low NKG2D, and defective cytotoxicity
	ITK	Defective tyrosine kinase function; defective cytotoxic T-cell expansion and cytolytic capacity; decreased iNKT cells
	CD27	CD27 expressed on T cells participates in costimulatory signaling, interacts with CD70; required for normal T-cell proliferation and triggering of cytotoxicity against EBV-infected B cells; decreased iNKT cells
	CD70	CD70 expressed by EBV-infected B cells interacts with CD27 on T cells; required for normal expansion and cytotoxicity of the T cells; decreased NKG2D, 2B4; decreased iNKT cells
	CTPS1	Enzyme involved in de novo synthesis of cytidine nucleotide triphosphate (critical precursor of nucleic acid metabolism); deficiency leads to impaired proliferation; decreased iNKT cells
	RASGRP1	Activates RAS, which leads to MAPK pathway activation; defects in T-cell activation, proliferation, and migration; decreased cytotoxicity; decreased iNKT cells

CTP, Cytidine triphosphate; *EBV,* Epstein-Barr virus; *FHLH,* familial hemophagocytic lymphohistiocytosis; *HLH,* hemophagocytic lymphohistiocytosis; *IL,* interleukin; *iNKT,* invariant natural killer T cells; *XLP,* X-linked lymphoproliferative disease.
From Canna SW, Marsh RA, Pediatric hemophagocytic lymphohistiocytosis. *Blood*, 2020. 135(16): pp. 1332-1343.

causes dysregulation of NLRP3 inflammasome function with overproduction of inflammatory IL-1β and IL-18.[41] The persistent high levels of IL-18 occurring in these patients likely contributes to the HLH susceptibility.[42] Another mechanism that can contribute to HLH in XIAP deficient patients is related to the direct inhibitory function of XIAP on caspase-3, caspase-7, and caspase-9 affecting regulation of cell death.[39] XIAP-deficient cells, including T cells, are more vulnerable to

cell death and the inefficient effector cell function may also contribute to HLH pathogenesis.[35] In XLP2, EBV infection acts as a trigger in 30% to 80% of cases.[43,44] Patients do not develop lymphoma but frequently develop inflammatory bowel disease, hypogammaglobulinemia, recurrent infections, and other more rare complications.[20]

In addition to XLP, there are several primary immunodeficiencies (PIDs) mainly related to mutations of

MAGT1, ITK, CD27, CD70, CTPS1, and *RASGRP1* genes, in which patients are at high risk of EBV infection, manifesting as severe EBV infection, EBV-HLH, chronic active EBV, and lymphoma (Table 52-1).[45]

A unifying process in these HLH conditions associated with EBV infection appears to be the failure to control viral replication in B cells[46,47] during severe primary EBV infection, caused by inability of CD8-positive T cells and NK cells to kill EBV-infected B cells (XLP1), resistance of EBV-specific T-cell cytolysis (XLP2), or impaired expansion of EBV-specific T-cell clones in the other genetic diseases with susceptibility to EBV-HLH. In all of these circumstances, persistent viral replication and sustained antigenic stimulation of T cells seems to drive HLH.[47]

Gain-of-function mutations in *NLRC4* and heterozygous mutations in *CDC42* represent other very uncommon genetic conditions predisposing to HLH.[48,49] Mutations of *NLRC4* can be dominantly inherited or happen as de novo germline or even as somatic mutations.[50] These lead to constitutive activation of the *NLRC4* inflammasome, resulting in high blood levels of IL-18, thought to be the main pathogenetic mechanism responsible for the disease, as also supported by the clinical response to recombinant IL-18BP, which decreases IL-18 activity.[51]

Heterozygous mutations of *CDC42* affecting the protein at C-terminal amino acids 186, 188, or 192 cause autoinflammation, including fatal HLH in some cases.[52,53] In addition, neonatal patients show facial dysmorphism, hepatosplenomegaly, recurrent fever, urticaria-like skin rashes, failure to thrive, cytopenias, high transaminases, and elevated inflammatory markers. It has been hypothesized that the *CDC42* mutations interfere with actin assembly, resulting in anomalies in several cell functions (e.g., cytoskeletal rearrangement, cell signaling, polarization, proliferation, migration, and cytotoxicity processes). The very high levels of IL-18 and increased production of IL-1β ex vivo support a dysregulated inflammasome function and the autoinflammatory nature of the disease.[52,53] The pathogenetic role of IL-1β is also supported by clinical response to IL-1β inhibitors.[53]

Numerous inborn errors of metabolism (e.g., multiple sulfatase deficiency, lysosomal acid lipase deficiency/Wolman disease, Gaucher disease [GD], Pearson syndrome, galactosialidosis, Niemann-Pick disease [NPD]) can also present with HLH but are not included in primary HLH. HLH particularly occurs in lysinuric protein intolerance caused by mutations in *SLC7A7*.[20,54] Lack of degradation of substrates results in their accumulation within macrophages and may lead to inflammasome and persistent macrophage activation, with subsequent development of HLH.

Secondary or Reactive Hemophagocytic Lymphohistiocytosis

A number of conditions are associated with SHLH, including viral infections (29%), other infections (20%), malignancies (27%), rheumatologic disorders (7%), immune deficiency syndromes (6%), and drugs.[55]

SHLH is predominantly driven by sustained immune activation rather than by an intrinsic defect in immune functions. The mechanisms leading to impaired host immunity and uncontrolled immune response are multifactorial. These include imbalance between infected cells and immune effector cells, transient immune dysfunction caused by immunosuppressive drugs or low NK-cell numbers, interference with cytotoxic function by viruses or cytokines, and single nucleotide polymorphisms in genes important in the immune response.[56] Notably, hypomorphic mutations in *PRF1, UNC13D,* and *STXBP2* have been found in 14% of adult patients with HLH,[57] suggesting that these mutations likely play a contributing role in development of HLH when patients face immune challenges such as EBV infection, autoimmune disorders, or malignant tumors.

Infection-associated HLH can be a sporadic event, or can be responsible for HLH occurring in other conditions.[4,10] EBV, CMV, and, less frequently, other members of the herpesvirus family are the most commonly reported causes of HLH.[55,58] Other DNA or RNA viruses belonging to different families may be associated with HLH,[55] including parvovirus B19,[59] all types of seasonal, avian, and swine influenza viruses, and severe acute respiratory syndrome coronavirus 2 (SARS-CoV-2).[60-62]

Bacteria (*Babesia, Bartonella, Borrelia,* and *Brucella* species, *Coxiella burnetii, Ehrlichia chaffeensis, Leptospira* spp., *Listeria* spp., *Mycoplasma pneumoniae, Mycobacterium avium, Mycobacterium bovis*–weakened form [Bacillus Calmette–Guérin, *Mycobacterium tuberculosis*]), protozoa (especially *Leishmania* spp., *Plasmodium* spp., and *Toxoplasma gondii*), and fungi (*Candida* spp., *Cryptococcus neoformans, Histoplasma capsulatum,* and *Penicillium marneffei*) have also been reported to cause HLH, in both immunocompetent and immunodeficient individuals.[55,63]

EBV triggers HLH, usually in the context of primary infection in young individuals with FHLH and primary immunodeficiency,[46,47] while in adults, HLH mostly depends on virus reactivation in immunocompromised patients.[10] EBV not only infects the B cells but also can infect T cells and NK cells, particularly in SHLH, in which infection of CD8-positive T cells results in a cytokine storm, leading to secondary activation of histiocytes and macrophages.[64] CMV causes HLH in both immunocompetent and immunocompromised patients.[58]

In addition to the genetic settings strongly associated with HLH (Table 52-1), HLH may also occur in severe combined immunodeficiency, chronic granulomatous disease, Wiskott-Aldrich syndrome, DiGeorge syndrome, X-linked agammaglobulinemia, and autoimmune lymphoproliferative syndrome (ALPS).[3,20] The host susceptibility to infection and the resulting abnormal immune responses caused by the underlying disease are likely responsible for HLH development, triggered by defective cytolysis during viral infections.[15]

Herpesviruses infections (primary or reactivation in the setting of immunosuppression) are the most common trigger of HLH developing in adults treated with chemotherapy for cancer or immunosuppressive drugs for inflammatory diseases.[3,10] Apart from susceptibility to infections, the pathogenesis of HLH in these conditions may also be related to drug-induced suppression of cytolytic activity.[4]

Patients with chronic human immunodeficiency virus (HIV) and hepatitis virus (B or C) infections can develop HLH during either the acute or chronic phase. In HIV, HLH can be triggered by opportunistic infections, especially intracellular pathogens such as *M. tuberculosis, Pneumocystis jiroveci,* and *Plasmodium* spp., and more rarely by other pathogens, neoplasms, or highly active antiretroviral therapy.[10,15]

HLH developing in patients with malignant neoplasms accounts for 40% to 70% of HLH cases.[12,65] It mainly occurs in adults, where it may complicate up to 1% of tumors,[10,66] but also occurs in infancy. There are a few plausible pathogenic mechanisms in malignancy-associated HLH, such as persistent antigen stimulation and hypersecretion of proinflammatory cytokines by the malignant cells, inherited immune defects such as *HAVCR2* mutation and XLP disease predisposing individuals to both cancer and HLH, and T-cell dysfunction and disruption of immune homeostasis related to cancer-directed therapy.[67] In cases of new onset HLH, it is possible that transformed cells are mainly responsible for HLH by the upregulation of IFN-γ and TNF-α production, especially in the presence of malignancy-associated EBV replication.[4]

Of SHLH occurring in adults, 50% is associated with a hematologic neoplasm. Lymphoma is the most common cause, especially NK-cell and peripheral T-cell lymphoma (35%), followed by B-cell lymphomas (32%), leukemias (6%), and Hodgkin lymphoma (6%).[67-69] Most large case series of lymphoma-associated HLH are from Asian centers, including China and South Korea for T-cell and NK-cell lymphoma, and Japan, where B-cell lymphoma is more prevalent.[67] Notably, HLH was found to have a 26% prevalence in the rare intravascular B-cell lymphoma, especially in Japan, and Asian compared with Western patients.[10,70] Not unexpectedly, HLH is frequently reported in histiocyte disorders,[67] and a retrospective study of HLH in Langerhans cell histiocytosis (LCH) showed a 9.3% 2-year cumulative incidence.[71]

HLH more rarely develops in patients with solid malignancies (3%), which include germ cell tumors, lung, prostate, colon and hepatocellular carcinoma, and neck squamous cell carcinoma.[72] HLH may develop before cancer treatment or during therapy; in the latter case, it is most probably caused by immunosuppression and associated infections.[66,73]

HLH occurring in in the context of rheumatologic disorders is also known as macrophage activation syndrome (MAS) or MAS-HLH.[2] Although MAS and HLH are very similar and should be viewed as the same disease,[3] there are notable differences in presentation, especially related to platelet and neutrophil counts and fibrinogen levels.[74] HLH occurs in approximately 10% of children with severe-onset juvenile idiopathic arthritis (so-JIA),[74] with subclinical presentations in 30% to 40% of cases and lethal complication in 20%.[75,76] In so-JIA, HLH presents at the onset of disease in 22% of cases and in roughly half of them in the context of active so-JIA without recognizable triggers, while infection and drugs have been associated with HLH in 30% and 4% of cases, respectively.[74] MAS in adults is most commonly seen in adult-onset Still disease (AOSD), reported in 15% up to 20% of cases.[77-79] MAS has also been reported in systemic lupus erythematosus (0.9%–4.6% of cases),[80] Kawasaki disease (1.1%–1.9%),[81] dermatomyositis, and rheumatoid arthritis.[82]

SHLH can be induced by immune-activating therapies for cancer and by drugs responsible for drug-induced hypersensitivity syndrome (DIHS).[4] Similarly to other forms of HLH, therapy-related HLH is likely driven by the aberrant and sustained activation of CD8-positive T cells. Immune checkpoint inhibitor therapies targeting PD-1, PD-L1, or CTLA-4 enhance antitumor T-cell activity, inducing CD8-positive T cell responses, which can result in inflammatory syndromes resembling HLH.[83,84] Similarly, genetically engineered autologous CD8-positive cytotoxic T cells expressing chimeric antigen receptors (CAR-T), especially applied for treating patients with hematologic and solid malignancies, frequently induce the IL-6–driven cytokine release syndrome, which can evolve into HLH.[85-87]

HLH can also be a complication of hematopoietic stem-cell transplantation (HSCT), with higher incidence in recipients of allogeneic HSCT and umbilical cord blood grafts containing mostly naïve T cells.[88-92] Posttransplant HLH can be difficult to diagnose, as clinical and laboratory signs overlap with recovering bone marrow.[55]

HLH occasionally occurs in the context of DIHS,[93] where molecular interactions occur between the drug and human leukocyte antigen (HLA) proteins encoded by DIHS-associated risk alleles, resulting in hyperstimulation of CD8-positive T cells.[4]

Clinical Features

The clinical features of HLH are widely variable; symptoms can manifest insidiously or arise quickly with critical illness that rapidly evolves into a shocklike clinical state.[4,5,10,15,57] Most patients with HLH are acutely ill and present with high, persistent fevers, multiple organ involvement with hepatosplenomegaly, skin rash, neurologic symptoms, liver dysfunction, and coagulopathy. Lymphadenopathy may occur in HLH, and when extensive or bulky it should prompt exclusion of an underlying lymphoma. Severe liver damage with synthetic dysfunction combined with endothelial activation and disseminated intravascular coagulation cause coagulopathy, with hemorrhage, petechiae, ecchymosis, and purpura.[4] Patients frequently have abdominal pain and non-specific gastrointestinal symptoms (diarrhea, nausea, vomiting, jaundice), or even gastrointestinal hemorrhage and pancreatitis.[10] Severe forms of HLH can involve lungs, heart, and kidney, with signs and symptoms requiring supportive care.[10,94] Central nervous system (CNS) involvement is more common in pediatric HLH, especially with FHLH, where it occurs in about one-third of cases. Symptoms are variable and include seizures, meningismus, ataxia, dysarthria, encephalopathy, and signs of cranial nerve involvement.[95,96] Notably, in rare cases HLH presents with isolated CNS inflammation, with minimal or even no systemic symptoms, thus causing irreparable delay in diagnosis.[97] Posterior reversible encephalopathy syndrome (PRES) may complicate HLH, particularly FHLH.[98]

HLH is typically associated with multiple laboratory abnormalities and their recognition as a full spectrum is important for diagnosis, since none alone is specific for HLH.[4] Most patients present with or develop a combination of cytopenia, signs of hepatocellular injury, coagulopathy, and in severe cases, biochemical evidence of organ failure. Blood cytopenia with combinations of leukopenia (including neutropenia), anemia, and thrombocytopenia are very frequent in children with HLH, while in adults it can be less severe.[15] Elevated liver aminotransferases occur during the early phases of the disease and often track its activity. The cytokine storm typically driving HLH is associated with high C-reactive protein levels and elevated erythrocyte sedimentation rates (ESR), the latter falling as disease progresses, while coagulation abnormalities (hypofibrinogenemia, elevated D-dimer, and prolonged prothrombin and partial thromboplastin time) increasingly worsen.

Ferritin is an indicator of macrophage activation and it is significantly increased in HLH, often 10 to 100 times higher than normal. Hyperferritinemia is found in essentially all pediatric HLH where it has a relevant diagnostic value (especially in so-JIA HLH); it is also increased in the vast majority of cases of adult-onset HLH,[3,14,15] but its specificity is lower,[4] since high ferritin levels have been reported in adults with variable diseases, such as infections, hematologic neoplasm, autoimmunity, and hepatocellular injury.[99] If both ferritin and sIL-2R are not significantly raised, the diagnosis of HLH should be questioned.[3] However, low percentages of ferritin glycosylation, indicating a macrophage origin, may be a unique finding of SHLH.[100]

HLH is almost always associated with high blood levels of sIL-2R (sCD25) and sCD163, respectively indicating activation of T cells and macrophages.[14-16] Reduced cytotoxic CD8-positive T cell and NK cell activity is often reported, reflecting either genetic deficiency or the effects of inflammation and immunosuppression.[10,18,101]

Early recognition of HLH is critical, because patients can decompensate rapidly and progress to multiorgan failure and death. The diagnosis of HLH requires awareness, but even when suspected, it is still challenging because there are no clinical, laboratory, or histopathologic findings pathognomonic for the disease. Over time, various criteria for HLH diagnosis have been proposed, some of them reserved for specific clinical conditions.

Diagnostic criteria for children with FHLH were developed in the early 90s (HLH 94)[1] and later updated (HLH 2004).[102] According to HLH 2004 criteria, diagnosis of FHLH requires five of the following eight features: fever; splenomegaly; cytopenias affecting ≥2 of 3 cell lineages and with defined thresholds for hemoglobin, platelets, and neutrophils; hypertriglyceridemia or hypofibrinogenemia; hemophagocytosis; hyperferritinemia; high sIL-2R levels; and low/absent NK cell activity (Box 52-1). Otherwise, the diagnosis of FLHL can be made by genetic testing, although this procedure, as well as NK cell activity and sIL-2R assays, are not always immediately available to most institutions.[102] Perforin and CD107a tests by flow cytometry assay are more sensitive and no less specific compared with NK cytotoxicity testing for screening for genetic HLH, and it has been suggested that these be added to current HLH diagnostic criteria.[103] It is worth mentioning that hemophagocytosis, despite featuring in the name of the disease, has limited diagnostic sensitivity and specificity, because it may not be always present or easily detected in bone marrow biopsies, and it can be observed in patients without HLH.[104-106] Lastly, hyperferritinemia is a sensitive criterion but has low specificity because it can be seen in many other inflammatory and noninflammatory conditions.[99] Although the HLH 2004 criteria are widely used to define and diagnose HLH, including forms other than FHLH, it has been recommended that all criteria, including hemophagocytosis, need not be met for initiating therapy in cases with strong suspicion of HLH.[3,4] Recently, an HLH-probability calculator (H-score) has been developed[107] (Box 52-2) showing higher sensitivity compared with HLH-2004 criteria but a lower, still-acceptable specificity.[107-109] The H-score is particularly useful to support the recognition of nonfamilial forms of HLH at initial presentation of the disease but has also been validated in adults with some differences in the cutoff values.[108] In a large cohort of patients with

---

Box 52-1 *Updated Diagnostic Hemophagocytic Lymphohistiocytosis—2004 Criteria*

Presence of either:
(A) Molecular diagnosis consistent with HLH
    or
(B) Presence of at least five of the eight following criteria:
1. Fever ≥38.5° C
2. Splenomegaly
3. Cytopenia affecting ≥2 of 3 lineages:
   • Hemoglobin <9 g/dL (infants <4 weeks: <10 g/dL)
   • Platelets <100 × 10³/mcL
   • Neutrophils <1 × 10³/mcL
4. Hypertriglyceridemia or hypofibrinogenemia
   • Fasting triglycerides ≥265 mg/dL
   • Fibrinogen ≤1.5 g/L
5. Hemophagocytosis in bone marrow or spleen or lymph nodes or liver
6. Low or absent natural killer cell activity
7. Ferritin ≥500 mcg/L
8. Soluble CD25 ≥2400 U/mL

Data from Griffin G, Shenoi S, Hughes GC, Hemophagocytic lymphohistiocytosis: an update on pathogenesis, diagnosis, and therapy. *Best Pract Res Clin Rheumatol*, 2020. 34(4): p. 101515. Henter JI., et al., HLH-2004: Diagnostic and therapeutic guidelines for hemophagocytic lymphohistiocytosis. *Pediatr Blood Cancer*, 2007. 48(2): pp. 124-131.

---

hematologic neoplasms, Zoref-Lorenz et al. showed that the simple combined elevation of soluble CD25 (>3999 U/mL) and ferritin (>1000 ng/mL) accurately identifies HLH, including cases missed by the HLH 2004 criteria, and at the same time is a potent predictor of mortality across diverse hematologic malignancies.[110] Specific scores to identify MAS/HLH associated with so-JIA have also been developed, including the "MS score," found to be particularly useful to distinguish so-JIA with MAS from active so-JIA without MAS, and a score helping to discriminate between FHLH and so-JIA-MAS/HLH.[74,111]

Morphology

The histologic counterpart of the mutual activation of lymphocytes and macrophages occurring in HLH is represented by prominent tissue accumulation of these cells, with macrophages exhibiting a variable degree of hemophagocytosis, consisting of the cytoplasmic engulfment of nucleated and nonnucleated red blood cells, neutrophils, lymphocytes, or their remains (Fig. 52-1).

Hemophagocytosis can be present in virtually all organs, but it typically occurs in the bone marrow, spleen, lymph nodes, liver, or body fluids.[9] It has also been found in the CNS,[112] skin, lungs, and rarely in the subcutaneous tissue.[113] The bone marrow is the tissue most commonly used for the identification of hemophagocytosis and aspirate morphology is often more effective than biopsies (84% versus 64%),[10] where the hemophagocytic cells may be very difficult to discern. Notably, in bone marrow biopsies the occurrence of abnormal clusters of red blood cells with pomegranate seed–like features should prompt to check for the presence of macrophages phagocytosing nucleated cells[114]; moreover, immunohistochemistry (IHC) stains for macrophage markers (such as CD68, CD163, or CD11c) significantly helps in their identification (Fig. 52-2).[62,105,115]

Box 52-2 *Diagnostic H-Score Criteria*

Known Underlying Immunosuppression:
- No = 0
- HIV-positive or receiving long-term immunosuppressive therapy (i.e., glucocorticoids, cyclosporine, azathioprine)= +18

Temperature (°C):
- <38.4 = 0
- 38.4–39.4 = +33
- >39.4 = +49

Organomegaly:
- No = 0
- Hepatomegaly or splenomegaly = +23
- Hepatomegaly and splenomegaly = +38

Number of Cytopenias (Defined as Hemoglobin ≤9.2 g/dL (≤5.71 mmol/L) or WBC ≤5000/mm³ or Platelets ≤110,000/mm³):
- 1 lineage = 0
- 2 lineage = +24
- 3 lineage = +34

Ferritin, ng/mL (or mcg/L):
- <2000 = 0
- 2000–6000 = +35
- 6000 = +50

Triglyceride, mmol/L
- <1.5 = 0
- 1.5–4 = +44
- >4 = +64

Fibrinogen, g/L:
- >2.5 = 0
- ≤2.5 = +30

AST U/L:
- <30 = 0
- ≥30 = +19

Hemophagocytosis Features on Bone Marrow Aspirate:
- No = 0
- Yes = +35

H-Scores higher than 169 are 93% sensitive and 86% specific for HLH. The H-scores can be calculated using the online H-Score calculator (http://saintantoine.aphp.fr/score/).
AST, Aspartate aminotransferase; *WBC,* white blood cell.
Data from Fardet L., et al., Development and validation of the HScore, a score for the diagnosis of reactive hemophagocytic syndrome. *Arthritis Rheumatol,* 2014. 66(9): pp. 2613-2620. Debaugnies F., et al., Performances of the H-Score for Diagnosis of Hemophagocytic Lymphohistiocytosis in Adult and Pediatric Patients. *Am J Clin Pathol,* 2016. 145(6): pp. 862-870.

The histiocytes have a mature appearance, and are commonly large with abundant cytoplasm, but occasionally can be small. They may occur in clusters or dispersed among the normal bone marrow cells, which tend to become progressively hypoplastic and, in severe cases, are completely replaced by the histiocytic infiltration.

In suspected SHLH, biopsies of the bone marrow, lymph nodes, and also skin and liver have been found to be useful to identify HLH triggers, mostly represented by hematologic neoplasms and infections (Fig. 52-3).[113,116] Liver involvement is characterized by Kupffer cell hyperplasia, and hemophagocytosis is generally detected in the sinusoids (Fig. 52-4A). Lymphocytes and histiocytes, with enrichment of CD3, CD8, and granzyme B–positive lymphocytes, involve the portal spaces, resembling chronic persistent hepatitis.[113,117] Massive liver involvement can lead to progressively altered liver function and acute liver failure.[118] More rarely, liver changes resemble leukemia, giant cell hepatitis, and storage diseases.[117] Examination of lymph nodes and spleen may show profound generalized lymphoid depletion with sinusoidal infiltration by hemophagocytic histiocytes (Fig. 52-4B), and in some patients a massive infiltration of histiocytes involves virtually the entire organ.[112] Rashes may correlate with lymphocyte infiltration on skin biopsy, where hemophagocytosis may also be found. In cases with CNS involvement, cerebrospinal fluid analysis shows pleocytosis, sometimes including hemophagocytic cells, and hyperproteinemia. Brain biopsy reveals T-cell and histiocytic infiltrates.[3,4]

As mentioned before, hemophagocytosis, despite featuring in the name of the disease, has limited diagnostic sensitivity and specificity, and because it is often cyclical, it may not be clearly apparent early in the disease process.[104] Moreover, the presence of rare histiocytes showing erythrophagocytosis in the bone marrow is a common finding, and increased hemophagocytosis may be encountered in patients without HLH, in the setting of sepsis, blood transfusions, hematopoietic transplantation, chemotherapy, and myelodysplastic syndromes (MDS).[104-106,119] Thus, there is no consensus on the differentiation of pathologic hemophagocytosis from the physiologic process,[104,106] and quantification of hemophagocytic cells in aspirates or in core biopsies does not correlate well with disease probability, even when present in high numbers.[105]

Notably, hemophagocytosis is the only HLH-2004 diagnostic criterion without a defined threshold value and no accepted diagnostic threshold or guidelines have been established. Gars et al.[120] studied the bone marrow aspirates of 78 patients presenting with clinical features suspicious for HLH, 40 with and 38 without HLH, and demonstrated that nonnucleated erythrophagocytosis alone is a non-specific finding, while hemophagocytosis of nucleated hematopoietic cells with quantitative thresholds for each of the lineages of ingested cell (at least one granulocyte, or four nucleated erythrocytes, or six cells from any four lineages among red blood cells, nucleated red blood cells, neutrophils, and lymphocytes in 1000 nucleated cells, or multiple nucleated cells in at least one hemophagocyte), revealed a strong association with HLH.

In anticipation of additional prospective studies for the validation of these data, at the present time it is reasonable to consider hemophagocytosis as neither necessary nor sufficient for diagnosing HLH. Its finding should not be overinterpreted in the absence of other clinical or biological features suggestive of HLH, and its absence should also not delay or even prevent the initiation of therapy whenever HLH is highly suspected.[3,4]

Immunophenotype

The hemophagocytic macrophages express various histiocytic markers and in some cases also show variable, generally weak expression of S100, in contrast to the histiocytes of Rosai-Dorfman disease (RDD), which are strongly positive.[121,122]

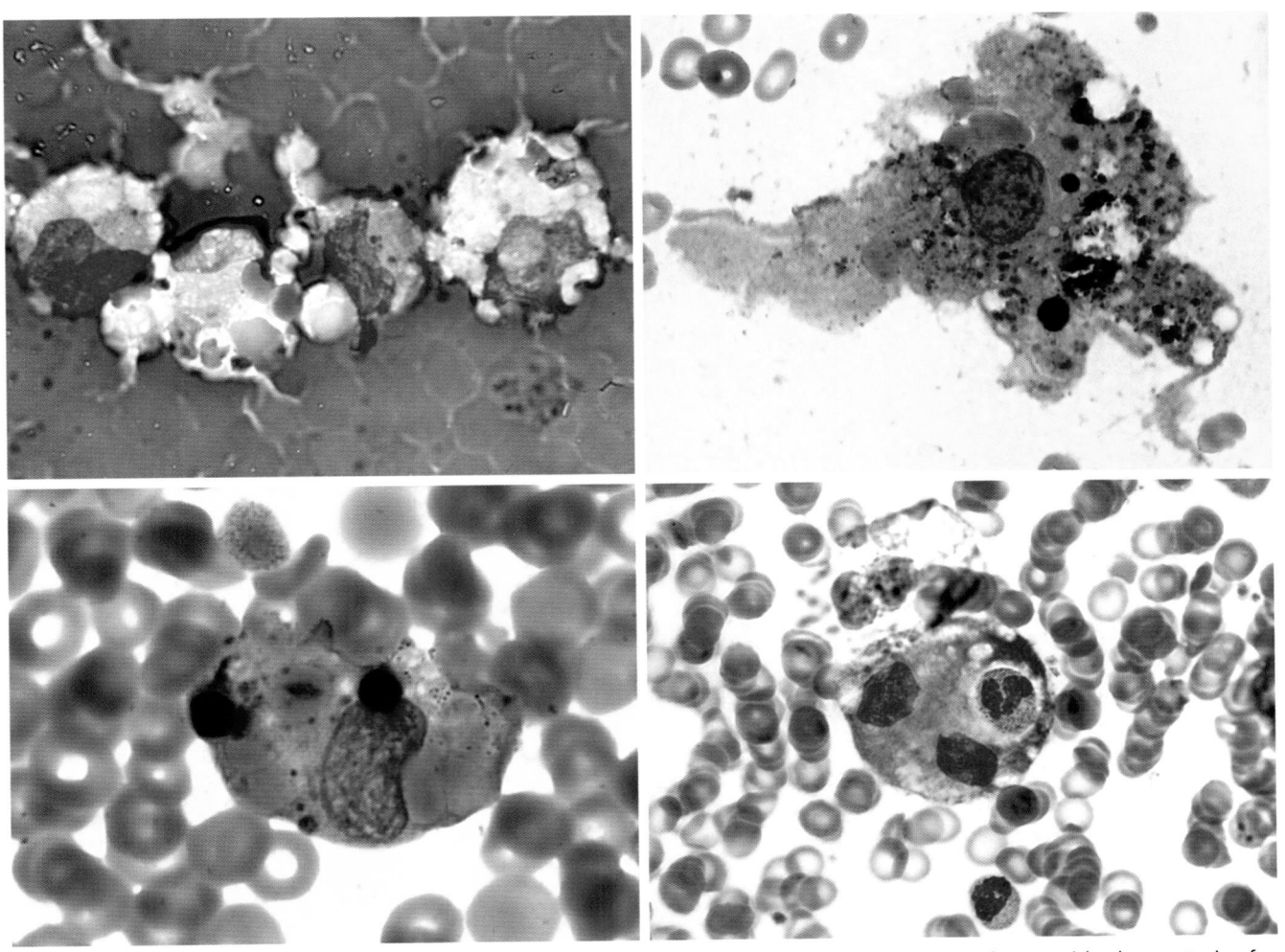

Figure 52-1. Hemophagocytic lymphohistiocytosis. Examples of bone marrow smears showing macrophages with phagocytosis of red blood cells, nucleated red cells, neutrophils, and cell debris. The upper left image is from a case of primary (familial) hemophagocytic lymphohistiocytosis (FHLH); the remaining are from secondary HLH (SHLH), all associated with lymphoma.

A CD14-dim, CD16-bright monocytic population has been described in one case: a phenotype associated with macrophages that secrete interleukin-1β, interleukin-6, and TNF-α.[123] Upregulation of CD163 (a receptor for hemoglobin-haptoglobin complexes) on monocyte-macrophages facilitates hemophagocytosis. The plasma levels of soluble CD163 in HLH are considerably higher than those found in infections, autoimmune diseases, and cancer.[124,125]

In individuals with perforin gene mutations, perforin intracellular staining by flow cytometry or IHC is significantly lower or totally absent in cytotoxic lymphocytes (NK cells, CD8-positive T cells, CD56-positive T cells), while it is normal in other forms of FHLH and EBV-associated HLH.[126,127] Downregulation of CD5 along with reduced CD7 expression by flow cytometry in circulating and bone marrow CD8-positive T cells has been described in some patients with FHLH and EBV-HLH,[128-130] and it may be used to distinguish EBV-positive from EBV-negative HLH.[131] Activated CD8-positive T cells in young patients with either FHLH or SHLH show high CD38 and HLA-DR expression and the presence of more than 7% of CD38-positive/HLA-DR-positive cells among CD8-positive T cells distinguishes HLH from early sepsis or healthy controls significantly.[132]

To protect the cytotoxic cell from preformed perforin and granzymes, the granules are lined with LAMP-1 (CD107a) protein, which can be measured by flow cytometry on the cell surface after degranulation. Decreased expression of CD107a has been reported to predict defects in genetic HLH, providing a useful screening tool.[103,133]

Clinical Course and Prognosis

HLH is typically lethal without intervention, and the initial goal consists of suppressing the hyperinflammatory process and treating the underlying trigger. Before the introduction of standardized therapeutic regimens, most patients with FHLH had a rapid downhill clinical course, and death within the first year of life was common. Clinical deterioration is characterized by hemorrhage, sepsis, and neurologic impairment. With the introduction of HLH-94[134] and HLH-2004[102] treatment protocols, the survival of children with FHLH markedly improved, with a 5-year survival rate of up to 54%.[95,135] However, FHLH survivors can develop long-term side effects, such as cognitive and growth delay, hearing impairment, and obstructive lung disease.[95]

In adults, the length and dosing of the HLH-94 treatment protocol has been adapted to the individual patient, taking

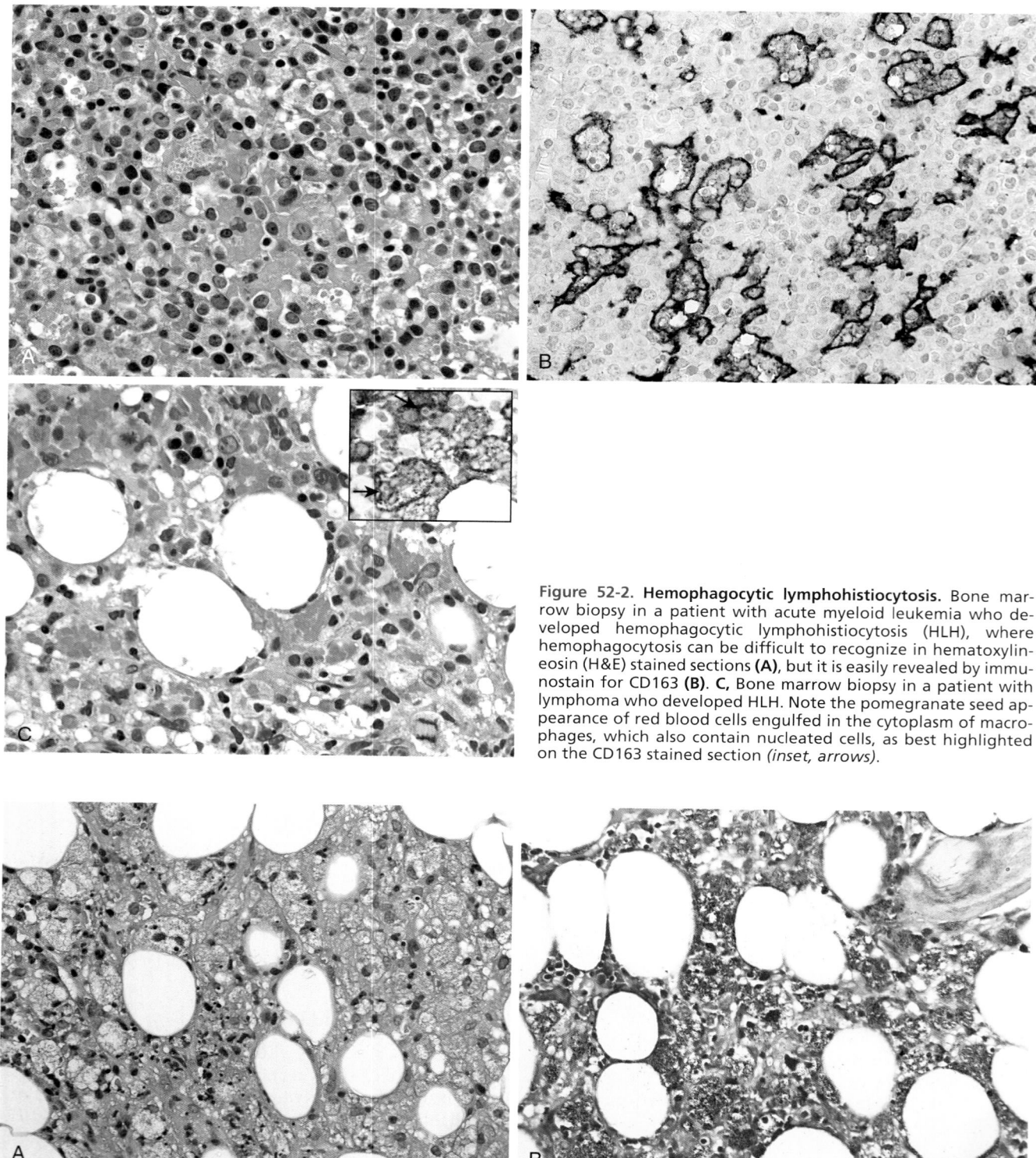

Figure 52-2. Hemophagocytic lymphohistiocytosis. Bone marrow biopsy in a patient with acute myeloid leukemia who developed hemophagocytic lymphohistiocytosis (HLH), where hemophagocytosis can be difficult to recognize in hematoxylin-eosin (H&E) stained sections **(A)**, but it is easily revealed by immunostain for CD163 **(B)**. **C,** Bone marrow biopsy in a patient with lymphoma who developed HLH. Note the pomegranate seed appearance of red blood cells engulfed in the cytoplasm of macrophages, which also contain nucleated cells, as best highlighted on the CD163 stained section *(inset, arrows).*

Figure 52-3. Hemophagocytic lymphohistiocytosis. Bone marrow biopsy in an immunosuppressed patient who developed hemophagocytic lymphohistiocytosis (HLH) syndrome secondary to disseminated mycobacteriosis: diffuse infiltration of large macrophages engulfing cells and nuclear debris in their cytoplasm **(A)**, which contains countless bacilli positive for Ziehl-Neelsen stain **(B)**.

into consideration the conditions acting as triggers and the associated morbidities.[73] Nevertheless, in adults, HLH prognosis remains poor, especially in elderly patients with comorbidities. Malignancy, particularly lymphoma, has been found to represent an adverse prognostic factor in several

studies, with worse outcome in T-cell lymphomas compared with B-cell lymphomas.[136,137] A retrospective review across three tertiary care centers identified 68 adults with HLH, with an average age of 53 years (range 18–77) and a predominance of males (63%). Underlying diseases included malignancy

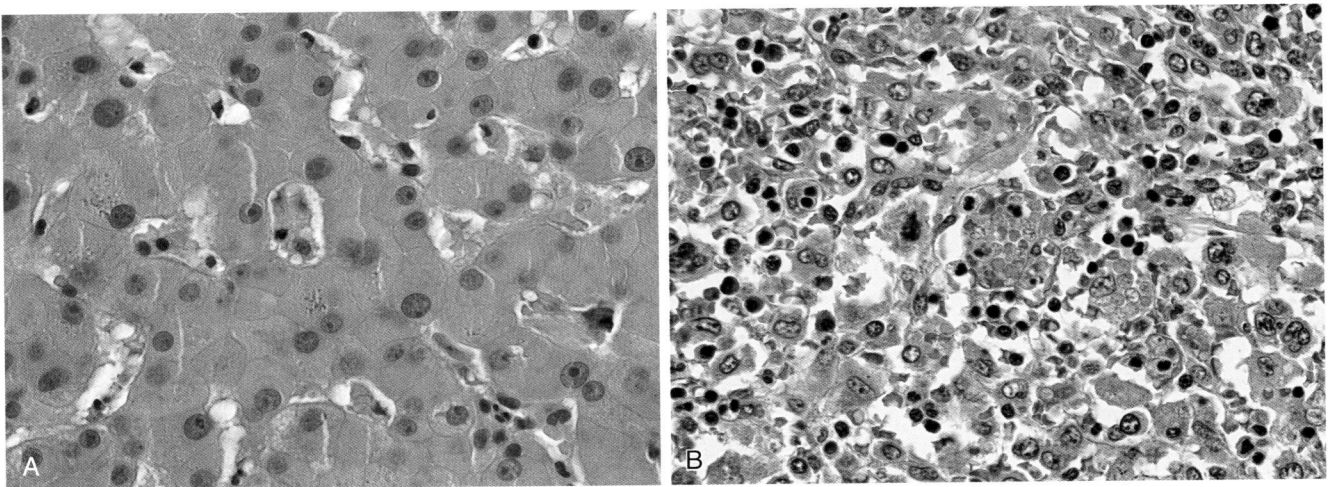

Figure 52-4. Hemophagocytic lymphohistiocytosis. Hemophagocytosis, including nucleated forms, is evident in the liver sinusoids of a patient with primary (familial) hemophagocytic syndrome **(A)** and in the spleen sinuses **(B)** from a patient with secondary hemophagocytic lymphohistiocytosis (HLH).

(33, 49%), infection (22, 33%), autoimmune disease (19, 28%) and idiopathic HLH (15, 22%). Forty-six (69%) patients died after a median follow-up of 32.2 months, and the median overall survival was 4 months. The presence of malignancy was a negative prognostic factor.[136] In a series of 162 adult patients with HLH, half of whom had an underlying malignancy, 31% were alive at a median follow-up of 32 months, with an overall mortality rate of 42%, and 20.4% mortality at 30 days. Negative prognostic factors were age, thrombocytopenia, underlying lymphoma, and no etoposide in the management.[13,138]

In a retrospective study of 120 adults with secondary nonmalignancy-associated HLH, HLH triggered by EBV had a worse 5-year overall survival (25.1%) compared with HLH occurring in autoimmune diseases (82.4%), non-EBV infections (78.7%), or of unknown origin (55.5%). Other factors associated with poor prognosis included age >45 years, hyperferritinemia, thrombocytopenia, and especially lack of response after 8 weeks of treatment.[139] In another large retrospective study including 260 adult patients, most (64%) with immunosuppression and with different HLH-associated triggers, the overall mortality rate was 57%, and it was unrelated to HLH etiology or the type of treatment, while factors associated with worse prognosis included age, bone marrow aspirate hemophagocytosis, organ failure at admission, and worsening during ICU hospitalization.[140]

Despite the development of standardized treatment protocols, the mortality rate of HLH is still high and research is underway in order to understand as a whole how to improve the diagnosis, better understand HLH pathogenetic mechanisms, and identify treatment strategies and new drugs that can improve the survival. The HLH-94 protocol remains the most commonly used treatment[141] and includes dexamethasone and etoposide, the latter having specific activity against activated T cells.[142] Etoposide can be avoided in patients with mild disease that may respond to corticosteroids alone. An alternative approach includes corticosteroids and antithymocyte globulin (ATG), a polyclonal antibody depleting human T cells, or etoposide and ATG, which has led to complete responses in 50% to 75% of patients.[143,144] HLH-specific treatment may be

postponed in patients with HLH caused by infections such as visceral leishmaniasis; histoplasmosis; atypical *Mycobacterium*, *Ehrlichia*, *Bartonella*, and *Brucella* species; and disseminated adenovirus or herpes simplex infections that can be controlled by antimicrobial therapy alone.[3,113] B-cell depletion treatments such as rituximab should be considered for EBV-associated HLH,[145] while HLH associated with malignancy may improve with oncologic-oriented treatments. Patients with MAS associated with autoimmune or autoinflammatory diseases are primarily treated with the IL1 inhibitor anakinra, high-dose corticosteroids, and cyclosporine, while etoposide is delivered only in cases where inflammation is insufficiently controlled by classical therapies.[101,146,147]

Allogeneic hematopoietic stem cell transplantation upon salvage treatment with full-intensity or reduced-intensity myeloablative protocols[113,148] is generally reserved for patients with severe genetic HLH disorders, patients with high-risk hematologic malignancy as consolidation treatment, and in refractory or relapsing HLH. Unrelated umbilical cord blood cells have been used successfully as an alternative to allo-HSCT.[149] Novel biological treatments have also been used to control HLH. The monoclonal antibody emapalumab targeting IFNγ has shown significant efficacy for refractory, recurrent, or progressive HLH, with responses in 63% of previously treated patients.[150]

Other approaches aimed at targeting specific immune cells, immune activation pathways, or cytokines include alemtuzumab, a monoclonal antibody against CD52[151]; the Janus kinase (JAK) inhibitor ruxolitinib, which blocks multiple cytokine signaling pathways[152,153]; anakinra, an IL1R antagonist effective in SHLH[154]; and monoclonal antibodies against IL-1, IL-6, and TNF-α, which have shown encouraging results in the treatment of acquired HLH[14] but could possibly be used in the management of FHLH as well, since these cytokines are also elevated in FHLH. The human recombinant IL18 binding protein tadekinig-α may be effective in pediatric patients with NLRC4-MAS and XIAP deficiency.[113,155] On the evidence of encouraging results in murine models, gene therapy targeting the genes involved in XLP1, FHL2, and FHL3 deficiency could open the way for future trials to evaluate the effectiveness of gene therapy as treatment of these forms of HLH.[113] Table 52-2 lists a number of features distinguishing FHLH and SHLH.

Differential Diagnosis

The diagnosis of HLH is a complex process that must be carried out rapidly, given the lethality of the disease, excluding mimicking conditions whose pathogenesis differs from that of authentic HLH, thus requiring alternative therapies.

A typical example is represented by sepsis, which significantly overlaps with many clinical features of HLH and can show hemophagocytosis, low NK-cell activity, and high sCD25.[156] Treatment of sepsis significantly differs from that of HLH, and in particular immunosuppression can be harmful in a patient with sepsis.[157] However, when patients with sepsis do not respond to antimicrobials and supportive measures, HLH should be considered and prompt the evaluation for HLH using the HLH-2004 diagnostic criteria.[73,113]

As HLH may be associated with an underlying lymphoma or leukemia, especially in adults, a search for a concurrent neoplasm should be conducted. Notably, in biopsy samples, the presence of a dense histiocytic reaction may obscure the recognition of the lymphoma.[158] There is evidence suggesting that a high sCD25 to ferritin ratio may point toward a lymphoma as an underlying cause for HLH rather than other secondary causes.[69]

LCH involving the bone marrow or visceral organs and multicentric Castleman disease, especially the TAFRO variant (thrombocytopenia, anasarca, myelofibrosis, renal dysfunction, and organomegaly) may closely resemble HLH. The treatment primarily addressing the underlying condition with or without additional corticosteroids can be effective in managing both of these diseases,[3] although disseminated LCH and TAFRO can, per se, be associated with a dismal prognosis.

Storage diseases in infants, such as Wolman disease (infantile lysosomal acid lipase deficiency) and GD, may present with extreme organomegaly or pancytopenia simulating HLH, even fulfilling the HLH-2004 criteria.[3,113] In most cases, however, these disorders develop features of HLH not caused by immune hyperactivation.[3] A correct diagnosis

is thus important because an HLH-oriented treatment is not indicated in both Wolman disease and GD. In contrast, patients with lysinuric protein intolerance and other metabolic disorders have been reported to develop authentic HLH,[3] with notable inflammatory features which may benefit from immune suppression.[159]

DIHS, also known as DRESS (drug reaction with eosinophilia and systemic symptoms), may present as HLH, with fever, liver function test abnormalities, and, rarely, hemophagocytosis, but generally lacks extremely high ferritin or cytopenias and shows skin rash and eosinophilia with temporal relationship with a drug, thus requiring withdrawal of the triggering drug and eventually corticosteroids.[160]

Certain uncommon clinical conditions can simulate HLH with restricted organ involvement, such as isolated CNS or liver HLH occurring in newborns. Isolated CNS HLH must be differentiated from viral encephalitis, autoimmune disseminated encephalomyelitis, CNS vasculitis, multiple sclerosis, Rasmussen encephalitis, febrile infection-related epilepsy syndrome (FIRES), and acute necrotizing encephalopathy, or interferonopathies.[3] Differential criteria are based on distinctive localization of the disease and imaging (e.g., single hemisphere in Rasmussen encephalitis, symmetric thalamic necrosis in acute necrotizing encephalopathy without marked matter changes, cerebral calcifications in interferonopathies),[3] while FIRES in some cases may really represent HLH.[161]

In newborns presenting with fulminant liver failure, HLH should be distinguished from gestational alloimmune liver disease, also known as neonatal hemochromatosis, associated with extrahepatic siderosis.[162] These patients can present with hyperferritinemia and coagulopathy, while hemophagocytosis and other signs of inflammation are absent.[163]

Increased histiocytes in the bone marrow may be associated with a chronic myeloproliferative disorder or MDS and may not represent HLH. Similarly, reactive lymph nodes with prominent sinus histiocytosis may occasionally exhibit hemophagocytosis. In the absence of the clinical and laboratory features of HLH, this diagnosis should not be proposed on the basis of biopsy findings. Hemophagocytosis can occur in histiocytic sarcoma (HS), but the presence of cell atypia and

Table 52-2 **Features Distinguish Primary and Secondary Hemophagocytic Lymphohistiocytosis**

Familial (Primary) HLH	Secondary HLH
Mendelian inherited conditions resulting in defects of immune regulation leading to hyperimmune states	Acquired conditions, except for rare cases in which an inherited condition is unknown; pathogenetic mechanisms causing the hyperimmune status poorly known
Familial involvement (autosomal recessive)	Not familial in most cases
Presentation in infancy	Presentation mostly in older individuals, except cases associated with autoimmunity
Usually not associated with immunodeficiency	Often associated with immunodeficiency
Onset may be triggered by a viral infection	Onset may be triggered by any infectious agent, malignant neoplasms, and allogenic HSCT
Not associated with autoimmunity	Can be associated with autoimmunity
Progressive disease, curable in about 50% of cases	Possible remission if the underlying cause can be eliminated; high mortality in cases associated with malignant neoplasms, especially lymphoma
Treatment mainly oriented toward hyperimmune state control	Treatment mainly oriented to elimination or control of the trigger
Perforin absent and mutations in perforin and other genes (30%)	Perforin expression and gene normal
Normal NK-cell numbers; absent NK-cell function	Normal or reduced NK-cell numbers and equivalent NK-cell function

HLH, Hemophagocytic lymphohistiocytosis; *HSCT*, hematopoietic stem cell transplantation; *NK*, natural killer.

mitoses easily permit identification of the neoplastic nature of the histiocytes.[164,165]

In RDD, nucleated cells are typically engulfed by macrophages, while phagocytosis of red blood cells is uncommon; in addition, numerous plasma cells are often present, and the macrophages strongly express S100.[166] Moreover, RDD very rarely involves the bone marrow and its clinical presentation is generally indolent. In contrast, a severe clinical onset classically occurs in newborns with ALK-positive histiocytosis, a rare disease often involving the bone marrow and sometimes associated with prominent hemophagocytosis.[167]

Extensive hemophagocytosis in the subcutaneous fat tissue is found in cytophagic histiocytic panniculitis, a rare disease associated with nonmalignant conditions, but more often representing the natural disease progression of subcutaneous panniculitis-like T-cell lymphoma.[168,169]

These patients rarely have the severe multiorgan involvement seen in HLH, but some cases evolve in HLH.[168,170,171]

Gaucher Disease

Definition

GD is the most common lysosomal storage disorder and it is inherited as an autosomal recessive trait. It is characterized by lipid storage and accumulation of glycosphingolipids in mononuclear phagocytes. There are three clinical subtypes of GD based on age of onset, disease progression rate, and absence or presence of early neurologic manifestations.[172]

Etiology

GD results from a deficiency in the lysosomal enzyme acid β-glucocerebrosidase, encoded by *GBA* on chromosome 1q21,[173,174] leading to the accumulation of the glycosphingolipids glucosylceramide and glucosylsphingosine in mononuclear phagocytes, primarily macrophages.[175] To date, more than 350 mutations have been reported involving the defective human gene *GBA*, the most common of which are p.N370S, p.L444P, and IVS2+1.[176,177] p.N370S and p.L444P account for the majority of mutant alleles in Ashkenazi Jews.[178,179] Type 1 disease is the most common lysosomal storage disorder and has a high incidence in this population.[180] Types 2 and 3 are pan-ethnic, although a variant of type 3 (Norrbottnian type) is reportedly more prevalent in Sweden.[181] A few patients have overlapping presentations that cannot be readily classified as a specific type.[177]

The accumulation of glucocerebrosides causes the release of various cytokines and lysosomal proteins from the activated macrophages, resulting in different presentations of the disease.[182] However, recent data indicate that the pathophysiology of GD is rather complex and may result from interconnection among different biological mechanisms, including oxidative stress, calcium dysregulation, mitochondrial dysfunction, autophagy defects, accumulation of α-synuclein aggregates, altered secretion and function of extracellular vesicles, and immunologic hyperactivity.[172]

Clinical Features

Type 1 GD is the most common variant. Although it is also referred to as "adult type," it may present clinically at any time between infancy and late adulthood, and it is diagnosed before the age of 20 in more than 50% of cases.[172] It has a wide range of severity, involving predominantly peripheral organs, such as the liver, spleen, skeletal muscle, and bone marrow, without neurologic involvement. Patients show hepatosplenomegaly, pancytopenia, osteolytic bone lesions, degenerative arthritis, and elevated risk of multiple myeloma.[175] Although GD type 1 is categorized as "nonneuropathic," middle-aged or elderly patients may develop peripheral neuropathy and symptomatic Lewy body–associated parkinsonism.[172]

Types 2 and 3 are typically neuropathic. Type 2 is acute and rapidly fatal within the first few years of life, whereas type 3 has a later onset and a chronic, progressive course, and it is more clinically heterogeneous than type 2 GD.[172,182] In type 2 GD, patients show limited psychomotor development; bulbar signs, including stridor and swallowing difficulty; stiffened opisthotonic posture; spasticity and trismus; and epilepsy.[175] In type 3 GD, the presenting symptoms include oculomotor apraxia, abnormal horizontal saccadic eye movements, and myoclonic or generalized epilepsy. Some individuals have an aggressive neurodegenerative disease and low life expectancy (6–20 years), while others may have negligible and nonprogressive neurologic symptoms and normal cognitive functions, and with the support of treatment, good quality of life until late middle age.[172,183] A perinatal lethal form of GD is the most severe variant and its complications can begin before birth or in early infancy; it is characterized by hepatosplenomegaly, pancytopenia, skin abnormalities, and nonimmune hydrops fetalis.[175]

Although initial studies of patients with GD demonstrated a 14.7-fold increased risk of cancer, especially hematologic malignant neoplasms,[184-186] more recent larger studies show no higher malignancy risk except for a reported 5.9-fold increased incidence of multiple myeloma.[187,188] Enzyme replacement therapy with recombinant enzyme is the current treatment; it is effective in reducing bone pain and hepatosplenomegaly but has a limited effect on neurologic symptoms.[175,188,189]

GD presents with a range of signs and symptoms that can hinder an early diagnosis, leading to significant delays and sometimes irreversible morbidities. Recently, the Gaucher Earlier Diagnosis Consensus (GED-C) Delphi project identified signs and covariables useful for early GD diagnosis and helping to increase the index of suspicion in recognizing patients suitable for diagnostic testing for GD.[190]

Morphology

The accumulated glucocerebrosides in the lysosomes of macrophages fill the cytoplasm, and on electron microscopy the storage material is composed of membrane-bound structures containing hollow tubules measuring 250 to 725 angstroms in diameter.[191] These macrophages, known as Gaucher cells, appear as large cells, 20 to 100 μm in diameter, with a single small nucleus and a cytoplasm showing a compactly striated or fibrillary pattern, with "wrinkled paper" appearance, reflecting the enlarged and deformed lysosomes, which are highlighted by CD68, recognizing lysosome-associated membrane glycoproteins. The cytoplasm of Gaucher cells stains positively with periodic acid–Schiff (PAS) and acid phosphatase techniques,[192] and pale blue to gray with Wright-Giemsa stain (Fig. 52-5).[191] Moreover, Gaucher cells show diffuse iron staining, in contrast to normal marrow histiocytes; this is probably secondary to phagocytosed red

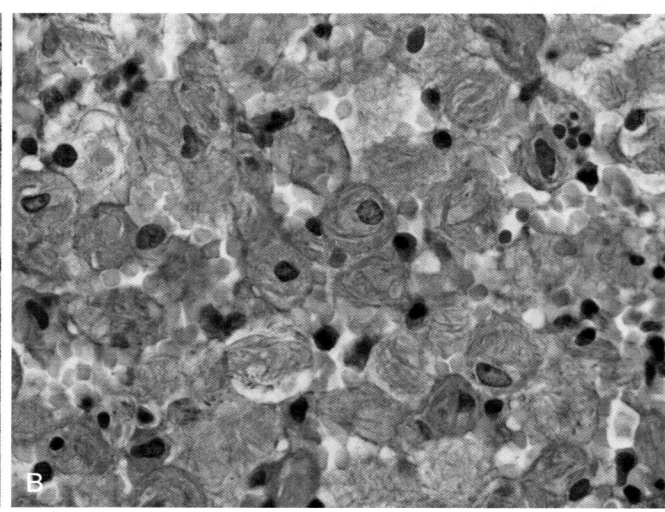

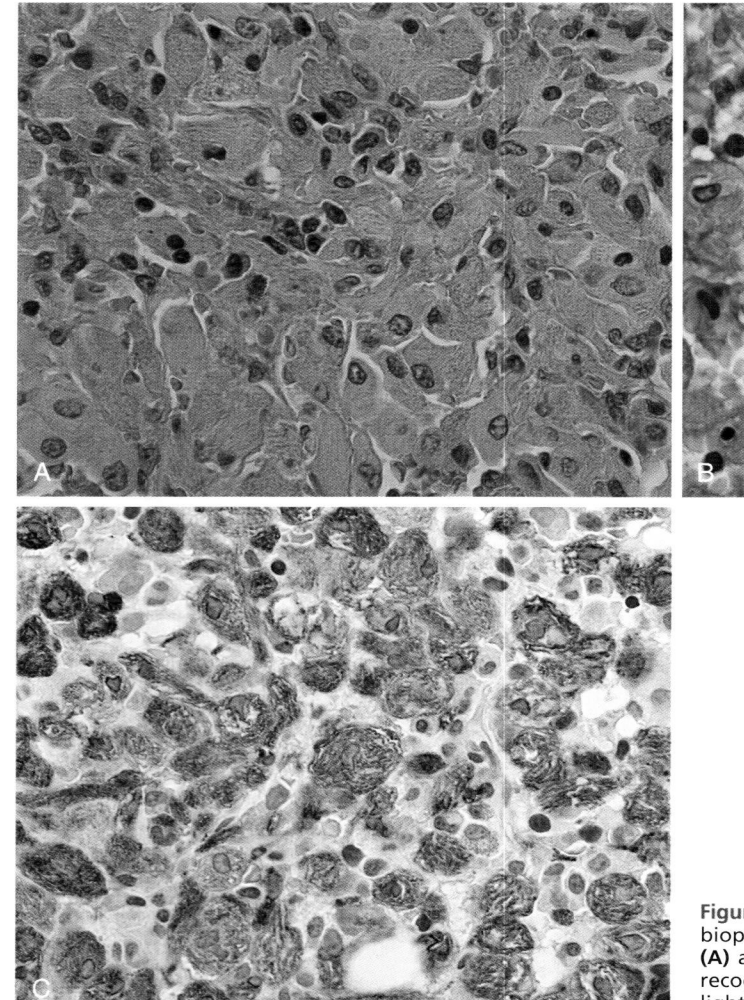

Figure 52-5. Gaucher disease. Gaucher cells in a bone marrow biopsy, showing the characteristic wrinkled paper cytoplasm **(A)** and positivity for periodic acid–Schiff (PAS) stain **(B)**. CD68, recognizing lysosome-associated membrane glycoproteins, highlights the peculiar structure of the cytoplasm of Gaucher cells **(C)**.

blood cells. In the bone marrow, these cells may diffusely replace the medullary cavity or form small aggregates and they are more recognizable in bone marrow biopsy than on smears.[191] The presence of histiocytes with diffuse iron uptake in the bone marrow suggests GD, and an appropriate clinical workup to rule out the disease should be initiated.[193]

Although an extensive infiltration of Gaucher cells in bone marrow biopsies strongly suggests GD, enzymatic assays for β-glucocerebrosidase activity in leukocytes and molecular analysis are the gold standard for GD diagnosis.[194,195] Plasma chitotriosidase levels, which are significantly elevated in GD, can also aid in establishing the diagnosis and can be used to monitor response to therapy as well.[177]

Currently clinical exome sequencing is extensively used in clinical practice[196] and multiplex ligation-dependent probe amplification has shown to be useful in the detection of *GBA* deletions and recombinations.[197,198]

Differential Diagnosis

Other disorders that cause the accumulation of histiocytes in tissues, such as other storage diseases, hemophagocytic syndromes, LCH, and infections are included in the differential diagnosis of GD. The most tricky differential diagnosis is represented by the occurrence of so-called "pseudo-Gaucher cells," which may be seen in various conditions characterized by increased cell turnover, especially in the bone marrow of patients with hematologic neoplasms, particularly chronic myelogenous leukemia.[199] They also occur in multiple myeloma, severe chronic hemolysis, congenital dyserythropoietic anemia, and other conditions.[191] These pseudo-Gaucher cells may have an identical cytologic appearance to true Gaucher cells, but generally are less prominently striated, are weakly PAS positive, and are positive for fat stains such as Sudan black B.[191]

In the spleen, red pulp histiocytosis can be prominent in patients with chronic idiopathic thrombocytopenic purpura, mimicking a storage disease. However, the identification of Gaucher cells with the characteristic cytoplasmic wrinkled paper appearance, in association with the typical clinical and laboratory findings, establishes a diagnosis of GD.

Niemann-Pick Disease

Definition

NPD is an autosomal recessive lipid storage disorder that is characterized by an accumulation of sphingomyelin and cholesterol in the lysosomes of cells of the macrophage-monocyte system, resulting in the accumulation of foamy histiocytes in the bone marrow, spleen, liver, and lymph nodes. NPD is classified into three main subtypes: NPD types A and B are caused by a congenital deficiency of sphingomyelinase, while NPD type C is pathophysiologically unrelated to types A and B and is caused by a defect in intracellular lipid transport.

Etiology

NPD types A and B are caused by a deficiency in acid sphingomyelinase activity resulting from mutations of the acid sphingomyelinase gene (*SMPD1*).[200] Three common missense mutations account for more than 90% of the mutant alleles in individuals of Ashkenazi Jewish ancestry in type A, whereas the most frequent mutation in type B is p.R608del.[201-203] Type C NPD is caused by a defect in the intracellular cholesterol transport from the lysosome to the cytosol because of either *NPC1* (intracellular cholesterol transporter 1) or *NPC2* mutations,[202,204] resulting in the overaccumulation of cholesterol and glycosphingolipids in late endosomal/lysosomal compartments. An *NPC1* mutation, mapped to chromosome 18q11, occurs in the majority of patients (95%),[205-207] whereas mutations in *NPC2*, mapped to chromosome 14q24.3, are rare.[175,206,208-210]

Dementia is a common symptom in patients with NPD type C, and postmortem studies of brains have shown many histopathologic features typically associated with late-onset Alzheimer disease, suggesting that the cell biology of NPD type C involves acceleration of processes typically found in this disease and associated with aging in the general population.[175]

Clinical Features

NPD type A patients present in early infancy with hepatosplenomegaly, failure to thrive, and a rapidly progressive neurologic course; death usually occurs within the first 2 years of life.[203] In contrast, patients with type B disease have a later onset of symptoms, and sometimes the diagnosis is made when they are adult. Patients present in late childhood with hepatosplenomegaly that eventually leads to liver cirrhosis and progressive pulmonary disease. Neurologic symptoms are lacking, the clinical course is more variable, and fatalities can occur in early adulthood.[203] The clinical severity and organ involvement in NPD types A and B are related to the level of residual SMPD1 activity, which is almost undetectable in patients with type A disease, whereas type B patients typically have 10% to 20% of normal activity, which presumably prevents the development of neurologic symptoms.

NPD type C patients exhibit a variable age at diagnosis and are clinically heterogeneous.[207,211] Hepatosplenomegaly is less prominent than in the other NPD types and may be absent. Three type C NPD clinical subtypes have been described, based on the age at onset of neurologic symptoms: infantile (including early-infantile and late-infantile), juvenile, and adolescent/adult-onset disease forms.[210] *NPC1* mutations are most commonly associated with the juvenile-onset form,[206,207] which typically presents with neonatal jaundice that eventually resolves, followed by an asymptomatic period, and subsequently by progressive neurologic deterioration. The age at onset of neurologic manifestations is an important parameter to assess, as patients with early-onset symptoms tend to have a more morbid clinical course and increased fatality rates.[210]

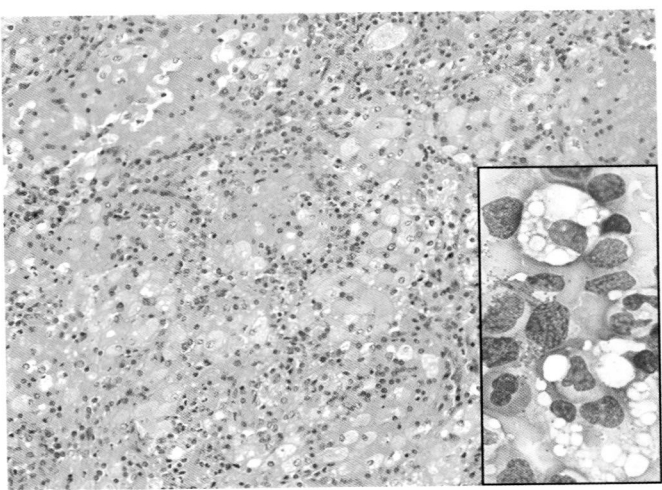

Figure 52-6. Niemann-Pick disease. Spleen from a patient with Niemann-Pick disease (NPD) showing aggregates of foam cells. The *inset* shows histiocytes in the bone marrow with distended cytoplasm caused by the presence of vacuoles that are characteristic of foam cells (Niemann-Pick cells). *(Inset courtesy Dr. Russell Brynes.)*

Morphology

In blood smears, lymphocytes with numerous sharply defined lipid vacuoles may be observed, while in bone marrow smears and biopsies two types of histiocytes are present: classic Niemann-Pick cells and sea-blue histiocytes.[191] The Niemann-Pick cells are enlarged macrophages with a single, often eccentric nucleus and abundant cytoplasm that is distended by vacuoles that contain sphingomyelin and cholesterol, resulting in the characteristic foamy cells (Fig. 52-6). The cytoplasm may also appear granular or partially vacuolated, and it is sometimes entirely occupied by large vacuoles. The presence of foam cells in the bone marrow space, red pulp sinusoids of the spleen, or intraparenchymal sinusoids of the liver is highly suggestive of NPD, but not pathognomonic. In advanced disease, aggregates of foam cells can replace the architecture of the organ involved. Sea-blue histiocytes are large histiocytes containing in their cytoplasm bright blue cytoplasmic granules of varying size. They may also contain vacuoles, and transitional forms between the foamy cells and sea-blue histiocytes can be observed.[191] In NPD type A, the "foamy" histiocytes predominate,[212] while in NPD types B and C, the sea-blue histiocytes are more often present and may predominate. Classic NPD cells stain with lipid stains such as Sudan black B and oil red O, and are weak or negative with PAS. Sea-blue histiocytes stain blue with May-Grünwald-Giemsa and are variably positive for PAS and Sudan black B.[191] On electron microscopy, the classic NPD cells contain lipid inclusions ranging from 0.5 to 50.0 μm in size, some with a lamellar appearance.

The diagnosis of NPD types A and B is confirmed by demonstration of reduced SMPD1 enzymatic activity in tissue samples, leukocyte extracts, or cultured skin fibroblasts.[200,213] In type C, NPD diagnosis is provided using filipin staining to demonstrate accumulated unesterified cholesterol in cultured fibroblasts or peripheral blood cells, and in positive cases by validation by DNA mutational analysis.[213,214] The measurement in plasma of 7-ketocholesterol and cholestanetriol have been reported to be useful screening tools, providing important diagnostic support for a disease that, because of its heterogeneous clinical phenotype, is often diagnosed with a delay of many years or even totally missed.[215,216]

Differential Diagnosis

The differential diagnosis of NPD includes any disorder in which histiocytes infiltrate and accumulate in tissues, such as infectious diseases, hemophagocytic syndrome, and other storage disorders. Hyperlipidemias can cause lipid accumulation in the cytoplasm of histiocytes, thus mimicking NPD cells; however, the presence of hepatosplenomegaly and bone marrow infiltration, along with identification of decreased sphingomyelinase activity in leukocytes, confirms the diagnosis of NPD. Sea-blue histiocytes may be present in variable numbers in high cell turnover states in which pseudo-Gaucher cells are also seen,[191] while marked infiltration of sea-blue histiocytes may occur in hyperlipidemic states and in patients receiving total parenteral nutrition containing lipid emulsions.[217] Foamy histiocytes are also found in Erdheim-Chester disease (ECD), but the association with progressive fibrosis and, especially, the markedly different clinical presentation easily allows its distinction from NPD.

Tangier Disease

Definition

Tangier disease (TD) is a rare autosomal recessive disorder characterized by severe deficiency or absence of high-density lipoprotein (HDL) in the circulation, and tissue accumulation of cholesteryl esters throughout the body, particularly in tissue macrophages.[218,219]

Etiology

TD is caused by pathogenic variants in the *ABCA1* gene, which encodes the ATP-binding cassette transporter A1,[220,221] which facilitates the efflux of cholesterol from cells to emerging HDL particles. Loss-of-function *ABCA1* variants result in reduced ABCA1 synthesis or activity and a diminished cholesterol efflux capacity. In homozygotes, the impaired efflux of free cholesterol from cells and the intracellular accumulation of cholesteryl esters prevent the conversion of lipid-poor apoA-I into preβ-HDL particles, while heterozygotes display an intermediate phenotype with low HDL-cholesterol and about 50% decrease in ABCA1-mediated cholesterol efflux.[218]

Most of the clinical manifestations of TD are largely because of the deposition of sterols in tissues.[220,222] Thrombocytopenia is caused by the sequestration of platelets in the enlarged spleen; in addition, altered platelet morphology and impaired platelet function and defective activation may be caused by reduced ABCA1 expression on platelets.[223]

Clinical Features

The main clinical features of TD include hyperplastic yellow-orange tonsils, hepatosplenomegaly, and peripheral neuropathy. Other complications include premature atherosclerotic coronary artery disease, corneal opacities, skin lesions, mild thrombocytopenia, reticulocytosis, stomatocytosis, or hemolytic anemia. In some individuals, the disease is clinically silent and only biochemical anomalies are recognizable. Peripheral neuropathies are found in 51% of patients, usually occur after the age of 15 years and consist of relapsing-remitting mononeuropathy or polyneuropathy.[224]

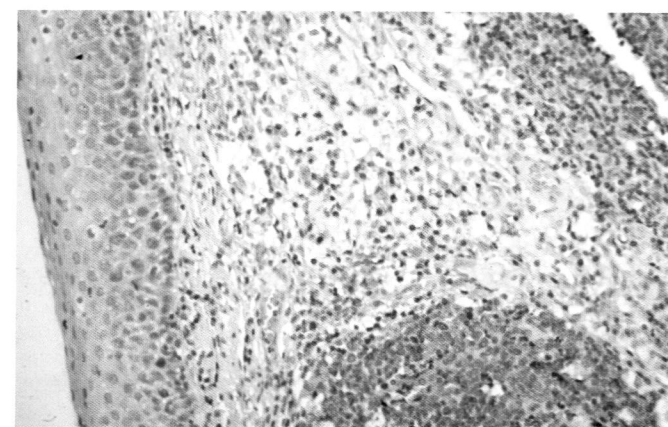

Figure 52-7. Tangier disease. Tonsil of a patient with Tangier disease showing accumulation of mature histiocytes in association with reactive lymphoid tissue. *(Courtesy Dr. Russell Brynes.)*

Despite patients with TD having very low or absent plasma HDL-cholesterol (<5 mg/dL) and very low or absent plasma apoA-I (<30 mg/dL),[218] 25% to 44% of them develop coronary artery disease,[225,226] perhaps owing to the partial protection offered by the coexistence of decreased low-density lipoprotein.[220] In a study including 185 patients with TD,[226] 25% had cardiovascular disease (about half of those aged 40–65 years), compared with 11% of age- and sex-matched controls.[226] Notably, premature atherosclerotic coronary artery disease is observed in TD patients but also in heterozygous carriers of *ABCA1* variants.[227] No effective treatment is currently available for this disorder, but glycosphingolipid inhibition represents a potential novel therapy for the neurologic complications.[228]

Morphology

Microscopically, the affected tissues demonstrate a marked accumulation of histiocytes with a large pale microvacuolar cytoplasm, containing lipid droplets and occasionally crystalline material. Lipid droplets are unbounded by membranes and are not present in lysosomes.[229,230] In tonsils and lymph nodes, the foamy histiocytes aggregate in clusters in the parafollicular area. Foamy histiocytes have also been detected in the thymus, skin, Schwann cells in peripheral nerves, and colonic and rectal mucosa, while they are scanty in the bone marrow and spleen.[229-231] Tissue accumulation of lipid-laden macrophages provides a clue to the diagnosis of TD but is not pathognomonic (Fig. 52-7). The clinical symptoms and the extremely low levels of HDL usually establishes the diagnosis, which is confirmed by detecting an *ABCA1* mutation.

HISTIOCYTIC AND DENDRITIC CELL NEOPLASMS

Introduction

Histiocytic/dendritic cell (H/DC) neoplasms, often collectively referred to as *histiocytoses*, are derived from the macrophages, dendritic cells, and monocytes of the mononuclear phagocyte system. The term *histiocyte* is a morphologic term, variably referring to a tissue-resident macrophage[2] or to the group of immune cells that includes macrophages and dendritic cells.[232]

Conventional (myeloid) dendritic cells and plasmacytoid dendritic cells are derived from bone marrow precursors[233] and Langerhans cells and tissue-resident macrophages, including microglia, are now thought to be long-lasting and self-renewing populations derived from fetal yolk sac erythro-myeloid progenitors.[234,235] However, it has been shown in mice models that bone marrow–derived myeloid precursors, including monocytes, can replenish these cell populations in an inflammatory context by differentiating into macrophages or Langerhans cells at sites of inflammation.[233,236] Thus, there is great heterogeneity and plasticity among the cells of the mononuclear phagocyte system, as well as complex cellular origins. Although follicular dendritic cell sarcomas (FDCSs) have been traditionally grouped under the category of *H/DC neoplasms*, unlike most other neoplasms in this category whose origins appear to be from bone marrow–derived precursor cells, these tumors are derived from follicular dendritic cells (FDCs) that are of mesenchymal origin.[237] FDCs have been intensively studied in lymph nodes, where they participate as antigen-presenting cells in the germinal center reaction,[238] but FDCS is not restricted to lymph nodes and may occur in extranodal sites as well.[239]

There are currently three systems used to classify neoplasms of histiocytic and dendritic cell lineages: the International Consensus Classification (ICC)[240] (Box 52-3); the World Health Organization (WHO) classification[241] (Box 52-4), which is currently in its 5th edition; and the 2016 revised classification of histiocytoses and neoplasms of the macrophage-dendritic cell lineages of the Histiocyte Society[2] (Box 52-5). The more recent ICC and WHO classifications include ALK-positive histiocytosis as a distinct disease type. Other changes in the WHO 5th edition classification are the inclusion of RDD and clonal plasmacytoid dendritic cell diseases in the *H/DC neoplasia* category and the moving of the mesenchymal stromal cell-derived FDCS and fibroblastic reticular cell tumor to a separate category. The revised classification from the histiocyte society divides the histiocytoses into five groups based on clinical, radiographic, pathologic, phenotypic, genetic, or molecular features while also incorporating hemophagocytic syndromes.[2]

Immunohistochemical and Molecular Evaluation of Histiocytic Disorders

IHC studies are essential in the diagnosis of histiocytic neoplasia and play a key role in distinguishing between the various subtypes. A basic IHC panel at diagnosis should include CD163, CD68, S100, CD1a, langerin (CD207), factor XIIIa, ALK, and cyclin D1. IHCs with *BRAF* p.V600E-specific antibody (VE1) is also recommended in suspected LCH and ECD, but negative or equivocal IHC for this antibody does not exclude mutated *BRAF* p.V600E[242] (Table 52-3).

Molecular evaluation by next-generating sequencing (NGS) and fusion testing has become increasingly important. The detection of activating alterations in RAS/RAF/MAPK/ERK and PI3K/AKT pathway genes not only aids in the diagnosis of histiocytic neoplasia, but also identifies potential targets for systemic therapy. NGS should assess for targetable somatic variants in common MAPK pathway genes such as *BRAF, MAP2K1, KRAS, NRAS, PIK3CA, ARAF, RAF1, MAP2K2, MAP3K1,* and *CSF1R*. Fusion testing should include *BRAF, ALK,* and *NTRK1* rearrangements.[242]

Box 52-3 *International Consensus Classification of Histiocytic and Dendritic Cell Neoplasms*

Histiocytic sarcoma
Langerhans cell histiocytosis
Langerhans cell sarcoma
Indeterminate dendritic cell histiocytosis
Interdigitating dendritic cell sarcoma
ALK-positive histiocytosis
Disseminated juvenile xanthogranuloma
Erdheim-Chester disease
Rosai-Dorfman-Destombes disease
Follicular dendritic cell sarcoma
Fibroblastic reticular cell sarcoma
Epstein-Barr virus-positive inflammatory follicular dendritic cell/fibroblastic reticular cell tumor

---

Box 52-4 *World Health Organization (5th Edition) Classification of Histiocytic and Dendritic Cell Neoplasms*

Plasmacytoid Dendritic Cell Neoplasms
Mature plasmacytoid dendritic cell proliferation associated with myeloid neoplasm
Blastic plasmacytoid dendritic cell neoplasm

Langerhans Cell and Other Dendritic Cell Neoplasms
Langerhans cell neoplasms
Langerhans cell histiocytosis
Langerhans cell sarcoma

Other Dendritic Cell Neoplasms
Indeterminate dendritic cell tumor
Interdigitating dendritic cell sarcoma

Histiocytic Neoplasms
Juvenile xanthogranuloma
Erdheim-Chester disease
Rosai-Dorfman disease
ALK-positive histiocytosis
Histiocytic sarcoma

Langerhans Cell Histiocytosis

Definition

Langerhans cell histiocytosis (LCH) is neoplastic H/DC disorder characterized by tissue infiltration by S100-positive/CD1a-positive/langerin (CD207)-positive cells and driven by activation of the MAPK pathway. *BRAF* p.V600E mutations are present in more than half of cases.[243]

Synonyms and Related Terms

Langerhans cell histiocytosis (ICC); Langerhans cell histiocytosis (WHO 5th ed.); Langerhans cell histiocytosis (WHO Revised 4th ed.); Langerhans cell histiocytosis (Revised Classification of the Histiocyte Society, 2016).

Background

Historical aspects of LCH have been detailed in a number of reviews.[244-246] One of the earliest descriptions in modern times has been attributed to Dr. Thomas Smith in 1865 who described a child with impetigo and three large holes in the calvarium, which he surmised to be congenital lesions.[247] A few decades later, a number of apparently separate diseases with characteristic clinical features emerged. In 1893, Dr. Alfred Hand reported a 3-year-old boy with exophthalmos

Box 52-5 *Revised Classification of Histiocytoses and Neoplasms of the Macrophage-Dendritic Cell Lineages (Histiocyte Society, 2016)*

L Group
Langerhans cell histiocytosis (LCH)
Indeterminate cell histiocytosis
Erdheim-Chester disease
Mixed Langerhans cell histiocytosis/Erdheim-Chester disease

C Group
Cutaneous non-Langerhans cell histiocytosis
- Nonxanthogranuloma family: cutaneous Rosai-Dorfman disease, necrobiotic xanthogranuloma, other (not otherwise specified, NOS)
- Xanthogranuloma family: juvenile xanthogranuloma, adult xanthogranuloma, solitary reticulohistiocytoma, benign cephalic histiocytosis, generalized eruptive histiocytosis, progressive nodular histiocytosis
Cutaneous non-LCH with a major systemic component

R Group
Familial Rosai-Dorfman disease (RDD)
Sporadic RDD
- Classical RDD
- Extranodal RDD
- RDD with neoplasia or immune disease
- Unclassified

M Group
Primary malignant histiocytoses
Secondary malignant histiocytoses (after or associated with another hematologic neoplasia)
- Histiocytic
- Interdigitating
- Langerhans
- Indeterminate cell

H Group
Primary hemophagocytic lymphohistiocytosis (HLH) (monogenic inherited conditions leading to HLH)
Secondary HLH (non-Mendelian HLH)
HLH of unknown/uncertain origin

who presented with polydipsia and polyuria and was found to have a skull lesion at autopsy.[248] Similar patients were also described in 1905 by Dr. Thomas W. Kay,[249] in 1915 by Dr. Artur Schüller,[250] and in 1920 by Dr. Henry Christian[251]; this co-occurrence of exophthalmos, diabetes insipidus, and bone lesions became known as Hand-Schüller-Christian disease. Letterer-Siwe disease, first named in 1936,[252] described a clinical syndrome of hepatosplenomegaly, lymphadenopathy, bone lesions, anemia, purpura, and hyperplasia of nonlipid-storing macrophages in various organs.[253,254] Isolated bone lesions with similar histologic features to Hand-Schüller-Christian disease were also observed,[255,256] termed *eosinophilic granuloma of the bone* by Jaffe and Lichtenstein.[257] By the early 1940s, overlap between these different disorders was noted, with eventual unification under the name *histiocytosis X*.[258] In 1973, Dr. Christian Nezelof observed similarities between the Langerhans cell and the cells of histiocytosis X, including the common presence of Birbeck granules on ultrastructural examination.[259] The term *Langerhans cell histiocytosis* as a name for the disorder followed,[260] and LCH was integrated into the recommended classification of histiocytosis in children from the Histiocyte Society, published in 1987.[261] Currently, LCH is

categorized within the L (Langerhans) group of disorders in the 2016 revised classification of histiocytoses and neoplasms of the macrophage-dendritic cell lineages from the Histiocyte Society.[2]

Epidemiology

LCH is predominantly a disease of children, with an incidence in the literature ranging from 2 to 9 per million children per year.[262,263] In a recent analysis, most cases reported over a 6-year period in the United States were in those under the age of five,[264] decreasing with age. There is a male predominance.[262-264] The exact incidence of adult LCH is not well established; currently figures stand at 1 to 1.5 cases per million population per year,[265] but this is likely to be an underestimate. In younger patients (0–20 years), the most common sites affected are bone and skin, whereas in older age groups (21–100 years), lung involvement increases dramatically while bone and skin involvement decreases.[264]

Etiology, Pathogenesis, and Cell of Origin

Studies on the pathogenesis of LCH have examined inflammatory and infectious mechanisms, including the role of viruses such as EBV, CMV, Merkel cell polyomavirus, and HHV8.[266,267] Evidence of the clonal nature of the disease was first shown using HUMARA gene assay,[268] and in 2010, recurrent *BRAF* p.V600E mutations were identified in 57% of archival LCH cases,[243] indicating the neoplastic nature of disorder. It was also shown that the cells in LCH had evidence of MAPK pathway activation regardless of mutational status, a finding also observed in other studies.[269,270] Since then, other non-p.V600E activating alterations have been described in *BRAF*[271] and in other genes of the MAPK pathway, including largely mutually exclusive mutations in *MAP2K1*[269,272] and mutations in *ARAF*.[273] Recurrent mutations in *NRAS*[270,274,275] have mostly been described in pulmonary LCH (PLCH), including concurrent *NRAS* and *BRAF* p.V600E mutations that occurred within distinct lesional cell populations.[270] *KRAS* mutations have been very rarely observed.[270,276]

In tandem with the discoveries related to molecular pathogenesis, there has been progress in the understanding of the cell of origin of the disease. Originally, differentiation from Langerhans cells was postulated because of the immunophenotype (CD1a-positive and langerin [CD207]-positive) and the presence of Birbeck granules in the cells of LCH on ultrastructural examination. Against this, langerin (CD207) expression was also observed in various other dendritic cell subsets,[277] and transcriptional studies showed that the neoplastic cell in LCH was more closely related to immature myeloid dendritic cells than to the hypothesized epidermal Langerhans cell.[278] Furthermore, in a subset of patients, the *BRAF* p.V600E mutation was detected in circulating CD14-positive monocytes and CD11c-positive myeloid dendritic cells, and also in CD34-positive bone marrow progenitors[279] in keeping with origin from a hematopoietic precursor. This led to the proposition of a model of misguided myeloid dendritic cell differentiation, whereby the stage of development of the hematopoietic cell in which the somatic mutation occurs determines the clinical severity of the disease and its distribution, such that somatic mutation in a hematopoietic stem cell or dendritic cell precursor may determine progression to high-risk disease and mutation in a tissue-restricted dendritic cell progenitor or differentiated dendritic cell may determine multifocal low-risk or single-site

Table 52-3 Typical Immunohistochemical Features of Histiocytic and Dendritic Cell Neoplasms

	Langerhans Cell Histiocytosis	Indeterminate Dendritic Cell Histiocytosis	Erdheim-Chester Disease	Juvenile Xanthogranuloma	ALK-Positive Histiocytosis	Rosai-Dorfman Disease	Histiocytic Sarcoma	Langerhans Cell Sarcoma	Interdigitating Dendritic Cell Sarcoma	Follicular Dendritic Cell Sarcoma
CD68	+	-/+	+	+	+	+	+	-/+	-/+	-/+
CD163	-	-	+	+	+	+	+	-/+	-/+	-/+
Factor XIIIa	-	*	+	+	+/-	+/-	*	*	*	-
S100	+	+/-	-/+	-/+	+/-	+	-/+	+/-	+	-
Langerin (CD207)	+	-	-	-	-	-	-	+/-	-	-
CD1a	+	+	-	-	-	-	-	+/-	-	-
BRAF p.V600E (VE1)	+/-	-/+	+/-	-	-	-	-/+	-/+	-/+	‡
ALK	-	-	-/+†	-	+	-	+	-	-	-
NTRK1	-	-	-	+†	-	-	+	-	-	+
CD21	-	-	-	-	-	-	-	-	-	+
CD23	-	-	-	-	-	-	-	-	-	+
CD35	-	-	-	-	-	-	-	-	-	+
Clusterin	-	-	-	-	-	-	-	-	-	+

*Not known.
†Fusion has been reported from one study.[511]
‡BRAF p.V600E genetic alteration reported from one study.[511]
+, Positive; −, negative; +/−, positive in a significant number of cases; −/+, negative in most cases.

Data from Go RS., et al., Histiocytic Neoplasms, Version 2.2021, NCCN Clinical practice guidelines in oncology. *J Natl Compr Canc Netw*, 2021. 19(11): pp. 1277-1303. Goyal G., et al., International expert consensus recommendations for the diagnosis and treatment of Langerhans cell histiocytosis in adults. *Blood*, 2022. 139(17): pp. 2601-2621. Davick JJ., et al., Indeterminate dendritic cell tumor: a report of two new cases lacking the ETV3-NCOA2 translocation and a literature review. *Am J Dermatopathol*, 2018. 40(10): pp. 736-748. Goyal G., et al., Erdheim-Chester disease: consensus recommendations for evaluation, diagnosis, and treatment in the molecular era. *Blood*, 2020. 135(22): p. 1929-1945. Kemps PG., et al., ALK-positive histiocytosis: a new clinicopathologic spectrum highlighting neurologic involvement and responses to ALK inhibition. *Blood*, 2022. 139(2): pp. 256-280. Zhou J., et al., Interdigitating dendritic cell sarcoma: analysis of two original extra-nodal cases and review of literature. *Virchows Arch*, 2022.

disease.[245] However, understanding remains imperfect. There is also evidence for an embryonic cell-of-origin shown by a mouse model in which targeted expression of *BRAF* p.V600E mutation in yolk sac erythro-myeloid progenitors and the resident macrophage lineage results in a neurodegenerative process similar to that of histiocytic disorders.[280]

Studies investigating the mechanisms through which ERK activation in myeloid dendritic cell precursors mediates LCH pathogenesis have identified *BRAF* p.V600E-induced senescence in hematopoietic progenitors as contributing to LCH pathophysiology[281] and show that extracellular signal-related kinase activity induced by *BRAF* p.V600E inhibits C-C motif chemokine receptor 7 (CCR7)-mediated dendritic cell migration, trapping dendritic cells in tissue lesions. Furthermore, *BRAF* p.V600E increases expression of BCL2-like protein 1 (*BCL2L1*) in dendritic cells, resulting in resistance to apoptosis.[282]

Clinical Features

LCH affects a wide age distribution from neonates to adults, and has a diverse clinical presentation depending on the affected organ systems, ranging from a self-limited course with a single site of involvement to a more aggressive disseminated, multisystem disease.[246]

Single-system LCH (SS-LCH) has one or more LCH lesions that are confined to a single tissue or organ. Multisystem LCH (MS-LCH) shows lesions in two or more organs/systems such as skin, bone, lung, lymph node, spleen, CNS, and liver. Involvement of the liver, spleen, and hematopoietic system in children is associated with an increased risk of mortality[283] and the presence or absence of this "risk organ" involvement further stratifies these patients into high and low risk categories. Recent consensus guidelines on the diagnosis and treatment of adult LCH do not differentiate risk-organ disease as a separate entity because of a lack of current data on prognostic and therapeutic implications in adults, and these guidelines have additionally proposed categories for SS-LCH of unifocal, single-system pulmonary (isolated lung involvement) and single-system multifocal (more than one lesion involving any organ) LCH in the adult age group.[265]

Involvement of the skin and skeletal system are frequent in LCH, and skeletal manifestations are present in 80% of cases.[144,284] Single-system bone disease in LCH may be unifocal or multifocal, and most often involves the skull vault in children, classically identified as punched-out lytic lesions on plain radiographs (Fig. 52-8). Other frequently involved sites include the vertebra, limbs, and pelvis.[285] Lesions may be asymptomatic or can have an associated soft tissue component that may encroach upon surrounding structures. Lesions of the frontal, ethmoid, occipital, sphenoid, zygomatic, and temporal bones have been considered CNS-risk lesions as they seem to be associated with a higher risk of developing CNS-LCH and diabetes insipidus.[283]

Skin involvement by LCH may present in the neonatal period as vesicles and pustules or crusted papulonodular lesions that mostly involve the scalp, face, and trunk and have a tendency to regress spontaneously within weeks or months (congenital self-healing LCH or Hashimoto-Pritzker syndrome). A significant subset of these patients have or will develop multisystem disease, necessitating careful evaluation and follow-up.[286] Other typical cutaneous presentations include an eczematous or seborrheic rash that may be mistaken for cradle cap or for fungal infection if involving intertriginous areas. Gingival lesions, ulceration, and tooth loss may be seen in oral cavity involvement.[287]

Lymphadenopathy related to LCH is most often evident in the cervical lymph nodes.[288] Lung involvement occurs in around 24% of children with multisystem disease[289] and there may be associated symptomatology, such as cough or shortness of breath, and imaging studies may show blebs, bullae, or fibrosis. Involvement of the hematopoietic system manifests clinically as cytopenias, usually anemia or thrombocytopenia.[283] Liver involvement presents with hepatomegaly (>3 cm below the costal margin at the midclavicular line confirmed by ultrasound) or liver dysfunction.[283] Other organ systems involved include the thyroid, thymus, and gastrointestinal tract. Some patients with MS-LCH may develop HLH.[71]

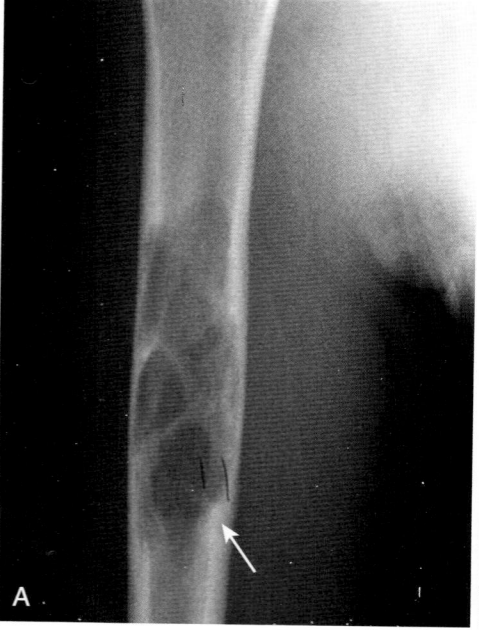
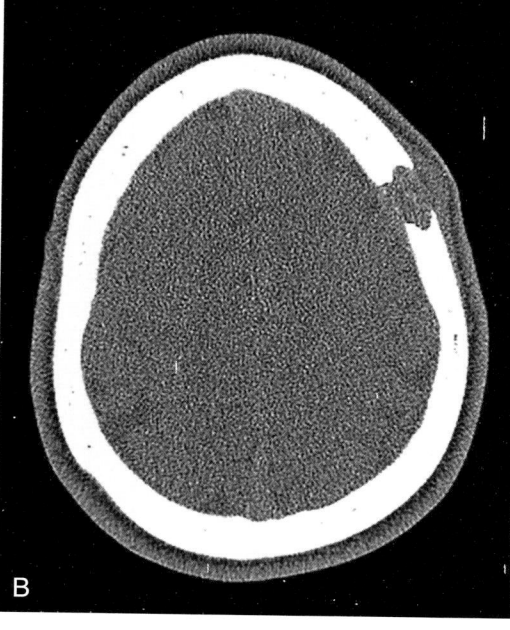

Figure 52-8. Langerhans cell histiocytosis in bone. A, Bones of the upper limb have extensive osteolytic changes on radiography. **B,** Computed tomography scan of the head reveals an osseous defect and adjacent soft tissue component.

Neurodegenerative LCH lesions (ND-LCH) are a late-onset complication of LCH manifesting as neurologic symptoms, particularly cerebellar ataxia, neurocognitive impairment, pyramidal signs, pseudobulbar palsy, and psychiatric disorders.[290] The median incidence of clinical ND-LCH is approximately 1 per year, and affected patients have typically been previously treated for a multisystem, risk-organ negative LCH. The presence of the *BRAF* p.V600E mutation is associated with a high risk of development of clinical ND-LCH in patients with pituitary, skull base, or orbit bone involvement.[290] LCH lesions may also present in the CNS, including in the hypothalamic-pituitary region with resultant diabetes insipidus, or as dural masses.[291]

Langerhans Cell Histiocytosis in Adults

LCH in adults presents with a similar symptomatology to childhood cases, although the likelihood of an alternative diagnosis is higher and prognostic stratification according to risk organ status is not currently considered relevant in the adult setting.[265,292] PLCH is commonly a single-system disease in adults, which has a very strong association with smoking and has a peak incidence of between 20 and 40 years of age.[293] There is also a higher incidence of oral and genital mucosa involvement in adults.[294]

Morphology

The histopathologic diagnosis of LCH requires a tissue biopsy showing a population of large (15–25 μm) histiocytic cells with ample eosinophilic cytoplasm and distinctive nuclear features with a complex, folded nuclear outline and often a nuclear groove ("coffee-bean nucleus") (Fig. 52-9; Fig. 52-10A). The cells are round-to-oval in shape and do not have the dendritic morphology of admixed inflammatory dendritic cells. Occasional multinucleated giant cells may be present. There is often an associated inflammatory milieu. Eosinophils are commonly present and may form microabscesses. Small lymphocytes and macrophages may be seen; however, plasma cells are typically rare.[2,295] Mitotic activity can be identified, as can focal necrosis; however, the presence of nuclear pleomorphism, frank cytologic atypia, and atypical mitoses should prompt consideration of Langerhans cell sarcoma (LCS), particularly in older patients.

Immunophenotype

The phenotype of LCH is characterized by the expression of S100 (nuclear and cytoplasmic), CD1a (surface and paranuclear), and langerin (CD207) (granular cytoplasmic), which correlates with Birbeck granule formation, replacing the requirement for ultrastructural examination (Fig. 52-10B; Fig. 52-11).[283] LCH cells show Golgi expression of CD68, but are usually negative for other monocytic and macrophage markers, including CD14, OCT2, and CD163.[265] Most cases show strong cyclin D1 expression in contrast to reactive Langerhans cell populations.[296]

In cases harboring a *BRAF* p.V600E mutation, IHC using the mutant-specific antibody clone VE1 shows moderate to strong cytoplasmic staining in mutated cells. However, the immunostaining has variable sensitivity and specificity in tissue biopsies based on the cellularity of the tumor and staining intensity; therefore, it is currently recommended to confirm any negative or equivocal results by molecular methods such as *BRAF* p.V600E allele-specific PCR.[242,265]

Histopathologic Features and Differential Diagnosis in Various Sites of Involvement

LCH can usually be separated from other forms of histiocytosis on the basis of histomorphology and immunophenotype, although care must be taken in small biopsies to avoid over-interpretation of perilesional macrophage infiltrates as non-LCH neoplasia (Table 52-3).

Bone

LCH in bone usually manifests as a lytic lesion composed of sheets of atypical cells with the diagnostic immunophenotype within an inflammatory background including eosinophils and osteoclast-like giant cells. There can be associated cortical destruction and necrosis and hemorrhage may be present. Some cases can show aneurysmal bone cyst-like features (Fig. 52-12).[297]

In long-standing lesions and lesions with an associated fracture, extensive fibrosis or xanthomatous changes may supervene and the LCH cells may be few or absent, precluding definitive diagnosis.[298] Distinction of LCH from reactive conditions such as chronic recurrent multifocal osteomyelitis may be challenging on the basis of histopathology in these

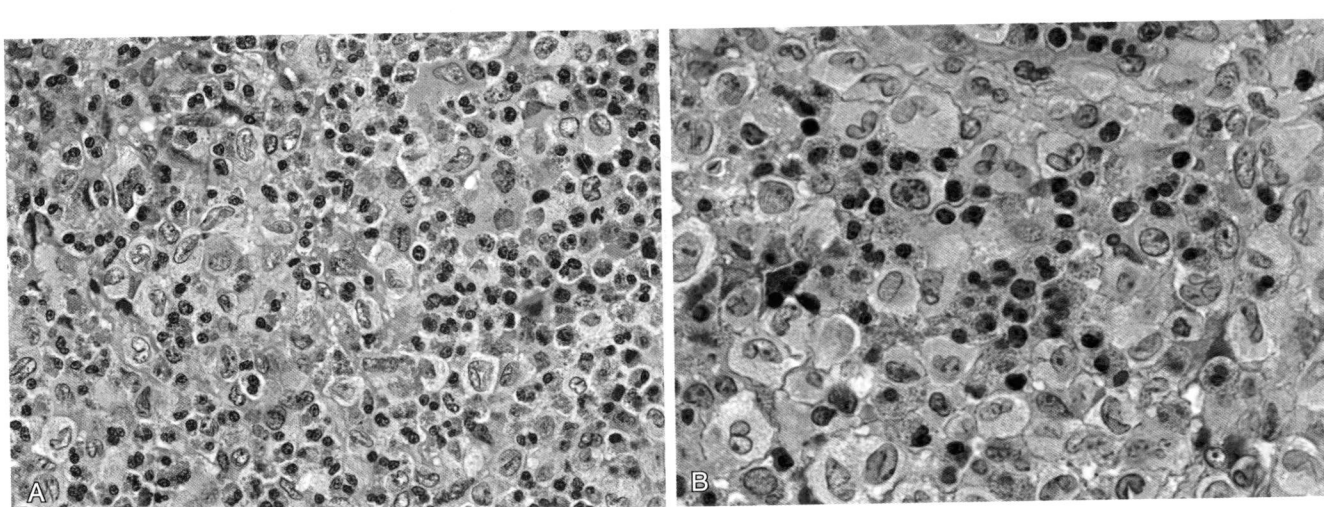

Figure 52-9. Langerhans cell histiocytosis. A–B, Langerhans cells have eosinophilic cytoplasm and distinctive nuclear features with a complex, folded nuclear outline and often a nuclear groove. Eosinophils are often abundant in the background and may form microabscesses.

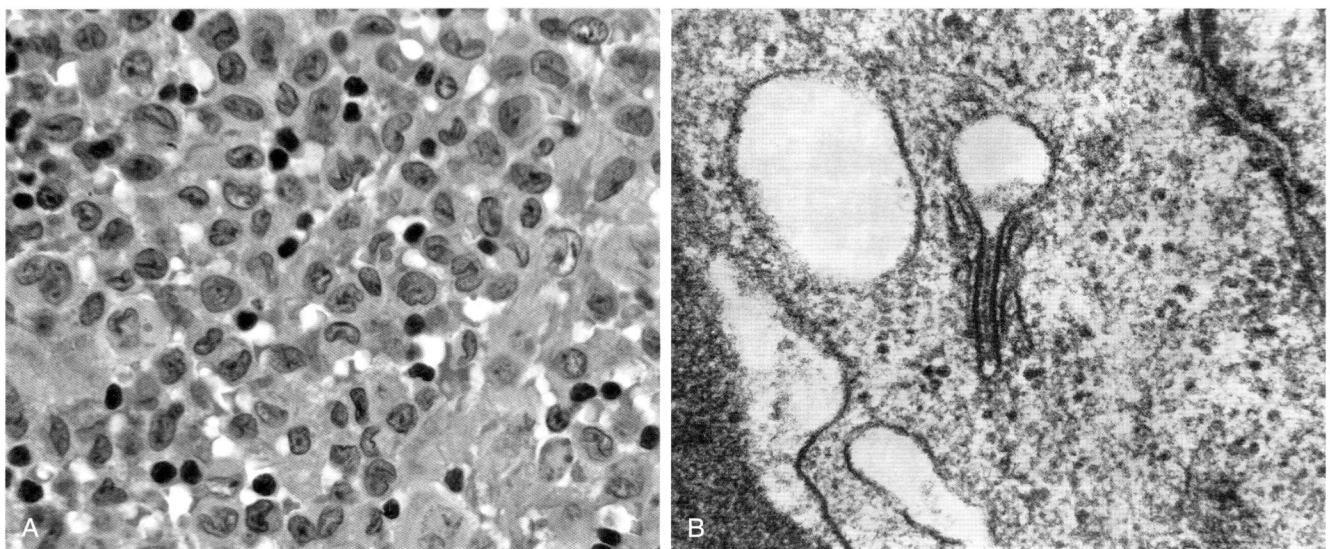

Figure 52-10. Langerhans cell histiocytosis in soft tissue. **A,** LCH cells have complex folded and grooved nuclei but limited pleomorphism. **B,** Electron microscopy reveals peripheral Birbeck granules, pentalaminar structures with a zipperlike appearance and a terminal bulbous swelling.

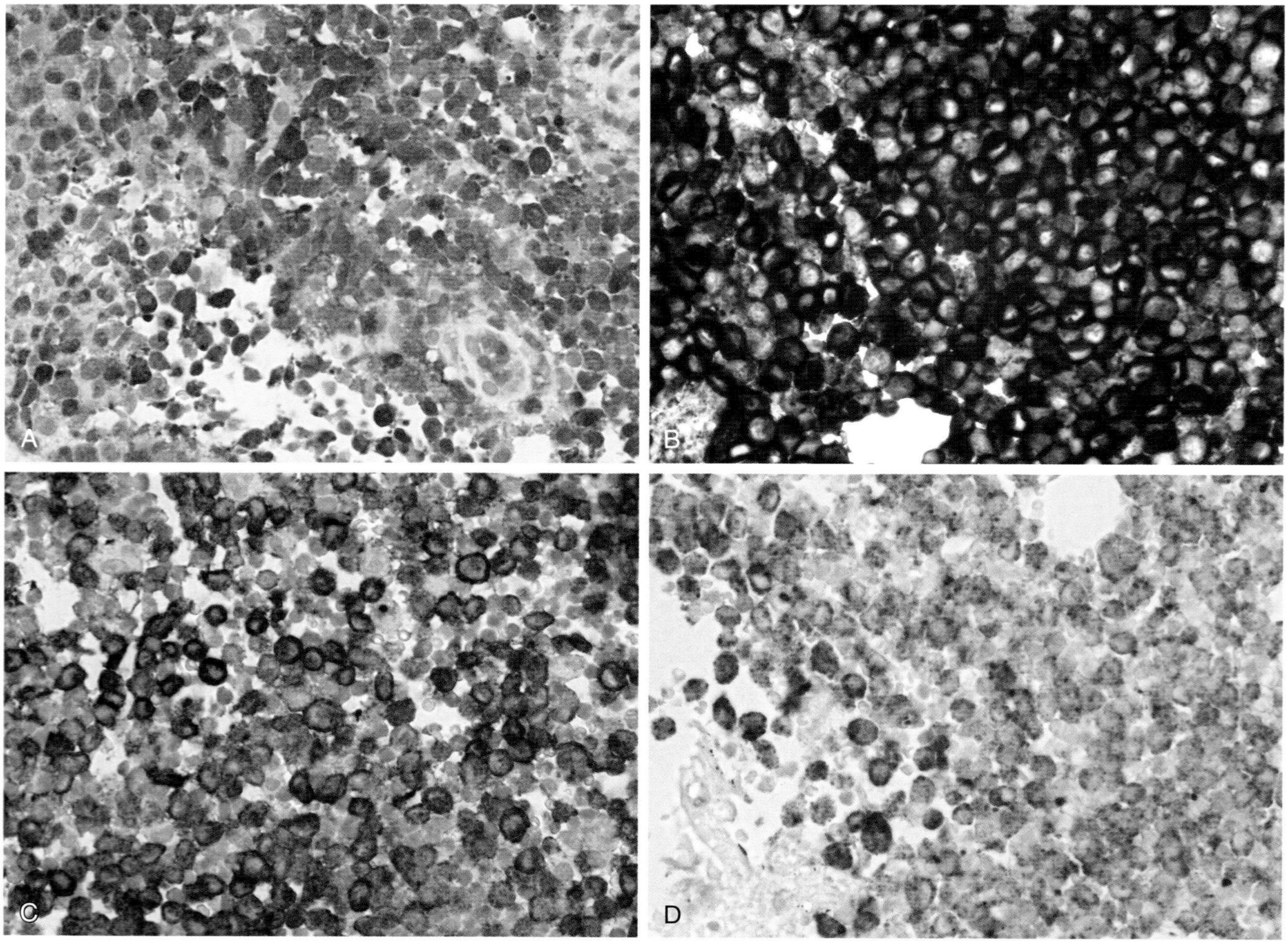

Figure 52-11. Langerhans cell histiocytosis. The cells express S100 **(A)**, CD1a **(B)**, and langerin **(C)**. Immunohistochemistry with *BRAF* p.V600E-specific antibody is also positive **(D)**.

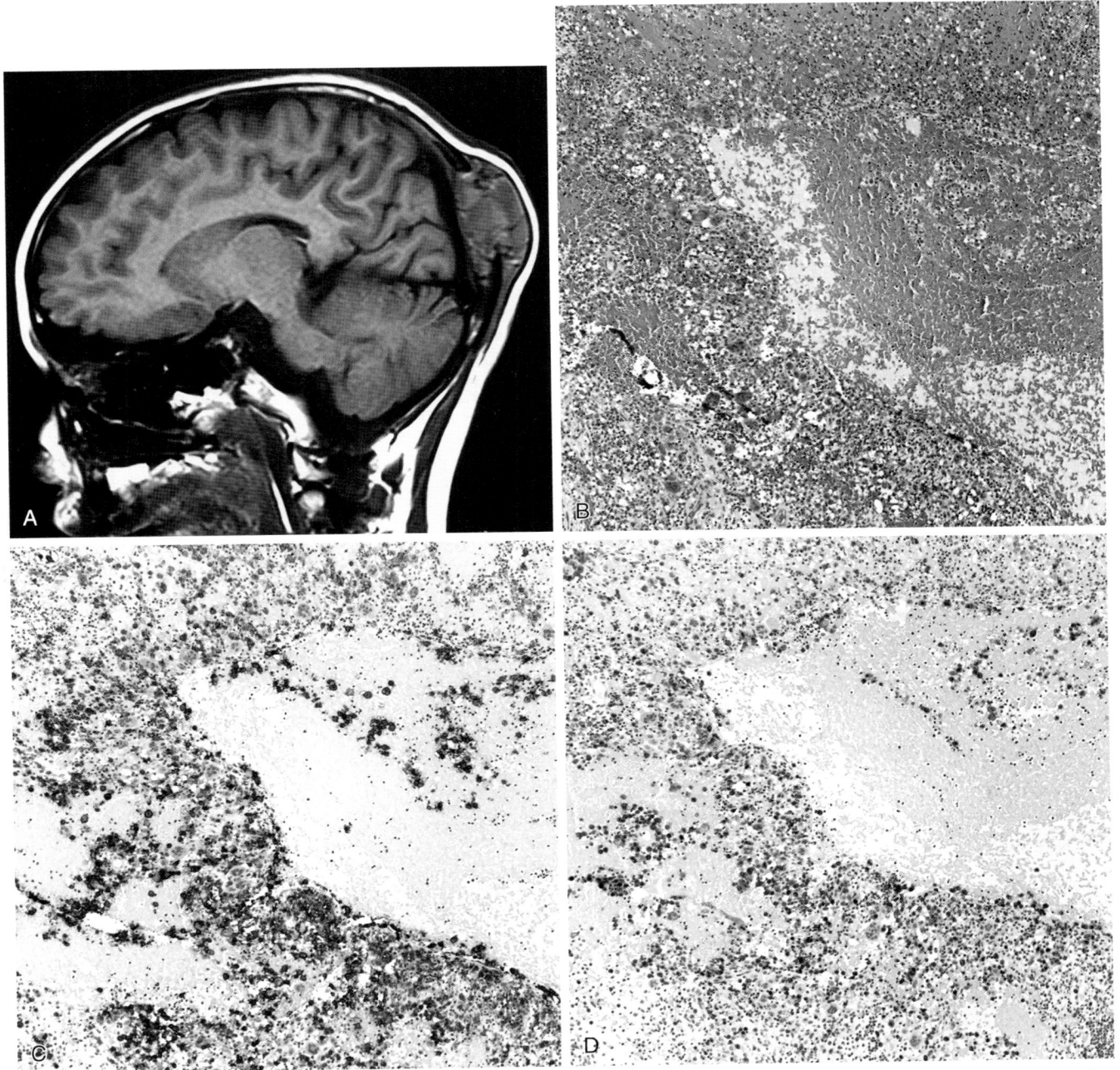

Figure 52-12. Bone Langerhans cell histiocytosis presenting as an aneurysmal bone cyst. A, Magnetic resonance imaging highlights a bone defect and variable soft tissue effect. **B,** Vascular spaces are lined in part with osteoclasts. **C,** The lining is rich in CD1a-positive LCH cells. **D,** Langerin (CD207) stains the same population.

cases; however, correlation with the entire clinical and radiologic picture should raise the suspicion of LCH. Prominent xanthomatous changes may raise the consideration of other histiocytic neoplasms, such as ECD. Radiologic findings may suggest other diagnoses. In children, other bone tumors, such as osteosarcoma or Ewing's sarcoma, may be considered and in adults, plasma cell neoplasia or metastatic tumor may be within the differential diagnosis.

Skin

Cutaneous involvement by LCH is characterized by infiltration of the upper papillary dermis by sheets of the atypical cells (Fig. 52-13). Epidermotropism with surface ulceration and epidermal inflammatory changes may be present, and there may be associated eosinophils. Xanthomatous changes are rare but may be seen in late LCH lesions and mimic juvenile xanthogranuloma (JXG).[299] The histologic differential diagnosis includes other neoplastic and inflammatory processes. Other types of cutaneous histiocytic lesions can generally be excluded on immunophenotypic grounds. Neoplasia of other lineages such as cutaneous melanocytic lesions or cutaneous mastocytosis can be differentiated by their negativity for CD1a and langerin (CD207) and expression of other markers such as MelanA and HMB45 (melanocytic lesions) or mast cell

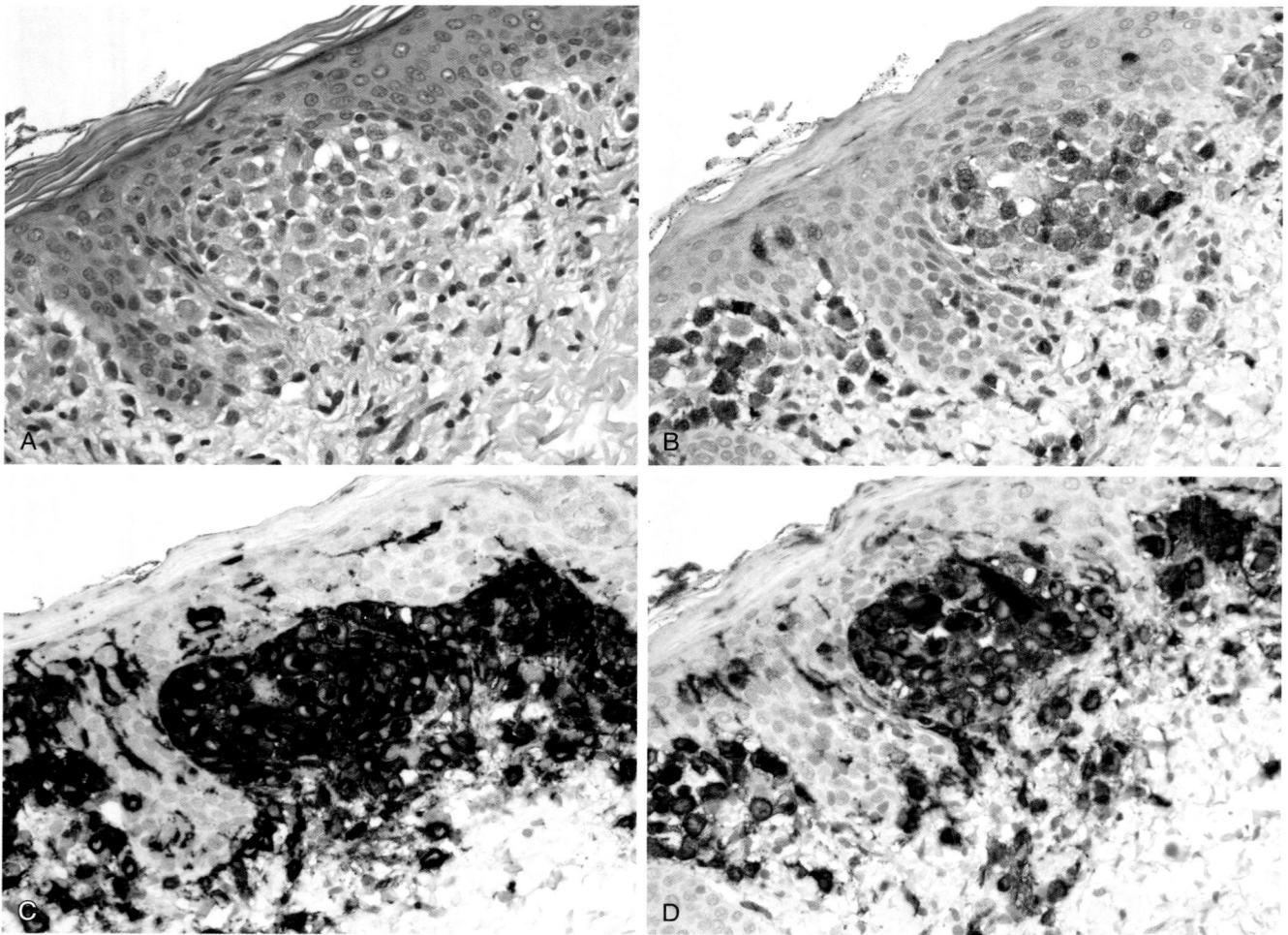

Figure 52-13. Langerhans cell histiocytosis in skin. There is infiltration of the upper papillary dermis by sheets of the atypical cells **(A)** that express S100 **(B)**, CD1a **(C)**, and langerin **(D)**.

tryptase and CD117 (mastocytosis). Cutaneous involvement by myelomonocytic neoplasms presents a potential pitfall,[300] as LCH can be associated with leukemic malignancy. Inflammatory dermatoses due to various causes may show hyperplasia of CD1a-positive dendritic cells, which can be distinguished from LCH by the spindled morphology of the cells and the more variable expression of langerin (CD207).

Lymph Node

Lymph nodes involved by LCH show sinusoidal infiltration by LCH cells, eosinophils, and other associated inflammatory cells (Fig. 52-14). Osteoclast-like multinucleated giant cells and small foci of necrosis can also be present. Occasionally, there may be total effacement of the nodal architecture with paracortical infiltration.[288] The sinusoidal pattern of involvement is key to the distinction of LCH from reactive nodal processes containing Langerhans cells, such as dermatopathic lymphadenitis.[301] Dermatopathic lymphadenitis shows prominent paracortical infiltration by a mixture of dendritic cells and Langerhans cells in contrast to the sinusoidal clusters of LCH cells that are present in LCH.[302] Nodal involvement by other types of neoplasia may also enter the differential diagnosis. Anaplastic large cell lymphoma can show an intrasinusoidal pattern of lymph node involvement; however, it can be distinguished by CD30 expression and negativity for

CD1a and langerin (CD207). LCH can co-occur with other neoplastic processes in lymph nodes; therefore, thorough evaluation is necessary so as not to overlook an associated second pathology such as classic Hodgkin lymphoma or metastatic thyroid carcinoma.

Lung

Early lesions of PLCH show cellular bronchiolocentric nodules composed of Langerhans cells and an admixed infiltrate of lymphocytes, eosinophils, plasma cells, and neutrophils associated with destruction of bronchiolar wall and adjacent lung parenchyma.[303] The differential diagnosis of PLCH includes respiratory bronchiolitis and desquamative interstitial pneumonia, hypersensitivity pneumonitis, and other histiocytosis, particularly ECD.

Late lesions of PLCH show bronchiolocentric stellate scars and cysts (Fig. 52-15). Langerhans cells might not be detectable in late lesions and histologic distinction from other causes of fibrosing cystic disease may not be possible, though LCH may be suspected based on imaging findings.

Central Nervous System

CNS disease can be tumorous or neurodegenerative, and the histopathologic diagnosis of CNS-LCH may be challenging because of difficulty in obtaining substantial tissue biopsies and

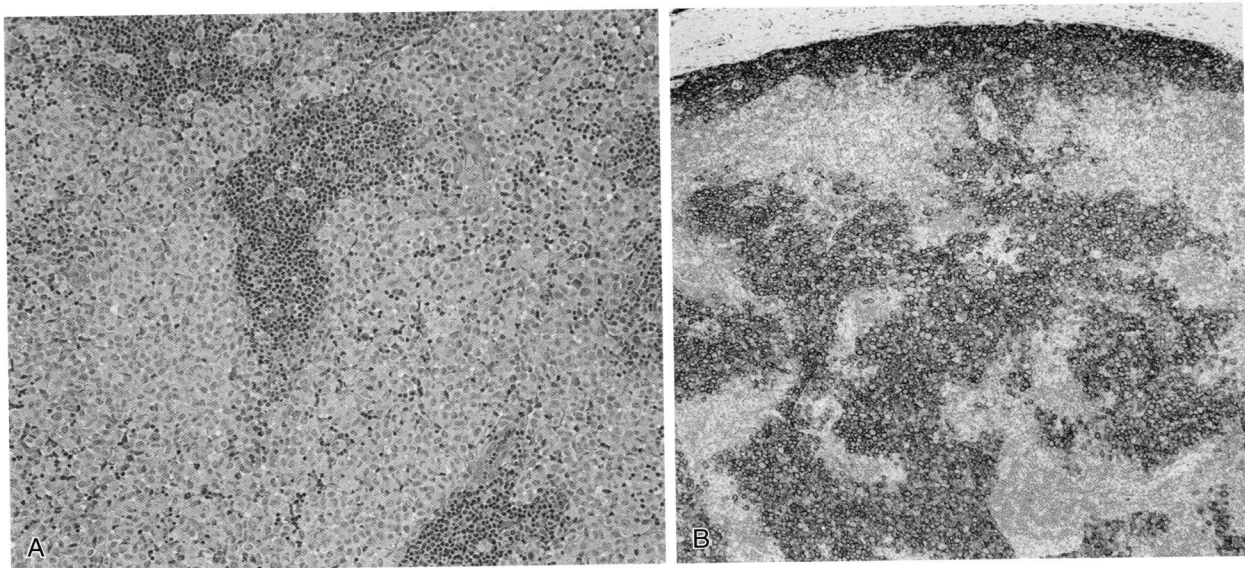

Figure 52-14. Langerhans cell histiocytosis, lymph node. A, When the node is replaced, the sinus pattern, characteristic of LCH involvement, is obscured. **B,** CD1a (and CD207) will generally reveal the sinus pattern. CD1a and CD207 can be absent or low on the infiltrating paracortical cells.

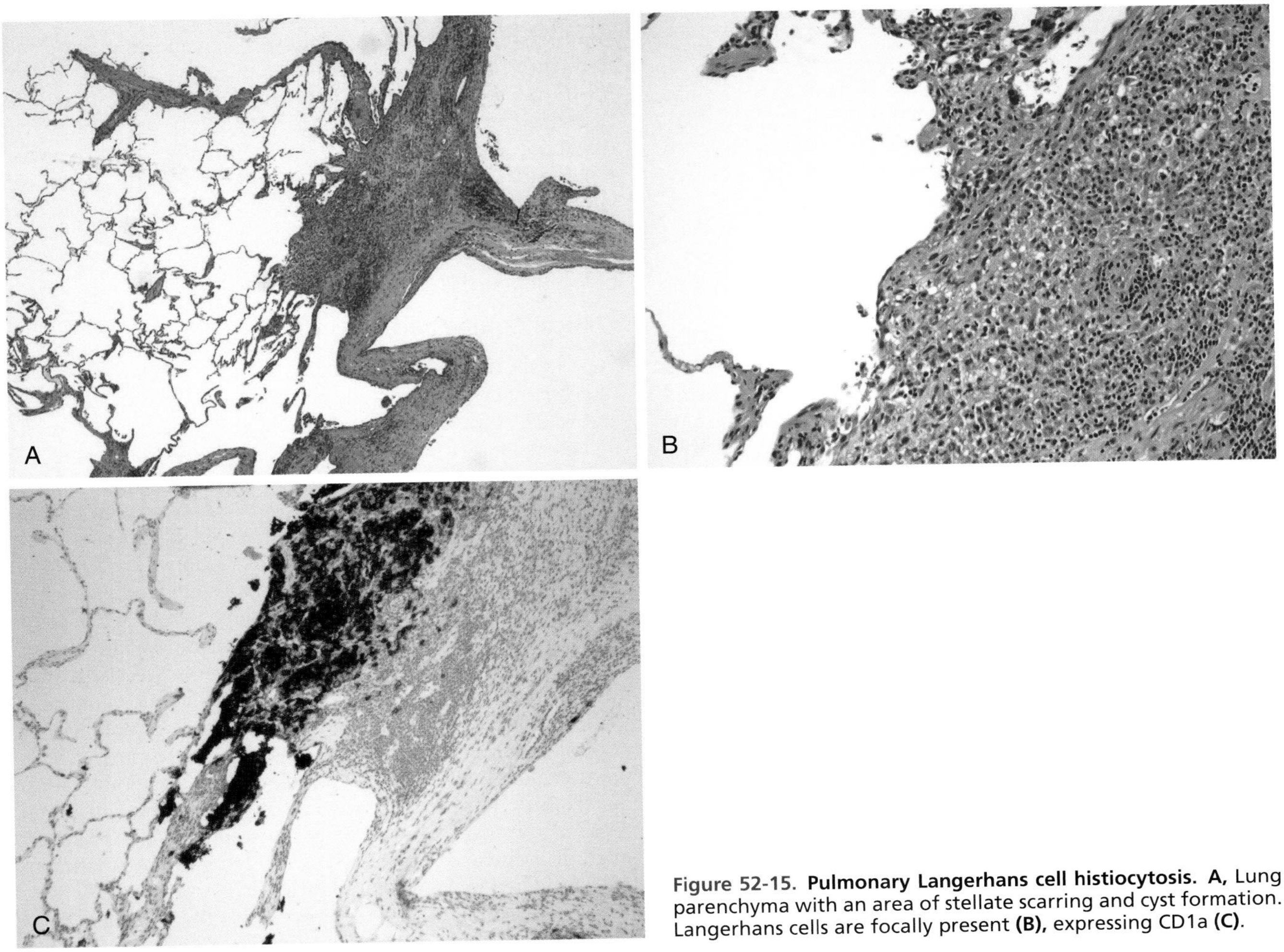

Figure 52-15. Pulmonary Langerhans cell histiocytosis. A, Lung parenchyma with an area of stellate scarring and cyst formation. Langerhans cells are focally present **(B)**, expressing CD1a **(C)**.

the potential to misinterpret adjacent perilesional inflammatory changes as other forms of histiocytosis. Tumor lesions involve the hypothalamic-pituitary axis and extraaxial sites including the meninges and choroid plexus. Intraparenchymal involvement is rare. Histopathology shows a mixed infiltrate of histiocytes, foamy macrophages, and multinucleated giant cells, as well as eosinophils, lymphocytes, and plasma cells.[304] The presence and number of CD1a-positive cells within lesions is variable, and these may be scarce. The differential diagnosis includes other histiocytic disorders such as JXG, ECD, and RDD, and also lymphoma, craniopharyngioma, and other metastatic lesions.

Neurodegenerative lesions mainly affect the cerebellum and are characterized by diffuse parenchymal inflammation associated with neuronal and axonal degeneration, and secondary myelin loss.[304] ND-LCH was originally considered a paraneoplastic process; however, migration of *BRAF* p.V600E mutated langerin/CD207-negative hematopoietic precursors to specific regions of the brain has recently been implicated in driving the neurodegenerative process.[305]

Liver

Liver biopsy taken at an early stage in the disease course may show a lobular infiltrate of LCH cells with the typical immunophenotype. These can form focal aggregates and are mixed with lymphocytes. Eosinophils and neutrophils may also be present. As the disease progresses, the bile ducts may be infiltrated and the appearance may resemble a sclerosing cholangitis. At this stage, LCH cells may not be easily identifiable, and the diagnosis of LCH may not be initially considered on histopathology without the appropriate clinical information.[306] The histologic findings of hepatic LCH may resemble primary sclerosing cholangitis or primary biliary cirrhosis. If granulomatous inflammation is present, an infectious etiology or sarcoidosis may be considered initially.

Bone Marrow

Involvement of the hematopoietic system or bone marrow is defined clinically by the detection of anemia or thrombocytopenia.[283] Histologic examination of the marrow has limited sensitivity, as CD1a-positive LCH cells are not often encountered, even in the presence of cytopenias,[307] although histiocytic aggregates and other features such as megakaryocyte hyperplasia and myelofibrosis may be present. A recent study has shown that measurable bone marrow disease may be detected more reliably by allele-specific ddPCR than by CD1a or *BRAF* p.V600E immunostaining.[308]

Thymus

LCH may involve the thymus as SS-LCH or as part of MS-LCH disease and presents with a solid or cystic mediastinal mass. The architecture of the gland can be replaced or disrupted by nodules of LCH with fibrosis, multinucleated giant cells, and eosinophils, or changes may be mostly confined to the medulla. There can be areas of necrosis and calcification. In rare cases, a mixed histiocytosis is present, including components of LCH and JXG.[309] Thymectomies may also show incidental small foci of Langerhans cell hyperplasia that are not sufficient to be diagnostic of LCH.[309]

Genetics and Molecular Findings

As previously noted, recurrent activating alterations in genes of the MAPK pathway are found in the majority of LCH cases. *BRAF* p.V600E[243,310] mutations are the most frequent,

identified in ~50% of cases, but other alterations in *BRAF*,[271] including *BRAF* p.N486_P490del[271,274,311] and alterations in *MAP2K1*,[269,272] are recurrently present. *BRAF* and *MAP2K1* alterations appear to be mostly mutually exclusive,[269] although rarely co-occur.[312] Mutations in *NRAS* are very rare outside of PLCH, and occasionally have been found to co-occur with *BRAF* p.V600E mutations in both PLCH and non-PLCH. In PLCH, it is suggested that the mutations are carried by different subclones of the tumor.[270] *KRAS* mutations are rare overall in LCH with only a very small number of cases reported.[274,275,311] Infrequently, mutations have also been found in *ARAF* and *CSF1R*[273,275] and a *PIK3CA* mutation was detected in a single case.[313]

Activating *BRAF* fusions have been identified with different partner genes (*BICD2, CSF2RA, PACSIN2, SPPL2A, LMTK2, FAM 73A*).[271,275,314] Case reports have also detailed single findings of other fusions in LCH including *PLEKHA6::NTRK3*[315] and *ETV3::NCOA2*,[311] which has also been identified in a small number of indeterminate dendritic cell histiocytosis (IDCH) cases.

Association With Malignancy

Solid cancers, lymphomas, and other hematologic malignancies seem to show a higher incidence in patients with LCH compared with the general population.[316] In children, most associated malignancies are leukemia (mainly acute myeloid leukemia) and myeloproliferative disorders, whereas in adults solid cancers and lymphoma are more common.[317] Lung, thyroid, and breast cancers are the most frequently occurring solid malignancies.[316,317] Synchronous *BRAF* p.V600E mutated papillary thyroid carcinoma and LCH has been reported.[318] Cases of LCH concomitant with or subsequent to classic Hodgkin lymphoma, T-lymphoblastic lymphoma, chronic lymphocytic leukemia/small lymphocytic lymphoma, and follicular lymphoma (FL) are also described. In some cases, a clonal relationship between the disorders has been shown; in others, the LCH population is postulated to be incidental.[319,320]

Clinical Course and Prognosis

LCH has a low overall mortality but a high relapse rate, with the disease course generally depending on the disease extent and sites of involvement. The clinical presentation appears to associated with the particular MAPK-activating mutation detected, with *BRAF* p.V600E mutated LCH presenting at a lower age and with a higher prevalence of MS-LCH, high-risk disease, and skin involvement, whereas *MAP2K1* alterations are associated with a higher prevalence of SS-bone LCH, and *BRAF* exon 12 deletions appear to correlate with lung involvement.[321]

Treatment decisions in LCH are made based on sites and extent of disease. For patients with SS-LCH disease and no involvement of critical organs such as the CNS, heart, liver, or spleen, treatment may be limited to observation or local therapy. Curettage or radiotherapy can be considered for localized bony lesions and topical therapies, oral methotrexate and 6-mercaptopurine may be used in isolated skin involvement.[242,265,322] Some cases of PLCH may resolve with smoking cessation, but others may benefit from treatment with high-dose prednisone or systemic therapy if disease is progressive.[242,265] Lung transplantation may be considered in advanced, refractory cases.

Systemic therapy can be required for the treatment of MS-LCH, multifocal SS-LCH, or unifocal LCH with critical organ involvement. Chemotherapy with vinblastine and prednisone is generally used in the pediatric setting.[322] Notably, pediatric chemotherapy regimens cause greater toxicities in adults, and initial treatment with cytarabine or cladribine may be preferable in adults.[242,265] In adults with LCH and CNS lesions, first-line treatment with MAP kinase inhibitors, cladribine or cytarabine (with methotrexate) is preferred.[242,265] Recent studies have reported on the use of targeted therapy, particularly BRAF inhibitors, in LCH in adults and in the setting of refractory LCH in children. Most patients have shown a good clinical response, but the majority experience disease reactivation upon discontinuing therapy.[323,324]

Indeterminate Dendritic Cell Histiocytosis

Definition

IDCH is an extremely rare tumor that shows immunophenotypic overlap with LCH (S100-positive/CD1a-positive), but does not express langerin (CD207) or contain Birbeck granules on ultrastructural examination.[325]

Synonyms and Related Terms

Indeterminate dendritic cell histiocytosis (ICC); Indeterminate dendritic cell tumor (WHO 5th ed.); Indeterminate dendritic cell tumor (WHO Revised 4th ed.); Indeterminate cell histiocytosis (Revised Classification of the Histiocyte Society, 2016); Primary/secondary malignant histiocytosis, indeterminate cell subtype (Revised Classification of the Histiocyte Society, 2016).

Epidemiology

IDCH is rare. In a review of ~85 cases published in the literature between 1985 and 2016, IDCH was found to affect all ages with a median age of 45 (range 0–87 years) and to show a slight male predominance (M:F ratio 1.2:1).[326]

IDCH has been observed either subsequent to or in association with diverse hematologic malignancies (reported as accounting for ~22% of cases in one review[327]), including angioimmunoblastic T-cell lymphoma (AITL),[328] mycosis fungoides,[329] FL,[325] T-lymphoblastic lymphoma,[330] B-lymphoblastic lymphoma,[331] chronic lymphocytic leukemia/small lymphocytic lymphoma,[332] and unspecified low-grade B-cell lymphoma,[333] as well as chronic myelomonocytic leukemia (CMML),[334-336] MDS,[337] acute myeloid leukemia,[338] and mast cell leukemia.[339] The IDCH may precede the diagnosis of a myeloid neoplasm by some time.[338,339] The nature of the relationship between the IDCH and associated hematologic malignancy has not been established in many cases.

Clinical Features

Most of the cases reported in the literature have shown cutaneous involvement, usually presenting with single to multiple skin nodules and papules, although patches or plaques may also occur and disseminated involvement may be present.[326,327,340] Extracutaneous involvement is very uncommon but has been reported with lymph node,[328] pancreatic,[341] bone,[342,343] and splenic[344] involvement. Rarely, multisystem disease can occur.[345]

Morphology

The tumor cells show a histiocytoid morphology with round-to-elongated nuclei and may show occasional nuclear

grooves, but eosinophils are not prominent, and cutaneous cases usually lack epidermotropism.[327] Cytologic appearances can be variable (Fig. 52-16A). Some cases, particularly those associated with CMML, may show marked atypia with blastic cytologic features.[336]

Immunophenotype

IDCH expresses CD1a and is usually positive for S100 with variable expression of CD68, but is negative for langerin (Fig. 52-16B–D).[327] CD163 may be rarely expressed, and CD56 positivity has been described in lesions with an IDCH immunophenotype, often in the setting of an associated myeloid neoplasm.[325,334,336]

Genetics and Molecular Findings

Molecular analysis has not been performed in most of the reported cases. An *ETV3::NCOA2* fusion has been documented in five cases[346-348] without a reported associated hematologic malignancy and a *BRAF* p.V600E mutation has been reported in another case.[343]

Some secondary cases of IDCH have been shown to be clonally related to the associated hematologic malignancy. A number of cases associated with CMML have shown shared mutations in both tumors, such as a shared *TET2* mutation,[349] shared *TET2, ASXL1,* and *ZRSR2* mutations,[350] and shared MAPK mutations, including in *KRAS* p.G12R[334] and *NRAS* p.G12V.[351]

Identical cytogenetic abnormalities have also been discovered in some cases, also supporting a common cell of origin. Trisomy 8 was detected in both CMML and IDCH samples in one report,[336] and a further case showed trisomy 12 in both T-ALL and IDCH components.[330] Another T-ALL–associated IDCH showed loss-of-heterozygosity on chromosome 9p with deletion of *CDKN2A* in both the T-ALL and IDCH, but also showed evidence of clonal divergence with the acquisition of a *KRAS* mutation in the IDCH component and a *TP53* mutation in the T-ALL, among other differing cytogenetic findings between the two lesions.[352]

BRAF p.V600E expression has been shown by IHC in a case associated with AITL[328] and has been found by sequencing in a case associated with both low-grade B-cell lymphoma and CMML, in addition to *TP53* and *RUNX1* mutations.[333] The t(14;18) was detected in an IDCH in which there was a previous history of FL.[325] A patient with unexplained systemic lymphadenopathy also had a clonal IG rearrangement detected in an excised IDCH.[325]

Clinical Course and Prognosis

The clinical behavior is variable. Isolated skin lesions usually have an indolent clinical course, and some cases may spontaneously regress[353]; however, a fatal clinical course has been described.[345] IDCH in the setting of CMML may exhibit more aggressive clinical behavior.[336,349]

Skin lesions have been managed with excision, UV-B phototherapy, or electron beam therapy. Some cases have been treated with thalidomide or methotrexate, and other chemotherapeutic agents have also been used, mainly in cases associated with hematologic malignancy.[326,327] A significant response to therapy with a BRAF inhibitor was obtained in one case.[343]

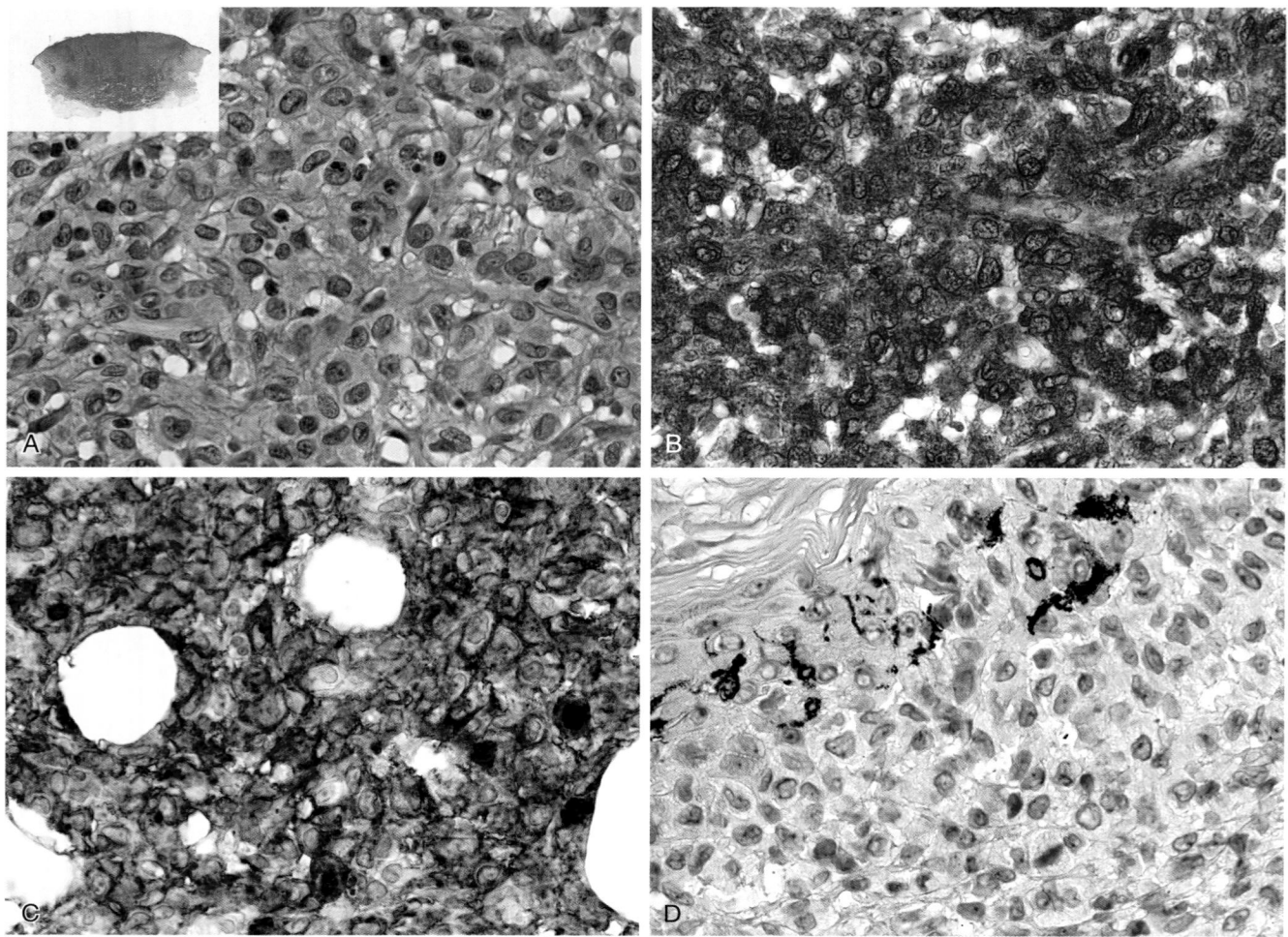

Figure 52-16. Indeterminate dendritic cell histiocytosis. The cytologic features may be variable. **A,** This is a skin lesion showing cells with a histiocytoid morphology with round-to-elongated nuclei and occasional nuclear grooves. Eosinophils are not prominent. They express S100 **(B)** and CD1a **(C),** but are negative for langerin **(D),** which highlights the intraepidermal Langerhans cells.

Differential Diagnosis

The major differential diagnosis is with other histiocytic tumors, which can be distinguished by IHC. Given the association with both lymphoid and myeloid neoplasms, further patient evaluation may be necessary to exclude systemic involvement by another hematologic malignancy.

Dermal infiltrates that are rich in indeterminate cells have also been described after tick or mosquito bites or post scabies infection, and may resolve spontaneously or with steroid therapy.[354]

Erdheim-Chester Disease

Definition

ECD is a rare multisystem clonal histiocytic disorder with distinct clinical and imaging features that is histologically characterized by a xanthomatous histiocytic infiltrate associated with variable inflammation and fibrosis, and driven by activating alterations in the MAPK pathway.

Synonyms and Related Terms

Erdheim-Chester disease (ICC); Erdheim-Chester disease (WHO 5th ed.); Erdheim-Chester disease (WHO Revised 4th ed.); Erdheim-Chester disease (Revised Classification of the Histiocyte Society, 2016).

Background and Pathogenesis

ECD was first described in 1930 as *Über Lipoidgranulomatose* by Jakob Erdheim and William Chester.[355] Since then, more than 1500 cases have been reported in the literature,[144] the majority in recent years, as greater awareness of the condition has led to an increase in diagnosis.

The pathogenesis of ECD has been a subject of debate, with initial discourse centered on whether it represented an inflammatory or neoplastic condition. Studies have described proinflammatory mediators and cytokine perturbations in the lesions and sera of ECD patients,[356,357] but the pathogenesis remained unclear until 2012 when *BRAF* p.V600E mutations were discovered in the majority of cases.[310,358] ECD was subsequently classified as a neoplasia by the WHO in 2016[295] and in the revised classification of histiocytoses and neoplasms of the macrophage-dendritic cell lineages from the Histiocyte Society[2] within the category of L type histiocytosis owing to the molecular overlap with LCH and the not-infrequent co-occurrence of the two disorders, so-called "mixed histiocytosis." Cases of extracutaneous JXG with MAPK pathway mutations and tumors with a JXG-like morphology harboring ALK fusions (ALK-positive histiocytosis) also fall under ECD in the revised classification of the Histiocyte Society; however, ALK-positive histiocytosis is now accepted as a distinct entity in the ICC[240] and in the WHO 5th edition.[241]

A complex cytokine and chemokine network is established within ECD lesions, resulting in the recruitment and activation of macrophages and T cells.[359] Studies using the BRAF p.V600E specific IHC antibody have shown that the oncogenic BRAF p.V600E mutation in the tissue infiltrate of ECD lesions localizes to a subset of the histiocytic population.[360] A number of mechanisms have been proposed as a link between the oncogenic mutation and the observed inflammatory activation, including oncogene-induced senescence, a major protective response against oncogenesis that is characterized by cell cycle arrest and upregulation of tumor suppressor proteins, including p16 and p21,[359-361] and oncogene-induced activation of trained immunity, a proinflammatory program.[362]

Epidemiology

ECD is primarily a disease of adults, with a male predominance of about 3:1 and mean ages at presentation of 46 and 56 years in two different cohorts.[363,364] Pediatric cases are described, but are rare.

Clinical Features and Imaging Findings

ECD is a chronic and multisystem disorder with a variety of clinical manifestations depending on the organ system involved. The vast majority of patients have bone involvement (80%–95%)[363,364] and many experience bone pain (40%–50%),[363] with the classic imaging appearance showing symmetric long bone osteosclerosis, often in the distal femur and tibia. In contrast to LCH, lesions are usually osteosclerotic rather than osteolytic, and involvement of the skull and axial skeleton occurs less frequently.[365] CNS disease has been reported in 37% to 40%,[363,364,366] and up to 90% of patients may experience neurologic symptoms.[363] ECD typically involves the posterior fossa brain parenchyma, but also occurs in the pituitary and dura. About 28% to 47% may have diabetes insipidus, which can have an onset prior to the diagnosis of ECD.[363,364] Retro-orbital involvement occurs in 22% to 30%.[363,364,366] Cardiac involvement in the form of right atrioventricular pseudotumor is reported in approximately 40%.[363,364] Circumferential encasement or soft tissue sheathing of the thoracic or abdominal aorta and its branches, so-called "coated aorta," can be detected on imaging in 46% to 62%,[363,364] and may be asymptomatic or result in vascular compromise such as arterial stenosis. Retroperitoneal and perinephric infiltration with the radiologic appearance of "hairy kidney" are also frequent (58%–65%) and may result in hydronephrosis. Cutaneous involvement most commonly occurs as xanthelasma around the eyelid region (27%–33%).[363,364] Pulmonary involvement can be apparent as interstitial fibrosis on CT scan, although patients are often asymptomatic.[363,367] ECD can also involve the bone marrow,

and there is a high prevalence of myeloid neoplasia in patients with ECD.[368,369]

Morphology

The classic histologic appearance of ECD is tissue infiltration by xanthomatous histiocytes with bland nuclear features and abundant foamy cytoplasm.[363] Touton-type giant cells are also present within the infiltrate and there may be an associated densely fibrotic stroma (Fig. 52-17A–B). There is often an admixed inflammatory infiltrate of plasma cells, lymphocytes, and occasional neutrophils.[370] The typical histopathology of ECD is indistinguishable from JXG.[371]

The pattern of histologic involvement varies depending on the site biopsied. Bone lesions typically show fibroxanthomatous replacement of the marrow spaces; however, in later fibrotic lesions, the histiocytes may be fewer in number, with an amorphous lipid-laden or granular appearance and lacking the typical xanthomatous morphology.[370] Retroperitoneal lesions may show a prominent plasma cell infiltrate that may be rich in IgG4-positive plasma cells, presenting a diagnostic pitfall.[365] Lesions of the CNS often do not show the characteristic morphologic features, instead showing perivascular lymphocytic infiltrates with a histiocytic component present as individual cells or small aggregates of nonlipidized cells with pale or eosinophilic cytoplasm and indistinct cell borders.[370] Lung involvement is typically characterized by thickening of the pleura, interlobular septa, and perivascular interstitium by fibrosis and a histiocytic infiltrate with a lymphangitic distribution.[370]

Immunophenotype

The histiocytes of ECD express CD68, CD163, CD14, and factor XIIIa,[363] and are negative for CD1a and langerin (CD207).[370] Variable S100 positivity may be seen[370] (Fig. 52-17C–E). IHC with BRAF p.V600E-specific antibody may be positive in BRAF p.V600E mutated cases; however, it may only stain scattered cells, therefore negative or equivocal results by IHC should be confirmed by molecular analysis[366,370] (Fig. 52-17F). PD-1 or PD-L1 are variably expressed in ECD, with PD-L1 positivity significantly associated with an absence of BRAF p.V600E mutation in one study.[372]

Diagnostic Criteria

Traditionally, the diagnosis of ECD has required the combination of the classic histologic appearances of a xanthomatous histiocytic infiltrate with the appropriate immunophenotype and the presence of the characteristic radiologic findings, namely symmetric osteosclerosis of the metadiaphysis of the lower-extremity bones on imaging studies.[365] However, the typical histiocyte morphology may not always be present,[370] and a small percentage of patients may not have the characteristic bone lesions on imaging[363,365]; thus, it is of paramount importance to consider the clinical, imaging, and molecular findings in their entirety to reach a final diagnosis. In the absence of bone lesions, ECD should only be considered in the setting of suggestive histopathology and highly characteristic nonosseous lesions on imaging studies, ideally with supportive mutational data. A diagnosis of ECD should also still be considered if characteristic clinical and radiologic features are present, even when tissue biopsy does not demonstrate classic morphologic features.[365]

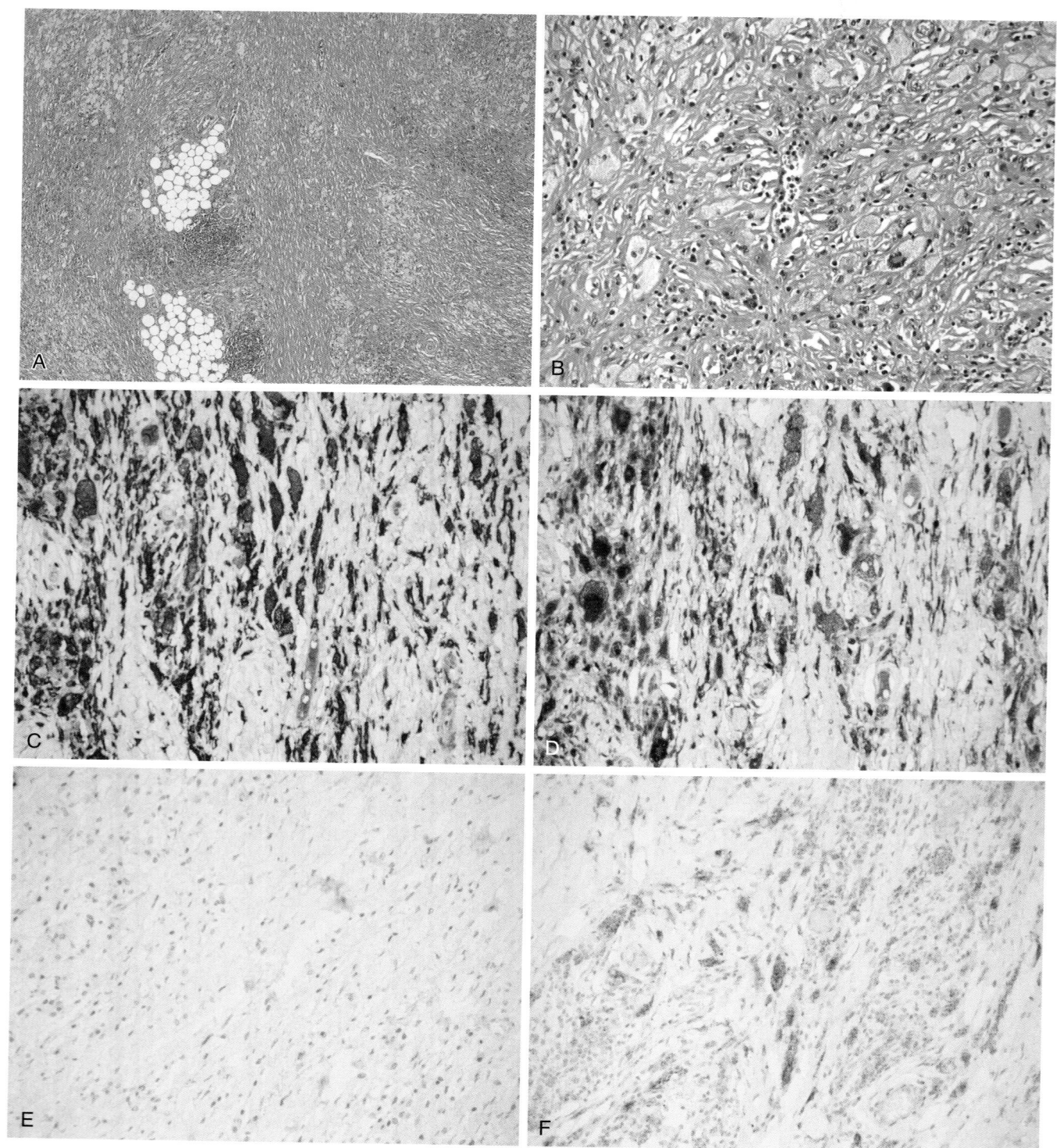

Figure 52-17. Erdheim-Chester disease. A–B, There is a densely fibrotic stroma with infiltration by xanthomatous histiocytes with bland nuclear features and abundant foamy cytoplasm. Touton-type giant cells are also present. The histiocytic cells express CD163 **(C)**, factor XIIIA **(D)**, and are negative for CD1a **(E)**. Immunohistochemistry for *BRAF* p.V600E-specific antibody is positive **(F)**.

Genetics and Molecular Findings

A breakthrough in the diagnosis and pathogenesis of ECD came with the discovery of *BRAF* p.V600E in over half of cases.[310,373] Further studies have confirmed additional alterations in the MAPK and phosphatidylinositol 3-kinase (PI3K)-AKT pathways, including in *BRAF* (non-p.V600E alterations),

MAP2K1,[275,373] *NRAS*,[313,374] *ARAF*,[275,373] *KRAS*,[275,375] and *PIK3CA*.[313] Recently, mutations in *CSF1R, RAF1*, and *MAP2K2* have also been described.[275] A minority of cases show fusions involving *BRAF* (*RNF11::BRAF, PICALM::BRAF, ANP32A::BRAF, UBTD2::BRAF*) and *NTRK1* (*LMNA::NTRK1*).[275,376] The novel group of tumors with a JXG-like morphology and harboring fusions involving the *ALK* gene have been previously regarded as a subgroup of ECD but are now the distinct entity of ALK-positive histiocytosis.[377]

Tissue biopsy is essential in all cases of ECD for histologic diagnosis and mutational analysis to allow therapeutic decision-making.[365] Reliable molecular assessment in ECD can be challenging because of low tumor cellularity. IHC with *BRAF* p.V600E-specific antibody is not sensitive or specific as the sole method for *BRAF* p.V600E mutational analysis, and negativity for *BRAF* p.V600E should be confirmed by another high-sensitivity molecular assay as the variant allele frequency may be low.[313] Where sufficient tumor tissue is difficult to obtain, analysis of cfDNA from the peripheral blood may be informative.[378]

Association With Other Conditions

There is a high prevalence of concomitant myeloid neoplasia in patients with ECD or mixed histiocytosis (~10.1%), including concurrent MDS, myeloproliferative neoplasms (MPNs), or MDS/MPN, particularly CMML.[369] Molecular analysis of these cases has shown driver mutations typical of myeloid neoplasia (for example *JAK2* p.V617F and *CALR* mutations) co-occurring with mutations that are commonly seen in histiocytosis (such as *BRAF* p.V600E and *MAP2K1* mutations).[369] The kinase mutations can be shared between both components or may be distinct with potential treatment implications, as paradoxical activation of cytokine signaling can occur in cells bearing kinase mutations other than *BRAF* p.V600E alterations upon exposure to BRAF inhibitors.[369] For this reason, bone marrow biopsy should be considered in ECD in the setting of unexplained cytopenias, cytosis, or monocytosis.[365]

The pathogenic mechanisms underlying development of myeloid neoplasia in ECD are not yet understood; however, a high frequency of clonal hematopoiesis has been reported in ECD patients (42.5%), with the most common mutations identified in *TET2* (22%), *ASXL1* (9%), and *DNMT3A* (8%).[379] Of these patients, 18 (15%) subsequently developed myeloid neoplasms, most often MDS, MPN, and CMML.

Approximately 20% of patients may have a mixed histiocytosis, characterized by co-occurring ECD, LCH, or RDD.[380]

Clinical Course and Prognosis

Most patients with ECD require systemic therapy, although a watch-and-wait approach can be considered in asymptomatic cases with noncritical organ involvement.[242] Targeted therapy with BRAF inhibitors such as vemurafenib or dabrafenib is effective in patients with *BRAF* p.V600E-mutated ECD. MEK inhibitors may be used in ECD associated with other MAPK pathway mutations, cases where a mutation is not detected, or in instances where testing is not available,[242] and there is potential for other targeted agents depending on the mutational profile.[242,365] A case report has described response to treatment with the *CSF1R* inhibitor pexidartinib in a patient with refractory ECD and an activating, in-frame deletion in the *CSF1R* gene.[381] Conventional therapies that have shown efficacy include IFN-α/PEG-IFN-α and cladribine. Anakinra may be considered in patients with low-volume disease in the bones or retroperitoneum.[365]

The prognosis of ECD is variable. One study of 165 patients has shown a median survival of 162 months with a 5-year survival of 82.7%. Retroperitoneal, lung, and CNS involvement were associated with a worse survival.[364]

Differential Diagnosis

The differential diagnosis varies depending on the age of the lesion and the site biopsied. In bone and retroperitoneum, histology may show extensive fibrosis without an obvious infiltrate of xanthomatous histiocytes, which may lead to the diagnosis of another process, such as osteomyelitis or retroperitoneal fibrosis. In such cases, radiologic correlation and molecular studies can aid in establishing the diagnosis of ECD.

ECD may coexist with other forms of histiocytosis, including LCH and RDD at different sites.[370] Dense lymphoplasmacytic infiltrates may raise the consideration of IgG4-related disease or extranodal marginal zone lymphoma, particularly in biopsies from orbital and retroperitoneal locations.[370] In biopsies from the CNS, areas of myelin loss associated with perivascular chronic inflammation could raise the consideration of multiple sclerosis.[370] Skin lesions showing features reminiscent of a dermatofibroma have been described,[370] as have panniculitis-like and granuloma annulare-like cutaneous presentations.[382]

Juvenile Xanthogranuloma

Definition

JXG is a non-LCH, forming part of a group of macrophage disorders that are characterized by a CD14-positive/CD163-positive/factor XIIIa-positive immunophenotype. In the revised classification of the Histiocyte Society,[2] the xanthogranuloma family of disorders mainly fall into the C group of cutaneous histiocytoses, with the exception of a subset of extracutaneous JXG harboring activating alterations in the MAPK pathway, which some consider as within the spectrum of ECD (L group).[2] The clinical presentation, imaging studies, and molecular findings are essential in the final classification of these lesions.

Synonyms and Related Terms

Disseminated juvenile xanthogranuloma (ICC Classification); Disseminated juvenile xanthogranuloma (WHO Revised 4th ed.); Juvenile xanthogranuloma (WHO 5th ed.); Juvenile xanthogranuloma (Revised Classification of the Histiocyte Society, 2016).

Background

Early descriptions of JXG have been attributed to Virchow in 1871,[383] to Adamson in 1905,[383,384] and to McDonagh in 1912, who postulated origin from the endothelium of the capillaries (nevoxanthoendothelioma).[383,385] In 1954, Helwig and Hackney noted the fibrohistiocytic nature of the lesion and originated the descriptive term of JXG.[386] Since then, origin from the indeterminate cell has been hypothesized[387] and consideration also given to the CD4-positive plasmacytoid "monocyte" as the principal element of JXG, though not further proven.[388] Based on the expression of factor XIIIa, the lesional cells have been postulated to be related to dermal dendritic cells[232,389] and, more recently, dermal macrophages.[390]

Epidemiology

JXG occurs predominantly in early childhood, most often within the first 2 years of life, and may present at birth.[384] There is a male predominance overall,[383,384] and an increased prevalence has been documented in children with neurofibromatosis type 1.[391]

A relationship between JXG and the development of juvenile myelomonocytic leukemia in children with neurofibromatosis type 1 has been postulated[392] although not confirmed in subsequent studies.[393] The exact incidence of JXG is not known as regressing, solitary lesions may not be reported, but the relative incidence of the disease was estimated at 0.52% (129 out of 24,600 patients) in the Kiel Pediatric Tumor Registry.[384] Approximately 4% of cases of JXG have systemic involvement,[383] although this figure is higher in neonatal patients and one review has shown a 3:1 female predominance among neonates with disseminated lesions.[394] Histologically similar lesions can also occur in adults (adult xanthogranuloma).

Clinical Features

Cutaneous JXG most commonly presents as a solitary nodule on the head and neck or trunk in a child under the age of 2 years, but may also present as multiple yellow or brown cutaneous papules.[395] Lesions can arise at any site on the body surface.[384] Systemic or disseminated JXG can involve multiple extracutaneous or visceral sites including deep soft tissue, liver, spleen, lung, eye/orbit, oropharynx, muscles, bone marrow, and CNS.[396] CNS JXG accounts for 1% to 2% of cases.[384] It mostly occurs in children <12 years of age and shows a male predominance.[397] Just over half of cases occurring in the CNS have multiple intracranial lesions or show concomitant systemic lesions,[397] and there is a higher mortality rate in CNS JXG (18.6%[397] compared with 1%–2% overall[384]). Ocular involvement by JXG is rare, occurs mainly in children <2 years of age, and is mostly unilateral and involving the iris and conjunctiva. Ocular involvement can be sight-threatening because of the development of complications such as hyphema and glaucoma.[398]

Similar lesions may also occur in adults ("adult xanthogranuloma"), with adults over the age of 20 years accounting for 27% of JXG cases in one single-center study.[399] Similarly to JXG in younger patients, cutaneous involvement of the head and neck predominates in the adult population, and systemic involvement is rare.[399]

Morphology

The histologic features of the xanthogranuloma family of lesions are variable and have been proposed to follow a time-dependent course with "early," "classic," and "late transitional" patterns representing time points in the continuous maturation of the lesional cells. A combination of these histologic patterns is often present within a single lesion.[384] JXG and ECD are morphologically and immunophenotypically similar, with the distinction between the disorders made on clinical, molecular, and radiologic grounds.

Early JXG is composed of a sheet-like infiltrate of small-to-intermediate-sized mononuclear histiocytes with sparse to moderate pale eosinophilic cytoplasm and small, round-to-ovoid and sometimes indented nuclei containing an inconspicuous nucleolus. Touton-type giant cells are generally absent. Mitotic figures are present and the mitotic activity is highest in this subtype, but nuclear atypia or atypical mitoses are lacking.

Classic JXG lesions contain histiocytes with more abundant and foamy cytoplasm and, in most cases, contain a population of irregularly distributed giant cells, including "early" Touton giant cells with multiple centrally grouped nuclei, but without surrounding foamy cytoplasm, and typical Touton giant cells with a rim of foamy cytoplasm surrounding a ring of nuclei and central eosinophilic core (Fig. 52-18A).

The late transitional pattern shows a predominance of spindle-shaped cells resembling benign fibrous histiocytoma but with focal foamy histiocytes and giant cells.

Cutaneous JXG involves the skin and the adjacent subcutaneous fat, but isolated lesions in deeper soft tissues, including skeletal muscles, are not uncommon, occurring in 14.7% to 16%.[383,384] Inflammatory cells, in particular eosinophils, may be present in the background with lymphocytes and, rarely, plasma cells. As mentioned, mitotic activity may be present, more often in soft tissue JXG than in the cutaneous form.[383]

Immunophenotype

Lesions of JXG show membranous staining for CD163 and CD14 and cytoplasmic staining for CD68 and factor XIIIa (Fig. 52-18B). Fascin and CD4 may be expressed.[388] S100 is typically negative, although positivity has been reported in a significant proportion.[383,388] CD1a and langerin (CD207) are not expressed.

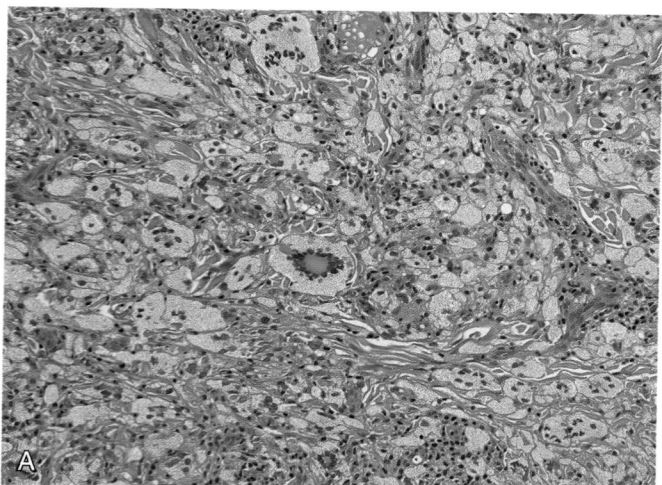
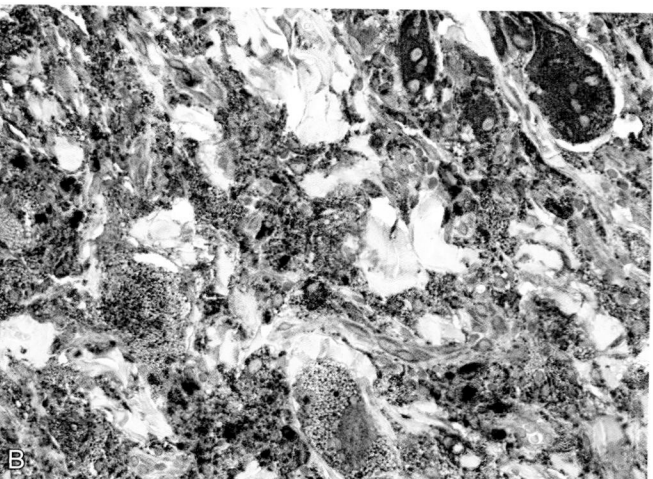

Figure 52-18. Juvenile xanthogranuloma. A, The lesion is composed of histiocyte with abundant foamy cytoplasm and Touton giant cells. There are occasional eosinophils. **B,** The lesional cells express CD68.

Genetics and Molecular Findings

The pathogenesis of JXG and related lesions has, until recently, been poorly understood. Studies using NGS have identified a role for MAPK and PI3K pathway activation in cutaneous, extracutaneous, and disseminated types with the discovery of recurrent mutations in *MAP2K1*, *CSF1R*, *NRAS*, *KRAS*, *ARAF*[275,373] and *MAPK1*,[400] and recurrent fusions involving *BRAF*,[376] *NTRK*, and *RET*.[275] A single case of JXG with a *MRC1::PDGFRB* fusion has been described.[401] The distinct subgroup of lesions with a JXG-like morphology that harbor ALK fusions are now classified as the separate entity of ALK-positive histiocytosis.[240,241,377]

The *BRAF* p.V600E mutation has rarely been described in a subgroup of intracranial JXG with a predilection for young males and aggressive/systemic disease.[402,403] These cases can show varying degrees of overlap with adult ECD: one patient had typical bone findings of ECD on imaging studies and was diagnosed as ECD; other cases have shown associated neurodegenerative changes in the absence of other features of ECD.[403] These findings raise the consideration as to whether intracranial JXG with *BRAF* p.V600E mutation could fall within an expanded spectrum of pediatric ECD, or whether this could represent a distinct subgroup of JXG.[403] The *BRAF* p.V600E mutation has also been found in cases of histiocytosis with a mixed LCH and JXG phenotype.[269]

Copy number analysis has indicated that genomic abnormalities are uncommon in solitary lesions of JXG.[404] JXG can also arise in the setting of neurofibromatosis with germline *NF1* mutations.[269]

Clinical Course and Prognosis

Cutaneous and solitary extracutaneous JXG typically follows a benign course with gradual regression of the lesions over months to years and a low rate of local recurrence if treated by excision.[383,384] Lesions in adults tend to persist rather than spontaneously regress.[2] Systemic JXG, including forms with ocular and CNS involvement, may result in significant morbidity[394] and require resection or chemotherapy for treatment. Very rarely, the disease can be fatal.[384]

Association With Hematologic Malignancies

Lesions with the morphology and immunophenotype of JXG have been seen in association with hematologic malignancies in both adults and children, though particularly in adults, including in B-ALL,[405,406] large B-cell lymphoma,[406] ATLL,[407] MDS,[408] CLL,[409] MGUS,[409] and MPNs.[410] Some lesions in this setting may show atypical features, including nuclear pleomorphism and an increase in proliferation index.[411] A clonal relationship between the JXG and hematologic malignancy was shown in a case with preceding T-ALL.[412]

Differential Diagnosis

JXG with a spindled morphology may raise the consideration of other cutaneous lesions such as dermatofibroma or blue nevus. ECD is within the histologic differential diagnosis, and warrants particular consideration in adults and in cases with detectable *BRAF* p.V600E mutation. Rarely, JXG can involve the bones, and needs to be distinguished from LCH with reparative and reactive inflammatory changes.

ALK-Positive Histiocytosis

Definition

ALK-positive histiocytosis is a rare histiocytic neoplasm characterized by the immunohistochemical expression of ALK within atypical histiocytes and associated with *ALK* fusions, particularly *KIF5B::ALK*.[377,413]

Synonyms and Related Terms

ALK-positive histiocytosis (ICC); ALK-positive histiocytosis (WHO 5th ed.); Not included (WHO Revised 4th ed); included within category of ECD (Revised Classification of the Histiocyte Society, 2016).

Background

ALK-positive histiocytosis was first described in 2008 by Chan et al.[414] in a case series of three infants who presented with massive hepatosplenomegaly, anemia, and thrombocytopenia with tissue infiltration by an atypical histiocytic population showing ALK immunoreactivity. A *TPM3::ALK* fusion was identified in one case. Since then, there have been sporadic case reports and small series of ALK-positive histiocytosis, showing that the clinical spectrum of the disorder is broader than first described and identifying the *KIF5B::ALK* fusion as a recurrent abnormality.[413] In the 2016 classification of the Histiocyte Society, the disease falls in the L group of histiocytic disorders within the spectrum of ECD.[2] Recent reports,[413,415] including a large case series,[377] have suggested that there is sufficient evidence for this to be recognized as a specific entity and it is now recognized as such in the ICC[240] and in the WHO 5th edition.[241]

Epidemiology

ALK-positive histiocytosis shows a female predilection and occurs over a wide age range (0–66 years),[377,413,416] but the majority of cases occur in childhood (79% in the largest study to date with a median age of 3 years).[377] One case has been described in association with CLL/SLL with identical immunoglobulin heavy-chain gene (IGH) rearrangements in both neoplasms.[417]

Clinical Features

ALK-positive histiocytosis has a varied clinical presentation. In accordance with the original description, it may manifest in young infants as liver and hematologic involvement with hepatomegaly, splenomegaly, anemia, and thrombocytopenia.[377,413,414] Other patients may present with a multisystem disease involving liver, lungs, bone nervous system, or lymph nodes. The disease may also involve a single system, often the central and peripheral nervous system with neurologic symptoms, but may be localized to lung, bone, breast, gastrointestinal tract, and skin.[377,413,415,418]

Morphology

The morphology is variable, but cases show a xanthogranulomatous morphology with foamy histiocytes and Touton-type giant cells, or are cellular and monomorphic without lipidized histiocytes.[377] Histiocytes can also have a spindled or epithelioid morphology, and nuclei are often slightly indented (Fig. 52-19A–B). In rare cases, the histiocytes can express S100 and show emperipolesis, strongly resembling RDD.[377]

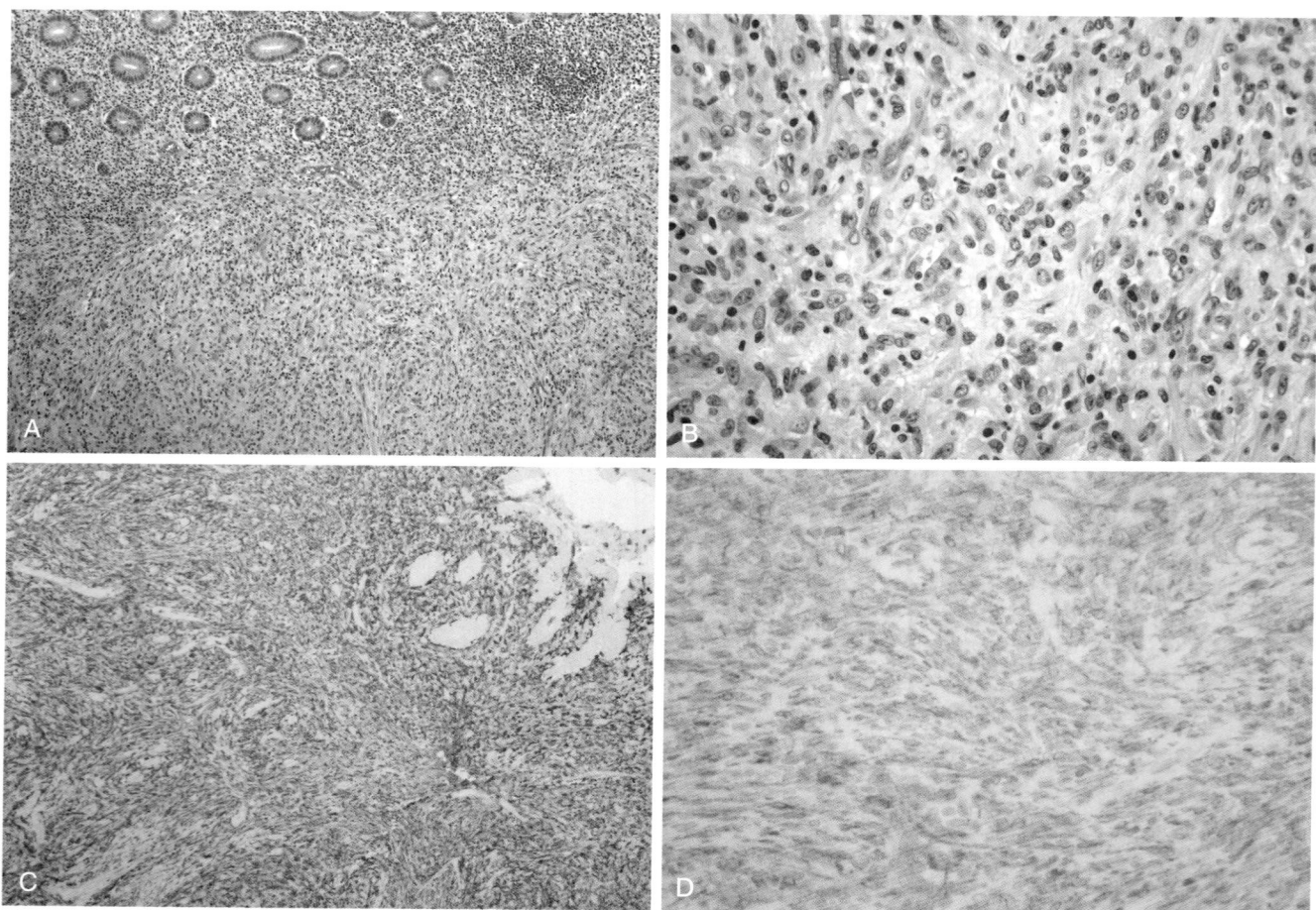

Figure 52-19. ALK-positive histiocytosis. A, An infiltrate with a spindled, histiocytoid morphology undermines the gastrointestinal tract mucosa. The cells have pale eosinophilic cytoplasm and oval to slightly indented nuclei **(B)** and express CD163 **(C)**. There is cytoplasmic positivity with ALK **(D)**.

The infiltrate may be focally subtle in involved liver biopsies and comprise only single cells or small aggregates in the sinusoids, though is more conspicuous in portal tracts. The histiocytes may be difficult to distinguish from hepatocytes, therefore ALK IHC may be required for identification.[413] Bone marrow involvement is typically focal and patchy,[377] though may be extensive.[413]

Immunophenotype

The tumor shows ALK immunoreactivity, usually with a cytoplasmic pattern with or without membranous staining; however, cases with exclusively dotlike Golgi positivity and cases with only focal weak staining are described. The pattern of ALK staining by IHC does not correlate with the underlying molecular alteration. The atypical cells express histiocytic markers CD163 and CD68, and are often positive for factor XIIIa (Fig. 52-19C–D). S100 and OCT2 are variably expressed, and cyclin D1 shows nuclear staining. CD1a is negative.[377,413]

Genetics and Molecular Findings

Most of the cases carry a recurrent fusion in *KIF5B::ALK*, usually with exon 24 of *KIF5B* fused to exon 20 of *ALK*.[377,413,415] Other ALK fusions have also been identified, including *COL1A2::ALK*,[413] *TRIM33::ALK*,[419] *CLTC::ALK*, *TPM3::ALK*, *TFG::ALK*, *EML4::ALK*, and *DCTN1::ALK*.[377,413]

If possible, the presence of an *ALK* rearrangement should be confirmed by molecular methods in order to confirm the diagnosis of ALK-positive histiocytosis. Cases with ALK staining but lacking *ALK* rearrangements may not benefit from ALK inhibition, and such cases may have other somatic activating alterations in the MAPK pathway.[377]

Clinical Course and Prognosis

The clinical course is diverse. Spontaneous resolution of disease can occur in infantile presentations, but progressive disease and death also occur. Although sustained complete responses have been seen with conventional chemotherapy in a few patients with multisystem disease, ALK inhibition has been found to induce significant and durable responses.[377,413,420,421]

Differential Diagnosis

ALK-rearranged tumors with prominent intermixed histiocytic infiltrates pose a particular diagnostic pitfall. A recent study[377] described a group of atypical *ALK*-rearranged histiocyte-rich tumors, in which the ALK-positive cells were within a histiocyte-rich background and often had a similar morphology to the atypical cells in ALK-positive histiocytosis; however, they did not express lineage-specific markers. Other *ALK*-rearranged entities, such as inflammatory myofibroblastic tumor and epithelioid fibrous histiocytoma, require exclusion.

ALK-positive histiocytosis and ECD may have a similar morphology and ALK-positive histiocytosis may present with bone involvement in a similar fashion to ECD. However, ECD patients are typically older than those with ALK-positive histiocytosis, and other characteristic imaging findings of ECD are generally absent. Furthermore, ALK immunoreactivity and *ALK* rearrangement can be demonstrated in ALK-positive histiocytosis but not in ECD, which may harbor the *BRAF* p.V600E or other MAPK pathway mutations. As noted previously, some cases may also show emperipolesis and resemble RDD; however, positivity for ALK will aid in its distinction from this entity.[377]

Rosai-Dorfman Disease

Definition

RDD, also known as Destombes disease[422] or sinus histiocytosis with massive lymphadenopathy,[423] is a rare non-Langerhans histiocytic disorder characterized by tissue infiltration of S100-positive, CD68-positive, and CD1a-negative macrophages typically engulfing living cells in their cytoplasm, a phenomenon termed *emperipolesis*. In the updated Histiocyte Society classification of histiocytoses,[2] RDD is categorized in the R group, which includes nodal classical RDD, extranodal RDD, immune-disease or neoplasia-associated RDD, and genetic-related RDD, while the exclusively cutaneous RDD is classified in the C group. Classical RDD typically occurs in young individuals, presenting with massive bilateral enlargement of cervical lymph nodes, often accompanied by fever and weight loss.[422,423] In most cases, RDD has an indolent course with spontaneous remission and excellent prognosis. Persistent disease is rare, and few patients have poor outcomes. Originally considered a reactive process, the occurrence of clonal mutations involving the MAPK pathway supports a neoplastic origin in at least a fraction of cases, and consequently it has been included in the *histiocytic and dendritic cell neoplasms* category in both the ICC of Mature Lymphoid Neoplasms[240] and in the WHO 5th edition Classification of Haematolymphoid Tumours.[241]

Synonyms and Related Terms

Rosai-Dorfman-Destombes disease (ICC); Rosai-Dorfman Disease (WHO 5th ed.).

Epidemiology

RDD can occur at any age but is most common in the 1st and 2nd decades of life (median age: 20.6 years), with a slight male preponderance[424] and predilection of African ancestry.[423] The cutaneous form is more frequent in women of White and Asian origin with a median age at onset of 43.5 years.[425,426]

Etiology

For a long time after its first description, RDD has been considered a benign reactive condition,[427] composed of macrophages activated by macrophage colony-stimulating factor.[428] A relationship with viral infections has been proposed without definite evidence. IgG4-positive plasma cells can be elevated in RDD, even reaching the cutoff values of IgG4-related diseases; however, the significance of this finding remains unclear and a definite relationship with

IgG4-related sclerosing diseases has not been established.[429,430] Nevertheless, it is recommended that all cases of RDD be evaluated for IgG4-positive plasma cells.[2]

Recent data reporting clonal somatic mutations in up to 33% of cases of RDD indicate that at least a fraction of RDD represent a neoplastic process.[373,424,431-433]

Associated Diseases

Two inherited conditions predispose to RDD: the "histiocytosis-lymphadenopathy plus syndrome" associated with germline biallelic mutations of the *SLC29A3* gene encoding for the equilibrative nucleoside transporter 3,[434,435] and ALPS type I, caused by mutations in the FAS gene *TNFRSF*.[436] The "histiocytosis-lymphadenopathy plus syndrome" encompasses H syndrome, Faisalabad histiocytosis, familial RDD, and pigmented hypertrichosis with insulin-dependent diabetes mellitus. These disorders have overlapping signs and symptoms[437,438] and in 20% of cases are characterized by accumulation of histiocytes with morphologic and phenotypical features of RDD, involving lymph nodes, skin, and nasal and oral mucosa.[434]

RDD-like lesions have been found to occur in 18 out of 44 (41%) lymph nodes of patients with ALPS type I and were associated with male predominance and early age of onset, without effect on the clinical course.[436] Notably, in 2 out of 18 cases, the histiocytic infiltrates were abundant and confluent, with distortion of the lymph node architecture, while in the remaining cases, the RDD-like lesions consisted of multifocal or isolated collections of S100-positive histiocytes with emperipolesis.

In 10% of cases, RDD occurs in patients with an immunologic disease, including systemic lupus erythematosus, idiopathic juvenile arthritis, and autoimmune hemolytic anemia.[424,439,440]

RDD has been reported in patients with myelodysplasia, acute leukemia, LCH, and ECD.[441,442] RDD and ECD can occur at diagnosis involving different sites, or the RDD lesions can develop later in time, with a peculiar predilection for the testis in elderly males.[443]

RDD-like lesions have been observed in patients with Hodgkin and non-Hodgkin lymphomas. In a few cases, the two diseases occurred in different sites at different times, while more frequently the RDD lesions were found in the same lymph node and mostly consisted of small collections of histiocytes showing emperipolesis.[167,444-447]

Clinical Features

RDD mostly involves single or multiple lymph nodes, which in 25% to 43% of cases are associated with at least one extranodal lesion, sometimes representing the initial manifestation of the disease.[439,440] In adult patients, however, skin involvement can be prevalent.[425,426,448] In 23% of cases, RDD occurs only in extranodal sites, especially skin, CNS, nasal cavity, and paranasal sinuses.[440,449] In 19% of cases, RDD has a multisystem spread.[440]

Patients with classical RDD are frequently young individuals (average age at onset of 20.6 years) with painless, massive bilateral cervical lymphadenopathy, sometimes accompanied by low-grade fever and weight loss.[422,423] Neutrophilic leukocytosis, mild normochromic normocytic anemia, polyclonal gammopathy, and elevated erythrocyte sedimentation rate can be observed in some cases.[440,448,450]

Inguinal, axillary, and mediastinal lymph nodes are more rarely involved, while retroperitoneal adenopathy is rare.

The extranodal sites more frequently involved include skin (10%, up to 52%),[448] nasal cavity and paranasal sinuses (11%), orbital tissues (11%), bones (5%–10%), CNS (5%), and kidneys (4%).[424,430] More rarely, RDD localizes in the oral cavity and salivary glands, larynx, pharynx, thyroid gland, lungs, thymus, liver, spleen, pancreas, breast, testis, and the gastrointestinal tract. Bone marrow is exceptionally involved by RDD.[424,440,448]

Cutaneous RDD can occur at any site, with prevalence of the extremities (54%) and trunk (47%), rarely with a generalized distribution; the lesions consist of reddish-brown papules, nodules, or large plaques measuring up to 30 cm, and can be asymptomatic or associated with tenderness or pruritus.[449,451] Sinonasal RDD causes nasal obstruction, epistaxis, or facial asymmetry, while oral cavity involvement manifests as soft and hard palate nodules, mucosal thickening, or tonsillitis.[440,452] Ophthalmic lesions mostly consist of expansive masses, uveitis, or compressive optic neuropathy.[424] RDD affecting bones is typically associated with nodal disease[440] and it mainly involves the metaphysis or diaphysis as osteolytic or mixed lytic/sclerotic lesions, causing pain and rarely pathologic fractures; it usually has a good prognosis with spontaneous involution of the lesions.[453] CNS RDD occurs as intracranial (75%) or spinal lesions (25%) associated with highly variable symptoms. The disease can be rapidly progressive and fatal, but patients eligible for surgical resection can have a favorable outcome.[454,455] Kidney involvement by RDD can manifest as a mass or diffuse infiltration, associated with pain, hematuria, renal failure, hypercalcemia, or nephrotic syndrome caused by amyloidosis or renal vein thrombosis, resulting in a mortality rate of 40%.[424,440]

Morphology

Lymph nodes involved by RDD are characterized by capsular sclerosis and follicular hyperplasia with significant dilatation of the sinuses by an infiltrate of large histiocytes, and accumulation of plasma cells in the medullary cords and intersinusoidal areas, the latter two findings resulting in a characteristic light and dark pattern of the parenchyma (Fig. 52-20A–B). In more advanced cases, the architecture is effaced by fibrosis and by a diffuse infiltrate of histiocytes, admixed with lymphocytes and plasma cells.

The histiocytes in RDD have an abundant pale eosinophilic cytoplasm; single or multiple large hypochromatic nuclei with a delicate nuclear membrane; and eosinophilic, often prominent, nucleoli (Fig. 52-20C). Emperipolesis consists of the occurrence of intact cells (lymphocytes, small macrophages, neutrophils, or plasma cells) within cytoplasmic vacuoles of the histiocytes, and it is highlighted on sections immunostained for S100 (Fig. 52-21B); emperipolesis is easily detectable on fine-needle aspiration cytologic specimens (Fig. 52-20D).

RDD identification in extranodal sites is sometimes difficult because the hallmark histiocytes can occur in small foci or as scattered cells and emperipolesis is less obvious; moreover, fibrosis can be prominent, plasma cells can be less numerous, and neutrophils are sometimes abundant, even forming microabscesses.[424,430] IHC is often necessary to identify the RDD cells and the diagnosis can require multiple biopsies (Fig. 52-22A–C).[448]

Immunophenotype

RDD histiocytes express multiple macrophage markers such as CD11c, CD14, CD68, CD163, and lysozyme, and are typically positive for the S100 protein[166,424,430,456,457] but negative for the dendritic cell markers CD1a, CD207, and ZBTB46.[333,458] In addition, they show diffuse expression of cyclin D1 and OCT2 and lack HLA-DR, in contrast to other histiocytic-derived tumors (Fig. 52-21A–C).[333,426,459]

Positivity for phosphorylated extracellular signal-regulated kinase (p-ERK) has been related to mutations activating the MAPK pathway[426,432,459] but found also in nonmutated cases.[460]

Genetics and Molecular Findings

Recurrent mutations affecting the mitogen-activated protein kinase/extracellular signal-regulated kinase (MAPK/ERK) pathway have been found in about one-third of RDD cases.[424] Mutations of KRAS[424,426,432,461,462] and MAP2K1[275,373,426,431,432,462] are the most frequently reported and are mutually exclusive.[432] Their occurrence is associated with younger age, head and neck region involvement, and multifocal presentation, but unrelated with the clinical outcome.[432] Other less-frequent mutations identified in RDD involve ARAF, CSF1R, NF1, PTPN11, SMARCA4, PTEN, and NRAS,[275,373,424,426,462] the latter especially found in the purely cutaneous forms of RDD.[463]

Notably, BRAF mutations, commonly encountered in other histiocytic disorders such as ECD and LCH, have been detected in cases of RDD associated with these diseases,[441,442] but only exceptionally in isolated RDD.[464] Notably, in the series of RDD cases associated with ECD, none of the RDD cases had BRAF mutations, the majority (9/12) having mutations of MAP2K1, which was identified also in the Erdheim-Chester histiocytes in only two cases.[443]

Clinical Course and Prognosis

Most cases with nodal and cutaneous disease have an indolent and often self-limited course with an excellent prognosis. Other patients experience alternating periods of remission and reactivation that may last years. In the series of Foucar et al.,[440] 17 out of 238 (7%) patients died because of disease-related complications, infections, or amyloidosis. In another study, disease-dependent death was reported in 10 out of 80 patients (12%).[465] Negative prognostic factors include extensive nodal disease, and multifocal and extranodal RDD, particularly involving the kidney, the liver, or the lower respiratory tract.[424,440] Patients with CNS involvement not eligible for surgical resection have an unfavorable prognosis.[454,455] Whether the occurrence of clonal mutations influence the clinical behavior is still controversial.[432,462]

A uniform treatment approach has not been defined for RDD, and it is generally tailored to the individual clinical circumstances, and particularly to the number and site of lesions, recurrences, presence of systemic symptoms, and life-threatening disease.[424,448,466] Thus, treatment can vary from a watch-and-wait approach to surgical resection of the primary and eventually relapsing localized disease, corticosteroids, radiation therapy, cladribine-based chemotherapy for multifocal disease, and immunomodulatory strategies (e.g., lenalidomide, thalidomide, sirolimus, or methotrexate).[424,448,466] Significant responses to MEK

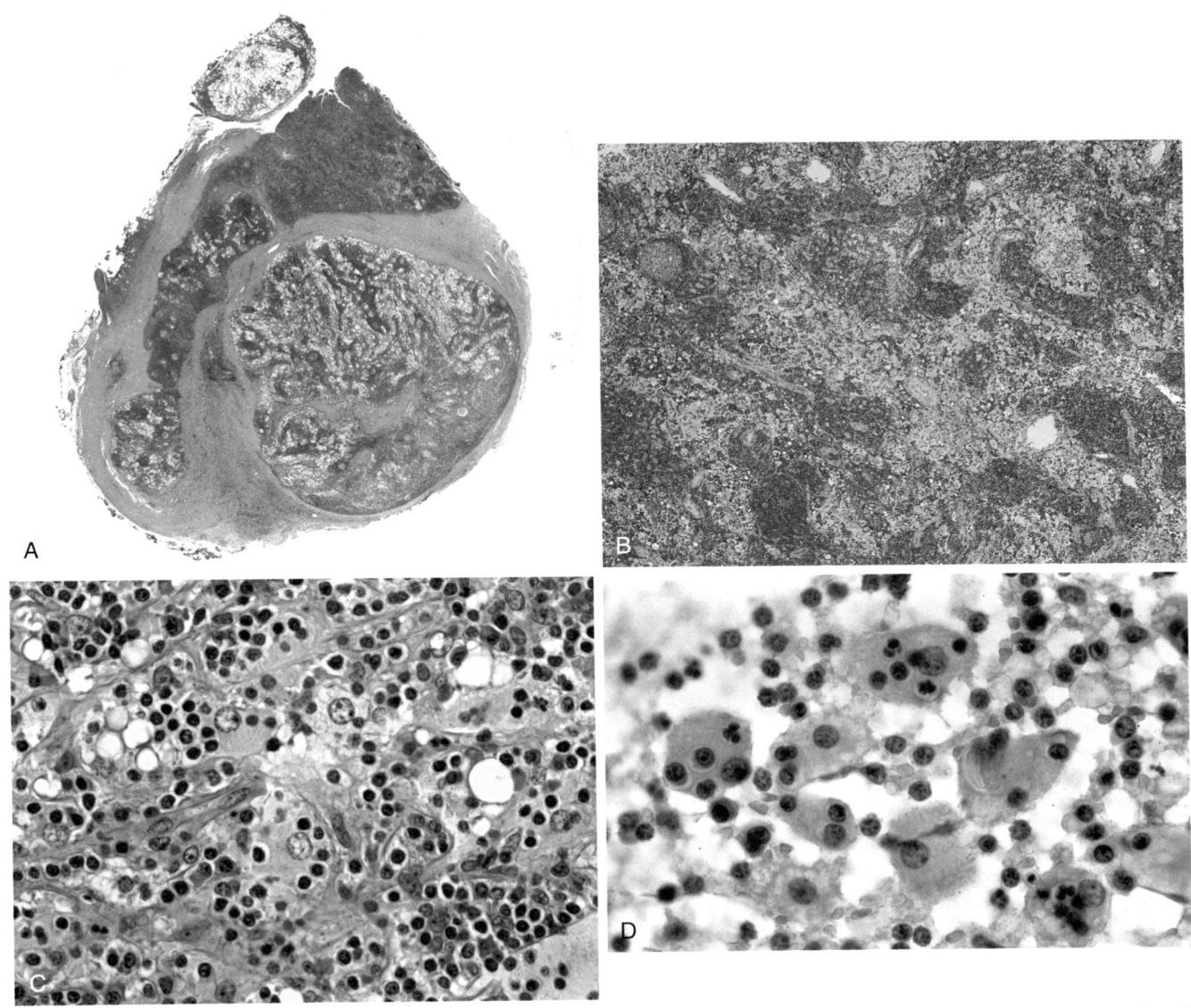

Figure 52-20. A–B, Rosai-Dorfman disease involving a lymph node: note the sclerotic capsule with septa and the parenchyma showing pale and dark zones, the former corresponding to dilated sinuses containing histiocytes, the latter to lymphocyte and plasma cell rich areas. **C,** The morphologic details of the histiocytes: large cells with pale eosinophilic cytoplasm engulfed by nucleated cells, some of which are surrounded by a clear halo; the nuclei of the histiocytes contain a prominent nucleolus. **D,** Fine-needle cytology showing marked emperipolesis.

inhibitors have been reported in cases with advanced and therapy refractory disease, independently from the occurrence of MAPK-activating mutations.[461,467-470]

Differential Diagnosis

In lymph nodes, marked sinusoidal involvement by S100-positive histiocyte-looking cells occurs in LCH,[333] but the distinctive cell morphology and phenotype of Langerhans cells, together with the presence of eosinophils and lack of significant plasmacytosis and emperipolesis easily allow the distinction from RDD. Hemophagocytic syndromes, especially the familial form occurring in early life, can mimic RDD because of the prominent sinus collection of phagocytizing macrophages. These macrophages, however, engulf many erythrocytes together with nucleated cells and are negative for S100. Moreover, these syndromes are characterized by disseminated disease and an aggressive

clinical course, which is quite uncommon in most RDD cases.

Although the prominent nucleoli of the histiocytes in RDD can give them an atypical appearance, the absence of mitotic activity is useful in ruling out malignancy, such as S100-positive melanomas and HS.[333]

Multiple or isolated RDD-like lesions may occur in lymph nodes involved by Hodgkin and non-Hodgkin lymphomas[167,444-447] and in lymph nodes from patients with ALPS.[436] These aggregates are distributed at the periphery of tumor nodules (Fig. 52-23A–B) or at the periphery of reactive follicles and in the expanded paracortex, admixed with numerous S100-positive interdigitating dendritic cells; sinuses are spared or minimally involved. Emperipolesis is generally focal and the S100 macrophages are negative for CD163.[447] These lesions are generally an incidental finding and not associated with overt RDD. According to the consensus

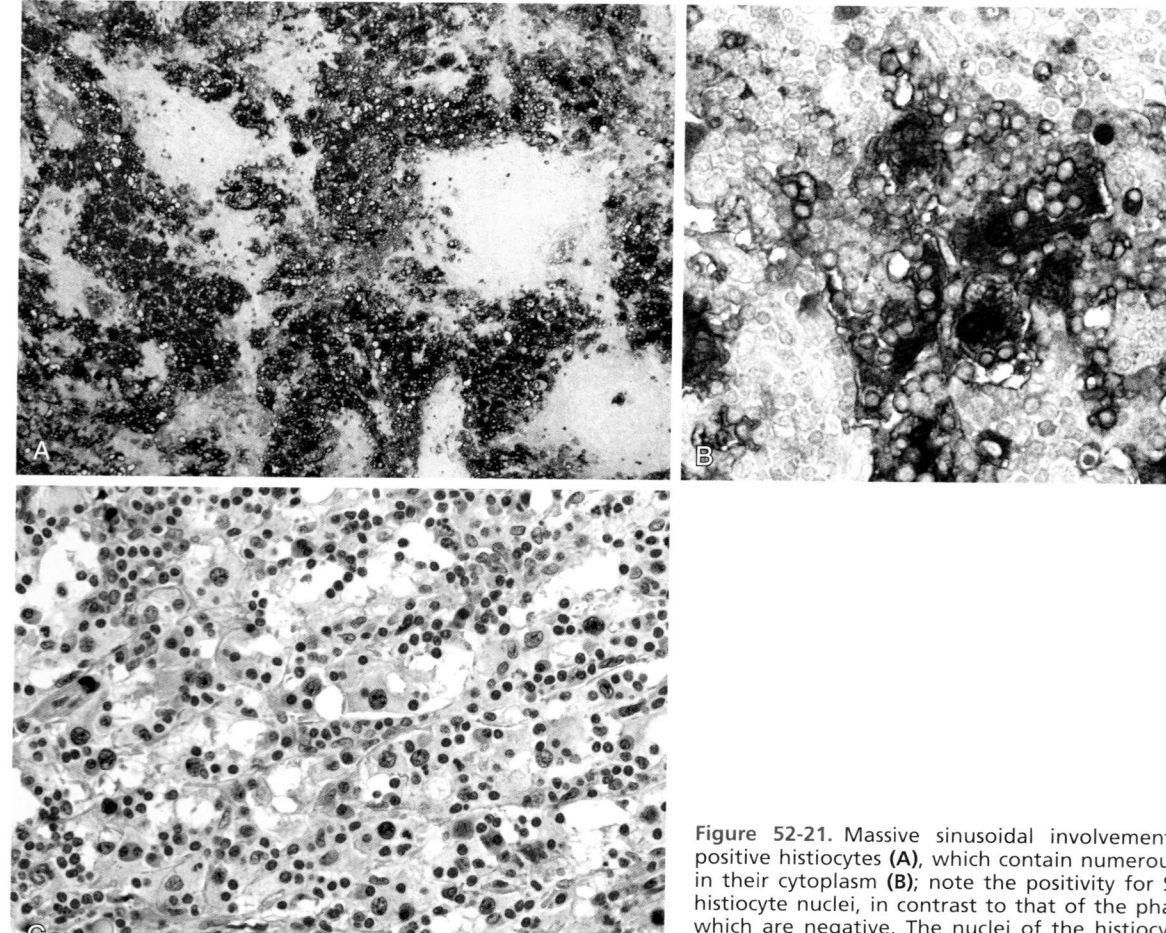

Figure 52-21. Massive sinusoidal involvement by the S100-positive histiocytes **(A)**, which contain numerous lymphoid cells in their cytoplasm **(B)**; note the positivity for S100 also of the histiocyte nuclei, in contrast to that of the phagocytosed cells, which are negative. The nuclei of the histiocytes are strongly positive for cyclin D1 **(C)**.

diagnostic recommendations, a RDD diagnosis should not be rendered when these foci involve less than 10% of the whole node.[424]

Nevertheless, the pathogenesis of these focal RDD-like lesions is intriguing. It has been suggested that they may result from abnormal monocyte recruitment and activation by cytokines occurring in lymphomas, or by the dysregulated immune environment taking place in ALPS.[436] The occurrence of numerous S100-positive interdigitating dendritic cells associated with these foci together with a morphologic spectrum ranging from S100-positive dendritic cells to S100-positive histiocytes with emperipolesis (Fig. 52-23B) suggested a possible derivation from activated interdigitating dendritic cells.[167] Notably, despite none of these cases showing mutations associated with classical RDD, the histiocytes are positive for cyclin D1 and p-ERK, suggesting that these focal RDD-like lesions might be the result of an autocrine or paracrine loop driving MAPK/ERK signaling.[447]

The distinction of RDD from other histiocytic diseases occurring in the skin and bones, such as ECD and JXG, can be challenging, because macrophages can focally express S100 and show emperipolesis. However, foamy cells and Touton-like multinucleated cells are very uncommon in RDD; moreover, OCT2 is generally negative in ECD.[459] In cases not easily resolved on the histologic and phenotypic basis, molecular evaluation and close clinical correlation is recommended.[424]

Macrophages occurring in ALK-positive histiocytosis can express S100 and show emperipolesis, strongly resembling RDD[167,333,414,471]; this advises to include stain for ALK in cases showing RDD features, especially when they occur in very young individuals with multifocal disease or in adults with CNS, skin, or breast lesions.

Combined (Mixed) Histiocytoses

Studies looking at the co-occurrence of LCH and non-LCH suggest that this phenomenon is a not infrequent finding. It most commonly occurs as a combination of LCH and ECD and mixed histiocytosis has been reported as accounting for up to 19% of the ECD cohort in one center.[380] The patients present with similar clinical findings to isolated LCH or ECD; however, at an age (~40 years) that is slightly older than that at typical presentation with LCH and younger than that with ECD. Patients are almost always diagnosed with LCH prior to or concurrent with ECD and there is an association with *BRAF* p.V600E.[380] Interestingly, a patient with LCH, ECD, and papillary thyroid carcinoma, all harboring *BRAF* p.V600E mutation, has been described.[472] LCH co-occurring with RDD and JXG has also been reported; however, the molecular relationship between these has mostly not been explored[473,474]; cases of histiocytosis showing a mixed LCH and JXG phenotype with *BRAF* p.V600E mutations have been described.[269]

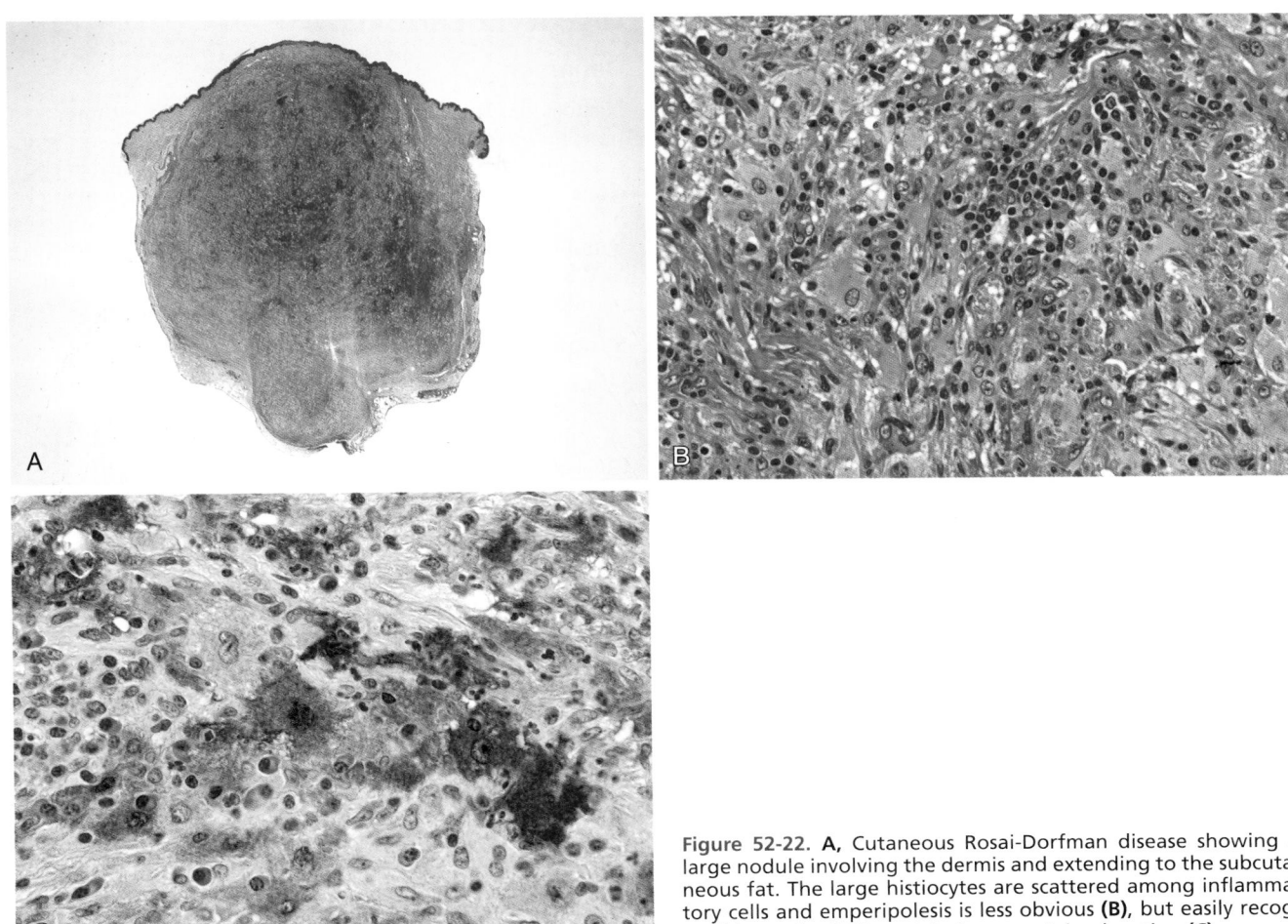

Figure 52-22. **A,** Cutaneous Rosai-Dorfman disease showing a large nodule involving the dermis and extending to the subcutaneous fat. The large histiocytes are scattered among inflammatory cells and emperipolesis is less obvious **(B)**, but easily recognizable on the S100-protein immunostained section **(C)**.

Figure 52-23. Small areas of Rosai-Dorfman disease–like histiocytes in a case of lymphocyte-predominant nodular Hodgkin lymphoma **(A)**; these cells are positive for S100, show emperipolesis, and many of them display a dendritic morphology **(B)**.

Biopsies from a subset of ECD patients with *MAP2K1* mutations may show histologic overlap with RDD and a predilection for testicular involvement.[443,475]

Malignant Histiocytic/Dendritic Cell Neoplasms

Malignant histiocytic/dendritic cell (H/DC) neoplasms are distinguished from other histiocytoses by a combination of atypical histologic features, including marked cellular pleomorphism and an increased mitotic rate, and a tendency to demonstrate aggressive clinical behavior.[2] Diagnosis and classification may be challenging as the minimum histologic criteria required for a diagnosis of malignancy are not established, and thresholds for antibody positivity when subtyping by IHC are not defined.

Evaluation of an IHC panel is central to final classification as HS, LCS, or interdigitating dendritic cell sarcoma (IDCS), although in the setting of immunophenotypic heterogeneity precise classification may be subjective and rely on the identification of a dominant component within the tumor.[333] The nomenclature of the ICC and WHO classifications does not distinguish a separate malignant tumor subtype with immunophenotypic features of IDCH; however, in the revised 2016 classification from the Histiocyte Society, malignant histiocytosis can be classified as indeterminate cell subtype, separate to the category of indeterminate cell histiocytosis.[2]

Malignant H/DC neoplasms are referred to as either primary (sporadic or occurring de novo), or as secondary (in which there is a clonally related associated malignancy). This is most often an associated lymphoid malignancy, with associated FL,[476,477] chronic lymphocytic leukemia/lymphoma,[478] T-lymphoblastic leukemia, B-lymphoblastic leukemia,[479] hairy cell leukemia,[480] and mantle cell lymphoma[481] described, among others. It is generally postulated that the secondary H/DC neoplasm arises through a poorly understood process termed *transdifferentiation*, whereby a mature cell of lymphoid lineage is converted to a mature myeloid lineage cell. In support of this theory, it has been shown in vitro that enforced expression of C/EBPα in B cells results in the downregulation of PAX5 and the activation of myeloid/macrophage differentiation programs.[482] The clonal relationship between the lymphoid malignancy and H/DC neoplasm has been well established in multiple reports through the demonstration of shared IG or TR rearrangements or shared cytogenetic abnormalities, such as the presence of the *IGH::BCL2*[476] rearrangements in both components. However, more recent comparative studies using NGS have yielded further insight into the nature of this clonal relationship with the discovery that the lymphoid and H/DC components harbor both shared and unique mutations, thus providing evidence in some cases for divergent evolution of each component from a common lymphoid precursor cell, and highlighting the acquisition of MAPK pathway–activating mutations as important in the pathogenesis of the H/DC neoplasm.[352,483-485]

Finally, the discovery of frequent activating alterations in the MAPK pathway has offered the potential of treatment with targeted therapeutic agents such as BRAF or MEK inhibitors in these aggressive neoplasms.[486,487]

Histiocytic Sarcoma

Definition

Histiocytic sarcoma (HS) is a malignant tumor with morphologic and immunophenotypic features of mature tissue histiocytes. It may arise de novo (primary HS) or clonally related to another hematologic malignancy, in particular low-grade B-cell lymphoma and lymphoblastic lymphoma (secondary HS). Recent studies have shown that MAPK pathway activation plays an important role in the pathogenesis of this disease.[488,489]

Synonyms and Related Terms

Histiocytic sarcoma (ICC) Histiocytic sarcoma (WHO 5th ed.); Histiocytic sarcoma (WHO Revised 4th ed.); Primary/secondary malignant histiocytosis, histiocytic subtype (Revised Classification of the Histiocyte Society, 2016).

Epidemiology

HS is rare. With advancements in IHC, many cases that were historically diagnosed as true histiocytic lymphoma or malignant histiocytosis have been reclassified as other forms of neoplasia, particularly diffuse large B-cell lymphoma (DLBCL) and anaplastic large cell lymphoma.[490-492]

In a study using data from the Surveillance, Epidemiology, and End Results (SEER) Program database (2000–2014) and including only adult patients, the overall incidence was calculated at 0.17 per 1000,000 individuals and the disease was more common in males than in females,[493] although notably some recent studies have shown a female predominance.[488,489] HS has a wide age range and occurs in both children and adults.[488,489,494]

Secondary HS accounts for ~20% of cases in some of the larger cohorts[489,494] and has been described in association with FL,[476] chronic lymphocytic leukemia,[478] marginal zone lymphoma,[495,496] hairy cell leukemia,[480] Burkitt lymphoma,[497] DLBCL,[494] mantle cell lymphoma,[481] B-lymphoblastic leukemia/lymphoma,[479,498] and T-lymphoblastic leukemia/lymphoma.[411,499] Rare cases have occurred in association with mediastinal germ cell tumors[500,501] and myeloid disorders including CMML,[351] MDS,[500] and biphenotypic/bilineal (B/myeloid) leukemia.[502] A case has also been reported in a patient with ALPS and RDD.[503]

Clinical Features

HS most commonly involves extranodal sites including the gastrointestinal tract, CNS, skin, soft tissue, spleen, bone,[504] and lymph nodes.[505] Patients present with symptoms related to the site of involvement including hepatosplenomegaly, lymphadenopathy, painful or painless masses, intestinal obstruction, or pancytopenia.[504,506] Systemic symptoms including fever, fatigue, and weight loss may also be present.[507]

Morphology

The atypical cells of HS have a varied appearance, but are usually medium-to-large in size with abundant eosinophilic cytoplasm. Some cells may have a foamy or xanthomatous appearance and cytoplasmic vacuolization may be present. There is often pronounced cytologic atypia with pleomorphic, bizarre, or folded nuclei (Fig. 52-24A–C). Multinucleated giant cells can be present and mitotic figures may be numerous with atypical forms (Fig. 52-24D). Hemophagocytosis by

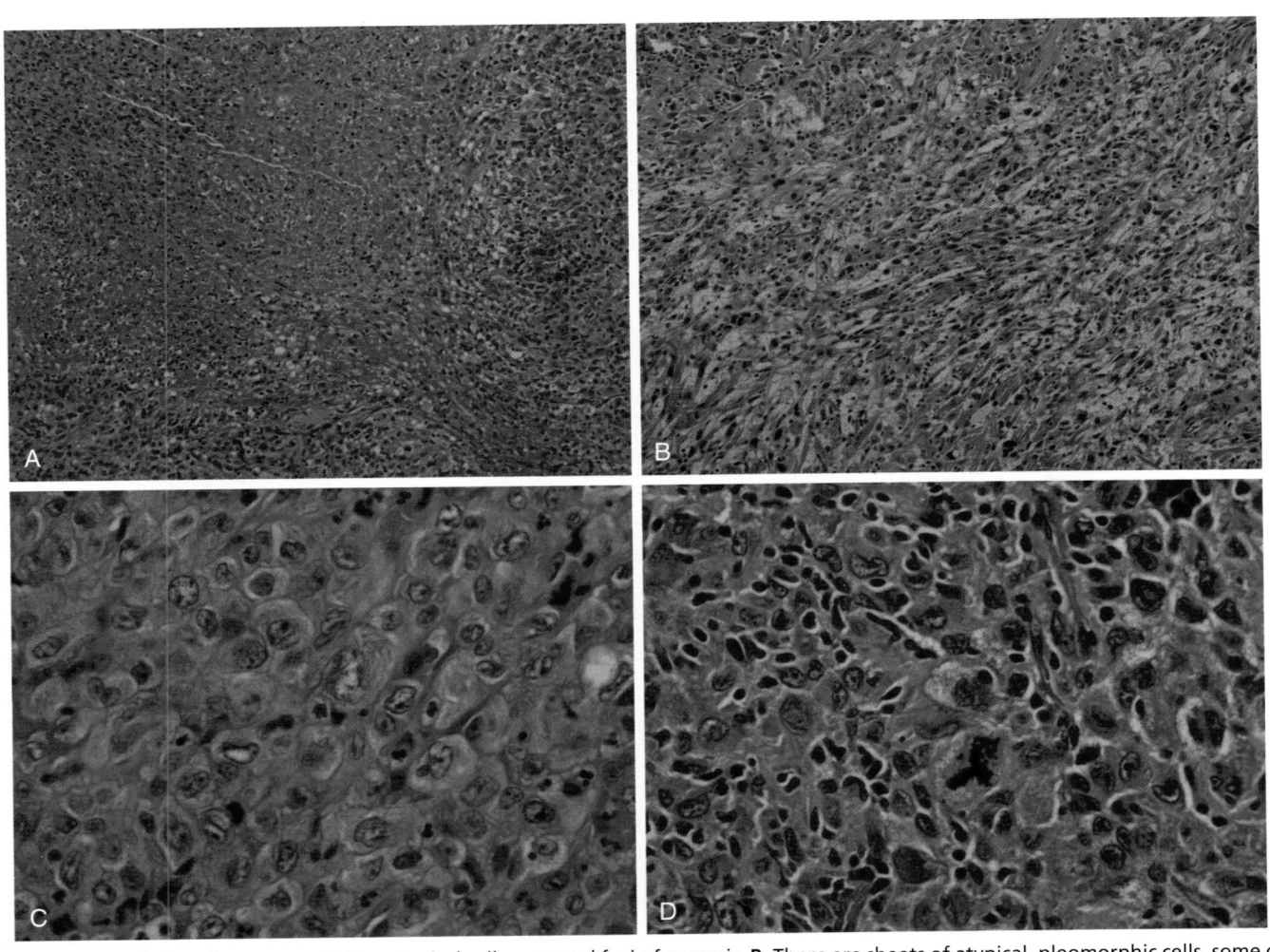

Figure 52-24. Histiocytic sarcoma. A, The atypical cells surround foci of necrosis. **B,** There are sheets of atypical, pleomorphic cells, some of which have foamy or xanthomatous cytoplasmic appearances. **C–D,** The neoplastic cells show marked cytologic atypia with pleomorphic, bizarre, or folded nuclei and atypical mitoses are present.

the neoplastic cells may be present.[164] The tumor cells can form diffuse sheets, and sarcomatoid areas with a storiform growth pattern have been described in some cases.[505] A prominent stromal inflammatory infiltrate is frequently present, most often composed of neutrophils or lymphocytes, but eosinophils or plasma cells may be present. There may be areas of necrosis. Sinusoidal involvement is frequently a feature in lymph node, bone marrow, and spleen biopsies.[504]

As HS may occur in association with a second hematologic malignancy, any lymphoid tissue in a biopsy should be carefully scrutinized to exclude a component of low-grade lymphoma.

Immunophenotype

The diagnosis of HS rests on the demonstration of immunophenotypic evidence of histiocytic derivation in tandem with the exclusion of tumors of other cell lineages such as carcinoma, melanoma, B and T cell lymphoma, anaplastic large cell lymphoma, and monocytic leukemia/myeloid sarcoma.

In general, there is expression of at least two histiocytic markers out of CD68, CD163, CD4, and lysozyme.[2] CD163 appears the more specific antibody for monocyte/macrophage lineage[508] as CD68 specificity depends on the antibody clone used. KP1 in particular is expressed in multiple tumor

types.[509] HS usually shows significant expression of multiple histiocytic markers. CD14 and CD11c may also be positive, and variable S100 expression is not uncommon.[506] HS is negative for markers of Langerhans cell lineage (CD1a and Langerin [CD207]), FDCs (CD21, CD23, and CD35), B cells (PAX5, CD20), T cells (CD3), CD30, and myeloperoxidase. PD-L1 expression has been found in a proportion of cases, raising the possibility of potential therapeutic targeting using immune checkpoint inhibitors.[510]

Genetics and Molecular Findings

Evidence implicating activating mutations of the MAPK pathway in the pathogenesis of HS began to emerge around 2014.[511] Since then, multiple studies have described activating alterations in MAPK pathway genes in both primary and secondary cases of the disease, including mutations in *BRAF* (both p.V600E and non-p.V600E mutations), *MAP2K1, KRAS, NRAS, PTPN11, NF1,* and *CBL*.[352,488,489,494] *BRAF* fusions are also known to occur with diverse gene partners[488,494] and a *TPM3::NTRK1* fusion has been identified.[489]

Co-occurring MAPK pathway mutations are not uncommon and have been described in both primary and secondary HS cases. These most often involve a noncanonical *BRAF* mutation in combination with a *KRAS* mutation,[489,494,512] or the presence of concurrent *MAP2K1* mutations,[488,489,494] but other co-occurring mutations such as in *NF1* and *PTPN11*,[488] *KRAS* mutations co-occurring with *MAP2K1, RAF1* or *CBL* mutations,[494] and *BRAF* mutations co-occurring with *NF1, PTPN11, NRAS, RAF1,* or *HRAS* mutations[489,494,513,514] have been described. In the case with both *HRAS* and *BRAF* mutations, the *BRAF* p.F959L mutation was shown to have intermediate signaling activity, requiring cooperation with mutated *HRAS* for maximal oncogenic activity.[514]

Copy number losses in *CDKN2A* occur relatively often in HS.[352,488,489,494] Alterations in TP53, and mutations and alterations in the AKT/PI3K pathway, including mutations in *PTEN*[488,489,494] and *PI3KCA*[489] or amplification of *PIK3CA*,[494] are less frequently present. A subset of cases also harbors mutations in *SETD2*; in a single study this was associated with mutations in *NF1, PTPN11,* and gastrointestinal tract involvement.[488]

Multiple studies of secondary HS have shown a clonal relationship between the HS and the associated lymphoid malignancy through the identification of identical IG or TR rearrangements in the lymphoid and histiocytic components,[478,479,515-517] the presence of shared cytogenetic alterations such as *IGH::BCL2* rearrangement in cases associated with FL,[476] *IGH::CCND1* rearrangement in cases associated with mantle cell lymphoma,[481,518] or other shared genetic alterations, such as *CDKN2A* deletion or *BRAF* p.V600E mutation.[411,480]

More recently, comparative NGS studies have confirmed this shared clonal origin and provided further insight into the evolution of these neoplasms, particularly those associated with FL. In addition to a shared *IGH::BCL2* translocation and clonal IG rearrangement, NGS studies on two cases with paired FL and HS samples[352,485] have shown that both FL and HS components shared mutations in genes that are implicated in the pathogenesis of FL (*CREBBP* or *KMT2D*), but there was evidence of clonal divergence, characterized by acquisition of an activating mutation in the MAPK pathway in the HS component (*MAP2K1* or *KRAS*), and also by the presence of other mutations and copy number alterations that were unique to both FL and HS components.

Similarly, cases of FL-associated HS for which matched FL samples were not available for comparison were shown to harbor activating mutations in genes of the MAPK pathway, as well as mutations in *CREBBP, KMT2D,* or both.[352,494] Taken together with the evidence of an aberrant somatic hypermutation signature,[489] or of somatic hypermutation[495] in analyzed cases of B-cell lymphoma–associated HS, this suggests that cases of secondary HS in this context originate from a late-stage common precursor B-cell.

Intriguingly, some cases of primary HS without a known history of B-cell lymphoma have been shown to harbor IG gene rearrangements, *IGH::BCL2* rearrangements, or mutations in genes associated with B-cell lymphoma, suggesting that a proportion of apparently sporadic/primary HS may also have a B-cell origin or that an occult or subclinical B-cell lymphoma may be present.[519] Rarely, the diagnosis of HS may precede the diagnosis of the associated B-cell lymphoma.[520]

Although NGS studies have greatly added to the understanding of the evolution of these tumors, complexities remain. MAPK pathway mutations have not been identified in all cases,[496] and limited studies of HS associated with B-ALL and T-ALL with available comparative samples have shown shared alterations, including IG or TR rearrangements, but also shared MAPK mutations in some cases,[352,499] indicating that the mechanisms and genetic events involved in transdifferentiation are likely diverse.

There are rare cases of HS associated with mediastinal germ cell tumor, most without molecular data, but a clonal relationship has been demonstrated in some instances, such as shared isochromosome 12p. Shared identical *TP53* and *BCOR* mutations were shown in a case of mediastinal germ cell tumor associated with MDS and subsequent HS.[500] A further report has shown clonal relatedness with evidence of a common precursor with *TP53* and *PIK3CD* mutations giving rise to GCT, CMML, HS, and AML. The GCT and AML evolved from a daughter precursor with 1q and 21q gain, and the CMML and HS evolved from a separate daughter precursor, with the HS acquiring an additional *NRAS* mutation.[501]

Clinical Course and Prognosis

HS has a poor prognosis with a median overall survival of 6 months.[493] Owing to its rarity, there are no established standard-of-care treatment regimens, and most cases with multisite disease have been treated by lymphoma chemotherapy regimens such as ifosfamide, carboplatin, and etoposide (ICE) or cyclophosphamide, doxorubicin, vincristine, and prednisone (CHOP). Surgery and radiotherapy have been used in the management of localized disease, or as part of a multimodal approach.[521]

More recently, case reports have detailed variable responses to novel, targeted therapeutic agents. BRAF and MEK inhibitors have been used in the treatment of cases with *BRAF* p.V600E and MAPK pathway mutations. While some cases have shown a good response to therapy, including to complete or near complete remission,[486,522] others have shown a good response but of limited duration.[523] Molecular evolution has been observed in a case after MAPK pathway inhibitor therapy, with loss of the *BRAF* p.V600E mutation and an *MTOR* mutation with an increasing allele frequency that was subsequently targeted with temsirolimus.[524] A clinical response of more than 1 year was also observed in a patient with *PTEN*-mutated HS treated with sirolimus.[525] Immune checkpoint inhibition with pembrolizumab and nivolumab has also been used in cases with PD-L1 expression with variable success.[526-528] Other agents that have been used in the therapy of HS include imatinib,[529] sorafenib, and bevacizumab.[522]

Differential Diagnosis

The differential diagnosis of HS is broad and requires careful assessment of morphology and immunohistochemical markers to establish histiocytic lineage and exclude other non-hematologic and hematologic tumors. Nonhematopoietic malignancies such as carcinoma and melanoma can be excluded by expression of cytokeratins or melanocytic markers. Anaplastic large cell lymphoma expresses CD30, and an expanded panel of B-cell and T-cell markers can be useful in the exclusion of B-cell and T-cell lymphoma. Extramedullary presentations of acute myeloid leukemia may be indistinguishable from HS on morphologic and immunophenotypic grounds; therefore, correlation with the clinical presentation, including bone marrow and peripheral blood findings, may be necessary, as well as with relevant molecular investigations.

Langerhans Cell Sarcoma

Definition

LCS is a rare malignant histiocytic/dendritic neoplasm that is characterized by malignant histologic features and immunophenotypic evidence of Langerhans cell differentiation. It has an aggressive clinical behavior and shows a poor prognosis, with a median overall survival of 19 months.[530]

Synonyms and Related Terms

Langerhans cell sarcoma (ICC); Langerhans cell sarcoma (WHO 5th ed.); Langerhans cell sarcoma (WHO Revised 4th ed.); Primary/secondary malignant histiocytosis, Langerhans cell subtype (Revised Classification of the Histiocyte Society, 2016).

Epidemiology

The overall incidence of the disease in the United States has been reported as 0.2 per 10,000,000 with a median age at diagnosis of 62 (range, 19–90) years.[530] Secondary cases have been described, usually after or concurrent with a diagnosis of lymphoid malignancy, including FL,[477,483,531] chronic lymphocytic leukemia,[478,532] hairy cell leukemia,[533] marginal zone lymphoma,[534] and T-lymphoblastic leukemia.[411] LCS has also been reported in the setting of chronic myeloid leukemia on imatinib, although the LCS did not have the *BCR::ABL1* fusion.[535] Rare cases have been reported after a diagnosis of LCH.[536] Notably, some cases were classified as LCS in the literature with CD1a expression alone, thus the possibility of indeterminate dendritic cell lineage is not excluded in these lesions.

Clinical Features

The most commonly affected sites are the connective tissue, bone marrow, lymph nodes, skin, liver, and spleen.[530,537] The disease can be localized and involve a single site or be widely disseminated.

Morphology

LCS is characterized by cytologic features of malignancy including nuclear pleomorphism and anaplasia, and a high mitotic rate with atypical mitoses.[2] The nuclear features may resemble cases of LCH with nuclear grooves, convoluted nuclei, and eosinophilic cytoplasm (Fig. 52-25A). Occasional eosinophils may be present, but accompanying inflammatory cells are usually few. Mitotic activity is usually conspicuous and the proliferation index in the atypical cells is moderate to high.

Immunophenotype

The atypical cells must show evidence of a Langerhans cell phenotype and demonstrate some expression of S100, CD1a, and langerin (CD207); however, this is often variable and the percentage of CD1a/langerin (CD207) positive cells needed to diagnose LCS is not well-defined (Fig. 52-25B). In some cases, these markers may only be present in a minor subset of the tumor cells. Expression can also differ between biopsies from the same patient and loss of some of the diagnostic markers can occur during the course of the disease.[411] LCS also variably expresses CD68, CD4, and lysozyme, and is negative for follicular dendritic cell markers CD21 and CD23.[538] Very rarely, expression of CD3,[539,540] CD30, and CD56,[541] as well as other T-cell markers,[540] has been reported. BCL6 expression has been reported in some secondary cases.[531]

Genetics and Molecular Findings

A recent molecular study of 10 cases of LCS (including three with a history of lymphoma) has shown frequent and apparently mutually exclusive mutations in *CDKN2A* (50%) and *TP53* (40%). Alterations in the MAPK pathway were also frequent, occurring in 90% of cases, and included mutations in *KRAS*, *BRAF* p.V600E, *MAP2K1*, and *PTPN11*. *PTEN* alterations were also identified in three MAPK pathway-mutated cases.[494] Case reports have also described *TP53* mutation co-occurring with both *PTPN11* and *NRAS* mutations, and with a *KRAS* mutation in primary LCS,[540,542] one of these also had a homozygous loss of *CDKN2A*.[540]

Other studies have confirmed MAPK pathway mutations in secondary LCS. A *BRAF* p.V600E[532] mutation has been described in LCS after CLL/SLL and a *KRAS* mutation has been reported in LCS after FL.[483] In both of these cases, the MAPK pathway activating mutation was only identified in the LCS component.[483,532] In a rare case of clonally related LCS that preceded the lymphoid malignancy (CLL/SLL),[543] both LCS and CLL/SLL components shared alterations in *MAP2K1*, *NRAS*, and *CDKN2A*.

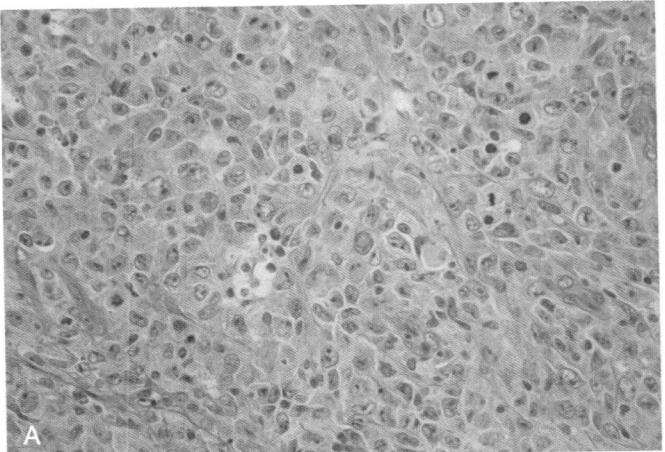
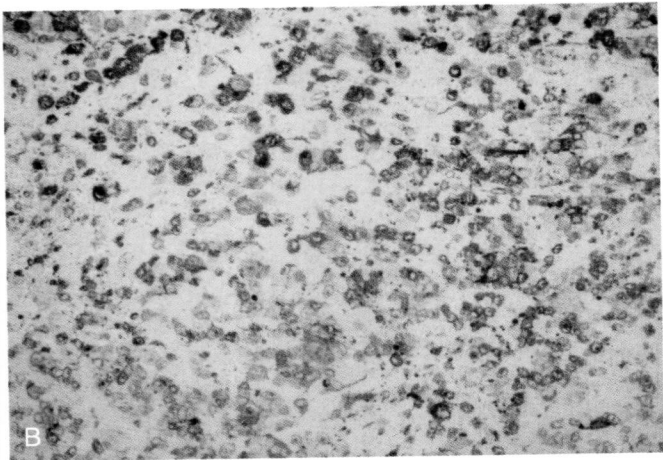

Figure 52-25. Langerhans cell sarcoma. A, The neoplastic cells have nuclear grooves, convoluted nuclei, and eosinophilic cytoplasm with atypical cytologic features and conspicuous mitotic activity. **B,** Langerin is expressed.

A common clonal origin has been shown in cases associated with lymphoid malignancy through shared IG or TR gene rearrangements[411,478,533,534] and shared cytogenetic abnormalities,[532,534] including shared *IGH::BCL2* rearrangements in cases associated with FL.[483,531] Furthermore, cases associated with low-grade B-cell lymphoma have also been shown to harbor mutations in genes that are typically mutated in B-cell lymphoma, such as *CREBBP, KMT2D,* and *TNFRSF14.*[494] Although comparative NGS studies have not been possible in all cases, at least some of these mutations may be common to both lymphoid and LCS components.[483]

Clinical Course and Prognosis

Treatment strategies are not well established and have included surgical excision of local disease or multimodality therapy, including radiotherapy and diverse chemotherapy regimens.[537] Recent case reports have shown variable success with novel agents including anti-PD1 therapy in the setting of PD-L1 expression, and BRAF or MEK inhibitors in *BRAF* p.V600E mutated cases.[487,542]

The prognosis is generally poor. A recent analysis has shown a 1-year overall survival rate of 62%, with a median overall survival of 19 months.[530] Previously, overall disease specific survival for all patients was estimated at 28% at 5 years in one study; in the case of single organ involvement (local disease), 5-year disease specific survival was 70%, dropping to 15% for loco-regional disease, and no patient with disseminated disease survived to 5 years.[537]

Differential Diagnosis

The immunophenotype of LCS is similar to that of LCH; however, LCS should show frank pleomorphism and cytologic atypia and an increased mitotic rate, allowing distinction. Expression of langerin aids in the distinction from other subtypes of histiocytic neoplasia.

Interdigitating Dendritic Cell Sarcoma

Definition

IDCS is a neoplasm derived from the interdigitating dendritic cells, the accessory cells found in the T-cell areas of peripheral lymphoid tissue, including the paracortical areas of lymph nodes and periarteriolar sheath of the spleen.[544]

Synonyms and Related Terms

Interdigitating dendritic cell sarcoma (ICC); Interdigitating dendritic cell sarcoma (WHO 5th ed.); Interdigitating dendritic cell sarcoma (WHO Revised 4th ed.); Primary/secondary malignant histiocytosis, interdigitating dendritic cell subtype (Revised Classification of the Histiocyte Society, 2016).

Epidemiology

IDCS is an extremely rare neoplasm, with 20 cases recorded in a retrospective review of data from the National Cancer Institute's SEER database spanning the period of 2001 to 2008. The mean age at diagnosis was 64 years, and there was a male predominance.[545] Another pooled analysis of 127 published cases showed a median age of 58 years and a slight male predominance.[546]

IDCS is associated with hematologic malignancy in ~12% of cases[546] and has occurred in patients with CLL/ SLL,[478,547,548] DLBCL,[549] FL,[476] NK/T cell lymphoma,[550] and B-lymphoblastic lymphoma.[494,551]

Other, non-hematologic malignancies have been reported in ~7% of patients with IDCS and include carcinoma (liver, gastric, breast, bladder, skin), leiomyosarcoma, and oligodendroglioma.[546]

Clinical Features

IDCS most often presents as isolated nodal involvement of cervical or axillary lymph nodes, but may also involve a variety of extranodal sites including the liver, spleen, skin, bone marrow, and gastrointestinal tract.[552] Some patients have systemic symptoms including fever, weight loss, night sweats, and fatigue.[552]

Morphology

The neoplastic cells are large in size with round, grooved, or indented nuclei and prominent nucleoli and abundant cytoplasm (Fig. 52-26A). Some cases may have pronounced nuclear pleomorphism with Reed-Sternberg–like cells; other cases may be composed of spindled cells with a whorled arrangement.[544] The background is rich in inflammatory cells, particularly small T lymphocytes, but neutrophils, macrophages, eosinophils, and plasma cells can be seen. Necrosis, fibrosis, hemorrhage, and hemosiderin deposition have been described in some cases. The mitotic count is variable and is often low (less than 5 per 10 high-power fields), although higher mitotic counts (>20 per 10 high-power fields) are also described.[552]

Immunophenotype

IDCS is positive with S100 (Fig. 52-26B) with variable positivity for CD68, CD163, lysozyme, and CD45 reported. Other specific markers for dendritic cells (CD1a, langerin), FDCs (CD23, CD21), B and T cells, melanoma, and carcinoma are generally negative[547,553] (Fig. 52-26C).

Genetics and Molecular Findings

The largest series of IDCS to date has found MAPK pathway alterations in 4 out of 7 (57%) of IDCS, including in *MAP2K1, NRAS, KRAS,* and a *CBL::USP2* fusion. Two cases also had *TP53* mutations.[494] One case in this series harbored both *NRAS* and *TP53* mutations and occurred after B-ALL, with both components showing shared clonal IG rearrangements. Another case report has also described IDCS associated with B-ALL with a *MAP2K1* mutation detected in the IDCS, but not in the previous B-ALL. Both components in this case showed identical clonal IG rearrangements and had several overlapping mutations by NGS confirming a clonal relationship.[551]

A common clonal origin has also been demonstrated in cases of IDCS associated with CLL/SLL by the presence of identical IG gene rearrangements and shared cytogenetic abnormalities between the two tumors, including trisomy 12 and 17p deletion.[478,547] The *IGH::BCL2* rearrangement has been found in both IDCS and an associated FL,[476] and a shared MYC rearrangement has also been shown in a case associated with DLBCL.[549]

The *BRAF* p.V600E mutation has been detected in a couple of cases,[328,554] one of which also showed clonal IG rearrangements without a known history of B-cell lymphoma. The *IGH::BCL2* rearrangement has also been detected in a case without a known history of associated lymphoma.[555]

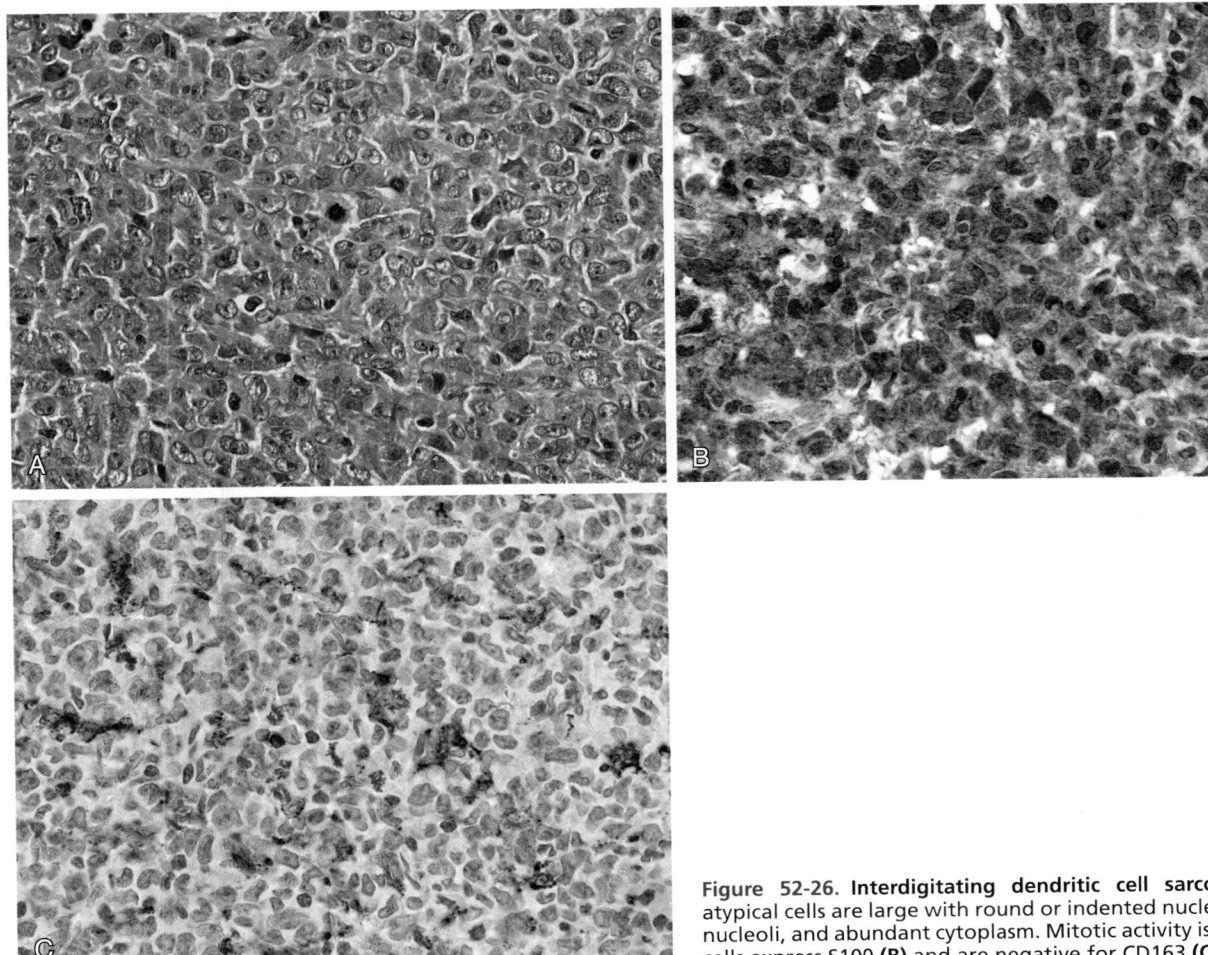

Figure 52-26. Interdigitating dendritic cell sarcoma. A, The atypical cells are large with round or indented nuclei, prominent nucleoli, and abundant cytoplasm. Mitotic activity is evident. The cells express S100 **(B)** and are negative for CD163 **(C).**

Clinical Course and Prognosis

Surgery has been the mainstay of treatment, with some patients receiving radiotherapy or systemic chemotherapy. Recurrence, both local and metastatic, occur in 50%.[546]

Cases are limited, but data suggests the overall prognosis is poor, particularly with disseminated disease. In one analysis, the median overall survival and progression-free survival of IDCS were 12 and 6 months with a disease-specific mortality rate of 36.4%. Mortality rates at 1 year were 21.1% for localized disease and 78.9% for disseminated disease.[546]

Differential Diagnosis

There is considerable overlap with spindle cell melanoma, with one study showing nearly equivalent IHC staining patterns and profiles in the tumors, leading to the question of whether these represent similar or identical processes.[556] Melanoma markers such as MelanA and HMB45 should be negative in IDCS, but a couple of studies have reported SOX10 expression in both diagnoses.[556,557] As distinction between these two entities may not be possible on immunophenotypic grounds, a recent study has noted that analysis of mutation signature by NGS to assess for a UV mutational signature may be helpful in difficult cases.[494]

FDCS may have overlapping morphologic features; however, IDCS is negative for follicular dendritic cell markers such as CD21, CD23, and CD35.[558]

Follicular Dendritic Cell Sarcoma and Epstein-Barr Virus–Positive Inflammatory Follicular Dendritic Cell/Fibroblastic Reticular Cell Tumor

Definition

Follicular dendritic cell sarcoma (FDCS) is a rare, malignant neoplasm of mesenchymal origin that shares histologic and immunohistochemical features, and a similar transcriptional profile, with FDCs.[237,559] This tumor, which may occur in nodal or extranodal sites, is considered to be a low-to-intermediate-grade sarcoma, although a significant number of cases may show locally aggressive or metastatic behavior.[560]

The related EBV-positive inflammatory follicular dendritic cell/fibroblastic reticular cell tumor (IFDCT) until recently was considered an EBV-associated variant of FDCS but is now considered a distinct clinicopathologic entity in the most current classifications schemes.[240,241,561] IFDCT is discussed together with typical FDCS.

Synonyms and Related Terms

Follicular dendritic cell sarcoma (ICC); Follicular dendritic cell sarcoma (WHO 5th ed.); Follicular dendritic cell sarcoma (WHO Revised 4th ed.).

Epstein-Barr virus-positive inflammatory follicular dendritic cell/fibroblastic reticular cell tumor (ICC); Epstein-Barr virus-positive inflammatory follicular dendritic cell sarcoma (WHO 5th ed.); Inflammatory pseudotumour-like follicular/fibroblastic dendritic cell sarcoma (WHO Revised 4th ed.).

Background

FDCS was first described by Monda et al. in 1986 in their seminal publication of four cases that presented with painless cervical lymphadenopathy.[562] The authors noted the morphologic, ultrastructural, and immunohistochemical similarities to normal lymph node "dendritic reticulum cells," which are today referred to as FDCs. FDCs are mesenchymal-derived antigen-presenting cells that play a critical role in the immune response and reside in the B-cell germinal center. (For comprehensive reviews of FDCs and their relationship to FDCS, the reader is referred to two recent reviews.[238,239]) Subsequently, in 1996, the same group reviewed the existing literature and reported an extended series of cases that they designated at that time as *Follicular Dendritic Cell Tumors*, and found that extranodal presentations accounted for 37% of cases.[563] The most recently updated information, published in 2021, reported that 79.4% (of 809 cases) were extranodal,[239] although this percentage may be high because of publication bias for unusual locations where this diagnosis is not expected. Nonetheless, it appears that extranodal locations account for the majority of cases.

IFDCT was first reported as a clinicopathologic variant of FDCS in 2001, characterized by frequent involvement of spleen and liver, a female predominance, an intense inflammatory infiltrate, and the presence of EBV in the tumor cells.[564] IFDCT was recognized as a distinct entity in 2016 in the WHO revised 4th edition.[561]

Epidemiology

FDCS occurs primarily in adults with a median age of 49 years,[552] but has been reported in children as young as 6 years of age.[565] There is no gender bias associated with the typical form of FDCS; however, there is a strong female prevalence in patients with IFDCT.[564] Although FDCS only accounts for 0.4% of all soft-tissue sarcomas,[566] it has been reported from nearly every geographic region in the world. Though the typical form has not been associated with known cancer viruses, IFDCT is characterized and defined by its association with EBV infection.[564]

Clinical Features

The clinical presentation of typical FDCS varies depending on the site of involvement, which can be both nodal or extranodal, as noted earlier.[239] The most common sites of lymph node disease are cervical, axillary, mediastinal, and abdominal. Patients with localized cervical or axillary lymphadenopathy commonly present with a slow growing, painless swelling of the affected region and are usually diagnosed early. Patients with mediastinal tumors may present with cough or difficulty swallowing, while patients with abdominal lymph node disease tend to present with vague abdominal pain and develop sizable tumor masses before a diagnosis is established. Patients with extranodal disease are more likely to present with generalized systemic symptoms including weight loss, lethargy, night sweats,

and fever, particularly those with IFDCT affecting liver or spleen.[552,567]

A subset (5%–10%) of typical FDCS has been associated with the hyaline vascular variant of Castleman disease.[568-572] These cases suggest a common link between the follicular dendritic cell component of Castleman disease and the tumor cells of FDCS, which is also supported by their shared transcriptional profile.[559] In addition, some cases with spatially coexisting diseases show clear transitions between the Castleman disease component and the FDCS component, often containing atypical dendritic cells that merge into regions of FDCS. Further evidence of a link between the two diseases is a recently reported case of FDCS with a *PDGFRB* p.N666S mutation,[494] a variant that has been reported in 10% to 20% of Castleman disease cases.[573]

Rare cases of FDCS have also been associated with paraneoplastic pemphigus and less commonly with myasthenia gravis.[574-580] FDCS should be seriously considered in patients presenting with pemphigus and a mass lesion.

In addition to the strong female gender bias and EBV involvement, IFDCT exclusively affects extranodal sites. Although the liver and spleen were the first sites of involvement to be recognized,[564] other visceral sites of involvement include bowel, bladder, and tonsils.[581-585] Despite its visceral location and frequent multiorgan involvement, IFDCT is generally indolent and has a low rate of recurrence after treatment, unlike typical FDCS.[567] These clinicopathologic differences have justified its classification as a distinctive clinicopathologic entity despite the apparent common cellular origin.

Morphology

FDCS grows as a solid, well-circumscribed mass and can reach a very large size, up to 20 cm or more, particularly in tumors that occur in the retroperitoneum or mediastinum. The tumors are generally described as firm, but the larger tumors may have areas of hemorrhage and necrosis.

Histologically, FDCS tumors are comprised of spindled-to-ovoid-shaped tumor cells that can show a variety of architectural growth patterns. Tumors may grow diffusely with little pattern, or more typically they may have a fascicular, storiform, or whirling growth pattern, the latter often described as resembling the growth pattern of meningioma (Fig. 52-27A–B).[562,586]

Cytologically, the tumor cells have eosinophilic cytoplasm with indistinct borders, and nuclei with finely dispersed chromatin containing small but distinct nucleoli (Fig. 52-27C). Although the tumor cells generally show little atypia and few mitoses, some tumors will display nuclear atypia and a higher number of mitoses. Binucleate and occasionally multinucleate cells may be present (Fig. 52-27D). These are reminiscent of the binucleated FDCs that are frequently seen in reactive germinal centers, and, when present, can be helpful in recognizing FDCS. Nearly all cases of typical FDCS will have a background of small lymphoid cells that are interspersed among the tumor cells. Cases that have large numbers of lymphocytes, particularly those that may present in the mediastinum, have been mistaken for thymomas.[586]

As its name suggests, IFDCT is notable for the very intense inflammatory cell infiltrate that, in addition to lymphocytes, may contain neutrophils and plasma cells (Fig. 52-28A). EBV is invariably present in the neoplastic tumor cells and is a requisite for this diagnosis (Fig. 52-28B). The inflammatory

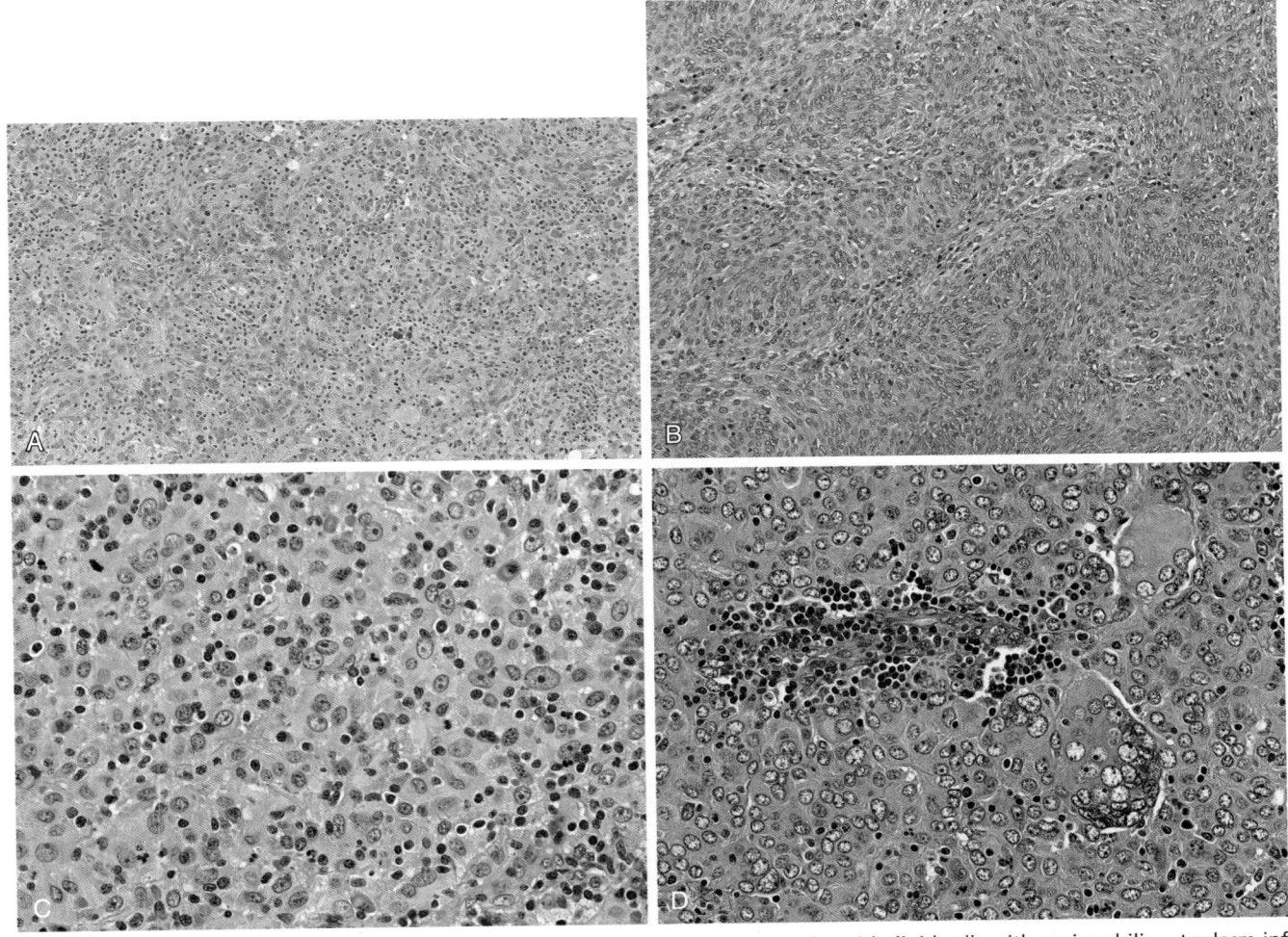

Figure 52-27. Typical follicular dendritic cell sarcoma. A, Case showing predominantly epithelioid cells with eosinophilic cytoplasm infiltrated by lymphocytes and with a rich vascular background. **B,** Case showing predominantly spindle cells arranged in bundles and whorls reminiscent of meningioma. **C,** High power showing indistinct cytoplasmic membranes, fine nuclear chromatin, and distinct nucleoli in a case of follicular dendritic cell sarcoma (FDCS) with epithelioid tumor cells. **D,** Multinucleated tumor cells in a case of FDCS. *(Photomicrograph [A] courtesy of Dr. Annapurna Saksena.)*

infiltrate may be so dense as to obscure the neoplastic spindle cell population and make its recognition difficult if this entity is not considered in the differential diagnosis, and result in its confusion with other types of inflammatory pseudotumors, or metastatic/ectopic thymoma. Once IFDCT enters into the differential diagnosis, it can be confirmed by IHC for FDC markers and detection of EBV.

Immunophenotype

The immunophenotype of FDCS is similar to that of normal FDCs.[333,504] The most useful and widely available markers in the clinical laboratory are CD21, CD23, and CD35, and a diagnosis of FDCS requires at least one of these markers to be positive (Fig. 52-29A–B). The majority of cases are also positive for CXCL13 (Fig. 52-29C),[333,587] clusterin,[588,589] and podoplanin.[590] More recently, two new markers, FDC-secreted protein (FDCSP) and serglycin (SRGN), were identified by whole transcriptome sequencing and found to be highly specific and sensitive for FDCS by IHC.[591] CD45 and the common lineage-specific B-cell and T-cell markers are negative.[504] Markers that are common in histiocytic tumors such as CD1a, lysozyme, langerin, and CD163 are usually

negative, although CD68 may be positive in some cases.[504] The immunophenotype of IFDCT is identical to that of typical FDC except for the presence of EBV-related markers such as LMP1 or EBV-encoded RNA, which are unique to IFDCT.

Genetics and Molecular Findings

There is limited information regarding the molecular pathogenesis of FDCS and virtually none regarding IFDCT. As expected in a tumor derived from a mesenchymal nonhematopoietic precursor cell, these tumors do not usually have immunoglobulin or T-cell receptor gene rearrangements, although there are occasional reports to the contrary.[519,592] Early studies using EBV terminal repeat analysis of IFDCT provided the first formal proof that these lesions were a clonal tumor[593] and subsequent cytogenetic studies in typical FDCS confirmed its clonal nature.[594-597] These later studies revealed complex alterations, some suggesting involvement of tumor suppressor gene loci; however, no recurrent cytogenetic abnormalities have been reported.

Molecular genetic studies are few in FDCS, but several themes appear to be emerging. Unlike most of the histiocytic tumors, mutations in the MAPK pathway are not common.

Although an initial early study reported *BRAF* p.V600E mutations in 5 out of 27 (28.5%) cases using droplet digital PCR technology,[511] subsequent studies using NGS technology have not confirmed this finding. Rather, these later NGS studies report frequent alterations within the NF-κB pathway, including *NFKB1A, BIRC3, TRAF3, SOCS3, CYLD,* and *TNFAIP3*[494,598,599]; alterations in MAPK pathway genes, including *BRAF* p.V600E, were not detected. Copy number losses at tumor suppressor gene loci (*CDKN2A, RB1, CYLD, BIRC3*)

have been recurrently reported in several of the referenced NGS studies, and by MIP array technology in additional cases.[600] Amplification of *CCND2* was reported in four patients from one study,[601] and focal copy gains in *CD274* (PD-L1) and *PDCD1LG* (PD-L2) were detected in three patients from a second study.[598] Intriguingly, a single case with a *PDGFRB* p.N666S variant was reported in the study of Massoth et al.[494] As previously mentioned, this variant has been reported in the hyaline vascular variant of Castleman disease, supporting the

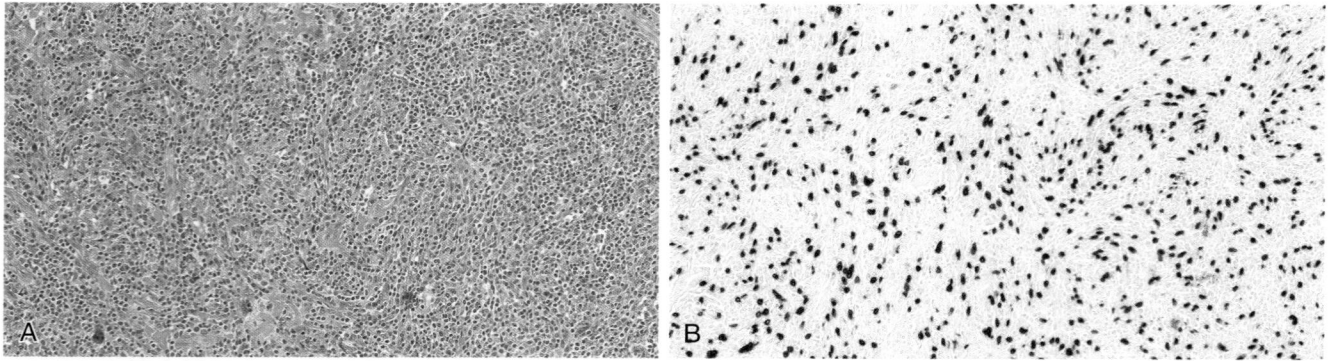

Figure 52-28. Epstein-Barr virus–positive inflammatory follicular dendritic cell sarcoma. A, Tumor cells are difficult to identify because of heavy inflammatory component consisting of lymphocytes and a few eosinophils. **B,** In situ hybridization for Epstein-Barr virus–encoded RNA assists identification of the positive tumor cells. *(Photomicrographs courtesy of Dr. Annapurna Saksena.)*

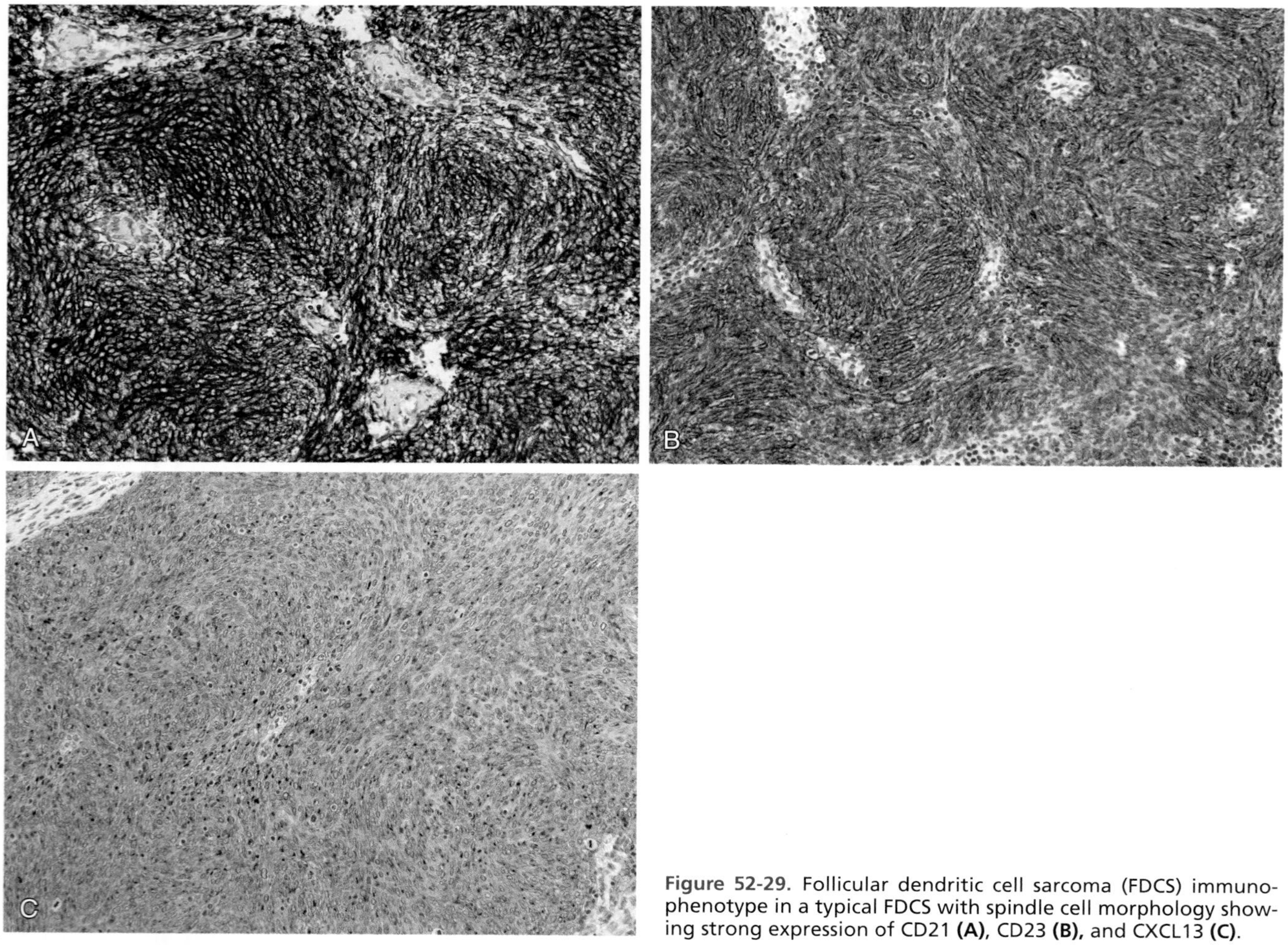

Figure 52-29. Follicular dendritic cell sarcoma (FDCS) immunophenotype in a typical FDCS with spindle cell morphology showing strong expression of CD21 **(A),** CD23 **(B),** and CXCL13 **(C).**

hypothesis that some cases of FDCS develop from the FDC component of Castleman disease.[573] No recurrent fusions have been identified, although several rare novel fusions of unknown significance have been reported, including *TYK2::ATPAF2*, *MAP3K1::GCOM1*, and *NTRK1::PDIA3*.[494]

The molecular profile of IFDCT is unknown. Bruehl et al. subjected two IFDCT cases to large-panel NGS sequencing and did not find pathogenic variants, including fusions.[602] This is consistent with our own experience as well (unpublished data). However, it should be noted that the inability to detect mutations may be because of the small number of tumor cells present, which may be beyond the resolving power of the NGS assays.

Clinical Course and Prognosis

Typical FDCS is generally considered a low-to-intermediate-grade tumor with unpredictable behavior.[240,241] They have a propensity for local recurrence if not excised completely, and a subset may metastasize.[560] Small lesions can be surgically removed, and the risk of recurrence is low. Lesions greater than 5 cm have a higher rate of recurrence and distant metastases.[560,603] There is no universally accepted staging system that predicts the behavior of these tumors; however, using retrospective data, Li et al. developed a risk assessment model for extranodal FDCS based on mitotic rate, tumor size, and histologic grade.[603] Lesions were defined as low, intermediate, and high risk and were associated with recurrence rates of 16%, 46%, and 73% and mortality rates of 0%, 4%, and 45%, respectively. This system has yet to be tested in a prospective trial but is a notable attempt to develop a histology-based system for predicting the biological behavior of these tumors.

There is no single treatment recommended for typical FDCS and the therapeutic approach is generally tailored to the presentation of the disease. As previously mentioned, localized tumors are surgically removed and may be accompanied by adjuvant chemotherapy or radiation therapy, while disseminated disease is generally treated with a combination of surgery, systemic chemotherapy, or radiation.[604,605] Newer biological therapies have been successful in rare cases but are anecdotal.[606,607] Interestingly, despite the visceral presentations of IFDCT, these cases tend to behave indolently, and therefore conservative approaches may be appropriate.[567]

Differential Diagnosis

The differential diagnosis of FDCS varies by location. Cases that are limited to lymph nodes have a narrower differential diagnosis and would include mainly primary tumors of lymph nodes such as IDCS and the very rare fibroblastic reticular cell sarcoma.[562,586] Once FDCS is considered, the characteristic FDC immunophenotypic profile is highly specific.

In extranodal sites, the differential diagnosis is broader, and, depending on the specific location, might include gastrointestinal stromal tumor, metastatic thymoma, ectopic/metastatic meningioma, spindle cell carcinoma, or other soft tissue sarcomas.[565,601]

IFDCT (as well as typical FDCS with large numbers of inflammatory cells) can be further confused with other tumors and conditions that have high percentages of inflammatory cells. These include ALK-positive histiocytosis, inflammatory myofibroblastic pseudotumor, and lymphocyte-rich metastatic thymomas.[585] A high degree of suspicion and the presence of

FDC markers CD21, CD23, or CD35 are key to distinguishing FDCS from other tumors, and the associated presence of EBV will further distinguish IFDCT.

Acknowledgment

The authors and editors dedicate this chapter to the memory of Ronald Jaffe, who wrote the Langerhans histiocytosis chapters in the two previous editions of this book.

Pearls and Pitfalls

Hemophagocytic Syndromes

- The clinical syndromes and morphology of primary and secondary hemophagocytic lymphohistiocytosis (HLH) are similar.
- A careful genetic history, testing for perforin expression and natural killer (NK)-cell number and function, and molecular analysis may be necessary to distinguish them.
- The presence of hemophagocytosis has limited diagnostic sensitivity and specificity, because it may not be always present and it can be observed in patients without HLH.
- The diagnosis of HLH is a complex process that must be carried out rapidly, given the lethality of the disease, excluding mimicking conditions whose pathogenesis differs from that of authentic HLH, thus requiring appropriate therapies.

Storage Disorders

- The diagnosis of Gaucher disease is established by identifying histiocytes with increased iron uptake and cytoplasmic wrinkled-paper appearance (Gaucher cells) in the bone marrow or any other tissue, in association with decreased activity of β-glucocerebrosidase in leukocytes.
- Histiocytes that mimic Gaucher cells can accumulate in the bone marrow of patients with disorders associated with high cell turnover, such as chronic myelogenous leukemia.
- The presence of splenomegaly and bone marrow infiltration by Niemann-Pick cells, as well as sea-blue histiocytes in association with decreased sphingomyelinase activity in leukocytes, confirms a diagnosis of Niemann-Pick disease.
- In Tangier disease, young individuals typically present with enlarged yellow-orange tonsils, and the identification of lipid-laden macrophages accumulated provides a clue for the diagnosis, but is not pathognomonic.

Histiocytic and Dendritic Cell Neoplasia

- The diagnosis of histiocytic and dendritic cell neoplasia can be challenging and requires the correlation of the clinical features, appearances on imaging studies, and histopathologic findings.
- Immunohistochemistry is an essential adjunct in the diagnosis of both histiocytic neoplasia and dendritic cell tumors, and plays a key role in distinguishing between the various subtypes of these tumors and excluding potential mimics.
- Molecular evaluation by next-generation sequencing studies and fusion testing allows the detection of activating alterations in MAPK, PI3K/AKT, and NF-κB pathway genes that not only aids in diagnosis but also identifies potential targets for systemic therapy.

KEY REFERENCES

4. Griffin G, Shenoi S, Hughes GC. Hemophagocytic lymphohistiocytosis: an update on pathogenesis, diagnosis, and therapy. *Best Pract Res Clin Rheumatol*. 2020;34(4):101515.
239. Facchetti F, Simbeni M, Lorenzi L. Follicular dendritic cell sarcoma. *Pathologica*. 2021;113(5):316–329.
243. Badalian-Very G, et al. Recurrent BRAF mutations in Langerhans cell histiocytosis. *Blood*. 2010;116(11):1919–1923.

265. Goyal G, et al. International expert consensus recommendations for the diagnosis and treatment of Langerhans cell histiocytosis in adults. *Blood*. 2022;139(17):2601–2621.

352. Egan C, et al. The mutational landscape of histiocytic sarcoma associated with lymphoid malignancy. *Mod Pathol*. 2021;34(2):336–347.

365. Goyal G, et al. Erdheim-Chester disease: consensus recommendations for evaluation, diagnosis, and treatment in the molecular era. *Blood*. 2020;135(22):1929–1945.

377. Kemps PG, et al. ALK-positive histiocytosis: a new clinicopathologic spectrum highlighting neurologic involvement and responses to ALK inhibition. *Blood*. 2022;139(2):256–280.

424. Abla O, et al. Consensus recommendations for the diagnosis and clinical management of Rosai-Dorfman-Destombes disease. *Blood*. 2018;131(26):2877–2890.

489. Shanmugam V, et al. Identification of diverse activating mutations of the RAS-MAPK pathway in histiocytic sarcoma. *Mod Pathol*. 2019;32(6):830–843.

494. Massoth LR, et al. Histiocytic and dendritic cell sarcomas of hematopoietic origin share targetable genomic alterations distinct from follicular dendritic cell sarcoma. *Oncol*. 2021;26(7):e1263–e1272.

Visit Elsevier eBooks+ for the complete set of references.

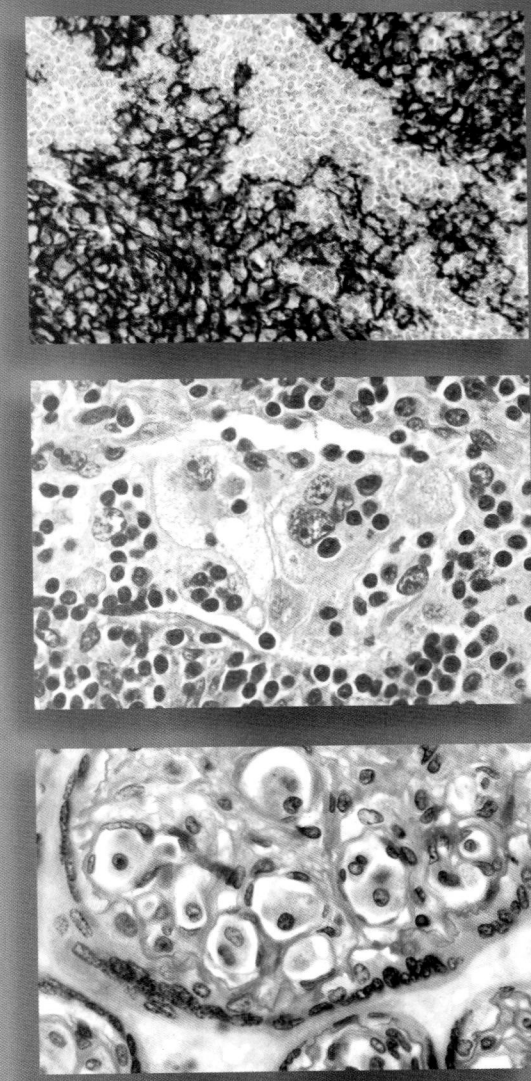

PART **V**

Immunodeficiency Disorders

Chapter 53

The Pathology of Primary Immunodeficiencies

Stefania Pittaluga, Kristian T. Schafernak, and Katherine R. Calvo

Primary immunodeficiencies (PIDs) are inborn errors of immunity and comprise 485 different genetic disorders at the time of the most recent interim update by the International Union of Immunological Societies (IUIS) Expert Committee.[1,2] PIDs often predispose to infection and tend to present early in life, with high morbidity and mortality if left untreated; in fact, they are often diagnosed because of severe, persistent, or recurrent infections during infancy that don't respond to therapy. However, it has become apparent that PIDs not only confer risk for developing infections, but increasingly they are associated with immune dysregulation, autoimmunity, autoinflammation, allergy, and susceptibility for developing malignancies, in particular lymphomas.[3] PIDs are monogenic, caused by a defect in a single gene, not necessarily with complete clinical penetrance, and in the majority of cases tend to cause loss of function (LOF) irrespective of autosomal dominant (AD), autosomal recessive (AR), or X-linked recessive (XR) inheritance. In recent years, gain-of-function mutations have also been described, predominantly in the AD group.[4] However, all mutations are *not* created equal; furthermore, great variability in clinical phenotype (i.e., age at onset, severity, and clinical presentation) can be observed even within the same family because of additional factors that come into play besides the specific characteristic of the causal mutation(s) involved, such as gene dosage; differential allelic expression; copy number variations and other modulatory influences; gene modifier (epigenetic changes);

and age, sex, and environmental factors.[1] The importance of the family history in the diagnosis of a possible PID cannot be overstated; however, a negative family history does not exclude PID, particularly for patients with XR disorders, who frequently harbor "new" mutations and do not have affected male relatives.

In the last 15 years, the number of PIDs has increased almost exponentially, largely because of the introduction in 2008 of next-generation sequencing (NGS), expanding the traditional approaches in classical genetics that used cytogenetic tools such as linkage analysis, positional cloning, and candidate gene approach with Sanger sequencing as the gold standard.[5-7] These new technologies, in particular whole-exome sequencing (WES), which detects mutations in protein-coding and RNA-coding genes, and whole-genome sequencing (WGS), which also analyzes intronic sequences, have also brought new challenges with the detection of many mutations in normal individuals, rendering it even more imperative to validate candidate genes with functional studies and in vivo models. In addition to the more traditional approach using transfection experiments with knockdown of candidate genes in primary cells and cell lines, new approaches using induced pluripotent stem (iPS) cells and gene editing with CRISPR/Cas9 have provided additional and more sophisticated tools to understand the role of candidate genes in the appropriate cellular context and to assess its relevance to the phenotype under study.[6]

As pathologists, it is important to be aware of these disorders and their pathologic features because an accurate and early diagnosis may not only save the life of the patient but that of his or her family members. Complete blood count (CBC) with differential, lymphocyte subset analysis, and quantitation of serum immunoglobulins (Ig) are a good jumping-off point in the diagnostic workup, but often the nature and location of a patient's infections tells a lot about the type of underlying immunodeficiency. This is illustrated well by the susceptibility of patients with phagocyte dysfunction like chronic granulomatous disease to staphylococcal infections, as they have an impaired ability to generate reactive oxygen species because of defects in the NADPH oxidase complex,[8] or *Neisseria meningitidis* meningitis revealing complement deficiency.[9] Humoral immunodeficiency often results in sinopulmonary infections with encapsulated bacteria or chronic diarrhea and is sometimes uncovered in infants after age 4 to 9 months, after maternal alloimmunity wanes. The T-cell arm of the immune system is not only important for controlling viral and fungal disease but also in helping B cells to be able to produce antibodies, so humoral immunodeficiency accompanies cellular immunodeficiency in diseases like severe combined immunodeficiency (SCID).

It may very well be the pathologist, aware of the systemic nature of these disorders, who puts everything together, recognizing other associated but sometimes overlooked clinical features suggesting a PID, like failure to thrive or rash in an infant. Besides the frequent involvement of not only immune organs (thymus, lymph nodes, bone marrow, and spleen), PIDs also have wide-ranging effects on target organs such as the lungs, gastrointestinal tract, skin, and central nervous system (CNS), either caused by infections (bacterial, fungal, viral, and parasitic), autoimmunity, allergic and inflammatory processes (e.g., vasculitis), or neoplasia. In some of these disorders, there are morphologic and phenotypic features we observe that are either unique or intrinsically related to the underlying genetic defect and lead us to a diagnosis; in other instances, the pathologic changes may be non-specific, but they can help by ruling out some of the other diagnostic possibilities. Lastly, understanding PIDs and their pathophysiology is important because it gives us clues about the functional aspects of the immune system, both innate and adaptive, and their intricate interrelationship, which will ultimately lead to the design and implementation of a more targeted therapeutic approach.

CLASSIFICATION

The classification of molecularly defined PIDs is formally updated every 2 years by the IUIS Expert Committee for Primary Immunodeficiency and provides a clinical and immunologic synopsis, genetic defect when known, and mode of inheritance in table format. In 2021 an interim report was issued and, just days after the 2019 update was published in early 2020, it had already become out of date, with 26 additional novel inborn errors of immunity.[1] The 2022 update added 29 novel gene defects, bringing the total number of inborn errors of immunity to 485—up from 191 in the 2011 biennial update.[2] Depending on the genetic defect, when known, or predominant symptom, it is divided into broad categories as follows: (1) immunodeficiencies affecting cellular and humoral immunity; (2) combined immunodeficiencies with associated or syndromic features; (3) predominantly antibody deficiencies; (4) diseases of immune dysregulation; (5) congenital defects of phagocyte number or function; (6) defects in intrinsic and innate immunity; (7) autoinflammatory disorders; (8) complement deficiencies; (9) bone marrow failure; and (10) phenocopies of inborn errors of immunity. Depending on the prevalent defect and symptoms, some of the inherited disorders are listed under multiple headings. The *phenocopies* category refers to patients (syndromes) presenting with characteristics that are similar to inherited PID but are not caused by a germline mutation, but rather arise from acquired mechanisms such as somatic mutations (see the discussion on somatic mutations in the section on autoimmune lymphoproliferative syndrome [ALPS] later in the chapter) or autoantibody production against cytokines, or immunologic factors leading to their depletion with subsequent development of PID-like symptoms. It is beyond the scope of this chapter to discuss the entire field of PIDs; our focus will be on a limited number of PIDs with particular emphasis on pathologic features and association with lymphoproliferation and lymphomas.

SYNONYMS AND RELATED TERMS

Inborn Errors of Immunity.

EPIDEMIOLOGY

The overall prevalence of monogenic PIDs is low; however, they vary greatly depending on ethnicity, consanguinity, and specific disorder. For instance, it ranges from 1 in 600 for selective IgA antibody deficiency to 1 in 100,000 for SCID or 1 in 1,000,000 males for X-linked lymphoproliferative syndrome-1 (XLP1). Interestingly, the introduction of newborn screening for the analysis of T-cell receptor excision circles (TRECs), a measure of thymic output, in 11 screening programs across the United States has provided more accurate data on SCID, with a prevalence of 1 in 58,000. As of December 2018, newborn screening for SCID has been implemented in all 50 states in the United States.[10]

SEVERE COMBINED IMMUNODEFICIENCY

SCID is an extreme form of T-cell deficiency. Depending on the gene defect, they are associated with the absence or presence of B cells and natural killer (NK) cells, and, in some instances, they are associated with nonimmunologic manifestations such as radiosensitivity and skeletal or neurologic abnormalities.[1] This is a very heterogeneous group involving several different genes important in T-cell development with deleterious mutations involving VDJ recombination (*RAG1* and *RAG2*, *DCLRE1C*, *PRKDC*, *NHEJ*, and *LIG4*) and with other severe maturation defects (*ADA*, *AK2*, and *PNP*).[11] In addition, profound genetic T-cell lymphopenias (combined immunodeficiency) may be considered within the spectrum of SCID because of their similar clinical presentation, and include mutations involving cytokine signaling (*IL2RG*, *IL7R*, and *JAK3*) and T-cell receptor signaling (*CD3D*, *CD3E*, and *CD3Z*) or motility (failure of thymic egression) (*CORO1A*). Leaky SCIDs result from hypomorphic mutations in some of these genes (including *RAG1* and *RAG2*), which allow some degree of T-cell development because of residual activity, but retain impaired T-cell–mediated immunity.[12,13] In typical SCID, the diagnosis is based on absence or a very low number of autologous T cells (less than 300/μL) and very low T-cell function (PHA stimulation less than 10%), frequently with T cells of maternal origin present (maternal engraftment); TREC levels are also undetectable or extremely low at birth.[14] Leaky SCID and some of the profound T-cell lymphopenias may have normal or even an increased number of circulating T cells associated with severe immune dysfunction leading to a similar clinical presentation, but often with a delayed onset and unusual symptoms such as autoimmunity, granulomatous inflammation, skin disease, and increased risk for lymphoproliferative malignancies.[15-18]

Infants with SCID, although normal at birth, present early in life with respiratory tract infections (*Pneumocystis jirovecii*, cytomegalovirus [CMV], adenovirus, parainfluenza type 3, and respiratory syncytial virus) that are often severe, prolonged, and complicated, or persistent bronchiolitis. Other symptoms include diarrhea, failure to thrive, or thrush. On physical examination, no lymph nodes are palpable, and imaging studies reveal lack of a thymic shadow. Adopting TREC analysis (originally used in HIV patients to monitor new T-cell output) for newborn screening was implemented in order to detect these disorders before symptoms develop so patients can rapidly receive appropriate medical treatment, avoid live vaccines and nonirradiated blood products, and ultimately reconstitute their

immune system with lifesaving allogeneic hematopoietic stem cell transplantation (HSCT), or gene therapy.[19-20] Untreated SCID is typically fatal before the patient's second birthday.

In general, despite some false positives (deemed acceptable given the severity of the disease being screened for), TREC analysis has been very successful in identifying typical SCID and most of the profound T-cell dysfunctions, but exceptions exist, including delayed-onset SCID, for which the diagnosis may be delayed.[21]

The Thymus in SCID, CID, and Leaky SCID

Histologic and immunophenotypic characterization of the thymus in these severe PIDs gives us clues to understand their pathophysiology. Various histologic patterns (i.e., dysplastic depleted, dysplastic nondepleted, and nondysplastic nondepleted) have been described based on the distribution of thymic epithelial cells (TECs), thymocytes, and their functional subsets including natural T-regulatory cells (nTregs), dendritic cells, and macrophages, and they correlate with the underlying genetic defect affecting T-cell development (Fig. 53-1).[16,22-25]

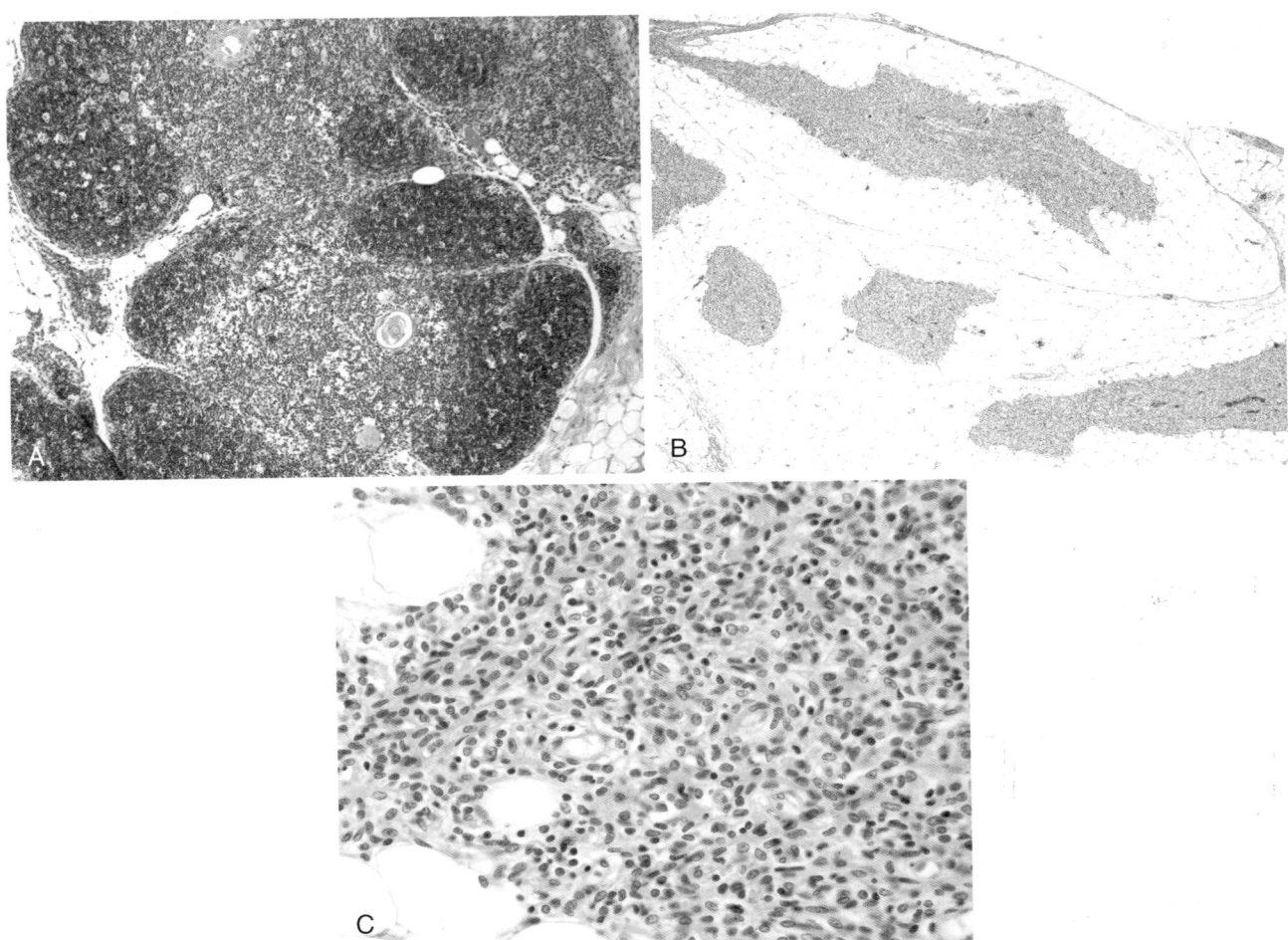

Figure 53-1. Example of thymus histology in primary immunodeficiency. A, Normal thymus showing normal lobular architecture with well-defined cortex and medulla with Hassall bodies. **B–C,** Hypomorphic "leaky" SCID with *RAG-1* mutation. Thymus showing fatty tissue infiltration of the lobules, loss of corticomedullary differentiation, and absence of Hassall bodies with a moderate number of thymocytes consistent with a dysplastic depleted thymus caused by a hypomorphic, partially permissive defect.

Omenn Syndrome

One of the exceptions that can be missed by TREC analysis is Omenn syndrome, in which T cells can be present in normal numbers or even increased because of hypomorphic mutations (leaky defect) occurring in a variety of genes involved in VDJ recombination (*RAG1, RAG2, DCLRE1C, LIG4, RMRP,* and *ADA*).[26] They allow some degree of maturation of a very limited number of thymic T cells with a limited repertoire reflected in oligoclonal expansion in the periphery.[27,28] Omenn syndrome was originally described by Gilbert Omenn in 1965 as a syndrome characterized by a profound immunodeficiency with severe erythroderma, lymphadenopathy, and eosinophilia.[29] Omenn syndrome shares a similar clinical presentation with typical SCID (i.e., presents in infancy with pneumonitis, chronic diarrhea, and failure to thrive); however, the presence of adenopathy, hepatosplenomegaly, and generalized erythroderma associated with increased IgE levels and eosinophilia are distinguishing features. In contrast to typical SCID, the persistent presence of inflammation leads to an increased number of circulating T cells with an activated phenotype and inability to proliferate in response to mitogens. Morphologically, lymph nodes show complete effacement of the architecture with a depleted appearance and increased numbers of dendritic cells and eosinophils; they usually lack primary and secondary B follicles. Phenotypically, CD3-positive T cells express CD45RO, CD4, GATA-3, and CD30 with a cytokine profile consistent with a Th2-type response (Figs. 53-2, 53-3).[30-32]

One of the protective effects of this type of response against persistent inflammation is the upregulation of nTregs; however, these are severely reduced because of thymic dysplasia with profound abnormalities of thymic epithelial cell differentiation affecting central tolerance. All these factors contribute to autoimmunity and inflammation in Omenn syndrome.[23,33,34]

Combined Immunodeficiency Generally Less Profound Than SCID

Class-switch recombination (CSR) deficiencies or hyper IgM (HIGM) syndromes are characterized by normal or elevated serum IgM and low or absent serum levels of other Ig classes. In the adaptive immune system, antibody-mediated immune responses are either T-cell independent, in which B cells proliferate upon encountering specific antigens and secrete IgM, or T-cell dependent, and to generate high affinity antibodies, B cells undergo clonal expansion, affinity maturation through somatic hypermutation (SHM), and CSR. These latter events take place within the germinal centers of secondary lymphoid organs upon T-cell–B-cell interaction mediated through CD40-ligand (CD40L) and CD40. Germline mutations can affect CD40/CD40L and CD40-signaling pathways, as well as enzymes involved in double-stranded DNA breaks and repair that occur during CSR.

CD40L Deficiency or Hyper IgM Type 1 Syndrome

CD40L deficiency (XL) or HIGM type 1 defect involves CD40L, which is expressed on activated T cells in a tightly controlled manner, but it is not lethal to T cells.[35,36] Originally thought to be a defect in isotype switching, it is now known to be a defect of T-cell priming, help, and function leading to impaired class switching, best classified as a combined immunodeficiency rather than a predominantly antibody deficiency.[37] About 200 cases have been described in the literature. It presents with recurrent upper and lower respiratory tract involvement caused by opportunistic infections (*P. jirovecii,* cytomegalovirus, *Cryptococcus, Histoplasma,* and *Candida*), diarrhea when infectious often caused by *Cryptosporidium parvum* (80%), and neutropenia before age 2 years. Subsequent complications involving the biliary tree

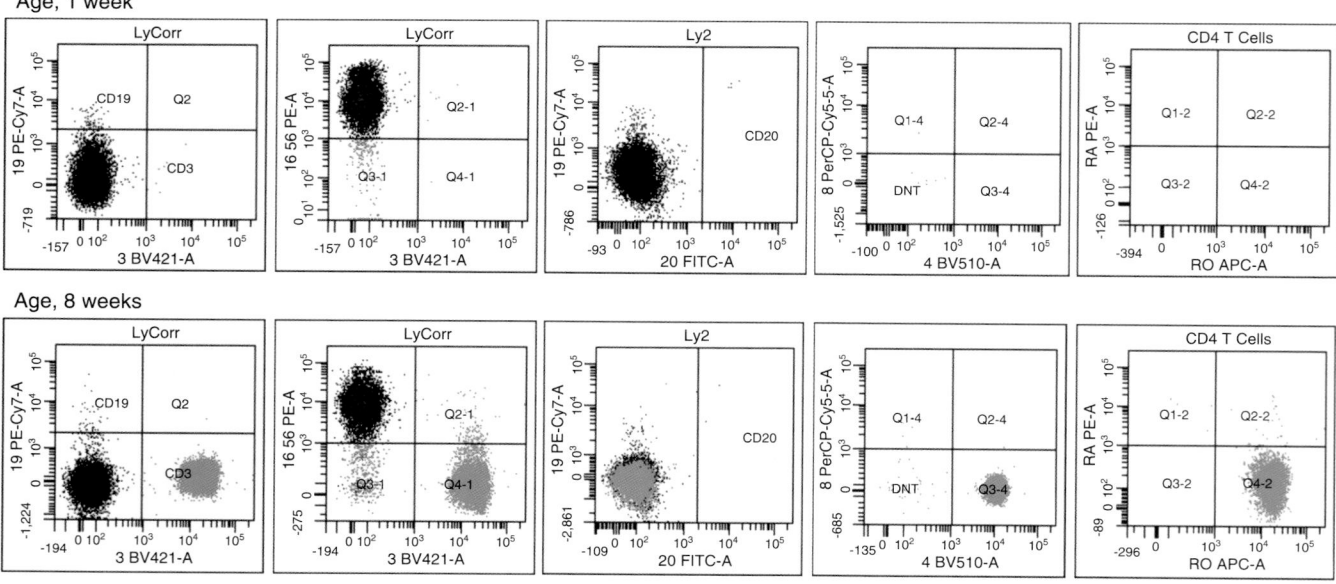

Figure 53-2. Omenn syndrome. Flow cytometry: Newborn baby with an abnormal TREC screen and absent T cells *(green)* and B cells *(blue)* and increased NK cells *(black)* developed a progressive rash, eosinophilia, and increased IgE and was ultimately diagnosed with Omenn syndrome with two mutations in *RAG1.* Lymphocyte subset analysis at age 8 weeks revealed engraftment of maternal T cells that were CD4-positive and expressed CD45RO.

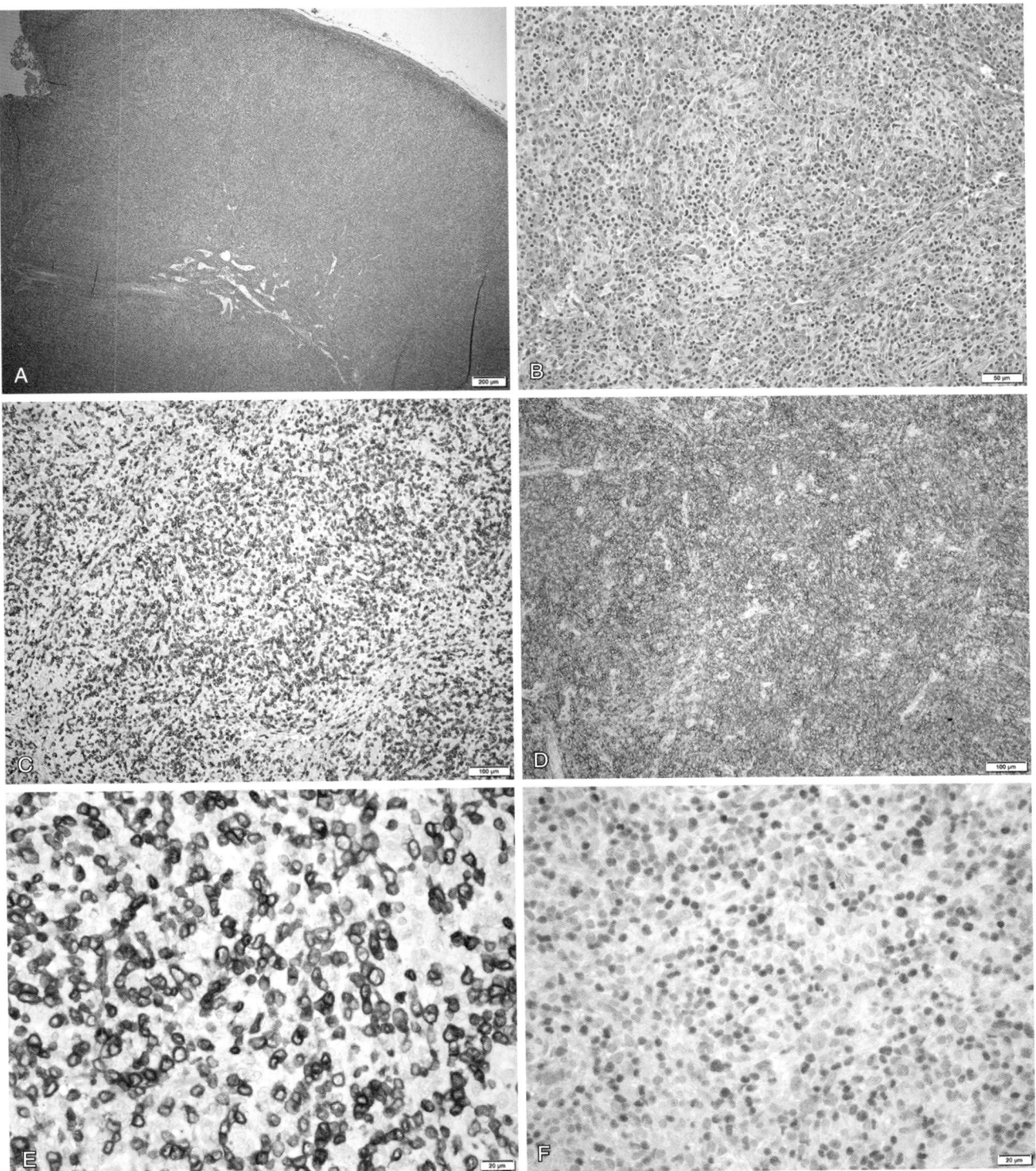

Figure 53-3. Lymph node biopsy from a 5-month-old baby boy diagnosed with Omenn syndrome carrying RAG-2 mutations. **A,** Paracortical hyperplasia with lack of B-follicles (hematoxylin and eosin [H&E], ×4). **B,** A polymorphic proliferation composed of small lymphocytes, immunoblast-like cells, and numerous eosinophils (H&E, ×20). The majority of the lymphoid cells is composed of CD3-positive T cells (**C,** CD3, ×10) with a predominance of CD4 (**D,** double-stain CD4/CD8, ×10). High magnification for CD3 (**E,** ×40) to highlight the cytologic atypia and typically positive for GATA-3 positive cells (**F,** ×40). TCR gamma gene rearrangement is polyclonal/oligoclonal.

and liver are often related to persistent *Cryptosporidium* and *Giardia* infections of the biliary system, leading to sclerosing cholangitis, hepatitis, cirrhosis, and increased gastrointestinal malignancies including cholangiocarcinoma. Immunologic features include very low serum levels of IgG and IgA with normal to increased IgM, decreased number of memory B cells, and limited-to-unswitched memory B cells (CD27 positive, IgM positive, IgD positive) in keeping with defects in CSR. Although the number and distribution of T-cell subsets is not affected, CD40L deficiency affects their costimulatory functions for T cells, B cells, and macrophages.[38] Dendritic cell signaling is also affected. Lymph nodes are usually small with IgM/IgD-positive B cells in the far cortex lacking secondary B follicles with minimal-to-absent dendritic meshworks, and well-preserved T-cell areas (Fig. 53-4). CD40 deficiency (AR) HIGM type 3 is similar in all respects to HIGM type 1.[37,39]

AID Deficiency or Hyper IgM Type 2 Syndrome

Patients with activation-induced cytidine deaminase (*AICDA* gene) AID deficiency (AR)/HIGM type 2 syndrome (HIGM2) present with lymphadenopathy, enlarged tonsils, and recurrent bacterial sinopulmonary infections, but no opportunistic infections. Morphologically, the lymph nodes are characterized by florid follicular hyperplasia with large, expanded germinal centers.[40] Similar to the other IGHM, they lack switched memory B cells and show profound defects also in SHM, reflecting the underlying genetic defect involving AID, which participates in both the CSR and SHM processes; however, not all AID mutants are associated with defects in SHM; AID C terminal defect (AD) is an example.[41] These observations have led to a better understanding of the complexity of the CSR mechanism. More recently, AID has been implicated not only in B-cell development through CSR and gene activation through demethylation, but also as a candidate gene in inducing genomic instability in other systems.[42]

Common Variable Immunodeficiency

Common variable immunodeficiency (CVID) represents a heterogeneous group of disorders with recurrent bacterial infections of the respiratory tract caused by antibody deficiency with severe reduction in at least two serum Ig isotypes with a normal number of or decreased B cells. The underlying genetic defect is unknown in most cases, and it remains a diagnosis of exclusion. Prevalence ranges from 1 in 10,000 to 1 in 50,000 (Europe/North America); males and females are affected equally.[43] Most individuals are diagnosed at between 20 and 40 years of age, making it the most common symptomatic PID in adults. Only 10% to 20% have a positive family history (AD greater than AR); most cases are sporadic. A diagnosis of CVID should not be entertained in very young patients, and it must be differentiated from transient hypogammaglobulinemia of infancy, so by definition the onset of immunodeficiency should be at greater than age 2 years; usually a cutoff of 4 years is used.[43] Underlying genetic defects (3% of cases cumulative) predisposing to CVID include defects in *ICOS* (inducible T-cell costimulator), B-cell receptor complex genes (CD19, CD81, and CD21), and CD20, which are monogenic defects. *TACI* (transmembrane activator, calcium modulator, and cyclophilin ligand interactor), found in 8% to 10%, *BAFFR*

(B-cell activating factor-receptor), and *MSH5* (mismatch repair gene) are now considered disease-associated rather than causative, because unaffected heterozygous patients have also been described, and the variants are also detected in normal individuals at a prevalence of 1% or more, and thus considered to represent polymorphisms.

Clinically, the symptoms are very heterogeneous, but two major groups can be broadly recognized based on predominant recurrent infections of the respiratory tract versus inflammatory complications with a variety of autoimmune disorders (22% to 48%), including cytopenias, granulomatous disease, and increased development of malignancy, mainly lymphomas. Splenomegaly is detected in 30% of patients and it is often associated with cytopenias, but hypersplenism is not considered sufficient to explain it, and other functional defects involving T cells and NK cells have been described.[44] Also, inflammatory bowel disease (IBD)-like symptoms are present in one-third of patients, and the liver is also commonly involved with hepatitis-like symptoms (43%) without evidence of viral infection. From a pathology standpoint, the lungs are the major target organ with acute bacterial infections and possible subsequent development of bronchiectasis and noninfectious immune-mediated changes with a lymphocytic interstitial infiltrate, follicular bronchiolitis, and follicular hyperplasia with often "naked" germinal centers and paucity or absence of plasma cells. In addition, a subset of patients may develop granulomatous lymphocytic interstitial lung disease (GLILD),[45,46] and these noninfectious patterns may coexist (Fig. 53-5). In the gastrointestinal tract, a celiac disease-like picture is often present with increased intraepithelial T cells, villous blunting, and, typically, absence of plasma cells. However, these changes do not respond to a gluten-free diet. In addition, prominent lymphoid aggregates consistent with nodular lymphoid hyperplasia are noted. In the liver, a periportal lymphocytic infiltrate of possible autoimmune origin can be seen, and it is often associated with nodular regenerative hyperplasia (NRH).[47-50] The frequency of NRH varies in different studies, ranging from as high as 50% based on the presence of portal hypertension, a known complication of NRH,[47] to as low as 12% or even 5%.[48,49]

Lymph node biopsies in patients with CVID show different patterns of follicular hyperplasia and a paucity of plasma cells, particularly in the medullary cords. Similar to extranodal sites (i.e., lung and gastrointestinal tract), the germinal centers may be more ill-defined, lack mantles, and show irregular outlines; occasionally, progressive transformation of germinal centers may be observed. The presence of ill-defined follicular structures may have led in the past to overdiagnosis of B-cell lymphomas because of the impression of a distorted architecture. Immunophenotypic studies and clonality studies are helpful in clarifying the diagnosis in such cases,[51-53] because these patients do in fact face an increased risk of B-cell lymphomas, ranging from 8.2% in the United States to less than 3.8% in Europe and the United Kingdom. These lymphomas, which tend to occur in the 4th to 7th decades of life, are mostly non-Hodgkin lymphomas of B-cell type including extranodal marginal zone lymphomas of mucosa-associated lymphoid tissue (MALT) type, and often are not associated with Epstein-Barr virus (EBV).[53,54] Risk of lymphoma seems to be the highest (29%) in patients with late-onset CVID associated with a severe T-cell defect,[55] and about 60% in this setting are EBV-associated. It is noteworthy that this subset of patients more frequently also has splenomegaly,

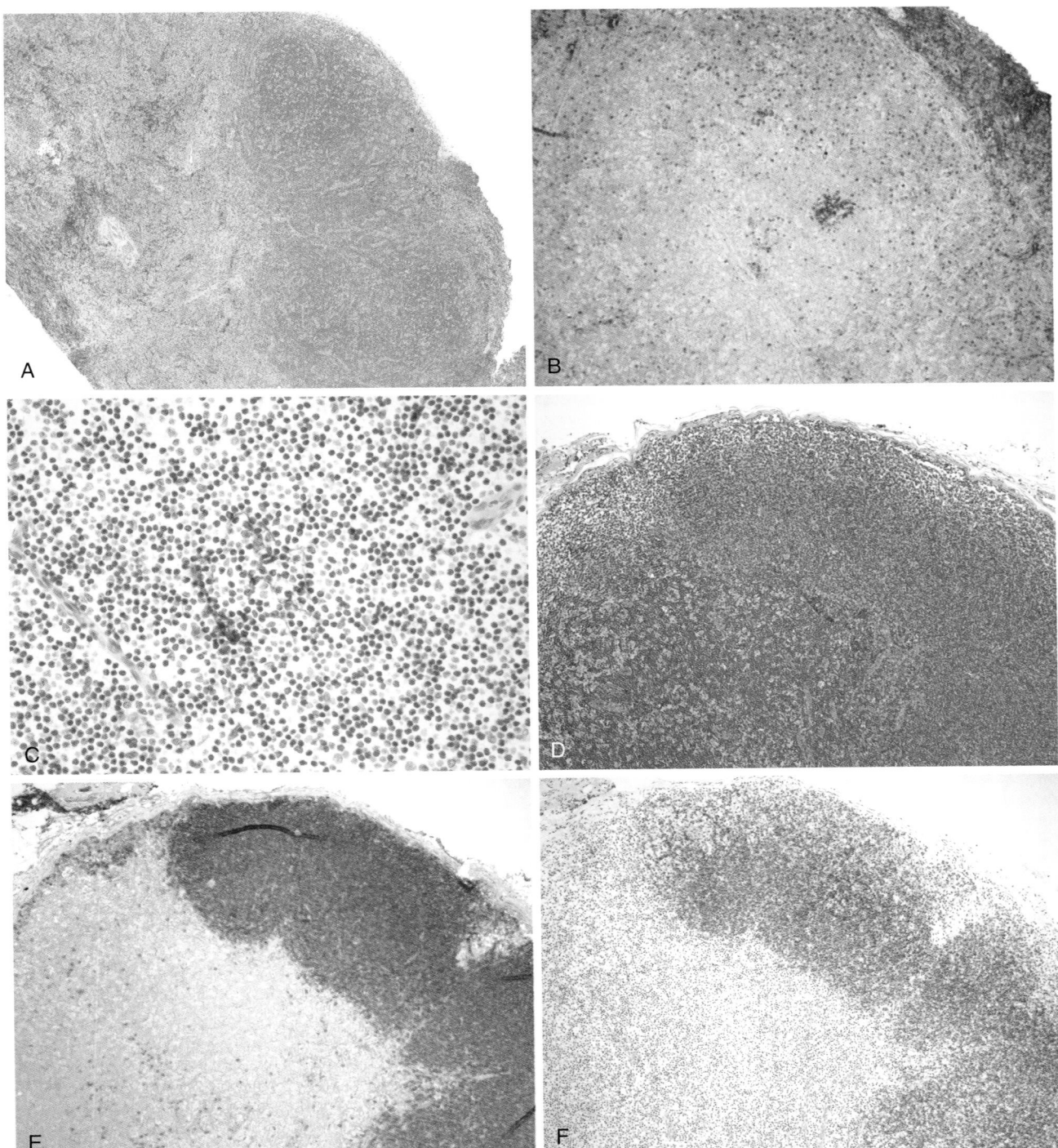

Figure 53-4. Two examples of hyper IgM syndrome related to CD40L deficiency. A, Small lymph node with prominent paracortical hyperplasia lacking secondary B follicles in the cortex. Note the fibrosis involving the rest of the node (×4). **B,** Only a few clusters of IgM-positive B cells are noted forming small aggregates with only rudimentary CD21-positive meshworks **(C).** Hematoxylin and eosin (H&E) uniform cortical areas lacking secondary B follicles adjacent to well-developed T-cell areas **(D)** are shown; the B cells in the cortex are uniformly positive for IGD and IgM, consistent with naïve B cells **(E),** and they are also positive for CD21 **(F),** but the follicular dendritic meshworks are still rudimentary.

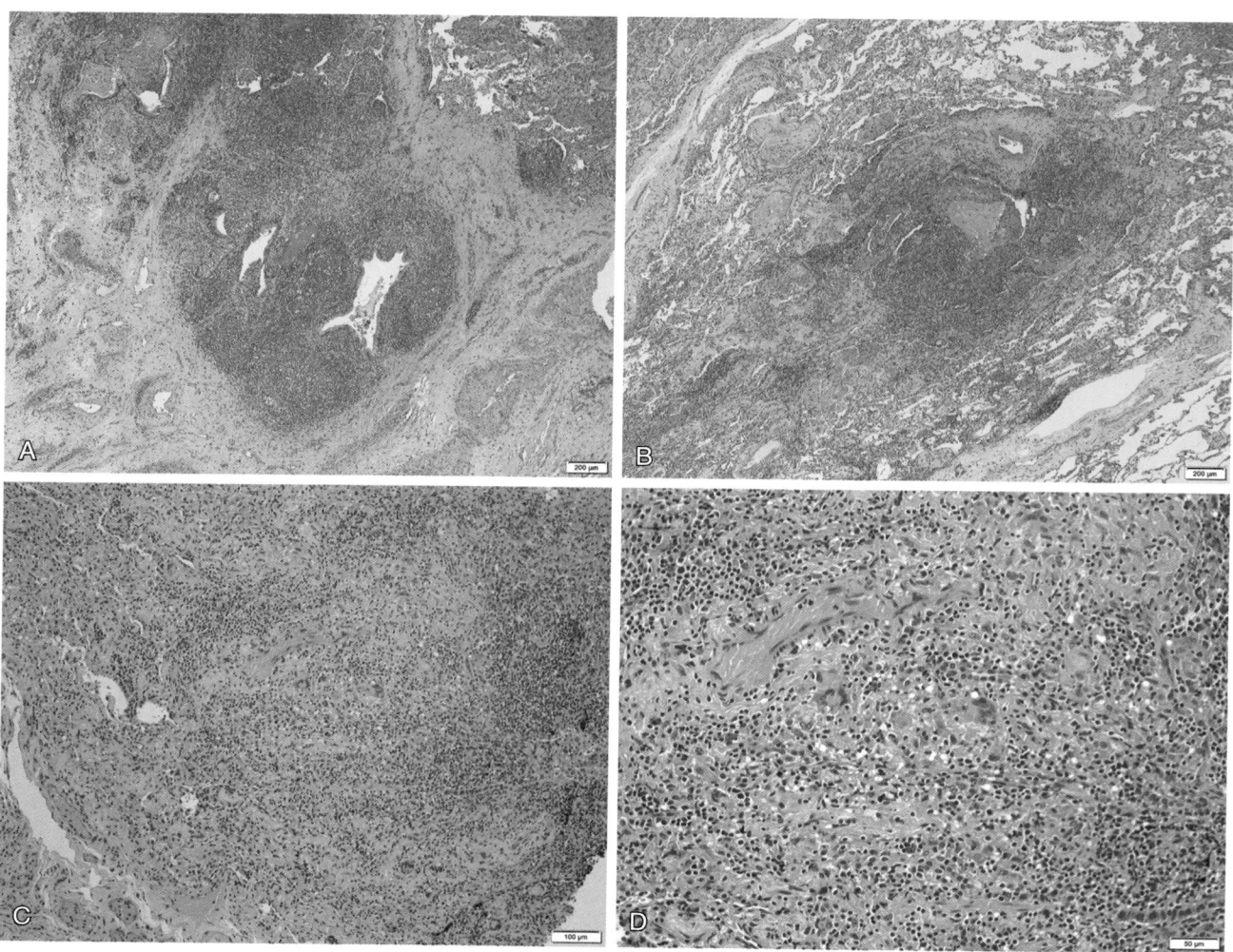

Figure 53-5. Lung wedge resection from a patient with a diagnosis of granulomatous lymphocytic interstitial lung disease (GLILD) in a patient with common variable immunodeficiency (CVID) on IV-Ig. **A,** At low power, a patchy peribronchial lymphocytic infiltrate with fibrosis associated with reactive follicles with naked germinal centers. **B,** Postobstructive changes, organizing pneumonia and areas of end-stage lung disease were noted (hematoxylin and eosin [H&E], ×2). **C–D,** Poorly formed granulomata and rare multinucleated giant cells are present (H&E, ×10 and ×40).

granulomatous disease, and enteropathy, all of which are associated with decreased overall survival.

Immunologic features include a marked decrease of IgG (two standard deviations below the normal age-adjusted range), a marked decrease of another isotype (IgA or IgM), an absolute decrease in number of naïve B cells and class-switched memory B cells (CD27 positive, IgM negative, IgD negative), and reduced IgM response to polysaccharide immunization. The decreased number of class-switched memory B cells is not unique or distinctive for CVID because it has been described in other PIDs, including X-linked HIGM syndrome, Wiskott-Aldrich syndrome (WAS), X-linked lymphoproliferative disease, idiopathic CD4 lymphopenia, chronic granulomatous disease, and, more recently, phosphatidylinositol 3-kinase (PI3K)-δ deficiency. An increase in transitional immature B cells (CD10 positive, CD38 high, IgM high) is often present in peripheral blood; a more mature population with CD21 low/CD38 low B cells is expanded in CVID, as well as in SLE.[56] The increase in transitional immature B cells is also a striking feature of PI3K-δ immunodeficiency, and it is of interest that several

of the patients with this mutation were originally diagnosed as CVID; it is, therefore, tempting to speculate that this particular subset of patients may indeed carry these mutations. In a subset of patients with granulomatous disease and splenomegaly, profound alteration of T-cell compartments is present, with low naïve CD4-positive T cells with an inverted CD4:CD8 ratio and T-cell activation markers[57]; also, low Tregs have been described in patients with more severe immunodeficiency, granulomatous disease, splenomegaly, and cytopenia. This latter phenomenon may account for the presence of autoreactive B cells (CD21 low/CD38 low); it is also of interest that a similar population is present in patients with haploinsufficiency for CTLA-4, and we can speculate that a subset of patients diagnosed with enteropathy and CVID may carry this genetic defect.

PI3K-RELATED IMMUNODEFICIENCIES

Primary immunodeficiencies caused by hyperactivation of the phosphatidylinositol 3-kinase (PI3K) signaling pathway were recently described either as heterozygous gain-of-function mutations in the *PIK3CD* gene encoding p110δ, the leukocyte-restricted catalytic subunit, (APDS1),[58-61] or involving p85α, one of the regulatory subunits that regulates the stability of p110 cellular localization, and function of class IA PI3K (APDS2).[62-65] Engagement of a variety of receptors (integrins, tyrosine kinase, B cells and T cells, cytokine, and G-protein) and other stimuli leads to the production of second-messenger phosphatidylinositol (3,4,5) triphosphates (PIP3) by PI3K kinase activity. These lipids serve as docking sites for proteins with a pleckstrin homology domain, including AKT and its upstream activator, PDK1. AKT plays a central role in proliferation, growth, survival, and metabolism in many cell types. PI3K signaling plays an important role in stages of B-cell and T-cell development, differentiation, function, and homeostasis.

With WES and retargeted Sanger sequencing, mutations were identified in different domains of the PI3K-δ subunit, with some recurring ones (hotspots) among different family members. Modeling of the mutations and functional studies confirmed the hyperactivation of PI3K function leading to sustained AKT/mTOR signaling.

Patients carrying PI3K-δ gain-of-function mutations (APDS1) present, often in childhood, with recurrent sinopulmonary infections; chronic CMV and EBV viremia; lymphadenopathy; lymphoid proliferation with nodular lymphoid hyperplasia involving respiratory and gastrointestinal systems; and increased lymphoma susceptibility, often EBV-associated.[58-61,66,67]

Some of these patients were initially diagnosed with CVID based on their clinical presentation and immunologic findings. In vivo analysis of their B-cell and T-cell populations revealed normal B-cell numbers, but with a decrease or absence of memory B cells (CD27 positive) and an increased number of transitional/immature B cells (CD10 positive, CD38 high, IgM high) with IgM and CD5 expression as seen in naïve B cells. Bone marrow evaluation reveals lymphocytosis with increased B-cell precursors (hematogones) with evidence of maturation arrest by flow cytometry analysis (Fig. 53-6). CD10-positive early-through-transitional hematogones are markedly increased with severely decreased to absent CD10-negative mature B-cells because of impaired class-switch recombination. These findings may raise

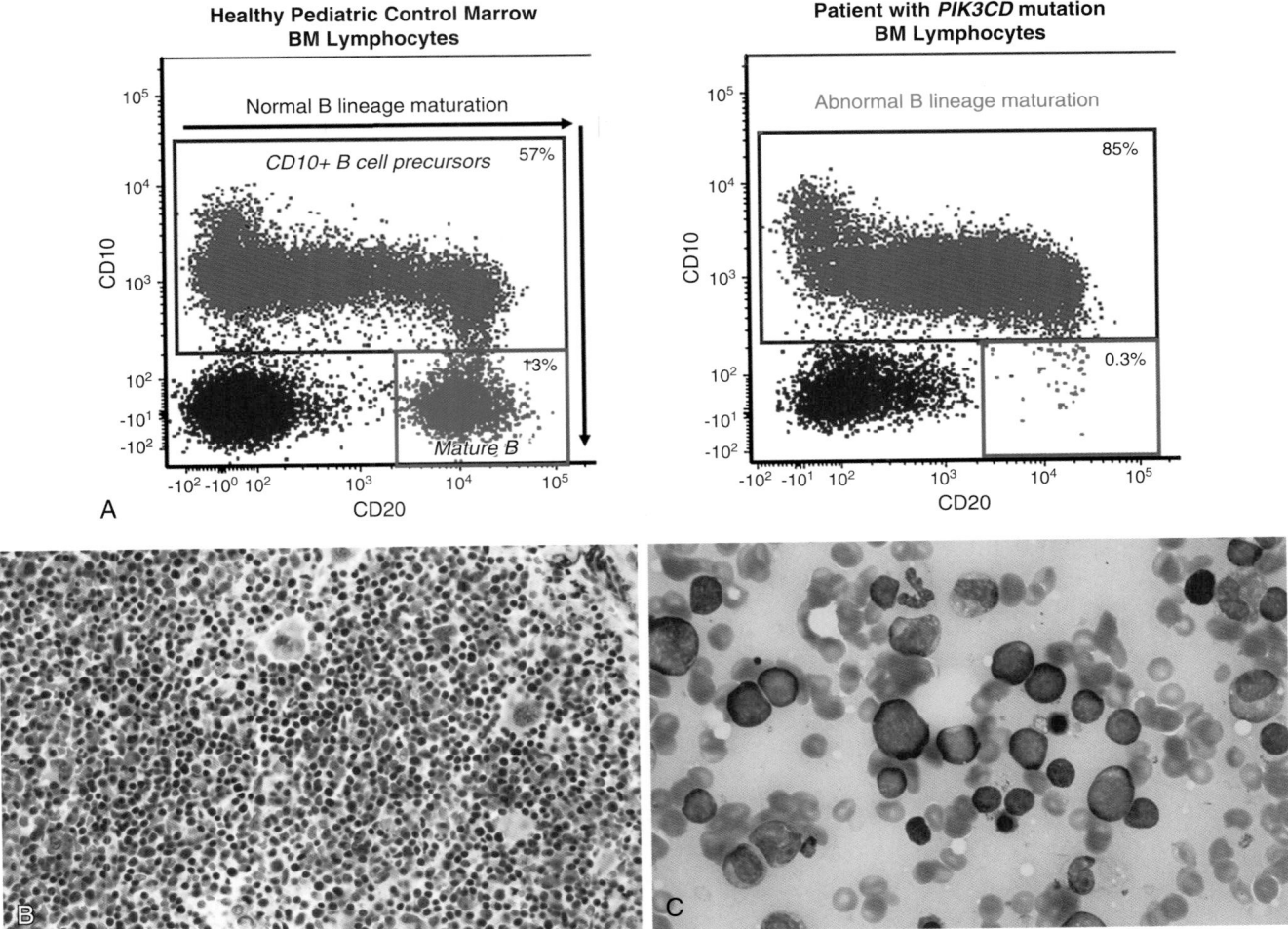

Figure 53-6. Hematogone hyperplasia with maturation block in PI3KCD immune deficiency (APDS1). **A,** Flow cytometry analysis of the PI3KCD marrow in comparison to a healthy pediatric control shows markedly abnormal B-cell maturation in the PIK3CD marrow characterized by increased early and transitional CD10 positive immature B-cells with a maturation block, resulting in near complete absence of mature B-cells (CD20 positive and CD10 negative). **B,** Bone marrow biopsy from a pediatric patient shows hypercellular marrow with lymphocytosis (hemotoxylin and eosin [H&E], ×500). **C,** Aspirate smear Wright-Giemsa stain.

concern for B-lymphoblastic leukemia. Immunoglobulin levels were variable (IgG), but usually high for IgM with low IgA; falling levels of IgG were observed over time in some patients. These observations were confirmed by in vitro studies where the B-cell proliferation was within normal limits, but the cells have impaired immunoglobulin production (defects in CSR). Interestingly, these findings were also mirrored in the sequential lymph nodes that we obtained from some of these patients, with a progressively increasing number of IgM-positive cells and a decline of IgG and IgA (Fig. 53-7). In vivo analysis of the T-cell compartment

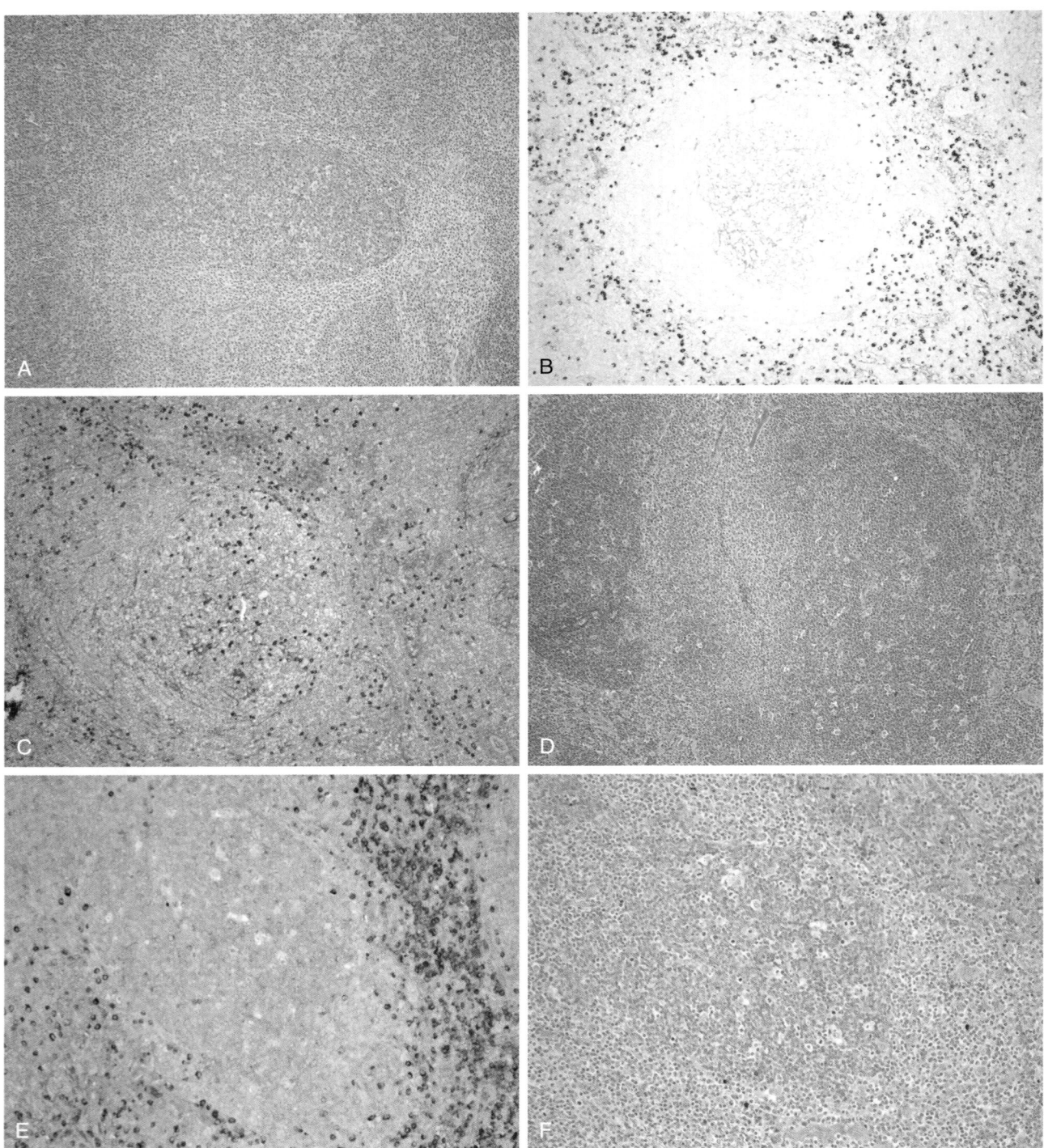

Figure 53-7. Lymph node biopsies from a patient with PI3KCD immune deficiency (APDS1). **A,** Low-power view showing typical features with "naked" reactive germinal centers and prominent monocytoid B-cell reaction. **B,** Numerous IgM-positive cells are in the parafollicular areas, and IgG-positive cells are also present within the germinal center **(C).** Subsequent biopsy (6-year interval) shows similar morphologic features, with large expanded naked germinal centers **(D)** surrounded by numerous IgM-positive cells **(E),** and extremely few IgG-positive cells **(F),** consistent with the serum immunoglobulin levels, simulating a hyper IgM syndrome.

revealed progressive CD4-positive T-cell lymphopenia and normal-to-high CD8-positive T cells, with an inverted CD4:CD8 ratio and greatly reduced naïve and central memory T cells with a corresponding increase in effector memory (CD45RA negative/CCR7 negative) T cells and terminally differentiated effector memory T cells (TEMRA, CD45RA positive) with a senescent phenotype, particularly in the CD8 subset, which may account for their chronic CMV and EBV viremia.[59]

Multiple and sequential lymph node biopsies from several members of different families with a gain-of-function mutation of *PIK3CD* were reviewed. Often these patients had prominent lymphadenopathy involving central and peripheral lymph nodes with compression of the airways in some patients. Lymph nodes showed similar features consisting of an atypical follicular hyperplasia with prominent naked germinal centers often with ill-defined outlines; in addition, a prominent monocytoid B-cell hyperplasia was almost invariably present (see Fig. 53-7). In some cases, the overall features resembled CMV lymphadenitis, and in some of these cases CMV infected cells were indeed present; however, in contrast to other cases of CMV lymphadenitis, the mantles were extremely diminished to absent. In some cases, the monocytoid B-cell reaction was more extensive, raising the possibility of involvement by nodal marginal zone lymphoma. However, most cases that were studied by immunoglobulin and T-cell receptor (TCR) gene rearrangements were polyclonal or oligoclonal. EBV, when present by in situ hybridization, was limited to a relatively small number of cells in these otherwise reactive lymph nodes. Plasma cells and plasmacytoid cells are easily identified in the medullary cords and parafollicular areas; in sequential cases over the course of several years, the IgG-positive cells decline in number, whereas the IgM-positive cells increase (see Fig. 53-7).[59] Another striking feature was the expansion of CD279-positive and CD57-positive cells in the T-cell areas consistent with the accumulation of terminally differentiated senescent T cells identified also in the peripheral blood.

In addition, these patients show prominent nodular lymphoid hyperplasia involving the respiratory and gastrointestinal tracts with prominent proliferation of B cells and T cells, often with germinal center formation. The degree of nodular lymphoid hyperplasia at the ileocecal junction can be quite pronounced and lead to intussusception (Fig. 53-8).

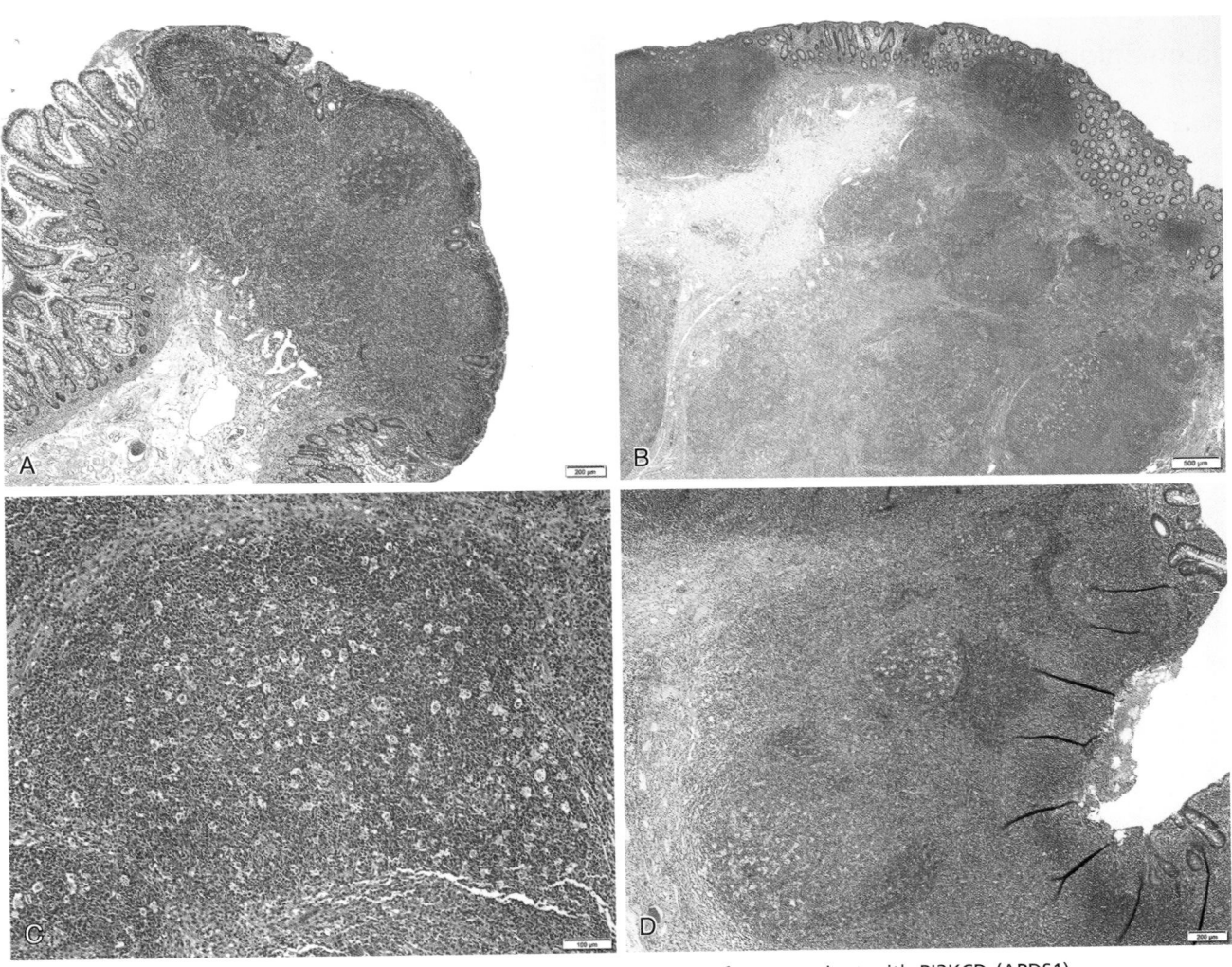

Figure 53-8. Ileocecal resection caused by intussusception from a patient with PI3KCD (APDS1). **A,** Prominent lymphoid infiltrate with naked germinal centers and monocytoid reaction adjacent to small intestine, consistent with exuberant Peyer's patches. **B,** Lymphoid proliferation with a nodular growth pattern and fibrosis involving the cecum. **C,** Reactive naked germinal centers are prominent. **D,** Similar features are also noted in the ulcerated areas. Lymph nodes from the ileocecal resection showed reactive changes as often seen in these patients.

APDS1 patients are also at risk of developing classic Hodgkin lymphoma (nodular sclerosis, EBV positive) and non-Hodgkin lymphoma, diffuse large B-cell lymphoma, and other EBV-positive and non-EBV–associated lymphomas.[59] One family had extensive involvement of the gastrointestinal tract by MALT lymphoma.[60]

With a similar approach (WES and Sanger retargeted), a homozygous mutation (G to A codon 298) with a premature stop codon of the p85α regulatory subunit of the *PIK3R1* gene was originally described in a female patient with IBD and no B cells with a developmental block at the very early B-cell precursors.[68] More recently, heterozygous splice site gain-of-function mutations involving the p85α regulatory subunit of the *PIK3R1* gene, leading to a shortened protein lacking inhibitory activity, have been described in several families.[62,64,65,69] Sequential lymph node biopsies from one patient with a gain-of-function mutation of the *PIK3R1* gene (unpublished) revealed similar changes as described in the *PIK3CD* patients with prominent atypical follicular hyperplasia and monocytoid B-cell reaction with no evidence of CMV- or EBV-infected cells; similar findings were also reported in a tonsil.[65,69]

Agammaglobulinemia

The most severe form of reduction of all serum Ig isotypes is found in agammaglobulinemia due to mutations that prevent signaling through the B-cell receptor, resulting in a block of B-cell differentiation and lack of mature B cells. The majority of these rare patients carries a mutation in the genes encoding Bruton's tyrosine kinase (BTK) (XL) (85%), adaptor BLNK (AR) (5%–7%), and in the pre-BCR chains (μ heavy chain, λ5 surrogate light chain) and Igα surrogate receptor (5%–7%).[70]

X-Linked Agammaglobulinemia

X-linked agammaglobulinemia (XLA) is a rare PID with an estimated minimal birth rate of 1 in 379,000 averaged over a 10-year period; as predicted, an increased susceptibility to infections is the most common initial clinical manifestation (86%). It is of interest that diagnosis is frequently delayed even in patients with a positive family history; regardless, nearly all patients become symptomatic before age 5 years. Most infections are because of encapsulated bacteria involving the upper and lower respiratory tract, but viral infections are also reported.[71] These patients have hypoplastic to absent tonsils, adenoids, and lymph nodes.

X-Linked Lymphoproliferative Disorder

Classic X-linked lymphoproliferative disorder (XLP1) is a prototypical PID associated with development of EBV-related lymphoproliferative processes caused by the inability to handle EBV infection. David Purtilo and colleagues described it in 1975 based on a study from a single generation of the Duncan family.[72] XLP1 is caused by a mutation in the *SH2D1A* gene, which encodes the signaling lymphocyte activation molecule (SLAM)-associated protein (SAP), while mutations in the *BIRC4* gene, encoding the X-linked inhibitor of apoptosis protein (XIAP), cause XLP2. There is a clinical overlap between the two genetic defects. It is a rare immunodeficiency with a prevalence of approximately 1 per 1 million males for XLP1 and 1 per 5 million males for XLP2. SAP is expressed in T cells and NK cells and is required for cytotoxicity of B cells.

In general, in affected male patients, EBV infection leads to an exaggerated and often fatal infectious mononucleosis–like syndrome with lymphadenopathy caused by polyclonal B-cell and CD8-positive T-cell expansions, often with involvement of liver, spleen, and bone marrow, leading to hemophagocytic lymphohistiocytosis (HLH) and bone marrow failure. Other symptoms include B-cell lymphoma and dysgammaglobulinemia. However, hypogammaglobulinemia and lymphomas can also develop independently of EBV infection in seronegative individuals and the underlying mechanism is poorly understood, but it implies that EBV is not necessary for the development of all clinical features. In rare instances, aplastic anemia, vasculitis, and lymphomatoid granulomatosis have been described in these patients.

From an immunologic standpoint, these patients have a reduced number of memory B cells, several cellular defects involving effector functions of CD8-positive/CD4-positive T cells and NK cells, and lack NKT cells.[73] The critical role of SAP in these different cellular subsets has been elucidated, with multiple elegant studies showing that the increased susceptibility to EBV infections is linked to decreased cytotoxicity of SAP-deficient CD8-positive T cells and NK cells, whereas the development of hypogammaglobulinemia is most likely caused by an intrinsic defect of CD4-positive T cells. Ninety-five percent of EBV-specific CTLs are indeed in the SAP-positive subset of CD8 T cells, whereas CMV and other virus-specific CTLs are equally present in SAP-positive and SAP-negative CD8 T cells; hence, the response to other viruses is not affected in XLP patients. Moreover, the lack of SAP in CD8-positive T cells also has an inhibitory effect by limiting the interaction with B cells through a defect in synapse formation and preventing the clearance of EBV-infected B cells.[74] The reduced cytotoxicity of SAP-deficient NK cells mediated through the 2B4 (CD244) receptor, part of the Ig superfamily together with SLAM, also plays a role in the poor handling of EBV infection, without affecting other NK-cell functions that are mediated through different receptors and do not require SAP as a second messenger. It is known that patients who lack NK cells or have severe functional NK-cell defects are susceptible to recurrent human herpesvirus infections with CMV, varicella-zoster virus (VZV), and EBV.[75] The absence/deficiency of NKT cells may also contribute to the susceptibility to EBV and the development of lymphoma, because other PIDs with similar clinical features caused by mutations involving *CD27*, *ITK*, *BIRC4*, and *CORO1A* also have low numbers of NKT cells. Lastly, the defective humoral immunity with subsequent development of hypogammaglobulinemia caused by poor antibody formation, and deficit in memory B cells has been shown to be related to intrinsic defects of CD4-positive T cells and impaired formation of follicular T-helper cells. To this extent, review of the pathology material from the XLP registry has revealed that some of these patients fail to form normal germinal centers, although some are present in gastrointestinal biopsies.

XLP2 is less common, with only about 70 cases reported since 2006. The main clinical features are increased susceptibility to EBV-HLH; recurrent splenomegaly; and IBD with Crohn's-like features. XLP2 is considered one of the underlying causes of IBD in infancy. XIAP consists of antiapoptotic molecules but is also involved in innate immunity and inflammation (as a negative regulator through the NOD pathway).[76]

Several other diseases with immune dysregulation, such as familial HLH syndromes leading to increased susceptibility of EBV infections, chronic active EBV, and EBV-driven lymphoproliferative disorders/lymphoma, are discussed in the chapters related to EBV (Chapters 28 and 29).

DEFECTS THAT AFFECT HOMEOSTASIS OF THE IMMUNE SYSTEM

The identification of PIDs that, as result of a single gene defect, give rise to multiple autoimmune phenomena has helped in understanding the immune dysregulation caused by a decreased ability in differentiating between self and foreign antigens. These disorders have offered the opportunity to better understand regulatory T-cell function both centrally and peripherally, how they develop, and how they maintain homeostasis.

Autoimmune polyendocrinopathy-candidiasis ectodermal dysplasia (APECED) is a monogenic autoimmune disease caused by biallelic LOF mutation in the autoimmune regulator *AIRE* gene, a transcription factor that promotes expression of tissue-restricted antigens[77] and that is expressed in a subset of medullary TECs.[78] It participates in the negative selection of self-reactive T cells and generation of self-antigen specific regulatory Tregs. AIRE deficiency is also associated with impaired B tolerance, resulting in the production of autoantibodies.[77] It has been shown that several patients have diminished and defective Tregs.[79]

APECED is clinically defined by chronic mucocutaneous candidiasis, hypoparathyroidism, and adrenal insufficiency; however, it is a multisystem autoimmune disease involving several endocrine and nonendocrine organs.[80,81]

Immune dysregulation, polyendocrinopathy, enteropathy, X-linked syndrome (IPEX) is a rare syndrome that presents with severe autoimmune enteropathy, eczema, early-onset endocrinopathy, and other autoimmune diseases. It is caused by mutation in the forkhead box protein P3 (*FOXP3*) gene. Allergic manifestations with eczema and food allergies are common with elevated IgE, hypereosinophilia, and TH2-skewing.[82] The mouse model—*Scurfy* mice, in which the lack of Tregs leads to lethal lymphoproliferative disorder with multiorgan infiltration—and IPEX patients share many similarities. Genotype/phenotype correlation has been demonstrated with some of the *FOXP3* mutations that maintain a near-normal protein expression and are associated with a milder clinical phenotype with normal number of Tregs, but with altered functionality.[83] Other genetic mutations may give rise to an IPEX-like syndrome including CD25 (IL2Ralpha) deficiency and STAT5b deficiency; in addition, some patients also with gain-of-function *STAT1* mutations have been reported.[84-86]

Autosomal Dominant Immune Dysregulation Syndrome With Heterozygous Germline Mutations of Cytotoxic T Lymphocyte–Associated Protein 4

This disease has been recently characterized.[87,88] Heterozygous mutations in CTLA4 lead to T-cell impairment with immune dysregulation with later onset compared with IPEX,

and incomplete penetrance. Several of these patients had a diagnosis of CVID caused by hypogammaglobulinemia, deficit in antibody production, and expansion of autoreactive B cells. Tregs constitutively express the inhibitory receptor CTLA4, which is an essential part of their suppressive functions. Upon antigen presentation by dendritic cells (or other specialized AP cells) in the presence of T-cell receptor, costimulatory molecule CD28 mediates T-cell effector function, T-cell activation, and generation of memory T cells, and provides helper function to B cells and antibody production. The inhibitory signals of these events are mediated by CTLA4. Both receptors share the same ligands CD80/CD86; it has been shown that CTLA4 not only recycles from the surface to the cytoplasm of T cells, where it can either be recycled to the surface or digested, but also has the ability to remove the ligands (CD80 and CD86) from the antigen-presenting cells (APCs) via transendocytosis.[89] Both mechanisms offer a way to regulate the availability of ligands and subsequently enhance or reduce T-cell activation and proliferation.

Patients present with recurrent respiratory tract infections, hypogammaglobulinemia, autoimmune cytopenias (thrombocytopenia resembling immune/idiopathic thrombocytopenic purpura [ITP], autoimmune hemolytic anemia), autoimmune enteropathy, and CNS lesions. Lymphadenopathy is present in about one-third of patients and in conjunction with cytopenias can prompt consideration of autoimmune lymphoproliferative syndrome (ALPS). Histologically, there are lymphocytic infiltrates involving the gastrointestinal tract with evidence of enterocolitis consistent with lymphocytic or neutrophilic (cryptitis) colitis, as well as lymphoid hyperplasia with a mixture of B cells and T cells; a full clinical spectrum of severity corresponding to underlying histology (not infectious) similar to the enterocolitis in patients treated with anti-CTLA4 antibody is observed.[90] Another distinguishing feature in these patients is the inflammatory infiltrate involving the CNS with supratentorial and infratentorial lesions, occasionally involving the brainstem or spine (Fig. 53-9). It is of interest that the degree of involvement by MRI does not correlate with severity of clinical symptoms.[91] Histologically, the infiltrate is either lymphohistiocytic with scattered plasma cells or mostly lymphoplasmacytic. There is no necrosis, granulomata, or tissue destruction; by immunophenotype, the majority of lymphocytes are T cells with a predominance of CD4-positive cells, plasma cells are often polyclonal, and in only one patient was there light chain restriction. Histology of the lymph node is more varied; in some cases follicular hyperplasia is present, and only one case showed an atypical T-cell proliferation not clonal in nature, but composed predominantly of CD8-positive T cells. One patient has been described with EBV-positive classic Hodgkin lymphoma.[87]

From an immunologic standpoint, quantitative deficiencies of CTLA4 are observed, leading to altered homeostasis with lymphopenia, but pronounced autoimmune phenomena with lymphocytic infiltrates in various organs. A progressive B-cell lymphopenia is also noted, with an increase of autoreactive B cells.[87,88]

There are several patterns of bone marrow pathology in CTLA4 deficiency. A subset of patients develops pancytopenia and has hypocellular marrow with prominent atypical lymphoid aggregates composed largely of T-cells with markedly decreased to absent B-cells (Fig. 53-10A–B). The T cells in the

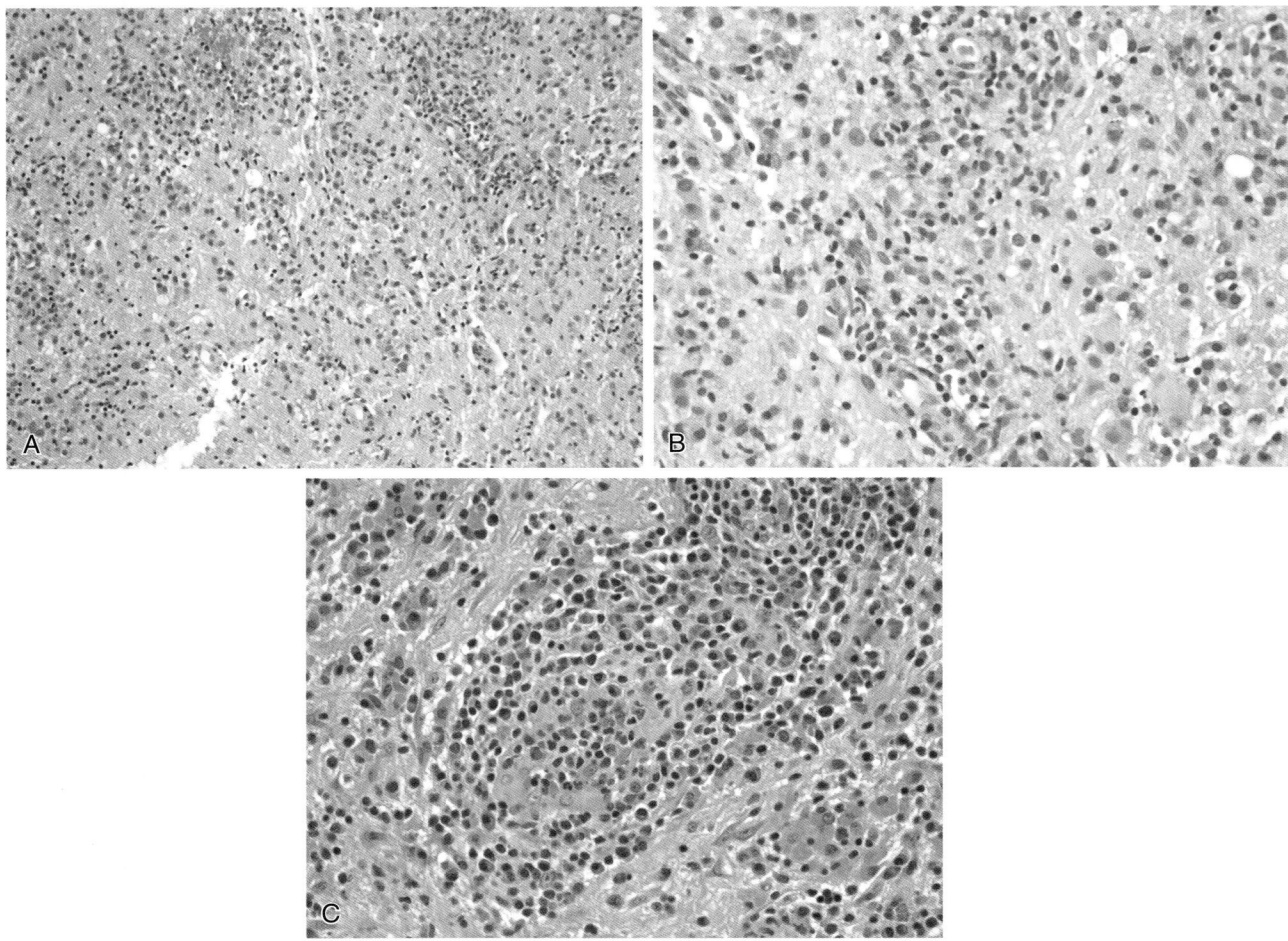

Figure 53-9. Brain biopsies from two different patients with CTLA4 deficiency. A–B, Lymphohistiocytic infiltrates involving the white matter with isolated plasma cells are shown. The lymphocytes are predominantly T cells. **C,** A dense plasmacytic perivascular infiltrate extending into the surrounding brain parenchyma; the plasma cells are polyclonal.

lymphoid aggregates are predominantly CD4 positive, while the T-cells scattered interstitially throughout the marrow are predominantly CD8 positive (Fig. 53-10C–F). In some patients, the marrow cellularity may be so low (<20%) that it raises concern for aplastic anemia. Other CTLA4 patients have hypercellular marrows with massive T-cell infiltration (Fig. 53-11), while a subset with thrombocytopenia and autoimmune hemolytic anemia may have hypercellular marrows with increased megakaryocytes and erythropoiesis, which may resemble ITP marrow (Fig. 53-11).

Autoimmune Lymphoproliferative Syndrome

ALPS, also known as Canale-Smith syndrome,[92] is a genetic disorder characterized by lymphoid proliferation caused by impaired apoptosis leading to the accumulation of TCRαβ positive CD4/CD8-double negative T (DNT) cells, both circulating and within lymph nodes; splenomegaly; multiple cytopenias; and increased risk for developing B-cell lymphomas of both Hodgkin and non-Hodgkin type.[93] In ALPS, lymphocyte homeostasis is disrupted because of defects in the FAS-mediated apoptotic pathway; the majority of patients

have deleterious heterozygous germline mutations involving the *FAS* gene or, less commonly, *FASLG* or *CASP10*. Somatic mutations involving the *FAS* gene have also been described.[94] An international workshop revised the diagnostic criteria for ALPS and proposed to divide them into two required criteria and six accessory criteria, further subdivided into primary and secondary (Box 53-1).[95] For a definitive diagnosis of ALPS, both required criteria have to be met, as well as one of the primary accessory criteria; a diagnosis of probable ALPS is based on both required criteria and one of the secondary accessory criteria. The two required criteria are the presence of noninfectious, nonmalignant chronic lymphadenopathy (>6 months) or splenomegaly and an elevated TCRαβ-positive DNT cells (≥1.5% of total lymphocyte count or 2.5% of CD3-positive lymphocytes in the setting of a normal or elevated lymphocyte count); the two primary accessory criteria are defective apoptosis and presence of germline or somatic mutations in *FAS, FASLG,* or *CASP10*. The presence of typical morphologic and immunophenotypic findings represents one of the secondary accessory criteria. A history of other autoimmune disorders like Hashimoto thyroiditis or type 1 diabetes can led to the diagnosis when considered together with waxing or waning lymphadenopathy or lymphocytosis.

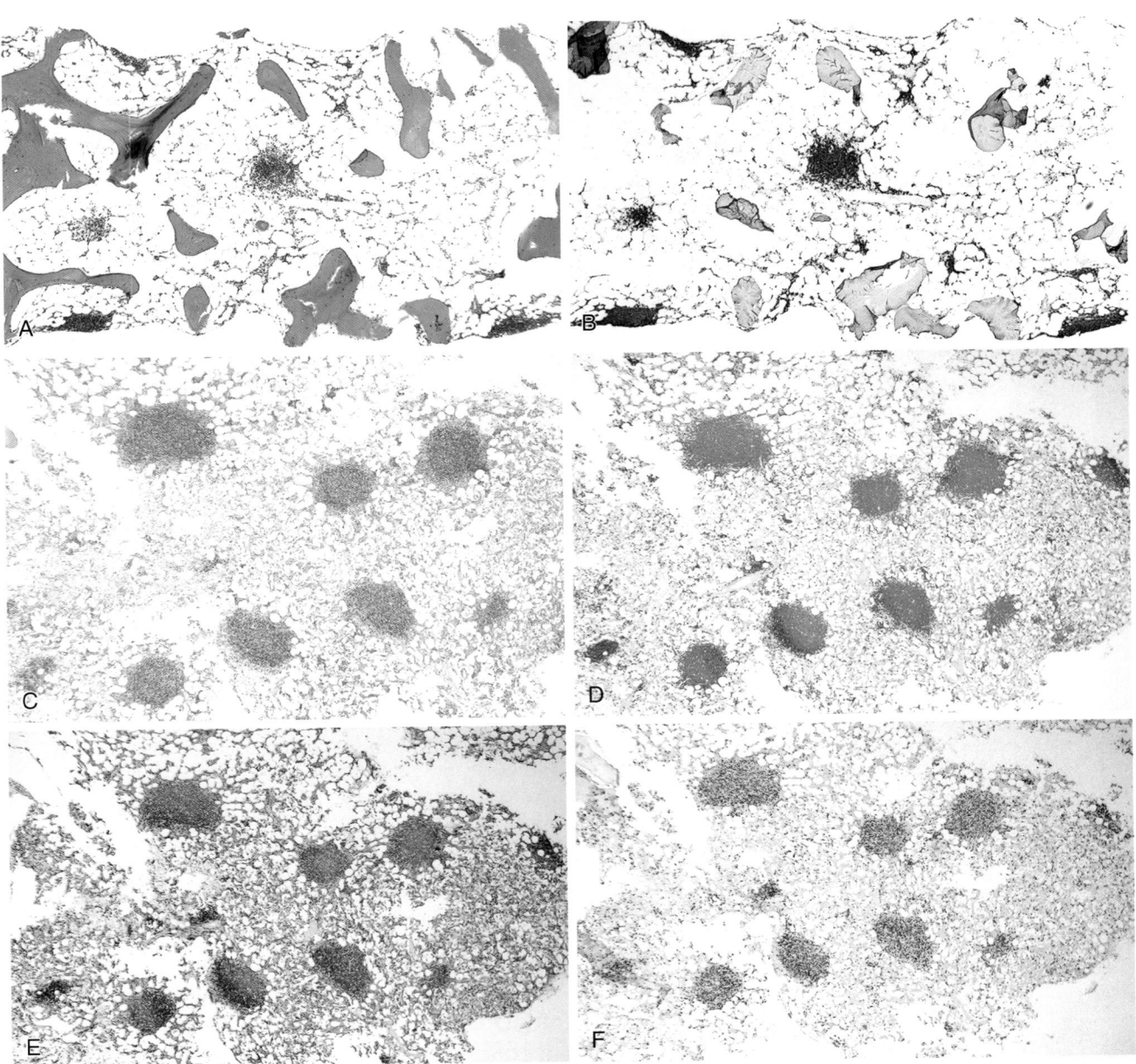

Figure 53-10. Bone marrow pathology in CTLA4 deficiency. **A–B,** Hypocellular marrow with atypical T-cell aggregates. Marrow from an 18-year-old male with pancytopenia and CTLA4 deficiency. The marrow was hypocellular for age with multiple atypical lymphoid aggregates **(A)**, which were positive for CD3 with T cells **(B)**. B-lineage cells were notably absent, demonstrated by CD79a (not shown). Karyotype was normal and TCRG PRC revealed polyclonal T cells. **C,** Marrow from a 44-year-old male with CTLA4 deficiency and marked pancytopenia. The marrow was hypercellular with a prominent nodular infiltrate composed largely of T cells **(D)** that were a mixture of CD4 positive cells **(E)** and CD8 positive cells **(F)**. B cells were decreased. Karyotype was normal and TRG PCR was polyclonal.

Note that lymphadenopathy and splenomegaly often resolve once patients reach adolescence or adulthood.

Recent studies on the natural history of ALPS based on long-term follow-up of over 200 patients showed a male predominance, a median age at onset of symptoms of approximately 3 years, and a *FAS* mutation in the intracellular domain in 70% to 83% of patients; in contrast, somatic *FAS* mutations more frequently occurred in the extracellular domain. In addition, only a 60% penetrance was found among family members carrying the same heterozygous gene mutation, indicating that other genetic differences or modifiers may exist. As expected, nearly all symptomatic patients had chronic adenopathy and splenomegaly. Laboratory findings revealed a median percentage of DNT cells of 5.9%; increased concentrations of vitamin B_{12}, IL10, and soluble FASL, all known biomarkers that are usually present in ALPS; hypergammaglobulinemia; and autoimmune cytopenias in 61% to 69% of patients. Risk for

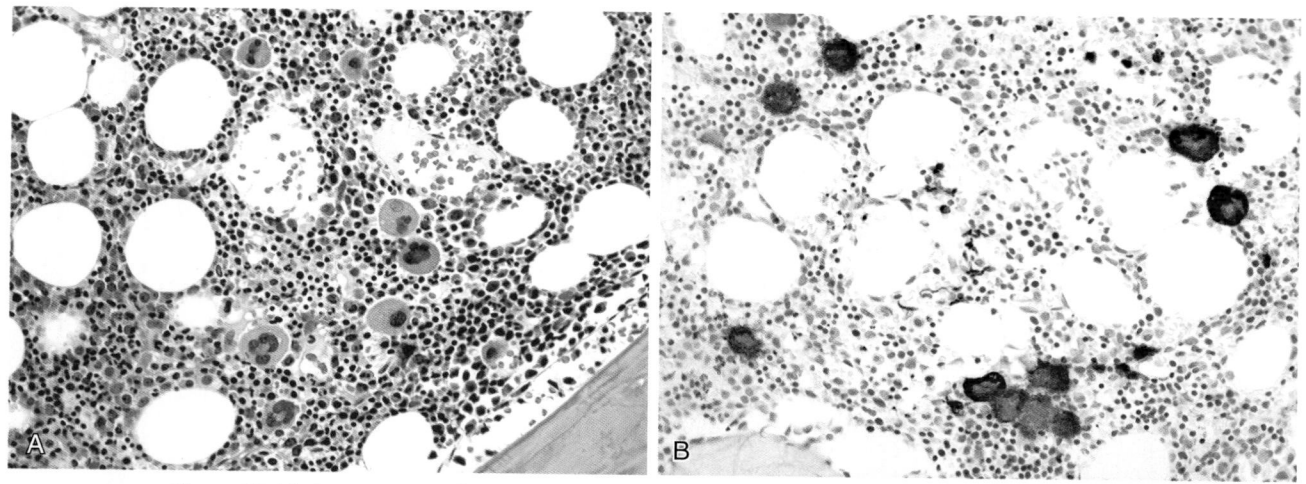

Figure 53-11. Bone marrow from a patient with CTLA4 presenting as immune/idiopathic thrombocytopenic purpura (ITP). **A,** Mild megakaryocytic hyperplasia (**B,** CD61 immunostain) in a bone marrow biopsy from an 8-year-old boy who presented with thrombocytopenia and high immature platelet fraction (accompanied by absolute neutropenia and mild anemia), whose initial response to IVIg suggested ITP.

Box 53-1 *Autoimmune Lymphoproliferative Syndrome (ALPS) Diagnostic Criteria (2009)*

Required
Chronic (>6 months), nonmalignant, noninfectious lymphadenopathy or splenomegaly
Elevated CD3-positive TCRαβ-positive CD4-CD8–double-negative T cells (≥1.5% of the total lymphocytes or 2.5% of the CD3-positive lymphocytes in the setting of normal or elevated lymphocyte counts)

Accessory
Primary
Defective lymphocyte apoptosis
Pathogenic mutations in *FAS, FASLG,* and *CASP10*

Secondary
Elevated biomarkers (sFASL, IL10, vitamin B_{12}, IL18)
Typical immunohistologic findings
Autoimmune cytopenias and increased IgG
Family history

For a definitive diagnosis: Both required criteria plus one primary accessory criterion. For a probable diagnosis: Both required criteria plus one secondary criterion.

---

sepsis was higher in patients who underwent splenectomy at an earlier age.[96-98]

Lymph node biopsies in ALPS type 1A (*FAS* mutations) patients reveal a preserved architecture, with often widely spaced secondary B follicles (some hyperplastic and some regressed) and a prominent paracortical hyperplasia characterized by a proliferation of lymphoid cells varying in cell size with more open chromatin and lacking the typical features of paracortical hyperplasia with small lymphocytes and condensed chromatin interspersed with macrophages and dendritic cells. Plasmacytosis in the medullary cords is also often present. A DNT cell population can be identified with immunohistochemical staining in a subset of cases, but flow cytometry is more sensitive and more accurate (Fig. 53-12). Abundant S100-positive dendritic cells are also present within the expanded paracortex. In a subset of patients, changes consistent with sinus histiocytosis with massive lymphadenopathy (SHML), also known as Rosai-Dorfman disease, can be observed either as focal or diffuse involvement. Because of the overlapping symptomatology between SHML and ALPS, the latter possibility should be excluded on clinical and immunologic grounds.[99] In ALPS patients, there is also an increased risk for lymphomas, which include both Hodgkin and non-Hodgkin B-cell lymphomas. A subset of these can be associated with EBV, particularly mixed cellularity classic Hodgkin lymphoma and Burkitt lymphoma.[96] Interestingly, some asymptomatic family members may also develop lymphoma, but it is unclear whether this is related to the underlying *FAS* mutation.

DEFECTS IN SYNAPSE FORMATION AND CROSSTALK BETWEEN ANTIGEN-PRESENTING CELLS AND T CELLS

Wiskott-Aldrich Syndrome

WAS is an X-linked PID characterized by eczema, thrombocytopenia with a decreased mean platelet volume, severe and often recurrent infections, and autoimmune disorders.[100] Prevalence in the United States is approximately 1 to 4 cases per 1,000,000 live male births and 1.2% of patients with identified primary immune defects.[101]

The *WAS* gene is located at Xp11.22-p11.23; the WAS protein (WASp) is involved in actin polymerization and plays a central role in TCR signaling to full T-cell activation, cytoskeletal remodeling, synapse formation, and migration. Mutations have been described along the entire *WAS* gene. The WASp family comprises eight members of actin regulatory proteins with different functions in various tissues[102,103]; WASp is exclusively present in hematopoietic cells. Variations in WASp expression or function correlate with the clinical spectrum, ranging from classic WAS with no protein expression to phenotypic variation of X-linked

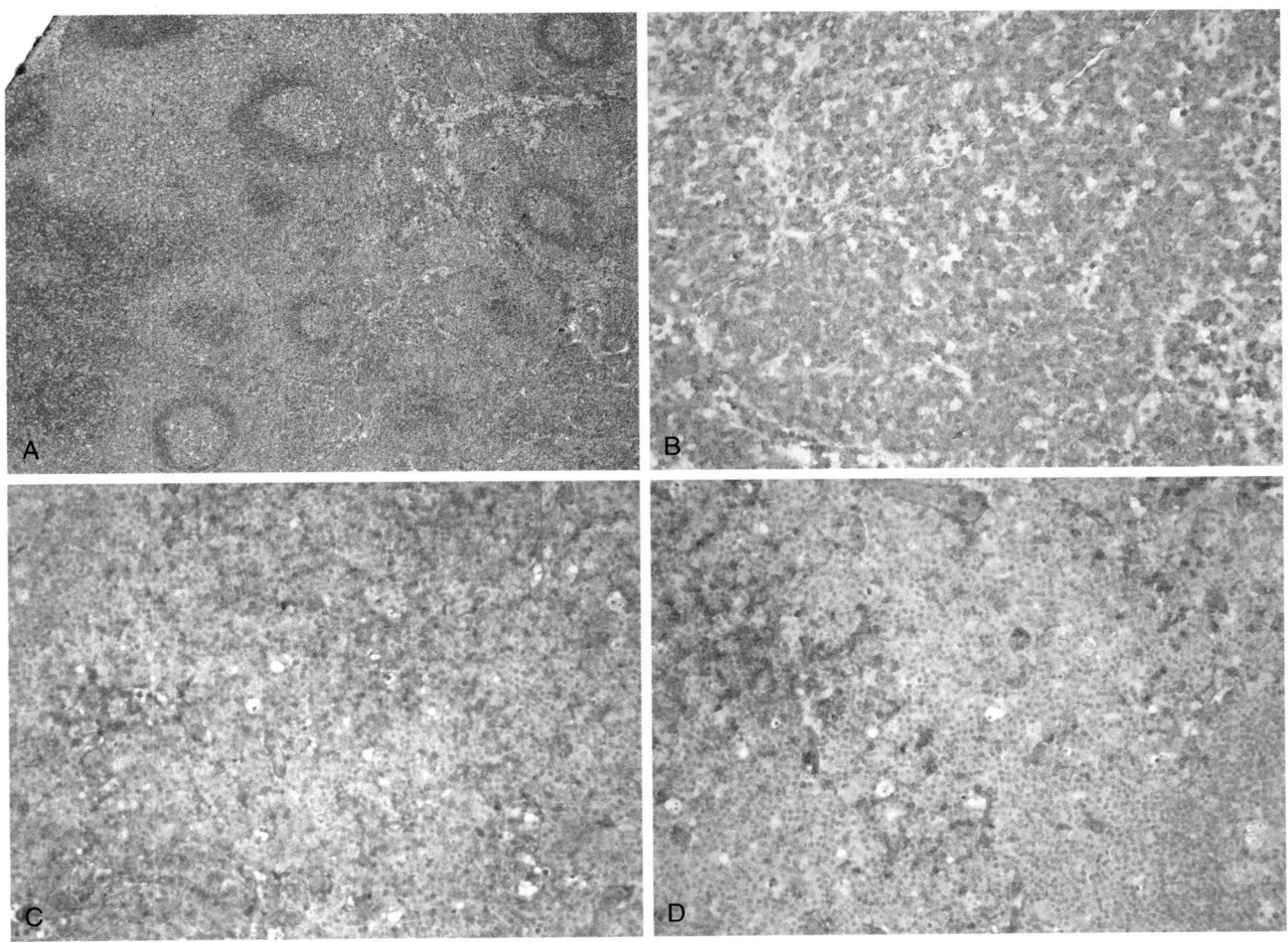

Figure 53-12. Lymph node biopsy from a patient with autoimmune lymphoproliferative syndrome (ALPS) type 1A (*FAS* mutations in the intracellular death domain). **A,** Hematoxylin and eosin (H&E) shows an atypical paracortical hyperplasia. **B,** CD3-positive T cells are shown. The majority lack CD4 **(C)** and CD8 **(D)** expression, consistent with double-negative T cells, typically seen in ALPS.

thrombocytopenia (XLT) with partial expression of the protein and X-linked neutropenia (XLN), caused by activating mutations. Female carriers are asymptomatic, with extreme rare symptomatic cases caused by deleterious mutations on the paternally derived X chromosome and non-random inactivation of the maternally derived X chromosome. When the mutation results in lack of WASp expression, the classical syndrome occurs. Spontaneous chimerism caused by genetic reversion, which may confer a selective advantage, has been observed in about 11% of patients, but the clinical significance of this finding is unclear.[104] A similar phenomenon has been observed in numerous other PIDs is not unique to WAS.

Clinically, patients present with skin rash (eczema) and bleeding (80%), such as petechiae and ecchymoses. Past medical history may also include mucosal or intracranial bleeding, recurrent sinopulmonary (otitis media, 64%; pneumonia, 25%), viral (herpes simplex virus 1 and 2, VZV, molluscum contagiosum), fungal, and opportunistic (*P. jirovecii*) infections. Autoimmune phenomena, seen in 40% of patients, include cytopenias (autoimmune hemolytic anemia in 14%), vasculitis (13%), IBD, arthritis (10%), and renal disease (IgA nephropathy, 12%). WAS patients are also at risk for developing lymphomas (13%) at a mean age of 9.5

years. EBV-positive non-Hodgkin lymphomas occur more frequently than classic Hodgkin lymphoma, and Burkitt lymphoma, lymphoblastic leukemia/lymphoma, and diffuse large B-cell lymphoma/lymphomatoid granulomatosis have been described in WAS patients. They can also develop myeloid disorders.[101]

Flow-cytometric analysis with quantification of intracytoplasmic WASp expression is used as a screening tool in suspected cases and allows for identification of various disease states.

Sequencing of the entire *WAS* gene (exons, intron and exon boundaries, and upstream regulatory regions) is recommended if diagnosis needs further confirmation; targeted sequencing is usually done in cases with family history and known mutations. Sequencing also has been used in the context of prenatal diagnosis in at-risk couples.

Laboratory findings confirm that all arms of the immune system are affected: adaptive, humoral, and innate. Quantitative immunoglobulins reveal variable IgM, with normal to high IgA and elevated IgG and IgE. Abnormal isohemagglutinin titers and diminished vaccine responses are present. Analysis of lymphocyte subsets reveals T-cell lymphopenia (lymphocyte count less than 1000/μL) with an abnormal response to mitogen. T-cell defects also lead to impaired antibody production by B cells, but intrinsic defects in B cells have also been described with hyper-responsiveness and autoantibody production.[105] Cytotoxic T cells and NK cells are also defective in their killing of targets because of the inefficient polarization of cytotoxic granules to the cell surface and inability to form synapses. This deficit in cytotoxic activity, in conjunction with the lymphopenia and intrinsic T-cell and B-cell defects, may be ultimately responsible for the inability to clear infectious agents and may contribute to the development of B-cell lymphomas.

Morphologically, in the spleen, depletion of the white pulp with diminished marginal zones and decreased numbers of B cells and T cells has been described.[106] Enlarged lymph nodes are often biopsied to monitor for the possible development of lymphomas; they usually show preserved architecture with prominent reactive secondary B follicles and expanded paracortex with prominent eosinophilia.

Warts, Hypogammaglobulinemia, Infections, and Myelokathexis

Warts, hypogammaglobulinemia, infections, and myeloka-thexis (WHIM) syndrome is caused by autosomal dominant mutations in *CXCR4*; this is a rare disorder that can affect both males and females and can also present with either B-cell or T-cell lymphopenia. CXCR4 is a G-protein–coupled trans-membrane receptor that is broadly expressed in leukocytes and other cells; its ligand, SDF-1 (CXCL-12), is secreted by many cells except blood cells. Most of the mutations abolish phosphorylation of CXCR4, inhibiting recycling of the receptor and leading to its prolonged activation.[107] Both chemokine and its receptor mediate the mobility and localization of T cells and APCs within secondary lymphoid organs and likely regulate their interaction, and ultimately confer stability to the T/APC synapses. Myelokathexis, a Greek neologism meaning bone marrow (*myelo-*) retention (*-kathexis*), refers to accumulation of mature neutrophils as they are unable to be released from the marrow. Bone marrow evaluation reveals hypercellularity with granulocytic hyperplasia and a right-shift with an abundance of mature neutrophils (Fig. 53-13). In aspirate smears, many of the neutrophils have a distinctive appearance, with pyknotic nuclear segments attached by long, wispy strands of chromatin, sometimes accompanied by cytoplasmic vacuoles (Fig. 53-13), though these cells are not seen in circulation. Use of CXCR4 inhibitors ameliorates neutropenia by allowing the release of neutrophils from the marrow.[108] Patients with WHIM syndrome also have a defect in high-affinity antibody maturation, likely because of defective CSR, with decreased antigen-specific memory responses.[109] These patients are also prone to EBV-related lymphomas.

Ataxia-Telangiectasia

Ataxia-telangiectasia (AT) is a rare autosomal recessively inherited disorder typically manifesting initially around age 2 years as progressive cerebellar degeneration (ataxia), with a later onset of oculocutaneous telangiectasias that first appear on the bulbar conjunctivae, ears, and nose; patients also suffer from defects in both cellular and humoral immunity (with thymic hypoplasia) predisposing them to sinopulmonary infection, and they face an increased risk of lymphoid

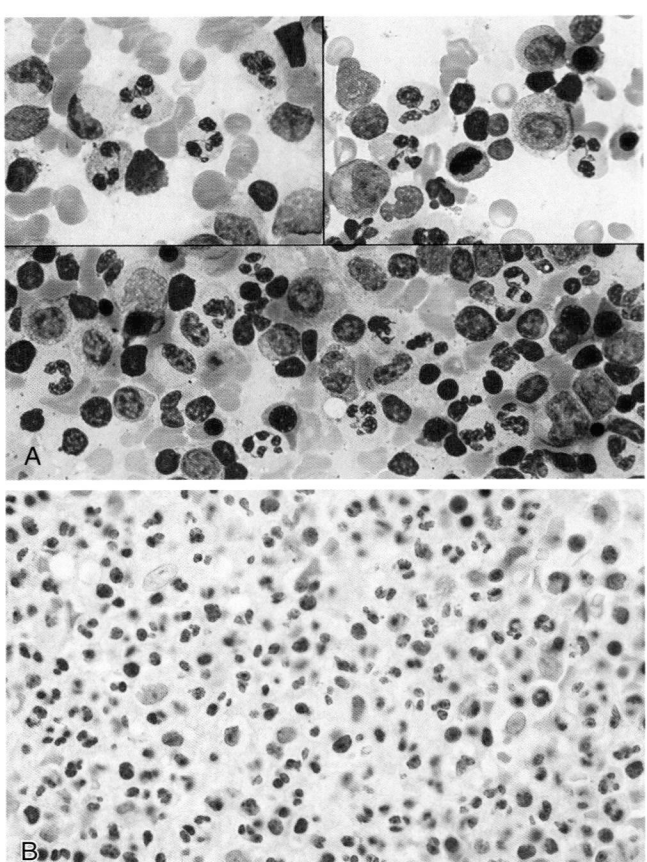

Figure 53-13. WHIM and myelokathexis. A, Marrow aspirate from a warts, hypogammaglobulinemia, infections, and myelokathexis (WHIM) patient showing a subset of characteristic WHIM neutrophils with pyknotic nuclear segments attached by thin chromatin strands (×1000, Wright-Giemsa). **B,** Bone marrow biopsy shows markedly hypercellular marrow with right-shifted myeloid hyperplasia and increased mature neutrophils demonstrating myelokathexis (×500, hematoxylin and eosin [H&E]).

and nonlymphoid tumors, the former developing earlier in life.[110] AT is caused by biallelic mutations in the *ATM* (ataxia-telangiectasia mutated) gene located on chromosome 11q22.3-23.1, which normally codes for a 350-kDa serine-threonine kinase, part of the PIK-related protein kinase family. ATM plays an important role in responding to DNA damage, which underlies the increased risk of malignancy in AT patients, and it is important to remember they are also hypersensitive to ionizing radiation: serious and sometimes fatal reactions can result when conventional doses of radiation therapy are used to treat those cancers. AT patients develop clonal T-cell proliferations with recurrent rearrangements involving chromosomes 7 and 14, where the TCR genes reside, that may evolve to T-prolymphocytic leukemia (T-PLL). Interestingly, T-lymphoblastic leukemia (T-ALL) and T-PLL occur less frequently than was previously thought. Acquired somatic mutations of the *ATM* gene are also detected in several lymphoproliferative disorders, including chronic lymphocytic leukemia and mantle cell lymphoma. A review from the French national registry of primary immune deficiencies reported cancer in 24.5% (69 of 279) of AT patients.[111] Of the patients, 38 developed non-Hodgkin lymphoma, mostly of aggressive B-cell type (median age, 9.7 years; 50% EBV positive), while 12 developed Hodgkin lymphoma (median age, 10.6 years; all EBV positive), with 8 patients each developing ALL (median age, 8.3 years, including 4 cases of T-ALL) or carcinoma (median age, 31.4 years; breast, gastric, liver, and thyroid), and 3 with T-PLL (median age, 24.2 years). Myeloid neoplasms are uncommon in AT, and as one would expect, overall survival is shorter in patients with AT who develop cancer.

Pearls and Pitfalls

- The concept of primary immunodeficiency (PID) has expanded over time and now includes 10 categories: combined immunodeficiencies, combined immunodeficiencies with syndromic features, predominantly antibody deficiencies, diseases of immune dysregulation, congenital defects of phagocytes, defects in intrinsic and innate immunity, autoinflammatory diseases, complement deficiencies, bone marrow failure, and phenocopies of inborn errors of immunity.
- With the use of modern technologies such as whole-exome sequencing (WES) and whole-genome sequencing (WGS), the number of PIDs with identified genetic defects has exploded from just over 100 to 485 in 20 years.
- Age of onset is commonly during but certainly not limited to infancy and early childhood; Common variable immunodeficiency (CVID) is a notable exception.
- The pathology should be interpreted in the context of the clinical presentation, family history, and appropriate immunologic workup.

KEY REFERENCES

2. Tangye SG, et al. Human inborn errors of immunity: 2022 update on the classification from the International Union of Immunological Societies Expert Committee. *J Clin Immunol.* 2022.

10. Puck JM. Newborn screening for severe combined immunodeficiency and T-cell lymphopenia. *Immunol Rev.* 2019;287(1):241–252.
13. Bosticardo M, Pala F, Notarangelo LD. RAG deficiencies: recent advances in disease pathogenesis and novel therapeutic approaches. *Eur J Immunol.* 2021;51(5):1028–1038.
18. Villa A, Notarangelo LD. RAG gene defects at the verge of immunodeficiency and immune dysregulation. *Immunol Rev.* 2019;287(1):73–90.
58. Angulo I, et al. Phosphoinositide 3-kinase delta gene mutation predisposes to respiratory infection and airway damage. *Science.* 2013;342(6160):866–871.
59. Lucas CL, et al. Dominant-activating germline mutations in the gene encoding the PI(3)K catalytic subunit p110delta result in T cell senescence and human immunodeficiency. *Nat Immunol.* 2014;15(1):88–97.
66. Coulter TI, et al. Clinical spectrum and features of activated phosphoinositide 3-kinase delta syndrome: a large patient cohort study. *J Allergy Clin Immunol.* 2017;139(2):597–606.e4.
87. Kuehn HS, et al. Immune dysregulation in human subjects with heterozygous germline mutations in CTLA4. *Science.* 2014;345(6204):1623–1627.
88. Schubert D, et al. Autosomal dominant immune dysregulation syndrome in humans with CTLA4 mutations. *Nat Med.* 2014;20(12):1410–1416.
97. Neven B, et al. A survey of 90 patients with autoimmune lymphoproliferative syndrome related to TNFRSF6 mutation. *Blood.* 2011;118(18):4798–4807.

Visit Elsevier eBooks+ for the complete set of references.

Chapter 54

Iatrogenic Immunodeficiency-Associated Lymphoproliferative Disorders

Steven H. Swerdlow and Sarah E. Gibson

DEFINITION

Lymphoproliferative disorders (LPDs) associated with iatrogenic immunodeficiency constitute a spectrum of lymphoid or plasmacytic proliferations, including a major subset that occurs after solid organ or hematopoietic stem cell transplantation (posttransplant lymphoproliferative disorders [PTLDs]). A smaller number of cases occur in other situations, such as in patients with rheumatoid arthritis treated with methotrexate, in young patients with Crohn's disease treated with tumor necrosis factor-α (TNF-α) antagonists along with antimetabolites, or rarely after some chemotherapeutic agents (other iatrogenic immunodeficiency-associated LPDs [OIIA-LPDs]). Many LPDs are associated with Epstein-Barr virus (EBV). They require further classification because of the great variation in their cytologic composition, degree of destructiveness, immunophenotype, cytogenetic and molecular findings, clinical behavior, and therapeutic approach.[1-7] Cases range from hyperplastic-appearing lesions to others that are indistinguishable from non-Hodgkin or Hodgkin lymphoma in immunocompetent hosts. Even the lymphoma-like cases are separately designated because reducing or discontinuing immunosuppression, when possible, or administering therapy that would be considered inadequate in immunocompetent hosts may lead to resolution.

SYNONYMS AND RELATED TERMS

WHO revised 4th ed.: Posttransplant lymphoproliferative disorders, other iatrogenic immunodeficiency-associated lymphoproliferative disorders

WHO proposed 5th ed.: Lymphoid proliferations and lymphomas associated with immune deficiency and dysregulation

CLASSIFICATION

The classification of immunodeficiency-associated LPDs is currently controversial (Box 54-1). The 2022 International Consensus Classification of Lymphoid Neoplasms (ICC) retains the categories of immunodeficiency-associated LPDs outlined in the World Health Organization (WHO) Revised 4th ed. classification.[5,8] The ICC classification preserves the category of PTLD because of the extensive literature regarding the clinicopathologic features of PTLD, which include therapeutic strategies that are not necessarily applicable to other immunodeficiency-associated LPDs.[8-18] Clinical guidelines published for managing patients with PTLD, and benchmark surveys about diagnosis, prevention, and treatment of PTLD are neither intended for nor tested in patients with OIIA-LPDs.[17,19] Thus, a proliferation like a diffuse large B-cell lymphoma, not otherwise specified

Box 54-1 *Current Classification Systems for Iatrogenic Immunodeficiency–Associated Lymphoproliferative Disorders (LPDs)*

2022 International Consensus Classification
Posttransplant Lymphoproliferative Disorders (PTLDs)
Nondestructive PTLDs
   Plasmacytic hyperplasia PTLD
   Infectious mononucleosis PTLD
   Florid follicular hyperplasia PTLD
Polymorphic PTLD
Monomorphic PTLDs*
   B-cell neoplasms
      Diffuse large B-cell lymphoma
      Burkitt lymphoma
      Multiple myeloma
      Plasmacytoma
      Other[†]
   T-cell neoplasms
      Peripheral T-cell lymphoma, not otherwise specified (NOS)
      Hepatosplenic T-cell lymphoma
      Other
Classic Hodgkin lymphoma PTLD

Other Iatrogenic Immunodeficiency-Associated
Lymphoproliferative Disorders[‡]

World Health Organization Classification, Proposed 5th Ed.
Lymphoid Proliferations and Lymphomas Associated With
Immune Deficiency and Dysregulation
Hyperplasias arising in immune deficiency/dysregulation
Polymorphic lymphoproliferative disorders arising in immune
   deficiency/dysregulation
Epstein-Barr virus (EBV)+ mucocutaneous ulcer
Lymphomas arising in immune deficiency/dysregulation
Inborn error of immunity-associated lymphoid proliferations and
   lymphomas

Three-Part Nomenclature Used by WHO Classification, Proposed 5th Ed. for Lymphoid Proliferations and Lymphomas Arising in the Setting of Immune Deficiency/Dysregulation
<u>Histologic Diagnosis:</u> Hyperplasia (specify type), Polymorphic lymphoproliferative disorder, Mucocutaneous ulcer, Lymphoma (classify as for immunocompetent patients)
<u>Viral Association:</u> EBV +/–, Kaposi sarcoma-associated herpesvirus/human herpesvirus 8 (KSHV/HHV8) +/–
<u>Immune Deficiency/Dysregulation Setting:</u> Inborn error of immunity (specify type), HIV infection, Posttransplant (specify: solid organ/bone marrow), Autoimmune disease, iatrogenic/therapy-related (specify), Immune senescence
*Classify according to the lymphoma/LPD in immunocompetent individuals they resemble.
[†]Small B-cell lymphomas arising in transplant patients are not considered PTLD, with the exception of EBV+ marginal zone lymphomas (see text and references 5, 156, and 160).
[‡]Classify in a fashion analogous to PTLD.
Data from Campo E, Jaffe ES, Cook JR, et al. The International Consensus Classification of Mature Lymphoid Neoplasms: a report from the Clinical Advisory Committee. *Blood.* 2022;140(11):1229-1253; and Alaggio R, Amador C, Anagnostopoulos I, et al. The 5th edition of the World Health Organization Classification of Haematolymphoid Tumours: Lymphoid Neoplasms. *Leukemia.* 2022;36(7):1720-1748.

(DLBCL, NOS) occurring in the posttransplant setting is viewed very differently from one occurring in a patient with HIV infection. Aside from the very different clinical settings, with therapeutic implications, biological differences including different prognostic implications have been documented between HIV-associated and PTLD DLBCL-type lesions.[20-22] Though difficult to be certain, Hodgkin type LPDs appear to be more common among the OIIA-LPDs than in the posttransplant setting, where they are very infrequent. In addition, while the diagnosis of PTLD is often made with great confidence, subclassification may be more problematic due in part to B-cell PTLDs forming a spectrum from nondestructive polymorphic proliferations to more destructive but polymorphic proliferations to proliferations that would fulfill the criteria for a conventional lymphoma, even if treatment strategies will differ. There remains a lack of consensus even on whether some of the subclassification matters clinically.[1,4,23] In contrast to this separate designation of PTLD, the proposed WHO 5th ed. includes a broad category of "lymphoid proliferations and lymphomas associated with immune deficiency and dysregulation" listed under the broader category of "mature B-cell neoplasms," even though some PTLD are of Hodgkin or T-cell type.[24-26] This category includes not only iatrogenic immunodeficiency-associated disorders, but also those associated with primary immunodeficiencies, termed "inborn errors of immunity."[26] The classification then uses a three-part unifying nomenclature (Box 54-1).[26] For these reasons, this chapter uses the 2022 ICC/WHO Revised 4th ed. nomenclature for PTLD and OIIA-LPDs.

POSTTRANSPLANT LYMPHOPROLIFERATIVE DISORDERS

The WHO Revised 4th ed. classification and 2022 ICC classification recognize four major categories of PTLD (Box 54-1).[5,8] Biopsies performed when there is a question of PTLD should be handled with a standard "rule out lymphoma" protocol that includes all the necessary ancillary techniques required for a complete diagnosis (Box 54-2). Although cytologic and fine-needle aspiration biopsy specimens can be useful in some circumstances, excisional biopsy is preferred because of the importance of assessing architectural features, the need for sufficient material for ancillary studies, and the intralesional heterogeneity present in a moderate number of PTLDs.

Epidemiology

PTLDs develop in approximately 2% of all transplant recipients, with significant variation in incidence based on the type of organ transplanted: kidney, 0.5% to 3%; bone marrow or stem cell, 1% to 2%; pancreas, 1% to 2%; liver, 1% to 4%; heart and lung, 1% to 10%; and intestinal and multivisceral, 5% to 20%.[5,27-39] Some report that the incidence of PTLD has decreased over time, possibly related to increased experience, improved immunosuppressive regimens, and increased use of molecular EBV monitoring with preemptive modulation of immunosuppressive therapy; however, others have found an increasing incidence, which may be related to a rising number of transplants, older age of donors and recipients, longer

Morphology
- Required for diagnosis and best accomplished with histologic sections
- Findings are extremely variable: lymphoplasmacytic proliferations with underlying architectural preservation; destructive polymorphic lymphoplasmacytic proliferations with moderately numerous transformed cells or immunoblasts; and lesions fulfilling the criteria for one of the non–small cell B-cell lymphomas, an Epstein-Barr virus (EBV)-positive marginal zone lymphoma, a plasma cell neoplasm, one of the T- or natural killer (NK)-cell lymphomas, or occasionally classic Hodgkin lymphoma

Immunophenotype
- Required for diagnosis
- Findings are extremely variable, including polytypic lesions, often with many admixed B and T cells, or lesions with the classic immunophenotypic features of one of the lymphoid or plasmacytic neoplasms
- Stains for EBV should be performed, with many, but not all, cases positive using EBV-encoded RNA (EBER) in situ hybridization or, in a somewhat smaller proportion of cases, using an EBV latent membrane protein 1 (LMP1) immunohistochemical stain

Molecular/Genetics
- Variably required
- Clonal B cells are demonstrable in most cases, except in plasmacytic hyperplasia, some infectious mononucleosis (IM) PTLDs, and T- or NK-cell PTLDs
- Clonal T cells are demonstrable in T-cell monomorphic PTLD and also in some other types of PTLD
- Various additional molecular cytogenetic and karyotypic findings are related to the type of PTLD, such as *MYC* rearrangements and *TP53* mutations
- These studies are most important in recognizing T-cell PTLD and classifying some of the B-cell monomorphic PTLDs

Clinical Features
- Assessment required for patient care
- PTLDs can present with an IM-type illness, like conventional lymphoid or plasmacytic neoplasms, or sometimes with vague or absent symptoms
- PTLDs are sometimes discovered only because of routine EBV monitoring or at autopsy
- Variable outcomes, ranging from indolent with only reduction in immunosuppression to very aggressive in spite of immunochemotherapy; many different factors affect outcome

survival of transplant recipients, and increasing diagnostic awareness of these LPDs.[9,28,31,40]

Many other factors have an effect on the incidence of PTLD. EBV seronegativity at the time of organ transplantation is an extremely important risk factor and explains in part the much higher incidence of PTLD in children than in adults.[5,31,34,38,39] Transplanting an organ from an EBV-seropositive donor into an EBV-seronegative recipient (EBV mismatch) increases the incidence of PTLD 10-fold to 75-fold.[41] Lack of previous exposure to cytomegalovirus (CMV) is also associated with an increased incidence of PTLD if the recipient is CMV negative and either the donor is CMV positive (CMV mismatch) or the recipient experiences a symptomatic primary CMV infection.[41]

The effects of EBV mismatch and CMV mismatch appear to be synergistic. Patients who undergo transplantation for hepatitis C-related cirrhosis reportedly have an increased incidence of PTLD, suggesting that hepatitis C may potentiate the oncogenicity of EBV.[42,43] Host factors, such as polymorphisms leading to lower expression of proinflammatory cytokines or greater expression of anti-inflammatory cytokines or HLA and other polymorphisms, may also influence the risk of selected PTLDs, although it has been noted that "it is currently not possible to predict which transplant patients will eventually develop PTLD."[32,44-49] Even after taking into consideration EBV and CMV serostatus, young age remains associated with an increased risk for development of PTLD, particularly early PTLD. The incidence increases again after the age of 50 years.[29,31] Overall, there is a higher incidence in males, especially for late-onset PTLD, but a higher incidence in females after small bowel transplantation.[29,40]

Another important risk factor for PTLD is the immunosuppressive regimen required to maintain or to prepare for the transplant or to treat graft-versus-host disease. The cumulative intensity of immunosuppressive therapy and the specific agents used are associated with the risk for development of early PTLD, whereas the overall duration of immunosuppression is associated with the risk for development of PTLD later.[41,50] Anti–T-cell antibody preparations, such as OKT3 and antithymocyte globulin (ATG), have been associated with an increased risk of PTLD.[41,50-53] In adults, the frequency of early PTLD is greater in patients receiving allogeneic hematopoietic stem cell transplantation than in those receiving solid organ transplants.[52] Some of the newer immunosuppressive strategies may be associated with a lower risk for PTLD.[40,51,54,55]

Etiology

Most PTLDs after solid organ transplantation are derived from recipient lymphoid cells, whereas those occurring after hematopoietic stem cell transplantation are most often donor derived.[56,57] PTLDs limited to the allograft after solid organ transplantation are more frequently of donor origin.[58,59] The majority of PTLDs are caused by EBV-infected lymphoid or plasmacytic cells that are not adequately controlled by the immune system because of immunosuppression or, in the case of stem cell and bone marrow transplants, myeloablative regimens.[50,60,61] EBV may be acquired from the donor or other sources as a primary infection, superinfection by a second strain of EBV in a seropositive recipient, or, especially in adults, reactivation of latent recipient EBV. EBV-associated PTLD shows variable latency patterns, and individual cells can express different sets of latency proteins.[62,63] Many cases have a type III latency pattern, similar to that seen in EBV-positive lymphoblastoid cell lines; some have a type II latency pattern; and fewer have a type I pattern.[50,64,65] Classic Hodgkin lymphoma (CHL) PTLD may demonstrate a type II pattern.[63,66,67]

Patients with EBV-positive PTLD lack an effective cytotoxic T-cell response to EBV infection, with decreased EBV-specific CD8-positive T cells and CD4-positive T cells.[68] Significantly fewer CD8-positive cytotoxic T cells have been observed in EBV-negative DLBCL-type monomorphic PTLD compared with EBV-negative DLBCL arising in immunocompetent individuals.[69,70] T-cell exhaustion, as indicated by increased expression of inhibitory receptors PD1/CD279 and

LAG3/CD223, may also play a role in PTLD development.[70-73] Similarly, natural killer (NK) cells show higher levels of PD1/CD279 expression and reduced levels of cytotoxicity and activation receptors in patients with PTLD.[73] Plasmacytoid dendritic cells, which function as antigen-presenting cells in the antiviral immune response, are decreased in polymorphic and monomorphic B-cell PTLDs compared with nondestructive lesions, as well as in DLBCL-type monomorphic PTLD compared with DLBCL in immunocompetent patients.[70,74,75] PDL1/CD274, which may be induced by EBV latent membrane protein 1 (LMP1) via the JAK/STAT pathway or by gain/amplification of 9p24.1 (*JAK2/PDL1/PDL2* locus), is expressed by at least 50% of PTLD, providing additional evidence that the PD1/PDL1 pathway affords a mechanism for immune escape in these LPDs.[71,73,76] Humoral responses to EBV are diminished after transplantation, but whether this plays a role in the development of PTLD is not known.[77] Patients with PTLD reportedly demonstrate a T-helper (Th) type 2 serum cytokine profile (interferon-γ [IFN-γ]/interleukin-2 negative; interleukin-4/interleukin-10 positive) that promotes EBV-induced B-cell proliferation.[41,78]

Genetic predisposition may play a role in the development of PTLD and in patients' response to therapy. A polymorphism in IFN-γ resulting in increased synthesis is associated with early-onset and pediatric PTLD, and a TNF gene polymorphism has been associated with the development of PTLD.[45,46,48] Polymorphic variants in the HLA system

have also been associated with PTLD development, possibly because of their role in interacting with NK cells and cytotoxic T lymphocytes.[47,49,79,80]

Although very few patients demonstrate a sequential development of PTLDs, they are thought to begin as polyclonal proliferations related to EBV or other stimuli, with the development over time of oligoclonal and then monoclonal B-cell or, much less frequently, T- or NK-cell proliferations (Fig. 54-1).[4,81,82] Genetic and epigenetic abnormalities of the types seen in conventional lymphoid or plasmacytic neoplasms also occur as the lesions progress, making them less responsive to immune regulation.[4,6,75,83,84] Advances in the understanding of the pathways involved in the pathogenesis of PTLD are not just of academic interest as they may suggest new therapeutic strategies, such as the use of JAK/STAT or immune checkpoint inhibitors.[76,85-87]

EBV cannot be demonstrated in approximately 20% to 40% of PTLDs, with the proportion of EBV-negative cases greater now than in the past.[81,88-93] At least some EBV-negative cases may represent EBV-related proliferations that have lost the virus after transformation (hit-and-run theory).[94] Others may reflect technical difficulties in the detection of EBV, represent lymphoid proliferations driven by other viral or infectious agents, or be related to chronic antigenic stimulation, possibly by the transplant itself. Gene-expression profiling studies have suggested a difference in pathobiology, with two studies showing viral-associated changes only in the

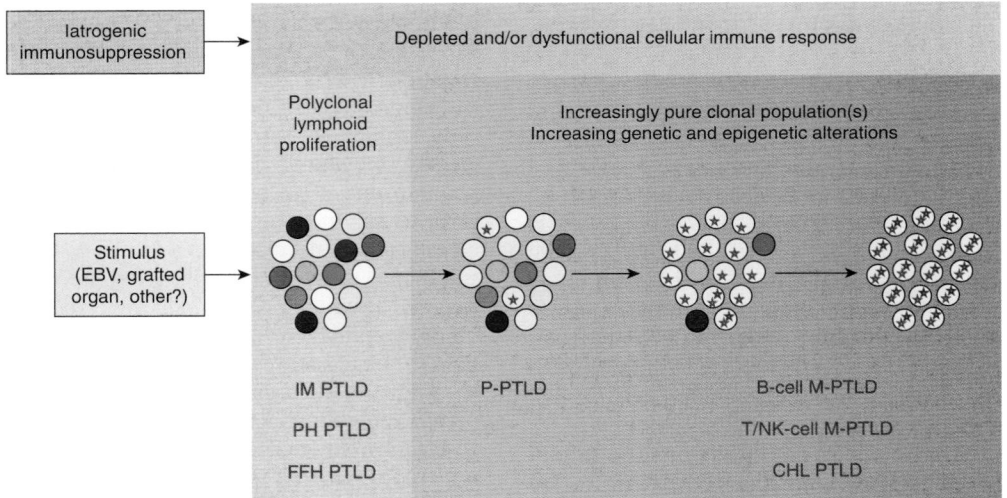

Figure 54-1. Model of posttransplant lymphoproliferative disorder development and correlation with clinicopathologic categories. This partially theoretical model is largely based on studies of B-cell posttransplant lymphoproliferative disorder (PTLD). Furthermore, documentation of progression through these varied stages is lacking in most cases, and the possibility that many lesions do not progress through all stages or that there may be nonlinear progression must be considered. Epstein-Barr virus (EBV) infection and, in a minority of cases, other stimuli (including chronic antigenic stimulation), in the presence of iatrogenic immunosuppression and an insufficient cellular immune response (caused by depleted or dysfunctional T cells, natural killer [NK] cells, and plasmacytoid dendritic cells), lead to a polyclonal lymphoid proliferation without causing significant destruction of the underlying tissue structures. Cases with few transformed cells fulfill the criteria for plasmacytic hyperplasia (PH); those with a more florid proliferation, including moderate numbers of transformed cells, are infectious mononucleosis (IM) PTLD. Some nondestructive PTLD also have the morphologic appearance of florid follicular hyperplasia (FFH). Increasingly pure clonal populations develop over time that are often, but not always, of B-cell origin. These may still be PH or IM PTLD, but often fulfill the criteria for a polymorphic (P-PTLD) or B-cell monomorphic PTLD (M-PTLD). If there is a pure plasma cell proliferation, a plasmacytoma-type or multiple myeloma-type M-PTLD is diagnosed; if there are clonal T cells, one of the T-cell M-PTLDs is usually diagnosed, particularly in the absence of a B-cell PTLD or other confounding features (see text). Occasional cases are T-cell rich, sometimes resembling either a T-cell/histiocyte–rich large B-cell lymphoma or classic Hodgkin lymphoma (CHL). Cytokine production by the PTLD and other cells in the tumor microenvironment may help foster the proliferation. Additional genetic alterations may accumulate, with *BCL6* mutations caused by aberrant somatic hypermutation seen in P-PTLDs and other abnormalities, such as *MYC* translocations, seen in some types of M-PTLD. Aberrant methylation of genes involved in B-cell activation, cell cycle regulation, apoptosis, and DNA damage repair is also common in P-PTLD and M-PTLDs. The *red stars* in the figure reflect earlier genetic/epigenetic abnormalities, such as some of the *BCL6* mutations, and the *green stars* represent later genetic/epigenetic alterations, such as *MYC* aberrations.

EBV-positive PTLDs, suggesting a possible nonviral etiology for the EBV-negative cases.[95,96] Genetic studies have shown fewer copy number alterations and gene mutations in EBV-positive PTLDs compared with EBV-negative cases, and one combined genomic and transcriptomic study found that EBV-negative DLBCL-type PTLDs segregated with DLBCL arising in immunocompetent patients.[21,76,96-99] However, two additional gene-profiling studies that included a broad spectrum of PTLDs failed to distinguish EBV-positive from EBV-negative PTLDs, and one study of DLBCL-type PTLD showed a mutational profile different from DLBCL in immunocompetent patients.[83,87,99]

Rare cases of human herpesvirus 8 (HHV8)-positive PTLD have been reported, including polymorphic lesions, multicentric Castleman disease-like lesions, and primary effusion lymphoma.[100-104] Other viral associations have been less frequently reported. A metagenomic analysis of DNA viruses identified anelloviruses in 52% of PTLDs, and other viruses in a lower percentage of cases.[105] In this exploratory series, the presence of anellovirus nucleic acid sequences was associated with worse patient survival; however, further validation is required, direct causality has not been established, and some consider the presence of anelloviruses to be a marker of immunosuppression intensity.[106]

Clinical Features

Although, historically, 80% of PTLDs occur within the first year, more recent studies have suggested a median time to PTLD of several years or longer, with a wide variation between studies and with up to 15% or 25% occurring more than 10 years after transplantation.[9,27,33,107-110] Some reports describe a decrease in the incidence of PTLD after an early phase and then a rise again at approximately 5 years, with the subsequent incidence remaining elevated.[31,33] Early-onset PTLD has been associated with younger patients; those presenting with an infectious mononucleosis (IM)–like syndrome; EBV positivity; PTLD after bone marrow, lung, heart-lung, and multivisceral transplantation; and hepatosplenic T-cell lymphoma PTLD.[9,11,32,33,52,111] Patients presenting after a longer interval reportedly are more likely to have localized extranodal disease and a worse prognosis.[16,89,112] Polymorphic PTLDs have been reported to have an earlier onset than monomorphic PTLDs; however, this could relate to the latter being more often EBV negative.[83] Monomorphic T-cell or NK-cell and CHL PTLDs are also more common among the PTLDs that occur later.[109,113] It is important to distinguish early-onset PTLD from what used to be termed "early lesions," which often occur later, with median times to occurrence of about 2 to 4 years.[114]

Patients with PTLD may have tumorous masses, often at extranodal sites; widely disseminated disease; an IM-like illness; vague, nonlocalized symptoms, such as fever; or no symptoms at all.[115] The most common sites of involvement include the gastrointestinal tract, lymph nodes, lung, and liver. Gastrointestinal tract involvement is often multifocal and may present with hemorrhage, obstruction, or perforation.[116] PTLDs may involve the central nervous system (CNS), with involvement often localized to that site.[117,118] PTLDs of the CNS are usually of monomorphic type, have a poor prognosis, and may occur relatively late after transplantation even though they are frequently EBV positive.[117,118] Nondestructive PTLDs often present with tonsil or adenoid enlargement, although

with nodal involvement in adults; and IM-like presentations are particularly common in younger patients.[114] Plasmacytoma PTLDs can be localized or disseminated, and may be associated with a paraprotein.[119,120] Approximately 20% of PTLDs occurring after solid organ transplantation are localized to the allograft.[30,121] Some PTLDs present with widely disseminated disease, including the multiple myeloma-type, which usually occurs in older patients and late after transplantation.[122-128]

EBV viral load often increases in the blood in association with PTLD, frequently before the development of overt disease, and has been proposed as a surveillance tool for high-risk patients.[17,46,129-133] Monitoring of EBV load has been suggested as one of the factors responsible for the recent decrease in incidence of some types of PTLD noted by some.[40,134] However, even EBV-positive PTLD can rarely develop in the setting of low viral loads; persistent high levels predict an increased risk of PTLD only in selected settings and may resolve spontaneously; and at least in some series, EBV loads relate more to the type of immunosuppressive regimen or the degree of iatrogenic immunosuppression.[135-140] Observation of trends in patients may be more useful than results from a single timepoint.

Morphology

The PTLDs form a morphologic spectrum from early, nondestructive polymorphic lesions to more infiltrative and destructive polymorphic or monomorphic proliferations (Boxes 54-1 and 54-2).[5,8] PTLDs are classified largely on the basis of their morphologic appearance, but doing so can be difficult and very subjective, in part because of frequent intralesional variability or variation between different sites of disease. Many studies report that about 60% to 80% of PTLDs are of monomorphic type, with some striking outliers at both ends of the spectrum.[9,13,33,107,109] Of the remaining cases, most studies report many more polymorphic PTLDs than nondestructive PTLD, with the latter usually making up less than 10% of cases.[13,33,107] Areas of geographic necrosis and vascular wall infiltration, and, at extranodal sites, neural infiltration are characteristic, but not required features.[2,7] Extranodal involvement may be masslike or more infiltrative, and parenchymal necrosis is sometimes present.[7] Areas adjacent to a main lesion may show more focal involvement, such as involvement of hepatic portal tracts or preservation of nodal sinuses.

Overt bone marrow involvement occurs in about 15% to 30% of patients with PTLD, and occasional patients may demonstrate peripheral blood involvement.[9,27,141-143] The bone marrow lesions, which can be either extensive or small and focal, are morphologically similar to those seen at other sites and can be found in patients with polymorphic and monomorphic types of PTLD.[141,143,144] Not uncommonly, children with PTLD may demonstrate an EBV-positive polyclonal-appearing plasmacytosis or small lymphoid or plasmacytic aggregates in the bone marrow that are of uncertain significance.[141]

Nondestructive Posttransplant Lymphoproliferative Disorders

Plasmacytic hyperplasia (PH) PTLD is usually diagnosed in biopsies of lymph nodes or sometimes tonsils in which the underlying architectural features are intact and there is a proliferation of small lymphocytes and plasma cells, with few transformed cells (Fig. 54-2).[6,7] These cases are not considered PTLD by all pathologists, and particularly when EBV is lacking, they are indistinguishable from non-specific lymphoid hyperplasia.

IM PTLD is also usually diagnosed in biopsies of lymph nodes or tonsils and adenoids (Fig. 54-3).[4,82] The specimens demonstrate changes associated with IM in the normal host, with a florid proliferation of small lymphocytes, plasma cells, and often very prominent transformed cells and immunoblasts. Although nodal sinuses may be obscured and hyperplastic follicles may appear indistinct, the basic architecture of the lymph node or tonsil is intact. In florid cases, it may be impossible to distinguish IM PTLD from a polymorphic PTLD. As long as the changes are acceptable for IM in the normal host, the former diagnosis is preferred. IM-like changes have also been identified in other extranodal sites, such as the liver; these are often considered to be more

like IM or simple EBV infection than PTLD; however, these changes may precede overt PTLD.[145] It is also important to rule out the possibility of partial nodal involvement by a monomorphic PTLD. Some nondestructive PTLDs have the morphologic appearance of florid follicular hyperplasia, without the interfollicular changes that characterize the other PTLDs of this type (Fig. 54-4).[5,8,114,146] Caution is advised in the absence of significant EBV positivity or a true mass lesion because otherwise the findings of florid follicular hyperplasia PTLD are totally non-specific.

As indicated, nondestructive PTLD are diagnosed in tonsils/adenoids and lymph nodes, but not generally at extranodal sites, where there may be some scattered EBV-positive cells in patients with EBV hepatitis or enteritis.[145,147,148] These may precede or be associated with PTLD at other sites, and sometimes they are treated like a PTLD. Unless there are large numbers of EBV-positive cells, the diagnosis of a nondestructive PTLD, especially at an extranodal site,

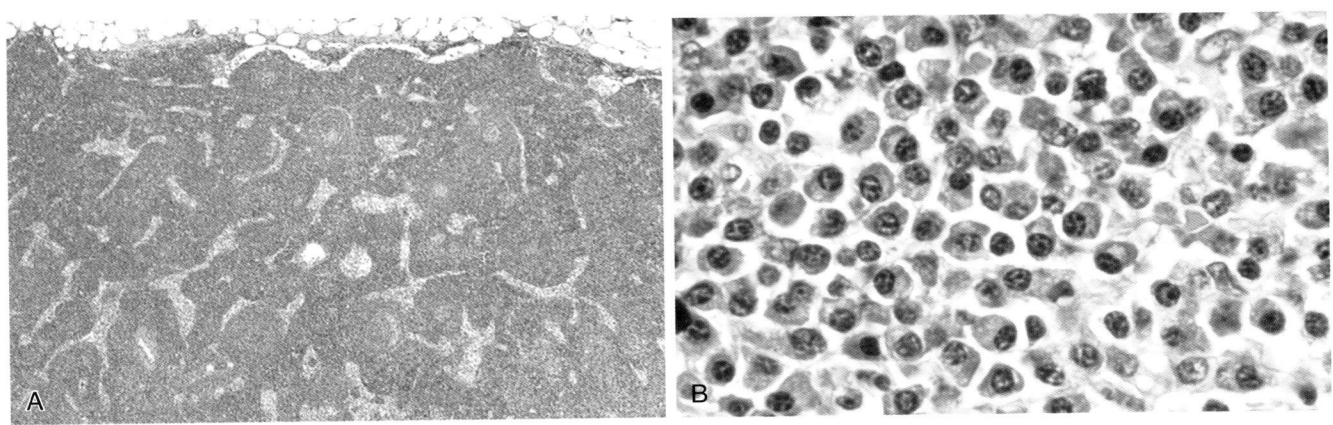

Figure 54-2. Plasmacytic hyperplasia in a perigastric lymph node. A, Normal architecture of the lymph node is preserved, with intact sinuses and occasional small follicles. **B,** Note the numerous plasma cells, which were shown to be polytypic with in situ hybridization stains for kappa and lambda. An Epstein-Barr virus–encoded RNA (EBER) in situ hybridization stain showed scattered positive cells.

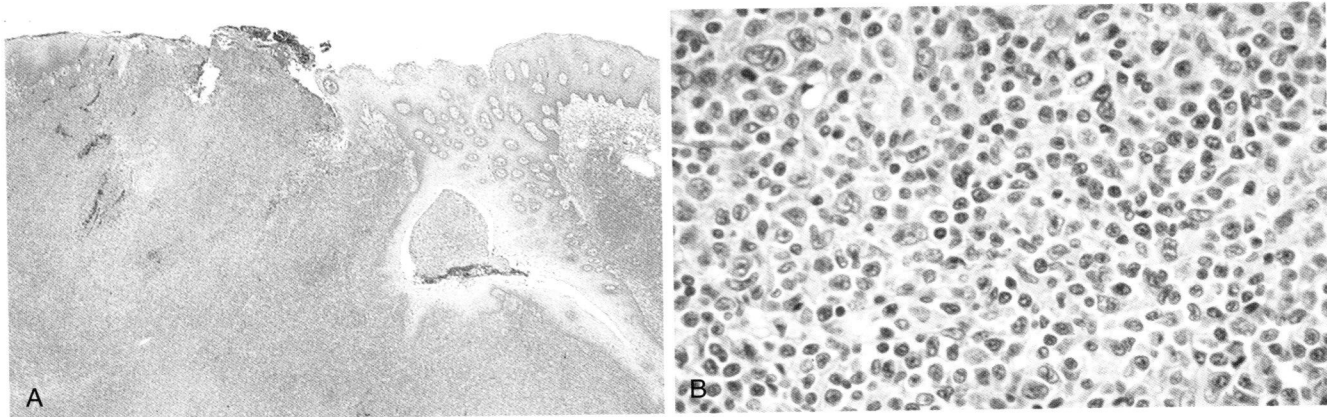

Figure 54-3. Infectious mononucleosis posttransplant lymphoproliferative disorder. Tonsil from an adolescent boy who presented with enlarged tonsils and adenoids and a sore throat several months after liver transplantation. The patient did well after reduction of tacrolimus immunosuppressive therapy and acyclovir treatment. **A,** Although the normal architecture of the tonsil is difficult to see, intact crypts are present. There is some superficial necrosis. **B,** The very polymorphic proliferation would be consistent with infectious mononucleosis in a normal host. Molecular clonality studies did not demonstrate evidence of B-cell clonality.

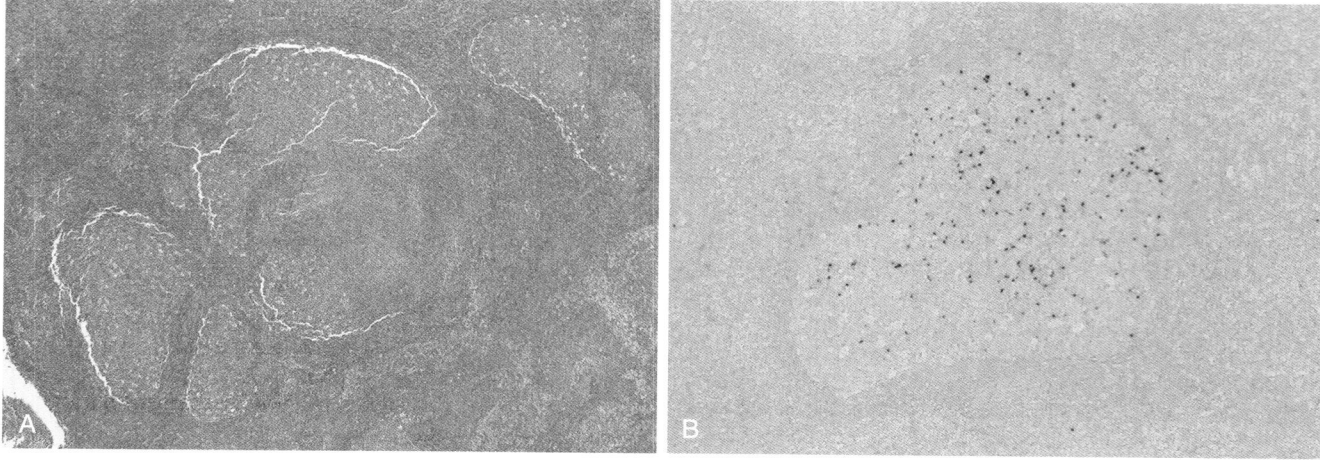

Figure 54-4. Florid follicular hyperplasia posttransplant lymphoproliferative disorder. Enlarged cervical lymph node from an adult man who was 8 years status post–renal transplantation. **A,** The lymph node architecture is preserved, with prominent follicular hyperplasia. **B,** An Epstein-Barr virus–encoded RNA (EBER) in situ hybridization stain shows scattered positive cells, which are particularly prominent in some germinal centers.

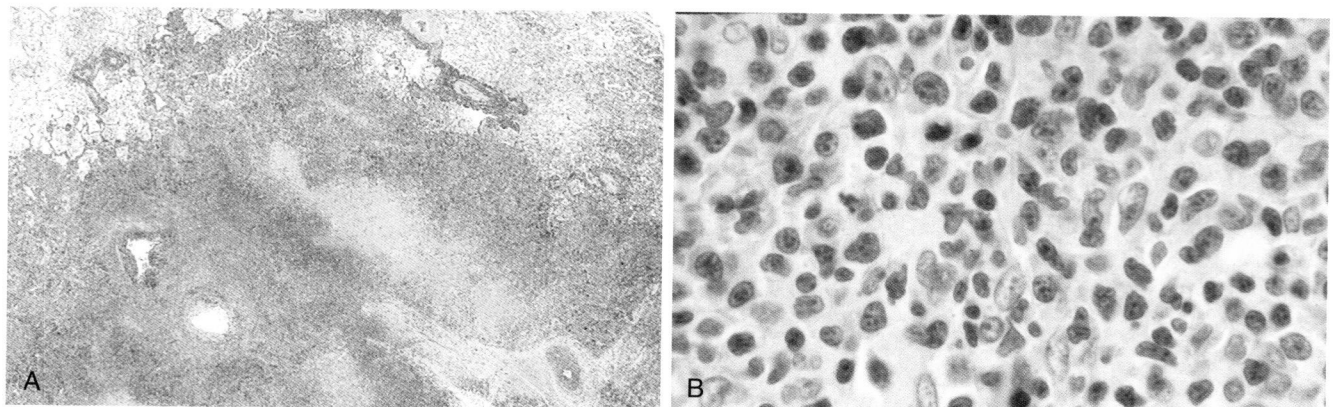

Figure 54-5. Polymorphic posttransplant lymphoproliferative disorder with numerous transformed cells focally. Lung from an adult man who presented with multiple pulmonary nodules 6 months after liver transplantation. **A,** Note the mass lesion, with infiltration of vascular and bronchial structures, as well as a large area of geographic necrosis. **B,** Most areas demonstrate a very polymorphic infiltrate composed of transformed cells and smaller lymphoid cells, including some with angulated nuclear contours.

should only be rendered with extreme caution. One study of gastrointestinal biopsies in children with small bowel transplants required more than 15 EBV-encoded small RNA (EBER)-positive cells per 0.065 mm² "field" before a diagnosis of PTLD was rendered.[148] Also remember that infiltrates in the allograft may have a differential diagnosis of rejection, which may be present in addition to a PTLD.

Polymorphic Posttransplant Lymphoproliferative Disorder

Polymorphic PTLD, the most morphologically characteristic type of PTLD, is a diffuse and destructive proliferation of variably sized and variably shaped lymphocytes, plasma cells, transformed cells, and immunoblasts (Fig. 54-5).[7] Many of the small lymphocytes may have angulated or clefted-appearing nuclei and were originally thought to resemble germinal center cells. The proportion of transformed cells/

immunoblasts varies, with some willing to make this diagnosis when they are very prominent (creating a "monomorphic appearance") and others describing them as "few."[32,149] The immunoblasts may be multinucleated, with very prominent nucleoli resembling Reed-Sternberg cells. Many cases previously diagnosed as Hodgkin-like PTLD (a category that is no longer recognized) probably represent polymorphic PTLD and require immunohistologic studies to distinguish from CHL PTLD. Some cases demonstrate large geographic areas of necrosis that are often associated with neutrophils and histiocytes and are surrounded by increased numbers of transformed cells or immunoblasts. Apoptosis may also be present. Pulmonary cases with prominent angioinvasion and geographic necrosis resemble lymphomatoid granulomatosis. Cases that would fulfill the criteria for a lymphoma in an immunocompetent host should be categorized as one of the lymphoma-like/monomorphic PTLDs. The diagnosis of polymorphic PTLD should therefore not be used in cases that demonstrate a predominance of transformed cells or immunoblasts even if they are pleomorphic, in cases that might appear polymorphic because there are prominent transformed cells with differentiation to mature plasma cells, in cases that would fulfill the criteria for a T-cell/histiocyte-rich large B-cell lymphoma, or in polymorphic-appearing lesions that fulfill the criteria for a T-cell lymphoma.[5] The broader spectrum of what is recognized today as a lymphoma in patients without iatrogenic immunosuppression and improved immunophenotypic studies has, in essence, diminished the frequency of polymorphic PTLD, although many still use this category for polymorphic lymphoma–like PTLD. Furthermore, one gene-expression profiling study did not show segregation of polymorphic PTLD from the non–germinal center B-cell (GCB) type of monomorphic PTLD, highlighting why this might be a difficult and somewhat arbitrary distinction to make.[83,91] At the other end of the spectrum of polymorphic PTLD are cases that overlap with florid IM PTLD where there can be some obscuring of normal architectural features, especially in some tonsillar lesions in children.[1] Some of these cases will be diagnosed as IM PTLD and others as polymorphic PTLD, largely based on pathologist preference, again highlighting the utility of being able to use PTLD as a diagnostic term rather than as only a qualifier of a specific histopathologic entity.

Some PTLDs fulfill the criteria for EBV-positive mucocutaneous ulcer (MCU).[5,150] These are variably polymorphic, well-circumscribed solitary oral or gastrointestinal tract ulcerations with prominent CD30-positive, CD20-positive, EBV-positive large B cells, often including some that resemble Reed-Sternberg cells, and with admixed T cells that often form a band at the base (Fig. 54-6). B-cell clonality is demonstrable in some but not all cases. Monoclonal or restricted T-cell populations are also found in the majority of MCUs,[151] although not reported in the three cases tested in the largest series of MCU PTLD.[150] These lesions have an excellent prognosis and resolve with decreased or altered immunosuppression with or without rituximab.[150] It is of interest that in contrast to most other patients with PTLD, individuals with MCU PTLD are reported to have undetectable or only very low levels of EBV DNA in their blood.[150,152]

Monomorphic Posttransplant Lymphoproliferative Disorders

Monomorphic PTLDs are lymphoid or plasmacytic proliferations that fulfill the criteria for one of the non-Hodgkin lymphomas (not of small B-cell type with the exception of EBV-positive marginal zone lymphomas) or plasma cell neoplasms that arise in immunocompetent hosts.[5] They must be further categorized on the basis of the type of neoplasm they most closely resemble.

Monomorphic B-Cell Posttransplant Lymphoproliferative Disorders

Many monomorphic PTLDs are composed of numerous transformed B cells that most commonly resemble DLBCL, NOS (Fig. 54-7); less commonly, Burkitt lymphoma (approximately 0%–5% of PTLDs) (Fig. 54-8); or more rarely, one of the other large B-cell lymphoma subtypes, such as plasmablastic lymphoma, primary DLBCL of the CNS,

or primary effusion lymphoma.[9,104,107,117,118] As with other DLBCLs, the transformed B cells may be very pleomorphic, and plasmacytic differentiation may create a variable degree of pleomorphism. Some cases are T-cell rich and therefore demonstrate only a minority of large, transformed B cells. It has also been reported that large B-cell lymphoma with 11q aberrations (formerly Burkitt-like lymphoma with 11q aberrations) makes up a higher proportion of "Burkitt lymphoma" in the posttransplant setting than in immunocompetent patients.[153] This diagnosis should be suspected in MYC rearrangement–negative lymphomas that resemble Burkitt lymphoma, although some are less Burkitt-like and more closely resemble a DLBCL.[8]

Distinguishing polymorphic PTLD from DLBCL-type monomorphic PTLD can be extremely difficult and, to some extent, arbitrary; there are no absolute guidelines for dealing with borderline lesions, and the clinical importance of this distinction may be limited. Some cases exhibit a definite polymorphic background but have either focal or extensive areas of numerous transformed B cells or immunoblasts. These cases are considered at least focally monomorphic in the WHO Revised 4th ed. and 2022 ICC classifications, but others have considered them polymorphic PTLD or polymorphic PTLD with numerous transformed cells.[4,5,8,149] Cases with admixed monotypic plasma cells and transformed cells or immunoblasts can also be problematic when the latter are not the dominant population; like polymorphic PTLD, such cases show a complete spectrum of B-cell maturation, but like monomorphic PTLD, these cases fulfill the criteria for a malignant lymphoma in a nonimmunocompromised host.[5]

The other major (but much less common) types of B-lineage monomorphic PTLDs include multiple myeloma and plasmacytoma-like lesions (Fig. 54-9). Multiple myeloma is a rare form of PTLD and should fulfill all the same criteria as in a normal host.[122-128] While most cases show a spectrum of cytologically mature to immature plasma cells, a subset may demonstrate a predominant plasmablastic cytology.[126,128] Such plasmablastic cases may have an inferior outcome.[126] Occasional cases may also have associated amyloid deposition.[126] Plasmacytoma-like lesions, which make up about 3% to 6% of PTLDs, occur most commonly in the gastrointestinal tract and skin or subcutaneous tissues, but also at nodal and other extranodal sites; they contain sheets of plasma cells that in most reports are usually "well differentiated" or mature, sometimes with occasional foci of lymphoid cells.[9,93,119,120,154,155] Some include cases with prominent nucleoli that have not been aggressive; however, these cases will have a differential diagnosis of a plasmablastic lymphoma-type monomorphic PTLD. The cutaneous and subcutaneous cases, which are reported to account for 38% of cutaneous B-cell PTLDs, may be similar to the EBV-positive extranodal marginal zone lymphomas of mucosa-associated lymphoid tissue (MALT lymphomas) with plasmacytic differentiation that have a predilection for the skin and subcutaneous tissues, occur late after transplantation, and usually follow an indolent clinical course.[156-158] These are currently considered a type of monomorphic PTLD.[5,8]

Among organ transplant recipients, whereas the standardized incidence ratio (SIR) for Burkitt lymphoma is 24.5 and for DLBCL is 13.5, it is not significantly increased for chronic lymphocytic leukemia/small lymphocytic lymphoma, follicular lymphoma, mantle cell lymphoma, or splenic/nodal

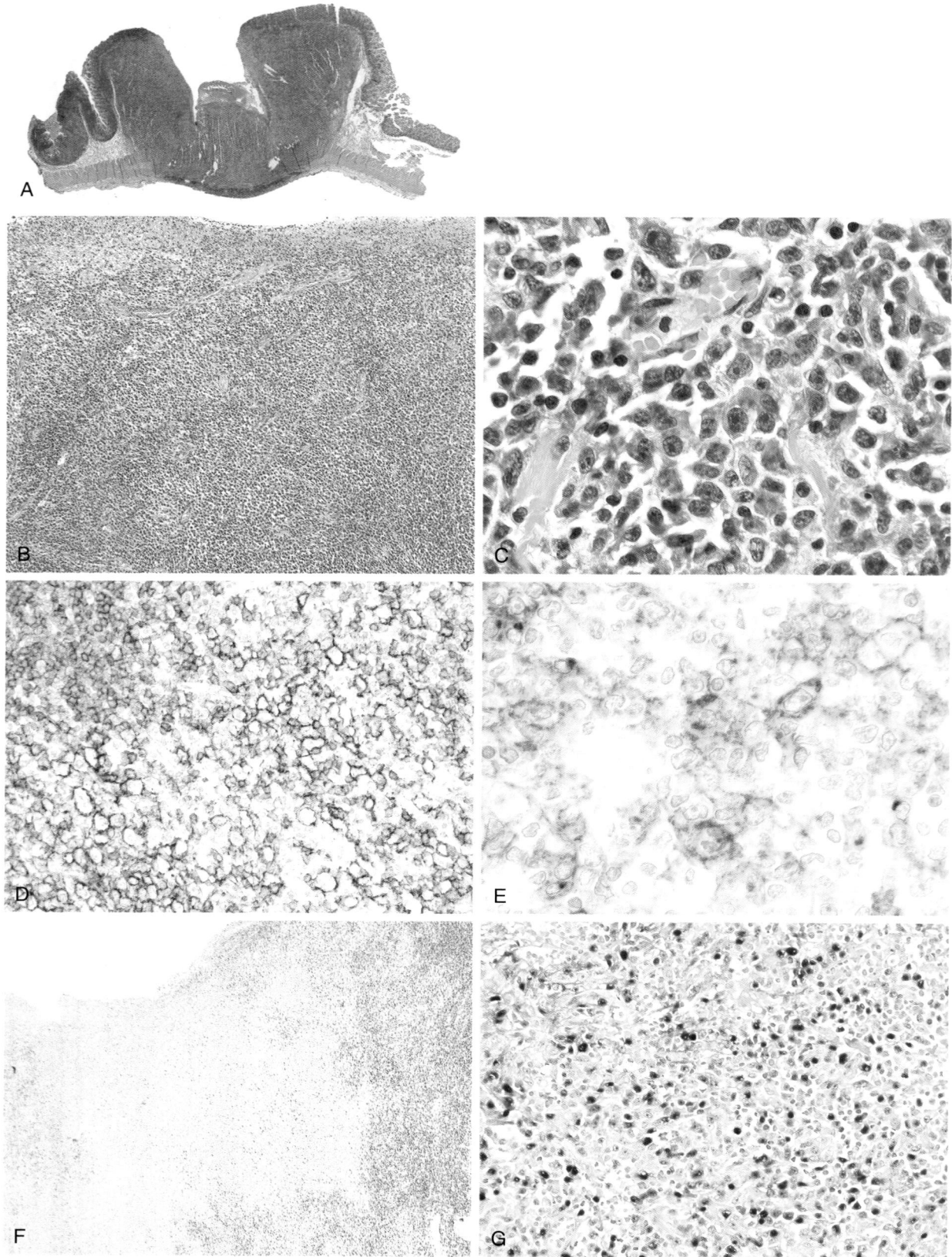

Figure 54-6. Posttransplant Epstein-Barr virus–positive mucocutaneous ulcer. Adult man 8 months after bilateral lung transplantation who presented with intussusception and was found to have a single 2.0 × 1.0 × 0.5 cm ileal ulcer with no disease at any other sites. Whole-blood Epstein-Barr virus (EBV) DNA quantification by polymerase chain reaction (PCR) was negative. The patient was treated with reduction of immunosuppression and four doses of weekly rituximab, followed by four courses of maintenance rituximab, with no recurrence of disease at 60 months of follow-up. **A,** Note the dense infiltrate in the ulcerated bowel. **B,** There is a polymorphic infiltrate beneath the ulcer base that particularly, in some areas, includes **(C)** many transformed/immunoblastic cells. The infiltrate includes **(D)** many CD20-positive cells including the large cells, **(E)** a moderate number of CD30-positive cells, and **(F)** many CD3-positive T cells concentrated at the periphery of the lesion. **G,** EBV-encoded RNA (EBER) in situ hybridization stain demonstrates many EBV-positive cells. *(Case and images A, D, E, and G courtesy Drs. R. McKenna and L. Moench; from Hart M, Thakral B, Yohe S, et al. EBV-positive mucocutaneous ulcer in organ transplant recipients: a localized indolent posttransplant lymphoproliferative disorder. Am J Surg Pathol. 2014;38(11):1522-1529.)*

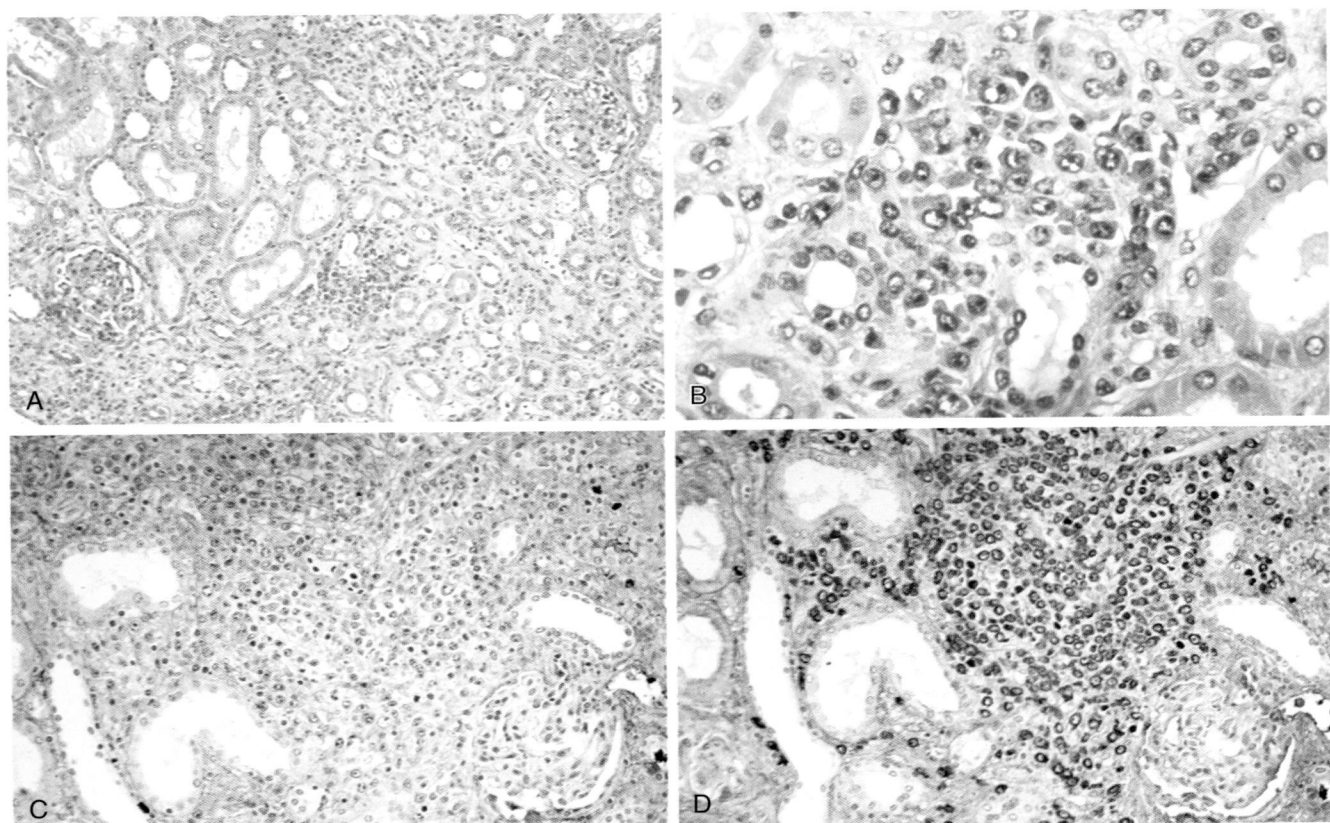

Figure 54-7. Diffuse large B-cell lymphoma-type monomorphic posttransplant lymphoproliferative disorder. A, Note the patchy infiltrate in the renal parenchyma of an adult man 4 months after renal transplantation. **B,** The infiltrate is composed predominantly of transformed and plasmacytoid-appearing large cells. In other areas, there was a prominent intravascular component. **C,** Kappa immunostain is essentially negative. **D,** Lambda immunostain is positive, supporting the monoclonality of this lesion.

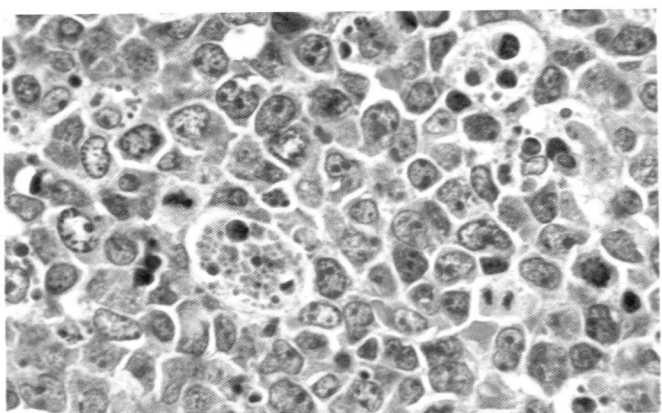

Figure 54-8. Monomorphic B-cell posttransplant lymphoproliferative disorder with *MYC* rearrangement. This example of posttransplant lymphoproliferative disorder (PTLD) in an adult woman after kidney transplantation is composed of intermediate-to-large-sized transformed cells. It has some Burkitt lymphoma features, with a high mitotic rate and tingible body macrophages, creating a starry-sky appearance.

marginal zone lymphoma.[159] The SIR is mildly increased for lymphoplasmacytic lymphoma and MALT lymphoma (both 2.8).[159] It has been specifically proposed that EBV-negative marginal zone lymphomas arising in the posttransplant setting should also be considered a form of monomorphic PTLD.[160] In one series of nine such cases, seven were of MALT lymphoma type and arose in the gastrointestinal tract.[160]

Monomorphic T-Cell or NK-Cell Posttransplant Lymphoproliferative Disorders

T-cell or the rare NK-cell PTLDs account for less than 15% of PTLDs and, by definition, are monomorphic.[5,9,33,107,109,113,161,162] In contrast to most monomorphic B-cell PTLDs, the T-cell cases are not necessarily composed of predominantly large transformed cells, but are morphologically similar to the spectrum of T-cell and NK-cell neoplasms seen in immunocompetent patients.[5,113,163] Particularly because some of these cases appear morphologically indistinguishable from polymorphic PTLDs, immunophenotypic and molecular studies are critical whenever the possibility of a T-cell PTLD is raised.[113] Most fulfill the criteria for a peripheral T-cell lymphoma (PTCL), NOS; others represent a variety of specific types of mature T-cell lymphomas (Fig. 54-10).[113,161-163] Approximately 15% of all hepatosplenic T-cell lymphomas occur in the posttransplant setting and make up slightly more than 10% of reported T-cell PTLDs (Fig. 54-11).[161,162,164] Very rare, aggressive true–NK-cell neoplasms also occur in this setting[163,165,166] and must be distinguished from indolent posttransplant T-cell large granular lymphocytic leukemia.[167,168] Posttransplant T-cell large granular lymphocytic leukemia is reported to have some clinical and laboratory features that differ from de novo cases, although

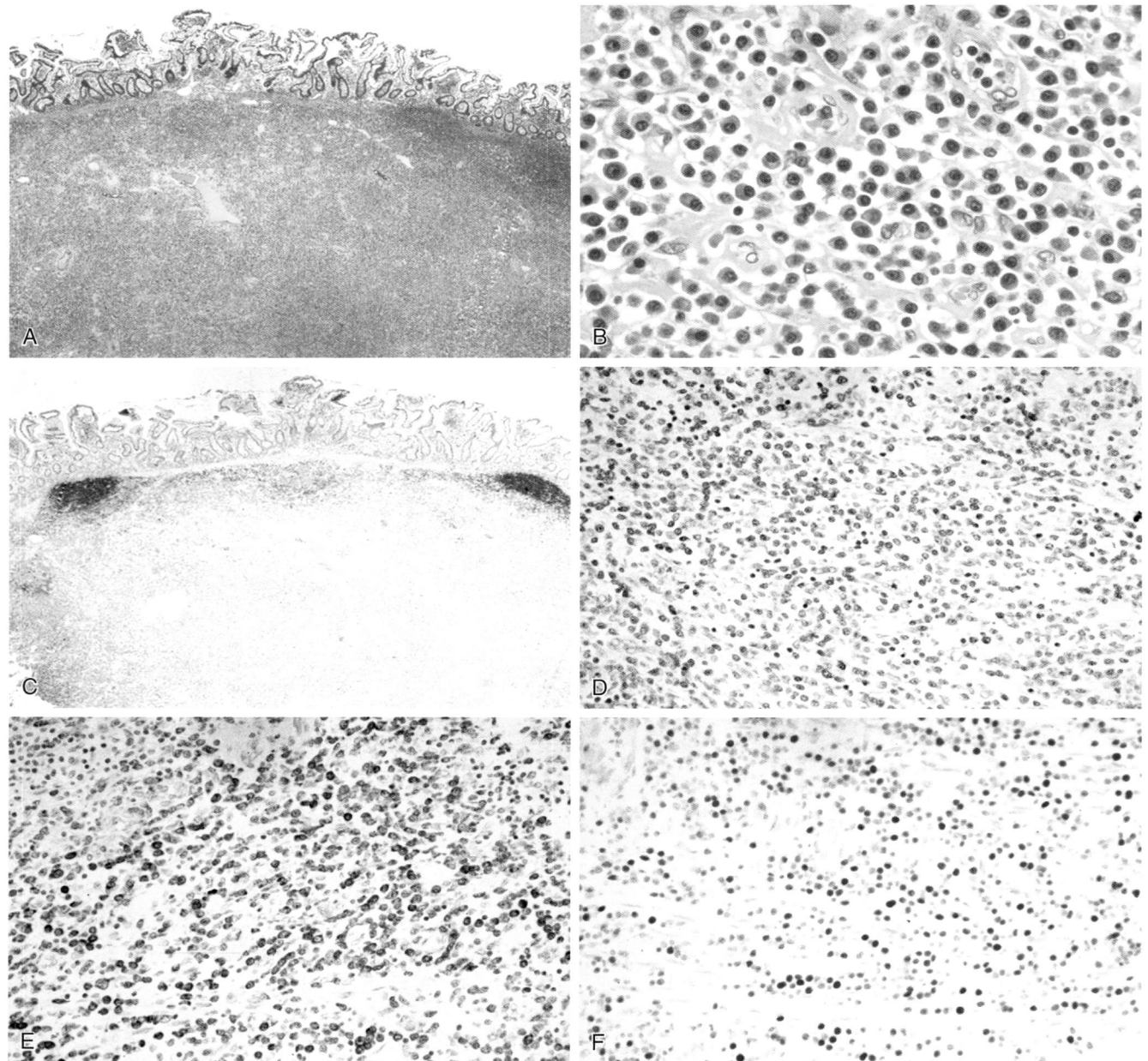

Figure 54-9. Plasmacytoma-type monomorphic posttransplant lymphoproliferative disorder in the small intestine. A, The mass lesion includes occasional lymphoid aggregates but otherwise demonstrates numerous plasma cells. **B,** There is a relatively homogeneous population of plasma cells. **C,** CD20 immunostain highlights the occasional lymphoid aggregates but is otherwise essentially negative. **D,** Kappa in situ hybridization stain is negative. **E,** Lambda in situ hybridization stain shows numerous positive cells, supporting the monoclonality of the plasma cells. **F,** Epstein-Barr virus–encoded RNA (EBER) in situ hybridization stain shows numerous positive nuclei.

there was not a significant difference in the frequency of *STAT3* mutations in one study.[169] Non-neoplastic oligoclonal increases in CD8-positive, CD57-positive T cells have been described after allogeneic hematopoietic stem cell transplantation,[170,171] and clonal CD8-positive T cells can also be seen in IM.[172] Rare cases of T-lymphoblastic leukemia/lymphoma have been reported, including some cases that could be clonally related to prior non–T-cell blastic neoplasms.[113,173] The concept that T-cell and NK-cell lymphoma-like proliferations are bona fide PTLD is supported by an overall SIR of 6.2, with a broad range depending on type, but with

most having a SIR significantly greater than 1.[159] Posttransplant hepatosplenic T-cell lymphoma has a reported SIR of 100.[159]

Classic Hodgkin Lymphoma Posttransplant Lymphoproliferative Disorder

CHL PTLD, the least common type, comprising 0% to 8% of PTLDs, often resembles mixed cellularity CHL.[2,9,66,107,109,174,175] These cases should fulfill both the

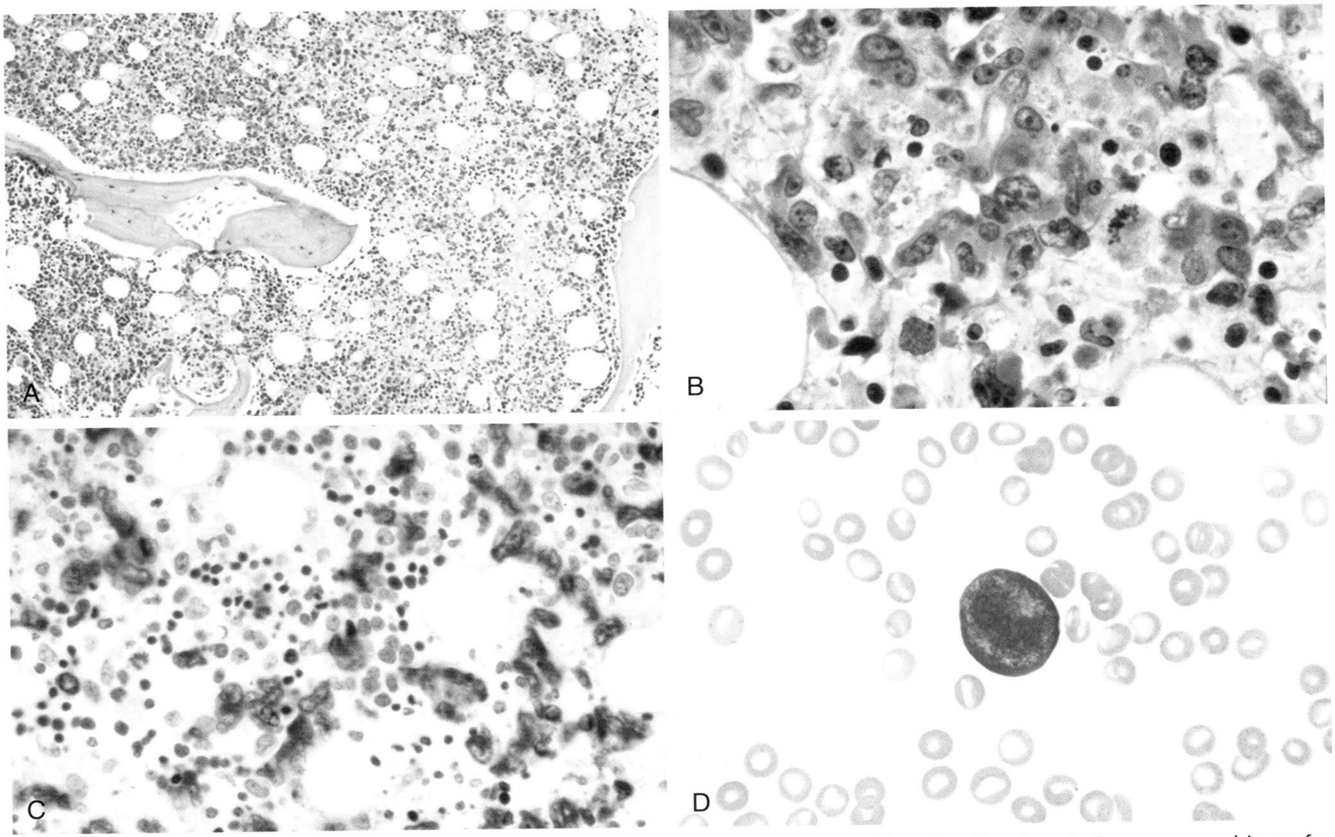

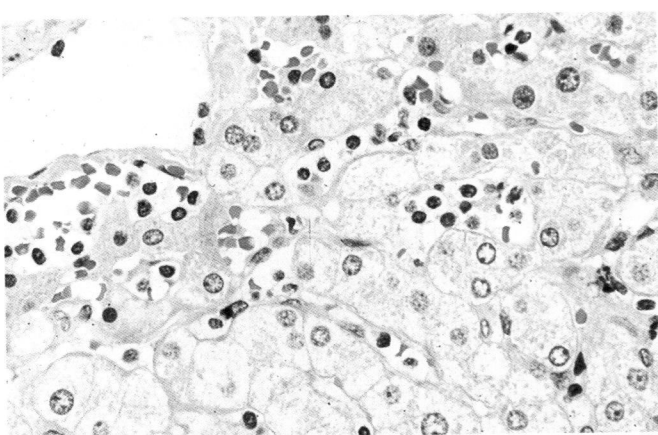

Figure 54-10. Peripheral T-cell lymphoma-type monomorphic posttransplant lymphoproliferative disorder. A, Bone marrow biopsy from a 39-year-old woman with pancytopenia, 4 years after kidney transplantation, shows a mostly interstitial large cell infiltrate admixed with hematopoietic elements, including an increased proportion of immature myeloid cells. There are also bone changes, consistent with hyperparathyroidism. **B,** The large abnormal cells have nucleoli and often irregular nuclear contours. Admixed hematopoietic elements are also seen. **C,** CD3 immunostain highlights the interstitial and scattered nature of the abnormal cells in many areas. The cells were also positive for TIA-1, indicating their cytotoxic nature, although CD4 and CD8 immunostains were both negative. The cells were negative for CD30 but positive for epithelial membrane antigen. Molecular studies demonstrated a clonal T-cell population. **D,** Peripheral blood demonstrates a small proportion of very large abnormal lymphoid cells, some of which have cytoplasmic granules.

Figure 54-11. Hepatosplenic T-cell lymphoma-type monomorphic posttransplant lymphoproliferative disorder (PTLD). Note the lymphoid cells infiltrating the hepatic sinuses. *(Courtesy Dr. Nancy Lee Harris.)*

morphologic and immunophenotypic criteria for CHL because atypical immunoblasts or Reed-Sternberg–like cells are commonly found in many PTLDs, and Hodgkin-like cases are not included in this category (Figs. 54-12 and 54-13).[5] The CHL PTLDs are more likely to express B-cell–associated

antigens (particularly OCT2, BOB1, and CD79a).[176] Some cases have occurred after non-Hodgkin lymphoma-type PTLDs.[82] They have a reported SIR of 3.6, again justifying their inclusion as a type of PTLD.[1]

Immunophenotype

The immunophenotype of PTLDs is variable, as would be expected for a spectrum of disorders that can resemble hyperplastic proliferations, B-cell or T-cell neoplasms, NK-cell neoplasms, CHL, or plasma cell neoplasms. In PH or IM PTLD, immunophenotypic studies do not demonstrate B-cell clonality, plasma cell clonality, or aberrant B-cell or T-cell phenotypes.[5] All types of PTLDs demonstrate variable numbers of admixed T cells, with the most numerous T cells described in IM, polymorphic, and CHL types.[177] Some cases not of clonal T-cell origin have more than 80% T cells.[178]

Polymorphic PTLDs demonstrate admixtures of B cells with variable pan–B-cell marker expression and heterogeneous T cells. Greater than 20% CD30-positive lesional cells are present in 94% of nondestructive/polymorphic PTLDs.[65] Paraffin section immunostains may demonstrate polytypic or monotypic light chain expression, and intralesional or interlesional heterogeneity with polytypic and monotypic areas or both kappa monotypic and lambda monotypic regions may be present.[7] Flow cytometric studies also show variable results.[179]

Monomorphic PTLDs have an immunophenotype consistent with that of the lymphomas in immunocompetent individuals which they resemble. Most DLBCL type monomorphic PTLDs have a non–GCB phenotype; a minority, especially EBV-negative cases, have a GCB phenotype.[83,110,180-182] CD30 positivity by more than 20% of cells is reported in 81% of DLBCL PTLDs.[65] A moderate number of T-cell PTLDs are composed of CD8-positive cytotoxic T cells that express TIA-1 and sometimes other cytotoxic granule proteins, although one meta-analysis found CD4-positive T-cell PTLDs to be slightly more common than CD8-positive cases.[113,161,183] Some PTLDs include both B-cell and T-cell components.[184]

CHL PTLD can be diagnosed with the greatest degree of confidence when CD15-positive, CD30-positive, CD45-negative Reed-Sternberg cells are present in an appropriate T-cell–rich background; however, as in an immunocompetent host, some CD15-negative cases can be expected. The Reed-Sternberg–like cells in other types of PTLDs are expected to be CD20-positive, CD45-positive, and CD15-negative. A CD30-negative immunophenotype makes CHL PTLD extremely

unlikely, but CD30 positivity cannot help in the distinction between CHL PTLD and other types of PTLD.[5]

About 60% to 80% of PTLDs are associated with EBV, as best demonstrated by EBER in situ hybridization, although some find a much higher proportion of EBV-negative cases.[9,32,81,88-90,92,93,107,185] EBER in situ hybridization is more sensitive than the immunohistochemical stain for EBV LMP1, but it is also somewhat more likely to be positive in the absence of a diagnosable PTLD and is dependent on preservation of RNA.[5,186] Most PTLDs have a latency type III EBV pattern and thus are positive for both LMP1 and EBNA2, a combination that suggests immunodeficiency. EBV-negative PTLDs are more often monomorphic compared with EBV-positive cases.[88,89] EBV is described in all other types of PTLDs, although multiple myeloma cases are often negative and CHL cases are almost always positive. Some also find nondestructive PTLD to be uniformly EBV positive.[114] Cases of EBV-negative PH or florid follicular hyperplasia are completely indistinguishable from a non-specific hyperplasia. About one-third of T-cell PTLDs are EBV positive, as are at least some of the rare NK-cell neoplasms.[113,161,162,166]

Genetics

Clonality Studies

Almost all polymorphic PTLDs and monomorphic B-cell PTLDs are monoclonal on the basis of immunoglobulin gene-rearrangement studies or EBV terminal repeat analysis.[6,102,187] With the very sensitive latter technique, even many IM PTLDs are demonstrably clonal, as are some cases of PH and even occasional hyperplastic lymph nodes in a nontransplantation setting.[188] Genotypic studies demonstrate occasional cases with more than one clone or with an oligoclonal B-cell proliferation. Monomorphic PTLDs usually have more dominant clones than polymorphic PTLDs.[189-191]

Distinct simultaneous or subsequent lesions in the same patient may show different B-cell clones or a monoclonal population at one site and a polyclonal population elsewhere.[6,7,189] The presence of numerous clonally distinct PTLDs is particularly well recognized in the gastrointestinal tract.[192] A recent study suggested that when multiple synchronous or metachronous PTLD are EBV positive, they

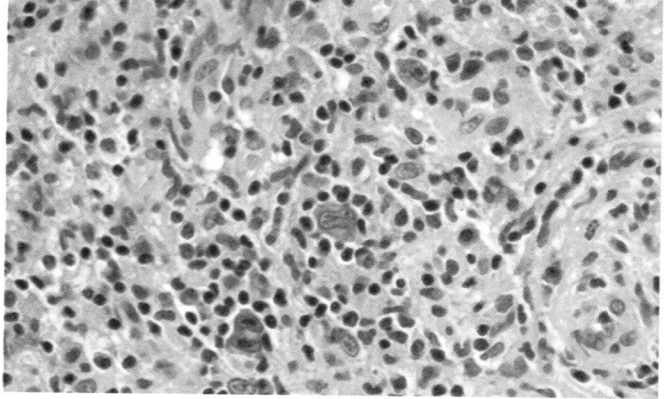

Figure 54-12. Mixed cellularity classic Hodgkin lymphoma post-transplant lymphoproliferative disorder (PTLD) in an adult man after kidney transplantation. Note the Reed-Sternberg and Reed-Sternberg variant cells admixed with numerous small lymphocytes, plasma cells, and histiocytes.

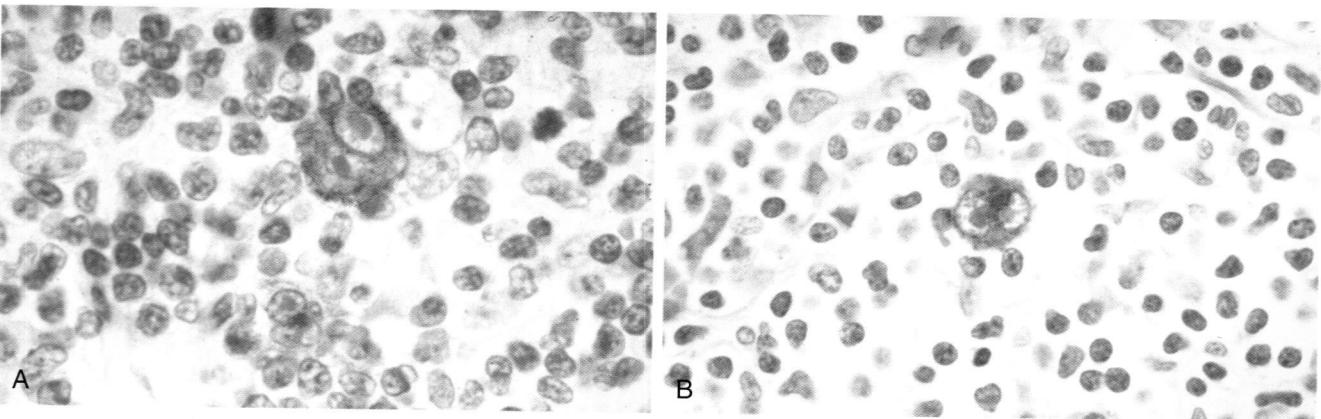

Figure 54-13. Classic Hodgkin lymphoma posttransplant lymphoproliferative disorder. A, CD30 stain highlights a Reed-Sternberg cell. **B,** Reed-Sternberg cells are also highlighted by an Epstein-Barr virus (EBV) latent membrane protein 1 immunostain.

are often clonally unrelated, but recurrent or multiple EBV-negative lesions appear to more often represent clonally related lesions.[193] Studies of IGHV gene usage and mutational patterns suggest that antigen selection may be important in the development or progression of PTLDs.[82,83,194] A minority of cases show crippling IGH mutations.[83] T-cell clonality is documented in the majority of monomorphic T-cell PTLDs. Occasional cases can be shown to have both clonal B cells and T cells either simultaneously or in different lesions.[184] Caution is advised, as one study reported half of B-cell PTLDs have monoclonal T-cell populations, usually in the absence of a recognizable T-cell PTLD, and especially in the presence of a predominance of CD8-positive T cells.[195]

Genetic and Epigenetic Studies

Classical cytogenetic studies document clonal abnormalities in a variable proportion of PTLDs; however, the limited published studies have not shown consistent recurrent abnormalities.[2,76,144,146,196] Abnormalities are most commonly found in monomorphic PTLDs, but are also reported in some polymorphic PTLDs and even occasional nondestructive PTLDs.[87,97,146,196] Some of the more commonly reported abnormalities in B-cell PTLDs include trisomy 9, trisomy 11, 8q24/MYC rearrangements (enriched in Burkitt lymphoma and plasmablastic lymphoma-type monomorphic PTLDs), 14q32 rearrangements, and breaks at 1q11-21.[146,153,197-199] Monomorphic PTLDs that often resemble Burkitt lymphoma but lack MYC rearrangements and demonstrate a chromosome 11q23 gain/11q24 loss pattern similar to that seen in immunocompetent patients have been reported.[153] BCL2 and BCL6, but not CCND1, gene rearrangements are described in rare PTLDs, as well as a small number of cases with MYC, BCL2, or BCL6 gains.[6,64,184,200,201] Comparative genomic hybridization/single nucleotide polymorphism analyses have demonstrated a variety of recurrent chromosomal gains and losses, as well as some high-level amplifications, with some similarities and differences from DLBCL in immunocompetent hosts; however, the precise findings are inconsistent.[20,21,97,98] A subset of DLBCL-type monomorphic PTLD and CHL PTLD have gains/amplification of chromosome 9p24.1, the JAK2/PDL1/PDL2 locus, which may have implications for potential checkpoint inhibitor therapy.[76,176] Karyotypic and fluorescence in situ hybridization analyses of multiple myeloma-type PTLDs demonstrate a spectrum of cytogenetic abnormalities typical for myelomas in immunocompetent individuals.[126-128]

BCL6 mutations are reported to be absent in PH and to be present in 43% of polymorphic PTLDs and 90% of monomorphic B-cell PTLDs.[84] Others, however, have found similar proportions of BCL6 mutations in polymorphic and monomorphic PTLDs.[83] Aberrant somatic hypermutation involving genes other than BCL6 is also reported to be more common in monomorphic than in polymorphic PTLDs, but is reported to be less frequent than in DLBCL arising in immunocompetent hosts.[83,96] A more recent high-throughput sequencing study showed fewer mutations in polymorphic and EBV-positive DLBCL-type monomorphic PTLD compared with both EBV-negative DLBCL PTLD and DLBCL occurring in normal hosts.[99] A low number of mutations and copy number alterations were also reported in a small series of EBV-positive MALT-type monomorphic PTLDs.[158] Mutations of TP53 and KMT2D were reported in 36% of DLBCL-type

monomorphic PTLDs in one study, as well as recurrent mutations of BTG1, MYC, MYD88, PIM1, and TET2 in more than 10% of cases.[99] Although a second study confirmed the relatively high prevalence of TP53 mutations in DLBCL-type PTLD, a more recent study did not and instead noted recurrent JAK3 mutations in both monomorphic and CHL PTLDs.[87,198] Alterations of TP53 and KMT2 family genes are also frequent in plasmablastic lymphoma-type monomorphic PTLDs.[199] Mutations of MAP kinase pathway genes, including NRAS, have been described in monomorphic B-cell PTLDs, including multiple myeloma and plasmablastic lymphoma types.[6,199] IFNA gene deletion has been reported in 44% of monomorphic PTLDs, but in 1.7% of other intermediate-to high-grade non-Hodgkin lymphomas.[202] Acquisition of mutations has also been associated with disease recurrence and progression in a limited number of patients with B-cell PTLD studied.[83]

Monomorphic T-cell and NK-cell PTLDs show similar genetic alterations as T-cell and NK-cell lymphomas arising in immunocompetent individuals.[163] TP53 and other oncogene mutations or deletions are reported in a high proportion of T-cell and NK-cell PTLDs, and JAK/STAT pathway genes are also commonly mutated.[163,203] Monomorphic T-cell and NK-cell PTLDs frequently exhibit complex copy number alterations.[163] Characteristic isochromosome 7q and trisomy 8 are found in hepatosplenic T-cell lymphoma-type monomorphic PTLD.[164]

In addition to genetic alterations, aberrant methylation as an epigenetic mechanism to silence tumor suppressor genes and initiate B-cell activation is implicated in the development of PTLDs.[32,75,204] Hypermethylation of genes involved in apoptosis, cell cycle regulation, and DNA damage repair is common in polymorphic and monomorphic PTLDs.[75] DAPK, which encodes a serine-threonine kinase that plays a role in apoptosis initiated by TNF-α, IFN-γ, and FAS, is hypermethylated in 76% of monomorphic PTLD.[75,205] Similarly, both polymorphic and monomorphic PTLD frequently show increased methylation of the DNA repair gene MGMT.[75,205] Approximately three-quarters of polymorphic and DLBCL-type PTLDs exhibit hypermethylation of PTPN6, which, under normal circumstances, functions as an inhibitor of the JAK/STAT pathway.[75] EBV modulates DNA methylation via LMP1 and EBNA proteins, and very likely contributes to the altered methylation pattern in at least a subset of PTLDs.[32,204]

Postulated Normal Counterparts

The postulated normal counterparts are mature follicular or postfollicular B cells, plasma cells, and postthymic T cells.

Clinical Course

PTLD is a serious complication of transplantation and can be associated with significant morbidity and mortality. Reported mortality rates vary widely, with many reports published before the current era of widespread rituximab use.[32] Recent cohorts report 3-year overall survivals ranging from 49% to 73%, with multiple factors influencing outcomes, including patient age, type of transplant, distribution of PTLD subtypes, and proportion of patients receiving rituximab.[9,13,33,107] With appropriate therapy, patients with lymphoma-type PTLD are reported to have survivals like those of patients in the general population with similar lymphomas.[11] However, a uniform PTLD treatment strategy does not exist, and it is an area with many controversies, in part because of the protean nature of these LPDs.[9,16,17,116,206-209] On one end of the spectrum, patients with nondestructive PTLDs often do very well with only surgery or with the addition of decreased immunosuppression; on the other end of the spectrum, monomorphic PTLDs, especially some types, often require some component of chemotherapy.[16,23,114,210] Most patients are treated, at least in part, with a decrease in their immunosuppressive regimens whenever possible, keeping in mind that the patient's well-being is dependent on the status of the allograft.[16]

Although decreased immunosuppressive therapy often remains the first line of treatment for PTLD, addition of other therapeutic modalities is a frequent practice either up-front or sequentially.[16,17,210] Surgical excision and sometimes radiation therapy for localized lesions are other important and frequently successful therapeutic strategies in appropriate cases.[18,210] Rituximab, used as monotherapy or in combination with chemotherapy, is an important component of treatment for polymorphic and monomorphic B-cell PTLDs. A commonly accepted treatment strategy for polymorphic and DLBCL-type monomorphic PTLDs arising in adults after solid organ transplantation is a sequential approach beginning with reduction of immunosuppression, if possible, with or without treatment with rituximab and followed by R-CHOP (rituximab, cyclophosphamide, doxorubicin hydrochloride, vincristine sulfate, and prednisone), if necessary.[10,210-212] The success of rituximab monotherapy in a significant number of patients with monomorphic B-cell PTLD highlights an important clinical difference from DLBCL, NOS in immunocompetent hosts, where rituximab alone would not be considered acceptable therapy. Although a sequential approach may be appropriate for many monomorphic B-cell PTLDs, upfront R-CHOP can be beneficial in selected high-risk patients in whom rapid attainment of response is desirable.[212] In the pediatric solid organ transplant setting, treatment of polymorphic and monomorphic B-cell PTLDs relies on low-dose chemotherapy (cyclophosphamide and either prednisone or methylprednisolone) combined with rituximab.[16,191,213] Preemptive rituximab therapy, based on EBV viremia and lack of T-cell reconstitution, may prevent the development of PTLD in the setting of allogeneic hematopoietic stem cell transplantation.[214] Less common subtypes of monomorphic PTLD, such as Burkitt lymphoma, primary CNS lymphoma, T-cell and NK-cell lymphomas, multiple myeloma, and CHL PTLD, are usually treated in a similar manner to these neoplasms arising in immunocompetent patients.[16,17,134,138,210,215,216] A trial of reduced immunosuppression is often omitted in the treatment of these rare PTLD subtypes.

Aside from reduced immunosuppression, rituximab, and chemotherapy, a variety of novel treatment strategies for PTLD, including other monoclonal antibodies and small molecule or checkpoint inhibitors, are under investigation.[16,18,213,217] Antiviral agents have been widely used, but with the possible exception of some newer strategies, they have not been very effective in PTLD.[206] Another strategy is the use of adoptive T-cell therapy with donor-derived unfractionated or EBV-specific cytotoxic T cells.[16,18,213,218-225] A variety of active

clinical trials are also underway evaluating chimeric antigen receptor T-cell therapy.[16,18,213]

Prognostic factors are another problematic area; the literature is inconsistent, and one must consider the specific type of PTLD and the clinical setting. The protean nature of PTLD and data primarily from single center analyses makes validation of prognostic factors challenging.[210] Nevertheless, several prognostic factors that are probably applicable in many PTLDs have been reported, although rigorous proof does not exist for many, and it is not always known which are independent prognostic indicators. One important predictor of outcome is response to a trial of decreased immunosuppression; however, the proportion of responding patients is variable, and those who fail to respond may still be cured of their disease.[116,206,208] Response to therapy in general is associated with a superior prognosis.[9] PTLD after allogeneic hematopoietic stem cell transplantation has a very poor prognosis, with reported survival rates of 8% to 20% and with long-term survival described as suboptimal.[57,226-228] Many solid organ transplant patients fare better, and those with PTLD of donor origin reportedly have better outcomes than those with the much more common PTLD of recipient origin.[58,59] PTLD localized to the allograft is usually associated with a good prognosis, with about three-quarters of patients surviving.[59,116,229] Although many patients who present with an IM syndrome have a good outcome, some go on to develop rapidly progressive PTLD that may be fatal.[230-232] CNS, bone marrow, and serous effusion involvement are all adverse prognostic indicators, as is hypoalbuminemia.[9,27,233-235] PTLD presenting as disseminated disease has been associated with a survival rate of less than 10%.[229] Elevated lactate dehydrogenase, organ dysfunction, CNS involvement, and multiorgan involvement adversely affect the likelihood of responding to decreased immunosuppression.[206,233] There is conflicting data regarding the value of the International Prognostic Index (IPI) in the setting of PTLD.[9,11,27,65,211,212,236-243] In pediatric patients, CD20 expression, age ≤16 years, and good performance status are associated with better survival, while a poor response to initial treatment and allograft rejection are associated with inferior survival.[243-245] The latter highlights how treatment of patients with PTLD must also take into consideration the implications for the transplanted organs, with loss of the allograft another cause of morbidity and, depending on the type of transplant, mortality.

Data concerning the prognostic implications of pathologic subtype are limited; however, some generalizations can be made. Patients with one of the nondestructive PTLD generally do well, whereas those with monomorphic PTLD appear to be less likely to respond to decreased immunosuppression and have a worse prognosis.[114,231,246,247] The degree to which patients with polymorphic PTLD do better than those with monomorphic PTLD, if at all, is controversial; some investigators report major differences, and others report no differences, sometimes with excellent survival even among those with monomorphic disease.[9,27,41,65,142,191,246,248-252] With modern therapies, the overall survival of post–solid organ transplant multiple myeloma is comparable to that in immunocompetent individuals.[6,122,126] Plasmacytoma PTLD appears to have a more variable outcome, but more recent publications emphasize how many of them do well, even oftentimes with limited treatment and sometimes with just a reduction in immunosuppression.[9,93,119,154,253] Nonetheless, some cases require more aggressive, often myeloma-type therapy.[120,154,254] Except for cases of indolent T-cell large granular lymphocytic leukemia, PTLDs of T-cell or NK-cell phenotype are often, but not invariably, associated with a poor prognosis, with the hepatosplenic T-cell lymphoma type doing extremely poorly.[113,161] Although data is limited, pediatric solid organ transplant recipients with CHL PTLD are reported to have good outcomes when treated with standard CHL regimens, with an overall survival ranging from 86% to 100% at 5 years.[255,256] A recent meta-analysis of adult solid organ transplant recipients with CHL PTLD suggested improved outcomes in this group since 2000, and a single institution study of patients with PTLD diagnosed between 1987 and 2017 reported CHL PTLD to have the best prognosis of all the PTLD, with a reported median survival of 197.1 months and a 100% 2-year overall survival.[107,257]

Although PTLDs with B-cell "clonality" demonstrated principally by immunophenotyping are more frequently resistant to decreased immunosuppression than are polyclonal-appearing PTLDs, a significant number of the former patients respond to this therapeutic strategy.[7,142] Secondary *NRAS* and *TP53* mutations and *MYC* translocations have also been associated with a poor prognosis.[6,189,196,197] Absence of detectable EBV is associated with a worse prognosis in some studies but not in others.[27,88,91,107,211,212]

Differential Diagnosis

The possibility of specific infectious or other inflammatory processes must always be ruled out when lymphoplasmacytic infiltrates are seen in posttransplant patients. These diagnoses may be based on the presence of viral inclusions or other organisms, the assessment of pathologic findings that suggest another specific diagnosis, and even the clinical situation, to some extent. Extensive EBV positivity or findings associated with any of the B-cell or T-cell lymphomas support the diagnosis of PTLD. Transplant patients may also have lymph node biopsies that show a completely non-specific hyperplasia, with architectural preservation and an absence of EBV. It is important to question whether such lymph nodes are representative of whatever is causing the clinical concern. Lymphadenopathy may also occur as an apparent allergic reaction to the therapeutic use of OKT3 and ATG.[258]

When allograft biopsies are being evaluated, the distinction from florid rejection can be difficult. The presence of expansile nodules or a mass lesion, numerous transformed cells, lymphoid atypia, a very B-cell–rich infiltrate, extensive serpiginous necrosis within the infiltrate, a high proportion of frank plasma cells, and evidence of many EBV-positive cells are among the features that support the diagnosis of PTLD rather than rejection.[90,259-261] Necrosis by itself and venous wall infiltration are not helpful findings. Significant arterial infiltration and variable numbers of eosinophils are among the features favoring rejection. Caution is advised, however, because PTLD can infiltrate arterial walls, have numerous T cells, and lack atypia. Conversely, some inflammatory processes, including in transplant patients, may have scattered (≤10%) EBV-positive cells.[148,260,262] Lesions not diagnostic of PTLD but with scattered EBV-positive cells may be associated with PTLD at another site or with an increased risk for development of PTLD.[145,148] Some allografts demonstrate evidence of both PTLD and rejection.

IATROGENIC IMMUNODEFICIENCY-ASSOCIATED LYMPHOPROLIFERATIVE DISORDERS IN NONTRANSPLANT SETTINGS

Outside the transplantation setting, OIIA-LPDs have been described in patients receiving a number of immunosuppressive/immunomodulatory agents or cytotoxic therapies.[5,263-271] Some of the implicated agents are the same as or similar to those used after transplantation, such as antimetabolites (azathioprine, 6-mercaptopurine, mycophenolate mofetil), calcineurin inhibitors (cyclosporine, tacrolimus), and corticosteroids.[264,270,272,273] Others include immunosuppressive/immunomodulatory agents used in therapy for autoimmune disorders or lymphoid neoplasms, such as methotrexate, TNF-α inhibitors, integrin antagonists, and fludarabine.[263,267,268,274-276] Rare cases associated with JAK or tyrosine kinase inhibitors are also described.[277-280] Assessment of whether a specific agent is responsible for an LPD is complicated by the fact that the patient's underlying disorder may be associated with an increased incidence of lymphoma, or oftentimes the patient is receiving more than one immunosuppressive/immunomodulatory agent.[265]

The best recognized OIIA-LPDs are those associated with methotrexate in patients being treated for rheumatoid arthritis, dermatomyositis, and, rarely, psoriasis.[5,14,265,268,281,282] These patients usually have long-standing rheumatic disease (often as long as 15 years), are receiving methotrexate at the time of diagnosis, and have been taking methotrexate for a median of 3 years.[14,268,283,284] About half the cases involve one or more extranodal sites.[14,281,284] Methotrexate-associated LPDs form a morphologic spectrum similar to that of the PTLDs, but with a different distribution among the morphologic subtypes.[5,269,281,283-285] Most commonly, cases fulfill the criteria for DLBCL (Fig. 54-14). Only a relatively small proportion of cases resemble polymorphic PTLD or are described as a lymphoplasmacytic infiltrate (Fig. 54-15).[269,285,286] Although an infrequent type of PTLD, approximately 25% of cases reportedly fulfill the criteria for CHL of mixed cellularity or another type.[270,285,286] Caution is advised because many "Hodgkin-like" lesions are also described in this setting. A small proportion of the monomorphic cases represent PTCLs, most commonly angioimmunoblastic T-cell lymphoma, with rare cases described as T-cell large granular lymphocytic leukemia.[287,288] Finally, some cases included in series of methotrexate-associated LPDs are small B-cell neoplasms of varied types.[283-286] Although series vary, about 40% of the methotrexate-associated LPDs are EBV positive, including some follicular lymphomas and marginal zone lymphomas; the CHL type have the highest proportion of EBV-positive cases.[5,157,265,269,270,281,284,285,287] EBV-positive nondestructive, reactive lymphoid hyperplasias are also reported in association with methotrexate, with most cases characterized by a follicular hyperplasia.[269,286]

Very little data exist about the genetic basis of methotrexate-associated LPDs; however, most appear to have a clonal immunoglobulin gene rearrangement, including polymorphic cases.[283,285,289] One study that performed copy number analysis of methotrexate-associated DLBCL showed a higher frequency of chromosome 3q, 12q, and 20p gains compared with DLBCL in immunocompetent patients.[289] Loss of *TNFRSF14* and *TNFAIP3* gene loci was found in 40% and 25%

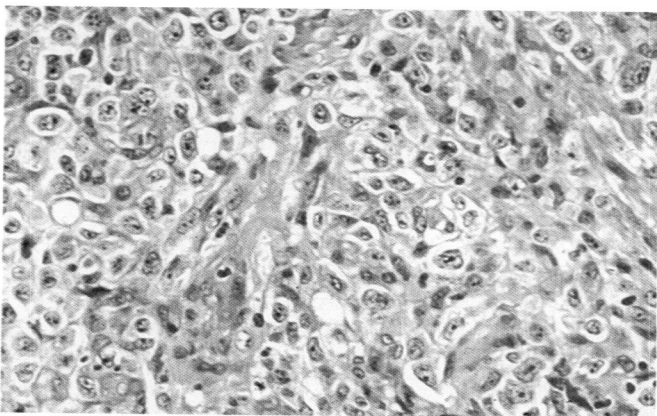

Figure 54-14. Diffuse large B-cell lymphoma methotrexate-associated lymphoproliferative disorder (Epstein-Barr virus [EBV]-positive) in a patient with rheumatoid arthritis. This relatively monomorphic proliferation of large, transformed B cells is indistinguishable from many diffuse large B-cell lymphomas in normal hosts. *(Courtesy Dr. Nancy Lee Harris.)*

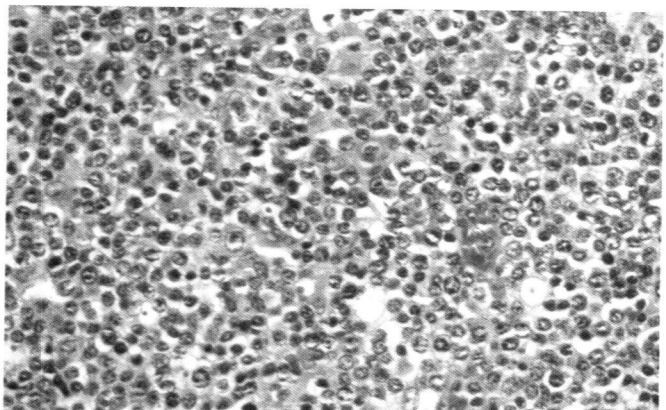

Figure 54-15. Polymorphic methotrexate-associated lymphoproliferative disorder (Epstein-Barr virus [EBV]-positive) that regressed after cessation of methotrexate therapy. There is a diffuse proliferation of very heterogeneous lymphoid cells. *(Courtesy Dr. Nancy Lee Harris.)*

of cases, respectively. EBV-positive methotrexate-associated DLBCLs also appeared to harbor fewer copy number alterations than EBV-negative cases.[289] A recent mutational analysis of methotrexate-associated DLBCLs showed frequent mutations of *KMT2D*, *TNFRSF14*, and *MYC*.[285] *TP53* mutations have been documented in 10% to 15% of cases.[285,290]

Recognition of methotrexate-associated LPD is important because approximately 60% of patients respond to withdrawal of methotrexate therapy.[5,269,283-285] EBV-positive methotrexate-associated LPDs are most likely to respond; however, some responses are seen with EBV-negative lesions.[281,283-285,291] CHL-type cases have also responded in some but not all reports.[284,285] Of the cases that show regression, approximately 20% will eventually recur and require conventional lymphoma therapies, although this percentage does vary between studies.[269,283,285] A small study using a simplified genetic algorithm that correlated with the LymphGen classifier reported that patients with methotrexate-associated DLBCL who had a clinical response to methotrexate withdrawal alone had fewer variants

than patients who required additional chemotherapy.[292] Although 83% of the LPDs in patients who did not require chemotherapy were unclassified by their genetic algorithm, 75% of LPDs from those who required chemotherapy could be categorized, with most cases falling within the MYD88 group (37.5%), and the remainder in the BCL2 (25%) and SGK1 (12.5%) groups.[292]

A subset of the methotrexate-associated LPDs have the features of EBV-positive MCU, which is considered a distinct entity in the WHO Revised 4th ed. and 2022 ICC classifications.[5,8,151,293] Other methotrexate-associated cutaneous LPDs, which may share some features with EBV-positive MCU, are also described. Not all of these are EBV positive, and they can look very worrisome, but often the patients do well with discontinuation of the methotrexate with or without other local therapies.[291,294]

Infliximab and other TNF-α antagonists have been associated with LPDs of varied types in patients with autoimmune diseases, with B-cell lymphoma–type lesions the most common and polymorphic lesions rare.[263,295] EBV has been associated with the B-cell and CHL-type lesions.[263] At least some of the nonlymphomatous lesions may respond to withdrawal of the immunomodulatory therapy.[263] Infliximab, in combination with azathioprine or mercaptopurine, has been specifically associated with hepatosplenic T-cell lymphomas in young patients with Crohn's disease; only rare cases have been associated with TNF-α inhibitor monotherapy.[5,266,267,296,297] The hepatosplenic T-cell lymphomas in these patients do not differ from those in immunocompetent hosts, do not respond to decreased immunosuppressive therapy, and are almost uniformly fatal. There are also a very small number of older and female patients who have developed hepatosplenic T-cell lymphoma in the setting of TNF-α inhibitors for inflammatory bowel disease or rheumatoid arthritis.[296] An increased risk for mycosis fungoides/Sézary syndrome is also reported in association with TNF-α inhibitor exposure.[296,298] Although many uncertainties still exist in terms of lymphoma risk,[296,299] it is well established that TNF-α inhibitors have a profound effect on the immune system and infliximab has been associated with EBV reactivation and an increased EBV viral load that reverses after discontinuation of the drug.[300-302] LPDs have also been reported in patients receiving other biological agents, such as rare CNS lymphomas associated with the integrin antagonist natalizumab used in the treatment of multiple sclerosis.[274]

Small molecule inhibitors used in the setting of autoimmune diseases and myeloid neoplasms have been associated with a variety of LPDs. Rare polymorphic or monomorphic EBV-positive B-cell LPDs may arise in association with the tyrosine kinase inhibitor imatinib, while EBV-positive reactive follicular hyperplasias and HHV8-negative effusion-based lymphomas are described in patients receiving dasatinib.[278,303-305] Aggressive B-cell and T-cell lymphomas are also reported in patients receiving JAK inhibitor therapy.[279,280] Although data is limited, at least a subset of these reported LPDs have shown regression after a withdrawal of therapy.[278,303,305] Fludarabine has been associated with the development of EBV-associated LPDs, most frequently in patients receiving treatment for a low-grade lymphoma.[275,276] The association between fludarabine therapy and LPD is more difficult to prove than with methotrexate because of the presence of a preexisting LPD and the difficulty encountered in reversing the immune defect.[306,307] The cases of EBV-positive LPD after fludarabine therapy include polymorphic B-cell LPDs, monomorphic B-cell lymphomas, and CHL-like proliferations; some do regress without antineoplastic therapy.[275,276,306,307] It is important in these cases to rule out a Richter-like transformation of the original neoplasm. EBV-positive LPD may also follow the use of other chemotherapeutic regimens, such as the LPD resembling lymphomatoid granulomatosis reported in a small number of children and rare adults after therapy for acute lymphoblastic leukemia.[271,308,309]

Pearls and Pitfalls

- Iatrogenic immunodeficiency-associated lymphoproliferative disorders (LPDs) are best described in patients after solid organ or allogeneic hematopoietic stem cell transplantation; in patients with rheumatoid arthritis after methotrexate therapy; and in young men with Crohn's disease treated with infliximab (and azathioprine or mercaptopurine). They can also occur after immunosuppression/immunomodulatory agents or immunosuppressive chemotherapeutic regimens in many other circumstances.
- Diagnosis of a posttransplant lymphoproliferative disorder (PTLD) rests heavily on the history of a prior transplantation; however, not every lymphoid proliferation in a transplant patient is a PTLD.
- Recognition of a PTLD is extremely important for clinical purposes, even if categorization is problematic. Absolute distinction between a "benign" and a "malignant" PTLD can be more of a philosophic problem than a practical one. Nondestructive PTLD can be fatal, and lymphoma-like lesions may regress with decreased immunosuppression. Small tissue biopsies may preclude a precise classification.
- Presence of a clonal lymphoid population does not indicate that a PTLD is a "lymphoma" type and should not be considered pathognomonic of PTLD.
- Patients with a nondestructive PTLD may have a polymorphic or monomorphic PTLD at other sites.
- Synchronous and metachronous PTLDs may or may not be clonally related.
- Before diagnosing a polymorphic PTLD, exclude a possible monomorphic T-cell PTLD, because morphologically, the latter may be very polymorphic.
- Even if not required for the diagnosis, the finding of numerous EBV-positive cells is very helpful in making the diagnosis of an iatrogenic immunodeficiency-associated LPD; however, their absence does not rule out the diagnosis, and the presence of small numbers of positive cells is not pathognomonic. EBV-positive cases should be distinguished from EBV-negative cases.
- Transplant patients can show both allograft rejection and PTLD at the same time.
- Always inquire about the use of immunosuppressive/immunomodulatory agents before diagnosing an overt lymphoma in patients with preexisting disorders that are often treated with these agents, such as rheumatoid arthritis.

KEY REFERENCES

10. Trappe R, Oertel S, Leblond V, et al. Sequential treatment with rituximab followed by CHOP chemotherapy in adult B-cell post-transplant lymphoproliferative disorder (PTLD): the prospective international multicentre phase 2 PTLD-1 trial. *Lancet Oncol.* 2012;13(2):196–206.

18. Toner K, Bollard CM. EBV+ lymphoproliferative diseases: opportunities for leveraging EBV as a therapeutic target. *Blood.* 2022;139(7):983–994.

19. Shah N, Eyre TA, Tucker D, et al. Front-line management of post-transplantation lymphoproliferative disorder in adult solid organ recipient patients—a British Society for Haematology Guideline. *Br J Haematol.* 2021;193(4):727–740.

23. Reshef R, Vardhanabhuti S, Luskin MR, et al. Reduction of immunosuppression as initial therapy for posttransplantation lymphoproliferative disorder. *Am J Transplant.* 2011;11(2):336–347.

33. Santarsieri A, Rudge JF, Amin I, et al. Incidence and outcomes of post-transplant lymphoproliferative disease after 5365 solid-organ transplants over a 20-year period at two UK transplant centres. *Br J Haematol.* 2022;197(3):310–319.

99. Menter T, Juskevicius D, Alikian M, et al. Mutational landscape of B-cell post-transplant lymphoproliferative disorders. *Br J Haematol.* 2017;178(1):48–56.

107. King RL, Khurana A, Mwangi R, et al. Clinicopathologic characteristics, treatment, and outcomes of post-transplant lymphoproliferative disorders: a single-institution experience using 2017 WHO diagnostic criteria. *Hemasphere.* 2021;5(10):e640.

163. Margolskee E, Jobanputra V, Jain P, et al. Genetic landscape of T- and NK-cell post-transplant lymphoproliferative disorders. *Oncotarget.* 2016;7(25):37636–37648.

210. Dierickx D, Habermann TM. Post-transplantation lymphoproliferative disorders in adults. *N Engl J Med.* 2018;378(6):549–562.

212. Burns DM, Clesham K, Hodgson YA, et al. Real-world outcomes with rituximab-based therapy for posttransplant lymphoproliferative disease arising after solid organ transplant. *Transplantation.* 2020;104(12):2582–2590.

285. Kaji D, Kusakabe M, Sakata-Yanagimoto M, et al. Retrospective analyses of other iatrogenic immunodeficiency-associated lymphoproliferative disorders in patients with rheumatic diseases. *Br J Haematol.* 2021;195(4):585–594.

Visit Elsevier eBooks+ for the complete set of references.

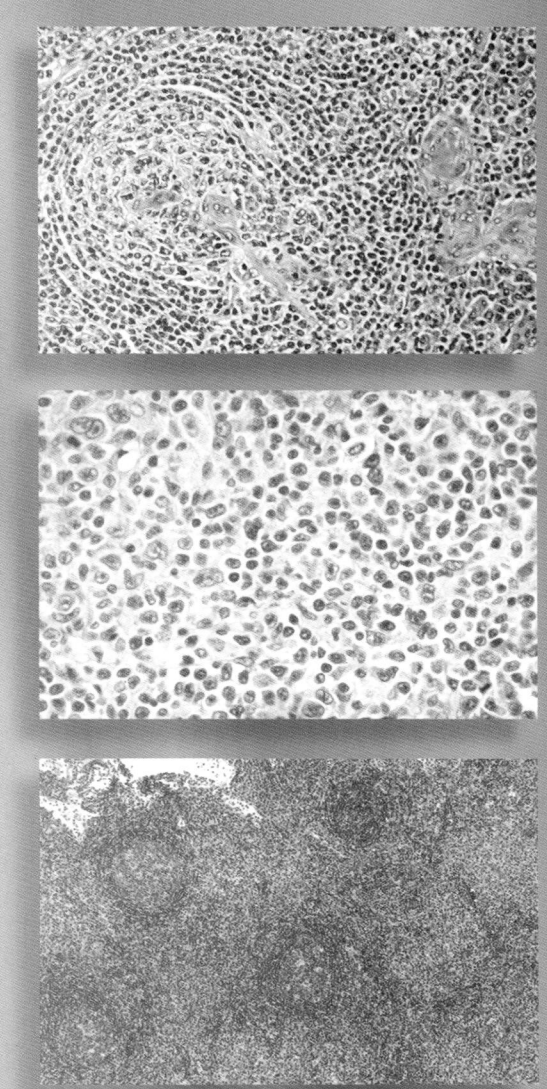

PART **VI**

Site-Specific Issues in the Diagnosis of Lymphoma and Leukemia

Chapter 55

Bone Marrow Evaluation for Lymphoma

Girish Venkataraman and Yi-Hua Chen

Bone marrow examination is an important part of the workup of patients with lymphoma. It is often performed for staging purposes and for follow-up to evaluate for response to therapy or recurrence.[1-3] In some patients, a diagnosis of lymphoma is initially made on a bone marrow biopsy obtained for evaluation for unexplained cytopenias, fevers of unknown origin, unexplained organomegaly, or mass lesions difficult to access for biopsy.[4,5]

Evaluation of bone marrow involvement by lymphoma can be challenging, particularly in patients without a prior diagnosis at an extramedullary site. For example, benign lymphoid infiltrates are frequently encountered in the bone marrow core biopsies in older individuals or patients with autoimmune diseases, and can be difficult to distinguish from lymphoma, even with the help of ancillary techniques.[6,7] In patients with an established diagnosis of lymphoma, the assessment of bone marrow involvement can be complicated by situations such as a discordant histologic type in the bone marrow compared with the extramedullary lesion.[8,9] Additionally, subclassification of lymphoma based on the bone

marrow findings is not always straightforward and requires not only the knowledge of the diagnostic features of various lymphoma subtypes but also the appropriate use of ancillary techniques. It is also important to recognize the limitations of classification of lymphoma based on bone marrow findings alone; biopsy of extramedullary lesions may be required.

The core biopsy is usually the most informative when evaluating bone marrow involvement by lymphoma. However, peripheral blood smear, bone marrow aspirate smear, particle clot section, and touch imprint also provide valuable complementary information and may be diagnostic in themselves. Therefore, all these preparations should be examined together and the findings correlated. An adequate bone marrow sampling is important to ensure the detection of focal lymphomatous infiltrates. It is recommended that the bone marrow core biopsy should be at least 1.5 to 2 cm long; the yield of lymphoma detection is significantly higher with bilateral than unilateral core biopsies (Fig. 55-1).[10,11] Additionally, sections from multiple levels of the core biopsy should be examined in order to increase the detection rate.

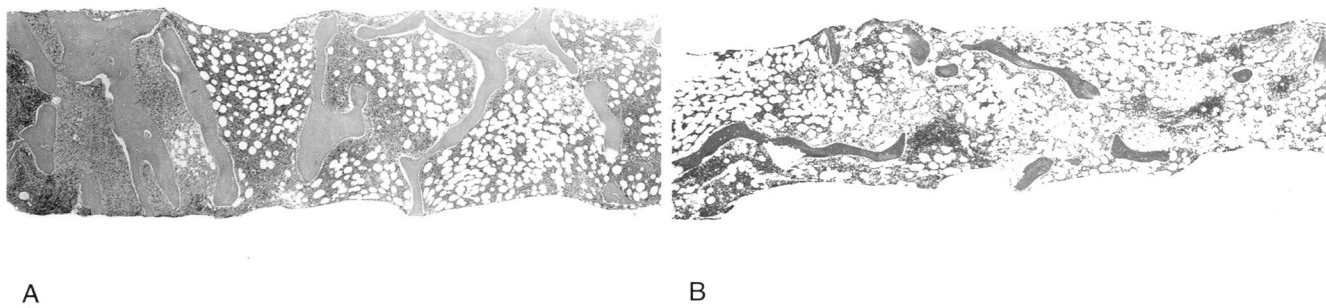

A   B

Figure 55-1. **Bilateral bone marrow core biopsy obtained for staging purposes from a patient with diffuse large B-cell lymphoma. A,** Only the *left side* core biopsy specimen is involved by lymphoma. The lymphomatous infiltrate is focal (involving only the left side of the core) but exhibits a diffuse growth pattern. **B,** The *right side* core biopsy specimen is uninvolved.

However, significant advances in PET imaging methodology have nearly obviated the need for routine staging marrow biopsies for diffuse large B-cell lymphoma (DLBCL) and Hodgkin lymphoma (HL) in cases with PET-positive disease in the marrow.[12,13]

Flow cytometric immunophenotyping, immunohistochemistry, cytogenetic analysis, and molecular testing are important in evaluation of bone marrow specimens for lymphoma, and should be used in a logical and cost-effective way based on the morphologic findings and clinical setting. Whenever ancillary techniques are employed, the results should be correlated with one another and with the morphologic findings. It is also worth noting that knowledge of each technique, including its limitations, is important in effective utilization of these techniques in bone marrow evaluation of lymphoma.

This chapter focuses on the distinction between benign and lymphomatous infiltrate and morphologic features of various subtypes of lymphoma in the bone marrow. In addition, nonlymphoid lesions mimicking lymphoma in the bone marrow are briefly discussed.

DISTINCTION BETWEEN BENIGN LYMPHOID AGGREGATES AND LYMPHOMA

Benign lymphoid aggregates frequently occur in the bone marrow in older individuals, as well as in various reactive conditions, such as systemic autoimmune disorders (rheumatoid arthritis, lupus, autoimmune hemolytic anemia, idiopathic thrombocytopenia, and Hashimoto thyroiditis), aplastic anemia, viral infection (HIV and hepatitis), and myeloproliferative neoplasms (MPNs) and myelodysplastic syndromes (MDSs).[6,14,15]

Morphology

The assessment of lymphoid infiltrates in the bone marrow is first based on the morphologic findings. However, other studies such as immunohistochemistry, flow cytometric immunophenotyping, or molecular analysis may be required for further evaluation. Although these techniques are usually informative, the nature of the lymphoid infiltrate may remain unknown in some cases. The extent of testing to analyze a lymphoid infiltrate in the bone marrow depends on the clinical setting and the degree of suspicion for lymphoma. Several morphologic features can be used in distinguishing benign lymphoid aggregates from lymphoma (Table 55-1).[6,7]

Benign lymphoid aggregates are usually single or few in number, small in size, well circumscribed, random, and nonparatrabecular (Fig. 55-2). The cells within the aggregates are often polymorphous and may include plasma cells and histiocytes. Reactive germinal centers may be present, which are more commonly seen in patients with autoimmune diseases. However, germinal centers are not exclusively seen in benign lymphoid infiltrates; non-Hodgkin lymphomas, particularly splenic marginal zone lymphoma (SMZL), may also contain reactive germinal centers in the bone marrow (see Fig. 55-15).[16] Additionally, lipogranulomas are often seen in the marrow and should not be confused with infectious granulomas or HL. These are, however, foamy and lymphocyte poor, allowing their distinction from other allied entities and lymphomas (Fig. 55-3).

In contrast to benign lymphoid aggregates, lymphomatous aggregates are more frequently multiple, larger in size, and have infiltrative borders. Paratrabecular lymphoid infiltrates are almost always neoplastic and most frequently associated with follicular lymphoma (FL), although this pattern is by no means exclusive to FL.[6,17] The presence of distinct intrasinusoidal lymphoid infiltrates is usually an indication of a neoplastic process and most commonly seen in SMZL, splenic diffuse red pulp small B-cell lymphoma (SDRPSBCL), intravascular large B-cell lymphoma, and hepatosplenic T-cell lymphoma.[18,19] Neoplastic lymphoid infiltrates generally exhibit a more homogeneous cellular composition than benign lymphoid infiltrates. However, a polymorphous infiltrate also characterizes some subtypes of lymphomas, most notably peripheral T-cell lymphoma and HL.[14,20] Importantly, the presence of morphologically abnormal lymphocytes and architectural features in the bone marrow core biopsy, such as paratrabecular localization and infiltrative borders, should raise the suspicion of a neoplastic process.

Table 55-1 Features Distinguishing Benign Lymphoid Aggregates From Lymphoma in Bone Marrow Biopsy

Benign	Malignant
Aggregates are few in number	Aggregates are variable in number and may be multiple
Aggregates with random distribution	Paratrabecular aggregates may be present
Aggregates are usually round, well-circumscribed	Aggregates are often irregularly shaped with infiltrative borders
Polymorphous cellular compositions	Usually homogeneous cellular composition except for some peripheral T-cell lymphomas and Hodgkin lymphoma; atypical cytologic features may be present
Intrasinusoidal infiltrates usually absent	Intrasinusoidal infiltrates may be present
Vascularity is often prominent	Vascularity is usually not prominent except in peripheral T-cell lymphomas
Benign germinal centers are occasionally present	Benign germinal centers are not present except for marginal zone lymphomas
No morphologically abnormal lymphocytes in bone marrow aspirate smears or imprints	Morphologically abnormal lymphocytes may be present in bone marrow aspirate smears or imprints
Immunohistochemical stains show a mixture of B and T cells, often with T-cell predominance (exceptions occur)	Immunohistochemical stains showing a predominance of B cells, aberrant phenotype, or monoclonal plasma cells suggest B-cell lymphoma; an aberrant T-cell phenotype suggests T-cell lymphoma
No monotypic B-cell population or phenotypically abnormal T-cell population identified by flow cytometry (exceptions occur)	Immunoglobulin light chain restriction or aberrant T-cell phenotype
No monoclonal IGH or TCR gene rearrangement by molecular analysis (exceptions occur)	Monoclonal IGH or TCR gene rearrangement are often identified by molecular analysis

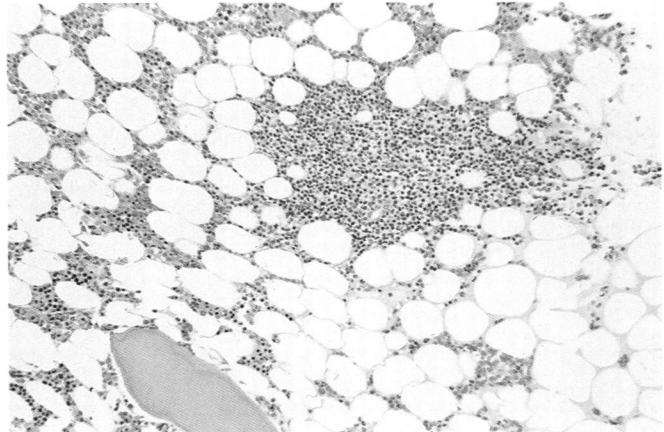

Figure 55-2. Benign lymphoid aggregate in a bone marrow core biopsy. The single lymphoid aggregate is small, well circumscribed, located between bony trabeculae, and composed predominantly of small, mature-appearing lymphocytes. A small blood vessel is present in the lymphoid aggregate.

Immunohistochemistry

A panel of immunohistochemical stains on the bone marrow core biopsy or particle clot section is often required to assist in the distinction between benign versus neoplastic lymphoid infiltrates. Immunohistochemical stains for B-cell markers (e.g., CD20, PAX5) and T-cell markers (e.g., CD3) are often used to determine the proportions of B and T cells within the lymphoid aggregates. Rarely, a cluster of plasmacytoid dendritic cells may resemble a lymphoid aggregate (Fig. 55-4), and appropriate immunohistochemical stains will help distinguish these from benign lymphoid aggregates. Benign lymphoid aggregates usually have a mixture of B and T cells, and T cells frequently predominate, whereas lymphoid infiltrates composed primarily of B cells, especially if multiple, are often neoplastic. However, some B-cell lymphomas may be accompanied by a significant number of reactive T cells, such as FL and T-cell/histiocyte-rich large B-cell lymphoma. Therefore, a mixture of B and T cells or a predominance of T cells in the lymphoid infiltrate does not completely exclude a diagnosis of B-cell lymphoma.[21]

Similar to extramedullary lymphomas, demonstration of an aberrant B-cell or T-cell phenotype by immunohistochemistry, such as expression of CD5 in B cells or loss of pan T-cell antigen in T cells, supports a diagnosis of B-cell or T-cell lymphoma, respectively. Demonstration of immunoglobulin light chain restriction in the plasma cells associated with an atypical B-cell infiltrate supports a diagnosis of B-cell lymphoma with plasmacytic differentiation, such as marginal zone lymphoma (MZL), lymphoplasmacytic lymphoma, and the more recently recognized primary cold agglutinin disease.[22] Immunohistochemical stains for markers associated with specific subtypes of lymphoid neoplasm, such as cyclin D1 in mantle cell lymphoma (MCL) and hairy cell leukemia (HCL), CD30/ALK1 in anaplastic large cell lymphoma, and LEF1 in chronic lymphocytic leukemia (CLL)/small lymphocytic lymphoma (SLL) (Fig. 55-5) not only help with diagnosis, but also subclassification and sometimes prognosis of lymphomas.

Special consideration should be given to patients who have been treated with an anti-CD20 agent and continue to exhibit lymphoid infiltrates in the bone marrow. In some cases, the lesions represent residual lymphoma, while in others, the lymphoma has likely been eliminated by anti-CD20 therapy, resulting in lymphoid infiltrates that are composed entirely of CD3-positive T cells.[23] These aggregates may mimic residual lymphoma because they can be large, multiple, or even paratrabecular (Fig. 55-6). When residual B-cell lymphoma remains in the bone marrow of patients treated with anti-CD20 therapy, immunohistochemical stains or flow cytometric immunophenotyping using B-cell markers other than CD20 (e.g., CD79a, PAX5) are necessary to evaluate post-therapy bone marrow.

It is also worth noting that in the early course of granulocyte colony-stimulating factor (G-CSF) therapy, the bone marrow frequently shows a marked myeloid shift to immaturity and

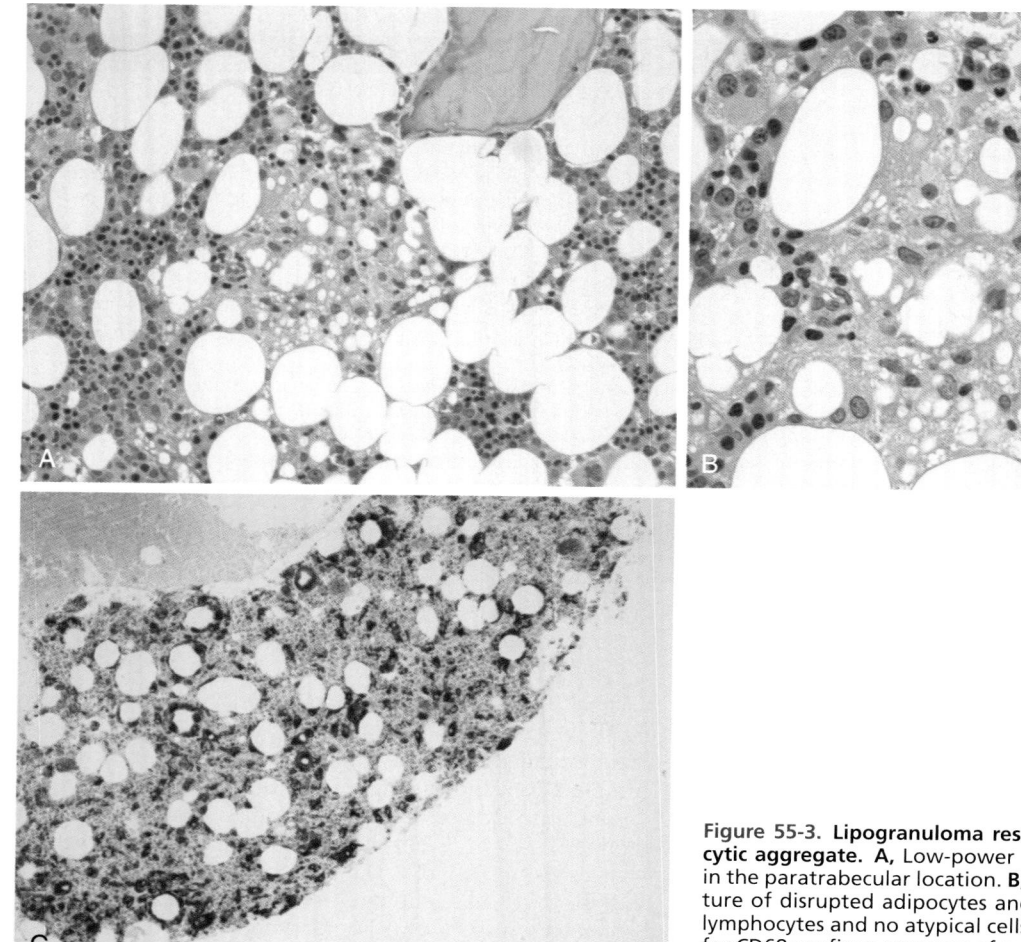

Figure 55-3. Lipogranuloma resembling atypical lymphohistiocytic aggregate. A, Low-power view showing a discrete cluster in the paratrabecular location. **B,** Higher power shows an admixture of disrupted adipocytes and foamy histiocytes with sparse lymphocytes and no atypical cells. **C,** Immunohistochemical stain for CD68 confirms presence of numerous histiocytes within these aggregates.

contains a significant number of promyelocytes, often in a paratrabecular location. The findings may mimic large cell lymphoma (Fig. 55-7). Knowledge of the history of G-CSF therapy can aid in the distinction from lymphoma. If the history is not provided, characteristic changes associated with G-CSF therapy, such as severe toxic changes and a shift to immaturity in granulocytes in the blood and bone marrow aspirate, can also alert one to this possibility. Well-prepared histologic sections that allow observation of the morphologic features of promyelocytes are essential. Immunohistochemical stains for myeloperoxidase, CD20, or CD3 may be required to make the distinction (Fig. 55-7).

Flow Cytometric Immunophenotyping

Flow cytometric immunophenotyping performed on the bone marrow aspirate or peripheral blood is an important part of the workup for bone marrow involvement by lymphoma, and the correlation with morphology is usually excellent.[24-26] However, discrepancies between the bone marrow core biopsy and the aspirate may occur because of small, focal paratrabecular lesions or bone marrow fibrosis preventing the aspiration of cells; thus a negative flow cytometric result does not exclude the possibility of lymphoma. Flow cytometric

immunophenotyping can be performed on a peripheral blood specimen when a bone marrow aspirate is not available, especially if the patient is known to have a lymphoma associated with a higher incidence of peripheral blood involvement, such as CLL/SLL, MCL, SMZL, and lymphoplasmacytic lymphoma (LPL). Occasionally, monotypic B cells are identified by flow cytometry without morphologic evidence of lymphoma. In these cases, it is prudent to evaluate whether the biopsy is of adequate size and quality, and examine multiple levels of sections (Fig. 55-8). It may also be appropriate to perform immunohistochemical stains to ensure that a subtle abnormal lymphoid infiltrate is not missed.

It is important to recognize that low levels of monoclonal B cells (<5.0 × 10⁹/L) can be identified in the blood in up to 7% of older individuals who are otherwise healthy and without clinical or morphologic evidence of lymphoma.[27-29] This finding is termed *monoclonal B lymphocytosis (MBL)*. MBL usually exhibits a CLL-like phenotype (CD5 positive, CD23 positive). Most patients with MBL also have lymphoid aggregates in the bone marrow, but they are not regarded as diagnostic for lymphoma.[30] Small monoclonal B-cell populations can also be initially identified in the bone marrow aspirate in patients without evidence of lymphoma, and these monoclonal B-cell populations are more commonly

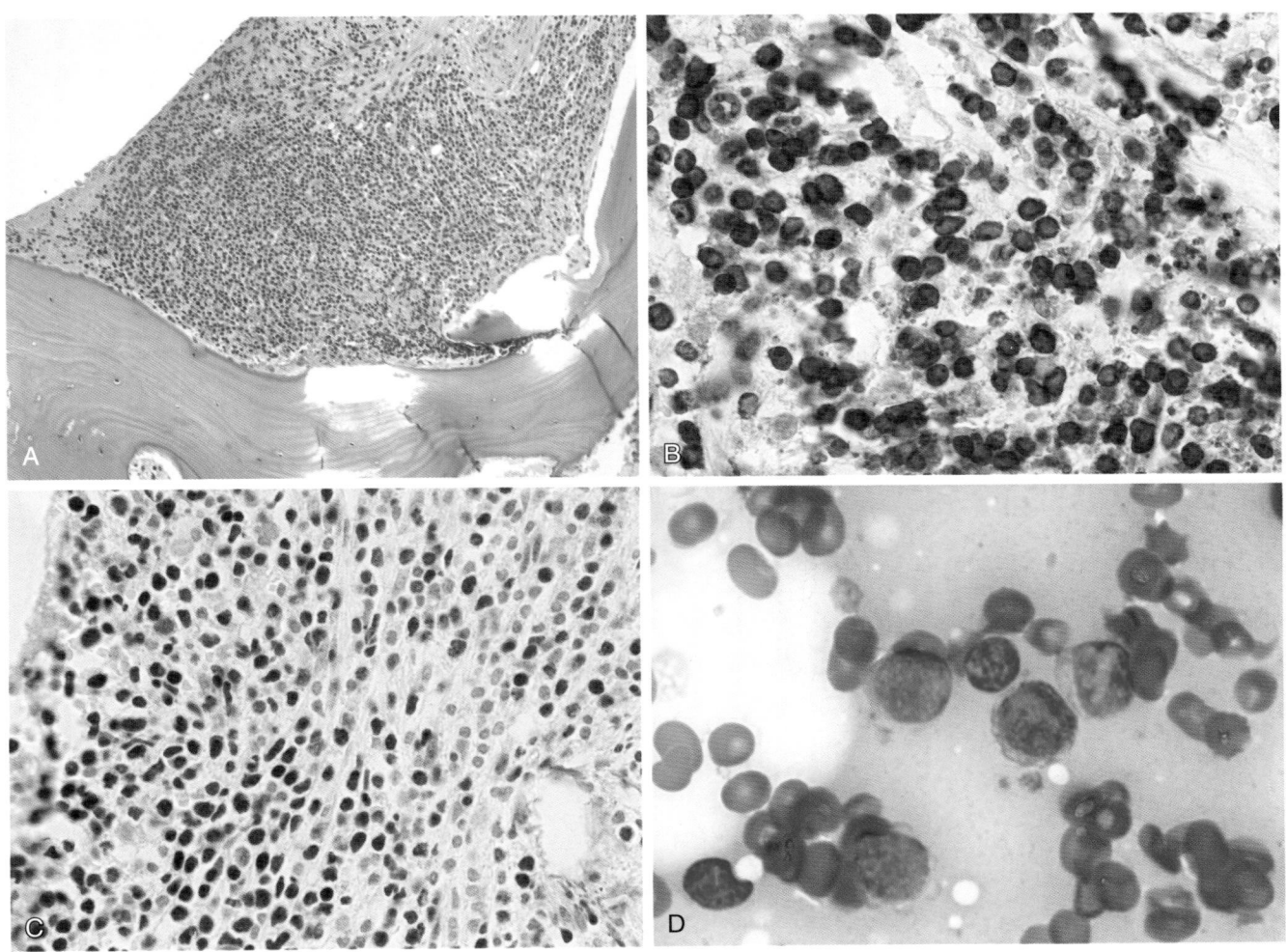

Figure 55-4. Plasmacytoid dendritic cells resembling lymphoid aggregate. A, Paratrabecular aggregate of lymphoid-appearing cells with infiltrative borders. **B–C,** Immunohistochemical stains for CD123 **(B)** and TCF4 **(C)** are both strongly positive in the atypical cells, confirming that these are plasmacytoid dendritic cells in a patient with treated blastic plasmacytoid dendritic cell neoplasm. **D,** Aspirate smears (Wright-Giemsa stain) show scattered plasmacytoid dendritic cells, which often have circumferential microvacuolations. Note the medium size of the atypical cells compared with the two small lymphocytes in the background.

CD5-negative than MBL in the peripheral blood.[31] In these CD5-negative cases, as well as cases with MCL-like phenotype, clinical and laboratory workup may be indicated to rule out lymphoma. Occasionally, aberrant T-cell populations of unclear significance can also be identified by flow cytometry in patients without evidence of lymphoma.[32] These findings emphasize the importance of correlating immunophenotypic results with the clinical and morphologic findings in bone marrow evaluation.

Molecular Diagnostic Studies

Molecular analysis plays an important adjunctive role, especially in cases where morphologic and immunohistochemical findings are uncertain.[33-38] Polymerase chain reaction (PCR) for immunoglobulin heavy chain (IGH) or T-cell receptor (TCR) gene rearrangement on paraffin-embedded bone marrow tissue or fresh aspirate is typically used to aid in the differentiation of benign versus neoplastic lymphoid infiltrate.

Clonal IGH or TCR gene rearrangements have been reported in about 65% to 85% and 60% to 70% of bone marrow specimens with morphologic and immunohistochemical evidence of B-cell or T-cell lymphoma, respectively.[33-35] Clonal IGH gene rearrangement has also been identified in about 15% to 65% of cases interpreted as suspicious for lymphoma and 10% to 40% of cases without morphologic evidence of lymphoma. Of importance, clonal TCR gene rearrangements were reportedly identified in morphologically negative bone marrow in over half of patients diagnosed with T-cell lymphomas.[36,38] Interestingly, one study reported that a clonal T-cell population was identified in about 13% of B-cell lymphomas and a clonal B-cell population in about 3% of T-cell lymphomas in the bone marrow.[34] It is also important to be aware that clonal B-cell or T-cell populations may be present in various reactive conditions such as inflammatory diseases, autoimmune disorders, and post–stem cell transplant.[39,40] Therefore, the results of molecular studies should be interpreted in context and correlated with additional information because monoclonality is not synonymous with

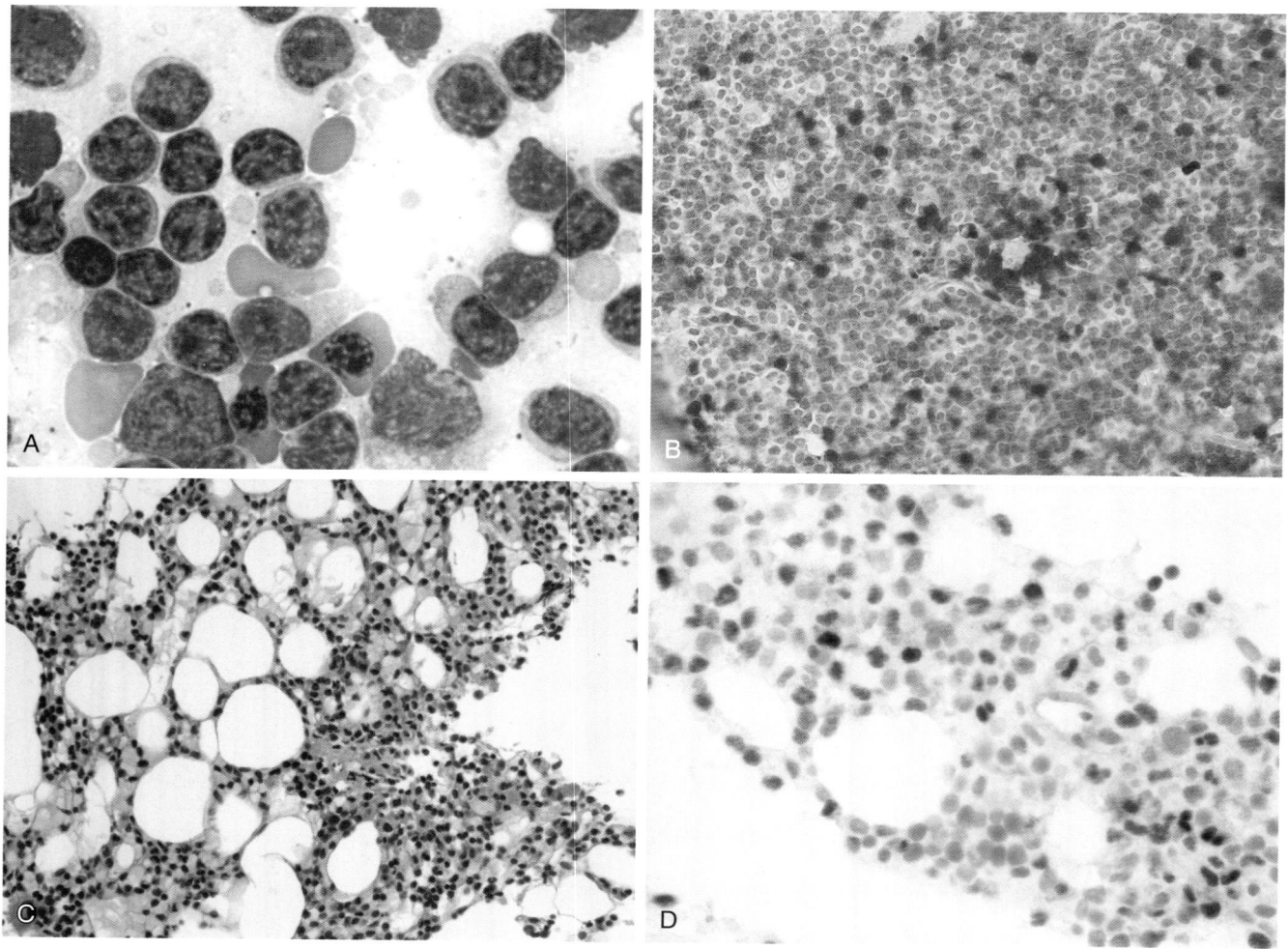

Figure 55-5. Diagnostic and prognostic value of immunohistochemical stains on bone marrow biopsy. A, Chronic lymphocytic leukemia (CLL) cells in the bone marrow aspirate smear. **B,** Immunohistochemical stain for ZAP70 on the bone marrow core biopsy of the same case shows weak staining in the CLL cells while a cluster of normal T cells in the center of the field shows strong ZAP70 staining that serves as an internal positive control. **C,** Seemingly normocellular marrow without apparent atypical lymphoid infiltrate in a patient with hairy cell leukemia. **D,** Immunostain for CD20 (not shown) highlights the abnormal infiltrate that is positive for cyclin D1, confirming the diagnosis. In addition to mantle cell lymphoma, cyclin D1 is positive in the majority cases of hairy cell leukemia and a subset of multiple myeloma cases. Normal endothelial cells and histiocytes service as internal positive controls for cyclin D1. Most bone marrow immunohistochemical stains have background internal control cells, which are probably the most appropriate cells to assess quality of staining.

malignancy, and failure to detect monoclonality does not rule out a lymphoma. Some molecular studies are important not only for distinguishing benign versus neoplastic process but also for subclassification and prognosis of certain lymphomas, such as assessment of *MYD88* and *CXCR4* mutations in LPL.[41]

NON-HODGKIN LYMPHOMA INVOLVING BONE MARROW

Incidence of Bone Marrow Involvement

Bone marrow involvement by lymphoma represents stage IV disease based on the Ann Arbor lymphoma staging system.[1] The overall incidence of lymphoma involving the bone marrow is 35% to 50%.[14] However, there is considerable variability

for different lymphoma subtypes. In general, indolent lymphoma, highly aggressive lymphoma, and the majority of peripheral T-cell lymphomas involve the bone marrow with high frequency. For example, FL, CLL/SLL, and MCL involve the bone marrow in up to 60%, 85%, and 90% of cases, respectively[14,42,43]; Burkitt lymphoma (BL) in about 30% to 60% of cases[14]; and DLBCLs in 20% to 30% of cases.[44,45]

The incidence of bone marrow involvement by specific subtypes of peripheral T-cell lymphomas has a wide range.[46,47] For example, virtually all hepatosplenic T-cell lymphoma and up to 70% of angioimmunoblastic T-cell lymphomas involve the bone marrow.[48,49] Anaplastic large cell lymphoma and extranodal natural killer (NK)/T--cell lymphoma, nasal type, involve the bone marrow in approximately 10% to 30% and 10% to 20% of cases,

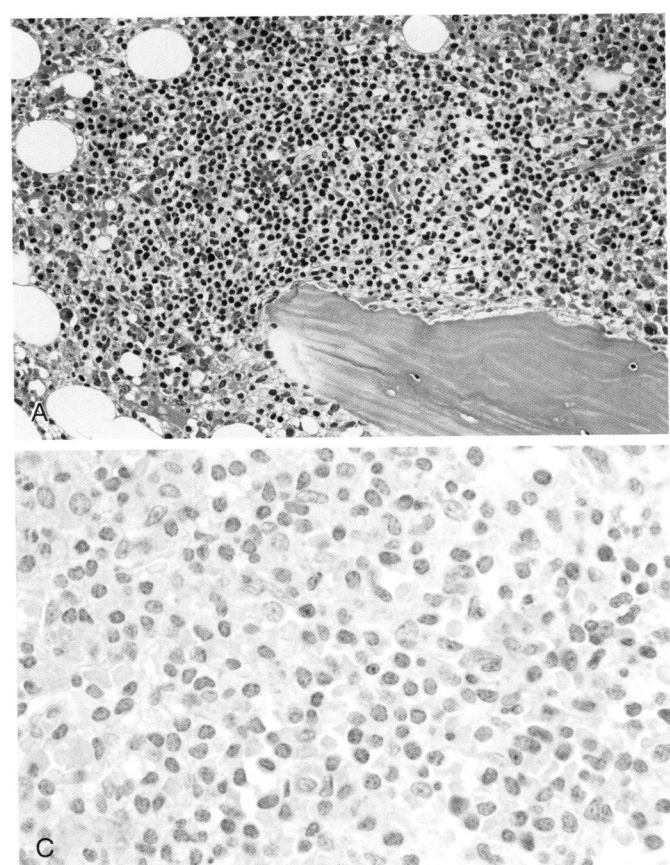
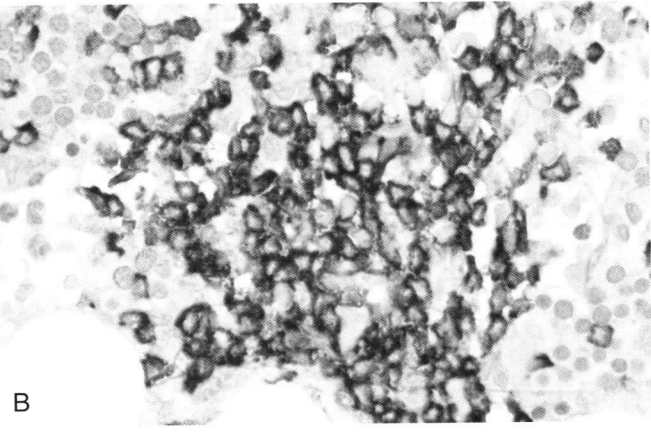

Figure 55-6. Paratrabecular lymphoid aggregate in bone marrow after rituximab therapy. A, This paratrabecular lymphoid aggregate after rituximab treatment for low-grade follicular lymphoma (FL) is composed of small lymphocytes, with rare histiocytes and stromal cells, mimicking residual FL. **B,** Immunohistochemical staining for CD3 shows that the lymphocytes are virtually all CD3-positive T cells. **C,** Immunohistochemical stains for PAX5 and CD79a (not shown) are both completely negative. Therefore, the lymphoid aggregate does not represent residual FL.

respectively.[46,47,50] Primary cutaneous T-cell lymphomas, such as mycosis fungoides (MF), are generally considered to spare the bone marrow until advanced stage. However, careful examination identifies marrow involvement in approximately 22% of patients with cutaneous T-cell lymphoma at diagnosis.[51]

Histologic Patterns of Bone Marrow Involvement

Non-Hodgkin lymphomas infiltrate the bone marrow in a variety of architectural patterns (Table 55-2), and more than one pattern is often seen in an individual patient.[9,10,17] Knowledge of these features is helpful in identifying neoplastic lymphoid infiltrates and in some cases facilitates lymphoma classification.

Lymphomatous infiltrates in the bone marrow can occur in five different patterns: focal random (nodular), focal paratrabecular, interstitial, diffuse, and intrasinusoidal (Fig. 55-9). Focal infiltrates are the most common and characterized by discrete collections of neoplastic lymphocytes. Even though they focally displace bone marrow and fat cells, they are usually associated with considerable sparing of normal hematopoietic tissue. Focal infiltrates are present in either random or paratrabecular locations. Focal random lymphoid infiltrates occupy space away from the bony trabeculae, whereas paratrabecular infiltrates preferentially grow along and "hug" the bony trabeculae. Random lymphoid infiltrates that expand and focally abut the bone are not considered

paratrabecular. In interstitial infiltrates, the neoplastic lymphocytes infiltrate between normal hematopoietic cells without significantly disrupting the bone marrow architecture. They usually do not replace large amounts of bone marrow tissue, even though there is generally widespread bone marrow involvement. Diffuse infiltrates completely replace the hematopoietic elements between the bony trabeculae in a portion or all of the bone marrow core biopsy section. Intrasinusoidal infiltration is characterized by collections of neoplastic lymphocytes within the sinusoids; these infiltrates are typically subtle and difficult to appreciate on hematoxylin and eosin (H&E)–stained sections but can be highlighted by immunohistochemical stains.

B-CELL LYMPHOMAS INVOLVING BONE MARROW

This section describes the characteristics of selected subtypes of B-cell lymphomas with emphasis on the morphologic features specific to bone marrow involvement. Other features such as immunophenotype and molecular cytogenetic features are briefly discussed, and more details can be found in the specific chapters on the disease entities.

Chronic Lymphocytic Leukemia/Small Lymphocytic Lymphoma

CLL is the leukemic manifestation, and SLL is the tissue counterpart of the same disease process. About 85% of

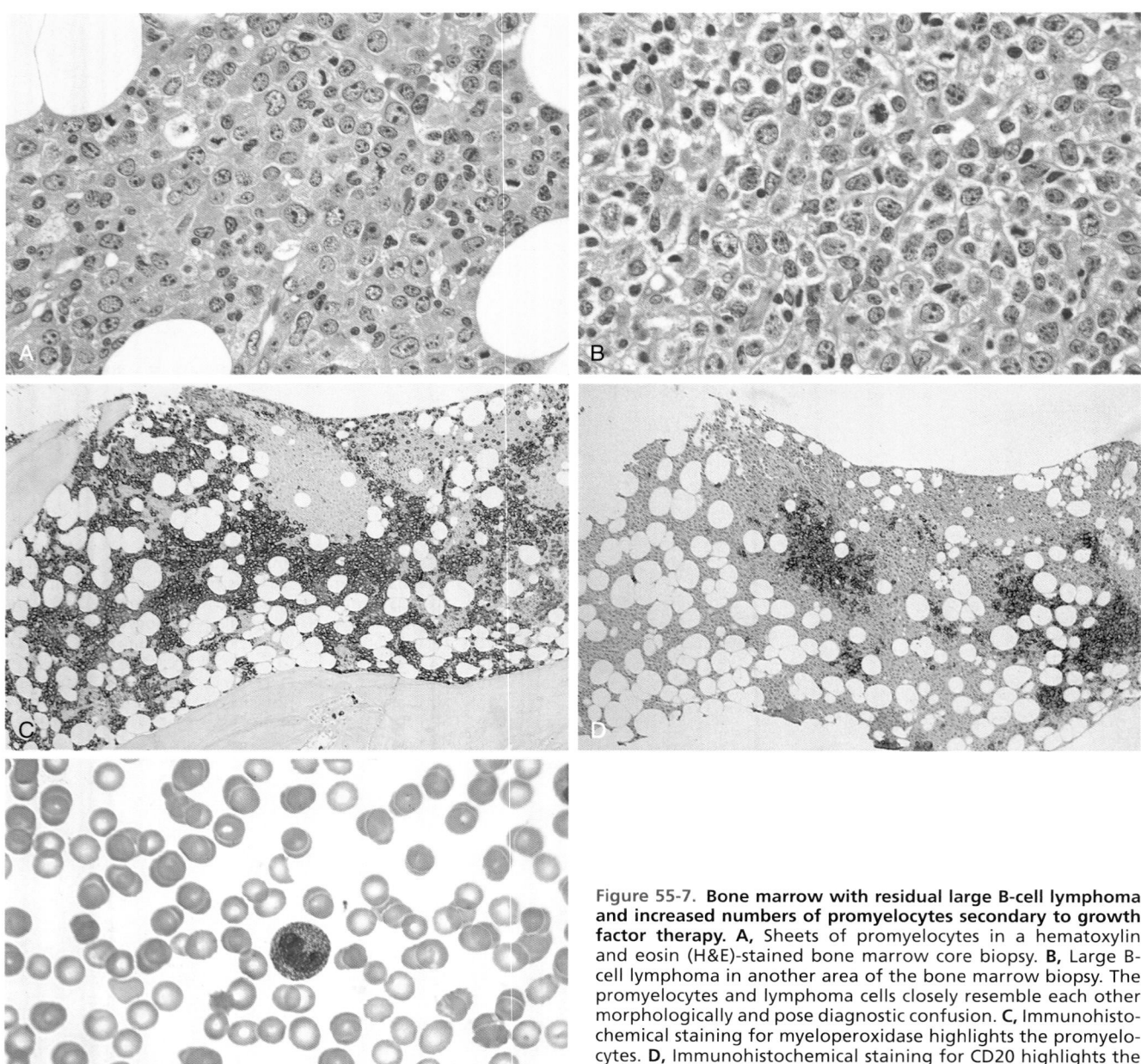

Figure 55-7. Bone marrow with residual large B-cell lymphoma and increased numbers of promyelocytes secondary to growth factor therapy. A, Sheets of promyelocytes in a hematoxylin and eosin (H&E)-stained bone marrow core biopsy. **B,** Large B-cell lymphoma in another area of the bone marrow biopsy. The promyelocytes and lymphoma cells closely resemble each other morphologically and pose diagnostic confusion. **C,** Immunohisto-chemical staining for myeloperoxidase highlights the promyelo-cytes. **D,** Immunohistochemical staining for CD20 highlights the lymphoma cells (note patchy multifocal infiltrative pattern sup-porting lymphoma). **E,** Neutrophil with prominent toxic granules and Döhle body because of colony-stimulating factor therapy.

patients with CLL/SLL have bone marrow involvement at diagnosis; rarely, patients may have isolated bone marrow involvement.[14,42] The patterns in which CLL/SLL infiltrates the bone marrow are focal random (Fig. 55-10), diffuse, interstitial, or mixed, and sometimes admixed with a transformed large cell component. Although focal random infiltrates can expand to touch the bony trabeculae, distinctly paratrabecular infiltrates are absent. When paratrabecular infiltrates are observed, the diagnosis of CLL/SLL should be questioned, and other types of lymphoma, such as FL and MCL, should be considered in the differential diagnosis. The neoplastic lymphocytes are small with round nuclei, condensed chromatin, and scant cytoplasm. Proliferation

centers, the characteristic morphologic finding of CLL/SLL in lymph node tissue, are occasionally encountered in the bone marrow core biopsy (Fig. 55-11).

The CLL/SLL is typically CD19+, dim CD20+, CD5+, CD10−, CD23+, FMC7−/dim+, CD79b−/dim+, CD200+, and dim surface immunoglobulin light chain restricted. Some cases of CLL/SLL may have overlapping morphologic and immunophenotypic features with MCL; however, negative immunohistochemical stains for cyclin D1 and SOX11 essentially rule out the latter possibility. CD200, an immunoglobulin superfamily membrane glycoprotein, is found to be highly expressed in virtually all cases of CLL/ SLL but absent or expressed at a low level in MCL. Thus

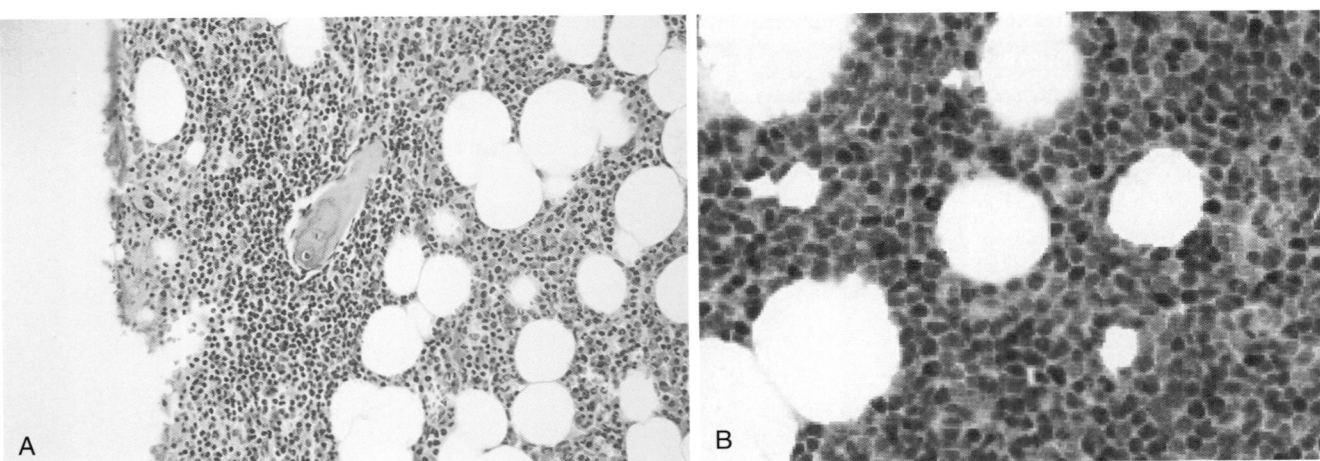

Figure 55-8. Mantle cell lymphoma (MCL) identified in the deeper section of bone marrow core biopsy from a patient with an established diagnosis of MCL. A, The initial bone marrow sections were negative for lymphoma. Deeper sections were obtained because CD5-positive monotypic B cells were identified by flow cytometry. Lymphoma cells were identified in the deeper sections surrounding a bony trabecula and infiltrating between fat cells. Flow cytometry is especially useful in MCL, and positive staining for cyclin D1 and SOX11 is valuable when flow cytometry immunophenotyping is not available. **B,** This image is from a different case demonstrating positive SOX11 staining in MCL.

Table 55-2 Histologic Features of Non-Hodgkin Lymphomas Involving Bone Marrow

Type of Lymphoma	Incidence of Involvement	Pattern of Involvement*	Cytology	Comments
Chronic lymphocytic leukemia/Small lymphocytic lymphoma (CLL/SLL)	85%	Focal random Diffuse Interstitial	Small, mature lymphocytes; proliferation centers may be present	Paratrabecular infiltrates indicate lymphoma of non-CLL/SLL type; proliferation centers may be present; positive for LEF1 and negative for cyclin D1 and SOX11; typical immunophenotypic profile in majority of cases
Lymphoplasmacytic lymphoma	80%–100%	Focal random Focal paratrabecular Interstitial Diffuse	Spectrum of cells including small lymphocytes, plasmacytoid lymphocytes, and plasma cells in variable proportions; Dutcher bodies are often present	Paratrabecular infiltrates may be present; plasma cells and plasmacytoid cells show the same light chain restriction as the B cells; serum IgM (rarely IgG) paraprotein; positive for *MYD88* L265P mutation
Mantle cell lymphoma	60%–90%	Focal random Interstitial Diffuse Focal paratrabecular	Small lymphocytes with irregular nuclei; may be blastoid or pleomorphic; rare cells with prominent nucleoli	Paratrabecular infiltrates may be present; circulating lymphoma cells may be present; positive for cyclin D1 and SOX11 and negative for LEF1 except for the indolent type (cyclin D1 positive, SOX11 negative)
Follicular lymphoma	Grade 1–2: 50%–70%; Grade 3: 15%–25%	Paratrabecular Focal random Diffuse Interstitial	Small cleaved lymphocytes usually predominate; large cleaved or noncleaved cells may be present	Distinct paratrabecular infiltrates are common; neoplastic follicles may be present; CD10 and BCL6 positivity in the lymphoma cells is lower in the bone marrow than in the lymph node; discordance in histologic types occurs in some cases, often with low-grade FL in the bone marrow and DLBCL in the extramedullary site
Splenic marginal zone lymphoma	100%	Intrasinusoidal Interstitial Focal random Diffuse	Small lymphocytes with slightly irregular nuclei, condensed chromatin, and moderate amounts of cytoplasm; variable plasmacytic differentiation	Intrasinusoidal infiltration is common; reactive germinal centers may be present; "villous lymphocytes" may be present in the blood smears; del(7q) in up to 40% of cases
Extranodal marginal zone lymphoma of mucosa-associated lymphoid tissue (MALT lymphoma)	5%–44%	Focal random Focal paratrabecular Interstitial Intrasinusoidal	Small lymphocytes with condensed chromatin and scant to moderate amounts of cytoplasm; occasional scattered large cells may be present	Extent of bone marrow infiltration usually minimal; overt blood involvement is uncommon

Continued

Table 55-2 Histologic Features of Non-Hodgkin Lymphomas Involving Bone Marrow—cont'd

Type of Lymphoma	Incidence of Involvement	Pattern of Involvement*	Cytology	Comments
Nodal marginal zone lymphoma	30%–50%	Focal random Interstitial Focal paratrabecular	Small cells with condensed chromatin and scant to moderate amounts of cytoplasm	
Diffuse large B-cell lymphoma	Common type: 10%–30%; Double-hit: 40%–90%	Focal random Paratrabecular Diffuse	Large cells with irregular nuclei, distinct or prominent nucleoli	Lymphomatous infiltrates can be heterogeneous with prominent T cells in T-cell/histiocyte-rich large B-cell lymphoma; immunohistochemistry for B-cell markers is essential in identifying the large B cells; rare cases of large cell lymphoma are intravascular
Burkitt lymphoma	30%–60%	Interstitial Diffuse	Medium-sized cells with reticular chromatin, multiple small nucleoli, and basophilic cytoplasm; cytoplasmic vacuoles are common	*MYC* gene rearrangement positive; starry-sky pattern may be present in the marrow; frequent mitoses and necrosis are common
Peripheral T-cell lymphoma, NOS	20%–40%	Focal random Diffuse	Polymorphous lymphoid population; nuclei are often hyperchromatic and irregular; large cells with nucleoli may be present; prominent reactive cell component may intermixed with lymphoma cells	Vascularity and reticulin fibrosis are often prominent
Anaplastic large cell lymphoma	10%–30%	Focal random Interstitial with scattered cells Diffuse	Large cells with horse shoe-shaped nuclei and abundant cytoplasm (hallmark cells)	Detection rate is higher with immunohistochemical staining for CD30 or ALK1
Hepatosplenic T-cell lymphoma	100%	Prominent intrasinusoidal infiltration Interstitial	Often medium-sized lymphocytes with cytologic atypia; may display blastic cytomorphology	Highly aggressive; lymphomatous infiltrates may be difficult to appreciate on H&E-stained slide; immunohistochemical staining for CD3 and cytotoxic proteins is helpful; typically TCRγδ+/CD3+/CD4−/CD8−/CD5−; a small subset of T-LGLL shows overlapping phenotype but different morphology; i7q is common in HSTCL
T-follicular helper cell lymphoma, angioimmunoblastic type	50%–80%	Focal random Paratrabecular	Polymorphous infiltrates; neoplastic cells with clear cytoplasm are uncommon	Positivity for CD10, BCL6, and CXCR13 is less common in the bone marrow than in the lymph node; EBER positive in majority cases; primary diagnosis based on the bone marrow findings alone is challenging
Extranodal NK/T-cell lymphoma	10%–20%	Interstitial, often with scattered single cells	Variably sized tumor cells or a mixture	CD56 and in situ hybridization for EBER help identify subtle bone marrow involvement

*The common patterns are listed; patterns may be mixed.
EBER, Epstein-Barr virus–encoded RNA; *HSTCL,* hepatosplenic T-cell lymphoma; *NK,* natural killer; *NOS,* not otherwise specified; *T-LGLL,* T-cell large granular lymphocytic leukemia.

positive staining for CD200 by flow cytometry helps distinguish CLL/SLL from MCL; however, it does not help the differential diagnosis between CLL/SLL from other B-cell lymphoproliferative disorders.[52] The nuclear overexpression of lymphoid-enhancer-binding factor 1 (LEF1) has also been found to be highly associated with CLL/SLL among small B-cell lymphomas and serves as a reliable immunohistochemical marker to differentiate CLL/SLL from other small B-cell lymphomas, including MCL and CD5-positive MZL (Fig. 55-12).[53-56] Care must be taken in interpreting cases with frequently admixed T cells, as LEF1 is normally expressed in the T cells.

Lymphoplasmacytic Lymphoma and Waldenström Macroglobulinemia

LPL is a B-cell neoplasm that commonly involves the bone marrow and, less frequently, lymph nodes. Most LPLs in the bone marrow represent Waldenström macroglobulinemia (WM), which is defined as LPL with bone marrow involvement and a serum IgM monoclonal protein of any concentration.[57,58] LPL infiltration in the bone marrow is commonly in a mixed pattern including focal random, paratrabecular, interstitial, or diffuse.[57,59] The infiltrates of LPL/WM consist of small lymphocytes, plasmacytoid lymphocytes, and

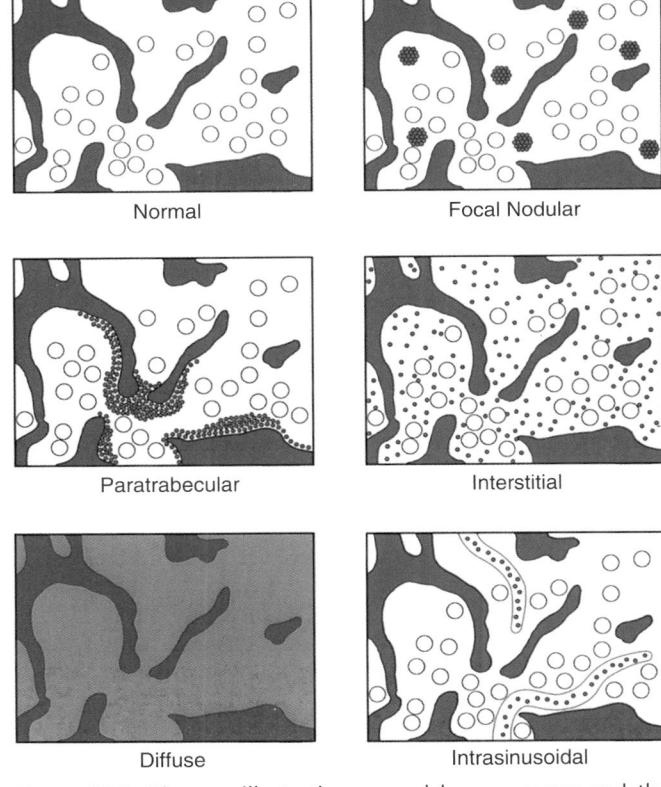

Figure 55-9. Diagram illustrating normal bone marrow and the five patterns of infiltration by lymphoma.

plasma cells at variable proportions (Fig. 55-13). The plasmacytoid lymphocytes are usually in the minority and may be inconspicuous. The number of plasma cells varies considerably, and they are usually a small component of the infiltrate but can be predominant in some cases. The plasma cells are often admixed within the neoplastic lymphoid infiltrate but are occasionally present as small clusters away from the lymphoid aggregates.[60] Intranuclear inclusions (Dutcher bodies) are often identified in the plasma cells (Fig. 55-13). Transformed lymphocytes with distinct nucleoli may be present, but are usually low in number. Additionally, mast cells and histiocytes are often increased in the bone marrow involved by LPL. The bone marrow aspirate contains lymphoma cells similar to those in the bone marrow core biopsy; peripheral blood may also be involved, but an absolute lymphocytosis is uncommon.[57,61]

LPL is typically CD19+, CD20+, CD23−, CD5−, CD10−, CD103−, surface IgM+, and surface immunoglobulin light chain–restricted, but expression of CD5 or CD23 may be observed in some cases.[57]

LPL/WM should be distinguished from other B-cell neoplasms with plasmacytic differentiation, such as SMZL. LPL may also mimic plasma cell myeloma when the plasma cell component predominates. The presence of both monotypic B cells and plasma cells with the same light chain restriction, lack of other atypical phenotype in the plasma cells (e.g., CD19 negative, CD56 positive), as well as other clinical and laboratory features such as a serum IgM paraprotein, hyperviscosity, lack of lytic bone lesions, and presence of lymphadenopathy, help distinguish LPL from plasma cell

myeloma. The distinction between LPL and SMZL in the bone marrow can be problematic because they share morphologic and immunophenotypic features and occasionally also clinical features.[62] LPL predominantly involves the bone marrow, but may also involve the lymph node or spleen in some cases. SMZL typically exhibits prominent splenomegaly and almost always involves blood and bone marrow, but peripheral lymph nodes are typically not involved. The most distinguishing features of LPL from SMZL in the bone marrow have been reported to include paratrabecular involvement, the presence of lymphoplasmacytic cells, Dutcher bodies, and increased numbers of mast cells,[59] while prominent intrasinusoidal infiltration and reactive germinal centers are more characteristic for SMZL.[63] However, the practical use of these distinguishing features may still be problematic when applied to an individual case.

There are no specific chromosomal abnormalities recognized in LPL.[57] The *MYD88* L265P mutation has been identified in over 90% of patients with LPL/WM; this mutation is uncommon in other B-cell lymphomas, including SMZL. Although not entirely specific, demonstration of *MYD88* L265P mutation is a valuable adjunct in the diagnosis of LPL/WM.[64]

Marginal Zone Lymphoma

MZL arises from post–germinal center B cells and consists of three distinct diseases: splenic MZL (SMZL), nodal MZL (NMZL), and extranodal MZL of mucosa-associated lymphoid tissue (MALT lymphoma).[65,66]

Splenic Marginal Zone Lymphoma

SMZL is an indolent B-cell lymphoma that typically presents with splenomegaly without lymphadenopathy. Patients may have a small monoclonal serum protein; however, marked hypergammaglobulinemia and hyperviscosity are uncommon.[65,66] SMZL involves the bone marrow and blood in nearly all cases, and the diagnosis is usually made based on the findings of the peripheral blood and bone marrow. The neoplastic cells of SMZL are small-to-medium-sized, with round to slightly irregular nuclei, condensed chromatin, and moderate amounts of pale-blue cytoplasm. Rare large lymphocytes with vesicular nuclei and visible nucleoli, as well as plasmacytoid cells with or without Dutcher bodies, may be admixed among the small neoplastic lymphocytes. Although an absolute lymphocytosis is not a constant feature, neoplastic lymphocytes can often be identified in the blood smears and may show short, polar villi on the cell surface in some cases.

SMZL infiltrates the bone marrow in one or more of the following patterns: intrasinusoidal, interstitial, focal random, and focal paratrabecular; diffuse involvement is uncommon. Intrasinusoidal infiltration is present in the majority of patients, often as one to a few layers of lymphocytes within the sinusoids (Fig. 55-14). This pattern of infiltration is difficult to appreciate on H&E-stained sections but can be highlighted by immunohistochemical staining for B-cell markers. Intrasinusoidal infiltration is not entirely specific for SMZL and may be seen, although often more subtly, in other B-cell lymphomas. Additionally, the presence of reactive germinal centers associated with the neoplastic infiltrate is a feature observed in about 30% of SMZL (Fig. 55-15).[63] Immunohistochemical staining for CD21 or CD23 can be

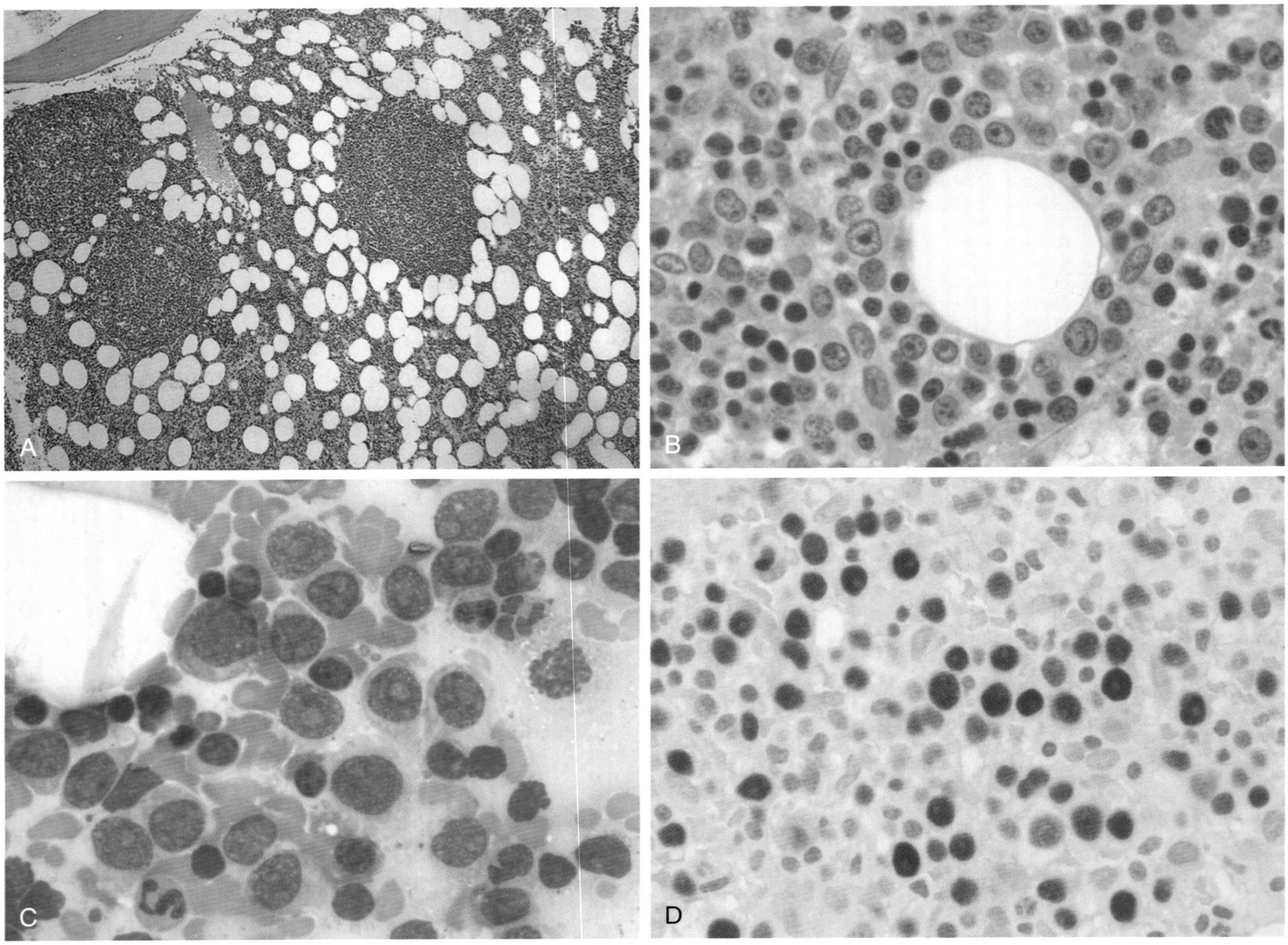

Figure 55-10. Chronic lymphocytic leukemia/small lymphocytic lymphoma in bone marrow core biopsy. A, Three focal nodular lymphoid infiltrates and interstitial infiltrates are demonstrated in this bone marrow core biopsy section. **B,** Increased numbers of large cells are admixed with the background small lymphocytes. The large cells have prominent nucleoli. **C,** The bone marrow aspirate smear of the same case shows prolymphocytes with centrally located, prominent nucleoli admixed with scattered small chronic lymphocytic leukemia (CLL) cells. **D,** Strong p53 staining is seen in the prolymphocytes in a patient with prolymphocytic transformation of preexisting CLL.

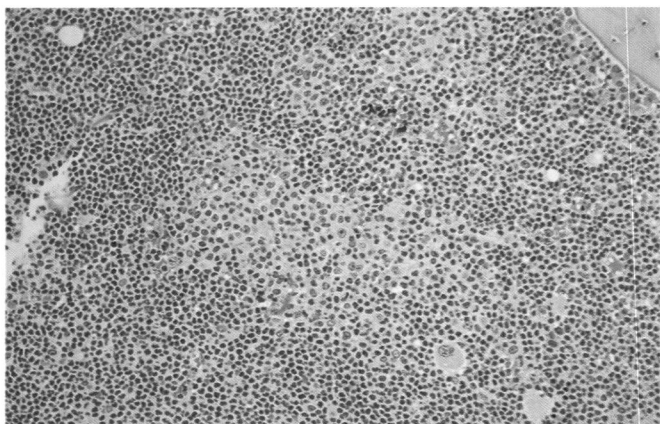

Figure 55-11. Proliferation centers of chronic lymphocytic leukemia/small lymphocytic lymphoma (CLL/SLL) in a bone marrow core biopsy. A proliferation center, an ill-defined pale area in the center of the image, in a background of small CLL cells. Proliferation centers contain prolymphocytes with an ample amount of pale cytoplasm and prominent central nucleoli.

used to highlight the follicular dendritic cell meshwork to confirm the germinal center nature of the lymphoid follicles. These reactive germinal centers should not be confused with foci of large cell transformation or neoplastic germinal centers in FL.

SMZL exhibits a "non-specific" immunophenotype, (i.e., CD19+, CD20+, CD5−, CD10−, CD23−, and surface immunoglobulin light chain restriction. This phenotype overlaps with several other B-cell lymphomas, including NMZL and LPL. Additionally, CD5 is positive in 5% to 10% of cases, CD11c and CD103 in a minority of cases, and CD25 is generally negative.[67-70]

The main differential diagnosis of SMZL in the bone marrow includes SDRPSBCL,[19] LPL, NMZL, and MALT lymphoma. Although the pattern of splenic involvement is distinct between SMZL (white pulp involvement) and SDRPSBCL (diffuse red pulp involvement), separating these two entities on the basis of a bone marrow biopsy is difficult because of overlapping bone marrow histology, immunophenotype, and clinical features. Similar to

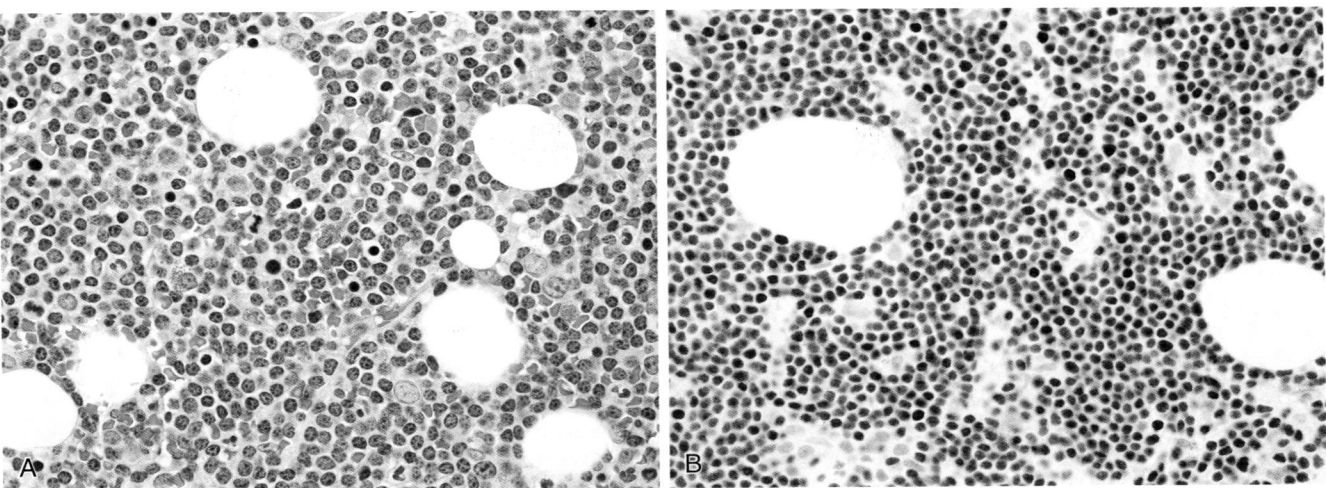

Figure 55-12. Chronic lymphocytic leukemia/small lymphocytic lymphoma (CLL/SLL) is positive for lymphoid-enhancer-binding factor 1 (LEF1). A, CLL/SLL infiltrates in the bone marrow core biopsy. **B,** Immunohistochemical staining shows strong nuclear staining for LEF1 in CLL/SLL cells.

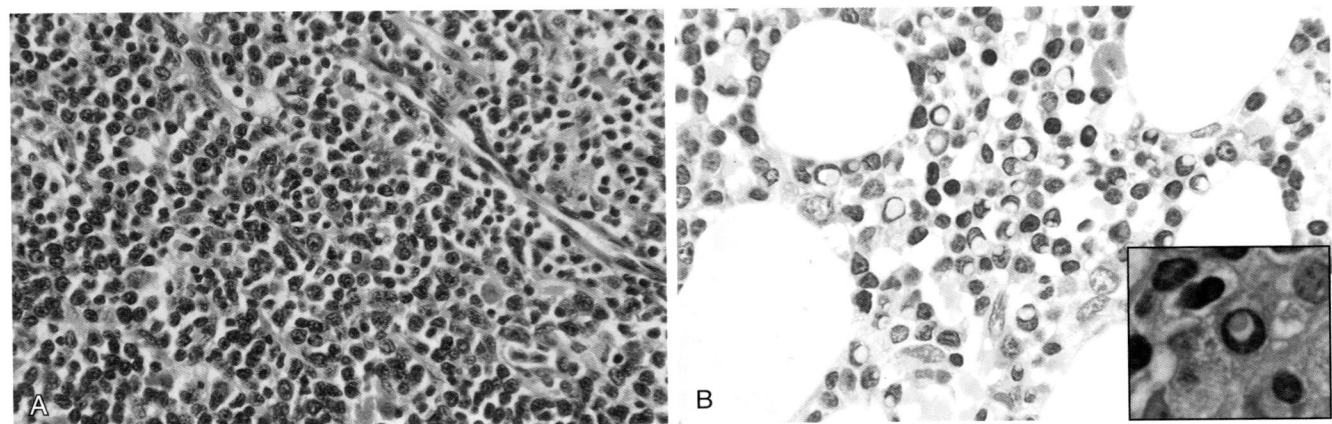

Figure 55-13. Lymphoplasmacytic lymphoma in a bone marrow core biopsy. A, The infiltrate is dense and contains small lymphocytes, plasmacytoid lymphocytes and plasma cells. **B,** Intranuclear inclusions (Dutcher bodies; *inset*) in the plasma cells are evident in this case.

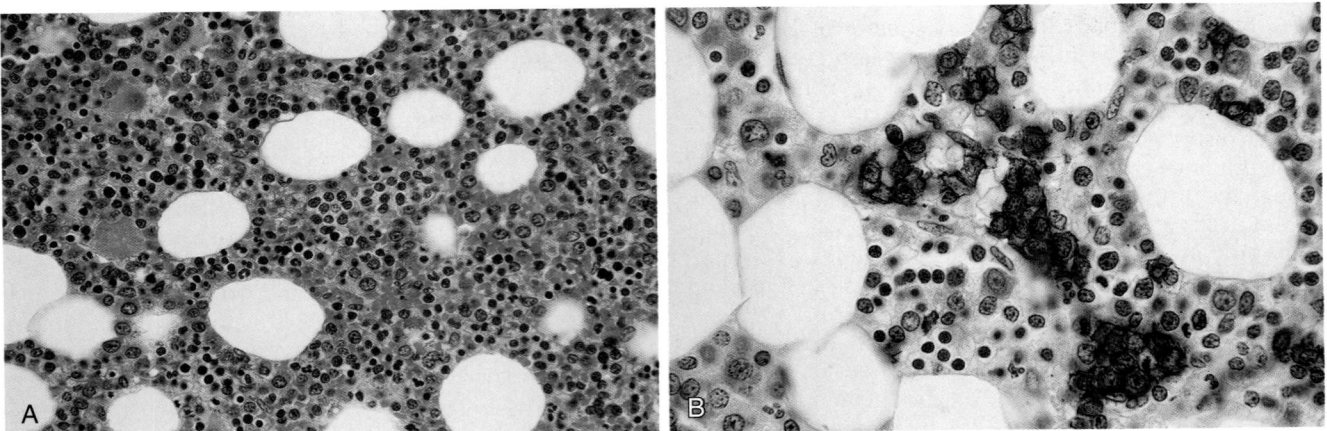

Figure 55-14. Splenic marginal zone lymphoma in a bone marrow core biopsy. A, The infiltrate blends in with the normal hematopoietic elements and is difficult to identify on the H&E-stained section in this case. **B,** Immunohistochemical staining for CD20 highlights the lymphoma cells with focal intrasinusoidal infiltration.

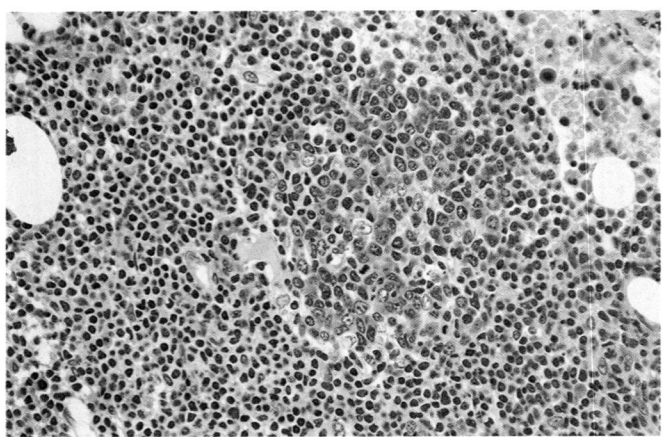

Figure 55-15. Splenic marginal zone lymphoma in a bone marrow core biopsy. Most of the lymphoma cells are small, with slightly irregular nuclei. A reactive germinal center is present in the neoplastic infiltrate.

SMZL, SDRPSBCL uniformly involves the bone marrow, frequently in intrasinusoidal and interstitial patterns. It has been suggested that an exclusive intrasinusoidal infiltration favors SDRPSBCL over MZL.[71] The distinction between SMZL and LPL has been discussed previously under "Lymphoplasmacytic Lymphoma and Waldenström Macroglobulinemia." SMZL also shares similar morphologic features with NMZL in the bone marrow, but intrasinusoidal infiltration is more prominent and reactive germinal centers are more frequent in SMZL than NMZL. Correlation with clinical features is important as SMZL does not involve peripheral lymph nodes or extranodal sites, in contrast to NMZL, and is often associated with HCV, as well as a small paraprotein, and hence testing may be appropriate in suspected SMZL.[72]

When villous lymphocytes are present in the blood smears or expression of CD103 or CD11c is seen in the neoplastic lymphocytes, HCL may come into the differential diagnosis. However, HCL typically shows interstitial or diffuse marrow infiltration and lacks prominent intrasinusoidal infiltration. The unique immunophenotype of HCL (i.e., increased side scatter, bright CD20 staining, and co-expression of CD103, CD11c, and CD25) usually easily discriminates HCL from SMZL. In questionable cases, demonstration of annexin-1, CD123, CD200, or cyclin D1 in the neoplastic cell by flow cytometric or immunohistochemical studies, or the presence of a *BRAF* V600E mutation, supports a diagnosis of HCL.[73-75] However, distinction of SMZL from HCL variant based on bone marrow findings can be difficult and sometimes impossible, although the distinction is prognostically relevant.[76]

SMZL lacks a characteristic genetic abnormality although the majority of cases harbor genomic aberrations.[77] Deletion of chromosome 7q31-32, a common abnormality in myeloid neoplasm, has been identified in up to 40% of patients with SMZL and is rarely seen in other types of lymphoma. Recurrent mutations in SMZL include *NOTCH2* mutations in up to 25% and *KLF2* mutations in up to 40% of patients, and these mutations are uncommon in other B-cell lymphomas.[78,79] More recent data indicate two distinct genetic clusters in SMZL: the NNK group (harboring *NF-κB, NOTCH,* and *KLF* mutations) and the DMT groups (harboring mutations in genes related to DNA damage response, MAPK and TLR), and NNK group has inferior survival.[80]

Nodal Marginal Zone Lymphoma

Bone marrow involvement by NMZL has been reported in about 30% to 50% of cases. Focal random or interstitial infiltration is relatively common; paratrabecular infiltration occurs less frequently, and diffuse infiltration is rare.[81-83] The neoplastic infiltrates include small centrocyte-like cells with irregular nuclei, condensed chromatin, and scant cytoplasm; plasma cells or plasmacytoid cells may be intermixed in variable numbers. NMZL only occasionally involves the peripheral blood; the cytology of the circulating lymphoma cells is similar to that observed in bone marrow specimens.

Extranodal Marginal Zone Lymphoma of Mucosa-Associated Lymphoid Tissue

MALT lymphoma typically involves the gastrointestinal tract and is usually localized at diagnosis. Salivary gland, lung, thyroid, and conjunctiva are other commonly involved sites. When dissemination occurs, MALT lymphoma preferentially spreads to other mucosal sites. The incidence of bone marrow involvement varies in the reports, ranging from 5% to 44%.[84,85] Most bone marrow infiltrates are focal random, although paratrabecular, interstitial, or intrasinusoidal infiltration may also occur. The extent of bone marrow involvement is variable but usually low. The infiltrates of MALT lymphoma in the bone marrow include a spectrum of cells, ranging from small lymphocytes with condensed chromatin to slightly larger lymphocytes with irregular nuclei and ample cytoplasm; admixed plasma cells may also be present. Overt peripheral blood involvement by MALT lymphoma is uncommon.

Follicular Lymphoma

Low-grade (grades 1–2) FL involves the bone marrow at a higher frequency (50%–70%) than high-grade (grade 3) FL (15%–25%).[86,87] Distinct paratrabecular infiltration is the morphologic characteristic of FL in the bone marrow (Fig. 55-16), and can be identified, at least focally, in greater than 90% of cases; exclusively, paratrabecular infiltration also occurs.[9,17] Focal random infiltration is the most common pattern accompanying the paratrabecular lesions; diffuse and interstitial infiltration are less frequent and occur in 5% to 10% of cases.[9,14] A follicular growth pattern in the bone marrow is uncommon, accounting for less than 5% of cases (Fig. 55-17). Similar to a lymph node, the follicular dendritic cell meshwork within the follicles can be highlighted by immunohistochemical staining for CD21 or CD23, and the neoplastic nature of the follicles can often be confirmed by positive staining for BCL2.[88] The bone marrow infiltrates are most frequently composed of small lymphocytes with condensed chromatin patterns and irregularly shaped nuclei (centrocytes). Large lymphocytes with prominent nucleoli (centroblasts) may be present, but usually are fewer in number. The lymphoma cells in the bone marrow aspirate smears are typically small-to-medium-sized with a deep nuclear cleft; similar cells are occasionally identified in the peripheral blood smear but are usually few in number. In a minority of cases, FL presents with an absolute lymphocytosis, and rarely, the lymphocytosis is marked (Fig. 55-18).[89] Rare FL may undergo

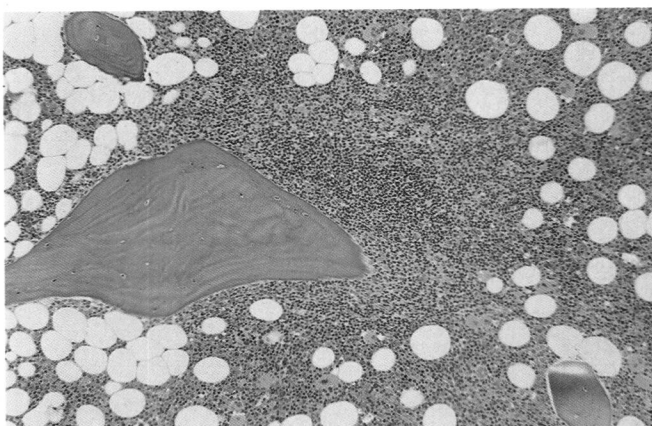

Figure 55-16. Follicular lymphoma with paratrabecular infiltration. The paratrabecular lymphoid infiltrates "hug" the bone and conform to its contour.

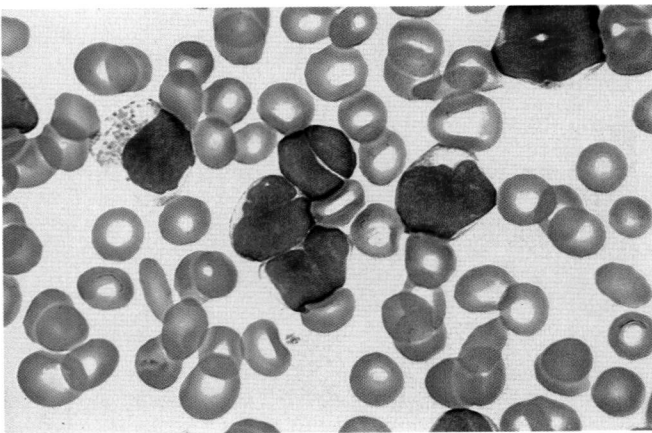

Figure 55-18. Follicular lymphoma cells in peripheral blood. The lymphoma cells are slightly larger than normal lymphocytes, and have slightly dispersed chromatin and deeply cleaved nuclei.

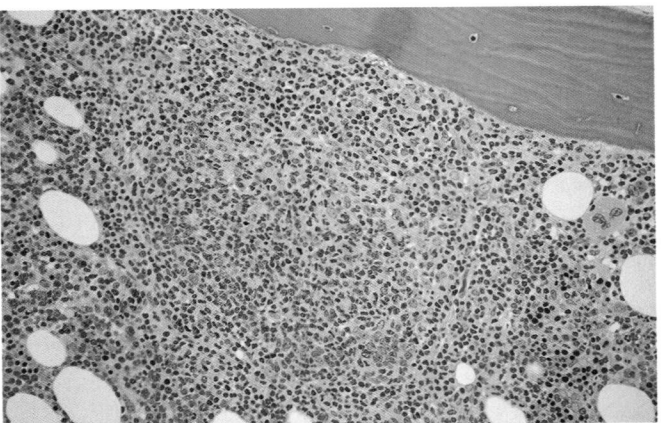

Figure 55-17. Follicular lymphoma with a follicular growth pattern. In this bone marrow core biopsy, the infiltrate is paratrabecular and contains a neoplastic follicle.

blastoid transformation and morphologically mimic acute lymphoblastic leukemia.[90-92] In these cases, flow cytometric analysis is important to make the distinction.

The classical immunophenotype of FL includes CD19+, CD20+, CD5-, CD10+, BCL6+, and BCL2+ with surface immunoglobulin light chain restriction. In the right morphologic context, identification of a CD10-positive monotypic B-cell population by flow cytometry, demonstration of CD10, or BCL6 expression support a diagnosis of FL. BCL2 is often positive in low-grade FL, but it should be interpreted in an architectural context because other types of small B-cell lymphomas frequently express BCL2.[93] It is noted that the frequency of CD10 positivity in the FL is lower in the bone marrow (~50%–60%) and peripheral blood (~40%) than in the primary site (~85%–95%) by both immunohistochemical and flow cytometric analysis.[93,94] Thus, CD10 negativity does not exclude FL, and a panel of immunohistochemical stains may be required for an accurate subclassification of lymphoma in the bone marrow. Additionally, flow cytometry may fail to identify a monotypic B-cell population when FL is exclusively paratrabecular, likely because of the difficulty in aspirating these cells in the paratrabecular location.

Distinguishing FL from other small B-cell lymphomas does not generally pose a diagnostic challenge because the majority cases demonstrate at least focal distinct paratrabecular infiltration. However, it is worth noting that paratrabecular infiltrate is not diagnostic for FL; for example, MCL may occasionally show prominent or rarely exclusive paratrabecular infiltration (see discussion in "Mantle Cell Lymphoma"). Caution should also be taken in the evaluation of post-therapy bone marrow from patients with FL because in some effectively treated patients the paratrabecular lymphoid aggregates are composed entirely of T cells that architecturally mimic residual FL (Fig. 55-6). Additionally, discordant histologic subtypes of lymphoma between the bone marrow and the extramedullary site occurs. In the majority of the cases, the bone marrow is involved by a low-grade FL, whereas the extramedullary site has a higher-grade FL or DLBCL (Fig. 55-19). It has been reported that patients with nodal DLBCL and discordant, low-grade FL in the bone marrow have more favorable prognosis than patients with concurrent large B-cell involving the marrow.[9,14,95] Additionally, discordant morphology may also occur between bilateral bone marrow core biopsies in rare cases (Fig. 55-20).

Mantle Cell Lymphoma

MCL involves the bone marrow in 60% to 90% of cases.[43,82,96-98] The most common pattern of marrow involvement is focal random and is seen in over 80% of cases; interstitial and diffuse infiltration are present in about 50% and 20% to 30% of cases, respectively.[43,99] Notably, paratrabecular infiltration occurs in up to 45% of patients; occasionally, the infiltrate may be exclusively paratrabecular, resembling FL (Fig. 55-21).[43,99] Rare cases with prominent intrasinusoidal infiltration have also been reported.[100] The lymphoma cells can exhibit a heterogeneous morphology, but in most cases, there is a uniform population of small-to-medium-sized lymphocytes with condensed chromatin and irregularly shaped nuclei. Occasionally the lymphoma cells are predominantly small with round nuclei and clumped chromatin, resembling CLL/SLL. The blastoid variant of MCL may mimic acute lymphoblastic leukemia in the peripheral blood and bone marrow (Fig. 55-22), and the pleomorphic

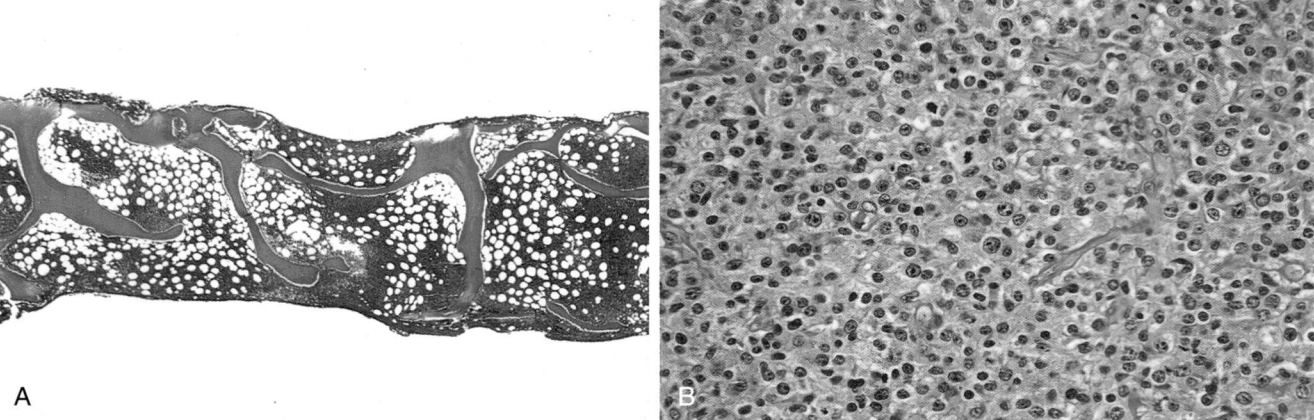

Figure 55-19. Diffuse large B-cell lymphoma with discordant morphology between lymph node and bone marrow. A, The bone marrow core biopsy contains several paratrabecular lymphoid aggregates composed of small lymphocytes. **B,** The lymph node biopsy shows diffuse large B-cell lymphoma.

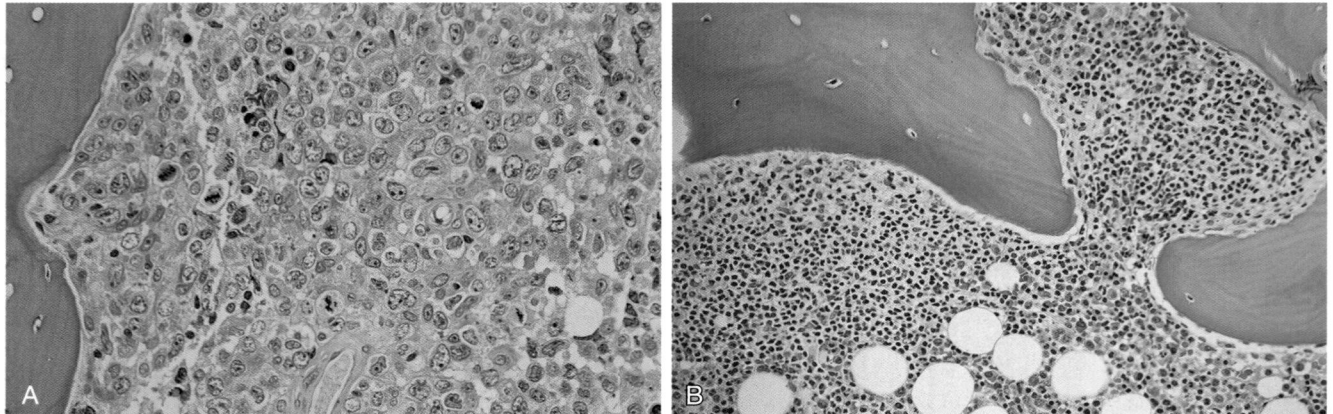

Figure 55-20. Lymphoma with discordant morphology in bilateral bone marrow core biopsies. A, Large B-cell lymphoma in the *right-sided* bone marrow core biopsy. **B,** Low-grade follicular lymphoma in the *left-sided* core biopsy. This patient has follicular lymphoma and diffuse large B-cell lymphoma in a lymph node biopsy.

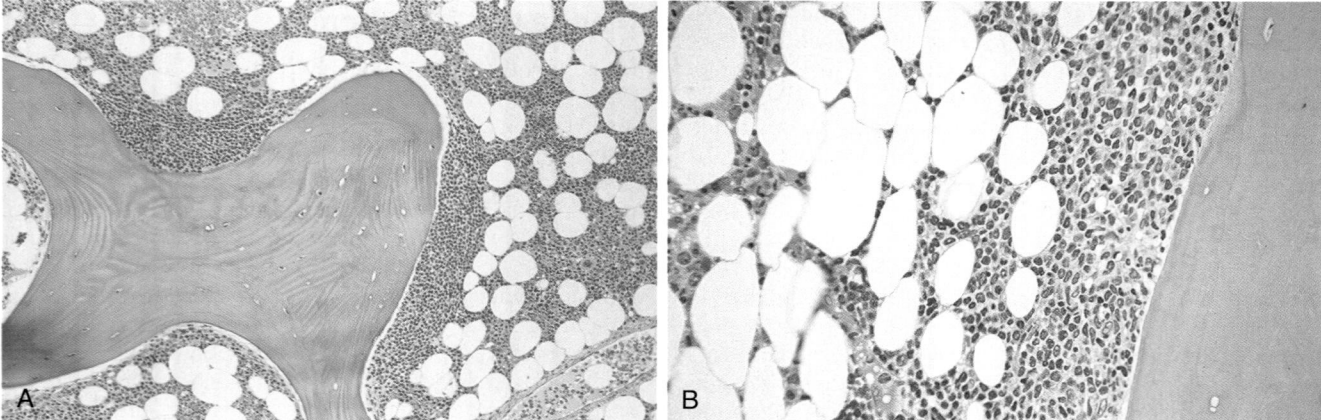

Figure 55-21. Mantle cell lymphoma with paratrabecular infiltration. A, The lymphomatous infiltrates are exclusively paratrabecular in this case. **B,** The lymphoma cells are small-to-medium-sized with condensed chromatin and round to irregular nuclei.

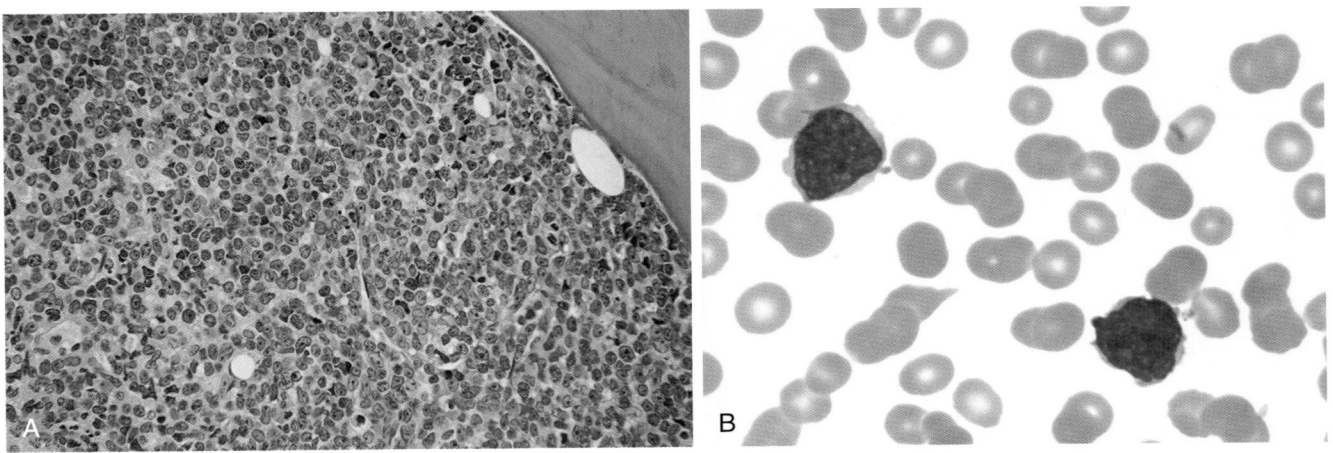

Figure 55-22. Mantle cell lymphoma, blastoid variant, in the bone marrow and peripheral blood. A, The infiltrate in the bone marrow core biopsy displays a diffuse infiltrative pattern and contains medium-to-large-sized cells with dispersed chromatin and one or more visible nucleoli. **B,** A blastoid lymphoma cell with cleaved nucleus, slightly dispersed chromatin, and scant cytoplasm is present in the peripheral blood.

variant of MCL resembles large B-cell lymphoma.[101,102] These variant MCLs tend to show interstitial or diffuse infiltration in the bone marrow.[101]

Circulating lymphoma cells are common in MCL, and can be identified by morphologic evaluation of the peripheral blood smears in about 35% to 80% of patients.[43,82,97,99] An absolute lymphocytosis is present in up to 28% of patients.[43,96] MCL cells show a spectrum of cytologic appearance in the blood smear, and can be confused with other types of lymphoma. They may be small with round nuclei, resembling CLL/SLL; small-to-medium-sized with cleaved nuclei, mimicking FL; or medium-to-large-sized with a central prominent nucleolus, resembling prolymphocytic leukemia (Fig. 55-23). A clinically indolent variant of MCL has been recognized, primarily characterized by a leukemic presentation with no or minimal nodal involvement and demonstrating morphologic features similar to CLL/SLL. In contrast to classical MCL, the indolent MCL is often positive for cyclin D1 but negative for SOX11 and harbors a mutated IGVH gene, indicating a post–germinal center origin.[103-105]

MCL and CLL/SLL are the two major CD5-positive small B-cell lymphomas that may display overlapping morphologic and immunophenotypic features. The presence of proliferation centers essentially rules out MCL, while distinct paratrabecular infiltration can occur in MCL but is absent in CLL/SLL. MCL is immunophenotypically characterized by bright CD20 and surface immunoglobulin light chain staining and is commonly CD23-, CD79b+, FMC7+, and CD200-, whereas CLL/SLL typically demonstrates dim CD20 and surface immunoglobulin light chain staining and is CD23+, CD79b-, FMC7-, and CD200+. However, variations in phenotype occur in MCL, including negative staining for CD5 and overlapping immunophenotype with CLL in the expression of CD23 and FMC7; rarely, MCL may express CD10.[106] Therefore, a diagnosis of MCL should not be solely based on the flow cytometric results.[107,108]

Overexpression of cyclin D1 (BCL1) serves as a convenient immunohistochemical marker for diagnosis of MCL. When immunohistochemical staining is equivocal, fluorescence in situ hybridization (FISH) analysis for t(11;14)-*CCND1/IGH*

may be required for confirmation (Fig. 55-24). It is worth mentioning that cyclin D1 is not exclusively overexpressed by MCL, as a majority of HCL and a subset of plasma cell myeloma are also positive for cyclin D1. Fortunately, these two diseases rarely enter into the differential diagnosis of MCL because of their distinct clinicopathologic features. SOX11 has been shown to be highly specific for MCL, and serves as an additional marker for MCL (Fig. 55-8).[109,110] It is particularly useful in the diagnosis of cyclin D1-negative MCL.[111,112] However, the indolent variant of MCL may lack overexpression of SOX11.[105,113] When used in combination, immunohistochemical stains for cyclin D1, SOX11, and LEF1 (discussed earlier in CLL/SLL) provide highly effective adjunct in diagnosis and differential diagnosis of small B-cell lymphomas.

Diffuse Large B-Cell Lymphoma

DLBCL is a heterogeneous group of tumors in terms of clinical, morphologic, and genetic features.[114] DLBCL, in general, infiltrates the bone marrow in about 10% to 30% of cases.[42,115-117] However, cases with both *MYC* and *BCL2* or *BCL6* gene rearrangement have a higher incidence of bone marrow involvement, ranging from 42% to 93%.[118-121] Focal random, diffuse, and mixed patterns of infiltration are common; paratrabecular infiltration occurs occasionally; and interstitial infiltration is uncommon.[9,17,122] The neoplastic cells may demonstrate a wide range of morphology but are typically large with one or more prominent nucleoli. DLBCL infiltrate is usually easily identified on H&E-stained bone marrow sections (Fig. 55-25). The aspirates or touch imprints occasionally contain lymphoma cells (Fig. 55-25). Peripheral blood involvement is uncommon but does occur.

As mentioned earlier, in approximately 20% to 45% of patients with DLBCL, the bone marrow and extramedullary site show discordant histology subtype, often characterized by a low-grade lymphoma, most commonly FL, in the bone marrow and DLBCL in the extramedullary site (Fig. 55-19).[9,42,116,117,122]

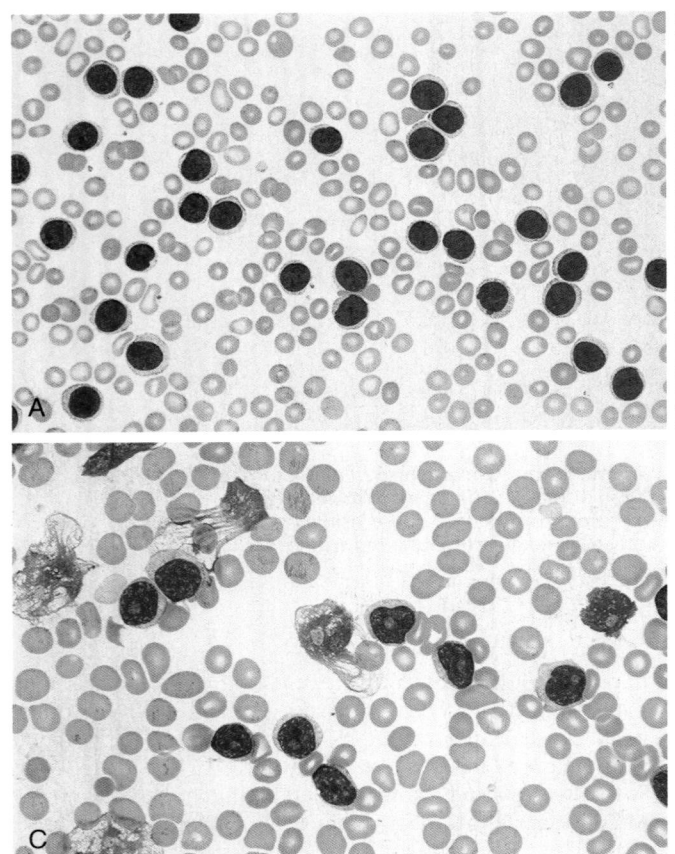

Figure 55-23. Leukemic phase of mantle cell lymphoma mimicking chronic lymphocytic leukemia (CLL) or prolymphocytic leukemia (PLL). A, The blood smear shows an absolute lymphocytosis (66 × 10⁹/L). The lymphoma cells are small with round or slightly irregular nuclei, condensed chromatin and scant cytoplasm that closely resemble CLL cells. **B,** This case shows an absolute lymphocytosis (134 × 10⁹/L) composed of variably sized lymphoma cells. Some cells are small with condensed chromatin, and others are medium-sized with slightly dispersed chromatin and prominent, central nucleolus, resembling CLL/PLL. **C,** The lymphoma cells in this case are medium-to-large-sized with ample cytoplasm, condensed chromatin, and a prominent central nucleolus, resembling PLL.

Molecular analysis of IGH or *BCL2* gene rearrangements in 16 discordant cases revealed that in two-thirds of the patients, the low-grade lymphoma in the marrow was clonally related to the DLBCL in the primary site, while in the remaining one-third of the patients, the two lymphoma subtypes were clonally unrelated.[123] It has been reported that patients with DLBCL who have a discordant, low-grade lymphoma in the bone marrow have an overall treatment response and survival similar to those without marrow involvement, but patients with concordant DLBCL in the bone marrow have a lower overall survival, and lower progression-free and disease-free survivals.[116,117,124-127]

Immunophenotypically, DLBCL is highly heterogeneous; however, a diagnosis of DLBCL can generally be made based on the morphologic findings and documentation of B-cell lineage of the large cells, such as expression of CD20, CD79a, or PAX5. When CD5 is expressed, immunohistochemical staining for cyclin D1 or SOX11 should be performed to exclude the possibility of a variant MCL. Rarely, CD20 can be aberrantly expressed in peripheral T-cell lymphoma or CD3 in DLBCL[128,129]; therefore, using additional B-cell and T-cell markers is necessary in these cases to accurately determine the lineage of the lymphoma; in some cases, molecular analysis for B-cell or T-cell clonality may be required.

There are a number of clinicopathologically distinct large B-cell lymphomas, such as T cell/histiocyte-rich large B-cell lymphoma (THRLBCL), EBV-positive large B-cell lymphoma, and primary mediastinal large B-cell lymphoma (PMLBCL).[65,66] THRLBCL exhibits abundant reactive T cells and histiocytes but only scattered large neoplastic B cells.[130]

When involving the bone marrow, THRLBCL may be difficult to distinguish from reactive infiltrates or other lymphomas that often have heterogeneous cellular compositions, such as HL or peripheral T-cell lymphoma (Fig. 55-26). Multiple levels of bone marrow sections may be necessary to confirm the presence of abnormal large lymphocytes within the infiltrates, and a panel of immunohistochemical stains is often required for diagnosis. The scattered large, abnormal cells in THRBCL are positive for CD45 and CD20, but negative for CD30, CD15, and CD3, which helps exclude classic Hodgkin lymphoma (CHL) and peripheral T-cell lymphoma. EBV-encoded RNA (EBER) staining is necessary to exclude EBV-positive large B-cell lymphoma. In most cases, however, an extramedullary tissue biopsy is indicated except for cases of isolated splenic micronodular THRLBCL that frequently show isolated marrow involvement without adenopathy.[131] PMLBCL is a subtype of large B-cell lymphoma that arises in the mediastinum and has a female predominance.[132] Bone marrow involvement by PMLBCL has been reported in 2% to 9% of cases, but the characteristics of marrow infiltration have not been described in detail, although extramediastinal involvement has been documented.

Intravascular Large B-Cell Lymphoma

Intravascular large B-cell lymphoma (IVLBCL) is an uncommon variant of extranodal large B-cell lymphoma that is localized within the small blood vessels, particularly capillaries. It is usually widely disseminated in extranodal sites,

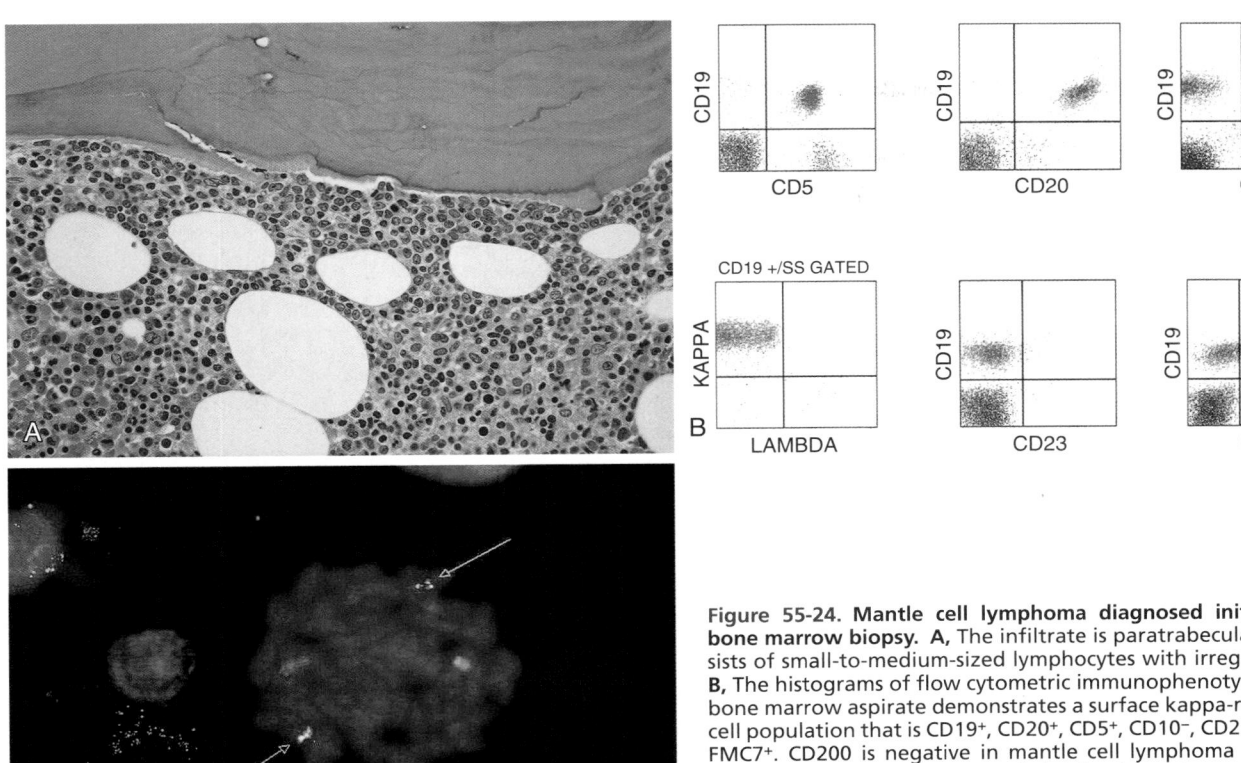

Figure 55-24. Mantle cell lymphoma diagnosed initially on a bone marrow biopsy. A, The infiltrate is paratrabecular and consists of small-to-medium-sized lymphocytes with irregular nuclei. **B,** The histograms of flow cytometric immunophenotyping of the bone marrow aspirate demonstrates a surface kappa-restricted B-cell population that is CD19+, CD20+, CD5+, CD10−, CD23−, and dim FMC7+. CD200 is negative in mantle cell lymphoma (MCL) (not shown). **C,** Fluorescence in situ hybridization using probes to the immunoglobulin heavy chain gene (IGH; *green*) and *CCND1* gene *(orange)* demonstrates a yellow fusion signal *(arrows)*, indicating t(11;14)-*CCND1::IGH* fusion. A subsequent lymph node biopsy confirmed the diagnosis of MCL. *(C, Courtesy of Dr. Gordon Dewald, Mayo Medical Laboratories, Rochester, MN.)*

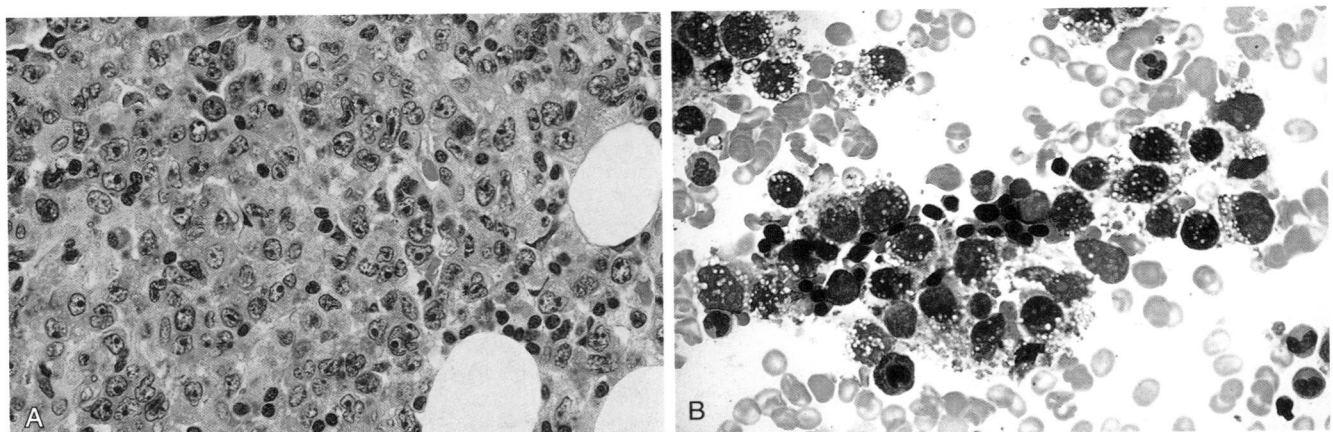

Figure 55-25. Diffuse large B-cell lymphoma in a bone marrow core biopsy and aspirate smear. A, Lymphoma cells in the bone marrow core biopsy are large with irregular nuclei, vesicular chromatin and distinct nucleoli. **B,** The lymphoma cells in the bone marrow aspirate contain cytoplasmic vacuoles in this case.

including bone marrow.[133-136] Because of the non-specific clinical features, bone marrow may be the initial diagnostic site for IVLBCL.[133,136] In a retrospective study of bone marrow biopsies performed for evaluation of fever of unknown origin or hemophagocytic syndrome, 12 of 146 (8.2%) patients were found to have IVLBCL in the bone marrow.[133] Morphologically, the neoplastic infiltrates in the marrow are predominantly confined to the sinusoids (Fig. 55-27); they may cause apparent distention of the sinusoids or may be subtle and difficult to appreciate on H&E-stained section. However, immunohistochemical staining for B-cell markers, such as CD20, CD79a, or PAX5, can highlight the lymphoma cells and delineate the intrasinusoidal pattern of infiltration (Fig. 55-27). IVLBCL exhibits heterogeneous immunophenotype

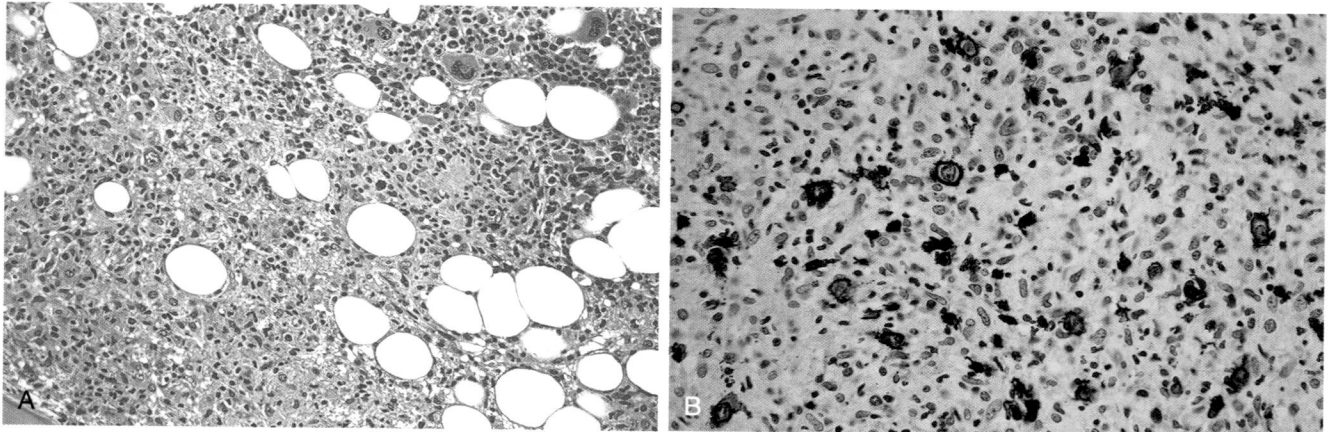

Figure 55-26. T-cell/histiocyte-rich large B-cell lymphoma involving the bone marrow. A, The infiltrate has poorly defined borders and contains many small lymphocytes, histiocytes, and scattered large, abnormal lymphocytes. **B,** Immunohistochemical staining for CD20 highlights the scattered large lymphoma cells. The majority of the cells are CD3-positive T cells (not shown). A micronodular pattern of involvement resembling nonnecrotizing granulomas may be seen in this lymphoma.

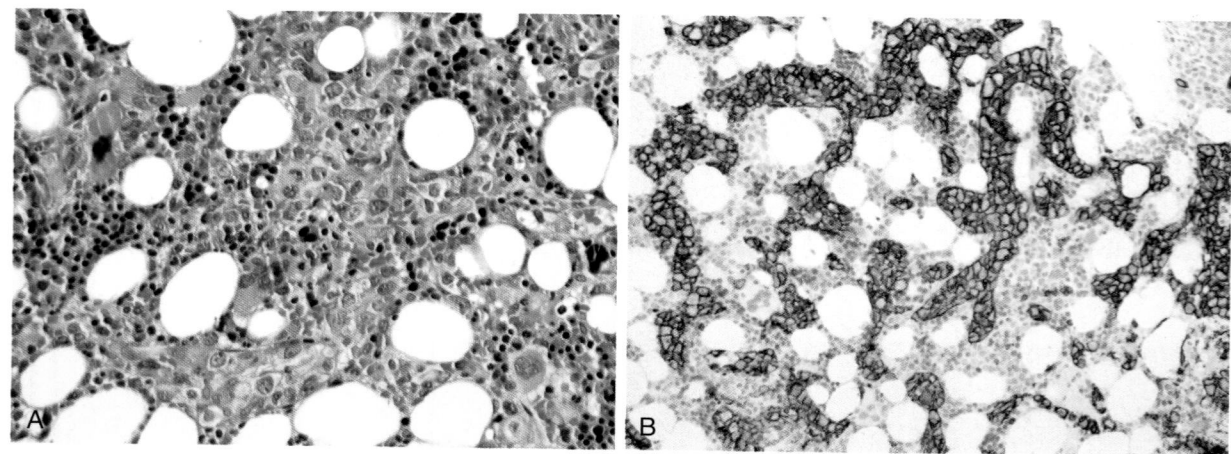

Figure 55-27. Intravascular large B-cell lymphoma in a bone marrow core biopsy. A, The lymphoma cells are present within the sinusoid, and can be missed in hematoxylin and eosin (H&E)-stained sections. **B,** Immunohistochemical staining for CD20 highlights the lymphoma cell in the sinusoids.

similar to other LBCLs; however, CD5 expression is reportedly more frequent than LBCLs in general.[133,136]

Primary Effusion Lymphoma

Primary effusion lymphoma (PEL) is a large B-cell lymphoma that most commonly occurs in HIV-infected patients, primarily involves body cavities, and presents as a lymphomatous effusion. Solid PEL occurring in extracavitary sites have also been reported.[137-139] PEL is universally associated with human herpesvirus 8 (HHV-8); EBV coinfection is common. Cytologically, the tumor cells may show plasmablastic, immunoblastic, or anaplastic appearance. Immunohistochemical staining to demonstrate HHV8 infection using antibody against HHV8-encoded latency-associated nuclear antigen (LANA) serves as a key diagnostic feature for PEL. PEL displays a phenotype of terminally differentiated B cells: positive for CD45, negative for pan B-cell markers, negative

for surface immunoglobulin, and positive for activation and plasma-cell associated markers (CD138, CD38, MUM-1, CD30, and EMA).[139,140] The data on bone marrow involvement by PEL are limited. In a study of 12 cases of PEL, bone marrow involvement was found in one of nine cases in the form of large sheets of tumor cells.[140]

Burkitt Lymphoma

BL involves the bone marrow in about 30% to 60% of cases, most often with a diffuse or interstitial pattern of infiltration.[14,141] The starry-sky pattern typically seen at extramedullary sites can also be present in the bone marrow biopsy; necrosis is common and can be extensive. Concurrent blood involvement is common, ranging from occasional lymphoma cells to overt lymphocytosis; however, a pure leukemic presentation is rare. Cytologically, BL cells are monotonous appearing, medium-sized, with reticular chromatin, multiple small nucleoli,

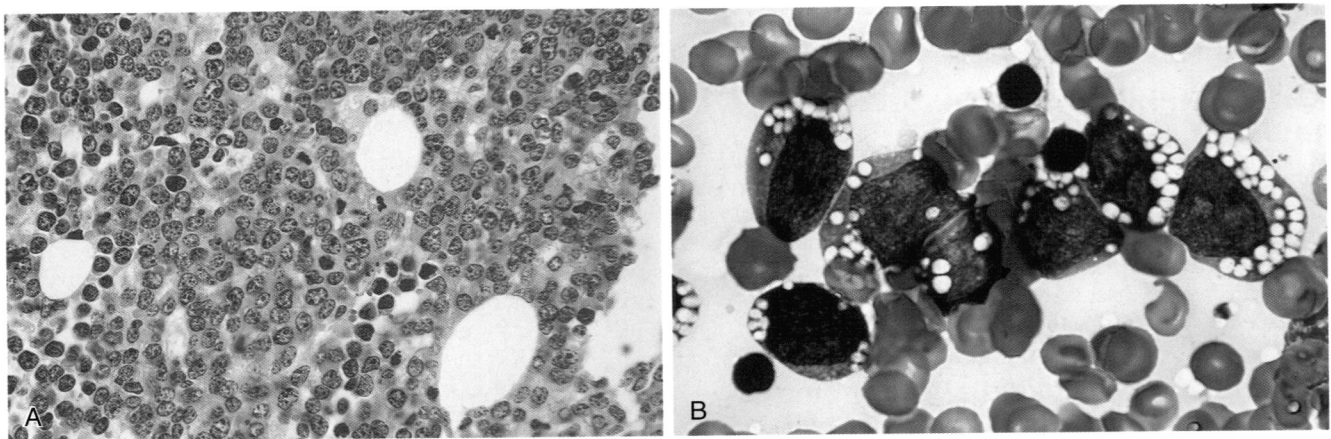

Figure 55-28. Burkitt lymphoma in the bone marrow core biopsy and aspirate smear. A, The bone marrow core biopsy contains a diffuse infiltration of monotonous, medium-sized lymphocytes with several small nucleoli, and scant to moderate amounts of cytoplasm. Frequent mitoses are present. **B,** The bone marrow aspirate contains lymphoma cells with basophilic cytoplasm and multiple cytoplasmic vacuoles.

deeply basophilic cytoplasm, and frequent mitoses. Abundant cytoplasmic vacuoles are common, and best appreciated in the bone marrow aspirate smears (Fig. 55-28), touch preparation, or peripheral blood smears. It has been reported that primary leukemic and marrow involvement ("Burkitt leukemia") at diagnosis has a better outcome compared with secondary marrow involvement by BL.[142]

BL is typically CD19+, CD20+, CD10+, and BCL6+; BCL2 is typically negative but may be weakly positive in occasional cases. BL has an extremely high proliferation rate with Ki67 positivity in virtually 100% of tumor cells. The genetic hallmark of BL is *MYC* gene rearrangement, which can be detected by FISH or conventional karyotyping.

BL should be differentiated from other aggressive B-cell neoplasms, such as B-lymphoblastic leukemia/lymphoma, blastoid MCL, and high-grade large B-cell lymphoma. In general, BL can be easily distinguished from B-lymphoblastic leukemia/lymphoma by flow cytometry immunophenotyping. B-lymphoblastic leukemia/lymphoma expresses one or more of the immature markers CD34 and TdT, and lacks surface immunoglobulin expression; additionally, *MYC* gene rearrangement is rare (~1%).[143] Blastoid MCL can be excluded by negative immunohistochemical staining for cyclin D1 and SOX11. P53 is often overexpressed in blastoid MCL. The distinction of BL from high-grade B-cell lymphoma is discussed later.

High-Grade B-Cell Lymphoma

High-grade B-cell lymphoma (HGBL) includes three subtypes based on the ICC classifications: HGBL with *MYC* and *BCL2* rearrangements (double-hit lymphoma [DHL]-*BCL2*); HGBL with *MYC* and *BCL6* rearrangements (DHL-*BCL6*; provisional entity); and HGBL, NOS.[65,66] DHL-*BCL2* is an aggressive B-cell lymphoma of germinal center origin with distinct biology from HGBL-*MYC/BCL6* and DLBCL-GCB, while DHL-*BCL6* is frequently of non-GCB origin with heterogenous molecular alterations and clinical behaviors. Some studies have demonstrated that *MYC/BCL6* rearrangements do not predict poorer survival in DLBCL patients.[144-146] HGBL, NOS,

is an aggressive B-cell lymphomas that often shows blastoid or Burkitt-like morphology without double-hit or triple-hit molecular alterations. HGBL involves the bone marrow at a higher frequency (42%–93%) than DLBCL in general (10%–25%).[118,119,121]

The distinction of HGBL types from BL can be challenging even in the lymph node biopsy because they can exhibit overlapping cytomorphology. Features favoring HGBL over BL include variations in cell or nuclear size, irregular nuclear contours, prominent nuclei, rearranged *BCL2* or *BCL6* gene, or complex karyotype. Additionally, expression of BCL2 or MUM1, Ki67 less than 95%, and absence of EBV also favor HGBL.[121,147]

B-Lymphoblastic Leukemia/Lymphoma

B-lymphoblastic leukemia/lymphoma is a neoplasm of precursor B cells. It commonly involves blood and bone marrow (B-acute lymphoblastic leukemia [B-ALL]), or occasionally primarily involves nodal or extranodal sites (B-lymphoblastic lymphoma [B-LBL]).[148] B-ALL often shows extensive, diffuse bone marrow infiltration, sometimes entirely replacing the marrow. B-LBL is defined arbitrarily as lymphomatous presentation with less than 25% bone marrow involvement.[149] In a study of 25 cases of B-LBL without concurrent B-ALL, the most common primary sites include skin, bone, soft tissue, and lymph node.[150] With aggressive chemotherapy, patients with B-LBL rarely develop leukemia and appear to have a better prognosis than patients with B-ALL.[150]

When bone marrow is involved, B-LBL infiltrate is usually focal random. The blasts are often uniformly small-to-medium-sized, with fine chromatin; scant, occasionally vacuolated cytoplasm; indistinct nucleoli; and frequent mitoses. B-LBL can be difficult to distinguish from some mature B-cell lymphomas, such as BL or blastoid MCL. Immunophenotypic analysis is crucial in making this distinction. Demonstration of TdT or CD34 expression in the neoplastic cells can essentially exclude a mature B-cell lymphoma. The subclassification of B-ALL/LBL is now largely based on the defining cytogenetic and molecular abnormalities that are discussed in detail in Chapter 41.

T-CELL LYMPHOMAS INVOLVING BONE MARROW

This section describes the characteristics of selected subtypes of T-cell lymphomas with emphasis on the morphologic features specific to the bone marrow involvement. Other features such as immunophenotype and molecular cytogenetic features are briefly discussed, and more details can be found in the specific chapters of these entities.

T-Lymphoblastic Leukemia/Lymphoma

Overall, T-lymphoblastic leukemia/lymphoma (T-ALL/LBL) more commonly has a lymphomatous presentation compared with B-ALL/LBL. Similar to its B-cell counterpart, the designation of T-LBL is used when bone marrow involvement is absent or less than 25%. When bone marrow is involved, the core biopsy shows focal random infiltrates of blasts with scant cytoplasm (Fig. 55-29). Blasts range from small to large cells with dispersed or condensed chromatin and may have convoluted nuclei. T-LBL is positive for cytoplasmic CD3, CD7, and expresses one or more of immature markers (CD34, TdT, CD1a, and CD99) and variably expresses CD4 or CD8, depending on the stage of maturation. It is worth noting that hematogones can also express TdT; therefore, it is important not to construe minimal T-ALL or B-ALL solely based on the TdT immunohistochemical staining (Fig. 55-29).[151]

Extranodal Natural Killer/T-Cell Lymphoma

Extranodal NK/T-cell lymphoma (ENKTL) frequently arises in the nasal cavity (80%), termed *ENKTL, nasal type*. It may also occur outside the nasal cavity (20%), commonly in the skin, gastrointestinal tract, and testis.[152,153] The cytology of the tumor cells varies from small, medium, to large-sized cells or a mixture of variably sized tumor cells. The incidence of bone marrow involvement by ENKTL has been reported from 8% to 23%.[46,47,50,154-157] Typically, singly distributed lymphoma cells are found in the interstitial areas of the bone marrow, and can be difficult to identify on H&E-stained sections. In contrast to nasal NKTCL that is localized to the upper aerodigestive tract at presentation, most patients with nonnasal type present with advanced disease involving multiple anatomic sites, including bone marrow involvement in 15% to 25% of cases.[50,153,158,159]

The ENKTL usually exhibits an NK cell phenotype, (i.e., negative for surface CD3 by flow cytometric analysis of surface-antigen expression, but positive for cytoplasmic CD3ε that can be detected by flow cytometric analysis with cytoplasmic CD3 staining or immunohistochemistry. The lymphoma cells are also typically CD56 positive and EBV positive. In situ hybridization for EBER or immunohistochemical staining for CD56 can highlight the isolated tumor cells in the bone marrow (Fig. 55-30). Hemophagocytic syndrome has been described in patients with ENKTL.[158-160]

Enteropathy-Associated T-Cell Lymphoma

Enteropathy-associated T-cell lymphoma (EATL) typically arises in the small intestine as a complication of long-standing celiac disease.[161] Bone marrow involvement is rare, and has been reported in 2% to 8% patients.[46,161,162] However, no details about the pattern of bone marrow involvement have been described.

Hepatosplenic T-Cell Lymphoma

Hepatosplenic T-cell lymphoma (HSTCL) is a rare, highly aggressive peripheral T-cell lymphoma, predominantly TCRγδ subtype, that occurs in adolescents, young adults, and older

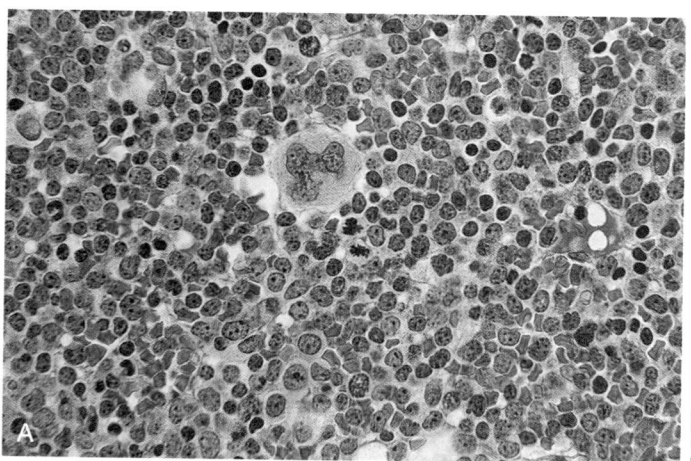
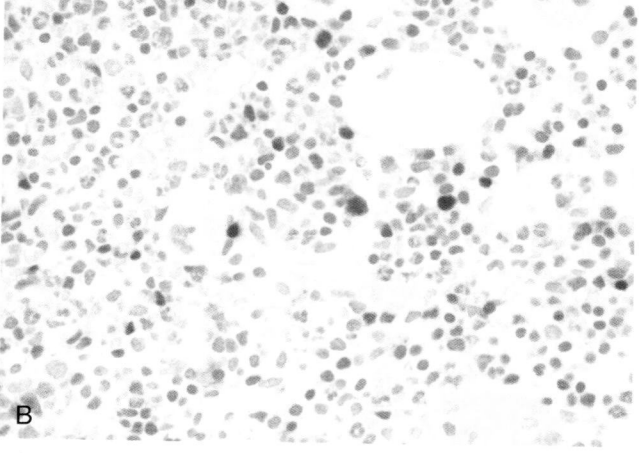

Figure 55-29. T-lymphoblastic leukemia/lymphoma involving the bone marrow. A, The bone marrow core biopsy demonstrates diffuse infiltration of neoplastic cells, replacing almost the entire bone marrow. The cells are small-to-medium-sized with slightly dispersed chromatin. A few mitotic figures are present. Flow cytometry immunophenotyping and immunohistochemical stains for CD3, TdT, CD1a, or CD99 are helpful for diagnosis (not shown). **B,** Image from a normal bone marrow showing occasional TdT-positive cells. It is important not to construe minimal T-lymphoblastic leukemia (T-ALL) solely based on the TdT immunohistochemical staining in the bone marrow as hematogones can also express TdT.

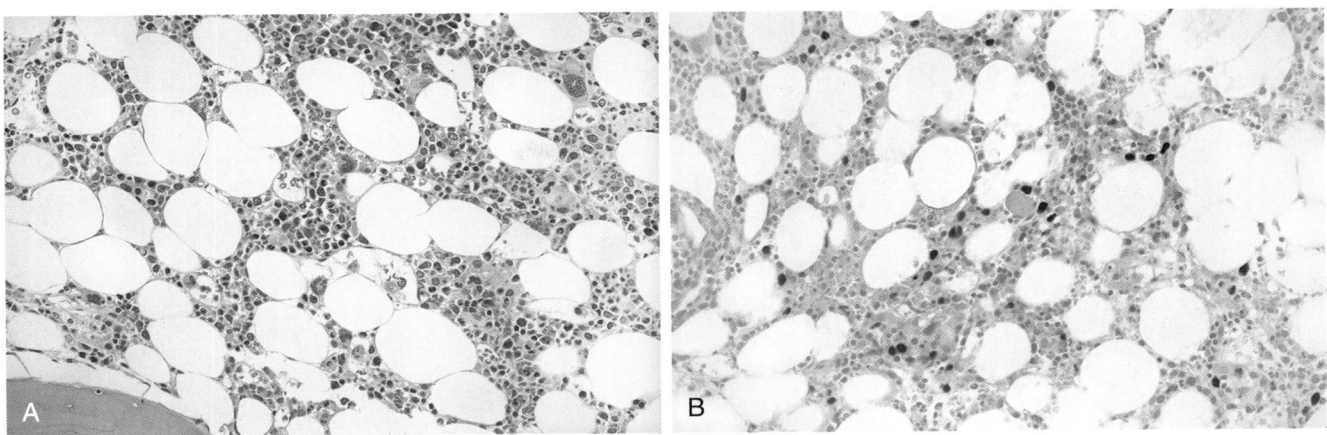

Figure 55-30. Natural killer/T-cell lymphoma, nasal type, involving the bone marrow. A, The tumor cells are difficult to appreciate on hematoxylin and eosin (H&E)–stained bone marrow core biopsy. **B,** In situ hybridization for Epstein-Barr virus–encoded RNA (EBER) highlights the scattered tumor cells.

individuals over the age of 60 years (about 50% of cases) with male predominance.[65] Patients often present with marked splenomegaly without lymphadenopathy, anemia, and marked thrombocytopenia.[48,65] HSTCL involves the peripheral blood or bone marrow in almost all cases, and the marrow involvement is characterized by a prominent intrasinusoidal infiltration associated with a hypercellular bone marrow with trilineage hyperplasia.[163] The infiltrate can be difficult to appreciate on H&E-stained sections, but immunohistochemical staining for CD3 highlights the intrasinusoidal lymphoma cells that often cause distension of the sinusoids (Fig. 55-31).[164,165] The lymphoma cells vary from small-to-medium-sized with condensed chromatin to blastic or pleomorphic cells (Fig. 55-31). The blastic-appearing lymphoma cells and the interstitial infiltration increase with the disease progression.[165]

Most cases of HSTCL arise from cytotoxic memory T cells, and the lymphoma cells are typically CD3+, TCR γδ+, CD4−, CD8−/+, CD5−, CD2+, CD7+, CD56+/−, CD57−, and have a nonactivated cytotoxic T-cell phenotype (i.e., TIA1+, granzyme M+, granzyme B−, and perforin).[48,164,165] A TCR αβ variant has been reported in a small number of cases and shows similar clinicopathologic features to γδ HSTCL.[166,167] EBV is consistently negative. Isochromosome 7q (i7q) is a recurrent genetic abnormality in HSTCL, often associated with trisomy 8.[149] The frequency of i7q varies in the reports. Approximately 70% of cases were positive in large series of studies, and the negative cases were mostly based on the conventional karyotyping rather than FISH.[48,168]

The differential diagnosis of HSTCL in the bone marrow is largely restricted to leukemia/lymphoma with propensity for sinusoidal infiltration. The B-cell lymphomas, such as intravascular large B-cell lymphoma and SMZL, can be easily excluded by positive staining for B-cell markers. Among T-cell leukemia/lymphoma, T-cell large granular lymphocytic leukemia (T-LGLL) is also associated with splenomegaly and has a predilection for an intrasinusoidal distribution in the bone marrow.[169] In particular, a rare variant of CD4−/CD8− γδ T-LGLL demonstrates an immunophenotype overlapping with HSTCL (CD3+, CD5−, CD4−, CD8−, TCR γδ+, and TIA1+), and may cause diagnostic confusion with HSTCL.[170-173] Clinically, γδ T-LGLL is an indolent disease primarily affecting older

individuals, similar to the common type of CD8-positive T-LGLL.[170,174] The pattern of bone marrow infiltration by CD4−/CD8− γδ T-LGLL is also similar to common T-LGLL (i.e., predominantly interstitial accompanied by a relatively small component of intrasinusoidal infiltration). The latter differs from HSTCL in that it rarely expands the sinusoids but takes the form of a short, linear array (often one-cell layer) of lymphocytes within the sinusoids (Fig. 55-32). The neoplastic cells in T-LGLL are morphologically indistinguishable from normal LGLs with no cytologic atypia. Additionally, i7q has not been reported in T-LGLL. It is important to include this rare variant of T-LGLL in the differential diagnosis because HSTCL is a highly aggressive lymphoma that requires chemotherapy, and bone marrow transplant may be considered; however, γδ T-LGLL is an indolent disease that may respond to immunomodulating agents, and bone marrow transplant is not indicated.

Other types of T or NK cell leukemia/lymphoma, such as aggressive NK cell leukemia, T-cell prolymphocytic leukemia (T-PLL), and adult T-cell leukemia and lymphoma (ATLL) often involve blood and bone marrow. However, these leukemia/lymphomas rarely show prominent intrasinusoidal infiltration in the bone marrow. Additionally, immunophenotyping can often discriminate HSTCL from these T or NK cell leukemia/lymphomas (e.g., aggressive NK cell leukemia exhibits an NK-cell phenotype and is always EBV positive; T-PLL and ATLL are both TCR αβ positive and predominantly CD4 positive.

Subcutaneous Panniculitis-Like T-Cell Lymphoma

Subcutaneous panniculitis-like T-cell lymphoma (SPTCL) is a rare neoplasm of cytotoxic (CD8 positive) T cells that has a predilection for subcutaneous tissue.[175,176] The diagnosis of SPTCL is now restricted to those expressing TCR αβ. SPTCL remains localized in the subcutaneous tissue and rarely involves the bone marrow.[177,178] A limited number of case reports described focal bone marrow involvement by SPTCL with morphologic features similar to the subcutaneous site (i.e., prominent rimming of the adipocytes by the

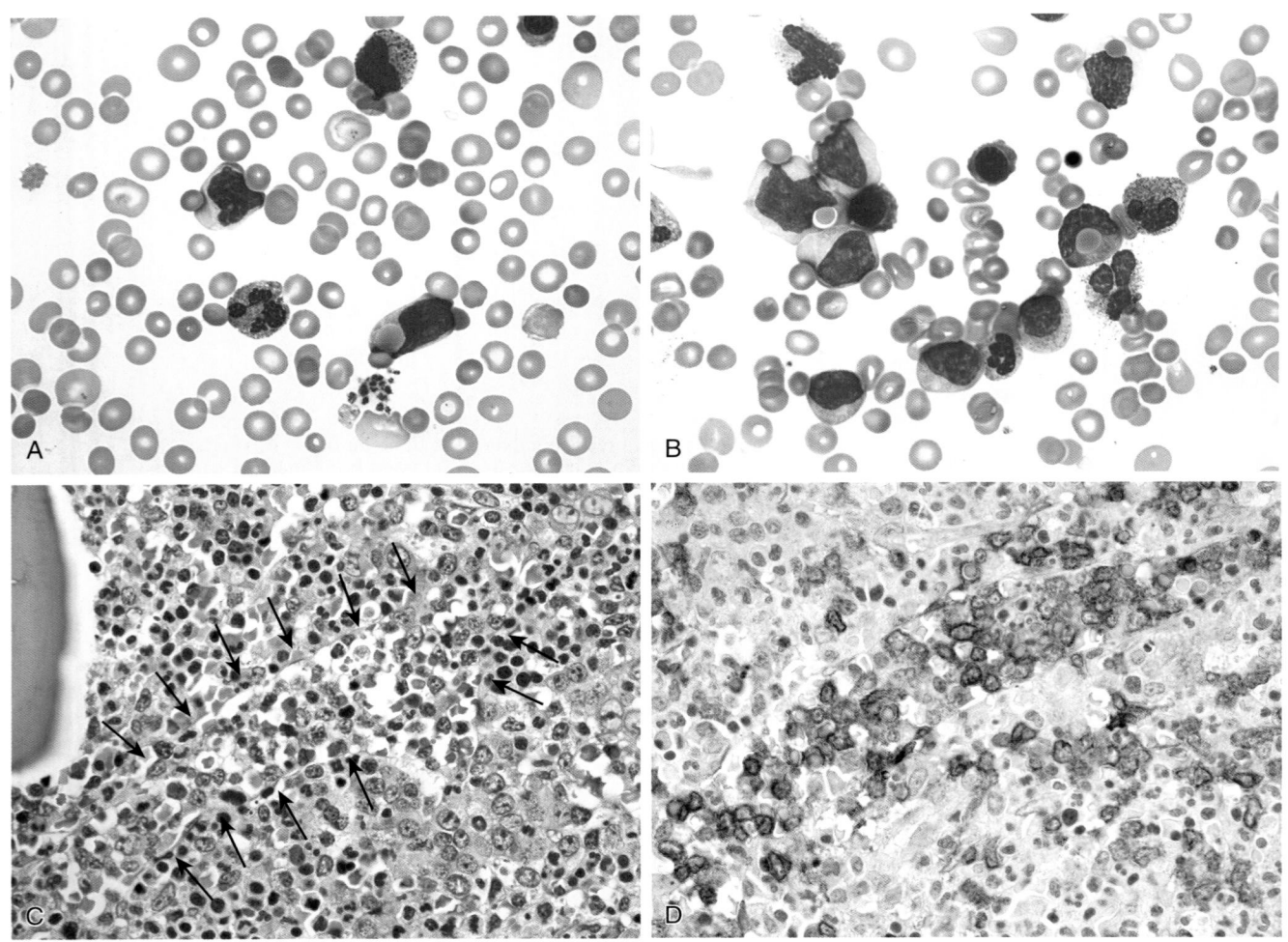

Figure 55-31. Hepatosplenic T-cell lymphoma involving peripheral blood and bone marrow. A, The lymphoma cells in the blood smears resemble blasts; some of the lymphoma cells show erythrophagocytosis. **B,** Lymphoma cells in the bone marrow aspirate smears show similar morphology to those in the peripheral blood smears. **C,** The bone marrow core biopsy shows intrasinusoidal infiltration of lymphoma cells that expand the sinusoids *(arrows).* **D,** Immunohistochemical staining for CD3 highlights the lymphoma cells within the sinusoids. This patient had a classical clinical presentation and characteristic immunophenotype for hepatosplenic T-cell lymphoma (HSTCL), and fluorescence in situ hybridization (FISH) was positive for isochromosome 7q.

neoplastic lymphocytes) (Fig. 55-33). These cells are small with condensed chromatin and scant cytoplasm, and are positive for CD3, CD8, βF1 and cytotoxic granule proteins (TIA1, granzyme B, and perforin). The recurrent germline mutations in *HAVCR2,* encoding T-cell immunoglobulin mucin 3, have been recently identified in 25% to 80% of patients with SPTCL and are associated with younger age and hemophagocytic lymphohistiocytosis (HLH) or HLH-like systemic illness.[179]

Mycosis Fungoides and Sézary Syndrome

MF is the most common primary cutaneous T-cell lymphoma that generally remains localized for years, and Sézary syndrome (SS) is a rare disorder characterized by diffuse erythroderma, lymphadenopathy, and circulating lymphoma cells (Sézary cells).[180] The incidence of bone marrow involvement by MF or SS has been reported from less than 2% to 25% at initial diagnosis.[51,181,182] The extent of bone

marrow infiltration is usually minimal to mild, and is focal random or interstitial, or both; paratrabecular and diffuse infiltrates are rare.[183] The infiltrates are composed primarily of variably sized abnormal lymphocytes with convoluted nuclei, and the infiltrates are often subtle and difficult to recognize on H&E-stained sections. Immunohistochemical stains for T-cell markers, such as CD3, aid in the recognition of lymphoma cells (Fig. 55-34). However, even with immunohistochemical stains, there is poor agreement between histologic-immunophenotypic detection of disease and molecular studies for T-cell clonality.[184]

The number of circulating lymphoma cells in SS is highly variable, ranging from occasional cells to a frankly leukemic picture. The neoplastic lymphocytes may be small or large with variable amounts of cytoplasm. The nuclei are characterized by striking convolutions that may give them a cerebriform appearance; nucleoli are absent or inconspicuous (Fig. 55-34). The lymphoma cells are typically CD3+, CD4+, CD8−, CD7−, and CD26− (Fig. 55-35).

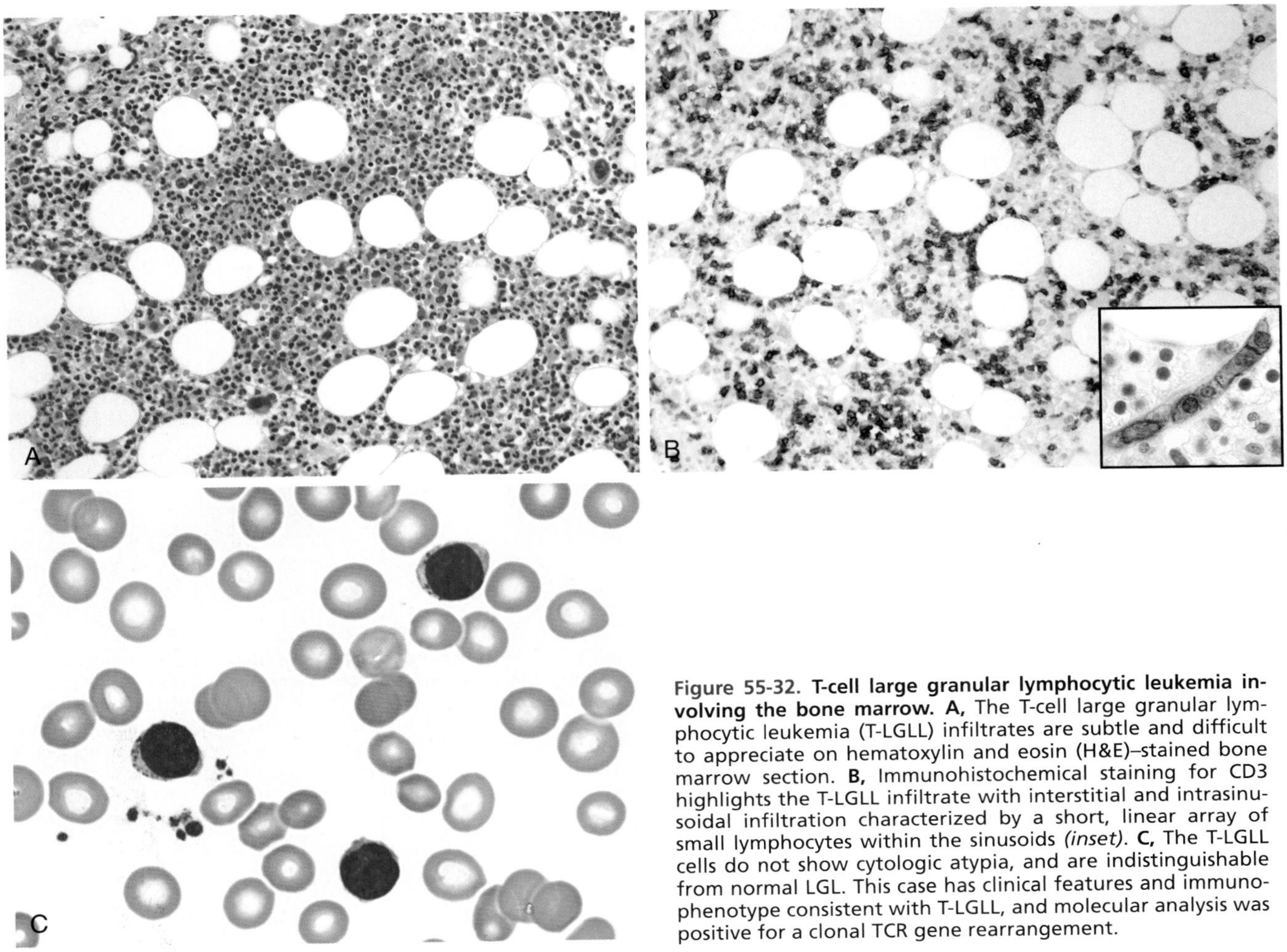

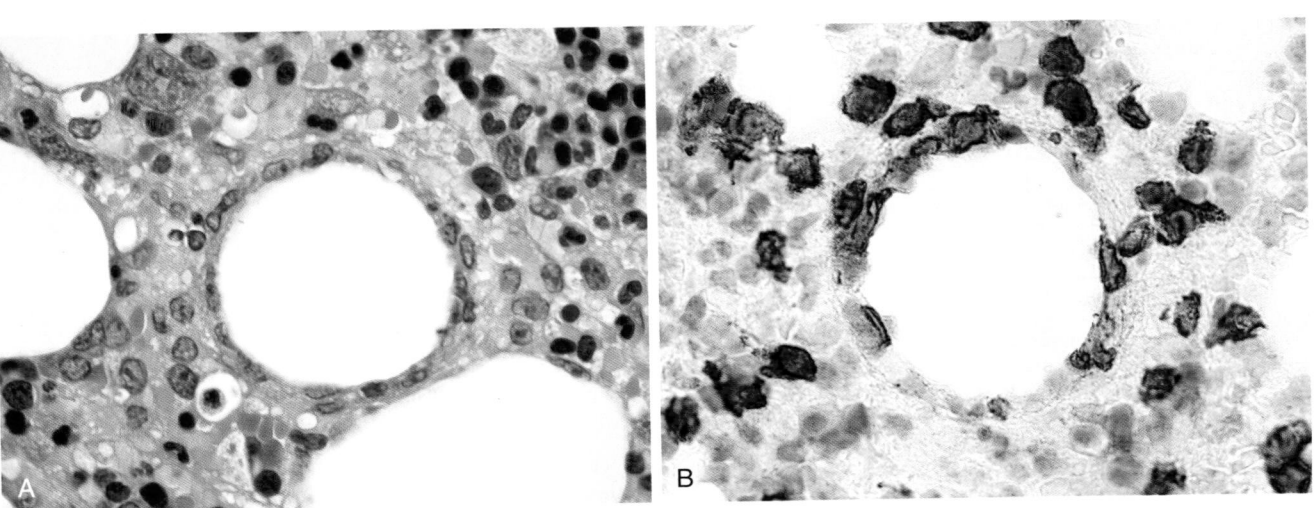

Figure 55-32. **T-cell large granular lymphocytic leukemia involving the bone marrow. A,** The T-cell large granular lymphocytic leukemia (T-LGLL) infiltrates are subtle and difficult to appreciate on hematoxylin and eosin (H&E)–stained bone marrow section. **B,** Immunohistochemical staining for CD3 highlights the T-LGLL infiltrate with interstitial and intrasinusoidal infiltration characterized by a short, linear array of small lymphocytes within the sinusoids *(inset)*. **C,** The T-LGLL cells do not show cytologic atypia, and are indistinguishable from normal LGL. This case has clinical features and immunophenotype consistent with T-LGLL, and molecular analysis was positive for a clonal TCR gene rearrangement.

Figure 55-33. **Subcutaneous panniculitis-like T-cell lymphoma involving the bone marrow. A,** The bone marrow core biopsy shows focal lymphoid infiltrates with prominent rimming of the fat cells, similar to the pattern in the subcutaneous site. **B,** Immunohistochemical staining for CD8 is positive in the neoplastic cells.

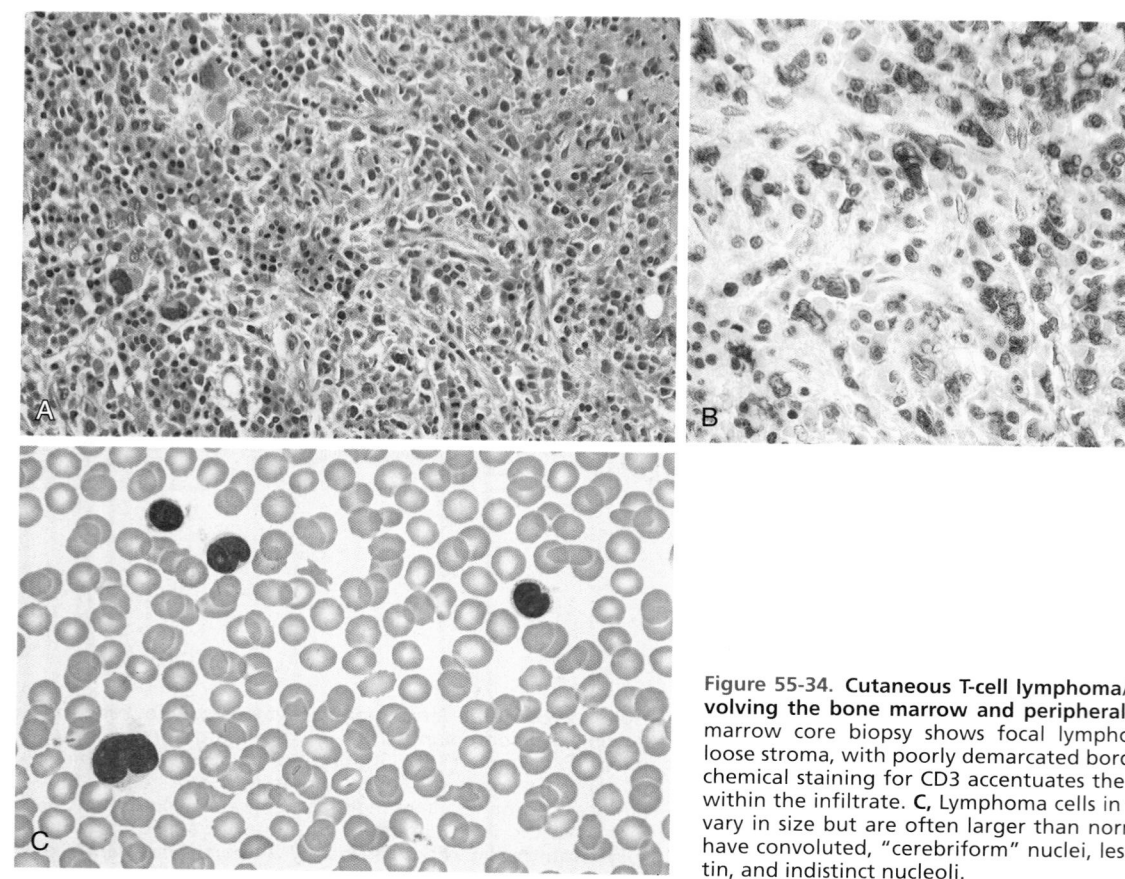

Figure 55-34. Cutaneous T-cell lymphoma/Sézary syndrome involving the bone marrow and peripheral blood. A, The bone marrow core biopsy shows focal lymphomatous infiltrate in loose stroma, with poorly demarcated borders. **B,** Immunohistochemical staining for CD3 accentuates the variably sized T cells within the infiltrate. **C,** Lymphoma cells in the peripheral blood vary in size but are often larger than normal lymphocytes and have convoluted, "cerebriform" nuclei, less condensed chromatin, and indistinct nucleoli.

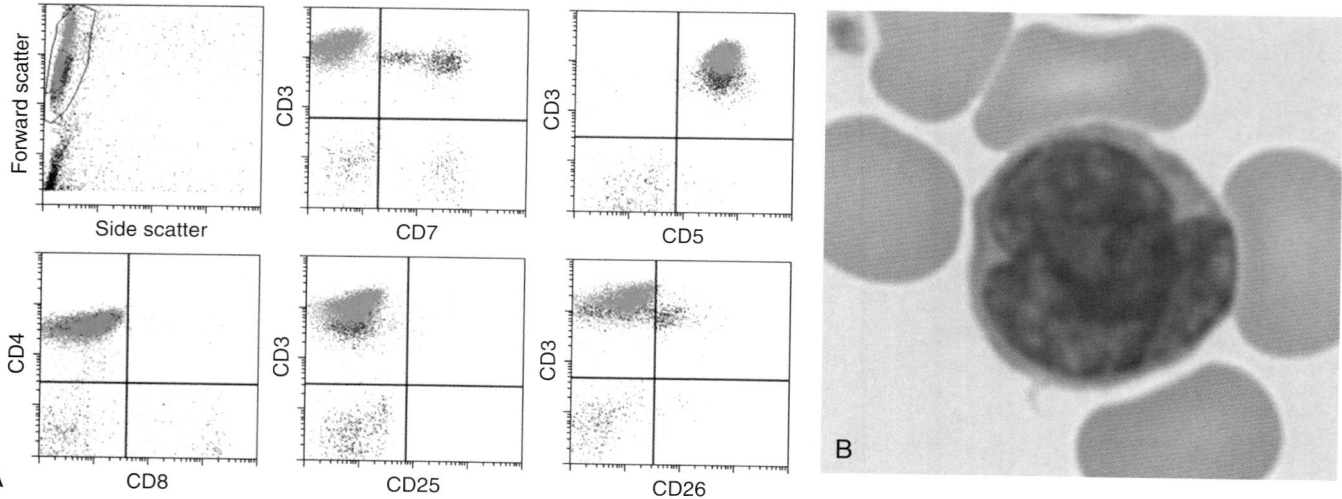

Figure 55-35. Sézary syndrome. A, Flow cytometric immunophenotyping demonstrates a CD3+ T-cell population *(red)* with an aberrant T-cell phenotype: CD3+, CD5+, CD7−, CD4+, CD8−, CD25−, and CD26−. **B,** High-power view of a Sézary cell in the peripheral blood smear.

T-Follicular Helper Cell Lymphoma

T-follicular helper (TFH) cell lymphoma include three subtypes: angioimmunoblastic, follicular, and not otherwise specified (NOS), which share a TFH cell immunophenotype and a common genetic landscape.[65,66] TFH-angioimmunoblastic type, previously designated angioimmunoblastic T-cell lymphoma (AITL), is the prototype of TFH cell lymphoma with well-defined morphologic, immunophenotypic, and molecular features. TFH-angioimmunoblastic type involves the bone marrow in about 50% to 80% of cases.[20,185,186] The infiltrates are generally identified by their hypocellularity in contrast to the surrounding hypercellular marrow. The lesions are typically focal random and multiple. Paratrabecular infiltration is also common, but diffuse infiltration is rare. The infiltrates are heterogeneous, consisting of a variable number of lymphocytes, plasma cells, immunoblasts, histiocytes, and eosinophils; small blood vessels may be prominent (Fig. 55-36). Neoplastic cells with clear cytoplasm typically seen in the extranodal sites are usually not common in the bone marrow biopsy. In some cases, the prominent plasmacytosis may obscure the neoplastic infiltrates.[185] Circulating plasma cells, plasmacytoid lymphocytes, or immunoblasts are present in about one-third of patients, but cytologically overt malignant cells are uncommon in the blood or bone marrow smears.

TFH cell lymphoma is derived from the T-follicular helper cells that normally reside in the germinal centers. Similar to their normal counterpart, the tumor cells are positive for CD3, CD4, CD10, BCL6, ICOS, PD-1, and CXCL13; EBV is positive in about 75% of cases.[65,66] However, immunohistochemical staining for these markers on a bone marrow biopsy is less helpful compared with lymph node because of different microenvironment and relatively small number of tumor cells (e.g., the expression of follicular T-helper–associated markers, CXCL13 and CD10, is much lower in the bone marrow than in the lymph node).

The differential diagnosis of TFH cell lymphoma in the bone marrow includes HL, THRLBCL, peripheral T-cell lymphoma,

NOS, and non-neoplastic lymphohistiocytic lesions. In general, HL and THRLBCL can be excluded by examining multiple levels of bone marrow section and immunohistochemical studies. Although bone marrow findings, in conjunction with clinical presentations, may suggest a diagnosis of TFH cell lymphoma, a primary diagnosis based on the bone marrow findings alone can be extremely challenging and should not be made without the right clinical context. Demonstration of a sCD3-negative/CD4-positive/CD10-positive T-cell aberrant population and common mutations seen in TFH cell lymphoma, such as *TET2* and *RHOA* mutations, are features that are relatively specific for a TFH cell neoplasm.[187,188] The details of morphologic features of three subtypes of TFH cell lymphoma and mutational profiles can be found in Chapter 35.

Peripheral T-Cell Lymphoma, Not Otherwise Specified

Peripheral T-cell lymphoma, not otherwise specified (PTCL, NOS) involves the bone marrow in about 20% to 40% of cases at diagnosis.[46,189-192] The bone marrow

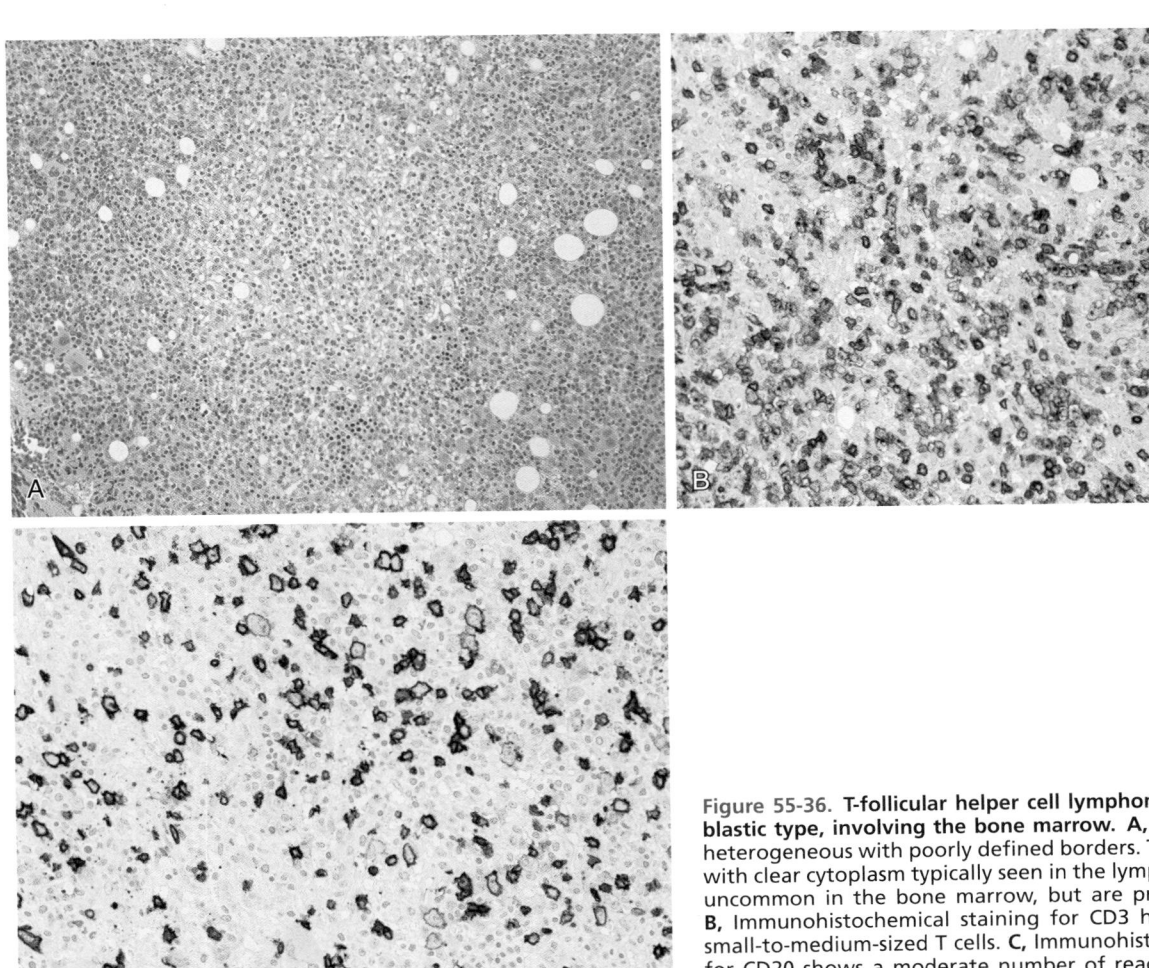

Figure 55-36. T-follicular helper cell lymphoma, angioimmunoblastic type, involving the bone marrow. A, The infiltrates are heterogeneous with poorly defined borders. The neoplastic cells with clear cytoplasm typically seen in the lymph node biopsy are uncommon in the bone marrow, but are present in this case. **B,** Immunohistochemical staining for CD3 highlights frequent small-to-medium-sized T cells. **C,** Immunohistochemical staining for CD20 shows a moderate number of reactive B cells, which vary from small to large, transformed cells (immunoblasts).

infiltrates are often diffuse or focal random.[163,193,194] As with many other PTCL, the lesions tend to be less sharply demarcated than B-cell lymphomas and intercalate into the surrounding bone marrow (Fig. 55-37). The bone marrow infiltrates are often polymorphous, containing abnormal lymphocytes admixed with reactive polymorphous infiltrates, including plasma cells, histiocytes, and eosinophils; prominent vascularity and reticulin fibrosis may also be present in the lesions.[193,194] The cytology of the neoplastic cells is variable but frequently similar to the primary site. They range from small-to-large in size, often with irregular and hyperchromatic nuclei. Occasional cases consisting of a monotonous population of medium-to-large cells or containing large, pleomorphic cells can also be seen.

Lymphoma cells are present in the aspirate smears in most cases (70%) when bone marrow is involved; they vary from occasional to numerous and are morphologically similar to those in the bone marrow core biopsy sections, with the exception of large lymphoma cells that are usually rare in the aspirate. Circulating lymphoma cells are present in about 30% of cases; rarely, a marked leukocytosis is present.[194]

Anaplastic Large Cell Lymphoma

Anaplastic large cell lymphoma (ALCL) involves the bone marrow in about 10% to 30% of cases.[46,47,190,192,195,196] The incidence of marrow involvement by ALK-positive and ALK-negative ALCL is 9% and 13%, respectively, in a large series.[46] The infiltrates are focal random, interstitial, intrasinusoidal, or occasionally diffuse. The lymphoma cells may also occur as small clusters or isolated single cells that are often difficult to identify on H&E-stained bone marrow sections, but immunohistochemical stains for CD30 and ALK1 can highlight these subtle infiltrates (Fig. 55-38). In one study, lymphoma cells were found by immunohistochemical staining in 23% of patients with negative bone marrow by routine histology.[195] It is important to identify bone marrow involvement by ALCL, even when subtle, because it is

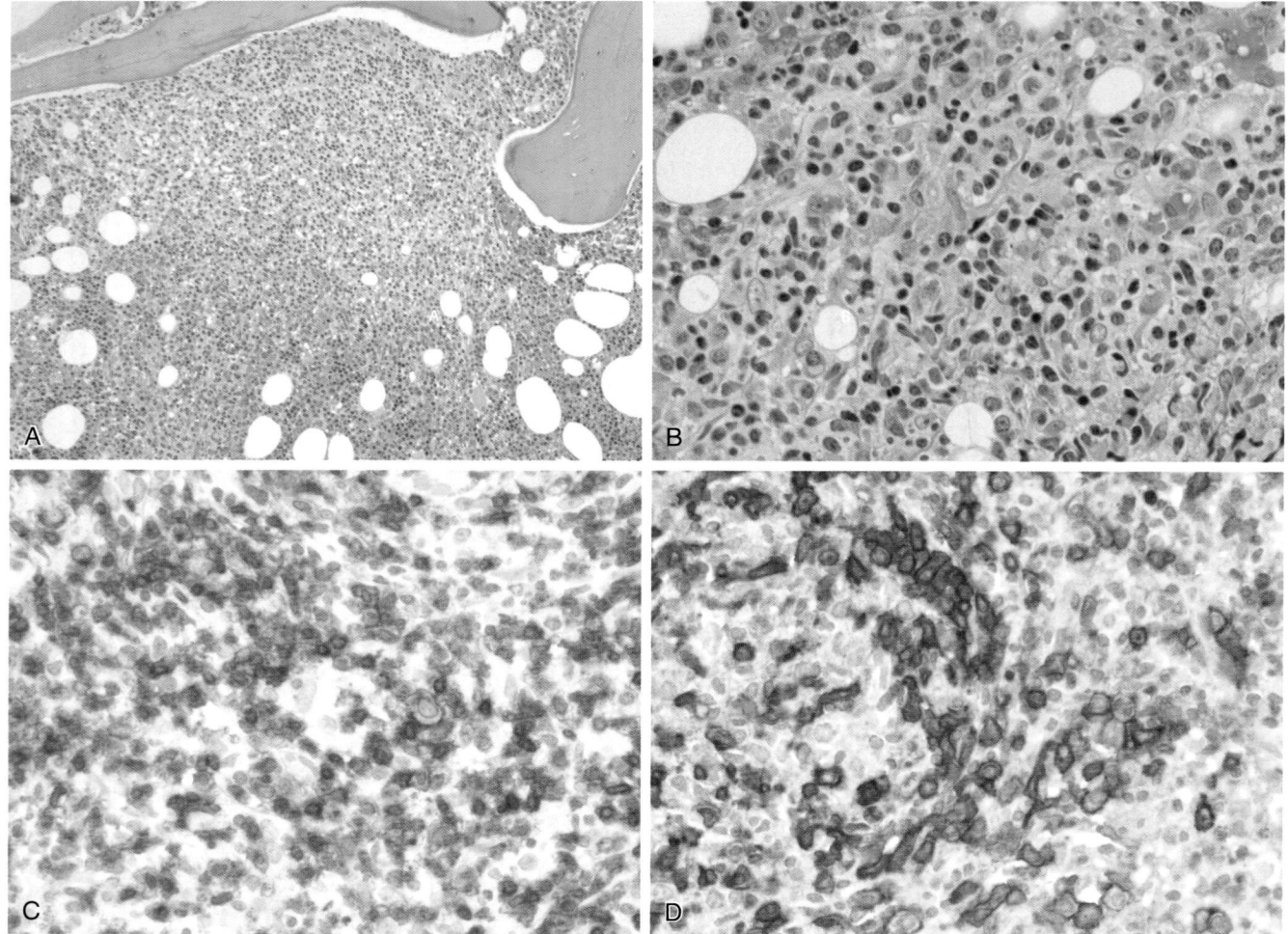

Figure 55-37. Peripheral T-cell lymphoma, not otherwise specified, involving the bone marrow. A–B, The hematoxylin and eosin (H&E)–stained bone marrow section demonstrates an abnormal lymphoid infiltrate with admixed inflammatory cells and many small blood vessels. **C,** Immunohistochemical staining for CD3 highlights the majority of lymphocytes within the infiltrate. **D,** PD1 is positive in number and distribution corresponding to CD3.

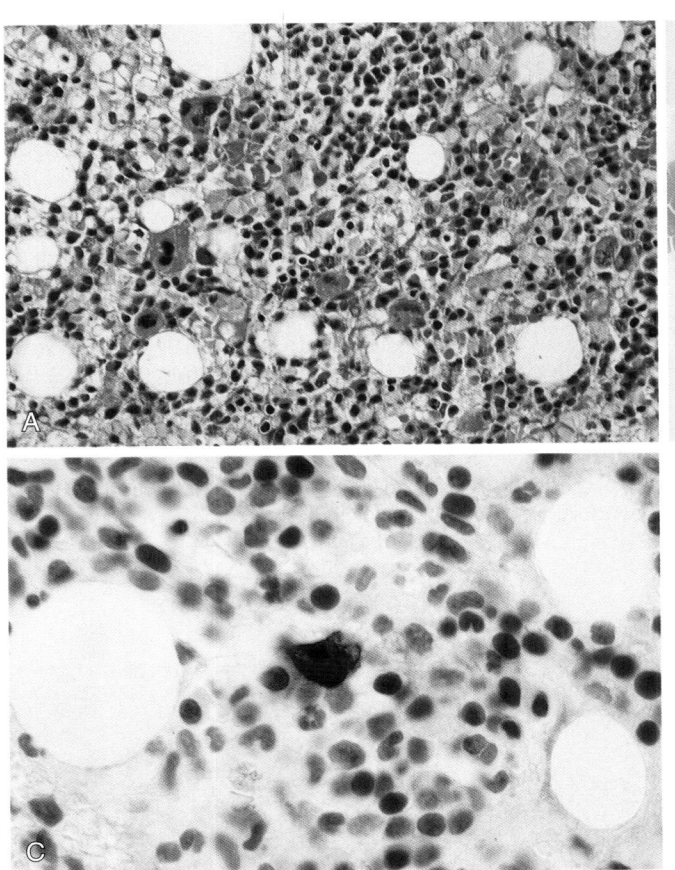

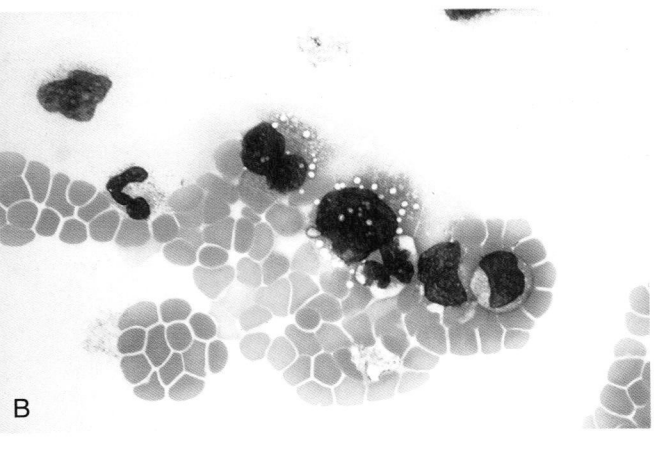

Figure 55-38. Anaplastic large cell lymphoma involving the bone marrow and peripheral blood. A, The lymphoma cells are not apparent on hematoxylin and eosin (H&E)–stained bone marrow core biopsy. **B,** Rare large lymphoma cells with cytoplasmic vacuoles are present at the feathered edge of the peripheral blood smear. **C,** One of the occasional lymphoma cells in the bone marrow highlighted by immunohistochemical staining for ALK1.

associated with a poor prognosis. The lymphoma cells are large but variably sized with irregular nuclei, dispersed chromatin, multiple prominent nucleoli, and abundant basophilic cytoplasm. In occasional cases, the lymphoma cells can be found in the peripheral blood (Fig. 55-38). Rare cases with numerous circulating lymphoma cells have also been reported.[197,198]

The differential diagnosis of ALCL in the bone marrow includes DLBCL, HL, and metastatic carcinoma. DLBCL can be easily excluded by negative staining for B-cell markers. In contrast to HL, ALCL usually lacks the inflammatory background and is negative for PAX5. ALCL may also mimic metastatic carcinoma when it forms cohesive clusters or sheets. A panel of immunohistochemical stains, such as cytokeratin, ALK1, and T-cell markers, will help in the distinction.

HODGKIN LYMPHOMA INVOLVING BONE MARROW

The overall incidence of bone marrow involvement by CHL is about 5% to 15% at diagnosis.[14,199,200] However, the frequency varies with the subtype. In a large study of 1161 patients with HL, the overall incidence of bone marrow involvement was 8%, but 19% in lymphocyte depleted, 14% in mixed cellularity, 4% in nodular sclerosis, and 2% in lymphocyte predominant type.[11] The study also showed that bilateral bone marrow biopsies increased the detection rate because the lymphoma cells were identified only in one of the bilateral biopsies in 35% (19 of 51) of patients.

In rare cases, bone marrow is the primary diagnostic site in HL. This occurs most frequently in patients with AIDS,[201-203] and HL is restricted to the bone marrow at diagnosis in approximately 14% of cases.[203] These patients usually lack lymphadenopathy and do not develop HL at extramedullary sites during the disease course.

If bone marrow is assessed, the bone marrow core biopsy is the procedure of choice for the diagnosis or staging of HL. The aspirate is insensitive for the detection of HL.[204] Reed-Sternberg cells are usually absent in the aspirate smears, although they can be identified in rare cases with extensive bone marrow involvement. HL in the bone marrow is characterized by discrete, space-occupying lesions that are usually clearly demarcated from the surrounding normal bone marrow. Focal involvement is present in about 30% of cases; the infiltrates may be single or multiple, random, or paratrabecular. Diffuse bone marrow involvement has been reported in about 70% of cases (Fig. 55-39).[14] The infiltrates are polymorphous and frequently contain a prominent component of small lymphocytes, and variable numbers of plasma cells, histiocytes, and eosinophils (Fig. 55-40). Reed-Sternberg cells or variants are almost always present, although in some cases, multiple sections must be examined to identify the neoplastic cells. Fibrosis is almost always present in the infiltrate and may be prominent, especially

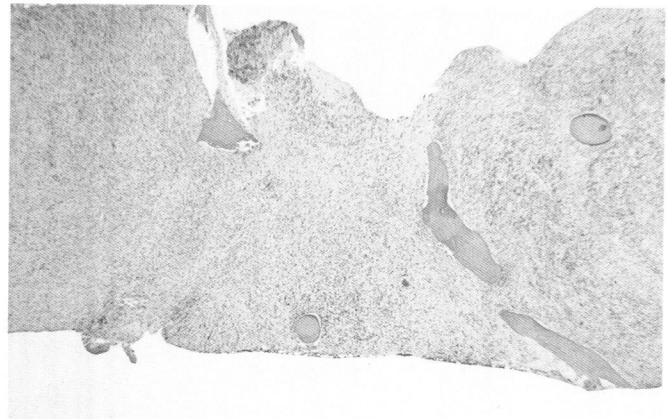

Figure 55-39. Hodgkin lymphoma involving the bone marrow. This case shows extensive bone marrow involvement by Hodgkin lymphoma that completely replaces the normal hematopoietic tissue.

in diffuse lesions. Necrosis may be present and is more common in treated patients.

Historically, the criteria for diagnosing HL in the bone marrow vary, depending on whether the bone marrow was the initial diagnostic site.[205,206] In current practice, when abnormal large cells with the characteristic immunophenotype of Hodgkin cells (CD30+, CD15+/−, CD45−, CD3−, CD20−/variably+, PAX5+, ALK1−) are identified in the bone marrow in a cellular background typical for HL, detection of morphologically classic Reed-Sternberg cells is not always necessary for a primary diagnosis of HL. However, subclassification of HL in a bone marrow biopsy is not encouraged as the small sample size and variability of histopathology between lymph node and bone marrow make subclassification unreliable.[205] The uninvolved bone marrow in patients with HL frequently exhibits reactive changes, including granulocytic hyperplasia, eosinophilia, and increased numbers of megakaryocytes. These findings can be confused with an MPN, particularly when the patient does not have an established diagnosis of HL.

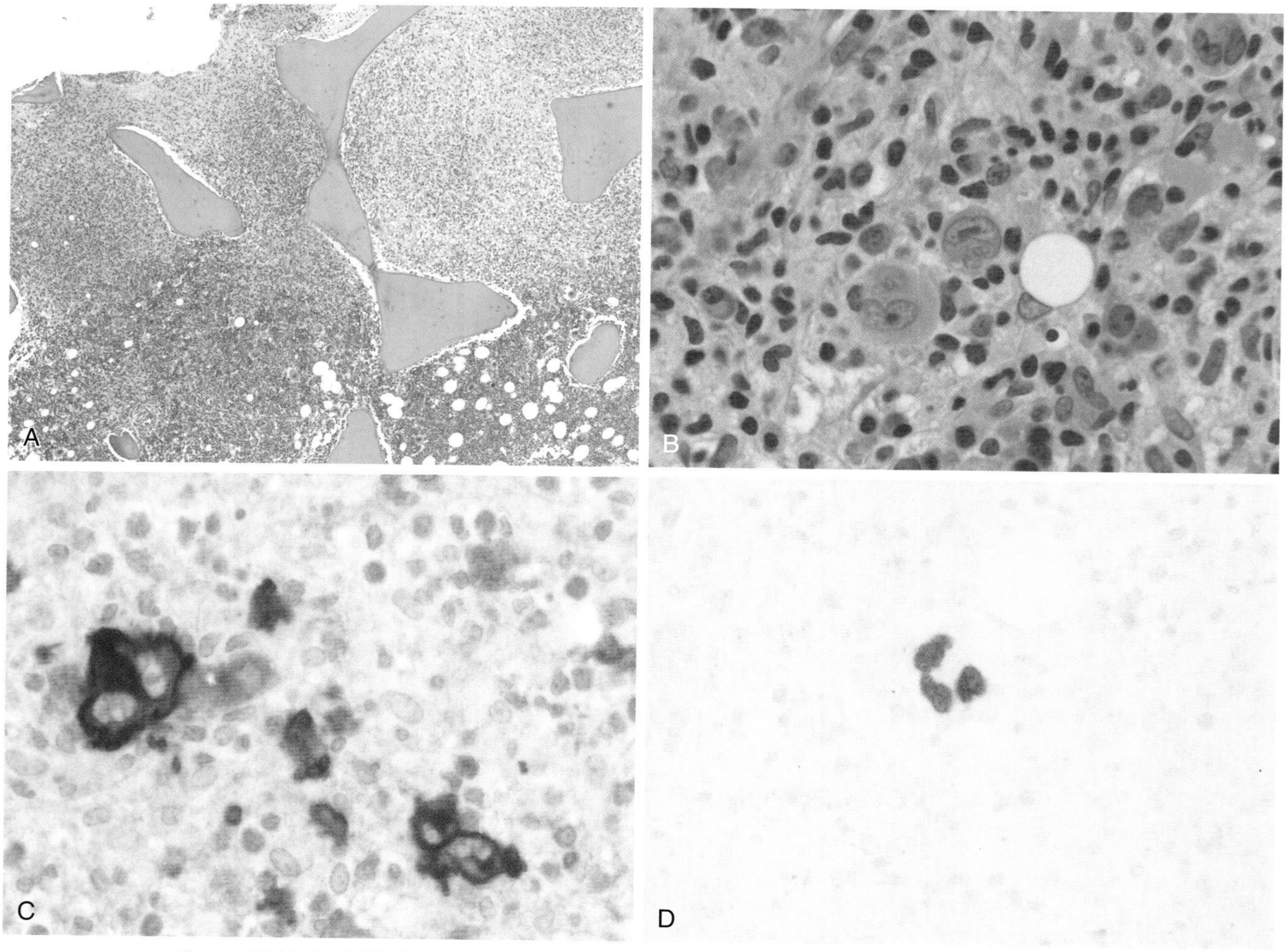

Figure 55-40. Hodgkin lymphoma involving the bone marrow. A–B, The bone marrow shows abnormal infiltrates that are polymorphous and contain Reed-Sternberg cells in a background of small lymphocytes, histiocytes, plasma cells, neutrophils, and occasional eosinophils. **C–D,** The neoplastic cells are positive for CD30 **(C)** and EBER **(D)**.

Nodular lymphocyte predominant HL (NLPHL) remains a subtype of HL in the 2022 WHO classification but is classified as a subtype of B-cell lymphoma, nodular lymphocyte predominant B-cell lymphoma (NLPBCL), in the ICC classification given its well-recognized germinal center B-cell origin.[65,66] NLPHL/NLPBCL rarely involves the bone marrow. In a large series of 275 patients with NLPHL of pure nodular pattern, bone marrow involvement was identified in 7 (2.5%) patients, including 4 (1.5%) at the initial diagnosis and 3 during therapy or at relapse.[207] The bone marrow was involved by large B cells (<10% cells) associated with a prominent T-cell and histiocytic infiltrate in the background, and the bone marrow involvement was associated with a poor prognosis.[207]

Non-Hodgkin lymphomas, such as ALCL, THRLBCL, and PTCL, may mimic HL in the bone marrow. In addition, granulomas may be present in HL infiltrates and could be mistaken for a benign infiltrative process. HL must be differentiated from reactive polymorphous lymphohistiocytic lesions, which are commonly encountered in the bone marrow of patients with immunodeficiency such as AIDS.[208,209] Appropriate immunohistochemical stains often allow this distinction. In equivocal cases, biopsy of lymph node or other tissue are necessary for a definite diagnosis.

NONLYMPHOID MALIGNANCIES THAT MIMIC LYMPHOMAS

Metastatic Tumors

Metastatic tumors in the bone marrow are usually easily distinguished from lymphoma because the malignant cells often occur as cohesive clusters (Fig. 55-41). However, tumor cells from small cell carcinoma and other small round blue cell tumors, such as embryonal rhabdomyosarcoma, neuroblastoma, retinoblastoma, and Ewing's sarcoma, can be present as discohesive cells in the aspirate smears and mimic lymphoma cells (Fig. 55-41).[210,211] Scanning the aspirate smear at low magnification is useful to identify cohesive clusters of tumor cells, even when they are rare. In the bone marrow core biopsy, foci of metastatic tumor are almost always sharply demarcated from normal hematopoietic cells. Rarely, they focally infiltrate as groups of cells between hematopoietic cells and resemble lymphoma (Fig. 55-42). In other cases, the metastatic carcinoma may be extensive and diffusely replace the normal bone marrow. When the carcinoma cells are large and anaplastic, they can resemble a large cell lymphoma or HL (Fig. 55-43). Immunohistochemical stains appropriate for the

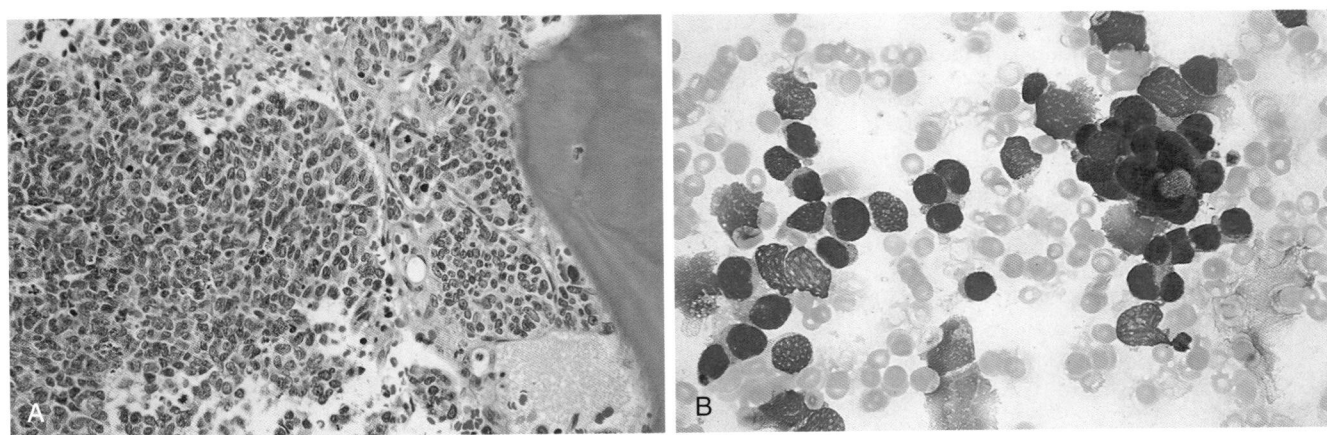

Figure 55-41. Metastatic neuroendocrine carcinoma in the bone marrow. A, Cohesive tumor cells in the bone marrow core biopsy. **B,** Discohesive, small carcinoma cells in the bone marrow aspirate smear resemble lymphoma cells; a small cohesive cluster of tumor cells, which is more typical of carcinoma, is also present.

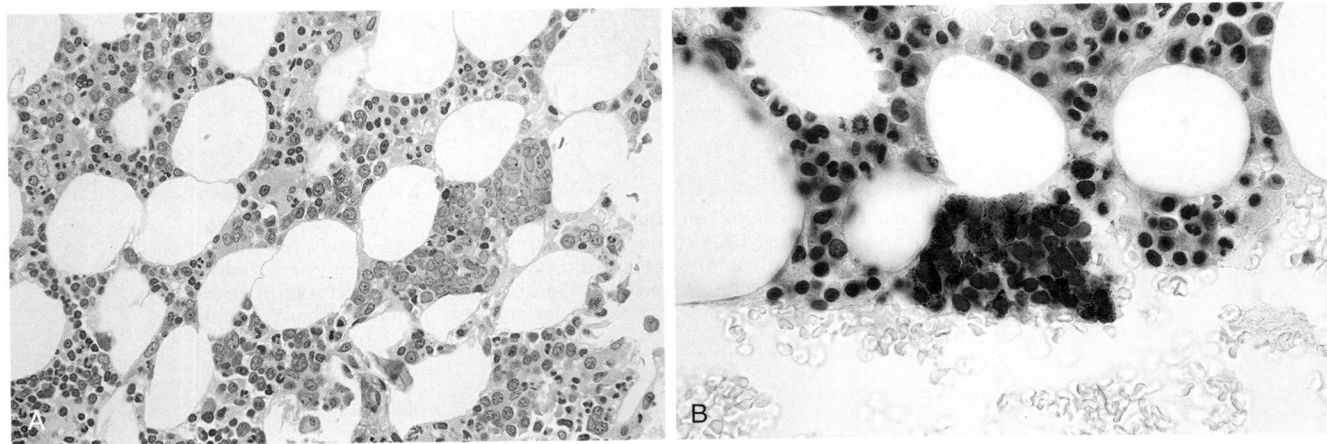

Figure 55-42. Metastatic neuroendocrine carcinoma in the bone marrow. A, Focal clusters of carcinoma cells with dispersed chromatin are nestled among the normal hematopoietic elements. The carcinoma cells superficially resemble a large cell lymphoma. **B,** Immunohistochemical staining for chromogranin is positive in the carcinoma cells.

tumor (e.g., cytokeratin, EMA, chromogranin, CD45, CD3, and CD20) performed on the bone marrow core biopsy or clot section can confirm the diagnosis of a metastatic tumor and exclude lymphoma.

Systemic Mastocytosis

Systemic mastocytosis involves the bone marrow in at least 90% of cases and shows similar patterns of infiltration as

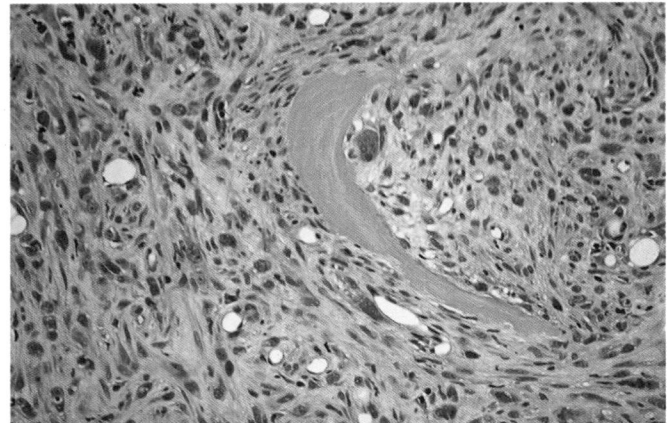

Figure 55-43. Metastatic carcinoma in the bone marrow. The metastatic carcinoma in this case is associated with marked fibrosis, and the tumor cells are large and anaplastic, resembling Hodgkin lymphoma. A cytokeratin stain (not shown) was positive in the tumor cells.

lymphoma, including paratrabecular, perivascular, random, or, rarely, diffuse infiltrates.[212] In most cases, the mast cell lesions in the bone marrow are polymorphous, and the mast cells are admixed with lymphocytes, eosinophils, neutrophils, histiocytes, endothelial cells, and fibroblasts in varying proportions. The polymorphous mast cell lesions can mimic lymphoma, particularly PTCL or HL. Occasionally, lymphocytes predominate and closely resemble non-Hodgkin lymphoma (Fig. 55-44). Recognition of mast cells in the bone marrow sections is critical to arrive at a diagnosis of systemic mastocytosis because they can look like foci of paratrabecular fibrosis. The mast cells show variable morphology and may have round, oval, spindle-shaped, or monocytoid nuclei with abundant, slightly eosinophilic cytoplasm. One helpful morphologic clue to recognizing systemic mast cell disease in the bone marrow is the frequent compartmentalization of cells, with clusters of small lymphocytes surrounded by mast cells, creating the classic "bull's eye" lesion.

The most specific immunohistochemical stain for identifying mast cells is tryptase (Fig. 55-44). In addition, mast cells express CD117, CD45, CD33, and CD68, but are negative for CD3, CD20, and CD15.[213] Neoplastic mast cells also aberrantly express CD30, CD25, or CD2, which can help distinguish them from reactive mast cell hyperplasia.[213,214] Somatic mutations of *KIT*, a proto-oncogene that encodes the tyrosine receptor for stem cell factor (CD117), is found in the mast cells from patients with systemic mastocytosis.[215]

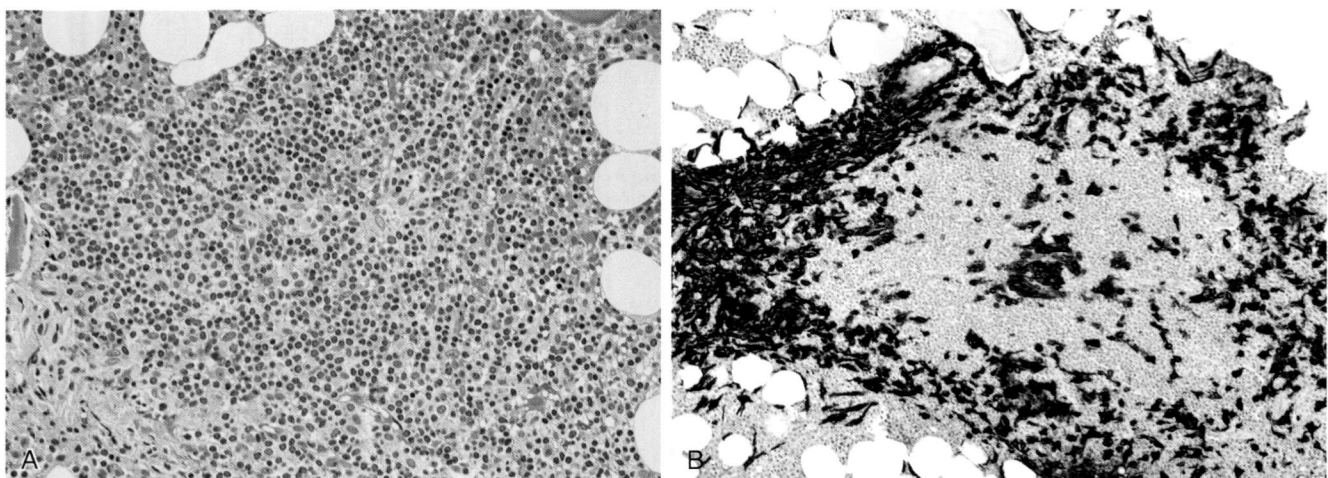

Figure 55-44. Systemic mastocytosis involving the bone marrow. A, The polymorphous infiltrates contain numerous small lymphocytes, occasional eosinophils, and small vessels, resembling a low-grade non-Hodgkin lymphoma. The mast cells are difficult to appreciate on hematoxylin and eosin (H&E)–stained section. Note the spindle-shaped mast cells with clear cytoplasm at the periphery of the lesion. **B,** Immunohistochemical staining for tryptase highlights the mast cells surrounding the lymphoid aggregate.

Pearls and Pitfalls

Pearls

- Benign lymphoid aggregates are usually small, well-circumscribed, and contain a heterogeneous cellular population.
- Reactive germinal centers usually indicate benign lymphoid infiltrate and are most commonly seen in patients with autoimmune diseases.
- Benign lymphoid aggregates often have a mixture of B and T cells, often with T-cell predominance.
- Distinct paratrabecular lymphoid infiltrates almost always indicate lymphoma, are most commonly associated with follicular lymphoma, and essentially exclude chronic lymphocytic leukemia (CLL)/small lymphocytic lymphoma (SLL).
- Intrasinusoidal lymphoid infiltrate usually indicates a neoplastic process and commonly associated with intravascular large B-cell lymphoma, splenic marginal zone B-cell lymphoma, hepatosplenic T-cell lymphoma, and T-cell large granular lymphocytic leukemia.
- Lymphoma-specific immunohistochemical markers (e.g., ALK1, LEF1, cyclin D1, and SOX11) and molecular cytogenetic abnormalities (e.g., *MYD88* mutation) are helpful in distinguishing benign versus neoplastic lymphoid infiltrate, as well as in subclassification of lymphoma.

Pitfalls

- Lymphoma, particularly T-cell types, can be morphologically heterogeneous and mimic a reactive process in the bone marrow.
- Reactive germinal centers are present in about 30% of splenic marginal zone lymphomas in the bone marrow.
- Exclusively paratrabecular lymphoid infiltrates can occasionally be present in mantle cell lymphoma.
- Paratrabecular lymphoid infiltrates may remain after anti-CD20 therapy for follicular lymphoma but may be composed entirely of T cells, which mimic residual follicular lymphoma.
- Intrasinusoidal infiltrates are difficult to appreciate on hematoxylin and eosin (H&E)–stained sections; immunohistochemical stains are helpful in highlighting the infiltrates.
- Anaplastic large cell lymphoma and nasal-type natural killer (NK)/T-cell lymphoma can infiltrate the bone marrow as isolated single cells; immunohistochemical stains can increase the detection rate.
- Diffuse large B-cell lymphoma may show a discordant lymphoma subtype in the bone marrow, often characterized by a low-grade lymphoma (most commonly follicular lymphoma).
- Low-level monoclonal B-cell populations may be identified in the peripheral blood or bone marrow in "healthy" individuals without evidence of lymphoma.
- Clonal T-cell populations can be detected in various benign conditions, particularly in autoimmune diseases.

KEY REFERENCES

6. Thiele J, Zirbes TK, Kvasnicka HM, Fischer R. Focal lymphoid aggregates (nodules) in bone marrow biopsies: differentiation between benign hyperplasia and malignant lymphoma—a practical guideline. *J Clin Pathol.* 1999;52:294–300.

9. Arber DA, George TI. Bone marrow biopsy involvement by non-Hodgkin's lymphoma: frequency of lymphoma types, patterns, blood involvement, and discordance with other sites in 450 specimens. *Am J Surg Pathol.* 2005;29:1549–1557.

14. McKenna RW, Hernandez JA. Bone marrow in malignant lymphoma. *Hematol Oncol Clin North Am.* 1988;2:617–635.

16. Kent SA, Variakojis D, Peterson LC. Comparative study of marginal zone lymphoma involving bone marrow. *Am J Clin Pathol.* 2002;117:698–708.

17. Sovani V, Harvey C, Haynes AP, McMillan AK, Clark DM, O'Connor SR. Bone marrow trephine biopsy involvement by lymphoma: review of histopathological features in 511 specimens and correlation with diagnostic biopsy, aspirate and peripheral blood findings. *J Clin Pathol.* 2014;67:389–395.

48. Weidmann E. Hepatosplenic T cell lymphoma. A review on 45 cases since the first report describing the disease as a distinct lymphoma entity in 1990. *Leukemia.* 2000;14:991–997.

53. Tandon B, Peterson L, Gao J, et al. Nuclear overexpression of lymphoid-enhancer-binding factor 1 identifies chronic lymphocytic leukemia/small lymphocytic lymphoma in small B-cell lymphomas. *Mod Pathol.* 2011;24:1433–1443.

111. Mozos A, Royo C, Hartmann E, et al. SOX11 expression is highly specific for mantle cell lymphoma and identifies the cyclin D1-negative subtype. *Haematologica.* 2009;94:1555–1562.

116. Chung R, Lai R, Wei P, et al. Concordant but not discordant bone marrow involvement in diffuse large B-cell lymphoma predicts a poor clinical outcome independent of the International Prognostic Index. *Blood.* 2007;110:1278–1282.

193. Gaulard P, Kanavaros P, Farcet JP, et al. Bone marrow histologic and immunohistochemical findings in peripheral. T-cell lymphoma: a study of 38 cases. *Hum Pathol.* 1991;22:331–338.

Visit Elsevier eBooks+ for the complete set of references.

Chapter 56

Evaluation of the Bone Marrow After Therapy

Heesun J. Rogers, Megan Nakashima, Sindhu Cherian, and Wayne Tam

Given the variety of therapies currently in use for hematologic diseases, knowledge of the many changes these therapies can induce in the bone marrow is necessary, both to determine therapy effectiveness and to avoid overinterpretation of reactive changes. Multiple therapies can cause changes in the marrow that may mimic malignancy, including chemotherapy with or without radiation, recombinant cytokines and colony stimulating factors, and bone marrow or hematopoietic stem cell transplantation. Serial bone marrow studies at prescribed intervals according to protocols during and after therapy are important for evaluation of residual disease, effectiveness of therapy, and regeneration of hematopoietic cells. After transplantation, an examination to confirm engraftment needs to be performed.

Optimal materials for evaluating post-therapy changes include a peripheral blood smear, bone marrow aspirate, touch preparations (imprints), and trephine biopsy sections. However, clot biopsy sections may also be useful, in particular if further molecular DNA or RNA studies are necessary. Extracted DNA and/or RNA or buffy coat preparations can also be used for further molecular genetic studies. An aspirate containing several marrow particles paired with core biopsies with a good length (greater than 1.5 cm or 10 partially preserved intertrabecular areas) are adequate material for a morphologic evaluation and ancillary tests.[1,2] Aspirate smears and touch imprints generally offer the best cytologic detail and are helpful in evaluating residual blasts after therapy. Biopsy material is useful for showing the pattern of blast distribution, once they are identified on the aspirate material, and the presence and pattern of residual lymphoma or solid tumor involvement. Ancillary studies are often of critical importance in the evaluation of post-therapy bone marrow specimens, particularly in the assessment of residual disease. These studies include flow cytometry, immunohistochemistry, and cytogenetic and molecular genetic studies. With the exception of immunohistochemistry and some molecular genetic tests, additional fresh bone marrow aspirate specimens are required to detect persistent or minimal residual disease. In addition, complete clinical information—including information about the primary disease process, type of treatment, and time interval since treatment—should be submitted with the bone marrow specimen.

This chapter describes the general effect of selected therapies, including hematopoietic stem cell transplantation, on the bone marrow and discusses the morphologic changes in the bone marrow at early and late intervals after therapy, including therapy-related neoplasms. The utility of ancillary studies, including flow cytometry, cytogenetics, and molecular genetic studies for follow-up of specific hematologic neoplasms post-therapy, is also covered.

EFFECTS OF SELECTED THERAPIES AND BONE MARROW TRANSPLANTATION

Chemotherapy

Several studies have evaluated bone marrow changes in acute leukemias after high-dose chemotherapy, with or without radiation, or after bone marrow or hematopoietic stem cell transplantation,[1,3-8] and there are many similarities in the findings (Box 56-1; Fig. 56-1). These changes are similar to the toxic changes resulting from drug/toxin injury of the bone marrow.[9,10] The extent and duration of changes can be influenced by various factors such as drugs, pharmacogenomics, dosage of drugs, or the neoplastic cells.

Morphologic changes in the marrow caused by chemotherapy are related to accelerated cell death in response to cytotoxic therapy and the subsequent reconstitution of hematopoietic cells.[2,3,6] Early changes expected in the first week after myeloablative treatment include decreased cellularity as a result of death of neoplastic and nonneoplastic cells to complete marrow aplasia. Peripheral cytopenias will occur at the same time. The marrow cellularity is often nearly zero, with an absence of normal marrow fat. There is prominent stromal edema, with dilated marrow sinuses. Scattered stromal cells, histiocytes, plasma cells, and lymphocytes may be present. Deposition of pink proteinaceous material may be seen, which can mimic fat serous atrophy (gelatinous transformation, discussed later in this chapter), but the presence of the eosinophilic gelatinous material of serous atrophy has only rarely been reported after chemotherapy. Normal hematopoietic cells, such as maturing granulocytes, nucleated red blood cells, and megakaryocytes, are often not identifiable. Phagocytic macrophages containing cellular debris are often present, and acellular areas of pink-staining

fibrin and fibrinoid necrosis often predominate. Rare cases may also show zonal areas of tumor cell necrosis or foci of residual tumor cells.[2,3]

Signs of early regenerating marrow begin with reappearance of fat cells, and development of mild transient reticulin fibrosis follow these changes.[2,3,8,11] The early fat in regenerating bone marrow is often loculated. Although the marrow remains markedly hypocellular, the fat is associated with focal areas of early hematopoiesis in the 2nd week after treatment. This may be represented by islands of erythroid cells, alone or in combination with areas of immature cells and left-shifted granulocytes (sheets of promyelocytes) in the paratrabecular area. Both elements are usually present after 2 weeks. Megakaryocytes, often occurring in clusters (groups of 3–5) with atypical or hypolobated nuclei, occur later in this process but are usually easily identified by the 3rd week.[4,8] In some patients, particularly children, early regeneration may be accompanied by an increase in precursor B cells, or hematogones. The features of these cells are discussed later in this chapter. As the bone marrow continues to repopulate and returns to normal age-adjusted cellularity, loss of the mild reticulin fibrosis of early regeneration and even a slightly increased marrow cellularity may be seen. All three normal marrow cell lines are present, although a left shift of granulocytes and erythroid cells and atypical megakaryocyte clustering may persist for some time. Distinguishing regenerative atypical changes after therapy from persistent neoplastic myelodysplastic features is always a diagnostic challenge for pathologists.[9]

In some cases, regeneration may be accompanied by findings such as transiently increased blasts or hematogones, marked increase in regenerating, left-shifted granulocytes (particularly in promyelocyte stage), and/or increased megakaryocytes. A prolonged delay in regeneration of bone marrow, particularly in elderly patients, can be seen after chemotherapy in some cases.[2,9,12,13]

Bone Marrow Transplantation

Some additional bone marrow changes may be observed in patients who have undergone bone marrow or hematopoietic stem cell transplantation after high-dose therapy (Box 56-2).[2,3,8,9]

The sequential morphologic changes from early transplantation until day 28 after transplantation typically show findings similar to those seen in the bone marrow after receiving high-dose chemotherapy; these include hypocellularity to marrow aplasia, extensive cellular necrosis, stromal damage and edema, fat necrosis, and hemophagocytic macrophages. Approximately 7 days after transplantation, foci of regeneration may be seen and can occur earlier in patients treated with stem cell infusion. Although clusters of regenerating marrow elements usually show a spectrum of maturation, these islands of cells may have a more monotonous appearance, without obvious maturation, after transplantation. This is most commonly seen with erythroid precursors. Early regeneration of marrow begins with appearance of small colonies of immature precursors (erythroid and granulocytic), often away from the bone (nonparatrabecular area) after transplantation. In comparison, immature granulocyte islands of blasts and promyelocytes usually occur adjacent to bony trabeculae (paratrabecular area)

Box 56-1 *Bone Marrow Changes in the 3 to 4 Weeks After Myeloablative Therapy*

Initial Changes
- Hypocellularity to marrow aplasia
- Absence of fat cells
- Edema
- Fibrinoid necrosis
- Dilated sinuses
- Rare stromal cells, histiocytes, lymphocytes, and perivascular plasma cells

Intermediate Changes
- Reappearance of fat, often lobulated
- Mild transient reticulin fibrosis
- Foci of left-shifted erythroid and granulocyte islands
- Increase in precursor B cells or hematogones on smears

Late Changes
- Resolution of reticulin fibrosis
- Appearance of small megakaryocytes in clusters
- Normal or slightly increased marrow cellularity

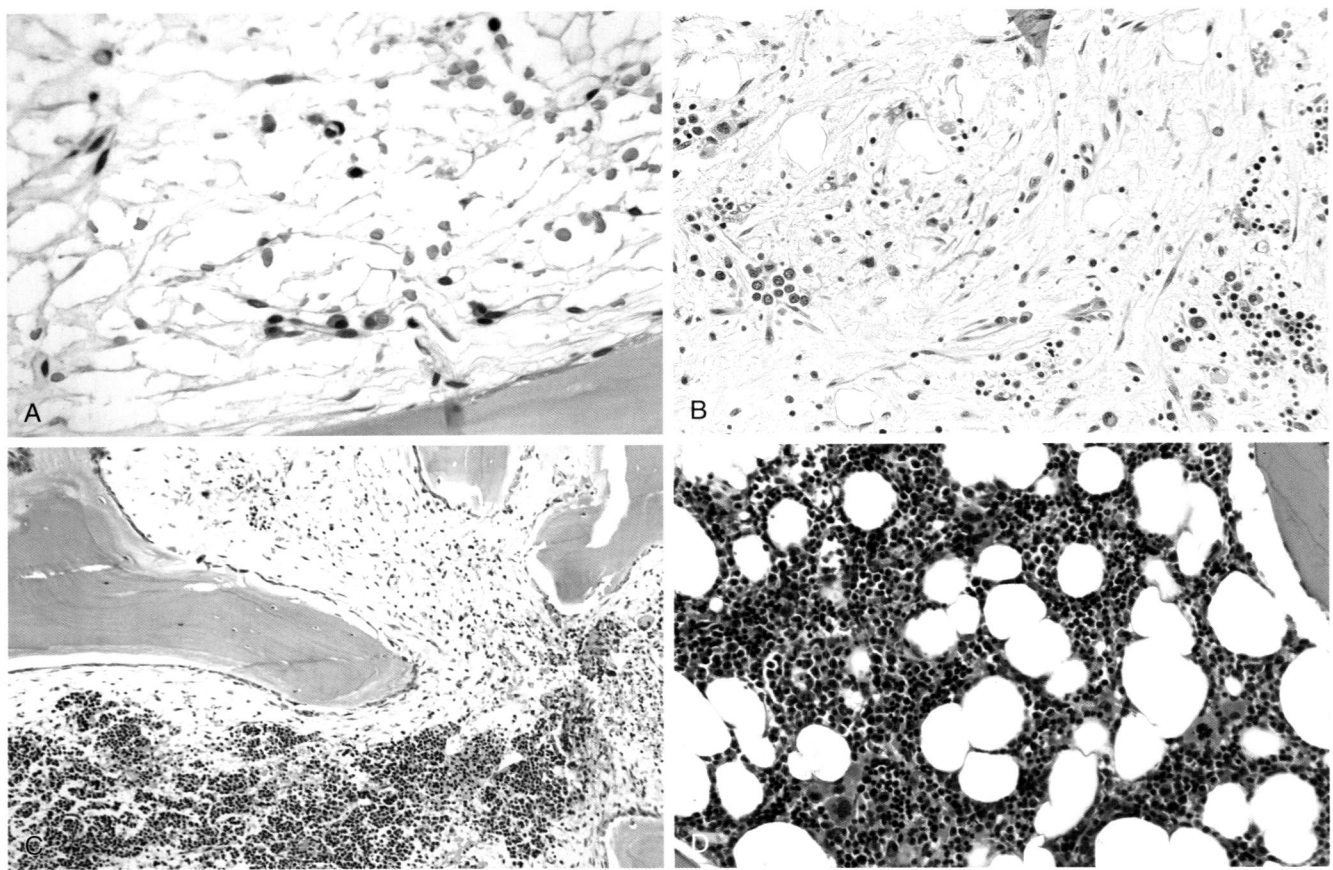

Figure 56-1. Bone marrow changes of myeloablative therapy. A, The marrow is initially acellular, with loss of fat cells. **B,** Islands of erythroid and granulocyte precursors then appear. **C,** The cellularity is often patchy, with acellular areas and areas of left-shifted cells. The hypocellular areas of this marrow still show mild fibrosis, which resolves as hematopoiesis returns. **D,** At 3 to 4 weeks, marrow cellularity returns.

Box 56-2 *Post-Therapy Bone Marrow Changes Unique to Hematopoietic Stem Cell Transplantation*

- Regenerative islands with a monotonous, immature appearance
- Localization of immature cell precursors away from bony trabeculae (nonparatrabecular area)
- Increased storage iron and siderotic iron with or without ring sideroblasts
- Prolonged variable cellularity with or without cytopenias
- Prolonged aplasia resulting from engraftment failure
- Increased large granular lymphocytes

in normal marrow and in regenerating marrow after cytotoxic therapy. The presence of such islands away from the bone is considered an abnormal feature, referred to as abnormal localization of immature precursors (ALIP), and is described as a feature of myelodysplastic syndrome (MDS) on biopsy sections. After hematopoietic stem cell transplantation, these immature cell islands often occur away from the bone, and this feature should not be considered evidence of recurrent or impending MDS (Fig. 56-2).[14,15]

Bone marrow cellularity approaches 50% to 100% of normal by day 21 to day 28. Although engraftment is affected by many variables, including dose of infused cells, source

of donor cells, and degree of HLA mismatch, engrafted trilineage hematopoiesis with normal cellularity is expected by day 28.[3,16] Transient dysplastic features in erythroid and granulocytic cells associated with chemotherapy may be seen.[9] Transient fibrosis and fibrinoid necrosis may be observed.[3] Increases in bone marrow iron storage or siderotic iron incorporation are also common findings after hematopoietic stem cell transplantation. This is usually apparent by an increase in hemosiderin-laden macrophages on both aspirate smears and trephine biopsy sections. Although the increase in siderotic iron is usually less uniform than that seen in refractory anemia with ring sideroblasts, in some cases, the pattern of iron staining may be similar or identical to that of sideroblastic anemia; therefore, iron stains must be interpreted with caution in post–marrow transplant patients.[17]

In some patients, bone marrow cellularity may never return to the normal range after hematopoietic stem cell transplantation. These patients frequently exhibit variability in marrow cellularity and often have a persistently hypocellular marrow that may be accompanied by mild peripheral blood cytopenias for many years. Prolonged impairment of hematopoiesis has been demonstrated after both standard and high-dose chemotherapy followed by bone marrow transplantation.[18,19] A hypocellular post-treatment marrow may result from bone marrow failure after solid

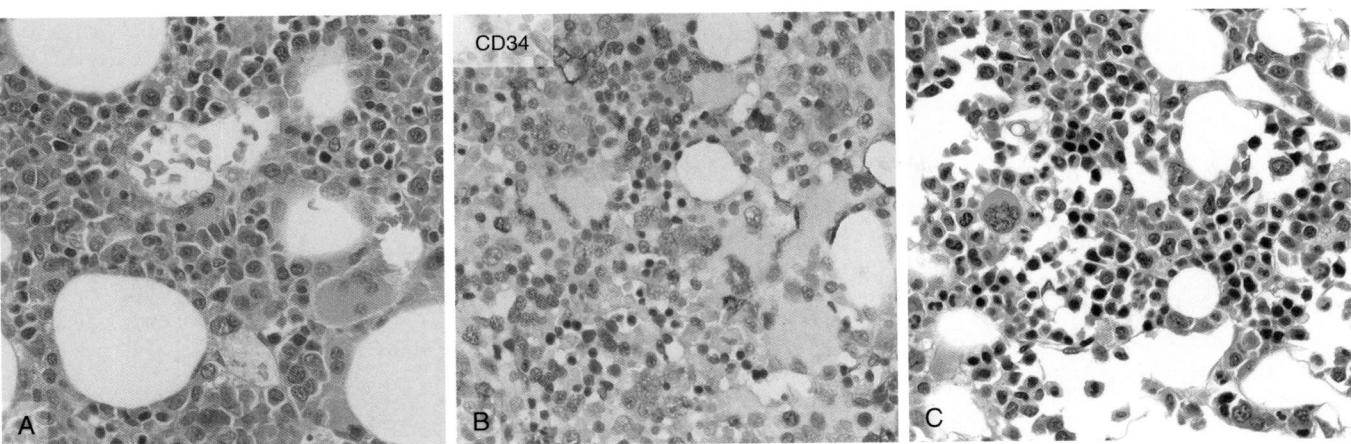

CD34

Figure 56-2. Although abnormal localization of immature precursors (ALIP) is a common neoplastic feature of myelodysplastic syndromes as shown by H&E (hematoxylin and eosin) in **(A)** and by CD34 immunostaining in **(B)**, in the case of patients after hematopoietic cell transplantation **(C)**, such myeloid maturation away from the bone is normal and should not be overinterpreted as evidence of myelodysplasia.

organ or hematopoietic stem cell transplantation, failure to engraft after transplantation, or delayed engraftment after transplantation. The bone marrow in these patients is similar and shows signs of aplasia, even after several weeks, with predominance of stromal cells, histiocytes, lymphocytes, and plasma cells. Delayed engraftment may occur in patients with marked marrow fibrosis before transplantation, and diffuse histiocytic proliferations.[20,21] Graft failure after hematopoietic stem cell transplantation or bone marrow failure after solid organ transplantation may occur secondary to viral infection, reactivation of a virus, or hemophagocytic syndrome.[22-25] Late marrow failure may also occur as a terminal event of post-therapy MDS. The immunodeficiency associated with chemotherapy or transplantation also increases these patients' risk of developing infectious diseases. If an infectious disease is suspected, fresh bone marrow aspirate material should be sent for microbiology studies. Histochemical stains for acid-fast and fungal organisms should be performed on all biopsy specimens containing granulomas.

Recombinant Cytokine Therapy

Recombinant human cytokine factors (granulocyte colony-stimulating factor [G-CSF], granulocyte-macrophage colony-stimulating factor [GM-CSF], interleukin [IL]2, IL3, IL11, erythropoietin, and thrombopoietin) are administered for a variety of reasons, including shortening cytopenic periods and enhancing bone marrow recovery after chemotherapy. In addition, such agents may be used to prime the marrow or peripheral blood before hematopoietic stem cell collection. It is essential that the administration of these agents be included in the clinical history of any patient undergoing bone marrow sampling.

The most commonly administered growth factors are human recombinant G-CSF and GM-CSF. Both peripheral blood and bone marrow alterations occur with these drugs (Box 56-3).[26-31] Both agents accelerate neutrophil recovery by 2 to 5 days and result in a peripheral blood leukocytosis with a left shift in granulocytes. Toxic granulation and Döhle bodies are often present and may give the appearance of a reactive proliferation. Enlarged neutrophils or neutrophils with vacuolated cytoplasm may also occur. The bone marrow shows a granulocytic hyperplasia (Fig. 56-3). Depending on the

Box 56-3 Changes Associated With Recombinant Granulocyte Colony-Stimulating Factor and Granulocyte-Macrophage Colony-Stimulating Factor Therapies

Peripheral Blood Changes
- Neutrophilia
- Granulocyte left shift
- Toxic granulation
- Döhle bodies
- Hypogranular neutrophils
- Vacuolated neutrophils
- Giant neutrophils
- Increase in large granular lymphocytes
- Eosinophilia
- Transient blast cells
- Circulating nucleated red blood cells

Early Bone Marrow Changes
- Granulocytic hyperplasia with an increased number of promyelocytes and myelocytes
- Transient blast-cell increase
- Toxic granulation of granulocytes
- Enlarged promyelocytes and myelocytes
- Increased macrophages (granulocyte-macrophage colony-stimulating factor [GM-CSF])
- Increased mitotic activity of granulocyte precursors
- Biopsy hypocellularity with left-shifted granulocytic precursors

Late Bone Marrow Changes
- Binucleated promyelocytes
- Marrow neutrophilia
- Marrow eosinophilia
- Toxic granulation
- Variable biopsy cellularity

timing of bone marrow examination, the marrow may exhibit the complete spectrum of granulocytic maturation, have the appearance of maturation arrest, or show a predominance of segmented neutrophils. The maturation arrest–type changes that occur just after administration of growth factor pose the greatest challenge because they may be indistinguishable from recurrent leukemia or MDS. A predominance of promyelocytes (enlarged binucleated form) and myelocytes is usually present. In rare cases, bone marrow and even peripheral blood blasts

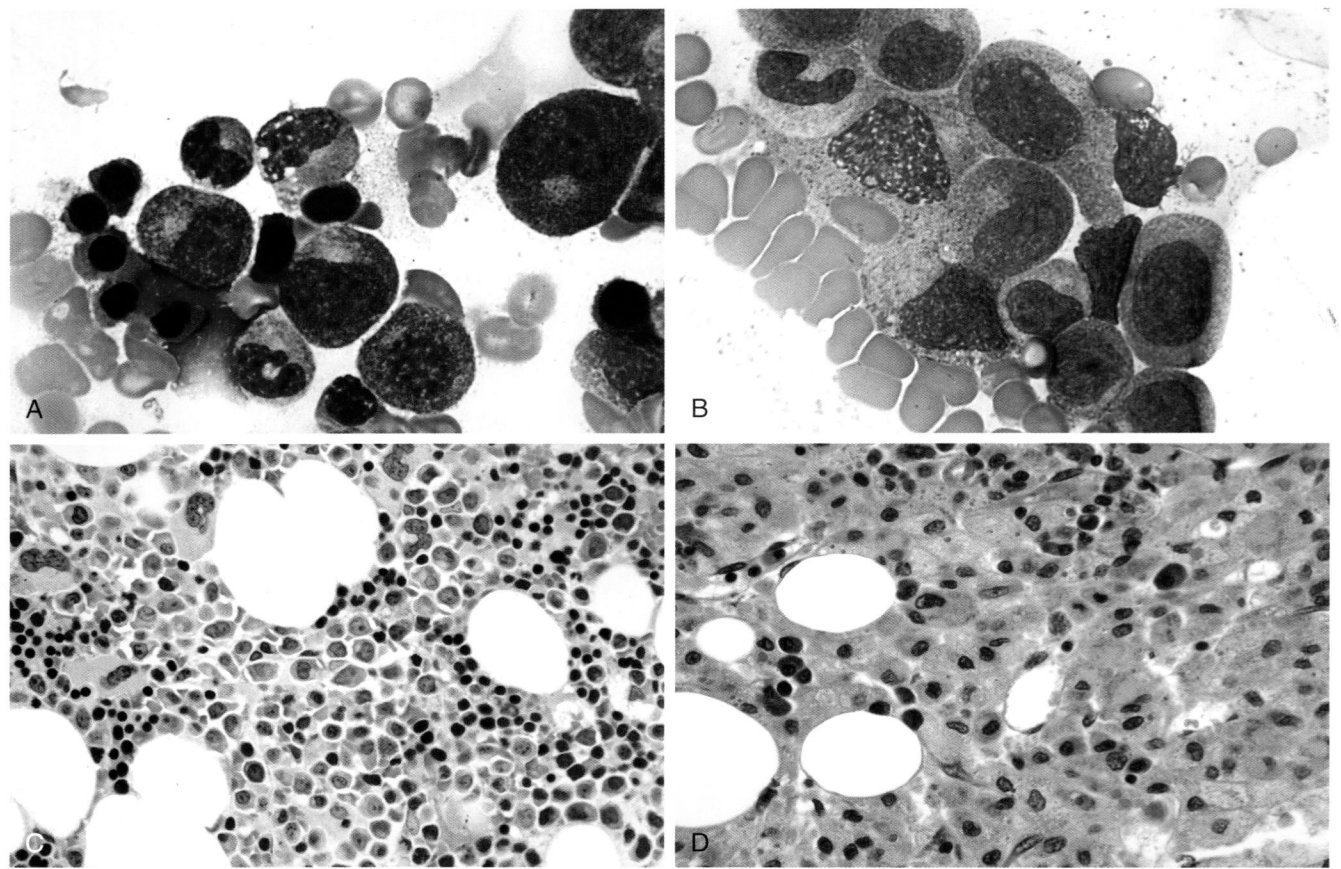

Figure 56-3. Bone marrow changes associated with granulocyte and granulocyte-macrophage colony-stimulating factors. A and **B,** Aspirate smears show an increase in promyelocytes with perinuclear hofs. **C,** Biopsy usually shows aggregates of left-shifted granulocytes. **D,** Rare cases show sheets of bone marrow histiocytes on the biopsy. These may be confused with metastatic tumor.

may exceed 5%,[31] but this increase is usually accompanied by an increase in promyelocytes.[32] The transient increase in blast cells from growth factor administration should result in even higher numbers of promyelocytes; thus, blast proliferations that are not accompanied by an increase in promyelocytes should be considered highly suspicious for leukemia and not simply attributed to growth factor–derived changes. In a patient with a history of acute myeloid leukemia (AML), it may not be possible to entirely exclude the possibility of residual leukemia in the setting of an increase in blasts, and flow cytometric evaluation for immunophenotypic aberrancies and/or cytogenetic studies may be useful in this setting. The promyelocytes that occur with G-CSF and GM-CSF therapy usually have prominent perinuclear hofs, and this feature should be a clue to the possibility of growth factor administration. These cells differ from those of acute promyelocytic leukemia,[33] which usually do not show perinuclear cytoplasmic clearing and demonstrate Auer rods, which are not present in reactive promyelocytes. Occasional giant tetraploid neutrophils are noted. In patients receiving GM-CSF, increased macrophages in the bone marrow and monocytosis in addition to hypercellular marrow involving trilineage hematopoietic cells may be present.[34] A repeat bone marrow examination 1 to 2 weeks after cessation of the growth factor usually demonstrates more complete granulocyte maturation, and such a study is advisable in cases suggestive of residual leukemia. If true leukemic blasts are present, they will

persist or increase during this brief interval, whereas reactive growth factor changes will resolve with time. Less common changes reported after G-CSF and GM-CSF therapy include marrow necrosis[35] and marrow histiocytic proliferation,[34,36] which may be confused with metastatic tumors.[37]

IL2 infusion appears to result in granulocyte recovery by stimulating the natural production of GM-CSF.[38] IL3 appears to stimulate differentiation of even earlier progenitor cells than those of G-CSF and GM-CSF, resulting in an increase of all lineage cells (granulocytes, erythroid precursors, lymphoid cells, and megakaryocytes) and marrow cellularity. This agent also results in eosinophilia and may cause bone marrow fibrosis.[39] IL11 also stimulates proliferation of earlier progenitor cells and synergizes with IL3 and erythropoietin to promote erythropoiesis and megakaryopoiesis.[40]

Changes related to erythropoietin usually do not cause as much diagnostic confusion, and bone marrow studies are less commonly performed in patients taking this drug. Erythropoietin, which is given for various causes of red cell aplasia, including renal disease and aplastic anemia, usually results in a relative increase in marrow cellularity owing to proliferation of red blood cell precursors and maturation.[41-46] This red blood cell increase may result in a normal or decreased myeloid-to-erythroid ratio in the marrow. Patients who have erythroid hyperplasia from erythropoietin may also show mild nuclear irregularities and a left shift of the maturing erythroid cells. The lack of dyspoietic changes in other cell lines is helpful in excluding MDS in this setting. Some patients with MDS treated with erythropoietin may actually show a relative decrease in erythropoiesis, presumably from a reduction in the degree of ineffective hematopoiesis.[45] Erythropoietin also stimulates megakaryopoiesis[46] and may result in megakaryocytic hyperplasia of the bone marrow. Rare patients who received erythropoietin have pure red cell aplasia caused by the development of anti-erythropoietin antibodies.[47]

Recombinant thrombopoietin may be given during or after chemotherapy, usually in combination with G-CSF or GM-CSF, to promote megakaryopoiesis and stimulate megakaryocyte precursors and platelet production.[48-50] Although peripheral blood platelets may increase to as high as $1000 \times 10^3/\mu L$, they are usually normal in appearance. Bone marrow cellularity increases in these patients, even compared with patients on GM-CSF alone, and the addition of thrombopoietin appears to increase the percentage of marrow granulocytes compared with GM-CSF alone. The megakaryocytic increase, however, is the most striking feature of thrombopoietin administration, with a subset of patients showing true megakaryocytic hyperplasia. The megakaryocytes are usually atypical, with a spectrum ranging from small hypolobated megakaryocytes with hyperchromatic nuclei to large megakaryocytes with hyperlobated nuclei. Intrasinusoidal megakaryocytes may also be present. The increase in megakaryocytes is usually associated with an increase in marrow fibrosis, and some patients have osteosclerosis. The atypical megakaryocytes may raise suspicion of MDS, but dysplastic changes are not seen in other cell lineages. A subset of patients may have leukoerythroblastosis, with circulating megakaryocyte nuclei and thrombocytosis. Because these patients may also exhibit marrow hypercellularity with atypical megakaryocytic hyperplasia and bony sclerosis, it may not be possible to distinguish the changes related to thrombopoietin therapy from a myeloproliferative neoplasm (MPN), particularly primary myelofibrosis, without adequate clinical information. The lack of splenomegaly and the rapid resolution of the changes after discontinuing thrombopoietin are useful in this differential diagnosis. The nonpeptide thrombopoietin receptor agonist eltrombopag stimulates megakaryopoiesis and contributes to differentiation and increased platelet numbers.[51]

Pegylated recombinant human megakaryocyte growth and development factor has also been shown to increase bone marrow megakaryocyte production in normal individuals and in patients with aplastic anemia, MDS, and AML.[52,53] The effects are significantly increased when used in combination with other growth factors. The morphologic features of the bone marrow after administration of this agent are not well described.

Other Selected Therapies

Lenalidomide and derivatives, immunomodulatory agents, are used to treat MDS, plasma cell neoplasms, and some lymphomas.[54,55] In MDS, cytologic dysplastic features in all trilineage cell lines, blast count, and ring sideroblast percentage are reduced after therapy. The dysplastic hypolobated or nonlobated megakaryocytes noted in isolated 5q deletion are particularly decreased after therapy. Lenalidomide therapy can also lead to degenerative changes in neoplastic plasma cells and increased apoptotic bodies and reduce neoplastic plasma cells. Lenalidomide is effective in treating some non-Hodgkin lymphomas as a single agent or in combination

therapy via T-cell/natural killer (NK)-cell enhancement and antiproliferative effects.[54]

The tyrosine kinase inhibitor (TKI) imatinib and second-generation TKIs are highly effective first-line therapies for chronic myeloid leukemia. TKIs bind to the ABL domain of the BCR::ABL fusion protein, thereby preventing adenosine triphosphate (ATP) binding and inhibiting the fusion protein. Response to therapy (hematologic, morphologic, cytogenetic, and molecular) is monitored according to the National Comprehensive Cancer Network® (NCCN) guidelines.[56] Response is determined by the normalization of parameters in peripheral blood counts, decrease in the number of Philadelphia (Ph)-positive metaphases on cytogenetics, and decrease in the number of BCR::ABL1 mRNA transcripts by quantitative polymerase chain reaction (qPCR). After TKI therapy, the bone marrow shows morphologic changes, including reduced overall cellularity, reduced myeloid precursors and megakaryocytes, reduced severity of myelofibrosis, and regeneration in erythroid precursors. However, it can cause bone marrow hypoplasia, gelatinous transformation, pseudo Gaucher cells, or benign transient lymphoid nodules.[57]

Janus kinase (JAK) inhibitors (ruxolitinib, fedratinib) target JAK-associated signaling pathways for erythropoietin-mediated and thrombopoietin-mediated signaling and are used to treat MPNs, many immune-mediated and inflammatory diseases, and graft-versus-host disease. Most patients with MPNs have *JAK2* mutations with upregulated JAK-STAT signaling. JAK inhibitors can reduce significant constitutional symptoms and splenomegaly and induce limited reversal of marrow fibrosis. Overall survival (OS) after JAK inhibitor therapy in primary myelofibrosis has improved. However, JAK inhibitors can often cause anemia and thrombocytopenia, which is most evident within the first 8 to 12 weeks of therapy.[58-61]

Rituximab, an anti-CD20 monoclonal antibody, is used to eradicate B cells in B-cell non-Hodgkin lymphomas or in some autoimmune or inflammatory disorders. It can be used as a single agent or in combination with other chemotherapeutic agents. The treatment is effective, particularly in a B-cell lymphoma expressing strong CD20.[62,63] However, after therapy with rituximab, bone marrow with involvement by a B-cell lymphoma may show lymphoid aggregates or lesions containing predominantly T cells.[64,65] Normal and neoplastic B cells can demonstrate a transient loss of CD20 expression after anti-CD20 therapy, and immunophenotypic evaluation after rituximab therapy (by flow cytometry or immunohistochemistry) will require other B-cell markers such as CD19, CD22, Pax5, or CD79a to find residual lymphoma. In some cases, a CD20-negative tumor subclone may emerge and lead to a CD20-negative relapse post–rituximab therapy. Rituximab can cause a self-limiting neutropenia with granulocytic maturation arrest, thrombocytopenia, and rarely, disseminate intravascular coagulation.[65-68] Additional markers such as CD19, CD22, and CD38 are now the targets of monoclonal antibodies, bispecific T-cell engaging antibodies, and CAR T cells. The effects of these will be discussed further in this chapter.

ACUTE LEUKEMIA OR MYELODYSPLASTIC SYNDROME

With effective chemotherapy, the marrow is completely ablated, and bone marrow studies may be performed to confirm obliteration of the neoplastic process. Once the bone marrow has begun to regain cellularity with normal hematopoietic cells, the pathologist is faced with the challenge of evaluating for residual or recurrent disease. It is well established that the presence of minimal/measurable residual disease (MRD) that is undetectable by morphologic methods is a powerful predictor of recurrence. Although different types of acute leukemia offer their own unique problems, some general features are common to all cases. A blast count of 5% in the bone marrow is the historical cutoff for delineating the presence of residual or recurrent leukemia. However, this cutoff is arbitrary, and the current goal is to detect the presence of neoplastic clones as early as possible. The use of multiparameter flow cytometry and molecular genetic techniques to detect MRD is redefining remission in many diseases.[26,69-71] A general overview of the sensitivity of the methods used to detect MRD is given in Table 56-1. Knowledge of the advantages and disadvantages of different methods and appropriate selection of the appropriate method requires considering turn-around time, cost, availability, and standardization.[72]

The common use of growth factors can cause regenerative blast to increase above 5% in some cases. In this setting, it may be difficult to differentiate regenerating blasts from leukemic blasts by morphology. Therefore, decisions regarding relapse or remission should not be based on blast counts alone. When a blast population in post-therapy bone marrow is suspicious for residual disease, comparison to the original acute leukemia is often helpful, and the presence of unique morphologic features such as Auer rods, distinctive cytoplasmic granules, prominent nucleoli, or nuclear irregularities that were identified in the original disease can be useful. In addition, the detection of an aberrant immunophenotype by flow cytometry is helpful. The immunohistochemical detection of immature CD34-positive or terminal deoxynucleotidyl transferase (TdT)-positive cells in clusters in a bone marrow biopsy is also helpful because immature cells in regenerating bone marrow do not normally show the clustering seen in recurrent leukemia specimens.

Surveillance of bone marrow is usually required to detect residual disease and recurrent disease, as most recurrence occurs within 1 to 3 years after the end of therapy. The detection of clonal cytogenetic abnormalities that were present in the patient's original leukemia can also be helpful in the evaluation of residual or recurrent disease.[26] Routine karyotype analysis or fluorescence in situ hybridization (FISH) studies are commonly used for this purpose. Ancillary

testing is not necessary on all follow-up specimens. If residual or recurrent disease is suspected in the absence of material for these tests, such suspicion should be relayed to the treating physician. A repeat bone marrow evaluation after 1 or 2 weeks is often helpful to determine a change in the number of blasts, which would be expected to increase with recurrent disease, and appropriate ancillary tests can be performed on the second specimen. In contrast, increased immature cells in an early phase of marrow regeneration would be expected to show more mature precursors in the second bone marrow study.

Two common approaches to detect MRD with high sensitivity are multiparameter flow cytometry and molecular tests including qPCR for specific targets and next-generation sequencing (NGS)-based technologies. Knowledge of the immunophenotypic and genetic characteristics of a leukemia at diagnosis may facilitate assessment for residual or recurrent disease post-therapy, though it is not critical in all settings. Assessment of MRD after cycle 1 or 2 of induction chemotherapy can allow earlier identification of poor responders.[73,74]

Acute Myeloid Leukemia and Myelodysplastic Syndrome

Morphologic Features

Early assessment of the bone marrow is considered the standard measure of response evaluation after induction chemotherapy in patients with AML, although the conventional measure of response after induction chemotherapy is to assess the blast counts on day 28.[26] Early blast clearance indicating adequate cytoreduction confers a good prognosis, irrespective of either the specific day of the bone marrow assessment or evaluation of blast clearance from the peripheral blood. The NCCN guidelines[27] recommend performing bone marrow aspiration and biopsy 14 to 21 days after starting induction therapy (commonly referred to as "day 14 marrow"). Those who have significant residual disease and do not achieve a hypoplastic marrow, defined as cellularity greater than 20% and blasts greater than 5%, are recommended to undergo an early second cycle of induction chemotherapy. Although blast counts on day 14 bone marrow are highly sensitive in predicting remission on day 28, there is increasing evidence of this measurement lacking specificity, as a significant proportion of patients with residual disease on day 14 bone marrow still achieve a complete remission of their disease without a second cycle of induction therapy. This lack of specificity may be explained by an inability of to identify covariates associated with resistance, slow responders in certain AML subtypes, and interobserver and intraobserver variability in assessing blast counts by morphology alone, particularly in the presence of hypoplastic changes induced by therapy.

Remission status is typically assessed from day 28 to 35, as the peripheral blood counts recover from induction chemotherapy. Published guidelines for the morphologic definition of complete remission in patients treated for AML require peripheral blood neutrophil counts of greater than 1.0×10^9/L, platelet counts of at least 100×10^9/L, less than 5% bone marrow blasts without Auer rods, no extramedullary disease, and independence from red cell transfusion.[27] Patients with MRD at the end of treatment or prior to transplantation have

Table 56-1 Sensitivity of Methods for Detecting Residual Disease

Method	Sensitivity (%)
Morphology	1–5
Cytogenetic karyotype analysis	3–5
FISH	1–5
Immunohistochemistry	0.1–5
Consensus primer PCR for gene rearrangements	0.1–1
Flow cytometry	0.01–1
Next-generation sequencing	0.0001–5
PCR and RT-PCR for specific translocations	0.001–0.01
Patient-specific PCR and RT-PCR	0.001

FISH, Fluorescence in situ hybridization; *PCR,* polymerase chain reaction; *RT-PCR,* reverse transcriptase polymerase chain reaction.

shown similar outcomes as those of patients who have bone marrow blasts >5%.[75] Therefore, more detailed evaluation of bone marrow and peripheral blood samples is needed than is suggested by the remission criteria.

The presence of an increased number of blasts with features similar to the original AML or MDS should be regarded with suspicion. Auer rods (rod-shaped cytoplasmic aggregates of granules) are not a feature of regenerating or nonneoplastic myeloblasts and should be considered evidence of residual disease. Auer rods may rarely be encountered in maturing granulocytes but are nevertheless considered abnormal. Regenerating blasts are usually admixed with promyelocytes and maturing granulocytes, and the presence of sheets of blasts on a smear is a sign of recurrent disease. In contrast, specimens with equal or fewer numbers of blasts compared with promyelocytes usually represent regeneration.[2,76] Clustering of blasts is often difficult to interpret on H&E (hematoxylin and eosin)-stained biopsy specimens, and aggregates of regeneration may be difficult to differentiate from leukemic blasts aggregates. Regeneration usually occurs adjacent to bony trabeculae, and the presence of immature cell aggregates away from the bone is considered abnormal. This abnormal localization of immature cell precursors has been used as a feature of myelodysplasia, but as mentioned, caution should be applied when these criteria are used in patients who have received hematopoietic stem cell transplants. After transplantation, the normal bone marrow architecture may change, and regenerating immature precursors may be present away from the bone on the biopsy specimens.

Cases previously considered AML with myelodysplasia-related changes and MDS may exhibit multilineage dysplasia before an increase in blasts at relapse. The features of the original multilineage dysplasia should be reviewed, and care should be taken not to overestimate multilineage dysplasia during or immediately after therapy. Dyserythropoietic changes are common during chemotherapy and often include a left shift of erythroid precursors and multinucleation or nuclear irregularity of erythroid cells (Fig. 56-4). In addition, some regenerating megakaryocytes can be small and can cluster during or immediately after chemotherapy; however, numerous megakaryocytes with separate nuclear lobes or a predominance and increase of small hypolobated megakaryocytes or micromegakaryocytes with absence of nuclear segmentation can be useful in identifying residual disease. Granulocyte changes after therapy are usually restricted to a left shift without the hypogranulation or nuclear abnormalities commonly seen in association with MDS. Therefore, dysplastic changes of maturing granulocytes are also more reliable in identifying recurrent AML with multilineage dysplasia during or immediately after chemotherapy than erythroid abnormalities alone (Fig. 56-5).

Currently, most patients with acute promyelocytic leukemia are treated with both standard chemotherapy and all-trans retinoic acid (ATRA) or combinations of ATRA with arsenic trioxide, and their bone marrow changes are usually similar to those seen in other AML samples. However, ATRA induces maturation of leukemic blasts/promyelocytes rather than their destruction; thus, morphologic remission can often be achieved without initial significant bone marrow hypoplasia or aplasia.[3,77] The bone marrow in these patients may remain hypercellular, with markedly elevated numbers of promyelocytes (Fig. 56-6). These cells usually undergo slow

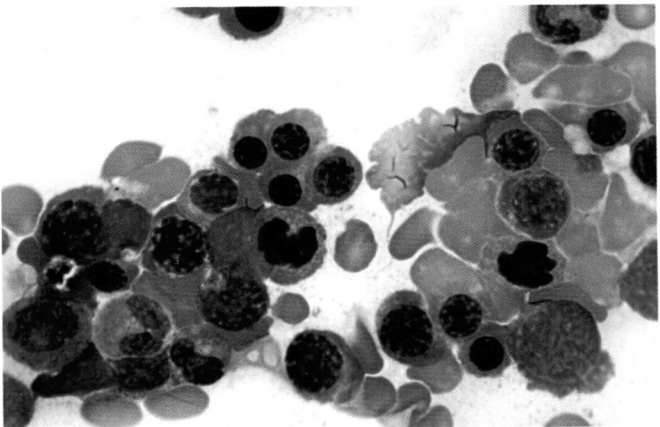

Figure 56-4. Post-therapy dyserythropoiesis associated with erythroid hyperplasia are common and should not be interpreted as myelodysplastic syndrome, which should exhibit dysplastic changes of other cell lines.

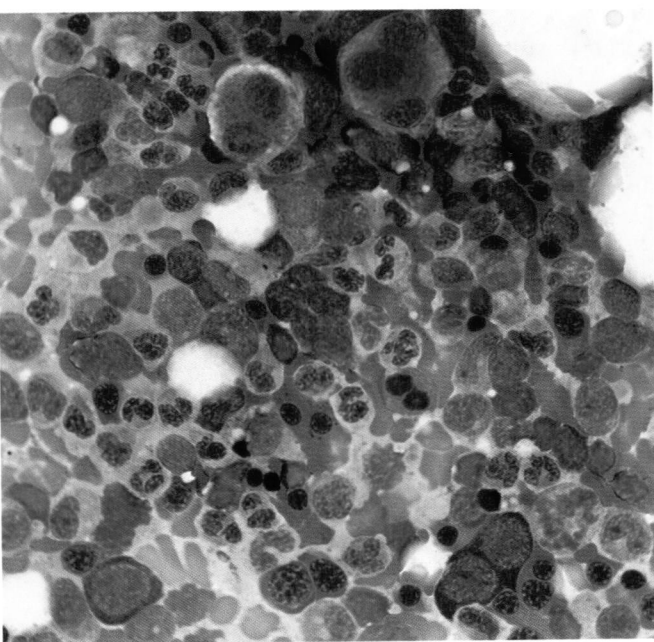

Figure 56-5. Relapse in a patient with previous acute myeloid leukemia with myelodysplasia-related changes. Although blasts are only slightly increased, dysplastic changes are clearly present in megakaryocytes, erythroid precursors, and myeloid cells.

maturation secondary to the therapy, with loss of the t(15;17) cytogenetic abnormality associated with acute promyelocytic leukemia. In this subgroup of patients, it should be understood that the presence of sheets of promyelocytes may not indicate treatment failure, and they should be followed closely with additional bone marrow examinations to confirm that maturational changes are occurring.

Immunophenotyping

Immunophenotyping by multiparametric flow cytometry is an extremely valuable tool in identification of residual disease post-therapy with proven prognostic significance in evaluating patients with AML post-therapy.[78] Flow cytometry is both

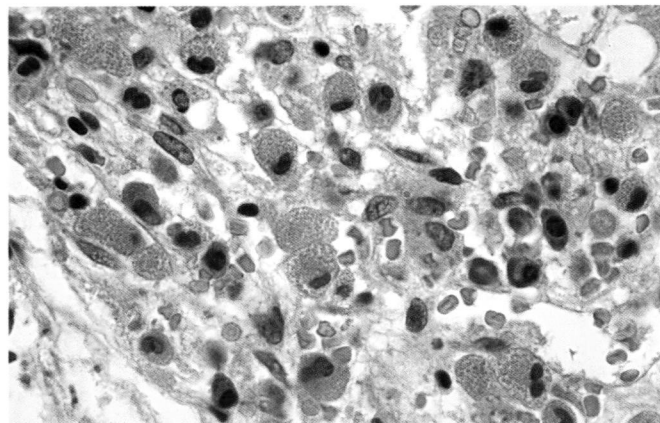

Figure 56-6. Residual promyelocytes during therapy for acute promyelocytic leukemia treated with all-trans retinoic acid. Follow-up bone marrow examination showed continued maturation of granulocytes without a change in therapy.

more sensitive and more specific for identifying abnormal blast populations than morphology, with some investigators suggesting that the morphologic blast percentage may provide limited data in the setting of high quality multiparametric flow cytometric data.[79] Normal regenerating marrow shows conserved and predictable changes in antigen expression with maturation, but residual blasts show immunophenotypic alterations that deviate from normal patterns, allowing identification as residual disease. Approaches to residual disease detection for AML by flow cytometry include a difference from normal (DfN) approach and the leukemia-associated immunophenotype approach (LAIP). When using both methods (events are collected, if adequate, and an adequate panel is used), abnormal myeloid blast populations can be reliably detected with a sensitivity of 0.1% (1 abnormal cell in 1000), a widely accepted level of clinical significance, and depending on the blast immunophenotype and assay characteristics, can sometimes be detected at lower levels. In the DfN approach, patterns of antigen expression on normal regenerating progenitors are defined using a standardized panel. Using these same panels, abnormal blast populations harbor immunophenotypic alterations that render them "different from normal," allowing their identification as persistent disease. In the LAIP approach, immunophenotypic abnormalities that characterize the leukemic blasts seen at diagnosis are characterized, and subsequent samples from the patient are evaluated for these same alterations. The abnormalities that characterize abnormal blasts in myeloid neoplasms can include abnormal intensity of antigen expression (i.e., increased or decreased expression; absence of an antigen; or homogeneous expression of an antigen normally expressed in a heterogenous fashion); asynchronous antigen expression (co-expression of a mature and immature antigen); and expression of an antigen of a lymphoid lineage.[80] Examples of MRD evaluation for AML by flow cytometry are shown in Figure 56-7. Both the DfN and LAIP approaches are associated with strengths and weaknesses, and the best approach involves incorporating both strategies in an evaluation for MRD. A combined approach is endorsed by the European Leukemia Net (ELN). The reader is referred to published comprehensive guidelines from the ELN for assessing MRD in AML.[81] Although flow cytometric MRD is applicable in

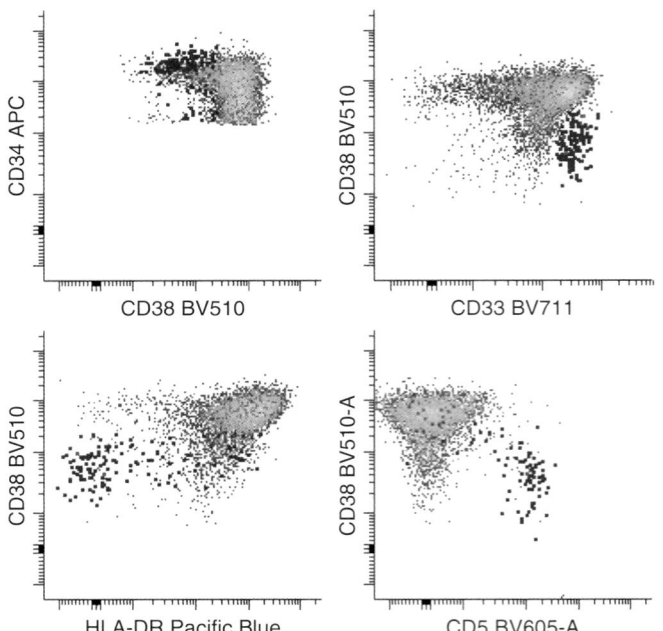

Figure 56-7. Example of minimal/measurable residual disease (MRD) in acute myeloid leukemia. All plots show CD34-positive myeloid blasts (1.2% of the total white blood cell count). Normal regenerating blasts are *colored aqua* (1.0% of the white blood cells), and residual leukemic blasts are *highlighted in red* (0.2% of the white blood cells). The residual leukemic blasts in this case have a stem-cell–like immunophenotype with bright CD34 and dim CD38 and show aberrant expression of CD5, CD33 (increased), CD38 (decreased), and HLA-DR (decreased to absent). Although the residual leukemic cells are difficult to distinguish from normal progenitors on the plot of CD34 versus CD38, the leukemic and normal blasts are well separated using other antigens and a multiparametric approach with evaluation of several informative projections allows confident identification of the abnormal population.

the vast majority of cases, it should be noted that sensitivity may be lower with some immunophenotypes (i.e., acute promyelocytic leukemia), which may benefit from alternative methods of MRD detection, including molecular-based studies. The ELN guidelines present a scheme for assessing AML MRD based on the genetic and immunophenotypic features of the acute leukemia at diagnosis.

Paraffin section immunohistochemistry may be of value in selected cases, particularly in the presence of left-shifted cell aggregates on H&E-stained sections. Immunophenotyping can show that the immature cell aggregates of regeneration represent a spectrum of left-shifted cells that are not exclusively blast cells, whereas in residual/recurrent leukemia, blast cell aggregates are a more uniform population of neoplastic cells. The identification of cohesive clusters of cells expressing the immature cell antigen CD34 and/or an aberrant combination of antigens may favor residual or recurrent disease. Immunohistochemistry has also been described as useful for identifying residual disease in cases of AML with an *NPM1* mutation, as immunohistochemistry for NPM1 may assist in identifying clusters of residual neoplastic cells.[82]

Cytogenetics and Molecular Studies

Cytogenetic studies are not performed on all post-therapy samples but may be of value in some situations. Although some cases of AML are associated with normal karyotypes, most show a clonal cytogenetic abnormality. However, an abnormal karyotype in the diagnostic bone marrow is an independent prognostic indicator that is predictive of induction success, cumulative incidence of relapse, and OS in adult patients with AML.[83-88] Identification of that abnormality in a follow-up sample is highly supportive of relapsed disease. Karyotype analysis routinely includes the study of 20 cells; therefore, this method is not optimal for the detection of MRD when blast cells are below 5%. Most cytogenetic laboratories also perform FISH, which allows the screening of several hundred cells for a specific abnormality. This method may increase the detection rate of residual disease over karyotype analysis alone, but it requires knowledge of the karyotypic abnormality of the original disease and probes specific for that abnormality. FISH probes are useful in identifying monosomies, trisomies, and masked 11q23.3 abnormalities, in addition to balanced chromosomal translocations. The detection of numerical chromosomal abnormalities by FISH during clinical remission has been shown to correlate with an increased risk of disease recurrence.[89] Another use of karyotype analysis and FISH is evaluation for XX/XY chimerism.[90] If a patient receives an allogeneic transplant from a donor of the opposite sex, karyotype and FISH studies can reveal the presence of residual host cells in the bone marrow, even if they are of a normal karyotype. In addition, human leukocyte antigen (HLA)-based chimerism studies are used in a similar fashion.[91] However, the detection of nondonor cells in the marrow is less predictive of recurrent disease than is the detection of a leukemia-specific abnormality.

The frequent presence of mutations in AML allows molecular monitoring of MRD. These methods generally use PCR and can potentially detect 1 tumor cell in 100,000 cells. Efforts have been made to standardize these procedures,[92] but there are still some differences in methodology and preferred targets of study among laboratories. In general, PCR testing for MRD requires knowledge of the original karyotypic or other molecular abnormalities and primers and probes for those abnormalities. However, not all markers are equally suitable for MRD monitoring. Currently, RUNX1::RUNX1T1 of t(8;21)(q22;q22.3), PML::RARA of t(15;17)(q24.1;q21.2), CBFB::MYH11 of inv(16)(p13.1q22)-t(16;16)(p13.1q22), and NPM1 mutations are thought to be the best molecular markers for MRD tracking.[81] The persistent presence of these molecular alterations after therapy is a strong predictor of relapse. These mutations can be determined accurately by real-time qPCR using cDNA as a template (Fig. 56-8). The assays for detecting these mutations are highly sensitive (10^{-4} to 10^{-6}) with excellent reproducibility, provided the sample is of good quality and the assay was carefully performed with appropriate controls. In addition, because of the unique translocations and insertions (in the case of NPM1), the assays for measuring these mutations are extremely specific with minimal background. This approach is applicable in about 40% to 50% of patients with AML harboring one of these mutations. The ELN has recommended molecular assessment of MRD in these groups of patients at clinically informative time points. These include at diagnosis, 2 months after standard induction/consolidation therapy, at the end of treatment, during follow-up, and every 3 months for 24 months after the end of treatment. The prognostic cutoff of MRD measurements differ among these groups of patients with AML harboring one of these mutations. Specifically, for

AML with CBFB::MYH11, MRD of ≥10 fusion copies per 10^5 ABL (control gene) copies at follow-up or end of therapy is associated with increased relapse risk but no difference in OS.[93] In AML with RUNX1::RUNXT1, MRD of ≥100 fusion copies per 10^5 ABL1 copies during follow-up is associated with a negative prognostic effect on relapse, but MRD negativity at earlier time points is prognostically irrelevant.[93,94] On the other hand, a >3 log reduction in levels of RUNX1::RUNXT1 fusion transcripts between the diagnosis and end of induction/consolidation therapy has a favorable prognostic effect with respect to relapse rate and OS.[94] It should be noted that low stable levels of CBFB::MYH11 and RUNX1::RUNX1T1 fusion transcripts may be detected by PCR years after the initial diagnosis without any evidence of disease relapse, suggesting other genetic or epigenetic aberrations are necessary for these types of leukemia to develop in addition to the translocations.[95] Thus, low levels of these fusion transcripts may not necessarily signify relapse, and consideration of the actual levels and dynamics of their abundance may be warranted. In APL, undetectable PML::RARA by sensitive PCR (at least 10^{-3}) at the end of consolation therapy is the most important MRD end point, associated with low risk of relapsed and better OS.[96,97] The presence of detectable NPM1 mutation after 2 cycles of cytotoxic therapy or at the end of therapy is associated with high risk of relapse.[98-100]

The qPCR approach described herein cannot be used for MRD assessment in the other AMLs without the aforementioned translocations or mutations. Molecular MRD must be determined using the other known mutations identified at the time of diagnosis based on the NGS approach. However, this approach may not be readily applicable because of two obstacles. First, the sensitivity of the current routine target sequencing platforms is ~1% to 5%, which is relatively low compared with that of the qPCR approach. In some cases, this level of sensitivity may not even be reached, depending on the library preparation protocol and bioinformatics pipeline. Second, many recurrently mutated genes found in AML are not suitable for use as molecular markers to track MRD. Some of the mutated genes, most commonly DNMT3A, TET2, and ASXL1 (so called "DTA genes"), persist at variable allele frequencies post-therapy despite achievement of complete morphologic remission (CR).[101-103] These mutations most likely represent postremission clonal hematopoiesis (CH) instead of residual AML and are present in the preleukemic founder clones. Postremission CH can persist long-term post-therapy and as a group is not correlated with increased relapse rate.[104] However, the persistence of non-DTA mutations during CR post-therapy (above a cutoff variant allele frequency [VAF] of 2.5%) has a negative prognostic effect with respect to the rates of relapse, relapse-free survival, and OS.[101-103] These findings support the utility of somatic mutations in non-preleukemic (non-DTA) genes as molecular MRD markers in AML. However, because of the tendency of these mutations to fluctuate as a result of clonal evolution, which results in gains or losses of these mutations at relapse, it is recommended that mutations in FLT3-ITD, FLT3-TKD, NRAS, KRAS, DNMT3A, ASXL1, IDH1, IDH2, and MLL-PTD not be used as single markers in MRD assessment. However, combination of two or more of these markers may be useful in determining MRD. For "hot-spot" mutations, for example, in codon 132 of IDH1; codons 140 and 172 of IDH2; and codons 12, 13, and 61 of KRAS, droplet digital PCR (ddPCR)

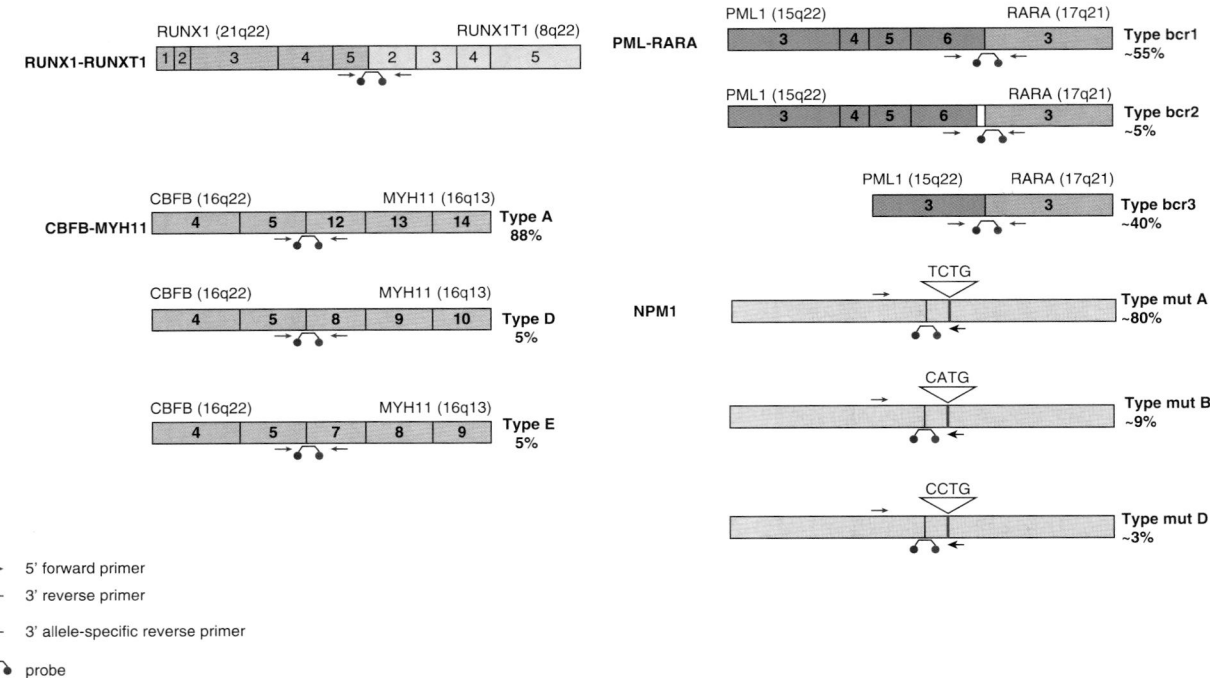

→   5′ forward primer

←   3′ reverse primer

←   3′ allele-specific reverse primer

⌒   probe

Figure 56-8. Real time quantitative polymerase chain reaction (PCR) measurement of four recommended biomarkers to measure minimal residual acute myeloid leukemia. The breakpoints of the reciprocal translocations and the types of insertions in *NPM1* mutations are indicated along with their respective frequencies: the forward primers, reverse primers (mutant-specific, if applicable), and probes are marked.

can be used to detect mutation at a sensitivity lower than that achieved by conventional target sequencing platforms. However, this approach is not feasible for the detection of other mutations that occur less frequently, as specific primers and probes need to be designed for individual patients. The detection of multiple mutations in different patients may be facilitated by the development of error-corrected NGS using unique molecular identifiers that enhance detection sensitivity and, in some cases, identify as few as 1 mutated cell in 1 million cells.[105,106]

In general, MRD assessment using these molecular markers requires periodic assessment of peripheral blood and bone marrow (e.g., every 3 months) for at least 2 years after the end of treatment. As discussed, the prognostic effect of MRD varies depending on its levels and the disease in question. Patients with complete molecular remission or molecular persistence at low levels below specific cutoffs may have a low risk of relapse. On the other hand, molecular progression, defined as an MRD increase of 1 log or more between any two positive samples, or molecular relapse, defined as an MRD increase of 1 log or more between any two positive samples in a patient with previously complete molecular remission, may signify increased risk of relapse. In summary, there is clear evidence that MRD is an independent prognostic indicator in AML that is important for risk stratification and treatment planning in conjunction with other well-established parameters and has the potential to serve as a surrogate end point for survival in clinical trials to facilitate drug approval.[81]

Acute Lymphoblastic Leukemia

Morphologic Features

Because of the morphologic overlap with myeloblasts, many of the features useful in distinguishing leukemic myeloblasts

from regenerating myeloblasts also apply to lymphoblasts. Comparison to the original leukemic blasts is useful to identify distinctive features, such as variation in blast cell size and cytoplasm, cytoplasmic vacuoles, nucleoli, and nuclear convolutions. Some lymphoblasts may contain cytoplasmic granules, but Auer rods are not seen. Distinguishing lymphoblasts from normal hematogones may create diagnostic difficulties and is discussed in detail herein. Not surprisingly, the early clearance of blast cells from peripheral blood (by day 7) and bone marrow (by day 14 or 15) in acute lymphoblastic leukemia (ALL) is associated with an improved prognosis in both adults and children.[107]

Bone marrow biopsy morphology can also help detect residual leukemia in ALL. As with leukemic myeloblasts, residual or recurrent lymphoblasts tend to cluster and form aggregates on biopsy material.

As noted, one of the most challenging problems in the evaluation of post-therapy ALL specimens is distinguishing residual or recurrent disease from hematogones. Hematogones are more frequent in children and may be the predominant cell type in bone marrow aspirates in some cases, such as in children with idiopathic thrombocytopenic purpura. They may also occur in children with other cytopenias, malignancies at other sites, or regenerating bone marrow after treatment for leukemia.[108-110] These cells also occur in adults, particularly after hematopoietic cell transplantation, but they may be seen in adults with lymphoma, autoimmune diseases, or acquired immunodeficiency syndrome.[111,112] Because of their monotonous lymphoid appearance and precursor B-cell lineage, they are easily misinterpreted as leukemic cells. Hematogones are predominantly small cells with scant cytoplasm, with smaller numbers of admixed large cells (Fig. 56-9). The small cells are uniform in size with round to oval nuclei but exhibit a spectrum of other nuclear

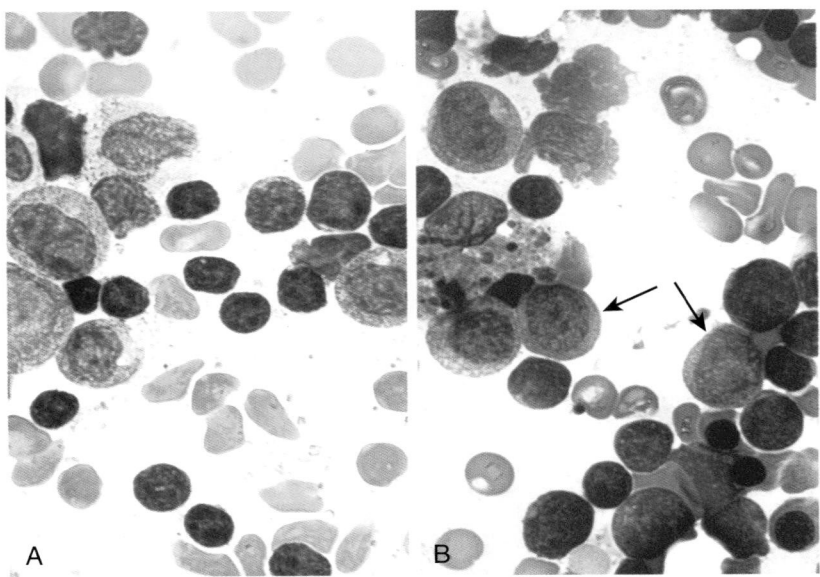

Figure 56-9. Hematogones after therapy. A, There is an increase in precursor cells, which are generally small and uniform in size and lack nucleoli. **B,** This similar population of cells also has larger blast cells *(arrows)* with nucleoli, in a specimen from an 8-month-old treated for *KMT2A*-rearranged pro–B-cell acute lymphoblastic leukemia. This sample shows an immunoglobulin kappa gene rearrangement by polymerase chain reaction analysis and a small population of *KMT2A*-rearranged cells by fluorescence in situ hybridization, consistent with minimal residual disease.

features, ranging from homogeneous, bland chromatin without nucleoli to mature, clumped chromatin. These cells differ from most lymphoblasts, which are usually larger and have more cytoplasm, more variation in size, irregular nuclear contours, distinct nucleoli, and no evidence of maturation. Although hematogones may be numerous in aspirate material, they are usually inconspicuous in biopsy material. Hematogones are usually found as interstitial infiltrates, whereas leukemic blasts often form aggregates in bone marrow biopsy specimens. Immunophenotyping provides a reliable method for distinguish hematogones from neoplastic blasts.

Immunophenotyping

Flow cytometry has been applied for MRD detection in B-lymphoblastic leukemia/lymphoma (B ALL) for many years and is considered standard of care for patients after therapy. The prognostic significance of flow cytometry for MRD detection has been described in numerous studies (summarized in a meta-analysis conducted by Berry and colleagues[113]) with some multivariate analyses suggesting MRD has the highest predictive value among prognostic inidcators.[114] Flow cytometry using an adequate panel and with collection of sufficient events can reliably be performed with a sensitivity allowing detection of an abnormal population at 0.01% (1 in 10,000 cells). Similar to AML MRD, detection of residual disease in B-ALL relies on identifying abnormal blast populations by virtue of the immunophenotypic aberrancies these abnormal cells harbor. Similar to myeloid maturation, B-lymphoid maturation takes place in the marrow; therefore, distinguishing abnormal blasts from normal background hematogones is critical.[115,116] This is particularly true because hematogone hyperplasia may be seen in the setting of marrow regeneration post-therapy or posttransplant, particularly in pediatric populations. An example of MRD detection by flow cytometry in the setting of B-ALL is illustrated in Figure 56-10.

Similar to AML, the abnormalities seen in B-ALL may include abnormal intensity of an antigen (for instance, CD9, CD10, CD34, and CD58 are often aberrantly overexpressed,

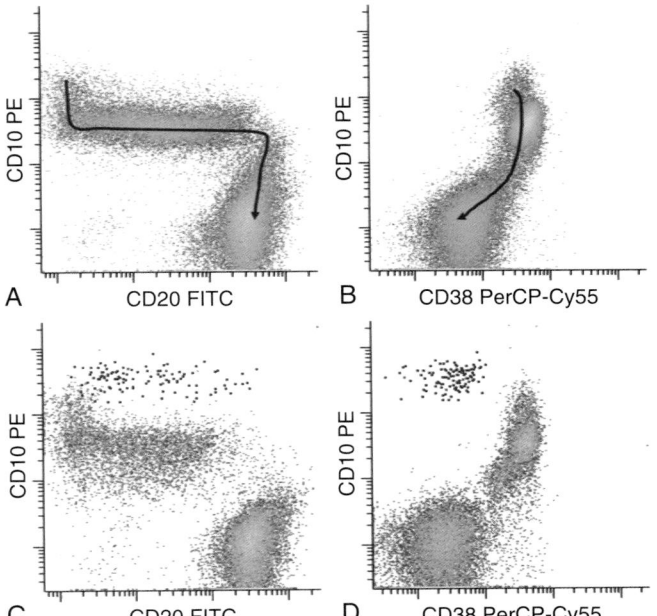

Figure 56-10. Example of minimal/measurable residual disease (MRD) in B-lymphoblastic leukemia. All plots show CD19-positive B cells. **A** and **B** plots demonstrate normal B-cell maturation with the *arrows* illustrating changes in antigen expression with B-cell maturation. Normal early hematogones have bright CD10 and express CD38 without CD20 and with dim CD45. With maturation, CD10 and CD38 decrease in intensity, and CD20 and CD45 increase. Normal hematogones may be increased post-therapy, particularly in children, but retain normal patterns of antigen expression. **C** and **D** plots illustrate CD19 positive B cells from a patient post-therapy for B-lymphoblastic leukemia with residual leukemic cells present. Normal background B cells and precursors are *colored aqua* and predominate; persistent leukemic cells account for 0.03% of the nucleated mononuclear cells and are *highlighted in red*. The leukemic cells can be differentiated from normal mature B cells and hematogones by aberrant expression of bright CD10 with variable CD20 and without CD38.

and CD38 and CD45 are often underexpressed on abnormal blasts) or expression of an antigen of a different lineage (with expression of CD13 and CD33 being relatively common).

Although not required, in some cases, knowledge of the diagnostic immunophenotype can be particularly helpful in confirming that a presumed abnormal population represents abnormal blasts.

A number of targeted immunotherapies are used in the setting of B-ALL, in particular in refractory/recurrent disease. Targeted therapies in common use include agents targeting CD19, including T cells genetically engineered to express a chimeric antigen receptor (CAR T cells) directed against CD19 and bispecific small molecules with specificity for CD3 and CD19 designed to engage the host T-cells against tumor CD19-positive B cells. Monoclonal antibodies directed against CD20 and CD22 are also in common use for treatment of B-ALL. The targets of such therapeutic agents may overlap with the antigens used for population identification or characterization, complicating immunophenotypic analysis. In the setting of targeted therapies, the immunophenotype of normal populations may be altered, and neoplastic blasts may become antigen negative or change lineage, a phenomenon that has been described in the setting of T-cell engaging anti-CD19 therapies.[117,118] Awareness of targeted therapies in use is critical for correct interpretation of data, and in some cases, alternative gating strategies (Fig. 56-11) may be required.[119]

As T-cell maturation takes place in the thymus, immature T cells should not be identified in the bone marrow, and the detection of cytoplasmic CD3-positive and TdT-positive populations are suggestive of residual T-lymphoblastic leukemia/lymphoma (T-ALL). Different flow cytometric approaches and panels for T-ALL MRD detection have been described in the literature.[116,120]

Immunohistochemical studies are also useful in the evaluation of immature cell aggregates in the bone marrow of patients treated for ALL. Though regenerating hematogones are typically present in an interstitial pattern, leukemic lymphoblasts tend to form clusters in the bone marrow, and the detection of clusters of TdT-positive and/or CD34-positive cells on biopsy material may be suggestive of residual disease (Fig. 56-12).[121]

Cytogenetics and Molecular Studies

Karyotype and FISH analyses offer results similar to those described for AML. Karyotype abnormalities are often detected at presentation with ALL, but a significant number of patients have normal karyotypes or abnormalities that are not easily followed by molecular methods. The specific abnormalities most often followed in patients with ALL are *BCR::ABL1* of t(9;22)(q34.1;q11.2), *TCF3::PBX1* of t(1;19) (q23.3;p13.3), *ETV6::RUNX1* of t(12;21)(p13.2;q22.1), and *KMT2A* translocations, particularly t(4;11).[122,123] PCR testing directed to a specific balanced cytogenetic translocation is very sensitive and can detect abnormal cells at a level of 1 translocated cell in 100,000 cells. Therefore, specific PCR testing against balanced translocations is the easiest and most sensitive method for identifying molecular genetic evidence of residual disease.[124] ALL cells also demonstrate T-cell and B-cell receptor gene rearrangements.[125] Such rearrangements are not entirely lineage-specific (dual immunoglobulin heavy chain [IGH] and T-cell receptor chain rearrangements are common in precursor B-cell ALL), but they can be used for residual disease testing. The European BIOMED-2 group has developed a series of PCR primers that are accurate and now widely used for establishing and monitoring B-cell and T-cell receptor gene rearrangements.[126] The sensitivity of the BIOMED-2 primer and PCR assay is about 1 mutated cell in 100 cells. This sensitivity is too low for detection of MRD; thus, regular BIOMED-2 PCR assay is not suitable for molecular detection of MRD. For many years, allele-specific oligonucleotide PCR (ASO-PCR) has been the gold standard to molecularly monitor residual disease in B-ALL and other B-cell neoplasms.[127] It requires the demonstration of a B-cell or T-cell immunoglobulin gene rearrangement in the pretreatment diagnostic acute leukemia sample. The junctional region of the rearrangement is then sequenced, and PCR primers and probes are designed specifically for the individual patient's abnormality. The follow-up samples are then tested with the patient-specific primers and probes for residual disease. This test can be performed in a quantitative manner.[128,129] This methodology is capable of detecting residual disease at a high sensitivity of 0.001% and is useful for predicting relapse in childhood ALL.[127,130,131] However, the technique is complex and labor-intensive, requiring extensive knowledge and experience, as the junctional regions of each leukemia have to be identified before the patient-specific real-time qPCR assays can be designed for MRD monitoring.

NGS is now the emerging modality used to detect MRD in lymphoid neoplasms, particularly in B-ALL. Briefly, the assay takes advantage of the unique *VDJ* gene rearrangement occurring on the genomic locus of the IgH gene in individual B-lymphoid cells (including B-lymphoid tumor cells) to track tumor loads by combining PCR and NGS-based deep sequencing technologies[132,133] (Fig. 56-13). The sensitivity of this assay is extremely high, reaching 1 in a million cells, provided adequate DNA input. The different modalities for MRD assessment in B-ALL are summarized in Table 56-2.

MRD determined by molecular means is an excellent prognostic tool to assess risk stratification in B-ALL. Studies of B-ALL patients demonstrate that molecular MRD is a powerful predictor for relapse and clinical outcome.[114,134-137] In adults with relapsed/refractory B-ALL, MRD negativity after salvage therapy is associated with significantly longer OS.[138]

In addition to prognostic significance, PCR-based MRD is playing an increasingly important role in tailoring individual risk-directed treatment decisions in B-ALL. A clinical trial of 778 pediatric patients with B-ALL showed that therapy intensification and reduction based on MRD levels significantly improved overall clinical outcome. Moreover, intensive chemotherapy or stem cell transplantation protocols of high risk patients designed on PCR and MRD-based readouts led to a fivefold increase (16%–78%) in the 5-year event-free survival (EFS) rate.[139] A study with 278 tested adult patients with B-ALL demonstrated that poor early MRD response, in contrast to conventional ALL risk factors, is an excellent tool to identify patients who may benefit from allogeneic stem cell transplantation in the context of intensified adult ALL therapy.[140] Among adult patients with B-ALL in complete hematologic remission with MRD $\geq 10^{-3}$ treated with blinatumomab, 78% achieved a complete MRD response after one cycle, and complete MRD response after blinatumomab treatment in this population was associated with significantly improved OS and relapse-free survival compared with that of MRD nonresponders.[141]

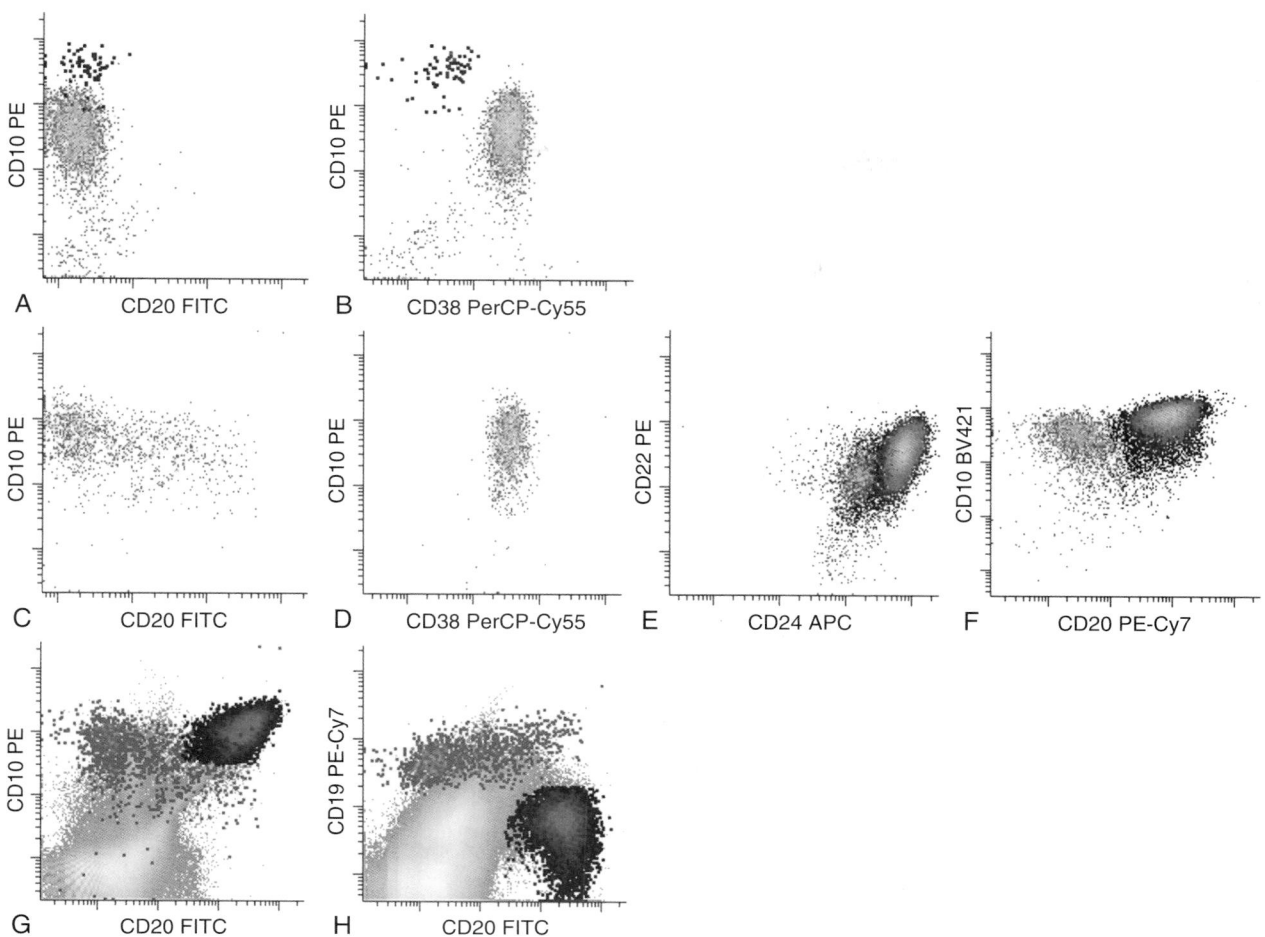

Figure 56-11. Effect of targeted therapy on flow cytometric studies. A and **B,** These plots show CD19-positive B cells from a patient with a history of B-lymphoblastic leukemia who has received a regimen including anti-CD20 therapy. This sample shows two distinct immature B-cell populations. Normal residual hematogones are *shown in aqua* and lack expression of CD20 as a result of prior anti-CD20 therapy. In addition, a small population of leukemic blasts is *highlighted in red* (0.02% of the nucleated mononuclear cells) and shows aberrant bright CD10 with dim to absent CD38. **C–H,** These dot plots show flow cytometric data from a patient with B-lymphoblastic leukemia who received an anti-CD19 targeted T-cell engaging therapy. **(C)** and **(D)** show CD19-positive B cells, which have left-shifted B-cell maturation with a predominance of early hematogones but with no immunophenotypic abnormalities. When using CD19 to identify B cells, no abnormal population is evident. In the setting of anti-CD19 therapy, it is critical that CD19 not be the only method used for identification of abnormal cells. **(E)** and **(F)** show B cells from this same sample expressing both CD22 and CD24. Using this alternative gating strategy, B cells include two subsets: a normal hematogone subset *(aqua)* and a population of leukemic blasts *(red)*, which accounts for 0.9% of the nucleated mononuclear cells. The abnormal blasts show bright expression of CD20 and CD24, co-expressed with CD10. **(G)** and **(H)** show all mononuclear cells. When looking at all mononuclear cells, the abnormal population *(highlighted in red)* is evident. The residual leukemic cells have lost CD19 expression post-therapy and can be distinguished from normal background hematogones, which retain CD19 expression *(highlighted in aqua)*.

CHRONIC MYELOID LEUKEMIA

Chronic MPNs have overlapping morphologic features and are generally diagnosed by a combination of morphologic, clinical, and genetic findings (see Chapter 47). Chronic myeloid leukemia (CML) is the most common chronic MPN and the one that most often requires post-therapy evaluation. A variety of therapies have historically been used for CML, including bone marrow transplantation and interferon-α therapy, but TKI therapy is now standard.

Morphologic Features

With treatment of the chronic phase of CML, the bone marrow becomes less cellular; with some therapies, it may become normocellular or even slightly hypocellular. The myeloid-to-erythroid (M/E) ratio, which is usually markedly elevated before treatment, usually returns to normal or may become decreased. In these cases, it is often difficult to determine by morphologic features alone whether leukemic cells persist in the bone marrow. The most common clues to residual disease are hypercellularity, the presence of clusters of atypical "dwarf" megakaryocytes, prominent basophilia,[142] and in some cases, the continued presence of clusters of Gaucher-like histiocytes.[143,144] Despite these clues, cytogenetic or molecular genetic studies to detect *BCR::ABL1* t(9;22)(q34.1;q11.2) are needed to definitively identify the continued presence of leukemia.

In the past, busulfan, hydroxyurea, and interferon-α therapies were used to treat CML, with some variation in the degree of bone marrow response. Some patients

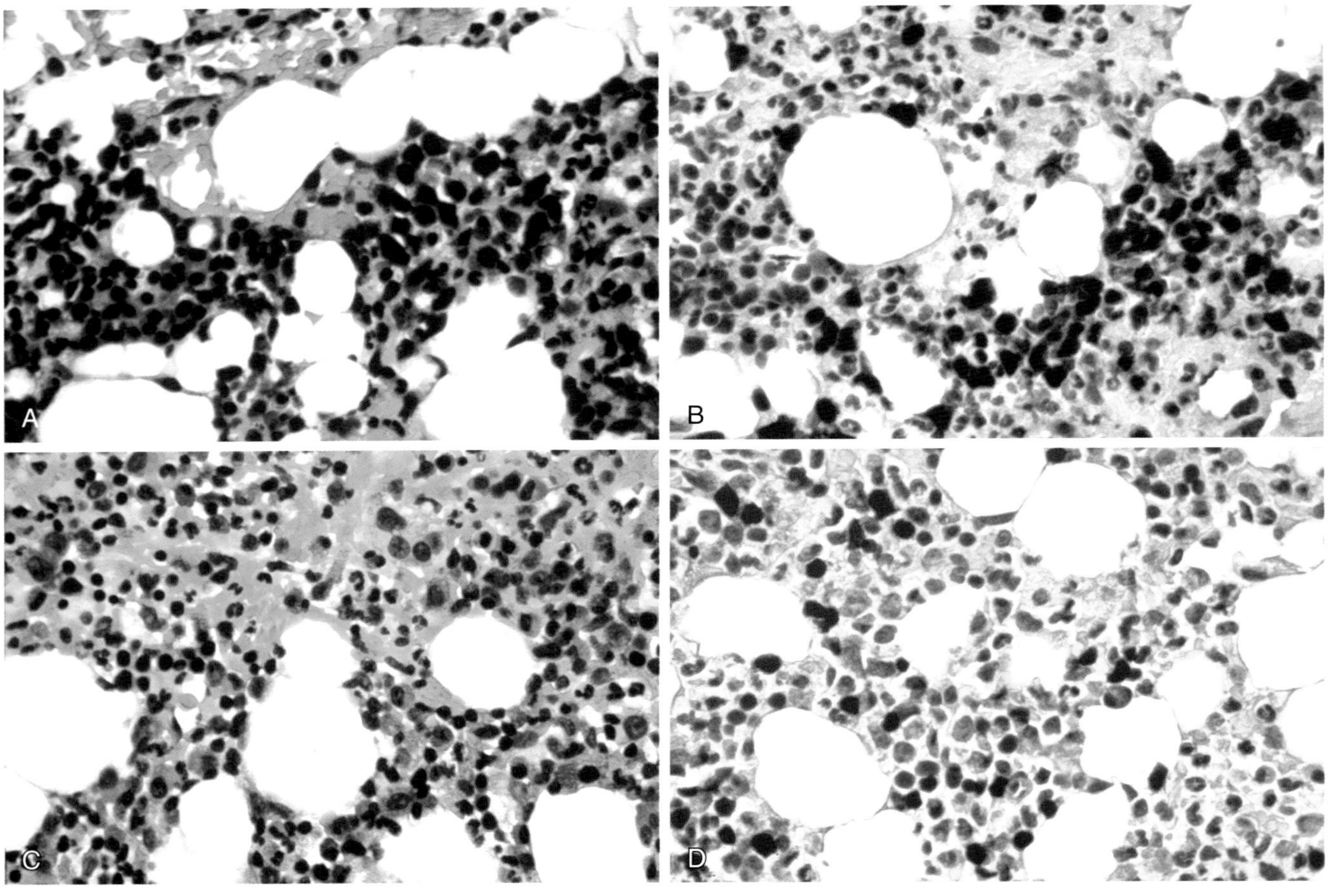

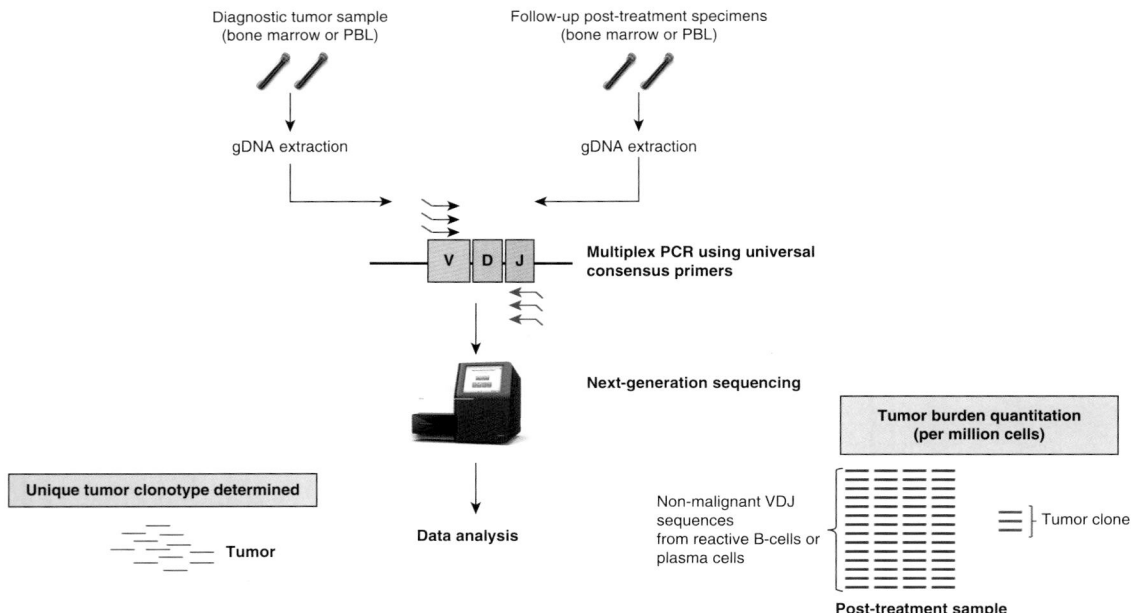

Figure 56-12. Immunohistochemical features of residual precursor B-cell acute lymphoblastic leukemia and normal precursor B cells (hematogones). A and **B,** This case of residual leukemia shows aggregates of terminal deoxynucleotidyl transferase (TdT)-positive cells. **C** and **D,** In this case, there is an increase in hematogones, which do not form distinct aggregates on the biopsy material, and only scattered individual TdT-positive cells.

Figure 56-13. Detection of minimal residual disease in B-cell neoplasms using deep sequencing of immunoglobulin heavy chain (IGH) genes. Briefly, genomic DNA extracted from tumor or post-treatment specimens are subjected to library preparation using multiplex primers. These libraries are then sequenced by next-generation sequencing (NGS). The tumor-specific VDJs are identified. The tumor burden is measured by the percentage of tumor-specific reads in a pool of VDJ reads.

Table 56-2 Summary of the Different Modalities for Minimal Residual Disease Assessment in B-Lymphoblastic Leukemia/Lymphoma (B-ALL)

Method	Applicability	Sensitivity	PROS	CONS
MFC	ALL: >90%	3 to 4 color: 10^{-3}–10^{-4} 6 to 9 color: 10^{-4}–10^{-5}	• Widely applicable and available • Standardized (EuroMRD) • Short turnaround time • Relatively inexpensive	• Clonal heterogeneity undetectable • Interpretation may be difficult
Real-time qPCR	ALL: 90%–95%	10^{-5}–10^{-6}	• Standardized (EuroMRD) • Fresh sample not necessary	• Clonal heterogeneity undetectable • Patient-specific primers necessary • Requires baseline sample • Time-consuming
Fusion transcript PCR	ALL: 25%–40%	10^{-4}–10^{-5}	• Rapid • Unequivocal link with leukemic/preleukemic clone • Stable target throughout therapy • Possible differences in expression levels (transcripts/cells) during the course of treatment	• RNA instability causes false negative • Limited to a subset of cases
NGS (IGH deep sequencing)	ALL: ~90%	10^{-6}	• Ultra-sensitive • Clonal heterogeneity detected	• Not yet standardized • Limited availability • Expensive, but costs decreasing • Requires baseline sample

ALL, Acute lymphoblastic leukemia; *IGH,* immunoglobulin heavy chain; *MFC,* multiparametric flow cytometry; *NGS,* next-generation sequencing; *PCR,* polymerase chain reaction; *qPCR,* quantitative PCR.

achieved clinical features of remission, with improvement in peripheral blood counts.[145,146] With busulfan, the bone marrow usually remains hypercellular, with an elevated M/E ratio. Megakaryocytes tend to be increased with therapy, and this increase is associated with an increase in bone marrow fibrosis. With hydroxyurea, the marrow cellularity decreases somewhat but usually remains above normal, with only a moderate correction in the M/E ratio. The number of megakaryocytes and degree of marrow fibrosis, however, tend to decrease with hydroxyurea. With interferon-α, complete normalization of peripheral blood counts may occur. The bone marrow remains slightly hypercellular in most patients, but approximately one-quarter of patients have normal bone marrow features on interferon-α.[146] Marrow megakaryocytes remain elevated, with associated fibrosis; bone marrow macrophages are reportedly increased in the marrow. Despite the improvement in marrow cellularity, most patients continue to show cytogenetic evidence of clonal bone marrow disease.

Bone marrow transplantation was the standard treatment for CML in the past and is still considered the only totally curative therapy.[147] After transplantation, the bone marrow undergoes the expected changes of aplasia, followed by regeneration. The majority of patients with CML treated with transplantation are cured and show normocellular or hypocellular bone marrow without specific abnormalities. Relapse specimens from patients treated with transplantation show changes similar to de novo disease, with granulocytic hyperplasia, basophilia, and hypercellularity, and are usually not diagnostic dilemmas.

At the time of this writing, most patients with all phases of CML are treated with a TKI that directly blocks the effects of the *BCR::ABL1* fusion gene.[148] The TKI most commonly used is imatinib, although newer-generation *BCR::ABL1* inhibitors (dasatinib, nilotinib) are available for patients who fail to respond, relapse, or experience intolerance to

imatinib. Imatinib therapy results in a clinical, morphologic, and at least partial or complete cytogenetic remission in most patients, with a reduction in marrow cellularity, normalization of the M/E ratio, and normalization of megakaryocyte number and morphology.[149-151] The peripheral blood is the first to respond to imatinib therapy; the white blood cell count returns to normal, basophils decrease, and the platelet count normalizes, with normal-appearing platelets occurring after about 2 months of therapy. The hemoglobin level tends to decrease slightly during therapy. A subset of patients may have neutropenia or thrombocytopenia while receiving the drug. The bone marrow hypercellularity gradually decreases, and by 8 to 11 months, the marrow is normocellular or hypocellular, with a normal or decreased M/E ratio in most patients. Even in the chronic phase, bone marrow blast cells and megakaryocytes decrease, the number of hypolobated megakaryocytes decreases, and megakaryocyte clustering becomes less common as the marrow cellularity decreases (Fig. 56-14). This therapy can also gradually eliminate the marrow fibrosis that is prominent is some cases of CML,[149,151,152] although progression of myelofibrosis has also been reported, mostly in cases with acceleration or blast phase.[150] Patients with accelerated or blast-phase CML, however, also show rapid decreases in peripheral blood and bone marrow blast cell counts.[149] After long-term treatment with imatinib, some patients may have increased pseudo-Gaucher cells and reactive lymphoid nodules.[150]

Relapse of CML may take the form of chronic or blast-phase disease and may result from natural evolution of the disease with cytogenetic evolution, from loss of responsiveness to imatinib therapy through the acquisition of mutations within the kinase domain of *BCR::ABL1* or amplification of the fusion gene, or through other mechanisms that are not yet clearly understood. Occasionally, patients have a myelodysplastic or blastic process in cells that are negative for the Philadelphia

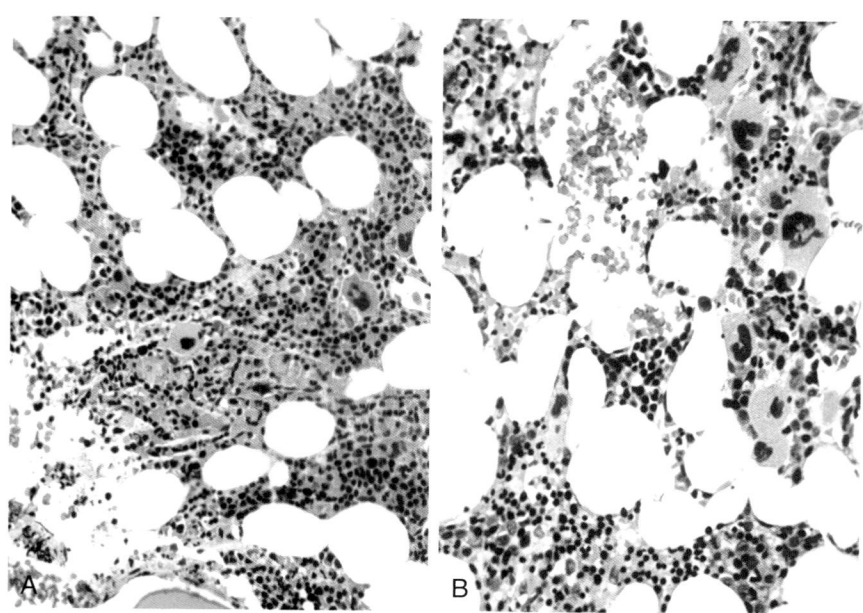

Figure 56-14. Post-therapy changes in chronic myeloid leukemia. After tyrosine kinase inhibitor (TKI) therapy, samples may be morphologically normal **(A)** or show residual clusters of atypical megakaryocytes **(B)**. Both samples remained positive for *BCR::ABL1* by reverse transcriptase polymerase chain reaction (RT-PCR).

(Ph) chromosome.[153] If the patient had a previous blast phase, comparison to the original material may be useful, similar to the evaluation of post-therapy acute leukemia specimens. Morphologic evaluation is of limited utility in predicting the type of blast crisis in CML, and immunophenotyping studies are required for accurate classification of the blast cell lineage.[154]

Immunophenotyping

Immunophenotyping studies generally are not useful in the follow-up of patients treated for CML in chronic phase. If an increase in blasts is noted during the course of therapy, flow cytometry can be used to determine the lineage of the blast population. Flow cytometry can be used in the follow-up of patients treated for CML in accelerated phase (with increased blasts) or in patients treated with induction for blast phase of CML. In this setting, the approach for identifying abnormal myeloid or lymphoid blasts is similar to that described for MRD assessment in acute leukemias.

Cytogenetics and Molecular Studies

The majority of patients treated with busulfan, hydroxyurea, and interferon-α have karyotypic evidence of disease during and after treatment. However, approximately 13% of patients treated with interferon-α, 63% or more of patients treated with imatinib for 60 months or longer, and most patients treated with hematopoietic cell transplantation have no karyotypic evidence of disease.[142,155,156] More sophisticated ultrasensitive methods, however, reveal the continued presence of very low levels of the Ph chromosome in the stem cells of patients treated with imatinib.[156] Many other patients receiving these therapies have partial cytogenetic responses.[148] The reversion to normal bone marrow morphology does not correlate with loss of t(9;22) in all cases, and molecular or cytogenetic confirmation is needed. Patients treated with

imatinib may develop a cytogenetic remission after only 2 months of therapy, but the time to achieve a cytogenetic response is variable. Patients who have early normalization of bone marrow cellularity by 2 to 5 months are reportedly more likely to have a complete cytogenetic response.

Various guidelines have been suggested for monitoring patients on therapy, particularly those receiving imatinib.[157-160] Most recommend routine karyotyping and real-time quantitative reverse transcriptase (RT)-PCR to measure *BCR::ABL1* transcripts be performed at regular intervals. FISH studies are generally not recommended for long-term follow-up, mainly because most FISH assays have background levels of up to 6%, limiting the ability to detect very low levels of disease. However, a highly sensitive interphase double-fusion assay, sometimes termed D-FISH, can detect very low levels of *BCR::ABL1* fusion and is much more sensitive than conventional karyotype analysis, although it does not allow the detection of additional chromosomal abnormalities.[161,162]

Measurement of *BCR::ABL1* transcript levels using real-time qPCR standardized to the international reporting scale (IS) is now the principal recommended monitoring strategy.[163] The introduction of the IS has allowed harmonization of testing processes, standardization of the nomenclature for reporting molecular response, and the development of reference material.[164-168] The incorporation of this molecular monitoring in the management of CML was initially recommended in 2013 by the ELN and is essential in monitoring patients receiving imatinib or other TKIs. Based on many clinical studies over the years, an optimal response was recommended by the ELN (2020) as follows: *BCR::ABL1* 10%, ≤1%, and ≤0.1% at 3, 6, and 12 months of TKI therapy, respectively.[163] A major molecular response (MMR), defined as ≤0.1% *BCR::ABL1* measured on the IS, is predictive of negligible risk for disease progression over 12 months[169,170] and is now considered a primary outcome measure in CML clinical trials. In addition, treatment of CML with TKIs has enabled many patients to achieve very low or undetectable levels of disease; some of these patients remain in sustained remission when treatment is withdrawn. Thus, accurate definition of deep molecular responses is increasingly important for optimal patient management and risk stratification.[164] A deep molecular response (DMR, *BCR::ABL1* ≤0.01% IS) represents an important second milestone, as achievement of a sustained DMR is a prerequisite for a trial of drug discontinuation with the aim of achieving treatment-free remission (TFR). Molecular response (MR)4, defined as ≤0.01% on the IS scale, maintained for at least 1 year is associated with stable DMR in CML, after which no MMR loss occurs if the patients are fully compliant and remain on a standard TKI dose.[171] MR4.5, defined as ≤0.0032% on the IS scale, is a new molecular predictor of superior long-term outcome. No patients who have achieved MR4.5 experienced progression of the disease.[172] In addition, a sustained MR4.5 prior to treatment discontinuation may be associated with a higher rate of TFR than with MR4.[173] It can be reached by a majority of patients treated with imatinib, although it takes, on average, 3 years longer to achieve MR4.5 than with MR4. However, the duration to achieve MR4.5 can be shortened with optimized high-dose imatinib. Achieving MMR or MR4 after 3 years of imatinib may be predictive of the likelihood of reaching MR4.5 at a later time point upon continuation of TKI therapy. Patients on imatinib for 3 years who have achieved MR4 have a higher probability of achieving MR4.5 with continued imatinib. On the other hand, patients without MMR at 3 years of imatinib therapy have a negligible probability of achieving MR4 or MR4.5 with up to 5 additional years of imatinib. Similarly, patients with MMR but not MR4 at 3 years of imatinib therapy have a significantly lower cumulative incidence of MR4.5 than that of patients with MR4.[163] These latter two groups of patients may benefit from a more potent TKI if achievement of MR4.5 is the ultimate goal. Thus, accurate and precise measurements of *BCR::ABL1* on the IS scale is critical to assess and correctly stratify molecular responses for patient prognosis and management (Fig. 56-15).

After transplantation, patients frequently remain *BCR::ABL1* positive by PCR for several months, with no clinical evidence of relapse in long-term clinical follow-up.[174] In part, the cause of these presumably false-positive PCR results is the presence of the fusion product in terminally differentiated cells, such as Gaucher-like histiocytes.[175] With time, these cells disappear, and the PCR test becomes negative. Therefore, PCR testing in the months immediately after transplantation may not have clinical relevance. Use of serial qPCR methods may be one means of avoiding overinterpretation of a positive PCR result, with an interval increase in the amount of *BCR::ABL1* transcripts presumably indicating residual or recurrent disease.[156] Performing qPCR tests 12 months and longer after transplantation is useful in predicting relapse.[176]

BCR::ABL1-NEGATIVE MYELOPROLIFERATIVE NEOPLASMS

BCR::ABL1–negative MPNs such as essential thrombocythemia (ET), primary myelofibrosis (PMF), and polycythemia vera (PV) may require post-therapy evaluation. Therapies for these MPNs are diverse and vary depending on disease stage. For instance, during the chronic phase of PV, phlebotomy is frequent, whereas patients with ET frequently take aspirin prophylactically and may also receive anagrelide. Hydroxyurea is a common cytoreductive therapy used in all

MPNs, and some patients may receive interferon-α. Newer targeted therapies, such as JAK2 inhibitors (ruxolitinib), may be used in patients with *JAK2* mutations, and some patients may undergo hematopoietic cell transplantation, particularly those with PMF. Each therapy confers specific changes to the bone marrow, which manifest morphologically and, in some cases, immunophenotypically; in others, the changes to the bone marrow affect cytogenetic and molecular data as well.

Morphologic Features

After therapy, each MPN may show different morphologic features. During the chronic phase of PV, patients are frequently treated with phlebotomy, which leads to a physiologic, responsive additional increase in marrow cellularity. Cytoreductive therapies such as hydroxyurea or busulfan result in decreased bone marrow cellularity across all three MPNs, though these chemotherapeutic agents do not significantly reduce marrow fibrosis.[177] Both interferon and busulfan reduce megakaryocyte numbers, whereas hydroxyurea may increase them. In some cases of ET, anagrelide is used to decrease platelet counts; common changes in megakaryopoiesis can be seen with increased numbers of immature small forms as a result of inhibition of both megakaryocyte maturation and endoreduplication.[178]

JAK pathway inhibitors (ruxolitinib) have been developed and are used to treat some patients with MPN with *JAK2* V617F mutations. Though significant morphologic marrow changes at 6 months or 1 year are generally not seen,[179,180] some patients with longer-term therapy (>2 years) have shown decreased bone marrow fibrosis and normalization of marrow cellularity with decreased megakaryocyte clustering.[181,182]

Finally, bone marrow transplantation may be performed in patients with MPN and, in particular, is more frequent in patients with PMF. After transplantation, if successful, marrow cellularity may return to normal with reestablishment of M/E ratios and slow resolution of fibrosis over the course of 3 months to more than 1 year.[183,184]

Immunophenotyping

In general, immunophenotyping has limited value in monitoring residual disease in *BCR::ABL1*-negative MPNs if the blast percentage is normal. A clear exception is the monitoring of blasts in MPNs with disease acceleration or when blast transformation has occurred. In these cases, blasts are most frequently of myeloid origin, though rare cases of ALL have been reported; however, unlike myeloid blast transformation, it is unclear whether these cases of ALL are clonally related to the underlying MPN.[185-187]

Cytogenetics and Molecular Studies

The majority of *BCR::ABL1*-negative MPNs have a normal karyotype, and cytogenetic abnormalities are detected in only a subset. When disease persists, these cytogenetic abnormalities generally persist.[188] In cases of ET and PV, though cytogenetic abnormalities are rare (~5% of patients), abnormalities of chromosomes 1, 8, 9, and 20 are the most frequently observed.[188-191] In PMF, abnormalities are more frequent (30%–40% of patients) and are seen in chromosomes 1, 8, 9, 13, and 20.[192] Again, these cytogenetic abnormalities

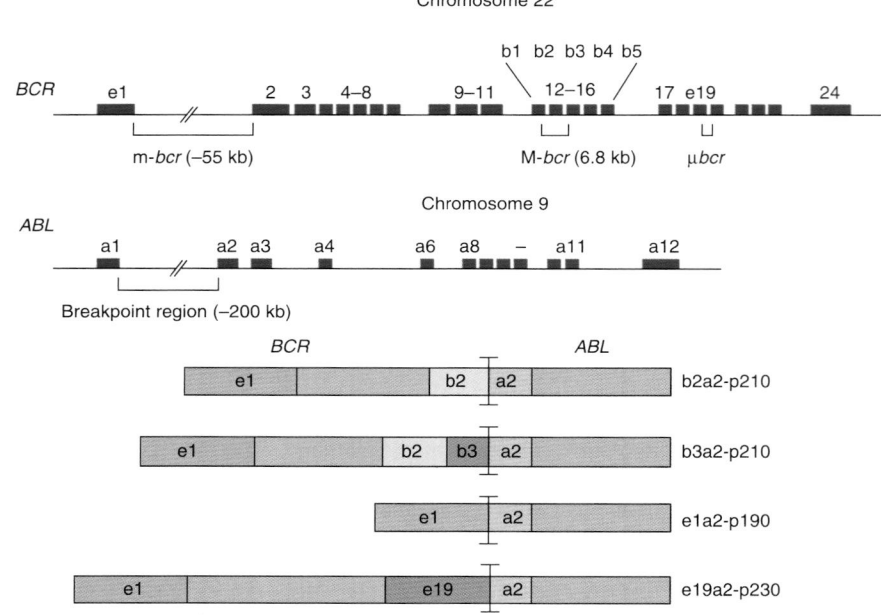

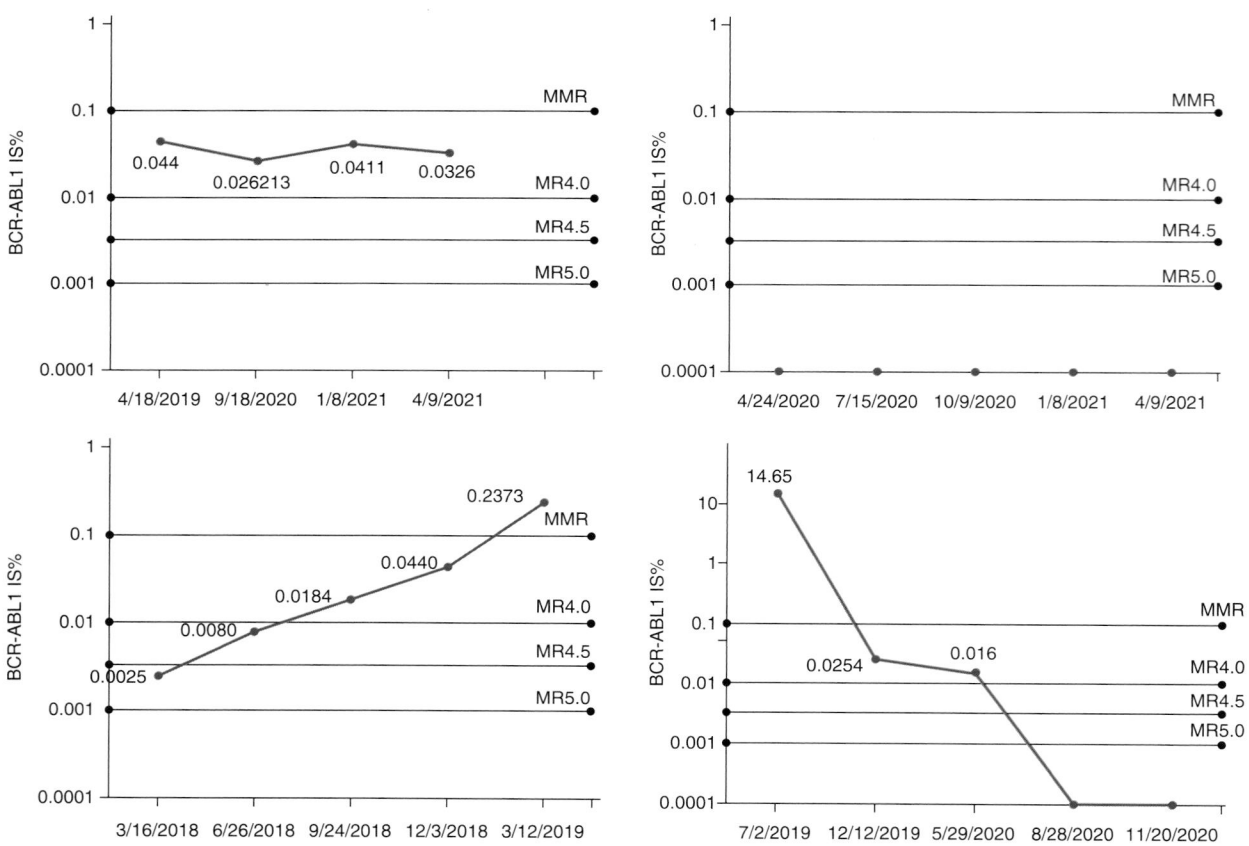

Figure 56-15. **Examples of different patterns of molecular responses in patients with chronic myeloid leukemia (CML) treated with tyrosine kinase inhibitors (TKIs).** The different breakpoints of *BCR::ABL1* and the primers and probes used for measurement of fusion transcripts are indicated. Persistent major molecular response (<0.1% international reporting scale ([IS]), *upper left*; persistent deep molecular response, *upper right*; molecular relapse, *lower left*; molecular remission achieved after TKI therapy, *lower right*.

can be followed during therapy with routine G-banding karyotype analysis. One caveat to be aware of in cytogenetic analyses is that marrow aspirate specimens in patients with fibrotic marrow may be hemodiluted and nonrepresentative of bone marrow constituents. In addition, during blast transformation, cytogenetic abnormalities may evolve, and in a subset, a complex karyotype may develop.[184,192] FISH studies, as in AML, can also be used to assess for more common cytogenetic abnormalities such as monosomies, trisomies, or translocations. These methods have inherent detection limits, as discussed previously. As in other transplant patients, HLA-based chimerism studies may be useful to assess for residual host marrow in patients with bone marrow transplants.

Molecular studies are routinely used in MPNs, as most patients with PV, ET, and PMF show a *JAK2* V617F mutation with general frequencies of greater than 95%, 50% to 60%, and 50% to 60%, respectively.[157,192-195] More recently, novel insertion and deletion mutations in calreticulin (*CALR*) exon 9 have been identified in patients with *JAK2*-negative ET and PMF (>30% of these patients).[196-198] In addition, a small subset of patients with ET and PMF has mutations in exon 10 of *MPL* (5%–10% of patients).[199,200] The presence of acquired mutations within the *JAK2*, *CALR*, and *MPL* driver genes in the majority of patients with MPNs permits use of these mutations as quantitative markers of MRD for additional evaluation of response to therapeutic intervention.[201] The reduction of *JAK2* V617F varies according to the treatment modalities used. Though hydroxyurea can result in partial reduction of at least 30% in *JAK2* V617F in about half of patients early in the disease course, prolonged treatment does not seem to cause further reduction in allele burden.[202-206] The majority of patients with PV and ET who are maintained on interferon therapy may experience sustained reduction in *JAK2* V617F and even complete MR in a few selected cases.[207-209] Busulfan, though less frequently used because of its leukemogenic potential, can induce substantial MRs, including complete molecular remission, in a subset of patients.[210] Though JAK2 inhibitors can be effective in improving clinical symptoms and prolonging OS, they have only modest effect in lowering the *JAK2* V617F mutation burden.[179,211] However, there is data suggesting long-term therapy may result in partial or complete MR in a small subset of patients.[212] Allogeneic stem cell transplantation (ASCT) is the only curative option for patients with advanced disease. MPN MRD assessment of *JAK2* V617F mutation by sensitive quantitative methods is a useful outcome and relapse predictor in ASCT, allowing preemptive intervention before overt relapse.[213-215] Similarly, interferon significantly reduced *CALR* exon 9 mutation burden in patients with *CALR*-mutated ET, with some achieving complete MR.[216] qPCR of *MPL* W515L and W515A mutations in individual patients has demonstrated clearance of MRD in patients with PMF after ASCT.[217,218] Although *MPL* exon 10 mutations are amenable to allele-specific qPCR approaches, their low frequency in ET and PMF, compared with that of *JAK2* V617F and *CALR* exon 9 mutations, has limited their wide clinical use as MRD markers.

A variety of allelic-specific qPCR approaches are available for quantitating *JAK2*. These tests have different performance characteristics, but all assays appear to have a sensitivity of ~0.1% to 0.5%.[219-222] About 2% to 5% of PV cases do not harbor *JAK2* V617F but do have exon 12 mutations in *JAK2*. Sensitive real-time qPCR has also been successfully designed

for some common exon 12 mutations.[223] *MPL* exon 10 hot spot and other mutations can also be detected by qPCR, but because of their low frequency in MPNs, their clinical utility as MRD markers has not been well established. Fragment length analysis (FLA) followed by capillary electrophoresis has been widely adopted for *CALR* exon 9 mutation detection. It displays a sensitivity compatible for MRD monitoring (approximately 1%) but remains semiquantitative.[224-226] The qPCR approach cannot detect the entire spectrum of *CALR* mutations, but it can be used to detect quantitatively and with higher sensitivity the most common *CALR* type 1 (52 bp deletion) and type 2 (5 bp insertion) mutations, which account for ~80% of *CALR* mutations.[227] Though earlier assays have analytical sensitivities of ~1% to 2%, the most sensitive qPCR assay was reported to reach a sensitivity of <0.1% for type 1 mutations and <0.01% for type 2 mutations.[228] ddPCR has also emerged as a useful technique for molecular MRD assessment in MPN. For *JAK2* V617F quantitation, ddPCR correlates well with qPCR, even for allele burden as low as 0.1%.[229-231] For *CALR* type 1 and type 2 mutations, ddPCR has a sensitivity of 0.025% and is capable of detecting MRD after ASCT and earlier detection of increasing MRD levels prior to clinical relapse.[232,233]

CHRONIC LYMPHOPROLIFERATIVE AND PLASMA CELL DISORDERS

Morphologic Features

Many lymphoproliferative disorders involve the bone marrow focally, forming aggregates of neoplastic cells. Because of the focal nature of the disease, it may be missed on a review of aspirate smears alone, and bone marrow trephine and clot sections are essential for a complete evaluation. Bilateral bone marrow biopsies increase the yield of detected focal lesions.[158] However, positron emission tomography with computed tomography (PET-CT) has largely replaced staging bone marrow biopsies for Hodgkin lymphoma and diffuse large B-cell lymphoma.[234] The finding of focal aggregates of atypical large lymphoid cells usually presents no diagnostic dilemma, but aggregates of small lymphoid cells of residual lymphoma must be distinguished from reactive lymphoid aggregates, which are common in older adults.[235,236] Even when the patient has a history of large cell lymphoma, discordant lymphoma morphology may occur, with only low-grade lymphoma present in the bone marrow aggregates.[237,238]

Reactive lymphoid aggregates are usually composed of predominantly small lymphocytes with admixed large cells; they may contain histiocytes and plasma cells as well. These aggregates are usually small and well circumscribed and may contain intervening small vessels. The reactive aggregates are nonparatrabecular in location.[236] The pattern of neoplastic aggregates of residual or recurrent lymphoma in the bone marrow varies by lymphoma type.[239,240] Follicular lymphoma characteristically involves the marrow in a paratrabecular pattern, with associated fibrosis and no fat spaces present between the lymphoid aggregate and the bone. After therapy, these aggregates may be less cellular, but they continue to exhibit lymphoid cells and fibrosis adjacent to bone.[241] In some cases, only T cells remain after therapy, and immunophenotyping by immunohistochemical studies and/or flow cytometry are necessary to determine whether aggregates contain neoplastic cells in this setting. The presence of any remaining B cells in the paratrabecular aggregates and/or an abnormal B-cell population by concurrent flow cytometry, however, is supportive of residual bone marrow involvement. Mantle cell lymphoma may show a mixed paratrabecular and nonparatrabecular pattern. An interstitial pattern of disease predominates in hairy cell leukemia and in some cases of chronic lymphocytic leukemia. Most other lymphomas show a predominantly nonparatrabecular pattern. Splenic marginal zone lymphoma may show an intrasinusoidal pattern of disease,[242,243] but this pattern does not appear to be specific for this disease, and patients who have undergone splenectomy for splenic marginal zone lymphoma may have nodular bone marrow involvement.[244] The most helpful morphologic clues for identifying bone marrow involvement by lymphoma are a paratrabecular pattern of involvement, the presence of a monotonous cell population within the aggregates, and large, irregularly shaped aggregates that show infiltration into the surrounding normal hematopoietic marrow. Small nonparatrabecular lymphoid aggregates in patients with a history of lymphoma usually require ancillary immunohistologic studies to determine the nature of the aggregates.[238,245]

Plasma cells can have a variety of atypical features in multiple myeloma, including binucleation or multinucleation, prominent nucleoli, and abnormally condensed chromatin. However, these can also be seen in reactive plasma cells. Standard response criteria for multiple myeloma incorporate both bone marrow findings and results of testing for paraproteins in the peripheral blood and serum. A complete response requires <5% plasma cells in bone marrow aspirates, absence of paraprotein by immunofixation of serum and urine, and lack of soft tissue plasmacytomas.[246] Detecting persistent or recurrent disease often requires ancillary testing (immunophenotyping and/or molecular methods).

Immunophenotyping

Immunophenotyping is the most common method of detecting residual disease in the bone marrow of patients with a history of lymphoma and can be performed by flow cytometry and/or immunohistochemistry. Immunohistochemistry allows the benefit of evaluating cells in the context of architecture, and flow cytometry allows for a multiparametric approach and, in most cases, a greater level of sensitivity. Sampling differences between bone marrow aspirate and biopsy material (particularly when abnormal cells are associated with fibrosis) may decrease the yield of flow cytometry. In such cases, flow cytometry can be performed on a disaggregated core biopsy.

When a suspicious lymphoid aggregate is present on the biopsy, immunohistochemical methods are useful. Because most lymphomas are of B-cell lineage and most bone marrow lymphocytes are T cells, the detection of aggregates or sheets of B cells in lymphoid aggregates is often good evidence of involvement by lymphoma (Fig. 56-16).[236,240] The primary exception to the correlation between an increase in aggregate B cells and lymphoma is when reactive germinal centers are present in the marrow. Bone marrow germinal centers are most common in patients with autoimmune diseases,[247] and these types of aggregates should not automatically be considered evidence of bone marrow involvement by lymphoma. Bone marrow evaluation can usually be accomplished with a relatively small panel of antibodies, including CD3 and CD20 (or PAX5 or CD79a if the patient has received anti-CD20 therapy), but more antibodies can be used if subclassification is needed. Aberrant expression of CD5 or CD43 in B cells is common in many lymphomas of small B cells in the marrow, and this finding is also useful to confirm bone marrow involvement by disease.[248]

Paraffin section immunophenotyping may cause confusion in cases of bone marrow involvement by follicular lymphoma. Follicular lymphoma at almost any site is usually accompanied by a relatively large number of T cells, and T cells may predominate in marrow involved by this type of lymphoma. Although CD10 expression is commonly seen with follicular lymphoma, this antigen is often lost in bone marrow lymphoma aggregates, and such antigen expression may be seen in non-neoplastic lymphocytes. Detection of BCL6 protein by immunohistochemistry may be useful in detecting follicular lymphoma, but this antigen is not restricted to germinal-center cells. For this reason, the morphologic feature of paratrabecular aggregates is considered the most reliable means of detecting follicular lymphoma in the marrow.[245] Cyclin D1 may be helpful in detecting persistent mantle cell lymphoma. LEF1 is positive in chronic lymphocytic leukemia/small lymphocytic lymphoma (CLL/SLL), but it is also positive in T cells and should only be interpreted in the context of T-cell and B-cell markers.

Antibodies directed against annexin A1 can been used to determine whether CD20-positive cells represent persistent/recurrent hairy cell leukemia; however, annexin A1 is positive in myeloid-lineage cells and may be difficult to interpret when small numbers of cells are present in a regenerating bone marrow. Antibodies specific to the *BRAF* V600E mutation have been developed that can be used to identify MRD with high specificity and sensitivity.[249,250]

For plasma cell disorders, CD138 can be used to quantitate plasma cells, and aberrant expression of cyclin D1, CD31, CD56, and CD117 on neoplastic plasma cells can be detected by immunohistochemistry.[251-253] Kappa and lambda staining also plays a role, as stringent complete response requires the lack of detectable paraprotein and <5% plasma cells on aspirate smears, plus a normal serum-free light chain ratio and absence of monotypic plasma cells in the bone marrow biopsy by immunohistochemistry.[246] However, widespread adoption of MRD testing, either by flow cytometry or molecular methods, may supplant these standard response criteria.

Flow cytometry is a useful modality to identify abnormal lymphoid cells or plasma cells in follow-up of post-therapy samples for lymphoid neoplasms and plasma cell neoplasms, respectively. In the setting of B-cell neoplasms, the utility of flow cytometry for residual disease detection has been established for a number of disease entities, including CLL/SLL[254,255] and hairy cell leukemia,[256] among others. Among mature lymphoid neoplasms, the data is perhaps strongest in CLL/SLL, where consensus guidelines exist and MRD has been established as a significant prognostic factor.[255,257] It should be noted, though, that the value of MRD data may vary based on therapeutic regimen.[254] In the setting of plasma cell neoplasms, post-therapy samples may be followed by flow cytometry and/or immunohistochemistry. Flow cytometry often underestimates plasma cell numbers because of factors such as hemodilution and preservation of plasma cells; therefore, immunohistochemistry for a

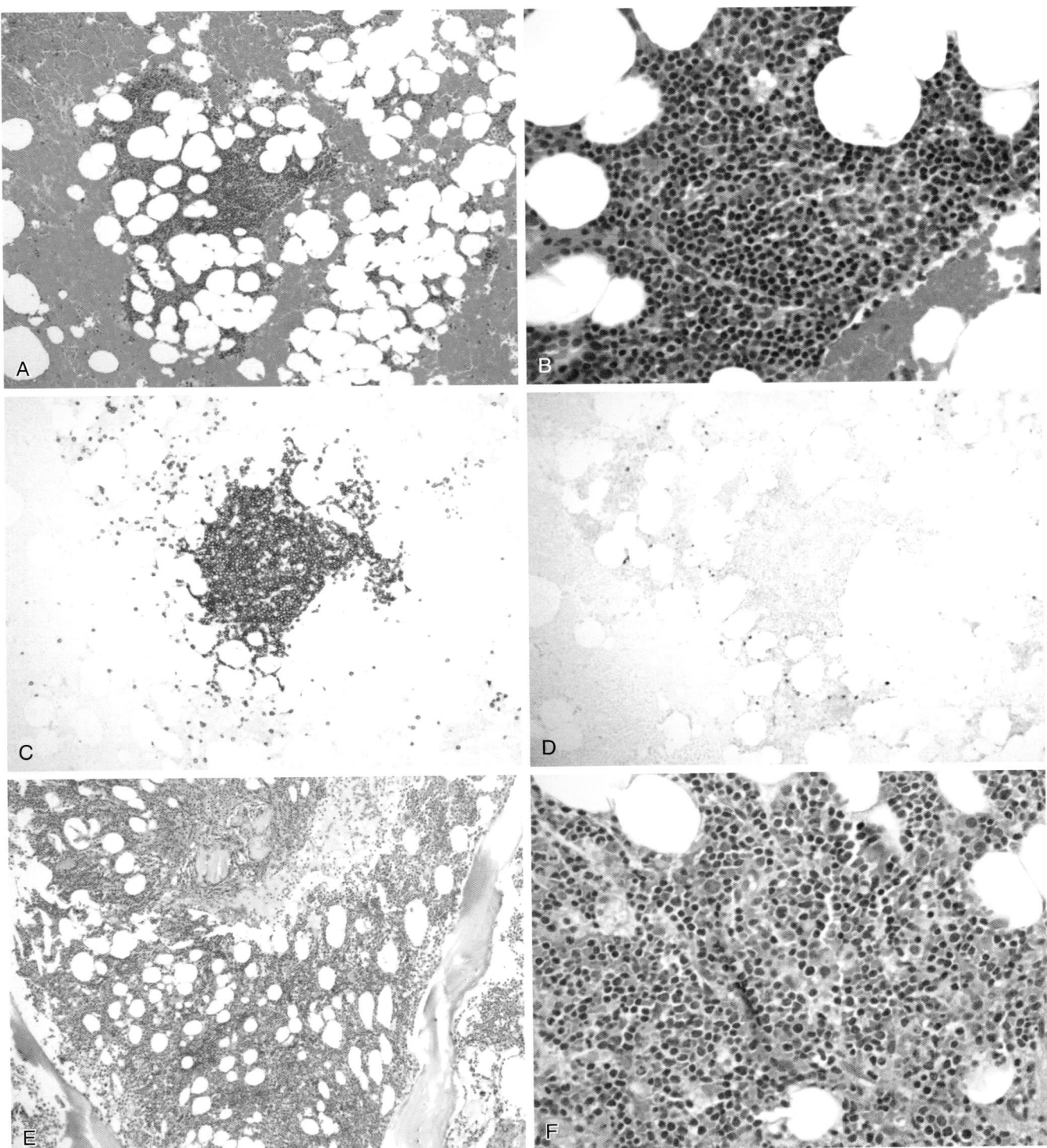

Figure 56-16. Morphologic and immunohistochemical features of reactive and neoplastic lymphoid aggregates. This reactive lymphoid aggregate in a patient treated for mantle cell lymphoma (**A** and **B**) is small, well circumscribed, and composed of CD3-positive T cells (**C**) with essentially no B cells detected by PAX5 staining (**D**). Cyclin D1 was also negative. In contrast, a recurrent mantle cell lymphoma shows diffuse marrow infiltration by small and intermediate-sized lymphoma cells (**E** and **F**), which are positive for cyclin D1.

plasma cell marker such as CD138 is helpful in accurately enumerating plasma cells. That being said, flow cytometry is effective in identifying abnormal plasma cell populations with high sensitivity and in distinguishing normal and abnormal plasma cells. As with other neoplasms, the potential effect

of targeted therapies on the immunophenotype of both normal cells and neoplastic plasma cells must be taken into consideration when interpreting flow cytometric data for residual myeloma in the post-therapy setting. Figure 56-17 illustrates MRD detection by flow cytometry for plasma cell

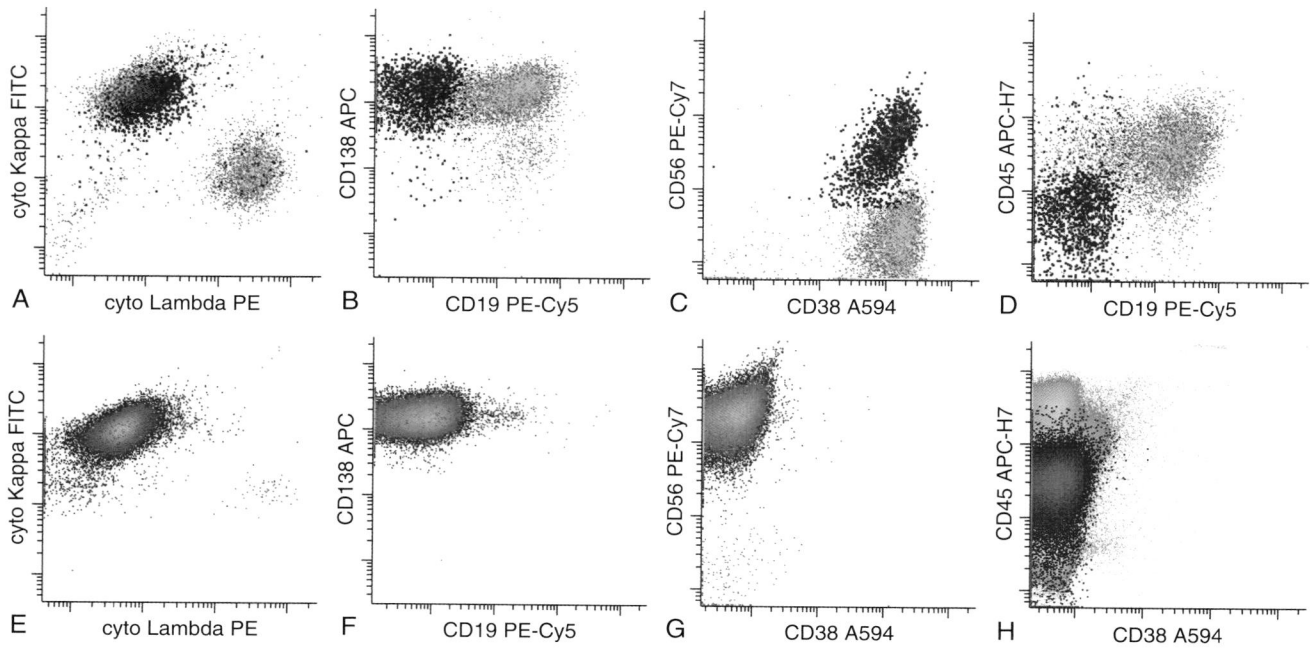

Figure 56-17. Example of residual disease post-therapy in a plasma cell neoplasm. A–D, All dot plots show plasma cells (cells expressing CD38 or CD138) in a bone marrow specimen from a patient with a history of plasma cell myeloma who presents for a pre-transplant evaluation. Plasma cells account for 0.8% of the white blood cells and include a minor subset of abnormal plasma cells *(highlighted in red)*, which account for 0.2% of the white blood cells, and a subset of normal background plasma cells *(colored aqua)*. The abnormal plasma cells have cytoplasmic kappa light chain expression, aberrantly express CD56, and lack CD19 and CD45; the normal plasma cells show polytypic cytoplasmic light chain expression and express normal levels of CD19 and CD45. Plots **E–G** show plasma cells (cells expressing CD38 or CD138) in a bone marrow specimen from a patient with a history of plasma cell myeloma who presents for a pre-transplant evaluation. The majority of plasma cells (6% of total white cell count) are abnormal plasma cells *shown in red* that express kappa cytoplasmic light chain with variable CD45, with CD56 and CD138, and without CD19 or CD38. This patient has received prior therapy, including the anti-CD38 monoclonal antibody daratumumab. Note, the dot plot illustrated in panel **H** shows all viable cells. (Abnormal plasma cells are *highlighted in red*; all other cells are *gray*.) No cells in this marrow specimen express CD38. As CD38 has an expected pattern of expression on several normal marrow populations (including normal myeloid progenitors and normal hematogones (Figs. 56-7 and 56-10), knowledge of the prior therapy is critical when evaluating antigen expression in these populations. Moreover, in this setting, it is critical that plasma cell identification include evaluation for antigens beyond the targeted CD38.

neoplasms. Several consensus guidelines exist for defining MRD by flow cytometry and for using this information for clinical decision making.[257-259] The prognostic value of MRD in plasma cell myeloma (PCM) is well established.[246,260,261] In fact, in one study, multiparametric flow cytometric detection of monotypic plasma cells on day 100 was the most relevant independent prognostic factor in PFS and OS among patients with myeloma undergoing autologous cell transplantation.[262]

Cytogenetics and Molecular Studies

Karyotype analysis of the bone marrow is useful when a clonal population similar to the patient's original neoplastic clone is identified, but the low mitotic rate of many low-grade lymphomas results in many false-negative results. The addition of interphase FISH is one method of overcoming this problem and is useful in detecting lymphoma-associated translocations. Neither karyotype nor FISH analysis can detect T-cell or B-cell–associated gene rearrangements that are not associated with translocations or other clonal abnormalities.

A subset of lymphomas has recurring cytogenetic abnormalities that make them ideal for evaluating residual disease by PCR.[125] PCR tests directed against specific translocations offer a sensitivity similar to that of patient-specific gene rearrangement testing but do not require the development of primers specific to an individual patient.

One of the most commonly studied translocations is the major breakpoint region of t(14;18)(q32.33;q21.3), involving the IGH gene of chromosome 14 and the BCL2 gene of chromosome 18. This translocation occurs most commonly in follicular lymphomas and a subset of large cell lymphomas. Approximately half of the translocations may be detected by PCR for this breakpoint, and a subset of other cases can be detected with primers directed against the other cluster regions of this translocation.[263] However, t(14;18) has been reported to occur in some normal individuals when very sensitive methods are used.[264,265] Therefore, serial qPCR methods may be more useful in monitoring patients for residual disease to determine whether the load of t(14;18)-positive cells is increasing.[266] The major translocation cluster of t(11;14) (q13;q32.33) is detectable in approximately 40% of cases of mantle cell lymphoma, but many mantle cell lymphomas have variant translocations that are not easily detected by PCR.[267,268] However, in cases with known major translocation clusters, the PCR test is a reliable method of following patients for early relapse and is superior to four-color flow cytometry in detecting MRD after immunochemotherapy.[268] The remaining patients can be followed using FISH studies. Although FISH analysis for t(11;14) does not detect the very low levels of disease detectable by PCR, it has a very low false-negative rate and is suitable for most patients with mantle cell lymphoma.[269] Similarly, the combined use of PCR and FISH analysis can be applied to the many other lymphoproliferative disorders with recurrent reciprocal translocations. The detection of residual molecular evidence of disease by FISH or qPCR in patients treated with autologous hematopoietic cell transplantation for follicular lymphoma is predictive of relapse.[270-272] However, some PCR-positive patients remain in remission, and quantitative assays are useful in better predicting disease behavior in these cases. In PCM, many patients have numerical chromosomal abnormalities or recurrent IGH-associated chromosomal abnormalities like t(11;14)(q13;q32), which can be monitored by FISH analysis[273,274]; however, this cannot detect very low levels of residual disease.

Molecular platforms that are more agnostic to the presence of specific translocations and therefore more universally applicable are being used more often to evaluate for residual disease in lymphoid and plasma cell disorders. Among the mature lymphoid neoplasms, molecular determination of MRD using these platforms has been most often used in CLL. Similar to B-ALL, the two most widely used molecular methodologies are allele-specific oligonucleotide (ASO), real-time qPCR, and high-throughput sequencing of the IGH gene. The former method is more labor-intensive and costly and has higher tendency to yield false-positive or false-negative results because of low-level amplification and potential emergence of a new clone or subclone.[275] The latter NGS MRD platform uses multiplex PCR followed by sequencing to identify and quantify the patient-specific leukemia signature immunoglobulin heavy and light chain rearrangement of CLL cells in the diagnostic and post-treatment samples.[276] Compared with ASO real-time qPCR, the NGS-based assay uses consensus primers without the need of customized patient-specific primers, resulting in even higher sensitivity (1 × 10^{-6}) and broader applicability. However, NGS-based assays may have a disadvantage in MRD determination in germinal or post–germinal center B-cell derived lymphoid neoplasms because, in a significant percentage of these patients, clonal rearrangements might not be detected with the consensus IGH gene primers that are commonly used because of the abundant somatic hypermutations.[277]

CLL MRD quantification has been shown to be an independent prognostic marker of PFS and OS after chemoimmunotherapy and after allogeneic transplantation.[276,278] Several clinical trials demonstrated that patients achieving U-MRD had a longer PFS compared with that of patients with detectable MRD, suggesting MRD may be a prognostic factor with some therapies.[279-281] MRD of ≥10^{-6} measured by high-throughput NGS IGH sequencing at multiple time points, including 9, 12, 18, and 24 months posttransplant, predicts relapse and inferior disease-free survival after reduced-intensity allogenic bone marrow transplantation.[282] However, the beneficial utility of MRD determination does not seem to apply to patients receiving Bruton tyrosine kinase (BTK)-inhibitors.[283] Less than 10% of these patients achieve MRD-negativity, but they demonstrate good PFS compared with that of patients receiving other therapies with higher rates of complete response and MRD-negativity. This suggests using only MRD test data for drug approvals may have limitations. Nevertheless, MRD is a useful prognostic tool to predict the outcome of patients with CLL in some settings and is now an accepted surrogate marker to assess treatment efficacy in randomized trials before clinical endpoints can be evaluated.[278] Despite this evidence, the role of MRD assessment in CLL is complex and multifactorial, and

it has yet to be used to influence treatment decisions in routine CLL clinical practice. There are, however, emerging studies that suggest MRD and its kinetics can be used to guide the decision of when to stop treatment, determine those who may safely stop therapy, and identify newly diagnosed patients with CLL who might require a longer duration of therapy or additional agents to achieve more durable U-MRD remissions.[283,284] Its potential as an important biomarker in CLL necessitates continuous evaluation and further standardization of methodology, nomenclature, and reporting.[255]

MRD determination can also be applied to other lymphomas and PCM using similar methodologies. There is accumulating evidence that MRD status is a strong prognostic factor for PFS and OS in mantle cell lymphoma.[255,285-287] In PCM, assessment of MRD status, either by NGS or MRD flow cytometry, can further stratify patients achieving a complete remission and is predictive of PFS and OS in all phases of the disease.[288] MRD negativity, defined as ≤1 tumor cell in 100,000 cells (10^{-5}), is associated with superior PFS and OS in newly diagnosed and relapsed/refractory PCM and appears to be independent of cytogenetics risk and depth of clinical response at the time of MRD measurement.[289-294] Numerous clinical trials are ongoing to address the question of how to use MRD as a surrogate endpoint to direct treatment.[295] Indeed, a new MRD status-based criteria to select patients with myeloma as transplant candidates has been proposed according to emerging clinical trial data.[296]

Increased understanding of the genomic landscape of chronic leukemias and lymphomas has prompted considerable interest in developing MRD tests based on detection and quantification of somatic mutations. Circulating tumor DNA (ctDNA) in plasma can serve as an important source of genetic materials for disease monitoring after therapy through this type of analysis. The sensitivity is limited by the error rates intrinsic to most conventional NGS techniques but can be enhanced through error correction using unique molecular identifiers (UMIs). ctDNA analysis allows a comprehensive genotyping of the disease from all the involved compartments, for a noninvasive serial analysis of clonal evolution, and possibly MRD investigation.[296] Its clinical utility has been demonstrated in several lymphoid malignancies, including CLL, diffuse large B-cell lymphoma, multiple myeloma, and other lymphomas.[297-301]

OTHER BONE MARROW CHANGES AFTER THERAPY

Necrosis

Bone marrow necrosis is a relatively uncommon finding, although the exact incidence is variable in the literature.[302,303] When present, however, it is most commonly associated with marrow involvement by malignancy and, less frequently, with infections, drugs, sickle cell disease, or other rare systemic abnormalities. The malignancies most often associated with marrow necrosis are acute leukemias, especially ALL, high-grade non-Hodgkin and Hodgkin lymphomas, and metastatic tumors. Bone marrow necrosis is more common after chemotherapy, especially in lymphoid lesions, but it should not be attributed to the chemotherapy alone, because cytotoxic agents induce apoptosis and not necrosis. The presence of necrosis was correlated to worse response rates in both AML and ALL and worse survival rates in AML in one study.[304] Post-therapy necrosis usually involves complete marrow replacement by nonviable "ghost cells" with pyknotic nuclei and degenerative cytoplasm (Fig. 56-18). A careful examination should be performed to exclude the possibility of foci of viable, residual tumor in these patients. Areas of necrosis may be replaced by normal regenerating elements on follow-up specimens or by fibrosis in subsequent biopsies.

Patients who have undergone prior therapy are also at high risk for infections, and infectious causes of bone marrow necrosis must be considered. Special stains for organisms should be performed, especially when focal areas of necrosis are present in the marrow, even in the absence of granulomatous inflammation. If special stains are negative for organisms, repeat bone marrow aspiration for bacterial, fungal, and viral cultures should be considered if unsuspected necrotic foci are found that are not associated with a necrotic tumor. Post-therapy bone marrow necrosis caused by specific drugs is even less common but has been reported with interferon-α, ATRA, fludarabine, and G-CSF.[34,302,304]

Fibrosis

Bone marrow fibrosis accompanies marrow involvement by a wide variety of malignant neoplasms, including chronic MPNs, Hodgkin lymphoma, mast cell disorders, metastatic carcinoma, hairy cell leukemia, and acute leukemias.[305] A mild reticulin fibrosis is often present in the markedly hypocellular post-therapy marrow, but this fibrosis quickly resolves as the marrow cellularity returns. Reticulin fibrosis is often slightly increased in association with acute leukemia.[306,307] Except for the development of fibrosis as part of the resolution of marrow necrosis, marrow fibrosis usually decreases or disappears after treatment of the primary disease by either chemotherapy or hematopoietic cell transplantation.[306] Bone marrow fibrosis secondary to CML is also significantly decreased by treatment with imatinib,[151] although increased marrow fibrosis after treatment can also be seen in some patients, particularly those in the accelerated or blast phase.[150]

Development of marrow fibrosis after therapy may represent recurrence of disease or metastasis, or it may be secondary to non-neoplastic sequelae of the therapy. These secondary causes are similar to the causes of marrow fibrosis in any

marrow,[305] such as fibrosis related to renal osteodystrophy, hypoparathyroidism or hyperparathyroidism, or vitamin D deficiency. Fibrosis may occur at the site of a prior biopsy or healing trauma. Patchy areas of fibrosis are also seen with bone marrow involvement by mast cell disease,[308,309] which may accompany other hematologic malignancies at diagnosis or relapse.

Serous Atrophy/Gelatinous Transformation

The predominance of gelatinous extracellular material with fat atrophy and associated marrow hypoplasia is termed serous atrophy or gelatinous transformation of the bone marrow. The material is light blue to pink with a mucoid or myxoid appearance, and residual hematopoietic elements may be present in chords. The gelatinous material is positive for Alcian blue, with staining eliminated after hyaluronidase treatment (Fig. 56-19).[310] This change is associated with starvation, wasting diseases, which include weight loss secondary to malignancies, and starch-free diets. The edema and deposition of fibrin and pink proteinaceous material in an aplastic marrow after myeloablative chemotherapy may mimic fat serous atrophy, but the presence of eosinophilic gelatinous material of serous atrophy has only rarely been reported after chemotherapy. When it does occur, it differs from the cachexia-associated form of serous atrophy in the lack of bone marrow fat atrophy. The gelatinous material differs from fibrin by its reactivity for Alcian blue, and it is a transient phenomenon in postchemotherapy marrow.[311]

Solid Tumors

Patients treated for solid tumors with or without prior bone marrow involvement may show transient aplasia and regeneration, similar to postchemotherapy changes in other diseases. If there was prior bone marrow involvement, foci of fibrosis or tumor necrosis may be present. Metastatic disease after therapy is usually detected by morphologic evaluation of bone marrow biopsy material (Fig. 56-20), which may be supplemented by immunohistochemistry.[312] Most metastatic tumors are associated with bone marrow fibrosis, and the detection of keratin-positive cells within these areas of fibrosis is useful to confirm the presence of metastatic carcinoma. Unusual patterns of recurrent disease include maturation of neuroblastoma with focal ganglion-like cells (differentiation) embedded in fibrosis and metastatic tumors that are not associated with marrow fibrosis. Identification of residual tumor cells may be difficult in the latter case. The most common metastatic tumors that involve the bone marrow without fibrosis are lobular breast carcinoma and neuroblastoma.[313] Recommendations for reporting bone marrow samples in patients being treated for neuroblastoma are that immunohistochemistry with at least two antibodies (e.g., synaptophysin and chromogranin A) be performed on at least three levels of bilateral core biopsies, which can help identify small areas of persistent disease (Fig. 56-20). Persistent tumor should be quantitated in intervals of 5% (0%, ≤5%, >5%–<10%, etc.).[314] The individual tumor cells of lobular carcinoma may have more abundant cytoplasm than normal bone marrow elements, and the presence of individual signet ring cells should raise suspicion for involvement by lobular carcinoma. Keratin immunohistochemistry is advised for all bone marrow biopsy specimens from patients with a

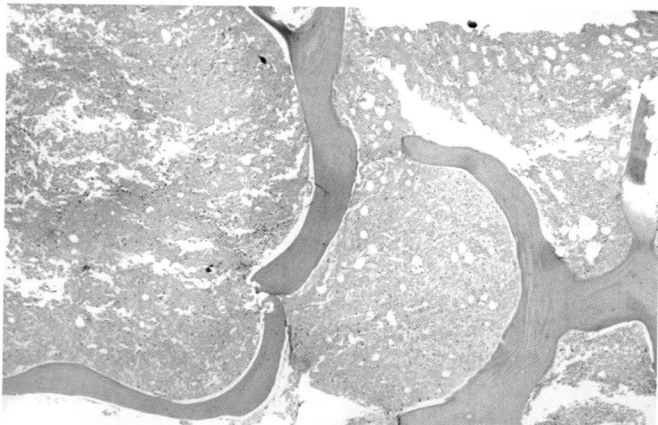

Figure 56-18. Extensive bone marrow necrosis after therapy for acute lymphoblastic leukemia.

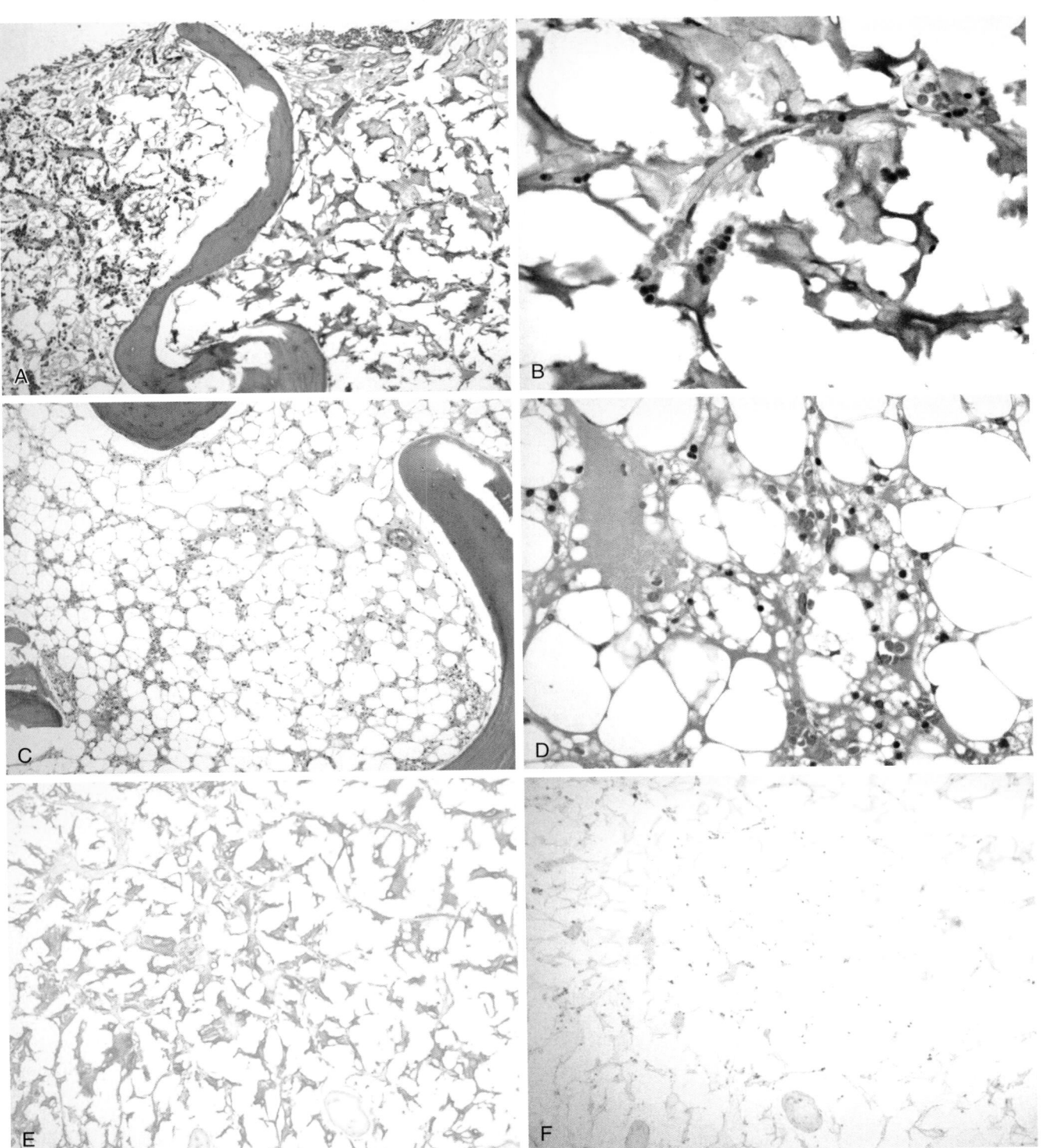

Figure 56-19. Serous atrophy/gelatinous transformation of bone marrow from an elderly patient with dementia (**A** and **B**) shows marrow hypocellularity and replacement by bluish acellular material when compared with the hypocellularity, edema, and fibrillary eosinophilic material (**C** and **D**) present in a patient post-induction chemotherapy for acute myeloid leukemia. Gelatinous transformation will stain positive for Alician blue (**E**), but stromal damage will not. Staining is decreased after hyaluronidase treatment (**F**).

history of lobular breast carcinoma to allow the detection of individual metastatic cells (Fig. 56-21).[315]

Several studies have evaluated the detection of occult metastatic disease in the bone marrow in tumors other than lobular breast carcinoma.[316-318] The detection of these occult tumor cells by immunohistochemistry has been associated with early relapse in several tumor types, including breast and ovarian carcinoma, and the detection of bone marrow disease in breast carcinoma may be of even more prognostic significance than the detection of lymph node metastasis.

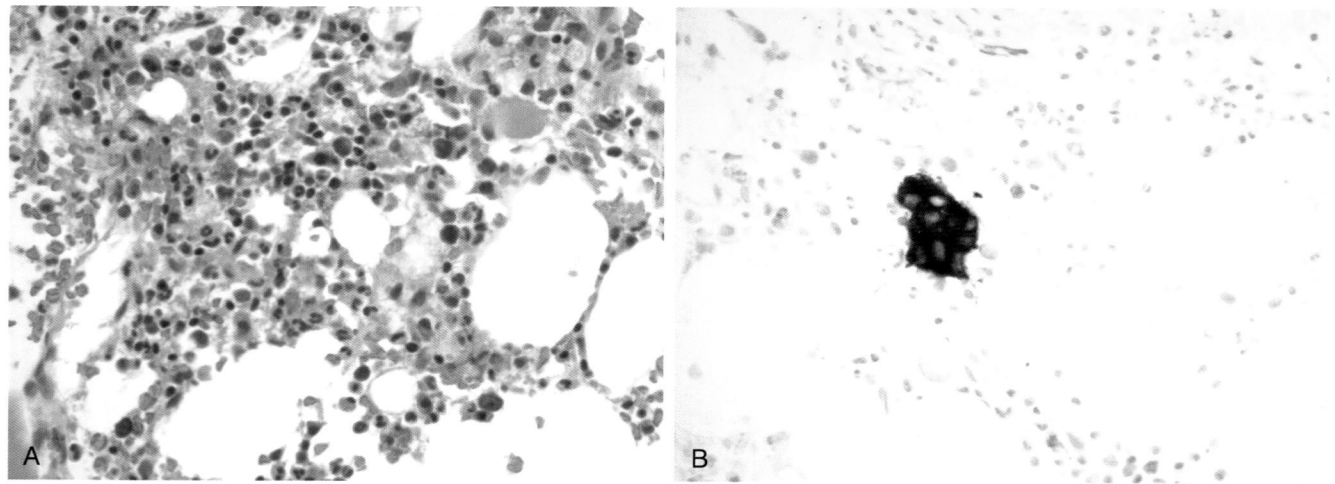

Figure 56-20. Small focus of recurrent neuroblastoma in the bone marrow **(A)**, highlighted by staining for synaptophysin **(B)**.

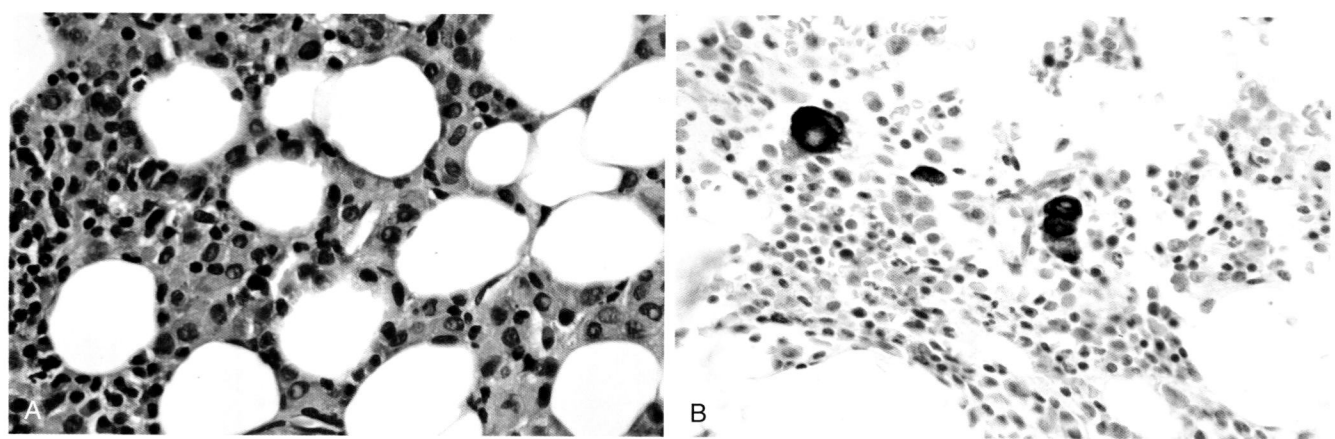

Figure 56-21. Metastatic lobular breast carcinoma forms less-obvious tumor aggregates in the bone marrow. A, Interstitial tumor infiltration is present in the upper portion of the specimen. **B,** Keratin immunohistochemistry of another case shows individual tumor cells in the marrow.

Late Effects of Therapy, Including Secondary Malignancies

In addition to disease recurrence, patients receiving high-dose chemotherapy and hematopoietic cell transplantation have other therapy-related complications. After allogeneic transplantation for leukemia or aplastic anemia, most patients are considered cured of the primary disease if they have not relapsed within 2 years.[319] However, they often experience other complications, such as graft-versus-host disease, veno-occlusive disease, sexual dysfunction, and impaired glucose tolerance and dyslipidemia.[319-324] Other than possible graft failure, however, these syndromes do not significantly affect the bone marrow.

A reactive peripheral blood lymphocytosis is common after transplantation. This lymphocytosis typically corresponds to large granular lymphocytes and can mimic T-cell large granular lymphocytic leukemia (T-LGL).[325,326] In the bone marrow, these reactive cells may be seen in an interstitial pattern. Unlike cases of T-LGL leukemia, this reactive proliferation of LGLs typically is not accompanied by cytopenias, and though

these LGLs correspond to CD8-positive/CD57-positive T cells, flow cytometry will not detect abnormalities in antigen expression. In many patients, these reactive LGLs can persist for years without significant consequence.

Patients who are treated with ibrutinib, a Bruton TKI, for CLL/SLL can have a transient large cell transformation if therapy is interrupted. This has been reported in the bone marrow and lymph nodes, and caution should be used in interpreting any new large cell proliferations in this setting.[327]

Secondary malignancies after solid organ transplantation, radiation therapy, or high-dose chemotherapy with hematopoietic cell transplantation are becoming increasingly common.[319,328-334] Although radiation-induced sarcomas may secondarily involve the bone marrow, such involvement is uncommon. However, therapy-related MDS, acute leukemia, and lymphoproliferative disorders may first be diagnosed on bone marrow examination.

Therapy-related myeloid neoplasms are fairly common in patients who have survived high-dose chemotherapy with hematopoietic cell transplantation (Fig. 56-22).

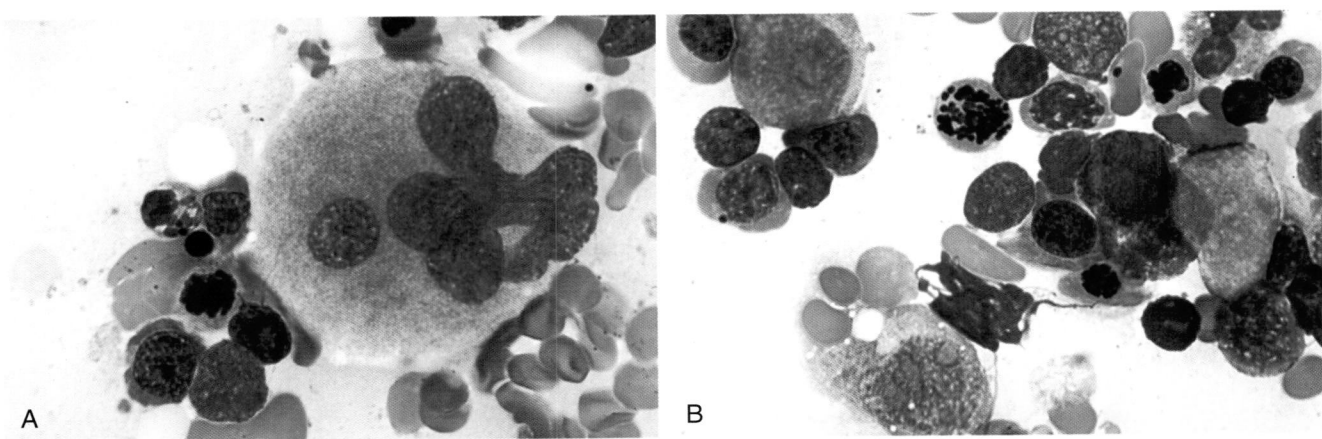

Figure 56-22. Therapy-related myelodysplastic syndrome. (A) and **(B)** are examples of cases that often show pronounced dyspoietic changes, including abnormal nuclear lobation of megakaryocytes and bizarre nuclear changes of erythroid precursors.

Approximately 10% to 20% of cases with AML, MDS, and myelodysplastic neoplasm/MPN are therapy-related.[335] The mechanisms of these neoplasms are thought to associate with a direct consequence of mutational events by cytotoxic therapy or via the selection of a myeloid clone with a mutator phenotype that has a markedly elevated risk for mutational events. These neoplasms are aggressive diseases with poor clinical outcomes, even in the case of therapy-related MDS without an increase in blast cells, and are frequently associated with an abnormal karyotype and a complex karyotype.

Two main causative cytotoxic agents associated with therapy-related AML and MDS are alkylating agents and topoisomerase II inhibitors.[330,335-339] Disease associated with alkylating agents usually has a long latency period of 5 to 10 years and may be associated with the development of cytopenias and MDS or AML with multilineage dysplasia. These cases are usually associated with deletion of a portion of chromosome 5 and/or 7, monosomy 5 and/or 7, or other unbalanced translocations. These chromosomal abnormalities may be detectable before the development of morphologic features of dysplasia, and cytogenetic studies should be performed on all cases of suspected therapy-related disease to detect this morphologically subtle presentation. Disease after topoisomerase II inhibitor therapy usually does not show changes of multilineage dysplasia and presents as an overt AML. Morphologically, most of these patients have monocytic or myelomonocytic features. These leukemias usually have a shorter latency period of 1 to 5 years and are associated with balanced cytogenetic translocations involving 11q23.3 (*KMT2A* gene) or 21q22.3 (*RUNX1* gene). A variety of other cytogenetic abnormalities may occur in therapy-related leukemia and MDS, including many different balanced translocations.[335,339] Patients with de novo AML with t(8;21), t(15;17) and inv(16) are known to have favorable prognosis. Although less frequent, these cytogenetic abnormalities account for approximately 10% of therapy-related myeloid neoplasms. Patients with t(8;21), t(15;17), and inv(16) in therapy-related myeloid neoplasms have poorer clinical outcomes than those of patients with the same abnormality in de novo disease.[338,340]

Mutational analysis using NGS has shown *TP53* mutations are more frequent in therapy-related myeloid neoplasms (20%–40%) than in de novo AML or MDS (5%–10%). Studies have reported this selective enrichment is a result of the preferential

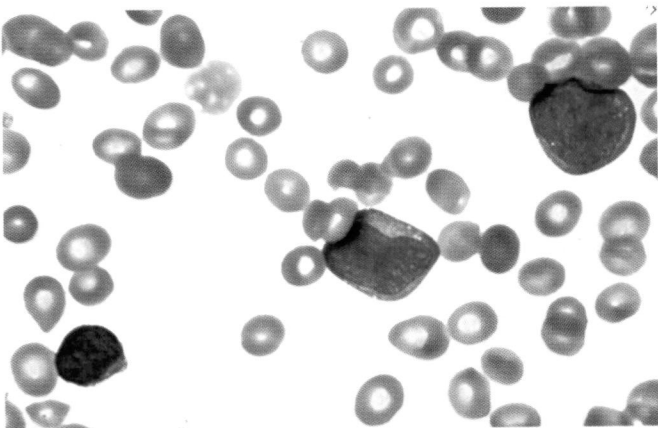

Figure 56-23. Therapy-related acute lymphoblastic leukemia. Blasts often show aberrant expression of the myeloid-associated antigens CD15 and CD65 and rearrangements of the *KMT2A* gene.

expansion of preleukemic clones harboring a somatic *TP53* mutation after cytotoxic therapy. *TP53* mutations are associated with complex karyotype and poor prognosis. Less frequent mutations observed included *TET2* (10%–37%) and *IDH1/IDH2* (around 7% and 12% in therapy-related MDS and AML, respectively). Other recurrent mutations found in a study of therapy-related myeloid neoplasms included mutations in *DNMT3A* (~20%), *FLT3* (8%–16%), and *NPM1* (18%).[335,341-344]

Other therapy-related leukemias are less common but include MDS or AML associated with 17p deletions and *TP53* mutations, which most often occur after hydroxyurea therapy for essential thrombocythemia.[342-344] There are prominent dysplastic changes of the neutrophil series, with pseudo–Pelger-Hüet cells, monolobated neutrophils, and prominent vacuolated cytoplasm. Similar morphologic and cytogenetic changes have been described in a subgroup of lymphoma patients with alkylating agent–related MDS and AML. Therapy-related ALL is also rare (Fig. 56-23),[345,346] but it occurs most often in patients treated with topoisomerase II inhibitors.[347] These leukemias are frequently of a pro–B-cell (CD10-negative) immunophenotype, with aberrant expression of the myeloid-associated antigens CD15 and CD65. They are usually associated with balanced translocations of the *KMT2A* gene, particularly t(4;11)(q21;q23); however, patients with amplification of *MLL* genes in addition to presence of complex karyotype have been reported.[348,349]

Donor-derived second malignancy after allogeneic hematopoietic stem cell transplantation is an extremely rare complication of transplantation.[275,276] Oncogenic transformation or premature senescence of transplanted donor cells in an immunosuppressed host and disruption of normal homeostasis after transplantation may be associated with donor-cell–derived malignancies. The incidence of donor-derived leukemia comprises less than 1% of cases. Reported cases have included acute myeloid or lymphoblastic leukemia, MDS, CML, and T-cell lymphoma.[241,350-353]

Posttransplant lymphoproliferative disorders (PTLDs), which are covered in detail in Chapter 54, may involve the bone marrow. Over half of patients who develop PTLDs after solid organ transplantation have bone marrow involvement, and bone marrow changes are more common in children than in adults with PTLDs.[354] Bone marrow involvement is associated with a poorer outcome. Aspirate smears tend to show an increased number of plasma cells. On the biopsy, the changes may range from aggregates of small lymphocytes or plasma cells without obvious atypia to aggregates of large, atypical cells, usually with plasmacytoid features. Atypical cell infiltrates may be associated with fibrosis. The cellular infiltrate is usually of B-cell lineage, but plasmacytoid cells may be underrecognized owing to their lack of immunoreactivity with antibodies directed against CD20. In situ hybridization studies for Epstein-Barr virus–encoded RNA (EBER) are positive in most cases. Although less common, PTLDs that occur after bone marrow transplantation are highly aggressive B-cell proliferations associated with Epstein-Barr virus and usually have a large-cell or immunoblastic morphology.[355] These proliferations are associated with T-cell–depleted transplantation, unrelated donor transplantation, or HLA-mismatched–related donor transplantation, and they usually occur within the 1st year after transplantation.[329]

Pearls and Pitfalls

- Bone marrow specimens must always be interpreted in the context of the clinical setting.
- Slight increases in blast cells (>5%) do not always mean residual disease.
- Residual disease can be present in patients with less than 5% blast cells.
- Flow cytometry is useful in separating regenerating progenitors (blasts) from leukemic cells.
- Residual or recurrent leukemia is favored over regeneration when sheets of blasts are present on smears or when blasts outnumber promyelocytes.
- Growth factor therapy may be a factor in patients with numerous promyelocytes with distinct perinuclear hofs.
- Aggregates of CD34-positive or TdT-positive cells on bone marrow biopsy material favor leukemia over regeneration or hematogones.
- Dyserythropoietic changes, including ring sideroblasts, during or shortly after chemotherapy are not sufficient for an interpretation of MDS.
- Hematogones should be considered when a small lymphoid cell proliferation is present in children.
- A spectrum of lymphoid cells that, by morphology or antigen expression, resemble precursor B-cell development is more characteristic of hematogones than leukemic cells.
- Hematogones do not show cytogenetic abnormalities or aberrant immunophenotypes.
- Never rely on a single feature to exclude the presence of disease.
- Consider the sensitivity and pitfalls of any test used, especially ancillary studies.
- Morphologically normal bone marrow may continue to show the Ph chromosome in patients treated for CML.

- MRD detection as measured by flow cytometry or molecular methods is emerging as an important modality in monitoring treatment response, prognostication of patients, and precise tailoring of therapy in acute leukemias, mature lymphoid neoplasms, and chronic myeloid neoplasms.
- By flow cytometry, separation of leukemic blasts from normal progenitors relies on recognizing differences in immunophenotype exhibited by leukemic cells compared with normal antigenic changes that characterize hematopoiesis.
- The best molecular markers for evaluating MRD in AML are *RUNX1::RUNXT1*, *CBF::MYH11*, *PML::RARA*, and mutated *NPM1*. Highly sensitive MRD detection using these markers can be achieved through real-time qPCR.
- Mutations in genes most frequently associated with clonal hematopoiesis (*DNMTA*, *TET2*, and *ASXL1*) are not suitable for MRD assessment in AML.
- NGS of immunoglobulin genes provides a highly sensitive platform to identify MRD in lymphoid neoplasms.
- Mutation profiling of cfDNA allows evaluation of residual disease, helps predict relapse, and offers a better evaluation of clonal heterogeneity and evolution. The molecular detection of very low levels of t(15;17), inv(16), and t(8;21) fusion transcripts at a single time point after therapy does not necessarily predict relapse, though sequential reading showing increasing levels of a fusion transcript do suggest relapse.
- Patients treated for multiple myeloma or CML may have small, decreasing but detectable populations of residual clonal disease for several months after transplantation, which may convert to molecular remission without additional therapy.

KEY REFERENCES

3. Riley RS, Idowu M, Chesney A, et al. Hematologic aspects of myeloablative therapy and bone marrow transplantation. *J Clin Lab Anal*. 2005;19(2):47–79.

26. Dohner H, Estey EH, Amadori S, et al. European LeukemiaNet. Diagnosis and management of acute myeloid leukemia in adults: recommendations from an international expert panel, on behalf of the European LeukemiaNet. *Blood*. 2010;115:453–474.

29. Ryder JW, Lazarus HM, Farhi DC. Bone marrow and blood findings after marrow transplantation and rhGM-CSF therapy. *Am J Clin Pathol*. 1992;97:631–637.

76. Dick FR, Burns CP, Weiner GJ, Heckman KD. Bone marrow morphology during induction phase of therapy for acute myeloid leukemia (AML). *Hematol Pathol*. 1995;9:95–106.

121. Rimsza LM, Viswanatha DS, Winter SS, Leith CP, Frost JD, Foucar K. The presence of CD34+ cell clusters predicts impending relapse in children with acute lymphoblastic leukemia receiving maintenance chemotherapy. *Am J Clin Pathol*. 1998;110:313–320.

132. Ladetto M, Bruggemann M, Monitillo L, et al. Next-generation sequencing and real-time quantitative PCR for MRD detection in B-cell disorders. *Leukemia*. 2014;28:1299–1307.

136. Wood B, Wu D, Crossley B, et al. Measurable residual disease detection by high-throughput sequencing improves risk stratification for pediatric B-ALL. *Blood.* 2018 Mar 22;131(12):1350–1359.

142. Braziel RM, Launder TM, Druker BJ, et al. Hematopathologic and cytogenetic findings in imatinib mesylate-treated chronic myelogenous leukemia patients: 14 months' experience. *Blood.* 2002;100:435–441.

181. Wilkins BS, Radia D, Woodley C, Farhi SE, Keohane C, Harrison CN. Resolution of bone marrow fibrosis in a patient receiving JAK1/JAK2 inhibitor treatment with ruxolitinib. *Haematologica.* 2013;98:1872–1876.

298. Kurtz DM, Scherer F, Jin MC, et al. Circulating tumor DNA measurements as early outcome predictors in diffuse large B-cell lymphoma. *J Clin Oncol.* 2018 Oct 1;36(28):2845–2853.

310. Seaman JP, Kjeldsberg CR, Linker A. Gelatinous transformation of the bone marrow. *Hum Pathol.* 1978;9:685–692.

Visit Elsevier eBooks+ for the complete set of references.

Chapter 57

Non-hematopoietic Neoplasms and Other Lesions of the Bone Marrow and Lymph Nodes

Lawrence R. Zukerberg[†] and Aliyah R. Sohani

INTRODUCTION

The bone marrow, the primary site of hematopoiesis, may contain hematopoietic or non-hematopoietic tumors and also frequently reflects metabolic disturbances. The occurrence of bone marrow metastases is strongly influenced by microenvironmental factors that favor the engraftment of certain malignancies.[1] Bone marrow involvement by metastatic tumor is often referred to as myelophthisis and

presents in the blood, usually subtly, as leukoerythroblastic anemia with left-shifted granulocytic precursors, nucleated red cells, teardrop red cells, and large platelets. Symptoms related to cytopenias, metabolic disturbances, and occupation of space (such as bone pain) may mimic leukemias and lymphomas. Imaging studies are often helpful, but a bone marrow examination is usually required to directly visualize the process. Bone marrow examination should include both aspiration and biopsy, and multiple sites (usually the bilateral iliac crests) may need sampling.

Similarly, nonlymphoid elements are frequently present in biopsied or excised lymph node specimens. This chapter

---

[†] Deceased. This chapter is dedicated to his memory and reflects the depth and breadth of his expertise as a diagnostic surgical pathologist.

Table 57-1 Differential Diagnosis of Poorly Differentiated Metastatic Tumors

Histologic Pattern	Tumor Types	Useful Diagnostic Tests and Clues
Small-cell tumors	Carcinoma (lobular breast, prostate)	Keratin
	Small-cell carcinoma, Merkel cell carcinoma	Synaptophysin, chromogranin; polyoma virus for Merkel cell carcinoma; keratin can be focal
	Neuroendocrine, carcinoid tumors	Synaptophysin, chromogranin, CD56, INSM1
	Neuroblastoma	NSE, neurofilament, NB84, PHOX2B, EM
	Lymphoblastic lymphoma	TdT, cytogenetics
	Ewing's sarcoma, other primitive sarcomas	PAS stain, CD99, NKX2-2, FLI1, PAX7, cytogenetics
	Rhabdomyosarcoma	Desmin, myogenin, MyoD1, EM, cytogenetics
Epithelioid tumors	Carcinoma (especially renal cell, prostate, breast)	Multiple keratin stains/cocktails often helpful
	Melanoma	S-100, SOX10, HMB45, tyrosinase, MART-1, Melan A
	Large-cell lymphoma	CD45/LCA, CD3, CD20
	Seminoma (especially retroperitoneum, mediastinum)	PLAP, PAS stain, OCT3/4, SALL4, LIN28, D2-40
	Extramedullary myeloid cell tumor	Myeloperoxidase, lysozyme, CD34, CD43, CD68, CD117/KIT
	Plasma cell myeloma	CD138, CD79a, CD38, immunoglobulins
Anaplastic tumors	Carcinoma (lung, bladder, breast, thyroid gland)	Focal keratinization or mucin
	Nasopharyngeal carcinoma	Epstein-Barr virus in situ hybridization
	Melanoma	S-100, SOX10, HMB45, melan A, tyrosinase, MiTF
	Anaplastic large-cell lymphoma	CD30, EMA, ALK, CD43 (often CD3⁻)
	Hodgkin lymphoma	CD15, CD30 (CD45/LCA⁻), MUM1, PAX5
	Dendritic cell neoplasms	CD21 (FDC), S-100 (IDC), EM
	Angiosarcoma	ERG, CD31, CD34, factor VIII–related antigen
	Leiomyosarcoma	Caldesmon, desmin (actins are less specific), EM
Spindle cell tumors	Sarcomatoid carcinoma	Keratins, especially high-molecular weight (often only focally positive)
	Desmoplastic melanoma	S-100, SOX10 (HMB45 and MART-1 often negative)
	Kaposi sarcoma	PAS, CD34, HHV-8 LANA-1, podoplanin, CD31, ERG
	Large-cell lymphoma with fibrosis (especially mediastinal)	CD20 (works in necrotic tumor areas as well), PAX5
	Syncytial variant of Hodgkin lymphoma	CD15, CD30 (CD43⁻, CD45/LCA⁻)
	FDC neoplasms	CD21, CD23, CD35, D2-40 (CD23 can be negative)
	Metastatic sarcoma (especially angiosarcoma, nerve sheath tumors, or myofibroblastic sarcoma)	EM and cytogenetics helpful
	Inflammatory pseudotumor	Admixed acute inflammatory cells, smooth muscle actin, ALK
	Infectious pseudotumor	AFB, fungal, spirochetes, and Gram stains

AFB, Acid-fast bacillus; *ALK,* anaplastic lymphoma kinase; *EM,* electron microscopy; *EMA,* epithelial membrane antigen; *FDC,* follicular dendritic cell; *HHV-8 LANA-1,* human herpesvirus 8 latency-associated nuclear antigen-1; *IDC,* interdigitating dendritic cell; *LCA,* leukocyte common antigen; *NSE,* neuron-specific enolase; *PAS,* periodic acid–Schiff; *PLAP,* placental alkaline phosphatase; *TdT,* terminal deoxynucleotidyl transferase.

reviews the most commonly encountered tumors and non-neoplastic lesions of bone marrow and lymph nodes and provides an update on studies useful in distinguishing them. Each section focuses on metastases because they present the most diagnostic difficulty and benign tumor-like lesions that may be in the differential diagnosis of metastatic tumors. Mesenchymal and vascular proliferations are also discussed, including those intrinsic to each organ.

METASTATIC TUMORS OF THE BONE MARROW

The most common metastatic tumors of the bone and bone marrow are carcinoma of the breast, lung, and prostate, together constituting two-thirds of cases.[2] Each of these is present in up to 20% of patients with the primary tumor. Other metastases seen at lower frequencies include adenocarcinoma of the stomach and colon, melanoma, renal cell carcinoma, ovarian and testicular carcinoma, transitional cell carcinoma, rhabdomyosarcoma, Ewing's sarcoma, and vascular tumors. Childhood tumors, including rhabdomyosarcoma, neuroblastoma, retinoblastoma, medulloblastoma, and Ewing's sarcoma, frequently involve the bone marrow.[3,4] Metastatic

tumors are best diagnosed and classified at their primary site; however, immunohistochemistry (IHC) provides an adjunct to morphology when the primary site is not known (Table 57-1). However, technical issues related to decalcification of bone marrow core biopsy specimens may lead to suboptimal staining.

Invasive Breast Carcinoma

In the 5th edition of the *World Health Organization (WHO) Classification of Tumours of the Breast,* invasive breast carcinoma is classified into a number of categories and subcategories.[5,6] By IHC, tumor cells stain for low–molecular-weight keratin, epithelial membrane antigen (EMA), and often for carcinoembryonic antigen (CEA), B72.3, and BCA-225.[7] Involved bone marrow may show abundant tumor nests, but areas of inconspicuous clusters and/or extensive fibrosis are also frequent (Fig. 57-1A–D). Microenvironmental factors strongly influence bone marrow involvement in this disease and may be altered by bisphosphonate drugs.[8] Detection of disseminated tumor cells in the bone marrow, most often by IHC, identifies high-risk patients and those who may benefit from bisphosphonate therapy.[9]

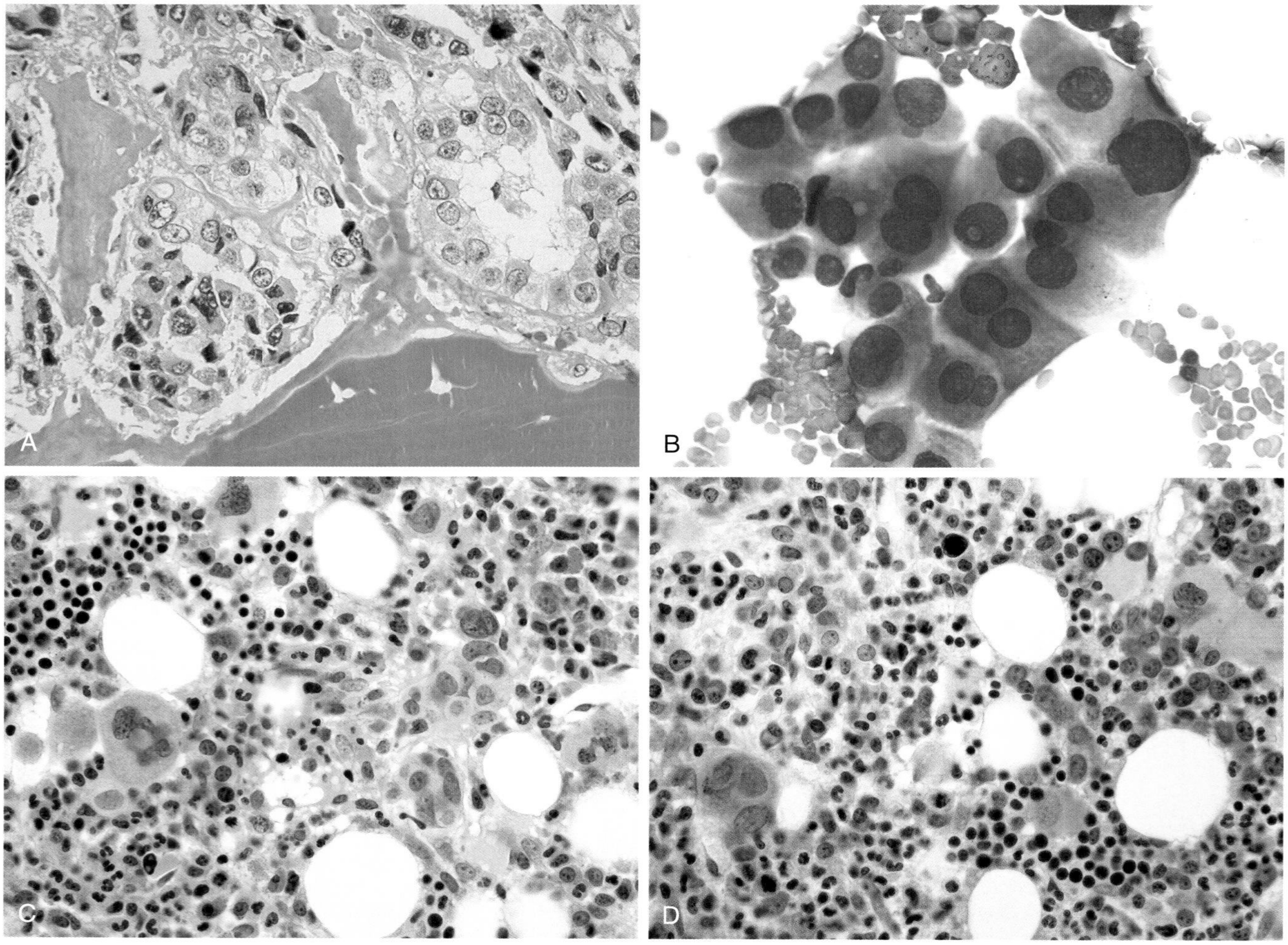

Figure 57-1. Metastatic adenocarcinoma of the breast in a bone marrow biopsy **(A)** and a bone marrow aspirate smear **(B)**. **C,** Another bone marrow biopsy shows inconspicuous involvement by metastatic breast carcinoma. **D,** The same biopsy shows the tumor cells highlighted by a pan-keratin stain.

Carcinoma of the Lung

Carcinoma of the lung involves the bone marrow, with frequency also varying by histologic type. Small-cell carcinoma most frequently metastasizes to the bone marrow (~20%), followed by squamous cell carcinoma (3%–15%) and adenocarcinoma (5%–10%).

Small-cell carcinoma cells resemble blasts but show frequent clustering and nuclear molding (Fig. 57-2). They label for pan-keratins, CK7, chromogranin, and synaptophysin. Patients frequently exhibit neuroendocrine syndromes.[7,10] Carcinoid tumors may also rarely metastasize to the bone marrow.

Squamous cell carcinoma is distinctive in the bone marrow biopsy but usually does not appear in aspirates, which may be acellular. Nests of cohesive tumor cells label for pan-keratins, CK7, CK5/6, and p63 and are often embedded in a fibrous background.

Adenocarcinomas (Fig. 57-3) are increasingly common in the lung and label for pan-keratins, CK7, napsin A, and TTF-1.[11,12] Morphologic classification; molecular and/or IHC determinations of *EGFR*, *KRAS*, and anaplastic lymphoma kinase *(ALK)* status; and assessment of PD-L1 expression by IHC are clinically indicated for assignment of

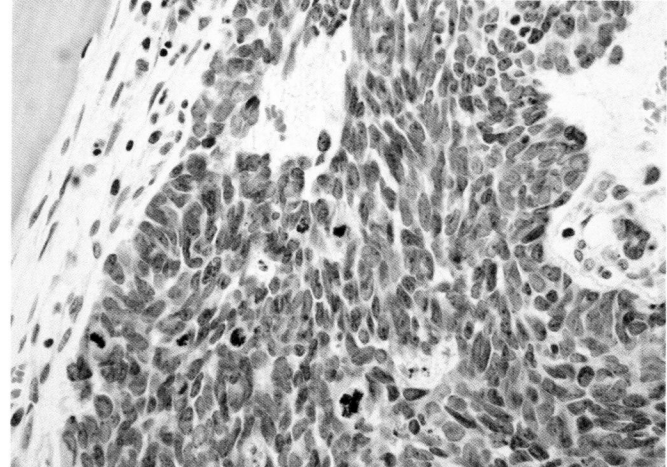

Figure 57-2. Small-cell carcinoma of the lung, metastatic to the bone marrow.

targeted therapy, usually from a primary site.[13] Detection in metastatic sites may be performed by IHC or fluorescence in situ hybridization (FISH), but there is significant intratumor

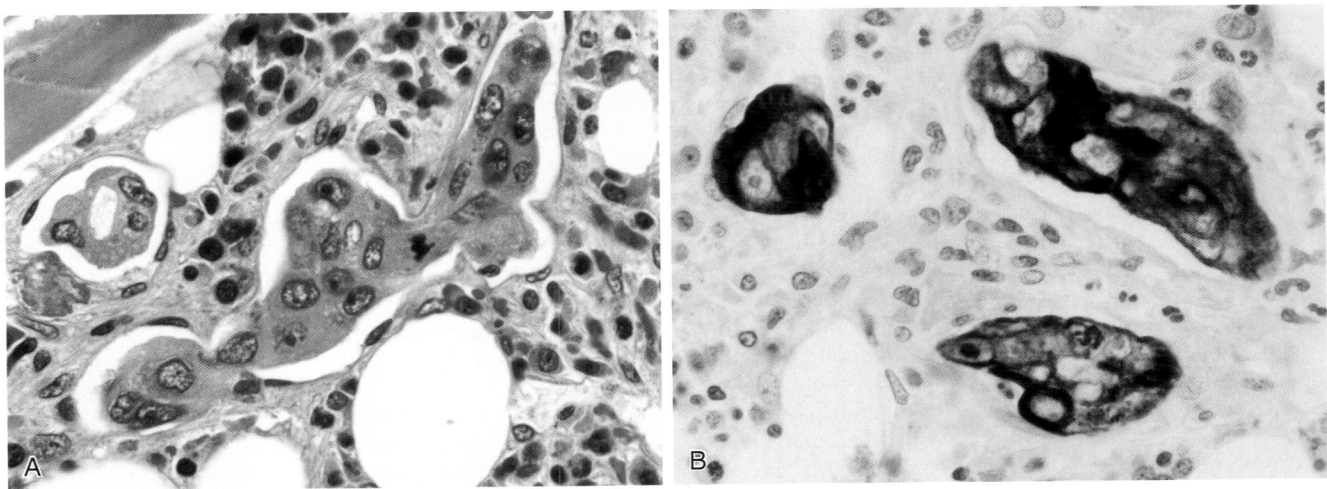

Figure 57-3. Metastatic adenocarcinoma of the lung in a bone marrow biopsy **(A)** expressing cytokeratin 7 **(B)**.

variability, with metastases often not reflecting the primary site.[2]

Metastatic Prostate Cancer

Metastatic prostate cancer most commonly involves bone marrow.[14] Although primary prostate tumors are frequently well-differentiated adenocarcinomas with small acinar formation, less well-differentiated forms tend to metastasize, particularly moderately differentiated forms with fused glands, cribriform or papillary formations, or loss of discernible gland formation (Fig. 57-4). Often, the diagnosis is suggested by serum screening for prostate-specific antigen (PSA) and confirmed by prostate biopsy, but it also appears as bone involvement by adenocarcinoma of unknown primary origin. IHC is usually positive for PSA, prostatic acid phosphatase, and pan-keratins. Poorly differentiated tumors negative for PSA and prostatic acid phosphatase may label for prostate-specific membrane antigen and prostein (P501S).[15]

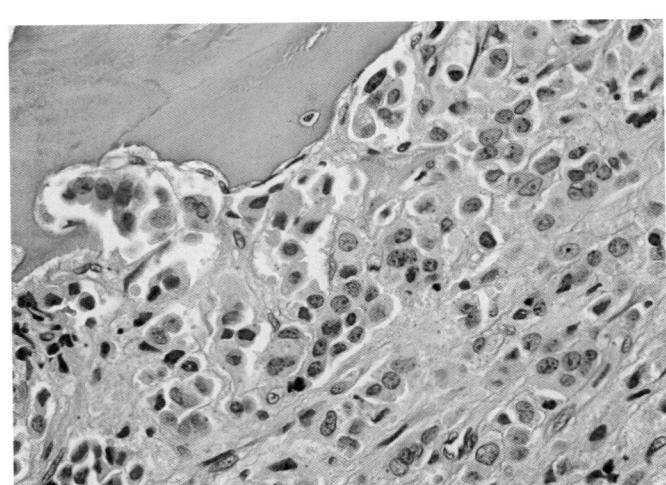

Figure 57-4. Metastatic prostate cancer in a bone marrow biopsy.

Carcinomas of the Stomach and Colon

Most carcinomas of the stomach are adenocarcinomas of intestinal or diffuse types, though they may include other variants and a lymphoepithelioma-like pattern with abundant lymphocytes may be seen.[16] IHC shows expression of pan-keratins, EMA, CEA, CK20, CK7, and CA19-9.

Most colorectal carcinomas are moderately differentiated adenocarcinomas (Fig. 57-5).[17] These tumors label for cytokeratins (typically positive for CK20 but negative for CK7), CEA, villin, CDX2, and tumor-associated glycoprotein (TAG-72).[7] A small-cell variant labels with neuron-specific enolase (NSE) and synaptophysin.[17]

Renal Cell Carcinoma

Renal cell carcinoma often involves bone in advanced stage, occurring in one-third of patients with renal cell carcinoma who are enrolled in clinical trials. Bisphosphonates have been used for treatment but may be supplanted by new targeted

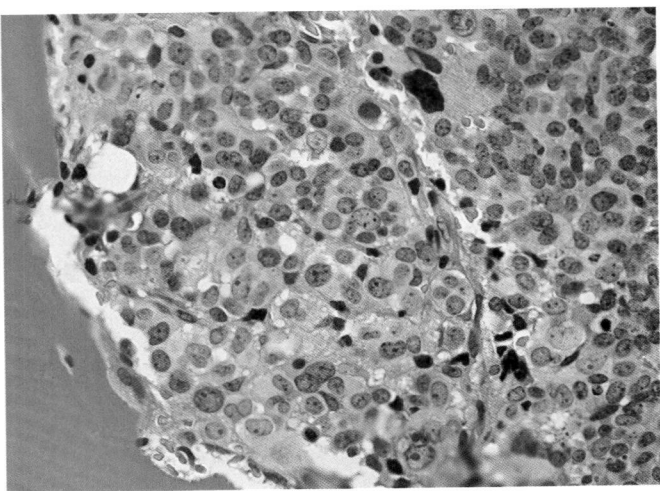

Figure 57-5. Bone marrow biopsy specimen extensively involved by metastatic colon carcinoma.

agents.[18] Diagnostic IHC includes pan-keratins, CD10, RCC, PAX2, and PAX8.[19]

Melanoma

Melanoma frequently mimics other metastatic tumors, and although melanin production is helpful, it is uncommon in bone marrow metastases. Tumor cells may resemble large-cell lymphoma with immunoblastic, plasmablastic, or anaplastic morphology; may mimic plasma cell myeloma, including plasmablastic plasma cell myeloma; or may exhibit sarcomatoid features. Therefore, melanoma should be in the differential diagnosis of any anaplastic or poorly differentiated tumor. IHC staining for S-100 protein, HMB-45, and melan-A (MART-1) is usually diagnostic, although HMB-45 is negative in desmoplastic melanoma.[20] *BRAF* V600 mutations in metastatic melanoma are targetable with anti-BRAF medications, and these may be detected in small biopsies by IHC.[21]

Pediatric Small Round Blue Cell Tumors

Pediatric small blue cell tumors generally require bone marrow examination for staging purposes, and results have significant effects on treatment and prognosis. Most of these tumors show highly variable patterns of involvement, sometimes with extensive disease at one site but undetectable involvement nearby.

Rhabdomyosarcoma, the most common soft-tissue sarcoma in children, is derived from skeletal muscle cells and bears myogenic proteins. Clinically relevant types include embryonal alveolar and rhabdomyosarcoma. Treatment and prognosis are based on age, stage, histology, and molecular or cytogenetic features, with a *FOXO1* translocation involving chromosome 13 accounting for poor prognosis in alveolar histology.[22] Bone marrow involvement is seen in 25% to 30% of patients, with an increased frequency of alveolar histology (50%).[23,24] Tumor cells in the bone marrow are often small to medium-sized blastoid cells, present singly or in small clusters, with an eosinophilic granular cytoplasm (Fig. 57-6). Hemophagocytosis and presentations resembling acute

leukemia may occur.[25-31] Tumor cells label for desmin, muscle-specific actin, myo-D1, and myogenin.[32]

Neuroblastoma and related differentiated tumors, ganglioneuroblastoma and ganglioneuroma, occur primarily in young children. Neuroblastomas are most commonly primary to the adrenal cortex, abdominal or thoracic sympathetic ganglia, neck, and pelvis, and they may be multifocal. Metastatic spread is both lymphatic and hematogenous, with bone marrow involvement common, seen in more than 50% of patients at diagnosis in some series.[33] Bilateral bone marrow biopsy and aspiration is recommended for staging. An adequate bone marrow specimen contains a biopsy of at least 1 cm in length and an aspirate containing spicules. Histology shows primitive neuroblasts, with varying Schwann and ganglion cells. Homer-Wright rosettes may be present and consist of neuroblasts surrounding a tangle of neuropil (Fig. 57-7). Fibrillary stroma is present in most cases, and Schwann cells with organized fascicles of neuritic processes and fibrosis are present in cases with ganglioneuromatous

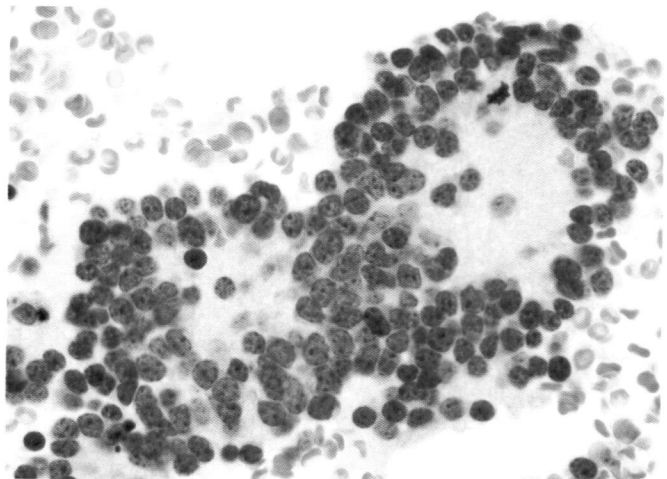

Figure 57-7. Rosettes of metastatic neuroblastoma in a clot section of bone marrow.

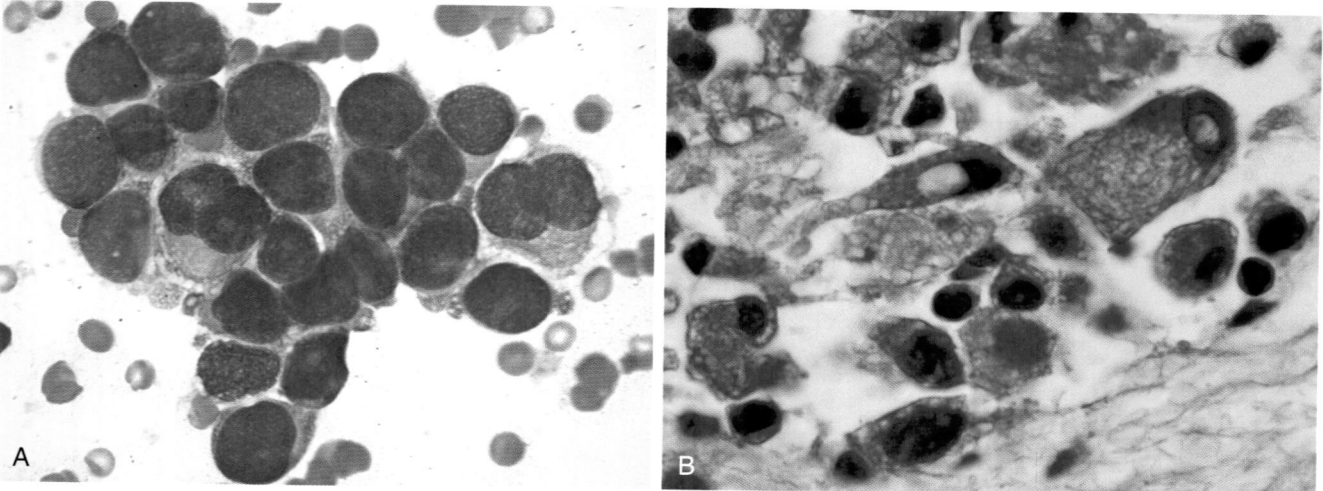

Figure 57-6. Metastatic rhabdomyosarcoma in bone marrow aspirate smears **(A)** and bone marrow biopsy **(B)**.

components. Aspirate smears should be carefully examined for small clusters of large blastoid cells.

IHC may be helpful in identifying tumor cells, particularly in small biopsies or cases with focal involvement. NSE and CD56 are usually positive, S-100 labels Schwann cells, synaptophysin labels differentiated neuroblasts and ganglion cells, and chromogranin labels ganglion cells. Myelofibrosis may be present at diagnosis, and neuroblastoma may morphologically resemble acute leukemia (Fig. 57-8). Presence of differentiating ganglion cells in bone marrow metastases may be prognostically favorable.[34] After chemotherapy, a differentiated tumor with ganglion cells and stroma without neuroblasts has no negative prognostic influence.[35]

Retinoblastoma is an aggressive childhood tumor of the eye.[36] It is one of the most common eye tumors and the most common in children. It is associated with mutations of the tumor suppressor retinoblastoma (*RB*) gene on chromosome 13q14 and usually presents before the age 5 years as a white light reflex. Disseminated disease usually presents in the bone marrow or central nervous system (CNS), but the actual incidence of marrow involvement is less than 10%, and the value of routine bone marrow examination is controversial.

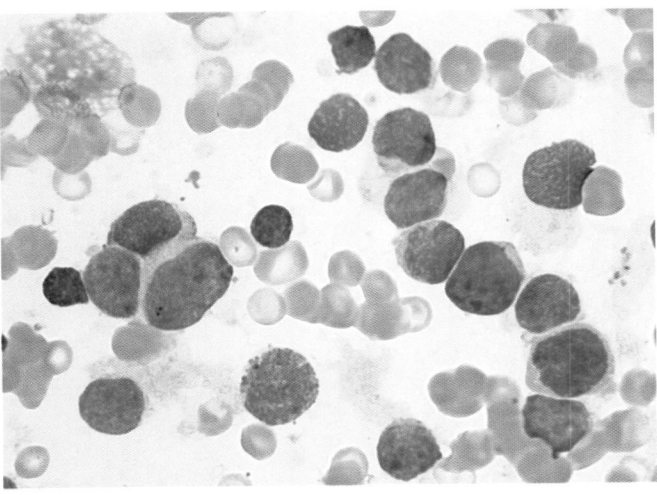

Figure 57-8. Neuroblastoma mimicking acute leukemia in the bone marrow aspirate; note the rare tumor cluster.

Histology varies from undifferentiated small blue cells to more differentiated forms with Homer-Wright and Flexner-Wintersteiner rosettes. By IHC, expression of rhodopsin, rhodopsin kinase, transducin, S antigen, GFAP, S-100, vimentin, and CD56 is seen.[37]

Medulloblastoma is a primitive neuroectodermal tumor of the cerebellum in children that sometimes metastasizes to the bone marrow. Advances in the underlying molecular pathogenesis have informed classification, prognostication, and targeted therapeutic approaches.[38] On histology, blastoid cells are present in sheets, often forming Homer-Wright rosettes, and sometimes present with features resembling neuroblastoma (neurofibrillary stroma and/or ganglionic differentiation). Tumors often are positive for synaptophysin and GFAP.

PRIMARY TUMORS OF BONE

Ewing's Sarcoma

Ewing's sarcoma is usually primary to bone, although extraskeletal forms occur. The median age is 13 years.[39] It is one of the most undifferentiated tumors and is composed of blastoid cells with interspersed small hyperchromatic cells resembling lymphocytes (Fig. 57-9). Mitoses are variable, and necrosis is often present, with pseudorosettes of tumor cells surrounding necrotic centers and perivascular tumor cuffing in necrotic areas. Some tumors show neuroectodermal differentiation, though the term "primitive neuroectodermal tumor" is no longer used and tumors are classified according to molecular characteristics, with Ewing's sarcoma most commonly associated with an *EWSR1::FLI1* fusion.[39] The IHC profile overlaps with that of neuroblastoma. Positive markers include vimentin, NSE, synaptophysin, CD56, and FLI1.[39] MIC2 (CD99) is characteristically present in Ewing's sarcoma but must be interpreted with caution because lymphoblasts and, sometimes, myeloblasts are also positive.

Bone and Cartilage–Forming Tumors

Bone-forming tumors (osteomas, osteoid osteomas, osteoblastomas, and osteosarcomas) are characterized by the presence of osteoid. Osteosarcoma is the most common

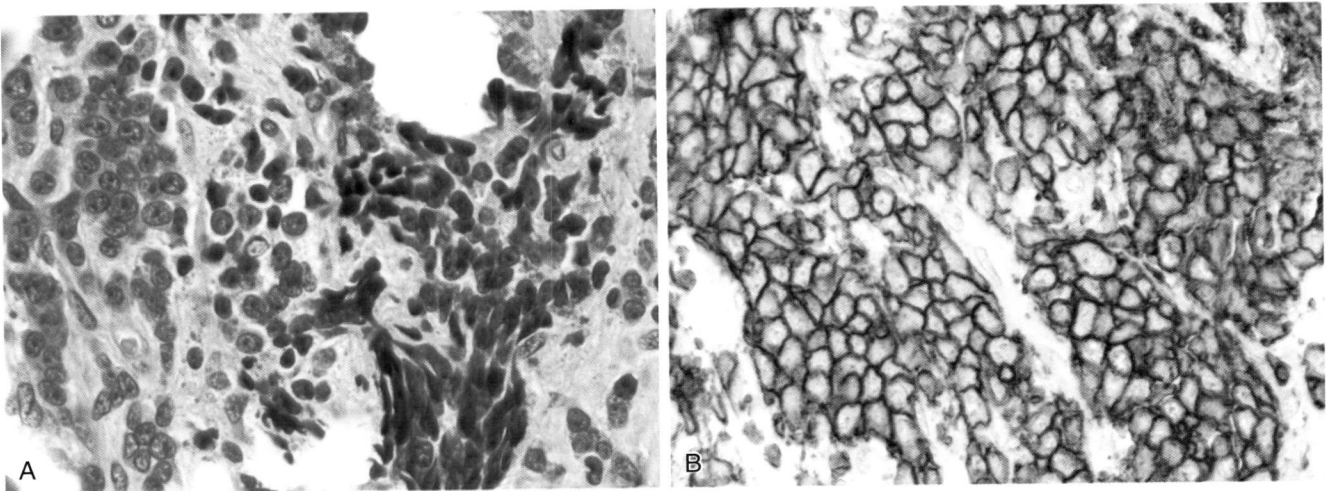

Figure 57-9. A, Appearance of Ewing's sarcoma in an H&E (hematoxylin-and-eosin)-stained bone marrow section. **B,** The same tumor expresses CD99.

primary bone tumor, usually occurring between ages 10 and 25 years or after 40 years. The incidence is increased in older patients with Paget's disease, after radiation or alkylating agent chemotherapy, and in the setting of pre-existing bone lesions, including fibrous dysplasia, osteochondromatosis, and chondromatosis. These sarcomas show a variety of histologic appearances, including fibroblastic and chondroblastic differentiation, but are diagnosed by the presence somewhere in the tumor of malignant osteoid formation.[40-42]

Cartilage-forming tumors include benign chondromas (those originating in the diaphyses are termed *enchondromas*) composed of mature lobules of hyaline cartilage, often with myxoid degeneration, calcification, and ossification. Osteochondromas are the most common benign bone tumor and have a characteristic radiologic appearance. Chondroblastomas are cellular and may contain giant cells; chondromyxoid fibromas are also cellular benign cartilaginous tumors. Chondrosarcomas, similar to osteosarcomas, show a wide variation in differentiation and may contain bone, but they lack malignant osteoid. Giant-cell tumors (osteoclastomas) are usually low-grade malignancies occurring in the long bones or skull.

VASCULAR TUMORS INVOLVING BONE

Hemangiomas

Hemangiomas of bone occur principally in flat bones of the skull and jaw and in vertebrae. They are benign vascular malformations consisting of lattice-like formations of endothelial-lined cavernous spaces containing blood. Lymphangiomas occur less commonly. Massive osteolysis (Gorham's disease) appears similar to hemangioma but is destructive, leading to resorption of bone and replacement by heavily vascularized fibrous tissue.

Epithelioid Hemangioendotheliomas

Epithelioid hemangioendotheliomas show vessels lined by plump eosinophilic epithelioid or histiocyte-like endothelial cells with large vesicular nuclei and often an inflammatory infiltrate rich in eosinophils. Tumor cells show a spectrum of cytologic atypia ranging from hemangioma to angiosarcoma. Endothelial cells express CD31, CD34, and von Willebrand factor antigen. This disorder may simulate Langerhans cell histiocytosis.

OTHER SOFT-TISSUE TUMORS INVOLVING BONE

A wide variety of additional soft-tissue tumors may present in bone and include desmoplastic fibromas, fibrosarcomas, undifferentiated pleomorphic sarcoma, leiomyomas, leiomyosarcomas, lipomas and liposarcomas, chordomas, and adamantinomas. For these and for details on primary bone tumors, refer to texts on the surgical pathology of bone tumors.[40-42]

MALIGNANT LYMPHOMAS INVOLVING BONE AND BONE MARROW

Malignant lymphomas may occur as tumors primary in the bone or bone marrow and are discussed in detail elsewhere in this volume. Most commonly, localized bone involvement by malignant lymphoma is a result of diffuse large B-cell lymphoma (Chapter 22). Those occurring in the tibia of young men may be a unique favorable variant.[43] Though uncommon, precursor B-cell lymphoblastic lymphoma (Chapter 41) may present as a localized tumor or in the bone or skin.

BENIGN LESIONS OF BONE

Benign Tumor-like Lesions

Benign tumor-like lesions of bone include solitary and aneurysmal bone cysts and ganglion cysts.[44] Radiographic changes are often characteristic. Solitary bone cysts occur most often in the proximal metaphysis of the humerus or femur of males younger than 20 years of age and consist of a membrane of well-vascularized fibrous tissue around a fluid-filled cyst. Aneurysmal bone cysts occur mostly in adolescents in vertebrae and flat bones. An eccentrically expanded, eroding hemorrhagic mass consists of blood-filled spaces separated by fibroblasts, myofibroblasts, and histiocytes. Septa also contain blood vessels, osteoid, bone, calcifying fibromyxoid stroma, and rows of osteoclasts. Ganglion cysts occur near a joint space and contain gelatinous material lined by a thin fibrous membrane and surrounded by condensed bone.

Metaphyseal Fibrous Defect (Nonossifying Fibroma) and Fibrous Dysplasia

Metaphyseal fibrous defect, also known as nonossifying fibroma, is a storiform fibrous lesion with scattered osteoclasts and hemosiderin-laden macrophages near the epiphyses of long bones in adolescents. Fibrous dysplasia is a benign lesion that consists of fusiform expansion of the medullary space with thinning of the cortex of long or flat bones. It consists of highly cellular fibrous tissue with irregular bone formations lined by abnormal fibroblast-like osteoblasts.

Paget's Disease

Paget's disease of the bone is a relatively common disorder in older adults usually involving multiple sites (polyostotic), most often the lumbosacral spine, pelvis, and skull. Pelvic involvement makes it likely to be seen in an iliac crest bone marrow biopsy. It is initially an osteoclastic lytic lesion in which there is irregular repair leading to thickened bony trabeculae with irregular cement lines demarcating successive layers of resorption and repair. More orderly cement lines are seen in reactive situations.

Chronic Osteomyelitis

Chronic osteomyelitis is characterized by increased inflammatory neutrophils, lymphocytes, and plasma cells, often in a fibrotic background with the presence of *sequestrum* (infected dead bone) and *involucrum* (a surrounding formation of new bone). In acute osteomyelitis, pus often perforates the periosteum and forms a sinus tract to the skin. With healing, the epithelium of the sinus tract may become entrapped within the bone and form inclusion cysts or even, over time, squamous cell carcinoma.

Epithelial inclusions may also be seen as artifacts in bone marrow biopsy specimens. If the central trocar of a biopsy needle is not firmly in place when the needle is pushed through skin overlying the biopsy site, fragments of skin or other dermal or subcutaneous structures may be sampled, appearing to be entrapped within the bone marrow space in histologic sections. Contaminants from other biopsies processed concurrently may be suspected when there is space between the unexpected tissue and the marrow space. Molecular characterization of suspected "floaters" may not be possible in bone marrow specimens as a result of prior decalcification, requiring repeat sampling.

Metabolic Bone Diseases

Patients with a history of normal skeletal development but with skeletal pain or fracture and radiologic evidence of osteopenia may have metabolic bone disease. Active osteoporosis (with accelerated bone turnover) shows increased osteoid formation with increased proportion (>20%) of trabeculae showing osteoid seams of normal width. Greater than four collagen layers of lamellae are present, and trabeculae are lined by plump osteoblasts. Increased osteoclasts (>1–2 per section and/or clustered) are also present. Peritrabecular fibrous tissue (osteitis fibrosa) similar to that of hyperparathyroidism may be seen. Inactive osteoporosis (with reduced turnover) shows thin osteoid seams, flattened osteoblasts, and reduced osteoclasts. There is both formation and resorption of bone; however, overall, there is loss of bone.

Osteomalacia and rickets (vitamin D deficiency) are abnormalities of calcification. Osteomalacia is histologically difficult to identify and may require fluorescence examination after tetracycline administration; positive results show decreased fluorescence. Rickets results in uncalcified masses of cartilage in the growth plate of a child. Hyperparathyroidism, either primary (from parathyroid adenoma) or secondary (from renal failure), results in increased osteoclastic and osteoblastic activity with peritrabecular fibrosis, known as osteitis fibrosa (Fig. 57-10). Scurvy (vitamin C deficiency) results in the inability to form osteoid because of abnormal collagen transformation. Calcified cartilage is seen with radiologic evidence of increased density at the growth plate.

METASTATIC TUMORS TO LYMPH NODES

The identification of metastatic solid tumors in lymph nodes is one of the most important tasks in diagnostic surgical pathology. Up to 5% of patients with cancer present with lymph node metastasis from an occult primary tumor. Most of these neoplasms are carcinomas; however, 2% of patients with melanoma and a smaller percentage of patients with germ cell tumors and sarcomas may initially present with lymph node metastasis. This section reviews the histologic features and ancillary tests that can be performed on a metastatic tumor to identify its site of origin.

Histologic Features of Metastatic Tumors

Most solid tumors metastasize to regional lymph nodes after invasion of peritumoral lymphatics, with sequential progression down the lymphatic chain. As a result, metastatic deposits in lymph nodes are initially located preferentially in the extranodal vessels and subcapsular sinuses. This localization pattern is diagnostically useful because it is uncommon in lymphoma, with the exception of anaplastic large-cell lymphoma. More extensive metastatic involvement is usually multifocal or geographic, but there is often a discrete boundary separating the tumor from uninvolved areas of the lymph node. Often, tumor nests or extranodal large vessel invasion in fat may be associated with a lymphoid response and mimic a lymph node, so attention to the presence of a capsule or subcapsular sinus and a circumscribed versus stellate appearance can be useful. Metastatic solid tumors usually have a cohesive appearance, forming sheets, nests, or islands, but undifferentiated carcinoma and melanoma often have a discohesive appearance, mimicking lymphoma.

Histologic clues to the site of origin of a metastatic tumor include keratinization or mucin production in carcinomas, rosette formation in neuroendocrine tumors, melanin pigment in melanomas, and abundant extracellular matrix or

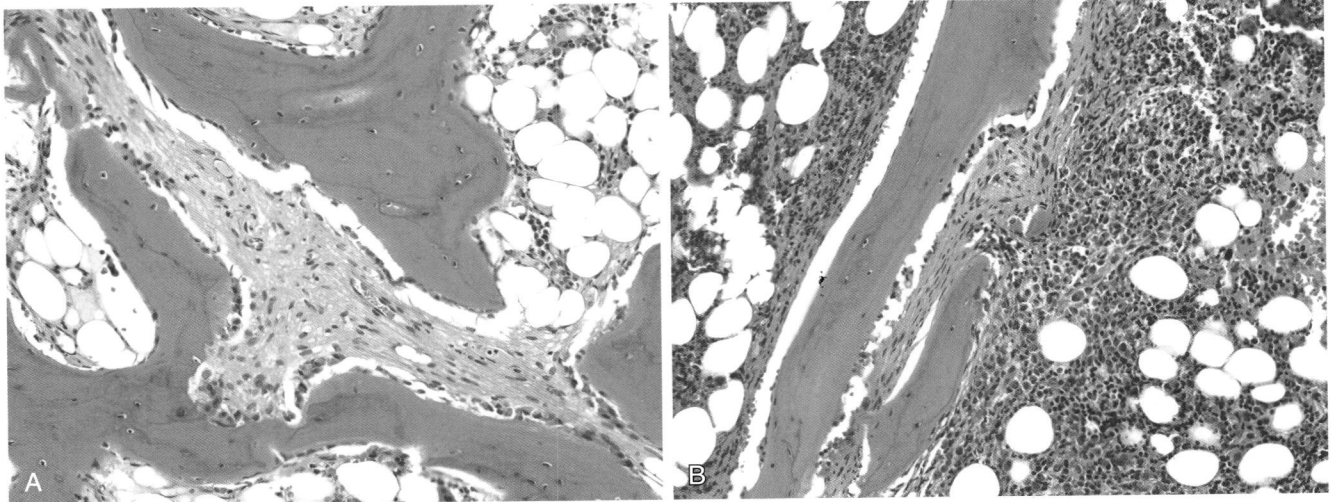

Figure 57-10. A–B, Osteitis fibrosa caused by secondary hyperparathyroidism in a patient with chronic renal insufficiency.

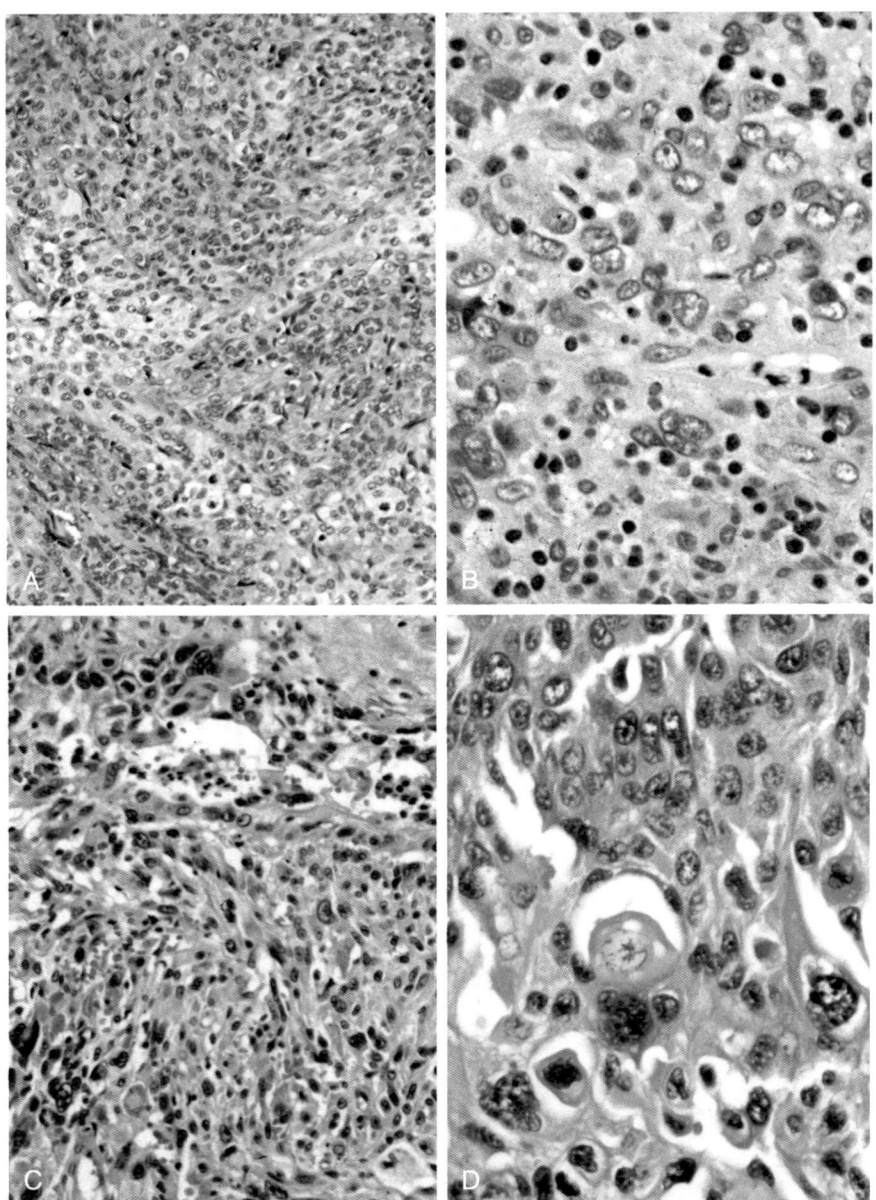

Figure 57-11. Histologic categories of metastatic tumor in lymph node. For the differential diagnosis to be simplified, metastatic tumors can be divided into those that have an epithelioid **(A)**, anaplastic **(B)**, or spindled **(C)** appearance. Areas of keratinization **(D)** can be useful in identifying carcinoma. All four cases shown are metastatic carcinoma.

a fibrillary-filamentous cytoplasmic appearance in sarcomas. Metastatic papillary tumors of the thyroid gland, kidney, ovary, or lung can show nuclear pseudoinclusions and psammoma bodies; carcinomas of lung and prostate origin often show evidence of partial neuroendocrine differentiation; and foci of necrosis (often with admixed neutrophils and debris) are common in colon adenocarcinoma. Cytochemical stains for mucin, neurosecretory granules (e.g., Grimelius and Fontana), or extracellular matrix proteins (e.g., reticulin and Masson trichrome) have largely been replaced by IHC in routine diagnosis.

Poorly differentiated metastatic tumors are common and can be classified preliminarily as epithelioid, anaplastic, spindled, or small cell (Fig. 57-11). Table 57-1 outlines the differential diagnosis of metastatic tumors in each of these morphologic categories. Because of their relatively small cell size and discohesive growth, small-cell tumors are among the most difficult to detect and distinguish from lymphoma;

in some instances, IHC is required for diagnosis. Lobular carcinoma of the breast (Fig. 57-12), carcinoid tumor, small-cell carcinoma, Merkel cell carcinoma, and neuroblastoma can all show subtle infiltration of the interfollicular nodal areas. Colonization of lymphoid follicles is also occasionally observed. In the mediastinum, occult lung metastasis of small-cell carcinoma can mimic lymphoblastic lymphoma but typically shows more prominent nuclear molding. Small-cell carcinomas of the lung also commonly have abundant coagulative necrosis and basophilic deposition of DNA within blood vessels (known as nuclear encrustation or the Azzopardi phenomenon). Zonal areas of necrosis may also be seen in neuroblastoma. Although rare, rhabdomyosarcoma (Fig. 57-13) and Ewing's sarcoma (Fig. 57-14) can both show subtle interfollicular infiltration of the lymph node and should be considered in younger patients.

Among epithelioid tumors, metastatic carcinoma and melanoma are the most common non-hematopoietic tumors

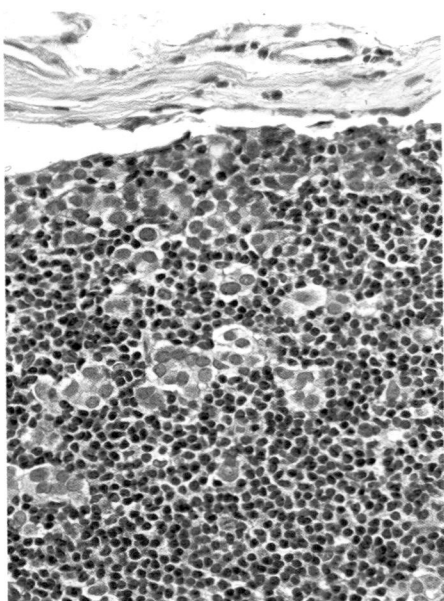

Figure 57-12. Metastatic lobular carcinoma of the breast. Subtle infiltration of the lymph node subcapsular sinus and paracortex by tumor cells in small nests is often observed.

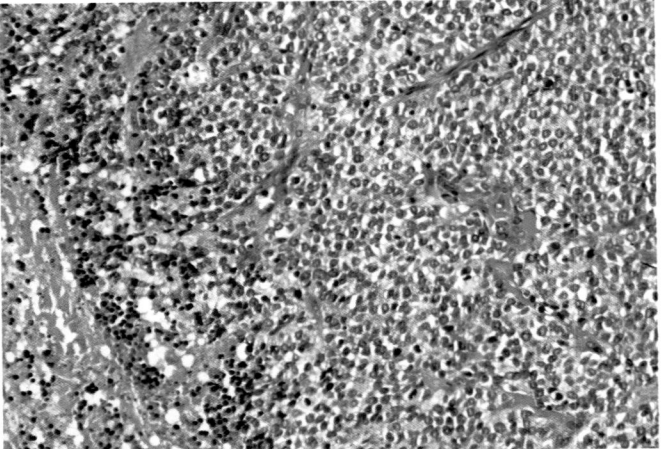

Figure 57-13. Metastatic rhabdomyosarcoma. Diffuse replacement of the lymph node by this small-cell neoplasm may be difficult to distinguish histologically from lymphoblastic lymphoma because diagnostic rhabdomyoblasts may be rare. A predominantly nested growth pattern can be a clue to the diagnosis.

encountered. Metastatic melanoma, in particular, may resemble a hematolymphoid neoplasm with immunoblastic, plasmablastic, or anaplastic morphology, including large-cell lymphoma or plasma cell myeloma (Fig. 57-15A). Other tumors with epithelioid morphology include metastatic seminoma (Fig. 57-16), especially in retroperitoneal lymph nodes, and large-cell lymphoma, cases of which may appear cohesive, particularly those with anaplastic morphology.

In general, anaplastic tumors presenting in a lymph node have a broad differential diagnosis and can show abnormal antigen-expression patterns (Fig. 57-15B–C). Moreover, antigen shedding from infiltrating lymphoid cells or histiocytes can mistakenly make the undifferentiated tumor appear positive for hematopoietic markers. While the presence of

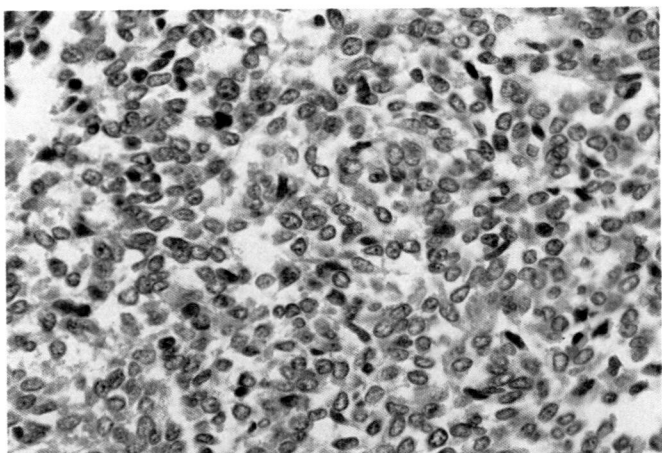

Figure 57-14. Metastatic Ewing's sarcoma. The fine nuclear chromatin (described as "smoky" or "dusty") of these small-cell tumors may mimic blastic hematopoietic malignancies, but they usually have more abundant cytoplasm with indistinct borders and large areas of necrosis *(not shown).* Pseudorosette formation is usually focal or absent in lymph node metastases.

so-called hallmark cells may suggest anaplastic large-cell lymphoma, similar cells can be seen in other anaplastic tumors, such as anaplastic thyroid carcinoma. Careful attention to cytoplasmic features is helpful: for example, focal mucin droplets may be present in poorly differentiated adenocarcinoma and intracellular lumens may be seen in vascular tumors.

Characteristic Biological Patterns of Metastasis

In addition to histologic features and patient demographic data, the location of an involved lymph node can narrow the possible sources of a metastatic tumor. In cervical lymph nodes, the most commonly encountered occult tumor is squamous cell carcinoma or undifferentiated carcinoma from a head or neck primary tumor.[45] The primary site can be located in approximately 40% of these cases by subsequent clinical examination and is usually at the base of the tongue or tonsillar fossa. Survival is determined by the extent of lymph node involvement at presentation. Occult carcinomas originating in the lung and esophagus are the next most commonly encountered metastatic tumors in cervical lymph nodes.[46]

In patients with supraclavicular lymphadenopathy as a result of metastasis, carcinoma is the most common pathologic finding.[47] Tumors of abdominal origin preferentially result in left supraclavicular (Virchow's) lymph node enlargement, whereas tumors of the head and neck, lung, and breast (in addition to lymphomas) can involve either side.[48] Metastatic tumors in axillary lymph nodes most often originate from the breast in women,[49,50] followed in frequency by melanoma, cutaneous squamous cell carcinoma, and lung cancers. In inguinal lymph nodes, the most common metastatic tumors are melanoma and prostate carcinoma in men and gynecologic malignancies in women.[51] Germ cell tumors, mostly seminoma, can present as metastases involving retroperitoneal lymph nodes and are frequently extensively necrotic.[52]

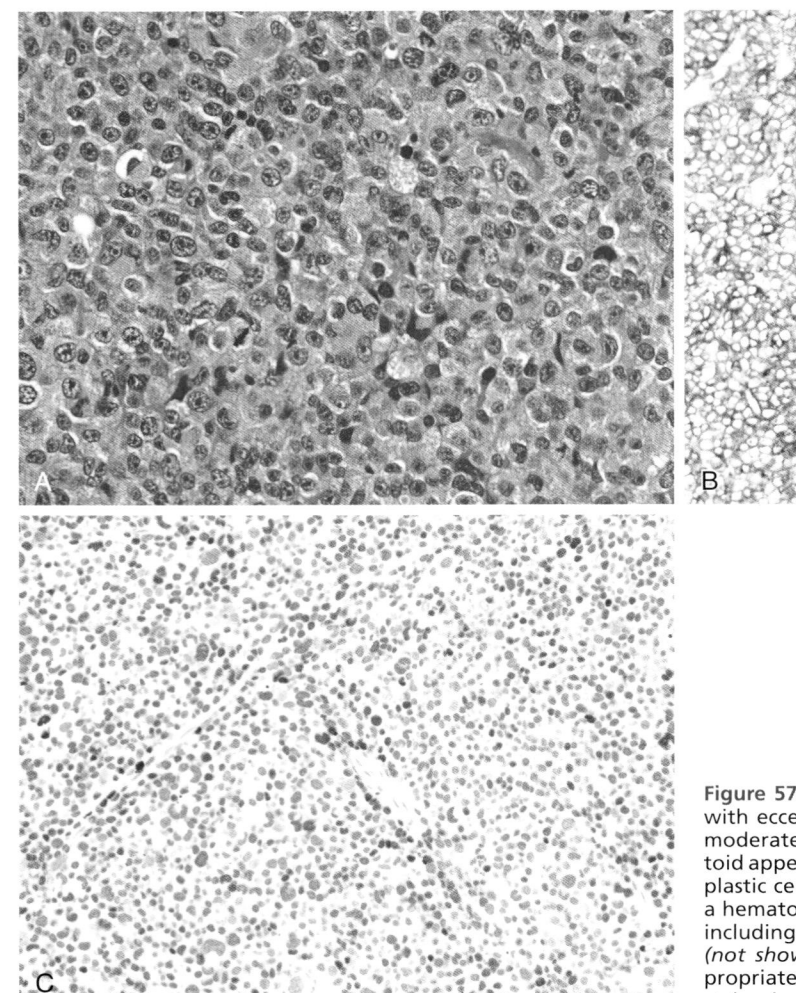

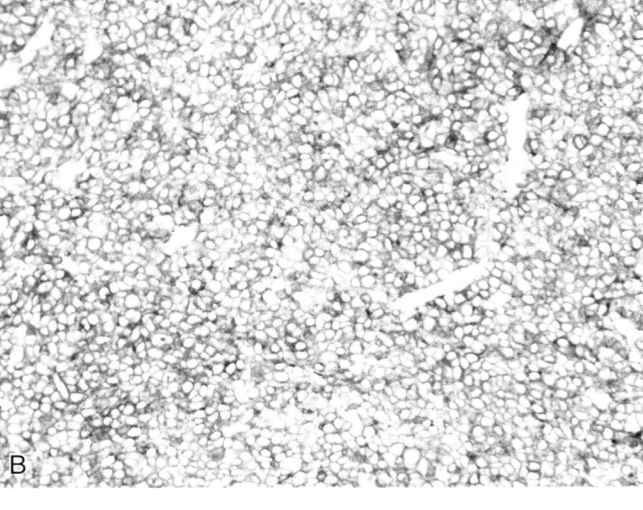

Figure 57-15. Metastatic melanoma. A, Discohesive tumor cells with eccentric nuclei, prominent nucleoli, open chromatin, and moderately abundant eosinophilic cytoplasm impart a plasmacy-toid appearance, mimicking plasmablastic lymphoma. **B,** The neo-plastic cells aberrantly express CD10, further raising concern for a hematopoietic neoplasm; however, B-lineage specific markers, including immunoglobin light chains, are not clearly expressed *(not shown).* Awareness of this diagnostic pitfall prompts ap-propriate immunohistochemical workup with melanoma-related stains, including SOX10 **(C)**, leading to the correct diagnosis.

Role of Immunohistochemistry in the Diagnosis of Metastatic Tumors

IHC stains for metastatic tumors are divided into those used for diagnosis and those used for prognostic or treatment purposes. A review of the prognostic markers is beyond the scope of this chapter, and they are constantly evolving. Suggested diagnostic IHC panels for different tumor categories are shown in Table 57-2.

In general, the commonly used first-tier diagnostic antibodies are highly specific but variably sensitive for the detection of particular tumor types.[53] However, aberrant or unrecognized patterns of staining with routine antibodies must always be considered. Most hematopoietic markers in common use are specific for hematopoietic cells, but some hematopoietic markers, such as CD5, CD7, CD10, CD43, CD56, and CD138/syndecan-1, are commonly expressed in neuroendocrine tumors or carcinomas from certain sites.[54-56] Also, CD30 is strongly expressed by embryonal germ cell tumors and sometimes by mesotheliomas,[57] and CD45 (leukocyte common antigen [LCA]) may be positive in the cytoplasm of breast carcinoma with rare membranous positivity in poorly differentiated carcinomas.[58] Conversely, S-100 protein and the vascular marker CD31 are variably expressed by monocytes and macrophages. VS38, CD138/

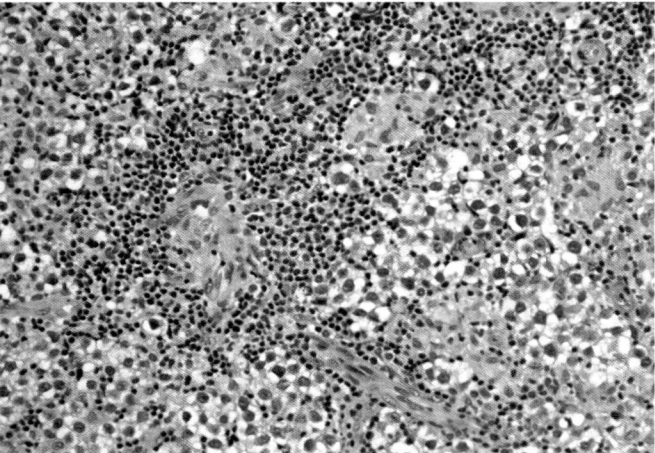

Figure 57-16. Seminoma metastatic to lymph node. The lymph node is infiltrated by large germ cells with abundant clear cyto-plasm and distinct cell borders. A helpful feature in distinguish-ing metastatic seminoma from large-cell lymphoma is the admixed granulomatous reaction and small lymphocytes.

syndecan-1, and CD38 are plasma cell markers. However, VS38 and CD138/syndecan-1 are expressed by many solid tumors,[59] whereas CD38 is more restricted to plasma cells and some lymphocytes and histiocytes. Finally, plasmacytomas are notorious for aberrant and false-positive immunoreactivity and can stain for cytokeratin, myeloperoxidase, and T-cell markers, among others.[60]

In metastatic carcinoma of unknown origin, a second group of immunohistochemical stains can complement the histologic appearance and clinical data, suggesting a possible primary site.[61] Currently, the most broadly useful antibodies are those that detect the cytokeratin expression pattern, particularly keratin 7 and keratin 20 (Fig. 57-17).[62,63] The overall patterns of these markers are summarized in Table 57-3, but it is important to note that variations may be seen among the more poorly differentiated tumors. Other markers can be helpful in identifying metastasis from less common primary sites. For example, hepatocellular carcinoma is typically negative for keratin 19 (in contrast to cholangiocarcinoma) but positive for low–molecular-weight keratin, as detected by CAM5.2.[64] The pattern of keratin positivity can also be helpful. A punctate or dotlike paranuclear cytoplasmic staining pattern is characteristically observed in Merkel cell carcinoma

and small-cell carcinoma but not completely specific for these tumor types. It should be noted that some lymphomas (approximately 2%) of both mature and lymphoblastic types can show some keratin positivity, most commonly keratin 8.[65,66]

The complex pattern of IHC expression of the classic serum tumor markers, including CEA, CA19-9, CA15-3, CA125, EMA/MUC1, β-human chorionic gonadotropin, and α fetoprotein, limits their role as diagnostic markers except in particular cases (e.g., canalicular CEA staining detected by polyclonal antiserum in hepatocellular carcinoma).[54,67] Similarly, polypeptide hormones and their receptors, such as testosterone, estrogen, and progesterone receptors, can be expressed by a wide variety of carcinomas and should be used cautiously as evidence of a particular cell lineage.

Molecular profiling with a limited array of transcripts of lineage-associated genes has shown great promise in accurate classification[68-70] and the selection of appropriate therapies.[71] Cytogenetic analysis, although technically demanding, can be highly useful in evaluating the poorly differentiated blastoid tumors; there are characteristic translocations that support the diagnosis of lymphoblastic lymphoma, neuroblastoma, rhabdomyosarcoma, Ewing's sarcoma, and other sarcoma types. Targeted FISH analysis for specific chromosomal translocations can routinely be performed on cytologic smears and touch imprints with high sensitivity. Although less sensitive, FISH is also frequently done on fixed, paraffin-embedded tissue sections. Next-generation sequencing (NGS)-based approaches on DNA extracted from paraffin-embedded tissue are increasingly being used to identify fusion proteins characteristic of certain tumors, even when only one gene partner is known.[72] Electron microscopy has a limited role in the differential diagnosis but can be helpful in the definitive diagnosis of poorly differentiated tumors, for example, by detecting melanosomes in poorly differentiated melanoma or cell junctions that would suggest a carcinoma or dendritic cell neoplasm. In small-cell tumors, electron microscopy is especially useful in detecting muscle filaments in rhabdomyosarcoma. Multigene expression profiling assays

Table 57-2 Routine Immunohistochemistry Panels for Diagnosis

Histologic Group	First Round of Staining	Second and Third Rounds of Staining
Small-cell tumors	Pan-keratin, TdT, LCA, desmin	Chromogranin, synaptophysin, CD56, CD34, CD99, NKX2.2, lymphoid markers, myogenin, myo-D1, calcitonin
Anaplastic and epithelioid tumors	Pan-keratin, S-100, CD30, LCA	EMA, PLAP, immunoglobulins, SOX10, HMB45, melan A, CD68, myeloperoxidase
Spindle cell tumors	Smooth muscle actin, desmin, S-100, pan-keratin	HHF35 actin, CD117/KIT, LCA, caldesmon, CD21, CD23, or CD35 (follicular dendritic cell sarcoma)

EMA, Epithelial membrane antigen; *FDC,* follicular dendritic cell; *LCA,* leukocyte common antigen; *PLAP,* placental alkaline phosphatase; *TdT,* terminal deoxynucleotidyl transferase.

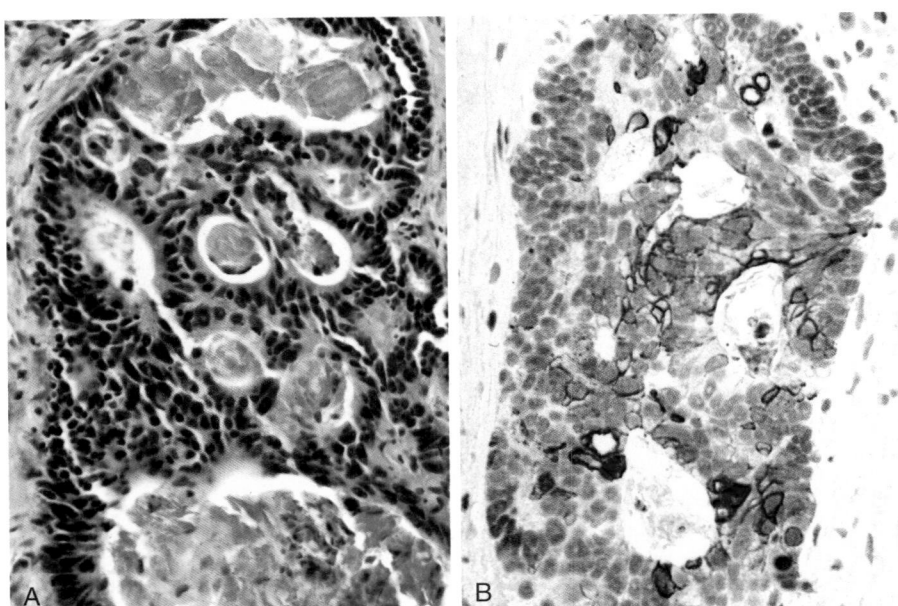

Figure 57-17. Keratin immunostaining of colon adenocarcinoma metastatic to lymph node. A, Columnar tumor cells that replace the nodal parenchyma exhibit gland formation with central necrosis, typical of colon adenocarcinoma. B, Tumor cells are positive for cytokeratin 20 but negative for cytokeratin 7 (not shown).

Table 57-3 Immunohistochemical Stains Used to Identify the Site of Origin of Metastatic Carcinoma

Marker	Specificity
Arginase	Liver
β-catenin	GI tract, ovarian
CDX2	GI tract
Calcitonin	Medullary thyroid carcinoma; rarely, other neuroendocrine tumors
Chromogranin	Neuroendocrine differentiation, including small-cell and Merkel cell carcinomas
Cytokeratin 7+, 20−	Lung, breast, transitional cell, endometrioid ovarian, some neuroendocrine and squamous cell carcinomas
Cytokeratin 7−, 20+	GI tract, mucinous ovarian, Merkel cell
Cytokeratin 7+, 20+	Transitional cell (bladder), cholangiocarcinoma
Cytokeratin 7−, 20−	Adrenocortical, hepatocellular, prostate, renal cell, small-cell carcinoma, squamous cell (esophageal), carcinoid, germ cell tumor
Fli-1	Ewing's sarcoma, vascular tumors
GATA3	Breast, salivary gland, urothelial tumors
GCDFP-15	Breast, salivary gland, some prostate tumors
HepPar1	Hepatocellular carcinoma, small subset (~5%) of other adenocarcinomas and neuroendocrine tumors
HMB45	Melanoma, lymphangioleiomyomatosis
Mammaglobin	Breast carcinoma, endometrial adenocarcinoma
MART-1/melan A	Melanoma, adrenocortical carcinoma, other steroid-producing tumors
Myogenin, MyoD1	Rhabdomyosarcoma
Napsin A	Lung adenocarcinoma, papillary renal cell carcinoma
Oct-4	Seminoma and embryonal carcinomas of testis
P63 and/or p40	Squamous cell carcinoma, urothelial carcinoma
PAP	Prostate, some carcinoids, apocrine breast and salivary tumors
PAX8	Endometrial adenocarcinoma, ovarian serous, renal cell carcinoma, thyroid carcinomas
PLAP	Germ cell tumors; occasional carcinomas of lung, GI, and Müllerian origin; some histiocytes
Podoplanin/D2-40	Kaposi sarcoma, some angiosarcomas, lymphangioma
PSA	Prostate carcinoma (decreased in poorly differentiated tumors), some breast carcinomas
pVHL	Renal clear cells in addition to clear cells of ovary and uterus
RCC	Renal cell carcinomas
Surfactant A	Lung adenocarcinomas
Synaptophysin	Neuroendocrine differentiation, including neuroblastoma, medulloblastoma, small-cell and Merkel cell carcinomas
Thyroglobulin	Thyroid tumors (not anaplastic or mucoepidermoid)
TTF-1	Lung and thyroid carcinomas and neuroendocrine tumors at these sites
Villin	GI tumors (brush border–type staining)
Vimentin	Negative in endometrial and low-grade renal carcinomas, positive in most other carcinomas

GCDFP, Gross cystic disease fluid protein; *GI,* gastrointestinal; *PAP,* prostatic acid phosphatase; *PLAP,* placental alkaline phosphatase; *PSA,* prostate-specific antigen; *TTF-1,* thyroid transcription factor-1.

can be used to identify tumors of uncertain origin using reverse transcription polymerase chain reaction (RT-PCR) for detecting mRNA or microRNA from frozen or paraffin tissue samples and are reported to have high diagnostic accuracy.[73-76]

Nonlymphoid Tumors With Prominent Reactive Lymphoid Components

In several neoplasms, the density of tumor-associated reactive lymphocytes can obscure the tumor cells. This is particularly common in seminoma, melanoma, and medullary carcinoma of the breast. In mediastinal biopsy specimens, thymoma should always be a diagnostic consideration when numerous small lymphocytes are associated with an epithelioid or spindle cell proliferation. The diagnosis of thymoma can be further complicated by the immature thymic immunophenotype of the reactive T-cell component, which can be indistinguishable from T-lymphoblastic lymphoma by flow-cytometric analysis. In such cases, IHC can easily detect the extensive cytokeratin-positive tumor meshwork.

Undifferentiated nasopharyngeal carcinoma (or undifferentiated carcinoma arising from other sites, such as urothelial tumors) is probably the solid tumor most frequently misdiagnosed as lymphoma.[77] This is because of its occasionally prominent inflammatory component and the fact that occult nodal presentations of nasopharyngeal carcinoma are common, occurring in up to 50% of cases. The keratinizing and nonkeratinizing squamous cell variants of nasopharyngeal carcinoma usually present few diagnostic difficulties (Fig. 57-18). However, in the lymphoepithelioma variant of undifferentiated nasopharyngeal carcinoma (also known as the Schmincke type), the neoplastic cells are often obscured by a dense lymphocyte infiltrate (Fig. 57-19). Other cases can be associated with numerous neutrophils and eosinophils and may mimic Hodgkin lymphoma (Fig. 57-20). Tumor cell cohesiveness and central necrosis within tumor cell aggregates are helpful clues. The most useful ancillary tests for the diagnosis of nasopharyngeal and undifferentiated

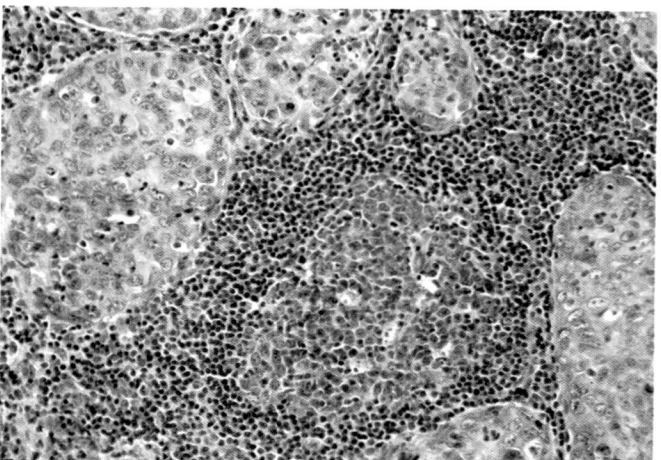

Figure 57-18. Metastatic nonkeratinizing squamous cell carcinoma of nasopharyngeal origin. Large nests of cohesive tumor cells are outlined by collagen bands and show multifocal nodal infiltration. In this field, a central reactive lymphoid follicle is surrounded by tumor.

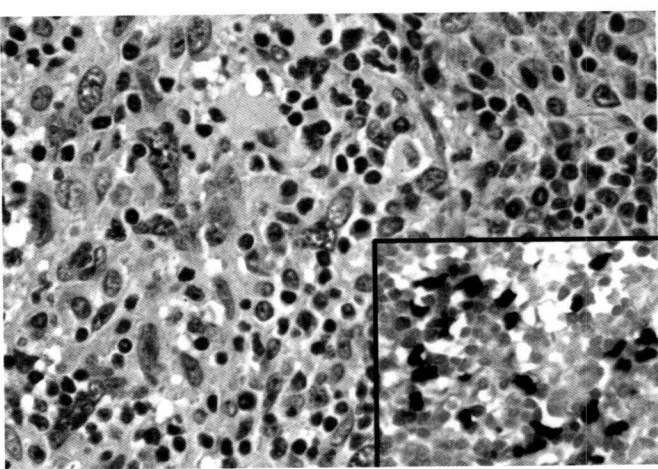

Figure 57-19. Metastatic undifferentiated nasopharyngeal carcinoma—Schmincke or lymphoepithelioma type. Anaplastic tumor cells are interspersed between numerous small lymphocytes. Keratin immunohistochemical stain and Epstein-Barr virus in situ hybridization *(inset)* were positive in tumor cells.

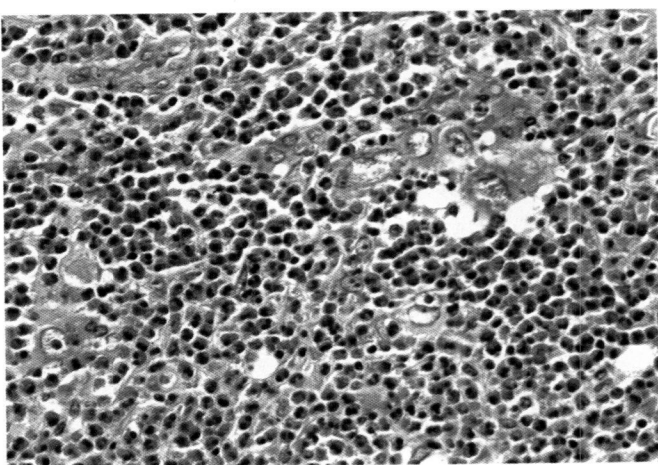

Figure 57-20. Metastatic undifferentiated nasopharyngeal carcinoma—eosinophil-rich variant. Large neoplastic tumor cells are interspersed between numerous eosinophils.

carcinomas are keratin IHC and Epstein-Barr virus–encoded small RNA (EBER) in situ hybridization.

BENIGN LYMPH NODE INCLUSIONS

Epithelial and Mesothelial Inclusions in Lymph Nodes

Müllerian inclusion cysts (MICs) are by far the most commonly encountered benign glandular inclusions, identified in up to 20% of lymph nodes excised from women. Such cysts may rarely be seen in men. Rare cases of florid MICs causing significant lymph node enlargement or ureteric obstruction have been reported.[78] MICs are most frequently located in the paraaortic lymph nodes and, less frequently, in the iliac lymph nodes. Inclusions have been reported in distant nodes such as axillary lymph nodes and can mimic breast cancer.[79,80] PAX8 IHC can be useful in the diagnosis of Müllerian epithelium but does not distinguish benign from malignant inclusions.[81]

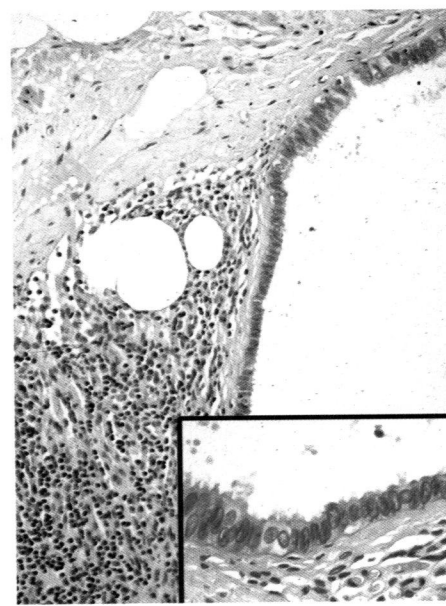

Figure 57-21. Endosalpingiosis of lymph node. A simple cyst in a subcapsular location, lined by cytologically bland cuboid and ciliated columnar epithelium *(inset)*.

MICs are usually simple cysts lined by serous-type (Müllerian) cuboidal to columnar epithelium that is cytologically bland (Fig. 57-21).[82] Histologic features distinguishing benign MICs from metastatic tumor deposits include an intertrabecular location in a lymph node, the presence of multiple types of benign lining cells, the lack of mitoses or cellular atypia, the presence of a periglandular basement membrane, and the absence of a desmoplastic stromal reaction. The increased incidence of MICs in patients with borderline ovarian tumors suggests neoplastic potential for benign-appearing MICs in rare cases.[83] IHC may be helpful in cases that architecturally resemble metastatic gynecologic cancers in that MICs are usually negative for CEA.[82]

Endometriosis in lymph nodes is usually seen only in patients with extensive peritoneal deposits; it shows benign-appearing glands with columnar epithelium, edematous endometrial-type stroma, and hemosiderin-laden macrophages (siderophages), as at other sites.[84] Estrogen and progesterone receptors and PAX8 staining can be detected by IHC.[81] Endosalpingiosis with associated psammoma bodies has been rarely reported in lymph nodes.

Benign epithelial inclusions resembling glands from nearly all solid organs have been reported in adjacent lymph nodes. Apparent neoplastic transformation of such benign inclusions has also been rarely reported.[85] Given the close proximity of many lymph nodes to the salivary glands, it is not surprising that these nodal groups often contain numerous salivary ducts and glands. In dense lymphoepithelial lesions of the salivary gland (e.g., lymphoepithelial cysts, acquired immunodeficiency syndrome [AIDS]-associated sialoadenitis, Sjögren syndrome), it may be difficult to distinguish salivary gland tissue from the adjacent lymph node. Salivary gland neoplasms, including Warthin's tumor and pleomorphic adenoma, have been reported to arise from heterotopic salivary gland ducts within lymph nodes. Similar collections of benign ducts and glands can be observed in perithyroidal, axillary, and perirenal lymph nodes. Rarely, squamous-type inclusion

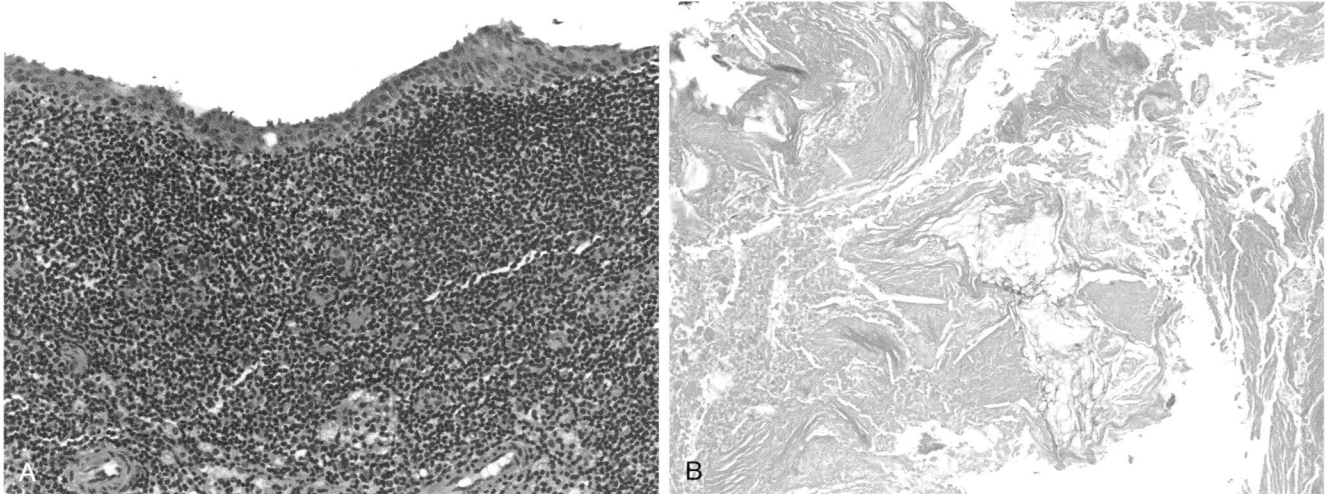

Figure 57-22. Nodal squamous-type inclusion cyst. A, An axillary lymph node core biopsy shows benign lymphoid tissue adjacent to a cyst wall composed of stratified squamous epithelium. **B,** Detached fragments of keratin debris are seen, consistent with cyst contents.

cysts may be identified in lymph nodes; clinical and radiologic correlation is necessary to exclude metastatic squamous cell carcinoma with cystic changes (Fig. 57-22).

Bland but occasionally enlarged mesothelial cells can occur as detached groups within the lymph node sinuses, usually in the mediastinum and rarely at other sites.[86] Lymph node sinus mesothelial cells are often increased and can be numerous after chest compression. These keratin-positive mesothelial inclusions are most problematic in crushed and fragmented mediastinal lymph node biopsy specimens obtained for the diagnosis of suspected malignancy. IHC positivity for mesothelial cell markers (e.g., calretinin, HMBE-1) and the absence of staining for pan-epithelial markers (e.g., Ber-EP4) can be helpful in problematic cases.

Keratin-Positive Fibroblastic Reticular Cells

In interpreting lymph node IHC, it is important to recognize that the fibroblastic reticular cell network can be variably positive for keratin. Fibroblastic reticular cells, usually identified by antibodies that detect keratins 8 and 18 (e.g., CAM5.2), have a spindled or dendritic morphology and usually present few diagnostic difficulties in tissue sections. However, their presence in cytologic preparations may be more confusing. In some reactive lymph node expansions, keratin-positive fibroblastic reticular cells may be quite numerous but still maintain their dispersed pattern of infiltration (Fig. 57-23). A rare sarcoma derived from these cells, termed *cytokeratin-positive interstitial reticulin cell (CIRC) sarcoma,* can easily be confused for metastatic carcinoma; these tumors stain for keratins 8 and 18, vimentin, and smooth muscle actin.

Nevus Cell Aggregates

Nevus cell aggregates are most commonly seen in axillary lymph node dissection specimens, where they may be mistaken for carcinoma, melanoma, and cervical and inguinal lymph nodes; nevus cell aggregates are rare in deep lymph nodes.[87] Nevus cells are present much more frequently in staging lymph nodes from patients with

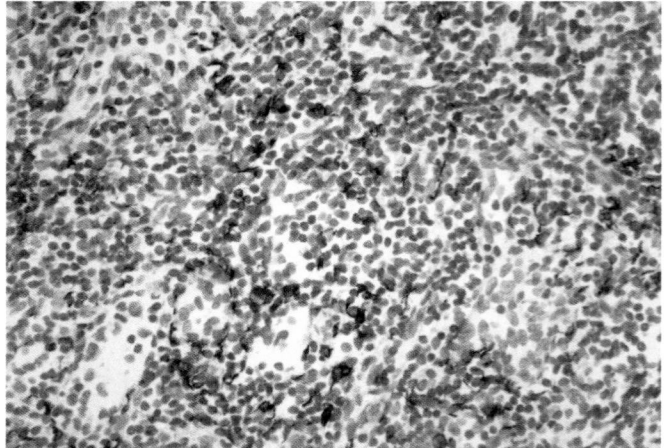

Figure 57-23. Keratin-positive fibroblastic reticular cells in lymph node. Cytologically benign nodal reticular cells with fine cytoplasmic cell processes are interspersed between lymphocytes (pan-keratin immunostain). Keratin-positive stromal cells are more commonly detected with low–molecular-weight keratin immunostains (e.g., CAM5.2) but may be seen with any cytokeratin antibody.

melanoma (up to 25%) than in lymph nodes excised for other reasons.[88] This finding, in addition to the increased frequency of nodal nevus aggregates in patients with congenital nevi, suggests aberrant developmental migration patterns of melanocytes in patients who subsequently develop melanocytic neoplasms.[89]

Nevus cell aggregates are most commonly embedded in the collagen of the lymph node capsule or trabeculae but can also be found within the subcapsular sinus or rarely in the lymphatics or surrounding small intranodal vessels.[88] These aggregates are usually composed of small, uniform melanocytes that resemble those seen in intradermal melanocytic nevi (Fig. 57-24). When melanin pigment is inconspicuous, IHC for S-100 protein or MART-1 can be used to confirm their identity; these aggregates are often negative for HMB-45, a useful marker in the differential diagnosis.[89] In addition, neural stem cell markers, Nestin and SOX2, are useful in distinguishing nodal

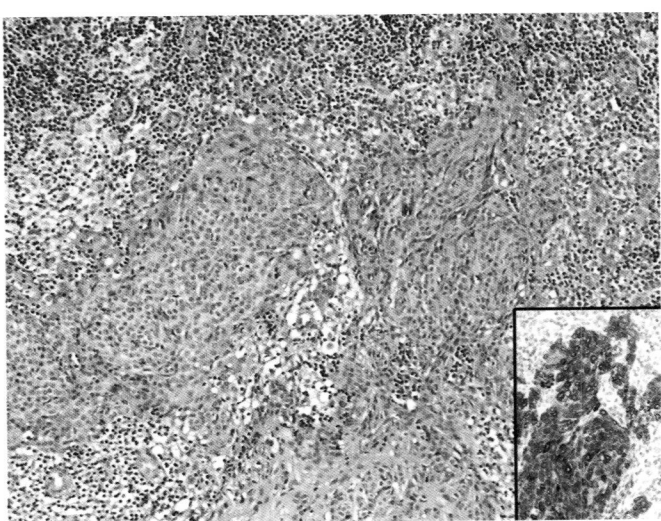

Figure 57-24. Nevus aggregates in lymph node. Variably pigmented nevus cells extend from lymph node trabeculae. MART-1 immunostain is diffusely positive *(inset). (Courtesy Dr. Victor Prieto.)*

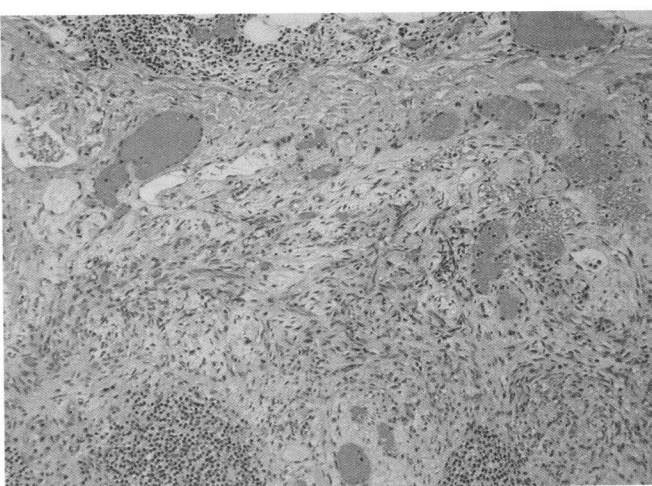

Figure 57-25. Vascular transformation of lymph node sinuses. Dilated sinuses show a proliferation of medium-sized and small-sized vascular spaces with red blood cells.

melanocytic nevi from metastatic melanoma, which expresses one or both markers, in contrast to nodal nevi.[90]

Lymph node metastasis from blue nevi and other cytologically bland melanocytic proliferations has been reported.[91] Clues to this occurrence would be more widespread intranodal distribution of nevus cells than commonly seen in benign nevus cell aggregates. Correlation with the presence of a large nevus in the area of the draining lymph node can help support a definitive diagnosis. The rarely reported primary nodal blue nevus usually represents similar capsular collections of spindle cells with abundant melanin pigment.[92]

MESENCHYMAL PROLIFERATIONS IN LYMPH NODES

A helpful and sensible approach to diagnosing stromal proliferations in lymph nodes is to identify the primary proliferating cell types. Benign proliferations of stroma intrinsic to the lymph node can arise from lymphatic vessels, blood vessels, fibroblastic stroma, dendritic cell types (covered in Chapter 52), or a combination of these types. In addition, the lymph node proliferation can be part of a (syndromic or sporadic) systemic mesenchymal disorder such as lymphangioleiomyomatosis or angiomatosis. Finally, both primary nodal sarcomas and metastatic sarcomas of all types must be considered.

Vascular Transformation of Lymph Node Sinuses and Lymphatic Proliferations

Vascular transformation of lymph node sinuses is probably the most commonly encountered reactive stromal lesion of lymph nodes. The overall architecture is preserved, but the lymph node sinuses are prominent and show complex anastomosing channels that may contain blood cells or fibrin or have a fibrotic appearance (Fig. 57-25). Some cases also show solid areas that resemble hemangiomas; others show mixed solid and sinusoidal, multinodular, and even plexiform patterns. Rare cases may involve the obliteration of sinuses by a proliferation of cytologically bland, plump fibroblasts and histiocytoid

cells.[93] In some cases, the proliferation raises the possibility of Kaposi sarcoma, which can be distinguished by IHC for human herpesvirus-8/Kaposi sarcoma herpesvirus (HHV-8/KSHV) latency-associated nuclear antigen-1 (LANA-1).

Vascular transformation of lymph node sinuses likely results from the effects of altered lymph flow caused by pressure changes or stasis secondary to venous or sinus obstruction.[94] Thus, it is common in lymph nodes compressed by adjacent solid tumors or in damaged lymphatic beds after surgery. The association of vascular transformation of lymph node sinuses and concurrent hemangiomas also suggests a role for angiogenic factors in inducing lymphatic proliferation or expansion. Similarly, vascular transformation–like changes can be seen in lymph node–draining lymphomas or inflammatory conditions that produce abundant cytokines.

In contrast, lymphangioma of lymph nodes is a proliferation of greatly distended, thin-walled lymphatic vessels with dense fibrotic stroma, resembling the cystic hygroma of infancy. In these benign proliferations, variably sized lymphatic spaces, filled with proteinaceous fluid and occasional lymphocytes, displace the normal nodal architecture and extend outside the lymph node.[95]

Mixed Smooth Muscle–Vascular Proliferations

Benign smooth muscle proliferations in lymph nodes are common and appear to be related to extrinsic effects; they occur most often in pelvic, inguinal, and abdominal sites, where gravitational effects on vascular or lymphatic drainage may contribute to their development. These cytologically bland lesions, which radiate out from the lymph node hilum, have been diagnosed as angiomyomatous hamartoma in cases with a mixed proliferation of smooth muscle and blood vessels (Fig. 57-26) in sclerotic stroma[96,97] or as leiomyomatous hamartoma when the smooth muscle component is more prominent.[97] Stromal cells in both these lesions are variably positive for smooth muscle actin, desmin, and vimentin but are negative for HMB-45. A variant of the lesion may have admixed lobules of adipose tissue and has been termed *angiomyolipomatous hamartoma of lymph node.*[98]

Palisaded myofibroblastoma (also known as hemorrhagic spindle cell tumor with amianthoid fibers) is a similar benign fibromuscular proliferation largely restricted to the pelvic lymph nodes.[99,100] These tumors are well demarcated and composed of a fascicular proliferation of spindle cells with focal nuclear palisading and acellular stellate or occasionally

calcified or ossified amianthoid collagen fibers (Fig. 57-27A–B). Thick-walled blood vessels and peripherally located hemorrhagic areas are admixed. Immunoreactivity for vimentin, α–smooth muscle actin (Fig. 57-27C), and muscle-specific actin (detected by the HHF35 antibody) and electron microscopic studies showing intracytoplasmic bundles of microfilaments support smooth muscle cell differentiation.[101] The differential diagnosis of this tumor includes schwannoma, which may contain similar amianthoid collagen but shows more prominent nuclear palisading and is positive for S-100.

Lymphangioleiomyomatosis is a systemic proliferation of abnormal smooth muscle and malformed blood vessels and lymphatics occurring in young women. This lesion, which is linked to inactivation of *TSC2*, can occur in association with tuberous sclerosis or sporadically in patients who may also have angiomyolipomas of the kidney. The primary site of disease is usually the lung, but lymph nodes are typically involved as well. Diagnosis is aided by the presence of HMB-45–positive plump smooth muscle proliferations underlying the anastomosing lymphovascular spaces.[102,103]

Inflammatory Pseudotumor of Lymph Nodes

Dense fibroblastic or myofibroblastic proliferations in lymph nodes have been variably diagnosed as inflammatory

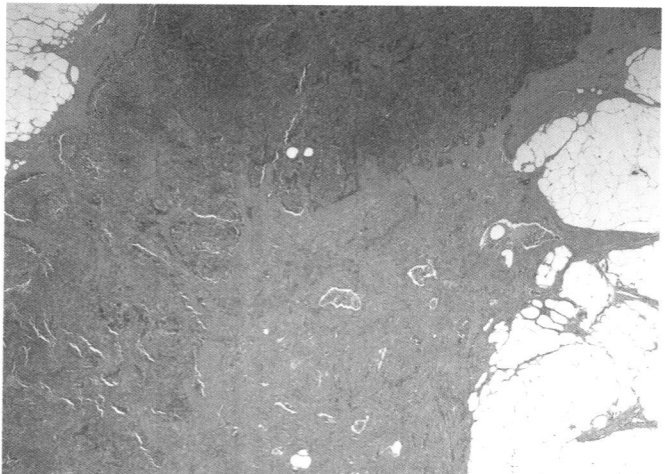

Figure 57-26. Angiomyomatous hamartoma of lymph node. A proliferation of smooth muscle with some large vessels fills the hilum and radiates into the lymph node cortex.

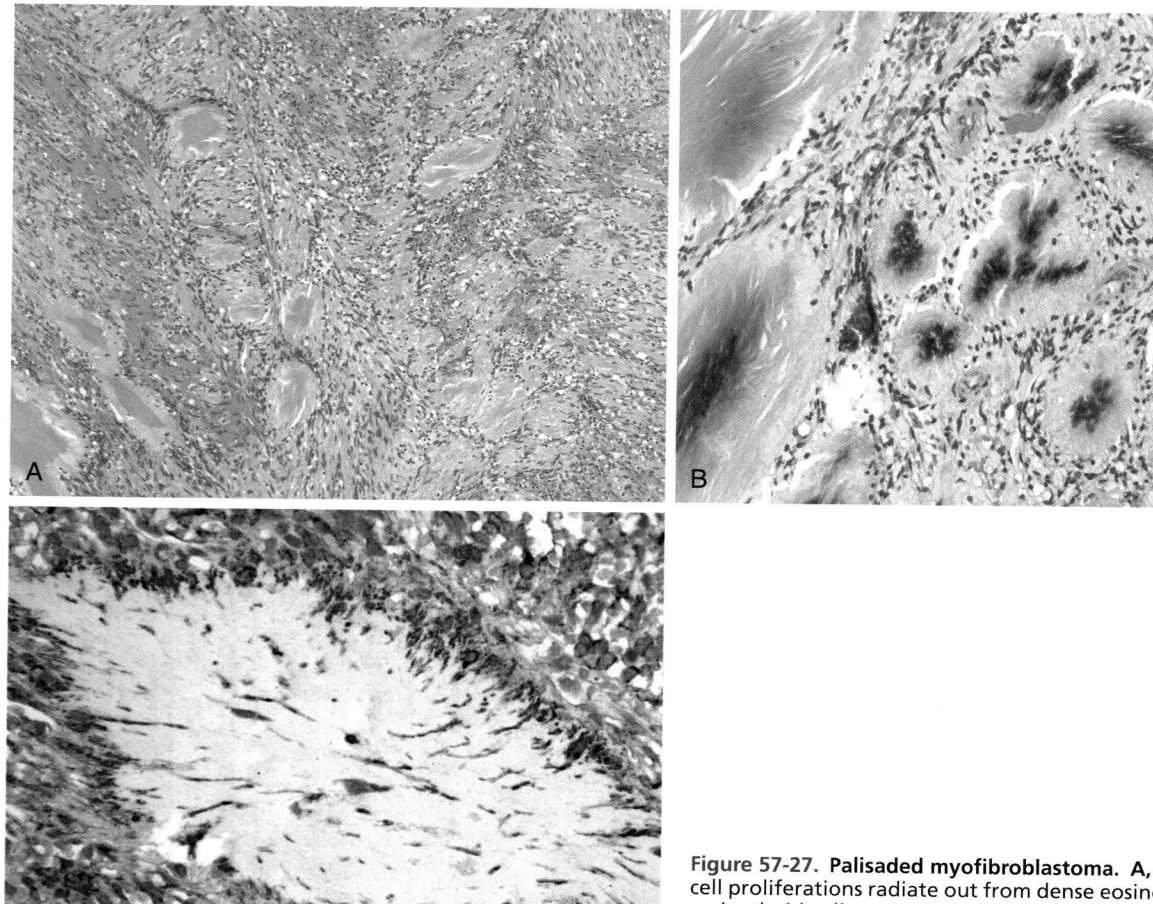

Figure 57-27. Palisaded myofibroblastoma. A, Stellate spindle cell proliferations radiate out from dense eosinophilic, sclerotic amianthoid collagen, some of which shows calcification **(B). C,** There is focal smooth muscle actin expression. *(C courtesy Dr. Mario Luna.)*

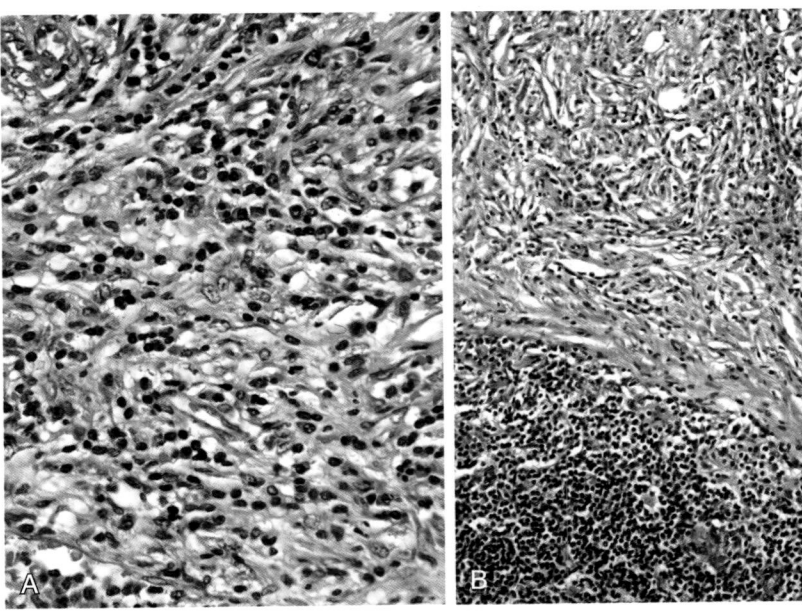

Figure 57-28. Inflammatory pseudotumor of lymph node. Various patterns have been described, including lesions rich in inflammatory cells **(A)** and other cellular or spindled lesions **(B)**. Differential diagnosis of the more cellular lesions includes myofibroblastic sarcoma, and underlying infection or IgG4-related disease should be excluded in lesions rich in inflammatory cells.

pseudotumor. The pathologic spectrum and cause of these changes have not been firmly established and are likely to be a reaction to a variety of processes or stimuli. Patients with inflammatory pseudotumor can have marked lymph node enlargement and prominent constitutional symptoms, and surgical resection usually leads to a dramatic resolution of symptoms.[104]

Inflammatory pseudotumor initially involves the paracortical areas and often the fibrous trabeculae of the lymph node, secondarily spreading into follicles and perinodal adipose tissue. Some cases are composed of a polymorphic infiltrate of acute or chronic inflammatory cells embedded in collagen-rich fibroblastic stroma (Fig. 57-28A). Other cases are composed of a dense, storiform proliferation of myofibroblasts (Fig. 57-28B). Unlike inflammatory pseudotumors of the liver or spleen, nodal cases are negative for Epstein-Barr virus.[105]

The diagnosis of inflammatory pseudotumor requires exclusion of entities in its differential diagnosis, which is broad and includes inflammatory myofibroblastic tumor; follicular dendritic cell sarcoma; lymphoproliferative disorders associated with a fibrohistiocytic response, including Hodgkin lymphoma and T-cell lymphomas; IgG4-related disease; and infectious lymphadenitis caused by mycobacteria, spirochetes, or fungi. Workup using ancillary histochemical and IHC studies may be helpful in this regard, including stains for microorganisms, Hodgkin/Reed-Sternberg cells, CD138 or IgG and IgG4, and follicular dendritic cell antigens. One study found evidence of luetic infection in four of nine cases of nodal inflammatory pseudotumor.[106] In contrast to some cases of inflammatory myofibroblastic tumor, inflammatory pseudotumors are negative for ALK by IHC.[105]

Kaposi Sarcoma

Kaposi sarcoma is a virally induced tumor characterized by a proliferation of vascular elements and stromal cells with variable myofibroblastic differentiation. It occurs in a variety of clinical settings, including immunosuppression (solid organ transplantation, human immunodeficiency virus [HIV] infection) and older age, particularly older adult patients who are living or have lived in Mediterranean or sub-Saharan African regions where HHV-8/KSHV is endemic. Epidemic variants of Kaposi sarcoma may also occur in these regions of the world, with a much younger age of onset.

Kaposi sarcoma often extends from the lymph node capsule along the fibrous trabeculae before completely replacing the nodal parenchyma. On histology, it is composed of curvilinear fascicles of bland-appearing spindle cells with characteristic cytoplasmic periodic acid-Schiff–positive hyaline globules (Fig. 57-29A–B) and admixed plasma cells, hemosiderin, and extravasated erythrocytes. In the less cellular areas, sieve-like vasoformative structures are easier to appreciate. Rare cases may show sinusoidal infiltration extending throughout the interfollicular areas in a pattern resembling vascular transformation of lymph node sinuses.

The pathogenetic role of HHV-8/KSHV in Kaposi sarcoma is now well established. IHC for HHV-8/KSHV LANA-1 is useful in confirming the diagnosis (Fig. 57-29C). Furthermore, Kaposi sarcoma may be found in lymph nodes adjacent to the regressed follicles of HHV-8/KSHV-associated multicentric Castleman disease.

Vascular Tumors

Benign hemangiomas of lymph nodes can show the full range of histologic variants seen at other anatomic sites. They are often centered in the hilum or medulla but can also completely efface the parenchyma. The most common types in lymph nodes are lobulated capillary hemangioma with myxoid stroma and cavernous hemangioma (Fig. 57-30). Cases of nodal cellular hemangioma have also been described. Rarely, lesions resembling epithelioid hemangioma or angiolymphoid hyperplasia with eosinophilia can be seen in lymph nodes.

Epithelioid hemangioendothelioma, which usually occurs in lymph nodes as a metastatic tumor, is characterized by sheets, nodules, or cords of plump, eosinophilic, vacuolated cells with small intracytoplasmic lumens that sometimes

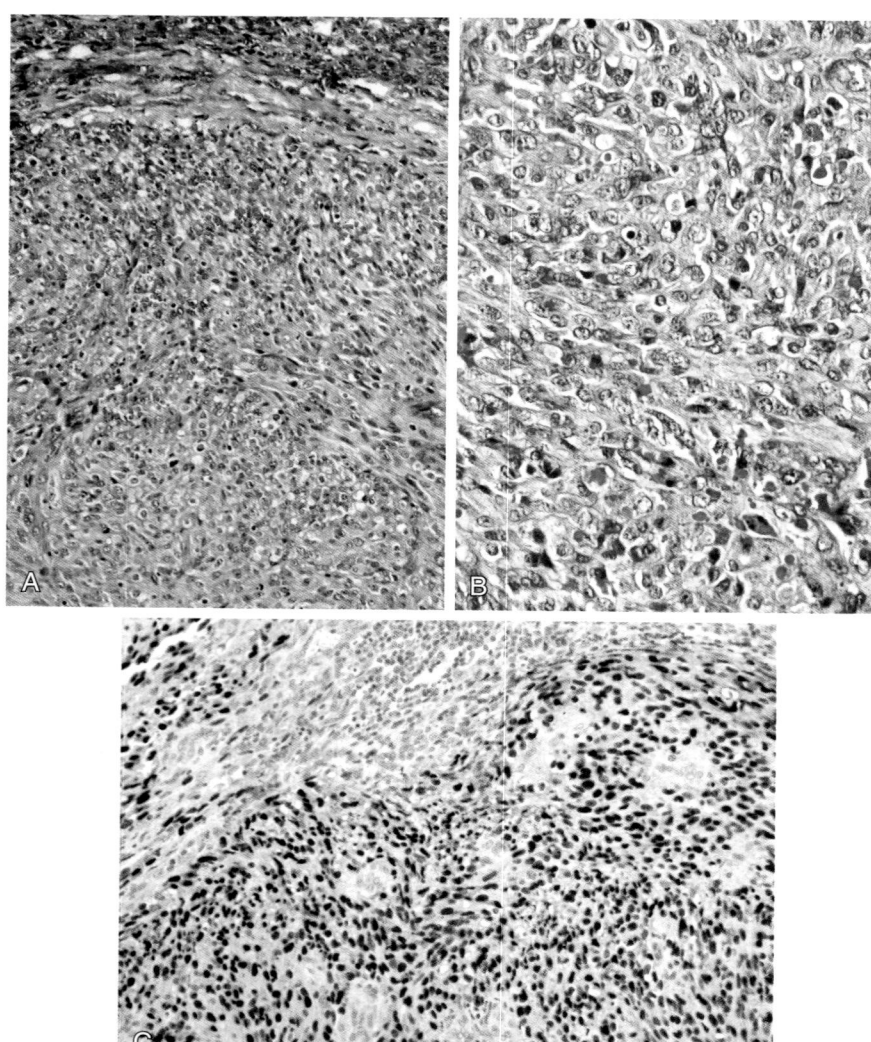

Figure 57-29. Kaposi sarcoma of lymph node. A, Hypervascular spindle cell and epithelioid cell proliferation centered on the lymph node capsule. **B,** Entrapped red blood cells and extracellular hyaline globules are diagnostic clues. **C,** IHC for human herpesvirus-8 (HHV-8) or Kaposi sarcoma herpesvirus (KSHV) LANA-1 is diffusely positive in proliferating spindle cells.

contain red blood cells in an abundant extracellular hyaline matrix (Fig. 57-31). The tumor cells are positive for vascular markers, including CD31 and factor VIII–associated protein. In nodal lesions of epithelioid hemangioendothelioma, central necrosis and dense fibrosis are frequently seen. Spindle cell hemangioendothelioma can be the sole histologic pattern but is more commonly a minor component of epithelioid hemangioendothelioma (Fig. 57-32).[107]

Nodal angiosarcoma appears to be an exceedingly rare primary neoplasm, but metastasis to lymph nodes from an occult tumor can occur. Angiosarcoma is distinguished from the lower-grade vascular tumors by marked atypia, a high mitotic rate, and multilayering of tumor cells in the vasoformative areas. Tumors can have a spindled, epithelioid, or anastomosing pattern or a mixture of all patterns (Fig. 57-33). Epithelioid angiosarcoma is more common in retroperitoneal lymph nodes (Fig. 57-34).

Metastatic Sarcomas of Other Types

Primary nodal sarcomas of follicular dendritic cell, interdigitating dendritic cell, and fibroblastic reticular cell origins are described in Chapter 52 and are not discussed here.

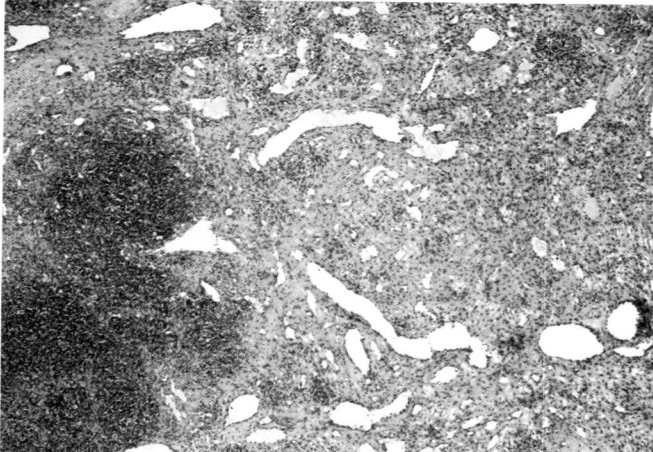

Figure 57-30. Hemangioma of lymph node. The nodal parenchyma is displaced by a proliferation of benign-appearing blood vessels of various sizes and dense sclerosis.

Although any histologic type of sarcoma can metastasize to lymph nodes, different sarcomas have different frequencies of lymph node metastasis. Among adult soft-tissue sarcomas, lymph

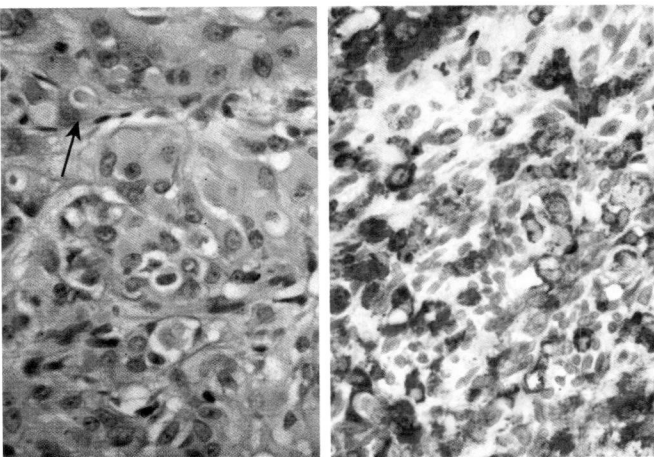

Figure 57-31. Epithelioid hemangioendothelioma involving lymph node. Large epithelioid cells with abundant pink cytoplasm show intracytoplasmic vacuolation *(left, arrow)*. Factor VIII–associated protein immunostain is positive *(right)*.

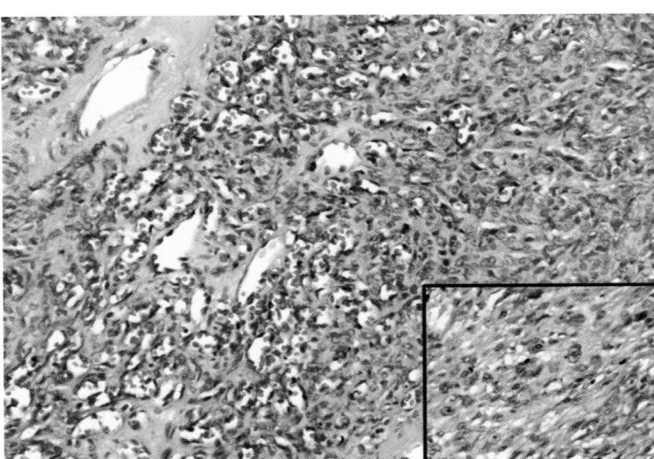

Figure 57-33. Angiosarcoma metastatic to lymph node. These tumors can have a wide variety of appearances, often with vasoformative areas mixed with cellular spindle cell areas *(inset)*.

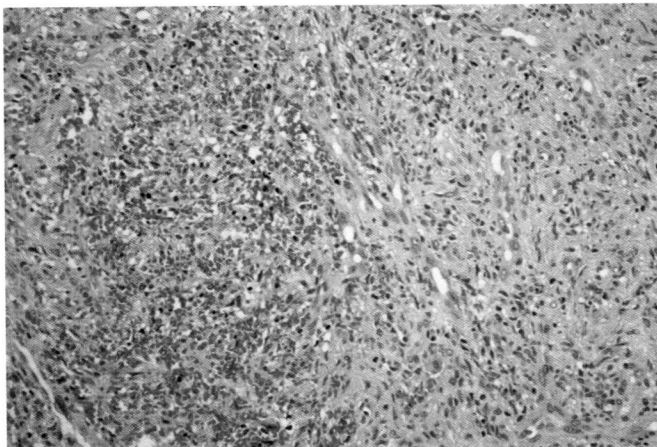

Figure 57-32. Hemangioendothelioma in lymph node with spindled and retiform growth patterns. A mixed pattern of solid collagenous areas *(right)* and anastomosing vasoformative areas *(left)* are common. The degree of atypia and number of mitoses are typically lower in epithelioid hemangioendothelioma than in angiosarcoma.

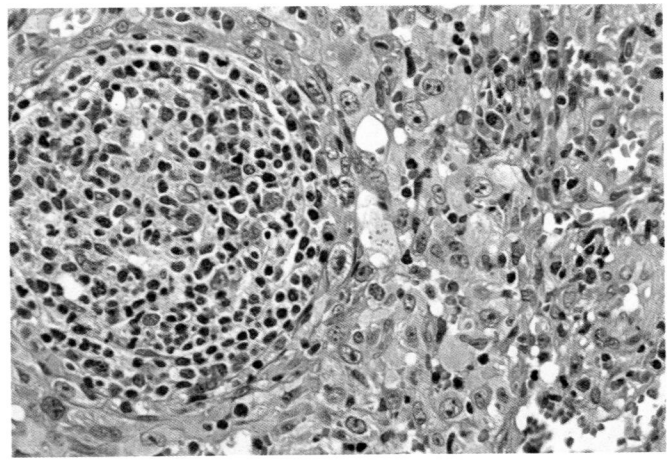

Figure 57-34. Epithelioid angiosarcoma metastatic to lymph node. An interfollicular pattern of tumor invasion is noted.

node metastases are most common with rhabdomyosarcoma, angiosarcoma, and hemangioendothelioma.[108,109] Liposarcomas rarely metastasize to lymph nodes. However, inflammatory liposarcomas can mimic lymphoma or dendritic cell neoplasms, and IHC for MDM2 and CDK4 should be performed in challenging cases. Among childhood sarcomas, rhabdomyosarcoma and Ewing's sarcoma most frequently metastasize to lymph nodes, with a 10% to 15% incidence over the course of the disease.[110] Ganglioneuroblastoma may metastasize to lymph nodes, particularly in the mediastinum (Fig. 57-35). Among bone tumors, both chondrosarcoma and osteosarcoma can metastasize to regional lymph nodes.

Bone Marrow Hematopoietic Elements and Tumors Involving Lymph Nodes

The presence of bone marrow hematopoietic elements in lymph nodes, also known as extramedullary hematopoiesis, occurs

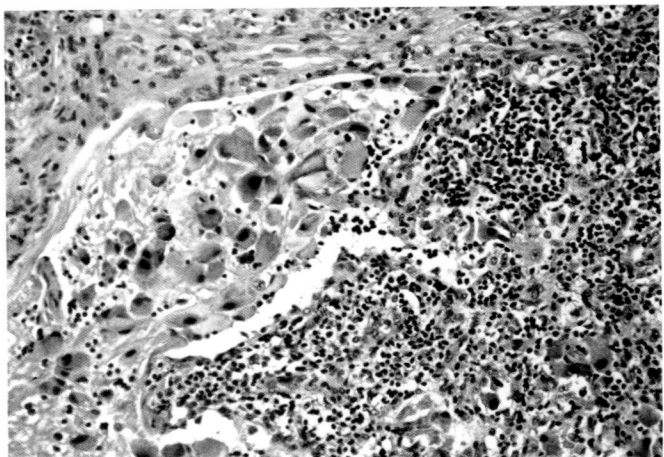

Figure 57-35. Metastatic ganglioneuroblastoma. Sinusoidal infiltration by spindled tumor cells with granular cytoplasm is noted. This patient had a history of a large posterior mediastinal mass.

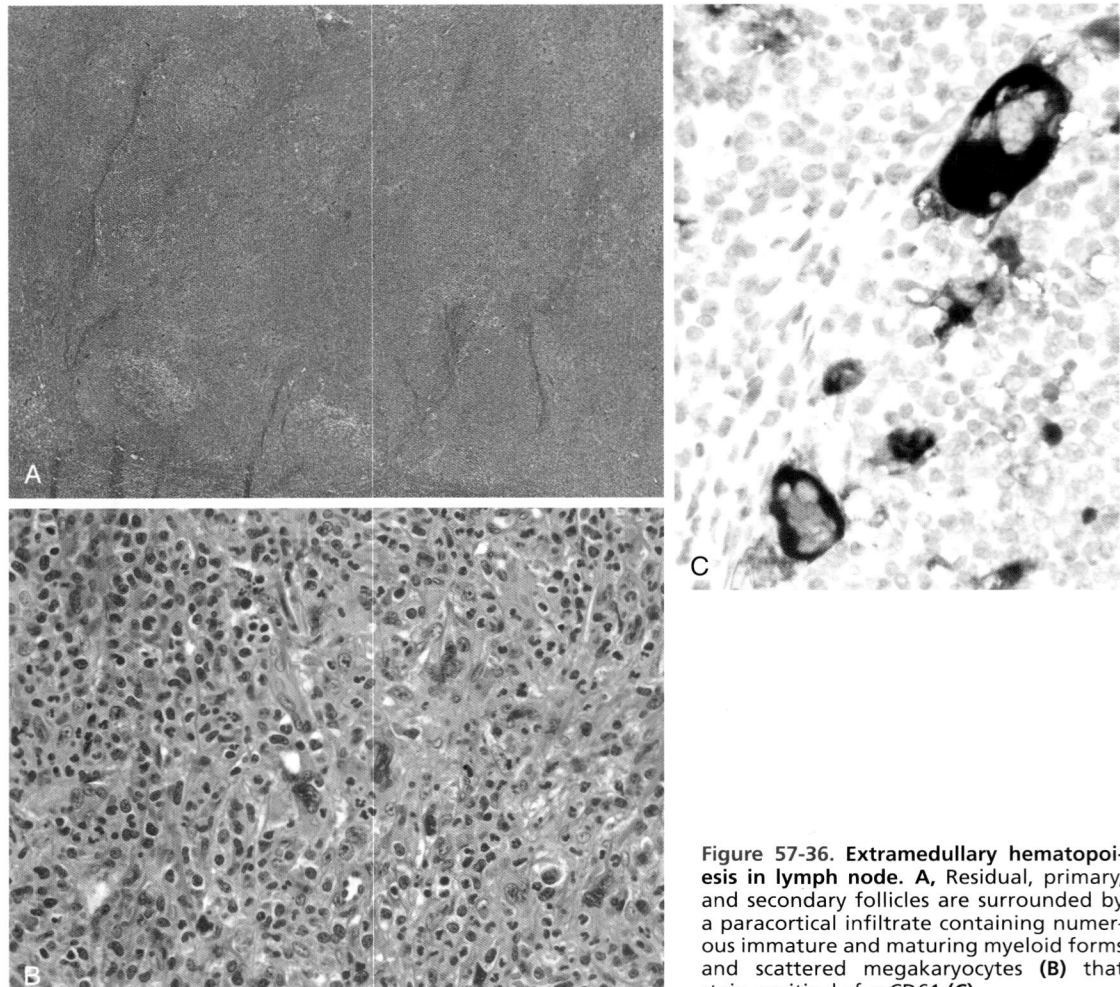

Figure 57-36. Extramedullary hematopoiesis in lymph node. A, Residual, primary, and secondary follicles are surrounded by a paracortical infiltrate containing numerous immature and maturing myeloid forms and scattered megakaryocytes **(B)** that stain positively for CD61 **(C).**

in a variety of settings, most commonly in association with myeloproliferative neoplasms with fibrosis, reflecting the altered bone marrow environment. In such cases, megakaryocytes and other bone marrow elements appear in great numbers in the interfollicular areas of lymph nodes (Fig. 57-36A–C).

Lymph nodes may be secondarily involved by acute leukemias and may be the first site of disease detection. Acute lymphoblastic leukemia involving lymph nodes resembles lymphoblastic lymphoma, as discussed in Chapter 41. An interfollicular pattern can be observed in lymphomas with early spread. Acute myeloid leukemia involving lymph nodes (myeloid sarcoma) is discussed in Chapter 46. The interfollicular pattern of infiltration in acute myeloid leukemia (Fig. 57-37) and the cytologic features, especially as seen on touch preparations, are clues to the correct diagnosis. The inclusion of CD45/LCA in routine immunohistochemical panels should detect most of these tumors, but the antibody is negative in a subset of cases. Other stains, such as myeloperoxidase, lysozyme, CD43, CD33, CD68, and CD117, are helpful for diagnosis.

Nodal involvement by mast cell disease is discussed in Chapter 49. Mast cell tumors in the lymph node are often associated with perivascular fibrosis and eosinophils—two clues to the correct diagnosis. Low-grade tumors can have abundant pale cytoplasm, resembling nodal marginal zone B-cell lymphoma. High-grade tumors can be difficult to distinguish from other poorly differentiated neoplasms. Metachromatic staining with Giemsa or toluidine blue and IHC stains for tryptase and CD117 are helpful in establishing the diagnosis.

Langerhans cell histiocytosis is a relatively common finding in lymph nodes and is discussed in Chapter 52. Rarely, these tumors can resemble poorly differentiated non-hematopoietic tumors and should be considered when the first round of IHC is negative. The strong, uniform immunoreactivity of tumor cells for CD1a and S-100 protein distinguishes these tumors from other histiocytic proliferations, which are negative or only focally positive.

CONCLUSION

The evaluation of non-hematopoietic disorders in the bone marrow and lymph nodes requires careful correlation with clinical, imaging, and other laboratory findings and communication with the patients' physicians. IHC stains may be used as an adjunct to diagnosis and may also be used for prognostic or therapeutic purposes with certain tumors. When evaluated properly, examination of these organs is a powerful tool for both hematopoietic and non-hematopoietic diagnoses.

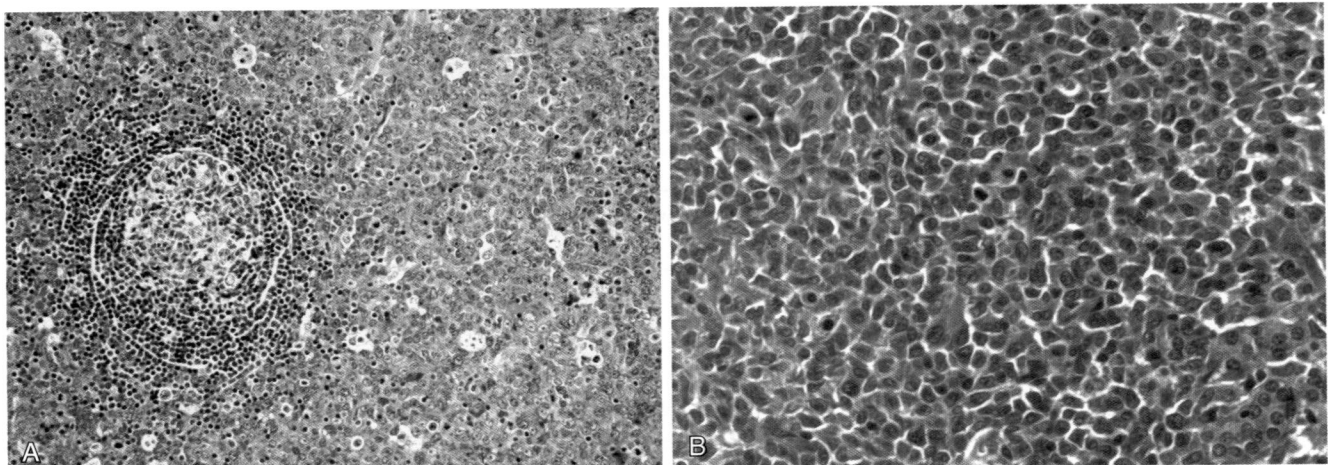

Figure 57-37. Acute myeloid leukemia in lymph node. A, The interfollicular areas are expanded by a neoplastic proliferation of immature myeloid forms. **B,** In this case of acute myeloid leukemia with inv(16) or *CBFB::MYH11* presenting as monoblastic sarcoma involving a lymph node, the blasts have folded or irregular nuclei consistent with monocytic differentiation, and numerous background eosinophils are present.

Pearls and Pitfalls

- Both the bone marrow biopsy and the aspirate are important in the evaluation of metastatic disease. Some tumors, such as neuroblastomas, may show only rare clusters on aspirates, even when there is extensive involvement.
- Request bone marrow biopsies, even in pediatric patients, when looking for metastatic disease. Bilateral bone marrow biopsies increase the likelihood of finding metastases.
- Biopsy of radiologically suspicious sites may be necessary to identify focal bone or bone marrow involvement.
- Lymph node location is often the most helpful clue to the primary site of origin of metastatic carcinoma. For instance, occult nasopharyngeal carcinoma commonly presents in neck lymph nodes.
- Sarcomatoid carcinoma should always be considered when a poorly differentiated spindle cell nodal metastasis is encountered.
- Anaplastic large-cell lymphoma can have a variety of appearances and exhibit the loss of nearly all lymphoid-associated markers. Perform CD30 IHC before ruling out a nodal large-cell malignancy.
- Follicular dendritic cell neoplasms often have an epithelioid or anaplastic morphology that mimics other tumors. A panel of follicular dendritic cell markers (CD21, CD23, CD35) is recommended because of partial differentiation. Residual nodal tissue may show colonization of lymphoid follicles by dysplastic follicular dendritic cells.
- Do not make a diagnosis based on subset of positive immunohistochemical stains; a variety of tumors may show lineage infidelity (e.g., melanoma can express CD10, and carcinomas outside the lung may be positive for TTF-1).
- When possible, use IHC controls that have been fixed and processed (e.g., decalcified) in the same way as the specimen being tested.
- Metastatic tumors are best classified based on the primary site, even though the bone marrow or a peripheral lymph node may be more accessible.
- Always correlate findings with the clinical history and radiologic findings and talk to clinicians; a skeptical clinician is a pathologist's best friend.
- Hesitate before making an unlikely diagnosis but realize that anything is possible.

KEY REFERENCES

2. Li S, Peng Y, Weinhandl ED, et al. Estimated number of prevalent cases of metastatic bone disease in the US adult population. *Clin Epidemiol.* 2012;4:87–93.
3. Brunning R, McKenna R. Tumors metastatic to the bone marrow. In: Brunning R, McKenna R, eds. *Tumors of the Bone Marrow.* Armed Forces Institute of Pathology; 1994:457–474.
7. Dabbs DJ. *Diagnostic Immunohistochemistry.* Elsevier Health Sciences; 2013.
13. Tan AC, Tan DSW. Targeted therapies for lung cancer patients with oncogenic driver molecular alterations. *J Clin Oncol.* 2022;40:611–625.
14. Bubendorf L, Schopfer A, Wagner U, et al. Metastatic patterns of prostate cancer: an autopsy study of 1,589 patients. *Hum Pathol.* 2000;31:578–583.
53. Park SY, Kim BH, Kim JH, et al. Panels of immunohistochemical markers help determine primary sites of metastatic adenocarcinoma. *Arch Pathol Lab Med.* 2007;131:1561–1567.
61. Chu P, Wu E, Weiss LM. Cytokeratin 7 and cytokeratin 20 expression in epithelial neoplasms: a survey of 435 cases. *Mod Pathol.* 2000;13:962–972.
72. Zheng Z, Liebers M, Zhelyazkova B, Cao Y, et al. Anchored multiplex PCR for targeted next-generation sequencing. *Nat Med.* 2014;20:1479–1484.
74. Lin F, Liu H. Immunohistochemistry in undifferentiated neoplasm/tumor of uncertain origin. *Arch Pathol Lab Med.* 2014;138:1583–1610.
87. Carson KF, Wen DR, Li PX, et al. Nodal nevi and cutaneous melanomas. *Am J Surg Pathol.* 1996;20:834–840.

Visit Elsevier eBooks+ for the complete set of references.

Chapter 58

Spleen: Normal Architecture and Neoplastic and Non-neoplastic Lesions

Attilio Orazi and Daniel A. Arber

Few hematologic malignancies arise primarily in the spleen; most conditions occurring at this site represent secondary involvement by diseases originating elsewhere in the body. The role of the pathologist in most cases is to confirm the known or suspected diagnosis and to exclude unsuspected pathology. Careful gross evaluation of the organ and optimal tissue fixation are essential for the successful interpretation of splenic pathology. Because of the amount of blood in the spleen, thin sections are particularly important. In addition, care must be exercised in isolating lymph nodes of the splenic hilum. Their examination can provide valuable additional information, particularly in the diagnosis of low-grade B-cell lymphomas. Obtaining adequate clinical information is often critical for the diagnostic

characterization of disorders that involve the spleen; this need cannot be overemphasized.

In this chapter, we present a comprehensive account of those aspects of splenic pathology likely to be encountered by diagnostic hematopathologists. We outline principles for a systematic histopathologic analysis that can be applied to achieve a specific diagnosis after the recognition of broad categories of abnormalities affecting individual splenic compartments. To avoid repetition of material covered elsewhere in this text, specific splenic disease entities, such as hepatosplenic T-cell lymphoma and splenic marginal zone lymphoma, are only mentioned briefly. The reader is directed to the specific chapters covering these entities and to chapters covering other hematopoietic tumors that may secondarily

Table 58-1 Normal Morphologic Compartments of the Spleen

Compartment	Elements	Description
White pulp	Follicles	
	Primary	Composed of small nodules of mantle-type B lymphocytes
	Secondary	Composed of a mixture of small, cleaved B lymphocytes (centrocytes) and large transformed cells (centroblasts), with intermixed dendritic cells and macrophages, as well as some T cells
	Mantle zone	Surrounds the germinal center; composed predominantly of small B lymphocytes with round to slightly irregular nuclei, condensed chromatin, and scant cytoplasm
	Periarteriolar lymphoid sheaths	Sheaths of predominantly small T lymphocytes that surround arterioles and arteries; other cells include larger transformed lymphocytes, natural killer (NK) cells, plasma cells, and B cells
Red pulp	Sinusoids	Lined by specialized endothelial cells with macrophage capacity; lack a continuous basal membrane
	Cords	Lie between the sinusoids; composed of extracellular space and cordal macrophages
Supporting stroma	Capsule and trabecular septa	Paucicellular dense fibrous tissue; thickened in reactive or chronic conditions

involve the spleen, such as Hodgkin lymphoma and the various non-Hodgkin lymphomas.

THE NORMAL SPLEEN

The characterization of disorders that involve the spleen can best be understood in light of the structure and function of that organ.[1-7] The spleen is composed of two anatomically and functionally distinct regions (Table 58-1). The lymphoid tissue of the spleen, called the *white pulp*, appears grossly as uniformly distributed white nodules. The white pulp is intimately associated with the splenic arterial circulation. The central arteries, which arise from trabecular arteries within the fibrous trabeculae, are surrounded by cylindrical cuffs of lymphocytes called *periarteriolar lymphoid sheaths.* The periarteriolar lymphoid sheaths contain an admixture of B cells and T cells, with a predominance of CD4-positive T lymphocytes. Periodically, splenic lymphoid follicles (Malpighian corpuscles) occur as outgrowths of the periarteriolar lymphoid sheaths. The morphology of the splenic white pulp varies with age and with its functional activity (e.g., presence of antigenic stimulation). Inactive or hypoplastic white pulp, in which no germinal centers are seen, is characteristic of infancy, senescence, and the immunologically unstimulated adult spleen. In the immunologically activated state, the splenic lymphoid follicle shows three distinct zones. The *germinal center,* structurally similar to germinal centers in

other lymphoid organs, is surrounded by a *mantle zone.* The mantle zone is encased by the outer *marginal zone,* a cellular layer at the interface between the white and red pulp. The marginal zone, composed of both B cells and T cells,[4] is the site of initial antigen trapping and processing (Fig. 58-1).

The red pulp contains the terminal branches of the splenic artery, which end in specialized capillaries known as *sheathed capillaries.* These unique capillaries simply terminate and outlet their contents into the surrounding red pulp, a functional arrangement known as *open splenic circulation.*[8] The *red pulp* of the spleen is mainly composed of splenic vascular sinuses and the splenic cords, also known as *cords of Billroth,* which are made up of splenic macrophages, scattered cord capillaries, venules, and stromal cells. All these cellular elements linked together, along with a relatively scanty amount of extracellular matrix, are responsible for the peculiar architecture of the red pulp. The splenic vascular sinuses provide the mechanism for filtration of the peripheral blood, one of the important functions of the spleen. The sinus-lining cells, also known as *littoral cells,* have long cytoplasmic processes that overlap and are closely apposed. However, because no tight junctions are present, circulating blood cells are able to squeeze through the interendothelial junctions and percolate through the splenic cords before entering the splenic sinuses, venules, and trabecular veins, eventually draining into the splenic vein, thus returning to the systemic circulation. The ability of circulating blood cells to enter the splenic sinuses and subsequently percolate through the cords depends on their deformability. Cells without the ability to deform cannot enter the sinuses and are destroyed in the acidotic, hypoxic environment of the cords of Billroth.[2,9,10]

The T cells found in the red pulp are predominantly CD8-positive small lymphocytes, which are rarely found in the periarteriolar lymphoid sheaths and are virtually absent in the germinal centers. Gamma-delta T cells also reside normally in the red pulp.[11] The distribution of immunoglobulin-containing B cells is comparable to that seen in the lymph nodes. The mantle zone B cells bear surface immunoglobulin, with co-expression of immunoglobulin (Ig) M and IgD. The marginal zone B cells predominantly express IgM, with only a small minority expressing IgD. IgG expression is lacking in these areas and is limited to scattered cells in the red pulp, where rare IgA-containing cells are also found. The red pulp contains numerous cells of monocyte-macrophage lineage, only a few of which are found in the white pulp. Natural killer (NK) cells are found scattered throughout the red pulp. The red pulp also contains granulocytes, monocytes, and lymphocytes that pass transiently through the red pulp circulation.

GROSS EXAMINATION

The initial evaluation of the spleen should consist of a gross examination of the organ. Three major patterns are recognized, based on involvement of the white pulp, red pulp, or more focal lesions (Table 58-2).

Diffuse Splenic Enlargement

White Pulp Involvement

Most proliferative disorders of the splenic lymphoid tissue produce a micronodular pattern owing to the abnormal

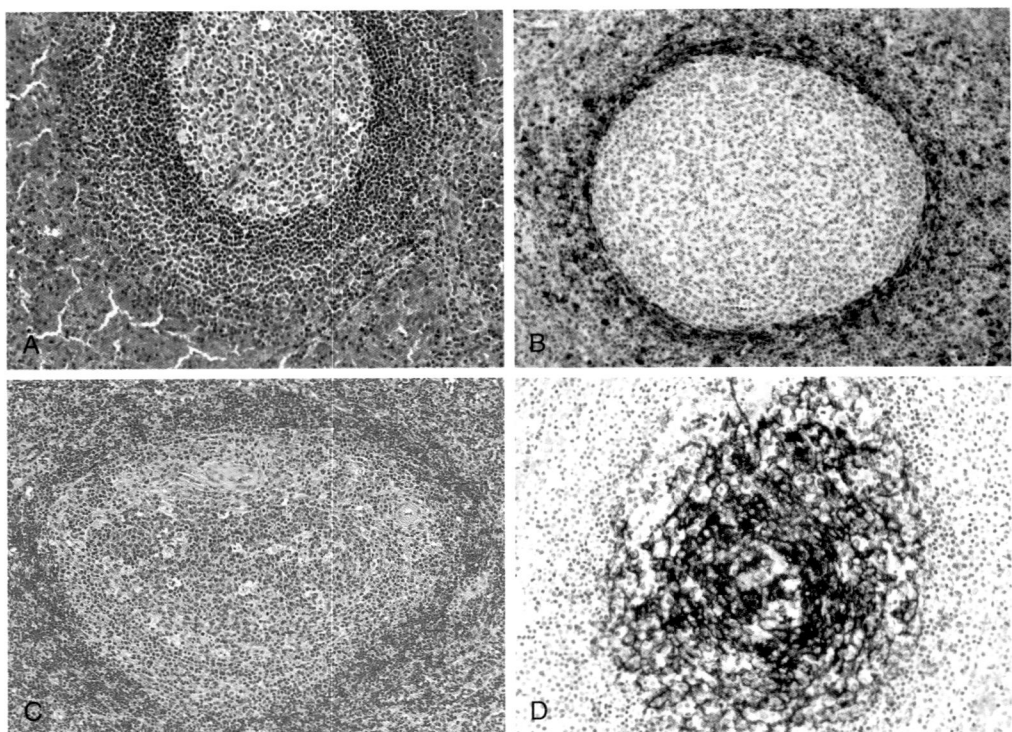

Figure 58-1. A, Splenic lymphoid follicle displaying its characteristic tripartite nature: germinal center, mantle zone, and well-defined marginal zone. **B,** DBA.44 immunohistochemical stain highlights mantle zone cells. Note negative staining in the follicle germinal center and rare positive cells within the predominantly negative marginal zone. **C,** Hyperplastic follicle, with less distinct mantle and marginal zones. **D,** CD21 immunohistochemical stain highlights the follicular dendritic cell network within a germinal center.

Table 58-2 Patterns of Involvement in Splenic Pathology

Pattern	Predominantly Red Pulp Based		Predominantly White Pulp Based	
	Neoplastic	Non-Neoplastic	Neoplastic	Non-Neoplastic
Diffuse	HCL and HCL variant Splenic diffuse red pulp small B-cell lymphoma Hepatosplenic T-cell lymphoma T-LGLL Acute leukemias MPN, other myeloid neoplasms CLL/SLL (rare) LPL (rare)	Hemolytic anemias Non-specific congestion Extramedullary hematopoiesis Storage diseases Cytokine effects HPS	Small B-cell lymphomas (CLL/SLL, LPL, SMZL, MCL) PTCL	Hyperplasia
Focal* or variable	Hodgkin lymphoma DLBCL T-PLL EBV-DCT Other dendritic cell tumors Mast cell disease Vascular tumors† Metastases	—	—	—

*Focal lesions may have considerable overlap, with both red pulp and white pulp involvement. At times, this division is arbitrary.
†Diffuse involvement is seen in systemic angiomatosis, as well as in some cases of littoral cell angioma.
CLL/SLL, Chronic lymphocytic leukemia/small lymphocytic lymphoma; *DLBCL,* diffuse large B-cell lymphoma; *EBV-DCT,* Epstein-Barr virus–positive inflammatory follicular dendritic cell/fibroblastic reticular cell tumor; *HCL,* hairy cell leukemia; *HPS,* hemophagocytic syndrome; *LPL,* lymphoplasmacytic lymphoma; *MCL,* mantle cell lymphoma; *MPN,* myeloproliferative neoplasm; *PTCL,* peripheral T-cell lymphoma; *SMZL,* splenic marginal zone lymphoma; *T-LGLL,* T-cell large granular lymphocytic leukemia; *T-PLL,* T-cell prolymphocytic leukemia.

expansion of preexisting splenic lymphoid structures (follicles and periarteriolar lymphoid sheaths). Grossly, multiple small, whitish nodules are noticeable on the cut surface, an appearance that is occasionally referred to as a *miliary pattern.* This pattern is most often seen in small B-cell lymphoid neoplasms, other than hairy cell leukemia, involving the spleen. The nodules occasionally become confluent or present as larger, dominant masses. Lymphoid malignancies that affect the white pulp are largely the same as those that affect lymph nodes. These disorders include classic Hodgkin lymphoma, nodular lymphocyte predominant B-cell lymphoma (World Health Organization [WHO]: nodular lymphocyte predominant Hodgkin lymphoma) and non-Hodgkin lymphomas, primarily of B-cell lineage.

Red Pulp Involvement

Red pulp involvement has a different gross appearance. Typically, expansion of the red pulp gives the spleen a more homogeneous red or "beefy" appearance. The normal nodularity of the white pulp is typically diminished or not seen. Microscopically, the white pulp is often atrophic or compressed by the expanded red pulp. Neoplastic proliferations that involve the red pulp include myeloid and lymphoid leukemias, myeloproliferative neoplasms, and a variety of nonhematopoietic tumors. In general, disorders with a large component of circulating cells (e.g., chronic lymphocytic leukemia, T-cell large granular lymphocytic leukemia, hairy cell leukemia, and acute leukemia) have significant red pulp involvement. However, some lymphomas (e.g., hepatosplenic T-cell lymphoma, intravascular large B-cell lymphoma, as well as other less well-defined lymphoid malignancies) also involve the red pulp.

Focal Splenic Pathology

Some benign and malignant proliferations produce focal lesions rather than more diffuse involvement of the red or white pulp. These include lesions that involve vascular, stromal, and hematolymphoid elements.

Splenic Rupture

Pathologic rupture of the spleen can be seen in a variety of hematologic disorders, both benign and malignant.[5] Spontaneous rupture of the spleen should always prompt a pathologic evaluation of the splenic tissue because various infectious causes (particularly infectious mononucleosis) have pathologic findings that are distinctive enough to make a presumptive diagnosis or suggest additional serologic studies. Other causes, such as storage diseases, present with characteristic findings as well. Splenic rupture as a primary presentation of hematologic malignancy is rare, but it has been reported with both low-grade and high-grade lymphoid malignancies. Acute and chronic myeloproliferative disorders and, rarely, acute lymphoblastic leukemia can present as splenic rupture. Nonhematopoietic lesions associated with splenic rupture include cysts, infarctions, vascular lesions or neoplasms, and metastatic malignancies.

LYMPHOID HYPERPLASIA

Various reactive conditions that affect the splenic white or red pulp can simulate hematopoietic malignancies (Box 58-1). Reactive follicular hyperplasia, with the formation of germinal centers, is usually easily recognized as benign (see Fig. 58-1).[2] However, follicular hyperplasia must occasionally be distinguished from follicular lymphoma. The finding of tingible body macrophages and a polymorphic lymphoid cell population within polarized splenic follicles points to the diagnosis of a reactive hyperplasia. A rare condition that may grossly simulate lymphoma is localized (nodular) reactive lymphoid hyperplasia. The area of nodular hyperplasia appears quite distinct from adjacent normal spleen and may raise the suspicion of lymphoma (Fig. 58-2). Histologically, this area is composed of a focal aggregation of hyperplastic follicles that have typical, benign features.[12]

- Immune reactions
  - Florid follicular hyperplasia
  - Marginal zone hyperplasia
- Congenital immunodeficiencies
- Autoimmune conditions
- Disorders of the reticuloendothelial system
  - Storage diseases
  - Hemophagocytic syndrome
- Castleman disease
- Reactive myeloid proliferations caused by cytokine treatment
- Nonhematopoietic lesions
  - Cyst
  - Hamartoma
  - Inflammatory pseudotumor

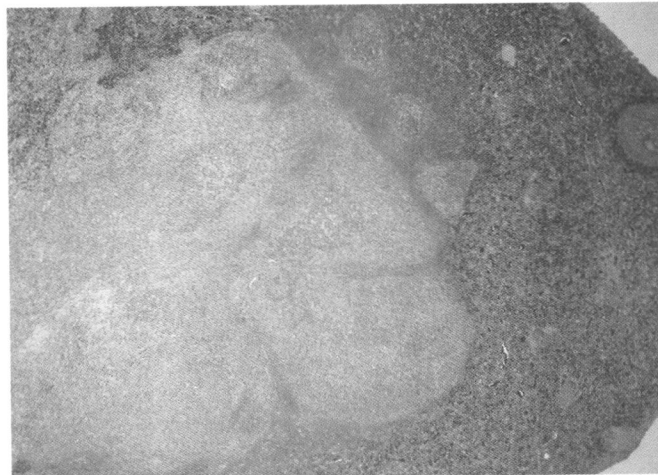

Figure 58-2. Nodular lymphoid hyperplasia of the spleen. Note the confluence of several hyperplastic follicles, which form a tumor-like lesion. This is surrounded by normal red pulp and other hyperplastic-appearing follicles. Although cytologically benign, this entity can mimic lymphoma or other focal splenic lesions.

In some cases, marginal zones may become widely expanded, a phenomenon referred to as *splenic marginal zone hyperplasia*.[2,5,13-15] This usually occurs in association with follicular hyperplasia, but such expansions may also occur with B-cell lymphomas other than splenic marginal zone lymphoma, particularly follicular lymphoma. It may be impossible to distinguish these reactive changes from cases of early marginal zone lymphoma on morphologic grounds alone,[16] although reactive marginal zone hyperplasia is usually not associated with an increase in red pulp B cells, which is common in true splenic marginal zone lymphoma.[14] Some autoimmune disorders can result in splenic marginal zone hyperplasia, including systemic lupus erythematosus or idiopathic thrombocytopenic purpura.

Reactive lymphoid hyperplasia without germinal center formation, which is characteristic of infectious mononucleosis, as well as herpes simplex and other viral infections, can simulate both Hodgkin and non-Hodgkin lymphoma.[2,17] The white pulp in these conditions lacks expanded follicles and, on low-power examination, resembles the immunologically unstimulated spleen.[2,5,7,18,19] This is the splenic equivalent of paracortical hyperplasia as seen in lymph nodes, being similarly characterized by an interfollicular T cell hyperplasia. Occasionally, reactive paracortical hyperplasia may take the appearance of small to large nodules composed of T cells. High-power examination reveals morphologic evidence of antigenic stimulation, characterized by the presence of lymphocytes in varying stages of transformation, including small and large lymphocytes, often with plasmacytoid features, and immunoblasts. Transformed lymphocytes and immunoblasts also proliferate around splenic arterioles and may infiltrate the subendothelial zones of the trabecular veins and the connective tissue framework, resulting in splenic rupture in extreme cases.[2] This pattern of lymphoid hyperplasia can also be seen in immunocompromised individuals, such as patients treated with steroids or other immunosuppressive therapies for conditions such as immune thrombocytopenic purpura or autoimmune hemolytic anemia.[20] Some peripheral T-cell lymphomas may produce a similar pattern of white pulp expansion. Nodular T-cell hyperplasia, simulating a peripheral T-cell lymphoma, can rarely be observed in patients with hypersensitivity reactions to phenytoin.[21] Abnormalities of the white pulp that may be worrisome for lymphoma can also be seen in patients with congenital conditions characterized by immunodeficiency or by abnormalities causing deregulated lymphoid production (e.g., autoimmune lymphoproliferative syndrome).

CASTLEMAN DISEASE

Occasional cases of Castleman disease of both the unicentric hyaline-vascular type and the multicentric type associated with human herpesvirus 8 (HHV-8)/Kaposi sarcoma-associated herpesvirus (KSHV) reportedly occur in the spleen.[22-25] Multicentric Castleman disease represents the majority of cases reported in more recent years. Splenic involvement is rare in the unicentric form, and most such reports are from the older literature, before cases were evaluated for HHV-8/KSHV; thus, the nature of these proliferations is not clearly established. The white pulp is expanded, with hypervascular germinal centers; the red pulp shows marked plasmacytosis. As seen in lymph nodes, immunoblastic cells expressing IgMλ are distributed in the perifollicular areas of the white pulp.[24] Multicentric Castleman disease is generally negative for Epstein-Barr virus (EBV), but rare cases resembling germinotropic lymphoproliferative disorders have been described. These tumors are coinfected with EBV and HHV-8/KSHV.[25]

AUTOIMMUNE LYMPHOPROLIFERATIVE SYNDROME

Autoimmune lymphoproliferative syndrome is a rare disorder that can mimic lymphoma in the spleen. It is a hereditary disorder, usually caused by mutations of the *FAS* (*CD95*) gene,[26,27] that presents in early childhood (younger than 2 years). Autoimmune lymphoproliferative syndrome is characterized by lymphoid hyperplasia, autoimmunity, and splenomegaly; the spleen frequently enlarges to more than 10 times its age-normal size. Histologically, the white pulp shows variable degrees of follicular hyperplasia, often with enlarged marginal zones. The periarteriolar lymphoid sheaths and red pulp are also expanded, owing to a markedly increased number of T cells (Fig. 58-3). These cells consist

of a mixture of small lymphocytes and immunoblasts. As in lymph nodes in this disorder, many of these T cells are negative for both CD4 and CD8. The pathologic picture of the spleen is complicated by the frequent association with immune cytopenias affecting red blood cells, granulocytes, and platelets, contributing to splenomegaly.[28,29] Patients with this disorder have an increased risk of having both Hodgkin and non-Hodgkin lymphomas.[30]

HODGKIN LYMPHOMA

Although the spleen is the most common extranodal organ involved by Hodgkin lymphoma,[31,32] primary Hodgkin lymphoma of the spleen is extremely rare.[2,33] The documentation of splenic involvement has therapeutic and prognostic implications, although these implications now appear to be less critical in light of the high rates of remission and cure obtained with current regimens of combination chemotherapy. Involvement of the liver and bone marrow is rarely found in the absence of splenic involvement.[31] All histologic subtypes of Hodgkin lymphoma can involve the spleen; nodular sclerosis and mixed cellularity are the most common,[31] and involvement by nodular lymphocyte predominant B-cell lymphoma (previously termed *nodular lymphocyte predominant Hodgkin lymphoma*) is less common.[34] On the contrary, widespread involvement, including of the subdiaphragmatic region, and splenic involvement have been associated with lymphocyte-depleted classic Hodgkin lymphoma.[35]

Hodgkin lymphoma produces either small miliary nodules or, more frequently, solitary or multiple tumor masses in the spleen (Fig. 58-4).[2,5] Splenic involvement is generally detectable grossly but may be subtle (Fig. 58-5). Foci of involvement may be only a few millimeters in size.[36,37] For this reason, the gross examination of the spleen must be meticulous in patients with Hodgkin lymphoma so that small foci of involvement are not missed. The early lesions of Hodgkin lymphoma in the spleen are found microscopically in the periarteriolar lymphoid sheaths or in the marginal zones.[5] As the disease progresses, the nodules expand to efface the lymphoid follicles and may involve the red pulp.

Sarcoid granulomas may be found in the spleens of patients with Hodgkin lymphoma, in addition to various other disorders associated with abnormal T-cell function.[38,39] The granulomas are not related to prior lymphangiography, and their origin is unknown. Several studies have suggested that granulomas occur more frequently in spleens uninvolved by Hodgkin lymphoma than in those involved by the disease.[40,41] Grossly, the granulomas may be so large as to mimic involvement by Hodgkin lymphoma. Microscopically, the granulomas are composed of clusters of epithelioid histiocytes that occur in the white pulp in close association with the arterial circulation. It has been suggested that patients with splenic sarcoid granulomas may have a better prognosis.[41]

The criteria for the diagnosis of Hodgkin lymphoma in the spleen are the same as those for other nonnodal sites (see Chapters 26 and 27). The subclassification of Hodgkin lymphoma in the spleen is sometimes difficult and is unnecessary in cases with a previous nodal diagnosis. However, the unique morphologic and immunophenotypic characteristics of nodular lymphocyte predominant B-cell

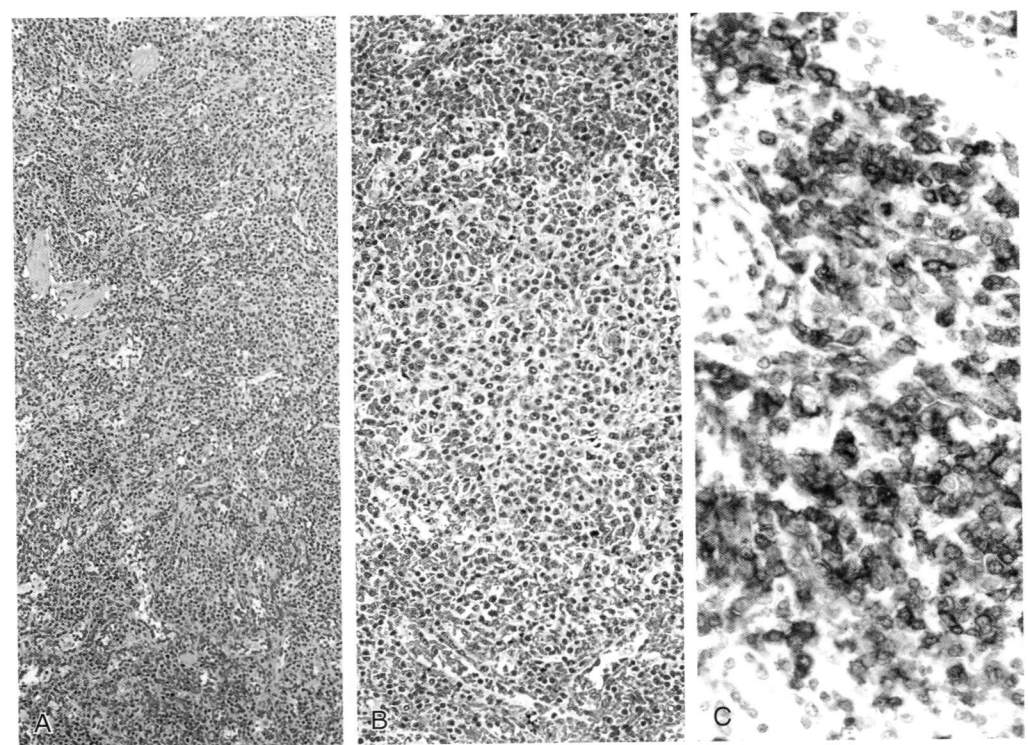

Figure 58-3. Splenic involvement in autoimmune lymphoproliferative syndrome. A, Low power shows atypical lymphoid hyperplasia that could easily be confused with lymphoma. Note the absence of reactive germinal centers, caused by prolonged steroid treatment. **B,** Higher magnification shows hyperplastic periarteriolar lymphoid sheaths and surrounding red pulp containing an increased number of atypical-appearing lymphocytes. **C,** CD3 stain demonstrates the T-cell nature of the proliferating lymphocytes.

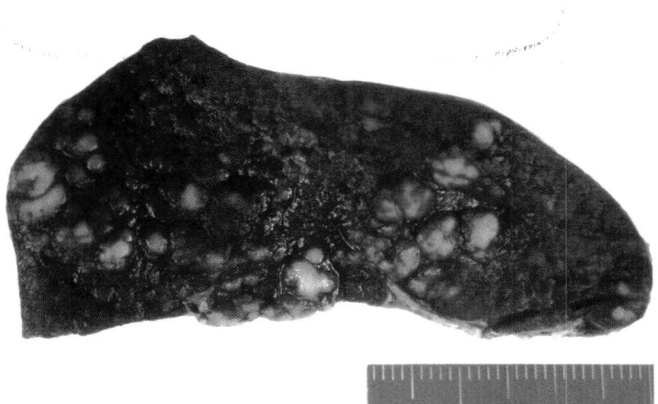

Figure 58-4. Gross photograph of Hodgkin lymphoma involving the spleen. Hodgkin lymphoma can present with a single mass or multiple discrete nodules. Thin sections after fixation are particularly valuable in detecting subtle involvement.

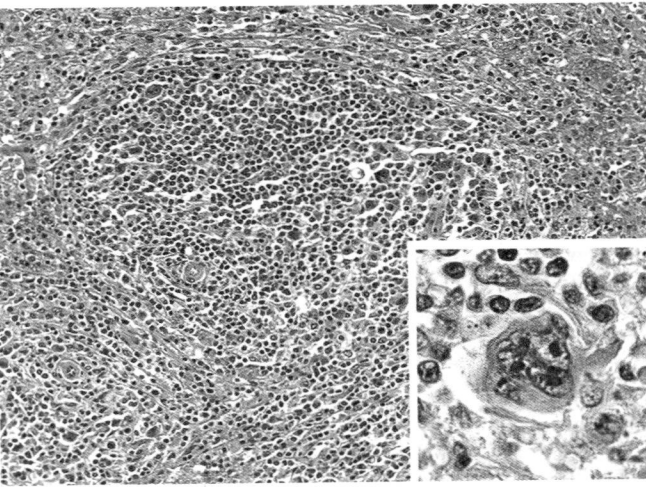

Figure 58-5. Early involvement of the spleen by Hodgkin lymphoma. Reed-Sternberg cells are seen within a polymorphic cellular background in perifollicular areas. *Inset,* Higher magnification shows classic Reed-Sternberg cells.

lymphoma allow its distinction from the classic Hodgkin lymphoma subtypes (see Chapter 26).

NON-HODGKIN LYMPHOMAS

Non-Hodgkin lymphomas may involve the spleen in three clinical settings. In the first and rarest setting, termed *true primary splenic lymphoma,* the tumor is confined to the spleen or splenic hilar lymph nodes, without evidence of involvement of other sites. In the second and most common setting, the organ is involved as part of generalized, systemic lymphomatous spread. In the third setting, the lymphomatous process is characterized by prominent or predominant splenomegaly and often distinctive clinicopathologic features.

Primary Splenic Lymphoma

Primary splenic lymphoma is rare, accounting for less than 1% of all lymphomas. Those primary to the spleen are described in separate chapters of this text and have been recently reviewed elsewhere.[42] Excluding lymphomas thought to arise in the spleen, such as splenic marginal zone lymphoma, most of these cases were described in the older literature and are not well defined.[43-53] Two cases occurred in HIV-positive patients,[44,45] and rare cases have been associated with hepatitis C infection.[52] Several studies of primary splenic lymphomas fulfilling the most stringent diagnostic criteria (i.e., tumor confined to the spleen and splenic hilar lymph nodes) include almost entirely adult patients with a slight male preponderance.[43,53] The most common presenting symptoms include left-sided abdominal pain and systemic symptoms such as fever, malaise, and weight loss. The gross findings and the histologic characteristics were similar to those observed in spleens secondarily involved by malignant lymphoma. Most reported cases are of B-cell lineage. Large B-cell lymphoma, some showing CD5 expression,[50,51] appears to be the most common subtype, with the remainder being mostly low-grade B-cell malignancies. A report of 32 patients presenting with follicular lymphoma first diagnosed in the spleen identified two variants: one with the t(14;18), high BCL2, and CD10 expression, similar to nodal follicular lymphoma, and a second subset that lacked t(14;18) and was of a higher histologic grade.[54] The majority of patients relapsed with systemic disease.

Secondary Splenic Involvement by Lymphoma

Clinical assessment of the likelihood of splenic involvement by malignant lymphomas may be difficult. The weights of involved spleens vary widely.[55] Although tumor involvement usually results in palpable splenomegaly, Goffinet and colleagues[56] found that approximately one-third of nonpalpable spleens were involved by lymphoma at staging laparotomy. Staging laparotomy has been replaced by imaging studies; positron emission tomography, in particular, provides an accurate determination.[57]

Non-Hodgkin lymphomas of different types involve the spleen with variable frequency. Splenic involvement is particularly frequent in low-grade B-cell lymphomas. As mentioned earlier, evaluation of splenic hilar lymph nodes is very important. Histologic findings of lymphoma that are ambiguous or incompletely diagnostic in splenic sections may be more distinctive in splenic hilar lymph nodes. Liver involvement by lymphoma is rare in the absence of splenic disease.

PRECURSOR LYMPHOID NEOPLASMS

Although enlargement of the spleen often occurs during the course of either B-lymphoblastic or T-lymphoblastic malignancies, it rarely approaches clinical significance. The histopathologic features are similar to those of other leukemic disorders, with diffuse infiltration of the red pulp by blast cells.[5]

SYSTEMIC OR SECONDARY MATURE B-CELL LYMPHOMAS AND LEUKEMIAS

Most B-cell lymphomas involve the spleen in one of two main patterns: with uniform nodular expansion of the white pulp, as seen in small B-cell lymphomas such as chronic lymphocytic leukemia/small lymphocytic lymphoma (CLL/SLL), splenic marginal zone lymphoma, mantle cell lymphoma, and follicular lymphoma (Fig. 58-6); or with the formation

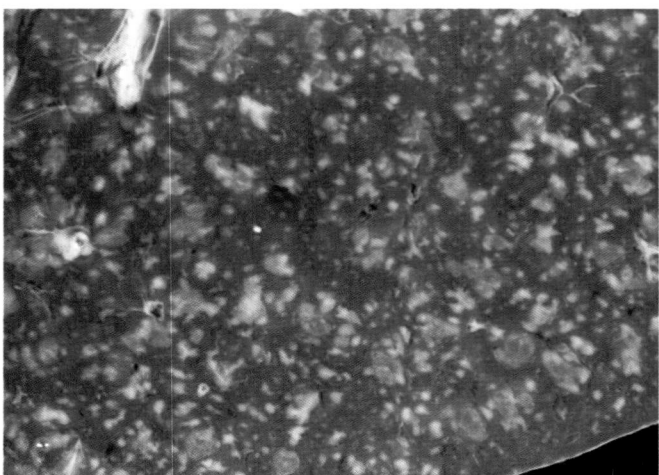

Figure 58-6. Gross photograph of miliary involvement of the spleen by low-grade B-cell lymphoma. This is an exaggeration of the normal white pulp appearance and is seen in lymphomas that preferentially involve the white pulp.

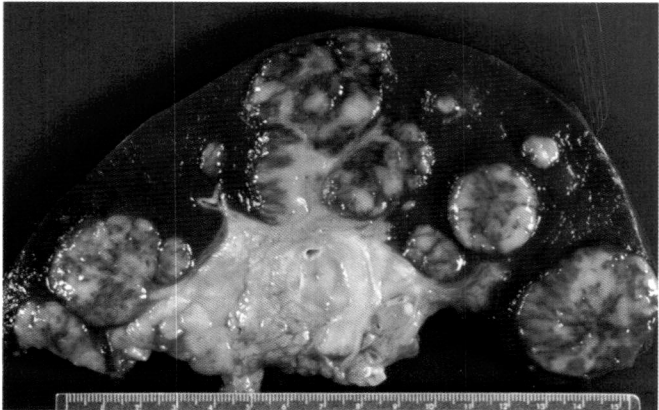

Figure 58-7. Gross photograph of diffuse large B-cell lymphoma involving the spleen. Large single or multiple tumor masses are not typically seen in low-grade lymphomas; they are more common in more aggressive lymphomas.

of single or multiple tumor masses, as seen in most cases of diffuse large B-cell lymphoma (DLBCL) (Fig. 58-7).[5,19] Occasionally, the spleen is the site of large-cell transformation of a low-grade B-cell lymphoma (Fig. 58-8).

Splenomegaly is often a common presenting feature for secondary involvement of the spleen by mature B-cell lymphoma and leukemia and is particularly common in patients with B-cell prolymphocytic leukemia and lymphoplasmacytic lymphoma. Although the gross and histologic patterns of splenic involvement of the various mature B-cell lymphomas and leukemia may vary, the morphologic and immunophenotypic features are similar to those described in other sites. The reader is referred to the various chapters specific to the mature B-cell lymphomas and leukemias elsewhere in this text, including the nonnodal type of mantle cell lymphoma[58] that is associated with prominent splenomegaly without adenopathy (see Chapter 21). Three fairly distinctive patterns of splenic infiltration have been described in DLBCL. DLBCL in the spleen characteristically produces solitary or multiple tumor masses that are usually

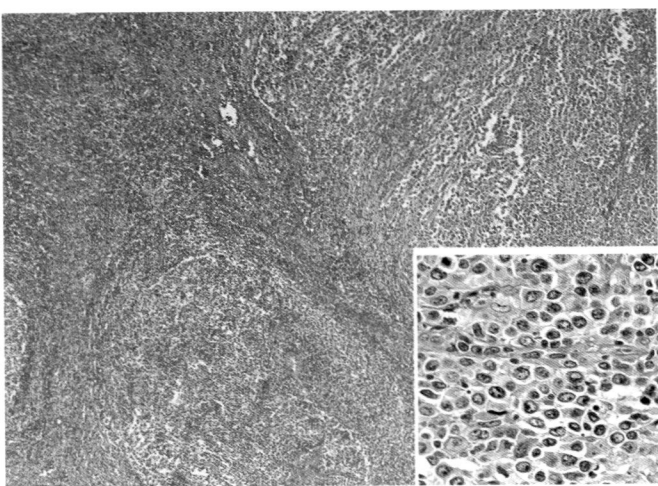

Figure 58-8. Low-power photomicrograph of follicular lymphoma *(lower left)* transforming to diffuse large B-cell lymphoma *(upper right)*. *Inset,* Higher magnification of the large-cell lymphoid component shows cytologic features consistent with a centroblastic subtype.

well demarcated and may show areas of necrosis. Predominant diffuse, red pulp involvement, however, may be observed in a small subset of cases,[47,59-62] with features similar to intravascular large B-cell lymphoma of other sites. Finally, a micronodular pattern of infiltration by T-cell/histiocyte-rich large B-cell lymphoma may occur and often mimics a reactive process. The spleen in these micronodular cases is markedly enlarged, but without distinct nodules. Small aggregates of lymphocytes and histiocytes are distributed in the red pulp and white pulp. The histiocytes are especially abundant, and neoplastic large B cells may be difficult to identify without the use of immunohistochemical studies.[60]

PRIMARY B-CELL LYMPHOID NEOPLASMS PRESENTING WITH PROMINENT SPLENOMEGALY

Several types of B-cell lymphoma/leukemia are primary to the spleen. These include splenic marginal zone lymphoma, splenic diffuse red pulp small B-cell lymphoma, hairy cell leukemia variant, and hairy cell leukemia. Because these disorders represent distinct clinical or provisional entities, such descriptions are not duplicated here; they are covered in specific chapters in this text that provide detailed descriptions of the splenic findings (see Chapters 15 and 16).

MATURE T-CELL AND NATURAL KILLER–CELL NEOPLASMS

Mature T-cell and NK-cell malignancies are relatively uncommon, and few studies have focused on the splenic pathology. Among the nonleukemic forms, splenic involvement is relatively common in cases of advanced-stage mycosis fungoides/Sézary syndrome. Splenic involvement in mycosis fungoides usually affects the white pulp and red pulp alike.[63] The marginal zones and the periarteriolar lymphoid sheaths are infiltrated by large, atypical cells, associated with both diffuse and patchy nodular involvement of the red pulp.[63,64] Not all cells have cerebriform nuclear contours, and a variable proportion of the tumor cells may appear blastic.

The node-based peripheral T-cell lymphomas (PTCLs) are perhaps the least-studied group of T-cell neoplasms that occur in the spleen. The pattern of splenic involvement in these diseases is different from that in B-cell lymphomas and is centered more on the red pulp.[18,65-67] We have seen a variety of patterns of involvement—some expanding the periarteriolar lymphoid sheath, some producing discrete masses, and one mimicking the pattern seen in mycosis fungoides. The lymphoepithelioid cell (Lennert) variant,[68] a cytologic subtype of PTCL, not otherwise specified, is characterized by a high content of epithelioid histiocytes. Early involvement usually occurs in the peripheral zones of follicles and the periarteriolar lymphoid sheaths, consistent with the T-cell origin of this lymphoma. The epithelioid histiocytes tend to localize in a ringlike arrangement at the periphery of the white pulp, but they occasionally form clusters.[68] Although originally thought to be characteristic of this type of lymphoma, the ringlike arrangement of epithelioid cells may be seen in other forms of both B-cell and T-cell lymphoma. The epithelioid cells may be difficult to differentiate from the sarcoid type of granulomas sometimes seen in the spleens of patients with Hodgkin lymphoma. Some cases of PTCL with marked splenomegaly have been associated with hemophagocytic syndrome.[69,70] In these cases, expansion of the red pulp predominates, and the erythrophagocytic histiocytes may overshadow the neoplastic T cells. A hemophagocytic syndrome may be seen with both T-cell and NK-cell malignancies, many of which are associated with EBV.

T-CELL LYMPHOID NEOPLASMS PRESENTING WITH PROMINENT SPLENOMEGALY

Several types of T-cell lymphomas and leukemias present with splenomegaly and distinct clinicopathologic characteristics, but these are discussed elsewhere in this text. Hepatosplenic T-cell lymphoma (see Chapter 33) and T-cell prolymphocytic leukemia (see Chapter 31) both present with pronounced splenomegaly and diffuse red pulp infiltration. T-cell large granular lymphocytic leukemia (see Chapter 30) also involves splenic red pulp but in contrast with the former two, spares the white pulp and often has less splenic enlargement.

MYELOID NEOPLASMS

Red pulp disease is characteristic of splenic involvement in leukemic processes (Fig. 58-9).[5,71] The leukemic cells usually appear localized to the cords of Billroth, with secondary involvement of the sinuses. Peritrabecular and subendothelial deposits may be seen early in the course of leukemic infiltration. Although splenic involvement is invariable in leukemic disorders, the degree of splenomegaly depends on the type of leukemia and the duration of the disease. The acute leukemias usually result in only mild-to-moderate splenic enlargement, but the chronic leukemias may produce prominent splenomegaly that often results in hypersplenism. Peripheral cytopenias may necessitate splenectomy, which may be effective in ameliorating the cytopenias but usually does not affect the course of the underlying disease. Splenic rupture is an occasional complication of leukemia. This is thought to result from tumor cells infiltrating the trabecular framework

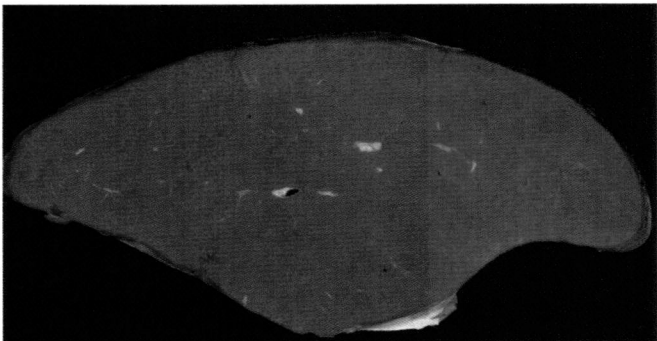

Figure 58-9. Leukemic involvement of the spleen. Disorders characterized by red pulp involvement, such as acute and chronic leukemias, produce a uniform red to purple appearance. The normal white pulp nodularity is typically absent.

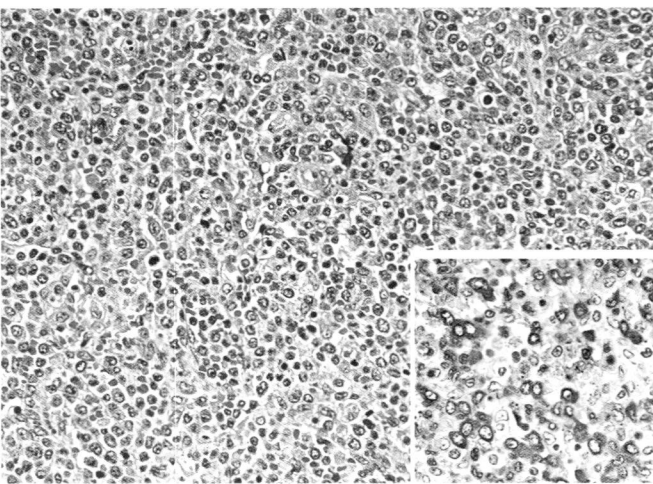

Figure 58-10. Left-shifted granulocytic hyperplasia in the spleen induced by granulocyte colony-stimulating factor. The red pulp is diffusely occupied by promyelocytes and other immature granulocytic forms, a finding that could be interpreted as evidence of acute myeloid leukemia. *Inset,* Myeloperoxidase immunostain highlights the myeloid cells.

and vascular structure of the organ or from infarction within the spleen. Rupture of the spleen is far more common in the chronic leukemias (particularly chronic myeloid leukemia) than in the acute forms.[72]

Splenectomy is rarely performed in patients with the various types of acute myeloid leukemia (AML) (see Chapter 46), and a primary diagnosis of AML is very unusual in that setting. Splenectomy caused by massive splenomegaly is relatively common, however, in patients with some myeloproliferative neoplasms (MPNs). For this reason, a more detailed description of the splenic changes in these disorders is provided.

Myeloproliferative Neoplasms

The MPNs are a group of chronic, interrelated clonal disorders of the hematopoietic stem cell.[73,74] These disorders include polycythemia vera, primary myelofibrosis, essential thrombocythemia, and chronic myeloid leukemia. A variable degree of splenomegaly occurs in all these disorders. Although each has its own somewhat distinctive "splenic" characteristics,[75] a precise diagnostic subtyping of the MPNs cannot be based on a morphologic examination of the spleen alone; this requires relevant clinical and laboratory data, as well as an examination of bone marrow and peripheral blood smears. The reader is directed to Chapter 47 for a more detailed description of the diagnostic criteria for each disorder.

Chronic Myeloid Leukemia

Chronic myeloid leukemia (CML) is frequently associated with massive splenomegaly. The cut surface of the spleen is deep red, without visible white pulp, because CML generally obliterates the lymphoid follicles, although small remnants of white pulp are occasionally seen.[5] Infarcts are common because of subendothelial invasion of the splenic trabecular veins, and fibrosis of the cords may be prominent. Histologic examination reveals a polymorphic cellular infiltrate in the red pulp, which includes myeloid cells at all stages of maturation.[5] The identification of immature myeloid cells (i.e., promyelocytes, myelocytes) can be facilitated with immunohistochemical stains for CD34, CD117, CD68 (or CD68R), and myeloperoxidase (or lysozyme) in combination with the enzymatic chloroacetate esterase reaction (Leder stain); the latter is particularly strongly expressed in promyelocytes. Localized collections of ceroid-containing

histiocytes (pseudo–Gaucher cells), similar to those seen in the bone marrow, may also be observed in the spleens of CML patients.

CML may terminate with the development of an accelerated or blastic phase that resembles de novo acute leukemia. Approximately one-third of cases of blast crisis arise in an extramedullary site, most commonly the spleen. Blast crisis in CML may result in a dramatic increase in spleen size.[76] Several studies have indicated that the myeloid cells in the spleen develop additional cytogenetic abnormalities before this occurs in such cells at other sites,[77-82] and they may proliferate in the spleen more rapidly than at other sites of blastic transformation.[82] Gross examination may reveal a homogeneous cut surface or, in some cases, discrete nodules that represent discrete collections of blasts.[5] Most often the blasts are myeloblasts, although they are lymphoblasts in approximately 25% of cases and megakaryoblasts or erythroblasts in rare cases. Immunohistochemistry with a panel of antibodies that includes both myeloid- and lymphoid-associated antigens (e.g., CD34, CD117, CD68, myeloperoxidase, CD42b [or CD61], TdT, CD79a [or PAX5], CD10, and CD3) may be helpful in confirming the presence of an increased number of blasts and in identifying their lineage.

Therapy with colony-stimulating factors (e.g., granulocyte colony-stimulating factor) may simulate splenic involvement with CML or another myeloid neoplasm (Fig. 58-10) or, occasionally, may even mimic extramedullary acute myeloid leukemia.[83] Rarely, the administration of this cytokine has been associated with splenic rupture.[83]

Polycythemia Vera

Splenomegaly occurs in the majority of patients with polycythemia vera. The degree of splenomegaly in the erythrocytotic phase of polycythemia vera is usually mild or moderate; the size of the spleen roughly correlates with the duration of the disease.[84-87] In approximately 15% of cases, however, polycythemia vera evolves to a spent phase, also called *postpolycythemic myeloid metaplasia,* in which the development of severe fibrosis in the bone marrow is accompanied by leukoerythroblastosis in the peripheral blood and marked splenomegaly.[75,88,89]

Although it was previously thought that splenic enlargement in polycythemia vera results from myeloid metaplasia, it has been demonstrated that extramedullary hematopoiesis is not a feature of this disease before the development of reticulin fibrosis in the bone marrow.[88] Spleens in the erythrocytotic phase show intense congestion of the cords of Billroth and the sinuses of the red pulp, accompanied by a proliferation of cordal macrophages without significant myeloid metaplasia. In contrast, spleens obtained from patients whose disease has evolved to postpolycythemic myeloid metaplasia show prominent myeloid metaplasia indistinguishable from that observed in cases of de novo primary myelofibrosis.[88,89]

Primary Myelofibrosis

The degree of splenomegaly seen in cases of primary myelofibrosis (PMF), formerly termed *agnogenic myeloid metaplasia* or *idiopathic myelofibrosis with myeloid metaplasia*, is most striking among the MPNs. In fibrotic phase PMF, splenomegaly is associated with fibrosis in the bone marrow (graded at least as MF2) and the presence of leukoerythroblastosis (circulating erythroblasts in association with immature myeloid cells—usually myelocytes or metamyelocytes) and teardrop erythrocytes in the peripheral blood.[89,90] Symptoms related to massive enlargement of the organ may be the presenting feature of this disorder. The degree of splenomegaly correlates with disease duration.[85,86,89] Increasing splenomegaly may be arrested, but only transiently, by splenic irradiation or chemotherapy. Spleen size can be decreased by *JAK2* inhibitory therapy.[91]

Splenomegaly in overt PMF results from the presence of clonal extramedullary hematopoiesis in the red pulp, also known as myeloid metaplasia. On gross examination, the spleen is enlarged and purple-red, with indistinct white pulp markings. Infarcts are common. In some cases, however, focal proliferations with grossly recognizable nodules, usually composed predominantly of one cell type, are observed.[5] Microscopic examination usually reveals multiple foci of extramedullary hematopoiesis distributed throughout the red pulp sinuses and in the splenic cords (Fig. 58-11; Table 58-3). Extramedullary hematopoiesis may be accompanied by a variable degree of fibrosis.

Histologically, although the hematopoiesis is always trilinear, one cell line may predominate in a given case.[75,82] Erythroid precursors occur in easily recognizable clusters, frequently in the sinuses. Megakaryocytes show the same atypical features as those seen in the bone marrow, with clusters of large, often bizarre forms. Although granulocytic precursors may be difficult to distinguish from cordal macrophages, they can be recognized in touch imprints or in tissue sections by using the immunoperoxidase technique with antibodies to myeloperoxidase or lysozyme.[75] Extramedullary hematopoiesis is accompanied by a proliferation of cordal macrophages, and phagocytosis of hematopoietic precursors may be seen.[5] The trilinear nature of the hematopoiesis seen in PMF aids in distinguishing this disorder from other types of myeloid neoplasms (e.g., CML). Blastic transformation in PMF may be heralded by an increase in immature cells. In these cases, the identification of an increased proportion of blasts can be facilitated by the use of appropriate immunohistochemical

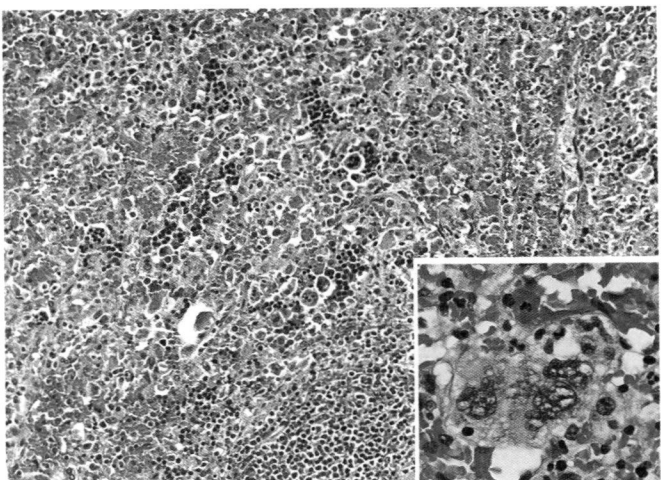

Figure 58-11. Extramedullary hematopoiesis in the spleen in a case of primary myelofibrosis. High-power photograph shows atypical megakaryocytes with cloudlike nuclear morphology and abnormally clumped chromatin *(inset).* When reactive versus hematopoietic neoplasm–associated extramedullary hematopoiesis is compared, the presence of atypical megakaryocytes favors a clonal hematopoietic process.

Table 58-3 Evaluation of Myeloid Metaplasia in the Spleen

	Etiology	Hematopoiesis
Benign	Hypersplenism caused by non-neoplastic causes	Typically trilineage, without atypia
	"Hematopoietic" hemolytic anemias and other anemias	Predominantly erythroid, with occasional megakaryocytes
	Cytokine induced (e.g., G-CSF)	Predominantly myeloid; may simulate acute myeloid leukemia (including acute promyelocytic leukemia)
	Lymphoma, other malignancies (carcinoma, sarcoma)	Variable degrees of trilineage, without atypia
Clonal	MPN	Usually trilineage; occasionally one lineage predominant; atypia seen in megakaryocytes; may represent initial site of blast transformation
	MDS/MPN	Overlapping findings of both MPN and MDS
	MDS	Usually trilineage, occasionally with increased monocytes-macrophages; dysplasia seen in megakaryocytes; increased immature myeloid blasts may herald blast transformation

G-CSF, Granulocyte colony-stimulating factor; *MDS,* myelodysplastic syndrome; *MPN,* myeloproliferative neoplasm.

stains, as previously described. In addition to CML, the differential diagnosis of myeloid metaplasia in the spleen includes various disorders associated with bone marrow fibrosis and peripheral blood leukoerythroblastosis. Metastatic carcinoma and infectious disorders that involve the bone marrow are well-known causes of bone marrow fibrosis that may mimic PMF to a certain extent. Others that are much less frequent include myelodysplastic syndrome (MDS),[92] myelodysplastic/myeloproliferative neoplasms (MDS/MPN) such as chronic myelomonocytic leukemia,[93] and juvenile myelomonocytic leukemia (Fig. 58-12).[94]

Essential Thrombocythemia

Essential thrombocythemia is characterized by a marked megakaryocytic proliferation in the bone marrow associated with thrombocytosis.[74,90] Clinical manifestations include hemorrhagic or, less commonly, thrombotic phenomena.[95] The degree of splenomegaly in essential thrombocythemia is usually less marked than that seen in the other chronic myeloproliferative disorders, and hypersplenism is not a common clinical manifestation. Because of the scarcity of splenectomy specimens, there are no large studies of the splenic pathology in essential thrombocythemia. In the few cases studied, the most notable finding was widening of the cords of Billroth, which may appear hypocellular at low power because of the presence of large masses of platelets, which may also be seen in the sinuses. Touch preparations of the spleen may be useful for demonstrating the sequestration of platelets. Although mild to moderate, splenomegaly is characteristic of most cases of essential thrombocythemia. In advanced cases, the spleen may become atrophic and nonfunctional, with atrophy probably resulting from infarction caused by the pooling of platelets.[96] The presence of fibrosis and microinfarcts (Gamna-Gandy bodies) may mimic the morphology of the spleen in advanced sickle cell disease. In our experience, no significant extramedullary hematopoiesis is seen. Occasionally, however, in the rare cases of essential thrombocythemia evolving to myelofibrosis, significant myeloid metaplasia reportedly occurs in the spleen.

Other Chronic Myeloid Neoplasms

Other types of myeloid neoplasms may produce splenomegaly. This complication is more likely to be associated with MDS/MPNs such as chronic myelomonocytic leukemia or juvenile myelomonocytic leukemia.[93,94] In these cases, the splenic red pulp contains an increased number of myelomonocytic cells (see Fig. 58-12). An increased number of blasts can be seen in cases undergoing acute transformation. Immunohistochemistry may be helpful to confirm the diagnosis and is necessary to confirm acute transformation. Aggregates of mature plasmacytoid dendritic cells (plasmacytoid monocytes) can also be observed in cases of chronic myelomonocytic leukemia[97,98] and in other types of myeloid neoplasms.

SYSTEMIC MASTOCYTOSIS

The spleen is usually involved in systemic mastocytosis (reviewed more completely in Chapter 49), although the degree of splenomegaly is frequently only mild to moderate.[99-102] The pattern of involvement of the spleen in mast cell disease is variable.[99-102] Early involvement may preferentially localize to paratrabecular areas or to the marginal zones of the white pulp. A characteristic fibroblastic reaction resulting in a concentric rimming of the lymphoid follicles may be observed (Fig. 58-13). Some investigators have reported a diffuse infiltration of the red pulp, and multinodular perivascular infiltrates have also been described.[102] Increased eosinophils are associated with the mast cell aggregates. Mast cells typically appear cuboid or spindle shaped, with pale nuclei and grayish cytoplasm. Mast cell granules can be demonstrated with chloroacetate esterase stain and are metachromatic with toluidine blue and Giemsa stains, although neoplastic mast cells are often hypogranular. Tryptase and CD117 positivity are helpful in confirming splenic involvement, particularly in cases associated with a marked fibroblastic reaction and relatively rare mast cells. Systemic mast cell disease may be associated with other clonal hematologic disorders, most notably chronic myelomonocytic leukemia, MPN, MDS, or acute myeloid leukemia,[103,104] which may be present concurrently in the spleen. Their identification within the splenic red pulp can be facilitated by immunohistology for myeloid-associated antigens.

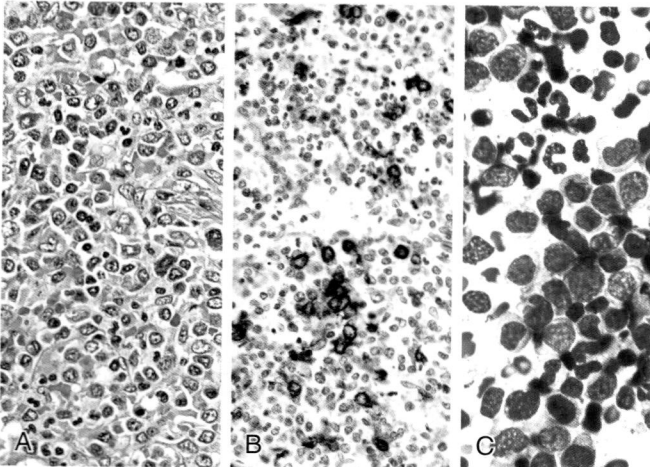

Figure 58-12. Juvenile myelomonocytic leukemia involving the spleen. A, The red pulp contains a polymorphic cellular population that includes blasts, other immature myeloid cells, monocytes, neutrophils, and eosinophils. **B,** CD34 stain highlights the presence of a variable proportion of blasts. **C,** Touch preparation of the spleen shows immature and mature granulocytic and monocytic cells (Wright-Giemsa stain).

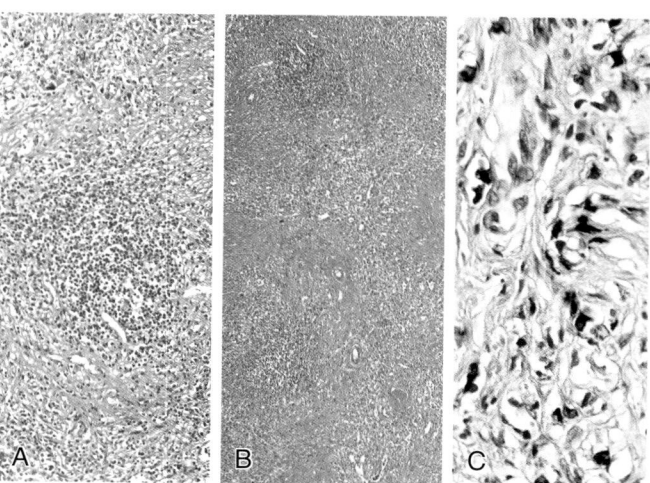

Figure 58-13. Systemic mastocytosis. A, Marked perifollicular fibrosis, with mast cells embedded in the fibrotic stroma. **B,** Perivascular, perifollicular, and trabecular fibrosis is often seen in mast cell disease in the spleen. **C,** Tryptase immunohistochemical stain highlights the mast cells entrapped in the sclerotic matrix.

PROLIFERATIONS OF THE MONOCYTE-MACROPHAGE SYSTEM

A variety of histiocytic and dendritic cell tumors may involve the spleen but have features similar to involvement in other sites. These are described in Chapters 51 and 52.

Hemophagocytic Syndromes

The hemophagocytic syndromes (HPSs) are a group of systemic disorders characterized by acute-onset pancytopenia caused by a proliferation of macrophages in lymphoreticular organs associated with prominent phagocytosis of hematopoietic elements (Box 58-2).[105,106] A familial (primary) form of HPS affecting infants and young children is termed *familial hemophagocytic lymphohistiocytosis.*[107] It is inherited in an autosomal recessive manner and is caused by the overwhelming activation of T lymphocytes and macrophages associated with defective triggering of apoptosis and reduced cytotoxic activity. Mutations in a variety of genes, including perforin *(PRF1)*, have been found in patients with familial hemophagocytic lymphohistiocytosis.[106,107] Most secondary cases of HPS are related to either infection or an NK-cell or T-cell neoplasm, most often EBV positive. These cases were once thought to represent malignant histiocytosis because of the acute clinical course culminating in death in many cases; the systemic distribution; and the striking proliferation of cells in all lymphoreticular organs. They are characterized by a proliferation of benign histiocytes demonstrating prominent hemophagocytosis. Patients exhibit fever and varying cytopenias in a clinical context of underlying viral infection or malignancy.[108,109] Cases associated with infection have been referred to as either viral-associated or, later, infection-associated HPS.[108]

The spleen in infection-associated HPS is moderately to markedly enlarged. The red pulp shows a proliferation of macrophages that display prominent hemophagocytosis, most characteristically of erythrocytes, but also of granulocytes, lymphocytes, and platelets. Fibrosis, focal infarctions, and gradual obliteration of the white pulp with B-cell depletion may occur.[5]

HPS-associated malignancies of the hematopoietic system differ morphologically because the spleen usually but not always contains a component of malignant cells. Lymphomas associated with HPS are most often of peripheral T-cell or NK-cell type.[109] Association with EBV is a major risk factor,

and HPS is a common complication of extranodal NK/T-cell lymphoma, aggressive NK-cell leukemia, and systemic EBV-positive lymphoproliferative disease of childhood associated with chronic active EBV infection. When only rare neoplastic T cells are found admixed with the numerous histiocytes, the resemblance to malignant histiocytosis may be marked (Fig. 58-14). The diagnosis of T-cell lymphoma in these cases usually requires molecular confirmation.

MESENCHYMAL TUMORS AND NON-NEOPLASTIC DISORDERS THAT MIMIC NEOPLASMS

Vascular tumors are the most common tumors of the spleen (Table 58-4) that typically involve the red pulp. They may be diffuse or form a tumor mass and are usually found incidentally on imaging.[110]

Splenic Hemangioma

Splenic hemangiomas may be capillary or cavernous and have morphologic features similar to those observed elsewhere. They are benign tumors that are usually asymptomatic; however, some cause splenomegaly, abdominal pain, and hypersplenism.[111-116] Localized hemangiomas are most common and form single or multiple tumor nodules that contain cystic blood-filled spaces lined by endothelial cells. Papillary projections and thrombi may occur. Localized hemangiomas form nodules that are usually surrounded by fibrosis and may show calcification. Most radiographic procedures, including computed tomographic scans and sonograms, are non-specific, but show discrete solid and cystic masses, and often show evidence of calcification. Diffuse hemangiomatosis of the spleen, which is less common, is often associated with systemic hemangiomatosis. Cases with massive splenomegaly are often associated with coagulopathies. Diffuse hemangiomatosis differs from peliosis by the presence of intervening fibrosis

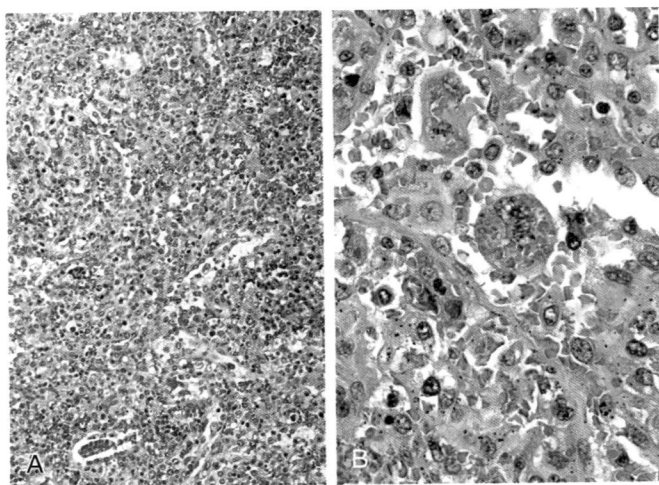

Figure 58-14. Peripheral T-cell lymphoma in the spleen associated with hemophagocytic syndrome. A, At low magnification, the findings are subtle. A variety of other disorders can be associated with hemophagocytosis in the spleen, most notably those with infectious or viral causes. **B,** Macrophage with ingested red blood cells *(center).* Also note the atypical-appearing lymphocytes, which proved to be T-cell lymphoma.

Box 58-2 *Disorders Associated With Hemophagocytosis in the Spleen*

Benign
- Storage diseases
- Congenital hemophagocytic syndromes
- Viral infections (Epstein-Barr, other viruses)
- Other infections (bacterial, fungal, rickettsial, parasitic)
- Autoimmune hemolytic anemia
- Drug-induced (e.g., fludarabine)

Malignant
- Histiocytic sarcoma (malignant histiocytosis)
- Hepatosplenic T-cell lymphoma
- Other peripheral T-cell lymphomas
- B-cell lymphomas

Table 58-4 Vascular and Other Nonhematopoietic Primary Splenic Tumors

Entity	Clinical Features	Pathologic Findings	Immunophenotype	Prognosis
Hamartoma	Rare, predominantly older adults, but all age groups affected; cytopenias are common	Nodular gross lesion, median size 5 cm. Numerous slitlike vascular channels lined by plump, flattened endothelial cells without white pulp	CD8+, vWF+, CD34+/–, CD21–, CD68–	Generally benign but possible risk for rupture in larger lesions
Hemangioma	Common benign tumor of the spleen, generally asymptomatic	Nonencapsulated <2 cm, vascular channels separated by red pulp and fibrous septae	CD31+, CD34+, vWF+, CD21–, CD68–, CD8–	Benign, but possible risk for rupture
Littoral cell angioma	Rare, often incidental finding	Numerous channel-like vascular spaces lined by plump cells that surround fibrovascular cores and luminal macrophages	CD31+, vWF+, ERG+, Langerin+, cyclin D1+, CD21+/–, CD68+/–, CD34–, CD8–	Benign, reported association with secondary malignancies
Lymphangioma	Rare, generally an isolated finding	Often subcapsular, variably sized cystic spaces with flat, bland endothelium filled with proteinaceous fluid	CD31+, CD34+/–, CD21–, CD8–, D2-40+	May recur if not completely excised
Hemangioendothelioma	Rare, controversial entity	Intermediate histology between benign hemangioma and angiosarcoma; the lining cells show mild to moderate atypia	CD31+, vWF+, CD34+/–, cytokeratin+/–	Generally indolent when resected
SANT	Rare, occurs in older adults (>50 years), generally asymptomatic; female-to-male ratio of 2:1	Red-tan, unencapsulated mass composed of nodules with slitlike round vascular spaces lined by plump endothelial cells and pericytes surrounded by densely collagenous fibrotic or fibrinoid granulomatous tissue	Three vascular patterns: CD34–, CD31+, CD8+ sinusoids; CD34+, CD31+, CD8– capillaries; CD34–, CD31+, CD8– veins. CD68 expression is variable	Indolent and benign with no tendency for recurrence after splenectomy
Angiosarcoma	Most common nonlymphoid malignancy of the spleen	Typically multifocal, with irregular anastomosing vascular channels with marked atypia, frequent mitoses, and invasion of surrounding stroma	CD31+, CD34+	Malignant lesion with high rate of dissemination
EBV-positive inflammatory follicular dendritic cell/fibroblastic reticular cell tumor	Rare, presents with fever and abdominal pain	Scarlike lesion composed of myofibroblastic spindle cells with mixed inflammatory cells (lymphocytes, plasma cells, eosinophils)	Spindle cells: EBV+, vimentin+, CD21+/–, CD34–, CD8–, ALK1–	Low-grade tumor that may recur or metastasize if not completely resected

EBV, Epstein-Barr virus; *SANT,* sclerosing angiomatoid nodular transformation.

in hemangiomatosis, whereas more normal splenic tissue is present between the vascular spaces of peliosis. The differential diagnosis of hemangioma includes lymphangioma and primary splenic cyst; however, localized lymphangiomas and primary splenic cysts of the spleen usually contain proteinaceous fluid rather than the blood of a hemangioma. In addition, diffuse lymphangiomatosis may be localized to the spleen, but is usually a systemic process and most commonly occurs in children and young adults with massive splenomegaly.

Cord capillary hemangiomas are splenic capillary hemangiomas displaying a proliferation of small vessels associated with increased numbers of histiocytes and fibrosis. They form circumscribed nodules displaying a lobular pattern both grossly and histologically. They can be differentiated

from other stromal proliferations by immunohistochemistry, highlighting the vascular nature of the lesion with expression of CD34, but not CD8.[117-119] This entity was first described by Krishnan and Frizzera[119] and was thought by these authors to represent a subtype of splenic hamartoma. More recently, however, clonality demonstrated in a few cases suggests that they represent true vascular tumors.[117]

Littoral Cell Angioma

Littoral cell angioma is a tumor that is unique to the spleen.[113,120] It may occur at any age and usually causes mild to moderate splenomegaly. As its name suggests, it is a tumor presumably derived from the littoral cells lining the sinus channels, but the tumor immunophenotype differs slightly from this presumed normal counterpart. Grossly, the spleen shows diffuse multinodularity with spongy, dark red nodules that can measure up to 9 cm in diameter. Rarely, it may present as a single, large mass. Histologically, the vascular spaces are lined by plump cells with nuclear enlargement and often show papillary areas with lining cells sloughing into the vascular spaces (Fig. 58-15). The lining cells of littoral cell angioma have a unique immunophenotype, expressing vascular, histiocytic, and dendritic-associated markers CD31, ERG, CD68, CD163, and at least focal CD21. Expression of Langerin and cyclin D1 have been described on the lining cells.[121] The actual lining cells are CD34 negative, and unlike normal splenic sinus lining cells, they do not express CD8. The differential diagnosis includes hemangioma and angiosarcoma. Hemangiomas of the spleen express CD34 and usually lack the nuclear enlargement of littoral cell angioma. Angiosarcomas show more cytologic atypia than littoral cell angiomas, as well as mitotic figures and necrosis, features that are not present in littoral cell angioma. Most cases of littoral cell angioma are treated with splenectomy without recurrence. Rare cases with foci containing a solid clear-cell proliferation have metastasized many years later, and such cases probably represent a rare controversial entity termed *littoral cell hemangioendothelioma*.[122,123] Other rare variants have also been reported (some are mostly pediatric).

Splenic Angiosarcoma

Splenic angiosarcoma is a rare tumor[113,124] that occurs most commonly in adults; fewer than 200 cases have been reported. It is usually associated with splenomegaly, abdominal pain, and cytopenias, and splenic rupture is seen in up to 30% of cases. Because most angiosarcomas involving the spleen are high-grade sarcomas with dissemination, it is often difficult to determine whether the splenic tumor is primary or secondary. The tumor typically forms a large infiltrating solid mass but can also form a network of anastomosing vascular channels (Fig. 58-16). Areas of cystic hemorrhage are sometimes present. Although the histologic appearance may be varied, angiosarcomas characteristically show atypical "hobnail" lining cells within vessels, high mitotic activity, and necrosis (Fig. 58-17). Many cases may be difficult to differentiate from other high-grade sarcomas, and immunohistochemical detection of vascular antigen expression, such as CD31, CD34, ERG, FLI1, VEGF, and von Willebrand factor, is necessary to diagnose such cases. The differential diagnosis includes cavernous hemangioma, normal splenic sinuses, or other sarcomas, including Kaposi sarcoma. Immunostains for CD34, CD8, or HHV-8 can usually distinguish angiosarcoma from littoral cell angioma and Kaposi sarcoma, and the presence of necrosis or mitotic activity essentially excludes littoral cell angioma. High-grade angiosarcomas involving the spleen have a generally poor prognosis, and most patients die of disease within 1 year of diagnosis; however, rare cares with long-term survival after splenectomy are reported.

Splenic Lymphangioma

Lymphangiomas of the spleen are uncommon tumors that often present as an isolated nodule or diffusely throughout the spleen, often in the setting of a patient with lymphangiomatosis.[125,126]

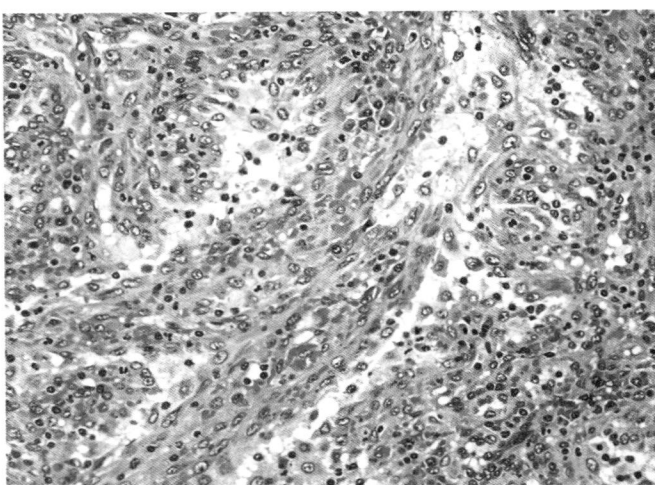

Figure 58-15. Littoral cell angioma with vascular spaces lined by plump endothelial cells lacking cytologic atypia. Sinus lining cells desquamate into the vascular lumens.

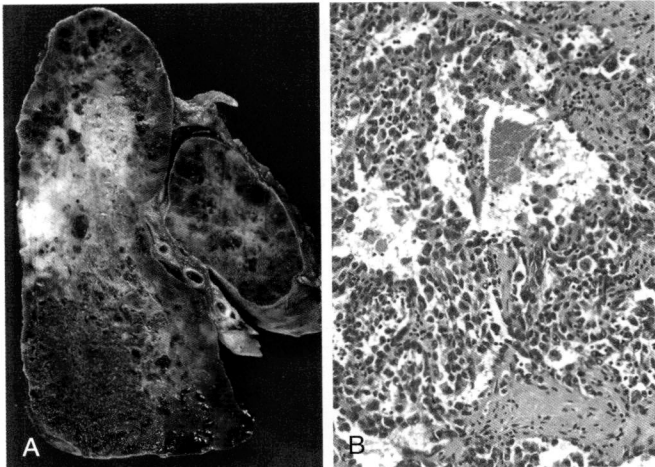

Figure 58-16. Gross **(A)** and microscopic **(B)** images of angiosarcoma of the spleen. Note the mixture of spongy, dark red cystic areas and more malignant-looking solid areas.

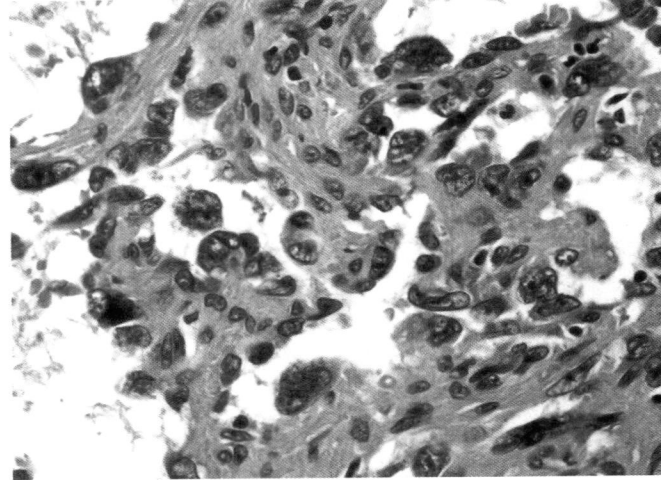

Figure 58-17. **Photomicrograph of splenic angiosarcoma.** The marked cellular pleomorphism is consistent with a diagnosis of angiosarcoma. Note the irregular, anastomosing appearance of the vascular channels.

The localized tumors are subcapsular, whereas diffuse proliferations may involve the entire spleen. Three histologic categories are recognized: cystic, cavernous, and simple or capillary. Cystic lymphangiomas are most common and show thin-walled cysts of variable size filled with serous fluid. The endothelial cells are positive for CD31 and D2-40 and often focally positive for CD34, but negative for CD21 and CD68. These are benign lesions that often are found incidentally and require no treatment.

Small, subcapsular cystic proliferations that are incidental findings in splenectomy specimens have been assumed to be localized lymphangiomas, but most are now known to have keratin-positive lining cells and represent small mesothelial primary cysts rather than lymphangiomas.[126]

Sclerosing Angiomatoid Nodular Transformation of the Spleen

Sclerosing angiomatoid nodular transformation (SANT) is a non-neoplastic vascular lesion of the spleen.[127-130] The median age at presentation is 54 years but ranges from 22 to 74 years. Most patients are asymptomatic, and a mass is only found incidentally; however, as many as 16% of patients complain of abdominal pain. A female predominance is seen with a female-to-male ratio of 2:1. A small subset of patients may have leukocytosis, an elevated erythrocyte sedimentation rate, and a polyclonal gammopathy.

The spleen is generally normal to slightly enlarged in size and on cut cross-section reveals a single red-tan, unencapsulated mass with a central stellate fibrous stroma and fibrous septa in areas surrounding multiple red-brown nodules. Although some nodules are outlined by densely collagenous fibrotic tissue, others are circumscribed by a fibrinoid rim that can give them a granulomatoid appearance (Fig. 58-18). Within the nodules, numerous slitlike round vascular spaces are seen that are lined by plump endothelial cells and pericytes. Rare mitoses can be seen, but cellular atypia should not be prominent. The fibrosclerotic internodular spaces are composed of myofibroblasts, and a mixed inflammatory infiltrate is commonly seen including lymphocytes, plasma cells, and macrophages.

The vessels of SANT show three staining patterns: a splenic sinusoidal immunophenotype with vessels lined by CD34⁻/CD31⁺/CD8⁺ endothelial cells, a capillary-like immunophenotype with vessels lined by CD34⁺/CD31⁺/CD8⁻ endothelial cells, and a venous immunophenotype with vessels lined by CD34⁻/CD31⁺/CD8⁻ endothelial cells. CD68 expression within nodules can also be demonstrated. These staining patterns are reminiscent of normal vasculature of red pulp vessels. The most sclerotic areas are often devoid of CD8-positive sinusoids. A background of scattered IgG4-positive plasma cells in the fibrosclerotic stroma is also seen.

The differential diagnosis of SANT includes other vascular lesions of the spleen, as well as nodular transformation of the splenic red pulp in response to metastatic carcinoma, and inflammatory pseudotumor. The nodular pattern with three different vessel types differentiates this proliferation from the others in the differential diagnosis. These proliferations are considered indolent, with no tendency for recurrence after splenectomy. Although many cases of SANT have admixed, IgG4-positive plasma cells,[130] SANT is not considered to be part of the spectrum of IgG4-related diseases.

Peliosis

Peliosis of the spleen is a rare proliferation of dilated blood-filled cavities.[131] Although it is more common in the liver, the spleen is occasionally a site of disease. Secondary conditions,

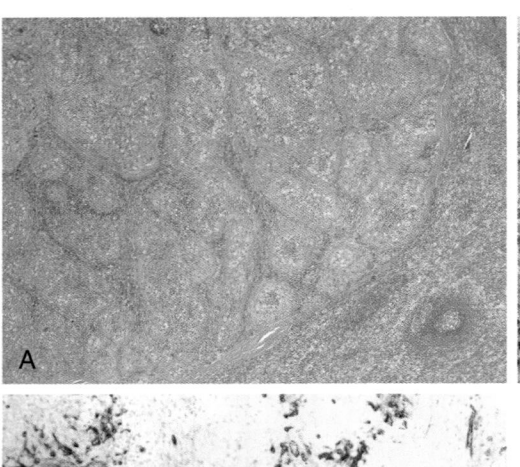
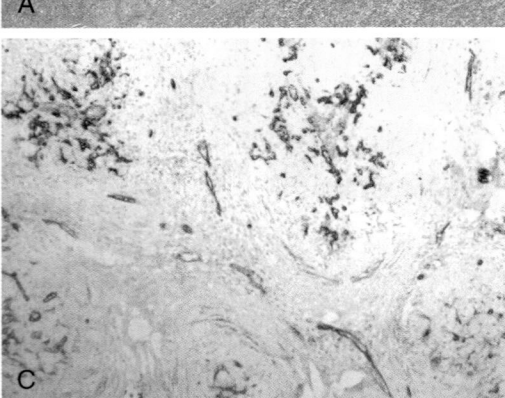
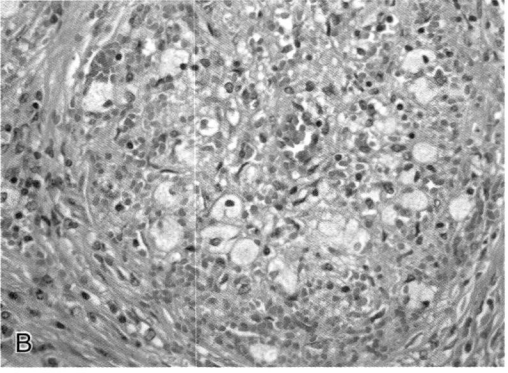

Figure 58-18. Sclerosing angiomatoid nodular transformation. A, The lesion is multinodular, with slitlike spacing surrounded by dense sclerosis. The gross appearance mimics inflammatory pseudotumor, but histologically, the distinction is usually not difficult. The lesion is sharply demarcated from adjacent spleen. **B,** Foam cells may be present in the nodules. **C,** The vascular slits within the nodules stain with CD34 and variably with CD31 and CD8 *(not shown).*

such as infections, particularly tuberculosis; malignant conditions, such as lymphomas and leukemias; and drug use, as in chemotherapy, can be associated with peliosis. Sections of the spleen demonstrate multiple round-to-oval, blood-filled cysts with or without sinusoidal endothelial lining cells. Peliosis differs from hemangiomas or hemangiomatosis by the lack of intervening fibrosis. In peliosis, the dilated vascular spaces are separated by normal-appearing splenic red pulp and white pulp. Peliosis may be associated with spontaneous splenic rupture.

Splenic Hamartoma

Hamartomas of the spleen are rare benign nodular lesions with an incidence of 0.13% and an equal occurrence in males and females.[113,132,133] It appears most commonly in older adults, but up to 20% of cases can occur in children. Clinically, patients may present with splenomegaly, thrombocytopenia, or with other symptoms of hypersplenism; however, 50% of cases will be asymptomatic. These lesions are generally less than 3 cm in size but rarely reach up to 18 cm in size, and they form a red bulging tumor on cut sections of the gross spleen (Fig. 58-19). By histology, they are indistinct lesions that mimic normal red pulp. They show numerous slitlike vascular channels lined by plump to flattened endothelial cells, with an absence of normal red pulp cords, lymphatic elements, or organized white pulp elements. The cells lining the spaces show an immunophenotype of normal sinusoids, with expression of CD8 and CD31; CD34 expression is variable. These cells lack CD21 and CD68. The differential diagnosis includes inflammatory pseudotumor, SANT, and benign vascular tumors, capillary hemangioma in particular; however, the lack of a distinct tumor nodule on histologic sections is a distinctive and characteristic finding only seen in splenic hamartoma. Although most cases are benign in behavior, with large lesions, there can be a risk for rupture. Splenectomy is the most frequent treatment for symptomatic hamartoma.

Although most authors consider splenic hamartoma to represent what is described earlier, Krishnan and Frizzera proposed four subtypes of splenic hamartoma: the classical type, cord capillary hemangioma, myoid angioendothelioma, and histiocyte-rich type.[119] They propose that each subtype presents with a dominant expression of one or more components of the splenic red pulp. The cord capillary type differs from the classical hamartoma because of its striking lobularity, bands of fibrosis, abundant plasma cells, and CD34-positive/CD8-negative phenotype of the vascular lining cells. This lesion may overlap with splenic capillary hemangioma with sclerosis. Clonality has been observed in some of these cases, which further suggests a true vascular origin for at least a subset of these cases.[117] The myoid angioendothelioma (originally described by Kraus and Dehner as benign vascular neoplasms of the spleen with myoid and angioendotheliomatous features) is a vascular lesion lined by CD34-positive cells, with prominent stromal cells positive for smooth muscle actin and muscle-specific actin.[134] The histiocyte-rich type has a predominance of histiocytes, including pseudosinuses lined by CD68-positive histiocytes, not endothelial cells. The latter two lesions are exceptionally rare. It is unclear whether the division into these subgroups has any clinical significance.

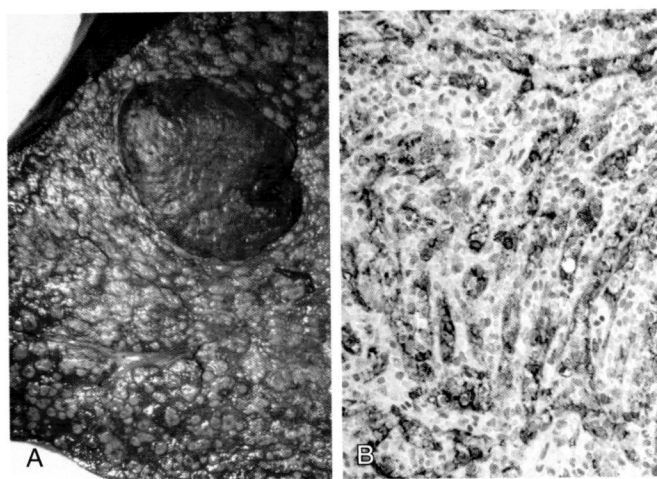

Figure 58-19. A, Gross photograph of a splenic hamartoma in a spleen removed for involvement by a low-grade B-cell lymphoma causing the background gross miliary pattern of infiltration. Note the well-circumscribed, bulging mass. The lesion consists of red pulp only and lacks white pulp. **B,** CD8 immunohistochemical stain highlights the splenic sinuses within the lesion.

EPSTEIN-BARR VIRUS—POSITIVE INFLAMMATORY FOLLICULAR DENDRITIC CELL/FIBROBLASTIC RETICULAR CELL TUMOR AND REACTIVE PSEUDOTUMORAL LESIONS OF THE SPLEEN

Epstein-Barr Virus–Positive Inflammatory Follicular Dendritic Cell/Fibroblastic Reticular Cell Tumor

Synonyms and Related Terms

WHO revised 4th ed.: Inflammatory Pseudotumor-Like Follicular/Fibroblastic Dendritic Cell Sarcoma

WHO proposed 5th ed.: EBV-Positive Inflammatory Follicular Dendritic Cell Sarcoma

Definition, Clinicopathologic Features, and Differential Diagnosis

Splenic and hepatic EBV-positive inflammatory follicular dendritic cell (FDC)/fibroblastic reticular cell (FRC) tumors (previously known as *inflammatory pseudotumor* or *inflammatory pseudotumor-like dendritic cell sarcoma*) are unique to these locations and differ from inflammatory pseudotumors or inflammatory myofibroblastic tumors at other sites.[135,136] They present predominantly in females as a fibroinflammatory process, often with fever and abdominal pain; a subset of cases are associated with a concomitant malignancy. The gross appearance of the spleen demonstrates a well-defined firm yellow-tan lesion without capsular extension; occasionally multiple nodules are seen (Fig. 58-20). Histologically it appears as a bland spindle cell myofibroblastic proliferation with interspersed variable amounts of collagenous stroma, and intervening abundant inflammatory cells including lymphocytes, plasma cells, histiocytes, and eosinophils. Foci of necrosis may be seen. The spindle cells in some, but not all, tumors express CD21, with other FDC markers including clusterin, CD23, and CD35 being more inconsistent. Unlike inflammatory pseudotumors in other organs, the spindled cells in the spleen are positive for EBV, and may express vimentin

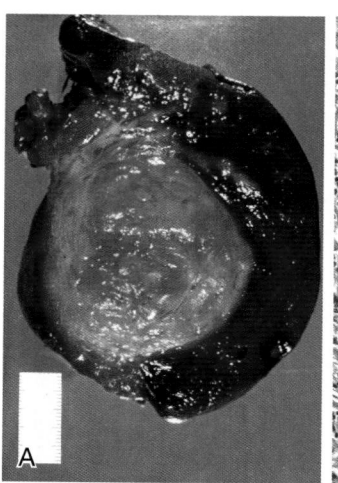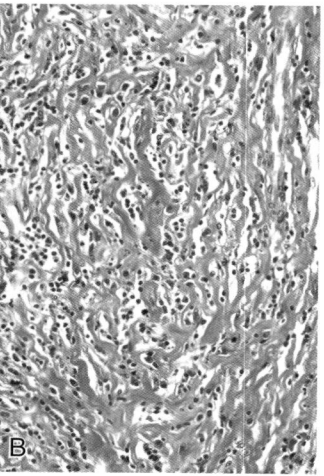

Figure 58-20. A, Gross photograph of an Epstein-Barr virus–positive inflammatory follicular dendritic cell/fibroblastic reticular cell tumor. The mass may mimic splenic involvement by a variety of malignancies, including Hodgkin and non-Hodgkin lymphomas. **B,** Microscopic appearance. This tumor has a predominance of fibrous bands, with a few spindle-shaped cells that are EBV positive *(not shown).* Mixed inflammatory cells and spindle cells may be more prominent in other cases.

and smooth muscle actin. The expression of smooth muscle actin may be indicative of a relationship to FRCs. Both FDCs and FRCs are mesenchymally derived stromal cells that may exhibit plasticity in their immunophenotype and function.[137] Thus, the spindle cells may express either FDC or FRC markers, but are always EBER positive. CD34 and CD8 are not expressed. All cases of EBV-positive inflammatory FDC/FRC tumor are negative for ALK1 in contrast to inflammatory myofibroblastic tumor of soft tissue, which is generally positive for ALK1. Splenectomy is curative for symptomatic cases, but cases that are partially resected may recur or rarely metastasize. Because most cases behave in a relatively indolent manner with resection, the International Consensus Classification (ICC) modified the name of this tumor to remove the "sarcoma" designation.[138]

Non-specific areas of fibrosis may mimic inflammatory pseudotumor in the spleen. Because they are generally reactive proliferations, it is important to distinguish them from EBV-positive inflammatory FDC/FRC tumor, which is a true neoplasm that may metastasize if not entirely resected. Areas of scarring after splenic infarction and hemorrhage (Gamna-Gandy bodies) are common in the spleens of children with sickle cell anemia, and fibrotic areas may occur after resolution of a splenic abscess or trauma.[139] SANTs often have areas of dense fibrosis with admixed (often IgG4-positive) plasma cells, but are EBV negative and do not contain FDC proliferations. Because of confusion caused by the term *inflammatory pseudotumor,* it is probably best to clarify that the reactive proliferations with fibrosis and inflammation are more inflammatory pseudotumor-like, with a clear statement that they do not represent a neoplastic proliferation.

SPLENIC CYSTS

One of the most common benign proliferations of the spleen is the splenic cyst.[140-142] These tumors have a male predominance and typically present in the 3rd decade of life. They are designated as primary (true) or secondary (false). Primary cysts represent approximately 20% of all splenic cysts. They

are unilocular and have a firm, fibrous, trabecular wall that is lined by mesothelial cells or squamous epithelium. Notably, the epithelial lining of primary cysts may be patchy, with denuded areas present that may simulate a secondary cyst. Primary cysts can be further subdivided into parasitic and nonparasitic types. Parasitic cysts, though uncommon, are typically attributable to *Echinococcus* and are readily identified by the presence of parasite scolices in the cyst contents. Nonparasitic primary cysts appear to arise from congenital inclusions of capsular mesothelium. Interestingly, patients with primary cysts may have elevations of CA19-9 and carcinoembryonic antigen (CEA). Treatment in symptomatic cases requires a complete splenectomy, as incomplete resection often leads to recurrence. Secondary cysts represent approximately 80% of splenic cysts and are often associated with a history of abdominal trauma. These are unilocular and thin walled and differ from primary cysts by the complete absence of an epithelial lining and are thus unlikely to recur even if only partially resected.

OTHER TUMORS

Primary sarcomas, other than angiosarcoma, and carcinomas of the spleen are extremely uncommon. Reported cases of sarcoma include malignant fibrous histiocytoma, fibrosarcoma, leiomyosarcoma, rhabdosarcoma, histiocytic sarcoma, interdigitating dendritic cell sarcoma, and FRC tumor.[141,143-149] Primary carcinomas reported include squamous cell carcinoma arising in a cyst, mucinous cystadenocarcinoma and carcinosarcoma, both possibly arising from peritoneal surface epithelium, and primary transitional cell carcinoma.[150-153] Although rare, carcinoma metastatic to the spleen or direct tumor extension are more common than primary disease. One-third of metastatic tumors are only identified on microscopic examination,[154] so the frequency of splenic involvement may be underestimated by imaging studies. Lung, gastric, ovarian, and breast carcinoma primaries are the most common to involve the spleen, and splenectomy may be performed for solitary splenic metastases.[155-157] Most metastases cause tumor masses, but some may infiltrate the organ diffusely (Fig. 58-21).

STORAGE DISEASES

The spleen is involved in many of the lysosomal storage diseases. These are predominantly autosomal recessive conditions whose diagnosis and classification are based on the enzymatic defect characteristic of each disease, often in combination with specific genetic testing. Although most of these conditions are rare, three of the lipid storage diseases are encountered (uncommonly) in surgical pathology practice. Gaucher and Niemann-Pick diseases, particularly in their nonneuronopathic forms, are the most common storage diseases encountered in removed spleens.[5,158,159] The significant splenomegaly observed in these cases may cause hypersplenism. Not uncommonly in these cases, the spleen is removed to confirm the diagnosis or to ameliorate cytopenias. Ceroid histiocytosis (sea-blue histiocytosis) can also be observed. Accumulation of sea-blue histiocytes may be seen in association with lipid disorders, infectious diseases, red blood cell disorders, and myeloproliferative disorders. However, it is also a prominent feature in spleens removed from patients with Hermansky-Pudlak syndrome, a rare, often fatal autosomal recessive condition that is currently

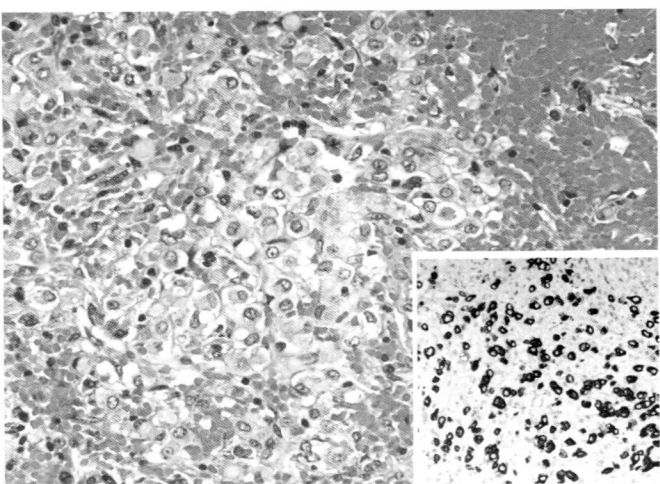

Figure 58-21. Signet ring carcinoma metastatic to the spleen. The malignant cells are strongly positive with a pan-cytokeratin immunostain *(inset).*

classified among the disorders of lysosome-related organelle biogenesis.[160]

In most storage disorders, affected spleens are usually pale and homogeneous in appearance. Rarely, areas of fibrosis are noted.[5] Microscopically, the red pulp is expanded because of the accumulation of numerous histiocytes in the splenic cords.[5]

Gaucher disease is the most common of the storage disorders. Gaucher cells range in size from 20 to 100 μm in diameter and have a fibrillar cytoplasm that appears brownish in hematoxylin and eosin (H&E)–stained preparations. Multinucleated cells may occur. The cytoplasm is intensely PAS positive, and this positivity is resistant to diastase digestion. The glucocerebroside in Gaucher cells is autofluorescent. Because Gaucher cells are macrophages and ingest red blood cells, they frequently stain positive for iron. Lipid stains are only weakly positive. Ultrastructural studies reveal numerous lysosomes containing characteristic lipid bilayers. Pseudo–Gaucher cells are often seen in the spleens of patients with CML.

Niemann-Pick cells are large, ranging from 20 to 100 μm in diameter, and appear foamy or bubbly because of numerous small vacuoles. They are clearer than Gaucher cells and usually stain only faintly with periodic acid–Schiff stain, but they contain neutral fat, as demonstrated by Sudan black B and oil red O stains. The lipid deposits are birefringent and, under ultraviolet light, display yellow-green fluorescence. Electron microscopy reveals lamellated structures resembling myelin figures within lysosomes.

In cases of ceroid histiocytosis, smaller histiocytes with more basophilic cytoplasm and vacuoles are characteristically seen. These cells can also be seen in Niemann-Pick disease. Ceroid-containing histiocytes measure up to 20 μm and contain cytoplasmic granules that measure 3 to 4 μm. The histiocytes show a variable degree of granulation. Foamy histiocytes with smaller, darker granules may also occur. Ceroid is composed of phospholipids and glycosphingolipids and is similar to lipofuscin in its physical and chemical properties. Histiocytes containing ceroid appear faintly yellow-brown in H&E–stained sections, but blue-green with Romanowsky

stains, resulting in the term *sea-blue histiocyte*. Ceroid is PAS-positive and resistant to diastase digestion and stains positive for lipid. It shows a strong affinity for basic dyes such as fuchsin and methylene blue. Ceroid is acid-fast and becomes autofluorescent with aging of the pigment. Ultrastructural studies reveal inclusions of lamellated membranous material with 4.5- to 5-nm periodicity.

None of the cell types identified in storage disorders is specific for a given disease, and their actual diagnosis should be based on biochemical or molecular genetic testing specific for these diseases.

Pearls and Pitfalls

- The most common primary splenic lymphomas—splenic marginal zone lymphoma and hepatosplenic T-cell lymphoma—tend to present with splenomegaly without peripheral lymphadenopathy and typically involve the bone marrow.
- Myeloid hyperplasia in the red pulp, which can mimic acute myeloid leukemia, may be caused by cytokines, particularly granulocyte colony-stimulating factor.
- Splenic hamartoma has distinct borders on gross examination, but the border of the lesion may be difficult to identify on microscopic examination.
- Littoral cell angioma has large lining cells with enlarged nucleoli, but fails to demonstrate mitotic activity or necrosis.
- Epstein-Barr virus (EBV)–positive inflammatory follicular dendritic cell/fibroblastic reticular cell tumor may mimic a reactive proliferation; extensive immunohistologic panels are usually necessary, as well as in situ hybridization for EBV.
- Careful interpretation of CD8, CD31, and CD34 stains is useful in assessing splenic vascular lesions (e.g., endothelial cells in hamartoma are CD8 positive).

KEY REFERENCES

42. Geyer JT, Prakash S, Orazi A. B-cell neoplasms and Hodgkin lymphoma in the spleen. *Sem Diagn Pathol.* 2021;38:125–134.

110. Arber DA. Tumors of the spleen. In: Means Jr RT, Dispenzieri A, Rodgers GM, et al., eds. *Wintrobe's Clinical Hematology.* 15th ed. Philadelphia: Wolters Kluwer; 2024.

113. Arber DA, Strickler JG, Chen Y-Y, et al. Splenic vascular tumors: a histologic, immunophenotypic, and virologic study. *Am J Surg Pathol.* 1997;21:827–835.

120. Falk S, Stutte HJ, Frizzera G. Littoral cell angioma. A novel splenic vascular lesion demonstrating histiocytic differentiation. *Am J Surg Pathol.* 1991;15:1023–1033.

127. Martel M, Cheuk W, Lombardi L, et al. Sclerosing Angiomatoid Nodular Transformation (SANT): report of 25 cases of a distinctive benign splenic lesion. *Am J Surg Pathol.* 2004;28:1268–1279.

132. Falk S, Stutte HJ. Hamartomas of the spleen: a study of 20 biopsy cases. *Histopathology.* 1989;14:603–612.

136. Sangiorgio A. Non-hematopoietic neoplastic and pseudoneoplastic lesions of the spleen. *Semin Diagn Pathol.* 2021;38:159–164.

141. Garvin DF, King FM. Cysts and nonlymphomatous tumors of the spleen. *Pathol Annu.* 1981;16:61–80.

Visit Elsevier eBooks+ for the complete set of references.

Chapter 59

Diagnosis of Lymphoma in Extranodal Sites Other Than Skin

Judith A. Ferry

The types of lymphoma encountered in extranodal sites differ from those encountered in lymph nodes. Many of the lymphomas that may involve extranodal sites are described as specific pathologic entities in other chapters. In this chapter, emphasis is placed on the types of lymphomas encountered in different extranodal sites, and on site-specific differences in clinical and pathologic features among these lymphomas.

LYMPHOMAS OF IMMUNE-PRIVILEGED SITES

Certain anatomic sites, including the central nervous system (CNS), the eyes, and the testes, are considered immune-privileged sites. Almost all of the lymphomas that arise in these sites are diffuse large B-cell lymphomas (DLBCLs) that share distinctive features: they almost all occur in adults over age 60, are characteristically Epstein-Barr virus (EBV)–negative DLBCLs with an activated B-cell immunophenotype, tend to spread to other immune-privileged sites, frequently have mutations of *MYD88* and *CD79B*, and frequently have genetic changes leading to immune evasion (inactivation of major histocompatibility complex [MHC] class I and II and β2 microglobulin).[1] They typically have a characteristic genomic signature by high-throughput sequencing (HTS), which has been variously designated as C5/MCD.[2] These cases were segregated under the above designation by the World Health Organization (WHO) 5th ed.[1] The International Consensus Classification (ICC) similarly identified the special features of primary DLBCL of the CNS and testis, segregating them from other subtypes of DBLCL.[3] However, the ICC deferred creation of this nosologic category, as the full scope of such cases is yet to be defined. For example, a subset of DLBCL of the breast and primary cutaneous DLBCL may share similar pathologic features.[4] Thus, it is likely that this designation may evolve over time.[1-4]

LYMPHOMA OF THE NERVOUS SYSTEM AND MENINGES

Primary Central Nervous System Lymphoma

Primary central nervous system lymphoma (PCNSL, almost all of which are DLBCLs) is defined as lymphoma confined to the CNS (brain, spinal cord, or leptomeninges) at presentation.[5] Vitreoretinal lymphoma (VRL) is closely related to PCNSL and, in the absence of prior or concurrent lymphoma outside the CNS, it is considered a subset of PCNSL (Table 59-1). VRL is considered separately.

Epidemiology and Etiology

Lymphoma may arise in the CNS in either immunocompetent patients or immunosuppressed patients. Those developing in immunocompromised patients are classified separately as *immunodeficiency-associated CNS lymphomas*.[6] Among immunocompetent patients, PCNSL makes up 1.5% to 3% of all brain tumors, 4% to 6% of all extranodal lymphomas, and 1% of all non-Hodgkin lymphomas.[7,8] PCNSL can occur at any age, but patients are predominantly older adults (median age, 55 to 66 years) with a male-to-female ratio of 3:2.[7,9-13]

Clinical Features

Symptoms are usually of short duration, and depending on the site of the lesion, include cognitive dysfunction, psychomotor slowing, speech disturbances, vertigo, weakness, hypothalamic dysfunction, ocular abnormalities, or disturbances of mobility such as ataxia, hemiparesis, hemiplegia, or abnormal gait. Patients may also have seizures or evidence of increased intracranial pressure such as headache, papilledema, nausea, or vomiting. Some present with personality changes, confusion, or dementia, mimicking a non-neoplastic disorder.[7,10,12,14,15] If the meninges are involved, symptoms related to cranial nerves may be seen.[7]

PCNSL usually presents as a supratentorial mass; cerebellar presentation is unusual and spinal cord presentation is rare. In immunocompetent patients, lesions are usually single. Though PCNSL in the brain or spinal cord may involve the leptomeninges secondarily, PCNSL rarely arises in the leptomeninges. The most common sites are the frontal, temporal, and parietal lobes, thalamus, basal ganglia, and corpus callosum. Presentation in the pituitary is rare (Fig. 59-1).[16] Lesions are often periventricular, so that cerebrospinal fluid (CSF) seeding may occur.[7,9,16-18] Imaging typically shows irregular, contrast-enhancing lesions with central hypodense areas, consistent with necrosis.[7]

Diagnosis is best established by stereotactic biopsy of the tumor. CSF for cytologic examination is relatively insensitive. Resection of the tumor does not improve survival and may lead to a greater neurologic deficit.[10,11,17]

Morphologic Features

Gross examination shows poorly circumscribed masses with replacement or displacement of normal structures, often with areas of necrosis or hemorrhage. Some patients have diffuse meningeal involvement resembling meningitis or, rarely, diffuse subependymal periventricular involvement by tumor.[19]

Table 59-1 Extranodal Lymphomas Arising in Sites Other Than Skin

Site	Lymphomas	Associations
Central Nervous System		
Brain	DLBCL	Subset HIV positive, EBV positive
Eyes (vitreo-retinal)	DLBCL	CNS involvement
Head and Neck		
Ocular adnexa	EMZL	*Chlamydia psittaci,* subset
	Follicular lymphoma	
	DLBCL	
Waldeyer's ring	DLBCL	GI involvement
	Follicular lymphoma	
	BL	Children
	Mantle cell lymphoma	Usually widespread
Nasal cavity	Extranodal NK/TCL	EBV positive
	DLBCL	
Paranasal sinuses	DLBCL	
Oral cavity	DLBCL	
	Follicular lymphoma	
	EMZL	
	Plasmablastic lymphoma	HIV positive, EBV positive
Salivary gland	EMZL	Sjögren syndrome
	Follicular lymphoma	Intra/periparotid nodes
	DLBCL	
Thyroid	DLBCL	Hashimoto thyroiditis
	EMZL	Hashimoto thyroiditis
	Follicular lymphoma	
Larynx	EMZL	
	DLBCL	
Thorax		
Lung	EMZL	Subset: autoimmune disease
	DLBCL	
	Lymphomatoid granulomatosis	Immunocompromise, EBV positive
Pleura	Primary effusion lymphoma	HIV-positive patients, KSHV/HHV8 positive, EBV positive
	Pyothorax-associated lymphoma	TB-positive patients, EBV positive
	Fluid overload–associated large BCL	Older patients with cardiac, hepatic, or renal disease
Thymus	Primary mediastinal large BCL	
	Classic Hodgkin lymphoma	
	Mediastinal gray-zone lymphoma	
	T-lymphoblastic lymphoma	
	EMZL	Usually IgA positive, autoimmune disease frequent
Heart	DLBCL	Subset: immunosuppressed
Breast	DLBCL	
	EMZL	
	Follicular lymphoma	
	BL	Pregnancy, lactation
	Breast implant–associated ALCL	Implants with textured surfaces
Gastrointestinal and Hepatobiliary Tract		
Stomach	DLBCL	
	EMZL	*Helicobacter pylori*
Small intestine	DLBCL	
	EMZL (rare subtype: IPSID)	
	BL	
	EATL	Celiac disease
	MEITL	
	Mantle cell lymphoma	Lymphomatous polyposis
	Follicular lymphoma	Duodenal, most cases
Large intestine	DLBCL	
	EMZL	
	Mantle cell lymphoma	Lymphomatous polyposis
	Follicular lymphoma	
	BL	

Table 59-1 Extranodal Lymphomas Arising in Sites Other Than Skin—cont'd

Site	Lymphomas	Associations
Anus	DLBCL	Subset HIV positive
	Plasmablastic lymphoma	HIV positive, EBV positive
Liver	DLBCL	
	BL	
	EMZL	
	Hepatosplenic TCL	Majority γδ positive; fewer αβ positive
Gallbladder	DLBCL	
	EMZL	
Pancreas	DLBCL	
Adrenal	DLBCL	
Genitourinary Tract		
Kidney	DLBCL	
	Follicular lymphoma	
	EMZL	
Urinary bladder	EMZL	Cystitis
	DLBCL	
Urethra	DLBCL	
	EMZL	
Testis	DLBCL	
	Follicular lymphoma	Children
	Extranodal NK/TCL	Asian men
Ovary	DLBCL	
	BL	
	Follicular lymphoma	
Uterus, cervix, vagina	DLBCL	
	Follicular lymphoma	
Skeleton		
Bone	DLBCL	
	Lymphoblastic lymphoma	Children
	ALK-positive and ALK-negative ALCL (rare)	

ALCL, Anaplastic large cell lymphoma; *BCL,* B-cell lymphoma; *BL,* Burkitt lymphoma; *CNS,* central nervous system; *DLBCL,* diffuse large B-cell lymphoma; *EATL,* enteropathy-associated T-cell lymphoma; *EBV,* Epstein-Barr virus; *EMZL,* extranodal marginal zone lymphoma; *GI,* gastrointestinal; *IPSID,* immunoproliferative small intestinal disease; *MEITL,* monomorphic epitheliotropic T-cell lymphoma; *NK,* natural killer; *TCL,* T-cell lymphoma.

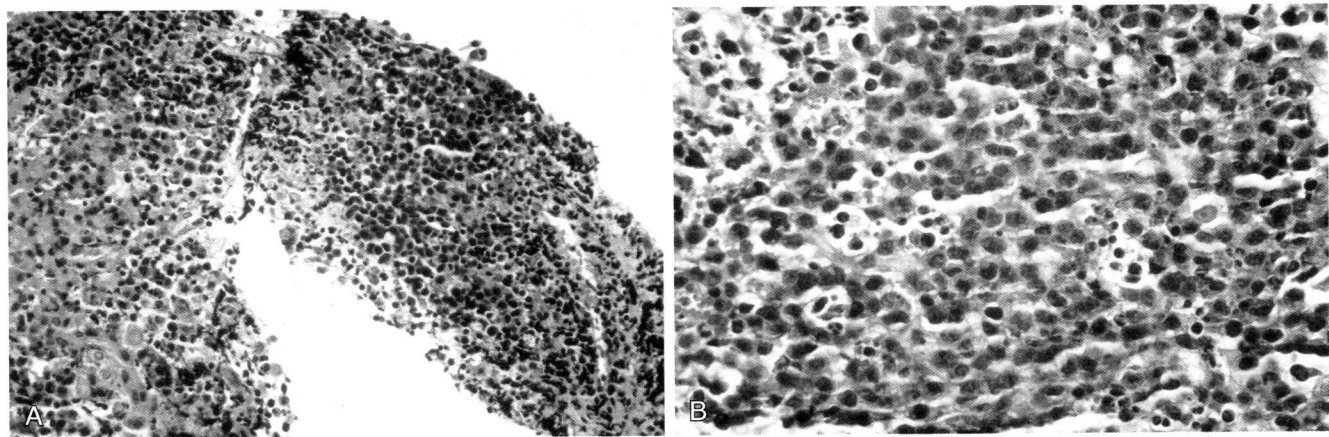

Figure 59-1. Diffuse large B-cell lymphoma, arising in the area of the pituitary. A, The biopsy fragments show a dense, diffuse lymphoid infiltrate, with a few residual bright red anterior pituitary parenchymal cells. **B,** High power shows large, atypical cells with interspersed tingible body macrophages.

The vast majority are DLBCLs. The characteristic microscopic appearance is a diffuse proliferation of centroblasts or immunoblasts, with peripheral areas of perivascular growth and, often, necrosis.[5,19] If steroids have been administered before biopsy, neoplastic cells may undergo extensive apoptosis and the tumor may temporarily shrink or even disappear, hindering diagnosis. The remainder are low-grade B-cell lymphomas sometimes classified as extranodal marginal zone lymphoma (EMZL),[20] Burkitt lymphoma (BL), and peripheral T-cell lymphoma, including rare cases of anaplastic large cell lymphoma.[21,22] Also, 1% to 2% of cases are intravascular large B-cell lymphoma.[7,19]

Immunophenotype

The DLBCLs express pan-B cell antigens and monotypic immunoglobulin (usually IgM, IgD).[7,23] They almost always have a non-GCB immunophenotype (CD10⁻, BCL6+/-, MUM1+).[24]

Genetic Features

Molecular genetic analysis shows monoclonal immunoglobulin gene rearrangements in DLBCL.[12,25] EBV is almost always negative, except in the setting of immune deficiency.[9,25] There is preferential use of certain VH families, as well as a high load of somatic mutations, in some cases accompanied by ongoing somatic hypermutation. Aberrant somatic hypermutation of genes that include BCL6, BCL2, MYC, PAX5, and others is common. Translocations involving immunoglobulin genes, BCL6, and ETV6 are frequent,[5,26] while translocations of MYC and BCL2 are rare to absent.[5,26] Gains of genetic material are common, most often affecting 18q21-q23 (including BCL2 and MALT1).[27] Losses of genetic material are also common; they most often involve chromosomal material at 6q21, 6p21 (including HLA class II–encoding HLA-DRB, HLA-DQA, and HLA-DQB), and 8q12.1-q12.2.[27] Accordingly, loss of expression of HLA proteins is common[28] and likely contributes to survival of the neoplastic cells through immune escape.[28,29] CDKN2A deletions, often biallelic, are common.[30,31]

The B-cell receptor, toll-like receptor, and NF-κB pathways are often activated because of mutations involving MYD88 (MYD88 L265P, found in the majority of cases), CD79B, PIM1, CDKN2A, INPP5D, CARD11, MALT1, and BCL2, which promote proliferation and cell survival.[27,30-35] Gene-expression profiling typically shows activated B-cell (ABC) DLBCL.[34,35]

Epigenetic changes likely also contribute to pathogenesis. Hypermethylation of DAPK1, CDKN2A, and MGMT are each seen in the majority of cases.[5,36] Neoplastic cells are believed to correspond to antigen-selected late germinal-center exit B cells.[5,12,23]

Staging, Treatment, and Outcome

Staging should be performed to exclude systemic lymphoma with secondary CNS involvement.[7] Primary CNS DLBCL is an aggressive neoplasm requiring prompt diagnosis and therapy.[23] Survival is only a few months without therapy. Therapy for PCNSL in years past was whole-brain radiation combined with steroids. This resulted in a complete remission in 90% of cases, but the lymphoma usually relapsed within a year, with a median survival of 12 to 18 months and 5-year survival of 3% to 4%.[10,11,17] More recently, therapy using methotrexate, an agent able to penetrate the blood-brain barrier, has improved survival.

Relapses usually involve the CNS. In a few cases, lymphoma spreads outside the CNS; these sites are usually extranodal, with frequent testicular involvement.[11] The prognosis is better for immunocompetent patients who are younger than 60 to 65 years.[10,11,14] The low-grade B-cell lymphomas have a relatively favorable prognosis.[9,19,20]

Differential Diagnosis

Sampling artifact or prior steroid therapy can result in a biopsy showing a predominance of small reactive T cells, mimicking a chronic inflammatory process.[5] Avoiding prebiopsy steroids and obtaining intraoperative frozen sections to be certain that tissue is representative in any case of suspected PCNSL are helpful in establishing a diagnosis. There may be a surrounding glial reaction that may mimic glioma. Other neoplasms, including small round cell tumors, undifferentiated carcinoma, melanoma, and certain gliomas can grow in sheets and mimic lymphoma.[19] Vasculitis can mimic areas of lymphoma with perivascular growth.

Immunodeficiency-Associated Central Nervous System Lymphomas

Immunologic abnormalities are important in the pathogenesis of a subset of CNS lymphomas.[6] Immunodeficient patients who develop PCNSL are mostly HIV positive, with risk previously estimated as high as 1000× that of immunocompetent individuals.[25] These patients are overall younger, with a prominent male preponderance. There is also an increased incidence of PCNSL with iatrogenic and congenital immunodeficiency. The increased risk posttransplant was seen mainly in older azathioprine-based regimens[37] and is much less with more recent regimens. The introduction of highly active antiretroviral therapy (HAART) for HIV-positive patients dramatically decreased the occurrence of PCNSL in this group.[38] Virtually all PCNSL in immunocompromised patients are EBV-positive DLBCL.[7,9,10,17,19,23,25] In contrast to the genetic changes seen in PCNSL in immunocompetent patients, EBV-positive PCNSL in immunodeficient patients typically harbors wild-type MYD88, CD79B, and PIM1 with a lower overall mutational burden, and also show different microenvironmental features, indicating striking differences in pathogenesis.[34,35]

Vitreoretinal Lymphoma

Clinical Features

VRL, also called *ocular lymphoma* or *intraocular lymphoma*—lymphoma of the eye itself—is uncommon.[39-41] It predominantly affects older adults,[42] although occasionally young adults[43] and, rarely, children[44] are affected. There is a female preponderance.[39,45] Most patients have no known predisposing conditions, but VRL has been described in HIV-infected patients[41] and in iatrogenically immunosuppressed allograft recipients.[40,44] As for PCNSL, these would be classified separately, as immunodeficiency-associated lymphomas.

Patients typically have decreased visual acuity, floating spots, or both.[46] Although symptoms are often unilateral, examination reveals bilateral involvement in about 80% of cases.[39] VRL arises beneath the retinal pigment epithelium (RPE) and above the Bruch membrane, and subsequently infiltrates the neuroretina, optic nerve head, and vitreous.[47-49] Whitish, yellow-white, or gray-white infiltrates or large masses may be seen beneath the RPE, in the uvea, suspended in the vitreous or invading the optic nerve, sometimes with edema, hemorrhage, necrosis, or retinal detachment. Other manifestations include increased intraocular pressure, keratic precipitates (deposits of cells on the posterior surface of the cornea), and anterior chamber cells and flare (presence of increased protein causing the normally clear fluid of the anterior chamber to become cloudy [flare] with tiny particles [cells] suspended in the fluid).[39,50]

VRL can mimic non-neoplastic conditions, including chronic idiopathic uveitis, retinal vasculitis, optic neuritis, amyloidosis, sarcoidosis, and infections, including toxoplasmosis, syphilis, tuberculosis, Whipple disease, and cytomegaloviral infection.[39] Poor response to steroids or antimicrobial therapy or onset of neurologic symptoms caused by CNS involvement can suggest lymphoma.[39]

Techniques used to establish a diagnosis include vitreous aspirate, vitrectomy, biopsy, or in patients with a blind, painful eye, ocular enucleation. The mode most commonly used is microscopic examination of vitreous, but the sensitivity of this procedure may be limited by admixed inflammatory cells or by prior steroid therapy, which may eliminate many tumor cells. Diagnostic yield may be improved by combining routine light microscopy with flow cytometry and molecular genetic analysis.[51] An elevated IL-10 level in the vitreous is strongly associated with VRL and could prompt rebiopsy if the initial specimen is nondiagnostic.[39]

Pathologic Features

Nearly all VRL are DLBCL.[41] Their morphologic, immunophenotypic, and genetic features are similar to primary CNS DLBCL.[52-54] DLBCL of nongerminal-center B-cell type (non-GCB) is more common than GCB type.[46] Rare cases of peripheral T-cell lymphoma presenting with ocular involvement have also been described.[43,45,55]

Staging, Treatment, and Outcome

Most VRL are associated with CNS lymphoma either at presentation or, without treatment, on follow-up; a minority are associated with systemic lymphoma or remain confined to the eye. Aggressive treatment of isolated VRL can decrease the risk of progression.[39,56]

VRL frequently responds to radiation therapy, but restoration of sight is not guaranteed, because the retina may already be irreversibly damaged and because radiation may be associated with retinopathy and cataracts. Patients treated with ocular radiation alone often develop ocular recurrence or progress to CNS or, less often, systemic involvement. Other therapeutic considerations include combined chemotherapy and radiation, chemotherapy alone, intensive chemotherapy with autologous stem cell transplant and intravitreal methotrexate. On follow-up, most patients are alive with lymphoma or succumb to lymphoma.[46]

Lymphoma of the Dura Mater

Clinical Features

Lymphoma arising in the dura mater is uncommon. Patients are mostly middle-aged and older adults. There are no known risk factors. They present with seizures, headache, cranial nerve abnormalities, radicular pain, syncope, or a combination of these findings.[57-61] Radiologic evaluation usually reveals a localized, expansile mass or plaque-like thickening of the dura over the brain[59,62,63] that is most often thought to be a meningioma or, less often, a nerve sheath tumor or a subdural hematoma preoperatively.[58,59]

Pathologic Features

Approximately half of cases are diffuse large cell lymphomas (B lineage when immunophenotyped). The remainder are mostly EMZLs of mucosa-associated lymphoid tissue.[59,61] EMZLs have histologic and immunohistologic features similar to those seen in other sites. They are composed of small lymphocytes and marginal zone cells, usually with prominent plasmacytic differentiation and admixed reactive follicles (Fig. 59-2).[20] An increased proportion of dural EMZLs contain monotypic plasma cells expressing IgG4,[64] although without evidence of associated IgG4-related disease. Entrapped meningothelial cells may be seen.[58,59,61] Dural EMZLs may arise in association with meningothelium, just as EMZLs often arise in association with epithelium in other sites.[58,59] Dural lymphomas are typically localized. The prognosis is excellent.[58,59,61]

Differential Diagnosis

Other low-grade B-cell lymphomas, such as lymphoplasmacytic lymphoma and chronic lymphocytic leukemia, can have histologic features mimicking EMZL, but the immunophenotype and localized nature of the lymphoma exclude other low-grade lymphomas. Some cases previously interpreted as dural plasmacytoma may represent EMZL with marked plasmacytic differentiation.[58,59] Some cases may raise the question of inflammatory pseudotumor or a chronic inflammatory process or lymphoplasmacyte-rich meningioma, but immunophenotyping or genotyping can help establish a diagnosis.

OCULAR ADNEXAL LYMPHOMA

Clinical Features

Primary ocular adnexal lymphoma is defined as lymphoma arising in orbital soft tissue, lacrimal gland, conjunctiva, or eyelids. The orbital soft tissue is the most common site, followed by the conjunctiva, the lacrimal gland, and then the eyelids.[65,66] The ocular adnexa is where 1% to 2% of all lymphomas[67] and approximately 8% of all extranodal lymphomas[68] arise. Lymphoid tumors compose 10% of orbital mass lesions, and lymphoma is the most common orbital malignancy.[67] Lymphomas in this site predominantly affect older women (M:F = 3:4) with a median age in the 60s.[69] Children are only rarely affected.[69] Occasionally, patients have a history of an autoimmune disorder,[69,70] another malignancy,[71] HIV infection,[70,72] or contact lens wear.[73] Some ocular adnexal lymphomas are associated with *Chlamydia psittaci* infection; a subset of lymphomas in such patients responds to antibiotic therapy.[74] However, this association has not been confirmed in other series, which may reflect geographic variation.[75]

Patients present with proptosis, ptosis, a palpable or visible mass, diplopia, limitation of movement, tearing, or discomfort.[69,70] High-grade lymphomas occasionally cause a rapid decrease in visual acuity.[46] Systemic symptoms are rare. Conjunctival lymphoma usually produces a salmon-colored plaque that is mobile over the surface of the eye. The orbital soft tissue is involved in the majority of cases, sometimes accompanied by lacrimal gland involvement. The conjunctiva is involved in up to approximately one-third of cases.[69] In 10% to 25% of cases,[69,76,77] there is bilateral involvement.

Pathologic Features

Lymphomas of many types can present with ocular adnexal involvement, but nearly all are B-cell lymphomas. Most (60%–75%) are EMZLs.[69,70,78,79] Most of the remainder are follicular lymphomas (FLs), followed by DLBCL. The DLBCLs

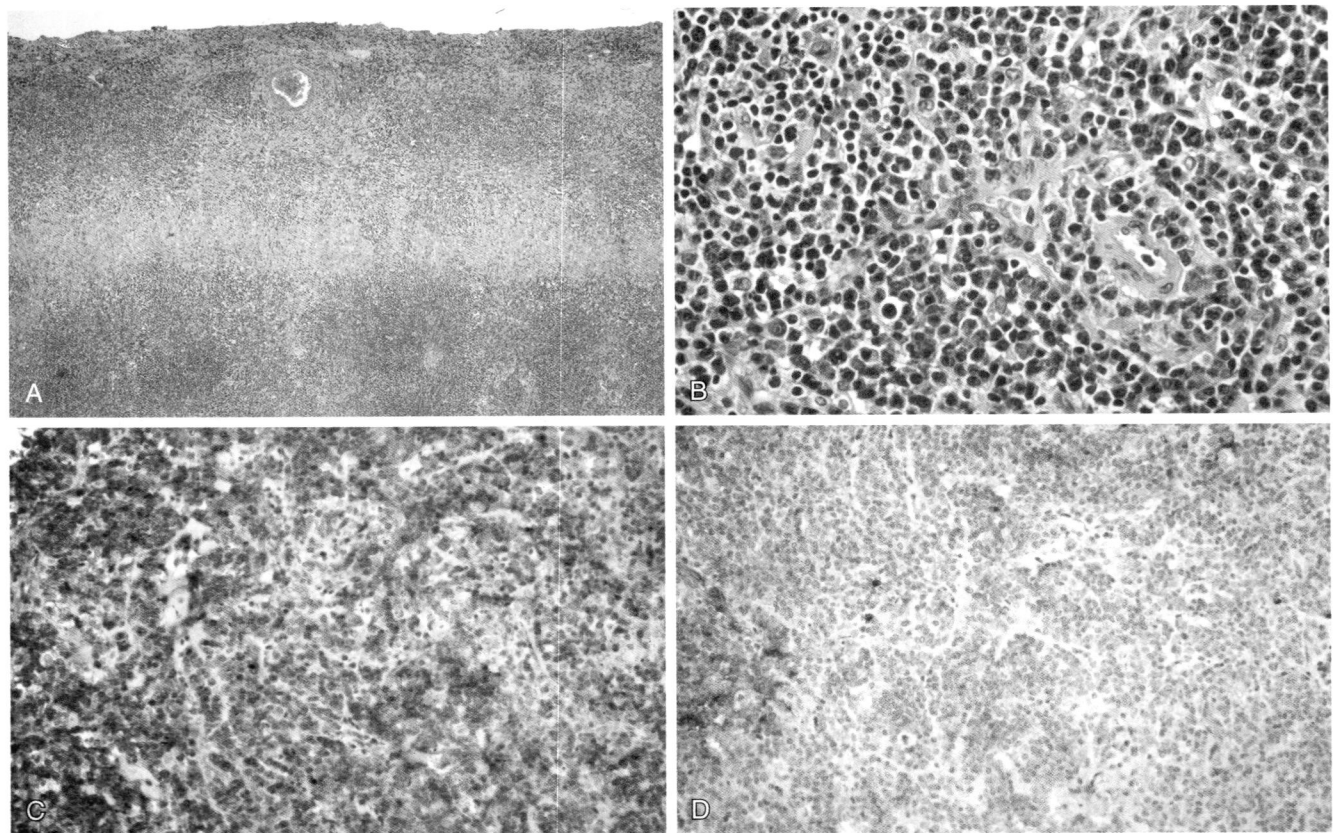

Figure 59-2. Extranodal marginal zone lymphoma of mucosa-associated lymphoid tissue, dura mater. A, The dura shows a dense lymphoid infiltrate. **B,** Higher power shows small lymphoid cells and aggregates of plasma cells. **C,** Plasma cells express monotypic cytoplasmic kappa light chain (immunoperoxidase technique on paraffin sections). **D,** Staining for cytoplasmic lambda light chain is negative (immunoperoxidase technique on paraffin sections).

are of GCB and non-GCB types, in roughly equal numbers.[46] Few cases of mantle cell lymphoma and rare cases of chronic lymphocytic leukemia, lymphoplasmacytic lymphoma, BL, plasmablastic lymphoma, and B lymphoblastic lymphoma present with ocular adnexal involvement.[69,80] The few primary ocular adnexal lymphomas encountered in children or in HIV-positive patients are usually high-grade B-cell lymphomas, either DLBCL or BL.[81,82] Rare cases of T-cell lymphoma and NK-cell lymphoma[69,70,79] have had ocular adnexal involvement at presentation. Hodgkin lymphoma is vanishingly rare.[70]

The immunophenotypic and genetic features are overall similar to those of the same types of lymphomas arising in other anatomic sites, although ocular adnexal EMZL shows a tendency for site-specific genetic changes. *TNFAIP3* mutation or deletion is common in ocular adnexal EMZL and uncommon in EMZL in other sites, while gains of 6p and loss of 6q are recurrently seen only in EMZL of the ocular adnexa.[1] Approximately one-quarter of ocular adnexal EMZL harbors t(14;18)(q32;q21)/*IGH::MALT1,* a translocation involving IGH and the *MALT1* gene; this translocation has also been found in EMZL arising in the liver, skin, and salivary glands, but is rare in EMZL in other sites.[83] Cases showing t(11;18)(q21;q21)/*BIRC3::MALT1* and t(3;14)(p14.1;q32)/*FOXP1::IGH* are also described.[70,84] In patients with bilateral ocular adnexal lymphoma, morphologic, immunophenotypic, and molecular genetic features are reported to be identical, consistent with a single neoplastic clone involving both sites, rather than two distinct, unrelated primary tumors.[72,73]

Staging, Treatment, and Outcome

Approximately 80% of patients have disease confined to the ocular adnexa, unilaterally or bilaterally.[71,77] In some studies, EMZLs are more likely to present with stage I disease than other types of lymphoma.[85] Localized low-grade lymphomas are usually treated with radiation. Intermediate or high-grade lymphoma, whether localized or widespread, are usually treated more aggressively.[65,70,79] Radiation therapy achieves excellent local control of disease; freedom from local recurrence is close to 100%.[85] Prevention and treatment of lymphoma away from the eye is not as successful, but the prognosis of ocular adnexal lymphoma is overall good. Overall survival (OS) at 5 years is approximately 90%, while the 5-year disease-free survival is approximately 70%.[77,85] When relapses occur, they involve lymph nodes, the opposite orbit, or other extranodal sites.[65,77]

Patients with disease localized to the ocular adnexa have a better prognosis than those with more widespread disease.[66,72,80,86] However, isolated bilateral ocular adnexal disease does not have a worse prognosis than unilateral disease.[77,87] In most reports, patients with high-grade lymphoma have had a worse outcome.[79,80,86,88,89]

Differential Diagnosis

Because most ocular adnexal lymphomas are low-grade lymphomas, the main differential diagnosis is with a reactive process, including inflammatory pseudotumor and reactive lymphoid hyperplasia. Inflammatory pseudotumor is a lesion with a variably cellular, polymorphous infiltrate of small lymphocytes, plasma cells, immunoblasts, and histiocytes, sometimes with eosinophils or neutrophils, in a stroma with areas that are hyalinized, edematous, or both. Immunohistochemical studies show a mixture of B cells, T cells, and polytypic plasma cells. In some instances, the plasma cells are predominantly IgG4 positive; these inflammatory pseudotumors are considered to represent IgG4-related sclerosing dacryoadenitis (if lacrimal gland is involved) and IgG4-related sclerosing orbital inflammation (if soft tissue is involved). Rare cases of lymphoma arising on a background of IgG4-positive inflammatory pseudotumor have been described.[90-92] Reactive lymphoid hyperplasia usually consists of follicular hyperplasia without a prominent diffuse lymphoid proliferation and without cytologic atypia. In favor of lymphoma is a dense, diffuse infiltrate composed predominantly of B cells. Such lesions usually express monotypic immunoglobulin and contain clonal B cells on molecular genetic analysis.

LYMPHOMAS OF WALDEYER'S RING

Waldeyer's ring is the circle of lymphoid tissue guarding the entrance to the alimentary and respiratory tracts. It consists of palatine tonsils, the nasopharynx, and the base of the tongue. Waldeyer's ring is the primary site for 5% to 10% of all non-Hodgkin lymphomas, accounting for more than half of all non-Hodgkin lymphomas primary in the head and neck.[93]

Clinical Features

Patients are mostly adults, and infrequently children, with a median age in the 50s, with a male-to-female ratio of 1:1 to 1:1.5.[93-96] A few patients are HIV positive or are iatrogenically immunosuppressed. Patients present with dysphagia, dyspnea, snoring, discomfort, foreign body sensation, or cervical lymphadenopathy. A minority have systemic symptoms.[96-98]

The tonsil is most frequently involved, accounting for more than half of Waldeyer's ring lymphomas, followed by the nasopharynx and the base of tongue.[93-95,99] Physical examination reveals a mass that is unilateral and exophytic in most cases, and may be smooth, polypoid, fungating, or ulcerated. The lymphoma is usually localized (stage I or II), but stage II disease (with cervical lymphadenopathy) is more common than stage I.[94,95]

Pathologic Features

Of cases, 60% to 84% are DLBCLs (Fig. 59-3). Other types are uncommon; they include FL, BL, mantle cell lymphoma (MCL), EMZL, and peripheral T-cell lymphoma.[93,94,98-100] MCL can present with involvement of Waldeyer's ring, but in contrast to DLBCL, MCL is usually widespread at the time of diagnosis. Among children with Waldeyer's ring lymphoma, BL is much more frequent than among adults (Fig. 59-4).[96] The lymphomas have pathologic features overall similar to those seen in other sites. The DLBCLs include GCB and non-GCB subtypes, with a modest excess of non-GCB DLBCL. The majority are double-expressors (MYC positive, BCL2 positive).[101] A subset of the DLBCL and grade 3 FL have IRF4 rearrangement (see Chapter 17).[95,102,103]

Hodgkin lymphoma, almost always classic type, rarely presents with involvement of Waldeyer's ring. In most cases, Hodgkin lymphoma involves other sites as well. In one study, among cases confined to Waldeyer's ring, lymphocyte-rich classic Hodgkin lymphoma (CHL) was the most common type.[104]

Treatment and Outcome

Patients respond well to therapy, with a high proportion achieving complete remission. A better prognosis is associated with a tonsillar primary, favorable International Prognostic Index (IPI), localized disease,[93,94] therapy including rituximab and CNS-directed therapy,[101] and favorable ECOG score.[95]

Differential Diagnosis

Reactive lymphoid hyperplasia often causes enlargement of one or more of the components of Waldeyer's ring, sometimes

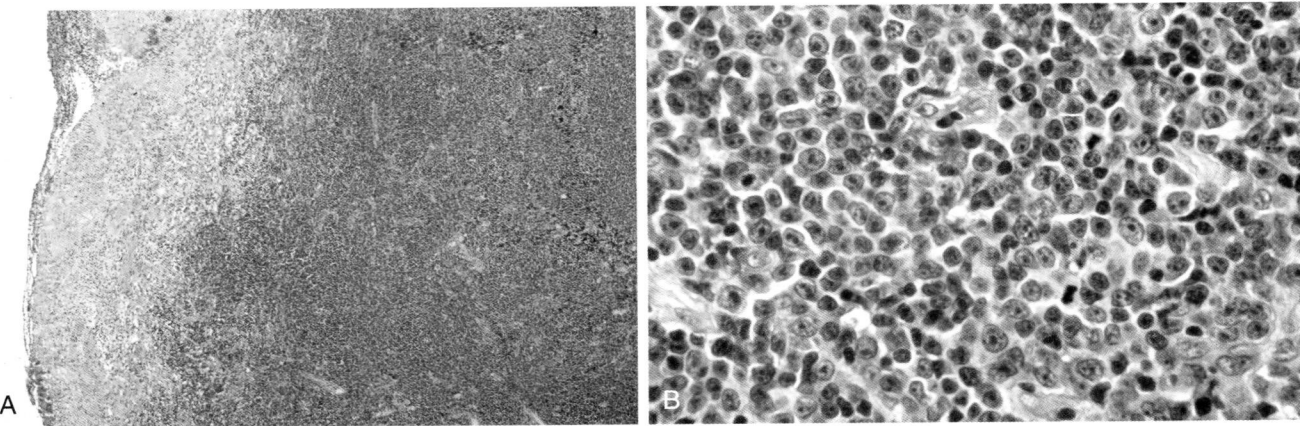

Figure 59-3. Diffuse large B-cell lymphoma, nasopharynx. A, The surface of the tissue is necrotic. The rest of the tissue is replaced by a dense lymphoid infiltrate. **B,** Higher power reveals a predominance of immunoblasts.

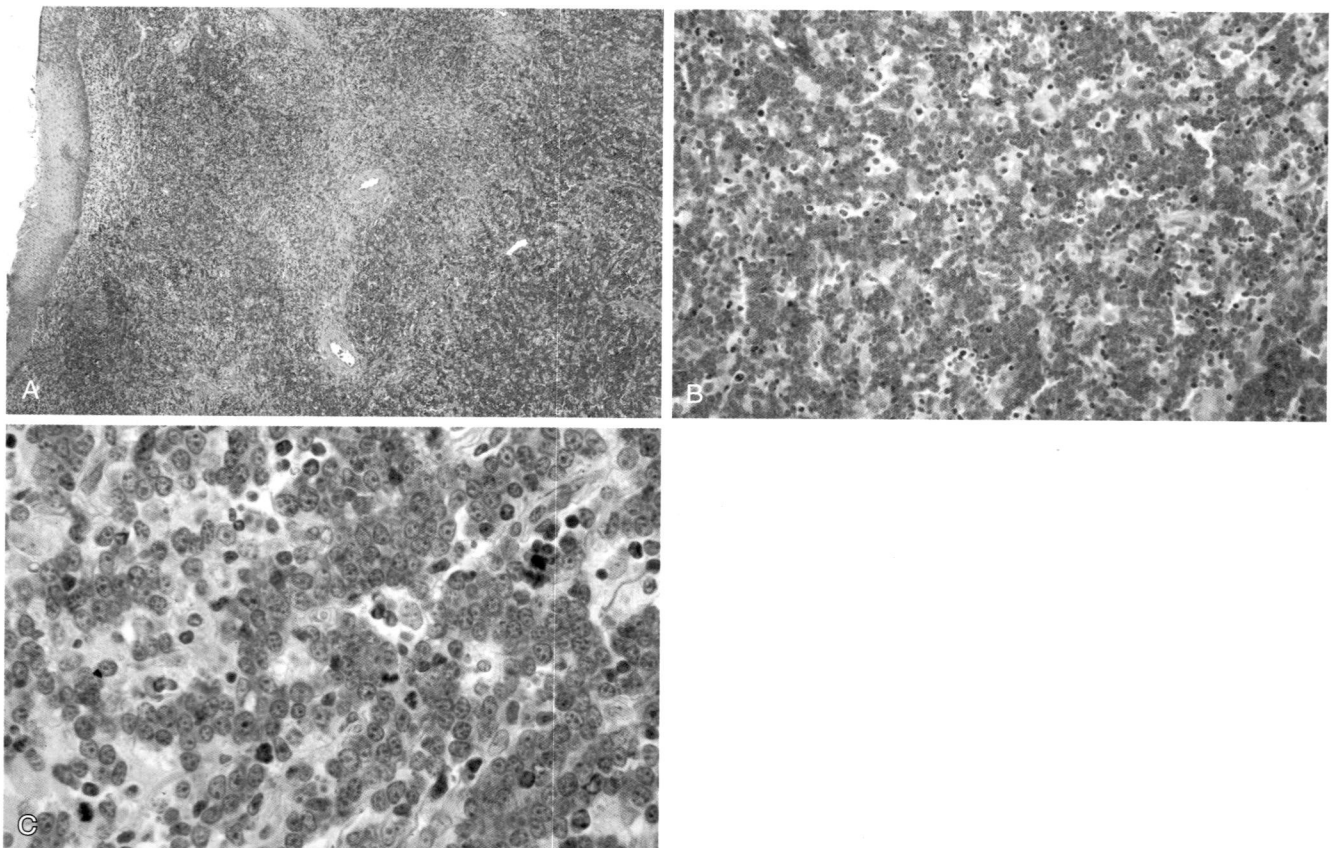

Figure 59-4. Burkitt lymphoma, tonsil of a child. A, A dense lymphoid infiltrate is seen beneath intact squamous epithelium. Normal crypt architecture has been obliterated. **B,** Medium power shows a striking starry-sky pattern. **C,** High power shows uniform medium-sized, round cells with finely stippled chromatin and small nucleoli with numerous mitotic figures and many admixed tingible body macrophages.

mimicking a neoplasm. Preservation of reactive follicles and of crypts favors a reactive process. Infectious mononucleosis caused by primary EBV infection can mimic DLBCL or CHL, but some architectural preservation, polymorphous composition, positive in situ hybridization for EBER, and clinical features, particularly age, can be helpful in differential diagnosis. Before making a diagnosis of DLBCL or CHL in Waldeyer's ring in a child or adolescent, evaluation for evidence of infectious mononucleosis is essential. Infiltration of crypt epithelium by lymphoid cells is normal and does not suggest EMZL. Atypical marginal zone hyperplasia with monotypic immunoglobulin light-chain expression in B cells that are polyclonal by molecular genetic analysis has been reported in Waldeyer's ring in rare children, and can mimic EMZL.[105] Nonkeratinizing nasopharyngeal squamous cell carcinoma, especially those cases with features of "lymphoepithelial carcinoma," and DLBCL may be difficult to distinguish on routine sections, but immunophenotyping readily establishes a diagnosis.

LYMPHOMAS OF THE NASAL CAVITY AND PARANASAL SINUSES

Among sinonasal malignancies, lymphoma is second in frequency only to squamous cell carcinoma.[106] Sinonasal lymphoma accounts for 0.2% to 2% of all lymphomas[107,108] and less than 5% of extranodal lymphomas.[99] The incidence of lymphoma in this anatomic site is higher in Asia and South America.[109,110] Two main types of lymphoma occur: DLBCL and extranodal NK/T-cell lymphoma, nasal type (ICC)/extranodal NK/T-cell lymphoma (WHO 5th edition) (ENKTCL). Lymphomas that arise in paranasal sinuses are almost always DLBCL, and lymphomas arising in the nasal cavity may be ENKTCL or DLBCL.[110-113] ENKTCL is discussed in Chapter 29. Other types of sinonasal lymphoma are discussed below.

Clinical Features

Paranasal sinus lymphoma affects men more often than women (M:F = 1.5 to 2:1). It predominantly affects middle-aged to older adults,[107,108,111] and occasionally children.[114] A few patients have been HIV positive[111,115] or iatrogenically immunosuppressed.[111,116] Symptoms include nasal obstruction or discharge, facial swelling, pain or numbness, epistaxis, sinus pressure, toothache, or headache. The lymphoma may invade adjacent structures including orbit, base of skull, CNS, pterygopalatine fossa, nasopharynx, and palate.[107,114,115] Patients may present with neurologic abnormalities, proptosis, diplopia, decreased visual acuity, and even blindness.[108,109,111,114,115,117] Patients occasionally have fever and night sweats.[111,115] The maxillary sinus is the sinus most often involved, followed by the ethmoid, sphenoid, and frontal sinus. Frequently, multiple sinuses are involved concurrently.[107,108,111,114,115,118]

Pathologic Features

In Western countries, the most common lymphoma is DLBCL, followed by ENKTCL. Other types are infrequent or rare, but BL, FL,[109,114,115,117,118] EMZL,[107,111] high-grade B-cell lymphoma, not otherwise specified (NOS), high-grade B-cell lymphoma with concurrent MYC and BCL2 rearrangement, plasmablastic lymphoma,[107] peripheral T-cell lymphoma, NOS, and adult T-cell leukemia/lymphoma[111] presenting with sinus involvement have been described. Lymphomas in HIV-positive patients have been DLBCL and BL.[115] Those in children are most often BL, followed by DLBCL.[111,119] Immunophenotypic features are similar to those in other sites. DLBCL of non-GCB subtype is more common than GCB subtype.[101] The proportion of sinonasal B cell lymphomas containing EBV varies among series[110,117,120]; in a study from Massachusetts General Hospital, EBV was only encountered in DLBCL in patients with underlying immunodeficiency.[111]

Staging, Treatment, and Outcome

Most lymphomas are localized at presentation.[111] Patients with stage IV case disease may have involvement of CNS, lung, bones, kidney, or gastrointestinal (GI) tract.[114,115] Most DLBCL patients receive radiation and chemotherapy, sometimes with CNS prophylaxis. When the lymphomas relapse or progress, they frequently involve lymph nodes, and may also involve a variety of extranodal sites, including the CNS, lung, bone, ovary, testis, marrow, liver, spleen, and skin.[107,108,113,117] In one series, sinonasal DLBCL had a 5-year progression-free survival (PFS) of 50% and a 5-year OS of 56%[107]; use of rituximab was associated with better outcome.[107].

Differential Diagnosis

DBLCL and ENKTCL may be difficult to distinguish on routine sections. Angioinvasion and angiocentric localization, prominent necrosis, epitheliotropism, and pseudoepitheliomatous hyperplasia favor ENKTCL. DLBCL more commonly arise in paranasal sinuses, while nasal localization and midfacial destructive disease favor ENK TCL.[111,118,121] Most DLBCLs are composed of a diffuse proliferation of large cells, so any other cellular composition with a diffuse pattern, especially a mixture of small and large cells or of medium-sized cells, should raise the question of ENKTCL.[121] B-cell and NK/T-cell lymphomas can be distinguished easily with immunophenotyping. Absence of EBV excludes ENKTCL.

SALIVARY GLAND LYMPHOMAS

Clinical Features

Lymphoma accounts for 2% to 5% of salivary gland malignancies.[40,122] The lymphomas arise in the parotid in at least 70% of cases, in the submaxillary gland in 10% to 25% of cases, and in the sublingual and minor salivary glands in <10% of cases. Patients are affected over a broad age range, but the vast majority are over age 50, with a slight female preponderance. Patients present with an enlarging mass that is usually painless, but that may be accompanied by facial nerve paralysis or cervical lymphadenopathy.[40,122-126]

Pathologic Features

EMZL of mucosa-associated lymphoid tissue (see Chapter 18) and DLBCL account for nearly all salivary gland lymphomas. EMZL is the most common lymphoma arising in salivary gland parenchyma. Of salivary gland EMZLs, 30% to 35% occur in patients with autoimmune disease, mainly Sjögren syndrome, and rarely, rheumatoid arthritis.[125,126] Salivary gland lymphomas in Sjögren syndrome patients are almost always EMZL.[126] EMZL predominantly affect females, in part because of the high ratio of women to men with Sjögren syndrome. EMZL usually arises in a background of lymphoepithelial sialadenitis (LESA) showing large, well-formed lymphoepithelial lesions (LELs). In contrast to LESA without lymphoma, LELs in EMZL are surrounded by large haloes and broad intersecting strands and sheets of monocytoid B cells, distorting and obliterating the salivary gland parenchyma. Also present are scattered reactive follicles and plasma cells, sometimes in large aggregates. In salivary glands other than the parotid, LELs may be less conspicuous, but histologic features are otherwise similar.

Salivary gland EMZL commonly harbor trisomy 3, which is especially frequent in patients without Sjögren syndrome.[125] A small minority have trisomy 18 or a rearrangement of *MALT1*. Most salivary gland EMZL express IgM with strong rheumatoid factor activity, so that IgG, likely in immune complexes in inflamed tissues, serves as the autoantigen that contributes to the chronic antigenic stimulation thought to drive the pathogenesis of some EMZL, including those arising in salivary glands.[127] Recurrent activating mutations in certain G-protein coupled receptors occur in EMZL; mutated *GPR34* and rarely t(X;14)(p11;q32)/*IGH::GPR34* appear specific for salivary gland EMZL.[128,129] Maintenance of GPR34 signaling in EMZL may be related to ligands produced by salivary gland LELs.[130] These changes may promote emergence and expansion of B-cell clones, particularly around LELs.

FL may also arise in the area of salivary glands but usually involves lymph nodes in the vicinity rather than salivary gland parenchyma. Pathologic features are similar to those of other nodal FLs (see Chapter 17). Salivary-gland DLBCL affects men and women equally[124] and has features similar to those of DLBCL in other sites (see Chapter 22). Some of the DLBCL may represent large-cell transformation of an underlying EMZL or FL.[40,122,123] Rare cases of BL,[122] peripheral T-cell lymphoma, NOS, anaplastic large cell lymphoma, and ENKTCL have been reported.[131]

Staging, Treatment, and Outcome

The majority of patients with salivary gland lymphoma, both EMZL and DLBCL, present with unilateral, localized disease.[124,125] EMZL occasionally spreads to lymph nodes or other MALT sites, but in general, prognosis is very favorable, with 5-year OS of >90%.[125] In a minority of cases, EMZL undergoes large cell transformation to DLBCL.[40,122,123] Improvements in therapy have improved the prognosis of salivary gland DLBCL; 5-year disease-specific survival among recently treated patients was 84%.[124]

Differential Diagnosis

In the differential diagnosis of EMZL and LESA, more extensive monocytoid B-cell proliferation outside LELs and more extensive glandular obliteration favor lymphoma. Monocytoid B cells confined to LELs and even discrete haloes around LELs can be seen in LESA, but broad intersecting bands of monocytoid B cells support a diagnosis of lymphoma. Demonstration of monotypic immunoglobulin in lymphoid cells or plasma cells supports lymphoma. Molecular genetic studies are not usually helpful because B-cell clones are reported in more than 50% of cases of LESA.[132] HIV-associated cystic lymphoid hyperplasia involves lymph nodes, is often bilateral, and typically consists of multiple dilated ducts surrounded by floridly hyperplastic follicles with attenuated mantles. LELs are not conspicuous, although large numbers of lymphoid cells may be found within the epithelium of dilated ducts. The differential diagnosis may also include IgG4-related sialadenitis, which typically involves submandibular glands.[133] These patients may have dry mouth and may carry a clinical diagnosis of Sjögren syndrome. IgG4-related sialadenitis may have prominent follicular hyperplasia and a dense lymphoid infiltrate with numerous plasma cells, but LELs are inconspicuous, and there is typically bandlike and storiform sclerosis.

LYMPHOMAS OF THE ORAL CAVITY

Clinical Features

Approximately 2% of all extranodal lymphomas arise in the oral cavity (i.e., palate, gingiva, tongue, buccal mucosa, floor of mouth, and lips).[68,134] Lymphoma arising in the bones of the jaw may present in the oral cavity.[135] Most patients are immunocompetent, middle-aged to older adults, with median age in the 6th or 7th decade and slight male preponderance.[134-138] Patients with HIV infection have a tendency to develop oral lymphomas.[137-139] HIV-infected patients are almost all males with an approximate median age of 40 years.[137,139,140] Oral lymphoma has also been reported rarely in transplant recipients.[138]

Patients present with soft tissue swelling, pain, mucosal ulceration or discoloration, paresthesias, anesthesia, or loosening of teeth.[135,138,139,141,142] The sites most often affected, in both HIV-positive and HIV-negative patients, are the palate/maxilla and gingiva, with tongue, buccal mucosa, floor of mouth, and lips affected less often.[134,135,137,139,140] Physical examination reveals an exophytic, often polypoid mass in the majority of cases. In a minority, the lymphoma is an infiltrative, ulcerated lesion with raised margins.[134]

Pathologic Features

A wide variety of lymphomas arise in the oral cavity, although nearly all are non-Hodgkin lymphoma.[143] Among immunocompetent patients, approximately half are DLBCL. Next most common is FL (Fig. 59-5), followed by EMZL, peripheral T-cell lymphoma, NOS, extranodal NK/T-cell lymphoma, BL, and others.[135-137] EMZL may arise in minor salivary glands. A predilection for FL to involve the palate is reported.[138] Mycosis fungoides occasionally involves the oral cavity. The majority of these cases are found in the setting of long-standing, advanced disease, but in exceptional cases, the first manifestation of mycosis fungoides is in the oral cavity. Aggressive epidermotropic CD8-positive cutaneous T-cell lymphoma may also involve the oral cavity.[144,145]

Oral lymphomas in HIV-infected individuals are less heterogeneous than those in immunocompetent patients; they are almost all diffuse high-grade lymphomas. Most are DLBCL, with rare BL.[40,137-140] Plasmablastic lymphoma is a distinctive type of DLBCL often arising in immunosuppressed individuals that typically occurs in the oral cavity and other extranodal sites; it is composed of cells with the appearance of immunoblasts or plasmablasts, with vesicular nuclei, prominent nucleoli, and scant to moderately abundant eccentrically placed cytoplasm with a paranuclear hof, high mitotic rate, frequent single cell necrosis, and scattered tingible-body macrophages. The immunophenotype is distinctive: neoplastic cells typically lack CD20 and have a plasma cell immunophenotype: CD138 positive, IRF4/MUM1 positive, CD79a variable, often with monotypic cytoplasmic immunoglobulin.[140,146]

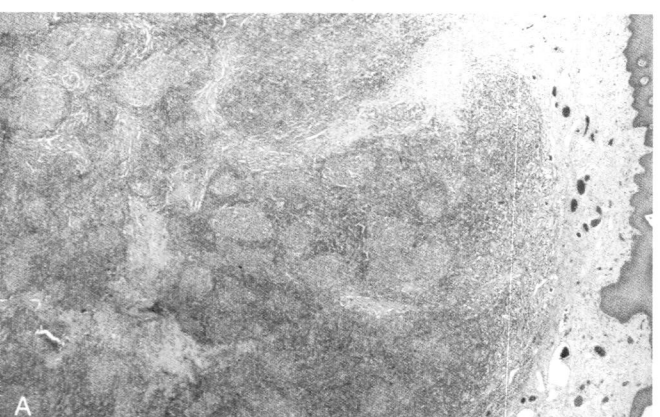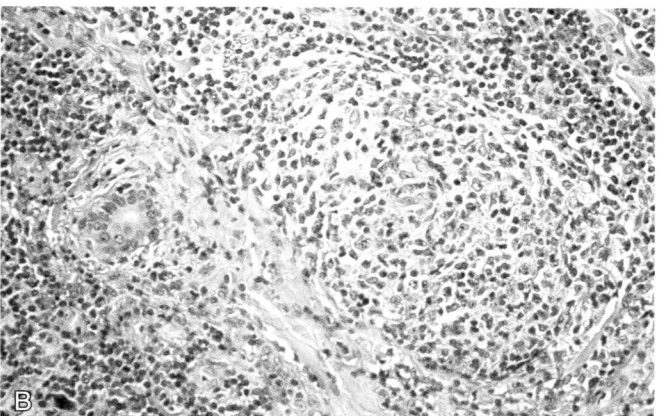

Figure 59-5. Follicular lymphoma, oral cavity. This lymphoma was a relapse from an orbital primary. **A,** Low power shows crowded follicles within soft tissue beneath squamous epithelium. **B,** Poorly circumscribed, neoplastic follicles predominantly contain centrocytes and are seen adjacent to small acini of minor salivary gland.

Most HIV-associated oral lymphomas, including plasmablastic lymphoma, contain EBV.[137-140] In contrast, only about 9% of oral lymphomas in nonimmunosuppressed patients are EBV positive.[137,138]

Staging, Treatment, and Outcome

Disease is localized in approximately 70% of cases.[135,140] The proportion with localized and disseminated disease is similar in HIV-positive and HIV-negative patients. Outcome depends on stage, type of lymphoma, type of treatment and HIV status, so that patients with localized, histologically low-grade lymphomas have an excellent outcome, while patients with high-grade lymphoma or disseminated disease have worse survival.[40,135,141,143] Improvements in therapy in recent years have been associated with improved outcome.[143]

Differential Diagnosis

Oral lymphoma can mimic dental conditions such as periodontal disease, acute necrotizing gingivitis, and dental infections.[139,142] Some lesions resemble carcinoma.[135] In HIV-positive patients, Kaposi sarcoma and deep fungal infections also enter the clinical differential diagnosis.[139]

THYROID LYMPHOMAS

Clinical Features

Primary lymphoma of the thyroid is uncommon. It accounts for 1% to 5% of all thyroidal malignancies and for 1% to 2.5% of all lymphomas.[147] Patients are affected over a wide age range, but most are older adults with a median age between 60 and 70 years. There is a female preponderance (3:1 to 4:1).[147-152] Most patients have Hashimoto thyroiditis. Patients with Hashimoto thyroiditis have an estimated 40-fold to 80-fold increased risk for lymphoma.[148,151] Patients complain of the presence of a mass, which may be rapidly enlarging. They may also have dysphagia, cough, dyspnea, and hoarseness, sometimes with tracheal compression.[147,151,152] A minority of patients with DLBCL have systemic symptoms.[153]

Pathologic Features

On gross examination, tumors range from 0.5 to 19 cm (mean, 4–7 cm) and form multinodular or diffuse, firm, or soft masses with smooth, pale tan or white-gray surfaces on sectioning.[151,153] DLBCL is the most common type, making up 50% to more than 90% of cases. DLBCL is bilateral in about 25% of cases, and it commonly involves adjacent soft tissue and other structures.[153] EMZL is next most common, accounting for 10% to 28% of cases. Lymphoma is bilateral in one-third of cases.[148] In a subset of the DLBCL there is a component of EMZL, consistent with transformation of the underlying low-grade lymphoma.[147,149,151,152,154] Of note, in some Asian series, EMZL is more common than DLBCL.[155,156] FL accounts for 2% to 10% of cases.[149,150,155,156] All other types of lymphoma are quite uncommon; among those reported are BL,[157] peripheral T-cell lymphomas, and Hodgkin lymphomas.[147,150,152,156] Most of the Hodgkin lymphomas are nodular sclerosis CHL.[158,159]

The histologic and immunophenotypic features are similar to those seen in other sites. DLBCL expresses pan–B-cell markers and includes GCB and non-GCB subtypes.[153,154] In one study, 29% were double-expressors (MYC positive, BCL2 positive).[153] Thyroidal EMZL has some distinctive characteristics, often containing a characteristic type of lymphoepithelial lesion showing round aggregates of marginal zone cells filling and expanding the lumens of thyroid follicles, so-called "MALT-ball" LELs.[151] Follicular colonization tends to be prominent, in some cases resulting in a follicular architecture so striking that it mimics FL. Blast transformation of neoplastic cells within colonized follicles is more common in the thyroid than elsewhere.[160] Changes of Hashimoto thyroiditis are often seen adjacent to the lymphoma (Fig. 59-6).[151] Approximately 50% of thyroid EMZL have a *FOXP1::IGH* translocation [(3;14)(p14.1;q32)] that results in upregulation of FOXP1, and that could play a role in the pathogenesis of EMZL.[84,154] This translocation is also found in a subset of thyroid DLBCL, all of non-GCB type, suggesting large cell transformation of an underlying EMZL. *FOXP1::IGH* is not found in FL or Hashimoto thyroiditis.[154] The majority of thyroid EMZL have pathogenic mutations of *TET2, CD274* (PD-L1), or *TNFRSF14*; many have mutated *TNFAIP3* and deletion of *CD274*.[128] The changes may deregulate interactions of neoplastic B cells with T cells, contributing to lymphomagenesis.

Although FL of the thyroid is uncommon, it has characteristic features. Immunostaining for BCL2 helps divide thyroid FL into two types: (1) BCL2+ FL, which is usually CD10+, BCL6+, low-grade, positive for *BCL2* translocation, often with widespread disease; and (2) BCL2− FL, which is usually CD10− or weak+, BCL6+, grade 3 or occasionally grade 2, lacks *BCL2* translocation, usually with disease confined to the thyroid.[161,162] FLs that are BCL2− and lack *IGH::BCL2* typically lack mutations of epigenetic modifiers such as *EZH2, KMT2D, ARID1A,* and others that are common in BCL2+ FLs with *IGH::BCL2*.[161]

Staging, Treatment, and Outcome

Most patients have localized disease at presentation; 50% to 70% of patients have stage I disease. Most of the remainder have stage II disease, usually with cervical or perithyroidal lymphadenopathy. A minority has more widespread nodal and extranodal involvement. Extranodal sites that may be involved include bone marrow, GI tract, lungs, liver, and bladder.[151,152] EMZL are almost always localized (stage I or II). Stage III and IV lymphomas are usually DLBCL.[147,151]

Patients are usually treated with radiation, chemotherapy, or both.[147,151] Median OS of DLBCL is 11 to 13 years, with a 5-year OS of 73% to 76%,[149,153] while EMZL has a 5-year OS of 94% and a median OS of 16 to 17 years, with only 1% to 4% dying of lymphoma.[148-150] Survival of DLBCL patients is better with combined radiation and chemotherapy, including rituximab.[153] Patients with EMZL often do well when treated with radiation alone.[149]

Differential Diagnosis

Both Hashimoto thyroiditis and EMZL have reactive lymphoid follicles and LELs, but in favor of EMZL are obliteration of thyroid parenchyma by a diffuse infiltrate of marginal zone B cells and lymphoid or plasma cells expressing monotypic immunoglobulin. LELs are larger and more numerous in EMZL. Cases of extramedullary plasmacytoma arising in

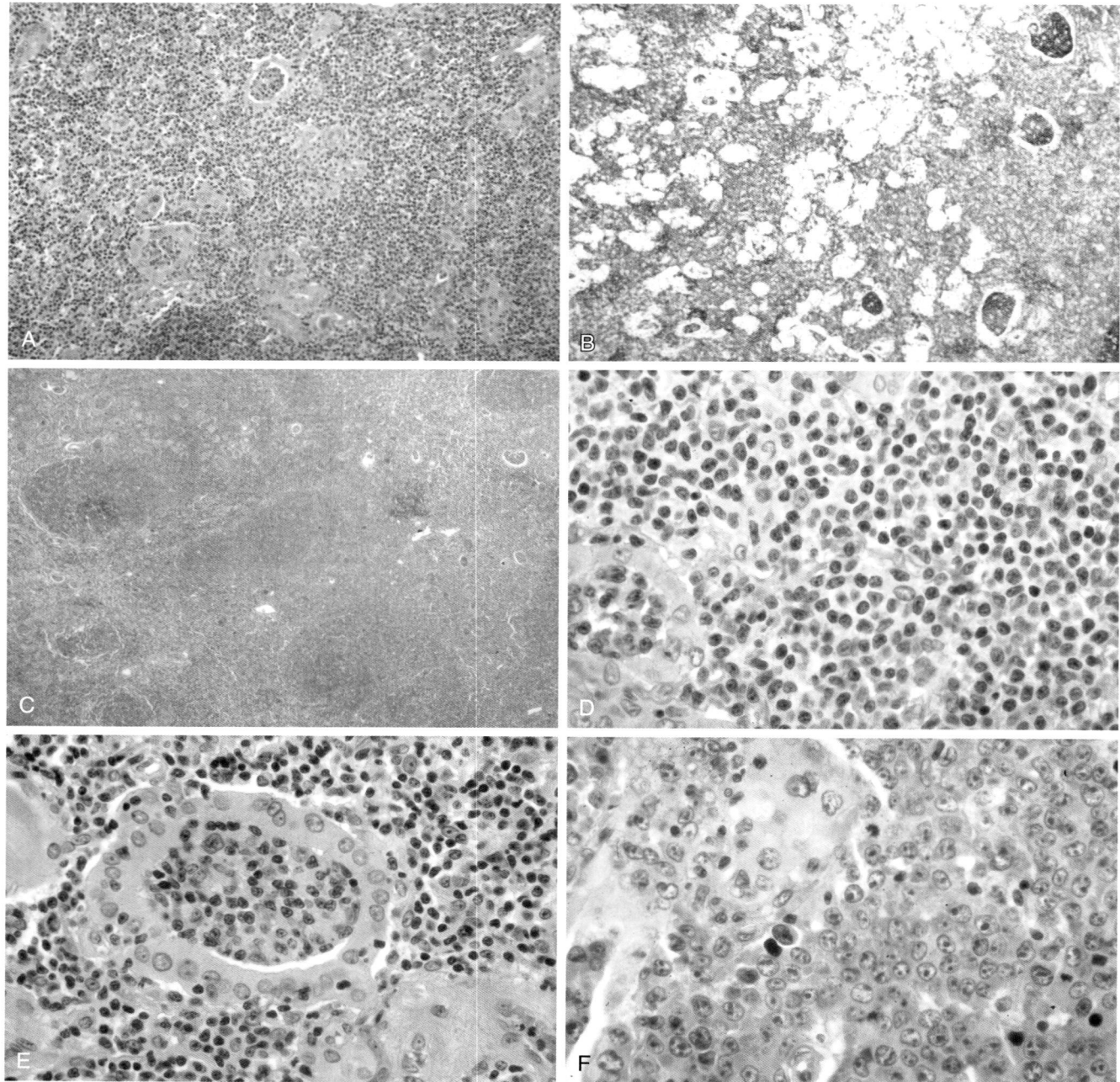

Figure 59-6. Thyroid gland with extranodal marginal zone lymphoma of mucosa-associated lymphoid tissue **(A–E)** with large cell transformation **(F)**. Other areas showed Hashimoto thyroiditis. **A,** Low power shows obliteration of the normal parenchyma. **B,** A stain for CD20 highlights the diffuse infiltrate of B cells; several rounded lymphoepithelial lesions are seen (immunoperoxidase technique on paraffin section). **C,** In areas there is vague nodularity, consistent with colonization of reactive lymphoid follicles by neoplastic marginal zone cells. **D,** The marginal zone cells are small, with oval-to-slightly-irregular nuclei and moderate amount of pale cytoplasm. **E,** MALT-ball lymphoepithelial lesion. The epithelium of the thyroid follicle shows oxyphil change. **F,** An area of large cell transformation. Many of the neoplastic cells are immunoblasts.

the thyroid have been described; some of these may represent EMZL with marked plasmacytic differentiation. Reactive follicles, an extrafollicular component of B cells, particularly with the morphology of marginal zone cells, and LELs make plasmacytoma unlikely. It may be difficult to distinguish undifferentiated carcinoma from DLBCL on routine sections, but diagnosis can be established using immunohistochemical studies.

LARYNGEAL LYMPHOMAS

Clinical Features

Primary laryngeal lymphoma is rare, accounting for fewer than 1% of laryngeal malignancies.[163,164] Patients are mostly middle-aged to older adults with few young adults and children affected. There is a slight male preponderance.[40,164-167] Several patients have had concurrent laryngeal squamous cell carcinoma or other malignancies.[166,167] Rarely, patients are HIV positive[40,165] or have another underlying immunodeficiency.[168]

Patients present with hoarseness, dyspnea, progressive or acute laryngeal obstruction, sore throat, foreign body sensation, or dysphagia.[40,164,166,167] The tumors are usually smooth-surfaced, submucosal, raised, often polypoid lesions.[165,166,169] Pedunculated tumors may prolapse into the airway.[165,167] Laryngeal lymphomas may arise from the lymphoid tissue that can be found in the larynx, mainly in the epiglottis and supraglottic larynx, correlating with the distribution of lymphomas.[169]

Pathologic Features

DLBCL and EMZL, together, account for approximately 80% of cases. Their pathologic features are similar to those in other sites.[164,166,167,169,170] Rare cases of FL[164] and peripheral T-cell lymphoma[166,171] are reported. Extranodal NK/T-cell lymphoma (see Chapter 29) is rare but is reported.[163,165,171] It is more common in Asians and Native Americans and accounts for about 2% of all extranodal NK/T-cell lymphomas.[163]

Staging, Treatment, and Outcome

In approximately 75% of cases, patients have Ann Arbor stage I disease; most of the remainder have stage II disease.[40,164-167] In a few EMZL, the larynx has been involved simultaneous with involvement of other extranodal sites in the head and neck.[40,172] Most patients with EMZL and DLBCL can be successfully treated with a combination of surgery and radiation or chemotherapy,[40,173] although laryngeal lymphoma rarely results in sudden death caused by acute airway obstruction.[169] When EMZL patients develop relapses, they tend to be isolated, extranodal tumors in the upper respiratory tract, stomach, orbit, and skin; when relapses occur, there may be long disease-free intervals, similar to EMZL in other sites.[40,166]

PULMONARY LYMPHOMAS

Primary pulmonary lymphoma is defined traditionally as lymphoma presenting as pulmonary lesion(s), with no clinical, pathologic, or radiographic evidence of lymphoma elsewhere in the past, at present, or for 3 months after presentation,[174,175] but others accept cases in which staging reveals disease outside the lung if pulmonary disease predominates.[176]

Clinical Features

Primary pulmonary lymphomas account for 0.3% of primary lung neoplasms,[175] <1% of all lymphomas,[177,178] and 3.6% of extranodal lymphomas.[175] Patients are typically adults (median age, about 60 years). It is uncommon before age 30,[174,176-180] although rare cases in younger patients are reported.[181,182] Most studies show a slight male predominance.[176-178]

Approximately 70% of cases are EMZL.[174,176,177,182] Pulmonary EMZL affects females more often in some reports[183] and affects males and females roughly equally in others[184,185] over a broad age range, with a median age in the 6th decade.[184,185] Many pulmonary lymphoma patients are asymptomatic at presentation. The remainder have pulmonary (cough, dyspnea, hemoptysis, or chest pain) or constitutional symptoms. Asymptomatic patients usually have EMZL.[174,176,179,180,182,186,187] Approximately one-third of patients have an associated autoimmune disease,[180,183] the most frequent of which is Sjögren syndrome.[176,177,180] Monoclonal paraproteins are relatively common,[174,176,183] being found in 10%[184] to 43% of cases.[180]

A small number of patients are HIV positive.[188] Lung allograft recipients may develop posttransplantation lymphoproliferative disorders (PTLD) involving the lung.[177]

Radiologic Features/Patterns of Involvement

Patients have single or multiple unilateral or bilateral lesions that can be nodules, masses, or infiltrates that may resemble consolidated lung.[174,176,177,179,180,186,187] Pulmonary EMZL involves the lungs unilaterally in 70% to 75% of cases, as single or multiple lesions.[183,184] Pulmonary lymphomas rarely show endobronchial or diffuse submucosal involvement.[177] Fewer than 10% are associated with a pleural effusion.[174,176]

Pathologic Features

Pulmonary EMZL has features similar to those of EMZL in other anatomic sites. Lymphoma spreads in a diffuse and interstitial pattern. Most cases have interspersed reactive lymphoid follicles and LELs formed with bronchial or bronchiolar epithelium (Fig. 59-7). Infiltration of the pleura is frequent.[176,180,189] Occasional cases are associated with amyloid deposition[179,180,184,189]; this seems to be more frequent in the lung than in other sites. A variety of genetic alterations are described. Among the most important is t(11;18)(q21;q21), a translocation almost exclusively found in EMZL, resulting in *BIRC3::MALT1* gene fusion, occurring in 30% to 50% of pulmonary EMZL.[83,183,190]

DLBCL is the next most common type of primary pulmonary lymphoma, accounting for approximately 20% of cases. Many have a component of EMZL, consistent with large-cell transformation of the EMZL.[174,176,180,182,183,187] Other types of lymphoma are uncommon; they include FL,[176,179,182] BL,[176] lymphomatoid granulomatosis (see Chapter 28),[182] peripheral T-cell lymphoma, NOS,[176,182] anaplastic large cell lymphoma,[175] and rarely, CHL.[177] Nearly all HIV-associated cases are diffuse, high-grade, EBV-positive B-cell lymphomas.[188,191]

Staging, Treatment, and Outcome

Lymphoma may be confined to the lungs, or may involve lymph nodes or other extranodal sites, especially so-called "MALT sites."[178,186] EMZL is stage I or II in about two-thirds of cases.[184] Patients with EMZL may develop relapses in the lung and other MALT sites, especially stomach and salivary glands, as well as lymph nodes, and some undergo transformation to DLBCL. Overall, patients do well, and survival is good with a variety of therapeutic approaches.[174,176,177,180,182,186,189] In one series of pulmonary EMZL, 15-year disease-specific survival was 95%, median PFS was 7.5 years and median OS was 15.7 years,[184] while in another, 5-year OS was 87% and 5-year PFS was 75%.[185] Inferior PFS has been associated with stage III or IV disease, MALT IPI of 2 or 3, involvement of MALT sites in addition to lung, and multifocal lung disease.[184] OS is inferior with older patient age.[185]

Pulmonary DLBCL have a prognosis similar to[180,182] or worse than[174,176] pulmonary EMZL. DLBCL patients usually receive more aggressive therapy; this could account for the lack of difference in outcome some have observed.

Differential Diagnosis

The main problem in differential diagnosis is distinguishing EMZL from chronic inflammatory processes with lymphoid hyperplasia, including nodular lymphoid hyperplasia, lymphocytic interstitial pneumonia, and IgG4-related disease.[183] In favor of lymphoma is a predominance of B cells with the morphology of marginal zone cells in a diffuse pattern outside follicles, CD43 co-expression by the B cells, monotypic immunoglobulin expression by lymphocytes or plasma cells, and clonal immunoglobulin gene rearrangement. In favor of a reactive process is a mixture of B and T cells, with B cells mostly confined to follicles. LELs are frequent in lymphoid hyperplasia, but they are less frequent than in EMZL, and the intraepithelial lymphocytes can be B or T cells, in contrast to the predominance of B cells seen in EMZL.[179]

LYMPHOMAS OF THE PLEURA AND PLEURAL CAVITY

Lymphomas rarely arise primarily in the pleural cavity and other body cavities. Several distinctive types have been described: *primary effusion lymphoma* (see Chapter 28), an aggressive HHV8-positive lymphoma mainly affecting HIV-positive individuals, *pyothorax-associated lymphoma* (see Chapter 28), a distinctive type of DLBCL with chronic inflammation, and HHV-8 and EBV-negative primary effusion-based lymphoma (ICC)/*fluid overload-associated large B-cell lymphoma* (WHO 5th edition), which presents as serous effusions, typically in older adults with cardiovascular, renal, or hepatic disease resulting in fluid overload.[192,193] Fluid overload-associated large B-cell lymphoma has been referred to by a variety of names, including PEL-like lymphoma and HHV8-unrelated PEL-like lymphoma.

By definition, they are negative for HHV8. In contrast to PEL, the majority are CD20 positive, a minority are EBV positive, and the prognosis is significantly more favorable.[1]

LYMPHOMAS OF THE THYMUS

Several types of lymphoma can arise in the anterior mediastinum, including the thymus: primary mediastinal large B-cell lymphoma (see Chapter 22), CHL and mediastinal gray zone lymphoma (Chapter 27), T-lymphoblastic leukemia/lymphoma (see Chapter 41), and EMZL of mucosa-associated lymphoid tissue (see Chapter 18). Thymic EMZLs are rare; they are distinctive in that they form LELs with Hassall corpuscles and usually express IgA (Fig. 59-8).[194]

CARDIAC LYMPHOMAS

Clinical Features

Primary cardiac lymphoma predominantly or exclusively involves the heart.[195,196] Primary cardiac lymphoma is rare; secondary cardiac involvement by lymphoma arising elsewhere is much more common[197] and is frequent among patients dying of lymphoma.[198] Primary cardiac tumors are uncommon; lymphoma accounts for 1% to 2% of primary cardiac neoplasms.[196,199,200] Primary cardiac lymphomas occur over a broad age range, but mainly occur in older adults (median, 7th decade), with males more affected than females.[195,198-205] They also occur in immunocompromised HIV-positive patients and allograft recipients (Figs. 59-9–59-10).[201,206] Those arising in HIV-positive individuals affect younger individuals with a pronounced male preponderance.[201] Children rarely develop cardiac lymphoma.[207,208] Patients present with chest pain, dyspnea, congestive heart failure, fatigue, syncope, or arrhythmias.[195,198,200,201] Pericardial effusion, sometimes with tamponade, and pleural effusion are common.[198,200,209] Complete atrioventricular block has been described.[209]

Primary cardiac lymphoma most often involves myocardium.[196] Valvular involvement is rare, but is described.[196,198] The lymphomas involve the right side of the heart more often than the left side.[197,198] Diagnosis may be

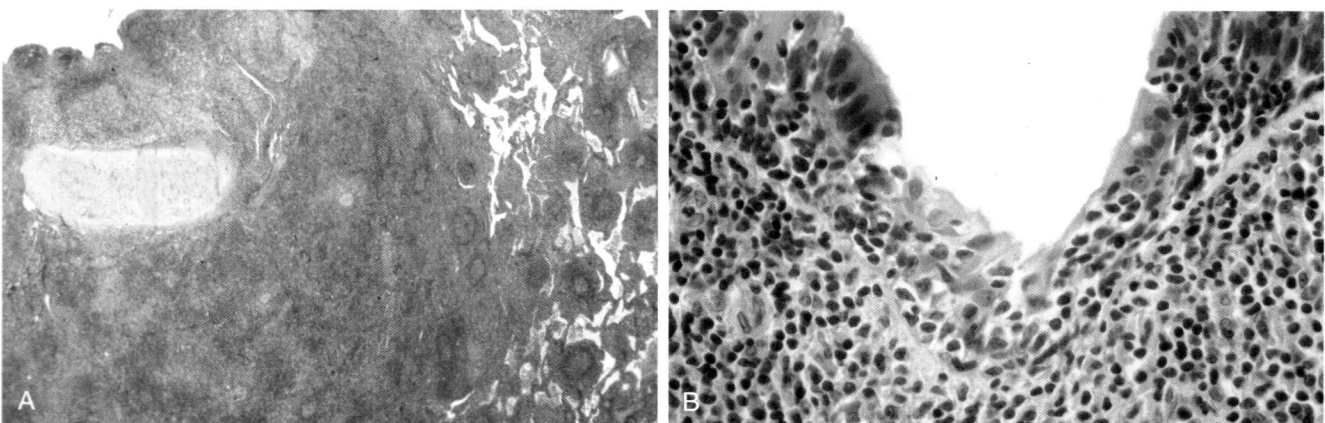

Figure 59-7. Extranodal marginal zone lymphoma of mucosa-associated lymphoid tissue, lung. A, A dense diffuse lymphoid infiltrate extends from the bronchial lumen *(upper left)*, past bronchial cartilage and into surrounding lung. At the periphery, there is an interstitial pattern. Reactive follicles are scattered evenly throughout the lymphoid infiltrate. **B,** Higher power shows bronchial epithelium with lymphoepithelial lesions; lymphoid cells are small with pale cytoplasm.

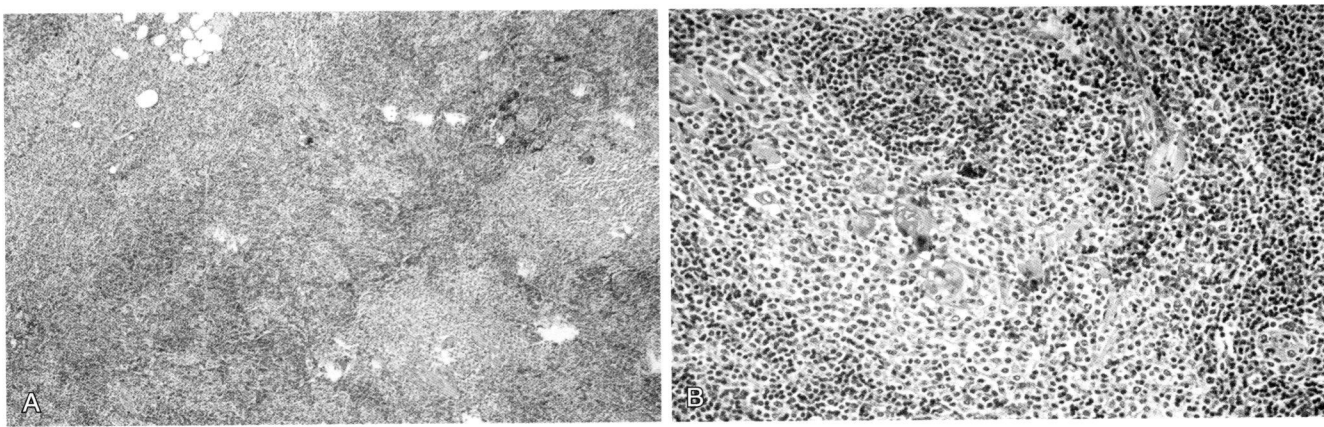

Figure 59-8. Extranodal marginal zone lymphoma of mucosa-associated lymphoid tissue, thymus. A, The normal thymic tissue is obliterated by a mottled pale and dark lymphoid infiltrate. **B,** Pale areas correspond to aggregates of marginal zone cells, shown here surrounding and invading a Hassall corpuscle.

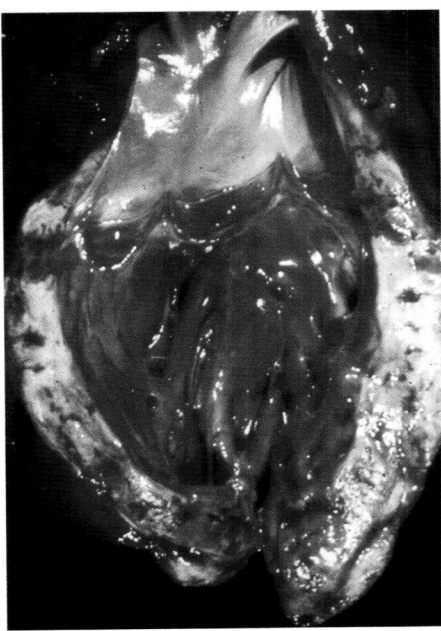

Figure 59-9. Cardiac lymphoma in a renal transplant recipient. Yellow tumor can be seen on cross-section, replacing normal myocardium.

based on biopsy or pericardial fluid cytology.[200,201,203,210,211] The prognosis has been poor, because diagnosis was often delayed and only made postmortem, and because fatal arrhythmias often accompanied chemotherapy.[195] Among more recent cases, prognosis appears better with earlier diagnosis and improvements in imaging and therapy, including careful monitoring of cardiac function. Optimally treated patients may attain a sustained complete remission.[196,199,200,212] Prognosis is worse with older age and advanced stage disease.[200,204,205]

Pathologic Features

Primary cardiac lymphomas are nearly exclusively (DLBCL) (Fig. 59-10).[195,201,209,211,212] Non-GCB immunophenotype is slightly more common than GCB type.[198] In one study, 53% of DLBCLs were double-expressors, co-expressing MYC

and BCL2.[200] Fibrin-associated DLBCL, often mimicking atrial myxoma, represents a subset of cases.[198,200] Rare cases of peripheral T-cell lymphoma, B and T lymphoblastic lymphoma, and BL are reported.[198,200,207,208] Primary cardiac extracavitary primary effusion lymphoma (HHV8 positive) has been reported in an HIV-positive male.[213] One double-hit high-grade B-cell lymphoma is reported.[198] Secondary cardiac lymphomas are pathologically much more heterogeneous.[197]

Differential Diagnosis

Because cardiac lymphomas are rare, lymphoma is rarely suspected prior to biopsy. Cardiac lymphoma can mimic much more common, non-neoplastic causes of cardiac dysfunction. The combination of right-sided tumor and high LDH, particularly in an immunocompromised patient, is suspicious for lymphoma.

LYMPHOMAS OF THE BREAST

Clinical Features

Primary lymphoma of the breast is usually defined as lymphoma confined to one or both breasts, with or without ipsilateral axillary lymph node involvement, but without disease elsewhere at presentation, in a patient without a history of lymphoma.[214] The breast is among the least-common primary sites for lymphoma, possibly correlating with sparse endogenous mammary lymphoid tissue. Only approximately 0.5% of primary breast malignancies are lymphomas.[214] Less than 1% of lymphomas arise in the breast.[215] Most patients are middle-aged to elderly women, although occasionally young adult or adolescent females and rare males are affected.[214-219] Occasionally lymphomas arise in pregnant or lactating women.[214,220] Patients often present with a palpable breast mass.[221] Occasional lymphomas are detected by mammography.[218,222,223] Constitutional symptoms are uncommon.[216] In 0% to 25% of cases in different series, patients present with bilateral disease.[214,216,219,224] Patients usually have discrete, mobile mass(es), without fixation to either superficial or deep structures. Involvement of the overlying skin is described[225]; the appearance can

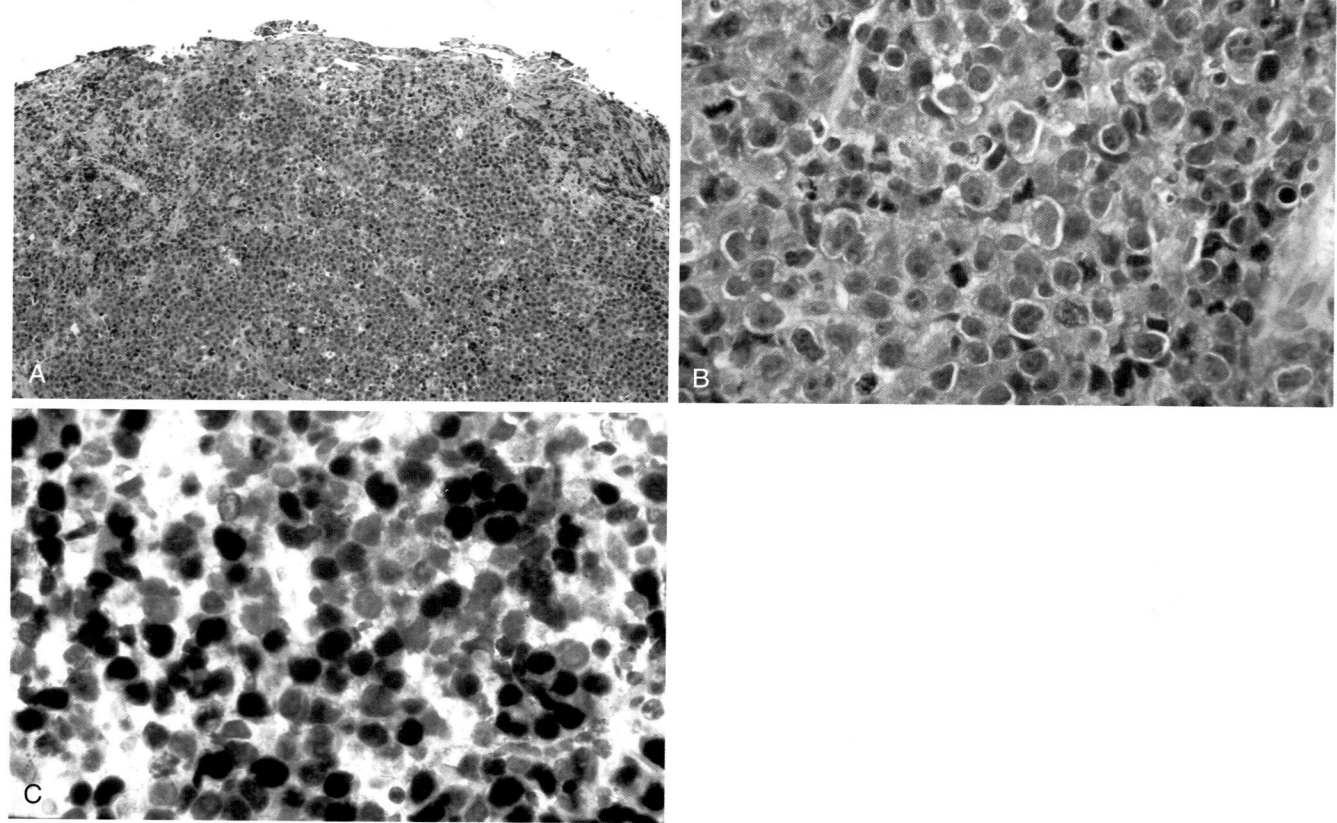

Figure 59-10. Cardiac diffuse large B-cell lymphoma in a HIV-positive male. A, A dense lymphoid infiltrate forms a mass involving the right side of the heart. **B,** Higher power shows large atypical lymphoid cells with frequent mitoses. **C,** Neoplastic cells contain Epstein-Barr virus (in situ hybridization on a paraffin section using a probe for EBER).

mimic inflammatory carcinoma.[226] Ipsilateral axillary lymphadenopathy involvement varies widely among series, from 11%[218] to ~50%.[216]

Breast implant-associated anaplastic large cell lymphoma (BI-ALCL) is a rare, distinctive, CD30-positive, ALK-negative T-cell neoplasm arising in association with breast implants (see Chapter 36).[227-229] Rare cases of fibrin-associated large B-cell lymphoma and DLBCL with chronic inflammation have also been reported in association with breast implants.[230,231]

Pathologic Features

The tumors vary greatly in size, from approximately 1 to 12 cm.[219] They are usually discrete but nonencapsulated, with a fleshy or soft consistency and white-gray or white-pink color. In some cases, there is more than one discrete mass.[214,218,226] Nearly all primary breast lymphomas are B-lineage (BI-ALCL being an exception). In most series, DLBCL is the most common type, comprising ~70% of cases (Fig. 59-11).[217,221,222,232] DLBCL of GCB is less common than DLBCL of non-GCB ABC type.[215,224] The DLBCLs are typically EBV negative.[233] Primary breast DLBCL of non-GCB type often have mutations of *MYD88* (MYD88 L265) and *CD79B*, resulting in activation of the NFκB pathway, contributing to lymphomagenesis.[234] Translocations of *BCL2, BCL6,* and *MYC* are absent or rare.[234]

Most of the remainder are either EMZL of mucosa-associated lymphoid tissue (Fig. 59-12) or FL. T-cell lymphomas are rare,[223,226] and are not well characterized except for BI-ALCL (see Chapter 36). Other lymphomas rarely arising in the breast include B-lymphoblastic lymphoma and CHL.[215,221]

DLBCL affects women over a wide age range. FL and EMZL affect middle-aged and older women. BL is mainly found in young women who may be pregnant or postpartum; a minority of DLBCL are also found in this clinical setting.[214,218,220,226,232,235] BL is more often synchronously bilateral than other breast lymphomas. Among African patients, a higher proportion of breast lymphomas are BL than in other geographic areas.[236]

Although breast lymphomas appear circumscribed grossly, they often show invasion into surrounding tissues at the periphery of the mass.[218] The neoplastic cells infiltrate around and within mammary ducts and lobules, sometimes with obliteration of these structures. FL of all grades (1–3) have been reported. EMZLs have an appearance similar to other sites, except that LELs are not usually found.[218,223,226]

Treatment and Outcome

The outcome of patients with lymphomas of the breast has improved over time. DLBCL of the breast is relatively aggressive. It can recur in the same breast or spread to lymph nodes and various extranodal sites including CNS, contralateral

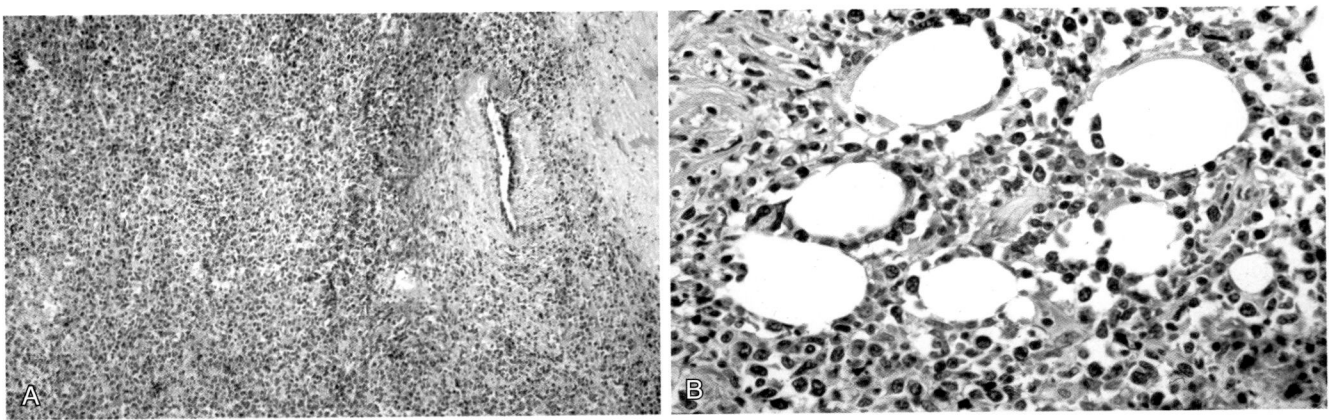

Figure 59-11. Diffuse large B-cell lymphoma, breast. A, Low power shows a dense, diffuse lymphoid infiltrate surrounding a ductule and replacing normal tissue. **B,** Large atypical lymphoid cells with irregular nuclei infiltrate fat.

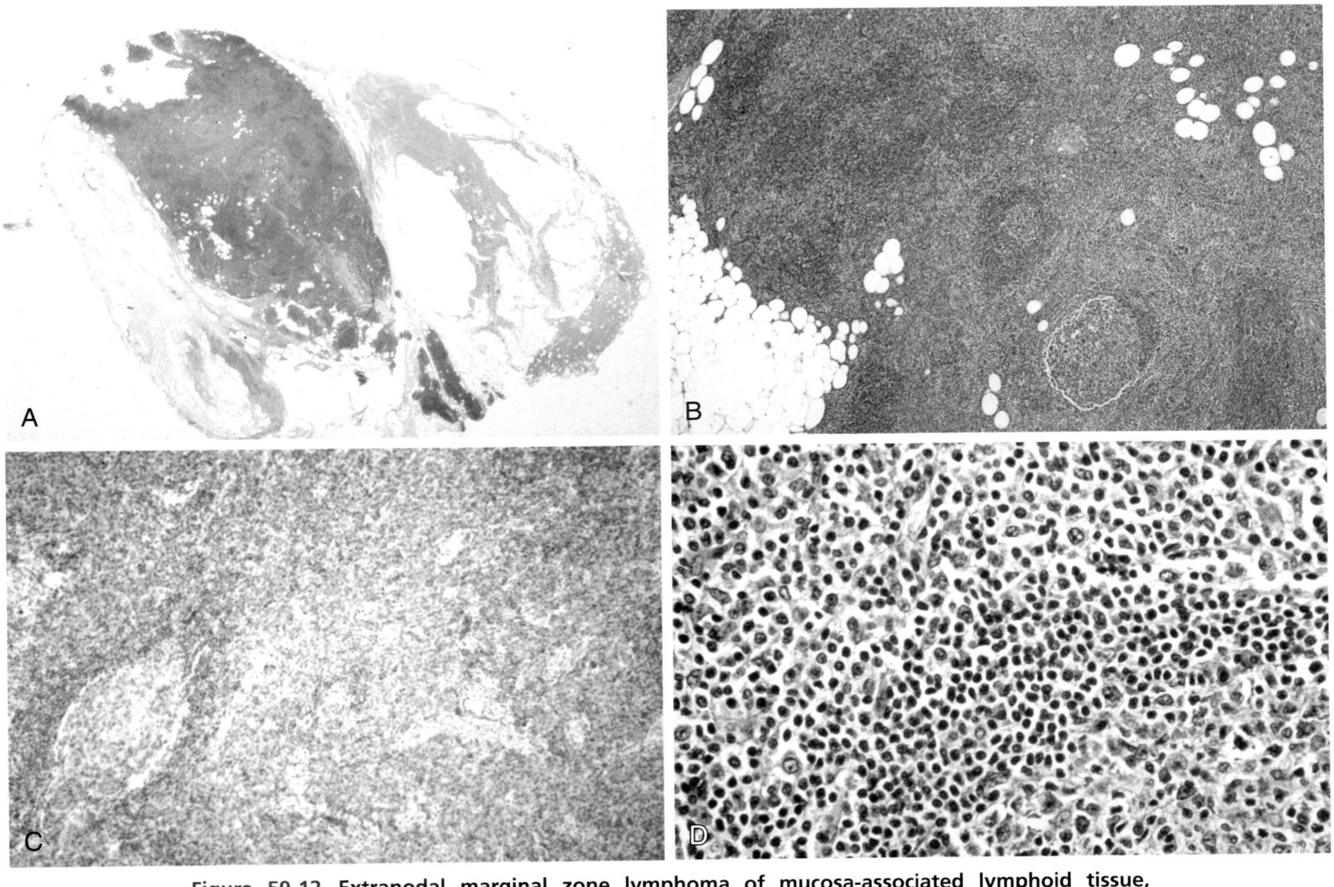

Figure 59-12. Extranodal marginal zone lymphoma of mucosa-associated lymphoid tissue, breast. A, Whole mount of the excisional biopsy specimen shows a well-delineated nodule of lymphoid tissue. **B,** Medium power shows a diffuse lymphoid infiltrate with scattered reactive follicles. **C,** A stain for CD20 shows staining of the follicle and of most extrafollicular lymphoid cells (immunoperoxidase technique on paraffin section). **D,** In the *lower right corner* is a portion of a reactive follicle with a mantle of small lymphocytes. The rest of the field is occupied by marginal zone cells.

breast, liver, spleen, and others.[214,217,219,224,232] EMZL patients typically remain well after treatment or develop relapses that are usually extranodal (subcutis, larynx, chest wall, parotid, orbit), but occasionally involving lymph nodes, although usually without generalized disease. Large cell transformation has been reported. Thus, mammary EMZL behaves in a manner similar to EMZL in other sites.[218,220,232] FL patients may develop generalized disease, similar to nodal FL.[218] With appropriate therapy, BL patients may attain long-term survival.[219]

Differential Diagnosis

As breast lymphoma is rare, that diagnosis is almost never suspected preoperatively. The clinical impression is usually carcinoma.[226] On pathologic grounds, the differential diagnosis includes carcinoma in cases of high-grade lymphoma and a reactive lymphoid infiltrate in cases of low-grade lymphoma. Lymphomas may be sampled via incisional or excisional biopsy, core needle biopsy, or fine-needle aspiration (Fig. 59-13). Careful attention to cytologic detail and to the discohesive nature of the lymphoid cells should lead to consideration of lymphoma. Diagnosis can then be confirmed by immunophenotyping. In the differential diagnosis of low-grade lymphoma and chronic inflammatory processes, in favor of EMZL are large numbers of B cells outside follicles, especially with the morphology of marginal zone cells, and monotypic immunoglobulin expression by B cells or plasma cells in the infiltrate. In distinguishing follicular hyperplasia from FL, criteria similar to those used in lymph nodes can be applied.

The uncommon reactive process known as *lymphocytic mastopathy, diabetic mastopathy,* or *autoimmune mastopathy* may be seen in patients with diabetes mellitus or immunologic disorders, or in women who are otherwise well. It usually presents as a palpable breast mass in young or middle-aged women.[236,237] Microscopic examination reveals a lobulocentric, sometimes also perivascular, lymphocytic infiltrate composed predominantly of B cells, sometimes with germinal-center formation, sometimes with lobular atrophy and sclerosis.[236,237] The tight perilobular distribution, lack of cytologic atypia, and lack of monotypic immunoglobulin help distinguish this disorder from lymphoma.

GASTROINTESTINAL LYMPHOMAS

The GI tract is the most common primary extranodal site for lymphoma; 30% to 40% of all extranodal lymphomas[238] and 4% to 20% of all non-Hodgkin lymphomas arise in this site. The stomach is most often involved, followed by the small intestine, the colon, and then, rarely, the esophagus.[238-241] Predisposing factors include infection, in particular by *Helicobacter pylori*; celiac disease; and possibly inflammatory bowel disease. The GI tract is one of the most common sites for lymphoma in patients with congenital immunodeficiency syndromes (see Chapter 53), HIV infection, and iatrogenic immunosuppression (see Chapter 54).

Findings include pain, anorexia, weight loss, bleeding, obstruction, palpable mass, diarrhea, nausea, vomiting, fever, and perforation. Intussusception may occur with bulky ileocecal lymphomas.[242-247]

GASTRIC LYMPHOMA

The stomach is the primary site in 55% to 75% of GI lymphomas. Of gastric malignancies, 1% to 7% are lymphoma.[241,248] DLBCL is the most common type, followed by EMZL (see Chapter 18). Other lymphomas are uncommon.

Gastric Diffuse Large B-Cell Lymphoma

Clinical Features

This is mainly a disease of older adults (median, 7th decade); younger adults are occasionally affected. There is a slight male preponderance.[249-251]

Pathologic Features

Gross examination reveals single or occasionally multiple large ulcerated or exophytic lesions that are usually transmurally invasive, sometimes associated with invasion of adjacent structures.[252] Microscopic examination reveals a diffuse proliferation of large cells with round, oval, irregular, or lobated nuclei, distinct nucleoli, and scant cytoplasm. An estimated one-third of cases have a concomitant component of EMZL consistent with large-cell transformation.[248] Immunophenotypic features are similar to DLBCL in other sites.[250,253]

Rearrangement of *BCL6* is more common, and *BCL2* rearrangement less common in gastric than in nodal DLBCL.[254] Despite the high frequency of t(11;18) (q21;q21)/*BIRC3*::MALT1 and trisomy 3 in EMZL, they are uncommon in DLBCL, implying that EMZL with these cytogenetic abnormalities are unlikely to undergo large-cell transformation.[253,255,256] Other trisomies (most often of chromosomes 12 and 18) are more common in DLBCL that

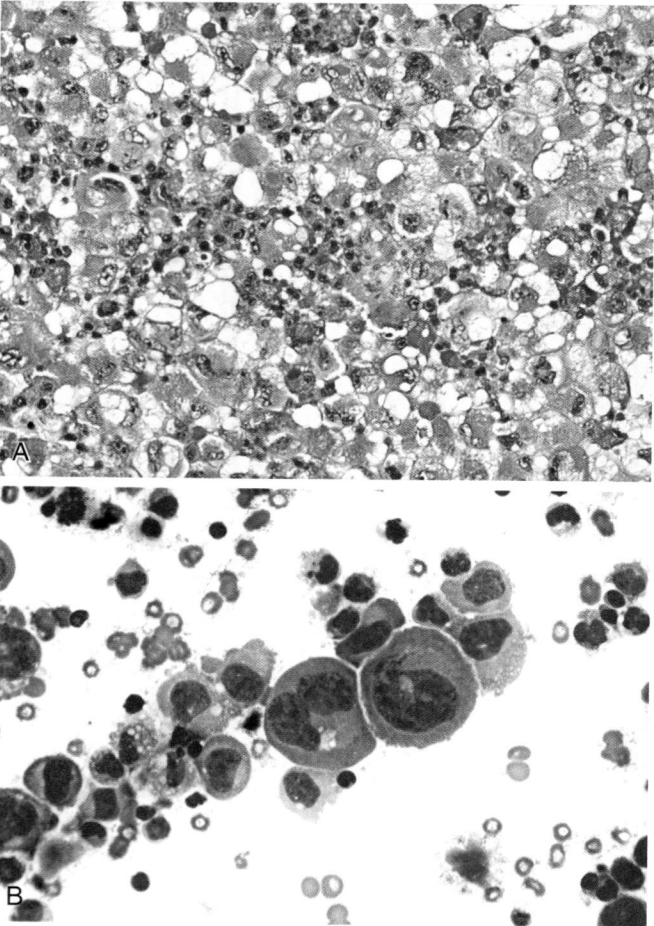

Figure 59-13. Breast implant associated anaplastic large cell lymphoma. **A,** Cell block from the seroma shows numerous large bizarre cells with large oval or indented nuclei, prominent nucleoli and abundant pink cytoplasm. **B,** Wright stained smear shows large atypical Uni nucleated and binucleated neoplastic cells in a background of scattered small lymphocytes and histiocytes. *(Images available through the courtesy of Dr. Elaine Jaffe.)*

have arisen through transformation of EMZL than in de novo large B-cell lymphomas.[257]

Staging, Treatment, and Outcome

In most cases (78%–95%), patients present with stage I or II disease.[249,250,253] A few have more distant spread to marrow, liver, or other sites.[248] Patients have been treated with surgery, radiation, chemotherapy, or a combination of these modalities. DLBCL associated with a component of EMZL is reported to have a better prognosis than de novo DLBCL.[249,250] Patients with stage Ie or IIe1 having a better outcome than those with IIe2 or higher.[250,253] A subset of gastric DLBCL is reported to respond to *H. pylori* eradication therapy.[256,258] Sensitivity or resistance to such therapy may be related to miRNA profile, mTOR pathway activation, and expression of Toll-like receptor 5.[259] An unknown factor may be overdiagnosis of DLBCL in cases of EMZL with "increased" large cells.

Differential Diagnosis

Poorly differentiated carcinomas may be composed of discohesive-appearing cells with little or no gland formation, and mimic DLBCL. Lymphoid cells may show artifactual vacuolar change and mimic signet ring cells. Immunohistochemical studies establish a diagnosis.

SMALL AND LARGE INTESTINAL LYMPHOMAS

The small intestine is the primary site in 15% to 35% of GI lymphomas.[241-243,248,260] The ileum/ileocecal region is more commonly affected than duodenum or jejunum.

Lymphoma accounts for ~25% of small intestinal neoplasms.[241] DLBCL is most common, followed by EMZL (including the distinctive subtype known as immunoproliferative small intestinal disease [IPSID]) (Chapter 18), BL (Chapter 23), T-cell lymphomas (Chapter 37), mantle cell lymphoma (Chapter 21), and FL (Chapter 17).[241,242,247,252,260]

Of GI lymphomas, 7% to 20% arise in the colon.[243,260] Lymphoma accounts for 0.5% of colonic malignancies.[241,261]

DLBCL is most common, followed by EMZL, mantle cell lymphoma, and rare cases of FL, BL, and peripheral T-cell lymphoma. Large intestinal lymphoma most often involves the cecum/ileocecal region, and the rectum is next most often involved; other portions of the colon are rarely affected.[241,262] Anal lymphomas are very rare; they are usually DLBCL.[263] Plasmablastic lymphoma may be primary in the large or small intestine, particularly the anal region.[264]

Intestinal Diffuse Large B-Cell Lymphoma

Clinical Features

Most patients are older adults, with a few cases occurring in younger adults or children. There is a slight male preponderance among adults; children are almost exclusively boys. Lymphoma in children is virtually only found in the ileocecal area.[245,247,261] Fewer than 1% of GI lymphomas arise in the setting of ulcerative colitis.[246] Ulcerative colitis–associated lymphomas, which are mostly DLBCL, are more often distally located in the colon, and almost always in sites of active inflammation. Compared with colonic lymphoma in the general population, in ulcerative colitis, lymphoma is more often multiple (38% vs. 10%).[265,266] These lymphomas have usually appeared in patients with long-standing ulcerative colitis,[265] although immunosuppressive/immunomodulatory therapy may accelerate lymphomagenesis.[267]

Pathologic Features

The gross and microscopic appearance is similar to gastric DLBCL (Fig. 59-14).[242,244,245,247,248] Some cases have a component of EMZL,[248] consistent with large-cell transformation of EMZL. The reported proportion of cases with an associated EMZL varies widely, from 10%[248] to >50% of DLBCL.[242,244,247] The immunophenotypic and genotypic features are similar to those of gastric DLBCL.

Staging, Treatment, and Outcome

In most cases, disease is confined to the intestine with or without regional lymph node involvement.[248] Treatment is usually surgical resection followed by chemotherapy. Five-year survival ranges from 25% to 67%.[252,255] DLBCL arising

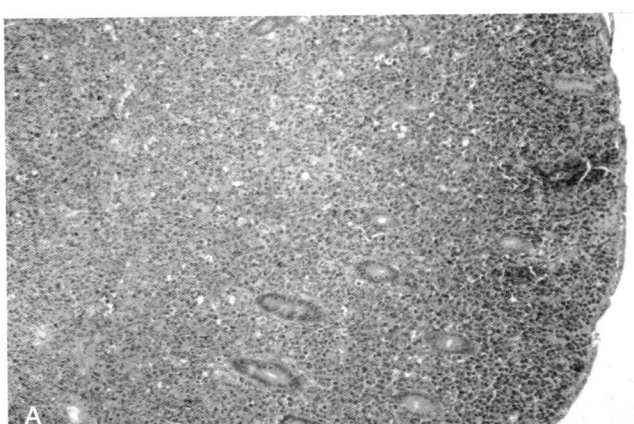
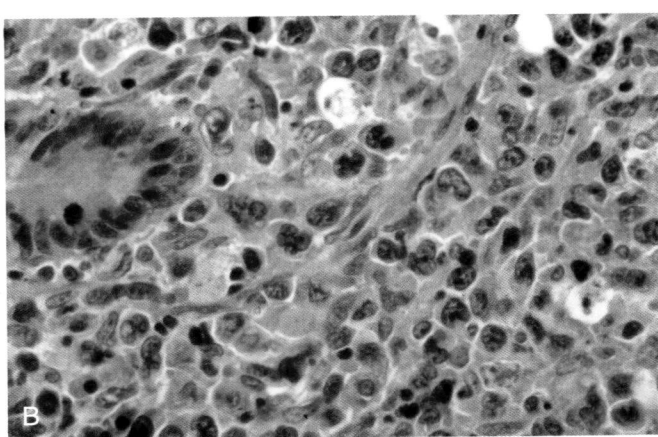

Figure 59-14. Diffuse large B-cell lymphoma, colon. A, Lymphoma invades deep into the wall of the bowel. **B,** The large, atypical neoplastic cells are highly irregular and often multilobated.

in association with EMZL may have a better prognosis than de novo DLBCL.[244]

Mantle Cell Lymphoma

Mantle cell lymphoma is discussed in Chapter 21. In the GI tract, it often manifests as lymphomatous polyposis, involving long segments of bowel,[244,255] usually with mesenteric lymph nodal involvement,[255] often with widespread disease away from the GI tract. The pathologic features and prognosis are similar to that of other cases of mantle cell lymphoma.

Follicular Lymphoma

FL accounts for 2% to 13% of all primary GI tract lymphomas[238,268]; any portion of the GI tract may be involved,[269] but the duodenum is the most common site.[260,268,270,271] Most GI tract FL are duodenal-type FL, a variant of FL with distinctive clinical and pathologic features, including limited stage disease, low histologic grade, and excellent prognosis (Chapter 17).

Burkitt Lymphoma

Clinical Features

Three clinical variants of BL are traditionally recognized: endemic, sporadic, and immunodeficiency-associated; however, more recent data suggest BL is better subdivided based on EBV status than on epidemiologic subtype, as the presence or absence of EBV separates BL into discrete biological groups based on their molecular features.[1] Involvement of the ileocecal region is the most common manifestation of sporadic BL. Ileocecal disease may also be seen in a minority of endemic and immunodeficiency-associated BL. BL rarely affects other portions of the GI tract, including the stomach[248] and more distal portions of the colon. BL most often affects children and young adults with a marked male preponderance.[242] In some cases, staging reveals disease beyond the GI tract.

Pathologic Features

The tumors are usually bulky exophytic lesions that may be associated with intussusception in the ileocecal area.[244] Histologic, immunophenotypic, and genetic features are similar to other sites. BL is discussed in Chapter 23.

T-Cell and Natural Killer–Cell Lymphomas

Gastrointestinal T-cell and NK-cell neoplasms are uncommon. Primary intestinal T-cell lymphomas, including enteropathy-associated T-cell lymphoma and monomorphic epitheliotropic intestinal T-cell lymphoma, and more recently recognized indolent disorders of the GI tract, including indolent clonal T-cell lymphoproliferative disorder of the gastrointestinal tract (ICC)/indolent T-cell lymphoma of the GI tract (WHO) (formerly *indolent T-cell lymphoproliferative disorder of the GI tract*)[1] and indolent NK-cell lymphoproliferative disorder of the GI tract (formerly *NK-cell enteropathy, lymphomatoid gastropathy*),[1,272] are discussed in Chapter 37. Other aggressive lymphomas, including anaplastic large-cell lymphoma and extranodal NK/T-cell lymphoma arising in the GI tract are described. Adult T-cell leukemia/lymphoma (HTLV1 positive) rarely presents with GI involvement. Acute-type and lymphoma-type adult T-cell lymphoma can involve the GI tract; involvement by chronic and smoldering forms of the disease is rare.[273]

Hodgkin Lymphoma

Clinical Features

Primary GI Hodgkin lymphoma is very rare, with fewer than 0.5% of cases of Hodgkin lymphoma arising in this site.[274] Given its rarity, careful evaluation to exclude other diseases is required. The differential diagnosis includes other aggressive lymphomas, poorly differentiated carcinoma, and EBV-positive mucocutaneous ulcer.[275]

LYMPHOMAS OF THE LIVER AND PANCREATOBILIARY TRACT

Hepatic Lymphomas

Clinical Features

Primary hepatic lymphoma is rare, representing an estimated 0.1% of hepatic malignancies, 0.4% of extranodal lymphomas, and 0.016% of all non-Hodgkin lymphomas.[276] Most patients are middle-aged and older adults with a wide age range (median, 50), and male-to-female ratio of ~2:1. Patients present with right upper quadrant or epigastric pain, nausea, vomiting, anorexia, or weakness. In ~50%, they have fever, night sweats, or weight loss, but jaundice is uncommon. Hepatomegaly is common.[277,278] Lactate dehydrogenase (LDH) is frequently elevated and hepatic transaminases may also be elevated; however, alpha fetoprotein (AFP) and carcinoembryonic antigen (CEA) levels are typically normal or only slightly elevated.[277-279] A minority of primary hepatic lymphomas are EMZL; hepatic EMZL is often an incidental finding.[276,280-282]

In up to 40% of cases, patients have another disorder such as an immunodeficiency, chronic infection, or autoimmune disease,[279,283] including hepatitis A, B, or C viral infection, HIV infection, organ transplantation, systemic lupus erythematosus, Felty syndrome, autoimmune cytopenias, primary biliary cirrhosis, active tuberculosis, and others.[278-280,283-289] HIV-positive patients are younger and are almost exclusively males.[288]

Pathologic Features

In ~50% of cases, the lymphoma forms a large solitary mass. In most of the remainder, there are multiple nodules that may become confluent. In ~5% of cases, there is diffuse hepatic enlargement without a discrete mass.[277-279,283] Most lymphomas are DLBCL. The remainder are BL, EMZL, lymphoplasmacytic lymphoma, FL, and peripheral T-cell lymphoma.[277,278,284-287] Almost all lymphomas in HIV-positive patients have been DLBCL or BL.[288] Necrosis is common; sclerosis is infrequent. Lymphomas with diffuse hepatic enlargement may show prominent sinusoidal involvement.[277] Some of these are DLBCL; some are hepatosplenic T-cell lymphomas (see Chapter 33). Immunohistochemical features are similar to those seen in the same types of lymphoma in other anatomic sites.

EMZL has histologic features similar to those seen in other sites. The neoplastic B cells markedly expand the portal tracts, form intersecting broad serpiginous bands entrapping nodules of hepatocytes, and in areas produce a diffuse, confluent infiltrate. Neoplastic cells form LELs with bile duct epithelium.[276,280-282] Neoplastic cells are CD20 positive, CD5 negative, CD10 negative, and cyclin D1 negative. BIRC3::MALT1 was reported in one case.[280]

Outcome

Most patients with hepatic EMZL have localized disease and are well on follow-up.[276,281,282,289,290] Prognosis for DLBCL patients is relatively good.[279]

Differential Diagnosis

The finding of one or more hepatic lesions can suggest hepatocellular carcinoma or metastatic carcinoma. The combination of high LDH and normal CEA and AFP, particularly in a patient with an underlying immunologic abnormality, can suggest lymphoma.[279]

Lymphomas of the Gallbladder

Rare cases of primary gallbladder lymphoma are reported.[291-293] Most patients are older adults. Rare patients are HIV positive.[294] Concurrent cholelithiasis is common.[295] Patients present with symptoms that often mimic cholecystitis, cholelithiasis, or choledocholithiasis, such as right-upper quadrant pain,[292] nausea, vomiting, or rarely, jaundice.[291] Gross inspection shows mural thickening or one or more discrete tumor nodules. DLBCL and EMZL are most common.[291,293,295,296]

Lymphomas of the Extrahepatic Biliary Tree

Lymphoma occasionally involves porta hepatis lymph nodes and compresses the extrahepatic biliary tree, resulting in jaundice. Lymphoma arising primarily from the extrahepatic biliary tree is rare. Patients present with obstructive jaundice. The clinical and radiographic features often suggest carcinoma or sclerosing cholangitis. The walls of the bile ducts appear thickened. DLBCL is the most common type.[295,297,298]

Pancreatic Lymphomas

Clinical Features

Primary pancreatic lymphoma is rare, accounting for <0.2% of pancreatic malignancies,[299] and <0.7% of non-Hodgkin lymphomas.[68] Patients are adults (3rd–9th decade of age; mean, 60) with male-to-female ratio of approximately 2:1.[300-303] Rare patients are HIV positive,[301] but with this exception, patients have not had conditions predisposing to lymphoma. Patients complain of abdominal pain, anorexia, weight loss, nausea, or vomiting.[300,302] Patients are often jaundiced and may have a palpable mass.[300] The clinical diagnosis is often pancreatic adenocarcinoma. Prognosis is difficult to assess because this tumor is rare and patients have not been treated uniformly.

Pathologic Features

The tumors take the form of large masses (generally >6 cm), most often involving the pancreatic head, although the lymphoma may involve the body, tail, or entire pancreas.[300,302,303] The majority are DLBCL.[302,304] Rare cases of EMZL[303] and peripheral T-cell lymphoma have been reported.[302]

Differential Diagnosis

The main entity in the clinical differential diagnosis is pancreatic adenocarcinoma. Lymphomas are larger than most carcinomas.[304] On ERCP, lymphoma may compress or distort ductal structures, but generally does not invade their walls, in contrast to carcinoma.[300] Establishing a diagnosis requires tissue for pathologic examination.

ADRENAL LYMPHOMAS

Clinical Features

Primary adrenal lymphomas are rare.[305,306] Patients are adults (median, ~60), with a male-to-female ratio of 1.5:1 to 3:1.[305-308] Rare patients are HIV positive,[307] and a few have had autoimmune disorders,[307] but there are no known specific predisposing factors. Patients commonly present with loss of appetite, abdominal pain, fatigue, fever, night sweats, weight loss, or fatigue.[305-307] Most have elevated LDH, β2 microglobulin, CRP, ferritin, and ESR.[308] In 60% to 80% of cases, both adrenals are involved. Adrenal insufficiency is common among patients with bilateral adrenal involvement.[305-308] Disease is commonly detected outside the adrenals, but adrenal lesion(s) should be the predominant site for a diagnosis of primary adrenal lymphoma.[305-308]

Pathologic Features

Diagnosis can be established on needle biopsy or resected adrenal. The lymphomas typically form bulky adrenal masses (median, 7–8 cm).[305,307,308] DLBCL is by far the most common type, accounting for up to ~90% of cases.[307,308] DLBCL of non-GCB subtype is much more common than GCB subtype. Other lymphomas, including peripheral T-cell lymphoma and extranodal NK/T-cell lymphoma, are described, but are rare.[305,307]

Staging, Treatment, and Outcome

Improved diagnostic techniques and combination chemotherapy have together resulted in improved outcomes in some reports.[305,306] In one study, the 2-year survival of patients treated with chemotherapy was 84%.[307] In other series, however, survival is very poor.[308]

URINARY TRACT LYMPHOMAS

Lymphomas arising in the urinary tract (i.e., kidneys, ureter, urinary bladder, urethra) are uncommon, accounting for less than 5% of extranodal lymphomas, with an annual incidence of about 1 per 1,000,000. Renal lymphomas are more common than those in other sites.[309] The peak age incidence is in the 70s.[310] DLBCL is most common, followed by EMZL, then FL; rare cases of BL and other types have been reported.[310] An inferior prognosis is associated with male sex, older age, DLBCL histology, and high-stage disease, while EMZL has the best cause-specific survival.[310]

Renal Lymphomas

Clinical Features

Most cases reported as primary renal lymphoma are lymphomas presenting with renal involvement, although they are not necessarily confined to the kidney. Approximately 0.2% of non-Hodgkin lymphomas[311] and 0.7% of extranodal lymphomas present in the kidney.[68] Primary renal lymphoma accounts for <1% of all renal masses.[311] In contrast, secondary renal involvement by lymphoma is common: up to 30% of all non-Hodgkin lymphomas involve the kidneys secondarily.[311] Primary renal lymphoma patients are affected over a broad age range but most are middle-aged or older adults (mean age, 7th decade) with a male-to-female ratio of 1.7:1.9.[310-321] A few cases are reported in children.[315,321] A few patients have been HIV-positive[315] or iatrogenically immunosuppressed allograft recipients. Patients with other malignancies, autoimmune diseases, or other disorders are described,[312,313,315,322,323] but no risk factors specific for renal lymphoma have been identified. Patients present with flank pain, loss of appetite, nausea, hematuria, weight loss, fever, renal insufficiency, or fatigue.[310,311,314-316,322,324] Rarely, the lymphoma is an incidental finding.[322]

Pathologic Features

Primary renal lymphoma is unilateral in approximately 75% to 95% of cases; the remainder are bilateral. Bilateral disease may be associated with renal insufficiency.[311,312,314-316,321,322] The lesions range from <5 cm to massive, with obliteration of the kidney. Frequently, the tumors invade adjacent tissues, including perinephric fat, psoas muscle, and even pancreas and duodenum. There may be vascular or ureteral encasement by the lymphoma. Occasional cases show extension into the renal vein and inferior vena cava, analogous to renal cell carcinoma.[314,315,322] Virtually all primary renal lymphomas are non-Hodgkin lymphoma, nearly all of which are B-lineage.[311,321] The most common renal lymphoma is DLBCL, accounting for slightly more than half of the cases. The remainder are of a variety of low-grade and high-grade types, including EMZL of mucosa-associated lymphoid tissue,[310,316,324] lymphoplasmacytic, follicular, lymphoblastic, BL, extranodal NK/T-cell, and very rare T-cell lymphomas,[310-312,314,315,317,319,321,320,322] including anaplastic large-cell lymphoma.[318] Lymphomas in HIV-positive patients have usually been DLBCL or BL.[315] Renal lymphoma in children is usually BL or, less often, lymphoblastic lymphoma.[315] Secondary renal lymphomas are less often DLBCL and are more often chronic lymphocytic leukemia/small lymphocytic lymphoma, compared with primary renal lymphoma.[325]

Staging, Treatment, and Outcome

Most patients presenting with renal lymphoma have more extensive disease on staging.[314-316,322] Five-year OS for all primary renal lymphoma patients is estimated at 64%, and that of DLBCL is reported as 58%.[321] The renal insufficiency found in some cases of bilateral renal lymphoma usually responds promptly to chemotherapy. A worse prognosis is associated with age over 60 years, male sex, advanced stage disease, and DLBCL or T-cell or NK-cell lymphoma.[311,321] Patients with EMZL have a better prognosis than other types of lymphoma.[321] Patients with bilateral disease tend to have a worse prognosis.[315,326]

Differential Diagnosis

Renal lymphomas, particularly when unilateral, may be mistaken clinically and radiographically for renal cell carcinomas.[313,315,323,324] Less often, they may mimic polycystic

kidney disease,[315] soft tissue tumors,[327] inflammatory lesions,[327] or Wilms' tumor.[315] Lymphoma can generally be readily distinguished from the other entities on microscopic examination.

Ureteral Lymphomas

Lymphomas occasionally involve the ureters. Manifestations include abdominal or flank pain, nausea and vomiting, dysuria, hematuria, fever, renal insufficiency, hydronephrosis, and hydroureter.[328] In most cases lymphoma is widespread at presentation, or the ureters are secondarily involved via extension from retroperitoneal disease. Lymphomas confined to the ureters at presentation are exceedingly unusual but have been described.[328] The majority are DLBCLs. The differential diagnosis includes idiopathic retroperitoneal fibrosis. Idiopathic retroperitoneal fibrosis can be associated with ureteral obstruction and a chronic inflammatory cell infiltrate, and retroperitoneal lymphomas can be associated with marked sclerosis and crush artifact, so differentiating the two may be difficult. Cytologic atypia of lymphoid cells and a diffuse, predominantly B-cell infiltrate support a diagnosis of lymphoma.

Lymphomas of the Urinary Bladder and Urethra

Clinical Features

Primary lymphomas of the urinary bladder are rare, accounting for <1% of bladder neoplasms.[309] Even less common are lymphomas arising in the urethra. Lymphomas arising in these sites share a number of clinical and pathologic features. They predominantly affect older adults, with a female preponderance.[310,329,330] Patients present with hematuria, urinary frequency, dysuria, recurrent urinary tract infections, or obstructive symptoms.[309,310,331] Analogous to the pathogenesis of EMZL at other sites, EMZL in the bladder may be related to prior inflammatory disease, with a number of patients having a history of chronic infectious cystitis,[330] or rarely chronic interstitial cystitis.[329]

Pathologic Features

The lesion(s) are single or occasionally multiple submucosal, exophytic, sessile nodules ranging from 1 to 15 cm. Sectioning usually reveals pale, firm tissue, although some tumors are soft and of variable color.[330] Most cases are EMZL.[331] Histologic features are similar to those in other sites. LELs may form in association with cystitis cystica, cystitis glandularis, or surface epithelium.[330] Associated follicular cystitis is sometimes seen. A minority are DLBCL. These are mostly DLBCL, NOS, although rare EBV-positive DLBCLs are reported.[309] Some may represent large-cell transformation of an underlying EMZL. The most common urethral lymphomas are DLBCL and EMZL.[332-334] Cytogenetic analysis has only rarely been performed, but one EMZL arising in the bladder harbored a t(11;18), corresponding to *BIRC3::MALT1*. That lymphoma also had trisomies of chromosomes 3 and 18.[330]

Staging, Treatment, and Outcome

Nearly all patients have localized disease at presentation.[309,315,335,336] Prognosis is favorable because the lymphomas are often localized and responsive to therapy.[315,335,337] The outlook for patients with EMZL is excellent. Rare patients have had complete regression of EMZL with antibiotics alone.[330] DLBCL may behave in a more aggressive manner.

Differential Diagnosis

The main entity in the differential diagnosis of DLBCL is poorly differentiated carcinoma.[309,315] Low-grade lymphomas may be mistaken for chronic inflammatory disorders.[315] Urothelial carcinoma may have a dense inflammatory infiltrate or undifferentiated neoplastic cells and may mimic either low-grade or high-grade lymphomas.[338]

MALE GENITAL TRACT LYMPHOMAS

Testicular and Epididymal Lymphomas

Clinical Features

Lymphoma accounts for ~5% of testicular tumors. Although uncommon, it is the most frequent testicular neoplasm in men over 50 years[339] (mean, late 50s or 60s in most series).[315,339-342] Children are rarely affected.[315,340,341,343,344] A few patients have been HIV positive,[345] but there is no known predisposing factor specific for testicular lymphoma. Patients typically present with a hard, painless scrotal mass; in a minority (14% in one series),[346] disease is bilateral. In a minority of cases, patients present with constitutional symptoms[315,345] or with symptoms related to extratesticular disease (e.g., neurologic abnormalities).[340] Lymphoma arising in the epididymis is much less common than testicular lymphoma, and lymphoma arising in the spermatic cord is extremely rare, but the clinical and pathologic features of lymphomas in these sites appear similar to those of testicular lymphoma.[340,347-352]

Pathologic Features

Orchiectomy specimens show a circumscribed, fleshy or firm, tan, gray, or white tumor ranging from a few millimeters to 16 cm in greatest dimension,[340] with a median of about 5 to 6 cm.[346,353] Lymphoma penetrates the tunica albuginea in about half of cases. The epididymis is often involved. The spermatic cord may also be involved.[340,353]

Lymphomas typically obliterate seminiferous tubules in at least some areas, with peripheral areas showing intertubular spread of tumor. In most cases, neoplastic cells invade seminiferous tubules, occupying the periphery of the tubules, displacing germ cells and Sertoli cells centrally, or filling the tubules completely.[340] Nearly all are DLBCL.[339-341,345,354] Most are composed of centroblasts, but some DLBCLs show a predominance of immunoblasts or multilobated lymphoid cells.[340] Immunohistochemical analysis reveals pan–B-antigen expression and, in >75% of cases, a non-GCB immunophenotype.[346,355] BCL2 protein expression is frequent[354]; a subset of cases co-express MYC and BCL2 ("double-expressors").[353]

Genetic features are similar to those of primary CNS DLBCL; primary testicular DLBCL is included in the category of primary large B-cell lymphoma of immune-privileged sites.[1] Gains and translocations of *PD-L1* and *PD-L2* and loss of major histocompatibility complex genes are common changes.[30,354,355] Somatic mutations of *MYD88*, *CD79B*, and other NF-κB pathway genes are often found.[30,354,355] Loss, often biallelic, of *CDKN2A* is common.[30] Gene-expression profiling typically shows activated B-cell (ABC) DLBCL.[354] Deregulated PI3K signaling may also play a role in the pathogenesis of primary testicular DLBCL.[355] *BCL6* translocation is found in up to 50% of cases, but translocations of *BCL2* and of *MYC* are uncommon.[354]

Most primary testicular lymphomas in childhood are FL (see Chapter 17). These lymphomas are usually confined to the testis, express pan–B-cell antigens and germinal-center markers, but are typically BCL2 protein-negative, with no *BCL2* gene rearrangement.[344,356] The prognosis is excellent. Rare cases of primary testicular T-lymphoblastic lymphoma and B-lymphoblastic lymphoma are described in children and young adults.[357] Rare BLs are reported.[346]

Only a few peripheral T-cell lymphomas, including peripheral T-cell lymphoma, NOS, and anaplastic large-cell lymphoma have been described.[358,359] Infrequent primary testicular extranodal NK/T-cell lymphomas are described, mainly in Asian men.[346,360] They account for <1% of all extranodal NK/T-cell lymphomas.[360] These are aggressive, CD56-positive, EBV-positive lymphomas associated with a poor prognosis (see Chapter 29).

Staging, Treatment, and Outcome

Approximately 70% to 80% of patients with primary testicular DLBCL have limited-stage disease.[315,339,346] Testicular lymphoma has a relatively poor prognosis. When relapses occur, they often involve extranodal sites, most often CNS[339,341,361,362] but also the opposite testis, bone, lung, skin, and other sites; relapses may also involve lymph nodes.[339-341,345] The best outcomes are associated with orchiectomy and Adriamycin-based combination chemotherapy with rituximab. Because of the high risk of relapse in the CNS and opposite testis, some authorities suggest that intrathecal chemotherapy and irradiation of the opposite testis should be considered.[339,346]

A number of clinical and pathologic features affect the prognosis of DLBCL patients. Patients with localized, unilateral disease have a better outcome than those with widespread disease.[339,340,346,362] IPI score 0 to 2 versus 3 to 5 is associated with a better OS.[346] Sclerosis is associated with a favorable prognosis. In one study, lymphomas with sclerosis had a much better outcome than those without sclerosis (72% vs. 16% 5-year disease-free survival for all patients; 90% vs. 34% 5-year disease-free survival for stage I patients).[340]

Differential Diagnosis

The most important entity in the differential diagnosis of testicular lymphoma is seminoma.[340] Compared with seminoma, lymphoma affects older patients, is more often bilateral, is more likely to involve the epididymis and spermatic cord, and is more likely to metastasize to sites such as bone or CNS.[340] Seminomas are composed of nests of neoplastic cells with abundant, glycogen-rich cytoplasm and uniform oval, euchromatic nuclei with prominent nucleoli delineated by fibrous septa that contain small lymphocytes and sometimes, granulomas. Seminomas express placental alkaline phosphatase (PLAP) and OCT4. Testicular DLBCL, particularly those with prominent sclerosis and large numbers of admixed non-neoplastic lymphocytes, may suggest a diagnosis of orchitis, including bacterial or viral infection or granulomatous orchitis. Acute inflammation with abscess formation and granulomas favors an inflammatory process.

Other unusual entities, including plasmacytoma[363] and rhabdomyosarcoma, can occasionally enter the differential diagnosis, but clinical and histologic features, augmented by immunophenotyping, establish a diagnosis.

Prostatic Lymphomas

Clinical Features

Primary prostatic lymphoma accounts for 0.1% of all non-Hodgkin lymphoma and 0.09% of prostatic neoplasms.[364] In a large series of prostatic biopsies, transurethral resection specimens, and prostatectomies, 0.17% of cases harbored primary prostatic lymphoma.[365] Secondary prostatic lymphoma is much more common than primary lymphoma; the most common type is chronic lymphocytic leukemia/small lymphocytic lymphoma.[331] Primary prostatic lymphoma affects patients over a broad age range, from childhood to advanced age (mean, ~60).[315,364,366-370] Patients present with bladder outlet obstruction, sometimes with hematuria.[365,366,368-371] Occasionally there is hydronephrosis,[368,370] sometimes with renal failure.[364] On physical examination, the prostate is usually diffusely enlarged and firm, but not as hard as with carcinoma.[367] Serum prostate-specific antigen (PSA) levels are often not significantly elevated, in contrast to carcinoma.[372] Patients are often thought to have benign prostatic hyperplasia,[315] and the diagnosis of lymphoma is only rarely suspected prospectively.

Pathologic Features

The lymphomas are of a variety of types, but DLBCL is most common.[366,367,372] Others have almost always been B cell lymphomas, including FL,[366,367] BL,[364,369,370] and several cases of EMZL of mucosa-associated lymphoid tissue (Fig. 59-15).[371,373] Microscopic examination reveals an atypical lymphoid infiltrate that is usually patchy, but that may be unifocal, extensive, and obliterative, or perivascular. Lymphoma infiltrates among fibromuscular bundles, and occasionally infiltrates glandular epithelium.[367]

Staging, Treatment, and Outcome

Staging has shown localized disease in most cases, although involvement of abdominal lymph nodes and of extranodal sites is not uncommon. The prognosis has been considered poor,[364] although patients treated in recent years with optimal therapy have had a better outcome.

Differential Diagnosis

The differential diagnosis includes poorly differentiated carcinoma and prostatitis. Even in poorly differentiated carcinoma, neoplastic cells at least focally form cords, cohesive sheets, and sometimes, glandular spaces. In the differential with prostatitis, a dense, monomorphous, cytologically atypical lymphoid infiltrate favors lymphoma.

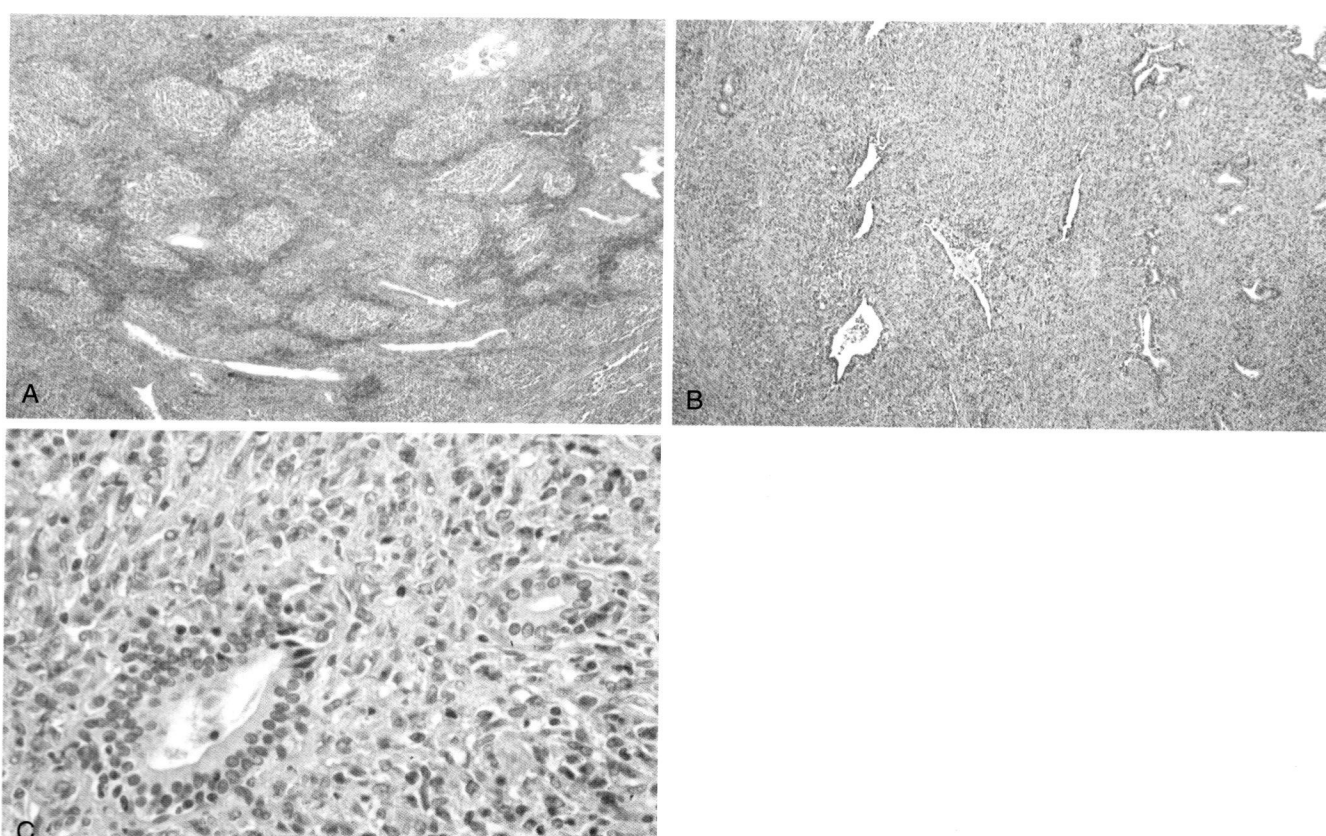

Figure 59-15. Diffuse large B-cell lymphoma with follicular lymphoma, primary in prostate. The lymphoma was an incidental finding at prostatectomy for carcinoma. **A,** An area of follicular lymphoma. **B,** Diffuse large B-cell lymphoma, adjacent to prostatic glands. **C,** An area of diffuse large B-cell lymphoma. Prostatic epithelial structures appear compressed and atrophic.

LYMPHOMAS OF THE FEMALE GENITAL TRACT

Lymphomas only rarely arise in the female genital tract, accounting for 1.5% of all extranodal lymphomas, with an annual incidence of 0.44/10[6] in the United States.[374] The ovaries are most commonly affected, followed by the uterine cervix, uterine corpus, vagina, vulva, and fallopian tube. Nearly all are non-Hodgkin lymphoma of B-lineage, with DLBCL being the most common type throughout the female genital tract. A subset of lymphomas arising in the uterine cervix and vagina share features with primary cutaneous follicle center lymphoma and have an excellent prognosis.[375] T-cell lymphoma is very uncommon and Hodgkin lymphoma is vanishingly rare.[315,374,376] Except for rare lymphomas arising in the setting of HIV infection or iatrogenic immunosuppression,[377,378] or endemic BL, there are no known predisposing factors for the development of female genital tract lymphoma. Secondary involvement of the female genital tract by lymphoma arising elsewhere is more common than primary female genital tract lymphoma.

Ovarian Lymphomas

Clinical Features

Most series of ovarian lymphoma include cases in which patients present with ovarian involvement but may also have extraovarian disease.[379,380] Less than 1% of lymphomas present with ovarian involvement.[68,315,381] In countries where BL is endemic, however, approximately 50% of childhood ovarian malignancies are BL.[382] Patients range from 18 months to 74 years[315,383] (peak incidence, 4th–5th decade).[315,381,384] Lymphoma may present during pregnancy.[315] Patients commonly have abdominal pain and increasing abdominal girth, sometimes with ascites.[380,381,384,385] Constitutional symptoms are common.[380]

Pathologic Features

Ovarian lymphomas range from microscopic (representing incidental findings)[384] to 25 cm in diameter (mean, 8–14 cm).[315,380,384] They typically have an intact external surface, which may be smooth or nodular. Their consistency ranges from soft and fleshy to firm and rubbery, depending on the degree of associated sclerosis. On sectioning, the tumors are usually white, tan, or gray pink. A minority have hemorrhage or necrosis.[315,383,386] Very rare cases of lymphoma arising from a teratoma have been described.[387]

DLBCL is most common, followed by BL and FL.[380,381] Rare anaplastic large-cell lymphomas and B- and T-lymphoblastic lymphomas are reported.[376,384] In contrast to adults, who develop lymphomas of various types, younger patients almost always have diffuse, aggressive lymphomas.

Ovarian lymphomas may be associated with sclerosis, with tumor cells growing in cords and nests, simulating carcinoma.[382] Neoplastic cells may be elongated and grow in a storiform pattern, mimicking a sarcoma. Ovarian lymphomas may preferentially spare a peripheral rim of cortical tissue, corpora lutea, corpora albicantia,[315] and follicles,[383] but otherwise typically obliterate normal parenchyma. Ovarian lymphomas have immunophenotypic features similar to those of the same lymphomas in other sites.[315,384] In one study, ovarian FLs were divided into two groups. In the first, BCL2 was negative or weakly expressed, *IGH::BCL2* fusion was absent, the lymphomas were grade 2 or grade 3A, and when stage was known, the lymphomas were confined to one ovary. In the second group, all lymphomas were low-grade, BCL2 was strongly expressed, *IGH::BCL2* fusion was present, and most had widespread disease. Outcome was more favorable for patients from the first group.[388]

Staging, Treatment, and Outcome

One or both ovaries are involved with approximately equal frequency.[383,386] Extraovarian spread is found in most cases, commonly to pelvic or paraaortic lymph nodes and occasionally to peritoneum, other portions of the female genital tract, or more distant sites.[315,381] Ovarian lymphoma has been considered prognostically unfavorable, although with aggressive combination chemotherapy the prognosis appears similar to that of nodal lymphomas of comparable stage and histologic type.[379,384] Patients with bilateral ovarian involvement, widespread disease on staging, and larger ovarian masses may have a worse prognosis.[380]

Differential Diagnosis

The differential diagnosis of ovarian lymphoma includes dysgerminoma, undifferentiated carcinoma, metastatic carcinoma (particularly from the breast),[383] primary small cell carcinoma, adult granulosa cell tumor,[385] sarcoma, and myeloid sarcoma.[315] Attention to cytologic detail and familiarity with the spectrum of histologic features of ovarian lymphoma are helpful in establishing a diagnosis.

Fallopian Tube Lymphomas

Primary fallopian tube lymphoma is very rare, but unilateral and fewer bilateral cases are described.[315,389-391] EMZL, DLBCL, and FL are reported. Among patients with ovarian lymphoma, secondary tubal involvement is found in >25%. DLBCL and BL are most common in this setting.[383,392]

Uterine Lymphomas

Clinical Features

Malignant lymphoma arising in the uterus is rare; <1% of extranodal lymphomas arise in this site.[68] Lymphomas arise much more often in the cervix than in the corpus, with a ratio of as high as 10:1 in one series.[393] Ages range from 20 to 80 years,[394] with a median in the 5th decade.[394-396] Patients usually present with abnormal vaginal bleeding.[315,392,394,395,397] Dyspareunia, or perineal, pelvic, or abdominal pain are less common. Constitutional symptoms are unusual.[315,396] Only a minority of cervical lymphomas yields a positive cervical smear, presumably because lymphomas are not usually ulcerated.[398]

Pathologic Features

Cervical lymphomas usually produce bulky lesions readily identifiable on pelvic examination.[397] The classic appearance is diffuse, circumferential enlargement of the cervix ("barrel-shaped" cervix). The lymphoma may also form a discrete submucosal tumor,[394] a polypoid or multinodular lesion,[394,399,400] or a fungating, exophytic mass; ulceration is unusual.[394] The tumors are fleshy, rubbery, or firm. They are usually homogeneous in color and white-tan to yellow.[394] Extensive local spread to vagina, parametria, or even pelvic side walls is common.[394,399] Ureteral obstruction with hydronephrosis is common.[315,394] Lymphomas of the uterine corpus are usually fleshy or soft, pale gray, yellow, or cream colored. They may form a polypoid mass or diffusely coat the endometrium, sometimes with deep invasion of the myometrium.[315,394]

The majority of lymphomas are DLBCL; they may be of GCB or non-GCB type (Fig. 59-16).[392,393,397,400] FL is next most common (Fig. 59-17). A few cases of BL[376] and small numbers of EMZL[315,376,392,393,401,402] are reported. Also described are rare B-lymphoblastic lymphomas,[376] peripheral T-cell lymphomas,[403,404] and extranodal NK/T-cell lymphomas.[392]

In the cervix, there is often a band of uninvolved tissue just beneath the epithelium, and the overlying epithelium is usually intact. Deep invasion of the cervical wall is common. Perivascular spread of tumor is common in FL.[394] Cervical lymphomas are frequently associated with prominent sclerosis,[400] which may be associated with a cord-like arrangement or spindle-shaped tumor cells.[394] Crush artifact is often prominent, hindering evaluation.[315,376,394,400]

A recent study described a series of follicle center lymphomas arising in the cervix or vagina with an excellent prognosis (5-year OS, 100%) and noted similarities to primary cutaneous follicle center lymphoma. The pattern was follicular or diffuse, with a frequent component of large centrocytes, lack of BCL2 expression and of *BCL2* rearrangement in nearly all, frequent mutation of *TNFRSF14,* lack of *CREBBP* and *KMT2D* mutations (which are common in nodal FL), presentation with localized disease, and absence of progression on follow-up.[375]

The rare primary endometrial EMZL have distinctive features.[401,402,405,406] They usually arise in postmenopausal women, often as an incidental finding. They are composed of nodules of small, monotonous lymphoid cells with clear cytoplasm scattered in the endometrium, typically with, at most, superficial myometrial invasion. The immunophenotype is similar to that of EMZL in other sites, except that CD43 is typically co-expressed by neoplastic B cells. One case had CD5 expression.[401]

Staging, Treatment, and Outcome

Although most uterine lymphomas are bulky and locally invasive, the majority are localized.[315,392] The prognosis of cervical DLBCL treated with immunochemotherapy is excellent.[397] There is not enough information to draw definite conclusions about the prognosis of the rare endometrial lymphomas. However, those with localized disease tend to do well, while those with advanced disease presenting with endometrial involvement tend to fare poorly.[394,402] Endometrial EMZL has an excellent prognosis.[405]

Vaginal and Vulvar Lymphomas

Lymphoma rarely arises in the vagina,[315,396,407] and even less often in the vulva.[315,378,408,409] Patients are affected over a wide age range. They present with vaginal bleeding, discharge, pain, dyspareunia, urinary frequency, or a mass. Surface epithelium is usually intact. Papanicolaou smears are generally negative.[410] Nearly all are DLBCL,[315,376,407,409,411] but rare cases of FL,[376,394] BL,[412] lymphoplasmacytic lymphoma,[376] and T-cell lymphoma[315,410] are reported. The vulva may also be affected by a variety of primary cutaneous lymphomas.[413,414] Vaginal lymphomas are often associated with sclerosis. Vaginal lymphoma usually presents with localized disease and has a favorable prognosis.[396,407,410,415] Vulvar lymphomas are relatively aggressive, but occasional patients have long disease-free survival.

Differential Diagnosis of Lower Female Genital Tract Lymphoma

Common entities in the differential diagnosis are poorly differentiated carcinoma and a reactive lymphoid infiltrate.[315,394] Unlike carcinoma, which tends to invade with obliteration of normal structures, lymphoma tends to infiltrate around them, with relative preservation of endometrial and endocervical glands and sparing of the most superficial subepithelial stroma.[315] Adjacent in situ squamous or adenocarcinoma favors carcinoma.

Marked chronic inflammation is common in the cervix, and occasionally seen in the endometrium, vagina, and vulva; infrequently it is so dense and extensive that it raises the question of lymphoma (so-called "lymphoma-like lesion").[416] In favor of an inflammatory process are absence of a mass, superficial location, association with erosion or ulceration of the overlying epithelium, and polymorphous composition with follicle center cells, immunoblasts, small lymphocytes,

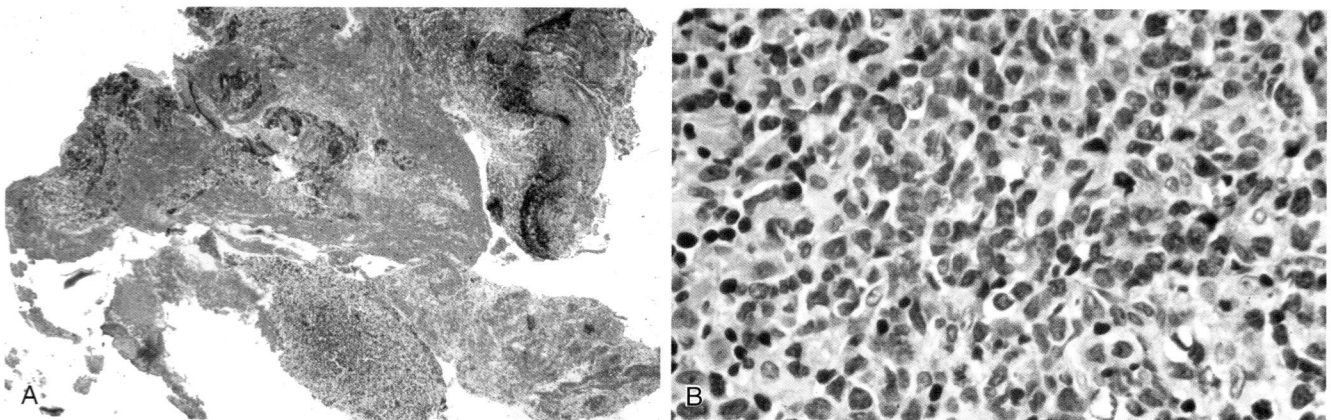

Figure 59-16. Diffuse large B-cell lymphoma, uterine cervix. A, Curetted fragments of lymphoma admixed with blood. **B,** Higher power shows large atypical lymphoid cells with irregular nuclei.

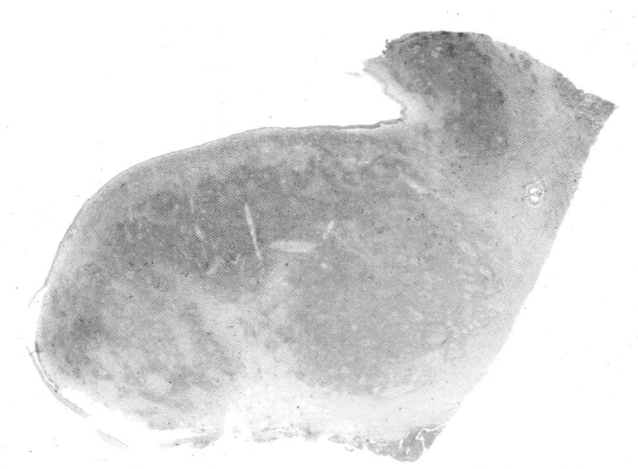

Figure 59-17. Follicular lymphoma, uterine cervix, whole mount. Neoplastic follicles invade deep into the wall of the cervix.

plasma cells, and neutrophils. Marked chronic inflammatory processes involving the endometrium are generally associated with areas of more typical-appearing chronic endometritis. Rarely, there is associated EBV infection.[417] In contrast, lymphoma usually produces a mass with extension into adjacent structures. Lymphomas tend to invade deeply, spare a narrow subepithelial zone, be composed of a monomorphous population of lymphoid cells (often with sclerosis), and spread in proximity to blood vessels.[417]

A rare entity that may suggest lymphoma is leiomyoma with lymphoid infiltration (i.e., uterine leiomyomas with a moderate-to-dense infiltrate of small lymphocytes with scattered larger lymphoid cells), occasionally with germinal centers, plasma cells, and rarely, eosinophils. The inflammatory cells are largely confined to the leiomyoma. The polymorphous nature of the infiltrate and its confinement to the leiomyoma help distinguish it from lymphoma. In all reported cases of leiomyoma with lymphoid infiltration, follow-up has been uneventful.[418]

LYMPHOMAS OF BONE

Clinical Features

Primary lymphomas of bone are defined as lymphomas arising in bone, with or without extension into adjacent soft tissue, without lymphoma elsewhere on staging. Some authorities accept cases with regional lymph node involvement, but not with more distant spread.[419-421] Primary lymphomas of bone account for 3% of primary osseous neoplasms,[422,423] <1% of all lymphomas,[419,424] and ~5% of extranodal non-Hodgkin lymphomas.[68] Among children, primary lymphomas of bone account for a higher proportion of non-Hodgkin lymphomas (2.8%–4.2%).[425] Etiology is unknown. Most patients have no known predisposing conditions, but rare patients with Paget disease of bone who developed primary lymphoma of bone are described.[426]

There is a slight male preponderance. Patients may be of any age, from young children to the elderly; however, most are adults (median, 5th–6th decades).[419,423,424,427-433] Patients present with localized pain.[419,420,423-425,434] A minority also

have swelling or a palpable mass or fracture.[422,424,427,434] Patients rarely present with constitutional symptoms.[424,425] Most commonly affected are the long bones of the extremities, with the femur involved most often, followed by the tibia and the humerus. Next most common are the flat bones of the shoulder and pelvis, followed by the remainder of the axial skeleton and the cranial and jaw bones.[423,424,427,430,431,434] Small bones of the hands and feet are rarely involved.[430] Disease is usually monostotic; in a minority of cases it is polyostotic.[419,420,425,427,431,434-437] Radiographic examination usually shows a lytic lesion with ill-defined margins. In a minority of cases the appearance is blastic or mixed blastic and lytic. Radiographs may demonstrate pathologic fracture or soft tissue extension with an associated periosteal reaction.[419,422,423,429,434]

Pathologic Features

In adults, nearly all primary lymphomas of bone are DLBCL. Many are composed of cells with large irregular or multilobated nuclei; others are composed of centroblasts with oval nuclei, immunoblasts, or bizarre pleomorphic cells.[423,428-432,434,438] Neoplastic cells may become elongated and resemble spindle cells.[423,439] Also reported are rare cases of BL, anaplastic large-cell lymphoma (ALK positive and ALK negative, Fig. 59-18),[438,440] B-lymphoblastic lymphoma,[441,442] low-grade lymphomas, peripheral T-cell lymphoma, NOS,[419] and adult T-cell lymphoma/leukemia.[443] Rare cases of CHL presenting in bone are reported.[422,444-446] Staging reveals lymph node involvement in most cases,[445] but some appear to represent true primary osseous Hodgkin lymphoma.[444,446]

In children, ~40% of bone lymphomas are lymphoblastic lymphoma, 10% are BL, and 50% are DLBCL. The DLBCLs may have a GCB or non-GCB-cell immunophenotype.[437,447] Like other extranodal DLBCL, and in contrast to nodal DLBCL, the *BCL2* translocation is uncommon.[431,437] PI3K/AKT/mTOR pathway activation is proposed to play a role in the pathogenesis of DLBCL with a non-GCB–like immunophenotype.[447]

Staging, Treatment, and Outcome

DLBCL is often localized; lymphoblastic lymphoma is more often associated with multifocal osseous disease and higher stage.[425,442,448] Staging may reveal more widespread disease, most often involving regional lymph nodes or other bones.[428,437] Primary lymphoma of bone has a better prognosis than other bony malignancies. In patients with localized disease who are optimally staged and treated, 5-year disease-free survival may be as high as 90%.[424,448] An inferior prognosis is associated with higher stage disease, polyostotic disease, extension into soft tissue, primary tumor in the pelvis or spine, and older age. Lymphomas arising in long bones have a better prognosis.[424-426,428,429,434] Among DLBCLs, a better outcome has been associated with treatment with chemotherapy,[426] cases composed of large irregular cells or multilobated cells,[429,432,438,449] and a GCB-like phenotype.[437]

Relapses are most often to other bones and lymph nodes.[419,420,423,431,438,448] Less common sites of relapse include adjacent soft tissue, lung, bone marrow, and CNS.[423,438]

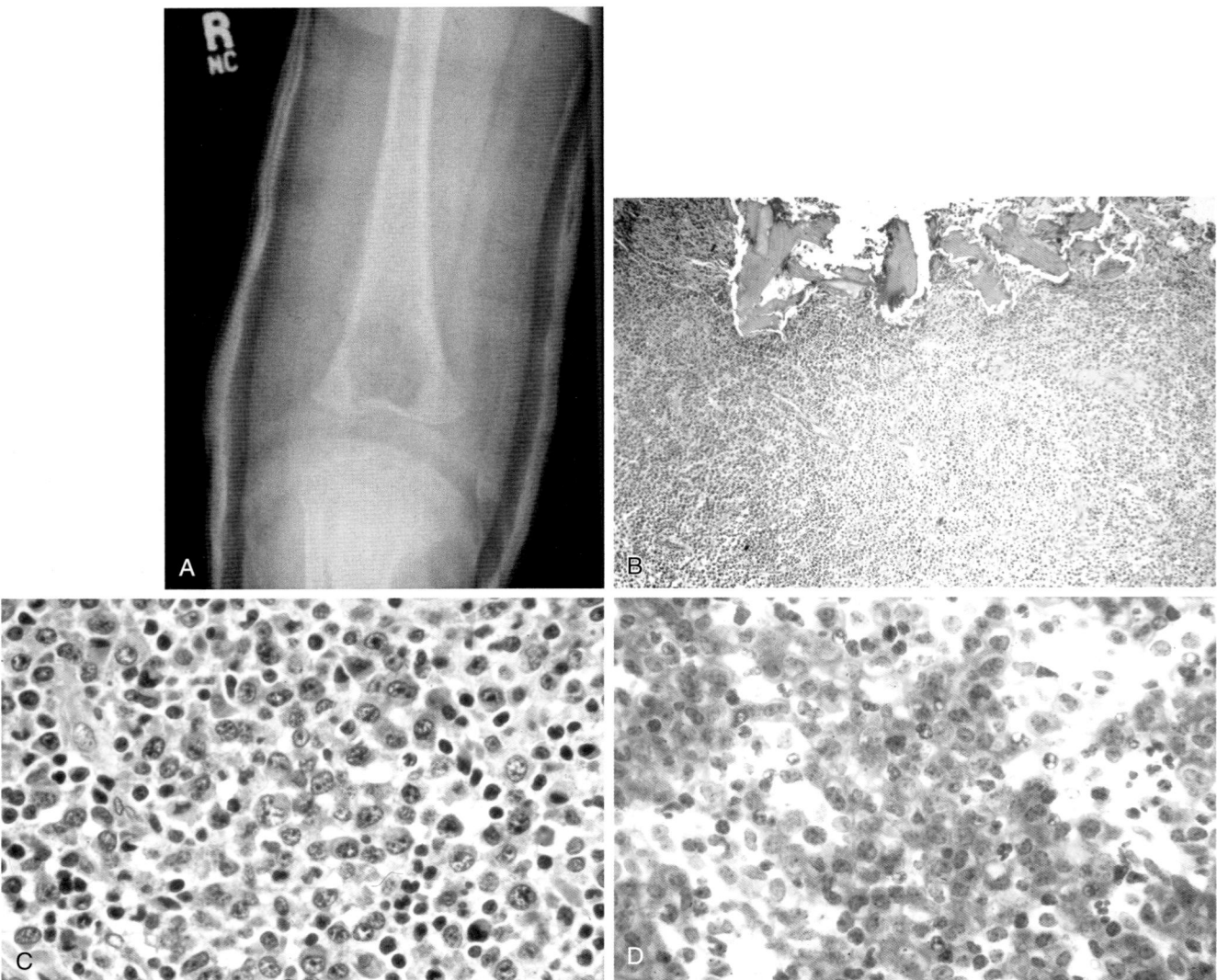

Figure 59-18. ALK-positive anaplastic large cell lymphoma in a child. A, A destructive lytic lesion involves the metaphysis of the distal femur. **B,** The lymphoma is associated with bony destruction. **C,** The lymphoma is composed of large, atypical cells with oval or indented nuclei and pink cytoplasm. **D,** Neoplastic cells are intensely positive for CD30 (immunoperoxidase technique on a paraffin section). ALK was also positive *(not shown)*.

Patients with lymphoblastic lymphoma may progress to acute lymphoblastic leukemia.[425,448]

Differential Diagnosis

Rendering the correct diagnosis may be difficult because of associated fibrosis, crush artifact, overdecalcification, small specimen size, and admixed reactive cells. The differential diagnosis of bone lymphoma is broad, and includes other types of neoplasms and inflammatory processes.[422,425,429,430,433] Bone lymphoma can be misdiagnosed as an inflammatory process such as chronic osteomyelitis[422,425,433] or as a simple fracture[422] if there is a large reactive component and if neoplastic cells are present in small numbers or are not well preserved. Because in some cases, particularly in association with sclerosis, neoplastic cells are elongate, spindle cell sarcoma can enter the differential.[423,433,439] Exuberant reactive woven bone may cause misinterpretation as osteosarcoma.

Langerhans cell histiocytosis and poorly differentiated plasmacytoma may enter the differential diagnosis, but cytologic features and immunophenotyping help establish a diagnosis. Myeloid sarcoma can mimic lymphoma, especially lymphoblastic lymphoma. If the myeloid sarcoma has a component of monocytes with irregular nuclei, the appearance can resemble diffuse DLBCL with large irregular or multilobated cells. Lymphoma may also raise consideration of a small round cell tumor, but Ewing sarcoma has cytoplasmic glycogen and a more cohesive growth pattern, and less pleomorphic nuclei than lymphoma. Neuroblastoma may present with bony metastases. The tumor cells may form rosettes; they are pear-shaped or carrot-shaped cells with denser chromatin than lymphoma. The differential of the rare Hodgkin lymphoma involving bone includes acute or chronic osteomyelitis, depending on the composition of the reactive population, particularly if large neoplastic cells are present in small numbers.[444]

Pearls and Pitfalls

- The types of lymphomas encountered in extranodal sites differ to some extent from those encountered in lymph nodes. These lymphomas vary by the specific extranodal site. Familiarity with the types of lymphomas arising in different extranodal sites facilitates diagnosis.
- Carcinomas are much more common than lymphomas in many extranodal sites, and this may lead to failure to consider a diagnosis of lymphoma. Lymphoma should be considered when the specimen shows an undifferentiated-appearing malignant neoplasm.
- In certain extranodal sites, such as bone and the lower female genital tract, crush artifact may be a significant barrier to establishing a diagnosis. In such cases, pathologists should request more tissue until an adequate specimen is obtained.
- Certain types of extranodal lymphomas tend to occur in certain age groups or ethnic groups or in association with an underlying immunodeficiency or autoimmune disorder. Clinical correlation is important in establishing the correct diagnosis.
- Infectious mononucleosis can mimic both classic Hodgkin lymphoma and diffuse large B-cell lymphoma; infectious mononucleosis should be considered in the differential diagnosis of atypical lymphoid proliferations in Waldeyer's ring, especially in young patients.
- Certain extranodal diffuse large B-cell lymphomas, such as primary effusion lymphoma and plasmablastic lymphoma, are characteristically CD20 negative. If morphology suggests lymphoma and CD20 is negative, the possibility of lymphoma should not be excluded until immunostaining with a broader panel of markers is performed.

KEY REFERENCES

1. Alaggio R, Amador C, Anagnostopoulos I, et al. The 5th edition of the World Health Organization classification of haematolymphoid tumours: lymphoid neoplasms. *Leukemia.* 2022;36(7):1720–1748.
2. de Leval L, Alizadeh AA, Bergsagel PL, et al. Genomic profiling for clinical decision making in lymphoid neoplasms. *Blood.* 2022;140(21):2193–2227.
3. Campo E, Jaffe ES, Cook JR, et al. The International Consensus Classification of mature lymphoid neoplasms: a report from the clinical advisory committee. *Blood.* 2022;140(11):1229–1253.
5. Deckert M, Batchelor T, Ferry J, et al. Primary diffuse large B-cell lymphoma of the CNS. In: Board EE, ed. *World Health Organization Histological Classification of Tumours of the Central Nervous System. World Health Organization Classification of Tumours.* 5th ed. Lyon: International Agency for Research on Cancer; 2021:351–355.
21. Ahrendsen JT, Ta R, Li J, et al. Primary central nervous system anaplastic large cell lymphoma, ALK positive. *Am J Clin Pathol.* 2022.
65. Ferry J, Fung C, Lucarelli M, Harris N, Hasserjian R. Ocular adnexal lymphoma: long-term outcome, patterns of failure and prognostic factors in 174 patients. *J Hematopathol.* 2021;14:41–52.
130. Korona B, Korona D, Zhao W, Wotherspoon AC, Du MQ. GPR34 activation potentially bridges lymphoepithelial lesions to genesis of salivary gland MALT lymphoma. *Blood.* 2022;139(14):2186–2197.
161. Hamamoto Y, Kukita Y, Kitamura M, et al. Bcl-2-negative IGH-BCL2 translocation-negative follicular lymphoma of the thyroid differs genetically and epigenetically from Bcl-2-positive IGH-BCL2 translocation-positive follicular lymphoma. *Histopathology.* 2021;79(4):521–532.
193. Alexanian S, Said J, Lones M, Pullarkat ST. KSHV/HHV8-negative effusion-based lymphoma, a distinct entity associated with fluid overload states. *Am J Surg Pathol.* 2013;37(2):241–249.
426. Wang HH, Dai KN, Li AB. A nomogram predicting overall and cancer-specific survival of patients with primary bone lymphoma: a large population-based study. *BioMed Res Int.* 2020;2020:4235939.

Visit Elsevier eBooks+ for the complete set of references.

Appendix A

The International Consensus Classification of Myeloid, Lymphoid, and Histiocytic Neoplasms

Myeloproliferative Neoplasms

Chronic myeloid leukemia

Polycythemia vera

Essential thrombocythemia

Primary myelofibrosis

  Early/prefibrotic primary myelofibrosis

  Overt primary myelofibrosis

Chronic neutrophilic leukemia

Chronic eosinophilic leukemia, not otherwise specified (NOS)

Myeloproliferative neoplasm, unclassifiable

Myeloid/Lymphoid Neoplasms With Eosinophilia and Tyrosine Kinase Gene Fusions

Myeloid/lymphoid neoplasm with *PDGFRA* rearrangement

Myeloid/lymphoid neoplasm with *PDGFRB* rearrangement

Myeloid/lymphoid neoplasm with *FGFR1* rearrangement

Myeloid/lymphoid neoplasm with *JAK2* rearrangement

Myeloid/lymphoid neoplasm with *FLT3* rearrangement

Myeloid/lymphoid neoplasm with *ETV6::ABL1*

Mastocytosis

Myelodysplastic/Myeloproliferative Neoplasms

Chronic myelomonocytic leukemia

  Clonal monocytosis of undetermined significance

Atypical chronic myeloid leukemia

Myelodysplastic/myeloproliferative neoplasm with *SF3B1* mutation and thrombocytosis

Myelodysplastic/myeloproliferative neoplasm with ring sideroblasts and thrombocytosis, NOS

Myelodysplastic/myeloproliferative neoplasm, NOS

  Myelodysplastic/myeloproliferative neoplasm with isolated isochromosome (17q)

Pre-malignant Clonal Cytopenias and Myelodysplastic Syndromes

Clonal cytopenia of undetermined significance and other clonal cytopenias

Myelodysplastic syndrome with mutated *SF3B1*

Myelodysplastic syndrome with del(5q)

Myelodysplastic syndrome with mutated *TP53*

Myelodysplastic syndrome, NOS (MDS, NOS)

  MDS, NOS without dysplasia

  MDS, NOS with single lineage dysplasia

  MDS, NOS with multilineage dysplasia

Myelodysplastic syndrome with excess blasts

Myelodysplastic syndrome/acute myeloid leukemia (MDS/AML)

  MDS/AML with mutated *TP53*

  MDS/AML with myelodysplasia-related gene mutations

  MDS/AML with myelodysplasia-related cytogenetic abnormalities

  MDS/AML, NOS

Pediatric and/or Germline Mutation–Associated Disorders

Juvenile myelomonocytic leukemia

Juvenile myelomonocytic leukemia-like neoplasms

Noonan syndrome–associated myeloproliferative disorder

Refractory cytopenia of childhood

Hematologic neoplasms with germline predisposition

Acute Myeloid Leukemias

Acute promyelocytic leukemia (APL) with t(15;17)(q24.1;q21.2)/*PML::RARA*

APL with other *RARA* rearrangements

AML with t(8;21)(q22;q22.1)/*RUNX1::RUNX1T1*

AML with inv(16)(p13.1q22) or t(16;16)(p13.1;q22)/*CBFB::MYH11*

AML with t(9;11)(p21.3;q23.3)/*MLLT3::KMT2A*

AML with other *KMT2A* rearrangements

AML with t(6;9)(p22.3;q34.1)/*DEK::NUP214*

AML with inv(3)(q21.3q26.2) or t(3;3)(q21.3;q26.2)/*GATA2; MECOM(EVI1)*

AML with other *MECOM* rearrangements

AML with other rare recurring translocations

AML with t(9;22)(q34.1;q11.2)/*BCR::ABL1*

AML with mutated *NPM1*

AML with in-frame bZIP *CEBPA* mutations

AML and MDS/AML with mutated *TP53*

AML and MDS/AML with myelodysplasia-related gene mutations

AML and MDS/AML with myelodysplasia-related cytogenetic abnormalities

AML and MDS/AML NOS

Myeloid sarcoma

Myeloid Proliferations Associated With Down Syndrome

Blastic Plasmacytoid Dendritic Cell Neoplasm

Acute Leukemia of Ambiguous Lineage

Acute undifferentiated leukemia

Mixed phenotype acute leukemia (MPAL) with t(9;22)(q34.1;q11.2); *BCR::ABL1*

MPAL, with t(v;11q23.3); *KMT2A* rearranged

MPAL, with *ZNF384* rearrangement

MPAL with *BCL11B* activation

MPAL, B/myeloid, NOS

MPAL, T/myeloid, NOS

B/T/myeloid MPAL

ALAL, NOS

B-Lymphoblastic Leukemia/Lymphoma (B-ALL)

B-ALL with recurrent genetic abnormalities

  B-ALL with t(9;22)(q34.1;q11.2)/*BCR::ABL1*

    with lymphoid only involvement

    with multilineage involvement

  B-ALL with t(v;11q23.3)/*KMT2A* rearranged

  B-ALL with t(12;21)(p13.2;q22.1)/*ETV6::RUNX1*

  B-ALL, hyperdiploid

  B-ALL, low hypodiploid

  B-ALL, near haploid

  B-ALL with t(5;14)(q31.1;q32.3)/*IL3::IGH*

  B-ALL with t(1;19)(q23.3;p13.3)/*TCF3::PBX1*

(Continued)

B-ALL, *BCR::ABL1*–like, ABL-1 class rearranged

B-ALL, *BCR::ABL1*–like, JAK-STAT activated

B-ALL, *BCR::ABL1*–like, NOS

B-ALL with iAMP21

B-ALL with *MYC* rearrangement

B-ALL with *DUX4* rearrangement

B-ALL with *MEF2D* rearrangement

B-ALL with *ZNF384* rearrangement

B-ALL with *NUTM1* rearrangement

B-ALL with *HLF* rearrangement

B-ALL with *UBTF::ATXN7L3/PAN3,CDX2* ("CDX2/UBTF")

B-ALL with mutated *IKZF1* N159Y

B-ALL with mutated *PAX5* P80R

Provisional entity: B-ALL, *ETV6::RUNX1*-like

Provisional entity: B-ALL, with *PAX5* alteration

Provisional entity: B-ALL, with mutated *ZEB2* (p.H1038R)/*IGH::CEBPE*

Provisional entity: B-ALL, *ZNF384* rearranged-like

Provisional entity: B-ALL, *KMT2A* rearranged-like

B-ALL, NOS

T-Lymphoblastic Leukemia/Lymphoma

Early T-cell precursor ALL with *BCL11B* rearrangement

Early T-cell precursor ALL, NOS

T-ALL, NOS

Provisional entities

Provisional Entity: Natural Killer (NK)–Cell ALL

Mature B-Cell Neoplasms

Chronic lymphocytic leukemia/small lymphocytic lymphoma

Monoclonal B-cell lymphocytosis

CLL type

Non-CLL type

B-cell prolymphocytic leukemia

Splenic marginal zone lymphoma

Hairy cell leukemia

Splenic B-cell lymphoma/leukemia, unclassifiable

Splenic diffuse red pulp small B-cell lymphoma

Hairy cell leukemia-variant

Lymphoplasmacytic lymphoma

Waldenström macroglobulinemia

IgM monoclonal gammopathy of undetermined significance (MGUS)

IgM MGUS, plasma cell type

IgM MGUS, NOS

Primary cold agglutinin disease

Heavy chain diseases

Mu heavy chain disease

Gamma heavy chain disease

Alpha heavy chain disease

Plasma cell neoplasms

Non-IgM monoclonal gammopathy of undetermined significance

Multiple myeloma (Plasma cell myeloma)

Multiple myeloma, NOS

Multiple myeloma with recurrent genetic abnormality

Multiple myeloma with *CCND* family translocation

Multiple myeloma with *MAF* family translocation

Multiple myeloma with *NSD2* translocation

Multiple myeloma with hyperdiploidy

Solitary plasmacytoma of bone

Extraosseous plasmacytoma

Monoclonal immunoglobulin deposition diseases

Immunoglobulin light chain amyloidosis (AL)

Localized AL amyloidosis

Light chain and heavy chain deposition disease

Extranodal marginal zone lymphoma of mucosa-associated lymphoid tissue (MALT lymphoma)

Primary cutaneous marginal zone lymphoproliferative disorder

Nodal marginal zone lymphoma

Follicular lymphoma

In situ follicular neoplasia

Duodenal-type follicular lymphoma

BCL2-R negative, CD23-positive follicle center lymphoma

Primary cutaneous follicle center lymphoma

Pediatric-type follicular lymphoma, with or without marginal zone differentiation

Testicular follicular lymphoma

Large B-cell lymphoma with *IRF4* rearrangement

Mantle cell lymphoma

In situ mantle cell neoplasia

Leukemic non-nodal mantle cell lymphoma

Diffuse large B-cell lymphoma (DLBCL), NOS

Germinal center B-cell subtype

Activated B-cell subtype

Large B-cell lymphoma with 11q aberration

Nodular lymphocyte predominant B-cell lymphoma

T cell/histiocyte rich large B-cell lymphoma

Primary DLBCL of the central nervous system

Primary DLBCL of the testis

Primary cutaneous DLBCL, leg type

Intravascular large B-cell lymphoma

HHV-8 and EBV–negative primary effusion-based lymphoma

EBV-positive mucocutaneous ulcer

EBV-positive DLBCL, NOS

DLBCL associated with chronic inflammation

Fibrin-associated DLBCL

Lymphomatoid granulomatosis

EBV-positive polymorphic B-cell lymphoproliferative disorder, NOS

ALK-positive large B-cell lymphoma

Plasmablastic lymphoma

HHV-8–associated lymphoproliferative disorder

Multicentric Castleman disease

HHV-8–positive germinotropic lymphoproliferative disorder

HHV-8–positive DLBCL, NOS

Primary effusion lymphoma

Burkitt lymphoma

High-grade B-cell lymphoma, with *MYC* and *BCL2* rearrangements

*High-grade B-cell lymphoma with MYC and BCL6 rearrangements**

High-grade B-cell lymphoma, NOS

Primary mediastinal large B-cell lymphoma

Mediastinal gray-zone lymphoma

Classic Hodgkin Lymphoma

Nodular sclerosis classic Hodgkin lymphoma

Lymphocyte-rich classic Hodgkin lymphoma

Mixed cellularity classic Hodgkin lymphoma

Lymphocyte-depleted classic Hodgkin lymphoma

Mature T-Cell and NK-Cell Neoplasms

T-cell prolymphocytic leukemia

T-cell large granular lymphocytic leukemia

Chronic lymphoproliferative disorder of NK cells

Adult T-cell leukemia/lymphoma

EBV-positive T/NK lymphoproliferative disorder (LPD) of childhood

Hydroa vacciniforme LPD

Classic

Systemic

(Continued)

Severe mosquito bite allergy

Chronic active EBV disease (T-cell and NK-cell phenotype)

Systemic EBV-positive T-cell lymphoma of childhood

Extranodal NK/T-cell lymphoma, nasal type

Aggressive NK cell leukemia

Primary nodal EBV-positive T/NK-cell lymphoma

Enteropathy-associated T-cell lymphoma

   Type II refractory celiac disease

Monomorphic epitheliotropic intestinal T-cell lymphoma

Intestinal T-cell lymphoma, NOS

Indolent clonal T-cell lymphoproliferative disorder of the gastrointestinal tract

Indolent NK cell lymphoproliferative disorder of the gastrointestinal tract

Hepatosplenic T-cell lymphoma

Mycosis fungoides

Sézary syndrome

Primary cutaneous CD30-positive T-cell lymphoproliferative disorders

   Lymphomatoid papulosis

   Primary cutaneous anaplastic large cell lymphoma

Primary cutaneous small/medium CD4-positive T-cell lymphoproliferative disorder

Subcutaneous panniculitis-like T-cell lymphoma

Primary cutaneous gamma-delta T-cell lymphoma

Primary cutaneous acral CD8-positive T-cell lymphoproliferative disorder

Primary cutaneous CD8-positive aggressive epidermotropic cytotoxic T-cell lymphoma

Peripheral T-cell lymphoma, NOS

Follicular helper T-cell lymphoma

   Follicular helper T-cell lymphoma, angioimmunoblastic type (Angioimmunoblastic T-cell lymphoma)

   Follicular helper T-cell lymphoma, follicular type

   Follicular helper T-cell lymphoma, NOS

Anaplastic large cell lymphoma, ALK-positive

Anaplastic large cell lymphoma, ALK-negative

Breast implant-associated anaplastic large cell lymphoma

Immunodeficiency-Associated Lymphoproliferative Disorders

Post-transplant lymphoproliferative disorders (PTLD)

   Plasmacytic hyperplasia PTLD

   Infectious mononucleosis PTLD

   Florid follicular hyperplasia PTLD

   Polymorphic PTLD

   Monomorphic PTLD (B-cell and T/NK-cell types)

   Classic Hodgkin lymphoma PTLD

Other iatrogenic immunodeficiency–associated lymphoproliferative disorders

Histiocytic and Dendritic Cell Neoplasms

Histiocytic sarcoma

Langerhans cell histiocytosis

Langerhans cell sarcoma

Indeterminate dendritic cell histiocytosis

Interdigitating dendritic cell sarcoma

ALK-positive histiocytosis

Disseminated juvenile xanthogranuloma

Erdheim-Chester disease

Rosai-Dorfman-Destombes disease

Follicular dendritic cell sarcoma

Fibroblastic reticular cell sarcoma

EBV-positive inflammatory follicular dendritic cell/fibroblastic reticular cell tumor

---

*Provisional entity.

Data from Daniel A. Arber, Attilio Orazi, Robert P. Hasserjian, et al; International Consensus Classification of Myeloid Neoplasms and Acute Leukemias: integrating morphologic, clinical, and genomic data. *Blood* 2022;140(11): 1200-1228; Campo E, Jaffe ES, Cook JR, et al. The International Consensus Classification of Mature Lymphoid Neoplasms: a report from the Clinical Advisory Committee. *Blood.* 2022;140(11):1229-1253.

Page numbers followed by *f* indicate figures; *t*, tables; *b*, boxes.

1274   Index

Nonlymphoid malignancies, mimicking
lymphoma, bone marrow involvement in,
1155–1156
Nonlymphoid tumors
LK-positive, 733, 734f
with prominent reactive lymphoid
components, of lymph nodes, 1200–
1201, 1200f–1201f
Noonan syndrome, juvenile myelomonocytic
leukemia associated with, 886
Noonan-syndrome-like disorders (CBL-
Syndrome), juvenile myelomonocytic
leukemia associated with, 886
Normochromic normocytic anemia, 211–215
high output, 217–224
underproduction, 215–217
NOTCH1, in T-cell lymphoblastic leukemia/
lymphoma, 818
NPM-ALK protein, 721
NPM1 gene, 36
NPM1 mutations, 96–97
acute myeloid leukemia with, 894f, 902–903
in myelodysplastic/myeloproliferative
neoplasms, 962
Nuclear factor-κB, in lymphocyte-predominant
cells, 550
Nuclear factor-κB pathway, activation of, 457
Nuclear factor of activated T cells (NFAT), in
lymphocyte-predominant cells, 550
Nucleic acid isolation, 65–66

O
Oct-1, in lymphocyte-predominant cells,
548t–549t, 550
Oct-2, in lymphocyte-predominant cells,
548t–549t, 550
Ocular adnexal lymphoma, 1233–1235
Ocular adnexal MALT lymphoma, 387
Ocular lymphoma, 1232
OKT3, posttransplant lymphoproliferative
disorders associated with, 1106
Omenn syndrome, 1088, 1088f–1089f
Oncogene abnormalities, in follicular lymphoma,
374t
Optical genome mapping (OGM), 75–76
Oral cavity, lymphoma of, 1238–1239, 1238f
Osmotic fragility studies, in hereditary
spherocytosis, 220
Osteitis fibrosa, 1195, 1195f
Osteochondroma, 1194
Osteoclastoma, 1194
Osteomyelitis, chronic, 1194–1195
Osteoporosis, 1195
Osteosarcoma, 1193–1194
Ovalocytosis, Southeast Asian, 220
Ovarian lymphoma, 1253
Overt primary myelofibrosis, 939–944, 941b
clinical course of, 943–944
clinical features of, 941
differential diagnosis of, 944, 944t, 945f–946f,
947t
epidemiology of, 941
in extramedullary tissues, 942–943, 943f
genetics of, 943
morphology of, 941–943

P
p27, in mantle cell lymphoma, 434, 438
p50, in lymphocyte-predominant cells, 550
p53
immunoreactivity for, in diffuse large B-cell
lymphoma, 454–455
in lymphocyte-predominant cells, 548t–549t, 551
in T-cell prolymphocytic leukemia, 661

p65, in lymphocyte-predominant cells,
548t–549t, 550
Pagetoid appearance, primary cutaneous T-cell
lymphomas and, 792–793, 793f
Pagetoid reticulosis, 769–770, 770f
Paget's disease, of bone, 1194
Pan-T-cell antigen(s), 688
Pancreas, lymphoma of, 1249
Pancreatobiliary tract, lymphoma of, 1248–1249
Papanicolaou stain
of fine-needle aspiration, 16
for lymph node biopsy specimen, 7–8
Paracortex, 142–144, 143f
Paracortical hyperplasia, 171–172
fine-needle aspiration of, 18
versus follicular helper T-cell, 713, 714t
Paracortical lymphoid nodules, 171–172
Paranasal sinuses, lymphoma of, 1236–1237
Parapsoriasis, 759
Parasitic infection, in bone marrow, 255
Paroxysmal nocturnal hemoglobinuria, 245,
246t, 247f
myelodysplastic syndrome *versus*, 862
Parvovirus B19
bone marrow findings in, 256
in pure red cell aplasia, 216, 216f
Patches, in mycosis fungoides, 759, 760f–762f,
762b
Pautrier's microabscesses, in mycosis fungoides,
761–762, 763f, 765–766
PCDLBCL, LT. *See* Primary cutaneous diffuse
large B-cell lymphoma, leg type
PCFCL. *See* Primary cutaneous follicle center
lymphoma
PCMZLPD. *See* Primary cutaneous marginal zone
lymphoproliferative disorder
PCNA, in lymphocyte-predominant cells,
548t–549t
PDGFRA, in myeloproliferative neoplasms,
unclassifiable, 951
PDGFRA rearrangement, myeloid/lymphoid
neoplasms with eosinophilia and, 835–837,
1002–1005
cell of origin of, postulated, 1004
clinical course of, 1004–1005
clinical features of, 1003
definition of, 1002
differential diagnosis of, 1005, 1005f, 1006t,
1013t
epidemiology of, 1003
etiology of, 1003
genetic/molecular findings of, 1003–1004,
1003b, 1005f
genetics of, 1003, 1003b
immunophenotype of, 1003
morphology of, 1003, 1004f–1005f
normal counterpart of, 1004
synonyms and related terms of, 1003
PDGFRB, in myeloproliferative neoplasms,
unclassifiable, 951
PDGFRB rearrangement, myeloid/lymphoid
neoplasms with eosinophilia and,
1005–1009
cell of origin of, postulated, 1008
clinical course of, 1008
clinical features of, 1006
definition of, 1005–1006
differential diagnosis of, 1006t, 1008–1009,
1013t
epidemiology of, 1006
etiology of, 1006
genetics/molecular findings of, 1003b, 1008
immunophenotype of, 1008
morphology of, 1006–1008, 1007f
normal counterpart of, 1008
synonyms and related terms of, 1006

Pearson marrow-pancreas syndrome, 213–215,
214f
Pearson's syndrome, 861
Pediatric-type follicular lymphoma (PTFL),
363–366, 365f, 366t
Pegylated recombinant human megakaryocyte
growth and development factor, bone
marrow changes after, 1163
Peliosis, of spleen, 1224–1225
Pentostatin, for T-cell prolymphocytic leukemia,
661
Perforin, in anaplastic large cell lymphoma, 719,
723f
Periarteriolar lymphoid sheaths, 1211, 1211t
Perifollicular blasts, in classic Hodgkin
lymphoma, 573
Periodic acid-Schiff (PAS) stain, for lymph node
biopsy specimen, 11
Peripheral blood findings
in adult T-cell leukemia/lymphoma, 667f
for anemia, evaluation of, 205
in bone marrow necrosis, 257–258, 260f
in chronic lymphocytic leukemia/small
lymphocytic lymphoma, 284–285, 284f
in chronic myeloid leukemia, 921, 921f
in chronic neutrophilic leukemia, 930, 931f
in cytomegalovirus, 255, 256f
in Epstein-Barr virus, 255, 257f
in essential thrombocythemia, 933, 935f
follicular lymphoma in, 363, 364f
in hantavirus, 256
in hepatic disease, 263, 264f
in histoplasmosis, 257–258, 259f
in lymphoplasmacytic lymphoma and
Waldenström macroglobulinemia, 311,
312f
in mantle cell lymphoma, 428, 431–432, 432f
in monoclonal B-cell lymphocytosis, 303–304
in myelodysplastic syndromes, 841–843, 843t
in myeloid neoplasms, 832, 833b
in neutropenia, 234t
in polycythemia vera, 946–947, 948f
in primary myelofibrosis
early/prefibrotic, 939, 940f
overt, 940f, 941
in reactive basophilia, 253
in reactive lymphocytosis, 251, 252f
in reactive monocytosis, 253
in reactive neutrophilia, 251f, 253
in splenic marginal zone lymphoma, 339, 342f
in T-cell large granular lymphocytic leukemia,
646
Peripheral blood smear, hairy cell leukemia in,
328–330, 329f
Peripheral T-cell lymphoma (PTCL)
versus classic Hodgkin lymphoma, 582, 583f
mycosis fungoides and, 768
not otherwise specified, 685–700.e5, 85t–87t,
88–89, 805
versus anaplastic large cell lymphoma, 731t
antigen receptor genes in, 690
bone marrow involvement in, 1151–1152,
1152f
CD30-positive, 699, 700t
cell-of-origin subgroups of, 694–695, 695f,
695t
clinical features of, 686
cytotoxic molecule-positive, 693, 694f
definition of, 685
diagnostic approach to, 697–699, 698f
epidemiology of, 685–686
etiology of, 686
extranodal, 693f, 695–696, 696f
fine-needle aspiration of, 26–27, 27f
versus follicular helper T-cell, 703, 714t
genetic abnormalities of, 690–692, 693f